A REFERENCE GUIDE TO FETAL AND NEONATAL RISK

Drugs in **Pregnancy** and **Lactation** Seventh Edition

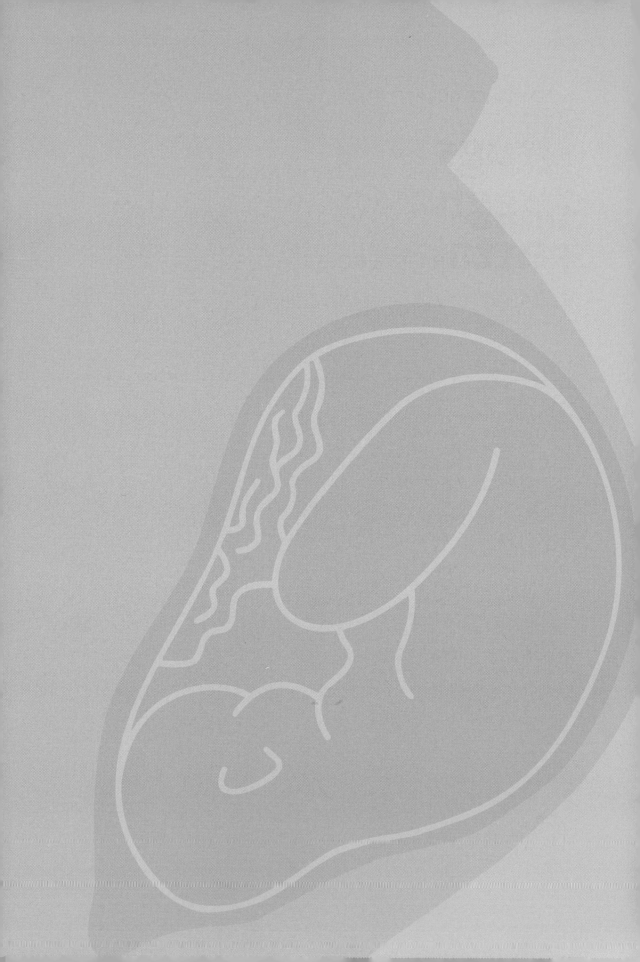

A REFERENCE GUIDE TO FETAL AND NEONATAL RISK

Drugs in Pregnancy and Lactation

Seventh Edition

Gerald G. Briggs, B.Pharm.
Pharmacist Clinical Specialist, Women's Pavilion
Miller Children's Hospital
Long Beach, California
Clinical Professor of Pharmacy
University of California, San Francisco
Adjunct Professor of Pharmacy Practice
University of Southern California, Los Angeles

Roger K. Freeman, M.D.
Director, Obstetrics/Gynecology/Normal Newborn Careline
Women's Pavilion
Miller Children's Hospital
Long Beach, California
Clinical Professor of Obstetrics and Gynecology
University of California, Irvine

Sumner J. Yaffe, M.D.
Visiting Professor
Department of Pediatrics
School of Medicine
University of California, Los Angeles

LIPPINCOTT WILLIAMS & WILKINS
A **Wolters Kluwer** Company
Philadelphia • Baltimore • New York • London
Buenos Aires • Hong Kong • Sydney • Tokyo

Acquisitions Editor: Anne M. Sydor
Developmental Editor: Holly Lukens
Production Manager: David Murphy
Senior Manufacturing Manager: Ben Rivera
Marketing Manager: Kathy Neely
Design Coordinator: Doug Smock
Production Service: TechBooks
Printer: Quebecor World-Taunton

530 Walnut Street
Philadelphia, PA 19106 USA
LWW.com

Printed in the USA

ISBN: 0-7817-5651-0

Care has been taken to confirm the accuracy of the information presented and to describe generally accepted practices. However, the authors, editors, and publisher are not responsible for errors or omissions or for any consequences from application of the information in this book and make no warranty, expressed or implied, with respect to the currency, completeness, or accuracy of the contents of the publication. Application of this information in a particular situation remains the professional responsibility of the practitioner.

The authors, editors, and publisher have exerted every effort to ensure that drug selection and dosage set forth in this text are in accordance with current recommendations and practice at the time of publication. However, in view of ongoing research, changes in government regulations, and the constant flow of information relating to drug therapy and drug reactions, the reader is urged to check the package insert for each drug for any change in indications and dosage and for added warnings and precautions. This is particularly important when the recommended agent is a new or infrequently employed drug.

Some drugs and medical devices presented in this publication have Food and Drug Administration (FDA) clearance for limited use in restricted research settings. It is the responsibility of the health care provider to ascertain the FDA status of each drug or device planned for use in their clinical practice.

10 9 8 7 6 5 4 3 2

Foreword

This book is now in its 7th edition, and has enjoyed great success with physicians and other professionals involved in the care of pregnant and lactating patients. There are about 130 additional drugs over the 6th edition, and updates are provided where indicated on all drugs in the book. The reviews are exhaustive, but pertinent to the management of pregnant and lactating patients who have already ingested a drug or who are in need of drug therapy where a cost-benefit analysis may be necessary for appropriate counseling. We also have added a new system to help those using this book assess the risk a drug represents to the embryo, fetus, or nursing infant.

There are seldom absolute answers to questions a woman may have when she ingests a drug while pregnant or nursing since human experience is usually, of necessity, somewhat anecdotal. Even though a drug may not show a problem among a large group of exposed patients, one can never rule out individual susceptibility, making the dictum of not using drugs in pregnancy without good cause still important. The effect or lack of effect in animals does not necessarily translate to human risks or safety, resulting in the persistent need to consider both animal and human studies when counseling exposed patients or selecting appropriate drugs for use in pregnant and lactating patients.

It is our hope that the 7th edition will continue to provide the practitioner appropriate assistance with questions regarding drugs in pregnancy and lactation.

Roger K. Freeman, M.D.
Director, Obstetrics/Gynecology/Normal Newborn Careline
Women's Pavilion
Miller Children's Hospital
Long Beach, California
Clinical Professor of Obstetrics and Gynecology
University of California, Irvine

Preface

In this edition, approximately 130 new drugs have been added and numerous drugs in the 6th edition have been revised. The impact of the new references on previous reviews is varied. In some cases, the new material is the drug's first reported human pregnancy experience, in others, it identified a previously unrecognized risk, and in still others, it confirmed the findings of previously limited data. Of course, no reference book of this type can include all the published material, so we have attempted (sometimes successfully and, undeniably, sometimes not) to cite the material that we thought had the most impact.

A new feature in this edition is the recommendations we have added for the pregnancy and lactation sections (see "Instructions for Use of the Reference Guide" for definitions of the recommendations). The level of risk to the embryo/fetus from exposure to a drug changes continuously throughout gestation. Almost all of the known human teratogens can be relatively benign in some portions of pregnancy. Consequently, in many cases, no short statement can adequately describe the potential adverse effects of a drug during pregnancy. Nevertheless, we understand the time constraints that confront healthcare professionals and our recommendations are intended to help them. When a woman of reproductive age requires drug therapy, the healthcare professional might not have time to conduct a review of the drug's effects on an unknown or unplanned pregnancy. The same may occur even when she is known to be pregnant. This is especially true if the toxicity profile in human pregnancy has not been adequately determined. In the ideal sequence of events, the healthcare professional would have studied sufficient material to make an informed opinion of the embryo/fetal risk, and would have the time to communicate this opinion to the patient in such a manner that she would fully understand. However, the time constraints placed on caregivers make it difficult to achieve this ideal scenario. Therefore, we have attempted to provide some indication of the risk level for each drug depending on the stage of pregnancy and the available human and animal data.

For the animal data, we based the level of risk on the relationship of the dose producing developmental toxicity (growth retardation, structural defects, functional/behavioral defects, or death) (in the absence of maternal toxicity) to the human dose. If the toxic dose in animals is greater than 10 times the human dose (based on body surface area or systemic exposure), than the drug appears to represent a low risk in humans (Scialli AR, et al. Birth Defects Res [Part A] 2004;70:7–12). Of course, risk assessment is much more complicated than just considering the animal data because it does not take into account other major factors, such as the route of administration, metabolism including the effects of active metabolites, species differences, type of defects, pharmacokinetics, or the embryo/fetal effects of untreated or under treated maternal disease. Therefore, these factors, if relevant, are included in our recommendations. However, there are unavoidable lapses, such as consideration of human metabolism.

It has become increasingly evident that a significant portion of the population has altered drug metabolism capability. The cytochrome P450 isoenzymes are involved in the intermediary metabolism of many drugs. In some individuals, perhaps as high as 10%, one or more of these important isoenzymes are missing or inactive (i.e., so called "poor metabolizers"). Currently, there is no simple method to identify these individuals before they take a drug. Thus, these persons will have much higher systemic concentrations of the drug and they will be present in the circulation for much longer times. In these cases, the embryo/fetus may be exposed to higher levels of the drug than embryo/fetuses of mothers with unaltered metabolism. Moreover, a number of inhibitors have been identified for specific isoenzymes that can result in clinically significant drug interactions. Fortunately, in these cases information is usually readily available. Because there is a dose-relationship with developmental toxicity and other adverse effects, this subject requires much more study.

The risks also change during breast-feeding because nearly all reported adverse effects in nursing infants have occurred in infants less than 6 months of age. The neonate and very young infant are most at risk for adverse effects from drugs present in breast milk. Some adverse effects are obvious, such as sedation, lethargy, diarrhea, etc., but long-term neurotoxicity is much more difficult to identify or predict. Balancing the well-known benefits of breast-feeding with this potential toxicity is a difficult task. A good general rule to consider is that long-term use of psychotropic medications by the mother represents an unknown risk of long-term neurobehavior abnormalities in her nursing infant. Our recommendations for breast-feeding risk reflect these considerations.

For some drugs, we have placed toll free telephone numbers at the end of the pregnancy section for the use of healthcare professionals to enroll patients in observational studies. These studies are an important method for gathering prospective data on pregnancy exposures for high-risk drugs. In fact, such studies are often the only published human pregnancy experience available for new drugs and new pharmacologic drug classes. These studies can be valuable in the early detection of major teratogens or showing that an agent is an unlikely major teratogen. Because their importance is so high, healthcare professionals are encouraged to call for information about patient enrollment.

As in past years, we take great pleasure in the opportunity to thank the many individuals who have helped us. To those who have sent us references know that your effort is sincerely appreciated. We also appreciate those who have commented on our work because it identifies areas that may need modification or topics that we need to cover in the next edition. In addition, the questions we received served to keep us informed of your information needs and often lead to the preparation of new reviews. Our appreciation also goes to Christina Chambers, PhD, MPH, for her helpful comments relating to Marijuana and Cigarette Smoking reviews. The medical library staff at Long Beach Memorial Medical Center continues to be a major source of assistance. Two staff members, Barbara Malinofsky and Elizabeth Mason-Renteria, have been particularly helpful in retrieving references and our thanks go to both of them. The staff (Drs. Susan Vancampen, Neepa Rai, Suk Lange, and Jennifer Chang) of Memorial's Drug Information Service, as in previous editions, has been supportive by sending us important references. My appreciation also goes to my wife, Susan, who has been a pillar of support and encouragement since the 1st edition in 1983.

Gerald G. Briggs, B.Pharm.
Pharmacist Clinical Specialist, Women's Pavilion
Miller Children's Hospital
Clinical Professor of Pharmacy
University of California, San Francisco
Adjunct Professor of Pharmacy Practice
University of Southern California, Los Angeles

Acknowledgment

We are pleased to acknowledge the assistance of our former students in the preparation of some of the reviews contained in this edition. The students came from three schools of pharmacy. During their clerkship training in obstetrics/gynecology, each researched and wrote one or two drug reviews. It was their first experience in how to assess the human reproductive toxicity of drugs and they did very well.

University of California, San Francisco
Kristan Aoki, Pharm.D.
Cyndi Cao, Pharm.D.
May Chan, Pharm.D.
Jessica Chen, Pharm.D.
Daisy Lee, Pharm.D.
Kristine McGill, Pharm.D.
Jenny Nguyen, Pharm.D.
Johnny Reyes, Pharm.D.
Lord Sarino, Pharm.D.
Yelena Slavina, Pharm.D.
Cecile Taylor, Pharm.D.
Quynhlam Tran, Pharm.D.

University of Southern California, Los Angeles
Armin Kasravi, Pharm.D.
Priscilla Luu, Pharm.D.
Carina Tea, Pharm.D.

Virginia Commonwealth University, Richmond
Phaneth Keo, Pharm.D.

In addition, we are also pleased to acknowledge the assistance of our colleague in Women's Pavilion, Stephanie Wan, Pharm.D. BCPS, Pharmacist Clinical Specialist, who also researched and wrote two drug reviews.

Contents

Introduction

Sumner J. Yaffe, M.D.

Until the middle of the 20th century, most physicians believed that the uterus provided a protected environment for the fetus and served as a shield from the external environment. This belief was questioned when an Australian physician, N.M. Gregg, observed that women who contracted rubella during the first trimester of pregnancy frequently gave birth to infants with specific anatomical defects, mainly in the heart, eyes, and ears. This finding forever shattered the concept held previously, and now it became clear that the external environment could affect fetal outcome. It is now generally accepted that the developing fetus may be adversely affected by exposure to drugs and environmental chemicals. The stage of development of the intrauterine host is a major determinant of the resultant effect, as well as the nature and the concentration of the drug or chemical agent. On a more positive side fetal therapy (i.e., treatment of fetal disease *in utero* by administering the drug to the mother or directly to the fetus) has been recognized recently as a rational approach to treat fetal disease.

With rare exception, all foreign compounds are transmitted across the placenta, and depending upon their lipid solubility and chemical structure, achieve varying concentrations in the embryo and fetus. Unfortunately, drug use during pregnancy continued unaffected by Gregg's observations. During the several decades following Gregg's report in 1941, most concern regarding drug effects upon the embryo and fetus had to do with the perinatal period, particularly with the effect of narcotics and analgesics on the ability of the new born infant to initiate and sustain respiration following delivery.

In 1948, Professor O. Smith at the Boston Lying in Hospital introduced diethylstilbestrol (DES; a synthetic estrogen) into medical practice as a treatment for the complications of early pregnancy. This therapy, although not validated, was widely adopted. Twenty three years later, the consequences of this unapproved therapy came to light with the establishment of a relationship between adenocarcinoma of the vagina and *in utero* exposure to DES. In many ways, the discovery of the adverse effects of DES was fortuitous. Since adenocarcinoma of the vagina in young females had been a rare disease, the causal role of DES was relatively readily elucidated. If maternal therapy with DES had been the cause of an increase in the incidence of some relatively more common adolescent disease, such as diabetes, the relationship would still be undetected today. The adverse effects of DES also serve as an example of long term delayed effects of *in utero* drug and chemical exposure, which are difficult to recognize but must always be considered when evaluating drugs and chemicals exposure during pregnancy.

Then, 40 years ago, the thalidomide catastrophe (limb defects) occurred when this drug was administered to pregnant women as an antianxiety agent during the first trimester. Thalidomide had been evaluated for safety in several animal species, had been given a clean bill of health, and had come to be regarded as a good pharmacologic agent (hypnotic/sedative). It is of interest that this drug is being reevaluated for use in leprosy and approval for this use has been given by the Food and Drug Administration (FDA).

It is important to note that, even though thalidomide induces a distinct cluster of anatomic defects that are virtually pathognomonic for this agent, it required several years of thalidomide use and the birth of many thousands of grossly malformed infants before the cause-and-effect relationship between thalidomide administration in early pregnancy and its harmful effects was recognized. This serves to emphasize the difficulties that exist in incriminating drugs and chemicals that are harmful when administered during pregnancy. Hopefully, we will never have another drug prescribed for use during pregnancy whose teratogenicity is as potent as thalidomide (about one-third of women taking this agent during the first trimester gave birth to infants with birth defects). Concern about the safety of foreign compounds administered to pregnant women has been increasingly evident since thalidomide. The direct response to this misadventure led to the promulgation of the drug regulations of 1962 in the United States. According to these regulations, a drug must be demonstrated to be safe and effective for the conditions of use prescribed in its labeling. The regulations concerning this requirement state that a drug should be investigated for the conditions of use specified in the labeling, including dosage levels and patient populations for whom the drug is intended. In addition, appropriate information must be provided in the labeling and be available when the drug is prescribed. The intent of the regulations is not only to ensure adequate labeling information for the safe and effective administration of the drug by the physician, but also to ensure that marketed drugs have an acceptable benefit:risk ratio for their intended uses.

In August of 1962, the same year as the congressional revision of the Food and Drugs Laws mentioned above, the Commission on Drug Safety was established with a grant from the Pharmaceutical Manufacturers Association. The commission represented the concern of the pharmaceutical industry for adverse effects of drugs administered to pregnant women. The commission served as an independent body of academicians to offer advice regarding the prenatal effects of drugs. Under the chairmanship of Dr. Lowell Coggeshiall, vice-president of the University of Chicago, 13 scientists reported in 1963 after subcommittee deliberation concerning methods to evaluate the safety of drugs administered to the pregnant woman. Their main conclusions are valid today. In general, they agreed that animal tests do not guarantee drug safety to the unborn child, but should not be abandoned because they do offer some insight into adverse effects in the human. They also strongly endorsed basic and analytical research to support the current (1963) existing empirical approaches to the evaluation of drug safety.

It is clear that any drug or chemical substance administered to the mother is able to cross the placenta to some extent unless it is destroyed or altered during passage or its molecular size and low lipid solubility limit transplacental transfer. Placental transport of maternal substrates to the fetus and of substances from the fetus to the mother is established at about the 5th week of fetal life. Substances of low molecular weight diffuse freely across the placenta, driven primarily by the concentration gradient. It is important to note, therefore, that almost every substance used for therapeutic purposes can and does pass from the mother to the fetus. Of greater importance is whether the rate and extent of transfer are sufficient to result in significant concentrations within the fetus. Today the concept of a placental barrier must be discarded.

Experiments with animals have provided considerable information concerning the teratogenic effects of drugs. Unfortunately, these experimental findings cannot be extrapolated from species to species, or even from strain to strain within the same species, much less from animals to humans. Research in this area and the prediction of toxicity in the human are further hampered by a lack of specificity between cause and effect.

Traditionally, teratogenic effects of drugs have been noted as anatomic malformations. It is clear that these are dose and time related and that the fetus is at greater risk during the first 3 months of gestation. However, it is possible for drugs and chemicals to exert their effects upon the fetus at other times during pregnancy. Functional and behavioral changes are much more difficult to identify as to cause and effect. Consequently, they are rarely recognized. A heightened awareness on the part of health providers and recipients will make this task easier.

The mechanisms by which drugs exert teratogenic effects are poorly understood, particularly in the human. Drugs may affect maternal receptors with indirect effects upon the fetus, or they may have a direct effect on embryonic development and result in specific abnormalities. Drugs may affect the nutrition of the fetus by interfering with the passage of nutrients across the placenta. Alterations in placental metabolism influence the development of the fetus since placental integrity is a major determinant of fetal growth. It is noteworthy that the National Institute of Child Health and Human Development (NICHD) has launched a major initiative regarding the molecular mechanisms responsible for deviations in normal development resulting in birth defects. This effort in 2000 combined with a previous (1998) initiative should lead to an in-depth understanding of drug- and chemical-induced malformations, and in turn enable preventive endeavors. Administration of a drug to a pregnant woman presents a unique problem for the physician. Not only must maternal pharmacologic mechanisms be taken into consideration when prescribing a drug, but the fetus must always be kept in mind as a potential recipient of the drug.

Recognition of the fact that drugs administered during pregnancy can affect the fetus should lead to decreased drug consumption. Nonetheless, studies conducted in the past few years indicate that drug consumption during pregnancy is increasing. This may be due to several reasons. Most people in the Western world are unaware of their drug and chemical exposure. Many are uninformed as to the potentially harmful effects of drugs on the fetus. Also, there are some who feel that many individuals in modern society are overly concerned with their own comfort, so that pregnant women seek pharmacologic solutions to the many symptoms that affect them. Although considerable attention has been given recently to illegal drug use during pregnancy, use of legal drugs, both prescription and over-the-counter, continues with little apparent diminution. "Most medicines taken by or administered to pregnant women cross the placenta and into the blood stream of the fetus. Thus, when a pregnant women takes medicine, she not only gives medicine to herself but is also giving the same medicine to her unborn baby. Since the not-fully-developed body systems of the fetus cannot process medicines as the mother's systems do, and since some medicines may effect normal development of the fetus, medicines that cross the placenta may have negative effects on the fetus and newborn. One only has to remember the thalidomide disaster to recognize the possible extent of the potential problems." (UNICEF: Drug Use in Pregnancy, *The Prescriber*, January 1992). The World Health Organization (WHO) has completed an international survey on drug utilization during pregnancy involving 14,778 pregnant women from 22 countries on four continents. Eighty-six percent of these women took medication during pregnancy, receiving an average of 2.9 (range 1–15) prescriptions. This survey did not take into account over-the-counter drugs purchased without the advice of the physician or a prescription. Of the total 37,309 prescriptions in the WHO survey, 73% were given by an obstetrician, 12% by a general practitioner, and only 5% by a midwife. This extremely high drug prescribing and utilization rate during pregnancy is then elevated by an increase in drug administration during the intrapartum period, wherein, according to the WHO survey, 79% of the women received an average 3.3 drugs. The WHO survey concludes: "There can be no doubt that at present some drugs are more widely used in pregnancy than is justified by the knowledge available. This may be one aspect of the medicalization of pregnancy, a process in which the use of a series of techniques and drugs is associated even with normal pregnancies, the employment of one technique or drug readily leading to the use of another. It would seem that whereas pregnancy is usually regarded as dangerous until proven safe, drugs may be regarded as safe in pregnancy provided they have not been proven dangerous, views which are often diametrically opposed to reality" (Collaborative Group on Drug Use in Pregnancy. An International Survey on Drug Utilization During Pregnancy. *International Journal of Risk and Safety in Medicine*, 1991;1:1). These recent pronouncements are quoted to demonstrate that drug use in pregnancy continues without let up and most often without a specific rationale, except to treat the many symptoms which accompany the normal pregnancy.

The FDA has proposed significant changes in pregnancy labeling. This will clarify for both the prescribing physician and the patient the risks associated with the administration of an individual drug and chemical to the pregnant woman. Much more information is needed to make pregnancy labeling more meaningful. To this end, the FDA has proposed a new regulation (2001) requiring drug manufactures to report safety data to a central registry. This regulation, currently under review, will provide the practitioner with significantly more drug safety information.

It is crucial that concern also be given to events beyond the narrow limits of congenital anatomic malformations; evidence exists that intellectual, social, and functional development also can be adversely affected by drug administration during pregnancy. There are examples that toxic manifestations of intrauterine exposure to environmental agents may be subtle, unexpected, and delayed. Concern for the delayed effects of drugs, following intrauterine exposure, was first raised following the tragic discovery that female fetuses exposed to diethylstilbestrol (DES) are at an increased risk for adenocarcinoma of the vagina (see above). This type of malignancy is not discovered until after puberty. Additional clinical findings indicate that male offspring were not spared from the effects of the drug. Some have abnormalities of the reproductive system, such as epididymal cysts, hypotrophic testes, capsular induration, and pathologic semen.

The concept of long-term latency has been confirmed by investigations conducted previously in our research laboratories at the Children's Hospital of Philadelphia. When the widely used hypnotic/sedative agent phenobarbital was administered to pregnant rats, the offspring were significantly smaller than normal and they experienced delays in vaginal opening. Sixty percent of the females exposed to phenobarbital in utero were infertile.

In male animals we found lower than normal testosterone levels in the brain and bloodstream of mate rats whose mothers were given low doses of phenobarbital late in pregnancy. Even at 120 days of age, these male rats showed abnormal testosterone synthesis, the mechanism responsible for the low concentrations. It is believed that phenobarbital exposure in fetal life may alter brain programming, resulting in permanent changes in sexual function. Phenobarbital is an old drug that is widely prescribed. It is also a component of many multi-ingredient pharmaceuticals whose use does not abate during pregnancy. The clinical significance of these experiments in animals is admittedly unknown, but the striking effects upon reproductive function warrant careful scrutiny of the safety of these agents during human pregnancy before prescribing them.

The physician is confronted with two imperatives in treating the pregnant woman: alleviate maternal suffering and do no harm to the fetus. Until now the emphasis has been on the amelioration of suffering, but the time has come to concentrate on not harming the fetus. The simple equation to be applied here is to weigh the therapeutic benefits of the drug to the mother against its risk potential to the developing fetus. Since fetal ova may also be exposed to drugs given to the mother, effects may be evident in future generations.

When one considers that more than 1.2 billion drug prescriptions are written each year, that there is unlimited self-administration of over-the-counter drugs, and that approximately 500 new pharmaceutical products are introduced annually, the need for prudence and caution in the administration of pharmaceuticals has reached a critical point. Pregnancy is a symptom-producing event. Pregnancy has the potential of causing women to increase their intake of drugs and chemicals, with the potential being that the fetus will be nurtured in a sea of drugs.

In today's society the physician cannot stand alone in the therapeutic decision-making process. It now has become the responsibility of each woman of childbearing age to consider carefully her use of drugs. In a pregnant woman, the decision to administer a drug should be made only after a collaborative appraisal between the woman and her physician of the risk:benefit ratio.

BREAST FEEDING AND DRUGS

Between 1930 and the late 1960s, there was a dramatic decline in the percentage of American mothers who breast-fed their babies. This was also accompanied by a reduction in the length of breast feeding for those who did nurse. The incidence of breast feeding declined from approximately 80% of the children born between 1926 and 1930 to 49% of children born some 25 years later. For children born between 1966 and 1970, 28% were breast-fed. Indeed, in 1972 only 20% of newborns were breast-fed. As data have become available for the following years, it is clear the decline has been reversed. By 1975, the percentage of first-born babies who were breast fed rose to 37%. At the present time in the United States, a number of surveys indicate that more than 50% of babies discharged from the hospital are breast-fed, and the number is increasing. Breast feeding is difficult to contemplate, since more than 50% of mothers work and return to work soon after delivery. New solutions must be found by employers to encourage breast feeding and develop the logistics to enable employees to breast-feed on the job.

Any number of hypotheses can be made regarding the decline and recent increase in breast feeding in this country. A fair amount of credit can be given to biomedical research of the past 15 years that has demonstrated and publicized the benefits of breast feeding.

Breast milk is known to possess nutritional and immunologic properties superior to those found in infant formulas. An American Academy of Pediatrics position paper emphasizes breast feeding as the best nutritional mode for infants for the first 6 months of life. In addition to those qualities, studies also suggest significant psychologic benefits of breast feeding for both the mother and the infant.

The upswing in breast feeding, together with a markedly increased concern about health needs on the part of parents, has led to increased questioning of the physician, pharmacist, and other health professionals about the safety and potential toxicity of drugs and chemicals that may be excreted in breast milk. Answers to these questions are not very apparent. Our knowledge concerning the long- and short-term effects and safety of maternally ingested drugs on the suckling infant is meager. We know more now than Soranus did in 150 AD, when he admonished wet nurses to refrain from the use of drugs and alcohol, lest it have an adverse effect on the nursing infant. We must know more! The knowledge to be acquired should be specific with respect to dose administered to the mother, amount excreted in breast milk, and amount absorbed by the suckling infant. In addition, effects on the infant should be determined (both acute and chronic).

It would be easy to recommend that the medicated mother not nurse, but it is likely that this recommendation would be ignored by the mother and may well offend many health providers, as well as their patients, on both psychosocial and physiologic grounds.

It must be emphasized that many of the investigations concerned with milk secretion and synthesis have been carried out in animals. The difficulty in studying human lactation using histologic techniques and the administration of radioactive isotopes is obvious. There are considerable differences in the composition of milk in different species. Some of these differences in composition would obviously bring about changes in drug elimination. Of great importance in this regard are the differences in the pH of human milk (pH usually >7.0) as contrasted to the pH of cow's milk (pH usually <6.8) where drug excretion has been extensively studied.

Human milk is a suspension of fat and protein in a carbohydrate-mineral solution. A nursing mother easily makes 600 mL of milk per day, which contains sufficient protein, fat, and carbohydrate to meet the nutritional demands of the developing infant. Milk proteins are fully synthesized from substrates delivered from the maternal circulation. The major proteins are casein and lactalbumin. The role of these proteins in the delivery of drugs into milk has not yet been completely elucidated. Drug excretion into milk may be accomplished by binding to the proteins or onto the surface of the milk fat globule.

There also exists the possibility for drug binding to the lipid, as well as to the protein components of the milk fat globule. It is also possible that lipid-soluble drugs may be sequestered within the milk fat globule. In addition to lipids and protein, carbohydrate is entirely synthesized within the breast. All of these nutrients achieve a concentration in human milk that is sufficient for the needs of the human infant for the first 6 months of life.

The transport of drugs into breast milk from maternal tissues and plasma may proceed by a number of different routes. In general, however, the mechanisms that determine the concentration of drug in breast milk are similar to those existing elsewhere within the organism. Drugs traverse membranes primarily by passive diffusion, and the concentration achieved will be dependent not only on the concentration gradient but also on the intrinsic lipid solubility of the drug and its degree of ionization, as well as on binding to protein and other cellular constituents.

A number of reviews give tables of the concentration of drugs in breast milk. Many times these tables also give the milk:plasma ratio. Most of the values from which the tables are derived consist of a single measurement of the drug concentration. Important information–such as the maternal dose, the frequency of dose, the time from drug administration to sampling, the frequency of nursing, and the length of lactation—is not given.

The significance of these concentration tables means only that the drug is present in the milk, and they offer no advice to the physician. Because the drug in the nursing infant's blood or urine is not measured, we have little information about the amount that is actually absorbed by the infant from the milk and, therefore, have no way of determining the possible pharmacologic effects on the infant. In fact, a critical examination of the tables that have been published reveals that much of the information was gathered decades ago when analytic methodology was not as sensitive as it is today. Since the discipline of pharmacokinetics was not developed until recently, many of the studies quoted in the tables of the review articles do not look precisely at the time relationship between drug administration and disposition.

Certain things are evident with regard to drugs administered during lactation. It is necessary that physicians become aware of the results of animal studies in this area and of the potential risk of maternal drug ingestion to the suckling infant. Many drugs prescribed to the lactating woman need to be thoroughly studied in order to assess their safety during lactation. It is clear that if the mother needs the drugs for therapeutic purposes, then she should consider not nursing. The ultimate decision must be individualized according to the specific illness and the therapeutic modality. Nursing should be avoided following the administration of radioactive pharmaceuticals that are usually given to the mother for diagnostic purposes.

The situation with the excretion of drugs into human breast milk might well be considered analogous to that of the prethalidomide era, when the effects on the fetus from maternally ingested drugs were recognized only as a result of a catastrophe. Objective evaluation of the efficacy and safety of drugs in breast milk must be undertaken. Until such data are available, the physician should always weigh the risk:benefit ratio when prescribing any maternal medication. It is also obligatory upon the nursing mother to become aware of the same factors and apply a measure of self-control before ingesting over-the-counter drugs. As stated before, it is quite evident that nearly all drugs will be present in breast milk following maternal ingestion. It is prudent to minimize maternal exposure, although very few drugs are currently known to be hazardous to the suckling child. If, after examining the risk:benefit factor, the physician decides that maternal medication is necessary, drug exposure to the infant may be minimized by scheduling the maternal dose just after a nursing period. More often than not just as in pregnancy, drugs are prescribed to the nursing mother for the relief of symptoms that do not require drug therapy. If mothers were apprised by their physicians of the potential risk to their infants, most would probably endure the symptoms, rather than take the drug and discontinue breast feeding.

CONCLUSIONS

Two basic situations are dealt with throughout this book: (a) risk potential to the fetus of maternal drugs ingested during the course of pregnancy and (b) risk potential to the infant of drugs taken by the mother while nursing.

The obvious solution to fetal and nursing infant risk avoidance is maternal abstinence. However, from a pragmatic standpoint, that would be impossible to implement. Another solution is to disseminate knowledge, in an authoritative manner, to all those involved in the pregnancy and breast-feeding processes: physician, mother, midwife, nurse, father, and pharmacist.

This book helps to fill a communication and information gap. We have carefully evaluated the research literature, animal and human, applied and clinical. We have established a risk factor for each of the nearly 900 drugs, in keeping with the FDA guidelines, that may be administered during pregnancy and lactation. This will be changed as new labelling guidelines are promulgated. We believe that this book will be helpful to all concerned parties in developing the risk:benefit decision.

This is but a beginning. It is our fervent hope that the information gained from the use of this book will cause the concerned parties to be more trenchant in their future decision making, either before prescribing or before ingesting drugs during pregnancy and lactation.

Instructions for Use of the Reference Guide

The Reference Guide is arranged so that the user can quickly locate a monograph. If the American generic name is known, go directly to the monographs, which are listed in alphabetical order. If only the trade or foreign name is known, refer to the Index for the appropriate American generic name. Foreign trade names have been included in the Index. To the best of our knowledge, all trade and foreign generic names are correct as shown, but because these may change, the reader should check other reference sources if there is any question as to the identity of an individual drug. Combination products are generally not listed in the Index. The user should refer to the manufacturer's product information for the specific ingredients, then use the Reference Guide as for single entities.

Each monograph contains six parts:

Generic Name (United States)
Pharmacologic Class
Risk Factor
Fetal Risk Summary and Recommendation
Breast Feeding Summary and Recommendation
References (if available)

FETAL RISK SUMMARY AND RECOMMENDATION

The Fetal Risk Summary is a brief review of the literature concerning the drug. The intent of the Summary is to provide clinicians and others with sufficient data to counsel patients and to arrive at conclusions on the risk:benefit ratio a particular drug poses for the fetus. The molecular weight of most drugs have been included in the reviews because they help determine if a drug can reach the embryo or fetus, but this value, by itself, may not predict the amount of transfer. The major determinant of the drug concentration in the embryo or fetus is the blood concentration of the drug in the mother. Other important factors include placental blood flow, the placental surface area available for transfer (i.e., correlated to the gestational age), and the lipid solubility, protein binding, and the amount of ionization of the drug at physiologic pH.

Because few absolutes are possible in the area of human teratology, the reader must carefully weigh the evidence, or lack thereof, before utilizing any drug in a pregnant woman. Readers who require more details than are presented should refer to the specific references listed at the end of the monograph. See Definitions for recommendations.

BREAST FEEDING SUMMARY AND RECOMMENDATION

The Breast Feeding Summary is a brief review of the literature concerning the passage of the drug into human breast milk and the effects, if any, on the nursing infant. In many studies of drugs in breast milk, infants were not allowed to breast feed. Readers should pay close attention to this distinction (i.e., excretion into milk vs. effects on the nursing infant) when using a Summary. Those who require more details than are presented should refer to the specific references listed at the end of the monograph. See Definitions for recommendations.

PREGNANCY AND BREAST FEEDING RECOMMENDATIONS

The pregnancy recommendations are intended to assist the reader in determining the level of risk of a specific drug. They apply only to the usual therapeutic dose of the drug in a typical patient. Because the genetic make-up of a specific patient may significantly alter the risk, the recommendations may not apply to the entire population. In addition to the animal reproduction data and known human pregnancy outcomes, the assessment of risk includes, when relevant, other major factors such as route of administration, metabolism to active metabolites, species differences, type of defects, pharmacokinetics, and the embryo/fetal effects of untreated or under treated maternal disease. Moreover, most drug exposures represent different levels of risk depending on the stage of pregnancy and, thus, timing of the exposure is critical in determining risk. Because short statements of risk may not always adequately assess the risk throughout the pregnancy, readers are encouraged to review the entire monograph before estimating the risk for a specific patient. Many reviews have a concluding paragraph that summarizes the findings and risks and readers may find it useful to refer to it. Recommendations appear in red throughout the text so that they can be found quickly and easily in the busy clinical setting.

The risks also change during breast-feeding because nearly all reported adverse effects in nursing infants have occurred in infants less than 6 months of age. The neonate and very young infant are most at risk for toxic effects from drugs present in breast milk. The recommendations for breast-feeding are based on the known toxicity of the drug or similar drugs in adults or children (when known) and the amount of drug excreted into breast milk (if known). Although most drugs taken by the mother are probably present in milk, the milk concentrations are usually unknown. Fortunately, the amounts are usually too low to cause toxicity. However, the therapeutic dose for infants of most drugs is rarely known. Therefore, we used a proposal from the literature (Ito S. N Engl J Med 2000;343:118–28) to classify exposures as clinically insignificant if, in the absence of data suggesting otherwise, the estimated dose ingested by a nursing infant was no more than 10% of the mother's weight-adjusted dose. In some cases, however, this classification may not be relevant. For example, the potential for neurotoxicity in a nursing infant from long-term maternal use of psychotropic medications continues to be a concern.

DEFINITIONS OF PREGNANCY RECOMMENDATIONS

COMPATIBLE

The human pregnancy experience, either for the drug itself or drugs in the same class or with similar mechanisms of action, is adequate to demonstrate that the embryo/fetal risk is very low or nonexistent. Animal reproduction data are not relevant.

NO (LIMITED) HUMAN DATA - PROBABLY COMPATIBLE

There may or may not be human pregnancy experience, but the characteristics of the drug suggest that it does not represent a significant risk to the embryo/fetus. For example, other drugs in the same class or with similar mechanisms are compatible or the drug does not obtain significant systemic concentrations. Any animal reproduction data are not relevant.

COMPATIBLE - MATERNAL BENEFIT >> EMBRYO/FETAL RISK

There may or may not be human pregnancy experience, but the potential maternal benefit far outweighs the known or unknown embryo/fetal risk. Animal reproduction data are not relevant.

HUMAN DATA SUGGEST LOW RISK

There is limited human pregnancy experience, either for the drug itself or drugs in the same class or with similar mechanisms of action, including the 1st trimester, suggesting that the drug does not represent a significant risk of developmental toxicity (growth retardation, structural defects, functional/behavioral defects, or death) at any time in pregnancy. The limited human pregnancy data outweighs any animal reproduction data.

NO (LIMITED) HUMAN DATA - ANIMAL DATA SUGGEST LOW RISK

Either there is no human pregnancy experience or the few pregnancy exposures have not been associated with developmental toxicity (growth retardation, structural defects, functional/behavioral defects, or death). The drug does not cause developmental toxicity (at doses that did not cause maternal toxicity) in all animal species studied at doses $\leq$10 times the human dose based on body surface area (e.g., mg/m^2) or AUC*.

NO (LIMITED) HUMAN DATA - ANIMAL DATA SUGGEST MODERATE RISK

Either there is no human pregnancy experience or the few pregnancy exposures have not been associated with developmental toxicity (growth retardation, structural defects, functional/behavioral defects, or death). The drug causes developmental toxicity (at doses that did not cause maternal toxicity) in one animal species at doses $\leq$10 times the human dose based on body surface area (e.g., mg/m^2) or AUC*.

NO (LIMITED) HUMAN DATA - ANIMAL DATA SUGGEST RISK

Either there is no human pregnancy experience or the few pregnancy exposures have not been associated with developmental toxicity (growth retardation, structural defects, functional/behavioral defects, or death). The drug causes developmental toxicity (at doses that did not cause maternal toxicity) in two animal species at doses $\leq$10 times the human dose based on body surface area (e.g., mg/m^2) or AUC*.

NO (LIMITED) HUMAN DATA - ANIMAL DATA SUGGEST HIGH RISK

Either there is no human pregnancy experience or the few pregnancy exposures have not been associated with developmental toxicity (growth retardation, structural defects, functional/behavioral defects, or death). The drug causes developmental toxicity (at doses

**AUC = area under the plasma concentration vs. time curve; a measure of the systemic exposure of a drug.*

that did not cause maternal toxicity) in three or more animal species at doses ≤ 10 times the human dose based on body surface area (e.g., mg/m^2) or AUC*.

CONTRAINDICATED - 1ST TRIMESTER

Human exposures in the 1st trimester, either to the drug itself or to drugs in the same class or with similar mechanisms of action, have been associated with developmental toxicity (growth retardation, structural defects, functional/behavioral defects, or death). The drug should not be used in the 1st trimester.

CONTRAINDICATED - 2ND AND 3RD TRIMESTERS

Human exposures in the 2nd and 3rd trimesters, either to the drug itself or to drugs in the same class or with similar mechanisms of action, have been associated with developmental toxicity (growth retardation, structural defects, functional/behavior defects, or death). The drug should not be used in the 2nd and 3rd trimesters.

CONTRAINDICATED

Human exposures at any time in pregnancy, either to the drug itself or to drugs in the same class or with similar mechanisms of action, have been associated with developmental toxicity (growth retardation, structural defects, functional/behavioral defects, or death). Animal reproduction data, if available, confirm the risk. The drug should not be used in pregnancy.

NO (LIMITED) HUMAN DATA - NO RELEVANT ANIMAL DATA

There is no human pregnancy data or relevant data in animals, or the human pregnancy experience, that may or may not include the 1st trimester, is limited. The risk in pregnancy cannot be assessed.

HUMAN DATA SUGGEST RISK IN 1ST AND 3RD TRIMESTERS

Evidence (for the drug or similar drugs) suggests that there may be an embryo/fetal risk for developmental toxicity (growth retardation, structural defects, functional/behavioral defects, or death) in the 1st and 3rd trimesters, but not in the 2nd trimester. The human pregnancy data outweigh any animal reproduction data.

HUMAN DATA SUGGEST RISK IN 2ND AND 3RD TRIMESTERS

Evidence (for the drug or similar drugs) suggests that there may be a fetal risk for developmental toxicity (growth retardation, structural defects, functional/behavioral defects, or death) in the 2nd and 3rd trimesters, but not in the 1st trimester. The human pregnancy data outweigh any animal reproduction data.

HUMAN DATA SUGGEST RISK IN 3RD TRIMESTER

Evidence (for the drug or similar drugs) suggests that there may be a fetal risk for developmental toxicity (growth retardation, structural defects, functional/behavioral defects, or death) in the 3rd trimester, or close to delivery, but not in the 1st or 2nd trimesters. The human pregnancy data outweigh any animal reproduction data.

HUMAN (AND ANIMAL) DATA SUGGEST RISK

The human data for the drug or drugs in the same class or with the same mechanism of action, and animal reproduction data if available, suggest there may be a risk for developmental toxicity (growth retardation, structural defects, functional/behavioral defects, or death) throughout pregnancy. Usually, pregnancy exposure should be avoided, but the risk may be acceptable if the maternal condition requires the drug.

DEFINITIONS OF BREAST FEEDING RECOMMENDATIONS

COMPATIBLE

Either the drug is not excreted in clinically significant amounts into human breast milk or its use during lactation does not, or is not expected to, cause toxicity in a nursing infant.

HOLD BREAST FEEDING

The drug may or may not be excreted into human breast milk, but the maternal benefit of therapy far outweighs the benefits of breast milk to an infant. Breast-feeding should be held until maternal therapy is completed and the drug has been eliminated (or reaches a low concentration) from her system.

NO (LIMITED) HUMAN DATA - PROBABLY COMPATIBLE

Either there is no human data or the human data are limited. The available animal or other data suggest that the drug does not represent a significant risk to a nursing infant.

NO (LIMITED) HUMAN DATA - POTENTIAL TOXICITY

Either there is no human data or the human data are limited. The characteristics of the drug suggest that it could represent a clinically significant risk to a nursing infant. Breast-feeding is not recommended.

NO (LIMITED) HUMAN DATA - POTENTIAL TOXICITY (MOTHER)

Either there is no human data or the human data are limited. The characteristics of the drug suggest that breast-feeding could represent a clinically significant risk to the mother (such as further loss of essential vitamins or nutrients). Breast-feeding is not recommended.

CONTRAINDICATED

There may or may not be human experience, but the combined data (including animal data if available) suggest that the drug may cause severe toxicity in a nursing infant, or breast-feeding is contraindicated because of the maternal condition for which the drug is indicated. Women should not breast-feed if they are taking the drug or have the condition.

RISK FACTORS

Risk Factors (A, B, C, D, X) have been assigned to all drugs, based on the level of risk the drug poses to the fetus. Risk Factors are designed to help the reader quickly classify a drug for use during pregnancy. They do not refer to breast-feeding risk. Because they tend to oversimplify a complex topic, they should always be used in conjunction with the Fetal Risk Summary. The definitions for the Factors are those used by the Food and Drug Administration (Federal Register 1980;44:37434–67). Many older drugs have not been given a letter rating by their manufacturers and the authors made the Risk Factor assignments. If the manufacturer rated its product in its professional literature, the Risk Factor will be shown with a subscript M (e.g., C_M). If the manufacturer and the authors differed in their assignment of a Risk Factor, our Risk Factor is marked with an asterisk and the manufacturer's rating is shown at the end of the Fetal Risk Summary. Other Risk Factors marked with an asterisk (e.g., sulfonamides, morphine, etc.) are drugs that present different risks to the fetus, depending on when or for how long they are used. In these cases, a second Risk Factor will be found with a short explanation at the end of the Fetal Risk Summary. We hope this will increase the usefulness of these ratings. The definitions used for the Risk Factors are presented below.

■ **Category A:** Controlled studies in women fail to demonstrate a risk to the fetus in the first trimester (and there is no evidence of a risk in later trimesters), and the possibility of fetal harm appears remote.

■ **Category B:** Either animal-reproduction studies have not demonstrated a fetal risk but there are no controlled studies in pregnant women or animal-reproduction studies have shown an adverse effect (other than a decrease in fertility) that was not confirmed in controlled studies in women in the first trimester (and there is no evidence of a risk in later trimesters).

■ **Category C:** Either studies in animals have revealed adverse effects on the fetus (teratogenic or embryocidal or other) and there are no controlled studies in women or studies in women and animals are not available. Drugs should be given only if the potential benefit justifies the potential risk to the fetus.

■ **Category D:** There is positive evidence of human fetal risk, but the benefits from use in pregnant women may be acceptable despite the risk (e.g., if the drug is needed in a life-threatening situation or for a serious disease for which safer drugs cannot be used or are ineffective).

■ **Category X:** Studies in animals or human beings have demonstrated fetal abnormalities or there is evidence of fetal risk based on human experience or both, and the risk of the use of the drug in pregnant women clearly outweighs any possible benefit. The drug is contraindicated in women who are or may become pregnant.

COMPARISON OF AGENTS WITHIN THE SAME PHARMACOLOGIC CLASS

The Appendix arranges the drugs by their pharmacologic category. This allows the reader to identify all of the drugs that have been reviewed within a specific category, thus allowing, if desired, a comparison of the drugs. For example, the subsection *Antihypertensives* lists together those agents used for this purpose under the general heading *Cardiovascular Drugs*. To assist the reader in locating an agent in the Appendix, page numbers (in parentheses) referring to the location in the Appendix have been added to the generic names (shown in **bold**) in the Index.

A

Name:	**ABACAVIR**	Risk Factor:	C_M
Class:	**Antiviral**		

FETAL RISK SUMMARY

RECOMMENDATION: Compatible - Maternal Benefit >> Embryo/Fetal Risk

Abacavir is a synthetic carbocyclic nucleoside analogue that is converted by cellular enzymes to the active metabolite, carbovir triphosphate. It is a nucleoside reverse transcriptase inhibitor (NRTI) used for the treatment of human immunodeficiency virus type 1 (HIV-1). Other drugs in this class are didanosine, lamivudine, stavudine, zalcitabine, and zidovudine.

In reproduction studies, doses of abacavir up to eight times the human therapeutic dose (HTD) based on body surface area comparisons had no effect on the fertility or mating performance of male and female rats (1). However, embryo toxicity (increased resorptions, decreased body weight) was observed. During organogenesis, doses up to 35 times the human exposure based on AUC (about 16 times the HTD) resulted in fetal growth retardation (reduced body weight and crown-rump length), and increased incidences of fetal anasarca and skeletal malformations. Offspring exposed from implantation through weaning had an increased incidence of stillbirth and, in survivors, decreased body weights throughout life. In contrast, no developmental toxicity or malformations were observed in rabbits at doses up to 8.5 times the human exposure based on AUC (1).

Abacavir is transferred across the rat placenta to the fetus (1). In an *ex vivo* human placental model, the antiviral agent also readily crossed to the fetal side with a high clearance index of about 50% that of antipyrine (2). This result is consistent with the relatively low molecular weight (about 671) and high lipophilic properties of the compound. No accumulation of the drug was found on the fetal side.

The Antiretroviral Pregnancy Registry reported, for the period January 1989 through January 2004, prospective data (reported to the Registry before the outcomes were known) involving 1,537 live births that had been exposed during the 1st trimester to one or more antiretroviral agents (3). Forty-seven of the newborns had congenital defects (3.1%, 95% confidence interval [CI] 2.3–4.1). In the 2407 live births with earliest exposure in the 2nd/3rd trimesters, there were 56 infants with defects (2.3%, 95% CI 1.8–3.0). The prevalence rates for the two periods did not differ significantly. There were 103 infants with birth defects among 3,944 live births with exposure anytime during pregnancy (2.6%, 95% CI 2.1–3.2). The prevalence rate did not differ significantly from the rate expected in a nonexposed population (3). There were 527 outcomes exposed to abacavir (223 in the 1st trimester and 304 in the 2nd/3rd trimesters) in combination with other antiretroviral agents. There were 9 (4.0%, 95% CI 1.9–7.5) birth defects among the 1st trimester exposures and 12 (3.9%, 95% CI 2.1–6.8) in those exposed in the 2nd/3rd trimesters (3).

In reviewing the birth defects of prospective and retrospective (pregnancies reported after the outcomes were known) registered cases, and clinical reports, the Registry concluded that there was no pattern of anomalies to suggest a common cause (3). (See Lamivudine for the required statement.)

In summary, the animal data suggest moderate embryo/fetal risk for toxicity and teratogenicity. Although limited, the human pregnancy experience does not suggest a risk of structural anomalies, but other developmental toxicities require study. Antiretroviral nucleosides have been shown to have a direct dose-related cytotoxic effect on preimplantation mouse embryos (see Didanosine, Stavudine, Zalcitabine, and Zidovudine). This toxicity has not been studied in humans. Mitochondrial dysfunction in offspring exposed *in utero* or postnatally to NRTIs has been reported (see Lamivudine and Zidovudine), but these findings are controversial and require confirmation.

Two reviews, one in 1996 and the other in 1997, concluded that all women currently receiving antiretroviral therapy should continue to receive therapy during pregnancy and that treatment of the mother with monotherapy should be considered inadequate therapy (4,5). In 1998, the Centers for Disease Control and Prevention (CDC) made a similar recommendation that antiretroviral therapy should be continued during pregnancy, but discontinuation of all therapy during the 1st trimester was a consideration (6). If indicated, therefore, abacavir should not be withheld in pregnancy (with the possible exception of the 1st trimester) because the expected benefit to the HIV-positive mother outweighs the unknown risk to the fetus. The efficacy and safety of combined therapy in preventing vertical transmission of HIV to the newborn, however, are unknown, and zidovudine remains the only antiretroviral agent recommended for this purpose (4,5).

BREAST FEEDING SUMMARY

RECOMMENDATION: Contraindicated

No reports have been located that describe the use of abacavir during human lactation. The molecular weight (about 671) is suggestive that the drug will be excreted into breast milk. The antiviral agent is excreted into the milk of lactating rats (1).

Reports on the use of abacavir during human lactation are unlikely because the drug is used in the treatment of HIV-1 infections. HIV-1 is transmitted in milk, and in developed countries, breast-feeding is not recommended (4,5,7–9). In developing countries, breast-feeding is undertaken, despite the risk, because there are no affordable milk substitutes available. Until 1999, no studies had been published that examined the effect of any antiretroviral therapy on HIV-1 transmission in milk. In that year, a study involving zidovudine was published that measured a 38% reduction in vertical transmission of HIV-1 infection in spite of breast-feeding when compared with controls (see Zidovudine).

References

1. Product information. Ziagen. Glaxo Wellcome, 2000.
2. Bawdon RE. The *ex vivo* human placental transfer of the anti-HIV nucleoside inhibitor abacavir and the protease inhibitor amprenavir. Infect Dis Obstet Gynecol 1998;6:244–6.
3. Antiretroviral Pregnancy Registry Steering Committee, Antiretroviral Pregnancy Registry International Interim Report for 1 January 1989 through 31 January 2004. Wilmington, NC: Registry Coordinating Center; 2004.
4. Carpenter CCJ, Fischi MA, Hammer SM, Hirsch MS, Jacobsen DM, Katzenstein DA, Montaner JSG, Richman DD, Saag MS, Schooley RT, Thompson MA, Vella S, Yeni PG, Volberding PA. Antiretroviral therapy for HIV infection in 1996. JAMA 1996;276;146–54.
5. Minkoff H, Augenbraun M. Antiretroviral therapy for pregnant women. Am J Obstet Gynecol 1997;176:478–89.
6. CDC. Public Health Service Task Force recommendations for the use of antiretroviral drugs in pregnant women infected with HIV-1 for maternal health and for reducing perinatal HIV-1 transmission in the United States. MMWR 1998;47:No. RR-2.
7. Brown ZA, Watts DH. Antiviral therapy in pregnancy. Clin Obstet Gynecol 1990;33:276–89.
8. de Martino M, Tovo P-A, Pezzotti P, Galli L, Massironi

E, Ruga E, Floreea F, Plebani A, Gabiano C, Zuccotti GV. HIV-1 transmission through breast-milk: appraisal of risk according to duration of feeding. AIDS 1992;6:991–7.

9. Van de Perre P. Postnatal transmission of human immunodeficiency virus type 1: the breast feeding dilemma. Am J Obstet Gynecol 1995;173:483–7.

Name:	**ABCIXIMAB**	Risk Factor:	C_M
Class:	**Hematologic Agent (Antiplatelet)**		

FETAL RISK SUMMARY

RECOMMENDATION: Compatible - Maternal Benefit >> Embryo/Fetal Risk

Abciximab, the Fab fragment of the chimeric human-murine monoclonal antibody 7E3, binds to the GP IIb/IIIa receptor on human platelets and inhibits platelet aggregation. It also binds to vessel wall endothelial and smooth muscle cells. Abciximab is indicated as an adjunct to percutaneous coronary intervention for the prevention of cardiac ischemic complications. It increases the risk of bleeding, especially when used with heparin and other anticoagulants or thrombolytics (1).

Animal reproduction studies have not been conducted with abciximab. No mutagenicity was observed with *in vitro* and *in vivo* tests, but long-term animal studies to detect carcinogenicity or adverse effects on fertility have not been conducted (1).

Using an *in vitro* perfused human placenta, researchers found that only pharmaceutically insignificant amounts of abciximab could be detected in the fetal circuit. Minute amounts of abciximab were found, however, on fetal platelets, but not on the endothelium or smooth muscle of fetal blood vessels, indicating that some transfer had taken place (2).

A 1998 case described the treatment of an acute myocardial infarction in a 30-year-old woman at 38 weeks' gestation (3). Since her condition did not improve with aspirin, heparin, nitrates, or balloon angioplasty after an abciximab infusion was started, a stent was placed in the partially occluded left anterior descending coronary artery. The drug infusion was continued for 12 hours. Adequate blood flow was re-established in the artery. Postoperatively, the woman was treated with ticlopidine, aspirin, and an unspecified β-blocker. Two weeks later, she delivered a healthy baby boy vaginally, with no evidence of bleeding and a normal ductus arteriosus. No excessive maternal bleeding was observed (3).

In summary, only one case report has described the use of abciximab during human pregnancy. In addition, the reproduction effects of the drug, if any, have not been studied in animals. However, the placental perfusion study above indicates that abciximab does not reach the fetus in clinically significant amounts. The primary risk, therefore, appears to be from maternal hemorrhage during drug administration. If this is adequately controlled, the benefits of the drug to the mother appear to far outweigh the unknown risks to the fetus.

BREAST FEEDING SUMMARY

RECOMMENDATION: Compatible

No reports describing the use of abciximab during lactation have been located. Because of the indications for abciximab, it is doubtful that such reports will be forthcoming. The very high molecular weight of the drug (about 48,000) suggests that it will not be excreted into milk in clinically significant amounts. Therefore, the risk to a nursing infant appears to be nil.

References

1. Product information. Reopro. Eli Lilly, 2004.
2. Miller RK, Mace K, Polliotti B, DeRita R, Hall W, Treacy G. Marginal transfer of ReoPro™ (abciximab) compared with immunoglobulin G (F105), inulin and water in the perfused human placenta in vitro. Placenta 2003;24:727–38.
3. Sebastian C, Scherlag M, Kugelmass A, Schechter E. Primary stent implantation for acute myocardial infarction during pregnancy: use of abciximab, ticlopidine, and aspirin. Cathet Cardiovasc Diagn 1998;45:275–9.

Name:	**ACARBOSE**	Risk Factor:	B_M
Class:	**Antidiabetic**		

FETAL RISK SUMMARY

RECOMMENDATION: Limited Human Data - Animal Data Suggest Low Risk

Acarbose is an oral α-glucosidase inhibitor that delays the digestion of ingested carbohydrates within the gastrointestinal tract, thereby reducing the rise in blood glucose after meals (1). It is used in the management of non-insulin-dependent diabetes mellitus (type II). Less than 2% of a dose is absorbed as active drug in adults, but the systemic absorption of metabolites is much higher (about 34% of the dose) (1).

Reproductive studies in rats found no evidence of impaired fertility or reproductive performance (1). Doses of acarbose up to 9 and 32 times the human dose in pregnant rats and rabbits, respectively, were not teratogenic in either species or, at 10 times the human dose, embryotoxic in rabbits (1).

A 1998 non-interventional observational cohort study described the outcomes of pregnancies in women who had been prescribed one or more of 34 newly marketed drugs by general practitioners in England (2). Data were obtained by questionnaires sent to the prescribing physicians one month after the expected or possible date of delivery. In 831 (78%) of the pregnancies, a newly marketed drug was thought to have been taken during the 1st trimester with birth defects noted in 14 (2.5%) singleton births of the 557 newborns (10 sets of twins). In addition, two birth defects were observed in aborted fetuses. However, few of the aborted fetuses were examined. Acarbose was taken during the 1st trimester in five pregnancies. The outcomes of these pregnancies included two spontaneous abortions and three normal newborns (one premature) (2).

A 2002 abstract reported the pregnancy outcomes (birth weight and gestational age at delivery) of 91 women at ≥20 weeks' gestation that were either treated with acarbose ($N = 45$) or insulin ($N = 46$) for gestational diabetes mellitus (3). The women had failed to achieve glucose goals with diet alone. In the oral group, 6% were changed to insulin because they were unable to tolerate acarbose (gastrointestinal complaints). There was no difference in the pregnancy outcomes between the groups.

A 2002 report described the use of acarbose (200 mg/day) in early pregnancy (4). A 35-year-old woman with several diseases (hypertension, diabetes mellitus, hypercholesterolemia, anxiety disorder, epilepsia, and morbid obesity) conceived while being treated with multiple drugs: rosiglitazone, gliclazide (a sulfonylurea), atorvastatin, spironolactone, hydrochlorothiazide, carbamazepine, thioridazine, amitriptyline, chlordiazepoxide, and pipenzolate bromide (an anti-spasmodic). Her pregnancy was diagnosed in the 8th week of gestation and all medications were stopped. She was treated with methyldopa and insulin for the remainder of her pregnancy. At 36 weeks' gestation, a repeat cesarean section delivered a healthy, 3.5-kg female infant with Apgar scores of 7 and 8 at 1 and 5 minutes, respectively. The infant was developing normally after 4 months (4).

In summary, less than 2% of acarbose is absorbed systemically, but several metabolites are absorbed in much greater proportions, and the embryo or fetal risk from any of these is unknown. Acarbose is normally used in combination with oral hypoglycemic agents, and these hypoglycemic drugs are not indicated for the pregnant diabetic as they may not provide good control in patients who cannot be controlled by diet alone (5). Carefully prescribed insulin therapy will provide better control of the mother's blood glucose, thereby preventing the fetal and neonatal complications that occur with this disease. High maternal glucose levels, as may occur in diabetes mellitus, are closely associated with a number of maternal and fetal effects, including fetal structural anomalies if the hyperglycemia occurs early in gestation. To prevent this toxicity, most experts, including the American College of Obstetricians and Gynecologists, recommend that insulin be used for types I and II diabetes occurring during pregnancy and, if diet therapy alone is not successful, for gestational diabetes (6,7).

BREAST FEEDING SUMMARY

RECOMMENDATION: No Human Data - Probably Compatible

Small amounts of acarbose, or its metabolites, are excreted in the milk of lactating rats (1). No studies describing the use of acarbose during human lactation have been located. Because the drug acts within the gastrointestinal tract to slow the absorption of ingested carbohydrates, and less than 2% of a dose is absorbed systemically, the amount of unmetabolized drug in the mother's circulation available for transfer to the milk is probably clinically insignificant. As with all drugs, however, the safest course while taking acarbose is not to breast-feed until data on its safety during lactation are available.

References

1. Product information. Precose. Bayer Corporation, 1997.
2. Wilton LV, Pearce GL, Martin RM, Mackay FJ, Mann RD. The outcomes of pregnancy in women exposed to newly marketed drugs in general practice in England. Br J Obstet Gynaecol 1998;105:882–9.
3. de Veciana M, Trail PA, Evans AT, Dulaney K. A comparison of oral acarbose and insulin in women with gestational diabetes mellitus (abstract). Obstet Gynecol 2002;99(Suppl):5S.
4. Yaris F, Yaris E, Kadioglu M, Ulku C, Kesim M, Kalyoncu NI. Normal pregnancy outcome following inadvertent exposure to rosiglitazone, gliclazide, and atorvastatin in a diabetic and hypertensive woman. Reprod Toxicol 2004;18:619–21.
5. Friend JR. Diabetes. Clin Obstet Gynecol 1981;8:353–82.
6. American College of Obstetricians and Gynecologists. Diabetes and pregnancy. *Technical Bulletin*. No. 200. December 1994.
7. Coustan DR. Management of gestational diabetes. Clin Obstet Gynecol 1991;34:558–64.

Name:	**ACEBUTOLOL**	Risk Factor:	$\mathbf{B_M}$*
Class:	**Sympatholytic (Antihypertensive)**		

FETAL RISK SUMMARY

RECOMMENDATION: Limited Human Data - Animal Data Suggest Low Risk

Acebutolol, a cardioselective β-adrenergic blocking agent, has been used for the treatment of hypertension occurring during pregnancy (1–5). The drug undergoes extensive first-pass hepatic metabolism after oral administration (absolute bioavailability about 40%) (6). The major metabolite, diacetolol, is equipotent to acebutolol (6).

In animal reproduction studies, no teratogenic effects were observed in pregnant rats and rabbits with doses up to about 32 times the maximum recommended human dose (MRHD) and up to about 7 times the MRHD, respectively (6). The maximum dose in rabbits produced slight intrauterine growth retardation (IUGR) that was thought to be secondary to maternal toxicity.

No human malformations attributable to acebutolol have been observed, but experience with the drug during the 1st trimester is lacking. In a study comparing three β-blockers, the mean birth weight of 56 newborns was slightly lower than 38 pindolol-exposed infants but higher than 31 offspring of atenolol-treated mothers (3160 g vs. 3375 g vs. 2745 g) (2). However, IUGR has been associated with β-blockers and the weight reduction may have been drug-induced (see last section below).

Acebutolol crosses the placenta, producing a maternal:cord ratio of 0.8 (3). The corresponding ratio for the active metabolite, diacetolol, was 0.6. Newborn serum levels of acebutolol and the metabolite were $<$5–244 ng/mL and 17–663 ng/mL, respectively (3). A cord:maternal ratio of 0.7 for acebutolol has also been reported (4).

In a comparison of 20 pregnant women treated with either acebutolol or methyldopa for mild to moderate hypertension, no differences between the drugs were found for pregnancy duration, birth weight, Apgar scores, or placental weight (5). In addition, no evidence of bradycardia, hypoglycemia, or respiratory problems was found in the acebutolol-exposed newborns. In an earlier study, however, 10 newborns exposed to acebutolol near term had blood pressures and heart rates significantly lower than similar infants exposed to methyldopa (7). The hemodynamic differences were still evident 3 days after birth. Mean blood glucose levels were not significantly lower than those of similar infants exposed to methyldopa, but transient hypoglycemia was present 3 hours after birth in four term newborns (5). The mean half-life of acebutolol in the serum of newborns has been calculated to be 10.1 hours, but the half-life based on urinary excretion was 15.6 hours (7). The manufacturer cites the elimination half-life of acebutolol in newborns as 6 to 14 hours, compared with a half-life for diacetolol of 24 to 30 hours during the first 24 hours, then 12 to 16 hours thereafter (6). Therefore, newborn infants of women consuming the drug near delivery should be closely observed for signs and symptoms of β-blockade for at least 3 to 4 days to allow for elimination of the parent and active metabolite from the infant. Long-term effects of *in utero* exposure to β-blockers have not been studied but warrant evaluation.

Some β-blockers may cause IUGR and reduced placental weight, especially those lacking intrinsic sympathomimetic activity (ISA) (i.e., partial agonist). Treatment beginning early in the 2nd trimester results in the greatest weight reductions, whereas treatment restricted to the 3rd trimester primarily affects only placental weight. Acebutolol does possess ISA. However, IUGR and reduced placental weight may potentially occur with all agents within this class. Although growth retardation is a serious concern, the benefits of maternal therapy with β-blockers in some cases might outweigh the risks to the fetus and must be judged on a case-by-case basis.

[*Risk Factor D if used in 2nd and 3rd trimesters.*]

BREAST FEEDING SUMMARY

RECOMMENDATION: Limited Human Data - Potential Toxicity

Acebutolol and its active metabolite, diacetolol, are excreted into breast milk (3,8). Milk:plasma ratios for the two compounds were 7.1 and 12.2, respectively (3). Absorption of both compounds was demonstrated in breast-feeding infants, but no adverse effects were mentioned (3). In a study of seven nursing, hypertensive mothers treated with 200–1200 mg/day within 13 days of delivery, milk:plasma acebutolol ratios in three varied from 2.3 to 9.2, whereas similar ratios of the metabolite ranged from 1.5 to 13.5 (8). The highest milk concentration of acebutolol, 4123 ng/mL, occurred in a mother taking 1200 mg/day. Two to three days after treatment was stopped, milk:plasma ratios of acebutolol and the metabolite in the seven women were 1.9–9.8 and 2.3–24.7, respectively (8). Symptoms of β-blockade (hypotension, bradycardia, and transient tachypnea) were observed in one nursing infant, although the time of onset of the adverse effects was not given. Neonatal plasma concentrations of the drug and metabolite (specific data not given), which were already high from *in utero* exposure, rose sharply after nursing commenced. The mother was taking 400 mg/day, and her milk:plasma ratios of acebutolol and metabolite during treatment were 9.2 and 13.5, respectively, the highest observed in this study. Breast-fed infants of mothers taking acebutolol should be closely observed for hypotension, bradycardia, and other signs or symptoms of β-blockade. Long-term effects of exposure to β-blockers from milk have not been studied but warrant evaluation. The American Academy of Pediatrics classifies acebutolol as a drug that has been associated with adverse effects in nursing infants (9).

References

1. Dubois D, Petitcolas J, Temperville B, Klepper A. Beta blockers and high-risk pregnancies. Int J Biol Res Pregnancy 1980;1:141–5.
2. Dubois D, Petitcolas J, Temperville B, Klepper A, Catherine P. Treatment of hypertension in pregnancy with B-adrenoceptor antagonists. Br J Clin Pharmacol 1982;13(Suppl):375S–8S.
3. Bianchetti G, Dubruc C, Vert P, Boutroy MJ, Morselli PL. Placental transfer and pharmacokinetics of acebutolol in newborn infants (abstract). Clin Pharmacol Ther 1981;29:233–4.
4. Boutroy MJ. Fetal and neonatal effects of the beta-adrenoceptor blocking agents. Dev Pharmacol Ther 1987;10:224–31.
5. Williams ER, Morrissey JR. A comparison of acebutolol with methyldopa in hypertensive pregnancy. Pharmatherapeutica 1983;3:487–91.
6. Product information. Sectral. Wyeth-Ayerst Pharmaceuticals, 2000.
7. Dumez Y, Tchobroutsky C, Hornych H, Amiel-Tison C. Neonatal effects of maternal administration of acebutolol. Br Med J 1981;283:1077–9.
8. Boutroy MJ, Bianchetti G, Dubruc C, Vert P, Morselli PL. To nurse when receiving acebutolol: is it dangerous for the neonate? Eur J Clin Pharmacol 1986;30:737–9.
9. Committee on Drugs, American Academy of Pediatrics. The transfer of drugs and other chemicals into human milk. Pediatrics 2001;108:776–89.

Name:	**ACETAMINOPHEN**	Risk Factor:	**B**
Class:	**Analgesic/Antipyretic**		

FETAL RISK SUMMARY

RECOMMENDATION: Compatible

Acetaminophen is routinely used during all stages of pregnancy for pain relief and to lower elevated body temperature. The drug crosses the placenta (1). In therapeutic doses, it is apparently safe for short-term use. However, continuous, high daily dosage in one mother probably caused severe anemia (possibly hemolytic) in her and fatal kidney disease in her newborn (2).

The pharmacokinetics of acetaminophen in pregnancy have been reported (3,4). In six healthy women who ingested a 1,000-mg dose at 36 weeks' gestation and again 6 weeks after delivery, the mean serum half-lives were similar, 3.7 hours and 3.1 hours, respectively (3). The absorption, metabolism, and renal clearance of the drug were similar in the pregnant and nonpregnant states. A 1994 study compared the pharmacokinetics of a single 650-mg acetaminophen oral dose in 10 nonpregnant women (controls) with eight women at a mean gestational age of 11.1 weeks (4). Among the pharmacokinetic parameters evaluated, significant differences between the pregnant vs. controls were found for elimination constant (0.431 vs. 0.348/hr), serum half-life (1.62 vs. 2.02 hours), and clearance (7.14 vs. 5.22 L/hr·kg).

The potential for acetaminophen-induced fetal liver toxicity after a toxic maternal dose was first suggested in 1979 (5). Two recent reports have described such toxicity (6,7). A woman, in her 27th–28th week of pregnancy, ingested 29.5 g of acetaminophen over less than 24 hours for severe dental pain (6). Fetal movements were last felt about 23 hours after the first dose, and on presentation to the hospital 16 hours later, no fetal heart beat was heard. The mother eventually recovered, although her serum levels of acetaminophen by extrapolation were thought to exceed 300 μg/mL, a toxic level. Autopsy of the 2190-g female fetus revealed a liver acetaminophen concentration of 250 μg/g of tissue. The extensive lysis of the fetal liver and kidneys, which may have been caused by autolysis before delivery (approximately 3 days after the mother last felt fetal movement), prevented documentation of the characteristic lesions observed in acetaminophen overdose (6).

A 1997 report described the fatal outcomes of a 38-year-old woman and her fetus at 31 weeks' gestation after she consumed an acute 35 g acetaminophen dose (7). The woman presented to the hospital 26 hours after the overdose with signs and symptoms of hepatorenal failure. On admission, she had a toxic acetaminophen serum level (40.43 μg/mL) which was predictive of a very high risk of hepatocellular damage and subsequent fulminant liver failure (7). IV administration of *N*-acetylcysteine was started 30 minutes after admission. Severe fetal distress was diagnosed 30 minutes later and a cesarean section under spinal anesthesia was performed to deliver a 1,620-g female infant who had Apgar scores of 0, 0, and 1 at 1, 5, and 10 minutes, respectively. The infant's acetaminophen serum level was 41.42 μg/mL. Despite intensive therapy, the infant died 34 hours after birth and the mother died 66 hours after the overdose. Although the infant's laboratory data indicated hepatorenal toxicity, the actual cause of death could not be determined as permission for autopsy was refused (7).

In four other cases of acute overdosage, acetaminophen-induced fetal liver toxicity was apparently not observed, although such damage may have resolved before delivery in some cases (8–11). One woman, at 36 weeks' gestation, consumed a single dose of 22.5 g of acetaminophen, producing toxic blood levels of 200 μg/mL (8). She was delivered of a normal infant approximately 6 weeks later. In another case, a woman at 20 weeks' gestation consumed a total of 25 g in two doses during a 10-hour period (9). She gave birth at 41 weeks to a normal infant with an occipital cephalohematoma as a result of birth position. At 24 hours of age, the infant had jaundice that responded to phototherapy. No evidence of permanent liver damage was observed. The jaundice was thought to have been caused by the cephalohematoma. A third case of acute maternal overdose occurred at 15.5 weeks of gestation when a mother ingested 64 g of the drug (10). Her acetaminophen level 10 hours after the ingestion was 198.5 μg/mL. Marked hepatic necrosis and adult respiratory distress syndrome (because of aspiration pneumonia) ensued and then gradually resolved. The patient was discharged home approximately 3 weeks after ingestion and subsequently was delivered of a healthy 2,000-g male infant at 32 weeks' gestation. The infant had physiologic hyperbilirubinemia with a peak level on the 4th day of life of 10.3 mg/dL, but phototherapy was not required. Follow-up evaluation at 4 months indicated normal development. One case involved a 22-year-old woman in her

31st week of pregnancy who consumed a 15-g dose, followed by a 50-g dose 1 week later (11). Fetal distress was observed 16 hours after the second overdose, as evidenced by a complete lack of fetal movements and breathing, a marked decrease in fetal heart rate beat-to-beat variability with no accelerations, and a falling baseline rate. Because of the fetal condition, labor was induced (cesarean section was excluded because of the mother's incipient hepatic failure). Eighty-four hours after the overdose, a healthy 2198-g female infant was delivered with Apgar scores at 1 and 5 minutes of 9 and 10, respectively. Except for hypoglycemia, mild respiratory disease, and mild jaundice, the newborn did well. Liver enzymes were always within the normal range, and the jaundice was compatible with immaturity. Acetaminophen was not detected in the cord blood. Follow-up examinations of the infant at 6 weeks and again at 6 months were normal. In each of these instances, protection against serious or permanent liver damage was probably afforded by the prompt administration of intravenous *N*-acetylcysteine.

A 1993 report described a 25-year-old woman at 27 weeks' gestation who consumed 12.5–15 g of acetaminophen as a single dose 36 hours before admission for premature labor (12). She had also consumed an unknown amount of the drug over a few days before the acute overdose. Because of severe fetal distress, a cesarean section was performed under general anesthesia before her preoperative laboratory tests indicating liver failure were available. A 1300-g male infant was delivered who had Apgar scores of 1, 4, and 4 at 1, 5, and 10 minutes, respectively. No mention was made of hepatic or other toxicity in the infant and his course was thought to be satisfactory for his gestational age. The mother was treated for progressive liver failure and eventually recovered.

The Rocky Mountain Poison and Drug Center reported the results of a nationwide study on acetaminophen overdose during pregnancy involving 113 women (13). Of the 60 cases that had appropriate laboratory and pregnancy outcome data, 19 occurred during the 1st trimester, 22 during the 2nd trimester, and 19 during the 3rd trimester. In those cases with a potentially toxic serum level of acetaminophen, early treatment with *N*-acetylcysteine was statistically associated with an improved pregnancy outcome by lessening the incidence of spontaneous abortion and fetal death. Only one congenital anomaly was observed in the series and that involved a 3rd trimester overdose with nontoxic maternal acetaminophen serum levels (13). Based on these observations, neither acetaminophen nor *N*-acetylcysteine were likely teratogens, although follow-up data on the infants were not available (13).

A Teratology Information Service in England conducted a prospective study of the pregnancy outcomes of 300 women who had consumed an overdose of acetaminophen, either alone, or as a combination product (14). The overdoses occurred in all trimesters: 118 (39.3%), 103 (34.3%), and 79 (26.3%) in the 1st, 2nd, and 3rd trimesters, respectively. Systemic antidote treatment consisted of *N*-acetylcysteine ($N = 33$), ipecac ($N = 52$), and methionine ($N = 16$). In the remaining 199 cases, treatment was not recorded or not given, or a variety of nonsystemic treatments (charcoal, gastric lavage, or miscellaneous) were used. The fetal outcomes included 219 (72%) normal infants (two sets of twins), 16 (5%) spontaneous abortions (10 within 3 weeks of the overdose), 2 (1%) late fetal deaths, 54 (18%) elective abortions (1 with a diaphragmatic hernia), and 11 (4%) newborns with malformations (exposed between 16 and 32 weeks' gestation). All of the spontaneous abortions and one late fetal death occurred after 1st trimester overdoses. The other late fetal death followed a 2nd trimester overdose. The majority of the elective abortions were conducted for "social," rather than medical reasons. Malformations included one each of systolic murmur, small port wine stain on occiput, cleft lip and palate, bilateral inguinal hernia, soft palate defect, spina bifida occulta/bilateral squint, hypospadias, and ptosis of left eye. There were three cases of talipes. The malformation rate was within the expected rate in England and none of the cases, including the one case of diaphragmatic hernia, can be related to acetaminophen (14). Seven full-term newborns had neonatal complications (all exposed during the 2nd or 3rd trimesters). The complications do not appear to be related to acetaminophen overdose (14). Moreover, evaluations up to at least 6 weeks of age did not demonstrate any clinical signs of renal or hepatotoxicity.

The Collaborative Perinatal Project monitored 50,282 mother-child pairs, 226 of whom had 1st trimester exposure to acetaminophen (15, pp. 286–295). Although no evidence was found to suggest a relationship to large categories of major or minor malformations, a possible association with congenital dislocation of the hip based on three cases was found, but independent confirmation is required (15, p. 471). For use anytime during pregnancy, 781 exposures were recorded (15, p. 434). As with the qualifications expressed for 1st trimester exposure, possible associations with congenital dislocation of the hip (eight cases) and clubfoot (six cases) were found (15, p. 484).

A 1982 report described craniofacial and digital anomalies in an infant exposed *in utero* to large daily doses of acetaminophen and propoxyphene throughout pregnancy (16). The infant also exhibited withdrawal symptoms as a result of the propoxyphene (see also Propoxyphene). The authors speculated with caution that the combination of propoxyphene with other drugs, such as acetaminophen, might have been teratogenic. In a study examining 6,509 women with live births, acetaminophen with or without codeine was used by 697 (11%) during the 1st trimester (17). No evidence of a relationship to malformations was observed.

In a surveillance study of Michigan Medicaid recipients conducted between 1985 and 1992 involving 229,101 completed pregnancies, 9,146 newborns had been exposed to acetaminophen during the 1st trimester (F. Rosa, personal communication, FDA, 1993). A total of 423 (4.6%) major birth defects were observed (416 expected). Specific data were available for six defect categories, including (observed/expected) 87/91 cardiovascular defects, 16/16 oral clefts, 4/7 spina bifida, 30/27 polydactyly, 14/16 limb reduction defects, and 16/22 hypospadias. These data do not support an association between the drug and the defects.

Using data from the North Jutland Pharmaco-Epidemiological Prescription Database in Denmark, investigators identified 123 women who had received a prescription for acetaminophen during pregnancy and/or 30 days before conception (18). The pregnancy outcomes of these women were compared with 13,329 controls who had received no prescriptions. Among the offspring of the 55 women who had received an acetaminophen prescription up to 30 days before conception and/or during the 1st trimester, there were six (10.9%) infants with congenital malformations compared with 697 (5.2%) from controls. The odds ratio (OR) for malformations was 2.3 (95% CI 1.0–5.4). The six malformations were ventricular septal defect, two congenital dislocations of the hip, stenosis of tear canal, diaphragmatic hernia, and megalocornea (keratoglobus). The nature of the defects do not indicate a causal relationship to acetaminophen (18). No increased risk of malformation was found when the analysis was restricted to primigravidas (OR 0.7, 95% CI 0.1–5.5) (18). In addition, no effect was observed on fetal growth.

Unlike aspirin, acetaminophen does not affect platelet function, and there is no increased risk of hemorrhage if the drug is given to the mother at term (19,20). In a study examining intracranial hemorrhage in premature infants, the incidence of bleeding after exposure of the fetus to acetaminophen close to birth was no different from that in nonexposed control infants (see also Aspirin) (21).

A 1993 study examined the effect of therapeutic levels of acetaminophen on prostacyclin (PGI_2) production by endothelial cells isolated from human umbilical veins in culture and during the 3rd trimester in women with either hypertension or various complications of pregnancy (22). The drug reduced the production of PGI_2 in culture and during pregnancy, but thromboxane (TxA_2) production was not affected in the women. A balance between PGI_2 and TxA_2 is thought to be critical during pregnancy. PGI_2, derived from endothelial cells, is vasodilatory and antiaggregatory, compared with the platelet-derived TxA_2, which is vasoconstrictive and proaggregatory (22). PGI_2 production increases normally during pregnancy, but this increase is markedly inhibited in pregnancy-induced hypertension (PIH) (22). Thus, a significant acetaminophen-induced reduction in PGI_2 production could adversely affect pregnancies complicated by PIH, including those treated with low-dose aspirin (see Aspirin). Because the effects of acetaminophen on PGI_2 are known to be tissue-specific, the authors of this study cautioned that additional studies, such as those measuring the effect of acetaminophen on placental PGI_2 and in patients being treated with low-dose aspirin for PIH, are required before the clinical significance of their findings can be determined (22).

In a prospective study of 1529 pregnant women studied in the mid-1970s, acetaminophen was used in the first half of pregnancy by 41% (23). Using a computerized system for stratifying on maternal alcohol and smoking histories, 421 newborns were selected for follow-up. Of this group, 43.5% had been exposed *in utero* to acetaminophen in the first half of pregnancy. After statistical control of numerous potentially confounding covariates, the data indicated that acetaminophen was not significantly related to child IQ at 4 years of age or to attention variables (see Aspirin for opposite results). Three physical growth parameters (height, weight, and head circumference) were also not significantly related to *in utero* acetaminophen exposure.

Acetaminophen has been used as an antipyretic just before delivery in women with fever secondary to chorioamnionitis (24). A significant improvement in fetal and newborn status, as measured by fetal heart rate tracings and arterial blood gases, was observed after normalization of the mother's temperature.

BREAST FEEDING SUMMARY

RECOMMENDATION: Compatible

Acetaminophen is excreted into breast milk in low concentrations (25–29). A single case of maculopapular rash on a breast-feeding infant's upper trunk and face was described in 1985 (25). The mother had taken 1 g of the drug at bedtime for 2 days before the onset of the symptoms. The rash resolved 24 hours after discontinuing acetaminophen. Two weeks later, the mother took another 1-g dose, and the rash recurred in the infant after breast feeding at 3, 8, and 12 hours after the dose. Milk levels at 2.25 and 3.25 hours after the dose were 5.78/7.10 μg/mL (right/left breasts) and 3.80/5.95 μg/mL (right/left breasts), respectively. These represented milk:plasma ratios of 0.76 and 0.50, respectively.

Unpublished data obtained from one manufacturer showed that after an oral dose of 650 mg, an average milk level of 11 μg/mL occurred (personal communication, McNeil Laboratories, 1979). Timing of the samples was not provided.

In 12 nursing mothers (nursing 2–22 months) given a single oral dose of 650 mg, peak levels of acetaminophen occurred at 1–2 hours in the range of 10–15 μg/mL (26). Assuming 90 mL of milk were ingested at 3-, 6-, and 9-hour intervals after ingestion, the amount of drug available to the infant was estimated to range from 0.04% to 0.23% of the maternal dose. After ingestion of a single analgesic combination tablet containing 324 mg of phenacetin, average milk levels of acetaminophen, the active metabolite, were 0.89 μg/mL (27). Milk:plasma ratios at 1 and 12 hours were 0.91 and 1.42, with a milk half-life of 4.7 hours, as compared with 3.0 hours in the serum. Repeated doses at 4-hour intervals were expected to result in a steady-state concentration of 2.69 μg/mL. In three lactating women, a mean milk:plasma ratio of 0.76 was reported after a single oral dose of 500 mg of acetaminophen (28). In this case, the mean serum and milk half-lives were 2.7 and 2.6 hours, respectively. Peak milk concentrations of 4.2 μg/mL occurred at 2 hours. In a more recent study, the calculated milk:plasma ratio was approximately 1.0 (29). Based on a dose of 1000 mg, the estimated maximum dose the infant could ingest was 1.85% of the maternal dose. Except for the single case of rash, no other adverse effects of acetaminophen ingestion via breast milk have been reported. The American Academy of Pediatrics classifies acetaminophen as compatible with breast-feeding (30).

References

1. Levy G, Garretson LK, Soda DM. Evidence of placental transfer of acetaminophen. Pediatrics 1975;55:895.
2. Char VC, Chandra R, Fletcher AB, Avery GB. Polyhydramnios and neonatal renal failure—a possible association with maternal acetaminophen ingestion. J Pediatr 1975;86:638–9.
3. Rayburn W, Shukla U, Stetson P, Piehl E. Acetaminophen pharmacokinetics: comparison between pregnant and nonpregnant women. Am J Obstet Gynecol 1986;155:1353–6.
4. Beaulac-Baillargeon L, Rocheleau S. Paracetamol pharmacokinetics during the first trimester of human pregnancy. Eur J Clin Pharmacol 1994;46:451–4.
5. Rollins DE, Von Bahr C, Glaumann H, Moldens P, Rane H. Acetaminophen: potentially toxic metabolite formed by human fetal and adult liver microsomes and isolated fetal liver cells. Science 1979;205:1414–6.
6. Haibach H, Akhter JE, Muscato MS, Cary PL, Hoffmann MF. Acetaminophen overdose with fetal demise. Am J Clin Pathol 1984;82:240–2.
7. Wang P-H, Yang M-J, Lee W-L, Chao H-T, Yang M-L, Hung J-H. Acetaminophen poisoning in late pregnancy. A case report. J Reprod Med 1997;42:367–71.
8. Byer AJ, Taylor TR, Semmer JR. Acetaminophen overdose in the third trimester of pregnancy. JAMA 1982;247:3114–5.
9. Stokes IM. Paracetamol overdose in the second trimester of pregnancy. Case report. Br J Obstet Gynaecol 1984;91:286–8.
10. Ludmir J, Main DM, Landon MB, Gabbe SG. Maternal acetaminophen overdose at 15 weeks of gestation. Obstet Gynecol 1986;67:750–1.
11. Rosevear SK, Hope PL. Favourable neonatal outcome following maternal paracetamol overdose and severe fetal distress: case report. Br J Obstet Gynaecol 1989;96:491–3.
12. Friedman S, Gatti M, Baker T. Cesarean section after maternal acetaminophen overdose. Anesth Analg 1993;77:632–4.
13. Riggs BS, Bronstein AC, Kulig K, Archer PG, Rumack BH. Acute acetaminophen overdose during pregnancy. Obstet Gynecol 1989;74:247–53.
14. McElhatton PR, Sullivan FM, Volans GN. Paracetamol overdose in pregnancy analysis of the outcomes of 300 cases referred to the teratology information service. Reprod Toxicol 1997;11:85–94.
15. Heinonen OP, Slone D, Shapiro S. *Birth Defects and Drugs in Pregnancy*. Littleton, MA:Publishing Sciences Group, 1977.
16. Golden NL, King KC, Sokol RJ. Propoxyphene and acetaminophen: possible effects on the fetus. Clin Pediatr 1982;21:752–4.
17. Aselton P, Jick H, Milunsky A, Hunter JR, Stergachis A. First-trimester drug use and congenital disorders. Obstet Gynecol 1985;65:451–5.
18. Thulstrup AM, Sorensen HT, Nielsen GL, Andersen L, Barrett D, Vilstrup H, Olsen J, and the EuroMap Study Group. Fetal growth and adverse birth outcomes in women receiving prescriptions for acetaminophen during pregnancy. Am J Perinatol 1999;16:321–6.
19. Pearson H. Comparative effects of aspirin and acetaminophen on hemostasis. Pediatrics 1978;62(Suppl):926–9.
20. Rudolph AM. Effects of aspirin and acetaminophen in pregnancy and in the newborn. Arch Intern Med 1981;141:358–63.
21. Rumack CM, Guggenheim MA, Rumack BH, Peterson RG, Johnson ML, Braithwaite WR. Neonatal intracranial hemorrhage and maternal use of aspirin. Obstet Gynecol 1981;58(Suppl):52S–6S.
22. O'Brien WF, Krammer J, O'Leary TD, Mastrogiannis DS. The effect of acetaminophen on prostacyclin production in pregnant women. Am J Obstet Gynecol 1993;168:1164–9.
23. Streissguth AP, Treder RP, Barr HM, Shepard TH, Bleyer WA, Sampson PD, Martin DC. Aspirin and acetaminophen use by pregnant women and subsequent child IQ and attention decrements. Teratology 1987;35:211–9.
24. Kirshon B, Moise KJ Jr, Wasserstrum N. Effect of acetaminophen on fetal acid-base balance in chorioamnionitis. J Reprod Med 1989;34:955–9.
25. Matheson I, Lunde PKM, Notarianni L. Infant rash caused by paracetamol in breast milk? Pediatrics 1985;76:651–2.
26. Berlin CM Jr, Yaffe SJ, Ragni M. Disposition of acetaminophen in milk, saliva, and plasma of lactating women. Pediatr Pharmacol 1980;1:135–41.
27. Findlay JWA, DeAngelis RL, Kearney MF, Welch RM, Findlay JM. Analgesic drugs in breast milk and plasma. Clin Pharmacol Ther 1981;29:625–33.
28. Bitzen PO, Gustafsson B, Jostell KG, Melander A, Wahlin Boll E. Excretion of paracetamol in human breast milk. Eur J Clin Pharmacol 1981;20:123–5.
29. Notarianni LJ, Oldham HG, Bennett PN. Passage of

paracetamol into breast milk and its subsequent metabolism by the neonate. Br J Clin Pharmacol 1987;24:63–7.
30. Committee on Drugs, American Academy of Pediatrics. The transfer of drugs and other chemicals into human milk. Pediatrics 2001;108:776–89.

Name:	**ACETAZOLAMIDE**	Risk Factor:	**C**
Class:	**Diuretic (Carbonic Anhydrase Inhibitor)**		

FETAL RISK SUMMARY

RECOMMENDATION: Compatible

Shepard reviewed six reproduction studies using acetazolamide in mice, rats, hamsters, and monkeys (1). Forelimb defects were observed in the fetuses of rodents, but not in those of monkeys. One of the studies found that potassium replacement reduced the risk of congenital defects in rats (1). A study with pregnant rabbits found that, with doses producing maternal acidosis and electrolyte changes, acetazolamide produced a dose-related increase in axial skeletal malformations (2). The combination of acetazolamide and amiloride was found to produce abnormal development of the ureter and kidney in fetal mice when given at the critical moment of ureter development (3).

Despite widespread usage, no reports linking the use of acetazolamide with congenital defects have been located. A single case of a neonatal sacrococcygeal teratoma has been described (4). The mother received 750 mg daily for glaucoma during the 1st and 2nd trimesters. A relationship between the drug and carcinogenic effects in the fetus has not been supported by other reports. Retrospective surveys on the use of acetazolamide during gestation have not demonstrated an increased fetal risk (5,6).

The Collaborative Perinatal Project monitored 50,282 mother-child pairs, 12 of whom had 1st trimester exposure to acetazolamide (7, p. 372). No anomalies were observed in the exposed offspring. For use anytime during pregnancy, 1,024 exposures were recorded (7, p. 441), and 18 infants were found to have malformations (18.06 expected). Thus, no evidence was found to suggest a relationship to large categories of major or minor malformations or to individual defects.

A woman with glaucoma was treated throughout pregnancy with acetazolamide, 250 mg twice daily, and topical pilocarpine and timolol (8). Within 48 hours of birth at 36 weeks' gestation, the infant's condition was complicated by hyperbilirubinemia and asymptomatic hypocalcemia, hypomagnesemia, and metabolic acidosis. The deficiencies of calcium and magnesium resolved quickly after treatment, as did the acidosis, even though the mother continued her medications while breast-feeding the infant. Mild hypertonicity of the lower limbs requiring physiotherapy was observed at 1-, 3-, and 8-month examinations (8). Two other healthy infants of an epileptic mother, treated throughout two pregnancies with acetazolamide 250 mg/day and carbamazepine, were delivered at term and showed no effects of exposure to the drugs (8).

BREAST FEEDING SUMMARY

RECOMMENDATION: Compatible

Acetazolamide is excreted into breast milk (9). A mother, 6 days postpartum, was given 500 mg (sustained-release formulation) twice daily for glaucoma, and she breast-fed her infant for the following week. Nursing was stopped after that time because of the mother's concerns about exposing the infant to the drug. However, no changes attributable to drug exposure were noted in the infant. Breast milk levels of acetazolamide on the 4th and 5th days of therapy, 1–9 hours after a maternal dose, varied between 1.3 and 2.1 μg/mL. A consistent relationship between concentration and time from last dose was not apparent. A milk:plasma ratio 1 hour after a dose was 0.25. Three plasma levels of acetazolamide in the infant were 0.2, 0.2, and 0.6 μg/mL. The authors estimated the infant ingested about 0.6 mg/day (i.e., 0.06% of the maternal dose) (9). The American Academy of Pediatrics classifies acetazolamide as compatible with breast-feeding (10).

References

1. Shepard TH. *Catalog of Teratogenic Agents*. 6th ed. Baltimore, MD: Johns Hopkins University Press, 1989:5–6.
2. Nakatsuka T, Komatsu T, Fujii T. Axial skeletal malformations induced by acetazolamide in rabbits. Teratology 1992;45:629–36.
3. Miller TA, Scott WJ Jr. Abnormalities in ureter and kidney development in mice give acetazolamide-amiloride or dimethadione (DMO) during embryogenesis. Teratology 1992;46:541–50.
4. Worsham GF, Beckman EN, Mitchell EH. Sacrococcygeal teratoma in a neonate. Association with maternal use of acetazolamide. JAMA 1978;240:251–2.
5. Favre-Tissot M, Broussole P, Robert JM, Dumont L. An original clinical study of the pharmacologic-teratogenic relationship. Ann Med Psychol 1964; 1:389. As cited in Nishimura H, Tanimura T, eds. *Clinical Aspects of The Teratogenicity of Drugs*. New York, NY: Excerpta Medica, 1976;210.
6. McBride WG. The teratogenic action of drugs. Med J Aust 1963;2:689–93.
7. Heinonen OP, Slone D, Shapiro S. *Birth Defects and Drugs in Pregnancy*. Littleton, MA: Publishing Sciences Group, 1977.
8. Merlob P, Litwin A, Mor N. Possible association between acetazolamide administration during pregnancy and metabolic disorders in the newborn. Eur J Obstet Gynecol Reprod Biol 1990;35:85–8.
9. Soderman P, Hartvig P, Fagerlund C. Acetazolamide excretion into human breast milk. Br J Clin Pharmacol 1984;17:599–60.
10. Committee on Drugs, American Academy of Pediatrics. The transfer of drugs and other chemicals into human milk. Pediatrics 2001;108:776–89.

Name:	**ACETOHEXAMIDE**	Risk Factor:	**C**
Class:	**Oral Hypoglycemic**		

FETAL RISK SUMMARY

RECOMMENDATION: Human Data Suggest Risk in 3rd Trimester

Acetohexamide is a sulfonylurea used for the treatment of adult-onset diabetes mellitus. It is not indicated for the pregnant diabetic. Shepard (1) and Schardein (2) cited a study in which acetohexamide was embryotoxic, but not teratogenic in rats.

When administered near term, acetohexamide crosses the placenta and may persist in the neonatal serum for several days (3). One mother, who took 1 g/day throughout pregnancy, was delivered of an infant whose serum level was 4.4 mg/dL at 10 hours of life (3). Prolonged symptomatic hypoglycemia because of hyperinsulinism lasted for 5 days. A 1971 reference briefly cited a case of prolonged hypoglycemia and convulsions in a newborn whose mother had taken acetohexamide during pregnancy (4).

Although teratogenic in animals, an increased incidence of congenital defects, other than that expected in diabetes mellitus, has not been found with acetohexamide (see also Chlorpropamide, Tolbutamide) (5–7). Insulin, however, is still the treatment of choice for this disease. Oral hypoglycemics are not indicated for the pregnant diabetic as they will not provide good control in patients who cannot be controlled by diet alone (8). Moreover, insulin, unlike acetohexamide, does not cross the placenta and, thus, eliminates the additional concern that the drug therapy itself is adversely affecting the fetus. Carefully prescribed insulin therapy will provide better control of the mother's blood glucose, thereby preventing the fetal and neonatal complications that occur with this disease. High maternal glucose levels, as may occur in diabetes mellitus, are closely associated with a number of maternal and fetal adverse effects, including fetal structural anomalies if the hyperglycemia occurs early in gestation. To prevent this toxicity, most experts, including the American College of Obstetricians and Gynecologists, recommend that insulin be used for types I and II diabetes occurring during pregnancy and, if diet therapy alone is not successful, for gestational diabetes (9,10). If acetohexamide is used during pregnancy, therapy should be changed to insulin and acetohexamide discontinued before delivery (the exact time before delivery is unknown) to lessen the possibility of prolonged hypoglycemia in the newborn.

BREAST FEEDING SUMMARY

RECOMMENDATION: No Human Data - Potential Toxicity

No reports describing the use of acetohexamide during lactation have been located. Other antidiabetic sulfonylurea agents are excreted into milk (e.g., see Chlorpropamide and Tolbutamide), and a similar excretion pattern for acetohexamide should be expected. The effect on the nursing infant from exposure to this drug via the milk is unknown, but hypoglycemia is a potential toxicity.

References

1. Shepard TH. *Catalog of Teratogenic Agents*. 8th ed. Baltimore, MD: Johns Hopkins University Press, 1995:4.
2. Schardein JL. *Chemically Induced Birth Defects*. 2nd ed. New York, NY: Marcel Dekker, 1993:417.
3. Kemball ML, McIver C, Milnar RDG, Nourse CH, Schiff D, Tiernan JR. Neonatal hypoglycaemia in infants of diabetic mothers given sulphonylurea drugs in pregnancy. Arch Dis Child 1970;45:696–701.
4. Harris EL. Adverse reactions to oral antidiabetic agents. Br Med J 1971;3:29–30.
5. Malins JM, Cooke AM, Pyke DA, Fitzgerald MG. Sulphonylurea drugs in pregnancy. Br Med J 1964; 2:187.
6. Adam PAJ, Schwartz R. Diagnosis and treatment: should oral hypoglycemic agents be used in pediatric and pregnant patients? Pediatrics 1968;42: 819–23.
7. Dignan PSJ. Teratogenic risk and counseling in diabetes. Clin Obstet Gynecol 1981;24:149–59.
8. Friend JR. Diabetes. Clin Obstet Gynaecol 1981;8: 353–82.
9. American College of Obstetricians and Gynecologists. Diabetes and pregnancy. *Technical Bulletin*. No. 200. December 1994.
10. Coustan DR. Management of gestational diabetes. Clin Obstet Gynecol 1991;34:558–64.

Name:	**ACETOPHENAZINE**	Risk Factor:	**C**
Class:	**Tranquilizer**		

FETAL RISK SUMMARY

RECOMMENDATION: No Human Data - No Relevant Animal Data

Acetophenazine is a piperazine phenothiazine in the same group as prochlorperazine (see Prochlorperazine). Phenothiazines readily cross the placenta (1). No specific information on the use of acetophenazine in pregnancy has been located. Although occasional reports have attempted to link various phenothiazine compounds with congenital malformations, the bulk of the evidence indicates that these drugs are safe for the mother and the fetus (see also Chlorpromazine).

A

BREAST FEEDING SUMMARY

RECOMMENDATION: No Human Data - Potential Toxicity

No data are available.

Reference

1. Moya F, Thorndike V. Passage of drugs across the placenta. Am J Obstet Gynecol 1962;84:1778–98.

Name:	**ACETYLCHOLINE**	Risk Factor:	**C**
Class:	**Parasympathomimetic (Cholinergic)**		

FETAL RISK SUMMARY

RECOMMENDATION: No Human Data - No Relevant Animal Data

Acetylcholine is used primarily in the eye. No reports of its use in pregnancy have been located. As a quaternary ammonium compound, it is ionized at physiologic pH, and transplacental passage in significant amounts would not be expected.

BREAST FEEDING SUMMARY

RECOMMENDATION: No Human Data - Probably Compatible

No data are available.

Name:	**ACETYLCYSTEINE**	Risk Factor:	**B_M**
Class:	**Respiratory Agent (Mucolytic), Antidote**		

FETAL RISK SUMMARY

RECOMMENDATION: Compatible - Maternal Benefits >> Embryo/Fetal Risk

Acetylcysteine (*N*-acetyl-L-cysteine) is a mucolytic agent indicated as adjuvant therapy in the treatment of abnormal, viscid, or inspissated mucous secretions in a variety of pulmonary conditions. It is also indicated as an antidote to prevent or lessen hepatic injury following the ingestion of potentially hepatic toxic doses of acetaminophen (1). Acetylcysteine has been used as an ophthalmic solution to treat keratoconjunctivitis sicca (dry eye) and as an enema for bowel obstruction due to meconium ileus (2), although these indications are not approved by the U. S. Food and Drug Administration. In mice, the agent has also demonstrated efficacy as a chelating agent to reduce organic mercury-induced developmental toxicity (3).

Reproductive studies with acetylcysteine have been conducted in rats and rabbits (1). Pregnant rabbits were given oral doses about three times the human mucolytic dose on days 6 to 16 of gestation. Additional pregnant rabbits were exposed to an aerosol of 10% acetylcysteine and 0.05% isoproterenol for 30 to 35 minutes twice daily from the 16th through the 18th day of gestation. No teratogenic effects were observed in either the oral or the aerosol studies. In pregnant rats, an aerosol combination of acetylcysteine and isoproterenol was given in a manner similar to that used in rabbits from the 6th through the 15th day of gestation. Other pregnant rats were exposed to the aerosol from the 15th through the 21st day of gestation. No teratogenic effects or maternal or fetal toxicity were observed in these studies (1).

Consistent with its low molecular weight (about 163), acetylcysteine crosses the human placenta. In a study of three pregnant women who delivered viable infants while undergoing treatment for acetaminophen toxicity, the mean acetylcysteine cord blood concentrations was 9.4 μg/mL (range 8.6–10.9 μg/mL) (4). The corresponding maternal serum concentrations (trough levels, 4 hours after a dose) ranged from 7.2 to 11.8 μg/mL. In a fourth nonviable infant, delivered at 22 weeks' gestation, the acetylcysteine level in a postmortem cardiac blood sample obtained 48 hours after death was 55.8 μg/mL. The mean cord blood level was within the range associated with therapeutic acetylcysteine doses in adults. No adverse effects attributable to acetylcysteine or acetaminophen were observed in the three viable infants, nor was there evidence of acetaminophen toxicity in the fourth infant (4).

The only published reports describing the use of acetylcysteine during human pregnancy involve the agent's use as an antidote following acute acetaminophen overdose (5–10). A case report published in 1982 described a woman at 36 weeks' gestation who took an overdose of acetaminophen (5). A few hours after the ingestion, acetylcysteine was administered (initial dose of 140 mg/kg IV, then 70 mg/kg IV every 4 hours for 17 doses). The mother made an uneventful recovery and 6 weeks later delivered a healthy 3.29-kg female infant with Apgar scores of 9 and 9 (5).

Two other case reports of maternal acetaminophen overdose, at 15 and 32 weeks' gestation, respectively, appeared in 1986 and 1989 (6,7). Both women were successfully treated with IV acetylcysteine. In the first case, a 2.00-kg male infant was eventually delivered at 32 weeks' gestation. He was developing normally at 4 months of age (6). Because of severe toxicity in the second woman and fetal distress, delivery was induced 84 hours after the overdose resulting in the birth of a healthy 2.198-kg female infant (7). Acetaminophen was not detected in the cord blood (no test for acetylcysteine was done). Except for hyperbilirubinemia of prematurity, the infant did well with no evidence of toxicity at follow-up examinations at 6 weeks and 6 months of age (7).

In a 1989 study from the Rocky Mountain Poison and Drug Center, covering 1976–1985, pregnancy outcomes were available for 60 of the 110 women who had an acute acetaminophen overdose during gestation (8). Of the 60 women, 24 were treated with IV acetylcysteine (4 in the 1st trimester) for toxic acetaminophen serum levels. The outcomes of the 24 cases were 14 viable infants (2 premature), 3 spontaneous abortions (SABs), 5 elective abortions, 1 stillbirth, and 1 maternal death. In the stillbirth case, the mother overdosed at 33 weeks' gestation with fetal death occurring 2 days later. An autopsy of the fetus revealed massive centrilobular hepatic necrosis that was consistent with acetaminophen-induced hepatotoxicity. Of the five potential independent variables evaluated, only two were significantly predictive of pregnancy outcome; time to start of acetylcysteine and gestational age. The probability of fetal death increased the longer it took to receive the antidote and the lower the gestational age. One infant was reported to have a mild positional deformity of the feet. No other congenital defects were reported (8).

A 1997 study from a Teratology Information Service in England reported the pregnancy outcomes of 300 cases of acute acetaminophen overdose (9). A total of 33 mothers

A

were treated with IV acetylcysteine. The outcomes of these cases were 24 normal infants, 3 SAB or fetal deaths, 5 elective terminations, and 1 infant with hypospadias. There was no relationship between the defect and either acetaminophen or acetylcysteine due to the timing of exposure. None of the other adverse outcomes were related to acetylcysteine (9).

In summary, acetylcysteine is not teratogenic or embryotoxic in experimental animals and, although the data are limited, does not appear to represent a risk to the human fetus when IV doses are used as an antidote for acute acetaminophen overdose. After IV administration, the drug crosses the placenta to achieve protective serum levels in the fetus. A 1999 report concluded that acetaminophen overdose in pregnant women should be managed the same way as in nonpregnant patients and that acetylcysteine therapy was protective to both the mother and the fetus (10). There is no reported human pregnancy experience after use of acetylcysteine as a mucolytic agent.

BREAST FEEDING SUMMARY

RECOMMENDATION: No Human Data - Probably Compatible

No reports have described the use of acetylcysteine during lactation. Although the molecular weight of the drug (about 163) is low enough for excretion into breast milk, the various conditions in which acetylcysteine is used suggests that the drug will rarely be prescribed during breast-feeding. Moreover, IV acetylcysteine has been administered directly to preterm neonates for therapeutic indications, at doses far above those that would be obtained from milk, without causing toxicity (11,12).

References

1. Product information. Acetylcysteine Solution, USP. Bedford Laboratories, 1999.
2. Acetylcysteine (*N*-Acetylcysteine). *Drug Facts and Comparisons*. St. Louis: Facts and Comparisons. January 2000.
3. Domingo JL. Developmental toxicity of metal chelating agents. Reprod Toxicol 1998;12:499–510.
4. Horowitz RS, Dart RC, Jarvie DR, Bearer CF, Gupta U. Placental transfer of *N*-acetylcysteine following human maternal acetaminophen toxicity. Clin Toxicol 1997;35:447–51.
5. Byer AJ, Traylor TR, Semmer JR. Acetaminophen overdose in the third trimester of pregnancy. JAMA 1982;247:3114–5.
6. Ludmir J, Main DM, Landon MB, Gabbe SG. Maternal acetaminophen overdose at 15 weeks of gestation. Obstet Gynecol 1986;67:750–1.
7. Rosevear SK, Hope PL. Favourable neonatal outcome following maternal paracetamol overdose and severe fetal distress. Case report. Br J Obstet Gynaecol 1989;96:491–3.
8. Riggs BS, Bronstein AC, Kulig K, Archer PG, Rumack BH. Acute acetaminophen overdose during pregnancy. Obstet Gynecol 1989;74:247–53.
9. McElhatton PR, Sullivan FM, Volans GN. Paracetamol overdose in pregnancy: analysis of the outcomes of 300 cases referred to the teratology information service. Reprod Toxicol 1997;11:85–94.
10. Zed PJ, Krenzelok EP. Treatment of acetaminophen overdose. Am J Health-Syst Pharm 1999;56:1081–91.
11. Ahola TM, Fellman V, Laaksonen R, Laitila J, Lapatto R, Neuvonen PJ, Raivio KO. Pharmacokinetics of intravenous N-acetylcysteine in preterm neonates (abstract). Pediatr Res 1998;43(Suppl 2):163.
12. Isbister GK, Bucens IK, Whyte IM. Paracetamol overdose in a preterm neonate. Arch Dis Child Fetal Neonat Ed 2001;85:F70–2.

Name:	**ACETYLDIGITOXIN**	Risk Factor:	**B**
Class:	**Cardiac Glycoside**		

See Digitalis.

Name:	**ACITRETIN**	Risk Factor:	X_M
Class:	**Vitamin/Psoralen**		

FETAL RISK SUMMARY

RECOMMENDATION: Contraindicated

Acitretin, an oral active synthetic retinoid and vitamin A derivative, is the active metabolite of etretinate (see also Etretinate). It is used for the treatment of severe psoriasis resistant to other forms of therapy and for severe congenital ichthyosis and keratosis follicularis (Darier's disease).

Similar to vitamin A and it derivatives, acitretin may cause congenital defects at human dosage levels in various animal species, including the mouse, rat, and rabbit (1). Fertility of rats was not impaired at the highest dose tested (3 mg/kg/day, or about 3 times the maximum recommended human dose). Chronic administration to male dogs (30 mg/kg/day) produced testicular changes: reversible mild to moderate spermatogenic arrest and the appearance of multinucleated giant cells (1).

After oral absorption, acitretin undergoes extensive metabolism and interconversion by simple isomerization to 13-*cis*-acitretin. When consumed with alcohol, acitretin may be converted back to etretinate, a retinoid with a very long elimination half-life (mean 120 days, but may be as long as 168 days). Because the prolonged elimination would increase the teratogenic potential for women of childbearing age (see also Etretinate), the manufacturer states that alcohol must not be ingested during therapy with acitretin and for 2 months after cessation of therapy because of the long elimination period of acitretin (1).

In a 1994 reference, the concentrations of etretinate, acitretin, and 13-*cis*-acitretin were measured in plasma and subcutaneous fat samples from 37 women of childbearing age (2). Twenty of the women were receiving acitretin and 17 had stopped. Sixteen of the 20 women who were current acitretin users had taken etretinate, but had stopped that drug a mean 45 ± 17 months before sampling, whereas four women had never received etretinate. Among current acitretin users, detectable etretinate levels in the plasma and subcutaneous fat were found in 45% and 83%, respectively. The 17 women who had stopped taking acitretin had been off the drug a mean 12 ± 10 months. Eleven of these women had also used etretinate but had stopped a mean 43 ± 14 months before sampling. The six women who had never taken etretinate stopped acitretin 17 ± 9 months before testing. Among these 17 women, etretinate was detected in 18% and 86%, respectively, of the plasma and subcutaneous fat samples. In some cases, acitretin and/or etretinate were detectable in plasma or subcutaneous fat up to 29 months after acitretin therapy had ceased. Thus, plasma concentrations correlated poorly with concentrations in fat. The findings led the authors to conclude that the recommended contraception period of 2 years after acitretin treatment (in 1994) was too short to avoid the risk of teratogenicity (2). Currently, the manufacturer recommends a contraception period of 3 years, but the human threshold concentration of acitretin below which the drug is not teratogenic has not been established (1).

A detailed case report of a pregnancy exposed to acitretin starting 10 days after conception and throughout the 1st trimester was published in 1995 (3). The 34-year-old woman was treated with acitretin (50 mg/day) for severe palmoplantar epidermolytic keratoderma. Pregnancy was diagnosed 6 weeks after stopping acitretin therapy. The pregnancy was terminated at 20 weeks' gestation with delivery of a stillborn, 210-g, 24-cm long male fetus with severe symmetric defects of the upper and lower limbs and craniofacial malformations (3). The extremity defects included bilateral short arms with pterygium formation in the elbows, shortened thumbs and little fingers without nails, contractures of both lower limbs in the groins and knees, irregularly thickened femora and tibiae, and point-shaped feet with only two small toes without nails (3). X-ray of the limbs revealed bilateral humeroradial synostosis and bone defects in the hands and feet. Craniofacial malformations included underdeveloped maxilla and mandibula, a small mouth with a high, arched and narrow palate, low-set ears, bilateral microtia, agenesis of the external ear canals, and bilateral preauricular tags (3). Except for an atrioventricular septal defect type II, no other anomalies were discovered on autopsy. Concentrations of acitretin, 13-*cis*-acitretin, and etretinate, in the maternal plasma, fetal brain and liver, and amniotic fluid 48 days after stopping therapy, were either undetectable (<0.3 ng/mL) or unquantifiable. An attempted chromosomal analysis of the fetus failed. Because the authors could find no other explanation for the malformations, including potential genetic defects, and the craniofacial malformations were similar to previous cases of retinoic acid embryopathy (e.g., see Isotretinoin), they concluded that the defects were caused by acitretin (3). In addition, the authors were aware of the poor correlation between plasma and fat concentrations of the vitamin A derivatives (see reference 2 above), so that the failure to detect the retinoids in the plasma did not affect their conclusion (3).

Authors of a study published in 1994 attempted to determine if there was a threshold dose or plasma concentration of acitretin below which there was no teratogenic risk in females (4). In various species, the highest non-teratogenic oral doses (mg/kg/day) were 1 (mouse), 7.5 (rat), and 0.2 (rabbit). No data were available for cynomolgus monkeys or humans. The authors also summarized the outcomes of pregnancies that had occurred during or after acitretin therapy and been reported to the manufacturer since human therapy with the drug began in 1983. A total of 75 women were either exposed to acitretin during pregnancy ($N = 8$) or before pregnancy ($N = 67$) (median time before pregnancy 5 months, range 6 weeks to 23 months). Among those exposed during pregnancy, there were four spontaneous abortions, one induced abortion (no information on the fetus), one induced abortion with typical malformations, one newborn with a non-typical anomaly, and one normal newborn. The mother of the fetus with typical malformations took 50 mg/day of acitretin during the first 19 weeks of gestation. Malformations in the fetus were microtia and defects of the face and extremities. The mother of the infant with a non-typical anomaly took acitretin (20 mg/day) during the first 8 months of pregnancy. The infant had a hearing impairment for high frequencies. The outcomes of the 67 pregnancies exposed before conception were 9 spontaneous abortions, 18 induced abortions (15 fetuses with no information, 3 normal fetuses), 4 newborns with non-typical abnormalities, and 36 normal newborns. One of the mothers who delivered an infant with non-typical malformations had received 1 week of acitretin, 25 mg/day, 18 months before conception. The abnormalities, considered incompatible with life, included macrocephaly, low-set ears, microphthalmia, low-inserted thumb, ventricular and atrial septal defects, total duodenal obstruction, and cystic kidneys. The malformations were thought to be due to a chromosomal abnormality (partial trisomy 1) and a history of maternal drug abuse (4). The non-typical abnormalities in the other three newborns were transitory neonatal icterus and hypocalcemia, left testis ectopia, and slight transitory hypotonia.

In 1999, a brief report from the manufacturer summarized the worldwide data relating to acitretin and human pregnancy exposures that had been reported to the manufacturer since acitretin became available (5). Some of these data may have also been reported in the study discussed above.

There were 123 reports of acitretin exposure either before or during pregnancy, 88 of which were prospective reports. Details on malformations were provided in only one case. Outcomes that did not involve congenital malformations were classified as "other abnormalities," defined as pregnancy-related, placental, perinatal, or neonatal disorders, such as hyperbilirubinemia, abnormal growth, and delayed motor skills (5). There were 11 exposures during pregnancy, five reported prospectively and six retrospectively. Among the prospective cases, there was one spontaneous abortion (no information on the fetus), three induced abortions (no information on the fetuses), and one newborn with malformations (no details provided, but reference #3 above was included whereas reference #4 was not). Among those reported retrospectively, there was one spontaneous abortion (no information), three induced abortions (two with malformations, and one with other adverse conditions), and two newborns with other adverse conditions. For exposures that occurred 0–2 years before pregnancy, there were 97 cases, 77 of them prospective. Outcomes in these cases were 8 spontaneous abortions (1 normal embryo/fetus, and 7 with no information), 25 induced abortions (3 normal, 2 with malformations, and 20 with no information), and 44 newborns (41 normal, 1 with an undescended testicle, 1 hypotonic, and 1 with hypocalcemia and jaundice). The outcomes in the 20 retrospective cases were 5 spontaneous abortions (no information), 4 induced abortions (1 normal, 1 with malformations, and 2 with no information), and 11 newborns (9 normal, 2 with malformations). Two of the five cases in which exposure occurred more than 2 years before pregnancy were prospective. Their outcomes were one spontaneous abortion (no information) and one normal newborn. The three retrospective cases all involved newborns with malformations. Finally, 10 cases involved exposure at an unknown time before conception, 4 of which were prospective. The outcomes were one spontaneous abortion (no information), one induced abortion (no information), and two normal neonates. For the six retrospective cases, there was one spontaneous abortion (no information), two induced abortions (one normal, one with no information), and three normal newborns.

An interaction between acitretin and a very low dose progestin contraceptive (levonorgestrel 0.03 mg) was observed in one woman undergoing treatment with acitretin 0.4 mg/kg/day (6). Her plasma progesterone level increased from 2.15 ng/mL before acitretin or contraceptive to 3.87–13.46 ng/mL while receiving both drugs. The increase in plasma concentration was thought to indicate failure of contraception and development of a corpus luteum after ovulation (6). No interaction, as evidenced by a rise in plasma progesterone concentration, was observed in nine other women who received combined oral contraceptives (normal or mini-dose).

Acitretin has been measured in the seminal fluid of men consuming either acitretin or etretinate (1). In men administered 30 to 50 mg/day for at least 12 weeks, the sperm count, concentration, motility, and morphology were unchanged. In addition, no adverse effects on testosterone production, LH, FSH, or on the hypothalamic-pituitary axis were observed (1). The maximum concentration of acitretin found in seminal fluid was 12.5 ng/mL. The amount of acitretin transferred in semen, assuming an ejaculate volume of 10 mL, would be 125 ng or 1/200,000 of a single 25 mg capsule (1). Of five pregnancies in which the father was receiving acitretin therapy, two ended in spontaneous abortion, one fetus had bilateral cystic hygromas and multiple cardiopulmonary anomalies, one normal newborn was delivered, and one was lost to follow-up (1). The relationship between acitretin and the fetal malformations is unknown (1). However, no teratogenicity was observed in the offspring of male rats treated with 5 mg/kg/day (about 5 times the maximum recommended human dose) for 10 weeks (approximate duration of one spermatogenic cycle) before and during mating with untreated females (1).

In summary, like all retinoids, acitretin, the active metabolite of etretinate, is a potent teratogen. It represents not only a significant fetal risk during pregnancy, but also a risk for an unknown time after therapy has ceased. This added fetal risk results because acitretin can be converted back to the parent drug, etretinate, which can persist, along with acitretin and 13-*cis*-acitretin, in subcutaneous fat for prolonged periods, perhaps for longer than 3 years. Measuring plasma levels of the retinoids does not appear to be beneficial in determining the risk of fetal harm. Effective contraception must be used for at least 1 month before beginning acitretin, during therapy, and for at least 3 years after acitretin therapy (1). Women of childbearing age who are considering treatment with acitretin must be informed of this very slow elimination and the possibility of adverse pregnancy outcome if they conceive within 3 years of therapy.

BREAST FEEDING SUMMARY

RECOMMENDATION: Limited Human Data - Potential Toxicity

Acitretin is excreted into the milk of lactating rats (1) and humans. A woman 8 months postpartum was treated with a single, daily, 40 mg dose of acitretin (0.65 mg/kg/day) for extensive plaque psoriasis and acral pustulosis (7). Nursing was stopped before the therapy was started. Milk was collected each day by an electric pump before the dose and again 12 hours later. At steady state, milk concentrations of the drug and its main metabolite were 30–40 ng/mL, corresponding to a milk:serum ratio of 0.18. The estimated infant dose was 1.5% of the maternal dose (7).

The plasma elimination half-lives of acitretin and 13-*cis*-acitretin may be as long as 96 and 157 hours, respectively (1). Because of storage in subcutaneous fat, the actual elimination of these compounds may take much longer. The manufacturer recommends a contraception period of 3 years after acitretin therapy is stopped, but a similar recommendation for breast-feeding has not been made. Although there is a potential for toxicity, the American Academy of Pediatrics classifies the drug as compatible with breast-feeding (8).

References

1. Product information. Soriatane. Roche Laboratories, 2000.
2. Sturkenboom MCJM, DeJong-Van Den Berg LTW, Van Voorst-Vader PC, Cornel MC, Stricker BHCH, Wesseling H. Inability to detect plasma etretinate and acitretin is a poor predictor of the absence of these teratogens in tissue after stopping acitretin treatment. Br J Clin Pharmacol 1994;38:229–35.
3. De Die-Smulders CEM, Sturkenboom MCJM, Veraart J, Van Katwijk C, Sastrowijoto P, Van Der Linden E. Severe limb defects and craniofacial anomalies in a fetus conceived during acitretin therapy. Teratology 1995;52:215–9.
4. Geiger JM, Baudin M, Saurat JH. Teratogenic risk with etretinate and acitretin treatment. Dermatology 1994;189:109–16.
5. Maradit H, Geiger JM. Potential risk of birth defects after acitretin discontinuation. Dermatology 1999;198:3–4.
6. Berbis Ph, Bun H, Geiger JM, Rognin C, Durand A, Serradimigni A, Hartmann D, Privat Y. Acitretin (RO10–1670) and oral contraceptives: interaction study. Arch Dermatol Res 1988;280:388–9.
7. Rollman O, Pihl-Lundin I. Acitretin excretion into human breast milk. Acta Derm Venereol (Stockh) 1990;70:487–90.
8. Committee on Drugs, American Academy of Pediatrics. The transfer of drugs and other chemicals into human milk. Pediatrics 2001;108:776–89.

Name:	ACYCLOVIR	Risk Factor:	B_M
Class:	Antiviral		

FETAL RISK SUMMARY

RECOMMENDATION: Compatible

Acyclovir is a synthetic acyclic purine nucleoside analogue used as an antiviral agent against the herpes viruses. Three studies observed no teratogenic effects in animals at nontoxic doses (1–3). One study, however, observed abnormal thymus development and functional deficits of the immune system in rats exposed *in utero* to acyclovir (4). Chromosome breaks were observed in some tests with cultured human lymphocytes, but only with prolonged exposure and at doses much higher than those obtainable in clinical use (5). A 1997 publication, however, cited studies that gave SC doses of 100 mg/kg once, twice, or three times to pregnant rats on day 10 of gestation (6). Altered development was observed in fetuses examined on day 11.5 (reduced grown-rump length, number of somites, and protein content) or on day 21 (skull, eye, and tail defects). The SC doses caused slight and reversible maternal nephropathia, but this was not thought to have induced the fetal anomalies (6).

Reproduction studies in mice, rats, and rabbits, as reported by the manufacturer, did not observe teratogenic effects (7). The doses used in the three species produced plasma levels that were the same as human levels, one to two times human levels, and four and nine times human levels, respectively.

Although there are no approved indications for acyclovir in pregnancy, the principal clinical use of acyclovir during this period is for the treatment of primary genital herpes simplex virus (HSV) type 2 infection and for the prophylaxis against recurrent genital HSV infection. The Acyclovir in Pregnancy Registry found that, of the American women reported to the Registry as exposed during pregnancy, 62% and 70% of their prospective and retrospective samples, respectively, had been treated for genital herpes (8). They estimated that as many as 7500 live-births per year in the United States may be exposed to acyclovir (8).

The treatment of genital herpes is intended to prevent the adverse outcomes on the fetus and newborn that the primary infection may cause, such as prematurity, intrauterine growth retardation (IUGR), and neonatal HSV infection, and to reduce the incidence of cesarean section with recurrent disease. Reviews evaluating the various indications for acyclovir in pregnancy concluded that life-threatening maternal HSV infection and varicella pneumonia were the most justifiable indications (9,10). Some evidence was cited that the benefits of treatment of primary genital herpes, under certain conditions, might outweigh the risks, but the lack of controlled studies prevented any conclusion (9,10). Similarly, the treatment of uncomplicated varicella infections and the prophylaxis against recurrent genital HSV were unproven indications because of the absence of supporting data (9,10). Some authors have proposed the use of acyclovir for the prophylaxis of genital HSV during pregnancy, although all qualify, their proposals with statements that controlled studies are needed to assess efficacy and safety (11–13).

A 1998 randomized, placebo controlled study was conducted to determine if oral acyclovir (800 mg/day) could reduce the rate of cesarean section in women with recurrent genital herpes infection at <36 weeks' gestation (14). A total of 63 women were enrolled (acyclovir $N = 31$, placebo $N = 32$) in the study. Except for a significant reduction in clinical recurrences (odds ratio [OR] 0.10, 95% confidence interval [CI] 0.00–0.86), the other outcome measures showed no significant difference from placebo:cesarean section (OR 0.44, 95% CI 0.09–1.59), and clinical recurrence or asymptomatic shedding (OR 0.32, 95% CI 0.05–1.56). None of the newborns were infected with herpes simplex virus and no abnormal findings were detected in the 19 exposed infants examined 1 year later. The investigators concluded that acyclovir should not be used for recurrent genital herpes infection during pregnancy outside of randomized controlled trials (14).

The Centers for Disease Control and Prevention (CDC) 1998 Sexually Transmitted Diseases Treatment Guidelines states, in part:

> The first clinical episode of genital herpes during pregnancy may be treated with oral acyclovir. In the presence of life-threatening maternal HSV infection (e.g., disseminated infection, encephalitis, pneumonitis, or hepatitis), acyclovir administered IV is indicated. Investigations of acyclovir use among pregnant women suggest that acyclovir treatment near term might reduce the rate of abdominal deliveries among women who have frequently recurring or newly acquired genital herpes by decreasing the incidence of active lesions. However, routine administration of acyclovir to pregnant women who have a history of recurrent genital herpes is not recommended at this time (15).

The drug readily crosses the placenta to the fetus (16–23). After intravenous dosing, acyclovir levels in cord blood were higher than those in maternal serum with ratios of 1.4 and 1.25 reported (16,17). A 1992 study concluded that the placental transfer of acyclovir was most consistent with a carrier-dependent, nucleobase-type uptake of the drug, but that the overall net transfer was passive and dependent on solubility characteristics (16).

The pharmacokinetics of oral acyclovir in term pregnant women was reported in 1991 (21). Fifteen women with a history of active recurrent genital HSV type 2 infection antedating and during pregnancy, but without currently active disease, were given either 200 mg ($N = 7$) or 400 mg ($N = 8$) orally every 8 hours from 38 weeks' gestation until delivery. The mean steady-state plasma peak and trough levels in the 200-mg group were 1.9 and 0.7 μmol/L, respectively; those in the 400-mg group were 3.3 and 0.8 μmol/L, respectively. Acyclovir was concentrated in the amniotic fluid with concentrations ranging from 1.87 to 6.06 μmol/L in the low-dose group compared with 4.20 to 15.5 μmol/L in the high-dose group. The maternal:cord plasma ratio was similar in both groups, with a mean of 1.3, a value comparable to that observed after intravenous dosing (21).

Acyclovir has been administered orally and intravenously during all stages of pregnancy (8,9,14,17–61). Topical acyclovir, which may produce low levels of the drug in maternal serum, urine, and vaginal excretions, has been used in pregnancy, and the manufacturer is aware of two women treated topically during the 3rd trimester who were delivered of normal infants (A. Clark, personal communication, Burroughs-Wellcome, 1985). However, no published reports of these cases have been located.

Favorable maternal and fetal outcomes were observed in two cases of isolated HSV encephalitis treated with IV and oral acyclovir (36,37). Treatment in the two mothers began at 29 and 26 weeks' gestation, respectively, and continued until term. In the only other reported cases occurring during pregnancy, none of whom were treated with acyclovir, four mothers and three fetuses died (37). The onset of the encephalitis in the mother of the surviving fetus was at term. A 1996 case report described the successful treatment with IV acyclovir of a woman with herpes simplex hepatitis at 24 weeks' gestation (38). A viable 1013-g male infant was delivered at 28 weeks' because of severe preeclampsia. Both the mother and her infant were doing well at the time of the report.

A 1991 case report and review cited data indicating that varicella pneumonia occurring during pregnancy resulted in a maternal mortality up to 44% (47). In 15 cases treated with IV acyclovir, however, only two (13%) mothers died, one fetus was stillborn, and one infant expired. Another 1991 reference added 5 new cases and a review of 16 cases from the literature to total 21 women treated during pregnancy with acyclovir for varicella pneumonia (48). Twelve women were treated during the 2nd trimester and nine during the 3rd trimester. The mean duration of acyclovir treatment was 7 days. Maternal mortality occurred in four cases, but two of the deaths occurred after delivery. One mother died of multi-organ failure 11 days after delivery, and one mother died after surgery for intestinal obstruction 1 month after delivery. The three maternal deaths directly attributable to varicella pneumonia were in the 3rd trimester at the onset of disease. Two fetal or infant deaths occurred, one from prematurity after birth at 26 weeks' gestation, and one stillborn at 34 weeks' (both cases also described in reference 47). No adverse effects were observed in the surviving infants. None of the infants had features of congenital varicella infection, nor did any develop active perinatal varicella infection. A 1993 abstract briefly described data collected retrospectively (1988–1992) on 14 pregnant women with varicella pneumonia, 11 of whom were treated with acyclovir (58). No specific information was given on the outcome of the 11 treated pregnancies. A 1998 case report described a woman at 32 weeks' gestation that was treated with IV acyclovir for varicella pneumonia (59). A healthy female infant was delivered approximately 3 days later because of fetal distress secondary to cord compression and prolapse into the right uterine segment. The infant was given varicella immunoglobulin and a 5 day course of IV acyclovir and was discharged home at 20 days of age without ever showing signs of varicella.

Data gathered for the period 1984–1999, by the Acyclovir in Pregnancy Registry, a group sponsored by the manufacturer and the CDC, were published in 2004 (8). Excluding 461 patients with exposure to topical acyclovir only, 1,234 pregnancies (12 sets of twins; 1,246 outcomes) with known outcomes were followed prospectively. The trimester of initial exposure was 1st—756 (7 sets of twins), 2nd—197 (2 sets of twins), 3rd—291 (3 sets of twins), and unknown—2. Among the 1st trimester exposures, there were 76 spontaneous abortions (SABs), 1 stillbirth, 83 elective abortions (EABs), 19 infants with birth defects, and 577 live births without birth defects. In the remaining exposures, there were no SABs, 2 EABs, 2 stillbirths, 9 infants with birth defects, and 477 live births without birth defects. For exposures during the 1st trimester with known outcomes (excluding SABs, EABs, and stillbirths), the rate of birth defects was 3.2% (19 of 596). For all trimesters, the rate was 2.6% (28 of 1,082). These rates are no different from the rates expected in a nonexposed population (8). As for pregnancies reported retrospectively (i.e., in which the outcome was known before reporting), there were 47 birth defects that, in general, were similar to those reported prospectively. There was no uniqueness or pattern among the malformations, reported prospectively or retrospectively, that suggested a common cause (8).

In a surveillance study of Michigan Medicaid recipients conducted between 1985 and 1992 involving 229,101 completed pregnancies, 478 newborns had been exposed to acyclovir during the 1st trimester (F. Rosa, personal communication, FDA, 1993). A total of 18 (3.8%) major birth defects were observed (20 expected). Specific data were available for six defect categories, including (observed/expected) 5/5 cardiovascular defects, 0/1 oral clefts, 0/0 spina bifida, 1/1 polydactyly, 1/1 limb reduction defects, and 2/1 hypospadia. These data do not support an association between the drug and the defects.

A 1998 non-interventional observational cohort study described the outcomes of pregnancies in women who had been prescribed one or more of 34 newly marketed drugs by general practitioners in England (60). Data were obtained by questionnaires sent to the prescribing physicians one month after the expected or possible date of delivery. In 831 (78%) of the pregnancies, a newly marketed drug was thought to had been taken during the 1st trimester with birth defects noted in 14 (2.5%) singleton births of the 557 newborns (10 sets of twins). In addition, two birth defects were observed in aborted fetuses. However, few of the aborted fetuses were examined. Acyclovir was taken during the 1st trimester in 24 pregnancies. The outcomes of these pregnancies included 1 spontaneous abortion, 5 elective abortions, and 18 normal term babies (60).

In summary, no adverse effects in the fetus or newborn attributable to the use of acyclovir during pregnancy have been reported. Congenital malformations have been reported in infants exposed during pregnancy, but these do not appear to be related to the drug. Systemic IV treatment is indicated for life-threatening disseminated HSV infections to reduce the maternal, fetal, and infant mortality of these infections. Oral acyclovir treatment of primary genital HSV infections also appears to be indicated to prevent adverse fetal outcomes, such as prematurity, IUGR, and neonatal HSV infection. In contrast, the benefit of therapy to prevent recurrent genital HSV infection and to reduce the need for cesarean section has not been established. At least one study has failed to find such a benefit, but additional controlled studies with larger subject populations are needed. Because there is more human pregnancy experience with acyclovir than with similar antiviral agents (e.g., valacyclovir or famciclovir) and this experience does not demonstrate a major risk, some authors consider acyclovir to be the drug of choice when indicated (62,63). However, long-term studies of children exposed *in utero* to acyclovir are needed.

BREAST FEEDING SUMMARY

RECOMMENDATION: Compatible

Acyclovir is concentrated in human milk with levels usually exceeding those found in maternal serum (64–68). In an *in vitro* experiment, the transfer of acyclovir from the plasma to breast milk was determined to be due to passive diffusion (64).

A woman, breast-feeding a 4-month-old infant, was treated with acyclovir 200 mg orally every 3 hours (five times daily) for presumed oral herpes (65). She had taken 15 doses of the drug before the study dose. Approximately 9 hours after her 15th dose, she was given another 200-mg dose and paired maternal plasma and breast milk samples were drawn at 0, 0.5, 1.5, 2.0, and 3.0 hours. Breast-feeding was discontinued during the study interval. Milk:plasma ratios ranged from 0.6 to 4.1. Milk concentrations were greater than those in maternal serum at all times except at 1.5 hours, the time of peak plasma concentration (4.23 μmol/L). (*Note:* 1 μmol/L = 0.225 μg/mL [9].) The initial level in the milk was 3.3 μmol/L, reflecting the doses taken prior to the study period. The highest level measured in milk was 5.8 μmol/L at 3.2 hours, but this was not the peak concentration because it was still rising at the time of sampling. Acyclovir was demonstrated in the infant's urine. Based on the poor lipid solubility of the drug, the pKa's, and other known pharmacokinetic parameters, the calculated theoretical milk:plasma ratio was 0.15. Because the actual measured ratio was much greater than this value, it was concluded that acyclovir entered the milk by an active or facilitated process that would make it unique from any other medicinal agent. The maximum ingested dose, based on 750 mL of milk/day, was calculated to be 1500 μg/day, approximately 0.2 mg/kg/day in the infant, or about 1.6% of the adult dose. This was thought not to represent an immediate risk to the infant, and, in fact, no adverse effects of the exposure were observed in the infant (65).

In a second case, a woman 1 year postpartum was treated with oral acyclovir, 200 mg five times a day, for presumed herpes zoster (66). The mean concentrations in the milk and serum were 1.06 μg/mL and 0.33 μg/mL, respectively, a milk:plasma ratio of 3.24. Detectable amounts were present in both serum and milk 48 hours after the last dose with an estimated half-life in the milk of 2.8 hours. The estimated amount of acyclovir ingested by the infant consuming 1000 mL/day of milk was about 1 mg (66).

Two recent studies measured the excretion of acyclovir in milk (67,68). In one, a woman 6 weeks postpartum suffering from eczema herpeticum received acyclovir IV 300 mg three times daily for 5 days (67). Breast-feeding was interrupted during the treatment. Serum and milk samples were collected after the last dose at 6-hour intervals for 4 days. Acyclovir levels in the milk exceeded those in the serum at every analysis and within the first 72 hours the milk concentration was 2.25 times higher than that in the serum. During the 88 hours that acyclovir was detectable in breast milk, a total of 4.448 mg was excreted (79% was recovered during the first 24 hours) (67).

In the other study, a woman was taking 800 mg 5 times daily for herpes zoster (68). She continued to breast-feed her 7-month-old infant. Three random milk samples were obtained (0.25–9.42 hours after a dose) with acyclovir levels ranging from 18.5 μmol/L (4.16 μg/mL) to 25.8 μmol/L (5.81 μg/mL). The highest level occurred 9.42 hours after a dose. No adverse effects were observed in the infant who had ingested from the milk, what was thought to be, a clinically insignificant amount of acyclovir (0.73 mg/kg/day or about 1% of the maternal dose in mg/kg/day) (68).

Because acyclovir has been used to treat herpes virus infections in the neonate, and because of the lack of adverse effects in the above cases, mothers undergoing treatment with acyclovir can probably breast-feed safely. The American Academy of Pediatrics classifies acyclovir as compatible with breast-feeding (69).

References

1. Moore HL, Szczech GM, Rodwell DE, Kapp RW Jr, deMiranda P, Tucker WE Jr. Preclinical toxicology studies with acyclovir: teratologic, reproductive, and neonatal tests. Fund Appl Toxicol 1983;3:560–8.
2. Stahlmann R, Klug S, Lewandowski C, Bochert G, Chahoud I, Rahm U, Merker HJ, Neubert D. Prenatal toxicity of acyclovir in rats. Arch Toxicol 1988;61:468–79.
3. Chahoud I, Stahlmann R, Bochert G, Dillmann I, Neubert D. Gross-structural defects in rats after acyclovir application on day 10 of gestation. Arch Toxicol 1988;62:8–14.
4. Stahlmann R, Korte M, Van Loveren H, Vos JG, Thiel R, Neubert D. Abnormal thymus development and impaired function of the immune system in rats after prenatal exposure to aciclovir. Arch Toxicol 1992;66: 551–9.
5. Clive D, Turner NT, Hozier J, Batson AGE, Tucker WE Jr. Preclinical toxicology studies with acyclovir: Genetic toxicity tests. Fund Appl Toxicol 1983;3:587–602.
6. Stahlmann R, Chahoud I, Thiel R, Klug S, Forster C. The developmental toxicity of three antimicrobial agents observed only in nonroutine animal studies. Reprod Toxicol 1997;11:1–7.
7. Product information. Zovirax. Glaxo Wellcome, 2000.
8. Stone KM, Reiff-Eldridge R, White AD, Cordero JF, Brown Z, Alexander ER, Andrews EB. Pregnancy outcomes following systemic prenatal acyclovir exposure: conclusions from the International Acyclovir Pregnancy Registry, 1984–1999. Birth Defects Res (Part A) 2004;70:201–7.
9. Brown ZA, Baker DA. Acyclovir therapy during pregnancy. Obstet Gynecol 1989;73:526–31.
10. Brown ZA, Watts DH. Antiviral therapy in pregnancy. Clin Obstet Gynecol 1990;33:276–89.
11. Arvin AM, Hensleigh PA, Prober CG, Au DS, Yasukawa LL, Wittek AE, Palumbo PE, Paryani SG, Yeager AS. Failure of antepartum maternal cultures to predict the infant's risk of exposure to herpes simplex virus at delivery. N Engl J Med 1986;315:796–800.
12. Carney O, Mindel A. Screening pregnant women for genital herpes. Br Med J 1988;296:1643.
13. Canadian Task Force on the Periodic Health Examination. Periodic health examination, 1989 update: 4. Intrapartum electronic fetal monitoring and prevention of neonatal herpes simplex. Can Med Assoc J 1989;141:1233–40.
14. Brocklehurst P, Kinghorn G, Carney O, Helsen K, Ross E, Ellis E, Shen R, Cowan F, Mindel A. A randomised placebo controlled trial of suppressive acyclovir in late pregnancy in women with recurrent genital herpes infection. Br J Obstet Gynaecol 1998;105:275–80.
15. CDC. 1998 Guideline for treatment of sexually transmitted diseases. MMWR 1998;47:25.
16. Henderson GI, Hu Z-Q, Johnson RF, Perez AB, Yang Y, Schenker S. Acyclovir transport by the human placenta. J Lab Clin Med 1992;120:885–92.

17. Landsberger EJ, Hager WD, Grossman JH III. Successful management of varicella pneumonia complicating pregnancy: a report of three cases. J Reprod Med 1986;31:311–4.
18. Utley K, Bromberger P, Wagner L, Schneider H. Management of primary herpes in pregnancy complicated by ruptured membranes and extreme prematurity: case report. Obstet Gynecol 1987;69:471–3.
19. Greffe BS, Dooley SL, Deddish RB, Krasny HC. Transplacental passage of acyclovir. J Pediatr 1986;108:1020–1.
20. Haddad J, Simeoni U, Messer J, Willard D. Transplacental passage of acyclovir. J Pediatr 1987;110:164.
21. Kingsley S. Fetal and neonatal exposure to acyclovir (abstract). Second World Congress on Sexually Transmitted Diseases, Paris, June 1986. As cited in Haddad J, Simeoni U, Messer J, Willard D. Transplacental passage of acyclovir. J Pediatr 1987;110:164.
22. Frenkel LM, Brown ZA, Bryson YJ, Corey L, Unadkat JD, Hensleigh PA, Arvin AM, Prober CG, Connor JD. Pharmacokinetics of acyclovir in the term human pregnancy and neonate. Am J Obstet Gynecol 1991;164:569–76.
23. Fletcher CV. The placental transport and use of acyclovir in pregnancy. J Lab Clin Med 1992;120:821–2.
24. Lagrew DC Jr, Furlow TG, Hager WD, Yarrish RL. Disseminated herpes simplex virus infection in pregnancy. JAMA 1984;252:2058–9.
25. Grover L, Kane J, Kravitz J, Cruz A. Systemic acyclovir in pregnancy: a case report. Obstet Gynecol 1985;65:284–7.
26. Berger SA, Weinberg M, Treves T, Sorkin P, Geller E, Yedwab G, Tomer A, Rabey M, Michaeli D. Herpes encephalitis during pregnancy: failure of acyclovir and adenine arabinoside to prevent neonatal herpes. Isr J Med Sci 1986;22:41–4.
27. Anderson H, Sutton RNP, Scarffe JH. Cytotoxic chemotherapy and viral infections: the role of acyclovir. J R Coll Physicians Lond 1984;18:51–5.
28. Hockberger RS, Rothstein RJ. Varicella pneumonia in adults: a spectrum of disease. Ann Emerg Med 1986;15:931–4.
29. Glaser JB, Loftus J, Ferragamo V, Mootabar H, Castellano M. Varicella-zoster infection in pregnancy. N Engl J Med 1986;315:1416.
30. Tschen EH, Baack B. Treatment of herpetic whitlow in pregnancy with acyclovir. J Am Acad Dermatol 1987;17:1059–60.
31. Kundsin RB, Falk L, Hertig AT, Horne HW Jr. Acyclovir treatment of twelve unexplained infertile couples. Int J Fertil 1987;32:200–4.
32. Chazotte C, Andersen HF, Cohen WR. Disseminated herpes simplex infection in an immunocompromised pregnancy: treatment with intravenous acyclovir. Am J Perinatol 1987;4:363–4.
33. Cox SM, Phillips LE, DePaolo HD, Faro S. Treatment of disseminated herpes simplex virus in pregnancy with parenteral acyclovir: a case report. J Reprod Med 1986;31:1005–7.
34. Bernuau J, Caujolle B, Rouzioux C, Degott C, Rueff B, Benhamou JP. Severe acute hepatitis due to herpes-simplex in the third trimester of pregnancy: combatting with acyclovir (abstract). Gastroenterol Clin Biol 1987;11:79.
35. Hankins GDV, Gilstrap LC III, Patterson AR. Acyclovir treatment of varicella pneumonia in pregnancy. Crit Care Med 1987;15:336–7.
36. Hankey GR, Bucens MR, Chambers JSW. Herpes simplex encephalitis in third trimester of pregnancy: successful outcome for mother and child. Neurology 1987;37:1534–7.
37. Frieden FJ, Ordorica SA, Goodgold AL, Hoskins IA, Silverman F, Young BK. Successful pregnancy with isolated herpes simplex virus encephalitis: case report and review of the literature. Obstet Gynecol 1990;75: 511–3.
38. Glorioso DV, Molloy PJ, Van Thiel DH, Kania RJ. Successful empiric treatment of HSV hepatitis in pregnancy. Case report and review of the literature. Dig Dis Sci 1996;41:1273–5.
39. Leen CLS, Mandal BK, Ellis ME. Acyclovir and pregnancy. Br Med J 1987;294:308.
40. Eder SE, Apuzzio JJ, Weiss G. Varicella pneumonia during pregnancy: treatment of two cases with acyclovir. Am J Perinatol 1988;5:16–8.
41. Boyd K, Walker E. Use of acyclovir to treat chickenpox in pregnancy. Br Med J 1988;296:393–4.
42. Key TC, Resnik R, Dittrich HC, Reisner LS. Successful pregnancy after cardiac transplantation. Am J Obstet Gynecol 1989;160:367–71.
43. Stray-Pedersen B. Acyclovir in late pregnancy to prevent neonatal herpes simplex. Lancet 1990;336:756.
44. Brocklehurst P, Carney O, Helson K, Kinghorn G, Mercey D, Mindel A. Acyclovir, herpes, and pregnancy. Lancet 1990;336:1594–5.
45. Stray-Pedersen B. Acyclovir, herpes, and pregnancy. Lancet 1990;336:1595.
46. Greenspoon JS, Wilcox JG, McHutchison LB. Does acyclovir improve the outcome of disseminated herpes simplex virus during pregnancy (abstract)? Am J Obstet Gynecol 1991;164:400.
47. Broussard RG, Payne DK, George RB. Treatment with acyclovir of varicella pneumonia in pregnancy. Chest 1991;99:1045–7.
48. Smego RA Jr, Asperilla MO. Use of acyclovir for varicella pneumonia during pregnancy. Obstet Gynecol 1991;78:1112–6.
49. Ciraru-Vigneron N, Nguyen Tan Lung R, Blondeau MA, Brunner C, Barrier J. Interest in the prescription acyclovir in the end of pregnancy in the case of genital herpes: a new protocol of the prevention of risks of herpes neonatal. Presse Med 1987;16:128.
50. Haddad J, Langer B, Astruc D, Messer J, Lokiec F. Oral acyclovir and recurrent genital herpes during late pregnancy. Obstet Gynecol 1993;82:102–4.
51. Esmonde TF, Herdman G, Anderson G. Chickenpox pneumonia: an association with pregnancy. Thorax 1989;44:812–5.
52. Horowitz GM, Hankins GDV. Early-second-trimester use of acyclovir in treating herpes zoster in a bone marrow transplant patient. A case report. J Reprod Med 1992;37:280–2.
53. Gilbert GL. Chickenpox during pregnancy. Br Med J 1993;306:1079–80.
54. Moling O, Mayr O, Gottardi H, Mian P, Zanon P, Oberkofler F, Gramegna M, Colucci G. Severe pneumonia in pregnancy three months after resolution of cutaneous zoster. Infection 1994;22:216–8.
55. Greenspoon JS, Wilcox JG, McHutchison LB, Rosen DJD. Acyclovir for disseminated herpes simplex virus

in pregnancy. A case report. J Reprod Med 1994;39: 311–7.
56. Randolph AG, Hartshorn RM, Washington AE. Acyclovir prophylaxis in late pregnancy to prevent neonatal herpes: a cost-effectiveness analysis. Obstet Gynecol 1996;88:603–10.
57. Scott LL, Sanchez PJ, Jackson GL, Zeray F, Wendel GD Jr. Acyclovir suppression to prevent cesarean delivery after first-episode genital herpes. Obstet Gynecol 1996;87:69–73.
58. Whitty JE, Renfroe YR, Bottoms SF, Isada NB, Iverson R, Cotton DB. Varicella pneumonia in pregnancy: clinical experience (abstract). Am J Obstet Gynecol 1993;168:427.
59. Chandra PC, Patel H, Schiavello HJ, Briggs SL. Successful pregnancy outcome after complicated varicella pneumonia. Obstet Gynecol 1998;92:680–2.
60. Wilton LV, Pearce GL, Martin RM, Mackay FJ, Mann RD. The outcomes of pregnancy in women exposed to newly marketed drugs in general practice in England. Br J Obstet Gynaecol 1998;105:882–9.
61. Anderson R, Lundqvist A, Bergstrom T. Successful treatment of generalized primary herpes simplex type 2 infection during pregnancy. Scand J Infect Dis 1999;31:210–2.
62. Balfour HH Jr. Antiviral drugs. N Engl J Med 1999;340:1255–68.
63. Smith JR, Cowan FM, Munday P. The management of herpes simplex virus infection in pregnancy. Br J Obstet Gynaecol 1998;105:255–60.
64. Bork K, Kaiser T, Benes P. Transfer of aciclovir from plasma to human breast milk. Drug Res 2000;50: 656–8.
65. Lau RJ, Emery MG, Galinsky RE. Unexpected accumulation of acyclovir in breast milk with estimation of infant exposure. Obstet Gynecol 1987;69: 468–71.
66. Meyer LJ, de Miranda P, Sheth N, Spruance S. Acyclovir in human breast milk. Am J Obstet Gynecol 1988;158:586–8.
67. Bork K, Benes P. Concentration and kinetic studies of intravenous acyclovir in serum and breast milk of a patient with eczema herpeticum. J Am Acad Dermatol 1995;32:1053–5.
68. Taddio A, Klein J, Koren G. Acyclovir excretion in human breast milk. Ann Pharmacother 1994;28: 585–7.
69. Committee on Drugs, American Academy of Pediatrics. The transfer of drugs and other chemicals into human milk. Pediatrics 2001;108:776–89.

Name:	**ADALIMUMAB**	Risk Factor:	**B_M**
Class:	**Immunologic Agent (Immunomodulator)**		

FETAL RISK SUMMARY

RECOMMENDATION: No Human Data - Animal Data Suggest Low Risk

Adalimumab is a recombinant immunoglobulin (IgG1) monoclonal antibody that binds specifically to human tumor necrosis factor-alpha (TNFα) to block its action on cell surface TNF receptors. It is administered by SC injection. Adalimumab is indicated for reducing the signs and symptoms and inhibiting the progression of structural damage in adult patients with moderate to severe active rheumatoid arthritis that have had an inadequate response to one or more disease-modifying anti-rheumatic drugs. The mean terminal elimination half-life is about 14 days (range 10–20 days) (1).

An animal reproduction study for perinatal development toxicity was conducted in pregnant cynomolgus monkeys (1). Doses up to 266 times the human AUC (40 mg SC with methotrexate every week) or 373 times the human AUC (40 mg SC without methotrexate) revealed no fetal harm (the timing of the exposure was not specified). No clastogenic or mutagenic effects were observed in various tests, but adalimumab has not been tested for carcinogenic or fertility effects (1).

It is not known if adalimumab crosses the human placenta. The molecular weight is very high (about 148,000), but immunoglobulin G (IgG) has been shown to cross the placenta late in pregnancy (see Immune Globulin Intravenous). Placental transfer of IgG was a function of dose, as well as gestational age.

No reports describing the use of adalimumab in human pregnancy have been located. The limited animal data suggest a low risk for the embryo/fetus, but the absence of pregnancy data prevents an assessment of the human risk. Theoretically, TNFα antagonists could interfere with implantation and ovulation, but this has not been shown clinically

(2). The potential maternal benefits from treatment with adalimumab appear to be great and, therefore, probably outweigh the unknown embryo/fetal risk. Until data are available, avoiding treatment during the 1st trimester is an option that should be discussed with the patient. However, the long elimination half-life suggests that inadvertent exposure in the 1st trimester of an unplanned pregnancy is probable. A pregnancy registry has been established to monitor fetal outcomes of pregnant women exposed to adalimumab for the treatment of rheumatoid arthritis. Health care providers are encouraged to register such patients by calling the toll free number 877–311–8972.

BREAST FEEDING SUMMARY

RECOMMENDATION: No Human Data - Probably Compatible

No reports describing the use of adalimumab during lactation have been located. The molecular weight is very high (about 148,000), but immunoglobulins are excreted into breast milk (1). Therefore, adalimumab is probably excreted into milk, but the amount in milk and the systemic bioavailability are not known. The effects of this exposure on a nursing infant are also unknown.

References

1. Product information. Humira. Abbott Laboratories, 2004.
2. Khanna D, McMahon M, Furst DE. Safety of tumour necrosis factor-α antagonists. Drug Saf 2004;27:307–24.

Name:	**ADAPALENE**	Risk Factor:	C_M
Class:	**Dermatologic Agent**		

FETAL RISK SUMMARY

RECOMMENDATION: Limited Human Data - Animal Data Suggest Low Risk

Adapalene is used topically (cream, gel, or solution) for the treatment of acne vulgaris. The agent is a retinoid-like compound that is a modulator of cellular differentiation, keratinization, and inflammatory processes. It binds to specific retinoic acid nuclear receptors. Plasma concentrations are very low after chronic topical application (<0.25 ng/mL) (1).

No teratogenic effects were noted in pregnant rats given oral doses up to 120 times the maximum daily human dose (MDHD). Topical application of adapalene to pregnant rats and rabbits up to 150 times the MDHD demonstrated no fetotoxicity and only minimal increases in supernumerary ribs in rats (1).

It is not known if adapalene crosses the human placenta. Although the molecular weight is approximately 413, the very low plasma concentrations suggest that minimal amounts of drug would be available to cross the placenta.

Only one report describing the use of adapalene during human pregnancy has been located (2). At 22 weeks' gestation, a small-for-date fetus with anophthalmia was detected by ultrasound examination and the pregnancy was terminated. Anophthalmia and agenesis of the optic chiasma were observed in the aborted fetus. The mother had been treated with adapalene gel (0.3 mg/day) from 1 month before conception until 13 weeks' gestation. The defects were not thought to be typical of retinoid-induced malformations (heart, central nervous system, thymus, limbs, and craniofacial) (2).

In summary, adapalene is not teratogenic in two experimental animal species. After chronic use in humans, trace amounts of adapalene have been detected in the systemic circulation. The adverse pregnancy outcome described above is the only report of adapalene exposure in human pregnancy. The combination of animal data and very low systemic bioavailability suggests that any risk to a fetus from inadvertent exposure would be very low, but the nearly complete absence of human data prevents further assessment. Until more experience in pregnancy has been reported, the safest course is to avoid use of this agent in the 1st trimester.

BREAST FEEDING SUMMARY

RECOMMENDATION: No Human Data - Probably Compatible

No reports describing the use of adapalene during lactation have been located. The systemic availability of this drug from topical administration is very low (<25 ng/mL) (1). The amount in breast milk, therefore, should also be very low. It is doubtful that this level, if it is excreted in milk, represents any risk to a nursing infant.

References

1. Product information. Differin. Galderma Laboratories, 2002.
2. Autret E, Berjot M, Jonville-Bera AP, Aubry MC, Moraine C. Anophthalmia and agenesis of optic chiasma associated with adapalene gel in early pregnancy. Lancet 1997;350:339.

Name:	**ADEFOVIR**	Risk Factor:	**C_M**
Class:	**Antiviral**		

FETAL RISK SUMMARY

RECOMMENDATION: No Human Data - Animal Data Suggest Low Risk

Adefovir, an acyclic nucleotide analog of adenosine monophosphate is used for the treatment of chronic hepatitis B, especially in patients with clinical evidence of lamivudine-resistant hepatitis B virus. The mechanism involves the inhibition of hepatitis B virus DNA polymerase (reverse transcriptase) (1). It has also been used in patients infected with the human immunodeficiency virus (HIV) (1,2). The antiviral agent is available as a prodrug, adefovir dipivoxil, that is rapidly converted to adefovir after oral administration (1). Adefovir is then phosphorylated to the active metabolite, adefovir diphosphate, by cellular kinases. Serum protein binding is very low (≤4%) and the terminal elimination half-life is about 7.5 hours (1).

Reproduction studies have been conducted in rats and rabbits. No evidence of embryotoxicity or teratogenicity was observed in rats after oral dosing that produced systemic exposures up to 23 times the human exposure achieved with the therapeutic dose of 10 mg/day (HE) or in rabbits at 40 times the HE. In rats given maternal toxic IV doses (systemic exposures 38 times the HE), embryotoxicity and an increase in the incidence of fetal malformations (anasarca, depressed eye bulge, umbilical hernia, and kinked tail) were observed. The no-effect exposure from IV doses in pregnant rats was 12 times the HE (1). Intraperitoneal doses of adefovir in mice resulted in dose-related resorptions, low birth weight, neonatal death, and severe lymphoid depletion of the thymus (3).

It is not known if adefovir crosses the human placenta. The molecular weight (about 501) of the prodrug, adefovir dipivoxil, the relative lack of protein binding, and the moderately long terminal elimination half-life suggest that the adefovir will cross to the fetal compartment.

The Antiretroviral Pregnancy Registry reported, for the period January 1989 through January 2004, prospective data (reported to the Registry before the outcomes were known) involving 1537 live births that had been exposed during the 1st trimester to one or more antiretroviral agents (4). Forty-seven of the newborns had congenital defects (3.1%, 95% confidence interval [CI] 2.3–4.1). In the 2407 live births with earliest exposure in the 2nd/3rd trimesters, there were 56 infants with defects (2.3%, 95% CI 1.8–3.0). The prevalence rates for the two periods did not differ significantly. There were 103 infants with birth defects among 3944 live births with exposure anytime during pregnancy (2.6%, 95% CI 2.1–3.2). The prevalence rate did not differ significantly from the rate expected in a nonexposed population (4). There were two outcomes exposed to adefovir in the 1st trimester in combination with other antiretroviral agents. There were no birth defects in these exposures. In reviewing the birth defects of prospective and retrospective (pregnancies reported after the outcomes were known) registered cases, and clinical reports, the Registry concluded that there was no pattern of anomalies to suggest a common cause (4). (See Lamivudine for required statement.)

No reports, other than the data above, describing the use of adefovir in human pregnancy have been located.

The animal data are suggestive of low embryo/fetal risk because the toxic effects in rats occurred at maternally toxic exposures. However, the near absence of human pregnancy experience prevents an assessment of the risk the drug represents to the embryo and/or fetus. If indicated, adefovir therapy should not be withheld because of pregnancy since chronic hepatitis B and HIV are diseases with significant morbidity and mortality and will result in poor pregnancy outcome. The manufacturer maintains a registry for adefovir pregnancy exposures; clinicians are encouraged to register patients by calling 1-800-258-4263.

BREAST FEEDING SUMMARY

RECOMMENDATION: No Human Data - Probably Compatible (Hepatitis B) Contraindicated (HIV)

No reports describing the use of adefovir during lactation have been located. The molecular weight (about 501) of the prodrug, adefovir dipivoxil, the relative lack of protein binding, and the moderately long terminal elimination half-life suggest that the adefovir will be excreted into breast milk. Although women infected with hepatitis B can breast-feed without additional risk for the transmission of hepatitis B, breast-feeding is contraindicated in those infected with HIV (5). Moreover, because of the risk of serious toxicity in a nursing infant (e.g., nephrotoxicity as seen in adults), women being treated with adefovir for any infection should not nurse.

References

1. Product information. Hepsera. Gilead Sciences, 2004.
2. Horowitz HW, Telzak EE, Sepkowitz KA, Wormser GP. Human immunodeficiency virus infection, Part II. Dis Mon 1998;44:677–716.
3. Lee JS, Mullaney S, Bronson R, Sharpe AH, Jaenisch R, Balzarini J, De Clercq E, Ruprecht RM. Transplacental antiretroviral therapy with 9-(2-phosphonylmethoxyethyl) adenine is embryotoxic in transgenic mice. J Acquir Immune Defic Syndr 1991;4:833–8.
4. Antiretroviral Pregnancy Registry Steering Committee. Antiretroviral Pregnancy Registry International Interim Report for 1 January 1989 through 31 January

2004. Wilmington, NC: Registry Coordinating Center; 2004.
5. American College of Obstetricians and Gynecologists. Breastfeeding: Maternal and infant aspects. *Educational Bulletin*. No. 258, July 2000.

Name: **ADENOSINE** Risk Factor: **C_M**
Class: **Antiarrhythmic**

FETAL RISK SUMMARY

RECOMMENDATION: Compatible - Maternal Benefit >> Embryo/Fetal Risk

Adenosine, an endogenous purine-based nucleoside found in all cells of the body, is used for the treatment of paroxysmal supraventricular tachycardia. Adenosine phosphate and adenosine triphosphate have been used as vasodilators. Ordinarily, adverse fetal effects secondary to adenosine would not be expected because of the widespread, natural distribution of this substance in the body and its very short (<10 seconds) half-life after IV administration. However, the maternal administration of large IV doses of adenosine may potentially produce fetal toxicity, as has been observed with other endogenous agents (e.g., see Epinephrine).

A reproduction study in chick embryos did not observe teratogenicity (1). Injection into the fourth cerebral ventricle of fetal sheep resulted in depressed fetal respiratory drive (2). In pregnant sheep, constant infusions and single injections of adenosine produced alterations in maternal heart rate and a decrease in diastolic pressure, but no changes in maternal systolic pressure or arterial blood gases, and had no effect on fetal heart rate, arterial pressure, or arterial blood gasses (3,4). Another experiment using near-term sheep demonstrated that angiotensin II-induced maternal-placental vasoconstriction could not be reversed by a high-dose infusion of adenosine (5).

Endogenous adenosine cord blood levels, measured in 14 fetuses of 19–34 weeks' gestation, were not related to gestational age, but were significantly increased in anemic fetuses and were positively associated with blood oxygen tension (6). The investigators concluded that the results were compatible with a fetal response to tissue hypoxia.

The first case describing the use of adenosine in human pregnancy appeared in 1991 (7). Recurrent narrow complex tachycardia occurred suddenly in a 40-year-old woman in her 39th week of gestation. She had been hospitalized 6 months before the current episode for a similar condition secondary to mitral valve prolapse and had been taking atenolol for tachyarrhythmia prophylaxis since that occurrence. Maternal blood pressure was 80 mm Hg systolic with a pulse of 240 beats/minute. Fetal heart rate was 140 beats/minute. Two IV bolus doses of adenosine (6 mg and 12 mg) were administered resulting in conversion to sinus rhythm with a rate of 80 beats/minute. A nonstress test, conducted after stabilization of the mother, was normal. Two weeks later, a healthy 3.6-kg infant was delivered. Both mother and baby were doing well 1 month postpartum.

Since the above case, a number of reports have described the safe use of adenosine to treat maternal or fetal supraventricular tachycardia (8–18) during all phases of gestation, including one woman in active labor (15), eight during the 1st trimester (16), and one case of direct fetal administration (18). The first three of the maternal reports and the fetal case are described below.

A 19-year-old woman was treated at 38 weeks' gestation for arrhythmia during labor (8). Conversion to a normal sinus rhythm required two IV bolus doses (6 and 12 mg).

No effect was observed on uterine contractions, fetal heart rate, or variability. A cesarean section was required for failure of the labor to progress. The second case occurred in a 34-year-old woman with onset of supraventricular tachycardia at 30 weeks' gestation (9). She responded within 30 seconds to a single 6-mg IV adenosine dose with no changes observed in the fetal heart rate tracing. A normal infant was delivered at term. The third woman was a 26-year-old patient with a history of Wolff-Parkinson-White syndrome who was initially treated successfully with 6 mg IV adenosine at 7 months' gestation (10). She was subsequently treated with atenolol and eventually admitted at term for labor induction. During labor the supraventricular tachycardia recurred and two doses (6 and 12 mg) of adenosine were required to convert to a normal sinus rhythm. During the mother's arrhythmia, fetal distress demonstrated by recurrent, deep variable decelerations with loss of short-term variability was observed, but fetal bradycardia resolved with a return to a fetal heart rate of 130 beats/minute on conversion of the mother. A third recurrence of the mother's tachycardia occurred shortly before a cesarean section and this was successfully converted with a 12-mg dose of adenosine. A male infant was delivered with Apgar scores of 1 and 5 at 1 and 5 minutes, respectively. No adverse effects in the fetus or newborn attributable to adenosine were observed in any of the above cases or in the other cited cases.

A 1995 reference described the direct fetal administration of adenosine for the treatment of persistent supraventricular tachycardia with massive hydrops at 28 weeks' gestation (18). Treatment with digoxin and flecainide for 5 weeks had not been successful in reversing the condition. Based on estimated fetal weight, 0.2 mg/kg of adenosine was given by bolus injection into the umbilical vein and a normal rhythm occurred within seconds. The umbilical serum levels of digoxin and flecainide were determined at the same time and further loading of the fetus with digoxin (0.05 mg/kg) and flecainide (1.0 mg/kg) were administered via the umbilical vein (18). After about 20 minutes of intermittent atrial arrhythmia and tachycardia, the fetal heart converted to a stable, normal rhythm. One week later, the fetus died *in utero* from what was thought to be a recurrence of the tachycardia or the onset of a drug-induced arrhythmia (18). Massive hydrops fetalis with a structurally normal heart was found at autopsy.

BREAST FEEDING SUMMARY

RECOMMENDATION: No Human Data - Probably Compatible

Because adenosine is used only by IV injection in acute care situations, it is doubtful that any reports will be located describing the use of adenosine during human lactation. Moreover, the serum half-life is so short, it is unlikely that any of the drug will pass into milk.

References

1. Shepard TH. *Catalog of Teratogenic Agents*. 6th ed. Baltimore, MD: Johns Hopkins University Press, 1989:194.
2. Bissonnette JM, Hohimer AR, Knopp SJ. The effect of centrally administered adenosine on fetal breath movements. Respir Physiol 1991;84:273–85.
3. Mason B, Ogunyemi D, Punla O, Koos B. Maternal and fetal cardiovascular effects of intravenous adenosine (abstract). Am J Obstet Gynecol 1993;168: 439.
4. Mason BA, Ogunyemi D, Punla O, Koos BJ. Maternal and fetal cardiorespiratory responses to adenosine in sheep. Am J Obstet Gynecol 1993;168:1558–61.
5. Landauer M, Phernetton TM, Rankin JHG. Maternal ovine placental vascular responses to adenosine. Am J Obstet Gynecol 1986;154:1152–5.
6. Ross Russell RI, Greenough A, Lagercrantz H, Dahlin I, Nicolaides K. Fetal anaemia and its relation with increased concentrations of adenosine. Arch Dis Child Fetal Neonatal 1993;68:35–6.

7. Podolsky SM, Varon J. Adenosine use during pregnancy. Ann Emerg Med 1991;20:1027–8.
8. Harrison JK, Greenfield RA, Wharton JM. Acute termination of supraventricular tachycardia by adenosine during pregnancy. Am Heart J 1992;123:1386–8.
9. Mason BA, Ricci-Goodman J, Koos BJ. Adenosine in the treatment of maternal paroxysmal supraventricular tachycardia. Obstet Gynecol 1992;80:478–80.
10. Afridi I, Moise KJ Jr, Rokey R. Termination of supraventricular tachycardia with intravenous adenosine in a pregnant woman with Wolff-Parkinson-White syndrome. Obstet Gynecol 1992;80:481–3.
11. Leffler S, Johnson DR. Adenosine use in pregnancy. Lack of effect on fetal heart rate. Am J Emerg Med 1992;10:548–9.
12. Propp DA, Broderick K, Pesch D. Adenosine during pregnancy. Ann Emerg Med 1992;21:453–4.
13. Adair RF. Fetal monitoring with adenosine administration. Ann Emerg Med 1993;22:1925.
14. Matfin G, Baylis P, Adams P. Maternal paroxysmal supraventricular tachycardia treated with adenosine. Postgrad Med J 1993;69:661–2.
15. Hagley MT, Cole PL. Adenosine use in pregnant women with supraventricular tachycardia. Ann Pharmacother 1994;28:1241–2.
16. Elkayam U, Goodwin TM Jr. Adenosine therapy for supraventricular tachycardia during pregnancy. Am J Cardiol 1995;75:521–3.
17. Hagley MT, Haraden B, Cole PL. Adenosine use in a pregnant patient with supraventricular tachycardia. Ann Pharmacother 1995;29:938.
18. Kohl T, Tercanli S, Kececioglu D, Holzgreve W. Direct fetal administration of adenosine for the termination of incessant supraventricular tachycardia. Obstet Gynecol 1995;85:873–4.

Name: **ALBENDAZOLE** Risk Factor: **C_M**

Class: **Anthelmintic**

FETAL RISK SUMMARY

RECOMMENDATION: Limited Human Data - Animal Data Suggest High Risk

Albendazole is an orally administered, benzimidazole class, broad-spectrum anthelmintic used in the treatment of parenchymal neurocysticerosis caused by larval forms of the pork tapeworm, *Taenia solium*. It is also active against the larval forms of *Echinococcus granulosus*. Plasma concentrations of albendazole are negligible or undetectable because of poor systemic absorption attributable to low water solubility and its rapid hepatic metabolism to the active metabolite, albendazole sulfoxide (1). However, administration of albendazole with a fatty meal will markedly increase the levels of the metabolite in human plasma (up to 5-fold on average) (1).

Reproduction studies have been conducted in mice, rats, and rabbits (1). In rats, albendazole did not adversely affect male or female fertility at oral doses 0.32 times the recommended human dose based on body surface area (RHD). The drug was embryotoxic and teratogenic (skeletal malformations) in pregnant rats given oral doses during organogenesis that were 0.10 and 0.32 times the RHD, respectively. Similar toxicity was observed in pregnant rabbits at 0.60 times the RHD. However, the dose in rabbits was maternally toxic (33% mortality). No teratogenicity was observed in mice given oral doses up to 0.16 times the RHD during organogenesis (1).

A reproductive study in rats examined the effect of oral albendazole (0, 10, or 20 mg/kg/day) administered on gestational days 9 to 11 (2). Compared to controls, the 10 mg/kg dose resulted in a decrease in grown-rump length, a small increase in resorptions, but no teratogenicity. The high dose, however, caused marked fetal growth retardation, an increase in the number of resorptions, and craniofacial and skeletal malformations. Because the severity of the toxic effects differed significantly among the litters, the results suggested that differences in maternal metabolism of albendazole might be involved (2).

In another report by the above researchers, pregnant rats were administered albendazole 0, 10, 20, or 30 mg/kg/day on gestational days 10 to 12 (3). Dose-related resorptions and growth retardation were observed in the three groups receiving albendazole. At 10 mg/kg/day, increased development delay of limb buds was observed, but less than 5% of the embryos had abnormal heads or shapes. At the two higher doses, however, more than 20% of the embryos had morphologic alterations in head shapes and in the development of forelimb buds, branchial bars, eyes, and telencephalon (3). As in their initial communication, the researchers concluded that differences in maternal metabolism may have accounted for the observed interlitter differences in adverse fetal outcomes (3).

It is not known if albendazole or its active metabolite, albendazole sulfoxide, crosses the placenta. The molecular weight of the parent compound (about 265) is low enough for transfer, but the poor oral bioavailability suggests that little, if any, of this agent reaches the plasma. No information is available on the metabolite other than that portions of it undergo further oxidative metabolism before elimination (1).

A brief 1993 publication reported the "accidental" exposure to "high doses" (specific doses not given) of albendazole for systemic infections during the 1st trimester in 10 women (4). The women were followed to term, and all delivered normal infants. Moreover, some of the offspring have been followed for up to 1 year without noting any adverse effects from the exposure (4).

In a randomized, placebo-controlled field trial in western Sierra Leone, anthelmintic treatment was studied as part of a strategy to control maternal anemia caused by parasitic infections (5). A single oral dose of albendazole (400 mg) was given to 61 pregnant women in the 2nd trimester. No adverse pregnancy outcomes attributable to the drug were observed.

In summary, albendazole is a broad-spectrum anthelmintic that is used both in humans and in mass treatments of farm animals (3,6). Although the human use of albendazole is apparently widespread (3), the published human pregnancy data are too limited to assess its fetal risk. The drug is embryo toxic and teratogenic in rats and rabbits, but not in mice at the dose tested. One source stated that the developmental toxicity of albendazole observed in animals was attributable to the active metabolite, albendazole sulfoxide (3). At least in rats, the oral bioavailability of albendazole is much higher than in humans: 1% in humans vs. 20% to 30% in rats (3). Because of the limb reduction defects observed at all doses in one animal study, the potential for much higher plasma concentrations of the metabolite if the drug is consumed with a fatty meal, and the very limited human pregnancy data, the use of albendazole during pregnancy is not recommended. If albendazole is required during pregnancy, avoiding the 1st trimester is strongly advised. A 1997 review also concluded that 1st trimester exposure to albendazole should be avoided (6).

BREAST FEEDING SUMMARY

RECOMMENDATION: No Human Data - Probably Compatible

No reports describing the use of albendazole during human lactation have been located. The anthelmintic is excreted in animal milk (1,7). Although the relatively low molecular weight (about 265) is low enough for excretion into breast milk, the negligible bioavailability of the parent drug suggests that excretion of clinically significant amounts of this compound do not occur. However, excretion of the active metabolite (albendazole sulfoxide) into breast milk may occur. Moreover, administration of albendazole with a fatty meal will markedly increase the plasma concentration of the metabolite (1) and, thus, may increase the amounts in milk. The effects of this exposure on a nursing infant are unknown.

References

1. Product information. Albenza. SmithKline Beecham Pharmaceuticals, 2001.
2. Mantovani A, Macri C, Stazi AV, Ricciardi C. Effects of albendazole on the early phases of rat organogenesis in vivo: preliminary results (abstract). Teratology 1992;46:25A.
3. Mantovani A, Ricciardi C, Stazi AV, Macri C. Effects observed on gestational day 13 in rat embryos exposed to albendazole. Reprod Toxicol 1995;9:265–73.
4. Horton J. The use of antiprotozoan and anthelmintic drugs during pregnancy and contraindications. J Infect 1993;26:104–5.
5. Torlesse H, Hodges M. Anthelminthic treatment and haemoglobin concentrations during pregnancy. Lancet 2000;356:1083.
6. de Silva N, Guyatt H, Bundy D. Anthelmintics. A comparative review of their clinical pharmacology. Drugs 1997;53:769–88.
7. Fletouris DJ, Botsoglou NA, Psomas IE, Mantis AI. Trace analysis of albendazole and its sulphoxide and sulphone metabolites in milk by liquid chromatography. J Chromatogr B Biomed Appl 1996;687:427–35.

Name:	**ALBUTEROL**	Risk Factor:	**C_M**
Class:	**Sympathomimetic (Adrenergic)**		

FETAL RISK SUMMARY

RECOMMENDATION: Compatible

Albuterol is a β-sympathomimetic used to prevent premature labor (see also Terbutaline and Ritodrine) (1–12). In twins, however, a double-blind, controlled study involving 144 women (74 treated with albuterol and 70 treated with placebo) observed no difference between the groups in the length of gestation, birth weight, or fetal outcome, except fewer infants in the albuterol group had respiratory distress syndrome (13).

In an *in vitro* experiment using perfused human placentas, 2.8% of infused drug crossed to the fetal side, but the method only used about 5% of the exchange area of the total placenta (14). Maternal serum concentrations during intravenous and oral albuterol therapy have been reported (15).

Reproduction studies in mice observed an increase in the incidence of cleft palate at a SC dose 0.4 times the maximum recommended human oral dose (MRHD) and higher (16). Cranioschisis was observed in 37% of the fetuses from pregnant rabbits treated with a dose 78 times the MRHD (16).

No published reports linking the use of albuterol to human congenital anomalies have been located, but the majority of reports do not involve 1st trimester exposures. However, in a surveillance study of Michigan Medicaid recipients conducted between 1985 and 1992 involving 229,101 completed pregnancies, 1,090 newborns had been exposed to albuterol during the 1st trimester (F. Rosa, personal communication, FDA, 1993). A total of 48 (4.4%) major birth defects were observed (43 expected). Specific data were available for six defect categories, including (observed/expected) 9/11 cardiovascular defects, 2/2 oral clefts, 2/0.6 spina bifida, 1/2 limb reduction defects, 0/3 hypospadias, and 6/3 polydactyly. Only with the latter defect is there a suggestion of a possible association, but other factors, including the mother's disease, concurrent drug use, and chance, may be involved.

A brief 1980 report described a patient who was treated with a continuous IV infusion of albuterol for 17 weeks via a catheter placed in the right subclavian vein (10,17,18). A normal male infant was delivered within a few hours of stopping the drug. A 1982 report described the use of albuterol in two women with incompetent cervix from the 14th week of gestation to near term (19). Both patients were delivered of normal infants.

Adverse reactions observed in the fetus and mother after albuterol treatment are secondary to the cardiovascular and metabolic effects of the drug. Albuterol may cause maternal and fetal tachycardia with fetal rates exceeding 160 beats/minute (1–3,12,20). Major decreases in maternal blood pressure have been reported, with both systolic and diastolic pressures dropping more than 30 mm Hg (2,4,6). Fetal distress after maternal hypotension was not mentioned. One study observed a maximum decrease in diastolic pressure of 24 mm Hg (34% decrease) but a rise in systolic pressure (20). Other maternal adverse effects associated with albuterol have been acute congestive heart failure, pulmonary edema, and death (21–29).

Like all β-mimetics, albuterol may cause transient fetal and maternal hyperglycemia followed by an increase in serum insulin (4,30–33). Cord blood levels of insulin are about twice those of untreated control infants and are not dependent on the duration of exposure, gestational age, or birth weight (32,33). These effects are more pronounced in diabetic patients, especially in juvenile diabetics, with the occurrence of significant increases in glycogenolysis and lipolysis (20,34,35). Maternal blood glucose should be closely monitored and neonatal hypoglycemia prevented with adequate doses of glucose.

A group of 20 women in premature labor, treated with oral albuterol (4 mg every 4 hours for several weeks), was matched with a control group of women who were not in premature labor (36). The mean gestational ages at delivery for the treated and nontreated patients were 36.4 and 37.0 weeks, respectively. No significant differences were found between the groups for cord blood concentrations of insulin, triiodothyronine (T_3), thyroxine (T_4), and thyroid-stimulating hormone (TSH). However, growth hormone levels were significantly higher in the treated group than in control patients (36.5 vs. 17.4 ng/mL, respectively, $p < 0.001$). The investigators did not determine the reason for the elevated growth hormone level but speculated that it could be caused by either the use of betamethasone for fetal lung maturation in some women of the albuterol group (and resulting fluctuations in fetal blood glucose and insulin levels) or direct adrenergic stimulation of the fetal pituitary (36). Of interest, of the 12 women who received betamethasone, cord blood growth hormone levels in 11 were compared with those of 8 untreated control women. Although the levels in the treated patients were higher (39.5 vs. 31.4 ng/mL), the difference was not significant.

Albuterol decreases the incidence of neonatal respiratory distress syndrome similar to the way that other β-mimetics do (13,37,38). Long-term evaluation of infants exposed to *in utero* β-mimetics has been reported, but not specifically for albuterol (39,40). No harmful effects were observed in these infants. However, a brief 1994 reference described the use of β-sympathomimetics (albuterol, $N = 1$; ritodrine $N = 7$) in eight infants from a group of 16 with retinopathy of prematurity (41). In a matched control group with retinopathy, only 1 of 16 infants was exposed to ritodrine ($p < 0.008$). The authors speculated that the β-sympathomimetics had compromised retinal perfusion *in utero* leading to ischemia and eventually to the ophthalmic complication (41).

The effects of inhaled albuterol on maternal and fetal hemodynamics were first published as an abstract (42) and then as a full report (43). Twelve pregnant asthmatic women between 33 and 39 weeks' gestation received two deep inhalations of a 0.05% solution as recommended by the manufacturer. No effects on the mean maternal, uterine, or fetal hemodynamics were observed.

In contrast to the above, a 1997 case report described fetal tachycardia from the inadvertent administration of a double dose of inhaled albuterol over 24 hours (44). The 34-year-old woman at 33 weeks' gestation received a metered-dose inhaler (two 90-μg actuations every 4–6 hours; 5 doses over 24 hours) and albuterol nebulizer treatment (2.5 mg) every 4 hours (5 doses over 24 hours). Three hours after the last dose, fetal tachycardia (>200 beats/minute) was detected (maternal heart rate was 90–100 beats/minute). Atrial flutter of 420 beats/minute was detected by fetal echocardiography with a predominate 2:1 conduction. Eight hours later, spontaneous conversion to a normal rate occurred. A normal infant was delivered at term and did well during the 4 days of hospitalization.

BREAST FEEDING SUMMARY

RECOMMENDATION: No Human Data - Probably Compatible

No reports describing the use of albuterol during human lactation have been located. Other drugs in the class (see Terbutaline) are considered compatible with breast-feeding and albuterol, most likely, is compatible.

References

1. Liggins GC, Vaughan GS. Intravenous infusion of salbutamol in the management of premature labor. J Obstet Gynaecol Br Commonw 1973;80:29–33.
2. Korda AR, Lynerum RC, Jones WR. The treatment of premature labor with intravenous administered salbutamol. Med J Aust 1974;1:744–6.
3. Hastwell G. Salbutamol aerosol in premature labour. Lancet 1975;2:1212–3.
4. Hastwell GB, Halloway CP, Taylor TLO. A study of 208 patients in premature labor treated with orally administered salbutamol. Med J Aust 1978;1:465–9.
5. Hastwell G, Lambert BE. A comparison of salbutamol and ritodrine when used to inhibit premature labour complicated by ante-partum haemorrhage. Curr Med Res Opin 1979;5:785–9.
6. Ng KH, Sen DK. Hypotension with intravenous salbutamol in premature labour. Br Med J 1974;3:257.
7. Pincus R. Salbutamol infusion for premature labour—the Australian trials experience. Aust NZ Obstet Gynaecol 1981;21:1–4.
8. Gummerus M. The management of premature labor with salbutamol. Acta Obstet Gynecol Scand 1981;60:375–7.
9. Crowhurst JA. Salbutamol, obstetrics and anaesthesia: a review and case discussion. Anaesth Intensive Care 1980;8:39–43.
10. Lind T, Godfrey KA, Gerrard J, Bryson MR. Continuous salbutamol infusion over 17 weeks to pre-empt premature labour. Lancet 1980;2:1165–6.
11. Kuhn RJP, Speirs AL, Pepperell RJ, Eggers TR, Doyle LW, Hutchison A. Betamethasone, albuterol, and threatened premature delivery: benefits and risks. Study of 469 pregnancies. Obstet Gynecol 1982;60:403–8.
12. Eggers TR, Doyle LW, Pepperell RJ. Premature labour. Med J Aust 1979;1:213–6.
13. Felicity Ashworth M, Spooner SF, Verkuyl DAA, Waterman R, Ashurst HM. Failure to prevent preterm labour and delivery in twin pregnancy using prophylactic oral salbutamol. Br J Obstet Gynaecol 1990;97:878–82.
14. Sodha RJ, Schneider H. Transplacental transfer of β-adrenergic drugs studied by an *in vitro* perfusion method of an isolated human placental lobule. Am J Obstet Gynecol 1983;147:303–10.
15. Haukkamaa M, Gummerus M, Kleimola T. Serum salbutamol concentrations during oral and intravenous treatment in pregnant women. Br J Obstet Gynaecol 1985;92:1230–3.
16. Product information. Proventil. Schering Corporation, 2000.
17. Boylan P, O'Discoll K. Long-term salbutamol or successful Shirodkar suture? Lancet 1980;2:1374.
18. Addis GJ. Long-term salbutamol infusion to prevent premature labor. Lancet 1981;1:42–3.
19. Edmonds DK, Letchworth AT. Prophylactic oral salbutamol to prevent premature labour. Lancet 1982;1:1310–1.
20. Wager J, Fredholm B, Lunell NO, Persson B. Metabolic and circulatory effects of intravenous and oral salbutamol in late pregnancy in diabetic and non-diabetic women. Acta Obstet Gynecol Scand 1982;Suppl 108:41–6.
21. Whitehead MI, Mander AM, Hertogs K, Williams RM, Pettingale KW. Acute congestive cardiac failure in a hypertensive woman receiving salbutamol for premature labour. Br Med J 1980;280:1221–2.
22. Poole-Wilson PA. Cardiac failure in a hypertensive woman receiving salbutamol for premature labour. Br Med J 1980;281:226.
23. Fogarty AJ. Cardiac failure in a hypertensive woman receiving salbutamol for premature labour. Br Med J 1980;281:226.
24. Davies PDO. Cardiac failure in a hypertensive woman receiving salbutamol for premature labour. Br Med J 1980;281:226–7.
25. Robertson M, Davies AE. Cardiac failure in a hypertensive woman receiving salbutamol for premature labour. Br Med J 1980;281:227.
26. Crowley P. Cardiac failure in a hypertensive woman receiving salbutamol for premature labour. Br Med J 1980;281:227.
27. Whitehead MI, Mander AM, Pettingale KW. Cardiac failure in a hypertensive woman receiving salbutamol for premature labour (reply). Br Med J 1980;281:227.

28. Davies AE, Robertson MJS. Pulmonary oedema after the administration of intravenous salbutamol and ergometrine-case report. Br J Obstet Gynaecol 1980;87:539–41.
29. Milliez, Blot Ph, Sureau C. A case report of maternal death associated with betamimetics and betamethasone administration in premature labor. Eur J Obstet Gynaecol Reprod Biol 1980;11:95–100.
30. Thomas DJB, Dove AF, Alberti KGMM. Metabolic effects of salbutamol infusion during premature labour. Br J Obstet Gynaecol 1977;84:497–9.
31. Wager J, Lunell NO, Nadal M, Ostman J. Glucose tolerance following oral salbutamol treatment in late pregnancy. Acta Obstet Gynecol Scand 1981;60:291–4.
32. Lunell NO, Joelsson I, Larsson A, Persson B. The immediate effect of a β-adrenergic agonist (salbutamol) on carbohydrate and lipid metabolism during the third trimester of pregnancy. Acta Obstet Gynecol Scand 1977;56:475–8.
33. Procianoy RS, Pinheiro CEA. Neonatal hyperinsulinism after short-term maternal beta sympathomimetic therapy. J Pediatr 1982;101:612–4.
34. Barnett AH, Stubbs SM, Mander AM. Management of premature labour in diabetic pregnancy. Diabetologia 1980;188:365–8.
35. Wager J, Fredholm BB, Lunell NO, Persson B. Metabolic and circulatory effects of oral salbutamol in the third trimester of pregnancy in diabetic and non-diabetic women. Br J Obstet Gynaecol 1981;88:352–61.
36. Desgranges M-F, Moutquin J-M, Peloquin A. Effects of maternal oral salbutamol therapy on neonatal endocrine status at birth. Obstet Gynecol 1987;69:582–4.
37. Hastwell GB. Apgar scores, respiratory distress syndrome and salbutamol. Med J Aust 1980;1:174–5.
38. Hastwell G. Salbutamol and respiratory distress syndrome. Lancet 1977;2:354.
39. Wallace RL, Caldwell DL, Ansbacher R, Otterson WN. Inhibition of premature labor by terbutaline. Obstet Gynecol 1978;51:387–92.
40. Freysz H, Willard D, Lehr A, Messer J, Boog G. A long term evaluation of infants who received a betamimetic drug while in utero. J Perinat Med 1977;5:94–9.
41. Michie CA, Braithwaite S, Schulenberg E, Harvey D. Do maternal β-sympathomimetics influence the development of retinopathy in the premature infant? Arch Dis Child 1994;71:F149.
42. Rayburn WF, Atkinson BD, Gilbert KA, Turnbull GL. Acute effects of inhaled albuterol (Proventil) on fetal hemodynamics (abstract). Teratology 1994;49:370.
43. Rayburn WF, Atkinson BD, Gilbert K, Turnbull GL. Short-term effects of inhaled albuterol on maternal and fetal circulations. Am J Obstet Gynecol 1994;171:770–3.
44. Baker ER, Flanagan MF. Fetal atrial flutter associated with maternal beta-sympathomimetic drug exposure. Obstet Gynecol 1997;89:861.

Name:	**ALENDRONATE**	Risk Factor:	**C_M**
Class:	**Bisphosphonate**		

FETAL RISK SUMMARY

RECOMMENDATION: Limited Human Data - Animal Data Suggest Risk

Bisphosphonates are synthetic analogs of pyrophosphate that bind to the hydroxyapatite found in bone. Alendronate, a specific inhibitor of osteoclast-mediated bone resorption, is indicated for the treatment and prevention of osteoporosis in postmenopausal women and men. Alendronate is also indicated for the treatment of Paget's disease of bone and for glucocorticoid-induced osteoporosis. The oral bioavailability, relative to an IV reference dose, is very low, with only about 0.6% absorbed under fasting conditions. Alendronate is not metabolized in animals or humans. Approximately 78% of the drug is bound to protein in human plasma. After an IV dose, the plasma half-life is about 1 hour (plasma concentrations fell by more than 95% within 6 hours). However, the terminal elimination half-life is greater than 10 years because of its slow release from bone (1).

In pregnant rats, a dose 0.26 times the maximum recommended human daily dose for Paget's disease of 40 mg based on body surface area (MRHD) caused decreased body weight in otherwise normal pups. Decreased post-implantation survival occurred at 0.52 times the MRHD. With higher doses (2.6 times the MRHD), there was an increase in the incidence of incomplete fetal ossification in vertebrae, skull, and sternebrae. *(Note: The daily doses for prevention and treatment of osteoporosis are 5 mg and 10 mg, respectively.)* None of these adverse effects was observed in pregnant rabbits treated with doses up to 10.3 times the MRHD (1).

Delays and failure of delivery secondary to maternal hypocalcemia (both total and ionized calcium) were observed in pregnant rats at 3.9 times the MRHD. Normal calcium levels were measured in the fetuses. Late maternal pregnancy deaths also were observed at this dose. When the rats were treated from before mating through gestation, doses as small as 0.13 times the MRHD resulted in protracted parturition. Oral calcium supplementation did not prevent the hypocalcemia or prevent maternal and fetal deaths secondary to delays in delivery. However, IV calcium did prevent maternal, though not fetal, deaths (1,2).

In a study published in 1999, pregnant rats were treated with a daily SC dose of alendronate (0.1 mg/kg) during days 11–20 of pregnancy (3). Based on body weight, the dose was comparable to a human oral dose of 10 mg/day, but the systemic bioavailability was much higher than that obtained in humans. The gestational period was chosen because it covered the time of active bone development in rat fetuses. Alendronate passed through the placenta and accumulated in the fetuses. A significant increase in fetal bone calcium content (i.e., bone mass) with an accompanying significant decrease in bone marrow volume was found (3).

It is not known if alendronate crosses the placenta to the human fetus, but the molecular weight (about 325) is low enough that fetal exposure should be expected. Although the low maternal plasma concentration and short plasma half-life should reduce the amount of drug available for passage to the fetus, any drug that crosses the placenta probably will accumulate in fetal bones, as it does in rat fetuses.

A single case report has described the use of alendronate in human pregnancy. A 49-year-old woman, who was amenorrheic and thought to be post-menopausal, was treated with oral alendronate 10 mg/day for osteoporosis (4). Treatment was begun before and continued throughout her gestation. She was unaware of the pregnancy until labor started. An apparently normal female infant with a birth weight of 2,390 g (50th percentile) was born at 36 weeks' gestation. Laboratory tests (phosphate, alkaline phosphatase, and ionized calcium) were within normal limits. X-ray studies of the skull and wrists revealed normal bone structure and density without abnormal calcifications (4). At 1 year of age, the girl's weight was 8 kg (10th percentile), her height was 73 cm (50th percentile), and her physical examination and psychomotor development were normal.

In summary, alendronate does not cause structural anomalies in animals but does produce dose-related maternal and fetal toxicity. Only one report has described its use in a human pregnancy. Although no apparent adverse effects were observed, the data are inadequate to determine the risk the drug presents to a human fetus. Alendronate does cross the rat placenta after SC injection. Because the oral bioavailability is very low and the plasma clearance is rapid, clinically significant amounts may not cross the human placenta. However, the drug is slowly released from bone so that use before pregnancy may result in low-level, continuous exposure throughout gestation. The use of alendronate in women who may become pregnant or during pregnancy is not recommended. However, inadvertent exposure during early pregnancy does not appear to present a major risk to the embryo or fetus. If alendronate is used in pregnancy, health care professionals are encouraged to call the toll free number (800–670–6126) for information about patient enrollment in the Motherisk study.

A

BREAST FEEDING SUMMARY

RECOMMENDATION: No Human Data - Probably Compatible

No reports describing the use of alendronate during nursing have been located. The molecular weight (about 325) is low enough for excretion into breast milk, but the low plasma concentrations and rapid plasma clearance suggest that minimal amounts will be excreted into milk. Moreover, since the oral bioavailability of this drug in the nonfasting state is negligible, so systemic levels in a nursing infant should also be negligible (1).

A 1998 case report described the use of alendronate in a postpartum patient suffering from transient osteoporosis of the hip associated with pregnancy. Treatment was started after delivery and the woman did not breast-feed (5).

References

1. Product information. Fosamax. Merck & Co, 2003.
2. Minsker DH, Manson JM, Peter CP. Effects of the bisphosphonate, alendronate, on parturition in the rat. Toxicol Appl Pharmacol 1993;121:217–23.
3. Patlas N, Golomb G, Yaffe P, Pinto T, Breuer E, Ornoy A. Transplacental effects of bisphosphonates on fetal skeletal ossification and mineralization in rats. Teratology 1999;60:68–73.
4. Rutgers-Verhage AR, deVries TW, Torringa MJL. No effects of bisphosphonates on the human fetus. Birth Defects Res (Part A) 2003;67:203–4.
5. Samdani A, Lachmann E, Nagler W. Transient osteoporosis of the hip during pregnancy: A case report. Am J Phys Med Rehabil 1998;77:153–6.

Name:	**ALFENTANIL**	Risk Factor:	$\mathbf{C_M}$*
Class:	**Narcotic Agonist Analgesic**		

FETAL RISK SUMMARY

RECOMMENDATION: Human Data Suggest Risk in 3rd Trimester

No reports linking the use of alfentanil during pregnancy with congenital abnormalities have been located, but experience in the 1st trimester has not been reported. The narcotic is not teratogenic in rats and rabbits (1,2). An embryocidal effect was observed with doses 2.5 times the upper human dose administered for 10–30 days, but this may have been related to maternal toxicity (1).

Alfentanil rapidly crosses the placenta to the fetus (3–5). A 1986 report described the pharmacokinetics and placental transfer of alfentanil after a single 30-μg/kg IV dose administered to five women scheduled for cesarean section (group A) and during a continuous epidural infusion (30-μg/kg loading dose followed by 30-μg/kg/hour infusion) given to five women for vaginal delivery (group B) (3). The ratio of total alfentanil in umbilical vein to maternal blood in the combined 10 women was 0.29 (0.31 and 0.28 for groups A and B, respectively). The fetal:maternal ratio of free (unbound) alfentanil, however, was 0.97, reflecting the decreased α_1-acid glycoprotein (the most important binding protein for the drug) levels in the fetuses compared with the mothers (3).

Alfentanil was administered as a continuous infusion (30 μg/kg/hour with as-needed bolus doses of 30 μg/kg) via an extradural catheter to 16 women undergoing vaginal delivery (4). The umbilical vein:maternal ratios in six patients varied between 0.221 and 0.576 (mean 0.33). For all 16 newborns, the mean (range) Apgar scores at 1, 3, and

5 minutes were 8.56 (range 7–10), 9.60 (range 8–10), and 9.80 (range 9–10), respectively, and were comparable to a control group. However, neurobehavioral assessment of the newborns using the Amiel-Tison score at 15–30 minutes of life indicated a significant decrease, compared with that of control newborns, in passive and active tone and total score. Primary reflexes and general assessment were not statistically different from those of control newborns. No abnormal feeding habits or behavior changes were noted on later evaluation, presumably after the effects of the narcotic had dissipated.

In 21 women scheduled for elective cesarean section, alfentanil (10 μg/kg IV) administered before the induction of anesthesia significantly decreased the pressor response to laryngoscopy and endotracheal intubation in comparison to 16 control patients ($p < 0.01$) (5). At delivery, the mean total alfentanil fetal:maternal ratio was 0.32, but based on the lower α_1-acid glycoprotein levels in the newborns (33% of maternal levels), the calculated unbound alfentanil concentrations in the newborns and mothers were approximately equal (5).

Other reports have described the use of IV alfentanil immediately before the induction of anesthesia for cesarean section to lessen the hypertensive effects of tracheal intubation in women with preeclampsia (6–8) or as a single epidural injection (1 mg) in combination with a continuous epidural infusion of bupivacaine before vaginal delivery (9). As with other opioid agonist analgesics, neonatal respiratory depression is a potential complication, but it can be quickly reversed with naloxone.

[**Risk Factor D if used for prolonged periods or in high doses at term.*]

BREAST FEEDING SUMMARY

RECOMMENDATION: Limited Human Data - Probably Compatible

Alfentanil is excreted into breast milk. Nine non-breast-feeding women undergoing postpartum tubal ligation were administered alfentanil, 50 μg/kg IV (10). An additional 10 μg/kg was given if needed. Colostrum was collected from the right breast 4 hours after the last injection of alfentanil and from the left breast at 28 hours. The mean level of alfentanil in the colostrum at 4 hours was 0.88 ng/mL (range 0.21–1.56 ng/mL), and the mean level at 28 hours was 0.05 ng/mL (range 0.11–0.26 ng/mL). The clinical significance of the drug level in milk to the nursing infant at either time is unknown but is probably nil.

References

1. Product information. Alfenta. Janssen Pharmaceutica, Inc., 1992.
2. Fujinaga M, Mazze RI, Jackson EC, Baden JM. Reproductive and teratogenic effects of sufentanil and alfentanil in Sprague-Dawley rats. Anesth Analg 1988;67:166–9.
3. Gepts E, Heytens L, Camu F. Pharmacokinetics and placental transfer of intravenous and epidural alfentanil in parturient women. Anesth Analg 1986;65:1155–60.
4. Heytens L, Cammu H, Camu F. Extradural analgesia during labour using alfentanil. Br J Anaesth 1987;59:331–7.
5. Cartwright DP, Dann WL, Hutchinson A. Placental transfer of alfentanil at caesarean section. Eur J Anaesthesiol 1989;6:103–9.
6. Ashton WB, James MFM, Janicki P, Uys PC. Attenuation of the pressor response to tracheal intubation by magnesium sulphate with and without alfentanil in hypertensive proteinuric patients undergoing caesarean section. Br J Anaesth 1991;67:741–7.
7. Rout CC, Rocke DA. Effects of alfentanil and fentanyl on induction of anaesthesia in patients with severe pregnancy-induced hypertension. Br J Anaesth 1990;65:468–74.
8. Batson MA, Longmire S, Csontos E. Alfentanil for urgent caesarean section in a patient with severe mitral stenosis and pulmonary hypertension. Can J Anaesth 1990;37:685–8.
9. Perreault C, Albert JF, Couture P, Meloche R. Epidural alfentanil during labor, in association with a continuous infusion of bupivacaine. Can J Anaesth 1990;37:S5.
10. Giesecke AH Jr, Rice LJ, Lipton JM. Alfentanil in colostrum. Anesthesiology 1985;63:A284.

Name:	**ALLOPURINOL**	Risk Factor:	**C_M**
Class:	**Miscellaneous**		

FETAL RISK SUMMARY

RECOMMENDATION: Limited Human Data - Probably Compatible

Allopurinol, a xanthine oxidase inhibitor, is used for the treatment of primary or secondary hyperuricemias, such as those occurring in gout or during cancer chemotherapy. Because these conditions are relatively rare in women of childbearing age, there are few reports describing the use of allopurinol during pregnancy. No adverse fetal outcomes attributable to allopurinol have been reported in humans. The manufacturer is aware of two unpublished reports of women receiving the drug during pregnancy who gave birth to normal infants (1). In a 1972 study, allopurinol produced cleft palate and skeletal defects in mice (2). However, in studies involving other animal species, no fetal harm was observed (1,3).

Allopurinol, in daily doses of 300–400 mg, was combined with cancer chemotherapeutic agents in four patients for the treatment of leukemia occurring during pregnancy (4–6). Treatment in each of these cases was begun in the 2nd or 3rd trimester. The outcomes of these pregnancies were as follows: two normal healthy infants (4); one intrauterine fetal death probably a result of severe preeclampsia (5); and one growth-retarded infant with absence of the right kidney, hydronephrosis of the left kidney, and hepatic subcapsular calcifications (6). The cause of the defects in the latter infant was unknown but because drug therapy was not started until the 20th week of gestation, any relationship to allopurinol can be excluded. The intrauterine growth retardation was thought to be caused by the chemotherapeutic agent, busulfan, that the mother received (6).

A 1976 case report described the use of allopurinol in a woman with type I glycogen storage disease (von Gierke's disease) (7). One of the characteristics of this inherited disease is hyperuricemia as a result of decreased renal excretion and increased production of uric acid (7). The woman was receiving allopurinol, 300 mg/day, at the time of conception and during the early portion of the 1st trimester (exact dates were not specified). The drug was stopped at that time. A term female infant was delivered by cesarean section for failed labor. Phenylketonuria, an autosomal recessive disorder, was subsequently diagnosed in the infant.

A woman with primary gout and gouty nephropathy was treated with 300 mg/day of allopurinol throughout gestation (8). She was delivered of an appropriate-for-gestational-age 2510-g healthy female infant at 35 weeks' gestation. The infant's weight gain was normal at 10 weeks of age, but other developmental milestones were not provided.

BREAST FEEDING SUMMARY

RECOMMENDATION: Limited Human Data - Probably Compatible

Allopurinol and the metabolite, oxipurinol, are excreted into human milk. A woman with hyperuricemia was taking allopurinol 300 mg/day for 4 weeks while breast-feeding her 5-week-old infant (9,10). Maternal plasma and milk samples were drawn 2 and 4 hours after a 300-mg dose. Her plasma levels of allopurinol and the metabolite, oxipurinol, at these times were 1.0 and 13.8 μg/mL, and 1.0 and 19.9 μg/mL, respectively. Milk levels of the drug and metabolite at 2 and 4 hours were 0.9 and 53.7 μg/mL, and 1.4 and 48.0 μg/mL, respectively, representing milk:plasma ratios of the active drug of 0.9 and

1.4, respectively. The mother breast-fed her infant 2 hours after her dose and a single infant plasma sample was taken 2 hours later. Allopurinol was not detected (detection limit 0.5 μg/mL) in the infant's plasma but the concentration of oxipurinol was 6.6 μg/mL. The average daily dose of allopurinol ingested by the infant from the milk was 0.14–0.20 mg/kg (10). No adverse effects in the nursing infant were observed. The American Academy of Pediatrics classifies allopurinol as compatible with breast-feeding (11).

References

1. Product information. Zyloprim. Burroughs Wellcome, 1990.
2. Fujii T, Nishimura H. Comparison of teratogenic action of substances related to purine metabolism in mouse embryos. Jpn J Pharmacol 1972;22:201–6.
3. Chaube S, Murphy ML. The teratogenic effects of the recent drugs active in cancer chemotherapy. In Woollam DHM, ed. *Advances in Teratology*. New York, NY: Academic Press, 1968;3:181–237. As cited in Shepard TH. *Catalog of Teratogenic Agents*. 6th ed. Baltimore, MD: Johns Hopkins University Press, 1989: 58.
4. Awidi AS, Tarawneh MS, Shubair KS, Issa AA, Dajani YF. Acute leukemia in pregnancy: report of five cases treated with a combination which included a low dose of Adriamcyin. Eur J Cancer Clin Oncol 1983;19: 881–4.
5. O'Donnell R, Costigan C, O'Connell LG. Two cases of acute leukaemia in pregnancy. Acta Haematol 1979;61:298–300.
6. Boros SJ, Reynolds JW. Intrauterine growth retardation following third-trimester exposure to busulfan. Am J Obstet Gynecol 1977;129:111–2.
7. Farber M, Knuppel RA, Binkiewicz A, Kennison RD. Pregnancy and von Gierke's disease. Obstet Gynecol 1976;47:226–8.
8. Coddington CC, Albrecht RC, Cefalo RC. Gouty nephropathy and pregnancy. Am J Obstet Gynecol 1979;133:107–8.
9. Kamilli I, Gresser U, Schaefer C, Zollner N. Allopurinol in breast milk. Adv Exp Med Biol 1991;309A:143–5.
10. Kamilli I, Gresser U. Allopurinol and oxypurinol in human breast milk. Clin Invest 1993;71:161–4.
11. Committee on Drugs, American Academy of Pediatrics. The transfer of drugs and other chemicals into human milk. Pediatrics 2001;108:776–89.

Name:	**ALMOTRIPTAN**	Risk Factor:	**C_M**
Class:	**Antimigraine**		

FETAL RISK SUMMARY

RECOMMENDATION: No Human Data - Animal Data Suggest Low Risk

Almotriptan is an oral selective serotonin (5-hydroxytryptamine; 5-$HT_{1B/1D}$) receptor agonist that has high affinity for 5-HT_{1B}, 5-HT_{1D}, and 5-HT_{1F} receptors. The drug is closely related to eletriptan, frovatriptan, naratriptan, rizatriptan, sumatriptan, and zolmitriptan (see also Eletriptan, Frovatriptan, Naratriptan, Rizatriptan, Sumatriptan, and Zolmitriptan). It is indicated for the acute treatment of migraine with or without aura in adults. Protein binding is minimal (about 35%). Almotriptan is metabolized to inactive metabolites, but about 40% is excreted unchanged in the urine. The mean elimination half-life is approximately 3–4 hours (1).

Reproduction studies have been conducted in rats and rabbits. Rats were given doses throughout organogenesis that produced maternal exposures up to about 958 times the human exposure from the maximum recommended daily human dose of 25 mg (MRHD) based on AUC (MRHD-AUC). At the highest dose (958 times the MRHD-AUC), increased embryo deaths were observed. Doses greater than 80 times the MRHD-AUC resulted in an increased incidence of fetal skeletal variations (decreased ossification). When almotriptan was administered to pregnant rats throughout gestation and lactation, a dose 160 times the MRHD based on body surface area (MRHD-BSA) caused an increase in gestational length and a decrease in litter size and pup birth weight. The decreased pup weight persisted throughout lactation. The no-observed-effect-level was 40 times the MRHD-BSA. In pregnant rabbits, a dose 50 times the MRHD-BSA resulted in an increase in embryo deaths (1).

It is not known if almotriptan crosses the human placenta to the fetus. The molecular weight (about 336 for the free base), however, is low enough that passage to the fetus should be expected. In addition, the minimal plasma protein binding, incomplete metabolism, and moderate elimination half-life suggest that substantial amounts of the drug will be available for transfer at the maternal:fetal interface.

No reports describing the use of almotriptan in human pregnancy have been located. The animal data are suggestive of low risk, but an assessment of the actual risk cannot be determined until human pregnancy experience is available.

BREAST FEEDING SUMMARY

RECOMMENDATION: No Human Data - Probably Compatible

No reports describing the use of almotriptan during human lactation have been located. Almotriptan was found in the milk of lactating rats. Milk and maternal plasma concentrations were approximately equal at 0.5 hours after dosing but, at 6 hours, milk levels were seven times higher than maternal levels (1). The molecular weight (about 336 for the free base) suggests that the drug will be excreted into breast milk. The effect of this exposure on a nursing infant is unknown.

Reference

1. Product information. Axert. Ortho-McNeil Pharmaceutical, 2004.

Name:	**ALOSETRON**	Risk Factor:	**B_M**
Class:	**Antidiarrheal/Antiemetic**		

FETAL RISK SUMMARY

RECOMMENDATION: No Human Data - Animal Data Suggest Low Risk

Alosetron is a selective antagonist of the serotonin 5-HT_3 receptor type. It is the same pharmacologic class as dolasetron, granisetron, ondansetron, and palonosetron. Although classified as an antiemetic, alosetron is indicated for the treatment of irritable bowel syndrome in women whose primary symptom is severe chronic diarrhea. Alosetron is extensively metabolized to metabolites with unknown biological activity. About 82% is bound to plasma proteins and the terminal elimination half-life is very short (about 1.5 hours) (1).

Reproduction studies have been conducted in rats and rabbits. In rats, doses up to about 160 times the recommended human dose based on body surface area (RHD) revealed no evidence of impaired fertility or fetal harm. Similar findings were observed in rabbits given doses up to about 240 times the RHD. In addition, doses up to about 160 times the RHD had no effect on reproductive performance in male or female rats (1).

It is not known if alosetron crosses the human placenta. The molecular weight of the free base (about 295) and moderate plasma protein binding suggest that the drug will cross to the embryo/fetus, but the very short terminal elimination half-life will limit the amount of drug at the maternal:fetal interface.

No reports describing the use of alosetron in human pregnancy have been located. Because the drug is restricted by the manufacturer to severe diarrhea-predominant irritable bowel syndrome, pregnancy exposures are probably infrequent. The animal data suggest low risk, but the absence of human pregnancy experience prevents an assessment of the embryo/fetal risk. Limited information for other agents in this class (e.g., see Ondansetron) do not suggest a risk of teratogenicity. Therefore, if indicated, alosetron should not be withheld because of pregnancy.

BREAST FEEDING SUMMARY

RECOMMENDATION: No Human Data - Potential Toxicity

No reports describing the use of alosetron during human lactation have been located. The drug and/or its metabolites are excreted into the milk of lactating rats. This is consistent with the low molecular weight of the free base (about 295) and moderate plasma protein binding. However, the very short terminal elimination half-life (about 1.5 hours) suggests that the amount of drug in milk will be minimal. The effects of this exposure on a nursing infant are unknown. However, because of the potential for severe toxicity (e.g., gastrointestinal symptoms which have caused deaths in adults), alosetron should probably not be used in women who are breast-feeding.

Reference

1. Product information. Lotronex. GlaxoSmithKline, 2004.

Name:	**ALPHAPRODINE**	Risk Factor:	**C_M***
Class:	**Narcotic Agonist Analgesic**		

FETAL RISK SUMMARY

RECOMMENDATION: Human Data Suggest Risk in 3rd Trimester

No reports linking the use of alphaprodine with congenital defects have been located. Characteristic of all narcotics used in labor, alphaprodine may produce respiratory depression in the newborn (1–8). Tissue pO_2 and pCO_2 were determined in nine women in active labor at term given intravenous alphaprodine (0.4 mg/kg prepregnancy weight) (9). Peak decreases in trancutaneous pO_2 ($tcpO_2$) occurred at 5 minutes after injection with peak increases of $tcpCO_2$ occurring at 20 minutes. Both changes were statistically significant variations from baseline values. The fetal heart rate fell from a mean predose rate of 139 to 132 beats/minute at 20 minutes, a significant change, with a consistent loss of variability occurring at 25 minutes. No adverse effects were noted in the mother or the fetus.

In a group of 40 women treated with alphaprodine during labor, sinusoidal fetal heart rate patterns were observed in 17 fetuses (42.5%) (10). The pattern occurred about 19 minutes after administration of the narcotic and persisted for about 60 minutes. No apparent harm resulted from the abnormal patterns.

Suppression of collagen-induced platelet aggregation has been demonstrated, but specific data were not given (11). Abnormal bleeding after use of this drug has not been reported, even though the magnitude of platelet dysfunction was comparable to that found in hemorrhagic states.

[**Risk Factor D if used for prolonged periods or in high doses at term.*]

BREAST FEEDING SUMMARY

RECOMMENDATION: No Human Data - Probably Compatible

No data are available.

References

1. Smith EJ, Nagyfy SF. A report on comparative studies of new drugs used for obstetrical analgesia. Am J Obstet Gynecol 1949;58:695–702.
2. Hapke FB, Barnes AC. The obstetric use and effect on fetal respiration of Nisentil. Am J Obstet Gynecol 1949;58:799–801.
3. Kane WM. The results of Nisentil in 1,000 obstetrical cases. Am J Obstet Gynecol 1953;65:1020–6.
4. Backner DD, Foldes FF, Gordon EH. The combined use of alphaprodine (Nisentil) hydrochloride and levallorphan (Lorfan) tartrate for analgesia in obstetrics. Am J Obstet Gynecol 1957;74:271–82.
5. Gillan JS, Hunter GW, Darner CB, Thompson GR. Meperidine hydrochloride and alphaprodine hydrochloride as obstetric analgesic agents. A double-blind study. Am J Obstet Gynecol 1958;75:1105–10.
6. Roberts H, Kuck MAC. Use of alphaprodine and levallorphan during labour. Can Med Assoc J 1960;83:1088–93.
7. Burnett RG, White CA. Alphaprodine for continuous intravenous obstetric analgesia. Obstet Gynecol 1966;27:472–7.
8. Anthinarayanan PR, Mangurten HH. Unusually prolonged action of maternal alphaprodine causing fetal depression. Q Pediatr Bull (Winter) 1977;3:14–6.
9. Miller FC, Mueller E, McCart D. Maternal and fetal response to alphaprodine during labor. A preliminary study. J Reprod Med 1982;27:439–42.
10. Gray JH, Cudmore DW, Luther ER, Martin TR, Gardner AJ. Sinusoidal fetal heart rate pattern associated with alphaprodine administration. Obstet Gynecol 1978;52:678–81.
11. Corby DG, Schulman I. The effects of antenatal drug administration on aggregation of platelets of newborn infants. J Pediatr 1971;79:307–13.

Name:	**ALPRAZOLAM**	Risk Factor:	**D_M**
Class:	**Sedative**		

FETAL RISK SUMMARY

RECOMMENDATION: Human and Animal Data Suggest Risk

Alprazolam, a member of the benzodiazepine class of agents, is used for the treatment of anxiety. Although no congenital anomalies have been attributed to the use of alprazolam during human pregnancies, other benzodiazepines (e.g., see Diazepam) have been suspected of producing fetal malformations after 1st trimester exposure. In pregnant rats, the drug produced thoracic vertebral anomalies and increased fetal death only at the highest dose (50 mg/kg) tested (1).

Researchers described the effects of alprazolam exposure on gestational day 18 (i.e., near term) on the neurodevelopment of mice in a series of reports (2–4). In one strain of mice, exposure induced persistent imbalance in the newborn and hind limb impairment in the adult offspring suggesting a defect in cerebellar development (2). In the second part of this study, *in utero* exposure to the drug (0.32 mg/kg orally) did not increase anxiety in adult offspring but did reduce motivation (3). A decrease in the tendency to engage in group activity and an increase in male aggression was observed in the third part of the study (4).

No data have been located on the placental passage of alprazolam. However, other benzodiazepines, such as diazepam, freely cross the placenta and accumulate in the fetus (see Diazepam). A similar distribution pattern should be expected for alprazolam.

One manufacturer has received 441 reports of *in utero* exposure to alprazolam or triazolam, two short-acting benzodiazepines, almost all of which occurred in the 1st trimester (5,6). Although most of the women discontinued the drugs when pregnancy was diagnosed, 24 continued to use alprazolam throughout their gestations (5). At the time of publication, about one-fifth of the 441 cases were still pregnant, one-sixth had been lost to follow-up, and one-sixth had been terminated by elective abortion for various reasons (5). Spontaneous abortion or miscarriage (no congenital anomalies were observed in the abortuses) occurred in 16 women; two pregnancies ended in stillbirths, and one newborn infant died within 24 hours of birth. Most of the remainder of the reported exposures ended with the delivery of a normal infant. The manufacturer also received two retrospective reports of congenital defects after alprazolam exposure (5). One of the cases involved an infant with Down's syndrome after maternal consumption of a single 5.5-mg dose of alprazolam and an unknown amount of doxepin during pregnancy (5). The second report involved a mother that had ingested 0.5 mg/day of alprazolam during the first 2 months of gestation. She was delivered of an infant with cat's eye with Pierre Robin syndrome. Neither of these outcomes can be attributed to alprazolam.

A 1992 reference reported the prospective evaluation of 542 pregnancies involving 1st trimester exposure to alprazolam gathered by a manufacturer from worldwide surveillance (7). These data were an extension of the data provided immediately above. Of the total, 131 (24.2%) were lost to follow-up. The outcome of the remaining 411 pregnancies was 42 (10.2%) spontaneous abortions, 5 (1.2%) stillbirths, 88 (21.4%) induced abortions, and 263 (64.0%) infants without and 13 (3.2%) infants with congenital anomalies. A total of 276 live births occurred, but two of these infants, both born prematurely, died shortly after birth. One, included in the group with congenital anomalies, had bilateral hydroceles and ascites, whereas the other died after intraventricular hemorrhage. The type and incidence of defects were comparable to those observed in the Collaborative Perinatal Project with no pattern of defects or excess of defects or spontaneous abortions apparent (7).

A second 1992 study reported on heavy benzodiazepine exposure during pregnancy from Michigan Medicaid data collected during 1980 to 1983 (8). Of the 2048 women, from a total sample of 104,339, who had received benzodiazepines, 80 had received 10 or more prescriptions for these agents. The records of these 80 women indicated frequent alcohol and substance abuse. Their pregnancy outcomes were 3 intrauterine deaths, 2 neonatal deaths in infants with congenital malformations, and 64 survivors. The outcome for 11 infants was unknown. Six of the surviving infants had diagnoses consistent with congenital defects. The investigators concluded that the high rate of congenital anomalies was suggestive of multiple alcohol and substance abuse. The outcome may not have been related to benzodiazepine exposure (8).

Single case reports of pyloric stenosis, moderate tongue-tie, umbilical hernia and ankle inversion, and clubfoot have been received by the manufacturer after *in utero* exposure to either alprazolam or triazolam (5). In addition, the manufacturer has received five reports of paternal use of alprazolam with pregnancy outcomes of two normal births, one elective abortion, one unknown outcome, and one stillbirth with multiple malformations (5). There is no evidence that the drug affected any of these outcomes.

Neonatal withdrawal after *in utero* exposure to alprazolam throughout gestation has been reported in three infants (5,9). In two cases involving maternal ingestion of 3 mg/day and 7–8 mg/day, mild withdrawal symptoms occurred at 2 days of age in the infant exposed to 3 mg/day (5). No details were provided on the onset or severity of the symptoms in the infant exposed to the higher dose. The third neonate was exposed to 1.0–1.5 mg/day (9). The mother continued this dosage in the postpartum interval while breast-feeding. Restlessness and irritability were noted in the infant during the 1st week. The symptoms worsened 2–3 days after the breast-feeding was stopped on the 7th day because of concerns over drug excretion into the milk. Short, episodic screams and bursts of crying were observed frequently. Treatment with phenobarbital was partially successful, allowing the infant to sleep for longer periods. However, on awakening, jerking movements of the extremities and crying continued to occur. The infant was lost to follow-up at approximately 3 weeks of age.

BREAST FEEDING SUMMARY

RECOMMENDATION: Limited Human Data - Potential Toxicity

Alprazolam is excreted into breast milk. Eight lactating women, who stopped breast-feeding their infants during the study, received a single 0.5-mg oral dose and multiple milk and serum samples were collected up to 36 hours after the dose (9). Transfer into milk was consistent with passive diffusion. The mean milk:serum concentrations ratio (using area under the drug concentration-time curve) was 0.36, indicating that a nursing infant would have received 0.3–5 μg/kg/day, or about 3% (body weight adjusted) of the maternal dose (9).

A brief 1989 report, citing information obtained from the manufacturer, described a breast-fed infant whose mother took alprazolam (dose not specified) for 9 months after delivery but not during pregnancy (10). The mother tapered herself off the drug over a 3-week period. Withdrawal symptoms consisting of irritability, crying, and sleep disturbances were noted in the nursing infant. The symptoms resolved without treatment after 2 weeks.

Because of the potent effects, the drug may have on a nursing infant's neurodevelopment, the case of probable alprazolam withdrawal, and the lethargy and loss of body weight observed with the chronic use of other benzodiazepines (see Diazepam), alprazolam should be avoided during lactation. The American Academy of Pediatrics classifies alprazolam as an agent for which the effect on a nursing infant is unknown but may be of concern (11).

References

1. Esaki K, Oshio K, Yanagita J. Effects of oral administration of alprazolam (TUS-1) on the rat fetus: experiment on drug administration during the organogenesis period. Preclin Rep Cent Inst Exp Anim 1981;7:65–77. As cited in Shepard TH. *Catalog of Teratogenic Agents.* 6th ed. Baltimore, MD: Johns Hopkins University Press, 1989:32.
2. Gonzalez C, Smith R, Christensen HD, Rayburn WF. Prenatal alprazolam induces subtle impairment in hind limb balance and dexterity in C57BL/6 mice (abstract). Teratology 1994;49:390.
3. Christensen HD, Pearce K, Gonzalez C, Rayburn WF. Does prenatal alprazolam exposure increase anxiety in adult mice offspring (abstract)? Teratology 1994;49:390.
4. Rayburn W, Gonzalez C, Christensen D. Social interactions of C57BL/6 mice offspring exposed prenatally to alprazolam (Xanax) (abstract). Am J Obstet Gynecol 1995;172:389.
5. Barry WS, St. Clair SM. Exposure to benzodiazepines *in utero*. Lancet 1987;1:1436–7.
6. Ayd FJ Jr, ed. Exposure to benzodiazepines in utero. *Int Drug Ther Newslett* 1987;22:37–8.
7. St. Clair SM, Schirmer RG. First-trimester exposure to alprazolam. Obstet Gynecol 1992;80:843–6.
8. Bergman U, Rosa FW, Baum C, Wiholm B-E, Faich GA. Effects of exposure to benzodiazepine during fetal life. Lancet 1992;340:694–6.
9. Oo CY, Kuhn RJ, Desai N, Wright CE, McNamara PJ. Pharmacokinetics in lactating women: prediction of alprazolam transfer into milk. Br J Clin Pharmacol 1995;40:231–6.
10. Anderson PO, McGuire GG. Neonatal alprazolam withdrawal—possible effects of breast-feeding. DICP Ann Pharmacother 1989;23:614.
11. Committee on Drugs, American Academy of Pediatrics. The transfer of drugs and other chemicals into human milk. Pediatrics 2001;108:776–89.

Name:	**ALTEPLASE**	Risk Factor:	C_M
Class:	**Thrombolytic**		

FETAL RISK SUMMARY

RECOMMENDATION: Compatible

Alteplase (tissue plasminogen activator; t-PA; rt-PA), an enzyme formed by recombinant DNA technology, is a thrombolytic agent used for the treatment of acute conditions such as myocardial infarction, pulmonary embolism, and ischemic stroke. The agent is a glycoprotein composed of 527 amino acids (1).

No maternal or fetal toxicity was observed in rats and rabbits dosed with 1 mg/kg approximately 0.65 times the human dose for acute myocardial infarction (HD) during organogenesis (1). An embryocidal effect was noted in rabbits administered an IV dose of 3 mg/kg (about 2 times the HD) (1). Shepard cited two studies in which no teratogenicity or other toxicity was observed in the offspring of pregnant rats and rabbits administered tissue plasminogen activator during organogenesis (2).

Eight case reports have described the use of alteplase in human pregnancy (3–10). A 27-year-old woman in premature labor at 31 weeks' gestation was treated with urokinase and heparin, supplemented with continuous dobutamine to maintain a stable hemodynamic state, for massive pulmonary embolism (3). Because she failed to improve, low-dose alteplase therapy was initiated at 10 mg/hour for 4 hours, followed by 2 mg/hour for 1.5 hours (total dose 43 mg). The patient's clinical condition markedly improved with complete reperfusion of the right upper and middle lobe and partial reperfusion of the left lower lobe. Coagulation tests (prothrombin time, partial thromboplastin time, and thrombin time) during alteplase therapy remained within or close to the normal range. A healthy, premature, 2100-g male infant was delivered 48 hours after thrombolysis. A 38-year-old woman at 32 weeks' gestation developed a superior vena caval thrombosis during total parenteral hyperalimentation (4). Treatment with alteplase, 2 mg/hour for 48 hours resulted in clinical resolution of her symptoms (swelling of face and arms) within 24 hours. No evidence of placental bleeding was observed. Labor was induced 2 days later, and a healthy premature infant was delivered. A 29-year-old woman with severe pulmonary embolism and congenital antithrombin III deficiency was treated at 35 weeks' gestation with 100 mg alteplase for 3 hours followed by IV heparin (5). Nearly complete reperfusion of the right lung and the lower two-thirds of the left lung was observed at the end of the alteplase infusion. No placental bleeding was noted. The male infant, delivered by cesarean section 20 hours later, died at 14 days of age secondary to intracranial hemorrhage, a complication thought to be caused by prematurity and unrelated to the thrombolytic therapy.

Brief details of a case (6) of t-PA therapy during pregnancy were described in a 1995 review (8). A 30-year-old woman in her 11th week of gestation was treated with alteplase for pulmonary embolism. No complications were observed, and she had a normal, term delivery (6). A 30-year-old woman at 21 weeks' gestation had an acute myocardial infarction that was treated with a total dose of 100 mg alteplase given IV for 90 minutes (7). Immediate relief of her chest pain occurred and the other effects of cardiac reperfusion (arrhythmias and hypotension) were successfully treated. A cesarean section was performed at 33 weeks' gestation for premature labor unresponsive to magnesium sulfate, and a 1640-g male infant who has done well was delivered. A 20% abruptio placentae was noted during surgery. The cause of the abruption was thought to be either alteplase or the aspirin (81 mg/day) the mother had received after her initial treatment (7).

A 32-year-old pregnant woman had two episodes of a thrombosed St. Jude mitral valve prosthesis (8). The first event, at 20 weeks' gestation, was successfully treated by clot removal under cardiopulmonary bypass. About 8 weeks later, another clot formed on the valve and it was treated with 50 mg alteplase. An anterior placental hematoma was noted on ultrasound during treatment, but it resolved spontaneously within 2 weeks. The patient eventually delivered vaginally a healthy girl with Apgar scores of 10 at 1 and 5 minutes at 38 weeks' gestation (8). A 31-year-old patient developed a pulmonary embolism at 12 weeks' gestation (9). The woman was initially treated with IV heparin. However, because of continued hemodynamic deterioration, IV alteplase 100 mg over 2 hours was administered with rapid clinical improvement. SC heparin was given for the remainder of the pregnancy. At 33 weeks' gestation, placental abruption was diagnosed and a cesarean section delivered a normal 2325-g female infant with Apgar scores of 7 and 8 at 1 and 5 minutes, respectively (9). The last case report involved a 28-year-old woman who underwent *in vitro* fertilization because of long-standing infertility (10). Approximately 7 days after embryo transfer, she experienced a middle cerebral artery thrombosis secondary to ovarian hyperstimulation syndrome induced by the fertility medications. Treatment with 15.5 mg of intra-arterial alteplase over 68 minutes dissolved the clot but a hematoma developed in the right basal ganglia resulting in worsening the stroke. She improved over the next 3 months with only mild residual effects of the stroke, and eventually delivered a healthy male infant by spontaneous vaginal delivery at term (10).

A 1995 review found no increased risk for preterm rupture of membranes, placental hemorrhage, or premature labor from thrombolytic agents (streptokinase, urokinase, or alteplase) (11). In seven women administered thrombolytic therapy before 14 weeks' gestation, pregnancy loss occurred in one case (11). Because of the small number of exposures, the concern that thrombolytics may interfere with placental implantation cannot be completely excluded and indeed, one such case has been reported, although the exact cause was not determined (11).

In summary, the limited use of alteplase during pregnancy does not suggest a significant fetal risk. Although none of the reported human exposures occurred during organogenesis, the high molecular weight probably precludes the transfer of alteplase to the embryo. Moreover, teratogenicity was not observed in animals. Hemorrhage is a risk of therapy at any time during gestation, but careful monitoring of the mother can prevent this from becoming a significant risk to the fetus. Therefore, it appears that alteplase may be used during gestation if the mother's condition requires this therapy.

BREAST FEEDING SUMMARY

RECOMMENDATION: Compatible

It is not known whether alteplase (t-PA) crosses into human milk. Because of the nature of the indications for this agent and its very short initial half-life (less than 5 minutes), the opportunities for its use during lactation or the possibility of exposure of a nursing infant are minimal.

References

1. Product information. Activase. Genentech, 2001.
2. Shepard TH. *Catalog of Teratogenic Agents*. 8th ed. Baltimore, MD: Johns Hopkins University Press, 1995:416.
3. Floβdorf Th, Breulmann M, Hopf H-B. Successful treatment of massive pulmonary embolism with recombinant tissue type plasminogen activator (rt-PA) in a pregnant woman with intact gravidity and preterm labour. Intensive Care Med 1990;16:454–6.
4. Barclay GR, Allen K, Pennington CR. Tissue plasminogen activator in the treatment of superior vena caval thrombosis associated with parenteral nutrition. Postgrad Med J 1990;66:398–400.
5. Baudo F, Caimi TM, Redaelli R, Nosari AM, Mauri M, Leonardi G, deCataldo F. Emergency treatment with recombinant tissue plasminogen activator of pulmonary embolism in a pregnant woman with antithrombin III deficiency. Am J Obstet Gynecol 1990; 163:1274–5.
6. Seifried E, Gabelmann A, Ellbrück D, et al. Thrombolytische Therapie einer Lungenarterienembolie in der Frühschwangerschaft mit rekombinantem Gewebe-Plasminogen-Aktivator. Geburtshilfe Frauenheilkd 1991;51:655. As cited in Turrentine MA, Braems G, Ramirez MM. Use of thrombolytics for the treatment of thromboembolic disease during pregnancy. Obstet Gynecol Surv 1995;50:534–41.
7. Schumacher B, Belfort MA, Card RJ. Successful treatment of acute myocardial infarction during pregnancy with tissue plasminogen activator. Am J Obstet Gynecol 1997;176:716–9.
8. Fleyfel M, Bourzoufi K, Huin G, Subtil D, Puech F. Recombinant tissue type plasminogen activator treatment of thrombosed mitral valve prosthesis during pregnancy. Can J Anaesth 1997;44:735–8.
9. Huang WH, Kirz DS, Gallee RC, Gordey K. First trimester use of recombinant tissue plasminogen activator in pulmonary embolism. Obstet Gynecol 2000;96:838.
10. Elford K, Leader A, Wee R, Stya PK. Stroke in ovarian hyperstimulation syndrome in early pregnancy treated with intra-arterial rt-PA. Neurology 2002;59:1270–2.
11. Turrentine MA, Braems G, Ramirez MM. Use of thrombolytics for the treatment of thromboembolic disease during pregnancy. Obstet Gynecol Surv 1995;50: 534–41.

Name:	**AMANTADINE**	Risk Factor:	C_M
Class:	**Antiviral/Antiparkinsonism**		

FETAL RISK SUMMARY

RECOMMENDATION: Contraindicated - 1st Trimester

Amantadine is used as an anti-Parkinson agent and as an antiviral drug for influenza A treatment and prophylaxis. In a 1975 correspondence, one author thought the drug was a potential human teratogen and the absence of published reports at the time had more to do with its infrequent use in pregnancy than to its teratogenic potency (1).

Amantadine was teratogenic in pregnant rats at 50 mg/kg/day (estimated human equivalent dose based on body surface area conversion [EHED] of 7.1 mg/kg/day) and embryotoxic at 100 mg/kg/day (EHED of 14.2 mg/kg/day) (2). No embryo or fetal harm was observed at 37 mg/kg/day (EHED of 5.3 mg/kg/day). No teratogenic or embryotoxic effects were seen in pregnant rabbits dosed with 32 mg/kg/day (EHED of 9.6 mg/kg/day) (2). The recommended human dose for antiviral indication is 200 mg/day and 100–200 mg/day for parkinsonism.

No reports describing the placental passage of amantadine in animals or humans have been located. The molecular weight of the drug (about 152 for the free base) is low enough, however, that passage to the fetus should be expected.

A cardiovascular defect (single ventricle with pulmonary atresia) has been reported in an infant exposed to amantadine during the 1st trimester (3). The mother was taking 100 mg/day for a parkinson-like movement disorder. The relationship between the drug and the defect is unknown.

In a surveillance study of Michigan Medicaid recipients conducted between 1985 and 1992, involving 229,101 completed pregnancies 51 newborns had been exposed to amantadine during the 1st trimester (F. Rosa, personal communication, FDA, 1993). A total of five (9.8%) major birth defects was observed (two expected). Among six categories of defects for which specific data were available, one cardiovascular defect (0.5 expected) and one limb reduction defect (0 expected) were observed. No cases of oral clefts, spina bifida, polydactyly, or hypospadias were recorded. Although the incidence of defects is high, the number of exposures is too small to draw any conclusions.

BREAST FEEDING SUMMARY

RECOMMENDATION: No Human Data - Potential Toxicity

Amantadine is excreted into breast milk in low concentrations. Although no reports of adverse effects in nursing infants have been located, the previous manufacturer recommended the drug be used with caution in nursing mothers because of the potential for urinary retention, vomiting, and skin rash (4). The current manufacturer recommends that amantadine should not be used in nursing mothers (2).

References

1. Coulson AS. Amantadine and teratogenesis. Lancet 1975;2:1044.
2. Product information. Symmetrel. Endo Pharmaceuticals, 2000.
3. Nora JJ, Nora AH, Way GL. Cardiovascular maldevelopment associated with maternal exposure to amantadine. Lancet 1975;2:607.
4. Product information. Symmetrel. Du Pont Pharmaceuticals, 1985.

Name:	**AMBENONIUM**	Risk Factor:	**C**
Class:	**Parasympathomimetic (Cholinergic)**		

FETAL RISK SUMMARY

RECOMMENDATION: Limited Human Data - No Relevant Animal Data

Ambenonium is a quaternary ammonium chloride with anticholinesterase activity used in the treatment of myasthenia gravis. It has been used in pregnancy, but too little information is available to analyze (1–3). In one case, the mother took ambenonium (60 mg/day), pyridostigmine (420 mg/day), and neostigmine (105 mg/day) throughout gestation without any apparently fetal harm (3).

Although it is ionized at physiologic pH, the molecular weight (about 609) is low enough that the nonionized fraction of ambenonium should cross the placenta to the fetus.

Some authors have cautioned that IV anticholinesterases should not be used in pregnancy because of the potential for inducing premature labor (1). Transient muscular weakness has been observed in about 20% of newborns of mothers with myasthenia gravis. The neonatal myasthenia is caused by transplacental passage of anti-acetylcholine receptor immunoglobulin G antibodies (see Pyridostigmine).

BREAST FEEDING SUMMARY

RECOMMENDATION: No Human Data - Probably Compatible

Although ambenonium is ionized at physiologic pH, the molecular weight (about 609) is low enough that excretion of the nonionized fraction into breast milk should occur. The amount of drug in milk, however, is probably small (4). The effect, if any, on a nursing infant from exposure to ambenonium from milk is unknown.

References

1. McNall PG, Jafarnia MR. Management of myasthenia gravis in the obstetrical patient. Am J Obstet Gynecol 1965;92:518–25.
2. Heinonen OP, Slone D, Shapiro S. *Birth Defects and Drugs in Pregnancy*. Littleton, MA: Publishing Sciences Group, 1977:345–56.
3. Lefvert AK, Osterman PO. Newborn infants to myasthenic mothers: a clinical study and an investigation of acetylcholine receptor antibodies in 17 children. Neurology 1983;33:133–8.
4. Wilson JT. Pharmacokinetics of drug excretion. In Wilson JT, ed. *Drugs in Breast Milk*. Australia: (Balgowlah), ADIS Press, 1981:17.

Name:	**AMIKACIN**	Risk Factor:	**C***
Class:	**Antibiotic (Aminoglycoside)**		

FETAL RISK SUMMARY

RECOMMENDATION: Human Data Suggest Low Risk

Amikacin is an aminoglycoside antibiotic. The drug causes dose-related nephrotoxicity in pregnant rats and their fetuses (1). Reproduction studies have been conducted in mice and rats and no evidence of impaired fertility or teratogenicity was observed (2).

The drug rapidly crosses the placenta into the fetal circulation and amniotic fluid (3–6). Studies in patients undergoing elective abortions in the 1st and 2nd trimesters indicate that amikacin distributes to most fetal tissues except the brain and cerebrospinal fluid (3,5). The highest fetal concentrations were found in the kidneys and urine. At term, cord serum levels were one-half to one-third of maternal serum levels whereas measurable amniotic fluid levels did not appear until almost 5 hours after injection (4).

No reports linking the use of amikacin to congenital defects have been located. Ototoxicity, which is known to occur after amikacin therapy in humans, has not been reported as an effect of *in utero* exposure. However, eighth cranial nerve toxicity in the human fetus is well known after exposure to other aminoglycosides (see Kanamycin and Streptomycin) and amikacin could potentially cause this.

[**Risk Factor D according to manufacturer's Astra USA and Elkins-Sinn.*]

BREAST FEEDING SUMMARY

RECOMMENDATION: Compatible

Amikacin is excreted into breast milk in low concentrations. After 100- and 200-mg IM doses, only traces of amikacin could be found for 6 hours in two of four patients (4,7). Because oral absorption of this antibiotic is poor, ototoxicity in the infant would not be expected. However, three potential problems exist for the nursing infant: modification of bowel flora, direct effects on the infant, and interference with the interpretation of culture results if a fever workup is required.

References

1. Mallie JP, Coulon G, Billerey C, Faucourt A, Morin JP. In utero aminoglycosides-induced nephrotoxicity in rat neonates. Kidney Inter 1988;33:36–44.
2. Product information. Amikacin. Elkins-Sinn, 2000.
3. Bernard B, Abate M, Ballard C, Wehrle P. Maternal-fetal pharmacology of BB-K8. Antimicrobial Agents and Chemotherapy 14th Annual Conference: Abstract 71, (Sep) 1974.
4. Matsuda C, Mori C, Maruno M, Shiwakura T. A study of amikacin in the obstetrics field. Jpn J Antibiot 1974;27:633–6.
5. Bernard B, Abate M, Thielen P, Attar H, Ballard C,

Wehrle P. Maternal-fetal pharmacological activity of amikacin. J Infect Dis 1977;135:925–31.
6. Flores-Mercado F, Garcia-Mercado J, Estopier-Jauregin C, Galindo-Hernandez E, Diaz-Gonzalez C. Clinical pharmacology of amikacin sulphate: blood, urinary and tissue concentrations in the terminal stage of pregnancy. J Int Med Res 1977;5;292–4.
7. Yuasa M. A study of amikacin in obstetrics and gynecology. Jpn J Antibiot 1974;27;377–81.

Name:	**AMILORIDE**	Risk Factor:	B_M*
Class:	**Diuretic**		

FETAL RISK SUMMARY

RECOMMENDATION: Limited Human Data - Animal Data Suggest Low Risk

Amiloride is a potassium-conserving diuretic. In general, diuretics are not recommended in the treatment of gestational hypertension because of the maternal hypovolemia characteristic of this disease.

Reproduction studies using amiloride alone in mice at 25 times the maximum recommended human dose (MRHD) and in rabbits at 20 times the MRHD found no evidence of fetal harm (1). The combination of acetazolamide and amiloride was found to produce abnormal development of the ureter and kidney in fetal mice when given at the critical moment of ureter development (2).

Amiloride crosses the placenta in modest amounts in mice and rabbits (1). No reports describing the human placenta passage of amiloride have been located. The molecular weight (about 302 for the dihydrate, monohydrochloride salt) is low enough, however, that passage to the human fetus should be expected.

Three reports of fetal exposure to amiloride have been located (3–5). In one case, a malformed fetus was discovered after voluntary abortion in a patient with renovascular hypertension (3). The patient had been treated during the 1st trimester with amiloride, propranolol, and captopril. The left leg of the fetus ended at midthigh without distal development and no obvious skull formation was noted above the brain tissue. The authors attributed the defects to captopril, but this agent is not thought to cause birth defects in the 1st trimester.

The second case involved a 21-year-old woman with Bartter's syndrome who was maintained on amiloride (20–30 mg/day) and potassium chloride (160–300 mEq/day) throughout pregnancy (4). Progressive therapy with the two agents was required to maintain normal potassium levels. Mild intrauterine growth retardation was detected at 30 weeks' gestation with eventual vaginal delivery of a 6-lb 2-ounce (about 2800-g) female infant at 41 weeks' gestation. No abnormalities were noted in the infant. A normal 3500-g female infant was delivered by cesarean section at 37 weeks' gestation from a mother who had been treated throughout pregnancy with amiloride, hydrochlorothiazide, and amiodarone for severe chronic atrial fibrillation (5).

In a surveillance study of Michigan Medicaid recipients conducted between 1985 and 1992, involving 229,101 completed pregnancies 28 newborns had been exposed to amiloride during the 1st trimester (F. Rosa, personal communication, FDA, 1993). Two (7.1%) major birth defects were observed (one expected), one of which was a hypospadias. No anomalies were observed in five other categories of defects (cardiovascular, oral clefts, spina bifida, polydactyly, and limb reduction defects) for which specific data were available.

[**Risk Factor D if used in gestational hypertension.*]

BREAST FEEDING SUMMARY

RECOMMENDATION: No Human Data - Probably Compatible

Amiloride is excreted in the milk of lactating rats at concentrations higher than that measured in blood (1). No reports describing the use of the diuretic in lactating humans have been located. The molecular weight (about 302 for the dihydrate, monohydrochloride salt) is low enough, however, that passage into milk should be expected.

References

1. Product information. Midamor. Merck, 2000.
2. Miller TA, Scott WJ Jr. Abnormalities in ureter and kidney development in mice given acetazolamide-amiloride or dimethadione (DMO) during embryogenesis. Teratology 1992;46:541–50.
3. Duminy PC, Burger PT. Fetal abnormality associated with the use of captopril during pregnancy. S Afr Med J 1981;60:805.
4. Almeida OD Jr, Spinnato JA. Maternal Bartter's syndrome and pregnancy. Am J Obstet Gynecol 1989;160:1225–6.
5. Robson DJ, Jeeva Raj MV, Storey GCA, Holt DW. Use of amiodarone during pregnancy. Postgrad Med J 1985;61:75–7.

Name: **AMINOCAPROIC ACID** Risk Factor: **C_M**

Class: **Hemostatic**

FETAL RISK SUMMARY

RECOMMENDATION: Limited Human Data - No Relevant Animal Data

Aminocaproic acid is used to enhance hemostasis when fibrinolysis contributes to bleeding. Animal reproduction studies have not been conducted with the drug (1).

No reports describing the placental passage of aminocaproic acid have been located. The molecular weight (about 131) is low enough, however, that passage to the fetus should be expected.

Aminocaproic acid was used during the 2nd trimester in a patient with subarachnoid hemorrhage as a result of multiple intracranial aneurysms (2). The drug was given for 3 days preceding surgery (dosage not given). No fetal toxicity was observed.

BREAST FEEDING SUMMARY

RECOMMENDATION: Hold Breast Feeding

No reports describing the use of aminocaproic acid during lactation have been located. Although the molecular weight (about 131) is low enough that excretion into breast milk should be expected, the indication for the drug probably implies that the chance of its use during nursing is very small.

References

1. Product information. Amicar. Immunex, 2000.
2. Willoughby JS. Sodium nitroprusside, pregnancy and multiple intracranial aneurysms. Anaesth Intensive Care 1984;12:358–60.

Name: **AMINOGLUTETHIMIDE** Risk Factor: **D_M**
Class: **Anticonvulsant/Anti-Adrenal**

FETAL RISK SUMMARY

RECOMMENDATION: Limited Human Data - No Relevant Animal Data

Aminoglutethimide is a weak anticonvulsant that is also used for the inhibition of the adrenal cortex to produce a "medical" adrenalectomy (1). It also inhibits peripheral aromatase to block the conversion of androgens to estrogen (1). No animal reproduction studies have been found.

No reports describing the placental transfer of aminoglutethimide have been located. The molecular weight (about 232) is low enough, however, that passage to the fetus should be expected.

Aminoglutethimide when given throughout pregnancy has been suspected of causing virilization (2,3). No adverse effect was seen when exposure was limited to the 1st and early 2nd trimesters (4,5). Virilization may be caused by inhibition of adrenocortical function.

BREAST FEEDING SUMMARY

RECOMMENDATION: No Human Data - Potential Toxicity

No reports describing the use of aminoglutethimide during lactation have been located. The molecular weight (about 232) is low enough, however, that excretion into breast milk should be expected.

References

1. Reynolds JEF, editor. *Martindate. The Extra Pharmacopoeia*. 31st ed. London: Royal Pharmaceutical Society, 1996:541.
2. Iffy L, Ansell JS, Bryant FS, Hermann WL. Nonadrenal female pseudohermaphroditism: an unusual case of fetal masculinization. Obstet Gynecol 1965;26;59–65.
3. Marek J, Horky K. Aminoglutethimide administration in pregnancy. Lancet 1970;2:1312–3.
4. Le Maire WJ, Cleveland WW, Bejar RL, Marsh JM, Fishman L. Aminoglutethimide: a possible cause of pseudohermaphroditism in females. Am J Dis Child 1972;124:421–3.
5. Hanson TJ, Ballonoff LB, Northcutt RC. Aminoglutethimide and pregnancy. JAMA 1974;230:963–4.

Name: **AMINOPHYLLINE** Risk Factor: **C**
Class: **Respiratory Drug (Bronchodilator)**

See Theophylline.

Name: **AMINOPTERIN** Risk Factor: **X**
Class: **Antineoplastic**

FETAL RISK SUMMARY

RECOMMENDATION: Contraindicated

Aminopterin is an antimetabolite antineoplastic agent. It is structurally similar to and has been replaced by methotrexate (amethopterin). Several reports have described fetal anomalies when the drug was used as an unsuccessful abortifacient (1–8). The malformations included:

- Meningoencephalocele
- Cranial anomalies
- Abnormal positioning of extremities
- Short forearms
- Anencephaly
- Talipes
- Incomplete skull ossification
- Cleft lip/palate
- Low-set ears
- Hypoplasia of thumb and fibula
- Brachycephaly
- Hydrocephaly
- Mental retardation
- Syndactyly
- Micrognathia or retrognathia

Use of aminopterin in the 2nd and 3rd trimesters has not been associated with congenital defects (8). Long-term studies of growth and mental development in offspring exposed to aminopterin during the 2nd trimester, the period of neuroblast multiplication, have not been conducted (9).

BREAST FEEDING SUMMARY

RECOMMENDATION: Contraindicated

No data are available.

References

1. Meltzer HJ. Congenital anomalies due to attempted abortion with 4-aminopteroylglutamic acid. JAMA 1956;161:1253.
2. Warkany J, Beaudry PH, Hornstein S. Attempted abortion with aminopterin (4-amino-pteroylglutamic acid). Am J Dis Child 1959;97:274–81.
3. Shaw EB, Steinbach HL. Aminopterin-induced fetal malformation. Am J Dis Child 1968;115:477–82.
4. Brandner M, Nussle D. Foetopathic due à l'aminoptérine avec sténose congénitale de l'escpace médullaire des os tubulaires longs. Ann Radiol 1969;12:705–10.
5. Shaw EB. Fetal damage due to maternal aminopterin ingestion: follow-up at age 9 years. Am J Dis Child 1972;124:93–4.
6. Reich EW, Cox RP, Becker MH, Genieser NB, McCarthy JG, Converse JM. Recognition in adult patients of malformations induced by folic acid antagonists. Birth Defects 1978;14:139–60.
7. Shaw EB, Rees EL. Fetal damage due to aminopterin ingestion: follow-up at 17 1/2 years of age. Am J Dis Child 1980;134:1172–3.
8. Nicholson HO. Cytotoxic drugs in pregnancy; review of reported cases. J Obstet Gynaecol Br Commonw 1968;75:307–12.
9. Dobbing J. Pregnancy and leukemia. Lancet 1977; 1:1155.

Name:	***PARA*-AMINOSALICYLIC ACID**	Risk Factor:	C_M
Class:	**Antitubercular**		

FETAL RISK SUMMARY

RECOMMENDATION: Human and Animal Data Suggest Risk

Para-aminosalicylic acid is a bacteriostatic agent used for the treatment of *Mycobacterium tuberculosis*. It is most frequently used in combination with other agents for the treatment of multi-drug resistant tuberculosis.

In reproduction studies with rats at doses within the human dose range, occipital malformations were observed (1). No adverse effects on the fetus were observed in rabbits treated with 5 mg/kg/day throughout gestation (1).

No reports describing the placental transfer of *para*-aminosalicylic acid have been located. The molecular weight (about 153) is low enough, however, that passage to the fetus should be expected.

The Collaborative Perinatal Project monitored 50,282 mother-child pairs, 43 of whom had 1st trimester exposure to *para*-aminosalicylic acid (4-aminosalicylic acid) (2). Congenital defects were found in five infants. This incidence (11.6%) was nearly twice the expected frequency. No major category of malformations or individual defects were identified. An increased malformation rate for ear, limb, and hypospadias has been reported for 123 patients taking 7–14 g/day of *para*-aminosalicylic acid with other antitubercular drugs (3). An increased risk of congenital defects has not been found in other studies (4–6).

BREAST FEEDING SUMMARY

RECOMMENDATION: Limited Human Data - Probably Compatible

Para-aminosalicylic acid is excreted into breast milk. In one non-breast-feeding patient given an oral 4-g dose of the drug, a peak milk concentration of 1.1 μg/mL was measured at 3 hours with an elimination half-life of 2.5 hours (7). The peak maternal plasma concentration, 70.1 μg/mL, occurred at 2 hours.

References

1. Product information. Paser. Jacobus Pharmaceutical, 2000.
2. Heinonen OP, Slone D, Shapiro S. *Birth Defects and Drugs in Pregnancy*. Littleton, MA: Publishing Sciences Group, 1977:299.
3. Varpela E. On the effect exerted by first line tuberculosis medicines on the foetus. Acta Tuberc Scand 1964;35:53–69.
4. Lowe CR. Congenital defects among children born to women under supervision or treatment for pulmonary tuberculosis. Br J Prev Soc Med 1964;18:14–6.
5. Wilson EA, Thelin TJ, Ditts PV. Tuberculosis complicated by pregnancy. Am J Obstet Gynecol 1973;115:526–9.
6. Scheinhorn DJ, Angelillo VA. Antituberculosis therapy in pregnancy. Risk to the fetus. West J Med 1977; 127:195–8.
7. Holdiness MR. Antituberculosis drugs and breast-feeding. Arch Intern Med 1984;144:1888.

Name: **AMIODARONE** Risk Factor: **D_M**

Class: **Antiarrhythmic**

FETAL RISK SUMMARY

RECOMMENDATION: Human and Animal Data Suggest Risk

Amiodarone is an antiarrhythmic agent used for difficult or resistant cases of arrhythmias. The drug contains about 75 mg of iodine per 200-mg dose (1–3).

Amiodarone was maternal and embryo toxic (increased fetal resorptions, decreased live litter size, growth retardation, and retarded sternum and metacarpal ossification) in rats administered an IV infusion about 1.4 times the maximum recommended human dose based on body surface area (MRHD) (4). Lower doses, about 0.4 and 0.7 times the MRHD, produced no embryo toxicity (4). In pregnant rabbits administered IV doses about 0.1, 0.3, and 0.7 times the MRHD, embryo toxicity was observed at 0.3 times the MRHD and above. At about 2.7 times the MRHD, more than 90% of the animals aborted. No teratogenic effects were observed in any of the rabbit groups (4).

Amiodarone and its metabolite, desethylamiodarone, cross the placenta to the fetus (1–3,5–9). In the 10 infants described in these reports, cord blood concentrations of the parent compound were 0.05–0.35 μg/mL, representing cord:maternal ratios of 0.10–0.28 in nine cases (1–3,5–9) and 0.6 in one case (9). Cord blood concentrations of the metabolite varied between 0.05 and 0.55 μg/mL, about one fourth of the maternal levels in 9 of the 10 cases. In one study, the amount of amiodarone crossing the placenta to the fetus was dependent on the degree of hydrops fetalis (10). The expected fetal concentrations of the drug were not achieved until substantial compensation of the fetus had occurred.

In 22 cases of amiodarone therapy during pregnancy, the antiarrhythmic was administered for maternal indications (1–3,5,7–9,11–16). One patient in the last 3 months of pregnancy was treated with 200 mg daily for resistant atrial tachycardia (1). She delivered a 2780-g female infant at 40 weeks' gestation. Both the mother and the infant had a prolonged QT interval on electrocardiogram (ECG). A second woman was also treated by these investigators under similar conditions. Both infants were normal (infant sex, weight, and gestational age were not specified for the second case), including having normal thyroid function. In another report, a woman was treated at 34 weeks' gestation when quinidine failed to control her atrial fibrillation (2). After an initial dose of 800 mg/day for 1 week, the dose was decreased to 400 mg/day and continued at this level until delivery at 41 weeks' gestation. The healthy 3220-g infant experienced bradycardia during labor induction (104–120 beats/minute) and during the first 48 hours after birth. No other adverse effects were observed in the infant, who had normal thyroid and liver function tests. A woman was treated during the 37th–39th weeks of pregnancy with daily doses of 600 mg, 400 mg, and 200 mg, each for 1 week, for atrial tachycardia that was resistant to propranolol, digoxin, and verapamil (3). No bradycardia or other abnormalities were noted in the newborn. The infant's thyroid-stimulating hormone (TSH) level on the 4th day was 9 mU/L, a normal value. Goiter was not observed and the infant was clinically euthyroid.

A 1985 report described the treatment of two women with amiodarone for maternal heart conditions (5). One of these patients, a 31-year-old woman with atrial fibrillation, was treated with amiodarone, 200 mg/day, and diuretics throughout gestation. She delivered a healthy 3500-g girl without goiter or corneal changes at 37 weeks' gestation. A cord blood thyroxine (T_4) level was elevated (209 nmol/L) and was still elevated 1 week later (207 nmol/L), but TSH concentrations at these times were 3.2 mU/L and <1 mU/L (both normal), respectively. The second woman, a 27-year-old primigravida, was treated with amiodarone, 400–800 mg/day, starting at 22 weeks' gestation. Fetal bradycardia, 100–120 beats/minute, was observed at approximately 33 weeks' gestation. Spontaneous labor ensued at 39 weeks with delivery of a healthy 2,900-g boy. Thyroid function studies were not reported, but the neonatal examinations were normal (5).

A woman in her 16th week of pregnancy presented with severe atrial fibrillation (7). She was treated with amiodarone, 800 mg/day for 1 week followed by 200 mg/day for the remainder of her pregnancy (7). She delivered a growth-retarded 2660-g male in the 39th week of gestation who had no goiter and whose free T_4 index, serum free triiodothyronine (T_3), and serum TSH concentrations were all within normal limits. An ECG at 1 day of age showed a prolonged QT interval. Follow-up of the infant at 6 months was normal.

A healthy 3650-g male infant was delivered at term from a mother who had taken 200–400 mg/day of amiodarone throughout gestation (8). The infant's thyroid function was normal at birth; no goiter or corneal deposits were noted; and subsequent growth and thyroid function remained within normal limits. In another case, a woman was treated with propranolol and amiodarone, 400 mg/day for 4 days each week, throughout gestation (11). A healthy 2670-g female infant was delivered, but the gestational age was not specified. No goiter or corneal microdeposits were present in the infant, and clinically she was euthyroid. The T_4 and TSH levels in cord blood were both normal although a total serum iodine level (290 μg/dL) was markedly elevated (normal 5.5–17.4 μg/dL).

A 1991 report described the use of amiodarone in one woman with a history of symptomatic ventricular arrhythmia, and mitral and tricuspid valve prolapse through two complete pregnancies (12). She also had a history of right upper lobectomy for drug-resistant pulmonary tuberculosis. She was treated with 400 mg/day of amiodarone during the first 12 weeks of gestation of one pregnancy before the dose was reduced to 200 mg/day. She continued this dose during the remainder of this pregnancy and through a successive pregnancy. One of the newborns was growth retarded, a 2500-g female delivered at 38 weeks' gestation. The second infant, a 2960-g male, was delivered prematurely at 35.5 weeks' gestation. Except for the growth retardation in the one infant, the newborns were physically normal and had no clinical or biochemical signs of hypothyroidism (12). The concentration of amiodarone and its metabolite, desethylamiodarone, were $<$0.3 μg/mL in the first-born infant (not determined in the second newborn).

In two other reports, treatment was begun at 25 and 32 weeks' gestation (13,14). Delivery occurred at 31 weeks in one case (sex and birth weight not given), and the infant died 2 days after delivery (13). In the second report, the infant (sex and birth weight not given) was born at 37 weeks' gestation (14). Amiodarone and desethylamiodarone concentrations in the cord blood were 0.1 and 0.2 μg/mL, respectively. The drug and its metabolite were not detected in the infant's serum at 3 and 6 days after birth. A prolonged QT interval was observed on the infant's ECG.

Five pregnancies in four women treated with amiodarone for various cardiac arrhythmias were described in a 1992 reference (9). The drug was used throughout gestation in four pregnancies and during the last 6 weeks in a fifth. One infant delivered at 34 weeks' gestation was growth retarded (birth weight, length, and head circumference were all at the 10th percentile or less), but the other four newborns were of normal size. No adverse effects—such as goiter, corneal microdeposits, pulmonary fibrosis, or dermatologic or neurologic signs—were observed (9). The infants were clinically euthyroid, but one of the five newborns had transient biochemical signs of hypothyroidism (low T_4 concentration) that responded to treatment. This latter infant, whose mother had taken the β-blocker, metoprolol, throughout gestation and amiodarone only during the last 6 weeks, had delayed motor development and impaired speech performance at 5 years of age. He had been delivered at 40 weeks' gestation with a birth weight of 2,880 g (10th percentile) and a length of 50 cm (50th percentile). The other four infants had normal follow-up examinations at periods ranging from 8 months to 5 years.

Congenital hypothyroidism with goiter was described in a growth-retarded 2450-g male newborn whose mother had taken 200 mg/day of amiodarone from the 13th week of gestation until delivery at 38 weeks for treatment of Wolff-Parkinson-White syndrome (15). The mother had no signs or symptoms of hypothyroidism. Thyroid tests of cord blood revealed a TSH level of $>$100 mU/L (normal 10–20 mU/L), a T_4 of 35.9 μg/L (normal 60–170 μg/L), and no thyroid antibodies. In addition to a homogeneous goiter, the newborn had persistent hypotonia and bradycardia, large anterior and posterior fontanels, and macroglossia, but no corneal microdeposits. The bradycardia resolved after several days. Greater than normal amounts of urinary iodine were measured from birth (144 μg/dL; normal $<$15 μg/dL) until the 6th week of life. The infant's plasma concentrations of amiodarone and desethylamiodarone on day 5 were 140 ng/mL and 260 ng/mL, respectively, and were still detectable after 1 month. His bone age at birth and at 20 months of age was estimated to be 28 weeks and 12 months, respectively. Treatment with levothyroxine during the first 20 months resulted in the complete disappearance of the goiter at about 3 months of age, but his psychomotor development was retarded.

A 1994 report described three pregnancies in two women who were being treated with amiodarone (16). Recurrent ventricular fibrillation was treated in one woman with an implanted defibrillator and amiodarone, 400 mg/day. She became pregnant 4 years after beginning this therapy and eventually delivered a premature, 2540-g male infant at 35 weeks' gestation with a holosystolic murmur and an umbilical hernia. At 2 weeks of age, the infant experienced mild congestive heart failure with labored breathing. A large midmuscular ventricular septal defect, with marked left ventricular and left atrial dilatation and left ventricular hypertrophy, was observed by echocardiogram (16). The defect was still present at 21 months of age. A second pregnancy in this woman, at the same amiodarone dose, was electively terminated at approximately 11 weeks' gestation. The thorax and limbs of the fetus were normal and contained 1.55 and 5.8 μg/g of amiodarone and desethylamiodarone, respectively. The second woman had been treated with amiodarone, 600 mg/day, for 2 years for recurrent sustained ventricular tachycardia (Chagas' disease) before conception. She eventually delivered a term 3300 g male infant with mild bradycardia (110 beats/minute) at birth. Both liveborn infants were clinically euthyroid without goiter or corneal changes.

Six cases of amiodarone therapy for refractory fetal tachycardia have been described in the literature (6,10,17–20). In the first of these, a fetus at 27 weeks' gestation experienced tachycardia, 260 beats/minute, that was unresponsive to digoxin and propranolol (17). Lidocaine and procainamide lowered the heart rate somewhat but were associated with unacceptable maternal toxicity. Amiodarone combined with verapamil was successful in halting the tachycardia and reversing the signs of congestive heart failure. An amiodarone maintenance dose of 400 mg/day was required for control. Spontaneous labor occurred after 39 days of therapy, with delivery of a 2700-g male infant at 33 weeks' gestation. Atrial flutter with a 2:1 block and a ventricular rate of 200 beats/minute were converted on the 3rd day by electrical cardioversion. No adverse effects from the drug therapy were mentioned.

A fetus with supraventricular tachycardia, 220 beats/minute, showed evidence of congestive heart failure at 32 weeks' gestation (6). Maternal therapy with digoxin alone or in combination with sotalol (a β-blocker) or verapamil failed to stop the abnormal rhythm. Digoxin was then combined with amiodarone, 1600 mg/day for 4 days, then 1200 mg/day for 3 days, then 800 mg/day for 6 weeks. The fetal heart rate fell to 140 beats/minute after 14 days of therapy, and the signs of congestive heart failure gradually resolved. Neonatal thyroid indices at birth (about 38 weeks' gestation) and at 1 month were as follows (normal values are shown in parentheses): free T_3 index, 3.4 and 5.6 pmol/L (4.3–8.6 pmol/L); free T_4 index, 5.4 and 25 pmol/L (9–26 pmol/L); T_3, 1.7 and 2.7 nmol/L (1.2–3.1 nmol/L); T_4, 196 and 300 nmol/L (70–175 nmol/L); and TSH, 30 and 4.12 mU/L (<5 mU/L). The elevated T4 level returned to normal at a later unspecified time. It was not mentioned whether a goiter was present at birth. At 10 months of age, all thyroid function tests were within normal limits.

A third case involved a fetus at 30 weeks' gestation with tachycardia, 220 beats/minute, with congestive heart failure that had not responded to digoxin and propranolol (18). At 32 weeks' gestation, digoxin and amiodarone lowered the rate to 110–180 beats/minute with improvement in the congestive failure. Amiodarone was given at 1200 mg/day for 3 days, then 600 mg/day until delivery 3 weeks later. The newborn had tachycardia of up to

200 beats/minute that was treated with digoxin, furosemide, and propranolol. Hypothyroidism was diagnosed based on the presence of a goiter and abnormal thyroid tests (normal values are in parentheses): T_4, 48 μg/mL (70–180 μg/mL); free T_4, 0.5 μg/mL (>1.5 μg/mL); and TSH, >240 mU/L (<30 mU/L). The infant was treated with 10 μg/day of T_4 until age 3 months, at which time his cardiac and thyroid functions were normal. Follow-up at 15 months was normal.

A 27-week fetus with refractory supraventricular tachycardia and hydrops fetalis was treated with repeated injections of amiodarone into the umbilical vein after maternal therapy with amiodarone and multiple other antiarrhythmic drugs failed to resolve the fetal condition (10). Subtherapeutic transplacental passage of amiodarone and digoxin was documented that did not improve until substantial resolution of the hydrops had occurred with direct administration of amiodarone to the fetus. A male infant was delivered at 37 weeks' gestation because of growth retardation, but thyroid function and other tests were within normal limits, and no corneal deposits were observed.

In a similar case, a 27-week fetus with severe hydrops secondary to congenital sinoatrial disease-induced sinus bradycardia and atrial flutter was treated with amiodarone via the intravenous, intraperitoneal, and transplacental routes (19). Prior maternal therapy with oral sotalol and flecainide had failed to reverse the worsening right heart failure. A 15-mg IV dose was administered to the fetus concurrently with initiation to the mother of 200 mg orally every 8 hours. Approximately 24 hours later, an additional 15-mg dose of amiodarone was given intraperitoneally to the fetus. The fetal ascites resolved over the next 3 weeks. A 2686-g female infant in good condition was eventually delivered at 37 weeks' gestation. Cardiac function was normal in the neonatal period and at 3-month follow-up, as were thyroid tests at 6 days of age.

A 1994 report described the use of amiodarone, 1600 mg/day (25 mg/kg/day), for the treatment of fetal supraventricular tachycardia that had failed to respond to flecainide at 33 weeks' gestation (20). The tachycardia recurred 2 weeks later and a cesarean section was performed under epidural anesthesia with lidocaine to deliver a 3380-g male infant (follow-up of the infant not specified).

A historic cohort study, first published as an abstract (21) and then as a full report (22), described the fetal effects of maternal treatment with amiodarone. Twelve women, with various heart conditions requiring amiodarone therapy, were treated with individualized therapeutic doses (mean dose 321 mg/day) during gestation. Seven patients were treated throughout their pregnancies, with one suffering a spontaneous abortion at 10 weeks. β-blockers were used concurrently in the six pregnancies that delivered live newborns, but in one the β-blocker was stopped after 14 weeks. In the other five women, treatment with amiodarone was begun in the 2nd or 3rd trimesters, and concurrent β-blockers were used in three for various intervals. The 11 infants were delivered at term (>37 weeks' gestation). Amiodarone was detected in two of three cord blood samples. The level in one was 0.2 μg/mL (maternal serum not detectable), and the cord blood level in the other was 21.3% of the maternal concentration. One of the newborns was hyperthyroid (asymptomatic, transient) and one was hypothyroid. Fetal bradycardia occurred in three of the infants, two of whom had been exposed to β-blockers (acebutolol and propranolol). Four infants were small for gestational age (<3rd percentile corrected for gestational age) and three of these had been exposed to β-blockers throughout pregnancy (22). Two infants had birth defects, only one of whom had been exposed during the 1st trimester. This infant had congenital jerk nystagmus with synchronous head titubation (exposed to amiodarone and propranolol throughout, quinidine during the 1st 3 weeks). The other newborn had hypotonia, hypertelorism, and micrognathia (exposed to amiodarone from the 20th week, atenolol from 18 to 20 weeks, and phenoxybenzamine during week 39), and delayed motor development assessed at 18 months (normal speech but milestone delay of about 3 months as indicated by lifting head, sitting unaided, crawling, standing, and walking) (22). The child's birth weight and Apgar scores had been normal for gestational age and his neonatal course, other than a meconium plug, had been unremarkable. Other than this case, the other exposed infants had normal development (mean age at follow-up 30 months, range 0 months to 11.5 years).

In summary, serious fetal adverse effects directly attributable to amiodarone have been observed. Congenital goiter/hypothyroidism and hyperthyroidism may occur after *in utero* exposure. Congenital defects have been observed in two newborns, but any association between amiodarone and the defects may be fortuitous. Ventricular septal defects reportedly occur at an incidence of 1–3/1000 live-births (16), and the cause of the neurotoxicity in the second case is unknown (22). The transient bradycardia and prolonged QT interval observed in some amiodarone-newborns are direct effects of the drug but apparently lack clinical significance. Intrauterine growth retardation occurs frequently in infants exposed *in utero* to amiodarone, but it is uncertain whether this is a consequence of amiodarone, the mother's disease, other drug therapy (such as β-blockers), or a combination of these and other factors. Growth retardation has also been observed in animal studies.

Because of the above outcomes and the limited data available, the drug should be used cautiously during pregnancy. As a result of the potential for fetal and newborn toxicity, it is not recommended as a first-line drug in uncomplicated cases of fetal supraventricular tachycardia (23).

Following chronic administration, amiodarone has a very long elimination half-life of 14–58 days (24). Therefore, the drug must be stopped several months before conception to avoid exposure in early gestation. A 1987 review of the management of cardiac arrhythmias during pregnancy recommends that amiodarone be restricted to refractory cases (25). Similarly, a 1992 review of maternal drug therapy for fetal disorders suggests caution, if it is used at all, before amiodarone is prescribed during pregnancy (26). Newborns exposed to amiodarone *in utero* should have thyroid function studies performed because of the large proportion of iodine contained in each dose.

BREAST FEEDING SUMMARY

RECOMMENDATION: Contraindicated

The effects on suckling rats of amiodarone obtained from breast milk were investigated in a study published in 1992 (27). No effect on neonatal weight gain was observed, but treatment did result in a decrease in maternal weight gain compared to controls. Accumulations of both amiodarone and its metabolite, desethylamiodarone, were demonstrated in neonatal lung and liver.

Amiodarone is excreted into breast milk (2,3,8,9). The drug contains about 75 mg of iodine/200-mg dose (2,3,5). One woman, consuming 400 mg/day, had milk levels of amiodarone and its metabolite, desethylamiodarone (activity unknown), determined at varying times between 9 and 63 days after delivery (2). Levels of the two substances in milk were highly variable during any 24-hour period. Peak levels of amiodarone and the metabolite ranged from 3.6–16.4 μg/mL and 1.3–6.5 μg/mL. The milk:plasma (M:P) ratio of the active drug at 9 weeks postpartum ranged from 2.3 to 9.1 and that of desethylamiodarone from 0.8 to 3.8. The authors calculated that the nursing infant received about

1.4–1.5 mg/kg/day of active drug. Plasma levels of amiodarone in the infant remained constant at 0.4 μg/mL (about 25% of maternal plasma) from birth to 63 days. In a second case, a mother taking 200 mg/day did not breast-feed, but milk levels of the drug and the metabolite on the 2nd and 3rd days after delivery were 0.5–1.8 μg/mL and 0.4–0.8 μg/mL, respectively (3). A mother taking 400 mg/day had milk concentrations of amiodarone and the metabolite during the first postpartum month ranging from 1.06–3.65 μg/mL and 0.50–1.24 μg/mL, respectively (8). No adverse effects were observed in her nursing infant.

Mothers of three breast-feeding infants had taken amiodarone, 200 mg/day, during pregnancy and continued the same dose in the postpartum period (9). Milk concentrations of the drug at various times after delivery in the three mothers were 1.70 μg/mL (2 days postpartum) and 3.04 μg/mL (3 weeks postpartum), 0.55 μg/mL (4 weeks postpartum) and 0.03 μg/mL (6 weeks postpartum), and 2.20 μg/mL (at birth), respectively. The milk:plasma ratios at these times varied widely from 0.4 to 13.0, as did the milk concentrations of the metabolite (0.002 to 1.81 μg/mL). Two of the infants had concentrations of amiodarone in their plasma of 0.01 to 0.03 μg/mL.

Although no adverse effects were observed in the one breast-fed infant, relatively large amounts of the drug and its metabolite are available through the milk. Amiodarone, after chronic administration, has a very long elimination half-life of 14–58 days in adults (24). Data in pediatric patients suggest a more rapid elimination, but the half-life in newborns has not been determined. The effects of chronic neonatal exposure to this drug are unknown. Because of this uncertainty and because of the high proportion of iodine contained in each dose (see also Potassium Iodide), breast-feeding is not recommended if the mother is currently taking amiodarone or has taken it chronically within the past several months. The American Academy of Pediatrics, noting that hypothyroidism is a potential complication, classifies amiodarone as a drug for which the effect on nursing infants is unknown but may be of concern (28).

References

1. Candelpergher G, Buchberger R, Suzzi GL, Padrini R. Trans-placental passage of amiodarone: electrocardiographic and pharmacologic evidence in a newborn. G Ital Cardiol 1982;12:79–82.
2. McKenna WJ, Harris L, Rowland E, Whitelaw A, Storey G, Holt D. Amiodarone therapy during pregnancy. Am J Cardiol 1983;51:1231–3.
3. Pitcher D, Leather HM, Storey GAC, Holt DW. Amiodarone in pregnancy. Lancet 1983;1:597–8.
4. Product information. Cordarone. Wyeth-Ayerst Laboratories, 2000.
5. Robson DJ, Jeeva Raj MV, Storey GAC, Holt DW. Use of amiodarone during pregnancy. Postgrad Med J 1985;61:75–7.
6. Arnoux P, Seyral P, Llurens M, Djiane P, Potier A, Unal D, Cano JP, Serradimigni A, Rouault F. Amiodarone and digoxin for refractory fetal tachycardia. Am J Cardiol 1987;59:166–7.
7. Penn IM, Barrett PA, Pannikote V, Barnaby PF, Campbell JB, Lyons NR. Amiodarone in pregnancy. Am J Cardiol 1985;56:196–7.
8. Strunge P, Frandsen J, Andreasen F. Amiodarone during pregnancy. Eur Heart J 1988;9:106–9.
9. Plomp TA, Vulsma T, de Vijlder JJM. Use of amiodarone during pregnancy. Eur J Obstet Gynecol Reprod Biol 1992;43:201–7.
10. Gembruch U, Manz M, Bald R, Rüddel H, Redel DA, Schlebusch H, Nitsch J, Hansmann M. Repeated intravascular treatment with amiodarone in a fetus with refractory supraventricular tachycardia and hydrops fetalis. Am Heart J 1989;118:1335–8.
11. Rey E, Bachrach LK, Burrow GN. Effects of amiodarone during pregnancy. Can Med Assoc J 1987;136: 959–60.
12. Widerhorn J, Bhandari AK, Bughi S, Rahimtoola SH, Elkayam U. Fetal and neonatal adverse effects profile of amiodarone treatment during pregnancy. Am Heart J 1991;122:1162–6.
13. Wladimiroff JW, Steward PA. Treatment of fetal cardiac arrhythmias. Br J Hosp Med 1985;34:134–40. As cited by Widerhorn J, Bhandari AK, Bughi S, Rahimtoola SH, Elkayam U. Fetal and neonatal adverse effects profile of amiodarone treatment during pregnancy. Am Heart J 1991;122:1162–6.
14. Foster CJ, Love HG. Amiodarone in pregnancy: case report and review of literature. Int J Cardiol 1988;20:307–16.
15. De Wolf D, De Schepper J, Verhaaren H, Deneyer M, Smitz J, Sacre-Smits L. Congenital hypothyroid goiter and amiodarone. Acta Paediatr Scand 1988;77: 616–8.
16. Ovadia M, Brito M, Hoyer GL, Marcus FI. Human

experience with amiodarone in the embryonic period. Am J Cardiol 1994;73:316–7.
17. Rey E, Duperron L, Gauthier R, Lemay M, Grignon A, LeLorier J. Transplacental treatment of tachycardia-induced fetal heart failure with verapamil and amiodarone: a case report. Am J Obstet Gynecol 1985;153:311–2.
18. Laurent M, Betremieux P, Biron Y, LeHelloco A. Neonatal hypothyroidism after treatment by amiodarone during pregnancy. Am J Cardiol 1987;60:942.
19. Flack NJ, Zosmer N, Bennett PR, Vaughan J, Fisk NM. Amiodarone given by three routes to terminate fetal atrial flutter associated with severe hydrops. Obstet Gynecol 1993;82:714–6.
20. Fulgencio JP, Hamza J. Anaesthesia for caesarean section in a patient receiving high dose amiodarone for fetal supraventricular tachycardia. Anaesthesia 1994;49:406–8.
21. Magee LA, Taddio A, Downar E, Sermer M, Boulton BC, Cameron D, Rosengarten M, Waxman M, Allen LC, Koren G. Pregnancy outcome following gestational exposure to amiodarone (abstract). Teratology 1994;49:398.
22. Magee LA, Downar E, Sermer M, Boulton BC, Allen LC, Koren G. Pregnancy outcome after gestational exposure to amiodarone in Canada. Am J Obstet Gynecol 1995;172:1307–11.
23. Ito S, Magee L, Smallhorn J. Drug therapy for fetal arrhythmias. Clin Perinatol 1994;21:543–72.
24. Sloskey GE. Amiodarone: a unique antiarrhythmic agent. Clin Pharm 1983;2:330–40.
25. Rotmensch HH, Rotmensch S, Elkayam U. Management of cardiac arrhythmias during pregnancy: current concepts. Drugs 1987;33:623–33.
26. Ward RM. Maternal drug therapy for fetal disorders. Semin Perinatol 1992;16:12–20.
27. Hill DA, Reasor MJ. Effects of amiodarone administration during lactation in Fischer-344 rats. Toxicol Lett 1992;62:119–25.
28. Committee on Drugs, American Academy of Pediatrics. The transfer of drugs and other chemicals into human milk. Pediatrics 2001;108:776–89.

Name:	**AMITRIPTYLINE**	Risk Factor:	**C_M**
Class:	**Antidepressant**		

FETAL RISK SUMMARY

RECOMMENDATION: Human Data Suggest Low Risk

Two reviews found reports of amitriptyline-induced teratogenicity in animals: encephaloceles and bent tails in hamsters (1) and skeletal malformations in rats (2). However, reproduction studies conducted by the manufacturer in mice, rats, or rabbits with oral doses up to 13 times the maximum recommended human dose revealed no evidence of teratogenicity (3). The manufacturer does cite the teratogenicity of amitriptyline in mice, hamsters, rats, and rabbits when higher doses were used (3).

The manufacturer states that amitriptyline crosses the placenta (3). The relatively low molecular weight (about 314) is consistent with this finding.

In humans, limb reduction anomalies have been reported with amitriptyline (4,5). However, analysis of 522,630 births, 86 with 1st trimester exposure to amitriptyline, did not confirm an association with this defect (6–13). Reported malformations other than limb reduction defects after therapeutic dosing included: micrognathia, anomalous right mandible, left pes equinovarus (1 case); swelling of hands and feet (1 case); hypospadias (1 case); and bilateral anophthalmia (1 case) (8,12–14).

A case of maternal suicide attempt with a combination of amitriptyline (725 mg) and perphenazine (58 mg) at 8 days' gestation was described in a 1980 abstract (15). An infant was eventually delivered with multiple congenital defects. The abnormalities included microcephaly, "cotton-like" hair with pronounced shedding, cleft palate, micrognathia, ambiguous genitalia, foot deformities, and undetectable dermal ridges (15).

Thanatophoric dwarfism was found in a stillborn infant exposed throughout gestation to amitriptyline (>150 mg/day), phenytoin (200 mg/day), and phenobarbital (300 mg/day) (16). The cause of the malformation could not be determined, but both drug and genetic etiologies were considered.

In a surveillance study of Michigan Medicaid recipients conducted between 1985 and 1992, involving 229,101 completed pregnancies 467 newborns had been exposed to amitriptyline during the 1st trimester (F. Rosa, personal communication, FDA, 1993). A total of 25 (5.4%) major birth defects were observed (20 expected). Specific data were available for six defect categories, including (observed/expected) 6/5 cardiovascular defects, 0/1 oral clefts, 0/0 spina bifida, 2/1 polydactyly, 2/1 limb reduction defects, and 1/1 hypospadias. These data do not support an association between the drug and the defects.

In a 1996 descriptive case series, the European Network of the Teratology Information Services (ENTIS) prospectively examined the outcomes of 689 pregnancies exposed to antidepressants (17). Multiple drug therapy occurred in about two-thirds of the mothers. Amitriptyline (118 exposures; 1 set of twins) was the second most commonly used tricyclic antidepressant. The outcomes of these pregnancies were 18 elective abortions, 10 spontaneous abortions, 2 stillbirths, 79 normal newborns (includes 7 premature infants), 5 normal infants with neonatal disorders, 4 infants with congenital defects, and 1 neonatal (premature plus other complications). The defects (all exposed in the 1st trimester or longer) were small ventricular septal defect; single palmar crease and small palpebral fissure; facial microangioma and right hydrocele (exposed also to clobazam and diphtheria, tetanus, typhoid vaccines); and facial muscle asymmetry and G6PD deficiency (exposed also to clonazepam and oxazepam) (17).

Neonatal withdrawal after *in utero* exposure to other antidepressants (see Imipramine), but not with amitriptyline, has been reported. However, the potential for this complication exists because of the close similarity among these compounds. Urinary retention in the neonate has been associated with maternal use of nortriptyline, an amitriptyline metabolite (see Nortriptyline) (18).

A 2002 prospective study compared two groups of mother-child pairs exposed to antidepressants throughout gestation (46 exposed to tricyclics—18 to amitriptyline; 40 to fluoxetine) to 36 nonexposed, not depressed controls (19). Offspring were studied between the ages 15 and 71 months for effects of antidepressant exposure in terms of IQ, language, behavior, and temperament. Exposure to antidepressants did not adversely affect the measured parameters, but IQ was significantly and negatively associated with the duration of depression, and language was negatively associated with the number of depression episodes after delivery (19).

In summary, although occasional reports have associated the therapeutic use of amitriptyline with congenital malformations, the bulk of the evidence indicates these widely used drugs are relatively safe during pregnancy. The single case of gross overdose is suggestive of an association between amitriptyline, perphenazine, or both, and malformations, but without confirming evidence no conclusions can be determined. Because of the experience with tricyclic antidepressants, one review recommended they were preferred during gestation over other antidepressants (2).

BREAST FEEDING SUMMARY

RECOMMENDATION: Limited Human Data - Potential Toxicity

Amitriptyline and its active metabolites are excreted into breast milk (20–24). A recent study has measured the amount of a second active metabolite, E-10-hydroxynortriptyline, in milk (23).

Serum and milk concentrations of amitriptyline in one patient were 0.14 and 0.15 μg/mL, respectively, a milk:plasma ratio of 1.0 (20). No drug was detected in the infant's serum. In another patient, it was estimated that the baby received about 1% of the mother's dose (22). No clinical signs of drug activity were observed in the infant.

In another study, the mother was treated with 175 mg/day of amitriptyline (23). Milk and maternal serum samples were analyzed for active drug and active metabolites on postpartum days 1–26. Amitriptyline serum levels ranged from 24 ng/mL (day 1) to 71 ng/mL (days 3–26), while those in the milk ranged from 24 ng/mL (day 1) to only 54% of the serum levels on days 2–26. Nortriptyline serum levels ranged from 17 ng/mL (day 1) to 87 ng/mL (day 26) with milk levels 74% of those in the serum. Mean concentration of the second metabolite, E-10-hydroxynortriptyline, was 127 ng/mL (days 1–26) in the serum and 70% of that in the milk. The total dose (parent drug plus metabolites) consumed by the male infant on day 26 was estimated to be 35 μg/kg (80 times lower than the mother's dose). The compounds were not detected in the nursing infant's serum on day 26 and no adverse effects, including sedation, were observed in him (23).

Ten nursing infants of mothers taking antidepressants (two with amitriptyline 100–175 mg/day) were compared to 15 bottle-fed infants of mothers with depression who did not breast-feed (24). Concentrations of clomipramine in fore- and hind-milk were 30 ng/mL (one patient) and 113 and 197 ng/mL (two patients), respectively. The milk:maternal plasma ratios were 0.2 and 0.9, respectively. One infant had a plasma level of 7.5 ng/mL when the mother was taking 100 mg/day. No toxic effects or delays in development were observed in the infants. The estimated daily dose consumed by the infants was about 1% of the mother's weight adjusted dose (24).

A 1996 review of antidepressant treatment during breast-feeding found no information that amitriptyline exposure of the infant during nursing caused adverse effects (25).

Although amitriptyline and its metabolite have not been detected in infant serum, the effects of exposure to small amounts in the milk are unknown (26). The American Academy of Pediatrics classifies amitriptyline as a drug whose effect on the nursing infant is unknown but may be of concern (27).

References

1. Shepard TH. *Catalog of Teratogenic Agents*. 6th ed. Baltimore, MD: Johns Hopkins University Press, 1989:44–5.
2. Elia J, Katz IR, Simpson GM. Teratogenicity of psychotherapeutic medications. Psychopharmacol Bull 1987;23:531–86.
3. Product information. Elavil. AstraZeneca, 2000.
4. McBride WG. Limb deformities associated with iminodibenzyl hydrochloride. Med J Aust 1972;1:492.
5. Freeman R. Limb deformities: possible association with drugs. Med J Aust 1972;1:606.
6. Australian Drug Evaluation Committee. Tricyclic antidepressants and limb reduction deformities. Med J Aust 1973;1:768–9.
7. Heinonen OP, Slone D, Shapiro S. *Birth Defects and Drugs in Pregnancy*. Littleton, MA: Publishing Sciences Group, 1977:336–7.
8. Idanpaan-Heikkila J, Saxen L. Possible teratogenicity of imipramine/chloropyramine. Lancet 1973;2:282–3.
9. Rachelefsky GS, Glynt JW, Ebbin AJ, Wilson MG. Possible teratogenicity of tricyclic antidepressants. Lancet 1972;1:838.
10. Banister P, Dafoe C, Smith ESO, Miller J. Possible teratogenicity of tricyclic antidepressants. Lancet 1972; 1:838–9.
11. Scanlon FJ. Use of antidepressant drugs during the first trimester. Med J Aust 1969;2:1077.
12. Crombie DL, Pinsent R, Fleming D. Imipramine in pregnancy. Br Med J 1972;1:745.
13. Kuenssberg EV, Knox JDE. Imipramine in pregnancy. Br Med J 1972;2:292.
14. Golden SM, Perman KI. Bilateral clinical anophthalmia: drugs as potential factors. South Med J 1980;73:1404–7.
15. Wertelecki W, Purvis-Smith SG, Blackburn WR. Amitriptyline/perphenazine maternal overdose and birth defects (abstract). Teratology 1980;21:74A.
16. Rafla NM, Meehan FP. Thanatophoric dwarfism: drugs and antenatal diagnosis. A case report. Eur J Obstet Gynecol Reprod Biol 1990;38:161–5.
17. McElhatton PR, Garbis HM, Elefant E, Vial T, Bellemin B, Mastroiacovo P, Arnon J, Rodriguez-Pinilla E, Schaefer C, Pexieder T, Merlob P, Dal Verme S. The outcome of pregnancy in 689 women exposed to therapeutic doses of antidepressants. A collaborative study of the European Network of Teratology Information Services (ENTIS). Reprod Toxicol 1996;10:285–94.
18. Shearer WT, Schreiner RL, Marshall RE. Urinary retention in a neonate secondary to maternal ingestion of nortriptyline. J Pediatr 1972;81:570–2.

19. Nulman I, Rovet J, Stewart DE, Wolpin J, Pace-Asciak P, Shuhaiber S, Koren G. Child development following exposure to tricyclic antidepressants or fluoxetine throughout fetal life: a prospective, controlled study. Am J Psychiatry 2002;159:1889–95.
20. Bader TF, Newman K. Amitriptyline in human breast milk and the nursing infants serum. Am J Psychiatry 1980;137;855–6.
21. Wilson JT, Brown D, Cherek DR, Dailey JW, Hilman B, Jobe PC, Manno BR, Manno JE, Redetzki HM, Stewart JJ. Drug excretion in human breast milk. Principles, pharmacokinetics and projected consequences. Clin Pharmacokinet 1980;5:1–66.
22. Brixen-Rasmussen L, Halgrener J, Jorgensen A. Amitriptyline and nortriptyline excretion in human breast milk. Psychopharmacology (Berlin) 1982; 76:94–5.
23. Breyer-Pfaff U, Nill K, Entenmann A, Gaertner HJ. Secretion of amitriptyline and metabolites into breast milk. Am J Psychiatry 1995;152:812–3.
24. Yoshida K, Smith B, Craggs M, Kumar RC. Investigation of pharmacokinetics and of possible adverse effects in infants exposed to tricyclic antidepressants in breast-milk. J Affect Disord 1997;43:225–37.
25. Wisner KL, Perel JM, Findling RL. Antidepressant treatment during breast-feeding. Am J Psychiatry 1996;153:1132–7.
26. Erickson SH, Smith GH, Heidrich F. Tricyclics and breast feeding. Am J Psychiatry 1979;136:1483.
27. Committee on Drugs, American Academy of Pediatrics. The transfer of drugs and other chemicals into human milk. Pediatrics 2001;108:776–89.

Name: **AMLODIPINE** Risk Factor: **C_M**

Class: **Calcium Channel Blocker**

FETAL RISK SUMMARY

RECOMMENDATION: No Human Data - Animal Data Suggest Moderate Risk

Amlodipine is a calcium channel blocking agent used in the treatment of hypertension and angina. The drug is not teratogenic or embryotoxic in rats and rabbits given doses up to 8 and 23 times, respectively, the maximum recommended human dose on a body surface area basis (MRHD) during their respective periods of major organogenesis (1). However, rats administered 8 times the MRHD for 14 days before mating and throughout gestation had a significant decrease in litter size (by about 50%), a significant increase in intrauterine deaths (about 5-fold), and prolonged labor and gestation (1). This dose, however, had no effect on fertility in the rat.

No reports describing the placental transfer of amlodipine in humans have been located. The molecular weight (about 567 for the besylate salt) is low enough, however, that passage to the fetus should be expected.

No reports on the use of amlodipine in human pregnancy have been located. If amlodipine is used in pregnancy, health care professionals are encouraged to call the toll free number (800-670-6126) for information about patient enrollment in the Motherisk study.

BREAST FEEDING SUMMARY

RECOMMENDATION: No Human Data - Probably Compatible

No reports describing the use of amlodipine during human lactation have been located. The molecular weight (about 567 for the besylate salt) is low enough, however, that excretion into breast milk should be expected. The effect of the drug on a nursing effect is unknown.

Reference

1. Product information. Norvasc. Pfizer, 2000.

A

Name: **AMMONIUM CHLORIDE** Risk Factor: **B**

Class: **Respiratory Drug (Expectorant)/ Urinary Acidifier**

FETAL RISK SUMMARY

RECOMMENDATION: Compatible

The Collaborative Perinatal Project monitored 50,282 mother-child pairs, 365 of whom had 1st trimester exposure to ammonium chloride as an expectorant in cough medications (1, pp. 378–381). For use anytime during pregnancy, 3,401 exposures were recorded (1, p. 442). In neither group was evidence found to suggest a relationship to large categories of major or minor malformations. Three possible associations with individual malformations were found but independent confirmation is required to determine the actual risk: inguinal hernia (1st trimester only) (11 cases); cataract (6 cases); and any benign tumor (17 cases) (1, pp. 478, 496).

When consumed in large quantities near term, ammonium chloride may cause acidosis in the mother and the fetus (2,3). In some cases, the decreased pH and pCO_2, increased lactic acid, and reduced oxygen saturation were as severe as those seen with fatal apnea neonatorum. However, the newborns did not appear in distress.

BREAST FEEDING SUMMARY

RECOMMENDATION: No Human Data - Probably Compatible

No data are available.

References

1. Heinonen OP, Slone D, Shapiro S. *Birth Defects and Drugs in Pregnancy*. Littleton, MA: Publishing Sciences Group, 1977.
2. Goodlin RC, Kaiser IH. The effect of ammonium chloride induced maternal acidosis on the human fetus at term. I. pH, hemoglobin, blood gases. Am J Med Sci 1957;233:666–74.
3. Kaiser IH, Goodlin RC. The effect of ammonium chloride induced maternal acidosis on the human fetus at term. II. Electrolytes. Am J Med Sci 1958;235:549–54.

Name: **AMOBARBITAL** Risk Factor: **D***

Class: **Sedative/Hypnotic**

FETAL RISK SUMMARY

RECOMMENDATION: Limited Human Data - No Relevant Animal Data

Amobarbital is a member of the barbiturate class. The drug crosses the placenta, achieving levels in the cord serum similar to those in the maternal serum (1,2). Single or continuous dosing of the mother near term does not induce amobarbital hydroxylation in the fetus as demonstrated by the prolonged elimination of the drug in the newborn (half-life 2.5 times maternal). An increase in the incidence of congenital defects in infants exposed *in utero* to amobarbital has been reported (3, 4, pp. 336, 344). One survey of 1369 patients exposed to multiple drugs found 273 who received amobarbital during the 1st trimester (3). Ninety-five of the exposed mothers delivered infants with major or minor abnormalities. Malformations associated with barbiturates, in general, were as follows:

Anencephaly
Congenital heart disease
Severe limb deformities
Cleft lip and palate
Intersex
Papilloma of the forehead
Hydrocele
Congenital dislocation of the hip
Soft-tissue deformity of the neck
Hypospadias
Accessory auricle
Polydactyly
Nevus

The Collaborative Perinatal Project monitored 50,282 mother-child pairs, 298 of whom had 1st trimester exposure to amobarbital (4, pp. 336, 344). For use anytime during pregnancy, 867 exposures were recorded (4, p. 438). A possible association was found between the use of the drug in the 1st trimester and the following:

Cardiovascular malformations (7 cases)
Polydactyly in blacks (2 cases in 29 blacks)
Genitourinary malformations other than hypospadias (3 cases)
Inguinal hernia (9 cases)
Clubfoot (4 cases)

In contrast to the above reports, a 1964 survey of 187 pregnant patients who had received various neuroleptics, including amobarbital, found a 3.1% incidence of malformations in the offspring (5). This is approximately the expected incidence of abnormalities in a nonexposed population. Arthrogryposis and multiple defects were reported in an infant exposed to amobarbital during the 1st trimester (6). The defects were attributed to immobilization of the limbs at the time of joint formation, multiple drug use, and active tetanus.

[**Risk Factor B according to the manufacturer, Eli Lilly & Co., 1985.*]

BREAST FEEDING SUMMARY

RECOMMENDATION: No Human Data - Potential Toxicity

No data are available.

References

1. Kraver B, Draffan GH, Williams FM, Calre RA, Dollery CT, Hawkins DF. Elimination kinetics of amobarbital in mothers and newborn infants. Clin Pharmacol Ther 1973;14:442–7.
2. Draffan GH, Dollery CT, Davies DS, Krauer B, Williams FM, Clare RA, Trudinger BJ, Darling M, Sertel H, Hawkins DF. Maternal and neonatal elimination of amobarbital after treatment of the mother with barbiturates during late pregnancy. Clin Pharmacol Ther 1976;19:271–5.
3. Nelson MM, Forfar JO. Associations between drugs administered during pregnancy and congenital abnormalities of the fetus. Br Med J 1971;1:523–7.
4. Heinonen OP, Slone D, Shapiro S. *Birth Defects and Drugs in Pregnancy*. Littleton, MA: Publishing Sciences Group, 1977.
5. Favre-Tissot M. An original clinical study of the pharmacologic-teratogenic relationship. Ann Med Psychol (Paris) 1967:389.
6. Jago RH. Arthrogryposis following treatment of maternal tetanus with muscle relaxants. Arch Dis Child 1970;45:277–9.

Name: **AMOXAPINE** Risk Factor: C_M
Class: **Antidepressant**

FETAL RISK SUMMARY

RECOMMENDATION: Limited Human Data - Animal Data Suggest Risk

No published reports linking the use of amoxapine with congenital defects have been located. Reproductive studies in mice, rats, and rabbits have found no teratogenicity, but embryotoxicity was observed in rats and rabbits given oral doses approximating the human dose (1). Intrauterine death, stillbirths, decreased weight, and decreased neonatal survival (days 0–4) were seen with oral doses at 3–10 times the human dose.

In a surveillance study of Michigan Medicaid recipients conducted between 1985 and 1992, involving 229,101 completed pregnancies 19 newborns had been exposed to amoxapine during the 1st trimester (F. Rosa, personal communication, FDA, 1993). Three (15.8%) major birth defects were observed (one expected). Data on the specific types of defects were not available, but no cases of cardiovascular defects, oral clefts, spina bifida, polydactyly, limb reduction defects, or hypospadias were observed. Although the total incidence of anomalies is high, the number of exposures is too small to draw a conclusion.

BREAST FEEDING SUMMARY

RECOMMENDATION: Limited Human Data - Potential Toxicity

Amoxapine and its metabolite are excreted into breast milk. A 29-year-old woman suffering from depression was treated with approximately 250 mg/day of amoxapine (2). She developed galactorrhea and oligomenorrhea. Milk samples were collected after 10 and 11 months of therapy and analyzed for amoxapine and the active metabolite, 8-hydroxyamoxapine. The levels of the parent compound at the sample collection times were both less than 20 ng/mL, but the metabolite was present in both samples, 45 minutes after the last dose at 10 months and 11.5 hours after the last dose at 11 months. Levels of the active metabolite at these times were 113 ng/mL and 168 ng/mL, respectively. A venous blood specimen obtained simultaneously with the first milk sample had concentrations of amoxapine and 8-hydroxyamoxapine of 97 ng/mL and 375 ng/mL, respectively. The American Academy of Pediatrics classifies amoxapine as a drug whose effect on the nursing infant is unknown but may be of concern (3).

References

1. Product information. Asendin. Lederle Laboratories, 1997.
2. Gelenberg AJ. Amoxapine, a new antidepressant, appears in human milk. J Nerv Ment Dis 1979;167:635–6.
3. Committee on Drugs, American Academy of Pediatrics. The transfer of drugs and other chemicals into human milk. Pediatrics 2001;108:776–89.

Name:	**AMOXICILLIN**	Risk Factor:	B_M
Class:	**Antibiotic (Penicillin)**		

FETAL RISK SUMMARY

RECOMMENDATION: Compatible

Amoxicillin is a penicillin antibiotic similar to ampicillin (see also Ampicillin). No reports linking its use to congenital defects have been located.

Reproduction studies have been conducted in mice and rats at doses up to 10 times the human dose (1). No effect on fertility or fetal harm was observed at this dose.

The Collaborative Perinatal Project monitored 50,282 mother-child pairs, 3546 of whom had 1st trimester exposure to penicillin derivatives (2, pp. 297–313). For use anytime during pregnancy, 7171 exposures were recorded (2, p. 435). In neither group was evidence found to suggest a relationship to large categories of major or minor malformations or to individual defects. Amoxicillin has been used as a single 3-g dose to treat bacteriuria in pregnancy without causing fetal harm (3,4).

In a surveillance study of Michigan Medicaid recipients conducted between 1985 and 1992, involving 229,101 completed pregnancies 8538 newborns had been exposed to amoxicillin during the 1st trimester (F. Rosa, personal communication, FDA, 1993). A total of 317 (3.7%) major birth defects were observed (363 expected). Specific data were available for six defect categories, including (observed/expected) 76/85 cardiovascular defects, 16/14 oral clefts, 6/7 spina bifida, 17/24 polydactyly, 9/16 limb reduction defects, and 22/22 hypospadias. These data do not support an association between the drug and the defects.

Amoxicillin depresses both plasma-bound and urinary excreted estriol (see also Ampicillin) (5). Urinary estriol was formerly used to assess the condition of the fetoplacental unit, but this is now done by measuring plasma unconjugated estriol, which is not usually affected by amoxicillin.

BREAST FEEDING SUMMARY

RECOMMENDATION: Compatible

Amoxicillin is excreted into breast milk in low concentrations. Following a 1-g oral dose given to six mothers, peak milk levels occurred at 4–5 hours, averaging 0.9 μg/mL (range 0.68–1.3 μg/mL) (6). Mean milk:plasma ratios at 1, 2, and 3 hours were 0.014, 0.013, and 0.043, respectively. Although no adverse effects have been observed, three potential problems exist for the nursing infant: modification of bowel flora, direct effects on the infant (e.g., allergy or sensitization), and interference with the interpretation of culture results if a fever workup is required. The American Academy of Pediatrics classifies amoxicillin as compatible with breast-feeding (7).

References

1. Product information. Amoxil. SmithKline Beecham Pharmaceuticals, 2000.
2. Heinonen OP, Slone D, Shapiro S. *Birth Defects and Drugs in Pregnancy*. Littleton, MA: Publishing Sciences Group, 1977.
3. Masterton RG, Evans DC, Strike PW. Single-dose amoxycillin in the treatment of bacteriuria in pregnancy and the puerperium—a controlled clinical trial. Br J Obstet Gynaecol 1985;92:498–505.
4. Jakobi P, Neiger R, Merzbach D, Paldi E. Single-dose antimicrobial therapy in the treatment of asymptomatic bacteriuria in pregnancy. Am J Obstet Gynecol 1987;156:1148–52.
5. Van Look PFA, Top-Huisman M, Gnodde HP. Effect of ampicillin or amoxycillin administration on plasma and urinary estrogen levels during normal pregnancy. Eur J Obstet Gynaecol Reprod Biol 1981;12:225–33.
6. Kafetzis D, Siafas C, Georgakopoulos P, Papadatos C. Passage of cephalosporins and amoxicillin into the breast milk. Acta Paediatr Scand 1981;70:285–8.
7. Committee on Drugs, American Academy of Pediatrics. The transfer of drugs and other chemicals into human milk. Pediatrics 2001;108:776–89.

Name:	**AMPHETAMINE**	Risk Factor:	**C_M**
Class:	**Central Stimulant**		

FETAL RISK SUMMARY

RECOMMENDATION: Human and Animal Data Suggest Risk

The amphetamines are a group of sympathomimetic drugs that are used to stimulate the central nervous system. Members of this group include amphetamine, dextroamphetamine, and methamphetamine. A number of studies have examined the possible relationship between amphetamines and adverse fetal outcome. Women were using these drugs for appetite suppression, narcolepsy, or illicit abuse purposes.

In near-term pregnant sheep administered IV doses at or below what is commonly regarded as abuse, methamphetamine rapidly crossed the placenta and accumulated in the fetus (1). Fetal blood pressure was increased 20%–37%, with a decrease in fetal oxyhemoglobin saturation and arterial pH. Approximately similar results were reported in a 1993 abstract that also used pregnant sheep (2). Fetal concentrations of the drug were approximately the same as maternal levels during a 6-hour interval.

The question as to whether amphetamines are teratogenic in humans has been examined in a number of studies and single-patient case histories. Cardiac malformations and other defects were produced in mice injected with very large doses (about 200 times the usual human dose) of dextroamphetamine (3). These same investigators then retrospectively and prospectively examined human infants whose mothers had ingested the drug (4). In the retrospective portion of the study, 219 infants and children under 2 years of age with congenital heart disease were compared with 153 similar-age infants and children without heart defects. Neither maternal exposure to dextroamphetamine during pregnancy nor exposure during the vulnerable period differed statistically between the groups. However, a positive family history of congenital heart disease occurred in 31.1% of the infants with the defects compared with only 5.9% of the control group ($p = 0.001$). The prospective study compared 52 mothers with a documented exposure to dextroamphetamine during the vulnerable period with 50 nonexposed mothers. Neither group produced an infant with congenital heart disease, and the numbers of other congenital abnormalities were similar (nine vs. seven). Thus, this study found no evidence for an association between congenital heart defects and dextroamphetamine. However, in a followup study published 3 years later, the investigators reported a significant relationship between dextroamphetamine exposure and heart defects (5). Comparing 184 infants under 1 year of age with congenital heart disease with 108 control infants, significant differences were found for maternal exposure to dextroamphetamine (18% vs. 8%, $p < 0.05$), exposure during the vulnerable period (11% vs. 3%, $p = 0.025$), and positive family history of congenital heart disease (27% vs. 6%, $p < 0.001$). Infants who were both exposed during the vulnerable period and had a positive family history were statistically similar for the groups (5% vs. 1%).

In a fourth study by the above investigative group, 240 women were followed prospectively during their pregnancies to determine exposure to medicinal agents, radiation, and other potential teratogens (6). Thirty-one (13%) consumed an appetite suppressant (usually dextroamphetamine) during the 1st trimester and an additional 34 (14%) were exposed later in pregnancy. Eight (3.3%) babies had a major congenital defect noted at birth, which is approximately the expected incidence in the United States. Three of the affected infants had been exposed during the 1st trimester to an appetite suppressant. Although the authors identified a wide range of maternal drug consumption during the 1st trimester, no conclusions as to the cause of the defects can be drawn from the data.

Four other reports have related various defects with amphetamine exposure (7–10). An infant with a bifid exencephalia was delivered from a mother who took 20–30 mg of dextroamphetamine daily throughout pregnancy (7). The infant died after an attempt was made at surgical correction. A second case involved a mother who ingested dextroamphetamine daily for appetite suppression and who delivered a full-term infant. The infant died 6 days later as a result of a congenital heart defect (8). Drug histories were obtained from mothers of 11 infants with biliary atresia and compared with the histories of 50 control mothers (9). Amphetamine exposure occurred in five women in the study group and in three of the controls. A 1966 report described a mother with two infants with microcephaly, mental retardation, and motor dysfunction (10). The mother had taken an appetite suppressant containing methamphetamine and phenobarbital during the 1st and 2nd trimesters of both pregnancies (pregnancy numbers 1 and 3). A spontaneous abortion occurred in pregnancy number 2, but no details were given of the mother's drug intake. Her fourth pregnancy, in which she did not take the appetite suppressant, resulted in the delivery of a normal child. There was no family history of developmental disorders, congenital defects, mental retardation, cerebral palsy, or epilepsy.

Fetal structural defects have been associated with maternal abuse of drugs in a large volume of literature (see also Ethanol, Cocaine, Heroin, Lysergic Acid Diethylamide [LSD], Marijuana, and Methadone). For example, in a 1972 case, multiple brain and eye anomalies were observed in an infant exposed *in utero* to amphetamines, LSD, meprobamate, and marijuana (11). In this and similar cases, the cause of the structural abnormalities is probably multifactorial, involving drug use, life-styles, infections, poor maternal health, and other factors.

In a retrospective study, 458 mothers who delivered infants with major ($N = 175$) or minor ($N = 283$) abnormalities were compared with 911 matched controls (12). Appetite suppressants were consumed during pregnancy by significantly more mothers of infants with anomalies than by controls (3.9% vs. 1.1%, $p < 0.01$). Dextroamphetamine consumption accounted for 13 of the 18 maternal exposures in the anomaly group. During the first 56 days of pregnancy, dextroamphetamine-containing compounds were used by 10 mothers in the anomaly group (2.2%) compared with only five of the controls (0.5%) ($p < 0.05$). The abnormalities (3 major and 7 minor) observed in the 10 infants were urogenital system defects (4 cases), congenital heart disease (1 case), cleft lip (1 case), severe limb deformity (1 case), accessory auricles (1 case), congenital dislocation of hip (1 case), and pilonidal sinus (1 case). Although statistically significant results were found in this study, the results must be interpreted cautiously due to the retrospective collection of drug histories and the lack of information pertaining to past and present maternal medical and obstetric histories.

A prospective study of 1824 white mothers who took anorectic drugs (primarily amphetamines) during pregnancy compared with 8989 white mothers who did not take such drugs measured rates of severe congenital defects of 3.7% and 3.4%, respectively, in infants with a gestational age of at least 37 weeks (13). When children of all known gestational ages were included, amphetamine usage occurred in 85% (1694 of 1992) of the group consuming anorectic drugs. The incidence of severe congenital defects in the amphetamine group was 3.4%. Fourteen infants were exposed in the first 84 days after the last menstrual period, and except for three infants with cleft lip and/or palate, no pattern of malformations was observed.

The effects of amphetamine abuse on fetal outcome and subsequent development were described in a series of reports from Sweden (14–18). Twenty-three women who ingested amphetamine during the 1st trimester were divided into two groups: 6 who claimed they stopped use of the drug after they became aware of their pregnancy or after the 1st trimester, and 17 who continued use of the drug throughout gestation (14). Two of the infants (group not specified) had congenital defects: a stillborn infant had myelomeningocele, and one had extensive telangiectasis (considered to be an inherited disorder). The outcome of the infants exposed throughout gestation included six preterm (<37 weeks), three small-for-gestational-age (all with poor prenatal care), one of whom had a seizure on the 1st day, and two full-term but extremely drowsy infants. In a later report, 66 infants born to amphetamine-addicted mothers were followed during their 1st year of life (16). Except for temporary drowsiness in the first few months, all children had normal somatic and psychomotor development at 12 months of age. In the final report from these investigators, the fetal outcome of 69 amphetamine-addicted women who delivered 71 children (one delivered twice and one delivered twins) was described (17). Seventeen of the women claimed to have stopped amphetamine ingestion as previously described, and 52 continued use of amphetamines throughout pregnancy. Three women in the first group and 17 in the second group were alcoholics (18). Four infants had congenital defects: intestinal atresia (two cases—both died and one also had hydrocephalus), congenital heart defect (one case), and epidermolysis bullosa without known heredity (one case). In one of the four cases, the mother was an alcoholic, but the particular case was not specified. Drowsiness was observed in 8 infants and jitteriness in 11 infants; 4 full-term infants required tube feedings. The four studies (14–17) were combined into a single article published in 1980 (18).

The Collaborative Perinatal Project monitored 50,282 mother-child pairs, 671 of whom had 1st trimester exposure to amphetamines (19, pp. 346–347). For use anytime during pregnancy, 1898 exposures were recorded (19, p. 439). In neither group was evidence found to suggest a relationship to large categories of major or minor malformations. Two case reports failed to observe any neonatal effects from the treatment of narcolepsy with large doses of amphetamine (20,21). A 1988 report described a mother who had used amphetamines, barbiturates, cocaine, LSD, alcohol, and marijuana during pregnancy who delivered a female infant with bilateral cerebrovascular accident and resulting porencephaly (22). The infant expired at 2.5 months of age. The fetal injury was thought to be caused by cocaine (see also Cocaine).

The effects of IV methamphetamine abuse on the fetus were evaluated in a 1988 report (23). Maternal use of the drug was identified by self-reporting before delivery in 52 women, and an equal number of controls were selected for comparison. Although self-reporting of illegal drug use is prone to underreporting, the drug histories were validated by social worker interviews and were thought to represent actual drug use in the study population. Other drugs used in the study and control groups were tobacco (24 vs. 6), marijuana (20 vs. 1), cocaine (14 vs. 0%), and one each in the study group for alcohol, lorazepam, dextroamphetamine, heroin, opium, LSD, and diazepam. No statistical differences were measured between the groups in the rate of obstetric complications (12% vs. 27%) or neonatal complications (21% vs. 17%). The latter category included meconium (10% vs. 12%), fetal heart rate decelerations (4% vs. 0) and tachycardia (2% vs. 0%), tachypnea (4% vs. 2%), and withdrawal symptoms (2% vs. 0%). Mean birth weight, length, and head circumference were all lower in the study infants compared to controls ($p = 0.001$). Six (12%) of the infants in the study group had a congenital defect compared with seven (14%) of the controls. Statistically, however, the investigators could only conclude that methamphetamine abuse does not cause a 12-fold or greater increase in congenital anomalies (23).

A 1992 abstract described the effects of methamphetamine abuse in 48 newborns in comparison to 519 controls (24). Offspring of women positive for opiates, cocaine, alcohol, and toluene were excluded from both groups. Except for a significantly lower birth weight, 3173 g vs. 3327 g ($p = 0.03$), all other parameters studied were similar, including birth length, head circumference, Apgar scores, gestational age at delivery, and the incidence of both major and minor malformations.

Intrauterine death occurred at 34 weeks' gestation in the fetus of a 29-year-old amphetamine addict who had injected 500 mg of amphetamine (25). The mother was exhibiting toxic signs and symptoms of amphetamine overdose when she was brought to the hospital. An initial fetal bradycardia of 90–100 beats/minute worsened over the next 50 minutes when the heart sounds became inaudible. Approximately 24 hours later, a 3000-g female stillborn infant without congenital abnormalities was delivered.

Amphetamine withdrawal has been described in newborns whose mothers were addicted to amphetamines during pregnancy (26–28). In a report of four mothers using methamphetamine, symptoms consisting of shrill cries, irritability, jerking, and sneezing were observed in two infants (26). One of the infants was evaluated at 4 months of age and appeared normal except for small size (weight 3rd percentile, head circumference 10th percentile). The author speculated that the symptoms in the newborns may have been caused by hidden narcotic addiction (26). Another report of four women with methamphetamine dependence described one newborn with marked drowsiness lasting for 4 days (27). The mother had not been taking narcotics. The third report of neonatal withdrawal involved an infant delivered from a mother who was a known amphetamine addict (28). Beginning 6 hours after birth, the female infant had diaphoresis, agitation alternating with periods of lassitude, apnea with feedings, a seizure on the 6th day, vomiting, miotic pupils, and a glassy-eyed stare. Her first 3 months were marked by slow development, but at 2.5 years of age, there was no evidence of neurologic disability and intelligence was considered above normal.

Methamphetamine withdrawal characterized by abnormal sleep patterns, poor feeding, tremors, and hypertonia was reported in a 1987 study (29). Infants exposed to methamphetamine or cocaine, either singly or in combination, were combined into a single group ($N = 46$) because of similar maternal and neonatal medical factors. Mothers in the drug group had a significantly greater incidence of prematurity compared to drug-free controls (28% vs. 9%, $p < 0.05$), and a greater incidence of placental hemorrhage and anemia compared with narcotic-using mothers and controls (13% vs. 2% vs. 2.2%, $p < 0.05$ and 13% vs. 2% vs. 0%, $p < 0.05$). Maternal methamphetamine abuse was significantly associated with lower gestational age, birth weight, length, and occipitofrontal circumference.

Echoencephalography (ECHO) was performed within 3 days of birth on 74 term (>37 weeks) infants who had tested positive for cocaine or methamphetamine, but who otherwise had uncomplicated perinatal courses (30). The infants had no other known risk factors for cerebral injury. The 74 newborns were classified into three groups: 24 (32%) exposed to methamphetamine, 32 (43%) exposed to cocaine, and 18 (24%) exposed to cocaine plus heroin, or methadone, or both. Two comparison groups were formed: a group of 87 term, drug-free infants studied by ECHO because of clinical concerns for hypoxic-ischemic encephalopathy, and a normal group of 19 drug-free term newborns. Both groups of comparison infants were also studied by ECHO within 3 days of birth. Only one structural anomaly, consisting of an absent septum pellucidum, was observed in the infants examined. The affected newborn, exposed to methamphetamine, was also found to have bilateral optic nerve atrophy and diffuse attenuation of the white matter. Twenty-six (35.1%) of the drug-exposed infants had cranial abnormalities detected by ultrasonography, which was similar to the 27.6% (24 of 87) incidence in the group suspected of encephalopathy ($p = 0.7$). The normal controls had an incidence of 5.3% (1 of 19) ($p < 0.01$ in comparison to both of the other groups). The lesions observed in the drug-exposed infants were intraventricular hemorrhage, echodensities known to be associated with necrosis, and cavitary lesions. Lesions were concentrated in the basal ganglion, frontal lobes, and posterior fossa (30). The ECHO abnormalities were not predicted by standard neonatal clinical assessment and were believed to be consistent with those observed in adult abusers of amphetamines and cocaine (30).

In summary, the use of amphetamines for medical indications does not pose a significant risk to the fetus for congenital anomalies. Amphetamines do not appear to be human teratogens (31–33). Mild withdrawal symptoms may be observed in the newborns, but the few studies of infant follow-up have not shown long-term sequelae, although more studies of this nature are needed. Illicit maternal use of amphetamines, on the other hand, presents significant risks to the fetus and newborn, including intrauterine growth retardation, premature delivery, and the potential for increased maternal, fetal, and neonatal morbidity. These poor outcomes probably reflect several factors, including multiple drug use, lifestyles, and poor maternal health. However, cerebral injuries occurring in newborns exposed *in utero* appear to be directly related to the vasoconstrictive properties of amphetamines (30).

BREAST FEEDING SUMMARY

RECOMMENDATION: **Limited Human Data - Potential Toxicity**
Contraindicated (Nonmedical Use)

Amphetamine, the racemic mixture of levo- and dextroamphetamine, is concentrated in breast milk (21). After continuous daily dosing of 20 mg, milk concentrations ranged from 55 to 138 ng/mL with milk:plasma ratios varying between 2.8 and 7.5. Amphetamine was found in the urine of the nursing infant. No adverse effects of this exposure were observed over a 24-month period. In a second study, no neonatal insomnia or stimulation was observed in 103 nursing infants whose mothers were taking various amounts of amphetamine (34). The American Academy of Pediatrics classifies amphetamines as contraindicated during breast-feeding (35).

References

1. Burchfield DJ, Lucas VW, Abrams RM, Miller RL, DeVane CL. Disposition and pharmacodynamics of methamphetamine in pregnant sheep. JAMA 1991;265:1968–73.
2. Stek A, Fisher B, Clark KE. Maternal and fetal cardiovascular responses to methamphetamine (abstract). Am J Obstet Gynecol 1993;168:333.
3. Nora JJ, Trasler DG, Fraser FC. Malformations in mice induced by dexamphetamine sulphate. Lancet 1965;2:1021–2.
4. Nora JJ, McNamara DG, Fraser FC. Dextroamphetamine sulphate and human malformations. Lancet 1967;1:570–1.
5. Nora JJ, Vargo T, Nora A, Love KE, McNamara DG. Dextroamphetamine: a possible environmental trigger in cardiovascular malformations. Lancet 1970;1:1290–1.
6. Nora JJ, Nora AH, Sommerville RJ, Hill RM, McNamara DG. Maternal exposure to potential teratogens. JAMA 1967;202:1065–9.
7. Matera RF, Zabala H, Jimenez AP. Bifid exencephalia: teratogen action of amphetamine. Int Surg 1968;50:79–85.
8. Gilbert EF, Khoury GH. Dextroamphetamine and congenital cardiac malformations. J Pediatr 1970;76:638.
9. Levin JN. Amphetamine ingestion with biliary atresia. J Pediatr 1971;79:130–1.
10. McIntire MS. Possible adverse drug reaction. JAMA 1966;197:62–3.
11. Bogdanoff B, Rorke LB, Yanoff M, Warren WS. Brain and eye abnormalities: possible sequelae to prenatal use of multiple drugs including LSD. Am J Dis Child 1972;123:145–8.
12. Nelson MM, Forfar JO. Associations between drugs administered during pregnancy and congenital abnormalities of the fetus. Br Med J 1971;1:523–7.

13. Milkovich L, van den Berg BJ. Effects of antenatal exposure to anorectic drugs. Am J Obstet Gynecol 1977;129:637–42.
14. Eriksson M, Larsson G, Winbladh B, Zetterstrom R. The influence of amphetamine addiction on pregnancy and the newborn infant. Acta Paediatr Scand 1978;67:95–9.
15. Larsson G, Eriksson M, Zetterstrom R. Amphetamine addiction and pregnancy: psycho-social and medical aspects. Acta Psychiatr Scand 1979;60: 334–45.
16. Billing L, Eriksson M, Larsson G, Zetterstrom R. Amphetamine addiction and pregnancy. III. One year follow-up of the children: psychosocial and pediatric aspects. Acta Paediatr Scand 1980;69:675–80.
17. Eriksson M, Larsson G, Zetterstrom R. Amphetamine addiction and pregnancy. II. Pregnancy, delivery and the neonatal period: socio-medical aspects. Acta Obstet Gynecol Scand 1981;60:253–9.
18. Larsson G. The amphetamine addicted mother and her child. Acta Paediatr Scand 1980;Suppl 278: 7–24.
19. Heinonen OP, Slone D, Shapiro S. *Birth Defects and Drugs in Pregnancy*. Littleton, MA: Publishing Sciences Group, 1977.
20. Briggs GG, Samson JH, Crawford DJ. Lack of abnormalities in a newborn exposed to amphetamine during gestation. Am J Dis Child 1975;129: 249–50.
21. Steiner E, Villen T, Hallberg M, Rane A. Amphetamine secretion in breast milk. Eur J Clin Pharmacol 1984;27:123–4.
22. Tenorio GM, Nazvi M, Bickers GH, Hubbird RH. Intrauterine stroke and maternal polydrug abuse: case report. Clin Pediatr 1988;27:565–7.
23. Little BB, Snell LM, Gilstrap LC III. Methamphetamine abuse during pregnancy: outcome and fetal effects. Obstet Gynecol 1988;72:541–4.
24. Ramin SM, Little BB, Trimmer KJ, Standard DI, Blakely CA, Snell LM. Methamphetamine use during pregnancy in a large urban population (abstract). Am J Obstet Gynecol 1992;166:353.
25. Dearlove JC, Betteridge T. Stillbirth due to intravenous amphetamine. Br Med J 1992;304:548.
26. Sussman S. Narcotic and methamphetamine use during pregnancy: effect on newborn infants. Am J Dis Child 1963;106:325–30.
27. Neuberg R. Drug dependence and pregnancy: a review of the problems and their management. J Obstet Gynaecol Br Commonw 1970;66: 1117–22.
28. Ramer CM. The case history of an infant born to an amphetamine-addicted mother. Clin Pediatr 1974;13:596–7.
29. Oro AS, Dixon SD. Perinatal cocaine and methamphetamine exposure: maternal and neonatal correlates. J Pediatr 1987;111:571–8.
30. Dixon SD, Bejar R. Echoencephalographic findings in neonates associated with maternal cocaine and methamphetamine use: incidence and clinical correlates. J Pediatr 1989;115:770–8.
31. Chernoff GF, Jones KL. Fetal preventive medicine: teratogens and the unborn baby. Pediatr Ann 1981;10:210–7.
32. Kalter H, Warkany J. Congenital malformations (second of two parts). N Engl J Med 1983;308: 491–7.
33. Zierler S. Maternal drugs and congenital heart disease. Obstet Gynecol 1985;65:155–65.
34. Ayd FJ Jr. Excretion of psychotropic drugs in human breast milk. Int Drug Ther News Bull 1973;8: 33–40.
35. Committee on Drugs, American Academy of Pediatrics. The transfer of drugs and other chemicals into human milk. Pediatrics 2001;108: 776–89.

Name:	**AMPHOTERICIN B**	Risk Factor:	**B_M**
Class:	**Antifungal Antibiotic**		

FETAL RISK SUMMARY

RECOMMENDATION: Compatible

No reports linking the use of amphotericin B with congenital defects have been located. Reproduction studies of amphotericin B liposome were conducted with maternal nontoxic doses in rats (0.16 to 0.8 times the recommended human clinical dose range of 1 to 5 mg/kg based on body surface area [RHCD]) and rabbits (0.2 to 1 times the RHCD) (1). Rabbits administered doses 0.5 to 2 times the RHCD had a higher rate of spontaneous abortions than did controls (1). No fetal harm was observed in reproduction studies of amphotericin B lipid complex in rats and rabbits at doses up to 0.64 the human dose (2).

The antibiotic crosses the placenta to the fetus with cord blood:maternal serum ratios ranging from 0.38–1.0 (3–5). In a term (42 weeks) infant whose mother was treated with amphotericin B 0.6 mg/kg every other day, cord and maternal blood levels at delivery were both 2.6 μg/mL, a cord blood:maternal serum ratio of 1.0 (3). Amniotic fluid concentration was 0.08 μg/mL at delivery. The time interval between the last dose and delivery was not specified. Concentrations in the cord blood and maternal serum of a woman treated with 16 mg of amphotericin B just before delivery (one fifth of a planned total dose of 80 mg had infused when delivery occurred) were 0.12 μg/mL and 0.32 μg/mL, respectively, a ratio of 0.38 (4). The woman's last dose before this time was 7 days previously when she had received 80 mg. In a third case, a mother was receiving 20 mg IV every other day (0.5 mg/kg) (5). The cord and maternal serum concentrations were 1.3 μg/mL and 1.9 μg/mL, respectively, a ratio of 0.68. The levels were determined 26 hours after her last dose.

The Collaborative Perinatal Project monitored 50,282 mother-child pairs, 9 of whom had 1st trimester exposure to amphotericin B (6). Numerous other reports have also described the use of amphotericin B during various stages of pregnancy, including the 1st trimester (4–22). No evidence of adverse fetal effects was found by these studies. Amphotericin B can be used during pregnancy in those patients who will clearly benefit from the drug.

BREAST FEEDING SUMMARY

RECOMMENDATION: No Human Data - Probably Compatible

No data are available.

References

1. Product information. Ambisome. Fujisawa Healthcare, 2000.
2. Product information. Abelcet. Liposome, 2000.
3. McCoy MJ, Ellenberg JF, Killam AP. Coccidioidomycosis complicating pregnancy. Am J Obstet Gynecol 1980;137:739–40.
4. Ismail MA, Lerner SA. Disseminated blastomycosis in a pregnant woman. Review of amphotericin B usage during pregnancy. Am Rev Respir Dis 1982;126: 350–3.
5. Hager H, Welt SI, Cardasis JP, Alvarez S. Disseminated blastomycosis in a pregnant woman successfully treated with amphotericin-B: a case report. J Reprod Med 1988;33:485–8.
6. Heinonen OP, Slone D, Shapiro S. *Birth defects and drugs in pregnancy*. Littleton, MA: Publishing Sciences Group, 1977:297.
7. Neiberg AD, Maruomatis F, Dyke J, Fayyad A. Blastomyces dermatitidis treated during pregnancy. Am J Obstet Gynecol 1977;128:911–2.
8. Philpot CR, Lo D. Cryptococcal meningitis in pregnancy. Med J Aust 1972;2:1005–7.
9. Aitken GWE, Symonds EM. Cryptococcal meningitis in pregnancy treated with amphotericin. A case report. Br J Obstet Gynaecol 1962;69:677–9.
10. Feldman R. Cryptococcosis (torulosis) of the central nervous system treated with amphotericin B during pregnancy. South Med J 1959;52:1415–7.
11. Kuo D. A case of torulosis of the central nervous system during pregnancy. Med J Aust 1962;1: 558–60.
12. Crotty JM. Systemic mycotic infections in Northern territory aborigines. Med J Aust 1965;1:184.
13. Littman ML. Cryptococcosis (torulosis). Current concepts and therapy. Am J Med 1959;27:976–8.
14. Mick R, Muller-Tyl E, Neufeld T. Comparison of the effectiveness of Nystatin and amphotericin B in the therapy of female genital mycoses. Wien Med Wochenschr 1975:125:131–5.
15. Silberfarb PM, Sarois GA, Tosh FE. Cryptococcosis and pregnancy. Am J Obstet Gynecol 1972;112:714–20.
16. Curole DN. Cryptococcal meningitis in pregnancy. J Reprod Med 1981;26:317–9.
17. Sanford WG, Rasch JR, Stonehill RB. A therapeutic dilemma: the treatment of disseminated coccidioidomycosis with amphotericin B. Ann Intern Med 1962;56:553–63.
18. Harris RE. Coccidioidomycosis complicating pregnancy. Report of 3 cases and review of the literature. Obstet Gynecol 1966;28:401–5.
19. Smale LE, Waechter KG. Dissemination of coccidioidomycosis in pregnancy. Am J Obstet Gynecol 1970;107:356–9.
20. Hadsall FJ, Acquarelli MJ. Disseminated coccidioidomycosis presenting as facial granulomas in pregnancy: a report of two cases and a review of the literature. Laryngoscope 1973;83:51–8.
21. Daniel L, Salit IE. Blastomycosis during pregnancy. Can Med Assoc 1984;131:759–61.
22. Peterson CW, Johnson SL, Kelly JV, Kelly PC. Coccidioidal meningitis and pregnancy: a case report. Obstet Gynecol 1989;73:835–6.

Name:	**AMPICILLIN**	Risk Factor:	**B**
Class:	**Antibiotic (Penicillin)**		

FETAL RISK SUMMARY

RECOMMENDATION: Compatible

Ampicillin is a penicillin antibiotic (see also Penicillin G). The drug rapidly crosses the placenta into the fetal circulation and amniotic fluid (1–6). Fetal serum levels can be detected within 30 minutes and equilibrate with maternal serum in 1 hour. Amniotic fluid levels can be detected in 90 minutes, reaching 20% of the maternal serum peak in about 8 hours. The pharmacokinetics of ampicillin during pregnancy have been reported (7,8).

Ampicillin depresses both plasma-bound and urinary excreted estriol by inhibiting steroid conjugate hydrolysis in the gut (9–13). Urinary estriol was formerly used to assess the condition of the fetoplacental unit, depressed levels being associated with fetal distress. This assessment is now made by measuring plasma unconjugated estriol, which is not usually affected by ampicillin. An interaction between ampicillin and oral contraceptives resulting in pregnancy has been suspected (14,15). Two studies, however, failed to confirm this interaction and concluded that alternate contraceptive methods were not necessary during ampicillin therapy (16,17).

The use of ampicillin in early pregnancy was associated with a prevalence ratio estimate of 3.3 (90% confidence limits [CI] 1.3–8.1, $p = 0.02$) for congenital heart disease in a retrospective study (18). A specific defect, transposition of the great arteries, had a risk of 7.7 (90% CI 1.3–38) based on exposure in 2 of the 29 infants with the anomaly. The investigators did note, however, that the results had to be viewed cautiously because the data were subject to recall bias (drug histories were taken by questionnaire or telephone up to a year after presumed exposure) and the study could not distinguish between the fetal effects of the drug versus those of the infectious agent(s) for which the drugs were used. Others have also shared this concern (19). Other reports linking the use of ampicillin with congenital defects have not been located.

The Collaborative Perinatal Project monitored 50,282 mother-child pairs, 3546 of whom had 1st trimester exposure to penicillin derivatives (20, pp. 297–313). For use anytime during pregnancy, 7171 exposures were recorded (20, p. 435). In neither group was evidence found to suggest a relationship to large categories of major or minor malformations or to individual defects. Based on these data, it is unlikely that ampicillin is teratogenic.

In a surveillance study of Michigan Medicaid recipients conducted between 1985 and 1992, involving 229,101 completed pregnancies 10,011 newborns had been exposed to ampicillin during the 1st trimester (F. Rosa, personal communication, FDA, 1993). A total of 441 (4.4%) major birth defects were observed (426 expected). Specific data were available for six defect categories, including (observed/expected) 116/100 cardiovascular defects, 13/16 oral clefts, 6/8 spina bifida, 36/29 polydactyly, 9/17 limb reduction defects, and 27/24 hypospadias. These data do not support an association between the drug and the defects.

Ampicillin is often used in the last half of pregnancies in which either the woman or her fetus is at risk for infections because of premature rupture of the membranes or other risk factors (21–23). In one report, a mother with ruptured membranes at 40 weeks' gestation had an anaphylactic reaction to ampicillin (24). A markedly distressed infant was delivered with severe metabolic acidosis (arterial cord blood pH 6.71). Multifocal clonic seizures and brain edema occurred during the neonatal period and pronounced neurologic abnormalities were evident at 6 months of age.

BREAST FEEDING SUMMARY

RECOMMENDATION: Compatible

Ampicillin is excreted into breast milk in low concentrations. Milk:plasma ratios have been reported up to 0.2 (25,26). Candidiasis and diarrhea were observed in one infant whose mother was receiving ampicillin (27). Other reports of this effect have not been located. Although adverse effects are apparently rare, three potential problems exist for the nursing infant: modification of bowel flora, direct effects on the infant (e.g., allergic response or sensitization), and interference with the interpretation of culture results if a fever workup is required.

References

1. Bray R, Boe R, Johnson W. Transfer of ampicillin into fetus and amniotic fluid from maternal plasma in late pregnancy. Am J Obstet Gynecol 1966;96:938–42.
2. MacAulay M, Abou-Sabe M, Charles D. Placental transfer of ampicillin. Am J Obstet Gynecol 1966;96:943–50.
3. Biro L, Ivan E, Elek E, Arr M. Data on the tissue concentration of antibiotics in man. Tissue concentrations of semi-synthetic penicillins in the fetus. Int Z Klin Pharmakol Ther Toxikol 1970;4:321–4.
4. Elek E, Ivan E, Arr M. Passage of penicillins from mother to foetus in humans. Int J Clin Pharmacol Ther Toxicol 1972;6:223–8.
5. Kraybill EN, Chaney NE, McCarthy LR. Transplacental ampicillin: inhibitory concentrations in neonatal serum. Am J Obstet Gynecol 1980;138:793–6.
6. Jordheim O, Hagen AG. Study of ampicillin levels in maternal serum, umbilical cord serum and amniotic fluid following administration of pivampicillin. Acta Obstet Gynecol Scand 1980;59:315–7.
7. Philipson A. Pharmacokinetics of ampicillin during pregnancy. J Infect Dis 1977;136:370–6.
8. Noschel VH, Peiker G, Schroder S, Meinhold P, Muller B. Untersuchungen zur pharmakokinetik von antibiotika und sulfanilamiden in der schwangerschaft und unter der geburt. Zentralbl Gynakol 1982;104:1514–8.
9. Willman K, Pulkkinen M. Reduced maternal plasma and urinary estriol during ampicillin treatment. Am J Obstet Gynecol 1971;109:893–6.
10. Boehn F, DiPietro D, Goss D. The effect of ampicillin administration on urinary estriol and serum estradiol in the normal pregnant patient. Am J Obstet Gynecol 1974;119:98–101.
11. Sybulski S, Maughan G. Effect of ampicillin administration on estradiol, estriol and cortisol levels in maternal plasma and on estriol levels in urine. Am J Obstet Gynecol 1976;124:379–81.
12. Aldercreutz H, Martin F, Lehtinen T, Tikkanen M, Pulkkinen M. Effect of ampicillin administration on plasma conjugated and unconjugated estrogen and progesterone levels in pregnancy. Am J Obstet Gynecol 1977;128:266–71.
13. Van Look PFA, Top Huisman M, Gnodde HP. Effect of ampicillin or amoxycillin administration on plasma and urinary estrogen levels during normal pregnancy. Eur J Obstet Gynecol Reprod Biol 1981;12:225–33.
14. Dossetor J. Drug interactions with oral contraceptives. Br Med J 1975;4:467–8.
15. DeSano EA Jr, Hurley SC. Possible interactions of antihistamines and antibiotics with oral contraceptive effectiveness. Fertil Steril 1982;37:853–4.
16. Friedman CI, Huneke AL, Kim MH, Powell J. The effect of ampicillin on oral contraceptive effectiveness. Obstet Gynecol 1980;55:33–7.
17. Back DJ, Breckenridge AM, MacIver M, Orme M, Rowe PH, Staiger C, Thomas E, Tjia J. The effects of ampicillin on oral contraceptive steroids in women. Br J Clin Pharmacol 1982;14:43–8.
18. Rothman KJ, Fyler DC, Goldblatt A, Kreidberg MB. Exogenous hormones and other drug exposures of children with congenital heart disease. Am J Epidemiol 1979;109:433–9.
19. Zierler S. Maternal drugs and congenital heart disease. Obstet Gynecol 1985;65:155–65.
20. Heinonen OP, Slone D, Shapiro S. *Birth defects and drugs in pregnancy*. Littleton, MA: Publishing Sciences Group, 1977.
21. Boyer KM, Gotoff SP. Prevention of early-onset neonatal group B streptococcal disease with selective intrapartum chemoprophylaxis. N Engl J Med 1986;314:1665–9.
22. Amon E, Lewis SV, Sibai BM, Villar MA, Arheart KL. Ampicillin prophylaxis in preterm premature rupture of the membranes: a prospective randomized study. Am J Obstet Gynecol 1988;159:539–43.
23. Morales WJ, Angel JL, O'Brien WF, Knuppel RA. Use of ampicillin and corticosteroids in premature rupture of membranes: a randomized study. Obstet Gynecol 1989;73:721–6.
24. Heim K, Alge A, Marth C. Anaphylactic reaction to ampicillin and severe complication in the fetus. Lancet 1991;337:859.
25. Wilson J, Brown R, Cherek D, Dailey JW, Hilman B,

Jobe PC, Manno BR, Manno JE, Redetzki HM, Stewart JJ. Drug excretion in human breast milk: principles, pharmacokinetics and projected consequences. Clin Pharmacokinet 1980;5:1–66.

26. Knowles J. Excretion of drugs in milk—a review. J Pediatr 1965;66:1068–82.
27. Williams M. Excretion of drugs in milk. Pharm J 1976;217:219.

Name:	**AMPRENAVIR**	Risk Factor:	**C_M**
Class:	**Antiviral**		

FETAL RISK SUMMARY

RECOMMENDATION: Compatible - Maternal Benefit >> Embryo/Fetal Risk

Amprenavir is an inhibitor of human immunodeficiency virus type 1 (HIV-1) protease (PI). Protease is an enzyme that is required for the cleavage of viral polyprotein precursors into active functional proteins found in infectious HIV. Amprenavir, in combination with other antiretroviral agents, is indicated for the treatment of HIV-1 infections. Other drugs in this class are indinavir, nelfinavir, ritonavir, and saquinavir.

In reproduction studies with amprenavir, doses two times the human clinical exposure based on AUC comparisons (HCE) in male and female rats had no effect on fertility or mating (1). During embryo and fetal development, doses one-half the HCE produced thymic elongation and incomplete ossification of bones. When administered from day 7 of gestation to day 22 of lactation, a dose two times the HCE was associated with reduced body weights. However, subsequent development of the offspring, including fertility and reproductive performance, was not affected (1). In rabbits, doses up to one-twentieth the HCE were associated with abortions and minor skeletal variations resulting from deficient ossification of the femur, humerus trochlea, and humerus (1).

Amprenavir is transferred across the rat and rabbit placentas to the fetus (1). In an *ex vivo* human placental model, the antiviral agent also readily crossed to the fetus but with a clearance index less than abacavir. No accumulation of the drug was measured (2). The placental transfer is consistent with the relatively low molecular weight of amprenavir (about 506).

The Antiretroviral Pregnancy Registry reported, for the period January 1989 through January 2004, prospective data (reported to the Registry before the outcomes were known) involving 1537 live births that had been exposed during the 1st trimester to one or more antiretroviral agents (3). Forty-seven of the newborns had congenital defects (3.1%, 95% confidence interval [CI] 2.3–4.1). In the 2407 live births with earliest exposure in the 2nd/3rd trimesters, there were 56 infants with defects (2.3%, 95% CI 1.8–3.0). The prevalence rates for the two periods did not differ significantly. There were 103 infants with birth defects among 3944 live births with exposure anytime during pregnancy (2.6%, 95% CI 2.1–3.2). The prevalence rate did not differ significantly from the rate expected in a nonexposed population (3). There were 25 outcomes exposed to amprenavir (18 in the 1st trimester and 7 in the 2nd/3rd trimesters) in combination with other antiretroviral agents. There was one birth defect among the 1st trimester exposures and none in those exposed in the 2nd/3rd trimesters (3). In reviewing the birth defects of prospective and retrospective (pregnancies reported after the outcomes were known) registered cases, and clinical reports, the Registry concluded that there was no pattern of anomalies to suggest a common cause (3). (See Lamivudine for required statement.)

A public health advisory has been issued by the Food and Drug Administration (FDA) on the association between protease inhibitors and diabetes mellitus (4). Because pregnancy is a risk factor for hyperglycemia, there was concern that these antiviral agents would exacerbate this risk. An abstract published in 2000 described the results of a study involving 34 pregnant women treated with protease inhibitors (none with amprenavir) who were compared with 41 controls that evaluated the association with diabetes (5). No association between protease inhibitors and an increased incidence of gestational diabetes was found.

In summary, the near absence of human data does not allow a prediction as to the safety of amprenavir during pregnancy. However, the developmental toxicity observed in animals at doses less than the human clinical dose is a potential concern for human pregnancies. Two reviews, one in 1996 and the other in 1997, however, concluded that all women currently receiving antiretroviral therapy should continue to receive therapy during pregnancy and that treatment of the mother with monotherapy should be considered inadequate therapy (6,7). In 1998, the Centers for Disease Control and Prevention (CDC) made a similar recommendation that antiretroviral therapy should be continued during pregnancy, but discontinuation of all therapy during the 1st trimester was a consideration (4). If indicated, therefore, protease inhibitors, including amprenavir, should not be withheld in pregnancy (with the possible exception of the 1st trimester) because the expected benefit to the HIV-positive mother probably outweighs the unknown risk to the fetus. However, one review suggested that during pregnancy ritonavir (see Ritonavir) was the drug of choice among the protease inhibitors (7). Pregnant women taking protease inhibitors should be monitored for hyperglycemia. The efficacy and safety of combined therapy in preventing vertical transmission of HIV to the newborn, however, are unknown, and zidovudine remains the only antiretroviral agent recommended for this purpose (6,7).

BREAST FEEDING SUMMARY

RECOMMENDATION: Contraindicated

No reports describing the use of amprenavir during human lactation have been located. The antiviral agent is excreted into the milk of lactating rats (1). In addition, the molecular weight (about 506) is low enough that excretion into human breast milk should be expected.

Reports on the use of amprenavir during human lactation are unlikely because the antiviral agent is used in the treatment of human immunodeficiency virus (HIV) infections. HIV-1 is transmitted in milk, and in developed countries, breast-feeding is not recommended (6–10). In developing countries, breast-feeding is undertaken, despite the risk, because there are no affordable milk substitutes available. Until 1999, no studies had been published that examined the effect of any antiretroviral therapy on HIV-1 transmission in milk. In that year, a study involving zidovudine was published that measured a 38% reduction in vertical transmission of HIV-1 infection in spite of breast-feeding when compared with controls (see Zidovudine).

References

1. Product information. Agenerase. Glaxo Wellcome, 2000.
2. Bawdon RE. The *ex vivo* human placental transfer of the anti-HIV nucleoside inhibitor abacavir and the protease inhibitor amprenavir. Infect Dis Obstet Gynecol 1998;6:244–6.
3. Antiretroviral Pregnancy Registry Steering Committee, Antiretroviral Pregnancy Registry International Interim Report for 1 January 1989 through 31 January 2004. Wilmington, NC: Registry Coordinating Center; 2004.
4. CDC. Public Health Service Task Force recommendations for the use of antiretroviral drugs in pregnant women infected with HIV-1 for maternal health and

A

for reducing perinatal HIV-1 transmission in the United States. MMWR 1998;47:No. RR-2.
5. Fassett M, Kramer F, Stek A. Treatment with protease inhibitors in pregnancy is not associated with an increased incidence of gestational diabetes (abstract). Am J Obstet Gynecol 2000;182:S97.
6. Carpenter CCJ, Fischi MA, Hammer SM, Hirsch MS, Jacobsen DM, Katzenstein DA, Montaner JSG, Richman DD, Saag MS, Schooley RT, Thompson MA, Vella S, Yeni PG, Volberding PA. Antiretroviral therapy for HIV infection in 1996. JAMA 1996;276;146–54.
7. Minkoff H, Augenbraun M. Antiretroviral therapy for pregnant women. Am J Obstet Gynecol 1997;176:478–89.
8. Brown ZA, Watts DH. Antiviral therapy in pregnancy. Clin Obstet Gynecol 1990;33:276–89.
9. de Martino M, Tovo P-A, Pezzotti P, Galli L, Massironi E, Ruga E, Floreea F, Plebani A, Gabiano C, Zuccotti GV. HIV-1 transmission through breast-milk: appraisal of risk according to duration of feeding. AIDS 1992;6:991–7.
10. Van de Perre P. Postnatal transmission of human immunodeficiency virus type 1: the breast feeding dilemma. Am J Obstet Gynecol 1995;173:483–7.

Name:	**AMRINONE**	Risk Factor:	C_M
Class:	**Cardiac Agent**		

FETAL RISK SUMMARY

RECOMMENDATION: Limited Human Data - Animal Data Suggest Low Risk

Amrinone is a cardiac inotropic agent that also has a vasodilatory effect (1). The drug is unrelated to cardiac glycosides or catecholamines. The principal indication for amrinone is the short-term management of congestive heart failure.

Amrinone is teratogenic in some animal species, producing skeletal and gross external malformations in one type of rabbits but not in other types, and having no effect on fetal rats (1). In pregnant baboons, amrinone infusion did not significantly affect uterine artery blood flow (2).

A single case report has described the use of amrinone in a human pregnancy (3). A 34-year-old woman at 18 weeks' gestation was treated with an amrinone IV infusion (0.5 mg/kg loading dose followed by 2 μg/kg/minute) for refractory congestive heart failure secondary to bacterial endocarditis. A higher dose was not used because of premature ventricular contractions. Although no fetal adverse effects attributable to the drug were noted, fetal death occurred 11 days after discontinuance of amrinone because of the deteriorating medical condition of the mother (3).

BREAST FEEDING SUMMARY

RECOMMENDATION: No Human Data - Probably Compatible

No reports describing the use of amrinone during lactation have been located. The molecular weight of amrinone (about 187) is low enough, however, that passage into milk should be expected.

References

1. Product information, Inocor. Sanofi Winthrop Pharmaceuticals, 1997.
2. Fishburne JI Jr, Dormer KJ, Payne GG, Gill PS, Ashrafzadeh AR, Rossavik IK. Effects of amrinone and dopamine on uterine blood flow and vascular responses in the gravid baboon. Am J Obstet Gynecol 1988;158:829–37.
3. Jelsema RD, Bhatia RK, Ganguly S. Use of intravenous amrinone in the short-term management of refractory heart failure in pregnancy. Obstet Gynecol 1991;78:935–6.

Name: **AMYL NITRITE** Risk Factor: **C**

Class: **Vasodilator**

FETAL RISK SUMMARY

RECOMMENDATION: Limited Human Data - No Relevant Animal Data

Amyl nitrite is a rapid-acting, short-duration vasodilator used primarily for the treatment of angina pectoris. Because of the nature of its indication, experience in pregnancy is limited. The Collaborative Perinatal Project recorded seven 1st trimester exposures to amyl nitrite and nitroglycerin plus eight other patients exposed to other vasodilators (1). From this small group of 15 patients, four malformed children were observed. It was not stated whether amyl nitrite was taken by any of the mothers of the affected infants. The number of cases is too small to assess the risk of amyl nitrite in pregnancy.

BREAST FEEDING SUMMARY

RECOMMENDATION: No Human Data - Probably Compatible

No data are available.

Reference

1. Heinonen OP, Slone D, Shapiro S. *Birth defects and drugs in pregnancy*. Littleton, MA: Publishing Sciences Group, 1977:371–3.

Name: **ANAGRELIDE** Risk Factor: **C_M**

Class: **Hematological Agent (Antiplatelet)**

FETAL RISK SUMMARY

RECOMMENDATION: Limited Human Data - Animal Data Suggest Low Risk

Anagrelide, an antiplatelet agent, is indicated for the reduction of elevated platelet counts and resulting risk of thrombosis in patients with thrombocythemia.

An animal teratology study observed no congenital abnormalities in pregnant rats given oral doses up to 730 times the maximum recommended human dose based on body surface area (MRHD) or in pregnant rabbits administered doses up to 32 times the MRHD (1). In a fertility and reproductive performance study of female rats, however, doses 49 times the MRHD or higher disrupted implantation and produced an adverse effect on embryo/fetal survival (1). The same dosage in a perinatal and postnatal study with pregnant rats caused a delay in parturition, deaths of undelivered dams and their fetuses, and increased mortality in pups that were born (1).

No reports describing the placental transfer of anagrelide in animals or humans have been located. The molecular weight of the drug (about 311 for the hydrochloride monohydrate salt) is low enough, however, that passage to the fetus should be expected.

The only reported human pregnancy exposure to anagrelide appears to be that described by the manufacturer in its product information (1). Five women became pregnant while receiving the drug at doses of 1 to 4 mg/day. Therapy was stopped when the pregnancies were diagnosed (timing not specified), and all the women delivered normal, healthy babies.

In summary, human pregnancy experience with anagrelide is limited to the above five cases, all apparently in early pregnancy. Although the outcomes were normal in each case, animal data appear to indicate a potential for embryo/fetal harm. The toxic dose in animals, however, was much higher than the dose used in humans, based on body surface area. The manufacturer recommends that women should not become pregnant while taking anagrelide, but the benefits of therapy must be weighed against the risks on a case-by-case basis. If therapy is started or continued during pregnancy, the woman should be fully informed of the potential risks to her embryo/fetus.

BREAST FEEDING SUMMARY

RECOMMENDATION: No Human Data - Potential Toxicity

No reports describing the use of anagrelide during lactation have been located. The molecular weight of the compound (about 311 for the hydrochloride monohydrate salt) is low enough, however, that passage into milk should be expected. The potential effects of this exposure on a nursing infant are unknown. Because the reduction in platelets is dose-related, thrombocytopenia, as well as other adverse effects, are potential complications.

Reference

1. Product information. Agrylin. Roberts Pharmaceutical, 2000.

Name:	**ANAKINRA**	Risk Factor:	**B_M**
Class:	**Immunologic Agent (Immunomodulator)**		

FETAL RISK SUMMARY

RECOMMENDATION: No Human Data - Animal Data Suggest Low Risk

Anakinra is a nonglycosylated form of the human cytokine interleukin-1 receptor antagonist (IL-1ra) produced by recombinant DNA technology. Anakinra (recombinant IL-1ra) is indicated for the reduction in signs and symptoms of moderately to severe rheumatoid arthritis. By binding to interleukin-1 receptors, IL-1ra competitively inhibits interleukin-1 activity, such as the stimulation of several inflammatory mediators. The terminal elimination half-life ranges from 4 to 6 hours (1).

Native IL-1ra is a normal constituent in the maternal, fetal, and amniotic fluid compartments (2,3). Endogenous IL-1ra has been measured in amniotic fluid and newborn urine. Fetal urine is a major source of the cytokine and is gender-dependent with the highest levels found in females. The investigators of one study concluded that the higher concentrations contributed to the better resistance of female fetuses against preterm birth and perinatal infections (3). Conversely, IL-1ra also has been shown to have partial agonist properties because it increases the prostaglandin E_2 (PGE_2) production of interleukin-1β in fetal membranes that is involved in the initiation of parturition at term (4).

Reproduction studies have been conducted in rats and rabbits. No evidence of impaired fertility or fetal harm was observed in either species at doses up to 100 times the human dose (*assumed to be based on weight*). Animal carcinogenic studies have not been conducted with anakinra, but it was not mutagenic in *in vitro* and *in vivo* tests (1).

In contrast to the above animal data, recombinant IL-1ra has been shown in mice to impair embryonic implantation by a direct inhibitory effect on transformation of the epithelial plasma membrane (5,6). Furthermore, the embryos were morphologically normal and were viable when transferred to pseudopregnant mice (6).

In a 1992 mouse study, interleukin-1-induced preterm delivery was blocked by IL-1ra (7). However, IL-1ra did not prevent preterm delivery or prolong pregnancy in mice with endotoxin-induced preterm labor (8).

A 2001 Australian study found evidence that polymorphisms in the gene encoding for endogenous IL-1ra was associated with recurrent miscarriage (three or more consecutive pregnancy losses before 20 weeks' gestation) (9). The study investigated 105 women with idiopathic recurrent miscarriage compared to 91 controls with a history of normal pregnancies and no pregnancy losses. Three alleles of IL-1ra polymorphisms were measured. Study subjects had a significantly higher level of polymorphic allele 2 suggesting that this was a genetic determinant of idiopathic recurrent miscarriage and that IL-1ra acted as a physiologic mediator. The study could not determine the degree of genetic IL-1ra deficiency that was associated with idiopathic recurrent miscarriage (9). In contrast, a 2003 Finish study found that significantly higher levels of polymorphic allele 3 were associated with recurrent spontaneous abortion, suggesting that the allele frequencies varied considerable in different ethnic groups (10).

Anakinra crosses the rabbit placenta. The cervixes of pregnant rabbits were inoculated with *Escherichia coli* and then the rabbits were given a 5-hour infusion of anakinra (10 mg/kg) (11). Although the treatment did not affect clinical or microbiological outcomes or amniotic fluid levels of tumor necrosis factor alpha or prostaglandins (PGE_2), amniotic fluid concentrations of anakinra were markedly elevated compared to controls (14.8 ng/mL vs. none detected) (11).

An *in vitro* study was conducted using term human placentas obtained at cesarean section from uncomplicated pregnancies to determine if recombinant IL-1ra crossed the placenta (12). Both maternal-to-fetal and fetal-to-maternal directions were studied. Minimal transfer occurred in either direction. The findings appear to be consistent with the high molecular weight (17,300) of the 153-amino acid protein.

No reports describing the use of anakinra in human pregnancy have been located. The animal data do not suggest a risk of structural defects, but the agent prevented embryo implantation in one study. Although the lack of data prevents an assessment of the risk for the human embryo/fetus, IL-1ra is a natural occurring cytokine that appears to have a role in the protection of the placenta/embryo/fetus from the maternal immune response mechanisms. Therefore, it is doubtful if recommended doses of recombinant IL-1ra will cause direct toxicity to the embryo or fetus. Until human pregnancy data are available, however, the safest course is to avoid anakinra during gestation. Planned or inadvertent pregnancy exposure appears to represent a low risk for the embryo and fetus. If anakinra is used in pregnancy for the treatment of rheumatoid arthritis, health care professionals are encouraged to call the toll free number (877-311-8972) for information about patient enrollment in the OTIS Rheumatoid Arthritis Study.

BREAST FEEDING SUMMARY

RECOMMENDATION: No Human Data - Probably Compatible

No reports describing the use of anakinra during human lactation have been located. Even though the molecular weight of the 153-amino acid cytokine is high (17,300), endogenous IL-1ra is excreted into colostrum and mature milk. In a 1996 study, concentrations of IL-1ra in colostrum were higher than in milk (13). Both colostrum and milk had significantly higher concentrations than did maternal serum or plasma. The measurements of another 1996 study mirrored these findings of IL-1ra in colostrum, transitional milk, and mature milk (14). In the first study, the high milk concentrations persisted over a sequential collection period of 2–6 months (13). It was thought that the presence of natural IL-1ra contributed to the known anti-inflammatory properties of breast milk (13). Indeed, in a 2001 study, milk levels of IL-1ra in eight lactating women with acute mastitis were markedly increased (15). Because of the presence of native IL-1ra in milk, there appears to be no risk to a nursing infant from maternal administration of anakinra.

References

1. Product information. Kineret. Amgen, 2004.
2. Romero R, Gomez R, Galasso M, Mazor M, Berry SM, Quintero RA, Cotton DB. The natural interleukin-1 receptor antagonist in the fetal, maternal, and amniotic fluid compartments: the effect of gestational age, fetal gender, and intrauterine infection. Am J Obstet Gynecol 1994;171:912–21.
3. Bry K, Lappalainen U, Waffarn F, Teramo K, Hallman M. Influence of fetal gender on the concentration of interleukin-1 receptor antagonist in amniotic fluid and in newborn urine. Pediatr Res 1994;35:130–4.
4. Brown NL, Alvi SA, Elder MG, Bennett PR, Sullivan MHF. Regulation of prostaglandin production in intact fetal membranes by interleukin-1 and its receptor antagonist. J Endocrinol 1998;159:519–26.
5. Simon C, Frances A, Piquette GN, El Danasouri I, Zurawski G, Dang W, Polan LM. Embryonic implantation in mice is blocked by interleukin-1 receptor antagonist. Endocrinology 1994;134:521–8.
6. Simon C, Valbuena D, Krussel J, Bernal A, Murphy CR, Shaw T, Pellicer A, Polan LM. Interleukin-1 receptor antagonist prevents embryonic implantation by a direct effect on the endometrial epithelium. Fertil Steril 1998;70:896–906.
7. Romero R, Tartakovsky B. The natural interleukin-1 receptor antagonist prevents interleukin-1-induced preterm delivery in mice. Am J Obstet Gynecol 1992;167:1041–5.
8. Fidel PL Jr, Romero R, Cutright J, Wolf N, Gomez R, Araneda H, Ramirez M, Yoon BH. Treatment with interleukin-1 receptor antagonist and soluble tumor necrosis factor receptor Fc fusion protein does not prevent endotoxin-induced preterm parturition in mice. J Soc Gynecol Invest 1997;4:22–6.
9. Unfried G, Tempfer C, Schneeberger C, Widmar B, Nagele F, Huber JC. Interleukin-1 receptor antagonist polymorphism in women with idiopathic recurrent miscarriage. Fertil Steril 2001;75:683–7.
10. Karhukorpi J, Laitinen T, Kivela H, Tiilikainen A, Hurme M. IL-1 receptor antagonist gene polymorphism in recurrent spontaneous abortion. J Reprod Immunol 2003;58:61–7.
11. McDuffie RS Jr, Davies JK, Leslie KK, Lee S, Sherman MP, Gibbs RS. A randomized controlled trial of interleukin-1 receptor antagonist in a rabbit model of ascending infection in pregnancy. Infect Dis Obstet Gynecol 2001;9:233–7.
12. Zaretsky MV, Alexander JM, Byrd W, Bawdon RE. Transfer of inflammatory cytokines across the placenta. Obstet Gynecol 2004;103:546–50.
13. Buescher ES, Malinowska I. Soluble receptors and cytokine antagonists in human milk. Pediatr Res 1996;40:839–44.
14. Srivastave MD, Srivastava A, Brouhard B, Saneto R, Groh-Wargo S, Kubit J. Cytokines in human milk. Res Commun Mol Pathol Pharmacol 1996;93:263–87.
15. Buescher ES, Hair PS. Human milk anti-inflammatory component contents during acute mastitis. Cell Immunol 2001;210:87–95.

Name: **ANILERIDINE** Risk Factor: **B***
Class: **Narcotic Agonist Analgesic**

FETAL RISK SUMMARY

RECOMMENDATION: Human Data Suggest Risk in 3rd Trimester

No reports linking the use of anileridine with congenital defects have been located. Usage in pregnancy is primarily confined to labor. Withdrawal may occur in infants exposed *in utero* to prolonged maternal treatment with anileridine. Respiratory depression in the neonate similar to that produced by meperidine or morphine should be expected (1).

[**Risk Factor D if used for prolonged periods or in high doses at term.*]

BREAST FEEDING SUMMARY

RECOMMENDATION: No Human Data - Probably Compatible

No data are available.

Reference

1. Bonica J. *Principles and Practice of Obstetric Analgesia and Anesthesia*. Philadelphia, PA: FA Davis, 1967:250.

Name:	**ANISINDIONE**	Risk Factor:	**D**
Class:	**Anticoagulant**		

FETAL RISK SUMMARY

RECOMMENDATION: Contraindicated

The indandione derivative, anisindione, is an oral anticoagulant. It is structurally related to phenindione, an anticoagulant not available in the United States.

In an investigation of the effects of occlusive thromboaortopathy (Takayasu's disease) on pregnancy, 4 of 27 women were maintained on anisindione throughout five pregnancies (1). No neonatal complications or anomalies were observed in the five infants. (See Coumarin Derivatives.)

BREAST FEEDING SUMMARY

RECOMMENDATION: No Human Data - Potential Toxicity

See Coumarin Derivatives.

Reference

1. Ishikawa K, Matsuura S. Occlusive thromboaortopathy (Takayasu's disease) and pregnancy: clinical course and management of 33 pregnancies and deliveries. Am J Cardiol 1982;50:1293–1300.

Name:	**ANISOTROPINE**	Risk Factor:	**C**
Class:	**Parasympatholytic**		

FETAL RISK SUMMARY

RECOMMENDATION: Limited Human Data - No Relevant Animal Data

Anisotropine is an anticholinergic quaternary ammonium methylbromide. In a large prospective study, 2323 patients were exposed to this class of drugs during the 1st trimester, 2 of whom took anisotropine (1). A possible association was found between the total group and minor malformations.

BREAST FEEDING SUMMARY

RECOMMENDATION: No Human Data - Probably Compatible

No data are available (see also Atropine).

Reference

1. Heinonen OP, Slone D, Shapiro S. *Birth defects and drugs in pregnancy*. Littleton, MA: Publishing Sciences Group, 1977:346–53.

Name:	**ANTAZOLINE**	Risk Factor:	**C**
Class:	**Antihistamine**		

See Diphenhydramine for representative agent in this class.

Name:	**ANTHRALIN**	Risk Factor:	**C_M**
Class:	**Dermatological Agent (Anti-Psoriatic)**		

FETAL RISK SUMMARY

RECOMMENDATION: No Human Data - No Relevant Animal Data

Anthralin (dithranol) is a synthetic product used in creams and ointments for the topical treatment of psoriasis. Systemic absorption of anthralin from human skin has not been studied. In addition, reproduction studies in animals have not been conducted (1).

Although the amount of drug that reaches the systemic circulation is not known, the molecular weight (about 226) is low enough for transfer across the placenta to the embryo/fetus.

No reports describing the use of anthralin in human pregnancy have been located. The lack of animal reproduction testing and human pregnancy experience prevents an assessment of the embryo/fetal risk.

BREAST FEEDING SUMMARY

RECOMMENDATION: No Human Data - Potential Toxicity

No reports describing the use of anthralin during human lactation have been located. In addition, the systemic absorption of anthralin from the skin has not been studied (1). The absence of this information prevents any assessment of the risk to a nursing infant from exposure of the drug in breast milk. Therefore, the safest course would be to avoid anthralin during lactation.

Reference

1. Product information. Psoriatec. Sirius Laboratories, 2004.

Name: **ANTIPYRINE** Risk Factor: **C**

Class: **Analgesic/Antipyretic**

FETAL RISK SUMMARY

RECOMMENDATION: Limited Human Data - No Relevant Animal Data

Because of its rare association with hemolytic anemia and agranulocytosis (1), antipyrine (phenazone), a prostaglandin synthesis inhibitor, is no longer available as a single agent. However, the drug is still available in some topical ear drops and in the prodrug, dichloralphenazone (see also Dichloralphenazone). This latter agent, a combination of chloral hydrate and antipyrine, is a component, along with isometheptene and acetaminophen, of several proprietary mixtures commonly used for tension and vascular (migraine) headaches (see also Isometheptene and Acetaminophen).

Although animal reproductive studies involving antipyrine have not been located, the drug has been used extensively in investigations of fetal metabolism in pregnant sheep as reviewed in a 1993 reference (2). This latter investigation found that antipyrine did not affect umbilical metabolism but did alter metabolism and blood flow distribution in the fetal lamb (2).

Eight cases of antipyrine exposure (presumably oral), among 27 women using a miscellaneous group of non-narcotic analgesics during the 1st trimester, were reported by the Collaborative Perinatal Project (3). From the 27 mother-child pairs, one infant had a congenital malformation (SRR 0.46), but the specific agent the mother had taken was not identified.

In a double-blind, randomized study of neonatal jaundice prophylaxis, either antipyrine ($N = 24$), 300 mg/day, or placebo ($N = 24$) was given from the 38th week of gestation until delivery (4). The average duration of treatment in both groups was 15.5 days. The mean bilirubin concentration in the infants 4 days after birth was 62.6 μmol/L in those exposed to antipyrine, compared with 111.5 μmol/L in the placebo group ($p < 0.005$). The authors attributed the decrease in bilirubin to the induction of glucuronyl transferase in the fetal liver, a known effect of antipyrine (4). No adverse effects in the newborns were observed.

BREAST FEEDING SUMMARY

RECOMMENDATION: No Human Data - Potential Toxicity

Antipyrine (phenazone), a nonelectrolyte with a molecular weight less than 200, freely diffuses into the aqueous phase of milk with a milk:plasma ratio of approximately 1.0 (5,6). No reports of its use during lactation have been located.

References

1. Swanson M, Cook R. *Drugs, Chemicals, and Blood Dyscrasias*. Hamilton, IL: Drug Intelligence Publications, 1977:88–9.
2. Gull I, Charlton V. Effects of antipyrine on umbilical and regional metabolism in late gestation in the fetal lamb. Am J Obstet Gynecol 1993;168:706–13.
3. Heinonen OP, Slone D, Shapiro S. *Birth defects and drugs in pregnancy*. Littleton, MA: Publishing Sciences Group, 1977:287.
4. Lewis PJ, Friedman LA. Prophylaxis of neonatal jaundice with maternal antipyrine treatment. Lancet 1979;1:300–2.
5. Hawkins DF. *Drugs and Pregnancy. Human Teratogenesis and Related Problems*. 2nd ed. New York, NY: Churchill Livingstone, 1987:312.

6. McNamara PJ, Burgio D, Yoo SD. Pharmacokinetics of acetaminophen, antipyrine, and salicylic acid in the lactating and nursing rabbit, with model predictions of milk to serum concentration ratios and neonatal dose. Toxicol Appl Pharmacol 1991;109:149–60.

Name:	**ANTITHROMBIN III (HUMAN)**	Risk Factor:	B_M
Class:	**Hematological Agents (Antithrombin)**		

FETAL RISK SUMMARY

RECOMMENDATION: Limited Human Data - Animal Data Suggest Low Risk

This product is prepared from pooled units of human plasma from screened normal plasma donors. Although the risk of transmitting infectious agents, such as viruses, has been reduced by measures taken during production, there is still a potential for transmitting disease (1). Antithrombin III is an α_2-glycoprotein that normally is present in human plasma at a concentration of approximately 12.5 mg/dL (1). It is the major plasma inhibitor of thrombin.

Reproduction studies have been conducted with antithrombin III in pregnant rats and rabbits. No evidence of impaired fertility or fetal harm was observed with doses up to four times the human dose (1).

It is not known whether there are physiologic processes that can carry maternal antithrombin to the embryo or fetus. The molecular weight of the protein, about 58,000, should prevent passive diffusion.

Two reports have described the use of antithrombin III in the treatment of preeclampsia (2,3). In both cases, the beneficial effects of antithrombin III were theorized to be related to the inhibition of thrombin resulting in a reduction in maternal hypertension and an increase in placental circulation (2,3). In a nonrandomized study, women with severe, early-onset preeclampsia (mean gestational age at onset 28–29 weeks) with intrauterine growth retardation were treated for 7 days with antithrombin III 1500 IU/day and heparin 5000 U/day ($N = 14$) or heparin 5000 U/day alone ($N = 15$) (2). None of the women received antihypertensive agents. The mean gestational age at the beginning of treatment was 30–31 weeks with delivery in both groups occurring at about 32 weeks' gestation. There was no difference in the mean birth weights (1280 g vs. 1135 g), but the estimated fetal weight gain (g/day) was higher in the antithrombin group (29.5 g vs. 15.3 g, $p < 0.05$). No information was provided on the status of the newborns, but there were no differences between the groups in the fetal biochemical profile score (2).

A total of 133 women with severe preeclampsia (24 to 35 weeks' gestation) were enrolled in a randomized, double-blind, placebo-controlled trial (3). The patients received either antithrombin III 3000 units once daily for 7 days ($N = 66$) or albumin once daily for 7 days ($N = 67$). The mean gestational age at the start of treatment was about 32 weeks in both groups. Treatment was interrupted in 23 and 29 patients in the antithrombin III and placebo groups, respectively, because of worsening of maternal and fetal findings. Patients in each group received antihypertensive agents and/or magnesium sulfate when indicated. There were no significant differences between the groups in the fetal biochemical profile score, but the antithrombin III group had a greater estimated fetal gain ($p = 0.029$). Pregnancy outcomes all favored the treatment group: gestational age at delivery (34.1 weeks vs. 33.0 weeks, $p = 0.007$), birth weight (1749 g vs. 1409 g, $p = 0.004$), and number of small for gestational age newborns (65.6% vs. 83.3%, $p = 0.020$). No adverse effects in the newborns were observed (3).

In summary, antithrombin III (Human) has been used in the 2nd and 3rd trimesters for the treatment of preeclampsia. Preliminary evidence suggests that this treatment may be beneficial, but further studies are needed to confirm these outcomes. Although the limited animal data is reassuring, there is no human 1st trimester experience with this agent.

BREAST FEEDING SUMMARY

RECOMMENDATION: No Human Data - Probably Compatible

No reports describing the use of antithrombin III during lactation have been located. The high molecular weight of the protein (about 58,000) suggests that it will not be excreted into breast milk. However, even if small amounts did enter the milk they likely would be digested in the infant's stomach. Therefore, the risk to a nursing infant from this agent appears to be nil.

References

1. Product information. Thrombate III. Bayer Corporation, Pharmaceutical Division, Biological Products, 2003.
2. Nakabayashi M, Asami M, Nakatani A. Efficacy of antithrombin replacement therapy in severe early-onset preeclampsia. Semin Thromb Hemost 1999;25:463–6.
3. Maki M, Kobayashi T, Terao T, Ikenoue T, Satoh K, Nakabayashi M, Sagara Y, Kajiwara Y, Urata M. Antithrombin therapy for severe preeclampsia. Results of a double-blind, randomized, placebo-controlled trial. Thromb Haemost 2000;84:583–90.

Name:	**APROBARBITAL**	Risk Factor:	**C**
Class:	**Sedative/Hypnotic**		

No data are available (see Amobarbital for related agent).

Name:	**APROTININ**	Risk Factor:	**B_M**
Class:	**Hemostatic**		

FETAL RISK SUMMARY

RECOMMENDATION: Limited Human Data - Animal Data Suggest Low Risk

Aprotinin, a polypeptide, is a natural, broad spectrum protease inhibitor obtained from bovine lung that is indicated for the prophylaxis of perioperative blood loss during cardiopulmonary bypass surgery. After IV administration, aprotinin undergoes rapid distribution into the total extracellular space and the plasma half-life, after the distribution phase, is about 150 minutes. The terminal half-life is about 10 hours (1).

Reproduction studies were conducted in rats with IV doses up to 200,000 KIU/kg/day for 11 days (2.4 times the human dose based on body weight [HD-BW]; 0.37 times the human dose based on body surface area [HD-BSA]) and in rabbits with IV doses up to 100,000 KIU/kg/day for 13 days (1.2 times the HD-BW; 0.36 times the HD-BSA). No effects on fertility or fetal harm were observed in either species.

No reports linking the use of aprotinin and congenital defects have been located. The drug crosses the placenta and decreases fibrinolytic activity in the newborn (2). The drug has been used safely in severe accidental hemorrhage with coagulation when labor was not established (3).

BREAST FEEDING SUMMARY

RECOMMENDATION: No Human Data - Probably Compatible

No reports have been located describing the use of aprotinin during lactation. Because of the indication for this drug, the opportunity for breast-feeding following its use is probably nil. The oral absorption of this polypeptide is unknown, but most likely poor.

References

1. Product information. Trasylol. Bayer, 2000.
2. Hoffhauer H, Dobbeck P. Untersuchungen uber die plactapassage des kallikrein-inhibitors. Klin Wochenschr 1970;48:183–4.
3. Sher G. Trasylol in cases of accidental hemorrhage with coagulation disorder and associated uterine inertia. S Afr Med J 1974;48:1452–5.

Name:	**ARGATROBAN**	Risk Factor:	B_M
Class:	**Hematologic Agent (Thrombin Inhibitor)**		

FETAL RISK SUMMARY

RECOMMENDATION: Compatible - Maternal Benefit >> Embryo/Fetal Risk

Argatroban, a synthetic reversible direct thrombin inhibitor derived from L-arginine, is indicated for anticoagulation in patients who cannot receive heparin because of heparin-induced thrombocytopenia. The drug is administered as a continuous IV infusion.

Reproduction studies with IV argatroban have been conducted in pregnant rats and rabbits at doses up to 0.3 and 0.2 times, respectively, the maximum recommended human dose based on body surface area (1). No evidence of impaired fertility or fetal harm was observed in either species.

It is not known if argatroban crosses the human placenta. The molecular weight (about 527 for the hydrated form), however, is low enough that exposure of the embryo/fetus should be expected.

No studies describing the use of argatroban during human pregnancy have been located. Although the animal studies are encouraging, human studies are required before an assessment can be made of the risk, including hemorrhage, that this drug represents to an embryo or fetus. If a pregnant woman requires argatroban therapy, however, the benefits to her appear to outweigh the theoretical risks.

BREAST FEEDING SUMMARY

RECOMMENDATION: No Human Data - Probably Compatible

No studies describing the use of argatroban during human lactation have been located. The drug is excreted in rat milk (1). The molecular weight (about 527 for the hydrated form) is low enough that excretion into breast milk should also be expected. The effects of this exposure on a nursing infant are unknown, but the oral absorption is probably poor.

Reference

1. Product information. Argatroban. GlaxoSmithKline, 2002.

Name: **ARIPIPRAZOLE** Risk Factor: **C_M**

Class: **Antipsychotic**

FETAL RISK SUMMARY

RECOMMENDATION: No Human Data - Animal Data Suggest Risk

Aripiprazole is an antipsychotic used in the treatment of schizophrenia. The drug is a partial agonist at dopamine D_2 and the serotonin 5-HT_{1A} receptors, and as an antagonist at serotonin 5-HT_{2A} receptor. Activity is due both to the parent drug and its active metabolite. Both are extensively (>99%) bound to serum proteins, primarily albumin. The mean elimination half-lives of aripiprazole and the active metabolite are about 75 and 94 hours, respectively (1,2).

Reproduction studies have been conducted in rats and rabbits. Female rats were treated for 2 weeks before mating through day 7 of gestation with doses up to 6 times the maximum recommended human dose based on body surface area (MRHD). Fertility was not impaired but increased pre-implantation loss was seen at 2 times the MRHD or greater and decreased fetal weight was noted at 6 times the MRHD. In pregnant rats, a dose 10 times the MRHD given during organogenesis caused a slightly prolonged gestation, and a slight delay in fetal development, as evidenced by decreased fetal weight, undescended testes, and delayed skeletal ossification. The latter effect was also seen at 3 times the MRHD. Some maternal toxicity was observed at 10 times the MRHD, but there was no evidence that the observed adverse effects were secondary to maternal toxicity (1,2). There were no effects on embryo, fetal, or pup survival, but offspring had decreased bodyweights (at 3 and 10 times the MRHD), and increased incidences of hepatodiaphragmatic nodules and diaphragmatic hernia (at 10 times the MRHD). Adverse effects in female offspring exposed *in utero* at 10 times the MRHD included delayed vaginal opening and impaired reproductive performance (decreased fertility rate, corpora lutea, implants, and live fetuses, and increased post-implantation loss). In peri- and postnatal rat studies, a dose 10 times the MRHD given from day 17 of gestation through postpartum day 21 resulted in slight maternal toxicity and prolongation of gestation, increases in stillbirths, and decreases in pup weight (persisting into adulthood) and survival. Disturbances in spermatogenesis and prostate atrophy, but not impaired fertility, were observed in male rats given doses 13 to 19 times the MRHD from 9 weeks before mating through mating (1,2).

In rabbits, a dose 11 times the human exposure at the maximum recommended human dose based on AUC (HE) (up to 65 times the MRHD) during organogenesis resulted in decreased maternal food consumption and increased abortions. Other adverse effects noted were increased fetal mortality (at 11 times the HE), decreased fetal weight (at 3 and 11 times the HE), and increased incidences of skeletal abnormalities (fused sternebrae at 3 and 11 times the HE) and minor skeletal variations (at 11 times the HE) (1,2).

It is not known if aripiprazole or its active metabolite crosses the human placenta. The molecular weight of the parent compound (about 448), combined with the prolonged elimination half-lives of aripiprazole and the metabolite, suggest that one or both will cross the placenta to the embryo and/or fetus. However, the extensive protein binding should limit this transfer.

No reports describing the use of aripiprazole in human pregnancy have been located. The animal data are suggestive of risk for developmental toxicity and possibly teratogenicity, but the absence of human pregnancy experience prevents an assessment of the risk for the embryo and fetus. Until such data are available, the safest course is to avoid the drug in pregnancy. However, if the mother's condition requires treatment with aripiprazole, the lowest effective dose, avoiding the 1st trimester if possible, should be used. In addition, long-term evaluation of the infant is warranted.

BREAST FEEDING SUMMARY

RECOMMENDATION: No Human Data - Potential Toxicity

No reports describing the use of aripiprazole during human lactation have been located. The drug is excreted in the milk of lactating rats (1,2). This is consistent with the molecular weight of the parent compound (about 448) combined with the prolonged elimination half-lives of aripiprazole (75 hours) and the active metabolite (94 hours). These factors suggest that one or both will be excreted into breast milk. However, the extensive serum protein binding of the parent compound and metabolite (both >99%) should limit this excretion. The effects of this exposure on a nursing infant are unknown. However, aripiprazole is a drug with potent central nervous system effects as well as sometimes rare, but potentially serious toxicities (e.g., orthostatic hypotension, seizures, dysphagia, nausea and vomiting, as seen in adults). If a woman chooses to breast-feed while taking this drug, the infant should be monitored for these and other potential adverse effects. Long-term evaluation of the infant is warranted.

References

1. Product information. Abilify. Bristol-Myers Squibb, 2004.
2. Product information. Abilify. Otsuka America Pharmaceutical, 2004.

Name:	**ASPARAGINASE**	Risk Factor:	C_M
Class:	**Antineoplastic**		

FETAL RISK SUMMARY

RECOMMENDATION: Human and Animal Data Suggest Risk

The antineoplastic agent asparaginase, which is used in the treatment of certain types of cancers, contains the enzyme, L-asparagine amidohydrolase, type EC-2, derived from *Escherichia coli* (1). The drug is teratogenic in rabbits, rats, and mice (1–3). In pregnant rabbits given 50 IU/kg (5% of the human dose), asparaginase crossed the placenta and produced malformations of the lung, kidney, and skeleton; spina bifida; abdominal extrusion; and missing tail (2). Doses of 1000 IU/kg (equal to the human dose) or more in rats and mice produced exencephaly and skeletal anomalies (3). Maternal and fetal growth retardation have also been observed in pregnant rats and mice treated with 1,000 IU/kg (1).

The reported use of asparaginase during human pregnancy is limited to six pregnancies, all in the 2nd trimester, resulting in the birth of seven infants (one set of twins) (4–9). In each case, multiple other chemotherapeutic agents were used with asparaginase for treatment of the acute leukemias. Therapy with asparaginase was initiated between 16.5 and 22 weeks of pregnancy. No congenital abnormalities were observed in any of the newborn infants, although two newborns had transient, drug-induced bone marrow hypoplasia (4,5). One 34-year-old mother, with acute lymphoblastic leukemia, was treated for 18 weeks, commencing at 22 weeks' gestation, with various combinations of asparaginase, daunorubicin, vincristine, cytarabine, cyclophosphamide, mercaptopurine, and methotrexate (9). Asparaginase, 5000 U/m^2/day, was administered on days 15–28 of therapy. She gave birth to a normal female infant after 40 weeks' gestation. The newborn had a normal karyotype (46,XX) but with gaps and a ring chromosome. The clinical significance of these findings is unknown, but because these abnormalities may persist for several years, the potential existed for an increased risk of cancer as well as for a risk of genetic damage in the next generation (9).

A number of reports have evaluated the reproductive histories of men and women who were exposed to asparaginase and multiple other antineoplastic agents before conception (10–15). Of the 13 men described, 9 fathered 15 children (10–13), including 1 who fathered a child while receiving therapy (10). Two congenital anomalies were observed; one infant had a birthmark (13), and one newborn had multiple anomalies (11). In the latter case, the man, who had been off therapy for at least 3.5 years, also fathered a normal child (11). No relationship between these outcomes and the fathers' exposure to either asparaginase or the other chemotherapeutic agents can be inferred from the two cases.

In 57 women treated with asparaginase and other agents 2 months to 15 years before conception, a total of 83 pregnancies occurred, resulting in 5 spontaneous abortions, 5 elective abortions, 2 stillbirths, and 71 liveborn infants (10,12–15). Among the liveborn infants, 4 were delivered prematurely, 1 was growth retarded, and 7 had congenital defects, 4 minor and 3 major. The minor abnormalities were an epidermal nevus (13), dark hair patch (14), ear tag (14), and congenital hip dysplasia (15). Infants with major defects were the offspring of women who had been treated 15–24 months before conception with asparaginase, chlorambucil, mercaptopurine, methotrexate, procarbazine, thioguanine, vinblastine, vincristine, and prednisone (14). The defects were hydrocephalus, tracheomalacia, and pelvic asymmetry. The authors concluded that the latter defect was most likely a deformation, resulting from the mother's scoliosis or from uterine scarring caused by radiation, rather than a mutagenic effect of drug therapy (14). Causes for the other two defects were not proposed, but they were not thought to be the result of germ cell damage.

In summary, based on limited reports in humans, the use of asparaginase, in combination with other antineoplastics, does not seem to pose a major risk to the fetus when used in the 2nd and 3rd trimesters, or when exposure occurs before conception in either women or men. No reports describing the use of only asparaginase in pregnancy have been located. Because of the teratogenicity observed in animals and the lack of human data after 1st trimester exposure, asparaginase should be used cautiously during this period, if at all.

A

BREAST FEEDING SUMMARY

RECOMMENDATION: No Human Data - Potential Toxicity

No data are available.

References

1. Product information. Elspar. Merck Sharpe & Dohme, 1993.
2. Adamson RH, Fabro S, Hahn MA, Creech CE, Whang-Peng J. Evaluation of the embryotoxic activity of L-asparaginase. Arch Int Pharmacodyn Ther 1970;186:310–20. As cited in Shepard TH. *Catalog of teratogenic agents,* 6th ed. Baltimore, MD: Johns Hopkins University Press, 1989:58–9.
3. Ohguro Y, Imamura S, Koyama K, Hara T, Miyagawa A, Hatano M, Kanda K. Toxicological studies on L-asparaginase. Yamaguchi Igaku 1969;18:271–92. As cited in Shepard TH. *Catalog of teratogenic agents,* 6th ed. Baltimore, MD: Johns Hopkins University Press, 1989:58–9.
4. Okun DB, Groncy PK, Sieger L, Tanaka KR. Acute leukemia in pregnancy: transient neonatal myelosuppression after combination chemotherapy in the mother. Med Pediatr Oncol 1979;7:315–9.
5. Khurshid M, Saleem M. Acute leukaemia in pregnancy. Lancet 1978;2:534–5.
6. Karp GI, Von Oeyen P, Valone F, Khetarpal VK, Israel M, Mayer RJ, Frigoletto FD, Garnick MB. Doxorubicin in pregnancy: possible transplacental passage. Cancer Treat Rep 1983;67:773–7.
7. Awidi AS, Tarawneh MS, Shubair KS, Issa AA, Dajani YF. Acute leukemia in pregnancy: report of five cases treated with a combination which included a low dose of Adriamycin. Eur J Cancer Clin Oncol 1983;19:881–4.
8. Turchi JJ, Villasis C. Anthracyclines in the treatment of malignancy in pregnancy. Cancer 1988;61:435–40.
9. Schleuning M, Clemm C. Chromosomal aberrations in a newborn whose mother received cytotoxic treatment during pregnancy. N Engl J Med 1987;317:1666–7.
10. Blatt J, Mulvihill JJ, Ziegler JL, Young RC, Poplack DG. Pregnancy outcome following cancer chemotherapy. Am J Med 1980;69:828–32.
11. Evenson DP, Arlin Z, Welt S, Claps ML, Melamed MR. Male reproductive capacity may recover following drug treatment with the L-10 protocol for acute lymphocytic leukemia. Cancer 1984;53:30–6.
12. Green DM, Hall B, Zevon MA. Pregnancy outcome after treatment for acute lymphoblastic leukemia during childhood or adolescence. Cancer 1989;64:2335–9.
13. Green DM, Zevon MA, Lowrie G, Seigelstein N, Hall B. Congenital anomalies in children of patients who received chemotherapy for cancer in childhood and adolescence. N Engl J Med 1991;325:141–6.
14. Mulvihill JJ, McKeen EA, Rosner F, Zarrabi MH. Pregnancy outcome in cancer patients: experience in a large cooperative group. Cancer 1987;60:1143–50.
15. Pajor A, Zimonyi I, Koos R, Lehoczky D, Ambrus C. Pregnancies and offspring in survivors of acute lymphoid leukemia and lymphoma. Eur J Obstet Gynecol Reprod Biol 1991;40:1–5.

Name: **ASPARTAME** Risk Factor: **B***

Class: **Artificial Sweetener**

FETAL RISK SUMMARY

RECOMMENDATION: Compatible

Aspartame is a nutritive sweetening agent used in foods and beverages. It contains 4 kcal/g and is about 180–200 times as sweet as sucrose. The product was discovered in 1965 and obtained final approval by the FDA as a food additive in certain dry foods in 1981 and in carbonated beverages in 1983 (1). Aspartame is probably the most extensively studied food additive ever approved by the FDA (2,3). Chemically, the compound is *N*-L-α-aspartyl-L-phenylalanine 1-methyl ester, the methyl ester of the amino acids L-phenylalanine and L-aspartic acid.

Aspartame is broken down in the lumen of the gut to methanol, aspartate, and phenylalanine (1–4). The major decomposition product when the parent compound is exposed to high temperatures or in liquids is aspartyl-phenylalanine diketopiperazine (DKP), a product formed by many dipeptides (3–5). The rate of conversion of aspartame to degradation products depends on pH and temperature (3). In addition to methanol, the two amino acids, and DKP, other degradation products are L,L-β-aspartame (aspartame is commercially available as the L,L-α isomer), three dipeptides (α-Asp-Phe, β-Asp-Phe, and Phe-Asp), and phenylalanine methyl ester (3). The dipeptide compounds are hydrolyzed to the individual amino acids in the gut, and these, along with methanol, will be evaluated in later sections. None of the other degradation products have shown toxic effects after extensive study (3). Moreover, the DKP compound and the β isomer of aspartame are essentially inactive biologically (3).

The projected maximum ingestion of aspartame has been estimated to be 22–34 mg/kg/day. The higher dose is calculated as the 99th percentile of projected daily ingestion (2). The 22–34 mg/kg dose range is equivalent to 2.4–3.7 mg/kg/day of methanol, 9.8 mg/kg/day of aspartate, and 12–19 mg/kg/day of phenylalanine (2). The FDA has set the allowable or acceptable daily intake (ADI) of aspartame at 50 mg/kg (1.5 times the 99th percentile of projected daily ingestion) (1,3). In Europe and Canada, the ADI is 40 mg/kg (3). The ADI is defined as an average daily ingestion that is considered harmless, even if continued indefinitely, but does not imply that amounts above this value are harmful (3).

The toxic effects of methanol ingestion are the result of its metabolism to formaldehyde and then to formic acid. Accumulation of this latter product is responsible for the acidosis and ocular toxicity attributable to methanol (1–3). The dose of methanol estimated to cause significant toxicity is estimated to be 200–500 mg/kg (4). Theoretically, since about 10% of aspartame is methanol, the toxic dose of aspartame, in terms only of methanol, would be about 2000 mg/kg, a dose considered far in excess of any possible ingestion (4). In 12 normal subjects, methanol plasma levels were below the level of detection (0.4 mg/dL) after ingestion of aspartame, 34 mg/kg (3). When abuse doses (100, 150, and 200 mg/kg) of aspartame were administered, statistically significant increases in methanol blood concentrations were measured with peak levels of 1.27, 2.14, and 2.58 mg/dL, respectively (3). Methanol was undetectable at 8 hours after the 100-mg/kg dose, but still present after the higher aspartame doses. Blood and urine formate concentrations were measured after ingestion of 200 mg/kg of aspartame in six healthy subjects (3). No significant increases in blood formate levels were measured, but urinary formate excretion did increase significantly. This indicated that the rate of formate synthesis did not exceed the rate of formate metabolism and excretion (3). No ocular changes or toxicity were observed in the test subjects (3). Moreover, the amount of methanol (approximately 55 mg/L) derived from aspartame-sweetened beverages, containing approximately 555 mg/L of aspartame, is much less than the average methanol content of fruit juices (140 mg/L) (2). Based on the above data, the risk to the fetus from the methanol component of aspartame is nil.

Aspartate is one of two dicarboxylic amino acids (glutamate is the other) that have caused hypothalamic neuronal necrosis in neonatal rodents fed large doses of either the individual amino acids or aspartame (2,5). In neonatal mice, plasma concentrations of aspartate and glutamate must exceed 110 μmol/dL and 75 μmol/dL, respectively, before brain lesions are produced (2). Concerns were raised that this toxicity could occur in humans, especially because glutamate is widespread in the food supply (e.g., monosodium glutamate [MSG]) (6). In addition, some aspartate is transaminated to glutamate, and the neural toxicity of the two amino acids is additive (6). However, brain lesions were not produced in nonhuman primates fed large doses of aspartame, aspartate, or monosodium glutamate (2).

In normal humans, ingestion of aspartame, 34 mg/kg, or equimolar amounts of aspartate, 13 mg/kg, did not increase plasma aspartate levels (7). Adults heterozygous for phenylketonuria (PKU) also metabolized aspartate normally as evidenced by insignificant increases in plasma aspartate concentrations and unchanged levels of those amino acids that could be derived from aspartate, such as glutamate, asparagine, and glutamine (8). When the dose of aspartame was increased to 50 mg/kg, again no increase in plasma aspartate levels was measured (9). When an abuse dose of aspartame, 100 mg/kg, was administered to adults heterozygous for PKU, plasma aspartate levels increased from a baseline of 0.49 μmol/dL to 0.80 μmol/dL (10). The increase was well within the range of normal postprandial levels. In normal adults given a higher abuse dose of aspartame (200 mg/kg), plasma levels of aspartate plus glutamate were increased from a baseline of 2.7 μmol/dL to 7 μmol/dL, still far below the estimated toxic human plasma level of 100 μmol/dL for aspartate and glutamate (7). Plasma aspartate levels at 2 hours after the 200-mg/kg dose were less than normal postprandial aspartate levels after a meal containing protein (1). Based on this data, subjects heterozygous for PKU metabolize aspartate normally (2). Moreover, neither aspartate nor glutamate is concentrated in the fetus, unlike most other amino acids (1,2,5,11,12). Human placentas perfused *in vitro* showed a fetal:maternal ratio of 0.13 for aspartic acid and 0.14 for glutamic acid (11). In pregnant monkeys infused with sodium aspartate, 100 mg/kg/hour, maternal plasma aspartate levels increased from 0.36 to 80.2 μmol/dL, whereas fetal levels changed from 0.42 to 0.98 μmol/dL (12). Thus, there is no evidence of a risk of fetal aspartate toxicity resulting from maternal ingestion of aspartame, either alone or in combination with glutamate.

High plasma levels of phenylalanine, such as those occurring in PKU, are known to affect the fetus adversely. Phenylalanine, unlike aspartate, is concentrated on the fetal side of the placenta with a fetal:maternal gradient of 1.2:1–1.3:1 (13). The fetus of a mother with PKU may either be heterozygous for PKU (i.e., those who only inherit one autosomal recessive gene and who are nonphenylketonuric) or homozygous for PKU (i.e., those who inherit two autosomal recessive genes and who are phenylketonuric). The incidence of phenylketonuria is approximately 1/15,000 persons (5). In contrast, individuals heterozygous for PKU are much more common, with an estimated incidence of 1:50 to 1:70 (8). In the former case of phenylketonuria, the fetus has virtually no (0.3% or less) phenylalanine hydroxylase activity and is unable to metabolize phenylalanine to tyrosine, thus allowing phenylalanine to accumulate to toxic levels (14). The heterozygous fetus does possess phenylalanine hydroxylase, although only about 10% of normal, with activity of the enzyme detected in the fetal liver as early as 8 weeks' gestation (13,14). Unfortunately, possession of some phenylalanine hydroxylase activity does not reduce the amount of phenylalanine transferred from the mother to the fetus (13). In a study of four families, evidence was found that the heterozygous fetus either did not metabolize the phenylalanine received from the mother or metabolism was minimal (13). This supported previous observations that the degree of mental impairment from exposure to high, continuous maternal levels of phenylalanine is often similar for both the nonphenylketonuric and phenylketonuric fetus (13). Moreover, the exact mechanism of mental impairment induced by elevated phenylalanine plasma levels has not yet been determined (4,15,16).

Offspring of women with PKU often are afflicted with mental retardation, microcephaly, congenital heart disease, and low birth weight (16). Pregnancies of these women are also prone to spontaneously abort (16). In one study, maternal phenylalanine plasma levels above 120 μmol/dL (classic PKU) were consistently associated with microcephaly, although true mental retardation was observed only when plasma levels exceeded 110 μmol/dL (16). However, research has not excluded the possibility that lower concentrations may be associated with less severe reductions in intelligence (16–18). For example, in the study cited above, maternal phenylalanine levels below 60 μmol/dL (mild hyperphenylalaninemia without urine phenylketones) were associated with normal intelligence in the infants (16). When maternal levels were in the range of 60–100 μmol/dL (atypical phenylketonuria), most of the infants also had normal intelligence, but their mean IQ was lower than that of the infants of mothers with mild hyperphenylalaninemia. Others have interpreted these and additional data as indicating a 10.5 point reduction in IQ for each 25.0 μmol/dL rise in maternal phenylalanine plasma concentration (19,20). A recent study, however, examined the nonhyperphenylalaninemic offspring of 12 mothers with untreated hyperphenylalaninemia (21). The results supported the contention that a maternal plasma phenylalanine threshold of 60 μmol/dL existed for an adverse effect on the intelligence of the offspring (21). The investigators, however, were unable to exclude the possibility that nonintellectual dysfunction, such as hyperactivity or attention deficit disorder, may occur at concentrations below the alleged threshold (21). Thus, although this latest study is evidence for a threshold effect, additional studies are needed before the concept of a linear relationship between offspring intelligence and maternal phenylalanine levels can be set aside (19,20,22–24).

In normal subjects, fasting and postprandial (after a meal containing protein) phenylalanine levels are approximately 6 and 12 μmol/dL, respectively (2,8). When normal adults were administered either a 34- or 50-mg/kg aspartame dose, the mean maximum phenylalanine concentrations were 9–12 and 16 μmol/dL, respectively, with levels returning to baseline 4 hours after ingestion (2,7–9). Single doses of 100–200 mg/kg, representing abuse ingestions of aspartame, resulted in peak phenylalanine plasma levels ranging from 20–49 μmol/dL (2,25). These elevated levels returned to near baseline values within 8 hours. Normal adults were also dosed with an aspartame-sweetened beverage, providing a 10-mg/kg dose of aspartame, at 2-hour intervals for three successive doses (2,26). Plasma levels of phenylalanine rose slightly after each dose, indicating that the phenylalanine load from the previous dose had not been totally eliminated. However, the increases were not statistically significant, and plasma phenylalanine levels never exceeded normal postprandial limits at any time (26). The results of the above studies suggest that even large doses of aspartame do not pose a fetal risk in the normal subject.

Humans heterozygous for the PKU allele metabolize phenylalanine slower than normal persons because of a decreased amount of liver phenylalanine hydroxylase (2). The conversion of phenylalanine to tyrosine is thus impaired, and potentially toxic levels of phenylalanine may accumulate. When adults with this genetic trait were administered aspartame, 34 mg/kg, the mean peak phenylalanine concentration was 15–16 μmol/dL, approximately 36%–45% higher than that measured in normal adults (11 μmol/dL) (2,8,27). To determine the effects of abuse doses, a dose of 100 mg/kg was administered, resulting in a mean peak plasma level of 42 μmol/dL, approximately 100% higher than observed in normal individuals (20 μmol/dL) (2,10). In both cases, phenylalanine plasma levels were well below presumed toxic levels and returned to baseline values within 8 hours.

A 1986 study examined the effects of a 10-mg/kg dose of aspartame obtained from a commercial product on the basal concentrations of several amino acids, including phenylalanine, in four types of patient: normal, PKU, hyperphenylalaninemic, and PKU carriers (28). One hour after ingestion, mean phenylalanine levels had increased 1.35 μmol/dL (+30%) in normal subjects and 1.35 μmol/dL (+20%) in PKU carriers, decreased 4.58 μmol/dL (−3%) in subjects with PKU, and remained unchanged in hyperphenylalaninemic individuals. The 10-mg/kg dose was selected because it represented, for a 60-kg adult, the dose received from three cans of an aspartame-sweetened soft drink or from approximately 1 quart of aspartame-sweetened Kool-Aid (28).

In summary, ingestion of aspartame-sweetened products during pregnancy does not represent a risk to the fetuses of normal mothers, or of mothers either heterozygous for or who have PKU. Elevated plasma levels of phenylalanine, an amino acid that is concentrated in the fetus, are associated with fetal toxicity. Whether a toxic threshold exists for neural toxicity or the toxicity is linear with phenylalanine plasma levels is not known. Women with PKU need to control their consumption of any phenylalanine-containing product. Because aspartame is a source of phenylalanine, although a minor source, this should be considered by these women in their dietary planning. The other components of aspartame methanol and aspartic acid and the various degradation products have no toxicity in doses that can be ingested by humans.

[**Risk Factor C in women with phenylketonuria.*]

BREAST FEEDING SUMMARY

RECOMMENDATION: Compatible (Excluding Those with Phenylketonuria)

Ingestion of aspartame, 50 mg/kg, by normal lactating women results in a small, but statistically significant, rise in overall aspartate and phenylalanine milk concentrations (9). Milk aspartate levels rose from 2.3 μmol/dL to 4.8 μmol/dL during a 4-hour fasting interval after the aspartame dose. The rise in phenylalanine milk levels during the same interval was approximately 0.5 μmol/dL to 2.3 μmol/dL. The investigators of this study concluded that these changes, even if spread over an entire 24-hour period, would have no effect on a nursing infant's phenylalanine intake (9). However, because mothers or infants with phenylketonuria need to monitor carefully their intake of phenylalanine, the American Academy of Pediatrics classifies aspartame as an agent to be used with caution during breast-feeding if the mother or infant has phenylketonuria (29).

References

1. Sturtevant FM. Use of aspartame in pregnancy. Int J Fertil 1985;30:85–7.
2. Stegink LD. The aspartame story: a model for the clinical testing of a food additive. Am J Clin Nutr 1987;46:204–15.
3. Stegink LD, Brummel MC, McMartin K, Martin-Amat G, Filer LJ Jr, Baker GL, Tephly TR. Blood methanol concentrations in normal adult subjects administered abuse doses of aspartame. J Toxicol Environ Health 1981;7:281–90.
4. Dews PB. Summary report of an international aspartame workshop. Food Chem Toxicol 1987;25:549–52.
5. London RS. Saccharin and aspartame: Are they safe to consume during pregnancy? J Reprod Med 1988;33:17–21.
6. Council on Scientific Affairs, American Medical Association. Aspartame: review of safety issues. JAMA 1985;254:400–2.
7. Stegink LD, Filer LJ Jr, Baker GL. Effect of aspartame and aspartate loading upon plasma and erythrocyte free amino acid levels in normal adult volunteers. J Nutr 1977;107:1837–45.
8. Stegink LD, Koch R, Blaskovics ME, Filer LJ Jr, Baker GL, McDonnell JE. Plasma phenylalanine levels in phenylketonuric heterozygous and normal adults administered aspartame at 34 mg/kg body weight. Toxicology 1981;20:81–90.
9. Stegink LD, Filer LJ Jr, Baker GL. Plasma, erythrocyte and human milk levels of free amino acids in lactating women administered aspartame or lactose. J Nutr 1979;109:2173–81.
10. Stegink LD, Filer LJ Jr, Baker GL, McDonnell JE. Effect of an abuse dose of aspartame upon plasma and erythrocyte levels of amino acids in phenylketonuric heterozygous and normal adults. J Nutr 1980;110:2216–24.
11. Schneider H, Mohlen KH, Challier JC, Dancis J. Transfer of glutamic acid across the human placenta perfused in vitro. Br J Obstet Gynaecol 1979;86:299–306.
12. Stegink LD, Pitkin RM, Reynolds WA, Brummel MC, Filer LJ Jr. Placental transfer of aspartate and its metabolites in the primate. Metabolism 1979;28:669–76.
13. Levy HL, Lenke RR, Koch R. Lack of fetal effect on blood phenylalanine concentration in maternal phenylketonuria. J Pediatr 1984;104:245–7.
14. Hilton MA, Sharpe JN, Hicks LG, Andrews BF. A simple method for detection of heterozygous carriers of the gene for classic phenylketonuria. J Pediatr 1986;109:601–4.
15. Perry TL, Hansen S, Tischler B, Bunting R, Diamond S. Glutamine depletion in phenylketonuria: a possible cause of the mental defect. N Engl J Med 1970;282:761–6.
16. Levy HL, Waisbren SE. Effects of untreated maternal phenylketonuria and hyperphenylalaninemia on the fetus. N Engl J Med 1983;309:1269–74.
17. Buist NRM, Tuerck J, Lis E, Penn R. Effects of

untreated maternal phenylketonuria and hyperphenylalaninemia on the fetus. N Engl J Med 1984;311:52–3.
18. Levy HL, Waisbren SE. Effects of untreated maternal phenylketonuria and hyperphenylalaninemia on the fetus. N Engl J Med 1984;311:53.
19. Pardridge WM. The safety of aspartame. JAMA 1986;256:2678.
20. Pardridge WM. The safety of aspartame. JAMA 1987;258:206.
21. Waisbren SE, Levy HL. Effects of untreated maternal hyperphenylalaninemia on the fetus: further study of families identified by routine cord blood screening. J Pediatr 1990;116:926–9.
22. Levy HL, Waisbren SE. The safety of aspartame. JAMA 1987;258:205.
23. Stegink LD, Krause WL. The safety of aspartame. JAMA 1987;258:205–6.
24. Hilton MA. Consumption of aspartame by heterozygotes for phenylketonuria. J Pediatr 1987;110:662–3.
25. Stegink LD, Filer LJ Jr, Baker GL. Plasma and erythrocyte concentrations of free amino acids in adult humans administered abuse doses of aspartame. J Toxicol Environ Health 1981;7:291–305.
26. Stegink LD, Filer LJ Jr, Baker GL. Effect of repeated ingestion of aspartame-sweetened beverages upon plasma aminograms in normal adults (abstract). Am J Clin Nutr 1983;37:704.
27. Stegink LD, Filer LJ Jr, Baker GL, McDonnell JE. Effect of aspartame loading upon plasma and erythrocyte amino acid levels in phenylketonuric heterozygotes and normal adult subjects. J Nutr 1979;109:708–17.
28. Caballero B, Mahon BE, Rohr FJ, Levy HL, Wurtman RJ. Plasma amino acid levels after single-dose aspartame consumption in phenylketonuria, mild hyperphenylalaninemia, and heterozygous state for phenylketonuria. J Pediatr 1986;109:668–71.
29. Committee on Drugs, American Academy of Pediatrics. The transfer of drugs and other chemicals into human milk. Pediatrics 2001;108:776–89.

Name:	**ASPIRIN**	Risk Factor:	**C***
Class:	**Nonsteroidal Anti-inflammatory**		

FETAL RISK SUMMARY

RECOMMENDATION: **Compatible (Low-Dose)**
Human Data Suggest Risk in 1st and 3rd Trimesters (Full-Dose)

Aspirin, a nonsteroidal anti-inflammatory agent (NSAID), is the most frequently ingested drug in pregnancy either as a single agent or in combination with other drugs (1). The terms "aspirin" and "salicylate" are used interchangeably in this monograph unless specifically separated. In eight surveys totaling more than 54,000 patients, aspirin was consumed sometime during gestation by slightly more than 33,000 (61%) (2–9). The true incidence is probably much higher than this because many patients either do not remember taking aspirin or consume drug products without realizing that they contain large amounts of salicylates (2,4,8). Evaluation of the effects of aspirin on the fetus is thus difficult because of this common, and often hidden, exposure. However, some toxic effects on the mother and fetus from large doses of salicylates have been known since 1893 (10).

Aspirin consumption during pregnancy may produce adverse effects in the mother: anemia, antepartum or postpartum hemorrhage, prolonged gestation, and prolonged labor (5,11–14). The increased length of labor and frequency of postmaturity result from the inhibition of prostaglandin synthesis by aspirin. Aspirin has been shown to significantly delay the induced abortion time in nulliparous (but not multiparous) patients by this same mechanism (15). In an Australian study, regular aspirin ingestion was also found to increase the number of complicated deliveries (cesarean sections, breech, and forceps) (5). Small doses of aspirin may decrease urinary estriol excretion (16).

Aspirin, either alone or in combination with β-mimetics, has been used to treat premature labor (17–19). Although adverse effects in the newborn were infrequent, maternal complications in one study included non-dose-related prolonged bleeding times and dose-related vertigo, tinnitus, headache, and hyperventilation (19).

Failure of intrauterine devices (IUDs) to prevent conception has been described in two patients who consumed frequent doses of aspirin (20). The anti-inflammatory action of aspirin was proposed as the mechanism of the failure.

Low-dose aspirin (about 85 mg/day) was used to treat maternal thrombocytopenia (platelet counts <60,000/mm^3) in 19 patients with either intrauterine growth retardation (IUGR) or toxemia (21). In five women who had a definite response to the aspirin, no improvement in plasma volume or fetal welfare was demonstrated.

In women with systemic lupus erythematosus complicated with either lupus anticoagulant or anticardiolipin antibody (i.e., antiphospholipid antibodies), low-dose aspirin (e.g., 80 mg/day) has been used in combination with prednisone to reduce the incidence of pregnancy loss (22–25) (see reference 22 for a review of this topic). This therapy has not been associated with drug-induced fetal or neonatal complications.

Several studies have investigated the effect of low-dose aspirin (e.g., 40–150 mg/day) on the prevention of gestational hypertension, preeclampsia, and eclampsia, and the associated fetal risks of IUGR and mortality (26–38) (see reference 36 for a review of this topic). Low-dose aspirin exerts its beneficial effects in these disorders by irreversible inactivation of platelet cyclo-oxygenase, resulting in a greater inhibition of thromboxane A_2 synthesis than of prostacyclin production. This inhibition restores the ratio of the two substances to a more normal value. Aspirin-induced fetal and neonatal toxicity has not been observed after the chronic use of low-dose aspirin for these indications. The lack of toxicity may be partially explained by the findings of a study published in 1989 (34). In that study, 60–80 mg of aspirin/day, starting 3 weeks before delivery and continuing until birth, inhibited maternal platelet cyclo-oxygenase, but not that of the newborn. These results were in agreement with other studies using 60–150 mg/day (34). Other toxicities associated with the use of full-dose aspirin near term, such as hemorrhage, premature closure of the ductus arteriosus, pulmonary hypertension, prolonged gestation, and prolonged labor, were not observed with low-dose aspirin therapy (34). Although these results are reassuring, in the opinion of some, too few studies have been reported to allow a true estimate of the fetal risk (36). However, other recent reports have observed no serious neonatal adverse effects, including hemorrhagic complications, in their series (39,40). In one of these studies, 33 women judged to be at risk for gestational hypertension were randomly assigned to either an aspirin ($N = 17$) or placebo ($N = 16$) group during the 12th week of gestation in a single-blind study (39). Patients in the aspirin group, treated with 60 mg/day from enrollment to delivery, had a longer duration of pregnancy (39 weeks vs. 35 weeks) and delivered heavier infants (2922 g vs. 2264 g). None of the aspirin-treated women developed gestational hypertension, whereas three of the placebo group did develop the complication. In a double blind study, 65 women with increased blood pressure during the rollover test administered during the 28th or 29th week of pregnancy were randomly divided into two groups: one group was treated with 100 mg/day of aspirin ($N = 34$) and the other with placebo ($N = 31$) (40). Four women (11.8%) of the aspirin-treated group developed gestational hypertension compared with 11 (35.5%) of the placebo group.

Fetal and newborn effects, other than congenital defects, from aspirin exposure *in utero*, may include increased perinatal mortality, IUGR, congenital salicylate intoxication, and depressed albumin-binding capacity (2,5,12,41–43). For the latter effect, no increase in the incidence of jaundice was observed (2). Perinatal mortality in the Australian study was a result of stillbirths more often than neonatal deaths (5,41). Some of the stillbirths were associated with antepartum hemorrhage and others may have been caused by closure of the ductus arteriosus *in utero* (44). Closure of the ductus has been shown in animals to be a result of aspirin inhibition of prostaglandin synthetase. In some early cases, *in utero* premature closure of the ductus arteriosus was probably caused by aspirin but not suspected (45). However, a large prospective American study involving 41,337 patients, 64% of whom used aspirin sometime during gestation, failed to show that aspirin was a cause of stillbirths, neonatal deaths, or reduced birth weight (46). The difference between these findings probably relates to the chronic or intermittent use of higher doses by the patients in the Australian study (44). Excessive use of aspirin was blamed for the stillbirth of a fetus in whom salicylate levels in the fetal blood and liver were 25–30 mg/dL and 12 mg/dL, respectively (47). Congenital salicylate intoxication was found in two newborns exposed to high aspirin doses before delivery (42,43). Although both infants survived, one infant exhibited withdrawal symptoms beginning on the 2nd neonatal day consisting of hypertonia, agitation, a shrill piercing cry, and increased reflex irritability (41). The serum salicylate level was 31 mg/dL. Most of the symptoms gradually subsided over 6 weeks, but some mild hypertonia may have persisted.

A 1996 case-control study investigated the relationship between aspirin and other NSAIDs and persistent pulmonary hypertension of the newborn (PPHN) (48). Case infants ($N = 103$) weighed at least 2500 g at birth and had no major congenital defects, whereas controls ($N = 298$) were full-term infants without congenital defects. Aspirin or other NSAIDs were used by mothers of 26 cases. Because 34% of the cases and all of the controls were born at one hospital (inborn), the investigators conducted two analyses, one for inborn infants and one for the total group. For the total group, the odds ratio and 95% confidence interval (CI) for the exposures and PPHN were aspirin 4.9 (1.6–15.3) and other NSAIDs 6.2 (1.8–21.8). For inborn cases, the findings were aspirin 9.6 (2.4–39.0) and other NSAIDs 17.5 (4.3–71.6). The timing of the exposures was earlier than expected, a median 3 months for aspirin and 1 month for NSAIDs. This result led to three potential conclusions: (a) the drugs caused early structural remodeling or functional alterations of the pulmonary vasculature, (b) the agents were also used in the 3rd trimester, or (c) there was another, unidentified primary cause of PPHN. Exposure in the 3rd trimester was the most likely conclusion because it would have been consistent with the presumed mechanism of *in utero* premature closure of the ductus arteriosus and resulting increased risk of PPHN. However, the investigators could not determine which of the choices was correct (48).

Aspirin given in doses of 325–650 mg during the week before delivery may affect the clotting ability of the newborn (49–55). In the initial study by Bleyer and Breckenridge (49), 3 of 14 newborns exposed to aspirin within 1 week of delivery had minor hemorrhagic phenomena vs. only 1 of 17 nonexposed controls. Collagen-induced platelet aggregation was absent in the aspirin group and, although of less clinical significance, factor XII activity was markedly depressed. A direct correlation was found between factor XII activity and the interval between the last dose of aspirin and birth. Neonatal purpuric rash with depressed platelet function has also been observed after maternal use of aspirin close to term (55). The use of salicylates other than aspirin may not be a problem because the acetyl moiety is apparently required to depress platelet function (56–58). In a 1982 study, 10 mothers consuming less than 1 g of aspirin within 5 days of delivery had excessive intrapartum or postpartum blood loss, resulting in hemoglobulin levels that were markedly lower than those of controls (13,14). One mother required a transfusion. Bleeding complications seen in 9 of the 10 infants included numerous petechiae over the presenting part, hematuria, a cephalohematoma, subconjunctival hemorrhage, and bleeding from a circumcision. No life-threatening hemorrhage, effect on Apgar scores, or increased hospital stay was found, nor was bleeding observed in seven mother-infant pairs when aspirin consumption occurred 6–10 days before delivery (13,14).

An increased incidence of intracranial hemorrhage (ICH) in premature or low-birth-weight infants may occur after maternal aspirin use near birth (59). Computed tomographic screening for ICH was conducted on 108 infants 3–7 days after delivery. All of the infants were either 34 weeks or less in gestation or 1500 g or less in birth weight. A total of 53 infants (49%) developed ICH, including 12 (71%) of the 17 aspirin-exposed newborns. This incidence was statistically significant when compared to the 41 (45%) non-aspirin-exposed infants who developed ICH. The conclusions of this study have been challenged and defended (60,61). In view of the potentially serious outcome, however, full doses of aspirin should be used with extreme caution by patients in danger of premature delivery.

Aspirin readily crosses the placenta (10). When given near term, higher concentrations are found in the neonate than in the mother (62). The kinetics of salicylate elimination in the newborn have been studied (62–64).

A 2003 population-based cohort study involving 1055 pregnant women investigated the prenatal use of aspirin, other NSAIDs, and acetaminophen (65). Fifty-three women (5%) reported used of NSAIDs around the time of conception or during pregnancy, 13 of whom had a spontaneous abortion (SAB). After adjustment, an 80% increased risk of SAB was found for other NSAIDs (adjusted hazard ratio 1.8, 95% CI 1.0–3.2). Moreover, the association was stronger if the initial use of drugs was around conception or if they were used longer than 1 week. A similar association was found with aspirin, but it was weaker because there were only 22 exposures (5 SAB). No association was observed with acetaminophen (65).

The relationship between aspirin and congenital defects is controversial. Several studies have examined this question with findings either supporting or denying a relationship. In two large retrospective studies, mothers of 1291 malformed infants were found to have consumed aspirin during pregnancy more frequently than had mothers of normal infants (66,67). In a retrospective survey of 599 children with oral clefts, use of salicylates in the 1st trimester by the mothers of children with this defect was almost three times more frequent than in the mothers of children without this defect (68). A reviewer of these studies noted several biases, including the fact that they were retrospective, that could account for the results (46). Three other reports of aspirin teratogenicity involving a total of 10 infants have been located (69–71). In each of these cases, other drugs and factors were present.

A 1985 study found a possible association between the use of aspirin in early pregnancy and congenital heart disease (72). The risk for defects in septation of the truncus arteriosus was increased about 2-fold over nonexposed controls. In an earlier retrospective case-control comparison of the relationship between maternal drug intake and congenital heart disease, aspirin was used by 80 of 390 mothers of infants with defects vs. 203 of 1254 mothers of control infants (73). Twelve of the exposed infants had transposition of the great arteries and six had tetralogy of Fallot, but the association between the drug and these defects was weak. The study could not distinguish between the effects of the drug and the underlying condition for which the drug was used (73). A brief review of this and other investigations that have examined the relationship between aspirin and congenital heart disease was published in 1985 (74). The review concluded that too few data existed to associate aspirin with cardiac defects.

A study published in 1989, however, concluded that 1st trimester use of aspirin did not increase the risk of congenital heart defects in relation to other structural anomalies (75). The interval examined encompassed the time of major cardiac development (i.e., from the 5th week after the onset of the last menstrual period to the 9th week of gestation). The data, from the Slone Epidemiology Unit Birth Defects Study, involved 1381 infants with any structural cardiac defect and five subgroups with selected cardiac defects (subgroups were not mutually exclusive): aortic stenosis ($N = 43$), coarctation of the aorta ($N = 123$), hypoplastic left ventricle ($N = 98$), transposition of the great arteries ($N = 210$), and conotruncal defects ($N = 791$). A control group of 6966 infants with other malformations was used for comparison. Infants with syndromes that included cardiac defects, such as Down's syndrome or Holt-Oram syndrome, were excluded from the data, as were mothers who were uncertain about 1st trimester aspirin use or its frequency. After adjustment for potentially confounding factors, the relative risks for the defects among aspirin users in comparison to controls were: 0.9 (95% CI 0.8–1.1) for any cardiac defect, 1.2 (95% CI 0.6–2.3) for aortic stenosis, 1.0 (95% CI 0.6–1.4) for coarctation of the aorta, 0.9 (95% CI 0.6–1.4) for hypoplastic left ventricle, 0.9 (95% CI 0.6–1.2) for transposition of the great arteries, and 1.0 (95% CI 0.8–1.2) for conotruncal defects. No dose-effect relationship was observed (75).

A 2003 case-control study was conducted to identify drug use in early pregnancy that was associated with cardiac defects (76). Cases (cardiovascular defects without known chromosome anomalies) were drawn from three Swedish health registers ($N = 5015$). Controls were all infants born in Sweden in 1995–2001 ($N = 577{,}730$). Associations were identified for several drugs, some of which were probably due to confounding from the underlying disease or complaint or multiple testing, but some were thought to be true drug effects (76). The total exposed, number of cases, and odds ratio (OR, 95% CI) for NSAIDs and aspirin were 7698, 80 cases, 1.24 (0.99–1.55) and 5920, 52 cases, 1.01 (0.76–1.33), respectively. These results demonstrated no association with cardiac defects (76).

In an FDA surveillance study of Michigan Medicaid recipients conducted between 1985 and 1992, involving 229,101 completed pregnancies 1709 newborns had been exposed to aspirin during the 1st trimester (F. Rosa, personal communication, FDA, 1993). A total of 83 (4.9%) major birth defects were observed (73 expected). Specific data were available for six defect categories, including (observed/expected) 19/17 cardiovascular defects, 2/3 oral clefts, 0/1 spina bifida, 3/5 polydactyly, 1/3 limb reduction defects, and 6/4 hypospadias. These data do not support an association between the drug and the defects.

The Collaborative Perinatal Project monitored 50,282 mother-child pairs, 14,864 of whom used aspirin during the 1st trimester (6). For use anytime during pregnancy, 32,164 (64%) aspirin exposures were recorded. This prospective study did not find evidence of a teratogenic effect with aspirin. However, the data did not exclude the possibility that grossly excessive doses of aspirin may be teratogenic. An Australian study of 144 infants of mothers who took aspirin regularly in pregnancy also failed to find an association between salicylates and malformations (41). Based on these studies and the fact that aspirin usage in pregnancy is so common, it is not possible to determine the teratogenic risk of salicylates, if indeed it exists.

A 1996 case-control study of gastroschisis found a significantly elevated risk with ibuprofen (see Ibuprofen) and other medications and exposures (77). A significant association also was found for aspirin ($N = 7$, OR 4.67, 95% CI 1.21–18.05). The data supported a vascular hypothesis for the pathogenesis of gastroschisis (77).

Full-dose aspirin has been reported to affect adversely the intelligence quotient (IQ) of children exposed *in utero* during the first half of pregnancy (78). In a longitudinal prospective study of the effects of prenatal alcohol exposure on child health and development conducted between 1974 and 1975, drug histories were obtained from 1529 women during the 5th month of pregnancy. At birth, 421 children were selected for later follow-up based on a system of prebirth criteria. Of these, 192 (45.6%) had been exposed to aspirin during the first half of pregnancy. A significant and negative association was discovered between aspirin and child IQ and the children's attentional decrements when they were examined at 4 years of age. The association was not changed after adjustment for a wide variety of potentially confounding covariates. Of interest, the data indicated that girls were significantly more affected than boys. The physical growth parameters, height, weight, and head circumference at 4 years of age, were not significantly related to maternal use of aspirin (78).

In a similar study, data were collected in 19,226 pregnancies by the Collaborative Perinatal Project; aspirin exposure during the first half of pregnancy was reported by 10,159 (52.8%) (79). In contrast to the earlier report, the mean child IQs at 4 years of age in the exposed and nonexposed groups were 98.3 and 96.1, respectively. Adjustment for multiple confounders reduced the difference between the groups to less than one point. No relationship between the amount of aspirin consumed and child IQ was found. The investigators concluded that an adverse effect of *in utero* aspirin exposure on child IQ was unlikely (79).

In summary, the use of aspirin during pregnancy, especially of chronic or intermittent high doses, should be avoided. The drug may affect maternal and newborn hemostasis mechanisms, leading to an increased risk of hemorrhage. High doses may be related to increased perinatal mortality, IUGR, and teratogenic effects. Low doses, such as 80 mg/day, appear to have beneficial effects in pregnancies complicated by systemic lupus erythematosus with antiphospholipid antibodies. In pregnancies at risk for the development of gestational hypertension and preeclampsia, and in fetuses with IUGR, low-dose aspirin (40–150 mg/day) may be beneficial, but more studies are required to assess accurately the risk:benefit ratio of such therapy. Near term, aspirin may prolong gestation and labor. Although aspirin has been used as a tocolytic agent, serious bleeding complications may occur in the newborn. Premature closure of the ductus arteriosus may occur in the latter part of pregnancy as a result of maternal consumption of full-dose aspirin. PPHN is a potential complication of the closure. If an analgesic or antipyretic is needed, acetaminophen should be considered.

Women attempting to conceive should not use any NSAID, including aspirin, because of the findings in a variety of animal models that indicate these agents block blastocyst implantation (80,81). Moreover, as noted above, NSAIDs have been associated with SABs in humans (see Ibuprofen for additional studies).

[**Risk Factor D if full-dose aspirin used in 3rd trimester.*]

BREAST FEEDING SUMMARY

RECOMMENDATION: Limited Human Data - Potential Toxicity

Aspirin and other salicylates are excreted into breast milk in low concentrations. Sodium salicylate was first demonstrated in human milk in 1935 (82). In one study of a mother taking sodium salicylate 4 g daily, no detectable salicylate in her milk or in her infant's serum was found, but the test sensitivity was only 50 μg/mL (83). Reported milk concentrations are much lower than this level. Following single or repeated oral doses, peak milk levels occurred at around 3 hours and ranged from 1.1–10 μg/mL (84,85). This represented a milk:plasma ratio of 0.03–0.08 at 3 hours. Because salicylates are eliminated more slowly from milk than from plasma, the ratio increased to 0.34 at 12 hours (84). Peak levels have also been reported to occur at 9 hours (86). Only one report has attributed infant toxicity to salicylates obtained in mother's milk (87). A 16-day-old female infant developed severe salicylate intoxication with a serum salicylate level of 24 mg/dL on the 3rd hospital day. Milk and maternal serum aspirin levels were not obtained, but the mother was taking aspirin 650 mg every 4 hours. Although the parents denied giving the baby aspirin or other salicylates, it is unlikely, based on the above reports, that she could have received the drug from the milk in the quantities found.

Adverse effects on platelet function in the nursing infant exposed to aspirin via the milk have not been reported but are a potential risk. The American Academy of Pediatrics recommends that aspirin should be used cautiously by the mother during lactation because of potential adverse effects in the nursing infant (88).

References

1. Corby DG. Aspirin in pregnancy: maternal and fetal effects. Pediatrics 1978;62(Suppl):930–7.
2. Palmisano PA, Cassady G. Salicylate exposure in the perinate. JAMA 1969;209:556–8.
3. Forfar JO, Nelson MM. Epidemiology of drugs taken by pregnant women: drugs that may affect the fetus adversely. Clin Pharmacol Ther 1973;14:632–42.
4. Finnigan D, Burry AF, Smith IDB. Analgesic consumption in an antenatal clinic survey. Med J Aust 1974;1:761–2.
5. Collins F, Turner G. Maternal effects of regular salicylate ingestion in pregnancy. Lancet 1975;2:335–7.
6. Slone D, Heinonen OP, Kaufman DW, Siskind V, Monson RR, Shapiro S. Aspirin and congenital malformations. Lancet 1976;1:1373–5.
7. Hill RM, Craig JP, Chaney MD, Tennyson LM, McCulley LB. Utilization of over-the-counter drugs during pregnancy. Clin Obstet Gynecol 1977;20:381–94.
8. Harrison K, Thomas I, Smith I. Analgesic use during pregnancy. Med J Aust 1978;2:161.
9. Bodendorfer TW, Briggs GG, Gunning JE. Obtaining drug exposure histories during pregnancy. Am J Obstet Gynecol 1979;135:490–4.
10. Jackson AV. Toxic effects of salicylate on the foetus and mother. J Pathol Bacteriol 1948;60:587–93.
11. Lewis RN, Schulman JD. Influence of acetylsalicylic acid, an inhibitor of prostaglandin synthesis, on the duration of human gestation and labour. Lancet 1973;2:1159–61.
12. Rudolph AM. Effects of aspirin and acetaminophen in pregnancy and in the newborn. Arch Intern Med 1981;141:358–63.
13. Stuart MJ, Gross SJ, Elrad H, Graeber JE. Effects of acetylsalicylic-acid ingestion on maternal and neonatal hemostasis. N Engl J Med 1982;307:909–12.
14. Stuart MJ. Aspirin and maternal or neonatal hemostasis. N Engl J Med 1983;308:281.
15. Niebyl JR, Blake DA, Burnett LS, King TM. The influence of aspirin on the course of induced midtrimester abortion. Am J Obstet Gynecol 1976;124:607–10.
16. Castellanos JM, Aranda M, Cararach J, Cararach V. Effect of aspirin on oestriol excretion in pregnancy. Lancet 1975;1:859.
17. Babenerd VJ, Kyriakidis K. Acetylsalicylic acid in the prevention of premature delivery. Fortschr Med 1979;97:463–6.
18. Wolff F, Bolte A, Berg R. Does an additional administration of acetylsalicylic acid reduce the requirement of betamimetics in tocolytic treatment? Geburtshilfe Frauenheilkd 1981;41:293–6.
19. Wolff F, Berg R, Bolte A. Clinical study of the labour inhibiting effects and side effects of acetylsalicylic acid (ASA). Geburtshilfe Frauenheilkd 1981;41:96–100.
20. Buhler M, Papiernik E. Successive pregnancies in women fitted with intrauterine devices who take antiinflammatory drugs. Lancet 1983;1:483.
21. Goodlin RC. Correction of pregnancy-related thrombocytopenia with aspirin without improvement in fetal outcome. Am J Obstet Gynecol 1983;146:862–4.
22. Gant NF. Lupus erythematosus, the lupus anticoagulant, and the anticardiolipid antibody. Supplement No. 6, May/June 1986, to Pritchard JA, MacDonald PC, Gant NF. *Williams Obstetrics*. 17th ed. Norwalk, CT: Appleton-Century-Crofts, 1985.
23. Branch DW, Scott JR, Kochenour NK, Hershgold E. Obstetric complications associated with the lupus anticoagulant. N Engl J Med 1985;313:1322–6.
24. Elder MG, DeSwiet M, Robertson A, Elder MA, Flloyd E, Hawkins DF. Low-dose aspirin in pregnancy. Lancet 1988;1:410.
25. Lockshin MD, Druzin ML, Qamar T. Prednisone does not prevent recurrent fetal death in women with antiphospholipid antibody. Am J Obstet Gynecol 1989;160:439–43.
26. Beaufils M, Uzan S, Donsimoni R, Colau JC. Prevention of pre-eclampsia by early antiplatelet therapy. Lancet 1985;1:840–2.
27. Beaufils M, Uzan S, Donsimoni R, Colau JC. Prospective controlled study of early antiplatelet therapy in prevention of preeclampsia. Adv Nephrol 1986;15:87–94.
28. Ylikorkala O, Makila U-M, Kaapa P, Viinikka L. Maternal ingestion of acetylsalicylic acid inhibits fetal and neonatal prostacyclin and thromboxane in humans. Am J Obstet Gynecol 1986;155:345–9.
29. Spitz B, Magness RR, Cox SM, Brown CEL, Rosenfeld CR, Gant NF. Low-dose aspirin. I. Effect on angiotensin II pressor responses and blood prostaglandin concentrations in pregnant women sensitive to angiotensin II. Am J Obstet Gynecol 1988;159:1035–43.
30. Wallenburg HCS, Rotmans N. Prevention of recurrent idiopathic fetal growth retardation by low-dose aspirin and dipyridamole. Am J Obstet Gynecol 1987;157:1230–5.
31. Wallenburg HCS, Rotmans N. Prophylactic low-dose aspirin and dipyridamole in pregnancy. Lancet 1988;1:939.
32. Uzan S, Beaufils M, Bazin B, Danays T. Idiopathic recurrent fetal growth retardation and aspirin-dipyridamole therapy. Am J Obstet Gynecol 1989;160:763.
33. Wallenburg HCS, Rotmans N. Idiopathic recurrent fetal growth retardation and aspirin-dipyridamole therapy. Reply. Am J Obstet Gynecol 1989;160:763–4.
34. Sibai BM, Mirro R, Chesney CM, Leffler C. Low-dose aspirin in pregnancy. Obstet Gynecol 1989;74:551–7.

35. Trudinger B, Cook CM, Thompson R, Giles W, Connelly A. Low-dose aspirin improves fetal weight in umbilical placental insufficiency. Lancet 1988;2:214–5.
36. Romero R, Lockwood C, Oyarzun E, Hobbins JC. Toxemia: new concepts in an old disease. Semin Perinatol 1988;12:302–23.
37. Lubbe WF. Low-dose aspirin in prevention of toxaemia of pregnancy. Does it have a place? Drugs 1987;34:515–8.
38. Wallenburg HCS, Dekker GA, Makovitz JW, Rotmans P. Low-dose aspirin prevents pregnancy-induced hypertension and pre-eclampsia in angiotensin-sensitive primigravidae. Lancet 1986;1:1–3.
39. Benigni A, Gregorini G, Frusca T, Chiabrando C, Ballerini S, Valcamonico A, Orisio S, Piccinelli A, Pinciroli V, Fanelli R, Gastaldi A, Remuzzi G. Effect of low-dose aspirin on fetal and maternal generation of thromboxane by platelets in women at risk for pregnancy-induced hypertension. N Engl J Med 1989;321:357–62.
40. Schiff E, Peleg E, Goldenberg M, Rosenthal T, Ruppin E, Tamarkin M, Barkai G, Ben-Baruch G, Yahal I, Blankstein J, Goldman B, Mashiach S. The use of aspirin to prevent pregnancy-induced hypertension and lower the ratio of thromboxane A_2 to prostacyclin in relatively high risk pregnancies. N Engl J Med 1989;321:351–6.
41. Turner G, Collins E. Fetal effects of regular salicylate ingestion in pregnancy. Lancet 1975;2:338–9.
42. Earle R Jr. Congenital salicylate intoxication-report of a case. N Engl J Med 1961;265:1003–4.
43. Lynd PA, Andreasen AC, Wyatt RJ. Intrauterine salicylate intoxication in a newborn. A case report. Clin Pediatr (Phila) 1976;15:912–3.
44. Shapiro S, Monson RR, Kaufman DW, Siskind V, Heinonen OP, Slone D. Perinatal mortality and birthweight in relation to aspirin taken during pregnancy. Lancet 1976;1:1375–6.
45. Arcilla RA, Thilenius OG, Ranniger K. Congestive heart failure from suspected ductal closure in utero. J Pediatr 1969;75:74–8.
46. Collins E. Maternal and fetal effects of acetaminophen and salicylates in pregnancy. Obstet Gynecol 1981;58(Suppl):57S–62S.
47. Aterman K, Holzbecker M, Ellenberger HA. Salicylate levels in a stillborn infant born to a drug-addicted mother, with comments on pathology and analytical methodology. Clin Toxicol 1980;16:263–8.
48. Van Marter LJ, Leviton A, Allred EN, Pagano M, Sullivan KF, Cohen A, Epstein MF. Persistent pulmonary hypertension of the newborn and smoking and aspirin and nonsteroidal antiinflammatory drug consumption during pregnancy. Pediatrics 1996;97:658–63.
49. Bleyer WA, Breckenridge RJ. Studies on the detection of adverse drug reactions in the newborn. II. The effects of prenatal aspirin on newborn hemostasis. JAMA 1970;213:2049–53.
50. Corby DG, Schulman I. The effects of antenatal drug administration on aggregation of platelets of newborn infants. J Pediatr 1971;79:307–13.
51. Casteels-Van Daele M, Eggermont E, de Gaetano G, Vermijlen J. More on the effects of antenatally administered aspirin on aggregation of platelets of neonates. J Pediatr 1972;80:685–6.
52. Haslam RR, Ekert H, Gillam GL. Hemorrhage in a neonate possible due to maternal ingestion of salicylate. J Pediatr 1974;84:556–7.
53. Ekert H, Haslam RR. Maternal ingested salicylate as a cause of neonatal hemorrhage. Reply. J Pediatr 1974;85:738.
54. Pearson H. Comparative effects of aspirin and acetaminophen on hemostasis. Pediatrics 1978; 62(Suppl):926–9.
55. Haslam RR. Neonatal purpura secondary to maternal salicylism. J Pediatr 1975;86:653.
56. O'Brien JR. Effects of salicylates on human platelets. Lancet 1968;1:779–83.
57. Weiss HJ, Aledort ML, Shaul I. The effect of salicylates on the haemostatic properties of platelets in man. J Clin Invest 1968;47:2169–80.
58. Bleyer WA. Maternal ingested salicylates as a cause of neonatal hemorrhage. J Pediatr 1974;85:736–7.
59. Rumack CM, Guggenheim MA, Rumack BH, Peterson RG, Johnson ML, Braithwaite WR. Neonatal intracranial hemorrhage and maternal use of aspirin. Obstet Gynecol 1981;58(Suppl):52S–6S.
60. Soller RW, Stander H. Maternal drug exposure and perinatal intracranial hemorrhage. Obstet Gynecol 1981;58:735–7.
61. Corby DG. Editorial comment. Obstet Gynecol 1981;58:737–40.
62. Levy G, Procknal JA, Garrettson LK. Distribution of salicylate between neonatal and maternal serum at diffusion equilibrium. Clin Pharmacol Ther 1975;18:210–4.
63. Levy G, Garrettson LK. Kinetics of salicylate elimination by newborn infants of mothers who ingested aspirin before delivery. Pediatrics 1974;53:201–10.
64. Garrettson LK, Procknal JA, Levy G. Fetal acquisition and neonatal elimination of a large amount of salicylate. Study of a neonate whose mother regularly took therapeutic doses of aspirin during pregnancy. Clin Pharmacol Ther 1975;17:98–103.
65. Li DK, Liu L, Odouli R. Exposure to non-steroidal anti-inflammatory drugs during pregnancy and risk of miscarriage: population based cohort study. Br Med J 2003;327:368–71.
66. Richards ID. Congenital malformations and environmental influences in pregnancy. Br J Prev Soc Med 1969;23:218–25.
67. Nelson MM, Forfar JO. Associations between drugs administered during pregnancy and congenital abnormalities of the fetus. Br Med J 1971;1:523–7.
68. Saxen I. Associations between oral clefts and drugs during pregnancy. Int J Epidemiol 1975;4:37–44.
69. Benawra R, Mangurten HH, Duffell DR. Cyclopia and other anomalies following maternal ingestion of salicylates. J Pediatr 1980;96:1069–71.
70. McNiel JR. The possible effect of salicylates on the developing fetus. Brief summaries of eight suggestive cases. Clin Pediatr (Phila) 1973;12:347–50.
71. Sayli BS, Asmaz A, Yemisci B. Consanguinity, aspirin, and phocomelia. Lancet 1966;1:876.
72. Zierler S, Rothman KJ. Congenital heart disease in relation to maternal use of Bendectin and other drugs in early pregnancy. N Engl J Med 1985;313:347–52.
73. Rothman KJ, Fyler DC, Goldblatt A, Kreidberg MB. Exogenous hormones and other drug exposures of children with congenital heart disease. Am J Epidemiol 1979;109:433–9.

74. Zierler S. Maternal drugs and congenital heart disease. Obstet Gynecol 1985;65:155–65.
75. Werler MM, Mitchell AA, Shapiro S. The relation of aspirin use during the first trimester of pregnancy to congenital cardiac defects. N Engl J Med 1989;321:1639–42.
76. Kallen BAJ, Olausson PO. Maternal drug use in early pregnancy and infant cardiovascular defect. Reprod Toxicol 2003;17:255–61.
77. Torfs CP, Katz EA, Bateson TF, Lam PK, Curry CJR. Maternal medications and environmental exposures as risk factors for gastroschisis. Teratology 1996;54:84–92.
78. Streissguth AP, Treder RP, Barr HM, Shepard TH, Bleyer WA, Sampson PD, Martin DC. Aspirin and acetaminophen use by pregnant women and subsequent child IQ and attention decrements. Teratology 1987;35:211–9.
79. Klebanoff MA, Berendes HW. Aspirin exposure during the first 20 weeks of gestation and IQ at four years of age. Teratology 1988;37:249–55.
80. Matt DW, Borzelleca JF. Toxic effects on the female reproductive system during pregnancy, parturition, and lactation. In Witorsch RJ, ed. *Reproductive Toxicology*. 2nd ed. New York, NY: Raven Press, 1995:175–93.
81. Daewood MY. Nonsteroidal antiinflammatory drugs and reproduction. Am J Obstet Gynecol 1993;169:1255–65.
82. Kwit NT, Hatcher RA. Excretion of drugs in milk. Am J Dis Child 1935;49:900–4.
83. Erickson SH, Oppenheim GL. Aspirin in breast milk. J Fam Pract 1979;8:189–90.
84. Weibert RT, Bailey DN. Salicylate excretion in human breast milk (abstract no.7). Presented at the 1979 Seminar of the California Society of Hospital Pharmacists, Los Angeles, October 13, 1979.
85. Findlay JWA, DeAngelis RL, Kearney MF, Welch RM, Findley JM. Analgesic drugs in breast milk and plasma. Clin Pharmacol Ther 1981;29:625–33.
86. Anderson PO. Drugs and breast feeding—a review. Drug Intell Clin Pharm 1977;11:208–23.
87. Clark JH, Wilson WG. A 16-day-old breast-fed infant with metabolic acidosis caused by salicylate. Clin Pediatr (Phila) 1981;20:53–4.
88. Committee on Drugs, American Academy of Pediatrics. The transfer of drugs and other chemicals into human milk. Pediatrics 2001;108:776–89.

Name:	**ASTEMIZOLE**	Risk Factor:	C_M
Class:	**Antihistamine**		

FETAL RISK SUMMARY

RECOMMENDATION: Limited Human Data - Animal Data Suggest Low Risk

Astemizole is a long-acting, nonsedating antihistamine that is used for the relief of symptoms caused by seasonal allergic rhinitis and chronic idiopathic urticaria. The lack of sedative action is a result of the drug's inability to reach H_1-receptors in the mother's brain, thus occupying only peripheral H_1-receptors (1). It is not known, however, if drug transfer is also blocked by the fetal blood-brain barrier. Because of the very long terminal half-life after chronic administration, about 19 days for the pharmacologically active fraction of parent drug and hydroxylated metabolites, it could take up to 4 months after the last dose to completely eliminate the metabolites from the mother's body (1). Conception during this interval, therefore, could result in exposure of the embryo and fetus.

Astemizole was not teratogenic in rats and rabbits at doses of 200 times the recommended human dose (RHD), but maternal toxicity in rabbits was evident at this dose (1). Maternal toxicity and embryocidal effects were seen at 100 times the RHD in rats. Neither maternal toxicity nor embryo toxicity was observed in either species at 50 times the RHD (1). The lack of teratogenicity in rats and rabbits was also discussed in a 1986 letter from the manufacturer (2).

The long-term behavioral and anatomic effects in rat pups have been examined after exposure throughout gestation to a maternal dose (10 mg/kg/day) that produced neither adverse maternal body weight changes nor other maternal toxicity (3). In comparisons between astemizole-exposed pups and controls, no difference was found in the average number of pups alive at birth. No gross malformations or pups dead at birth were found in either group. The mean birth weight, however, was significantly less ($p < 0.05$) in the exposed group than in controls, and stayed significantly less throughout the 21-day lactation period. Compared with controls, two landmark and reflex development parameters, the appearance of pinna detachment and auditory startle reflex, were significantly ($p < 0.05$) delayed in astemizole-exposed pups. Five other parameters, incisor eruption, eyes opening, vaginal opening, testes descent, and negative geotaxis, did not differ between the groups. In open field tests of locomotion, rearing frequencies, immobility duration, and defecation, the two groups were similar. When the locomotion test results were compared by sexes, however, exposed male pups were delayed compared with male controls, whereas exposed females were faster than their controls. Finally, prenatally exposed male rats exhibited significantly less ($p < 0.05$) reproductive behavior than controls and had a significant reduction in testis wet weight. No differences in the sexual behavior tests were observed in the two groups of female rats. Although the exact cause of the above differences was not determined, the authors proposed that the mechanism may have been interference with the hormonal mechanism regulating central nervous system masculinization or a direct action on the pups during development (3).

No studies have been located that describe the placental transfer of astemizole in animals or humans. The molecular weight of the drug (about 459) is low enough that transfer to the fetus would normally be expected and the fetal effects noted above indicate that transfer did occur.

In a prospective, controlled, observational study, two teratogen information services compared the pregnancy outcomes of 114 women who took astemizole during the 1st trimester of pregnancy to the outcomes of 114 control women, matched for age, smoking, and alcohol use, who had consulted one of the services after exposure to nonteratogen agents (4). The mean dose ingested (10 mg/day) was taken by 76 women up to 16 weeks' gestation, 38 women took it for longer periods. A final follow-up interview was conducted at least 6 months after delivery. No statistically significant differences were recorded between the groups in prepregnancy weight, weight gain during pregnancy, mode of delivery, gestational age at birth, or number of live births, spontaneous abortions, elective abortions, or stillbirths. Two major malformations were observed in each group (1.9% in each). In the astemizole-exposed group, one case of hypospadias and one of spina bifida occulta were observed. Both infants had been exposed throughout the 1st trimester. In the control group, one infant had a ventricular septal defect and the other had ocular myopathy. The authors concluded that their results suggested that the drug could be used safely during pregnancy (4).

A 1998 letter, however, challenged the above conclusion because the letter's authors calculated the upper value of the 95% confidence interval of the drug's relative risk to be 7.5 (5). They claimed, therefore, that the sample size was too small to detect an increased incidence of birth defects.

A brief 1997 review on the use of H_1-receptor blocking antihistamines concluded that first generation antihistamines were preferred over second generation agents (6). In particular, the authors recommended chlorpheniramine as the preferred oral agent and diphenhydramine as the preferred parenteral antihistamine. They also concluded that if a second-generation drug (e.g., astemizole) is required, exposure during organogenesis should be avoided except when the expected benefit is large (6). For pregnant patients with daily symptoms of allergic rhinitis, they recommended intranasal cromolyn or, if that is not successful, then intranasal beclomethasone supplemented, if necessary, with antihistamines. Antihistamines were recommended for pregnant patients with intermittent symptoms (6).

In summary, limited data on the use of astemizole during animal and human pregnancy, including the 1st trimester, do not support a major teratogenic risk for this antihistamine.

Although H_1-receptor occupying antihistamines, in general, are considered relatively safe during pregnancy (7), the number of human exposures to astemizole are too small to exclude such a risk completely. Moreover, the subtle behavioral and anatomic changes noted in one animal study are of concern and need to be addressed in future human research of offspring exposed *in utero* to this agent. Until more data are available in these and related areas, the safest course is to avoid the use of astemizole during the period of organogenesis.

BREAST FEEDING SUMMARY

RECOMMENDATION: No Human Data - Probably Compatible

No reports describing the use of astemizole during human lactation have been located. The molecular weight of astemizole (about 459) is low enough, however, that passage into breast milk should be expected. The effects of this potential exposure on a nursing infant are unknown.

References

1. Product information. Hismanal. Janssen Pharmaceutica, 1998.
2. Whyatt PL. Astemizole in pregnancy. Aust Fam Physician 1986;15:382, 384.
3. Almeida RG, Massoco CO, Spinosa HS, Bernardi MM. Perinatal astemizole exposure in the rat throughout gestation: long-term behavioral and anatomic effects associated with reproduction. Comp Biochem Physiol 1996;114C:123–7.
4. Pastuszak A, Schick B, D'Alimonte D, Donnenfeld A, Koren G. The safety of astemizole in pregnancy. J Allergy Clin Immunol 1996;98:748–50.
5. Kelso JM, Schatz M. Astemizole use in pregnancy. J Allergy Clin Immunol 1998;101:144.
6. Schatz M, Petitti D. Antihistamines and pregnancy. Ann Allergy Asthma Immunol 1997;78:157–9.
7. Seto A, Einarson T, Koren G. Pregnancy outcome following first trimester exposure to antihistamines: meta-analysis. Am J Perinatol 1997;14:119–24.

Name:	**ATAZANAVIR**	Risk Factor:	**B_M**
Class:	**Antiviral**		

FETAL RISK SUMMARY

RECOMMENDATION: Compatible - Maternal Benefit >> Embryo/Fetal Risk

Atazanavir is an azapeptide human immunodeficiency virus type 1 (HIV-1) protease inhibitor. The agent selectively inhibits the virus-specific processing viral Gag and Gag-Pol polyproteins in HIV-1 infected cells, thereby preventing formation of mature virions (1). The hepatic metabolites of atazanavir are inactive. Plasma protein binding is 86% with about equal amounts bound to albumin and α_1-glycoprotein. The mean elimination half-life is about 7 hours (1).

Reproduction studies have been conducted in rats and rabbits. In rats, doses producing systemic drug exposures that were two times the human exposure from the clinical dose of 400 mg once daily (HE) had no adverse effect on mating or fertility and were not teratogenic or embryotoxic. However, in pre- and postnatal rat development studies, the dose resulted in body weight loss or decreased weight gain in offspring and maternal toxicity. No effects on offspring were observed when the maternal exposure was equivalent to the HE. No teratogenic effects were observed in rabbits at doses producing maternal exposures equal to the HE.

It is not known if atazanavir crosses the human placenta. The molecular weight (about 705 for the free base) and moderately long elimination half-life suggest that passage to the embryo and fetus may occur.

The Antiretroviral Pregnancy Registry reported, for the period January 1989 through January 2004, prospective data (reported to the Registry before the outcomes were known) involving 1537 live births that had been exposed during the 1st trimester to one or more antiretroviral agents (2). Forty-seven of the newborns had congenital defects (3.1%, 95% confidence interval [CI] 2.3–4.1). In the 2407 live births with earliest exposure in the 2nd/3rd trimesters, there were 56 infants with defects (2.3%, 95% CI 1.8–3.0). The prevalence rates for the two periods did not differ significantly. There were 103 infants with birth defects among 3944 live births with exposure anytime during pregnancy (2.6%, 95% CI 2.1–3.2). The prevalence rate did not differ significantly from the rate expected in a nonexposed population (2). There were 13 outcomes exposed to atazanavir (nine in the 1st trimester and four in the 2nd/3rd trimesters) in combination with other antiretroviral agents. There was one birth defect in the 1st trimester exposures. In reviewing the birth defects of prospective and retrospective (pregnancies reported after the outcomes were known) registered cases, and clinical reports, the Registry concluded that there was no pattern of anomalies to suggest a common cause (2). (See Lamivudine for required statement.)

No reports, other than the data above, describing the use of atazanavir in human pregnancy have been located. Although the near absence of human data prevents an assessment of the safety of atazanavir during pregnancy, the animal data suggests that the drug may represent a low risk to the developing fetus. Of note, though, the systemic exposures in two animal species were very close to those obtained clinically. Past reviewers have concluded that all women currently receiving antiretroviral therapy, including protease inhibitors, should continue to receive therapy during pregnancy (3–5). Discontinuing all therapy until after 10–12 weeks' gestation, however, is an option (5,6). If indicated, therefore, atazanavir should not be withheld in pregnancy, except possibly in the 1st trimester, because the expected benefit for the HIV-positive mother appears to outweigh the unknown risks to the fetus. The efficacy and safety of combined therapy in preventing vertical transmission of HIV to the newborn, however, are unknown, and zidovudine remains the only antiretroviral agent recommended for this purpose (6).

Hyperbilirubinemia is a common adverse effect with atazanavir, but it is not known if this will worsen physiologic hyperbilirubinemia in the newborn or young infant and lead to kernicterus. In the prepartum period, additional monitoring and alternative therapy to atazanavir should be considered (1).

BREAST FEEDING SUMMARY

RECOMMENDATION: Contraindicated

No reports describing the use of atazanavir during human lactation have been located. The molecular weight (about 705 for the free base) and the moderately long elimination half-life (about 7 hours) suggest that the drug will be excreted into breast milk. The effect on a nursing infant from this exposure is unknown. However, reports on the use of atazanavir during lactation are unlikely because of the potential toxicity, especially hyperbilirubinemia, and because the drug is indicated in the treatment of patients with HIV. HIV type 1 (HIV-1) is transmitted in milk, and in developed countries, breast-feeding is not recommended

(3,4,7–10). In developing countries, breast-feeding is undertaken, despite the risk, because there are no affordable milk substitutes available.

References

1. Product information. Reyataz. Bristol-Myers Squibb, 2004.
2. Antiretroviral Pregnancy Registry Steering Committee. Antiretroviral Pregnancy Registry International Interim Report for 1 January 1989 through 31 January 2004. Wilmington, NC: Registry Coordinating Center; 2004.
3. Carpenter CCJ, Fischl MA, Hammer SM, Hirsch MS, Jacobsen DM, Katzenstein DA, Montaner JSG, Richman DD, Saag MS, Schooley RT, Thompson MA, Vella S, Yeni PG, Volberding PA. Antiretroviral therapy for HIV infection in 1996. JAMA 1996;276:146–54.
4. Minkoff H, Augenbraun M. Antiretroviral therapy for pregnant women. Am J Obstet Gynecol 1997;176:478–89.
5. Centers for Disease Control and Prevention. Public Health Service Task Force recommendations for the use of antiretroviral drugs in pregnant women infected with HIV-1 for maternal health and for reducing perinatal HIV-1 transmission in the United States. MMWR 1998;47:NO. RR-2.
6. Public Health Service Task Force Perinatal HIV Guidelines Working Group. Summary of the updated recommendations from the Public Health Service Task Force to reduce perinatal human immunodeficiency virus-1 transmission in the United States. Obstet Gynecol 2002;99:1117–26.
7. Brown ZA, Watts DH. Antiviral therapy in pregnancy. Clin Obstet Gynecol 1990;33:276–89.
8. de Martino M, Tovo P-A, Pezzotti P, Galli L, Massironi E, Ruga E, Floreea F, Plebani A, Gabiano C, Zuccotti GV. HIV-1 transmission through breast-milk: appraisal of risk according to duration of feeding. AIDS 1992;6:991–7.
9. Van de Perre P. Postnatal transmission of human immunodeficiency virus type 1: the breast feeding dilemma. Am J Obstet Gynecol 1995;173:483–7.
10. American College of Obstetricians and Gynecologists. Breast-feeding: Maternal and infant aspects. *Educational Bulletin*. No. 258, July 2000.

Name:	**ATENOLOL**	Risk Factor:	**D_M**
Class:	**Sympatholytic (Antihypertensive)**		

FETAL RISK SUMMARY

RECOMMENDATION: Human Data Suggest Risk in 2nd and 3rd Trimesters

Atenolol is a cardioselective β_1-adrenergic blocking agent used for the treatment of hypertension. The drug did not cause structural anomalies in pregnant rats and rabbits, but a dose-related increase in embryo and fetal resorptions in rats was observed at doses equal to or greater than 25 times the maximum recommended human antihypertensive dose based on 100 mg/day in a 50-kg patient (MRHD). This effect was not seen in rabbits at doses up to 12.5 times the MRHD (1).

In contrast with propranolol and sotalol, atenolol exposure during gestation did not increase motor activity or cause poor performance in rat offspring (2). The adverse effects observed with propranolol and sotalol, but not atenolol, were attributed to the β_2-blocking activity of propranolol and sotalol.

A 2002 abstract, reviewing both published and non-published sources to assess atenolol developmental toxicity, found that fetal growth restriction occurred in both animals and humans (3). The animal-human concordance was thought to result from the reduced placental and fetal circulation induced by atenolol.

Atenolol readily crosses the placenta to the fetus producing steady state fetal levels approximately equal to those in the maternal serum (4–11). When 11 pregnant patients were treated with 100 mg/day, the serum half-life (8.1 hours) and the 24-hour urinary excretion (52 mg) were similar to those values in nonpregnant women (8). In nine women treated with atenolol for cardiac disease, the average maternal and cord drug concentrations at delivery were 133 and 126 ng/mL, respectively (11). No evidence of altered atenolol pharmacokinetics during pregnancy was found. Atenolol transfer was one-third to one-fourth the transfer of the more lipid-soluble β-blockers propranolol, timolol, and labetalol in an *in vitro* experiment using perfused human placentas (12).

In a surveillance study of Michigan Medicaid recipients conducted between 1985 and 1992, involving 229,101 completed pregnancies 105 newborns had been exposed to atenolol during the 1st trimester (F. Rosa, personal communication, FDA, 1993). A total of 12 (11.4%) major birth defects were observed (4 expected). Specific data were available for six defect categories, including (observed/expected) 3/1 cardiovascular defects, 1/0 oral clefts, 0/0 spina bifida, 0/0 polydactyly, 1/0 limb reduction defects, and 4/0 hypospadias. Only with the latter defect is there a suggestion of a possible association, but other factors, including the mother's disease, concurrent drug use, and chance, may be involved.

A 1997 abstract (13) and later full report (14) described a case of retroperitoneal fibromatosis in a fetus exposed *in utero* to atenolol from the 2nd month of gestation through delivery at 37 weeks. The obese (134 kg at term), 25-year-old mother, in her third pregnancy, was treated for hypertension with 100 mg atenolol daily until giving birth to the 3790-g male infant. Other drug therapy included magnesium supplements and occasional metoclopramide. The mother had no familial history of cancer and both of her other children were normal. Treatment of the tumor with chemotherapy during the first 3 months of life was successful, but a severe scoliosis was present in the child at 4 years of age. The authors attributed the rare tumor to the drug because, among other reasons, the location of the mass was similar to that of fibroses reported in adults exposed to atenolol (13,14).

The use of atenolol for the treatment of hypertension in pregnant women has been described frequently (7,10,15–28). No fetal malformations attributable to atenolol have been reported in these trials, but in most cases, the treatment with atenolol did not occur during the 1st trimester.

Thirteen women, 11 in the 3rd trimester and 2 in the 2nd trimester, were treated for gestational hypertension with atenolol 100 mg/day until delivery in a 1981 study (15). The birth weights of 12 of the 13 newborns were less than the 50th percentile (3 were less than the 10th percentile), but the authors thought they were consistent with severe preeclampsia. The pharmacokinetic profiles of atenolol in the pregnant subjects were similar to those measured in nonpregnant women (15).

A 1982 study described the pregnancy outcomes of 10 women with chronic hypertension who were treated with atenolol 100–200 mg/day beginning at 11–32 weeks (16). One woman delivered a stillborn infant at 41+ weeks' gestation, but the remaining nine women delivered at a median of 39 weeks. The median birth weight was 82% of the gestational mean with placental weights ranging from 235 g to 795 g.

A 1983 retrospective study examined the effects of atenolol ($N = 87$) and metoprolol ($N = 2$), either alone or in combination with other antihypertensives, for the treatment of hypertension (chronic or preeclampsia) in pregnancy (17). Birth weights were not given. There were three stillbirths, but the maternal therapy in these cases was not specified.

A randomized, double-blind study published in 1983 compared atenolol ($N = 46$) with placebo ($N = 39$) for the treatment of mild to moderate gestational hypertension (18). Treatment was started at a mean 34 weeks' gestation in both groups. The mean gestational ages at delivery were 38 weeks (placebo) and 39 weeks (atenolol) ($p < 0.05$). No differences in the incidence of hypoglycemia, respiratory distress syndrome, or hyperbilirubinemia were observed between the groups. Although not statistically significant, both the mean birth weights (2961 g vs. 3017 g) and placental weights (549 g vs. 608 g) were lower in those treated with atenolol. However, significantly more atenolol-exposed newborns had bradycardia, 39% (18 of 46) vs. 10% (4 of 39) ($p < 0.01$). None of the infants required treatment for the lowered heart rate. Three intrauterine deaths occurred, two in the placebo group and one in the atenolol group (18). In the same year, the authors of this study and a previous report (16) commented briefly on the benefits of β-blockers in the management of hypertension during pregnancy (19).

A 1992 study evaluated the effectiveness of atenolol in three groups of pregnant women having chronic hypertension ($N = 12$), gestational hypertension without proteinuria ($N = 52$), or preeclampsia ($N = 6$) (20). The mean doses in the three groups were 62.5, 70.0, and 100.0 mg, respectively. The drug was started at a mean gestational age of 24.5, 29.8, and 31.0 weeks, respectively. The mean birth weights observed were approximately 2902, 3059, and 2431 g, respectively.

The effect of β-blockers in pregnancy was reviewed in a 1988 article. Citing only three reports, the authors concluded that atenolol was safe and effective therapy during pregnancy (21).

Antihypertensive therapy with atenolol has been associated with fetal growth retardation in a number of studies (7,10,22–27). A nonrandomized 1983 study compared atenolol ($N = 28$; enrolled before May 1981) with labetalol ($N = 28$; enrolled after May 1981) in the treatment of chronic ($N = 6$) or gestational hypertension ($N = 50$) (7). The average daily doses were 144.6 mg (atenolol) and 614 mg (labetalol). Newborn weights were significantly higher in those exposed to labetalol, 3280 g vs. 2750 g, respectively ($p < 0.001$). Two newborns were premature (<37 weeks) in the atenolol group compared with one in the labetalol group. In addition, two mothers treated with atenolol delivered stillborn infants at 29 and 38 weeks, respectively (7).

A 1984 case report described the pregnancy outcome of a woman treated with atenolol (50 mg/day increased to 100 mg/day at 33 weeks' gestation) throughout a 36-week gestation (10). Intrauterine growth retardation (IUGR) was diagnosed by ultrasound and a small (weight not given) but otherwise normal baby girl was delivered with Apgar scores of 5, 7, and 9 at 1, 5, and 10 minutes, respectively. The maternal plasma and cord blood atenolol concentrations were 510 and 380 ng/mL, respectively. Other than a transient decrease in heart rate to 100 beats per minute at 16 hours of age, the infant had no complications (10).

A 1980 report described 60 pregnancy outcomes from 59 women treated with β-blockers for hypertension (22). The agents used were atenolol ($N = 10$; daily dose 100–200 mg), acebutolol ($N = 28$; daily dose 200–600 mg), pindolol ($N = 21$; daily dose 10–20 mg), and propranolol ($N = 1$; daily dose 40 mg). Although the birth weights were not differentiated by drug, 9 newborns weighed <2500 g, 11 weighed 2500–2800 g, and 40 weighed >2800 g (21). Two years later, this research group compared atenolol ($N = 31$), acebutolol ($N = 56$), and pindolol ($N = 38$) in a nonrandomized study for the treatment of hypertension during pregnancy (23). One year later, the researchers increased the number of atenolol cases to 37 (24). The mean birth weights of the three groups were 2.82, 3.16, and 3.38 kg, respectively (23,24).

In a prospective, randomized, double-blind study, women with mild essential hypertension were given either atenolol (50–200 mg/day) or placebo starting at a mean gestational age of 15.9 weeks (25). The 15 newborns in the treated group had a significantly lower birth weight than the 14 untreated controls (2620 g vs. 3530 g; $p < 0.001$). In the treated group, 5 of the newborns had weights below the 5th percentile and 10 were below the 10th percentile, compared with 1 newborn below the 25th percentile in controls. In addition, the atenolol group had significantly smaller placentas (442 g vs. 635 g; $p < 0.002$) (25).

A 1992 report described the outcomes of 29 women with pregnancy-induced hypertension in the 3rd trimester (26). The women were randomized to receive either atenolol ($N = 13$) or pindolol ($N = 16$). The decrease in mean maternal arterial blood pressure in the two groups was similar. In comparing the women's status before and after therapy, several significant changes were measured in fetal hemodynamics with atenolol but, except for fetal heart rate, no significant changes were measured with pindolol. The atenolol-induced changes included a decrease in fetal heart rate; increases in the pulsatility indices (and thus, the peripheral vascular resistance) of the fetal thoracic descending aorta, the abdominal aorta, and the umbilical artery; and a decrease in the umbilical venous blood flow (26). Although no difference in birth weights was observed in the two groups, the placental weight in atenolol-treated pregnancies was significantly less, 529 g vs. 653 g ($p = 0.03$).

A 1997 report described an open, retrospective survey on the use of antihypertensives in 398 consecutive pregnant women who attended an antenatal hypertension clinic in the years from 1980 to 1995 (27). The 76 women who used atenolol were compared with those using calcium channel blockers ($N = 22$), diuretics ($N = 26$), methyldopa ($N = 17$), other β-blockers ($N = 12$), or no drug therapy ($N = 235$). The mean birth weights/placental weights in the groups were atenolol 2.19 kg/390 g ($p < 0.001$), other β-blockers 2.36 kg/450 g, calcium channel blockers 2.50 kg/385 g ($p = 0.001$), diuretics 2.53 kg/500 g; methyldopa 2.70 kg/500 g, and no drug treatment 2.78 kg/535 g. The ponderal index (kg/m^3 $\times$ 10^4), an indirect measure of impaired placental function in some forms of IUGR, also was calculated for each group: 2.21 ($p < 0.001$), 2.44, 2.22, 2.33, 2.67, and 2.39, respectively. The authors concluded that atenolol was associated with IUGR and reduced placental weights and should be avoided in women who are trying to conceive or are in the early stages of gestation (27).

A 1999 retrospective cohort study reported the outcomes of 312 pregnancies in 223 women treated for gestational hypertension ($N = 80$), preeclampsia ($N = 19$), chronic hypertension ($N = 179$), or superimposed preeclampsia on chronic hypertension ($N = 34$) (28). The women were treated with atenolol monotherapy ($N = 78$), other monotherapy ($N = 53$), combination therapy ($N = 90$; atenolol in 57), or no treatment ($N = 91$). The atenolol outcomes were statistically significant when compared with other monotherapy or with no treatment. (Combination therapy implied more-severe disease and consistently had the worst outcomes.) Birth weights were atenolol 2372 g vs. other monotherapy 2756 g or no treatment 3068 g ($p < 0.05$), and combination therapy 2220 g; birth lengths were atenolol 47.9 cm vs. other monotherapy 48.3 cm, no treatment 50.4 cm ($p < 0.05$), and combination therapy 46.3 cm. There were two nonsignificant trends: (a) higher prevalence of preterm delivery (<37 weeks)—atenolol 33% vs. other monotherapy 26%, no treatment 15%, and combination therapy 46%; and (b) higher prevalence of small for gestational age (<10th percentile)—atenolol 49% vs. other monotherapy 34%, no treatment 21%, and combination therapy 52%. The adverse fetal effects of atenolol were more pronounced when the therapy was started early in pregnancy, and were duration-dependent (28).

A prospective randomized study compared 24 atenolol-treated women with 27 pindolol-treated women (29). No differences between the groups were found in gestational length, birth weight, Apgar scores, rates of cesarean section, or umbilical cord blood glucose levels. Treatment in both groups started at about 33 weeks' gestation. Placentas in the atenolol group weighed less than those from pindolol-treated women, 440 g vs.533 g, $p < 0.02$.

A 1987 study used Doppler ultrasound to evaluate maternal and fetal circulation during atenolol therapy in 14 women (9 nulliparous) with pregnancy-induced hypertension at a mean gestational age of 35 weeks (range 33–38 weeks) (30). The studies were conducted before and during the first and third days of treatment. During treatment, the volume of blood flow remained unchanged in the fetal descending aorta and the umbilical vein. In contrast, the pulsatility index increased in the fetal descending aorta and the maternal arcuate artery, suggesting that peripheral vascular resistance had increased on both the maternal and fetal sides of the placenta. No effect on placental or fetal weight occurred because of the short treatment period (delivery occurred a mean 18 days after the start of the study) (30). The study design and techniques were criticized based on concerns for reproducibility, including day-to-day variability in Doppler measurements, the lack of controls, and the uncertainty of the clinical significance of velocity waveform measurements (31).

A 1995 randomized study examined the short-term effects of IV 15- to 20-minute infusions of atenolol or pindolol in 24 women with gestational hypertension (32). Comparisons were made for uterine and umbilicoplacental vascular impedance, fetal hemodynamics, and cardiac function. Both drugs significantly decreased maternal blood pressure and maternal heart rate immediately after infusion, but the effect of atenolol was still evident 30 minutes after the end of the infusion. Pindolol produced no changes in uteroplacental or umbilicoplacental vascular impedance, whereas atenolol increased vascular impedance in the nonplacental uterine artery. The umbilical artery pulsatility indices, an indication of increased vascular resistance, were higher after atenolol than after pindolol. Pindolol had no effects on fetal hemodynamics whereas atenolol decreased pulsatility indices in the fetal renal artery. In addition, atenolol significantly decreased peak systolic velocity in the fetal pulmonary trunk. The investigators concluded that both drugs were equally effective in lowering maternal blood pressure, that atenolol increased utero-placental vascular impedance, and that atenolol had direct effects on fetal hemodynamics. Based on these findings, pindolol was the preferred agent (32).

A 1995 review of vasoactive drugs in pregnancy stated that pregnancy-induced hypertension (now known as gestational hypertension) was associated with increased vascular resistance that could reduce uteroplacental blood flow by 40%–70% (33). In addition, atenolol treatment was associated with increased resistance in uterine arteries and decreased peak velocity in the fetal pulmonary trunk, but that pindolol lacked these effects (32). They concluded that the use of vasoconstricting β-blockers during pregnancy should be reconsidered (33).

Normotensive women at risk for preeclampsia (cardiac output >7.4 L/minute before 24 weeks' gestation) were enrolled in a 1999 double blind, randomized, controlled trial to determine if atenolol could reduce this risk (34). The treatment groups were nulliparous: atenolol ($N = 21$) or placebo ($N = 19$); diabetics: atenolol ($N = 7$) or placebo ($N = 9$); and controls: no treatment ($N = 18$). A significant decrease ($p = 0.04$) in the incidence of preeclampsia was noted in the atenolol-treated women, but their offspring had a birth weight 440 g less than that of placebo infants ($p = 0.02$). However, no increase in the rate of small for gestational age fetuses was observed. Previous research by these investigators had suggested that in women with hypertension, fetal growth retardation occurred primarily when increased vascular resistance was present but not when hypertension was mediated by increased cardiac output (34). They concluded that a change in therapy was indicated if the maternal cardiac output was less than the mean for gestational age or if peripheral resistance was greater than 1150 dyne·sec·cm^{-5}. If these guidelines had been followed, atenolol therapy would have been changed in seven subjects, including four cases involving the smallest infants (34).

A 2001 retrospective review of pregnancies ($N = 235$) at risk for preeclampsia that were treated with atenolol (25–100 mg/day) early in gestation was reported by the same authors as those of the above study (35). The goals of therapy were to reduce cardiac output to one standard deviation above the mean for gestational age and to lower mean arterial pressure to <90 mm Hg. To maintain fetal growth, this was modified to maintaining cardiac output above the mean for gestational age and maintaining peripheral vascular resistance at <1150 dyne-sec-cm^5. Low birth weight was associated with: (a) prior pregnancy with IUGR ($p = 0.001$); (b) failure to adjust the dose properly for cardiac output and peripheral vascular resistance ($p < 0.001$); and (c) a pregnancy in an earlier year of the investigator's experience ($p < 0.001$). In the study population, the birth weight increased from the 20th percentile at the beginning of the study period (1991) to the 40th percentile by the end (1999) ($p = 0.002$) (35).

In a group of pregnant women with symptomatic mitral valve stenosis, 11 were treated with atenolol and 14 with propranolol (36). The mean birth weight of the 25 infants was 2.8 kg (range 2.1–3.5 kg). Atenolol, 25 mg twice daily, was administered from 18 weeks' gestation to term in a normotensive woman who had suffered a myocardial infarction (37). She delivered a 2720-g infant with normal Apgar scores and blood gasses.

Intrauterine fetal deaths have been observed in women with severe hypertension treated with atenolol, but this also has occurred with other β-blockers and in hypertensive women not treated with drugs (7,16–18,38). Four cases of fetal death (at 18, 29, and 33 weeks) or neonatal death (at 6.5 days) have been reported when the mothers were treated with atenolol combined with either angiotensin-converting enzyme inhibitors (39–41) or a selective angiotensin II receptor antagonist (42).

In eight women treated with atenolol or pindolol, a decrease in the basal fetal heart rate was noted only in atenolol-exposed fetuses (43). Before and during treatment, fetal heart rates in the atenolol patients were 136 and 120 beats per minute, respectively, whereas the rates for the pindolol group were 128 and 132 beats per minute, respectively. In 60 patients treated with atenolol for pregnancy-induced hypertension, no effect on fetal heart rate pattern in response to uterine contractions was observed (44). Accelerations, variables, and late decelerations all were easily distinguishable.

Persistent β-blockade was observed in a newborn whose mother was treated with atenolol, 100 mg/day, for hypertension (5). At 15 hours of age, the otherwise-normal infant developed bradycardia at rest and when crying, and hypotension. The serum atenolol concentration was 0.24 μg/mL. Urinary excretion of the drug during the first 7 days ranged from 0.085–0.196 μg/mL.

A 1992 case report described a pregnant woman who was diagnosed with a pheochromocytoma at 28 weeks' gestation (45). She was treated with atenolol (100 mg/day) and phenoxybenzamine (30 mg/day) to control her blood pressure. An elective cesarean section was performed at 37 weeks to deliver a normal female infant (birth weight not given).

A woman with a renal transplant was treated with cyclosporine, prednisolone, and atenolol (50 mg/day) throughout a normotensive pregnancy without proteinuria (46). An 820-g (below the 3rd percentile) male infant was delivered at 30 weeks' gestation because of severe IUGR. The authors attributed the growth retardation to cyclosporine, but atenolol and prednisolone probably contributed to the condition.

A review published in 2002 examined the pharmacokinetic and pharmacodynamic issues relevant to the toxic effects of atenolol exposure during pregnancy (47). The authors concluded that: (a) maternal hypertension can potentiate the adverse effects of atenolol on placental and fetal circulation, resulting in decreased placental and birth weight; (b) decreased placental weight has been significantly associated with IUGR and lower birth weight independent of gestational age; (c) the effects of atenolol are duration-dependent;

and (d) several other agents have a more-favorable effect on birth weight, including labetalol, pindolol, acebutolol, and calcium channel blockers (47).

In summary, atenolol may cause IUGR and reduce placental weight. The drug does not possess intrinsic sympathomimetic activity (ISA) (i.e., partial agonist). The reduced fetal growth appears to be related to increased vascular resistance in both the mother and fetus, and is a function of the length of drug exposure. Treatment starting early in the 2nd trimester is associated with the greatest decrease in fetal and placental weights, whereas treatment restricted to the 3rd trimester primarily affects only placental weight. The duration of treatment, rather than the dose used, appears to be a critical factor in causing atenolol-induced fetal growth retardation (48). At one center, adjustment of the dose for maternal cardiac output and peripheral vascular resistance has reduced these toxic effects. Although growth retardation is a serious concern, the benefits of maternal therapy with β-blockers, in some cases, might outweigh the risks to the fetus and must be judged on a case-by-case basis. Infant behavior is apparently not affected by atenolol exposure, as no differences were noted in the development at 1 year of age of offspring from mothers treated during the 3rd trimester for mild to moderate pregnancy-induced hypertension with either bed rest alone or rest combined with atenolol (49). The mean duration of therapy in the atenolol-treated patients was 5 weeks. Because only one case has been reported, an association between atenolol and fetal retroperitoneal fibromatosis requires confirmation.

Newborns exposed to atenolol near delivery should be closely observed during the first 24–48 hours for signs and symptoms of β-blockade. Although the results of the study cited above are reassuring, the long-term effects of prolonged *in utero* exposure to this class of drugs have not been studied but warrant evaluation.

BREAST FEEDING SUMMARY

RECOMMENDATION: Limited Human Data - Potential Toxicity

Atenolol is excreted into breast milk (6,8,10,47,50–54). The drug is a weak base, and when used during lactation, accumulation in the milk will occur with concentrations significantly greater than corresponding plasma levels (6,8,47,50–53). Peak milk concentrations after single-dose (50 mg) and continuous-dosing (25–100 mg/day) regimens were 3.6 and 2.9 times greater, respectively, than simultaneous plasma levels (52). Atenolol has been found in the serum and urine of breast-fed infants (6,8,10,50). Other studies have been unable to detect the drug in the infant serum (test limit 10 ng/mL) (51,52).

Symptoms consistent with β-adrenergic blockade were observed in a breast-fed, 5-day-old, full-term female infant, including cyanosis, hypothermia (35.5°C rectal), and bradycardia (80 beats per minute) (54). Blood pressure was 80/40 mm Hg. Except for these findings, physical examination was normal and bacterial cultures from various sites were negative. The mother had been treated orally with atenolol, 50 mg every 12 hours, for postpartum hypertension. Breast-feeding was stopped 3 days after onset of the symptoms and 6 hours later, the infant's symptoms had resolved. A milk sample, collected 10 days postpartum and 1.5 hours after a 50-mg dose, contained 469 ng/mL of atenolol. Concentrations in the infant's serum, 48 and 72 hours after breast-feeding, were 2010 ng/mL and 140 ng/mL, respectively. The calculated serum half-life in the infant was 6.4 hours. By extrapolation, the minimum daily dose absorbed by the infant was estimated to be 8.97 mg, approximately 9% of the mother's daily dose (54). (These calculations have been questioned and defended [55,56].)

Except for the single case cited above, adverse reactions in infants have not been reported. However, because milk accumulation occurs with atenolol, nursing infants must be closely monitored for bradycardia and other signs and symptoms of β-blockade. Moreover, one author has recommended that water-soluble, low-protein-bound, renally excreted β-blockers, such as atenolol, should not be used during lactation (57). Because of the availability of safer alternatives, this seems to be good advice. Long-term effects on infants exposed to β-blockers from breast milk have not been studied but warrant evaluation.

The American Academy of Pediatrics classifies atenolol as a drug that has been associated with significant effects in nursing infants (cyanosis and bradycardia) and should be used by nursing mothers with caution (58).

References

1. Product information. Tenormin. Zeneca Pharmaceuticals, 2003.
2. Speiser Z, Gordon I, Rehavi M, Gitter S. Behavioral and biochemical studies in rats following prenatal treatment with β-adrenoceptor antagonists. Eur J Pharmacol 1991;195:75–83.
3. Tabacova SA, Kimmel CA, Wall K, McCloskey CA. Animal-human concordance in the developmental toxicity of two antihypertensive agents (abstract). Teratology 2002;65:304.
4. Melander A, Niklasson B, Ingemarsson I, Liedholm H, Schersten B, Sjoberg NO. Transplacental passage of atenolol in man. Eur J Clin Pharmacol 1978;14:93–4.
5. Woods DL, Morrell DF. Atenolol: side effects in a newborn infant. Br Med J 1982;285:691–2.
6. Liedholm H. Transplacental passage and breast milk accumulation of atenolol in humans. Drugs 1983;25(Suppl 2):217–8.
7. Lardoux H, Gerard J, Blazquez G, Chouty F, Flouvat B. Hypertension in pregnancy: evaluation of two beta blockers, atenolol and labetalol. Eur Heart J 1983;4(Suppl G):35–40.
8. Thorley KJ. Pharmacokinetics of atenolol in pregnancy and lactation. Drugs 1983;25(Suppl 2):216–7.
9. Boutroy MJ. Fetal and neonatal effects of the beta-adrenoceptor blocking agents. Dev Pharmacol Ther 1987;10:224–31.
10. Fowler MB, Brudenell M, Jackson G, Holt DW. Essential hypertension and pregnancy: successful outcome with atenolol. Br J Clin Pract 1984;38:73–4.
11. Hurst AK, Shotan A, Hoffman K, Johnson J, Goodwin TM, Koda R, Elkayam U. Pharmacokinetic and pharmacodynamic evaluation of atenolol during and after pregnancy. Pharmacotherapy 1998;18:840–6.
12. Schneider H, Proegler M. Placental transfer of B-adrenergic antagonists studied in an *in vitro* perfusion system of human placental tissue. Am J Obstet Gynecol 1988;159:42–7.
13. Satge D, Sasco AJ, Col JY, Lemonnier PG, Hemet J, Robert E. Antenatal exposure to atenolol and retroperitoneal fibromatosis (abstract). Teratology 1997;55:103.
14. Satge D, Sasco AJ, Col J-Y, Lemonnier PG, Hemet J, Robert E. Antenatal exposure to atenolol and retroperitoneal fibromatosis. Reprod Toxicol 1997;11:539–41.
15. Thorley KJ, McAinsh J, Cruickshank JM. Atenolol in the treatment of pregnancy-induced hypertension. Br J Clin Pharmacol 1981;12:725–30.
16. Rubin PC, Butters L, Low RA, Reid JL. Atenolol in the treatment of essential hypertension during pregnancy. Br J Clin Pharmacol 1982;14:279–81.
17. Liedholm H. Atenolol in the treatment of hypertension of pregnancy. Drugs 1983;25(Suppl 2):206–11.
18. Rubin PC, Butters L, Clark DM, Reynolds B, Sumner DJ, Steedman D, Low RA, Reid JL. Placebo-controlled trial of atenolol in treatment of pregnancy-associated hypertension. Lancet 1983;1:431–4.
19. Rubin PC, Butters L, Low RA, Clark DC, Reid JL. Atenolol in the management of hypertension during pregnancy. Drugs 1983;25(Suppl 2):212–4.
20. Fabregues G, Alvarez L, Varas Juri P, Drisaldi S, Cerrato C, Moschettoni C, Pituelo D, Baglivo HP, Esper RJ. Effectiveness of atenolol in the treatment of hypertension during pregnancy. Hypertension 1992;19(Suppl II):II129–II31.
21. Frishman WH, Chesner M. Beta-adrenergic blockers in pregnancy. Am Heart J 1988;115:147–52.
22. Dubois D, Petitcolas J, Temperville B, Klepper A. Beta blockers and high-risk pregnancies. Int J Biol Res Pregnancy 1980;1:141–5.
23. Dubois D, Petitcolas J, Temperville B, Klepper A, Catherine P. Treatment of hypertension in pregnancy with β-adrenoceptor antagonists. Br J Clin Pharmacol 1982;13(Suppl):375S–8S.
24. Dubois D, Peticolas J, Temperville B, Klepper A. Treatment with atenolol of hypertension in pregnancy. Drugs 1983;25(Suppl 2):215–8.
25. Butters L, Kennedy S, Rubin PC. Atenolol in essential hypertension during pregnancy. Br Med J 1990;301:587–9.
26. Montan S, Ingemarsson I, Marsal K, Sjoberg N-O. Randomized controlled trial of atenolol and pindolol in human pregnancy: effects on fetal haemodynamics. Br Med J 1992;304:946–9.
27. Lip GYH, Beevers M, Churchill D, Shaffer LM, Beevers DG. Effect of atenolol on birth weight. Am J Cardiol 1997;79:1436–8.
28. Lydakis C, Lip GYH, Beevers M, Beevers DG. Atenolol and fetal growth in pregnancies complicated by hypertension. Am J Hypertens 1999;12:541–7.
29. Tuimala R, Hartikainen-Sorri A-L. Randomized comparison of atenolol and pindolol for treatment of hypertension in pregnancy. Curr Ther Res 1988;44:579–84.
30. Montan S, Liedholm H, Lingman G, Marsal K, Sjöberg N-O, Solum T. Fetal and uteroplacental haemodynamics during short-term atenolol treatment of

hypertension in pregnancy. Br J Obstet Gynaecol 1987;94:312–7.
31. Rubin PC. Beta blockers in pregnancy. Br J Obstet Gynaecol 1987;94:292–3.
32. Rasanen J, Jouppila P. Uterine and fetal hemodynamics and fetal cardiac function after atenolol and pindolol infusion. A randomized study. Eur J Obstet Gynecol Reprod Biol 1995;62:195–201.
33. Jouppila P, Rasanen J, Alahuhta S, Jouppila R. Vasoactive drugs in obstetrics: a review of data obtained by Doppler and color Doppler methods. Hypertens Pregnancy 1995;14:261–75.
34. Easterling TR, Brateng D, Schmucker B, Brown Z, Millard SP. Prevention of preeclampsia: a randomized trial of atenolol in hyperdynamic patients before onset of hypertension. Obstet Gynecol 1999;93:725–33.
35. Easterling TR, Carr DB, Brateng D, Diederichs C, Schmucker B. Treatment of hypertension in pregnancy: effect of atenolol on maternal disease, preterm delivery, and fetal growth. Obstet Gynecol 2001;98:427–33.
36. Al Kasab SM, Sabag T, Al Zaibag M, Awaad M, Al Bitar I, Halim MA, Abdullah MA, Shahed M, Rajendran V, Sawyer W. β-Adrenergic receptor blockade in the management of pregnant women with mitral stenosis. Am J Obstet Gynecol 1990;163:37–40.
37. Soderlin MK, Purhonen S, Haring P, Hietakorpi S, Koski E, Nuutinen LS. Myocardial infarction in a parturient. Anaesthesia 1994;49:870–2.
38. Lubbe WF. More on beta-blockers in pregnancy. N Engl J Med 1982;307:753.
39. Knott PD, Thorpe SS, Lamont CA. Congenital renal dysgenesis possibly due to Captopril. Lancet 1989;1:451.
40. Mehta N, Modi N. ACE inhibitors in pregnancy. Lancet 1989;2:96.
41. Smith AM. Are ACE inhibitors safe in pregnancy? Lancet 1989;2:750–1.
42. Briggs GG, Nageotte MP. Fatal fetal outcome with the combined use of valsartan and atenolol. Ann Pharmacother 2001;35:859–61.
43. Ingemarsson I, Liedholm H, Montan S, Westgren M, Melander A. Fetal heart rate during treatment of maternal hypertension with beta-adrenergic antagonists. Acta Obstet Gynecol Scand 1984;118(Suppl): 95–7.
44. Rubin PC, Butters L, Clark D, Sumner D, Belfield A, Pledger D, Low RAL, Reid JL. Obstetric aspects of the use in pregnancy-associated hypertension of the β-adrenoceptor antagonist atenolol. Am J Obstet Gynecol 1984;150:389–92.
45. Bakri YN, Ingemansson SE, Ali A, Parikh S. Pheochromocytoma and pregnancy: report of three cases. Acta Obstet Gynecol Scand 1992;71:301–4.
46. Pickrell MD, Sawers R, Michael J. Pregnancy after renal transplantation: severe intrauterine growth retardation during treatment with cyclosporin A. Br Med J 1988;296:825.
47. Tabacova SA, Kimmel CA. Atenolol: pharmacokinetic/dynamic aspects of comparative developmental toxicity. Reprod Toxicol 2002;16:1–7.
48. Sibai BM. Chronic hypertension in pregnancy. In reply. Obstet Gynecol 2002;100:1358–9.
49. Reynolds B, Butters L, Evans J, Adams T, Rubin PC. First year of life after the use of atenolol in pregnancy associated hypertension. Arch Dis Child 1984;59:1061–3.
50. Liedholm H, Melander A, Bitzen PO, Helm G, Lonnerholm G, Mattiasson I, Nilsson B, Wahlin-Boll E. Accumulation of atenolol and metoprolol in human breast milk. Eur J Clin Pharmacol 1981;20:229–31.
51. Kulas J, Lunell NO, Rosing U, Steen B, Rane A. Atenolol and metoprolol. A comparison of their excretion into human breast milk. Acta Obstet Gynecol Scand 1984;118(Suppl):65–9.
52. White WB, Andreoli JW, Wong SH, Cohn RD. Atenolol in human plasma and breast milk. Obstet Gynecol 1984;63:42S–4S.
53. White WB. Management of hypertension during lactation. Hypertension 1984;6:297–300.
54. Schmimmel MS, Eidelman AJ, Wilschanski MA, Shaw D Jr, Ogilvie RJ, Koren G. Toxic effects of atenolol consumed during breast-feeding. J Pediatr 1989;114:476–8.
55. Diamond JM. Toxic effects of atenolol consumed during breast-feeding. J Pediatr 1989;115:336.
56. Koren G. Toxic effects of atenolol consumed during breast-feeding. J Pediatr 1989;115:336–7.
57. Anderson PO. Drugs and breast milk. Pediatrics 1995;95:957.
58. Committee on Drugs, American Academy of Pediatrics. The transfer of drugs and other chemicals into human milk. Pediatrics 2001;108:776–89.

Name:	**ATOMOXETINE**	Risk Factor:	**C_M**
Class:	**Psychotherapeutic (Miscellaneous)**		

FETAL RISK SUMMARY

RECOMMENDATION: Limited Human Data - Animal Data Suggest Risk

Atomoxetine is used for the treatment of Attention-Deficit/Hyperactivity Disorder (ADHD). Atomoxetine has an equipotent active metabolite, but the plasma concentration is only 1% (in normal metabolizers) of the parent drug. A second active metabolite has much less activity and its plasma levels are 5% (in normal metabolizers) of the parent drug. The plasma elimination half-life in normal (extensive) metabolizers is about 5 hours. In persons who are "poor metabolizers" (7% of Caucasians and 2% of African Americans), the drug plasma levels are much higher and the plasma elimination half-life is 24 hours. The plasma protein binding is 98%, primarily to albumin (1).

Reproduction studies have been conducted in rats and rabbits. No effects on rat fertility were observed at doses up to about six times the maximum human dose based on a body surface area (MHD). In one of two studies in which rats were treated in the diet for 2 weeks prior to mating through organogenesis and lactation with doses up to about six times the MHD, a decrease in pup weight (female only) and pup survival (also seen at three times the MHD) was observed. The no-effect dose for pup survival was about two times the MHD. A diet dose about five times the MHD given throughout the period of organogenesis resulted in a decrease in fetal weight and an increase in the incidence of incomplete ossification of the vertebral arch in fetuses. The no-effect dose for these effects was about 2.5 times the MHD. No adverse fetal effects were observed when rats were gavage fed with doses up to 17 times the MHD throughout organogenesis (1).

In pregnant rabbits given atomoxetine by gavage, a dose about 23 times the MHD resulted in an increase in early absorptions and a decrease in live fetuses in one of three studies. In addition, slight increases in the incidences of atypical origin of carotid artery and absence subclavian artery were observed, as was slight maternal toxicity. The no-effect dose was about 7 times the MHD. The high dose produced plasma levels (AUC) in rabbits that were about 3.3 times (normal metabolizers) or 0.4 times (poor metabolizers) those in humans receiving the maximum human dose. The no-effect dose for these effects was about 7 times the MHD (1).

It is not known if atomoxetine or its active metabolites cross the human placenta. The molecular weight for the parent drug (about 256 for the free base) combined with elimination half-life suggest that atomoxetine will cross to the embryo and/or fetus. The extensive protein binding, however, will limit the amount available for transfer.

In a brief correspondence, representatives of the manufacturer and others stated that there had been three pregnancies in adult clinical trials with atomoxetine (2). Two resulted in healthy newborns, but the third pregnancy was lost to follow-up. No other details were provided.

In summary, although the animal data are suggestive of risk, the absence of detailed human pregnancy experience prevents an assessment of the embryo/fetal risk. Until such data are available, the safest course is to avoid the drug in pregnancy. If the mother's condition requires atomoxetine, the lowest effective dose, avoiding the 1st trimester, if possible, should be used. However, inadvertent exposure in the 1st trimester does not appear to represent a major risk. Long-term follow-up of exposed offspring may be warranted.

BREAST FEEDING SUMMARY

RECOMMENDATION: No Human Data - Potential Toxicity

No reports describing the use of atomoxetine during human lactation have been located. The drug and/or its metabolites were excreted in the milk of lactating rats (1). This is consistent with the molecular weight of the parent drug (about 256 for the free base) and the relatively long elimination half-life (5 hours for normal metabolizers; 24 hours for poor metabolizers). These factors suggest that atomoxetine and/or its metabolites will be excreted into breast milk. The effects of this exposure on a nursing infant are unknown. If a mother chooses to breast-feed while taking atomoxetine, the infant should be monitored for potential toxicity (e.g., such as upper abdominal pain, constipation, or dyspepsia).

References

1. Product information. Strattera. Eli Lilly, 2004.
2. Heiligenstein J, Michelson D, Wernicke J, Milton D, Kratochvil CJ, Spencer TJ, Newcorn JH. Atomoxetine and pregnancy. J Am Acad Child Adolesc Psychiatry 2003;42:884–5.

Name: **ATORVASTATIN**	Risk Factor: **X_M**
Class: **Antilipemic Agent**	

FETAL RISK SUMMARY

RECOMMENDATION: Contraindicated

Atorvastatin, a 3-hydroxy-3-methylglutaryl-coenzyme A (HMG-CoA) reductase inhibitor (a 'statin') that is lipophilic, is indicated as an adjunct to diet to reduce total cholesterol, low-density lipoprotein (LDL) cholesterol, apolipoprotein B, and triglyceride levels in patients with primary hypercholesterolemia and mixed dyslipidemia. It has the same mechanism of action as cerivastatin, fluvastatin, lovastatin, pravastatin, and simvastatin. Atorvastatin is extensively metabolized and some of the metabolites are as pharmacologically active as the parent compound. Atorvastatin is highly bound (≥98%) to plasma proteins and it has a mean plasma elimination of about 14 hours. However, because of the active metabolites, the half-life of inhibitory activity for HMG-CoA reductase is 20–30 hours (1,2).

In reproduction studies with pregnant rats and rabbits, doses that were about 30 and 20 times, respectively, the human exposure based on body surface area, were not teratogenic. With maternal dosing in rats from gestation day 7 through lactation day 21 (weaning), at a dose 22 times the human exposure based on area under the plasma concentration curve (HE-AUC), there was decreased pup survival at birth, during the neonatal period, at weaning, and at maturity, and decreased pup weight at birth, during nursing, and at maturity. In addition, pup development was inhibited at this dose (1–3). A 1994 report described developmental toxicity of atorvastatin at maternally toxic doses in pregnant rats and rabbits (4). There was evidence, however, of teratogenicity in either species (4).

It is not known if atorvastatin or its active metabolites cross the human placenta. The relatively high molecular weight (about 1161 for the non-hydrated form) and extensive protein binding suggest that transfer across the placenta will be inhibited. In pregnant rats, however, fetal liver levels of atorvastatin are equivalent to maternal levels (1–3).

A 2002 report described the use of atorvastatin in early pregnancy (5). A 35-year-old woman with several diseases (hypertension, diabetes mellitus, hypercholesterolemia, anxiety disorder, epilepsia, and morbid obesity) conceived while being treated with multiple drugs: atorvastatin (40 mg/day), rosiglitazone, gliclazide (a sulfonylurea), acarbose, spironolactone, hydrochlorothiazide, carbamazepine, thioridazine, amitriptyline, chlordiazepoxide, and pipenzolate bromide (an anti-spasmodic). Her pregnancy was diagnosed in the 8th week of gestation and all medications were stopped. She was treated with methyldopa and insulin for the remainder of her pregnancy. At 36 weeks' gestation, a repeat cesarean section delivered a healthy, 3.5-kg female infant with Apgar scores of 7 and 8 at 1 and 5 minutes, respectively. The infant was developing normally after 4 months (5).

A 2004 report described the outcomes of pregnancy that had been exposed to statins and reported to the FDA (see Lovastatin).

The interruption of cholesterol-lowering therapy during pregnancy should have no effect on the long-term treatment of hyperlipidemia. Moreover, because cholesterol and products synthesized by cholesterol are important during fetal development, the use of atorvastatin is contraindicated during pregnancy. If atorvastatin is used in pregnancy, health care professionals are encouraged to call the toll free number (800-670-6126) for information about patient enrollment in the Motherisk study.

BREAST FEEDING SUMMARY

RECOMMENDATION: Contraindicated

No reports describing the use of atorvastatin in human lactation have been located. The relatively high molecular weight (about 1161 for the non-hydrated form) suggests that excretion into milk would be inhibited. However, the drug is excreted into the milk of lactating rats, resulting in plasma and liver levels that were 50% and 40%, respectively, of the mother's milk (1–3). Thus, some excretion into human breast milk should be expected. Because of the potential for adverse effects in a nursing infant, women who are taking atorvastatin should not breast-feed.

References

1. Product information. Lipitor. Parke-Davis, 2004.
2. Product information. Lipitor. Pfizer, 2004.
3. Henck JW, Craft WR, Black A, Colgin J, Anderson JA. Pre- and postnatal toxicity of the HMG-CoA reductase inhibitor, atorvastatin in rats. Toxicol Sci 1998;41:88–99.
4. Dostal LA, Schardein JL, Anderson JA. Developmental toxicity of the HMG-CoA reductase inhibitor, atorvastatin, in rats and rabbits. Teratology 1994;50:387–94.
5. Yaris F, Yaris E, Kadioglu M, Ulku C, Kesim M, Kalyoncu NI. Normal pregnancy outcome following inadvertent exposure to rosiglitazone, gliclazide, and atorvastatin in a diabetic and hypertensive woman. Reprod Toxicol 2004;18:619–21.

Name:	**ATOVAQUONE**	Risk Factor:	C_M
Class:	**Antiprotozoal**		

FETAL RISK SUMMARY

RECOMMENDATION: Compatible - Maternal Benefit >> Embryo/Fetal Risk

Atovaquone is an analog of ubiquinone that is indicated for the prevention and treatment of *Pneumocystis carinii* pneumonia in patients intolerant of trimethoprim-sulfamethoxazole (1). The agent, when combined with proguanil, is also indicated for the prevention and treatment of malaria due to *Plasmodium falciparum* (2,3). Unlabeled uses include the treatment of babesiosis (in combination with quinine and/or clindamycin and/or azithromycin), and toxoplasmosis (in combination with pyrimethamine) (4). The drug undergoes little, if any, metabolism, and is extensively bound (99.9%) to plasma proteins (1). Elimination is almost exclusively in the feces with less than 0.6% of a dose excreted in the urine. The elimination half-life is long, ranging from about 67 to 78 hours (1).

Reproduction studies have been conducted in rats and rabbits (1,2). In rats, no teratogenicity or reproductive toxicity was observed at plasma concentrations 2–3 times the estimated human exposure (HE) for *P. carinii* (1) or 5–6.5 times the HE for malaria (2). In rabbits, plasma concentrations about 0.5 times the HE for *P. carinii* (1) and 0.6–1.3 times the HE for malaria (2) were maternally toxic. At these exposures, mean fetal body weights and lengths were decreased, and there were higher numbers of early resorption and post-implantation losses. These effects may have been due to the maternal toxicity (1,2). The combination of atovaquone and proguanil was not teratogenic in rats (1.7 and 0.10 times the HE for malaria, respectively) or rabbits (0.34 and 0.82 times the HE for malaria, respectively). There was also no embryotoxicity in rabbits at these exposures (2).

Atovaquone was not carcinogenic in rats, but hepatocellular adenoma and carcinoma were observed with all doses tested in mice (1.4–3.6 times the average plasma concentrations in humans). In other tests, there was no evidence of atovaquone-induced mutagenicity or genotoxicity (1).

It is not known if atovaquone crosses the human placenta. The anti-infective does cross the rat and rabbit placentas (1). In rats, fetal levels were 18% (middle gestation) and 60% (late gestation) of concurrent maternal plasma concentrations. Fetal levels in rabbits averaged 30% of concurrent maternal plasma levels (1). The molecular weight (about 367), absence of metabolism, and long elimination half-life suggest that atovaquone will cross the human placenta to the embryo/fetus. However, the extensive plasma protein binding should limit the amount that is transferred.

Only one report describing the use of atovaquone in human pregnancy has been located. In an antenatal clinic in Thailand, 24 pregnant women who had tested positive for malaria were treated with atovaquone (20 mg/kg/day) plus proguanil (8 mg/kg/day) plus artesunate (4 mg/kg/day) for 3 days (4). The study was conducted to determine the pharmacokinetic properties of the drugs in pregnancy. The median estimated gestational age at the start of treatment was 28.5 weeks (range 19.1–35.9 weeks). No adverse effects of the therapy were observed in the fetuses or newborns (4).

In summary, the lack of toxicity in animals when there is no maternal toxicity, is reassuring, but the doses used were very close to those used in humans. However, the limited human pregnancy experience, including the absence of 1st trimester exposures, prevents an assessment of the risk this anti-infective presents to an embryo or fetus. A 1999 review stated that atovaquone should not be used in pregnancy (5). In contrast, a 2004 review concluded that the combination of atovaquone/proguanil, while not recommended, could be used if no other alternative was available (3). In either case, the maternal benefit appears to exceed the unknown embryo/fetal risk, so the agent should not be withheld because of pregnancy.

BREAST FEEDING SUMMARY

RECOMMENDATION: No Human Data - Potential Toxicity

No reports describing the use of atovaquone during lactation have been located. The molecular weight (about 367), absence of metabolism, and long elimination half-life (about 67–78 hours) suggest that the drug will be excreted into breast milk. However, the extensive plasma protein binding (99.9%) should limit the amount in milk. In lactating rats, milk concentrations were about 30% of the concurrent maternal plasma levels (1). The effects, if any, of exposure to atovaquone via the milk on a nursing infant are unknown. The severity of the mother's illness, such as infection with human immunodeficiency virus (HIV), may preclude breast-feeding. In addition, the potential for severe adverse effects in a nursing infant, such as gastrointestinal symptoms, rash, fever, headache, hepatic toxicity, and carcinogenicity, suggests that even women who do not have HIV should not breast-feed if they are taking this drug.

References

1. Product information. Mepron. GlaxoSmithKline, 2004.
2. Product information. Malarone. GlaxoSmithKline, 2004.
3. Taylor WRJ, White NJ. Antimalarial drug toxicity: a review. Drug Saf 2004;27:25–61.
4. McGready R, Stepniewska K, Edstein MD, Cho T, Gilveray G, Looareesuwan S, White NJ, Nosten F. The pharmacokinetics of atovaquone and proguanil in pregnant women with acute falciparum malaria. Eur J Clin Pharmacol 2003;59:545–52.
5. Rosenblatt JE. Antiparasitic agents. Mayo Clin Proc 1999;74:1161–75.

Name:	**ATRACURIUM**	Risk Factor:	**C_M**
Class:	**Skeletal Muscle Relaxant**		

FETAL RISK SUMMARY

RECOMMENDATION: Limited Human Data - Probably Compatible

The competitive (nondepolarizing) neuromuscular blocking agent, atracurium besylate, provides muscle relaxation during surgery or mechanical ventilation. The drug undergoes rapid, nonenzymatic, spontaneous degradation in the plasma (Hofmann elimination) that is independent of hepatic or renal mechanisms (1,2).

In reproduction studies in rabbits with SC doses of 0.15 mg/kg once daily or 0.10 mg/kg twice daily (human IV bolus doses vary from 0.08 to 0.5 mg/kg), an increased incidence of spontaneously occurring visceral or skeletal anomalies was observed in both treatment groups when compared to nontreated controls (3). Moreover, in comparison to controls, a lower percentage of male fetuses (41% vs. 51%) and a higher percentage of postimplantation losses (15% vs. 8%) were observed in the 0.15 mg/kg-once-daily group (3).

In a study conducted by the manufacturer and published in 1983, SC doses of atracurium, identical to those above, were injected into rabbits on days 6–18 of pregnancy (4). Rabbits, and cats in the perinatal study below, were used because the pharmacokinetics of atracurium in these species are similar to humans, whereas the kinetics in rats are markedly different from humans. No teratogenicity or adverse effects were observed in the rabbit fetuses (4).

Theoretically, the relatively high molecular weight (about 1244) of atracurium besylate and its high degree of ionization at physiologic pH should inhibit the placental passage of atracurium. In the perinatal portion of the study cited above, six pregnant cats, 1–3 days before term, were given a single dose of atracurium, 0.6 mg/kg IV (4). No atracurium was detected in fetal blood, leading to the conclusion that the drug did not cross the placenta (4). Moreover, no depression of respiratory activity was observed when a dose of 0.6 mg/kg was injected directly into the fetuses. A brief 1985 report described the failure to detect placental transfer of atracurium during a 60-minute interval after a 0.5 mg/kg IV dose in five pregnant sheep (5). Small amounts of laudanosine, the major metabolite, crossed the placenta and were detected in some of the fetuses. The metabolite, however, is considered to be inactive at the doses of parent drug used clinically (1). In contrast to the above animal data, human placental transfer of atracurium has been documented (6,7).

In five women, from a total group of 26 undergoing cesarean section, average venous concentrations of the drug, following a 0.3 mg/kg IV dose, ranged from 3.34 μg/mL at 3 minutes to 0.7 μg/mL at 10 minutes (6). Venous cord blood concentrations of atracurium ranged from undetectable to 0.23 μg/mL, suggesting that the cord:maternal ratio varied from 5% to 20% (6). In the second report by these authors, 53 women, delivered by cesarean section, received atracurium 0.3 mg/kg IV followed by increments of 0.1–0.2 mg/kg IV as necessary to maintain surgical relaxation (7). Concentrations of the drug in 16 women at delivery ranged from 0.54 to 3.34 μg/mL. Only 1 patient received a second IV dose (0.2 mg/kg). Venous cord concentrations in 7 newborns were undetectable (<0.1 μg/mL in 2, <0.05 μg/mL in 5), 1 cord blood sample was contaminated, and in 8 newborns, concentrations ranged from 0.05 to 0.23 μg/mL. The cord:maternal blood ratio varied from 0.03 to 0.33 (mean 0.12). Newborn neuromuscular activity was reported as normal in all newborns. Furthermore, no adverse effects on Apgar scores or on the time to sustained respiration attributable to atracurium were observed in these two studies (6,7) or in an earlier report by the same authors (8).

A number of reports have described the safe use of atracurium during human pregnancy (9–13). A woman scheduled for a cesarean section had a low plasma concentration of cholinesterase activity. Atracurium, which does not depend on plasma cholinesterase for its metabolism, was successfully used for neuromuscular blockade in a dose of 0.4 mg/kg IV bolus (9). A healthy newborn with Apgar scores of 8 and 10 at 1 and 5 minutes, respectively, was delivered 10 minutes after the IV bolus. In another case, an IV infusion of atracurium was used during a 16-hour interval to maintain maternal muscle paralysis in a patient with pneumococcal pneumonia who required mechanical ventilation (10). In addition to other anesthetic agents, the woman received 520 mg of atracurium over 16 hours or an average of 32.5 mg/hour until vaginal delivery of a 1800-g female infant. No neuromuscular blockade was observed in the newborn that had Apgar scores of 7, 10, and 10 at 1, 5, and 10 minutes, respectively. Neuromuscular blockade with atracurium was used in a pregnant woman at 24 weeks' gestation that underwent resection of a pheochromocytoma (11). She eventually delivered a healthy, 2977-g male infant at 39 weeks' gestation. Normal newborns were also described in two other reports following the use of atracurium prior to cesarean section (12,13). Moreover, a 1986 review on obstetrical anesthesia concluded that atracurium was safe to use in obstetric patients (14).

Three studies have described the direct human fetal administration of atracurium to achieve neuromuscular blockade (15–17). In one study, atracurium (0.4 mg/kg) was used in 11 fetuses during 18 intrauterine transfusions and compared to pancuronium (0.1 mg/kg, 12 fetuses, 19 transfusions); (gestational ages not specified in either group) (15). The two agents were similar in onset of neuromuscular blockade. Atracurium, however, was statistically superior to pancuronium in terms of return of fetal movements (22 vs. 67 minutes), more fetal movements, fetal movements/minute, and more heart accelerations than pancuronium after transfusion (15). The authors concluded that atracurium was the preferred drug if fetal paralysis was required. A 1988 reference also used a 0.4 mg/kg IV fetal dose after determining that a 0.2 mg/kg dose was inadequate to arrest fetal activity during intrauterine transfusions (16). Atracurium was used in 6 women undergoing 12 transfusion procedures for fetal Rh isoimmunization. Onset of paralysis occurred within 1–5 minutes and fetal activity returned between 20 and 130 minutes. One fetus developed bradycardia and died 1 hour after transfusion of severe erythroblastosis fetalis and rupture of the spleen.

Atracurium, 1.0 mg/kg IM (fetal gluteal muscle), was used in 5 fetuses for various intrauterine procedures conducted between 32 and 38 weeks' gestation (17). In comparison to 5 fetuses treated with pancuronium, 0.15 mg/kg IM, neuromuscular blockade was achieved slightly faster (mean 4.7 vs. 5.8 minutes) and fetal movements returned sooner (mean 36 vs. 92 minutes) with atracurium. One fetus with peritonitis given pancuronium was stillborn, one fetus with peritonitis given atracurium was born alive with a gastrointestinal perforation, and one fetus given atracurium for ascites drainage and albumin transfusion died after birth. Although the authors did not discuss these outcomes, they do not appear to be related to the neuromuscular blocking agents. No evidence of soft tissue, nerve, or muscle damage at the sites of injection was observed in the newborns.

In summary, no adverse effects in the fetus or newborn attributable to *in utero* atracurium exposure have been reported. Because of the drug's high molecular weight and ionization at physiologic pH, only small amounts cross the human placenta, thus limiting the exposure of the embryo or fetus. Moreover, direct administration to the fetus in the latter part of pregnancy has not been associated with fetal harm. Human fetal exposures early in pregnancy, however, have not been reported. Animal reproduction studies have only been conducted in rabbits, and although the drug may be a potential teratogen in this species, further studies are required to determine the magnitude of this potential. Based on the above data, the use of atracurium during the latter portion of human pregnancy appears to represent little, if any, risk.

BREAST FEEDING SUMMARY

RECOMMENDATION: No Human Data - Probably Compatible

No reports describing the use of atracurium during human lactation have been located. Atracurium undergoes rapid, spontaneous degradation in plasma (Hofmann elimination) with an elimination half-life of approximately 20 minutes. The metabolites are not biologically active. In addition, the drug has a relatively high molecular weight (about 1244) and is highly ionized at physiologic pH, both factors that would markedly reduce transfer into milk. Although usage in lactating women is possible, at least several hours (and most likely much more time) would pass after use of atracurium before lactation was resumed. The rapid breakdown of atracurium that occurs in plasma would also be expected in milk, even though the latter medium is slightly more acidic than plasma. Thus, any amounts that were transferred into milk would most likely be rapidly degraded. Based on these data, nursing can probably be safely resumed, especially after single-dose use, following recovery from atracurium-induced neuromuscular blockade. A 1994 review of anesthetic agents also concluded that nursing could be allowed as soon as feasible after surgery (18).

References

1. Drenck NE, Viby-Mogensen J, Ostergaard D, Seraj M. Atracurium (tracrium). Middle East J Anesthesiol 1988;9:457–65.
2. Anonymous. Atracurium. Lancet 1983;1:394–5.
3. Product information. Tracrium. Glaxo Wellcome, 1998.
4. Skarpa M, Dayan AD, Follenfant M, James DA, Moore WB, Thomson PM, Lucke JN, Morgan M, Lovell R, Medd R. Toxicity testing of atracurium. Br J Anaesth 1983;55:27S–9S.
5. Mandel MD, Stiller RL, Kennedy RL, Tyler IL, Edelmann CA, Cook DR. Placental transfer of atracurium and

laudanosine in the pregnant ewe (abstract). Anesthesiology 1985;63:A429.
6. Frank M, Flynn PJ, Hughes R. Atracurium in obstetric anaesthesia. A preliminary report. Br J Anaesth 1983;55:113S–4S.
7. Flynn PJ, Frank M, Hughes R. Use of atracurium in caesarean section. Br J Anaesth 1984;56:599–0604.
8. Flynn PJ, Frank M, Hughes R. Evaluation of atracurium in caesarian section using train-of-four responses (abstract). Anesthesiology 1982;57:A286.
9. Baraka A, Jaude CA. Atracurium in a parturient with atypical cholinesterase. Br J Anaesth 1984;56:930–1.
10. Thomas D, Windsor JPW. Prolonged sedation and paralysis in a pregnant patient. Delivery of an infant with a normal Apgar score. Anaesthesia 1985;40:465–7.
11. Mitchell SZ, Freilich JD, Brant D, Flynn M. Anesthetic management of pheochromocytoma resection during pregnancy. Anesth Analg 1987;66:478–80.
12. Hardy PAJ. Atracurium and bradycardia. Anaesthesia 1985;40:504–5.
13. Stuart JC, Kan AF, Rowbottom SJ, Yau G, Gin T. Acid aspiration prophylaxis for emergency caesarean section. Anaesthesia 1996;51:415–21.
14. Biehl D, Palahniuk RJ. Update on obstetrical anaesthesia. Can Anaesth Soc J 1986;33:238–45.
15. Mouw RJC, Hermans J, Brandenburg HCR, Kanhai HHH. Effects of pancuronium or atracurium on the anemic fetus during and directly after intrauterine transfusion (IUT): a double blind randomized study (abstract). Am J Obstet Gynecol 1997;176:S18.
16. Bernstein HH, Chitkara U, Plosker H, Gettes M, Berkowitz RL. Use of atracurium besylate to arrest fetal activity during intrauterine intravascular transfusions. Obstet Gynecol 1988;72:813–6.
17. Fan SZ, Huang FY, Lin SY, Wang YP, Hsieh FJ. Intrauterine neuromuscular blockade in fetus. Acta Anaesth Sin 1990;28:31–4.
18. Spigset O. Anaesthetic agents and excretion in breast milk. Acta Anaesthesiol Scand 1994;38:94–103.

Name:	**ATROPINE**	Risk Factor:	**C**
Class:	**Parasympatholytic**		

FETAL RISK SUMMARY

RECOMMENDATION: Human Data Suggest Low Risk

Atropine, an anticholinergic, rapidly crosses the placenta (1–4). Atropine exposure in the 1st, 2nd, and 3rd trimesters was estimated in one study to be 11.3, 6.7, and 6.3/1,000 women, respectively (5). The drug has been used to test placental function in high-risk obstetric patients by producing fetal vagal blockade and subsequent tachycardia (6).

Intravenous atropine (0.5 mg) caused a decrease of 10% to 100% in fetal breathing in 13 of 15 fetuses, an increase of 300% in one fetus, and no effect in another (7). The decrease in fetal breathing occurred approximately 2 minutes after administration of the drug and lasted 5–10 minutes. No fetal hypoxia was observed, nor was there an effect on fetal heart rate or beat-to-beat variability.

The Collaborative Perinatal Project monitored 50,282 mother-child pairs, 401 of whom used atropine in the 1st trimester (8, pp. 346–353). For use anytime during pregnancy, 1198 exposures were recorded (8, p. 439). In neither group was evidence found for an association with malformations. However, when the group of parasympatholytics were taken as a whole (2323 exposures), a possible association with minor malformations was found (8, pp. 346–353).

In a surveillance study of Michigan Medicaid recipients conducted between 1985 and 1992, involving 229,101 completed pregnancies 381 newborns had been exposed to atropine during the 1st trimester (F. Rosa, personal communication, FDA, 1993). A total of 18 (4.7%) major birth defects were observed (16 expected). Specific data were available for six defect categories, including (observed/expected) 4/4 cardiovascular defects, 0/0.5 oral clefts, 1/0 spina bifida, 2/0 polydactyly, 1/1 hypospadias, and 2/0 limb reduction defects. Only with the latter defect is there a suggestion of a possible association, but other factors, such as the mother's disease, concurrent drug use, and chance may be involved.

Atropine has been used to reduce gastric secretions before cesarean section without producing fetal or neonatal effects (9,10). In a study comparing atropine and glycopyrrolate, 10 women in labor received 0.01 mg/kg of atropine IV (11). No statistically significant changes were noted in fetal heart rate or variability nor was there any effect on uterine activity.

A single case of a female infant born at 36 weeks' gestation with multiple defects, including Ebstein's anomaly, was described in a 1989 report (12). In addition to the cardiac defect, other abnormalities noted were hypertelorism, epicanthal folds, low-set, posteriorly rotated ears, a cleft uvula, medially rotated hands, deafness, and blindness. The mother had taken Lomotil (diphenoxylate and atropine) for diarrhea during the 10th week of gestation. Because exposure was beyond the susceptible stages of development for these defects, the drug combination was not considered causative. However, a possible viremia in the mother as a cause of the diarrhea could not be excluded as playing a role in the infant's anomalies.

BREAST FEEDING SUMMARY

RECOMMENDATION: Limited Human Data - Probably Compatible

The passage of atropine into breast milk is controversial (13). It has not been adequately documented whether measurable amounts are excreted or, if excretion does occur, whether it may affect the nursing infant. Although neonates are particularly sensitive to anticholinergic agents, no adverse effects have been reported in nursing infants whose mothers were taking atropine and the American Academy of Pediatrics classifies the agent as compatible with breast-feeding (14).

References

1. Nishimura H, Tanimura T. *Clinical Aspects of The Teratogenicity of Drugs*. New York, NY: American Elsevier, 1976:63.
2. Kivalo I, Saarikoski S. Placental transmission of atropine at full-term pregnancy. Br J Anaesth 1977;49:1017–21.
3. Kanto J, Virtanen R, Iisalo E, Maenpaa K, Liukko P. Placental transfer and pharmacokinetics of atropine after a single maternal intravenous and intramuscular administration. Acta Anaesth Scand 1981;25: 85–8.
4. Onnen I, Barrier G, d'Athis Ph, Sureau C, Olive G. Placental transfer of atropine at the end of pregnancy. Eur J Clin Pharmacol 1979;15:443–6.
5. Piper JM, Baum C, Kennedy DL, Price P. Maternal use of prescribed drugs associated with recognized fetal adverse drug reactions. Am J Obstet Gynecol 1988;159:1173–7.
6. Hellman LM, Fillisti LP. Analysis of the atropine test for placental transfer in gravidas with toxemia and diabetes. Am J Obstet Gynecol 1965;91:797–805.
7. Roodenburg PJ, Wladimiroff JW, Van Weering HK. Effect of maternal intravenous administration of atropine (0.5 mg) on fetal breathing and heart pattern. Contrib Gynecol Obstet 1979;6:92–7.
8. Heinonen OP, Slone D, Shapiro S. *Birth defects and drugs in pregnancy*. Littleton, MA: Publishing Sciences Group, 1977.
9. Diaz DM, Diaz SF, Marx GF. Cardiovascular effects of glycopyrrolate and belladonna derivatives in obstetric patients. Bull N Y Acad Med 1980;56: 245–8.
10. Roper RE, Salem MG. Effects of glycopyrrolate and atropine combined with antacid on gastric acidity. Br J Anaesth 1981;53:1277–80.
11. Abboud T, Raya J, Sadri S, Grobler N, Stine L, Miller F. Fetal and maternal cardiovascular effects of atropine and glycopyrrolate. Anesth Analg 1983;62: 426–30.
12. Siebert JR, Barr M Jr, Jackson JG, Benjamin DR. Ebstein's anomaly and extracardiac defects. Am J Dis Child 1989;143:570–2.
13. Stewart JJ. Gastrointestinal drugs. In Wilson JT, ed. *Drugs in Breast Milk*. (Balgowlah), Australia: ADIS Press, 1981:65–71.
14. Committee on Drugs, American Academy of Pediatrics. The transfer of drugs and other chemicals into human milk. Pediatrics 2001;108:776–89.

Name:	**AUROTHIOGLUCOSE**	Risk Factor:	C_M
Class:	**Immunologic Agent (Antirheumatic)**		

FETAL RISK SUMMARY

RECOMMENDATION: Limited Human Data - Animal Data Suggest Low Risk

Aurothioglucose is a sterile suspension administered by IM injection for the adjunctive treatment of early active rheumatoid arthritis. The manufacturer recommends against its use in pregnancy because of the potential nephrotoxicity of gold superimposed on the normal physiologic renal changes that occur in pregnancy (1).

Gold sodium thiomalate, administered by SC injection, is teratogenic in rats and rabbits (See Gold Sodium Thiomalate). The administration of oral gold to pregnant rabbits from days 6 through 18 of pregnancy, in doses that produced both maternal and embryo toxicity, also resulted in multiple congenital malformations (1). The malformations observed included abdominal wall defects (gastroschisis and umbilical hernia), anomalies of the brain, heart, lung, and skeleton, and microphthalmia.

See Gold Sodium Thiomalate for the clinical use of gold compounds in pregnant humans. If aurothioglucose is used in pregnancy for the treatment of rheumatoid arthritis, health care professionals are encouraged to call the toll free number (877-311-8972) for information about patient enrollment in the OTIS Rheumatoid Arthritis study.

BREAST FEEDING SUMMARY

RECOMMENDATION: Limited Human Data - Probably Compatible

See Gold Sodium Thiomalate.

Reference

1. Product information. Solganal. Schering, 2000.

Name:	**AZATADINE**	Risk Factor:	B_M
Class:	**Antihistamine**		

FETAL RISK SUMMARY

RECOMMENDATION: Limited Human Data - Animal Data Suggest Low Risk

Azatadine is not teratogenic in rats and rabbits given doses much higher than human doses (1). Published reports of exposure during human pregnancy have not been located. (See also Diphenhydramine for a representative agent in this class.)

In a surveillance study of Michigan Medicaid recipients conducted between 1985 and 1992, involving 229,101 completed pregnancies 127 newborns had been exposed to azatadine during the 1st trimester (F. Rosa, personal communication, FDA, 1993). A total of six (4.7%) major birth defects were observed (five expected). Among the six types of defects for which specific data were available, one oral cleft (none expected) and one limb reduction defect (none expected) were observed. No cases of cardiovascular defects, spina bifida, polydactyly, or hypospadias were reported. These data do not support an association between the drug and the defects.

BREAST FEEDING SUMMARY

RECOMMENDATION: No Human Data - Probably Compatible

No data are available.

Reference

1. Product information. Optimine. Schering Corporation, 1993.

Name:	**AZATHIOPRINE**	Risk Factor:	**D_M**
Class:	**Immunologic Agent (Immunosuppressant)**		

FETAL RISK SUMMARY

RECOMMENDATION: Human and Animal Data Suggest Risk

Azathioprine is used primarily in patients with organ transplants or in those with inflammatory bowel disease as an immunosuppressant. Prednisone is commonly combined with azathioprine in these patients. The drug readily crosses the placenta, and trace amounts of its active metabolite, 6-mercaptopurine, have been found in fetal blood (see also Mercaptopurine) (1).

Azathioprine is teratogenic in rabbits, producing limb reduction defects after small doses, but not in mice and rats (2). The manufacturer, however, has reproduction data on file indicating that azathioprine, in doses equivalent to the human dose (5 mg/kg/day), was teratogenic in both mice and rabbits (3). Malformations included skeletal defects and visceral anomalies.

In a surveillance study of Michigan Medicaid recipients conducted between 1985 and 1992, involving 229,101 completed pregnancies 7 newborns had been exposed to azathioprine during the 1st trimester (F. Rosa, personal communication, FDA, 1993). One (14.3%) major birth defect was observed (none expected), but information on the type of malformation is not available. No cases were observed in six defect categories, including cardiovascular defects, oral clefts, spina bifida, polydactyly, limb reduction defects, and hypospadias.

Most investigators have found azathioprine to be relatively safe in pregnancy (4–25). Several references have described the use of azathioprine during pregnancy in women who have received renal transplants (22,25–29), liver transplants (30–32), or a heart transplant (33). The drug has not been associated with congenital defects in these reports.

Sporadic anomalies have been reported but these are not believed to be related to the drug therapy (22,26). Defects observed include pulmonary valvular stenosis (34), preaxial polydactyly (thumb polydactyly type) (35), hypothyroidism and atrial septal defect (azathioprine therapy started in 2nd trimester) (36), hypospadias (mother also had severe diabetes mellitus) (19), plagiocephaly with neurologic damage (13), congenital heart disease (mild mitral regurgitation) (13), bilateral pes equinovarus (13), cerebral palsy (frontal hemangioma) and cerebral hemorrhage (died at 2 days of age) in twins (13), hypospadias (13), and congenital cytomegalovirus infection (13). The latter infection has also been reported in another infant whose mother was taking azathioprine (10). Chromosomal aberrations were noted in three infants after *in utero* exposure to the drug, but the relationship to azathioprine and the clinical significance of the findings are questionable (13,37).

Immunosuppression of the newborn was observed in one infant whose mother received 150 mg of azathioprine and 30 mg of prednisone daily throughout pregnancy (10). The suppression was characterized by lymphopenia, decreased survival of lymphocytes in culture, absence of immunoglobulin M, and reduced levels of immunoglobulin G. Recovery occurred at about 15 weeks of age. An infant exposed to 125 mg of azathioprine plus 12.5 mg of prednisone daily during pregnancy was born with pancytopenia and severe combined immune deficiency (38). The infant died at 28 days of complications brought on by irreversible bone marrow and lymphoid hypoplasia. To avoid neonatal leukopenia and thrombocytopenia, maternal doses of azathioprine were reduced during the 3rd trimester in a 1985 study (39). The investigators found a significant correlation between maternal leukocyte counts at 32 weeks' gestation and at delivery and cord blood leukocyte count. If the mother's count was at or below 1 SD for normal pregnancy, her dose of azathioprine was halved. Before this technique was used, several newborns had leukopenia and thrombocytopenia, but no low levels were measured after institution of the new procedure.

Intrauterine growth retardation may be related to the use of azathioprine in pregnancy. Based on animal experiments and analysis of human exposures, one investigator concluded that growth retardation was associated with the drug (40). Reports that are more recent have also supported this association (41). The incidence of small for gestational age infants from women who have undergone renal transplants and who are maintained on azathioprine and corticosteroids is approximately 20% (20,22), but some centers have rates as high as 40% (41). However, the effects of the underlying disease, including hypertension, vascular disease, and renal impairment, as well as the use of multiple medications other than azathioprine, cannot be excluded as major or sole contributors to the growth retardation.

Azathioprine has been reported to interfere with the effectiveness of intrauterine contraceptive devices (IUDs) (22,42). Two renal transplant patients, maintained on azathioprine and prednisone, received a copper IUD (Cu-7) and both became pregnant with the IUD in place (42). At another institution, 6 of 20 renal transplant patients have became pregnant with IUD devices in place (22). Because of these failures, additional or other methods of contraception should be considered in sexually active women receiving azathioprine and prednisone. If azathioprine is used in pregnancy for the treatment of rheumatoid arthritis, health care professionals are encouraged to call the toll free number (877-311-8972) for information about patient enrollment in the OTIS Rheumatoid Arthritis study.

BREAST FEEDING SUMMARY

RECOMMENDATION: No Human Data - Potential Toxicity

No data are available.

References

1. Sarrikoski S, Seppala M. Immunosuppression during pregnancy. Transmission of azathioprine and its metabolites from the mother to the fetus. Am J Obstet Gynecol 1973;115:1100–6.
2. Tuchmann-Duplessis H, Mercier-Parot L. Foetopathes therapeutiques: production experimentale de malformations des membres. Union Med Can 1968;97:283–8. As cited in Shepard TH. *Catalog of teratogenic agents,* 6th ed. Baltimore, MD: Johns Hopkins University Press, 1989:63.
3. Product information. Imuran. FARO Pharmaceuticals, 2000.

4. Gillibrand PN. Systemic lupus erythematosus in pregnancy treated with azathioprine. Proc R Soc Med 1966;59:834.
5. Board JA, Lee HM, Draper DA, Hume DM. Pregnancy following kidney homotransplantation from a non-twin: report of a case with concurrent administration of azathioprine and prednisone. Obstet Gynecol 1967;29:318–23.
6. Kaufmann JJ, Dignam W, Goodwin WE, Martin DC, Goldman R, Maxwell MH. Successful, normal childbirth after kidney homotransplantation. JAMA 1967;200:338–41.
7. Anonymous. Eleventh annual report of human renal transplant registry. JAMA 1973;216:1197.
8. Nolan GH, Sweet RL, Laros RK, Roure CA. Renal cadaver transplantation followed by successful pregnancies. Obstet Gynecol 1974;43:732–8.
9. Sharon E, Jones J, Diamond H, Kaplan D. Pregnancy and azathioprine in systemic lupus erythematosus. Am J Obstet Gynecol 1974;118:25–7.
10. Cote CJ, Meuwissen HJ, Pickering RJ. Effects on the neonate of prednisone and azathioprine administered to the mother during pregnancy. J Pediatr 1974;85:324–8.
11. Erkman J, Blythe JG. Azathioprine therapy complicated by pregnancy. Obstet Gynecol 1972;40:708–9.
12. Price HV, Salaman JR, Laurence KM, Langmaid H. Immunosuppressive drugs and the foetus. Transplantation 1976;21:294–8.
13. The Registration Committee of the European Dialysis and Transplant Association. Successful pregnancies in women treated by dialysis and kidney transplantation. Br J Obstet Gynaecol 1980;87:839–45.
14. Golby M. Fertility after renal transplantation. Transplantation 1930;10:201–7.
15. Rabau-Friedman E, Mashiach S, Cantor E, Jacob ET. Association of hypoparathyroidism and successful pregnancy in kidney transplant recipient. Obstet Gynecol 1982;59:126–8.
16. Myers RL, Schmid R, Newton JJ. Childbirth after liver transplantation. Transplantation 1980;29:432.
17. Williams PF, Johnstone M. Normal pregnancy in renal transplant recipient with history of eclampsia and intrauterine death. Br Med J 1982;285:1535.
18. Westney LS, Callender CO, Stevens J, Bhagwanani SG, George JPA, Mims OL. Successful pregnancy with sickle cell disease and renal transplantation. Obstet Gynecol 1984;63:752–5.
19. Ogburn PL Jr, Kitzmiller JL, Hare JW, Phillippe M, Gabbe SG, Miodovnik M, Tagatz GE, Nagel TC, Williams PP, Goetz FC, Barbosa JJ, Sutherland DE. Pregnancy following renal transplantation in class T diabetes mellitus. JAMA 1986;255:911–5.
20. Marushak A, Weber T, Bock J, Birkeland SA, Hansen HE, Klebe J, Kristoffersen K, Rasmussen K, Olgaard K. Pregnancy following kidney transplantation. Acta Obstet Gynecol Scand 1986;65:557–9.
21. Key TC, Resnik R, Dittrich HC, Reisner LS. Successful pregnancy after cardiac transplantation. Am J Obstet Gynecol 1989;160:367–71.
22. Davison JM, Lindheimer MD. Pregnancy in renal transplant recipients. J Reprod Med 1982;27:613–21.
23. Symington GR, Mackay IR, Lambert RP. Cancer and teratogenesis: infrequent occurrence after medical use of immunosuppressive drugs. Aust NZ J Med 1977;7:368–72.
24. Alstead EM, Ritchie JK, Lennard-Jones JE, Farthing MJG, Clark ML. Safety of azathioprine in pregnancy in inflammatory bowel disease. Gastroenterology 1990;99:443–6.
25. Haugen G, Fauchald P, Sødal G, Halvorsen S, Oldereid N, Moe N. Pregnancy outcome in renal allograft recipients: influence of ciclosporin A. Eur J Obstet Gynecol Reprod Biol 1991;39:25–9.
26. Kossoy LR, Herbert CM III, Wentz AC. Management of heart transplant recipients: guidelines for the obstetrician-gynecologist. Am J Obstet Gynecol 1988;159:490–9.
27. Cararach V, Carmona F, Monleón FJ, Andreu J. Pregnancy after renal transplantation: 25 years experience in Spain. Br J Obstet Gynaecol 1993;100:122–5.
28. Sturgiss SN, Davison JM. Perinatal outcome in renal allograft recipients: prognostic significance of hypertension and renal function before and during pregnancy. Obstet Gynecol 1991;78:573–7.
29. Sturgiss SN, Davison JM. Effect of pregnancy on long-term function of renal allografts. Am J Kidney Dis 1992;19:167–72.
30. Laifer SA, Darby MJ, Scantlebury VP, Harger JH, Caritis SN. Pregnancy and liver transplantation. Obstet Gynecol 1990;76:1083–8.
31. Zaballos J, Perez-Cerda F, Riao D, Davila P, Martinez P, Sevillano A, Garcia I, de Andres A, Moreno E. Anesthetic management of liver transplantation in a pregnant patient with fulminant hepatitis. Transplant Proc 1991;23:1994–5.
32. Ville Y, Fernandez H, Samuel D, Bismuth H, Frydman R. Pregnancy in liver transplant recipients: course and outcome in 19 cases. Am J Obstet Gynecol 1993;168:896–902.
33. Kirk EP. Organ transplantation and pregnancy. A case report and review. Am J Obstet Gynecol 1991;164:1629–34.
34. Nishimura H, Tanimura T. *Clinical Aspects of The Teratogenicity of Drugs*. New York, NY: American Elsevier, 1976:106–7.
35. Williamson RA, Karp LE. Azathioprine teratogenicity: review of the literature and case report. Obstet Gynecol 1981;58:247–50.
36. Burleson RL, Sunderji SG, Aubry RH, Clark DA, Marbarger P, Cohen RS, Scruggs BF, Lagraff S. Renal allotransplantation during pregnancy. Successful outcome for mother, child, and kidney. Transplantation 1983;36:334.
37. Leb DE, Weisskopf B, Kanovitz BS. Chromosome aberrations in the child of a kidney transplant recipient. Arch Intern Med 1971;128:441–4.
38. DeWitte DB, Buick MK, Cyran SE, Maisels MJ. Neonatal pancytopenia and severe combined immunodeficiency associated with antenatal administration of azathioprine and prednisone. J Pediatr 1984;105:625–8.
39. Davison JM, Dellagrammatikas H, Parkin JM. Maternal azathioprine therapy and depressed haemopoiesis in the babies of renal allograft patients. Br J Obstet Gynaecol 1985;92:233–9.
40. Scott JR. Fetal growth retardation associated with maternal administration of immunosuppressive drugs. Am J Obstet Gynecol 1977;128:668–76.

41. Pirson Y, Van Lierde M, Ghysen J, Squifflet JP, Alexandre GPJ, van Ypersele De Strihou C. Retardation of fetal growth in patients receiving immunosuppressive therapy. N Engl J Med 1985;313:328.

42. Zerner J, Doil KL, Drewry J, Leeber DA. Intrauterine contraceptive device failures in renal transplant patients. J Reprod Med 1981;26:99–102.

Name:	**AZELASTINE**	Risk Factor:	**C_M**
Class:	**Antihistamine**		

FETAL RISK SUMMARY

RECOMMENDATION: No Human Data - Animal Data Suggest Low Risk

The antihistamine azelastine is formulated for intranasal and ophthalmic administration. It is a phthalazinone derivative that has histamine H_1-receptor antagonist activity. Azelastine nasal spray is indicated for the treatment of the symptoms of seasonal allergic rhinitis such as rhinorrhea, sneezing, and nasal pruritus, and for the treatment of the symptoms of vasomotor rhinitis, such as rhinorrhea, nasal congestion, and postnasal drip (1). The ophthalmic preparation is indicated for the treatment of itching of the eye associated with allergic conjunctivitis (2).

The systemic bioavailability, after nasal administration, is 40% with peak plasma concentrations obtained in 2–3 hours (1). In contrast, very small amounts are absorbed after ophthalmic administration (2). The plasma concentrations of the major active metabolite desmethylazelastine range from 20–50% of the parent drug concentrations (1). The elimination half-life of azelastine and the active metabolite are 22 and 54 hours, respectively.

Reproduction studies have been conducted in mice, rats, and rabbits. In pregnant mice, an oral dose about 280 times the maximum recommended daily intranasal dose in adults based on body surface area (MRDID) caused embryo-fetal death, malformations (cleft palate; short or absent tail; fused, absent, or branched ribs), delayed ossification, and decreased fetal weight. However, the dose also was maternal toxic (decreased weight). Neither maternal nor fetal toxicity were noted at a dose 10 times the MRDID (1). In rats, a dose about 240 times the MRDID was not maternal toxic but did cause fetal malformations (oligo- and brachydactylia), and delayed and skeletal variations. A maternal toxic dose (560 times the MRDID) resulted in embryo-fetal death and decreased fetal weight. A dose 25 times the MRDID caused no toxicity in the mother or fetus (1,3). In rabbits, doses greater than 500 times the MRDID caused severe maternal toxicity and resulted in abortions, delayed ossification, and reduced fetal weight. Neither maternal nor fetal adverse effects were observed with a dose 5 times the MRDID (1,3). In peri- and postnatal studies with rats, doses 25–240 times the MRDID were not associated with toxicity in the pups in terms of physical growth, reflexive behavior, activity, motor coordination, learning, and reproductive performance (3).

No carcinogenic effects in mice and rats were observed in 2-year studies at doses 100 and 240 times the MRDID, respectively. In addition, studies with azelastine for genotoxicity also were negative, as were fertility tests in rats at 240 times the MRDID (1).

It is not known if azelastine crosses the human placenta. The molecular weight (about 382 for the free base) and prolonged elimination half-life suggest that the drug could cross to the embryo and fetus. However, the low systemic concentrations of the parent drug and major active metabolite suggest that the amount available at the maternal:fetal interface will be clinically insignificant.

A

No reports describing the use of azelastine in human pregnancy have been located. The animal data suggest that the risk to the embryo-fetus is low. Moreover, the systemic bioavailability of the antihistamine after intranasal administration is only 40% and it is much lower after ocular administration. Nevertheless, the complete absence of human pregnancy experience prevents a full assessment of the risk. A 2000 review of the use of newer asthma and allergy medications in pregnancy stated that, based on the animal studies, there were better choices available than azelastine (4).

BREAST FEEDING SUMMARY

RECOMMENDATION: No Human Data - Probably Compatible

No reports describing the use of azelastine during human lactation have been located. The relative low molecular weight (about 382 for the free base) and the prolonged elimination half lifes of the parent drug and major active metabolite suggest that the drugs will be excreted into breast milk. However, the systemic bioavailability after intranasal administration is only 40% and it is much lower after ocular administration. Therefore, it is doubtful if clinically significant amounts will be excreted into milk.

References

1. Product information. Astelin. MedPointe Pharmaceuticals, 2004.
2. Product information. Optivar. MedPointe Pharmaceuticals, 2004.
3. Suzuki Y, Okada F, Mikami T, Goto M, Hasegawa H, Chiba T. Teratology and reproduction studies of azelastine, a novel antiallergic agent, in rats and rabbits. Arzneimittelforschung 1981;31:1225–30.
4. Joint Committee of the American College of Obstetricians and Gynecologists (ACOG) and the American College of Allergy, Asthma and Immunology (ACAAI). The use of newer asthma and allergy medications during pregnancy. Ann Allergy Asthma Immunol 2000;84:475–80.

Name: **AZITHROMYCIN** Risk Factor: B_M

Class: **Antibiotic**

FETAL RISK SUMMARY

RECOMMENDATION: Limited Human Data - Animal Data Suggest Low Risk

Azithromycin, an azalide antibiotic that is categorized as a member of the macrolides, is derived from erythromycin. Animal studies using mice and rats treated with doses up to maternal toxic levels revealed no impairment of fertility or harm to the fetus (1).

Azithromycin crosses the human placenta at term (2,3). In 20 women scheduled for elective cesarean section, a single 1-g oral dose of azithromycin was given 6 ($N = 2$), 12 ($N = 7$), 24 ($N = 5$), 72 ($N = 5$), or 168 ($N = 1$) hours before delivery. The mean maternal concentrations at delivery for the five groups were 311, 144, 63, 60, and <10 ng/mL, respectively, whereas the corresponding mean cord serum levels were 19, 26, 27, 19, and <10 ng/mL, respectively. Cerebrospinal fluid levels in the mothers (all had spinal anesthesia) were undetectable (<16 ng/mL) in each group.

In an *ex vivo* experiment with term human placentas utilizing a single placental cotyledon model, the mean transplacental transfer of three macrolide antibiotics (azithromycin, erythromycin, and roxithromycin) were 2.6%, 3.0%, and 4.3%, respectively (3). The percentages were calculated as the ratio between the steady state level in fetal venous and maternal arterial sides (3).

A number of reports have described the use of azithromycin in human pregnancy, but in only one of the studies (11) was the drug used early in gestation (4–11). A 1994 abstract reported that 16 pregnant patients with cervicitis caused by *chlamydia* had been treated with a single 1-g oral dose of the antibiotic in a comparison trial with erythromycin (4). Fifteen of the women had negative tests for *chlamydia* after treatment. No data were given on gestational age at the time of treatment or on the pregnancy outcomes. In a second, similar report, also comparing efficacy with erythromycin, 15 pregnant women with chlamydial cervicitis were treated with a single 1-g oral dose (5). All of the women had negative cervical swabs for *chlamydia* as analyzed by direct DNA assay 14 days after the dose. Three more recent reports have also documented the efficacy of azithromycin in the treatment of pregnant women with *chlamydia* (6–8). Of the five reports, only the last study (8) indicated the gestational age at treatment (about 24 weeks'), but none provided information on fetal outcome. In contrast to the effectiveness of azithromycin for *chlamydia* infections, a single 1-g oral dose of the antibiotic was ineffective in reducing lower genital colonization with *ureaplasma* in pregnant women between 22 and 34 weeks' gestation with ruptured membranes or preterm labor (9). Two women with scrub typhus (tsutsugamushi disease) in the 2nd trimester were treated successfully with 3-day courses of azithromycin (10). Both delivered healthy infants.

A 1998 non-interventional observational cohort study described the outcomes of pregnancies in women who had been prescribed one or more of 34 newly marketed drugs by general practitioners in England (11). Data were obtained by questionnaires sent to the prescribing physicians one month after the expected or possible date of delivery. In 831 (78%) of the pregnancies, a newly marketed drug was thought to have been taken during the 1st trimester, with birth defects were noted in 14 (2.5%) singleton births of the 557 newborns (10 sets of twins). In addition, two birth defects were observed in aborted fetuses. However, few of the aborted fetuses were examined. Azithromycin was taken during the 1st trimester in 11 pregnancies. The outcomes of these pregnancies were 1 elective abortion and 10 normal, term babies (11).

Although no congenital malformations were observed in the above study, the data are too limited to assess the safety of azithromycin. Moreover, the study lacked sensitivity to identify minor anomalies because of the absence of standardized examinations. Late appearing major defects may also have been missed due to the timing of the questionnaires. However, macrolide antibiotics are not considered to be major human teratogens.

BREAST FEEDING SUMMARY

RECOMMENDATION: Limited Human Data - Probably Compatible

Azithromycin accumulates in breast milk (12). A woman, in the 1st week after a term vaginal delivery, was treated with a single 1-g oral dose of azithromycin for a wound infection following a bilateral tubal ligation and then, because of worsening symptoms, given 48 hours of IV gentamicin and clindamycin. She was discharged from the hospital on a 5-day course of azithromycin, 500 mg daily, but only took three doses because she wanted to resume breast-feeding that had been stopped during azithromycin therapy. The patient continued pumping her breasts during this time to maintain milk flow and resumed breast-feeding 24 hours after the third dose of the antibiotic. Drug doses and approximate time from the first dose were 1 g (0 hours), 500 mg (59 hours), 500 mg (83 hours), and

500 mg (107 hours). Milk concentrations of azithromycin and times from the first dose were 0.64 μg/mL (48 hours), 1.3 μg/mL (60 hours), and 2.8 μg/mL (137 hours) (maternal serum concentrations were not determined). The authors attributed the antibiotic's milk accumulation to its lipid solubility and ion trapping of a weak base (12).

References

1. Product information. Zithromax. Pfizer Labs, 1994.
2. Ramsey PS, Vaules MB, Vasdev GM, Andrews WW, Ramin KD. Maternal and transplacental pharmacokinetics of azithromycin. Am J Obstet Gynecol 2003;188:714–8.
3. Heikkinen T, Laine K, Neuvonen PJ, Ekblad U. The transplacental transfer of the macrolide antibiotics erythromycin, roxithromycin and azithromycin. Br J Obstet Gynaecol 2000;107:770–5.
4. Edwards M, Rainwater K, Carter S, Williamson F, Newman R. Comparison of azithromycin and erythromycin, for *Chlamydia cervicitis* in pregnancy (abstract). Am J Obstet Gynecol 1994;170:419.
5. Bush MR, Rosa C. Azithromycin and erythromycin in the treatment of cervical chlamydial infection during pregnancy. Obstet Gynecol 1994;84:61–3.
6. Rosenn M, Macones GA, Silverman N. A randomized trial of erythromycin and azithromycin for the treatment of chlamydia infection in pregnancy (abstract). Am J Obstet Gynecol 1996;174:410.
7. Wehbeh H, Ruggiero R, Ali Y, Lopez G, Shahem S, Zarou D. A randomized clinical trial of a single dose of zithromycin in the treatment of chlamydia among pregnant women (abstract). Am J Obstet Gynecol 1996;174:361.
8. Wehbeh HA, Ruggeirio RM, Shahem S, Lopez G, Ali Y. Single-dose azithromycin for chlamydia in pregnant women. J Reprod Med 1998;43:509–14.
9. Ogasawara KK, Goodwin TM. Efficacy of azithromycin in reducing lower genital ureaplasma colonization in women at risk for preterm delivery (abstract). Am J Obstet Gynecol 1997;176:S57.
10. Choi EK, Pai H. Azithromycin therapy for scrub typhus during pregnancy. Clin Infect Dis 1998;27:1538–9.
11. Wilton LV, Pearce GL, Martin RM, Mackay FJ, Mann RD. The outcomes of pregnancy in women exposed to newly marketed drugs in general practice in England. Br J Obstet Gynaecol 1998;105:882–9.
12. Kelsey JJ, Moser LR, Jennings JC, Munger MA. Presence of azithromycin breast milk concentrations: a case report. Am J Obstet Gynecol 1994;170:1375–6.

Name:	**AZTREONAM**	Risk Factor:	**B_M**
Class:	**Antibiotic**		

FETAL RISK SUMMARY

RECOMMENDATION: No Human Data - Animal Data Suggest Low Risk

Aztreonam is a synthetic, monocyclic β-lactam antibiotic that is structurally different from other β-lactam antibiotics, such as the penicillins and cephalosporins. Administration of high IV doses of the drug to pregnant rats (15 times the maximum recommended human dose [MRHD] and rabbits (5 times the MRHD) did not produce embryotoxic, fetotoxic, or teratogenic effects (1–5).

Single 1-g IV doses of aztreonam administered 2 to 8 hours before elective termination produced detectable concentrations of the antibiotic in fetal serum and amniotic fluid (6). No reports describing the therapeutic use of the antibiotic in human pregnancy have been located.

BREAST FEEDING SUMMARY

RECOMMENDATION: Limited Human Data - Probably Compatible

Aztreonam is excreted into breast milk (7). Twelve lactating women received a single 1-g dose of the antibiotic either by IM injection ($N = 6$) or by the IV route ($N = 6$). Infants were not allowed to breast-feed during the study. Milk and serum samples were collected at scheduled intervals for 8 hours after the dose. In the IM group, the mean peak milk concentration was estimated to be 0.3 μg/mL, corresponding to a milk:serum ratio of 0.007. Similar calculations for the IV group yielded a peak value of 0.2 μg/mL and a ratio of 0.002. The low milk concentrations measured in the study were compatible with the acidic nature of the drug and its very low lipid solubility (7). These data, combined with the poor oral absorption of the antibiotic, indicate that direct systemic effects from the antibiotic in nursing infants are unlikely (7). The American Academy of Pediatrics classifies aztreonam as compatible with breast-feeding (8).

References

1. Furuhashi T, Kato I, Igarashi Y, Nakayoshi H. Toxicity study of azthreonam. fertility study in rats. Chemotherapy 1985;33:190–202. As cited in Shepard TH. *Catalog of teratogenic agents,* 6th ed. Baltimore, MD. Johns Hopkins University Press, 1989:66.
2. Furuhashi T, Ushida K, Sato K, Nakayoshi H. Toxicity study on azthreonam: Teratology study in rats. Chemotherapy 1985;33:203–18. As cited in Shepard TH. *Catalog of teratogenic agents,* 6th ed. Baltimore, MD: Johns Hopkins University Press, 1989:66.
3. Furuhashi T, Ushida K, Kakei A, Nakayoshi H. Toxicity study on azthreonam: Perinatal and postnatal study in rats. Chemotherapy 1985;33:219–31. As cited in Shepard TH. *Catalog of teratogenic agents,* 6th ed. Baltimore, MD: Johns Hopkins University Press, 1989:66.
4. Singhvi SM, Ita CE, Shaw JM, Keim GR, Migdalof BH. Distribution of aztreonam into fetuses and milk of rats. Antimicrob Agents Chemother 1984;26:132–5.
5. Product information. Azactam. E. R. Squibb & Sons, 1994.
6. Hayashi R, Devlin RG, Frantz M, Stern M. Concentration of aztreonam in body fluids in mid-pregnancy (abstract). Clin Pharmacol Ther 1984,35:246.
7. Fleiss PM, Richwald GA, Gordon J, Stern M, Frantz M, Devlin RG. Aztreonam in human serum and breast milk. Br J Clin Pharmacol 1985;19:509–11.
8. Committee on Drugs, American Academy of Pediatrics. The transfer of drugs and other chemicals into human milk. Pediatrics 2001;108:776–89.

B

Name:	**BACAMPICILLIN**	Risk Factor:	B_M
Class:	**Antibiotic (Penicillin)**		

FETAL RISK SUMMARY

RECOMMENDATION: Compatible

Bacampicillin, a penicillin antibiotic, is converted to ampicillin during absorption from the gastrointestinal tract (see Ampicillin for use in human pregnancy).

Reproduction studies have been conducted with bacampicillin in mice and rats at doses up to greater than 25 times the recommended human dose based on body weight (1). No evidence of impaired fertility or fetal harm was found.

In a surveillance study of Michigan Medicaid recipients conducted between 1985 and 1992 involving 229,101 completed pregnancies, 30 newborns had been exposed to bacampicillin during the 1st trimester (F. Rosa, personal communication, FDA, 1993). Two (6.7%) major birth defects were observed (one expected). Specific information on the defects was not available, but no anomalies were observed in six categories (cardiovascular defects, oral clefts, spina bifida, polydactyly, limb reduction defects, and hypospadias). The number of exposures is too small to draw any conclusions.

BREAST FEEDING SUMMARY

RECOMMENDATION: Compatible

See Ampicillin.

Reference

1. Product information. Spectrobid. Pfizer, 2000.

Name:	**BACITRACIN**	Risk Factor:	C
Class:	**Antibiotic**		

FETAL RISK SUMMARY

RECOMMENDATION: Compatible (Topical)

No reports linking the use of bacitracin with congenital defects have been located. The drug is primarily used topically, although the injectable form is available. One study listed 18 patients exposed to the drug in the 1st trimester (1). The route of administration was not specified. No association with malformations was found.

B

BREAST FEEDING SUMMARY

RECOMMENDATION: Compatible (Topical)

No data are available.

Reference

1. Heinonen OP, Slone D, Shapiro S. *Birth Defects and Drugs in Pregnancy*. Littleton, MA: Publishing Sciences Group, 1977:297, 301.

Name:	**BACLOFEN**	Risk Factor:	**C**
Class:	**Muscle Relaxant**		

FETAL RISK SUMMARY

RECOMMENDATION: Limited Human Data - Animal Data Suggest Low Risk

Only two reports have been located that describe the use of the muscle relaxant, baclofen, in human pregnancy. Because of its specialized indication to control spasticity secondary to multiple sclerosis and other spinal cord diseases and injuries, its use in pregnancy is anticipated to be limited.

When baclofen doses 7–13 times the recommended human dose were administered to pregnant rats and rabbits, increased incidences of omphalocele and incomplete sternebral ossification were observed in rat fetuses and an increased incidence of unossified phalangeal nuclei of the fetal limbs was noted in rabbits (1). Shepard reviewed three studies involving rats, mice, and rabbits in which the drug was administered during organogenesis, and all reported negative teratogenic findings (2). In contrast, a 1995 study in pregnant rats using 30 or 60 mg/kg on day 10 of gestation observed vertebral arch widening at the lower dose, similar to that produced by valproic acid in rats (3). The author concluded that baclofen could produce spina bifida or other neural tube defects in rats. Interestingly, the 60-mg/kg dose did not produce this effect, causing speculation that the dose caused a greater severity of neural tube defects, and thus a greater number of unrecorded early fetal deaths (3).

Two reports, involving three pregnancies, have been located that describe the use of baclofen in pregnant humans (4,5). A 29-year-old woman with quadriplegia due to an incomplete cervical C6–7 spinal cord lesion following discitis after discography was treated with a continuous intrathecal infusion of baclofen (1000 μg/24 hours) for 15 months to control her intractable spasticity (4). Conception occurred after ovulation stimulation with clomiphene. The baclofen dose was gradually increased to 1200 μg/24 hours to maintain control of her spasticity as the pregnancy progressed. Because of severe symptoms of autonomic dysfunction and loss of spasticity control (even at 1400 μg/24 hours), a cesarean section was conducted under epidural bupivacaine anaesthesia in the 35th week of gestation. A 2040-g, healthy female infant was delivered with Apgar scores of 9 and 10 (timing not specified).

A second case report, similar to the one above, was published in 2000 (5). A 38-year-old woman became pregnant after approximately 3.5 years of continuous intrathecal

B

baclofen infusion to control severe spasticity resulting from a complete fifth cervical vertebra (C5)-level medullar injury. Good control of her spasticity was obtained with intrathecal baclofen (140 μg/day) throughout her pregnancy. A healthy, 2155-g, male infant was delivered by cesarean section at 36 weeks' gestation with Apgar scores of 9 and 10 at one and five minutes, respectively. The birth weight, length (47 cm), and head circumference (33 cm) were appropriate for gestational age (5). No major or minor malformations were noted on physical and ultrasonography examinations and the child was developing normally at 24 months of age. Three months after delivery of her first infant, the woman became pregnant a second time and again received continuous intrathecal baclofen (140 μg/day) throughout the gestation. A repeat cesarean section was performed at 34 weeks' gestation with delivery of another healthy, 2240-g, male infant with Apgar scores of 8 and 10 at one and five minutes, respectively. The weight, length (46 cm), and head circumference (32 cm) were appropriate for gestational age. No abnormalities were noted in the infant and he was developing normally at 12 months of age (5).

BREAST FEEDING SUMMARY

RECOMMENDATION: Limited Human Data - Probably Compatible

In an animal study, the γ-aminobutyric acid agonist, baclofen, was a potent inhibitor of suckling-induced prolactin release from the anterior pituitary (6). The drug had no effect on milk ejection. Because prolactin release is required to maintain lactation, the potential for decreased milk production with chronic use may exist. However, no human studies on this topic have been located.

Small amounts of baclofen are excreted into human milk. A 20-year-old woman with spastic paraplegia, who was 14 days postpartum, was given a single 20-mg (94 μmol) dose of baclofen (7). No mention was made as to whether her infant was nursing. Serum samples were drawn at 1, 3, 6, and 20 hours after the dose, and milk samples were obtained at 2, 4, 8, 14, 20, and 26 hours. The highest serum concentration measured, 1.419 μmol/L, occurred at 3 hours, whereas the highest milk level, 0.608 μmol/L, was obtained at 4 hours. The total amount of drug recovered from the milk during the 26-hour sampling period was 22 μg (0.10 μmol), or about 0.1% of the mother's dose. The authors speculated that this amount would not lead to toxic levels in a nursing infant (7). The American Academy of Pediatrics classifies baclofen as compatible with breast-feeding (8).

References

1. Product information. Lioresal. Geigy Pharmaceuticals, 1993.
2. Shepard TH. *Catalog of Teratogenic Agents*. 6th ed. Baltimore, MD: Johns Hopkins University Press, 1989: 66.
3. Briner W. Muscimol- and baclofen-induced spina bifida in the rat. Med Sci Res 1995;24:639–40.
4. Delhaas EM, Verhagen J. Pregnancy in a quadriplegic patient treated with continuous intrathecal baclofen infusion to manage her severe spasticity. Case report. Paraplegia 1992;30:527–8.
5. Munoz FC, Marco DG, Perez AV, Camacho MM. Pregnancy outcome in a woman exposed to continuous intrathecal baclofen infusion. Ann Pharmacother 2000;34:956.
6. Lux VA, Somoza GM, Libertun C. Beta-(-4 chlorophenyl) GABA (baclofen) inhibits prolactin and thyrotropin release by acting on the rat brain. Proc Soc Exp Biol Med 1986;183:358–62.
7. Eriksson G, Swahn C-G. Concentrations of baclofen in serum and breast milk from a lactating woman. Scand J Clin Lab Invest 1981;41:185–7.
8. Committee on Drugs, American Academy of Pediatrics. The transfer of drugs and other chemicals into human milk. Pediatrics 2001;108:776–89.

Name:	**BALSALAZIDE**	Risk Factor:	B_M
Class:	**Anti-inflammatory Bowel Disease Agent**		

B

FETAL RISK SUMMARY

RECOMMENDATION: No Human Data - Animal Data Suggest Low Risk

The oral prodrug balsalazide is enzymatically cleaved in the colon to produce mesalamine (5-aminosalicylic acid) (see also Mesalamine). It is indicated for the treatment of mildly to moderately active ulcerative colitis. A very small portion of a balsalazide dose is absorbed intact into the systemic circulation where it is extensively (≥99%) protein bound.

Reproduction studies have been conducted in rats and rabbits. In pregnant rats and rabbits, doses up to 2.4 and 4.7 times the recommended human dose based on body surface area, respectively, revealed no evidence of impaired fertility or fetal harm (1). In addition, studies with mesalamine in these species did not observe fetal toxicity or teratogenicity (see Mesalamine).

It is not known if balsalazide crosses the human placenta. The molecular weight (about 437) is low enough but the very small amounts in the plasma and extensive plasma protein binding suggest that little if any drug crosses to the embryo/fetus. Moreover, only small amounts of mesalamine are absorbed into the systemic circulation and then are rapidly excreted in the urine.

No reports describing the use of balsalazide in human pregnancy have been located. The animal data do not suggest a major risk but the doses used were close to those used in humans. However, mesalamine is the primary active drug produced by metabolism of balsalazide and it has not been associated, except for one unconfirmed report, with adverse fetal effects. Moreover, a 2002 review concluded that mesalamine is safe to use during pregnancy (2). Therefore, the maternal benefits of balsalazide appear to outweigh the unknown risks to the fetus.

BREAST FEEDING SUMMARY

RECOMMENDATION: No Human Data - Potential Toxicity

No reports describing the use of the prodrug balsalazide during human lactation have been located. Only small amounts of balsalazide and its active metabolite mesalamine are absorbed into the systemic circulation. Moreover, the parent drug is extensively (≥99%) bound to plasma proteins. A 2002 review concluded that mesalamine was safe to use by nursing mothers (2). However, a possible allergic reaction (diarrhea) was observed in a nursing infant whose mother was using mesalamine rectal suppositories. Because of this adverse effect, nursing infants should be closely observed for changes in bowel function if the mother is taking balsalazide.

References

1. Product information. Colazal. Salix Pharmaceuticals, 2004.
2. Schroeder KW. Role of mesalazine in acute and long-term treatment of ulcerative colitis and its complications. Scand J Gastroentrol Suppl 2002;236: 42–7.

B

Name: **BECLOMETHASONE** Risk Factor: C_M
Class: **Corticosteroid**

FETAL RISK SUMMARY

RECOMMENDATION: Compatible

Beclomethasone dipropionate is given by inhalation for the chronic treatment of bronchial asthma in patients requiring corticosteroid therapy for the control of symptoms. It is also available for intranasal use and, outside of the United States, for topical application.

Beclomethasone was embryocidal (increased fetal resorption) and teratogenic when administered by SC injection to mice and rabbits at approximately 10 times the human dose (1,2). Congenital malformations observed included cleft palate, agnathia, microstomia, absence of the tongue, delayed ossification, and agenesis of the thymus. Similar toxic effects in both species were observed with SC injections that were approximately one-half the maximum recommended adult daily inhalation dose based on body surface area (3). In the rat, no embryo or fetal harm was found with inhaled (at 10 times the human dose) or oral (at 1000 times the human dose) beclomethasone (1,2).

No human reports associating the use of beclomethasone with human congenital anomalies have been found. A 1975 report briefly mentioned seven healthy babies born from mothers who had used beclomethasone aerosol for over 6 months (4). In another report, beclomethasone was used during 45 pregnancies in 40 women (5). Dosage ranged between 4 and 16 inhalations/day (mean 9.5), with each inhalation delivering 42 μg of drug. Three of the 33 prospectively studied pregnancies ended in abortion that was not thought to be caused by the maternal asthma. Forty-three living infants resulted from the remaining 42 pregnancies. Six infants had low birth weights, including two of the three premature newborns (less than 37 weeks' gestation). There was no evidence of neonatal adrenal insufficiency. One full-term infant had cardiac malformations (double ventricular septal defect, patent ductus arteriosus, and subaortic stenosis). However, the mother's asthma was also treated with prednisone, theophylline, and epinephrine. In addition, she had schizophrenia and diabetes mellitus for which she took fluphenazine and insulin. Cardiac malformations are known to occur with diabetes mellitus (see Insulin).

In a surveillance study of Michigan Medicaid recipients conducted between 1985 and 1992 involving 229,101 completed pregnancies, 395 newborns had been exposed to beclomethasone during the 1st trimester (F. Rosa, personal communication, FDA, 1993). A total of 16 (4.1%) major birth defects were observed (16 expected). Specific information was not available on the defects, but no anomalies were observed in six categories (cardiovascular defects, oral clefts, spina bifida, polydactyly, limb reduction defects, and hypospadias). These data do not support an association between the drug and congenital defects.

A 2004 prospective, double-blind, double placebo-controlled, randomized study compared inhaled beclomethasone (194 women) to theophylline (191 women) for the treatment of moderate asthma during pregnancy (6). The mean gestational age at randomization was about 20 weeks' in both groups. There was no significant difference in the rate of asthma exacerbations between the groups, but significantly fewer discontinued beclomethasone because of adverse effects. There also were no differences in maternal or perinatal outcomes (6).

In a position statement from a joint committee of the American College of Obstetricians (ACOG) and the American College of Allergy, Asthma, and Immunology (ACAAI) published in 2000, either beclomethasone or budesonide were considered the inhaled steroids of choice for use during pregnancy (7).

BREAST FEEDING SUMMARY

RECOMMENDATION: Limited Human Data - Probably Compatible

It is not known whether beclomethasone is excreted into breast milk. Other corticosteroids are excreted into milk in low concentrations (see Prednisone) and the passage of beclomethasone into milk should be expected. One report has been located that notes three cases of maternal beclomethasone use during breast-feeding (4). Effects on the nursing infants were not mentioned.

References

1. Product information. Beconase. Glaxo Wellcome, 2000.
2. Product information. Vancenase; Vanceril. Schering, 2000.
3. Product information. Beclovent. Glaxo Wellcome, 2000.
4. Brown HM, Storey G. Treatment of allergy of the respiratory tract with beclomethasone dipropionate steroid aerosol. Postgrad Med J 1975;51(Suppl 4):59–64.
5. Greenberger PA, Patterson R. Beclomethasone dipropionate for severe asthma during pregnancy. Ann Intern Med 1983;98.478–80.
6. Dombrowski MP, Schatz M, Wise R, Thom EA, Landon M, Mabie W, Newman RB, McNellis D, Hauth JC, Lindheimer M, Caritis SN, Leveno KJ, Meis P, Miodovnik M, Wapner RJ, Varner MW, O'Sullivan MJ, Conway DL, for the National Institute of Child Health and Human Development Maternal-Fetal Medicine Units Network, and the National Heart, Lung, and Blood Institute. Randomized trial of inhaled beclomethasone dipropionate versus theophylline for moderate asthma during pregnancy. Am J Obstet Gynecol 2004;190:737–44.
7. Joint Committee of the American College of Obstetricians (ACOG) and the American College of Allergy, Asthma, and Immunology (ACAAI). Position statement. The use of newer asthma and allergy medications during pregnancy. Ann Allergy Asthma Immunol 2000;84:475–80.

Name:	**BELLADONNA**	Risk Factor:	**C**
Class:	**Parasympatholytic**		

FETAL RISK SUMMARY

RECOMMENDATION: Limited Human Data - No Relevant Animal Data

Belladonna is an anticholinergic agent. The Collaborative Perinatal Project monitored 50,282 mother-child pairs, 554 of whom used belladonna in the 1st trimester (1, pp. 346–353). Belladonna was found to be associated with malformations in general and with minor malformations. Specifically, increased risks (standardized relative risk greater than 1.5) were observed for respiratory tract anomalies, hypospadias, and eye and ear malformations. The association between belladonna and eye and ear malformations was statistically significant. Interpretation of these data is difficult, however, because the authors of the study emphasized that even though some agents had elevated risks and significant associations did occur, a cause-and-effect relationship could not be inferred. For use anytime during pregnancy, 1355 exposures were recorded (1, p. 439). No association was found in this group.

B

BREAST FEEDING SUMMARY

RECOMMENDATION: No Human Data - Probably Compatible

See Atropine.

Reference

1. Heinonen OP, Slone D, Shapiro S. *Birth Defects and Drugs in Pregnancy*. Littleton, MA: Publishing Sciences Group, 1977.

Name:	**BENAZEPRIL**	Risk Factor:	$\mathbf{C_M}$*
Class:	**Antihypertensive**		

FETAL RISK SUMMARY

RECOMMENDATION: Human Data Suggest Risk in 2nd and 3rd Trimesters

Benazepril is an angiotensin-converting enzyme (ACE) inhibitor. It is indicated for the treatment of hypertension. The molecular weight of the free base is about 425.

Reproduction studies have been conducted in mice, rats, and rabbits. No teratogenic effects were observed at doses that were 9, 60, and more than 0.8 times, respectively, the maximum recommended human dose based on body surface area (assuming a 50-kg woman) (1).

A 1997 report described the use of benazepril (40 mg/day) in a 35-year-old woman with chronic hypertension (2). Treatment had begun several years before conception. Anhydramnios was noted at 27 weeks' gestation and the drug was discontinued. Twelve days later, complete resolution of the severe oligohydramnios was documented and the woman eventually delivered a healthy, 2600-g (10th percentile) male infant at 38 weeks' gestation. No signs or symptoms of impaired renal function were observed in the healthy infant (2).

Use of ACE-inhibitors in the 1st trimester does not represent a significant risk to the fetus, but fetal exposure after this time has been associated with structural anomalies and severe toxicity in the fetus and newborn, including death. See Captopril or Enalapril for a summary of fetal and neonatal effects from these agents. If benazepril is used in pregnancy, healthcare professionals are encouraged to call the toll free number (800-670-6126) for information about patient enrollment in the Motherisk study.

[*Risk Factor D_M if used in 2nd or 3rd trimesters.*]

BREAST FEEDING SUMMARY

RECOMMENDATION: No Human Data - Probably Compatible

No reports describing the use of benazepril during lactation have been located. Because of its relatively low molecular weight (about 461), passage into milk should be expected. Other agents in this class are excreted into milk and, because the amounts are low and no adverse effects have been observed in nursing infants, are classified as compatible with breast-feeding (see Captopril and Enalapril).

References

1. Product information. Lotensin. Novartis Pharmaceuticals, 2004.
2. Chisholm CA, Chescheir NC, Kennedy M. Reversible oligohydramnios in a pregnancy with angiotensin-converting enzyme inhibitor exposure. Am J Perinatol 1997;14:511–3.

Name: **BENDROFLUMETHIAZIDE** Risk Factor: C_M*

Class: **Diuretic**

FETAL RISK SUMMARY

RECOMMENDATION: Limited Human Data - No Relevant Animal Data

Bendroflumethiazide is a thiazide diuretic. Animal reproduction studies during the period of organogenesis have not been conducted with this agent.

In a study reported in 1964, 1011 women received bendroflumethiazide, 5 mg/day, from the 30th week of gestation until delivery, in an attempt to prevent preeclampsia and eclampsia (1). No fetal adverse effects were noted.

See Chlorothiazide for other reports of the clinical use of thiazide diuretics in pregnancy and the potential fetal and newborn toxicity of these agents. In general, diuretics are not recommended in the treatment of gestational hypertension because of the maternal hypovolemia characteristic of this disease.

[*Risk Factor D if used in gestational hypertension.*]

BREAST FEEDING SUMMARY

RECOMMENDATION: No Human Data - Probably Compatible

Bendroflumethiazide has been used to suppress lactation (see Chlorothiazide) (2). The American Academy of Pediatrics classifies bendroflumethiazide as compatible with breast-feeding (3).

References

1. Cuadros A, Tatum HJ. The prophylactic and therapeutic use of bendroflumethiazide in pregnancy. Am J Obstet Gynecol 1964;89:891–7.
2. Healy M. Suppressing lactation with oral diuretics. Lancet 1961;1:1353–4.
3. Committee on Drugs, American Academy of Pediatrics. The transfer of drugs and other chemicals into human milk. Pediatrics 2001;108:776–89.

Name: **BENZPHETAMINE** Risk Factor: X_M

Class: **Anorexiant**

FETAL RISK SUMMARY

RECOMMENDATION: Contraindicated

The sympathomimetic amine, benzphetamine, is chemically and pharmacologically related to the amphetamines. The primary pharmacologic actions include central nervous system stimulation and elevation of blood pressure. The drug is contraindicated in patients with

B

moderate to severe hypertension and several other conditions. Benzphetamine is indicated in the management of obesity in combination with a regimen of weight reduction based on caloric restriction. As with all agents in this class, tolerance and tachyphylaxis may develop. Animal reproduction studies have not been conducted (1).

It is not known if benzphetamine crosses the human placenta to the fetus. The relatively low molecular weight (about 276), however, suggests that exposure of the embryo/fetus will occur.

No reports describing the use of benzphetamine in human pregnancy have been located. There are no animal reproductive data, but because of its close relationship to amphetamines, the manufacturer classes the drug as contraindicated during pregnancy. Although this drug should not be used in pregnancy, inadvertent exposure to benzphetamine does not appear to represent a significant risk to the embryo or fetus (see Amphetamines).

BREAST FEEDING SUMMARY

RECOMMENDATION: Contraindicated

No reports describing the use of benzphetamine during lactation have been located. The relatively low molecular weight (about 276) suggests that the drug will be excreted in breast milk. The effects on a nursing infant from exposure via the milk are unknown, but there is potential for severe toxicity. Benzphetamine is chemically and pharmacologically related to the amphetamines. As such, it is contraindicated during nursing. (See Amphetamines.)

Reference

1. Product information. Didrex. Pharmacia, 2000.

Name:	**BENZTHIAZIDE**	Risk Factor:	**C***
Class:	**Diuretic**		

See Chlorothiazide. In general, diuretics are not recommended in the treatment of gestational hypertension because of the maternal hypovolemia characteristic of this disease.

[**Risk Factor D if used in gestational hypertension.*]

Name:	**BENZTROPINE**	Risk Factor:	**C**
Class:	**Parasympatholytic**		

FETAL RISK SUMMARY

RECOMMENDATION: Limited Human Data - No Relevant Animal Data

Benztropine is an anticholinergic agent structurally related to atropine (see also Atropine). It also has antihistaminic activity. In a large prospective study, 2323 patients were exposed to this class of drugs during the 1st trimester, 4 of whom took benztropine (1). A possible association was found in the total group between benztropine and minor malformations.

In a surveillance study of Michigan Medicaid recipients conducted between 1985 and 1992 involving 229,101 completed pregnancies, 84 newborns had been exposed to

benztropine during the 1st trimester (F. Rosa, personal communication, FDA, 1993). Four (4.8%) major birth defects were observed (three expected), three of which were cardiovascular defects (one expected). No anomalies were observed in five other categories of defects (oral clefts, spina bifida, polydactyly, limb reduction defects, and hypospadias) for which specific data were available. Based on a small number of exposures, a possible association is suggested with cardiovascular defects.

Paralytic ileus has been observed in two newborns exposed to chlorpromazine and benztropine at term (2). In one of these infants, other anticholinergic drugs may have contributed to the effect (see Doxepin). The small left colon syndrome was characterized by decreased intestinal motility, abdominal distention, vomiting, and failure to pass meconium. The condition cleared rapidly in both infants after a Gastrografin enema.

BREAST FEEDING SUMMARY

RECOMMENDATION: No Human Data - Probably Compatible

No data are available (see Atropine).

References

1. Heinonen OP, Slone D, Shapiro S. *Birth Defects and Drugs in Pregnancy*. Littleton, MA: Publishing Sciences Group, 1977:346–53.
2. Falterman CG, Richardson CJ. Small left colon syndrome associated with maternal ingestion of psychotropic drugs. J Pediatr 1980;97:308–10.

Name:	**BEPRIDIL**	Risk Factor:	**C_M**
Class:	**Calcium Channel Blocker**		

FETAL RISK SUMMARY

RECOMMENDATION: No Human Data - Animal Data Suggest Low Risk

Bepridil is a calcium channel blocking agent used in the treatment of angina. No teratogenic effects were observed in rats and rabbits, but at doses 37 times the maximum recommended human dose, reduced litter sizes and decreased pup survival were observed (1). No reports describing the use of bepridil during human pregnancy have been located.

BREAST FEEDING SUMMARY

RECOMMENDATION: No Human Data - Probably Compatible

Bepridil is excreted into breast milk with a maximum milk:plasma ratio of approximately 0.33 (1). No reports on the use of bepridil during nursing have been located.

Reference

1. Product information. Vascor. McNeil Pharmaceutical, 1993.

B

Name: **β-CAROTENE** Risk Factor: **C**
Class: **Vitamin**

FETAL RISK SUMMARY

RECOMMENDATION: Compatible

β-carotene, a natural precursor to vitamin A found in green and yellow vegetables as well as being commercially available, is partially converted in the small intestine to vitamin A (1). Even with therapeutic doses of the drug, serum levels of vitamin A do not rise above normal. Studies in animals have failed to show a teratogenic effect (see also Vitamin A) (2).

A single case describing the therapeutic use of this vitamin in human pregnancy has been located. A 35-year-old woman at 6.5 weeks' gestation was seen because of her daily intake of 180 mg (300,000 IU) of β-carotene for the past year for the treatment of skin lesions of porphyria (3). She had stopped taking the vitamin at 4.5 weeks' gestation because of the pregnancy, but her skin still had a yellow-orange tinge. Serum levels of β-carotene and retinol (vitamin A) were determined 2 weeks after her last dose. The β-carotene level was markedly elevated (0.403 mg/dL; normal: 0.05–0.2 mg/dL), whereas the retinol concentration was low normal (0.069 mg/dL; normal: 0.05–0.2 mg/dL) (3). At 18 weeks' gestation, her β-carotene level had fallen to 0.22 mg/dL. She delivered a healthy, normal-appearing, 3910-g, male infant without skin discoloration at term, who was developing normally at 6 weeks of age.

BREAST FEEDING SUMMARY

RECOMMENDATION: Compatible

No data are available (see Vitamin A).

References

1. American Hospital Formulary Service. *Drug Information 1997*. Bethesda, MD: American Society of Health-System Pharmacists, 1997:2806–7.
2. Nishimura H, Tanimura T. *Clinical Aspects of the Teratogenicity of Drugs*. New York, NY: American Elsevier, 1978:252.
3. Polifka JE, Dolan CR, Donlan MA, Friedman JM. Clinical teratology counseling and consultation report: high dose β-carotene use during early pregnancy. Teratology 1996;54:103–7.

Name: **BETAMETHASONE** Risk Factor: **C***
Class: **Corticosteroid**

FETAL RISK SUMMARY

RECOMMENDATION: Compatible - Maternal Benefit >> Embryo/Fetal Risk

Betamethasone is often used in patients with premature labor at about 26–34 weeks' gestation to stimulate fetal lung maturation (1–15). The benefits of this therapy are:

Reduction in incidence of respiratory distress syndrome (RDS)
Decreased severity of RDS if it occurs

Decreased incidence of, and mortality from, intracranial hemorrhage
Increased survival of premature infants

Betamethasone crosses the placenta to the fetus (16). The drug is partially metabolized (47%) by the perfused placenta to its inactive 11-ketosteroid derivative, but less so than other corticosteroids, although the differences are not statistically significant (17).

In patients with premature rupture of the membranes (PROM), administration of betamethasone to the mother does not always reduce the frequency of RDS or perinatal mortality (18–22). An increased risk of maternal infection has also been observed in patients with PROM treated with corticosteroids (19,20). In a study comparing betamethasone therapy with nonsteroid management of women with PROM, neonatal sepsis was observed in 23% (5 of 22) of steroid-exposed newborns vs. only 2% (1 of 46) of the nonsteroid-exposed group (21). A 1985 study also found increased neonatal sepsis in exposed newborns who were delivered more than 48 hours after PROM, 18.6% (14 of 75) vs. 7.4% (4 of 54) of nonexposed controls (22). In addition, moderate to severe respiratory morbidity was increased over that in controls, 21.3% vs. 11.1%, as well as overall mortality, 8% vs. 1.8% (22). Other reports, however, have noted beneficial effects of betamethasone administration to patients with PROM with no increase in infectious morbidity (15,23,24). In women colonized with group B streptococci, the combined use of betamethasone and ampicillin improved the outcome of preterm pregnancies with PROM (25).

Betamethasone therapy is less effective in decreasing the incidence of RDS in male infants than in female infants (23,26,27). The reasons for this difference have not been discovered. Slower lung maturation in male fetuses has been cited as a major contributing factor to the sex differential noted in neonatal mortality (28). Therapy is also less effective in multiple pregnancies (27,29), even when doses have been doubled (27). In twins, only the first-born seems to benefit from antenatal steroid therapy (27).

An increased incidence of hypoglycemia in newborns exposed *in utero* to betamethasone has been reported (30). Although other investigators have not observed this effect, maternal betamethasone-induced hyperglycemia is a possible explanation if the drug was given shortly before delivery.

In the initial study examining the effect of betamethasone on RDS, investigators reported an increased risk of fetal death in patients with severe preeclampsia (1). They proposed that the corticosteroid had an adverse effect on placentas already damaged by vascular disease. A second study did not confirm these findings (7).

A case of suspected betamethasone-induced leukemoid reaction was observed in an 880-g, 30-weeks'-gestation female infant whose mother received 12 mg of betamethasone 4 hours prior to delivery (31). A second case, involving a female infant born at 25–26 weeks' gestation and 71 hours after betamethasone was administered, was published in 1997 (32). Within about 7–10 days, the white blood cell count had returned to normal in both infants. A 1984 study examined the effect of betamethasone on leukocyte counts in mothers with PROM or premature labor (33). No effect, as compared to untreated controls, was found in either group.

A case of acute, life-threatening exacerbation of muscular weakness requiring intubation and mechanical ventilation was reported in a 24-year-old woman who was treated with betamethasone, 12 mg IM, to enhance fetal lung maturity at 32 weeks' gestation (34). The onset of symptoms occurred 30 minutes after the corticosteroid dose. The authors attributed the crisis to betamethasone (adrenocorticosteroids are known to aggravate myasthenia) after other potential causes were ruled out. The infant was delivered by emergency cesarean section and, except for the typical problems related to prematurity, he had a normal hospital course.

Hypertensive crisis associated with the use of ritodrine and betamethasone has been reported (35). Systolic blood pressure was above 300 mm Hg with a diastolic pressure of 120 mm Hg. Although the hypertension was probably caused by ritodrine, it is not known whether the corticosteroid was a contributing factor.

The effect of betamethasone administration on patent ductus arteriosus (PDA) was investigated in premature infants with a birth weight of less than 2000 g (36). Infants of nontreated mothers had a PDA incidence of 44% vs. 6.5% for infants of treated mothers ($p < 0.01$). This reduction in the incidence of PDA after betamethasone therapy has also been observed in other studies (25). A study published in 1989 indicated that betamethasone caused transient, mild constriction of the ductus arteriosus (37). Eleven women with placenta previa with a mean gestational age of 31.7 weeks (range 27.3–37.3 weeks) were given two 12-mg IM doses of the drug, 24 hours apart, to promote fetal lung maturation. Fetal Doppler echocardiography of the ductus arteriosus was conducted just before the first dose, then at 5 and 30 hours after the dose. Two of the fetuses showed mild constriction of the ductus 4–5 hours after the first injection, but the tests were normal when performed at 30 hours. No evidence of tricuspid regurgitation was observed (37). The authors concluded that the changes were probably not clinically significant.

A 1984 article discussed the potential benefits of combining thyroid hormones with corticosteroids to produce an additive or synergistic effect on fetal lung phosphatidylcholine synthesis (38). The therapy may offer advantages over corticosteroid therapy alone, but it is presently not possible because of the lack of commercially available thyroid stimulators that cross the placenta. The thyroid hormones, T_4 and T_3, are poorly transported across the placenta and thus would not be effective.

Five premature infants (three males and two females), exposed *in utero* to two 8-mg IM doses of betamethasone administered to the mother 48 and 24 hours before birth, were evaluated to determine the effect of the drug on endogenous progesterone, mineralocorticoid, and glucocorticoid activity (39). Plasma levels of the mineralocorticoids, aldosterone and 11-deoxycorticosterone, were not significantly decreased in the newborns at birth or during the next few days. Glucocorticoid activity in the newborns, as measured by levels of corticosterone, cortisol, cortisone, and 11-deoxycortisol, was significantly depressed at birth but rebounded above normal values when the subjects were 2 hours of age, then returned to normal ranges shortly after this time. Progesterone and 17-hydroxyprogesterone levels in the fetuses and neonates were not affected by betamethasone.

A 1994 case report described a pregnancy in which seven weekly courses (two 12.5 mg IM doses every 12 hours) of betamethasone were given between 24 weeks' gestation and delivery at 34.5 weeks' (40). The 2625-g male infant had a "moon facies" appearance and a "buffalo hump" of apparent excess adipose deposition in the upper back. Tests in the mother and infant shortly after delivery were consistent with hypothalamic-pituitary-adrenal axis suppression with low basal serum cortisol levels (40). At 10 months of age, the infant's motor development and cognitive function were normal for age, length, and head circumference were at the 20th percentile, and weight was slightly less than the 5th percentile. The cushingoid features had completely resolved (40). Two more recent reports have also described adrenal suppression in women secondary to multiple antenatal betamethasone courses (41,42), and in newborns exposed to ($\geq$3 courses (43). A 1999 study, however, did not observe adrenal suppression in nine infants whose mothers had received a mean of 4.8 treatment courses of betamethasone (44).

Although human studies have usually shown a benefit, the use of corticosteroids in animals is associated with several toxic effects (45,46):

Reduced fetal head circumference
Reduced fetal adrenal weight
Increased fetal liver weight
Reduced fetal thymus weight
Reduced placental weight

None of these effects has been observed in human investigations with single courses of betamethasone. However, multiple courses of betamethasone have been associated with lower birth weights and reduced head circumference at birth (43,47,48).

In children born of mothers treated with betamethasone for premature labor, studies of children conducted at 4 and 6 years of age have found no differences from controls in cognitive and psychosocial development (49,50). Two studies published in 1990 evaluated children at 10–12 years of age who had been exposed *in utero* to betamethasone in a randomized, double-blind, placebo-controlled trial of the effects of the corticosteroid on fetal lung maturity (51,52). No differences were found between the exposed and placebo groups in terms of intellectual and motor development, school achievement, and social-emotional functioning (51). Concerning physical development, no differences between the groups were measured in terms of physical growth, neurologic and ophthalmologic development, and lung function (52). However, during the first few years of life, the corticoid-exposed group had significantly more hospital admissions relating to infections than did those in the placebo group (52).

Studies conducted on very-low-birth-weight infants (500–1500 g) at 2 years of age indicated that, compared to nonexposed controls, exposed infants received antenatal betamethasone therapy that was associated with a significant improvement in survival, improved growth, and a decrease in early respiratory morbidity (53). Further study of the children at 5 years of age, but limited to those with birth weights of 500–999 g, found significantly improved survival but without significantly improved growth or decrease in early respiratory morbidity (54).

A study published in 1999 (55), with an accompanying editorial (54), reported a decrease in the incidence of cystic periventricular leukomalacia (PL) with prenatal betamethasone, but not with dexamethasone. Among 883 live-born infants, with gestational ages ranging from 24 to 31 weeks', the rates of cystic PL in infants of mothers given betamethasone ($N = 361$), dexamethasone ($N = 165$), or no prenatal corticosteroids ($N = 357$), were 4.4%, 11.0%, and 8.4%, respectively. Cystic PL (necrosis of the white matter adjacent to the lateral ventricles resulting in the formation of cysts [56]), is the most frequent cause of cerebral palsy in premature infants (55).

A 1999 study reported a modest reduction in the risk of cerebral white matter damage (echolucency) and intraventricular hemorrhage (IVH), but a significant reduction in ventriculomegaly in premature infants weighing 500 to 1500 g (57). Significant reductions in the risk for echolucency and ventriculomegaly were seen in the gestationally youngest infants and in those with IVH, hypothyroxinemia, or vasculitis of the umbilical cord or chorionic plate of the placenta (57). In addition to this study, three other reports have also shown that the risk of IVH is reduced in preterm infants by the administration of antenatal betamethasone (58–60).

Another study on the reduction of PL with betamethasone appeared in 2001 (61). In 1161 neonates born at gestational ages of 24–34 weeks', 400 were exposed to antenatal betamethasone and 761 were not exposed (controls). The effects of antenatal betamethasone compared to controls were: PL or IVH 23% vs. 31%, $p = 0.005$, PL with IVH 5% vs. 11%, $p = 0.001$, and isolated PL 3% vs. 7%, $p = 0.009$. The investigators concluded that antenatal betamethasone therapy was associated with a greater than 50% decrease in PL in preterm infants (61).

Among the miscellaneous effects of antenatal betamethasone, decreased fetal heart rate variability has been demonstrated (62,63). In addition, a 1999 report described three newborns that developed various degrees of transient hypertrophic cardiomyopathy after multiple courses of antenatal betamethasone (64).

Although no reports linking the use of betamethasone with birth defects have been located, four large epidemiologic studies have associated the use of corticosteroids during the 1st trimester with orofacial clefts. Betamethasone was not specifically identified in these studies, but only one study listed the corticosteroids used (see Hydrocortisone for details).

[*Risk Factor D if used in 1st trimester.*]

BREAST FEEDING SUMMARY

RECOMMENDATION: No Human Data - Probably Compatible

No reports describing the use of betamethasone during human lactation have been located. The molecular weight (about 435 for the acetate salt and about 517 for the sodium phosphate salt) are low enough, however, that excretion into milk should be expected.

References

1. Liggins GC, Howie RN. A controlled trial of antepartum glucocorticoid treatment for prevention of the respiratory distress syndrome in premature infants. Pediatrics 1972;50:515–25.
2. Gluck L. Administration of corticosteroids to induce maturation of fetal lung. Am J Dis Child 1976;130:976–8.
3. Ballard RA, Ballard PL. Use of prenatal glucocorticoid therapy to prevent respiratory distress syndrome: a supporting view. Am J Dis Child 1976;130:982–7.
4. Mead PB, Clapp JF III. The use of betamethasone and timed delivery in management of premature rupture of the membranes in the preterm pregnancy. J Reprod Med 1977;19:3–7.
5. Block MF, Kling OR, Crosby WM. Antenatal glucocorticoid therapy for the prevention of respiratory distress syndrome in the premature infant. Obstet Gynecol 1977;50:186–90.
6. Ballard RA, Ballard PL, Granberg JP, Sniderman S. Prenatal administration of betamethasone for prevention of respiratory distress syndrome. J Pediatr 1979;94:97–101.
7. Nochimson DJ, Petrie RH. Glucocorticoid therapy for the induction of pulmonary maturity in severely hypertensive gravid women. Am J Obstet Gynecol 1979;133:449–51.
8. Eggers TR, Doyle LW, Pepperell RJ. Premature labour. Med J Aust 1979;1:213–6.
9. Doran TA, Swyer P, MacMurray B, et al. Results of a double-blind controlled study on the use of betamethasone in the prevention of respiratory distress syndrome. Am J Obstet Gynecol 1980;136:313–20.
10. Schutte MF, Treffers PE, Koppe JG, Breur W. The influence of betamethasone and orciprenaline on the incidence of respiratory distress syndrome in the newborn after preterm labour. Br J Obstet Gynaecol 1980;87:127–31.
11. Dillon WP, Egan EA. Aggressive obstetric management in late second-trimester deliveries. Obstet Gynecol 1981;58:685–90.
12. Johnson DE, Munson DP, Thompson TR. Effect of antenatal administration of betamethasone on hospital costs and survival of premature infants. Pediatrics 1981;68:633–7.
13. Bishop EH. Acceleration of fetal pulmonary maturity. Obstet Gynecol 1981;58(Suppl):48S–51S.
14. Ballard PL, Ballard RA. Corticosteroids and respiratory distress syndrome: status 1979. Pediatrics 1979;63:163–5.
15. Gamsu HR, Mullinger BM, Donnai P, Dash CH. Antenatal administration of betamethasone to prevent respiratory distress syndrome in preterm infants: report of a UK multicentre trial. Br J Obstet Gynaecol 1989;96:401–10.
16. Ballard PL, Granberg P, Ballard RA. Glucocorticoid levels in maternal and cord serum after prenatal betamethasone therapy to prevent respiratory distress syndrome. J Clin Invest 1975;56:1548–54.
17. Levitz M, Jansen V, Dancis J. The transfer and metabolism of corticosteroids in the perfused human placenta. Am J Obstet Gynecol 1978;132:363–6.
18. Eggers TR, Doyle LW, Pepperell RJ. Premature rupture of the membranes. Med J Aust 1979;1:209–13.
19. Garite TJ, Freeman RK, Linzey EM, Braly PS, Dorchester WL. Prospective randomized study of corticosteroids in the management of premature rupture of

the membranes and the premature gestation. Am J Obstet Gynecol 1981;141:508–15.

20. Garite TJ. Premature rupture of the membranes: the enigma of the obstetrician. Am J Obstet Gynecol 1985;151:1001–5.
21. Nelson LH, Meis PJ, Hatjis CG, Ernest JM, Dillard R, Schey HM. Premature rupture of membranes: a prospective, randomized evaluation of steroids, latent phase, and expectant management. Obstet Gynecol 1985;66:55–8.
22. Simpson GF, Harbert GM Jr. Use of β-methasone in management of preterm gestation with premature rupture of membranes. Obstet Gynecol 1985;66: 168–75.
23. Kuhn RJP, Speirs AL, Pepperell RJ, Eggers TR, Doyle LW, Hutchison A. Betamethasone, albuterol, and threatened premature delivery: benefits and risks. Obstet Gynecol 1982;60:403–8.
24. Schmidt PL, Sims ME, Strassner HT, Paul RH, Mueller E, McCart D. Effect of antepartum glucocorticoid administration upon neonatal respiratory distress syndrome and perinatal infection. Am J Obstet Gynecol 1984;148:178–86.
25. Morales WJ, Angel JL, O'Brien WF, Knuppel RA. Use of ampicillin and corticosteroids in premature rupture of membranes: a randomized study. Obstet Gynecol 1989;73:721–6.
26. Ballard PL, Ballard RA, Granberg JP, et al. Fetal sex and prenatal betamethasone therapy. J Pediatr 1980;97:451–4.
27. Avery ME, Aylward G, Creasy R, Little AB, Stripp B. Update on prenatal steroid for prevention of respiratory distress: report of a conference—September 26–28, 1985. Am J Obstet Gynecol 1986;155: 2–5.
28. Khoury MJ, Marks JS, McCarthy BJ, Zaro SM. Factors affecting the sex differential in neonatal mortality: the role of respiratory distress syndrome. Am J Obstet Gynecol 1985;151:777–82.
29. Turrentine MA, Dupras-Wilson P, Wilkins IA. A retrospective analysis of the effect of antenatal steroid administration on the incidence of respiratory distress syndrome in preterm twin pregnancies. Am J Perinatol 1996;13:351–4.
30. Papageorgiou AN, Desgranges MF, Masson M, Colle E, Shatz R, Gelfand MM. The antenatal use of betamethasone in the prevention of respiratory distress syndrome: a controlled double-blind study. Pediatrics 1979;63:73–9.
31. Bielawski D, Hiatt IM, Hegyi T. Betamethasone-induced leukaemoid reaction in pre-term infant. Lancet 1978;1:218–9.
32. Hoff DS, Mammel MC. Suspected betamethasone-induced leukemoid reaction in a premature infant. Pharmacotherapy 1997;17:1031–4.
33. Ferguson JE, Hensleigh PA, Gill P. Effects of betamethasone on white blood cells in patients with premature rupture of the membranes and preterm labor. Am J Obstet Gynecol 1984;150:439–41.
34. Catanzarite VA, McHargue AM, Sandberg EC, Dyson DC. Respiratory arrest during therapy for premature labor in a patient with myasthenia gravis. Obstet Gynecol 1984;64:819–22.
35. Gonen R, Samberg I, Sharf M. Hypertensive crisis associated with ritodrine infusion and betamethasone administration in premature labor. Eur J Obstet Gynecol Reprod Biol 1982;13:129–32.
36. Waffarn F, Siassi B, Cabal LA, Schmidt PL. Effect of antenatal glucocorticoids on clinical closure of the ductus arteriosus. Am J Dis Child 1983;137:336–8.
37. Wasserstrum N, Huhta JC, Mari G, Sharif DS, Willis R, Neal NK. Betamethasone and the human fetal ductus arteriosus. Obstet Gynecol 1989;74: 897–900.
38. Ballard PL. Combined hormonal treatment and lung maturation. Semin Perinatol 1984;8:283–92.
39. Dorr HG, Versmold HT, Sippell WG, Bidlingmaier F, Knorr D. Antenatal betamethasone therapy: effects on maternal, fetal, and neonatal mineralocorticoids, glucocorticoids, and progestins. J Pediatr 1986;108: 990–3.
40. Bradley BS, Kumar SP, Mehta PN, Ezhuthachan SG. Neonatal cushingoid syndrome resulting from serial courses of antenatal betamethasone. Obstet Gynecol 1994;83:869–72.
41. McKenna DS, Wittber GM, Nagaraja HN, Samuels P. The effects of repeated doses of antenatal corticosteroids on maternal adrenal function. Am J Obstet Gynecol 2000;183:669–73.
42. Helal KJ, Gordon MC, Lightner CR, Barth WH Jr. Adrenal suppression induced by betamethasone in women at risk for premature delivery. Obstet Gynecol 2000;96:287–90.
43. Banks BA, Cnaan A, Morgan MA, Parer JT, Merrill JD, Ballard PL, Ballard RA, and the North American Thyrotropin-Releasing Hormone Study Group. Multiple courses of antenatal corticosteroids and outcome of premature neonates. Am J Obstet Gynecol 1999;181:709–17.
44. Terrone DA, Rinehart BK, Rhodes PG, Roberts WE, Miller RC, Martin JN Jr. Multiple courses of betamethasone to enhance fetal lung maturation do not suppress neonatal adrenal response. Am J Obstet Gynecol 1999;180:1349–53.
45. Taeusch HW Jr. Glucocorticoid prophylaxis for respiratory distress syndrome: a review of potential toxicity. J Pediatr 1975;87:617–23.
46. Johnson JWC, Mitzner W, London WT, Palmer AE, Scott R. Betamethasone and the rhesus fetus: multisystemic effects. Am J Obstet Gynecol 1979;133: 677–84.
47. French NP, Hagan R, Evans SF, Godfrey M, Newnham JP. Repeated antenatal corticosteroids: size at birth and subsequent development. Am J Obstet Gynecol 1999;180:114–21.
48. Abbasi S, Hirsch D, Davis J, Tolosa J, Stouffer N, Debbs R, Gerdes JS. Effect of single versus multiple courses of antenatal corticosteroids on maternal and neonatal outcome. Am J Obstet Gynecol 2000;182: 1243–9.
49. MacArthur BA, Howie RN, Dezoete JA, Elkins J. Cognitive and psychosocial development of 4-year-old children whose mothers were treated antenatally with betamethasone. Pediatrics 1981;68:638–43.
50. MacArthur BA, Howie RN, Dezoete JA, Elkins J. School progress and cognitive development of 6-year-old children whose mothers were treated antenatally with betamethasone. Pediatrics 1982;70:99–105.
51. Schmand B, Neuvel J, Smolders-de Haas H, Hoeks J, Treffers PE, Koppe JG. Psychological development of

B

children who were treated antenatally with corticosteroids to prevent respiratory distress syndrome. Pediatrics 1990;86:58–64.
52. Smolders-de Haas H, Neuvel J, Schmand B, Treffers PE, Koppe JG, Hoeks J. Physical development and medical history of children who were treated antenatally with corticosteroids to prevent respiratory distress syndrome: a 10- to 12-year follow-up. Pediatrics 1990;85:65–70.
53. Doyle LW, Kitchen WH, Ford GW, Rickards AL, Lissenden JV, Ryan MM. Effects of antenatal steroid therapy on mortality and morbidity in very low birth weight infants. J Pediatr 1986;108:287–92.
54. Doyle LW, Kitchen WH, Ford GW, Rickards AL, Kelly EA. Antenatal steroid therapy and 5-year outcome of extremely low birth weight infants. Obstet Gynecol 1989;73:743–6.
55. Baud O, Foix-L'Helias L, Kaminski M, Audibert F, Jarreau PH, Papiernik E, Huon C, Leperco J, Dehan M, Lacaze-Masmonteil T. Antenatal glucocorticoid treatment and cystic periventricular leukomalacia in very premature infants. N Engl J Med 1999;341:1190–6.
56. Fanaroff AA, Hack M. Periventricular leukomalacia—prospects for prevention. N Engl J Med 1999;341: 1229–31.
57. Leviton A, Dammann O, Allred EN, Kuban K, Pagano M, Van Marter L, Paneth N, Reuss ML, Susser M, for The Developmental Epidemiology Network Investigators. Antenatal corticosteroids and cranial ultrasonographic abnormalities. Am J Obstet Gynecol 1999;181:1007–17.
58. Ment LR, Oh W, Ehrenkranz RA, Philip AGS, Duncan CC, Makuch RW. Antenatal steroids, delicry mode, and intraventricular hemorrhage in preterm infants. Am J Obstet Gynecol 1995;172:795–800.
59. Garland JS, Buck R, Leviton A. Effect of maternal glucocorticoid exposure on risk of severe intraventricular hemorrhage in surfactant-treated preterm infants. J Pediatr 1995;126:272–9.
60. Chen B, Basil JB, Schefft GL, Cole FS, Sadovsky Y. Antenatal steroids and intraventricular hemorrhage after premature rupture of membranes at 24–28 weeks' gestation. Am J Perinatol 1997;14:171–6.
61. Canterino JC, Verma U, Visintainer PF, Elimian A, Klein SA, Tejani N. Antenatal steroids and neonatal periventricular leukomalacia. Obstet Gynecol 2001;97: 135–9.
62. Ville Y, Vincent Y, Tordjman N, Hue MV, Fernandez H, Frydman R. Effect of betamethasone on the fetal heart rate pattern assessed by computerized cardiotocography in normal twin pregnancies. Fetal Diagn Ther 1995;10:301–6.
63. Senat MV, Minoui S, Multon O, Fernandez H, Frydman R, Ville Y. Effect of dexamethasone and betamethasone on fetal heart rate variability in preterm labour: a randomised study. Br J Obstet Gynaecol 1998;105:749–55.
64. Yunis KA, Bitar FF, Hayek P, Mroueh SM, Mikati M. Transient hypertrophic cardiomyopathy in the newborn following multiple doses of antenatal corticosteroids. Am J Perinatol 1999;16:17–21.

Name:	**BETAXOLOL**	Risk Factor:	**C_M***
Class:	**Sympatholytic (Antihypertensive)**		

FETAL RISK SUMMARY

RECOMMENDATION: Human Data Suggest Risk in 2nd and 3rd Trimesters

Betaxolol is a cardioselective β_1-adrenergic blocking agent used in the treatment of hypertension and topically in the therapy of glaucoma. Betaxolol is teratogenic in rats producing skeletal and visceral anomalies at maternally toxic doses (600 times the maximum recommended human dose [MRHD]) (1). At this dose, postimplantation loss and reduced litter size and weight were also noted. At doses 6 and 60 times the MRHD, a possible increased incidence of incomplete descent of testes and sternebral reductions were observed (1). No teratogenic effects were observed in rabbits, but an increase in postimplantation loss occurred at the highest dose tested (54 times the MRHD) (1).

No reports describing the use of betaxolol in human pregnancy have been located. Some β-blockers may cause intrauterine growth retardation (IUGR) and reduced placental weight, especially those lacking intrinsic sympathomimetic activity (ISA) (i.e., partial agonist). Treatment beginning early in the 2nd trimester results in the greatest weight reductions, whereas treatment restricted to the 3rd trimester primarily affects only placental weight. Betaxolol does not possess ISA. However, IUGR and reduced placental weight may potentially occur with all agents within this class. Although growth retardation is a serious

B

concern, the benefits of maternal therapy with β-blockers, in some cases, might outweigh the risks to the fetus and must be judged on a case-by-case basis.

If used near delivery, the newborn infant should be closely monitored for 24–48 hours for signs and symptoms of β-blockade. Long-term effects of *in utero* exposure to β-blockers have not been studied but warrant evaluation.

[**Risk Factor D if used in 2nd or 3rd trimesters.*]

BREAST FEEDING SUMMARY

RECOMMENDATION: Limited Human Data - Potential Toxicity

Betaxolol is excreted into human milk in quantities sufficient to produce β-blockade in a nursing infant (1). No reports have been located that describe the use of this agent during nursing. If used during nursing, the infant should be closely observed for hypotension, bradycardia, and other signs or symptoms of β-blockade. Long-term effects of exposure to β-blockers from milk have not been studied but warrant evaluation.

Reference

1. Product information. Kerlone. G. D. Searle & Co., 1997.

Name:	**BETHANECHOL**	Risk Factor:	**C_M**
Class:	**Parasympathomimetic (Cholinergic)**		

FETAL RISK SUMMARY

RECOMMENDATION: Limited Human Data - No Relevant Animal Data

Bethanechol is indicated for the treatment of nonobstructive urinary retention and neurogenic atony of the urinary bladder with retention. Reproduction studies in animals have not been conducted (1).

The use of bethanechol in human pregnancy has been reported, but too little data are available to analyze (2).

BREAST FEEDING SUMMARY

RECOMMENDATION: Limited Human Data - Potential Toxicity

Specific data on the excretion of bethanechol into breast milk are lacking. The molecular weight (about 197) is low enough, however, that excretion into milk should be expected. One author cautioned that mothers receiving regular therapy with this drug should not breast-feed (3). Abdominal pain and diarrhea have been reported in a nursing infant exposed to bethanechol in milk (4).

References

1. Product information. Urecholine. Merck, 2000.
2. Heinonen OP, Slone D, Shapiro S. *Birth Defects and Drugs in Pregnancy*. Littleton, MA: Publishing Sciences Group, 1977:345–56.
3. Platzker ACD, Lew CD, Stewart D. Drug "administration" via breast milk. Hosp Pract 1980;15:111–22.
4. Shore MF. Drugs can be dangerous during pregnancy and lactations. Can Pharm J 1970;103:358. As cited in: Committee on Drugs, American Academy of Pediatrics. The transfer of drugs and other chemicals into human breast milk. Pediatrics 1983;72:375–383.

B

Name: **BEXAROTENE** Risk Factor: X_M

Class: **Antineoplastic**

FETAL RISK SUMMARY

RECOMMENDATION: Contraindicated

Bexarotene is a member of a subclass of retinoids that selectively binds and activates retinoid X receptor subtypes (RXRα, RXRβ, and RXRγ). These subtypes then interact with various receptor partners to function as transcription factors that regulate the expression of genes that control cellular differentiation and proliferation. Bexarotene is indicated for the treatment of refractory cutaneous manifestations of cutaneous T-cell lymphoma. Four active metabolites have been identified (1).

In reproduction studies with pregnant rats during organogenesis, an oral dose approximately one-third of the area under the plasma concentration curve in humans at the recommended human dose (RHD) caused incomplete ossification (1). When a dose about 1.33 times the RHD was given, cleft palate, depressed eye bulge/microphthalmia, and small ears were observed. Doses greater than about 0.8 times the RHD caused embryo and fetal death. The no-effect dose was one-sixth the RHD (1). Studies on fertility and carcinogenicity have not been conducted, but tests for mutagenicity or clastogenicity were negative (1).

It is not known if bexarotene crosses the human placenta. The molecular weight (about 348) is low enough, however, that transfer to the fetus should be expected.

Bexarotene is contraindicated in pregnancy. No reports describing its use during human pregnancy have been located. Pregnancy should be excluded and the use of effective contraception (two reliable forms used simultaneously) confirmed before bexarotene therapy is started in women of childbearing age. If these criteria are met, therapy should be initiated on the second or third day of a normal menstrual cycle. The contraceptive methods should be used for 1 month before therapy, during therapy, and for 1 month after stopping therapy. The manufacturer also recommends that pregnancy tests be repeated monthly during treatment (1). In addition, male patients with sexual partners who are pregnant, possibly pregnant, or who could become pregnant, should use condoms during sexual intercourse during therapy and for 1 month after therapy has been stopped (1).

BREAST FEEDING SUMMARY

RECOMMENDATION: No Human Data - Potential Toxicity

No reports describing the use of bexarotene in human lactation have been located. The molecular weight (about 348) is low enough that excretion into breast milk should be expected. Because of the unknown amounts present in milk and the potential for serious adverse effects in a nursing infant, women receiving bexarotene should probably not breast-feed.

Reference

1. Product information. Targretin. Ligand Pharmaceuticals, 2001.

Name:	**BIPERIDEN**	Risk Factor:	C_M
Class:	**Parasympatholytic**		

FETAL RISK SUMMARY

RECOMMENDATION: No Human Data - No Relevant Animal Data

Biperiden is an anticholinergic agent used in the treatment of parkinsonism. Animal reproduction studies have not been conducted with this drug. It is not known if the drug crosses the placenta to the fetus, but the molecular weight (about 312 for the free base) is low enough that placental transfer should be expected. No reports of its use in pregnancy have been located (see also Atropine).

BREAST FEEDING SUMMARY

RECOMMENDATION: No Human Data - Probably Compatible

No reports describing the use of biperiden during lactation have been located. The molecular weight (about 312 for the free base) is low enough, however, that excretion into milk should be expected. Neonates may be sensitive to anticholinergics and this should be considered if a nursing woman is taking the drug.

Name:	**BISMUTH SUBSALICYLATE**	Risk Factor:	C
Class:	**Antidiarrheal**		

FETAL RISK SUMMARY

RECOMMENDATION: Human Data Suggest Low Risk

Bismuth subsalicylate (bismuth salicylate) is hydrolyzed in the gastrointestinal tract to bismuth salts and sodium salicylate (1,2). Two tablets or 30 mL suspension of the compound yields 204 mg and 258 mg, respectively, of salicylate. Inorganic bismuth salts, in contrast to organic complexes of bismuth, are relatively water-insoluble and poorly absorbed systemically, but significant absorption of salicylate does occur (1,2). A brief 1992 study found minimal absorption of bismuth (exact serum concentrations not specified) from bismuth subsalicylate in 12 healthy subjects as opposed to a peak serum level of 0.050 μg/mL after a dose of 216-mg colloidal bismuth subcitrate in a single patient (3). Some bismuth absorption was documented across the normal gastric mucosa, but the primary absorption occurred from the duodenum (3). Others believe, however, that the design of the study produced the observed results, and that bismuth absorption occurs only in the gastric antrum, not in the gastric body or duodenum (4).

Although absorption of inorganic bismuth salts is negligible, in a study of chronic administration of bismuth tartrate 5 mg/kg/day, one of four lambs born of treated ewes was stunted, hairless, and exophthalmic, and a second was aborted (5). Moreover, in one case report, the use of an extemporaneously compounded antidiarrheal mixture containing bismuth subsalicylate was associated with bismuth encephalopathy in a 60-year-old man who took an unknown amount of the preparation for a period of 1 month (6). Encephalopathy was diagnosed by an electroencephalogram characteristic of bismuth toxicity and a blood bismuth level of 72 ng/mL (upper limit of normal is 5 ng/mL).

B

No reports of adverse fetal outcome after the use of commercially available bismuth subsalicylate have been located for humans. The Collaborative Perinatal Project recorded 15 1st trimester exposures to bismuth salts (bismuth subgallate $N = 13$, bismuth subcarbonate $N = 1$, and milk of bismuth $N = 1$), but none to bismuth subsalicylate (7, pp. 384–7). These numbers are small, but no evidence was found to suggest any association with congenital abnormalities. For use anytime during pregnancy, 144 mother-child pairs were exposed to bismuth subgallate and 5 of the *in utero* exposed infants had inguinal hernia, a hospital standardized relative risk (SRR) of 2.6 (7, pp. 442, 497). A causal relationship, however, cannot be determined from these data.

In contrast to bismuth, salicylate is rapidly absorbed with more than 90% of the dose recovered in the urine. Data on the use of salicylates in human pregnancy, primarily acetylsalicylic acid (aspirin), is extensive. The main concerns from exposure to this drug during pregnancy include congenital defects, increased perinatal mortality from premature closure of the ductus arteriosus *in utero*, intrauterine growth retardation, and salicylate intoxication (see Aspirin). An increased risk of intracranial hemorrhage in premature or low-birth-weight infants is a potential complication of aspirin exposure near delivery, but other salicylates, including sodium salicylate, probably do not present a risk because the presence of the acetyl moiety seems to be required to suppress platelet function (8–10).

In summary, inorganic bismuth salts, formed from metabolism of bismuth subsalicylate in the gastrointestinal tract, apparently present little or no risk to the fetus from normal therapeutic doses, but the data available for bismuth in pregnancy are poor and the actual fetal risk cannot be determined (11). On the other hand, the potential actions of salicylates on the fetus are complex. Although the risk for toxicity may be small, significant fetal adverse effects have resulted from chronic exposure to salicylates. Because of this, the use of bismuth subsalicylate during gestation should be restricted to the first half of pregnancy, and then only in amounts that do not exceed the recommended doses.

BREAST FEEDING SUMMARY

RECOMMENDATION: No Human Data - Potential Toxicity

The excretion of significant amounts of bismuth obtained from bismuth subsalicylate into breast milk is not expected because of the poor absorption of bismuth into the systemic circulation. Salicylates, however, are excreted in milk and are eliminated more slowly from milk than from plasma with milk:plasma ratios rising from 0.03–0.08 at 3 hours to 0.34 at 12 hours (12). Because of the potential for adverse effects in the nursing infant, the American Academy of Pediatrics recommends that salicylates should be used cautiously during breast-feeding (13). A 1991 review stated that bismuth subsalicylate should be avoided during lactation because of systemic salicylate absorption (14).

References

1. Pickering LK, Feldman S, Ericsson CD, Cleary TG. Absorption of salicylate and bismuth from a bismuth subsalicylate-containing compound (Pepto-Bismol). J Pediatr 1981;99:654–6.
2. Feldman S, Chen S-L, Pickering LK, Cleary TG, Ericsson CD, Hulse M. Salicylate absorption from a bismuth subsalicylate preparation. Clin Pharmacol Ther 1981;29:788–92.
3. Menge H, Brosius B, Lang A, Gregor M. Bismuth absorption from the stomach and small intestine. Gastroenterology 1992;102:2192.
4. Nwokolo CU, Pounder RE. Bismuth absorption from the stomach and small intestine. Reply. Gastroenterology 1992;102:2192–3.
5. James LF, Lazar VA, Binns W. Effects of sublethal doses of certain minerals on pregnant ewes and fetal development. Am J Vet Res 1966;27:132–5.
6. Hasking GJ, Duggan JM. Encephalopathy from bismuth subsalicylate. Med J Aust 1982;2:167.
7. Heinonen OP, Slone D, Shapiro S. *Birth Defects and Drugs in Pregnancy*. Littleton, MA: Publishing Sciences Group, 1977.

8. O'Brien JR. Effects of salicylates on human platelets. Lancet 1968;1:779–83.
9. Weiss HJ, Aledort ML, Shaul I. The effect of salicylates on the haemostatic properties of platelets in man. J Clin Invest 1968;47:2169–80.
10. Bleyer WA. Maternal ingested salicylates as a cause of neonatal hemorrhage. J Pediatr 1974;85: 736–7.
11. Friedman JM, Little BB, Brent RL, Cordero JF, Hanson JW, Shepard TH. Potential human teratogenicity of frequently prescribed drugs. Obstet Gynecol 1990;75:594–9.
12. Findlay JWA, DeAngelis RL, Kearney MF, Welch RM, Findley JM. Analgesic drugs in breast milk and plasma. Clin Pharmacol Ther 1981;29:625–33.
13. Committee on Drugs, American Academy of Pediatrics. The transfer of drugs and other chemicals into human milk. Pediatrics 2001;108:776–89.
14. Anderson PO. Drug use during breast feeding. Clin Pharm 1991;10:594–624.

Name:	**BISOPROLOL**	Risk Factor:	**C_M***
Class:	**Sympatholytic (Antihypertensive)**		

FETAL RISK SUMMARY

RECOMMENDATION: Human Data Suggest Risk in 2nd and 3rd Trimesters

Bisoprolol is a cardioselective β_1-adrenergic blocking agent used in the management of hypertension. In animal reproduction studies, bisoprolol was not teratogenic in rats at doses up to 375 and 77 times the maximum recommended human dose (MRHD) based on weight and body surface area, respectively, but fetotoxicity (increased late resorptions) was observed (1). No teratogenic effects were observed in rabbits at doses up to 31 and 12 times the MRHD based on body weight and surface area, respectively (1). Embryo lethality (increased early resorptions) was observed in rabbits.

A 2004 case report described a 24-year-old woman who took bisoprolol (5 mg/day), naproxen (550 mg about twice a week), and sumatriptan (100 mg about once a week) for migraine headaches during the first 5 weeks of pregnancy (2). An elective cesarean section was performed at 37 weeks' gestation for breech presentation to deliver a 3125-g male infant. The infant had a wide bilateral cleft lip/palate, marked hypertelorism, a broad nose, and bilateral but asymmetric toe abnormalities (missing and hypoplastic phalanges) (2).

Some β-blockers may cause intrauterine growth retardation (IUGR) and reduced placental weight, especially those lacking intrinsic sympathomimetic activity (ISA) (i.e., partial agonist). Treatment beginning early in the 2nd trimester results in the greatest weight reductions, whereas treatment restricted to the 3rd trimester primarily affects only placental weight. However, IUGR and reduced placental weight may potentially occur with all agents within this class. Although growth retardation is a serious concern, the benefits of maternal therapy with β-blockers, in some cases, might outweigh the risks to the fetus and must be judged on a case-by-case basis.

Newborn infants of mothers consuming the drug near delivery should be closely observed for 24–48 hours for signs and symptoms of β-blockade. Long-term effects of *in utero* exposure to β-blockers have not been studied but warrant evaluation.

[**Risk Factor D if used in 2nd or 3rd trimesters.*]

BREAST FEEDING SUMMARY

RECOMMENDATION: No Human Data - Potential Toxicity

Bisoprolol is excreted into the milk of lactating rats (<2% of the dose) (1), but reports describing the use in lactating women have not been located. Nursing infants of mothers consuming bisoprolol should be closely observed for hypotension, bradycardia, and other signs or symptoms of β-blockade. Long-term effects of exposure to β-blockers from milk have not been studied but warrant evaluation.

References

1. Product information. Zebeta. Lederle Laboratories, 1997.
2. Kajantie E, Somer M. Bilateral cleft lip and palate, hypertelorism and hypoplastic toes. Clin Dysmorphol 2004;13:195–6.

Name:	**BIVALIRUDIN**	Risk Factor:	**B_M**
Class:	**Thrombin Inhibitor**		

FETAL RISK SUMMARY

RECOMMENDATION: Compatible - Maternal Benefit >> Embryo/Fetal Risk

The reversible direct thrombin inhibitor bivalirudin is a synthetic 20-amino acid peptide. It is indicated, in combination with aspirin, for use as an IV anticoagulant in patients undergoing percutaneous transluminal coronary angioplasty. In patients with normal renal function, bivalirudin has a very short half-life (25 minutes) but may be as long as 3.5 hours for dialysis-dependent patients. Bivalirudin is not bound to plasma proteins (other than thrombin) or to red blood cells (1).

Reproduction studies have been conducted in rats and rabbits. In rats, SC doses up to 1.6 times the maximum recommended human dose based on body surface area (MRHD) revealed no evidence of impaired fertility or fetal harm. Similar findings were observed in rabbits with SC doses up to 3.2 times the MRHD (1).

It is not known if bivalirudin crosses the human placenta. The molecular weight (about 2180 for the anhydrous free base) and the very short elimination half-life in patients with normal renal function suggest that little, if any, of the peptide will cross the placenta.

No reports describing the use of bivalirudin in human pregnancy have been located. The animal data suggest low risk but the doses used are close to those used in humans. Presumably, higher doses were maternal toxic. The absence of human data prevents an assessment of the embryo/fetal risk. However, the manufacturer recommends that bivalirudin should always be used with aspirin (300–325 mg/day) and aspirin may be toxic if used in the 3rd trimester (see Aspirin). In addition, maternal bleeding secondary to both agents is a potential complication, especially in the 3rd trimester, and in the newborn, bleeding secondary to both agents is a potential complication if exposure has occurred within a week of delivery. If indicated, however, the maternal benefit appears to outweigh the potential, but unknown, embryo/fetal risk.

BREAST FEEDING SUMMARY

RECOMMENDATION: No Human Data - Probably Compatible

No reports describing the use of bivalirudin during human lactation have been located. The molecular weight (about 2180 for the anhydrous free base) and short elimination half-life (25 minutes in patients with normal renal function) suggest that little, if any, drug will be excreted into milk. The indication for the drug suggests that women would not breast-feed while receiving bivalirudin. Waiting 3 hours or longer for patients with impaired renal function after the last dose would assure that the exposure of a nursing infant was minimal or nil. In addition, bivalirudin is a peptide that should be digested in the nursing infant's gastrointestinal tract.

Reference

1. Product information. Angiomax. The Medicines Company, 2004.

Name:	**BLEOMYCIN**	Risk Factor:	D_M
Class:	**Antineoplastic**		

FETAL RISK SUMMARY

RECOMMENDATION: Human and Animal Data Suggest Risk

Bleomycin is an antineoplastic agent whose mechanism of action is thought to be inhibition of DNA synthesis and lesser inhibition of RNA and protein synthesis (1). The drug is teratogenic in rats. Skeletal malformations, shortened innominate artery, and hydroureter were observed at an intraperitoneal dose about 1.6 times the recommended human dose based on body surface area (RHD) given on days 6–15 of gestation (1). An IV dose about 2.4 times the RHD administered to rabbits on gestational days 6–18 resulted in abortions, but no teratogenic effects.

No reports linking the use of bleomycin with congenital defects in humans have been located. Chromosomal aberrations in human marrow cells have been reported, but the significance to the fetus is unknown (2). Two separate cases of non-Hodgkin's lymphoma in pregnancy were treated during the 2nd and 3rd trimesters with bleomycin and other antineoplastic agents (3,4). Normal infants without anomalies or chromosomal changes were delivered. In another case, a 21-year-old woman with a Ewing's sarcoma of the pelvis was treated with bleomycin and four other antineoplastic agents at approximately 25 weeks' gestation (5). Nine weeks later, recurrence of tumor growth necessitated delivery of the normal infant by cesarean section to allow for more definitive treatment of the tumor. The child was reported to be developing normally at 4 years of age.

A 1989 case report described the effect of maternal chemotherapy on a premature newborn delivered at approximately 27 weeks' gestation (6). The mother was treated with bleomycin (30 mg), etoposide (165 mg), and cisplatin (55 mg) (all given daily for 3 days), 1 week before delivery, for an unknown primary cancer with metastases to the eye and liver. The mother developed profound neutropenia just before delivery. On the 3rd day after delivery, the 1190-g female infant also developed a profound leukopenia with neutropenia 10 days after *in utero* exposure to the antineoplastic agents. The condition resolved after 10 days. At 10 days of age, the infant began losing her scalp hair and experienced a rapid loss of lanugo (6). Etoposide was thought to be the most likely cause of the neutropenia and the alopecia (6). By 12 weeks of age, substantial hair regrowth had occurred, and at 1 year follow-up, the child was developing normally except for moderate bilateral hearing loss. The investigators could not determine whether the sensorineural deafness was caused by the maternal and/or neonatal gentamicin therapy, or by the maternal cisplatin chemotherapy (6).

B

A 25-year-old woman underwent surgery at 25 weeks' gestation for an endodermal sinus tumor of the ovary (7). A chemotherapy cycle consisting of bleomycin (50 mg), cisplatin (75 mg/m^2), and vinblastine (0.25 mg/kg) was started 9 days later. Approximately 3 weeks later she received a second cycle of therapy. A normal, healthy 1900-g male infant was delivered by scheduled cesarean section at 32 weeks' gestation. The infant was alive and growing normally at the time of the report.

Combination chemotherapy with bleomycin was used for teratoma of the testis in two men (8). In both cases, recovery of spermatogenesis with apparently successful fertilization occurred, but the possibility of alternate paternity could not be excluded.

The long-term effects of combination chemotherapy on menstrual and reproductive function were described in a 1988 report (9). Only 7 of 40 women treated for malignant ovarian germ cell tumors received bleomycin. The results of this study are discussed in the monograph for cyclophosphamide (see Cyclophosphamide).

Occupational exposure of the mother to antineoplastic agents during pregnancy may present a risk to the fetus. A position statement from the National Study Commission on Cytotoxic Exposure and a research article involving some antineoplastic agents are presented in the monograph for cyclophosphamide (see Cyclophosphamide).

BREAST FEEDING SUMMARY

RECOMMENDATION: No Human Data - Potential Toxicity

No data are available.

References

1. Product information. Blenoxane. Bristol-Myers Squibb Oncology/Immunology Division, 2000.
2. Bornstein RS, Hungerford DA, Haller G, Engstrom PF, Yarbro JW. Cytogenic effects of bleomycin therapy in man. Cancer Res 1971;31:2004–7.
3. Ortega J. Multiple agent chemotherapy including bleomycin of non-Hodgkin's lymphoma during pregnancy. Cancer 1977;40:2829–35.
4. Falkson HC, Simson IW, Falkson G. Non-Hodgkin's lymphoma in pregnancy. Cancer 1980;45:1679–82.
5. Haerr RW, Pratt AT. Multiagent chemotherapy for sarcoma diagnosed during pregnancy. Cancer 1985;56:1028–33.
6. Raffles A, Williams J, Costeloe K, Clark P. Transplacental effects of maternal cancer chemotherapy: case report. Br J Obstet Gynaecol 1989;96:1099–1100.
7. Malone JM, Gershenson DM, Creasy RK, Kavanagh JJ, Silva EG, Stringer CA. Endodermal sinus tumor of the ovary associated with pregnancy. Obstet Gynecol 1986;68(Suppl):86S–9S.
8. Rubery ED. Return of fertility after curative chemotherapy for disseminated teratoma of testis. Lancet 1983;1:186.
9. Gershenson DM. Menstrual and reproductive function after treatment with combination chemotherapy for malignant ovarian germ cell tumors. J Clin Oncol 1988;6:270–5.

Name:	BLUE COHOSH	Risk Factor:	C
Class:	Herb		

FETAL RISK SUMMARY

RECOMMENDATION: Human and Animal Data Suggest Risk

Blue cohosh (*Caulophyllum thalictroides* Michx., family Berberidaceae [barberries]) is found throughout damp woodlands of the eastern part of North America, especially in the Allegheny Mountains (1,2). It is an early spring, leafy perennial herb with yellowish-green flowers that mature into bitter, bright blue seeds. The medicinal parts, collected in the autumn, are the matted, knotty rootstock (rhizomes) (1,2). A species found in Asia (*C. robustum* Maxim.), is also used for medicine (1).

Blue cohosh is often used to stimulate labor. In a survey of nurse-midwives, blue cohosh was the most frequently used herbal preparation for this purpose (65% of respondents), usually administered prior to or instead of oxytocin (3). Native Americans used blue cohosh for menstrual cramps and suppression of profuse menstruation (1). It has also been used as an emmenagogue, antispasmodic, antirheumatic, laxative, or for colic, sore throat, hiccups, epilepsy, hysterics, and uterine inflammation (1,4). The roasted seeds have been used as a coffee substitute (4).

The chemical composition of blue cohosh has been investigated since 1863 (5). Because early Native Americans used the herb to facilitate childbirth, researchers in 1954 described a technique to isolate a crystalline glycoside from blue cohosh rhizome and roots that demonstrated marked activity as a smooth muscle stimulant. Increased tone and rate of contraction were observed in rat, rabbit, and guinea pig uteruses, as well as in other smooth muscle preparations (5).

A number of chemical constituents have been isolated from blue cohosh rhizomes. These include anagyrine, baptifoline, 5,6-dehydro-α-islupanine, α-isolupanine, lupanine, sparteine, and *N*-methylcytisine (all are quinolizidine alkaloids), aporphine alkaloids (magnoflorine and taspine), caulophyllosaponin (also known as caluosaponin, a triterpene saponin), and caulosapogenin (1,2,6). In addition, a novel alkaloid, thalictroidine, has been recently found (6). *N*-methylcytisine (also known as caulophylline) is a nicotinic agonist in animals (1,2).

Citing previously published data, a 1999 study listed the concentrations of the quinolizidine alkaloids found in some blue cohosh-containing dietary supplements: *N*-methylcytisine 5–850 ppm, anagyrine, 2–390 ppm, and baptifoline, 9–900 ppm (the lower concentrations were found in liquid-extract products) (6). In contrast, the level of magnoflorine in the *C. thalictroides* rhizomes was 11,000 ppm (6).

N-methylcytisine was teratogenic in a rat embryo culture, but thalictroidine, anagyrine, and α-isolupanine were not teratogenic in this system at the concentrations tested (6). Marked embryo toxicity, without evidence of teratogenicity, was shown for taspine (6).

In an animal reproduction test, pregnant rats were administered either a low or high potency of *Caulophyllum* extract (homeopathic concentrations) on day 1 to day 5 of pregnancy (7). The lower potency prevented implantation by disrupting the site of implantation. In contrast, the high potency preparation caused no adverse effect compared with controls, but did increase the average number of young per litter (8 vs. 5 for controls) (7).

Anagyrine is teratogenic in ruminants, such as cattle, causing "crooked calf syndrome" (8–13). The severity of the malformations has been shown to be dose-related (11,12). Malformations include bowed or twisted limbs, spinal or neck curvature, and cleft palate. The defects may result from decreased normal fetal movements, which are required for normal skeletal development, secondary to the action of the alkaloid on fetal muscarinic and nicotinic receptors.

In an experiment with rats, a low potency extract of blue cohosh (homeopathic concentration) administered between estrus cycles, immediately before estrus, and during estrus was shown to be an effective inhibitor of ovulation and also inhibited physiologic changes in the uterus (14). A high potency extract (also homeopathic concentration) had no effect on ovulation or uterine changes.

No studies describing the placental crossing of any constituent of blue cohosh have been located. Based on the animal studies above, however, some or all of the alkaloids and other chemicals isolated from the herb probably cross the placenta.

A brief 1996 case report described an adverse newborn outcome after a woman with an uneventful pregnancy was given a combination of black and blue cohosh (dosage not specified) for labor induction (15). After a normal labor, a 3840-g female infant was born with Apgar scores of 1, 4, and 5 at 1, 5, and 10 minutes, respectively. No spontaneous breathing was observed, but resuscitation efforts were successful with the onset of breathing noted at 30 minutes. Mechanical ventilation was required during the hospital course, which was complicated by seizures and acute tubular necrosis. Computed tomography revealed basal ganglia and parasagittal hypoxic injury. Lower limb spasticity was apparent at 3 months of age, and the infant required nasogastric tube feeding. Although the cause of the neurologic toxicity in the newborn was unknown, the authors could not rule out a possible role for the herbal preparation. Citing published data, they speculated that black cohosh may have caused peripheral vasodilation and hypotension, whereas blue cohosh may have caused increased uterine activity. The combination of these actions may have led to a reduction of placental perfusion and caused hypoxia in the infant (15). The accuracy of this assessment has been challenged (16), but the case report below lends credibility to the concept that the use of blue cohosh in pregnancy may cause toxicity (17,18).

A 1998 case report described profound neonatal congestive heart failure in a newborn that was thought to have been caused by the mother's use of blue cohosh to promote uterine contractions (19). The 36-year-old woman had hypothyroidism but was euthyroid on replacement therapy. Except for this one condition, she had an uncomplicated pregnancy. One month before term, she was instructed by a midwife to take one tablet prepared from blue cohosh daily. Instead, for the next 5 weeks, the woman took one tablet three times daily. During this period, she reported increased uterine contractions and a decrease in fetal movements. A precipitous delivery occurred 1 hour after the onset of spontaneous labor, 15 minutes after spontaneous rupture of membranes. There was slight meconium-stained amniotic fluid. The 3.66-kg male infant had Apgar scores of 6 and 9 (presumably at 1 and 5 minutes, respectively), but cyanosis and poor perfusion developed within minutes of birth that required intubation and mechanical ventilation. At 1 hour of age, on 100% oxygen, umbilical arterial blood pH was 7.07, P_{CO_2} 40 mm Hg, and P_{O_2} 38 mm Hg. A chest X-ray revealed cardiomegaly and pulmonary edema, and an electrocardiogram showed acute myocardial infarction. Hepatomegaly was present in addition to the cardiac abnormalities. The infant's condition gradually improved and he was discharged home after 31 days. At 2 years of age, the child was progressing well with normal growth and development and good exercise tolerance, but continued to receive digoxin therapy. There was persistent cardiomegaly and his left ventricular function remained mildly reduced. The authors attributed the toxicity to blue cohosh because it contains vasoactive glycosides and it is known to cause toxic effects on the heart of animals (19).

A 2004 case report described a stroke in a female, full-term infant (birth weight 3860-g) 26 hours after birth (20). The mother, on advice of her physician, had consumed a tea made from blue cohosh to induce labor. A cesarean section was performed because of a failed attempt at vaginal delivery. Focal motor seizures of the right arm began at 26 hours of age. At 2 days of age, a computed tomographic scan revealed an evolving infarct in the distribution of the left middle cerebral artery. Laboratory tests in the infant for thrombophilia were normal and a family history for clotting disorders was negative. A cocaine metabolite, benzoylecgonine, was detected in the urine, meconium, the mother's bottle of blue cohosh, and the contents of a sealed bottle of a different preparation of the herb. Although cocaine contamination of the products could not be excluded, a blue cohosh preparation ("Inca Tea") contains coca leaves and can cause a positive test for cocaine exposure (20). In addition, among the natural constituents of blue cohosh, caulophyllosaponin can cause uterine contraction and coronary-artery constriction in animals (20), and methylcytisine is a nicotine agonist.

In summary, blue cohosh is an herbal product that has uterine stimulant properties. Some of its constituents have been shown to be teratogenic and toxic in various animal species. The herb should be avoided in the 1st trimester because of the animal teratogenicity data and its estrogenic effect demonstrated in humans (2). It is used in human pregnancy to induce labor, but the potential fetal and newborn toxicity appears to outweigh any medical benefit (1,4). In addition, preparations of blue cohosh are not standardized as to content or purity.

BREAST FEEDING SUMMARY

RECOMMENDATION: No Human Data - Potential Toxicity

No reports describing the use of blue cohosh during lactation have been located. It is not known if the constituents of the herb are excreted into breast milk. Depending on the maternal serum concentration of the various chemicals, however, some excretion should be expected. The effects of this exposure on a nursing infant are unknown, but the potential toxicity and estrogenic effects are substantial reasons to avoid blue cohosh ingestion during breast-feeding. At least one source states that its use during this period is likely unsafe (4).

References

1. Blue Cohosh. *The Review of Natural Products*. St. Louis: Facts and Comparisons, April 2000.
2. Blue Cohosh. *PDR for Herbal Medicines*. 2nd ed. Montvale, NJ: Medical Economics, 2000:109–10.
3. McFarlin BL, Gibson MH, O'Rear J, Harman P. A national survey of herbal preparation use by nurse-midwives for labor stimulation. Review of the literature and recommendations for practice. J Nurse-Midwifery 1999;44:205–16.
4. Blue Cohosh. *Natural Medicines Comprehensive Database*. Stockton, CA: Therapeutic Research Faculty, 1999:160–1.
5. Ferguson HC, Edwards LD. A pharmacological study of a crystalline glycoside of *Caulophyllum thalictroides*. J Am Pharm Assoc 1954;43:16–21.
6. Kennelly EJ, Flynn TJ, Mazzola EP, Roach JA, McClud TG, Danford DE, Betz JM. Detecting potential teratogenic alkaloids from blue cohosh rhizomes using an *in vitro* rat embryo culture. J Nat Prod 1999;62:1385–9.
7. Chandrasekhar K, Rao Vishwanath C. Studies on the effect of *Caulophyllum* on implantation in rats (abstract). J Reprod Fertil 1974;38:245–6.
8. Shupe JL, Binns W, James LF, Keeler RF. Lupine, a cause of crooked calf disease. J Am Vet Med Assoc 1967;151:198–203.
9. Keeler RF. Lupin alkaloids from teratogenic and nonteratogenic lupins. I. Correlation of crooked calf disease incidence with alkaloid distribution determined by gas chromatography. Teratology 1973;7:23–30.
10. Keeler RF. Lupin alkaloids from teratogenic and nonteratogenic lupins. II. Identification of the major alkaloids by tandem gas chromatography-mass spectrometry in plants producing crooked calf disease. Teratology 1973;7:31–35.
11. Keeler RF. Lupin alkaloids from teratogenic and nonteratogenic lupins. III. Identification of anagyrine as the probable teratogen by feeding trials. J Toxicol Environ Health 1976;1:887–98.
12. Keeler RF, Cronin EH. Lupin alkaloids from teratogenic and nonteratogenic lupins. IV. Concentration of total alkaloids, individual major alkaloids, and the teratogen anagyrine as a function of plant part and stage of growth and their relationship to crooked calf disease. J Toxicol Environ Health 1976;1:899–908.
13. Keeler RF. Teratogens in plants. J Animal Sci 1984;58:1029–39.
14. Chandrasekhar K, Sarma GHR. Observations on the effect of low and high doses of *Caulophyllum* on the ovaries and the consequential changes in the uterus and thyroid in rats (abstract). J Reprod Fertil 1974;38:236–7.
15. Gunn TR, Wright IMR. The use of black and blue cohosh in labour. Lancet 1996;109:410–1.
16. Baillie N, Rasmussen P. Black and blue cohosh in labour. Lancet 1997;110:20–1.
17. Wright IMR. Neonatal effects of maternal consumption of blue cohosh. J Pediatr 1999;134:384.
18. Jones TK. Neonatal effects of maternal consumption of blue cohosh. Reply. J Pediatr 1999;134:384–5.
19. Jones TK, Lawson BM. Profound neonatal congestive heart failure caused by maternal consumption of blue cohosh herbal medication. J Pediatr 1998;132:550–2.
20. Finkel RS, Zarlengo KM. Blue cohosh and perinatal stroke. N Engl J Med 2004;351:302–3.

B

Name: **BOSENTAN**
Class: **Vasodilator**

Risk Factor: X_M

FETAL RISK SUMMARY

RECOMMENDATION: No Human Data - Animal Data Suggest Moderate Risk

The endothelin receptor antagonist bosentan is indicated for the treatment of pulmonary arterial hypertension. It is a neurohormone that binds specifically to endothelin receptor types ET_A and ET_B. After oral administration, bosentan has one active (contributes 10%–20% of the total activity) and two inactive metabolites. Bosentan is highly (98%) bound to plasma albumin (1). It has an elimination half-life of about 5 hours (1,2).

Reproduction studies have been conducted in rats and rabbits. In rats, daily doses equal to or greater than two times the maximum recommended human daily dose based on body surface area (MRHDD) showed dose-related teratogenicity (defects of the head, mouth, face, and large blood vessels). Increased stillbirths and pup mortality were observed at doses two times the MRHDD or higher. Birth defects were not observed in rabbits given doses up to 1500 mg/kg/day (relationship to MRHDD not specified), but plasma concentrations were lower than those obtained in rats. The malformations observed in rats were similar to those observed in animals with other endothelin receptor antagonists and were thought to represent a class effect of these drugs (1).

Bosentan showed dose-related carcinogenicity in mice and rats given the agent over a 2-year period but no mutagenic or clastogenic activity. Short-duration studies showed no effect on fertility in male or female rats (1).

In near-term rats, closure of the fetal ductus arteriosus by indomethacin, *N*-nitro-L-arginine monomethyl ester (L-Name), or dexamethasone was prevented by the simultaneous administration of bosentan (3). An investigational selective endothelin receptor (ET_A) blocker (CI-1020) also was effective in preventing ductus closure (3).

The effects of bosentan on uteroplacental and maternal renal blood flow in pregnant rats were described in a 2002 report (4). On gestational day 19 (term 23 days), bosentan increased uteroplacental blood flow significantly higher than the normal physiologic increase but had no effect on renal blood flow. On gestational days 20 and 21, bosentan had no effect on uteroplacental blood flow but decreased renal blood flow by 20% (4).

It is not known if bosentan or its active metabolite crosses the human placenta to the fetus. The molecular weight (about 570) of bosentan, however, is low enough that passage to the fetal compartment should be expected.

Bosentan is an isoenzymes-inducer and is metabolized by the isoenzymes CYP2C9 and CYP3A4. Because many hormonal contraceptives are metabolized by CYP3A4, treatment with bosentan could cause decreased plasma concentrations and failure of these agents. Therefore, women should not rely on hormonal contraceptives alone (oral, injectable, or implantable) for contraception (1,2).

No reports describing the use of bosentan during human pregnancy have been located. Based only on the animal data, the manufacturer states that pregnancy must be excluded and that reliable contraceptive methods should be before the drug is prescribed. It also recommends monthly pregnancy tests during treatment (1). Therefore, pregnant women should not take this drug unless the severity of pulmonary arterial hypertension warrants the risk.

B

BREAST FEEDING SUMMARY

RECOMMENDATION: No Human Data - Potential Toxicity

No reports describing the use of bosentan during lactation have been located. The molecular weight (about 570) is low enough that excretion into breast milk should be expected. In addition, bosentan has an active metabolite that accounts for 10%–20% of the total activity and excretion of this agent into milk also is possible. The effects of this exposure on a nursing infant are unknown, but there is a potential for severe toxicity. Therefore, women taking bosentan should probably not breast-feed.

References

1. Cheng JWM. Bosentan. Heart Dis 2003;5:161–9.
2. Product information. Tracleer. Actelion Pharmaceuticals, 2004.
3. Momma K, Nakanishi I, Imamura S. Inhibition of *in vivo* constriction of fetal ductus arteriosus by endothelin receptor blockage in rats. Pediatr Res 2003;53:479–85.
4. Ajne G, Nisell H, Wolff K, Jansson I. The role of endogenous endothelin in the regulation of uteroplacental and renal blood flow during pregnancy in conscious rats. Placenta 2003;24:813–8.

Name: **BOTULINUM TOXIN TYPE A** Risk Factor: **C_M**

Class: **Central Nervous System Agent (Physical Adjunct)**

FETAL RISK SUMMARY

RECOMMENDATION: Limited Human Data - Animal Data Suggest Low Risk

Botulinum toxin Type A is produced by fermentation of the anaerobic bacterium *Clostridium botulinum* Type A. One unit (U) of the commercial preparation corresponds to the calculated median intraperitoneal lethal dose (LD_{50}) in mice. Botulinum toxin type A causes paralysis by binding to acceptor sites on motor nerve terminals, entering the nerve terminals, and inhibiting the release of acetylcholine (1). The toxin is not expected to enter the systemic circulation following IM injection. Botox is indicated for the treatment of cervical dystonia to decrease the severity of abnormal head position and neck associated with the disorder. It is also indicated for the treatment of strabismus and blepharospasm associated with dystonia, including benign essential blepharospasm or cranial VII nerve disorders (1). Botox Cosmetic is indicated for the temporary improvement in the appearance of moderate to severe glabellar lines associated with corrugator or procerus muscle activity (2).

Reproduction studies have been conducted in mice, rats, and rabbits. In mice and rats given IM injections during organogenesis, the developmental no-observed-effect-level (NOEL) was 4 U/kg. Doses of 8 U/kg or 16 U/kg were associated with decreased fetal body weights and/or delayed ossification. Doses above 8 U/kg impaired fertility in female rats by altering the estrous cycle. In rabbits, IM doses of 0.125 U/kg/day (gestational days 6–18) or 2 U/kg/day (gestational days 6 and 13) resulted in severe maternal toxicity, abortions, and fetal malformations. Higher doses caused maternal death (1). Interestingly, a 1965 study provided indirect evidence that botulinum toxin Type A crossed the placentas of pregnant mice, even though the toxin has a very high molecular weight (3).

It is not known if botulinum toxin Type A crosses the human placenta. It is a large protein with a very high molecular weight. In addition, it is not expected to enter the systemic circulation and, therefore, would not be present at the maternal:fetal interface. Moreover, the case reports below provide indirect evidence that botulinum toxins do not cross to the fetus in clinically significant amounts.

The first reported case of botulism in a pregnant woman appeared in 1975 (4). The case report involved a 32-year-old woman at 34 weeks' gestation that developed botulism and required assisted ventilation. Botulinum toxin type A was detected in her serum and she was treated with trivalent botulism antitoxin, but with limited success. Fetal heart tones were 140–160 beats per minute. On the fifth day of illness, she precipitously delivered a 1538-g male infant that was cyanotic with shallow respirations. No botulinum toxin was detected in the infant's serum obtained within 4 hours of birth. The infant's 42-day hospital course included aspiration pneumonia, anemia, seizures, and a probable intraventricular hemorrhage. The infant developed hydrocephalus several months after discharge but the condition resolved spontaneously. At 20 months of age, he was nearly totally blind (probable optic atrophy) and developmentally retarded. The infant's condition was attributed to hypoxia, a precipitous delivery, and intraventricular hemorrhage (4).

A 30-year-old woman at about 27 weeks' gestation was admitted to a hospital with signs and symptoms of botulism (5). She had been "skin popping" black tar heroin and had developed multiple abscesses on her left leg. Because botulism was suspected, she received two vials of antitoxin. The abscesses were excised and culture revealed *C. botulinum* Type A. Ten days before she was discharged from the hospital, at 34 weeks' gestation, her baby was delivered by cesarean section. No details regarding the infant were provided other than the fact that the infant remained in intensive care at 24-days of age (5).

A 1996 case report described a 37-year-old woman at 23 weeks' gestation that developed botulism from home-produced green beans (6). She eventually required assisted ventilation because of near complete paralysis. At the peak of the disease, fetal movement was the visible motion. Although she was treated with botulism antitoxin, she required tracheotomy and ventilation for 2 months. Throughout the woman's 3-month hospitalization, repeated surveillance revealed normal fetal development. Four months after the onset of the poisoning, a normal infant was delivered spontaneously (sex and other details of the infant not provided) (6).

A second 1996 case report involved a 24-year-old Alaskan Native at 16 weeks' gestation that was poisoned by consumption of fermented whitefish (7). Both *C. botulinum* Types A and E were cultured from her stool and type E organisms and toxin were detected in the whitefish. Ultrasonography revealed a fetus with normal breathing and movements. The woman was treated with trivalent botulinum antitoxin and rapidly recovered. At 42 weeks' gestation, she spontaneously delivered a healthy, 4300-g male infant. The child's growth and development during the first year were normal (7).

In an *in vitro* study, botulinum toxin Type A has been demonstrated to inhibit or completely arrest myometrial activity (8). The investigators thought that the toxin might eventually have application in the prevention of preterm labor after fetal surgery. Moreover, the effects were potentially reversible (8).

In summary, no reports describing the use of commercially prepared botulinum toxin type A in human pregnancy have been located. The animal data are suggestive of low risk, but the absence of human pregnancy experience prevents a full assessment of the embryo/fetal risk. However, the commercially prepared and wild toxins should be identical. Moreover, the case reports above suggest that the wild toxins do not cross the human placenta in the last half of pregnancy. In addition, the appearance in the systemic circulation of botulinum toxin type A is not expected after IM injections. Therefore, although the safety of use of the commercial toxin in pregnancy is unknown (9,10), the risk of embryo or fetal harm appears to be very low or nonexistent.

BREAST FEEDING SUMMARY

RECOMMENDATION: No Human Data - Probably Compatible

No reports describing the use of botulinum toxin type A during human lactation have been located. Because the toxin is not expected to appear in the systemic circulation, it would not be available for excretion into breast milk. Therefore, the risk to a nursing infant is probably nil.

References

1. Product information. Botox. Allergan, 2004.
2. Product information. Botox Cosmetic. Allergan, 2002. As cited by *Facts and Comparisons*. St. Louis, MO: Walters Kluwer Health, 2002:1997–98a.
3. Hart LG, Dixon RL, Long JP, Mackay B. Studies using *Clostridium botulinum* toxin—Type A. Toxicol Appl Pharmacol 1965;7:84–9.
4. St. Clair EH, DiLiberti JH, O'Brien ML. Observations of an infant born to a mother with botulism. J Pediatr 1975;87:658.
5. Centers for Disease Control and Prevention. Wound botulism - California 1995. MMWR 1995;44:889–92.
6. Polo JM, Martin J, Berciano J. Botulism and pregnancy. Lancet 1996;348:195.
7. Robin L, Herman D, Redett R. Botulism in a pregnant woman. N Engl J Med 1996;335:823–4.
8. Garza JJ, Downard CD, Clayton N, Maher TJ, Fauza DO. *Clostridium botulinum* toxin inhibits myometrial activity *in vitro*: possible application on the prevention of preterm labor after fetal surgery. J Pediatr Surg 2003;38:511–3.
9. Anonymous. Botulinum toxin. Consensus Statement 1990;8:1–20.

Name:	BRETYLIUM	Risk Factor:	C
Class:	Antiarrhythmic		

FETAL RISK SUMMARY

RECOMMENDATION: No Human Data - No Relevant Animal Data

Bretylium, a quaternary ammonium compound, is an adrenergic blocker used as an antiarrhythmic agent. No information on its use in pregnancy has been located. Hypotension has been observed in 50% of patients after they had taken bretylium (1). Although reports are lacking, reduced uterine blood flow with fetal hypoxia (bradycardia) is a potential risk.

BREAST FEEDING SUMMARY

RECOMMENDATION: Hold Breast Feeding

No data are available.

Reference

1. Product information. Bretylol. Du Pont Critical Care, 1988.

B

Name: **BROMIDES** Risk Factor: **D**
Class: **Anticonvulsant/Sedative**

FETAL RISK SUMMARY

RECOMMENDATION: Human and Animal Data Suggest Risk

The Collaborative Perinatal Project monitored 50,282 mother-child pairs, 986 of whom had 1st trimester exposure to bromides (1, pp. 402–406). For use anytime during pregnancy, 2610 exposures were recorded (1, p. 444). In neither group was evidence found to suggest a relationship to large categories of major or minor malformations. Four possible associations with individual malformations were found, but independent confirmation is required: polydactyly (14 cases), gastrointestinal anomalies (10 cases), clubfoot (7 cases), and congenital dislocation of hip (use anytime) (92 cases).

Two infants with intrauterine growth retardation from a mother who chronically ingested a proprietary product containing bromides (Bromo-Seltzer) have been described (2). Both male infants were microcephalic (one at the 2nd percentile and one at less than the 2nd percentile) and one had congenital heart disease (atrial septal defect with possible pulmonary insufficiency). The mother did not use the product in three other pregnancies, two before and one after the affected children, and all three of these children were of normal height. In a similar case, a woman chronically ingested tablets containing bromides throughout gestation and eventually gave birth to a female infant who was growth retarded (all parameters below the 10th percentile) (3). Follow-up of the infant at 2.5 years of age indicated persistent developmental delay.

Neonatal bromide intoxication from transplacental accumulation has been described in four infants (4–7). In each case, the mother had either taken bromide-containing medications (three cases) or was exposed from employment in a photographic laboratory (one case). Bromide concentrations in three of the four infants were 3650, 2000, and 2420 μg/mL on days 6, 5, and 5, respectively (4–6). In the fourth case, a serum sample, not obtained until 18 days after birth, contained 150 μg/mL (7). All four infants exhibited symptoms of neonatal bromism consisting of poor suck, weak cry, diminished Moro reflex, lethargy, and hypotonia. One of the infants also had cyanosis and a large head with dysmorphic face (7). Subsequent examinations of three of the above infants revealed normal growth and development after several months (4–6). One infant, however, had mild residual hypotonia of the neck muscles persisting at 6 and 9.5 months (7).

Cord serum bromide levels were determined on 1267 newborn infants born in Rochester, NY, during the first half of 1984 (8). Mean bromide concentrations were 8.6 μg/mL (range 3.1–28.5 μg/mL), well below the serum bromide level (>720 μg/mL) that is considered toxic (8). The measured concentrations were not related to Apgar scores, neonatal condition, or congenital abnormalities. None of the mothers was taking bromide-containing drugs (most of which have been removed from the market), and the concentrations in cord blood were thought to have resulted from occupational exposure to photographic chemicals or from the low levels encountered in food and water.

BREAST FEEDING SUMMARY

RECOMMENDATION: Limited Human Data - Potential Toxicity

The excretion of bromides into breast milk has been known since at least 1907 (9). A 1938 report reviewed this topic and demonstrated the presence of bromides in milk in an additional 10 mothers (9). A 1935 report measured milk concentrations of 1666 μg/mL in two patients treated with 5 g daily for 1 month (10). Rash and sedation of varying degrees in several nursing infants have been reported as a result of maternal consumption of bromides during lactation (9–11). Although bromide-containing medications are no longer available in the United States, these drugs may be available in other countries. In addition, high maternal serum levels may be obtained from close, frequent exposure to chemicals used in photographic developing. Women who are breast-feeding and are exposed to such chemicals should be alert for symptoms of sedation or drowsiness and unexplained rashes in their infants. Monitoring of bromide levels in these women may be beneficial. Nursing is not recommended for women receiving bromide-containing medications, although the American Academy of Pediatrics classifies bromides as compatible with breast-feeding (12).

References

1. Heinonen OP, Slone D, Shapiro S. *Birth Defects and Drugs in Pregnancy*. Littleton, MA: Publishing Sciences Group, 1977.
2. Opitz JM, Grosse RF, Haneberg B. Congenital effects of bromism? Lancet 1972;1:91–2.
3. Rossiter EJR, Rendel-Short TJ. Congenital effects of bromism? Lancet 1972;2:705.
4. Finken RL, Robertson WO. Transplacental bromism. Am J Dis Child 1963;106:224–6.
5. Mangurten HH, Ban R. Neonatal hypotonia secondary to transplacental bromism. J Pediatr 1974;85:426–8.
6. Pleasure JR, Blackburn MG. Neonatal bromide intoxication: prenatal ingestion of a large quantity of bromides with transplacental accumulation in the fetus. Pediatrics 1975;55:503–6.
7. Mangurten HH, Kaye CI. Neonatal bromism secondary to maternal exposure in a photographic laboratory. J Pediatr 1982;100:596–8.
8. Miller ME, Cosgriff JM, Roghmann KJ. Cord serum bromide concentration: variation and lack of association with pregnancy outcome. Am J Obstet Gynecol 1987;157:826–30.
9. Tyson RM, Shrader EA, Perlman HH. Drugs transmitted through breast milk. III. Bromides. J Pediatr 1938;13:91–3.
10. Kwit NT, Hatcher RA. Excretion of drugs in milk. Am J Dis Child 1935;49:900–4.
11. Van der Bogert F. Bromin poisoning through mother's milk. Am J Dis Child 1921;21:167.
12. Committee on Drugs, American Academy of Pediatrics. The transfer of drugs and other chemicals into human milk. Pediatrics 2001;108:776–89.

Name: **BROMOCRIPTINE** Risk Factor: B_M

Class: **Miscellaneous**

FETAL RISK SUMMARY

RECOMMENDATION: Compatible

Bromocriptine has been used during all stages of pregnancy. In 1982, Turkalj and coworkers (1) reviewed the results of 1410 pregnancies in 1,335 women exposed to bromocriptine during gestation. The drug, used for the treatment of infertility as a result of hyperprolactinemia or pituitary tumors including acromegaly, was usually discontinued as soon as pregnancy was diagnosed. The mean duration of exposure after conception was 21 days. The review included all reported cases from 1973, the year bromocriptine was introduced, through 1980. Since then, 11 other studies have reported the results of treatment in 121 women with 145 pregnancies (2–12). The results of the pregnancies in the combined studies are:

Total patients/pregnancies: 1456/1555
Liveborn infants: 1369 (88%)
Stillborn infants: 5 (0.3%)

Multiple pregnancies (30 twins/3 triplets) 33 (2.1%)
Spontaneous abortions: 66 (10.7%)
Elective abortions: 26 (1.7%)
Extrauterine pregnancies: 12 (0.8%)
Hydatidiform moles (2 patients) 3 (0.2%)
Pregnant at time of report, outcome unknown: 10

[**Two women with twins were also treated with clomiphene or gonadotropin.*]

A total of the 1374 liveborn and stillborn infants, had detectable anomalies at birth (1–12). This incidence is similar to the expected rate of congenital defects found in the general population. In the review by Turkalj and co-workers, the mean duration of fetal exposure to bromocriptine was similar between children with congenital abnormalities and normal children. No distinguishable pattern of anomalies was found. The malformations detected in 36 infants (number of infants shown in parentheses) were as follows:

Down's syndrome (2)
Hydrocephalus and multiple atresia of esophagus and intestine (1)
Microcephalus/encephalopathy (1)
Omphalocele/talipes (1)
Pulmonary artery atresia (1)
Reduction deformities (4)
Renal agenesis (1)
Pierre Robin syndrome (1)
Bat ear and plagiocephalus (1)
Cleft palate (1)
Ear lobe deformity (1)
Head posture constrained (1)
Hip dislocation (aplasia of cup) (9)
Hydrocele (3)
Hydrocele/omphalocele (1)
Hypospadias (1)
Inguinal hernia (2)
Skull soft and open fontanella (1)
Single palmar crease (1)
Single umbilical artery (1)
Syndactyly (2)
Talipes (5)
Umbilical hernia (1)
Cutaneous hemangioma (4)
Testicular ectopia (1) (spontaneous correction occurred at age 7 months)

Long-term studies on 213 children followed up to 6 years of age have shown normal mental and physical development (1,2).

In a surveillance study of Michigan Medicaid recipients conducted between 1985 and 1992 and involving 229,101 completed pregnancies, 50 newborns had been exposed to bromocriptine during the 1st trimester (F. Rosa, personal communication, FDA, 1993). Three (6.0%) major birth defects were observed (two expected). Specific information was not available on the malformations, but no anomalies were observed in six categories of defects (cardiovascular defects, oral clefts, spina bifida, polydactyly, limb

B

reduction defects, and hypospadias) for which data were available. Based on a small number of exposures, the data do not support an association between the drug and congenital defects.

In summary, bromocriptine apparently does not pose a significant risk to the fetus. The pattern and incidence of anomalies are similar to those expected in a nonexposed population.

BREAST FEEDING SUMMARY

RECOMMENDATION: Contraindicated

Since bromocriptine is indicated for the prevention of physiologic lactation, breastfeeding is not possible during therapy (13,14). However, in one report, a mother taking 5 mg/day for a pituitary tumor was able to breast-feed her infant successfully (3). No effects on the infant were mentioned. Because bromocriptine suppresses lactation, the American Academy of Pediatrics classifies bromocriptine as a drug that should be given to nursing women with caution (15).

References

1. Turkalj I, Braun P, Krupp P. Surveillance of bromocriptine in pregnancy. JAMA 1982;247:1589–91.
2. Konopka P, Raymond JP, Merceron RE, Seneze J. Continuous administration of bromocriptine in the prevention of neurological complications in pregnant women with prolactinomas. Am J Obstet Gynecol 1983;146:935–8.
3. Canales ES, Garcia IC, Ruiz JE, Zarate A. Bromocriptine as prophylactic therapy in prolactinoma during pregnancy. Fertil Steril 1981;36:524–6.
4. Bergh T, Nillius SJ, Larsson SG, Wide L. Effects of bromocriptine-induced pregnancy on prolactin-secreting pituitary tumors. Acta Endocrinol 1981;98:333.
5. Yuen BH, Cannon W, Sy L, Booth J, Burch P. Regression of pituitary microadenoma during and following bromocriptine therapy: persistent defect in prolactin regulation before and throughout pregnancy. Am J Obstet Gynecol 1982;142:634–9.
6. Maeda T, Ushiroyama T, Okuda K, Fujimoto A, Ueki M, Sugimoto O. Effective bromocriptine treatment of a pituitary macroadenoma during pregnancy. Obstet Gynecol 1983;61:117–21.
7. Hammond CB, Haney AF, Land MR, van der Merwe JV, Ory SJ, Wiebe RH. The outcome of pregnancy in patients with treated and untreated prolactin-secreting pituitary tumors. Am J Obstet Gynecol 1983;147:148–57.
8. Cundy T, Grundy EN, Melville H, Sheldon J. Bromocriptine treatment of acromegaly following spontaneous conception. Fertil Steril 1984;42:134–6.
9. Randall S, Laing I, Chapman AJ, Shalet SM, Beardwell CG, Kelly WF, Davies D. Pregnancies in women with hyperprolactinaemia: obstetric and endocrinological management of 50 pregnancies in 37 women. Br J Obstet Gynaecol 1982;89:20–33.
10. Andersen AN, Starup J, Tabor A, Jensen HK, Westergaard JG. The possible prognostic value of serum prolactin increment during pregnancy in hyperprolactinaemic patients. Acta Endocrinol 1983;102:1–5.
11. van Roon E, van der Vijver JCM, Gerretsen G, Hekster REM, Wattendorff RA. Rapid regression of a suprasellar extending prolactinoma after bromocriptine treatment during pregnancy. Fertil Steril 1981;36:173–77.
12. Crosignani P, Ferrari C, Mattei AM. Visual field defects and reduced visual acuity during pregnancy in two patients with prolactinoma: rapid regression of symptoms under bromocriptine. Case reports. Br J Obstet Gynaecol 1984;91:821–3.
13. Product information. Parlodel. Sandoz Pharmaceuticals, 1985.
14. Thorbert G, Akerlund M. Inhibition of lactation by cyclofenil and bromocriptine. Br J Obstet Gynaecol 1983;90:739–42.
15. Committee on Drugs, American Academy of Pediatrics. The transfer of drugs and other chemicals into human milk. Pediatrics 2001;108:776–89.

Name:	**BROMODIPHENHYDRAMINE**	Risk Factor:	**C**
Class:	**Antihistamine**		

Bromodiphenhydramine is a derivative of diphenhydramine (see Diphenhydramine).

B

Name: **BROMPHENIRAMINE** Risk Factor: **C_M**
Class: **Antihistamine**

FETAL RISK SUMMARY

RECOMMENDATION: Limited Human Data - No Relevant Animal Data

The Collaborative Perinatal Project monitored 50,282 mother-child pairs, 65 of whom had 1st trimester exposure to brompheniramine (1, pp. 322–325). Based on 10 malformed infants, a statistically significant association ($p < 0.01$) was found between this drug and congenital defects. This relationship was not found with other antihistamines. For use anytime during pregnancy, 412 exposures were recorded (1, p. 437). In this group, no evidence was found for an association with malformations.

The use of antihistamines in general (specific agents and dose not given) during the last 2 weeks of pregnancy has been associated with an increased risk of retrolental fibroplasia in premature infants (2). Infants weighing less than 1750 g, who had no detectable congenital anomalies and who survived for at least 24 hours after birth, were enrolled in the multicenter National Collaborative Study on Patent Ductus Arteriosus in Premature Infants conducted between 1979 and 1981 (2). After exclusions, 3026 infants were available for study. Exposures to antihistamines and other drugs were determined by interview and maternal record review. The incidence of retrolental fibroplasia in infants exposed to antihistamines during the last 2 weeks of gestation was 22% (19 of 86) vs. 11% (324 of 2940) in infants not exposed during this interval. Adjustment for severity of disease did not change the estimated rate ratio.

BREAST FEEDING SUMMARY

RECOMMENDATION: Limited Human Data - Probably Compatible

A single case report has been located describing adverse effects in a 3-month-old nursing infant of a mother consuming a long-acting preparation containing 6 mg of dexbrompheniramine and 120 mg of *d*-isoephedrine (3). The mother had begun taking the preparation on a twice-daily schedule about 1 or 2 days before the onset of symptoms in the infant. Symptoms consisted of irritability, excessive crying, and disturbed sleeping patterns, which resolved spontaneously within 12 hours when breast-feeding was stopped. One manufacturer considers the drug to be contraindicated for nursing mothers (4). The American Academy of Pediatrics noted the above adverse effects observed with dexbrompheniramine plus *d*-isoephedrine, but classified the combination as usually compatible with breast-feeding (5).

References

1. Heinonen OP, Slone D, Shapiro S. *Birth Defects and Drugs in Pregnancy*. Littleton, MA: Publishing Sciences Group, 1977.
2. Zierler S, Purohit D. Prenatal antihistamine exposure and retrolental fibroplasia. Am J Epidemiol 1986;123:192–6.
3. Mortimer EA Jr. Drug toxicity from breast milk? Pediatrics 1977;60:780–1.
4. Product information. Dimetane. AH Robins Company, 1990.
5. Committee on Drugs, American Academy of Pediatrics. The transfer of drugs and other chemicals into human milk. Pediatrics 2001;108:776–89.

Name:	**BUCLIZINE**	Risk Factor:	**C**
Class:	**Antihistamine/Antiemetic**		

FETAL RISK SUMMARY

RECOMMENDATION: Limited Human Data - Animal Data Suggest Risk

Buclizine is a piperazine antihistamine that is used as an antiemetic (see Cyclizine and Meclizine for closely related drugs). The drug is teratogenic in animals, but its effects on the human fetus have not been thoroughly studied.

The Collaborative Perinatal Project monitored 50,282 mother-child pairs, 44 of whom had 1st trimester exposure to buclizine (1, pp. 323–324). No evidence was found to suggest a relationship to large categories of major or minor malformations. For use anytime during pregnancy, 62 exposures were recorded (1, p. 437). A possible association with congenital defects, based on the report of three malformed children, was found from this exposure. The manufacturer considers the drug to be contraindicated in early pregnancy (2).

An association between exposure during the last 2 weeks of pregnancy to antihistamines in general and retrolental fibroplasia in premature infants has been reported. See Brompheniramine for details.

BREAST FEEDING SUMMARY

RECOMMENDATION: No Human Data - Probably Compatible

No data are available.

References

1. Heinonen OP, Slone D, Shapiro S. *Birth Defects and Drugs in Pregnancy*. Littleton, MA: Publishing Sciences Group, 1977.
2. Product information. Bucladin. Stuart Pharmaceuticals, 1990.

Name:	**BUDESONIDE**	Risk Factor: **B_M/C_M***
Class:	**Respiratory Drug (Corticosteroid), Corticosteroid**	

FETAL RISK SUMMARY

RECOMMENDATION: Compatible - Maternal Benefit >> Embryo/Fetal Risk (Inhaled/Nasal) No Human Data - Animal Data Suggest Risk (Oral)

Budesonide is an anti-inflammatory corticosteroid used in the maintenance treatment of asthma as prophylactic therapy (Pulmicort Turbuhaler) or for the management of symptoms of allergic rhinitis (Rhinocort Nasal Inhaler). Pulmicort Turbuhaler delivers approximately 160 μg of micronized budesonide per actuation, whereas Rhinocort Nasal Inhaler delivers approximately 32 μg of micronized budesonide per actuation (1,2). The latter dose is suspended in a mixture of propellants (dichlorodifluoromethane, trichloromonofluoromethane, and dichlorotetrafluoroethane) and sorbitan trioleate.

Budesonide has potent glucocorticoid but weak mineralocorticoid, activity. Compared to hydrocortisone (cortisol), budesonide is 40 times more potent when administered SC and 25 times more potent when given orally (1,2). Approximately 34% of the delivered dose of Pulmicort and 21% of Rhinocort are absorbed systemically (1,2).

Similar to other glucocorticoid agents, budesonide administered to pregnant rabbits at a SC dose about 0.33 times the maximum recommended human daily inhalation dose based on body surface area (MRHD) produced fetal loss, intrauterine growth retardation (IUGR), and skeletal anomalies (mostly delayed ossification of the vertebra and skull) (1–3). In pregnant rats, a SC dose about 3 times the MRHD resulted in similar outcomes (1,2). No teratogenic or embryocidal effects were observed in pregnant rats administered inhalation doses up to about 2 times the MRHD (1,2).

No reports describing the placental transfer of budesonide have been located. The relatively low molecular weight (about 431 for the butyraldehyde formulation) and high lipid solubility predict substantial placental transfer. The actual amount of active budesonide reaching the fetus, however, may be small because of the low systemic bioavailability after inhalation (see above) and the observation that other corticosteroids undergo extensive placental metabolism to inactive compounds (e.g., see Hydrocortisone, Betamethasone, and Dexamethasone).

Data from the Swedish Medical Birth Registry involving 2014 infants whose mothers had inhaled budesonide for asthma during early pregnancy were reported in 1999 (4). Drug exposures were identified prospectively, before the pregnancy outcomes were known. Among the mothers of the 2014 infants, 1675 also used β_2-adrenergic agonists, 16 used other inhaled corticosteroids in addition to budesonide, and 316 used no other antiasthmatic drug. A total of 76 infants (3.8%) in the exposed group had a congenital malformation, compared with 3.5% for all infants born in 1995–1997. Major structural defects were observed in 41 of the infants, whereas 35 infants had a minor and/or variable conditions. Five of the major defects were chromosomal anomalies. It is unlikely that these were due to drug therapy (4). Four (expected 3.3) of the major anomaly group had an orofacial cleft (median cleft palate [$N = 2$], unilateral cleft lip [$N = 1$], and unilateral cleft lip and palate [$N = 1$]) (relative risk 1.2, 95% (Confidence Interval 0.3–3.1) (4). Among the major and minor defects, 18 (expected 17–18) involved the heart, including two premature infants with patent ductus arteriosus (both categorized as minor defects). The other cardiac malformations were: ventricular septal defects (VSD) with or without other anomalies ($N = 11$); atrial septal defects with or without other anomalies ($N = 4$); and unspecified cardiac defect ($N = 1$). Only two of the cases with VSD, one with transposition of the great vessels and another with tricuspidal atresia (both successfully repaired), were reported to the Swedish Child Cardiology Registry (expected number 5.6). Because the other 16 cases were not reported, the authors concluded that the defects were mild and of little clinical significance (4).

Twenty-one pregnancies in which the woman received an active drug were reported to the manufacturer during clinical trials of Pulmicort Turbuhaler (A. Marants, personal communication, Astra Pharmaceuticals, 1999). Two of the pregnancies were terminated voluntarily, one woman had a miscarriage, three had unknown outcomes, 13 delivered normal infants, and two delivered infants with congenital malformations. In one case, the 27-year-old mother was receiving budesonide 1600 μg/day at conception. She was also taking prednisone 10 mg/day and a combination oral contraceptive (levonorgestrel + ethinyl estradiol). Although the reason for early delivery was not specified, a female infant with coarctation of the aorta was delivered by cesarean section at 30 weeks' gestation. The infant was scheduled for surgical repair of the defect. In the second case, a 41-year-old mother used budesonide inhaler for 22 days (dosage unknown) before discontinuing it because of her pregnancy. Seven months later, she delivered a female infant with double-sided maxillary clefts, double digits of the left hand, and persistent fetal circulation (i.e., patent ductus arteriosus). The infant died at 8 days of age.

The infant outcomes of five asthmatic women who used budesonide during pregnancy were described in retrospective postmarketing reports to the manufacturer (A. Marants, personal communication, Astra Pharmaceuticals, 1999). Only limited data were available for each pregnancy. The first case involved a 36-year-old woman, treated with an unknown dose of budesonide combined with a β_2-adrenergic agonist (albuterol), who delivered an anencephalic infant. In the second case, a 32-year-old woman administering budesonide 1600 μg/day gave birth to a healthy, 2.65-kg baby. A 33-year-old woman was treated with four antiasthmatic agents during gestation, including budesonide 1600 μg/day, an oral corticosteroid (name not specified), a β_2-adrenergic agonist (not specified), and theophylline. She gave birth to a female infant with agenesis of the left foot who was otherwise healthy. Another 33-year-old woman being treated with budesonide 1600 μg/day, phenobarbital, and terbutaline (a β_2-adrenergic agonist) delivered an infant with cleft palate, an unspecified cardiac defect, and hydrocephalus. Finally, IUGR and oligohydramnios were noted in a pregnancy of a 36-year-old woman who was being treated with budesonide 400 μg/day, salmeterol (an inhaled β_2-adrenergic agonist), and terfenadine (an antihistamine). She gave birth to a growth-retarded infant (2.0 Kg) who had multiple malformations, including a diaphragmatic hernia, renal hypoplasia, and a VSD. The infant died on the day of birth.

A 2003 case-control study, using data from three Swedish health registers, was conducted to identify drug use in early pregnancy that was associated with cardiac defects (5). Cases (cardiovascular defects without known chromosome anomalies) (N = 5015) were compared to controls consisting of all infants born in Sweden (1995–2001) (N = 577,730). Associations were identified for several drugs, some of which were probably due to confounding from the underlying disease or complaint or multiple testing, but some were thought to be true drug effects (5). For all inhaled corticosteroids, there were 66 cases in 7404 (odds ratio [OR] 1.05, 95% confidence interval [CI] 0.82–1.34). For inhaled budesonide, there were 16 cases in 6557 exposures (OR 1.12, 95% CI 0.87–1.44). For all nasal corticosteroids, there were 31 cases among 2872 exposures (1.24, 95% CI 0.87–1.78), but 28 of the cases involved nasal budesonide (2230 exposures) (1.45, 95% CI 0.99–2.10). Restricting the analysis of nasal budesonide to less severe defects increased the probability of an association (OR 1.58, 95% CI 1.02–2.46), as also was seen with unspecified cardiovascular defects (OR 2.39, 95% CI 0.96–4.92). The risk for ventricular and atrial septum defects were 1.67 (95% CI 0.99–2.81) and 2.18 (95% CI 0.71–5.08), respectively (5).

In summary, parenteral budesonide causes teratogenicity and toxicity in animals, but in humans, inhaled budesonide does not appear to represent a significant risk for congenital defects. However, a small risk may exist between nasal budesonide and cardiac defects. A small, but statistically significant, increased risk for cleft lip with or without cleft palate has been reported for corticosteroids (see Hydrocortisone). A similar risk for orofacial clefts was observed with inhaled budesonide, but the number of exposed infants was too small for statistical significance. The data from the manufacturer's postmarketing surveillance do not show a clustering of defects and thus in themselves cannot be used as evidence of an increased risk for birth defects. Surveillance reports of this type are important for detecting early signals of major teratogens, but they have several difficulties. The primary problems with these voluntary reports are their retrospective nature (reported after the outcome is known), their selection bias (mainly adverse outcomes are reported), and their lack of sufficient details on the mother, her family history, her disease, and her pregnancy. Moreover, these data cannot be used to determine true rates of outcomes.

B

During pregnancy, the benefits of treating allergic rhinitis with any product, including budesonide, must be carefully weighed against the potential risks of therapy. Consideration should be given to limiting corticosteroid exposure, especially during the 1st trimester. In contrast, poorly controlled asthma may result in adverse maternal, fetal, and neonatal outcomes (6). Maternal complications include an increased risk of preeclampsia, pregnancy-induced hypertension, hyperemesis gravidarum, vaginal hemorrhage, and induced and difficult labors. Fetal and neonatal adverse effects may be an increased risk of perinatal mortality, IUGR, prematurity, lower birth weight, and neonatal hypoxia. Because controlling maternal asthma can ameliorate or prevent all of these complications (6), the benefits of therapy outweigh the potential risks of drug-induced teratogenicity or toxicity. Therefore, pregnant women who require an inhaled corticosteroid, such as budesonide, for control of their asthma should be counseled as to the risks and benefits of therapy, but treatment should not be withheld because of their pregnancy.

[*Inhaled formulation Risk Factor B_M; oral formulation Risk Factor C_M.*]

BREAST FEEDING SUMMARY

RECOMMENDATION: No Human Data - Probably Compatible

No reports describing the use of inhaled budesonide during human lactation have been located. The relatively low molecular weight (about 431 for the butyraldehyde formulation) and the high lipid solubility predict substantial excretion of systemic budesonide into milk. However, the systemic bioavailability of budesonide following inhalation therapy is relatively low (see section above), so that the actual amount in milk also may be low. Small amounts of other corticosteroids are excreted into milk (e.g., see Prednisone), and if the mother is inhaling budesonide, the presence of the corticosteroid in her milk should be anticipated. Because of the oral potency of budesonide (about 25 times more glucocorticoid activity than hydrocortisone), the clinical significance of this potential exposure on a nursing infant is unknown. The manufacturer recommends stopping breast-feeding if the mother must use the Pulmicort Turbuhaler (1).

References

1. Product information. Pulmicort Turbuhaler. AstraZeneca, 2000.
2. Product information. Rhinocort. AstraZeneca, 2000.
3. Kihlstrom I, Lundberg C. Teratogenicity study of the new glucocorticosteroid budesonide in rabbits. Arzneimittelforschung/Drug Res 1987;37:43–6.
4. Kallen B, Rydhstroem H, Aberg A. Congenital malformations after the use of inhaled budesonide in early pregnancy. Obstet Gynecol 1999;93:392–5.
5. Kallen BAJ, Olausson PO. Maternal drug use in early pregnancy and infant cardiovascular defect. Reprod Toxicol 2003;17:255–61.
6. Report of the Working Group on Asthma and Pregnancy, National Institutes of Health. *Management of Asthma During Pregnancy*. NIH Publication No. 93–3279, September 1993.

Name: **BUMETANIDE** Risk Factor: **C_M***

Class: **Diuretic**

FETAL RISK SUMMARY

RECOMMENDATION: Limited Human Data - Animal Data Suggest Low Risk

Bumetanide is a potent loop diuretic that is similar in action to furosemide; it shares the same indications and precautions for use during gestation as this latter diuretic (Also see Furosemide). The drug is not teratogenic in rats, mice, hamsters, or rabbits (1,2). In rats, doses 3400 times the maximum therapeutic human dose (MTHD) had a slight embryocidal effect, produced fetal growth retardation, and increased the incidence of delayed ossification of sternebrae (2). In rabbits, which are more sensitive to the effects of bumetanide than other test species, doses 3.4 times the MTHD were slightly embryocidal (2). At doses 10 times the MTHD, an increased embryocidal effect was observed, as well as an increased incidence of delayed ossification of sternebrae (2).

In a surveillance study of Michigan Medicaid recipients conducted between 1985 and 1992 involving 229,101 completed pregnancies, 44 newborns had been exposed to bumetanide during the 1st trimester (F. Rosa, personal communication, FDA, 1993). Two (4.5%) major birth defects were observed (two expected), both of which were cardiovascular defects (0.4 expected).

No published reports on the use of bumetanide in human pregnancy have been located, but the diuretic has been recommended for the treatment of the nephrotic syndrome occurring during pregnancy (3). However, diuretics are not recommended for the treatment of gestational hypertension because of the maternal hypovolemia characteristic of this disease.

[**Risk Factor D if used in gestational hypertension.*]

BREAST FEEDING SUMMARY

RECOMMENDATION: No Human Data - Probably Compatible

No data are available. Bumetanide and other diuretics should be used cautiously during nursing because they may suppress lactation.

References

1. McClain RM, Dammers KD. Toxicologic evaluation of bumetanide, a potent diuretic agent. J Clin Pharmacol 1981;21:543–54. As cited in Shepard TH. *Catalog of Teratogenic Agents*. 6th ed. Baltimore, MD: Johns Hopkins University Press, 1989:92.
2. Product information. Bumex. Roche Laboratories, 1993.
3. Wood SM, Blainey JD. Hypertension and renal disease. In Wood SM, Beeley L, eds. Prescribing in pregnancy. Clin Obstet Gynaecol 1981;8:439–53.

Name:	**BUPRENORPHINE**	Risk Factor:	**C_M**
Class:	**Narcotic Agonist-Antagonist Analgesic**		

FETAL RISK SUMMARY

RECOMMENDATION: Limited Human Data - Animal Data Suggest Low Risk

Buprenorphine, an analgesic that possesses both narcotic agonist and antagonist activity, is approximately 33 times more potent than morphine (0.3 mg buprenorphine is equivalent to 10 mg morphine in analgesic and respiratory depressant effects). Although a sublingual formulation is available in other countries, only parenteral buprenorphine has been approved for general use in the United States. The human adult dose is 0.3–0.6 mg IM or IV repeated up to every 6 hours (0.017–0.034 mg/kg/day for a 70-kg person).

Buprenorphine is currently under investigation as an alternative to methadone maintenance treatment of narcotic dependence (1–3). The drug has also been studied as an alternative to cocaine, but it is apparently not effective for this use (2). Although these trials have not yet included pregnant women, the advantages of buprenorphine over methadone during gestation may include less respiratory depression at high doses, less toxicity from overdose, less severe withdrawal after abrupt discontinuance of the drug, and potentially less abuse liability (1,2). Of interest, however, abuse of buprenorphine, often concurrently with opiates, has been reported outside of the United States (4,5). One of these latter citations reported frequent abuse of buprenorphine by pregnant women but provided no outcome data (4).

Reproduction studies in rats and rabbits have been conducted (6–12). No fetal adverse effects were observed in rats and rabbits when their mothers were administered doses up to 5 mg/kg IM during organogenesis (6). Shepard cited a study in which fetal growth retardation, but not congenital defects, was observed in rats exposed to maternal doses of >0.05–5 mg/kg/day (about 3–300 times the recommended human dose [RHD]) given after implantation through delivery (7). Rat fetuses exposed to 5 mg/kg/day in the last week of pregnancy had a reduced survival rate after delivery (7). As reported by the manufacturer, no major congenital malformations were observed in rats given doses of 10–1000 times (SC or IM) or 160 times (IV) the RHD, but significant increases in postimplantation losses and early fetal deaths were noted with IM doses of 10 and 100 times the RHD (8). A slight increase in postimplantation losses was also observed with IV doses of 40 and 160 times the RHD. In rabbits, IM doses produced a dose-related increase in extra rib formation that was statistically significant at 1000 times the RHD (8). Rats pups exposed *in utero* throughout gestation to maternal doses of buprenorphine, 1 and 2 mg/kg/day SC, had reduced survival. Minimal effects were observed on the endogenous opioid system, however, as determined by a comparison of the brain enkephalin levels of buprenorphine-exposed pups to those in methadone-exposed pups (9).

In a study involving pregnant rats, buprenorphine was administered by a continuous infusion in doses of 0.3, 1.0, and 3.0 mg/kg/day from day 8 of gestation through parturition (10). At these doses, no evidence of significant maternal toxicity was observed, nor were there any significant effects on the offspring in terms of morbidity and mortality, birth weight, and postnatal growth (up to 60 days) (10). In a second publication by these researchers, using the same drug-administration technique and animal type described above, no disruption in the rest-activity cycle was observed in the exposed offspring at 22 and 30 days of age (11).

The long-term effects on sexual differentiation in rats exposed *in utero* to maternal injections of buprenorphine, 0.3 or 0.6 mg/kg every 48 hours from day 6 to day 20 of gestation, were described in a study published in 1997 (12). Compared with controls and the lower dose group, spontaneous parental behavior (at 23–28 days of age) and the expected sex difference in the consumption of a 0.25% saccharin solution (at 42–55 days of age) were impaired in the 0.6-mg/kg-exposed offspring. The authors concluded that the higher dose of buprenorphine produced long-term adverse effects on behavior (12).

As suggested by the molecular weight of the free base (about 468), buprenorphine crosses the placenta to the fetus. In a 1997 case report, a 24-year-old woman was treated with buprenorphine 4 mg/day for heroin addiction, starting in the 4th month of pregnancy (13). Frequent tests during the remainder of the pregnancy and at delivery confirmed her rapid withdrawal from heroin. Except for buprenorphine, all tests were negative for opiates, cocaine, cannabis, and amphetamines. An apparently normal female infant (birth weight not specified) was delivered at 39 weeks' gestation. Apgar scores were 10 and 10 at 1 and 10 minutes, respectively. High levels of buprenorphine and its metabolite were measured in the newborn approximately 20 hours after birth. Maternal trough serum concentrations of buprenorphine and the metabolite, norbuprenorphine, obtained a few days before delivery were 0.3 and 2.3 ng/mL, respectively. Parent drug and metabolite concentrations in the meconium were 107 and 295 ng/g, respectively. Levels of drug and metabolite were, respectively, 1.9 and 1.7 ng/mL and in the newborn's serum and 36.8 and 61.1 ng/mL in the newborn's urine. The estimated cord:maternal serum ratio was 6.3, whereas the ratio for the metabolite was 0.7. A weak withdrawal syndrome was observed at 48 hours of age with an adapted Finnegan score (used to evaluate the intensity of withdrawal syndromes; range 0–40) of 12 (13). Symptoms, which resolved without therapy, consisted of agitation, sleep disturbance, tremor, yawning, noisy breathing, and a slight fever (13). The Finnegan score fell to 8 at 3 days of age and was normal by 6 days of age.

The effect of epidural buprenorphine combined with bupivacaine has been compared with epidural combinations of bupivacaine and morphine, fentanyl, sufentanil, and oxymorphone for analgesia during and after cesarean section (14–17). The analgesic effects of the narcotic agents were similar, but buprenorphine caused a significant increase in maternal vomiting (14–16). No adverse neonatal effects were observed in the two studies that used buprenorphine before delivery (14,17).

The use of sublingual buprenorphine for labor pain in 34 primigravida women was described in a 1992 report (18). Each patient received a single 6-μg/kg dose during the first stage of labor. No effects were observed on the progression of labor and none of the women had nausea or vomiting. Similarly, no changes in fetal heart rate (range 138–150 beats/minute) were observed. Buprenorphine produced no neonatal depression as evidenced by the average Apgar scores (range not specified) at 1 and 5 minutes of 9.71 and 9.94, respectively.

In summary, buprenorphine is a potent narcotic agonist and antagonist that has been used during human pregnancy for analgesia immediately prior to delivery in a small number of cases. Only one pregnancy case has been located in which the drug was given as a narcotic substitute for heroin dependency. Neonatal withdrawal was observed, but the symptoms were less than that expected with methadone. Animal studies have demonstrated dose-related maternal, embryo, and fetal toxicity, and dose-related behavioral changes in offspring, but no congenital malformations. Although the lack of congenital anomalies is reassuring, the behavioral changes in animals combined with the absence of published early human pregnancy experience prevent an assessment of the risk this drug presents to the embryo or fetus. Because there is substantially more published human pregnancy experience for other narcotic analgesics, they are preferred to buprenorphine, especially during early gestation. Buprenorphine may have a role as substitution therapy for maternal heroin addiction, but additional reports are needed to define its pregnancy safety profile before this use can be recommended.

BREAST FEEDING SUMMARY

RECOMMENDATION: Limited Human Data - Potential Toxicity

Buprenorphine is excreted into human milk. In a 1997 case report (see above), a 24-year-old former heroin addict on buprenorphine maintenance therapy (4 mg/day) gave birth to an apparently normal female infant at 39 weeks' gestation (13). She continued taking buprenorphine while nursing her infant. At 4 weeks of age, buprenorphine and its metabolite, norbuprenorphine, were determined in her milk at each feeding over a 24-hour period. The volume of milk drunk was estimated by weighing the infant before and after the feedings. Although the specific milk concentrations were not provided, the authors estimated that the total doses of drug and metabolite ingested by the infant over the 24-hour period were 3.28 and 0.33 μg, respectively. No withdrawal symptoms in the infant were observed when lactation was abruptly interrupted at 8 weeks of age.

A study published in 1997 described the effects of continuous extradural bupivacaine and buprenorphine on analgesia and breast-feeding in 20 healthy women who had undergone a cesarean section at term (19). The study group ($N = 10$) received a 5-mL bolus of bupivacaine 0.25% with 200 μg of buprenorphine extradurally at cord clamping, followed by a continuous extradural infusion of bupivacaine (0.25%) and buprenorphine (12 μg/mL) infused at 0.7 mL/hour for 3 days. The control group ($N = 10$) received the same bolus and continuous infusion, but without the buprenorphine. There were no significant differences in visual analogue pain scores between the groups at 2 hours, 1 day, and 2 days, but the controls received significantly more supplemental diclofenac (a nonsteroidal anti-inflammatory agent) during the 2-day period (mean 25 mg vs. 5 mg, $p < 0.05$). The weight of breast milk ingested at each feeding was estimated by weighing the infant before and after each feeding. Compared with the control group, the buprenorphine group ingested significantly less milk each day (starting at day 3), and the infant's daily weight as a percentage of birth weight was significantly less starting at day 7. In both effects, the significant differences continued up to 11 days, near the time of discharge from the hospital. The investigators speculated that the differences between the two groups might be due to central nervous system depression in the mother and infant. Although one author thought the stress of the prolonged hospital stay may have depressed the breast-feeding (20), the investigators responded that long hospital stays are normal in Japan and, if stress is a factor, would have affected both groups similarly (19).

Because buprenorphine is excreted into milk and because depression of the nursing infant resulting in lower weight gain is a possibility, mothers receiving buprenorphine should probably not breast-feed. If breast-feeding is undertaken, the mother should be advised of the potential risk to her infant.

References

1. Vocci F, Chiang CN, Cummings L, Hawks R. Overview: medications development for the treatment of drug abuse. NIDA Res Monogr 1995;149:4–15.
2. Schottenfeld RS. Clinical trials of pharmacologic treatments in pregnant women—methodologic considerations. NIDA Res Monogr 1995;149:201–23.
3. O'Connor PG, Oliveto AH, Shi JM, Triffleman EG, Carroll KM, Kosten TR, Rounsaville BJ, Pakes JA, Schottenfeld RS. A randomized trial of buprenorphine maintenance for heroin dependence in a primary care clinic for substance users versus a methadone clinic. Am J Med 1998;105:100–5.
4. Stewart MJ. Effect of scheduling of buprenorphine (Temgesic) on drug abuse patterns in Glasgow. BMJ 1991;302:969.
5. Strang J. Abuse of buprenorphine (Temgesic) by snorting. BMJ 1991;302:969.
6. Heel RC, Brogden RN, Speight TM, Avery GS. Buprenorphine: a review of its pharmacological properties and therapeutic efficacy. Drugs 1979;17:81–110.
7. Mori N, Sakanoue M, Kamata S, Takeuchi M, Shimpo K, Tamagawa M. Toxicological studies of buprenorphine teratogenicity, perinatal and postnatal studies in the rat. Iyaku Kenkyu 1982;13:509–44. As cited in Shepard TH. *Catalog of Teratogenic Agents.* 8th ed. Baltimore, MD: Johns Hopkins University Press, 1995:58–9.
8. Product information. Buprenex. Reckitt & Colman Pharmaceuticals, 1998.
9. Tiong GK, Olley JE. Effects of exposure in utero to methadone and buprenorphine on enkephalin levels in the developing rat brain. Neurosci Lett 1988;93:101–6.
10. Hutchings DE, Zmitrovich AC, Hamowy AS, Liu P-YR. Prenatal administration of buprenorphine using the osmotic minipump: a preliminary study of maternal and offspring toxicity and growth in the rat. Neurotoxicol Teratol 1995;17:419–23.
11. Hutchings DE, Hamowy AS, Williams EM, Zmitrovich AC. Prenatal administration of buprenorphine in the rat: effects on the rest-activity cycle at 22 and 30 days of age. Pharmacol Biochem Behav 1996;55:607–13.
12. Barron S, Chung VM. Prenatal buprenorphine exposure and sexually dimorphic nonreproductive behaviors in rats. Pharmacol Biochem Behav 1997;58:337–43.
13. Marquet P, Chevrel J, Lavignasse P, Merle L, Lachatre G. Buprenorphine withdrawal syndrome in a newborn. Clin Pharmacol Ther 1997;62:569–71.
14. Celleno D, Costantino P, Emanuelli M, Capogna G,

Muratori F, Sebastiani M, Cipriani G. Epidural analgesia during and after cesarean delivery. Comparison of five opioids. Reg Anesth 1991;16:79–83.
15. Cohen S, Amar D, Pantuck CB, Pantuck EJ, Weissman AM, Landa S, Singer N. Epidural patient-controlled analgesia after cesarean section: buprenorphine-0.015% bupivacaine with epinephrine versus fentanyl-0.015% bupivacaine with and without epinephrine. Anesth Analg 1992;74:226–30.
16. Cohen S, Amar D, Pantuck CB, Pantuck EJ, Weissman AB. Adverse effects of epidural 0.03% bupivacaine during analgesia after cesarean section. Anesth Analg 1992;75:753–6.
17. Lehmann KA, Stern S, Breuker KH. Obstetrical peridural anesthesia with bupivacaine and buprenorphine. A randomized double-blind study in comparison with untreated controls. Anaesthesist 1992;41:414–22.
18. Roy S, Basu RK. Role of sublingual administration of tablet buprenorphine hydrochloride on relief of labour pain. J Indian Med Assoc 1992;90:151–3.
19. Hirose M, Hosokawa T, Tanaka Y. Extradural buprenorphine suppresses breast feeding after caesarean section. Br J Anaesth 1997;79:120–1.
20. Celebioglu B. Extradural buprenorphine and breast feeding after caesarean section. Br J Anaesth 1998;80:271.

Name: **BUPROPION** Risk Factor: B_M
Class: **Antidepressant**

FETAL RISK SUMMARY

RECOMMENDATION: Limited Human Data - Animal Data Suggest Low Risk

Bupropion is a unique antidepressant of the aminoketone class that differs from other antidepressants in that it does not inhibit monoamine oxidase and does not alter the reuptake of norepinephrine or serotonin (1). Anticholinergic effects are much less frequent and less severe than those observed with other antidepressants (1). No published reports on the use of bupropion in human pregnancy have been located, but data from a surveillance study and a pregnancy registry are presented below.

Reproduction studies in rats and rabbits at doses up to 15 to 45 times the human dose revealed no definitive evidence of impaired fertility or fetal harm (2). A slight increase in nonspecific fetal abnormalities, however, was observed in two studies with rabbits (2).

In a surveillance study of Michigan Medicaid recipients conducted between 1985 and 1992 involving 229,101 completed pregnancies, three newborns had been exposed to bupropion during the 1st trimester (F. Rosa, personal communication, FDA, 1993). No major birth defects were observed (none expected).

Over about a 7-year period (September 1997 through February 2004), the manufacturer's pregnancy registry prospectively (before the pregnancy outcome was known) enrolled 956 pregnancies exposed to bupropion (3). In these cases, 125 were still pregnant, 302 were lost to follow-up, and there were 534 known outcomes (includes 5 sets of twins). The number of outcomes involving earliest exposure in the 1st, 2nd, or 3rd trimester were 426, 81, and 27, respectively. The outcomes of those with earliest exposure in the 1st trimester included 53 spontaneous abortions (SABs), 18 elective abortions (EABs), 1 fetal death, 12 fetuses/live births with birth defects, and 342 live births without reported birth defects. Of the 12 cases of birth defects (the possibility of additional birth defects could not be excluded), there was one fetal death (21 weeks' gestation; pulmonary lymphangiectasis in one lung, atrial septal defect (ASD), cleft palate, protuberant maxilla, low-set ears, flattened pinnae with left malformed, pectus excavatum, and kyphosis) and one EAB (Down's syndrome). Defects in the remaining 10 cases were: bilateral clubfeet; abnormal aortic valve thickening with secondary mild aortic insufficiency; Klinefelter's syndrome with no physical abnormalities; ventricular septal defect (VSD); trivial valvular pulmonic stenosis with tiny ASD; heart defect (coarctation) and VSD; premature infant with thickened heart muscle; pulmonary stenosis; coarctation of the aorta; and trisomy 21. All of the 2nd and

B

3rd trimester exposures ended with live births with no reported defects, but there was one SAB and one EAB in the 2nd trimester group. (See required statement below.)

There were 16 outcomes, all with earliest exposure in the 1st trimester, with birth defects reported retrospectively (after the pregnancy outcome was known) (3). Although retrospective reports are usually biased, reporting adverse outcomes and not normal infants, seven of the defects involved the heart and great vessels. The Registry has noted the increased number of cardiac defects in the prospective and retrospective groups. However, the relatively small sample size, the potential bias from the large percentage of cases lost to follow-up, and the incomplete descriptions of the defects prevented determining if the data reflects a potential drug effect on the developing cardiovascular system (3). Health care providers are encouraged to report exposures by calling the toll free number (800) 336-2176 (United States and Canada) or by calling collect (910) 256-0549 (International).

Required statement: Committee consensus. After reviewing the 534 prospectively reported pregnancy outcomes, the Bupropion Pregnancy Registry Advisory Committee concludes that this sample is of insufficient size to reliably compute a birth defect risk, and no conclusions can be made regarding the possible teratogenic risk of bupropion. This sample size does not allow for a formal comparison of the frequency of birth defects.

BREAST FEEDING SUMMARY

RECOMMENDATION: Limited Human Data - Potential Toxicity

Bupropion is excreted into breast milk. A 37-year-old lactating woman was treated with the drug, 100 mg three times daily (4). She was nursing her 14-month-old infant twice daily at times corresponding to 9.5 and 7.5 hours after a dose. Peak milk concentrations of bupropion occurred 2 hours after a 100-mg dose with a value of 0.189 μg/mL, but the peak plasma level measured, 0.072 μg/mL, occurred at 1 hour. The milk:plasma ratios at 0, 1, 2, 4, and 6 hours after a dose were 7.37, 2.49, 4.31, 8.72, and 6.24, respectively. Two metabolites, hydroxybupropion and threohydrobupropion, were also measured with peak concentrations of both occurring at 2 hours in milk and plasma. The ranges of milk levels and milk:plasma ratios for the metabolites were 0.093–0.132 μg/mL and 0.366–0.443 μg/mL, respectively, and 0.09–0.11 and 1.23–1.57, respectively. The levels of a third metabolite, erythrohydrobupropion, were too low to be measured in breast milk (test sensitivity 0.02 μg/mL). No adverse effects were observed in the infant nor was any drug or metabolite found in his plasma, an indication that accumulation had not occurred (4).

A 1996 review of antidepressant treatment during breast-feeding found no information that bupropion exposure during nursing resulted in quantifiable amounts in an infant or that the exposure caused adverse effects (5). However, the American Academy of Pediatrics classifies bupropion as a drug whose effect on the nursing infant is unknown but may be of concern (6).

References

1. Weintraub M, Evan P. Bupropion: a chemically and pharmacologically unique antidepressant. Hosp Form 1989;24:254–9.
2. Product information. Wellbutrin. Burroughs Wellcome Co., 1993.
3. Bupropion Pregnancy Registry. Interim Report, 1 September 1887 through 29 February 2004. Issued: June 2004.
4. Briggs GG, Samson JH, Ambrose PJ, Schroeder DH. Excretion of bupropion in breast milk. Ann Pharmacother 1993;27:431–3.
5. Wisner KL, Perel JM, Findling RL. Antidepressant treatment during breast-feeding. Am J Psychiatry 1996;153:1132–7.
6. Committee on Drugs, American Academy of Pediatrics. The transfer of drugs and other chemicals into human milk. Pediatrics 2001;108:776–89.

B

Name: **BUSPIRONE** Risk Factor: **B_M**

Class: **Sedative**

FETAL RISK SUMMARY

RECOMMENDATION: Limited Human Data - Animal Data Suggest Low Risk

Buspirone is an antianxiety agent that is unrelated chemically and pharmacologically to other sedative and anxiolytic drugs. Reproduction studies in rats and rabbits at doses approximately 30 times the maximum recommended human dose revealed no fertility impairment or fetal adverse effects (1).

A 1993 report described the use of buspirone, in combination with four other agents, all started before conception, in a pregnant woman with major depression, a coexisting panic disorder, and migraine headaches (2). The pregnancy was electively terminated after 12 weeks, resulting in the delivery of a male fetus with normal organ formation and a normal placenta. No dysmorphology was observed during the complete macroscopic and microscopic examination, including a normal 46,XY karyotype.

In a surveillance study of Michigan Medicaid recipients conducted between 1985 and 1992 involving 229,101 completed pregnancies, 42 newborns had been exposed to buspirone during the 1st trimester (F. Rosa, personal communication, FDA, 1993). One (2.4%) major birth defect was observed (two expected). The anomaly was not included in six defect categories for which specific data were available (cardiovascular defects, oral clefts, spina bifida, polydactyly, limb reduction defects, and hypospadias).

A 1998 non-interventional observational cohort study described the outcomes of pregnancies in women who had been prescribed one or more of 34 newly marketed drugs by general practitioners in England (3). Data were obtained by questionnaires sent to the prescribing physicians one month after the expected or possible date of delivery. In 831 (78%) of the pregnancies, a newly marketed drug was thought to have been taken during the 1st trimester with birth defects noted in 14 (2.5%) singleton births of the 557 newborns (10 sets of twins). In addition, two birth defects were observed in aborted fetuses. However, few of the aborted fetuses were examined. Buspirone was taken during the 1st trimester in 16 pregnancies. The outcomes of these pregnancies included 2 elective abortions, 1 intrauterine death, 12 normal term babies, and 1 newborn with a genetic defect (cystic fibrosis) (3).

In a 1998 case report, a 32-year-old woman with bipolar disorder took buspirone, fluoxetine, and carbamazepine (see Breast Feeding Summary for doses and further details) throughout gestation (4). At 42 weeks' gestation she gave birth to a healthy 3940-g, normally developed female infant. The mother continued her medications for 3 weeks while exclusively breast-feeding the infant. She reported seizure-like activity in her infant at 3 weeks, 4 months, and 5.5 months of age.

Although no drug-induced congenital malformations have been observed after 1st trimester exposure to buspirone, the data are too limited to assess the safety of the drug in human pregnancy. The cause of the intrauterine death cited above is unknown. Moreover, that study lacked the sensitivity to identify minor anomalies because of the absence of standardized examinations. Late appearing major defects, including neurobehavior effects, may also have been missed as a consequence of the timing of the questionnaires.

B

BREAST FEEDING SUMMARY

RECOMMENDATION: Limited Human Data - Potential Toxicity

Buspirone and its metabolites, at least one of which is pharmacologically active, are excreted into the milk of lactating rats (1). Only one report has investigated the excretion of buspirone into human milk. In a 1998 case report, a 32-year-old woman with bipolar disorder took buspirone (45 mg/day), fluoxetine (20 mg/day), and carbamazepine (600 mg/day) throughout pregnancy and during the first 3 weeks postpartum (4). She reported seizure-like activity in the infant at 3 weeks, 4 months, and 5.5 months of age. Breast milk, maternal serum, and infant serum were evaluated for buspirone on postpartum day 13, but the drug was not detected in any of the samples (test sensitivity not reported). Similar evaluations were conducted for fluoxetine, norfluoxetine, and carbamazepine on days 13 and 21 postpartum (see Fluoxetine and Carbamazepine for results). A neurologic examination of the infant, that included electroencephalography, was within normal limits. The authors were unable to determine the cause of the seizure-like activity, if it had indeed occurred (none of the episodes had been observed by medical personnel) (4).

Although buspirone was not detected in breast milk or maternal and infant serum in the above case, the timing of the samples in relation to the mother's ingestion of the drug and the test sensitivity were not specified. Therefore, because other agents in this pharmacologic class are excreted into milk (e.g., see Diazepam), the excretion of buspirone, at least to some degree, should still be expected.

Because of the potential for central nervous system impairment in a nursing infant, maternal use of the drug, especially for prolonged periods, should be undertaken cautiously, if at all. The American Academy of Pediatrics classifies other antianxiety agents as drugs whose effects on the nursing infant are unknown, but may be of concern because effects on the developing brain may not be apparent until later in life (5).

References

1. Product information. Buspar. Mead Johnson Pharmaceuticals, 1994.
2. Seifritz E, Holsboer-Trachsler E, Haberthur F, Hemmeter U, Pöldinger W. Unrecognized pregnancy during citalopram treatment. Am J Psychiatry 1993;150:1428–9.
3. Wilton LV, Pearce GL, Martin RM, Mackay FJ, Mann RD. The outcomes of pregnancy in women exposed to newly marketed drugs in general practice in England. Br J Obstet Gynaecol 1998;105:882–9.
4. Brent NB, Wisner KL. Fluoxetine and carbamazepine concentrations in a nursing mother/infant pair. Clin Pediatr 1998;37:41–4.
5. Committee on Drugs, American Academy of Pediatrics. The transfer of drugs and other chemicals into human milk. Pediatrics 2001;108:776–89.

Name: **BUSULFAN** Risk Factor: **D_M**

Class: **Antineoplastic**

FETAL RISK SUMMARY

RECOMMENDATION: Contraindicated - 1st Trimester

Busulfan is an alkylating antineoplastic agent. Reproductive studies in pregnant rats revealed that the drug produced sterility in both male and female offspring due to the absence of germinal cells in testes and ovaries (1).

The use of busulfan has been reported in at least 49 human pregnancies, of which 31 were treated in the 1st trimester (2–10). One of these references reviewed eight earlier cases that are included in the above totals (9). Malformations in six infants were unspecified malformations, aborted at 20 weeks; anomalous deviation of left lobe liver, bilobar spleen, pulmonary atelectasis; pyloric stenosis; cleft palate, microphthalmia, cytomegaly, hypoplasia of ovaries and thyroid gland, corneal opacity, intrauterine growth retardation (IUGR); myeloschisis, aborted at 6 weeks; IUGR, left hydronephrosis and hydroureter, absent right kidney and ureter, hepatic subcapsular calcifications (2,4–6).

Data from one review indicated that 40% of the infants exposed to anticancer drugs were of low birth weight (2). This finding was not related to the timing of the exposure. One mother with chronic granulocytic leukemia was treated with busulfan and allopurinol beginning at 20 weeks' gestation (8). A growth-retarded infant was delivered at 39 weeks with absence of the right kidney, hydronephrosis of the left kidney, and hepatic subcapsular calcifications. The kidney and liver defects predated the onset of drug therapy, but their cause was unknown. The growth retardation, however, was thought to be caused by busulfan.

Long-term studies of growth and mental development in offspring exposed to busulfan during the 2nd trimester, the period of neuroblast multiplication, have not been conducted (11). However, a few infants have been studied for periods of up to 10 years without evidence of adverse outcome (3,9,10). Moreover, a 1994 review concluded that although there were insufficient data to assess the fetal risk from busulfan, use after the 1st trimester would reduce the risk of birth defects (12).

Chromosomal damage has been associated with busulfan therapy, but the clinical significance of this to the fetus is unknown (13). Irregular menses and amenorrhea, with the latter at times permanent, have been reported in women receiving busulfan (14,15). Reversible ovarian failure with delivery of a normal infant has also been reported after busulfan therapy (16).

Occupational exposure of the mother to antineoplastic agents during pregnancy may present a risk to the fetus. A position statement from the National Study Commission on Cytotoxic Exposure and a research article involving some antineoplastic agents are presented in the monograph for cyclophosphamide (see Cyclophosphamide).

BREAST FEEDING SUMMARY

RECOMMENDATION: Contraindicated

No studies describing the use of busulfan during human lactation or measuring the amount, if any, excreted into milk have been located. Because of the potential for serious toxicity in a nursing infant, the use of the drug during lactation should be considered contraindicated.

References

1. Product information. Myleran. Glaxo Wellcome Oncology/HIV, 1997.
2. Nicholson HO. Cytotoxic drugs in pregnancy: review of reported cases. J Obstet Gynaecol Br Commonw 1968;75:307–12.
3. Lee RA, Johnson CE, Hanlon DG. Leukemia during pregnancy. Am J Obstet Gynecol 1962;84:455–8.
4. Diamond I, Anderson MM, McCreadie SR. Transplacental transmission of busulfan (Myleran) in a mother with leukemia: production of fetal malformation and cytomegaly. Pediatrics 1960;25:85–90.
5. Abramovici A, Shaklai M, Pinkhas J. Myeloschisis in a six weeks embryo of a leukemic woman treated by busulfan. Teratology 1978;18:241–6.
6. Gililland J, Weinstein L. The effects of cancer chemotherapeutic agents on the developing fetus. Obstet Gynecol Surv 1983;38:6–13.
7. Ozumba BC, Obi GO. Successful pregnancy in a

patient with chronic myeloid leukemia following therapy with cytotoxic drugs. Int J Gynecol Obstet 1992;38:49–53.
8. Boros SJ, Reynolds JW. Intrauterine growth retardation following third-trimester exposure to busulfan. Am J Obstet Gynecol 1977;129:111–2.
9. Dugdale M, Fort AT. Busulfan treatment of leukemia during pregnancy. JAMA 1967;199:131–3.
10. Zuazu J, Julia A, Sierra J, Valentin MG, Coma A, Sanz MA, Batlle J, Flores A. Pregnancy outcome in hematologic malignancies. Cancer 1991;67:703–9.
11. Dobbing J. Pregnancy and leukaemia. Lancet 1977;1:1155.
12. Wiebe VJ, Sipila PEH. Pharmacology of antineoplastic agents in pregnancy. Crit Rev Oncol Hematol 1994;16:75–112.
13. Gebhart E, Schwanitz G, Hartwich G. Chromosomal aberrations during busulphan therapy. Dtsch Med Wochenschr 1974;99:52–6.
14. Galton DAG, Till M, Wiltshaw E. Busulfan: summary of clinical results. Ann NY Acad Sci 1958;68:967–73.
15. Schilsky RL, Lewis BJ, Sherins RJ, Young RC. Gonadal dysfunction in patients receiving chemotherapy for cancer. Ann Intern Med 1980;93:109–14.
16. Shalev O, Rahav G, Milwidsky A. Reversible busulfan-induced ovarian failure. Eur J Obstet Gynecol Reprod Biol 1987;26:239–42.

Name: **BUTALBITAL** Risk Factor: **C***
Class: **Sedative**

FETAL RISK SUMMARY

RECOMMENDATION: Limited Human Data - No Relevant Animal Data

Butalbital is a short-acting barbiturate that is contained in a number of analgesic mixtures. In a large prospective study, 112 patients were exposed to this drug during the 1st trimester (1). No association with malformations was found. Severe neonatal withdrawal was described in a male infant whose mother took 150 mg of butalbital daily during the last 2 months of pregnancy in the form of a proprietary headache mixture (Esgic-butalbital 50 mg, caffeine 40 mg, and acetaminophen 325 mg/dose) (2). The infant was also exposed to oxycodone, pentazocine, and acetaminophen during the 1st trimester, but apparently these had been discontinued before the start of the butalbital product. Onset of withdrawal occurred within 2 days of birth.

In a surveillance study of Michigan Medicaid recipients conducted between 1985 and 1992 involving 229,101 completed pregnancies, 1124 newborns had been exposed to butalbital during the 1st trimester (F. Rosa, personal communication, FDA, 1993). A total of 53 (4.7%) major birth defects were observed (45 expected). Specific data were available for six defect categories, including (observed/expected) 10/11 cardiovascular defects, 1/2 oral clefts, 0/0.5 spina bifida, 1/3 polydactyly, 2/2 limb reduction defects, and 2/3 hypospadias. These data do not support an association between the drug and congenital defects.

[*Risk Factor D if used for prolonged periods or in high doses at term.*]

BREAST FEEDING SUMMARY

RECOMMENDATION: No Human Data - Potential Toxicity

No data are available (see Pentobarbital).

References

1. Heinonen OP, Slone D, Shapiro S. *Birth Defects and Drugs in Pregnancy*. Littleton, MA: Publishing Sciences Group, 1977:336–7.
2. Ostrea EM. Neonatal withdrawal from intrauterine exposure to butalbital. Am J Obstet Gynecol 1982;143:597–9.

Name: **BUTAPERAZINE** Risk Factor: **C**
Class: **Tranquilizer**

FETAL RISK SUMMARY

RECOMMENDATION: No Human Data - No Relevant Animal Data

Butaperazine is a piperazine phenothiazine in the same group as prochlorperazine (see Prochlorperazine). The phenothiazines readily cross the placenta (1). No specific information on the use of butaperazine in pregnancy has been located. Although occasional reports have attempted to link various phenothiazine compounds with congenital malformations, the bulk of the evidence suggests that these drugs represent a low risk for embryo/fetal harm (see also Chlorpromazine).

BREAST FEEDING SUMMARY

RECOMMENDATION: No Human Data - Potential Toxicity

No reports describing the use of butaperazine during human lactation have been located. Because other phenothiazines appear in human milk (e.g., chlorpromazine), excretion of butaperazine should be expected. Sedation is a potential effect in the nursing infant.

Reference

1. Moya F, Thorndike V. Passage of drugs across the placenta. Am J Obstet Gynecol 1962;84:1778–98.

Name: **BUTOCONAZOLE** Risk Factor: **C_M**
Class: **Antifungal**

FETAL RISK SUMMARY

RECOMMENDATION: Limited Human Data - Probably Compatible

Butoconazole, an imidazole derivative, is available as a topical cream for the treatment of vaginal fungal infections. The agent is teratogenic in some animal species, but only when large oral doses are administered (1).

An average 5.5% of a vaginal dose is absorbed systemically with peak plasma levels appearing at about 24 hours (1). No data are available on the placental transfer of this agent, but the low molecular weight (about 475) indicates that transfer to the fetus probably occurs.

No published reports of butoconazole use in the 1st trimester have been located. However, butoconazole is one of several agents that have been approved for 2nd and 3rd trimester use in the treatment of vulvovaginal mycotic infections (2–4). Therapy for 6 days is recommended if this antifungal is used.

In a surveillance study of Michigan Medicaid recipients conducted between 1985 and 1992 involving 229,101 completed pregnancies, 444 newborns had been exposed to vaginal butoconazole during the 1st trimester (F. Rosa, personal communication, FDA, 1993). A total of 16 (3.6%) major birth defects were observed (17 expected). Specific data

B

were available for six defect categories, including (observed/expected) 4/4 cardiovascular defects, 0/1 oral clefts, 1/0 spina bifida, 0/0.5 polydactyly, 0/1 limb reduction defects, and 0/1 hypospadias. These data do not support an association between the vaginal use of the drug and congenital defects.

BREAST FEEDING SUMMARY

RECOMMENDATION: No Human Data - Probably Compatible

No data are available.

References

1. Product information. Femstat. Syntex, 1993.
2. Weisberg M. Treatment of vaginal candidiasis in pregnant women. Clin Ther 1986;8:563–7.
3. Hagler L, Brett L. Treatment of vaginal candidiasis in pregnant women. Clin Ther 1987;9:559–60.
4. Weisberg M. Treatment of vaginal candidiasis in pregnant women. Clin Ther 1987;9:561.

Name:	**BUTORPHANOL**	Risk Factor:	**C_M***
Class:	**Narcotic Agonist-Antagonist Analgesic**		

FETAL RISK SUMMARY

RECOMMENDATION: Human Data Suggest Risk in 3rd Trimester

No reports linking the use of butorphanol with congenital defects have been located. Because it has both narcotic agonist and antagonist properties, prolonged use during gestation may result in fetal addiction with subsequent withdrawal in the newborn (see also Pentazocine). The drug is commercially available as injection and nasal spray formulations.

No teratogenic effects were observed in reproduction studies in rats and rabbits administered butorphanol during organogenesis (1). An increased frequency of stillbirth was observed in rats given 1 mg/kg (5.9 mg/m^2) SC and in rabbits dosed orally with 30 mg/kg (360 mg/m^2) and 60 mg/kg (720 mg/m^2).

At term, butorphanol rapidly crosses the placenta, producing cord serum levels averaging 84% of maternal concentrations (2,3). Depressant effects on the newborn from *in utero* exposure during labor are similar to those seen with meperidine (2–4).

The use of 1 mg of butorphanol combined with 25 mg of promethazine administered intravenously to a woman in active labor was associated with a sinusoidal fetal heart rate pattern (5). Onset of the pattern occurred 6 minutes after drug injection and persisted for approximately 58 minutes. The newborn infant showed no effects from the abnormal heart pattern. A subsequent study to determine the incidence of sinusoidal fetal heart rate pattern after butorphanol administration was published in 1986 (6). Fifty-one women in labor who received butorphanol, 1 mg IV, were compared with a control group of 55 women who did not receive narcotic analgesia. Sinusoidal fetal heart rate pattern was observed in 75% (38 of 51) of the treated women vs. 13% (7 of 55) of controls ($p < 0.001$). The mean time of onset of the abnormal tracing was 12.74 minutes after butorphanol with a duration of 31.26 minutes. This duration was significantly longer than that observed in the nontreated controls (13.86 minutes; $p < 0.02$). Because no short-term maternal or neonatal adverse effects were observed, the investigators concluded that, in the absence of other signs, the abnormal heart rate pattern was not indicative of fetal hypoxia (6).

A study comparing the effects of maternal analgesics on neonatal neurobehavior was conducted in 135 patients during their 1st day of life (7). Maternal analgesia consisted of 1 mg of butorphanol ($N = 68$) or 40 mg of meperidine ($N = 67$). No difference between the drugs was observed.

[**Risk Factor D if used for prolonged periods or in high doses at term.*]

BREAST FEEDING SUMMARY

RECOMMENDATION: Limited Human Data - Probably Compatible

Butorphanol passes into breast milk in concentrations paralleling levels in maternal serum (3). Milk:plasma ratios after intramuscular (12 mg) or oral (8 mg) doses were 0.7 and 1.9, respectively. Using 2 mg intramuscularly or 8 mg orally four times per day would result in 4 μg excreted in the full daily milk output (1000 mL). Although it has not been studied, this amount is probably insignificant. The American Academy of Pediatrics classifies butorphanol as compatible with breast-feeding (8).

References

1. Product information. Stadol NS. Bristol-Myers Squibb, 2000.
2. Maduska AL, Hajghassemali M. A double-blind comparison of butorphanol and meperidine in labour: maternal pain relief and effect on the newborn. Can Anaesth Soc J 1978;25:398–404.
3. Pittman KA, Smyth RD, Losada M, Ziqhelboim I, Maduska AL, Sunshine A. Human perinatal distribution of butorphanol. Am J Obstet Gynecol 1980;138:797–800.
4. Quilligan EJ, Keegan KA, Donahue MJ. Double-blind comparison of intravenously injected butorphanol and meperidine in parturients. Int J Gynaecol Obstet 1980;18:363–7.
5. Angel JL, Knuppel RA, Lake M. Sinusoidal fetal heart rate pattern associated with intravenous butorphanol administration: a case report. Am J Obstet Gynecol 1984;149:465–7.
6. Hatjis CG, Meis PJ. Sinusoidal fetal heart rate pattern associated with butorphanol administration. Obstet Gynecol 1986;67:377–80.
7. Hodgkinson R, Huff RW, Hayashi RH, Husain FJ. Double-blind comparison of maternal analgesia and neonatal neurobehaviour following intravenous butorphanol and meperidine. J Int Med Res 1979;7:224–30.
8. Committee on Drugs, American Academy of Pediatrics. The transfer of drugs and other chemicals into human milk. Pediatrics 2001;108:776–89.

Name:	**BUTRIPTYLINE**	Risk Factor:	**C**
Class:	**Antidepressant**		

No data are available (see Imipramine).

C

Name:	**CABERGOLINE**	Risk Factor:	B_M
Class:	**Miscellaneous**		

FETAL RISK SUMMARY

RECOMMENDATION: Human Data Suggest Low Risk

Cabergoline is a synthetic ergot derivative that is a long-acting dopamine receptor (D_2) agonist with low affinity for other dopamine (D_1), adrenergic (α_1 and α_2), and serotonin (5-HT_1 and 5-HT_2) receptors. The drug has a direct inhibitory effect on prolactin secretion from the anterior pituitary gland. Cabergoline is indicated for the treatment of hyperprolactinemic disorders, either idiopathic or caused by pituitary adenomas (1).

Animal reproduction studies have been conducted in mice, rats, and rabbits with daily oral doses (comparisons to human doses are made with the total weekly animal dose and the maximum recommended weekly human dose for a 50-kg human [MRHD], both based on body surface area) (1). In mice, doses up to about 55 times the MRHD caused maternal toxicity but no teratogenic effects in the offspring. In rats, a dose about 1/7th the MRHD caused an increase in post-implantation embryo and fetal losses, an effect that was thought to be a result of the prolactin inhibitory effects of cabergoline (1). Conception in female rats was inhibited at a dose 1/28th the MRHD given 2 weeks before mating and throughout the mating period. A similar dose given to pregnant rats from 6 days before delivery throughout the lactation period caused growth retardation and death in offspring because of decreased milk secretion. In rabbits, a dose approximately 19 times the MRHD during organogenesis caused maternal toxicity (decreased food consumption and weight loss). An increased occurrence of various malformations was observed in one rabbit study using a dose 150 times the MRHD, but no increase in defects was observed in a second study at 300 times the MRHD (1).

A 1996 reproduction study in mice, rats, and rabbits concluded that cabergoline did not impair male rat fertility, was not teratogenic in mice and rabbits, had no effects on the latter phase of gestation or parturition in rats, and caused no toxicity in neonatal rats (2). The study also found that cabergoline could inhibit egg nidation in mice and rats and prevent conception (2). However, this effect has no relevance to humans because egg nidation in these species, but not in humans, is regulated by prolactin through a luteotrophic effect. A 1997 study in rats demonstrated that cabergoline-inhibited prolactin release resulted in the inhibition of ovarian progesterone biosynthesis, thereby preventing implantation and terminating pregnancy (3).

No reports describing the placental crossing of cabergoline in humans have been located. The molecular weight (about 452) is low enough, however, that exposure of the embryo and/or fetus should be expected.

In a group of 56 women with amenorrhea secondary to hyperprolactinemia (serum prolactin levels >20 μg/L), 17 (81% of pregnancy-seeking women) became pregnant while under treatment with cabergoline (4). Women were instructed to discontinue cabergoline immediately after a positive pregnancy test. Of the 17 pregnancies, there was 1 spontaneous abortion, 10 normal-term outcomes, and 6 outcomes pending. All 10 children have had normal physical and mental development (4).

A 1994 case report described the outcome of a pregnancy exposed to cabergoline (5). A 38-year-old woman with a microadenoma of the pituitary gland was treated for hyperprolactinemia with a stable cabergoline dose of 0.5 mg twice weekly. She had a 17-year history of infertility and was intolerant to bromocriptine therapy. The prolactin level 2 days after a dose, was 1133 mU/L (normal range 60–550 mU/L). After return of her menstrual cycles, she became pregnant but had a spontaneous abortion at 17 weeks' gestation (not mentioned if cabergoline was stopped when pregnancy was diagnosed). Approximately 5 months later (2 months after restarting cabergoline), she again became pregnant and cabergoline was stopped (gestational age not specified). Labor was induced at 38 weeks' gestation for intrauterine growth retardation. A 2.26-kg male infant without malformations was delivered with Apgar scores of 3 and 8 at 1 and 5 minutes, respectively. The placenta weight was 370 g. He was discharged home with his mother at 6 days of age (5).

A multinational French study published in 1996 described the outcomes of 226 pregnancies (all singletons) in 205 women who had been receiving cabergoline treatment (0.125–4.0 mg/wk) before gestation (6). The women were from a group of 1,650 premenopausal hyperprolactinemic women who had been treated with the drug. In seven cases, pregnancy occurred during the first cycle after discontinuation of cabergoline. The time of exposure could not be determined in 18 other cases. In the remaining 201 pregnancies, embryo-fetal exposure to cabergoline was thought to have ranged between 1 and 144 days. The 226 outcomes included early pregnancy loss ($N = 56$), live births ($N = 148$), ongoing pregnancies ($N = 16$), and lost to followup ($N = 6$). Among the 56 early pregnancy losses, there were 28 elective abortions (EABs), 23 spontaneous abortions (SABs), 1 intrauterine death (a cord accident at 25 weeks), 1 tubal pregnancy, and 3 EABs for the following major anomalies (dose and time of exposure shown in parentheses): Down's syndrome, maternal age 42 years, woman later conceived on another cycle and gave birth to a normal infant (0.5 mg/wk; exposure for 2 weeks after conception); limb-body wall defect—large abdominal wall defect, deformed left leg, and proximal phocomelia of right lower limb (0.5 mg/wk; exposure for 2 weeks after conception); and hydrocephalus, cerebral atrophy, and facial dysmorphic (0.5 mg/wk; exposure for 7 weeks after conception).

Among the 148 live births, 17 were preterm, and 2 cases had an unknown length of gestation (6). Birth weights ranged from 1600 to 4350 g, with 10 infants below 2500 g (6.8%, 95% confidence intervals [CI] 3%–12%). In addition to the three cases above, seven infants had birth defects, but only two of them were major defects. The major defects were (dose and exposure times not specified) left megaureter and craniosynostosis and scaphocephaly. Thus, there were 5 infants with major malformations among 151 outcomes (3.3%, 95% CI 1.0%–7.6%). The postnatal development of 148 infants was known for various periods after birth, of whom 107 were followed up for 1 to 72 months. All the infants showed normal physical and mental development (6).

In a 1997 report, nine women became pregnant (from a group of 47) against medical advice after a mean of 12.4 months (range 1–37 months) of cabergoline therapy for hyperprolactinemia (7). The doses ranged from 0.25 to 3.5 mg/wk. Cabergoline was discontinued as soon as pregnancy was diagnosed. One pregnancy aborted spontaneously, and one woman underwent elective abortion at 8 weeks' gestation. In the remaining cases, all the pregnancies were brought to term without complication. The infants were healthy

C

at birth and all had normal development during long-term follow-up (8 years) that was still ongoing (7).

A 2002 study reported the outcomes of 61 pregnancies in 50 women who had been treated with cabergoline for hyperprolactinemia (8). Pregnancy began during treatment in 60 cases and immediately after stopping treatment in 1 case. The median duration of treatment before pregnancy was 42.5 weeks (range 1–236 weeks) and the mean dose was 1.1 mg/week (range 0.25–7.0 mg/week). The pregnancy outcomes were five EABs (one for a suspected malformation; specific details not available), six SABs, one hydatidiform mole, and 49 livebirths. Among the livebirths, there was one minor defect and one major defect (trisomy 18) (8).

In summary, cabergoline does not exhibit direct embryo or fetal toxicity or teratogenicity in animals. Because it inhibits prolactin release, the agent can prevent or abort pregnancies in mice and rats, but this has no human relevance because human egg nidation is not regulated by prolactin. A 2002 review stated that cabergoline was the current treatment of choice for the majority of patients with hyperprolactinemia (9). In addition, the review recommended that once ovulatory cycles were established, women should stop treatment 1 month before they intend to conceive. Hyperprolactinemia is a frequent cause of infertility (6). In many of these women, the partial or complete resolution of this condition will result in conception (6). When pregnancy is diagnosed, cabergoline should be discontinued. However, there is no evidence that exposure to cabergoline in pregnancy is harmful.

BREAST FEEDING SUMMARY

RECOMMENDATION: Contraindicated

Although it is not an approved indication, cabergoline suppresses lactation because of its inhibition of prolactin release from the anterior pituitary gland. This action is similar to that of bromocriptine, another prolactin-inhibiting agent. A number of studies have examined this effect (10–15). The oral doses ranged from 0.4 mg to 1 mg, usually given as a single dose within 24 hours of delivery, but sometimes given as a divided dose over 2 days. The 1-mg dose appeared to be the most effective for long-term suppression of lactation.

The manufacturer states that cabergoline should not be used to suppress physiologic lactation because of the known toxicities associated with bromocriptine, when used for this purpose (1). These toxicities include hypertension, stroke, and seizures.

References

1. Product information. Dostinex. Pharmacia & Upjohn, 2001.
2. Beltrame D, Longo M, Mazue G. Reproductive toxicity of cabergoline in mice, rats, and rabbits. Reprod Toxicol 1996;10:471–83.
3. Negishi H, Koide SS. Prevention and termination of pregnancy in rats by cabergoline, a dopamine agonist. J Reprod Fertil 1997;109:103–7.
4. Ferrari C, Paracchi A, Mattei AM, de Vincentiis S, D'Alberton A, Grosignani PG. Cabergoline in the long-term therapy of hyperprolactinemic disorders. Acta Endocrinol (Copenh) 1992;126:489–94.
5. Jones TH, Fraser RB. Cabergoline treated hyperprolactinaemia results in pregnancy in a bromocriptine intolerant patient after seventeen years of infertility. Br J Obstet Gynaecol 1994;101:349–50.
6. Robert E, Musatti L, Piscitelli G, Ferrari CI. Pregnancy outcome after treatment with the ergot derivative, cabergoline. Reprod Toxicol 1996;10: 333–7.
7. Ciccarelli E, Grottoli S, Razzore P, Gaia D, Bertagna A, Cirillo S, Cammarota T, Camanni M, Camanni F. Long-term treatment with cabergoline, a new long-lasting ergoline derivative, in idiopathic or tumorous hyperprolactinaemia and outcome of drug-induced pregnancy. J Endocrinol Invest 1997;20:547–51.
8. Ricci E, Parazzini F, Motta T, Ferrari CI, Colao A, Clavenna A, Rocchi F, Gangi E, Paracchi S, Gasperi M, Lavezzari M, Nicolosi AE, Ferrero S, Landi ML, Beck-Peccoz P, Bonati M. Pregnancy outcome after cabergoline treatment in early weeks of gestation. Reprod Toxicol 2002;16:791–3.

9. Colao A, di Sarno A, Pivonello R, di Somma C, Lombardi G. Dopamine receptor agonists for treating prolactinomas. Expert Opin Investig Drugs 2002;11:787–800.
10. Melis GB, Gambacciani M, Paoletti AM, Beneventi F, Mais V, Baroldi P, Fioretti P. Dose-related prolactin inhibitory effect of the new long-acting dopamine receptor agonist cabergoline in normal cycling, puerperal, and hyperprolactinemic women. J Clin Endocrinol Metab 1987;65:541–5.
11. Melis GB, Mais V, Paoletti AM, Beneventi F, Gambacciani M, Fioretti P. Prevention of puerperal lactation by a single oral administration of the new prolactin-inhibiting drug, cabergoline. Obstet Gynecol 1988;71:311–4.
12. Giorda G, de Vincentiis S, Motta T, Casazza S, Fadin M, D'Alberton A. Cabergoline versus bromocriptine in suppression of lactation after cesarean delivery. Gynecol Obstet Invest 1991;31:93–6.
13. Rolland R, Piscitelli G, Ferrari C, Petroccione A, and the European Multicentre Study Group for Cabergoline in Lactation Inhibition. Single dose cabergoline versus bromocriptine in inhibition of puerperal lactation: randomised, double blind, multicentre study. BMJ 1991;302:1367–71.
14. Caballero-Gordo A, Lopez-Nazareno N, Calderay M, Caballero JL, Mancheno E, Sghedoni D. Oral cabergoline. Single-dose inhibition of puerperal lactation. J Reprod Med 1991;36:717–21.
15. Ferrari C, Piscitelli G, Grosignani PG. Cabergoline: a new drug for the treatment of hyperprolactinaemia. Hum Reprod 1995;10:1647–52.

Name: **CAFFEINE** Risk Factor: **B**
Class: **Central Stimulant**

FETAL RISK SUMMARY

RECOMMENDATION: Compatible

Caffeine is one of the most popular drugs in the world (1). It is frequently used in combination products containing aspirin, phenacetin, and codeine and is present in a number of commonly consumed beverages, such as coffee, teas, and colas, as well as many food items. The mean caffeine content in the usual servings of some common beverages was reported as caffeinated coffee (66–146 mg), nonherbal tea (20–46 mg), and caffeinated soft drinks (47 mg) (2), but these amounts may vary widely. (For example, see also reference 26 in which it is reported that the average caffeine content in two cups of regular coffee totaled 454 mg, and the average content in a similar amount of decaffeinated coffee totaled 12 mg.)

Caffeine crosses the placenta, and fetal blood and tissue levels similar to maternal concentrations are achieved (1,3–5). Cord blood levels of 1–1.6 μg/mL have been measured (3). Caffeine has also been found in newborns exposed to theophylline *in utero* (6).

The mutagenicity and carcinogenicity of caffeine have been evaluated in more than 50 studies involving laboratory animals, human and animal cell tissue cultures, and human lymphocytes *in vivo* (1,3). The significance of mutagenic and carcinogenic effects found in nonmammalian systems has not been established in humans. The drug is an animal teratogen only when doses high enough to cause toxicity in the mother have been given (1).

The Collaborative Perinatal Project (CPP) monitored 50,282 mother-child pairs, 5378 of whom had 1st trimester exposure to caffeine (7, pp. 366–370). No evidence of a relationship to congenital defects was found. For use anytime during pregnancy, 12,696 exposures were recorded (7, pp. 493–494). In this group, slightly increased relative risks were found for musculoskeletal defects, hydronephrosis, adrenal anomalies, and hemangiomas or granulomas, but the results are uninterpretable without independent confirmation (7, pp. 493–494). A follow-up analysis by the CPP on 2030 malformed infants and maternal use of caffeine-containing beverages did not support caffeine as a teratogen (8). Other reports have also found no association between the use of caffeine during pregnancy and congenital malformations (9–12).

Several authors have associated high caffeine consumption (6–8 cups of coffee/day) with decreased fertility, increased incidence of spontaneous abortion, and low birth weights (3,13–17). Unfortunately, few of these studies have isolated the effects of caffeine from cigarette or alcohol use, both of which are positively associated with caffeine consumption (3). One German study has observed that high coffee use alone is associated with low birth weights (18). In an American study of more than 12,400 women, low birth weights and short gestations occurred more often among offspring of women who drank four or more cups of coffee/day and who smoked (12). No relationship between low birth weights or short gestation and caffeine was found after controlling for smoking, alcohol intake, and demographic characteristics. However, other investigators have questioned whether this study accurately assessed the total caffeine intake of the women (19,20). A Canadian study retrospectively investigated 913 newborn infants for the effects of caffeine and cigarette smoking on birth weight and placental weight (21). Significant caffeine-cigarette interactions were found when daily consumption of caffeine was 300 mg or more. Compared to nonsmokers, cigarette smoking significantly lowered mean birth weight. When caffeine use was considered, daily consumption of 300 mg or more combined with smoking 15 cigarettes or more caused an additional significant reduction in weight. Head circumference and body length were not affected by any level of caffeine consumption. Placental weight, which normally increases with cigarette smoking, an effect hypothesized to be caused by compensatory hypertrophy induced by chronic fetal hypoxia, was found to decrease significantly in women smoking 15 cigarettes or more/day and ingesting 300 mg or more of caffeine/day (21).

A prospective cohort study examined the relationship between caffeine intake and the incidence of late spontaneous abortion in 3,135 predominantly white, educated, professional women (22). Of this population, 2,483 (79%) used caffeine during pregnancy. Caffeine consumption was calculated based on the intake of coffee (107 mg/serving), tea (34 mg/serving), colas (47 mg/serving), and drugs. Moderate to heavy consumption, defined as 151 mg or more of caffeine intake/day, occurred in 28% (879) and was associated with a 2-fold increased risk of late 1st and 2nd trimester spontaneous abortion (relative risk 1.95, $p = 0.07$). Consumption of greater than 200 mg/day did not increase this risk. In women who had a spontaneous abortion in their last pregnancy, light use of caffeine (0–150 mg/day) was associated with a 4-fold increase in late pregnancy loss (relative risk: 4.18, $p = 0.04$). The data were adjusted for such factors as demographic characteristics, obstetric and medical histories, contraceptive use, smoking, and alcohol exposure. The investigators cautioned, however, that other independent epidemiologic studies were required to confirm their findings because spontaneous abortion is of multifactorial etiology (22,23).

No increased risk for spontaneous abortion, intrauterine growth retardation, or microcephaly was found in a study that was able to identify all abortions that occurred 21 or more days after conception (24). The mean 1st-trimester caffeine consumption was statistically similar in those who aborted compared to those who delivered liveborn infants, 125.9 ± 123.1 mg vs. 111.6 ± 107.0 mg. After adjustment for other risk factors, notably smoking, the adjusted odds ratios for growth retardation and microcephaly were 1.11 (95% confidence interval [CI] 0.88–1.40) and 1.09 (95% CI 0.86–1.37), respectively (24).

A publication, evaluating studies published between 1981 and 1986, reviewed the effects of caffeine consumption on human pregnancies in terms of congenital malformations, low birth weight, preterm birth, spontaneous abortions, and behavior in *in utero* exposed children (25). Based on this evaluation of the literature, the author concluded that moderate intake of caffeine was not related to any adverse pregnancy outcome. A second article (120 references) reviewed the effect of caffeine on pregnancy outcome in both animals and humans (26). This author also concluded that modest amounts of caffeine present no proven risk to the fetus, but that limitation of daily amounts to less than 300 mg/day may lessen the possibility of growth retardation.

Research on the effects of caffeine consumption on human fecundability (i.e., the probability of becoming clinically pregnant in a given menstrual cycle) was reported in 1988 (27). Drawing from women they had enrolled in a study of very early pregnancy loss, the investigators chose 104 women who had not become pregnant in the first 3 months. Data were recorded daily by the women on menstrual bleeding, intercourse, and caffeine and other substance exposures. Caffeine consumption was calculated by assuming brewed coffee contained 100 mg, instant coffee contained 65 mg, tea contained 50 mg, and soft drinks contained 40 mg. The subjects were primarily white, college educated, and in their late 20s or early 30s. Caffeinated beverages were consumed by 93% (97 of 104) of the women. The women were divided into lower caffeine consumers (less than 3150 mg/month, or about one cup of brewed coffee/day) and higher consumers (using more than 3150 mg/month). Based on this division, the higher consumers were consistently less likely to become pregnant than the lower consumers, with a weighted mean of fecundability ratios across 13 menstrual cycles of 0.59. (The fecundability ratio was determined in each cycle by dividing the number of women who became pregnant by the total number of woman-cycles at risk, which was divided by the fraction obtained in the higher caffeine consumption group by the fraction obtained for the lower consumption group.) The ratio was less than 1.0 in every cycle. For cycles occurring after 6 months, the ratio was 0.53, indicating a slightly stronger association between higher caffeine consumption and the inability to become pregnant (27). Statistical adjustment of the data for age, frequency of intercourse, age at menarche, cigarette smoking, vitamin and analgesic intake, alcohol and marijuana use, and the mother's weight and height did not significantly change these findings. Moreover, when caffeine consumption was further subdivided, a partial dose-response relationship was observed with a ratio of 0.26 for women consuming more than 7000 mg/month (i.e., more than 70 cups of coffee/month). Unadjusted data on infertility (defined as women who failed to achieve pregnancy after 1 year) indicated that only 6% of the lower consumption group met this definition compared with 28% of the higher consumption group, an estimated relative risk of 4.7 ($p < 0.005$) (27). Evidence was also found to suggest that the effects of caffeine on fertility were short-acting because recent consumption was far more important than previous consumption. Although the study attempted to include all related factors, the investigators did caution that they could not exclude the possibility that some unknown factor or condition might have accounted for these results and that independent confirmation was required (27,28). Partial confirmation of this study was reported in 1989 (29). In a retrospective analysis of data collected from 1959 to 1967 on 6303 pregnancies, a dose–response relationship was found between caffeine consumption and difficulty in becoming pregnant. Using data adjusted for ethnicity (white, black), parity (0,1), and smoking, the relative risk of decreased fertility for less than 1 cup of coffee/day was 1.00, 1–3 cups/day 1.20, 4–6 cups/day 1.88, and more than 7 cups/day 1.96 (29).

Some investigators have expressed concern over the altering of catecholamine levels in the fetus by caffeine (30). Two cups of regular coffee containing a total of 454 mg of caffeine have been shown to increase maternal epinephrine levels significantly but not

C

norepinephrine or dopamine concentrations (31). Decaffeinated coffee (12 mg of caffeine in two cups) does not affect these catecholamine levels.

A 1989 single-blind, crossover study of eight women at 32–36 weeks of gestation investigated the effects of 2 cups of caffeinated (regular) or decaffeinated coffee on fetal breathing movements and heart rate (31). Administration of the test beverages, containing a total of 454 mg and 12 mg of caffeine, respectively, were separated by 1 week, and in each case, were consumed over a 15-minute period. Fetal breathing movements increased significantly during the 3rd hour after regular coffee, rising from 144 breaths/hour to 614 breaths/hour ($p < 0.01$). Fetal heart rate fell 9% ($p < 0.05$) at 1–1.5 hours after the regular coffee, and then slowly rose toward control levels at 2 and 4 hours. However, the mean number, amplitude, and duration of fetal heart rate accelerations did not differ statistically from the control period. Decaffeinated coffee also caused a significant increase in fetal breathing movements, rising to 505 breaths/hour during the 2nd hour, but this beverage caused only a slight, nonsignificant lowering of the fetal heart rate. In an earlier study using 200-mg tablets of caffeine, no increase in fetal breathing rates was observed (32). The differences between the two studies may have been related to the lower dose and/or the dosage form of caffeine.

Cardiac arrhythmias and other symptoms in newborn infants were associated with maternal caffeine use of more than 500 mg/day ($N = 16$) in comparison to the offspring of women who used less than 250 mg/day ($N = 56$) of caffeine (33). The percentages of observed symptoms in the infants of the high and low caffeine groups were tachyarrhythmias (supraventricular tachycardia and atrial flutter) 25% vs. 1.7% ($p < 0.01$), premature atrial contraction 12.5% vs. 0 ($p < 0.01$), fine tremors 100% vs. 10.7% ($p < 0.001$), and tachypnea (resting respiratory rate >60 respirations/minute) 25% vs. 3.5% ($p < 0.01$), respectively. The authors attributed the symptoms to caffeine withdrawal after birth (33).

Two reports have described adverse fetal outcomes, including teratogenic effects, in the offspring of two mothers taking migraine preparations consisting of ergotamine and caffeine (34,35). Complete details of these cases are provided under Ergotamine.

A 1993 reference compared the effects of maternal caffeine greater than 500 mg/day with those of less than 200 mg/day on fetal behavior in the 3rd trimester (36). Long-term consumption of high amounts of caffeine apparently modulated fetal behavior in terms of quiet sleep (infrequent body movements, regular breathing patterns, and little variability in fetal heart rate [FHR]), active sleep (rapid eye movements, increased body activity, irregular breathing, and increased FHR variability), and arousal (rapid eye movements, frequent body movements, highly irregular FHR baseline, and breathing activity). Fetuses of mothers in the high caffeine group spent less mean time in active sleep, similar mean time in quiet sleep, and much greater mean time in arousal than did low caffeine-exposed fetuses (36). It could not be determined if the modulation of behavior had any clinical significance to the newborn or in later life.

In summary, although the amount of caffeine in commonly used beverages varies widely, caffeine consumption in pregnancy in moderate amounts apparently does not pose a measurable risk to the fetus. When used in moderation, no association with congenital malformations, spontaneous abortions, preterm birth, or low birth weight has been proven. A 2001 review concluded that in those who do not smoke or drink alcohol, moderate caffeine consumption (<5–6 mg/kg/day spread throughout the day) did not increase any reproductive risks (37). Use of high doses may be associated with spontaneous abortions, difficulty in becoming pregnant, and infertility. A dose-response relationship may exist for the latter two problems. However, confirmation of these findings is needed before any firm conclusions can be drawn. The consumption of high caffeine doses with cigarette smoking may increase the risk for delivery of infants with lower birth weight than that induced by smoking alone. Moreover, consumption of large amounts of caffeine may be associated with becoming a smoker and excessive alcohol drinking (37).

BREAST FEEDING SUMMARY

RECOMMENDATION: Compatible

Caffeine is excreted into breast milk (38–45). Milk:plasma ratios of 0.5 and 0.76 have been reported (39,40). Following ingestion of coffee or tea containing known amounts of caffeine (36–335 mg), peak milk levels of 2.09–7.17 μg/mL occurred within 1 hour (41). An infant consuming 90 mL of milk every 3 hours would ingest 0.01–1.64 mg of caffeine over 24 hours after the mother drank a single cup of caffeinated beverage (41). In another study, peak milk levels after a 100-mg dose were 3.0 μg/mL at 1 hour (40). In this and an earlier study, the authors estimated a nursing infant would receive 1.5–3.1 mg of caffeine after a single cup of coffee (39,40).

Nine breast-feeding mothers consumed a measured amount of caffeine (750 mg/day) added to decaffeinated coffee for 5 days, then abstained from all caffeine ingestion for the next 4 days (44). In six women, 24-hour pooled aliquots of milk samples from each feeding were collected on days 5 and 9. In another mother, pooled aliquots were collected daily for 9 days. The average milk caffeine concentrations from these seven mothers on day 5 were 4.3 μg/mL (range <0.25–15.7 μg/mL). Caffeine was not detected (i.e., <0.25 μg/mL) in any of the seven samples on day 9. Serum levels in the infants of these seven mothers on day 5 averaged 1.4 μg/mL (range 0.8–2.8 μg/mL in five infants, not detectable in two). On day 9, caffeine was only detectable in the sera of two infants, decreasing from 0.8 μg/mL on day 5 to 0.6 μg/mL on day 9 in one, and decreasing from 2.8 to 2.4 μg/mL in the other. The remaining two mothers collected milk samples with each feeding for the entire 9 days of the study but did not pool the samples. These mothers were breast-feeding infants aged 79 and 127 days, and their mean daily milk caffeine levels on days 1–5 ranged from 4.0 to 28.6 μg/mL. Caffeine could not be detected in any of the milk samples after 5 days. The two infant's sera contained <0.25 μg/mL (mother's milk 13.4 μg/mL) and 3.2 μg/mL (mother's milk 28.6 μg/mL) on day 5, and both were <0.25 μg/mL on day 9. The wide variance in milk concentrations of caffeine was attributed to the mother's ability to metabolize caffeine (44). Based on the average level of 4.3 μg/mL, and assuming an infant consumed 150–180 mL/kg/day, the author calculated the infant would receive 0.6–0.8 mg/kg/day of caffeine (44).

In an extension of the above study, the effect of 500 mg of caffeine consumption/day on infant heart rate and sleep time was evaluated in 11 mother-infant pairs (45). Mothers consumed decaffeinated coffee daily for 5 days and then decaffeinated coffee with added caffeine for another 5-day period. Milk caffeine levels on the last day of the caffeine period ranged from 1.6 to 6.2 μg/mL, providing an estimated 0.3–1.0 mg/kg/day of caffeine to the infants. No significant difference in 24-hour heart rate or sleep time was observed between the two phases of the study.

The elimination half-life of caffeine is approximately 80 hours in term newborns and 97.5 hours in premature babies (42). A 1987 study investigated the metabolism of caffeine in breast-fed and formula-fed infants given oral doses of caffeine citrate (46). The serum

C

half-lives of caffeine were greater than three times as long in the breast-fed infants as compared with the formula-fed infants (76 vs. 21 hours at 47–50 weeks postconceptional age; 54 vs. 16 hours at 51–54 weeks postconceptional age). The investigators attributed the findings to inhibition or suppression of caffeine metabolism by the hepatic cytochrome P450 system by some element of breast milk (46).

The amounts of caffeine in breast milk after maternal ingestion of caffeinated beverages are probably too low to be clinically significant. However, accumulation may occur in infants when mothers use moderate to heavy amounts of caffeinated beverages. Irritability and poor sleeping patterns have been observed in nursing infants during periods of heavy maternal use of caffeine (43). The American Academy of Pediatrics classifies usual amounts of caffeinated beverages as compatible with breast-feeding (47).

References

1. Soyka LF. Effects of methylxanthines on the fetus. Clin Perinatol 1979;6:37–51.
2. Bunker ML, McWilliams M. Caffeine content of common beverages. J Am Diet Assoc 1979;74:28–32.
3. Soyka LF. Caffeine ingestion during pregnancy: in utero exposure and possible effects. Semin Perinatol 1981;5:305–9.
4. Goldstein A, Warren R. Passage of caffeine into human gonadal and fetal tissue. Biochem Pharmacol 1962;17:166–8.
5. Parsons WD, Aranda JV, Neims AH. Elimination of transplacentally acquired caffeine in full term neonates. Pediatr Res 1976;10:333.
6. Brazier JL, Salle B. Conversion of theophylline to caffeine by the human fetus. Semin Perinatol 1981;5:315–20.
7. Heinonen OP, Slone D, Shapiro S. *Birth Defects and Drugs in Pregnancy*. Littleton, MA: Publishing Sciences Group, 1977.
8. Rosenberg L, Mitchell AA, Shapiro S, Slone D. Selected birth defects in relation to caffeine-containing beverages. JAMA 1982;247:1429–32.
9. Van't Hoff W. Caffeine in pregnancy. Lancet 1982;1:1020.
10. Kurppa K, Holmberg PC, Kuosma E, Saxen L. Coffee consumption during pregnancy. N Engl J Med 1982;306:1548.
11. Curatolo PW, Robertson D. The health consequences of caffeine. Ann Intern Med 1983;98(Part 1):641–53.
12. Linn S, Schoenbaum SC, Monson RR, Rosner B, Stubblefield PG, Ryan KJ. No association between coffee consumption and adverse outcomes of pregnancy. N Engl J Med 1982;306:141–5.
13. Weathersbee PS, Olsen LK, Lodge JR. Caffeine and pregnancy. Postgrad Med 1977;62:64–9.
14. Anonymous. Caffeine and birth defects—another negative study. Pediatr Alert 1982;7:23–4.
15. Hogue CJ. Coffee in pregnancy. Lancet 1981;2:554.
16. Weathersbee PS, Lodge JR, Caffeine: its direct and indirect influence on reproduction. J Reprod Med 1977;19:55–63.
17. Lechat MF, Borlee I, Bouckaert A, Misson C. Caffeine study. Science 1980;207:1296–7.
18. Mau G, Netter P. Kaffee— und alkoholkonsum-riskofaktoren in der schwangerschaft? Geburtshilfe Frauenheilkd 1974;34:1018–22.
19. Bracken MB, Bryce-Buchanan C, Silten R, Srisuphan W. Coffee consumption during pregnancy. N Engl J Med 1982;306:1548–9.
20. Luke B. Coffee consumption during pregnancy. N Engl J Med 1982;306:1549.
21. Beaulac-Baillargeon L, Desrosiers C. Caffeine-cigarette interaction on fetal growth. Am J Obstet Gynecol 1987;157:1236–40.
22. Srisuphan W, Bracken MB. Caffeine consumption during pregnancy and association with late spontaneous abortion. Am J Obstet Gynecol 1986;154:14–20.
23. Bracken MB. Caffeine consumption during pregnancy and association with late spontaneous abortion: reply. Am J Obstet Gynecol 1986;155:1147.
24. Mills JL, Holmes LB, Aarons JH, Simpson JL, Brown ZA, Jovanovic-Peterson LG, Conley MR, Graubard BI, Knopp RH, Metzger BE. Moderate caffeine use and the risk of spontaneous abortion and intrauterine growth retardation. JAMA 1993;269:593–7.
25. Leviton A. Caffeine consumption and the risk of reproductive hazards. J Reprod Med 1988;33:175–8.
26. Berger A. Effects of caffeine consumption on pregnancy outcome: a review. J Reprod Med 1988;33:945–56.
27. Wilcox A, Weinberg C, Baird D. Caffeinated beverages and decreased fertility. Lancet 1988;2:1453–6.
28. Wilcox AJ. Caffeinated beverages and decreased fertility. Lancet 1989;1:840.
29. Christianson RE, Oechsli FW, van den Berg BJ. Caffeinated beverages and decreased fertility. Lancet 1989;1:378.
30. Bellet S, Roman L, DeCastro O, Kim KE, Kershbaum A. Effect of coffee ingestion on catecholamine release. Metabolism 1969;18:288–91.
31. Salvador HS, Koos BJ. Effects of regular and decaffeinated coffee on fetal breathing and heart rate. Am J Obstet Gynecol 1989;160:1043–7.
32. McGowan J, Devoe LD, Searle N, Altman R. The effects of long- and short-term maternal caffeine ingestion on human fetal breathing and body movements in term gestations. Am J Obstet Gynecol 1987;157:726–9.
33. Hadeed A, Siegel S. Newborn cardiac arrhythmias

associated with maternal caffeine use during pregnancy. Clin Pediatr 1993;32:45–7.
34. Graham JM Jr, Marin-Padilla M, Hoefnagel D. Jejunal atresia associated with Cafergot® ingestion during pregnancy. Clin Pediatr 1983;22:226–8.
35. Hughes HE, Goldstein DA. Birth defects following maternal exposure to ergotamine, beta blockers, and caffeine. J Med Genet 1988;25:396–9.
36. Devoe LD, Murray C, Youssif A, Arnaud M. Maternal caffeine consumption and fetal behavior in normal third-trimester pregnancy. Am J Obstet Gynecol 1993;168:1105–12.
37. Christian MS, Brent RL. Teratogen update: evaluation of the reproductive and developmental risks of caffeine. Teratology 2001;64:51–78.
38. Jobe PC. Psychoactive substances and antiepileptic drugs. In Wilson JT, ed. *Drugs in Breast Milk*. Balgowlah, Australia: ADIS Press, 1981:40.
39. Tyrala EE, Dodson WE. Caffeine secretion into breast milk. Arch Dis Child 1979;54:787–800.
40. Sargraves R, Bradley JM, Delgado MJM, Wagner D, Sharpe GL, Stavchansky S. Pharmacokinetics of caffeine in human breast milk after a single oral dose of caffeine (abstract). Drug Intell Clin Pharm 1984;18:507.
41. Berlin CM Jr, Denson HM, Daniel CH, Ward RM. Disposition of dietary caffeine in milk, saliva, and plasma of lactating women. Pediatrics 1984;73:59–63.
42. Berlin CM Jr. Excretion of the methylxanthines in human milk. Semin Perinatol 1981;5:389–94.
43. Hill RM, Craig JP, Chaney MD, Tennyson LM, McCulley LB. Utilization of over-the-counter drugs during pregnancy. Clin Obstet Gynecol 1977;20:381–94.
44. Ryu JE. Caffeine in human milk and in serum of breast-fed infants. Dev Pharmacol Ther 1985;8:329–37.
45. Ryu JE. Effect of maternal caffeine consumption on heart rate and sleep time of breast-fed infants. Dev Pharmacol Ther 1985;8:355–63.
46. Le Guennec J-C, Billon B. Delay in caffeine elimination in breast-fed infants. Pediatrics 1987;79:264–8.
47. Committee on Drugs, American Academy of Pediatrics. The transfer of drugs and other chemicals into human milk. Pediatrics 2001;108:776–89.

Name:	**CALCIFEDIOL**	Risk Factor:	**C***
Class:	**Vitamin**		

FETAL RISK SUMMARY

RECOMMENDATION: Compatible

Calcifediol is converted in the kidneys to calcitriol, one of the active forms of vitamin D. See Vitamin D.

[**Risk Factor D if used in doses above the recommended daily allowance.*]

BREAST FEEDING SUMMARY

RECOMMENDATION: Compatible

See Vitamin D.

Name:	**CALCITONIN-SALMON**	Risk Factor:	$\mathbf{C_M}$
Class:	**Calcium Regulation Hormone**		

FETAL RISK SUMMARY

RECOMMENDATION: No Human Data - Probably Compatible

Calcitonin-salmon is a synthetic polypeptide of 32 amino acids in the same linear sequence that is found in the hormone from salmon. The hormone does not cross the placenta (1).

A decrease in fetal birth weights in rabbits has been observed when calcitonin-salmon was administered in doses 14–56 times the recommended human dose (1). The fetal weight reduction may have been a result of metabolic effects on the mother (1).

No reports linking the use of calcitonin-salmon with congenital defects have been located. Marked increases of calcitonin concentrations in fetal serum greater than maternal levels have been demonstrated at term (2). The significance of this finding is unknown.

C

BREAST FEEDING SUMMARY

RECOMMENDATION: No Human Data - Probably Compatible

No reports describing the use of calcitonin-salmon during lactation have been located. Because it is a polypeptide, excretion into milk would not be expected. However, calcitonin-salmon has been shown to inhibit lactation in animals. Mothers wishing to breast-feed should be informed of this potential complication (1).

References

1. Product information. Miacalcin. Novartis Pharmaceuticals, 2000.
2. Kovarik J, Woloszczuk W, Linkesch W, Pavelka R. Calcitonin in pregnancy. Lancet 1980;1:199–200.

Name:	**CALCITRIOL**	Risk Factor:	C_M*
Class:	**Vitamin**		

FETAL RISK SUMMARY

RECOMMENDATION: Compatible

Calcitriol is one of three physiologically active forms of vitamin D (see Vitamin D). Calcitriol is teratogenic in rabbits dosed with 0.08 and 0.3 μg/kg (about 2 and 6 times the maximum recommended human dose based on body surface area [MRHD]) (1). Defects observed included external and skeletal malformations. The higher dose (0.3 μg/kg/day) given on gestation days 7 to 18 also increased maternal mortality, decreased mean fetal body weight, and reduced the number of newborn surviving to 24 hours. No teratogenic effects were observed in rats treated with doses up to 0.45 μg/kg (about 5 times the MRHD) (1). However, hypercalcemia was measured in the offspring of rats given 0.08 and 0.3 μ/kg/day (about 1 and 3 times the MRHD) (1).

The manufacturer cites a case of mild hypercalcemia during the first 2 days of life in an infant who was exposed to a maternal dose of 17 to 36 μg/day (approximately 17 to 36 times the maximum recommended dose) during pregnancy (1). The hypercalcemia resolved by the third day.

[*Risk Factor D if used in doses above the recommended daily allowance.*]

BREAST FEEDING SUMMARY

RECOMMENDATION: Compatible

See Vitamin D.

Reference

1. Product information. Rocaltrol. Roche Laboratories, 2000.

Name:	**CAMPHOR**	Risk Factor:	**C**
Class:	**Antipruritic/Local Anesthetic**		

FETAL RISK SUMMARY

RECOMMENDATION: Compatible (Topical)

Camphor is a natural product obtained from the subtropical tree *Cinnamomum camphora* in the form of d-camphor and also is produced synthetically in the optically inactive racemic form. In reproductive studies in rats and rabbits with oral doses, no evidence of embryotoxicity or teratogenicity was observed even at maternally toxic doses (1).

No reports linking the use of topically applied camphor with congenital defects have been located. Camphor is toxic and potentially a fatal poison if taken orally in sufficient quantities. Four cases of fetal exposure after accidental ingestion, including a case of fetal death and neonatal respiratory failure, have been reported (2–5). The drug crosses the placenta (3). A 1997 case report described a 16-year-old girl at 6 weeks' gestation who ingested 30 g of camphor dissolved in 250 mL of wine in an unsuccessful attempt to induce abortion (6). After successful treatment of the symptoms of camphor poisoning, her pregnancy was electively terminated a few weeks later. An autopsy of the embryo was not done.

The Collaborative Perinatal Project monitored 50,282 mother-child pairs, 168 of whom had 1st trimester exposure to topical camphor (7, pp. 410–412). No association was found with congenital malformations. For use anytime during pregnancy, 763 exposures were recorded and, again, no relationship to defects was noted (7, pp. 444, 499).

BREAST FEEDING SUMMARY

RECOMMENDATION: No Human Data - Probably Compatible

No data are available.

References

1. Leuschner J. Reproductive toxicity studies of d-Camphor in rats and rabbits. Arzneim-Forsch/Drug Res 1997;47:124–8.
2. Figgs J, Hamilton R, Homel S, McCabe J. Camphorated oil intoxication in pregnancy. Report of a case. Obstet Gynecol 1965;25:255–8.
3. Weiss J, Catalano P. Camphorated oil intoxication during pregnancy. Pediatrics 1973;52:713–4.
4. Blackman WB, Curry HB. Camphor poisoning: report of case occurring during pregnancy. J Fla Med Assoc 1957;43:99.
5. Jacobziner H, Raybin HW. Camphor poisoning. Arch Pediatr 1962;79:28.
6. Rabl W, Katzgraber F, Steinlechner M. Camphor ingestion for abortion (case report). Forensic Sci Int 1997;89:137–40.
7. Heinonen OP, Slone D, Shapiro S. *Birth Defects and Drugs in Pregnancy*. Littleton, MA: Publishing Sciences Group, 1977.

Name:	**CANDESARTAN CILEXETIL**	Risk Factor:	C_M*
Class:	**Antihypertensive**		

FETAL RISK SUMMARY

RECOMMENDATION: Human Data Suggest Risk in 2nd and 3rd Trimesters

The prodrug candesartan cilexetil is hydrolyzed to the active drug candesartan during absorption from the gastrointestinal tract. Candesartan is a selective angiotensin II

C

receptor antagonist that is used, either alone or in combination with other antihypertensive agents, for the treatment of hypertension. It blocks the vasoconstrictor and aldosterone-secreting effects of angiotensin II by preventing angiotensin II from binding to AT_1 receptors (1).

Reproduction studies have been conducted with candesartan cilexetil in mice, rats, and rabbits at oral doses up to approximately 138, 2.8, and 1.7 times the maximum recommended human dose of 32 mg based on body surface area (MRHD), respectively (1). Rat offspring, exposed to the drug during late gestation and through lactation, had decreased survival and an increased incidence of hydronephrosis, whereas no maternal toxicity or fetal harm were observed in pregnant mice. In pregnant rabbits, maternal toxicity (decreased body weight and death) was noted but, in the offspring of surviving dams, no adverse effects were seen on fetal survival, fetal weight, or on external, visceral, or skeletal development (1). No effects on fertility or reproductive performance were observed in male and female rats given oral doses up to 83 times the MRHD (1).

It is not known if candesartan crosses the human placenta to the fetus. The molecular weight of candesartan (about 440 after hydrolysis of the prodrug, candesartan cilexetil) is low enough, however, that passage to the fetus should be expected.

In a 2001 case report, candesartan (7 mg/day) was used for mild hypertension throughout gestation (2). Amniotic fluid was reduced at term. The female infant (birth weight not given) had left-sided facial palsy, plexus paresis, and was anuric. On ultrasound, the kidneys were hyperechogenic with poor corticomedullary differentiation. Urine production started at 5 days of age and the sonographic appearance of the kidneys normalized during the following month. At 8 months of age, the infant was developing normally and only a discrete facial and plexus palsy remained (2).

The antihypertensive mechanisms of action of candesartan and angiotensin-converting enzyme (ACE) inhibitors are very close; that is, the former selectively blocks the binding of angiotensin II to AT_1 receptors, whereas the latter prevents the formation of angiotensin II itself. Therefore, use of this drug during the 2nd and 3rd trimesters may cause teratogenicity and severe fetal and neonatal toxicity that is identical to that seen with ACE inhibitors (e.g., see Captopril or Enalapril). Fetal toxic effects may include anuria, oligohydramnios, fetal hypocalvaria, intrauterine growth retardation, prematurity, and patent ductus arteriosus. Anuria-associated oligohydramnios may produce fetal limb contractures, craniofacial deformation, and pulmonary hypoplasia. Severe anuria and hypotension, that is resistant to both pressor agents and volume expansion, may occur in the newborn following *in utero* exposure to candesartan cilexetil. Newborn renal function and blood pressure should be closely monitored. If candesartan is used in pregnancy, healthcare professionals are encouraged to call the toll free number (800–670–6126) for information about patient enrollment in the Motherisk study.

[**Risk factor* D_M *if used in 2nd or 3rd trimesters.*]

BREAST FEEDING SUMMARY

RECOMMENDATION: No Human Data - Probably Compatible

No reports describing the use of candesartan cilexetil during human lactation have been located. The drug is excreted into rat milk (1). Because the molecular weight of the active drug, candesartan, is about 440, excretion into human breast milk should also be expected. The effects of this exposure on a nursing infant are unknown. The American Academy of

Pediatrics, however, classifies ACE inhibitors, a closely related group of antihypertensive agents, as compatible with breast-feeding (see Captopril or Enalapril).

References

1. Product information. Atacand. AstraZeneca LP, 2000.
2. Hinsberger A, Wingen AM, Hoyer PF. Angiotensin-II-receptor inhibitors in pregnancy. Lancet 2001;357:1620.

Name:	CAPREOMYCIN	Risk Factor:	C_M
Class:	Antibiotic (Antituberculosis)		

FETAL RISK SUMMARY

RECOMMENDATION: No Human Data - No Relevant Animal Data

Capreomycin is a polypeptide antibiotic isolated from *Streptomyces capreolus*. The antibiotic is a mixture of four active components consisting of capreomycin IA and IB (combined total at least 90% of the product), and capreomycin IIA and IIB. Capreomycin is given by IM injection. Less than 1% is absorbed orally. It is indicated, in combination with other antituberculosis agents, as an alternate drug when the primary agents are ineffective or cannot be used because of toxicity. Because the toxicity of capreomycin is similar to aminoglycosides (e.g., cranial nerve VIII and renal), it should not be used with these agents.

Capreomycin caused a low incidence of wavy ribs in rats given doses 3.5 times the human dose (1). No studies have been conducted on the effects of the antibiotic on fertility, carcinogenicity, or mutagenicity (1).

No reports describing the use of capreomycin during human pregnancy have been located. A 1992 review of tuberculosis and pregnancy stated that the safety of capreomycin in pregnancy was not established, but cited no references of its use (2). Two other sources, one published in 1995 and the other in 1996, concluded that capreomycin should be avoided, if possible, because of the potential for ototoxicity and deafness (3,4). Neither source cited pregnancy data involving capreomycin.

BREAST FEEDING SUMMARY

RECOMMENDATION: No Human Data - Probably Compatible

No reports describing the use of capreomycin in lactation have been located. Because most antibiotics are excreted, however, the presence of the antibiotic in milk should be assumed. The effects on a nursing infant from this exposure are unknown. However, less than 1% of an oral dose is absorbed by the mother systemically, so the risk, if any, to a nursing infant appears to be minimal.

References

1. Product information. Capastat. 1990.
2. Hamadeh MA, Glassroth J. Tuberculosis and pregnancy. Chest 1992;101:1114–20.
3. Davidson PT. Managing tuberculosis during pregnancy. Lancet 1995;346:199–200.
4. Robinson CA, Rose NC. Tuberculosis: current implications and management in obstetrics. Obstet Gynecol Surv 1996;51:115–24.

Name:	**CAPTOPRIL**	Risk Factor:	**C_M***
Class:	**Antihypertensive**		

C

FETAL RISK SUMMARY

RECOMMENDATION: Human Data Suggest Risk in 2nd and 3rd Trimesters

Captopril, a competitive inhibitor of angiotensin I-converting enzyme (ACE), is used for the treatment of hypertension and in the management of heart failure. The drug is embryocidal in animals and has been shown to cause an increase in stillbirths in some species (1–3). In pregnant sheep and rabbits, the use of captopril was associated with a decrease in placental blood flow and oxygen delivery to the fetus (4,5).

Because of the toxicity identified in early animal studies, a committee of the National Institutes of Health recommended in 1984 that captopril be avoided during pregnancy (6). A 1985 review on the treatment of hypertension in pregnancy also stated the opinion that captopril should not be used in pregnancy because of the animal toxicity (7). However, use of captopril limited to the 1st trimester does not appear to present a significant risk to the fetus. Fetal exposure after this time has been associated with teratogenicity and severe toxicity in the fetus and newborn, including death.

A number of reports have described the use of captopril, usually in combination with other antihypertensive agents and often after the failure of other medications, for the treatment of resistant hypertension during human pregnancy (8–28). Included among these is a 1991 review that summarized those cases of captopril-exposed pregnancies published before January 1, 1990 (28). Some of these reports are reviewed below.

In a surveillance study of Michigan Medicaid recipients conducted between 1985 and 1992 involving 229,101 completed pregnancies, 86 newborns had been exposed to captopril during the 1st trimester (Franz Rosa, personal communication, FDA, 1993). Four (4.7%) major birth defects were observed (three expected). Specific data were available for six defect categories, including (observed/expected) 1/1 cardiovascular defects, 0/0 oral clefts, 0/0 spina bifida, 1/0 polydactyly, 1/0 limb reduction defects, and 1/0 hypospadias. These data do not support an association between 1st trimester use of captopril and congenital defects.

One pregnancy treated with captopril was reported in a 1997 study of 19 pregnancies exposed to ACE inhibitors (8). Captopril therapy was stopped at 8 weeks' gestation. No congenital anomalies or renal dysfunction was noted in the newborn (8).

A malformed fetus was discovered after voluntary abortion in a patient with renovascular hypertension (9). The patient had been treated during the 1st trimester with captopril, propranolol, and amiloride. The left leg ended at midthigh without distal development, and no obvious skull formation was noted above the brain tissue. However, because of the very small size of the fetus (1.5 cm), the pathologist could not be certain that the defects were not a result of the abortion (10).

A mother with a history of renal artery stenosis and malignant hypertension was treated throughout gestation with captopril, minoxidil, and propranolol (11). Three of her four previous pregnancies had ended in midgestation stillbirths. The most recent stillbirth, her fourth pregnancy, involved a 500-g male infant with low-set ears but no gross anomalies. The mother had been treated with the above regimen plus furosemide. In her second pregnancy, she had been treated only with hydrochlorothiazide and she had delivered a normal term infant. No information was available on the first and third pregnancies, both of which ended in stillbirths. In her latest pregnancy, daily doses of the three drugs were 50 mg, 10 mg, and 160 mg, respectively. The infant, delivered by cesarean section at 38 weeks, had multiple abnormalities including an omphalocele (repaired on the 2nd day), pronounced hypertrichosis of the back and extremities, depressed nasal bridge, low-set ears, micrognathia, bilateral fifth finger clinodactyly, undescended testes, a circumferential midphallic constriction, a large ventriculoseptal defect, and a brain defect consisting of slightly prominent sulci, especially the basal cisterns and interhemispheric fissure. Growth retardation was not evident, but the weight (3170 g, 60th percentile), length (46 cm, 15th percentile), and head circumference (32.5 cm, 25th percentile) were disproportionate. Neurologic examinations, as well as examinations of the skeleton and kidneys, were normal. Marked hypotension (30–50 mm Hg systolic) was present, which resolved after 24 hours. Heart rate, blood glucose, and renal function were normal. The infant's hospital course was marked by failure to thrive, congestive heart failure, prolonged physiologic jaundice, and eight episodes of hyperthermia (>38.5°C without apparent cause) between 2 and 6 weeks of age. The hypertrichosis, which was much less prominent at 2 months of age, is a known adverse effect of minoxidil therapy in both children and adults, and the condition in this infant was thought to be caused by that drug. The cause of the other defects could not be determined, but a chromosomal abnormality was excluded based on a normal male karyotype (46,XY), determined after a midgestation amniocentesis (11).

One case involved a mother with polyarteritis nodosa treated throughout gestation with captopril, hydralazine, and furosemide (12). The pregnancy was electively terminated at approximately 31 weeks' gestation because of worsening maternal disease. A normal, non-growth-retarded infant was delivered who did well in the neonatal period (12).

Oligohydramnios developed after 3 weeks of therapy with captopril in a woman who was treated at 25 weeks' gestation (13). Cesarean section at 29 weeks' gestation produced a 1040-g infant with dehydration, marked peripheral vasodilation, severe hypotension, respiratory distress, and anuria. Epidermolysis of the trunk and extremities appeared after birth. Diagnostic studies indicated a normal bladder, but neither kidney was perfused. ACE activity was reported as very low. The infant died on day 8 as a result of persistent anuria. At autopsy, hemorrhagic foci were discovered in the renal cortex and medulla, but nephrogenesis was adequate for the gestational age.

A woman was treated at 27 weeks' gestation with daily doses of captopril (200 mg), labetalol (1600 mg), and furosemide (80 mg) (14). Fourteen days after treatment was begun, signs of fetal distress, attributed to the maternal hypertension, appeared and the infant was delivered by cesarean section. No adverse effects of the drug treatment were observed in the infant (14).

Captopril and acebutolol were used throughout pregnancy to treat a woman with nephrotic syndrome and arterial hypertension (15). Intrauterine growth retardation (IUGR), most probably because of the severe maternal disease (although a contribution from drug therapy could not be excluded), was identified early in the 2nd trimester and became progressively worse. The growth-retarded male infant was delivered prematurely at 34 weeks by cesarean section. Captopril was found in the cord blood with levels in the mother and fetus less than 100 ng/mL, 4 hours after the last dose. Angiotensin-converting enzyme activity was below normal limits in both the mother and the newborn. Neonatal respiratory arrest occurred 15 minutes after delivery with varying degrees of hypotension persisting over the first 10 days. A patent ductus arteriosus was also present (15).

A woman with hypertension secondary to bilateral renal artery stenosis was treated with captopril, 150 mg/day, beginning 6 weeks before conception (16). Daily drug therapy during pregnancy consisted of captopril (600 mg), methyldopa (750 mg), and furosemide

(80 mg). Oligohydramnios and IUGR were diagnosed at 35 weeks' gestation, at which time a cesarean section was performed to deliver the 2120-g male infant. Some of the abnormalities in the infant, such as pulmonary hypoplasia, small skull circumference (28.5 cm, <3rd percentile), hypoplastic skull bones with wide sutures, and contractures of the extremities, were probably caused by captopril-induced oligohydramnios and fetal hypotension. The severe neonatal hypotension (27/20 mm Hg), which slowly resolved over 5 days despite volume expansion and pressor agents, and the anuria were also most likely caused by captopril. The infant was anuric for 7 days, then oliguric with 7–10 mL/day output for the next 12 days. All diagnostic tests during the first 10 days after birth indicated apparently normal kidneys. Peritoneal dialysis was commenced on the 20th day, but the infant died at 1 month of age (16).

A 1985 case report described a woman with twins treated throughout pregnancy with captopril (75–100 mg/day), hydralazine (75 mg/day), metoprolol (200 mg/day), and chlorthalidone (25 mg/day; stopped after 3 months) (17). Three previous pregnancies complicated by severe hypertension had ended with one term, mentally retarded infant and two spontaneous abortions, one at 5 months and one at 7 months. Two weeks before term the dose of captopril was reduced to 37.5 mg/day. Other than their small size (weight and length of both were less than the 10th percentile), both infants were normal and had normal mental and physical growth at 10 months (17).

In another case report, a woman who had had a renal transplant was treated throughout gestation with daily doses of captopril (75 mg), cyclosporine (200 mg), atenolol (200 mg), cimetidine, and amoxicillin (18). Oligohydramnios was diagnosed at 18 weeks' gestation and IUGR with gross oligohydramnios was discovered at 26 weeks. Ultrasound scanning at 27 weeks indicated renal dysplasia. Intrauterine fetal death occurred at 29 weeks. No congenital anomalies were found at autopsy. The kidneys appeared normal, but no urine was found in the ureters or bladder. The authors attributed the renal dysgenesis to the captopril therapy (18).

An 18-year-old woman with severe chronic hypertension became pregnant while taking captopril, hydralazine, and propranolol (19). Captopril and hydralazine were discontinued on presentation at 10 weeks' gestation. Because her subsequent blood pressure control was poor, her therapy was changed at 20 weeks' gestation to captopril (37.5–75 mg/day), atenolol (100 mg/day), and nifedipine (40 mg/day). IUGR was identified by serial scanning. A healthy, 1590-g female infant was delivered by cesarean section at 30 weeks' gestation. No other additional information was provided, other than that the infant survived (19).

Two abstracts described two pregnancies terminating with newborns exhibiting characteristic patterns of captopril-induced fetotoxicity and malformations (24,25). The fetopathy consisted of fetal hypotension, severe anuria and oligohydramnios, IUGR, hypocalvaria, renal tubular dysplasia, and pulmonary hypoplasia. Both infants died.

The result of a survey on the use of captopril during pregnancy was published in 1988 (26). The outcomes of therapy in the 37 pregnancies (38 fetuses, 1 set of twins) were 3 stillbirths, 11 premature births, 4 small-for-gestational-age infants, 4 cases of patent ductus arteriosus, and 2 neonatal deaths secondary to anuria (26).

A 1992 reference described the effects of ACE inhibitors on pregnancy outcome (27). Among 106,813 women enrolled in the Tennessee Medicaid program who delivered either a liveborn or stillborn infant, 19 had taken either captopril, enalapril, or lisinopril during gestation. One premature newborn, exposed *in utero* to captopril, had microcephaly, a large occipital encephalocele, and was probably blind (27).

Investigators at the FDA summarized some of the known cases of captopril-induced neonatal anuria in a 1989 report (29). These cases have been described above (13,15,16).

The FDA authors cautioned that if captopril was used during pregnancy, then preparations should be made for neonatal hypotension and renal failure (29). Of interest, a 1991 review concluded that fetal and neonatal renal dysfunction was more common after maternal use of enalapril than with captopril (28).

A 1991 report presented two cases of fetopathy and hypocalvaria in newborns exposed *in utero* to ACE inhibitors, including one case in which captopril, prednisone, atenolol, and furosemide were used throughout pregnancy (same case as described in reference 24) and one case caused by lisinopril (30). Twelve other cases of hypocalvaria or acalvaria were reviewed, three of which were thought to be caused by captopril ($N = 2$) or enalapril ($N = 1$) and nine others with causes that were either not drug-related or unknown. The authors speculated that the underlying pathogenetic mechanism in these cases is fetal hypotension (30).

In a 1991 article examining the teratogenesis of ACE inhibitors, the authors cited evidence linking fetal calvarial hypoplasia with the use of these agents after the 1st trimester (31). They speculated that the mechanism was related to drug-induced oligohydramnios that allowed the uterine musculature to exert direct pressure on the fetal skull. This mechanical insult, combined with drug-induced fetal hypotension, could inhibit peripheral perfusion and ossification of the calvaria (31).

Investigators in a study published in 1992 examined microscopically the kidneys of nine fetuses exposed to ACE inhibitors, one of which was enalapril (32). The researchers concluded that the renal defects associated with ACE inhibitors were caused by decreased renal perfusion and are similar to the defects seen in other conditions related to reduced fetal renal blood flow (32).

In a retrospective 2000 study, the outcomes of 10 pregnant women treated with low-dose captopril (12.5–25 mg/day) for severe, unresponsive vasoconstricted hypertension were reviewed (33). Maternal hemodynamics improved without fetal or neonatal complications. Assuming an expected complication rate of 5%–10%, however, the number of exposed pregnancies may have been too small to identify adverse effects (33).

In summary, captopril and other ACE inhibitors appear to be human teratogens when used in the 2nd and 3rd trimesters, producing fetal hypocalvaria and renal defects. The cause of the defects and other toxicity associated with angiotensin-converting enzyme inhibitors is probably related to fetal hypotension and decreased renal blood flow.

The use of captopril during the 1st trimester does not appear to present a risk to the fetus. Use during the 2nd and 3rd trimesters, however, may compromise the fetal renal system and result in severe, and at times fatal, anuria, both in the fetus and in the newborn. Anuria-associated oligohydramnios may produce pulmonary hypoplasia, limb contractures, persistent patent ductus arteriosus, craniofacial deformation, and neonatal death (34,35). IUGR, prematurity, and severe neonatal hypotension may also be observed. Two reviews of fetal and newborn renal function indicated that both renal perfusion and glomerular plasma flow are low during gestation and that high levels of angiotensin II may be physiologically necessary to maintain glomerular filtration at low perfusion pressures (36,37). Captopril prevents the conversion of angiotensin I to angiotensin II and, thus, may lead to *in utero* renal failure. In those cases in which captopril must be used to treat the mother's disease, the lowest possible dose should be used, combined with close monitoring of amniotic fluid levels and fetal well-being. Newborn renal function and blood pressure should also be closely monitored. If oligohydramnios occurs, stopping captopril may resolve the problem but may not improve infant outcome because of irreversible fetal damage (34). Guidelines for counseling exposed pregnant patients have been published and should be of benefit to health professionals faced with this task (31,34). If captopril is used in pregnancy, healthcare professionals are encouraged to call the toll free number (800-670-6126) for information about patient enrollment in the Motherisk study.

[*Risk Factor D_M if used in the 2nd or 3rd trimesters.]

C

BREAST FEEDING SUMMARY

RECOMMENDATION: Compatible

Captopril is excreted into breast milk in low concentrations. In 12 mothers given 100 mg three times/day, average peak milk levels were 4.7 ng/mL at 3.8 hours after their last dose (38,39). This represented an average milk:plasma ratio of 0.012. No differences were found in captopril levels in milk before and after the drug. No effects on the nursing infants were observed. The American Academy of Pediatrics classifies captopril as compatible with breast-feeding (40).

References

1. Broughton Pipkin F, Turner SR, Symonds EM. Possible risk with captopril in pregnancy: some animal data. Lancet 1980;1:1256.
2. Broughton Pipkin F, Symonds EM, Turner SR. The effect of captopril (SQ14,225) upon mother and fetus in the chronically cannulated ewe and in the pregnant rabbit. J Physiol 1982;323:415–22.
3. Keith IM, Will JA, Weir EK. Captopril: association with fetal death and pulmonary vascular changes in the rabbit (41446). Proc Soc Exp Biol Med 1982;170:378–83.
4. Lumbers ER, Kingsford NM, Menzies RI, Stevens AD. Acute effects of captopril, an angiotensin-converting enzyme inhibitor, on the pregnant ewe and fetus. Am J Physiol 1992;262 (Regul Integrative Comp Physiol 31):R754–R60.
5. Binder ND, Faber JJ. Effects of captopril on blood pressure, placental blood flow and uterine oxygen consumption in pregnant rabbits. J Pharmacol Exp Ther 1992;260:294–9.
6. Anonymous. The 1984 report of the Joint National Committee on Detection, Evaluation, and Treatment of High Blood Pressure. Arch Intern Med 1984;144:1045–6.
7. Lindheimer MD, Katz AI. Current concepts. Hypertension in pregnancy. N Engl J Med 1985;313:675–80.
8. Lip GYH, Churchill D, Beevers M, Auckett A, Beevers DG. Angiotensin-converting-enzyme inhibitors in early pregnancy. Lancet 1997;350:1446–7.
9. Duminy PC, Burger PT. Fetal abnormality associated with the use of captopril during pregnancy. S Afr Med J 1981;60:805.
10. Broude AM. Fetal abnormality associated with captopril during pregnancy. S Afr Med J 1982;61:68.
11. Kaler SG, Patrinos ME, Lambert GH, Myers TF, Karlman R, Anderson CL. Hypertrichosis and congenital anomalies associated with maternal use of minoxidil. Pediatrics 1987;79:434–6.
12. Owen J, Hauth JC. Polyarteritis nodosa in pregnancy: a case report and brief literature review. Am J Obstet Gynecol 1989;160:606–7.
13. Guignard JP, Burgener F, Calame A. Persistent anuria in a neonate: a side effect of captopril. (abstract)? Int J Pediatr Nephrol 1981;2:133.
14. Millar JA, Wilson PD, Morrison N. Management of severe hypertension in pregnancy by a combined drug regimen including captopril: case report. NZ Med J 1983;96:796–8.
15. Boutroy MJ, Vert P, Hurault de Ligny B, Miton A. Captopril administration in pregnancy impairs fetal angiotensin converting enzyme activity and neonatal adaptation. Lancet 1984;2:935–6.
16. Rothberg AD, Lorenz R. Can captopril cause fetal and neonatal renal failure? Pediatr Pharmacol 1984;4:189–92.
17. Coen G, Cugini P, Gerlini G, Finistauri D, Cinotti GA. Successful treatment of long-lasting severe hypertension with captopril during a twin pregnancy. Nephron 1985;40:498–500.
18. Knott PD, Thorpe SS, Lamont CAR. Congenital renal dysgenesis possibly due to captopril. Lancet 1989;1:451.
19. Smith AM. Are ACE inhibitors safe in pregnancy? Lancet 1989;2:750–1.
20. Fiocchi R, Lijnen P, Fagard R, Staessen J, Amery A, Van Assche F, Spitz B, Rademaker M. Captopril during pregnancy. Lancet 1984;2:1153.
21. Caraman PL, Miton A, Hurault de Ligny B, Kessler M, Boutroy MJ, Schweitzer M, Brocard O, Ragage JP, Netter P. Grossesses sous captopril. Therapie 1984; 39:59–63.
22. Plouin PF, Tchobroutsky C. Angiotensin converting-enzyme inhibition during human pregnancy: fifteen cases. Presse Méd 1985;14:2175–8.
23. Ducret F, Pointet Ph, Lauvergeon B, Jacoulet C, Gagnaire J. Grossesse sous inhibiteur de l'enzyme de conversion. Presse Méd 1985;14:897.
24. Barr M. Fetal effects of angiotensin converting enzyme inhibitor (abstract). Teratology 1990;41:536.
25. Pryde PG, Nugent CE, Sedman AB, Barr M Jr. ACE inhibitor fetopathy (abstract). Am J Obstet Gynecol 1992;166:348.
26. Kreft-Jais C, Plouin P-F, Tchobroutsky C, Boutroy J. Angiotensin-converting enzyme inhibitors during pregnancy: a survey of 22 patients given captopril and nine given enalapril. Br J Obstet Gynaecol 1988;95:420–2.
27. Piper JM, Ray WA, Rosa FW. Pregnancy outcome

following exposure to angiotensin-converting enzyme inhibitors. Obstet Gynecol 1992;80:429–32.
28. Hanssens M, Keirse MJNC, Vankelecom F, Van Assche FA. Fetal and neonatal effects of treatment with angiotensin-converting enzyme inhibitors in pregnancy. Obstet Gynecol 1991;78:128–35.
29. Rosa FW, Bosco LA, Graham CF, Milstien JB, Dreis M, Creamer J. Neonatal anuria with maternal angiotensin-converting enzyme inhibition. Obstet Gynecol 1989;74:371–4.
30. Barr M Jr, Cohen MM Jr. ACE inhibitor fetopathy and hypocalvaria: the kidney-skull connection. Teratology 1991;44:485–95.
31. Brent RL, Beckman DA. Angiotensin-converting enzyme inhibitors, an embryopathic class of drugs with unique properties: information for clinical teratology counselors. Teratology 1991;43:543–6.
32. Martin RA, Jones KL, Mendoza A, Barr M Jr, Benirschke K. Effect of ACE inhibition on the fetal kidney: decreased renal blood flow. Teratology 1992;46:317–21.
33. Easterling TR, Carr DB, Davis C, Diederichs C, Brateng DA, Schmucker B. Low dose, short acting, angiotensin-converting enzyme inhibitors as rescue therapy in pregnancy. Obstet Gynecol 2000;96:956–61.
34. Barr M Jr. Teratogen Update: angiotensin-converting enzyme inhibitors. Teratology 1994;50:399–409.
35. Shotan A, Widerhorn J, Hurst A, Elkayam U. Risks of angiotensin-converting enzyme inhibition during pregnancy: experimental and clinical evidence, potential mechanisms, and recommendations for use. Am J Med 1994;96:451–6.
36. Robillard JE, Nakamura KT, Matherne GP, Jose PA. Renal hemodynamics and functional adjustments to postnatal life. Semin Perinatol 1988;12:143–50.
37. Guignard JP, Gouyon JB. Adverse effects of drugs on the immature kidney. Biol Neonate 1988;53:243–52.
38. Devlin RG, Fleiss PM. Selective resistance to the passage of captopril into human milk. Clin Pharmacol Ther 1980;27:250.
39. Devlin RG, Fleiss PM. Captopril in human blood and breast milk. J Clin Pharmacol 1981;21:110–3.
40. Committee on Drugs, American Academy of Pediatrics. The transfer of drugs and other chemicals into human milk. Pediatrics 2001;108:776–89.

Name:	**CARBACHOL**	Risk Factor:	**C**
Class:	**Parasympathomimetic (Cholinergic)**		

FETAL RISK SUMMARY

RECOMMENDATION: No Human Data - Probably Compatible

Carbachol is used in the eye. No reports of its use in pregnancy have been located. As a quaternary ammonium compound, it is ionized at physiologic pH and transplacental passage in significant amounts would not be expected.

BREAST FEEDING SUMMARY

RECOMMENDATION: No Human Data - Probably Compatible

No data are available.

Name:	**CARBAMAZEPINE**	Risk Factor:	**D_M**
Class:	**Anticonvulsant**		

FETAL RISK SUMMARY

RECOMMENDATION: Compatible - Maternal Benefit >> Embryo/Fetal Risk

Carbamazepine, a tricyclic anticonvulsant, has been in clinical use since 1962. The drug is teratogenic in rats at doses 10 to 25 times the maximum human daily dose (MHDD) of 1200 mg/day or 1.5 to 4 times the MHDD based on body surface area (1). Anomalies observed included kinked ribs, cleft palate, talipes, and anophthalmos.

The drug crosses the placenta with highest concentrations found in fetal liver and kidneys (2–4). Fetal levels are approximately 50%–80% of maternal serum levels (4).

Placental function in women taking carbamazepine has been evaluated (5). No effect was detected from carbamazepine as measured by serum human placental lactogen, 24-hour urinary total estriol excretion, placental weight, and birth weight.

In a surveillance study of Michigan Medicaid recipients conducted between 1985 and 1992 involving 229,101 completed pregnancies, 172 newborns had been exposed to carbamazepine during the 1st trimester (F. Rosa, personal communication, FDA, 1993). A total of 13 (7.6%) major birth defects were observed (7 expected), including 4 cardiovascular defects (2 expected) and 1 spina bifida (none expected). No anomalies were observed in four other categories of defects (oral clefts, polydactyly, limb reduction defects, and hypospadias) for which specific data were available. Although the above data have not yet been analyzed to distinguish between combination and monotherapy (F. Rosa, personal communication, FDA, 1993), the total number of malformations suggests an association between the drug and congenital defects (see also discussion of reference 25 below).

Additional reports to the FDA involved five cases of holoprosencephaly in which carbamazepine was used either alone (two cases) or in combination with valproic acid and phenytoin (one case), phenytoin and primidone (one case), or gabapentin (one case) (6). Because of the lack of family histories, an association with familial holoprosencephaly or maternal neurologic problems could not be excluded (6).

A number of reports have described the use of carbamazepine during the 1st trimester (5,7–23,27,33–40). Multiple anomalies were found in one stillborn infant in whom carbamazepine was the only anticonvulsant used by the mother (15). These included closely set eyes, flat nose with single nasopharynx, polydactylia, atrial septal defect, patent ductus arteriosus, absent gallbladder and thyroid, and collapsed fontanel. Individual defects observed in this and other cases include talipes, meningomyelocele, anal atresia, ambiguous genitalia, congenital heart disease, hypertelorism, hypoplasia of the nose, cleft lip, congenital hip dislocation, inguinal hernia, hypoplasia of the nails, and torticollis (7–18). One infant, also exposed to lithium during the 1st trimester, had hydrocephalus and meningomyelocele (18). Decreased head circumference, 7 mm less than controls, has been observed in infants exposed only to carbamazepine during gestation (19). The head size was still small by 18 months of age with no catch-up growth evident. Dysmorphic facial features, combined with physical and mental retardation, were described in an infant girl exposed during gestation to 500–1700 mg/day of carbamazepine monotherapy (23). Maternal carbamazepine serum levels had been monitored frequently during gestation and all were reported to be in the therapeutic range (23).

In a 1982 review, Janz (24) stated that nearly all possible malformations had been observed in epileptic patients. Minor malformations, such as those seen in the fetal hydantoin syndrome (FHS) (see Phenytoin), have also been observed with carbamazepine monotherapy, causing Janz to conclude that the term FHS was misleading (24). Because carbamazepine was thought to present a lower risk to the fetus, the drug has been recommended as the treatment of choice for women who may become pregnant and who require anticonvulsant therapy for the first time (25). However, a 1989 report has indicated that carbamazepine is also probably a human teratogen (22).

Eight children were identified retrospectively after *in utero* exposure to carbamazepine either alone ($N = 4$), or in combination with other anticonvulsants (phenobarbital $N = 2$, primidone $N = 1$, or phenobarbital and clonazepam $N = 1$) (22). In six mothers, daily carbamazepine doses ranged from 600 to 1600 mg (dosage unknown in two). The following defects were noted in the children: intrauterine growth retardation (two cases), poor neonatal performance (three cases), postnatal growth deficiency (three cases, not determined in four), developmental delay (three cases, not determined in four), microcephaly (three cases, not determined in four), upslanting palpebral fissures (two cases), short nose with long philtrum (two cases), hypoplastic nails (four cases), and cardiac defect (two cases).

Concurrently with the above evaluations, a prospective study involving 72 women treated with carbamazepine in early pregnancy was conducted (22). Fifty-four liveborn children were evaluated from the 72 mothers with the remaining 18 excluded for various reasons (seven spontaneous abortions, five therapeutic abortions, and six lost to follow-up before delivery). A control group of 73 pregnant women was prospectively selected for comparison. Anticonvulsant drug therapy in the study group consisted of carbamazepine either alone ($N = 50$) or in combination with phenobarbital ($N = 12$), phenobarbital and valproic acid ($N = 4$), primidone ($N = 3$), valproic acid ($N = 1$), ethosuximide ($N = 1$), and primidone and ethosuximide ($N = 1$). Carbamazepine dosage varied from 200 to 1200 mg/day. Seizures occurred at least once during pregnancy in 59% of the women, but they did not correlate with either malformations or developmental delay in the offspring (22). Of the 54 liveborn children, 48 were examined by the study investigators. Five (10%) of these children had major anomalies consisting of lumbosacral meningomyelocele ($N = 1$), multiple ventricular septal defects ($N = 1$), indirect inguinal hernia ($N = 1$) (all three exposed to carbamazepine alone), and cleft uvula ($N = 2$) (exposed to carbamazepine and phenobarbital). Five (7%) of the control infants also had major anomalies. The incidence of children with two minor malformations was statistically similar for the study and control groups, 23% (11 of 48) vs. 13% (9 of 70), respectively. Those presenting with three or more minor anomalies, however, were more frequent in the exposed group (38%, 18 of 48) than in controls (6%, 4 of 70) ($p = 0.001$). Based on the combined results from the retrospective and prospective studies, the investigators concluded that carbamazepine exposure was associated with a pattern of congenital malformations whose principal features consisted of minor craniofacial defects, fingernail hypoplasia, and developmental delay. Because these defects were similar to those observed with the fetal hydantoin syndrome, and because both carbamazepine and phenytoin are metabolized through the arene oxide pathway, a mechanism was proposed that attributed the teratogenicity to the epoxide intermediates rather than to the specific drugs themselves (22).

In later correspondence concerning the above study, the investigators cited unofficial data obtained from the FDA involving 1307 pregnancies in which the maternal use of carbamazepine was not confounded by the concomitant use of valproic acid (26). Eight infants with spina bifida were identified in the offspring of these mothers. The incidence of 0.6% (1 in 163) represented a 9-fold relative risk for the neural tube defect (26).

A 1991 report cited data accumulated by the FDA on 237 infants with spina bifida born to women taking antiepileptic drugs during gestation (27). Carbamazepine was part of the anticonvulsant regimen in at least 64 of the women, 36 without valproic acid and 28 with valproic acid. The author noted that substantial underreporting was likely in these data, and an accurate assessment of the risk of spina bifida with carbamazepine could not be determined from voluntarily reported cases (27). To overcome these and other biases, the pregnancy outcomes of all Medicaid recipients in Michigan who gave birth in the period from 1980 through 1988, and who took anticonvulsants during the 1st trimester, were examined. Four cases of spina bifida were identified from 1490 women, including 107 who had taken carbamazepine. Three of the infants with spina bifida had been exposed to carbamazepine *in utero*, one of whom was also exposed to valproic acid, and two of whom were also exposed to phenytoin, barbiturates, or primidone alone or in combination.

Combined with other published studies, the author concluded that *in utero* exposure to carbamazepine during the 1st trimester, without concurrent exposure to valproic acid, results in a 1% risk of spina bifida (27). The relative risk (RR) was estimated to be about 13.7 (95% confidence limits [CI], 5.6–33.7) times the expected rate.

The above study generated several published comments involving the risk of spina bifida after 1st trimester exposure to carbamazepine (28–32). The last reference described an infant with closed spina bifida resulting from a pregnancy in which the mother took 600 mg of carbamazepine alone throughout gestation (32). The 3400-g female infant, delivered at 36 weeks' gestation, had a lumbosacral myelomeningocele covered with skin and no sensory loss. The authors of this report commented on four other cases of spina bifida after exposure to carbamazepine, either alone or in combination with valproic acid (32).

The effects of exposure at any time during the 2nd or 3rd month after the last menstrual period to folic acid antagonists on embryo/fetal development were evaluated in a large, multicenter, case-control surveillance study published in 2000 (33). The report was based on data collected between 1976 and 1998 from 80 maternity or tertiary care hospitals. Mothers were interviewed within 6 months of delivery about their use of drugs during pregnancy. Folic acid antagonists were categorized into two groups: group I—dihydrofolate reductase inhibitors (aminopterin, methotrexate, sulfasalazine, pyrimethamine, triamterene, and trimethoprim); group II - agents that affect other enzymes in folate metabolism, impair the absorption of folate, or increase the metabolic breakdown of folate (carbamazepine, phenytoin, primidone, and phenobarbital). The case subjects were 3870 infants with cardiovascular defects, 1962 with oral clefts, and 1100 with urinary tract malformations. Infants with defects associated with a syndrome were excluded as were infants with coexisting neural tube defects (NTDs; known to be reduced by maternal folic acid supplementation). Too few infants with limb-reduction defects were identified to be analyzed. Controls ($N = 8387$) were infants with malformations other than oral clefts and cardiovascular, urinary tract, limb-reduction, and NTDs, but included infants with chromosomal and genetic defects. The risk of malformations in control infants would not have been reduced by vitamin supplementation, and none of the controls used folic acid antagonists. For group I cases, the RRs of cardiovascular defects and oral clefts were 3.4 (95% CI 1.8–6.4) and 2.6 (95% CI 1.1–6.1), respectively. For group II cases, the RRs of cardiovascular, urinary tract defects, and oral clefts were 2.2 (95% CI 1.4–3.5), 2.5 (95% CI 1.2–5.0), and 2.5 (95% CI 1.5–4.2), respectively. Maternal use of multivitamin supplements with folic acid (typically 0.4 mg) reduced the risks in group I cases, but not in group II cases (33).

A 2001 case-control study, using the same database as in the above study, compared 1242 infants with NTDs (spina bifida, anencephaly, and encephalocele) to a control group of 6660 infants with congenital defects not related to vitamin supplements (34). Based on six exposed cases, the adjusted odds ratio (OR) for carbamazepine was 6.9%, 95% CI 1.9–25.7. For all folic acid antagonists (carbamazepine, phenobarbital, phenytoin, primidone, sulfasalazine, triamterene, and trimethoprim), based on 27 cases, the adjusted OR was 2.9, 95% CI 1.7–4.6 (34).

A 1996 study described typical dysmorphic facial features in 6 of 47 children (ages 6 months–6 years) who had been exposed to carbamazepine monotherapy during pregnancy (35). Moreover, the average cognitive score for the 47 children was significantly lower than that of a control group. The authors concluded that the facial features and mild mental retardation were consistent with a carbamazepine syndrome that had been described earlier (see reference 22) (35).

In a 2000 study, a group of 100 Swedish children who had been exposed to antiepileptic drugs (carbamazepine most frequently) *in utero* was compared to 100 matched controls at 9 months of age (36). Exposed children had a significant increase in the number of minor anomalies, 31 vs. 18, and, after carbamazepine exposure, an increased number of facial anomalies, 11 vs. 6. A blinded assessment of psychomotor development using Griffiths' test (gross motor function, personal and social behavior, hearing and speech, eye and hand coordination, and performance), however, found that antiepileptic drug exposure did not influence the results (36).

The effect of *in utero* exposure to antiepileptic drugs on fetal growth was described for 977 newborns in another 2000 Swedish study (37). Birth data was collected from 1973 to 1997, during which time the frequency of antiepileptic monotherapy increased from 46% to 88%. As expected, the most marked effects on body weight, length, and head circumference were found with polytherapy. For monotherapy, however, only carbamazepine had a negative influence on these measurements (37).

A 1997 study, using the General Practice Research Database in the United Kingdom, reported an increased prevalence of major malformations in infants of epileptic mothers treated with antiepileptic drugs (3.4%, 10 of 297) compared with matched controls (1.0%, 6 of 594), RR 3.3, 95% CI 1.2–9.2 (38). Eight of the 10 congenital anomalies involved carbamazepine (7 with monotherapy): ventricular septal defect; pulmonary stenosis; cleft palate, hare lip; Pierre Robin syndrome with cleft palate (also alcohol abuse); sensorineural deafness; congenital megaureter, hydronephrosis syndrome; vesicoureteric reflux; and Marcus Gunn ptosis (combined with sodium valproate) (38).

A 2000 study, using data from the MADRE (an acronym for MAlformation and DRug Exposure) surveillance project, assessed the human teratogenicity of anticonvulsants (39). Among 8005 malformed infants, cases were defined as infants with a specific malformation, whereas controls were infants with other anomalies. Of the total group, 299 were exposed in the 1st trimester to anticonvulsants. Among these, exposure to monotherapy occurred in the following: phenobarbital ($N = 65$), mephobarbital ($N = 10$), carbamazepine ($N = 46$), valproic acid ($N = 80$), phenytoin ($N = 24$), and other agents ($N = 16$). A statistically significant association was found between carbamazepine monotherapy and spina bifida ($N = 4$). When all 1st trimester exposures (mono- and polytherapy) were evaluated, a significant association was found between carbamazepine and hypertelorism with localized skull defects ($N = 3$). Although the study confirmed some previously known associations, several new associations with anticonvulsants were discovered and require independent confirmation (see Mephobarbital, Phenobarbital, Phenytoin, and Valproic Acid) (39).

A prospective study published in 1999 described the outcomes of 517 pregnancies of epileptic mothers identified at one Italian center from 1977 (40). Excluding genetic and chromosomal defects, malformations were classified as severe structural defects, mild structural defects, and deformations. Minor anomalies were not considered. Spontaneous ($N = 38$) and early ($N = 20$) voluntary abortions were excluded from the analysis, as were 7 pregnancies that delivered at other hospitals. Of the remaining 452 outcomes, 427 were exposed to anticonvulsants of which 313 involved monotherapy: carbamazepine ($N = 113$), phenobarbital ($N = 83$), valproate ($N = 44$), primidone ($N = 35$), phenytoin ($N = 31$), clonazepam ($N = 6$), and other ($N = 1$). There were no defects in the 25 pregnancies not exposed to anticonvulsants. Of the 42 (9.3%) outcomes with malformations, 24 (5.3%) were severe, 10 (2.2%) were mild, and 8 (1.8%) were deformities. There were 12 malformations with carbamazepine monotherapy: 7 (6.2%) were severe (spina bifida, hydrocephalus, diaphragmatic hernia, esophagus atresia, pyloric stenosis, omphalocele, renal dysplasia, and hydronephrosis), 1 (0.9%) was mild (inguinal hernia and valgus/varus foot), and 4 (3.5%) were deformations (club foot and hip dislocation). The investigators concluded that the anticonvulsants were the primary risk factor for an increased incidence of congenital malformations (see Clonazepam, Phenobarbital, Phenytoin, Primidone, and Valproic Acid) (40).

A 2001 prospective cohort study, conducted from 1986 to 1993 at five maternity hospitals, was designed to determine if anticonvulsant agents or other factors (e.g., genetic) were responsible for the constellation of abnormalities seen in infants of mothers treated with anticonvulsants during pregnancy (41). A total of 128,049 pregnant women were screened at delivery for exposure to anticonvulsant drugs. Three groups of singleton infants were identified: (a) exposed to anticonvulsant drugs, (b) not exposed to anticonvulsant drugs but with a maternal history of seizures, and (c) not exposed to anticonvulsant drugs and with no maternal history of seizures (control group). After applying exclusion criteria, including exposure to other teratogens, 316, 98, and 508 infants, respectively, were analyzed. Anticonvulsant monotherapy occurred in 223 women: phenytoin ($N = 87$), phenobarbital ($N = 64$), carbamazepine ($N = 58$); there were too few cases for analysis with valproic acid, clonazepam, diazepam, and lorazepam. Ninety-three infants were exposed to two or more anticonvulsant drugs. All infants were examined systematically (blinded as to group in 93% of the cases) for embryopathy associated with anticonvulsant exposure (major malformations, hypoplasia of the midface and fingers, microcephaly, and intrauterine growth retardation). Compared to controls, significant associations between anticonvulsants and anticonvulsant embryopathy were: phenytoin monotherapy 20.7% (18/87), phenobarbital monotherapy 26.6% (17/64), any monotherapy 20.6% (46/223), exposure to two or more anticonvulsants 28.0% (26/93), and all infants exposed to anticonvulsants (mono- and polytherapy) 22.8% (72/316). Nonsignificant associations were found for carbamazepine monotherapy 13.8% (8/58), nonexposed infants with a maternal history of seizures 6.1% (6/98), and controls 8.5% (43/508). The investigators concluded that the distinctive pattern of physical abnormalities observed in infants exposed to anticonvulsants during gestation was caused by the drugs, rather than by epilepsy itself (41).

In a study designed to evaluate the effect of *in utero* exposure to anticonvulsants on intelligence, 148 Finnish children of epileptic mothers were compared with 105 controls (21). Previous studies had shown intellectual impairment from either this exposure or no effect. Of the 148 children of epileptic mothers, 129 were exposed to anticonvulsant therapy during the first 20 weeks of pregnancy, 2 were only exposed after 20 weeks, and 17 were not exposed. In those mothers treated during pregnancy, 42 received carbamazepine (monotherapy in 9 cases) during the first 20 weeks, and 1 received the drug after 20 weeks. The children were evaluated at 5.5 years of age for both verbal and nonverbal measures of intelligence. A child was considered mentally deficient if the results of both tests were less than 71. Two of the 148 children of epileptic mothers were diagnosed as mentally deficient and 2 others had borderline intelligence (the mother of one of these latter children had not been treated with anticonvulsant medication). None of the controls was considered mentally deficient. One child with profound mental retardation had been exposed *in utero* to carbamazepine monotherapy, but the condition was compatible with dominant inheritance and was not thought to be caused by drug exposure. Both verbal and nonverbal intelligence scores were significantly lower in the study group children than in controls. In both groups, intelligence scores were significantly lower when seven or more minor anomalies were present. However, the presence of hypertelorism and digital hypoplasia, two minor anomalies considered typical of exposure to some anticonvulsants (e.g., phenytoin), was not predictive of low intelligence (21).

A prospective, controlled, blinded, observational 1994 study compared the global IQ and language development of children exposed *in utero* to either carbamazepine ($N =$ 34) or phenytoin ($N =$ 36) monotherapy to their respective matched controls (42). The cognitive tests were administered to the children between the ages of 18 and 36 months. The maternal IQ scores and socioeconomic status in the carbamazepine subjects and their controls were similar, 96.5 vs. 96.0, and 44.7 vs. 46.1, respectively, as they were in the phenytoin subjects and controls, 90.0 vs. 93.9, and 40.8 vs. 40.9, respectively. Compared to controls, no significant differences were measured in either IQ or language development scores between carbamazepine-exposed children and their matched controls. In contrast, phenytoin-exposed children had both lower mean global IQ and language development scores than their matched controls (see Phenytoin). No correlation between the daily dose (mg/kg) of either anticonvulsant and global IQ was found. Major malformations were observed in two carbamazepine-exposed children (missing last joint of right index finger and nail hypoplasia; hypospadias), one carbamazepine control (pulmonary atresia), and two phenytoin-exposed children (42). In subsequent correspondence relating to the above study (43,44), various perceived problems were cited and were addressed in a reply (45).

A possible teratogenic mechanism for carbamazepine in combination with other anticonvulsants was proposed in 1984 to account for the higher than expected adverse pregnancy outcome that is observed with combination therapy (46). Accumulation of the toxic oxidative metabolite, carbamazepine-10,11-epoxide, was shown when the drug was combined with other antiepileptic agents, such as phenobarbital, valproic acid, and phenytoin. These last two agents are also known to produce toxic epoxide metabolites that can bind covalently to macromolecules and may produce mutagenic or teratogenic effects (see Phenytoin) (46).

A case of attempted suicide with carbamazepine, possibly resulting in a neural tube defect, has been reported (47). A 44-year-old nonepileptic woman at 3–4 weeks after conception (i.e., during the period of neural tube closure) ingested approximately 4.8 g of the drug as a single dose. Her serum carbamazepine levels for 2 days after the ingestion were more than twice the recommended maximum therapeutic level. Subsequently, a large thoracolumbar spinal defect was observed on sonographic examination and her pregnancy was terminated at 20 weeks' gestation. Fetal autopsy of the male infant revealed an open myeloschisis and a hypoplastic left cerebral hemisphere, the latter defect thought to be the result of focal necrosis (47).

A case of neuroblastoma was described in a developmentally normal 2.5-year-old male infant who had been exposed throughout gestation to carbamazepine and phenytoin (48). The tumor was attributed to phenytoin exposure.

The effect of carbamazepine on maternal and fetal vitamin D metabolism was examined in a 1984 study (49). In comparison to normal controls, several significant differences were found in the level of various vitamin D compounds and in serum calcium, but the values were still within normal limits. No alterations were found in alkaline phosphatase and phosphate concentrations. The observed differences were not thought to be of major clinical significance (49).

In summary, carbamazepine use in pregnancy is associated with an increased incidence of major and minor malformations, including NTDs. A fetal carbamazepine syndrome that consists of minor craniofacial defects, fingernail hypoplasia, and developmental delay, has been proposed. The latter abnormality, however, is controversial; some studies have found mild mental retardation and some have not. Although pregnant women should be advised of these potential adverse outcomes, if the drug is required during pregnancy it should not be withheld because the benefits of preventing seizures outweigh the potential fetal harm.

C

BREAST FEEDING SUMMARY

RECOMMENDATION: Compatible

Carbamazepine is excreted into breast milk, producing milk:plasma ratios of 0.24–0.69 (2,4,9,14,50–52). The amount of carbamazepine measured in infant serum is low, with typical levels around 0.4 μg/mL, but levels may be as high as 0.5–1.8 μg/mL (2,51). In one case, infant serum levels were 15% and 20% of the maternal total and free carbamazepine concentrations, respectively (51). Accumulation does not seem to occur.

In a 1998 case report, seizures were reported by the mother in a nursing infant (52). The mother had bipolar disorder that was being treated with fluoxetine (20 mg/day), buspirone (45 mg/day), and carbamazepine (600 mg/day) (see Fluoxetine and Buspirone). Carbamazepine was detected in breast milk and the infant's serum (both 0.5 ng/mL). A neurologic examination of the infant that included electroencephalography was within normal limits. The cause of the seizure-like activity could not be determined, if, indeed, it had occurred (none of the episodes had been observed by medical personnel) (52).

The American Academy of Pediatrics classifies carbamazepine as compatible with breast-feeding (53).

References

1. Product information. Tegretol. Novartis Pharmaceuticals, 2000.
2. Pynnonen S, Kanto J, Sillanpae M, Erkkola R. Carbamazepine: placental transport, tissue concentrations in the foetus and newborns, and level in milk. Acta Pharmacol Toxicol 1977;41:244–53.
3. Rane A, Bertilsson L, Palmer L. Disposition of placentally transferred carbamazepine (Tegretol) in the newborn. Eur J Clin Pharmacol 1975;8:283–4.
4. Nau H, Kuhnz W, Egger HJ, Rating D, Helge H. Anticonvulsants during pregnancy and lactation: transplacental, maternal and neonatal pharmacokinetics. Clin Pharmacokinet 1982;7:508–43.
5. Hiilesmaa VK. Evaluation of placental function in women on antiepileptic drugs. J Perinat Med 1983; 11:187–92.
6. Rosa F. Holoprosencephaly and antiepileptic exposures. Teratology 1995;51:230.
7. Geigy Pharmaceuticals. Tegretol in epilepsy. In Monograph 319–80950, Ciba-Geigy, Ardsley, 1978:18–19.
8. McMullin GP. Teratogenic effects of anticonvulsants. Br Med J 1971;4:430.
9. Pynnonen S, Sillanpae M. Carbamazepine and mothers milk. Lancet 1975;2:563.
10. Lander CM, Edwards VE, Endie MJ, Tyrer JH. Plasma anticonvulsant concentrations during pregnancy. Neurology 1977;27:128–31.
11. Nakane Y, Okuma T, Takahashi R, et al. Multi-institutional study on the teratogenicity and fetal toxicity to antiepileptic drugs: a report of a collaborative study group in Japan. Epilepsia 1980;21: 633–80.
12. Janz D. The teratogenic risk of antiepileptic drugs. Epilepsia 1975;16:159–69.
13. Meyer JG. Teratogenic risk of anticonvulsants and the effects on pregnancy and birth. Eur Neurol 1979; 10:179–90.
14. Niebyl JR, Blake DA, Freeman JM, Luff RD. Carbamazepine levels in pregnancy and lactation. Obstet Gynecol 1979;53:139–40.
15. Hicks EP. Carbamazepine in two pregnancies. Clin Exp Neurol 1979;16:269–75.
16. Thomas D, Buchanan N. Teratogenic effects of anticonvulsants. J Pediatr 1981;99:163.
17. Niesen M, Froscher W. Finger- and toenail hypoplasia after carbamazepine monotherapy in late pregnancy. Neuropediatrics 1985;16:167–8.
18. Jacobson SJ, Jones K, Johnson K, Ceolin L, Kaur P, Sahn D, Donnenfeld AE, Rieder M, Santelli R, Smythe J, Pastuszak A, Einarson T, Koren G. Prospective multicentre study of pregnancy outcome after lithium exposure during first trimester. Lancet 1992;339:530–3.
19. Hiilesmaa VK, Teramo K, Granstrom ML, Bardy AH. Fetal head growth retardation associated with maternal antiepileptic drugs. Lancet 1981;2:165–7.
20. Hiilesmaa VK, Bardy A, Teramo K. Obstetric outcome in women with epilepsy. Am J Obstet Gynecol 1985;152:499–504.
21. Gaily E, Kantola-Sorsa E, Granstrom M-L. Intelligence of children of epileptic mothers. J Pediatr 1988;113: 677–84.
22. Jones KL, Lacro RV, Johnson KA, Adams J. Pattern of malformations in the children of women treated with carbamazepine during pregnancy. N Engl J Med 1989;320:1661–6.
23. Vestermark V, Vestermark S. Teratogenic effect of carbamazepine. Arch Dis Child 1991;66:641–2.
24. Janz D. Antiepileptic drugs and pregnancy: altered utilization patterns and teratogenesis. Epilepsia 1982; 23(Suppl 1):S53–S63.

25. Paulson GW, Paulson RB. Teratogenic effects of anticonvulsants. Arch Neurol 1981;38:140–3.
26. Jones KL, Johnson KA, Adams J, Lacro RV. Teratogenic effects of carbamazepine. N Engl J Med 1989;321:1481.
27. Rosa FW. Spina bifida in infants of women treated with carbamazepine during pregnancy. N Engl J Med 1991;324:674 7.
28. Anonymous. Teratogenesis with carbamazepine. Lancet 1991;337:1316–7.
29. Hughes RL. Spina bifida in infants of women taking carbamazepine. N Engl J Med 1991;325:664.
30. Hesdorffer DC, Hauser WA. Spina bifida in infants of women taking carbamazepine. N Engl J Med 1991;325:664.
31. Rosa F. Spina bifida in infants of women taking carbamazepine. N Engl J Med 1991;325:664–5.
32. Oakeshott P, Hunt GM. Carbamazepine and spina bifida. BMJ 1991;303:651.
33. Hernandez-Diaz S, Werler MM, Walker AM, Mitchell AA. Folic acid antagonists during pregnancy and the risk of birth defects. N Engl J Med 2000;343:1608–14.
34. Hernandez-Diaz S, Werler MM, Walker AM, Mitchell AA. Neural tube defects in relation to use of folic acid antagonists during pregnancy. Am J Epidemiol 2001;153:981–8.
35. Ornoy A, Cohen E. Outcome of children born to epileptic mothers treated with carbamazepine during pregnancy. Arch Dis Child 1996;75:517–20.
36. Wide K, Winbladh B, Tomson T, Sars-Zimmer K, Berggren E. Psychomotor development and minor anomalies in children exposed to antiepileptic drugs in utero: a prospective population-based study. Dev Med Child Neurol 2000;42:87–92.
37. Wide K, Winbladh B, Tomson T, Kallen B. Body dimensions of infants exposed to antiepileptic drugs in utero: observations spanning 25 years. Epilepsia 2000;41:854–61.
38. Jick SS, Terris BZ. Anticonvulsants and congenital malformations. Pharmacotherapy 1997;17:561–4.
39. Arpino C, Brescianini S, Robert E, Castilla EE, Cocchi G, Cornel MC, de Vigan C, Lancaster PAL, Merlob P, Sumiyoshi Y, Zampino G, Renzi C, Rosano A, Mastroiacovo P. Teratogenic effects of antiepileptic drugs: use of an international database on malformations and drug exposure (MADRE). Epilepsia 2000;41:1436–43.
40. Canger R, Battino D, Canevini MP, Fumarola C, Guidolin L, Vignoli A, Mamoli D, Palmieri C, Molteni F, Granata T, Hassibi P, Zamperini P, Pardi G, Avanzini G. Malformations in offspring of women with epilepsy: a prospective study. Epilepsia 1999;40:1231–6.
41. Holmes LB, Harvey EA, Coull BA, Huntington KB, Khoshbin S, Hayes AM, Ryan LM. The teratogenicity of anticonvulsant drugs. N Engl J Med 2001;344:1132–8.
42. Scolnik D, Nulman I, Rovet J, Gladstone D, Czuchta D, Gardner HA, Gladstone R, Ashby P, Weksberg R, Einarson T, Koren G. Neurodevelopment of children exposed in utero to phenytoin and carbamazepine monotherapy. JAMA 1994;271:767–770.
43. Jeret JS. Neurodevelopment after in utero exposure to phenytoin and carbamazepine. JAMA 1994;272:850.
44. Loring DW, Meador KJ, Thompson WO. Neurodevelopment of children exposed in utero to phenytoin and carbamazepine. JAMA 1994;272:850–1.
45. Koren G. Neurodevelopment of children exposed in utero to phenytoin and carbamazepine. JAMA 1994;272:851.
46. Lindhout D, Höppener RJEA, Meinardi H. Teratogenicity of antiepileptic drug combinations with special emphasis on epoxidation (of carbamazepine). Epilepsia 1984;25:77–83.
47. Little BB, Santos-Ramos R, Newell JF, Maberry MC. Megadose carbamazepine during the period of neural tube closure. Obstet Gynecol 1993;82:705–8.
48. Al-Shammri S, Guberman A, Hsu E. Neuroblastoma and fetal exposure to phenytoin in a child without dysmorphic features. Can J Neurol Sci 1992;19:243–5.
49. Markestad T, Ulstein M, Strandjord RE, Aksnes L, Aarskog D. Anticonvulsant drug therapy in human pregnancy: effects on serum concentrations of vitamin D metabolites in maternal and cord blood. Am J Obstet Gynecol 1984;150:254–8.
50. Kok THHG, Taitz LS, Bennett MJ, Holt DW. Drowsiness due to clemastine transmitted in breast milk. Lancet 1982;1:914–5.
51. Wisner KL, Perel JM. Serum levels of valproate and carbamazepine in breast-feeding mother-infant pairs. J Clin Psychopharmacol 1998;18:167–9.
52. Brent NB, Wisner KL. Fluoxetine and carbamazepine concentrations in a nursing mother/infant pair. Clin Pediatr 1998;37:41–4.
53. Committee on Drugs, American Academy of Pediatrics. The transfer of drugs and other chemicals into human milk. Pediatrics 2001;108:776–89.

Name: **CARBARSONE** Risk Factor: **D**

Class: **Amebicide**

FETAL RISK SUMMARY

RECOMMENDATION: Contraindicated

No reports linking the use of carbarsone with congenital defects have been located. However, carbarsone contains approximately 29% arsenic, which has been associated with lesions of the central nervous system (1). In view of potential tissue accumulation and reported fetal fatalities secondary to arsenic poisonings, carbarsone is not recommended during pregnancy (1,2).

BREAST FEEDING SUMMARY

RECOMMENDATION: Contraindicated

No data are available.

References

1. Arnold W. Morphologic und pathogenese der Salvarsan-schadigungen des zentralnervensystems. Virchows Arch (Pathol Anat) 1944;311:1.
2. Lugo G, Cassady G, Palmisano P. Acute maternal arsenic intoxication with neonatal death. Am J Dis Child 1969;117:328.

Name:	**CARBENICILLIN**	Risk Factor:	**B**
Class:	**Antibiotic (Penicillin)**		

FETAL RISK SUMMARY

RECOMMENDATION: Compatible

Carbenicillin is a penicillin antibiotic (see also Penicillin G). Reproduction studies conducted in mice (200 mg/kg), rats (500 or 1000 mg/kg), and monkeys (500 mg/kg) observed no fetal harm (1).

The drug crosses the placenta and distributes to most fetal tissues (2,3). After a 4-g IM dose, mean peak concentrations in cord and maternal serums at 2 hours were similar. Amniotic fluid levels averaged 7%–11% of maternal peak concentrations.

No published reports linking the use of carbenicillin with congenital defects have been located. The Collaborative Perinatal Project monitored 50,282 mother-child pairs, 3546 of whom had documented 1st trimester exposure to penicillin derivatives (4, pp. 297–313). For use anytime during pregnancy, 7171 exposures were recorded (4, p. 435). In neither group was evidence found to suggest a relationship to large categories of major or minor malformations or to individual defects.

In a surveillance study of Michigan Medicaid recipients conducted between 1985 and 1992 involving 229,101 completed pregnancies, 31 newborns had been exposed to carbenicillin during the 1st trimester (F. Rosa, personal communication, FDA, 1993). A total of five (16.1%) major birth defects were observed (one expected), one of which was a cardiovascular defect (0.5 expected). No anomalies were observed in five other categories of defects (oral clefts, spina bifida, polydactyly, limb reduction defects, and hypospadias) for which specific data were available. The number of exposures is too small to draw any conclusions.

BREAST FEEDING SUMMARY

RECOMMENDATION: Compatible

No reports describing the use of carbenicillin during lactation have been located. Because other penicillins are excreted in milk in low concentrations (see Ampicillin and Penicillin G), the presence of carbenicillin should also be expected. Although adverse effects from other penicillins in breast milk are rare, three potential problems exist for the nursing infant: modification of bowel flora, direct effects on the infant (e.g., allergic response), and interference with the interpretation of culture results if a fever workup is required.

References

1. Product information. Geocillin. Pfizer, 2000.
2. Biro L, Ivan E, Elek E, Arr M. Data on the tissue concentration of antibiotics in man. Tissue concentrations of semi-synthetic penicillins in the fetus. Int Z Pharmakol Ther Toxikol 1970;4:321–4.
3. Elek E, Ivan E, Arr M. Passage of penicillins from mother to foetus in humans. Int J Clin Pharmacol Ther Toxicol 1972;6:223–8.
4. Heinonen OP, Slone D, Shapiro S. *Birth Defects and Drugs in Pregnancy*. Littleton, MA: Publishing Sciences Group, 1977.

Name: **CARBIDOPA** Risk Factor: **C_M**
Class: **Antiparkinsonian Agent**

FETAL RISK SUMMARY

RECOMMENDATION: Limited Human Data - Animal Data Suggest Low Risk

This antiparkinsonian agent has no pharmacologic effect when given alone and is almost always used in conjunction with levodopa (see also Levodopa). Carbidopa (α-methyldopa hydrazine; MK-486) inhibits decarboxylation of extracerebral levodopa. When used in combination with this latter agent, lower doses of levodopa can be administered, resulting in fewer adverse effects, and more levodopa is available for passage to the brain and eventual conversion in that organ to the active metabolite, dopamine.

Combinations of carbidopa and levodopa, as well as levodopa alone, have caused visceral and skeletal malformations in rabbits (1). However, carbidopa, 10 or 100 mg/kg/day given orally to rats from day 1 through day 21 of gestation, did not have a teratogenic effect but did cause a significant dose-related increase in brown fat (interscapular brown adipose tissue) hemorrhage and vasodilation in the newborn pups (2). The hemorrhage, 4.6% and 12.1%, respectively, for the two doses, was thought to be related to dopamine. Combining carbidopa and levodopa resulted in a lower incidence of hemorrhage.

A study published in 1978 examined the effect of carbidopa (20 mg/kg SC every 12 hours for 7 days) and levodopa plus carbidopa (200/20 mg/kg SC every 12 hours for 7 days) on the length of gestation in pregnant rats (3). Only the combination had a statistically significant effect on pregnancy duration, causing a delay in parturition of 12 hours. The results were thought to be consistent with dopamine inhibition of oxytocin release.

In pregnant rats, small amounts of carbidopa cross the placenta and can be detected in amniotic fluid and fetal tissue (4). Carbidopa concentrations were measured at 1, 2, and 4 hours after a 20-mg/kg IV dose administered near the end of gestation (19th day). The highest levels in the maternal plasma, placenta, amniotic fluid, and fetus (time of maximum concentration shown in parentheses) were 9.9 μg/mL (1 hour), 2.35 μg/g (1 hour), 0.32 μg/mL (2 and 4 hours), and 0.65 μg/g (2 hours), respectively.

Human placental transfer of carbidopa, although the amounts were very small, was documented in a study published in 1995 (5). A 34-year-old woman with juvenile Parkinson's disease was treated with carbidopa/levodopa (200/800 mg/day) during two pregnancies (see also Levodopa). Both pregnancies were electively terminated, one at 8 weeks' gestation and the other at 10 weeks' gestation. Mean concentrations of carbidopa (expressed as ng/mg protein from 2 fetuses) in the maternal serum, placental tissue (including umbilical cord), fetal peripheral organs (heart, kidney, muscle), and fetal neural tissue (brain and spinal cord) were 2.05, 8.0, 0.14, and <0.15, respectively. The low concentrations of carbidopa in the fetus, compared with those in the mother and placenta, were interpreted as evidence for an effective placental barrier to the transport of carbidopa (5).

Because Parkinson's disease is relatively uncommon in women of childbearing age, only four reports have been located that describe the use of carbidopa, always in combination with levodopa, in human pregnancy (6–9). A woman with at least a 7-year history of parkinsonism conceived while being treated with carbidopa/levodopa (five 25/250-mg tablets/day) and amantadine (100 mg twice/day) (6). She had delivered a normal male infant approximately 6 years earlier, but no medical treatment had been given during that pregnancy. Amantadine was immediately discontinued when the current pregnancy was diagnosed. Other than slight vaginal bleeding in the 1st trimester, there were no maternal or fetal complications. She gave birth to a normal term infant (sex and weight not specified) who was doing well at 1.5 years of age.

A 1987 retrospective report described the use of carbidopa/levodopa, starting before conception in five women during seven pregnancies, one of which was electively terminated during the 1st trimester (7). All of the other pregnancies went to term (newborn weights and sexes not specified). Maternal complications in three pregnancies included slight 1st-trimester vaginal bleeding, nausea and vomiting during the 8th and 9th months (only one patient reported nausea and vomiting after the 1st trimester) and depression that resolved postpartum, and preeclampsia. One infant, whose mother took amantadine and carbidopa/levodopa and whose pregnancy was complicated by preeclampsia, had an inguinal hernia. No adverse effects or congenital anomalies were noted in the other five newborns, and all remained healthy at follow-up (approximately 1–5 years of age).

A 27-year-old woman with a history of chemotherapy and radiotherapy for non-Hodgkin's lymphoma occurring approximately 4 years earlier had developed a progressive parkinsonism syndrome that was treated with a proprietary preparation of carbidopa/levodopa (co-careldopa; Sinemet Plus; 375 mg/day) (8). She conceived 5 months after treatment began and eventually delivered a healthy, 3540-g male infant at term. Apgar scores were 9 at both 1 and 10 minutes, respectively. Co-careldopa was continued throughout her pregnancy.

A brief case report, published in 1997, described a normal outcome in the third pregnancy of a woman with levodopa-responsive dystonia (Segawa's type) who was treated throughout gestation with 500 mg/day of levodopa alone (9). The male infant weighed 2350 g at birth and was developing normally at the time of the report. Two previous pregnancies had occurred while the woman was being treated with daily doses of levodopa 100 mg and carbidopa 10 mg. Spontaneous abortions had occurred in both pregnancies; one at 6 weeks and the other at 12 weeks. An investigation failed to find any cause for the miscarriages.

In summary, although the number of reports describing the use of carbidopa (in combination with levodopa) during human pregnancy are few, which is as expected because of the relatively rarity of this condition in women of childbearing age, exposure to this agent during gestation does not appear to present a major risk to the fetus. Limited studies have not found teratogenicity in animals with carbidopa, except when combined with levodopa, and this outcome may be related to the latter drug. The cause of the two miscarriages described above is unknown, but requires further study. Brown fat hemorrhage observed in newborn rats treated during the 1st week of gestation was dose-related, and the toxicity has not been reported in humans. Moreover, the placental passage of carbidopa in animals and humans is limited. Based on the above data and the fact that lower doses of levodopa can be used if carbidopa is added to the mother's regimen, therapy with carbidopa, if indicated, should not be withheld during gestation.

BREAST FEEDING SUMMARY

RECOMMENDATION: No Human Data - Probably Compatible

No reports describing the use of carbidopa during human lactation have been located. In at least two cases, breast-feeding was held because of concerns with other drug therapy (levodopa or amantadine) that the mother was taking with carbidopa (6,8). Small amounts of carbidopa, probably from nonionic diffusion, were measured in the milk of five rats (15 days postpartum) 2 hours after a 20-mg/kg IV dose (4). The average milk and plasma concentrations were 0.5 μg/mL and 6.1 μg/mL, respectively, representing a milk:plasma ratio of 0.08. The relationship of these amounts to those that might occur in humans is unknown.

References

1. Product information. Sinemet. DuPont Pharma, 2000.
2. Kitchin KT, DiStefano V. L-Dopa and brown fat hemorrhage in the rat pup. Toxicol Appl Pharmacol 1976; 38:251–63.
3. Seybold VS, Miller JW, Lewis PR. Investigation of a dopaminergic mechanism for regulating oxytocin release. J Pharmacol Exp Ther 1978;207:605–10.
4. Vickers S, Stuart EK, Bianchine JR, Hucker HB, Jaffe ME, Rhodes RE, Vandenheuvel WJA. Metabolism of carbidopa [L-(−)-α-hydrazino-3,4-dihydroxy-α-methylhydrocinnamic acid monohydrate], an aromatic amino acid decarboxylase inhibitor, in the rat, dog, rhesus monkey, and man. Drug Metab Dispos 1974;2:9–22.
5. Merchant CA, Cohen G, Mytilineou C, DiRocco A, Moros D, Molinari S, Yahr MD. Human transplacental transfer of carbidopa/levodopa. J Neural Transm Park Dis Dement Sect 1995;9:239–42.
6. Cook DG, Klawans HL. Levodopa during pregnancy. Clin Neuropharmacol 1985;8:93–5.
7. Golbe LI. Parkinson's disease and pregnancy. Neurology 1987;37:1245–9.
8. Ball MC, Sagar HJ. Levodopa in pregnancy. Mov Disord 1995;10:115.
9. Nomoto M, Kaseda S, Iwata S, Osame M, Fukuda T. Levodopa in pregnancy. Mov Disord 1997;12:261.

Name:	**CARBIMAZOLE**	Risk Factor:	**D**
Class:	**Antithyroid**		

Carbimazole is converted *in vivo* to methimazole. See Methimazole.

Name:	**CARBINOXAMINE**	Risk Factor:	**C**
Class:	**Antihistamine**		

No data are available. See Diphenhydramine for representative agent in this class.

Name:	**CARBOPLATIN**	Risk Factor:	**D_M**
Class:	**Antineoplastic**		

C

FETAL RISK SUMMARY

RECOMMENDATION: Contraindicated - 1st Trimester

The antineoplastic agent carboplatin is indicated for the treatment of ovarian cancer. It is closely related to cisplatin, another cancer chemotherapeutic agent. Carboplatin and cisplatin share the same cell-cycle nonspecific mechanism of action, producing inter-strand DNA cross-links. Carboplatin is not protein bound (1).

Carboplatin is mutagenic both *in vitro* and *in vivo*. Its carcinogenic potential has not been studied but drugs with similar mechanisms of action are carcinogenic. Carboplatin is embryotoxic and teratogenic in rats given the drug during organogenesis (dose not specified) (1).

A 1989 study reported dose-related embryo lethality and teratogenicity in rats treated in the early phase of organogenesis (2). Previous work by these researchers had found no teratogenicity at a dose of 4 mg/kg/day (relationship to human dose not stated). In their current study, however, a dose of 6 mg/kg/day produced a significant increase in embryo deaths and multiple malformations (e.g., gastroschisis, dilation of cerebral ventricles, cleft sternum, fused ribs, and malformed thoracic vertebrae) (2).

It is not known if carboplatin crosses the placenta to the fetus. The molecular weight (about 371) is low enough that passage to the fetal compartment should be expected. A 2002 review of cancer chemotherapy stated that carboplatin was widely distributed throughout all body tissues, including, presumably, the amniotic fluid (3).

Three reports (two pregnancies) have described the use of carboplatin in human pregnancy (4–6). A 40-year-old woman was treated for ovarian cancer at 20 weeks' gestation with cisplatin (100 mg/m^2) and cyclophosphamide (600 mg/m^2) (4). A second course of these agents was given a few weeks later. Further cisplatin doses were discontinued because the woman developed ototoxicity. At 30 weeks' gestation carboplatin (300 mg/m^2) and cyclophosphamide (1000 mg/m^2) were given. A normal-appearing 3600-g male infant was delivered by cesarean section 7 weeks later. Apgar scores were 9 and 9 at 1 and 5 minutes, respectively. The infant was developing normally, including normal audiograms and neurologic findings, at 12 months of age (4).

In a followup report to the above case, researchers used a modified cisplatin-DNA enzyme-linked immunosorbent assay (ELISA) test to determine if platinum-DNA adducts could be detected in amniotic fluid obtained at 36 weeks or in cord blood at 37 weeks (5). Platinum-DNA adducts were not detected in either sample, but insufficient DNA was extracted from the samples to assay at the limit of ELISA sensitivity. Atomic absorbance spectrometry (AAS), a less-sensitive assay, also failed to detect platinum drug binding to DNA in amniotic fluid or cord blood. In contrast, DNA from the placenta was positive for platinum-DNA adducts in both the ELISA and AAS assays (5).

A 2003 report described the pregnancy outcome of a 30-year-old woman treated with carboplatin and paclitaxel during the 2nd and 3rd trimesters (6). She was diagnosed with an advanced stage of serous papillary adenocarcinoma of the ovary in the 1st trimester. The woman underwent an exploratory laparotomy at 7.5 weeks' gestation and then consented to chemotherapy beginning at 16–17 weeks. She received six cycles of carboplatin (dose specified as AUC 5) and paclitaxel (175 mg/m^2), and was delivered by cesarean hysterectomy 3 weeks after the last cycle at 35.5 weeks. The newborn (sex not specified) had Apgar scores of 9, 9, and 9 at 1, 5, and 10 minutes, respectively. Birth weight was 2500 g (44th percentile), and the physical examination and laboratory tests were normal. In addition, the placenta appeared grossly normal. The infant was doing well at 15 months of age with no evidence of neurologic, renal, growth, or hematologic effects from the exposure (6).

A number of pregnancies with successful outcomes have been documented after previous treatment with carboplatin (7–11). A 28-year-old woman delivered a normal male infant (birth weight 3.88 kg) 4 years after treatment of a bilateral ovarian dysgerminoma (7). Treatment consisted of a laparotomy to remove the right tube and ovary and carboplatin (dose 735 mg). A 29-year-old woman conceived with the assistance of a donated ovum that had been fertilized *in vitro* followed by embryo transfer (8). Five years earlier, both ovaries had been removed for stage III borderline ovarian adenocarcinoma. Her last course of carboplatin chemotherapy was given approximately 4 years before the pregnancy (8). In a retrospective study, the postsurgical reproductive histories of 50 women with ovarian cancer treated with unilateral oophorectomy from 1965 to 2000 were analyzed (9). Twenty-four women had attempted pregnancy and 17 (71%) had conceived 32 pregnancies. Six of the 17 had received prior chemotherapy (carboplatin or cisplatin plus paclitaxel in three; cisplatin plus cyclophosphamide in two; melphalan in one). The pregnancy outcomes were 1 on-going pregnancy, 5 spontaneous abortions (SABs), and 26 term gestations. There were no congenital anomalies in any of the offspring (9).

A large cohort study published in 2000 compared the pregnancy outcomes in survivors of various childhood cancers based on the type of treatment received (10). Among the total group of women, 340 had 594 pregnancies. The pregnancies were divided into five groups: 165 (non-sterilizing surgery or no treatment), 113 (chemotherapy with various agents, including an unknown number treated with carboplatin and cisplatin), 97 (abdominal-pelvic radiation), 53 (chemotherapy plus abdominal-pelvic radiation), and 166 (other treatments). The incidence of SABs and perinatal deaths did not differ among the groups. The proportion of live births with low birth weight (excluding preterm births) or congenital anomalies was highest in those treated only with radiation (16.0%) and those treated only with surgery (9.5%), respectively. The rates of low birth weight (excluding preterm births) and congenital defects in the two chemotherapy groups were 2.3% and 2.3% (chemotherapy only) and 7.1% and 2.4% (chemotherapy plus radiation) (10).

In a novel case report, a 21-year-old woman was diagnosed with metastatic ovarian cancer that was initially treated with surgery that left her uterus, right fallopian tube and ovary *in situ* (11). She then was enrolled into a phase I transplant protocol and received three cycles of carboplatin (dose specified as AUC 6) and paclitaxel (225 mg/m^2). Subsequent high-dose chemotherapy was then given (carboplatin, paclitaxel, and/or cyclophosphamide). After her chemotherapy, the woman received a successful transplant of autologous peripheral blood stem cells. Approximately 16 months after the transplant she conceived but had a 1st trimester miscarriage. She conceived again several months later and eventually delivered a healthy full-term, 3000-g female infant. The child was developing normally at 17 months of age (11).

In summary, carboplatin exhibits dose-related embryo toxicity and teratogenicity in one animal species. Treatment during human gestation has been reported in only two cases, both of which were treated in the 2nd and 3rd trimesters. The absence of human exposures during organogenesis prevents an assessment of the actual teratogenic risk but, based on the animal data and the pharmacology of the drug, the risk appears to be high. Therefore,

C

pregnant women should not be treated with this agent during the 1st trimester. Moreover, carboplatin is mutagenic and probably carcinogenic in experimental systems, but these effects have not been studied in human pregnancy. Based on very limited data, however, women who have been treated with carboplatin before pregnancy appear to be able to conceive and to carry natural or surrogate pregnancies to normal outcomes.

BREAST FEEDING SUMMARY

RECOMMENDATION: Contraindicated

No reports describing the use of carboplatin during lactation have been located. The relatively low molecular weight (about 371) suggests that carboplatin will be excreted into breast milk. A related drug, cisplatin, has a molecular weight of 300 and is excreted into milk (see Cisplatin.) Because of the mutagenic and probable carcinogenic properties, women receiving carboplatin should not nurse.

References

1. Product information. Paraplatin. Bristol-Myers Squibb, 2004.
2. Kai S, Kohmura H, Ishikawa K, Makihara Y, Ohta S, Kawano S, Takahashi N. Teratogenic effects of carboplatin, an oncostatic drug, administered during the early organogenetic period in rats. J Toxicol Sci 1989;14:115–30.
3. Leslie KK. Chemotherapy and pregnancy. Clin Obstet Gynecol 2002;45:153–64.
4. Henderson CE, Elia G, Garfinkel D, Poirier MC, Shamkhani H, Runowicz CD. Platinum chemotherapy during pregnancy for serous cystadenocarcinoma of the ovary. Gynecol Oncol 1993;49:92–4.
5. Shamkhani H, Anderson LM, Henderson CE, Moskal TJ, Runowicz CD, Dove LF, Jones AB, Chaney SG, Rice JM, Poirier MC. DNA adducts in human and patas monkey maternal and fetal tissues induced by platinum drug chemotherapy. Reprod Toxicol 1994;8:207–16.
6. Méndez LE, Mueller A, Salom E, González-Quintero VH. Paclitaxel and carboplatin chemotherapy administered during pregnancy for advanced epithelial ovarian cancer. Obstet Gynecol 2003;102:1200–2.
7. Hudson CN, Slevin ML, Tebbutt H. Successful pregnancy after treatment of stage III bilateral ovarian dysgerminoma. Br J Obstet Gynaecol 1995;102:1015–6.
8. Lawal AH, Lynch CB. Borderline ovarian cancer, bilateral surgical castration, chemotherapy and a normal delivery after ovum donation and in vitro fertilisation-embryo transfer. Br J Obstet Gynaecol 1996;103:931–2.
9. Schilder JM, Thompson AM, DePriest PD, Ueland FR, Cibull ML, Kryscio RJ, Modesitt SC, Lu KH, Geisler JP, Higgins RV, Magtibay PM, Cohn DE, Powell MA, Chu C, Stehman FB, van Nagell J. Outcome of reproductive age women with stage 1A or 1C invasive epithelial ovarian cancer treated with fertility-sparing therapy. Gynecol Oncol 2002;87:1–7.
10. Chiarelli AM, Marrett LD, Darlington GA. Pregnancy outcomes in females after treatment for childhood cancer. Epidemiology 2000;11:161–6.
11. Seiden MV, Spitzer TR, McAfee S, Fuller AF. Successful pregnancy after high-dose cyclophosphamide, carboplatinum, and Taxol with peripheral blood stem cell transplant in a young woman with ovarian cancer. Gynecol Oncol 2001;83:412–4.

Name:	**CARISOPRODOL**	Risk Factor:	**C**
Class:	**Muscle Relaxant**		

FETAL RISK SUMMARY

RECOMMENDATION: Limited Human Data - No Relevant Animal Data

Carisoprodol is a centrally acting muscle relaxant. The reproductive effect of this drug in animals has not been studied. No published studies describing the use of this agent in human pregnancy, other than the one shown below, have been located.

The Collaborative Perinatal Project monitored 50,282 mother-child pairs, 14 of whom were exposed in the 1st trimester to carisoprodol (1). No association of the drug with large classes of malformations or to individual defects was found.

In a surveillance study of Michigan Medicaid recipients conducted between 1985 and 1992 involving 229,101 completed pregnancies, 326 newborns had been exposed to carisoprodol during the 1st trimester (F. Rosa, personal communication, FDA, 1993). Twenty (6.1%) major birth defects were observed (14 expected), including (observed/expected) 3/3 cardiovascular defects, 2/0.5 oral clefts, and 1/1 hypospadias. No anomalies were observed in three other categories of defects (spina bifida, polydactyly, and limb reduction defects) for which data were available. Only with the two cases of oral clefts is there a suggestion of a possible association, but other factors, including the mother's disease, concurrent drug use, and chance, may be involved.

BREAST FEEDING SUMMARY

RECOMMENDATION: Limited Human Data - Potential Toxicity

Carisoprodol is concentrated in human milk with concentrations two to four times those in the maternal plasma (2). The American Academy of Pediatrics classifies another centrally acting skeletal muscle relaxant as compatible with breast-feeding (see Baclofen). However, because of the high concentrations of carisoprodol that appear in milk and the absence of reports describing its use during lactation, the drug should be used cautiously, if at all, during lactation. Women taking this drug and who elect to nurse should closely monitor their infants for sedation and other changes in behavior or functions.

References

1. Heinonen OP, Slone D, Shapiro S. *Birth Defects and Drugs in Pregnancy*. Littleton, MA: Publishing Sciences Group, 1977:357–65.
2. Product information. Soma. Wallace Laboratories, 1994.

Name:	**CARMUSTINE**	Risk Factor:	**D_M**
Class:	**Antineoplastic**		

FETAL RISK SUMMARY

RECOMMENDATION: Human and Animal Data Suggest Risk

Carmustine (BCNU) is an alkylating agent that is chemically classified as a nitrosourea. Other antineoplastics in this group include lomustine (CCNU) and streptozocin. Carmustine is indicated for the palliative therapy of certain brain tumors, multiple myeloma, Hodgkin's disease, and non-Hodgkin's lymphoma. The drug alkylates deoxyribonucleic acid (DNA) and ribonucleic acid (RNA), in addition to inhibiting some enzymes by carbamoylation of amino acids in proteins. Carmustine undergoes rapid degradation in the plasma with a terminal half-life of 22 minutes after an IV dose. The antineoplastic and toxic properties of carmustine are thought to be secondary to metabolites. The most severe toxicities are delayed bone marrow suppression and pulmonary toxicity (1,2).

Carmustine is carcinogenic in mice and rats at doses less than the recommended human dose based on body surface area (RHD). The agent was mutagenic in *in vitro* assays and clastogenic in both *in vivo* and *in vitro* tests (2). Reproduction studies have been conducted with carmustine in pregnant rats and rabbits (1,2). A dose about 0.17 times the RHD in rats caused embryotoxicity and fetal malformations (anophthalmia, micrognathia, and omphalocele). In rabbits, increased embryo lethality was observed at approximately 1.2 times the RHD (1,2). In another animal study, pregnant rats were given an intraperitoneal dose of 20 mg/kg on embryonic day 15 (3). (*Note: This dose is approximately 3.4 times the RHD.*) Exposed offspring had histologic alterations suggestive of cortical dysplasia (laminar disorganization, cytomegalic neurons, and neuronal heterotopias). Of interest, cortical dysplasia is associated with epilepsy in children and adults (3).

It is not known if carmustine or its metabolites crosses the placenta. The molecular weight (about 214), however, is low enough that exposure of the embryo or fetus should be expected. Two characteristics of carmustine, its high lipid solubility and its relatively lack of ionization at physiologic pH, will promote transfer of the drug across the placenta. The very short plasma half-life may lessen the transfer of the parent drug, but the pharmacology and pharmacokinetics of the active metabolites have not been fully elucidated.

A 1984 report described a 21-year-old woman with diffuse histiocytic lymphoma who received carmustine and procarbazine for 5 months before conception and throughout the first 24 weeks of pregnancy (4). A second nitrosourea agent, streptozocin, replaced carmustine and procarbazine in the 2nd trimester. Before pregnancy, the patient had received multiple courses of chemotherapy including cyclophosphamide, doxorubicin, vincristine, bleomycin, methotrexate, cytarabine, and etoposide, in addition to radiation therapy to the neck. Because of the failure of the previous therapy, she was started on carmustine 110 mg IV on day 1 and procarbazine 100 mg orally for 10 days every 4 weeks. She conceived after five monthly cycles of this latter therapy. The woman refused pregnancy termination and received five more cycles of therapy at 4-week intervals starting at 4 weeks' gestation. Three courses of streptozocin, 800 mg IV for 3 days every 4 weeks, were started at 24 weeks' gestation because of disease progression. She received the last dose of streptozocin 2 weeks before delivery at 35 weeks' gestation. The woman's normal-appearing male infant weighed 2.34 kg with a head circumference of 32.5 cm and a length of 51.5 cm. The Apgar scores were 7 and 9 at 1 and 5 minutes, respectively. The initial blood test revealed normal hemoglobin, white blood cell, and platelet counts. All other clinical tests were within normal limits, including electrolytes, multiple chemistry, urinalysis, renal ultrasound, and chromosome studies (4).

In a second case report, a 27-year-old woman with a history of malignant melanoma was admitted to the hospital at 14 weeks' gestation for progressive weight loss and persistent headache (5). Approximately 9 months earlier an enlarged nevus had been removed from her left shoulder and the pathology had revealed the melanoma. The work-up for metastatic disease was negative and she was discharged home. Two months later, the woman was readmitted for severe back pain, which was attributed to diffuse metastatic disease of the spine. At 23 weeks' gestation, she was started on chemotherapy consisting of carmustine 150 mg/m^2 IV on day 1, tamoxifen 80 mg orally twice daily for 7 days, cisplatin 25 mg/m^2 IV on days 1 to 3, and dacarbazine 220 mg/m^2 on days 1 to 3. Approximately 3 weeks later, she received a second course of these agents. Corticosteroids were administered for fetal lung maturity and as an antiemetic for chemotherapy. Because the woman continued to deteriorate, a 1520-g female infant was delivered by cesarean section at 30 weeks' gestation. The 325-g placenta had malignant melanoma in the intervillous space and melanin pigment granules in villous Hofbauer cells and syncytial trophoblasts. The mother died 1 month later. At 17 months of age the child's weight was 6.6 kg (5th percentile), length 74.5 cm (<5th percentile), and head circumference 47 cm (10th percentile). Examination revealed age-appropriate evaluations for mental age, motor age, and language scores (5).

A number of reports have described pregnancy outcomes after the use of carmustine before conception (6–11). In four studies, the outcomes of 16 pregnancies (12 women) were 14 normal newborns, one stillbirth (twins), and one elective abortion (6–9). In one case, a man treated earlier with carmustine fathered a normal infant (7). A 2000 study analyzed the pregnancy outcomes of 340 cancer survivors who had one or more pregnancies after treatment with carmustine and 11 other alkylating agents (10). The cases were divided into five mutually exclusive treatment groups: non-sterilizing surgery, chemotherapy with alkylating agents, abdominal-pelvic radiation, alkylating agents plus abdominal-pelvic radiation, and all other treatments. The study found no evidence of an increased risk of birth defects or spontaneous abortions (10). In a 2002 study, 1915 women had 4029 pregnancies after chemotherapy with or without radiation (11). No statistical differences in pregnancy outcomes (live births and spontaneous abortions) by treatment group were found, including the 126 pregnancies in women treated with carmustine.

In summary, typical of many chemotherapeutic agents, carmustine is carcinogenic, mutagenic, clastogenic, embryotoxic, and teratogenic in experimental animals. However, only two reports have described the use of carmustine in human pregnancy. In one case, a woman was treated with carmustine before and during the first two trimesters. She gave birth to a normal infant. In the other case, a woman who was not treated until late in the 2nd trimester was electively delivered prematurely because of her disease. Her infant was growth retarded 17 months after birth but had apparently normal mental and motor development. As with other cancer chemotherapeutic agents, treatment after the 1st trimester does not appear to result in newborn toxicity, although bone marrow suppression has been reported when multiple agents were used close to delivery (e.g., see Cyclophosphamide). Several alkylating agents are thought to be human teratogens (e.g., busulfan, chlorambucil, and cyclophosphamide), but few infants have been exposed to these drugs in the 1st trimester. Until proven otherwise, carmustine should be considered a potential teratogen if used during the period of organogenesis. Therefore, a woman whose condition requires treatment during organogenesis, or who conceives while under treatment, should be informed of the potential risk to her embryo.

BREAST FEEDING SUMMARY

RECOMMENDATION: Contraindicated

No reports describing the use of carmustine during lactation have been located. The low molecular weight (about 214), high lipid solubility, and relative lack of ionization at physiologic pH suggest that carmustine will be excreted into breast milk. The short elimination half-life in the plasma may limit the amount of parent drug in milk, but the pharmacology and pharmacokinetics of the active metabolites have not been adequately characterized. Because there is substantial risk of harm for a nursing infant, women who are being treated with carmustine should not nurse.

References

1. Product information. BiCNU. Bristol-Myers Squibb, 1998.
2. Product information. Gliadel Wafer. Guilford Pharmaceuticals, 2003.
3. Benardete EA, Kriegstein AR. Increase excitability and decreased sensitivity to GABA in an animal model of dysplastic cortex. Epilepsia 2002;43:970–82.
4. Schapira DV, Chudley AE. Successful pregnancy

C

following continuous treatment with combination chemotherapy before conception and throughout pregnancy. Cancer 1984;54:800–3.
5. DiPaola RS, Goodin S, Ratzell M, Florczyk M, Karp G, Ravikumar TS. Chemotherapy for metastatic melanoma during pregnancy. Gynecol Oncol 1997;66:526–30.
6. Blatt J, Mulvihill JJ, Ziegler JL, Young RC, Poplack DG. Pregnancy outcome following cancer chemotherapy. Am J Med 1980;69:828–32.
7. Green DM, Zevon MA, Lowrie G, Seigelstein N, Hall B. Congenital anomalies in children of patients who received chemotherapy for cancer in childhood and adolescence. N Engl J Med 1991;325:141–6.
8. Bierman PJ, Bagin RG, Jagannath S, Vose JM, Spitzer G, Kessinger A, Dicke KA, Armitage JO. High dose chemotherapy followed by autologous hematopoietic rescue in Hodgkin's disease: long-term follow-up in 128 patients. Ann Oncol 1993;4:767–73.
9. Brice P, Pautier P, Marolleau JP, Castaigne S, Gisselbrecht C. Pregnancy after autologous bone marrow transplantation for malignant lymphomas. Nouv Rev Fr Hematol 1994;36:387–8.
10. Chiarelli AM, Marrett LD, Darlington GA. Pregnancy outcomes in females after treatment for childhood cancer. Epidemiology 2000;11:161–6.
11. Green DM, Whitton JA, Stovall M, Mertens AC, Donaldson SS, Ruymann FB, Pendergrass TW, Robison LL. Pregnancy outcome of female survivors of childhood cancer: a report from the Childhood Cancer Survivor study. Am J Obstet Gynecol 2002;187: 1070–80.

Name: **CARPHENAZINE** Risk Factor: **C**

Class: **Tranquilizer**

FETAL RISK SUMMARY

RECOMMENDATION: No Human Data - No Relevant Animal Data

Carphenazine is a piperazine phenothiazine in the same group as prochlorperazine (see Prochlorperazine). Phenothiazines readily cross the placenta (1). No specific information on the use of carphenazine in pregnancy has been located. Although occasional reports have attempted to link various phenothiazine compounds with congenital malformations, the bulk of the evidence indicates that these drugs are safe for the mother and fetus (see also Chlorpromazine).

BREAST FEEDING SUMMARY

RECOMMENDATION: No Human Data - Potential Toxicity

No data are available.

Reference

1. Moya F, Thorndike V. Passage of drugs across the placenta. Am J Obstet Gynecol 1962;84:1778–98.

Name: **CARTEOLOL** Risk Factor: **C_M***

Class: **Sympatholytic (Antihypertensive)**

FETAL RISK SUMMARY

RECOMMENDATION: Human Data Suggest Risk in 2nd and 3rd Trimesters

Carteolol is a nonselective β_1/β_2-adrenergic blocking agent used in the treatment of hypertension and topically in the therapy of glaucoma. No teratogenic effects were observed in pregnant mice and rabbits treated with doses much higher than the maximum recommended human dose (1–3). A dose-related increase in the incidence of wavy ribs was noted in fetal rats whose mothers were given doses 212 times the maximum recommended human dose (MRHD) (3). Fetotoxicity (increased resorptions and decreased fetal weight) was observed in rats and rabbits at doses up to 5264 and 1052 times the MRHD (3). These effects were not noted in mice at doses up to 1052 times the MRHD (3).

No studies describing the use of carteolol in human pregnancies have been located. If used near delivery, the newborn infant should be closely observed for 24–48 hours for signs and symptoms of β-blockade. Long-term effects of *in utero* exposure to β-blockers have not been studied but warrant evaluation.

Some β-blockers may cause intrauterine growth retardation (IUGR) and reduced placental weight, especially those lacking intrinsic sympathomimetic activity (ISA) (i.e., partial agonist). Treatment beginning early in the 2nd trimester results in the greatest weight reductions, whereas treatment restricted to the 3rd trimester primarily affects only placental weight. Carteolol does possess ISA. However, IUGR and reduced placental weight may potentially occur with all agents within this class. Although growth retardation is a serious concern, the benefits of maternal therapy with β-blockers, in some cases, might outweigh the risks to the fetus and must be judged on a case-by-case basis.

[**Risk Factor D if used in the 2nd or 3rd trimesters.*]

BREAST FEEDING SUMMARY

RECOMMENDATION: No Human Data - Potential Toxicity

Carteolol is excreted into the milk of lactating rats (3), but human studies describing the use of the drug during lactation have not been located. If carteolol is used during nursing, the infant should be closely observed for hypotension, bradycardia, and other signs or symptoms of β-blockade. Long-term effects of exposure to β-blockers from milk have not been studied but warrant evaluation.

References

1. Tanaka N, Shingai F, Tamagawa M, Nakatsu I. Reproductive study of carteolol hydrochloride in mice, part 1. Fertility and reproductive performance. J Toxicol Sci 1979;4:47–58. As cited in Shepard TH. *Catalog of Teratogenic Agents*. 6th ed. Baltimore, MD: Johns Hopkins University Press, 1989:119.
2. Tamagawa M, Namoto T, Tanaka N, Hishino H. Reproduction study of carteolol hydrochloride in mice, part 2. Perinatal and postnatal toxicity. J Toxicol Sci 1979;4:59–78. As cited in Shepard TH. *Catalog of Teratogenic Agents*. 6th ed. Baltimore, MD: Johns Hopkins University Press, 1989:119.
3. Product information. Cartrol. Abbott Laboratories, 1997.

Name:	**CARVEDILOL**	Risk Factor:	**C_M***
Class:	**Sympatholytic (Antihypertensive)**		

FETAL RISK SUMMARY

RECOMMENDATION: Human Data Suggest Risk in 2nd and 3rd Trimesters

Carvedilol is a combined α/β-adrenergic blocking agent that is used for the treatment of hypertension and mild to moderate heart failure. The α_1-adrenoreceptor blocking activity has been associated with vasodilation and a reduction in peripheral vascular resistance (1). Some of the metabolites of carvedilol have greater β-receptor blocking activity than the parent drug. No reports of its use in human pregnancy have been located.

Reproduction studies in rats and rabbits at 50 and 25 times the maximum recommended human dose based on body surface area (MRHD), respectively, revealed post-implantation loss in both species (1). The dose in rats, which was maternally toxic, was also associated with a decrease in fetal weight and an increase in frequency of fetuses with delayed skeletal development (missing or stunted 13th rib). The no-observed-effect levels for developmental toxicity in the test animals was 10 times the MRHD for rats and 5 times the MRHD for rabbits (1). Toxicity (sedation, reduced weight gain) and impaired fertility were observed in adult rats at $\geq$32 times the MRHD, including a reduced number of successful matings, prolonged mating time, fewer implants per dam, and complete resorption of 18% of the litters (1).

It is not known if carvedilol crosses the human placenta. The molecular weight (about 407) is low enough, however, that passage to the fetus should be expected. The drug and/or its metabolites cross the placenta in rats (1).

In summary, the lack of human pregnancy experience limits any assessment of fetal risk that might occur with the use of carvedilol (2). Based on animal studies and the experience with other, similar agents, the risk of teratogenicity appears to be low. Intrauterine growth retardation (IUGR), however, has been reported with another α/β-blocker (see Labetalol) when the drug was used for the treatment of mild preeclampsia. Some β-blockers have caused IUGR and reduced placental weight, especially those lacking intrinsic sympathomimetic activity (ISA) (i.e., partial agonist). Treatment beginning early in the 2nd trimester results in the greatest weight reductions, whereas treatment restricted to the 3rd trimester primarily affects only placental weight. Carvedilol does not possess ISA. However, IUGR and reduced placental weight may potentially occur with all agents within this class. Although growth retardation is a serious concern, the benefits of maternal therapy with carvedilol (or other α/β-blockers), in some cases, might outweigh the risks to the fetus and must be judged on a case-by-case basis.

[**Risk Factor D if used in 2nd or 3rd trimesters.*]

BREAST FEEDING SUMMARY

RECOMMENDATION: No Human Data - Potential Toxicity

No reports describing the use of carvedilol during human lactation have been located. The molecular weight (about 407) is low enough that excretion into breast milk should be expected. The drug and/or its metabolites are found in the milk of lactating rats. Increased pup mortality at 1 week postpartum was observed when pregnant rats were treated with carvedilol at $\geq$10 times the MRHD during the last trimester and continued through day 22 of lactation (1).

Although there are no reports of human exposure during lactation, nursing infants of women who are consuming carvedilol should be closely monitor for bradycardia, hypotension, and other symptoms of α/β-blockade. A similar agent is classified by the American Academy of Pediatrics as compatible with breast-feeding (see Labetalol).

References

1. Product information. Coreg. SmithKline Beecham Pharmaceuticals, 2000.
2. Frishman WH. Carvedilol. N Engl J Med 1998;339: 1759–65.

Name: **CASANTHRANOL** Risk Factor: **C**
Class: **Purgative**

FETAL RISK SUMMARY

RECOMMENDATION: Compatible

Casanthranol is an anthraquinone purgative. In a large prospective study, 109 patients were exposed to this agent during pregnancy, 21 in the 1st trimester (1). No evidence of an increased risk for malformations was found (see also Cascara Sagrada).

In a surveillance study of Michigan Medicaid recipients conducted between 1985 and 1992 involving 229,101 completed pregnancies, 96 newborns had been exposed to casanthranol during the 1st trimester (F. Rosa, personal communication, FDA, 1993). Four (4.2%) (four expected) major birth defects were observed. Specific data were available for six defect categories, including (observed/expected) 2/1 cardiovascular defects, 1/0 spina bifida, and 1/0.5 polydactyly. No anomalies were observed in the other three categories (oral clefts, limb reduction defects, and hypospadias. These data do not support an association between the drug and congenital defects.

BREAST FEEDING SUMMARY

RECOMMENDATION: No Human Data - Probably Compatible

See Cascara Sagrada.

Reference

1. Heinonen OP, Slone D, Shapiro S. *Birth Defects and Drugs in Pregnancy*. Littleton, MA: Publishing Sciences Group, 1977:384–7, 442.

Name: **CASCARA SAGRADA** Risk Factor: **C**
Class: **Purgative**

FETAL RISK SUMMARY

RECOMMENDATION: Limited Human Data - Probably Compatible

Cascara sagrada is an anthraquinone purgative. In a large prospective study, 53 mother-child pairs were exposed to cascara sagrada during the 1st trimester (1, pp. 384–387). Although the numbers are small, no evidence for an increased risk of malformations was found. For anytime use during pregnancy, 188 exposures were recorded (1, pp. 438, 442, 497). The relative risk for benign tumors was higher than expected, but independent confirmation is required (1, pp. 438, 442, 497).

A 1977 study found that more than 50% of the women taking laxatives during pregnancy had taken a laxative of the anthraquinone type (2). Danthron (1:8 dihydroxyanthraquinone) was administered to nine women shortly before induction of labor. Presence of the laxative and/or its metabolite was documented in the amniotic fluid and in the urine of the newborns. No fetal adverse effects were noted (2).

BREAST FEEDING SUMMARY

RECOMMENDATION: Limited Human Data - Probably Compatible

C

Most reviewers acknowledge the presence of anthraquinones (e.g., cascara and danthron) in breast milk and warn of the consequences for the nursing infant (3–5). A comprehensive review described the excretion of laxatives into human milk, but little is known about the presence of these agents in breast milk (6). Two reports suggest an increased incidence of diarrhea in infants when nursing mothers are given cascara sagrada or senna for postpartum constipation (7,8). However, the American Academy of Pediatrics classifies cascara and danthron as compatible with breast-feeding (9).

References

1. Heinonen OP, Slone D, Shapiro S. *Birth Defects and Drugs in Pregnancy*. Littleton, MA: Publishing Sciences Group, 1977.
2. Blair AW, Burdon M, Powell J, Gerrard M, Smith R. Fetal exposure to 1:8 dihydroxyanthraquinone. Biol Neonate 1977;31:289–93.
3. Knowles JA. Breast milk: a source of more than nutrition for the neonate. Clin Toxicol 1974;7:69–82.
4. O'Brien TE. Excretion of drugs in human milk. Am J Hosp Pharm 1974;31:844–54.
5. Edwards A. Drugs in breast milk—a review of the recent literature. Aust J Hosp Pharm 1981;11:27–39.
6. Stewart JJ. Gastrointestinal drugs. In Wilson JT, ed. *Drugs in Breast Milk*. Balgowlah, Australia: ADIS Press, 1981:65–71.
7. Tyson RM, Shrader EA, Perlman HH. Drugs transmitted through breast milk. Part I. Laxatives. J Pediatr 1937;11:824–32.
8. Greenleaf JO, Leonard HSD. Laxatives in the treatment of constipation in pregnant and breast-feeding mothers. Practitioner 1973;210:259–63.
9. Committee on Drugs, American Academy of Pediatrics. The transfer of drugs and other chemicals into human milk. Pediatrics 2001;108:776–89.

Name: **CASPOFUNGIN** Risk Factor: **C_M**

Class: **Antifungal**

FETAL RISK SUMMARY

RECOMMENDATION: No Human Data - Animal Data Suggest Risk

Caspofungin inhibits the synthesis of glucan, an integral component of the fungal cell wall and is the first antifungal agent in this class. It is a semisynthetic lipopeptide (echinocandin) compound that is synthesized from a fermentation product of the fungus *Glarea lozoyensis*. Caspofungin is approved for the treatment of *Candida* infections and for invasive aspergillosis in patients who cannot be treated with other antifungals. Caspofungin is extensively bound to albumin (about 97%). Plasma clearance of caspofungin is primarily from distribution, rather than by excretion or metabolism. The γ-phase half-life is 40–50 hours (1).

Reproduction studies have been conducted in rats and rabbits. In rats, doses producing exposures similar to those obtained in humans treated with a 70-mg dose (HE) were embryotoxic, resulting in increased resorptions and peri-implantation losses. Other effects included incomplete ossification of the skull and torso and an increased incidence of cervical ribs. The agent was also embryotoxic in rabbits causing increased resorptions at doses similar to the HE. In addition, incomplete ossifications of the talus/calcaneus were observed in rabbits (1).

Caspofungin crosses the placenta in rats and rabbits (gestational age not specified) and the drug could be detected in fetal plasma (1). It is not known if the agent crosses the human placenta. The molecular weight (about 1213 for the acetate salt) and extensive plasma protein binding should limit the amount crossing the placenta, but the long β-phase half-life should provide substantial amounts of the drug available for transfer.

No reports describing the use of caspofungin in human pregnancy have been located. A 2003 review of antifungal agents was also unable to find such reports (2). The animal data are suggestive of human risk, especially if exposure occurs in the 1st trimester. However, the absence of human pregnancy experience prevents an assessment of the embryo/fetal risk. If indicated, maternal treatment should avoid the 1st trimester, if possible.

BREAST FEEDING SUMMARY

RECOMMENDATION: No Human Data - Probably Compatible

No reports describing the use of caspofungin during human lactation have been located. The drug is excreted in the milk of lactating rats. The high molecular (about 1213 for the acetate salt) and extensive plasma protein binding (about 97%) should limit the amount of drug excreted in breast milk, but the long γ-phase half-life may allow for some drug in the milk. The effects of this exposure on a nursing infant are unknown. However, other drugs from different classes of antifungal agents, such as fluconazole and ketoconazole, are classified as compatible with breast-feeding by the American Academy of Pediatrics (see Fluconazole and Ketoconazole). The risk of harm from exposure to caspofungin also appears to be low and women being treated with caspofungin should be allowed to breast-feed. Their infants should be monitored for signs and symptoms of histamine release (e.g., rash, facial swelling, pruritus, etc.) and gastrointestinal complaints.

References

1. Product information. Cancidas. Merck, 2004.
2. Moudgal VV, Sobel JD. Antifungal drugs in pregnancy: a review. Expert Opin Drug Saf 2003;2:475–83.

Name:	**CEFACLOR**	Risk Factor:	B_M
Class:	**Antibiotic (Cephalosporin)**		

FETAL RISK SUMMARY

RECOMMENDATION: Compatible

Cefaclor is an oral, semisynthetic cephalosporin antibiotic. Reproduction studies in mice, rats, and ferrets found no evidence of impaired fertility or fetal harm at doses up to 12, 12, and 3 times, respectively, the human dose (1). Cephalosporins are usually considered safe to use during pregnancy (see other cephalosporins for published human experience).

In a surveillance study of Michigan Medicaid recipients conducted between 1985 and 1992 involving 229,101 completed pregnancies, 1325 newborns had been exposed to the antibiotic during the 1st trimester (F. Rosa, personal communication, FDA, 1993). A total of 75 (5.7%) major birth defects were observed (56 expected). Specific data were available for six defect categories, including (observed/expected) 19/13 cardiovascular defects, 8/2 oral clefts, 1/0.7 spina bifida, 1/4 polydactyly, 2/2 limb reduction defects, and 3/3 hypospadias. The data for all defects, cardiovascular defects, and oral clefts are suggestive of an association between cefaclor and congenital defects, but other factors, such as the mother's disease, may be involved. However, similar findings were measured for another cephalosporin antibiotic with more than a thousand exposures (see Cephalexin). Positive

C

results were also suggested for cephradine (339 exposures) but not for cefadroxil (722 exposures) (see Cephradine and Cefadroxil). In contrast, other anti-infectives with large cohorts (see Ampicillin, Amoxicillin, Penicillin G, Erythromycin, and Tetracycline) were not associated with congenital defects.

No detectable teratogenic risk with cefaclor and other cephalosporin antibiotics was found in a large 2001 study (see Cephalexin).

BREAST FEEDING SUMMARY

RECOMMENDATION: Compatible

Cefaclor is excreted into breast milk in low concentrations. Following a single 500-mg oral dose, average milk levels ranged from 0.16–0.21 μg/mL during a 5-hour period (2). Only trace amounts of the antibiotic could be measured at 1 and 6 hours. Even though these levels are low, three potential problems exist for the nursing infant: modification of bowel flora, direct effects on the infant, and interference with the interpretation of culture results if a fever workup is required. Although not specifically listing cefaclor, the American Academy of Pediatrics classifies other cephalosporin antibiotics as compatible with breast-feeding (for example, see Cefadroxil and Cefazolin).

References

1. Product information. Ceclor. Eli Lilly and Company, 1997.
2. Takase Z, Shirafuji H, Uchida M. Clinical and laboratory studies of cefaclor in the field of obstetrics and gynecology. Chemotherapy (Tokyo) 1979;27(Suppl):666–72.

Name:	**CEFADROXIL**	Risk Factor:	**B_M**
Class:	**Antibiotic (Cephalosporin)**		

FETAL RISK SUMMARY

RECOMMENDATION: Compatible

Cefadroxil is an oral, semisynthetic cephalosporin antibiotic. Reproduction studies in mice and rats found no evidence of impaired fertility or fetal harm at doses up to 11 times the human dose (1). Cephalosporins are usually considered safe to use during pregnancy (see other cephalosporins for published human experience).

At term, a 500-mg oral dose produced an average peak cord serum level of 4.6 μg/mL at 2.5 hours (about 40% of maternal serum) (2). Amniotic fluid levels achieved a peak of 4.4 μg/mL at 10 hours. No infant data were given.

In a surveillance study of Michigan Medicaid recipients conducted between 1985 and 1992 involving 229,101 completed pregnancies, 722 newborns had been exposed to cefadroxil during the 1st trimester (F. Rosa, personal communication, FDA, 1993). A total of 27 (3.7%) major birth defects were observed (30 expected). Specific data were available for six defect categories, including (observed/expected) 1/1 cardiovascular defects, 0/1 oral clefts, 0/0.5 spina bifida, 2/2 polydactyly, 2/1 limb reduction defects, and 1/2 hypospadias. These data do not support an association between the drug and congenital defects (see also Cefaclor, Cephalexin, and Cephradine for contrasting results).

Cefadroxil, 500 mg twice daily for 10 days following an IV dose of ceftazidime, was used in 12 women for the treatment of asymptomatic bacteriuria during the

1st trimester (see also Ceftazidime) (3). No adverse effects of the treatment were observed.

BREAST FEEDING SUMMARY

RECOMMENDATION: Compatible

Cefadroxil is excreted into breast milk in low concentrations. Following a single 500-mg oral dose, peak milk levels of about 0.6–0.7 μg/mL occurred at 5–6 hours (2). A 1-g oral dose given to six mothers produced peak milk levels averaging 1.83 μg/mL (range 1.2–2.4 μg/mL) at 6–7 hours (4). In this latter group, milk:plasma ratios at 1, 2, and 3 hours were 0.009, 0.011, and 0.019, respectively. Although these levels are low, three potential problems exist for the nursing infant: modification of bowel flora, direct effects on the infant, and interference with the interpretation of culture results if a fever workup is required. The American Academy of Pediatrics classifies cefadroxil as compatible with breast-feeding (5).

References

1. Product information. Duricef. Bristol-Myers Squibb Company, 1997.
2. Takase Z, Shirafuji H, Uchida M. Experimental and clinical studies of cefadroxil in the treatment of infections in the field of obstetrics and gynecology. Chemotherapy (Tokyo) 1980;28(Suppl 2):424–31.
3. Nathorst-Boos J, Philipson A, Hedman A, Arvisson A. Renal elimination of ceftazidime during pregnancy. Am J Obstet Gynecol 1995;172:163–6.
4. Kafetzi DA, Siafas CA, Georgakopoulos PA, Papdatos CJ. Passage of cephalosporins and amoxicillin into the breast milk. Acta Paediatr Scand 1981;70:285–8.
5. Committee on Drugs, American Academy of Pediatrics. The transfer of drugs and other chemicals into human milk. Pediatrics 2001;108:776–89.

Name:	**CEFAMANDOLE**	Risk Factor:	B_M
Class:	**Antibiotic (Cephalosporin)**		

FETAL RISK SUMMARY

RECOMMENDATION: Compatible

Cefamandole is a parenteral, semisynthetic cephalosporin antibiotic. Reproduction studies in rats found no evidence of impaired fertility or fetal harm, including testicular toxicity, at doses up to approximately 5 times the human dose (1).

Although pregnant patients were excluded from clinical trials of cefamandole, one patient did receive the drug in the 1st trimester (J.T. Anderson, personal communication, Lilly Research Laboratories, 1981). No apparent adverse effects were noted in the newborn. Cephalosporins are usually considered safe to use during pregnancy (see other cephalosporins for published human experience).

No detectable teratogenic risk with cefamandole and other cephalosporin antibiotics was found in a large 2001 study (see Cephalexin).

BREAST FEEDING SUMMARY

RECOMMENDATION: Compatible

Cefamandole is excreted into breast milk in low concentrations. Following a 1-g IV dose, average milk levels in four patients ranged from 0.46 (1 hour) to 0.19 μg/mL (6 hours)

(J. T. Anderson, personal communication. Lilly Research Laboratories, 1981). The milk: plasma ratio at 1 hour was 0.02. No neonate information was given. Even though these levels are low, three potential problems exist for the nursing infant: modification of bowel flora, direct effects on the infant, and interference with the interpretation of culture results if a fever workup is required. Although not specifically listing cefamandole, the American Academy of Pediatrics classifies other cephalosporin antibiotics as compatible with breast-feeding (e.g., see Cefadroxil and Cefazolin).

Reference

1. Product information. Mandol. Eli Lilly and Company, 1997.

Name:	**CEFATRIZINE**	Risk Factor:	B_M
Class:	**Antibiotic (Cephalosporin)**		

FETAL RISK SUMMARY

RECOMMENDATION: Compatible

Cefatrizine is a cephalosporin antibiotic. No controlled studies on its use in pregnancy have been located. Transplacental passage of cefatrizine has been demonstrated in women undergoing elective therapeutic surgical abortion in the 1st and 2nd trimesters (1). None of the fetuses from prostaglandin $F_{2\alpha}$-induced abortions revealed evidence of cefatrizine.

BREAST FEEDING SUMMARY

RECOMMENDATION: Compatible

No reports describing the use of cefatrizine during human lactation have been located. However, most cephalosporins are excreted into breast milk in low concentrations. The American Academy of Pediatrics classifies other cephalosporin antibiotics as compatible with breast-feeding (e.g., see Cefadroxil and Cefazolin).

Reference

1. Bernard B, Thielen P, Garcia-Cazares SJ, Ballard CA. Maternal-fetal pharmacology of cefatrizine in the first 20 weeks of pregnancy. Antimicrob Agents Chemother 1977;12:231–6.

Name:	**CEFAZOLIN**	Risk Factor:	B_M
Class:	**Antibiotic (Cephalosporin)**		

FETAL RISK SUMMARY

RECOMMENDATION: Compatible

Cefazolin is a parenteral, semisynthetic cephalosporin antibiotic. Reproduction studies in mice, rats, and rabbits found no evidence of impaired fertility or fetal harm at doses up to 25 times the human dose (1).

Cefazolin crosses the placenta into the cord serum and amniotic fluid (2–6). In early pregnancy, distribution is limited to the body fluids and these concentrations are considerably lower than those found in the 2nd and 3rd trimesters (3). At term, 15–70 minutes after a 500-mg dose, cord serum levels range from 35% to 69% of maternal serum (4). The maximum concentration in amniotic fluid after 500 mg was 8 μg/mL at 2.5 hours (5). No data on the newborns were given. Following a 2-g IV dose to seven women between 23 and 32 weeks' gestation, the mean serum concentration of cefazolin in hydropic and nonhydropic fetuses was 18.04 and 21.02 μg/mL, respectively, providing evidence that the presence of hydrops did not significantly impair the transfer of the antibiotic (6).

Cephalosporins are usually considered safe to use during pregnancy. Cefazolin, 2 g IV every 8 hours, has been used in the treatment of pyelonephritis occurring in the second half of pregnancy (7). No adverse fetal outcomes attributable to the drug were observed.

BREAST FEEDING SUMMARY

RECOMMENDATION: Compatible

Cefazolin is excreted into breast milk in low concentrations. Following a 2-g IV dose, average milk levels ranged from 1.2 to 1.5 μg/mL over 4 hours (milk:plasma ratio 0.02) (8). When cefazolin was given as a 500-mg IM dose, one to three times daily, the drug was not detectable (5). Although these levels are low, three potential problems exist for the nursing infant: modification of bowel flora, direct effects on the infant, and interference with the interpretation of culture results if a fever workup is required. The American Academy of Pediatrics classifies cefazolin as compatible with breast-feeding (9).

References

1. Product information. Ancef. SmithKline Beecham Pharmaceuticals, 1997.
2. Dekel A, Elian I, Gibor Y, Goldman JA. Transplacental passage of cefazolin in the first trimester of pregnancy. Eur J Obstet Gynecol Reprod Biol 1980;10:303–7.
3. Bernard B, Barton L, Abate M, Ballard CA. Maternal-fetal transfer of cefazolin in the first twenty weeks of pregnancy. J Infect Dis 1977;136:377–82.
4. Cho N, Ito T, Saito T, et al. Clinical studies on cefazolin in the field of obstetrics and gynecology. Chemotherapy (Tokyo) 1970;18:770–7.
5. von Kobyletzki D, Reither K, Gellen J, Kanyo A, Glocke M. Pharmacokinetic studies with cefazolin in obstetrics and gynecology. Infection 1974;2(Suppl):60–7.
6. Brown CEL, Christmas JT, Bawdon RE. Placental transfer of cefazolin and piperacillin in pregnancies remote from term complicated by Rh isoimmunization. Am J Obstet Gynecol 1990;163:938–43.
7. Sanchez-Ramos L, McAlpine KJ, Adair CD, Kaunitz AM, Delke I, Briones DK. Pyelonephritis in pregnancy: once-a-day ceftriaxone versus multiple doses of cefazolin. Am J Obstet Gynecol 1995;172:129–33.
8. Yoshioka H, Cho K, Takimoto M, Maruyama S, Shimizu T. Transfer of cefazolin into human milk. J Pediatr 1979;94:151–2.
9. Committee on Drugs, American Academy of Pediatrics. The transfer of drugs and other chemicals into human milk. Pediatrics 2001;108:776–89.

Name:	**CEFDINIR**	Risk Factor:	$\mathbf{B_M}$
Class:	**Antibiotic (Cephalosporin)**		

FETAL RISK SUMMARY

RECOMMENDATION: Compatible

Cefdinir is an oral, semisynthetic, third generation cephalosporin antibiotic. The molecular weight (about 395) is low enough that passage to the fetus should be expected.

C

Reproduction studies have been conducted in pregnant rats and rabbits (1). In pregnant rats, oral doses up to 11 times the human dose based on body surface area (HD) were not teratogenic, but decreased fetal weight occurred at doses ≥1.1 times the HD. No effects on maternal reproductive performance or offspring survival, behavior, development, or reproductive function. In rabbits, oral doses up to 0.23 times the HD were not teratogenic, but maternal toxicity (decreased body weight) was noted at the highest dose. No adverse effects on offspring were observed (1).

Although no published reports on the use of cefdinir during human pregnancy have been located, cephalosporin antibiotics are usually considered safe to use during gestation.

BREAST FEEDING SUMMARY

RECOMMENDATION: Compatible

No published reports describing the use of cefdinir in human lactation have been located. The molecular weight (about 395) is low enough that excretion into breast milk should be expected. However, the drug was not detected in breast milk after a single, 600-mg oral dose (1). Multiple dosing during lactation has apparently not been studied. If excretion does occur, three potential problems exist for the nursing infant: modification of bowel flora, direct effects on the infant, and interference with the interpretation of culture results if a fever workup is required. The American Academy of Pediatrics classifies other cephalosporins as compatible with breast-feeding (e.g., see Cefadroxil and Cefazolin).

Reference

1. Product information. Omnicef. Abbott Laboratories, 2001.

Name:	**CEFDITOREN**	Risk Factor:	**B_M**
Class:	**Antibiotic (Cephalosporin)**		

FETAL RISK SUMMARY

RECOMMENDATION: Compatible

Cefditoren pivoxil is a prodrug that is hydrolyzed during absorption to the active drug, cefditoren. It is an oral, semisynthetic cephalosporin antibiotic similar to other agents in this class.

Reproduction studies have been conducted with cefditoren pivoxil in rats and rabbits. In pregnant rats and rabbits, doses up to about 24 and 4 times, respectively, the human dose of 200 mg twice daily based on body surface area (HD) were not teratogenic. In addition, rat fertility and reproduction were not affected by the highest dose. However, in rabbits the highest dose caused severe maternal toxicity, resulting in fetal toxicity and abortions. In a postnatal study in rats, a dose 18 times the HD produced no adverse effects on postnatal survival, physical and behavioral development, learning abilities, and reproductive capability at sexual maturity (1).

Although no reports have been located describing the use of cefditoren in human gestation, other cephalosporins have been used frequently in pregnancy without any evidence of fetal harm. Cefditoren probably crosses the placenta similar to other antibiotics in the class. Because this class of antibiotics does not appear to cause fetal toxicity, cefditoren can be used during gestation.

BREAST FEEDING SUMMARY

RECOMMENDATION: Compatible

No reports describing the use of cefditoren in human lactation have been located. The drug is excreted into the milk of lactating rats (1). Small amounts of antibiotic have been found in breast milk for all cephalosporins that have been studied, so the presence of cefditoren in milk should be expected. In most cases, the effects of this exposure will be insignificant. However, three potential problems exist for the nursing infant exposed to cefditoren in milk: modification of bowel flora, direct effects on the infant, and interference with the interpretation of culture results if a fever workup is required. The American Academy of Pediatrics classifies other cephalosporins as compatible with breast-feeding (e.g., see Cefadroxil and Cefazolin).

Reference

1. Product information. Spectracef. Purdue Pharmaceutical Products, 2004.

Name:	**CEFEPIME**	Risk Factor:	B_M
Class:	**Antibiotic (Cephalosporin)**		

FETAL RISK SUMMARY

RECOMMENDATION: Compatible

Cefepime is a parenteral, semisynthetic cephalosporin antibiotic. No adverse effects on fertility or reproduction, including embryo toxicity and teratogenicity, were observed in mice, rats, and rabbits dosed at one to four times the recommended maximum human daily dose on a mg/m^2/day basis (1).

No reports describing the use of cefepime in human pregnancy have been located. Cephalosporins are usually considered safe to use during pregnancy (see other cephalosporins for published human experience).

BREAST FEEDING SUMMARY

RECOMMENDATION: Compatible

Cefepime is excreted in human milk. The manufacturer reports that very low concentrations (0.5 μg/mL) were measured in milk, but the maternal dose was not provided (1). In spite of these low levels, three potential problems exist for the nursing infant exposed to cefepime in milk: modification of bowel flora, direct effects on the infant, and interference with the interpretation of culture results if a fever workup is required. Although not specifically listing cefepime, the American Academy of Pediatrics classifies other cephalosporin antibiotics as compatible with breast-feeding (e.g., see Cefadroxil and Cefazolin).

Reference

1. Product information. Maxipime. Bristol-Myers Squibb Company, 1997.

C

Name: **CEFIXIME** Risk Factor: **B_M**

Class: **Antibiotic (Cephalosporin)**

FETAL RISK SUMMARY

RECOMMENDATION: Compatible

Cefixime is an oral, semisynthetic cephalosporin antibiotic. Reproduction studies found no evidence in rats of impaired fertility or reproductive performance at doses up to 125 times the adult therapeutic dose or, in mice and rats, of teratogenicity at doses up to 400 times the human dose (1).

A 1998 non-interventional observational cohort study described the outcomes of pregnancies in women who had been prescribed one or more of 34 newly marketed drugs by general practitioners in England (2). Data were obtained by questionnaires sent to the prescribing physicians one month after the expected or possible date of delivery. In 831 (78%) of the pregnancies, a newly marketed drug was thought to have been taken during the 1st trimester with birth defects noted in 14 (2.5%) singleton births of the 557 newborns (10 sets of twins). In addition, two birth defects were observed in aborted fetuses. However, few of the aborted fetuses were examined. Cefixime was taken during the 1st trimester in 11 pregnancies. The outcomes of these pregnancies included two spontaneous abortions, one elective abortion, seven normal newborns (one premature), and one unknown outcome (2).

No other reports describing the use of cefixime in human pregnancy have been located. Cephalosporins are usually considered safe to use during pregnancy (see also other cephalosporins).

BREAST FEEDING SUMMARY

RECOMMENDATION: Compatible

No reports describing the use of cefixime during human lactation have been located. Low concentrations of other cephalosporins have been measured, however, and the presence of cefixime in milk should be expected. Three potential problems exist for the nursing infant exposed to cefixime in milk: modification of bowel flora, direct effects on the infant, and interference with the interpretation of culture results if a fever workup is required. The American Academy of Pediatrics classifies other cephalosporin antibiotics as compatible with breast-feeding (e.g., see Cefadroxil and Cefazolin).

References

1. Product information. Suprax. Lederle Laboratories, 1997.
2. Wilton LV, Pearce GL, Martin RM, Mackay FJ, Mann RD. The outcomes of pregnancy in women exposed to newly marketed drugs in general practice in England. Br J Obstet Gynaecol 1998;105:882–9.

C

Name: **CEFMETAZOLE**	Risk Factor:	**B**
Class: **Antibiotic (Cephalosporin)**		

FETAL RISK SUMMARY

RECOMMENDATION: Compatible

Cefmetazole is an injectable, second-generation cephalosporin antibiotic. Structurally it is similar to cefamandole (*N*-methylthiotetrazole side chain) and may cause similar adverse effects (hypoprothrombinemia and bleeding, and a disulfiram-like reaction with alcohol) (1).

Shepard reviewed three reproduction studies that had been conducted in pregnant rats and dogs (2). No adverse effects or teratogenicity were observed when the antibiotic was administered during organogenesis or other stages of gestation.

It is not known if cefmetazole crosses the human placenta. The molecular weight (about 494 for the sodium salt) is low enough that transfer to the fetus should be expected.

Although no published reports on the use of cefmetazole during human pregnancy have been located, cephalosporin antibiotics are usually considered safe to use during gestation.

BREAST FEEDING SUMMARY

RECOMMENDATION: Compatible

No reports describing the use of cefmetazole during human lactation have been located. The molecular weight (about 494 for the sodium salt) is low enough that excretion into breast milk should be expected. If excretion does occur, three potential problems exist for the nursing infant: modification of bowel flora, direct effects on the infant, and interference with the interpretation of culture results if a fever workup is required. The American Academy of Pediatrics classifies other cephalosporins as compatible with breast-feeding (e.g., see Cefadroxil and Cefazolin).

References

1. Reynolds JEF, editor. *Martindale. The Extra Pharmacopoeia*. 31st ed. London, England: Royal Pharmaceutical Society, 1996:187.
2. Shepard TH. *Catalog of Teratogenic Agents*. 9th ed. Baltimore, MD: The Johns Hopkins University Press, 1998:85.

Name: **CEFONICID**	Risk Factor:	**B_M**
Class: **Antibiotic (Cephalosporin)**		

FETAL RISK SUMMARY

RECOMMENDATION: Compatible

Cefonicid is a parenteral, semisynthetic cephalosporin antibiotic. Reproduction studies in mice, rats, and rabbits found no evidence of impaired fertility or fetal harm, including testicular toxicity, at doses up to 40 times usual adult human dose (1).

No studies on the use of cefonicid in human pregnancy have been located. Cephalosporins are usually considered safe to use during pregnancy (see other cephalosporins for published human experience).

C

BREAST FEEDING SUMMARY

RECOMMENDATION: Compatible

Cefonicid is excreted into breast milk in low concentrations. Milk levels 1 hour after a 1-g IM dose were equal to or less than 0.3 μg/mL, averaging 0.16 μg/mL (2). Even though these concentrations are low, three potential problems exist for the nursing infant: modification of bowel flora, direct effects on the infant, and interference with the interpretation of culture results if a fever workup is required. Although not specifically listing cefonicid, the American Academy of Pediatrics classifies other cephalosporin antibiotics as compatible with breast-feeding (e.g., see Cefadroxil and Cefazolin).

References

1. Product information. Monocid. SmithKline Beecham Pharmaceuticals, 1997.
2. Lou MA Sr, Wu YH, Jacob LS, Pitkin DH. Penetration of cefonicid into human breast milk and various body fluids and tissues. Rev Infect Dis 1984;6(Suppl 4):S816–20.

Name:	**CEFOPERAZONE**	Risk Factor:	**B_M**
Class:	**Antibiotic (Cephalosporin)**		

FETAL RISK SUMMARY

RECOMMENDATION: Compatible

Cefoperazone is a parenteral, semisynthetic cephalosporin antibiotic. Reproduction studies in mice, rats, and monkeys have found no evidence of impaired fertility, reproductive performance, or fetal harm at doses up to 10–20 times the human dose (1).

Following a 1-g IV or IM dose of cefoperazone, cord blood levels averaged 34.4% and 33.2%, respectively, of the maternal serum (2). Peak concentrations occurred at about 1 hour after both IV and IM doses. Amniotic fluid levels were 3–4 μg/mL within 6 hours of administration. Continuous IV dosing (1 g given two to four times every 12 hours) produced higher levels, with cord blood averaging 40%–48% of maternal serum and amniotic fluid levels increasing to 3.8–8.8 μg/mL. In a second study, 1 g IV produced peak cord blood concentrations averaging about 45% of maternal serum (25 μg/mL vs. 56.1 μg/mL) at 70 minutes, with amniotic fluid concentrations varying between 2.8 and 4.8 μg/mL at 180 minutes (3). No effects on the newborns were reported in either study. In an *in vitro* experiment, placental transfer of cefoperazone was shown to occur only by simple diffusion (4). Cephalosporins are usually considered safe to use during pregnancy.

The placental transfer of cefoperazone and ceftizoxime were studied in an *in vitro* perfused human placental system (5). The mean clearance indices for the two antibiotics were 0.037 and 0.126, respectively. The steady-state fetal concentrations of the two agents were 4 μg/mL and 4–5 μg/mL, respectively.

No detectable teratogenic risk with cefoperazone and other cephalosporin antibiotics was found in a large 2001 study (see Cephalexin).

BREAST FEEDING SUMMARY

RECOMMENDATION: Compatible

Cefoperazone is excreted into breast milk in low concentrations. An IV dose of 1 g produced milk levels ranging from 0.4 to 0.9 μg/mL (C.E. Jacobson, personal communication, Roerig, 1985). Even though these concentrations are low, three potential problems exist for the nursing infant: modification of bowel flora, direct effects on the infant, and interference with the interpretation of culture results if a fever workup is required. Although not specifically listing cefoperazone, the American Academy of Pediatrics classifies other cephalosporin antibiotics as compatible with breast-feeding (e.g., see Cefadroxil and Cefazolin).

References

1. Product information. Cefobid. Pfizer, 1997.
2. Matsuda S, Tanno M, Kashiwagura T, Furuya H. Placental transfer of cefoperazone (T-1551) and a clinical study of its use in obstetrics and gynecological infections. Curr Chemo Infect Dis 1979;2:167–8.
3. Shimizu K. Cefoperazone: absorption, excretion, distribution, and metabolism. Clin Ther 1980;3(Special Issue):60–79.
4. Fortunato SJ, Bawdon RE, Baum M. Placental transfer of cefoperazone and sulbactam in the isolated in vitro perfused human placenta. Am J Obstet Gynecol 1988;159:1002–6.
5. Fortunato SJ, Bawdon RE, Maberry MC, Swan KF. Transfer of ceftizoxime surpasses that of cefoperazone by the isolated human placental perfused in vitro. Obstet Gynecol 1990;75:830–3.

Name:	**CEFORANIDE**	Risk Factor:	B_M
Class:	**Antibiotic (Cephalosporin)**		

FETAL RISK SUMMARY

RECOMMENDATION: Compatible

Ceforanide is a cephalosporin antibiotic. No data on its use in pregnancy have been located.

BREAST FEEDING SUMMARY

RECOMMENDATION: Compatible

No studies on the excretion of ceforanide into breast milk have been located. Like other cephalosporins, however, excretion should be expected. The American Academy of Pediatrics classifies other cephalosporin antibiotics as compatible with breast-feeding (e.g., see Cefadroxil and Cefazolin).

Name:	**CEFOTAXIME**	Risk Factor:	B_M
Class:	**Antibiotic (Cephalosporin)**		

FETAL RISK SUMMARY

RECOMMENDATION: Compatible

Cefotaxime is a parenteral, semisynthetic cephalosporin antibiotic. Reproduction studies in mice and rats have found no evidence of impaired fertility or fetal harm at doses up to

20 times the human dose (1). Cephalosporins are usually considered safe to use during pregnancy.

During the 2nd trimester, the drug readily crosses the placenta (2). The half-life of cefotaxime in fetal serum and in amniotic fluid is 2.3 and 2.8 hours, respectively. Five women with chorioamnionitis and in labor received cefotaxime (dose not specified) (3). The maternal and cord blood concentrations were nearly equivalent at 8.90 and 8.60 μg/mL, respectively, but the placental tissue:maternal blood ratio was 0.2 (dose to delivery interval not specified).

No detectable teratogenic risk with cefotaxime and other cephalosporin antibiotics was found in a large 2001 study (see Cephalexin).

BREAST FEEDING SUMMARY

RECOMMENDATION: Compatible

Cefotaxime is excreted into breast milk in low concentrations. Following a 1-g IV dose, mean peak milk levels of 0.33 μg/mL were measured at 2–3 hours (2,4). The half-life in milk ranged from 2.36 to 3.89 hours (mean: 2.93 hours). The milk:plasma ratios at 1, 2, and 3 hours were 0.027, 0.09, and 0.16, respectively. Although these levels are low, three potential problems exist for the nursing infant: modification of bowel flora, direct effects on the infant, and interference with the interpretation of culture results if a fever workup is required. The American Academy of Pediatrics classifies cefotaxime as compatible with breast-feeding (5).

References

1. Product information. Claforan. Hoechst Marion Roussel, 1997.
2. Kafetzis DA, Lazarides CV, Siafas CA, Georgakopoulos PA, Papadatos CJ. Transfer of cefotaxime in human milk and from mother to foetus. J Antimicrob Chemother 1980;6 (Suppl A):135–41.
3. Maberry MC, Trimmer KJ, Bawdon RE, Sobhi S, Dax JB, Gilstrap LC III. Antibiotic concentration in maternal blood, cord blood and placental tissue in women with chorioamnionitis. Gynecol Obstet Invest 1992;33:185–6.
4. Kafetzis DA, Siafas CA, Georgakopoulos PA, Papadatos CJ. Passage of cephalosporins and amoxicillin into the breast milk. Acta Paediatr Scand 1981;70:285–8.
5. Committee on Drugs, American Academy of Pediatrics. The transfer of drugs and other chemicals into human milk. Pediatrics 2001;108:776–89.

Name:	**CEFOTETAN**	Risk Factor:	B_M
Class:	**Antibiotic (Cephalosporin)**		

FETAL RISK SUMMARY

RECOMMENDATION: Compatible

Cefotetan is a parenteral, semisynthetic cephalosporin antibiotic. Reproduction studies in rats and monkeys found no evidence of impaired fertility or fetal harm at doses up to 20 times the human dose (1). Cephalosporins are usually considered safe to use during pregnancy.

A 1985 study measured the placental passage of the drug when administered just prior to cesarean section (2). Twenty women received a single, 1-g IV bolus dose of the antibiotic at intervals of 1–4 hours before surgery. The peak maternal plasma level obtained was 28 μg/mL. Cord blood concentrations progressively increased depending on the length of time after a mother received a dose and were highest (12.5 μg/mL) when she received the drug 4 hours prior to surgery. Similarly, a progressive increase in amniotic fluid concentrations was observed with values of 5.1, 7.5, and 8.1 μg/mL measured at 2, 3, and 4 hours, respectively. The increases in the level of antibiotic in the amniotic fluid paralleled those in the cord blood.

Three Japanese studies reported placental passage of cefotetan (3–5). Cord blood levels of 24.7 μg/mL, almost double those measured above, were reported 1 hour after a 1.0-g IV dose (3). This value was 15.4% of the peak maternal serum level, indicating that the peak maternal level was about 160 μg/mL. The amniotic fluid concentration was 12.3% of the mother's level, or approximately 20 μg/mL. A confirming study also found high cord blood levels after a single 1-g IV dose with the highest value of 29.0 μg/mL measured 3.6 hours after the maternal dose (4). The highest amniotic fluid level, however, was 8.6 μg/mL, which was also observed at 3.6 hours. The third study measured cord serum concentrations of 15, 31.4, and 3.5 μg/mL at 0.85, 3.75, and 16 hours, respectively, after a 1-g IV dose (5). Amniotic fluid concentrations ranged from 1.18 to 13.6 μg/mL up to 16 hours after a dose.

BREAST FEEDING SUMMARY

RECOMMENDATION: Compatible

Small amounts of cefotetan are excreted into human breast milk (5,6). A 1982 reference reported milk levels ranging from 0.22 to 0.34 μg/mL 1–6 hours after a 1-g IV dose (5). In six women treated with cefotetan 1 g IM every 12 hours, mean milk levels 4–10 hours after a dose varied from 0.29 to 0.59 μg/mL (6). No accumulation in the milk was observed as evidenced by a steady milk:plasma ratio. The mean ratio 10 hours after the first dose was 0.05, compared to 0.07 at 10 hours after the fifth dose.

Even though the amounts of antibiotic are very small, and no reports of adverse effects in a nursing infant have been located, three potential problems exist for the infant exposed to cefotetan in milk: modification of bowel flora, direct effects on the infant, and interference with the interpretation of culture results if a fever workup is required. Although not specifically listing cefotetan, the American Academy of Pediatrics classifies other cephalosporin antibiotics as compatible with breast-feeding (e.g., see Cefadroxil and Cefazolin).

References

1. Product information. Cefotan. Zeneca Pharmaceuticals, 1997.
2. Bergogne-Berezin E, Berthelot O, Ravina JH, Yernant D. Study of placental transfer of cefotetan (abstract). Program and Abstracts of the 25th Interscience Conference on Antimicrobial Agents and Chemotherapy, Minneapolis, MN, September 29–October 2, 1985, p. 144.
3. Takase Z, Fujiwara M, Kawamoto Y, Seto M, Shirafuji H, Uchida M. Laboratory and clinical studies of cefotetan (YM09330) in the field of obstetrics and gynecology (English abstract). Chemotherapy (Tokyo) 1982;30(Suppl 1):869–81.
4. Motomura R, Teramoto C, Souda Y, Fujita A, Chiyoda R, Mori H, Yamabe T. Fundamental and clinical study of cefotetan (YM09330) in the field of obstetrics and gynecology (English abstract). Chemotherapy (Tokyo) 1982;30(Suppl 1):882–7.
5. Cho N, Fukunaga K, Kunii K. Fundamental and clinical studies on cefotetan (YM09330) in the field of obstetrics and gynecology (English abstract). Chemotherapy (Tokyo) 1982;30(Suppl 1):832–42.
6. Novelli A, Mazzei T, Ciuffi M, Nicoletti P, Buzzoni P, Reali EF, Periti P. The penetration of intramuscular cefotetan disodium into human extra-vascular fluid and maternal milk secretion. Chemioterapia 1983;2:337–42.

Name: **CEFOXITIN**	Risk Factor: B_M
Class: **Antibiotic (Cephalosporin)**	

C

FETAL RISK SUMMARY

RECOMMENDATION: Compatible

Cefoxitin is a parenteral, semisynthetic cephalosporin antibiotic. Reproduction studies found no evidence in rats of impaired fertility or reproductive performance at doses three times the maximum recommended human dose (MRHD) or, in mice and rats, fetal harm (other than a slight decrease in fetal weight) or teratogenesis at doses up to approximately 7.5 times the MRHD (1).

Multiple reports have described the transplacental passage of cefoxitin (2–14). Two patients were given 1 g IV just prior to therapeutic abortion at 9 and 10 weeks' gestation (10). At 55 minutes, the serum level in one woman was 10.5 μg/mL, whereas none was found in the fetal tissues. In the second patient, at 4.25 hours the maternal serum was "nil," whereas the fetal tissue level was 35.7 μg/mL.

At term, following IM or rapid IV doses of 1 or 2 g, cord serum levels up to 22 μg/mL (11%–90%) of maternal levels have been measured (7–10). Amniotic fluid concentrations peaked at 2–3 hours in the 3 to 15 μg/mL range (7,8,10,11,14). No apparent adverse effects were noted in any of the newborns. Cephalosporins are usually considered safe to use during pregnancy.

BREAST FEEDING SUMMARY

RECOMMENDATION: Compatible

Cefoxitin is excreted into breast milk in low concentrations (6,10,12,13,15). Up to 2 μg/mL has been detected in the milk of women receiving therapeutic doses (J.J. Whalen, personal communication, Merck, Sharpe & Dohme, May 13, 1981). No data on the infants were given. Following prophylactic administration of 2–4 g of cefoxitin to 18 women during and following cesarean section, milk samples were collected a mean 25 hours (range 9–56 hours) after the last dose of antibiotic (15). Only one sample, collected 19 hours after the last dose, contained measurable concentrations of cefoxitin (0.9 μg/mL). Although these levels are low, three potential problems exist for the nursing infant: modification of bowel flora, direct effects on the infant, and interference with the interpretation of culture results if a fever workup is required. The American Academy of Pediatrics classifies cefoxitin as compatible with breast-feeding (16).

References

1. Product information. Mefoxin. Merck & Company, 1997.
2. Bergone-Berezin B, Kafe H, Berthelot G, Morel O, Benard Y. Pharmacokinetic study of cefoxitin in bronchial secretions. In *Current Chemotherapy: Proceedings of The 10th International Congress of Chemotherapy, Zurich, Switzerland, September 18–23,1977*. Washington, DC: American Society for Microbiology, 1978.
3. Aokawa H, Minagawa M, Yamamiohi K, Sugiyama A. Studies on cefoxitin. Chemotherapy (Tokyo) 1977;(Suppl):394.
4. Matsuda S, Tanno M, Kashiwakura S, Furuya H. Basic and clinical studies on cefoxitin. Chemotherapy (Tokyo) 1977;(Suppl):396.
5. Berthelot G, Bergogne-Berezin B, Morel O, Kafe H, Benard Y. Cefoxitin: pharmacokinetic study in bronchial secretions—transplacental diffusion (abstract

No. 80). Paper presented at 10th International Congress of Chemotherapy, Zurich, Switzerland, September 18–23, 1977.
6. Mashimo K, Mihashi S, Fukaya I, Okubo B, Ohgob M, Saito A. New drug symposium IV. Cefoxitin. Chemotherapy (Tokyo) 1978;26:114–9.
7. Matsuda S, Tanno M, Kashiwakura T, Furuya H. Laboratory and clinical studies on cefoxitin in the field of obstetrics and gynecology. Chemotherapy (Tokyo) 1978;26(Suppl 1):460–7.
8. Cho N, Ubhara K, Suigizaki K, et al. Clinical studies of cefoxitin in the field of obstetrics and gynecology. Chemotherapy (Tokyo) 1978;26(Suppl 1): 468–75.
9. Seiga K, Minagawa M, Yamaji K, Sugiyama Y. Study on cefoxitin. Chemotherapy (Tokyo) 1978;26(Suppl 1): 491–501.
10. Takase Z, Shirafuji H, Uchida M. Clinical and laboratory studies on cefoxitin in the field of obstetrics and gynecology. Chemotherapy (Tokyo) 1978;26(Suppl 1): 502–5.
11. Bergogne-Berezin B, Lambert-Zeohovsky N, Rouvillois JL. Placental transfer of cefoxitin (abstract No.314). Paper presented at the 18th Interscience Conference on Antimicrobial Agents and Chemotherapy, Atlanta, Georgia, October 1–4, 1978.
12. Brogden RN, Heel RC, Speight TM, Avery GS. Cefoxitin: a review of its antibacterial activity, pharmacological properties and therapeutic use. Drugs 1979;17: 1–37.
13. Dubois M, Delapierre D, Demonty J, Lambotte R, Dresse A. Transplacental and mammary transfer of cefoxitin (abstract No. 118). Paper presented at 11th International Congress of Chemotherapy and 19th Interscience Conference on Antimicrobial Agents and Chemotherapy, Boston, Massachusetts, October 1–5, 1979.
14. Bergogne-Berezin B, Morel O, Kafe H, et al. Pharmacokinetic study of cefoxitin in man: diffusion into the bronchi and transfer across the placenta. Therapie 1979;34:345–54.
15. Roex AJM, van Loenen AC, Puyenbroek JI, Arts NFT. Secretion of cefoxitin in breast milk following short-term prophylactic administration in caesarean section. Eur J Obstet Gynecol Reprod Biol 1987;25:299–302.
16. Committee on Drugs, American Academy of Pediatrics. The transfer of drugs and other chemicals into human milk. Pediatrics 2001;108:776–89.

Name:	**CEFPODOXIME**	Risk Factor:	B_M
Class:	**Antibiotic (Cephalosporin)**		

FETAL RISK SUMMARY

RECOMMENDATION: Compatible

Cefpodoxime is an oral, semisynthetic cephalosporin antibiotic. Reproduction studies found no evidence in rats of impaired fertility or reproductive performance or, in rats and rabbits, of embryo toxicity or teratogenicity, at doses up to two times the human dose on a mg/m^2 basis (1).

No reports describing the use of cefpodoxime during human pregnancy have been located. Cephalosporins are usually considered safe to use during pregnancy (see other cephalosporins for published human experience).

BREAST FEEDING SUMMARY

RECOMMENDATION: Compatible

According to the manufacturer, low concentrations of cefpodoxime are excreted into human milk (1). Following 200-mg oral doses administered to three women, milk concentrations, as a percentage of concomitant serum levels, 4 hours after the dose were 0%, 2%, and 6%, respectively, and at 6 hours, were 0%, 9%, and 16%, respectively. Although not specifically stated for these three women, mean serum concentrations in fasted adults after a 200-mg dose were 2.2 μg/mL at 2 and 3 hours (peak levels), 1.8 μg/mL at 4 hours, and 1.2 μg/mL at 6 hours (1).

In spite of these low levels, three potential problems exist for the nursing infant exposed to cefpodoxime in milk: modification of bowel flora, direct effects on the infant, and interference with the interpretation of culture results if a fever workup is required. Although not specifically listing cefpodoxime, the American Academy of Pediatrics classifies other cephalosporin antibiotics as compatible with breast-feeding (e.g., see Cefadroxil and Cefazolin).

C

Reference

1. Product information. Vantin. Pharmacia & Upjohn Company, 1997.

Name:	CEFPROZIL	Risk Factor:	B_M
Class:	Antibiotic (Cephalosporin)		

FETAL RISK SUMMARY

RECOMMENDATION: Compatible

Cefprozil is an oral, semisynthetic cephalosporin antibiotic. Reproduction studies found no evidence in animals of impaired fertility or, in mice, rats, and rabbits, of fetal harm at doses of 8.5, 18.5, and 0.8 times, respectively, the maximum human daily dose on a mg/m^2 basis (1).

No reports describing the use of cefprozil in human pregnancy have been located. Cephalosporins are usually considered safe to use during pregnancy (see other cephalosporins for published human experience).

BREAST FEEDING SUMMARY

RECOMMENDATION: Compatible

Low concentrations of cefprozil are excreted in human milk. In a study published in 1992, nine healthy, lactating women were given a single 1000-mg oral dose of cefprozil consisting of *cis* and *trans* isomers in an approximately 90:10 ratio (2). The mean peak plasma concentrations of the *cis* and *trans* isomers were 14.8 μg/mL and 1.9 μg/mL, respectively. For the *cis* isomer, the mean milk concentration over a 24-hour period ranged from 0.25 to 3.36 μg/mL, whereas the average maximum concentration in milk of the *trans* isomer was <0.26 μg/mL. Less than 0.3% of the maternal dose was excreted into milk for the two isomers. The investigators estimated that an infant receiving 800 mL/day of milk would ingest a maximum of 3 mg of cefprozil, an amount they assessed as clinically insignificant.

Three potential problems exist for the nursing infant exposed to cefprozil in milk: modification of bowel flora, direct effects on the infant, and interference with the interpretation of culture results if a fever workup is required. The American Academy of Pediatrics classifies cefprozil as compatible with breast-feeding (3).

References

1. Product information. Cefzil. Bristol-Myers Squibb Company, 2000.
2. Shyu WC, Shah VR, Campbell DA, Venitz J, Jaganathan V, Pittman KA, Wilber RB, Barbhaiya RH. Excretion of cefprozil into human breast milk. Antimicrob Agents Chemother 1992;36:938–41.
3. Committee on Drugs, American Academy of Pediatrics. The transfer of drugs and other chemicals into human milk. Pediatrics 2001;108:776–89.

Name:	**CEFTAZIDIME**	Risk Factor:	B_M
Class:	**Antibiotic (Cephalosporin)**		

FETAL RISK SUMMARY

RECOMMENDATION: Compatible

Ceftazidime is a parenteral, semisynthetic cephalosporin antibiotic. Reproduction studies in mice and rats found no evidence of impaired fertility or fetal harm at doses up to 40 times the human dose (1). Cephalosporins are usually considered safe to use during pregnancy.

Ceftazidime administered at various stages of gestation, including the 1st trimester, crosses the placenta to the fetus and appears in the amniotic fluid (2–4). A brief English abstract of a 1983 Japanese report stated that levels in the cord blood and amniotic fluid following a 1-g IV dose exceeded the minimum inhibitory concentrations for most causative organisms but did not give specific values (2).

Nine women, undergoing abortion for fetuses affected by β-thalassemia major between 19 and 21 weeks' gestation, were given ceftazidime 1 g IM three times a day (3). At least three doses of the antibiotic were administered prior to abortion. The average concentrations of the drug in maternal serum at 2 and 4 hours after the last dose were 19.5 μg/mL (range 14–25 μg/mL) and 1.5 μg/mL (range 1.4–1.6 μg/mL), respectively. The simultaneous levels in amniotic fluid were 2.7 μg/mL (range 1.3–4 μg/mL) and 3.1 μg/mL (range 2.2–3.9 μg/mL), respectively, corresponding to approximately 14% and 207% of the maternal concentrations, respectively.

In a 1987 report, 30 women received a single, 2-g IV bolus dose of ceftazidime over 3 minutes between 1 and 4 hours prior to undergoing abortion of a fetus at a mean gestational age of 10 weeks' gestation (range 7–12 weeks) (4). Antibiotic concentrations were determined in maternal plasma, placental tissue, and amniotic fluid. In maternal plasma, mean levels ranged from 76 μg/mL at 1 hour to 16.5 μg/mL at 4 hours. Placental tissue concentrations were constant over this time interval, 12 mg/kg at 1 hour and 13 mg/kg at 4 hours, whereas the amniotic fluid concentration increased from 0.5 μg/mL to 2.8 μg/mL, respectively.

Increased renal elimination of ceftazidime was found in 12 women with asymptomatic bacteriuria treated with a 400-mg bolus dose followed by a continuous infusion of 1 g for 4 hours (5). The initial treatment occurred during the 1st trimester, followed by treatments approximately 2 weeks before delivery at term and after cessation of breast-feeding. The mean renal clearances of the antibiotic during the three administrations were 143, 170, and 103 mL/minute, respectively.

BREAST FEEDING SUMMARY

RECOMMENDATION: Compatible

Low concentrations of ceftazidime are excreted into breast milk (6). Eleven women were treated with 2 g of ceftazidime IV every 8 hours for endometritis following cesarean section. No mention was made as to whether the women were breast-feeding during treatment. Plasma and milk samples were collected between 2 and 4 days of therapy (total number of doses received averaged 12.6). The mean maternal plasma levels of the antibiotic just prior to a dose and 1 hour after a dose were 7.6 μg/mL and 71.8 μg/mL, respectively. The mean concentrations in breast milk before a dose and at 1 and 3 hours after a dose were 3.8, 5.2, and 4.5 μg/mL, respectively. No accumulation of the antibiotic in milk was observed.

C

Three potential problems exist for the nursing infant exposed to ceftazidime in milk: modification of bowel flora, direct effects on the infant, and interference with the interpretation of culture results if a fever workup is required. The American Academy of Pediatrics classifies ceftazidime as compatible with breast-feeding (7).

References

1. Product information. Fortaz. Glaxo Wellcome, 1997.
2. Cho N, Suzuki H, Mitsukawa M, Tamura T, Yamaguchi Y, Maruyama M, Aoki K, Fukunaga K, Kuni K. Fundamental and clinical evaluation of ceftazidime in the field of obstetrics and gynecology (English abstract). Chemotherapy (Tokyo) 1983;31(Suppl 3): 772–82.
3. Giamarellou H, Gazis J, Petrikkos G, Antsaklis A, Aravantinos D, Daikos GK. A study of cefoxitin, moxalactam, and ceftazidime kinetics in pregnancy. Am J Obstet Gynecol 1983;147:914–9.
4. Jørgensen NP, Walstad RA, Molne K. The concentrations of ceftazidime and thiopental in maternal plasma, placental tissue and amniotic fluid in early pregnancy. Acta Obstet Gynecol Scand 1987;66:29–33.
5. Nathorst-Boos J, Philipson A, Hedman A, Arvisson A. Renal elimination of ceftazidime during pregnancy. Am J Obstet Gynecol 1995;172:163–6.
6. Blanco JD, Jorgensen JH, Castaneda YS, Crawford SA. Ceftazidime levels in human breast milk. Antimicrob Agents Chemother 1983;23:479–80.
7. Committee on Drugs, American Academy of Pediatrics. The transfer of drugs and other chemicals into human milk. Pediatrics 2001;108:776–89.

Name: **CEFTIBUTEN** Risk Factor: **B_M**

Class: **Antibiotic (Cephalosporin)**

FETAL RISK SUMMARY

RECOMMENDATION: Compatible

Ceftibuten is an oral, semisynthetic cephalosporin antibiotic. Reproduction studies in rats found no evidence of impaired fertility at doses up to approximately 43 times the human dose on a mg/m^2 basis (1). No teratogenesis or fetal harm was found in studies with rats and rabbits at doses up to approximately 8.6 and 1.5 times, respectively, the human dose on a mg/m^2 basis.

No reports describing the use of ceftibuten in human pregnancy have been located. Cephalosporins are usually considered safe to use during pregnancy (see other cephalosporins for published human experience).

No detectable teratogenic risk with ceftibuten and other cephalosporin antibiotics was found in a large 2001 study (see Cephalexin).

BREAST FEEDING SUMMARY

RECOMMENDATION: Compatible

No reports describing the use of ceftibuten during human lactation have been located. Low concentrations of other cephalosporins are excreted into milk, however, and the presence of ceftibuten in milk should be expected. Three potential problems exist for the nursing infant exposed to ceftibuten in milk: modification of bowel flora, direct effects on the infant, and interference with the interpretation of culture results if a fever workup is required. The American Academy of Pediatrics classifies other cephalosporin antibiotics as compatible with breast-feeding (e.g., see Cefadroxil and Cefazolin).

Reference

1. Product information. Cedax. Schering Corporation, 1997.

C

Name:	**CEFTIZOXIME**	Risk Factor:	B_M
Class:	**Antibiotic (Cephalosporin)**		

FETAL RISK SUMMARY

RECOMMENDATION: Compatible

Ceftizoxime is a parenteral, semisynthetic cephalosporin antibiotic. Reproduction studies in rats found no evidence of impaired fertility at doses up to approximately two times the maximum human daily dose based on body surface area or, in rats and rabbits, of fetal harm (1).

The placental transfer of ceftizoxime and cefoperazone were studied in an *in vitro* perfused human placental system (2). The mean clearance indices for the two antibiotics were 0.126 and 0.037, respectively. The steady-state fetal concentrations of the two agents were 4–5 μg/mL and 4 μg/mL, respectively.

Following 1- or 2-g IV doses administered to women at term, peak cord blood levels occurred at 1–2 hours, with concentrations ranging between 12 and 30 μg/mL (3–7). Amniotic fluid concentrations were lower with peak levels of 10–20 μg/mL at 2–3 hours. The mean fetal:maternal ratio reported in one group of patients after a 2-g IV dose was 0.28 (7). In a different study, maternal, fetal, and amniotic concentrations were measured in women who had received at least three doses of ceftizoxime 2 g at 8-hour intervals (8). Mean levels at delivery in the various compartments were 11.96, 24.54, and 43.45 μg/mL, respectively. Cord blood levels averaged 1.6 times higher than maternal levels with average amniotic fluid concentrations 2.9 times those in the maternal serum (8). No adverse fetal or newborn effects were noted in any of the trials.

A 1993 report found that protein binding of ceftizoxime was significantly less in fetal blood than in maternal blood (9). The mean binding to fetal proteins was 21.9% compared with maternal protein binding of 57.8%.

An abstract of a multicenter, double-blind, randomized study published in 1993 found no difference between ceftizoxime (2 g IV every 8 hours) ($N = 154$) and placebo ($N = 152$) in the percentage of women with preterm premature rupture of the membranes who were undelivered at 7 days (10). Only noninfected women who were not in labor were enrolled in the study. A prospective, double-blind, placebo-controlled study published in 1995 found that ceftizoxime (2 g IV every 8 hours) had no effect on the interval to delivery or duration of pregnancy in women, with intact membranes and without chorioamnionitis, who were in preterm (<37 weeks' gestation) labor (11).

No fetal or newborn adverse effects following exposure to ceftizoxime during pregnancy have been reported. Cephalosporins are usually considered safe to use during pregnancy.

BREAST FEEDING SUMMARY

RECOMMENDATION: Compatible

Ceftizoxime is excreted into breast milk in low concentrations (7,12). Mean levels following single doses of 1 and 2 g were less than 0.5 μg/mL. Even though these levels are low, three potential problems exist for the nursing infant: modification of bowel flora, direct effects on the infant, and interference with the interpretation of culture results if a fever workup is required. Although not specifically listing ceftizoxime, the American Academy of Pediatrics classifies other cephalosporin antibiotics as compatible with breast-feeding (e.g., see Cefadroxil and Cefazolin).

References

1. Product information. Cefizox. Fujisawa USA, 1997.
2. Fortunato SJ, Bawdon RE, Maberry MC, Swan KF. Transfer of ceftizoxime surpasses that of cefoperazone by the isolated human placental perfused in vitro. Obstet Gynecol 1990;75:830–3.
3. Cho N, Fukunaga K, Kunii K. Studies on ceftizoxime (CZX) in the field of obstetrics and gynecology. Chemotherapy (Tokyo) 1980;28(Suppl 5):821–30.
4. Matsuda S, Seida A. Clinical use of ceftizoxime in obstetrics and gynecology. Chemotherapy (Tokyo) 1980;28(Suppl 5):812–20.
5. Okada E, Kawada A, Shirakawa N. Clinical studies on transplacental diffusion of ceftizoxime into fetal blood and treatment of infections in obstetrics and gynecology. Chemotherapy (Tokyo) 1980;28(Suppl 5): 874–87.
6. Seiga K, Minagawa M, Egawa J, Yamaji K, Sugiyama Y. Clinical and laboratory studies on ceftizoxime (CZX) in the field of obstetrics and gynecology. Chemotherapy (Tokyo) 1980;28(Suppl 5):845–62.
7. Motomura R, Kohno M, Mori H, Yamabe T. Basic and clinical studies of ceftizoxime in obstetrics and gynecology. Chemotherapy (Tokyo) 1980;28(Suppl 5): 888–99.
8. Fortunato SJ, Bawdon RE, Welt SI, Swan KF. Steady-state cord and amniotic fluid ceftizoxime levels continuously surpass maternal levels. Am J Obstet Gynecol 1988;159:570–3.
9. Fortunato SJ, Welt SI, Stewart JT. Differential protein binding of ceftizoxime in cord versus maternal serum. Am J Obstet Gynecol 1993;168:914–5.
10. Blanco J, Iams J, Artal R, Baker D, Hibbard J, McGregor J, Cetrulo C. Multicenter double-blind prospective random trial of ceftizoxime vs. placebo in women with preterm premature ruptured membranes (PPROM). Am J Obstet Gynecol 1993;168:378.
11. Gordon M, Samuels P, Shubert P, Johnson F, Gebauer C, Iams J. A randomized, prospective study of adjunctive ceftizoxime in preterm labor. Am J Obstet Gynecol 1995;172:1546–52.
12. Gerding DN, Peterson LR. Comparative tissue and extravascular fluid concentrations of ceftizoxime. J Antimicrob Chemother 1982;10(Suppl C): 105–16.

Name:	**CEFTRIAXONE**	Risk Factor:	$\mathbf{B_M}$
Class:	**Antibiotic (Cephalosporin)**		

FETAL RISK SUMMARY

RECOMMENDATION: Compatible

Ceftriaxone is a parenteral, semisynthetic cephalosporin antibiotic. Reproduction studies in rats found no evidence of impaired fertility or reproduction performance at a dose approximately 20 times the recommended human dose or, in mice, rats, and nonhuman primates, of embryotoxicity, fetotoxicity, or teratogenicity at doses approximately 20, 20, and 3 times, respectively, the recommended human dose (1).

A 1993 report described the pharmacokinetics of ceftriaxone, 2 g IV once daily for about 10 days, in nine women at 28 to 40 weeks' gestation who were being treated for chorioamnionitis or pyelonephritis (2). No accumulation of the antibiotic was noted and the pharmacokinetic profile was similar to healthy, nonpregnant adults. No adverse effects in fetuses or newborns were observed.

Peak levels in cord blood following 1- or 2-g IV doses occurred at 4 hours with concentrations varying between 19.6 and 40.6 μg/mL (1–8 hours) (3–5). Amniotic fluid levels over 24 hours ranged from 2.2 to 23.4 μg/mL with peak levels occurring at 6 hours (3–5). Ceftriaxone concentrations in the first voided newborn urine were highly variable, ranging from 6 to 92 μg/mL. Elimination half-lives from cord blood (7 hours), amniotic fluid

(6.8 hours), and placenta (5.4 hours) were nearly identical to maternal serum (3,4,6). No adverse effects in the newborns were mentioned.

In a surveillance study of Michigan Medicaid recipients conducted between 1985 and 1992 involving 229,101 completed pregnancies, 60 newborns had been exposed to ceftriaxone during the 1st trimester (F. Rosa, personal communication, FDA, 1993). Four (6.7%) major birth defects were observed (three expected), including three cardiovascular defects (one expected). No anomalies were observed in five other categories of defects (oral clefts, spina bifida, polydactyly, limb reduction defects, and hypospadias) for which specific data were available. A possible association between ceftriaxone and cardiovascular defects is suggested, but other factors, such as the mother's disease, concurrent drug use, and chance, may be involved. However, other cephalosporin antibiotics from this study have shown possible associations with congenital malformations (see also Cefaclor, Cephalexin, and Cephradine).

Cephalosporins are usually considered safe to use during pregnancy. Ceftriaxone, 1 g IV daily, has been used in the treatment of pyelonephritis occurring in the second half of pregnancy (7). No adverse fetal outcomes attributable to the drug were observed.

Ceftriaxone 1 g IV has been used for preoperative prophylaxis prior to emergency cesarean section (8). Amniotic fluid and fetal serum levels ranged from 0.016 to 0.25 μg/mL (mean: 0.085 μg/mL) and from 0.66 to 18.4 μg/mL (mean: 4.6 μg/mL), respectively.

In a study published in 1993, gonorrhea infecting 114 pregnant women in the 2nd trimester was treated with a single, 250-mg IM dose of ceftriaxone (9). The treatment was compared with approximately similar numbers of pregnant women treated with spectinomycin or amoxicillin with probenecid. Ceftriaxone and spectinomycin were similar in efficacy and both were superior to the amoxicillin/probenecid regimen. A 20-year-old woman with endocarditis caused by *Neisseria sicca* was treated for 4 weeks with ceftriaxone, 2 g IV every 12 hours, late in the 3rd trimester (10). She eventually delivered a term, small-for-gestational-age female infant, whose low weight was attributed to the mother's chronic disease state.

BREAST FEEDING SUMMARY

RECOMMENDATION: Compatible

Ceftriaxone is excreted into breast milk in low concentrations. Following either 1- or 2-g IV or IM doses, peak levels of 0.5–0.7 μg/mL occurred at 5 hours, approximately 3%–4% of maternal serum (3,4). High protein binding in maternal serum probably limited transfer to the milk (3,4). The antibiotic was still detectable in milk at 24 hours (3). Elimination half-lives after IV and IM doses were 12.8 and 17.3 hours, respectively (3). Chronic dosing would eventually produce calculated steady-state levels in 1.5–3 days in the 3- to 4-μg/mL range (4). Although these levels are low, three potential problems exist for the nursing infant: modification of bowel flora, direct effects on the infant, and interference with the interpretation of culture results if a fever workup is required. The American Academy of Pediatrics classifies ceftriaxone as compatible with breast-feeding (11).

References

1. Product information. Rocephin. Roche Laboratories, 1997.
2. Bourget P, Fernandez H, Quinquis V, Delouis C. Pharmacokinetics and protein binding of ceftriaxone during pregnancy. Antimicrob Agents Chemother 1993;37:54–9.
3. Kafetzis DA, Brater DC, Fanourgakis JE, Voyatzis J, Georgakopoulos P. Placental and breast-milk transfer

of ceftriaxone (C). In Proceedings of the 22nd Intersci Conf on Antimicrob Ag Chemother, Miami, Florida, October 4–6, 1982:155. New York: Academic Press, 1983.
4. Kafetzis DA, Brater DC, Fanourgakis JE, Voyatzis J, Georgakopoulos P. Ceftriaxone distribution between maternal blood and fetal blood and tissues at parturition and between blood and milk postpartum. Antimicrob Agents Chemother 1983;23:870–3.
5. Cho N, Kunii K, Fukunago K, Komoriyama Y. Antimicrobial activity, pharmacokinetics and clinical studies of ceftriaxone in obstetrics and gynecology. In Proceedings of the 13th Inter Cong Chemother, Vienna, Austria, August 28 to September 2, 1983:100/64–66. Princeton: Excerpta Medica, 1984.
6. Graber H, Magyar T. Pharmacokinetics of ceftriaxone in pregnancy. Am J Med 1984;77:117–8.
7. Sanchez-Ramos L, McAlpine KJ, Adair CD, Kaunitz AM, Delke I, Briones DK. Pyelonephritis in pregnancy: once-a-day ceftriaxone versus multiple doses of cefazolin. Am J Obstet Gynecol 1995;172:129–33.
8. Lang R, Shalit I, Segal J, Arbel Y, Markov S, Hass H, Fejgin M. Maternal and fetal and tissue levels of ceftriaxone following preoperative prophylaxis in emergency cesarean section. Chemotherapy 1993;39:77–81.
9. Cavenee MR, Farris JR, Spalding TR, Barnes DL, Castaneda YS,Wendel GD Jr. Treatment of gonorrhea in pregnancy. Obstet Gynecol 1993;81:33–8.
10. Deger R, Ludmir J. Neisseria sicca endocarditis complicating pregnancy. A case report. J Reprod Med 1992;37:473–5.
11. Committee on Drugs, American Academy of Pediatrics. The transfer of drugs and other chemicals into human milk. Pediatrics 2001;108:776–89.

Name: **CEFUROXIME** Risk Factor: **B_M**
Class: **Antibiotic (Cephalosporin)**

FETAL RISK SUMMARY

RECOMMENDATION: Compatible

Cefuroxime is an oral and parenteral, semisynthetic cephalosporin antibiotic. Reproduction studies in rats have found no evidence of impaired fertility at doses up to 9 times the maximum recommended human dose based on body surface area (MRHD) or, mice and rats, of fetal harm at doses up to 23 times the MRHD (1).

Cefuroxime readily crosses the placenta in late pregnancy and labor, achieving therapeutic concentrations in fetal serum and amniotic fluid (2–7). Therapeutic antibiotic levels in infants can be demonstrated up to 6 hours after birth with measurable concentrations persisting for 26 hours. The pharmacokinetics of cefuroxime in pregnancy have been reported (8). The antibiotic has been used for the treatment of pyelonephritis in pregnancy (9). Adverse effects in the newborn after *in utero* exposure have not been observed. Cephalosporins are usually considered safe to use during pregnancy.

In women at 15–35 weeks' gestation, a single 750-mg IV dose produced mean serum concentrations in mothers, hydropic fetuses, and fetuses with oligohydramnios of 7.4, 6.2, and 4.9 μg/mL, respectively (10). The concentrations did not correlate with gestational age. Nine women with premature rupture of the membranes at 27–33 weeks' gestation received 1.5 g IV of cefuroxime three times daily (11). The mean concentrations of the antibiotic in the mothers (1 hour after a dose), umbilical cord plasma, placenta, and membranes were 35.0 μg/mL, 3.0 μg/mL, 11.2 μg/g, and 35.6 μg/g, respectively.

In a surveillance study of Michigan Medicaid recipients conducted between 1985 and 1992 involving 229,101 completed pregnancies, 143 newborns had been exposed to cefuroxime during the 1st trimester (F. Rosa, personal communication, FDA, 1993). Three (2.1%) major birth defects were observed (six expected), but no anomalies were observed in six categories of defects for which specific data were available (cardiovascular defects, oral clefts, spina bifida, polydactyly, limb reduction defects, and hypospadias). These data do not support an association between the drug and congenital defects (see also Cefaclor, Cephalexin, and Cephradine for contrasting results).

The pregnancy outcomes of 106 women exposed in the 1st trimester to cefuroxime were described in a 2000 study (12). Compared to 106 matched controls, there was no difference in pregnancy outcomes in terms of live births, spontaneous abortions, gestational age at birth, prematurity, birth weight, fetal distress, method of delivery, and major or minor malformations. Induced abortions, however, occurred in significantly more cefuroxime-exposed women than in controls, possibly as a consequence of misinformation and misperception of the risk the antibiotic posed to a pregnancy (12).

No detectable teratogenic risk with cefuroxime and other cephalosporin antibiotics was found in a large 2001 study (see Cephalexin).

BREAST FEEDING SUMMARY

RECOMMENDATION: Compatible

Cefuroxime is excreted into breast milk in low concentrations (1). Even though the levels are low, three potential problems exist for the nursing infant exposed to cefuroxime in milk: modification of bowel flora, direct effects on the infant, and interference with the interpretation of culture results if a fever workup is required. Although not specifically listing cefuroxime, the American Academy of Pediatrics classifies other cephalosporin antibiotics as compatible with breast-feeding (e.g., see Cefadroxil and Cefazolin).

References

1. Product information. Ceftin. Glaxo Wellcome, 1997.
2. Craft I, Mullinger BM, Kennedy MRK. Placental transfer of cefuroxime. Br J Obstet Gynaecol 1981;88:141 5.
3. Bousfield P, Browning AK, Mullinger BM, Elstein M. Cefuroxime: potential use in pregnant women at term. Br J Obstet Gynaecol 1981;88:146–9.
4. Bergogne-Berezin E, Pierre J, Even P, Rouvillois JL, Dumez Y. Study of penetration of cefuroxime into bronchial secretions and of its placental transfer. Therapie 1980;35:677–84.
5. Tzingounis V, Makris N, Zolotas J, Michalas S, Aravantinos D. Cefuroxime prophylaxis in caesarean section. Pharmatherapeutica 1982;3:140–2.
6. Coppi G, Berti MA, Chehade A, Franchi I, Magro B. A study of the transplacental transfer of cefuroxime in humans. Curr Ther Res 1982;32:712–6.
7. Bousefield PF. Use of cefuroxime in pregnant women at term. Res Clin Forums 1984;6:53–8.
8. Philipson A, Stiernstedt G. Pharmacokinetics of cefuroxime in pregnancy. Am J Obstet Gynecol 1982;142:823–8.
9. Faro S, Pastorek JG II, Plauche WC, Korndorffer FA, Aldridge KE. Short-course parenteral antibiotic therapy for pyelonephritis in pregnancy. S Med J 1984;77:455–7.
10. Holt DE, Fisk NM, Spencer JAD, de Louvlis J, Hurley R, Harvey D. Transplacental transfer of cefuroxime in uncomplicated pregnancies and those complicated by hydrops or changes in amniotic fluid volume. Arch Dis Child 1993;68:54–7.
11. De Leeuw JW, Roumen FJME, Bouckaert PXJM, Cremers HMHG, Vree TB. Achievement of therapeutic concentrations of cefuroxime in early preterm gestations with premature rupture of the membranes. Obstet Gynecol 1993;81:255–60.
12. Berkovitch M, Segal-Socher I, Greenberg R, Bulkowshtein M, Arnon J, Perlob P, Or-Noy A. First trimester exposure to cefuroxime: a prospective cohort study. Br J Clin Pharmacol 2000;50:161–5.

Name:	**CELECOXIB**	Risk Factor:	C_M*
Class:	**Nonsteroidal Anti-Inflammatory**		

FETAL RISK SUMMARY

RECOMMENDATION: Human Data Suggest Risk in 1st and 3rd Trimesters

Celecoxib is a second-generation nonsteroidal anti-inflammatory drug (NSAID) that inhibits prostaglandin synthesis via the inhibition of cyclooxygenase-2 (COX-2). It is in the same NSAID subclass (COX-2 inhibitors) as rofecoxib and valdecoxib. In therapeutic concentrations, it does not inhibit, as do first-generation NSAIDs, the cyclooxygenase-1 (COX-1) isoenzyme. Celecoxib is indicated for the relief of the signs and symptoms of osteoarthritis and rheumatoid arthritis (1).

Celecoxib was not mutagenic or clastogenic in Chinese hamster ovary cells or clastogenic in an *in vivo* micronucleus test in rat bone marrow (1). Administration to female rats of oral doses ≥50 mg/kg/day (about 6 times the maximum recommended human dose [MRHD] based on AUC at 200 mg twice a day) resulted in pre-implantation and post-implantation losses and reduced embryo/fetal survival, a natural consequence of its inhibition of prostaglandin synthesis (1).

Teratogenicity studies have been conducted in rats and rabbits (1). In pregnant rats, a dose-related increase in diaphragmatic hernias was observed in one of two studies at doses of ≥30 mg/kg/day (about 6 times the MRHD). No teratogenic effects occurred in pregnant rabbits dosed at 60 mg/kg/day (equal to the MRHD), but at ≥150 mg/kg/day (approximately 2 times the MRHD), an increased incidence of fetal alterations (fused ribs and fused, misshapen sternebrae) was observed (1). No evidence of delayed labor or parturition at doses up to 100 mg/kg (approximately 7 times the MRHD) was observed in rats (1).

Two studies in pregnant rabbits were designed to test the hypothesis that celecoxib was effective in preventing preterm delivery and did not adversely effect fetal ductus arteriosus patency (2,3). In the first study, the rabbits received celecoxib 30 mg/kg/day for differing periods starting at day 13 of gestation (2). Concentrations of prostanoids, cytokines, and nitric oxide were altered by the treatment resulting in a decrease in the incidence compared to controls of preterm parturition. In the second study, no adverse effect on the fetal ductus arteriosus was observed (3).

No reports describing the placental transfer of celecoxib have been located. The molecular weight (about 381), however, is low enough that passage to the fetus should be expected. Celecoxib metabolism is mediated by the cytochrome P450 2C9 enzyme, resulting in at least three inactive metabolites (1). Women in whom metabolism by this enzyme is known or suspected to be deficient may have abnormally high plasma levels of celecoxib and, thus, more of the drug will be available for placental transfer.

A combined 2001 population-based observational cohort study and a case-control study estimated the risk of adverse pregnancy outcome from the use of NSAIDs (4). The use of NSAIDs during pregnancy was not associated with congenital malformations, preterm delivery, or low birth weight, but a positive association was discovered with spontaneous abortions (SABs). A similar study, also published in 2001, failed to find a relationship, in general, between NSAIDs and congenital malformations, but did find a significant association with cardiac defects and orofacial clefts (5). In addition, a 2003 study found a significant association between exposure to NSAIDs in early pregnancy and SABs (6) (see Ibuprofen for details on these three studies).

An *in vitro* study demonstrated that celecoxib had significant uterine relaxant effects (7). Celecoxib was more potent, in this regard, than nimesulide or meloxicam. A 2002 randomized, double-blind, placebo-controlled study compared the tocolytic effects of celecoxib (100 mg orally every 12 hours for 4 doses) and indomethacin (100 mg rectally, then 50 mg orally every 6 hours for 7 doses) (8). The subjects, 12 in each group, were in preterm labor at 24 to 34 weeks' gestation. Partial premature constriction of the fetal ductus arteriosus occurred in the indomethacin group, but not in the celecoxib group. A transient decrease in amniotic fluid volume was observed in both groups, but more so with indomethacin. Both drugs were equally effective in the maintenance of tocolysis, but the authors concluded that the safety of celecoxib was superior to that of indomethacin (8).

In summary, no reports describing the use of celecoxib in human pregnancy have been located. The animal data are suggestive of a low risk for congenital malformations. Moreover, a brief 2003 editorial on the potential for NSAID-induced developmental toxicity concluded that NSAIDs, and specifically those with greater COX-2 affinity, had a lower risk of this toxicity in humans than aspirin (9).

The use of first-generation NSAIDs during the latter half of pregnancy has been associated with oligohydramnios and premature closure of the ductus arteriosus (e.g., see Indomethacin) (10). Persistent pulmonary hypertension of the newborn may occur if NSAIDs are used in the 3rd trimester close to delivery (10,11). These drugs also inhibit labor and prolong pregnancy, both in humans (12) and in animals (13). Similar effects should be expected if celecoxib is used during the 3rd trimester or close to delivery. Women attempting to conceive should not use any prostaglandin synthesis inhibitor, including celecoxib, because of the findings in a variety of animal models that indicate these agents block blastocyst implantation (14,15). Moreover, as noted above, NSAIDs are associated with SABs and congenital malformations. If celecoxib is used in pregnancy for the treatment of rheumatoid arthritis, health care professionals are encouraged to call the toll free number (877–311–8972) for information about patient enrollment in the OTIS Rheumatoid Arthritis Study.

[*Risk Factor D if used in 3rd trimester or near delivery.*]

BREAST FEEDING SUMMARY

RECOMMENDATION: Limited Human Data - Potential Toxicity

Celecoxib is excreted in the milk of lactating rats in concentrations similar to those measured in plasma (1). The drug is also excreted into the milk of humans (16). A 40-year-old woman who was breast-feeding her 5-month-old daughter was admitted to the hospital for surgery to remove a gangrenous appendix (16). In the post-operative period, she received four doses of celecoxib (100 mg twice/day) in addition to other medications. Starting about 5 hours after her last dose, four milk samples were obtained by hand expression over a 24-hour interval. The area under the concentration curve was 1751 and 1445 μg/L-hour for the left and right breasts, respectively. The elimination half-life range was 4.0–6.5 hours. These data suggest that celecoxib would be eliminated from breast milk about 24 hours after the last dose (16). Although maternal plasma was not obtained, the estimated milk:plasma$_{auc}$ ratios (based on reported adult plasma levels) were 0.27–0.59. The infant did not resume breast-feeding until 48 hours after the last dose. If she had nursed, the estimated maximum dose she would have received was about 40 μg/kg/day. The authors concluded that this small amount probably would not cause adverse effects in a nursing infant (16).

Several first-generation NSAIDs are considered low-risk during nursing (e.g., see Diclofenac, Fenoprofen, Flurbiprofen, Ibuprofen, Ketoprofen, Ketorolac, and Tolmetin) and, based on the single report, celecoxib can probably be similarly classified. However, additional data are needed. Until such data are available, the safest course is to avoid breast-feeding during continuous celecoxib therapy. If the mother chooses to nurse, the infant should be closely monitored for potential toxicity, such as abdominal pain, diarrhea, nausea, headache, and dizziness.

References

1. Product information. Celebrex. G.D. Searle, 1999.
2. Hausman N, Beharry KD, Nishihara KC, Akmal Y, Asrat T. Effect of the antenatal administration of celecoxib during the second and third trimesters of pregnancy on prostaglandin, cytokine, and nitric oxide levels in rabbits. Am J Obstet Gynecol 2003;189:1737–43.
3. Hausman N, Beharry K, Nishihara K, Akmal V, Stavitsky Y, Asrat T. Response of fetal prostanoids, nitric oxide, and ductus arteriosus to the short- and long-term antenatal administration of celecoxib, a selective cyclooxygenase-2 inhibitor, in the pregnant rabbit. Am J Obstet Gynecol 2003;189:1744–50.
4. Nielsen GL, Sorensen HT, Larsen H, Pedersen L. Risk of adverse birth outcome and miscarriage in pregnant users of non-steroidal anti-inflammatory drugs: population based observational study and case-control study. BMJ 2001;322:266–70.
5. Ericson A, Kallen BAJ. Nonsteroidal anti-inflammatory drugs in early pregnancy. Reprod Toxicol 2001;15:371–3.
6. Li DK, Liu L, Odouli R. Exposure to non-steroidal anti-inflammatory drugs during pregnancy and risk of miscarriage: population based cohort study. BMJ 2003;327:368–71.
7. Slatterm MM, Friel AM, Healy DG, Morrison JJ. Uterine relaxant effects of cyclooxygenase-2 inhibitors in vitro. Obstet Gynecol 2001;98:563–9.
8. Stika CS, Gross GA, Leguizamon G, Gerber S, Levy R, Mathur A, Bernhard LM, Nelson DM, Sadovsky Y. A prospective randomized safety trial of celecoxib for treatment of preterm labor. Am J Obstet Gynecol 2002;187:653–60.
9. Tassinari MS, Cook JC, Hunt ME. NSAIDs and development toxicity. Birth Defects Res Part B Dev Reprod Toxicol 2003;68:3–4.
10. Levin DL. Effects of inhibition of prostaglandin synthesis on fetal development, oxygenation, and the fetal circulation. Semin Perinatol 1980;4:35–44.
11. Van Marter LJ, Leviton A, Allred EN, Pagano M, Sullivan KF, Cohen A, Epstein MF. Persistent pulmonary hypertension of the newborn and smoking and aspirin and nonsteroidal antiinflammatory drug consumption during pregnancy. Pediatrics 1996;97:658–63.
12. Fuchs F. Prevention of prematurity. Am J Obstet Gynecol 1976;126:809–20.
13. Powell JG, Cochrane RL. The effects of a number of non-steroidal anti-inflammatory compounds on parturition in the rat. Prostaglandins 1982;23:469–88.
14. Matt DW, Borzelleca JF. Toxic effects on the female reproductive system during pregnancy, parturition, and lactation. In Witorsch RJ, ed. *Reproductive Toxicology*. 2nd ed. New York, NY: Raven Press, 1995:175–93.
15. Dawood MY. Nonsteroidal antiinflammatory drugs and reproduction. Am J Obstet Gynecol 1993;169:1255–65.
16. Knoppert DC, Stempak D, Baruchel S, Koren G. Celecoxib in human milk: a case report. Pharmacotherapy 2003;23:97–100.

Name: **CELIPROLOL** Risk Factor: **B***

Class: **Sympatholytic (Antihypertensive)**

FETAL RISK SUMMARY

RECOMMENDATION: Human Data Suggest Risk in 2nd and 3rd Trimesters

Celiprolol is a third-generation, cardioselective β-adrenergic blocking agent used in the treatment of hypertension and angina. The drug is available in some foreign countries and is approved for the treatment of pregnancy-induced hypertension (1), but clinical studies in pregnant women have not been located. It is expected to be approved for use in the United States in the near future.

Reproductive studies in rats before conception, during organogenesis, and in the perinatal period up to a maximum dose of 320 mg/kg revealed no evidence of teratogenicity or adverse effects in the offspring (2–4). Similarly, no teratogenic effects were observed in a reproductive study with rats and rabbits (5).

A study using an *in vitro* perfusion system of human placental tissue demonstrated that celiprolol crossed to the fetal side of the preparation (6). Although the diffusion rate of the hydrophilic celiprolol was three to four times less than those of the lipid-soluble β-blockers labetalol, propranolol, and timolol, this degree of difference has not been observed in *in vivo* measurements (see Labetalol and Propranolol). A study published in 1993 measured the placental passage of celiprolol in four pregnant women with hypertension who were administered an oral 200-mg dose once daily (1). Fetal plasma concentrations were

25%–50% of maternal concentrations. No mention was made if any effects on the newborn were observed.

Some β-blockers may cause intrauterine growth retardation (IUGR) and reduced placental weight, especially those lacking intrinsic sympathomimetic activity (ISA) (i.e., partial agonist). Treatment beginning early in the 2nd trimester results in the greatest weight reductions, whereas treatment restricted to the 3rd trimester primarily affects only placental weight. Celiprolol does possess ISA. Although growth retardation is a serious concern, the benefits of maternal therapy with β-blockers, in some cases, might outweigh the risks to the fetus and must be judged on a case-by-case basis.

[**Risk Factor D if used in 2nd or 3rd trimesters.*]

BREAST FEEDING SUMMARY

RECOMMENDATION: No Human Data - Potential Toxicity

Studies describing the measurement of celiprolol in milk have not been located. Because other β-blockers are excreted into milk, the appearance of celiprolol in milk should be expected. As a consequence, nursing infants of mothers consuming this agent should be closely monitored for bradycardia and other signs and symptoms of β-blockade.

References

1. Kotahl B, Henke D, Hettenbach A, Mutschler E. Studies on placental transfer of celiprolol. Eur J Clin Pharmacol 1993;44:381–2.
2. Nimomiya H, Akitsuki S, Kondo J, Nishikawa K, Yamashita Y, Watanabe M, Nagawawa H, Sumi N, Nomura A. Reproduction study of celiprolol: (1) fertility study in rats. Oyo Yakuri 1989;37:201–13. As cited in Shepard TH. *Catalog of Teratogenic Agents*. 7th ed. Baltimore, MD: Johns Hopkins University Press, 1992:77.
3. Nimomiya H, Akitsuki S, Kondo J, Nishikawa K, Yamashita Y, Watanabe M, Nagasawa H, Sumi N, Nomura A. Reproduction study of celiprolol: (2) teratogenicity study in rats. Oyo Yakuri 1989;37:215–29. As cited in Shepard TH. *Catalog of Teratogenic Agents*. 7th ed. Baltimore, MD: Johns Hopkins University Press, 1992:77.
4. Ninomiya H, Akitsui S, Kondo J, Nishikawa K, Watanabe M, Nagasawa H, Sumi N, Nomura A. Reproduction study of celiprolol: (3) peri- and postnatal study in rats. Oyo Yakuri 1989;37:231–42. As cited in Shepard TH. *Catalog of Teratogenic Agents*. 7th ed. Baltimore, MD. Johns Hopkins University Press, 1992:77.
5. Wendtlandt W, Pittner H. Toxicological evaluation of celiprolol, a cardioselective beta-adrenergic blocking agent. Arzneimittelforschung 1983;33:41–9. As cited in Schardein JL. *Chemically Induced Birth Defects*. 2nd ed. New York, NY: Marcel Dekker, 1993:89.
6. Schneider H, Proegler M. Placental transfer of β-adrenergic antagonists studied in an in vitro perfusion system of human placental tissue. Am J Obstet Gynecol 1988;159:42–7.

Name:	**CEPHALEXIN**	Risk Factor:	$\mathbf{B_M}$
Class:	**Antibiotic (Cephalosporin)**		

FETAL RISK SUMMARY

RECOMMENDATION: Compatible

Cephalexin is an oral, semisynthetic cephalosporin antibiotic. Reproduction studies found no evidence in rats, at doses up to 500 mg/kg, of impaired fertility or reproductive performance or, in mice and rats, of fetal harm (1).

Several published reports have described the administration of cephalexin to pregnant patients in various stages of gestation (2–12). None of these have linked the use of cephalexin with congenital defects or toxicity in the newborn. However, even though

C

cephalosporins are usually considered safe to use during pregnancy, the surveillance study described below found results contrasting to the published data.

In a surveillance study of Michigan Medicaid recipients conducted between 1985 and 1992 involving 229,101 completed pregnancies, 3,613 newborns had been exposed to cephalexin during the 1st trimester (F. Rosa, personal communication, FDA, 1993). A total of 176 (4.9%) major birth defects were observed (154 expected). Specific data were available for six defect categories, including (observed/expected) 44/36 cardiovascular defects, 11/5 oral clefts, 3/2 spina bifida, 3/10 polydactyly, 1/6 limb reduction defects, and 8/9 hypospadias. The data for total defects, cardiovascular defects, and oral clefts are suggestive of an association between cephalexin and congenital defects, but other factors, such as the mother's disease, concurrent drug use, and chance, may be involved. However, similar findings were measured for another cephalosporin antibiotic with more than a thousand exposures (see Cefaclor). Positive results were also suggested for cephradine (339 exposures) but not for cefadroxil (722 exposures) (see Cephradine and Cefadroxil). In contrast, other anti-infectives with large cohorts (see Ampicillin, Amoxicillin, Penicillin G, Erythromycin, and Tetracycline) had negative findings.

Transplacental passage of cephalexin has been demonstrated only near term (2,3). Following a 1-g oral dose, peak concentrations for maternal serum, cord serum, and amniotic fluid were about 34 (1 hour), 11 (4 hours), and 13 μg/mL (6 hours), respectively (3). Patients in whom labor was induced were observed to have falling concentrations of cephalexin in all samples when labor was prolonged beyond 18 hours (4). In one report, all fetal blood samples gave a negative Coombs' reaction (2).

The effect of postcoital prophylaxis with a single oral dose of either cephalexin (250 mg) or nitrofurantoin macrocrystals (50 mg) starting before or during pregnancy in 33 women (39 pregnancies) with a history of recurrent urinary tract infections was described in a 1992 reference (11). A significant decrease in the number of infections was documented without fetal toxicity.

The manufacturer has unpublished information on 46 patients treated with cephalexin during pregnancy (C. L. Lynch, personal communication, Dista Products, 1981). Two of these patients received the drug from 1–2 months prior to conception to term. No effects on the fetus attributable to the antibiotic were observed. Follow-up examination on one infant at 2 months was normal.

A 2001 study used the Hungarian Case-Control Surveillance of Congenital Abnormalities (1980–1996) database to examine the association between cephalosporins (cephalexin, cefaclor, cefamandole, cefoperazone, cefotaxime, ceftibuten, and cefuroxime) and birth defects (12). Cases were drawn from 22,865 pregnant women who had fetuses or newborn infants with congenital abnormalities. Matched controls were obtained from pregnant women who had infants without defects. Most of the 308 case women were treated with cephalexin. No detectable teratogenic risk was found.

BREAST FEEDING SUMMARY

RECOMMENDATION: Compatible

Cephalexin is excreted into breast milk in low concentrations. A 1-g oral dose given to six mothers produced peak milk levels at 4–5 hours averaging 0.51 μg/mL (range 0.24–0.85 μg/mL) (13). Mean milk:plasma ratios at 1, 2, and 3 hours were 0.008, 0.021, and 0.14, respectively. Even though these levels are low, three potential problems exist for the nursing infant: modification of bowel flora, direct effects on the infant, and interference with the interpretation of culture results if a fever workup is required. Although not specifically listing cephalexin, the American Academy of Pediatrics classifies other cephalosporin antibiotics as compatible with breast-feeding (e.g., see Cefadroxil and Cefazolin).

C

References

1. Product information. Keflex. Dista Products, 1997.
2. Paterson ML, Henderson A, Lunan CB, McGurk S. Transplacental transfer of cephalexin. Clin Med 1972;79:22–4.
3. Creatsas G, Pavlatos M, Lolis D, Kaskarelis D. A study of the kinetics of cephapirin and cephalexin in pregnancy. Curr Med Res Opin 1980;7:43–6.
4. Hirsch HA. Behandlung von harnwegsinfektionen in gynakologic und geburtshilfe mit cephalexin. Int J Clin Pharmacol 1969;2(Suppl):121–3.
5. Brumfitt W, Pursell R. Double-blind trial to compare ampicillin, cephalexin, co-trimoxazole, and trimethoprim in treatment of urinary infection. Br Med J 1972;2:673–6.
6. Mizuno S, Metsuda S, Mori S. Clinical evaluation of cephalexin in obstetrics and gynaecology. In Proceedings of a Symposium on the Clinical Evaluation of Cephalexin, Royal Society of Medicine, London, June 2 and 3, 1969.
7. Guttman D. Cephalexin in urinary tract infections—preliminary results. In Proceedings of a Symposium on the Clinical Evaluation of Cephalexin, Royal Society of Medicine, London, June 2 and 3, 1969.
8. Soto RF, Fesbre F, Cordido A, et al. Ensayo con cefalexina en el tratamiento de infecciones urinarias en pacientes embarazadas. Rev Obstet Ginecol Venez 1972;32:637–41.
9. Campbell-Brown M, McFadyen IR. Bacteriuria in pregnancy treated with a single dose of cephalexin. Br J Obstet Gynaecol 1983;90:1054–9.
10. Jakobi P, Neiger R, Merzbach D, Paldi E. Single-dose antimicrobial therapy in the treatment of asymptomatic bacteriuria in pregnancy. Am J Obstet Gynecol 1987;156:1148–52.
11. Pfau A, Sacks TG. Effective prophylaxis for recurrent urinary tract infections during pregnancy. Clin Infect Dis 1992;14:810–4.
12. Czeizel AE, Rockenbauer M, Sorensen HT, Olsen J. Use of cephalosporins during pregnancy and in the presence of congenital abnormalities: a population-based, case-control study. Am J Obstet Gynecol 2001;184:1289–96.
13. Kafetzis D, Siafas C, Georgakopoulos P, Papadatos CJ. Passage of cephalosporins and amoxicillin into the breast milk. Acta Paediatr Scand 1981;70:285–8.

Name:	**CEPHALOTHIN**	Risk Factor:	B_M
Class:	**Antibiotic (Cephalosporin)**		

FETAL RISK SUMMARY

RECOMMENDATION: Compatible

Cephalothin is a parenteral, semisynthetic cephalosporin antibiotic. The drug has been used during all stages of gestation (1–3). Cephalosporins are usually considered safe to use during pregnancy.

No reports linking the use of cephalothin with congenital defects or toxicity in the newborn have been located. The drug crosses the placenta and distributes in fetal tissues (4–10). Following a 1-g dose, average peak cord serum levels were 2.8 μg/mL (16% of maternal peak) at 1–2 hours for the intramuscular route and 12.5 μg/mL (41% of maternal peak) 10 minutes after IV administration (4–6). In amniotic fluid, cephalothin was slowly concentrated reaching an average level of 21 μg/mL at 4–5 hours (5).

BREAST FEEDING SUMMARY

RECOMMENDATION: Compatible

Cephalothin is excreted into breast milk in low concentrations. A 1-g IV bolus dose given to six mothers produced peak milk levels at 1–2 hours averaging 0.51 μg/mL (range

C

0.36–0.62 μg/mL) (11). Mean milk:plasma ratios at 1, 2, and 3 hours were 0.073, 0.26, and 0.50, respectively. Even though these levels are low, three potential problems exist for the nursing infant: modification of bowel flora, direct effects on the infant, and interference with the interpretation of culture results if a fever workup is required. Although not specifically listing cephalothin, the American Academy of Pediatrics classifies other cephalosporin antibiotics as compatible with breast-feeding (12).

References

1. Cunningham FG, Morris GB, Mickal A. Acute pyelonephritis of pregnancy: a clinical review. Obstet Gynecol 1973;42:112–7.
2. Harris RE, Gilstrap LC. Prevention of recurrent pyelonephritis during pregnancy. Obstet Gynecol 1974;44:637–41.
3. Moro M, Andrews M. Prophylactic antibiotics in cesarean section. Obstet Gynecol 1974;44:688–92.
4. MacAulay MA, Charles D. Placental transfer of cephalothin. Am J Obstet Gynecol 1968;100:940–5.
5. Sheng KT, Huang NN, Promadhattavedi V. Serum concentrations of cephalothin in infants and children and placental transmission of the antibiotic. Antimicrob Agents Chemother 1964:200–6.
6. Fukada M. Studies on chemotherapy during the perinatal period with special reference to such derivatives of Cephalosporin C as cefazolin, cephaloridine and cephalothin. Jpn J Antibiot 1973;26:197–212.
7. Paterson L, Henderson A, Lunan CB, McGurk S. Transfer of cephalothin sodium to the fetus. J Obstet Gynaecol Br Commonw 1970;77:565–6.
8. Morrow S, Palmisano P, Cassady G. The placental transfer of cephalothin. J Pediatr 1968;73:262–4.
9. Stewart KS, Shafi M, Andrews J, Williams JD. Distribution of parenteral ampicillin and cephalosporins in late pregnancy. J Obstet Gynaecol Br Commonw 1973;80:902–8.
10. Corson SL, Bolognese RJ. The behavior of cephalothin in amniotic fluid. J Reprod Med 1970;4:105–8.
11. Kafetzis D, Siafas C, Georgakopoulos P, Papadatos CJ. Passage of cephalosporins and amoxicillin into the breast milk. Acta Paediatr Scand 1981;70: 285–8.
12. Committee on Drugs, American Academy of Pediatrics. The transfer of drugs and other chemicals into human milk. Pediatrics 2001;108:776–89.

Name:	**CEPHAPIRIN**	Risk Factor:	B_M
Class:	**Antibiotic (Cephalosporin)**		

FETAL RISK SUMMARY

RECOMMENDATION: Compatible

Cephapirin is a parenteral cephalosporin antibiotic. At term, following a 1-g IM dose, peak concentrations for maternal serum, cord serum and amniotic fluid were about 17 (0.5 hour), 10 (4 hours), and 13 μg/mL (6 hours), respectively (1). No data on the newborns were given. Cephalosporins are usually considered safe to use during pregnancy.

BREAST FEEDING SUMMARY

RECOMMENDATION: Compatible

Cephapirin is excreted into breast milk in low concentrations. A 1-g intravenous bolus dose given to six mothers produced peak milk levels at 1–2 hours averaging 0.49 μg/mL (range 0.30–0.64 μg/mL) (2). Mean milk:plasma ratios at 1, 2, and 3 hours were 0.068, 0.250, and 0.480, respectively. Even though these levels were low, three potential problems exist for the nursing infant: modification of bowel flora, direct effects on the infant, and interference with the interpretation of culture results if a fever workup is required. Although not specifically listing cephapirin, the American Academy of Pediatrics classifies other cephalosporin antibiotics as compatible with breast-feeding (3).

References

1. Creatsas G, Pavlatos M, Lolis D, Kasharelis D. A study of the kinetics of cephapirin and cephalexin in pregnancy. Curr Med Res Opin 1980;7:43–6.
2. Kafetzis D, Siafas C, Georgakopoulos P, Papadatos CJ. Passage of cephalosporins and amoxicillin into the breast milk. Acta Paediatr Scand 1981;70:285–8.
3. Committee on Drugs, American Academy of Pediatrics. The transfer of drugs and other chemicals into human milk. Pediatrics 2001;108:776–89.

C

Name:	**CEPHRADINE**	Risk Factor:	B_M
Class:	**Antibiotic (Cephalosporin)**		

FETAL RISK SUMMARY

RECOMMENDATION: Compatible

Cephradine is an oral and parenteral cephalosporin antibiotic. The drug rapidly crosses the placenta throughout gestation (1–4). In the 1st and 2nd trimesters, IV or oral doses produce amniotic fluid levels in the 1 μg/mL range or less. Between 15 and 30 weeks of gestation, a 1-g IV dose produces therapeutic fetal levels, peaking in 40–50 minutes (1). At term, oral doses of 2 g/day for 2 days or more allowed cephradine to concentrate in the amniotic fluid, producing levels in the range of 3–15 μg/mL (2,3). A 2-g IV dose 17 minutes prior to delivery produced high cord serum levels (29 μg/mL) but low amniotic fluid concentrations (1.1 μg/mL) (4). Serum samples taken from two of the newborns within 20 hours of birth indicated cephradine is excreted by the neonate (4). No other infant data were given in any of the studies. Cephalosporins are usually considered safe to use during pregnancy.

In a surveillance study of Michigan Medicaid recipients conducted between 1985 and 1992 involving 229,101 completed pregnancies, 339 newborns had been exposed to cephradine during the 1st trimester (F. Rosa, personal communication, FDA, 1993). A total of 27 (8.0%) major birth defects were observed (14 expected). Specific data were available for six defect categories, including (observed/expected) 9/3 cardiovascular defects, 0/0.5 oral clefts, 0/0 spina bifida, 1/1 polydactyly, 0/0.5 limb reduction defects, and 1/1 hypospadias. The data for all defects and cardiovascular defects are suggestive of an association between cephradine and congenital defects, but other factors, such as the mother's disease, may be involved. However, similar findings were measured for cefaclor and cephalexin (see Cefaclor and Cephalexin). In contrast, other anti-infectives with large cohorts (see Ampicillin, Amoxicillin, Penicillin G, Erythromycin, and Tetracycline) were not associated with defects.

BREAST FEEDING SUMMARY

RECOMMENDATION: Compatible

Cephradine is excreted into breast milk in low concentrations. After 500 mg orally every 6 hours for 48 hours, constant milk concentrations of 0.6 μg/mL were measured during 6 hours, a milk:plasma ratio of about 0.2 (2,3). Even though these levels are low, three potential problems exist for the nursing infant: modification of bowel flora, direct effects on the infant, and interference with the interpretation of culture results if a fever workup is required. Although not specifically listing cephradine, the American Academy of Pediatrics classifies other cephalosporin antibiotics as compatible with breast-feeding (5).

References

1. Lange IR, Rodeck C, Cosgrove R. The transfer of cephradine across the placenta. Br J Obstet Gynaecol 1984;91:551–4.
2. Mischler TW, Corson SL, Bolognese RJ, Letocha MJ, Neiss ES. Presence of cephradine in body fluids of lactating and pregnant women. Clin Pharmacol Ther 1974;15:214.
3. Mischler TW, Corson SL, Larranaga A, Bolognese RJ, Neiss ES, Vukovich RA. Cephradine and epicillin in body fluids of lactating and pregnant women. J Reprod Med 1978;21:130–6.
4. Craft I, Forster TC. Materno-fetal cephradine transfer in pregnancy. Antimicrob Agents Chemother 1978;14:924–6.
5. Committee on Drugs, American Academy of Pediatrics. The transfer of drugs and other chemicals into human milk. Pediatrics 2001;108:776–89.

Name:	**CERIVASTATIN**[§]	Risk Factor:	**X_M**
Class:	**Antilipemic Agent**		

FETAL RISK SUMMARY

RECOMMENDATION: Contraindicated

Cerivastatin, a 3-hydroxy-3-methylglutaryl-coenzyme A (HMG-CoA) reductase inhibitor (a "statin") that is lipophilic, is indicated as an adjunct to diet to reduce total cholesterol, low-density lipoprotein (LDL) cholesterol, apolipoprotein B, and triglyceride levels in patients with primary hypercholesterolemia and mixed dyslipidemia. It has the same mechanism of action as atorvastatin, fluvastatin, lovastatin, pravastatin, and simvastatin. The parent drug and some of the metabolites are pharmacologically active in humans (1).

Reproduction studies have been conducted in pregnant rats and rabbits (1). At doses producing plasma levels about 6 and 3 times, respectively, the human exposure at a dose of 0.8 mg (HE), a significant increase in incomplete ossification of the lumbar center of the vertebrae was observed in rats, but no malformations were seen in rabbits.

It is not known if cerivastatin crosses the human placenta. The molecular weight (about 482) is low enough that transfer to the fetus should be expected. Cerivastatin crossed the rat placenta and was found in the fetal liver, gastrointestinal tract, and kidneys after a single maternal dose that resulted in about 17 times the HE (1).

A 2004 report described the outcomes of pregnancy that had been exposed to statins and reported to the FDA (see Lovastatin).

The interruption of cholesterol-lowering therapy during pregnancy should have no effect on the long-term treatment of hyperlipidemia. Moreover, because cholesterol and products synthesized by cholesterol are important during fetal development, and because of the human pregnancy data reported with a similar drug (see Lovastatin), the use of cerivastatin is contraindicated during pregnancy.

[[§]*Withdrawn from the market in 2001.*]

BREAST FEEDING SUMMARY

RECOMMENDATION: Contraindicated

Cerivastatin is excreted into human breast (1). The milk:plasma ratio is 1.3 (1). Because of the potential for adverse effects in a nursing infant, women who are taking cerivastatin should not breast-feed.

Reference

1. Product information. Baycol. Bayer, 2001.

Name:	**CETIRIZINE**	Risk Factor:	B_M
Class:	**Antihistamine**		

FETAL RISK SUMMARY

RECOMMENDATION: Limited Human Data - Animal Data Suggest Low Risk

The antihistamine, cetirizine, is a second-generation, orally active, selective peripheral H_1-receptor antagonist. It is indicated for the relief of seasonal and perennial allergic rhinitis and for the treatment of chronic urticaria. The agent is a human metabolite of hydroxyzine.

Reproduction studies in mice, rats, and rabbits at oral doses up to 40, 180, and 220 times the maximum recommended human daily dose on a body surface area basis (MRHD), respectively, revealed no teratogenic effects (1).

It is not known if cetirizine crosses the human placenta to the fetus. The molecular weight (about 462 for the dihydrochloride salt) is low enough, however, that transfer to the fetus should be expected.

A prospective controlled study published in 1997 evaluated the teratogenic risk of cetirizine and hydroxyzine (see also Hydroxyzine) in human pregnancy (2). A total of 120 pregnancies (2 sets of twins) exposed to either cetirizine ($N = 39$) or hydroxyzine ($N = 81$) during pregnancy were identified and compared to 110 controls. The control group was matched for maternal age, smoking, and alcohol use. The drugs were taken during the 1st trimester in 37 (95%) of the cetirizine exposures and in 53 (65%) of the hydroxyzine cases for a variety of indications (e.g., rhinitis, urticaria, pruritic urticarial papules and plaques of pregnancy, sedation, and other nonspecified reasons). Fourteen spontaneous abortions (cetirizine 6, hydroxyzine 3, controls 5) and 11 induced abortions (hydroxyzine 6, controls 5) occurred in the three groups. Among the live births, there were no statistical differences among the groups in birth weight, gestational age at delivery, rate of cesarean section, or neonatal distress. Two minor anomalies were observed in liveborn infants exposed to cetirizine during organogenesis; one had an ectopic kidney and one had undescended testes. No major abnormalities were seen in this group. In the hydroxyzine group, two of the live births had major malformations; one had a ventricular septal defect and one a complex congenital heart defect (also exposed to carbamazepine). A third infant, exposed after organogenesis, also had a ventricular septal defect. Minor abnormalities were observed in four hydroxyzine-exposed infants: one case each of hydrocele, inguinal hernia, hypothyroidism (mother also taking propylthiouracil), and strabismus. In the control group, no major malformations were observed, but five infants had minor defects (dislocated hip, growth hormone deficiency, short lingual frenulum, and two unspecified defects). Statistically, there were no differences between the groups in outcome (2).

A recent review compared the published pregnancy outcomes in terms of congenital malformations of various first and second generation antihistamines (3). Based on the one study above, the authors calculated a relative risk for cetirizine of 1.2 (95% confidence interval 0.1-11.7). They concluded that in pregnancy, chlorpheniramine is the oral antihistamine of choice and that diphenhydramine should be used if a parenteral antihistamine is required (3).

A 1998 non-interventional observational cohort study described the outcomes of pregnancies in women who had been prescribed one or more of 34 newly marketed drugs by general practitioners in England (4). Data were obtained by questionnaires sent to the

C

prescribing physicians one month after the expected or possible date of delivery. In 831 (78%) of the pregnancies, a newly marketed drug was thought to have been taken during the 1st trimester with birth defects noted in 14 (2.5%) singleton births of the 557 newborns (10 sets of twins). In addition, two birth defects were observed in aborted fetuses. However, few of the aborted fetuses were examined. Cetirizine was taken during the 1st trimester in 20 pregnancies. The outcomes of these pregnancies included 4 spontaneous abortions, 1 elective abortion, and 16 normal, term infants (1 set of twins) (4). Although this study found no major birth defects, it lacked the sensitivity to identify minor anomalies because of the absence of standardized examinations. Furthermore, late-appearing major defects may also have been missed because of the timing of the questionnaires.

A 2000 publication reported the antiemetic effects of cetirizine in 60 women who were using the antihistamine (10 mg/day) for the treatment of allergies during pregnancy (5). A control group of pregnant women, matched for the use of pyridoxine (vitamin B_6) but who were not taking an antihistamine, was used for comparison. The cetirizine group had a significantly lower rate of nausea and vomiting (7% vs. 37%, $p = 0.0001$). No pregnancy outcome data were provided.

In summary, cetirizine is not an animal teratogen, and there is no evidence in human pregnancy that the antihistamine presents a significant risk to the fetus. However, the number of human pregnancy exposures is too few to adequately assess the potential risk. Although cetirizine appears unlikely to be a major human teratogen, an oral first generation agent, such as chlorpheniramine or tripelennamine, should be considered if antihistamine therapy during pregnancy (especially in the 1st trimester) is required. Cetirizine or loratadine were considered acceptable alternatives, except during the 1st trimester, if a first generation agent was not tolerated (6–8). The use of cetirizine as an antiemetic needs further study.

BREAST FEEDING SUMMARY

RECOMMENDATION: No Human Data - Probably Compatible

No published reports describing the use of cetirizine during human lactation have been located, but the manufacturer states that the antihistamine is excreted into human milk. This is consistent with the relatively low molecular weight (about 462 for the dihydrochloride salt). Retarded pup weight gain was observed when lactating mice were given an oral dose (approximately 40 times the MRHD) of cetirizine (1). Moreover, in beagle dogs, about 3% of a cetirizine dose was excreted into milk (1). The effects, if any, on a nursing infant exposed to cetirizine in milk are unknown, but sedation is a possibility.

References

1. Product information. Zyrtec. Pfizer, 2001.
2. Einarson A, Bailey B, Jung G, Spizzirri D, Baillie M, Koren G. Prospective controlled study of hydroxyzine and cetirizine in pregnancy. Ann Allergy Asthma Immunol 1997;78:183–6.
3. Schatz M, Petitti D. Antihistamines and pregnancy. Ann Allergy Asthma Immunol 1997;78:157–9.
4. Wilton LV, Pearce GL, Martin RM, Mackay FJ, Mann RD. The outcomes of pregnancy in women exposed to newly marketed drugs in general practice in England. Br J Obstet Gynaecol 1998;105:882–9.
5. Einarson A, Levichek Z, Einarson TR, Koren G. The antiemetic effect of cetirizine during pregnancy. Ann Pharmacol 2000;34:1486–7.
6. Mazzotta P, Loebstein R, Koren G. Treating allergic rhinitis in pregnancy. Safety considerations. Drug Saf 1999;20:361–75.
7. Horak F, Stubner UP. Comparative tolerability of second generation antihistamines. Drug Saf 1999;20:385–401.
8. Position statement of a joint committee of the American College of Obstetricians and Gynecologists and the American College of Allergy, Asthma and Immunology. The use of newer asthma and allergy medications during pregnancy. Ann Allergy Asthma Immunol 2000;84:475–80.

Name:	**CEVIMELINE**	Risk Factor:	C_M
Class:	**Parasympathomimetic (Cholinergic)**		

FETAL RISK SUMMARY

RECOMMENDATION: No Human Data - No Relevant Animal Data

Cevimeline is an oral cholinergic agonist indicated for the treatment of dry mouth in patients with Sjögren's syndrome.

In reproduction studies with rats, a dose, approximately 5 times the recommended human dose for a 60-kg person on a body surface area basis, given from 14 days before mating through day 7 of gestation, caused a reduction in the mean number of implantations. This effect may have been a result of maternal toxicity (1).

No studies examining the placental transfer of cevimeline have been located. The molecular weight (about 245 for the hydrated salt form) is low enough, however, that passage to the fetus should be expected.

No studies describing the use of cevimeline during human pregnancy have been located. The very limited animal data that did not include exposure during organogenesis, and the lack of any reported human pregnancy experience prevents an assessment of the risk that this drug presents to a fetus.

BREAST FEEDING SUMMARY

RECOMMENDATION: No Human Data - Potential Toxicity

No reports describing the use of cevimeline in human lactation have been located. The molecular weight (about 245 for the hydrated salt form) suggests that excretion into breast milk should be expected. Because the effects of this exposure on a nursing infant are unknown, combined with the lack of data on the amount of drug that may be in milk, women who are taking cevimeline should probably not breast-feed

Reference

1. Product information. Evoxac. Daiichi Pharmaceutical, 2001.

Name:	**CHENODIOL**	Risk Factor:	X_M
Class:	**Gastrointestinal Agent (Gallstone Solubilizing Agent)**		

FETAL RISK SUMMARY

RECOMMENDATION: Contraindicated

Chenodiol (chenodeoxycholic acid) is a naturally occurring bile acid used orally to dissolve gallstones. No reports on the use of this drug during human pregnancy have been located.

Chenodiol is not teratogenic in animals, but fetotoxicity has occurred in some species. Studies with pregnant rats, mice, and baboons did not observe congenital malformations after *in utero* exposure to the agent during organogenesis (1–3). In one study using three

C

dosage levels, dose-related hepatotoxicity was observed in dams but not in newborn rats (4). No fetal hepatotoxicity was observed in a study of rats in which the drug composed 0.25% of the maternal diet during pregnancy (5). Hepatotoxicity was observed, however, in newborn baboons and rhesus monkeys exposed to chenodiol during gestation (3,6). Extensive hemorrhagic necrosis of the adrenal glands and interstitial hemorrhage of the kidneys were also noted in the newborn rhesus monkeys (6). Theoretically, the main hepatotoxic property of chenodiol in animals is due to its principal bacterial metabolite, lithocholic acid (7). In contrast to humans that readily metabolize lithocholic acid to poorly absorbed, nontoxic compounds, animals such as rabbits, rhesus monkeys, and baboons are unable to fully form sulfate conjugates to detoxify the metabolite, and thus are susceptible to liver damage (7).

One study concluded that dihydroxy bile acids, such as chenodiol, are transferred, at least in rats, from the mother to the fetus (5). Based on the observed hepatotoxicity of this agent, the use of chenodiol is contraindicated during pregnancy.

BREAST FEEDING SUMMARY

RECOMMENDATION: No Human Data - Potential Toxicity

No data are available on the excretion of chenodiol into breast milk.

References

1. Kitao T, Kamishita S, Yoshikawa H, Sakaguchi M. Teratogenicity studies of chenodeoxycholic acid in rats. Yakuri to Chiryo 1982;10:3887–3901 as cited in Shepard TH. *Catalog of Teratogenic Agents*. 6th ed. Baltimore, MD: Johns Hopkins University Press, 1989:127.
2. Takahashi H, Miyashita T, Tozuka K. Effects of chenodeoxycholic acid, administered in the organogenetic period, on the pre- and post-natal development of rat's and mouse's offsprings. Oyo Yakuri (Pharmacometrics) 1978;15:1047–55.
3. McSherry CK, Morrissey KP, Swarm RL, May PS, Niemann WH, Glenn F. Chenodeoxycholic acid induced liver injury in pregnant and neonatal baboons. Ann Surg 1976;184:490–9.
4. Celle G, Cavanna M, Bocchini R, Robbiano L. Chenodeoxycholic acid (CDCA) versus ursodeoxycholic acid (UDCA): a comparison of their effects in pregnant rats. Arch Int Pharmacodyn Ther 1980;246:149–58.
5. Sprinkle DJ, Hassan AS, Subbiah MTR. Effect of chenodeoxycholic acid feeding during gestation in the rat on bile acid metabolism and liver morphology. Proc Soc Exp Biol Med 1984;175:386–97.
6. Heywood R, Palmer AK, Foll CV, Lee MR. Pathological changes in fetal rhesus monkey induced by oral chenodeoxycholic acid. Lancet 1973;2:1021.
7. Allan RN, Thistle JL, Hofmann AF, Carter JA. Lithocholate metabolism during chemotherapy for gallstone dissolution. 1. Serum levels of sulphated and unsulphated lithocholates. Gut 1976;17:405–12.

Name:	**CHLORAL HYDRATE**	Risk Factor:	C_M
Class:	**Sedative/Hypnotic**		

FETAL RISK SUMMARY

RECOMMENDATION: Limited Human Data - No Relevant Animal Data

No reports linking the use of chloral hydrate with congenital defects have been located. The drug has been given in labor and demonstrated to be in cord blood at concentrations similar to maternal levels (1). Sedative effects on the neonate have not been studied.

The Collaborative Perinatal Project recorded 71 1st trimester exposures to chloral hydrate (2, pp. 336–44). From this group, 8 infants with congenital defects were observed (standardized relative risk [SRR] 1.68). When only malformations with uniform rates by hospital were examined, the SRR was 2.19. Neither of these relative risks reached statistical significance. Moreover, when chloral hydrate was combined with all tranquilizers and nonbarbiturate sedatives, no association with congenital malformations was found (SRR 1.13; 95% confidence interval [CI] 0.88–1.44). For use anytime during pregnancy, 358 exposures to chloral hydrate were discovered (2, p. 438). The 9 infants with anomalies yielded a SRR of 0.98 (95% CI 0.45–1.84).

BREAST FEEDING SUMMARY

RECOMMENDATION: Limited Human Data - Probably Compatible

Chloral hydrate and its active metabolite are excreted into breast milk. Peak concentrations of about 8 μg/mL were obtained about 45 minutes after a 1.3-g rectal dose (3). Only trace amounts are detectable after 10 hours.

Mild drowsiness was observed in the nursing infant of a mother taking 1300 mg of dichloralphenazone every evening (4). The mother was also consuming chlorpromazine 100 mg three times daily. Dichloralphenazone is metabolized to trichloroethanol, the same active metabolite of chloral hydrate. Milk levels of trichloroethanol were 60%–80% of the maternal serum. Infant growth and development remained normal during the exposure and at follow-up 3 months after the drug was stopped. The American Academy of Pediatrics classifies the drug as compatible with breast-feeding (5).

References

1. Bernstine JB, Meyer AE, Hayman HB. Maternal and fetal blood estimation following the administration of chloral hydrate during labor. J Obstet Gynecol Br Emp 1954;61:683–5.
2. Heinonen OP, Slone D, Shapiro S. *Birth Defects and Drugs in Pregnancy*. Littleton, MA: Publishing Sciences Group, 1977.
3. Bernstine JB, Meyer AE, Bernstine RL. Maternal blood and breast milk estimation following the administration of chloral hydrate during the puerperium. J Obstet Gynecol Br Emp 1956;63:228–31.
4. Lacey JH. Dichloralphenazone and breast milk. Br Med J 1971;4:684.
5. Committee on Drugs, American Academy of Pediatrics. The transfer of drugs and other chemicals into human milk. Pediatrics 2001;108:776–89.

Name:	**CHLORAMBUCIL**	Risk Factor:	**D_M**
Class:	**Antineoplastic**		

FETAL RISK SUMMARY

RECOMMENDATION: Contraindicated - 1st Trimester

The use of the alkylating agent, chlorambucil, during pregnancy has resulted in both normal and deformed infants (1–5). Two reports observed unilateral agenesis of the left kidney and ureter in male fetuses following 1st trimester exposure to chlorambucil (3,4). Similar defects have been found in animals exposed to the drug (6). In a third case, a pregnant patient was treated with chlorambucil at the 10th week of gestation (5). A full-term infant was delivered, but died 3 days later of multiple cardiovascular anomalies.

Chlorambucil is mutagenic as well as carcinogenic (7–11). These effects have not been reported in newborns following *in utero* exposure. Data from one review indicated that 40% of the infants exposed to anticancer drugs were of low birth weight (12). Long-term studies of growth and mental development in offspring exposed to chlorambucil during the 2nd trimester, the period of neuroblast multiplication, have not been conducted (13).

Amenorrhea and reversible azoospermia with high doses have been reported (14–18). Long-term follow-up of menstrual and reproductive function in women treated with various antineoplastic agents was reported in 1988 (18). Only two of the 40 women studied, however, may have been exposed to chlorambucil (see Cyclophosphamide).

C

Occupational exposure of the mother to antineoplastic agents during pregnancy may present a risk to the fetus. A position statement from the National Study Commission on Cytotoxic Exposure and a research article involving some antineoplastic agents are presented in the monograph for cyclophosphamide (see Cyclophosphamide).

BREAST FEEDING SUMMARY

RECOMMENDATION: Contraindicated

No reports describing the use of chlorambucil during lactation have been located. Because of the potential for severe adverse effects in a nursing infant, women receiving this alkylating agent should not breast-feed.

References

1. Sokal JE, Lessmann EM. Effects of cancer chemotherapeutic agents on the human fetus. JAMA 1960;172:1765–71.
2. Jacobs C, Donaldson SS, Rosenberg SA, Kaplan HS. Management of the pregnant patient with Hodgkin's disease. Ann Intern Med 1981;95:669–75.
3. Shotton D, Monie IW. Possible teratogenic effect of chlorambucil on a human fetus. JAMA 1963;186:74–5.
4. Steege JF, Caldwell DS. Renal agenesis after first trimester exposure to chlorambucil. South Med J 1980;73:1414–5.
5. Thompson J, Conklin KA. Anesthetic management of a pregnant patient with scleroderma. Anesthesiology 1983;59:69–71.
6. Monie IW. Chlorambucil-induced abnormalities of urogenital system of rat fetuses. Anat Rec 1961;139:145.
7. Lawler SD, Lele KP. Chromosomal damage induced by chlorambucil and chronic lymphocytic leukemia. Scand J Haematol 1972;9:603–12.
8. Westin J. Chromosome abnormalities after chlorambucil therapy of polycythemia vera. Scand J Haematol 1976;17:197–204.
9. Catovsky D, Galton DAG. Myelomonocytic leukaemia supervening on chronic lymphocytic leukaemia. Lancet 1971;1:478–9.
10. Rosner R. Acute leukemia as a delayed consequence of cancer chemotherapy. Cancer 1976;37:1033–6.
11. Reimer RR, Hover R, Fraumeni JF, Young RC. Acute leukemia after alkylating-agent therapy of ovarian cancer. N Engl J Med 1977;297:177–81.
12. Nicholson HO. Cytotoxic drugs in pregnancy: review of reported cases. J Obstet Gynaecol Br Commonw 1968;75:307–12.
13. Dobbing J. Pregnancy and leukaemia. Lancet 1977;1:1155.
14. Freckman HA, Fry HL, Mendex FL, Maurer ER. Chlorambucil-prednisolone therapy for disseminated breast carcinoma. JAMA 1964;189:111–4.
15. Richter P, Calamera JC, Morganfeld MC, Kierszenbaum AL, Lavieri JC, Mancinni RE. Effect of chlorambucil on spermatogenesis in the human malignant lymphoma. Cancer 1970;25:1026–30.
16. Morgenfeld MC, Goldberg V, Parisier H, Bugnard SC, Bur GE. Ovarian lesions due to cytostatic agents during the treatment of Hodgkin's disease. Surg Gynecol Obstet 1972;134:826–8.
17. Schilsky RL, Lewis BJ, Sherins RJ, Young RC. Gonadal dysfunction in patients receiving chemotherapy for cancer. Ann Intern Med 1980;93:109–14.
18. Gershenson DM. Menstrual and reproductive function after treatment with combination chemotherapy for malignant ovarian germ cell tumors. J Clin Oncol 1988;6:270–5.

Name:	**CHLORAMPHENICOL**	Risk Factor:	**C**
Class:	**Antibiotic**		

FETAL RISK SUMMARY

RECOMMENDATION: Compatible

No reports linking the use of chloramphenicol with congenital defects have been located. The drug crosses the placenta at term, producing cord serum concentrations 30%–106% of maternal levels (1,2).

The Collaborative Perinatal Project monitored 50,282 mother-child pairs, 98 of whom had 1st trimester exposure to chloramphenicol (3, pp. 297–301). For use anytime in pregnancy, 348 exposures were recorded (3, p. 435). In neither group was evidence found to suggest a relationship to large categories of major or minor malformations or to individual defects. A 1977 case report described a 14-day course of IV chloramphenicol, 2 g daily, given to a patient with typhoid fever in the 2nd trimester (4). A normal infant was delivered at term. Twenty-two patients, in various stages of gestation, were treated with chloramphenicol for acute pyelonephritis (5). No difficulties in the newborn could be associated with the antibiotic. In a controlled study, 110 patients received one to three antibiotics during the 1st trimester for a total of 589 weeks (6). Chloramphenicol was given for a total of 205 weeks. The incidence of birth defects was similar to that in controls.

A 1998 report described the use of chloramphenicol for the treatment of Rocky Mountain spotted fever in a woman at 28 weeks' gestation (7). She was treated with IV chloramphenicol (3 g/day) and ceftriaxone (2 g/day) for 1 week, followed by oral amoxicillin for 3 weeks. She eventually delivered a full-term, healthy, 3916-g infant.

Although apparently nontoxic to the fetus, chloramphenicol should be used with caution at term. Specific details were not provided, but one report claimed that cardiovascular collapse (gray syndrome) developed in babies delivered from mothers treated with chloramphenicol during the final stage of pregnancy (8). Additional reports of this severe adverse effect have not been located. It is well known that newborns exposed directly to high doses of chloramphenicol may develop the gray syndrome (9,10). Because of this risk, some authors consider the drug to be contraindicated during pregnancy (11).

BREAST FEEDING SUMMARY

RECOMMENDATION: Limited Human Data - Potential Toxicity

Chloramphenicol is excreted into breast milk. Two milk samples, separated by 24 hours in the same patient, were reported as 16 and 25 μg/mL, representing milk:plasma ratios of 0.51 and 0.61, respectively (12). Both active drug and inactive metabolite were measured. No effect on the infant was mentioned. No infant toxicity was mentioned in a 1964 report that found peak levels occurring in milk 1–3 hours after a single 1-g oral dose (13). In a similar study, continuous excretion of chloramphenicol into breast milk was established after the 1st day of therapy (14). Minimum and maximum milk concentrations were determined for five patients receiving 250 mg orally every 6 hours (0.54 and 2.84 μg/mL) and for five patients receiving 500 mg orally every 6 hours (1.75 and 6.10 μg/mL). No infant data were given.

The safety of maternal chloramphenicol consumption and breast-feeding is unknown. The American Academy of Pediatrics classifies the antibiotic as an agent whose effect on the nursing infant is unknown but may be of concern because of the potential for idiosyncratic bone marrow suppression (15). Another publication recommended that chloramphenicol not be used in the lactating patient (16). Milk levels of this antibiotic are too low to precipitate the gray syndrome, but a theoretical risk does exist for bone marrow depression. Two other potential problems of lesser concern involve the modification of bowel flora and possible interference with the interpretation of culture results if a fever workup is required. Several adverse effects were reported in 50 breast-fed infants whose mothers were being treated with chloramphenicol, including refusal of the breast, falling asleep during feeding, intestinal gas, and heavy vomiting after feeding (17).

C

References

1. Scott WC, Warner RF. Placental transfer of chloramphenicol (Chloromycetin). JAMA 1950;142:1331–2.
2. Ross S, Burke RG, Sites J, Rice EC, Washington JA. Placental transmission of chloramphenicol (Chloromycetin). JAMA 1950;142:1361.
3. Heinonen OP, Slone D, Shapiro S. *Birth Defects and Drugs in Pregnancy*. Littleton, MA: Publishing Sciences Group, 1977.
4. Schiffman P, Samet CM, Fox L, Neimand KM, Rosenberg ST. Typhoid fever in pregnancy—with probable typhoid hepatitis. N Y State J Med 1977;77:1778–9.
5. Cunningham FG, Morris GB, Mickal A. Acute pyelonephritis of pregnancy: a clinical review. Obstet Gynecol 1973;42:112–7.
6. Ravid R, Roaff R. On the possible teratogenicity of antibiotic drugs administered during pregnancy. In Klingberg MA, Abramovici H, Chemke J, eds. *Drugs and Fetal Development*. New York, NY: Plenum Press, 1972:505–10.
7. Markley KC, Levine AB, Chan Y. Rocky Mountain spotted fever in pregnancy. Obstet Gynecol 1998;91:860.
8. Oberheuser F. Praktische Erfahrungen mit Medikamenten in der Schwangerschaft. Therapiewoche 1971;31:2200. As reported in Manten A. Antibiotic drugs. In Dukes MNG, ed. *Meyler's Side Effects of Drugs*. Volume VIII. New York, NY: American Elsevier, 1975:604.
9. Sutherland JM. Fatal cardiovascular collapse of infants receiving large amounts of chloramphenicol. J Dis Child 1959;97:761–7.
10. Weiss CV, Glazko AJ, Weston JK. Chloramphenicol in the newborn infant. A physiologic explanation of its toxicity when given in excessive doses. N Engl J Med 1960;262:787–94.
11. Schwarz RH, Crombleholme WR. Antibiotics in pregnancy. South Med J 1979;72:1315–8.
12. Smadel JE, Woodward TE,Ley HL Jr, Lewthwaite R. Chloramphenicol (Chloromycetin) in the treatment of Tsutsugamushi disease (scrub typhus). J Clin Invest 1949;28:1196–215.
13. Prochazka J, Havelka J, Hejzlar M. Excretion of chloramphenicol by human milk. Cas Lek Cesk 1964; 103:378–80.
14. Havelka J, Hejzlar M, Popov V, Viktorinova D, Prochazka J. Excretion of chloramphenicol in human milk. Chemotherapy 1968;13:204–11.
15. Committee on Drugs, American Academy of Pediatrics. The transfer of drugs and other chemicals into human milk. Pediatrics 2001;108:776–89.
16. Anonymous. Update: drugs in breast milk. Med Lett Drugs Ther 1979;21:21–4.
17. Havelka J, Frankova A. Contribution to the question of side effects of chloramphenicol therapy in newborns. Cesk Pediatr 1972;21:31–3.

Name:	**CHLORCYCLIZINE**	Risk Factor:	**C**
Class:	**Antihistamine**		

No data are available. See Meclizine for representative agent in this class.

Name:	**CHLORDIAZEPOXIDE**	Risk Factor:	**D**
Class:	**Sedative**		

FETAL RISK SUMMARY

RECOMMENDATION: Human Data Suggest Risk in 1st and 3rd Trimesters

Chlordiazepoxide is a benzodiazepine (see also Diazepam). The drug has antianxiety, sedative, appetite-stimulating, and weak analgesic actions (1).

No teratogenic effects were observed in rats given doses of 10–80 mg/kg/day through one or two matings (1). At 100 mg/kg/day, maternal toxicity (decreased interest in mating and nursing) and marked decreases in offspring viability and body weight were attributed to sedative effects of the drug (1). Moreover, at this dose, one newborn in each of two matings had major skeletal abnormalities.

In a study evaluating 19,044 live births, the use of chlordiazepoxide was associated with a greater than 4-fold increase in severe congenital anomalies (2). In 172 patients exposed to the drug during the first 42 days of gestation, the following defects were observed: mental deficiency, spastic diplegia and deafness, microcephaly and retardation, duodenal atresia, and Meckel's diverticulum (2). Although not statistically significant, an increased fetal death rate was also found with maternal chlordiazepoxide ingestion (2). A survey of 390 infants with congenital heart disease matched with 1,254 normal infants found a higher rate of exposure to several drugs, including chlordiazepoxide, in the offspring with defects (3).

In contrast, other studies have not confirmed a relationship with increased defects or mortality (4–8). The Collaborative Perinatal Project monitored 50,282 mother-child pairs, 257 of whom were exposed in the 1st trimester to chlordiazepoxide (5,8). No association with large classes of malformations or to individual defects was found.

In a surveillance study of Michigan Medicaid recipients conducted between 1985 and 1992 involving 229,101 completed pregnancies, 788 newborns had been exposed to chlordiazepoxide during the 1st trimester (F. Rosa, personal communication, FDA, 1993). A total of 44 (5.6%) major birth defects were observed (34 expected). Specific data were available for six defect categories, including (observed/expected) 10/7 cardiovascular defects, 2/1 oral clefts, 0/0.5 spina bifida, 3/2 polydactyly, 1/1 limb reduction defects, and 2/2 hypospadias. These data do not support an association between the drug and congenital defects.

A 1992 study reported on heavy benzodiazepine exposure during pregnancy from Michigan Medicaid data collected during 1980 to 1983 (9). Of the 2048 women, from a total sample of 104,339, who had received benzodiazepines, 80 had received 10 or more prescriptions for these agents. The records of these 80 women indicated frequent alcohol and substance abuse. Their pregnancy outcomes were 3 intrauterine deaths, 2 neonatal deaths in infants with congenital malformations, and 64 survivors. The outcome for 11 infants was unknown. Six of the surviving infants had diagnoses consistent with congenital defects (9). The investigators concluded that the high rate of congenital anomalies was suggestive of multiple alcohol and substance abuse and may not have been related to benzodiazepine exposure (9).

Neonatal withdrawal consisting of severe tremulousness and irritability has been attributed to maternal use of chlordiazepoxide (10). The onset of withdrawal symptoms occurred on the 26th day of life. Chlordiazepoxide readily crosses the placenta at term in an approximate 1:1 ratio (11–13). The drug has been used to reduce pain during labor, but the maternal benefit was not significant (14,15). Marked depression was observed in three infants whose mothers received chlordiazepoxide within a few hours of delivery (13). The infants were unresponsive, hypotonic, hypothermic, and fed poorly. Hypotonicity persisted for up to a week. Other studies have not seen depression (11,12).

BREAST FEEDING SUMMARY

RECOMMENDATION: No Human Data - Potential Toxicity

No reports describing the use of chlordiazepoxide during human lactation have been located. The molecular weight (about 300) is low enough, however, that passage into milk should be expected. Moreover, other benzodiazepines are excreted into milk and have produced adverse effects in nursing infants (see Diazepam). Because of the potential for drug accumulation and toxicity in nursing infants, chlordiazepoxide should be avoided during breast-feeding.

C

References

1. Product information. Librium. ICN Pharmaceuticals, 2000.
2. Milkovich L, van den Berg BJ. Effects of prenatal meprobamate and chlordiazepoxide hydrochloride on human embryonic and fetal development. N Engl J Med 1974;291:1268–71.
3. Rothman KJ, Fyler DC, Golblatt A, Kreidberg MB. Exogenous hormones and other drug exposures of children with congenital heart disease. Am J Epidemiol 1979;109:433–9.
4. Crombie DL, Pinsent RJ, Fleming DM, Rumeau-Rouguette C, Goujard J, Huel G. Fetal effects of tranquilizers in pregnancy. N Engl J Med 1975;293:198–9.
5. Hartz SC, Heinonen OP, Shapiro S, Siskind V, Slone D. Antenatal exposure to meprobamate and chlordiazepoxide in relation to malformations, mental development, and childhood mortality. N Engl J Med 1975;292:726–8.
6. Bracken MB, Holford TR. Exposure to prescribed drugs in pregnancy and association with congenital malformations. Obstet Gynecol 1981;58:336–44.
7. Committee on Drugs, American Academy of Pediatrics. Psychotropic drugs in pregnancy and lactation. Pediatrics 1982;69:241–4.
8. Heinonen OP, Slone D, Shapiro S. *Birth Defects and Drugs in Pregnancy*. Littleton, MA: Publishing Sciences Group, 1977:336–7.
9. Bergman U, Rosa FW, Baum C, Wiholm B-E, Faich GA. Effects of exposure to benzodiazepine during fetal life. Lancet 1992;340:694–6.
10. Athinarayanan P, Pierog SH, Nigam SK, Glass L. Chlordiazepoxide withdrawal in the neonate. Am J Obstet Gynecol 1976;124:212–3.
11. Decancq HG Jr, Bosco JR,Townsend EH Jr. Chlordiazepoxide in labour: its effect on the newborn infant. J Pediatr 1965;67:836–40.
12. Mark PM, Hamel J. Librium for patients in labor. Obstet Gynecol 1968;32:188–94.
13. Stirrat GM, Edington PT, Berry DJ. Transplacental passage of chlordiazepoxide. Br Med J 1974;2:729.
14. Duckman S, Spina T, Attardi M, Meyer A. Double-blind study of chlordiazepoxide in obstetrics. Obstet Gynecol 1964;24:601–5.
15. Kanto JH. Use of benzodiazepines during pregnancy, labour and lactation, with particular reference to pharmacokinetic considerations. Drugs 1982;23:354–80.

Name:	**CHLORHEXIDINE**	Risk Factor:	**B**
Class:	**Anti-infective**		

FETAL RISK SUMMARY

RECOMMENDATION: Compatible

Chlorhexidine, a bisbiguanide antiseptic and disinfectant, is effective against most bacteria, and against some fungi and viruses (including HIV). In addition to its topical use on the skin and intravaginally, it has been used for gingivitis and the prevention of dental plaque. Chlorhexidine has also been used as a spermicide (1). No adverse fetal effects were observed in pregnant rats administered chlorhexidine by gastric intubation on days 6 through 15 of gestation (2).

A number of studies have documented the safety and possible effectiveness of vaginal disinfection with chlorhexidine prior to delivery, primarily to prevent colonization of newborns with group B streptococci (3–15). Application to the groin and perineum, to the abdomen prior to cesarean section, and whole body washing have also been effective in preventing fetal and maternal infection (3,16–19). However, two double-blinded, placebo-controlled, randomized studies published in 1997, one using a single intravaginal wash with 20 mL of a 0.4% chlorhexidine solution (20) and the other a 200 mL vaginal irrigation with a 0.2% solution (21), with both groups in active labor, did not find a significant reduction in maternal infection rates compared with sterile water or saline. No adverse effects in the newborns were observed.

One author, hypothesizing an etiological connection between sudden infant death syndrome (SIDS) and toxigenic *Escherichia coli* or *Chlamydia* species, has suggested that decontamination of the birth canal with chlorhexidine during labor might reduce infant mortality from this disease (22), but a temporal relationship is speculative. In contrast to the real and theoretical benefits realized by the newborn from maternal chlorhexidine use, a single vaginal washing with a 0.4% chlorhexidine solution did not decrease the incidence of intra-amniotic infection or endometritis (23).

In one study involving nonpregnant women, swabbing of the entire vagina for 1 minute with gauze sponges soaked in 4% chlorhexidine gluconate did not result in detectable blood concentrations (sensitivity 0.1 μg/mL) of the agent (24). A second study, using a method ten times more sensitive (sensitivity: 0.01 μg/mL), was able to detect chlorhexidine in maternal blood from 34 of 96 women following vaginal washing with a 0.2% solution (25). Mean blood chlorhexidine concentrations obtained using two different methods of washing were 0.0146 μg/mL and 0.0104 μg/mL, respectively (range 0.01–0.083 μg/mL). No accumulation of chlorhexidine in maternal blood was observed after a second vaginal washing at 6 hours in 14 patients or after a third washing, 6 hours later, in 3. The disinfectant was not detected in 62 of the women.

One writer has cautioned that the potential long-term effects (not specified) in the newborn from exposure to respiratory and other epithelial surfaces following vaginal use of chlorhexidine during labor have not been investigated (26). However, no reports of adverse effects in newborns have been reported even though chlorhexidine is used commonly during labor and in the neonate. Moreover, only very small amounts of disinfectant reach the maternal circulation and, presumably, the fetus. Although the agent is an effective disinfectant, single vaginal applications of chlorhexidine solutions do not appear to offer any advantage over sterile water or saline in the prevention of maternal infections during labor or in the postpartum period.

BREAST FEEDING SUMMARY

RECOMMENDATION: No Human Data - Probably Compatible

No reports describing the excretion of chlorhexidine into milk have been located. The presence of the drug in breast milk is probably clinically insignificant because of the very small amounts absorbed into the maternal circulation following vaginal washing. As a general precaution, the mother's nipples should be rinsed thoroughly with water if chlorhexidine is used on them as a disinfectant, even though absorption of the agent from the gastrointestinal tract is poor.

References

1. Editorial. Multipurpose spermicides. Lancet 1992;340:211–3.
2. Gilman MR, De Salva SJ. Teratology studies of benzethonium chloride, cetyl pyridinium chloride and chlorhexidine in rats (Abstract). Toxicol Appl Pharmacol 1979;48:A35.
3. Vorherr H, Ulrich JA, Messer RH, Hurwitz EB. Antimicrobial effect of chlorhexidine on bacteria of groin, perineum and vagina. J Reprod Med 1980;24:153–7.
4. Christensen KK, Christensen P, Dykes AK, Kahlmeter G, Kurl DN, Linden V. Chlorhexidine for prevention of neonatal colonization with group B streptococci. I. In vitro effect of chlorhexidine on group B streptococci. Eur J Obstet Gynecol Reprod Biol 1983;16:157–65.
5. Dykes AK, Christensen KK, Christensen P, Kahlmeter G. Chlorhexidine for prevention of neonatal colonization with group B streptococci. II. Chlorhexidine concentrations and recovery of group B streptococci following vaginal washing in pregnant women. Eur J Obstet Gynecol Reprod Biol 1983;16:167–72.
6. Christensen KK, Christensen P. Chlorhexidine for prevention of neonatal colonization with GBS. Antibiot Chemother 1985;35:296–302.
7. Christensen KK, Christensen P, Dykes AK, Kahlmeter G. Chlorhexidine for prevention of neonatal colonization with group B streptococci. III. Effect of vaginal washing with chlorhexidine before rupture of the membranes. Eur J Obstet Gynecol Reprod Biol 1985;19:231–6.
8. Christensen KK, Dykes AK, Christensen P. Reduced colonization of newborns with group B streptococci following washing of the birth canal with chlorhexidine. J Perinat Med 1985;13:239–43.
9. Easmon CSF. Group B streptococcus. Infect Control 1986;7(Suppl 2):135–7.
10. Dykes AK, Christensen KK, Christensen P. Chlorhexidine for prevention of neonatal colonization with

C

group B streptococci. IV. Depressed puerperal carriage following vaginal washing with chlorhexidine during labour. Eur J Obstet Gynecol Reprod Biol 1987;24:293–7.
11. Burman LG, Christensen P, Christensen K, Fryklund B, Helgesson AM, Svenningsen NW, Tullus K, and the Swedish Chlorhexidene Study Group. Prevention of excess neonatal morbidity associated with group B streptococci by vaginal chlorhexidine disinfection during labour. Lancet 1992;340:65–9.
12. Burman LG, Tullus K. Vaginal chlorhexidine disinfection during labour. Lancet 1992;340:791–2.
13. Lindemann R, Henrichsen T, Svenningsen L, Hjelle K. Vaginal chlorhexidine disinfection during labour. Lancet 1992;340:792.
14. Henrichsen T, Lindemann R, Svenningsen L, Hjelle K. Prevention of neonatal infections by vaginal chlorhexidine disinfection during labour. Acta Paediatr 1994; 83:923–6.
15. Kollée LAA, Speyer I, van Kuijck MAP, Koopman R, Dony JM, Bakker JH, Wintermans RGF. Prevention of group B streptococci transmission during delivery by vaginal application of chlorhexidine gel. Eur J Obstet Gynecol Reprod Biol 1989;31:47–51.
16. Vorherr H, Vorherr UF, Moss JC. Comparative effectiveness of chlorhexidine, povidone-iodine, and hexachlorophene on the bacteria of the perineum and groin of pregnant women. Am J Infect Control 1988;16:178–81.
17. Brown TR, Ehrlich CE, Stehman FB, Golichowski AM, Madura JA, Eitzen HE. A clinical evaluation of chlorhexidine gluconate spray as compared with iodophor scrub for preoperative skin preparation. Surg Gynecol Obstet 1984;158:363–6.
18. Sanderson PJ, Haji TC. Transfer of group B streptococci from mothers to neonates: effect of whole body washing of mothers with chlorhexidine. J Hosp Infect 1985;6:257–64.
19. Frost L, Pedersen M, Seiersen E. Changes in hygienic procedures reduce infection following caesarean section. J Hosp Infect 1989;13:143–8.
20. Sweeten KM, Ericksen NL, Blanco JD. Chlorhexidine versus sterile water vaginal wash during labor to prevent peripartum infection. Am J Obstet Gynecol 1997;176:426–30.
21. Rouse DJ, Hauth JC, Andrews WW, Mills BB, Maher JE. Chlorhexidine vaginal irrigation for the prevention of peripartal infection: a placebo-controlled randomized clinical trial. Am J Obstet Gynecol 1997;176:617–22.
22. Elfast RA. Chlorhexidine prophylaxis at labor. Prevention of sudden infant death? Lakartidningen 1993;90:3771–2.
23. Eriksen NL, Blanco JD. Chlorhexidine versus sterile water vaginal wash during labor to prevent peripartum infection (Abstract). Am J Obstet Gynecol 1995;172:304.
24. Vorherr H, Vorherr UF, Mehta P, Ulrich JA, Messer RH. Antimicrobial effect of chlorhexidine and povidone-iodine on vaginal bacteria. J Infect 1984;8:195–9.
25. Nilsson G, Larsson L, Christensen KK, Christensen P, Dykes AK. Chlorhexidine for prevention of neonatal colonization with group B streptococci. V. Chlorhexidine concentrations in blood following vaginal washing during delivery. Eur J Obstet Gynecol Reprod Biol 1989;31:221–6.
26. Feldman R, van Oppen C, Noorduyn A. Vaginal chlorhexidine disinfection during labour. Lancet 1992;340:791.

Name: **CHLOROQUINE** Risk Factor: **C**

Class: **Antimalarial/Amebicide**

FETAL RISK SUMMARY

RECOMMENDATION: Compatible - Maternal Benefit >> Embryo/Fetal Risk

Chloroquine is the drug of choice for the prophylaxis and treatment of sensitive malaria species during pregnancy (1–4). The drug is also indicated for the treatment of extraintestinal invasion by the protozoan parasite *Entamoeba histolytica* (5). Chloroquine is generally considered safe for these purposes by most authorities (1–7). However, the antimalarial is embryotoxic and teratogenic in rats given a 1000-mg/kg dose, causing embryonic death in 27% and producing anophthalmia and microphthalmia in 47% of the surviving fetuses (8).

Chloroquine crosses the placenta to the fetus with fetal concentrations approximating those in the mother (9). In seven mothers at term in the second stage of labor, chloroquine, 5 mg/kg IM, produced mean levels in maternal blood, cord venous blood, and cord arterial blood that were all about 0.7 μg/mL. The time interval from administration to sampling averaged 5.3 hours (range 2.4–10.5 hours). In the pregnant monkey, an ^{125}I-labeled chloroquine analogue crossed the placenta and concentrated in the fetal adrenal cortex and retina (10). Chloroquine rapidly crosses the placenta in pregnant mice and selectively accumulates in the melanin structures of the fetal eyes (11). The drug was retained in the ocular structures for 5 months after elimination from the rest of the body.

The risks of complications from malarial infection occurring during pregnancy are increased, especially in women not living in endemic areas (i.e., nonimmune women) (12–14). Infection is associated with a number of severe maternal and fetal outcomes, including anemia, abortion, stillbirth, prematurity, low birth weight, fetal distress, and congenital malaria (12–14). However, it is not yet clear if all of these are related to malarial infection (13). For example, prevention of low birth weight and the resulting risk of infant mortality by antimalarial chemoprophylaxis has not yet been proven (13). Increased maternal morbidity and mortality includes adult respiratory distress syndrome, massive hemolysis, disseminated intravascular coagulation, acute renal failure, and hypoglycemia, with the latter symptom occurring in up to 50% of women in whom quinine is used (14). Severe *Plasmodium falciparum* malaria in pregnant nonimmune women has a poor prognosis and may be associated with asymptomatic uterine contractions, intrauterine growth retardation, fetal tachycardia, fetal distress, hypoglycemia, and placental insufficiency because of intense parasitization (13). Because of the severity of this disease in pregnancy, chemoprophylaxis is recommended for women of child-bearing age traveling in areas where malaria is present (12–14).

Congenital malaria may occur in up to 10% of infants born to mothers not living in endemic areas (14). In most cases, clinical malaria manifests 3–8 weeks after birth, probably as a result of exchange of infected maternal erythrocytes at birth, and is characterized by fever, hepatosplenomegaly, jaundice, and thrombocytopenia (14). In areas of hyperendemicity, transplacental passage of maternal IgG may protect the newborn against development of clinical malaria (14).

Congenital defects have been reported in three infants delivered from one mother who was treated during pregnancy with 250–500 mg/day of chloroquine for discoid lupus erythematosus (15). This woman also had two normal infants who had not been exposed to chloroquine during gestation, and one normal infant who had been exposed. Anomalies in the three infants were Wilms' tumor at age 4 years, left-sided hemihypertrophy (one infant), and cochleovestibular paresis (two infants).

A 1985 report summarized the results of 169 infants exposed *in utero* to 300 mg of chloroquine base once weekly throughout pregnancy (16). The control group consisted of 454 nonexposed infants. Two infants (1.2%) in the study group had anomalies (tetralogy of Fallot and congenital hypothyroidism) compared to four control infants who had defects (0.9%). Based on these data, the authors concluded that chloroquine is not a major teratogen, but a small increase in birth defects could not be excluded (16).

BREAST FEEDING SUMMARY

RECOMMENDATION: Compatible

Chloroquine is excreted into breast milk (9,17). When chloroquine, 5 mg/kg intramuscular, was administered to six nursing mothers 17 days postpartum, mean milk and serum concentrations 2 hours later were 0.227 μg/mL (range 0.163–0.319 μg/mL) and 0.648 μg/mL (range 0.46–0.95 μg/mL), respectively. The mean milk:blood ratio was 0.358

C

(range 0.268–0.462). Based on an average consumption of 500 mL of milk/day, an infant would have received about 114 μg/day of chloroquine, an amount considered safe by the investigators (9). In an earlier study, three women were given a single dose of 600 mg of chloroquine 2–5 days postpartum (17). Serum and milk samples were collected up to 227 hours after administration. The milk:plasma area under the concentration time curve ratios for chloroquine and the principal metabolite, desethylchloroquine, ranged from 1.96 to 4.26 and from 0.54 to 3.89, respectively. Based on a daily milk intake of 1000 mL, the nursing infants would have ingested between 2.2% and 4.2% of the maternal doses over a 9-day period (17).

Although the amounts of chloroquine excreted into milk are not considered to be harmful to a nursing infant, they are insufficient to provide adequate protection against malaria (12). The American Academy of Pediatrics classifies chloroquine as compatible with breast-feeding (18).

References

1. Gilles HM, Lawson JB, Sibelas M, Voller A, Allan N. Malaria, anaemia and pregnancy. Ann Trop Med Parasitol 1969;63:245–63.
2. Diro M, Beydoun SN. Malaria in pregnancy. South Med J 1982;75:959–62.
3. Anonymous. Malaria in pregnancy. Lancet 1983;2: 84–5.
4. Strang A, Lachman E, Pitsoe SB, Marszalek A, Philpott RH. Malaria in pregnancy with fatal complications: case report. Br J Obstet Gynaecol 1984;91:399–403.
5. D'Alauro F, Lee RV, Pao-In K, Khairallah M. Intestinal parasites and pregnancy. Obstet Gynecol 1985;66:639–43.
6. Ross JB, Garatsos S. Absence of chloroquine induced ototoxicity in a fetus. Arch Dermatol 1974;109:573.
7. Lewis R, Lauresen NJ, Birnbaum S. Malaria associated with pregnancy. Obstet Gynecol 1973;42:698–700.
8. Udalova LD. The effect of chloroquine on the embryonal development of rats. Pharmacol Toxicol (Russian) 1967;2:226–8. As cited in Shepard TH. *Catalog of Teratogenic Agents*. 6th ed. Baltimore, MD: Johns Hopkins University Press, 1989;140–1.
9. Akintonwa A, Gbajumo SA, Biola Mabadeje AF. Placental and milk transfer of chloroquine in humans. Ther Drug Monit 1988;10:147–9.
10. Dencker L, Lindquist NG, Ulberg S. Distribution of an I-125 labeled chloroquine analogue in a pregnant Macaca monkey. Toxicology 1975;5:255–64. As cited in Shepard TH. *Catalog of Teratogenic Agents*. 6th ed. Baltimore, MD: Johns Hopkins University Press, 1989;140–1.
11. Product information. Aralen. Sanofi Pharmaceuticals, 2000.
12. CDC. Recommendations for the prevention of malaria among travelers. MMWR 1990;39:1–10.
13. World Health Organization. Practical chemotherapy of malaria. WHO Tech Rep Ser 1990;805:1–141.
14. Subramanian D,Moise KJ Jr,White AC Jr. Imported malaria in pregnancy: report of four cases and review of management. Clin Infect Dis 1992;15:408–13.
15. Hart CW, Naunton RF. The ototoxicity of chloroquine phosphate. Arch Otolaryngol 1964;80:407–12.
16. Wolfe MS, Cordero JF. Safety of chloroquine in chemosuppression of malaria during pregnancy. Br Med J 1985;290:1466–7.
17. Edstein MD, Veenendaal JR, Newman K, Hyslop R. Excretion of chloroquine, dapsone and pyrimethamine in human milk. Br J Clin Pharmacol 1986;22: 733–5.
18. Committee on Drugs, American Academy of Pediatrics. The transfer of drugs and other chemicals into human milk. Pediatrics 2001;108:776–89.

Name: **CHLOROTHIAZIDE** Risk Factor: **C_M***
Class: **Diuretic**

FETAL RISK SUMMARY

RECOMMENDATION: Compatible

Chlorothiazide is a member of the thiazide group of diuretics. The information in this monograph applies to all members of the group, including the pharmacologically and structurally related diuretics, chlorthalidone, indapamide, metolazone, and quinethazone.

Reproduction studies in mice (500 mg/kg/day), rats (60 mg/kg/day), and rabbits (50 mg/kg/day) revealed no external malformations or growth impairment, and no effect on fetal survival (1). However, these studies did not include a thorough examination for visceral anomalies and skeletal defects (1).

Data from published reports indicate that thiazide and related diuretics are infrequently administered during the 1st trimester. In the past, when these drugs were routinely given to prevent or treat toxemia, therapy was usually begun in the 2nd or 3rd trimester and adverse effects in the fetus were rare (2–11). No increases in the incidence of congenital defects were discovered, and thiazides were considered nonteratogenic (12–15).

In contrast, the Collaborative Perinatal Project monitored 50,282 mother-child pairs, 233 of whom were exposed in the 1st trimester to thiazide or related diuretics (16, pp. 371–373). All of the mothers had cardiovascular disorders, which makes interpretation of the data difficult. However, an increased risk for malformations was found for chlorthalidone (20 patients) and miscellaneous thiazide diuretics (35 patients, excluding chlorothiazide and hydrochlorothiazide). For use anytime during pregnancy, 17,492 exposures were recorded and only polythiazide showed a slight increase in risk (16, p. 441). The statistical significance of these findings is unknown and independent confirmation is required.

In a surveillance study of Michigan Medicaid recipients conducted between 1985 and 1992 involving 229,101 completed pregnancies, a number of newborns had been exposed to this class of diuretics during the 1st trimester: 20 (chlorothiazide), 48 (chlorthalidone), and 567 (hydrochlorothiazide) (Franz Rosa, personal communication, FDA, 1993). The number of major birth defects observed, the number expected, and the incidence for each drug were 2/1/10.0%, 2/2/4.2%, and 24/22/4.2%, respectively. Specific data were available for six defect categories (observed/expected), including cardiovascular defects 0/0, 1/0.5, and 7/6; oral clefts 0/0, 0/0, and 0/1; spina bifida, 0/0, 0/0, and 0/0.5; polydactyly, 0/0, 0/0, and 1/2; limb-reduction defects 0/0, 0/0, and 0/1; and hypospadias 1/0, 0/0, and 1/1, respectively. Although the number of exposures is small for two of the diuretics, these data do not support an association between the drug and congenital defects.

Many investigators consider diuretics contraindicated in pregnancy, except for patients with heart disease or chronic hypertension, because they do not prevent or alter the course of toxemia and they may decrease placental perfusion (8,17–21). A 1984 study determined that the use of diuretics for hypertension in pregnancy prevented normal plasma volume expansion and did not change perinatal outcome (22). In 4035 patients treated for edema in the last half of the 3rd trimester (hypertensive patients were excluded), higher rates were found for induction of labor, stimulation of labor, uterine inertia, meconium staining, and perinatal mortality (20). All except perinatal mortality were statistically significant compared with 13,103 controls. In another study, a decrease in endocrine function of the placenta as measured by placental clearance of estradiol was found in three patients treated with hydrochlorothiazide (23).

Chlorothiazide readily crosses the placenta at term, and fetal serum levels may equal those of the mother (24). In 10 women following 2 weeks of hydrochlorothiazide, 50 mg/day, the cord:maternal plasma ratio determined 2–13 hours after the last dose ranged from 0.10 to 0.80 (25). Chlorthalidone also crosses the placenta (26). Other diuretics probably cross to the fetus in similar amounts, although specific data are lacking.

Thiazides are considered mildly diabetogenic because they can induce hyperglycemia (18). Several investigators have noted this effect in pregnant patients treated with thiazides (27–30). Other studies have failed to show maternal hyperglycemia (31,32). Although apparently a low risk, newborns exposed to thiazide diuretics near term should be observed closely for symptoms of hypoglycemia resulting from maternal hyperglycemia (30).

Neonatal thrombocytopenia has been reported following the use near term of chlorothiazide, hydrochlorothiazide, and methyclothiazide (15,27,33–38). Other studies have not found a relationship between thiazide diuretics and platelet counts (39,40). The positive reports involve only 11 patients; however, although the numbers are small, 2 of the affected infants died (27,34). The mechanism of the thrombocytopenia is unknown, but the transfer of antiplatelet antibody from the mother to the fetus has been demonstrated (38). Thiazide-induced hemolytic anemia in 2 newborns was described in 1964 following the use of chlorothiazide and bendroflumethiazide at term (33). Thiazide diuretics may induce severe electrolyte imbalances in the mother's serum, in amniotic fluid, and in the newborn (41–43). In one case, a stillborn fetus was attributed to electrolyte imbalance and/or maternal hypotension (41). Two hypotonic newborns were discovered to be hyponatremic, a condition believed to have resulted from maternal diuretic therapy (42). Fetal bradycardia, 65–70 beats/minute, was shown to be secondary to chlorothiazide-induced maternal hypokalemia (43). In a 1963 study, no relationship was found between neonatal jaundice and chlorothiazide (44). Maternal and fetal deaths in two cases of acute hemorrhagic pancreatitis were attributed to the use of chlorothiazide in the 2nd and 3rd trimesters (45).

In summary, the published experience with 1st trimester use of thiazides and related diuretics does not indicate that these agents are teratogenic. One large study (the Collaborative Perinatal Project) did find an increased risk of defects when diuretics were used during the 1st trimester in women with cardiovascular disorders, but causal relationships cannot be inferred from these data without independent confirmation.

Diuretics are not recommended for the treatment of gestational hypertension because of the maternal hypovolemia characteristic of this disease. Other risks to the fetus or newborn include hypoglycemia, thrombocytopenia, hyponatremia, hypokalemia, and death from maternal complications. Moreover, thiazide diuretics may have a direct effect on smooth muscle and inhibit labor.

[**Risk Factor D if used in gestational hypertension.*]

BREAST FEEDING SUMMARY

RECOMMENDATION: Compatible

Chlorothiazide is excreted into breast milk in low concentrations (46). Following a single, 500-mg oral dose, milk levels were less than 1 μg/mL at 1, 2, and 3 hours. The authors speculated that the risks of pharmacologic effects in nursing infants would be remote. However, it has been stated that thrombocytopenia can occur in the nursing infant if the mother is taking chlorothiazide (47). Documentation of this is needed (48). Chlorthalidone has a very low milk:plasma ratio of 0.05 (26).

In one mother taking 50 mg of hydrochlorothiazide (HCTZ) daily, peak milk levels of the drug occurred 5–10 hours after a dose and were about 25% of maternal blood concentrations (49). The mean milk concentration of HCTZ was about 80 ng/mL. An infant consuming 600 mL of milk/day would thus ingest about 50 μg of the drug, probably an insignificant amount (49). The diuretic could not be detected in the serum of the nursing

1-month-old infant, and measurements of serum electrolytes, blood glucose, and blood urea nitrogen were all normal.

Thiazide diuretics have been used to suppress lactation (50,51). However, the American Academy of Pediatrics classifies bendroflumethiazide, chlorothiazide, chlorthalidone, and hydrochlorothiazide as compatible with breast-feeding (52).

C

References

1. Product information. Diuril. Merck, 2000.
2. Finnerty FA Jr, Buchholz JH, Tuckman J. Evaluation of chlorothiazide (Diuril) in the toxemias of pregnancy. Analysis of 144 patients. JAMA 1958;166:141–4.
3. Zuspan FP, Bell JD, Barnes AC. Balance-ward and double-blind diuretic studies during pregnancy. Obstet Gynecol 1960;16:543–9.
4. Sears RT. Oral diuretics in pregnancy toxaemia. Br Med J 1960;2:148.
5. Assoli NS. Renal effects of hydrochlorothiazide in normal and toxemic pregnancy. Clin Pharmacol Ther 1960;1:48–52.
6. Tatum H, Waterman EA. The prophylactic and therapeutic use of the thiazides in pregnancy. GP 1961;24: 101–5.
7. Flowers CE, Grizzle JE, Easterling WE, Bonner OB. Chlorothiazide as a prophylaxis against toxemia of pregnancy. Am J Obstet Gynecol 1962;84:919–29.
8. Weseley AC, Douglas GW. Continuous use of chlorothiazide for prevention of toxemia of pregnancy. Obstet Gynecol 1962;19:355–8.
9. Finnerty FA Jr. How to treat toxemia of pregnancy. GP 1963;27:116–21.
10. Fallis NE, Plauche WC, Mosey LM, Langford HG. Thiazide versus placebo in prophylaxis of toxemia of pregnancy in primigravid patients. Am J Obstet Gynecol 1964;88:502–4.
11. Landesman R, Aguero O, Wilson K, LaRussa R, Campbell W, Penaloza O. The prophylactic use of chlorthalidone, a sulfonamide diuretic, in pregnancy. J Obstet Gynaecol Br Commonw 1965;72:1004–10.
12. Cuadros A, Tatum H. The prophylactic and therapeutic use of bendroflumethiazide in pregnancy. Am J Obstet Gynecol 1964;89:891–7.
13. Finnerty FA Jr, Bepko FJ Jr. Lowering the perinatal mortality and the prematurity rate. The value of prophylactic thiazides in juveniles. JAMA 1966;195:429–32.
14. Kraus GW, Marchese JR, Yen SSC. Prophylactic use of hydrochlorothiazide in pregnancy. JAMA 1966;198: 1150–4.
15. Gray MJ. Use and abuse of thiazides in pregnancy. Clin Obstet Gynecol 1968;11:568–78.
16. Heinonen OP, Slone D, Shapiro S. *Birth Defects and Drugs in Pregnancy*. Littleton, MA: Publishing Sciences Group, 1977.
17. Watt JD, Philipp EE. Oral diuretics in pregnancy toxemia. Br Med J 1960;1:1807.
18. Pitkin RM, Kaminetzky HA, Newton M, Pritchard JA. Maternal nutrition: a selective review of clinical topics. Obstet Gynecol 1972;40:773–85.
19. Lindheimer MD, Katz AI. Sodium and diuretics in pregnancy. N Engl J Med 1973;288:891–4.
20. Christianson R, Page EW. Diuretic drugs and pregnancy. Obstet Gynecol 1976;48:647–52.
21. Lammintausta R, Erkkola R, Eronen M. Effect of chlorothiazide treatment of renin-aldosterone system during pregnancy. Acta Obstet Gynecol Scand 1978;57:389–92.
22. Sibai BM, Grossman RA, Grossman HG. Effects of diuretics on plasma volume in pregnancies with long-term hypertension. Am J Obstet Gynecol 1984;150: 831–5.
23. Shoemaker ES, Grant NF, Madden JD, MacDonald PC. The effect of thiazide diuretics on placental function. Tex Med 1973;69:109–15.
24. Garnet J. Placental transfer of chlorothiazide. Obstet Gynecol 1963;21:123–5.
25. Beermann B, Fahraeus L, Groschinsky-Grind M, Lindstrom B. Placental transfer of hydrochlorothiazide. Gynecol Obstet Invest 1980;11:45–8.
26. Mulley BA, Parr GD, Pau WK, Rye RM, Mould JJ, Siddle NC. Placental transfer of chlorthalidone and its elimination in maternal milk. Eur J Clin Pharmacol 1978;13:129–31.
27. Menzies DN. Controlled trial of chlorothiazide in treatment of early pre-eclampsia. Br Med J 1964;1: 739–42.
28. Ladner CN, Pearson JW, Herrick CN, Harrison HE. The effect of chlorothiazide on blood glucose in the third trimester of pregnancy. Obstet Gynecol 1964;23: 555–60.
29. Goldman JA, Neri A, Ovadia J, Eckerling B, DeVries A. Effect of chlorothiazide on intravenous glucose tolerance in pregnancy. Am J Obstet Gynecol 1969;105:556–60.
30. Senior B, Slone D, Shapiro S, Mitchell AA, Heinonen OP. Benzothiadiazides and neonatal hypoglycaemia. Lancet 1976;2:377.
31. Lakin N, Zeytinoglu J, Younger M, White P. Effect of chlorothiazide on insulin requirements of pregnant diabetic women. JAMA 1960;173:353–4.
32. Esbenshade JH Jr, Smith RT. Thiazides and pregnancy: a study of carbohydrate tolerance. Am J Obstet Gynecol 1965;92:270–1.
33. Harley JD, Robin H, Robertson SEJ. Thiazide-induced neonatal haemolysis? Br Med J 1964;1:696–7.
34. Rodriguez SU, Leikin SL, Hiller MC. Neonatal thrombocytopenia associated with ante-partum administration of thiazide drugs. N Engl J Med 1964;270:881–4.
35. Leikin SL. Thiazide and neonatal thrombocytopenia. N Engl J Med 1964;271:161.
36. Prescott LF. Neonatal thrombocytopenia and thiazide drugs. Br Med J 1964;1:1438.
37. Jones JE, Reed JF Jr. Renal vein thrombosis and thrombocytopenia in the newborn infant. J Pediatr 1965;67: 681–2.
38. Karpatkin S, Strick N, Karpatkin MB, Siskind GW. Cumulative experience in the detection of antiplatelet

antibody in 234 patients with idiopathic thrombocytopenic purpura, systemic lupus erythematosus and other clinical disorders. Am J Med 1972;52:776–85.
39. Finnerty FA Jr, Assoli NS. Thiazide and neonatal thrombocytopenia. N Engl J Med 1964;271:160–1.
40. Jerkner K, Kutti J, Victoria L. Platelet counts in mothers and their newborn infants with respect to antepartum administration of oral diuretics. Acta Med Scand 1973;194:473–5.
41. Pritchard JA, Walley PJ. Severe hypokalemia due to prolonged administration of chlorothiazide during pregnancy. Am J Obstet Gynecol 1961;81:1241–4.
42. Alstatt LB. Transplacental hyponatremia in the newborn infant. J Pediatr 1965;66:985–8.
43. Anderson GG, Hanson TM. Chronic fetal bradycardia: possible association with hypokalemia. Obstet Gynecol 1974;44:896–8.
44. Crosland D, Flowers C. Chlorothiazide and its relationship to neonatal jaundice. Obstet Gynecol 1963;22:500–4.
45. Minkowitz S, Soloway HB, Hall JE, Yermakov V. Fatal hemorrhagic pancreatitis following chlorothiazide administration in pregnancy. Obstet Gynecol 1964;24:337–42.
46. Werthmann MW Jr, Krees SV. Excretion of chlorothiazide in human breast milk. J Pediatr 1972;81:781–3.
47. Anonymous. Drugs in breast milk. Med Lett Drugs Ther 1976;16:25–7.
48. Dailey JW. Anticoagulant and cardiovascular drugs. In Wilson JT, ed. *Drugs in Breast Milk*. Balgowlah, Australia: ADIS Press, 1981:61–4.
49. Miller ME, Cohn RD, Burghart PH. Hydrochlorothiazide disposition in a mother and her breast-fed infant. J Pediatr 1982;101:789–91.
50. Healy M. Suppressing lactation with oral diuretics. Lancet 1961;1:1353–4.
51. Catz CS, Giacoia GP. Drugs and breast milk. Pediatr Clin North Am 1972;19:151–66.
52. Committee on Drugs, American Academy of Pediatrics. The transfer of drugs and other chemicals into human milk. Pediatrics 2001;108:776–89.

Name: **CHLOROTRIANISENE** Risk Factor: **X_M**
Class: **Estrogenic Hormone**

FETAL RISK SUMMARY

RECOMMENDATION: Contraindicated

No data are available. Use of estrogenic hormones during pregnancy is contraindicated (see Oral Contraceptives).

BREAST FEEDING SUMMARY

RECOMMENDATION: No Human Data - Probably Compatible

See Oral Contraceptives.

Name: **CHLORPHENIRAMINE** Risk Factor: **B**
Class: **Antihistamine**

FETAL RISK SUMMARY

RECOMMENDATION: Compatible

The Collaborative Perinatal Project monitored 50,282 mother-child pairs, 1070 of whom had 1st trimester exposure to chlorpheniramine (1, pp. 322–334). For use anytime during pregnancy, 3931 exposures were recorded (1, pp. 437, 488). In neither group was evidence found to suggest a relationship to large categories of major or minor malformations. Several possible associations with individual malformations were found, but independent confirmation is required to determine the actual risk.

Polydactyly in blacks (7 cases in 272 blacks)
Gastrointestinal defects (13 cases)

Eye and ear defects (7 cases)
Inguinal hernia (22 cases)
Hydrocephaly (8 cases)
Congenital dislocation of the hip (16 cases)
Malformations of the female genitalia (6 cases)

A 1971 study found that significantly fewer infants with malformations were exposed to antihistamines in the 1st trimester as compared to controls (2). Chlorpheniramine was the sixth most commonly used antihistamine.

In a surveillance study of Michigan Medicaid recipients conducted between 1985 and 1992 involving 229,101 completed pregnancies, 61 newborns had been exposed to chlorpheniramine during the 1st trimester (F. Rosa, personal communication, FDA, 1993). Most of the exposures involved decongestant combinations including adrenergics. Two (3.3%) major birth defects were observed (three expected), including one case of polydactyly (none expected). No anomalies were observed in five other categories of defects (cardiovascular defects, oral clefts, spina bifida, limb reduction defects, and hypospadias) for which specific data were available. These data do not support an association between the drug and congenital defects.

A case of infantile malignant osteopetrosis was described in a 4-month-old boy exposed *in utero* on several occasions to Contac (chlorpheniramine, phenylpropanolamine, and belladonna alkaloids), but this is a known genetic defect (3). The boy also had a continual "stuffy" nose.

An association between exposure during the last 2 weeks of pregnancy to antihistamines in general and retrolental fibroplasia in premature infants has been reported. See Brompheniramine for details.

BREAST FEEDING SUMMARY

RECOMMENDATION: No Human Data - Probably Compatible

No data are available.

References

1. Heinonen OP, Slone D, Shapiro S. *Birth Defects and Drugs in Pregnancy*. Littleton, MA: Publishing Sciences Group, 1977.
2. Nelson MM, Forfar JO. Associations between drugs administered during pregnancy and congenital abnormalities of the fetus. Br Med J 1971;1:523–7.
3. Golbus MS, Koerper MA, Hall BD. Failure to diagnose osteopetrosis *in utero*. Lancet 1976;2:1246.

Name:	**CHLORPROMAZINE**	Risk Factor:	**C**
Class:	**Tranquilizer**		

FETAL RISK SUMMARY

RECOMMENDATION: Compatible

Chlorpromazine is a propylamino phenothiazine. The drug readily crosses the placenta (1–4). Reproductive studies in rodents have shown a potential for embryotoxicity, increased neonatal mortality, and decreased offspring performance (5). In animals, selective accumulation and retention occur in the fetal pigment epithelium (6). Although delayed ocular damage from high, prolonged doses in pregnancy has not been reported in humans, concern has been expressed for this potential toxicity (6,7).

Chlorpromazine has been used for the treatment of nausea and vomiting of pregnancy during all stages of gestation, including labor, since the mid-1950s (8–10). The drug seems to be safe and effective for this indication. Its use in labor to promote analgesia and amnesia is usually safe, but some patients, up to 18% in one series, have a marked unpredictable fall in blood pressure that could be dangerous to the mother and the fetus (11–15). Use of chlorpromazine during labor should be discouraged because of this adverse effect.

One psychiatric patient, who consumed 8,000 mg of chlorpromazine in the last 10 days of pregnancy, delivered a hypotonic, lethargic infant with depressed reflexes and jaundice (4). The adverse effects resolved within 3 weeks.

An extrapyramidal syndrome, which may persist for months, has been observed in some infants whose mothers received chlorpromazine near term (16–20). This reaction is characterized by tremors, increased muscle tone with spasticity, and hyperactive deep tendon reflexes. Hypotonicity was observed in one newborn and paralytic ileus in two newborns after exposure at term to chlorpromazine (4,21). However, most reports describing the use of chlorpromazine in pregnancy have concluded that it does not adversely affect the fetus or newborn (22–27).

The Collaborative Perinatal Project (CPP) monitored 50,282 mother-child pairs, 142 of whom had 1st trimester exposure to chlorpromazine (28). For use anytime during pregnancy, 284 exposures were recorded. No evidence was found in either group to suggest a relationship to malformations or an effect on perinatal mortality rate, birth weight, or intelligence quotient scores at 4 years of age. Opposite results were found in a prospective French study that compared 315 mothers exposed to phenothiazines during the 1st trimester with 11,099 nonexposed controls (29). Malformations were observed in 11 exposed infants (3.5%) and in 178 controls (1.6%) ($p < 0.01$). In the phenothiazine group, 57 women took chlorpromazine and four infants had malformations: syndactyly; microcephaly, clubfoot/hand, muscular abdominal aplasia (also exposed to acetylpromazine); endocardial fibroelastosis, brachymesophalangy, clinodactyly (also exposed to pipamazine); and microcephaly (also exposed to promethazine).

The case of microcephaly, although listed as a possible drug-induced malformation, was considered by the authors to be more likely a genetic defect because the mother had already delivered two previous children with microcephaly (29). However, even after exclusion of this case, the association between phenothiazines and malformations remained significant (29). In another report, a stillborn fetus delivered at 28 weeks with ectromelia and omphalocele was attributed to the combined use of chlorpromazine and meclizine in the 1st trimester (30).

In a surveillance study of Michigan Medicaid recipients conducted between 1985 and 1992 involving 229,101 completed pregnancies, 36 newborns had been exposed to chlorpromazine during the 1st trimester (F. Rosa, personal communication, FDA, 1993). No major birth defects were observed (two expected).

In an *in vitro* study, chlorpromazine was shown to be a potent inhibitor of sperm motility (31). A concentration of 53 μmol/L produced a 50% reduction in motility.

Using data from the CPP, researchers discovered that offspring of psychotic/neurotic mothers who had consumed chlorpromazine or other neuroleptics for more than 2 months during gestation, whether or not they were breast-fed, were significantly taller than nonexposed controls at 4 months, 1 year, and 7 years of age (32). At 7 years of age, the difference between the exposed and nonexposed groups was approximately 3 cm. The mechanisms behind these effects were not clear, but may have been related to the dopamine receptor-blocking action of the drugs.

In summary, although one survey found an increased incidence of defects and a report of ectromelia exists, most studies have found chlorpromazine to be safe for both mother and fetus if used occasionally in low doses. Other reviewers have also concluded that the phenothiazines are not teratogenic (26,33). Another review concluded that because of its extensive clinical experience, chlorpromazine should be included among the treatments of choice if antipsychotic therapy was required during pregnancy (34). However, use near term should be avoided because of the danger of maternal hypotension and adverse effects in the newborn.

BREAST FEEDING SUMMARY

RECOMMENDATION: Limited Human Data - Potential Toxicity

Chlorpromazine is excreted into breast milk in very small concentrations. Following a 1200 mg oral dose (20 mg/kg), peak milk levels of 0.29 μg/mL were measured at 2 hours (35). This represented a milk:plasma ratio of less than 0.5. The drug could not be detected following a 600 mg oral dose. In a study of four lactating mothers consuming unspecified amounts of the neuroleptic, milk concentrations of chlorpromazine ranged from 7–98 ng/mL with maternal serum levels ranging from 16–52 ng/mL (36). In two mothers, more of the drug was found in the milk than in the plasma. Only two of the mothers breast-fed their infants. One infant, consuming milk with a level of 7 nq/mL, showed no ill effects, but the second took milk containing 92 ng/mL and became drowsy and lethargic.

With the one exception described above, there has been a lack of reported adverse effects in breast-fed babies whose mothers were ingesting chlorpromazine (26). Based on this report, however, nursing infants exposed to the agent in milk should be observed for sedation. The American Academy of Pediatrics classifies chlorpromazine as an agent whose effect on the nursing infant is unknown but may be of concern because of the drowsiness and lethargy observed in the infant described above, and because of the galactorrhea induced in adults (37).

References

1. Franchi G, Gianni AM. Chlorpromazine distribution in maternal and fetal tissues and biological fluids. Acta Anaesthesiol (Padava) 1957;8:197–207.
2. Moya F, Thorndike V. Passage of drugs across the placenta. Am J Obstet Gynecol 1962;84:1778–98.
3. O'Donoghue SEF. Distribution of pethidine and chlorpromazine in maternal, foetal and neonatal biological fluids. Nature 1971;229:124–5.
4. Hammond JE, Toseland PA. Placental transfer of chlorpromazine. Arch Dis Child 1970;45:139–40.
5. Product information. Thorazine. SmithKline Beecham Pharmaceuticals, 2000.
6. Ullberg S, Lindquist NG, Sjostrand SE. Accumulation of chorio-retinotoxic drugs in the foetal eye. Nature 1970;227:1257–8.
7. Anonymous. Drugs and the fetal eye. Lancet 1971;1:122.
8. Karp M, Lamb VE, Benaron HBW. The use of chlorpromazine in the obstetric patient: a preliminary report. Am J Obstet Gynecol 1955;69:780–5.
9. Benaron HBW, Dorr EM, Roddick WJ, et al. Use of chlorpromazine in the obstetric patient: a preliminary report I. In the treatment of nausea and vomiting of pregnancy. Am J Obstet Gynecol 1955;69: 776–9.
10. Sullivan CL. Treatment of nausea and vomiting of pregnancy with chlorpromazine. A report of 100 cases. Postgrad Med 1957;22:429–32.
11. Harer WB. Chlorpromazine in normal labor. Obstet Gynecol 1956;8:1–9.

C

12. Lindley JE, Rogers SF, Moyer JH. Analgesic-potentiation effect of chlorpromazine during labor; a study of 2093 patients. Obstet Gynecol 1957;10:582–6.
13. Bryans CI Jr, Mulherin CM. The use of chlorpromazine in obstetrical analgesia. Am J Obstet Gynecol 1959;77:406–11.
14. Christhilf SM Jr, Monias MB, Riley RA Jr, Sheehan JC. Chlorpromazine in obstetric analgesia. Obstet Gynecol 1960;15:625–9.
15. Rodgers CD, Wickard CP, McCaskill MR. Labor and delivery without terminal anesthesia. A report of the use of chlorpromazine. Obstet Gynecol 1961;17:92–5.
16. Hill RM, Desmond MM, Kay JL. Extrapyramidal dysfunction in an infant of a schizophrenic mother. J Pediatr 1966;69:589–95.
17. Ayd FJ Jr, ed. Phenothiazine therapy during pregnancy—effects on the newborn infant. Int Drug Ther Newslett 1968;3:39–40.
18. Tamer A, McKay R, Arias D, Worley L, Fogel BJ. Phenothiazine-induced extrapyramidal dysfunction in the neonate. J Pediatr 1969;75:479–80.
19. Levy W, Wisniewski K. Chlorpromazine causing extrapyramidal dysfunction in newborn infant of psychotic mother. NY State J Med 1974;74:684–5.
20. O'Connor M, Johnson GH, James DI. Intrauterine effect of phenothiazines. Med J Aust 1981;1:416–7.
21. Falterman CG, Richardson J. Small left colon syndrome associated with maternal ingestion of psychotropic drugs. J Pediatr 1980;97:308–10.
22. Kris EB, Carmichael DM. Chlorpromazine maintenance therapy during pregnancy and confinement. Psychiatr Q 1957;31:690–5.
23. Kris EB. Children born to mothers maintained on pharmacotherapy during pregnancy and postpartum. Recent Adv Biol Psychiatry 1962;4:180–7.
24. Kris EB. Children of mothers maintained on pharmacotherapy during pregnancy and postpartum. Curr Ther Res 1965;7:785–9.
25. Sobel DE. Fetal damage due to ECT, insulin coma, chlorpromazine, or reserpine. Arch Gen Psychiatry 1960;2:606–11.
26. Ayd FJ Jr. Children born of mothers treated with chlorpromazine during pregnancy. Clin Med 1964;71:1758–63.
27. Loke KH, Salleh R. Electroconvulsive therapy for the acutely psychotic pregnant patient: a review of 3 cases. Med J Malaysia 1983;38:131–3.
28. Slone D, Siskind V, Heinonen OP, Monson RR, Kaufman DW, Shapiro S. Antenatal exposure to the phenothiazines in relation to congenital malformations, perinatal mortality rate, birth weight, and intelligence quotient score. Am J Obstet Gynecol 1977;128:486–8.
29. Rumeau-Rouquette C, Goujard J, Huel G. Possible teratogenic effect of phenothiazines in human beings. Teratology 1976;15:57–64.
30. O'Leary JL, O'Leary JA. Nonthalidomide ectromelia; report of a case. Obstet Gynecol 1964;23:17–20.
31. Levin RM, Amsterdam JD, Winokur A, Wein AJ. Effects of psychotropic drugs on human sperm motility. Fertil Steril 1981;36:503–6.
32. Platt JE, Friedhoff AJ, Broman SH, Bond RN, Laska E, Lin SP. Effects of prenatal exposure to neuroleptic drugs on children's growth. Neuropsychopharmacology 1988;1:205–12.
33. Ananth J. Congenital malformations with psychopharmacologic agents. Compr Psychiatry 1975;16:437–45.
34. Elia J, Katz IR, Simpson GM. Teratogenicity of psychotherapeutic medications. Psychopharmacol Bull 1987;23:531–86.
35. Blacker KH, Weinstein BJ, Ellman GL. Mothers milk and chlorpromazine. Am J Psychol 1962;114:178–9.
36. Wiles DH, Orr MW, Kolakowska T. Chlorpromazine levels in plasma and milk of nursing mothers. Br J Clin Pharmacol 1978;5:272–3.
37. Committee on Drugs, American Academy of Pediatrics. The transfer of drugs and other chemicals into human milk. Pediatrics 2001;108:776–89.

Name:	**CHLORPROPAMIDE**	Risk Factor:	C_M
Class:	**Oral Hypoglycemic**		

FETAL RISK SUMMARY

RECOMMENDATION: Human Data Suggest Risk in 3rd Trimester

Chlorpropamide is a sulfonylurea used for the treatment of adult-onset diabetes mellitus. It is not the treatment of choice for the pregnant diabetic patient.

In a study using neurulating mouse embryos in whole-embryo culture, chlorpropamide produced malformations and growth retardation at concentrations similar to therapeutic levels in humans (1). The defects were not a result of hypoglycemia or of chlorpropamide metabolites.

When administered near term, chlorpropamide crosses the placenta and may persist in the neonatal serum for several days (2–4). One mother, who took 500 mg/day throughout pregnancy, delivered an infant whose serum level was 15.4 mg/dL at 77 hours of life (2). Infants of three other mothers, who were consuming 100–250 mg/day at term, had serum levels varying between 1.8 and 2.8 mg/dL 8–35 hours after delivery (3). All four infants had prolonged symptomatic hypoglycemia secondary to hyperinsulinism lasting for 4–6 days. Another newborn, whose mother had been taking chlorpropamide, had severe, prolonged hypoglycemia and seizures (4). In other reports, totaling 69 pregnancies, chlorpropamide in doses of 100–200 mg or more/day either gave no evidence of neonatal hypoglycemia and hyperinsulinism or no constant relationship between daily maternal dosage and neonatal complications (5,6). One reviewer, however, thought that chlorpropamide should be stopped at least 48 hours before delivery to avoid this potential complication (7).

In an abstract (8), and later in a full report (9), the *in vitro* placental transfer, using a single-cotyledon human placenta, of four oral hypoglycemic agents was described. As expected, molecular weight was the most significant factor for drug transfer, with dissociation constant (pKa) and lipid solubility providing significant additive effects. The cumulative percent placental transfer at 3 hours of the four agents and their approximate molecular weights (shown in parenthesis) were tolbutamide (270) 21.5%, chlorpropamide (277) 11.0%, glipizide (446) 6.6%, and glyburide (494) 3.9%.

Although teratogenic in animals, an increased incidence of congenital defects, other than that expected in diabetes mellitus, was not found with chlorpropamide in several studies (10–19). Four malformed infants have been attributed to chlorpropamide but the relationship is unclear: hand and finger anomalies (10); stricture of lower ileum, death (10); preauricular sinus (10); and microcephaly and spastic quadriplegia (13).

In a surveillance study of Michigan Medicaid recipients conducted between 1985 and 1992 involving 229,101 completed pregnancies, 18 newborns had been exposed to chlorpropamide during the 1st trimester (F. Rosa, personal communication, FDA, 1993). No major birth defects were observed (one expected).

A 1991 report described the outcomes of pregnancies in 21 non–insulin-dependent diabetic women who were treated with oral hypoglycemic agents (17 sulfonylureas, 3 biguanides, and 1 unknown type) during the 1st trimester (20). The duration of exposure ranged from 3–28 weeks, but all patients were changed to insulin therapy at the first prenatal visit. Forty non-insulin-dependent diabetic women matched for age, race, parity, and glycemic control served as a control group. Eleven (52%) of the exposed infants had major or minor congenital malformations as compared to six (15%) of the controls. Moreover, ear defects, a malformation that is observed, but uncommonly, in diabetic embryopathy, occurred in six of the exposed infants and in none of the controls (20). Six of the 11 infants with defects had been exposed *in utero* to chlorpropamide (length of exposure during pregnancy is in parentheses): severe microtia right ear, multiple tags left ear (22 weeks); bilateral auricular tags (8 weeks); single umbilical artery (14 weeks); ear tag (10 weeks); facial, auricular, and vertebral defects, deafness, ventricular septal defect (15 weeks); and multiple vertebral anomalies, ventricular septal defect, severe aortic coarctation; bilateral ear tags and posterior rotated ears (14 weeks) (20).

Sixteen livebirths occurred in the exposed group compared to 36 in controls (20). The groups did not differ in the incidence of hypoglycemia at birth (53% vs. 53%), but three of the exposed newborns had severe hypoglycemia lasting 2, 4, and 7 days, even though the mothers had not used oral hypoglycemics (two women had used chlorpropamide) close to delivery. The authors attributed this to irreversible β-cell hyperplasia that may have been increased by exposure to oral hypoglycemics (20). Hyperbilirubinemia was noted in 10 (67%) of 15 exposed newborns as compared to 13 (36%) of controls ($p < 0.04$), and polycythemia and hyperviscosity requiring partial exchange transfusions were observed in 4 (27%) of 15 exposed vs. 1 (3.0%) control ($p < 0.03$) (one exposed infant not included in these data because the infant presented after completion of study).

A study published in 1995 assessed the risk of congenital malformations in infants of mothers with non-insulin-dependent diabetes during a 6-year period (21). Women were included in the study if, during the first 8 weeks of pregnancy, they had not participated in a preconception care program and had been treated either with diet alone (group 1), diet and oral hypoglycemic agents (predominantly chlorpropamide, glyburide, or glipizide) (group 2), or diet and exogenous insulin (group 3). The 302 women eligible for analysis gave birth to 332 infants (five sets of twins and 16 with two or three separate singleton pregnancies during the study period). Of the infants, 56 (16.9%) had one or more congenital malformations, 39 (11.7%) of which were classified as major anomalies (defined as those that were either lethal, caused significant morbidity, or required surgical repair). The major anomalies were divided among those involving the central nervous system, face, heart and great vessels, gastrointestinal, genitourinary, and skeletal (includes caudal regression syndrome) systems. Minor anomalies included all of these, except those of the central nervous system, and a miscellaneous group composed of sacral skin tags, cutis aplasia of the scalp, and hydroceles. The number of infants in each group and the number of major and minor anomalies observed were group 1: 125 infants, 18 (14.4%) major, 6 (4.8%) minor; group 2: 147 infants, 14 (9.5%) major, 9 (6.1%) minor; group 3: 60 infants, 7 (11.7%) major, 2 (3.3%) minor. There were no statistical differences among the groups. Six (4.1%) of the infants exposed *in utero* to oral hypoglycemic agents and four other infants in the other two groups had ear anomalies (included among those with face defects). Other than the incidence of major anomalies, two other important findings of this study were the independent associations between the risk of major anomalies (but not minor defects) and poor glycemic control in early pregnancy, and a younger maternal age at the onset of diabetes (21). Moreover, the study did not find an association between the use of oral hypoglycemics during organogenesis and congenital malformations because the observed anomalies appeared to be related to poor maternal glycemic control (21).

In summary, although the use of chlorpropamide during human gestation does not appear to be related to structural anomalies, insulin is still the treatment of choice for this disease. Oral hypoglycemics are not indicated for the pregnant diabetic because they will not provide good control in patients who cannot be controlled by diet alone (7). Moreover, insulin, unlike chlorpropamide, does not cross the placenta and, thus, eliminates the additional concern that the drug therapy itself is adversely affecting the fetus. Carefully prescribed insulin therapy will provide better control of the mother's blood glucose, thereby preventing the fetal and neonatal complications that occur with this disease. High maternal glucose levels, as may occur in diabetes mellitus, are closely associated with a number of maternal and fetal adverse effects, including fetal structural anomalies if the hyperglycemia occurs early in gestation. To prevent this toxicity, most experts, including the American College of Obstetricians and Gynecologists, recommend that insulin be used for types I and II diabetes occurring during pregnancy and, if diet therapy alone is not successful, for gestational diabetes (22,23). If chlorpropamide is used during pregnancy, therapy should be changed to insulin and chlorpropamide discontinued before delivery (the exact time before delivery is unknown) to lessen the possibility of prolonged hypoglycemia in the newborn.

C

BREAST FEEDING SUMMARY

RECOMMENDATION: Limited Human Data - Potential Toxicity

Chlorpropamide is excreted into breast milk. Following a 500-mg oral dose, the milk concentration in a composite of two samples obtained at 5 hours was 5 μg/mL (G.G. D'Ambrosio, personal communication, Pfizer Laboratories, 1982). The effects on a nursing infant from this amount of drug are unknown, but hypoglycemia is a potential toxicity.

References

1. Smoak IW. Embryopathic effects of the oral hypoglycemic agent chlorpropamide in cultured mouse embryos. Am J Obstet Gynecol 1993;169:409–14.
2. Zucker P, Simon G. Prolonged symptomatic neonatal hypoglycemia associated with maternal chlorpropamide therapy. Pediatrics 1968;42:824–5.
3. Kemball ML, McIver C, Milnar RDG, Nourse CH, Schiff D, Tiernan JR. Neonatal hypoglycaemia in infants of diabetic mothers given sulphonylurea drugs in pregnancy. Arch Dis Child 1970;45:696–701.
4. Harris EL. Adverse reactions to oral antidiabetic agents. Br Med J 1971;3:29–30.
5. Sutherland HW, Stowers JM, Cormack JD, Bewsher PD. Evaluation of chlorpropamide in chemical diabetes diagnosed during pregnancy. Br Med J 1973;3: 9–13.
6. Sutherland HW, Bewsher PD, Cormack JD, et al. Effect of moderate dosage of chlorpropamide in pregnancy on fetal outcome. Arch Dis Child 1974;49:283–91.
7. Friend JR. Diabetes. Clin Obstet Gynecol 1981;8: 353–82.
8. Elliott B, Schenker S, Langer O, Johnson R, Prihoda T. Oral hypoglycemic agents: profound variation exists in their rate of human placental transfer. Society of Perinatal Obstetricians Abstract. Am J Obstet Gynecol 1992;166:368.
9. Elliott BD, Schenker S, Langer O, Johnson R, Prihoda T. Comparative placental transport of oral hypoglycemic agents in humans: a model of human placental drug transfer. Am J Obstet Gynecol 1994;171:653–60.
10. Soler NG, Walsh CH, Malins JM. Congenital malformations in infants of diabetic mothers. Q J Med 1976;45:303–13.
11. Adam PAJ, Schwartz R. Diagnosis and treatment: should oral hypoglycemic agents be used in pediatric and pregnant patients? Pediatrics 1968;42: 819–23.
12. Dignan PSJ. Teratogenic risk and counseling in diabetes. Clin Obstet Gynecol 1981;24:149–59.
13. Campbell GD. Chlorpropamide and foetal damage. Br Med J 1963;1:59–60.
14. Jackson WPU, Campbell GD, Notelovitz M, Blumsohn D. Tolbutamide and chlorpropamide during pregnancy in human diabetes. Diabetes 1962;11(Suppl):98–101.
15. Jackson WPU, Campbell GD. Chlorpropamide and perinatal mortality. Br Med J 1963;2:1652.
16. Macphail I. Chlorpropamide and foetal damage. Br Med J 1963;1:192.
17. Malins JM, Cooke AM, Pyke DA, Fitzgerald MG. Sulphonylurea drugs in pregnancy. Br Med J 1964;2: 187.
18. Moss JM, Connor EJ. Pregnancy complicated by diabetes. Report of 102 pregnancies including eleven treated with oral hypoglycemic drugs. Med Ann DC 1965;34:253–60.
19. Douglas CP, Richards R. Use of chlorpropamide in the treatment of diabetes in pregnancy. Diabetes 1967;16:60–1.
20. Piacquadio K, Hollingsworth DR, Murphy H. Effects of in-utero exposure to oral hypoglycaemic drugs. Lancet 1991;338:866–9.
21. Towner D, Kjos SL, Leung B, Montoro MM, Xiang A, Mestman JH, Buchanan TA. Congenital malformations in pregnancies complicated by NIDDM. Diabetes Care 1995;18:1446–51.
22. American College of Obstetricians and Gynecologists. Diabetes and pregnancy. *Technical Bulletin*. No. 200. December 1994.
23. Coustan DR. Management of gestational diabetes. Clin Obstet Gynecol 1991;34:558–64.

Name:	**CHLORPROTHIXENE**	Risk Factor:	**C**
Class:	**Tranquilizer**		

FETAL RISK SUMMARY

RECOMMENDATION: No Human Data - Probably Compatible

Chlorprothixene is structurally and pharmacologically related to chlorpromazine and thiothixene. No specific data on its use in pregnancy have been located (see also Chlorpromazine).

C

BREAST FEEDING SUMMARY

RECOMMENDATION: Limited Human Data - Potential Toxicity

Chlorprothixene is excreted into breast milk (1). Serum and milk concentrations of chlorprothixene and its metabolite, chlorprothixene sulfoxide, were determined in two women consuming 200 mg/day. In one woman, plasma concentrations of the parent drug and the metabolite, 1.5–24 hours after the 200-mg dose, ranged from 13 to 51 nmol/L and 75 to 130 nmol/L, respectively. Simultaneously obtained milk levels ranged from 6 to 60 nmol/L and 42 to 96 nmol/L, respectively. The second patient had a single determination drawn 30 hours after a 200-mg dose with levels in the plasma and milk for the parent compound and metabolite of 38 and 98 nmol/L (plasma) and 115 and 54 nmol/L (milk), respectively. The milk:plasma ratio for chlorprothixene varied between 1.2 and 2.6, whereas that of the metabolite varied from 0.5 to 0.8. The test method used was able to recover 90%–100% of the drugs from the plasma but only 60%–70% from the milk. No adverse effects were noted in the nursing infants. The investigators calculated that a nursing infant consuming 800 mL of milk/day would ingest no more than 15 μg of chlorprothixene/day. The American Academy of Pediatrics classifies chlorprothixene as an agent whose effect on the nursing infant is unknown but may be of concern (2).

References

1. Matheson I, Evang A, Fredricson Overo K, Syversen G. Presence of chlorprothixene and its metabolites in breast milk. Eur J Clin Pharmacol 1984;27:611–3.
2. Committee on Drugs, American Academy of Pediatrics. The transfer of drugs and other chemicals into human milk. Pediatrics 2001;108:776–89.

Name:	**CHLORTETRACYCLINE**	Risk Factor:	**D**
Class:	**Antibiotic (Tetracycline)**		

FETAL RISK SUMMARY

RECOMMENDATION: Contraindicated in 2nd and 3rd Trimesters

See Tetracycline.

BREAST FEEDING SUMMARY

RECOMMENDATION: Compatible

Chlortetracycline is excreted into breast milk. Eight patients were given 2–3 g orally/day for 3–4 days (1). Average maternal and milk concentrations were 4.1 and 1.25 μg/mL, respectively, producing a milk:plasma ratio of 0.4. Infant data were not given.

Theoretically, dental staining and inhibition of bone growth could occur in breast-fed infants whose mothers were consuming chlortetracycline. However, this theoretical possibility seems remote because in infants exposed to a closely related antibiotic, tetracycline, serum levels were undetectable (less than 0.05 μg/mL) (2). The American Academy of Pediatrics classifies tetracycline as compatible with breast-feeding (3). Three potential problems may exist for the nursing infant, even though there are no reports in this regard: modification of bowel flora, direct effects on the infant, and interference with the interpretation of culture results if a fever workup is required.

References

1. Guilbeau JA, Schoenbach EB, Schuab IG, Latham DV. Aureomycin in obstetrics; therapy and prophylaxis. JAMA 1950;143:520–6.
2. Posner AC, Prigot A, Konicoff NG. Further observations on the use of tetracycline hydrochloride in prophylaxis and treatment of obstetric infections. In *Antibiotics Annual 1954–55*. New York, NY: Medical Encyclopedia, 1955:594–8.
3. Committee on Drugs, American Academy of Pediatrics. The transfer of drugs and other chemicals into human milk. Pediatrics 2001;108:776–89.

Name:	**CHLORTHALIDONE**	Risk Factor:	B_M*
Class:	**Diuretic**		

FETAL RISK SUMMARY

RECOMMENDATION: Compatible

Chlorthalidone is structurally related to the thiazide diuretics (see Chlorothiazide). In general, diuretics are not recommended for the treatment of gestational hypertension because of the maternal hypovolemia characteristic of this disease.

Reproduction studies in rats and rabbits at doses up to 420 times the human dose have observed no evidence of fetal harm (1).

[**Risk Factor D if used in gestational hypertension.*]

BREAST FEEDING SUMMARY

RECOMMENDATION: Compatible

See Chlorothiazide.

Reference

1. Product information. Thalitone. Monarch Pharmaceuticals, 2000.

Name:	**CHLORZOXAZONE**	Risk Factor:	C
Class:	**Muscle Relaxant**		

FETAL RISK SUMMARY

RECOMMENDATION: Limited Human Data - No Relevant Animal Data

The reproductive effects of the centrally acting muscle relaxant, chlorzoxazone, have not been studied in animals. Moreover, no published reports of its use in human pregnancy have been located.

No reports describing the placental transfer of chlorzoxazone have been located. The molecular weight (about 170), however, is low enough that transfer to the fetus should be expected.

In a surveillance study of Michigan Medicaid recipients conducted between 1985 and 1992 involving 229,101 completed pregnancies, 42 newborns had been exposed to chlorzoxazone during the 1st trimester (F. Rosa, personal communication, FDA, 1993). One

(2.4%) major birth defect was observed (two expected), a cardiovascular defect (0.5 expected). Earlier data, obtained from the same source between 1980 and 1983, totaled 264 1st trimester exposures with 17 defects observed (17 expected). These combined data do not support an association between the drug and congenital defects.

BREAST FEEDING SUMMARY

RECOMMENDATION: No Human Data - Potential Toxicity

No reports describing the use of chlorzoxazone during lactation have been located. The molecular weight (about 170), however, is low enough that excretion in milk should be expected. The effects of this potential exposure on a nursing infant are unknown.

Name:	**CHOLECALCIFEROL**	Risk Factor:	**C***
Class:	**Vitamin**		

FETAL RISK SUMMARY

RECOMMENDATION: Compatible

Cholecalciferol (vitamin D_3) is converted in the liver to calcifediol, which, in turn, is converted in the kidneys to calcitriol, one of the active forms of vitamin D (see Calcitriol and Vitamin D).

[**Risk Factor D if used in doses above the recommended daily allowance.*]

BREAST FEEDING SUMMARY

RECOMMENDATION: Compatible

See Vitamin D.

Name:	**CHOLESTYRAMINE**	Risk Factor:	**B**
Class:	**Antilipemic**		

FETAL RISK SUMMARY

RECOMMENDATION: Compatible

Cholestyramine is a resin used to bind bile acids in a nonabsorbable complex. In a reproductive study involving rats and rabbits, the resin was given in doses up to 2 g/kg/day without evidence of fertility impairment or adverse fetal effects (1). In a comparison between pregnant and nonpregnant rats, administration of cholestyramine failed to lower the plasma cholesterol concentration or to increase bile acid synthesis (2). The drug therapy had no effect, in comparison to control animals, on maternal weight gain, number of fetuses, and fetal weight.

Cholestyramine has been used for the treatment of cholestasis of pregnancy (3–7). Except for the case described below, no adverse fetal effects were observed in these studies. One review recommended the resin as first-line therapy for the pruritus that accompanies intrahepatic cholestasis of pregnancy (6). Cholestyramine also binds fat-soluble vitamins, and long-term use could result in deficiencies of these agents in either the mother or the fetus (8). In one study, treatment with 9 g daily up to a maximum duration of 12 weeks was not associated with fetal or maternal complications (3).

A 31-year-old woman in her third pregnancy was treated with cholestyramine (8 g/day) beginning at 19 weeks' gestation for intrahepatic cholestasis of pregnancy (7). At 22 weeks' gestation, the dose was increased to 16 g/day. Four weeks later, she was clinically jaundiced and at 29 weeks' gestation, she was admitted to the hospital for reduced fetal movements. Fetal ultrasound scans over the next week revealed expanding bilateral subdural hematomas with hydrocephalus, an enlarged liver, and bilateral pleural effusions (7). The mother's prothrombin ratio was markedly elevated but responded to two doses of IV vitamin K. One week later, following labor induction for fetal distress, a 1660-g infant was delivered who died at 15 minutes of age. It was thought that the fetal subdural hematomas were the result of vitamin K deficiency caused by the cholestyramine, cholestasis, or both (7).

A 1989 report described the use of cholestyramine and other agents in the treatment of inflammatory bowel disease during pregnancy (9). Seven patients were treated during gestation with the resin. One of the seven delivered prematurely (<37 weeks' gestation) and one of the newborns was small for gestational age (<10th percentile for gestational age). Both of these outcomes were probably related to the mother's disease, rather than to the therapy.

In a surveillance study of Michigan Medicaid recipients conducted between 1985 and 1992 involving 229,101 completed pregnancies, 4 newborns had been exposed to cholestyramine during the 1st trimester (10). Thirty-three other newborns were exposed after the 1st trimester. None of the infants had congenital malformations.

BREAST FEEDING SUMMARY

RECOMMENDATION: Compatible

Cholestyramine is a nonabsorbable resin. No reports describing its use during lactation have been located. Because it binds fat-soluble vitamins, prolonged use may result in deficiencies of these vitamins in the mother and her nursing infant.

References

1. Koda S, Anabuki K, Miki T, Kahi S, Takahashi N. Reproductive studies on cholestyramine. Kiso to Rinsho 1982;16:2040–94. As cited in Shepard TH. *Catalog of Teratogenic Agents*. 7th ed. Baltimore, MD: Johns Hopkins University Press, 1992:90.
2. Innis SM. Effect of cholestyramine administration during pregnancy in the rat. Am J Obstet Gynecol 1983;146:13–6.
3. Lutz EE, Margolis AJ. Obstetric hepatosis: treatment with cholestyramine and interim response to steroids. Obstet Gynecol 1969;33:64–71.
4. Heikkinen J, Maentausta O, Ylostalo P, Janne O. Serum bile acid levels in intrahepatic cholestasis of pregnancy during treatment with phenobarbital or cholestyramine. Eur J Obstet Gynecol Reprod Biol 1982;14:153–62.
5. Shaw D, Frohlich J, Wittmann BAK, Willms M. A prospective study of 18 patients with cholestasis of pregnancy. Am J Obstet Gynecol 1982;142:621–5.
6. Schorr-Lesnick B, Lebovics E, Dworkin B, Rosenthal WS. Liver disease unique to pregnancy. Am J Gastroenterol 1991;86:659–70.
7. Sadler LC, Lane M, North R. Severe fetal intracranial haemorrhage during treatment with cholestyramine for intrahepatic cholestasis of pregnancy. Br J Obstet Gynaecol 1995;102:169–70.
8. American Hospital Formulary Service. *Drug Information 1997*. Bethesda, MD: American Society of Health-System Pharmacists, 1997:1330–4.
9. Fedorkow DM, Persaud D, Nimrod CA. Inflammatory bowel disease: a controlled study of late pregnancy outcome. Am J Obstet Gynecol 1989;160:998–1001.
10. Rosa F. Anti-cholesterol agent pregnancy exposure outcomes. Presented at the 7th International Organization for Teratogen Information Services, Woods Hole, MA, April 1994.

C

Name: **CICLOPIROX** Risk Factor: B_M

Class: **Antifungal**

FETAL RISK SUMMARY

RECOMMENDATION: No Human Data - Probably Compatible

Ciclopirox is a synthetic anti-infective agent used topically for its antifungal properties. Very small amounts (1.3% of the dose with occlusive dressings) are absorbed systemically from the skin (1).

There was no evidence of teratogenic effects or other fetal harm in animals (mice, rats, rabbits, and monkeys) given doses of 10 times or more the topical human dose by various routes of administration (1).

No reports of its use in human pregnancy have been located. The manufacturer has no case reports of congenital abnormalities occurring after use of ciclopirox (C.K. Whitmore, personal communication, Hoechst-Roussel Pharmaceuticals, Inc., 1987).

BREAST FEEDING SUMMARY

RECOMMENDATION: No Human Data - Probably Compatible

No reports describing the use of ciclopirox during lactation have been located. The very small amounts (1.3%) absorbed systemically with occlusive dressings probably indicates that infant exposure via the milk is negligible, if it occurs at all.

Reference

1. Product information. Loprox. MEDICIS, The Dermatology Company, 2000.

Name: **CIDOFOVIR** Risk Factor: C_M

Class: **Antiviral**

FETAL RISK SUMMARY

RECOMMENDATION: Compatible - Maternal Benefit >> Embryo/Fetal Risk

Cidofovir (HPMPC) is used in the treatment of cytomegalovirus (CMV) retinitis in patients with acquired immunodeficiency syndrome. The antiviral agent is converted to the active metabolite, cidofovir diphosphate, by intracellular enzymes. In animals, cidofovir is carcinogenic, embryotoxic, and teratogenic.

Cidofovir was carcinogenic in female rats, producing mammary adenocarcinoma at doses as low as 0.6 mg/kg/week, about 0.04 times the recommended human dose based on an area under the plasma concentration curve (RHD-AUC). Reproductive studies with cidofovir have been conducted with rats and rabbits (1). Both maternal toxicity and embryotoxicity (reduced fetal body weights) were observed at IV doses of 1.5 mg/kg/day in rats and 1.0 mg/kg/day in rabbits, administered during organogenesis. The no-observable-effect doses for embryotoxicity in rats and rabbits were 0.5 and 0.25 mg/kg/day, respectively, approximately 0.04 and 0.05 times the RHD-AUC, respectively. Teratogenic effects, consisting of external, soft tissue, and skeletal malformations (meningocele, short snout, and short maxillary bones), were observed in the fetuses of rabbits given 1.0 mg/kg/day during organogenesis.

Pregnant mice inoculated intranasally with equine herpesvirus 1 in the 2nd or 3rd week of gestation, were treated with a single dose of cidofovir 50 mg/kg SC 1 day prior to inoculation (2). A noninfected, control group of pregnant mice was also treated at a similar gestational time with the same dose of cidofovir. In the infected group, cidofovir significantly reduced the incidence of virus transfer to the fetus and subsequent abortion, a predictable effect of the virus. No obvious toxic effects were observed in either group.

No reports describing the use of cidofovir during human pregnancy have been located. It is not known whether the drug crosses the placenta to the fetus, but because of its relatively low molecular weight of approximately 315, passage to the fetus should be expected.

Because of the lack of human data, the risk to the human embryo and fetus cannot be assessed. Some risk may exist because of the adverse effects observed at very low doses in the limited animal studies. Despite this risk, the use of cidofovir after the 1st trimester in a pregnant HIV-positive woman with sight-threatening CMV retinitis may be a rational decision.

BREAST FEEDING SUMMARY

RECOMMENDATION: Contraindicated

No reports describing the use of cidofovir during lactation have been located. This antiviral agent should not be used during breast-feeding because of the potential severe toxicity in a nursing infant. Moreover, although no studies have been reported in lactating humans, cidofovir has induced mammary cancer with very low doses in female rats.

In addition, the mother's clinical status will usually preclude the use of cidofovir during breast-feeding. Cidofovir's only approved indication is for the treatment of CMV retinitis in patients infected with human immunodeficiency virus type 1 (HIV-1). Because HIV-1 is transmitted in milk, breast-feeding is not recommended in developed countries where there are available affordable milk substitutes (3–5).

References

1. Product information. Vistide. Gilead Sciences, 1997.
2. Awan AR, Field HJ. Effects of phosphonylmethoxyalkyl derivatives studied with a murine model for abortion induced by equine herpesvirus 1. Antimicrob Agents Chemother 1993;37:2478–82.
3. Brown ZA, Watts DH. Antiviral therapy in pregnancy. Clin Obstet Gynecol 1990;33:276–89.
4. de Martino M, Tovo P-A, Pezzotti P, Galli L, Massironi E, Ruga E, Floreea F, Plebani A, Gabiano C, Zuccotti GV. HIV-1 transmission through breast-milk: appraisal of risk according to duration of feeding. AIDS 1992;6:991–7.
5. Van de Perre P. Postnatal transmission of human immunodeficiency virus type 1: the breast-feeding dilemma. Am J Obstet Gynecol 1995;173:483–7.

Name: **CIGARETTE SMOKING** Risk Factor: **X**

Class: **Stimulant**

FETAL RISK SUMMARY

RECOMMENDATION: Contraindicated

Cigarette smoking during pregnancy is a significant health hazard to the mother, embryo, fetus, infant, and adolescent. Cigarette smoke contains more than 3000 different compounds, including nicotine, carbon monoxide, ammonia, polycyclic aromatic hydrocarbons, hydrogen cyanide, and vinyl chloride (1–5). Although these and other chemical constituents of cigarette smoke represent a risk to the pregnancy, the principal concerns relate to nicotine and carbon monoxide. Nicotine has a plasma half-life of about 40 minutes, whereas its primary inactive metabolite, cotinine, has a half-life of 15–30 hours (4). Nicotine releases epinephrine that results in a marked reduction in uterine blood flow and an increase in uterine vascular resistance (1–4).

Although the frequency of cigarette smoking during pregnancy is declining, the self-reported overall prevalence ranges from about 13% to 20% (3,4,6,7). The prevalence is dependent on a number of factors, primarily ethnic group, age, and education. The highest frequency is among American Indian and Alaskan Native women (20.2%) and white women (16.2%), whereas it is lower in Black (9.6%), Hispanic (4%), and Asian and Pacific Islander women (3.1%) (5). The highest prevalence of smoking during pregnancy is among women age 18–24 years (5,7) and more women with 12 years of education or less (11.7% to 25.5%) smoke than do women with 13–15 years (9.6%) or ≥16 years (2.2%) of education (5). However, these self-reported rates, whether based on questionnaires, interviews, or birth certificate data, probably underestimate the actual frequency of smoking (5,6,8). The high rates of nondisclosure have led some to recommend that biochemical validation of smoking status should be a part of all studies involving pregnant women (6).

Nicotine and carbon monoxide rapidly cross the placenta (1–5). Nicotine and carboxyhemoglobin fetal concentrations are about 10%–15% higher than those in the mother.

Cigarette smoking before and during pregnancy is associated with a number of adverse reproductive effects. These toxic effects can be classified as:

- Subfertility and ectopic pregnancy
- Pregnancy complications
  - Spontaneous abortions
  - Premature delivery
  - Placental abruption/placenta previa
  - Placental previa
  - Premature rupture of membranes
- Embryo/fetal complications
  - Growth retardation
  - Perinatal mortality
  - Congenital malformations
- Neonatal complications
  - Neonatal intensive care unit admissions
  - Retinal abnormalities
- Adolescent complications
  - Neurodevelopment
  - Sudden infant death syndrome
  - Childhood morbidity

Subfertility and Ectopic Pregnancy

Cigarette smoking adversely effects female fertility (4,9,10–12). A 1986 review explored this topic in depth and concluded that cigarette smoking adversely affects the ability to conceive during a given menstrual cycle (i.e., reduced fecundity) (11). One mechanism of smoking-induced reduced fecundity might be related to altered uterine tubal function (increased uterotubal amplitude and tonus). This could also explain the higher incidence of ectopic tubal pregnancies in women who smoke (11). Other potential contributing mechanisms are effects on the preimplantation embryo, implantation, gamete maturation and function, and adverse effects on sperm density, motility, and morphology induced by paternal smoking (11).

Pregnancy Complications

Spontaneous Abortions

Cigarette smoking is associated with an increased risk of spontaneous abortions (SABs) of fetuses with normal karyotype (1–5,8–11,13,14). Compared to nonsmokers, the risk of abortion may be increased by as much as 20%–80% (2–4,9). An estimated 19,000–141,000 SABs annually may be caused by tobacco (5). However, adjustment for confounding factors, such as a previous history of SAB and alcohol consumption, may reduce the association (9). The mechanism of smoking-induced SAB is unknown but may be a result of interference with placentation or implantation (11).

Premature Delivery

Preterm delivery is increased in women who smoke (1,4,5,7,9,10,14,15). Smoking may be responsible for 14%–15% of all premature births (5,10). The effect of smoking is most pronounced in infants born at less than 33 weeks' gestation (7). The risk increases with the number of cigarettes smoked (9).

Placental Abruption/Placenta Previa

An increased risk of vaginal bleeding secondary to placental abruption or previa has been shown with smoking (2–4,6,9,10,12,13,14,16). There is a dose-dependent association with these complications (2,3,10,13). The risk of abruption and previa in those smoking less than one-pack/day was 23% and 25%, respectively, greater than that of nonsmokers, whereas the risk in those smoking one-pack/day or more was increased 86% and 92%, respectively (3). Moreover, a smoking history of more than 6 years was associated with an increased incidence of placenta previa of 14.3% and of placental abruption of 72% (4). The estimated annual number of infant deaths from these two complications is 1900–4800 (5).

Premature Rupture of Membranes

Premature rupture of membranes (PROM) is an adverse effect of maternal smoking (1,2,4,5,9). Similar to other complications, a dose-dependent relationship has been found (2,4). One cited study found that the incidence of PROM was 1.4% in women smoking 20 or more cigarettes/day, 0.6% in those smoking 1–5 cigarettes/day, and 0.3% in nonsmokers (4).

Embryo/Fetal Complications

Growth Retardation

Intrauterine growth retardation (IUGR) at any gestational age is a well-known complication of cigarette smoking during pregnancy (1–7,10–16). Growth retardation is typically symmetrical IUGR, but aspects of asymmetrical IUGR may be present in the last trimester (7). The negative effects of smoking on fetal growth include weight, length, and head, chest, and shoulder circumference, and involve a dose-dependent relationship. The infants of women who smoke, on average, weigh 200 g less than infants of women who do not smoke (2–4). Moreover, compared with nonsmokers, the risk of having an infant weighing less than 2500 g is 52% greater in those smoking less than one-pack/day and 130% greater in those smoking one-pack/day or more (3). Overall, the relative risk (smokers vs. nonsmokers) of giving birth to an infant weighing less than 2500 g is approximately 2.0 (13). In 1993, it was estimated that smoking was responsible for 40,000 low-birth-weight (LBW) infants (4). Smoking during pregnancy may account for 20%–30% of LBW infants (5). Quitting smoking before or during pregnancy decreases the risk of delivering a LBW infant to a level of risk equivalent to that of nonsmokers (5,7,13). The primary cause of the growth retardation is thought to be chronic fetal hypoxia secondary to nicotine and carbon monoxide (1,5,10,12). Nicotine-induced vasoconstriction causes reduced placental blood flow. Carbon monoxide binds to hemoglobin, both maternal and fetal, with an affinity that is more than 200 times that of oxygen (5).

Mortality

An increase in perinatal deaths (fetal deaths after 20 weeks' gestation and infant deaths within 28 days of birth) is frequently associated with cigarette smoking during pregnancy (1–3,5,8–11,13,14,16). Increased rates of perinatal death have been reported, with the highest risk found in smoking women who had had multiple pregnancies, were of low socioeconomic class, and were anemic (2,3). A dose-dependent relationship between maternal smoking and perinatal mortality is evident. The increased perinatal mortality is secondary to stillbirths, prematurity, respiratory distress syndrome, pneumonia, placental abruption, and placenta previa. The risk of perinatal mortality from cigarette smoking is about 10% and most deaths occur in infants with IUGR (9). Of interest, heavy tobacco chewing is associated with decreased birth weight (100–200 g; primarily as a consequence of prematurity) and a three-fold increase in the stillbirth rate (2,17).

Congenital Malformations

The relationship between cigarette smoking during pregnancy and structural malformations is controversial (2–5,9,11,14,15). Several reports found low associations between smoking and various birth defects, but the studies relied on self-reported smoking prevalence. A 2003 statement from the Teratology Society on the benefits of smoking cessation during pregnancy concluded that smoking is not associated with major congenital malformations (5).

Cardiovascular Defects

In addition to the references cited in this section, see reference 24.

In a brief 1971 correspondence using data from the 1958 British Perinatal Mortality Survey, a statistically significant association was found for congenital heart disease between smokers (at least one cigarette/day after the fourth month of pregnancy) and non-smokers (18). Congenital heart disease was determined by medical examination or autopsy. The incidence of congenital heart disease per 1,000 births in smokers and nonsmokers was 7.3 and 4.7, respectively. After adjustment, the smoking effect was independent of maternal age, parity, and social class (18).

A 1978 case-control study found a significant increase in congenital defects in women who smoked 21 or more cigarettes/day (19). There were 1,370 cases (41% smoked) and 2,968 controls (39% smoked). There was a significant increase in the estimated relative risk (RR) for congenital defects in smokers when compared to nonsmokers, 1.6 vs. 1.0, respectively. Defects with RR estimates of 2.0 or higher were heart valves (2.0), inguinal hernia (2.8), pyloric stenosis (3.3), and defects of the digestive system (2.9) (19). A 1978 study, using data from a previous study on the effects of exposure to trace anesthetic agents on the health of health care professionals, discovered a significant association between smoking and an increase in the risk of SABs and congenital defects (20). Compared to nonsmokers, there was an increase for cardiovascular, gastrointestinal, and urogenital malformations. For all defects, smokers had a risk as high as 2.3 times that of nonsmokers (20).

A case-control study conducted in California involved 207 cases with conotruncal heart defects, 246 with neural tube defects (NTDs), 178 with limb deficiencies, and 481 controls delivered during 1987–1988 (21). The confirmed heart defects in infants included tetralogy of Fallot; *d*-transposition of the great arteries; truncus arteriosus communis; double-outlet right ventricle; pulmonary valve atresia with ventricular septal defect (VSD); subaortic VSD type 1; and aorticopulmonary window (21). Confirmed cases of NTDs and limb deficiencies in infants and fetuses (spontaneous and elective abortions) included anencephaly, spina bifida cystica, craniorrhachischisis, iniencephaly, and longitudinal, transverse, or amniotic band limb deficiency defects of the upper and/or lower limbs (21). Moderately elevated associations, but only when both parents smoked, were found for conotruncal heart defects (odds ratio [OR] 1.9 [95% confidence interval (CI) 1.2–3.1]) and limb deficiencies (OR 1.7 [95% CI 0.96–2.9]), but parenteral smoking was not associated with increased risks for NTDs (21).

Data relating to risk factors for *l*-transposition of the great arteries obtained from the Baltimore-Washington Infant Study (1981–1989), a population-based case-control study, were published in 2003 (22). *l*-Transposition of the great arteries is an uncommon congenital cardiovascular malformation. Among 3377 cases of congenital cardiovascular malformations, 36 (1.1%) had the targeted defect. The majority of the cases had multiple cardiovascular anomalies and 47% had a single ventricle. Seventy-five percent of the cases came from two regions (clusters) within the study's boundaries that were characterized by the release of toxic chemicals into the air and hazardous waste sites (22). For the two clusters, the case-control OR of the targeted defect was 13.4 (95% CI 4.7–37.8). Three other possible associations with *l*-transposition of the great arteries were identified: maternal smoking (OR 1.6, 95% CI 1.1–2.4), maternal use of hair dye (OR 3.0, 95% CI 0.9–9.7), and paternal exposure to laboratory chemicals (OR 8.2, 95% CI 1.7–40.1) (22).

Neural Tube Defects

In addition to the references cited in this section, see references 21 and 37.

A 1979 case-control study examined the effects of cigarette smoking on closure defects of the central nervous system (CNS) (anencephaly, myelomeningocele, and encephalocele; 66 cases) and oral clefts (cleft lip or cleft palate; 66 cases) (23). Smoking frequency was determined from hospital records. Although significantly more case women smoked than did control women (83% vs. 39%), there was no association between smoking and CNS closure defects (33% vs. 39%) (23). Another 1979 study found no association, compared with nonsmokers, between smoking and congenital malformations (2.8% vs. 2.8%) (24). Similarly, no associations with specific defects (cardiovascular, gastrointestinal, genitourinary, musculoskeletal, or oral clefts) were found. After adjustment for socioeconomic class, a possible dose-dependent association with NTDs (anencephaly and spina bifida) was found. However, even if smoking was causal, it was thought to have only modest importance in the etiology of NTDs (24). In addition, women might have understated the number of cigarettes smoked because they were aware of medical opposition to smoking, especially during pregnancy. Information was more likely to be accurate for nonsmokers and heavy smokers (24).

A 1998 Swedish study found a protective effect of maternal smoking on the incidence of NTDs: total NTDs OR 0.75 (95% CI 0.61–0.91); anencephaly OR 0.49 (95% CI 0.28–0.85); and spina bifida OR 0.76 (95% CI 0.61–0.95) (25). Although the exact cause for this unexpected finding was unknown, one logical reason could have been an excess in early losses of embryos with NTDs (25).

Limb Defects

In addition to the references cited in this section, see reference 21.

A 1994 case-control study used the Hungarian Congenital Abnormality Registry (1975–1984) and three other sources of ascertainment (1,575,904 births) to examine the association between smoking and isolated congenital limb deficiencies (six types) (26).

After adjustment, the relative odds (RO) 1.48 (95% CI 0.98–2.23) of cases of terminal transverse limb deficiencies (but not five other types of limb deficiencies) were higher among smoking mothers. A causal relationship could not be proven because of unadjusted potential confounders. However, the data did support the hypothesis of vascular disruption as a cause of the defects (26). A 1997 study used data from Swedish Health registries to identify 610 cases of limb reduction defects among 1,109,299 infants born between 1983 and 1993 (27). The OR for an association between any maternal smoking and all cases of limb reductions was 1.2, 95% CI 1.06–1.50. Of the various types of defects, only transverse limb reductions had an OR and 95% CI above unity (27).

Craniosynostosis

An increased risk of craniosynostosis (premature ossification of the skull and obliteration of the sutures resulting in a misshapen head) in mothers who smoked was reported in 1994 (28). In the Colorado Craniosynostosis Registry (1986–1989), 212 cases confirmed by an independent radiologist were identified and participated in the study. Cases and controls were interviewed between 1989 and 1991. The types of craniosynostosis were lambdoid ($N = 86$), sagittal ($N = 69$), coronal ($N = 25$), metopic ($N = 18$), and multiple suture synostosis ($N = 14$). Smoking was associated with craniosynostosis RO 1.7 (95% CI 1.2–2.6). For mothers who smoked more than one pack/day, the association for all types of craniosynostosis combined was RO 3.5 (95% CI 1.5–8.4) and for coronal synostosis it was RO 5.6 (95% CI 2.1–15.3). No significant association was noted for drinking (28). A 1999 study found a significant association between isolated craniosynostosis and smoking (29). For any smoking, the adjusted OR was 1.67 (95% CI 1.27–2.19), but a dose-dependent association also was found: OR 1.45 (95% CI 1.04–2.02) for $<$10 cigarettes/day and OR 2.12 (95% CI 1.50–2.99) for $\geq$10 cigarettes/day. Among the different types of craniosynostosis, only premature closure of the sagittal suture OR 1.48 (95% CI 1.02–2.14) reached statistical significance. Male sex had the strongest association with the defects (29). A 2000 study reported evidence that supported the conclusion of the above studies that smoking was associated with craniosynostosis (30). Using data gathered by the Centers for Disease Control and Prevention's (CDC) population-based surveillance system (1968–1980), 61 mothers of infants with craniosynostosis and 3029 mothers of normal infants were interviewed. After exclusions, 44 cases of isolated craniosynostosis remained, 27 of which were sagittal synostosis. The association between maternal smoking and isolated craniosynostosis was OR 1.92 (95% CI 1.01–3.66) and for sagittal craniosynostosis OR 1.71 (95% CI 0.75–3.89). As with previous studies, male infants were predominantly affected. A limitation of this study was that smoking exposure was only identified for the first 3 months of pregnancy. Smoking frequency may have changed in the last part of pregnancy that is the most critical period for the development of craniosynostosis (30).

Oral Clefts

In addition to the references cited in this section, see references 23 and 24.

Several studies and one review have examined the relationship between smoking and isolated oral clefts. In a 1983 Finish study that appeared to be well controlled for many potential confounders, no significant associations between smoking ($\geq$5 cigarettes/day) and oral clefts, central nervous system defects, or musculoskeletal anomalies were found (31). Using data from the Atlanta Birth Defects Case-Control Study (1968–1980), 238 cases of cleft lip $\pm$ cleft palate and 107 cases of cleft palate were compared to 2,809 match controls (32). Smoking was ascertained by structured questionnaire and exposure was defined as maternal smoking during the period 3 months before conception to 3 months after pregnancy began. After adjustment, significant associations were found between smoking and offspring with isolated cleft lip ± palate (OR 1.55 [95% CI 1.10–2.18]), and isolated cleft palate (OR 1.96 [95% CI 1.10–3.50]) (32).

A 1999 case-control study used data from the Slone Epidemiology Unit Births Defect Study (1976–1992) to examine the relationship between smoking in the first 13 weeks of pregnancy and isolated cleft lip and palate (33). Four control groups, all with other malformations, were selected from the database. The OR and 95% CI were nearly identical in the four groups: 1.5–1.6 (95% CI 1.1–1.3, 1.8–2.7). The investigators concluded that infants with malformations other than the defect of interest were suitable controls (33). Using the same database, the investigators examined the relationship between smoking and oral clefts (34). Cases were isolated oral clefts (cleft lip alone [*N* = 334], cleft lip and palate [*N* = 494], or cleft palate [*N* = 244]), and oral clefts with other malformations (cleft lip [*N* = 58], cleft lip and palate [*N* = 140], or cleft palate [*N* = 209]). Controls had other malformations, but not oral clefts or defects possibly associated with smoking. There were no associations between smoking and any oral cleft group. However, a positive dose-response was found in infants with cleft lip and palate and other malformations: 1–14 cigarettes/day OR 1.09 (95% CI 0.6–1.9), 15–24 cigarettes/day OR 1.84 (95% CI 1.2–2.9), and >24 cigarettes/day OR 1.85 (95% CI 1.0–3.5). This finding might have been related to the presence of malformations associated with smoking (34). The authors also reviewed 16 other published studies on the association between smoking and oral clefts.

A 1999 study was conducted in Denmark to determine the relationship between smoking and infant transforming growth factor alpha (TGFα) locus mutations and isolated cleft lip and/or palate (35). A second objective was to determine if there was a synergistic effect of these two risk factors. Smoking was associated with a slightly increased risk of cleft lip ± palate (OR 1.40 [95% CI 0.88–2.00]), but not with isolated cleft palate. The TGFα allele is elevated in the Danish population, occurring in 25% of both cases and controls. It was not associated with either type of oral cleft and no synergistic effect with smoking was observed (35).

The 1996 United States Natality database involving 3,891,494 live births was used in a 2000 case-control study (36). Four states were excluded because they did not collect smoking data. A total of 2207 live births with cleft lip and palate were compared to 4,414 normal controls. After adjustment for maternal age, race, education levels, and maternal conditions (diabetes and gestational hypertension), a significant association was found between smoking and the defect (OR 1.34 [95% CI 1.16–1.54]). Moreover, compared to no smoking, a dose response was found: 1–10 cigarettes/day OR 1.50 (95% CI 1.28–1.76), 11–20 cigarettes/day OR 1.55 (95% CI 1.23–1.95); and 21 or more cigarettes/day OR 1.78 (95% CI 1.22–2.59) (36).

A 2002 case-control study examined the status of a biotransformation enzyme *N*-acetyltransferase 2 (NAT2) in 45 case mothers who had a child with an oral cleft, 39 case mothers who had a child with spina bifida, and 73 control mothers (37). NAT2 is involved in the inactivation of toxic compounds in cigarette smoke and some drugs. The maternal phenotype, either slow or fast NAT2 acetylators, was determined for case and control mothers. Compared to fast NAT2 acetylators, slow acetylators had no increased risk for oral clefts (OR 1.0 [95% CI 0.4–2.3]) or spina bifida (OR 0.7 [95% CI 0.3–1.7]). In the oral cleft group, significantly more mothers smoked and used medications than controls (36% vs. 18% and 38% vs. 19%, respectively). In the spina bifida group, case mothers were similar to controls for smoking, but significantly more used medications during pregnancy (23% vs. 18% and 44% vs. 19%) (37).

A 1996 review examined the relationship between potentially teratogenic environmental exposures and nonsyndromic oral clefts (38). The origin of oral clefts is multifactorial and involves both genetic and environmental factors, one of which is believed to be cigarette smoking. Several studies, some of which are discussed above, were reviewed that found negative and positive associations between smoking and oral clefts. Although not arriving at any conclusions as to specific causes of isolated oral clefts (none were possible), the review did identify common misclassifications and confounding bias that could distort a study's findings (38).

Genitourinary Defects

In addition to the references cited in this section, see references 20 and 24.

A 1996 case-control study assessed the association between smoking and urinary tract anomalies (39). There were 112 cases and 354 controls. After adjustment, a significant association between smoking and urinary tract defects was found (OR 2.3 [95% CI 1.2–4.5]). Significant associations also were found for mothers who smoked 1 to 1,000 cigarettes (light smoking) during the entire pregnancy (OR 3.7 [95% CI 1.7–8.6]) or during the 1st trimester (OR 2.9 [95% CI 1.4–6.7]). When analyzed by infant sex, the associations were significant for females (OR 6.1 [95% CI 2.0–18.4] and OR 5.7 [95% CI 2.0–16.5], respectively), but not for males (OR 2.5 [95% CI 0.8–7.6] and OR 1.7 [95% CI 0.7–4.5], respectively). No significant associations were found for heavy smoking (>1000 cigarettes) either in the entire pregnancy or in the 1st trimester. The authors hypothesized that the lack of a dose response might have been a result of a greater prevalence of fetal loss from SAB or stillbirth and that these fetuses may have had major congenital defects that involved the urinary tract (39). A 1997 study used Swedish health registries to identify 483 infants with kidney malformations and 719 infants with other urinary organ malformations with no involvement of the kidneys from 1,117,021 infants born during the period 1983–1993 with known smoking exposure in early pregnancy (40). A moderate significant association with kidney malformations (agenesis/hypoplasia, dysplasia, or unspecified cystic disease) was found (OR 1.22 [95% CI 1.00–1.48]), but there was no dose-response association ($<$10 cigarettes/day vs. $\geq$10 cigarettes/day). No association with other urinary organ malformations was observed (40).

A negative association was found between cigarette smoking and hypospadias in a 2002 case-control study (41). Data from the Swedish health registries provided 3262 cases among 1,413,811 infants born during the period 1983–1996. The association between any smoking ($N = 715$) and the defect was OR 0.83 (95% CI 0.76–0.90). The results were similar for those $<$10 cigarettes/day ($N = 450$) or $\geq$10/day ($N = 265$). Because the negative association was only found in those cases where the mother's parity was 1 or >4, confounding was suspected (41).

Foot Defects

Several studies have discovered positive associations between maternal smoking and foot deformities. A brief 1998 report described an association between maternal smoking and foot defects (adjusted OR 1.21 [95% CI 1.14–1.29]) (42). The authors also cited six other studies examining the relationship between foot defects and smoking, four of which had ORs ranging from 1.0 to 2.6 with 95% CI above 1.0 (42). In a 2000 study, 346 infants with isolated clubfoot were identified from the Atlanta Birth Defects Case-Control (1968–1980) database (43). Case infants and normal controls ($N = 3029$) were born during the period 1968–1980 and the mothers were interviewed in 1982–1983. The adjusted OR and 95% CI were smoking only: 1.34 (1.04–1.72); family history only:

6.52 (2.95–14.41); and smoking and family history: 20.30 (7.90–52.17). The findings suggested a potentially important gene–environmental factor interaction (43). A 2002 report compared 239 cases of congenital idiopathic clubfoot (talipes equinovarus) to 365 unmatched controls in a population-based study of the relationship between maternal smoking and the foot anomaly (44). The OR for smoking and talipes equinovarus was 2.2 (95% CI 1.5–3.3). A dose-dependent response was seen and, in addition, female infants had a higher risk than in males (OR 2.8 vs. 1.8). For isolated clubfoot, the OR for smoking was 2.4 (95% CI 1.6–3.6) (44).

Poland Syndrome

A 1999 case-control study examined data from the Hungarian Congenital Abnormality Registry (HCAR) (population-based) and the Spanish Collaborative Study of Congenital Malformations (ECEMC) (hospital-based, case-control) to determine if there was an association between maternal cigarette smoking and isolated Poland sequence (45). Poland syndrome, or sequence, is thought to be caused by interruption of the early embryonic blood supply in the subclavian arteries and is characterized by pectoral muscle defect and ipsilateral hand deficiencies of various types and severity (45). In the HCAR database, 20 cases were identified from 1,575,904 births (prevalence 0.13 per 10,000 births), whereas in the ECEMC database, there were 32 cases among 1,405,392 births (prevalence 0.23 per 10,000 births). Logistic regression analyses (after controlling for maternal age, birth weight, gestational age, and pregnancy order) revealed that maternal smoking was associated with an increased risk of Poland sequence in both the HCAR (OR 2.72) and ECEMC (OR 2.61) databases. When combined, the OR was 1.83. The investigators concluded that the results suggested a two-fold increase in the risk of Poland sequence from *in utero* exposure to cigarette smoking. Although the number of cases were small, the results were similar in two programs with different methodologies and possibly different uncontrolled confounding factors. However, confirmation of the findings is required (45).

Gastroschisis

The cause of gastroschisis is unknown but vascular disruption during early embryonic development has been suggested. No association between cigarette smoking and the abdominal wall defect was found in two studies published in the 1990s (46,47). A 2000 review cited 10 case-control studies that reported various associations with gastroschisis, two of which associated the defect with cigarette smoking, in addition to other factors (48). In one of the studies, smoking ascertainment was obtained from birth certificates, a source known to underestimate maternal smoking, so the significant OR 4.1 (95% CI 1.4–12) is suspect. In the second study, the source was a 2nd trimester interview and the result was OR 2.1 (95% CI 0.9–4.8) (48).

A 2002 abstract examined gastroschisis and small intestine atresia, two defects believed to arise from vascular disruption (49). Maternal smoking and use of vasoconstrictive drugs (pseudoephedrine, phenylpropanolamine, ephedrine, and ecstasy [methylenedioxymethamphetamine]) was ascertained by retrospective interview. The number of cases and controls were 205 gastroschisis, 127 small intestine atresia, 381 malformed controls, and 416 normal controls. In the four groups, the reported use of a vasoconstrictive drug in the first 2 months of pregnancy was 20%, 21%, 13%, and 12%, respectively, whereas maternal smoking was present in 48%, 24%, 34%, and 34%, respectively. The OR for vasoconstrictive drug use or smoking were gastroschisis, −1.7 (95% CI 1.0–2.8) and 1.5 (95% CI 1.1–2.2), and small intestine atresia, −2.0 (95% CI 1.0–3.7) and 1.0 (95% CI 0.6–1.7), respectively. Combined exposure to the drugs and smoking increased the gastroschisis risk 2.1-fold and the small intestine atresia risk 2.8-fold. Vasoconstrictive drug use and smoking 20 or more cigarettes/day increased the risks 3.6-fold and 4.2-fold, respectively (49).

Neonatal Complications

Neonatal Intensive Care Unit Admissions

Infants of smoking mothers have an increased risk of admission to a neonatal intensive care unit (NICU) (5). Approximately 14,000 to 26,000 admissions annually may be attributable to smoking.

Retinal Abnormalities

A 2000 study investigated the relationship between maternal cigarette smoking and retinal abnormalities in neonates (50). The infants, both cases and controls (162 each), were grouped by birth weight: small for gestational age (SGA), appropriate for gestational age (AGA), and large for gestational age (LGA). All infants were delivered at term, had clear amniotic fluid, had Apgar scores of 7 or higher, and were healthy with no signs of fetal distress either at birth or during the first 3 days after birth. Smoking was determined by maternal interview. Infants of mothers who had stopped smoking during pregnancy were excluded. Eye examinations were conducted on the 2nd or 3rd day of life by one ophthalmologist who was blinded to the maternal smoking history. Compared to infants of nonsmoking mothers, a highly significant increase in the incidence of retinal arterial narrowing and straightening (RANS) was observed in the eyes of infants of smoking mothers, 52 vs. 10 eyes, respectively. Significant increases in the incidences of RANS also were observed when the results where analyzed by birth weight: SGA 22 vs. 2, AGA 26 vs. 8, and LGA 4 vs. 0 eyes, respectively. In addition, eyes of infants in the smoking exposure group had a significant increase in the incidence of retinal venous dilatation and tortuosity (RVDT), 100 vs. 36, respectively. The results for RVDT were significant in SGA (38 vs. 10 eyes) and AGA (56 vs. 24 eyes) infants, but not in LGA infants (6 vs. 2 eyes). The hematocrit of the infants was significantly higher in the total smoking group and in each birth weight subgroup. Intraretinal hemorrhage (IH), in association with elevated hematocrit and RVDT, was found in the total smoking group, 61 vs. 31 eyes, respectively. When analyzed by birth weight, only the incidence in AGA infants was significantly increased, 39 vs. 18 eyes, respectively. No IH was observed when RANS was present. The IH resolved within 3 months and the other retinal abnormalities (RANS, RVDT) resolved by 6 months of age. The rapid resolution of the IH and other considerations suggested that it would not lead to amblyopia. However, concern was expressed that the vascular retinal abnormalities could be a sign that the exposed infants were predisposed to vascular disease early in adult life (50).

Infant/Adolescent Complications

Neurodevelopment

Smoking during pregnancy may have long-term effects on the cognitive performance, emotional development, perceptual motor abilities, and behavior of offspring (1–3,5,8,10–13,14,16,51–53). Similar findings have been found in experimental animal studies (5,14). Negative effects on learning, such as reading, mathematics, and general ability, have been detected in children as old as 11 years (2,11,13,51). In addition, behavior problems and attention deficit hyperactivity disorder (ADHD) have been observed (3,8,13,51,52). Mean decreases in IQ of 5 points for each 100 g weight decrement have been reported (3). A 1996 study of 10-year-olds with idiopathic mental retardation (most had mild retardation with an IQ between 50 and 70) found, after adjustment for multiple factors including LBW and alcohol, that maternal smoking was associated with a 44% increase in the prevalence of mental retardation (52). When mothers smoked at least 1 pack/day, the increase was 70% after adjustment. Some of the adverse neurodevelopment outcomes cannot be completely separated from potential confounding factors such as the actual amount of smoking, socioeconomic status, education, and passive smoking (11), but the experimental animal studies support the findings. Moreover, more recent studies have controlled for social and family history factors and have found consistent patterns of deficits (15). For example, a 1996 study and subsequent correspondence found, after adjustment for socioeconomic status, parental IQ and ADHD status, and alcohol, a significant association between maternal smoking and ADHD as well as a nearly significant association with decreased IQ (53–55).

Sudden Infant Death Syndrome

An increased risk of sudden infant death syndrome (SIDS) has been associated with maternal cigarette smoking (3–5,7–9,12,13,14,16). Approximately 24% (1200 to 2200 cases) of SIDS/year may be a result of smoking (5). Prenatal and postnatal smoking doubles the risk of SIDS from a baseline of 2.3 per 1,000 births in nonsmokers to 4.6 per 1,000 births (4). The greatest risk appears to be for infants exposed both prenatally and postnatally (9). The risk is also dose-dependent, increasing with the number of cigarettes smoked per day (4,13).

Childhood Morbidity

An increased risk of other diseases and complications has been associated with prenatal and postnatal exposure to cigarette smoke. Separating the effects of these exposure periods on childhood morbidity is very difficult because most infants exposed during gestation will also be exposed postnatally. For example, data from 1988 estimated that only 1.2% of United States children exposed to cigarette smoking *in utero* were not exposed after birth (9). Exposed infants have increased incidences of pneumonia and bronchitis (2,5), childhood asthma (5,12), other respiratory illnesses (7,12), childhood obesity (5), and otitis media (7). Not surprisingly, they also have more hospital admissions for pneumonia and bronchitis (5,12).

Smoking Cessation

Women that are attempting to conceive and those that are pregnant should be encouraged to stop smoking (5,6–8,56). In addition to the obvious health benefits for the woman, smoking cessation can significantly decrease the known risks to the embryo, fetus, newborn, infant, and adolescent. For example, women who quit smoking in the first three or four months of pregnancy can lower the risk of a LBW infant to that of nonsmoking women (5). Smoking cessation also reduces the risk of prematurity and perinatal deaths, and results in fewer infant/adolescent complications (5). Many different strategies have been developed to promote smoking cessation (5,6–8,56). A nonpharmacologic approach is preferred, but many women may be heavily addicted to smoking and require nicotine replacement products and other agents. Nicotine replacement products, such as gums and transdermal patches, however, have not been adequately studied in pregnancy. One concern is the potential for nicotine-induced decreased uterine blood flow and increased uterine vascular resistance that could result in impaired fetal growth and other complications. Transdermal systems appear to more effective than chewing gum because of improper use and taste of the latter (6). On the other hand, transdermal patches may actually deliver more nicotine to the embryo/fetus because continuous blood levels of nicotine, in contrast to periodic levels from episodic smoking, are available to cross the placenta (8). Therefore, nonpharmacologic approaches are the safest for the embryo/fetus, but transdermal patches and gums should be used if other measures fail. At least, these products will avoid exposure to carbon monoxide and the other toxic components of cigarette smoke.

Summary

Maternal and paternal cigarette smoking before pregnancy is associated with reduced fertility and ectopic tubal pregnancies. During pregnancy, maternal smoking is related to increased risks for SABs, premature delivery, placental abruption, placenta previa, and PROM. Symmetrical and asymmetrical fetal growth retardation that involves weight, length, and head, chest, and shoulder circumference, is a consistent finding of numerous studies. Up to 30% of low-birth-weight infants may be caused by maternal smoking. A major consequence of smoking-induced toxicity is a significantly increased perinatal mortality rate, in addition to the losses from SABs. Maternal smoking is also a risk for increased neonatal, infant, and adolescent complications. These include increased admissions to NICU, abnormal neurobehavioral development, SIDS, and childhood diseases such as asthma, respiratory infections, and obesity. Vascular retinal abnormalities in infants are another complication. Although reversible, the abnormalities might be a harbinger of later vascular disease.

Cigarette smoking appears to be associated with small increases (usually less than twofold) in major birth defects and possible deformations. The defects with positive associations involve the heart and great vessels, limbs, skull, genitourinary system, feet, abdominal wall, small bowel, and muscles. Dose-dependent relationships, gene-smoking interactions, and synergistic combinations with some medications have been noted. However, the prevalence and frequency of maternal cigarette smoking are based on self-reports that typically underestimate the actual amount of smoking. This and the failure to adjust for other confounders may have biased the results of some studies. Biochemical validation should be, but rarely is, a component of studies on the effects of smoking during pregnancy.

BREAST FEEDING SUMMARY

RECOMMENDATION: Contraindicated

Nicotine is excreted into breast milk. Nursing infants of mothers who smoke will be exposed to nicotine by inhalation and orally (13,57). Cigarette smoking may also decrease the volume of milk (57). In addition, smoking decreases the duration of breast-feeding. A 1998 review cited data from an earlier survey that found that the duration of breast-feeding was significantly decreased in women who smoked when compared with those that did not smoke (58). In nonsmokers, the duration was 145.0 days, whereas the duration of breast-feeding in those that smoked ≤1 pack/day or >1 pack/day was 99.5 and 77.9 days, respectively. Women who are breast-feeding should be urged to quit because cigarette smoking is a significant risk to their health and to their infant's health (see the above sections on Neonatal Complications and Infant/Adolescent Complications). If a woman cannot stop smoking, at least she should try not to smoke in the same room with the infant or during nursing. The American Academy of Pediatrics encourages smoking cessation during lactation, but makes no recommendation for or against nicotine replacement products because of insufficient data (59).

References

1. Longo LD. Environmental pollution and pregnancy: risks and uncertainties for the fetus and infant. Am J Obstet Gynecol 1980;137:162–73.
2. Report of Committee Appointed by Action on Smoking and Health. Mothers who smoke and their children. Practitioner 1980;224:735–9.
3. Longo LD. Some health consequences of maternal smoking: issues without answers. Birth Defects Orig Artic Ser 1982;18:13–31.
4. Lee MJ. Marihuana and tobacco use in pregnancy. Obstet Gynecol Clin North Am 1998;25:65–83.

5. Adams J. Statement of the Public Affairs Committee of the Teratology Society on the importance of smoking cessation during pregnancy. Birth Defects Res Part A Clin Mol Teratol 2003;67:895–9.
6. Kendrick JS, Merritt RK. Women and smoking: an update for the 1990s. Am J Obstet Gynecol 1996;175:528–35.
7. Floyd RL, Rimer BK, Giovino GA, Mullen PD, Sullivan SE. A review of smoking in pregnancy: effects on pregnancy outcomes and cessation efforts. Annu Rev Publ Health 1993;14:379–411.
8. Slotkin TA. Fetal nicotine or cocaine exposure: which one is worse? J Pharmacol Exp Ther 1998;285:931–45.
9. Werler MM. Teratogen update: smoking and reproductive outcomes. Teratology 1997;55:382–8.
10. Merritt TA. Smoking mothers affect little lives. Am J Dis Child 1981;135:501–2.
11. Stillman RJ, Rosenberg MJ, Sachs BP. Smoking and reproduction. Fertil Steril 1986;46:545–66.
12. Mercelina-Roumans PEAM, Ubachs JMH, van Wersch JWJ. Smoking and pregnancy. Eur J Obstet Gynecol Reprod Biol 1997;75:113–4.
13. King JC, Fabro S. Alcohol consumption and cigarette smoking: effect on pregnancy. Clin Obstet Gynecol 1983;26:437–48.
14. Landesman-Dwyer S, Emanuel I. Smoking during pregnancy. Teratology 1979;19:119 26.
15. Hill RM, Craig JP, Chaney MD, Tennyson LM, McCulley LB. Utilization of over-the-counter drugs during pregnancy. Clin Obstet Gynecol 1977;20:381–94.
16. Niebury P, Marks JS, McLaren NM, Remington PL. The fetal tobacco syndrome. JAMA 1985;253:2998–9.
17. Krishna K. Tobacco chewing in pregnancy. Br J Obstet Gynaecol 1978;85:726–8.
18. Fedrick J, Alberman ED, Goldstein H. Possible teratogenic effect of cigarette smoking. Nature 1971;231:529–30.
19. Kelsey JL, Dwyer T, Holford TR, Bracken MB. Maternal smoking and congenital malformations: an epidemiological study. J Epidemiol Comm Health 1978;32:102–7.
20. Himmelberger DU,Brown BW Jr, Cohen EN. Cigarette smoking during pregnancy and the occurrence of spontaneous abortion and congenital abnormality. Am J Epidemiol 1978;108;470–9.
21. Wasserman CR, Shaw GM, O'Malley CD, Tolarova MM, Lammer EJ. Parental cigarette smoking and risk for congenital anomalies of the heart, neural tube, or limb. Teratology 1996;53:261–7.
22. Kuehl KS, Loffredo CA. Population-based study of l-transposition of the great arteries: possible associations with environmental factors. Birth Defects Res Part A Clin Mol Teratol 2003;67:162–7.
23. Ericson A, Kallen B, Westerholm P. Cigarette smoking as an etiologic factor in cleft lip and palate. Am J Obstet Gynecol 1979;135:348–51.
24. Evans DR, Newcombe RG, Campbell H. Maternal smoking habits and congenital malformations: a population study. Br Med J 1979;2:171–3.
25. Kallen K. Maternal smoking, body mass index, and neural tube defects. Am J Epidemiol 1998;147:1103–11.
26. Czeizel AE, Kodaj I, Lenz W. Smoking during pregnancy and congenital limb deficiency. BMJ 1994;308:1473–6.
27. Kallen K. Maternal smoking during pregnancy and limb reduction malformations in Sweden. Am J Public Health 1997;87:29–32.
28. Alderman BW, Bradley CM, Greene C, Fernbach SK, Baron AE. Increase risk of craniosynostosis with maternal cigarette smoking during pregnancy. Teratology 1994;50:13–8.
29. Kallen K. Maternal smoking and craniosynostosis. Teratology 1999;60:146–50.
30. Honein MA, Rasmussen SA. Further evidence for an association between maternal smoking and craniosynostosis. Teratology 2000;62:145–6.
31. Hemminki K, Mutanen P, Saloniemi I. Smoking and the occurrence of congenital malformations and spontaneous abortions: multivariate analysis. Am J Obstet Gynecol 1983;145:61–6.
32. Khoury MJ, Gomez-Farias M, Mulinare J. Does maternal cigarette smoking during pregnancy cause cleft lip and palate in offspring? Am J Dis Child 1989;143:333–7.
33. Lieff S, Olshan AF, Werler M, Savitz DA, Mitchell AA. Selection bias and the use of controls with malformations in case-control studies of birth defects. Epidemiology 1999;10:238–41.
34. Lieff S, Olshan AF, Werler M, Strauss RP, Smith J, Mitchell A. Maternal cigarette smoking during pregnancy and risk of oral clefts in newborns. Am J Epidemiol 1999;150:683–94.
35. Christensen K, Olsen J, Norgaard-Pedersen B, Basso O, Stovring H, Milhollin-Johnson L, Murray JC. Oral clefts, transforming growth factor alpha gene variants, and maternal smoking: a population-based case-control study in Denmark, 1991–1994. Am J Epidemiol 1999;149:248–55.
36. Chung KC, Kowalski CP, Kim HM, Buchman SR. Maternal cigarette smoking during pregnancy and the risk of having a child with cleft lip/palate. Plast Reconstr Surg 2000;105:485–91.
37. van Rooij IALM, Groenen PMW, van Drongelen M, Te Morsche RHM, Peters WHM, Steegers-Theunissen RPM. Orofacial clefts and spina bifida: *N*-acetyltransferase phenotype, maternal smoking, and medication use. Teratology 2002;66:260–6.
38. Wyszynski DF, Beaty TH. Review of the role of potential teratogens in the origin of human nonsyndromic oral clefts. Teratology 1996;53:309–17.
39. Li DK, Mueller BA, Hickok DE, Daling JR, Fantel AG, Checkoway H, Weiss NS. Maternal smoking during pregnancy and the risk of congenital urinary tract anomalies. Am J Public Health 1996;86:249–53.
40. Kallen K. Maternal smoking and urinary organ malformations. Int J Epidemiol 1997;26:571–4.
41. Kallen K. Role of maternal smoking and maternal reproductive history in the etiology of hypospadias in the offspring. Teratology 2002;66:185–91.
42. Reefhuis J, de Walle HEK, Cornel MC, EUROCAT Working Group. Maternal smoking and deformities of the foot: results of the EUROCAT study. Am J Public Health 1998;88:1554–5.
43. Honein MA, Paulozzi LJ, Moore CA. Family history, maternal smoking, and clubfoot: an indication of a gene-environment interaction. Am J Epidemiol 2000;152:658–65.

44. Skelly AC, Holt VL, Mosca VS, Alderman BW. Talipes equinovarus and maternal smoking: a population-based case-control study in Washington State. Teratology 2002;66:91–100.
45. Martinez-Frias ML, Czeizel AE, Rodriguez-Pinilla E, Bermejo E. Smoking during pregnancy and Poland sequence: results of a population-based registry and a case-control registry. Teratology 1999;59:35–8.
46. Torfs CP, Velie EM, Oechsli FW, Bateson TF, Curry CJR. A population-based study of gastroschisis: demographic, pregnancy, and lifestyle risk factors. Teratology 1994;50:44–53.
47. Penman DG, Fisher RM, Noblett HR, Soothill PW. Increase in incidence of gastroschisis in the south west of England in 1995. Br J Obstet Gynaecol 1998;105:328–31.
48. Curry JI, McKinney P, Thornton JG, Stringer MD. The aetiology of gastroschisis. Br J Obstet Gynaecol 2000;107:1339–46.
49. Werler MM, Mitchell AA. Case-control study of vasoconstrictive exposures and risks of gastroschisis and small intestinal atresia (abstract). Teratology 2002;65:298.
50. Beratis NG, Varvarigou A, Katsibris J, Gartaganis SP. Vascular retinal abnormalities in neonates of mothers who smoked during pregnancy. J Pediatr 2000;136:760–6.
51. Tong S, McMichael AJ. Maternal smoking and neuropsychological development in childhood: a review of the evidence. Dev Med Child Neurol 1992;34:191–7.
52. Drews CD, Murphy CC, Yeargin-Allsopp M, Decoufle P. The relationship between idiopathic mental retardation and maternal smoking during pregnancy. Pediatrics 1996;97:547–53.
53. Milberger S, Biederman J, Faraone SV, Chen L, Jones J. Is maternal smoking during pregnancy a risk factor for attention deficit hyperactivity disorder in children? Am J Psychiatry 1996;153:1138–42.
54. Chabrol H, Peresson G. ADHD and maternal smoking during pregnancy. Am J Psychiatry 1997;154:1177.
55. Milberger S, Biederman J, Faraone SV. ADHD and maternal smoking during pregnancy. Reply. Am J Psychiatry 1997;154:1177–8.
56. American College of Obstetricians and Gynecologists. Smoking cessation during pregnancy. Educational Bulletin. No. 260. September 2000.
57. U.S. Department of Health and Human Services. *HHS Blueprint for Action on Breastfeeding*. Washington, DC: Office on Women's Health, 2000.
58. Howard CR, Lawrence RA. Breast-feeding and drug exposure. Obstet Gynecol Clin North Am 1998;25:195–217.
59. American Academy of Pediatrics. The transfer of drugs and other chemicals into human milk. Pediatrics 2001;108:776–89.

Name:	**CIGUATOXIN**	Risk Factor:	**X**
Class:	**Toxin**		

FETAL RISK SUMMARY

RECOMMENDATION: Human Data Suggest Risk

Ciguatoxin is a marine toxin produced by the blue-green algae, *Gambierdiscus toxicus* that is concentrated in the fish food chain (1). The toxin is stable to cooking, freezing, drying, or salting and results in ciguatera poisoning when infected tropical fish are ingested (1). Other toxins that may be present with ciguatoxin include scaritoxin and maitotoxin (2,3).

Eight cases of ciguatera poisoning during pregnancy have been published (1–4). An Australian woman at term developed symptoms of poisoning within 4 hours of ingesting the toxin from a reef fish (1). Fetal symptoms of poisoning, beginning simultaneously with the mother's symptoms, consisted of "tumultuous fetal movements, and an intermittent peculiar fetal shivering" (1). The unusual fetal movements continued for 18 hours, then gradually subsided over the next 24 hours. A cesarean section performed 2 days later delivered a 3800-g male infant with meconium aspiration and left-sided facial palsy. At 1 day of age, possible myotonia of the muscles of the hands was noted. Pulmonary signs and symptoms of the meconium aspiration resolved with time. At 6 weeks of age, the baby had not yet smiled, but he was otherwise normal (1). The mother was unable to breast feed because of excruciating hyperesthesia of the nipples.

Six cases of ciguatera poisoning during pregnancy (gestational ages not provided) were described by researchers from the San Francisco Bay area in an abstract published in 1991 (2). The women had neurologic, neuromuscular, and cardiovascular signs and symptoms of poisoning, and all experienced increased fetal activity in conjunction with their symptoms. One fetus was aborted during the acute phase of the poisoning (2). The other five women were delivered, at or near term, of apparently normal infants without sequelae from the exposure. The exposure-delivery intervals for the latter five cases were not specified.

In another case from California, a woman in her 16th week of gestation developed ciguatera poisoning 4 hours after eating a meal of cooked barracuda (4). This case may have been briefly mentioned in another reference (3). Increased fetal movements persisted only for a few hours. A cesarean section, performed 19 days past term, delivered a normal, 3630-g male infant who was developing normally at 10 months of age.

Of the cases described, none of the liveborn infants appeared to have had lasting sequelae from exposure to the toxin. However, long-term adverse effects could not be completely excluded in the one infant exposed shortly before birth. The timing of the exposure in relation to delivery may have been a factor in this case. The association between the toxin and the abortion cannot be determined from the available data. Transplacental passage of the toxin has not been studied, but its high molecular weight (1112) presumably limits its transfer, at least early in gestation before thinning of the placental membranes has occurred.

BREAST FEEDING SUMMARY

RECOMMENDATION: Contraindicated

Ciguatoxin is apparently excreted in breast milk. A 4-month-old infant was breast-fed 1 hour and 3 hours after his mother consumed a portion of a presumed ciguatera-infected fish (5). The mother's symptoms of poisoning developed within a few hours of ingesting the fish meal and resolved by 3 weeks. She continued to nurse her infant throughout the entire course of her illness. Approximately 10 hours after the first nursing following the mother's fish meal, the baby became colicky, irritable, and developed diarrhea lasting 48 hours, followed by a fine maculopapular rash. The signs and symptoms in the infant, which were considered compatible with ciguatera toxicity by the authors, completely resolved within 2 weeks (5).

Ciguatoxin was thought to be the cause of green stools in a nursing 3-month-old infant who was breast-fed 12 hours after the mother had developed symptoms of ciguatera poisoning (6). The infant was changed to formula and then rechallenged with breast milk a few days later, resulting in the reappearance of the green stools. Prompt cessation of breast-feeding again resolved the problem. No other symptoms were observed in the infant.

References

1. Pearn J, Harvey P, De Ambrosis W, Lewis R, McKay R. Ciguatera and pregnancy. Med J Austr 1982;1:57–8.
2. Rivera-Alsina ME, Payne C, Pou A, Payne S. Ciguatera poisoning in pregnancy (Abstract). Am J Obstet Gynecol 1991;164:397.
3. Geller RJ, Olson KR, Senecal PE. Ciguatera fish poisoning in San Francisco, California, caused by imported barracuda. West J Med 1991;155:639–42.
4. Senecal PE, Osterloh JD. Normal fetal outcome after maternal ciguateric toxin exposure in the second trimester. J Toxicol Clin Toxicol 1991;29:473–8.
5. Blythe DG, de Sylva DP. Mother's milk turns toxic following fish feast. JAMA 1990;264:2074.
6. Thoman M. Letters to the editor. Vet Hum Toxicol 1989;31:71.

C

Name:	**CILOSTAZOL**	Risk Factor:	**C_M**
Class:	**Hematologic Agent (Antiplatelet)**		

FETAL RISK SUMMARY

RECOMMENDATION: No Human Data - Animal Data Suggest Risk

Cilostazol, an antiplatelet agent, is an inhibitor of cellular phosphodiesterase III. It is indicated for the reduction of symptoms of intermittent claudication. The drug undergoes extensive hepatic metabolism. Two of the metabolites are active.

Reproduction studies have been conducted with cilostazol in rats and rabbits (1). No effects on fertility or mating performance were observed in male and female rats at oral doses up to 1000 mg/kg/day. The highest dose produced systemic exposures less than 1.5 times in males, and about 5 times in females, the human systemic exposure based on the area under the plasma concentration curve of unbound cilostazol at the maximum recommended human dose. In pregnant rats, the 1000 mg/kg/day dose resulted in decreased fetal weights and an increased incidence of congenital malformations in the cardiovascular (ventricular septal, aortic arch, and subclavian artery defects), renal (renal pelvic dilation), and skeletal (14th rib; retarded ossification) systems. Increased incidences of ventricular septal defects and retarded ossification were also observed at 150 mg/kg/day. This same dose administered to rats in late pregnancy was associated with stillbirths and decreased birth weight. In pregnant rabbits, a dose of 150 mg/kg/day was associated with an increased incidence of retarded ossification of the sternum (1).

It is not known if cilostazol crosses the human placenta to the fetus. The molecular weight (about 369) is low enough that transfer to the fetus should be expected. Moreover, transfer of the two active metabolites may also occur.

In summary, no reports describing the use of cilostazol during human pregnancy have been located. The drug is teratogenic and toxic in two animal species, but the complete lack of human data prevents any assessment of the risk that cilostazol presents to a human fetus.

BREAST FEEDING SUMMARY

RECOMMENDATION: No Human Data - Potential Toxicity

No reports describing the use of cilostazol during human lactation have been located. The drug is excreted into the milk of lactating rats (1). This is consistent with the relatively low molecular weight (about 369) of the drug and excretion into breast milk should be expected. The effect on a nursing infant from exposure to cilostazol in milk is unknown. Because of the potential for severe adverse effects, breast-feeding while receiving cilostazol is not recommended.

Reference

1. Product information. Pletal. Otsuka America Pharma, 2000.

Name:	**CIMETIDINE**	Risk Factor:	B_M
Class:	**Gastrointestinal Agent (Antisecretory)**		

C

FETAL RISK SUMMARY

RECOMMENDATION: Compatible

Cimetidine is an H_2-receptor antagonist that inhibits gastric acid secretion. In pregnancy, the antihistamine is primarily used for the treatment of peptic ulcer disease and for the prevention of gastric acid aspiration (Mendelson's syndrome) prior to delivery.

In studies with multiple animal species, no evidence of impaired fertility or teratogenesis was observed with doses up to 40 times higher than the usual human dose (1). Cimetidine does have weak antiandrogenic effects in animals, as evidenced by a reduction in the size of testes, prostatic glands, and seminal vesicles (2,3), and in humans, by reports of decreased libido and impotence (4). Conflicting reports on the antiandrogenic activity in animals exposed *in utero* to cimetidine have been published (5–9).

Three references, all from the same research group, described the effects on male rats of exposure to cimetidine from gestation up to the time of weaning (5–7). The rats had decreased weights of testicles, prostate gland, and seminal vesicles at 55 and 110 days of age as compared to nonexposed controls. Exposed animals also had reduced testosterone serum levels, lack of sexual motivation, and decreased sexual performance, but normal luteinizing hormone levels. The observed demasculinization effects were still present 35 days after discontinuation of the drug, indicating that exposure may have modified both central and end-organ androgen receptor activity or responsiveness (5–7). In contrast, researchers from the manufacturer treated rats similarly to rats in the above reports and found no effect on any of the parameters described previously (8). Another group found no effect of cimetidine exposure during gestation and lactation on masculine sexual development, except for an insensitivity of the pituitary gland to androgen regulation, and no effect at all on female pups (9). These authors concluded that cimetidine was not an animal teratogen.

Cimetidine crosses the placenta to the fetus by simple diffusion (10–14). In an *in vitro* study, the placental transfer of cimetidine across human and baboon placentas was similar (10). Cimetidine is not metabolized by the placenta (11). At term, cimetidine crosses the placenta, resulting in a peak mean fetal:maternal ratio of 0.84 at 1.5–2 hours (12). In an earlier study, 20 women were administered a single, 200-mg bolus injection of cimetidine prior to delivery (19 vaginal, 1 cesarean section) (13). The drug was detected in all but two cord blood samples with levels ranging from 0.05–1.22 μg/mL. The injection-to-delivery intervals in the two patients with no cimetidine in cord blood were prolonged, 435 and 780 minutes. A 1983 study measured a peak mean fetal:maternal ratio of about 0.5 at 2.5 hours (14).

The manufacturer has received a number of reports of women who took the drug during pregnancy, including throughout gestation (B. Dickson, personal communication, Smith Kline & French Laboratories, 1986). They are aware of three isolated incidences of congenital defects, apparently unrelated to cimetidine therapy, including congenital heart disease, mental retardation detected later in life, and clubfoot.

The drug has been used throughout pregnancy in a case ending in intrauterine fetal death, but the adverse outcome was believed to be caused by severe maternal disease and captopril therapy (see Captopril) (15). Three pregnant women with gastric hemorrhage secondary to peptic ulcer disease were described in a 1982 report (16). The women, at 16, 12, and 31 weeks' gestation, were treated for various lengths of time with cimetidine and other standard therapy and all delivered healthy newborns without congenital defects or metabolic disturbances. Transient liver impairment has been described in a newborn exposed to cimetidine at term (17). However, other reports have not confirmed this toxicity (13,18–35).

In a surveillance study of Michigan Medicaid recipients conducted between 1985 and 1992 involving 229,101 completed pregnancies, 460 newborns had been exposed to cimetidine during the 1st trimester (F. Rosa, personal communication, FDA, 1993). A total of 20 (4.3%) major birth defects were observed (20 expected). Specific data were available for six defect categories, including (observed/expected) 8/5 cardiovascular defects, 0/1 oral clefts, 0/0 spina bifida, 1/1 polydactyly, 0/1 limb reduction defects, and 1/1 hypospadias. These data do not support an association between the drug and congenital defects.

Cimetidine has been used at term either with or without other antacids to prevent maternal gastric acid aspiration pneumonitis (Mendelson's syndrome) (13,14,19–35). No neonatal adverse effects were noted in these studies.

Data from the Swedish Medical Birth Registry were presented in 1998 (36). A total of 553 infants (6 sets of twins) were delivered from 547 women who had used acid-suppressing drugs early in pregnancy. A number of other pharmaceutical agents, identified only by drug category, were also used by these women. Seventeen infants with birth defects were identified (3.1%; 95% confidence interval [CI] 1.8–4.9) compared with the crude malformation rate of 3.9% in the Registry. The odds ratio (OR) for a congenital malformation, stratified for birth year, maternal age, parity, and smoking was 0.72 (95% CI 0.41–1.24) (36). The OR for malformations after proton pump blocker exposure was 0.91 (95% CI 0.45–1.84), compared with 0.46 (95% CI 0.17–1.20) for H_2-receptor antagonists (OR 0.86, 95% CI 0.33–2.23; $p = 0.13$). Of the 17 infants with birth defects, 10 had been exposed to proton pump blockers, 6 to H_2 antagonists, and 1 to both classes of drug. Cimetidine was the only acid-suppressing drug exposure in 35 infants. Three other offspring were exposed *in utero* to cimetidine combined either with famotidine (one infant) or with omeprazole (two infants). Two birth defects (5.7%) were observed in the group where cimetidine was the only acid-suppressing agent used. The defects were an encephalocele and an unstable hip (36).

Two databases, one from England and the other from Italy, were combined for a study published in 1999 that was designed to assess the incidence of congenital malformations in women who had received a prescription during the 1st trimester for an acid-suppressing drug (cimetidine, ranitidine, and omeprazole) (37). Nonexposed women were selected from the same databases to form a control group. Spontaneous abortions and elective abortions (except two cases for anomalies that were grouped with stillbirths) were excluded from the analysis. Stillbirths were defined as any pregnancy loss occurring at 28 weeks' gestation or later. Cimetidine was taken in 233 pregnancies, resulting in 234 live births (14 [6.0%] premature), 3 stillbirths, and 1 neonatal death. Eleven (4.7%) of the newborns had a congenital malformation (shown by system): craniofacial (cleft lip and palate), musculoskeletal (dysplastic hip/dislocation/clicking hip $N = 3$; polydactyly), genital and urinary (hypospadias $N = 2$; congenital hydrocele/inguinal hernia, ovarian cyst, renal defects/hydronephrosis), and gastrointestinal (pyloric stenosis). In addition, two newborns had a small head circumference for gestational age. In comparison, the outcomes of 1547 nonexposed pregnancies included 1560 live births (115 [7.4%] premature), 15 stillbirths (includes 2 elective abortions for anomalies), and 10 neonatal deaths. Sixty-four

(4.1%) of the newborns had malformations involving the following: central nervous system ($N = 2$), head/face ($N = 13$), eye ($N = 2$), heart ($N = 7$), muscle/skeleton ($N = 13$), genital/urinary ($N = 18$), gastrointestinal ($N = 2$), and those of polyformation ($N = 3$) or known genetic defects ($N = 4$). Twenty-one newborns were small for gestational age and 78 had a small head circumference for gestational age. The relative risk of malformation (adjusted for mother's age and prematurity) associated with cimetidine was 1.3 (95% CI 0.7–2.6), with omeprazole 0.9 (95% CI 0.4–2.4), and with ranitidine 1.5 (95% CI 0.9–2.6) (37).

In summary, no increased risk of congenital malformations attributable to cimetidine in humans have been reported. One group of reviewers has recommended that the drug not be used during pregnancy because of the possibility for feminization, as observed in some animals and in nonpregnant humans (38). Apparently, this potential toxicity has not been studied in humans exposed *in utero* to cimetidine, but research in this area is warranted.

BREAST FEEDING SUMMARY

RECOMMENDATION: Compatible

In a study using lactating mice, drug-metabolizing enzymes in nursing pups were inhibited to a greater extent by cimetidine than those in the mother (39). Mouse dams were treated with cimetidine from the delivery date to 6 weeks, the time of weaning. Male pups were adversely affected from 4 weeks of age to 8 weeks, 2 weeks after cessation of exposure, whereas female pups were affected for a longer time, commencing at 2 weeks of age and continuing up to 8–10 weeks. The effects on enzyme activity were completely resolved in both sexes at 10 weeks of age.

Cimetidine is excreted into breast milk and may accumulate in concentrations greater than that found in maternal plasma (40). Following a single 400-mg oral dose, a theoretical milk:plasma ratio of 1.6 was calculated (40). Multiple oral doses of 200 and 400 mg result in milk:plasma ratios of 4.6 to 7.44, respectively. An estimated 6 mg of cimetidine per liter of milk could be ingested by the nursing infant. The results of a study published in 1995 suggested that cimetidine was actively transported into milk (41). Using single oral doses of 100, 600, or 1200 mg in healthy lactating volunteers, the average of the mean milk:serum ratios for the three doses was 5.77 (range 5.65–5.84), much higher than that predicted by diffusion (41).

The clinical significance of an infant ingesting cimetidine from milk is unknown. Theoretically, the drug could adversely affect the nursing infant's gastric acidity, inhibit drug metabolism, and produce central nervous system stimulation, but these effects have not been reported. The American Academy of Pediatrics classifies cimetidine as compatible with breast-feeding (42).

References

1. Product information. Tagamet. SmithKline Beecham Pharmaceuticals, 2000.
2. Finkelstein W, Isselbacher KJ. Cimetidine. N Engl J Med 1978;299:992–6.
3. Pinelli F, Trivulzio S, Colombo R, Cocchi D, Faravelli R, Caviezel F, Galmozzi G, Cavallaro R. Antiprostatic effect of cimetidine in rats. Agents Actions 1987;22:197–201.
4. Sawyer D, Conner CS, Scalley R. Cimetidine: adverse reactions and acute toxicity. Am J Hosp Pharm 1981;38:188–97.
5. Anand S, Van Thiel DH. Prenatal and neonatal exposure to cimetidine results in gonadal and sexual dysfunction in adult males. Science 1982;21:493–4.
6. Parker S, Udani M, Gavaler JS, Van Thiel DH. Pre- and neonatal exposure to cimetidine but not ranitidine

C

adversely affects adult sexual functioning of male rats. Neurobehav Toxicol Teratol 1984;6:313–8.
7. Parker S, Schade RR, Pohl CR, Gavaler JS, Van Thiel DH. Prenatal and neonatal exposure of male rat pups to cimetidine but not ranitidine adversely affects subsequent adult sexual functioning. Gastroenterology 1984;86:675–80.
8. Walker TF, Bott JH, Bond BC. Cimetidine does not demasculinize male rat offspring exposed in utero. Fundam Appl Toxicol 1987;8:188–97.
9. Shapiro BH, Hirst SA, Babalola GO, Bitar MS. Prospective study on the sexual development of male and female rats perinatally exposed to maternally administered cimetidine. Toxicol Lett 1988;44: 315–29.
10. Dicke JM, Johnson RF, Henderson GI, Kuehl TJ, Schenker S. A comparative evaluation of the transport of H_2-receptor antagonists by the human and baboon placenta. Am J Med Sci 1988;295:198–206.
11. Schenker S, Dicke J, Johnson RF, Mor LL, Henderson GI. Human placental transport of cimetidine. J Clin Invest 1987;80:1428–34.
12. Howe JP, McGowan WAW, Moore J, McCaughey W, Dundee JW. The placental transfer of cimetidine. Anaesthesia 1981;36:371–5.
13. McGowan WAW. Safety of cimetidine in obstetric patients. J R Soc Med 1979;72:902–7.
14. Johnston JR, Moore J, McCaughey W, Dundee JW, Howard PJ, Toner W, McClean E. Use of cimetidine as an oral antacid in obstetric anesthesia. Anesth Analg 1983;62:720–6.
15. Knott PD, Thorpe SS, Lamont CAR. Congenital renal dysgenesis possibly due to captopril. Lancet 1989;1:451.
16. Corazza GR, Gasbarrini G, Di Nisio Q, Zulli P. Cimetidine (Tagamet) in peptic ulcer therapy during pregnancy: a report of three cases. Clin Trials J 1982; 19:91–3.
17. Glade G, Saccar CL, Pereira GR. Cimetidine in pregnancy: apparent transient liver impairment in the newborn. Am J Dis Child 1980;134:87–8.
18. Zulli P, DiNisio Q. Cimetidine treatment during pregnancy. Lancet 1978;2:945–6.
19. Husemeyer RP, Davenport HT. Prophylaxis for Mendelson's syndrome before elective caesarean sections. A comparison of cimetidine and magnesium trisilicate mixture regimens. Br J Obstet Gynaecol 1980;87: 565–70.
20. Pickering BG, Palahniuk RJ, Cumming M. Cimetidine premedication in elective caesarean section. Can Anaesth Soc J 1980;27:33–5.
21. Dundee JW, Moore J, Johnston JR, McCaughey W. Cimetidine and obstetric anaesthesia. Lancet 1981;2: 252.
22. McCaughey W, Howe JP, Moore J, Dundee JW. Cimetidine in elective caesarean section. Effect on gastric acidity. Anaesthesia 1981;36:167–72.
23. Crawford JS. Cimetidine in elective caesarean section. Anaesthesia 1981;36:641–2.
24. McCaughey W, Howe JP, Moore J, Dundee JW. Cimetidine in elective caesarean section. Anaesthesia 1981;36:642.
25. Hodgkinson R, Glassenberg R, Joyce TH III, Coombs DW, Ostheimer GW, Gibbs CP. Safety and efficacy of cimetidine and antacid in reducing gastric acidity before elective cesarean section. Anesthesiology 1982;57:A408.
26. Ostheimer GW, Morrison JA, Lavoie C, Sepkoski C, Hoffman J, Datta S. The effect of cimetidine on mother, newborn and neonatal neurobehavior. Anesthesiology 1982;57:A405.
27. Hodgkinson R, Glassenberg R, Joyce TH III, Coombs DW, Ostheimer GW, Gibbs CP. Comparison of cimetidine (Tagamet) with antacid for safety and effectiveness in reducing gastric acidity before elective cesarean section. Anesthesiology 1983;59:86–90.
28. Qvist N, Storm K. Cimethidine pre-anesthetic: a prophylactic method against Mendelson's syndrome in cesarean section. Acta Obstet Gynecol Scand 1983;62:157–9.
29. Okasha AS, Motaweh MM, Bali A. Cimetidine-antacid combination as premedication for elective caesarean section. Can Anaesth Soc J 1983;30:593–7.
30. Frank M, Evans M, Flynn P, Aun C. Comparison of the prophylactic use of magnesium trisilicate mixture B.P.C., sodium citrate mixture or cimetidine in obstetrics. Br J Anaesth 1984;56:355–62.
31. McAuley DM, Halliday HL, Johnston JR, Moore J, Dundee JW. Cimetidine in labour: absence of adverse effect on the high-risk fetus. Br J Obstet Gynaecol 1985;92:350–5.
32. Johnston JR, McCaughey W, Moore J, Dundee JW. Cimetidine as an oral antacid before elective caesarean section. Anaesthesia 1982;37:26–32.
33. Johnston JR, McCaughey W, Moore J, Dundee JW. A field trial of cimetidine as the sole oral antacid in obstetric anaesthesia. Anaesthesia 1982;37: 33–8.
34. Thorburn J, Moir DD. Antacid therapy for emergency caesarean section. Anaesthesia 1987;42:352–5.
35. Howe JP, Dundee JW, Moore J, McCaughey W. Cimetidine: Has it a place in obstetric anaesthesia? Anaesthesia 1980;35:421–2.
36. Kallen B. Delivery outcome after the use of acid-suppressing drugs in early pregnancy with special reference to omeprazole. Br J Obstet Gynaecol 1998;105:877–81.
37. Ruigomez A, Rodriguez LAG, Cattaruzzi C, Troncon MG, Agostinis L, Wallander MA, Johansson S. Use of cimetidine, omeprazole, and ranitidine in pregnant women and pregnancy outcomes. Am J Epidemiol 1999;150:476–81.
38. Smallwood RA, Berlin RG, Castagnoli N, Festen HPM, Hawkey CJ, Lam SK, Langman MJS, Lundborg P, Parkinson A. Safety of acid-suppressing drugs. Dig Dis Sci 1995;40(Suppl):63S–80S.
39. Kwanashie HO, Osuide G, Wambebe C, Ikediobi CO. Effects of maternally administered cimetidine during lactation on the development of drug metabolizing enzymes in mouse pups. Biochem Pharmacol 1989;38:204–6.
40. Somogyi A, Gugler R. Cimetidine excretion into breast milk. Br J Clin Pharmacol 1979;7:627–9.
41. Oo CY, Kuhn RJ, Desai N, McNamara PJ. Active transport of cimetidine into human milk. Clin Pharmacol Ther 1995;58:548–55.
42. Committee on Drugs, American Academy of Pediatrics. The transfer of drugs and other chemicals into human milk. Pediatrics 2001;108:776–89.

C

Name:	**CINNARIZINE**	Risk Factor:	**C**
Class:	**Antihistamine**		

No data are available. See Meclizine for representative agent in this class.

Name:	**CINOXACIN**	Risk Factor:	**C_M**
Class:	**Urinary Germicide (Quinolone)**		

FETAL RISK SUMMARY

RECOMMENDATION: No Human Data - Animal Data Suggest Low Risk

Cinoxacin is a synthetic, oral quinolone antibacterial agent indicated for the treatment of urinary tract infections. Its actions and uses are similar to nalidixic acid. No evidence of impaired fertility or fetal harm was observed in reproduction studies in rats and rabbits at doses up to 10 times the daily human dose (1).

It is not known if cinoxacin crosses the placenta. The molecular weight (about 262) is low enough, however, that transfer to the fetus should be expected.

No reports describing the use of cinoxacin during human pregnancy have been located. Because of the potential for cinoxacin-induced arthropathy in the fetus and newborn, the manufacturer recommends that it not be used in pregnancy (1).

BREAST FEEDING SUMMARY

RECOMMENDATION: No Human Data - Probably Compatible

No reports describing the use of cinoxacin during human lactation have been located. In immature dogs, a single 250-mg/kg dose caused lameness secondary to cartilage lesions of the weight-bearing joints (1). Because of the potential for this type of toxicity in a nursing infant, the manufacturer recommends that it not be used in lactating women (1).

Reference

1. Product information. Cinobac. Oclassen Pharmaceuticals, 1998.

Name:	**CIPROFLOXACIN**	Risk Factor:	**C_M**
Class:	**Anti-infective (Quinolone)**		

FETAL RISK SUMMARY

RECOMMENDATION: Human Data Suggest Low Risk

Ciprofloxacin is a synthetic, broad-spectrum antibacterial agent. As a fluoroquinolone, it is in the same class as enoxacin, levofloxacin, lomefloxacin, norfloxacin, ofloxacin, and sparfloxacin. Nalidixic acid and Cinoxacin are also quinolone drugs.

Ciprofloxacin did not impair fertility and was not embryotoxic or teratogenic in mice and rats at doses up to 6 times the usual human daily dose (1). A similar lack of embryo and fetal toxicity was observed in rabbits. As with other quinolones, multiple doses of ciprofloxacin produced permanent lesions and erosion of cartilage in weight-bearing joints leading to lameness in immature rats and dogs (1).

A number of reports have described the use of ciprofloxacin during human gestation (2–10). In a 1993 reference, data on 103 pregnancies exposed to the drug were released by the manufacturer (2). Of these cases, there were 63 normal, live newborns (52 exposed during 1st trimester, 7 during the 2nd or 3rd trimesters, and 4 in which the exposure time was unknown), 18 terminations, 10 spontaneous abortions (all 1st trimester), 4 fetal deaths (3 during 1st trimester, 1 in 3rd trimester), and 8 infants with congenital defects (7 exposed between 2 and 12 weeks postmenstruation and 1 on a single day of her last menstrual period; these defects are included among those shown in reference 9 below).

No congenital malformations were observed in the infants of 38 women who received either ciprofloxacin ($N = 10$) or norfloxacin ($N = 28$) during pregnancy (35 in the 1st trimester) (3). Most ($N = 35$) received the drugs for the treatment of urinary tract infections. Matched to a control group, the fluoroquinolone-exposed pregnancies had a significantly higher rate of cesarean section for fetal distress and their infants were significantly heavier. No differences were found between the groups in infant development or in the musculoskeletal system.

A 1995 letter described seven pregnant women with multidrug resistant typhoid fever who were treated with ciprofloxacin during the 2nd and 3rd trimesters (4). All delivered healthy infants who were doing well at 5 years of age without evidence of cartilage damage. The authors also described the healthy outcome of another pregnant woman treated with ciprofloxacin during the 1st trimester. That infant was doing well at 6 months of age. A subsequent letter, also in women with typhoid fever, described three pregnant women in the 2nd and 3rd trimesters who were treated with ciprofloxacin (5). A normal outcome occurred in one patient and the pregnancies of the other two were progressing satisfactorily.

A surveillance study on the use of fluoroquinolones during pregnancy was conducted by the Toronto Motherisk Program among members of the Organization of Teratology Information Services (OTIS) and briefly reported in 1995 (6). Pregnancy outcome data were available for 134 cases, of which 68 involved ciprofloxacin, 61 were exposed to norfloxacin, and 5 were exposed to both drugs. Most (90%) were exposed during the first 13 weeks postconception. Fluoroquinolone-exposed pregnancies were compared to matched controls and there were no differences in live births (87% vs. 86%), terminations (3% vs. 5%), miscarriages (10% vs. 9%), abnormal outcomes (7% vs. 4%), cesarean section rate (12% vs. 22%), fetal distress (15% vs. 15%), and pregnancy weight gain (15 kg vs. 16 kg). The mean birth weight of the exposed infants was 162 g higher than those in the control group, and their gestations were a mean 1 week longer.

An abstract, published in 1996, described six pregnancies exposed to ciprofloxacin during the 1st trimester (7). Five healthy babies (one set of twins) had been born and two pregnancies were progressing normally. In a 1997 reference, a pregnant woman with Q fever (*Coxiella burnetii*) at 28 weeks' gestation was treated with ciprofloxacin for 3 weeks (8). Because her symptoms did not resolve, a cesarean section was performed at 32 weeks' with delivery of a healthy, female infant. No evidence of transplacental spread of the infection, which is known to cause stillbirth and abortion in animals and humans, was found (8).

In a prospective follow-up study conducted by the European Network of Teratology Information Services (ENTIS), data on 549 pregnancies exposed to fluoroquinolones (70 to ciprofloxacin) were described in a 1996 report (9). Data on another 116 prospective and 25 retrospective pregnancy exposures to the antibiotics were also included. From the

549 follow-up cases, 509 were treated during the 1st trimester, 22 after the 1st trimester, and in 18 cases the exposure occurred at an unknown gestational time. The live-born infants were delivered at a mean gestational age of 39.4 weeks and had a mean birth weight of 3302 g, length of 50.3 cm, and head circumference of 34.9 cm. Of the 549 pregnancies, there were 415 live-born infants (390 exposed during the 1st trimester), 356 of whom were normal term deliveries (including one set of twins); 15 were premature; 6 were small-for-gestational age (IUGR, <10th percentile); 20 had congenital anomalies (19 from mothers exposed during the 1st trimester; 4.9%); and 18 had postnatal disorders unrelated to either prematurity, low birth weight, or malformations (9). Of the remaining 135 pregnancies, there were 56 spontaneous abortions or fetal deaths (none late) (1 malformed fetus), and 79 elective abortions (4 malformed fetuses). A total of 116 (all involving ciprofloxacin) prospective cases were obtained from the manufacturer's registry (9). Among these, there were 91 live-born infants, 6 of whom had malformations. Of the remaining 25 pregnancies, 15 were terminated (no malformations reported), and 10 aborted spontaneously (one embryo with acardia, no data available on a possible twin). Thus, of the 666 cases with known outcome, 32 (4.8%) of the embryos, fetuses, or newborns had congenital malformations. Based on previous epidemiologic data, the authors concluded that the 4.8% frequency of malformations did not exceed the background rate (9). Finally, 25 retrospective reports of infants with anomalies who had been exposed *in utero* to fluoroquinolones were analyzed, but no specific patterns of major congenital malformations were detected.

The defects observed in the 10 infants followed prospectively and in the 8 infants reported retrospectively, all with 1st trimester ciprofloxacin exposure, were (9):

Source: Prospective ENTIS
Angioma right lower leg
Hip dysplasia left side
Trisomy, unspecified (pregnancy terminated)

Source: Prospective Manufacturer's Registry
Hypospadias
Auricle indentation, hip dysplasia
Cerebellum hypoplasia, oculomotor palsy, development retardation
Hooded foreskin
Amputation right forearm
Hypospadias, bilateral hernia inguinalis
Acardia (spontaneous abortion)

Source: Retrospective Reports
Teeth discoloration
Hypoplastic auricle, absence external auditory canal
Rubinstein-Taybi syndrome
Femur aplasia
Femur-fibula-ulna complex
Ectrodactyly
Defects of heart, trachea, esophagus, urethra, anus, gallbladder, skeleton, heterotopic gastric mucosa, mucosa
Heart defect

The authors of the above study concluded that pregnancy exposure to quinolones was not an indication for termination, but that this class of antibacterials should still be considered contraindicated in pregnant women because safer alternatives are usually available (9). Because of their own and previously published findings, they further recommended that the focus of future studies should be on malformations involving the abdominal wall and urogenital system, and limb reduction defects. Moreover, this study did not address the issue of cartilage damage from quinolone exposure and the authors recognized the need for follow-up studies of this potential toxicity in children exposed *in utero*.

In a surveillance study of Michigan Medicaid recipients conducted between 1985 and 1992 involving 229,101 completed pregnancies, 132 newborns had been exposed to ciprofloxacin during the 1st trimester (F. Rosa, personal communication, FDA, 1993). Three (2.3%) major birth defects were observed (six expected), one of which was a case of spina bifida (none expected). No anomalies were observed in five other categories of defects (cardiovascular defects, oral clefts, polydactyly, limb reduction defects, and hypospadias) for which specific data were available. These data do not support an association between the drug and congenital defects.

A 1998 prospective multicenter study reported the pregnancy outcomes of 200 women who had been exposed to fluoroquinolones as compared with 200 matched controls (10). Subjects were pregnant women who had called one of four teratogen information services concerning their exposure to fluoroquinolones. The agents, number of subjects, and daily doses were ciprofloxacin ($N = 105$; 500–1000 mg), norfloxacin ($N = 93$; 400–800 mg), and ofloxacin ($N = 2$; 200–400 mg). The most common infections involved the urinary tract (69.4%) or the respiratory tract (24%). The fewer live births in the fluoroquinolone group (173 vs. 188, $p = 0.02$) was attributable to the greater number of spontaneous abortions (18 vs. 10, *ns*) and induced abortions (9 vs. 2, *ns*). There were no differences between the groups in terms of premature birth, fetal distress, method of delivery, low birth weight (<2500 g), or birth weight. Among the liveborn infants exposed during organogenesis, major malformations were observed in 3 of 133 subjects and 5 of 188 controls (*ns*). The defects in subject infants were two cases of ventricular septal defect and one case of patent ductus arteriosus, whereas those in controls were two cases of ventricular septal defect, one case of atrial septal defect with pulmonic valve stenosis, one case of hypospadias, and one case of displaced hip. There were also no differences between the children of the groups in gross motor development milestone achievements (musculoskeletal functions: lifting, sitting, crawling, standing, or walking) as measured by the Denver Developmental Scale (10).

In a study investigating the pharmacokinetics of ciprofloxacin, 20 pregnant women, between 19 and 25 weeks' gestation (mean: 21.16 weeks), were scheduled for pregnancy termination because the fetuses were affected by β-thalassemia major (11). Two doses of ciprofloxacin, 200 mg IV every 12 hours, were given prior to abortion. Serum and amniotic fluid concentrations were drawn concomitantly at 4, 8, and 12 hours after dosing. Mean maternal serum concentrations at these times were 0.28, 0.09, and 0.01 μg/mL, respectively, compared to mean amniotic fluid levels of 0.12, 0.13, and 0.10 μg/mL, respectively. The amniotic fluid:maternal serum ratios were 0.43, 1.44, and 10.0, respectively.

In summary, the use of ciprofloxacin during human gestation does not appear to be associated with an increased risk of major congenital malformations. Although a number of birth defects have occurred in the offspring of women who had taken this drug during pregnancy, the lack of a pattern among the anomalies is reassuring. However, a causal relationship with some of the birth defects cannot be excluded. Because of this and the available animal data, the use of ciprofloxacin during pregnancy, especially during the 1st trimester, should be used with caution, but the overall risk appears to be low. A 1993 review on the safety of fluoroquinolones concluded that these antibacterials should be avoided during pregnancy because of the difficulty in extrapolating animal mutagenicity results to humans and because interpretation of this toxicity is still controversial (12). The authors of this review were not convinced that fluoroquinolone-induced fetal cartilage damage and subsequent arthropathies were a major concern, even though this effect had been demonstrated in several animal species after administration to both pregnant and immature animals and in occasional human case reports involving children (12). Others have also concluded that fluoroquinolones should be considered contraindicated in pregnancy, because safer alternatives are usually available (9).

BREAST FEEDING SUMMARY

RECOMMENDATION: Limited Human Data - Probably Compatible

When first marketed, the administration of ciprofloxacin during breast-feeding was not recommended because of the potential for arthropathy (based on animal data) and other serious toxicity in the nursing infant (1). Phototoxicity has been observed with some members of the quinolone class of drugs when exposure to excessive sunlight (i.e., ultraviolet light) has occurred (1). Well-differentiated squamous cell carcinomas of the skin have been produced in mice who were exposed chronically to some quinolones and periodic ultraviolet light (e.g., see Lomefloxacin), but studies to evaluate the carcinogenicity of ciprofloxacin in this manner have not been conducted.

Ciprofloxacin is excreted into human milk (11,13,14). Ten lactating women were given three oral doses, 750 mg each, of ciprofloxacin (11). Six simultaneous serum and milk samples were drawn between 2 and 24 hours after the third dose of the antibacterial. The mean peak serum level occurred at 2 hours (2.06 μg/mL), then steadily fell to 0.02 μg/mL at 24 hours. Milk concentrations exhibited a similar pattern with a mean peak level measured at 2 hours (3.79 μg/mL) and the lowest amount at 24 hours (0.02 μg/mL). The mean milk:serum ratio varied from 0.85–2.14, with the highest ratio occurring 4 hours after the last dose.

A 24-year-old woman, 17 days postpartum, was given a single 500-mg dose of the antibacterial to treat a urinary tract infection (13). She was also suffering from acute renal failure and had undergone her final hemodialysis treatment 7 days prior to administration of ciprofloxacin. Her serum creatinine and blood urea nitrogen at the time of the dose were 740 mmol/L and 26.8 mmol/L, respectively. Milk samples, 40 mL each, were collected at 4, 8, 12, and 16 hours. Concentrations of ciprofloxacin at these times were 9.1, 9.1, 9.1, and 6.0 μmol/L, respectively. (*Note:* 9.1 and 6.0 μmol/L are approximately 3.0 and 2.0 μg/mL, respectively.) Based on the volume of milk and concentrations, the potential cumulative dose for the infant, who was not allowed to breast-feed, was 1.331 μmol.

The only published case involving a woman consuming ciprofloxacin who was breast-feeding appeared in 1992 (14). The 4-month-old female infant was being exclusively breast-fed six times/day. The mother had taken a single nighttime dose (500 mg) of the antibacterial for 10 days prior to the collection of simultaneous samples of milk, maternal serum, and infant serum approximately 11 hours after a dose. On the day of sampling, breast-feeding occurred 8 hours after the mother's dose. Maternal serum, milk, and infant serum ciprofloxacin concentrations were 0.21 μg/mL, 0.98 μg/mL, and undetectable (<0.03 μg/mL), respectively. The authors estimated the infant was consuming 0.92 mg/day (0.15 mg/kg/day) of ciprofloxacin (14). No adverse effects were observed in the infant.

In unpublished studies available to the manufacturer, peak milk levels occurred approximately 4 hours after a ciprofloxacin dose and were about the same as serum levels (personal communication, Miles Pharmaceutical, June 1990). Levels of the antibacterial were

C

undetectable 36–48 hours after a dose. Based on these data, the manufacturer recommends that 48 hours elapse after the last dose of ciprofloxacin before breast-feeding is resumed (personal communication, Miles Pharmaceutical, June 1990).

In an unusual report, follow-up of infants who had been treated as neonates with ciprofloxacin for severe *Klebsiella pneumoniae* revealed two of five infants with greenish colored teeth on eruption (15). The teeth were stained uniformly with dyscalcification at the cervical part. The investigators could not determine the cause of the condition. Other reports of this condition have not been located and the clinical significance of this to a nursing infant exposed to fluoroquinolones via the milk is unknown.

Although the data are limited, the amount of ciprofloxacin in breast milk does not appear to represent a significant risk to a nursing infant. The American Academy of Pediatrics classifies ciprofloxacin as compatible with breast-feeding (16).

References

1. Product information. Cipro. Miles Pharmaceutical, 1993.
2. Bomford JAL, Ledger JC, O'Keeffe BJ, Reiter CH. Ciprofloxacin use during pregnancy. Drugs 1993;45 (Suppl 3):461–2.
3. Berkovitch M, Pastuszak A, Gazarian M, Lewis M, Koren G. Safety of the new quinolones in pregnancy. Obstet Gynecol 1994;84:535–8.
4. Koul PA, Wani JI, Wahid A. Ciprofloxacin for multiresistant enteric fever in pregnancy. Lancet 1995;346: 307–8.
5. Leung D, Venkatesan P, Boswell T, Innes JA, Wood MJ. Treatment of typhoid in pregnancy. Lancet 1995;346:648.
6. Pastuszak A, Andreou R, Schick B, Sage S, Cook L, Donnenfeld A, Koren G. New postmarketing surveillance data supports a lack of association between quinolone use in pregnancy and fetal and neonatal complications. Reprod Toxicol 1995;9:584.
7. Baroncini A, Calzolari E, Calabrese O, Zanetti A. First-trimester exposure to ciprofloxacin (abstract). Teratology 1996;53:24A.
8. Ludlam H, Wreghitt TG, Thornton S, Thomson BJ, Bishop NJ, Coomber S, Cunniffe J. Q fever in pregnancy. J Infect 1997;34:75–8.
9. Schaefer C, Amoura-Elefant E, Vial T, Ornoy A, Garbis H, Robert E, Rodriguez-Pinilla E, Pexieder T, Prapas N, Merlob P. Pregnancy outcome after prenatal quinolone exposure. Evaluation of a case registry of the European Network of Teratology Information Services (ENTIS). Eur J Obstet Gynecol Reprod Bio 1996;69:83–9.
10. Loebstein R, Addis A, Ho E, Andreou R, Sage S, Donnenfeld AE, Schick B, Bonati M, Mortetti M, Lalkin A, Pastuszak A, Koren G. Pregnancy outcome following gestational exposure to fluoroquinolones: a multicenter prospective controlled study. Antimicrob Agents Chemother 1998;42:1336–9.
11. Giamarellou H, Kolokythas E, Petrikkos G, Gazis J, Aravantinos D, Sfikakis P. Pharmacokinetics of three newer quinolones in pregnant and lactating women. Am J Med 1989;87(Suppl 5A):49S–51S.
12. Norrby SR, Lietman PS. Safety and tolerability of fluoroquinolones. Drugs 1993;45(Suppl 3):59–64.
13. Cover DL, Mueller BA. Ciprofloxacin penetration into human breast milk: a case report. Ann Pharmacother 1990;24:703–4.
14. Gardner DK, Gabbe SG, Harter C. Simultaneous concentrations of ciprofloxacin in breast milk and in serum in mother and breast-fed infant. Clin Pharm 1992;11:352–4.
15. Lumbiganon P, Pengsaa K, Sookpranee T. Ciprofloxacin in neonates and its possible effect on the teeth. Pediatr Infect Dis J 1991;10:619–20.
16. Committee on Drugs, American Academy of Pediatrics. The transfer of drugs and other chemicals into human milk. Pediatrics 2001;108:776–89.

Name: **CISAPRIDE** Risk Factor: C_M

Class: **Gastrointestinal Stimulant**

FETAL RISK SUMMARY

RECOMMENDATION: Limited Human Data - Animal Data Suggest Low Risk

Cisapride, an oral gastrointestinal prokinetic agent, was withdrawn from the market in the United States in July 2000 because of the risk of serious cardiac arrhythmias and death. The drug is available only through an investigational, limited access program sponsored by the manufacturer.

In female rats, doses of ≥40 mg/kg/day (25 times the maximum recommended human dose [MRHD]) impaired fertility by prolonging the breeding interval required for conception (1). Similar fertility impairment was observed at maturity in female rats exposed *in utero* to maternal doses of ≥10 mg/kg/day. Cisapride was embryotoxic and fetotoxic at doses 12 and 100 times the MRHD in rabbits and rats, respectively (1). Intrauterine growth retardation and increased neonatal mortality were also observed.

A 1998 non-interventional observational cohort study described the outcomes of pregnancies in women who had been prescribed one or more of 34 newly marketed drugs by general practitioners in England (2). Data were obtained by questionnaires sent to the prescribing physicians one month after the expected or possible date of delivery. In 831 (78%) of the pregnancies, a newly marketed drug was thought to have been taken during the 1st trimester with birth defects noted in 14 (2.5%) singleton births of the 557 newborns (10 sets of twins). In addition, two birth defects were observed in aborted fetuses. However, few of the aborted fetuses were examined. Cisapride was taken during the 1st trimester in 12 pregnancies. The outcomes of these pregnancies included 2 elective abortions, 1 lost to follow-up, and 10 normal, term babies (one set of twins). In two other cases, cisapride was taken during the 2nd and/or 3rd trimesters (2).

A 1997 prospective multicenter compared the pregnancy outcomes of 129 subjects who had taken cisapride during pregnancy with two groups of matched controls (3). Outcomes included major and minor malformations, birth weight (including birth weight <2500 g), live births (including premature births), spontaneous or induced abortions, fetal distress, and gestational age at birth. All of the subjects and controls had contacted one of 10 antenatal counseling services. The mean daily cisapride dose was 25 mg (range 5–120 mg), and the mean length of exposure was 4.6 weeks (range 0.14–41 weeks). Among 113 (87.6%) subjects who had taken cisapride during the 1st trimester, 88 (68.2%) had taken it during the period of organogenesis. There were no significant differences in outcomes between the subjects and controls (3).

In summary, cisapride is not an animal teratogen in two species, although embryo and fetal toxicity were observed at doses greater than 10 times the maximum human dose, and it does not appear to be a major human teratogen. However, the data are still too limited to adequately assess the safety of cisapride. Moreover, the studies lacked sensitivity to identify minor anomalies because of the absence of standardized examinations. Late-appearing major defects may also have been missed because of the timing of the questionnaires.

BREAST FEEDING SUMMARY

RECOMMENDATION: Limited Human Data - Probably Compatible

Cisapride is excreted into human milk (4). Ten women in the immediate postpartum period (mean: 1.2 days after delivery), who had elected not to breast-feed their infants, were administered the drug 20 mg orally every 8 hours for 4 days. Milk samples were collected on the 3rd and 4th days before and 1 hour after a dose. A single serum sample was obtained on the 4th day 1 hour after a dose. The mean milk concentrations just before a dose on days 3 and 4 were 4.2 ng/mL and 4.8 ng/mL, respectively, whereas on both days the mean concentrations in the 1-hour samples were 6.2 ng/mL. The serum level at this time was 137 ng/mL, yielding a milk:serum ratio of 0.063. The investigators estimated that a breast-feeding infant would have ingested 1 μg/kg/day of the drug, about 0.1% of the mother's dose, an amount 600 to 800 times lower than the usual therapeutic dose for an infant (4).

C

References

1. Product information. Propulsid. Janssen Pharmaceutical, 1994.
2. Wilton LV, Pearce GL, Martin RM, Mackay FJ, Mann RD. The outcomes of pregnancy in women exposed to newly marketed drugs in general practice in England. Br J Obstet Gynaecol 1998;105:882–9.
3. Bailey B, Addis A, Lee A, Sanghvi K, Mastroiacovo P, Mazzone T, Bonati M, Paolini C, Garbis H, Val T, De Souza CFM, Matsui D, Schechtman AS, Conover B, Lau M, Koren G. Cisapride use during human pregnancy. A prospective, controlled multicenter study. Dig Dis Sci 1997;42:1848–52.
4. Hofmeyr GJ, Sonnendecker EWW. Secretion of the gastrokinetic agent cisapride in human milk. Eur J Clin Pharmacol 1986;30:735–6.

Name: **CISPLATIN** Risk Factor: D_M
Class: **Antineoplastic**

FETAL RISK SUMMARY

RECOMMENDATION: Contraindicated - 1st Trimester

Cisplatin is an antineoplastic used in the treatment of various cancers. This agent is mutagenic in bacteria, produces chromosomal aberrations in animal cells in tissue culture, and is teratogenic and embryotoxic in mice (1). Cisplatin is also a transplacental carcinogen in rats, producing tumors in the liver, lung, nervous system, and kidneys of adult offspring (2). The mechanism for the production of these tumors is probably the result of DNA damage in fetal rat tissues (3). A 1994 review also reviewed the animal teratogenicity of cisplatin (4).

Only seven cases of cisplatin usage during pregnancy have been located (5–11). In one case, the mother, in her 10th week of gestation, received a single intravenous dose of 50 mg/kg for carcinoma of the uterine cervix (5). Two weeks later, a radical hysterectomy was performed. The male fetus was morphologically normal for its developmental age.

A 25-year-old woman underwent surgery at 25 weeks' gestation for an endodermal sinus tumor of the ovary (6). The chemotherapy cycle consisting of cisplatin (75 mg/m^2), vinblastine (0.25 mg/kg), and bleomycin (50 mg) was started 9 days later. Approximately 3 weeks later she received a second cycle of therapy. A normal, healthy 1900-g male infant was delivered by scheduled cesarean section at 32 weeks' gestation. The infant was alive and growing normally at the time of the report.

A 1989 case report described the effect of maternal chemotherapy on a premature newborn delivered at approximately 27 weeks' gestation (7). The mother had been treated with cisplatin (55 mg), bleomycin (30 mg), and etoposide (165 mg) (all given daily for 3 days) 1 week prior to delivery for an unknown primary cancer with metastases to the eye and liver. The mother developed profound neutropenia just prior to delivery. On the 3rd day after birth, 10 days after *in utero* exposure to the antineoplastic agents, the 1190-g female infant also developed a profound leukopenia with neutropenia. The condition resolved after 10 days. At 10 days of age, the infant began losing her scalp hair along with a rapid loss of lanugo. Etoposide was thought to be the most likely cause of the neutropenia and the alopecia (7). By 12 weeks of age, substantial hair regrowth had occurred, and at 1 year follow-up, the child was developing normally except for moderate bilateral hearing loss. The investigators could not determine whether the sensorineural deafness was a consequence of the maternal and/or neonatal gentamicin therapy or of the maternal cisplatin chemotherapy (7).

A third case of cisplatin usage during pregnancy involved a 28-year-old woman with advanced epithelial ovarian carcinoma (8). Following surgical treatment at 16 weeks' gestation, the patient was treated with cisplatin, 50 mg/m^2, and cyclophosphamide, 750 mg/m^2, every 21 days for seven cycles. Labor was induced at 37–38 weeks' gestation, resulting in the delivery of a healthy, 3275-g male infant. Height, weight, and head circumference were in the 75th–90th percentile. No abnormalities of the kidneys, liver, bone-marrow, or auditory-evoked potential were found at birth and the infant's physical, and neurologic growth was normal at 19 months of age.

In a report similar to that above, a 24-year-old woman was treated during the 2nd trimester of pregnancy for epithelial ovarian carcinoma (9). Surgery was performed at 15.5 weeks' gestation, followed by five courses of chemotherapy consisting of cisplatin (100 mg/m^2) and cyclophosphamide (600 mg/m^2 × 2,1000 mg/m^2 × 3). Spontaneous rupture of membranes occurred just prior to the sixth course of chemotherapy at 36.5 weeks' gestation, and she delivered a normal-appearing, 3060-g male infant who, except for initial mild respiratory distress, had developed normally as of 28 months of age.

A 21-year-old woman with a dysgerminoma was treated surgically at 26 weeks' gestation, followed approximately 1 week later with cisplatin, 20 mg/m^2, and etoposide, 100 mg/m^2, daily for 5 days at 3–4 week intervals (10). A healthy, 2320-g female infant was delivered at 38 weeks. The infant was developing normally at 9 months of age.

Three treatments of cisplatin (75 mg/m^2; total dose 330 mg) were administered at 22, 25, and 28 weeks' gestation to a 34-year-old woman with a rapidly progressing cervical cancer (11). A cesarean section was performed at 32 weeks' with delivery of a normal, 2120-g male infant, who was doing well at 12 months of age.

The long-term effects of cisplatin and other antineoplastic agents on menstrual function in females and reproductive function in females and males after treatment of various cancers have been described (12–14). Of the 76 women studied, cisplatin was used in 9, and of the 25 men studied, cisplatin had been given to 4. The results of one of these studies (12) are discussed in the monograph for cyclophosphamide (see Cyclophosphamide). In the second report, a normal, term infant was delivered from a woman who had been treated for choriocarcinoma with cisplatin, etoposide, dactinomycin, and intrathecal methotrexate 2 years prior to conception (13). Similarly, no congenital malformations were observed in seven liveborn offspring of four males and two females treated with cisplatin during childhood or adolescence (14).

A 1996 report described successful pregnancy outcomes in 14 women who had been treated prior to conception for ovarian germ cell tumors with a chemotherapy regimen (POMB/ACE) consisting of cisplatin (120 mg/m^2), vincristine, methotrexate, bleomycin, dactinomycin, cyclophosphamide, and etoposide (15). No congenital malformations were observed.

Reversible azoospermia occurred in a male treated for teratoma of the testis with cisplatin, vinblastine, bleomycin, surgery, and radiation (16). Fifteen months after the end of therapy, the sperm count was $<$50,000 sperm/μL with 70% motile and a high percentage of abnormal forms. Three months later the patient and his wife reported a pregnancy, which was terminated at their request.

A significant reduction in reproductive organ weights, sperm counts, sperm motility, fertility, and levels of testosterone, LH, and FSH occurred in male rats treated with cisplatin 1 week prior to mating (17). After mating, a significant preimplantation loss and lower fetal weights in comparison to controls were observed.

C

Occupational exposure of the mother to antineoplastic agents during pregnancy may present a risk to the fetus. A position statement from the National Study Commission on Cytotoxic Exposure and a research article involving some antineoplastic agents are presented in the monograph for cyclophosphamide (see Cyclophosphamide).

BREAST FEEDING SUMMARY

RECOMMENDATION: Contraindicated

Three studies, two with opposite results from the third, have examined the excretion of cisplatin into human milk. In a 1985 study, a 31-year-old woman, 7 months postpartum with ovarian cancer, was treated with doxorubicin and cisplatin (18). Doxorubicin (90 mg) was given intravenously over 15 minutes, followed by intravenous cisplatin (130 mg, 100 mg/m^2) infused over 26 hours. Blood and milk samples were collected frequently for cisplatin determination from 0.25–71.25 hours after the start of the infusion. Peak plasma concentrations of platinum reached 2.99 μg/mL, but platinum was undetectable (sensitivity 0.1 μg/mL) in the milk.

Opposite results were obtained in a 1989 study (19). A 24-year-old woman with an entodermal sinus tumor of the left ovary was treated with cisplatin, 30 mg/m^2 IV for 4 hours daily, for 5 consecutive days. Etoposide and bleomycin were also administered during this time. On the 3rd day of therapy, milk and serum samples were collected 30 minutes before the cisplatin dose was administered. Cisplatin concentrations in the milk and plasma were 0.9 and 0.8 μg/mL, respectively, a milk:plasma ratio of 1.1. The infant was not allowed to breast-feed.

In the third study, cisplatin was measured in breast milk in the range of 0.1–0.15 μg/mL (over 2 hours), with a milk:plasma ratio of about 0.1 over an 18-hour sampling period (20). The woman, who was still lactating 2 years after her last delivery, was treated with six courses of cisplatin (100 mg/course) and cyclophosphamide (1600 mg/course) for ovarian cancer.

The American Academy of Pediatrics did not cite either of these latter two studies and classifies cisplatin as compatible with breast-feeding (21). However, based on the two reports, breast-feeding during cisplatin therapy should be considered contraindicated.

References

1. Product information. Platinol. Bristol-Myers Squibb Oncology/Immunology Division, 1997.
2. Diwan BA, Anderson LM, Ward JM, Henneman JR, Rice JM. Transplacental carcinogenesis by cisplatin in F344/NCr rats: promotion of kidney tumors by postnatal administration of sodium barbital. Toxicol Appl Pharmacol 1995;132:115–21.
3. Giurgiovich AJ, Diwan BA, Lee KB, Anderson LM, Rice JM, Poirier MC. Cisplatin-DNA adduct formation in maternal and fetal rat tissues after transplacental cisplatin exposure. Carcinogenesis 1996;17:1665–9.
4. Wiebe VJ, Sipila PEH. Pharmacology of antineoplastic agents in pregnancy. Crit Rev Oncol Hematol 1994;16:75–112.
5. Jacobs AJ, Marchevsky A, Gordon RE, Deppe G, Cohen CJ. Oat cell carcinoma of the uterine cervix in a pregnant woman treated with cis-diamminedichloroplatinum. Gynecol Oncol 1980;9:405–10.
6. Malone JM, Gershenson DM, Creasy RK, Kavanagh JJ, Silva EG, Stringer CA. Endodermal sinus tumor of the ovary associated with pregnancy. Obstet Gynecol 1986;68(Suppl):86S–9S.
7. Raffles A, Williams J, Costeloe K, Clark P. Transplacental effects of maternal cancer chemotherapy: case report. Br J Obstet Gynaecol 1989;96:1099–1100.
8. Malfetano JH, Goldkrand JW. Cis-platinum combination chemotherapy during pregnancy for advanced epithelial ovarian carcinoma. Obstet Gynecol 1990;75:545–7.
9. King LA, Nevin PC, Williams PP, Carson LF. Treatment of advanced epithelial ovarian carcinoma in pregnancy with cisplatin-based chemotherapy. Gynecol Oncol 1991;41:78–80.
10. Buller RE, Darrow V, Manetta A, Porto M, DiSaia PJ. Conservative surgical management of dysgerminoma concomitant with pregnancy. Obstet Gynecol 1992;79:887–90.
11. Giacalone P-L, Laffargue F, Benos P, Rousseau O, Hedon B. Cis-platinum neoadjuvant chemotherapy

in a pregnant woman with invasive carcinoma of the uterine cervix. Br J Obstet Gynaecol 1996;103: 932–4.
12. Gershenson DM. Menstrual and reproductive function after treatment with combination chemotherapy for malignant ovarian germ cell tumors. J Clin Oncol 1988;6:270–5.
13. Bakri Y, Pedersen P, Nassar M. Normal pregnancy after curative multiagent chemotherapy for choriocarcinoma with brain metastases. Acta Obstet Gynecol Scand 1991;70:611–3.
14. Green DM, Zevon MA, Lowrie G, Seigelstein N, Hall B. Congenital anomalies in children of patients who received chemotherapy for cancer in childhood and adolescence. N Engl J Med 1991;325:141–6.
15. Bower M, Fife K, Holden L, Paradinas FJ, Rustin GJS, Newlands ES. Chemotherapy for ovarian germ cell tumours. Eur J Cancer 1996;32A:593–7.
16. Rubery ED. Return of fertility after curative chemotherapy for disseminated teratoma of testis. Lancet 1983;1:186.
17. Kinkead T, Flores C, Carboni AA, Menon M, Seethalakshmi L. Short term effects of cis-platinum on male reproduction, fertility and pregnancy outcome. J Urol 1992;147:201–6.
18. Egan PC, Costanza ME, Dodion P, Egorin MJ, Bachur NR. Doxorubicin and cisplatin excretion into human milk. Cancer Treat Rep 1985;69:1387–9.
19. De Vries EGE, Van Der Zee AGJ, Uges DRA, Sleijfer DTH. Excretion of platinum into breast milk. Lancet 1989;1:497.
20. Ben-Baruch G, Menczer J, Goshen R, Kaufman B, Gorodetsky R. Cisplatin excretion in human milk. J Natl Cancer Inst 1992;84:451–2.
21. Committee on Drugs, American Academy of Pediatrics. The transfer of drugs and other chemicals into human milk. Pediatrics 2001;198:776–89.

Name:	**CITALOPRAM**	Risk Factor:	C_M
Class:	**Antidepressant**		

FETAL RISK SUMMARY

RECOMMENDATION: Human Data Suggest Risk in 3rd Trimester

The antidepressant, citalopram, is a selective serotonin reuptake inhibitor (SSRI) that has a chemical structure unrelated to those of other antidepressants (1). All the antidepressant agents in this class (citalopram, escitalopram, fluoxetine, fluvoxamine, paroxetine, and sertraline) share a similar mechanism of action, although they have different chemical structures. These differences could be construed as evidence against any conclusion that they share similar effects on the embryo, fetus, or newborn. In the mouse embryo, however, craniofacial morphogenesis appears to be regulated, at least in part, by serotonin. Interference with serotonin regulation by chemically different inhibitors produces similar craniofacial defects (2). Regardless of the structural differences, therefore, some of the potential adverse effects on the pregnancy may also be similar.

Both mating and fertility were reduced in male and female rats at oral doses approximately five times the maximum recommended human daily dose of 60 mg/day based on body surface area (MRHD). The duration of gestation was increased at approximately eight times the MRHD.

Citalopram demonstrated dose-related embryo and fetal growth retardation, reduced survival, and teratogenicity in rats dosed during organogenesis at about 18 times the MRHD (1). Fetal malformations included cardiovascular and skeletal defects, but the dose was maternal toxic (clinical signs, decreased weight gain). The developmental no-effect dose was about nine times the MRHD. In contrast, no developmental adverse effects were observed in the offspring of pregnant rabbits given doses up to about five times the MRHD (1).

Increased offspring mortality during the first 4 days after birth and persistent growth retardation were observed when pregnant rats were dosed at about five times the MRHD throughout gestation and early lactation. Similar effects were observed with doses about four times the MRHD in late gestation through weaning. The no-effect dose in this group was about twice the MRHD (1).

In an *in vitro* experiment using a single placental cotyledon, both citalopram and its metabolite desmethylcitalopram crossed to the fetal side (3). The mean steady-state placental transfer for the two compounds was 9.1% and 5.6%, respectively. A 2003 study of the placental transfer of antidepressants found cord blood:maternal serum ratios for citalopram and its metabolite that ranged from 0.17–1.42 and 0.50–1.00, respectively (4). The dose-to-delivery interval was 14–48 hours with the highest ratio for the parent drug and metabolite occurring at 48 hours.

In a 2002 study, 11 women took citalopram (20–40 mg/day) during pregnancy; 10 throughout gestation and 1 starting at 20 weeks' gestation (5). The mean ratio of two metabolites was significantly higher during pregnancy than at 2 months postdelivery, indicating induction of the cytochrome P450 (CYP) 2D6 isoenzyme (5). The trough plasma concentrations of citalopram, desmethylcitalopram, and didesmethylcitalopram in the normal newborns were 64%, 66%, and 68% of the maternal concentrations, respectively. The neurodevelopment of the infants up to the age of 1 year was normal (5). All infants were breast-fed (see Breast-Feeding Summary).

Citalopram is at least eight times more potent in the inhibition of serotonin reuptake than its four metabolites (1). It has an elimination half-life of approximately 35 hours. This is in the same general range as the other SSRI agents with weakly active or inactive metabolites (elimination half-life of parent compound in parentheses): fluvoxamine (15.6 hours), paroxetine (21 hours), and sertraline (26 hours). All have a much shorter elimination half-life than either fluoxetine (4–6 days) or fluoxetine's active metabolite (4–16 days).

A brief 1993 case report described a woman who was treated with citalopram for major depression during the first 6 weeks of an undiagnosed pregnancy (6). She received 40 mg/day during the first 3 weeks, and then the dose was increased to 60 mg/day. She also took several other drugs for coexisting panic disorder and migraine headaches. All medication was stopped in the sixth week of gestation when the pregnancy was diagnosed. Because of her deteriorating mental status and anxiety concerning fetal development, she requested an abortion, which was performed at 12 weeks' gestation. At autopsy, a thorough macroscopic and microscopic evaluation, including a detailed neuropathological examination, found no evidence of malformation (6).

In 1999, the Swedish Medical Birth Registry published the results of a study on the use of antidepressants in early pregnancy and delivery outcome for the years 1995–1997 (7). During the period, 281,728 infants were registered, 531 of whom had been exposed *in utero* to SSRI antidepressants, 15 to SSRIs plus a non-SSRI antidepressant, and 423 to non-SSRI antidepressants. Of the 376 women who used citalopram, 364 used it alone, 1 used it in combination with sertraline, and 11 used it in combination with non-SSRI antidepressants (clomipramine, amitriptyline, or imipramine). There were no significant differences in relative risk (RR = observed/expected) for birth defects between those exposed to any depressant (total 39; RR 1.13), SSRIs only (total 21; RR 1.12), and non-SSRIs only (total 18; RR 1.15). Similarly, no significant differences in infant survival were observed among the groups. A shorter gestational duration (<37 weeks) was observed for any antidepressant exposure (odds ratio [OR] 1.43, 95% Confidence Interval [CI] 1.14–1.80), but no difference between SSRI and non-SSRI antidepressants was observed. Moreover, antidepressant exposure was not associated with an increased risk of low birth weight (defined as <2500 g) among singletons as the crude OR 1.32 (95% CI 0.96–1.80) decreased to 1.03 after adjustment for confounders. Fifteen (4.0%) of the citalopram-exposed infants had anomalies, but one was a trisomy 13 syndrome and five were classified as uncertain anomalies (laryngeal/bronchial anomaly [$N = 1$]; undescended testicle [$N = 4$]). No signals of teratogenicity or patterns of defects were observed in the other 10 citalopram-exposed infants (7).

Five male infants exposed to citalopram (30 mg/day), paroxetine (10–40 mg/day), or fluoxetine (20 mg/day) during gestation exhibited withdrawal symptoms at or within a few days of birth and lasting up to 1 month (8). Symptoms included irritability, constant crying, shivering, increased tonus, eating and sleeping problems and convulsions. The four infants exposed to paroxetine and fluoxetine required treatment with chlorpromazine.

A 2004 prospective study examined the effect of four SSRIs (citalopram, fluoxetine, paroxetine, and sertraline) on newborn neurobehavior, including behavioral state, sleep organization, motor activity, heart rate variability, tremulousness, and startles (9). Seventeen SSRI-exposed, healthy, full-birth-weight newborns and 17 nonexposed, full-birth-weight newborns were matched for maternal cigarette use, social class, and maternal age. A wide range of disrupted neurobehavioral outcomes were shown in the infants exposed *in utero* to SSRIs. After adjustment for gestational age, the exposed infants were found to differ significantly from controls in terms of tremulousness, behavioral states, and sleep organization. Although the effects observed on motor activity, startles, and heart rate variability were not significant after adjustment, the investigators thought they might be mediated through the effects of SSRI exposure on gestational age (9).

In summary, citalopram does not appear to be a major human teratogen, although the data are limited. The above studies observed no increase in defects or pattern of major anomalies over that expected in a nonexposed population. An increase in minor malformations and severe perinatal complications has been observed with another SSRI, fluoxetine. Moreover, other studies have documented disruption of newborn neurobehavior and withdrawal by other SSRIs, including citalopram.

A 1999 review of SSRI antidepressants concluded that if therapy was required during pregnancy, the SSRIs were a good choice because of their side-effect profile and safety in overdose (10). Additional research, however, is needed on all SSRIs, including citalopram, to better define their relationship to minor malformations and perinatal morbidity. In addition, more investigations are needed on the potential of SSRIs for neurobehavior teratogenicity that might not become evident for years after birth.

BREAST FEEDING SUMMARY

RECOMMENDATION: Limited Human Data - Potential Toxicity

Citalopram is excreted into human milk. A 1997 report described breast milk concentrations of the antidepressant in two lactating women who were being treated for depression and one healthy lactating volunteer (11). All three subjects were extensive metabolizers of citalopram with respect to the liver enzymes (CYP2C19 and CYP2D6) involved in the metabolism of the drug. The two women with depression were being treated with 20 mg/day and 40 mg/day at 2 and 4 months postpartum, respectively. The healthy volunteer was given a single dose of 40 mg at 10 months postpartum. The milk:serum ratio in the two women ranged from 1.16 to 1.88, whereas in the volunteer, the ratio was 1.00, based on the area-under-the-time-concentration curve (AUC). The dose ingested by an infant was calculated to range from 4.3 to 17.6 μg/kg/day (0.7%–5.9% of the weight-adjusted maternal dose) in the two women on chronic therapy, and 11.2 μg/kg/day (1.8% of the weight-adjusted maternal dose based on AUC) in the volunteers. The two mothers on chronic therapy observed no adverse effects in their nursing infants. Compared with other SSRI antidepressants, the relative dose to the infant from citalopram (0.7%–5.9%) was comparable to fluoxetine and its active metabolite (1.2%–6.5%), but higher than that for fluvoxamine (0.5%), sertraline (0.45%), and paroxetine (0.34%). Based on these data, the authors recommended that caution should be used with the administration of citalopram during lactation (11).

In a second 1997 report, a 21-year-old mother developed severe depression 2 months after delivery of a female infant and was begun on citalopram (12). Blood and milk samples were collected after 15 days of treatment following 8 days of a continuous 20 mg/day dose. The mean milk:serum ratio over a 24-hour period was approximately 3 for both citalopram and its inactive metabolite. The investigators estimated that the weight-adjusted dose of citalopram received by the infant was 4.8% of the mother's dose. After 3 weeks of therapy, a blood sample was obtained from the infant. The serum concentration of citalopram in the infant (the concentration of the metabolite was too low to measure) was about 1/15th of the mother's level just before a dose. These low levels indicate that no accumulation of citalopram or the metabolite occurred in the baby. Furthermore, no immediate adverse effects or unusual behavior was observed in the infant (12).

A 2000 report measured citalopram concentrations in the milk and plasma of seven women who were nursing their infants (mean age: 4.1 months) (13). The median citalopram dose was 0.36 mg/kg/day. The mean milk:plasma ratios of citalopram and the metabolite, desmethylcitalopram, were 1.8 (range 1.2–3) and 1.8 (range 1.0–2.5), respectively. Citalopram was detected in the plasma of three infants (2.0–2.3 ng/mL), two of whom also had detectable levels of the metabolite (2.2 ng/mL). The mean combined dose of citalopram and metabolite (expressed as a percentage of the maternal weight-normalized dose) was 4.4% to 5.1%. No adverse effects were observed in the infants and all had normal Denver Developmental Scale quotients. Because the dose was less than the 10% notional level of concern and because there was an absence of adverse effects, the authors concluded that citalopram was safe to use during breast-feeding (13).

A 29-year-old woman, 4 weeks after delivery, was started on citalopram (40 mg/day) for postpartum depression (14). Eight days later, at steady state, single samples of milk and serum (time from last dose not specified) yielded concentrations of 205 ng/mL and 98.9 ng/mL, respectively. Uneasy sleep was noted in the breast-fed infant starting about 2 to 3 days after initiation of drug therapy. The citalopram concentration in the infant's serum after 16 days of maternal therapy was 12.7 ng/mL. Reducing the dose to 20 mg/day and substituting two breast-feedings with artificial nutrition normalized the infant's sleeping. One week later, the serum concentrations of citalopram in the mother and infant were 49.0 ng/mL and 4.5 ng/mL, respectively (14).

In their product information, the manufacturer describes two infants with excessive somnolence, decreased feeding, and weight loss associated with nursing from mothers receiving citalopram (1). Both cases involved reports to the manufacturer that apparently were not published. Although the information is incomplete, the manufacturer was able to obtain partial details of these cases (G. Fagen, personal communication, Forrest Pharmaceuticals, 2000). One full-term infant was born to a Danish woman who had been started on citalopram, 40 mg/day, shortly before delivery. The infant was presumably breast-fed. When the adverse effects were noted 3 to 4 days after birth, the mother stopped the drug. The infant made a full recovery. The second case involved an 8-day-old Swedish baby who developed tiredness, weight loss, and decreased suckling. The mother had started taking citalopram, 20 mg/day, approximately 1 year earlier. She was also taking an antihistamine. Five days before the onset of the adverse symptoms, without medical advice, she increased her dose to 30 mg/day. A single milk sample (timing in relationship to the dose not specified) yielded a drug concentration of 377 nmol/L (about 0.122 μg/mL) (1 mol of citalopram = 324.4 g [11]). The concentration of the metabolite was 111 nmol/L. These amounts are very close to those reported in the above published cases. No other details of the case were available, although it is known that the infant was doing well at 4 years of age.

Nine women treated with citalopram during pregnancy (see Fetal Risk Summary) continued to use the antidepressant while nursing their infants (5). Maternal plasma concentrations of the parent compound and metabolites demonstrated a tendency to rise at 2 weeks and 2 months postpartum. The milk:plasma ratios for citalopram, desmethylcitalopram, and didesmethylcitalopram ranged from 1.2–3.3, 1.3–4.1, and 1.1–4.6, respectively. In contrast, the infant plasma concentrations of the parent compound and two metabolites at various intervals up to 2 months of age all declined from those measured at birth. The weight and neurodevelopment of the infants up to 1 year of age were normal (5).

A prospective, observational cohort study designed to determine the frequency of adverse effects in nursing infants exposed to citalopram in milk was published in 2004 (15). Three groups of nursing women were formed: 31 women who were depressed and taking citalopram; 12 women who were depressed but who were taking other SSRI antidepressants; and 31 healthy women matched to the first group by maternal age and parity. There was no statistically significant difference in the rate of adverse events among the nursing infants in the three groups (3/31 events, 0/12 events, and 1/31 events, respectively) (14). In the citalopram group, two of the events were colic and decreased feeding, but both were considered nonspecific and insignificant and did not require intervention. The third event involved irritability and restlessness that were observed in the infant when the mother started citalopram at 2 months postpartum. Breast-feeding was stopped after 2 weeks and the symptoms resolved (15).

A 1999 review of SSRI agents concluded that if there were compelling reasons to treat a mother for postpartum depression, a condition in which a rapid antidepressant effect is important, the benefits of therapy with SSRIs would most likely outweigh the risks (16). Based on the data cited previously, however, nursing women receiving citalopram, in particular those taking doses >20 mg/day or concurrently with other sedative agents, should be warned of the potential for toxicity in their infants. Moreover, the long-term consequences of exposure to SSRI antidepressants in breast milk on the infant's neurobehavior development are unknown (no such adverse effects have been reported to date, but additional research is needed). Avoiding nursing around the time of peak maternal concentrations (about 4 hours after a dose) may limit infant exposure. However, the long elimination half-life of all SSRIs and their weakly basic properties, which are conducive to ion trapping in the relatively acidic milk, probably will lessen the effectiveness of this strategy. The American Academy of Pediatrics classifies other SSRIs as drugs whose effect on the nursing infant is unknown but may be of concern (see Fluoxetine, Fluvoxamine, Paroxetine, and Sertraline).

References

1. Product information. Celexa. Forest Pharmaceuticals, 2000.
2. Shuey DL, Sadler TW, Lauder JM. Serotonin as a regulator of craniofacial morphogenesis: site specific malformations following exposure to serotonin uptake inhibitors. Teratology 1992;46: 367–78.
3. Heikkinen T, Ekblad U, Laine K. Transplacental transfer of citalopram, fluoxetine and their primary demethylated metabolites in isolated perfused human placenta. BJOG 2002;109:1003–8.
4. Hendrick V, Stowe ZN, Altshuler LL, Hwang S, Lee E, Haynes D. Placental passage of antidepressant medications. Am J Psychiatry 2003;160:993–6.
5. Heikkinen T, Ekblad U, Kero P, Ekblad S, Laine K. Citalopram in pregnancy and lactation. Clin Pharmacol Ther 2002;72:184–91.
6. Seifritz E, Holsboer-Trachsler E, Haberthur F,

Hemmeter U, Poldinger W. Unrecognized pregnancy during citalopram treatment. Am J Psychiatry 1993;150:1428–9.
7. Ericson A, Kallen B, Wiholm BE. Delivery outcome after the use of antidepressants in early pregnancy. Eur J Clin Pharmacol 1999;55:503–8.
8. Nordeng H, Lindemann R, Perminov KV, Reikvam A. Neonatal withdrawal syndrome after *in utero* exposure to selective serotonin reuptake inhibitors. Acta Paediatr 2001;90:288–91.
9. Zeskind PS, Stephens LE. Maternal selective serotonin reuptake inhibitor use during pregnancy and newborn neurobehavior. Pediatrics 2004;113:368–75.
10. Masand PS, Gupta S. Selective serotonin-reuptake inhibitors: an update. Harvard Rev Psychiatry 1999;7:69–84.
11. Spigset O, Carleborg L, Ohman R, Norstrom A. Excretion of citalopram in breast milk. Br J Clin Pharmacol 1997;44:295–8.
12. Jensen PN, Olesen OV, Bertelsen A, Linnet K. Citalopram and desmethylcitalopram concentrations in breast milk and in serum of mother and infant. Therap Drug Monitor 1997;19:236–9.
13. Rampono J, Kristensen JH, Hackett LP, Paech M, Kohan R, Ilett KF. Citalopram and demethylcitalopram in human milk; distribution, excretion and effects in breast-fed infants. Br J Clin Pharmacol 2000;50:263–8.
14. Schmidt K, Olesen OV, Jensen PN. Citalopram and breast-feeding: serum concentration and side effects in the infant. Biol Psychiatry 2000;47:164–5.
15. Lee A, Woo J, Ito S. Frequency of infant adverse events that are associated with citalopram use during breast-feeding. Am J Obstet Gynecol 2004;190:218–21.
16. Edwards JG, Anderson I. Systematic review and guide to selection of selective serotonin reuptake inhibitors. Drugs 1999;57:507–33.

Name: **CLARITHROMYCIN** Risk Factor: **C_M**
Class: **Antibiotic**

FETAL RISK SUMMARY

RECOMMENDATION: Limited Human Data - Animal Data Suggest High Risk

Clarithromycin, a semisynthetic antibiotic structurally related to erythromycin, belongs to the same macrolide class of anti-infectives as azithromycin, dirithromycin, erythromycin, and troleandomycin (the triacetyl ester of oleandomycin).

The effects of clarithromycin on fertility and reproduction in rats, mice, rabbits, and monkeys have been reported by the manufacturer. Doses up to 1.3 times the recommended maximum human dose based on body surface area (MRHD) (serum levels approximately 2 times the levels in humans) in male and female rats produced no adverse effects on the estrous cycle, fertility, parturition, or fetal outcome. No teratogenic effects were observed in four studies involving one rat strain using oral and IV doses up to 1.3 times the MRHD, but a low incidence of cardiovascular anomalies were seen in two studies with a second rat strain at an oral dose about 1.2 times the MRHD. A variable incidence of cleft palate occurred in mice given oral doses about 2–4 times the MRHD (1).

In rabbits, IV doses 17 times less than the MRHD resulted in fetal death, but teratogenic effects were not observed with various oral or IV doses (1). Embryonic loss attributed to maternal toxicity occurred in monkeys administered oral doses 2.4 times the MRHD (serum levels three times the levels in humans). In monkeys, an oral dose approximately equal to the MRHD (serum levels about twice those obtained in humans) caused fetal growth retardation.

Clarithromycin crosses the human placenta (2). In an *in vitro* experiment using perfused term placentas, the mean transplacental transfer of clarithromycin was 6.1%.

At a 1996 meeting, a teratogen information service (TIS) reported the outcomes of 34 exposures to clarithromycin during pregnancy (3). All of the exposures occurred during the 1st and early 2nd trimesters for the treatment of upper respiratory infections. Among the 29 known pregnancy outcomes (5 were pending), there were 8 (28%) abortions (4 spontaneous/4 voluntary), 20 (69%) normal newborns, and 1 (3%) infant with a 0.5 cm brown mark on the temple. One of the normal newborns, delivered at 26 weeks, died from complications of prematurity. Although follow-up of the remaining newborns had not been long enough to completely exclude the presence of congenital malformations, these outcomes do not appear to be different from those expected in a nonexposed population.

Case reports of clarithromycin and congenital anomalies available to the FDA through June 1996 were limited to six diverse birth defects: cystic head, pregnancy terminated; craniofacial anomalies, absent clavicles, bilateral hip deformities, and underdeveloped left heart; spina bifida; cleft lip; pulmonary hypoplasia, anomalous infradiaphragmatic venous return; and CHARGE syndrome (F. Rosa, personal communication, FDA, 1996). By definition, infants having CHARGE association or syndrome must have two or more of the following: coloboma of the eye or eye defects, heart disease, choanal atresia, and retarded growth and development with or without CNS anomalies, genital hypoplasia, and ear anomalies with or without deafness (4). The diversity of the malformations lessens the probability of an association with clarithromycin and any or all of these outcomes may have occurred by chance.

A 1998 prospective controlled multicenter study compared the outcomes of 157 pregnancies exposed to clarithromycin to an equal number of matched controls (5). All of the women had called a TIS. The most common indications for use of the antibiotic were respiratory infections. Of the subjects, 122 (78%) were exposed during the 1st trimester. The outcomes of subjects and controls were spontaneous abortions (22 vs. 11, $p = 0.04$), elective abortions (11 vs. 3, $p = 0.04$), live births (123 vs. 143, $p = 0.003$), stillbirths (1 vs. 0, *ns*), major malformations (3 vs. 2, *ns*), and minor malformations (7 vs. 7, *ns*). The major anomalies (exposure occurred in the 3rd trimester in one case) in the study group were hydrocephalus, Turner's syndrome, and stenosis uteropelvic junction and cranial synostosis. The minor malformations were a large birth mark, a reflux valve problem, an enlarged right ventricle (brain), a minor ventricular septal defect, undescended testes, a blocked tear duct defect, and excess breast tissue on the right. The types of malformations in controls were comparable, with no pattern of defects apparent in either group. Although the increased number of spontaneous abortions in exposed women was within the expected background rate and may have been affected by confounding factors, the investigators concluded that it warranted further study (5).

Three pregnant women with documented *Helicobacter pylori* infections, persistent nausea and vomiting, and epigastric pain were treated in the 2nd trimester with a 2-week course of clarithromycin combined with amoxicillin and either famotidine, omeprazole, or ranitidine (6). The therapy was effective in eliminating the conditions. No adverse effects on the pregnancy outcomes were noted.

BREAST FEEDING SUMMARY

RECOMMENDATION: No Human Data - Probably Compatible

No reports describing the use of this macrolide antibiotic during lactation have been located. Because other antibiotics in this class are excreted into milk (e.g., see Erythromycin), the passage of clarithromycin into milk should be expected. Clarithromycin is excreted in the milk of rats with milk concentrations higher than those measured in the plasma (1). Exposure of the pups to the antibiotic via milk for 3 weeks produced no adverse effects. Based on experience with other antibiotics, including erythromycin, the risk to a nursing infant from clarithromycin in breast milk is probably minimal, but because this is a new drug, caution should be exercised until the effects of this exposure, if any, have been studied.

C

References

1. Product information. Biaxin. Abbott Laboratories, 1996.
2. Witt A, Sommer EM, Cichna M, Postlbauer K, Widhalm A, Gregor H, Reisenberger K. Placental transfer of clarithromycin surpasses other macrolide antibiotics. Am J Obstet Gynecol 2003;188:816–9.
3. Schick B, Hom M, Librizzi R, Donnenfeld A. Pregnancy outcome following exposure to clarithromycin (abstract). Abstracts of the Ninth International Conference of the Organization of Teratology Information Services, May 2–4, 1996, Salt Lake City, Utah. Reprod Toxicol 1996;10:162.
4. Escobar LF, Weaver DD. Charge Association. In Buyse ML, ed. *Birth Defects Encyclopedia*. Volume 1. Dover, MA: Center for Birth Defects Information Services, 1990:308–9.
5. Einarson A, Phillips E, Mawji F, D'Alimonte D, Schick B, Addis A, Mastroiacova P, Mazzone T, Matsui D, Koren G. A prospective controlled multicentre study of clarithromycin in pregnancy. Am J Perinatol 1998;15: 523–5.
6. Jacoby EB, Porter KB. *Helicobacter pylori* infection and persistent hyperemesis gravidarum. Am J Perinatol 1999;16:85–8.

Name: **CLAVULANATE, POTASSIUM** Risk Factor: B_M

Class: **Anti-infective**

FETAL RISK SUMMARY

RECOMMENDATION: Compatible

Clavulanic acid is a β-lactamase inhibitor produced by *Streptomyces clavuligerus* that is combined, as the potassium salt, with the penicillin antibiotics, amoxicillin or ticarcillin, to broaden their antibacterial spectrum of activity. No adverse fetal effects were observed in mice, rats, and pigs administered potassium clavulanate in combination with amoxicillin or ticarcillin during gestation (1–5).

Following a single oral dose of amoxicillin (250 mg) and potassium clavulanate (125 mg) in humans, both agents crossed the placenta to the fetus (6,7). Cord blood levels were found 1 hour after the dose with peak levels occurring at 2–3 hours. In one study, the mean peak maternal serum and umbilical cord blood levels occurred at 2 hours with values of 2.20 and 1.23 μg/mL, respectively (fetal:maternal ratio 0.56) (7). Both amoxicillin and potassium clavulanate have been demonstrated in the amniotic fluid (6–8), with peak concentrations of clavulanate (0.44 μg/mL) measured 5.5 hours after administration (7). A study using *in vitro* perfused human placentas demonstrated the transfer of potassium clavulanate when concentrations on the maternal side were 10–13 μg/mL, but not at 2–6 μg/mL (8). A fetal/maternal gradient of 1:1 was obtained at the higher concentrations.

Several studies have described the use of amoxicillin and potassium clavulanate for various infections in pregnant women (7,9–11). No adverse effects in the fetus or newborn attributable to the combination were observed (see also Amoxicillin and Ticarcillin).

In a surveillance study of Michigan Medicaid recipients conducted between 1985 and 1992 involving 229,101 completed pregnancies, 556 newborns had been exposed to clavulanic acid (presumably in combination with penicillins) during the 1st trimester (F. Rosa, personal communication, FDA, 1993). A total of 24 (4.3%) major birth defects were observed (24 expected). Specific data were available for six defect categories, including (observed/expected) 5/6 cardiovascular defects, 2/1 oral clefts, 1/2 polydactyly, 0/1 limb reduction defects, 1/1 hypospadias, and 2/0.3 spina bifida. Only with the latter defect is there a suggestion of a possible association, but other factors, including the mother's disease, concurrent drug use, and chance may be involved.

BREAST FEEDING SUMMARY

RECOMMENDATION: No Human Data - Probably Compatible

Both amoxicillin and ticarcillin are excreted into breast milk (see Amoxicillin and Ticarcillin), but data pertaining to potassium clavulanate have not been located. Excretion probably occurs because of the low molecular weight (about 237). The effects of the β-lactamase inhibitor on the nursing infant are unknown.

References

1. Baldwin JA, Schardein JL, Koshima Y. Reproduction studies of BRL14151K and BRL25000. I. Teratology studies in rats. Chemotherapy (Tokyo) 1983;31(Suppl 2):238–51.
2. Baldwin JA, Schardein JL, Koshima Y. Reproduction studies of BRL14151K and BRL25000. II. Peri- and post-natal studies in rats. Chemotherapy (Tokyo) 1983;31(Suppl 2):252–62.
3. Hirakawa T, Suzuki T, Sano Y, Tamura K, Koshima Y, Hiura KI, Fujita K, Hardy TL. Reproduction studies of BRL14151K and BRL25000. III. Fertility studies in rats. Chemotherapy (Tokyo) 1983;31(Suppl 2):263–72.
4. James PA, Hardy TL, Koshima Y. Reproduction studies of BRL 25000. IV. Teratology in pig. Chemotherapy (Tokyo) 1983;31(Suppl 2):274–9.
5. Tasker TCG, Cockburn A, Jackson D, Mellows G, White D. Safety of ticarcillin/potassium clavulanate. J Antimicrob Chemother 1986;17:225–32.
6. Matsuda S, Tanno M, Kashiwagura T, Seida A. Fundamental and clinical studies on BRL25000 (clavulanic acid-amoxicillin) in the field of obstetrics and gynecology. Chemotherapy (Tokyo) 1982;30(Suppl 2): 538–47.
7. Takase Z, Shirafuji H, Uchida M. Clinical and laboratory studies on BRL25000 (clavulanic acid-amoxicillin) in the field of obstetrics and gynecology. Chemotherapy (Tokyo) 1982;30(Suppl 2):579–86.
8. Fortunato SJ, Bawdon RE, Swan KF, Bryant EC, Sobhi S. Transfer of Timentin (ticarcillin and clavulanic acid) across the in vitro perfused human placenta: comparison with other agents. Am J Obstet Gynecol 1992;167:1595–9.
9. Matsuda S. Augmentin treatment in obstetrics and gynaecology. Augmentin: Proceedings of an International Symposium, Montreux, Switzerland. July 1981 Leigh DA, Robinson OPW, ed. Excerpta Medica 1982:179–91.
10. Mayer HO, Jeschek H, Kowatsch A. Augmentin in the treatment of urinary tract infection in pregnant women and pelvic inflammatory disease. Proceedings of the European Symposium on Augmentin, Scheveningen, June 1982,1983:207–17.
11. Pedler SJ, Bint AJ. Comparative study of amoxicillin-clavulanic acid and cephalexin in the treatment of bacteriuria during pregnancy. Antimicrob Agents Chemother 1985;27:508–10.

Name:	**CLEMASTINE**	Risk Factor:	**B_M**
Class:	**Antihistamine**		

FETAL RISK SUMMARY

RECOMMENDATION: Compatible

Reproductive studies with the antihistamine, clemastine, in rats and rabbits have revealed no evidence of teratogenic effects (1). No published reports describing the use of clemastine in human pregnancy have been located.

In a surveillance study of Michigan Medicaid recipients conducted between 1985 and 1992 involving 229,101 completed pregnancies, 1617 newborns had been exposed to clemastine during the 1st trimester (F. Rosa, personal communication, FDA, 1993). A total of 71 (4.4%) major birth defects were observed (68 expected). Specific data were available for six defect categories, including (observed/expected) 13/16 cardiovascular defects, 3/3 oral clefts, 3/1 spina bifida, 4/5 polydactyly, 4/4 hypospadias, and 5/1.9 limb reduction defects. Only with the latter defect is there a suggestion of a possible association, but other factors, including the mother's disease, concurrent drug use, and chance, may be involved.

A 2002 study found no increased risk of teratogenicity or other pregnancy or newborn complications for antihistamines when used in early pregnancy for the treatment of nausea and vomiting ($N = 12,394$) and allergy ($N = 5,041$) (2). Clemastine was used by 1,230 women.

An association between exposure during the last 2 weeks of pregnancy to antihistamines and retrolental fibroplasia in premature infants has been reported. See Brompheniramine for details.

BREAST FEEDING SUMMARY

RECOMMENDATION: Limited Human Data - Potential Toxicity

Clemastine is excreted into breast milk (3). A 10-week-old girl developed drowsiness, irritability, refusal to feed, neck stiffness, and a high-pitched cry 12 hours after the mother began taking the antihistamine, 1 mg twice daily. The mother also was also taking phenytoin and carbamazepine. Twenty hours after the last dose, clemastine levels in maternal plasma and milk were 20 and 5–10 ng/mL, respectively, a milk:plasma ratio of 0.25–0.5. The drug could not be detected in the infant's plasma. Symptoms in the baby resolved within 24 hours after the drug was stopped, although breast-feeding was continued. Examination 3 weeks later was also normal. Because of the above case report, the American Academy of Pediatrics states that the drug should be used with caution during breast-feeding (4).

References

1. Product information. Tavist. Sandoz Pharmaceuticals, 1993.
2. Kallen B. Use of antihistamine drugs in early pregnancy and delivery outcome. J Matern Fetal Neonatal Med 2002;11:146–52.
3. Kok THHG, Taitz LS, Bennett MJ, Holt DW. Drowsiness due to clemastine transmitted in breast milk. Lancet 1982;1:914–5.
4. Committee on Drugs, American Academy of Pediatrics. The transfer of drugs and other chemicals into human milk. Pediatrics 2001;108:776–89.

Name:	**CLIDINIUM**	Risk Factor:	**C**
Class:	**Parasympatholytic**		

FETAL RISK SUMMARY

RECOMMENDATION: Limited Human Data - No Relevant Animal Data

Clidinium is an anticholinergic quaternary ammonium bromide. In a large prospective study, 2323 patients were exposed to this class of drugs during the 1st trimester, 4 of whom took clidinium (1). A possible association was found between the total group and minor malformations.

BREAST FEEDING SUMMARY

RECOMMENDATION: No Human Data - Probably Compatible

No data are available (see also Atropine).

Reference

1. Heinonen OP, Slone D, Shapiro S. *Birth Defects and Drugs in Pregnancy*. Littleton, MA: Publishing Sciences Group, 1977:346–53.

Name: **CLINDAMYCIN**	Risk Factor: B_M
Class: **Antibiotic**	

FETAL RISK SUMMARY

RECOMMENDATION: Compatible

No reports linking the use of clindamycin with congenital defects have been located. Reproduction studies in mice and rats with oral doses up to about 1.1 and 2.1 times the maximum recommended human adult dose based on body surface area (MRHD), respectively, revealed no evidence of teratogenicity. In addition, SC doses in the two species up to 0.5 and 0.9 times the MRHD, respectively, failed to show teratogenicity (1).

The drug crosses the placenta, achieving maximum cord serum levels of approximately 50% of the maternal serum (2,3). Levels in the fetus were considered therapeutic for susceptible pathogens. A study published in 1988 measured a mean cord:maternal ratio of 0.15 in three women given an unknown amount of clindamycin in labor for the treatment of chorioamnionitis (4). At the time of sampling, mean maternal blood, cord blood, and placental membrane concentrations of the antibiotic were 1.67 μg/mL, 0.26 μg/mL, and 1.86 μg/g, respectively (placenta:maternal ratio 1.11). Fetal tissue levels increase following multiple dosing with the drug concentrating in the fetal liver (2). Maternal serum levels after dosing at various stages of pregnancy were similar to those of nonpregnant patients (3,5). Clindamycin has been used as prophylactic therapy prior to cesarean section (6).

In a surveillance study of Michigan Medicaid recipients conducted between 1985 and 1992 involving 229,101 completed pregnancies, 647 newborns had been exposed to clindamycin during the 1st trimester (includes both maternal systemic and nonsystemic administration) (F. Rosa, personal communication, FDA, 1993). A total of 31 (4.8%) major birth defects were observed (28 expected). Specific data were available for six defect categories, including (observed/expected) 5/6 cardiovascular defects, 0/1 oral clefts, 1/0.5 spina bifida, 1/2 polydactyly, 0/1 limb reduction defects, and 3/2 hypospadias. These data do not support an association between the drug and congenital defects.

BREAST FEEDING SUMMARY

RECOMMENDATION: Compatible

Clindamycin is excreted into breast milk. In two patients receiving 600 mg IV every 6 hours, milk levels varied from 2.1 to 3.8 μg/mL (0.2–3.5 hours after drug) (7). When the patients were changed to 300 mg orally every 6 hours, levels varied from 0.7 to 1.8 μg/mL (2–7 hours after drug). Maternal serum levels were not given.

Two grossly bloody stools were observed in a nursing infant whose mother was receiving clindamycin and gentamicin (8). No relationship to either drug could be established. However, the condition cleared rapidly when breast-feeding was stopped. Except for this one case, no other adverse effects in nursing infants have been reported.

Three potential problems that may exist for the nursing infant are modification of bowel flora, direct effects on the infant, and interference with the interpretation of culture results if a fever workup is required. The American Academy of Pediatrics classifies clindamycin as compatible with breast-feeding (9).

C

References

1. Product information. Cleocin. Pharmacia & Upjohn, 2000.
2. Philipson A, Sabath LD, Charles D. Transplacental passage of erythromycin and clindamycin. N Engl J Med 1973;288:1219–21.
3. Weinstein AJ, Gibbs RS, Gallagher M. Placental transfer of clindamycin and gentamicin in term pregnancy. Am J Obstet Gynecol 1976;124:688–91.
4. Gilstrap LC III, Bawdon RE, Burris J. Antibiotic concentration in maternal blood, cord blood, and placental membranes in chorioamnionitis. Obstet Gynecol 1988;72:124–5.
5. Philipson A, Sabath LD, Charles D. Erythromycin and clindamycin absorption and elimination in pregnant women. Clin Pharmacol Ther 1976;19:68–77.
6. Rehu M, Jahkola M. Prophylactic antibiotics in caesarean section: effect of a short preoperative course of benzyl penicillin or clindamycin plus gentamicin on postoperative infectious morbidity. Ann Clin Res 1980;12:45–8.
7. Smith JA, Morgan JR, Rachlis AR, Papsin FR. Clindamycin in human breast milk. Can Med Assoc J 1975;112:806.
8. Mann CF. Clindamycin and breast-feeding. Pediatrics 1980;66:1030–1.
9. Committee on Drugs, American Academy of Pediatrics. The transfer of drugs and other chemicals into human milk. Pediatrics 2001;108:776–89.

Name: **CLOFAZIMINE** Risk Factor: **C_M**

Class: **Anti-infective (Leprostatic)**

FETAL RISK SUMMARY

RECOMMENDATION: Limited Human Data - Animal Data Suggest Low Risk

Clofazimine, a bright-red dye with antibacterial properties against *Mycobacterium leprae*, is used for the treatment of lepromatous leprosy. Animal studies involving mice and rats with doses up to 50 mg/kg/day, and rabbits with doses of 15 mg/kg/day, found no evidence of teratogenicity (1). Fetotoxicity in mice at doses 12–25 times the human dose, however, included retardation of fetal skull ossification, increased incidence of abortions and stillbirths, and decreased neonatal survival (2).

A number of studies have reported the use of clofazimine throughout human pregnancies (3–9). In 13 pregnancies, three exposed newborns died shortly after birth, but none of the outcomes could be attributed to clofazimine. The causes of death were unspecified (died 3 hours after birth), prematurity and antemortem hemorrhage, and gastroenteritis (5,7). The mother of the newborn who died at 3 hours was steroid dependent, but she had stopped her prednisolone 4 weeks before delivery (5). No congenital anomalies were observed in any of the 13 infants, although some of the infants were pigmented at birth. In at least 3 infants (data not provided in 10 infants), the pigmentation gradually resolved over a 1-year period (8).

A 1982 case report described the effects of clofazimine exposure during pregnancy on two newborns (10). The first case involved a woman with erythema nodosum leprosum who was treated throughout gestation with clofazimine, 300 mg/day, and prednisone. Rifampin was also used early in pregnancy. Oligohydramnios developed just prior to delivery after a gestation of uncertain dates. Thick, foul-smelling, meconium-stained fluid was present, and the placenta showed signs of acute severe amnionitis. A 2575-g male infant was delivered vaginally who appeared normal except for his skin, which was "not excessively pigmented." Bilateral hydrocele and iron deficiency anemia were diagnosed at 14 days of age with fever of unknown origin occurring then and again at 5 months of age. The infant was doing well at 12 months of age. In the second case, a woman was treated throughout pregnancy with clofazimine, 300 mg/day, for tuberculoid leprosy. A normal, healthy 3070-g female infant was delivered vaginally at an unspecified gestational age, and she was growing and developing normally at 3 years of age. Skin pigmentation was not mentioned.

A 1984 reference examined the results of 79 pregnancies from 76 women with lepromatous leprosy, of whom 4 (5 pregnancies) were treated with clofazimine (300 mg/week) (11). No information was given on the outcome of these pregnancies, although the authors stated that clofazimine was the best drug available, if given after the 1st trimester, to prevent transient relapses and to prevent or treat erythema nodosum leprosy (11).

BREAST FEEDING SUMMARY

RECOMMENDATION: Limited Human Data - Potential Toxicity

Clofazimine is excreted into breast milk and pigmentation of the nursing infant may result. In one case, a mother was ingesting clofazimine, between 100 and 300 mg/day (exact dose not specified), 6 days/week, for a 6-month period (3). Her nursing infant became "ruddy and then slightly hypermelanotic." The baby's skin returned to a normal color 5 months after the mother's medication was stopped.

The American Academy of Pediatrics classifies clofazimine as a drug whose effect on the nursing infant is unknown (other than the skin pigmentation) but may be of concern (12).

References

1. Stenger EG, Aeppli L, Peheim E, Thomann PE. Zur toxikologie des leprostaticums 3-(*p*-chloranilino)-10-(*p*-chlorophenyl)-2–10-dihydro 2(isopropyl-amino) phenazin (G-30320). Arzneimittelforschung 1970;20: 794–9. As cited in Shepard TH. *Catalog of Teratogenic Agents*. 6th ed. Baltimore, MD: Johns Hopkins University Press, 1989:157.
2. Product information. Lamprene. Ciba-Geigy Corp, 1992.
3. Browne SG, Hogerzeil LM. "B 663" in the treatment of leprosy. Preliminary report of a pilot trial. Lepr Rev 1962;33:6–10.
4. Imkamp FMJH. A treatment of corticosteroid-dependent lepromatous patients in persistent erythema nodosum leprosum. A clinical evaluation of G.30320 (B663). Lepr Rev 1968;39:119–25.
5. Plock H, Leiker DL. A long term trial with clofazimine in reactive lepromatous leprosy. Lepr Rev 1976;47: 25–34.
6. De las Aguas JT. Treatment of leprosy with Lampren (B.663 Geigy). Int J Lepr Other Mycobact Dis 1971;39:493–503.
7. Schulz EJ. Forty-four months' experience in the treatment of leprosy with clofazimine (Lamprene [Geigy]). Lepr Rev 1972;42:178–187.
8. Karat AB. Long-term follow-up of clofazimine (Lamprene) in the management of reactive phases of leprosy. Lepr Rev 1975;46(Suppl):105–9.
9. Waters MFR. Symposium on B.663 (Lamprene, Geigy) in the treatment of leprosy and leprosy reactions. Int J Lepr 1968;36:560–1.
10. Farb H, West DP, Pedvis-Leftick A. Clofazimine in pregnancy complicated by leprosy. Obstet Gynecol 1982;59:122–3.
11. Duncan ME, Pearson JMH. The association of pregnancy and leprosy. III. Erythema nodosum leprosum in pregnancy and lactation. Lepr Rev 1984;55:129–42.
12. Committee on Drugs, American Academy of Pediatrics. The transfer of drugs and other chemicals into human milk. Pediatrics 2001;108:776–89.

Name: **CLOFIBRATE** Risk Factor: **C_M**

Class: **Antilipemic Agent**

FETAL RISK SUMMARY

RECOMMENDATION: No Human Data - No Relevant Animal Data

No reports linking the use of clofibrate with congenital defects have been located. Animal reproduction studies have not been conducted with clofibrate (1).

There is pharmacologic evidence that clofibrate crosses the rat placenta and reaches measurable levels, but data in humans are lacking (2). The low molecular weight (about

243), however, indicates that the drug probably crosses the human placenta to the fetus. The drug is metabolized by glucuronide conjugation. Because this system is immature in the newborn, accumulation may occur. Consequently, the use of clofibrate near term is not recommended.

BREAST FEEDING SUMMARY

RECOMMENDATION: No Human Data - Potential Toxicity

No reports describing the use of clofibrate during human lactation have been located. Animal studies suggest that the drug is excreted into milk (2). The low molecular weight (about 243) also suggests that the drug is excreted into human milk. Moreover, the manufacturer states that an active metabolite has been measured in breast milk (1). Because of the potential for severe adverse effects in the nursing infant, mother's using clofibrate probably should not breast-feed.

References

1. Product information. Atromid-S. Wyeth-Ayerst Pharmaceuticals, 2000.
2. Chabra S, Kurup CKR. Maternal transport of chlorophenoxyisobutyrate at the foetal and neonatal stages of development. Biochem Pharmacol 1978;27:2063–5.

Name:	**CLOMIPHENE**	Risk Factor:	X_M
Class:	**Fertility Agent (Nonhormonal)**		

FETAL RISK SUMMARY

RECOMMENDATION: Contraindicated

Clomiphene is used to induce ovulation and is contraindicated after conception has occurred. Multiple pregnancies, most often twins, may be a complication of ovulation induction with clomiphene (1).

Shepard reviewed five animal reproduction studies involving the use of clomiphene in mice, rats, and monkeys (2). Hydramnios, cataracts, dose-related fetal mortality, and multiple abnormalities of the genital tract were observed in fetal mice and rats, but no congenital anomalies resulted after exposure of monkeys during the embryonic period. In mice, preovulatory administration of clomiphene produced a decrease in implantation rates, and growth retardation and an increased incidence of exencephaly in surviving fetuses (3). The decreased rate of implantation and growth retardation, which were most pronounced when the drug was given immediately before ovulation, apparently were caused by impairment of uterine function, rather than by a direct effect on the embryo itself (3).

Several case reports of neural tube defects have been reported after stimulating ovulation with clomiphene (4–8). However, an association between the drug and these defects has not been established (9–17). In one review, the percentage of congenital anomalies after clomiphene use was no greater than in the normal population (9). Similarly, another study involving 1034 pregnancies after clomiphene-induced ovulation found no association with the incidence or type of malformation (18). Recent studies have also failed to find an association between ovulation induction with clomiphene and neural tube defects (19–25) or any defects (19,23). Congenital malformations reported in patients who received clomiphene before conception include the following (8,9,26–40):

Hydatidiform mole
Syndactyly
Pigmentation defects
Congenital heart defects
Down's syndrome
Hypospadias
Hemangioma
Persistent hyperplastic primary vitreous
Retinal aplasia
Clubfoot
Microcephaly
Cleft lip/palate
Ovarian dysplasia
Polydactyly
Anencephaly

A 1996 prospective study examined the possible relationship between clomiphene and spontaneous abortions (41). The outcomes of 1744 clomiphene-induced pregnancies were compared with the outcomes of 3245 spontaneous pregnancies. The incidence of spontaneous abortion (clinical and preclinical) was higher in clomiphene-induced pregnancies than in spontaneous pregnancies (23.7% vs. 20.4%, $p < 0.01$).

Acardius acephalus in a monozygotic twin was observed in a pregnancy occurring after ovulation induced with clomiphene (42). Because monozygotic twining is associated with an increased incidence of congenital defects, and because clomiphene-induced ovulation increases the incidence of multiple gestation and possibly of monozygotic twins, the investigators thought that the drug may have had a causative role, either directly or indirectly, in the defect. Another case of acardius acephalus similar to the one above was published in 1995 (43). The authors also mentioned a third case that had been published in 1990 (44). However, they concluded that there was insufficient evidence to establish a relationship between clomiphene and acardiac twinning (43).

A single case of hepatoblastoma in a 15-month-old female was thought to be caused by the use of clomiphene and follicle-stimulating/luteinizing hormone prior to conception (45).

Inadvertent use of clomiphene early in the 1st trimester has been reported in two patients (32,38). A ruptured lumbosacral meningomyelocele was observed in one infant exposed during the 4th week of gestation (32). There was no evidence of neurologic defect in the lower limbs or of hydrocephalus. The second infant was delivered with esophageal atresia with fistula, congenital heart defects, hypospadias, and absent left kidney (38). The mother also took methyldopa throughout pregnancy for mild hypertension.

In a surveillance study of Michigan Medicaid recipients conducted between 1985 and 1992 involving 229,101 completed pregnancies, 41 newborns may have been exposed to clomiphene during the 1st trimester (F. Rosa, personal communication, FDA, 1993). Three (7.3%) (two expected) major birth defects were observed, one of which was a cardiovascular defect (0.5 expected). No anomalies were observed in five other categories of defects (oral clefts, spina bifida, polydactyly, limb reduction defects, and hypospadias) for which specific data were available. Although the number of exposures is small, these data do not support an association between the drug and congenital defects.

Patients requiring the use of clomiphene should be cautioned that each new course of the drug should be started only after pregnancy has been excluded.

BREAST FEEDING SUMMARY

RECOMMENDATION: No Human Data - Potential Toxicity

No reports describing the use of clomiphene during lactation have been located. The drug may reduce lactation in some patients (46).

References

1. Product information. Serophene. Serono Laboratories, 1993.
2. Shepard TH. *Catalog of Teratogenic Agents*. 6th ed. Baltimore, MD: Johns Hopkins University Press, 1989:158–9.
3. Dziadek M. Preovulatory administration of clomiphene citrate to mice causes fetal growth retardation and neural tube defects (exencephaly) by an indirect maternal effect. Teratology 1993;47: 263–73.
4. Barrett C, Hakim C. Anencephaly, ovulation stimulation, subfertility, and illegitimacy. Lancet 1973;2: 916–7.
5. Dyson JL, Kohler HG. Anencephaly and ovulation stimulation. Lancet 1973;1:1256–7.
6. Field B, Kerr C. Ovulation stimulation and defects of neural tube closure. Lancet 1974;2:1511.
7. Sandler B. Anencephaly and ovulation stimulation. Lancet 1973;2:379.
8. Biale Y, Leventhal H, Altaras M, Ben-Aderet N. Anencephaly and clomiphene-induced pregnancy. Acta Obstet Gynecol Scand 1978;57:483–4.
9. Asch RH, Greenblatt RB. Update on the safety and efficacy of clomiphene citrate as a therapeutic agent. J Reprod Med 1976;17:175–80.
10. Harlap S. Ovulation induction and congenital malformations. Lancet 1976;2:961.
11. James WH. Clomiphene, anencephaly, and spina bifida. Lancet 1977;1:603.
12. Ahlgren M, Kallen B, Rannevik G. Outcome of pregnancy after clomiphene therapy. Acta Obstet Gynecol Scand 1976;55:371–5.
13. Elwood JM. Clomiphene and anencephalic births. Lancet 1974;1:31.
14. Czeizel A. Ovulation induction and neural tube defects. Lancet 1989;2:167.
15. Cuckle H, Wald N. Ovulation induction and neural tube defects. Lancet 1989;2:1281.
16. Cornel MC, Ten Kate LP, Graham Dukes MN, De Jong-V D Berg LTW, Meyboom RHB, Garbis H, Peters PWJ. Ovulation induction and neural tube defects. Lancet 1989;1:1386.
17. Cornel MC, Ten Kate LP, Te Meerman GJ. Ovulation induction, in-vitro fertilisation, and neural tube defects. Lancet 1989;2:1530.
18. Kurachi K, Aono T, Minagawa J, Miyake A. Congenital malformations of newborn infants after clomiphene-induced ovulation. Fertil Steril 1983;40: 187–9.
19. Mills JL, Simpson JL, Rhoads GG, Graubard BI, Hoffman H, Conley MR, Lassman M, Cunningham G. Risk of neural tube defects in relation to maternal fertility and fertility drug use. Lancet 1990;336:103–4.
20. Rosa F. Ovulation induction and neural tube defects. Lancet 1990;336:1327.
21. Mills JL. Clomiphene and neural-tube defects. Lancet 1991;337:853.
22. Van Loon K, Besseghir K, Eshkol A. Neural tube defects after infertility treatment: a review. Fertil Steril 1992;58:875–84.
23. Shoham Z, Zosmer A, Insler V. Early miscarriage and fetal malformations after induction of ovulation (by clomiphene citrate and/or human menotropins), in vitro fertilization, and gamete intrafallopian transfer. Fertil Steril 1991;55:1–11.
24. Werler MM, Louik C, Shapiro S, Mitchell AA. Ovulation induction and risk of neural tube defects. Lancet 1994;344:445–6.
25. Greenland S, Ackerman DL. Clomiphene citrate and neural tube defects: a pooled analysis of controlled epidemiologic studies and recommendations for future studies. Fertil Steril 1995;64:936–41.
26. Miles PA, Taylor HB, Hill WC. Hydatidiform mole in a clomiphene related pregnancy: a case report. Obstet Gynecol 1971;37:358–9.
27. Schneiderman CI, Waxman B. Clomid therapy and subsequent hydatidiform mole formation: a case report. Obstet Gynecol 1972;39:787–8.
28. Wajntraub G, Kamar R, Pardo Y. Hydatidiform mole after treatment with clomiphene. Fertil Steril 1974;25:904–5.
29. Berman P. Congenital abnormalities associated with maternal clomiphene ingestion. Lancet 1975;2:878.
30. Drew AL. Letter to the editor. Dev Med Child Neurol 1974;16:276.
31. Hack M, Brish M, Serr DM, Insler V, Salomy M, Lunenfeld B. Outcome of pregnancy after induced ovulation. Follow-up of pregnancies and children born after clomiphene therapy. JAMA 1972;220:1329–33.
32. Ylikorkala O. Congenital anomalies and clomiphene. Lancet 1975;2:1262–3.
33. Laing IA, Steer CR, Dudgeon J, Brown JK. Clomiphene and congenital retinopathy. Lancet 1981;2:1107–8.
34. Ford WDA, Little KET. Fetal ovarian dysplasia possibly associated with clomiphene. Lancet 1981;2:1107.
35. Kistner RW. Induction of ovulation with clomiphene citrate. Obstet Gynecol Surv 1965;20:873–99.
36. Goldfarb AF, Morales A, Rakoff AE, Protos P. Critical review of 160 clomiphene-related pregnancies. Obstet Gynecol 1968;31:342–5.
37. Oakely GP, Flynt IW. Increased prevalence of Down's syndrome (mongolism) among the offspring of women treated with ovulation-inducing agents. Teratology 1972;5:264.
38. Singhi M, Singhi S. Possible relationship between clomiphene and neural tube defects. J Pediatr 1978;93:152.
39. Mor-Joseph S, Anteby SO, Granat M, Brzezinsky A, Evron S. Recurrent molar pregnancies associated with clomiphene citrate and human gonadotropins. Am J Obstet Gynecol 1985;151:1085–6.
40. Bishai R, Arbour L, Lyons C, Koren G. Intrauterine exposure to clomiphene and neonatal persistent hyperplastic primary vitreous. Teratology 1999;60:143–5.
41. Dickey RP, Taylor SN, Curole DN, Rye PH, Pyrzak R. Incidence of spontaneous abortion in clomiphene pregnancies. Hum Reprod 1996;11:2623–8.
42. Haring DAJP, Cornel MC, Van Der Linden JC, Van Vugt JMG, Kwee ML. Acardius acephalus after induced ovulation: a case report. Teratology 1993;47:257–62.
43. Martinez-Roman S, Torres PJ, Puerto B. Acardius acephalus after ovulation induction by clomiphene. Teratology 1995;51:231–2.
44. Sceusa DK, Klein PE. Ultrasound diagnosis of an acardius acephalic monster in a quintuplet pregnancy. JDMS 1990;2:109–12. As cited by Martinez-Roman S,

Torres PJ, Puerto B. Acardius acephalus after ovulation induction by clomiphene. Teratology 1995;51:231–2.
45. Melamed I, Bujanover Y, Hammer J, Spirer Z. Hepatoblastoma in an infant born to a mother after hormonal treatment for sterility. N Engl J Med 1982;307:820.
46. Product information. Clomid. Hoechst Marion Roussel, 2000.

Name: **CLOMIPRAMINE** Risk Factor: **C_M**
Class: **Antidepressant**

FETAL RISK SUMMARY

RECOMMENDATION: Human Data Suggest Risk in 1st and 3rd Trimesters

Clomipramine is a tricyclic antidepressant in the same class as amitriptyline, doxepin, imipramine, and trimipramine. No teratogenic effects were observed after dosing with clomipramine via the oral (mice and rats), SC (mice and rats), and IV (mice and rabbits) routes (1). Congenital malformations (2,3) and toxic symptoms (caused by apparent drug withdrawal) (4–10) have been reported in human fetuses exposed to clomipramine.

In a 1996 descriptive, large, case series, the European Network of the Teratology Information Services (ENTIS) prospectively examined the outcomes of 689 pregnancies exposed to antidepressants (2). Multiple-drug therapy occurred in about two-thirds of the mothers. Clomipramine (134 exposures) was the most commonly used tricyclic antidepressant. The outcomes of these pregnancies were 20 elective abortions, 22 spontaneous abortions, 4 stillbirths, 76 normal newborns (including 2 premature infants), 9 normal infants with neonatal disorder (primarily withdrawal symptoms), and 3 infants with congenital defects. The defects (all exposed in the 1st trimester or longer) were Down's syndrome, bilateral talipes (also exposed to prazepam), and Harlequin syndrome with multiple anomalies (exposed to multiple other agents).

A 2003 case-control study, using data from three Swedish health registers, was conducted to identify drug use in early pregnancy that was associated with cardiac defects (3). Cases (cardiovascular defects without known chromosome anomalies) ($N = 5015$) were compared to controls consisting of all infants born in Sweden (1995–2001) ($N = 577,730$). Associations were identified for several drugs, some of which were probably a result of confounding from the underlying disease or complaint or multiple testing, but some were thought to be true drug effects (2). For all antidepressants, there were 40 cases in 4068 exposures (odds ratio [OR] 1.14, 95% confidence interval [CI] 0.83–1.56). There was an increased OR for the tricyclic/tetracyclic antidepressants (16 cases, 1018 exposures; OR 1.77, 95% CI 1.07–2.91), but the association was caused by clomipramine (15 cases, 838 exposures; OR 2.03, 95% CI 1.22–3.40). The lack of an association with other antidepressants suggested to the investigators that it was unlikely that the underlying disease itself caused the association with clomipramine (3).

A mother took clomipramine 25 mg three times daily throughout a normal pregnancy (4). Twelve hours after birth, the 3140-g male infant became dusky and was hypothermic (rectal temperature 35.4°C). Hypothermia persisted for 4 days and was aggravated by feeding and handling. Jitteriness, attributed to drug withdrawal, developed on the 2nd day and persisted for 48 hours. The symptoms were controlled with phenobarbital. Plasma levels of clomipramine and its metabolite, chlordesipramine, were <20 ng/mL and 116 ng/mL, respectively, at 1 day of age, and <20 ng/mL and 96 ng/mL, respectively, at age 3 days. Recovery was uneventful and normal development was noted at 3 and 6 months of age (4).

Drug withdrawal was observed in two newborns exposed throughout gestation to clomipramine (5). A 3550-g infant, exposed to clomipramine 200 mg/day, appeared normal at birth but became lethargic, cyanotic, and tachypneic with moderate respiratory acidosis within a few hours. Oxygen therapy corrected the cyanosis and respiratory acidosis. Jitteriness and tremors developed by the end of the 1st day, followed by intermittent hypertonia and hypotonia, tachypnea, and feeding problems. Phenobarbital was used to control the symptoms, which resolved completely in 1 week. A 4020-g newborn, whose mother had taken 100 mg/day of clomipramine, had symptoms similar to those observed in the first infant. Oxygen and phenobarbital therapy were used, and although the neurologic symptoms had resolved within a few days, tachypnea and feeding difficulties persisted for 16 days. Both infants were developing normally at 5 months of age (5).

Neonatal convulsions were observed in two male infants after *in utero* exposure to clomipramine (maternal doses not specified) (6). The onset of seizures occurred at 8 and 7 hours. The first infant, a 3420-g newborn whose mother had been treated with clomipramine during the last 7 weeks of gestation, had persistent intermittent convulsions, despite treatment with phenobarbital and paraldehyde, until 53 hours of age, after which he remained hypertonic and jittery with ankle clonus until the 11th day. The second infant, exposed throughout gestation to clomipramine and flurazepam (dose not specified), delivered at 33 weeks' gestation with a birth weight of 2360 g, had convulsions that were unresponsive to phenobarbital. At 24 hours of age, 0.4 mg of clomipramine was given intravenously over 2 hours, resulting in complete cessation of the symptoms for 11 hours. Upon their recurrence, a dose of 0.5 mg over 2 hours was given, followed by a continuous tapering infusion until age 12 days when oral therapy was started (doses not given). No additional convulsions were observed, but he remained jittery. All therapy was stopped at age 17 days without adverse effects. No follow-up of either infant was mentioned. The combined concentrations of drug and metabolite in the mothers were 610 ng/mL and 549 ng/mL, respectively, both higher than the suggested therapeutic range of 200–500 ng/mL. Although exact values could not be obtained from the graphs used in the reference, the initial combined serum levels of clomipramine and metabolite in the infants appear to be in the range of 250–400 ng/mL. The authors attributed the convulsions to the initial steep decline in serum drug levels, with clomipramine therapy in the second infant permitting a more gradual decline in concentrations and, thus, control of the infant's symptoms. Neurologic symptoms in the infants did not resolve completely until the concentration of clomipramine was <10 ng/mL (6).

Six cases of fetal exposure to clomipramine were described in a 1991 report (7). One infant, with meconium-stained fluid in the trachea, had mild respiratory distress with acidosis, mild hypotonia, and a tremor at birth. At 12 hours of age, the newborn developed jitteriness that resolved spontaneously, along with the other symptoms, by 6 days of age. At birth, clomipramine concentrations were 474.4 ng/mL in the maternal serum and 266.6 ng/mL in the neonatal plasma (ratio 1.8). Levels of the metabolite were not determined. The mother's dose at this time was 125 mg/day. The elimination half-life of clomipramine in the infant during the first week, when the male infant was not breastfeeding, was 92.8 hours. Among the other five cases, one woman had a therapeutic abortion at 9 weeks' gestation, one stopped clomipramine therapy when she realized she was pregnant, and the remaining three continued therapy with daily doses between 75 and 250 mg throughout gestation. Mild hypotonia, persisting for several weeks, was observed in one of the four liveborn infants, and transient tachypnea requiring oxygen therapy was observed in another. No other symptoms or signs of toxicity were noted (7).

Three additional cases of drug withdrawal to clomipramine have been reported (8–10). A short 1990 case report described symptoms of drug withdrawal in a newborn exposed during the last 8–9 weeks of gestation to daily doses of 125 mg of clomipramine and 3 mg of lorazepam (8). The 3900-g infant was normal until 8 hours of age, when tachypnea, with a respiratory rate of 100–120 breaths/minute, and recessions developed. Other symptoms noted in the infant over the next 10 days were intermittent hypertonia and marked diaphoresis. Treatment consisted of intravenous fluids, oxygen, and empiric antibiotic therapy. No follow-up of the infant was reported (8). In the second case, a 33-year-old woman with an obsessive-compulsive disorder was treated with clomipramine, 100–150 mg/day, from the 12th through the 32nd week of gestation (9). At that time, the mother decided on her own to discontinue the drug; 4 days later she presented in premature labor and imminent delivery, and a 2.7-kg infant was delivered by cesarean section. Repetitive seizures, rigidity, irritability, and decerebrate-like posturing that was unresponsive to phenobarbital and phenytoin occurred 10 minutes after birth. After 3 days of convulsions, 0.5 mg of clomipramine was given via gastric tube with resolution of the seizures within 30 minutes. When the seizures recurred 10 hours later, clomipramine, 0.5 mg three times daily, was started and the phenobarbital discontinued. The clomipramine was gradually tapered over the next 20 days. An EEG shortly after birth showed a left temporal epileptogenic focus, but was normal after 20 days of clomipramine therapy. The infant was discharged home at the age of 1 month with no signs or symptoms of neurological damage (9). The third case involved a term male infant who had been exposed throughout gestation to 100 mg/day (10). Generalized, stimulant-sensitive status myoclonus developed at age 2 days (clomipramine serum level <10 ng/mL) that was successfully treated with 0.5 mg clomipramine. Previous treatment with clonazepam and phenobarbital was unsuccessful. At 3 weeks of age, only mild jitteriness in response to touch was noted (10).

A 2002 prospective study compared two groups of mother-child pairs exposed to antidepressants throughout gestation (46 exposed to tricyclics: 7 to clomipramine; 40 to fluoxetine) to 36 nonexposed, not depressed controls (11). Offspring were studied between the ages 15 and 71 months for effects of antidepressant exposure in terms of IQ, language, behavior, and temperament. Exposure to antidepressants did not adversely affect the measured parameters, but IQ was significantly and negatively associated with the duration of depression, and language was negatively associated with the number of depression episodes after delivery (11).

In summary, clomipramine was not teratogenic in animals, but a statistically significant association between clomipramine and cardiac defects was found in a human study. These results require confirmation. In addition, newborn toxicity may occur due to apparent drug withdrawal. In two cases, *in utero* exposure to a benzodiazepine sedative may have contributed to the observed symptoms. Although the data are very limited, no long-term effects of *in utero* exposure to clomipramine have been observed.

BREAST FEEDING SUMMARY

RECOMMENDATION: Limited Human Data - Potential Toxicity

Clomipramine is excreted into human milk (7). A woman taking 125 mg/day of the antidepressant had milk and plasma concentrations determined on the 4th and 6th postpartum days. Her infant was not breast feeding during this time. Milk levels were 342.7 and

215.8 ng/mL, respectively, compared to plasma levels of 211.0 and 208.4 ng/mL, respectively. The milk:plasma ratios on the 4th and 6th days were 1.62 and 1.04, respectively. Neonatal plasma concentrations of clomipramine, from drug obtained *in utero*, declined from 266.6 ng/mL at birth to 94.8 ng/mL on the 6th day. The baby was allowed to breast-feed commencing at 7 days of age; at the same time, the mother's dose was increased to 150 mg/day. Repeat determinations of milk and plasma clomipramine concentrations were made between 10 and 14 hours after the daily dose on the 10th, 14th, and 35th days after delivery. Milk levels ranged from 269.8–624.2 ng/mL compared to plasma concentrations of 355.0–509.8 ng/mL, corresponding to milk:plasma ratios of 0.76–1.22. The highest concentrations for both the milk and the plasma occurred on the 35th day, but neonatal drug levels continued to decline from 45.4 ng/mL on the 10th day to 9.8 ng/mL on the 35th day. No adverse effects were noted in the infant during breast-feeding (7).

A 1996 review of antidepressant treatment during breast-feeding found no information that clomipramine exposure during nursing resulted in quantifiable amounts in an infant or that the exposure caused adverse effects (12).

Ten nursing infants of mothers taking antidepressants (two with clomipramine 75–125 mg/day) were compared to 15 bottle-fed infants of mothers with depression who did not breast-feed (13). Concentrations of clomipramine in fore-milk and hind-milk ranged from 32–212 ng/mL and 32–436 ng/mL, respectively. The milk:maternal plasma ratios were 0.4–1.2 and 0.4–3.0, respectively. One infant had plasma levels of 3.2 ng/mL when the mother was taking 75 mg/day and 5.5 ng/mL when the dose was increased to 125 mg/day. No toxic effects or delays in development were observed in the infants. The estimated daily dose consumed by the infants was about 1% of the mother's weight adjusted dose (13).

The American Academy of Pediatrics classifies clomipramine as a drug whose effect on the nursing infant is unknown but may be of concern (14).

References

1. Watanabe N, Nakai T, Iwanami K, Fujii T. Toxicological studies of clomipramine hydrochloride. Kiso to Rinsho 1970;4:2105–24. As cited in Shepard TH. *Catalog of Teratogenic Agents*. 6th ed. Baltimore, MD: Johns Hopkins University Press, 1989:159–60.
2. McElhatton PR, Garbis HM, Elefant E, Vial T, Bellemin B, Mastroiacovo P, Arnon J, Rodriguez-Pinilla E, Schaefer C, Pexieder T, Merlob P, Dal Verme S. The outcome of pregnancy in 689 women exposed to therapeutic doses of antidepressants. A collaborative study of the European Network of Teratology Information Services (ENTIS). Reprod Toxicol 1996;10:285–94.
3. Kallen BAJ, Olausson PO. Maternal drug use in early pregnancy and infant cardiovascular defect. Reprod Toxicol 2003;17:255–61.
4. Ben Muza A, Smith CS. Neonatal effects of maternal clomipramine therapy. Arch Dis Child 1979;54:405.
5. Ostergaard GZ, Pedersen SE. Neonatal effects of maternal clomipramine treatment. Pediatrics 1982;69:233–4.
6. Cowe L, Lloyd DJ, Dawling S. Neonatal convulsions caused by withdrawal from maternal clomipramine. Br Med J 1982;284:1837–8.
7. Schimmell MS, Katz EZ, Shaag Y, Pastuszak A, Koren G. Toxic neonatal effects following maternal clomipramine therapy. J Toxicol Clin Toxicol 1991;29:479–84.
8. Singh S, Gulati S, Narang A, Bhakoo ON. Non-narcotic withdrawal syndrome in a neonate due to maternal clomipramine therapy. J Pediatr Child Health 1990;26:110.
9. Bromiker R, Kaplan M. Apparent intrauterine fetal withdrawal from clomipramine hydrochloride. JAMA 1994;272:1722–3.
10. Bloem BR, Lammers GJ, Roofthooft DWE, De Beaufort AJ, Brouwer OF. Clomipramine withdrawal in newborns. Arch Dis Child Fetal Neonatal Ed 1999;81:F77.
11. Nulman I, Rovet J, Stewart DE, Wolpin J, Pace-Asciak P, Shuhaiber S, Koren G. Child development following exposure to tricyclic antidepressants or fluoxetine throughout fetal life: a prospective, controlled study. Am J Psychiatry 2002;159:1889–95.
12. Wisner KL, Perel JM, Findling RL. Antidepressant treatment during breast-feeding. Am J Psychiatry 1996;153:1132–7.
13. Yoshida K, Smith B, Craggs M, Kumar RC. Investigation of pharmacokinetics and of possible adverse effects in infants exposed to tricyclic antidepressants in breast-milk. J Affect Disord 1997;43:225–37.
14. Committee on Drugs, American Academy of Pediatrics. The transfer of drugs and other chemicals into human milk. Pediatrics 2001;108:776–89.

Name:	**CLOMOCYCLINE**	Risk Factor:	**D**
Class:	**Antibiotic (Tetracycline)**		

C

See Tetracycline.

Name:	**CLONAZEPAM**	Risk Factor:	**D_M**
Class:	**Anticonvulsant**		

FETAL RISK SUMMARY

RECOMMENDATION: Human Data Suggest Low Risk

Clonazepam is a benzodiazepine anticonvulsant that is chemically and structurally similar to diazepam (1). The drug is used either alone or in combination with other anticonvulsants.

Reproduction studies in mice and rats during organogenesis at doses up to 4 and 20 times, respectively, the maximum recommended human dose of 20 mg/day for seizures (MRHD-S), and 20 and 100 times, respectively, the maximum recommended human dose of 4 mg/day for panic disorders (MRHD-P), based on body surface area, revealed no evidence of embryo or fetal effects (2). In rabbits administered doses that were 0.2 to 10 times the MRHD-S and 1–50 times the MRHD-P, a low, non-dose-related incidence of a similar pattern of malformations (cleft palate, open eyelid, fused sternebrae, and limb defects) was observed in all dosage groups (2). At the highest dose (twice the dose that produced reductions in maternal weight gain), intrauterine growth retardation was also observed.

In a small series of patients (*N* = 150) matched with nonepileptic controls, anticonvulsant therapy, including five women using clonazepam, had no effect on the incidence of gestational hypertension, albuminuria, premature contractions, premature labor, bleeding in pregnancy, duration of labor, blood loss at delivery, cesarean sections, and vacuum extractions (3).

In a surveillance study of Michigan Medicaid recipients conducted between 1985 and 1992 involving 229,101 completed pregnancies, 19 newborns had been exposed to clonazepam during the 1st trimester (F. Rosa, personal communication, FDA, 1993). Three (15.8%) major birth defects were observed (one expected), two of which were cardiovascular defects (0.2 expected). No anomalies were observed in five other categories of defects (oral clefts, spina bifida, polydactyly, limb reduction defects, and hypospadias) for which specific data were available.

A prospective study published in 1999 described the outcomes of 517 pregnancies of epileptic mothers identified at one Italian center from 1977 (4). Excluding genetic and chromosomal defects, malformations were classified as severe structural defects, mild structural defects, and deformations. Minor anomalies were not considered. Spontaneous (*N* = 38) and elective (*N* = 20) abortions were excluded from the analysis, as were 7 pregnancies that delivered at other hospitals. Of the remaining 452 outcomes, 427 were exposed to anticonvulsants of which 313 involved the following monotherapies: clonazepam (*N* = 6), carbamazepine (*N* = 113), phenobarbital (*N* = 83), valproate (*N* = 44), primidone (*N* = 35), phenytoin (*N* = 31), and other (*N* = 1). There were no defects in the 25 pregnancies not exposed to anticonvulsants. Of the 42 (9.3%) outcomes with malformations, 24 (5.3%) were severe, 10 (2.2%) were mild, and 8 (1.8%) were deformities. There were no malformations with clonazepam monotherapy. The investigators concluded that the

C

anticonvulsants were the primary risk factor for an increased incidence of congenital malformations (see also Carbamazepine, Phenobarbital, Phenytoin, Primidone, and Valproic Acid) (4).

A 2001 report described the pregnancy outcomes of 38 women treated during gestation with clonazepam for panic disorder (5). Twenty-nine of the women were taking clonazepam at the time of conception and 27 were taking the drug at delivery. The Apgar scores were within normal limits. Hospital records were available for 27 infants, 17 of whom were exposed to the agent at delivery. In the 27 infants, there was no evidence of neonatal withdrawal or congenital anomalies, but 2 infants had minor defects—hydrocele and two-vessel umbilical cord. One infant had cardiac disease (no specific details) but was not exposed to clonazepam in the 1st trimester (5).

The database of the Hungarian Case-Control Surveillance of Congenital Abnormalities (1980–1996) was used in a 2002 report that evaluated the teratogenicity of five benzodiazepines: clonazepam, alprazolam, medazepam, nitrazepam, and tofisopam (6). Of the 22,865 women who delivered infants with congenital abnormalities, 57 (0.25%) had used one of the benzodiazepines in pregnancy. Clonazepam was used throughout gestation in four cases (cleft lip and/or palate, cardiovascular defect, hypospadias, and multiple defects). Although the data were limited, no teratogenic risk was found for clonazepam or the other agents (6).

In a 2004 report, the medical records of 28,565 infants were surveyed to identify cases exposed to anticonvulsants (7). Of 166 cases, 52 had been exposed to clonazepam, 43 as monotherapy. Thirty-three of the monotherapy cases had been exposed in the 1st trimester. Congenital defects were noted in one (3.0%) infant: dysmorphic facial features (small eyes, ptosis, and external auditory canal stenosis), tetralogy of Fallot, 11 pair of ribs, and growth retardation (length and head circumference <5th percentile). As with other case series, the data are limited but no increase in congenital malformations was observed (7).

Toxicity in the newborn, apparently related to clonazepam, has been reported. Apnea, cyanosis, lethargy, and hypotonia developed at 6 hours of age in an infant of 36 weeks' gestational age exposed throughout pregnancy to an unspecified amount of clonazepam (8). There was no evidence of congenital defects in the 2750-g newborn. Cord and maternal serum levels of clonazepam were 19 and 32 ng/mL, respectively, a ratio of 0.59. Both levels were within the therapeutic range (5–70 ng/mL). At 18 hours of age, the clonazepam level in the infant's serum measured 4.4 ng/mL. Five episodes of prolonged apnea (16–43 seconds/occurrence) were measured by pneumogram over the next 12 hours. Hypotonia and lethargy resolved within 5 days, but overt clinical apnea persisted for 10 days. Followup pneumograms demonstrated apnea spells until 10 weeks of age, but the presence of the drug in breast milk may have contributed to the condition (see Breast Feeding Summary). The authors concluded that apnea as a consequence of prematurity was not a significant factor. Neurologic development was normal at 5 months (8).

A 1995 case report described paralytic ileus of the small bowel in a fetus at 32 weeks' gestation associated with polyhydramnios (9). The fetal stomach was enlarged (more than 2 standard deviations above the mean). The mother had been treated with clonazepam (4 mg/day) and carbamazepine (1800 mg/day) for epilepsy throughout gestation. A 2420-g male infant was delivered by cesarean section at 36 weeks' gestation. Normal bowel movements started after three Gastrografin enemas. No evidence of cystic fibrosis or Hirschsprung's disease was found, and the child was developing normally at 20 months of age. The ileus was attributed to clonazepam (9).

In summary, clonazepam was teratogenic in one animal species but not in another. Published human pregnancy experience in the 1st trimester is limited to 71 cases (including reference 10 below). In these exposures, one major congenital defect was observed. Fetal and neonatal toxicity also has been reported. Although the true incidence of teratogenicity and toxicity cannot be determined, the risk of adverse pregnancy outcome appears to be low but additional study is needed. Until such data are available, the safest course is to avoid the 1st trimester. However, if clonazepam is indicated, it should not be withheld because of pregnancy.

BREAST FEEDING SUMMARY

RECOMMENDATION: Limited Human Data - Potential Toxicity

Clonazepam is excreted into breast milk. In a woman treated with an unspecified amount of the anticonvulsant, milk concentrations remained constant between 11 and 13 ng/mL (8). The milk:maternal serum ratio was approximately 0.33. After 7 days of nursing, the infant, described above, had a serum concentration of 2.9 ng/mL. A major portion of this probably resulted from *in utero* exposure because the elimination half-life of clonazepam in neonates is thought to be prolonged. No evidence of drug accumulation after breast-feeding was found. Persistent apneic spells, lasting until 10 weeks of age, were observed, but it was not known whether breast-feeding contributed to the condition. Based on this case, the authors recommended that infants exposed *in utero* or during breast-feeding to clonazepam should have serum levels of the drug determined and be closely monitored for central nervous system depression or apnea (8).

A 1988 report described a woman who was treated with clonazepam (4 mg/day) and phenytoin (400 mg/day) throughout gestation and during nursing (10). The healthy, 3930-g infant was delivered at term. Maternal serum and milk samples were collected several times over postpartum days 2–4 at 0–11 hours after a dose. The concentrations of clonazepam in the serum ranged from 51–104 nmol/L (about 16–33 ng/mL), whereas those in the milk ranged from <10–34 nmol/L (about 3–11 ng/mL). The infant's serum level of clonazepam in the pooled sample from days 2–4 was 15 nmol/L (about 5 ng/mL). The study could not determine the proportions of the infant drug level that resulted from placental transfer and ingestion from milk. No effects on the infant were mentioned (10).

References

1. Reith H, Schafer H. Antiepileptic drugs during pregnancy and the lactation period. Pharmacokinetic data. Dtsch Med Wochenschr 1979;104:818–23.
2. Product information. Klonopin. Roche Laboratories, 2000.
3. Hiilesmaa VK, Bardy A, Teramo K. Obstetric outcome in women with epilepsy. Am J Obstet Gynecol 1985;152:499–504.
4. Canger R, Battino D, Canevini MP, Fumarola C, Guidolin L, Vignoli A, Mamoli D, Palmieri C, Molteni F, Granata T, Hassibi P, Zamperini P, Pardi G, Avanzini G. Malformations in offspring of women with epilepsy: a prospective study. Epilepsia 1999;40:1231–6.
5. Weinstock L, Cohen LS, Bailey JW, Blatman R, Rosenbaum JF. Obstetrical and neonatal outcome following clonazepam use during pregnancy: a case series. Psychother Psychosom 2001;70:158–62.
6. Eros E, Czeizel AE, Rockenbauer M, Sorensen HT, Olsen J. A population-based case-control teratology study of nitrazepam, medazepam, tofisopam, alprazolam, and clonazepam treatment during pregnancy. Eur J Obstet Gynecol Reprod Biol 2002;101:147–54.
7. Lin AE, Peller AJ, Westgate MN, Houde K, Franz A, Holmes LB. Clonazepam use in pregnancy and the risk of malformations. Birth Defects Res Part A Clin Mol Teratol 2004;70:534–6.
8. Fisher JB, Edgren BE, Mammel MC, Coleman JM. Neonatal apnea associated with maternal clonazepam therapy: a case report. Obstet Gynecol 1985;66(Suppl):34S–5S.
9. Haeusler MC, Hoellwarth ME, Holzer P. Paralytic ileus in a fetus-neonate after maternal intake of benzodiazepine. Prenat Diagn 1995;15:1165–7.
10. Soderman P, Matheson I. Clonazepam in breast milk. Eur J Pediatr 1988;147:212–3.

Name:	**CLONIDINE**	Risk Factor:	C_M
Class:	**Antihypertensive/Central Analgesic**		

C

FETAL RISK SUMMARY

RECOMMENDATION: Limited Human Data - Animal Data Suggest Risk

No reports linking the use of clonidine with congenital defects have been located. The drug has been used during all trimesters, but experience during the 1st trimester is very limited. Adverse fetal effects attributable to clonidine have not been observed (1–8).

Reproduction studies in rats at doses as low as 1/3 the oral maximum recommended daily human dose MRDHD-W (based on weight) or 1/15 times the MRDHD-BSA (based on body surface area), started before gestation, resulted in increased resorptions (9). Decreased embryo/fetal survival was not observed when these doses were used on gestation days 6–15, but did occur in both mice and rats at doses 40 times the MRDHD-W or 4 to 8 times the MRDHD-BSA. No embryo or fetal toxicity or teratogenicity was observed in rabbits given doses up to 3 times the MRDHD-W (9).

In a surveillance study of Michigan Medicaid recipients conducted between 1985 and 1992 involving 229,101 completed pregnancies, 59 newborns had been exposed to clonidine during the 1st trimester (F. Rosa, personal communication, FDA, 1993). Three (5.1%) major birth defects were observed (three expected), two of which were cardiovascular defects (0.6 expected). No anomalies were observed in five other categories of defects (oral clefts, spina bifida, polydactyly, limb reduction defects, and hypospadias) for which specific data were available. The number of exposures is too small to draw any conclusions.

The pharmacokinetics of clonidine during pregnancy have been reported (10). The mean maternal and cord serum concentrations in 10 women were 0.46 and 0.41 ng/mL, respectively, corresponding to a cord:maternal ratio of 0.89. The mean amniotic fluid concentration was 1.50 ng/mL. The mean maternal dose was 330 μg/day. Results of neurologic examinations and limited blood chemistry tests in the exposed infants were similar to those in untreated controls. No neonatal hypotension was observed.

BREAST FEEDING SUMMARY

RECOMMENDATION: Limited Human Data - Probably Compatible

Clonidine is secreted into breast milk (8,10). Following a 150-μg oral dose, milk concentrations of 1.5 ng/mL may be achieved (milk:plasma ratio 1.5) (P. A. Bowers, personal communication, Boehringer Ingelheim, Ltd., 1981). In a study of nine nursing women taking mean daily doses of 391.7 μg (postpartum days 1–5), 309.4 μg (postpartum days 10–14), and 241.7 μg (postpartum days 45–60), milk concentrations were approximately twice those in maternal serum (10). Mean milk levels were close to 2 ng/mL or higher during the three sampling periods. Hypotension was not observed in the nursing infants, although clonidine was found in the serum of the infants (mean levels less than maternal). The long-term significance of this exposure is not known.

References

1. Turnbull AC, Ahmed S. Catapres in the treatment of hypertension in pregnancy, a preliminary study. In *Catapres in Hypertension*. Symposium of the Royal College of Surgeons. London, 1970:237–45.
2. Johnston CI, Aickin DR. The control of high blood pressure during labour with clonidine. Med J Aust 1971;2:132.
3. Raftos J, Bauer GE, Lewis RG, Stokes GS, Mitchell AS, Young AA, Maclachlan I. Clonidine in the treatment of severe hypertension. Med J Aust 1973;1:786–93.
4. Horvath JS, Phippard A, Korda A, Henderson-Smart DJ, Child A, Tiller DJ. Clonidine hydrochloride—a safe and effective antihypertensive agent in pregnancy. Obstet Gynecol 1985;66:634–8.
5. Horvath JS, Korda A, Child A, Henderson-Smart D, Phippard A, Duggin GC, Hall BM, Tiller DJ. Hypertension in pregnancy: a study of 142 women presenting before 32 weeks' gestation. Med J Aust 1985;143:19–21.
6. NG Wingtin L, Frelon JH, Beaute Y, Pellerin M, Guillaumin JP. Clonidine et traitement de l'hypertension arterielle de la femme enceinte. Cah Anesthesiol 1986;34:389–93.
7. Ng-Wing Tin L, Frelon JH, Beaute Y, Pellerin M, Guillaumin JP, Bazin C. Clonidine et traitement de l'hypertension arterielle de la femme enceinte. Rev Franc Gynecol Obstet 1986;81:563–6.
8. Wing-Tin LNG, Frelon JH, Hardy F, Bazin C. Clonidine et traitement des urgences hypertensives de la femme enceinte. Rev Franc Gynecol Obstet 1987;82:519–22.
9. Product information. Catapres. Boehringer Ingelheim Pharmaceuticals, 2000.
10. Hartikainen-Sorri A-L, Heikkinen JE, Koivisto M. Pharmacokinetics of clonidine during pregnancy and nursing. Obstet Gynecol 1987;69:598–600.

Name:	**CLOPIDOGREL**	Risk Factor:	**B_M**
Class:	**Hematologic Agent (Antiplatelet)**		

FETAL RISK SUMMARY

RECOMMENDATION: Limited Human Data - Animal Data Suggest Low Risk

Clopidogrel is a direct inhibitor of adenosine diphosphate (ADP)-induced platelet aggregation. It is a prodrug that must be biotransformed to an active metabolite to inhibit platelet aggregation. Neither clopidogrel nor its main circulating metabolite has platelet-inhibiting activity. The active metabolite, which has not been identified, acts by irreversibly inhibiting ADP binding to its receptor and the subsequent ADP-mediated activation of the glycoprotein GPIIb/IIIa complex. Clopidogrel is indicated for the reduction of atherosclerotic events (myocardial infarction, stroke, and vascular death) in patients with atherosclerosis documented by recent occurrences of myocardial infarction, stroke, or established peripheral arterial disease (1).

Reproduction studies have been conducted in pregnant rats and rabbits at doses up to 65 and 78 times, respectively, the recommended daily human dose based on body surface area (1). No evidence of impaired fertility or fetotoxicity was seen in either species.

It is not known if clopidogrel, or its active and inactive metabolites, cross the human placenta. The molecular weight of the inactive parent drug (about 420 for the bisulfate) is low enough that some drug probably crosses to the embryo or fetus. The identity and characteristics of the active metabolite, however, have not been determined.

Only one case of exposure to clopidogrel during a human pregnancy has been located (2). The woman had a history of essential thrombocythemia and an anterior wall myocardial infarction. She received treatment with chemotherapy (details not specified) to normalize her platelet count and then cardiac bypass surgery. After surgery, she conceived while taking aspirin (300 mg/day) and ticlopidine (500 mg/day) but aborted the pregnancy in the 2nd trimester (6 months after surgery). Her treatment was then changed to clopidogrel (150 mg/day) combined with intermittent low molecular weight heparin (dalteparin), which she took throughout a second pregnancy. Clopidogrel was discontinued 10 days before vaginal delivery of a healthy, 3170-g female infant. The Apgar scores were 9, 10, 10, and 10 at 1, 5, 10, and 60 minutes, respectively. The mother had no unusual bleeding at delivery and the repair of a mediolateral episiotomy was uneventful. There was no evidence of infarcts or areas of fibrin deposits in the normal placenta. The bottle-fed infant was discharged home with her mother 5 days after delivery (2).

In summary, clopidogrel is not teratogenic in two animal species, but the human pregnancy experience is limited to one case report. Moreover, it is not known if the inactive parent drug, or its active or inactive metabolites, cross the placenta, although the relatively low molecular weight suggests that some passage should be expected. This lack of human information prevents an accurate assessment, but the known benefits to a woman appear to outweigh the unknown fetal risks. Therefore, if a patient's condition requires clopidogrel, the treatment should not be withheld because of pregnancy.

BREAST FEEDING SUMMARY

RECOMMENDATION: No Human Data - Probably Compatible

No reports describing the use of clopidogrel during human lactation have been located. The drug and/or its metabolites, however, are excreted into the milk of lactating rats (1). The molecular weight of the inactive parent drug (about 420 for the bisulfate) suggests that some drug is excreted into breast milk. The effect of this possible exposure on a nursing infant is unknown.

References

1. Product information. Plavix, Bristol-Myers Squibb, 2002.
2. Klinzing P, Markert UR, Liesaus K, Peiker G. Case report: successful pregnancy and delivery after myocardial infarction and essential thrombocythemia treated with clopidogrel. Clin Exp Obstet Gynecol 2001;28:215–6.

Name:	**CLORAZEPATE**	Risk Factor:	**D**
Class:	**Sedative**		

FETAL RISK SUMMARY

RECOMMENDATION: Human Data Suggest Risk

Clorazepate is a member of the benzodiazepine class of agents. No teratogenic effects were observed in two species of animals fed large doses of the drug during gestation. However, cases of congenital malformations in humans after *in utero* exposure to other benzodiazepines (e.g., see Chlordiazepoxide and Diazepam) have been reported.

One report described multiple anomalies in an infant exposed to clorazepate during the 1st trimester (1). Exposure may have commenced as early as the 3rd week of gestation (5th week after the last menstrual period). The woman reportedly consumed 23 doses of the drug during the 1st trimester. Deformities present in the infant at birth were distended abdomen; oval mass in the suprapubic area; skin tag at site of penis without a urethral opening; absent scrotum and anus; marked shortening of the right thigh; bifid distal part of left foot; left great toe abnormality; right foot with four toes and an abnormal great toe; short digit attached to right finger in place of the thumb on left hand; deformities of the sacrum and fourth and fifth lumbar vertebrae with a narrowed pelvis; underdeveloped right femur; absent right fibula; absence of two left metacarpal bones; hypoplasia of first right metacarpal bone; patent ductus arteriosus; absence of right lung lobe, cecum, rectum, and right kidney; and the presence of several supernumerary spleens. The infant expired 24 hours after birth.

In an unconfirmed, retrospective report of oral contraceptive drug interactions, one woman became pregnant while taking a combination tablet of ethinyl estradiol 80 μg/norethindrone 1 mg (2). The only other medications consumed immediately prior to the pregnancy were clorazepate and an unidentified cold tablet. The authors speculated that a possible interaction may have occurred between the antihistamine in the cold tablet and the contraceptive. Although the woman claimed she did not miss any doses of the oral contraceptive, there was no confirmation of compliance. Interpretation of this interaction, if it exists, is not possible.

BREAST FEEDING SUMMARY

RECOMMENDATION: No Human Data - Potential Toxicity

No reports describing the use of clorazepate during human lactation have been located. Other benzodiazepines accumulate in human milk, and adverse effects in the nursing infant have been reported (see Diazepam). The excretion of clorazepate in milk should be expected. The American Academy of Pediatrics classifies other benzodiazepines as drugs whose effect on the nursing infant is unknown but may be of concern (e.g., see Diazepam).

References

1. Patel DA, Patel AR. Clorazepate and congenital malformations. JAMA 1980;244:135–6.
2. DeSano EA Jr, Hurley SC. Possible interactions of antihistamines and antibiotics with oral contraceptive effectiveness. Fertil Steril 1982;37:853–4.

Name:	**CLOTRIMAZOLE**	Risk Factor:	**B**
Class:	**Antifungal Antibiotic**		

FETAL RISK SUMMARY

RECOMMENDATION: Compatible

No reports linking the use of clotrimazole with congenital defects have been located. The topical use of the drug in pregnancy has been studied (1–4). No adverse effects attributable to clotrimazole were observed. Absorption of the agent from the skin and vagina is minimal (5).

Suspected birth defect diagnoses occurred in 6564 offspring of 104,339 women in a retrospective analysis of women who had delivered in Michigan hospitals during 1980–1983 (6). First trimester vaginitis treatment with clotrimazole occurred in 74 of the 6,564 deliveries linked to birth defect diagnoses and in 1012 of the 97,775 cases not linked to such diagnoses. The estimated relative risk of birth defects when clotrimazole was used was 1.09 (95% confidence interval [CI] 0.9–1.4). Although an increased relative risk was not found, this study could not exclude the possibility of an association with a specific birth defect (6).

C

In a surveillance study of Michigan Medicaid recipients conducted between 1985 and 1992 involving 229,101 completed pregnancies, 2,624 newborns had been exposed to clotrimazole (maternal vaginal use) during the 1st trimester (F. Rosa, personal communication, FDA, 1993). A total of 118 (4.5%) major birth defects were observed (112 expected). Specific data were available for six defect categories, including (observed/expected) 27/26 cardiovascular defects, 4/4 oral clefts, 3/1 spina bifida, 9/7 polydactyly, 1/4 limb reduction defects, and 6/6 hypospadias. These data do not support an association between vaginal use of clotrimazole and congenital defects.

Data from the Hungarian Case-Control Surveillance of Congenital Abnormalities (1980–1992) were used to examine the potential teratogenic effects of vaginal and/or topical use of clotrimazole (7). Although clotrimazole use was not associated with an increase in the prevalence of any birth defect (fetal and live births), there was a suggestion that it was associated with a decrease in the prevalence of undescended testis (prevalence odds ratio 0.72, 95% CI 0.54–0.95) (7).

BREAST FEEDING SUMMARY

RECOMMENDATION: Compatible

The absorption of clotrimazole from the skin and vagina is minimal (5). Therefore, it is doubtful if measurable amounts of the antifungal agent appear in milk.

References

1. Tan CG, Good CS, Milne LJR, Loudon JDO. A comparative trial of six-day therapy with clotrimazole and nystatin in pregnant patients with vaginal candidiasis. Postgrad Med 1974;50(Suppl 1):102–5.
2. Frerich W, Gad A. The frequency of Candida infections in pregnancy and their treatment with clotrimazole. Curr Med Res Opin 1977;4:640–4.
3. Haram K, Digranes A. Vulvovaginal candidiasis in pregnancy treated with clotrimazole. Acta Obstet Gynecol Scand 1978;57:453–5.
4. Svendsen E, Lie S, Gunderson TH, Lyngstad-Vik I, Skuland J. Comparative evaluation of miconazole, clotrimazole and nystatin in the treatment of candidal vulvovaginitis. Curr Ther Res 1978;23:666–72.
5. Product information. Lotrimin. Schering, 2000.
6. Rosa FW, Baum C, Shaw M. Pregnancy outcomes after first-trimester vaginitis drug therapy. Obstet Gynecol 1987;69:751–5.
7. Czeizel AE, Toth M, Rockenbauer M. No teratogenic effect after clotrimazole therapy during pregnancy. Epidemiology 1999;10:437–40.

Name:	**CLOXACILLIN**	Risk Factor:	**B_M**
Class:	**Antibiotic (Penicillin)**		

FETAL RISK SUMMARY

RECOMMENDATION: Compatible

Cloxacillin is a penicillin antibiotic (see also Penicillin G). No published reports linking its use with congenital defects have been located. The Collaborative Perinatal Project monitored 50,282 mother-child pairs, 3546 of which had 1st trimester exposure to penicillin derivatives (1, pp. 297–313). For use anytime during pregnancy, 7171 exposures were recorded (1, p. 435). In neither group was evidence found to suggest a relationship to large categories of major or minor malformations or to individual defects.

In a surveillance study of Michigan Medicaid recipients conducted between 1985 and 1992 involving 229,101 completed pregnancies, 46 newborns had been exposed to

cloxacillin during the 1st trimester (F. Rosa, personal communication, FDA, 1993). Three (6.5%) major birth defects were observed (two expected), including three cardiovascular defects (0.5 expected) and one hypospadias (none expected). Only with the former defect is there a suggestion of a possible association, but other factors, including the mother's disease, concurrent drug use, and chance, may be involved.

C

BREAST FEEDING SUMMARY

RECOMMENDATION: Compatible

No reports describing the use of cloxacillin during lactation have been located. Because other penicillins are excreted in milk in low concentrations (see Ampicillin and Penicillin G) the presence of cloxacillin should also be expected. Although adverse effects from penicillins in breast milk are rare, three potential problems exist for the nursing infant: modification of bowel flora, direct effects on the infant (e.g., allergic response), and interference with the interpretation of culture results if a fever workup is required.

Reference

1. Heinonen OP, Slone D, Shapiro S. *Birth Defects and Drugs in Pregnancy*. Littleton, MA: Publishing Sciences Group, 1977.

Name:	**CLOZAPINE**	Risk Factor:	**B_M**
Class:	**Tranquilizer**		

FETAL RISK SUMMARY

RECOMMENDATION: Limited Human Data - Animal Data Suggest Low Risk

Clozapine is an antipsychotic drug used in the treatment of schizophrenia. Reproduction studies in rats and rabbits at doses two to four times the human dose have found no evidence of impaired fertility or fetal harm (1,2).

A brief 1993 report described a woman who was treated prior to and throughout gestation with clozapine (dose not given) for treatment-resistant chronic undifferentiated schizophrenia (3). An apparently healthy, male, 8 lb 2 oz (about 3689 g) infant was delivered at term. The authors cited information on 14 other women who had taken clozapine during gestation apparently without fetal adverse effects (4).

Another reference on the use of clozapine during pregnancy appeared in 1994 (5). A woman was maintained on 100 mg/day prior to and during the first 32 weeks of gestation. The dose was then lowered to 50 mg/day until she delivered a normal female infant at 41 weeks' gestation. No psychomotor abnormalities were observed up to 6 months of age. Clozapine plasma levels, measured in the mother throughout her pregnancy, ranged from 38–55 ng/mL (100 mg/day) to 14.1–15.4 ng/mL (50 mg/day). At birth, the cord blood concentration was 27 ng/mL (maternal 14.1 ng/mL), representing a ratio of approximately 2. The amniotic fluid concentration was 11.6 ng/mL.

Nine diverse case reports of adverse pregnancy outcomes involving the use of clozapine during pregnancy have been reported to the FDA (F. Rosa, personal communication, FDA, 1995). In the absence of a cohort denominator, the cases do not suggest a fetal risk and

C

may have been caused by chance. The cases were neonatal hypocalcemia and convulsions; asymmetry of buttock crease; Turner's syndrome (chromosomal abnormality); spontaneous abortion (SAB) and hydropic villous degeneration (chromosomal abnormality); SAB in 8th week (abnormal gestational sac); multiple congenital defects (unspecified) (pregnancy terminated); congenital blindness; clinodactyly thumbs and big toes; and neonatal cerebral hemorrhage.

A case report in 1996 described an otherwise healthy male infant, exposed throughout gestation to clozapine (200–300 mg/day) and lorazepam (7.5–12.5 mg/day), who developed transient, mild, floppy infant syndrome after delivery at 37 weeks' gestation (6). The mother had taken the combination therapy for the treatment of schizophrenia. The hypotonia, attributed to lorazepam because of the absence of such reports in pregnancies exposed to clozapine alone, resolved 5 days after birth.

BREAST FEEDING SUMMARY

RECOMMENDATION: Limited Human Data - Potential Toxicity

Clozapine is concentrated in breast milk (5). While taking clozapine 50 mg/day, a mother (described above), on her first postpartum day, had a plasma concentration of 14.7 ng/mL and a concentration of 63.5 ng/mL from the first portion of her breast milk (milk:plasma ratio 4.3). One week postpartum, 4 days after the dose was increased to 100 mg/day, the two concentrations were 41.4 and 115.6 ng/mL (milk:plasma ratio 2.8), respectively. The infant was not allowed to breast-feed.

The American Academy of Pediatrics classifies clozapine as a drug whose effect on the nursing infant is unknown but may be of concern (7).

References

1. Product information. Clozaril. Novartis Pharmaceuticals, 2000.
2. Lindt S, Lauener E, Eichenberger E. The toxicology of 8-chloro-11-(4-methyl-1-piperazinyl)-5H-dibenzo[1,4]-diazepine (clozapine). Farmaco (Sci) 1971;26:585–602. As cited in Shepard TH. *Catalog of Teratogenic Agents*. 7th ed. Baltimore, MD: Johns Hopkins University Press, 1992:99.
3. Walderman MD, Safferman AZ. Pregnancy and clozapine. Am J Psychiatry 1993;150:168–9.
4. Lieberman J, Safferman AZ. Clinical profile of clozapine: adverse reactions and agranulocytosis. In: Lapierre Y, Jones B, eds. *Clozapine in Treatment Resistant Schizophrenia: A Scientific Update*. London: Royal Society of Medicine, 1992. As cited in Walderman MD, Safferman AZ. Pregnancy and clozapine. Am J Psychiatry 1993;150:168–9.
5. Barnas C, Bergant A, Hummer M, Saria A, Fleischhacker WW. Clozapine concentrations in maternal and fetal plasma, amniotic fluid, and breast milk. Am J Psychiatry 1994;151:945.
6. Di Michele V, Ramenghi LA, Sabatino G. Clozapine and lorazepam administration in pregnancy. Eur Psychiatry 1996;11:214.
7. Committee on Drugs, American Academy of Pediatrics. The transfer of drugs and other chemicals into human milk. Pediatrics 2001;108:776–89.

Name:	**COCAINE**	Risk Factor:	**C_M***
Class:	**Sympathomimetic**		

FETAL RISK SUMMARY

RECOMMENDATION: Contraindicated (Systemic); Compatible (Topical)

Cocaine, a naturally occurring alkaloid, is legally available in the United States as a topical anesthetic, but its illegal use as a central nervous system stimulant far exceeds any medicinal market for the drug. Cocaine is a sympathomimetic, producing hypertension and vasoconstriction as a result of its direct cardiovascular activity. The increasing popularity of cocaine is because of its potent ability to produce euphoria, an effect that is counterbalanced by the strong addictive properties of the drug (1). As of 1985, an estimated 30 million Americans had used cocaine and 5 million were believed to be using it regularly (1). Although the exact figures are unknown, current usage probably exceeds these estimates. Preliminary results of a study conducted between July 1984 and June 1987 in the Boston area indicated that 117 (17%) of 679 urban women used cocaine at least once during pregnancy as determined by prenatal and postpartum interviews and urine assays for cocaine metabolites (2). Final results from this study, now involving 1,226 mothers, found that 216 (18%) used cocaine during pregnancy, but that only 165 (76%) of these women would have been detected by history alone (3). Fifty-one women who had denied use of cocaine had positive urine assays for cocaine metabolites. Other investigators have reported similar findings (4). Of 138 women who had positive urine screens for cocaine at delivery, only 59 (43%) would have been identified by drug history alone. In this same study, the increasing prevalence of maternal cocaine abuse was demonstrated (4). Over a 24-month period (September 1986 to August 1988), the incidence of positive urine screens for cocaine in women at delivery rose steadily, starting at 4% in the first 6-month quarter and increasing to 12% in the final quarter. The total number of women (1776) was approximately equally divided among the four quarters.

Illicitly obtained cocaine varies greatly in purity, and it is commonly adulterated with such substances as lactose, mannitol, lidocaine, and procaine (5). Cocaine is detoxified by liver and plasma cholinesterases (1,5). Activity of the latter enzyme system is much lower in the fetus and in infants and is decreased in pregnant women, resulting in slower metabolism and elimination of the drug (1,5). Moreover, most studies have found a correlation between cocaine use and the use of other abuse drugs such as heroin, methadone, methamphetamine, marijuana, tobacco, and alcohol. Compared to drug-free women, this correlation was highly significant ($p < 0.0001$) and, furthermore, users were significantly more likely to be heavy abusers of these substances ($p < 0.0001$) (2).

Research on the effects of maternal and fetal cocaine exposure has focused on several different areas. It reflects the wide-ranging concerns for fetal safety this drug produces:

- Placental transfer of cocaine
- Pregnancy complications
  - Placental receptor function
  - Premature labor and delivery
  - Spontaneous abortions
  - Premature rupture of membranes (PROM)
  - Placenta previa
  - Gestational hypertension
  - Abruptio placentae
  - Ruptured ectopic pregnancy
- Maternal mortality
- Fetal complications
  - Growth retardation
  - Fetal distress

Cerebrovascular accidents
Congenital anomalies

C

Infant complications
Neurobehavior
Mortality
Hospitalizations

Placental Transfer

Although the placental transfer of cocaine has not been quantified in humans, cocaine metabolites are frequently found in the urine of *in utero*-exposed newborns. Because cocaine has high water and lipid solubility, low molecular weight (about 340), and low ionization at physiologic pH, it should freely cross to the fetus (5). In pregnant sheep given IV cocaine, 0.5 mg/kg, to produce plasma levels similar to those observed in humans, fetal plasma levels at 5 minutes were 46.8 ng/mL compared to simultaneous maternal levels of 405 ng/ml (fetus 12% of mother) (6). At 30 minutes, the levels for fetal and maternal plasma had decreased to 11.8 and 83 ng/ml, respectively (fetus 14% of mother). Uterine blood flow was decreased in a dose-dependent manner by 36% after the above dose (6). Decreases in uterine blood flow of similar magnitude have also been observed in other studies with pregnant sheep (7,8). In one report, the reduction was accompanied by fetal hypoxemia, hypertension, and tachycardia, which were more severe then when cocaine was administered directly to the fetus (8).

Pregnancy Complications

Placental Receptor Function

In a study examining the effects of prenatal cocaine exposure on human placental tissue, significant decreases, as compared to nonexposed controls, were found for the total number of β-adrenergic receptor-binding sites (202 vs. 313 fmol/mg, $p < 0.01$), μ-opiate receptor-binding sites (77 vs. 105 fmol/mg, $p < 0.05$), and δ-opiate receptor-binding sites (77 vs. 119 fmol/mg, $p < 0.01$) (9). These effects were interpreted as a true downregulation of the receptor population and may be associated with increased levels of adrenergic compounds (9,10). The authors speculated that if a similar down-regulation of the fetal adrenergic receptor-binding sites also occurred, it could result in disruption of synaptic development of the fetal nervous system. However, the clinical significance of these findings has not yet been determined (9).

Premature Labor/Delivery

The effect of maternal cocaine use on the duration of gestation has been included in several research papers (3,4,11–25). When compared with non-drug-using controls, *in utero* cocaine exposure invariably resulted in significantly shortened mean gestational periods ranging up to 2 weeks. A statistically significant mean shorter (1.9 weeks) gestational period was also observed when cocaine-polydrug users (20% used heroin) were compared with noncocaine-polydrug users (26% used heroin) (13). Two other studies, comparing cocaine/amphetamine (18) or cocaine/methadone (17) consumption with noncocaine heroin/methadone-abusing women, found nonsignificant shorter gestational lengths, 37.9 vs. 38.3 weeks and 37.2 vs. 38.1 weeks, respectively. A third study classified some of its subjects into two subgroups: cocaine only ($N = 24$) and cocaine plus polyabuse drugs ($N = 46$) (20). No statistical differences were measured for gestational age at delivery (36.6 vs. 37.4 weeks) or for the incidence of preterm (<37 weeks) delivery (25.0% vs. 23.9%).

When included as part of the research format, the incidence of premature labor and delivery was significantly increased in comparison to that in drug-free women (4,11,18–25). When comparisons were made with noncocaine opiate abusers, the incidences were higher, but not significant. One investigation also found that cocaine use significantly increased the incidence of precipitous labor (11). Although objective data were not provided, a 1985 report mentioned that several cocaine-exposed women had noted uterine contractions and increased fetal activity within minutes of using cocaine (26). In 1989, this same group reported that infants who had been exposed to cocaine throughout pregnancy ($N = 52$) (average maternal dose/use = 0.5 g) had a significantly shorter mean gestational age than did infants of drug-free women ($N = 40$), 38.0 weeks vs. 39.8 weeks ($p < 0.001$), respectively (24). The gestational period of those who used cocaine only during the 1st trimester was a mean 38.9 weeks, which was not significantly different from that of either of the other two groups. The incidence of preterm delivery (defined as <38 weeks) in the three groups was 17% (4 of 23; 1st trimester use only), 31% (16 of 52; cocaine use throughout pregnancy), and 3% (1 of 40; drug-free controls) (24). Only the difference between the latter two groups was statistically significant ($p < 0.003$). In another 1989 study, bivariate comparisons of 114 cocaine users (as determined by positive urine assays) with 1,010 nonusers (as determined by interview and negative urine assays) indicated the difference in gestational length to be statistically significant (38.8 weeks vs. 39.3 weeks, $p < 0.05$) (3). However, multivariate analyses to control the effect of other substances and maternal characteristics known to affect pregnancy outcome adversely resulted in a loss of significance, thus demonstrating that, in this population, cocaine exposure alone did not affect the duration of gestation (3).

Spontaneous Abortions

A 1985 report found an increased rate of spontaneous abortions (SABs) in previous pregnancies of women using cocaine either alone or with narcotics when compared with women using only narcotics and women not abusing drugs (26). These data were based on patient recall so the authors were unable to determine whether a causal relationship existed. In a subsequent report on this patient population, the incidence of previous abortions (not differentiated between elective and spontaneous) was significantly greater in women who predominantly used cocaine either alone or with opiates when compared to those who used only opiates or to non–drug-using controls (25). A statistically significant ($p < 0.05$) higher incidence of one or more SABs was found in 117 users (30%), compared with 562 nonusers (21%) (2). Other studies examining cocaine consumption in current pregnancies found no correlation between the drug and SABs (5,15–17,22).

Premature Rupture of Membranes

Premature rupture of membranes (PROM) was observed in 2% of 46 women using cocaine and/or methamphetamine vs. 10% of 49 women using narcotics vs. 4.4% of 45 drug-free controls (differences not significant) (18). Similarly, no difference in PROM rates were noted between two groups of women admitted in labor without previous prenatal care (cocaine group, $N = 124$; noncocaine group, $N = 218$) (23). However, a 1989 report found a statistically significant increase in the incidence of PROM in women with a positive urine screen for cocaine (29 of 138, 21%) in comparison to non-cocaine-using controls (3 of 88, 3%) ($p < 0.0005$) (4). Although not statistically significant, the risk of PROM was higher in women who predominantly used cocaine either alone (10%, 6 of 63) or with opiates (14%, 4 of 28) than in drug-free controls (2%, 3 of 123) (26). The incidence of placenta previa was also not increased by cocaine use in this study (22). In contrast, 33% of 50 "crack" (alkaloidal cocaine that is smoked) users had PROM, compared with

18% of non-drug-using controls ($p = 0.05$) (21). Drug abuse patterns in both groups were determined by interview, which may have introduced classification error into the results, but the authors reasoned that any error would have underestimated the actual effect of the cocaine exposure (21).

Gestational Hypertension

Two studies have measured the incidence of gestational hypertension in their patients (22,23). In one, the rate of this complication in cocaine-exposed and nonexposed women was too low to report (22). In the second, 25% (13 of 53) of cocaine-exposed women vs. 4% (4 of 100) of nonexposed controls had the disorder ($p < 0.05$) (23). Such other factors as maternal age, race, use of multiple abuse drugs, small numbers, and self-reported cocaine exposure may have accounted for this difference.

Abruptio Placentae

Two cases of abruptio placentae after IV and intranasal cocaine use were reported in 1983 (27). Since this initial observation, a number of similar cases of this complication have been described (1,4,5,11,14,18,19,21,24–26,28–30), although some investigators either did not observe any cases (31) or the number of cases in the studied patients was too low to report (22). The findings of one study indicated that abruptio placentae-induced stillbirths in cocaine users ($N = 50$), multiple drug users (some of whom used cocaine) ($N = 110$), and drug-free controls ($N = 340$) were 8%, 4.5%, and 0.8%, respectively (5). The difference between the cocaine-only group and the controls was significant ($p < 0.001$). The four mothers in the cocaine group suffered placental abruption after IV and intranasal administration (one case each) and smoking (two cases). Two of the five mothers in the multiple drug use group suffered the complication after injection of a "speed ball" (heroin plus cocaine) (5). Thus, 6 of the 12 cases were associated with cocaine use. Onset of labor with abruptio placentae was observed in 4 of 23 women after the use of IV cocaine (25). Additional information was provided by these investigators in a series of papers extending into 1989 (11,14,20,24,25). The latest data indicated that in women who had used cocaine during pregnancy ($N = 75$, 23 of whom used cocaine only during the 1st trimester), 10 (13.3%) had suffered abruptio placentae compared with none of the 40 drug-free controls ($p < 0.05$) (24). Retroplacental hemorrhages, including placental abruption, were significantly increased in a cocaine and/or methamphetamine group (13% of 46) in comparison with either opiate users (2% of 49) or drug-free controls (2.2% of 45) ($p < 0.05$) (18). Two cases of abruptio placentae were observed in 55 women using "crack" (none in 55 drug-free controls) (21) and one case in a woman using cocaine in 102 consecutive deliveries at a Texas hospital (28). Three additional cases of sonographically diagnosed abruption probably related to cocaine use were described in a 1988 report (29). While the exact mechanism of cocaine-induced abruptio placentae is still unknown, the pharmacologic effects of the drug offer a reasonable explanation. Cocaine prevents norepinephrine reuptake at nerve terminals, producing peripheral and placental vasoconstriction, reflex tachycardia with acute hypertension, and uterine contractions. The net effect of these actions in some cases may be abruptio placentae (1,5,11,18,24, 26,27,32).

Ruptured Ectopic Pregnancy

Two cases of rupture of ectopic pregnancies were reported in 1989 (33). In both incidences, the women described severe abdominal pain immediately after consuming cocaine (smoking in one, nasally in the other). While the authors of this report could not totally exclude spontaneous rupture of the tubal pregnancies, they concluded that the short time interval between cocaine ingestion and the onset of symptoms made the association appear likely (33).

Maternal Mortality

Fatalities following adult cocaine use have been reported frequently, but only two cases have been located that involve pregnant women (34,35). A 24-year-old woman, who smoked "crack" daily, presented at 34 weeks' gestation with acute onset of severe headache and photophobia (34). Her symptoms were determined to be caused by subarachnoid hemorrhage resulting from a ruptured aneurysm. Following surgery to relieve intracranial pressure and an unsuccessful attempt to isolate the aneurysm, the patient gave birth to a normal 2400-g male infant. Her condition subsequently worsened on postpartum day 21 and she expired 4 days later from recurrent intracranial hemorrhage. The second case involved a 21-year-old in approximately her 16th week of pregnancy (35). She was admitted to the hospital in a comatose condition after about 1.5 g of cocaine had been placed in her vagina. She was maintained on life support systems and eventually delivered, by cesarean section, a female infant at 33 weeks' gestation with severe brain abnormalities. The infant died at 10 days of age, and the mother expired approximately 4 months later.

Fetal Complications

Growth Retardation

Fetal complications reported after exposure to cocaine include growth retardation, fetal distress, cerebrovascular accidents, and congenital anomalies. A large number of studies have examined the effect of *in utero* cocaine exposure on fetal growth parameters (birth weight, length, and head circumference) (2–5,11–26,36–39). The majority of these studies found, after correcting for confounding variables, that cocaine exposure, when compared to non-drug-abuse populations, was associated with reduced fetal growth. This reduction was comparable, in most cases, to that observed in fetuses exposed to opiates, such as heroin or methadone. A survey of 117 users compared to 562 nonusers discovered that 14% of the former had given birth to a low-birth-weight infant vs. 8% of the nonexposed women ($p < 0.05$) (2). In one investigation, when maternal drug use included both cocaine (or amphetamines) and narcotics, the infants ($N = 9$) had a significant reduction in birth weight, length, and head circumference compared to either stimulant or narcotic use alone (18). In an earlier report, no significant differences were observed in fetal growth parameters between groups of women consuming cocaine ($N = 12$), cocaine plus methadone ($N = 11$), methadone ($N = 15$), and noncocaine/nonmethadone controls ($N = 15$) (26). However, in a subsequent publication from these researchers, women who used cocaine throughout gestation (as opposed to those who only used it during the 1st trimester) were significantly more likely than drug-free controls to deliver low-birth-weight infants—25% (13 of 52) vs. 5% (2 of 40) ($p < 0.003$), respectively (24). Fetal growth parameters (birth weight, length, and head circumference) were also significantly ($p < 0.001$) depressed, compared with those of controls, if the woman used cocaine throughout pregnancy (24). Exposure during the 1st trimester only resulted in reduced growth but the difference was not significant. Some investigators have suggested that the decrease in fetal growth in two studies may have been a result of poor nutrition or alcohol intake (40,41). In both instances, however, women abusing alcohol either had been excluded or their exclusion would not have changed the findings (42,43). In one study that found no statistical difference in birth weights between infants of cocaine users and noncocaine users, only 10 cocaine-exposed newborns were involved (28). The cocaine group had been identified from obstetric records of 102 consecutively delivered women. However, the sample size is very small and the character of cocaine use (e.g., dose, frequency) could not always be determined. In addition, recent research has shown that self-reporting of cocaine use probably underestimates actual usage (3,4).

A single case of oligohydramnios at 17 weeks' gestation with two increased serum α-fetoprotein levels (125 μg/L and 168 μg/L) has been described, but any relationship between these events and the mother's history of cocaine abuse is unknown (44). Intrauterine growth retardation was diagnosed at 26 weeks' gestation followed shortly thereafter by fetal death *in utero*. Analysis of fetal whole blood showed a cocaine level of 1 μg/mL, within the range associated with fatalities in adults (44).

In a prospective 1989 study involving 1226 mothers, 18% used cocaine as determined by interview or urine assay (3). After controlling for potentially confounding variables and other substance abuse, infants of women with positive urine assay for cocaine, compared to infants of nonusers, had lower birth weights (93 g less, $p = 0.07$), lengths (0.7 cm less, $p = 0.01$), and head circumferences (0.43 cm less, $p = 0.01$). The effect of cocaine on birth weight was even greater if prepregnancy weight and pregnancy weight gain were not considered. The mean reduction in infant birth weight was now 137 g vs. 93 g when these factors were considered ($p < 0.01$). In those cases where the history of cocaine use was positive but the urine assay was negative, no significant differences were found by multivariate analyses. The authors concluded that cocaine impaired fetal growth but also that urine assays (or another biologic marker) were important to show the association (3).

Multiple ultrasound examinations (two to four) were used to evaluate fetal growth in a series of 43 women with primary addiction to cocaine (45). An additional 24 women were studied, but their ultrasound examinations were incomplete in one aspect or another and they were not included in the analysis. Careful attention was given to establishing gestational age. Complete ultrasonic parameters included biparietal diameter, femur length, and head and abdominal circumferences. The number of addicted infants with birth weight, head circumference, and femur length at the equal to or <50th, equal to or <25th, and equal to or <10th percentile ranks did not differ significantly from expected standard growth charts. However, the number of examinations yielding values for biparietal diameter and abdominal circumference at the equal to or <50th and equal to or <25th percentile ranks was significantly more than expected ($p = 0.001$). Because biparietal diameter and head circumference are not independent parameters, each being an indicator of fetal head size, the authors speculated that the most logical explanation for their findings was late-onset dolichocephalia (45). Based on these findings, the study concluded that maternal cocaine use had adversely affected fetal growth. If only birth weight had been used as a criterion, this effect may have been missed (45).

Fetal Distress

Several studies included measurements of fetal distress in their research findings (11,15–21,23,26,31,37,39). In some reports, perinatal distress was significantly ($p < 0.05$) increased in cocaine abusers, as compared with women using heroin/methadone (11,12) and drug-free controls (19). Perinatal distress was also noted more frequently in other studies comparing cocaine users to drug-free controls (10% vs. 5.7% and 11.1% vs. 3.7%, respectively), but the differences were not significant (20,21). Compared to nondrug users, higher rates of fetal tachycardia (2% vs. 0%) and bradycardia (17% vs. 6%) have been observed, but, again, the differences were not significant (18). One-minute Apgar scores were lower after *in utero* cocaine exposure in several studies (4,15–17,20,23,37) but only statistically significant in some (15–17,23) and no different in another (25). In contrast, only two studies, one a series of three reports on the same group of patients, found a significant lowering of the 5-minute Apgar score (15–17,25). Other studies observed no difference in this value (4,20,23,26,31,37,39). Significantly more ($p < 0.05$) meconium-stained infants were observed in studies comparing cocaine users to methadone-maintained women (25% vs. 8.2%) (10) and to noncocaine/other drug-exposed subjects (25% vs. 4%) (23).

Three other studies observed nonsignificant increased rates of meconium staining or passage (22% vs. 17%, 29% vs. 23%, and 73% vs. 58%) (18,20,25), and a fourth reported a lower incidence (22% vs. 27%), compared to non–drug-using controls (21).

Cerebrovascular Accidents

Eight reports described perinatal or newborn cerebrovascular accidents and resulting brain damage in infants exposed *in utero* to cocaine (11,14,18,46–50). The first report of this condition was published in 1986 (46). A mother who had used an unknown amount of cocaine intranasally during the first 5 weeks of pregnancy and approximately 5 g during the 3 days before delivery, gave birth to a full-term, 3660-g male infant. The last dose of approximately 1 g had been consumed 15 hours before delivery. Fetal monitoring during the 12 hours before delivery showed tachycardia (180–200 beats/minute) and multiple variable decelerations. At birth, the infant was limp, he had a heart rate of 80 beats/minute, and thick meconium staining (without aspiration) was noted. Apnea, cyanosis, multiple focal seizures, intermittent tachycardia (up to 180 beats/minute), hypertension (up to 140 mm Hg by palpation), abnormalities in tone (both increased and decreased depending on the body part), and miotic pupils were noted beginning at 16 hours of age. Noncontrast computed tomographic scan at 24 hours of age showed an acute infarction in the distribution of the left middle cerebral artery. Repeat scans showed a persistent left-sided infarct with increased gyral density (age 7 days) and a persistent area of focal encephalomalacia at the site of the infarction (age 2.5 months). One other infant with perinatal cerebral infarction associated with maternal cocaine use in the 48–72 hours prior to delivery has been mentioned by these investigators (11,14,24). A separate report described a mother who had used cocaine and multiple other abuse drugs during gestation who delivered a female infant (gestational age not specified) with bilateral cerebrovascular accident and resulting porencephaly (47). The infant expired at 2.5 months of age. In another study of 55 infants exposed to cocaine (with or without opiates), one infant with perinatal asphyxia had a cerebral infarction (18). A severely depressed male infant delivered at 38 weeks' gestation had an electroencephalogram and cranial ultrasound suggestive of hemorrhagic infarction (48). Follow-up during the neonatal period indicated mild to moderate neurodevelopmental abnormalities. Brain lesions were described in 39% (11 of 28) of infants with a positive urine assay for cocaine and in 33% (5 of 15) of newborns with a positive assay for methamphetamine (49). The brain injuries, which were not differentiated by drug type, were hemorrhagic infarction in the deep brain (six cases; three around the internal capsule/basal ganglion), cystic lesions in the deep brain (four cases), large posterior fossa hemorrhage (three cases), absent septum pellucidum with atrophy (one case), diffuse atrophy (one case), and brain edema (one case) (49). In a control group of 20 term infants with severe asphyxia, only one had a similar brain lesion. A second report also described brain lesions in infants exposed *in utero* to cocaine (50). The 11 infants all had major central nervous system (CNS) anomalies, and 10 of the infants also had craniofacial defects (described later). The CNS defects were hydranencephaly (one case), porencephaly (two cases), hypoplastic corpus callosum with unilateral parietal lobe cleft and heterotopias (one case), intraparenchymal hemorrhage (five cases), unilateral three-vessel hemispheric infarction (one case), and encephalomalacia (one case). In addition, three infants had arthrogryposis multiplex congenita of central origin (50). Four of the infants died, and the other seven had serious neurodevelopmental disabilities (50).

Echoencephalography (ECHO) was performed within 3 days of birth on 74 term (>37 weeks' gestation) infants who had tested positive for cocaine or methamphetamine but who otherwise had uncomplicated perinatal courses (51). The infants had no other known risk factors for cerebral injury. The 74 newborns were classified into three groups: 32 (43%)

cocaine exposed, 24 (32%) methamphetamine exposed, and 18 (24%) exposed to cocaine plus heroin or methadone, or both. Two comparison groups were formed: a group of 87 term, drug-free infants studied by ECHO because of clinical concerns for hypoxic–ischemic encephalopathy, and a normal group of 19 drug-free term newborns. Both groups of comparison infants were also studied by ECHO within 3 days of birth. Only one structural anomaly—an absent septum pellucidum—was observed in the infants examined. The affected newborn, exposed to methamphetamine, was also found to have bilateral optic nerve atrophy and diffuse attenuation of the white matter. Twenty-six (35.1%) of the drug-exposed infants had cranial abnormalities detected by ultrasonography, which was similar to the 27.6% (24 of 87) incidence in the comparison group with possible hypoxic–ischemic encephalopathy ($p = 0.7$). The normal controls had an incidence of 5.3% (1 of 19) ($p < 0.01$ in comparison to both of the other groups). The lesions observed in the drug-exposed infants were intraventricular hemorrhage, echo densities known to be associated with necrosis, and cavitary lesions. Lesions were concentrated in the basal ganglion, frontal lobes, and posterior fossa (51). Cerebral infarction was found in two cocaine-exposed infants. The ECHO abnormalities were not predicted by standard neonatal clinical assessment and were believed to be consistent with those observed in adult abusers of cocaine and amphetamines (51).

Congenital Anomalies

Maternal cocaine abuse is associated with numerous other congenital malformations. In a series of publications extending from 1985–1989, a group of investigators described the onset of ileal atresia (with bowel infarction in one) within the first 24 hours after birth in two infants and genitourinary tract malformations in nine infants (11,13,20,24,26). The abnormalities in the nine infants were prune belly syndrome with urethral obstruction; bilateral cryptorchidism (one also had absence of third and fourth digits on the left hand and a second-degree hypospadias) (two males); female pseudohermaphroditism (one case) (defects included hydronephrosis, ambiguous genitalia with absent uterus and ovaries, anal atresia, absence of third and fourth digits on the left hand, and clubfoot), secondary hypospadias (two cases); hydronephrosis (three cases); and unilateral hydronephrosis with renal infarction of the opposite kidney (one case). Data from the metropolitan Atlanta Birth Defects Case-Control study, involving 4,929 liveborn and stillborn infants with major defects who were compared to 3,029 randomly selected controls, showed a statistically significant association between cocaine use and urinary tract malformations (adjusted odds ratio 4.81, 95% CI 1.15–20.14) (52,53). The adjusted risk for anomalies of the genitalia was 2.27 (*ns*). Cocaine exposure for this analysis was based on self-reported use any time from 1 month before conception through the first 3 months of pregnancy (52,53).

The rates of major congenital malformations in a study involving 50 cocaine-only users, 110 cocaine plus polydrug users, and 340 drug-free controls were 10% (five cases), 4.5% (five cases), and 2% (seven cases), respectively (4). The groups were classified by history and infant urine assays, and chronic alcohol abusers were excluded. The difference between the first and last groups was significant ($p < 0.01$). The incidence of minor abnormalities (e.g., hypertelorism, epicanthal folds, and micrognathia) was similar among the groups (5). Congenital heart defects were observed in all three groups as follows: cocaine-only, transposition of the great arteries (one case) and hypoplastic right heart syndrome (one case); cocaine plus polydrug, ventricular septal defects (three cases); controls, ventricular septal defect (one case), patent ductus arteriosus (one case), and pulmonary stenosis (one case). Skull defects were observed in three infants in the cocaine-only group: exencephaly (stillborn), interparietal encephalocele, and parietal bone defects without herniation of meninges or cerebral tissue. One infant in the cocaine plus polydrug group had microcephalia. Significantly more major and minor malformations were seen in a group of cocaine-exposed infants ($N = 53$) (five major/four minor) than in a matched nonexposed sample ($N = 100$) (two major/four minor) ($p < 0.05$) (23). Congenital heart defects occurred in four of the cocaine-exposed infants: atrial septal defect (one case), ventricular septal defects (two cases), and cardiomegaly (one case). None of the infants born from controls had heart defects ($p < 0.01$). The authors noted, however, that their findings were weakened by the self-reported nature of the drug histories (23).

A 1989 report of 138 women at delivery with positive urine cocaine tests found 10 (7%) infants with congenital anomalies: ventricular septal defect (two), atrial septal defect (one), complete heart block (one), inguinal hernia (two), esophageal atresia (one), hypospadias (one), cleft lip and palate with trisomy 13 (one), and polydactyly (one) (4). Only two (2%) of 88 non-cocaine-using controls had congenital defects, but the difference between the two groups was not significant. When the cocaine group was divided into cocaine only (114 women) and cocaine plus other abuse drugs (24 women), five infants in each group were found to have a malformation. The difference between these subgroups was highly significant ($p < 0.005$).

Necrotizing enterocolitis has been described in two infants after *in utero* cocaine exposure (48). One infant was also exposed to heroin and methamphetamine. The proposed mechanism for the injuries was cocaine-induced ischemia of the fetal bowel followed by invasion of anaerobic bacteria (48). In another report, three newborns (two may have been described immediately above) presented with intestinal defects: one each with midcolonic atresia, ileal atresia, and widespread infarction of the bowel distal to the duodenum (54). Five other infants plus one of those with intestinal disruption had congenital limb reduction defects: unilateral terminal transverse defect (three), Poland sequence (one) (i.e., unilateral defect of pectoralis muscle and syndactyly of hand [55]), bilateral upper limb anomalies including ulnar ray deficiencies (one), and bilateral radial ray defects (two) (54). The defects were thought to be caused by cocaine-induced vascular disruption or hypoperfusion (54).

Facial defects seen in 10 of 11 infants exposed either to cocaine alone (6 of 11) or to cocaine plus other abuse drugs (5 of 11) included blepharophimosis (two), ptosis and facial diplegia (one), unilateral oro-orbital cleft (one), Pierre Robin anomaly (one), cleft palate (one), cleft lip and palate (one), skin tags (two), and cutis aplasia (one) (50). All of the infants had major brain abnormalities, which were described above.

Ocular defects consisting of persistent hyperplastic primary vitreous in one eye and changes similar to those observed in retinopathy of prematurity in the other eye were described in a case report of an infant exposed throughout gestation to cocaine and multiple other abuse drugs (56). The association of the two defects was thought to be coincidental and not likely a consequence of cocaine use (56). Thirteen newborns with cocaine toxicity (each infant with multiple symptoms and positive urine assay) had a complete ophthalmic examination; six were discovered to have marked dilation and tortuosity of the iris vasculature (57). The five infants who were most severely affected were followed for at least 3 months and all showed a gradual resolution of the defects without apparent visual impairment. The transient iris vasculature defects have also been found in infants of diabetic mothers (both gestational and insulin-dependent) (58) and in non-cocaine-exposed controls (57,59). However, the vascular changes have not yet been observed in infants of mothers abusing methadone, heroin, amphetamines, marijuana, or a combination of these drugs (specific data on the number of infants examined in these categories were not given) (58).

Two mothers who had used cocaine during the 1st trimester produced infants with unusual abnormalities (60,61). Both mothers used other abuse drugs, heroin in one case and marijuana and methaqualone in the other case. The anomalies observed were chromosomal aneuploidy 45,X, bilaterally absent fifth toes, and features consistent with Turner's syndrome in one (60) and multiple defects including hypothalamic hamartoblastoma in the other (61). Hydrocephaly was noted in one infant (from a group of 10) exposed *in utero* to cocaine, marijuana, and amphetamines (28). No major anomalies were seen in 8 infants exposed to cocaine (all had positive urine assays for cocaine) and other abuse drugs, but two infants had minor defects, consisting of a sacral exostosis and capillary hemangioma in one and a capillary hemangioma in the other (37). In the latter case, the mother claimed to have used cocaine only during the month preceding delivery. Cocaine was not considered a causative agent in any of these cases (28,37,60,61).

In contrast to the above reports, no congenital abnormalities were observed in several series of cocaine-exposed women, totaling 55 (21), 39 (31), 56 (39), and 38 (62) subjects. A prospective 1989 study mentioned previously found cocaine metabolites in the urine assays from 114 (9.3%) of 1226 women (3). After controlling for the effects of other substances and maternal characteristics known to affect pregnancy outcome adversely, no significant association was found between cocaine and one or more minor anomalies, a constellation of three minor anomalies, or one major anomaly (3). An association with the latter two, however, was suggested by the data ($p = 0.10$) (3). Although animal data cannot be directly extrapolated to humans, administration of cocaine to pregnant rats and mice did not increase the incidence of congenital abnormalities (63).

Infant Complications

Neurobehavior

Newborn infants who have been exposed *in utero* to cocaine may have significant neurobehavior impairment in the neonatal period. An increased degree of irritability, tremulousness, and muscular rigidity has been observed by a number of researchers (4,11, 15–19,21,23,26,62,64). Gastrointestinal symptoms (vomiting, diarrhea) have also been observed (4,21). The onset of these symptoms usually occurs 1–2 days after birth with peak severity of symptoms occurring on days 2 and 3 (19,21,62,64). Seizures, which might have been related to withdrawal, have been observed (14,23). The overall incidence of severe withdrawal symptoms, however, is apparently not increased over that expected in opiate-addicted newborns (15–17). In one report that identified 138 infants whose mothers tested positive for cocaine, 24 (17%) of the mothers also tested positive for other abuse substances, usually opiates (4). The incidence of withdrawal in infants of the cocaine-only group was 25% (28 of 114) vs. 54% (13 of 24) in infants of the multiple abuse drug group ($p < 0.005$).

The Neonatal Behavior Assessment Scale (NBAS) has been used in several studies to quantify the observed symptoms (11,24,26,64). In a blinded study comparing infants of methadone-maintained women to those of cocaine-exposed women, the latter group had a significantly increased degree of irritability, tremulousness, and state lability ($p < 0.03$) (11). Expansion of this study to include drug-free controls and cluster analysis of the NBAS revealed that the cocaine group had significant impairment in state organization compared to either the opiate group infants or controls (24,26). The NBAS was used to evaluate 16 term, newborn infants with cocaine-positive urine assays (65). All demonstrated no to very poor visual attention and tracking, abnormal state regulation, and mild to moderate hypertonicity with decreased spontaneous movement (65). Flash evoked visual potentials were abnormal in 11 of 12 infants studied, and the disturbances remained in six infants studied at 4–6 months (65).

Ultrasound was used in a study published in 1989 to evaluate the behavior of 20 fetuses exposed to cocaine as a predictor of neonatal outcome (66). All fetuses were exposed to cocaine during the 1st trimester; 4 during the 1st trimester only, 7 during the 1st and 2nd trimesters, and 9 throughout gestation. The investigators were able to document that fetal state organization was predictive of newborn neurobehavioral well-being and state organization. In this study, the most frequent indicators of neurobehavioral well-being were excessive tremulousness of the extremities, unexplained tachypnea, or both (66). Abnormal state organization was shown by hyperresponsiveness and difficulty in arousal (66).

Electroencephalographic (EEG) abnormalities indicative of cerebral irritation have been documented in cocaine-exposed neonates (31,64,65). Normalization of the EEG abnormalities may require up to 12 months (31,64).

Mortality

Increased perinatal mortality was observed in a study published in 1989, although in comparison to controls, the higher incidence was not significant (4). Seven (5%) of 140 infants (138 mothers, two sets of twins) whose mothers tested positive for cocaine at delivery died, compared with none of 88 infants whose mothers did not test positive for cocaine at delivery. The seven cases included three intrauterine fetal deaths and four neonatal deaths.

Three studies suggest an increased risk of sudden infant death syndrome (SIDS) (11,17,67). Two infants, from a group of 50 exposed *in utero* to cocaine and methadone, died of SIDS, one at 1 month of age and the other at 3 months (17). It could not be determined whether a relationship existed between the deaths and maternal cocaine use (17). In one study, 10 of 66 infants (15%) exposed to cocaine *in utero* died of SIDS over a 9–180-day interval (mean 46 days) following birth (11). This incidence was estimated to be approximately 30 times that observed in the general population and almost 4 times that seen in the infants of opiate-abusing women (11). Based on this experience, a prospective study was commenced and the results were reported in 1989 (67). Thirty-two infants of cocaine-using mothers were compared to 18 infants of heroin/methadone-addicted mothers. Eight of the mothers in the cocaine group also used heroin/methadone. The mothers of both groups received similar prenatal care, and they used similar amounts of alcohol, cigarettes, and marijuana. Infants in both groups were delivered at a gestational age of 38 weeks or more, and mean birth weight, length, and head circumference were identical. Cardiorespiratory recordings (pneumograms), conducted in most cases at 8–14 days of age, were abnormal in 13 infants, 12 cocaine exposed and 1 opiate exposed ($p < 0.05$). Five of the cocaine-exposed infants had an episode of life-threatening apnea of infancy requiring home resuscitation before the pneumograms could be performed. The 13 infants were treated with theophylline until age 6 months, or longer if the pneumogram had not yet normalized. No cases of SIDS were observed in any of the 50 infants. In an earlier study, pneumograms were used to quantify abnormal sleeping ventilatory patterns in infants of substance-abusing mothers (68). Of three cocaine-exposed infants, one had an abnormal pneumogram. Apnea and/or abnormal pneumograms were observed in 20 (14%) of 138 infants whose mothers tested positive for cocaine at delivery (4). None of the 88 control infants whose mothers tested negative for cocaine at delivery had apnea or abnormal pneumograms ($p < 0.0005$). In a large study examining the relationship between SIDS and cocaine exposure, one infant of 175 exposed to cocaine died of SIDS compared to four infants of 821 who were not exposed (36). The risks per 1000 in the two groups were similar, 5.6 and 4.9, respectively, corresponding to a relative risk for SIDS among infants of cocaine-abusing women of 1.17 (95% CI 0.13–10.43) (36). Based on these data, the study concluded that the increased rates reported previously probably reflected other risk factors that were independently associated with SIDS (36). However, because the study relied on self-reported cocaine use and urine screens (only detects recent exposure), some of the women may have been misclassified as nonusers (69). Analysis of the hair, where the drug accumulates for months, has been advocated as a technique to ensure accurate assessment of past exposure (69).

C

Hospitalization

Increased neonatal hospitalization in infants whose mothers tested positive for cocaine at delivery has been reported (4). In 137 infants (138 mothers, two sets of twins, three fetal deaths excluded), the mean number of days hospitalized was 19.2 compared to 5.1 for 88 infants of mothers who tested negative for cocaine at delivery ($p < 0.0001$). Moreover, the incidences of neonatal hospitalization for longer than 3 and 10 days were both significantly greater for the cocaine group (80% vs. 24%, respectively, $p < 0.00001$; 35% vs. 10%, respectively, $p < 0.0005$). The implications of these findings on the limited resources available to hospitals are, obviously, very important.

Summary

The widespread abuse of cocaine has resulted in major toxicity in the mother, the fetus, and the newborn. The use of cocaine is often significantly correlated with the heavy use of other abuse drugs. Many of the studies reviewed here were unable completely to separate this usage in their patient populations or were unable to verify self-reported usage of cocaine, thus resulting in the possible misclassification of patients into the various groups. Whether the reported consequences of maternal cocaine exposure are a consequence of these biases, to cocaine itself, to other drugs acting independently or in conjunction with cocaine, to poor lifestyles, or to other maternal characteristics, is not presently clear. It is clear, however, that women who use cocaine during pregnancy are at significant risk for shorter gestations, premature delivery, spontaneous abortions, abruptio placentae, and death. The drug decreases uterine blood flow and induces uterine contractions. An increased risk may exist for premature rupture of the membranes, but apparently not for placenta previa. The unborn children of these women may be growth retarded or severely distressed, and they are at risk for increased mortality. *In utero* cerebrovascular accidents with profound morbidity and mortality may occur. Congenital abnormalities involving the genitourinary tract, heart, limbs, and face may occur, and cocaine abuse should be considered teratogenic. Bowel atresias have also been observed in newborn infants, which may be a result of intrauterine bowel infarctions. The exact mechanism of cocaine-induced malformation is presently uncertain, but it may be related to the placental vasoconstriction and fetal hypoxia produced by the drug with the resulting intermittent vascular disruptions and ischemia actually causing the fetal damage. Interactions with other drugs, however, may play a role. In addition to the above toxicities, the newborn child exposed to cocaine during gestation is at risk for severe neurobehavior and neurophysiologic abnormalities that may persist for months. An increased incidence of sudden infant death syndrome in the first few months after birth also may be a consequence of maternal cocaine abuse in conjunction with other factors. Long-term studies of cocaine-exposed children need to be completed before a true assessment of the damage caused by this drug can be determined.

[**Risk Factor X if nonmedicinal use.*]

BREAST FEEDING SUMMARY

RECOMMENDATION: Contraindicated (Systemic); Compatible (Topical)

Milk:plasma ratios of cocaine in breast milk have not been determined. In one case, the urine of a normal, breast-fed, 6-week-old boy was positive for a cocaine metabolite (70). The mother was using an unspecified amount of cocaine. In another patient, a milk sample

12 hours after the last dose of approximately 0.5 g taken intranasally over 4 hours contained measurable levels (specific data not given) of cocaine and the metabolite, benzoylecgonine, that persisted until 36 hours after the dose (71). The 14-day-old infant was breast-fed five times over the 4-hour period during which the mother ingested the cocaine. Approximately 3 hours after the first dose, the child became markedly irritable with onset of vomiting and diarrhea. Other symptoms observed on examination were tremulousness, increased startle response, hyperactive Moro reaction, increased symmetrical deep tendon reflexes with bilateral ankle clonus, and marked lability of mood (71). The irritability and tremulousness steadily improved over the next 48 hours. Large amounts of cocaine and the metabolite were found in the infant's urine 12 hours after the mother's last dose, which persisted until 60 hours postdose. On discharge (time not specified), the physical and neurologic examinations were normal. Additional follow-up of the infant was not reported.

In an unusual case report, a mother applied cocaine powder to her nipples to relieve soreness shortly before breast-feeding her 11-day-old infant (72). Although a breast shield was used, the unsheathed nipple protruded to allow feeding. Three hours after feeding, the infant was found gasping, choking, and blue. Seizures, which occurred with other symptoms of acute cocaine ingestion, stopped 2 hours after admission to the hospital. The mother's milk was negative for cocaine and metabolites but the infant's urine was positive. Physical and neurologic examinations were normal on discharge 5 days later and again at 6 months. Computed tomography (CT) scan during hospitalization showed a small area of lucency in the left frontal lobe and an EEG at this time was abnormal. A repeat CT scan and EEG were normal at 2 months of age.

Based on the toxicity exhibited in the infant after exposure via the milk, maternal cocaine use during breast-feeding should be strongly discouraged and considered contraindicated. Obviously, mothers should also be warned against using the drug topically for nipple soreness. The American Academy of Pediatrics classifies the use of cocaine as contraindicated during breast-feeding (73).

References

1. Cregler LL, Mark H. Special report. medical complications of cocaine abuse. N Engl J Med 1986;315:1495–500.
2. Frank DA, Zuckerman BS, Amaro H, Aboagye K, Bauchner H, Cabral H, Fried L, Hingson R, Kayne H, Levenson SM, Parker S, Reece H, Vinci R. Cocaine use during pregnancy: prevalence and correlates. Pediatrics 1988;82:888–95.
3. Zuckerman B, Frank DA, Hingson R, Amaro H, Levenson SM, Kayne H, Parker S, Vinci R, Aboagye K, Fried LE, Cabral H, Timperi R, Bauchner H. Effects of maternal marijuana and cocaine use on fetal growth. N Engl J Med 1989;320:762–8.
4. Neerhof MG, MacGregor SN, Retzky SS, Sullivan TP. Cocaine abuse during pregnancy: peripartum prevalence and perinatal outcome. Am J Obstet Gynecol 1989;161:633–8.
5. Bingol N, Fuchs M, Diaz V, Stone RK, Gromisch DS. Teratogenicity of cocaine in humans. J Pediatr 1987;110:93–6.
6. Moore TR, Sorg J, Miller L, Key TC, Resnik R. Hemodynamic effects of intravenous cocaine on the pregnant ewe and fetus. Am J Obstet Gynecol 1986;155:883–8.
7. Foutz SE, Kotelko DM, Shnider SM, Thigpen JW, Rosen MA, Brookshire GL, Koike M, Levinson G, Elias-Baker B. Placental transfer and effects of cocaine on uterine blood flow and the fetus (Abstract). Anesthesiology 1983;59:A422.
8. Woods JR Jr, Plessinger MA, Clark KE. Effect of cocaine on uterine blood flow and fetal oxygenation. JAMA 1987;257:957–61.
9. Wang CH, Schnoll SH. Prenatal cocaine use associated with down regulation of receptors in human placenta. Neurotoxicol Teratol 1987;9:301–4.
10. Wang CH, Schnoll SH. Prenatatal cocaine use associated with down regulation of receptors in human placenta. Natl Inst Drug Abuse Res Monogr Ser 1987;76:277.
11. Chasnoff IJ, Burns KA, Burns WJ. Cocaine use in pregnancy: perinatal morbidity and mortality. Neurotoxicol Teratol 1987;9:291–3.
12. Chasnoff IJ. Cocaine- and methadone-exposed infants: a comparison. Natl Inst Drug Abuse Res Monogr Ser 1987;76:278.
13. Chasnoff IJ, Chisum GM, Kaplan WE. Maternal cocaine use and genitourinary tract malformations. Teratology 1988;37:201–4.
14. Chasnoff I, MacGregor S. Maternal cocaine use and neonatal morbidity (Abstract). Pediatr Res 1987;21:356A.
15. Ryan L, Ehrlich S, Finnegan L. Outcome of infants born

C

to cocaine using drug dependent women (Abstract). Pediatr Res 1986;20:209A.
16. Ryan L, Ehrlich S, Finnegan LP. Cocaine abuse in pregnancy: effects on the fetus and newborn. Natl Inst Drug Abuse Res Monogr Ser 1987;76:280.
17. Ryan L, Ehrlich S, Finnegan L. Cocaine abuse in pregnancy: effects on the fetus and newborn. Neurotoxicol Teratol 1987;9:295–9.
18. Oro AS, Dixon SD. Perinatal cocaine and methamphetamine exposure: maternal and neonatal correlates. J Pediatr 1987;111:571–8.
19. Dixon SD, Oro A. Cocaine and amphetamine exposure in neonates: perinatal consequences (Abstract). Pediatr Res 1987;21:359A.
20. MacGregor SN, Keith LG, Chasnoff IJ, Rosner MA, Chisum GM, Shaw P, Minogue JP. Cocaine use during pregnancy: adverse perinatal outcome. Am J Obstet Gynecol 1987;157:686–90.
21. Cherukuri R, Minkoff H, Feldman J, Parekh A, Glass L. A cohort study of alkaloidal cocaine ("crack") in pregnancy. Obstet Gynecol 1988;72:147–51.
22. Chouteau M, Namerow PB, Leppert P. The effect of cocaine abuse on birth weight and gestational age. Obstet Gynecol 1988;72:351–4.
23. Little BB, Snell LM, Klein VR, Gilstrap LC III. Cocaine abuse during pregnancy: maternal and fetal implications. Obstet Gynecol 1989;73:157–60.
24. Chasnoff IJ, Griffith DR, MacGregor S, Dirkes K, Burns KA. Temporal patterns of cocaine use in pregnancy: perinatal outcome. JAMA 1989;261:1741–4.
25. Keith LG, MacGregor S, Friedell S, Rosner M, Chasnoff IJ, Sciarra JJ. Substance abuse in pregnant women: recent experience at the Perinatal Center for Chemical Dependence of Northwestern Memorial Hospital. Obstet Gynecol 1989;73:715–20.
26. Chasnoff IJ, Burns WJ, Schnoll SH, Burns KA. Cocaine use in pregnancy. N Engl J Med 1985;313:666–9.
27. Acker D, Sachs BP, Tracey KJ, Wise WE. Abruptio placentae associated with cocaine use. Am J Obstet Gynecol 1983;146:220–1.
28. Little BB, Snell LM, Palmore MK, Gilstrap LC III. Cocaine use in pregnant women in a large public hospital. Am J Perinatol 1988;5:206–7.
29. Townsend RR, Laing FC, Jeffrey RB Jr. Placental abruption associated with cocaine abuse. AJR Am J Roentgenol 1988;150:1339–40.
30. Collins E, Hardwick RJ, Jeffery H. Perinatal cocaine intoxication. Med J Aust 1989;150:331–4.
31. Doberczak TM, Shanzer S, Senie RT, Kandall SR. Neonatal neurologic and electroencephalographic effects of intrauterine cocaine exposure. J Pediatr 1988;113:354–8.
32. Finnegan L. The dilemma of cocaine exposure in the perinatal period. Natl Inst Drug Abuse Res Monogr Ser 1988;81:379.
33. Thatcher SS, Corfman R, Grosso J, Silverman DG, DeCherney AH. Cocaine use and acute rupture of ectopic pregnancies. Obstet Gynecol 1989;74:478–9.
34. Henderson CE, Torbey M. Rupture of intracranial aneurysm associated with cocaine use during pregnancy. Am J Perinatol 1988;5:142–3.
35. Greenland VC, Delke I, Minkoff HL. Vaginally administered cocaine overdose in a pregnant woman. Obstet Gynecol 1989;74:476–7.
36. Bauchner H, Zuckerman B, McClain M, Frank D, Fried LE, Kayne H. Risk of sudden infant death syndrome among infants with in utero exposure to cocaine. J Pediatr 1988;113:831–4.
37. Madden JD, Payne TF, Miller S. Maternal cocaine abuse and effect on the newborn. Pediatrics 1986;77:209–11.
38. Fulroth R, Phillips B, Durand DJ. Perinatal outcome of infants exposed to cocaine and/or heroin in utero. Am J Dis Child 1989;143:905–10.
39. Hadeed AJ, Siegel SR. Maternal cocaine use during pregnancy: effect on the newborn infant. Pediatrics 1989;84:205–10.
40. Bauchner H, Zuckerman B, Amaro H, Frank DA, Parker S. Teratogenicity of cocaine. J Pediatr 1987;111:160–1.
41. Donvito MT. Cocaine use during pregnancy: adverse perinatal outcome. Am J Obstet Gynecol 1988;159:785–6.
42. Bingol N, Fuchs M, Diaz V, Stone RK, Gromisch DS. Teratogenicity of cocaine (reply). J Pediatr 1987;111:161.
43. MacGregor SN. Cocaine use during pregnancy: adverse perinatal outcome (reply). Am J Obstet Gynecol 1988;159:786.
44. Critchley HOD, Woods SM, Barson AJ, Richardson T, Lieberman BA. Fetal death *in utero* and cocaine abuse: case report. Br J Obstet Gynaecol 1988;95:195–6.
45. Mitchell M, Sabbagha RE, Keith L, MacGregor S, Mota JM, Minoque J. Ultrasonic growth parameters in fetuses of mothers with primary addiction to cocaine. Am J Obstet Gynecol 1988;159:1104–9.
46. Chasnoff IJ, Bussey ME, Savich R, Stack CM. Perinatal cerebral infarction and maternal cocaine use. J Pediatr 1986;108:456–9.
47. Tenorio GM, Nazvi M, Bickers GH, Hubbird RH. Intrauterine stroke and maternal polydrug abuse. Clin Pediatr 1988;27:565–7.
48. Telsey AM, Merrit TA, Dixon SD. Cocaine exposure in a term neonate: necrotizing enterocolitis as a complication. Clin Pediatr 1988;27:547–50.
49. Dixon SD, Bejar R. Brain lesions in cocaine and methamphetamine exposed neonates (Abstract). Pediatr Res 1988;23:405A.
50. Kobori JA, Ferriero DM, Golabi M. CNS and craniofacial anomalies in infants born to cocaine abusing mothers (Abstract). Clin Res 1989;37:196A.
51. Dixon SD, Bejar R. Echoencephalographic findings in neonates associated with maternal cocaine and methamphetamine use: incidence and clinical correlates. J Pediatr 1989;115:770–8.
52. Chavez GF, Mulinare J, Cordero JF. Maternal cocaine use and the risk for genitourinary tract defects: an epidemiologic approach (Abstract). Am J Hum Genet 1988;43(Suppl):A43.
53. Chavez GF, Mulinare J, Cordero JF. Maternal cocaine use during early pregnancy as a risk factor for congenital urogenital anomalies. JAMA 1989;262:795–8.
54. Hoyme HE, Jones KL, Dixon SD, Jewett T, Hanson JW, Robinson LK, Msall ME, Allanson J. Maternal cocaine use and fetal vascular disruption (Abstract). Am J Hum Genet 1988;43(Suppl):A56.
55. Smith DW, Jones KL. *Recognizable Patterns of Human Malformations*. 3rd ed. Philadelphia, PA: WB Saunders, 1982:224.
56. Teske MP, Trese MT. Retinopathy of prematurity-like

fundus and persistent hyperplastic primary vitreous associated with maternal cocaine use. Am J Ophthalmol 1987;103:719–20.
57. Isenberg SJ, Spierer A, Inkelis SH. Ocular signs of cocaine intoxication in neonates. Am J Ophthalmol 1987;103:211–4.
58. Ricci B, Molle F. Ocular signs of cocaine intoxication in neonates. Am J Ophthalmol 1987;104:550–1.
59. Isenberg SJ, Inkelis SH, Spierer A. Ocular signs of cocaine intoxication in neonates (reply). Am J Ophthalmol 1987;104:551.
60. Kushnick T, Robinson M, Tsao C. 45,X chromosome abnormality in the offspring of a narcotic addict. Am J Dis Child 1972,124.772–3.
61. Huff DS, Fernandes M. Two cases of congenital hypothalamic hamartoblastoma, polydactyly, and other congenital anomalies (Pallister-Hall syndrome). N Engl J Med 1982;306:430–1.
62. LeBlanc PE, Parekh AJ, Naso B, Glass L. Effects of intrauterine exposure to alkaloidal cocaine ("crack"). Am J Dis Child 1987;141:937–8.
63. Fantel AG, MacPhail BJ. The teratogenicity of cocaine. Teratology 1982;26:17–9.
64. Doberczak TM, Shanzer S, Kandall SR. Neonatal effects of cocaine abuse in pregnancy (Abstract). Pediatr Res 1987;21:359A.
65. Dixon SD, Coen RW, Crutchfield S. Visual dysfunction in cocaine-exposed infants (Abstract). Pediatr Res 1987;21:359A.
66. Hume RF Jr, O'Donnell KJ, Staner CL, Killam AP, Gingras JL. In utero cocaine exposure: observations of fetal behavioral state may predict neonatal outcome. Am J Obstet Gynecol 1989;161:685–90.
67. Chasnoff IJ, Hunt CE, Kletter R, Kaplan D. Prenatal cocaine exposure is associated with respiratory pattern abnormalities. Am J Dis Child 1989;143:583–7.
68. Davidson Ward SL, Schuetz S, Krishna V, Bean X, Wingert W, Wachsman L, Keens TG. Abnormal sleeping ventilatory pattern in infants of substance-abusing mothers. Am J Dis Child 1986;140:1015–20.
69. Graham K, Koren G. Maternal cocaine use and risk of sudden infant death. J Pediatr 1989;115:333.
70. Shannon M, Lacouture PG, Roa J, Woolf A. Cocaine exposure among children seen at a pediatric hospital. Pediatrics 1989;83:337–42.
71. Chasnoff IJ, Lewis DE, Squires L. Cocaine intoxication in a breast-fed infant. Pediatrics 1987;80:836–8.
72. Chaney NE, Franke J, Wadlington WB. Cocaine convulsions in a breast-feeding baby. J Pediatr 1988;112:134–5.
73. Committee on Drugs, American Academy of Pediatrics. The transfer of drugs and other chemicals into human milk. Pediatrics 2001;108:776–89.

Name:	**CODEINE**	Risk Factor:	**C***
Class:	**Narcotic Agonist Analgesic, Respiratory Drug (Antitussive)**		

FETAL RISK SUMMARY

RECOMMENDATION: Human Data Suggest Risk in 3rd Trimester

The Collaborative Perinatal Project monitored 50,282 mother-child pairs, 563 of whom had 1st trimester exposure to codeine (1, pp. 287–295). No evidence was found to suggest a relationship to large categories of major or minor malformations. Associations were found with six individual defects (1, pp. 287–295, 471) (independent confirmation is required for all associations found in this study): respiratory (8 cases); genitourinary (other than hypospadias) (7 cases); Down's syndrome (1 case); tumors (4 cases); umbilical hernia (3 cases); and inguinal hernia (12 cases). For use anytime during pregnancy, 2522 exposures were recorded (1, p. 434). With the same qualifications, possible associations with four individual defects were found (1, p. 484): hydrocephaly (7 cases); pyloric stenosis (8 cases); umbilical hernia (7 cases); and inguinal hernia (51 cases).

In an investigation of 1427 malformed newborns compared to 3001 controls, 1st trimester use of narcotic analgesics (codeine most common) was associated with inguinal hernias, cardiac and circulatory system defects, cleft lip and palate, dislocated hip, and other musculoskeletal defects (2). Second trimester use was associated with alimentary tract defects. In a large retrospective Finnish study, the use of opiates (mainly codeine) during the 1st trimester was associated with an increased risk of cleft lip and palate (3,4). Finally, a survey of 390 infants with congenital heart disease matched with 1254 normal infants found a higher rate of exposure to several drugs, including codeine, in the offspring

C

with defects (5). Although all four of these studies contain several possible biases that could have affected the results, the data serve as a possible warning that indiscriminate use of codeine may present a risk to the fetus.

In a surveillance study of Michigan Medicaid recipients conducted between 1985 and 1992 involving 229,101 completed pregnancies, 7,640 newborns had been exposed to codeine during the 1st trimester (F. Rosa, personal communication, FDA, 1993). A total of 375 (4.9%) major birth defects were observed (325 expected). Specific data were available for six defect categories, including (observed/expected) 74/76 cardiovascular defects, 14/13 oral clefts, 4/4 spina bifida, 25/22 polydactyly, 15/13 limb reduction defects, and 14/18 hypospadias. Only with the total number of defects is there a suggestion of an association between codeine and congenital defects, but other factors, including the mother's disease, concurrent drug use, and chance may be involved.

Use of codeine during labor produces neonatal respiratory depression to the same degree as other narcotic analgesics (6). The first known case of neonatal codeine addiction was described in 1965 (7). The mother had taken analgesic tablets containing 360 to 480 mg of codeine/day for 8 weeks prior to delivery.

A second report described neonatal codeine withdrawal in two infants of nonaddicted mothers (8). The mother of one infant began consuming a codeine cough medication 3 weeks prior to delivery. Approximately 2 weeks before delivery, analgesic tablets with codeine were taken at a frequency of up to six tablets/day (48 mg of codeine/day). The second mother was treated with a codeine cough medication, consuming 90–120 mg of codeine/day for the last 10 days of pregnancy. Apgar scores of both infants were 8–10 at 1 and 5 minutes. Typical symptoms of narcotic withdrawal were noted in the infants shortly after birth but not in the mothers.

[**Risk Factor D if used for prolonged periods or in high doses at term.*]

BREAST FEEDING SUMMARY

RECOMMENDATION: Limited Human Data - Probably Compatible

Codeine passes into breast milk in very small amounts that are probably insignificant (9–11). The American Academy of Pediatrics classifies codeine as compatible with breast-feeding (12).

References

1. Heinonen OP, Slone D, Shapiro S. *Birth Defects and Drugs in Pregnancy*. Littleton, MA: Publishing Sciences Group, 1977.
2. Bracken MB, Holford TR. Exposure to prescribed drugs in pregnancy and association with congenital malformations. Obstet Gynecol 1981;58:336–44.
3. Saxen I. Associations between oral clefts and drugs taken during pregnancy. Int J Epidemiol 1975;4;37–44.
4. Saxen I. Epidemiology of cleft lip and palate: an attempt to rule out chance correlations. Br J Prev Soc Med 1975;29:103–10.
5. Rothman KJ, Fyler DC, Goldblatt A, Kreidberg MB. Exogenous hormones and other drug exposures of children with congenital heart disease. Am J Epidemiol 1979;109:433–9.
6. Bonica JJ. *Principles and Practice of Obstetric Analgesia and Anesthesia*. Philadelphia, PA: FA Davis, 1967: 245.
7. Van Leeuwen G, Guthrie R, Stange F. Narcotic withdrawal reaction in a newborn infant due to codeine. Pediatrics 1965;36;635–6.
8. Mangurten HH, Benawra R. Neonatal codeine withdrawal in infants of nonaddicted mothers. Pediatrics 1980;65:159–60.
9. Kwit NT, Hatcher RA. Excretion of drugs in milk. Am J Dis Child 1935;49:900–4.
10. Horning MG, Stillwell WG, Nowlin J, Lertratanangkoon K, Stillwell RN, Hill RM. Identification and quantification of drugs and drug metabolites in human breast milk using GC-MS-COM methods. Mod Probl Paediatr 1975;15:73–9.
11. Anonymous. Drugs in breast milk. Med Lett Drugs Ther 1974;16:25–7.
12. Committee on Drugs, American Academy of Pediatrics. The transfer of drugs and other chemicals into human milk. Pediatrics 2001;108:776–89.

Name:	COLCHICINE	Risk Factor:	D_M
Class:	Miscellaneous (Metaphase Inhibitor)		

C

FETAL RISK SUMMARY

RECOMMENDATION: Limited Human Data - Animal Data Suggest Risk

Colchicine is used in the treatment of gout and familial Mediterranean fever. Seven animal studies, reviewed by Shepard in 1989, indicated that colchicine and its derivative, demecolcine (desacetylmethylcolchicine), were teratogenic in mice and rabbits at low doses and embryocidal in mice, rats, and rabbits at higher doses (1). Mutagenic effects were also observed in rabbit blastocysts. No adverse fetal effects were observed in limited studies with pregnant monkeys (1).

No congenital malformations have been reported in a small number of human fetuses exposed to colchicine (2–7). A 1960 review of the effects of cancer chemotherapy on the fetus cited three cases in which demecolcine had been used for the treatment of leukemia (2). In one of these cases, the mother was treated with 6-mercaptopurine, aminopterin, and high-dose (10 mg four times) demecolcine. The colchicine derivative was administered, along with 6-mercaptopurine, during the 6th month of gestation, shortly before an infant, without malformations, was delivered prematurely. The infant expired at 19 hours. The other two mothers were treated throughout gestation with doses ranging between 1.5 and 7.5 mg/day. Both newborns were normal at birth, and one was developing normally at 2 years of age. The second child died at 2 years of age of postnecrotic cirrhosis, probably secondary to undiagnosed hepatitis (2). A double renal artery and a large calculus in the left kidney were found at autopsy.

A woman conceived while being treated with colchicine for familial Mediterranean fever (FMF) and continued the drug during the first 5 weeks of pregnancy (3,4). A healthy infant was eventually delivered. Four other reports briefly described the results of 10 pregnancies conceived while mothers were being treated with colchicine for FMF (5–8). Seven of the women continued therapy throughout gestation and six gave birth to normal infants, but the status of the seventh infant was not mentioned (5,7). Of the seven who stopped colchicine after pregnancy detection, three gave birth to healthy newborns, three were still pregnant, and one, with nephrotic syndrome as a result of amyloidosis, aborted in the 2nd month (5).

The known mutagenic effects of colchicine and the possible relationship of this drug to sperm abnormalities and the production of congenital malformations were the subjects of a number of publications (9–16). A 1965 report described three pregnancies occurring in a woman between the ages of 24 and 27 years, two of which ended abnormally (9). Her first pregnancy resulted in the spontaneous abortion of a macerated fetus at 4.5 months, her second in the delivery of a normal girl, and her third in the delivery of a male with atypical Down's syndrome, who died 24 hours after birth. The infant had palmar transverse folds on the hands, inner epicanthic folds, unspecified cardiac malformations, trigger thumbs, syndactyly in the second and third toes, hypognathous, cleft palate, low-set ears, and an incompletely developed scapha helix (9). The father was 27 to 30 years of age during these pregnancies and was being treated for gout, on an intermittent basis with 1–2 mg/day of colchicine. Cultures of leukocytes obtained from him demonstrated mutagenic changes when exposed to colchicine, but blood and sperm samples, collected 3 months after the end of colchicine therapy, were normal. The investigators theorized that the colchicine therapy may have caused diploid spermatozoa that resulted in the production of triploid children (9).

A brief report from the same laboratory as the reference above described the analysis of lymphocyte cultures from three male patients being treated with colchicine (10). Compared to controls, a significant increase in the number of cells with abnormal numbers of chromosomes was found in the colchicine-exposed men. The investigators proposed that this finding indicated that these men were at higher risk of producing trisomic offspring than were nonexposed men (10). Of 54 children with Down's syndrome (trisomy 21) in their clinic, two had been fathered by men being treated with colchicine. The validity of this proposed association between colchicine and Down's syndrome was the subject of several references (11–14). One of the arguments against the association included the high possibility of Down's syndrome and colchicine therapy occurring at the same time in an older population (12). Moreover, several references have described healthy children fathered by men who were being treated with colchicine (3–5,15,16).

Colchicine may induce azoospermia. Hamsters and mice treated chronically with subcutaneous injections of demecolcine developed extensive damage to the germinal epithelium, resulting in azoospermia within 35–45 days (17). One study observed azoospermia in a 36-year-old patient induced by 1.2 mg/day of colchicine, but not with 0.6 mg/day (18). A second study, however, using 1.8–2.4 mg/day in seven healthy men 20–25 years old, measured no effect on sperm production or on serum levels of testosterone, luteinizing hormone, or follicle-stimulating hormone (19). The authors of this second report, however, could not exclude the fact that some men may be unusually sensitive to the drug, resulting in testicular toxicity (19).

In summary, the indications for colchicine therapy in pregnancy are few; thus, the number of exposures to this drug during gestation are also few. Although no cases of congenital malformations or other toxicity resulting from maternal consumption of colchicine have been located, the drug should be used cautiously during pregnancy because of the limited data available in humans and the teratogenicity observed in animals. The use of colchicine by the father prior to conception does not seem to present a significant reproductive risk, but azoospermia may be a rare complication.

BREAST FEEDING SUMMARY

RECOMMENDATION: Limited Human Data - Probably Compatible

Colchicine is excreted into breast milk (6–8). A 31-year-old woman, receiving long-term therapy with colchicine, 0.6 mg twice daily, for familial Mediterranean fever (FMF), was treated throughout a normal pregnancy, labor, and delivery (6). Milk, urine, and serum samples were obtained from her between 16 and 21 days after delivery. Colchicine was detected in three of five milk samples collected on days 16–20 with levels ranging from 1.2–2.5 ng/mL (test sensitivity 0.5 ng/mL). However, the authors could not determine whether their analysis method was recovering all of the drug in the milk because of the high lipid content of the samples (6). Two serum samples collected on days 19 and 21 measured 0.7 and 1.0 ng/mL of the drug, indicating that the milk:plasma ratio exceeded 1.0. Daily urine colchicine concentrations (days 16–20) ranged from 70–390 ng/mL. No apparent effects were observed in the nursing infant over the first 6 months of life.

In four lactating women on long-term colchicine therapy (at least 7 years) for FMF, 1–1.5 mg/day, serum and milk samples were drawn before a dose and at 1, 3, and 6 hours after a dose (7). Maximum breast milk drug concentrations ranged between 1.9 and

8.6 ng/mL, whereas maximum serum concentrations ranged from 3.6 to 6.46 ng/mL. The peak concentrations in milk and serum both occurred at 1 hour and the colchicine concentration time curves for milk and serum were parallel. No apparent effects in the nursing infants were observed over a 10-month period. The authors concluded that nursing was safe for women taking colchicine, but that waiting 12 hours after a dose to breast-feed would minimize exposure of the nursing infant (7).

Much higher colchicine milk concentrations were measured in a second study. A 21-year-old woman had taken colchicine, 1 mg/day, throughout gestation and continued while breast-feeding her normal infant (8). On postpartum days 5 and 15, colchicine concentrations in the mother's 24-hour urine sample were 276,000 and 123,000 ng/24 hours, respectively, while none was detected (test sensitivity 5 ng/mL) in the infant's 12-hour urine collection. Milk samples were collected four times each on day 5 (2, 4, 15, and 21 hours after a dose) and day 15 (0, 4, 7, and 11 hours after a dose). Colchicine concentrations in the 2- and 4-hour samples on day 5 were 31 and 24 ng/mL, respectively, and below the level of detection at 15 and 21 hours. On day 15, levels at 0 and 11 hours were below detection, while those at 4 and 7 hours were 27 and 10 ng/mL, respectively. Assuming 100% of the dose in milk was absorbed, the estimated dose per kg the infant was receiving, during the 8 hour-period after a dose, was 10% of the mother's dose per kg (8). Although no adverse effects were observed in the infant, the authors recommended that a mother could minimize drug exposure from her milk by taking her dose at bedtime and waiting 8 hours to breast-feed (8).

Because of the absence of infant toxicity observed during nursing in one of the above cases (6), the American Academy of Pediatrics classifies colchicine as compatible with breast-feeding (20).

References

1. Shepard TH. *Catalog of Teratogenic Agents*. 6th ed. Baltimore, MD: Johns Hopkins University Press, 1989: 164–6.
2. Sokal JE, Lessmann EM. Effects of cancer chemotherapeutic agents on the human fetus. JAMA 1960; 172:1765–72.
3. Cohen MM, Levy M, Eliakim M. A cytogenetic evaluation of long-term colchicine therapy in the treatment of familial Mediterranean fever (FMF). Am J Med Sci 1977;274:147–52.
4. Levy M, Yaffe C. Testicular function in patients with familial Mediterranean fever on long-term colchicine treatment. Fertil Steril 1978;29: 667–8.
5. Zemer D, Pras M, Sohar E, Gafni J. Colchicine in familial Mediterranean fever. N Engl J Med 1976;294: 170–1.
6. Milunsky JM, Milunsky A. Breast-feeding during colchicine therapy for familial Mediterranean fever. J Pediatr 1991;119:164.
7. Ben-Chetrit E, Scherrmann JM, Levy M. Colchicine in breast milk of patients with familial Mediterranean fever. Arthritis Rheum 1996;39:1213–7.
8. Guillonneau M, Aigrain EJ, Galliot M, Binet M-H, Darbois Y. Colchicine is excreted at high concentrations in human breast milk. Eur J Obstet Gynecol Reprod Biol 1995;61:177–8.
9. Cestari AN, Botelho Vieira Filho JP, Yonenaga Y, Magnelli N, Imada J. A case of human reproductive abnormalities possibly induced by colchicine treatment. Rev Bras Biol 1965;25:253–6.
10. Ferreira NR, Buoniconti A. Trisomy after colchicine therapy. Lancet 1968;2:1304.
11. Walker FA. Trisomy after colchicine therapy. Lancet 1969;1:257–8.
12. Timson J. Trisomy after colchicine therapy. Lancet 1969;1:370.
13. Hoefnagel D. Trisomy after colchicine therapy. Lancet 1969;1:1160.
14. Ferreira NR, Frota-Pessoa O. Trisomy after colchicine therapy. Lancet 1969;1:1160–1.
15. Yu TF, Gutman AB. Efficacy of colchicine prophylaxis in gout. Prevention of recurrent gouty arthritis over a mean period of five years in 208 gouty subjects. Ann Intern Med 1961;55:179–92.
16. Goldfinger SE. Colchicine for familial Mediterranean fever: possible adverse effects. N Engl J Med 1974;290:56.
17. Poffenbarger PL, Brinkley BR. Colchicine for familial Mediterranean fever: possible adverse effects. N Engl J Med 1974;290:56.
18. Merlin HE. Azoospermia caused by colchicine—a case report. Fertil Steril 1972;23:180–1.
19. Bremer WJ, Paulsen CA. Colchicine and testicular function in man. N Engl J Med 1976;294:1384–5.
20. Committee on Drugs, American Academy of Pediatrics. The transfer of drugs and other chemicals into human milk. Pediatrics 2001;108:776–89.

C

Name:	**COLESEVELAM**	Risk Factor:	B_M
Class:	**Antilipemic Agent**		

FETAL RISK SUMMARY

RECOMMENDATION: Compatible

This non-absorbed, polymeric, lipid-lowering agent binds bile acids to prevent their absorption. Because cholesterol is the sole precursor of bile acids, this action eventually results in the lowering of low-density lipoprotein (LDL) cholesterol levels in the blood. It is indicated, either alone or in combination with a HMG-CoA reductase inhibitor (atorvastatin, cerivastatin, fluvastatin, lovastatin, pravastatin, or simvastatin), as adjunctive therapy to diet and exercise for the reduction of elevated LDL cholesterol in patients with primary hypercholesterolemia (1). Because the drug is not absorbed, no direct embryo or fetal exposure will occur.

Reproduction studies have been conducted in pregnant rats and rabbits (1). Doses that were about 50 and 17 times, respectively, the maximum human dose based on body weight (MHD), revealed no evidence of fetal harm. In addition, no effect on rat fertility was seen at 50 times the MHD (1). In rats, doses greater than 30 times the MHD caused vitamin K deficiency and hemorrhage, but the absorption of fat soluble vitamins (A, D, E, and K) was not significantly impaired (1).

The effect of colesevelam on the absorption of vitamins and other nutrients from the gastrointestinal tract in pregnant women has not been studied (1). Fat soluble vitamin deficiency, especially vitamin K (see above), is a potential complication if this agent is used during pregnancy.

BREAST FEEDING SUMMARY

RECOMMENDATION: Compatible

No reports describing the use of colesevelam in lactation have been located. The drug is not absorbed after oral administration so no drug exposure of a nursing infant via breast milk will occur. However, maternal deficiency of fat soluble vitamins, especially vitamin K (see above), is a potential complication. This may result in lower fat soluble vitamin concentrations in milk because these vitamins are natural constituents of breast milk.

Reference

1. Product information. WelChol. Sankyo Pharma, 2001.

Name:	**COLESTIPOL**	Risk Factor:	**B**
Class:	**Antilipemic Agent**		

FETAL RISK SUMMARY

RECOMMENDATION: Compatible

The anion exchange resin, colestipol, is used to bind bile acids in the intestine into a nonabsorbable complex that is excreted in the feces. The prevention of the systemic reabsorption of the bile acids lowers the total amount of cholesterol in the patient. Because less than 0.17% of a dose is absorbed systemically, it is not expected to cause fetal harm when administered during pregnancy in recommended doses (1).

In a reproductive study with rats and rabbits, doses up to 1000 mg/kg/day produced no adverse effects on the fetuses (2). No published or unpublished cases involving the use of colestipol during human pregnancy have been located. Rosa also reported finding no recipients of this drug in his 1994 presentation on the outcome of pregnancies following exposure to anticholesterol agents (3).

The actions of colestipol are similar to those of cholestyramine, another exchange resin (see also Cholestyramine). Because it is not absorbed into the systemic circulation, it should have no direct effect on the fetus. However, as with cholestyramine, prolonged use of colestipol may result in reduced intestinal absorption of the fat-soluble vitamins, A, D, E, and K. Because the interruption of cholesterol lowering therapy during pregnancy should have no effect on the long-term treatment of hyperlipidemia, the use of colestipol should probably be halted during gestation.

BREAST FEEDING SUMMARY

RECOMMENDATION: Compatible

Because colestipol is poorly absorbed (less than 0.17% of a dose) into the systemic circulation, its use by the lactating woman should have no direct effect on the nursing infant. Prolonged use of the exchange resin, however, may result in decreased maternal absorption of the fat-soluble vitamins, A, D, E, and K. The resulting deficiencies in the mother would lessen the amounts of these vitamins in her milk.

References

1. Product information. Colestid. Pharmacia & Upjohn, 2000.
2. Webster HD, Bollert JA. Toxicologic, reproductive and teratologic studies of colestipol hydrochloride: A new bile acid sequestrant. Toxicol Appl Pharmacol 1974;28:57–65. As cited in Shepard TH. *Catalog of Teratogenic Agents*. 7 th ed. Baltimore, MD: Johns Hopkins University Press, 1992:105.
3. Rosa F. Anti cholesterol agent pregnant exposure out comes. Presented at the 7th International Organization for Teratogen Information Services, Woods Hole, MA, April 1994.

Name:	**COLISTIMETHATE**	Risk Factor:	**C_M**
Class:	**Antibiotic**		

FETAL RISK SUMMARY

RECOMMENDATION: Limited Human Data - Animal Data Suggest Moderate Risk

No reports linking the use of colistimethate with congenital defects have been located. The drug crosses the placenta at term (1).

Colistimethate was not teratogenic in rats at IM doses about 0.13 and 0.30 times the maximum recommended human dose based on body surface area (MRHD) (2). The same weight doses in rabbits (about 0.25 and 0.55 times the MRHD) resulted in talipes varus in 2.6% and 2.9% of the fetuses, respectively. Increased resorption of rabbit embryos occurred at the highest dose.

C

BREAST FEEDING SUMMARY

RECOMMENDATION: Limited Human Data - Probably Compatible

Colistimethate is excreted into breast milk. The milk:plasma ratio is 0.17–0.18 (3). Although this level is low, three potential problems exist for the nursing infant: modification of bowel flora, direct effects on the infant, and interference with the interpretation of culture results if a fever workup is required.

References

1. MacAulay MA, Charles D. Placental transmission of colistimethate. Clin Pharmacol Ther 1967;8:578–86.
2. Product information. Coly-Mycin. Monarch Pharmaceuticals, 2000.
3. Wilson JT. Milk/plasma ratios and contraindicated drugs. In Wilson JT, ed. *Drugs in Breast Milk*. Balgowlah, Australia: ADIS Press, 1981:78–9.

Name:	**CORTICOTROPIN/COSYNTROPIN**	Risk Factor:	**C**
Class:	**Corticosteroid Stimulating Hormone**		

FETAL RISK SUMMARY

RECOMMENDATION: Limited Human Data - No Relevant Animal Data

Studies reporting the use of corticotropin in pregnancy have not demonstrated adverse fetal effects (1–4). However, corticosteroids have been suspected of causing malformations (see Hydrocortisone). Because corticotropin stimulates the release of endogenous corticosteroids, this relationship should be considered when prescribing the drug to women in their reproductive years.

BREAST FEEDING SUMMARY

RECOMMENDATION: No Human Data - Probably Compatible

No data are available.

References

1. Johnstone FD, Campbell S. Adrenal response in pregnancy to long-acting tetracosactin. J Obstet Gynaecol Br Commonw 1974;81:363–7.
2. Simmer HH, Tulchinsky D, Gold EM, et al. On the regulation of estrogen production by cortisol and ACTH in human pregnancy at term. Am J Obstet Gynecol 1974;119:283–96.
3. Aral K, Kuwabara Y, Okinaga S. The effect of adrenocorticotropic hormone and dexamethasone, administered to the fetus in utero, upon maternal and fetal estrogens. Am J Obstet Gynecol 1972;113:316–22.
4. Potert AJ. Pregnancy and adrenalcortical hormones. Br Med J 1962;2:967–72.

Name:	**CORTISONE**	Risk Factor:	**C***
Class:	**Corticosteroid**		

FETAL RISK SUMMARY

RECOMMENDATION: Human Data Suggest Risk

Cortisone (Compound E) is an inactive corticosteroid precursor that is secreted by the adrenal cortex. It is converted by reduction to hydrocortisone, primarily in the liver. See Hydrocortisone.

[*Risk factor D if used in 1st trimester.*]

BREAST FEEDING SUMMARY

RECOMMENDATION: No Human Data - Probably Compatible

See Hydrocortisone.

Name:	**COUMARIN DERIVATIVES**	Risk Factor:	**D***
Class:	**Anticoagulant**		

FETAL RISK SUMMARY

RECOMMENDATION: Contraindicated - 1st Trimester

Coumarin derivatives (dicumarol, ethyl biscoumacetate, and warfarin) are oral anticoagulants, as are the indandione derivatives (anisindione and phenindione). Use of any of these agents during pregnancy may result in significant problems for the fetus and newborn. Since the first case of fetal coumarin embryopathy described by DiSaia in 1966 (1), a large volume of literature has accumulated. Hall and co-workers (2) reviewed this subject in 1980 (167 references). In the 3 years following this review, a number of other reports appeared (3–12). The principal problems confronting the fetus and newborn are:

Embryopathy (fetal warfarin syndrome)
Central nervous system defects
Spontaneous abortion
Stillbirth
Prematurity
Hemorrhage

First trimester use of coumarin derivatives may result in the fetal warfarin syndrome (FWS) (1–4). The common characteristics of the FWS are nasal hypoplasia, because of failure of development of the nasal septum, and stippled epiphyses. The bridge of the nose is depressed, resulting in a flattened, upturned appearance. Neonatal respiratory distress occurs frequently because of upper airway obstruction. Other features that may be present are:

Birth weight less than 10th percentile for gestational age
Eye defects (blindness, optic atrophy, microphthalmia) when drug also used in 2nd and 3rd trimesters

Hypoplasia of the extremities (ranging from severe rhizomelic dwarfing to dystrophic nails and shortened fingers)
Developmental retardation
Seizures
Scoliosis
Deafness/hearing loss
Congenital heart disease
Death

The critical period of exposure, based on the work of Hall and coworkers (2), seems to be the 6th–9th weeks of gestation. All of the known cases of FWS were exposed during at least a portion of these weeks. Exposure after the 1st trimester carries the risk of central nervous system (CNS) defects. No constant grouping of abnormalities was observed, nor were there an apparent correlation between time of exposure and the defects, except that all fetuses were exposed in the 2nd and/or 3rd trimesters. After elimination of those cases that were probably caused by late fetal or neonatal hemorrhage, the CNS defects in 13 infants were thought to represent deformations that occurred as a result of abnormal growth arising from an earlier fetal hemorrhage and subsequent scarring (2). Two patterns were recognized: (a) dorsal midline dysplasia characterized by agenesis of corpus callosum, Dandy-Walker malformations, and midline cerebellar atrophy (encephaloceles may be present) and (b) ventral midline dysplasia characterized by optic atrophy (eye anomalies).

Other features of CNS damage in the 13 infants were (number of infants shown in parenthesis):

Mental retardation (13)
Blindness (7)
Spasticity (4)
Seizures (3)
Deafness (1)
Scoliosis (1)
Growth failure (1)
Death (3)

Long-term effects in the children with CNS defects were more significant and debilitating than those from the fetal warfarin syndrome (2).

Fetal outcomes for the 471 cases of *in utero* exposure to coumarin derivatives reported through 1983 are summarized below (2–12):

1st Trimester Exposure (263):
Normal infants—167 (63%)
Spontaneous abortions—41 (16%)
Stillborn/neonatal death—17 (6%)
FWS—27 (10%)
CNS/other defects—11 (4%)

2nd Trimester Exposure (208):
Normal infants—175 (84%)
Spontaneous abortions—4 (2%)
Stillborn/neonatal death—19 (9%)
CNS/other defects—10 (5%)

Total Infants Exposed (471):

Normal infants—342 (73%)
Spontaneous abortions—45 (10%)
Stillborn/neonatal death—36 (8%)
FWS/CNS/other defects—48 (10%)

Hemorrhage was observed in 11 (3%) of the normal newborns (premature and term). Two of the patients in the 2nd and 3rd trimester groups were treated with the coumarin derivatives phenprocoumon and nicoumalone. Both infants were normal.

Congenital abnormalities that did not fit the pattern of the FWS or CNS defects were reported in 10 infants (2,9). These were thought to be incidental malformations that were probably not related to the use of coumarin derivatives (see also three other cases, in which the relationship to coumarin derivatives is unknown, described in the text below at references 16, 20, and 22). The congenital abnormalities reported for each infant were as follows:

Asplenia, two-chambered heart, agenesis of pulmonary artery
Anencephaly, spina bifida, congenital absence of clavicles
Congenital heart disease, death
Fetal distress, focal motor seizures
Bilateral polydactyly
Congenital corneal leukoma
Nonspecified multiple defects
Asplenia, congenital heart disease, incomplete rotation of gut, short broad phalanges, hypoplastic nails
Single kidney, toe defects, other anomalies, death
Cleft palate

A 1984 study examined 22 children, with a mean age of 4.0 years, who were exposed *in utero* to warfarin (13). Physical and mental development of the children was comparable to that of matched controls.

Since publication of the above data, a number of additional reports and studies have appeared describing the outcomes of pregnancies treated at various times with coumarin derivatives (14–25). The largest series involved 156 women with cardiac valve prostheses who had 223 pregnancies (14). During a period of 19 years, the women were grouped based on evolving treatment regimens: group I—68 pregnancies treated with acenocoumarol until the diagnosis of pregnancy was made, and then treated with dipyridamole or aspirin, or both; group II—128 pregnancies treated with acenocoumarol throughout gestation; group III—12 pregnancies treated with acenocoumarol, except when heparin was substituted from pregnancy diagnosis to the 13th week of gestation, and again from the 38th week until delivery; and group IV—15 pregnancies in women with biologic prostheses who were not treated with anticoagulant therapy. The fetal outcomes in the four groups were spontaneous abortions 10.3% vs. 28.1% vs. 0% vs. 0% ($p < 0.0005$); stillbirths 7.4% vs. 7.1% vs. 0% vs. 6.7%; and neonatal deaths 0% vs. 2.3% vs. 0% vs. 0%. (See references for maternal outcomes in the various groups.) Of the 38 children examined in group II, 3 (7.9%) had features of the FWS.

In a subsequent report from these investigators, the outcomes of 72 pregnancies studied prospectively were described in 1986 (15). The pregnancies were categorized into three groups according to the anticoagulant therapy: group I—23 pregnancies treated with acenocoumarol except for heparin from the 6th–12th weeks of gestation; group II—12 pregnancies treated the same as group I except that heparin treatment was started after the 7th week; and group III—37 pregnancies treated with acenocoumarol throughout gestation (pregnancies in this group were not detected until after the 1st trimester). In most patients, heparin was substituted for the coumarin derivative after the 38th week of gestation. The fetal outcomes in the three groups were spontaneous abortions 8.7% vs. 25% vs. 16.2%; and stillbirths 0% vs. 8.3% vs. 0%. Not all of the infants born to the mothers were examined, but of those that were, the FWS was observed in 0% of group I (0 of 19), 25.0% of group II (2 of 8), and 29.6% of group III (8 of 27). Thus, 10 (28.6%) of the 35 infants examined who were exposed at least during the first 7 weeks of gestation had warfarin embryopathy.

A 1983 report described 14 pregnancies in 13 women with a prosthetic heart valve who were treated throughout pregnancy with warfarin (16). Two patients had spontaneous abortions, two delivered premature stillborn infants (one infant had anencephaly), and two newborns died during the neonatal period. The total fetal and neonatal mortality in this series was 43%. Other defects noted were corneal changes in two, bradydactyly and dysplastic nails in two, and nasal hypoplasia in one.

In 18 pregnancies of 16 women with an artificial heart valve, heparin was substituted for warfarin when pregnancy was diagnosed (between 6 and 8 weeks after the last menstrual period) and continued until the 13th week of gestation (17). Nine of the 18 pregnancies aborted, but none of the nine liveborn infants had congenital anomalies or other complications.

Three recent reports have described the pregnancy outcomes in mothers with prosthetic heart valves and who were treated with anticoagulants (18–20). A study published in 1991 described the outcomes of 64 pregnancies in 40 women with cardiac valve replacement, 34 of whom had mechanical valves (18). Warfarin was used in 47 pregnancies (23 women), heparin in 11 pregnancies (11 women), and no anticoagulation was given in 6 pregnancies (6 women). Fetal wastage (spontaneous abortions, neonatal death after preterm delivery, and stillbirths) occurred in 25 (53%) of the warfarin group, 4 (36%) of those treated with heparin, and 1 (17%) of those not treated. Two infants, both exposed to warfarin, had congenital malformations: single kidney and toe, and finger defects in one; cleft lip and palate in the other.

Two groups of pregnant patients with prosthetic heart valves were compared in a study published in 1992 (19). In Group 1 ($N = 40$), all treated with coumarin-like drugs until near term when therapy was changed to heparin, 34 (85%) had mechanical valves, whereas none of those in Group 2 ($N = 20$) were treated with anticoagulation and all had biological valves. The pregnancy outcomes of the two groups were spontaneous abortions 7 vs. 0, prematurity 14 vs. 2 ($p < 0.05$), low birth weight 15 vs. 2 ($p < 0.05$), stillbirth 1 vs. 0, neonatal mortality 5 vs. 0, and birth defects 4 vs. 0, respectively. The four infants from Group 1 with birth defects included three with typical features of the fetal warfarin syndrome (one with low birth weight and upper airway obstruction) and one with left ventricular hypoplasia and aortic atresia (died in neonatal period). The other four neonatal deaths involved three from respiratory distress syndrome and one from a cerebral hemorrhage.

A 1994 reference compared retrospectively two groups of pregnant women: Group 1 (56 pregnancies in 31 women) with mechanical valve replacements, all of whom were treated with warfarin; and Group 2 (95 pregnancies in 57 women) with porcine tissue valves, none of whom received anticoagulation. Twenty women in Group 1 either continued the warfarin throughout delivery ($N = 12$) or discontinued the drug ($N = 8$) 1–2 days before delivery. The pregnancy outcomes of the two groups were induced abortion 9 vs. 22, fetal loss before 20 weeks' gestation 7 vs. 8, fetal loss after 20 weeks' gestation: 6 vs. 1 ($p < 0.01$), total fetal loss 13 vs. 9 ($p < 0.05$), and live births 34 vs. 64 ($p < 0.05$).

Two infants, both in Group 1 had birth defects, a ventricular septal defect in one and a hypoplastic nose in the other.

Five reports have described single cases of exposure to warfarin during pregnancy (21–25). A woman with Marfan's syndrome had replacement of her aortic arch and valve combined with coronary artery bypass performed during the 1st week of her pregnancy (1–8 days after conception) (21). She was treated with warfarin throughout gestation. A normal female infant was delivered by elective cesarean section at 34 weeks' gestation. Warfarin was used to treat a deep vein thrombosis during the 3rd trimester in a 34-year-old woman because of heparin-induced maternal thrombocytopenia (22). A normal infant was delivered at term. In another case involving a woman with a deep vein thrombosis that had occurred before the present pregnancy, warfarin therapy was continued through the first 14 weeks of gestation (23). At term, a 3660 g infant was delivered who did not breathe and who died after 35 minutes. At autopsy, an almost total agenesis of the left diaphragm and hypoplasia of both lungs were noted. The relationship between warfarin and the defect is unknown.

The use of warfarin to treat a deep vein thrombosis associated with circulating lupus anticoagulant during pregnancy has been described (24). Therapy was started after the 9th week of gestation. Because of severe pregnancy-induced hypertension, a 1830-g female infant was delivered by cesarean section at 31 weeks. No information was provided about the condition of the infant.

A woman with a mitral valve replacement 8 months before pregnancy was treated continuously with warfarin until 6 weeks after her last menstrual period (25). Warfarin was then stopped and except for cigarette smoking, no other drugs were taken during the pregnancy. A growth-retarded (2340 g, 3rd percentile; 50 cm length, 50th percentile; 35 cm head circumference, 50th percentile) female infant was delivered at term. Congenital abnormalities noted in the infant were triangular face with broad forehead, micrognathia, microglossia, hypoplastic fingernails and toenails, and hypoplasia of the distal phalanges. No epiphyseal stippling was seen on a skeletal survey. A normal female karyotype, 46,XX, was found on chromosomal analysis. Psychomotor development was normal at 1 year of age but physical growth remained retarded (3rd percentile). The authors concluded that the pattern of defects represented the earliest teratogenic effects of warfarin, but they could not exclude a chance association with the drug.

In a surveillance study of Michigan Medicaid recipients conducted between 1985 and 1992 involving 229,101 completed pregnancies, 22 newborns had been exposed to warfarin during the 1st trimester (Franz Rosa, personal communication, FDA, 1993). One (4.5%) major birth defect was observed (one expected), a cardiovascular defect (0.2 expected).

A report published in 1994 assessed the neurological, cognitive, and behavioral development of 21 children (8 to 10 years of age) who had been exposed *in utero* to coumarin derivatives (26). A control group of 17 children was used for comparison. Following examination, 32 of the children were classified as normal (18 exposed and 14 control children), 5 had minor neurological dysfunction (2 exposed and 3 control children), and one child had severe neurological abnormalities which were thought to be a consequence of oral anticoagulants. Although no significant differences were measured between the groups, the children with the lowest neurological assessments and the lowest IQ-scores had been exposed to coumarin derivatives.

In summary, the use of coumarin derivatives during the 1st trimester carries with it a significant risk to the fetus. For all cases, only about 70% of pregnancies are expected to result in a normal infant. Exposure in the 6th–9th weeks of gestation may produce a pattern of defects termed *fetal warfarin syndrome*, with an incidence up to 25% or greater in some series. Infants exposed before and after this period have had other congenital anomalies, but the relationship between warfarin and these defects is unknown. Infrequent central nervous system defects, which have greater clinical significance to the infant than the defects of the fetal warfarin syndrome, may be deformations related to hemorrhage and scarring with subsequent impaired growth of brain tissue. Spontaneous abortions, stillbirths, and neonatal deaths may also occur. If the mother's condition requires anticoagulation, the use of heparin from the start of the 6th gestational week through the end of the 12th gestational week, and again at term, may lessen the risk to the fetus of adverse outcome.

[**Risk Factor X according to manufacturer—DuPont Pharma, 2000.*]

BREAST FEEDING SUMMARY

RECOMMENDATION: Compatible; Contraindicated (Phenindione)

Excretion of coumarin (dicumarol, ethyl biscoumacetate, and warfarin) and indandione (anisindione and phenindione) derivatives into breast milk is dependent on the agent used. Three reports on warfarin have been located totaling 15 lactating women (27–29). Doses ranged between 2 and 12 mg/day in 13 patients (7 nursing, 6 not nursing) with serum levels varying from 1.6–8.5 μmol/L (27,28). Warfarin was not detected in the milk of any of the 13 patients or in the plasma of the 7 nursing infants. No anticoagulant effect was found in the plasma of the three infants tested (27,28). In another report, the warfarin doses in two breast-feeding women were not specified nor were maternal plasma drug levels determined (29). However, no spectrophotometric evidence for the drug was found in the milk of one mother and no anticoagulant effect was measured in either nursing infant (29).

Exposure to ethyl biscoumacetate in milk resulted in bleeding in 5 of 42 exposed infants in one report (30). The maternal dosage was not given. An unidentified metabolite was found in the milk that may have led to the high complication rate. A 1959 study measured ethyl biscoumacetate levels in 38 milk specimens obtained from four women taking 600–1200 mg/day (31). The drug was detected in only 13 samples with levels varying from 0.09–1.69 μg/mL. No correlation could be found between the milk concentrations and the dosage or time of administration. Twenty-two infants were breast-fed from these and other mothers receiving ethyl biscoumacetate. No adverse effects were observed in the infants, but coagulation tests were not conducted.

More than 1600 postpartum women were treated with dicumarol to prevent thromboembolic complications in a 1950 study (32). Doses were titrated to adjust the prothrombin clotting time to 40%–50% of normal. No adverse effects or any change in prothrombin times were noted in any of the nursing infants.

Phenindione use in a lactating woman resulted in a massive scrotal hematoma and wound oozing in a 1.5-month-old breast-fed infant shortly after a herniotomy was performed (33). The mother was taking 50 mg every morning and alternating between 50 and 25 mg every night for suspected pulmonary embolism that developed postpartum. Milk levels varying from 1–5 μg/mL have been reported after 50- or 75-mg single doses of phenindione (34). When the dose was 25 mg, only 18 of 68 samples contained detectable amounts of the anticoagulant.

In summary, maternal warfarin consumption apparently does not pose a significant risk to normal, full-term, breast-fed infants. Other oral anticoagulants should be avoided by the lactating woman. The American Academy of Pediatrics classifies phenindione (which is not used in the United States) as contraindicated during breast-feeding because of the risk of hemorrhage in the infant (35). Both warfarin and dicumarol (bishydroxycoumarin) are classified by the Academy as compatible with breast-feeding (35).

C

References

1. DiSaia PJ. Pregnancy and delivery of a patient with a Starr-Edwards mitral valve prosthesis. Obstet Gynecol 1966;28:469–71.
2. Hall JG, Pauli RM, Wilson KM. Maternal and fetal sequelae of anticoagulation during pregnancy. Am J Med 1980;68:122–40.
3. Baillie M, Allen ED, Elkington AR. The congenital warfarin syndrome: a case report. Br J Ophthalmol 1980;64:633–5.
4. Harrod MJE, Sherrod PS. Warfarin embryopathy in siblings. Obstet Gynecol 1981;57:673–6.
5. Russo R, Bortolotti U, Schivazappa L, Girolami A. Warfarin treatment during pregnancy: a clinical note. Haemostasis 1979;8:96–8.
6. Biale Y, Cantor A, Lewenthal H, Gueron M. The course of pregnancy in patients with artificial heart valves treated with dipyridamole. Int J Gynaecol Obstet 1980;18:128–32.
7. Moe N. Anticoagulant therapy in the prevention of placental infarction and perinatal death. Obstet Gynecol 1982;59:481–3.
8. Kaplan LC, Anderson GG, Ring BA. Congenital hydrocephalus and Dandy-Walker malformation associated with warfarin use during pregnancy. Birth Defects 1982;18:79–83.
9. Chen WWC, Chan CS, Lee PK, Wang RYC, Wong VCW. Pregnancy in patients with prosthetic heart valves: an experience with 45 pregnancies. Q J Med 1982;51:358–65.
10. Vellenga E, Van Imhoff GW, Aarnoudse JG. Effective prophylaxis with oral anticoagulants and low-dose heparin during pregnancy in an antithrombin III deficient woman. Lancet 1983;2:224.
11. Michiels JJ, Stibbe J, Vellenga E, Van Vliet HHDM. Prophylaxis of thrombosis in antithrombin III-deficient women during pregnancy and delivery. Eur J Obstet Gynecol Reprod Biol 1984;18:149–53.
12. Oakley C. Pregnancy in patients with prosthetic heart valves. Br Med J 1983;286:1680–3.
13. Chong MKB, Harvey D, De Swiet M. Follow-up study of children whose mothers were treated with warfarin during pregnancy. Br J Obstet Gynaecol 1984;91:1070–3.
14. Salazar E, Zajarias A, Gutierrez N, Iturbe I. The problem of cardiac valve prostheses, anticoagulants, and pregnancy. Circulation 1984;70(Suppl 1):I169–77.
15. Iturbe-Alessio I, Fonseca MDC, Mutchinik O, Santos MA, Zajarias A, Salazar E. Risks of anticoagulant therapy in pregnant women with artificial heart valves. N Engl J Med 1986;315:1390–3.
16. Sheikhzadeh A, Ghabusi P, Hakim S, Wendler G, Sarram M, Tarbiat S. Congestive heart failure in valvular heart disease in pregnancies with and without valvular prostheses and anticoagulant therapy. Clin Cardiol 1983;6:465–70.
17. Lee P-K, Wang RYC, Chow JSF, Cheung K-L, Wong VCW, Chan T-K. Combined use of warfarin and adjusted subcutaneous heparin during pregnancy in patients with an artificial heart valve. J Am Coll Cardiol 1986;8:221–4.
18. Ayhan A, Yapar EG, Yuce K, Kisnisci HA, Nazli N, Ozmen F. Pregnancy and its complications after cardiac valve replacement. Int J Gynecol Obstet 1991;35:117–22.
19. Born D, Martinez EE, Almeida PAM, Santos DV, Carvalho ACC, Moron AF, Miyasaki CH, Moraes SD, Ambrose JA. Pregnancy in patients with prosthetic heart valves: the effects of anticoagulation on mother, fetus, and neonate. Am Heart J 1992;124:413–7.
20. Lee C-N, Wu C-C, Lin P-Y, Hsieh F-J, Chen H-Y. Pregnancy following cardiac prosthetic valve replacement. Obstet Gynecol 1994;83:353–60.
21. Cola LM, Lavin JP Jr. Pregnancy complicated by Marfan's syndrome with aortic arch dissection, subsequent aortic arch replacement and triple coronary artery bypass grafts. J Reprod Med 1985;30:685–8.
22. Copplestone A, Oscier DG. Heparin-induced thrombocytopenia in pregnancy. Br J Haematol 1987;65:248.
23. Normann EK, Stray-Pedersen B. Warfarin-induced fetal diaphragmatic hernia: case report. Br J Obstet Gynaecol 1989;96:729–30.
24. Campbell JM, Tate G, Scott JS. The use of warfarin in pregnancy complicated by circulating lupus anticoagulant; a technique for monitoring. Eur J Obstet Gynecol Reprod Biol 1988;29:27–32.
25. Ruthnum P, Tolmie JL. Atypical malformations in an infant exposed to warfarin during the first trimester of pregnancy. Teratology 1987;36:299–301.
26. Olthof E, De Vries TW, Touwen BCL, Smrkovsky M, Geven-Boere LM, Heijmans HSA, Van der Veer E. Late neurological, cognitive and behavioural sequelae of prenatal exposure to coumarins: a pilot study. Early Hum Dev 1994;38:97–109.
27. Orme ML, Lewis PJ, De Swiet M, Serlin MJ, Sibeon R, Baty JD, Breckenridge AM. May mothers given warfarin breast-feed their infants? Br Med J 1977;1:1564–5.
28. De Swiet M, Lewis PJ. Excretion of anticoagulants in human milk. N Engl J Med 1977;297:1471.
29. McKenna R, Cole ER, Vasan U. Is warfarin sodium contraindicated in the lactating mother? J Pediatr 1983;103:325–7.
30. Gostof, Momolka, Zilenka. Les substances derivees du tromexane dans le lait maternal et leurs actions paradoxales sur la prothrombine. Schweiz Med Wochenschr 1952;30:764–5. As cited in Daily JW. Anticoagulant and cardiovascular drugs. In Wilson JT, ed. *Drugs in Breast Milk*. Balgowlah, Australia: ADIS Press, 1981:63.
31. Illingworth RS, Finch E. Ethyl biscoumacetate (Tromexan) in human milk. J Obstet Gynaecol Br Commonw 1959;66:487–8.
32. Brambel CE, Hunter RE. Effect of dicumarol on the nursing infant. Am J Obstet Gynecol 1950;59:1153–9.

33. Eckstein HB, Jack B. Breast-feeding and anticoagulant therapy. Lancet 1970;1:672–3.
34. Goguel M, Noel G, Gillet JY. Therapeutique anticoagulante et allaitement: etude du passage de la phenyl-2-dioxo,1,3 indane dans le lait maternal. Rev Fr Gynecol Obstet 1970;65:409–12. As cited in Anderson PO. Drugs and breast feeding—a review. Drug Intell Clin Pharm 1977;11:208–23.
35. Committee on Drugs, American Academy of Pediatrics. The transfer of drugs and other chemicals into human milk. Pediatrics 2001;108:776–89.

Name:	**CROMOLYN SODIUM**	Risk Factor:	B_M
Class:	**Respiratory Drug (Anti-inflammatory)**		

FETAL RISK SUMMARY

RECOMMENDATION: Compatible

Cromolyn sodium is an inhaled anti-inflammatory agent used for the prevention of bronchial asthma. The drug is generally considered safe for use during pregnancy (1–6). Although small amounts are absorbed systemically from the lungs, it is not known whether the drug crosses the placenta to the fetus (6).

Reproductive studies using SC doses of cromolyn in mice and rats, and both SC and IV doses in rabbits, have not revealed teratogenicity (7,8). In one source, the doses used in the three animal species were 27, 16, and 98 times the maximum recommended human dose, respectively, on a mg/m^2 basis (8). Increased resorptions and decreased fetal weight were observed only with high parenteral doses that were associated with maternal toxicity (8).

A 1984 study, cited by Shepard, reported over 300 pregnancies in which cromolyn was used in combination with other drugs, most often with isoproterenol, without a link with congenital defects (9).

Congenital malformations were noted in four (1.35%) newborns in a 1982 study of 296 women treated throughout gestation with cromolyn sodium (10). This incidence is less than the expected rate of 2%–3% in a nonexposed population. The defects observed were patent ductus arteriosus, clubfoot, nonfused septum, and harelip alone. The author concluded that there was no association between the defects and cromolyn sodium (10).

As of 1983, the manufacturer had reports of 185 women treated during all or parts of pregnancy, but the small number probably reflects underreporting of the actual usage (personal communication, Fisons Corporation, 1983). From these cases, 10 infants had been born with congenital defects, at least 3 of which appeared to be genetic in origin. Multiple-drug exposure was common. In none of the 10 cases was there evidence to link the defects with cromolyn sodium.

In a surveillance study of Michigan Medicaid recipients conducted between 1985 and 1992 involving 229,101 completed pregnancies, 191 newborns had been exposed to cromolyn during the 1st trimester (F. Rosa, personal communication, FDA, 1993). Seven (3.7%) major birth defects were observed (eight expected). Specific data were available for six defect categories, including (observed/expected) 1/2 cardiovascular defects, 1/0.5 oral clefts, 0/0 spina bifida, 1/0.5 polydactyly, 0/0.5 limb reduction defects, and 0/0.5 hypospadias. These data do not support an association between the drug and congenital defects.

BREAST FEEDING SUMMARY

RECOMMENDATION: No Human Data - Probably Compatible

No reports describing the use of cromolyn sodium during lactation have been located.

References

1. Dykes MHM. Evaluation of an antiasthmatic agent cromolyn sodium (Aarane, Intal). JAMA 1974;227:1061–2.
2. Greenberger P, Patterson R. Safety of therapy for allergic symptoms during pregnancy. Ann Intern Med 1978;89:234–7.
3. Weinstein AM, Dubin BD, Podleski WK, Spector SL, Farr RS. Asthma and pregnancy. JAMA 1979;241:1161–5.
4. Pratt WR. Allergic diseases in pregnancy and breast feeding. Ann Allergy 1981;47:355–60.
5. Mawhinney H, Spector SL. Optimum management of asthma in pregnancy. Drugs 1986;32:178–87.
6. Niebyl JR. *Drug Use in Pregnancy*. Philadelphia, PA: Lea & Febiger, 1982:53.
7. Cox JSG, Beach JE, Blair AMJN, Clarke AJ. Disodium cromoglycate (Intal). Adv Drug Res 1970;5:135–6. As cited in Shepard TH. *Catalog of Teratogenic Agents*. 6th ed. Baltimore, MD: Johns Hopkins University Press, 1989:174.
8. Product information. Intal. Rhone-Poulenc Rorer Pharmaceuticals, 2000.
9. Shepard TH. *Catalog of Teratogenic Agents*. 6th ed. Baltimore, MD: Johns Hopkins University Press, 1989:174.
10. Wilson J. Use of sodium cromoglycate during pregnancy: results on 296 asthmatic women. Acta Therap 1982;8(Suppl):45–51.

Name:	**CYCLACILLIN**	Risk Factor:	**B_M**
Class:	**Antibiotic (Penicillin)**		

FETAL RISK SUMMARY

RECOMMENDATION: Compatible

Cyclacillin is a penicillin antibiotic (see Penicillin G). No published reports linking its use with congenital defects have been located. The Collaborative Perinatal Project monitored 50,282 mother-child pairs, 3546 of whom had 1st trimester exposure to penicillin derivatives (1, pp. 297–313). For use anytime during pregnancy, 7171 exposures were recorded (1, p. 435). In neither case was evidence found to suggest a relationship to large categories of major or minor malformations or to individual defects.

In a surveillance study of Michigan Medicaid recipients conducted between 1985 and 1992 involving 229,101 completed pregnancies, nine newborns had been exposed to cyclacillin during the 1st trimester (F. Rosa, personal communication, FDA, 1993). Two (22.2%) major birth defects were observed (0.4 expected), both of which were cardiovascular defects (0.1 expected). The number of exposures is too small to draw any conclusions.

BREAST FEEDING SUMMARY

RECOMMENDATION: Compatible

No reports describing the use of cyclacillin during lactation have been located. Because other penicillins are excreted in milk in low concentrations (see Ampicillin and Penicillin G) the presence of cyclacillin should also be expected. Although adverse effects from other penicillins in breast milk are rare, three potential problems exist for the nursing infant: modification of bowel flora, direct effects on the infant (e.g., allergic response), and interference with the interpretation of culture results if a fever workup is required.

Reference

1. Heinonen OP, Slone D, Shapiro S. *Birth Defects and Drugs in Pregnancy*. Littleton, MA: Publishing Sciences Group, 1977.

C

Name: **CYCLAMATE** Risk Factor: **C**
Class: **Artificial Sweetener**

FETAL RISK SUMMARY

RECOMMENDATION: Limited Human Data - Probably Compatible

Controlled studies on the effects of cyclamate on the fetus have not been found. The drug crosses the placenta to produce fetal blood levels of about 25% of maternal serum (1). Cyclamate has been suspected of having cytogenetic effects in human lymphocytes (2). One group of investigators attempted to associate these effects with an increased incidence of malformations and behavioral problems, but a causal relationship could not be established (3).

BREAST FEEDING SUMMARY

RECOMMENDATION: No Human Data - Probably Compatible

No data are available.

References

1. Pitkin RM, Reynolds WA, Filer LJ. Placental transmission and fetal distribution of cyclamate in early human pregnancy. Am J Obstet Gynecol 1970;108:1043–50.
2. Bauchinger M. Cytogenetic effect of cyclamate on human peripheral lymphocytes in vivo. Dtsch Med Wochenschr 1970;95:2220–3.
3. Stone D, Matalka E, Pulaski B. Do artificial sweeteners ingested in pregnancy affect the offspring? Nature 1971;231:53.

Name: **CYCLANDELATE** Risk Factor: **C**
Class: **Vasodilator**

FETAL RISK SUMMARY

RECOMMENDATION: No Human Data - No Relevant Animal Data

No data are available.

BREAST FEEDING SUMMARY

RECOMMENDATION: No Human Data - Probably Compatible

No data are available.

Name: **CYCLAZOCINE** Risk Factor: **D**
Class: **Narcotic Antagonist**

FETAL RISK SUMMARY

C

RECOMMENDATION: No Human Data - No Relevant Animal Data

Cyclazocine is not available in the United States. In addition to its ability to reverse narcotic overdose, it has been used in the treatment of narcotic dependence (1). Its actions are similar to those of nalorphine (see also Nalorphine).

BREAST FEEDING SUMMARY

RECOMMENDATION: No Human Data - Probably Compatible

No data are available.

Reference

1. Wade A, ed. Martindale: The Extra Pharmacopoeia. 27th ed. London: Pharmaceutical Press, 1977:985.

Name:	**CYCLIZINE**	Risk Factor:	**B**
Class:	**Antihistamine/Antiemetic**		

FETAL RISK SUMMARY

RECOMMENDATION: Compatible

Cyclizine is a piperazine antihistamine that is used as an antiemetic (see Buclizine and Meclizine for closely related drugs). The drug is teratogenic in animals but apparently not in humans. In 111 patients given cyclizine during the 1st trimester, no increased malformation rate was observed (1). Similarly, the Collaborative Perinatal Project found no association between 1st trimester cyclizine use and congenital defects, although the number of exposed patients ($N = 15$) was small compared to the total sample (2). The Food and Drug Administration's OTC Laxative Panel acting on this data concluded that cyclizine is not teratogenic (3). In 1974, investigators searching for an association between antihistamines and oral clefts found no relationship between this defect and the cyclizine group (4). Finally, a 1971 retrospective study found that significantly fewer infants with malformations were exposed to antihistamines/antiemetics in the 1st trimester as compared to controls (5). Cyclizine was the fifth most commonly used antiemetic.

An association between exposure during the last 2 weeks of pregnancy to antihistamines in general and retrolental fibroplasia in premature infants has been reported. See Brompheniramine for details.

BREAST FEEDING SUMMARY

RECOMMENDATION: No Human Data - Probably Compatible

No data are available.

References

1. Milkovich L, Van den Berg BJ. An evaluation of the teratogenicity of certain antinauseant drugs. Am J Obstet Gynecol 1976;125:244–8.
2. Heinonen OP, Slone D, Shapiro S. *Birth Defects and Drugs in Pregnancy*. Littleton, MA: Publishing Sciences Group, 1977:323.
3. Anonymous. Meclizine; cyclizine not teratogenic. Pink Sheets. FDC Rep 1974:T&G-2.

4. Saxen I. Cleft palate and maternal diphenhydramine intake. Lancet 1974;1:407–8.
5. Nelson MM, Forfar JO. Associations between drugs administered during pregnancy and congenital abnormalities of the fetus. Br Med J 1971;1:523–7.

C

Name: **CYCLOBENZAPRINE** Risk Factor: **B_M**
Class: **Skeletal Muscle Relaxant**

FETAL RISK SUMMARY

RECOMMENDATION: Limited Human Data - Animal Data Suggest Low Risk

Cyclobenzaprine is a centrally acting skeletal muscle relaxant that is closely related to the tricyclic antidepressants (e.g., imipramine). The agent is not teratogenic or embryotoxic in mice, rats, and rabbits given doses up to 20 times the human dose (1). No published reports of its use in human pregnancy have been located.

In a surveillance study of Michigan Medicaid recipients conducted between 1985 and 1992 involving 229,101 completed pregnancies, 545 newborns had been exposed to cyclobenzaprine during the 1st trimester (F. Rosa, personal communication, FDA, 1993). A total of 24 (4.4%) major birth defects were observed (23 expected), including (observed/expected) 5/5 cardiovascular defects, 1/1 oral clefts, and 2/2 polydactyly. No anomalies were observed in three other categories of defects (spina bifida, limb reduction defects, and hypospadias) for which data were available. Earlier data, obtained from the same source between 1980 and 1983, totaled 168 1st trimester exposures with 12 defects observed (10 expected). These combined data do not support an association between the drug and congenital defects.

BREAST FEEDING SUMMARY

RECOMMENDATION: No Human Data - Potential Toxicity

No reports have been located on the excretion of cyclobenzaprine into milk. The molecular weight (about 276 for the free base), however, is low enough that excretion into milk should be expected. In addition, the closely related tricyclic antidepressants (e.g., see Imipramine) are excreted into milk, which should be considered before cyclobenzaprine is used during lactation.

Reference

1. Product information. Flexeril. Merck Sharpe & Dohme, 1993.

Name: **CYCLOPENTHIAZIDE** Risk Factor: **C***
Class: **Diuretic**

See Chlorothiazide.

[**Risk Factor D if used in gestational hypertension.*]

Name: **CYCLOPHOSPHAMIDE**	Risk Factor: **D_M**
Class: **Antineoplastic**	

FETAL RISK SUMMARY

RECOMMENDATION: Contraindicated - 1st Trimester

Cyclophosphamide is an alkylating antineoplastic agent. Both normal and malformed newborns have been reported following the use in pregnancy of cyclophosphamide (1–33). Ten malformed infants have resulted from 1st trimester exposure (1–8). Radiation therapy was given to most of the mothers, and at least one patient was treated with other antineoplastics (1,2,4). Defects observed in four of the infants are shown in the list below, and three other infants are described in the text that follows:

Flattened nasal bridge, palate defect, skin tag, four toes each foot, hypoplastic middle phalanx fifth finger, bilateral inguinal hernia sacs
Toes missing, single coronary artery
Hemangioma, umbilical hernia
Imperforate anus, rectovaginal fistula, growth retarded

A newborn exposed *in utero* to cyclophosphamide during the 1st trimester presented with multiple anomalies (6). The mother, who was being treated for a severe exacerbation of systemic lupus erythematosus, received two IV doses of 200 mg each between 15 and 46 days' gestation. Except for prednisone, 20 mg daily, no other medication was given during the pregnancy. The 3150-g female infant was delivered at 39 weeks' gestational age with multiple abnormalities, including dysmorphic facies; multiple eye defects, including bilateral blepharophimosis with left microphthalmos; abnormally shaped, low-set ears; cleft palate; bilaterally absent thumbs; and dystrophic nails. Borderline microcephaly, hypotonia, and possible developmental delay were observed at 10 months of age.

A 1993 publication reported a 29-year-old woman with twins who was treated for acute lymphocytic leukemia throughout gestation with cyclophosphamide (200 mg/day) and intermittent prednisone (7). Therapy was stopped at 33 weeks' gestation and she delivered 4 weeks later. Both infants recovered from their severe respiratory distress syndromes. The 1250-g female twin has developed normally and is now 22 years of age. Except for strabismus repair at age 9 years, she has not required any further hospitalizations (7). In contrast, the 1190-g male twin required hospitalization until 10 months of age because of multiple congenital anomalies: dyschondrosteosis (Madelung's deformity) of the right arm, esophageal atresia, abnormal inferior vena cava, abnormal renal collecting system later diagnosed as cross-renal atopia, and a rudimentary left testicle (found later) (7). Chromosomal analysis of the child revealed a normal karyotype (46,XY). Developmental and neurological problems were diagnosed at about 8 years of age and an IQ test performed at 11 years of age was in the low average range (full-scale IQ of 81) with even lower verbal skills (7). At 14 years of age, a stage III neuroblastoma arising from the left adrenal gland was diagnosed and was treated with surgery and radiation. At 16 years of age, metastatic papillary thyroid cancer was found and this was treated with surgery. In addition, three courses of radioactive iodine were administered to treat the primary cancer and two recurrences (7). The authors speculated that the different outcomes in the twins might have been a result of differences in metabolism, either by the individual placentas or by the hepatic cytochrome P-450 activity of the fetuses (7). In either case, two cyclophosphamide active metabolites, phosphoramide mustard and acrolein, may have actually caused the malformations. Moreover, because of the timing of the two malignancies in the boy, the authors also thought it was possible that they were the result of *in utero* exposure to cyclophosphamide (7).

A 23-year-old woman with hypertension and lupus nephritis received four IV doses of cyclophosphamide (20 mg/kg/dose), three of which were given before conception and one during the 6th week of gestation (8). She delivered a female, 1705-g (<5th percentile) infant at 37 weeks' gestation with Apgar scores of 5 and 7 at 1 and 5 minutes, respectively. The infant's length was 46 cm (5th–10th percentile) and the head circumference 30.2 cm (<5th percentile). Other medications received throughout gestation were prednisone, nifedipine, atenolol, clonidine, potassium chloride, and aspirin. In addition to respiratory distress syndrome, multiple anomalies were noted, including microbrachycephaly, coronal craniosynostosis, blepharophimosis, shallow orbits, proptosis, hypertelorism, broad, flat nasal bridge, bulbous nasal tip, overfolded small ears, left preauricular pit, microstomia, high-arched palate, micrognathia, hypoplastic thumbs, 5th finger clinodactyly, and absent 4th and 5th toes bilaterally (8). Other malformations were detected in the skeleton and central nervous system during diagnostic workups. Growth delay (<3rd percentile in all growth parameters) and gross motor skills continued to be impaired at age 17.5 months. Based on their comparisons to previous cases of cyclophosphamide-induced congenital defects, the authors concluded that cyclophosphamide was a human teratogen and that a distinct phenotype existed (8).

A case report of a 16-year-old woman with ovarian endodermal sinus tumor presenting in two pregnancies was published in 1979 (19). Conservative surgery, suction curettage to terminate a pregnancy estimated to be at 8–10 weeks' gestation, and chemotherapy with cyclophosphamide, dactinomycin, and vincristine (VAC) produced a complete clinical response for 12 months. The patient then refused further therapy and presented a second time, 6 months later, with tumor recurrence and a pregnancy estimated at 18–20 weeks' gestation. She again refused chemotherapy, but her disease progressed to the point where she allowed VAC chemotherapy to be reinstated 4 weeks later. At 33 weeks' gestation, 2 weeks after her last dose of chemotherapy, she spontaneously delivered a normal 2213-g female infant. The infant was developing normally when last seen at 8 months of age. In a similar case, a woman, treated with surgery and chemotherapy in her 15th week of pregnancy for an ovarian endodermal sinus tumor, delivered a normal 2850-g male infant at 37 weeks' gestation (20). Chemotherapy, begun during the 16th gestational week, included six courses of VAC chemotherapy. The last course was administered 5 days prior to delivery. No information was provided on the subsequent growth and development of the infant.

Following surgical treatment at 16 weeks' gestation, a 28-year-old woman with advanced epithelial ovarian carcinoma was treated with cyclophosphamide, 750 mg/m^2, and cisplatin, 50 mg/m^2, every 21 days for seven cycles (21). Labor was induced at 37–38 weeks' gestation resulting in the delivery of a healthy, 3275-g male infant. Height, weight, and head circumference were in the 75th–90th percentiles. No abnormalities of the kidneys, liver, bone-marrow, or audiometry-evoked potential were found at birth, and the infant's physical and neurologic growth was normal at 19 months of age.

Pancytopenia occurred in a 1000-g male infant who had been exposed to cyclophosphamide and five other antineoplastic agents in the 3rd trimester (14). In a similar case, maternal treatment for leukemia was begun at 12.5 weeks' gestation and eventually included cyclophosphamide, five other antineoplastic agents, and whole brain radiation (25).

A normally developed, premature female infant was delivered at 31 weeks, who subsequently developed transient severe bone marrow hypoplasia in the neonatal period. The myelosuppression was probably caused by mercaptopurine therapy.

In a brief 1997 report, three pregnant women with breast cancer were successfully treated with two or three courses of vinorelbine (20–30 mg/m^2) and fluorouracil (500–750 mg/m^2) at 24, 28, and 29 weeks' gestation, respectively (33). Delivery occurred at 34, 41, and 37 weeks' gestation, respectively. One patient also required six courses of epidoxorubicin and cyclophosphamide. Her infant developed transient anemia at 21 days of age that resolved spontaneously. No adverse effects were observed in the other two newborns. All three infants were developing normally at about 2–3 years of age (33).

A 1999 report from France described the outcomes of pregnancies in 20 women with breast cancer who were treated with antineoplastic agents (34). The first cycle of chemotherapy occurred at a mean gestational age of 26 weeks with delivery occurring at a mean 34.7 weeks. A total of 38 cycles were administered during pregnancy with a median of two cycles per woman. None of the women received radiation therapy during pregnancy. The pregnancy outcomes included two spontaneous abortions (SABs) (both exposed in the 1st trimester), one intrauterine death (exposed in the 2nd trimester), and 17 live births, one of whom died at 8 days of age without apparent cause. The 16 surviving children were developing normally at a mean follow-up of 42.3 months (34). Cyclophosphamide (C), in combination with various other agents (doxorubicin [D], epirubicin [E], fluorouracil [F], or mitoxantrone [M]) was administered to 13 of the women at a mean dose of 600 mg/m^2 (range 300–1200 mg/m^2). The outcomes were one SAB (CEF; 1st trimester), one stillbirth (one cycle of CE at 23 weeks'), one neonatal death (one cycle of CEF 32 days before birth), and 11 surviving liveborn infants (one CE, six CEF, two CDF, and two CFM; all in the 3rd trimester). One of the infants who had been exposed to two cycles of CEF, with the second exposure at 25 days before birth, had transient leukopenia and another was growth retarded (1460-g, born at 33 weeks' gestation after two cycles of CFM) (34).

Data from one review indicated that 40% of the patients exposed to anticancer drugs during pregnancy delivered low-birth-weight infants (35). This finding was not related to the timing of exposure. Use of cyclophosphamide in the 2nd and 3rd trimesters does not seem to place the fetus at risk for congenital defects. Except in a few individual cases, long-term studies of growth and mental development in offspring exposed to cyclophosphamide during the 2nd trimester, the period of neuroblast multiplication, have not been conducted (36).

Cyclophosphamide is one of the most common causes of chemotherapy-induced menstrual difficulties and azoospermia (37–45). Permanent secondary amenorrhea with evidence of primary ovarian damage has been observed after long-term (20 months) use of cyclophosphamide (45). In contrast, successful pregnancies have been reported following high-dose therapy (39,40,46–50). Moreover, azoospermia appears to be reversible when the drug is stopped (41–44,51).

One report associated paternal use of cyclophosphamide and three other antineoplastics prior to conception with congenital anomalies in an infant (52). Defects in the infant included syndactyly of the first and second digits of the right foot and tetralogy of Fallot. In a group of men treated over a minimum of 3.5 years with multiple chemotherapy for acute lymphocytic leukemia, one man fathered a normal child while a second fathered two children, one with multiple anomalies (53). Any relationship between these outcomes and paternal use of cyclophosphamide is doubtful because of the lack of experimental evidence and confirming reports.

Cyclophosphamide-induced chromosomal abnormalities are also of doubtful clinical significance but have been described in some patients after use of the drug. A study published in 1974 reported chromosome abnormalities in patients treated with cyclophosphamide for rheumatoid arthritis and scleroderma (54). In contrast, chromosomal studies were normal in a mother and infant treated during the 2nd and 3rd trimesters in another report (16). In another case, a 34-year-old woman with acute lymphoblastic leukemia was treated with multiple antineoplastic agents from 22 weeks' gestation until delivery of a healthy female infant 18 weeks later (22). Cyclophosphamide was administered three times between the 26th and 30th weeks of gestation. Chromosomal analysis of the newborn revealed a normal karyotype (46,XX), but with gaps and a ring chromosome. The clinical significance of these findings is unknown, but because these abnormalities may persist for several years, the potential existed for an increased risk of cancer, as well as for a risk of genetic damage in the next generation (22).

The long-term effects of cyclophosphamide on female and male reproductive function have been reported (55,56). In a 1988 publication, 40 women who had been treated with combination chemotherapy for malignant ovarian germ cell tumors (median age at diagnosis 15 years; range 6–29 years) were evaluated approximately 10 years later (median age 25.5 years; range 14–40 years) (55). Cyclophosphamide had been used in 33 (83%) of the women. Menstrual function in these women after chemotherapy was as follows: premenarchal ($N = 1$), regular menses ($N = 27$), irregular menses ($N = 5$), oligomenorrhea ($N = 2$), amenorrhea ($N = 4$), and premature menopause ($N = 1$). Of the 12 women with menstrual difficulties, only 3 were considered serious or persistent. Evaluation of the reproductive status after chemotherapy revealed that 24 women had not attempted to become pregnant, 9 had problem-free conceptions, 3 had initial infertility followed by conceptions, and 4 had chronic infertility. Of the 12 women who had conceived on one or more occasions, 1 had an elective abortion at 10 weeks' gestation, and 11 had delivered 22 healthy infants, although 1 had amelogenesis imperfecta.

A study published in 1985 examined 30 men to determine the effect of cyclophosphamide on male hormone levels and spermatogenesis (56). The men had been treated at a mean age of 9.4 years for a mean duration of 280 days. The mean age of the men at the time of the study was 22 years with a mean interval from end of treatment to evaluation of 12.8 years. Four of the men were azoospermic, 9 were oligospermic, and 17 were normospermic. Compared to normal controls, however, the 17 men classified as normospermic had lower ejaculate volumes (3.1 mL vs. 3.3 mL), lower sperm density (54.5×10^6/mL vs. 79×10^6/mL), decreased sperm motility (42% vs. 61%, $p < 0.05$), and less normal sperm forms (61% vs. 70%, $p < 0.05$). Concentrations of testosterone, dehydroepiandrosterone sulfate, and prolactin were not significantly different between patients and controls. One oligospermic man (sperm density 12×10^6/mL) had fathered a child.

The effect of occupational exposure to antineoplastic agents on pregnancy outcome was examined in a 1985 case-control study involving 124 nurses in 17 Finnish hospitals who were compared to 321 matched controls (57). The cases involved nurses working in 1979 and 1980 in hospitals that used at least 100 g of cyclophosphamide (the most commonly administered antineoplastic agent in Finland) per year or at least 200 g of all antineoplastic drugs per year. The average total antineoplastic drug use for all hospitals was 1,898 g, but a lower total use, 887 g, occurred for intravenous drugs (58). Moreover, the nurses had to be 40 years of age or younger in 1980 and had to work in patient areas where antineoplastic agents were mixed and administered (57). The agents were prepared without the use of vertical-airflow biologic-safety hoods or protective clothing (58). Exposure to these agents during the 1st trimester was significantly associated with early fetal loss (odds ratio [OR] 2.30, 95% confidence interval [CI] 1.20–4.39) ($p = 0.01$) (57). Cyclophosphamide, one of four individual antineoplastic agents to which at least 10 women had been exposed, had an OR for fetal loss of 2.66 (95% CI 1.25–5.71). Other significant associations were found for doxorubicin (OR 3.96, 95% CI 1.31–11.97) and vincristine (OR 2.46, 95% CI 1.13–5.37). The association between fluorouracil and fetal loss (OR 1.70, 95% CI 0.55–5.21) was not significant. Based on the results of their study and data from previous studies, the investigators concluded that nursing personnel should exercise caution in handling these agents (57).

Although there is no current consensus on the danger posed to pregnant women from the handling of antineoplastic agents (e.g., the above study generated several letters that questioned the observed association [59–62]), pharmacy and nursing personnel should take precautions to avoid exposure to these potent agents. The National Study Commission on Cytotoxic Exposure published a position statement on this topic in January 1987 (63). Because of the importance of this issue, the statement is quoted in its entirety below:

> *The Handling of Cytotoxic Agents by Women Who Are Pregnant, Attempting to Conceive, or Breast Feeding*
>
> There are substantial data regarding the mutagenic, teratogenic and abortifacient properties of certain cytotoxic agents both in animals and humans who have received therapeutic doses of these agents. Additionally, the scientific literature suggests a possible association of occupational exposure to certain cytotoxic agents during the first trimester of pregnancy with fetal loss or malformation. These data suggest the need for caution when women who are pregnant or attempting to conceive, handle cytotoxic agents. Incidentally, there is no evidence relating male exposure to cytotoxic agents with adverse fetal outcome.
>
> There are no studies which address the possible risk associated with the occupational exposure to cytotoxic agents and the passage of these agents into breast milk. Nevertheless, it is prudent that women who are breast feeding should exercise caution in handling cytotoxic agents.
>
> If all procedures for safe handling, such as those recommended by the Commission are complied with, the potential for exposure will be minimized.
>
> Personnel should be provided with information to make an individual decision. This information should be provided in written form and it is advisable that a statement of understanding be signed.
>
> It is essential to refer to individual state right-to-know laws to insure compliance.

BREAST FEEDING SUMMARY

RECOMMENDATION: Contraindicated

Cyclophosphamide is excreted into breast milk (64). Although the concentrations were not specified, the drug was found in milk up to 6 hours after a single 500-mg IV dose. The mother was not nursing. A brief 1977 correspondence from investigators in New Guinea described neutropenia in a breast-fed infant whose mother received weekly injections of 800 mg of cyclophosphamide, 2 mg of vincristine, and 30-mg daily oral doses of prednisolone for 6 weeks (65). Absolute neutropenia was present 9 days after breast-feeding had been stopped, which persisted for at least 12 days (65). Serial determinations of the infant's white cell and neutrophil counts were begun 2 days after the last exposure to breast milk. The lowest measured absolute lymphocyte count was 4750/μL. Except for the neutropenia and a brief episode of diarrhea, no other adverse effects were observed in the infant.

A 1979 report involved a case of an 18-year-old woman with Burkitt's lymphoma diagnosed in the 26th week of gestation (66). She was treated with a 7-day course of cyclophosphamide, 10 mg/kg IV, as a single daily dose (total dose 3.5 g). Six weeks after the last chemotherapy dose, she delivered a normal, 2160-g male infant. Analysis of the newborn's blood counts was not conducted. The tumor recurred in the postpartum period and treatment with cyclophosphamide, 6 mg/kg/day IV, was started 20 days after delivery. Although she was advised not to nurse her infant, she continued to do so until her sudden death after the third dose of cyclophosphamide. Blood counts were conducted on both the mother and the infant during therapy. Immediately prior to the first dose, the infant's leukocyte and platelet counts were 4800/mm^3 (abnormally low for age) and 270,000/mm^3, respectively. After the third maternal dose, the infant's counts were 3200/mm^3 and 47,000/mm^3, respectively. Both counts were interpreted by the investigator as signs of cyclophosphamide-induced toxicity. It was concluded that breast-feeding should be stopped during therapy with the agent (66).

The American Academy of Pediatrics classifies cyclophosphamide as a drug that may interfere with cellular metabolism of the nursing infant (67). Because of the reported cases of neutropenia and thrombocytopenia, and the potential for adverse effects relating to immune suppression, growth, and carcinogenesis, women receiving this drug should not nurse.

References

1. Greenberg LH, Tanaka KR. Congenital anomalies probably induced by cyclophosphamide. JAMA 1964;188:423–6.
2. Toledo TM, Harper RC, Moser RH. Fetal effects during cyclophosphamide and irradiation therapy. Ann Intern Med 1971;74:87–91.
3. Coates A. Cyclophosphamide in pregnancy. Aust N Z J Obstet Gynaecol 1970;10:33–4.
4. Murray CL, Reichert JA, Anderson J, Twiggs LB. Multimodal cancer therapy for breast cancer in the first trimester of pregnancy. JAMA 1984;252:2607–8.
5. Sweet DL, Kinzie J. Consequences of radiotherapy and antineoplastic therapy for the fetus. J Reprod Med 1976;17:241–6.
6. Kirshon B, Wasserstrum N, Willis R, Herman GE, McCabe ERB. Teratogenic effects of first-trimester cyclophosphamide therapy. Obstet Gynecol 1988;72:462–4.
7. Zemlickis D, Lishner M, Erlich R, Koren G. Teratogenicity and carcinogenicity in a twin exposed in utero to cyclophosphamide. Teratog Carcinog Mutagen 1993;13:139–43.
8. Enns GM, Roeder E, Chan RT, Catts ZA-K, Cox VA, Golabi M. Apparent cyclophosphamide (Cytoxan) embryopathy: a distinct phenotype? Am J Med Genet 1999;86:237–41.
9. Lasher MJ, Geller W. Cyclophosphamide and vinblastine sulfate in Hodgkin's disease during pregnancy. JAMA 1966;195:486–8.
10. Lergier JE, Jimenez E, Maldonado N, Veray F. Normal pregnancy in multiple myeloma treated with cyclophosphamide. Cancer 1974;34:1018–22.
11. Garcia V, San Miguel J, Borrasca AL. Doxorubicin in the first trimester of pregnancy. Ann Intern Med 1981;94:547.
12. Lowenthal RM, Funnell CF, Hope DM, Stewart IG, Humphrey DC. Normal infant after combination chemotherapy including teniposide for Burkitt's lymphoma in pregnancy. Med Pediatr Oncol 1982;10:165–9.
13. Daly H, McCann SR, Hanratty TD, Temperley IJ. Successful pregnancy during combination chemotherapy for Hodgkin's disease. Acta Haematol 1980;64:154–6.
14. Pizzuto J, Aviles A, Noriega L, Niz J, Morales M, Romero F. Treatment of acute leukemia during pregnancy: presentation of nine cases. Cancer Treat Rep 1980;64:679–83.
15. Sears HF, Reid J. Granulocytic sarcoma: local presentation of a systemic disease. Cancer 1976;37:1808–13.
16. Falkson HC, Simson IW, Falkson G. Non-Hodgkin's lymphoma in pregnancy. Cancer 1980;45:1679–82.
17. Webb GA. The use of hyperalimentation and chemotherapy in pregnancy: a case report. Am J Obstet Gynecol 1980;137:263–6.
18. Gililland J, Weinstein L. The effects of cancer chemotherapeutic agents on the developing fetus. Obstet Gynecol Surv 1983;38:6–13.
19. Weed JC Jr, Roh RA, Mendenhall HW. Recurrent endodermal sinus tumor during pregnancy. Obstet Gynecol 1979;54:653–6.
20. Kim DS, Park MI. Maternal and fetal survival following surgery and chemotherapy of endodermal sinus tumor of the ovary during pregnancy: a case report. Obstet Gynecol 1989;73:503–7.

21. Malfetano JH, Goldkrand JW. Cis-platinum combination chemotherapy during pregnancy for advanced epithelial ovarian carcinoma. Obstet Gynecol 1990;75:545–7.
22. Schleuning M, Clemm C. Chromosomal aberrations in a newborn whose mother received cytotoxic treatment during pregnancy. N Engl J Med 1987;317: 1666–7.
23. Haerr RW, Pratt AT. Multiagent chemotherapy for sarcoma diagnosed during pregnancy. Cancer 1985;56: 1028–33.
24. Turchi JJ, Villasis C. Anthracyclines in the treatment of malignancy in pregnancy. Cancer 1988;61: 435–40.
25. Okun DB, Groncy PK, Sieger L, Tanaka KR. Acute leukemia in pregnancy: transient neonatal myelosuppression after combination chemotherapy in the mother. Med Pediatr Oncol 1979;7:315–9.
26. Ortega J. Multiple agent chemotherapy including bleomycin of non-Hodgkin's lymphoma during pregnancy. Cancer 1977;40:2829–35.
27. Hardin JA. Cyclophosphamide treatment of lymphoma during third trimester of pregnancy. Obstet Gynecol 1972;39:850–1.
28. Khurshid M, Saleem M. Acute leukaemia in pregnancy. Lancet 1978;2:534–5.
29. Yankowitz J, Kuller JA, Thomas RL. Pregnancy complicated by Goodpasture syndrome. Obstet Gynecol 1992;79:806–8.
30. Barry C, Davis S, Garrard P, Ferguson IT. Churg-Strauss disease: deterioration in a twin pregnancy. Successful outcome following treatment with corticosteroids and cyclophosphamide. Br J Obstet Gynaecol 1997;104:746–7.
31. Mavrommatis CG, Daskalakis GJ, Papageorgiou IS, Antsaklis AJ, Michalas SK. Non-Hodgkin's lymphoma during pregnancy—case report. Eur J Obstet Gynecol Reprod Biol 1998;79:95–7.
32. Dayoan ES, Dimen LL, Boylen CT. Successful treatment of Wegener's granulomatosis during pregnancy. A case report and review of the medical literature. Chest 1998;113:836–8.
33. Cuvier C, Espie M, Extra JM, Marty M. Vinorelbine in pregnancy. Eur J Cancer 1997;33:168–9.
34. Giacalone PL, Laffargue F, Benos P. Chemotherapy for breast carcinoma during pregnancy. Cancer 1999;86:2266–72.
35. Nicholson HO. Cytotoxic drugs in pregnancy: review of reported cases. J Obstet Gynaecol Br Commonw 1968;75:307–12.
36. Dobbing J. Pregnancy and leukaemia. Lancet 1977;1:1155.
37. Schilsky RL, Lewis BJ, Sherins RJ, Young RC. Gonadal dysfunction in patients receiving chemotherapy for cancer. Ann Intern Med 1980;93:109–14.
38. Stewart BH. Drugs that cause and cure male infertility. Drug Ther 1975;5:42–8.
39. Schwartz PE, Vidone RA. Pregnancy following combination chemotherapy for a mixed germ cell tumor of the ovary. Gynecol Oncol 1981;12:373–8.
40. Bacon C, Kernahan J. Successful pregnancy in acute leukaemia. Lancet 1975;2:515.
41. Qureshji MA, Pennington JH, Goldsmith HJ, Cox PE. Cyclophosphamide therapy and sterility. Lancet 1972;2:1290–1.
42. George CRP, Evans RA. Cyclophosphamide and infertility. Lancet 1972;1:840–1.
43. Sherins RJ, DeVita VT Jr. Effect of drug treatment for lymphoma on male reproductive capacity. Ann Intern Med 1973;79:216–20.
44. Lendon M, Palmer MK, Hann IM, Shalet SM, Jones PHM. Testicular histology after combination chemotherapy in childhood for acute lymphoblastic leukaemia. Lancet 1978;2:439–41.
45. Uldall PR, Feest TG, Morley AR, Tomlinson BE, Kerr DNS. Cyclophosphamide therapy in adults with minimal-change nephrotic syndrome. Lancet 1972;2: 1250–3.
46. Card RT, Holmes IH, Sugarman RG, Storb R, Thomas D. Successful pregnancy after high dose chemotherapy and marrow transplantation for treatment of aplastic anemia. Exp Hematol 1980;8:57–60.
47. Deeg HJ, Kennedy MS, Sanders JE, Thomas ED, Storb R. Successful pregnancy after marrow transplantation for severe aplastic anemia and immunosuppression with cyclosporine. JAMA 1983;250:647.
48. Javaheri G, Lifchez A, Valle J. Pregnancy following removal of and long-term chemotherapy for ovarian malignant teratoma. Obstet Gynecol 1983;61:8S–9S.
49. Rustin GJS, Booth M, Dent J, Salt S, Rustin F, Bagshawe KD. Pregnancy after cytotoxic chemotherapy for gestational trophoblastic tumours. Br Med J 1984;288:103–6.
50. Lee RB, Kelly J, Ely SA, Benson WL. Pregnancy following conservative surgery and adjunctive chemotherapy for stage III immature teratoma of the ovary. Obstet Gynecol 1989;73:853–5.
51. Hinkes E, Plotkin D. Reversible drug-induced sterility in a patient with acute leukemia. JAMA 1973;223: 1490–1.
52. Russell JA, Powles RL, Oliver RTD. Conception and congenital abnormalities after chemotherapy of acute myelogenous leukaemia in two men. Br Med J 1976;1:1508.
53. Evenson DP, Arlin Z, Welt S, Claps ML, Melamed MR. Male reproductive capacity may recover following drug treatment with the L-10 protocol for acute lymphocytic leukemia. Cancer 1984;53:30–6.
54. Tolchin SF, Winkelstein A, Rodnan GP, Pan SF, Nankin HR. Chromosome abnormalities from cyclophosphamide therapy in rheumatoid arthritis and progressive systemic sclerosis (scleroderma). Arthritis Rheum 1974;17:375–82.
55. Gershenson DM. Menstrual and reproductive function after treatment with combination chemotherapy for malignant ovarian germ cell tumors. J Clin Oncol 1988;6:270–5.
56. Watson AR, Rance CP, Bain J. Long term effects of cyclophosphamide on testicular function. Br Med J 1985;291:1457–60.
57. Selevan SG, Lindbohm M-L, Hornung RW, Hemminki K. A study of occupational exposure to antineoplastic drugs and fetal loss in nurses. N Engl J Med 1985;313:1173–8.
58. Selevan SG, Hornung RW. Antineoplastic drugs and spontaneous abortion in nurses. N Engl J Med 1986; 314:1050–1.
59. Kalter H. Antineoplastic drugs and spontaneous abortion in nurses. N Engl J Med 1986;314:1048–9.
60. Mulvihill JJ, Stewart KR. Antineoplastic drugs and

C

spontaneous abortion in nurses. N Engl J Med 1986;314:1049.
61. Chabner BA. Antineoplastic drugs and spontaneous abortion in nurses. N Engl J Med 1986;314:1049–50.
62. Zellmer WA. Antineoplastic drugs and spontaneous abortion in nurses. N Engl J Med 1986;314:1050.
63. Jeffrey LP, Chairman, National Study Commission on Cytotoxic Exposure. Position statement. The handling of cytotoxic agents by women who are pregnant, attempting to conceive, or breast feeding. January 12, 1987.
64. Wiernik PH, Duncan JH. Cyclophosphamide in human milk. Lancet 1971;1:912.
65. Amato D, Niblett JS. Neutropenia from cyclophosphamide in breast milk. Med J Aust 1977;1:383–4.
66. Durodola JI. Administration of cyclophosphamide during late pregnancy and early lactation: a case report. J Natl Med Assoc 1979;71:165–6.
67. Committee on Drugs, American Academy of Pediatrics. The transfer of drugs and other chemicals into human milk. Pediatrics 2001;108:776–89.

Name: **CYCLOSERINE** Risk Factor: **C_M**

Class: **Antituberculosis Agent**

FETAL RISK SUMMARY

RECOMMENDATION: Limited Human Data - Animal Data Suggest Moderate Risk

Cycloserine is a broad-spectrum antibiotic used primarily for active pulmonary and extrapulmonary tuberculosis. No teratogenic effects were observed in rats given doses up to 100 mg/kg/day through two generations (1).

The Collaborative Perinatal Project monitored 50,282 mother-child pairs, 3 of whom had 1st trimester exposure to cycloserine (2). No evidence of adverse fetal effects was suggested by the data. The American Thoracic Society recommends avoidance of cycloserine during pregnancy, if possible, because of the lack of information on the fetal effects of the drug (3).

BREAST FEEDING SUMMARY

RECOMMENDATION: Limited Human Data - Probably Compatible

Cycloserine is excreted into breast milk. Milk concentrations in four lactating women taking 250-mg of the drug four times daily ranged from 6 to 19 μg/mL, an average of 72% of serum levels (4). Approximately 0.6% of the mother's daily dose was estimated to be in the milk (5). No adverse effects were observed in the nursing infants (4). The American Academy of Pediatrics classifies cycloserine as compatible with breast-feeding (6).

References

1. Product information. Seromycin. Dura Pharmaceuticals, 2000.
2. Heinonen OP, Slone D, Shapiro S. *Birth Defects and Drugs in Pregnancy*. Littleton, MA: Publishing Sciences Group, 1977:297.
3. American Thoracic Society. Medical Section of the American Lung Association: Treatment of tuberculosis and tuberculosis infection in adults and children. Am Rev Respir Dis 1986;134:355–63.
4. Morton RF, McKenna MH, Charles E. Studies on the absorption, diffusion, and excretion of cycloserine. Antibiot Annu 1955–1956;3:169–72. As cited by Snider DE Jr, Powell KE. Should women taking antituberculosis drugs breast-feed? Arch Intern Med 1984;144:589–90.
5. Vorherr H. Drug excretion in breast milk. Postgrad Med 1974;56:97–104. As cited by Snider DE Jr, Powell KE. Should women taking antituberculosis drugs breast-feed? Arch Intern Med 1984;144:589–90.
6. Committee on Drugs, American Academy of Pediatrics. The transfer of drugs and other chemicals into human milk. Pediatrics 2001;108:776–89.

Name:	**CYCLOSPORINE**	Risk Factor:	**C_M**
Class:	**Immunologic Agent (Immunosuppressant)**		

FETAL RISK SUMMARY

RECOMMENDATION: Limited Human Data - Animal Data Suggest Risk

Cyclosporine (cyclosporin A), an antibiotic produced by certain fungi, is used as an immunosuppressive agent to prevent rejection of kidney, liver, or heart allografts.

In reproduction studies, cyclosporine produced embryo and fetal toxicity only at maternally toxic dose levels in rats (0.8 times the human transplant dose of 6 mg/kg corrected for body surface area) and in rabbits (5.4 times the human dose) (1). Toxic effects included increased pre- and postnatal mortality, and reduced fetal weight and related skeletal retardation. No teratogenic effects were observed.

Cyclosporine readily crosses the placenta to the fetus (2–6). In a 1983 study, the cord blood:maternal plasma ratio at delivery was 0.63 (2). In a second study, cord blood and amniotic fluid levels 8 hours after a 325 mg dose were 57 and 234 ng/mL, respectively (3). Concentrations in the newborn fell to 14 ng/mL at 14 hours and were undetectable (<4 ng/mL) at 7 days. Cord blood:maternal plasma ratios in twins delivered at 35 weeks' gestation were 0.35 and 0.57, respectively (4). A similar ratio of 0.40 was reported in a case delivered at 31 weeks' gestation (5).

Several case reports describing the use of cyclosporine throughout gestation have been published (2–13). Maternal doses ranged between 260 and 550 mg/day (2–4,7,9,10,13). Cases usually involved maternal renal transplantation (2–4,6–12), but one report described a successful pregnancy in a woman after heart transplantation (5), one involved a combined transplant of a kidney and paratrophic segmental pancreas in a diabetic woman (10), and one involved a patient with a liver transplant (13). In addition, a report has described a successful pregnancy in a woman with aplastic anemia who was treated with bone marrow transplantation (14). In this case, however, cyclosporine therapy had been stopped prior to conception. Guidelines for counseling heart transplant patients who wish to become pregnant have been published (15).

As of October 1987, the manufacturer had knowledge of 34 pregnancies involving cyclosporine (A. Poploski and D. A. Colasante, personal communication, Sandoz Pharmaceuticals Corporation, 1987) (15). Some of these cases are described above. These pregnancies resulted in six abortions (one after early detection of anencephaly, three elective, and two spontaneous abortions, one at 20 weeks' gestation), one pregnancy that was still ongoing, and 27 live births. One of the newborns died at age 3 days. Autopsy revealed a complete absence of the corpus callosum. Other problems observed in individual newborns exposed *in utero* to cyclosporine were thrombocytopenia (thought to be caused by hydralazine taken by the mother for hypertension) (7); a hydrocele that resolved spontaneously (9); asphyxia and intracerebral bleeding in an extremely premature infant (A. Poploski and D. A. Colasante, personal communication, 1987); physiologic jaundice (A. Poploski and D. A. Colasante, personal communication); leukopenia (4) (A. Poploski and D. A. Colasante, personal communication, 1987); hypoglycemia and mild disseminated intravascular coagulation that resolved spontaneously (A. Poploski and D. A. Colasante, personal communication, 1987); and bilateral cataracts (A. Poploski and D. A. Colasante, personal communication, 1987). A 1989 case report described an infant with hypoplasia of the right leg and foot after *in utero* exposure to cyclosporine (11). The right leg was 2 cm shorter than the left. Hypoplasia of the muscles and subcutaneous tissue of the right leg was also present. The authors proposed a possible mechanism for the defect, which involved cyclosporine inhibition of lymphocytic interleukin-2 release and subsequent interference with the differentiation of osteoclasts (11).

Many of the liveborn infants were growth retarded (3,7,9–13). Birth weights of full-term newborns ranged from 2160–3200 g (12,13) (A. Poploski and D. A. Colasante, personal communication, 1987). A 1985 review article observed that growth retardation was common in the offspring of renal transplant patients, occurring in 8%–45% of reported pregnancies (16). Although the specific cause of the diminished growth could not be determined, the most likely processes involved were considered to be maternal hypertension, renal function, and immunosuppressive drugs (16).

Followup of children exposed *in utero* to cyclosporine has been conducted in a few cases (4,10) (A. Poploski and D. A. Colasante, personal communication, 1987). In 15 of 27 surviving neonates, early postnatal development was normal except for one infant with slight growth retardation (4,10) (A. Poploski and D. A. Colasante, personal communication, 1987). Postnatal development of 10 children followed from 1–13 months revealed normal physical and mental development (4,10) (A. Poploski and D. A. Colasante, personal communication, 1987). No abnormal renal or liver function has been reported in the exposed newborns.

In summary, based on relatively small numbers, the use of cyclosporine during pregnancy apparently does not pose a major risk to the fetus. Cyclosporine is not an animal teratogen (1,17), and the limited experience in women indicates that it is unlikely to be a human teratogen. No pattern of defects has emerged in the few newborns with anomalies. Skeletal defects, other than the single case of osseous malformation, have not been observed. The disease process itself, for which cyclosporine is indicated, makes these pregnancies high risk and subject to numerous potential problems, of which the most common is growth retardation. This latter problem is probably related to the mother's disease rather than to her drug therapy, but a contribution from cyclosporine and corticosteroids cannot be excluded. Long-term followup studies are warranted, however, to detect latent effects including those in subsequent generations. If cyclosporine is used in pregnancy for the treatment of rheumatoid arthritis, health care professionals are encouraged to call the toll free number (877–311–8972) for information about patient enrollment in the OTIS Rheumatoid Arthritis study.

BREAST FEEDING SUMMARY

RECOMMENDATION: Limited Human Data - Potential Toxicity

Cyclosporine is excreted into breast milk. In a patient taking 450 mg of cyclosporine/day, milk levels on postpartum days 2, 3, and 4 were 101, 109, and 263 ng/mL, respectively (2). No details were given about the relationship of maternal doses with these levels. In another patient, milk concentrations 22 hours after a dose of 325 mg were 16 ng/mL, whereas maternal blood levels were 52 ng/mL, a milk:plasma ratio of 0.31 (3). A milk:plasma ratio of 0.40 was reported in one study (5) and a ratio of approximately 0.17 was measured in another (6). Breast-feeding was not allowed in any of these studies and has been actively discouraged by most sources because of concerns for potential toxicity in the nursing infant (12,13,15,17) (A. Poploski and D. A. Colasante, personal communication, 1987).

A 2001 study reported the use of cyclosporin in a woman who was breast-feeding (18). The woman had a simultaneous kidney-pancreas transplant 13 months before conception. She was treated before, during, and after pregnancy with cyclosporine (300 mg twice daily), azathioprine (100 mg/day), and prednisone (10 mg/day). At 34 weeks' gestation, she delivered an 1800-g male infant with Apgar scores of 5 and 8 at 1 and 5 minutes, respectively. Mild hyperbilirubinemia, treated with phototherapy, was the infant's only complication. The mother's cyclosporine levels during pregnancy were 75–173 ng/mL (therapeutic range 100–125 ng/mL in whole blood) but were not determined at birth. The cord blood cyclosporine concentration was 67 ng/mL. Breast-feeding was initiated 2 hours after birth and continued exclusively for the first 10.5 months of life. Random cyclosporine levels in the infant's serum were <25 ng/mL at approximately 1, 1.5, 2.5, 4, and 10.5 months of age. Maternal serum cyclosporine levels at approximately 1, 1.5, and 2.5 months were 193, 273, and 123 ng/mL, respectively, and breast milk levels were 160, 286, and 79 ng/mL, respectively. No adverse effects from exposure to cyclosporine were observed in the infant. At 12 months of age, his weight and height were at the 46th and 55th percentile, respectively. The mother subsequently delivered a second child that was also breast-fed (18).

In a 2003 report, infant cyclosporine exposure was quantified in five mother-infant pairs (19). The five mothers had taken cyclosporine throughout pregnancy and continued the drug while nursing their infants. In two cases, the milk:maternal blood ratios were 0.45 and 1.4 (not specified in the other three cases). In the latter case, the infant's dose from milk was about 1% of the therapeutic dose (weight basis). The infant's blood levels were as high as 78% of the corresponding maternal trough concentrations that were in the therapeutic range. Cyclosporine was not detected in the blood of three other infants (not tested in one infant). In the five cases, the estimated infant dose from milk, based on a milk consumption of 150 mL/kg/day, ranged from 0.2% to 2.1% of the mother's weight-adjusted dose. No adverse effects in the infants were observed, but specific immunologic effects were not investigated (19).

The American Academy of Pediatrics classifies cyclosporine as a drug that may interfere with cellular metabolism in the nursing infant (20).

References

1. Product information. Neoral. Novartis Pharmaceuticals, 2000.
2. Lewis GJ, Lamont CAR, Lee HA, Slapak M. Successful pregnancy in a renal transplant recipient taking cyclosporin A. Br Med J 1983;286:603.
3. Flechner SM, Katz AR, Rogers AJ, Van Buren C, Kahan BD. The presence of cyclosporine in body tissues and fluids during pregnancy. Am J Kidney Dis 1985;5:60–3.
4. Burrows DA, O'Neil TJ, Sorrells TL. Successful twin pregnancy after renal transplant maintained on cyclosporine A immunosuppression. Obstet Gynecol 1988;72:459–61.
5. Lowenstein BR, Vain NW, Perrone SV, Wright DR, Boullon FJ, Favaloro RG. Successful pregnancy and vaginal delivery after heart transplantation. Am J Obstet Gynecol 1988;158:589–90.
6. Ziegenhagen DJ, Grombach G, Dieckmann M, Zehnter E, Wienand P, Baldamus CA. Pregnancy under cyclosporine administration after renal transplantation. Dtsch Med Wochenschr 1988;113:260–3.
7. Klintmalm G, Althoff P, Appleby G, Segerbrandt E. Renal function in a newborn baby delivered of a renal transplant patient taking cyclosporine. Transplantation 1984;38:198–9.
8. Grischke E, Kaufmann M, Dreikorn K, Linderkamp O, Kubli F. Successful pregnancy after kidney transplantation and cyclosporin A. Geburtshilfe Frauenheilkd 1986;46:176–9.
9. Pikrell MD, Sawers R, Michael J. Pregnancy after renal transplantation: severe intrauterine growth retardation during treatment with cyclosporin A. BMJ 1988;296:825.
10. Calne RY, Brons IGM, Williams PF, Evans DB, Robinson RE, Dossa M. Successful pregnancy after paratrophic segmental pancreas and kidney transplantation. BMJ 1988;296:1709.
11. Pujals JM, Figueras G, Puig JM, Lloveras J, Aubia J, Masramon J. Osseous malformation in baby born to woman on cyclosporin. Lancet 1989;1:667.
12. Al-Khader AA, Absy M, Al-Hasani MK, Joyce B, Sabbagh T. Successful pregnancy in renal transplant recipients treated with cyclosporine. Transplantation 1988;45:987–8.
13. Sims CJ, Porter KB, Knuppel RA. Successful pregnancy after a liver transplant. Am J Obstet Gynecol 1989;161:532–3.

14. Deeg HJ, Kennedy MS, Sanders JE, Thomas ED, Storb R. Successful pregnancy after marrow transplantation for severe aplastic anemia and immunosuppression with cyclosporine. JAMA 1983;250:647.
15. Kossoy LR, Herbert CM III, Wentz AC. Management of heart transplant recipients: guidelines for the obstetrician - gynecologist. Am J Obstet Gynecol 1988;159:490–9.
16. Lau RJ, Scott JR. Pregnancy following renal transplantation. Clin Obstet Gynecol 1985;28:339–50.
17. Product information. Sandimmune. Sandoz Pharmaceutical Corporation, 1986.
18. Thiagarajan (Munoz-Flores) KD, Easterling T, Davis C, Bond EF. Breast-feeding by a cyclosporin-treated mother. Obstet Gynecol 2001;97:816–8.
19. Moretti ME, Sgro M, Johnson DW, Sauve RS, Woolgar MJ, Taddio A, Verjee Z, Giesbrecht E, Koren G, Ito S. Cyclosporin excretion into breast milk. Transplantation 2003;75:2144–6.
20. Committee on Drugs, American Academy of Pediatrics. The transfer of drugs and other chemicals into human milk. Pediatrics 2001;108:776–89.

Name:	**CYCLOTHIAZIDE**	Risk Factor:	**C***
Class:	**Diuretic**		

See Chlorothiazide.

[**Risk Factor D if used in gestational hypertension.*]

Name:	**CYCRIMINE**	Risk Factor:	**C**
Class:	**Parasympatholytic**		

FETAL RISK SUMMARY

RECOMMENDATION: No Human Data - No Relevant Animal Data

Cycrimine is an anticholinergic agent used in the treatment of parkinsonism. No reports of its use in pregnancy have been located (see Atropine).

BREAST FEEDING SUMMARY

RECOMMENDATION: No Human Data - Probably Compatible

No data are available (see Atropine).

Name:	**CYPROHEPTADINE**	Risk Factor:	**B_M**
Class:	**Antihistamine/Antiserotonin**		

FETAL RISK SUMMARY

RECOMMENDATION: Limited Human Data - Animal Data Suggest Low Risk

Cyproheptadine has been used as a serotonin antagonist to prevent habitual abortion in patients with increased serotonin production (1,2). No congenital defects were observed when the drug was used for this purpose.

Reproductive studies in mice, rats, and rabbits with oral or SC doses up to 32 times the maximum recommended human dose found no evidence of impaired fertility or fetal harm (3,4). In contrast, Shepard cited a 1982 study that observed dose-related fetotoxicity characterized by skeletal retardation, hydronephrosis, liver and brain toxicity, and increased mortality in fetuses of rats administered 2–50 mg/kg/day intraperitoneally during organogenesis (5).

Two patients, who were being treated with cyproheptadine for Cushing's syndrome, conceived while taking the drug (6,7). Therapy was stopped at 3 months in one patient but continued throughout gestation in the second. Apparently healthy infants were delivered prematurely (33–34 weeks and 36 weeks) from both mothers. Fatal gastroenteritis developed at 4 months of age in the 33–34 week gestational infant who was exposed throughout pregnancy to the drug (6). The use of cyproheptadine to treat a pregnant woman with Cushing's syndrome secondary to bilateral adrenal hyperplasia was described in a 1990 reference (8). Specific details were not provided on the case, except that the fetus was delivered prematurely at 33 weeks' gestation. In a separate case, a woman with Cushing's was successfully treated with cyproheptadine; 2 years after stopping the drug, she conceived and eventually delivered a healthy male infant (9).

In a surveillance study of Michigan Medicaid recipients conducted between 1985 and 1992 involving 229,101 completed pregnancies, 285 newborns had been exposed to cyproheptadine during the 1st trimester (F. Rosa, personal communication, FDA, 1993). A total of 12 (4.2%) major birth defects were observed (12 expected), including (observed/expected) 2/3 cardiovascular defects, 2/0.6 oral clefts, and 2/0.7 hypospadias. Only with the latter two defects is there a suggestion of an association, but other factors, including the mother's disease, concurrent drug use, and chance, may be involved. No anomalies were observed in three other categories of anomalies (spina bifida, polydactyly, and limb reduction defects) for which specific data were available.

BREAST FEEDING SUMMARY

RECOMMENDATION: No Human Data - Probably Compatible

No reports describing the use of cyproheptadine during lactation have been located. Chronic use of cyproheptadine will lower serum prolactin levels and it has been used in the management of galactorrhea (10). No studies have been found, however, that evaluated its potential to interfere with the normal lactation process. Because of the increased sensitivity of newborns to antihistamines and the potential for adverse reactions, the manufacturer considers cyproheptadine to be contraindicated in nursing mothers (3).

References

1. Sadovsky E, Pfeifer Y, Polishuk WZ, Sulman FG. A trial of cyproheptadine in habitual abortion. Isr J Med Sci 1972;8:623–5.
2. Sadovsky E, Pfeifer Y, Sadovsky A, Sulman FG. Prevention of hypothalamic habitual abortion by Periactin. Harefuah 1970;78:332–4. As cited in Anonymous. References and reviews. JAMA 1970;212:1253.
3. Product information. Periactin. Merck & Co., 1997.
4. Pfeifer Y, Sadovsky E, Sulman FG. Prevention of serotonin abortion in pregnant rats by five serotonin antagonists. Obstet Gynecol 1969;33:709–14.
5. Shepard TH. *Catalog of Teratogenic Agents*. 8th ed. Baltimore, MD: Johns Hopkins University Press, 1995: 121–2.
6. Kasperlik-Zaluska A, Migdalska B, Hartwig W, Wilczynska J, Marianowski L, Stopinska-Gluszak U, Lozinska D. Two pregnancies in a woman with Cushing's syndrome treated with cyproheptadine. Br J Obstet Gynaecol 1980;87:1171–3.
7. Khir ASM, How J, Bewsher PD. Successful pregnancy after cyproheptadine treatment for Cushing's disease. Eur J Obstet Gynecol Reprod Biol 1982;13:343–7.
8. Aron DC, Schnall AM, Sheeler LR. Cushing's syndrome and pregnancy. Am J Obstet Gynecol 1990;162: 244–52.
9. Griffith DN, Ross EJ. Pregnancy after cyproheptadine treatment for Cushing's disease. N Engl J Med 1981;305:893–4.
10. Wortsman J, Soler NG, Hirschowitz J. Cyproheptadine in the management of the galactorrhea-amenorrhea syndrome. Ann Intern Med 1979;90:923–5.

Name:	**CYTARABINE**	Risk Factor:	D_M
Class:	**Antineoplastic**		

C

FETAL RISK SUMMARY

RECOMMENDATION: Human Data Suggest Risk

Cytarabine is an antineoplastic agent used in the treatment of various types of leukemia. The drug is teratogenic in the hamster and rat (1).

Normal infants have resulted following *in utero* exposure to cytarabine during all stages of gestation (2–27). Follow-up of seven infants exposed *in utero* during the 2nd trimester to cytarabine revealed normal infants at 4–60 months (20,22–26). Two cases of intrauterine fetal death after cytarabine combination treatment have been located (20,23). In one case, maternal treatment for 5 weeks starting at the 15th week of gestation ended in intrauterine death at 20 weeks' gestation of a fetus without abnormalities or leukemic infiltration (20). The second case also involved a woman treated from the 15th week who developed severe pregnancy-induced hypertension at 29 weeks' gestation (23). An apparently normal fetus died 1 week later, most likely as a consequence of the preeclampsia.

Use during the 1st and 2nd trimesters is associated with congenital and chromosomal abnormalities (21,28–30). One leukemic patient treated during the 2nd trimester elected to have an abortion at 24 weeks' gestation (21). The fetus had trisomy for group C autosomes without mosaicism. A second pregnancy in the same patient with identical therapy ended normally. In another case, a 34-year-old woman with acute lymphoblastic leukemia was treated with multiple antineoplastic agents from 22 weeks' gestation until delivery of a healthy female infant 18 weeks later (28). Cytarabine was administered only during the 27th week of gestation. Chromosomal analysis of the newborn revealed a normal karyotype (46,XX), but with gaps and a ring chromosome. The clinical significance of these findings is unknown, but because these abnormalities may persist for several years, the potential existed for an increased risk of cancer as well as for a risk of genetic damage in the next generation (28). Two women, one treated during the 1st trimester and the other treated throughout pregnancy, delivered infants with multiple anomalies:

Bilateral microtia and atresia of external auditory canals, right hand lobster claw with three digits, bilateral lower limb defects (29)

Two medial digits of both feet missing, distal phalanges of both thumbs missing with hypoplastic remnant of the right thumb (30)

Congenital anomalies have also been observed after paternal use of cytarabine plus other antineoplastics prior to conception (31). The investigators suggested that the antineoplastic agents may have damaged the sperm without producing infertility in the two fathers. The relationship between use of the chemotherapy in these men and the defects observed is doubtful because of the lack of experimental evidence and confirming reports. The results of these pregnancies were tetralogy of Fallot, syndactyly of first and second digits of right foot, and a stillborn with anencephaly. Cytarabine may produce reversible azoospermia (32,33). However, male fertility has been demonstrated during maintenance therapy with cytarabine (34).

Pancytopenia was observed in a 1000-g male infant exposed to cytarabine and five other antineoplastic agents during the 3rd trimester (12).

Data from one review indicated that 40% of the mothers exposed to antineoplastic drugs during pregnancy delivered low-birth-weight infants (35). This finding was not related to the timing of exposure. Except for the few cases noted above, long-term studies of growth and mental development in offspring exposed to cytarabine during the 2nd trimester, the period of neuroblast multiplication, have not been conducted (36).

Occupational exposure of the mother to antineoplastic agents during pregnancy may present a risk to the fetus. A position statement from the National Study Commission on Cytotoxic Exposure and a research article involving some antineoplastic agents are presented in the monograph for cyclophosphamide (see Cyclophosphamide).

BREAST FEEDING SUMMARY

RECOMMENDATION: Contraindicated

No reports describing the use of cytarabine during lactation have been located. Because of the potential for serious adverse effects in nursing infants, women receiving this drug should not breast-feed.

References

1. Product information. Cytosar-U. Pharmacia & Upjohn, 2000.
2. Pawliger DF, McLean FW, Noyes WD. Normal fetus after cytosine arabinoside therapy. Ann Intern Med 1971;74:1012.
3. Au-Yong R, Collins P, Young JA. Acute myeloblastic leukemia during pregnancy. Br Med J 1972;4:493–4.
4. Raich PC, Curet LB. Treatment of acute leukemia during pregnancy. Cancer 1975;36:861–2.
5. Gokal R, Durrant J, Baum JD, Bennett MJ. Successful pregnancy in acute monocytic leukaemia. Br J Cancer 1976;34:299–302.
6. Sears HF, Reid J. Granulocytic sarcoma: local presentation of a systemic disease. Cancer 1976;37:1808–13.
7. Durie BGM, Giles HR. Successful treatment of acute leukemia during pregnancy. Arch Intern Med 1977;137:90–1.
8. Lilleyman JS, Hill AS, Anderton KJ. Consequences of acute myelogenous leukemia in early pregnancy. Cancer 1977;40:1300–3.
9. Moreno H, Castleberry RP, McCann WP. Cytosine arabinoside and 6-thioguanine in the treatment of childhood acute myeloblastic leukemia. Cancer 1977;40:998–1004.
10. Newcomb M, Balducci L, Thigpen JT, Morrison FS. Acute leukemia in pregnancy: successful delivery after cytarabine and doxorubicin. JAMA 1978;239:2691–2.
11. Manoharan A, Leyden MJ. Acute non-lymphocytic leukaemia in the third trimester of pregnancy. Aust N-Z J Med 1979;9:71–4.
12. Pizzuto J, Aviles A, Noriega L, Niz J, Morales M, Romero F. Treatment of acute leukemia during pregnancy: presentation of nine cases. Cancer Treat Rep 1980;64:679–83.
13. Colbert N, Najman A, Gorin NC, Blum F, Treisser A, Lasfargues G, Cloup M, Barrat H, Duhamel G. Acute leukaemia during pregnancy: favourable course of pregnancy in two patients treated with cytosine arabinoside and anthracyclines. Nouv Presse Med 1980;9:175–8.
14. Tobias JS, Bloom HJG. Doxorubicin in pregnancy. Lancet 1980;1:776.
15. Taylor G, Blom J. Acute leukemia during pregnancy. South Med J 1980;73:1314–5.
16. Dara P, Slater LM, Armentrout SA. Successful pregnancy during chemotherapy for acute leukemia. Cancer 1981;47:845–6.
17. Plows CW. Acute myelomonocytic leukemia in pregnancy: report of a case. Am J Obstet Gynecol 1982;143:41–3.
18. De Souza JJL, Bezwoda WR, Jetham D, Sonnendecker EWW. Acute leukaemia in pregnancy: a case report and discussion on modern management. S Afr Med J 1982;62:295–6.
19. Feliu J, Juarez S, Ordonez A, Garcia-Paredes ML, Gonzalez-Baron M, Montero JM. Acute leukemia and pregnancy. Cancer 1988;61:580–4.
20. Volkenandt M, Buchner T, Hiddemann W, Van De Loo J. Acute leukaemia during pregnancy. Lancet 1987;2:1521–2.
21. Maurer LH, Forcier RJ, McIntyre OR, Benirschke K. Fetal group C trisomy after cytosine arabinoside and thioguanine. Ann Intern Med 1971;75:809–10.
22. Lowenthal RM, Marsden KA, Newman NM, Baikie MJ, Campbell SN. Normal infant after treatment of acute myeloid leukaemia in pregnancy with daunorubicin. Aust N Z J Med 1978;8:431–2.
23. O'Donnell R, Costigan C, O'Donnell LG. Two cases of acute leukaemia in pregnancy. Acta Haematol 1979;61:298–300.
24. Doney KC, Kraemer KG, Shepard TH. Combination chemotherapy for acute myelocytic leukemia during pregnancy: three case reports. Cancer Treat Rep 1979;63:369–71.
25. Cantini E, Yanes B. Acute myelogenous leukemia in pregnancy. South Med J 1984;77:1050–2.
26. Alegre A, Chunchurreta R, Rodrigueq-Alarcon J, Cruz E, Prada M. Successful pregnancy in acute promyelocytic leukemia. Cancer 1982;49:152–3.
27. Hamer JW, Beard MEJ, Duff GB. Pregnancy

C

complicated by acute myeloid leukaemia. N Z Med J 1979;89:212–3.
28. Schleuning M, Clemm C. Chromosomal aberrations in a newborn whose mother received cytotoxic treatment during pregnancy. N Engl J Med 1987;317:1666–7.
29. Wagner VM, Hill JS, Weaver D, Baehner RL. Congenital abnormalities in baby born to cytarabine treated mother. Lancet 1980;2:98–9.
30. Schafer AI. Teratogenic effects of antileukemic chemotherapy. Arch Intern Med 1981;141:514–5.
31. Russell JA, Powles RL, Oliver RTD. Conception and congenital abnormalities after chemotherapy of acute myelogenous leukaemia in two men. Br Med J 1976;1:1508.
32. Lendon M, Palmer MK, Hann IM, Shalet SM, Jones PHM. Testicular histology after combination chemotherapy in childhood for acute lymphoblastic leukaemia. Lancet 1978;2:439–41.
33. Lilleyman JS. Male fertility after successful chemotherapy for lymphoblastic leukaemia. Lancet 1979;2:1125.
34. Matthews JH, Wood JK. Male fertility during chemotherapy for acute leukemia. N Engl J Med 1980;303:1235.
35. Nicholson HO. Cytotoxic drugs in pregnancy: review of reported cases. J Obstet Gynaecol Br Commonw 1968;75:307–12.
36. Dobbing J. Pregnancy and leukaemia. Lancet 1977;1:1155.

D

Name: **DACARBAZINE** Risk Factor: **C_M**

Class: **Antineoplastic**

FETAL RISK SUMMARY

RECOMMENDATION: No Human Data - Animal Data Suggest Moderate Risk

No reports describing the use of dacarbazine in human pregnancy have been located. Single intraperitoneal doses of 800 or 1000 mg/kg in pregnant rats produced skeletal reduction defects, cleft palates, and encephaloceles in their offspring (1).

No congenital malformations were observed in four liveborn offspring of one male and one female treated with dacarbazine during childhood or adolescence (2).

Occupational exposure of the mother to antineoplastic agents during pregnancy may present a risk to the fetus. A position statement from the National Study Commission on Cytotoxic Exposure and a research article involving some antineoplastics agents are presented in the monograph for cyclophosphamide (see Cyclophosphamide).

BREAST FEEDING SUMMARY

RECOMMENDATION: No Human Data - Potential Toxicity

No reports describing the use of dacarbazine during lactation have been located. Because of the potential for severe adverse effects, such as hemopoietic depression, in a nursing infant, the drug should not be used during breast-feeding.

References

1. Chaube S. Protective effects of thymidine, and 5-aminoimidazolecarboxamide and riboflavin against fetal abnormalities produced in rats by 5-(3,3-dimethyl-1-triazeno)imidazole-4-carboxamide. Cancer Res 1973;33:2231–40. As cited in Shepard TH. *Catalog of Teratogenic Agents*. 6th ed. Baltimore, MD: Johns Hopkins University Press, 1989:189.
2. Green DM, Zevon MA, Lowries G, Seigelstein N, Hall B. Congenital anomalies in children of patients who received chemotherapy for cancer in childhood and adolescence. N Engl J Med 1991;325:141–6.

Name: **DACTINOMYCIN** Risk Factor: **C_M**

Class: **Antineoplastic**

FETAL RISK SUMMARY

RECOMMENDATION: Limited Human Data - Animal Data Suggest High Risk

Dactinomycin is an antimitotic antineoplastic agent. Reproduction studies in the rat, rabbit, and hamster at IV doses 3 to 7 times the maximum recommended human dose have shown embryo and fetal toxicity and teratogenic effects (1).

D

Normal pregnancies have followed the use of this drug prior to conception (2–10). Women, however, were less likely to have a live birth following treatment with this drug than with other antineoplastics (6).

Eight women who were treated with dactinomycin in childhood or adolescence subsequently produced 20 liveborn offspring, 3 (15%) of whom had congenital anomalies (11). This rate was the highest among 14 antineoplastic agents studied. Another report, however, observed no major congenital malformations in 52 offspring born to 11 men and 25 women who had been treated with dactinomycin during childhood or adolescence, suggesting that the results of the initial study occurred by chance (12).

Reports on the use of dactinomycin in six pregnancies have been located (13–18). In these cases, dactinomycin was administered during the 2nd and 3rd trimesters and apparently normal infants were delivered. The infant from one of the pregnancies was continuing to do well 4 years after birth (15). Two of the other pregnancies (16,17) are discussed in more detail in the monograph for cyclophosphamide (see Cyclophosphamide).

Data from one review indicated that 40% of the infants exposed to anticancer drugs were of low birth weight (13). This finding was not related to the timing of exposure. Long-term studies of growth and mental development in offspring exposed to dactinomycin during the 2nd trimester, the period of neuroblast multiplication, have not been conducted (19).

The long-term effects of combination chemotherapy on menstrual and reproductive function were described in a 1988 report (20). Thirty-two of the 40 women treated for malignant ovarian germ cell tumors received dactinomycin. The results of this study are discussed in the monograph for cyclophosphamide (see Cyclophosphamide).

Occupational exposure of the mother to antineoplastic agents during pregnancy may present a risk to the fetus. A position statement from the National Study Commission on Cytotoxic Exposure and a research article involving some antineoplastic agents are presented in the monograph for cyclophosphamide (see Cyclophosphamide).

BREAST FEEDING SUMMARY

RECOMMENDATION: No Human Data - Potential Toxicity

No reports describing the use of dactinomycin during human lactation or measuring the amount, if any, of the drug excreted into milk have been located. Although its relatively high molecular weight (about 1255) should impede the transfer into milk, women receiving this drug should not breast-feed because of the potential risk of severe adverse reactions in the nursing infant.

References

1. Product information. Cosmegen. Merck, 2000.
2. Ross GT. Congenital anomalies among children born of mothers receiving chemotherapy for gestational trophoblastic neoplasms. Cancer 1976;37:1043–7.
3. Walden PAM, Bagshawe KD. Pregnancies after chemotherapy for gestational trophoblastic tumours. Lancet 1979;2:1241.
4. Schwartz PE, Vidone RA. Pregnancy following combination chemotherapy for a mixed germ cell tumor of the ovary. Gynecol Oncol 1981;12:373–8.
5. Pastorfide GB, Goldstein DP. Pregnancy after hydatidiform mole. Obstet Gynecol 1973;42:67–70.
6. Rustin GJS, Booth M, Dent J, Salt S, Rustin F, Bagshawe KD. Pregnancy after cytotoxic chemotherapy for gestational trophoblastic tumours. Br Med J 1984;288:103–6.
7. Evenson DP, Arlin Z, Welt S, Claps ML, Melamed MR. Male reproductive capacity may recover following drug treatment with the L-10 protocol for acute lymphocytic leukemia. Cancer 1984;53:30–6.
8. Sivanesaratnam V, Sen DK. Normal pregnancy after successful treatment of choriocarcinoma with cerebral metastases: a case report. J Reprod Med 1988;33:402–3.
9. Lee RB, Kelly J, Elg SA, Benson WL. Pregnancy following conservative surgery and adjunctive chemotherapy

for stage III immature teratoma of the ovary. Obstet Gynecol 1989;73:853–5.
10. Bakri YN, Pedersen P, Nassar M. Normal pregnancy after curative multiagent chemotherapy for choriocarcinoma with brain metastases. Acta Obstet Gynecol Scand 1991;70:611–3.
11. Green DM, Zevon MA, Lowrie G, Seigelstein N, Hall B. Congenital anomalies in children of patients who received chemotherapy for cancer in childhood and adolescence. N Engl J Med 1991;325:141–6.
12. Byrne J, Nicholson HS, Mulvihill JJ. Absence of birth defects in offspring of women treated with dactinomycin. N Engl J Med 1992;326:137.
13. Nicholson HO. Cytotoxic drugs in pregnancy: review of reported cases. J Obstet Gynaecol Br Commonw 1968;75:307–12.
14. Gilliland J, Weinstein L. The effects of cancer chemotherapeutic agents on the developing fetus. Obstet Gynecol Surv 1983;38:6–13.
15. Haerr RW, Pratt AT. Multiagent chemotherapy for sarcoma diagnosed during pregnancy. Cancer 1985; 56:1028–33.
16. Weed JC Jr, Roh RA, Mendenhall HW. Recurrent endodermal sinus tumor during pregnancy. Obstet Gynecol 1979;54:653–6.
17. Kim DS, Park MI. Maternal and fetal survival following surgery and chemotherapy of endodermal sinus tumor of the ovary during pregnancy: a case report. Obstet Gynecol 1989;73:503–7.
18. Kim DS, Moon H, Lee JA, Park MI. Anticancer drugs during pregnancy: are we able to discard them? Am J Obstet Gynecol 1992;166:265.
19. Dobbing J. Pregnancy and leukaemia. Lancet 1977; 1:1155.
20. Gershenson DM. Menstrual and reproductive function after treatment with combination chemotherapy for malignant ovarian germ cell tumors. J Clin Oncol 1988;6:270–5.

Name:	**DALTEPARIN**	Risk Factor:	**B_M**
Class:	**Anticoagulant**		

FETAL RISK SUMMARY

RECOMMENDATION: Compatible

Dalteparin is a low molecular weight heparin prepared by depolymerization of heparin obtained from porcine intestinal mucosa. The molecular weight of dalteparin varies from <3000 to >8000, but 65%–78% is in the 3000 to 8000 range (1). Reproduction studies found no evidence of impaired fertility in male and female rats or fetal harm in rats and rabbits (1).

Because of its relatively high molecular weight, dalteparin is not expected to cross the placenta to the fetus (2). Thirty women undergoing elective pregnancy termination in the 2nd trimester ($N = 15$) or 3rd trimester ($N = 15$) for fetal malformations or chromosomal abnormalities were administered a single subcutaneous dose of 2500 IU or 5000 IU, respectively, of dalteparin immediately prior to the procedure (3). Heparin activity was not evident in fetal blood, demonstrating the lack of transplacental passage at this stage of gestation.

Dalteparin was administered as a continuous IV infusion at 36 weeks' gestation in a woman who was being treated for a deep vein thrombosis that had occurred during the 1st trimester (4). During the 1st trimester, she had been treated with IV heparin and then, maintained on SC doses for 4 weeks before developing an allergic reaction. Skin testing revealed immediate type allergic reactions to heparin and some other derivatives, but not to dalteparin. She was changed to warfarin therapy at 14 weeks' gestation, and this therapy was continued until the change to dalteparin at 36 weeks. Following stabilization of the anti-Factor Xa plasma levels with a continuous infusion (400 anti-Factor Xa U/hour), dalteparin therapy was changed to SC dosing and this was continued until delivery at 38.5 weeks of a healthy, 3010-g female infant. No anti-Factor Xa activity was detected in the cord blood.

A 1992 report described the use of dalteparin in seven women at 16–23 weeks' gestation just before undergoing therapeutic termination of pregnancy (5). Dalteparin was given subcutaneously 15 and 3 hours before pregnancy termination. Heparin activity (anti-Factor Xa) was detected in all mothers but not in any of the fetuses. In the second part of the study, 11 pregnant women with a history of severe thromboembolic tendency, as evidenced by recurrent miscarriages, were treated throughout gestation with SC dalteparin (5). All of the women gave birth to healthy infants without complication. As with heparin, maternal osteoporosis may be a complication resulting from the use of low molecular weight heparins, including dalteparin, during pregnancy (see also Heparin and Vitamin D). However, all of the 11 patients described above had normal mineral mass as determined by bone density scans performed shortly after delivery (5). Moreover, a study published in 1996, compared two groups of pregnant women receiving dalteparin, either 5000 IU SC daily ($N = 9$) or 5000 IU SC daily in the 1st trimester, then twice daily thereafter ($N = 8$), both starting in the 1st trimester, to a control group ($N = 8$) that did not receive heparin (6). Lumbar spine bone density fell by similar amounts in all pregnancies, and the normal physiological change of pregnancy was not increased by dalteparin.

The use of dalteparin in 184 pregnant women for thromboprophylaxis was reviewed in a brief 1994 report (7). No placental passage of the drug was found in the 9 patients investigated. Congenital malformations were observed in 3.3% of the outcomes, a rate believed to be normal for this population. Another 1994 letter reference described the use of dalteparin in five pregnant women starting between 15 and 18 weeks' gestation (8). Apparently normal infants were delivered.

Dalteparin was used for thromboembolic prophylaxis in 24 pregnant women with a risk of thromboembolic disease (9). The women received total daily doses of 2500 (16 mg) to 10,000 (32 mg) anti-Factor Xa IU. Anti-Factor Xa activity was demonstrated in the blood samples from the mothers but not in the normal newborns, indicating the lack of placental transfer of the drug.

A 1997 case report described the successful use of dalteparin in the 3rd trimester of a pregnant woman with iliofemoral vein thrombosis who was resistant to unfractionated heparin (10). She was treated with 7000 U (100 U/kg) every 12 hours from 30 weeks' gestation until 24 hours before an uncomplicated vaginal delivery at 38 weeks.

In a randomized 1999 trial, unfractionated heparin ($N = 55$; mean 20,569 IU/day) and dalteparin ($N = 50$; mean 4631 IU/day) were compared in 105 pregnant women with previous or current thromboembolism (11). There were no recurrences of thromboembolism or cases of thrombocytopenia in either group, but there were more bleeding complications in the patients receiving unfractionated heparin. The pregnancy outcomes in terms of blood loss at delivery, number of cesarean sections, birth weight, and Apgar scores were similar.

In a 2000 trial, a prophylactic dalteparin dose of 5000 IU/day given during pregnancy was adequate for 25 women (mean weight 70.2 kg), but the dose was decreased in 6 women (mean 58.0 kg) and increased in 2 (mean 102.5 kg) after the first anti-Xa activity measurement (12). An adjusted-weight therapeutic dose (100 IU/kg twice daily) was appropriate during pregnancy based on measured anti-Xa activity.

In summary, the use of dalteparin during pregnancy appears to present no greater risk to the fetus or newborn, and perhaps less, than that from standard, unfractionated heparin or from no therapy.

BREAST FEEDING SUMMARY

RECOMMENDATION: Compatible

No reports describing the use of dalteparin during lactation have been located. Dalteparin, a low molecular weight heparin, still has a relatively high molecular weight (65%–78%

in the range of 3000–8000) and, as such, should not be expected to be excreted into human milk. Because the drug would be inactivated in the gastrointestinal tract, the risk to a nursing infant from ingestion of dalteparin from milk appears to be negligible.

References

1. Product information. Fragmin. Pharmacia & Upjohn Company, 1997.
2. Nelson-Piercy C. Low molecular weight heparin for obstetric thromboprophylaxis. Br J Obstet Gynaecol 1994;101:6–8.
3. Forestier F, Solé Y, Aiach M, Alhenc Gélas M, Daffos F. Absence of transplacental passage of Fragmin (Kabi) during the second and the third trimesters of pregnancy. Thromb Haemost 1992;67:180–1.
4. de Boer K, Heyboer H, ten Cate JW, Borm JJJ, van Ginkel CJW. Low molecular weight heparin treatment in a pregnant woman with allergy to standard heparins and heparinoid. Thromb Haemost 1989;61:148.
5. Melissari E, Parker CJ, Wilson NV, Monte G, Kanthou C, Pemberton KD, Nicolaides KH, Barrett JJ, Kakkar VV. Use of low molecular weight heparin in pregnancy. Thromb Haemost 1992;68:652–6.
6. Shefras J, Farquharson RG. Bone density studies in pregnant women receiving heparin. Eur J Obstet Gynecol Reprod Biol 1996;65:171–4.
7. Wahlberg TB, Kher A. Low molecular weight heparin as thromboprophylaxis in pregnancy. Haemostasis 1994;24:55–6.
8. Manoharan A. Use of low molecular weight heparin during pregnancy. J Clin Pathol 1994;47:94–5.
9. Rasmussen C, Wadt J, Jacobsen B. Thromboembolic prophylaxis with low molecular weight heparin during pregnancy. Int J Gynecol Obstet 1994;47:121–5.
10. Anand SS, Brimble S, Ginsberg JS. Management of iliofemoral thrombosis in a pregnant patient with heparin resistance. Arch Intern Med 1997;157:815–6.
11. Pettila V, Kaaja R, Leinonen P, Ekblad U, Kataja M, Ikkala E. Thromboprophylaxis with low molecular weight heparin (dalteparin) in pregnancy. Thromb Res 1999;96:275–82.
12. Rey E, Rivard GE. Prophylaxis and treatment of thromboembolic diseases during pregnancy with dalteparin. Int J Gynecol Obstet 2000;71:19–24.

Name:	**DANAPAROID**	Risk Factor:	D_M
Class:	**Anticoagulant**		

FETAL RISK SUMMARY

RECOMMENDATION: Limited Human Data - Probably Compatible

Danaparoid is a low molecular weight heparinoid extracted from porcine mucosa. It has an average molecular weight of about 5500 (1). Reproduction studies in pregnant rats and rabbits have found no evidence of impaired fertility or fetal harm (1).

A 1991 report described the use of a low molecular weight heparinoid (Org-10172) in a woman at about 11 weeks' gestation with lupus anticoagulant and a history of heparin-induced thrombocytopenia (2). She was initially treated with aspirin, prednisone, and the heparinoid at 750 U SC every 12 hours, which was increased to 1500 Units every 12 hours. At 25 weeks' gestation, the dose was increased to 1250 Units SC every 8 hours because of a suspected subclinical thrombotic event. Severe thrombocytopenia was diagnosed 4 days later and the heparinoid and aspirin discontinued and warfarin begun. Because of progressive growth retardation and increasing fetal distress, a cesarean section was performed at 28 weeks' gestation with delivery of a 510-g male infant, who died of prematurity complications 2 days later. Approximately 30% of the placenta was found to be infarcted. This was the probable cause of the growth retardation, not the drugs.

Four other case reports involving five outcomes (one set of twins) have described the use of danaparoid in pregnancies complicated by heparin-induced thrombocytopenia (3–6). In three of the cases, the platelet count normalized after initiation of danaparoid.

In the fourth case, danaparoid was started at 20 weeks' gestation because of the development of heparin allergy while on prophylactic dalteparin (6). No fetal or newborn complications attributable to danaparoid were noted. In addition, there was no evidence of anti-factor Xa activity in the cord blood samples (3–5) or in the colostrum (6).

BREAST FEEDING SUMMARY

RECOMMENDATION: Compatible

No reports describing the use of danaparoid during lactation or breast-feeding have been located. Danaparoid has an average molecular weight of about 5500 and, as such, should not be expected to be excreted into human milk (see reference #6 above). Because the drug would be inactivated in the gastrointestinal tract, the risk to a nursing infant from ingestion of danaparoid from milk appears to be negligible.

References

1. Product information. Orgaran. Organon, 1997.
2. van Besien K, Hoffman R, Golichowski A. Pregnancy associated with lupus anticoagulant and heparin induced thrombocytopenia: management with a low molecular weight heparinoid. Thromb Res 1991;62:23–9.
3. Henny ChP, ten Cate H, ten Cate JW, Prummel MF, Peters M, Buller HR. Thrombosis prophylaxis in an AT III deficient pregnant woman: application of a low molecular weight heparinoid. Thromb Haemost 1986;55:301.
4. Greinacher A, Eckhardt Th, MuBmann J, Mueller-Eckhardt C. Pregnancy complicated by heparin associated thrombocytopenia: management by a prospectively *in vitro* selected heparinoid (ORG 10172). Thromb Res 1993;71:123–6.
5. Gill J, Kovacs MJ. Successful use of danaparoid in treatment of heparin-induced thrombocytopenia during twin pregnancy. Obstet Gynecol 1997;90:648–50.
6. Myers B, Westby J, Strong J. Prophylactic use of danaparoid in high-risk pregnancy with heparin-induced thrombocytopenia-positive skin reaction. Blood Coagul Fibrinolysis 2003;14:485–7.

Name:	**DANAZOL**	Risk Factor:	X_M
Class:	**Androgen**		

FETAL RISK SUMMARY

RECOMMENDATION: Contraindicated

Danazol is a synthetic androgen derived from ethisterone that is used in the treatment of various conditions, such as endometriosis, fibrocystic breast disease, and hereditary angioedema. No fetal harm was observed in reproduction studies with pregnant rats at doses 7 to 15 times the human dose, but fetal development was inhibited in rabbits at doses 2 to 4 times the human dose (1).

Early studies with this agent had examined its potential as an oral contraceptive (2–4). This use was abandoned, however, because low doses (e.g., 50–100 mg/day) were associated with pregnancy rates up to 10% and higher doses were unacceptable to the patient because of adverse effects (2,4).

In experimental animals, danazol crosses the placenta to the fetus, but human data are lacking. However, it is reasonable to assume that it does reach the human fetus. Because danazol is used to treat endometriosis, frequently in an infertile woman, a barrier (nonhormonal) contraception method is recommended to prevent accidental use during pregnancy.

A number of reports have described the inadvertent use of danazol during human gestation resulting in female pseudohermaphroditism (5–14). This teratogenic condition is characterized by a normal XX karyotype and internal female reproductive organs, but ambiguous external genitalia. No adverse effects in male fetuses are associated with danazol.

The first published report of female pseudohermaphroditism appeared in 1981 (5). A woman was treated for endometriosis with a total danazol dose of 81 g divided over 101 days. Subsequent evaluation revealed that the treatment period corresponded to approximately the first 14 weeks of pregnancy. The female infant, whose length and weight were at the 5th percentile, had mild clitoral enlargement and a urogenital sinus evident at birth. Physical findings at 2 years of age were normal except for clitoromegaly, empty, darkened, rugated labia majora, and a complete urogenital sinus formation. Studies indicated the child had a normal vagina, cervix, fallopian tubes, and ovaries. The mother had no evidence of virilization.

A second case reported in 1981 involved a woman with endometriosis who was inadvertently treated with danazol, 800 mg/day, during the first 20 weeks of gestation (6). The mother went into premature labor at 27 weeks and delivered a female infant with a birth weight of 980 g. Ambiguous genitalia were evident at birth, consisting of marked clitoromegaly with fusion of the labia scrotal folds. A urogenital sinus, with well-developed vagina and uterus, was noted on genitogram. Bilateral inguinal hernias with palpable gonads were also present. At 4 days of age, clinical and laboratory findings compatible with a salt-losing congenital adrenal hyperplasia were observed. The infant was successfully treated for this complication, which was thought to be caused by a transitory block of the steroid 21- and 11β-monooxygenases (6). At 1 year of age, the infant was asymptomatic, and no signs of progressive virilization were observed.

The authors of the above report cited knowledge of 27 other pregnancies in which danazol had been accidentally used (6). Seven of these pregnancies were terminated by abortion. Of the remaining 20 pregnancies, 14 delivered female infants and 5 (36%) of these had evidence of virilization with ambiguous genitalia.

A 1982 case report described female pseudohermaphroditism in an infant exposed to a total danazol dose of 96 g administered over 120 days, corresponding to approximately the first 16 weeks of gestation (7). The infant, weighing 3100 g (5th percentile) with a length of 53.5 cm (25th–50th percentile), had fused labia with coarse rugations, mild clitoromegaly, and a urogenital sinus opening below the clitoris. An 8-cm mass, eventually shown to be a hydrometrocolpos, was surgically drained because of progressive obstructive uropathy. A balanced somatic chromosomal translocation was an incidental finding in this case, most likely inherited from the mother. Growth and development were normal at 6 months of age with no further masculinization.

Two brief 1982 communications described infants exposed *in utero* to danazol (8,9). In one, a 2400-g term female infant with ambiguous genitalia had been exposed to danazol (dose not specified) during the first 4 months of pregnancy (8). The infant's phallus measured 0.75 cm and complete posterior labial fusion was observed. The second case involved a woman treated with danazol, 200 mg/day, during the first 6 weeks of gestation, who eventually delivered a female infant with normal external genitalia (9). The absence of virilization of the infant's genitalia, as evidenced by a normal clitoris and no labial fusion, indicates the drug was stopped prior to the onset of fetal sensitivity to androgens.

British investigators reported virilization of the external genitalia consisting of clitoromegaly, a fused, scrotalized labia with a prominent median raphe, and a urogenital sinus in a female infant exposed *in utero* to danazol, 400 mg/day, during the first 18 weeks of pregnancy (10). The mother showed no signs of virilization.

A summary of known cases of danazol exposure during pregnancy was reported in 1984 by F. Rosa, an investigator from the Epidemiology Branch of the Food and Drug Administration (FDA) (11). A total of 44 cases of pregnancy exposure, all to 800 mg/day, were known as of this date, but this number was considered to be understated since normal outcomes were unlikely to be reported (11). Each of the cases of exposure was thought to have occurred after conception had taken place. Of the 44 cases, 7 (16%) aborted and the outcome in 14 others was unknown. Seven males and 15 females resulted from the 22 pregnancies that had been completed. Ten (67%) of the females had virilization and one male infant had multiple congenital abnormalities (details not given). No cases of virilization were observed when the drug was discontinued prior to the 8th gestational week, the onset of androgen receptor sensitivity (11).

An Australian case of an infant with masculinized external genitalia secondary to danazol was reported in 1985 (12). The mother had been treated with 400 mg/day, without evidence of virilization, until the 19th week of gestation. The infant was developing normally at 6 months of age except for a minimally enlarged clitoris, rugose and fused labia with a thick median raphe, and a urogenital sinus opening at the base of the phallus.

A 1985 case report described a female fetus exposed *in utero* to 800 mg/day of danazol until pregnancy was terminated at 20 weeks' gestation (13). A urogenital sinus was identified in the aborted fetus but the external genitalia were normal except for a single opening in the vulva. Citing a personal communication from the manufacturer, the authors noted a total of 74 cases of danazol exposure during pregnancy (13). Among these cases were 29 term females, 9 (31%) of whom had clitoromegaly and labial fusion.

A retrospective review of fetal exposure to danazol included cases gathered from multiple sources, including individual case reports, data from the Australian Drug Reactions Advisory Committee, the FDA, and direct reports to the manufacturers (14). Of the 129 total pregnancies that were exposed to danazol, 23 were electively terminated and 12 miscarried. Among the 94 completed pregnancies there were 37 normal males, 34 nonvirilized females, and 23 virilized females. All of the virilized female offspring were exposed beyond 8 weeks' gestation. The lowest daily dose that resulted in virilization was 200 mg.

In a surveillance study of Michigan Medicaid recipients conducted between 1985 and 1992 involving 229,101 completed pregnancies, 10 newborns had been exposed to danazol during the 1st trimester (F. Rosa, personal communication, FDA, 1993). No major birth defects were observed.

There is no conclusive evidence of fetal harm when conception occurs in a menstrual cycle shortly after cessation of danazol therapy (15–17). A 1978 publication noted 4 intrauterine fetal deaths occurring from a total of 39 pregnancies following danazol treatment, presumably after elimination of the drug from the mother (18). The stillbirths, two each in the 2nd and 3rd trimesters, occurred in women who had conceived within 0–3 cycles of stopping danazol. However, one of the fetal deaths was caused by cord torsion and a second death in a twin was caused by placental insufficiency, neither of which can be attributed to danazol.

No long-term follow-up studies of children exposed *in utero* to danazol have been located. A 1982 reference, however, did describe this type of evaluation in 12 young women, age 16–27 years, who had been exposed to *in utero* synthetic androgenic progestins resulting in the virilization of the external genitalia in 11 of them (19). Despite possible virilization of early behavior with characterization as "tomboys" (e.g., increased amounts of "rough-and-tumble play" and "an avid interest in high school sports"), all of the women eventually "displayed stereotypically feminine sexual behavior" without any suggestion of behavior abnormalities (19).

BREAST FEEDING SUMMARY

RECOMMENDATION: Contraindicated

No reports describing the use of danazol during lactation have been located. Because of the potential for severe adverse effects in a nursing infant, women taking this drug should not breast-feed.

D

References

1. Product information. Danocrine. Sanofi Pharmaceuticals, 2000.
2. Greenblatt RB, Oettinger M, Borenstein R, Bohler CSS. Influence of danazol (100 mg) on conception and contraception. J Reprod Med 1974;13:201–3.
3. Colle ML, Greenblatt RB. Contraceptive properties of danazol. J Reprod Med 1976;17:98–102.
4. Lauersen NH, Wilson KH. Evaluation of danazol as an oral contraceptive. Obstet Gynecol 1977;50:91–6.
5. Duck SC, Katayama KP. Danazol may cause female pseudohermaphroditism. Fertil Steril 1981;35:230 1.
6. Castro-Magana M, Cheruvanky T, Collipp PJ, Ghavami-Maibodi Z, Angulo M, Stewart C. Transient adrenogenital syndrome due to exposure to danazol in utero. Am J Dis Child 1981;135:1032–4.
7. Peress MR, Kreutner AK, Mathur RS, Williamson HO. Female pseudohermaphroditism with somatic chromosomal anomaly in association with in utero exposure to danazol. Am J Obstet Gynecol 1982;142: 708–9.
8. Schwartz RP. Ambiguous genitalia in a term female infant due to exposure to danazol in utero. Am J Dis Child 1982;136:474.
9. Wentz AC. Adverse effects of danazol in pregnancy. Ann Intern Med 1982;96:672–3.
10. Shaw RW, Farquhar JW. Female pseudohermaphroditism associated with danazol exposure in utero. Case report. Br J Obstet Gynecol 1984;91: 386–9.
11. Rosa FW. Virilization of the female fetus with maternal danazol exposure. Am J Obstet Gynecol 1984;149:99–100.
12. Kingsbury AC. Danazol and fetal masculinization: a warning. Med J Aust 1985;143:410–1.
13. Quagliarello J, Greco MA. Danazol and urogenital sinus formation in pregnancy. Fertil Steril 1985;43: 939–42.
14. Brunskill PJ. The effects of fetal exposure to danazol. Br J Obstet Gynaecol 1992;99:212–5.
15. Daniell JF, Christianson C. Combined laparoscopic surgery and danazol therapy for pelvic endometriosis. Fertil Steril 1981;35:521–5.
16. Fayez JA, Collazo LM, Vernon C. Comparison of different modalities of treatment for minimal and mild endometriosis. Am J Obstet Gynecol 1988;159: 927–32.
17. Butler L, Wilson E, Belisle S, Gibson M, Albrecht B, Schiff I, Stillman R. Collaborative study of pregnancy rates following danazol therapy of stage I endometriosis. Fertil Steril 1984;41:373–6.
18. Dmowski WP, Cohen MR. Antigonadotropin (danazol) in the treatment of endometriosis. Evaluation of posttreatment fertility and three-year follow-up data. Am J Obstet Gynecol 1978;130:41–8.
19. Money J, Mathews D. Prenatal exposure to virilizing progestins: an adult follow-up study of twelve women. Arch Sex Behav 1982;11:73–83.

Name:	**DANTHRON**	Risk Factor:	**C**
Class:	**Purgative**		

FETAL RISK SUMMARY

RECOMMENDATION: Limited Human Data - Probably Compatible

Danthron is an anthraquinone purgative (see Cascara Sagrada).

BREAST FEEDING SUMMARY

RECOMMENDATION: Limited Human Data - Probably Compatible

See Cascara Sagrada.

Name:	**DANTROLENE**	Risk Factor:	C_M
Class:	**Muscle Relaxant**		

FETAL RISK SUMMARY

RECOMMENDATION: Limited Human Data - No Relevant Animal Data

In obstetrics, the only documented use of dantrolene, a hydantoin derivative used as a direct-acting skeletal muscle relaxant, is to prevent or treat malignant hyperthermia. The syndrome of malignant hyperthermia is a potentially lethal complication of anesthesia induced with halogenated anesthetics and depolarizing skeletal muscle relaxants. References describing the use of dantrolene in pregnant patients for chronic spasticity or during the 1st or 2nd trimesters have not been located. The agent is embryocidal in animals and, in some species, produced minor skeletal variations at the highest dose tested (1–3).

Three studies have described the transfer of dantrolene across the human placenta to the fetus with cord:maternal serum ratios of 0.29–0.69 (4–6). Two women, who were considered to be malignant hyperthermia susceptible (MHS), were treated with oral doses of the drug prior to cesarean section (4). One woman received 100 mg twice daily for 3 days prior to elective induction of labor. The second patient received 150 mg on admission in labor and a second dose of 100 mg six hours later. Both women were delivered by cesarean section because of failure to progress in labor. Neither were exposed to malignant hyperthermia-triggering agents and neither developed the complication. The cord and maternal blood concentrations in the two cases were 0.40 and 1.38 μg/mL (ratio 0.29), and 1.39 and 2.70 μg/mL (ratio 0.51), respectively. The timing of the doses in relationship to delivery was not specified by the author. No adverse effects of the drug exposure were noted in the infants.

A second report described the prophylactic use of dantrolene, administered as a 1-hour IV infusion (2.2 mg/kg) 7.5 hours prior to vaginal delivery, under epidural anesthesia, of a healthy, vigorous infant (5). The mother had been confirmed to be MHS by previous muscle biopsy. At the time of delivery, the cord and maternal blood dantrolene concentrations were 2.1 and 4.3 μg/mL, respectively, a ratio of 0.48. The mother did not experience malignant hyperthermia. No respiratory depression or muscle weakness was noted in the newborn.

A study published in 1988 treated 20 pregnant women diagnosed as MHS with oral dantrolene, 100 mg/day, for 5 days prior to delivery and for 3 days following delivery (6). Three of the patients were delivered by cesarean section. Known anesthetic malignant hyperthermia-triggering agents were avoided and no cases of the syndrome were observed. All fetuses had reactive nonstress tests and normal biophysical profiles before and after the onset of dantrolene administration. The mean maternal predelivery dantrolene serum concentration was 0.99 μg/mL compared to a mean cord blood level of 0.68 μg/mL, a ratio of 0.69. The mean serum half-life of dantrolene in the newborns was 20 hours (6). Extensive neonatal testing up to 3 days after delivery failed to discover any adverse effects of the drug.

Prophylactic dantrolene, 600 mg given as escalating oral doses over 3 days, was administered to a woman with biopsy-proven MHS 3 days prior to a repeat cesarean section (7). The woman had experienced malignant hyperthermia during her first cesarean section but did not during this surgery. No adverse effects were noted in the newborn.

Although no dantrolene-induced complications have been observed in fetuses or newborns exposed to the drug shortly before birth, some investigators do not recommend prophylactic use of the agent because safety in pregnancy has not been sufficiently documented, and the incidence of malignant hyperthermia in the anesthetized patient is very low (8–10). (A recent reference cited incidences of 1:12,000 anesthesias in children and 1:40,000 in adults [11].) They recommend avoidance of those anesthetic agents that might trigger the syndrome, careful monitoring of the patient during delivery, and preparation to treat the complication if it occurs.

In summary, dantrolene has been used in a limited number of pregnant patients shortly before delivery. No fetal or newborn adverse effects have been observed, but a risk:benefit ratio has not yet been defined. Moreover, published 1st and 2nd trimester experience with this drug is completely lacking.

BREAST FEEDING SUMMARY

RECOMMENDATION: Hold Breast Feeding

Dantrolene is excreted into human breast milk. A 37-year-old woman undergoing an urgent cesarean section with general anesthesia (succinylcholine, thiopental, nitric oxide, oxygen, and isoflurane) developed tachycardia, respiratory acidosis, and hyperthermia (12). After delivery of the infant and cord clamping, IV dantrolene (160 mg) was administered. Over the next 3 days, she received decreasing total doses of IV dantrolene: 560 mg on day 1, 320 mg on day 2, and 80 mg on day 3. The infant was not allowed to nurse during this time. Seven breast milk samples were obtained (volume of milk samples and collection method not specified) over an 84-hour interval after the first dose. Milk concentrations of dantrolene ranged from a maximum of 1.2 μg/mL (day 2, 36 hours after the first dose with a total dose of 720 mg at the time) to 0.05 μg/mL on day 3 (total dose 1120 mg received at the time). The estimated elimination half-life from milk was 9.02 hours (12). Thus waiting 2 days after the last dantrolene dose to breast-feed would assure that the exposure of the nursing infant would be negligible.

References

1. Nagaoka T, Osuka F, Hatano M. Reproductive studies of dantrolene. Teratogenicity study in rabbits. Clinical Report 1977;11:2212–17. As cited in Shepard TH. *Catalog of Teratogenic Agents*. 6th ed. Baltimore, MD: Johns Hopkins University Press, 1989: 549.
2. Nagaoka T, Osuka F, Shigemura T, Hatano M. Reproductive test of dantrolene. Teratogenicity test on rats. Clinical Report 1977;11:2218–30. As cited in Shepard TH. *Catalog of Teratogenic Agents*. 6th ed. Baltimore, MD: Johns Hopkins University Press, 1989: 549.
3. Product information. Dantrium. Norwich Eaton Pharmaceuticals, 1993.
4. Morison DH. Placental transfer of dantrolene. Anesthesiology 1983;59:265.
5. Glassenberg R, Cohen H. Intravenous dantrolene in a pregnant malignant hyperthermia susceptible (MHS) patient (Abstract). Anesthesiology 1984;61: A404.
6. Shime J, Gare D, Andrews J, Britt B. Dantrolene in pregnancy: lack of adverse effects on the fetus and newborn infant. Am J Obstet Gynecol 1988;159: 831–4.
7. Cupryn JP, Kennedy A, Byrick RJ. Malignant hyperthermia in pregnancy. Am J Obstet Gynecol 1984; 150:327–8.
8. Khalil SN, Williams JP, Bourke DL. Management of a malignant hyperthermia susceptible patient in labor with 2-chloroprocaine epidural anesthesia. Anesth Analg 1983;62:119–21.
9. Kaplan RF, Kellner KR. More on malignant hyperthermia during delivery. Am J Obstet Gynecol 1985;152: 608–9.
10. Sorosky JI, Ingardia CJ, Botti JJ. Diagnosis and management of susceptibility to malignant hyperthermia in pregnancy. Am J Perinatol 1989;6:46–8.
11. Sessler DI. Malignant hyperthermia. J Pediatr 1986; 109:9–14.
12. Fricker RM, Hoerauf KH, Drewe J, Kress HG. Secretion of dantrolene into breast milk after acute therapy of a suspected malignant hyperthermia crisis during cesarean section. Anesthesiology 1998;89: 1023–5.

Name:	**DAPSONE**	Risk Factor:	**C_M**
Class:	**Leprostatic/Antimalarial**		

D

FETAL RISK SUMMARY

RECOMMENDATION: Compatible - Maternal Benefit >> Embryo/Fetal Risk

Dapsone (DDS), a sulfone antibacterial agent, is used in the treatment of leprosy and dermatitis herpetiformis, and for various other unlabeled indications, including antimalarial prophylaxis, the treatment of *Pneumocystis carinii* pneumonia, inflammatory bowel disease, rheumatic and connective tissue disorders, and relapsing polychondritis. Because the drug is known to cause blood dyscrasias in adults, some of which have been fatal, close patient monitoring is required during use.

Although reproduction studies in animals have not been conducted (1), a 1980 reference described a study investigating carcinogenicity that was conducted in pregnant and lactating mice and rats (2). A maximum maternally tolerated dose, 100 mg/kg (usual human dose 50–300 mg/day), was administered twice in late gestation and 5 times a week during lactation and then was continued in the offspring after weaning. A small but significant increase in tumors was noted.

A number of studies have described the use of dapsone during all stages of human pregnancy. A few fetal or newborn adverse effects directly attributable to dapsone have been reported, but no congenital anomalies thought to be due to the drug have been observed. The indications for use of dapsone during pregnancy have included dermatologic conditions, leprosy, malaria, and *P. carinii*.

A brief 1968 reference described Heinz-body hemolytic anemia in a mother and her newborn during therapy with dapsone (3). The mother had been diagnosed with herpes gestationis at 22 weeks' gestation, for which she was treated with sulfapyridine for 1 week. At 26 weeks, treatment with dapsone was begun at 400 mg/day for 1 week, 300 mg/day during weeks 2 and 3, 200 mg/day in week 4, 100 mg/day in week 5, followed by 200 mg/day beginning in week 6 until delivery of a male infant at 36 weeks' gestation. She developed well-compensated Heinz body hemolytic anemia 6 days after starting dapsone. The anemia in the infant, who had a normal glucose-6-phosphate dehydrogenase (G6PD) level, completely resolved within 10 days, and he has remained hematologically normal.

In three cases, dapsone was used for the treatment of dermatitis herpetiformis or its variant, herpes gestationis (4,5). In two other reports of herpes gestationis (also referred to as pemphigoid gestationis) occurring during pregnancy, dapsone was not started until after delivery (6,7). A 26-year-old pregnant woman with recurrent herpes gestationis was treated with dapsone and other nonspecific therapy from the 24th week of gestation until delivery of a normal male infant at 38 weeks (4). A 25-year-old woman with dermatitis herpetiformis was treated with dapsone, 100–150 mg/day, during the first 3 months of pregnancy (5). The drug was discontinued briefly during the 4th month of pregnancy because of concerns of teratogenicity, then resumed at 50 mg/day because of worsening of her disease. She eventually gave birth to a full-term, normal infant who developed dapsone-induced hemolytic anemia while breast feeding (see Breast Feeding Summary below). A 33-year-old woman, treated with dapsone, 25–50 mg/day, throughout pregnancy for dermatitis herpetiformis delivered a healthy full-term infant (8).

A 1978 paper described the clinical courses of 62 pregnancies in 26 women treated for leprosy (Hansen's disease) (9). All of the patients received therapy, with sulfone drugs (specific drugs not mentioned) being used in 58 (94%) of the pregnancies. Two (3.6%) infants (about the expected rate) among the 56 pregnancies with infants who reached an age of viability had congenital anomalies. One infant had a cleft palate, and another had a congenital hip dislocation. A review, published in 1993, discussed the adverse association of leprosy and pregnancy (10). Although dapsone was not thought to cause adverse toxic effects or teratogenicity in the fetus, resistance to dapsone monotherapy has become a problem, and combination therapy, such as dapsone, clofazimine, and rifampin, is recommended for all forms of leprosy (10). Normal pregnancy outcomes of 15 women treated for leprosy were noted in a 1996 letter ($N = 13$) (11) and in a 1997 report ($N = 2$) (12). The patients had been treated throughout gestation with dapsone, 100 mg/day, plus rifampin, 600 mg once monthly (11), or with dapsone alone (12). In addition, two had also received clofazimine, and two had taken intermittent prednisolone (11).

Neonatal hyperbilirubinemia, suspected of being due to displacement of bilirubin from albumin binding sites, has been attributed to the use of dapsone during gestation (13). A 25-year-old woman with leprosy was treated with dapsone, 300 mg/week, until 3 months before delivery. At that time, her dose was decreased to 50 mg/week and then was discontinued 1 week prior to a normal, spontaneous, vaginal delivery of a 3740-g male infant. The infant, who was not breast-fed and had no evidence of ABO incompatibility, developed hyperbilirubinemia that was attributed to dapsone. In a subsequent pregnancy, dapsone therapy was stopped 1 month prior to delivery of a healthy 4070-g male infant who did not develop hyperbilirubinemia.

The combination of dapsone and pyrimethamine (Maloprim) has been frequently used during pregnancy for the chemoprophylaxis of malaria (14–21). Most consider the benefits of this combination in the prevention of maternal malaria to outweigh the risks to the fetus (16–21), but two authors classified the combination as contraindicated in pregnancy (14,15). The adverse effects of the combination were reviewed in a 1993 reference (22). Because of the potential for significant dose-related toxicity, the authors considered the drug combination to be a second-line choice for use in areas where the risk of malaria was high. Folic acid supplements should be given when pyrimethamine is used (21). (See also Pyrimethamine).

A study published in 1990 compared chlorproguanil plus dapsone ($N = 44$), chloroquine alone ($N = 58$), and pyrimethamine plus sulfadoxine ($N = 54$) in a group of pregnant women with falciparum malaria parasitemia (23). A single dose of chlorproguanil plus dapsone during the 3rd trimester cleared the parasitemia in all women within 1 week, compared with 84% and 94%, respectively, in the other two groups. Six weeks after treatment, the proportion of those with parasitemia in each group was 81%, 84%, and 23%, respectively. No adverse effects of the therapy in the fetuses or newborns were mentioned.

An adverse pregnancy outcome in a mother who received malarial chemoprophylaxis with three drugs was the subject of a brief 1983 communication (24). During the 1st month of pregnancy the 31-year-old woman had taken chloroquine (100 mg/day) and Maloprim (dapsone 100 mg plus pyrimethamine 12.5 mg) on days 10, 20, and 30 after conception. The stillborn male infant was delivered at 26 weeks' gestation with a defect of the abdominal and thoracic wall with exteriorization of most of the abdominal viscera, the heart, and the lungs (a variant of ectopia cordis?) and a missing left arm. The authors concluded that the defects were due to pyrimethamine, but others have questioned this conclusion (see Pyrimethamine).

Dapsone, either alone or in combination with pyrimethamine or trimethoprim, has been suggested as having utility in the prophylaxis of *P. carinii* during pregnancy (25,26).

Although the efficacy of these therapeutic options has not been confirmed, the risks of the disease to the mother far outweigh the risks to the fetus (26).

A 1992 report described an attempted suicide with dapsone and alcohol in a 29-year-old pregnant woman (length of gestation not specified) under treatment for dermatitis herpetiformis (27). The woman had ingested 50 tablets (100 mg each) of dapsone plus six alcoholic drinks. She developed severe methemoglobinemia and hemolytic anemia, treated successfully with methylene blue (total dose about 7 mg/kg) and other therapy, and splenomegaly that resolved spontaneously. No mention was made of the pregnancy outcome.

In summary, the use of dapsone during pregnancy does not appear to present a major risk to the fetus or the newborn. The agent has been used extensively for malarial treatment or chemoprophylaxis and for the treatment of leprosy and certain other dermatologic conditions without producing major fetotoxicity or causing birth defects. If used in combination with pyrimethamine (a folic acid antagonist) for malaria prophylaxis, folic acid supplements (5 mg/day) or folinic acid (leucovorin, 5 mg/week) should be given (21,28).

BREAST FEEDING SUMMARY

RECOMMENDATION: Limited Human Data - Potential Toxicity

Dapsone and its primary metabolite, monoacetyldapsone, are excreted into human milk (5,29,30). A 25-year-old woman with dermatitis herpetiformis was treated with dapsone throughout most of her pregnancy and continued this therapy while breast-feeding her infant (5). During the latter two-thirds of her pregnancy and during lactation she took dapsone, 50 mg/day. Approximately 6 weeks after delivery, mild hemolytic anemia was diagnosed in the mother and her infant. Measurements of dapsone and the metabolite were conducted on the mother's serum and milk and on the infant's serum. Dapsone concentrations were 1622, 1092, and 439 ng/mL, respectively, whereas those of the metabolite were 744 ng/mL, none detected, and 204 ng/mL, respectively. The milk:plasma ratio of dapsone was 0.67. The investigators noted that the weak base properties of dapsone, its high lipid solubility, and its long serum half-life (about 20 hours) all favored excretion and entrapment of the drug in milk (5). Moreover, both the mother and her infant appeared to be rapid acetylator phenotypes because of the relatively high ratios of metabolite to parent drug in both (0.459 in the mother, 0.465 in the infant) (5). Neither patient was tested for G6PD deficiency, although persons with this genetic defect are especially susceptible to dapsone-induced hemolytic anemia. Dose-related hemolytic anemia is the most common toxicity reported with dapsone and occurs in patients with or without G6PD deficiency (1).

A 1952 reference studied the excretion into breast milk of dapsone (diaminodiphenylsulfone) and another sulfone antibacterial agent in one and five women, respectively, with leprosy (29). Although stating that dapsone was excreted in the mother's milk and absorbed and excreted in the infant's urine, the investigator did not quantify the amount in the milk.

Three women, 2–5 days postpartum, who were not breast-feeding were given a single dose of dapsone (100 mg) plus pyrimethamine (12.5 mg; Maloprim) and a single dose of chloroquine (300 mg base) (30). Milk and serum samples for dapsone analysis were collected at intervals up to 52, 102, and 124 hours, yielding milk:plasma ratios, based on area under the concentration-time curve, of 0.38, 0.45, and 0.22, respectively. The authors calculated that the amounts of dapsone excreted into milk, based on 1000 mL/day, were 0.31, 0.85, and 0.59 mg, respectively, which are too small to afford malarial chemoprophylaxis to a nursing infant (30).

Although not citing the case of dapsone-induced hemolytic anemia in a nursing infant described above, the American Academy of Pediatrics classifies dapsone as compatible with breast-feeding (31).

References

1. Product information. Dapsone. Jacobus Pharmaceutical, 1997.
2. Griciute L, Tomatis L. Carcinogenicity of dapsone in mice and rats. Int J Cancer 1980;25:123–9.
3. Hocking DR. Neonatal haemolytic disease due to dapsone. Med J Aust 1968;1:1130–1.
4. Diamond WJ. Herpes gestationis. S Afr Med J 1976;50:739–40.
5. Sanders SW, Zone JJ, Foltz RL, Tolman KG, Rollins DE. Hemolytic anemia induced by dapsone transmitted through breast milk. Ann Intern Med 1982;96:465–6.
6. Sills ES, Mabie WC. A refractory case of herpes gestationis. J Tenn Med Assoc 1992;85:559–60.
7. Kirtschig G, Collier PM, Emmerson RW, Wojnarowska F. Severe case of pemphigoid gestationis with unusual target antigen. Br J Dermatol 1994;131:108–11.
8. Tuffanelli DL. Successful pregnancy in a patient with dermatitis herpetiformis treated with low-dose dapsone. Arch Dermatol 1982;118:876.
9. Maurus JN. Hansen's disease in pregnancy. Obstet Gynecol 1978;52:22–5.
10. Duncan ME. An historical and clinical review of the interaction of leprosy and pregnancy: a cycle to be broken. Soc Sci Med 1993;37:457–72.
11. Bhargava P, Kuldeep CM, Mathur NK. Antileprosy drugs, pregnancy and fetal outcome. Int J Lepr Other Mycobact Dis 1996;64:457.
12. Lyde CB. Pregnancy in patients with Hansen disease. Arch Dermatol 1997;133:623–7.
13. Thornton YS, Bowe ET. Neonatal hyperbilirubinemia after treatment of maternal leprosy. South Med J 1989;82:668.
14. Sturchler D. Malaria prophylaxis in travelers: the current position. Experientia 1984;40:1357–62.
15. Brown GV. Chemoprophylaxis of malaria. Med J Aust 1986;144:696–702.
16. Anonymous. Prevention of malaria in pregnancy and early childhood. Br Med J 1984;289:1296–7.
17. Greenwood AM, Armstrong JRM, Byass P, Snow RW, Greenwood BM. Malaria chemoprophylaxis, birth weight and child survival. Trans R Soc Trop Med Hyg 1992;86:483–5.
18. Greenwood AM, Menendez C, Todd J, Greenwood BM. The distribution of birth weights in Gambian women who received malaria chemoprophylaxis during their first pregnancy and in control women. Trans R Soc Trop Med Hyg 1994;88:311–2.
19. Menendez C, Todd J, Alonso PL, Lulat S, Francis N, Greenwood BM. Malaria chemoprophylaxis, infection of the placenta and birth weight in Gambian primigravidae. J Trop Med Hyg 1994;97:244–8.
20. Kahn G. Dapsone is safe during pregnancy. J Am Acad Dermatol 1985;13:838–9.
21. Spracklen FHN, Monteagudo FSE. Malaria prophylaxis. S Afr Med J 1986;70:316.
22. Luzzi GA, Peto TEA. Adverse effects of antimalarials. An update. Drug Saf 1993;8:295–311.
23. Keuter M, van Eijk A, Hoogstrate M, Raasveld M, van de Ree M, Ngwawe WA, Watkins WM, Were JBO, Brandling-Bennett AD. Comparison of chloroquine, pyrimethamine and sulfadoxine, and chlorproguanil and dapsone as treatment for falciparum malaria in pregnant and non-pregnant women, Kakamega district, Kenya. BMJ 1990;301:466–70.
24. Harpey J-P, Darbois Y, Lefebvre G. Teratogenicity of pyrimethamine. Lancet 1983;2:399.
25. Connelly RT, Lourwood DL. *Pneumocystis carinii* pneumonia prophylaxis during pregnancy. Pharmacotherapy 1994;14:424–9.
26. American College of Obstetricians and Gynecologists. Human immunodeficiency virus infections in pregnancy. *Educational Bulletin*. No. 232, January 1997.
27. Erstad BL. Dapsone-induced methemoglobinemia and hemolytic anemia. Clin Pharm 1992;11:800–5.
28. Spracklen FHN. Malaria 1984 Part I. Malaria prophylaxis. S Afr Med J 1984;65:1037–41.
29. Dreisbach JA. Sulphone levels in breast milk of mothers on sulphone therapy. Lepr Rev 1952;23:101–6.
30. Edstein MD, Veenendaal JR, Newman K, Hyslop R. Excretion of chloroquine, dapsone and pyrimethamine in human milk. Br J Clin Pharmacol 1986;22:733–5.
31. Committee on Drugs, American Academy of Pediatrics. The transfer of drugs and other chemicals into human milk. Pediatrics 2001;108:776–89.

Name: **DARBEPOETIN ALFA** Risk Factor: **C_M**

Class: **Hematopoietic**

FETAL RISK SUMMARY

RECOMMENDATION: Compatible - Maternal Benefit >> Embryo/Fetal Risk

Darbepoetin is an erythropoiesis 165-amino acid protein produced by recombinant DNA technology in Chinese hamster ovary cells. It is indicated for the treatment of anemia and is closely related to epoetin alfa. The half-life after SC administration is 49 hours (range 27–89 hours) that is reflective of its slow absorption, whereas after IV administration the terminal half-life is 21 hours.

Reproduction studies have been conducted in pregnant rats and rabbits. No evidence of direct embryotoxic, fetotoxic, or teratogenic effects was observed at IV doses up to 20 μg/kg/day. (*Note: Dose is about 300 times the recommended human dose of 0.45μg/kg once weekly based on body weight in patients with chronic renal failure [RHD-CRF] or about 60 times the recommended human dose of 2.25 μg/kg once weekly based on body weight in cancer patients receiving chemotherapy [RHD-C]*). A slight reduction in fetal weight was observed at doses that were ≥1 μg/kg/day (≥15 times RHD-CRF; ≥3 times RHD-C) but this was a maternal toxic dose. In rats, IV doses of ≥2.5 μg/kg every other day (about ≥20 times the RHD-CRF or about ≥4 times the RHD-C) from day 6 of gestation through day 23 of lactation caused decreased body weights and delayed eye opening and preputial separation. Darbepoetin had no adverse effect on uterine implantation in rats or rabbits. However, an increase in post implantation fetal loss was observed in rats given doses ≥0.5 μg/kg three times weekly (about ≥3 times the RHD-CRF; about ≥0.7 times the RHD-C) (1).

It is not known if darbepoetin alfa crosses the human placenta. The drug does not cross the rat placenta (1). The very high molecular weight (about 37,000) of this glycoprotein argues against transfer across the placenta. A closely related drug, epoetin alfa, has a lower molecular weight (about 30,000) and it does not cross to the fetus. (See Epoetin Alfa.)

No reports describing the use of darbepoetin alfa in human pregnancy. The absence of major toxicity in animals and the experience with epoetin alfa (see Epoetin Alfa) suggest that darbepoetin does not represent a significant embryo or fetal risk. However, the increase in abortions observed in rats warrant further study. In addition, severe maternal hypertension, including a case of abruptio placentae, and worsening renal disease have been noted in pregnant women receiving epoetin alfa. If these adverse effects were caused by epoetin alfa, similar effects should be expected with darbepoetin. Because anemia and the need for frequent blood transfusions also present significant risks to the mother and fetus, the benefits derived from darbepoetin probably outweigh the known risks.

BREAST FEEDING SUMMARY

RECOMMENDATION: No Human Data - Probably Compatible

No reports describing the use of darbepoetin in human lactation have been located. Darbepoetin is a 165-amino acid glycoprotein with a molecular weight of 37,000. Passage into milk is not expected, but in the event that some transfer did occur, digestion in the nursing infant's gastrointestinal tract would occur. Moreover, preterm infants have been treated with epoetin alfa, a closely related agent. (See Epoetin Alfa.) Thus, the risk to a nursing infant from ingestion of the drug via the milk appears to be nonexistent.

Reference

1. Product information. Aranesp. Amgen, 2004.

Name:	**DAUNORUBICIN**	Risk Factor:	D_M
Class:	**Antineoplastic**		

FETAL RISK SUMMARY

RECOMMENDATION: Human and Animal Data Suggest Risk

Daunorubicin is a cytotoxic antibiotic used as an antineoplastic agent. In animal reproduction studies, exposure to daunorubicin during pregnancy produced teratogenic and toxic effects in rabbits, rats, and mice (1). In rabbits, a dose of 0.05 mg/kg/day (about 1/100th of the maximum recommended human dose on a body surface area basis) resulted in an increased incidence of abortions and fetal anomalies (parieto-occipital cranioschisis, umbilical hernias, or rachischisis). Malformations in rats administered doses of 4 mg/kg/day (about 1/2 the human dose) included esophageal, cardiovascular, and urogenital malformations, as well as fused ribs. Retarded fetal and neonatal growth was observed in mice after maternal administration of daunorubicin (1).

The use of daunorubicin during pregnancy has been reported in 29 patients, four during the 1st trimester (2–19). No congenital defects were observed in the 22 (one set of twins) liveborns, but one of these infants was anemic and hypoglycemic and had multiple serum electrolyte abnormalities (8). Two infants had transient neutropenia at 2 months of age (4). Severe, transient, drug-induced bone marrow hypoplasia occurred in one newborn after *in utero* exposure to daunorubicin and five other antineoplastic agents (18). The myelosuppression was probably secondary to mercaptopurine. The infant made an uneventful recovery. Results of the remaining pregnancies were three elective abortions (one with enlarged spleen), three intrauterine deaths (one probably a result of severe pregnancy-induced hypertension), one stillborn with diffuse myocardial necrosis, and one maternal death (8,9,15,17). Thirteen of the infants (including one set of twins) were studied for periods ranging from 6 months to 9 years and all showed normal growth and development (4,9–11,14,15,17–19).

Data from one review indicated that 40% of the infants exposed to anticancer drugs were of low birth weight (20). This finding was not related to timing of the exposure. Except for the infants noted above, long-term studies of growth and mental development in offspring exposed to daunorubicin during the 2nd trimester, the period of neuroblast multiplication, have not been conducted (21).

In one report, the use of daunorubicin and other antineoplastic drugs in two males was thought to be associated with congenital defects in their offspring (22). The defects observed were tetralogy of Fallot and syndactyly of the first and second digits of the right foot, and an anencephalic stillborn. Although the authors speculated that the drugs damaged the germ cells without producing infertility and thus were responsible for the defects, any relationship to paternal use of daunorubicin is doubtful due to the lack of experimental evidence and other confirming reports. In a third male, fertilization occurred during treatment with daunorubicin and resulted in the birth of a healthy infant (23). Successful pregnancies have also been reported in two women after treatment with daunorubicin (24).

Chromosomal aberrations were observed in the fetus of a 34-year-old woman with acute lymphoblastic leukemia who was treated with multiple antineoplastic agents (12). Daunorubicin was administered for approximately 3 weeks beginning at 22 weeks'

D

gestation. A healthy female infant was delivered 18 weeks after the start of therapy. Chromosomal analysis of the newborn revealed a normal karyotype (46,XX) but with gaps and a ring chromosome. The clinical significance of these findings is unknown, but since these abnormalities may persist for several years, the potential existed for an increased risk of cancer as well as for a risk of genetic damage in the next generation (12).

Occupational exposure of the mother to antineoplastic agents during pregnancy may present a risk to the fetus. A position statement from the National Study Commission on Cytotoxic Exposure and a research article involving some antineoplastic agents are presented in the monograph for cyclophosphamide (see Cyclophosphamide).

BREAST FEEDING SUMMARY

RECOMMENDATION: Contraindicated

No reports describing the use of daunorubicin during lactation have been located. Because of the potential for severe toxicity in a nursing infant, the use of this agent is contraindicated during breast-feeding.

References

1. Product information. Cerubidine. Bedford Laboratories, 2000.
2. Sears HF, Reid J. Granulocytic sarcoma: local presentation of a systemic disease. Cancer 1976;37:1808–13.
3. Lilleyman JS, Hill AS, Anderton KJ. Consequences of acute myelogenous leukemia in early pregnancy. Cancer 1977;40:1300–3.
4. Colbert N, Najman A, Gorin NC, Blum F. Acute leukaemia during pregnancy: favourable course of pregnancy in two patients treated with cytosine arabinoside and anthracyclines. Nouv Presse Med 1980;9: 175–8.
5. Tobias JS, Bloom HJG. Doxorubicin in pregnancy. Lancet 1980;1:776.
6. Sanz MA, Rafecas FJ. Successful pregnancy during chemotherapy for acute promyelocytic leukemia. N Engl J Med 1982;306:939.
7. Alegre A, Chunchurreta R, Rodriguez-Alarcon J, Cruz E, Prada M. Successful pregnancy in acute promyelocytic leukemia. Cancer 1982;49:152–3.
8. Gililand J, Weinstein L. The effects of cancer chemotherapeutic agents on the developing fetus. Obstet Gynecol Surv 1983;38:6–13.
9. Feliu J, Juarez S, Ordonez A, Garcia-Paredes ML, Gonzalez-Baron M, Montero JM. Acute leukemia and pregnancy. Cancer 1988;61:580–4.
10. Volkenandt M, Buchner T, Hiddemann W, Van De Loo J. Acute leukaemia during pregnancy. Lancet 1987;2:1521–2.
11. Turchi JJ, Villasis C. Anthracyclines in the treatment of malignancy in pregnancy. Cancer 1988;61: 435–40.
12. Schleuning M, Clemm C. Chromosomal aberrations in a newborn whose mother received cytotoxic treatment during pregnancy. N Engl J Med 1987;317:1666–7.
13. Gokal R, Durrant J, Baum JD, Bennett MJ. Successful pregnancy in acute monocytic leukaemia. Br J Cancer 1976;34:299–302.
14. Lowenthal RM, Marsden KA, Newman NM, Baikie MJ, Campbell SN. Normal infant after treatment of acute myeloid leukaemia in pregnancy with daunorubicin. Aust N Z J Med 1978;8:431–2.
15. O'Donnell R, Costigan C, O'Connell LG. Two cases of acute leukaemia in pregnancy. Acta Haematol 1979; 61:298–300.
16. Hamer JW, Beard MEJ, Duff GB. Pregnancy complicated by acute myeloid leukaemia. N Z Med J 1979;89:212–3.
17. Doney KC, Kraemer KG, Shepard TH. Combination chemotherapy for acute myelocytic leukemia during pregnancy: three case reports. Cancer Treat Rep 1979;63:369–71.
18. Okun DB, Groncy PK, Sieger L, Tanaka KR. Acute leukemia in pregnancy: transient neonatal myelosuppression after combination chemotherapy in the mother. Med Pediatr Oncol 1979;7:315–9.
19. Cantini E, Yanes B. Acute myelogenous leukemia in pregnancy. South Med J 1984;77:1050–2.
20. Nicholson HO. Cytotoxic drugs in pregnancy: review of reported cases. J Obstet Gynaecol Br Commonw 1968;75:307–12.
21. Dobbing J. Pregnancy and leukaemia. Lancet 1977; 1:1155.
22. Russell JA, Powles RL, Oliver RTD. Conception and congenital abnormalities after chemotherapy of acute myelogenous leukaemia in two men. Br Med J 1976; 1:1508.
23. Matthews JH, Wood JK. Male fertility during chemotherapy for acute leukemia. N Engl J Med 1980; 303:1235.
24. Estiu M. Successful pregnancy in leukaemia. Lancet 1977;1:433.

Name:	**DECAMETHONIUM**	Risk Factor:	**C**
Class:	**Muscle Relaxant**		

FETAL RISK SUMMARY

RECOMMENDATION: No Human Data - No Relevant Animal Data

Decamethonium is no longer manufactured in the United States. No reports linking the use of decamethonium with congenital defects have been located. The drug has been used at term for maternal analgesia (1).

BREAST FEEDING SUMMARY

RECOMMENDATION: No Human Data - Potential Toxicity

No data are available.

Reference

1. Moya F, Thorndyke V. Passage of drugs across the placenta. Am J Obstet Gynecol 1962;84:1778–98.

Name:	**DEFEROXAMINE**	Risk Factor:	**C_M**
Class:	**Antidote/Chelating Agent**		

FETAL RISK SUMMARY

RECOMMENDATION: Compatible

Deferoxamine is used for the treatment of acute iron intoxication and chronic iron overload. Animal reproduction studies have shown delayed ossification in mice and skeletal anomalies in rabbits with daily doses up to 4.5 times the maximum daily human dose (1). No fetal adverse effects were observed in rats administered similar doses (1).

In another animal reproduction study, pregnant mice were administered intraperitoneal doses of deferoxamine (44, 88, 176, and 352 mg/kg/day) on gestational days 6 through 15 and then sacrificed on gestational day 18 (2). On a weight basis, the lower two doses are comparable to the therapeutic human dose. The NOAEL (no observed adverse effect level) for maternal toxicity (reduced body weight) was <44 mg/kg/day, whereas the NOAEL for fetal developmental toxicity was 176 mg/kg/day (2). The only fetal toxic effect was a decrease in the number of live fetuses that was observed at 352 mg/kg/day.

A number of reports have described the use of deferoxamine in human pregnancy either for acute iron overdose or for transfusion-dependent thalassemia (3–8). Brief mention of three other pregnant patients treated with deferoxamine for acute overdose appeared in an earlier report, but no details were given except that all of the infants were normal (9). The authors knew of a seventh patient treated in the 3rd trimester for overdose with normal outcome (S. M. Lovett, unpublished data, 1985).

In a thalassemia patient, deferoxamine was given by continuous subcutaneous infusion pump, 2 g every 12 hours, for the first 16 weeks of pregnancy (3). A cesarean section

D

was performed at 33 weeks' gestation for vaginal bleeding and premature rupture of the membranes, with delivery of a normal preterm male infant. The neonatal period was complicated by hypoglycemia and prolonged jaundice lasting 6 weeks, but neither problem was thought to be related to deferoxamine. A 1999 report described the use of deferoxamine in a 18-year-old pregnant woman with hemoglobin E beta zero thalassemia, chronic hepatitis C, and iron overload (4). She conceived while receiving a SC dose of 40 mg/kg four days a week plus an additional 50 mg/kg IV every month with a transfusion. Therapy was stopped when the pregnancy was diagnosed, but then restarted at 18 weeks' gestation because of increased iron accumulation. The dose was increased in increments in response to her high ferritin levels, eventually reaching 50 mg/kg/day IV. She delivered an approximate 2298-g, normal male infant at 38 weeks' gestation. The boy was developing normally at 10 months of age and no toxic effects on bone formation, auditory, or ocular systems were found (4).

Several pregnant women have received deferoxamine therapy for iron overdose that occurred at 15 to 38 weeks' gestation (5–8). The women were treated with IM deferoxamine, and one also received the drug nasogastrically. Spontaneous labor with rupture of the membranes occurred 8 hours after iron ingestion in a 34-week gestation patient, resulting in the vaginal delivery 6 hours later of a normal male infant (5). The cord blood iron level was 121 μg/dL (normal 106–227 μg/dL) but fell to 21 μg/dL at 12 hours. The infant's clinical course was normal except for low iron levels requiring iron supplementation. The authors suggested that the low neonatal iron levels were due to chelation of iron by transplacentally transferred deferoxamine. In another case, a normal term male infant was delivered without evidence of injury from deferoxamine (6). Normal infants were delivered also in the other two cases, both at times distant from the use of deferoxamine (7,8).

In summary, deferoxamine produces toxicity and teratogenicity in various animal species. Although the number of published human pregnancy exposures to deferoxamine are limited, none of the reports have observed adverse human developmental effects. In one of the reports discussed above, the authors reviewed more than 65 cases of human pregnancy exposure to the agent that occurred during the management of thalassemia or iron overdose (4). No toxic or teratogenic effects were documented. A 1998 review of metal chelating agents also failed to find any published evidence of human developmental toxicity (10).

BREAST FEEDING SUMMARY

RECOMMENDATION: No Human Data - Probably Compatible

No reports describing the use of deferoxamine in lactation have been located. The molecular weight (about 657) is low enough that some excretion into breast milk probably occurs. The effects, if any, on a nursing infant from this exposure are unknown.

References

1. Product information. Desferal. Novartis Pharmaceuticals, 2000.
2. Bosque MA, Domingo JL, Corbella J. Assessment of the developmental toxicity of deferoxamine in mice. Arch Toxicol 1995;69:467–71.
3. Thomas RM, Skalicka AE. Successful pregnancy in transfusion-dependent thalassaemia. Arch Dis Child 1980;55:572–4.
4. Singer ST, Vichinsky EP. Deferoxamine treatment during pregnancy: is it harmful? Am J Hematol 1999;60:24–26.
5. Rayburn WF, Donn SM, Wulf ME. Iron overdose during pregnancy: successful therapy with deferoxamine. Am J Obstet Gynecol 1983;147:717–8.
6. Blanc P, Hryhorczuk D, Danel I. Deferoxamine treatment of acute iron intoxication in pregnancy. Obstet Gynecol 1984;64:12S–4S.
7. Van Ameyde KJ, Tenenbein M. Whole bowel

irrigation during pregnancy. Am J Obstet Gynecol 1989;160:646–7.
8. Lacoste H, Goyert GL, Goldman LS, Wright DJ, Schwartz DB. Acute iron intoxication in pregnancy: case report and review of the literature. Obstet Gynecol 1992;80:500–1.
9. Strom RL, Schiller P, Seeds AE, Ten Bensel R. Fatal iron poisoning in a pregnant female: case report. Minn Med 1976;59:483–9.
10. Domingo JL. Developmental toxicity of metal chelating agents. Reprod Toxicol 1998;12:499–510.

Name: **DELAVIRDINE** Risk Factor: C_M
Class: **Antiviral**

FETAL RISK SUMMARY

RECOMMENDATION: Compatible - Maternal Benefit >> Embryo/Fetal Risk

The synthetic non-nucleoside reverse transcriptase inhibitor (nnRTI), delavirdine, is used in the treatment of the human immunodeficiency virus type 1 (HIV-1). Because resistant viruses emerge rapidly with delavirdine monotherapy, the drug should always be used in combination with other antiretroviral agents (1). Other drugs in this class are efavirenz and nevirapine.

Reproductive studies with delavirdine have been conducted in rats and rabbits. Ventricular septal defects were produced when pregnant rats were administered the agent during organogenesis at doses producing systemic levels equal to or lower than the expected human exposure at the recommended dose (1). Reduced pup survival on the day of birth was also noted at this dose. At doses producing 5 times the expected human exposure at the recommended dose, marked maternal toxicity, embryo toxicity, fetal developmental delay, and reduced pup survival were observed. Delavirdine administered during organogenesis to rabbits caused maternal toxicity, embryo toxicity, and abortions (1). The lowest dose producing these effects was about 6 times the expected human exposure at the recommended dose. No malformations were observed in the surviving rabbit offspring, but only a few were available for examination (1).

It is not known if delavirdine crosses the human placenta. The molecular weight (about 553 for the mesylate salt) is low enough, however, that passage to the fetus should be expected.

During premarketing clinical studies, seven unplanned pregnancies occurred resulting in three ectopic pregnancies, three healthy live births, and one premature infant with a birth defect (1). The infant, exposed early in gestation to about 6 weeks of delavirdine and zidovudine, had a small muscular ventricular septal defect.

The Antiretroviral Pregnancy Registry reported, for the period January 1989 through January 2004, prospective data (reported to the Registry before the outcomes were known) involving 1537 live births that had been exposed during the 1st trimester to one or more antiretroviral agents (2). Forty-seven of the newborns had congenital defects (3.1%, 95% confidence interval [CI] 2.3–4.1). In the 2407 live births with earliest exposure in the 2nd/3rd trimesters, there were 56 infants with defects (2.3%, 95% CI 1.8–3.0). The prevalence rates for the two periods did not differ significantly. There were 103 infants with birth defects among 3944 live births with exposure anytime during pregnancy (2.6%, 95% CI 2.1–3.2). The prevalence rate did not differ significantly from the rate expected in a nonexposed population (2). There were eight outcomes exposed to delavirdine (seven in the 1st trimester and one in the 2nd/3rd trimesters) in combination with other antiretroviral agents. There were no birth defects in either exposure group. In reviewing the birth defects of prospective and retrospective (pregnancies reported after the outcomes were known) registered cases, and clinical reports, the Registry concluded that there was no pattern of anomalies to suggest a common cause (2). (See Lamivudine for required statement.)

In summary, the limited human data do not allow a prediction as to the safety of delavirdine during pregnancy. However, the animal data indicates that the drug may represent a risk to the developing human fetus. Moreover, one exposed newborn had a ventricular septal defect, an anomaly identical to that seen in rats. Two reviews, one in 1996 and the other in 1997, concluded that all women currently receiving antiretroviral therapy should continue to receive therapy during pregnancy and that treatment of the mother with monotherapy should be considered inadequate therapy (3,4). In 1998, the Centers for Disease Control and Prevention (CDC) made a similar recommendation that antiretroviral therapy should be continued during pregnancy, but discontinuation of all therapy during the 1st trimester was a consideration (5). Whether these recommendations to continue therapy apply to delavirdine, however, is unknown. If possible, another agent should be substituted for delavirdine if pregnancy is planned or occurs while the mother is undergoing treatment with this agent. However, if combination therapy with delavirdine is mandatory, it should not be withheld (with the possible exception of the 1st trimester) because the expected benefit to the HIV-positive mother probably outweighs the unknown risk to the fetus. The mother should be counseled on the risk to her fetus. The efficacy and safety of combined therapy in preventing vertical transmission of HIV to the newborn are unknown, and zidovudine remains the only antiretroviral agent recommended for this purpose (3,4).

BREAST FEEDING SUMMARY

RECOMMENDATION: Contraindicated

No reports describing the use of delavirdine during lactation have been located. The molecular weight (about 553 for the mesylate salt) is low enough that excretion into breast milk should be expected. Delavirdine is concentrated (3–5 times the maternal plasma level) in the milk of lactating rats (1).

Reports on the use of delavirdine during human lactation are unlikely, however, because the antiviral agent is used in the treatment of human immunodeficiency virus (HIV) infections. HIV-1 is transmitted in milk, and in developed countries, breast-feeding is not recommended (3,4,6–8). In developing countries, breast-feeding is undertaken, despite the risk, because there are no affordable milk substitutes available. Until 1999, no studies had been published that examined the effect of any antiretroviral therapy on HIV-1 transmission in milk. In that year, a study involving zidovudine was published that measured a 38% reduction in vertical transmission of HIV-1 infection despite breast feeding when compared to controls (see Zidovudine).

References

1. Product information. Rescriptor. Agouron Pharmaceuticals, 2001.
2. Antiretroviral Pregnancy Registry Steering Committee. *Antiretroviral Pregnancy Registry International Interim Report for 1 January 1989 through 31 January 2004.* Wilmington, NC: Registry Coordinating Center, 2004.
3. Carpenter CCJ, Fischi MA, Hammer SM, Hirsch MS, Jacobsen DM, Katzenstein DA, Montaner JSG, Richman DD, Saag MS, Schooley RT, Thompson MA, Vella S, Yeni PG, Volberding PA. Antiretroviral therapy for HIV infection in 1996. JAMA 1996;276;146–54.
4. Minkoff H, Augenbraun M. Antiretroviral therapy for pregnant women. Am J Obstet Gynecol 1997;176: 478–89.

5. CDC. Public Health Service Task Force recommendations for the use of antiretroviral drugs in pregnant women infected with HIV-1 for maternal health and for reducing perinatal HIV-1 transmission in the United States. MMWR 1998;47:No. RR-2.
6. Brown ZA, Watts DH. Antiviral therapy in pregnancy. Clin Obstet Gynecol 1990;33:276–89.
7. de Martino M, Tovo P-A, Pezzotti P, Galli L, Massironi E, Ruga E, Floreea F, Plebani A, Gabiano C, Zuccotti GV. HIV-1 transmission through breast-milk: appraisal of risk according to duration of feeding. AIDS 1992;6:991–7.
8. Van de Perre P. Postnatal transmission of human immunodeficiency virus type 1: the breast feeding dilemma. Am J Obstet Gynecol 1995;173:483–7.

D

Name: **DEMECARIUM** Risk Factor: **C***

Class: **Parasympathomimetic (Cholinergic)**

FETAL RISK SUMMARY

RECOMMENDATION: No Human Data - No Relevant Animal Data

Demecarium, a reversible, long-acting cholinesterase inhibitor, is used in the eye for the treatment of open-angle glaucoma. Apparently, no animal reproduction studies have been conducted with demecarium.

The manufacturer states that the drug is contraindicated in women who are or who may become pregnant because of the general toxicity of cholinesterase inhibitors (1). However, other agents with similar anticholinesterase activity have been used during human pregnancy without apparent complications (see Edrophonium, Neostigmine, and Physostigmine).

No reports of the use of demecarium in pregnancy have been located. As a quaternary ammonium compound, it is ionized at physiologic pH and transplacental passage in significant amounts would not be expected (see also Neostigmine).

[**Risk Factor X according to one manufacturer, Merck, 2000.*]

BREAST FEEDING SUMMARY

RECOMMENDATION: No Human Data - Potential Toxicity

No reports describing the use of demecarium during lactation have been located. The manufacturer states that the drug should not be used during breast-feeding because of the potential for severe adverse effects in a nursing infant (1).

Reference

1. Product information. Humorsol. Merck, 2000.

Name: **DEMECLOCYCLINE** Risk Factor: **D**

Class: **Antibiotic (Tetracycline)**

See Tetracycline.

Name:	**DESFLURANE**	Risk Factor:	B_M
Class:	**General Anesthetic**		

FETAL RISK SUMMARY

RECOMMENDATION: Limited Human Data - Animal Data Suggest Low Risk

Desflurane, a general inhalation anesthetic agent administered via vaporizer, is indicated for the induction and/or maintenance of anesthesia during surgery. It is a nonflammable, volatile liquid that is in the same class of halogenated agents as enflurane, halothane, isoflurane, methoxyflurane, and sevoflurane. Desflurane is closely related chemically to enflurane and isoflurane. The only difference between desflurane and isoflurane is the substitution of fluorine in desflurane for the single chlorine atom in isoflurane. This small change, however, produces marked pharmacokinetic and clinical effects. The potency of desflurane is 20% that of isoflurane, the blood-gas partition coefficient is reduced (i.e., reduced solubility in blood) (0.42 vs. 1.46) as is tissue solubility (brain-blood partition coefficient 1.3 vs. 1.6), and recovery from anesthesia is faster (1).

Three mutagenic tests with desflurane found no evidence of genotoxicity (2). No teratogenic effects were observed in reproduction tests with rats and rabbits at doses of approximately 10 and 13 cumulative MAC-Hour exposures at 1 MAC-Hour per day, respectively, during organogenesis (2). (*Note: the minimum alveolar anesthetic concentration [MAC] is the concentration that causes immobility in 50% of patients exposed to a noxious stimulus such as a surgical incision; it represents the* ED_{50} [3]). However, an approximately 6% decrease in the body weight of male rat pups delivered prematurely by cesarean section was noted at this dose. No treatment-related behavioral changes or other toxicity (dystocia; decreased body weight) were observed in rat offspring exposed to desflurane 1 MAC-Hour per day from gestation day 15 to lactation day 21 (2).

The low molecular weight (about 168) and desflurane's presence in the brain suggest that it will cross the placenta to the fetus. Two reviews have concluded that, in general, inhalational anesthetic agents are freely transferred to fetal tissues (4,5) and, in most cases, the maternal and fetal blood concentrations are approximately equivalent (5). The relatively low human blood-gas partition coefficient and the rapid clearance from the maternal blood also suggest that desflurane will be rapidly cleared from the fetus, thus reducing the potential for neurobehavior depression of the newborn.

A brief 1993 report compared the closely related anesthetic agents, desflurane and enflurane (10 patients in each group), during cesarean delivery (6). Uterine tone increased significantly over time (a potential risk factor for maternal bleeding), but there were no differences between the groups. The mean umbilical vein:maternal artery ratios were 0.69 and 0.51, respectively. No differences between the groups were measured in the Neurological and Adaptive Capacity Scores (NACS) at 2 and 24 hours, 1- and 5-minute Apgar scores (8.0 and 8.9 vs. 7.5 and 9.0, respectively), and cord arterial blood gasses or pH (6).

Two end-tidal concentrations of desflurane (3% and 6%) were compared to enflurane (0.6%) for cesarean section delivery in a 1995 study (7). The MACs for the three groups were 0.45,0.90, and 0.40, respectively, thus representing sub-anesthetic concentrations. A 50–50 mixture of nitrous oxide and oxygen was administered with the anesthetic agents (25 patients in each group). Maternal blood loss was similar among the groups. In the newborns, the time-to-sustained-respiration was greater than 90 seconds in one (4%), seven (28%), and five (20%), respectively. The increased incidence in the 6% desflurane group was significantly longer than the 3% desflurane group ($p < 0.05$). There were no significant differences in the NACS at 2 and 24 hours, but some depression was noted: NACS <35 at 2 hours—four (16%), seven (28%), and six (24%); and at 24 hours—one (4%), one (4%), and none, respectively. The incidence of low Apgar scores (<7) at 1 and 5 minutes were at 1 minute, three (12%), seven (28%), and six (24%), respectively (*ns*); at 5 minutes, none, one (4%), and one (4%), respectively (*ns*) (7).

D

A 1995 study compared desflurane (1.0%–4.5%) and oxygen ($N = 40$) with nitrous oxide (30%–60%) in oxygen ($N = 40$) for analgesia during vaginal delivery (8). Maternal analgesia scores and blood loss were similar between the groups. Four (10%) of the desflurane group had a NACS less than 35 at 2 hours compared with seven (18%) of those exposed to nitrous oxide (*ns*). At 24 hours, none of desflurane group had a NACS less than 35 compared with three (8%) in the nitrous oxide group (*ns*). Apgar scores <7 at 1 minute occurred in 13% and 8% (*ns*), respectively, but all Apgar scores were 7 or greater at 5 minutes. However, nine patients in the desflurane group had amnesia for delivery, a potentially undesirable effect in an obstetrical patient (8).

A study published in 1998 evaluated the exposure of nine nurses in a post-anesthesia care unit (PACU) to exhaled desflurane and isoflurane and compared these exposures with the National Institute of Occupational Safety and Health (NIOSH) recommended exposure limits (9). The NIOSH recommendation for volatile anesthetics (without concomitant nitrous oxide exposure) is a maximum of 2 parts per million, but it has not been adopted by the Occupational Safety and Health Administration. Moreover, the recommended limit is controversial and is thought by some to be inappropriately low (9). However, a potential for reproductive risk (spontaneous abortion and infertility) is thought to exist for some anesthetic agents. The study involved exposure in the PACU to exhaled anesthetic gases from 50 adult patients (desflurane $N = 31$, isoflurane $N = 19$) over an approximate 1 hour recovery time. About half the patients were extubated in the PACU. Exposure was continuously measured from the shoulders (i.e., breathing-zone) of the nurses. Breathing-zone anesthetic concentrations of desflurane and isoflurane exceeded the NIOSH limits in 87% and 37% of the cases, respectively. These exposures were above the limit 49% of the time for desflurane and 12% of the time for isoflurane. The investigators listed several limitations to their study and concluded that the results might represent a "worst-case analysis" (9).

A 2004 study found a significant association between maternal occupational exposure to waste anesthetic gases during pregnancy and developmental deficits in their children, including gross and fine motor ability, inattention/hyperactivity, and IQ performance (see Nitrous Oxide).

In summary, desflurane is not teratogenic in rats and rabbits, but there are no reports of its use early in human gestation. The animal data is reassuring, but the absence of human data during organogenesis precludes an estimation of the risk for structural anomalies. In addition, general anesthesia usually involves the use of several pharmacological agents. Although no teratogenicity has been observed with three other halogenated general anesthetic agents (halothane, isoflurane, and methoxyflurane), only halothane has 1st trimester human exposure data (4). The use of desflurane during cesarean section does not appear to affect the newborn any differently than other general anesthetic agents. All such agents can cause depression in the newborn that may last for 24 hours or more. The potential reproductive toxicity (spontaneous abortion and infertility) of occupational exposure to desflurane has not been studied but is a concern based on the exposure concentration found in one study. In addition, occupational exposure to nitrous oxide also was measured in that study, and indicated that the nurses were exposed to both nitrous oxide and volatile anesthetic agents at the same time.

BREAST FEEDING SUMMARY

D

RECOMMENDATION: No Human Data - Probably Compatible

Although desflurane has been administered during labor and delivery, the effects of this exposure on the infant that begins nursing immediately after birth have not been described. Desflurane is probably excreted into colostrums and milk as suggested by its presence in the maternal blood and its low molecular weight (about 168), but the toxic potential of this exposure for the infant is unknown. However, the risk to a nursing infant from exposure to desflurane is probably very low (10). Moreover, the concentrations in milk should be less than other halogenated anesthetic agents because of the decreased blood and tissue solubility of desflurane and its rapid washout from the mother's system. The manufacturer states that excretion in milk was not clinically important 24 hours after anesthesia (2). Another halogenated inhalation anesthetic, halothane, is classified as compatible with breast-feeding (see Halothane).

References

1. Eger EI II. Desflurane animal and human pharmacology: aspects of kinetics, safety, and MAC. Anesth Analg 1992;75:S3–9.
2. Product information. Suprane. Baxter Healthcare Corporation, Anesthesia & Critical Care, 2002.
3. Trevor AJ, Miller RD. General anesthetics. In Katzung BG, ed. *Basic and Clinical Pharmacology*. 8th ed. New York: McGraw-Hill, 2001:426.
4. Friedman JM. Teratogen update: anesthetic agents. Teratology 1988;37:69–77.
5. Kanto J. Risk-benefit assessment of anaesthetic agents in the puerperium. Drug Saf 1991;6:285–301.
6. Wallace DH, Armstrong A, Darras A, Gajraj N, Gambling D, White P. The effect of desflurane or low-dose enflurane on uterine tone at cesarean delivery: placental transfer and recovery (abstract). Anesthesiology 1993;79:A1019.
7. Abboud TK, Zhu J, Richardson M, Peres Da Silva P, Donovan M. Desflurane: a new volatile anesthetic for cesarean section. Maternal and neonatal effects. Acta Anaesthesiol Scand 1995;39:723–6.
8. Abboud TK, Swart F, Zhu J, Donovan MM, Peres Da Silva E, Yakal K. Desflurane analgesia for vaginal delivery. Acta Anaethesiol Scan 1995;39:259–61.
9. Sessler DI, Badgwell JM. Exposure of postoperative nurses to exhaled anesthetic gases. Anesth Analg 1998;87:1083–8.
10. Spigset O. Anaesthetic agents and excretion in breast milk. Acta Anaesthesiol Scand 1994;38:94–103.

Name:	**DESIPRAMINE**	Risk Factor:	**C**
Class:	**Antidepressant**		

FETAL RISK SUMMARY

RECOMMENDATION: Human Data Suggest Low Risk

Desipramine is an active metabolite of imipramine (see also Imipramine). Desipramine is a tricyclic antidepressant in the same class as amoxapine, nortriptyline, and protriptyline. No reports linking the use of desipramine with congenital defects have been located. Neonatal withdrawal symptoms, including cyanosis, tachycardia, diaphoresis, and weight loss, were observed after desipramine was taken throughout pregnancy (1).

In a surveillance study of Michigan Medicaid recipients conducted between 1985 and 1992 involving 229,101 completed pregnancies, 31 newborns had been exposed to desipramine during the 1st trimester (F. Rosa, personal communication, FDA, 1993). One

(3.2%) major birth defect was observed (one expected). No anomalies were observed in six defect categories (cardiovascular defects, oral clefts, spina bifida, polydactyly, limb reduction defects, and hypospadias) for which specific data were available. The number of exposures is too small for comment.

In a 1996 descriptive case series, the European Network of the Teratology Information Services (ENTIS) prospectively examined the outcomes of 689 pregnancies exposed to antidepressants (2). Multiple drug therapy occurred in about two-thirds of the mothers. Desipramine was used in one pregnancy and the outcome was a spontaneous abortion.

In an *in vitro* study, desipramine was shown to be a potent inhibitor of sperm motility (3). A concentration of 27 μmol/L produced a 50% reduction in motility.

A 2002 prospective study compared two groups of mother-child pairs exposed to antidepressants throughout gestation (46 exposed to tricyclics: 3 to desipramine; 40 to fluoxetine) to 36 nonexposed, not depressed controls (4). Offspring were studied between the ages 15 and 71 months for effects of antidepressant exposure in terms of IQ, language, behavior, and temperament. Exposure to antidepressants did not adversely affect the measured parameters, but IQ was significantly and negatively associated with the duration of depression, and language was negatively associated with the number of depression episodes after delivery (4).

BREAST FEEDING SUMMARY

RECOMMENDATION: Limited Human Data - Potential Toxicity

Desipramine is excreted into breast milk (5–7). No reports of adverse effects have been located. In one patient, milk:plasma ratios of 0.4–0.9 were measured with milk levels ranging between 17 and 35 μg/mL (5). A 35-year-old mother in her 9th postpartum week took 300 mg of desipramine daily at bedtime for depression (7). One week later, simultaneous milk and serum samples were collected about 9 hours after a dose. Concentrations of desipramine in the milk and serum were 316 and 257 ng/mL (ratio 1.2), respectively, whereas levels of the metabolite, 2-hydroxydesipramine, were 381 and 234 ng/mL (ratio 1.6), respectively. The measurements were repeated 1 week later, 10.33 hours after the dose, and milk levels of the parent drug and metabolite were 328 and 327 ng/mL, respectively. No drug was detected in the infant's serum nor were any clinical signs of toxicity observed in the infant after 3 weeks of maternal treatment (7).

A 1996 review of antidepressant treatment during breast-feeding found no information that desipramine exposure during nursing resulted in quantifiable amounts in an infant or that the exposure caused adverse effects (8). The American Academy of Pediatrics classifies desipramine as a drug whose effect on the nursing infant is unknown but may be of concern (9).

References

1. Webster PA. Withdrawal symptoms in neonates associated with maternal antidepressant therapy. Lancet 1973;2:318–9.
2. McElhatton PR, Garbis HM, Elefant E, Vial T, Bellemin B, Mastroiacovo P, Arnon J, Rodriguez-Pinilla E, Schaefer C, Pexieder T, Merlob P, Dal Verme S. The outcome of pregnancy in 689 women exposed to therapeutic doses of antidepressants. A collaborative study of the European Network of Teratology Information Services (ENTIS). Reprod Toxicol 1996;10:285–94.
3. Levin RM, Amsterdam JD, Winokur A, Wein AJ. Effects of psychotropic drugs on human sperm motility. Fertil Steril 1981;36:503–6.
4. Nulman I, Rovet J, Stewart DE, Wolpin J, Pace-Asciak P, Shuhaiber S, Koren G. Child development following exposure to tricyclic antidepressants or fluoxetine

throughout fetal life: a prospective, controlled study. Am J Psychiatry 2002;159:1889–95.
5. Sovner R, Orsulak PJ. Excretion of imipramine and desipramine in human breast milk. Am J Psychiatry 1979;136:451–2.
6. Erickson SH, Smith GH, Heidrich F. Tricyclics and breast-feeding. Am J Psychiatry 1979;136:1483.
7. Stancer HC, Reed KL. Desipramine and 2-hydroxydesipramine in human breast milk and the nursing infant's serum. Am J Psychiatry 1986;143: 1597–1600.
8. Wisner KL, Perel JM, Findling RL. Antidepressant treatment during breast-feeding. Am J Psychiatry 1996;153:1132–7.
9. Committee on Drugs, American Academy of Pediatrics. The transfer of drugs and other chemicals into human milk. Pediatrics 2001;108:776–89.

Name: **DESLANOSIDE** Risk Factor: **C**
Class: **Cardiac Glycoside**

See Digitalis.

Name: **DESMOPRESSIN** Risk Factor: **B_M**
Class: **Pituitary Hormone, Synthetic**

FETAL RISK SUMMARY

RECOMMENDATION: No Human Data - Animal Data Suggest Low Risk

Desmopressin is a synthetic polypeptide structurally related to vasopressin. See Vasopressin. Reproduction studies with desmopressin in rats and rabbits at doses up to approximately 0.1 times and 38 times, respectively, the maximum systemic human exposure based on body surface area, did not reveal fetal harm (1).

BREAST FEEDING SUMMARY

RECOMMENDATION: Compatible

See Vasopressin.

Reference

1. Product information. DDAVP. Rhone-Poulenc Rorer Pharmaceuticals, 2000.

Name: **DEXAMETHASONE** Risk Factor: **C***
Class: **Corticosteroid**

FETAL RISK SUMMARY

RECOMMENDATION: Compatible - Maternal Benefit >> Embryo/Fetal Risk

Although most sources have not linked the use of dexamethasone with congenital defects, four large epidemiologic studies have found positive associations between systemic corticosteroids and nonsyndromic orofacial clefts. Specific corticosteroids were not identified in three of these studies (see Hydrocortisone for details), but dexamethasone and other agents were listed in a 1999 study discussed below.

In a case-control study, the California Birth Defects Monitoring Program evaluated the association between selected congenital anomalies and the use of corticosteroids 1 month before to 3 months after conception (periconceptional period) (1). Case infants or fetal deaths diagnosed with orofacial clefts, conotruncal defects, neural tubal defects (NTD), and limb anomalies were identified from a total of 552,601 births that occurred from 1987 through the end of 1989. Controls, without birth defects, were selected from the same data base. Following exclusion of known genetic syndromes, mothers of case and control infants were interviewed by telephone, an average of 3.7 years (cases) or 3.8 years (controls) after delivery, to determine various exposures during the periconceptional period. The number of interviews completed were orofacial cleft case mothers ($N = 662$, 85% of eligible), conotruncal case mothers ($N = 207$, 87%), NTD case mothers ($N = 265$, 84%), limb anomaly case mothers ($N = 165$, 82%), and control mothers ($N = 734$, 78%) (1). Orofacial clefts were classified into four phenotypic groups: isolated cleft lip with or without cleft palate (ICLP, $N = 348$), isolated cleft palate (ICP, $N = 141$), multiple cleft lip with or without cleft palate (MCLP, $N = 99$), and multiple cleft palate (MCP, $N = 74$). A total of 13 mothers reported using corticosteroids during the periconceptional period for a wide variety of indications. Six case mothers of ICLP and 3 of ICP used corticosteroids (unspecified corticosteroid $N = 1$, prednisone $N = 2$, cortisone $N = 3$, triamcinolone acetonide $N = 1$, dexamethasone $N = 1$, and cortisone plus prednisone $N = 1$). One case mother of an infant with NTD used cortisone and an injectable unspecified corticosteroid, and three controls used corticosteroids (hydrocortisone $N = 1$ and prednisone $N = 2$). The odds ratio for corticosteroid use and ICLP was 4.3 (95% confidence interval [CI] 1.1–17.2), whereas the odds ratio for ICP and corticosteroid use was 5.3 (95% CI 1.1–26.5). No increased risks were observed for the other anomaly groups. Commenting on their results, the investigators thought that recall bias was unlikely because they did not observe increased risks for other malformations, and it was also unlikely that the mothers would have known of the suspected association between corticosteroids and orofacial clefts (1).

Maternal free estriol and cortisol are significantly depressed after dexamethasone therapy, but the effects of these changes on the fetus have not been studied (2–4).

Dexamethasone has been used in patients with premature labor at about 26–34 weeks' gestation to stimulate fetal lung maturation (5–15). Although this therapy is supported by many clinicians, its use is still controversial because the beneficial effects of steroids are greatest in singleton pregnancies with female fetuses (16–19). These benefits are:

Reduction in incidence of respiratory distress syndrome (RDS)
Decreased severity of RDS if it occurs
Decreased incidence of and mortality from intracranial hemorrhage
Increased survival of premature infants

Toxicity in the fetus and newborn following the use of dexamethasone is rare.

In studies of women with premature rupture of the membranes (PROM), administration of corticosteroids does not always reduce the frequency of RDS or perinatal mortality (20–22). In addition, an increased risk of maternal infection has been observed in patients with PROM treated with corticosteroids (21,22). A recent report, however, found no difference in the incidence of maternal complications between treated and nontreated patients (23).

Dexamethasone crosses the placenta to the fetus (24,25). The drug is partially metabolized (54%) by the perfused placenta to its inactive 11-ketosteroid derivative, more so than betamethasone, but the difference is not statistically significant (25).

Leukocytosis has been observed in infants exposed antenatally to dexamethasone (26,27). The white blood cell counts returned to normal in about a week.

The use of corticosteroids, including dexamethasone, for the treatment of asthma during pregnancy has not been related to a significantly increased risk of maternal or fetal complications (28). A slight increase in the number of premature births was found, but it could not be determined whether this was an effect of the corticosteroids. An earlier study also recorded a shortening of gestation with chronic corticosteroid use (29).

In Rh-sensitized women, the use of dexamethasone may have prevented intrauterine fetal deterioration and the need for fetal transfusion (30). Five women, in the 2nd and 3rd trimesters, were treated with 24 mg of the steroid weekly for 2–7 weeks, resulting, in each case, in a live newborn.

Dexamethasone, 4 mg/day for 15 days, was administered to a woman late in the 3rd trimester for the treatment of autoimmune thrombocytopenic purpura (31). Therapy was given in an unsuccessful attempt to prevent fetal/neonatal thrombocytopenia due to the placental transfer of antiplatelet antibody. Platelet counts in the newborn were 38,000–49,000/mm^3, but the infant made an uneventful recovery.

The use of dexamethasone for the pharmacologic suppression of the fetal adrenal gland was described in two women with 21-hydroxylase deficiency (32,33). This deficiency results in the overproduction of adrenal androgens and the virilization of female fetuses. Dexamethasone, in divided doses of 1 mg/day, was administered from early in the 1st trimester (5th week and 10th week) to term. Normal female infants resulted from both pregnancies.

Although human studies have usually shown a benefit, the use of corticosteroids in animals has been associated with several toxic effects (34,35):

Reduced fetal head circumference
Reduced fetal adrenal weight
Increased fetal liver weight
Reduced fetal thymus weight
Reduced placental weight

Fortunately, none of these effects has been observed in human investigations. Long-term follow-up evaluations of children exposed *in utero* to dexamethasone have shown no adverse effects from this exposure (36,37).

[**Risk factor D if used in 1st trimester.*]

BREAST FEEDING SUMMARY

RECOMMENDATION: No Human Data - Probably Compatible

No reports describing the use of dexamethasone during lactation have been located. The molecular weight (about 516) is low enough for passage into breast milk. Moreover, trace amounts of other corticosteroids are excreted into milk (e.g., see

Hydrocortisone and Prednisone) and the excretion of dexamethasone into milk should be expected.

References

1. Carmichael SL, Shaw GM. Maternal corticosteroid use and risk of selected congenital anomalies. Am J Med Genet 1999;86:242–4.
2. Reck G, Nowostawski, Bredwoldt M. Plasma levels of free estriol and cortisol under ACTH and dexamethasone during late pregnancy. Acta Endocrinol 1977;84:86–7.
3. Kauppilla A. ACTH levels in maternal, fetal and neonatal plasma after short term prenatal dexamethasone therapy. Br J Obstet Gynaecol 1977;84:128–34.
4. Warren JC, Cheatum SG. Maternal urinary estrogen excretion: effect of adrenal suppression. J Clin Endocrinol 1967;27:436–8.
5. Caspi I, Schreyer P, Weinraub Z, Reif R, Levi I, Mundel G. Changes in amniotic fluid lecithin sphingomyelin ratio following maternal dexamethasone administration. Am J Obstet Gynecol 1975;122:327–31.
6. Spellacy WN, Buhi WC, Riggall FC, Holsinger KL. Human amniotic fluid lecithin/sphingomyelin ratio changes with estrogen or glucocorticoid treatment. Am J Obstet Gynecol 1973;115:216–8.
7. Caspi E, Schreyer P, Weinraub Z, Reif R, Levi I, Mundel G. Prevention of the respiratory distress syndrome in premature infants by antepartum glucocorticoid therapy. Br J Obstet Gynaecol 1976;83:187–93.
8. Ballard RA, Ballard PL. Use of prenatal glucocorticoid therapy to prevent respiratory distress syndrome. Am J Dis Child 1976;130:982–7.
9. Thornfeldt RE, Franklin RW, Pickering NA, Thornfeldt CR, Amell G. The effect of glucocorticoids on the maturation of premature lung membranes: preventing the respiratory distress syndrome by glucocorticoids. Am J Obstet Gynecol 1978;131:143–8.
10. Ballard PL, Ballard RA. Corticosteroids and respiratory distress syndrome: status 1979. Pediatrics 1979; 63:163–5.
11. Taeusch HW Jr, Frigoletto F, Kitzmiller J, Avery ME, Hehre A, Fromm B, Lawson E, Neff RK. Risk of respiratory distress syndrome after prenatal dexamethasone treatment. Pediatrics 1979;63:64–72.
12. Caspi E, Schreyer P, Weinraub Z, Lifshitz Y, Goldberg M. Dexamethasone for prevention of respiratory distress syndrome: multiple perinatal factors. Obstet Gynecol 1981;57:41–7.
13. Bishop EH. Acceleration of fetal pulmonary maturity. Obstet Gynecol 1981;58(Suppl):48S–51S.
14. Farrell PM, Engle MJ, Zachman RD, Curet LB, Morrison JC, Rao AV, Poole WK. Amniotic fluid phospholipids after maternal administration of dexamethasone. Am J Obstet Gynecol 1983;145:484–90.
15. Ruvinsky ED, Douvas SG, Roberts WE, Martin JN Jr, Palmer SM, Rhodes PG, Morrison JC. Maternal administration of dexamethasone in severe pregnancy-induced hypertension. Am J Obstet Gynecol 1984; 149:722–6.
16. Avery ME. The argument for prenatal administration of dexamethasone to prevent respiratory distress syndrome. J Pediatr 1984;104:240.
17. Sepkowitz S. Prenatal corticosteroid therapy to prevent respiratory distress syndrome. J Pediatr 1984;105: 338–9.
18. Avery ME. Prenatal corticosteroid therapy to prevent respiratory distress syndrome (reply). J Pediatr 1984;105:339.
19. Levy DL. Maternal administration of dexamethasone to prevent RDS. J Pediatr 1984;105:339.
20. Eggers TR, Doyle LW, Pepperell RJ. Premature rupture of the membranes. Med J Aust 1979;1:209–13.
21. Garite TJ, Freeman RK, Linzey EM, Braly PS, Dorchester WL. Prospective randomized study of corticosteroids in the management of premature rupture of the membranes and the premature gestation. Am J Obstet Gynecol 1981;141:508–15.
22. Garite TJ. Premature rupture of the membranes: the enigma of the obstetrician. Am J Obstet Gynecol 1985;151:1001–5.
23. Curet LB, Morrison JC, Rao AV. Antenatal therapy with corticosteroids and postpartum complications. Am J Obstet Gynecol 1985;152:83–4.
24. Osathanondh R, Tulchinsky D, Kamali H, Fencl MdeM, Taeusch HW Jr. Dexamethasone levels in treated pregnant women and newborn infants. J Pediatr 1977;90: 617–20.
25. Levitz M, Jansen V, Dancis J. The transfer and metabolism of corticosteroids in the perfused human placenta. Am J Obstet Gynecol 1978;132:363–6.
26. Otero L, Conlon C, Reynolds P, Duval-Arnould B, Golden SM. Neonatal leukocytosis associated with prenatal administration of dexamethasone. Pediatrics 1981;68:778–80.
27. Anday EK, Harris MC. Leukemoid reaction associated with antenatal dexamethasone administration. J Pediatr 1982;101:614–6.
28. Schatz M, Patterson R, Zeitz S, O'Rourke J, Melam H. Corticosteroid therapy for the pregnant asthmatic patient. JAMA 1975;233:804–7.
29. Jenssen H, Wright PB. The effect of dexamethasone therapy in prolonged pregnancy. Acta Obstet Gynecol Scand 1977;56:467–73.
30. Navot D, Rozen E, Sadovsky E. Effect of dexamethasone on amniotic fluid absorbance in Rh-sensitized pregnancy. Br J Obstet Gynaecol 1982;89:456–8.
31. Yin CS, Scott JR. Unsuccessful treatment of fetal immunologic thrombocytopenia with dexamethasone. Am J Obstet Gynecol 1985;152:316–7.
32. David M, Forest MG. Prenatal treatment of congenital adrenal hyperplasia resulting from 21-hydroxylase deficiency. J Pediatr 1984;105:799–803.
33. Evans MI, Chrousos GP, Mann DW, Larsen JW Jr, Green I, McCluskey J, Loriaux L, Fletcher JC, Koons G, Overpeck J, Schulman JD. Pharmacologic suppression of the fetal adrenal gland in utero. JAMA 1985;253:1015–20.
34. Taeusch HW Jr. Glucocorticoid prophylaxis for respiratory distress syndrome: a review of potential toxicity. J Pediatr 1975;87:617–23.

35. Johnson JWC, Mitzner W, London WT, Palmer AE, Scott R. Betamethasone and the rhesus fetus: multisystemic effects. Am J Obstet Gynecol 1979;133:677–84.
36. Wong YC, Beardsmore CS, Silverman M. Antenatal dexamethasone and subsequent lung growth. Arch Dis Child 1982;57:536–8.
37. Collaborative Group on Antenatal Steroid Therapy. Effects of antenatal dexamethasone administration in the infant: long-term follow-up. J Pediatr 1984;104:259–67.

D

Name:	**DEXBROMPHENIRAMINE**	Risk Factor:	**C**
Class:	**Antihistamine**		

FETAL RISK SUMMARY

RECOMMENDATION: No Human Data - Probably Compatible

Dexbrompheniramine is the *dextro*-isomer of brompheniramine (see Brompheniramine). No reports linking its use with congenital defects have been located.

BREAST FEEDING SUMMARY

RECOMMENDATION: Limited Human Data - Probably Compatible

See Brompheniramine.

Name:	**DEXCHLORPHENIRAMINE**	Risk Factor:	**B_M**
Class:	**Antihistamine**		

FETAL RISK SUMMARY

RECOMMENDATION: Limited Human Data - Probably Compatible

Dexchlorpheniramine is the *dextro*-isomer of chlorpheniramine (see also Chlorpheniramine). No reports linking its use with congenital defects have been located. One study recorded 14 exposures in the 1st trimester without evidence for an association with malformations (1). Animal studies for chlorpheniramine have not shown a teratogenic effect (2).

In a surveillance study of Michigan Medicaid recipients conducted between 1985 and 1992 involving 229,101 completed pregnancies, 1080 newborns had been exposed to dexchlorpheniramine during the 1st trimester (F. Rosa, personal communication, FDA, 1993). A total of 50 (4.6%) major birth defects were observed (43 expected). Specific data were available for six defect categories, including (observed/expected) 10/11 cardiovascular defects, 2/2 oral clefts, 0/0.5 spina bifida, 3/3 polydactyly, 0/2 limb reduction defects, and 4/3 hypospadias. These data do not support an association between the drug and congenital defects.

An association between exposure during the last 2 weeks of pregnancy to antihistamines in general and retrolental fibroplasia in premature infants has been reported. See Brompheniramine for details.

BREAST FEEDING SUMMARY

RECOMMENDATION: No Human Data - Probably Compatible

No data are available.

References

1. Heinonen OP, Slone D, Shapiro S. *Birth Defects and Drugs in Pregnancy*. Littleton, MA: Publishing Sciences Group, 1977:323.
2. Product information. Polaramine. Schering Corporation, 1990.

D

Name:	**DEXFENFLURAMINE**	Risk Factor:	**C_M**
Class:	**Anorexiant**		

FETAL RISK SUMMARY

RECOMMENDATION: Limited Human Data - Animal Data Suggest Low Risk

Dexfenfluramine, the dextrorotatory isomer of fenfluramine, is a serotonin reuptake inhibitor and releasing agent used for the treatment of obesity. In reproductive studies with pregnant rats and rabbits at doses up to 10 times the daily human dose based on body surface area (DHD), no treatment-related embryotoxicity or teratogenicity was observed (1). In a three-generation study of pregnant rats given a dose 2.5 and 5 times the DHD, a dose-related significant reduction in maternal body weight and weight gain throughout pregnancy was noted. There were also a reduced number of placental implantations, fetuses, and live young, and delayed ossification in the fetuses (1). No significant treatment-related adverse effects or abnormalities were observed in second- and third-generation rats.

A 1992 report described the effects on brain serotonin of a continuous SC infusion of either 6 or 12 mg/kg/day of dexfenfluramine during the last week of pregnancy in pregnant rats and their offspring (2). Compared to controls, treated mothers had blunted weight gain, but no effect was observed on the number or the birth weight of their offspring. In contrast to the mothers, who had large depletions of serotonin when measured 3 weeks after birth, the amount of brain serotonin of the pups was either not affected or had returned to pretreatment levels within 24 hours.

The fatal course of a 30-year-old woman who had been treated with dexfenfluramine for 6 months immediately prior to pregnancy was described in a 1992 reference (3). She was delivered by cesarean section at 34 weeks' gestation because of premature labor. She died 4 days later of irreversible primary pulmonary hypertension. The authors concluded that the drug treatment, plus a short stay at an altitude of approximately 2400 feet (800 m) above sea level, and her subsequent pregnancy were the cause of the condition. The condition of the newborn was not mentioned.

Two birth defects were reported by the WHO International Drug Monitoring System following use of dexfenfluramine during pregnancy (F. Rosa, personal communication, FDA, 1997). One involved a malformation of the hand in 1989 and the second, in 1995, of an infant with multiple birth defects including anencephaly, a spinal anomaly, and a ventricular septal defect. No other details of these cases were available.

Except for the above, no published studies have reported the use of dexfenfluramine during human pregnancy and the limited animal data appear to indicate a minimal fetal risk. Use of the anorexiant during gestation, however, is not recommended. If weight loss is needed during gestation, then nonpharmacologic methods such as diet control combined with professional assistance should be used.

D

BREAST FEEDING SUMMARY

RECOMMENDATION: No Human Data - Potential Toxicity

No studies describing the use of dexfenfluramine during human lactation or measuring the amount of drug, if any, excreted into milk have been located. Dexfenfluramine is excreted into rat milk (1). Because of its low molecular weight, about 268, passage into human milk in measurable quantities should be expected.

The use of dexfenfluramine during lactation is not recommended because of its unknown effect on serotonin parameters within the nursing infant's brain and the potential for long-term adverse changes.

References

1. Product information. Redux. Wyeth-Ayerst Laboratories, 1997.
2. Rowland NE, Robertson RM. Administration of dexfenfluramine in pregnant rats: effect on brain serotonin parameters in offspring. Pharmacol Biochem Behav 1992;42:855–8.
3. Atanassoff PG, Weiss BM, Schmid ER, Tornic M. Pulmonary hypertension and dexfenfluramine. Lancet 1992;339:436.

Name:	**DEXMETHYLPHENIDATE**	Risk Factor:	**C_M**
Class:	**Central Stimulant**		

FETAL RISK SUMMARY

RECOMMENDATION: No Human Data - Animal Data Suggest Low Risk

Dexmethylphenidate is a central nervous system stimulant that is indicated for the treatment of Attention Deficit/Hyperactivity Disorder (ADHD). There are no active metabolites. The mean plasma elimination half-life is about 2.2 hours (1).

Reproduction studies have been conducted in rats and rabbits. No evidence of teratogenicity was observed in rats treated during organogenesis with doses resulting in maternal plasma levels (AUC) up to five times the levels (AUC) obtained in adult humans taking the recommended dose of 20 mg/day (RHD). However, at the highest dose, delayed skeletal ossification was seen. When doses resulting in plasma levels up to five times the RHD were given throughout gestation and lactation, the highest dose resulted in decreased post-weaning body weight in male offspring. In rabbits, no evidence of teratogenicity was observed at plasma levels up to one time the RHD (1).

It is not known if dexmethylphenidate crosses the human placenta. The molecular weight (about 234 for the free base) suggests that the drug will cross to the embryo and/or the fetus. The relatively short half-life, however, should limit the amount crossing the placenta.

No reports describing the use of dexmethylphenidate in human pregnancy have been located. No teratogenicity was observed in two animal species, but the maximum maternal systemic exposures obtained were very close to those measured in humans clinically.

Reported pregnancy exposures to methylphenidate, a closely related agent, are limited, but have not shown a major risk for embryo/fetal harm (see also Methylphenidate). Until human data are available for dexmethylphenidate, the safest course is to avoid the drug in pregnancy. If the mother's condition requires the drug, the lowest effective dose, avoiding the 1st trimester if possible, should be used. Long-term follow-up of exposed offspring may be warranted.

BREAST FEEDING SUMMARY

RECOMMENDATION: No Human Data - Potential Toxicity

No reports describing the use of dexmethylphenidate during human lactation have been located. The molecular weight (about 234 for the free base) is low enough that excretion into breast milk should be expected. However, the relatively short plasma elimination half-life should limit the amount of the drug in milk. The effects of this exposure on a nursing infant are unknown. If a mother chooses to breast-feed while taking dexmethylphenidate, the infant should be monitored for adverse effects observed in children and adults (e.g., abdominal pain, fever, anorexia, nausea, etc.).

Reference

1. Product information. Focalin. Novartis Pharmaceuticals, 2003.

Name:	**DEXTROAMPHETAMINE**	Risk Factor:	C_M
Class:	**Central Stimulant**		

See Amphetamine.

Name:	**DEXTROMETHORPHAN**	Risk Factor:	**C**
Class:	**Respiratory Drug (Antitussive)**		

FETAL RISK SUMMARY

RECOMMENDATION: Compatible

Dextromethorphan, a derivative of the narcotic analgesic levorphanol (see also Levorphanol) that is widely used as a cough suppressant in over-the-counter (OTC) preparations, produces little or no central nervous system depression. Although it is an antitussive without expectorant, analgesic, or addictive characteristics, abuse of the liquid product, possibly because of the ethanol vehicle used in some proprietary mixtures, is a potential complication (see case below). The agent is available either alone (as capsules, lozenges, or oral solutions) or in combination with a large variety of other compounds used for upper respiratory tract symptoms. Combination products containing ethanol should be avoided during pregnancy (see also Ethanol).

No information is available on the placental transfer of dextromethorphan. The molecular weight (about 271), however, is low enough that transfer to the fetus should be expected.

Only one published animal reproduction study involving dextromethorphan has been located (see reference 3 for unpublished data). A 1998 report examined the effects of dextromethorphan on chick embryos (1). The authors hypothesized that *N*-methyl-D-aspartate (NMDA) receptor antagonists, such as ethanol and dextromethorphan, induced neural crest (craniofacial and cardiac septal defects) and neural tube defects (NTD). Dextromethorphan, a NMDA receptor antagonist that acts as a channel blocker at the receptor, was injected into chick embryos *in ovo* for 3 consecutive days at doses of 0.5, 5, 50, and 500 nmol/embryo/day. The embryos were examined 24 hours after the third dose (none of the embryos were allowed to hatch). Dextromethorphan caused a dose-related increase in embryo mortality with rates of 14.1% with the 50-nmol dose ($p < 0.05$ versus controls) and 56.7% with the 500-nmol dose ($p < 0.001$ versus controls). Seven (1.2%) of the 595 control embryos injected only with vehicle (normal saline) had anomalies (spinal defect [$N = 1$], craniofacial defects [$N = 4$], and multiple defects [$N = 2$]), whereas 30 (8.0%) of all dextromethorphan-treated embryos had anomalies (spinal defect [$N = 1$], craniofacial defects [$N = 12$], multiple defects [$N = 16$], and other defects [$N = 1$]). Only the number of defects (about 15%) in the 500-nmol group, however, was significantly increased ($p < 0.001$) over the number in the control group. The authors cited published evidence that the receptors blocked by dextromethorphan in the chick embryos are analogous to receptors in other animals, including humans, during early development and that the drug would also block these receptors, resulting in similar malformations (1).

Interpretation of the results of the above study have been criticized (2–4) and defended (5). The primary concerns raised were the inappropriateness of the chick embryo model for determining human teratogenicity and the design of the study (3,4). Of particular concern, none of the embryos were allowed to hatch (the doses used were lethal) so it could not be determined if dextromethorphan was actually teratogenic. In addition, one author cited unpublished animal reproduction data from a drug manufacturer showing that in pregnant rats and rabbits, daily doses up to 20 and 100 times the human therapeutic dose on a body weight basis, respectively, caused no embryo or fetal harm in comparison with controls (3).

Metabolism of dextromethorphan has been shown to be primarily a result of O-demethylation to dextrorphan (6). The ability to metabolize many drugs, including O-demethylation of dextromethorphan, is genetically determined in adults. In this study of 155 adult volunteers, 144 (93%) metabolized dextromethorphan rapidly, and 11 (7%) were poor metabolizers, but the poor (slow) drug metabolizer phenotype has been reported in 5–10% of whites (6). In poor metabolizers, unmetabolized drug was the main excretion product, implying that these individuals had much higher and more prolonged plasma concentrations of dextromethorphan than did those who were extensive metabolizers. Moreover, using microsomal preparations obtained from aborted 10–30-week-old human fetuses and live newborn infants, the average activity of O-demethylation was less than 1% of the adult value and did not begin to rise until after birth (6). Thus, accumulation of unmetabolized dextromethorphan in the fetal compartment is a potential result of maternal ingestion of the drug during pregnancy (6).

The Collaborative Perinatal Project monitored 50,282 mother-child pairs, 300 of whom took dextromethorphan during the 1st trimester (7, p. 378). Twenty-four of the infants exposed *in utero* had a congenital malformation, a standardized relative risk (SRR) of 1.18. When only malformations showing uniform rates by hospital were considered, 17 (SRR 1.21) infants had a congenital defect (7, p. 379). Of these 17, 9 had major defects (SRR

1.10), and 8 had minor defects (SRR 1.30) (7, p. 382). For use anytime during pregnancy, 580 exposures were recorded, 15 of which had a malformation (SRR 1.39) (7, pp. 438,442). Ten of these defects were inguinal hernias (7, p. 496). The SSR do not support a relationship between the drug and congenital malformations.

A case report published in 1981 described a woman who consumed 480–840 mL/day of a cough syrup throughout pregnancy (8). The potential maximum daily doses based on 840 mL of syrup were 1.68 g of dextromethorphan, 16.8 g of guaifenesin, 5.0 g of pseudoephedrine, and 79.8 mL of ethanol. The infant had facial features of the fetal alcohol syndrome (bilateral epicanthal folds, short palpebral fissures, short, upturned nose, hypoplastic philtrum and upper lip with thinned vermilion, and a flattened midface) (8) (see also Ethanol). Other defects noted were an umbilical hernia and labia that appeared hypoplastic. The infant displayed irritability, tremors, and hypertonicity. It is not known if dextromethorphan or the drugs other than ethanol were associated with the adverse effects observed in the infant.

The use of dextromethorphan in four of five cases of a rare and distinct malformation complex was reported in 1984 (9). The complex of defects included absence of external genitalia, urinary, genital, and anal orifices, and persistence of the cloaca (9).

Chromosome analysis in four of the cases was normal and genetics did not appear to be a cause of the defects. Although a causative relationship could not be determined, the authors noted that three of the pregnancies, possibly all five, were exposed to doxylamine during the first 50 days of pregnancy (9). Dextromethorphan, however, was not thought to be related to the outcomes because only four of the mothers had symptoms of respiratory infection or took dextromethorphan during the critical period.

A surveillance study published in 1985 examined the prevalence of certain major birth defects among live-born infants of 6509 mothers (10). Dextromethorphan was assumed to have been used by 59 of the mothers, only one of whom gave birth to an infant with a major anomaly. This study found no strong association between any of the commonly used drugs and the congenital malformations surveyed (10).

Data from the Spanish Collaborative Study of Congenital Malformations (ECEMC) evaluating prenatal exposure to cough medicines containing dextromethorphan were published in 2001 (11). Using standardized methods, all newborn infants born in more than 77 hospitals throughout Spain were examined during the first 3 days of life for major and/or minor congenital defects. The case-control study was conducted between 1976 and 1998 and included 1,575,388 liveborn infants, 27,864 of whom had congenital defects detected during the first 3 days. Each case infant (those with defects) and its control (the next non-malformed, same sex infant born) were obtained from the same hospital. Among the case and control mothers, 0.26% ($N = 70$) and 0.18% ($N = 48$), respectively, had taken cough medicines containing dextromethorphan during the 1st trimester. The data were primarily analyzed for NTD and cardiac defects to test the hypothesis raised in the chick embryo study cited above (reference 1), but about 600 different categories of defects were also examined. Most of these categories, however, had no cases or controls. The adjusted (for maternal age, fever, drugs other than dextromethorphan, flu/cold, first-degree relatives with the same defects) odds ratio and 95% confidence intervals for selected anomalies were NTD 0.67 (0.09–4.94), central nervous system defects 1.36 (0.39–4.72), hydrocephaly 3.39 (0.38–30.35), congenital heart defects 0.92 (0.13–6.61), oral clefts 4.72 (0.55–40.24), and cleft palate 3.26 (0.35–30.34). When data on the amount consumed were available, the estimated total dextromethorphan dose and duration for cases and controls was about 101 mg/2.69 days and 117 mg/3.96 days, respectively. The investigators concluded that the use of dextromethorphan during the 1st trimester was not associated with an increase in congenital defects (11).

A 1984 review on the effect of over-the-counter drugs on human pregnancy concluded that dextromethorphan was safe to use during this period (12). Other reference sources (13–16) have also concluded that this antitussive does not pose a risk to the human fetus, and a 1998 source states that dextromethorphan is one of the drugs of choice during pregnancy for cough (17). Two of these references recommended a combination of guaifenesin plus dextromethorphan as the preferred antitussive in pregnant asthmatic patients (15,16).

A study published in 2001 described the outcomes of 184 pregnancies exposed to dextromethorphan, 128 of which were exposed in the 1st trimester, compared to 184 matched controls (18). The subjects were women who had called a teratogen information service concerning their use of dextromethorphan during pregnancy. There were six major birth defects (type not specified) in the subject group. One was a chromosomal abnormality and two were born to women who had used the antitussive after the 1st trimester. Among controls, there were five major birth defects (type not specified), one of which was a chromosomal abnormality. There were also no statistical differences between all subjects and controls in other outcomes: live births (172 vs. 174), spontaneous abortions (10 vs. 8), therapeutic abortions (1 vs. 2), stillbirths (1 vs. 0), minor malformations (10 vs. 8), and birth weight (3381 g vs. 3446 g) (18).

In summary, the available human data on the reproductive effects of dextromethorphan do not demonstrate a major teratogenic risk. Except for one study involving chick embryos, there are no published animal reproductive studies. Unpublished pregnant rat and rabbit data have been cited, though, that indicated there was no embryo or fetal harm with the doses used. Extrapolation of the chick embryo data to humans is not possible because of the lethal dose used and the absence of maternal and placental metabolizing systems. Moreover, prior teratology studies have not shown agreement between the chick and mammalian models (3). Fetuses of women with the phenotype for slow dextromethorphan metabolism should have higher concentrations of the drug than fetuses of mothers with normal metabolism, but this may not be clinically significant in the absence of a demonstrated dose effect. Use of liquid preparations of dextromethorphan that contain ethanol, however, should be avoided during pregnancy because ethanol is a known teratogen.

Many authors consider dextromethorphan to be safe for consumption during pregnancy. This opinion appears to have been based on the low incidence of congenital defects reported in surveillance studies and its wide appeal as a cough suppressant, rather than on evidence derived from human pregnancy research with dextromethorphan or from studies in any animal model. The latest data, however, provides more assurance that dextromethorphan is not a major teratogen.

BREAST FEEDING SUMMARY

RECOMMENDATION: Compatible

No reports describing the use of dextromethorphan during human lactation or measuring the amount, if any, excreted into milk have been located. The relatively low molecular weight of dextromethorphan, about 271, indicates that passage into milk probably occurs. Many preparations containing dextromethorphan also contain ethanol. These products should be avoided during nursing (see Ethanol). Preparations without ethanol, however, are probably safe to use during breast-feeding.

References

1. Andaloro VJ, Monaghan DT, Rosenquist TH. Dextromethorphan and other *N*-methyl-D-aspartate receptor antagonists are teratogenic in the avian embryo model. Pediatr Res 1998;43:1–7.
2. Polifka JE, Shepard TH. Studies of the fetal effects of dextromethorphan *in ovo*. Teratology 1999;60:56–7. (Originally published as an untitled letter to the editior: Pediatr Res 1998;44:415.)
3. Brent RL. Studies of the fetal effects of dextromethorphan *in ovo*. Teratology 1999;60:57–8. (Originally published as an untitled letter to the editor: Pediatr Res 1998;44:415–6.)
4. Brent RL, Shepard TH, Polifka JE. Response to Dr. Rosenquist's comments pertaining to the paper by Andaloro et al ('98) "Dextromethorphan and other *N*-methyl-D-aspartate receptor antagonists are teratogenic in the avian embryo model" and letters to the editor by Polifka JE and Shepard TH ('98) and Brent RL ('98). Teratology 1999;60:61–2.
5. Rosenquist TH. Studies of the fetal effects of dextromethorphan *in ovo*. Teratology 1999;60:56–60. (Originally published as an untitled author's response: Pediatr Res 1998;44:416–7.)
6. Jacqz-Aigrain E, Cresteil T. Cytochrome P450-dependent metabolism of dextromethorphan: fetal and adult studies. Dev Pharmacol Ther 1992;18:161–8.
7. Heinonen OP, Slone D, Shapiro S. *Birth Defects and Drugs in Pregnancy*. Littleton, MA: Publishing Sciences Group, 1977.
8. Chasnoff IJ, Diggs G, Schnoll SH. Fetal alcohol effects and maternal cough syrup abuse. Am J Dis Child 1981;135:968.
9. Robinson HBJr, Tross K. Agenesis of the cloacal membrane. A probable teratogenic anomaly. Perspect Pediatr Pathol 1984;8:79–96.
10. Aselton P, Jick H, Milunsky A, Hunter JR, Stergachis A. First-trimester drug use and congenital disorders. Obstet Gynecol 1985;65:451–5.
11. Martinez-Frias ML, Rodriguez-Pinilla E. Epidemiologic analysis of prenatal exposure to cough medicines containing dextromethorphan: no evidence of human teratogenicity. Teratology 2001;63:38–41.
12. Rayburn WF. OTC drugs and pregnancy. Perinatol Neonatol 1984;8:21–7.
13. Berglund F, Flodh H, Lundborg P, Prame B, Sannerstedt R. Drug use during pregnancy and breast-feeding. A classification system for drug information. Acta Obstet Gynecol Scand Suppl 1984;126:1–55.
14. Onnis A, Grella P. *The Biochemical Effects of Drugs in Pregnancy*. Volume 2. West Sussex, England: Ellis Harwood Limited, 1984:62–3.
15. Clark SL. Asthma in Pregnancy. National Asthma Education Program Working Group on Asthma and Pregnancy, National Institutes of Health, National Heart, Lung, and Blood Institute. Obstet Gynecol 1993;82:1036–40.
16. Report of the Working Group on Asthma and Pregnancy. Executive Summary: Management of asthma during pregnancy. J Allergy Clin Immunol 1994;93:139–62.
17. Koren G, Pastuszak A, Ito S. Drugs in pregnancy. N Engl J Med 1998;338:1128–37.
18. Einarson A, Lyszkiewicz D, Koren G. The safety of dextromethorphan in pregnancy. Results of a controlled study. Chest 2001;119:466–9.

Name:	**DEXTROTHYROXINE**	Risk Factor:	**C**
Class:	**Antilipemic**		

FETAL RISK SUMMARY

RECOMMENDATION: No Human Data - Probably Compatible

Dextrothyroxine is the *dextro*-isomer of levothyroxine (see also Levothyroxine). Although formerly used to treat hypothyroidism, the drug is now used exclusively for the therapy of hyperlipidemia. In a study of placental passage of dextrothyroxine, approximately 9% of a radiolabeled dose given 2–8 hours before delivery was found in the cord blood (1). Except for this one report, no mention of its use in human pregnancy has been located.

BREAST FEEDING SUMMARY

RECOMMENDATION: No Human Data - Probably Compatible

No data are available.

Reference

1. Kearns JE, Hutson W. Tagged isomers and analogues of thyroxine (their transmission across the human placenta and other studies). J Nucl Med 1963;4:453–61.

Name:	**DIATRIZOATE**	Risk Factor:	**D**
Class:	**Diagnostic**		

FETAL RISK SUMMARY

RECOMMENDATION: Human Data Suggest Risk in 2nd and 3rd Trimesters

The use of diatrizoate for amniography has been described in several studies (1–10). Except for inadvertent injection of the contrast media into the fetus during amniocentesis, the use of diatrizoate was not thought to result in fetal harm. More recent studies have examined the effect of the drug on fetal thyroid function.

All of the various preparations of diatrizoate contain a high concentration of organically bound iodine. Twenty-eight pregnant women received intra-amniotic injections (50 mL) of diatrizoate for diagnostic indications (11). When compared to nontreated controls, no effect was observed on cord blood levothyroxine (T4) and liothyronine resin uptake values regardless of the time interval between injection and delivery. The authors concluded that the iodine remained organically bound until it was eliminated in 2–4 days from the amniotic fluid.

In another report, seven patients within 13 days or less of term were injected intra-amniotically with a mixture of ethiodized oil (12 mL) and diatrizoate (30 mL) (12). Thyrotropin (TSH) levels were determined in the cord blood of five newborns and in the serum of all seven infants on the 5th day of life. TSH was markedly elevated in three of five cord samples and six of seven neonatal samples. Three of the infants had signs and symptoms of hypothyroidism:

Elevated TSH/normal T4; apathy and jaundice clearing immediately with thyroid therapy (1 infant)
Elevated TSH/decreased T4 (1 infant)
Elevated TSH/decreased T4 with goiter (1 infant)

In contrast to the initial report, the severity of thyroid suppression seemed greater the longer the time interval between injection and delivery. The explanation offered for these different results was the use of the more sensitive TSH serum test and the use of only water-soluble contrast media in the first study.

In summary, diatrizoate may suppress the fetal thyroid when administered by intra-amniotic injection. Appropriate measures should be taken to diagnose and treat neonatal hypothyroidism if amniography with diatrizoate is performed.

BREAST FEEDING SUMMARY

RECOMMENDATION: Limited Human Data - Probably Compatible

Diatrizoate was not detected in breast milk in one study. A woman, 7 weeks postpartum, received the contrast medium for urography (13). Nine hours after the dose, no measurable drug was identified by spectrophotometer. Based on this report, the American Academy of Pediatrics classifies diatrizoate as compatible with breast-feeding (14). (See Potassium Iodide.)

References

1. McLain CR Jr. Amniography studies of the gastrointestinal motility of the human fetus. Am J Obstet Gynecol 1963;86:1079–87.
2. McLain CR Jr. Amniography, a versatile diagnostic procedure in obstetrics. Obstet Gynecol 1964;23:45–50.
3. McLain CR Jr. Amniography for diagnosis and management of fetal death in utero. Obstet Gynecol 1965;26:233–6.
4. Ferris EJ, Shapiro JH, Spira J. Roentgenologic aspects of intrauterine transfusion. JAMA 1966;196:127–8.
5. Wiltchik SG, Schwarz RH, Emich JP Jr. Amniography for placental localization. Obstet Gynecol 1966;28:641–5.
6. Misenhimer HR. Fetal hemorrhage associated with amniocentesis. Am J Obstet Gynecol 1966;94:1133–5.
7. Blumberg ML, Wohl GT, Wiltchik S, Schwarz R, Emich JP. Placental localization by amniography. AJR 1967;100:688–97.
8. Berner HW Jr. Amniography, an accurate way to localize the placenta. Obstet Gynecol 1967;29:200–6.
9. Creasman WT, Lawrence RA, Thiede HA. Fetal complications of amniocentesis. JAMA 1968;204:949–52.
10. Bottorff MK, Fish SA. Amniography. S Med J 1971;64:1203–6.
11. Morrison JC, Boyd M, Friedman BI, Bucovaz ET, Whybrew WD, Koury DN, Wiser WL, Fish SA. The effects of Renografin-60 on the fetal thyroid. Obstet Gynecol 1973;42:99–103.
12. Rodesch F, Camus M, Ermans AM, Dodion J, Delange F. Adverse effect of amniofetography on fetal thyroid function. Am J Obstet Gynecol 1976;126:723–6.
13. FitzJohn TP, Williams DG, Laker MF, Owen JP. Intravenous urography during lactation. Br J Radiol 1982;55:603–5.
14. Committee on Drugs, American Academy of Pediatrics. The transfer of drugs and other chemicals into human milk. Pediatrics 2001;108:776–89.

Name:	DIAZEPAM	Risk Factor:	D
Class:	Sedative		

FETAL RISK SUMMARY

RECOMMENDATION: Human Data Suggest Risk in 1st and 3rd Trimesters

Shepard reviewed six studies of the reproductive effects of the benzodiazepine, diazepam in rats and mice in 1989 (1). Cleft palates in mice and delayed neurobehavior development and postnatal malignancies in rats were the only adverse effects noted (1).

Diazepam and its metabolite, desmethyldiazepam, freely cross the placenta and accumulate in the fetal circulation with newborn levels about 1 to 3 times greater than maternal serum levels (2–13). Transfer across the placenta has been demonstrated as early as 6 weeks' gestation (12). Of interest, fetal drug levels were independent of maternal serum concentrations and time from drug administration to sampling. These data suggest that diazepam accumulates in the fetal circulation and tissues during organogenesis (12). At term, equilibrium between mother and fetus occurs in 5–10 minutes after IV administration (11). The maternal and fetal serum binding capacity for diazepam is reduced in pregnancy and is not correlated with albumin (14,15). The plasma half-life in newborns is significantly increased due to a decreased clearance of the drug. Because the transplacental passage is rapid at term, timing of the IV administration with uterine contractions will greatly reduce the amount of drug transferred to the fetus (7).

In a case of gross overdose, a mother who took 580 mg of diazepam as a single dose on about the 43rd day of gestation delivered an infant with cleft lip and palate, craniofacial asymmetry, ocular hypertelorism, and bilateral periauricular tags (16). The authors concluded that the drug ingestion was responsible for the defects. An association between diazepam and an increased risk of cleft lip or palate has been suggested by several studies (17–20). The findings indicated that 1st or 2nd trimester use of diazepam, and selected other drugs, is significantly greater among mothers of children born with oral clefts. However, a review of these studies, published in 1976, concluded that a causal relationship between diazepam and oral clefts had not yet been established, but even if it had, the actual risk was only 0.2% for cleft palate and only 0.4% for cleft lip with or without cleft palate (21). In addition, large retrospective studies showing no association between diazepam and cleft lip/palate have been published (22–25). The results of one of these studies has been criticized and defended (26,27). Although no association was found with cleft lip/palate, a statistically significant association was discovered between diazepam and inguinal hernia (27). This same association, along with others, was found in another investigation (28).

In 1427 malformed newborns compared to 3,001 controls, 1st trimester use of tranquilizers (diazepam most common) was associated with inguinal hernia, cardiac defects, and pyloric stenosis (28). Second trimester exposure was associated with hemangiomas and cardiac and circulatory defects. The combination of cigarette smoking and tranquilizer use increased the risk of delivering a malformed infant by 3.7-fold as compared to those who smoked but did not use tranquilizers (28). A survey of 390 infants with congenital heart disease matched with 1254 normal infants found a higher rate of exposure to several drugs, including diazepam, in the offspring with defects (29). Other congenital anomalies reported in infants exposed to diazepam include absence of both thumbs (two cases), spina bifida (one case), and absence of left forearm and syndactyly (one case) (30–32). Any relationship between diazepam and these defects is unknown.

A 1989 report described dysmorphic features, growth retardation, and central nervous system defects in eight infants exposed either to diazepam, 30 mg/day or more, or oxazepam, 75 mg/day or more throughout gestation (33). Three of the mothers denied use of drugs during pregnancy, but diazepam and its metabolite were demonstrated in their plasma in early pregnancy. The mothers did not use alcohol or street drugs, had regular prenatal care, and had no record of criminality or prostitution. The mean birth weight of the infants was 1.2 standard deviations below the Swedish average, only one having a weight above the mean, and one was small for gestational age. Six of the newborns had low Apgar scores primarily as a consequence of apnea, five needed resuscitation, all were hypotonic at birth, and all had neonatal drug withdrawal with episodes of opisthotonos and convulsions. Seven of the eight infants had feeding difficulties caused by a lack of rooting and sucking reflexes. Craniofacial defects observed in the infants (number of infants with defect shown in parenthesis) were short nose with low nasal bridge (six); uptilted nose (six); slanted eyes (eight); epicanthic folds (eight); telecanthus (two); long eyelashes (three); highly arched palate (four); cleft hard palate and bifid uvula (two); low-set/abnormal ears (four); webbed neck (three); flat upper lip (five); full lips (four); hypoplastic mandible (five); and microcephaly (two). Other defects present were small, wide-spaced nipples (two), renal defect (one), inguinal hernia (two), and cryptorchidism (two). An infant with severe psychomotor retardation died of possible sudden infant death syndrome at 11 weeks of age. Microscopic examination of the brain demonstrated slight cortical dysplasia and an increased number of single-cell neuronal heterotopias in the white matter. Six other children had varying degrees of mental retardation, some had severely disturbed visual perception, all had gross motor disability, and hyperactivity and attention deficits were common. Extensive special examinations were conducted to identify other possible etiologies, but the only common factor in the eight cases was maternal consumption of benzodiazepines (33). Based on the apparent lack of other causes, the investigators concluded that the clinical characteristics observed in the infants probably represented a teratogenic syndrome caused by benzodiazepines.

A 1992 study reported on heavy benzodiazepine exposure during pregnancy from Michigan Medicaid data collected during 1980 to 1983 (34). Of the 2048 women, from a total sample of 104,339, who had received benzodiazepines, 80 had received 10 or more prescriptions for these agents. The records of these 80 women indicated frequent alcohol and substance abuse. Their pregnancy outcomes were three intrauterine deaths, two neonatal deaths in infants with congenital malformations, and 64 survivors. The outcome for 11 infants was unknown. Six of the 64 surviving infants had diagnoses consistent with congenital defects and neurological abnormalities. No cases of oral clefts were found in 1,354 1st trimester benzodiazepine exposures. The investigators concluded that the high rate of congenital anomalies was suggestive of multiple alcohol and substance abuse and may not have been related to benzodiazepine exposure. However, subtle defects, developmental abnormalities, and retardations may not have been included in the records (34).

A 1992 letter correspondence suggested that the Möbius syndrome observed in a 3-week-old infant was the result of *in utero* exposure to benzodiazepines (diazepam and oxazepam) (35). The mother had been treated for hypertension starting at 16 weeks' gestation with methyldopa. Diazepam (20 mg/day) was added at 25 weeks', and shortly thereafter, hyoscine butylbromide, oxazepam (20 mg/day), and ritodrine were added. The infant had normal weight, length, and head circumference but was markedly hypotonic at birth. In addition to an expressionless face, malformations observed were epicanthal folds, short palpebral fissures, convergent strabismus, low nasal bridge, short upturned nose, hypertelorism, and high arched palate (35). An electromyogram confirmed bilateral cranial nerve VII palsy. The authors speculated that the Möbius syndrome and the strabismus were caused by the benzodiazepine therapy based on previous reports. At least one mechanism of Möbius syndrome (VI and VII nerve palsy), however, was thought to be a result of mechanical trauma induced by uterine contractions early in gestation that results in ischemia in the cranial nuclei VI and VII (see Shepard, 1995, in Misoprostol).

The pregnancy outcomes of five women who had attempted suicide with diazepam combined with other drugs early in gestation were described in a 1997 report (36). The gestational ages when the overdoses occurred were 3–4 weeks and the diazepam doses ranged from 90–200 mg. All five of the infants were delivered at term and, except for an infant with bilateral undescended testis, were normal. The undescended testis were not thought to have been related to the self-poisoning (36).

A meta-analysis of cohort and case-control studies involving the association of 1st trimester exposure to benzodiazepines and major malformations was published in 1998 (37). Analysis of nine cohort studies (non-epileptic patients) showed no relationship to major malformations (odds ratio [OR] 0.90, 95% confidence interval [CI] 0.61–1.35) or to oral clefts (OR 1.19, 95% CI 0.34–4.15). Two cohort studies involving epileptic patients were also negative. In contrast, pooled data from nine case-control studies showed an association with major defects (OR 3.01, 95% CI 1.32–6.84) or to oral clefts alone (OR 1.79, 95% CI 1.13–2.82) (37). In correspondence concerning this study, objections were raised as to the exclusion of certain studies and to the statistical methods used (38–40).

Another 1998 study described the outcomes of 460 pregnancies (subjects) exposed to benzodiazepines, 98% during the 1st trimester, compared to 424 control pregnancies (41). Subjects and controls had called the Israeli Teratogen Information Service concerning

D

either exposure to benzodiazepines (subjects) or various other nonteratogenic exposures (controls). Diazepam was used by 89 women, but several subjects in the total group used more than one type of benzodiazepine. Subjects were older (31.7 vs. 29.4 years, $p = 0.001$) and called earlier in pregnancy (10.3 vs. 12.9 weeks, $p = 0.001$) than controls. There were also more spontaneous and induced abortions in subjects, 8.7% vs. 5.2%, $p = 0.047$, and 14.1% vs. 4.7%, $p = 0.001$, respectively. None of the induced abortions involved major congenital defects. The higher rates of spontaneous and induced abortions were thought to be related to the lower gestational ages at calling and to the counseling of the callers, respectively (41). The gestational ages and birth weights of the two groups were similar. Major malformations were observed in 11 of the 355 subject live births (3.1%) and in 10 of 382 control live births (2.6%) (*ns*). The birth defects in infants of subjects were four cases of congenital heart disease (ventricular septal defect, pulmonic stenosis, and two unspecified with one neonatal death; carbamazepine used in two cases), two cases of polydactyly, two cases of hydronephrosis, and one each of esophageal atresia, cerebral palsy, and Down's syndrome (41).

Several investigators have observed that the use of diazepam during labor is not harmful to the mother or her infant (42–49). A dose response is likely as the frequency of newborn complications rises when doses exceed 30–40 mg or when diazepam is taken for extended periods, allowing accumulation to occur (50–56). Two major syndromes of neonatal complications have been observed:

Floppy infant syndrome:
- Hypotonia
- Lethargy
- Sucking difficulties

Withdrawal syndrome:
- Intrauterine growth retardation
- Tremors
- Irritability
- Hypertonicity
- Diarrhea/vomiting
- Vigorous sucking

Under miscellaneous effects, diazepam may alter thermogenesis, cause loss of beat-to-beat variability in the fetal heart rate, and decrease fetal movements (33,57–62).

In summary, the effects of benzodiazepines, including diazepam, on the human embryo and fetus are controversial. Although a number of studies have reported an association with various types of congenital defects, other studies have not found such associations. Maternal denial of exposure, as reported in one study, and the concurrent exposure to other toxic drugs and substances (e.g., alcohol and smoking) may be confounding factors. However, the risk appears to be low, if indeed diazepam and the other agents do cause birth defects. Continuous use during gestation has resulted in neonatal withdrawal and a dose-related syndrome is apparent if diazepam is used close to delivery. Consequently, if the maternal condition requires the use of diazepam during pregnancy, the lowest possible dose should be taken. Moreover, abrupt discontinuance of benzodiazepines should be avoided. Severe withdrawal symptoms (physical and psychological) may occur in the mother and, in some cases, result in the substitution of other substances (e.g., alcohol) to treat the symptoms (63). Fetal withdrawal, such as that observed with narcotics, has not been reported, but should be considered.

D

BREAST FEEDING SUMMARY

RECOMMENDATION: Limited Human Data - Potential Toxicity

Diazepam and its metabolite, *n*-demethyldiazepam, enter breast milk (61,62,64–69). Lethargy and loss of weight have been reported (67,69). Milk:plasma ratios varied between 0.2 and 2.7 (66).

A mother who took 6–10 mg daily throughout pregnancy delivered a full-term, normally developed male infant (69). The infant was breast fed and the mother continued to take her diazepam. Sedation was noted in the infant if nursing occurred less than 8 hours after taking a dose. Paired samples of maternal serum and breast milk were obtained on five occasions between 1 and 4 months after delivery. Milk concentrations of diazepam and desmethyldiazepam varied between 7.5 and 87 ng/mL and 19.2 and 77 ng/mL, respectively. The milk:serum ratios for diazepam varied between 0.14 and 0.21 in four samples but was 1.0 in one sample. The ratio for desmethyldiazepam varied from 0.10 to 0.18 in four samples and was 0.53 in the sample with the high diazepam ratio. A serum level was drawn from the infant on one occasion, revealing levels of diazepam and the metabolite of 0.7 and 46 ng/mL, respectively (69).

Diazepam may accumulate in breast-fed infants, and its use in lactating women is not recommended. The American Academy of Pediatrics classifies the effects of diazepam on the nursing infant as unknown but may be of concern (70).

References

1. Shepard TH. *Catalog of Teratogenic Agents*. 6th ed. Baltimore, MD: Johns Hopkins University Press, 1989:203–6.
2. Erkkola R, Kanto J, Sellman R. Diazepam in early human pregnancy. Acta Obstet Gynecol Scand 1974;53:135–8.
3. Kanto J, Erkkola R, Sellman R. Accumulation of diazepam and *n*-demethyldiazepam in the fetal blood during labor. Ann Clin Res 1973;5:375–9.
4. Idanpaan-Heikkila JE, Jouppila PI, Puolakka JO, Vorne MS. Placental transfer and fetal metabolism of diazepam in early human pregnancy. Am J Obstet Gynecol 1971;109:1011–6.
5. Mandelli M, Morselli PL, Nordio S, Pardi G, Principi N, Sereni F, Tognoni G. Placental transfer of diazepam and its disposition in the newborn. Clin Pharmacol Ther 1975;17:564–72.
6. Gamble JAS, Moore J, Lamke H, Howard PJ. A study of plasma diazepam levels in mother and infant. Br J Obstet Gynaecol 1977;84:588–91.
7. Haram K, Bakke DM, Johannessen KH, Lund T. Transplacental passage of diazepam during labor: influence of uterine contractions. Clin Pharmacol Ther 1978;24:590–9.
8. Bakke OM, Haram K, Lygre T, Wallem G. Comparison of the placental transfer of thiopental and diazepam in caesarean section. Eur J Clin Pharmacol 1981;21:221–7.
9. Haram K, Bakke OM. Diazepam as an induction agent for caesarean section: a clinical and pharmacokinetic study of fetal drug exposure. Br J Obstet Gynaecol 1980;87:506–12.
10. Kanto JH. Use of benzodiazepines during pregnancy, labour and lactation, with particular reference to pharmacokinetic considerations. Drugs 1982;23:354–80.
11. Bakke OM, Haram K. Time course of transplacental passage of diazepam: influence of injection-delivery interval on neonatal drug concentrations. Clin Pharmacokinet 1982;7:353–62.
12. Jauniaux E, Jurkovic D, Lees C, Campbell S, Gulbis B. In-vivo study of diazepam transfer across the first trimester human placenta. Hum Reprod 1996;11:889–92.
13. Jorgensen NP, Thurmann-Nielsen E, Walstad RA. Pharmacokinetics and distribution of diazepam and oxazepam in early pregnancy. Acta Obstet Gynecol Scand 1988;67:493–7.
14. Lee JN, Chen SS, Richens A, Menabawey M, Chard T. Serum protein binding of diazepam in maternal and foetal serum during pregnancy. Br J Clin Pharmacol 1982;14:551–4.
15. Ridd MJ, Brown KF, Nation RL, Collier CB. Differential transplacental binding of diazepam: causes and implications. Eur J Clin Pharmacol 1983;24:595–601.
16. Rivas F, Hernandez A, Cantu JM. Acentric craniofacial cleft in a newborn female prenatally exposed to a high dose of diazepam. Teratology 1984;30:179–80.
17. Safra JM, Oakley GP Jr. Association between cleft lip with or without cleft palate and prenatal exposure to diazepam. Lancet 1975;2:478–80.
18. Saxen I. Epidemiology of cleft lip and palate: an attempt to rule out chance correlations. Br J Prev Soc Med 1975;29:103–10.
19. Saxen I. Associations between oral clefts and drugs taken during pregnancy. Int J Epidemiol 1975;4:37–44.

20. Saxen I, Saxen L. Association between maternal intake of diazepam and oral clefts. Lancet 1975;2:498.
21. Safra MJ, Oakley GP Jr. Valium: an oral cleft teratogen? Cleft Palate J 1976;13:198–200.
22. Czeizel A. Diazepam, phenytoin, and etiology of cleft lip and/or cleft palate. Lancet 1976;1:810.
23. Rosenberg L, Mitchell AA, Parsells JL, Pashayan H, Louik C, Shapiro S. Lack of relation of oral clefts to diazepam use during pregnancy. N Engl J Med 1983;309:1282–5.
24. Shiono PH, Mills JL. Oral clefts and diazepam use during pregnancy. N Engl J Med 1984;311:919–20.
25. Lakos P, Czeizel E. A teratological evaluation of anticonvulsant drugs. Acta Paediatr Acad Sci Hung 1977;18:145–53.
26. Entman SS, Vaughn WK. Lack of relation of oral clefts to diazepam use in pregnancy. N Engl J Med 1984;310:1121–2.
27. Rosenberg L, Mitchell AA. Lack of relation of oral clefts to diazepam use in pregnancy. N Engl J Med 1984;310:1122.
28. Bracken MB, Holford TR. Exposure to prescribed drugs in pregnancy and association with congenital malformations. Obstet Gynecol 1981;58:336–44.
29. Rothman KJ, Fyler DC, Goldblatt A, Kreidberg MB. Exogenous hormones and other drug exposures of children with congenital heart disease. Am J Epidemiol 1979;109:433–9.
30. Istvan EJ. Drug-associated congenital abnormalities. Can Med Assoc J 1970;103:1394.
31. Ringrose CAD. The hazard of neurotrophic drugs in the fertile years. Can Med Assoc J 1972;106:1058.
32. Fourth Annual Report of the New Zealand Committee on Adverse Drug Reactions. N Z Med J 1969;70: 118–22.
33. Laegreid L, Olegard R, Walstrom J, Conradi N. Teratogenic effects of benzodiazepine use during pregnancy. J Pediatr 1989;114:126–31.
34. Bergman U, Rosa FW, Baum C, Wiholm B-E, Faich GA. Effects of exposure to benzodiazepine during fetal life. Lancet 1992;340:694–6.
35. Courtens W, Vamos E, Hainaut M, Vergauwen P. Moebius syndrome in an infant exposed in utero to benzodiazepines. J Pediatr 1992;121:833–4.
36. Czeizel AE, Mosonyi A. Monitoring of early human fetal development in women exposed to large doses of chemicals. Environ Mol Mutagen 1997;30:240–4.
37. Dolovich LR, Addis A, Vaillancourt JMR, Power JDB, Koren G, Einarson TR. Benzodiazepine use in pregnancy and major malformations or oral cleft: meta-analysis of cohort and case-controlled studies. BMJ 1998;317:839–43.
38. Game E, Bergman U. Benzodiazepine use in pregnancy and major malformations or oral clefts. BMJ 1999;319:918.
39. Cates C. Pooled results are sensitive to zero transformation used. BMJ 1999;319:918–9.
40. Khan KS, Wukes C, Gee H. Quality of primary studies must influence inferences made from meta-analyses. BMJ 1999;319:919.
41. Ornoy A, Arnon J, Shechtman S, Moerman L, Lukashova I. Is benzodiazepine use during pregnancy really teratogenic? Reprod Toxicol 1998;12:511–5.
42. Greenblatt DJ, Shader RI. Effect of benzodiazepines in neonates. N Engl J Med 1975;292:649.
43. Modif M, Brinkman CR, Assali NS. Effects of diazepam on uteroplacental and fetal hemodynamics and metabolism. Obstet Gynecol 1973;41:364–8.
44. Toaff ME, Hezroni J, Toaff R. Effect of diazepam on uterine activity during labor. Isr J Med Sci 1977;13:1007–9.
45. Shannon RW, Fraser GP, Aitken RG, Harper JR. Diazepam in preeclamptic toxaemia with special reference to its effect on the newborn infant. Br J Clin Pract 1972;26:271–5.
46. Yeh SY, Paul RIT, Cordero L, Hon EH. A study of diazepam during labor. Obstet Gynecol 1974;43: 363–73.
47. Kasturilal D, Shetti RN. Role of diazepam in the management of eclampsia. Curr Ther Res 1975;18: 627–30.
48. Eliot BW, Hill JG, Cole AP, Hailey DM. Continuous pethidine/diazepam infusion during labor and its effects on the newborn. Br J Obstet Gynaecol 1975;82:126–31.
49. Lean TH, Retnam SS, Sivasamboo R. Use of benzodiazepines in the management of eclampsia. J Obstet Gynaecol Br Commonw 1968;75:856–62.
50. Scanlon JW. Effect of benzodiazepines in neonates. N Engl J Med 1975;292:649.
51. Gillberg C. "Floppy infant syndrome" and maternal diazepam. Lancet 1977;2:244.
52. Haram K. "Floppy infant syndrome" and maternal diazepam. Lancet 1977;2:612–3.
53. Speight AN. Floppy-infant syndrome and maternal diazepam and/or nitrazepam. Lancet 1977;1:878.
54. Rementeria JL, Bhatt K. Withdrawal symptoms in neonates from intrauterine exposure to diazepam. J Pediatr 1977;90:123–6.
55. Thearle MJ, Dunn PM. Exchange transfusions for diazepam intoxication at birth followed by jejunal stenosis. Proc R Soc Med 1973;66:13–4.
56. Backes CR, Cordero L. Withdrawal symptoms in the neonate from presumptive intrauterine exposure to diazepam: report of case. J Am Osteopath Assoc 1980;79:584–5.
57. Cree JE, Meyer J, Hailey DM. Diazepam in labour: its metabolism and effect on the clinical condition and thermogenesis of the newborn. Br Med J 1973;4: 251–5.
58. McAllister CB. Placental transfer and neonatal effects of diazepam when administered to women just before delivery. Br J Anaesth 1980;52:423–7.
59. Owen JR, Irani SF, Blair AW. Effect of diazepam administered to mothers during labour on temperature regulation of neonate. Arch Dis Child 1972;47: 107–10.
60. Scher J, Hailey DM, Beard RW. The effects of diazepam on the fetus. J Obstet Gynaecol Br Commonw 1972;79:635–8.
61. van Geijn HP, Jongsma HW, Doesburg WH, Lemmens WA, deHaan J, Eskes TK. The effect of diazepam administration during pregnancy or labor on the heart rate variability of the newborn infant. Eur J Obstet Gynaecol Reprod Biol 1980;10: 187–201.
62. Birger M, Homberg R, Insler V. Clinical evaluation of fetal movements. Int J Gynaecol Obstet 1980;18: 377–82.
63. Einarson A, Selby P, Koren G. Abrupt discontinuation

of psychotropic drugs during pregnancy: fear of teratogenic risk and impact on counseling. J Psychiatry Neurosci 2001;26:44–8.
64. van Geijn HP, Kenemans P, Vise T, Vanderkleijn E, Eskes TK. Pharmacokinetics of diazepam and occurrence in breast milk. In Proceedings of the Sixth International Congress of Pharmacology, Helsinki 1975:514.
65. Hill RM, Nowlin J, Lertratanangkoon K, Stillwell WG, Stillwell RN, Horning MG. The identification and quantification of drugs in human breast milk. Clin Res 1974;22:77A.
66. Cole AP, Hailey DM. Diazepam and active metabolite in breast milk and their transfer to the neonate. Arch Dis Child 1975;50:741–2.
67. Patrick MJ, Tilstone WJ, Reavey P. Diazepam and breast-feeding. Lancet 1972;1:542–3.
68. Catz CS. Diazepam in breast milk. Drug Ther 1973; 3:72–3.
69. Wesson DR, Camber S, Harkey M, Smith DE. Diazepam and desmethyldiazepam in breast milk. J Psychoactive Drugs 1985;17:55–6.
70. Committee on Drugs, American Academy of Pediatrics. The transfer of drugs and other chemicals into human milk. Pediatrics 2001;108:776–89.

Name:	**DIAZOXIDE**	Risk Factor:	C_M
Class:	**Antihypertensive**		

FETAL RISK SUMMARY

RECOMMENDATION: Human Data Suggest Risk in 3rd Trimester

Diazoxide readily crosses the placenta and reaches fetal plasma concentrations similar to maternal levels (1). The drug has been used for the treatment of severe hypertension associated with pregnancy (1–12). Daily doses of 30, 21, and 10 mg/kg in rats, rabbits, and dogs, respectively, were associated with reduced fetal and pup survival, and reduced fetal growth (13).

Some investigators have cautioned against the use of diazoxide in pregnancy (14,15). In one study, the decrease in maternal blood pressure was sufficient to produce a state of clinical shock and endanger placental perfusion (14). Transient fetal bradycardia has been reported in other studies following a rapid, marked decrease in maternal blood pressure (7,16). Fatal maternal hypotension has been reported in one patient after diazoxide therapy (17). Recommendations have been made that the infusion technique, rather than rapid IV boluses, is preferred to prevent maternal and fetal complications (18). However, small IV boluses at frequent intervals (30 mg every 1–2 minutes) have successfully controlled maternal hypertension without producing fetal toxicity (19).

Diazoxide is a potent relaxant of uterine smooth muscle and may inhibit uterine contractions if given during labor (2,3,5–7,20–22). The degree and duration of uterine inhibition are dose dependent (21). Augmentation of labor with oxytocin may be required in patients receiving diazoxide.

Hyperglycemia in the newborn (glucose 500–700 mg/dL) secondary to IV diazoxide therapy in a mother just prior to delivery has been observed to persist for up to 3 days (23). In some series, all of the mothers and newborns had hyperglycemia without ketoacidosis (14). The glucose levels returned to near normal within 24 hours.

The use of oral diazoxide for the last 19–69 days of pregnancy has been associated with alopecia, hypertrichosis lanuginosa, and decreased ossification of the wrist (1). However, long-term oral therapy has not caused similar problems in other newborns exposed *in utero* (4).

Because other antihypertensive drugs are available for severe maternal hypertension and the long-term effects on the infant have not been evaluated, diazoxide should be used with caution, if at all, during pregnancy. If diazoxide is needed after other therapies have failed, small doses are recommended.

BREAST FEEDING SUMMARY

RECOMMENDATION: No Human Data - Potential Toxicity

No reports describing the use of diazoxide during lactation have been located. The molecular weight (about 231) is low enough, however, that passage into milk should be expected.

References

1. Milner RDG, Chouksey SK. Effects of fetal exposure to diazoxide in man. Arch Dis Child 1972;47:537–43.
2. Finnerty FA Jr, Kakaviatos N, Tuckman J, Magill J. Clinical evaluation of diazoxide: a new treatment for acute hypertension. Circulation 1963;28:203–8.
3. Finnerty FA Jr. Advantages and disadvantages of furosemide in the edematous states of pregnancy. Am J Obstet Gynecol 1969;105:1022–7.
4. Pohl JEF, Thurston H, Davis D, Morgan MY. Successful use of oral diazoxide in the treatment of severe toxaemia of pregnancy. Br Med J 1972;2:568–70.
5. Pennington JC, Picker RH. Diazoxide and the treatment of the acute hypertensive emergency in obstetrics. Med J Aust 1972;2:1051–4.
6. Koch-Weser J. Diazoxide. N Engl J Med 1976;294:1271–4.
7. Morris JA, Arce JJ, Hamilton CJ, Davidson EC, Maidman JE, Clark JH, Bloom RS. The management of severe preeclampsia and eclampsia with intravenous diazoxide. Obstet Gynecol 1977;49:675–80.
8. Keith TA III. Hypertension crisis: recognition and management. JAMA 1977;237:1570–7.
9. MacLean AB, Doig JR, Aickin DR. Hypovolaemia, pre-eclampsia and diuretics. Br J Obstet Gynaecol 1978;85:597–601.
10. Barr PA, Gallery ED. Effect of diazoxide on the antepartum cardiotocograph in severe pregnancy-associated hypertension. Aust N Z J Obstet Gynaecol 1981;21:11–5.
11. MacLean AB, Doig JR, Chatfield WR, Aickin DR. Small-dose diazoxide administration in pregnancy. Aust N Z J Obstet Gynaecol 1981;21:7–10.
12. During VR. Clinical experience obtained from use of diazoxide (Hypertonalum) for treatment of acute intrapartum hypertensive crisis. Zentralbl Gynakol 1982;104:89–93.
13. Product information. Hyperstat. Schering, 2000.
14. Neuman J, Weiss B, Rabello Y, Cabal L, Freeman RK. Diazoxide for the acute control of severe hypertension complicating pregnancy: a pilot study. Obstet Gynecol 1979;53(Suppl):50S–5S.
15. Perkins RP. Treatment of toxemia of pregnancy. JAMA 1977;238:2143–4.
16. Michael CA. Intravenous diazoxide in the treatment of severe preeclamptic toxaemia and eclampsia. Aust N Z J Obstet Gynaecol 1973;13:143–6.
17. Henrich WL, Cronin R, Miller PD, Anderson RJ. Hypotensive sequelae of diazoxide and hydralazine therapy. JAMA 1977;237:264–5.
18. Thien T, Koene RAP, Schijf C, Pieters GFFM, Eskes TKAB, Wijdeveld PGAB. Infusion of diazoxide in severe hypertension during pregnancy. Eur J Obstet Gynaecol Reprod Biol 1980;10:367–74.
19. Dudley DKL. Minibolus diazoxide in the management of severe hypertension in pregnancy. Am J Obstet Gynecol 1985;151:196–200.
20. Barden TP, Keenan WJ. Effects of diazoxide in human labor and the fetus-neonate (abstract). Obstet Gynecol 1971;37:631–2.
21. Landesman R, Adeodato de Souza FJ, Countinho EM, Wilson KH, Bomfim de Sousa FM. The inhibitory effect of diazoxide in normal term labor. Am J Obstet Gynecol 1969;103:430–3.
22. Paulissian R. Diazoxide. Int Anesthesiol Clin 1978;16:201–36.
23. Milsap RL, Auld PAM. Neonatal hyperglycemia following maternal diazoxide administration. JAMA 1980;243:144–5.

Name:	**DIBENZEPIN**	Risk Factor:	**C**
Class:	**Antidepressant**		

No data are available. See Imipramine.

Name:	**DICHLORALPHENAZONE**	Risk Factor:	**B**
Class:	**Sedative**		

FETAL RISK SUMMARY

RECOMMENDATION: Limited Human Data - Probably Compatible

Dichloralphenazone is a sedative hypnotic composed of two molecules of chloral hydrate (a sedative/hypnotic) (see also Chloral Hydrate) bound together with the analgesic/antipyretic, phenazone (see also Antipyrine) (1). Antipyrine and chloral hydrate are derived from dichloralphenazone and the latter drug is metabolized to the active agent, trichloroethanol. Little information is available on the reproductive effects of antipyrine, chloral hydrate, or the prodrug, dichloralphenazone, a component, along with isometheptene and acetaminophen, of several proprietary mixtures commonly used for tension and vascular (migraine) headaches (see also Isometheptene and Acetaminophen).

Two studies have been located that examined the effect of dichloralphenazone in pregnant rats (1,2). No teratogenic or other adverse fetal effects were observed when doses ranging from 50 to 500 mg/kg/day were fed to rats throughout gestation.

No published reports describing the use of dichloralphenazone in human pregnancy have been located, although one reference commented that the drug has been "widely used" during pregnancy (3). The Collaborative Perinatal Project recorded 71 1st trimester exposures to chloral hydrate (4, pp. 336–44), one of the drugs derived from dichloralphenazone. From this group, eight infants with congenital defects were observed (standardized relative risk [SRR] 1.68). When only malformations with uniform rates by hospital were examined, the SRR was 2.19. Neither of these relative risks reached statistical significance. Moreover, when chloral hydrate was combined with all tranquilizers and nonbarbiturate sedatives, no association with congenital malformations was found (SRR 1.13; 95% confidence interval [CI] 0.88–1.44). For use anytime during pregnancy, 358 exposures to chloral hydrate were discovered (4, p. 438). The nine infants with anomalies yielded a SRR of 0.98 (95% CI 0.45–1.84). (See also Antipyrine for additional information.)

BREAST FEEDING SUMMARY

RECOMMENDATION: Limited Human Data - Probably Compatible

Dichloralphenazone is a prodrug composed of the sedative/hypnotic, chloral hydrate, bound together with the analgesic/antipyretic, phenazone. Trichloroethanol, an active metabolite of chloral hydrate, is excreted into human breast milk as is phenazone (see Antipyrine).

Mild morning drowsiness was observed in a nursing infant of a woman taking 1300 mg (13 times the dose per capsule in the proprietary headache products mentioned above) of dichloralphenazone at bedtime (5). The mother was also taking chlorpromazine, 100 mg 3 times daily. Milk concentrations of trichloroethanol were 60% to 80% of the maternal serum levels. The metabolite was not detected in the infant's plasma 20 hours after a dose. Infant growth and development remained normal during the exposure and at follow-up 3 months after the drug was stopped. Apparently, no attempt was made in this study to determine the milk concentration of phenazone, the other component of dichloralphenazone. The American Academy of Pediatrics classifies chloral hydrate as compatible with breast-feeding (see Chloral Hydrate).

References

1. McColl JD, Globus M, Robinson S. Effect of some therapeutic agents on the developing rat fetus. Toxicol Appl Pharmacol 1965;7:409–17. As cited in Shepard TH. *Catalog of Teratogenic Agents*. 7th ed. Baltimore, MD: Johns Hopkins University Press, 1992:131.
2. Onnis A, Grella P. *The Biochemical Effects of Drugs in*

Pregnancy. Volume 1. West Sussex, England: Ellis Harwood Limited, 1984:60.
3. Lewis PJ, Friedman LA. Prophylaxis of neonatal jaundice with maternal antipyrine treatment. Lancet 1979;1:300–2.
4. Heinonen OP, Slone D, Shapiro S. *Birth Defects and Drugs in Pregnancy*. Littleton, MA: Publishing Sciences Group, 1977.
5. Lacey JH. Dichloralphenazone and breast milk. Br Med J 1971;4:684.

D

Name:	**DICHLORPHENAMIDE**	Risk Factor:	**C_M**
Class:	**Diuretic (Carbonic Anhydrase Inhibitor)**		

FETAL RISK SUMMARY

RECOMMENDATION: No Human Data - No Relevant Animal Data

Dichlorphenamide is a carbonic anhydrase inhibitor used in the treatment of glaucoma. Its mechanism of action is similar to, but much more potent than, acetazolamide or methazolamide (see also Acetazolamide and Methazolamide). The drug is teratogenic in chicks, mice, and rats, producing otolith deficits and forelimb deformities in the fetuses of the latter two species, respectively (1). Skeletal anomalies were observed in rats at a dose 100 times the human dose (2). No reports of human use of dichlorphenamide during pregnancy have been located.

BREAST FEEDING SUMMARY

RECOMMENDATION: No Human Data - Probably Compatible

No reports describing the use of dichlorphenamide during lactation have been located. The molecular weight (about 305) is low enough, however, that excretion into milk should be expected.

References

1. Shepard TH. *Catalog of Teratogenic Agents*. 6th ed. Baltimore, MD: Johns Hopkins University Press, 1989:213.
2. Product information. Daranide. Merck, 2000.

Name:	**DICLOFENAC**	Risk Factor:	**B_M***
Class:	**Nonsteroidal Anti-inflammatory**		

FETAL RISK SUMMARY

RECOMMENDATION: Human Data Suggest Risk in 1st and 3rd Trimesters

Diclofenac is a nonsteroidal anti-inflammatory drug (NSAID) used for the treatment of arthritis, acute and chronic pain, and primary dysmenorrhea. Similar to other agents in this class, it also has antipyretic activity. Diclofenac is in the same subclass (acetic acids) as three other NSAIDs (indomethacin, sulindac, and tolmetin).

In reproduction studies in mice, rats and rabbits, the drug was not teratogenic with doses up to those that produced maternal and fetal toxicity (1). Maternal toxic doses, however, were associated with dystocia, prolonged gestation, decreased fetal survival (1), and intrauterine growth retardation (1,2).

A 1990 report described an investigation on the effects of several nonsteroidal anti-inflammatory agents on mouse palatal fusion both *in vivo* and *in vitro* (3). The compounds, including diclofenac, were found to induce cleft palate. In the rat, diclofenac, presumably by inhibiting prostaglandin synthesis, has been shown to inhibit implantation and placentation (2).

The tocolytic effect of diclofenac was demonstrated in a study that used mifepristone (RU 486) to induce preterm labor in rats (4). Diclofenac inhibited preterm delivery but had no effect on mifepristone-induced cervical maturation.

Diclofenac crosses the human placenta. In a 2000 study, 30 women undergoing termination of pregnancy at a mean gestational age of 10.2 weeks (range 8–12 weeks) were given two 50 mg oral doses at a mean 13.5 and 2.5 hours before the procedure (5). Diclofenac was detected in all maternal serum (mean 183.9 ng/mL) and fetal tissue (mean 279.2 ng/mL) samples, producing a mean maternal serum:fetal tissue ratio of 0.95 (range 0.05–4.26). Only 7 of the 30 amniotic fluid samples contained detectable diclofenac (range 0.6–3.5 ng/mL), whereas 17 of 30 coelomic fluid samples contained the drug (range 1.1–33.4 ng/mL) (5).

In a surveillance study of Michigan Medicaid recipients conducted between 1985 and 1992 involving 229,101 completed pregnancies, 51 newborns had been exposed to diclofenac during the 1st trimester (F. Rosa, personal communication, FDA, 1993). One unspecified major birth defect was observed (two expected). No anomalies were observed in six defect categories (cardiovascular defects, oral clefts, spina bifida, polydactyly, limb reduction defects, and hypospadias) for which specific data were available. Although the number of exposures is small, these data do not support an association between the drug and congenital defects.

A 29-year-old woman at 33 weeks' gestation was diagnosed by clinical symptoms and ultrasound as having a spontaneous rupture of the right renal pelvis with a small amount of perinephric extravasation of urine (6). She was treated conservatively with diclofenac while hospitalized (50 mg twice daily; duration not specified) and delivered a healthy female infant 5 weeks later. A follow-up examination of her kidney by ultrasonography 5 days postpartum was normal.

A combined 2001 population-based observational cohort study and a case-control study estimated the risk of adverse pregnancy outcome from the use of NSAIDs (7). The use of NSAIDs during pregnancy was not associated with congenital malformations, preterm delivery, or low birth weight, but a positive association was discovered with spontaneous abortions (SABs). A similar study, also published in 2001, failed to find a relationship, in general, between NSAIDs and congenital malformations, but did find a significant association with cardiac defects and orofacial clefts (8). In addition, a 2003 study found a significant association between exposure to NSAIDs in early pregnancy and SABs (9). (See Ibuprofen for details on these three studies.)

A brief 2003 editorial on the potential for NSAID-induced developmental toxicity concluded that NSAIDs, and specifically those with greater COX-2 affinity, had a lower risk of this toxicity in humans than aspirin (10).

A 2003 case-control study was conducted to identify drug use in early pregnancy that was associated with cardiac defects (11). Cases (cardiovascular defects without known chromosome anomalies) were drawn from three Swedish health registers ($N = 5015$) and controls consisting of all infants born in Sweden (1995–2001) ($N = 577,730$). Among the

NSAIDs, only naproxen had a positive association with the defects (see Naproxen). For diclofenac, there were 1362 pregnant women exposed and 15 cases of cardiac defects (odds ratio 1.30, 95% confidence interval 0.78–2.16) (11).

Premature closure of the ductus arteriosus in a fetus who was exposed to diclofenac, 50 mg twice daily, for 2 weeks from the 34th week of gestation was reported in 1998 (12). The mother had taken the drug for musculoskeletal back pain and carpal tunnel syndrome. At 41 weeks' gestation, a fetal echocardiogram revealed the ductus defect, enlargement of the right side of the heart, and early cardiac failure. An emergency cesarean section was performed and the baby was successfully resuscitated (12). Another 1998 case described the effects of diclofenac in late gestation (13). The woman, in the 35th week of pregnancy, was treated for thrombophlebitis with a 5-day course of diclofenac (75 mg twice daily) and heparin. Thirteen days after completion of therapy, she delivered a 3200-g female infant with Apgar scores of 6 and 2 at 1 and 5 minutes, respectively. The infant was treated for severe pulmonary hypertension secondary to intrauterine ductal closure. Normal motor and mental development was noted at 2 years of age, but the infant still had cardiac dysfunction (13).

A 1999 report described constriction of the fetal ductus following a single 75-mg IM dose of diclofenac administered at 36 weeks' gestation (14). The constriction resolved within 24 hours and 32 hours after the dose, the mother delivered a 2780-g female infant with an Apgar score of 9 at 1 minute.

In another 1999 case, a woman took diclofenac (50 mg twice daily) for severe arthritis of the hands for 10 days during gestational weeks 34 and 35 (15). She also was occasionally taking Chinese herbs in what was thought to be homeopathic doses. Fetal distress was noted at 41 weeks' gestation and an ultrasound revealed hydrops fetalis with cardiomegaly and right atrial and right ventricular dilatation. An emergency cesarean section delivered a 3980-g female infant with Apgar scores of 6, 7, and 9, at 1, 5, and 10 minutes, respectively. The infant was flaccid with profound bradycardia requiring resuscitation. An echocardiogram within 30 minutes of birth revealed a severely dilated, poorly contractile right ventricle, dilated right atrium, a patent foramen ovale with right to left shunt, moderate tricuspid regurgitation, and a closed ductus arteriosus. The findings were compatible with pulmonary hypertension. The infant markedly improved over the next 4 weeks and was asymptomatic with normal growth and intellectual development at 18 months of age (15).

A 2004 case report described severe pulmonary hypertension in a newborn exposed *in utero* to diclofenac near delivery (16). The mother, at about 38 weeks' gestation, had been prescribed diclofenac (25 mg three times daily for 3 days) for flu-like symptoms. Immediately after completion of the prescribed course, fetal bradycardia was detected and the mother was delivered of a 3.4-kg male infant by cesarean section. The nonhydropic infant was cyanotic with respiratory distress and required mechanical ventilation. An echocardiogram was consistent with severe neonatal pulmonary hypertension and transient right-sided hypertrophic cardiomyopathy caused by premature closure of the ductus arteriosus. The condition was thought to have resulted from diclofenac. By 40 days of age, the pulmonary hypertension had resolved and the right ventricular hypertrophy had markedly regressed (16).

Constriction of the ductus arteriosus *in utero* is a pharmacologic consequence arising from the use of prostaglandin synthesis inhibitors during pregnancy, as is inhibition of labor, prolongation of pregnancy, and suppression of fetal renal function (see also Indomethacin) (17). As indicated above and published cases with other NSAIDs, persistent pulmonary hypertension of the newborn may occur if these agents are used in the 3rd trimester close to delivery (17,18). Women attempting to conceive should not use any prostaglandin synthesis inhibitor, including diclofenac, because of the findings in a variety of animal models that indicate these agents block blastocyst implantation (19,20). Moreover, as noted above, NSAIDs have been associated with SABs and congenital malformations.

[**Risk Factor D if used in 3rd trimester or near delivery.*]

D

BREAST FEEDING SUMMARY

RECOMMENDATION: No Human Data - Probably Compatible

No reports describing the use of diclofenac during lactation have been located. The manufacturer states that diclofenac is excreted into the milk of nursing mothers but does not cite quantitative data (1). One reviewer classified diclofenac as one of several low-risk alternatives, because of its short adult serum half-life (1.1 hours) and toxicity profile compared with other similar agents, if a NSAID was required while nursing (21). Other reviewers have also stated that diclofenac can be safely used during breast-feeding (22,23). Another NSAID in the same subclass as diclofenac is classified as compatible with breast-feeding by the American Academy of Pediatrics (see Indomethacin).

References

1. Product information. Voltaren. Geigy Pharmaceuticals, 1995.
2. Carp HJA, Fein A, Nebel L. Effect of diclofenac on implantation and embryonic development in the rat. Eur J Obstet Gynecol Reprod Biol 1988;28:273–7.
3. Montenegro MA, Palomino H. Induction of cleft palate in mice by inhibitors of prostaglandin synthesis. J Craniofac Genet Del Biol 1990;10:83–94.
4. Cabrol D, Carbonne B, Bienkiewicz A, Dallot E, Alj AE, Cedard L. Induction of labor and cervical maturation using mifepristone (RU 486) in the late pregnant rat. Influence of a cyclooxygenase inhibitor (diclofenac). Prostaglandins 1991;42:71–9.
5. Siu SSN, Yeung JHK, Lau TK. A study on placental transfer of diclofenac in first trimester of human pregnancy. Hum Reprod 2000;15:2423–5.
6. Royburt M, Peled Y, Kaplan B, Hod M, Friedman S, Ovadia J. Non-traumatic rupture of kidney in pregnancy - case report and review. Acta Obstet Gynecol Scan 1994;73:663–7.
7. Nielsen GL, Sorensen HT, Larsen H, Pedersen L. Risk of adverse birth outcome and miscarriage in pregnant users of non-steroidal anti-inflammatory drugs: population based observational study and case-control study. BMJ 2001;322:266–70.
8. Ericson A, Kallen BAJ. Nonsteroidal anti-inflammatory drugs in early pregnancy. Reprod Toxicol 2001;15:371–5.
9. Li DK, Liu L, Odouli R. Exposure to non-steroidal anti-inflammatory drugs during pregnancy and risk of miscarriage: population based cohort study. BMJ 2003;327:368–71.
10. Tassinari MS, Cook JC, Hurtt ME. NSAIDs and developmental toxicity. Birth Defects Res Part B Dev Reprod Toxicol 2003;68:3–4.
11. Kallen BAJ, Olausson PO. Maternal drug use in early pregnancy and infant cardiovascular defect. Reprod Toxicol 2003;17:255–61.
12. Adverse Drug Reactions Advisory Committee. Premature closure of the fetal ductus arteriosus after maternal use of non-steroidal anti-inflammatory drugs. Med J Aust 1998;169:270–1.
13. Zenker M, Klinge J, Kruger C, Singer H, Scharf J. Severe pulmonary hypertension in a neonate caused by premature closure of the ductus arteriosus following maternal treatment with diclofenac: a case report. J Perinat Med 1998;26:231–4.
14. Rein AJJT, Nadjari M, Elchalal U, Nir A. Contraction of the fetal ductus arteriosus induced by diclofenac. Fetal Diagn Ther 1999;14:24–5.
15. Mas C, Menahem S. Premature in utero closure of the ductus arteriosus following maternal ingestion of sodium diclofenac. Aust N Z J Obstet Gynaecol 1999;39:106–7.
16. Siu KL, Lee WH. Maternal diclofenac sodium ingestion and severe neonatal pulmonary hypertension. J Paediatr Child Health 2004;40:152–3.
17. Levin DL. Effects of inhibition of prostaglandin synthesis on fetal development, oxygenation, and the fetal circulation. Semin Perinatol 1980;4:35–44.
18. Van Marter LJ, Leviton A, Allred EN, Pagano M, Sullivan KF, Cohen A, Epstein MF. Persistent pulmonary hypertension of the newborn and smoking and aspirin and nonsteroidal antiinflammatory drug consumption during pregnancy. Pediatrics 1996;97:658–63.
19. Matt DW, Borzelleca JF. Toxic effects on the female reproductive system during pregnancy, parturition, and lactation. In Witorsch RJ, editor. *Reproductive Toxicology*. 2nd ed. New York, NY: Raven Press, 1995: 175–93.
20. Dawood MY. Nonsteroidal antiinflammatory drugs and reproduction. Am J Obstet Gynecol 1993;169: 1255–65.
21. Anderson PO. Medication use while breast feeding a neonate. Neonatal Pharmacol Q 1993;2:3–14.
22. Goldsmith DP. Neonatal rheumatic disorders. View

of the pediatrician. Rheum Dis Clin North Am 1989;15:287–305.

23. Needs CJ, Brooks PM. Antirheumatic medication during lactation. Br J Rheumatol 1985;24:291–7.

D

Name: **DICLOXACILLIN**	Risk Factor: B_M
Class: **Antibiotic (Penicillin)**	

FETAL RISK SUMMARY

RECOMMENDATION: Compatible

Dicloxacillin is a penicillin antibiotic (see also Penicillin G). The drug crosses the placenta into the fetal circulation and amniotic fluid. Levels are low compared to other penicillins because of the high degree of maternal protein binding (1,2). Following a 500-mg IV dose, the fetal peak serum level of 3.4 μg/mL occurred at 2 hours (8% of maternal peak) (2). A peak of 1.8 μg/mL was obtained at 6 hours in the amniotic fluid.

No reports linking the use of dicloxacillin with congenital defects have been located. The Collaborative Perinatal Project monitored 50,282 mother-child pairs, 3546 of whom had 1st trimester exposure to penicillin derivatives (3, pp. 297–313). For use anytime in pregnancy, 7171 exposures were recorded (3, p. 435). In neither case was evidence found to suggest a relationship to large categories of major or minor malformations or to individual defects.

In a surveillance study of Michigan Medicaid recipients conducted between 1985 and 1992 involving 229,101 completed pregnancies, 46 newborns had been exposed to dicloxacillin during the 1st trimester (F. Rosa, personal communication, FDA, 1993). One (2.2%) major birth defect was observed (two expected). No anomalies were observed in six defect categories (cardiovascular defects, oral clefts, spina bifida, polydactyly, limb reduction defects, and hypospadias) for which specific data were available. Although the number of exposures is small, these data do not support an association between the drug and congenital defects.

BREAST FEEDING SUMMARY

RECOMMENDATION: Compatible

No reports describing the use of dicloxacillin during lactation have been located. Because other penicillins are excreted in breast milk in low concentrations (e.g., see Ampicillin and Penicillin G) the presence of dicloxacillin should also be expected. Although adverse effects from other penicillins in breast milk are rare, three potential problems exist for the nursing infant: modification of bowel flora, direct effects on the infant (e.g., allergic response), and interference with the interpretation of culture results if a fever workup is required.

References

1. MacAulay M, Berg S, Charles D. Placental transfer of dicloxacillin at term. Am J Obstet Gynecol 1968; 102:1162–8.
2. Depp R, Kind A, Kirby W, Johnson W. Transplacental passage of methicillin and dicloxacillin into the fetus and amniotic fluid. Am J Obstet Gynecol 1970;107:1054–7.
3. Heinonen OP, Slone D, Shapiro S. *Birth Defects and Drugs in Pregnancy*. Littleton, MA: Publishing Sciences Group, 1977.

Name:	**DICUMAROL**	Risk Factor:	**D**
Class:	**Anticoagulant**		

See Coumarin Derivatives.

Name:	**DICYCLOMINE**	Risk Factor:	**B_M**
Class:	**Parasympatholytic**		

FETAL RISK SUMMARY

RECOMMENDATION: Compatible

This anticholinergic/antispasmodic agent was a component of a proprietary mixture (Bendectin, others) used for the treatment and prevention of pregnancy-induced nausea and vomiting from 1956 until 1976, when the product was reformulated. Dicyclomine was removed at that time because it was discovered that it did not contribute to the effectiveness of the mixture as an antiemetic (see also Doxylamine).

Animal studies conducted with dicyclomine alone, and in combination with doxylamine and pyridoxine (i.e., Bendectin), have found no evidence of impaired fertility or adverse fetal effects (1,2).

In the Collaborative Perinatal Project, 1024 mother-child pairs of the 50,282 studied were exposed to dicyclomine during the 1st trimester (3, pp. 346–50). It was the most common parasympatholytic agent consumed by the women studied. A statistically significant association (standardized relative risk [SRR] 1.46) was discovered for minor malformations with 21 malformed children (3, p. 353). Other defects with an SRR greater than 1.5, and the number of affected newborns, were polydactyly in blacks (SRR 1.89; $N = 6$; 277 black mothers), macrocephaly (SRR 8.8; $N = 3$), diaphragmatic hernia (SRR 12.0; $N = 3$), and clubfoot (SRR 1.8; $N = 7$) (3, pp. 353, 477). For use anytime during pregnancy, 1593 women consumed dicyclomine and an increased SRR was measured for macrocephaly (6.2; $N = 3$) and pectus excavatum (1.8; $N = 9$) (3, p. 492). The authors of this study, however, strongly cautioned that a causal relationship could not be inferred from any of these data, especially when the drug was used after the 1st trimester, and that independent confirmation was required with other studies.

A retrospective study published in 1971, involving more than 1200 mothers, examined the relationship between drugs and congenital malformations (4). This investigation found that significantly fewer mothers of infants with major anomalies, as compared to normal controls, took antiemetics during the first 56 days of pregnancy. Dicyclomine was the fourth most frequently ingested antiemetic.

In a surveillance study of Michigan Medicaid recipients conducted between 1985 and 1992 involving 229,101 completed pregnancies, 642 newborns had been exposed to dicyclomine during the 1st trimester (F. Rosa, personal communication, FDA, 1993). A total of 31 (4.8%) major birth defects were observed (27 expected). Specific data were available for six defect categories, including (observed/expected) 5/6 cardiovascular defects, 1/1 oral clefts, 0/0.5 spina bifida, 0/1 limb reduction defects, 0/2 hypospadias, and 3/1 hypospadias. Only with the latter defect is there a suggestion of a possible association, but other factors, including the mother's disease, concurrent drug use, and chance may be involved.

In summary, the use of dicyclomine during human pregnancy does not appear to represent a risk to the fetus or newborn. A 1990 review on the teratogenic risk of commonly used drugs categorized the risk from dicyclomine as "none" (5).

BREAST FEEDING SUMMARY

RECOMMENDATION: Limited Human Data - Potential Toxicity

No published reports on the excretion of dicyclomine into breast milk have been located. The manufacturer has received a case report of apnea in a breast-fed 12-day-old infant whose mother was receiving dicyclomine (N. G. Dahl, personal communication, Marion Merrell Dow, Inc., 1992). Following the adverse event, the mother was administered a single, 20-mg dose of the drug and breast-feeding was suspended for 24 hours. Plasma and milk concentrations of dicyclomine 2 hours after the dose were 59 ng/mL and 131 ng/mL (milk:plasma ratio 2.2), respectively. Although a causal relationship between dicyclomine and apnea was not established, similar adverse reactions have occurred when the drug was administered directly to infants (1). Consequently, dicyclomine should not be given to nursing women.

References

1. Product information. Bentyl. Marion Merrell Dow, Inc. 1992.
2. Gibson JP, Staples RE, Larson EJ, Kuhn WL, Holtkamp DE, Newberne JW. Teratology and reproduction studies with an antinauseant. Toxicol Appl Pharmacol 1968;13:439–47.
3. Heinonen OP, Slone D, Shapiro S. *Birth Defects and Drugs in Pregnancy*. Littleton, MA: Publishing Sciences Group, 1977.
4. Nelson MM, Forfar JO. Associations between drugs administered during pregnancy and congenital abnormalities of the fetus. Br Med J 1971;1:523–7.
5. Friedman JM, Little BB, Brent RL, Cordero JF, Hanson JW, Shepard TH. Potential human teratogenicity of frequently prescribed drugs. Obstet Gynecol 1990;75:594–9.

Name:	**DIDANOSINE**	Risk Factor:	**B_M**
Class:	**Antiviral**		

FETAL RISK SUMMARY

RECOMMENDATION: Compatible - Maternal Benefit >>Embryo/Fetal Risk

Didanosine (2′,3′-dideoxyinosine; ddI) inhibits viral reverse transcriptase and DNA synthesis. It is classified as a nucleoside reverse transcriptase inhibitor (NRTI) used for the treatment of human immunodeficiency virus (HIV) infections. Its mechanism of action is similar to that of five other nucleoside analogues: abacavir, lamivudine, stavudine, zalcitabine, and zidovudine. Didanosine is converted by intracellular enzymes to the active metabolite, dideoxyadenosine triphosphate (ddATP).

No evidence of teratogenicity or toxicity was observed in pregnant rats and rabbits administered doses of didanosine up to 12 and 14.2 times the human dose, respectively (1). In another report, didanosine was given to pregnant mice in doses ranging from 10–300 mg/kg/day, through all or part of gestation, without resulting in teratogenic effects or other toxicity (2).

The reproductive toxicity of 2′,3′-dideoxyadenosine (ddA; the unphosphorylated active metabolite of didanosine) in rats was compared in a combined *in vitro/in vivo* experiment with four other nucleoside analogues (vidarabine-phosphate, ganciclovir, zalcitabine, and zidovudine), and these results were then compared to previous data obtained under identical conditions with acyclovir (3). Using various concentrations of the drug in a whole-embryo culture system and direct administration to pregnant females (200 mg/kg subcutaneously every 4 hours for three doses) during organogenesis, *in vitro* vidarabine showed the highest potential to interfere with embryonic development, whereas *in vivo* acyclovir had the highest teratogenic potential. In this study, the *in vitro* reproductive toxicity of ddA was less than that of the other agents, except for zidovudine. The *in vivo* toxicity was less than that of acyclovir, vidarabine, and ganciclovir, and equal to that observed with zalcitabine and zidovudine.

Antiretroviral nucleosides have been shown to have a direct dose-related cytotoxic effect on preimplantation mouse embryos. A 1994 report compared this toxicity among zidovudine and three newer compounds, didanosine, stavudine, and zalcitabine (4). Whereas significant inhibition of blastocyst formation occurred with a 1 μmol/L concentration of zidovudine, stavudine, and zalcitabine toxicity was not detected until 100 μmol/L, and no toxicity was observed with didanosine up to 100 μmol/L. Moreover, postblastocyst development was severely inhibited in those embryos that did survive exposure to 1 μmol/L zidovudine. As for the other compounds, stavudine, at a concentration of 10 μmol/L (2.24 μg/mL), inhibited postblastocyst development, but no effect was observed with concentrations up to 100 μmol/L of didanosine or zalcitabine. An earlier study found no cytotoxicity in preimplantation mouse embryos exposed to didanosine concentrations up to 500 μmol/L (2). Although there are no human data, the authors of the 1994 study concluded that the three newer agents may be safer than zidovudine to use in early pregnancy (4).

A 1995 report described the effect of exposure to a relatively high concentration of didanosine (20 μmol/L vs. recommended therapeutic concentrations of 3–5 μmol/L) for prolonged periods (2–11 days) on trophoblasts from term and 1st-trimester placentas (5). No significant effects on trophoblast function, as measured by human chorionic gonadotropin secretion, protein synthesis, progesterone synthesis, and glucose consumption, were observed.

A 1999 study also investigated the effects of a single 24 hour exposure of zidovudine (AZT) or didanosine on human trophoblast cells using a human choriocarcinoma cell line that exhibited many characteristics of the early placenta (6). Two drug concentrations (7.6 mM or 0.076 mM) were studied for their effects on trophoblast cell proliferation and hormone production (human chorionic gonadotropin [hCG], estradiol [E_2], and progesterone [P_4]). The higher concentrations of AZT or ddI resulted in significant decreases in cell numbers and growth rate (38% and 51% of control values, respectively), but increased production of hCG, E_2, and P_4. The decrease in trophoblast cell proliferation may have been the mechanism for the increased incidence of rodent embryo loss observed with AZT (6). In contrast, the lower concentrations of AZT and ddI did not cause changes in cell numbers, producing only significant increases in E_2 production. Because of these findings, the researchers concluded that high therapeutic doses of either AZT or ddI during early human gestation were potentially embryo toxic (6).

Didanosine crosses the placenta to the fetus in both animals and humans (1,7–13). In pregnant macaques (*Macaca nemestrina*), didanosine was administered by constant infusion at a dose of either 42.5 μg/minute/kg or 425 μg/minute/kg (7). The compound crossed the placenta by simple diffusion, resulting in fetal:maternal concentration ratios for both doses of approximately 0.5. In near-term rhesus monkeys, a single IV bolus (2.0 mg/kg) of didanosine resulted in mean fetal concentrations of unmetabolized drug of 33% of the maternal plasma concentrations (8). Concentrations of didanosine were 20% of those in the fetal plasma by 3 hours. However, ddATP was not found in any fetal tissue.

Using a perfused term human placenta, investigators concluded in a 1992 publication that the placental transfer of didanosine was most likely a result of passive diffusion (9). Two other studies, again using perfused human placenta, found that only about 50% of the drug would be passively transferred to the fetal circulation (10), and at approximately half the rate of zidovudine (11). In contrast to zidovudine (see Zidovudine), no metabolite was detected in the placenta (10).

Two HIV-positive women, at 21 and 24 weeks' gestation, respectively, were given a single 375-mg oral dose of didanosine immediately prior to pregnancy termination (12). Drug concentrations in the maternal blood, fetal blood, and amniotic fluid at slightly more than 1 hour after the dose were 295, 42, and <5 ng/mL, respectively, in the first woman, and 629, 121, and 135 ng/mL, respectively, in the second woman. The fetal:maternal blood ratios were 0.14 and 0.19, respectively. Although single drug level determinations are difficult to interpret, a study published in 1993 found that human placental first-pass metabolism was not the reason for these low fetal and amniotic fluid levels (13).

Three experimental *in vitro* models using perfused human placentas to predict the placental transfer of NRTIs (didanosine, stavudine, zalcitabine, and zidovudine) were described in a 1999 publication (14). For each drug, the predicted fetal:maternal plasma drug concentration ratios at steady state with each of the three models were close to those actually observed in pregnant macaques. Based on these results, the authors concluded that their models would accurately predict the mechanism, relative rate, and the extent of *in vivo* human placental transfer of NRTIs (14).

The pharmacokinetics of IV (1.6 mg/kg/hr) and oral (200 mg twice daily) didanosine have been studied in pregnant women with HIV infection at 31 weeks' gestation, during labor, and 6 weeks postpartum (15). This study also described the pharmacokinetics of oral didanosine (60 mg/m^2) in infants at day 1 and at week 6 after birth.

The Antiretroviral Pregnancy Registry reported, for the period January 1989 through January 2004, prospective data (reported to the Registry before the outcomes were known) involving 1537 live births that had been exposed during the 1st trimester to one or more antiretroviral agents (16). Forty-seven of the newborns had congenital defects (3.1%, 95% confidence interval [CI] 2.3–4.1). In the 2407 live births with earliest exposure in the 2nd/3rd trimesters, there were 56 infants with defects (2.3%, 95% CI 1.8–3.0). The prevalence rates for the two periods did not differ significantly. There were 103 infants with birth defects among 3944 live births with exposure anytime during pregnancy (2.6%, 95% CI 2.1–3.2). The prevalence rate did not differ significantly from the rate expected in a nonexposed population (16). There were 332 outcomes exposed to didanosine (166 in the 1st trimester and 166 in the 2nd/3rd trimesters) in combination with other antiretroviral agents. There were 11 birth defects among the 1st trimester exposures and 1 in those exposed in the 2nd/3rd trimesters. In reviewing the birth defects of prospective and retrospective (pregnancies reported after the outcomes were known) registered cases, and clinical reports, the Registry concluded that there was no pattern of anomalies to suggest a common cause (16). (See Lamivudine for required statement.)

A case of life-threatening anemia following *in utero* exposure to antiretroviral agents was described in 1998 (17). A 30-year-old woman with HIV infection was treated with zidovudine, didanosine, and trimethoprim/sulfamethoxazole (three times weekly) during the 1st trimester. Vitamin supplementation was also given. Because of an inadequate response, didanosine was discontinued and lamivudine and zalcitabine were started in the 3rd trimester. Two weeks before delivery the HIV viral load was undetectable. At term, a pale, male infant was delivered who developed respiratory distress shortly after birth. Examination revealed a hyperactive precordium and hepatomegaly without evidence of hydrops. The hematocrit was 11% with a reticulocyte count of zero. An extensive work-up of the mother and infant failed to determine the cause of the anemia. Bacterial and viral infections, including HIV, parvovirus B19, cytomegalovirus, were excluded. The infant received a transfusion and was apparently doing well at 10 weeks of age. Because no other cause of the anemia could be found, the authors attributed the condition to bone marrow suppression, most likely to zidovudine (17). A contribution of the other agents to the condition, however, could not be excluded.

A 2000 case report described the adverse pregnancy outcomes, including neural tube defects (NTDs), of two pregnant women with HIV infection who were treated with the anti-infective combination, trimethoprim/sulfamethoxazole, for prophylaxis against *Pneumocystis carinii*, concurrently with antiretroviral agents (18). Exposure to didanosine occurred in one of these cases. A 31-year-old woman presented at 15 weeks' gestation. She was receiving trimethoprim/sulfamethoxazole, didanosine, stavudine, nevirapine, and vitamin B supplements (specific vitamins and dosage not given) that had been started before conception. A fetal ultrasound at 19 weeks' gestation revealed spina bifida and ventriculomegaly. The patient elected to terminate her pregnancy. The fetus did not have HIV infection. Defects observed at autopsy included ventriculomegaly, an Arnold-Chiari malformation, sacral spina bifida, and a lumbo-sacral meningomyelocele. The authors attributed the NTDs in both cases to the antifolate activity of trimethoprim (18).

No data are available on the advisability of treating pregnant women who have been exposed to HIV via occupational exposure, but one author discourages this use (19).

In summary, although the limited human data does not allow an assessment as to the safety of didanosine during pregnancy, the animal data and the human experience with other similar antiretroviral agents suggests that didanosine is a low risk to the developing fetus. Theoretically, exposure to didanosine at the time of implantation could result in impaired fertility due to embryonic cytotoxicity, but this has not been studied in humans. Mitochondrial dysfunction in offspring exposed *in utero* or postnatally to NRTIs has been reported (see Lamivudine and Zidovudine).

Two reviews, one in 1996 and the other in 1997, concluded that all women currently receiving antiretroviral therapy should continue to receive therapy during pregnancy and that treatment of the mother with monotherapy should be considered inadequate therapy (20,21). In 1998, the Centers for Disease Control and Prevention (CDC) made a similar recommendation that antiretroviral therapy should be continued during pregnancy, but discontinuation of all therapy during the 1st trimester was a consideration (22). If indicated, therefore, didanosine should not be withheld in pregnancy (with the possible exception of the 1st trimester) because the expected benefit to the HIV-positive mother probably outweighs the unknown risk to the fetus. The efficacy and safety of combined therapy in preventing vertical transmission of HIV to the newborn, however, are unknown, and zidovudine remains the only antiretroviral agent recommended for this purpose (20,21).

BREAST FEEDING SUMMARY

RECOMMENDATION: Contraindicated

No reports describing the use of didanosine during lactation have been located. The molecular weight (about 236) is low enough that excretion into milk should be expected. Both didanosine and its metabolites are excreted into the milk of lactating rats (1).

Reports on the use of didanosine during human lactation are unlikely because the antiviral agent is used in the treatment of human immunodeficiency virus (HIV) infections. HIV-1 is transmitted in milk, and in developed countries, breast-feeding is not recommended (20,21,23–25). In developing countries, breast-feeding is undertaken, despite the risk, because there are no affordable milk substitutes available. Until 1999, no studies had been published that examined the effect of any antiretroviral therapy on HIV-1 transmission in milk. In that year, a study involving zidovudine was published that measured a 38% reduction in vertical transmission of HIV-1 infection despite breast-feeding when compared to controls (see Zidovudine).

D

References

1. Product information. Videx. Bristol-Myers Squibb, 2001.
2. Sieh E, Coluzzi ML, Cusella de Angelis MG, Mezzogiorno A, Floridia M, Canipari R, Cossu G, Vella S. The effects of AZT and DDI on pre- and postimplantation mammalian embryos: an *in vivo* and *in vitro* study. AIDS Res Hum Retroviruses 1992;8:639–49.
3. Klug S, Lewandowski C, Merker H-J, Stahlmann R, Wildi L, Neubert D. *In vitro* and *in vivo* studies on the prenatal toxicity of five virustatic nucleoside analogues in comparison to acyclovir. Arch Toxicol 1991;65:283–91.
4. Toltzis P, Mourton T, Magnuson T. Comparative embryonic cytotoxicity of antiretroviral nucleosides. J Infect Dis 1994;169:1100–2.
5. Esterman AL, Rosenberg C, Brown T, Dancis J. The effect of zidovudine and 2'3'-dideoxyinosine on human trophoblast in culture. Pharmacol Toxicol 1995;76:89–92.
6. Plessinger MA, Miller RK. Effects of zidovudine (AZT) and dideoxyinosine (ddl) on human trophoblast cells. Reprod Toxicol 1999;13:537–46.
7. Pereira CM, Nosbisch C, Winter HR, Baughman WL, Unadkat JD. Transplacental pharmacokinetics of dideoxyinosine in pigtailed macaques. Antimicrob Agents Chemother 1994;38:781–6.
8. Sandberg JA, Binienda Z, Lipe G, Rose LM, Parker WB, Ali SF, Slikker W Jr. Placental transfer and fetal disposition of 2'3'-dideoxycytidine and 2'3'-dideoxyinosine in the rhesus monkey. Drug Metab Dispos 1995;23:881–4.
9. Bawdon RE, Sobhi S, Dax J. The transfer of anti-human immunodeficiency virus nucleoside compounds by the term human placenta. Am J Obstet Gynecol 1992;167:1570–4.
10. Dancis J, Lee JD, Mendoza S, Liebes L. Transfer and metabolism of dideoxyinosine by the perfused human placenta. J Acquir Immune Defic Syndr 1993;6:2–6.
11. Henderson GI, Perez AB, Yang Y, Hamby RL, Schenken RS, Schenker S. Transfer of dideoxyinosine across the human isolated placenta. Br J Clin Pharmacol 1994;38:237–42.
12. Pons JC, Boubon MC, Taburet AM, Singlas E, Chambrin V, Frydman R, Papiernik E, Delfraissy JF. Fetoplacental passage of 2',3'-dideoxyinosine. Lancet 1991;337:732.
13. Dalton JT, Au JL-S. 2'3'-Dideoxyinosine is not metabolized in human placenta. Drug Metab Dispos 1993;21:544–6.
14. Tuntland T, Odinecs A, Pereira CM, Nosbisch C, Unadkat JD. *In vitro* models to predict the *in vivo* mechanism, rate, and extent of placental transfer of dideoxynucleoside drugs against human immunodeficiency virus. Am J Obstet Gynecol 1999;180:198–206.
15. Wang Y, Livingston E, Patil S, McKinney RE, Bardeguez AD, Gandia J, O'Sullivan MJ, Clax P, Huang S, Unadkat JD. Pharmacokinetics of didanosine in antepartum and postpartum human immunodeficiency virus-infected pregnant women and their neonates: an AIDS Clinical Trials Group study. J Infect Dis 1999;180:1536–41.
16. Antiretroviral Pregnancy Registry Steering Committee. *Antiretroviral Pregnancy Registry International Interim Report for 1 January 1989 through 31 January 2004.* Wilmington, NC: Registry Coordinating Center, 2004.
17. Watson WJ, Stevens TP, Weinberg GA. Profound anemia in a newborn infant of a mother receiving antiretroviral therapy. Pediatr Infect Dis J 1998;17:435–6.
18. Richardson MP, Osrin D, Donaghy S, Brown NA, Hay, Sharland M. Spinal malformations in the fetuses of HIV infected women receiving combination antiretroviral therapy and co-trimoxazole. Eur J Obstet Gynecol Reprod Biol 2000;93:215–7.
19. Gerberding JL. Management of occupational exposures to blood-borne viruses. N Engl J Med 1995;332:444–51.
20. Carpenter CCJ, Fischi MA, Hammer SM, Hirsch MS, Jacobsen DM, Katzenstein DA, Montaner JSG, Richman DD, Saag MS, Schooley RT, Thompson MA, Vella S, Yeni PG, Volberding PA. Antiretroviral therapy for HIV infection in 1996. JAMA 1996;276:146–54.
21. Minkoff H, Augenbraun M. Antiretroviral therapy for pregnant women. Am J Obstet Gynecol 1997;176:478–89.
22. CDC. Public Health Service Task Force recommendations for the use of antiretroviral drugs in pregnant women infected with HIV-1 for maternal health and for reducing perinatal HIV-1 transmission in the United States. MMWR 1998;47:No. RR-2.
23. Brown ZA, Watts DH. Antiviral therapy in pregnancy. Clin Obstet Gynecol 1990;33:276–89.
24. de Martino M, Tovo P-A, Tozzi AE, Pezzotti P, Galli L, Livadiotti S, Caselli D, Massironi E, Ruga E, Fioredda F, Plebani A, Gabiano C, Zuccotti GV. HIV-1 transmission through breast-milk: appraisal of risk according to duration of feeding. AIDS 1992;6:991–7.
25. Van de Perre P. Postnatal transmission of human immunodeficiency virus type 1: the breast-feeding dilemma. Am J Obstet Gynecol 1995;173:483–7.

Name: **DIENESTROL** Risk Factor: X_M
Class: **Estrogenic Hormone**

D

FETAL RISK SUMMARY

RECOMMENDATION: Contraindicated

Dienestrol is used topically. Estrogens are readily absorbed, and intravaginal use can lead to significant concentrations of estrogen in the blood (1,2). The Collaborative Perinatal Project monitored 614 mother-child pairs with 1st trimester exposure to estrogenic agents, including 36 with exposure to dienestrol (3, pp. 389, 391). An increase in the expected frequency of cardiovascular defects, eye and ear anomalies, and Down's syndrome was found for estrogens as a group but not for dienestrol (3, pp. 389, 391, 395). Use of estrogenic hormones during pregnancy is contraindicated.

BREAST FEEDING SUMMARY

RECOMMENDATION: No Human Data - Probably Compatible

No reports of adverse effects of dienestrol on the nursing infant have been located. It is possible that decreased milk volume and decreased nitrogen and protein content could occur (see Mestranol and Ethinyl Estradiol).

References

1. Gilman AG, Goodman LS, Gilman A. *The Pharmacological Basis of Therapeutics*. New York, NY: Macmillan, 1980:1428.
2. Rigg LA, Hermann H, Yen SSC. Absorption of estrogens from vaginal creams. N Engl J Med 1978;298:195–7.
3. Heinonen OP, Slone D, Shapiro S. *Birth Defects and Drugs in Pregnancy*. Littleton, MA: Publishing Sciences Group, 1977.

Name: **DIETHYLPROPION** Risk Factor: B_M
Class: **Central Stimulant/Anorexiant**

FETAL RISK SUMMARY

RECOMMENDATION: Human Data Suggest Low Risk

No reports linking the use of diethylpropion with congenital defects have been located. The drug has been studied as an appetite suppressant in 28 pregnant patients and, although adverse effects were common in the women, no problems were observed in their offspring (1). A retrospective survey of 1232 patients exposed to diethylpropion during pregnancy found no difference in the incidence of defects (0.9%) when compared to a matched control group (1.1%) (2). No impairment of fertility, teratogenicity, or fetotoxicity was observed in animal studies with doses up to 9-times those used in humans (3,4).

BREAST FEEDING SUMMARY

RECOMMENDATION: Limited Human Data - Potential Toxicity

Diethylpropion and its metabolites are excreted into breast milk (4). No reports of adverse effects in a nursing infant have been located.

References

1. Silverman M, Okun R. The use of an appetite suppressant (diethylpropion hydrochloride) during pregnancy. Curr Ther Res 1971;13:648–53.
2. Bunde CA, Leyland HM. A controlled retrospective survey in evaluation of teratogenicity. J New Drugs 1965;5:193–8.
3. Schardein JL. *Drugs as Teratogens*. Cleveland: CRC Press, 1976:73–5.
4. Product information. Tenuate. Marion Merrell Dow, Inc., 1992.

Name: DIETHYLSTILBESTROL	Risk Factor: X_M
Class: Estrogenic Hormone	

FETAL RISK SUMMARY

RECOMMENDATION: Contraindicated

Between 1940 and 1971, an estimated 6 million mothers and their fetuses were exposed to diethylstilbestrol (DES) to prevent reproductive problems such as miscarriage, premature delivery, intrauterine fetal death, and toxemia (1–4). Controlled studies have since proven that DES was not successful in preventing these disorders (5,6). This use has resulted, however, in significant complications of the reproductive system in both female and male offspring (1–12). Two large groups have been established to monitor these complications: the Registry for Research on Hormonal Transplacental Carcinogenesis and the Diethylstilbestrol Adenosis (DESAD) Project (4). The published findings and recommendations of the DESAD project through 1980 plus a number of other studies including the Registry were reviewed in a 1981 National Institutes of Health booklet available from the National Cancer Institute (4). This information was also reprinted in a 1983 journal article (13). The complications identified in female and male children exposed *in utero* to DES are:

Female
- Lower müllerian tract
  - Vaginal adenosis
  - Vaginal and cervical clear cell adenocarcinoma
  - Cervical and vaginal fornix defects (10)
  - Cock's comb (hood, transverse ridge of cervix)
  - Collar (rim, hood, transverse ridge of cervix)
  - Pseudopolyp
  - Hypoplastic cervix (immature cervix)
  - Altered fornix of vagina
  - Vaginal defects (exclusive of fornix) (10)
  - Incomplete transverse septum
  - Incomplete longitudinal septum
- Upper müllerian tract
- Uterine structural defects
- Fallopian tube structural defects

Male
- Reproductive dysfunction
- Altered semen analysis
- Infertility

The Registry was established in 1971 to study the epidemiologic, clinical, and pathologic aspects of clear cell adenocarcinoma of the vagina and cervix in DES-exposed women (2). More than 400 cases of clear cell adenocarcinoma have been reported to the registry. Additional reports continue to appear in the literature (14). The risk of carcinoma is apparently higher when DES treatment was given before the 12th week of gestation and is estimated to be 0.14–1.4/1000 for women younger than 25 years of age (2,4).

D

The first known case of adenosquamous carcinoma of the cervix in an exposed patient was described in 1983 (15). In a second case, a fatal malignant teratoma of the ovary developed in a 12-year-old exposed girl (16). The relationship between these tumors and DES is unknown.

The frequency of dysplasia and carcinoma in situ (CIS) of the cervix and vagina in 3980 DESAD Project patients was significantly increased over controls with an approximately 2- to 4-fold increase in risk (11). These results were different from earlier studies of these same women which had indicated no increased risk for dysplasia and CIS (17,18). Researchers speculated that the increased incidence now observed was related to the greater amount of squamous metaplasia found in DES-exposed women (11). Scanning electron microscopy of the cervicovaginal transformation zone has indicated that maturation of epithelium is slowed or arrested at the stage of immature squamous epithelium in some DES-exposed women (19). This process may produce greater susceptibility to such factors as herpes and papillomavirus obtained through early coitus with multiple partners and result in the observed increased rates of dysplasia/CIS (11). Of interest in this regard, a 1983 article reported detectable papillomavirus antigen in the cervical-vaginal biopsies of 16 (43%) of 37 DES-exposed women (20).

The incidence of cervical or vaginal structural changes has been reported to occur in up to 85% of exposed women, although most studies place the incidence in the 22%–58% range (2,3,5,7,12,21–24). The structural changes are outlined above. The DESAD Project reported an incidence of approximately 25% in 1655 women (10). Selection bias was eliminated by analyzing only those patients identified by record review. Patients referred by physicians and self-referrals had much higher rates of defects, about 49% and 43%, respectively. Almost all of the defects were confined to the cervical-vaginal fornix area, with only 14 patients having vaginal changes exclusive of the fornix and nearly all of these being incomplete transverse septums (10).

Reports linking the use of DES with major congenital anomalies have not been located. The Collaborative Perinatal Project monitored 614 mother-child pairs with 1st trimester exposure to estrogens, including 164 with exposure to DES (25, pp. 389, 391). Evidence for an increase in the expected frequency for cardiovascular defects, eye and ear anomalies, and Down's syndrome was found for estrogens as a group, but not for DES (25, pp. 389, 391, 395). Re-evaluation of these data in terms of timing of exposure, vaginal bleeding in early pregnancy, and previous maternal obstetric history, however, failed to support an association between estrogens and cardiac malformations (26). An earlier study also failed to find any relationship with nongenital malformations (27).

Alterations in the body of the uterus have led to concern regarding increased pregnancy wastage and premature births (8,22,28–31). Increased rates of spontaneous abortions, premature births and ectopic pregnancies are well established by these latter reports, although the relationship to the abnormal changes of the cervix and/or vagina is still unclear (8). Serial observations of vaginal epithelial changes indicate that the frequency of such changes decreases with age (4,17,24).

Spontaneous rupture of a term uterus has been described in a 25-year-old primigravid with DES-type changes in her vagina, cervix and uterus (32). Other reports of this type have not been located.

In a 1984 study, DES exposure had no effect on the age at menarche, first coitus, pregnancy, or live birth, or on a woman's ability to conceive (33). One group of investigators found that although anomalies in the upper genital tract increased the risk for poor pregnancy outcome, they could not relate specific changes to specific types of outcomes (34).

Hirsutism and irregular menses were found in 72% and 50%, respectively, of 32 DES-exposed women (35). The degree of hirsutism was age related, with the mean ages of severely and mildly hirsute women being 28.8 and 24.7 years, respectively. Based on various hormone level measurements, the authors concluded that *in utero* DES exposure might result in hypothalamic-pituitary-ovarian dysfunction (35). However, other studies in much larger exposed populations have not observed disturbances of menstruation or excessive hair growth (36).

Data on DES-exposed women who had undergone major gynecologic surgical procedures, excluding cesarean section, were reported in a 1982 study (37). Of 309 exposed women, 33 (11%) had a total of 43 procedures. The authors suggested that DES exposure resulted in an increased incidence of adnexal disease involving adhesions, benign ovarian cysts, and ectopic pregnancies (37). Surgical manipulation of the cervix (cryocautery or conization) in DES-exposed patients results in a high incidence of cervical stenosis and possible development of endometriosis (38,39). Both studies concluded, however, that the causes of infertility in these patients were comparable to those in a non-DES-exposed population.

Adverse effects in male offspring attributable to *in utero* DES exposure have been reported (1,5,40–46). Abnormalities thought to occur at greater frequencies include:

Epididymal cysts
Hypotrophic testis
Microphallus
Varicocele
Capsular induration
Altered semen (decreased count, concentration, motility, and morphology)

An increase in problems with passing urine and urogenital tract infections has also been observed (40).

DES exposure has been proposed as a possible cause of infertility in male offspring (1). However, in a controlled *in vitro* study, no association was found between exposure to DES and reduced sperm penetration of zona-free hamster eggs (46). In addition, a study of 828 exposed males found no increase over controls for risk of genitourinary abnormalities, infertility, or testicular cancer (47). Based on their data, the authors proposed that previous studies showing a positive relationship might have had selection biases, differences in DES use, or both.

Testicular tumors have been reported in three DES-exposed patients (6,48). In one case, a teratoma was discovered in a 23-year-old male (6). Two patients, 27 and 28 years of age, were included in the second report (48). Both had left-sided anaplastic seminomas, and one had epididymal cysts. A male sibling of one of the patients, also DES exposed, had severe oligospermia, and two exposed sisters had vaginal adenosis and vaginal adenocarcinoma.

Changes in the psychosexual performance of young boys have been attributed to *in utero* exposure to DES and progesterone (49,50). The mothers received estrogen/

progestogen regimens for diabetes. A trend to less heterosexual experience and fewer masculine interests than controls was shown. A 2-fold increase in psychiatric disease, especially depression and anxiety, has been observed in both male and female exposed offspring (6).

D

BREAST FEEDING SUMMARY

RECOMMENDATION: Contraindicated

No data are available. Decreased milk volume and nitrogen-protein content may occur if diethylstilbestrol is used during lactation (see Mestranol and Ethinyl Estradiol).

References

1. Stenchever MA, Williamson RA, Leonard J, Karp LE, Ley B, Shy K, Smith D. Possible relationship between in utero diethylstilbestrol exposure and male fertility. Am J Obstet Gynecol 1981;140:186–93.
2. Herbst AL. Diethylstilbestrol and other sex hormones during pregnancy. Obstet Gynecol 1981;58(Suppl):35s–40s.
3. Nordquist SAB, Medhat IA, Ng AB. Teratogenic effects of intrauterine exposure to DES in female offspring. Compr Ther 1979;5:69–74.
4. Robboy SJ, Noller KL, Kaufman RH, Barnes AB, Townsend D, Gundersen JH, Nash S. *Information for physicians. Prenatal diethylstilbestrol (DES) exposure: recommendations of the Diethylstilbestrol-Adenosis (DESAD) Project for the identification and management of exposed individuals*. NIH Publication No. 81–2049, 1981.
5. Stillman RJ. *In utero* exposure to diethylstilbestrol: adverse effects on the reproductive tract and reproductive performance in male and female offspring. Am J Obstet Gynecol 1982;142:905–21.
6. Vessey MP, Fairweather DVI, Norman-Smith B, Buckley J. A randomized double-blind controlled trial of the value of stilboestrol therapy in pregnancy: long-term follow-up of mothers and their offspring. Br J Obstet Gynaecol 1983;90:1007–17.
7. Prins RP, Morrow P, Townsend DE, Disaia PJ. Vaginal embryogenesis, estrogens, and adenosis. Obstet Gynecol 1976;48:246–50.
8. Sandberg EC, Riffle NL, Higdon JV, Getman CE. Pregnancy outcome in women exposed to diethylstilbestrol in utero. Am J Obstet Gynecol 1981;140:194–205.
9. Noller KL, Townsend DE, Kaufman RH, Barnes AB, Robboy SJ, Fish CR, Jefferies JA, Bergstralh EJ, O'Brien PC, McGorray SP, Scully R. Maturation of vaginal and cervical epithelium in women exposed in utero to diethylstilbestrol (DESAD Project). Am J Obstet Gynecol 1983;146:279–85.
10. Jefferies JA, Robboy SJ, O'Brien PC, Bergstralh EJ, Labarthe DR, Barnes AB, Noller KL, Hatab PA, Kaufman RH, Townsend DE. Structural anomalies of the cervix and vagina in women enrolled in the Diethylstilbestrol Adenosis (DESAD) Project. Am J Obstet Gynecol 1984;148:59–66.
11. Robboy SJ, Noller KL, O'Brien P, Kaufman RH, Townsend D, Barnes AB, Gundersen J, Lawrence WD, Bergstrahl E, McGorray S, Tilley BC, Anton J, Chazen G. Increased incidence of cervical and vaginal dysplasia in 3,980 diethylstilbestrol-exposed young women. Experience of the National Collaborative Diethylstilbestrol Adenosis Project. JAMA 1984;252:2979–83.
12. Chanen W, Pagano R. Diethylstilboestrol (DES) exposure in utero. Med J Aust 1984;141:491–3.
13. NCI DES Summary. Prenatal diethylstilbestrol (DES) exposure. Clin Pediatr 1983;22:139–43.
14. Kaufman RH, Korhonen MO, Strama T, Adam E, Kaplan A. Development of clear cell adenocarcinoma in DES-exposed offspring under observation. Obstet Gynecol 1982;59(Suppl):68S–72S.
15. Vandrie DM, Puri S, Upton RT, Demeester LJ. Adenosquamous carcinoma of the cervix in a woman exposed to diethylstilbestrol in utero. Obstet Gynecol 1983;61(Suppl):84S–7S.
16. Lazarus KH. Maternal diethylstilboestrol and ovarian malignancy in offspring. Lancet 1984;1:53.
17. O'Brien PC, Noller KL, Robboy SJ, Barnes AB, Kaufman RH, Tilley BC, Townsend DE. Vaginal epithelial changes in young women enrolled in the National Cooperative Diethylstilbestrol Adenosis (DESAD) Project. Obstet Gynecol 1979;53:300–8.
18. Robboy SJ, Kaufman RH, Prat J, Welch WR, Gaffey T, Scully RE, Richart R, Fenoglio CM, Virata R, Tilley BC. Pathologic findings in young women enrolled in the National Cooperative Diethylstilbestrol Adenosis (DESAD) Project. Obstet Gynecol 1979;53:309–17.
19. McDonnell JM, Emens JM, Jordan JA. The congenital cervicovaginal transformation zone in young women exposed to diethylstilboestrol in utero. Br J Obstet Gynaecol 1984;91:574–9.
20. Fu YS, Lancaster WD, Richart RM, Reagan JW, Crum CP, Levine RU. Cervical papillomavirus infection in diethylstilbestrol-exposed progeny. Obstet Gynecol 1983;61:59–62.
21. Ben-Baruch G, Menczer J, Mashiach S, Serr DM. Uterine anomalies in diethylstilbestrol-exposed women with fertility disorders. Acta Obstet Gynecol Scand 1981;60:395–7.
22. Pillsbury SG Jr. Reproductive significance of changes in the endometrial cavity associated with exposure in utero in diethylstilbestrol. Am J Obstet Gynecol 1980;137:178–82.
23. Professional and Public Relations Committee of the Diethylstilbestrol and Adenosis Project of the Division of Cancer Control and Rehabilitation. Exposure in utero to diethylstilbestrol and related synthetic

hormones. Association with vaginal and cervical cancers and other abnormalities. JAMA 1976;236: 1107–9.
24. Burke L, Antonioli D, Friedman EA. Evolution of diethylstilbestrol-associated genital tract lesions. Obstet Gynecol 1981;57:79–84.
25. Heinonen OP, Slone D, Shapiro S. *Birth Defects and Drugs in Pregnancy*. Littleton, MA: Publishing Sciences Group, 1977.
26. Wiseman RA, Dodds-Smith IC. Cardiovascular birth defects and antenatal exposure to female sex hormones: a reevaluation of some base data. Teratology 1984;30:359–70.
27. Wilson JG, Brent RL. Are female sex hormones teratogenic? Am J Obstet Gynecol 1981;141:567–80.
28. Herbst AL, Hubby MM, Blough RR, Azizi F. A comparison of pregnancy experience in DES-exposed daughters. J Reprod Med 1980;24:62–9.
29. Barnes AB, Colton T, Gundersen J, Noller KL, Tilley BC, Strama T, Townsend DE, Hatab P, O'Brien PC. Fertility and outcome of pregnancy in women exposed in utero to diethylstilbestrol. N Engl J Med 1980;302:609–13.
30. Veridiano NP, Dilke I, Rogers J, Tancer ML. Reproductive performance of DES-exposed female progeny. Obstet Gynecol 1981;58:58–61.
31. Mangan CE, Borow L, Burnett-Rubin MM, Egan V, Giuntoli RL, Mikuta JJ. Pregnancy outcome in 98 women exposed to diethylstilbestrol in utero, their mothers, and unexposed siblings. Obstet Gynecol 1982;59:315–9.
32. Williamson HO, Sowell GA, Smith HE. Spontaneous rupture of gravid uterus in a patient with diethylstilbestrol-type changes. Am J Obstet Gynecol 1984;150:158–60.
33. Barnes AB. Menstrual history and fecundity of women exposed and unexposed in utero to diethylstilbestrol. J Reprod Med 1984;29:651–5.
34. Kaufman RH, Noller K, Adam E, Irwin J, Gray M, Jefferies JA, Hilton J. Upper genital tract abnormalities and pregnancy outcome in diethylstilbestrol-exposed progeny. Am J Obstet Gynecol 1984;148:973–84.
35. Peress MR, Tsai CC, Mathur RS, Williamson HO. Hirsutism and menstrual patterns in women exposed to diethylstilbestrol in utero. Am J Obstet Gynecol 1982;144:135–40.
36. Verkauf BS. Discussion. Am J Obstet Gynecol 1982;144:139–40.
37. Schmidt G, Fowler WC Jr. Gynecologic operative experience in women exposed to DES in utero. South Med J 1982;75:260–3.
38. Haney AF, Hammond MG. Infertility in women exposed to diethylstilbestrol in utero. J Reprod Med 1983;28:851–6.
39. Stillman RJ, Miller LC. Diethylstilbestrol exposure in utero and endometriosis in infertile females. Fertil Steril 1984;41:369–72.
40. Henderson BE, Benton B, Cosgrove M, Baptista J, Aldrich J, Townsend D, Hart W, Mack TM. Urogenital tract abnormalities in sons of women treated with diethylstilbestrol. Pediatrics 1976;58:505–7.
41. Gill WB, Schumacher GFB, Bibbo M. Pathological semen and anatomical abnormalities of the genital tract in human male subjects exposed to diethylstilbestrol in utero. J Urol 1977;117:477–80.
42. Gill WB, Schumacher GFB, Bibbo M, Strous FH, Schoenberh HW. Association of diethylstilbestrol exposure *in utero* with cryptorchidism, testicular hypoplasia and semen abnormalities. J Urol 1979;122:36–9.
43. Gill WB, Schumacher GFB, Bibbo M. Structural and functional abnormalities in the sex organs of male offspring of mothers treated with diethylstilbestrol (DES). J Reprod Med 1976;16:147–53.
44. Driscoll SG, Taylor SM. Effects of prenatal maternal estrogen on the male urogenital system. Obstet Gynecol 1980;56:537–42.
45. Bibbo M, Gill WB, Azizi F, Blough R, Fang VS, Rosenfield RL, Schaumacher GFB, Sleeper K, Sonek MG, Wied GL. Follow-up study of male and female offspring of DES-exposed mothers. Obstet Gynecol 1977;49:1–8.
46. Shy KK, Stenchever MA, Karp LE, Berger RE, Williamson RA, Leonard J. Genital tract examinations and zona-free hamster egg penetration tests from men exposed in utero to diethylstilbestrol. Fertil Steril 1984;42:772–8.
47. Leary FJ, Resseguie LJ, Kurland LT, O'Brien PC, Emslander RF, Noller KL. Males exposed in utero to diethylstilbestrol. JAMA 1984;252:2984–9.
48. Conley GR, Sant GR, Ucci AA, Mitcheson HD. Seminoma and epididylmal cysts in a young man with known diethylstilbestrol exposure in utero. JAMA 1983;249:1325–6.
49. Yalom ID, Green R, Fisk N. Prenatal exposure to female hormones. Effect on psychosexual development in boys. Arch Gen Psychiatry 1973;28:554–61.
50. Burke L, Apfel RJ, Fischer S, Shaw J. Observations on the psychological impact of diethylstilbestrol exposure and suggestions on management. J Reprod Med 1980;24:99–102.

Name: **DIFLUNISAL** Risk Factor: **C_M***
Class: **Nonsteroidal Anti-inflammatory**

FETAL RISK SUMMARY

RECOMMENDATION: Human Data Suggest Risk in 1st and 3rd Trimesters

Diflunisal is a nonsteroidal anti-inflammatory agent (NSAID) used in the treatment of mild to moderate pain, osteoarthritis, and rheumatoid arthritis. The drug is teratogenic and embryotoxic in rabbits administered 40–60 mg/kg/day, the highest dose equivalent to 2 times the maximum human dose (1). Similar results were not observed in mice and rats treated with 45–100 mg/kg/day (1,2) or in monkeys treated with 80 mg/kg during organogenesis (3). No published reports describing the use of this drug in human pregnancy have been located.

In a surveillance study of Michigan Medicaid recipients conducted between 1985 and 1992 involving 229,101 completed pregnancies, 258 newborns had been exposed to diflunisal during the 1st trimester (F. Rosa, personal communication, FDA, 1993). A total of 19 (7.4%) major birth defects were observed (10 expected). Specific data were available for six defect categories, including (observed/expected) 1/3 cardiovascular defects, 1/0.4 oral clefts, 0/0 spina bifida, 1/1 polydactyly, 0/0 limb reduction defects, and 1/1 hypospadias. It remains to be investigated whether an unusual frequency distribution of the other 15 defects is in the overall excess of birth defects.

A combined 2001 population-based observational cohort study and a case-control study estimated the risk of adverse pregnancy outcome from the use of NSAIDs (4). The use of NSAIDs during pregnancy was not associated with congenital malformations, preterm delivery, or low birth weight, but a positive association was discovered with spontaneous abortions (SABs). A similar study, also published in 2001, failed to find a relationship, in general, between NSAID and congenital malformations, but did find a significant association with cardiac defects and orofacial clefts (5). In addition, a 2003 study found a significant association between exposure to NSAIDs in early pregnancy and SABs (6). (See Ibuprofen for details on these three studies.)

A brief 2003 editorial on the potential for NSAID-induced developmental toxicity concluded that NSAIDs, and specifically those with COX-2 affinity, had a lower risk of this toxicity in humans than aspirin (7).

Constriction of the ductus arteriosus *in utero* is a pharmacologic consequence arising from the use of prostaglandin synthesis inhibitors during pregnancy (see also Indomethacin) (8). Persistent pulmonary hypertension of the newborn may occur if these agents are used in the 3rd trimester close to delivery (8,9). These drugs also have been shown to inhibit labor and prolong pregnancy, both in humans (10) (see also Indomethacin), and in animals (11). Women attempting to conceive should not use any prostaglandin synthesis inhibitor, including diflunisal, because of the findings in a variety of animal models that indicate these agents block blastocyst implantation (12,13). Moreover, as noted above, NSAIDs have been associated with SABs and congenital malformations.

[**Risk Factor D if used in 3rd trimester or near delivery.*]

BREAST FEEDING SUMMARY

RECOMMENDATION: Limited Human Data - Probably Compatible

Diflunisal is excreted into human milk. Milk concentrations range from 2% to 7% of the levels in the mother's plasma (1). No reports describing the use of this agent during lactation have been located.

References

1. Product information. Dolobid. Merck Sharpe & Dohme, 1993.
2. Nakatsuka T, Fujii T. Comparative teratogenicity study of diflunisal (MK-647) and aspirin in the rat. Oyo Yakuri 1979;17:551–7. As cited in Shepard TH. *Catalog of Teratogenic Agents*. 6th ed. Baltimore, MD: Johns Hopkins University Press, 1989:222.
3. Rowland JM, Robertson RT, Cukierski M, Prahalada S, Tocco D, Hendrickx AG. Evaluation of the teratogenicity and pharmacokinetics of diflunisal in cynomolgus

monkeys. Fund Appl Toxicol 1987;8:51–8. As cited in Shepard TH. *Catalog of Teratogenic Agents*. 6th ed. Baltimore, MD: Johns Hopkins University Press, 1989:222.
4. Nielsen GL, Sorensen HT, Larsen H, Pedersen L. Risk of adverse birth outcome and miscarriage in pregnant users of non-steroidal anti-inflammatory drugs: population based observational study and case-control study. BMJ 2001;322:266–70.
5. Ericson A, Kallen BAJ. Nonsteroidal anti-inflammatory drugs in early pregnancy. Reprod Toxicol 2001;15:371–5.
6. Li DK, Liu L, Odouli R. Exposure to non-steroidal anti-inflammatory drugs during pregnancy and risk of miscarriage: population based cohort study. BMJ 2003;327:368–71.
7. Tassinari MS, Hurtt ME. NSAIDs and developmental toxicity. Birth Defects Res Part B Dev Reprod Toxicol 2003;68:3–4.
8. Levin DL. Effects of inhibition of prostaglandin synthesis on fetal development, oxygenation, and the fetal circulation. Semin Perinatol 1980;4:35–44.
9. Van Marter LJ, Leviton A, Allred EN, Pagano M, Sullivan KF, Cohen A, Epstein MF. Persistent pulmonary hypertension of the newborn and smoking and aspirin and nonsteroidal antiinflammatory drug consumption during pregnancy. Pediatrics 1996;97:658–663.
10. Fuchs F. Prevention of prematurity. Am J Obstet Gynecol 1976;126:809–20.
11. Powell JG, Cochrane RL. The effects of a number of non-steroidal anti-inflammatory compounds on parturition in the rat. Prostaglandins 1982;23:469–88.
12. Matt DW, Borzelleca JF. Toxic effects on the female reproductive system during pregnancy, parturition, and lactation. In Witorsch RJ, editor. *Reproductive Toxicology*. 2nd ed. New York, NY: Raven Press, 1995: 175–93.
13. Dawood MY. Nonsteroidal antiinflammatory drugs and reproduction. Am J Obstet Gynecol 1993;169:1255–65.

Name:	**DIGITALIS**	Risk Factor:	**C**
Class:	**Cardiac Glycoside**		

FETAL RISK SUMMARY

RECOMMENDATION: Compatible

No reports linking digitalis or the various digitalis glycosides with congenital defects have been located. Animal studies have failed to show a teratogenic effect (1).

Rapid passage to the fetus has been observed after digoxin and digitoxin (2–9). One group of investigators found that the amount of digitoxin recovered from the fetus was dependent on the length of gestation (2). In the late 1st trimester, only 0.05%–0.10% of the injected dose was recovered from three fetuses. Digitoxin metabolites accounted for 0.18%–0.33%. At 34 weeks of gestation, digitoxin recovery was 0.85% and metabolite recovery was 3.49% from one fetus. Average cord concentrations of digoxin in three reports were 50%, 81%, and 83% of the maternal serum (3,4,9). The highest fetal concentrations of digoxin in the second half of pregnancy were found in the heart (5). The fetal heart has only a limited binding capacity for digoxin in the first half of pregnancy (5). In animals, amniotic fluid acts as a reservoir for digoxin, but no data are available in humans after prolonged treatment (5). The pharmacokinetics of digoxin in pregnant women have been reported (10,11).

Digoxin has been used for both maternal and fetal indications (e.g., congestive heart failure and supraventricular tachycardia) during all stages of gestation without causing fetal harm (12–25). Direct administration of digoxin to the fetus by periodic IM injections has been used to treat supraventricular tachycardia when indirect therapy via the mother failed to control the arrhythmia (26).

In a surveillance study of Michigan Medicaid recipients conducted between 1985 and 1992 involving 229,101 completed pregnancies, 34 newborns had been exposed to digoxin during the 1st trimester (F. Rosa, personal communication, FDA, 1993). One (2.9%) major birth defect was observed (one expected), an oral cleft. Although the number of exposures is small, these data are supportive of previous experience for a lack of association between the drug and congenital defects.

Fetal toxicity resulting in neonatal death has been reported after maternal overdose (27). The mother, in her 8th month of pregnancy, took an estimated 8.9 mg of digitoxin as a single dose. Delivery occurred 4 days later. The baby demonstrated digitalis cardiac effects until death at age 3 days from prolonged intrauterine anoxia.

In a series of 22 multiparous patients maintained on digitalis, spontaneous labor occurred more than 1 week earlier than in 64 matched controls (28). The first stage of labor in the treated patients averaged 4.3 hours vs. 8 hours in the control group. In contrast, others found no effect on duration of pregnancy or labor in 122 patients with heart disease (29).

BREAST FEEDING SUMMARY

RECOMMENDATION: Compatible

Digoxin is excreted into breast milk. Data for other cardiac glycosides have not been located. Digoxin milk:plasma ratios have varied from 0.6–0.9 (4,7,30,31). Although these amounts seem high, they represent very small amounts of digoxin due to significant maternal protein binding. No adverse effects in the nursing infant have been reported. The American Academy of Pediatrics classifies digoxin as compatible with breast-feeding (32).

References

1. Shepard TH. *Catalog of Teratogenic Agents.* 3rd ed. Baltimore, MD: Johns Hopkins University Press, 1980: 116–7.
2. Okita GT, Plotz EF, Davis ME. Placental transfer of radioactive digitoxin in pregnant women and its fetal distribution. Circ Res 1956;4:376–80.
3. Rogers MC, Willserson JT, Goldblatt A, Smith TW. Serum digoxin concentrations in the human fetus, neonate and infant. N Engl J Med 1972;287: 1010–3.
4. Chan V, Tse TF, Wong V. Transfer of digoxin across the placenta and into breast milk. Br J Obstet Gynaecol 1978;85:605–9.
5. Saarikoski S. Placental transfer and fetal uptake of ^{3}H-digoxin in humans. Br J Obstet Gynaecol 1976;83:879–84.
6. Allonen H, Kanto J, Lisalo E. The foeto-maternal distribution of digoxin in early human pregnancy. Acta Pharmacol Toxicol 1976;39:477–80.
7. Finley JP, Waxman MB, Wong PY, Lickrish GM. Digoxin excretion in human milk. J Pediatr 1979;94: 339–40.
8. Soyka LF. Digoxin: placental transfer, effects on the fetus, and therapeutic use in the newborn. Clin Perinatol 1975;2:23–35.
9. Padeletti L, Porciani MC, Scimone G. Placental transfer of digoxin (beta-methyl-digoxin) in man. Int J Clin Pharmacol Biopharm 1979;17:82–3.
10. Marzo A, Lo Cicero G, Brina A, Zuliani G, Ghirardi P, Pardi G. Preliminary data on the pharmacokinetics of digoxin in pregnancy. Boll Soc Ital Biol Sper 1980;56:219–23.
11. Luxford AME, Kellaway GSM. Pharmacokinetics of digoxin in pregnancy. Eur J Clin Pharmacol 1983;25:117–21.
12. Lingman G, Ohrlander S, Ohlin P. Intrauterine digoxin treatment of fetal paroxysmal tachycardia: case report. Br J Obstet Gynaecol 1980;87:340–2.
13. Kerenyi TD, Gleicher N, Meller J, Brown E, Steinfeld L, Chitkara U, Raucher H. Transplacental cardioversion of intrauterine supraventricular tachycardia with digitalis. Lancet 1980;2:393–4.
14. Harrigan JT, Kangos JJ, Sikka A, Spisso KR, Natarajan N, Rosenfeld D, Leiman S, Korn D. Successful treatment of fetal congestive heart failure secondary to tachycardia. N Engl J Med 1981;304:1527–9.
15. Diro M, Beydoun SN, Jaramillo B, O'Sullivan MJ, Kieval J. Successful pregnancy in a woman with a left ventricular cardiac aneurysm: a case report. J Reprod Med 1983;28:559–63.
16. Heaton FC, Vaughan R. Intrauterine supraventricular tachycardia: cardioversion with maternal digoxin. Obstet Gynecol 1982;60:749–52.
17. Simpson PC, Trudinger BJ, Walker A, Baird PJ. The intrauterine treatment of fetal cardiac failure in a twin pregnancy with an acardiac, acephalic monster. Am J Obstet Gynecol 1983;147:842–4.
18. Spinnato JA, Shaver DC, Flinn GS, Sibai BM, Watson DL, Marin-Garcia J. Fetal supraventricular tachycardia: in utero therapy with digoxin and quinidine. Obstet Gynecol 1984;64:730–5.
19. Bortolotti U, Milano A, Mazzucco A, Valfre C, Russo R, Valente M, Schivazappa L, Thiene G, Gallucci V. Pregnancy in patients with a porcine valve bioprosthesis. Am J Cardiol 1982;50:1051–4.
20. Rotmensch HH, Rotmensch S, Elkayam U. Management of cardiac arrhythmias during pregnancy: current concepts. Drugs 1987;33:623–33.
21. Tamari I, Eldar M, Rabinowitz B, Neufeld HN. Medical treatment of cardiovascular disorders during pregnancy. Am Heart J 1982;104:1357–63.
22. Dumesic DA, Silverman NH, Tobias S, Golbus MS.

Transplacental cardioversion of fetal supraventricular tachycardia with procainamide. N Engl J Med 1982; 307:1128–31.
23. Gleicher N, Elkayam U. Cardiac problems in pregnancy. II. Fetal aspects: advances in intrauterine diagnosis and therapy. JAMA 1984;252:78–80.
24. Golichowski AM, Caldwell R, Hartsough A, Peleg D. Pharmacologic cardioversion of intrauterine supraventricular tachycardia. A case report. J Reprod Med 1985;30:139–44.
25. Reece EA, Romero R, Santulli T, Kleinman CS, Hobbins JC. In utero diagnosis and management of fetal tachypnea. A case report. J Reprod Med 1985;30:221–4.
26. Weiner CP, Thompson MIB. Direct treatment of fetal supraventricular tachycardia after failed transplacental therapy. Am J Obstet Gynecol 1988;158:570–3.
27. Sherman JL Jr, Locke RV. Transplacental neonatal digitalis intoxication. Am J Cardiol 1960;6:834–7.
28. Weaver JB, Pearson JF. Influence of digitalis on time of onset and duration of labour in women with cardiac disease. Br Med J 1973;3:519–20.
29. Ho PC, Chen TY, Wong V. The effect of maternal cardiac disease and digoxin administration on labour, fetal weight and maturity at birth. Aust N Z J Obstet Gynaecol 1980;20:24–7.
30. Levy M, Granit L, Laufer N. Excretion of drugs in human milk. N Engl J Med 1977;297:789.
31. Loughnan PM. Digoxin excretion in human breast milk. J Pediatr 1978;92:1019–20.
32. Committee on Drugs, American Academy of Pediatrics. The transfer of drugs and other chemicals into human milk. Pediatrics 2001;108:776–89.

Name: **DIGITOXIN** Risk Factor: **C_M**
Class: **Cardiac Glycoside**

See Digitalis.

Name: **DIGOXIN** Risk Factor: **C_M**
Class: **Cardiac Glycoside**

See Digitalis.

Name: **DIGOXIN IMMUNE FAB (OVINE)** Risk Factor: **C_M**
Class: **Antidote**

FETAL RISK SUMMARY

RECOMMENDATION: Compatible - Maternal Benefit >> Embryo/Fetal Risk

Digoxin immune fab (ovine) is administered IV for the treatment of potentially life-threatening digoxin intoxication. It is composed of antigen binding fragments (fab) derived from specific antibodies raised in sheep. After papain-digestion, the digoxin-specific fab fragments are isolated and purified. Digoxin immune fab binds digoxin, thereby preventing the cardiac agent from binding to cells. The fab-digoxin complex is then excreted in the urine. The elimination half-life is approximately 15–20 hours. Reproduction studies in animals have not been conducted with digoxin immune fab (ovine) (1).

It is not known if digoxin immune fab (ovine) can cross the human placenta to the fetus. The antibody fragments probably do not cross because of their high molecular weight (about 46,000), but some antibodies are able to cross the placenta (e.g., see Immune Globulin Intravenous).

A 31-year-old woman at 25.5 weeks' gestation with severe preeclampsia was treated with two doses (10 mg each, 12 hours apart) digoxin immune fab (ovine) because of high, endogenous digitalis-like factor (serum digoxin level 0.3 ng/mL) (2). A marked decline in blood pressure and serum digoxin level (<0.1–0.2 ng/mL) accompanied each dose. Urine output also increased, but this was thought to be secondary to IV albumin that had also been given. The patient refused further therapy, and she was delivered by cesarean section. The 734-g female infant died shortly after birth. The high digoxin level in cord blood (0.7 ng/mL) suggested that digoxin immune fab (ovine) did not cross the placenta in effective amounts (2).

A 1996 case report described the use of digoxin immune fab (ovine) in pregnancy (3). A 23-year-old woman with twins at 19.5 weeks' gestation was hospitalized for worsening preeclampsia. She had hypertension, proteinuria (4.4 g/24 hours), and hand and facial edema. Serum digoxin was reported to be 0.4 ng/mL (normal is undetectable), even though she had no chronic medical illnesses and was not taking digoxin. The investigators speculated that the digoxin level was related to digoxin-like immune factors. Because the woman refused termination, therapy with digoxin immune fab (ovine) was offered. A total dose of 30 mg was administered by IV infusion over 24 hours. (The long infusion period was chosen to prevent hypotension.) Although the patient's condition improved markedly (decreased mean arterial pressure, increased creatinine clearance, and a doubling of the urinary output), her proteinuria worsened (≥9 g/day) and she then agreed to medical termination of the nonviable female twins (3).

No other cases of the use of digoxin immune fab (ovine) in pregnancy have been located. Although an embryo/fetal risk assessment cannot be made, the maternal benefits of therapy, in cases of digoxin overdose, should outweigh the unknown embryo/fetal risks. If indicated, therapy with this product should not be withheld because of pregnancy (4).

BREAST FEEDING SUMMARY

RECOMMENDATION: Compatible

No reports describing the use of digoxin immune fab (ovine) during lactation have been located. It is doubtful that clinically significant amounts are excreted into breast milk. Even if some excretion did occur, it would be digested in the nursing infant's stomach. Therefore, the risk to a nursing infant appears to be nil. In addition, the maternal benefits of therapy in cases of digoxin overdose should outweigh the unknown risk to a nursing infant.

References

1. Product information. Digibind. GlaxoSmithKline, 2004.
2. Goodlin RC. Antidigoxin antibodies in eclampsia. N Engl J Med 1988;318:518–9.
3. Adair CD, Buckalew V, Taylor K, Ernest JM, Frye AH, Evans C, Veille JC. Elevated endoxin-like factor complicating a multifetal second trimester pregnancy: treatment with digoxin-binding immunoglobulin. Am J Nephrol 1996;16:529–31.
4. Bailey B. Are there teratogenic risks associated with antidotes used in the acute management of poisoned pregnant women? Birth Defects Res Part A Clin Mol Teratol 2003;67:133–40.

Name:	**DIHYDROCODEINE BITARTRATE**	Risk Factor:	**B***
Class:	**Narcotic Agonist Analgesic**		

FETAL RISK SUMMARY

RECOMMENDATION: Human Data Suggest Risk in 3rd Trimester

No reports linking the use of dihydrocodeine with congenital defects have been located. Usage in pregnancy is primarily confined to labor. Respiratory depression in the newborn has been reported to be less than with meperidine, but depression is probably similar when equianalgesic doses are compared (1–3).

[*Risk Factor D if used for prolonged periods or in high doses at term.*]

D

BREAST FEEDING SUMMARY

RECOMMENDATION: No Human Data - Probably Compatible

No reports describing the use of dihydrocodeine bitartrate during lactation have been located. Because other opiates are excreted into milk (e.g., see Morphine) and the molecular weight (about 452) of dihydrocodeine bitartrate is low enough, the presence of the narcotic in milk should be expected. The long-term effects on neurobehavior and development in a nursing infant are unknown but warrant study.

References

1. Ruch WA, Ruch RM. A preliminary report on dihydrocodeine-scopolamine in obstetrics. Am J Obstet Gynecol 1957;74:1125–7.
2. Myers JD. A preliminary clinical evaluation of dihydrocodeine bitartrate in normal parturition. Am J Obstet Gynecol 1958;75:1096–100.
3. Bonica JJ. *Principles and Practice of Obstetric Analgesia and Anaesthesia*. Philadelphia, PA: FA Davis, 1967:245.

Name:	**DIHYDROERGOTAMINE**	Risk Factor:	X_M
Class:	**Sympatholytic (Antimigraine)**		

FETAL RISK SUMMARY

RECOMMENDATION: Contraindicated

Dihydroergotamine is the hydrogenated derivative of ergotamine (see also Ergotamine). It is available only in formulations for injection and nasal spray because oral absorption is poor. Both preparations are indicated for the acute treatment of migraine headaches with or without aura. In addition, the injectable formulation is indicated for the acute treatment of cluster headaches. The mean bioavailability of the nasal spray is 32% relative to the injectable administration. Plasma protein binding is 93% and the elimination half-life is about 9 hours (1,2). Another source, however, states that elimination is biphasic with half-lives of about 1–2 hours and 22–32 hours, respectively (3).

The oxytocic properties of ergotamine have been known since the early 1900s; producing a prolonged and marked increase in uterine tone that may lead to fetal hypoxia (4). The pharmacologic properties of dihydroergotamine are different then ergotamine as it is a much more potent sympatholytic (4). In a 1952 study, the oxytocic and toxic effects of dihydroergotamine were demonstrated (5). Twenty women at term were given 1 mg of dihydroergotamine in 500 ml distilled water IV over a period of 2–4 hours to induce labor. Labor induction was successful in eight women (40%), but in six other women the outcomes were four stillborns, one neonatal death 1.25 hours after delivery, and one severely depressed infant that developed seizures 3 days after delivery (progressing satisfactorily at 3 months of age with no abnormal neurological signs). The investigators concluded that dihydroergotamine should not be used to induce labor (5).

Reproduction studies have been conducted in rats and rabbits. In rats, intranasal administration throughout the period of organogenesis at doses producing maternal plasma exposures (AUC) about 0.4–1.2 times the human exposure (AUC) from the maximum recommended daily dose of 4 mg (MRDD) or greater resulted in decreased fetal body weights and/or skeletal ossification. Administration of the dose throughout pregnancy and lactation resulted in reduced body weights and impaired reproductive function in the offspring. The no-effect level for rat embryo-fetal toxicity was not established. In rabbits administered the nasal spray during organogenesis, maternal exposures at about 7 times the MRDD also resulted in delayed skeletal ossification. The no-effect dose for rabbit embryo-fetal toxicity was about 2.5 times the MRDD. The embryo-fetal toxic doses in both species did not cause maternal toxicity. The *in utero* growth retardation in the animal studies was thought to have resulted from reduced uteroplacental blood flow and/or increased myometrial tone (1,2).

A study in guinea pigs quantified the effect of dihydroergotamine on uteroplacental blood flow (6). Pregnant guinea pigs were given the drug (14 μg/kg/day) days 30–60 of pregnancy (*gestational length for guinea pigs is 64–68 days*). At term, placental blood flow was decreased by 51% and, fetal weight and fetal weight/placental weight ratio were significantly decreased compared to controls (6).

It is not known if dihydroergotamine crosses the human placenta. The molecular weight of the free base (about 584) and long elimination half-life suggest that the drug will cross the placenta, but the extensive protein binding will limit passage.

The Collaborative Perinatal Project monitored 50,282 mother-child pairs, 32 of whom were exposed to ergot derivatives (three to dihydroergotamine) other than ergotamine during the 1st trimester (7). Three malformed children were observed from this group, but the numbers are too small to draw any conclusion.

A brief 1993 report described a 31-year-old woman with depression, panic disorder, and migraine headaches who was exposed to a number of drugs in the first 6 weeks of pregnancy, including dihydroergotamine, citalopram, buspirone, thioridazine, and etilefrine (a sympathomimetic agent) (8). An elective abortion was performed at 12 weeks' gestation. A thorough macroscopic and microscopic examination of the intact, 38-g, 8.5-cm long male fetus revealed no evidence of malformation. A detailed neuropathological examination and chromosome analysis (46,XY karyotype) was normal (8).

In summary, dihydroergotamine is a potent semi-synthetic ergot alkaloid that has oxytocic and sympatholytic properties. The animal data suggest a risk of intrauterine growth retardation probably resulting from reduced uteroplacental blood flow and/or increased myometrial tone. Although there is no evidence that it is a teratogen, dihydroergotamine is contraindicated in pregnancy, especially near term. Inadvertent exposure early in gestation, however, does not appear to represent a major risk.

BREAST FEEDING SUMMARY

RECOMMENDATION: Contraindicated

No reports describing the use of dihydroergotamine during human lactation have been located. The molecular weight of the free base (about 584) and long elimination half-life (may be as long as 22 hours) suggest that the drug will be excreted into breast milk, but the high protein binding (about 93%) will limit this excretion. The closely related agent ergotamine is excreted into milk (see Ergotamine). An ergot product has been associated with symptoms of ergotism (vomiting, diarrhea, and convulsions) in nursing infants of mothers taking the agent for the treatment of migraine (see Ergotamine). Moreover, dihydroergotamine is a member of the same chemical family as bromocriptine, an agent that is used to suppress lactation. Although no specific information has been located relating to the effects of dihydroergotamine on lactation, ergot alkaloids may hinder lactation by inhibiting maternal pituitary prolactin secretion (9).

D

References

1. Product information. D. H. E. 45. Novartis Pharmaceuticals, 2001.
2. Product information. Migranal. Novartis Pharmaceuticals, 2001.
3. Parfitt K, Editor. *Martindale. The Complete Drug Reference*. 32nd ed. London: Pharmaceutical Press, 1999: 444–5.
4. Gill RC, Farrar JM. Experiences with di-hydroergotamine in the treatment of primary uterine inertia. J Obstet Gynaecol Br Emp 1951;58:79–91.
5. Altman SG, Waltman R, Lubin S, Reynolds SRM. Oxytocic and toxic actions of dihydroergotamine-45. Am J Obstet Gynecol 1952;64:101–9.
6. Hohmann M, Künzel W. Dihydroergotamine causes fetal growth retardation in guinea pigs. Arch Gynecol Obstet 1992;251:187–92.
7. Heinonen OP, Sloan D, Shapiro S. *Birth Defects and Drugs in Pregnancy*. Littleton, MA: Publishing Sciences Group, 1977:358–9.
8. Seifritz E, Holsboer-Trachsler E, Haberthur F, Hemmeter U, Poldinger W. Unrecognized pregnancy during citalopram treatment. Am J Psychiatry 1993;150:1428–9.
9. Vorherr H. Contraindications to breast-feeding. JAMA 1974;227:676.

Name:	**DIHYDROTACHYSTEROL**	Risk Factor:	**A***
Class:	**Vitamin**		

FETAL RISK SUMMARY

RECOMMENDATION: Compatible

Dihydrotachysterol is a synthetic analogue of vitamin D. It is converted in the liver to 25-hydroxydihydrotachysterol, an active metabolite. See Vitamin D.

[**Risk Factor D if used in doses above the recommended daily allowance.*]

BREAST FEEDING SUMMARY

RECOMMENDATION: Compatible

See Vitamin D.

Name:	**DILTIAZEM**	Risk Factor:	**C_M**
Class:	**Calcium Channel Blocker**		

FETAL RISK SUMMARY

RECOMMENDATION: Limited Human Data - Animal Data Suggest High Risk

Diltiazem is a calcium channel inhibitor used for the treatment of angina. Reproductive studies in mice, rats, and rabbits at doses up to 5–10 times (on a mg/kg basis) the daily recommended human dose found increased mortality in embryos and fetuses. These doses also produced abnormalities of the skeletal system. An increased incidence of stillbirths were observed in perinatal animal studies at 20 times the human dose or greater (1). In fetal sheep, diltiazem, like ritodrine and magnesium sulfate, inhibited bladder contractions, resulting in residual urine (2).

A 34-year-old woman, in her 1st month of pregnancy, was treated with diltiazem, 60 mg 4 times/day, and isosorbide dinitrate, 20 mg 4 times/day, for symptomatic myocardial ischemia (3). Both medications were continued throughout the remainder of gestation. Normal twins were delivered by repeat cesarean section at 37 weeks' gestation. Both infants were alive and well at 6 months of age.

In a surveillance study of Michigan Medicaid recipients conducted between 1985 and 1992 involving 229,101 completed pregnancies, 27 newborns had been exposed to diltiazem during the 1st trimester (F. Rosa, personal communication, FDA, 1993). Four (14.8%) major birth defects were observed (one expected), two of which were cardiovascular defects (0.3 expected). No anomalies were observed in five other categories of defects (oral clefts, spina bifida, polydactyly, limb reduction defects, and hypospadias) for which data were available. Although the number of exposures is small, the total number of defects and the number of cardiovascular defects are suggestive of an association, but other factors, including the mother's disease, concurrent drug use, and chance may be involved.

A prospective, multicenter cohort study of 78 women (81 outcomes; 3 sets of twins) who had 1st trimester exposure to calcium channel blockers, including 13% to diltiazem, was reported in 1996 (4). Compared to controls, no increase in the risk of major congenital malformations was found.

Diltiazem has been used as a tocolytic agent (5). In a prospective randomized trial, 22 women treated with the agent were compared with 23 treated with nifedipine. No differences between the groups in outcomes or maternal effects were observed. If diltiazem is used in pregnancy, healthcare professionals are encouraged to call the toll free number (800-670-6126) for information about patient enrollment in the Motherisk study.

BREAST FEEDING SUMMARY

RECOMMENDATION: Limited Human Data - Probably Compatible

Diltiazem is excreted into human milk (6). A 40-year-old woman, 14 days postpartum, was unsuccessfully treated with diltiazem, 60 mg 4 times/day, for resistant premature ventricular contractions. Her infant was not allowed to breast-feed during the treatment period. Simultaneous serum and milk levels were drawn at several times on the 4th day of therapy. The peak level in milk was approximately 200 ng/mL, almost the same as the peak serum concentration. Milk and serum concentrations were nearly the same during the measurement interval, with changes in the concentrations closely paralleling each other. The data indicated that diltiazem freely diffuses into milk (6). In a separate case described above, a mother nursed twins for at least 6 months while being treated with diltiazem and isosorbide dinitrate (3). Milk concentrations were not determined, but both infants were alive and well at 6 months of age. The American Academy of Pediatrics classifies diltiazem as compatible with breast-feeding (7).

References

1. Product information. Cardizem. Hoechst Marion Roussel, 1997.
2. Kogan BA, Iwamoto HS. Lower urinary tract function in the sheep fetus: studies of autonomic control and pharmacologic responses of the fetal bladder. J Urol 1989;141:1019–24.
3. Lubbe WF. Use of diltiazem during pregnancy. N Z Med J 1987;100:121.

4. Magee LA, Schick B, Donnenfeld AE, Sage SR, Conover B, Cook L, McElhatton PR, Schmidt MA, Koren G. The safety of calcium channel blockers in human pregnancy: A prospective, multicenter cohort study. Am J Obstet Gynecol 1996;174:823–8.
5. El-Sayed Y, Holbrook RH Jr. Diltiazem (D) for the maintenance tocolysis of preterm labor (PTL): a prospective randomized trial (abstract). Am J Obstet Gynecol 1996;174:468.
6. Okada M, Inoue H, Nakamura Y, Kishimoto M, Suzuki T. Excretion of diltiazem in human milk. N Engl J Med 1985;313:992–3.
7. Committee on Drugs, American Academy of Pediatrics. The transfer of drugs and other chemicals into human milk. Pediatrics 2001;108:776–89.

D

Name: **DIMENHYDRINATE** Risk Factor: B_M
Class: **Antihistamine/Antiemetic**

FETAL RISK SUMMARY

RECOMMENDATION: Compatible

Dimenhydrinate is the chlorotheophylline salt of the antihistamine diphenhydramine. A prospective study in 1963 compared dimenhydrinate usage in three groups of patients: 266 with malformed infants and two groups of 266 each without malformed infants (1). No difference in usage of the drug was found between the three groups.

The Collaborative Perinatal Project monitored 50,282 mother-child pairs, 319 of whom had 1st trimester exposure to dimenhydrinate (2, pp. 367–370). For use anytime in pregnancy, 697 exposures were recorded (2, p. 440). In neither case was evidence found to suggest a relationship to large categories of major or minor malformations. Two possible associations with individual malformations were found: cardiovascular defects (five cases) and inguinal hernia (eight cases). Independent confirmation is required to determine the actual risk for these anomalies (2, p. 440).

A number of reports have described the oxytocic effect of IV dimenhydrinate (3–13). When used either alone or with oxytocin, most studies found a smoother, shorter labor. However, in one study of 30 patients who received a 100-mg dose during 3.5 minutes, some (at least two, but exact number not specified) also showed evidence of uterine hyperstimulation and fetal distress (e.g., bradycardia and loss of beat-to-beat variability) (13). Due to these effects, dimenhydrinate should not be used for this purpose.

Dimenhydrinate has been used for the treatment of hyperemesis gravidarum (14). In 64 women presenting with the condition prior to 13 weeks' gestation, all were treated with dimenhydrinate followed by various other antiemetics. Three of the newborns had integumentary abnormalities consisting of one case of webbed toes with an extra finger, and two cases of skin tags (one preauricular and one sacral). The defects were not thought to be related to the drug therapy (14).

An association between exposure during the last 2 weeks of pregnancy to antihistamines in general and retrolental fibroplasia in premature infants has been reported. See Brompheniramine for details.

BREAST FEEDING SUMMARY

RECOMMENDATION: No Human Data - Probably Compatible

No reports describing the use of dimenhydrinate during lactation have been located. The molecular weight (about 470) is low enough, however, that excretion into milk should be expected. For a closely related product, see Diphenhydramine.

References

1. Mellin GW, Katzenstein M. Meclozine and fetal abnormalities. Lancet 1963;1:222–3.
2. Heinonen OP, Slone D, Shapiro S. *Birth Defects and Drugs in Pregnancy*. Littleton, MA: Publishing Sciences Group, 1977.
3. Watt LO. Oxytocic effects of dimenhydrinate in obstetrics. Can Med Assoc J 1961;84:533–4.
4. Rotter CW, Whitaker JL, Yared J. The use of intravenous Dramamine to shorten the time of labor and potentiate analgesia. Am J Obstet Gynecol 1958:75:1101–4.
5. Scott RS, Wallace KH, Badley DN, Watson BH. Use of dimenhydrinate in labor. Am J Obstet Gynecol 1962;83:25–8.
6. Humphreys DW. Safe relief of pain during labor with dimenhydrinate. Clin Med (Winnetka) 1962;69: 1165–8.
7. Cooper K. Failure of dimenhydrinate to shorten labor. Am J Obstet Gynecol 1963;86:1041–3.
8. Harkins JL, Van Praagh IG, Irwin NT. A clinical evaluation of intravenous dimenhydrinate in labor. Can Med Assoc J 1964;91:164–6.
9. Scott RS. The use of intravenous dimenhydrinate in labor. New Physician 1964;13:302–7.
10. Klieger JA, Massart JJ. Clinical and laboratory survey into the oxytocic effects of dimenhydrinate in labor. Am J Obstet Gynecol 1965;92:1–10.
11. Hay TB, Wood C. The effect of dimenhydrinate on uterine contractions. Aust N Z J Obstet Gynaecol 1967;1:81–9.
12. Shephard B, Cruz A, Spellacy W. The acute effects of Dramamine on uterine contractibility during labor. J Reprod Med 1976;16:27–8.
13. Hara GS, Carter RP, Krantz KE. Dramamine in labor: potential boon or a possible bomb? J Kans Med Soc 1980;81:134–6,155.
14. Gross S, Librach C, Cecutti A. Maternal weight loss associated with hyperemesis gravidarum: a predictor of fetal outcome. Am J Obstet Gynecol 1989;160:906–9.

Name: **DIMERCAPROL** Risk Factor: **C_M**

Class: **Antidote**

FETAL RISK SUMMARY

RECOMMENDATION: Compatible - Maternal Benefit >> Embryo/Fetal Risk

Dimercaprol is a chelating agent indicated in the treatment of arsenic, gold, and acute mercury poisoning, and for lead poisoning when used concomitantly with edetate calcium disodium. It is not very effective for chronic mercury poisoning. Dimercaprol is administered by IM injection. The mechanism of action involves dimercaprol sulfhydryl groups forming complexes with certain heavy metals, thereby preventing or reversing the metal from binding sulfhydryl-containing enzymes (1).

A 1998 review cited five studies that evaluated the reproductive toxicity of dimercaprol in animals (2). The antidote was given to pregnant mice in doses of 15–60 mg/kg/day for 4 days to protect against methylmercury-induced developmental toxicity. Similar single or multiple doses given to mice daily did not alleviate arsenate-induced fetal toxicity, but no dimercaprol-induced developmental toxicity was noted (2). In another study, SC dimercaprol (125 mg/kg/day) in mice on gestational days 9–12 resulted in embryotoxicity (growth retardation, increased mortality) and teratogenicity (digits with abnormal direction and situation, cleft palate, and cerebral hernia) (2). (*Note: the human IM dose, depending on the type of poisoning, varies from 2.5 mg/kg/day to 18 mg/kg/day with up to 13-day courses.)*

It is not known if dimercaprol can cross the human placenta. The low molecular weight (about 124), however, suggests that the drug does cross to the embryo/fetal compartment.

Apparently, the first reported case of dimercaprol in a human pregnancy appeared in 1948 (3). An 18-year-old woman at about 26 weeks' gestation was given dimercaprol for arsenical encephalopathy. The woman had received several arsenic-containing injections for vaginal and perineal warts 10 days earlier. She was given a total dose of 5440 mg over 13 days. Labor was induced at about 36 weeks' gestation because of eclampsia, and she delivered a 5.5-lb male infant who required resuscitation but was otherwise healthy. Long-term follow-up of the infant was not reported (3).

A 1969 case report detailed the pregnancy outcome of a 17-year-old patient at 30 weeks' gestation who had ingested approximately 30 mL of arsenic trioxide containing 1.32% of total elemental arsenic (4). About 24 hours after ingestion, she was treated with 150 mg of IM dimercaprol but developed renal failure over the next 72 hours. Spontaneous labor occurred, and she delivered a 1.1-kg female infant with an Apgar score of 4 at 1 minute. A qualitative test for arsenic on the baby's plasma was negative. The infant died 11 hours later of respiratory distress syndrome. At autopsy, toxicologic analysis for arsenic (reported as arsenic trioxide per 100 g of wet tissue) revealed that the metal had crossed the placenta to the fetus with the following concentrations: 0.740 mg (liver), 0.150 mg (kidneys), and 0.0218 mg (brain). The arsenic levels in the infant were all significantly higher than those measured in adult autopsy material (4). The authors could locate only one other similar case of inorganic arsenic poisoning in pregnancy. In that case, published in 1928 in a French journal, both the mother and infant died. Arsenic levels for the infant were not reported, but the level in the maternal liver was 0.56 g/100 g, less than the level found in the current infant (4).

A 2002 report described the use of IV edetate and IM dimercaprol (dose not specified) in a woman at 30 weeks' gestation with a high blood lead concentration (5.2 μmol/L; goal $\leq$0.48 μmol/L) (5). Twenty-four hours after initiation of chelation therapy, her lead level was 2.3 μmol/L. Twelve hours later labor was induced because of uterine hemorrhage and she gave birth to a 1.6-kg (75th percentile) female infant. Lead concentration in the cord blood was 7.6 μmol/L. The Apgar scores were 4 and 6 (presumably at 1 and 5 minutes, respectively). The newborn was flaccid with absent reflexes, no movement to noxious stimuli, and no gag reflex, but she did have spontaneous eye movement. Bilateral diaphragmatic palsy was confirmed by fluoroscopy. During her 7 months of hospitalization, the infant received multiple courses of chelation to treat the intrauterine lead intoxication. In spite of this therapy, she had right sensorineural deafness and neurodevelopment delay at discharge. Oral succimer was continued at home because the blood lead level was still elevated (0.95 μmol/L). The mother's lead source was identified as herbal tablets that had been prescribed for a gastrointestinal complaint. She had taken the tablets periodically over the past 9 years and throughout her pregnancy. Mercury also was present in some of the tablets. The lead intake during pregnancy was estimated to be 50 times the average weekly intake of Western populations (5).

Although the limited animal data suggest low embryo/fetal risk, there are no reports of dimercaprol use during organogenesis in humans. This absence of data prevents an assessment of the human embryo risk. However, the maternal benefit, and indirect embryo/fetal benefit, appears to far outweigh the unknown embryo/fetal risk. Therefore, if indicated, dimercaprol should not be withheld because of pregnancy (6).

BREAST FEEDING SUMMARY

RECOMMENDATION: Contraindicated

No reports describing the use of dimercaprol during human lactation have been located. The molecular weight (about 124) and the typical prolonged therapy (i.e., 13 days) suggest that the antidote will be excreted into breast milk. The effect, if any, of this exposure on a nursing infant is unknown. Because the use of dimercaprol implies poisoning with arsenic, gold, mercury, or lead, these metals also will be excreted into milk and are toxic to a nursing infant. Therefore, breast-feeding is contraindicated in women receiving dimercaprol.

References

1. Product information. BAL in Oil. Akorn, 2004.
2. Domingo JL. Developmental toxicity of metal chelating agents. Reprod Toxicol 1998;12:499–510.
3. Kantor HI, Levin PM. Arsenical encephalopathy in pregnancy with recovery. Am J Obstet Gynecol 1948;56:370–4.
4. Lugo G, Cassady G, Palmisano P. Acute maternal arsenic intoxication with neonatal death. Am J Dis Child 1969;117:328–30.
5. Tait PA, Vora A, James S, Fitzgerald DJ, Pester BA. Severe congenital lead poisoning in a preterm infant due to a herbal remedy. Med J Aust 2002;177:193–5.
6. Bailey B. Are there teratogenic risks associated with antidotes used in the acute management of poisoned pregnant women? Birth Defects Res Part A Clin Mol Teratol 2003;67:133–40.

Name:	DIMETHINDENE	Risk Factor:	B
Class:	Antihistamine		

FETAL RISK SUMMARY

RECOMMENDATION: Limited Human Data - Probably Compatible

Reproductive toxicity studies using dimethindene in rats (up to 200 mg/kg/day orally or 16 mg/kg/day IV) and rabbits (up to 50 mg/kg/day orally) revealed no embryo lethality or teratogenicity (G. J. Golden, personal communication, Zyma Switzerland, 1995). Embryotoxicity (decreased fetal weight and slight retarded ossification) was observed in rats at the highest dose, but not in rabbits.

The Collaborative Perinatal Project monitored 113 pregnancies that were exposed to a miscellaneous group of antihistamines during the 1st trimester (1). Two patients in the group took dimethindene. No association was found between the drug exposure in the total group and congenital defects.

BREAST FEEDING SUMMARY

RECOMMENDATION: No Human Data - Probably Compatible

Very small amounts of dimethindene are excreted in the milk of lactating rats (G. J. Golden, personal communication, Zyma Switzerland, 1995). One source states that the drug is contraindicated during lactation, but no reasons for this statement were given (2). No studies describing the use of dimethindene during human lactation or measuring the amount of drug in human milk have been located.

References

1. Heinonen OP, Slone D, Shapiro S. *Birth Defects and Drugs in Pregnancy*. Littleton, MA: Publishing Sciences Group, 1977:323.
2. Onnis A, Grella P. *The Biochemical Effects of Drugs in Pregnancy. Volume 1: Drugs Active on the Nervous, Cardiovascular and Haemopoietic Systems*. West Sussex, England: Ellis Harwood, 1984:248.

D

Name:	**DIMETHOTHIAZINE**	Risk Factor:	**C**
Class:	**Antihistamine**		

No data are available. See Promethazine for representative agent in this class.

Name:	**DIOXYLINE**	Risk Factor:	**C**
Class:	**Vasodilator**		

FETAL RISK SUMMARY

RECOMMENDATION: No Human Data - No Relevant Animal Data

No data are available.

BREAST FEEDING SUMMARY

RECOMMENDATION: No Human Data - Probably Compatible

No data are available.

Name:	**DIPHEMANIL**	Risk Factor:	**C**
Class:	**Parasympatholytic**		

FETAL RISK SUMMARY

RECOMMENDATION: No Human Data - No Relevant Animal Data

Diphemanil is an anticholinergic quaternary ammonium methylsulfate. No reports of its use in pregnancy have been located (see also Atropine).

BREAST FEEDING SUMMARY

RECOMMENDATION: No Human Data - Probably Compatible

No data are available (see also Atropine).

Name:	**DIPHENADIONE**	Risk Factor:	**D**
Class:	**Anticoagulant**		

See Coumarin Derivatives.

Name:	**DIPHENHYDRAMINE**	Risk Factor:	**B_M**
Class:	**Antihistamine**		

FETAL RISK SUMMARY

RECOMMENDATION: Compatible

Diphenhydramine is a first generation antihistamine agent. Reproductive studies with diphenhydramine in rats and rabbits at doses up to 5 times the human dose revealed no evidence of impaired fertility or fetal harm (1). Rapid placental transfer of diphenhydramine has been demonstrated in pregnant sheep with a fetal:maternal ratio of 0.85 (2). Peak fetal concentrations occurred within 5 minutes of a 100-mg IV dose.

The Collaborative Perinatal Project monitored 50,282 mother-child pairs, 595 of whom had 1st trimester exposure to diphenhydramine (3, pp. 323–337). For use anytime during pregnancy, 2948 exposures were recorded (3, p. 437). In neither case was evidence found to suggest a relationship to large categories of major or minor malformations. Several possible associations with individual malformations were found, but independent confirmation is required to determine the actual risk: genitourinary (other than hypospadias) (5 cases); hypospadias (3 cases); eye and ear defects (3 cases); syndromes (other than Down's syndrome) (3 cases); inguinal hernia (13 cases); clubfoot (5 cases); any ventricular septal defect (open or closing) (5 cases); and malformations of diaphragm (3 cases) (3, pp. 323–337, 437, 475).

Cleft palate and diphenhydramine usage in the 1st trimester were statistically associated in a 1974 case-control study (4). A group of 599 children with oral clefts was compared to 590 controls without clefts. *In utero* exposures to diphenhydramine in the groups were 20 and 6, respectively, a significant difference. However, in a 1971 report significantly fewer infants with malformations were exposed to antihistamines in the 1st trimester as compared to controls (5). Diphenhydramine was the second most commonly used antihistamine. In addition, a 1985 study reported 1st trimester use of diphenhydramine in 270 women from a total group of 6509 (6). No association between the use of the drug and congenital abnormalities was found.

In a surveillance study of Michigan Medicaid recipients conducted between 1985 and 1992 involving 229,101 completed pregnancies, 1461 newborns had been exposed to diphenhydramine during the 1st trimester (F. Rosa, personal communication, FDA, 1993). A total of 80 (5.5%) major birth defects were observed (62 expected). Specific data were available for six defect categories, including (observed/expected) 14/14 cardiovascular defects, 3/2 oral clefts, 0/1 spina bifida, 9/4 polydactyly, 1/2 limb reduction defects, and 3/4 hypospadias. Possible associations with congenital defects are suggested for the total number of anomalies and for polydactyly, but other factors, including the mother's disease, concurrent drug use, and chance may be involved.

Diphenhydramine withdrawal was reported in a newborn infant whose mother had taken 150 mg/day during pregnancy (7). Generalized tremulousness and diarrhea began on the 5th day of life. Treatment with phenobarbital resulted in the gradual disappearance of the symptoms.

A stillborn, full-term, 1000-g female infant was exposed during gestation to high doses of diphenhydramine, theophylline, ephedrine, and phenobarbital, all used for maternal asthma (8). Except for a ventricular septal defect, no other macroscopic internal or external anomalies were observed. However, complete triploidy was found in lymphocyte cultures, which is unusual because very few such infants survive until term (8). No relationship between the chromosome abnormality or the congenital defect and the drug therapy can be inferred from this case.

A 1996 report described the use of diphenhydramine, droperidol, metoclopramide, and hydroxyzine in 80 women with hyperemesis gravidarum (9). The mean gestational age at the start of treatment was 10.9 ± 3.9 weeks. The patients received 200 mg/day IV of diphenhydramine for 2–3 days and 12 (15%) required a second course of therapy when their symptoms recurred. Three of the mothers (all treated in the 2nd trimester) delivered offspring with congenital defects: Poland's syndrome, fetal alcohol syndrome, and hydrocephalus and hypoplasia of the right cerebral hemisphere. Only the latter anomaly is a potential drug effect, but the most likely cause was thought to be the result of an *in utero* fetal vascular accident or infection (9).

A 2001 study, using a treatment method similar to the above study, described the use of droperidol and diphenhydramine in 28 women hospitalized for hyperemesis gravidarum (10). Pregnancy outcomes in the study group were compared to a historical control of 54 women who had received conventional antiemetic therapy. Oral metoclopramide and hydroxyzine were used after discharge from the hospital. Therapy was started in the study and control groups at mean gestational ages of 9.9 and 11.1 weeks', respectively. The study group appeared to have more severe disease than controls as suggested by a greater mean loss from the pre-pregnancy weight, 2.07 kg vs. 0.81 kg (*n.s.)*, and a slightly lower serum potassium level, 3.4 vs. 3.5 mmol/L (*n.s.)*. Compared to controls, the droperidol group had a shorter duration of hospitalization (3.53 vs. 2.82 days, $p = 0.023$), fewer readmissions (38.9% vs. 14.3%, $p = 0.025$), and lower average daily nausea and vomiting scores (both $p < 0.001$). There were no statistical differences ($p > 0.05$) in outcomes (study vs. controls) in terms of spontaneous abortions ($N = 0$ vs. $N = 2$ [4.3%]), elective abortions ($N = 3$ [12.0%] vs. $N = 3$ [6.5%]), Apgar scores at 1, 5, and 10 minutes, age at birth (37.3 vs. 37.9 weeks), and birth weight (3114 vs. 3347 g) (10). In controls, there was one (2.4%) major malformation of unknown cause, an acardiac fetus in a set of triplets, and one newborn with a genetic defect (Turner syndrome). There was also one unexplained major birth defect (4.4%) in the droperidol group (bilateral hydronephrosis), and two genetic defects (translocation of chromosomes 3 and 7; tyrosinemia) (10).

A potential drug interaction between diphenhydramine and temazepam resulting in the stillbirth of a term female infant has been reported (11). The mother had taken diphenhydramine 50 mg for mild itching of the skin, and approximately 1.5 hours later, took 30 mg of temazepam for sleep. Three hours later she awoke with violent intrauterine fetal movements, which lasted several minutes and then abruptly stopped. The stillborn infant was delivered approximately 4 hours later. Autopsy revealed no gross or microscopic anomalies. In an experiment with pregnant rabbits, neither of the drugs alone caused fetal mortality but when combined, 51 (81%) of 63 fetuses were stillborn or died shortly after birth (11). No definite mechanism could be established for the suggested interaction.

A 1980 report described the oxytocic properties of diphenhydramine when used in labor (12). Fifty women were given 50 mg IV over 3.5 minutes in a study designed to compare its effect with dimenhydrinate (see also Dimenhydrinate). The effects on the uterus were similar to those of dimenhydrinate but not as pronounced. Although no uterine hyperstimulation or fetal distress was observed, the drug should not be used for this purpose due to these potential complications.

Regular (every 1–2 minutes with intervening uterine relaxation), painful uterine contractions were observed in a 19-year-old woman at 26 week's gestation, following ingestion of about 35 capsules of diphenhydramine and an unknown amount of acetaminophen in a suicide attempt (13). The uterine contractions responded promptly to IV magnesium sulfate tocolysis and 5 hours later, after treatment with oral activated charcoal for the overdose, no further contractions were observed. The eventual outcome of the pregnancy was not mentioned.

An association between exposure during the last 2 weeks of pregnancy to antihistamines in general and retrolental fibroplasia in premature infants has been reported. See Brompheniramine for details.

In summary, both the animal data and the published human experience suggest that diphenhydramine is safe for use in human pregnancy. The exception is the case-control study showing an association with cleft palate. In addition, premature infants exposed within 2 weeks of birth may be at risk for toxicity. At least one review has concluded that diphenhydramine is the drug of choice if parenteral antihistamines are indicated in pregnancy (14).

BREAST FEEDING SUMMARY

RECOMMENDATION: Limited Human Data - Probably Compatible

Diphenhydramine is excreted into human breast milk, but levels have not been reported (15). Although the levels are not thought to be sufficiently high to affect the infant after therapeutic doses, the manufacturer considers the drug contraindicated in nursing mothers (1). The reason given for this is the increased sensitivity of newborn or premature infants to antihistamines.

References

1. Product information. Benadryl. Parke-Davis, 1997.
2. Yoo GD, Axelson JE, Taylor SM, Rurak DW. Placental transfer of diphenhydramine in chronically instrumented pregnant sheep. J Pharm Sci 1986;75:685–7.
3. Heinonen OP, Sloan D, Shapiro S. *Birth Defects and Drugs in Pregnancy*. Littleton, MA: Publishing Sciences Group, 1977.
4. Saxen I. Cleft palate and maternal diphenhydramine intake. Lancet 1974;1:407–8.
5. Nelson MM, Forfar JO. Associations between drugs administered during pregnancy and congenital abnormalities of the fetus. Br Med J 1971;1:523–7.
6. Aselton P, Jick H, Milunsky A, Hunter JR, Stergachis A. First-trimester drug use and congenital disorders. Obstet Gynecol 1985;65:451–5.
7. Parkin DE. Probable Benadryl withdrawal manifestations in a newborn infant. J Pediatr 1974;85:580.
8. Halbrecht I, Komlos L, Shabtay F, Solomon M, Bock JA. Triploidy 69,XXX in a stillborn girl. Clin Genet 1973;4:210–2.
9. Nageotte MP, Briggs GG, Towers CV, Asrat T. Droperidol and diphenhydramine in the management of hyperemesis gravidarum. Am J Obstet Gynecol 1996;174:1801–6.
10. Turcotte V, Ferreira E, Duperron L. Utilité du dropéridol et de la diphenhydramine dans l'hyperemesis gravidarum. J Soc Obstet Gynaecol Can 2001;23:133–9.
11. Kargas GA, Kargas SA, Bruyere HJ Jr, Gilbert EF, Opitz JM. Perinatal mortality due to interaction of diphenhydramine and temazepam. N Engl J Med 1985;313:1417.
12. Hara GS, Carter RP, Krantz KE. Dramamine in labor: potential boon or a possible bomb? J Kans Med Soc 1980;81:134–6, 155.
13. Brost BC, Scardo JA, Newman RB. Diphenhydramine overdose during pregnancy: lessons from the past. Am J Obstet Gynecol 1996;175:1376–7.
14. Schatz M, Petitti D. Antihistamines and pregnancy. Ann Allergy Asthma Immunol 1997;78:157–9.
15. O'Brien TE. Excretion of drugs in human milk. Am J Hosp Pharm 1974;31:844–54.

Name:	**DIPHENOXYLATE**	Risk Factor:	C_M
Class:	**Antidiarrheal**		

D

FETAL RISK SUMMARY

RECOMMENDATION: Limited Human Data - Animal Data Suggest Low Risk

Diphenoxylate is a narcotic related to meperidine. It is available only in combination with atropine (to discourage overdosage) for the treatment of diarrhea. Diphenoxylate is rapidly metabolized to diphenoxylic acid (difenoxin), a biologically active metabolite (1).

Reproduction studies have been conducted in mice, rats, and rabbits with oral doses of 0.4 to 20 mg/kg/day (1). Because of the experimental design and small numbers of litters, embryotoxic, fetotoxic, and teratogenic effects could not be adequately assessed, but examination of the available fetuses did not reveal any evidence of teratogenicity (1).

No reports describing the placental transfer of diphenoxylate to the fetus have been located. The molecular weight of the active, major metabolite difenoxin (461 for the hydrochloride salt) is low enough that the presence of this agent in the fetus should be expected.

In one study, no malformed infants were observed after 1st trimester exposure in seven patients (2). A single case of a female infant born at 36 weeks' gestation with multiple defects, including Ebstein's anomaly, was described in a 1989 report (3). In addition to the cardiac defect, other abnormalities noted were hypertelorism; epicanthal folds; low-set, posteriorly rotated ears; a cleft uvula; medially rotated hands; deafness; and blindness. The mother had taken Lomotil (diphenoxylate and atropine) for diarrhea during the 10th week of gestation. Because exposure was beyond the susceptible stages of development for these defects, the drug combination was not considered causative. A possible viremia in the mother as a cause of the diarrhea and the defects could not be excluded.

In a surveillance study of Michigan Medicaid recipients conducted between 1985 and 1992 involving 229,101 completed pregnancies, 179 newborns had been exposed to diphenoxylate (presumably combined with atropine) during the 1st trimester (F. Rosa, personal communication, FDA, 1993). Nine (5.0%) major birth defects were observed (seven expected). Specific data were available for six defect categories, including (observed/expected) 3/2 cardiovascular defects, 0/0.3 oral clefts, 1/0 spina bifida, 1/0.5 polydactyly, 1/0.3 limb reduction defects, and 1/0.4 hypospadias. These data do not support an association between the drug and congenital defects.

BREAST FEEDING SUMMARY

RECOMMENDATION: Limited Human Data - Potential Toxicity

The manufacturer reports that the active metabolite, diphenoxylic acid (difenoxin), is probably excreted into breast milk, and the effects of that drug and atropine may be evident in the nursing infant (1). One source recommends that the drug should not be used in lactating mothers (4). However, the American Academy of Pediatrics classifies atropine (diphenoxylate was not listed) as compatible with breast-feeding (5).

References

1. Product information. Lomotil. G. D. Searle and Company, 2000.
2. Heinonen OP, Slone D, Shapiro S. *Birth Defects and Drugs in Pregnancy*. Littleton, MA: Publishing Sciences Group, 1977:287.
3. Siebert JR, Barr M Jr, Jackson JC, Benjamin DR. Ebstein's anomaly and extracardiac defects. Am J Dis Child 1989;143:570–2.
4. Stewart JJ. Gastrointestinal drugs. In Wilson JT, ed. *Drugs in Breast Milk*. Balgowlah, Australia: ADIS Press, 1981:71.
5. Committee on Drugs, American Academy of Pediatrics. The transfer of drugs and other chemicals into human milk. Pediatrics 2001;108:776–89.

Name:	DIPYRIDAMOLE	Risk Factor:	D_M
Class:	**Hematological Agent (Antiplatelet)**		

FETAL RISK SUMMARY

RECOMMENDATION: Limited Human Data - Animal Data Suggest Low Risk

Dipyridamole is a platelet inhibitor that is indicated as an adjunct to coumarin anticoagulants in the prevention of postoperative thromboembolic complications of cardiac valve replacement. The drug has a terminal elimination half-life of about 10 hours and is highly bound to plasma proteins (1).

Reproduction studies have been conducted in mice, rats, and rabbits at doses up to 1.3, 20, and 1.6 times the maximum recommended daily human dose based on body surface area, respectively. No evidence of fetal harm was found in these studies (1).

No reports linking the use of dipyridamole with congenital defects have been located. The drug has been used in pregnancy (2–9). A single IV 30-mg dose of dipyridamole was shown to increase uterine perfusion in the 3rd trimester in 10 patients (10). In one pregnancy, a malformed infant was delivered, but the mother was also taking warfarin (2). The multiple defects in the infant were consistent with the fetal warfarin syndrome (see Coumarin Derivatives).

In a randomized, nonblinded study to prevent preeclampsia, 52 high-risk patients treated from the 13th week of gestation through delivery with daily doses of 300 mg of dipyridamole plus 150 mg of aspirin were compared to 50 high-risk controls (11). Four treated patients were excluded from analysis (spontaneous abortions before 16 weeks) vs. five controls (two lost to follow-up plus three spontaneous abortions). Hypertension occurred in 41 patients—19 treated and 22 controls. The outcome of pregnancy was significantly better in treated patients in three areas: preeclampsia (none vs. 6), fetal and neonatal loss (none vs. 5), and severe intrauterine growth retardation (none vs. 4). No fetal malformations were observed in either group. Other reports and reviews have documented the benefits of this therapy, namely a reduction in the incidence of stillbirth, placental infarction, and intrauterine growth retardation (12–18).

BREAST FEEDING SUMMARY

RECOMMENDATION: Limited Human Data - Probably Compatible

Dipyridamole is excreted into breast milk (1). The effects of this exposure on a nursing infant are unknown.

D

References

1. Product information. Persantine. Boehringer Ingelheim Pharmaceuticals, 2004.
2. Tejani N. Anticoagulant therapy with cardiac valve prosthesis during pregnancy. Obstet Gynecol 1973;42:785–93.
3. Del Bosque MR. Dipiridamol and anticoagulants in the management of pregnant women with cardiac valvular prosthesis. Ginecol Obstet Mex 1973;33: 191–8.
4. Littler WA, Bonnar J, Redman CWG, Beilin LJ, Lee GD. Reduced pulmonary arterial compliance in hypertensive patients. Lancet 1973;1:1274–8.
5. Biale Y, Lewenthal H, Gueron M, Beu-Aderath N. Caesarean section in patient with mitral-valve prosthesis. Lancet 1977;1:907.
6. Taguchi K. Pregnancy in patients with a prosthetic heart valve. Surg Gynecol Obstet 1977;145: 206–8.
7. Ahmad R, Rajah SM, Mearns AJ, Deverall PB. Dipyridamole in successful management of pregnant women with prosthetic heart valve. Lancet 1976;2:1414–5.
8. Biale Y, Cantor A, Lewenthal H, Gueron M. The course of pregnancy in patients with artificial heart valves treated with dipyridamole. Int J Gynaecol Obstet 1980;18:128–32.
9. Salazar E, Zajarias A, Gutierrez N, Iturbe I. The problem of cardiac valve prostheses, anticoagulants, and pregnancy. Circulation 1984;70(Suppl 1): I169–77.
10. Lauchkner W, Schwarz R, Retzke U. Cardiovascular action of dipyridamole in advanced pregnancy. Zentralbl Gynaekol 1981;103:220–7.
11. Beaufils M, Uzan S, Donsimoni R, Colau JC. Prevention of pre-eclampsia by early antiplatelet therapy. Lancet 1985;1:840–2.
12. Beaufils M, Uzan S, Donsimoni R, Colau JC. Prospective controlled study of early antiplatelet therapy in prevention of preeclampsia. Adv Nephrol 1986;15:87–94.
13. Wallenburg HCS, Rotmans N. Prevention of recurrent idiopathic fetal growth retardation by low-dose aspirin and dipyridamole. Am J Obstet Gynecol 1987;157:1230–5.
14. Uzan S, Beaufils M, Bazin B, Danays T. Idiopathic recurrent fetal growth retardation and aspirin-dipyridamole therapy. Am J Obstet Gynecol 1989;160: 763.
15. Wallenburg HCS, Rotmans N. Idiopathic recurrent fetal growth retardation and aspirin-dipyridamole therapy. Reply. Am J Obstet Gynecol 1989;160: 763–4.
16. Wallenburg HCS, Rotmans N. Prophylactic low-dose aspirin and dipyridamole in pregnancy. Lancet 1988;1:939.
17. Capetta P, Airoldi ML, Tasca A, Bertulessi C, Rossi E, Polvani F. Prevention of pre-eclampsia and placental insufficiency. Lancet 1986;1:919.
18. Romero R, Lockwood C, Oyarzun E, Hobbins JC. Toxemia: new concepts in an old disease. Semin Perinatol 1988;12:302–23.

Name: **DIRITHROMYCIN** Risk Factor: **C_M**

Class: **Antibiotic**

FETAL RISK SUMMARY

RECOMMENDATION: No Human Data - Animal Data Suggest Moderate Risk

Dirithromycin, a semi-synthetic antibiotic structurally related to erythromycin, belongs to the same macrolide class of anti-infectives as azithromycin, clarithromycin, erythromycin, and troleandomycin (the triacetyl ester of oleandomycin). Dirithromycin is a prodrug that is converted by nonenzymatic hydrolysis in the intestinal tract to the active form of the antibiotic, erythromycylamine.

No teratogenic effects were observed in the offspring of pregnant mice given a dose eight times the recommended maximum human dose based on body surface area (MRHD). A significant increase in the incidence of fetal growth retardation was observed at this dose, as well as an increased occurrence of incomplete ossification (a result of retarded development). Doses up to 21 and 4 times the MRHD in rats and rabbits, respectively, revealed no evidence of impaired fertility or fetal harm (1).

No reports describing the use of dirithromycin in human pregnancy have been located. The antibiotic was approved in 1995 by the FDA for use in the United States.

BREAST FEEDING SUMMARY

RECOMMENDATION: No Human Data - Probably Compatible

No reports describing the use dirithromycin during lactation have been located. The antibiotic is excreted into the milk of rodents (1). Because other antibiotics in this class appear in milk (e.g., see Erythromycin), the passage of dirithromycin into human milk should be expected. Based on experience with other antibiotics, including erythromycin, risk to a nursing infant from dirithromycin in breast milk is probably minimal but because there is no data, caution should be exercised until the effects, if any, of this exposure have been studied.

D

Reference

1. Product information. Dynabac. Sanofi Pharmaceutcials, 2000.

Name:	**DISOPYRAMIDE**	Risk Factor:	C_M
Class:	**Antiarrhythmic**		

FETAL RISK SUMMARY

RECOMMENDATION: Human Data Suggest Risk in 3rd Trimester

No reports linking the use of disopyramide with congenital defects in humans or animals have been located. Maternal toxicity (decreased food consumption and weight gain), embryotoxicity (decreased number of implantation sites), and fetotoxicity (decreased growth and pup survival) were observed in pregnant rats dosed at 250 mg/kg/day (20 or more times the recommended human dose of 12 mg/kg/day, assuming a patient weighing at least 50 kg [RHD]) (1). Increased resorption rates occurred in rabbits dosed at 60 mg/kg/day (5 or more times the RHD), but implantation rates, fetal growth, and offspring survival were not evaluated.

At term, a cord blood level of 0.9 μg/mL (39% of maternal serum) was measured 6 hours after a maternal 200-mg dose (2). A 27-year-old woman took disopyramide throughout a full-term gestation, 1350 mg/day for the last 16 days, and delivered a healthy, 2920-g female infant (2). Concentrations of disopyramide and the metabolite N-monodesalkyl disopyramide in the cord and maternal serum were 0.7 and 0.9 μg/mL, and 2.7 and 2.1 μg/mL, respectively. The cord:maternal ratios for the parent drug and metabolite were 0.26 and 0.43, respectively (3). In a separate study, the mean fetal:maternal total plasma ratio was 0.78 when the mother's plasma concentration was within the therapeutic range of 2.0–5.0 μg/mL (4).

Disopyramide has been used throughout other pregnancies without evidence of congenital abnormalities or growth retardation (2,5,6) (M. S. Anderson, personal communication, G. D. Searle and Company, 1981). Early onset of labor was reported in one patient (7). The mother, in her 32nd week of gestation, was given 300 mg orally, followed by 100 or 150 mg every 6 hours for posterior mitral leaflet prolapse. Uterine contractions, without vaginal bleeding or cervical changes, and abdominal pain occurred 1–2 hours after each dose. When disopyramide was stopped, symptoms subsided over the next 4 hours. Oxytocin induction 1 week later resulted in the delivery of a healthy infant. The oxytocic

D

effect of disopyramide was studied in 10 women at term (8). Eight of the 10 women, treated with 150 mg every 6 hours for 48 hours, delivered within 48 hours, compared to none in a placebo group. In one patient, use of 200 mg twice daily during the 18th and 19th weeks of pregnancy was not associated with uterine contractions or other observable adverse effects in the mother or fetus (9). Most reviews of antiarrhythmic drug therapy consider the drug probably safe during pregnancy (5,10), but one does not recommend it for routine therapy (11), and one warns of its oxytocic effects (12).

BREAST FEEDING SUMMARY

RECOMMENDATION: Limited Human Data - Probably Compatible

Disopyramide is excreted into breast milk (3,6,13,14). In a woman taking 200 mg 3 times daily, samples obtained on the 5th–8th days of treatment revealed a mean milk:plasma ratio of 0.9 for disopyramide and 5.6 for the active metabolite (13). Neither drug was detected in the infant's plasma. In a second case, a mother was taking 450 mg of disopyramide every 8 hours 2 weeks postpartum (3). Milk and serum samples were obtained at 0, 2, 4, and 8 hours after the dose following an overnight fast. Milk concentrations of disopyramide and its metabolite, N-monodesalkyl disopyramide, ranged from 2.6–4.4 μg/mL and from 9.6–12.3 μg/mL, respectively. In both cases, the lowest levels occurred at the 8-hour sampling time. The mean milk:plasma ratios for the two were 1.06 and 6.24, respectively. Disopyramide was not detected in the infant's serum (test sensitivity 0.45 μg/mL), but both disopyramide and the metabolite were found in the infant's urine, 3.3 and 3.7 μg/mL, respectively. A brief 1985 report described a woman taking 100 mg five times a day throughout pregnancy who delivered a normal female infant (6). On the 2nd postpartum day and 2 hours after a dose, paired milk and serum samples were obtained. The concentrations of disopyramide in the aqueous phase of the milk and the serum were 4.0 and 10.3 μmol/L, respectively, a milk:serum ratio of 0.4. The same ratio was obtained 2 weeks later with samples drawn 3 hours after a dose and levels of 5.0 and 11.5 μmol/L, respectively. No disopyramide was found in the infant's serum (limit of test accuracy 1.5 μmol/L) during the second sampling. A woman taking 200 mg twice daily had milk and serum samples drawn before and 3.5 hours after a dose (14). The concentrations in the serum were 3.7 and 5.5 μmol/L, and those in the milk were 1.7 and 2.9 μmol/L, respectively. The milk:serum ratios were 0.46 before and 0.53 after the dose. No adverse effects were noted in the nursing infants in any of the above cases. The American Academy of Pediatrics classifies disopyramide as compatible with breast-feeding (15).

References

1. Product information. Norpace. G. D. Searle and Company, 2000.
2. Shaxted EJ, Milton PJ. Disopyramide in pregnancy: a case report. Curr Med Res Opin 1979;6:70–2.
3. Ellsworth AJ, Horn JR, Raisys VA, Miyagawa LA, Bell JL. Disopyramide and N-monodesalkyl disopyramide in serum and breast milk. Drug Intell Clin Pharm 1989;23:56–7.
4. Echizen H, Nakura M, Saotome T, Minoura S, Ishizaki T. Plasma protein binding of disopyramide in pregnant and postpartum women, and in neonates and their mothers. Br J Clin Pharmacol 1990;29:423–30.
5. Rotmensch HH, Elkayam U, Frishman W. Antiarrhythmic drug therapy during pregnancy. Ann Intern Med 1983;98:487–97.
6. MacKintosh D, Buchanan N. Excretion of disopyramide in human breast milk. Br J Clin Pharmacol 1985;19:856–7.
7. Leonard RF, Braun TE, Levy AM. Initiation of uterine contractions by disopyramide during pregnancy. N Engl J Med 1978;299:84–5.
8. Tadmor OP, Keren A, Rosenak D, Gal M, Shaia M, Hornstein E, Yaffe H, Graff E, Stern S, Diamant YZ. The effect of disopyramide on uterine contractions during pregnancy. Am J Obstet Gynecol 1990;162:482–6.
9. Stokes IM, Evans J, Stone M. Myocardial infarction and cardiac arrest in the second trimester followed by assisted vaginal delivery under epidural analgesia at 38 weeks gestation. Case report. Br J Obstet Gynaecol 1984;91:197–8.

10. Tamari I, Eldar M, Rabinowitz B, Neufeld HN. Medical treatment of cardiovascular disorders during pregnancy. Am Heart J 1982;104:1357–63.
11. Rotmensch HH, Rotmensch S, Elkayam U. Management of cardiac arrhythmias during pregnancy: current concepts. Drugs 1987;33:623–33.
12. Ward RM. Maternal drug therapy for fetal disorders. Semin Perinatol 1992;16:12 20.
13. Barnett DB, Hudson SA, McBurney A. Disopyramide and its N-monodesalkyl metabolite in breast milk. Br J Clin Pharmacol 1982;14:310–2.
14. Hoppu K, Neuvonen PJ, Korte T. Disopyramide and breast feeding. Br J Clin Pharmacol 1986;21:553.
15. Committee on Drugs, American Academy of Pediatrics. The transfer of drugs and other chemicals into human milk. Pediatrics 2001;108:776–89.

Name:	DISULFIRAM	Risk Factor:	C
Class:	Miscellaneous		

FETAL RISK SUMMARY

RECOMMENDATION: Limited Human Data - No Relevant Animal Data

Disulfiram is used to prevent alcohol consumption in patients with a history of alcohol abuse. In animals, disulfiram is embryotoxic, possibly due to copper chelation, but it is not teratogenic (1).

No reports describing the placental transfer of disulfiram have been located. The molecular weight (about 297) is low enough that transfer to the fetus probably occurs.

Published reports describing the use of disulfiram in gestation involve 36 pregnancies (2–9). Eleven of the 38 exposed fetuses (two sets of twins) had congenital defects, 6 pregnancies were terminated electively, a spontaneous abortion occurred in 1 case, 1 was stillborn, 5 were lost to follow-up, and 14 newborns were normal. No congenital malformations were observed in autopsies conducted on three of the elective terminations (4). The malformations observed, some of which were or may have been related to alcohol exposure or other causes, were:

Clubfoot (two cases) (2)
Multiple anomalies with VACTERL syndrome (radial aplasia, vertebral fusion, tracheo-esophageal fistula) (twin) (3)
Phocomelia of lower extremities (one case) (3)
Microcephaly, mental retardation (possible fetal alcohol syndrome) (one case) (5)
Pierre-Robin sequence, pulmonary atresia (one case) (6)
Cleft soft palate, short palpebral fissure (twin) (8)
Limb reduction right forearm (radius and ulna), 2 rudimentary fingers without nails, short palpebral fissure (twin) (8)
Fetal alcohol syndrome (two cases; both mothers continued to drink) (9)
Fetal hydantoin syndrome (mother also took phenytoin) (one case) (9)

In a surveillance study of Michigan Medicaid recipients conducted between 1985 and 1992 involving 229,101 completed pregnancies, 25 newborns had been exposed to disulfiram during the 1st trimester (F. Rosa, personal communication, FDA, 1993). One (4.0%) major birth defect was observed (one expected), a cardiovascular defect.

In summary, the lack of teratogenicity in animals and the absence of a clustering of similar birth defects in human pregnancies exposed to disulfiram suggests that this drug is not a major human teratogen. Obviously, women taking disulfiram should not drink alcohol, but this is occasionally the case because of the findings of fetal alcohol syndrome and defects that are suggestive of fetal alcohol exposure.

BREAST FEEDING SUMMARY

RECOMMENDATION: No Human Data - Potential Toxicity

No reports describing the use of disulfiram during lactation have been located. Because of the relatively low molecular weight (about 297), excretion into milk should be expected. The potential effects of this exposure on a nursing infant are unknown.

D

References

1. Shepard TH. *Catalog of Teratogenic Agents*. 6th ed. Baltimore, MD: Johns Hopkins University Press, 1989:239–40.
2. Favre-Tissot M, Delatour P. Psychopharmacologie et teratogenese a propos du sulfirame: essal experimental. Annales Medico-psychogiques 1965;1:735–40. As cited in Shepard TH. *Catalog of Teratogenic Agents*. 6th ed. Baltimore, MD: Johns Hopkins University Press, 1989:239–40.
3. Nora AH, Nora JJ, Blu J. Limb-reduction anomalies in infants born to disulfiram-treated alcoholic mothers. Lancet 1977;2:664.
4. Hamon B, Soyez C, Jonville AP, Autret E. Grossesse chez les malades traitées par le disulfirame. Presse Med 1991;20:1092.
5. Gardner RJM, Clarkson JE. A malformed child whose previously alcoholic mother had taken disultiram. N Z Med J 1981;93:184–6. As cited in Reitnauer PJ, Callanan NP, Farber RA, Aylsworth AS. Prenatal exposure to disulfiram implicated in the cause of malformations in discordant monozygotic twins. Teratology 1997;56:358–62.
6. Dehaene P, Titran M, Dubois D. Syndrome de Pierre Robin et malformations cardiaques chez un nouveaune. Presse Med 1984;13:1394–5. As cited in Reitnauer PJ, Callanan NP, Farber RA, Aylsworth AS. Prenatal exposure to disulfiram implicated in the cause of malformations in discordant monozygotic twins. Teratology 1997;56:358–62.
7. Helmbrecht GD, Hoskins IA. First trimester disulfiram exposure: report of two cases. Am J Perinatol 1993;10:5–7.
8. Reitnauer PJ, Callanan NP, Farber RA, Aylsworth AS. Prenatal exposure to disulfiram implicated in the cause of malformations in discordant monozygotic twins. Teratology 1997;56:358–62.
9. Johnson KA, Jones KL, Chambers CC, Hames C, Emery M. The effect of disulfiram on the unborn baby (abstract). Teratology 1991;43:438.

Name:	**DOBUTAMINE**	Risk Factor:	B_M
Class:	**Sympathomimetic (Adrenergic)**		

FETAL RISK SUMMARY

RECOMMENDATION: Limited Human Data - Animal Data Suggest Low Risk

Dobutamine, an inotropic agent, is structurally related to dopamine. Reproduction studies in rats (at doses up to the normal human dose of 10 μg/kg/min for 24 hours for a total daily dose of 14.4 mg/kg [NHD]) and rabbits (at doses up to twice the NHD) did not reveal any evidence of fetal harm (1).

No reports describing the placental transfer of dobutamine or studying its effects during human pregnancy have been located (see also Dopamine). The relatively low molecular weight (about 301), however, probably indicates that transfer to the fetus occurs. Short-term use in one patient with a myocardial infarction at 18 weeks' gestation was not associated with any known adverse effects (2).

BREAST FEEDING SUMMARY

RECOMMENDATION: No Human Data - Probably Compatible

No data are available.

References

1. Product information. Dobutrex. Eli Lilly and Company, 2000.
2. Stokes IM, Evans J, Stone M. Myocardial infarction and cardiac arrest in the second trimester followed by assisted vaginal delivery under epidural analgesia at 38 weeks' gestation. Case report. Br J Obstet Gynaecol 1984;91:197–8.

D

Name:	**DOCUSATE CALCIUM**	Risk Factor:	**C**
Class:	**Laxative**		

See Docusate Sodium.

Name:	**DOCUSATE POTASSIUM**	Risk Factor:	**C**
Class:	**Laxative**		

See Docusate Sodium.

Name:	**DOCUSATE SODIUM**	Risk Factor:	**C**
Class:	**Laxative**		

FETAL RISK SUMMARY

RECOMMENDATION: Compatible

No reports linking the use of docusate sodium (DSS) with congenital defects have been located. DSS is a common ingredient in many laxative preparations available to the public. In a large prospective study, 116 patients were exposed to this drug during pregnancy (1). No evidence for an association with malformations was found. Similarly, no evidence of fetal toxicity was noted in 35 women treated with a combination of docusate sodium and dihydroxyanthraquinone (2).

In a surveillance study of Michigan Medicaid recipients conducted between 1985 and 1992 involving 229,101 completed pregnancies, 232 newborns had been exposed to a docusate salt during the 1st trimester (F. Rosa, personal communication, FDA, 1993). Nine (3.9%) major birth defects were observed (nine expected), including one cardiovascular defect (two expected) and one polydactyly (one expected). No anomalies were observed in four other categories of defects (oral clefts, spina bifida, limb reduction defects, and hypospadias) for which specific data were available. These data do not support an association between the drug and congenital defects.

Chronic use of 150–250 mg/day or more of docusate sodium throughout pregnancy was suspected of causing hypomagnesemia in a mother and her newborn (3). At 12 hours of age, the neonate exhibited jitteriness, which resolved spontaneously. Neonatal serum magnesium levels ranged from 0.9–1.1 mg/dL between 22 and 48 hours of age with a maternal level of 1.2 mg/dL on the 3rd postpartum day. All other laboratory parameters were normal.

BREAST FEEDING SUMMARY

RECOMMENDATION: Compatible

A combination of docusate sodium and dihydroxyanthraquinone (Normax) was given to 35 postpartum women in a 1973 study (2). One infant developed diarrhea, but the relationship between the symptom and the laxative is unknown.

D

References

1. Heinonen OP, Slone D, Shapiro S. *Birth Defects and Drugs in Pregnancy*. Littleton, MA: Publishing Sciences Group, 1977:442.
2. Greenhalf JO, Leonard HSD. Laxatives in the treatment of constipation in pregnant and breast-feeding mothers. Practitioner 1973;210:259–63.
3. Schindler AM. Isolated neonatal hypomagnesaemia associated with maternal overuse of stool softener. Lancet 1984;2:822.

Name:	**DOFETILIDE**	Risk Factor:	C_M
Class:	**Antiarrhythmic**		

FETAL RISK SUMMARY

RECOMMENDATION: No Human Data - Animal Data Suggest Risk

Dofetilide is an antiarrhythmic agent with Class III (cardiac action potential duration prolongation) properties that is indicated for the maintenance of normal sinus rhythm in patients with atrial fibrillation/flutter. Only about 20% of the drug is metabolized.

In reproduction studies in mice and rats, oral doses of dofetilide equal to or greater than 4 and 2 times, respectively, the maximum likely human exposure (based on the 24-hour area under the plasma concentration curve) (MHE), caused sternebral and vertebral anomalies in both species (1). In addition, an increased incidence of unossified calcaneum was noted in mice. In rats given doses approximately equal to the MHE, an increased incidence of unossified metacarpal and the occurrence of hydroureter and hydronephroses were observed. When the dose was doubled (2 times the MHE) in rats, additional defects noted were cleft palate, adactyly, levocardia, and dilation of cerebral ventricles. The no effect adverse effect dose in mice was approximately equal to the MHE, whereas in rats it was about one-half the MHE (1).

Dofetilide had no effect on mating and fertility in rats at doses up to 3 times the MHE (1). It was also not mutagenic in *in vitro* and *in vivo* tests, nor was it carcinogenic in tests with mice and rats. Chronic administration of dofetilide did cause testicular atrophy, decreased testicular weight, and/or epididymal oligospermia in mice, rats, and dogs at doses greater than 3, 4, and 1.3 times, respectively, the MHE (1).

In a 1996 study, the embryo toxicity and teratogenicity of dofetilide in rats were shown to be gestational-age related and resulted from dose-dependent bradycardia in *in vitro* (rat embryo culture) and *in vivo* (pregnant rat) experiments (2). In the embryo cultures, the minimum effective concentration for significant bradycardia (22 ng/mL) was about 6 times the human peak plasma concentration achieved after an oral dose of 12 μg/kg (3.5 ng/mL) (2). An embryo culture dose twice the minimum effective dose caused an almost complete cessation of the heart beat. In pregnant rats, single oral doses of various concentrations were given on different gestational days. On gestational day (GD) 10, a high incidence of resorptions occurred, but no malformations except one fetus with a short tail. Defects and/or toxicity seen on other days included GD 11 (right-sided cleft lip), GD 12 (small number of defects; 100% lethality at highest dose), and GD 13 (most sensitive day; hind limb defects; resorptions at higher doses). The defects were preceded by hemorrhage, but the investigators could not determine if the hemorrhage caused the defect or if the hemorrhage and defect were caused by the bradycardia-induced hypoxia (2).

D

It is not known if dofetilide crosses the human placenta. The molecular weight (about 442) is low enough that transfer to the fetus should be expected.

No reports describing the use of dofetilide during human pregnancy have been located. Although the antiarrhythmic is teratogenic and toxic in animals at exposures slightly above those expected in humans, the lack of human data prevents an assessment of the potential embryo/fetal risk. However, if dofetilide therapy is required in a pregnant woman, the benefits appear to outweigh the unknown risk.

BREAST FEEDING SUMMARY

RECOMMENDATION: No Human Data - Potential Toxicity

No reports describing the use of dofetilide in human lactation have been located. The molecular weight (about 442) is low enough that excretion in breast milk should be expected. The effects of this exposure on a nursing infant are unknown. Until the pharmacokinetics of dofetilide in milk have been determined, and until the effects on a nursing infant from exposure to the drug in milk have been clarified, women receiving this agent should probably not breast-feed.

References

1. Product information. Tikosyn. Pfizer, 2001.
2. Webster WS, Brown-Woodman PDC, Snow MD, Danielsson BRG. Teratogenic potential of almokalant, dofetilide, and d-sotalol: drugs with potassium channel blocking activity. Teratology 1996;53:168–75.

Name:	**DOLASETRON**	Risk Factor:	B_M
Class:	**Antiemetic**		

FETAL RISK SUMMARY

RECOMMENDATION: No Human Data - Animal Data Suggest Low Risk

Dolasetron is a specific and selective serotonin subtype 3 (5-HT_3) receptor antagonist that is used for the treatment and prevention of nausea and vomiting in the postoperative period and after chemotherapy. The drug has no effect on plasma prolactin levels (1).

Dolasetron had no effect on fertility and reproductive performance in female rats at doses up to 8 times the recommended human dose based on body surface area (RHD) or in male rats at doses up to 32 times the RHD. No evidence of impaired fertility or fetal harm was observed in pregnant rats and rabbits at oral doses up to 8 and 16 times, respectively, the RHD (1). In 24-month carcinogenicity studies there was a dose-related significant increase in combined hepatocellular adenomas and carcinomas in male mice, but not in female mice or in male and female rats. No mutagenicity was observed in various tests (1).

It is not known if dolasetron crosses the human placenta. The molecular weight of the free base (about 325) is low enough that transfer to the fetus should be expected.

No reports describing the use of dolasetron during human pregnancy have been located. Among other agents with similar mechanisms of actions and indications (see Granisetron and Ondansetron), only ondansetron has published human pregnancy experience. Based on this experience and the lack of embryo/fetal toxicity in two animal species, dolasetron appears to represent a minimal, if any, risk to a human fetus.

BREAST FEEDING SUMMARY

RECOMMENDATION: No Human Data - Probably Compatible

No reports describing the use of dolasetron in human lactation have been located. The molecular weight (about 325 for the free base) is low enough that excretion into breast milk should be expected. The effects on a nursing infant are unknown.

Reference

1. Product information. Anzemet. Aventis Pharmaceuticals, 2001.

Name:	**DOMPERIDONE**	Risk Factor:	**C**
Class:	**Antiemetic/Gastrointestinal Stimulant**		

FETAL RISK SUMMARY

RECOMMENDATION: No Human Data - Animal Data Suggest Risk

Domperidone is a dopamine antagonist that is used for the short-term treatment of nausea and vomiting and for its prokinetic activity in disorders of gastrointestinal motility (e.g., diabetic gastroparesis). It also has been used to stimulate milk production. The actions of domperidone are similar to metoclopramide. The bioavailability after oral administration is low, about 15% with fasting conditions, higher when taken with food. It undergoes extensive first-pass metabolism by the liver and more than 90% of the drug reaching the systemic circulation is bound to plasma proteins. The elimination half-life is about 7.5 hours (1).

Shepard reviewed a 1980 study on the effects of domperidone in mice, rats, and rabbits (2). Oral doses of 1 mg/kg decreased the percent of successful matings. *(Note: The recommended human oral dose is 10–20 mg every 4–8 hours.)* During organogenesis, an oral dose of 70 mg/kg was maternally toxic (reduced body weight) and reduced fetal survival and teratogenicity (displacement of the subclavian artery, skeletal and eye defects) occurred at 200 mg/kg. The only postnatal effect noted was retarded genital development with doses greater than 70 mg/kg. Dosing by the IV or IP routes caused impaired fertility (0.2 mg/kg), and growth retardation and skeletal defects (15–30 mg/kg) but, in rabbits, only reduced fetal survival was noted (2).

It is not known if domperidone crosses the human placenta. The drug does not readily cross the blood-brain barrier (1). However, the molecular weight (about 426), availability of unbound drug, and prolonged elimination half-life suggest that some drug will cross to the embryo/fetus.

Neither the oral nor the injectable formulations of domperidone are available in the United States. The agent is available in other countries, but the parenteral formulation was withdrawn from the market in the United Kingdom because of serious toxicity secondary to high-dose IV domperidone (ventricular arrhythmias, cardiac arrest, sudden death) (1). Other reported toxicities associated with domperidone are gynecomastia, galactorrhea, mastalgia, extrapyramidal reactions, and seizures.

D

No reports describing the use of domperidone in human pregnancy have been located. The combination of limited animal data and absence of human pregnancy experience prevents an assessment of the embryo/fetal risk. However, severe dose-related toxicity has been reported in adults and the drug is not approved by the Food and Drug Administration for use in the United States. The use of safer agents during pregnancy is advised.

BREAST FEEDING SUMMARY

RECOMMENDATION: Limited Human Data - Probably Compatible

Consistent with the molecular weight (about 426), availability of unbound drug, and prolonged elimination half-life, small amounts of domperidone are excreted into breast milk. Excretion is probably limited by the extensive first-pass hepatic metabolism.

Domperidone has been used to stimulate breast milk production because of its action to increase prolactin levels (3–6). Two women that were not breast-feeding were given domperidone 10 mg every 8 hours for 4 days. Maternal serum samples ($N = 5$) were drawn 1.75–3 hours after a dose and milk samples ($N = 30$) were collected four times a day (timing in relationship to the doses not stated) (3). The mean serum and milk levels were 10 and 2.6 ng/mL, respectively, a milk:serum ratio of 0.25. The investigators repeated the study with a single 20-mg dose (4). Serum and milk levels 2 hours after the dose were 8.0 and 0.24 ng/mL, respectively, a milk:serum ratio of 0.03. The milk level rose to 1.1 ng/mL at 4 hours (4). In both studies, milk samples were obtained by manual expression. Moreover, the increasing milk concentration indicates that the level had not yet reached steady state.

A 1985 double-blind study described the effects of domperidone in two groups of postpartum women with defective lactogenesis: eight subjects—10 mg three times daily for 3 days; nine subjects—10 mg three times daily for 10 days (5). Both study groups had a significant increase in daily milk yield compared to women given placebos. No adverse effects were noted in the subjects or controls or their infants (5).

In a 2001 randomized, double-blind, placebo-controlled study, women with insufficient milk production to meet the daily oral feeding requirements of their premature infants were either given domperidone (10 mg three times daily) or placebo for 7 days (6). Four domperidone subjects were excluded (three with inadequate records or no milk samples and one infant death shortly after enrollment). The mean gestational age at delivery was 29.1 weeks in both groups. After collection by a mechanical pump, the milk was fed to the infants through a nasogastric tube. The mean daily milk production in the subjects (112.8 mL) was much higher than controls (48.2 mL). Compared to the baseline, the mean increase in daily milk production was significantly higher in the domperidone group (49.5 vs. 8.0 mL). Maternal serum and milk samples for drug analysis were obtained on day 5. The mean milk:serum ratio was 0.4. The investigators estimated that the amount of drug ingested by an infant was 0.2 μg/kg/day, a clinically insignificant amount. No adverse effects were noted in the infants (6).

In summary, domperidone increases daily milk production in lactating women with insufficient milk production. Small amounts of domperidone are excreted into breast milk, but no adverse effects in nursing infants have been reported. The American Academy of Pediatrics classifies the drug as compatible with breast-feeding (7). However, because of the potential for serious toxicity in the mother, safer alternatives are advised.

D

References

1. Parfitt K, editor. *Martindale. The Complete Drug Reference*. 32nd ed. London, UK: Pharmaceutical Press, 1999:1190–1.
2. Hara T, Nishikawa S, Miyazaki E, Ogura T. Toxicologic studies on KW-5338 reproductive studies. Yakuri to Chiryo 1980;8:4045–60. As cited by Shepard TH. *Catalog of Teratogenic Agents*. 10th ed. Baltimore: The Johns Hopkins University Press, 2001:184–5.
3. Hofmeyr GJ, Van Iddekinge. Domperidone and lactation. Lancet 1983;1:647.
4. Hofmeyr GJ, Van Iddekinge B, Blott JA. Domperidone: secretion in breast milk and effect on puerperal prolactin levels. Br J Obstet Gyaencol 1985;92:141–4.
5. Petraglia F, De Leo V, Sardelli S, Pieroni ML, D'Antona N, Genazzani AR. Domperidone in defective and insufficient lactation. Eur J Obstet Gynecol Reprod Biol 1985;19:281–7.
6. da Silva OP, Knoppert DC, Angelini MM, Forret PA. Effect of domperidone on milk production in mothers of premature newborns: a randomized, double-blind, placebo-controlled trial. CMAJ 2001;164: 17–21.
7. Committee on Drugs, American Academy of Pediatrics. The transfer of drugs and other chemicals into human milk. Pediatrics 2001;108:776–89.

Name:	**DONEPEZIL**	Risk Factor:	**C_M**
Class:	**Cholinesterase Inhibitor (CNS Agent)**		

FETAL RISK SUMMARY

RECOMMENDATION: No Human Data - Animal Data Suggest Low Risk

Donepezil (known previously as E2020) is a reversible cholinesterase inhibitor that is indicated for the treatment of mild to moderate dementia of the Alzheimer's type. Two metabolites of donepezil are known to be active. The drug is extensively protein bound (about 96%) in the plasma, primarily to albumin (about 75%) and α_1-acid glycoprotein. The plasma elimination half-life is about 70 hours (1,2).

Reproduction studies have been conducted in rats and rabbits. In rats, doses up to about 13 times the maximum recommended human dose based on body surface area (MRHD) were not teratogenic. At 8 times the MRHD given from gestational day 17 through postpartum day 20, there was a slight increase in stillbirths and a slight decrease in pup survival through postpartum day 4. Donepezil had no effect on rat fertility at doses up to about 8 times the MRHD. In rabbits, no teratogenic effects were observed at a dose 16 times the MRHD (1,2).

It is not known if donepezil or its active metabolites cross the human placenta. The molecular weight of the parent compound (about 416) and its long plasma elimination half-life suggest that the drug will cross to the embryo/fetus, but the extensive protein binding will limit this transfer.

No reports describing the use of donepezil in human pregnancy have been located. Because of its indication, such reports should be rare. Moreover, the animal data suggest that the risk to the embryo and/or fetus is low. Therefore, inadvertent exposure to donepezil during pregnancy should not be a reason for pregnancy termination.

BREAST FEEDING SUMMARY

RECOMMENDATION: No Human Data - Potential Toxicity

No reports describing the use of donepezil during human lactation have been located. Because of its indication, such reports should be rare. Donepezil has two active metabolites. The molecular weight of the parent compound (about 416) and its long plasma elimination half-life (about 70 hours) suggest that donepezil, and possible the active metabolites, will be excreted into breast milk. The extensive protein binding (about 96%), however, should limit this excretion. The effects of this exposure on a nursing infant are unknown.

References

1. Product information. Aricept. Eisai, 2004.
2. Product information. Aricept. Pfizer, 2004.

Name:	**DOPAMINE**	Risk Factor:	**C**
Class:	**Sympathomimetic (Adrenergic)**		

FETAL RISK SUMMARY

RECOMMENDATION: Compatible - Maternal Benefit >> Embryo/Fetal Risk

Experience with dopamine in human pregnancy is limited. Because dopamine is indicated only for life-threatening situations, chronic use would not be expected. Animal studies have shown both increases and decreases in uterine blood flow (1,2). In a study in pregnant baboons, dopamine infusion increased uterine vascular resistance and thus impaired uteroplacental perfusion (1). Because of this effect, the investigators concluded that the drug should not be used in patients with severe preeclampsia or eclampsia (1). However, although human studies on uterine perfusion have not been conducted, the use in women with severe toxemia has not been associated with fetal harm. The drug has been used to prevent renal failure in nine oliguric or anuric eclamptic patients by re-establishing diuresis (3). In another study of six women with severe preeclampsia and oliguria, low-dose dopamine (1–5 μg/kg/minute) infusion produced a significant rise in urine and cardiac output (4). No significant changes in blood pressure, central venous pressure, or pulmonary capillary wedge pressure occurred. Dopamine has also been used to treat hypotension in 26 patients undergoing cesarean section (2). No adverse effects attributable to dopamine were observed in the fetuses or newborns of the mothers in these studies.

BREAST FEEDING SUMMARY

RECOMMENDATION: No Human Data - Probably Compatible

No data are available.

References

1. Fishburne JI Jr, Dormer KJ, Payne GG, Gill PS, Ashrafzadeh AR, Rossavik IK. Effects of amrinone and dopamine on uterine blood flow and vascular responses in the gravid baboon. Am J Obstet Gynecol 1988;158:829–37.
2. Clark RB, Brunner JA III. Dopamine for the treatment of spinal hypotension during cesarean section. Anesthesiology 1980;53:514–7.
3. Gerstner G, Grunberger W. Dopamine treatment for prevention of renal failure in patients with

severe eclampsia. Clin Exp Obstet Gynecol 1980;7:219–22.
4. Kirshon B, Lee W, Mauer MB, Cotton DB. Effects of low-dose dopamine therapy in the oliguric patient with preeclampsia. Am J Obstet Gynecol 1988;159:604–7.

D

Name:	**DOTHIEPIN**	Risk Factor:	**C**
Class:	**Antidepressant**		

FETAL RISK SUMMARY

RECOMMENDATION: Limited Human Data - No Relevant Animal Data

Dothiepin is a tricyclic antidepressant (not available in the United States). The drug is metabolized to an active metabolite desmethyldothiepin (also known as northiaden) (1). Dothiepin has a molecular weight of about 296 (free base) and probably crosses the placenta to the embryo/fetus.

In a 1996 descriptive case series, the European Network of the Teratology Information Services (ENTIS) prospectively examined the outcomes of 689 pregnancies exposed to antidepressants (2). Multiple drug therapy occurred in about two-thirds of the mothers. Dothiepin was used in nine pregnancies (one set of twins) with the following outcomes: three elective abortions, six normal newborns (one premature), and one infant with a congenital defect. In the pregnancy with twins exposed to dothiepin in the first 6 weeks, one twin was normal and one had defects (esophageal atresia with tracheoesophageal fistula) (2).

BREAST FEEDING SUMMARY

RECOMMENDATION: Limited Human Data - Potential Toxicity

Dothiepin is excreted into breast milk (3,4). In one patient treated with dothiepin, 25 mg three times a day for 3 months, milk and maternal serum concentrations 3 hours after the second dose of the day were 11 and 33 ng/mL (ratio 0.33), respectively (3). A second woman, treated intermittently over a 6-day period with a total dose of 300 mg, had a milk level of 10 ng/mL. Effects of this exposure in the nursing infants were not mentioned (3).

Milk concentrations of dothiepin and three metabolites were measured in eight postpartum women being treated for depression with dothiepin, 25–225 mg/day (4). Some of the women had apparently taken the drug during pregnancy but details of the treatment and pregnancy outcome were not given. The ages of the nursing infants ranged from 0.13 to 12.5 months. Milk samples were collected from the women just before and immediately after breast-feeding. Plasma samples were collected at periods ranging from 2.8 to 15.8 hours after a dose. The mean milk:plasma ratios before feeding for dothiepin, nordothiepin, dothiepin-S-oxide, and nordothiepin-S-oxide were 0.78, 0.85, 1.18, and 1.86, respectively. The milk:plasma ratios for the metabolites in the post-feed samples were similar to those before feeding, but dothiepin was significantly higher (1.59; $p < 0.05$). The authors calculated that a nursing infant would ingest approximately 0.58% of the mother's daily dothiepin dose and amounts varying from 0.23% to 2.47% of the metabolites. No adverse effects were observed in the infants (4).

A 1995 study found no difference in either cognitive scores or, after adjustment, in child behavior in children 3–5 years of age who had been exposed to dothiepin ($N = 15$) during breast-feeding compared to nonexposed infants of depressed mothers and normal controls (5). Milk levels of the parent drug and its metabolite northiaden were 0–138 ng/mL and 0–88 ng/mL, respectively.

A 1996 review of antidepressant treatment during breast-feeding found no information that dothiepin exposure during nursing resulted in quantifiable amounts in the infant or that the exposure caused adverse effects (6).

Ten nursing infants taking antidepressants during breast-feeding (two with dothiepin 50–225 mg/day) were compared to 15 bottle-fed infants of mothers with depression who did not breast-feed (7). Concentrations of dothiepin in fore- and hind-milk ranged from 54–988 ng/mL and 121–1250 ng/mL, respectively. The milk:maternal plasma ratios were 1.2–2.7 and 1.8–4.5, respectively. One infant had a plasma level of 4.1 ng/mL when the mother was taking 225 mg/day. No toxic effects or delays in development were observed in the infants. The estimated daily dose consumed by the infants was about 1% of the mother's weight-adjusted dose (7).

The American Academy of Pediatrics classifies dothiepin as an agent whose effect on the nursing infant is unknown but may be of concern, especially if therapy is prolonged (8).

References

1. Parfitt K, Editor. *Martindale. The Complete Drug Reference*. 32nd ed. London, UK: Pharmaceutical Press, 1999:283.
2. McElhatton PR, Garbis HM, Elefant E, Vial T, Bellemin B, Mastroiacovo P, Arnon J, Rodriguez-Pinilla E, Schaefer C, Pexieder T, Merlob P, Dal Verme S. The outcome of pregnancy in 689 women exposed to therapeutic doses of antidepressants. A collaborative study of the European Network of Teratology Information Services (ENTIS). Reprod Toxicol 1996;10:285–94.
3. Rees JA, Glass RC, Sporne GA. Serum and breast milk concentrations of dothiepin. Practitioner 1976;217:686.
4. Ilett KF, Lebedevs TH, Wojnar-Horton RE, Yapp P, Roberts MJ, Dusci LJ, Hackett LP. The excretion of dothiepin and its primary metabolites in breast milk. Br J Clin Pharmacol 1992;33:635–9.
5. Buist A, Janson H. Effect of exposure to dothiepin and northiaden in breast milk on child development. Br J Psychiatry 1995;167:370–3.
6. Wisner KL, Perel JM, Findling RL. Antidepressant treatment during breast-feeding. Am J Psychiatry 1996;153:1132–7.
7. Yoshida K, Smith B, Craggs M, Kumar RC. Investigation of pharmacokinetics and of possible adverse effects in infants exposed to tricyclic antidepressants in breast-milk. J Affect Disord 1997;43:225–37.
8. Committee on Drugs, American Academy of Pediatrics. The transfer of drugs and other chemicals into human milk. Pediatrics 2001;108:776–89.

Name:	**DOXAPRAM**	Risk Factor:	B_M
Class:	**Central Stimulant**		

FETAL RISK SUMMARY

RECOMMENDATION: No Human Data - Animal Data Suggest Low Risk

Doxapram is a short-acting respiratory stimulant. It is administered IV to stimulate respiration in acute situations such as postanesthesia, mild to moderate respiratory and central nervous system depression as a consequence of drug overdosage, and hypercapnia in patients with chronic obstructive pulmonary disease. The duration of effect varies from 5–12 minutes (1). Doxapram is extensively metabolized by the liver after IV injection (2).

Reproduction studies have been conducted in mice and rats. In rats, doses up to 1.6 times the human dose revealed no evidence of impaired fertility or fetal harm. The dose, assumed to be based on weight, was given by the IM and oral routes, but the human dose (either a single dose of 1–2 mg/kg, or an IV infusion of 1–3 mg/kg/hr) are given IV (1).

D

In another study, no teratogenicity was observed in rats (3). In pregnant mice, a dose of 144 mg/kg/day was given intraperitoneal during organogenesis (4). No gross defects were observed, but fetal death and growth retardation were noted. In addition, minor skeletal defects occurred in the fetuses of one pregnancy (4).

Doxapram crosses the sheep placenta and stimulates fetal breathing (5). Doxapram was infused into a maternal vein over 2–5 minutes and peak fetal plasma levels occurred between 0.08 and 0.17 hours after the start of the infusion. The increase in fetal breathing, up to about 41% during the infusion, was dose-related (5).

It is not known if doxapram crosses the human placenta. The drug does cross the placenta in dogs (1) and sheep (5). The molecular weight of the free base (about 379) is low enough for transfer, but the very short duration of action suggests that limited amounts will be available at the maternal:fetal interface after single injections. However, continuous infusions of doxapram probably allows for placental passage to the embryo/fetus.

In an *in vitro* study, doxapram was shown to undergo substantial metabolism by the human fetal liver (6). The fetal livers were obtained from elective abortions conducted at 10–20 weeks' gestation.

No reports describing the use of doxapram in human pregnancy have been located. The animal data are limited but do not suggest a major risk for the embryo and/or fetus. Moreover, although the elimination half-life of the drug is unknown, the duration of effect is very short and the agent is extensively metabolized. Thus, the embryo and/or fetal exposure are probably limited except when continuous infusions are administered. The commercial product contains 0.9% benzyl alcohol as a preservative. Because benzyl alcohol can cross the placenta, the use of doxapram near term, especially continuous infusions, should be avoided because of the potential for toxicity in the newborn. However, if indicated, the maternal benefit from single injections of doxapram at any time in pregnancy appears to outweigh the unknown embryo/fetal risk.

BREAST FEEDING SUMMARY

RECOMMENDATION: No Human Data - Potential Toxicity

No reports describing the use of doxapram during human lactation have been located. In addition, the indications for the drug suggest that such reports will be rare. However, doxapram has been given to newborns at risk for respiratory depression when narcotic analgesics or general anesthetics were used during delivery (7). No adverse effects attributable to doxapram were observed. The molecular weight of the free base (about 379) suggests that the drug will be excreted into breast milk. The maternal plasma elimination half-life is unknown, but the relatively short duration of effect combined with the extensive hepatic metabolism, probably indicates a short half-life, at least for the parent compound. Of note, though, doxapram is a basic drug and accumulation in the relatively acidic breast milk by ion trapping is a potential concern, especially if continuous infusions are used. An additional concern involves benzyl alcohol, the preservative used in the commercial preparation that is known to be toxic in newborns.

References

1. Product information. A. H. Robins, 1986.
2. Parfitt K, Editor. *Martindale. The Complete Drug Reference*. 32nd ed. London, UK: Pharmaceutical Press, 1999:1480.
3. Imai K. Effect of Doxapram hydrochloride administered to pregnant rats on pre- and post-natal development of their offspring. Oyo Yakuri 1974;8:237–43. As cited by Shepard TH. *Catalog of Teratogenic Agents*. 10th ed. Baltimore: The Johns Hopkins University Press, 2001:186.

4. Imai K. Effect of Doxapram hydrochloride administered to pregnant mice on pre- and post-natal development of their offspring. Oyo Yakuri 1974;8:229–36. As cited by Shepard TH. *Catalog of Teratogenic Agents*. 10th ed. Baltimore: The Johns Hopkins University Press, 2001:186.
5. Hogg MIJ, Golding RH, Rosen M. The effect of doxapram on fetal breathing in the sheep. Br J Obstet Gynaecol 1977;84:48–50.
6. Bairam A, Branchaud C, Beharry K, Rex J, Laudignon N, Papageorgiou A, Aranda JV. Doxapram metabolism in human fetal hepatic organ culture. Clin Pharmacol Ther 1991;50:32–8.
7. Gupta PK, Moore J. The use of doxapram in the newborn. J Obstet Gynaecol Br Commonw 1973;80:1002–6.

D

Name: **DOXAZOSIN** Risk Factor: C_M
Class: **Sympatholytic (Antiadrenergic)**

FETAL RISK SUMMARY

RECOMMENDATION: No Human Data - Animal Data Suggest Low Risk

Doxazosin is a peripherally acting α_1-adrenergic blocking agent used in the treatment of hypertension. No adverse fetal effects were observed when pregnant rats and rabbits were given oral doses 4 and 10 times the human serum levels achieved with a 12 mg/day therapeutic dose (HD), respectively (1). However, reduced fetal survival occurred in rabbits dosed at 20 times the HD and delayed postnatal development was observed in rat pups whose mothers were given doses 8 times the HD during the perinatal and postnatal periods (1). Doxazosin crosses the placenta in rats (1).

No reports describing the use of doxazosin in human pregnancy have been located.

BREAST FEEDING SUMMARY

RECOMMENDATION: No Human Data - Potential Toxicity

Doxazosin is concentrated in the milk of lactating rats given a single oral dose of 1 mg/kg with peak levels about 20 times those achieved in the maternal serum (1). No reports describing the use of doxazosin during human lactation have been located. However, the presence and possible accumulation in human milk should be anticipated based on the animal study.

Reference

1. Product information. Cardura. Pfizer, 2000.

Name: **DOXEPIN** Risk Factor: **C**
Class: **Antidepressant**

FETAL RISK SUMMARY

RECOMMENDATION: Human Data Suggest Low Risk

Doxepin is a tricyclic antidepressant in the same class as amitriptyline, clomipramine, imipramine, and trimipramine. It was not teratogenic in rats, rabbits, monkeys, and dogs

D

(1–3). At the highest doses used, however, an increase in neonatal death was observed in rats and rabbits (1,2).

No published reports linking the use of doxepin with human congenital malformations have been located. Because of the relatively low molecular weight (316 for the hydrochloride salt), placental transfer of the drug to the fetus should be expected.

In a surveillance study of Michigan Medicaid recipients conducted between 1985 and 1992 involving 229,101 completed pregnancies, 118 newborns had been exposed to doxepin during the 1st trimester (F. Rosa, personal communication, FDA, 1993). A total of 12 (10.2%) major birth defects were observed (4.5 expected), including (observed/expected) cardiovascular defects (2/1), oral clefts (2/0.2), and polydactyly (2/0.3). No anomalies were observed in three other categories of malformations (spina bifida, limb reduction defects, and hypospadias) for which specific data were available. The total number of major birth defects and the cases of polydactyly are suggestive of an association, but other factors, including concurrent drug use and chance may be involved.

In a 1996 descriptive case series, the European Network of the Teratology Information Services (ENTIS) prospectively examined the outcomes of 689 pregnancies exposed to antidepressants (4). Multiple drug therapy occurred in about two-thirds of the mothers. Doxepin was used in 14 pregnancies. The outcomes of these pregnancies were four elective abortions, one spontaneous abortion, one stillbirth, and eight normal newborns.

Paralytic ileus has been observed in an infant exposed to doxepin at term (5). The condition was thought to be due primarily to chlorpromazine, but the authors speculated that the anticholinergic effects of doxepin worked synergistically with the phenothiazine.

A 2002 prospective study compared two groups of mother-child pairs exposed to antidepressants throughout gestation (46 exposed to tricyclics—2 to doxepin; 40 to fluoxetine) to 36 nonexposed, not depressed controls (6). Offspring were studied between the ages of 15 and 71 months for effects of antidepressant exposure in terms of IQ, language, behavior, and temperament. Exposure to antidepressants did not adversely affect the measured parameters, but IQ was significantly and negatively associated with the duration of depression, and language was negatively associated with the number of depression episodes after delivery (6).

BREAST FEEDING SUMMARY

RECOMMENDATION: Limited Human Data - Potential Toxicity

Doxepin and its active metabolite, N-desmethyldoxepin, are excreted into breast milk (7–9). A 36-year-old woman was treated with doxepin, 10 mg daily, for approximately 5 weeks starting 2 weeks after the birth of her daughter (7). The dose was increased to 25 mg three times daily 4 days before the wholly breast-fed 8-week-old infant was found pale, limp, and near respiratory arrest. Although drowsiness and shallow respirations continued on admission to the hospital, the baby made a rapid recovery and was normal in 24 hours. A peak milk concentration of doxepin, 29 ng/mL, was measured 4–5 hours after a dose, while two levels obtained just prior to a dose (12 hours after the last dose in each case) were 7 and 10 ng/mL, respectively. Milk concentrations of the metabolite ranged from "not detectable" (lower limit of detection 7 ng/mL) to 11 ng/mL. The averages of nine determinations for doxepin and the metabolite in the milk were 18 and 9 ng/mL, respectively. Maternal serum doxepin and N-desmethyldoxepin levels ranged from trace to 21 ng/mL (average 15 ng/mL) and 33–66 ng/mL (average 57 ng/mL), respectively. The milk:serum ratio for doxepin on two determinations was 0.9, whereas ratios for the metabolite were 0.12 and 0.17. Doxepin was almost undetectable (estimated to be 3 ng/mL) in the infant's serum, but the levels of the metabolite on two occasions were 58 and 66 ng/mL, demonstrating marked accumulation in the infant's serum. The initial infant urine sample contained 39 ng/mL of the metabolite (7).

A 26-year-old woman, 30 days postpartum, was treated with doxepin (150 mg/day) (8). Blood samples were obtained a mean 18 hours after a dose on days 7, 14, 22, 28, 36, 43, 50, and 99 days of treatment. On the same days that blood specimens were drawn, milk samples were collected at the start of feeding (17.2 hours after the last dose) and at the end of feeding (17.7 hours after the last dose). Plasma concentrations of doxepin varied between 35 and 68 ng/mL, with a mean value of 46 ng/mL. Levels for the metabolite, N-desmethyldoxepin, ranged from 65 to 131 ng/mL, with a mean of 90 ng/mL. Mean pre- and post-feed milk:plasma ratios for doxepin were 1.08 (range 0.51–1.44) and 1.66 (range 0.79–2.39), respectively, and for the metabolite, 1.02 (range 0.54–1.45) and 1.53 (range 0.85–2.35), respectively. A plasma sample drawn from the infant on day 43 showed no detectable doxepin (sensitivity 5 ng/mL) and 15 ng/mL of the metabolite. No adverse effects of the exposure to doxepin were observed in the infant (8).

Muscle hypotonia, drowsiness, poor sucking and swallowing, and vomiting were reported in a 9-day-old breast-fed, 2950-g male baby whose mother was taking doxepin 35 mg/day (9). The mother had started doxepin in the 3rd trimester and continued it postpartum. The normal, full-term, 3030-g infant had Apgar scores of 10 and 10 at 1 and 5 minutes, respectively. Breast-feeding began 8 hours after birth. Hyperbilirubinemia (indirect bilirubin 17 mg/dL) was diagnosed at age 3 days. He was discharged at age 5 days with a bilirubin of 9 mg/dL and a weight of 3100 g. At presentation 9 days after birth, jaundice was again present (indirect bilirubin 18 mg/dL) and was treated with 24 hours of phototherapy. The concentrations of doxepin and metabolite in the infant's serum at 11 days of age, 2 hours after breast-feeding, were about 10 ng/mL and <10 ng/mL, respectively. The milk:plasma ratio, 13–15 hours after the last dose, was estimated to be 1.0–1.7 (doxepin plus metabolite). The calculated infant dose, based on 150–200 mL milk/kg/day, was 10–20 μg/kg/day, or about 2.5% of the weight-adjusted maternal dose. Breast-feeding was stopped at age 14 days because of persistent drowsiness and vomiting and, about 24 hours later, his symptoms resolved. He was asymptomatic when discharged home 2 days later (9).

Adverse effects were observed in two of the three cases cited above and were potentially lethal to one infant. Based on these reports, doxepin should be avoided during lactation. The American Academy of Pediatrics classifies doxepin as an agent whose effect on the nursing infant is unknown but may be of concern (10).

References

1. Owaki Y, Momiyama H, Onodera N. Effects of doxepin hydrochloride administered to pregnant rats upon the fetuses and their postnatal development. Oyo Yakuri 1971;5:913–24. As cited in Shepard TH. *Catalog of Teratogenic Agents*. 6th ed. Baltimore, MD: Johns Hopkins University Press, 1989:243.
2. Owaki Y, Momiyama H, Onodera N. Effects of doxepin hydrochloride administered to pregnant rabbits upon the fetuses. Oyo Yakuri 1971;5:905–12. As cited in Shepard TH. *Catalog of Teratogenic Agents*. 6th ed. Baltimore, MD: Johns Hopkins University Press, 1989:243.
3. Product information. Sinequan. Pfizer, 2000.
4. McElhatton PR, Garbis HM, Elefant E, Vial T, Bellemin B, Mastroiacovo P, Arnon J, Rodriguez-Pinilla E, Schaefer C, Pexieder T, Merlob P, Dal Verme S. The outcome of pregnancy in 689 women exposed to therapeutic doses of antidepressants. A collaborative study of the European Network of Teratology Information Services (ENTIS). Reprod Toxicol 1996;10:285–94.
5. Falterman CG, Richardson CJ. Small left colon syndrome associated with maternal ingestion of psychotropic drugs. J Pediatr 1980;97:308–10.
6. Nulman I, Rovet J, Stewart DE, Wolpin J, Pace-Asciak P, Shuhaiber S, Koren G. Child development following exposure to tricyclic antidepressants or fluoxetine throughout fetal life: a prospective, controlled study. Am J Psychiatry 2002;159:1889–95.

7. Matheson I, Pande H, Alertsen AR. Respiratory depression caused by N-desmethyldoxepin in breast milk. Lancet 1985;2:1124.
8. Kemp J, Ilett KF, Booth J, Hackett LP. Excretion of doxepin and N-desmethyldoxepin in human milk. Br J Clin Pharmacol 1985;20:497–9.
9. Frey OR, Scheidt P, von Brenndorff AI. Adverse effects in a newborn infant breast-fed by a mother treated with doxepin. Ann Pharmacother 1999;33:690–3.
10. Committee on Drugs, American Academy of Pediatrics. The transfer of drugs and other chemicals into human milk. Pediatrics 2001;108:776–89.

D

Name:	**DOXORUBICIN**	Risk Factor:	D_M
Class:	**Antineoplastic**		

FETAL RISK SUMMARY

RECOMMENDATION: Contraindicated - 1st Trimester

Doxorubicin is an antineoplastic agent used for the treatment of various types of cancer. The drug is embryotoxic and teratogenic in rats and embryotoxic and abortifacient in rabbits (1).

Several reports have described the use of doxorubicin in pregnancy, including three during the 1st trimester (2–18). One of the fetuses exposed during the 1st trimester to doxorubicin, cyclophosphamide, and unshielded radiation was born with an imperforate anus and rectovaginal fistula (15). At about 3 months of age, the infant was small with a head circumference of 46 cm (<5th percentile) but was doing well after two corrective surgeries (15). A 1983 report described the use of doxorubicin and other antineoplastic agents in two pregnancies, one of which ended in fetal death 36 hours after treatment had begun (18). Other than maceration, no other fetal abnormalities were observed. The investigators could not determine the exact cause of the outcome but concluded that the chemotherapy was probably not responsible. The only other complication observed in exposed infants was transient polycythemia and hyperbilirubinemia in one subject. Infants who have been evaluated have shown normal growth and development.

A 1999 report from France described the outcomes of pregnancies in 20 women with breast cancer who were treated with antineoplastic agents (18). The first cycle of chemotherapy occurred at a mean gestational age of 26 weeks with delivery occurring at a mean 34.7 weeks. A total of 38 cycles were administered during pregnancy with a median of two cycles per woman. None of the women received radiation therapy during pregnancy. The pregnancy outcomes included two spontaneous abortions (both exposed in the 1st trimester), one intrauterine death (exposed in the 2nd trimester), and 17 live births, one of whom died at 8 days of age without apparent cause. The 16 surviving children were developing normally at a mean follow-up of 42.3 months (18). Doxorubicin (D), in combination with cyclophosphamide (C), fluorouracil (F), or vincristine (V), was administered to four of the women at a mean dose of 68.7 mg/m^2 (range 50–100 mg/m^2). The outcomes were four surviving liveborn infants (two exposed to DCF and one each to DF and DV in the 2nd or 3rd trimesters).

Three studies have investigated the placental passage of doxorubicin (2,19,20). In one, the drug was not detected in the amniotic fluid at 20 weeks of gestation, which suggested that the drug was not transferred in measurable amounts to the fetus (2). Placental transfer was demonstrated in a 17-week-old aborted fetus, however, using high-performance liquid chromatography (HPLC) (20). High concentrations were found in fetal liver, kidney, and lung. The drug was not detected in amniotic fluid (<1.66 ng/mL), brain, intestine, or gastrocnemius muscle. A third study examined the placental passage of doxorubicin in two pregnancies, one resulting in the birth of a healthy infant at 34 weeks' gestation and one ending with a stillborn fetus at 31 weeks' gestation (19). Using HPLC, doxorubicin was demonstrated in the first case, 48 hours after a 45 mg/m^2 dose (total cumulative dose, 214 mg/m^2), on both sides of the placenta and in the umbilical cord, but not in cord blood plasma. In the stillborn, doxorubicin was not detected in any fetal tissue, 36 hours after a single dose of 45 mg/m^2. However, a substance was detected in all fetal tissues analyzed that the investigators concluded may have represented an unknown doxorubicin metabolite.

Long-term studies of growth and mental development of offspring exposed to doxorubicin and other antineoplastic agents in the 2nd trimester, the period of neuroblast multiplication, have not been conducted (21).

Doxorubicin may cause reversible testicular dysfunction (22,23). Similarly, normal pregnancies have occurred in women treated before conception with doxorubicin (24). In 436 long-term survivors treated with chemotherapy for gestational trophoblastic tumors between 1958 and 1978, 33 (8%) received doxorubicin as part of their treatment regimens (24). Of the 33 women, five (15%) had at least one live birth (data given in parentheses refer to mean/maximum doxorubicin dose in milligrams) (100/100), two (6%) had no live births (150/200), one (3%) failed to conceive (100/100), and 25 (76%) did not try to conceive (140/400). Additional details, including congenital anomalies observed, are described in the monograph for methotrexate (see Methotrexate).

The long-term effects of combination chemotherapy on menstrual and reproductive function were described in a 1988 report (25). Only one of the 40 women treated for malignant ovarian germ cell tumors received doxorubicin. The results of this study are discussed in the monograph for cyclophosphamide (see Cyclophosphamide).

Occupational exposure of the mother to antineoplastic agents during pregnancy may present a risk to the fetus. A position statement from the National Study Commission on Cytotoxic Exposure and a research article involving some antineoplastic agents, including doxorubicin, are presented in the monograph for cyclophosphamide (see Cyclophosphamide).

BREAST FEEDING SUMMARY

RECOMMENDATION: Contraindicated

Doxorubicin is excreted into human milk. A 31-year-old woman, 7 months postpartum, was given doxorubicin (70 mg/m^2), infused over 15 minutes, for the treatment of ovarian cancer (26). Both doxorubicin and the metabolite, doxorubicinol, were detected in the plasma and the milk. Peak concentrations of the two substances in the plasma occurred at the first sampling time (0.5 hour) and were 805 and 82 ng/mL, respectively. In the milk, the peak concentrations occurred at 24 hours with levels of 128 and 111 ng/mL, respectively. The area under concentration time curves (AUC) of the parent compound and metabolite in the plasma were 8.3 and 1.7 μmol/L × hours, respectively, while the AUC in the milk were 9.9 and 16.5 μmol/L × hours, respectively. The highest milk:plasma ratio, 4.43, was measured at 24 hours. Although milk concentrations often exceeded those in the plasma, the total amount of active drug available in the milk was only 0.24 μg/mL (26). If the infant consumed 150 mL/kg/day, the estimated dose would be 0.036 mg/kg/day.

Although the above amounts might be considered negligible, the American Academy of Pediatrics classifies doxorubicin as a drug that may interfere with cellular metabolism of the nursing infant (27).

D

References

1. Product information. Adriamycin. Pharmacia & Upjohn, 2000.
2. Roboz J, Gleicher N, Wu K, Kerenyi T, Holland J. Does doxorubicin cross the placenta? Lancet 1979;2:1382–3.
3. Khursid M, Saleem M. Acute leukaemia in pregnancy. Lancet 1978;2:534–5.
4. Newcomb M, Balducci L, Thigpen JT, Morrison FS. Acute leukemia in pregnancy: successful delivery after cytarabine and doxorubicin. JAMA 1978;239:2691–2.
5. Hassenstein E, Riedel H. Zur teratogenitat von Adriamycin ein fallbericht. Geburtshilfe Frauenheilkd 1978;38:131–3.
6. Cervantes F, Rozman C. Adriamycina y embarazo. Sangre (Barc) 1980;25:627.
7. Pizzuto J, Aviles A, Noriega L, Niz J, Morales M, Romero F. Treatment of acute leukemia during pregnancy: presentation of nine cases. Cancer Treat Rep 1980;64:679–83.
8. Tobias JS, Bloom HJG. Doxorubicin in pregnancy. Lancet 1980;1:776.
9. Garcia V, San Miguel J, Borrasca AL. Doxorubicin in the first trimester of pregnancy. Ann Intern Med 1981;94:547.
10. Garcia V, San Miguel IJ, Borrasca AL. Adriamycin and pregnancy. Sangre (Barc) 1981;26:129.
11. Dara P, Slater LM, Armentrout SA. Successful pregnancy during chemotherapy for acute leukemia. Cancer 1981;47:845–6.
12. Lowenthal RM, Funnell CF, Hope DM, Stewart IG, Humphrey DC. Normal infant after combination chemotherapy including teniposide for Burkitt's lymphoma in pregnancy. Med Pediatr Oncol 1982;10:165–9.
13. Webb GA. The use of hyperalimentation and chemotherapy in pregnancy: a case report. Am J Obstet Gynecol 1980;137:263–6.
14. Gililland J, Weinstein L. The effects of cancer chemotherapeutic agents on the developing fetus. Obstet Gynecol Surv 1983;38:6–13.
15. Murray CL, Reichert JA, Anderson J, Twiggs LB. Multimodal cancer therapy for breast cancer in the first trimester of pregnancy. A case report. JAMA 1984;252:2607–8.
16. Haerr RW, Pratt AT. Multiagent chemotherapy for sarcoma diagnosed during pregnancy. Cancer 1985;56:1028–33.
17. Turchi JJ, Villasis C. Anthracyclines in the treatment of malignancy in pregnancy. Cancer 1988;61:435–40.
18. Giacalone PL, Laffargue F, Benos P. Chemotherapy for breast carcinoma during pregnancy. Cancer 1999;86:2266–72.
19. Karp GI, Von Oeyen P, Valone F, Khetarpal VK, Israel M, Mayer RJ, Frigoletto FD, Garnick MB. Doxorubicin in pregnancy: possible transplacental passage. Cancer Treat Rep 1983;67:773–7.
20. D'Incalci M, Broggini M, Buscaglia M, Pardi G. Transplacental passage of doxorubicin. Lancet 1983;1:75.
21. Dobbing J. Pregnancy and leukaemia. Lancet 1977;1:1155.
22. Lendon M, Palmer MK, Hann IM, Shalet SM, Jones PHM. Testicular histology after combination chemotherapy in childhood for acute lymphoblastic leukaemia. Lancet 1978;2:439–41.
23. Schilsky RL, Lewis BJ, Sherins RJ, Young RC. Gonadal dysfunction in patients receiving chemotherapy for cancer. Ann Intern Med 1980;93:109–14.
24. Rustin GJS, Booth M, Dent J, Salt S, Rustin F, Bagshawe KD. Pregnancy after cytotoxic chemotherapy for gestational trophoblastic tumours. Br Med J 1984;288:103–6.
25. Gershenson DM. Menstrual and reproductive function after treatment with combination chemotherapy for malignant ovarian germ cell tumors. J Clin Oncol 1988;6:270–5.
26. Egan PC, Costanza ME, Dodion P, Egorin MJ, Bachur NR. Doxorubicin and cisplatin excretion into human milk. Cancer Treat Rep 1985;69:1387–9.
27. Committee on Drugs, American Academy of Pediatrics. The transfer of drugs and other chemicals into human milk. Pediatrics 2001;108:776–89.

Name:	**DOXYCYCLINE**	Risk Factor:	**D_M**
Class:	**Antibiotic (Tetracycline)**		

FETAL RISK SUMMARY

RECOMMENDATION: Contraindicated in 2nd and 3rd Trimesters

See Tetracycline.

BREAST FEEDING SUMMARY

RECOMMENDATION: Compatible

Doxycycline is excreted into breast milk. Oral doxycycline, 200 mg followed after 24 hours by 100 mg, was given to 15 nursing mothers (1). Milk:plasma ratios determined at 3 and 24 hours after the second dose were 0.3 and 0.4, respectively. Mean milk concentrations were 0.77 and 0.38 μg/mL.

Theoretically, dental staining and inhibition of bone growth could occur in breast-fed infants whose mothers were consuming doxycycline. However, this theoretical possibility seems remote, because in infants exposed to a closely related antibiotic, tetracycline, serum levels were undetectable (less than 0.05 μg/mL) (2).

The American Academy of Pediatrics classifies tetracycline as compatible with breastfeeding (3). Three potential problems may exist for the nursing infant even though there are no reports in this regard: modification of bowel flora, direct effects on the infant, and interference with the interpretation of culture results if a fever workup is required.

References

1. Morganti G, Ceccarelli G, Ciaffi EG. Comparative concentrations of a tetracycline antibiotic in serum and maternal milk. Antibiotica 1968;6:216–23.
2. Posner AC, Prigot A, Konicoff NG. Further observations on the use of tetracycline hydrochloride in prophylaxis and treatment of obstetric infections. *Antibiotics Annual 1954–55*. New York, NY: Medical Encyclopedia, 1955:594–8.
3. Committee on Drugs, American Academy of Pediatrics. The transfer of drugs and other chemicals into human milk. Pediatrics 2001;108:776–89.

Name:	**DOXYLAMINE**	Risk Factor:	**A**
Class:	**Antihistamine/Antiemetic**		

FETAL RISK SUMMARY

RECOMMENDATION: Compatible

Doxylamine, an antihistamine of the ethanolamine class, is approved for use as a sedative, either alone or in combination with other agents in cough and cold preparations. It is not used in the United States for the symptomatic relief of hypersensitivity reactions, most likely because of its pronounced sedative effects.

The antihistamine was a component of the proprietary product, Bendectin, which contained equal concentrations of doxylamine, pyridoxine (vitamin B_6), and dicyclomine (an antispasmodic). Bendectin was marketed in 1956 for the prevention and treatment of nausea and vomiting during pregnancy. The product was reformulated in 1976 to eliminate dicyclomine because that component was not found to contribute to the antiemetic effectiveness. A similar Canadian two-drug formulation (doxylamine and pyridoxine), Diclectin, was marketed in 1978. More than 30 million women have taken this product during pregnancy, making it one of the most heavily prescribed drugs for this condition. The United States manufacturer ceased producing the drug combination in 1983 because of litigation and adverse media coverage over its alleged association with congenital limb defects. The fixed two-drug combination, although no longer available in the United States, continues to be produced in Canada and the individual components are marketed worldwide by various manufacturers.

D

Six studies in rodents and nonhuman primates have not observed teratogenic effects with Bendectin or its components (1–6), but dose-related toxicity was observed in three studies. In a 1968 publication, the reproductive effects of dicyclomine, doxylamine, and Bendectin (the three-drug combination of doxylamine [10 mg], dicyclomine [10 mg], and pyridoxine [10 mg]) in rats and rabbits were reported (1). Dicyclomine and doxylamine were given as pure compounds, whereas Bendectin was administered as pulverized tablets. In rats, dicyclomine and doxylamine (10–100 mg/kg/day) (15–150 times the maximum recommended human dose [four tablets] for a 60-kg human [MRHD]) were given orally for 80 days or more before pregnancy and continued during one (dicyclomine) or two (doxylamine) successive liters. The Bendectin group received 3–60 mg/kg/day (5–90 times the MRHD) orally beginning on the first day of gestation and continued throughout the remainder of the study. First-generation male and female offspring from the control and 60 mg/kg/day groups were then bred (nonsibling matings) and their progeny examined. Compared with nonexposed controls, no increase in congenital malformations or other adverse effects were noted in the pregnancy outcomes of the three drug groups. The one exception appeared to be a small dose-related decrease in fetal weight that was observed in the dicyclomine and doxylamine groups. Pregnant rabbits were administered 10–100 mg/kg/day (15–150 times the MRHD) orally of dicyclomine or doxylamine, or 3–30 mg/kg/day (5–45 times the MRHD) orally of Bendectin on days 9 through 16 of gestation (1). Similar to the study with rats, no adverse effects in pregnancy outcomes were noted when compared with controls except when toxic (100 mg/kg/day) doses were used in the pure drug groups (1).

A 1993 reference studied the effects of three antiemetic histamine H_1 antagonists, doxylamine, chlorcyclizine, and promethazine, on the skeletons of rat fetuses exposed during organogenesis (days 7–13) (2). Doxylamine was given orally at doses of 500 and 750 mg/kg (750 and 1125 times the MRHD). Compared with controls, a dose-dependent loss of skeletal integrity and marked fragility occurred with each antihistamine (2). The investigators concluded that the fragility was due to a defect in joint development rather than to intrauterine growth retardation.

No increase in malformations was observed in rats given Bendectin (two-drug combination) during organogenesis in doses of 0, 200, 500, and 800 mg/kg/day (3). Both maternal and fetal toxicity were evident at the two highest doses. Developmental toxicity observed was reduced prenatal viability (800 mg/kg/day) and reduced fetal body weight/litter (500 and 800 mg/kg/day).

Three of the reproduction studies involved nonhuman primates (4–6). In an unpublished study, rhesus monkeys were given a dose of 7 mg/kg/day (10 times the MRHD) without producing malformations (4). A second study, published in 1985, administered pulverized Bendectin (10 mg doxylamine plus 10 mg pyridoxine) to pregnant cynomolgus monkeys, rhesus monkeys, and baboons (5). A commercial preparation of doxylamine (Decapryn) was used in some baboons to reduce the total amount of drug if they would not take Bendectin. Nonexposed controls were used in each species. Most animals received the study drugs daily from gestation days 22 to 50, the major period of organogenesis (5). Cynomolgus and rhesus monkeys were given doses 10–40 times the MRHD, whereas baboons received doses 1–10 times the MRHD of Bendectin or 10 times the MRHD of doxylamine. A few cynomolgus monkeys (short-term exposure group) received Bendectin doses 20 times the MRHD for 4 consecutive days on gestation days 22–25, 26–29, 30–33, 34–37, or 38–41. Some of the long-term exposure monkey groups, all of the short-term exposure groups, and all of the baboon fetuses were removed by hysterotomy prenatally at day

100 of gestation. The remaining monkey fetuses were delivered at term (150–160 days). In the offspring examined prenatally, the incidence of ventricular septal defect (VSD) was 40% (6 of 15) in cynomolgus monkeys, 0% (0 of 8) in cynomolgus monkey short-term exposure groups, 18% (2 of 11) in rhesus monkeys, 23% (3 of 13) in Bendectin-exposed baboons, and 20% (1 of 5) in doxylamine-exposed baboons. The VSD was restricted to the muscular portion of the septum in 91% (11 of 12). No other defects were observed in the monkeys and no dose response was evident among the long-term treated groups. In addition to the VSD, one baboon fetus (drug group not specified) had exophthalmia, micrognathia, reduction of first and fifth digits on both hands, facial hemangioma, and ambiguous genitalia, and was small for gestational age. The cause of the multiple defects was unknown, but a genetic basis for the anomalies could not be excluded (karyotyping was not available at that time) (5). At term, no cases of VSD were found in nine cynomolgus and four rhesus monkey offspring, but one cynomolgus monkey had a mitral valve defect. Data from the author's laboratory indicated a very low incidence of spontaneous VSD in the three species: 0.3% (1 of 297) cynomolgus monkeys; 0% (0 of 1692) rhesus monkeys; 1.6% (1 of 61) baboons (5). The authors concluded, therefore, that the results suggested a delay in closure of the ventricular septum but that closure would occur before birth (5).

In the second part of the above investigation, daily Bendectin (doxylamine plus pyridoxine) doses 2, 5, and 20 times the MRHD were administered double-blind to cynomolgus monkeys ($N = 69$) from gestational days 22 through 50 (6). A control group ($N = 21$) received placebo tablets containing inert excipients and coatings similar to those in Bendectin. The doses for the four groups (three active, one placebo) were prepared by the manufacturer, and their identity was unknown to the researchers. Delivery occurred at term (approximately 155 days of gestation). No congenital malformations were noted, and no evidence of embryo, fetal, or maternal toxicity was observed.

More than 160 cases of congenital defects have been reported in the literature or to the FDA as either "Bendectin-induced" or associated with use of the drug in the 1st trimester (7–12). Defects observed included skeletal, limb, and cardiac anomalies, as well as cleft lip or palate. A 1983 study found an association between Debendox (three-drug formulation) and clefts of the lip, palate, or both, although the authors stated that the association may have been a result of chance alone (13).

In a 1989 study, the association between maternal use of marijuana and childhood acute nonlymphoblastic leukemia (ANLL) was investigated (see Marijuana) (14). An incidental finding was that the relative risk (RR) for ANLL in offspring of case mothers who used antinauseant medication was 1.75 (95% confidence interval [CI] 0.98–3.20) ($p = 0.06$). A statistically significant dose-response relationship was observed when the RR increased to 2.81 if the use of antinauseant medication continued for more than 10 weeks. Although not all of the mothers used Bendectin, most of them specifically named the product (14). However, several factors make a causal relationship between Bendectin and ANLL unlikely, including the possibility of recall bias between cases and controls, the absence of biological plausibility, the likelier possibility that the leukemia was induced by other toxins (e.g., marijuana, herbicides, or pesticides), and the lack of other reports of such an association.

A possible association between doxylamine-pyridoxine and diaphragmatic hernia was reported in 1983 and was assumed to reflect earlier findings of a large prospective study (12). Authors of the latter study, however, cautioned that their results could not be interpreted, even when apparently strong associations existed, without independent confirmation (15,16). In a large case-control study, infants exposed to the combination *in utero* had a slightly greater RR of 1.40 for congenital defects (17). The risk was more than doubled (RR 2.91) if the mother also smoked. An increased risk for heart valve anomalies (RR 2.99) was also found. A minimal relationship was found between congenital heart disease and doxylamine (Bendectin) use in early pregnancy in another 1985 report comparing 298 cases with 738 controls (18). The authors went to great efforts to establish that their drug histories were accurate. Their findings provided evidence that if an association existed, it was very small.

In one of the above studies, an association was discovered between Bendectin and pyloric stenosis (RR 4.33 to 5.24), representing about a 4-fold increase in risk for this anomaly (17). Similarly, the Boston Collaborative Drug Surveillance Programs reported preliminary findings to the FDA indicating a 2.7-fold increase in risk (19). A 1983 case-control study, however, found no association between Bendectin use and the anomaly (20). In evaluating these three reports, the FDA considered them the best available information on the topic but concluded that no definite causal relationship had been shown between Bendectin and pyloric stenosis (19). In addition, the FDA commented that even if there were evidence for an association between the drug and the defect, it did not necessarily constitute evidence of a causal relationship since the nausea and vomiting themselves, or the underlying disease causing the condition, could be responsible for the increased risk (19). A 1984 study, which was not included in the above FDA evaluation, found a possible association with pyloric stenosis but could not eliminate the possibility that it was due to other factors (21). Compared with a control group, the odds ratio (OR) for pyloric stenosis in the offspring of mothers using Bendectin was 2.5 (95% CI 1.2–5.2). However, the authors stated that a conclusion supporting a causal association was not warranted because of the absence of a plausible biologic basis for the defect and conflicting results from other studies (21). Of interest, the *Birth Defects Encyclopedia* describes the etiology of pyloric stenosis (i.e., congenital hypertrophic pyloric stenosis) as probably polygenic and sex-modified, with an occurrence rate of 1:250 births (1:200 males; 1:1000 females) (22).

The evidence indicating that doxylamine-pyridoxine is safe in pregnancy is impressive. A number of large studies, many reviewed in a 1983 article (23), have not discovered a relationship between the drug combination and birth weight or length, head circumference, gestational age, congenital malformations, or other adverse fetal outcomes (24–40). An editorial accompanying the review article pointed out that Bendectin met none of the criteria for judging that a drug was a teratogen (41). One study was unable to observe chromosomal abnormalities associated with the drug combination, whereas a second study found that use of the drugs was not related to the Poland anomaly (unilateral absence of the pectoralis major muscle with or without ipsilateral hand defect) (42,43).

The Northern California Kaiser Permanente Birth Defects Study, published in 1989, prospectively studied the occurrence of 58 categories of major congenital defects in 31,564 newborns in relation to maternal Bendectin use (44). The OR for any major anomaly and Bendectin was 1.0 (95% CI 0.8–1.4). Three categories of defects were statistically associated with the drug: microcephaly (OR 5.3, 95% CI 1.8–15.6); congenital cataract (OR 5.3, 95% CI 1.2–24.3); and lung malformations (OR 4.6, 95% CI 1.9–10.9). However, this was the exact number of associations that would have been expected by chance alone (44). The authors then reviewed an earlier independent study that did not involve Bendectin and found strong positive associations of microcephaly and congenital cataract with vomiting in pregnancy (44). They concluded that Bendectin use during the 1st trimester was not associated with an increase in congenital malformations and that the associations found were unlikely to be causal (44).

A meta-analysis of 17 studies involving the use of Bendectin in pregnancy was published in 1988 (45). The OR 1.01 (95% CI 0.66–1.55) for all studies indicated that Bendectin was not related to congenital defects. The studies were then separated by study type (cohort and case-control studies), and again, no relationship to birth defect outcomes was found (45). Another meta-analysis, published in 1994, examined 16 cohort and 11 case-control studies that had reported birth defects in pregnancies exposed to Bendectin during the 1st trimester (46). The RR of any birth defect in association with exposure to Bendectin was 0.95 (95% CI 0.88–1.04). The RR and 95% CI intervals for specific defects were cardiac (0.90, 0.77–1.05), central nervous system (1.00, 0.83–1.20), neural tube (0.99, 0.76–1.29), limb reduction (1.12, 0.83–1.48), genital tract (0.98, 0.79–1.22), oral clefts (0.81, 0.64–1.03), and pyloric stenosis (1.04, 0.85–1.29). These results indicate that the use of Bendectin during the 1st trimester is unlikely to be associated with congenital malformations (46).

A five-part analysis of the medical literature involving Bendectin and pregnancy outcomes, published in 1995, was used as a demonstration of methodology to determine if a drug presented a human reproductive hazard (47). Some of the legal history surrounding Bendectin's alleged reproductive hazards was also reviewed. The analysis included (a) analysis of human epidemiologic studies, (b) the relationship between the secular trend of birth defects and the population exposure to drugs, (c) the ability to develop an animal model, (d) analysis of dose-response relationships and pharmacokinetics of the drug in animals and humans, and (e) the biological plausibility for the alleged teratogenicity (47). The author reviewed eight *in vitro* studies that examined the toxicity, mutagenicity, teratogenicity, and other toxicities of doxylamine. None of these studies found toxicity at serum concentrations obtainable in humans. Moreover, the author emphasized the fact that *in vitro* studies, by themselves, cannot establish human teratogenicity (47). Based on the total data presented in this analysis, a strong case was made for the contention that Bendectin has no measurable teratogenic effects. In response to this and other publications, however, an intense debate in the scientific literature has developed between some who contend that Bendectin is safe and a proponent of the view that Bendectin induces limb reduction defects (48–53).

Interestingly, a population-based case-control study conducted in 1982–1983 by the Atlanta Birth Defects Case-Control Study and published in 1999 found a protective effect from Bendectin for congenital heart defects (54). The use of antiemetic medication, particularly Bendectin (two- and three-drug combinations), in early moderate to severe nausea during pregnancy was associated with a lower risk for heart defects compared with the absence of nausea (OR 0.67, 95% CI 0.50–0.92) and nausea without medication use (OR 0.70, 95% CI 0.50–0.94). The authors concluded that the results suggested that pregnancy hormones, other factors, or a component of Bendectin (most likely pyridoxine) may be important for normal heart development (54).

In spite of the abundant evidence supporting the safety of doxylamine-pyridoxine in pregnancy, the adverse media publicity and litigation proceedings surrounding Bendectin have affected the use of the combination in other countries. A 1995 article briefly reviewed the history of Bendectin in the United States and compared it with a similar Canadian product, Diclectin (55). Diclectin is the drug of choice for the treatment of emesis in pregnancy as specified by a Canadian Department of Health and Welfare task force, and is labeled for this indication. It is used less frequently, however, than another antihistamine, dimenhydrinate (Gravol; Dramamine in the United States), that is not specifically labeled for pregnancy use. The reason for this appears to be a fear of possible teratogenicity and subsequent litigation (55).

A 2003 ecological analyses of Bendectin found no evidence of a teratogenic effect (56). This study was accompanied by a historical review of the drug and a recommendation that the combination be re-introduced in the American market (57).

In summary, the preponderance of *in vivo* data supports the assessment that the fixed combination of doxylamine-pyridoxine is safe in human pregnancy, including the 1st trimester. Positive associations with congenital malformations have been observed but probably reflect outcomes that have occurred by chance or are the consequences of nausea and vomiting itself. Moreover, these reports do not consistently describe a specific syndrome or group of malformations. Therefore, pregnant women who request medication for nausea and vomiting can be offered this drug combination, but, as with any treatment during pregnancy, the available evidence should be reviewed with them to obtain their informed consent before initiating therapy.

BREAST FEEDING SUMMARY

RECOMMENDATION: No Human Data - Probably Compatible

No reports describing the use of doxylamine or the fixed combination of doxylamine-pyridoxine during human lactation have been located. Both components of the fixed combination, however, are available as single agents. Pyridoxine is excreted into breast milk but presents no risk to a nursing infant (see Pyridoxine). Doxylamine is an antihistamine that is used not only as an antiemetic, but also as a hypnotic and in cough and common cold preparations. The molecular weight of doxylamine succinate, about 389, is low enough that passage into breast milk should be expected. The effects on a nursing infant, if any, are unknown, but sedative and other antihistamine actions are a potential concern. The manufacturer of at least one doxylamine preparation states that the drug is contraindicated during nursing (58).

References

1. Gibson JP, Staples RE, Larson EJ, Kuhn WL, Holtkamp DE, Newberne JW. Teratology and reproduction studies with an antinauseant. Toxicol Appl Pharmacol 1968;13:439–47.
2. Sturman G, Freeman P, Bailey AR, Meade HM, Seeley NA. Loss of skeletal integrity in rat fetuses from dams treated with histamine H_1 antagonists. Agents Actions 1993;38:C185–7.
3. Tyl RW, Price CJ, Marr MC, Kimmel CA. Developmental toxicity evaluation of Bendectin in CD rats. Teratology 1988;37:539–52.
4. McClure HM. Research and development studies relative to the experimental induction of oral facial malformation in the Rhesus monkey. No. 1 DE52452 Final report, May 1975 - July 1981, August 1982. As cited in Brent RL. Bendectin: review of the medical literature of a comprehensively studied human nonteratogen and the most prevalent tortogen-litigen. Reprod Toxicol 1995;9:337–49.
5. Hendrickx AG, Cukierski M, Prahalada S, Janos G, Rowland J. Evaluation of Bendectin embryotoxicity in nonhuman primates: I. Ventricular septal defects in prenatal macaques and baboon. Teratology 1985;32:179–89.
6. Hendrickx AG, Cukierski M, Prahalada S, Janos G, Booher S, Nyland T. Evaluation of Bendectin embryotoxicity in nonhuman primates: II. Double-blind study in term cynomolgus monkeys. Teratology 1985;32:191–4.
7. Korcok M. The Bendectin debate. Can Med Assoc J 1980;123:922–8.
8. Soverchia G, Perri PF. Two cases of malformations of a limb in infants of mothers treated with an antiemetic in a very early phase of pregnancy. Pediatr Med Chir 1981;3:97–9.
9. Donaldson GL, Bury RG. Multiple congenital abnormalities in a newborn boy associated with maternal use of fluphenazine enanthate and other drugs during pregnancy. Acta Paediatr Scand 1982;71:335–8.
10. Grodofsky MP, Wilmott RW. Possible association of use of Bendectin during early pregnancy and congenital lung hypoplasia. N Engl J Med 1984;311:732.
11. Fisher JE, Nelson SJ, Allen JE, Holsman RS. Congenital cystic adenomatoid malformation of the lung.

A unique variant. Am J Dis Child 1982;136:1071–4.
12. Bracken MB, Berg A. Bendectin (Debendox) and congenital diaphragmatic hernia. Lancet 1983;1:586.
13. Golding J, Vivian S, Baldwin JA. Maternal antinauseants and clefts of lip and palate. Human Toxicol 1983;2:63–73.
14. Robison LL, Buckley JD, Daigle AE, Wells R, Benjamin D, Arthur DC, Hammond GD. Maternal drug use and risk of childhood nonlymphoblastic leukemia among offspring: an epidemiologic investigation implicating marijuana (a report from the Children's Cancer Study Group). Cancer 1989;63:1904–11.
15. Heinonen OP, Slone D, Shapiro S. *Birth Defects and Drugs in Pregnancy*. Littleton, MA: Publishing Sciences Group, 1977:474–5.
16. Ohga K, Yamanaka R, Kinumaki H, Awa S, Kobayashi N. Bendectin (Debendox) and congenital diaphragmatic hernia. Lancet 1983;1:930.
17. Eskenazi B, Bracken MB. Bendectin (Debendox) as a risk factor for pyloric stenosis. Am J Obstet Gynecol 1982;144:919–24.
18. Zierler S, Rothman KJ. Congenital heart disease in relation to maternal use of Bendectin and other drugs in early pregnancy. N Engl J Med 1985;313:347–52.
19. Bendectin and pyloric stenosis. FDA Drug Bull 1983; 13:14–5.
20. Mitchell AA, Schwingl PJ, Rosenberg L, Louik C, Shapiro S. Birth defects in relation to Bendectin use in pregnancy. II. Pyloric stenosis. Am J Obstet Gynecol 1983;147:737–42.
21. Aselton P, Jick H, Chentow SJ, Perera DR, Hunter JR, Rothman KJ. Pyloric stenosis and maternal Bendectin exposure. Am J Epidemiol 1984;120:251–6.
22. Pyloric stenosis. In Buyse ML, ed. *Birth Defects Encyclopedia*. Volume II. Cambridge, MA: Blackwell Scientific Publications, 1990:1448.
23. Holmes LB. Teratogen update: Bendectin. Teratology 1983;27:277–81.
24. Aselton P, Jick H, Milunsky A, Hunter JR, Stergachis A. First-trimester drug use and congenital malformations. Obstet Gynecol 1985;65:451–5.
25. Milkovich L, van den Berg BJ. An evaluation of the teratogenicity of certain antinauseant drugs. Am J Obstet Gynecol 1976;125:244–8.
26. Shapiro S, Heinonen OP, Siskind V, Kaufman DW, Monson RR, Slone D. Antenatal exposure to doxylamine succinate and dicyclomine hydrochloride (Bendectin) in relation to congenital malformations, perinatal mortality rate, birth weight, intelligence quotient score. Am J Obstet Gynecol 1977;128:480–5.
27. Rothman KJ, Flyer DC, Goldblatt A, Kreidberg MB. Exogenous hormones and other drug exposures of children with congenital heart disease. Am J Epidemiol 1979;109:433–9.
28. Bunde CA, Bowles DM. A technique for controlled survey of case records. Curr Ther Res 1963;5:245–8.
29. Gibson GT, Collen DP, McMichael AJ, Hartshorne JM. Congenital anomalies in relation to the use of doxylamine/dicyclomine and other antenatal factors. An ongoing prospective study. Med J Aust 1981;1:410–4.
30. Correy JF, Newman NM. Debendox and limb reduction deformities. Med J Aust 1981;1:417–8.
31. Clarke M, Clayton DG. Safety of Debendox. Lancet 1981;2:659–60.
32. Harron DWG, Griffiths K, Shanks RG. Debendox and congenital malformations in Northern Ireland. Br Med J 1980;4:1379–81.
33. Smithells RW, Sheppard S. Teratogenicity testing in humans: a method demonstrating safety of Bendectin. Teratology 1978;17:31–5.
34. Morelock S, Hingson R, Kayne H, et al. Bendectin and fetal development: a study at Boston City Hospital. Am J Obstet Gynecol 1982;142:209–13.
35. Cordero JF, Oakley GP, Greenberg F, James LM. Is Bendectin a teratogen? JAMA 1981;245:2307–10.
36. Mitchell AA, Rosenberg L, Shapiro S, Slone D. Birth defects related to Bendectin use in pregnancy: I. Oral clefts and cardiac defects. JAMA 1981;245:2311–4.
37. Fleming DM, Knox JDE, Crombie DL. Debendox in early pregnancy and fetal malformation. Br Med J 1981;283:99–101.
38. Greenberg G, Inman WHW, Weatherall JAC, Adelstein AM, Haskey JC. Maternal drug histories and congenital abnormalities. Br Med J 1977;2:853–6.
39. Aselton PJ, Jick H. Additional follow-up of congenital limb disorders in relation to Bendectin use. JAMA 1983;250:33–4.
40. McCredie J, Kricker A, Elliott J, Forrest J. The innocent bystander: doxylamine/dicyclomine/pyridoxine and congenital limb defects. Med J Aust 1984;140:525–7.
41. Brent RR. Editorial. The Bendectin saga: another American tragedy. Teratology 1983;27:283–6.
42. Hughes DT, Cavanagh N. Chromosomal studies on children with phocomelia, exposed to Debendox during early pregnancy. Lancet 1983;2:399.
43. David TJ. Debendox does not cause the Poland anomaly. Arch Dis Child 1982;57:479–80.
44. Shiono PH, Klebanoff MA. Bendectin and human congenital malformations. Teratology 1989;40:151–5.
45. Einarson TR, Leeder JS, Koren G. A method for meta-analysis of epidemiological studies. Drug Intell Clin Pharm 1988;22:813–24.
46. McKeigue PM, Lamm SH, Linn S, Kutcher JS. Bendectin and birth defects: I. A meta-analysis of the epidemiologic studies. Teratology 1994;50:27–37.
47. Brent RL. Bendectin: review of the medical literature of a comprehensively studied human nonteratogen and the most prevalent tortogen-litigen. Reprod Toxicol 1995;9:337–49.
48. Newman SA. Bendectin—birth defects controversy. JAMA 1990;264:569.
49. Skolnick A. Bendectin—birth defects controversy. Reply. JAMA 1990;264:569–70.
50. Scialli AR. Editor's note. Reprod Toxicol 1999;13:239.
51. Newman SA. Dr. Brent and scientific debate. Reprod Toxicol 1999;13:241–4.
52. Brent RL. Response to Dr. Stuart Newman's commentary on an article entitled "Bendectin: review of the medical literature of a comprehensively studied human nonteratogen and the most prevalent tortogen-litigen." Reprod Toxicol 1999;13:245–53.
53. Newman SA. Response to Dr. Brent's commentary on "Dr. Brent and scientific debate." Reprod Toxicol 1999;13:255–60.
54. Boneva RS, Moore CA, Botto L, Wong L-Y, Erickson JD. Nausea during pregnancy and congenital heart defects: a population-based case-control study. Am J Epidemiol 1999;149:717–25.
55. Ornstein M, Einarson A, Koren G. Bendectin/Diclectin

for morning sickness: a Canadian follow-up of an American tragedy. Reprod Toxicol 1995;9:1–6.
56. Kutcher JS, Engle A, Firth J, Lamm SH. Bendectin and birth defects II: ecological analyses. Birth Defects Res Part A Clin Mol Teratol 2003;67:88–97.
57. Brent R. Bendectin and birth defects: hopefully, the final chapter. Birth Defects Res Part A Clin Mol Teratol 2003;67:79–87.
58. Product information. Unisom SleepTabs. Pfizer Inc, 1999.

Name:	**DROPERIDOL**	Risk Factor:	C_M
Class:	**Tranquilizer/Antiemetic**		

FETAL RISK SUMMARY

RECOMMENDATION: Compatible

Droperidol is a butyrophenone derivative structurally related to haloperidol (see also Haloperidol). The agent is not teratogenic in animals, but has produced a slight increase in the mortality of newborn rats (1). After IM administration, the increased pup mortality was attributed to central nervous system depression of the dams resulting in their failure to remove the placentae from the offspring (1).

The relatively low molecular weight of droperidol (about 379) suggests that the drug crosses the placenta to the fetus. In humans, the placental transfer of droperidol is slow (2).

Droperidol promotes analgesia for patients undergoing cesarean section without affecting the respiration of the newborn (2,3). The drug was also administered during labor as a sedative in a study comparing 48 women treated with droperidol with 52 women receiving promethazine (4). These investigators noted eight other reports in which the drug was used in a similar manner. No serious maternal or fetal adverse effects were observed.

Droperidol has been used for the treatment of severe nausea and vomiting occurring during pregnancy (5,6). A 1996 report described the use of droperidol and other drugs (diphenhydramine, metoclopramide and hydroxyzine) in 80 women with hyperemesis gravidarum (6). The mean gestational age at the start of treatment was 10.9 $\pm$ 3.9 weeks and the mean total dose received for the approximately 2 days of therapy was 49.6 mg. Twelve (15%) of the women required a second hospitalization and were again treated with the same therapy. Three of the mothers (all treated in the 2nd trimester) delivered offspring with congenital defects: Poland's syndrome, fetal alcohol syndrome, and hydrocephalus and hypoplasia of the right cerebral hemisphere. Only the latter anomaly is a potential drug effect, but the most likely cause was thought to be the result of an *in utero* fetal vascular accident or infection (6).

A 2001 study, using a treatment method similar to the above study, described the use of droperidol and diphenhydramine in 28 women hospitalized for hyperemesis gravidarum (7). Pregnancy outcomes in the study group were compared to a historical control of 54 women who had received conventional anti-emetic therapy. Oral metoclopramide and hydroxyzine were used after discharge from the hospital. Therapy was started in the study and control groups at mean gestational ages of 9.9 and 11.1 weeks, respectively. The study group appeared to have more severe disease then controls as suggested by a greater mean loss from the pre-pregnancy weight, 2.07 kg vs. 0.81 kg (*n.s.)*, and a slightly lower serum potassium level, 3.4 vs. 3.5 mmol/L (*n.s.)*. Compared to controls, the droperidol group had a shorter duration of hospitalization (3.53 vs. 2.82 days, $p = 0.023$), fewer readmissions (38.9% vs. 14.3%, $p = 0.025$), and lower average daily nausea and vomiting scores (both

$p < 0.001$). There were no statistical differences ($p < 0.05$) in outcomes (study vs. controls) in terms of spontaneous abortions ($N = 0$ vs. $N = 2$ [4.3%]), elective abortions ($N = 3$ [12.0%] vs. $N = 3$ [6.5%]), Apgar scores at 1, 5, and 10 minutes, age at birth (37.3 vs. 37.9 weeks'), and birth weight (3114 vs. 3347 g) (7). In controls, there was one (2.4%) major malformation of unknown cause, an acardiac fetus in a set of triplets, and one newborn with a genetic defect (Turner syndrome). There was also one unexplained major birth defect (4.4%) in the droperidol group (bilateral hydronephrosis), and two genetic defects (translocation of chromosomes 3 and 7; tyrosinemia) (7).

In summary, the limited animal and human data suggest that droperidol does not represent a significant risk to the fetus for major anomalies. The drug is a potent antiemetic that is effective for the treatment of severe nausea and vomiting of pregnancy.

BREAST FEEDING SUMMARY

RECOMMENDATION: No Human Data - Potential Toxicity

No reports describing the use of droperidol during lactation have been located. The molecular weight (about 379), however, is low enough that excretion into human milk should be expected. Because the drug is only available as an injectable formulation, the opportunity for exposure of a nursing infant appears to be limited. The effect of exposure, if any, is unknown.

References

1. Product information. Inapsine. Akorn, 1997.
2. Zhdanov GG, Ponomarev GM. The concentration of droperidol in the venous blood of the parturients and in the blood of the umbilical cord of neonates. Anesteziol Reanimatol 1980;4:14–6.
3. Smith AM, McNeil WT. Awareness during anesthesia. Br Med J 1969;1:572–3.
4. Pettit GP, Smith GA, McIlroy WL. Droperidol in obstetrics: a double-blind study. Mil Med 1976;141:316–7.
5. Martynshin MYA, Arkhengel'skii AE. Experience in treating early toxicoses of pregnancy with metoclopramide. Akush Ginekol 1981;57:44–5.
6. Nageotte MP, Briggs GG, Towers CV, Asrat T. Droperidol and diphenhydramine in the management of hyperemesis gravidarum. Am J Obstet Gynecol 1996;174:1801–6.
7. Turcotte V, Ferreira E, Duperron L. Utilité du dropéridol et de la diphenhydramine dans l'hyperemesis gravidarum. J Soc Obstet Gynaecol Can 2001;23:133–9.

Name:	**DROTRECOGIN ALFA (Activated)**	Risk Factor:	C_M
Class:	**Hematologic Agent (Thrombolytic)**		

FETAL RISK SUMMARY

RECOMMENDATION: Compatible - Maternal Benefit >> Embryo/Fetal Risk

Drotrecogin alfa (activated), a serine protease, is a recombinant (from a human cell line) form of human activated protein C. This glycoprotein is indicated for the reduction of mortality in adult patients with severe sepsis who have a high risk of death. It is administered as a continuous IV infusion because of its very short elimination half-life. The antithrombotic action of drotrecogin alfa (activated) is a result of inhibition of factors Va and VIIIa. The agent is inactivated by endogenous plasma protease inhibitors. Animal reproduction studies have not been conducted with drotrecogin alfa (activated) (1).

It is not known if drotrecogin alfa (activated) crosses the human placenta to the embryo or fetus, but the molecular weight (about 55,000) of this glycoprotein should inhibit transfer. In addition, because the fetus can synthesize coagulation factors from early in gestation, there are no known physiologic processes in which endogenous maternal activated protein C would be actively transported across the placenta (2). Furthermore, *in vitro* studies have found no evidence that endogenous protein C crosses the placenta or that it is metabolized by the placenta (2). However, the effect on these processes from high maternal plasma concentrations of activated protein C resulting from infusion of the drug has not been studied.

Drotrecogin alfa (activated) has been recommended for the treatment of preeclampsia because this disease is similar in some ways to severe sepsis: diffuse effects on the maternal vascular endothelium resulting in multiple organ dysfunctions (2,3). A 2002 publication reviewed previous reports on the pathogenesis of preeclampsia to determine whether administration of drotrecogin alfa (activated) could be beneficial in the treatment of this disease (2). The authors of this in-depth assessment concluded that, although the data were limited, there was adequate evidence to support phase II clinical studies in women with early onset preeclampsia (before 33 weeks' gestation) or severe or worsening postpartum disease (2).

A preliminary report of a phase II study describing the use of human activated protein C for the treatment of disseminated intravascular coagulation (DIC) was published in 1999. A total of 16 women with moderate to severe placental abruption were treated over a 2-day period (4). The activated protein C was prepared by extracting protein C from human plasma and activating it with human thrombin. Clinical signs were markedly improved and all coagulation/fibrinolysis parameters, except for the number of platelets, demonstrated significant changes toward normal values. No adverse effects attributable to the treatment were observed (4).

The complete absence of human and animal experience with drotrecogin alfa (activated) during organogenesis prevents an assessment of the risk that this thrombolytic agent presents in human pregnancy. The drug does not appear to cross the placenta so that a direct risk to the embryo or fetus seems unlikely. However, drotrecogin alfa (activated) has been associated with a nonsignificant trend to more maternal hemorrhage and this would be a major risk to both the mother and fetus (2).

BREAST FEEDING SUMMARY

RECOMMENDATION: No Human Data - Probably Compatible

No reports describing the use of drotrecogin alfa (activated) during lactation (human or animal) have been located. It is doubtful if a nursing infant would have access to the breast milk of a woman treated with this drug because of its indication for severe, life-threatening disease. The very high molecular weight of this glycoprotein (about 55,000) should inhibit excretion into milk, but even if such excretion occurred, the drug would most likely be digested in the infant's gut.

References

1. Product information. Xigris. Eli Lilly and Company, 2003.
2. von Dadelszen P, Magee LA, Lee SK, Stewart SD, Simone C, Koren G, Walley KR, Russell JA. Activated protein C in normal human pregnancy and pregnancies complicated by severe preeclampsia: a therapeutic opportunity? Crit Care Med 2002;30:1883–92.
3. Lapinsky SE, Mehta S. Activated protein C for preeclampsia: tailoring the disease to the therapy. Crit Care Med 2002;30:1929–30.
4. Kobayashi T, Terao T, Maki M, Ikenoue T. Activated protein C is effective for disseminated intravascular coagulation associated with placental abruption. Thromb Haemost 1999;82:1363.

Name: **DYPHYLLINE** Risk Factor: **C_M**

Class: **Respiratory Drug (Bronchodilator)**

D

FETAL RISK SUMMARY

RECOMMENDATION: Limited Human Data - No Relevant Animal Data

Animal reproductive studies have not been conducted with dyphylline. This xanthine derivative is closely related to theophylline (see also Theophylline).

No published reports of its use in human pregnancy have been located. In a surveillance study of Michigan Medicaid recipients conducted between 1985 and 1992 involving 229,101 completed pregnancies, 97 newborns had been exposed to dyphylline during the 1st trimester (F. Rosa, personal communication, FDA, 1993). Seven (7.2%) major birth defects were observed (four expected), including (observed/expected) cardiovascular defects (3/1), and polydactyly (1/0.3). No anomalies were observed in four other categories of defects (oral clefts, spina bifida, limb reduction defects, and hypospadias) for which specific data were available. Only with cardiovascular defects is there a suggestion of a possible association, but other factors, including the mother's disease, concurrent drug use, and chance may be involved.

BREAST FEEDING SUMMARY

RECOMMENDATION: Limited Human Data - Probably Compatible

Dyphylline is excreted into breast milk. In 20 normal lactating women a single 5 mg/kg IM dose produced an average milk:plasma ratio of 2.08 (1). The milk and serum elimination rates were equivalent. Although the drug accumulates in milk, the American Academy of Pediatrics classifies dyphylline as compatible with breast-feeding (2).

References

1. Jarboe CH, Cook LN, Malesic I, Fleischaker J. Dyphylline elimination kinetics in lactating women: blood to milk transfer. J Clin Pharmacol 1981;21:405–10.
2. Committee on Drugs, American Academy of Pediatrics. The transfer of drugs and other chemicals into human milk. Pediatrics 2001;108:776–89.

E

Name:	**ECHINACEA**	Risk Factor:	**C**
Class:	**Herb**		

FETAL RISK SUMMARY

RECOMMENDATION: Limited Human Data - No Relevant Animal Data

The traditional uses of echinacea are as a topical agent to enhance wound healing and systemically as an immunostimulant (1). It was used by the American Indians before colonization of the continent and was a common medicine in the United States in the late nineteenth and early twentieth centuries (2). The herb is available orally as capsules, as expressed, fresh juice, and as tinctures. In Germany, an intravenous preparation is also available (3). Specific indications for systemic echinacea listed in one publication were prophylaxis and treatment of viral upper respiratory tract infections and combined with conventional anti-infective agents in the treatment of more severe infections (2). Specific topical indications listed were the treatment of eczema, psoriasis, and herpes simplex (2). Another publication listed antiseptic and antiviral indications (4).

Echinacea angustifolia, the plant most commonly used for medicinal purposes, is a perennial herb of the Compositae family that grows to a height of 3 feet, terminating in a single colorful flower head. The plant is indigenous to the central United States. Related species that have been used in traditional medicine include *E. purpurea* and *E. pallida* (1,5). Because *E. angustifolia* and *E. pallida* closely resemble each other, preparations of echinacea may be mislabeled or contain mixtures of the two species. The Germans recommend the use of the above-ground parts (not the roots) of *E. purpurea* or the roots of *E. angustifolia* for medicinal purposes (5).

The principal anti-inflammatory and immunostimulant compounds are found in the hydrophilic and lipophilic fractions of the root, leaves, and flowers (1,2). The specific active ingredients accounting for the medicinal effects of the herb have not been identified. The water-soluble polysaccharides in the roots, however, appear to be a major component of the anti-inflammatory and immune-stimulating properties (2). Essential oil from the root also contains unsaturated alkyl ketones and isobutylamides. Although not all components from the various parts of the plant have been identified, the chemical compounds that have been isolated include echinacoside (a caffeic acid glycoside), a volatile germacrene alcohol (not usually found in dried plant material), echinacein (an isobutylamide responsible for the pungent odor), echinacin B, chicoric acid, cyanrine, chlorogenic acid, caftaric acid, (z)-1,8-pentadecadiene (also known as Z-pentadeca-1,8-diene), and arabinogalactan (1,2).

No animal studies examining the reproductive effects of any of the species of echinacea or their components have been located. One prospective report, however, has described the use of this herb in human pregnancies (6). Between 1996 and 1998, 206 women contacted a teratogen information service regarding their exposure to echinacea products (primarily *E. angustifolia* and *E. purpurea*) during gestation. Of these, 112 used echinacea during the 1st trimester. The total cohort was disease-matched to 206 women exposed to nonteratogenic agents by maternal age, alcohol, and cigarette use. There were three sets of twins in the study group, none in the control group. Both groups were followed prospectively to determine pregnancy outcomes. No statistically significant differences between the study and control women were found for the following outcomes: live birth (94.7% vs. 96.1%); spontaneous abortion (6.3% vs 3.4%); induced abortion (0.5% vs. 0.5%); vaginal delivery (83.1% vs. 81.3%); maternal weight gain (15.2 vs. 14.4 kg); gestational age at delivery (39.2 vs. 39.2 weeks); birth weight (3466 vs. 3451 g) (excluding twins); fetal distress (23.6% vs. 21.1%); major malformations (in total group) (3.6% vs. 3.5%); and minor malformations (3.6% vs. 3.5%). Among the 98 newborns exposed during the 1st trimester, there were four (4.1%) major defects: left inguinal hernia requiring surgical repair; bilateral hydronephrosis; syndactyly 2nd and 3rd toes; and duplicate left renal pelvis. The authors concluded there was no increased risk for major anomalies (6).

An *in vitro* study using *E. purpura* reported adverse effects in human sperm (7). In a sperm penetration assay, zona-free hamster oocytes were incubated for 1 hour with two concentrations of *E. purpua*, 0.8 mg/mL and 8 mg/mL, dissolved in HEPES-buffered synthetic human tubal fluid (modified HTF). Fresh human donor sperm was suspended in the modified HTF and then mixed with the oocytes for 3 hours. Modified HTF served as the control. At the 0.8 mg/mL concentration, 5 of 9 (56%) oocytes were penetrated, whereas at 8 mg/mL, only 1 of 8 (13%) oocytes was penetrated. The decrease in penetration was not associated with a decrease in sperm motility. In the second part of the study, sperm were incubated with the herbal solutions for 7 days (7). Both concentrations caused significant sperm DNA denaturation concomitant with decreases in sperm viability compared with controls. Extrapolation of these data to the reproductive risk of echinacea in males is difficult, in part because the concentration of echinacea in semen or sperm has not been studied (7). Moreover, although the doses used in this study are small fractions of the actual recommended human dose, there is no published evidence that the adverse effects observed have occurred *in vivo*.

In summary, echinacea is an ancient preparation that has recently undergone resurgence in usage. Use during pregnancy creates the potential for exposure of the embryo and fetus to multiple chemical compounds that have not undergone reproductive toxicity testing in animals or humans. Moreover, standardization of any herbal product as to its constituents, concentrations, and the presence of contaminants is generally lacking. Two sources recommend that parenteral administration of the herb (product form not available in the United States) should not be used in pregnancy (8,9). Another source states echinacea should be avoided during pregnancy because of the lack of information (10). There is only one published report describing human pregnancy exposure. Although this study found no increased risk for major malformations, it was limited by its small sample size, the self-selection of the study group, and the lack of dosage standardization (6). Therefore, the safety of echinacea products during pregnancy remains to be established and, until such additional evidence is published, pregnant women should be counseled of such.

BREAST FEEDING SUMMARY

RECOMMENDATION: No Human Data - Potential Toxicity

No reports describing the use of echinacea during lactation have been located. For the reasons discussed above, and because of the immaturity of an infant's metabolic and elimination systems, use of this herb should probably be avoided during nursing.

E

References

1. Echinacea. *The Review of Natural Products*. St. Louis, MO: Facts and Comparisons. December, 1996.
2. Pepping J. Alternative therapies: Echinacea. Am J Health-Syst Pharm 1999;56:121–2.
3. Zink T, Chaffin J. Herbal "health" products: What family physicians need to know. Am Fam Physician 1998;58:1133–40.
4. Ernst E. Harmless herbs? A review of the recent literature. Am J Med 1998;104:170–8.
5. Miller LG. Herbal medicinals. Selected clinical considerations focusing on known or potential drug-herb interactions. Arch Intern Med 1998;158: 2200–11.
6. Gallo M, Sarkar M, Au W, Pietrzak K, Comas B, Smith M, Jaeger TV, Einarson A, Koren G. Pregnancy outcome following gestational exposure to echinacea. A prospective controlled study. Arch Intern Med 2000;160:3141–3.
7. Ondrizek RR, Chan PJ, Patton WC, King A. An alternative medicine study of herbal effects on the penetration of zona-free hamster oocytes and the integrity of sperm deoxyribonucleic acid. Fertil Steril 1999;71:517–22.
8. Blumenthal M, ed. Echinacea purpurea herb. *The Complete German Commission E Monographs: Therapeutic Guide to Herbal Medicines*. Austin, TX: American Botanical Council, 1998:122–3.
9. *PDR for Herbal Medicines*. Montvale, NJ: Medical Economics Company, 1998:816–23.
10. *Natural Medicines Comprehensive Database*. 3rd ed. Stockton, CA: Therapeutic Research Faculty, 2000: 388–90.

Name: **ECHOTHIOPHATE** Risk Factor: **C**

Class: **Parasympathomimetic (Cholinergic)**

FETAL RISK SUMMARY

RECOMMENDATION: No Human Data - Probably Compatible

Echothiophate is a long-acting, relatively irreversible organophosphate that is used in the eye for its anticholinesterase activity. No reports of its use in pregnancy have been located. As a quaternary ammonium compound, it is ionized at physiologic pH and transplacental passage in significant amounts would not be expected (see also Neostigmine).

BREAST FEEDING SUMMARY

RECOMMENDATION: No Human Data - Probably Compatible

No data are available.

Name: **ECONAZOLE** Risk Factor: **C_M**

Class: **Antifungal**

FETAL RISK SUMMARY

RECOMMENDATION: Compatible

The imidazole antifungal agent econazole is available only in a topical cream formulation. Vaginal suppositories, spray powder, lotion, and spray solution are available outside the United States. Econazole is indicated for the treatment of dermatologic fungal infections including candidiasis. The antimicrobial activity is similar to that of ketoconazole. Systemic absorption from the skin or vagina is minimal, with less than 1% of a dose absorbed and recovered in the urine and feces (1–3).

In reproduction studies with oral econazole, no evidence of teratogenicity was observed in mice, rats, or rabbits. Oral doses 10 to 80 times the human dermal dose, however, did cause embryo and fetal toxicity in some or all members of these species. In addition, prolonged gestation was observed in rats (1). SC doses have also been studied in pregnant mice and rabbits (4). Although no teratogenicity was observed, prolonged gestation and/or fetal death were noted.

It is not known if econazole nitrate crosses the human placenta. The molecular weight (about 445) is low enough, but the amount of drug in the systemic circulation is very low. It is doubtful that clinically significant amounts of the antifungal agent reach the embryo or fetus.

A 1979 report described the use of econazole vaginal suppositories (150 mg at bedtime for 3 days) for the treatment of vaginal candidiasis (5). Some patients required a second course of therapy. Among the patients treated, 24 were pregnant, but the gestational timing of the treatment and pregnancy outcomes were not provided. In a 1981 study, 33 women in various phases of gestation used the same dose and route of administration (6). A second 3-day course of treatment was given to nine of these patients. No details on pregnancy outcomes were reported.

Pregnancy outcome after treatment with a 3-day regimen of econazole vaginal suppositories for vaginal candidiasis was detailed in a 1985 open study (7). Treated were 117 pregnant women with a mean gestational age of 30 weeks (range 10–42 weeks), 44.4% at or after the 36th week of gestation. The number of patients in each trimester was not specified. In 106 pregnancies for which outcome data were available (107 infants, one set of twins), 13 deliveries were premature. No prolongation of gestation was observed. There were three stillbirths among the 107 infants: one twin; one after intrauterine infection (no fungus recovered); and one death *in utero*. No congenital defects were observed in the 104 healthy newborns. The mean weight and height were 3301 g and 50.3 cm, respectively. One newborn developed oral thrush, but the mother was still infected at delivery (7).

In summary, topical econazole does not appear to represent a risk to the human fetus. No teratogenic effects were observed in three animal species following oral and SC dosing that produced systemic exposures far greater than those obtained in humans. The very low systemic bioavailability of this antifungal agent after topical or vaginal application prevents clinically significant amounts from reaching the maternal circulation. Although details of the available human pregnancy experience are incomplete, the risk to an embryo or fetus from the maternal use of econazole probably is nil.

BREAST FEEDING SUMMARY

RECOMMENDATION: No Human Data - Probably Compatible

Although no reports describing the use of topical or vaginal econazole during lactation have been located, the very low systemic bioavailability after topical use suggests that little, if any, of this antifungal will be excreted into breast milk. Therefore, the risk of this exposure to a nursing infant appears to be nil.

References

1. Product information. Spectazole. Ortho-McNeil Pharmaceuticals, 2001.
2. Parfitt K, editor. *Martindale. The Complete Drug Reference*. 32nd edition. London, UK: Pharmaceutical Press, 1999:377.
3. *Drug Facts and Comparisons*. Econazole nitrate. 2000:1612.
4. Maruoka H, Kadota Y, Upshima M, Uesako T, Takemoto Y, Sato H. Toxicological studies on econazole nitrate. 4. Teratological studies in mice and rabbits. Iyakuhin Kenkyu 1978;9:955–70. As cited in Shepard TH. *Catalog of Teratogenic Agents*. 10th ed. Baltimore, MD: The Johns Hopkins University Press, 2001:189.
5. Lecart C, Claerhout F, Franck R, Godts P, Lilien C, Macours L, Schuerwegh, Longree H, Mine M, Strebelle P,

Van Gijsegem M, Wesel S. A new treatment of vaginal candidiasis: three-day treatment with econazole. Eur J Obstet Gynecol Reprod Biol 1979;9:125–7.

6. Karoussos K, Carvalho A, Coelho P, Gomes V, Graca L, Carvalho J, Bacelar Autunes A, Andrade C, Filipe G, Helena Pereira M. Gyno-Pevaryl 150: A new drug for the treatment of vaginal candidosis. J Int Med Res 1981;9:165–7.

7. Goormans E, Beck JM, Declercq JA, Loendersloot EW, Roelofs HJM, van Zanten A. Efficacy of econazole ("Gyno-Pevaryl" 150) in vaginal candidosis during pregnancy. Curr Med Res Opin 1985;9:371–7.

E

Name: **ECSTASY** Risk Factor: **C**

Class: **Central Stimulant**

FETAL RISK SUMMARY

RECOMMENDATION: Contraindicated

In the United States, ecstasy ("Adam"), a central stimulant, is an illicit substance of abuse that is used for its mind-altering properties. It is associated with dance events known as "raves" (1). Chemically, ecstasy is a member of the amphetamine (3,4-methylenedioxymethamphetamine; MDMA) class of drugs (see also Amphetamines) (1,2).

A brief 2000 publication reported the results of a chemical analysis of 107 pills of ecstasy that were voluntarily and anonymously donated to the authors for analysis after a nationwide solicitation (1). However, because the donors were required to pay a fee for the analysis, the findings may not represent what is actually available. Of the total, only 67 pills (63%) contained some MDMA or a closely related analogue (either 3,4-methylenedioxy-ethyl-amphetamine or 3,4-methylenedioxyamphetamine) (1). Forty (37%) contained no MDMA or related amphetamine. Of these, 23 (58%) contained the antitussive dextromethorphan (see also Dextromethorphan) and 9 (23%) contained no identifiable drug. Other substances identified were caffeine, ephedrine, pseudoephedrine, and salicylates (1).

MDMA was not teratogenic in pregnant rats at oral doses of 2.5 or 10 mg/kg/day administered on alternate days from gestational day 6 to day 18 (3). The drug had no effect on gestational duration, litter sizes, or birth weights. Although most pup neurobehavior parameters were unaffected, olfactory discrimination was enhanced in both males and females, and negative geotaxis was delayed in females. However, the density of brain serotonin uptake sites and levels of brain serotonin and 5-hydroxyindoleacetic acid (5-HIAA; metabolite of serotonin) were not affected. There was a significant reduction of maternal weight and a dose-dependent decrease in maternal brain serotonin (5-HT) (3).

In another study with pregnant rats, MDMA 20 mg/kg SC was administered twice daily on days 14–17 of gestation (4). Marked, long-lasting maternal hyperthermia was observed after the first dose, but the response was attenuated with further doses. The body weight of the dams decreased during treatment and there was a 20% decrease in litter size. There was a slight reduction in pup weights on postnatal day 7, but the difference was not statistically significant compared with controls. In the dams, a significant decrease in the concentration of 5-HT and 5-HIAA in the hippocampus, striatum, and cortex of the brain were measured 1 week after parturition (i.e., nearly 2 weeks after the last dose). In contrast, neither the 5-HT or 5-HIAA level in the dorsal telencephalon of the pups was different from that of controls. The lack of MDMA-induced toxicity in the fetal brains suggested that either MDMA was not being metabolized to free radical-producing entities or the fetal brains were more efficient than adult brains in eliminating the toxic free radical metabolites (4).

Although there is no information on the placental passage of MDMA, other amphetamines rapidly cross the human placenta (see Amphetamines). Moreover, the relatively low molecular weight of MDMA (about 179, compared with about 135 for amphetamine), suggests that it also rapidly crosses to the fetus.

An abstract published in 1998 described the pregnancy outcomes of 49 women who had called a Teratology Information Service (TIS) in Holland concerning their exposure to pure MDMA or to closely related amphetamines (methylene dioxyamphetamine, MDA; methylene dioxyethylamphetamine, MDEA; or other) (5). In 47 cases, the exposure occurred during the 1st trimester; the other 2 cases were in the 2nd trimester. The mean age of the women was 26 years (range 17–44 years). Other abuse drugs, usually cocaine or marijuana, were taken by 43%; 34% drank alcohol and 63% smoked cigarettes. Eleven pregnancies were still ongoing. The outcomes of the remaining 38 pregnancies were 2 spontaneous abortions, 2 elective abortions (1 fetus with a defect suggestive of an omphalocele), and 36 live-born infants (6 premature including 1 set of triplets). One term newborn, exposed *in utero* to ecstasy alone, had a congenital heart defect and died a few hours after birth (5).

A 1999 report from the United Kingdom National TIS cited 302 inquiries from pregnant women concerning ecstasy from January 1989 to June 1998 (6). Of the total, 31 pregnancies were ongoing and 135 were lost to follow-up. Outcome data were available for 136 pregnancies (1 set of twins). Among this group, 74 women took only ecstasy, and 62 took ecstasy with other drugs, including amphetamines ($N = 37$), cocaine ($N = 20$), marijuana ($N = 16$), alcohol ($N = 13$), and/or lysergic acid diethylamide (LSD) ($N = 9$). Exposure to ecstasy was limited to the 1st trimester in 127 pregnancies (71 to ecstasy alone, 56 to ecstasy plus other drugs of abuse), to the 1st and 2nd trimesters in 2, to the 2nd trimester in 2, to the 3rd trimester in 1, and throughout gestation in 4. Thus, 133 of the pregnancies (98%) were exposed to ecstasy in the 1st trimester. The outcomes included 11 spontaneous abortions (8%) and 48 elective abortions (35%). One elective abortion occurred at 22 weeks' gestation because of a fetus with absent upper limbs, left scapula, and clavicles, and hypoplasticity of the first rib pair. The mother said she had taken only ecstasy during the 1st trimester. No data were available on the other aborted fetuses. There were 12 infants with congenital defects among the 78 born live infants (15.4%, 95% confidence interval [CI] 8.2–25.4). One newborn (without apparent birth defects), who was exposed *in utero* to ecstasy, heroin, and methadone throughout pregnancy died from an unknown cause. The birth defects and drug exposures (all in the 1st trimester except one case) were ecstasy only (6 cases): left 4th toe underlying 3rd toe; right-sided plagiocephaly; 2 with unilateral talipes; bilateral talipes; pyloric stenosis; ecstasy and amphetamine (2 cases): clicking hips; intrauterine growth retardation, ambiguous sex (1 of twins born at 25 weeks' gestation); ecstasy, amphetamine, and gamma-hydroxybutyric acid (1 case): ventricular septal defect (VSD) (possibly atrial and ventricular), bilateral hydronephrosis, bilateral clinodactyly; ecstasy and alcohol (3 cases): VSD; pigmentation of the right thigh; and ptosis of left eye (exposed in 2nd trimester). There were 3 female infants with talipes (3.8%, 95% CI 8–109) compared with the expected rate of 0.1% (6). In addition, in Great Britain, there is a 3:1 male predominance of idiopathic talipes equinovarus (6). Neither the sex ratio nor birth weights of term infants (specific data not provided) were adversely affected by the exposures (6).

In summary, the use of amphetamines under controlled conditions, such as MDMA in the animal studies above and as amphetamines in the treatment of human disease (see

Amphetamines), suggests that these agents are not teratogenic when used alone and do not cause clinically significant fetal toxicity. Other abuse drugs (e.g., LSD and marijuana) are also not teratogenic (see Lysergic Acid Diethylamide and Marijuana), but alcohol and cocaine are well-known teratogens and/or fetal toxins (see Cocaine and Ethanol). However, ecstasy is not used under controlled conditions. Neither the dosage nor the actual chemical consumed is usually known and, in many cases, the product is taken with other abuse drugs. Because both human studies involved voluntary reporting, a true incidence of major congenital defects cannot be determined, but there does not appear to be a clustering of similar anomalies. If ecstasy is used in pregnancy, healthcare professionals are encouraged to call the toll free number (800-670-6126) for information about patient enrollment in the Motherisk study.

BREAST FEEDING SUMMARY

RECOMMENDATION: Contraindicated

No reports describing the use of ecstasy or MDMA during human lactation have been located. The molecular weight (about 179) is low enough, however, that excretion into milk should be expected. The closely related drug amphetamine is concentrated in breast milk with milk:plasma ratios ranging from 2.8 to 7.5 (see Amphetamine). The American Academy of Pediatrics classifies amphetamines as contraindicated during breast-feeding (7).

References

1. Baggott M, Heifets B, Jones RT, Mendelson J, Sferios E, Zehnder J. Chemical analysis of ecstasy pills. JAMA 2000;284:2190.
2. Plessinger MA. Prenatal exposure to amphetamines. Risks and adverse outcomes in pregnancy. Obstet Gynecol Clin North Am 1998;25:119–38.
3. St. Omer VEV, Ali SF, Holson RR, Duhart HM, Scalzo FM, Slikker W Jr. Behavioral and neurochemical effects of prenatal methylenedioxymethamphetamine (MDMA) exposure in rats. Neurotoxicol Teratol 1991;13:13–20.
4. Colado MI, O'Shea E, Granados R, Misra A, Murray TK, Green AR. A study of the neurotoxic effect of MDMA ("ecstasy") on 5-HT neurones in the brains of mothers and neonates following administration of the drug during pregnancy. Br J Pharmacol 1997;121:827–33.
5. van Tonningen MR, Garbis H, Reuvers M. Ecstasy exposure during pregnancy (abstract). Teratology 1998;58:33A.
6. McElhatton PR, Bateman DN, Evans C, Pughe KR, Thomas SHL. Congenital anomalies after prenatal ecstasy exposure. Lancet 1999;354:1441–2.
7. Committee on Drugs, American Academy of Pediatrics. The transfer of drugs and other chemicals into human milk. Pediatrics 2001;108:776–89.

Name:	**EDETATE CALCIUM DISODIUM**	Risk Factor:	B_M
Class:	**Antidote**		

FETAL RISK SUMMARY

RECOMMENDATION: Compatible - Maternal Benefit >> Embryo/Fetal Risk

The chelating agent edetate calcium disodium (edetate) is the calcium chelate of disodium ethylenediaminetetra acetate. It is indicated for the reduction of blood levels and depot stores of lead in acute or chronic lead poisoning and lead encephalopathy. Edetate also forms stable chelates with other divalent or trivalent metals that can displace calcium, such as cadmium, iron, manganese, mercury, and zinc, but not copper. However, insignificant amounts of iron and manganese are chelated, and mercury is either too tightly bound to be chelated or is stored in inaccessible body compartments. In contrast, the excretion of zinc is significantly increased. Edetate must be given by injection (IM preferred but also by IV) because it is poorly absorbed from the gastrointestinal (GI) tract. The drug is not metabolized and is excreted by the kidneys with an elimination half-life of 20–60 minutes (1).

Reproduction studies have been conducted in pregnant rats. In one study, doses (route not stated but presumed to be oral) up to 13 times the human dose (assumed to be based on body weight) revealed no evidence of impaired fertility or fetal harm. In a second study, doses up to about 25–40 times the human dose caused fetal malformations, but the anomalies were prevented by simultaneous supplementation of dietary zinc (1).

A 1998 review summarized the developmental toxicity of metal chelating agents, including ethylenediaminetetraacetic acid (EDTA) and its salts (disodium, trisodium, calcium disodium, and tetrasodium edetate) (2). The author cited several animal studies showing teratogenicity that was proven to be secondary to EDTA-induced zinc deficiency. Different incidences of teratogenicity were observed depending on the route of administration (IV, SC, gavage, or diet) and dose. In one study, oral administration of EDTA and its salts, even at maternally toxic doses, had little or no teratogenic effects in rats. The different outcomes were thought to be partially caused by poor absorption of the compounds after oral administration (2).

It is not known if edetate crosses the human placenta to the embryo or fetus. The molecular weight (about 374) is low enough for transfer to the fetus. In addition, small amounts of the drug cross the blood-brain barrier as about 5% of the plasma concentration can be found in spinal fluid. However, the very short elimination half-life will limit the amount of drug at the maternal-fetal interface.

The first known case of lead poisoning treated with edetate in a pregnant woman was reported in 1964 (3). A family of six (father, mother, and four male siblings) was diagnosed with lead poisoning caused by using battery cases as fuel in the living room stove for several months. The mother, who was 8 months pregnant, had a blood lead level of 0.24 mg/dL. She was treated with a 7-day course of edetate (75 mg/kg/day). Four weeks later, she delivered an apparently healthy 3.2-kg male infant. The cord blood lead level was undetectable (<0.06 mg/dL). At follow-up, the physical and neurologic examination and developmental assessment were normal at 4.25 years (3).

An unusual case of lead poisoning in a 17-year-old pregnant woman was apparently reported by two different groups of authors from the same New York hospital (4,5). The patient had eaten paint from the walls of her apartment for several months during pregnancy. She was hospitalized at about 38 weeks' gestation because of abdominal pain, paresthesias in her feet, and calf pain. A blood sample yielded a lead level of 86 μg/mL, whereas the amniotic fluid lead level was 90 μg/mL. She was treated with IV edetate 1 g twice daily for 3 days. Two days after chelation therapy, her blood level was 41 μg/mL. Six days later, she delivered a 2665-g female infant spontaneously. The cord blood lead concentration was 60 μg/mL, whereas the maternal level at discharge was 26 μg/mL. The small-for-date infant's head circumference was 32 cm (10th percentile), and the length was 45 cm (25th percentile). Radiographs revealed a dense skull with delayed deciduous dental development and abnormal long bones. At about 2 years of age, the girl's growth and development were normal (4,5).

A 2002 report described the use of IV edetate (dose not specified) and IM dimercaprol in a woman at 30 weeks' gestation with a high blood lead concentration (5.2 μmol/L; goal ≤0.48 μmol/L) (6). Twenty-four hours after initiation of chelation therapy, her lead level was 2.3 μmol/L. Twelve hours later, labor was induced because of uterine hemorrhage, and she gave birth to a 1.6-kg (75th percentile) female infant. Lead concentration in the cord blood was 7.6 μmol/L. The Apgar scores were 4 and 6 (presumably at 1 and 5 minutes, respectively). The newborn was flaccid with absent reflexes, no movement to noxious stimuli, and no gag reflex, but she did have spontaneous eye movement. Bilateral diaphragmatic palsy was confirmed by fluoroscopy. During her 7 months of hospitalization, the infant received multiple courses of chelation to treat the intrauterine lead intoxication. In spite of this therapy, she had right sensorineural deafness and neurodevelopment delay at discharge. Oral succimer was continued at home because the blood lead level was still elevated (0.95 μmol/L). The mother's lead source was identified as herbal tablets that had been prescribed for a gastrointestinal complaint. She had taken the tablets periodically over the past 9 years and throughout pregnancy. Mercury also was present in some of the tablets. The lead intake during pregnancy was estimated to be 50 times the average weekly intake of Western populations (6).

In summary, there are only two reports of human pregnancy experience with edetate, both involving a short course in late gestation. Moreover, interpretation of the rat study is hindered by the presumed oral administration of edetate, a drug that is poorly absorbed from the GI tract. That study did suggest, however, that the observed fetal malformations were induced by zinc deficiency. The human cases and limited animal data are insufficient to assess the risk for the human embryo and fetus. Dietary zinc supplementation might be an option if prolonged treatment with edetate calcium disodium were required during pregnancy, but this has not been studied. In addition, hypotension is a reported adverse effect in adults, and in a pregnant patient, this could jeopardize placental perfusion and the fetus. However, lead is a well-known reproductive toxicant that has significant associations with preterm birth, reduced birth weight and postnatal growth, minor congenital anomalies, and deficits in postnatal neurological or neurobehavioral status (7). Therefore, if indicated, the maternal, and possibly the embryo/fetal, benefit of therapy appear to outweigh any unknown direct or indirect risks (8).

BREAST FEEDING SUMMARY

RECOMMENDATION: Contraindicated

No reports describing the use of edetate calcium disodium (edetate) during lactation have been located. The molecular weight (about 374) suggests that the drug will be excreted into breast milk, but the very short elimination half-life will limit the amount excreted. Moreover, edetate is poorly absorbed after oral dosing, at least from the adult gastrointestinal tract. The risk to a nursing infant from exposure to the drug in milk is unknown but appears to be very low or nonexistent. However, because the use of edetate implies poisoning with lead, this metal also will be excreted into milk and is toxic to a nursing infant. Therefore, breast-feeding is contraindicated in women receiving edetate.

References

1. Product information. Calcium Disodium Versenate. Eli Lilly and Company, 2004.
2. Domingo JL. Developmental toxicity of metal chelating agents. Reprod Toxicol 1998;12:499–510.
3. Angle CR, McIntire MS. Lead poisoning during pregnancy. Fetal tolerance of calcium disodium edetate. Am J Dis Child 1964;108:436–9.
4. Timpo AE, Amin JS, Casalino MB, Yuceoglu AM. Congenital lead intoxication. J Pediatr 1979;94:765–7.
5. Pearl M, Boxi LM. Radiographic findings in congenital lead poisoning. Radiology 1980;136:83–4.
6. Tait PA, Vora A, James S, Fitzgerald DJ, Pester BA. Severe congenital lead poisoning in a preterm infant due to a herbal remedy. Med J Aust 2002;177:193–5.
7. Schardein JL. Metals. In *Chemically Induced Birth Defects*. 3rd ed. New York, NY: Marcel Dekker, 2000:879.
8. Bailey B. Are there teratogenic risks associated with antidotes used in the acute management of poisoned pregnant women? Birth Defects Res Part A Clin Mol Teratol 2003;67:133–40.

Name: **EDROPHONIUM** Risk Factor: **C**
Class: **Parasympathomimetic (Cholinergic)**

E

FETAL RISK SUMMARY

RECOMMENDATION: Human Data Suggest Risk in 3rd Trimester

Edrophonium is a short-acting quaternary ammonium chloride with anticholinesterase activity used in the diagnosis of myasthenia gravis. The drug has been used in pregnancy without producing fetal malformations (1–7).

Because it is ionized at physiologic pH, edrophonium would not be expected to cross the placenta in significant amounts. The molecular weight (about 202 for edrophonium chloride) is low enough, however, that placental transfer of the nonionized fraction probably occurs.

Caution has been advised against the use during pregnancy of IV anticholinesterases because they may cause premature labor (1,3). This effect on the pregnant uterus increases near term. IM neostigmine has been recommended as an alternative to IV edrophonium if diagnosis of myasthenia gravis is required in a pregnant patient (3). However, vaginal bleeding and abortion have occurred with IM neostigmine and are potential complications (see Neostigmine). In one report, IV edrophonium was given to a woman in the 2nd trimester in an unsuccessful attempt to treat tachycardia secondary to Wolff-Parkinson-White syndrome (6). No effect on the uterus was mentioned and she continued with an uneventful full-term pregnancy.

Transient muscular weakness has been observed in about 20% of newborns of mothers with myasthenia gravis (8). The neonatal myasthenia is caused by transplacental passage of anti-acetylcholine receptor immunoglobulin G antibodies (8).

BREAST FEEDING SUMMARY

RECOMMENDATION: No Human Data - Probably Compatible

No reports describing the use of edrophonium during lactation have been located. Edrophonium is ionized at physiologic pH and is not expected to be excreted into breast milk (9). The molecular weight (about 202 for edrophonium chloride) is low enough, however, that excretion of the nonionized fraction into milk may occur. The effects, if any, on a nursing infant from this exposure are unknown (9).

References

1. Foldes FF, McNall PG. Myasthenia gravis: a guide for anesthesiologists. Anesthesiology 1962;23:837–72.
2. Plauche WG. Myasthenia gravis in pregnancy. Am J Obstet Gynecol 1964;88:404–9.
3. McNall PG, Jafarnia MR. Management of myasthenia gravis in the obstetrical patient. Am J Obstet Gynecol 1965;92:518–25.
4. Hay DM. Myasthenia gravis in pregnancy. J Obstet Gynaecol Br Commonw 1969;76:323–9.
5. Heinonen OP, Slone D, Shapiro S. *Birth Defects and Drugs in Pregnancy*. Littleton, MA: Publishing Sciences Group, 1977:345–56.
6. Gleicher N, Meller J, Sandler RZ, Sullum S. Wolff-Parkinson-White syndrome in pregnancy. Obstet Gynecol 1981;58:748–52.
7. Blackhall MI, Buckley GA, Roberts DV, Roberts JB, Thomas BH, Wilson A. Drug-induced neonatal myasthenia. J Obstet Gynaecol Br Commonw 1969;76:157–62.
8. Plauche WC. Myasthenia gravis in pregnancy: an update. Am J Obstet Gynecol 1979;135:691–7.
9. Wilson JT. Pharmacokinetics of drug excretion. In Wilson JT, ed. *Drugs in Breast Milk*. Balgowlah, Australia: ADIS Press, 1981:17.

Name:	**EFAVIRENZ**	Risk Factor:	C_M
Class:	**Antiviral**		

FETAL RISK SUMMARY

RECOMMENDATION: Compatible - Maternal Benefit >> Embryo/Fetal Risk

E

Efavirenz is an orally active, nonnucleoside reverse transcriptase inhibitor (nnRTI) that is specific for human immunodeficiency virus, type 1 (HIV-1). It is indicated, in combination with other antiretroviral agents, for the treatment of HIV-1 infections. Other drugs in this class are delavirdine and nevirapine. Efavirenz has a terminal half-life of 52–76 hours after a single dose, and 40–55 hours after multiple dosing (1). The shorter elimination time after chronic dosing is a result of P450 enzyme induction that induces its own metabolism.

In reproduction studies, cynomolgus monkeys were administered oral efavirenz (60 mg/kg/day) throughout pregnancy (post-coital days 20–150) (1). This dose produced plasma drug concentrations similar to those achieved in humans with 600 mg/day. Three of 20 exposed newborns had major congenital malformations, compared with 0 of 20 in nonexposed control monkeys. The defects observed were 1 case each of anencephaly and unilateral anophthalmia, microphthalmia, and cleft palate. In pregnant rats, doses producing plasma concentrations similar to those in humans resulted in an increase in fetal resorptions (1). Neither mating nor fertility was impaired in rats at these doses. No teratogenic or toxic effects were observed in rabbits given doses producing plasma concentrations similar to those in humans (1).

It is not known if efavirenz crosses the human placenta to the fetus. The relatively low molecular weight (about 316), however, suggests that the drug is transferred to the fetus. Placental transfer of efavirenz has been documented in cynomolgus monkeys, rats, and rabbits, with fetal blood concentrations approximately the same as maternal plasma concentrations (1).

The Antiretroviral Pregnancy Registry reported, for the period January 1989 through January 2004, prospective data (reported to the Registry before the outcomes were known) involving 1537 live births who had been exposed during the 1st trimester to one or more antiretroviral agents (2). Forty-seven of the newborns had congenital defects (3.1%, 95% confidence interval [CI] 2.3–4.1). In the 2407 live births with earliest exposure in the 2nd/3rd trimesters, there were 56 infants with defects (2.3%, 95% CI 1.8–3.0). The prevalence rates for the two periods did not differ significantly. There were 103 infants with birth defects among 3944 live births with exposure anytime during pregnancy (2.6%, 95% CI 2.1–3.2). The prevalence rate did not differ significantly from the rate expected in a nonexposed population (2). There were 171 outcomes exposed to efavirenz (159 in the 1st trimester and 12 in the 2nd/3rd trimesters) in combination with other antiretroviral agents. There were five birth defects among the 1st trimester exposures and none in those exposed in the 2nd/3rd trimesters. In reviewing the birth defects of prospective and retrospective (pregnancies reported after the outcomes were known) registered cases, and clinical reports, the Registry concluded that there was no pattern of anomalies to suggest a common cause (2). (See Lamivudine for required statement.)

In summary, the limited human data do not allow a prediction as to the safety of efavirenz during pregnancy. However, the teratogenicity observed in cynomolgus monkeys and the embryo toxicity in rats suggests that there is a potential for risk in the developing human. Moreover, exposure of the human embryo/fetus is likely to occur because the agent was found to easily cross the placenta of all animal species tested. Two reviews, one in 1996 and the other in 1997, concluded that all women receiving antiretroviral therapy should continue to receive therapy during pregnancy and that treatment of the mother with monotherapy should be considered inadequate (3,4). In 1998, the Centers for Disease Control and Prevention (CDC) made a similar recommendation that antiretroviral therapy be continued during pregnancy, but discontinuation of all therapy during the 1st trimester was a consideration (5). Whether these recommendations to continue therapy apply to efavirenz, however, is unknown, especially in light of the animal data. If possible, another agent should be substituted for efavirenz if pregnancy is planned or occurs while the mother is undergoing treatment with this agent. However, if combination therapy with efavirenz is mandatory, it should not be withheld (with the possible exception of during the 1st trimester) because the expected benefit to the HIV-positive mother probably outweighs the potential risk to the fetus. The mother should be counseled on the risk to her fetus. The efficacy and safety of combined therapy in preventing vertical transmission of HIV to the newborn are unknown, and zidovudine remains the only antiretroviral agent recommended for this purpose (3,4).

BREAST FEEDING SUMMARY

RECOMMENDATION: Contraindicated

No reports describing the use of efavirenz during human lactation have been located. The molecular weight (about 316) is low enough that excretion into breast milk should be expected. In lactating rats, efavirenz is excreted into milk (1).

Reports on the use of efavirenz during human lactation are unlikely because the antiviral agent is used in the treatment of human immunodeficiency virus (HIV) infections. HIV-1 is transmitted in milk, and in developed countries, breast-feeding is not recommended (3,4,6–8). In developing countries, breast-feeding is undertaken, despite the risk, because there are no affordable milk substitutes available. Until 1999, no studies had been published that examined the effect of any antiretroviral therapy on HIV-1 transmission in milk. In that year, a study involving zidovudine was published that measured a 38% reduction in vertical transmission of HIV-1 infection despite breast-feeding when compared with controls (see Zidovudine).

References

1. Product information. Sustiva. DuPont Pharma, 2000.
2. Antiretroviral Pregnancy Registry Steering Committee. *Antiretroviral Pregnancy Registry International Interim Report for 1 January 1989 through 31 January 2004*. Wilmington, NC: Registry Coordinating Center, 2004.
3. Carpenter CCJ, Fischi MA, Hammer SM, Hirsch MS, Jacobsen DM, Katzenstein DA, Montaner JSG, Richman DD, Saag MS, Schooley RT, Thompson MA, Vella S, Yeni PG, Volberding PA. Antiretroviral therapy for HIV infection in 1996. JAMA 1996;276;146–54.
4. Minkoff H, Augenbraun M. Antiretroviral therapy for pregnant women. Am J Obstet Gynecol 1997;176: 478–89.
5. CDC. Public Health Service Task Force recommendations for the use of antiretroviral drugs in pregnant women infected with HIV-1 for maternal health and for reducing perinatal HIV-1 transmission in the United States. MMWR 1998;47:No. RR-2.
6. Brown ZA, Watts DH. Antiviral therapy in pregnancy. Clin Obstet Gynecol 1990;33:276–89.
7. de Martino M, Tovo P-A, Pezzotti P, Galli L, Massironi E, Ruga E, Floreea F, Plebani A, Gabiano C, Zuccotti GV. HIV-1 transmission through breast milk: appraisal of risk according to duration of feeding. AIDS 1992;6: 991–7.
8. Van de Perre P. Postnatal transmission of human immunodeficiency virus type 1: the breast-feeding dilemma. Am J Obstet Gynecol 1995;173:483–7.

Name:	**ELECTRICITY**	Risk Factor:	**D**
Class:	**Miscellaneous**		

FETAL RISK SUMMARY

RECOMMENDATION: Human Data Suggest Risk

Published reports have described the exposure of pregnant women to electric currents through five different means: accidental electric injury in the home, lightning strikes, electroconvulsive therapy, antiarrhythmic direct-current cardioversion, and from a Taser weapon. Dramatically different fetal outcomes have occurred based on the type of exposure.

Four reports involved 14 women described accidental electric shock with alternating current, either 110 volts or 220 volts, from appliances or wiring in the home (1–4). In each case, the electric current took an assumed hand-to-foot pattern through the body and, thus, probably through the uterus. Gestational ages varied from 12–40 weeks. Although none of the mothers was injured or even lost consciousness, in these otherwise harmless events, fetal death occurred in 10 (71%) cases. In at least five of the cases, immediate cessation of fetal movements was noted. One mother, who received the shock at about 28 weeks' gestation, subsequently developed hydramnios and delivered an infant 4 weeks later (1). Burn marks were evident on the newborn, who died 3 days after birth. A second growth-retarded infant was stillborn at 33 weeks' gestation, 12 weeks after the electrical injury (4). In most cases, no specific clinical or pathologic signs could be noted (4). However, oligohydramnios was observed in two cases in which the fetuses survived (4). The accidents occurred at 20 and 32 weeks' gestation, with injury-to-delivery intervals of 6 and 21 weeks, respectively. The specific cause of fetal damage has not been determined. It may be a result of changes in fetal heart conduction resulting in cardiac arrest (3,4) or by lesions in the uteroplacental bed (4).

A 1997 paper described 20 cases from the literature of electric shock during pregnancy with healthy newborn outcomes occurring in only 5 cases (5). The authors of this report then described the outcomes of 31 women studied prospectively after exposure to home appliances with 110 V ($N = 26$) or 220 V ($N = 2$), or to high voltage (2000 and 8000 V) from electrified fences ($N = 2$), or to a low-voltage (12 V) telephone line ($N = 1$). (An abstract of their preliminary findings was published in 1995 [6].) An additional 16 women who had received electric shocks during pregnancy were either lost to follow-up ($N = 10$) or had not yet given birth ($N = 6$). Of the 31 outcomes, there were 2 spontaneous abortions, one of which may have been caused by the electric shock. In that case, the abortion occurred 2 weeks after the mother had received the shock. One of the live newborns had a ventricular septal defect that eventually closed spontaneously. In comparison to the group of 20 cases from the literature, there were significant differences discovered in the number of live births (94% vs. 25%), voltage involved (77% to 110 V vs. 76% to 220 V), and current crossing the uterus (i.e., hand-to-foot transmission suggesting that the current crossed the uterus) (10% vs. 62%).

Lightning strikes of pregnant women are rare, with only 12 cases described since 1833 (1,7–11). All mothers survived the event, but 6 (50%) of the fetuses died. A 1965 reference reported a lightning strike of a woman in approximately the 11th week of gestation (1). The woman briefly lost consciousness, but other than transient nausea and anxiety that decreased as the pregnancy progressed, she was unhurt. She subsequently delivered a healthy term infant who was developing normally at 5 months of age. This report also described five other cases of lightning strikes of pregnant women that occurred between 1833 and 1959 with two fetal deaths. In one of the latter cases, the electrical injury caused uterine rupture in a mother at 6 months' gestation requiring an immediate cesarean section that was unable to save the fetus. Two cases of lightning strikes in term pregnant women were reported in 1972 (7). Both women were in labor when examined shortly after the events. One infant was delivered 12.5 hours after the maternal injury but died 15.5 hours after birth apparently secondary to congestive heart failure. In the other case, a healthy infant was delivered 14 hours after the lightning strike. A 1979 report described a near-fatal lightning strike in the chest of a 21-year-old woman at 34 weeks' gestation (8). Successful cardiopulmonary resuscitation was performed on the mother, but fetal heart tones were absent on initial examination. A stillborn fetus was delivered 48 hours after admission while the mother was still comatose. No fetal movements were felt by a 12-year-old mother at term after awakening from a lightning strike (9). She went into labor 9 days after the accident and delivered a macerated male fetus. Both the fetus and the placenta appeared grossly normal. A case of a woman in her 7th month of pregnancy who was struck in the right arm by lightning was published in 1982 (10). She apparently did not lose consciousness. Examination revealed minimal maternal injury and normal fetal heart tones. A healthy infant was delivered 10 weeks later who is developing normally at 19 months of age. Finally, the picture and brief description of a 41-year-old woman, in her 26th week of pregnancy, who was struck by lightning was presented in 1994 (11). The woman, but not the fetus, survived. Interestingly, the direction of the lightning strike in the mother was discussed in later correspondence (12,13).

Electroconvulsive therapy (ECT) for depression and psychosis in pregnant patients has been the subject of a large number of references (14–39). The procedure has been used in all trimesters of pregnancy and is considered safe for the fetus. One report described mental retardation in a 32-month-old child whose mother had received 12 ECT treatments in the 2nd and 3rd trimesters for schizophrenia, but the investigators did not believe the treatments were responsible (37). A 1955 reference examined 16 children who had been exposed *in utero* to maternal ECT between the 9th and 21st weeks of pregnancy (38). The age of the children at examination ranged from 14 to 81 months and all exhibited normal mental and physical development. Transient (2.5 minutes) fetal heart rate deceleration was observed in a twin pregnancy in which the mother was receiving ECT under general anesthesia (39). A total of eight ECT treatments were given, two before the observed deceleration and five afterwards.

General guidelines for ECT established by the National Institutes of Health (NIH) were published in 1985 (34). The NIH report recommended that ECT, instead of drug therapy, be considered for pregnant patients with severe depression or psychosis in their 1st trimester but did not mention use in the other phases of gestation. Guidelines for the use of ECT in pregnant women were first proposed in 1978 (29), and expanded in 1984 (33). The combined guidelines from these two sources are: (a) thorough physical examination, including a pelvic examination, if not completed earlier; (b) the presence of an obstetrician; (c) endotracheal intubation; (d) low-voltage, nondominant ECT with EEG monitoring; (e) electrocardiographic monitoring of the mother; (f) evaluation of arterial blood gases during and immediately after ECT; (g) Doppler ultrasonography of fetal heart rate; (h) tocodynamometer recording of uterine tone; (i) administration of glycopyrrolate (see Glycopyrrolate) as the anticholinergic of choice during anesthesia; and (j) weekly nonstress tests.

Only one report has been located that described arterial blood gas analyses during ECT in a pregnant patient (28). As observed in previous studies, maternal blood pressure (average systolic blood pressure increase 10 mm Hg) and heart rate (average pulse increase 15 beats/minute) rose slightly immediately after the shock, but no maternal hypoxia was measured. A fetal arrhythmia lasting about 15 minutes occurred that was apparently unrelated to oxygen changes in the mother (28).

Transient maternal hypotension after ECT was described in a 1984 case report (32). The adverse effect was attributed to decreased intravascular volume. IV hydration preceded subsequent ECT treatments in the patient, and no further episodes of hypotension were observed.

A 1991 report noted mild, bright red vaginal bleeding and uterine contractions after each of seven weekly ECT treatments between 30 and 36 weeks' gestation (35). A cesarean section, performed at 37 weeks' gestation because of bleeding, confirmed a diagnosis of abruptio placentae. The authors attributed the complication to the transient marked hypertension caused by the ECT. Only one other report, however, has described vaginal bleeding after ECT (26). Three women, all in the 8th or 9th month of pregnancy, complained either of severe recurrent abdominal pain ($N = 2$) or vaginal bleeding ($N = 1$) after ECT. Therapy was stopped in these cases, and normal infants were eventually delivered.

Antiarrhythmic, direct-current cardioversion is considered a safe procedure during gestation (40–43). Cardioversion has been used in the 2nd trimester in a woman with atrial fibrillation after mitral valvulotomy (40), in the 1st trimester in a patient with atrial flutter in 1:1 atrioventricular conduction (41), 7 times during three pregnancies in one patient for atrial tachycardia resistant to drug therapy (42), and twice in a single patient in two pregnancies for atrial fibrillation (43). No fetal harm was noted from the procedure in any of these cases. Two review articles on cardiac arrhythmias during pregnancy considered cardioversion (with energies of 10–50 J [44]) to be safe and usually effective in this patient population (44,45).

A 1992 reference described the effect from using a Taser (an electronic immobilization and defense weapon) on a pregnant woman at an estimated 8–10 weeks' gestation (46). The subject, in custody at the time because of drug abuse, was struck by one dart above the uterus and by a second dart in the left thigh, thereby establishing a current path through the uterus (46). Vaginal spotting began the next day and heavy vaginal bleeding began 7 days after the Taser incident. Uterine curettage performed 7 days later confirmed the presence of an incomplete spontaneous abortion.

In summary, exposure of the pregnant woman to electric current may produce dramatically different fetal outcomes depending on the source and type of current. Based on published reports previous to 1997, otherwise harmless maternal exposure to household alternating current was usually fatal to the fetus. In contrast, a 1997 prospective controlled cohort study cited above described live births in 94% of their cases (5). The difference between this latter report and the previous published experience is most likely caused by selective reporting of adverse outcomes, the level of voltage involved (i.e., 110 V vs. 220 V), and whether the current passed through the uterus. Although the new data should lessen a woman's concern for her fetus after electric shock, pregnant women who have experienced this type of injury, even when deemed to be minor, should be advised to consult their health care provider. Oligohydramnios, intrauterine growth retardation, and fetal death may be late effects of exposure to alternating current (4). Lightning strikes of any human are often fatal, but in those rare cases in which the victim is pregnant and survives, about half of the fetuses will also survive. ECT and direct-current cardioversion do not seem to pose a significant risk to the fetus. However, abruptio placentae has been observed in at least one and possibly two cases after ECT. Based on one report, the use of a Taser weapon on a pregnant woman may result in spontaneous abortion.

BREAST FEEDING SUMMARY

RECOMMENDATION: No Human Data - Potential Toxicity (Mother)

No data are available.

E

References

1. Rees WD. Pregnant woman struck by lightning. Br Med J 1965;1:103–4.
2. Peppler RD, Labranche FJ, Comeaux JJ. Intrauterine death of a fetus in a mother shocked by an electric current: a case report. J La State Med Soc 1972;124:37–8.
3. Jaffe R, Fejgin M, Aderet NB. Fetal death in early pregnancy due to electric current. Acta Obstet Gynecol Scand 1986;65:283.
4. Leiberman JR, Mazor M, Molcho J, Haiam E, Maor E, Insler V. Electrical accidents during pregnancy. Obstet Gynecol 1986;67:861–3.
5. Einarson A, Bailey B, Inocencion G, Ormond K, Koren G. Accidental electric shock in pregnancy: a prospective cohort study. Am J Obstet Gynecol 1997;176:678–81.
6. Einarson A, Innocencion G, Koren G. Accidental electric shock in pregnancy: a prospective cohort study (abstract). Reprod Toxicol 1995;9:581.
7. Chan Y-F, Sivasamboo R. Lightning accidents in pregnancy. J Obstet Gynaecol Br Commonw 1972;79:761–2.
8. Weinstein L. Lightning: a rare cause of intrauterine death with maternal survival. South Med J 1979;72:632–3.
9. Guha-Ray DK. Fetal death at term due to lightning. Am J Obstet Gynecol 1979;134:103–5.
10. Flannery DB, Wiles H. Follow-up of a survivor of intrauterine lightning exposure. Am J Obstet Gynecol 1982;142:238–9.
11. Zehender M. Images in Clinical Medicine: Struck by lightning. N Engl J Med 1994;330:1492.
12. Bourke DL, Harrison CM, Sprung J. Direction of a lightning strike. N Engl J Med 1994;331:953.
13. Zehender M, Wiesinger J. Direction of a lightning strike. N Engl J Med 1994;331:954.
14. Goldstein HH, Weinberg J, Sankstone MI. Shock therapy in psychosis complicating pregnancy; a case report. Am J Psychiatry 1941;98:201–2.
15. Thorpe FT. Shock treatment in psychosis complicating pregnancy. Br Med J 1942;2:281.
16. Polatin P, Hoch P. Electroshock therapy in pregnant mental patients. N Y J Med 1945;45:1562–3.
17. Sands DE. Electro-convulsion therapy in 301 patients in a general hospital. Br Med J 1946;2:289–93.
18. Gralnick A. Shock therapy in psychoses complicated by pregnancy; report of two cases. Am J Psychiatry 1946;102:780–2.
19. Turner CC, Wright LD. Shock therapy in psychoses during pregnancy; report of one case. Am J Psychiatry 1947;103:834–6.
20. Moore MT. Electrocerebral shock therapy; a reconsideration of former contraindications. Arch Neurol Psychiatry 1947;57:693–711.
21. Simon JL. Electric shock treatment in advanced pregnancy. J Nerv Ment Dis 1948;107:579–80.
22. Block S. Electric convulsive therapy during pregnancy. Am J Psychiatry 1948;104:579.
23. Charatan FB, Oldham AJ. Electroconvulsive treatment in pregnancy. J Obstet Gynaecol Br Emp 1954;61:665–7.
24. Laird DM. Convulsive therapy in psychoses accompanying pregnancy. N Engl J Med 1955;252:934–6.
25. Smith S. The use of electroplexy (E.C.T.) in psychiatric syndromes complicating pregnancy. J Ment Sci 1956;102:796–800.
26. Sobel DE. Fetal damage due to ECT, insulin coma, chlorpromazine, or reserpine. Arch Gen Psychiatry 1960;2:606–11.
27. Impastato DJ, Gabriel AR, Lardaro HH. Electric and insulin shock therapy during pregnancy. Dis Nerv Syst 1964;25:542–6.
28. Levine R, Frost EAM. Arterial blood-gas analyses during electroconvulsive therapy in a parturient. Anesth Analg 1975;54:203–5.
29. Remick RA, Maurice WL. ECT in pregnancy. Am J Psychiatry 1978;135:761–2.
30. Fink M. Convulsive and drug therapies of depression. Annu Rev Med 1981;32:405–12.
31. Loke KH, Salleh R. Electroconvulsive therapy for the acutely psychotic pregnant patient: a review of 3 cases. Med J Malaysia 1983;38:131–3.
32. Repke JT, Berger NG. Electroconvulsive therapy in pregnancy. Obstet Gynecol 1984;63(Suppl):39S–41S.
33. Wise MG, Ward SC, Townsend-Parchman W, Gilstrap LC III, Hauth JC. Case report of ECT during high-risk pregnancy. Am J Psychiatry 1984;141:99–101.
34. Office of Medical Applications of Research, National Institutes of Health. Electroconvulsive therapy. JAMA 1985;254:2103–8.
35. Sherer DM, D'Amico ML, Warshal DP, Stern RA, Grunert HF, Abramowicz JS. Recurrent mild abruptio placentae occurring immediately after repeated electroconvulsive therapy in pregnancy. Am J Obstet Gynecol 1991;165:652–3.
36. Yellowlees PM, Page T. Safe use of electroconvulsive therapy in pregnancy. Med J Aust 1990;153:679–80.
37. Yamamoto J, Hammes EM, Hammes EM Jr. Mental deficiency in a child whose mother was given electric convulsive therapy during gestation. A case report. Minn Med 1953;36:1260–1.
38. Forssman H. Follow-up study of sixteen children whose mothers were given electric convulsive

therapy during gestation. Acta Psychiatr Neurol Scand 1955;30:437–41.
39. Livingston JC, Johnstone WM Jr, Hadi HA. Electroconvulsive therapy in a twin pregnancy: a case report. Am J Perinatol 1994;11:116–8.
40. Vogel JHK, Pryor R, Blount SG Jr. Direct-current defibrillation during pregnancy. JAMA 1965;193:970–1.
41. Sussman HF, Duque D, Lesser ME. Atrial flutter with 1:1 A-V conduction; report of a case in a pregnant woman successfully treated with DC countershock. Dis Chest 1966;49:99–103.
42. Schroeder JS, Harrison DC. Repeated cardioversion during pregnancy; treatment of refractory paroxysmal atrial tachycardia during 3 successive pregnancies. Am J Cardiol 1971;27:445–6.
43. McKenna WJ, Harris L, Rowland E, Whitelaw A, Storey G, Holt D. Amiodarone therapy during pregnancy. Am J Cardiol 1983;51:1231–3.
44. Brown CEL, Wendel GD. Cardiac arrhythmias during pregnancy. Clin Obstet Gynecol 1989;32:89–102.
45. Rotmensch HH, Rotmensch S, Elkayam U. Management of cardiac arrhythmias during pregnancy. Current concepts. Drugs 1987;33:623–33.
46. Mehl LE. Electrical injury from tasering and miscarriage. Acta Obstet Gynecol Scand 1992;71:118–23.

Name: **ELETRIPTAN** Risk Factor: **C_M**
Class: **Antimigraine**

FETAL RISK SUMMARY

RECOMMENDATION: No Human Data - Animal Data Suggest Moderate Risk

Eletriptan is an oral selective serotonin (5-hydroxytryptamine; $5HT_{1B/1D}$) receptor agonist that has high affinity for $5HT_{1B}$, $5HT_{1D}$, and $5HT_{1F}$ receptors. The drug is closely related to almotriptan, frovatriptan, naratriptan, rizatriptan, sumatriptan, and zolmitriptan (see also Almotriptan, Frovatriptan, Naratriptan, Rizatriptan, Sumatriptan, and Zolmitriptan). It is indicated for the acute treatment of migraine with or without aura in adults. Protein binding is moderate (about 85%). One active metabolite has been identified. The elimination half-life of eletriptan is about 4 hours, whereas the half-life of the active metabolite is about 13 hours (1).

Reproduction studies have been conducted in rats and rabbits. In rats, eletriptan was given during organogenesis at doses ranging from about 1.2 to 12 times the maximum recommended human daily dose of 80 mg based on body surface area (MRHDD). At 12 times the MRHDD, fetal weights were decreased and the incidence of vertebral and sternebral variations were increased, but this dose was also maternal toxic (decreased body weight gain during pregnancy). The no-effect-dose for developmental toxicity in rats was about 4 times the MRHDD. When rabbits were administered doses ranging from about 1.2 to 12 times the MRHDD throughout organogenesis, fetal weights were reduced at the highest dose. All doses were associated with increased incidences of fused sternebrae and vena cava deviations. Maternal toxicity was not observed with the doses used. A no-effect-dose for development toxicity in rabbits was not determined (1).

It is not known if eletriptan or its active metabolite crosses the human placenta to the fetus. The molecular weight of the parent compound (about 382 for the free base), however, is low enough that passage to the fetus should be expected. In addition, the moderate protein binding and elimination half-life suggest that the drug will be available for transfer at the maternal-fetal interface.

No reports describing the use of eletriptan in human pregnancy have been located. The animal data are suggestive of moderate risk, but an assessment of the actual risk cannot be determined until human pregnancy experience is available.

BREAST FEEDING SUMMARY

RECOMMENDATION: Compatible

Eletriptan is excreted into human breast milk. In a study conducted by the manufacturer, eight women were given a single oral dose of 80 mg (1). The mean amount of drug recovered from milk over a 24-hour period was approximately 0.02% of the maternal dose. The mean milk:plasma ratio was 1:4, but there was great variability. At 18–24 hours after the dose, the drug was still present in milk in low concentrations (mean 1.7 ng/mL). The active metabolite was not measured in the milk (1).

The effects of this exposure on a nursing infant are unknown. However, the very low concentrations measured in milk suggest that eletriptan is compatible with breast-feeding.

Reference

1. Product information. Relpax. Pfizer, 2004.

Name: **EMTRICITABINE**	Risk Factor: B_M
Class: **Antiviral**	

FETAL RISK SUMMARY

RECOMMENDATION: Compatible - Maternal Benefit >> Embryo/Fetal Risk

Emtricitabine is a synthetic nucleoside analogue reverse transcriptase inhibitor. It is indicated, in combination with other antiretroviral agents, for the treatment of human immunodeficiency virus type 1 (HIV-1) infections. Emtricitabine is in the same antiviral class as abacavir, didanosine, lamivudine, stavudine, tenofovir, zalcitabine, and zidovudine. Plasma protein binding of emtricitabine is <4% and the plasma elimination half-life is about 10 hours (1).

Reproduction studies have been conducted in mice, rats, and rabbits. In mice and rabbits, no evidence of fetal variations or congenital malformations was observed at systemic exposures (AUC_{0-24}) about 60 and 120 times, respectively, the human exposure at the recommended human daily dose of 200 mg based on AUC_{0-24} (HE). Fertility was normal in mice offspring exposed *in utero* through sexual maturity at about 60 times the HE. In addition, no effects on fertility were observed in male rats exposed to about 140 times the HE, or in male and female mice exposed to about 60 times the HE (1,2).

Emtricitabine crosses the placenta to the fetus in mice and rabbits. The average fetal plasma:maternal plasma ratio was about 0.40 in mice and 0.50 in rabbits (2). The placental passage is consistent with the relatively low molecular weight (about 247), low plasma protein binding, and long plasma elimination half-life of the antiviral. These factors suggest also that the agent will cross the human placenta.

The Antiretroviral Pregnancy Registry reported, for the period January 1989 through January 2004, prospective data (reported to the Registry before the outcomes were known) involving 1537 live births who had been exposed during the 1st trimester to one or more antiretroviral agents (3). Forty-seven of the newborns had congenital defects (3.1%, 95% confidence interval [CI] 2.3–4.1). In the 2407 live births with earliest exposure in the 2nd/3rd trimesters, there were 56 infants with defects (2.3%, 95% CI 1.8–3.0). The prevalence rates for the two periods did not differ significantly. There were 103 infants with birth defects among 3944 live births with exposure anytime during pregnancy (2.6%, 95% CI 2.1–3.2). The prevalence rate did not differ significantly from the rate expected in a nonexposed population (3). There were seven outcomes exposed to emtricitabine in the 1st trimester in combination with other antiretroviral agents. There were no birth defects in this group. In reviewing the birth defects of prospective and retrospective (pregnancies reported after the outcomes were known) registered cases, and clinical reports, the Registry concluded that there was no pattern of anomalies to suggest a common cause (3). (See Lamivudine for required statement.)

No reports, other than the data above, describing the use of emtricitabine in human pregnancy have been located. Although the animal data are suggestive of low risk, the absence of human pregnancy experience prevents an assessment of the embryo/fetal risk. Animal data suggest that substantial amounts of the agent will cross the placenta to the fetus. Past reviewers concluded that all women currently receiving antiretroviral therapy should continue to receive therapy during pregnancy (4–6). Discontinuing all therapy, however, until after 10–12 weeks' gestation is an option (6,7). If indicated, therefore, emtricitabine should not be withheld in pregnancy, except possibly in the 1st trimester, because the expected benefit for the HIV-positive mother appears to outweigh the unknown risks to the fetus. The efficacy and safety of combined therapy in preventing vertical transmission of HIV to the newborn, however, are unknown, and zidovudine remains the only antiretroviral agent recommended for this purpose (7).

BREAST FEEDING SUMMARY

RECOMMENDATION: Contraindicated

No reports describing the use of emtricitabine during human lactation have been located. The relatively low molecular weight (about 247), low plasma protein binding (<4%), and long plasma elimination half-life (about 10 hours) suggest that the agent will be excreted into human breast milk. The effects of this exposure on a nursing infant are unknown.

However, reports on the use of emtricitabine during lactation are unlikely because the drug is indicated in the treatment of patient's with HIV infection. HIV type 1 (HIV-1) is transmitted in milk, and in developed countries, breast-feeding is not recommended (4,5,8–11). In developing countries, breast-feeding is undertaken, despite the risk, because there are no affordable milk substitutes available.

References

1. Product information. Emtriva. Gilead Sciences, 2004.
2. Szczech GM, Wang LH, Walsh JP, Rousseau FS. Reproductive toxicology profile of emtricitabine in mice and rabbits. Reprod Toxicol 2003;17:95–108.
3. Antiretroviral Pregnancy Registry Steering Committee. *Antiretroviral Pregnancy Registry International Interim Report for 1 January 1989 through 31 January 2004*. Wilmington, NC: Registry Coordinating Center, 2004.
4. Carpenter CCJ, Fischi MA, Hammer SM, Hirsch MS, Jacobsen DM, Katzenstein DA, Montaner JSG, Richman DD, Saag MS, Schooley RT, Thompson MA, Vella S, Yeni PG, Volberding PA. Antiretroviral therapy for HIV infection in 1996. JAMA 1996;276:146–54.
5. Minkoff H, Augenbraun M. Antiretroviral therapy for pregnant women. Am J Obstet Gynecol 1997;176:478–89.
6. Centers for Disease Control and Prevention. Public Health Service Task Force recommendations for the use of antiretroviral drugs in pregnant women infected with HIV-1 for maternal health and for reducing perinatal HIV-1 transmission in the United States. MMWR 1998;47:No. RR-2.
7. Public Health Service Task Force Perinatal HIV Guidelines Working Group. Summary of the updated recommendations from the Public Health Service Task Force to reduce perinatal human immunodeficiency virus-1 transmission in the United States. Obstet Gynecol 2002;99:1117–26.
8. Brown ZA, Watts DH. Antiviral therapy in pregnancy. Clin Obstet Gynecol 1990;33:276–89.
9. de Martino M, Tovo P-A, Pezzotti P, Galli L, Massironi E, Ruga E, Floreea F, Plebani A, Gabiano C,

Zuccotti GV. HIV-1 transmission through breast-milk: appraisal of risk according to duration of feeding. AIDS 1992;6:991–7.
10. Van de Perre P. Postnatal transmission of human immunodeficiency virus type 1: the breast-feeding dilemma. Am J Obstet Gynecol 1995;173: 483–7.
11. American College of Obstetricians and Gynecologists. Breastfeeding: Maternal and infant aspects. *Educational Bulletin*. No. 258, July 2000.

Name:	**ENALAPRIL**	Risk Factor:	**C_M***
Class:	**Antihypertensive**		

FETAL RISK SUMMARY

RECOMMENDATION: Human Data Suggest Risk in 2nd and 3rd Trimesters

Enalapril, a competitive inhibitor of angiotensin I-converting enzyme (ACE inhibitor), is used for the treatment of hypertension (see also Captopril). Following oral administration, the prodrug enalapril is bioactivated by hydrolysis to the active agent, enalaprilat. Use of the drug in pregnant rats produced fetal growth retardation and, in two fetuses, incomplete skull ossification (1).

Enalaprilat crosses the human placenta. In an *in vitro* experiment using a human placental lobe, enalaprilat crossed from to the fetal side with a mean transfer of 2.99% (2). The maximum concentration on the fetal side was about 20–48 ng/mL.

A number of references on the use of enalapril during pregnancy have appeared (3–22). A 1991 review summarized the cases of enalapril-exposed pregnancies published prior to January 1, 1990 (23). Use of enalapril limited to the 1st trimester does not appear to present a significant risk to the fetus, but fetal exposure after this time has been associated with teratogenicity and severe toxicity in the fetus and newborn, including death. Of interest, an apparent autosomal recessive syndrome of renal tubular dysplasia with fetal/neonatal anuric renal failure, intrauterine growth retardation, and skull ossification defects, but without exposure to ACE inhibitors, has been described in five infants from two separate kindreds (24).

In a surveillance study of Michigan Medicaid recipients conducted between 1985 and 1992 involving 229,101 completed pregnancies, 40 newborns had been exposed to enalapril during the 1st trimester (F. Rosa, personal communication, FDA, 1993). Four (10.0%) major birth defects were observed (two expected), including (observed/expected) 2/0.4 cardiovascular defects, and 1/0.1 polydactyly. No anomalies were observed in four other categories of defects (oral clefts, spina bifida, limb reduction defects, and hypospadias) for which specific data were available.

A European survey on the use of ACE inhibitors in pregnancy briefly reviewed the results obtained in nine mother-child pairs (3). Two spontaneous abortions occurred: one at 7 weeks in a 44-year-old woman and one at 11 weeks in a 41-year-old diabetic patient. Enalapril, 20 mg/day, had been used from conception until abortion in the first case and from conception until 6 weeks' gestation in the second. In both cases, factors other than the drug therapy were probably responsible for the pregnancy losses. In a third case, enalapril (30 mg/day) was started at 24 weeks; the patient, with severe glomerulopathy, delivered a stillborn infant 2 weeks later. It is not known whether enalapril therapy was associated with the adverse outcome. The remaining six women were being treated at the time of conception with 10–20 mg/day for essential hypertension or lupus-induced hypertension. Therapy was discontinued by 7 weeks' gestation in four pregnancies, and at 28 weeks in one, and enalapril was continued throughout gestation (40 weeks) in one.

Two infants were small for gestational age; one had been exposed only during the first 4 weeks, and one was exposed throughout (40 weeks). No anomalies were mentioned, nor were any other problems in the exposed liveborn infants. The growth retardation was probably a result of the severe maternal disease (3).

A 1988 case report described a woman with pregnancy-induced hypertension who was treated with methyldopa and verapamil for 6 weeks with poor control of her blood pressure (4). At 32 weeks' gestation, methyldopa was discontinued and enalapril (20 mg/day) was combined with verapamil (360 mg/day), resulting in good control. An elective cesarean section was performed after 17 days of combination therapy. Oligohydramnios was noted, as was meconium staining. The 2100-g female infant was anuric during the first 2 days, although tests indicated normal kidneys without obstruction. A renal biopsy showed hyperplasia of the juxtaglomerular apparatus. She began producing urine on the 3rd day (2 mL within a period of 24 hours), 12 hours after the onset of peritoneal dialysis. She remained oliguric when dialysis was stopped at age 10 days, producing only 30 mL of urine in a period of 24 hours. By the 19th postnatal day, her urine output had reached 125 mL/24 hours. The plasma enalaprilat concentration was 28 ng/mL before dialysis and then fell to undetectable (<0.16 ng/mL) levels after dialysis. Angiotensin-converting enzyme levels (normal 95 nmol/mL minute) were <1 (days 2 and 3), 2.1 (day 5), 15.6 (day 8), 127 (day 31), and >130 (day 90). Angiotensin II concentrations (normal 182 fmol/mL) were still suppressed (39.8) on day 31; plasma renin activity, active renin, and total renin were all markedly elevated until day 90. By this time, renal function had returned to normal. Clinical follow-up at 1 year of age was normal (4).

A renal transplant patient was treated with enalapril, azathioprine, atenolol, and prednisolone (doses not given) throughout pregnancy (5). Ultrasound at 32 weeks' gestation indicated oligohydramnios and asymmetrical growth retardation. A 1280-g (10th percentile) male infant with a head circumference of 25.7 cm (3rd percentile) was delivered by cesarean section. Severe hypotension (mean 25 mm Hg), present at birth, was resistant to volume expansion and pressor agents. The newborn was anuric for 72 hours, then oliguric, passing only 2.5 mL during the next 36 hours. Ultrasonography revealed a normal-sized kidney and a normal urinary tract. Peritoneal dialysis was commenced on day 8, but the infant died 2 days later. Defects secondary to oligohydramnios were squashed facies, contractures of the extremities, and pulmonary hypoplasia. Ossification of the occipital skull was absent. A chromosomal abnormality was excluded based on a normal male karyotype (46,XY). The renal failure and skull hypoplasia were probably caused by enalapril (5).

A 24-year-old woman with malignant hypertension and familial hypophosphatemic rickets was treated from before conception with enalapril (10 mg/day), furosemide (40 mg/day), calciferol, and slow phosphate (6). Blood pressure was normal at 15 weeks' gestation as was fetal growth. However, oligohydramnios developed 2 weeks later; by 20 weeks' gestation, virtually no fluid was present. Fetal growth retardation was also evident at this time. Enalapril and furosemide therapy were slowly replaced by labetalol over the next week, and a steady improvement in amniotic fluid volume was noted by 24 weeks. Volume was normal at 27 weeks' gestation, but shortly thereafter, abruptio placentae occurred, requiring an emergency cesarean section. A 720-g (below 3rd percentile) male infant was delivered who died on day 6. A postmortem examination indicated a normal urogenital tract (6).

An 18-year-old woman with severe chronic hypertension had four pregnancies over an approximately 4-year period, all while taking ACE inhibitors and other antihypertensives (7). During her first pregnancy, she had been maintained on captopril and she delivered a premature, growth-retarded, but otherwise healthy female infant who survived. In the postpartum period, captopril was discontinued and enalapril (10 mg/day) was started while continuing atenolol (100 mg/day) and nifedipine (40 mg/day). She next presented in the 13th week of her second pregnancy with unchanged antihypertensive therapy. Fetal death occurred at 18 weeks' gestation. The 340-g male fetus was macerated but otherwise normal. Her third and fourth pregnancies, again with basically unchanged antihypertensive therapy except for the addition of aspirin (75 mg/day) at the 10th week, resulted in the delivery of an 1170-g female and a 1540-g male, both at 29 weeks (7).

The case of a 27-year-old woman with scleroderma renal disease who was treated with both enalapril and captopril at different times in her pregnancy was published in 1989 (8). Treatment with enalapril (10 mg/day) and nifedipine (60 mg/day) had begun approximately 4 years before the woman presented at an estimated 29 weeks' gestation. Because of concerns for the potential fetal harm induced by the current treatment, therapy was changed to methyldopa. This agent failed to control the woman's hypertension and therapy with captopril (150 mg/day) was initiated at approximately 33 weeks' gestation, 4 weeks prior to delivery of a normal male infant weighing 1740 g. No evidence of renal impairment was observed in the infant (8).

A woman with active systemic lupus erythematosus became severely hypertensive at 22 weeks' gestation (9). Therapy included prednisone, phenytoin (for one episode of tonic clonic seizure activity), and the antihypertensive agents enalapril, hydralazine (used only briefly), clonidine, nitroprusside, nifedipine, and propranolol. A 600-g male infant with hyaline membrane disease was delivered by cesarean section at 26 weeks' gestation. Severe, persistent hypotension (mean blood pressure during first 24 hours was 18–23 mm Hg) that was resistant to volume expansion and dopamine was observed. Both kidneys were normal by ultrasonography but no urine was visualized in the bladder. The infant died on the 7th day. Gross and microscopic examination of the kidneys at autopsy revealed no abnormalities. Nephrogenesis was appropriate for gestational age (9).

A 1710-g male infant, delivered by cesarean section for fetal distress at 35 weeks' gestation, had been exposed to enalapril (20 mg/day) and diazepam (5 mg/day) from the 32nd week of pregnancy for the treatment of maternal hypertension (10). Prior to this, treatment had consisted of a 2-week course of methyldopa and amiloride plus hydrochlorothiazide. Except for a few drops, the growth-retarded infant produced no urine, and peritoneal dialysis was started at 86 hours of age. Renal ultrasonography indicated normal kidneys without evidence of obstruction. Renal function slowly improved following dialysis, but some impairment was still present at 18 months of age (10).

Investigators at the FDA reviewed five cases of enalapril-induced neonatal renal failure, one of which had been published previously in a 1989 report (11). Enalapril doses ranged from 10-45 mg/day. Two of the mothers were treated throughout gestation, one was treated from 27–34 weeks' gestation, and one was treated during the last 3 weeks only. All of the infants required dialysis for anuria. Renal function eventually recovered in two infants, it was still abnormal 1 month after birth in one, and tubular acidosis occurred in the fourth infant 60 days after delivery. Hypotension was reported in three of the four newborns. The authors cautioned that if enalapril was used during pregnancy, then preparations should be made for neonatal hypotension and renal failure (11).

In a 1991 abstract, the FDA investigators updated their previous report on ACE inhibitors and perinatal renal failure by listing a total of 29 cases: 18 were caused by enalapril, 9 captopril, and 2 lisinopril (12). Of the 29 cases, 12 (41%) were fatal (another fatal case was listed but it was apparently not caused by renal failure), 9 recovered, and 8 had persistent renal impairment. Only 2 deaths occurred among dialyzed patients. Two cases of oligohydramnios resolved when therapy was stopped before delivery, but one of the infants was stillborn (12).

A 1990 case report suggested that structural kidney defects may be a consequence of enalapril therapy (13). A 22-year-old mother, with systemic lupus erythematosus and severe chronic hypertension, was treated throughout gestation with enalapril 20 mg/day, propranolol 40 mg/day, and hydrochlorothiazide 50 mg/day. Blood pressure was well controlled on this regimen, and no evidence of active lupus occurred during pregnancy. Normal amniotic fluid volume was documented at 16 weeks' gestation followed by severe oligohydramnios at 27 weeks' gestation. Although normal fetal growth was observed, the male infant was delivered at 34 weeks' gestation by emergency cesarean section because thick meconium was found on amniocentesis. No meconium was found below the vocal cords. The profound neonatal hypotension induced by enalapril required aggressive treatment with fluids and pressor agents. The newborn had the characteristic features of the oligohydramnios sequence. Both kidneys were morphologically normal by renal ultrasonogram, but no urine output was observed, and no urine was found in the bladder. The infant died at about 25 hours of age. Pulmonary hypoplasia, a condition secondary to oligohydramnios, was found at autopsy. Except for their large size, approximately 1.5 times the expected weight, the kidneys were grossly normal with normal vessels and ureters and a contracted bladder. Microscopic examination revealed a number of kidney abnormalities: irregular corticomedullary junctions; glomerular maldevelopment with a decreased number of lobulations in many of the glomeruli, and some congested glomeruli; a reduced number of tubules in the upper portion of the medulla with increased mesenchymal tissue; and tubular distension in the cortex and medulla. The investigators could not determine whether the renal defects were caused by reduced renal blood flow secondary to enalapril, a direct teratogenic effect of the drug, or by an effect of the specific drug combination. However, no renal anomalies have been reported after use of the other two drugs (see Hydrochlorothiazide and Propranolol), and similar renal defects have not been reported as a complication of maternal lupus (13).

Three cases of *in utero* exposure to ACE inhibitors, one of which was enalapril, were reported in a 1992 abstract (14). The infant, delivered at 32 weeks' gestation because of severe oligohydramnios and fetal distress, had growth retardation, hypocalvaria, short limbs, and renal tubular dysplasia. Profound neonatal hypotension and anuria was observed at birth and improved only with dialysis, but the infant died at 9 days of age as a consequence of the renal failure (14).

A woman took enalapril (10 mg/day) and furosemide (80 mg/day) throughout gestation for hypertension and delivered a 2.76-g male infant at 37 weeks' gestation (19). An ultrasound at 20 weeks' had noted oligohydramnios, multicystic kidneys, a small thorax, and no visible bladder. The newborn died a few minutes after birth. Autopsy revealed low set ears, small epicanthic folds, bilateral talipes, a markedly bell-shaped thorax, grossly cystic kidneys, and no apparent normal renal tissue. The karyotype was normal (19).

A 1997 case report described the pregnancy outcome of a woman who was treated with enalapril (20 mg/day) for gestational hypertension from about 28 weeks' gestation to delivery at 36 weeks' (20). Severe oligohydramnios had developed shortly before delivery. The growth retarded, 2000-g male infant had hypocalvaria, anuria, and profound hypotension. Peritoneal dialysis was started at age 3 days. Before dialysis, the serum ACE level was 7.4 μmol/mL (normal 20–30 μmol/mL). After dialysis, the level was 20.5 μmol/mL, whereas enalaprilat concentrations in the infant's serum and dialysate were 6.92 and 3.3 μg/mL, respectively. Blood pressure normalized after 4 days of dialysis but chronic renal failure persisted. At 8 months of age, expansion of the calvarial bones with gradual closing of the fontanelles was evident and development, other than growth, was normal. However, the renal failure had worsened and the infant was on the waiting list for a renal transplant (20).

Ten pregnancies treated with enalapril were reported in a 1997 study of 19 pregnancies exposed to ACE inhibitors (21). Enalapril therapy was stopped in the 1st trimester in eight pregnancies, and at 14 and 15 weeks' gestation, respectively, in the others. No congenital anomalies or renal dysfunction were noted in the 10 neonates (21).

The outcomes of 21 pregnancies exposed to ACE inhibitors between 1991 and 1996 were reported using data from the Danish birth registry (22). Exposure to the agents occurred at a median of 8 weeks' gestation (range 5–15 weeks). No fetal or neonatal complications attributable to the drug therapy were discovered (22).

A 1992 reference described the effects of ACE inhibitors on pregnancy outcome (25). Among 106,813 women enrolled in the Tennessee Medicaid program who delivered either a liveborn or stillborn infant, 19 had taken either enalapril, captopril, or lisinopril during gestation. One newborn, exposed *in utero* to enalapril, was delivered at 29 weeks' gestation for severe oligohydramnios, intrauterine growth retardation, and fetal distress. Gradual resolution of the infant's renal failure occurred following dialysis (25).

Fourteen cases of fetal hypocalvaria or acalvaria were reviewed in a 1991 reference, one of which was caused by enalapril (26). The authors speculated that the underlying pathogenetic mechanism in these cases was fetal hypotension.

In an article examining the teratogenesis of ACE inhibitors, the authors cited evidence linking fetal calvarial hypoplasia with the use of these agents after the 1st trimester (27). They speculated that the mechanism was related to drug-induced oligohydramnios that allowed the uterine musculature to exert direct pressure on the fetal skull. This mechanical insult, combined with drug-induced fetal hypotension, could inhibit peripheral perfusion and ossification of the calvaria (27).

Investigators in a study published in 1992 examined microscopically the kidneys of nine fetuses from chronically hypertensive mothers, one of whom was taking enalapril (28). The researchers concluded that the renal defects associated with ACE inhibitors were a consequence of decreased renal perfusion and are similar to the defects seen in other conditions related to reduced fetal renal blood flow.

The severe enalapril-induced fetal/neonatal renal failure and neonatal hypotension are a consequence of its pharmacologic effect in the fetus (see also Captopril). Two reviews of fetal and newborn renal function, published in 1988, indicated that both renal perfusion and glomerular plasma flow are low during gestation and that high levels of angiotensin II may be physiologically necessary to maintain glomerular filtration at low perfusion pressures (29,30). Enalapril prevents the conversion of angiotensin I to angiotensin II and, thus, may lead to *in utero* renal failure. Because the primary means of removal of the drug is renal, the impairment of this system in the newborn prevents elimination of the drug and its active metabolite, enalaprilat, resulting in prolonged hypotension.

In summary, enalapril and other ACE inhibitors appear to be teratogenic when used in the 2nd and 3rd trimesters, producing fetal hypocalvaria and renal defects. The cause of the defects and other toxicity associated with ACE inhibitors is probably related to fetal hypotension and decreased renal blood flow. The use of enalapril during pregnancy may compromise the fetal renal system and result in severe, and at times fatal, anuria, both in the fetus and in the newborn. Anuria-associated oligohydramnios may produce pulmonary hypoplasia, limb contractures, persistent patent ductus arteriosus, craniofacial deformation, and neonatal death (31,32). Intrauterine growth retardation, prematurity, and severe neonatal hypotension have also been observed after use of these drugs. Because of these effects, some investigators have stated that ACE inhibitors should not be used in pregnancy (31–34). In those cases when enalapril must be used to treat the mother's disease, close monitoring of amniotic fluid levels, and fetal well-being are required. Newborn renal function and blood pressure should also be monitored. If oligohydramnios occurs, stopping the drug may resolve the problem but may not improve infant outcome because of irreversible fetal damage (31). Guidelines for counseling exposed pregnant patients have been published and should be of benefit to health professionals faced with this task (27,31). If enalapril or enalaprilat are used in pregnancy, healthcare professionals are encouraged to call the toll free number (800-670-6126) for information about patient enrollment in the Motherisk study.

[*Risk Factor D_M if used in the 2nd or 3rd trimesters.*]

BREAST FEEDING SUMMARY

RECOMMENDATION: Limited Human Data - Probably Compatible

A study published in 1989 was unable to demonstrate the excretion of enalapril and enalaprilat in breast milk (35). Direct concentrations of enalapril, however, were not measured in this study. Three women, 3–45 days postpartum, were treated with enalapril for hypertension. One woman had chronic glomerulonephritis and slightly impaired renal function and was treated with 5 mg twice daily for 40 days before the study. The other two women, both with essential hypertension and normal renal function, were treated with 10 mg (duration not specified). ACE activity in the serum of the women was markedly depressed 4 hours after treatment with activity dropping from 18.7–24.0 U/mL to 0.4–0.7 U/mL (reference value in controls 28.0 U/mL). ACE activity in milk samples was not affected—11.7–18.6 U/mL before the dose vs. 12.4–15.4 U/mL 4 hours after the dose (reference value in controls 9.1–22.6 U/mL)—indicating that little, if any, of the drug was excreted into milk. Concentrations of enalaprilat in maternal serum ranged from 23.9 to 48.0 ng/mL in the two women with normal renal function and 179 ng/mL in the woman with renal impairment. Milk levels were all <0.2 ng/mL, the level of sensitivity for the assay (35).

In contrast to the above study, concentrations of both enalapril and enalaprilat were measured in a study published in 1991 (36). A woman, 12 months postpartum, had been treated with enalapril (10 mg/day) for essential hypertension for 11 months. Twenty-four hours after her last dose, she was given 10 mg, and milk samples were drawn at 0, 4, 8.75, and 24 hours. Serum samples were also drawn at various times over the next 24 hours. The total amount of the enalapril and enalaprilat measured in the milk over the 24-hour sample period was 81.9 ng and 36.1 ng, respectively. These values corresponded to 1.44 ng/mL and 0.63 ng/mL, respectively. The peak concentration of enalapril, 2.05 ng/mL, occurred in the 4-hour sample, whereas that of enalaprilat, 0.75 ng/mL, occurred in the 8.75-hour sample. When milk levels were compared to serum concentrations at these sampling times, the milk:serum ratios were 0.14 and 0.02, respectively (36).

In a third study, milk and serum concentrations of enalapril and enalaprilat were measured in five women at 0, 4, 6, and 24 hours after a single 20-mg dose (37). The mean maximum milk concentration of enalapril was 1.74 ng/mL, whereas that of enalaprilat was 1.72 ng/mL. No enalapril was measured in the milk of one patient. The milk:serum ratio for the parent compound and the metabolite varied from 0–0.043 and 0.021–0.031, respectively (37).

Based on the above data, the amount of enalapril and enalaprilat that could potentially be ingested by a breast-feeding infant appears to be negligible and is probably clinically insignificant.

The American Academy of Pediatrics classifies enalapril as compatible with breast-feeding (38).

References

1. Valdés G, Marinovic D, Falcón C, Chuaqui R, Duarte I. Placental alterations, intrauterine growth retardation and teratogenicity associated with enalapril use in pregnant rats. Biol Neonate 1992;61:124–30.
2. Reisenberger K, Egarter C, Sternberger B, Eckenberger P, Eberle E, Weissenbacher ER. Placental passage of angiotensin-converting enzyme inhibitors. Am J Obstet Gynecol 1996;174:1450–5.
3. Kreft-Jais C, Plouin P-F, Tchobroutsky C, Boutroy M-J. Angiotensin-converting enzyme inhibitors during pregnancy: a survey of 22 patients given captopril and nine given enalapril. Br J Obstet Gynaecol 1988;95:420–2.
4. Schubiger G, Flury G, Nussberger J. Enalapril for pregnancy-induced hypertension: acute renal failure in a neonate. Ann Intern Med 1988;108:215–6.
5. Mehta N, Modi N. ACE inhibitors in pregnancy. Lancet 1989;2:96.
6. Broughton Pipkin F, Baker PN, Symonds EM. ACE inhibitors in pregnancy. Lancet 1989;2:96–7.
7. Smith AM. Are ACE inhibitors safe in pregnancy? Lancet 1989;2:750–1.
8. Baethge BA, Wolf RE. Successful pregnancy with scleroderma renal disease and pulmonary hypertension in a patient using angiotensin converting enzyme inhibitors. Ann Rheum Dis 1989;48:776–8.
9. Scott AA, Purohit DM. Neonatal renal failure: a complication of maternal antihypertensive therapy. Am J Obstet Gynecol 1989;160:1223–4.
10. Hulton SA, Thomson PD, Cooper PA, Rothberg AD. Angiotensin-converting enzyme inhibitors in pregnancy may result in neonatal renal failure. S Afr Med J 1990;78:673–6.
11. Rosa FW, Bosco LA, Graham CF, Milstien JB, Dreis M, Creamer J. Neonatal anuria with maternal angiotensin-converting enzyme inhibition. Obstet Gynecol 1989;74:371–4.
12. Rosa FW, Bosco L. Infant renal failure with maternal ACE inhibition (abstract 92). Am J Obstet Gynecol 1991;164:273.
13. Cunniff C, Jones KL, Phillipson J, Benirschke K, Short S, Wujek J. Oligohydramnios sequence and renal tubular malformation associated with maternal enalapril use. Am J Obstet Gynecol 1990;162:187–9.
14. Pryde PG, Nugent CE, Sedman AB, Barr M Jr. ACE inhibitor fetopathy (abstract). Am J Obstet Gynecol 1992;166:348.
15. Neerhof MG, Shlossman PA, Poll DS, Ludomirsky A, Weiner S. Idiopathic aldosteronism in pregnancy. Obstet Gynecol 1991;78:489–91.
16. Boutroy M-J. Fetal effects of maternally administered clonidine and angiotensin-converting enzyme inhibitors. Dev Pharmacol Ther 1989;13:199–204.
17. Svensson A, Andersch B, Dahlof B. ACE-hammare i samband med graviditet kan medfora risker for fostret. Lakartidningen 1986;83:699–700.
18. Scanferla F, Coli U, Landini S, et al. Treatment of pregnancy-induced hypertension with ACE inhibitor enalapril (abstract). Clin Exp Hypertens Pregn 1987;B6:45.
19. Thorpe-Beeston JG, Armar NA, Dancy M, Cochrane GW, Ryan G, Rodeck CH. Pregnancy and ACE inhibitors. Br J Obstet Gynaecol 1993,100:692–3.
20. Lavoratti G, Seracini D, Fiorini P, Cocchi C, Materassi M, Donzelli G, Pela I. Neonatal anuria by ACE inhibitors during pregnancy. Nephron 1997;76:235–6.
21. Lip GYH, Churchill D, Beevers M, Auckett A, Beevers DG. Angiotensin-converting-enzyme inhibitors in early pregnancy. Lancet 1997;350:1446–7.
22. Steffensen FH, Nielsen GL, Sorensen HT, Olesen C, Olsen J. Pregnancy outcome with ACE-inhibitor use in early pregnancy. Lancet 1998;351:596.
23. Hanssens M, Keirse MJNC, Vankelecom F, Van Assche FA. Fetal and neonatal effects of treatment with angiotensin-converting enzyme inhibitors in pregnancy. Obstet Gynecol 1991,78:128–35.
24. Kumar D, Moss G, Primhak R, Coombs R. Congenital renal tubular dysplasia and skull ossification defects similar to teratogenic effects of angiotensin converting enzyme (ACE) inhibitors. J Med Genet 1997;34:541–5.
25. Piper JM, Ray WA, Rosa FW. Pregnancy outcome following exposure to angiotensin-converting enzyme inhibitors. Obstet Gynecol 1992;80:429–32.
26. Barr M Jr, Cohen MM Jr. ACE inhibitor fetopathy and hypocalvaria: the kidney-skull connection. Teratology 1991;44:485–95.
27. Brent RL, Beckman DA. Angiotensin-converting enzyme inhibitors, an embryopathic class of drugs with unique properties: information for clinical teratology counselors. Teratology 1991;43:543–6.
28. Martin RA, Jones KL, Mendoza A, Barr M Jr, Benirschke K. Effect of ACE inhibition on the fetal kidney: decreased renal blood flow. Teratology 1992;46: 317–21.
29. Robillard JE, Nakamura KT, Matherne GP, Jose PA. Renal hemodynamics and functional adjustments to postnatal life. Semin Perinatol 1988;12:143–50.
30. Guignard J-P, Gouyon J-B. Adverse effects of drugs on the immature kidney. Biol Neonate 1988;53: 243–52.
31. Barr M Jr. Teratogen update: angiotensin-converting enzyme inhibitors. Teratology 1994;50:399–409.
32. Shotan A, Widerhorn J, Hurst A, Elkayam U. Risks of angiotensin-converting enzyme inhibition during pregnancy: experimental and clinical evidence, potential mechanisms, and recommendations for use. Am J Med 1994;96:451–6.

33. Lindheimer MD, Katz AI. Hypertension in pregnancy. N Engl J Med 1985;313:675–80.
34. Lindheimer MD, Barron WM. Enalapril and pregnancy-induced hypertension. Ann Intern Med 1988;108:911.
35. Huttunen K, Gronhagen-Riska C, Fyhrquist F. Enalapril treatment of a nursing mother with slightly impaired renal function. Clin Nephrol 1989;31:278.
36. Rush JE, Snyder BA, Barrish A, Hichens M. Comment. Clin Nephrol 1991;35:234.
37. Redman CWG, Kelly JG, Cooper WD. The excretion of enalapril and enalaprilat in human breast milk. Eur J Clin Pharmacol 1990;38:99.
38. Committee on Drugs, American Academy of Pediatrics. The transfer of drugs and other chemicals into human milk. Pediatrics 2001;108:776–89.

Name:	**ENCAINIDE**	Risk Factor:	B_M
Class:	**Antiarrhythmic**		

FETAL RISK SUMMARY

RECOMMENDATION: Compatible - Maternal Benefit >> Embryo/Fetal Risk

Encainide is a cardiac agent used for the treatment of ventricular arrhythmias. Neither animal nor human teratogenicity has been observed, but human experience is very limited.

The parent compound and its two active metabolites (more potent than encainide on a per milligram basis), *o*-demethylencainide and 3-methoxy-*o*-demethylencainide, cross the placenta to the fetus (B. D. Quart, personal communication, Bristol-Myers Company, 1988). Concentrations of encainide and its metabolites in fetal plasma have ranged from 30%–300% of simultaneously collected maternal serum levels (B. D. Quart, personal communication, Bristol-Myers Company, 1988). Excessive accumulation of the drug or its metabolites in the fetal plasma apparently does not occur. Amniotic fluid levels of the three compounds in one case were 2–3 times greater than in fetal plasma (B. D. Quart, personal communication, Bristol-Myers Company, 1988).

Encainide has been successfully used to treat a fetal cardiac arrhythmia *in utero*, but a high maternal dose, 50 mg four times a day, was required to control the abnormality (B. D. Quart, personal communication, Bristol-Myers Company, 1988). The gestational age of the fetus was not given nor was the length of therapy. In this case, encainide could not be found in fetal plasma, and concentrations of the two metabolites were less than 100 ng/mL. Very high concentrations of the metabolites were measured in the newborn's first several urine samples.

BREAST FEEDING SUMMARY

RECOMMENDATION: No Human Data - Probably Compatible

Encainide and its active metabolites are excreted in breast milk. In one patient taking 50 mg four times a day, milk levels of encainide and one metabolite, *o*-demethylencainide, were 200–400 ng/mL and 100–200 ng/mL, respectively (B. D. Quart, personal communication, Bristol-Myers Company, 1988). These levels were comparable to maternal peak plasma levels. A third metabolite, 3-methoxy-*o*-demethylencainide, evidently was not produced by the mother because it was not found in her plasma or milk. However, based on animal experiments, it is also expected to cross into the milk if present in the maternal plasma (B. D. Quart, personal communication, Bristol-Myers Company, 1988).

Name:	**ENFLURANE**	Risk Factor:	**B**
Class:	**General Anesthetic**		

E

FETAL RISK SUMMARY

RECOMMENDATION: Limited Human Data - Animal Data Suggest Low Risk

Enflurane, a nonflammable general inhalation anesthetic agent administered via vaporizer, is indicated for the induction and/or maintenance of anesthesia during surgery. It also provides analgesia for vaginal delivery and, in low concentrations, is used to supplement other general anesthetic agents during delivery by cesarean section. Enflurane is in the same class of volatile liquid halogenated agents as desflurane, halothane, isoflurane, methoxyflurane, and sevoflurane. It is closely related chemically to desflurane and isoflurane (1). The blood-gas partition coefficient is 1.9 (1). This is higher (i.e., increased solubility in blood) than either isoflurane (1.46) or desflurane (0.42) (see Desflurane or Isoflurane).

Studies in animals have not revealed evidence of carcinogenic or mutagenic effects. Reproduction studies, conducted in rats and rabbits at doses up to four times the human dose, revealed no evidence of impaired fertility or fetal harm (1).

In a 1981 study with mice, chronic exposure to subanesthetic and anesthetic concentrations of enflurane was evaluated. High exposures, about 100 times greater than the level of human occupational exposure in unscavenged operating rooms, were associated with minor developmental variations (lumbar ribs and increased pelvic cavitation) and defects (cleft palate, minor skeletal and visceral anomalies). The effects were greater than those observed with methoxyflurane, but less than those with halothane (2).

In a second study by the authors of the above report, the effects of four general anesthetic agents were compared in pregnant rats (3). The doses and agents used were nitrous oxide (75%; 0.55 MAC), enflurane (1.65%; 0.75 MAC), halothane (0.8%; 0.75 MAC), and isoflurane (1.05%; 0.75 MAC). (*Note: the minimum alveolar anesthetic concentration [MAC] is the concentration that causes immobility in 50% of patients exposed to a noxious stimulus such as a surgical incision; it represents the* ED_{50} *[4].*) Each agent was administered for 6 hours on each of three consecutive days in one of three gestational periods: pregnancy days 8–10, 11–13, or 14–16. Compared with controls, significantly decreased maternal weight gain was observed in three of the groups (nitrous oxide, isoflurane, and enflurane) after exposure on days 14–16. Exposure on those days resulted in significantly decreased fetal weight in all four groups, and when exposure occurred on days 8–10, in three groups (all except nitrous oxide). Nitrous oxide exposure during days 14–16 resulted in significant increases in total fetal wastage and resorptions (3-fold increases). However, no major or minor teratogenic effects were observed in any of the groups (3).

The teratogenic potential of isoflurane, enflurane, and sevoflurane was studied by evaluating the effect of each agent on the proliferation and differentiation of cells exiting from the G1-phase of the cell cycle (5). The theory behind the study was that normal development during embryogenesis, organogenesis, and histogenesis depended upon the proliferation and differentiative processes of cell migration (5). For example, valproate, a known human teratogen, is a potent G1-phase inhibitor of the *in vitro* proliferation rate at concentrations less than two times the therapeutic plasma concentration. At anesthetic concentrations less than two times the MAC, the antiproliferative potency of the three agents was isoflurane = enflurane >> sevoflurane. However, in the growth-arrested cell population, there was no specific accumulation of any cell cycle phase and no specific effect on the G1 phase. The investigators concluded that the three agents lacked the specific *in vitro* characteristics of valproate (5).

In a 1990 study, mice were exposed for 8 hours to sevoflurane and enflurane combined with three different concentrations of oxygen (6). Both anesthetic agents caused cleft palate, but the incidence was lower than that observed with halothane. Increasing the concentrations of oxygen lowered the incidence of the defect (6).

Reviews have concluded that, in general, inhalational anesthetics are freely transferred to fetal tissues (7,8) and, in most cases, the maternal and fetal concentrations are equivalent (8). The low molecular weight (about 185) and the presence of enflurane in the maternal brain support this assertion.

Two reports described the use of enflurane in 100 women for anesthesia for cesarean section (9,10). No increase in newborn adverse effects was observed.

A small 1983 study compared the neonatal outcomes in four groups (10 patients each) of women receiving general anesthesia for cesarean section: 50% nitrous oxide and 50% oxygen, either alone or combined with 0.5% halothane, 1.0% enflurane, or 0.75% isoflurane (11). One newborn had an Apgar score less than 7 at 1 minute (enflurane group), but all newborns in all groups had scores of 7 or greater at 5 minutes. There were no significant differences between the groups in neonatal neurobehavior assessment 2–4 hours after delivery or in maternal or umbilical blood gas analysis at delivery (11).

In a 1977 *in vitro* study, enflurane was shown to have a statistically significant depressive effect on myometrial strips from non-gravid and gravid uteri (12). Three anesthetic agents, isoflurane, enflurane, and halothane, were studied at three concentrations (0.5, 1.0, and 1.5 MAC). The amount of depression was dose-related for each agent and was similar with all agents (12).

In a study to determine if pregnancy decreases the MAC, enflurane and halothane were administered to 16 women (8 with each agent) scheduled for pregnancy termination at 8–13 weeks' gestation (13). A comparison group of 16 nonpregnant women undergoing laparoscopic sterilization received either enflurane or halothane (8 in each group). In pregnant women, the median MAC of 1.15 volume% (range 0.95–1.25) was less than that in nonpregnant women, 1.65% volume% (range 1.45–1.75) ($p = 0.0007$). The percentage decrease (95% confidence interval) for pregnant women was 30% (24% to 36%). Similar results were found with halothane (13).

Chronic occupational exposure to anesthetic gases in operating rooms during pregnancy has raised concerns that such exposure could cause birth defects and spontaneous abortions (14). The concentration of enflurane in an operating-room environment was stated to 5–46 parts per million (ppm) near the anesthesiologist and 1–8 ppm near the surgeon. A 1988 review cited a number of studies investigating the possible association between occupational exposure to anesthetic gases and adverse pregnancy outcomes (7). The reviewer concluded that serious methodological weaknesses in these studies precluded arriving at a firm conclusion, but a slightly increased risk of miscarriage was a possibility. However, there was no evidence of an association between occupational exposure and congenital anomalies (7).

In a 1982 study, the infants of mothers who had received analgesia before vaginal delivery consisting of either enflurane, nitrous oxide (both mixed with oxygen), or no inhalation agent were evaluated for neurobehavior during the first 24 hours (15). The infants were tested with the Neurologic and Adaptive Capacity Score at 15 minutes, 2 hours, and 24 hours, and with the Early Neonatal Neurobehavioral Scale at 2 and 24 hours. For all groups, scores were the lowest at 2 hours, but no significant differences were measured between the groups (15).

A 2004 study, however, found a significant association between maternal occupational exposure to waste anesthetic gases during pregnancy and developmental deficits in their children, including gross and fine motor ability, inattention/hyperactivity, and IQ performance (see Nitrous Oxide).

In summary, enflurane is teratogenic in mice but not in rats. No reports of its use early in human gestation have been located. The absence of human experience during organogenesis prevents an assessment of the risk for structural anomalies. In addition, general anesthesia usually involves the use of multiple pharmacological agents. Although no teratogenicity has been observed with other halogenated general anesthetic agents, only halothane has 1st trimester human exposure data (see Halothane). Enflurane has been used immediately prior to delivery for analgesia and anesthesia. This use does not appear to affect the newborn any differently than other general anesthetic agents. The uterine effects of enflurane (relaxation and increased blood loss) also appear to be similar to other agents in this class, but the low concentrations used clinically minimize these actions (16). All anesthetic agents can cause depression in the newborn that may last for 24 hours or more but, again, this is lessened by the low doses. The potential reproductive toxicity (spontaneous abortion and infertility) of occupational exposure to halogenated general anesthetic agents has not been adequately studied.

BREAST FEEDING SUMMARY

RECOMMENDATION: No Human Data - Probably Compatible

Although enflurane has been administered during labor and delivery, the effects of this exposure on the infant that begins nursing immediately after birth have not been described. Enflurane is probably excreted into colostrum and milk as suggested by its presence in the maternal blood and its low molecular weight (about 185), but the toxic potential of this exposure for the infant is unknown. However, the risk to a nursing infant from exposure to enflurane via milk is probably very low (17,18). Another halogenated inhalation anesthetic, halothane, is classified as compatible with breast-feeding by the American Academy of Pediatrics (see Halothane).

References

1. Product information. Ethrane. Abbott Laboratories (NZ), 1999.
2. Wharton RS, Mazze RI, Wilson AI. Reproduction and fetal development in mice chronically exposed to enflurane. Anesthesiology 1981;54:505–10.
3. Mazze RI, Fujinaga M, Rice SA, Harris SB, Baden JM. Reproductive and teratogenic effects of nitrous oxide, halothane, isoflurane, and enflurane in Sprague-Dawley rats. Anesthesiology 1986;64:339–44.
4. Trevor AJ, Miller RD. General anesthetics. In Katzung BG, ed. *Basic and Clinical Pharmacology*. 8th ed. New York: McGraw-Hill, 2001:426.
5. O'Leary G, Bacon CL, Odumeru O, Fagan C, Fitzpatrick T, Gallagher HC, Moriarty DC, Regan CM. Antiproliferative actions of inhalational anesthetics: comparisons to the valproate teratogen. Int J Dev Neurosci 2000;18:39–45.
6. Natsume N, Miura S, Sugimoto S, Nakamura T, Horiuchi R, Kondo S, Furukawa H, Inagaki S, Kawai T, Yamada M, Arai T, Hosoda R. Teratogenicity caused by halothane, enflurane, and sevoflurane, and changes depending on O_2 concentration (abstract). Teratology 1990;42:30A.
7. Friedman JM. Teratogen update: anesthetic agents. Teratology 1988;37:69–77.
8. Kanto J. Risk-benefit assessment of anaesthetic agents in the puerperium. Drug Saf 1991;6:285–301.
9. Coleman AJ, Downing JW. Enflurane anesthesia for cesarean section. Anesthesiology 1975;43: 354–7.
10. Dick W, Knoche E, Traub E. Clinical investigations concerning the use of Ethrane for cesarean section. J Perinat Med 1979;7:125–33.
11. Warren TM, Datta S, Ostheimer GW, Naulty JS, Weiss JB, Morrison JA. Comparison of the maternal and neonatal effects of halothane, enflurane, and isoflurane for cesarean section. Anesth Analg 1983;62:516–20.
12. Munson ES, Embro WJ. Enflurane, isoflurane, and halothane and isolated human uterine muscle. Anesthesiology 1977;46:11–4.
13. Chan MTV, Mainland P, Gin T. Minimum alveolar

concentration of halothane and enflurane are decreased in early pregnancy. Anesthesiology 1996;85: 782–6.
14. Corbett TH. Cancer and congenital anomalies associated with anesthetics. Ann N Y Acad Sci 1976;271:58–66.
15. Stefani SJ, Hughes SC, Shnider SM, Levinson G, Abboud TK, Henriksen EH, Williams V, Johnson J. Neonatal neurobehavioral effects of inhalation analgesia for vaginal delivery. Anesthesiology 1982;56: 351–5.
16. Quail AW. Modern inhalational anaesthetic agents: a review of halothane, isoflurane and enflurane. Med J Aust 1989;150:95–102.
17. Lee JJ, Rubin AP. Breast feeding and anaesthesia. Anaesthesia 1993;48:616–25.
18. Spigset O. Anaesthetic agents and excretion in breast milk. Acta Anaesthesiol Scand 1994;38:94–103.

Name:	**ENFUVIRTIDE**	Risk Factor:	**B_M**
Class:	**Antiviral**		

FETAL RISK SUMMARY

RECOMMENDATION: Compatible - Maternal Benefit >> Embryo/Fetal Risk

Enfuvirtide, a linear 36-amino acid synthetic peptide administered by SC injection, is an inhibitor of the fusion of human immunodeficiency virus type 1 (HIV-1) with CD4+ cells. It is indicated, in combination with other antiretroviral agents, for the treatment of HIV-1 infection in treatment-experienced patients with evidence of HIV-1 replication despite ongoing antiretroviral therapy. Plasma protein binding of enfuvirtide is about 92%, primarily to albumin and, to a lesser extent, to α_1-acid glycoprotein. The agent is thought to undergo catabolism to the constituent amino acids with subsequent recycling of the amino acids in the body pool. The mean elimination half-life is 3.8 hours (1).

Reproduction studies have been conducted in rats and rabbits. In these species, SC doses up to 27 and 3.2 times, respectively, the human dose based on body surface area (HD) revealed no evidence of fetal harm. In male and female rats, SC doses up to 1.6 times the HD had no effect on fertility (1).

It is not known if enfuvirtide crosses the human placenta. The high molecular weight (4492) and protein binding suggest that placental transfer will be inhibited but may not be prevented.

The Antiretroviral Pregnancy Registry reported, for the period January 1989 through January 2004, prospective data (reported to the Registry before the outcomes were known) involving 1537 live births that had been exposed during the 1st trimester to one or more antiretroviral agents (2). Forty-seven of the newborns had congenital defects (3.1%, 95% confidence interval [CI] 2.3–4.1). In the 2407 live births with earliest exposure in the 2nd/3rd trimesters, there were 56 infants with defects (2.3%, 95% CI 1.8–3.0). The prevalence rates for the two periods did not differ significantly. There were 103 infants with birth defects among 3944 live births with exposure anytime during pregnancy (2.6%, 95% CI 2.1–3.2). The prevalence rate did not differ significantly from the rate expected in a nonexposed population (2). The Registry reported no outcomes exposed to enfuvirtide. In reviewing the birth defects of prospective and retrospective (pregnancies reported after the outcomes were known) registered cases, and clinical reports, the Registry concluded that there was no pattern of anomalies to suggest a common cause (2). (See Lamivudine for required statement.)

No reports describing the use of enfuvirtide in human pregnancy have been located. Although the animal data are suggestive of low risk, the absence of human pregnancy experience prevents an assessment of the embryo/fetal risk. Enfuvirtide belongs to a new antiviral class, but past reviewers have concluded that all women currently receiving antiretroviral therapy should continue to receive therapy during pregnancy (3–5). Discontinuing all therapy, however, until after 10–12 weeks' gestation is an option (5,6). If indicated, therefore, enfuvirtide should not be withheld in pregnancy, except possibly in the 1st trimester, because the expected benefit for the HIV-positive mother appears to outweigh the unknown risks to the fetus. The efficacy and safety of combined therapy in preventing vertical transmission of HIV to the newborn, however, are unknown, and zidovudine remains the only antiretroviral agent recommended for this purpose (6).

E

BREAST FEEDING SUMMARY

RECOMMENDATION: Contraindicated

No reports describing the use of enfuvirtide during human lactation have been located. The high molecular weight (4492) and protein binding (92%) should inhibit, but may not prevent, excretion into human breast milk. The effects of this exposure on a nursing infant are unknown. However, enfuvirtide is a 36-amino acid peptide and any amounts that enter milk should be digested by the nursing infant. In addition, reports on the use of enfuvirtide during lactation are unlikely because the drug is indicated in the treatment of patients with HIV infection. HIV type 1 (HIV-1) is transmitted in milk, and in developed countries, breast-feeding is not recommended (3,4,7–10). In developing countries, breast-feeding is undertaken, despite the risk, because there are no affordable milk substitutes available.

References

1. Product information. Fuzeon. Roche Pharmaceuticals, 2004.
2. Antiretroviral Pregnancy Registry Steering Committee. *Antiretroviral Pregnancy Registry International Interim Report for 1 January 1989 through 31 January 2004.* Wilmington, NC: Registry Coordinating Center, 2004.
3. Carpenter CCJ, Fischi MA, Hammer SM, Hirsch MS, Jacobsen DM, Katzenstein DA, Montaner JSG, Richman DD, Saag MS, Schooley RT, Thompson MA, Vella S, Yeni PG, Volberding PA. Antiretroviral therapy for HIV infection in 1996. JAMA 1996;276:146–54.
4. Minkoff H, Augenbraun M. Antiretroviral therapy for pregnant women. Am J Obstet Gynecol 1997;176:478–89.
5. Centers for Disease Control and Prevention. Public Health Service Task Force recommendations for the use of antiretroviral drugs in pregnant women infected with HIV-1 for maternal health and for reducing perinatal HIV-1 transmission in the United States. MMWR 1998;47:No. RR-2.
6. Public Health Service Task Force Perinatal HIV Guidelines Working Group. Summary of the updated recommendations from the Public Health Service Task Force to reduce perinatal human immunodeficiency virus-1 transmission in the United States. Obstet Gynecol 2002;99:1117–26.
7. Brown ZA, Watts DH. Antiviral therapy in pregnancy. Clin Obstet Gynecol 1990;33:276–89.
8. de Martino M, Tovo P-A, Pezzotti P, Galli L, Massironi E, Ruga E, Floreea F, Plebani A, Gabiano C, Zuccotti GV. HIV-1 transmission through breast-milk: appraisal of risk according to duration of feeding. AIDS 1992;6:991–7.
9. Van de Perre P. Postnatal transmission of human immunodeficiency virus type 1: the breast-feeding dilemma. Am J Obstet Gynecol 1995;173:483–7.
10. American College of Obstetricians and Gynecologists. Breastfeeding: Maternal and infant aspects. *Educational Bulletin*. No. 258, July 2000.

Name:	**ENOXACIN**	Risk Factor:	C_M
Class:	**Anti-infective (Quinolone)**		

FETAL RISK SUMMARY

RECOMMENDATION: Human Data Suggest Low Risk

Enoxacin is an oral, synthetic, broad-spectrum antibacterial agent. As a fluoroquinolone, it is in the same class of agents as ciprofloxacin, levofloxacin, lomefloxacin, norfloxacin, ofloxacin, and sparfloxacin. Nalidixic acid is also a quinolone drug.

No effects on fertility were observed in female rats at a dose of 1000 mg/kg, approximately 13 times the maximum human clinical daily dose on a mg/m^2 basis (1). Decreased spermatogenesis and subsequent impaired fertility were observed in male rats at this dose. No evidence of teratogenicity was observed in either mice or rats following administration of oral enoxacin (dose not specified) (1). In pregnant rabbits, however, an intravenous infusion of 10–50 mg/kg enoxacin produced maternal and fetal toxicity, the latter at the highest dose tested (maximum recommended human dose is 800 mg/day, or 16 mg/kg for a 50-kg individual). Fetal toxicity consisted of increased postimplantation loss and stunted fetuses and, in the presence of maternal and fetal toxicity, a significant increase in the incidence of congenital malformations (type not specified). As with other quinolones, multiple doses of enoxacin produced permanent lesions and erosion of cartilage in weight-bearing joints leading to lameness in immature rats and dogs (1).

It is not known if enoxacin crosses the placenta to the human fetus, but the molecular weight (about 320) is low enough that transfer to the fetus should be expected. Only one report describing the use of the antibiotic in human gestation has been located.

In a prospective follow-up study conducted by the European Network of Teratology Information Services (ENTIS), data on 549 pregnancies exposed to fluoroquinolones (1 to enoxacin) were described in a 1996 reference (see Ciprofloxacin for full details of this study) (2). Data on another 116 prospective and 25 retrospective pregnancy exposures to the antibacterials were also included. Of the 666 cases with known outcome, 32 (4.8%) of the embryos, fetuses, or newborns had congenital malformations. None of the outcomes with congenital anomalies had been exposed to enoxacin. Based on previous epidemiologic data, the authors concluded that the 4.8% frequency of malformations did not exceed the published background rate (2). Finally, data on 25 retrospective pregnancies that had been exposed *in utero* to fluoroquinolones were described, but no specific patterns of major congenital malformations were detected.

The authors of the above study concluded that pregnancy exposure to quinolones was not an indication for termination, but that this class of antibacterials should still be considered contraindicated in pregnant women because there were several, safer alternatives that could be used in pregnancy (2). Because of their own and previously published findings, they further recommended that the focus of future studies should be on malformations involving the abdominal wall and urogenital system, and on limb reduction defects. Moreover, this study did not address the issue of cartilage damage from quinolone exposure and the authors recognized the need for follow-up studies of this potential toxicity in children exposed *in utero*.

In summary, only one report describing the use of enoxacin during human gestation has been located, but the available evidence for other members of this class indicates that a causal relationship with birth defects cannot be excluded (see also Ciprofloxacin, Norfloxacin, or Ofloxacin). Because of this and the available animal data, the use of enoxacin during pregnancy, especially during the 1st trimester, should be used with caution. A 1993 review on the safety of fluoroquinolones concluded that these antibacterials should be avoided during pregnancy because of the difficulty in extrapolating animal mutagenicity results to humans and because interpretation of this toxicity is still controversial (3). The authors of this review were not convinced that fluoroquinolone-induced fetal cartilage damage and subsequent arthropathies were a major concern, even though this effect had been demonstrated in several animal species after administration to both pregnant and immature animals and in occasional human case reports involving children (3). Others have also concluded that fluoroquinolones should be considered contraindicated in pregnancy, because safer alternatives are usually available (2).

BREAST FEEDING SUMMARY

RECOMMENDATION: No Human Data - Probably Compatible

When first marketed, the administration of enoxacin during breast-feeding was not recommended because of the potential for arthropathy and other serious toxicity in the nursing infant (1). Phototoxicity has been observed with quinolones, including enoxacin, when exposure to excessive sunlight (i.e., UV light) has occurred (1). Well-differentiated squamous cell carcinomas of the skin has been produced in mice who were exposed chronically to some quinolones and periodic UV light (e.g., see Lomefloxacin), but studies to evaluate the carcinogenicity of enoxacin in this manner have not been conducted.

No reports describing the use of enoxacin in human lactation have been located. The antibacterial is excreted into the milk of lactating rats (1). Other quinolones are excreted into human milk and, because of its relatively low molecular weight (about 320), the passage of enoxacin into milk should be expected. The American Academy of Pediatrics classifies two other fluoroquinolones as compatible with breast-feeding (see Ciprofloxacin and Ofloxacin).

References

1. Product information. Penetrex. Rhône-Poulenc Rorer, 1997.
2. Schaefer C, Amoura-Elefant E, Vial T, Ornoy A, Garbis H, Robert E, Rodriguez-Pinilla E, Pexieder T, Prapas N, Merlob P. Pregnancy outcome after prenatal quinolone exposure. Evaluation of a case registry of the European Network of Teratology Information Services (ENTIS). Eur J Obstet Gynecol Reprod Biol 1996;69:83–9.
3. Norrby SR, Lietman PS. Safety and tolerability of fluoroquinolones. Drugs 1993;45(Suppl 3):59–64.

Name: ENOXAPARIN	Risk Factor: B_M
Class: **Anticoagulant**	

FETAL RISK SUMMARY

RECOMMENDATION: Compatible

Enoxaparin is a low molecular weight heparin (LMWH) product prepared from porcine intestinal mucosa heparin. The anticoagulant is not teratogenic or embryotoxic in rats and rabbits (1).

Enoxaparin has an average molecular weight of about 4500 (1). Because this is a relatively large molecule, it does not cross the placenta (2,3) and, thus, presents a low risk to the fetus.

Several reports have described the use of enoxaparin during pregnancy without maternal or fetal complications (4–15).

A woman with an extensive lower limb venous thrombosis was treated with unfractionated heparin for 2 weeks starting at 11 weeks' gestation and then changed to enoxaparin (4). She was continued on enoxaparin until delivery of a healthy infant at 34 weeks' gestation.

A 1992 reference described the use enoxaparin in six pregnant women for the treatment and prophylaxis of thromboembolism (5). In two women treated from the 8th or 9th gestational week, one ended with a healthy term infant and the other was progressing normally at 18 weeks (outcome was not available at time of the report). Three other women were treated during the 2nd and/or 3rd trimesters and had normal term deliveries. In the remaining case, a woman with Sjögren's syndrome and a history of deep venous thrombosis (DVT) and pulmonary embolism, developed a DVT at 18 weeks' gestation. She was treated for 10 days with IV heparin and then started on enoxaparin 40 mg twice daily. The DVT recurred at 25 weeks' gestation and she was again treated with a course of IV heparin followed by SC heparin. Because of severe fetal distress after 5 days of SC heparin, an emergency cesarean section was performed. The infant died a few minutes after birth, but permission for an autopsy was refused. An examination of the placenta showed multiple hemorrhages (5).

The use of enoxaparin for the achievement of successful thromboprophylaxis in 16 women during 18 pregnancies was described in a 1994 communication (6). The mean gestational age at the start of therapy was 10 weeks. Eight women had a history of thromboembolism, six had thrombophilia, and two had systemic lupus erythematosus. A 20 mg SC dose once daily was used in the first 11 women, but because of low anti-factor Xa levels, the dose was increased to 40 mg SC once daily in the last 7 pregnancies. From the 18 pregnancies, there were 2 missed abortions and 2 mid-trimester abortions, all in pregnancies of women with anticardiolipin syndrome (6).

The thromboprophylaxis of 41 pregnancies (34 women), most with 40 mg enoxaparin SC daily, was described in a 1996 report (7). Some of these cases had been reported earlier in a 1995 abstract (8). Only one thromboembolic event occurred, a hepatic infarction in a woman treated with 20 mg/day SC. No maternal hemorrhages were observed even though the therapy was continued throughout labor, delivery, and the immediate postpartum period. Nineteen of the women underwent 24 surgical procedures while receiving enoxaparin, including cervical cerclage ($N = 2$), amniocentesis ($N = 5$), 2nd trimester terminations ($N = 4$), and cesarean section ($N = 13$). Epidural anesthesia during labor was used in nine women. No abnormal bleeding was observed in any of these cases and there were no reports of intraventricular hemorrhage in the neonates (7).

Enoxaparin, usually 40 mg SC daily starting in the 1st trimester, was used for prophylaxis in 61 women (69 pregnancies) at high risk for thromboembolism in a prospective study published in 1997 (9). Some of these patients ($N = 18$) had been reported earlier (6). Mean steady-state plasma heparin levels, as determined by anti-factor Xa assay, following a 40 mg dose were three times as high as those with 20 mg, 0.09 U/mL vs. 0.03 U/mL, respectively, but were not affected by gestational age. No increased bleeding risk during pregnancy was observed and no episodes of thromboembolism in pregnancy occurred, although one patient, treated with 20 mg, had a postpartum pulmonary embolus. Furthermore, no cases of epidural hematomas were observed in the 43 patients receiving regional analgesia or anesthesia. Six pregnancy losses were recorded, four described earlier (6) and two new cases of fetal deaths at 18 and 26 weeks, both in women with lupus anticoagulant and previous fetal loss. Other than seven preterm deliveries, none of which were attributable to drug therapy, the remaining fetal and newborn outcomes were normal. Decreased bone density after delivery (lumbar spine or hip; 1 SD below the mean for nonpregnant age-matched women) was measured in 9 of 26 women after 28 pregnancies.

In seven of these cases, unfractionated heparin had been used previously. Based on other published studies, the investigators could not determine whether the low bone density was present before treatment with enoxaparin, or if it was caused by pregnancy and breast feeding, but a previous study with another LMWH (see Dalteparin) found no effect on bone density (9).

A 1997 case report described the use of enoxaparin (dose not specified) throughout most of the gestation, including labor, in a woman with congenital hypofibrinogenemia and protein S deficiency (10). A male infant with hypofibrinogenemia was delivered by cesarean section at 38 week's gestation.

A number of other studies (11–15) and reviews (3,16–22) have described the safe use of enoxaparin and other LMWH agents during pregnancy. Use of LMWH within 2 hours prior to cesarean section, however, was associated with an increase in wound hematoma (23). Also, lower maximum enoxaparin concentrations and anti-factor Xa activity levels occur during pregnancy compared to the nonpregnant state, thus requiring dose adjustments (24).

In summary, the use of enoxaparin during pregnancy appears to present no more fetal and/or newborn risk, and perhaps less, than that from standard, unfractionated heparin or from no therapy. An opinion of the American College of Obstetricians and Gynecologists (ACOG) states that LMWH is at least as effective in pregnant patients with venous thrombosis, pulmonary embolism, or thrombophilic disorders as unfractionated heparin (25). Moreover, LMWHs have the advantages of ease of administration and less frequent laboratory monitoring. LMWHs may also reduce maternal complications, compared to standard heparin, such as bleeding, osteoporosis, and thrombocytopenia (3). However, there is inadequate information to recommend the use of LMWH in a pregnant woman with a mechanical heart valve (25).

BREAST FEEDING SUMMARY

RECOMMENDATION: Compatible

No reports describing the use of enoxaparin during lactation have been located. However, because of the relatively high molecular weight of this drug and its inactivation in the gastrointestinal tract if it was ingested orally, its passage into milk and subsequent risk to a nursing infant should be considered negligible.

References

1. Product information. Lovenox. Rhone-Poulenc Rorer, 1993.
2. Nelson-Piercy C. Low molecular weight heparin for obstetric thromboprophylaxis. Br J Obstet Gynaecol 1994;101:6–8.
3. American College of Obstetricians and Gynecologists. Thromboembolism in pregnancy. *ACOG Practice Bulletin*. No. 19, August 2000.
4. Priollet P, Roncato M, Aiach M, Housset E, Poissonnier MH, Chavinie J. Low-molecular-weight heparin in veinous thrombosis during pregnancy. Br J Haematol 1986;63:605–6.
5. Gillis S, Shushan A, Eldor A. Use of low molecular weight heparin for prophylaxis and treatment of thromboembolism in pregnancy. Int J Gynecol Obstet 1992;39:297–301.
6. Sturridge F, de Swiet M, Letsky E. The use of low molecular weight heparin for thromboprophylaxis in pregnancy. Br J Obstet Gynaecol 1994;101:69–71.
7. Dulitzki M, Pauzner R, Langevitz P, Pras M, Many A, Schiff E. Low-molecular-weight heparin during pregnancy and delivery: preliminary experience with 41 pregnancies. Obstet Gynecol 1996;87:380–3.
8. Dulitzki M, Seidman DS, Sivan E, Horowitz A, Barkai G, Schiff E. Low-molecular-weight heparin in pregnancy and delivery: experience with 24 cases. Society of Perinatal Obstetricians Abstracts. Am J Obstet Gynecol 1995;172:363.
9. Nelson-Piercy C, Letsky EA, de Swiet M. Low-molecular-weight heparin for obstetric thromboprophylaxis: experience of sixty-nine pregnancies in

sixty-one women at high risk. Am J Obstet Gynecol 1997;176:1062–8.
10. Funai EF, Klein SA, Lockwood CJ. Successful pregnancy outcome in a patient with both congenital hypofibrinogenemia and protein S deficiency. Obstet Gynecol 1997;89:858.
11. Casele H, Laifer S. Prospective evaluation of bone density changes in pregnant women on low molecular weight heparin (abstract). Am J Obstet Gynecol 1998;178:S65.
12. Laifer SA, Stiller RJ, Dunston-Boone G, Whetham JCG. Low-molecular weight heparin for treatment of pulmonary embolism in a pregnant woman. Thromb Haemost 1999;82:1361–2.
13. Ellison J, Walker ID, Greer IA. Antenatal use of enoxaparin for prevention and treatment of thromboembolism in pregnancy. Br J Obstet Gynaecol 2000;107:1116–21.
14. Magdelaine A, Verdy E, Coulet F, Berkane N, Girot R, Uzan S, Soubrier F. Deep vein thrombosis during enoxaparin prophylactic treatment in a young pregnant woman homozygous for factor V Leiden and heterozygous for the G127-A mutation in the thrombomodulin gene. Blood Coagul Fibrinolysis 2000;11:761–5.
15. Younis JS, Ohel G, Brenner B, Haddad S, Lanir N, Ben-Ami M. The effect of thrombophylaxis on pregnancy outcome in patients with recurrent pregnancy loss associated with factor V Leiden mutation. Br J Obstet Gynaecol 2000;107:415–9.
16. Schulman S. Long-term prophylaxis in venous thromboembolism: LMWH or oral anticoagulation? Haemostasis 1998;(Suppl 3):17–21.
17. Conard J, Horellou MH, Samama MM. Management of pregnancy in women with thrombophilia. Haemostasis 1999;29(Suppl 1):98–104.
18. Bates SM. Optimal management of pregnant women with acute venous thromboembolism. Haemostasis 1999;29(Suppl 1):107–11.
19. Chan WS, Ray JG. Low molecular weight heparin use during pregnancy: issues of safety and practicality. Obstet Gynecol Sur 1999;54:649–54.
20. Robin F, Lecuru F, Desfeux P, Boucaya V, Taurelle R. Anticoagulant therapy in pregnancy. Eur J Obstet Gynecol Reprod Biol 1999;83:171–7.
21. Sanson BJ, Lensing AWA, Prins MH, Ginsberg JS, Barkagan ZS, Lavenne-Pardonge E, Brenner B, Dulitzky M, Nielsen JD, Boda Z, Turi S, MacGillavry MR, Hamulyak K, Theunissen IM, Hunt BJ, Buller HR. Safety of low-molecular-weight heparin in pregnancy: a systematic review. Thromb Haemost 1999;81:668–72.
22. Ensom MHH, Stephenson MD. Low-molecular-weight heparin in pregnancy. Pharmacotherapy 1999;19:1013–25.
23. Wolf H, Piek JMJ, van Wijk FH, Buller HR. Administration of low molecular weight heparin within two hours prior to cesarean section increases the prevalence of wound hematoma (abstract). Am J Obstet Gynecol 2000;182:S158.
24. Casele HL, Laifer SA, Woelkers DA, Venkataramanan R. Changes in the pharmacokinetics of the low-molecular-weight heparin enoxaparin sodium during pregnancy. Am J Obstet Gynecol 1999;181:1113–7.
25. American College of Obstetricians and Gynecologists. Anticoagulation with low-molecular-weight heparin during pregnancy. *Committee Opinion*. No. 211, November 1998.

Name:	**ENTACAPONE**	Risk Factor:	C_M
Class:	**Antiparkinsonian Agent**		

FETAL RISK SUMMARY

RECOMMENDATION: No Human Data - Animal Data Suggest Moderate Risk

Entacapone is indicated as an adjunct to levodopa/carbidopa in patients experiencing end-of-dose "wearing off" effect. The agent is a selective and reversible inhibitor of catechol-*O*-methyltransferase (COMT), an enzyme involved in the metabolism of levodopa. Inhibition of COMT by entacapone allows for more sustained plasma levels of levodopa resulting in greater beneficial effects on the signs and symptoms of Parkinson's disease. Entacapone is nearly completely metabolized and elimination is biphasic with elimination half-life's of 0.4–0.7 hours (β-phase; serum) and 2.4 hours (γ-phase; tissue) (1).

Entacapone did not impair fertility or general reproductive performance in rats at doses producing systemic exposures up to 28 times the human exposure based on AUC from a maximum recommended daily dose of 1600 mg (HE-MRDD), but did delay mating at the highest dose. In addition, entacapone was mutagenic and clastogenic in one *in vitro* mouse assay but not in other assays (1).

Reproduction tests have been conducted in rats and rabbits. In pregnant rats treated during organogenesis, systemic exposure 34 times the HE-MRDD, without producing overt maternal toxicity, caused increased incidences of variations in fetal development. There was no evidence of impaired development in the offspring when this dose was given during late gestation and throughout lactation. When doses producing systemic exposures 7 times the HE-MRDD or greater were given before mating and during early gestation, an increased incidence of fetal eye anomalies (microphthalmia, anophthalmia) was observed. In pregnant rabbits, systemic exposure 0.4 times the HE-MRDD or greater during organogenesis resulted in increased incidences of abortions, late/total resorptions, and decreased fetal weights. However, these doses were maternal toxic in rabbits. No teratogenic effects were observed in rabbits (1).

Although entacapone is always combined with levodopa/carbidopa, and levodopa is known to cause fetal toxicity and visceral and skeletal malformations in rabbits (see Levodopa), the potential reproductive toxicity and teratogenicity of combined entacapone-levodopa/carbidopa has not been studied in animals (1).

It is not known if entacapone crosses the human placenta to the fetus. The molecular weight (about 305), however, is low enough that embryo and fetal exposure probably occur, but the short elimination half-life will limit the degree of exposure.

No reports describing the use entacapone in human pregnancy have been located. The drug is teratogenic in rats at plasma exposures close to those observed in humans, but no teratogenicity was seen in rabbits. Entacapone is always used with levodopa/carbidopa and, although the data are very limited, these latter agents do not appear to present a major risk to the human fetus. (See Levodopa). Moreover, conditions requiring the use of levodopa/carbidopa during the childbearing years are relatively uncommon and, thus, the use of entacapone should also be uncommon. Although the lack of human pregnancy experience prevents an assessment of the risk to an embryo or fetus, inadvertent exposure to entacapone during early gestation does not appear to represent a significant risk and should not be a reason for pregnancy termination.

BREAST FEEDING SUMMARY

RECOMMENDATION: No Human Data - Potential Toxicity

No reports describing the use of entacapone during human lactation have been located. The drug is excreted into the milk of lactating rats (1). The molecular weight (about 305) is low enough that excretion into milk should be expected, but the relatively short elimination half-life should limit the amount in milk. Entacapone is always given with levodopa/carbidopa. Even though levodopa inhibits prolactin release, normal lactation has been reported while women were being treated with the drug, and levodopa is excreted into breast milk. In addition, the effect of entacapone on levodopa metabolism will increase the amount of plasma levodopa available for transfer into milk. The use of carbidopa during lactation has also been described (see Carbidopa). It is also excreted into rat milk but the amount in human milk has not been measured. Therefore, a nursing infant will probably be exposed to all three drugs via the milk. The effects of this multiple exposure on a nursing infant are unknown but warrant investigation.

Reference

1. Product information. Comtan. Novartis Pharmaceuticals, 2003.

Name:	**EPHEDRINE**	Risk Factor:	**C**
Class:	**Sympathomimetic (Adrenergic)**		

E

FETAL RISK SUMMARY

RECOMMENDATION: Compatible

Ephedrine is a sympathomimetic used widely for bronchial asthma, allergic disorders, hypotension, and the alleviation of symptoms caused by upper respiratory infections. It is a common component of proprietary mixtures containing antihistamines, bronchodilators, and other ingredients. Thus it is difficult to separate the effects of ephedrine on the fetus from other drugs, disease states and viruses. Ephedrine-like drugs are teratogenic in some animal species, but human teratogenicity has not been suspected (1,2).

The Collaborative Perinatal Project monitored 50,282 mother-child pairs, 373 of whom had 1st trimester exposure to ephedrine (3, pp. 345–356). For use anytime during pregnancy, 873 exposures were recorded (3, p. 439). No evidence for a relationship to large categories of major or minor malformations or to individual defects was found. However, an association in the 1st trimester was found between the sympathomimetic class of drugs as a whole and minor malformations (not life-threatening or major cosmetic defects), inguinal hernia, and clubfoot (3, pp. 345–356).

Ephedrine is routinely used to treat or prevent maternal hypotension following spinal anesthesia (4–7). Significant increases in fetal heart rate and beat-to-beat variability may occur, but these effects may have been the result of normal reflexes following hypotension-associated bradycardia. A recent study, however, has demonstrated the placental passage of ephedrine with fetal levels at delivery approximately 70% of the maternal concentration (8). The presence of ephedrine in the fetal circulation is probably a major cause of the fetal heart rate changes.

BREAST FEEDING SUMMARY

RECOMMENDATION: Limited Human Data - Potential Toxicity

A single case report has been located describing adverse effects in a 3-month-old nursing infant of a mother consuming a long-acting preparation containing 120 mg of *d*-isoephedrine and 6 mg of dexbrompheniramine (9). The mother had begun taking the preparation on a twice daily schedule 1 or 2 days prior to onset of the infant's symptoms. The infant exhibited irritability, excessive crying, and disturbed sleeping patterns that resolved spontaneously within 12 hours when breast-feeding was stopped.

References

1. Nishimura H, Tanimura T. *Clinical Aspects of The Teratogenicity of Drugs*. New York, NY: American Elsevier, 1976:231.
2. Shepard TH. *Catalog of Teratogenic Agents*. 3rd ed. Baltimore, MD: Johns Hopkins University Press, 1980: 134–5.
3. Heinonen OP, Slone D, Shapiro S. *Birth Defects and Drugs in Pregnancy*. Littleton, MA: Publishing Sciences Group, 1977.
4. Wright RG, Shnider SM, Levinson G, Rolbin SH, Parer JT. The effect of maternal administration of ephedrine on fetal heart rate and variability. Obstet Gynecol 1981;57:734–8.
5. Antoine C, Young BK. Fetal lactic acidosis with

epidural anesthesia. Am J Obstet Gynecol 1982;142:55–9.
6. Datta S, Alper MH, Ostheimer GW, Weiss JB. Method of ephedrine administration and nausea and hypotension during spinal anesthesia for cesarean section. Anesthesiology 1982;56:68–70.
7. Antoine C, Young BK. Fetal lactic acidosis with epidural anesthesia. Am J Obstet Gynecol 1982;142:55–9.
8. Hughes SC, Ward MG, Levinson G, Shnider SM, Wright RG, Gruenke LD, Craig JC. Placental transfer of ephedrine does not affect neonatal outcome. Anesthesiology 1985;63:217–9.
9. Mortimer EA Jr. Drug toxicity from breast milk? Pediatrics 1977;60:780–1.

E

Name: **EPINEPHRINE** Risk Factor: **C**

Class: **Sympathomimetic (Adrenergic)**

FETAL RISK SUMMARY

RECOMMENDATION: Human Data Suggest Risk

Epinephrine is a sympathomimetic that is widely used for conditions such as shock, glaucoma, allergic reactions, bronchial asthma, and nasal congestion. Because it occurs naturally in all humans, it is difficult to separate the effects of its administration from effects on the fetus induced by endogenous epinephrine, other drugs, disease states, and viruses.

The drug readily crosses the placenta (1). Epinephrine is teratogenic in some animal species, but human teratogenicity has not been suspected (2,3). The Collaborative Perinatal Project monitored 50,282 mother-child pairs, 189 of whom had 1st trimester exposure to epinephrine (4, pp. 345–356). For use anytime during pregnancy, 508 exposures were recorded (4, p. 439). A statistically significant association was found between 1st trimester use of epinephrine and major and minor malformations. An association was also found with inguinal hernia after both 1st trimester and anytime use (4, pp. 477, 492). Although not specified, these data may reflect the potentially severe maternal status for which epinephrine administration is indicated.

In a surveillance study of Michigan Medicaid recipients conducted between 1985 and 1992 involving 229,101 completed pregnancies, 35 newborns had been exposed to epinephrine (route not specified) during the 1st trimester (F. Rosa, personal communication, FDA, 1993). No major birth defects were observed (1.5 expected).

Theoretically, epinephrine's α-adrenergic properties might lead to a decreased in uterine blood flow. A large intravenous dose of epinephrine, 1.5 mL of a 1:1000 solution during a 1-hour period to reverse severe hypotension secondary to an allergic reaction, may have contributed to intrauterine anoxic insult to a 28-week-old fetus (5). Decreased fetal movements occurred after treatment and the infant, delivered at 34 weeks' gestation, had evidence of intracranial hemorrhage at birth and died 4 days later. Thus, in situations such as maternal hypotension where a pressor agent is required, use of ephedrine may be a better choice.

BREAST FEEDING SUMMARY

RECOMMENDATION: No Human Data - Potential Toxicity

No data are available.

References

1. Morgan CD, Sandler M, Panigel M. Placental transfer of catecholamines in vitro and in vivo. Am J Obstet Gynecol 1972;112:1068–75.
2. Nishimura H, Tanimura T. *Clinical Aspects of The Teratogenicity of Drugs*. New York, NY: American Elsevier, 1976:231.
3. Shepard TH. *Catalog of Teratogenic Agents*. 3rd ed. Baltimore, MD: Johns Hopkins University Press, 1980: 134–5.
4. Heinonen OP, Slone D, Shapiro S. *Birth Defects and Drugs in Pregnancy*. Littleton, MA: Publishing Sciences Group, 1977.
5. Entman SS, Moise KJ. Anaphylaxis in pregnancy. S Med J 1984;77:402.

Name: **EPIRUBICIN**	Risk Factor: **D_M**
Class: **Antineoplastic**	

FETAL RISK SUMMARY

RECOMMENDATION: Contraindicated - 1st Trimester

Epirubicin is a cell cycle phase non-specific anthracycline in the same antineoplastic class as daunorubicin, doxorubicin, idarubicin, and valrubicin. It is used as adjuvant therapy in patients with breast cancer. The mechanism of action includes the inhibition of nucleic acid (DNA and RNA), protein synthesis, and DNA helicase activity.

In reproduction studies, epirubicin was embryolethal (increased resorptions and post-implantation loss) in pregnant rats administered an IV dose about 0.04 times the maximum recommended single human dose on a body surface basis (MRHD) during days 5 to 15 of gestation (1). Intrauterine growth retardation (IUGR), but not teratogenicity, was also observed up to this dose. Doses as low as 0.005 times the MRHD resulted in embryo lethality, and IUGR was evident at a dose 0.0015 times the MRHD. At a dose approximately 2.5 times the MRHD given on days 9 and 10 of gestation, fetal deaths, reduced placental weight, and multiple congenital malformations (external: anal atresia, misshapen tail, abnormal genital tubercle; visceral: gastrointestinal, urinary, and cardiovascular systems; skeletal: deformed long bones and girdles, rib abnormalities, irregular spinal ossification) were observed (1). In contrast, a dose 0.02 times the MRHD during days 6 to 18 of gestation in rabbits was not embryotoxic or teratogenic (1). Administration of maternally toxic doses in rabbits caused abortions and delayed ossification, but no teratogenicity. In fertility studies with male and female rats, mice, rabbits, and dogs, various low doses of epirubicin were associated with atrophy of the testes and epididymis, reduced spermatogenesis, or uterine atrophy (1).

It is not known if epirubicin crosses the placenta. The molecular weight (about 580) is low enough, however, that transfer to the human fetus should be expected.

The manufacturer's product information describes two human pregnancies in which epirubicin was administered (1). In the first case, a 34-year-old woman at 28 weeks' gestation, who was diagnosed with breast cancer, was treated with epirubicin and cyclophosphamide every 3 weeks for three cycles. The last dose was given at 34 weeks' gestation and she delivered a healthy baby 1 week later. No follow-up of the infant after birth was mentioned. The second case involved a 34-year-old woman with breast cancer metastatic to the liver who was randomized to the FEC-50 regimen (epirubicin, 5-fluorouracil, and cyclophosphamide). She was removed from the study because of pregnancy, but the gestational age and number of doses received were not specified. The pregnancy ended with a spontaneous abortion (1).

A 30-year-old woman at about 25 weeks' gestation was treated with four courses of epirubicin (100 mg) and vincristine (2 mg) for non-Hodgkin's lymphoma (2). Prednisolone was also given during each treatment and then tapered. Her disease responded well to the therapy. Labor was induced at 34 weeks' gestation and she gave birth to a normal 2.32-kg, 44.5-cm long, female infant with Apgar scores of 8 at 1 and 5 minutes. The mother remained in complete remission and her child appeared to be doing well at 4 years of age.

A 1996 report described the case of a 39-year-old woman with extensive metastatic breast cancer who had a unilateral mastectomy and axillary dissection at 29 weeks' gestation (3). After surgery, she was started on combination chemotherapy with epirubicin (50 mg/m^2), 5-fluorouracil (600 mg/m^2), and cyclophosphamide (600 mg/m^2). At 35 weeks' gestation, a few days after receiving her second course of therapy, she developed eclamptic tonic-clonic seizures. She subsequently delivered a healthy but growth-retarded (1650-g; $<$10th percentile) infant. Although hypertension and proteinuria were not detected before the seizures, both were documented in the postpartum period. No follow-up of the infant after delivery was reported.

A 1999 report from France described the outcomes of pregnancies in 20 women with breast cancer who were treated with antineoplastic agents (4). The first cycle of chemotherapy occurred at a mean gestational age of 26 weeks with delivery occurring at a mean 34.7 weeks. A total of 38 cycles were administered during pregnancy with a median of two cycles per woman. None of the women received radiation therapy during pregnancy. The pregnancy outcomes included two spontaneous abortions (SAB) (both exposed in the 1st trimester), one intrauterine death (exposed in the 2nd trimester), and 17 live births, one of whom died at 8 days of age without apparent cause. The 16 surviving children were developing normally at a mean follow-up of 42.3 months (4). Epirubicin (E), in combination with various other agents (cyclophosphamide [C], fluorouracil [F], methotrexate [M], or vincristine [V]) was administered to 10 of the women at a mean dose of 70 mg/m^2 (range 50–100 mg/m^2). The outcomes were two SABs (ECF, EMV; 1st trimester), one stillbirth (one cycle of EC at 23 weeks' gestation), one neonatal death (one cycle of ECF 32 days before birth), and six surviving liveborn infants (one EC, five ECF; all in the 3rd trimester). One of the infants, exposed to two cycles of ECF with the last at 25 days before birth, had transient leukopenia (4).

Occupational exposure of the mother to antineoplastic agents during pregnancy may present a risk to the fetus. A position statement from the National Study Commission on Cytotoxic Exposure and a research article involving some antineoplastic agents are presented in the monograph for cyclophosphamide (see Cyclophosphamide).

BREAST FEEDING SUMMARY

RECOMMENDATION: Contraindicated

No reports describing the use of epirubicin during human lactation have been located. The antineoplastic agent is excreted into the milk of lactating rats receiving 0.5 mg/kg/day (2). The molecular weight (about 580) is low enough that excretion into breast milk should be expected. In addition, another anthracycline (see Doxorubicin) is excreted into human milk. Because of the potential for serious adverse effects, such as immune suppression, carcinogenesis, neutropenia, and unknown effects on growth, women receiving epirubicin should not breast-feed.

References

1. Product information. Ellence. Pharmacia & Upjohn, 2001.
2. Goldwasser F, Pico JL, Cerrina J, Fernandez H, Pons JC, Cosset JM, Hayat M. Successful chemotherapy including epirubicin in a pregnant non-Hodgkin's lymphoma patient. Leuk Lymphoma 1995;20:173–6.
3. Muller T, Hofmann J, Steck T. Eclampsia after polychemotherapy for nodal-positive breast cancer during pregnancy. Eur J Obstet Gynecol Reprod Biol 1996;67:197–8.
4. Giacalone PL, Laffargue F, Benos P. Chemotherapy for breast carcinoma during pregnancy. Cancer 1999;86:2266–72.

Name: **EPOETIN ALFA** Risk Factor: **C_M**
Class: **Hematopoietic**

FETAL RISK SUMMARY

RECOMMENDATION: Compatible - Maternal Benefit >> Embryo/Fetal Risk

Recombinant human erythropoietin (epoetin alfa), a 165-amino acid glycoprotein produced by a recombinant DNA method with the same biologic effects as endogenous erythropoietin, is used to stimulate red blood cell production.

Fetal toxicity (decreased growth, delays in appearance of abdominal hair, delayed eyelid opening, delayed ossification, and decreases in the number of caudal vertebrae) was observed in the offspring of pregnant rats dosed with 500 U/kg (five times the human dose) (1). In addition, a trend toward increased fetal wastage occurred in pregnant rats dosed with 100 and 500 U/kg. No fetal adverse effects were seen in rabbits at doses up to 500 U/kg from days 6 to 18 of gestation (1).

Epoetin alfa crosses the placenta in significant amounts to the fetus in pregnant mice (2) but not from the mother to the fetus (3) or from the fetus to the mother in sheep (4). Another study also found no transfer of recombinant epoetin alfa to the fetus in sheep and monkeys, in spite of high maternal concentrations (5). The question of human placental transfer of endogenous erythropoietin and epoetin alfa was examined in a 1993 review (6). Five reasons arguing against transfer were presented: poor correlation between maternal and fetal levels; high correlation between fetal plasma and amniotic fluid levels; high molecular weight; animal studies; and one human *in vitro* study (6). Since then, several studies have investigated whether or not epoetin alfa is transferred across the human placenta (7,10–15).

A 1992 study measured an elevated cord erythropoietin level (62 mIU/mL; normal <19) in an infant whose mother was receiving 150 U/kg/week (9000 U/week) of the drug (7). However, because the mother had insulin-dependent diabetes, a disease known to display elevated cord levels of erythropoietin (8–10), the investigators could not determine whether the cord concentrations were a result of exogenous or endogenous erythropoietin (7). The lack of correlation between maternal and fetal erythropoietin concentrations, at least between 19 and 28 weeks' gestation, suggests that endogenous maternal erythropoietin does not cross the placenta to the fetus (10). At 7–12 weeks' gestation, however, mean maternal and extraembryonic coelomic fluid concentrations of endogenous erythropoietin were nearly identical, 15.4 mU/mL (range 6.8–32.1 mU/mL) compared to

15.45 mU/mL (range 5.6–29.4 mU/mL), respectively (11). Passage of maternal erythropoietin to the coelomic fluid via the decidualized endometrium was offered as a possible explanation for the identical levels. This latter study also found low amniotic fluid levels of erythropoietin, mean 5.0 mU/mL (range <5.0–5.8 mU/mL), at 7–12 weeks of gestation, but their samples may have been contaminated with coelomic fluid (11). An earlier study was unable to find endogenous erythropoietin in amniotic fluid before the 11th week of gestation (12). More recent investigations have demonstrated the lack of placental passage of recombinant epoetin alfa across the human placenta (13–15).

E

In the fetus, erythropoietin is primarily produced by the fetal liver during most of pregnancy (16). Erythropoietin binding sites have been found in the 1st trimester of pregnancy in the human fetal liver and lung (17) and in cultures of umbilical vein endothelial cells derived at cesarean section (18). A 1994 report compared the levels of endogenous erythropoietin measured in the umbilical serum in normal women at term and in premature labor, and in those with preeclampsia or diabetes (19). Women with preeclampsia had the highest concentrations (95.8 mU/mL), followed by those with diabetes (38.0 mU/mL), women in premature labor (25.2 mU/mL) and normal women (21.1 mU/mL), demonstrating that fetal hypoxia was not the only factor that determines levels of this glycoprotein (19).

The first published report on the use of epoetin alfa in human pregnancy appeared in a 1990 abstract (20). A 28-year-old Japanese woman with chronic glomerulonephritis became pregnant 8 years after the start of dialysis and approximately 22 months after the initiation of weekly doses of epoetin alfa. She had been amenorrheic prior to epoetin alfa therapy; her menses returned 17 months after start of treatment. The duration of her dialysis treatments (in hours per week) was gradually increased throughout gestation. She received 4500–9000 U/week of epoetin alfa from the 20th gestational week (doses prior to this time were not specified) until delivery at 36 weeks' gestation. Her blood pressure was normal throughout pregnancy, as was intrauterine fetal growth. The 2396-g, healthy, male infant was normal at birth with Apgar scores of 9 and 9 at 1 and 5 minutes, respectively. He was discharged with his mother 12 days after birth.

A report published in 1991 described a 32-year-old hypertensive woman with end-stage renal disease of unknown origin, who had been on hemodialysis for 4 years (21). She was started on epoetin alfa early in the 1st trimester and continued until delivery (36 weeks by dates, 34 weeks by ultrasound). No transfusions were required during pregnancy. An emergency cesarean section was performed because of fetal distress secondary to severe maternal hypertension. The 1140-g male infant had Apgar scores of 7 and 8 at 1 and 5 minutes, respectively. No congenital malformations were noted in the infant, who was discharged home at 35 days of age.

A second 1991 publication involved a 37-year-old woman who was treated throughout pregnancy with escalating doses of epoetin alfa (22). The patient had received a renal transplant 9 years before pregnancy because of reflux nephropathy, but the onset of chronic rejection caused progressive renal failure. Because of persistent anemia, she was started on a regimen of epoetin alfa, 4000 U/week, and supplemental iron shortly before conception. The dose was increased at 18 weeks' gestation to 8000 U/week, and then to 12,000 U/week at 27 weeks' gestation. Hemodialysis was started during the 25th week of pregnancy because of severe renal failure, polyhydramnios, and fetal intrauterine growth retardation. Her blood pressure was controlled with atenolol and nifedipine. Severe intrauterine growth retardation and fetal distress were diagnosed at 31 weeks and, after betamethasone therapy for fetal lung maturation, a cesarean section was performed to deliver a 780-g female infant. Birth weight was below the 3rd percentile for gestational age. Although the growth retardation was attributed to the mother's renal disease, the use of atenolol was probably a factor (see Atenolol). Except for transient coagulopathy and thrombocytopenia found at birth, both thought to be caused by the mother's condition or premature delivery, the infant progressed normally and was discharged home at 66 days of age with a weight of 2140 g.

A 1992 report described the use of epoetin alfa combined with supplemental oral iron in three human pregnancies that resulted in the birth of four (one set of twins) infants (7). The birth weights of the newborns were all at approximately the 50th percentile for gestational age (7). Two of the women developed polyhydramnios after starting treatment with epoetin alfa, and all developed preeclampsia or worsening renal impairment, but the authors could not determine whether these were effects of the drug treatment or the underlying disease (7). Hematocrit values were maintained in the targeted 30%–33% range, and no coagulation problems or significant changes in platelet counts were observed. The three pregnancies are described below.

A 30-year-old woman, with onset of renal disease secondary to immunoglobulin A nephropathy and chronic hypertension before pregnancy, was treated with epoetin alfa 50–65 U/kg/week starting in the 20th gestational week (7). Polyhydramnios was noted at 32 weeks' gestation. Because of worsening renal failure, labor induction was initiated at 35 weeks resulting in the delivery of a 2570-g male infant with Apgar scores of 8 and 8 at 1 and 5 minutes, respectively. The newborn had mild hyperbilirubinemia and required oxygen, but no other problems were noted. He was doing well at 3 months.

The second patient, a 33-year-old woman with hypertension, diabetes, and renal impairment, was treated with 150 U/kg/week of epoetin alfa beginning at 26 weeks' gestation (7). Polyhydramnios developed, and labor was induced at 32 weeks because of worsening renal function and superimposed preeclampsia. After maternal betamethasone therapy to accelerate fetal lung maturity, a 2020-g male infant was delivered, with Apgar scores of 4 and 7 at 1 and 5 minutes, respectively. The infant had mild hypoglycemia and hyperbilirubinemia, and initially required oxygen therapy. He was discharged home at 2 weeks of age.

The third patient was a 26-year-old with renal disease secondary to crescentic segmental necrotizing glomerulonephritis following streptococcal pharyngitis (7). She was treated with azathioprine and prednisone throughout a twin gestation to control her renal disease. Beginning at 14 weeks' gestation, she was treated with epoetin alfa, 85–160 U/kg/week, continuously until 33 weeks' gestation, except for a 4-week period at weeks 23–27. Therapy was halted during that time because of a low ferritin level, and therapy was discontinued when it recurred at 33 weeks' gestation. Labor was induced at 35 weeks' gestation for worsening renal function. A cesarean section was required because of failure to descend, resulting in the delivery of a 2220-g female (Apgar scores of 4 and 8, respectively) and a 2410-g male (Apgar scores of 2 and 5, respectively). The infants were developing normally at 7 months of age (7).

The pregnancies of six women who became pregnant while on dialysis for end-stage renal disease and who were treated with epoetin alpha have been described (23,24). No effects on the mothers' blood pressure control were observed in these cases, and in one of the reports, the investigators found no evidence that the drug crossed the placenta to the fetuses (24).

A number of additional studies have been published describing the use of epoetin alfa during human pregnancy (25–32). In most of the studies or reports, the drug was used to treat the maternal anemia associated with severe renal disease (25–29), but in three reports, epoetin alfa was used in women with either heterozygous β-thalassemia (30), hypoproliferative anemia and a low serum erythropoietin level (31), or acute promyelocytic leukemia (32). Except for a single complication in which abruptio placentae with resulting fetal death occurred at 23 weeks' gestation for which drug therapy could not be excluded as a contributing factor (28), no other fetal and/or newborn adverse effects attributable to epoetin alfa were observed.

In summary, the use of recombinant human erythropoietin (epoetin alfa) does not seem to present a major risk to the fetus. The glycoprotein does not cross the human placenta to the fetus. The severe maternal hypertension or worsening of renal disease requiring delivery of the fetus that occurred in four pregnancies may be an adverse effect of the drug therapy, a consequence of the preexisting renal disease or current pregnancy, or a combination of these factors. The contribution of epoetin alfa to the case of abruptio placentae in a woman with severe hypertension and chronic renal insufficiency is unknown. No cases of thrombosis were reported in the pregnant women treated with epoetin alfa, but this is a potentially serious complication. Because anemia and the need for frequent blood transfusions also present significant risks to the mother and fetus, it appears that the benefits derived from the use of epoetin alfa outweigh the known risks.

BREAST FEEDING SUMMARY

RECOMMENDATION: Compatible

Epoetin is a 165-amino acid glycoprotein produced by recombinant DNA technology that has the same biologic activity as endogenous erythropoietin. No reports describing its use during lactation have been located. Passage into milk is not expected, but in the event that some transfer did occur, digestion in the nursing infant's gastrointestinal system would occur. Moreover, preterm infants have been treated directly with the drug (33). Thus, the risk to a nursing infant from ingestion of the agent via the milk appears to be nonexistent.

References

1. Product information. Epogen. Amgen, 2000.
2. Koury MJ, Bondurant MC, Graber SE, Sawyer ST. Erythropoietin messenger RNA levels in developing mice and transfer of $^{125-}$I-erythropoietin by the placenta. J Clin Invest 1988;82:154–9.
3. Widness JA, Sawyer ST, Schmidt RL, Chestnut DH. Lack of maternal to fetal transfer of $^{125-}$I-labelled erythropoietin in sheep. J Dev Physiol 1991;15: 139–43.
4. Widness JA, Malone TA, Mufson RA. Impermeability of the ovine placenta to ^{35}S-recombinant erythropoietin. Pediatr Res 1989;25:649–51.
5. Zanjani ED, Pixley JS, Slotnick N, MacKintosh ER, Ekhterae D, Clemons G. Erythropoietin does not cross the placenta into the fetus. Pathobiology 1993;61: 211–5.
6. Huch R, Huch A. Maternal and fetal erythropoietin: physiological aspects and clinical significance. Ann Med 1993;25:289–93.
7. Yankowitz J, Piraino B, Laifer SA, Frassetto L, Gavin L, Kitzmiller JL, Crombleholme W. Erythropoietin in pregnancies complicated by severe anemia of renal failure. Obstet Gynecol 1992;80:485–8.
8. Widness JA, Teramo KA, Clemons GK, Voutilainen P, Stenman UH, McKinlay SM, Schwartz R. Direct relationship of antepartum glucose control and fetal erythropoietin in human type 1 (insulin-dependent) diabetic pregnancy. Diabetologia 1990;33:378–83.
9. Salvesen DR, Brudenell JM, Snijders RJM, Ireland RM, Nicolaides KH. Fetal plasma erythropoietin in pregnancies complicated by maternal diabetes mellitus. Am J Obstet Gynecol 1993;168:88–94.
10. Thomas RM, Canning CE, Cotes PM, Linch DC, Rodeck CH, Rossiter CE, Huehns ER. Erythropoietin and cord blood haemoglobin in the regulation of human fetal erythropoiesis. Br J Obstet Gynaecol 1983;90: 795–800.
11. Campbell J, Wathen N, Lewis M, Fingerova H, Chard T. Erythropoietin levels in amniotic fluid and extraembryonic coelomic fluid in the first trimester of pregnancy. Br J Obstet Gynaecol 1992;99:974–6.
12. Zivny J, Kobilkova J, Neuwirt J, Andrasova V. Regulation of erythropoiesis in fetus and mother during normal pregnancy. Obstet Gynecol 1982;60: 77–81.
13. Malek A, Sager R, Eckardt K-U, Bauer C, Schneider H. Lack of transport of erythropoietin across the human placenta as studied by an in vitro perfusion system. Pflügers Arch 1994;427:157–61.
14. Santolaya-Forgas J, Meyer W, Gauthier D, Vengalil S, Duval J, Gottmann D. Transplacental passage of erythropoietin (EPO-Alfa): a case control study. Society of

Perinatal Obstetricians Abstract. Am J Obstet Gynecol 1997;176:S83.
15. Reisenberger K, Egarter C, Kapiotis S, Sternberger B, Gregor H, Husslein P. Transfer of erythropoietin across the placenta perfused in vitro. Obstet Gynecol 1997;89:738–42.
16. Finne PH, Halvorsen S. Regulation of erythropoiesis in the fetus and newborn. Arch Dis Child 1972;47: 683–7.
17. Pekonen F, Rosenlof K, Rutanen EM, Fyhrquist F. Erythropoietin binding sites in human foetal tissues. Acta Endocrinol 1987;116:561–7.
18. Anagnostou A, Lee ES, Kessimian N, Levinson R, Steiner M. Erythropoietin has a mitogenic and positive chemotactic effect on endothelial cells. Proc Natl Acad Sci U S A 1990;87:5978–82.
19. Mamopoulos M, Bili H, Tsantali C, Assimakopoulos E, Mantalenakis S, Farmakides G. Erythropoietin umbilical serum levels during labor in women with preeclampsia, diabetes, and preterm labor. Am J Perinatol 1994;11:427–9.
20. Fujimi S, Hori K, Miijima C, Shigematsu M. Successful pregnancy and delivery in a patient following rHuEPO therapy and on long-term dialysis (abstract). J Am Soc Nephrol 1990;1:391.
21. Barri YM, Al-Furayh O, Qunibi WY, Rahman F. Pregnancy in women on regular hemodialysis. Dial Transplant 1991;20:652–4, 656, 695.
22. McGregor E, Stewart G, Junor BJR, Rodger RSC. Successful use of recombinant human erythropoietin in pregnancy. Nephrol Dial Transplant 1991;6:292–3.
23. Gadallah MF, Ahmad B, Karubian F, Campese VM. Pregnancy in patients with chronic ambulatory peritoneal dialysis. Am J Kidney Dis 1992;20:407–10.
24. Hou S, Orlowski J, Pahl M, Ambrose S, Hussey M, Wong D. Pregnancy in women with end-stage renal disease: treatment of anemia and premature labor. Am J Kidney Dis 1993;21:16–22.
25. Barth W Jr, Lacroix L, Goldberg M, Greene M. Recombinant human erythropoietin (rHEpo) for severe anemia in pregnancies complicated by renal disease. Society of Perinatal Obstetricians Abstract. Am J Obstet Gynecol 1994;170:329.
26. Scott LL, Ramin SM, Richey M, Hanson J, Gilstrap LC III. Erythropoietin use in pregnancy: two cases and review of the literature. Am J Perinatol 1995;12:22–4.
27. Amoedo ML, Fernandez E, Borras M, Pais B, Montoliu J. Successful pregnancy in a hemodialysis patient treated with erythropoietin. Nephron 1995;70:262–3.
28. Braga J, Marques R, Branco A, Goncalves J, Lobato L, Pimentel JP, Flores MM, Goncalves E, Jorge CS. Maternal and perinatal implications of the use of human recombinant erythropoietin. Acta Obstet Gynecol Scand 1996;75:449–53.
29. Pascual J, Liano F, Ortuno J. Pregnancy in an anephric woman. Am J Obstet Gynecol 1995;172:1939.
30. Junca J, Vela D, Orts M, Riutort N, Feliu E. Treating the anaemia of a pregnancy with heterozygous β thalassaemia with recombinant human erythropoietin (r-HuEPO). Eur J Haematol 1995;55:277–8.
31. Harris SA, Payne G Jr, Putman JM. Erythropoietin treatment of erythropoietin-deficient anemia with renal disease during pregnancy. Obstet Gynecol 1996;87: 812–4.
32. Lin C-P, Huang M-J, Liu H-J, Chang IY, Tsai C-H. Successful treatment of acute promyelocytic leukemia in a pregnant Jehovah's Witness with all-trans retinoic acid, rhG-CSF, and erythropoietin. Am J Hematol 1996;51:251–2.
33. Emmerson AJB, Coles HJ, Stern CMM, Pearson TC. Double blind trial of recombinant human erythropoietin in preterm infants. Arch Dis Child 1993;68:291–6.

Name: **EPOPROSTENOL** Risk Factor: **B_M**
Class: **Vasodilator**

FETAL RISK SUMMARY

RECOMMENDATION: Compatible - Maternal Benefit >> Embryo/Fetal Risk

The naturally occurring prostaglandin, epoprostenol (prostacyclin, PGI_2, PGX), is a metabolite of arachidonic acid. Available in the United States since 1995, it is a potent direct vasodilator of pulmonary and systemic arterial vascular beds and an inhibitor of platelet aggregation. Epoprostenol is indicated for the long-term IV treatment of primary pulmonary hypertension (1).

Reproduction studies have revealed no evidence of impaired fertility or fetal harm in pregnant rats and rabbits at 2.5 and 4.8 times the recommended human dose based on body surface area, respectively (1).

In animals, epoprostenol causes dose-related changes on the heart rate: bradycardia at low doses and reflex tachycardia secondary to vasodilation and hypotension at higher doses. Other pharmacologic effects in animals include bronchodilation, inhibition of gastric acid secretion, and decreased gastric emptying (1).

No reports describing the placental transfer of epoprostenol have been located. The molecular weight (about 374) of the drug is low enough for placental transfer, but the clinical significance of this is unknown because the agent is rapidly hydrolyzed and undergoes enzymatic degradation in the plasma. In addition, other factors (e.g., ionization, placental metabolism) may limit transfer to the fetus. Continuous infusions of the prostaglandin, which reach steady-state plasma levels within 15 minutes in animals and are proportional to infusion rates, could potentially provide a reservoir to allow placental transfer. But the *in vivo* plasma half-life of tritium-labeled epoprostenol in animals is very short (2.7 minutes) (1). In humans, the *in vitro* half-life in blood is slightly longer, approximately 6 minutes, and the *in vivo* half-life, although it has not yet been determined, is expected to be no longer than this time (1). Thus, even if placental transfer does occur the amounts reaching the fetus may be clinically insignificant. The effects of adding to the endogenous concentrations of the prostaglandin in the fetus are unknown.

In an *in vitro* study, prostacyclin was shown to be a potent inhibitor of human fetal and maternal platelet aggregation and more potent than *S*-nitroso-*N*-acetylpenicillamine (a releaser of nitric oxide) (2). Moreover, fetal platelets were more sensitive to both agents than were maternal platelets.

The effects of various drugs on the production of maternal and fetal endogenous prostacyclin have been studied in *in vivo* and *in vitro* systems. For ritodrine, one study found an increase in the synthesis of the prostaglandin (3), whereas a second study reported no effect (4). Ethanol was shown to decrease prostacyclin synthesis in a dose-related manner (5). No effect on prostacyclin production was shown with aspirin (6–8) or magnesium sulfate (9).

The enzymes involved in the synthesis of prostacyclin (PGI_2) and thromboxane A_2 (TXA_2) were studied in maternal and fetal platelets and venous endothelium in a 1991 publication (10). Three groups of pregnant women were studied: normal controls; mild preeclampsia; and severe preeclampsia. Based on their findings, the authors concluded that the production of both PGI_2 and TXA_2 was equal in mild preeclampsia, but in severe preeclampsia, the rise in TXA_2 exceeded that of PGI_2.

A number of reports have described the use of epoprostenol for the treatment of severe preeclampsia (11–17) or pulmonary hypertension (18–20). In a 1980 case report, a 29-year-old woman at 27 weeks' gestation with hypertension uncontrolled with oral methyldopa (3 g/day) and hydralazine (150 mg/day) was started on a continuous infusion of epoprostenol at 8 ng/kg/minute (11). Diastolic pressure fell from 140 mm Hg to 80 mm Hg and remained at or below 95 mm Hg during the next 3 days. Adverse effects in the mother included flushing, tachycardia (95–100 beats per minute [bpm]), and transient, nonspecific chest and abdominal pain. On day 4 of therapy, prolonged (1–2 minutes) fetal bradycardia occurred (60 bpm) and delivery by cesarean section was initiated. During the induction phase of anesthesia, the epoprostenol infusion was stopped for 4 minutes. During this interval, the blood pressure rose to 200/100 mm Hg but returned to 130/80 mm Hg when the infusion was restarted. More than normal bleeding occurred during the procedure and the infusion was discontinued. The 730-g newborn was alive and making good progress at 3 weeks of age.

A continuous IV infusion of epoprostenol was started at 25 weeks' gestation in a 27-old-woman with preeclampsia only partially responsive to methyldopa, aspirin (300 mg every other day), and hydralazine (12). The woman had a history of two previous pregnancies complicated by pregnancy-induced hypertension, severe intrauterine growth retardation, and fetal death at 27 weeks' gestation. Epoprostenol was chosen because of a rise in her diastolic pressure to 90 mm Hg, a slowing of fetal growth, and a falling maternal plasma concentration of 6-oxo-$PGF_{1\alpha}$ (6-keto-prostaglandin $F_{1\alpha}$), the hydrolyzed product of epoprostenol (12). Mild nausea, facial flushing, and headache limited the dose tolerated by the patient to 4 ng/kg/minute. The maternal diastolic blood pressure stabilized at or below 85 mm Hg and her pulse rate increased from 69 bpm to 84 bpm, but the FHR remained unchanged. In spite of almost continuous FHR monitoring, the fetus died on the 4th day of the infusion, after which a macerated 430-g female fetus was delivered. The authors speculated that intervention with epoprostenol came to late to save the pregnancy (12).

E

A study published in 1985 examined the effect of IV infusions of epoprostenol in five women (gestational ages 24 to 30 weeks) with severe preeclampsia that was unresponsive to various combinations of other antihypertensive therapy (methyldopa, hydralazine, labetalol, and atenolol) (13). The maximum continuous IV infusion doses tolerated by the patients ranged from 1 to 6 ng/kg/minute with durations varying from 5 hours to 11 days. Facial flushing, nausea and vomiting, and headache were dose-limiting adverse effects. Four infants were delivered by cesarean section when the infusions (duration 5 hours to 7 days) were stopped, but one newborn (mother treated for 4 days) died 5 hours after delivery (birth weight 480 g). Another fetus (600 g) was stillborn at 26 weeks' gestation on the 11th day of epoprostenol (2.5 ng/kg/minute). Ultrasound and FHR monitoring did not detect any significant changes in the fetus prior to death. The authors thought that the two deaths were not related to the drug. The blood pressures of the mothers were reduced, but dose-limiting adverse effects prevented satisfactory control in one patient. Epoprostenol had no effect on uterine activity in any of the cases (13).

No significant changes in placental (intervillous) and umbilical vein blood flow were measured in a study of 13 women (gestational ages 28–38 weeks) with either superimposed preeclampsia ($N = 6$) or preeclampsia ($N = 7$) (14). The infusion dose was increased in four increments (1, 2, 4, and 8 ng/kg/minute), each given for 20 minutes. All women experienced facial flushing and two complained of headache. Significant decreases in maternal blood pressure and consistent increases in maternal plasma or urinary 6-keto-prostaglandin $F_{1\alpha}$ levels were measured. In contrast, no changes in maternal or fetal pulse rates or uterine activity were observed. The fetuses were delivered 1 to 13 days after the study. Except for one 850-g newborn delivered at 30 weeks' who died at age 2 days from respiratory distress syndrome, the other newborns (birth weights 980 g to 2840 g) were well at birth and survived (14).

Two vasodilators, epoprostenol ($N = 22$) or dihydralazine ($N = 25$), were compared in a prospective randomized study of women with proteinuria and acute diastolic blood pressures >110 mm Hg immediately before delivery (15). The mean gestational age in both groups was 36 weeks (range 32–40 weeks). The epoprostenol infusion was started at 0.5 ng/kg/minute and was increased to a maximum of 10 ng/kg/minute within 120 minutes, if needed to control the blood pressure. The initial dihydralazine dose was 0.5 mg/kg/minute and increased to a maximum of 1.5 mg/kg/minute, if needed. Both drugs were continued for 24 hours after delivery and during delivery for those requiring cesarean section. Increases in maternal pulse rate occurred in both groups, but the rise in the epoprostenol patients (6 bpm) was significantly less than the rise with dihydralazine (22 bpm) ($p = 0.0024$). Blood pressures were reduced in both groups, but the difference between them was not significant. Cesarean sections were performed in 13 (60%) (11 for FHR decelerations) of the epoprostenol group and in 20 (80%) (14 for FHR decelerations) of those receiving dihydralazine (*ns*). One neonatal death occurred in each group, but neither was related to the drug therapy (15).

A brief 1992 communication reported the treatment of a 35-year-old woman with thrombotic microangiopathy superimposed on preeclampsia at about 26 weeks' gestation (16). Epoprostenol was started at 2 ng/kg/minute and increased to 20 ng/kg/minute over 24 hours with reduction of her blood pressure and a rise in the platelet count. After stabilization, therapy was stopped but restarted later when her condition worsened. Improvement was again achieved, but she was delivered at 28 weeks' because of oligohydramnios and growth retardation. The baby girl died a week later from respiratory arrest. In addition, the authors described, without details, the successful treatment of a 27-year-old patient with HELLP (hemolysis, elevated liver enzymes, and low platelets) syndrome (16). Epoprostenol has also been used to treat a severe case of HELLP syndrome in the immediate postpartum period (17).

A 1999 publication described the use of epoprostenol for the treatment of pulmonary hypertension in three women in the 3rd trimester (18). One patient, at 28 weeks' gestation, died from severe disease within hours of the diagnosis. The other two women delivered newborns of 3333 g and 2905 g, respectively, but the condition and status of the newborns was not mentioned.

In another case of primary pulmonary hypertension, a 34-year-old woman became pregnant with twins after 1.5 years of continuous IV infusion of epoprostenol (40 ng/kg/hour) (19). She was also taking warfarin, digoxin, furosemide, spironolactone, and ferrous sulfate. She first presented at 15 weeks' gestation at which time the warfarin was discontinued. An ultrasound examination 2 weeks later revealed the death of twin A and hydrocephalus and bilateral clubfeet in twin B. She refused pregnancy termination. She was treated twice for central catheter-related septicemia with vancomycin and gentamicin. The dose of epoprostenol was increased as pregnancy progressed, eventually reaching a dose of 60 ng/kg/hour. Betamethasone was given for lung maturity. Nitric oxide via nasal cannula was started just prior to cesarean section for breech presentation. A live, 2155-g male infant was delivered with Apgar scores of 7 and 8 at 1 and 5 minutes, respectively. The infant had severe hydrocephalus and facial anomalies consistent with fetal warfarin syndrome (19). He was alive but still hospitalized at the time of the report. The nitric oxide was discontinued after 40 days and the mother was discharged home 43 days after delivery on epoprostenol 77 ng/kg/hour.

A 2004 case report described the use of IV and inhaled epoprostenol for the treatment of severe primary pulmonary hypertension (20). The woman was started on the IV drug at 26 weeks' gestation. Because of concern that systemic administration could inhibit platelet aggregation and place the patient at risk during epidural catheter placement for labor, she was changed to inhaled epoprostenol at 35 weeks' gestation. A healthy, 2250-g male infant was delivered vaginally with Apgar scores of 7 and 9 at 1 and 5 minutes, respectively. The infant was doing well at 6 months of age (20).

In summary, epoprostenol is not teratogenic in animals but the human data are too limited—only one human case of exposure during early gestation has been reported—to assess. The placental transfer of the prostaglandin has not been characterized, but it is unlikely if clinically significant amounts of exogenous epoprostenol reach the fetus. Because the prostaglandin occurs naturally in the fetus, it is also unlikely that maternal administration would produce a direct adverse effect on the embryo or fetus. The adverse fetal outcomes that have been noted (bradycardia, FHR decelerations, and death) were most likely caused by severe maternal disease or other factors. Although the maternal benefits obtained from use of epoprostenol for severe preeclampsia have not been well documented, its use for pulmonary hypertension is beneficial and appear to far outweigh any potential risks to the fetus.

BREAST FEEDING SUMMARY

RECOMMENDATION: No Human Data - Probably Compatible

No reports describing the use of epoprostenol during lactation have been located. There is potential for its use during breast-feeding, such as in postpartum women with pulmonary hypertension on long-term infusions of the drug. However, this situation must be exceedingly rare. Because of its rapid degradation at physiologic pH and probably in the gut, the clinical significance of any transfer into milk to a nursing infant is probably nil. Moreover, the prostaglandin has been given directly by inhalation to a premature neonate with beneficial effects (21).

References

1. Product information. Flolan. Glaxo Wellcome, 2000.
2. Varela AF, Runge A, Ignarro LJ, Chaudhuri G. Nitric oxide and prostacyclin inhibit fetal platelet aggregation: a response similar to that observed in adults. Am J Obstet Gynecol 1992;167:1599–604.
3. Jouppila P, Kirkinen P, Koivula A, Ylikorkala O. Ritodrine infusion during late pregnancy: effects on fetal and placental blood flow, prostacyclin, and thromboxane. Am J Obstet Gynecol 1985;151:1028–32.
4. Ekblad U, Erkkola R, Uotila P, Kanto J, Palo P. Ritodrine infusion at term: effects on maternal and fetal prostacyclin, thromboxane and prostaglandin precursor fatty acids. Gynecol Obstet Invest 1988;25:106–12.
5. Randall CL, Saulnier JL. Effect of ethanol on prostacyclin, thromboxane, and prostaglandin E production in human umbilical veins. Alcohol Clin Exp Res 1995;19: 741–6.
6. Martin C, Varner MW, Brance DW, Rodgers G, Mitchell MD. Dose-related effects of low dose aspirin on hemostasis parameters and prostacyclin/thromboxane ratios in late pregnancy. Prostaglandins 1996;51:321–30.
7. Tulppala M, Marttunen M, Soderstrom-Anttila V, Foudila T, Ailus K, Palosuo T, Ylikorkala O. Low-dose aspirin in prevention of miscarriage in women with unexplained or autoimmune related recurrent miscarriage: effect on prostacyclin and thromboxane A_2 production. Hum Reprod 1997;12:1567–72.
8. Vainio M, Maenpaa J, Riutta A, Ylitalo P, Ala-Fossi SL, Tuimala R. In the dose range of 0.5–2.0 mg/kg, acetylsalicylic acid does not affect prostacyclin production in hypertensive pregnancies. Acta Obstet Gynecol Scand 1999;78:82–8.
9. Walsh SW, Romney AD, Wang Y, Walsh MD. Magnesium sulfate attenuates peroxide-induced vasoconstriction in the human placenta. Am J Obstet Gynecol 1998;178:7–12.
10. Satoh K, Seki H, Sakamoto H. Role of prostaglandins in pregnancy-induced hypertension. Am J Kidney Dis 1991;17:133–8.
11. Fidler J, Bennett MJ, De Swift M, Ellis C, Lewis PJ. Treatment of pregnancy hypertension with prostacyclin. Lancet 1980;2:31–2.
12. Lewis PJ, Shepherd GL, Ritter J, Chan SMT, Bolton PJ, Jogee M, Myatt L, Elder MG. Prostacyclin and preeclampsia. Lancet 1981;1:559.
13. Belch JJF, Thorburn J, Greer IA, Sarfo S, Prentice CRM. Intravenous prostacyclin in the management of pregnancies complicated by severe hypertension. Clin Exp Hypertens Preg 1985;B4:75–86.
14. Jouppila P, Kirkinen P, Koivula A, Ylikorkala O. Failure of exogenous prostacyclin to change placental and fetal blood flow in preeclampsia. Am J Obstet Gynecol 1985;151:661–5.
15. Moodley J, Gouws E. A comparative study of the use of epoprostenol and dihydralazine in severe hypertension in pregnancy. Br J Obstet Gynaecol 1992;99: 727–30.
16. De Belder AJ, Weston MJ. Epoprostenol infusions in thrombotic microangiopathy of pregnancy. Lancet 1992;339:741–2.
17. Huber W, Schweigart U, Classen M. Epoprostenol and plasmapheresis in complicated HELLP syndrome with pancreatitis. Lancet 1994;343:848.
18. Easterling TR, Ralph DD, Schmucker BC. Pulmonary hypertension in pregnancy: treatment with pulmonary vasodilators. Obstet Gynecol 1999;93:494–8.
19. Badalian SS, Silverman RK, Aubry RH, Longo J. Twin pregnancy in a woman on long-term epoprostenol therapy for primary pulmonary hypertension. A case report. J Reprod Med 2000;45:149–52.
20. Bildirici I, Shumway JB. Intravenous and inhaled epoprostenol for primary pulmonary hypertension during pregnancy and delivery. Obstet Gynecol 2004; 103:1102–5.
21. Soditt V, Aring C, Groneck P. Improvement of oxygenation induced by aerosolized prostacyclin in a preterm infant with persistent pulmonary hypertension of the newborn. Intensive Care Med 1997;23: 1275–8.

Name:	**EPROSARTAN**	Risk Factor:	C_M*
Class:	**Antihypertensive**		

E

FETAL RISK SUMMARY

RECOMMENDATION: Human Data Suggest Risk in 2nd and 3rd Trimesters

Eprosartan is a selective angiotensin II receptor antagonist that is used, either alone or in combination with other antihypertensive agents, for the treatment of hypertension. Eprosartan blocks the vasoconstrictor and aldosterone-secreting effects of angiotensin II by preventing angiotensin II from binding to AT_1 receptors.

Reproduction studies have been conducted in rats and rabbits (1). No teratogenic effects were observed in either species, but dose-related toxicity occurred in pregnant rabbits. In pregnant rats, no adverse effects on the fetus or on the postnatal development and maturation of offspring were observed at oral doses up to approximately 0.6 times the human exposure (based on area under the plasma concentration curve) at the maximum recommended human dose or 800 mg/day (MRHD). Similarly, a dose approximately 0.8 times the MRHD did not result in fetal or maternal toxicity in pregnant rabbits. Increasing the dose to approximately 2.7 times the MRHD in pregnant rabbits, however, caused both maternal (reduced body weight, decreased food consumption, and death) and embryo/fetal (resorptions, abortions, and litter loss) toxicity (1).

It is not known if eprosartan crosses the human placenta. The molecular weight (about 521) is low enough that passage to the fetus should be expected.

No reports describing the use of eprosartan during human pregnancy have been located. The antihypertensive mechanisms of action of eprosartan and angiotensin converting enzyme (ACE) inhibitors are very close. That is, the former selectively blocks the binding of angiotensin II to AT_1 receptors, whereas the latter blocks the formation of angiotensin II itself. Therefore, use of this drug during the 2nd and 3rd trimesters may cause teratogenicity and severe fetal and neonatal toxicity that is identical to that seen with ACE inhibitors (e.g., see Captopril or Enalapril). Fetal toxic effects may include anuria, oligohydramnios, fetal hypocalvaria, intrauterine growth retardation, prematurity, and patent ductus arteriosus. Anuria-associated oligohydramnios may produce fetal limb contractures, craniofacial deformation, and pulmonary hypoplasia. Severe anuria and hypotension, that is resistant to both pressor agents and volume expansion, may occur in the newborn following *in utero* exposure to eprosartan. Newborn renal function and blood pressure should be closely monitored. If eprosartan is used in pregnancy, healthcare professionals are encouraged to call the toll free number (800-670-6126) for information about patient enrollment in the Motherisk study.

[*Risk factor D_M if used in 2nd or 3rd trimesters.*]

BREAST FEEDING SUMMARY

RECOMMENDATION: No Human Data - Probably Compatible

No reports describing the use of eprosartan during human lactation have been located. The drug is excreted into animal milk (1). The molecular weight (about 521) is low enough that excretion into breast milk should also be expected. The effects of this exposure on a nursing infant are unknown. The American Academy of Pediatrics, however, classifies

ACE inhibitors, a closely related group of antihypertensive agents, as compatible with breast-feeding (see Captopril and Enalapril).

Reference

1. Product information. Teveten. Unimed Pharmaceuticals, 2001.

Name:	**EPTIFIBATIDE**	Risk Factor:	B_M
Class:	**Hematologic Agent (Antiplatelet)**		

FETAL RISK SUMMARY

RECOMMENDATION: No Human Data - Animal Data Suggest Low Risk

The cyclic heptapeptide, eptifibatide, is indicated for the treatment of acute coronary syndrome in patients who will be managed medically or in those undergoing percutaneous coronary intervention. Eptifibatide acts as a reversible inhibitor of platelet aggregation by blocking the GP IIb/IIIa receptor on the platelet surface (1).

Reproduction studies with eptifibatide have been conducted in rats and rabbits. In pregnant rats and rabbits, continuous daily IV infusions at total daily doses up to about 4 times the maximum recommended human daily dose based on body surface area (MRHDD) revealed no evidence of fetal harm. Although long-term studies in animals for carcinogenicity have not been conducted, no evidence of mutagenicity was found in several tests. Similarly, no evidence of impaired fertility or reproductive performance was observed in rats given daily doses up to about 4 times the MRHDD (1).

It is not known if eptifibatide crosses the human placenta to the fetus. The molecular weight (about 832), however, is low enough that transfer to the fetus should be expected. Moreover, the drug is given as a continuous IV infusion for periods up to 72 hours, thus allowing for prolonged contact at the maternal-fetal interface.

No reports describing the use of eptifibatide in human pregnancy have been located. The animal data are reassuring but human data are required to assess the risk this agent presents to a fetus. The primary risk, however, appears to be from maternal hemorrhage during drug administration. If this is adequately controlled, the benefits of the drug to the mother appear to far outweigh the unknown risks to the fetus.

BREAST FEEDING SUMMARY

RECOMMENDATION: Hold Breast Feeding

No reports describing the use of eptifibatide during lactation have been located. Because of the indications for eptifibatide, it is doubtful if such reports will forthcoming. The molecular weight (about 832) and the potentially long IV infusions of the drug, however, suggest that some drug will be excreted into breast milk. The effect of this exposure for a nursing infant is unknown, but most likely the risk is very low or nil because the drug should be digested in the infant's gastrointestinal tract. Until data are available, however, the safest course is to hold breast-feeding while the drug is being infused.

References

1. Product information. Integrilin. Millenium Pharmaceuticals, 2004.
2. Product information. Integrilin. Schering, 2004.

Name:	**ERGOCALCIFEROL**	Risk Factor:	**A***
Class:	**Vitamin**		

FETAL RISK SUMMARY

RECOMMENDATION: Compatible

Ergocalciferol (vitamin D_2) is converted in the liver to 25-hydroxyergocalciferol, which in turn is converted in the kidneys to 1,25-dihydroxyergocalciferol, one of the active forms of vitamin D. See Vitamin D.

[**Risk Factor D if used in doses above the recommended daily allowance.*]

BREAST FEEDING SUMMARY

RECOMMENDATION: Compatible

See Vitamin D.

Name:	**ERGOTAMINE**	Risk Factor:	**X_M**
Class:	**Sympatholytic (Antimigraine)**		

FETAL RISK SUMMARY

RECOMMENDATION: Contraindicated

Ergotamine is a naturally occurring ergot alkaloid that is used in the prevention or treatment of vascular headaches such as migraine. The oxytocic properties of ergotamine have been known since the early 1900s, but because it produces a prolonged and marked increase in uterine tone that may lead to fetal hypoxia, it is not used for this purpose (1). A semisynthetic derivative, dihydroergotamine, has also been abandoned as an oxytocic for the same reason (2). (See Dihydroergotamine.) Small amounts of ergotamine have been reported to cross the placenta to the fetus (3).

Ergotamine is not an animal teratogen (4). In pregnant mice, rats, and rabbits, however, doses sufficient to affect maternal weight gain were fetotoxic, producing increased prenatal mortality and growth retardation. The mechanism proposed for these effects was an impairment of blood supply to the uterus and placenta (4). Another study demonstrating fetal death in pregnant rats arrived at the same conclusion (5). Ergotamine (0.25%) fed to pregnant sheep produced severe ergotism, fetal death and abortions (6).

Most authorities consider ergotamine in pregnancy to be either contraindicated or to be used sparingly and with caution, because of the oxytocic properties of the drug (7–10). Fortunately, the frequency of migraine attacks decreases during pregnancy, thus lessening the need for any medication (8–10).

The Collaborative Perinatal Project monitored 50,282 mother-child pairs, 25 of whom were exposed to ergotamine during the 1st trimester (11). Two malformed children were observed from this group, but the numbers are too small to draw any conclusion.

In a surveillance study of Michigan Medicaid recipients conducted between 1985 and 1992 involving 229,101 completed pregnancies, 59 newborns had been exposed to ergotamine during the 1st trimester (F. Rosa, personal communication, FDA, 1993). A total of nine (15.3%) major birth defects were observed (two expected). Specific data were available for six defect categories, including (observed/expected) 1/0.6 cardiovascular defects, 0/0 oral clefts, 0/0 spina bifida, 1/0 polydactyly, 0/0 limb reduction defects, and 1/0 hypospadias. The total number of defects is suggestive of an association, but other factors, such as the mother's disease, concurrent drug use, and chance may be involved.

A retrospective study published in 1978 evaluated the reproductive outcome of women attending a migraine clinic (12). The study group was composed of 777 women enrolling in the clinic for the first time. A control group composed of 182 wives of new male patients at the clinic was formed for comparison. Of the women with migraine, 450 (58%) had been pregnant vs. 136 (75%) of the women without migraine. The difference in the percentage of pregnancies may have been because all of the control women were married while the marriage status of the study women was not known (12). The incidence of at least one spontaneous abortion or stillbirth, 27% vs. 29%, including 1st trimester loss, and the occurrence of toxemia, 18% vs. 18%, were similar for the groups. The total number of pregnancies was 1142 in the study patients and 342 in the controls, with a mean number of pregnancies per patient of 2.54 vs. 2.51, respectively. The migraine group had 924 (81%) live births compared to 277 (81%) for the control women. Congenital defects observed among the live births totaled 31 (3.4%) for the study group vs. 11 (4.0%) for the controls (*ns*). Major abnormalities, found in 20 (2.2%) of the infants from the women with migraine compared to 7 (2.5%) of the infants from controls, were of similar distribution to those found in the geographic area of the clinic (12). Moreover, the incidence of defects was similar to the expected frequency for that location (12). Although the investigators were unable to document reliable and accurate drug histories during the pregnancies because of the retrospective nature of the study, 70.8% of the women with migraine indicated they had used ergotamine in the past. They concluded, therefore, that ergotamine exposure during pregnancy, especially early in gestation, was highly likely, and that this drug and others used for the prevention or treatment of the disease were probably not teratogenic (12).

In contrast to the above study, six case reports have described adverse fetal outcomes attributable to ergotamine (13–17,19). An infant, who expired at 4 weeks of age, was delivered at 24 weeks' gestation with a large rugated, perineal mass, no external genitalia or anal orifice, and a small, polycystic left kidney (13). Two separate sacs made up the mass, one of which resembled a urinary bladder with two ureteral and a vaginal orifice, and the other containing bowel, left ovary, uterus and right kidney (13). The mother had used an ergotamine inhaler once or twice weekly during the first 8 weeks of pregnancy for migraine headaches. The inhaler delivered 0.36 mg of ergotamine per inhalation and she received two or three inhalations during each headache for a total dose of 0.72–1.08 mg once or twice weekly. The mother also smoked about 10 cigarettes daily.

A female infant with multiple congenital malformations was delivered from a woman who had used a proprietary preparation containing ergotamine, caffeine, belladonna, and pentobarbital during the 2nd month of pregnancy for migraine (14). Two other similar cases in pregnant women who did not receive an ergotamine preparation were included in the report. The birth defects included hydrocephalus, sacral or coccygeal agenesis, digital and muscle hypoplasia, joint contractures, short stature, short perineum, and pilonidal sinus. Because of the similarity of the cases, the authors thought it might be a new syndrome, which they termed *cerebroarthrodigital syndrome*, in which the primary pathogenetic event is a neural tube-neural crest dysplasia (14). Although they could not determine the cause, they considered an environmental agent, such as ergotamine, or a genetic cause as possibilities (14).

A 1983 report described a 27-year-old woman with migraine headaches who consumed up to 8 tablets/day of a preparation containing 1 mg of ergotamine tartrate and 100 mg of caffeine throughout a total of six pregnancies (15). The 1st pregnancy resulted in the birth of a 2200-g female infant, whose subsequent growth varied between the 3rd and 10th percentiles. She had no medical problems other than enuresis and hay fever. The woman's 2nd, 4th, 5th, and 6th pregnancies all ended in spontaneous abortions. A male infant was delivered in the 3rd pregnancy at 35 weeks' gestation. His birth weight (1892 g) and length (43 cm) were at the 20th percentile for gestational age. The infant died at 25 days of age secondary to hyaline membrane disease and after two surgical attempts to correct jejunal atresia. At autopsy, a short small intestine with portions of incomplete or absent muscular coat around the bowel lumen was found. The authors could not exclude a hereditary cause for the anomaly, but they believed the most likely cause was a disruptive vascular mechanism resulting from an interruption of the superior mesenteric arterial supply to the affected organ (15).

In a suicide attempt, a 17-year-old pregnant woman, at 35 weeks' gestation, took a single dose of 10 ergotamine tablets (20 mg) (16). Five hours after ingestion, the fetal heart rate was 165 beats/minute with fetal movement. Uterine contractions were mild but frequent, with little relaxation between contractions. Fetal death occurred approximately 8.5 hours later, about 13.5 hours after ingestion. The most likely mechanism for the fetal death was impairment of placental perfusion by the uterine contractions resulting in fetal hypoxia (16). However, the authors considered two other possible mechanisms: arterial spasm causing decreased uterine arterial perfusion, and altered peripheral resistance and venous return resulting in fetal myocardial ischemia (16).

A 1988 case report described the result of a pregnancy complicated by severe migraine headaches (17). The mother consumed a variety of drugs, including 1–4 rectal suppositories/week during the first 14 weeks of gestation, with each dose containing ergotamine (2 mg), belladonna (0.25 mg), caffeine (100 mg), and phenobarbital (60 mg). Other medications, frequency of ingestion, and gestational weeks of exposure were propranolol (40 mg; 2/day; 0–20 weeks), acetaminophen/codeine (325 mg/8 mg; 6–20/day; 0–16 weeks), and dimenhydrinate (75 mg; 0–3/week; 0–12 weeks). The term, female infant was a breech presentation weighing 2860 g, with a length of 46 cm. The infant was microcephalic and paraplegic with underdeveloped and hypotonic lower limbs. The anal, knee, and ankle reflexes were absent. Sensation was absent to the level of the knees and variably absent on the thighs. This pattern was suggestive of a spinal cord defect in the upper lumbar region (17). Other abnormalities apparent were dislocated hips and marked bilateral talipes equinovarus. Computed tomography of the brain revealed a small organ with lissencephaly, a primitive Sylvian fissure, and ventriculomegaly (17). The above findings were compatible with arrest of cerebral development that occurred after 10–13 weeks (17). The authors concluded that the most likely etiology was a disruptive vascular mechanism, and that the combination of ergotamine, caffeine, and propranolol may have potentiated the vasoconstriction (17).

In response to the case report above, a 1989 letter cited prospective and retrospective data from the Hungarian Case-Control Surveillance of Congenital Anomalies, 1980–1986 system (18). Among controls (normal infants, but including those with Down's syndrome), 0.11% (18 of 16,477) had used ergotamine during pregnancy whereas 0.14% (13 of 9,460) of pregnancies with a birth defect had been exposed to the drug (*ns*). Four of the index cases, however, involved neural tube defects compared to none of the controls ($p < 0.01$), a finding that prompted the author to state that further study was required.

A female infant, the smaller of dizygotic twins, was born at 32 weeks' gestation (19). Paraplegia and arthrogryposis multiplex was present at birth and thought to be a consequence of prenatal cord trauma. The mother had had a severe reaction (intractable nausea, vertigo and dizziness requiring bed rest for 3 days) following the use of one rectal suppository containing ergotamine, caffeine, belladonna, and butalbital at 4.5 months' gestation. Because of this reaction, the authors speculated that ergotamine may have caused vascular spasm of a fetal medullary artery that resulted in spinal cord ischemia and neuronal loss (19).

The accidental use at 38 weeks' gestation of a rectal suppository containing ergotamine (2 mg) and caffeine (100 mg) in a woman with nonproteinuric hypertension produced sudden fetal distress that led to an emergency cesarean section (20). A growth-retarded, 2660-g female infant was delivered with Apgar scores of 4 and 8 at 1 and 5 minutes, respectively. The obstetrician, who was unaware of the drug administration, noted the strikingly small amount (100 mL) of blood loss during the procedure. The infant was doing well at 10 years of age.

A 1995 reference reviewed the teratogenicity of ergotamine (21). Because many of the reports of adverse outcomes following the use of the drug during pregnancy are consistent with vascular injury, and because ergotamine toxicity is known to cause vasospasm, the author recommended that the drug should be avoided during all parts of pregnancy (21). The use of the agent in small, appropriate doses, however, was thought to have a low teratogenic potential because ergotamine appeared to be teratogenic only at higher doses, or possibly in those cases involving idiosyncratic susceptibility (21). Recommendations for counseling of exposed women included not only determining the dosage and timing of exposure, but also asking questions relating to the presence or absence of signs and symptoms of ergotism, past usage, and possible continuing abuse (21).

In summary, small, infrequent doses of ergotamine used for migraine headaches do not appear to be fetotoxic or teratogenic, but idiosyncratic responses may occur that endanger the fetus. Larger doses or frequent use, however, may cause fetal toxicity or teratogenicity that is probably a result of maternal and/or fetal vascular disruption. Based on one report, the combination of ergotamine, caffeine, and propranolol may represent an added risk. Because the risk has not been adequately defined, and because of the oxytocic properties of the agent, ergotamine should be avoided during pregnancy.

BREAST FEEDING SUMMARY

RECOMMENDATION: Contraindicated

Ergotamine is excreted into breast milk, but data quantifying this excretion have not been located. A 1934 study reported that 90% of nursing infants of mothers using an ergot preparation for migraine therapy had symptoms of ergotism (22). Because of the vomiting, diarrhea, and convulsions observed in this study, the American Academy of Pediatrics classifies ergotamine as a drug that has been associated with significant effects on some nursing infants and should be given to nursing mothers with caution (23). Moreover, ergotamine is a member of the same chemical family as bromocriptine, an agent that is used to suppress lactation. Although no specific information has been located relating to the effects of ergotamine on lactation, ergot alkaloids may hinder lactation by inhibiting maternal pituitary prolactin secretion (24).

References

1. Gill RC, Farrar JM. Experiences with di-hydro-ergotamine in the treatment of primary uterine inertia. J Obstet Gynaecol Br Emp 1951;58:79–91.
2. Altman SG, Waltman R, Lubin S, Reynolds SR. Oxytocic and toxic actions of dihydroergotamine-45. Am J Obstet Gynecol 1952;64:101–9.
3. Griffith RW, Grauwiler J, Holdel CH, et al. Toxicologic considerations. In Berde B, Schild HO, eds. *Ergot Alkaloids and Related Compounds. Handbook of Experimental Pharmacology*. Volume 49. Berlin: Springer Verlag, 1979:805–51. As cited in Hughes HE, Goldstein DA. Birth defects following maternal exposure to ergotamine, beta-blockers, and caffeine. J Med Genet 1988;25:396–9.
4. Grauwiler J, Schon H. Teratological experiments with ergotamine in mice, rats, and rabbits. Teratology 1973;7:227–36.
5. Schon H, Leist KH, Grauwiler J. Single-day treatment of pregnant rats with ergotamine (abstract). Teratology 1975;11:32A.
6. Greatorex JC, Mantle PG. Effect of rye ergot on the pregnant sheep. J Reprod Fertil 1974;37:33–41.
7. Foster JB. Migraine-traditional uses of ergot compounds. Postgrad Med J 1976;52(Suppl 1):12–4.
8. Massey EW. Migraine during pregnancy. Obstet Gynecol Surv 1977;32:693–6.
9. Lance JW. The pharmacotherapy of migraine. Med J Aust 1986;144:85–8.
10. Reik L Jr. Headaches in pregnancy. Semin Neurol 1988;8:187–92.
11. Heinonen OP, Sloan D, Shapiro S. *Birth Defects and Drugs in Pregnancy*. Littleton, MA: Publishing Sciences Group, 1977:358–60.
12. Wainscott G, Sullivan FM, Volans GN, Wilkinson M. The outcome of pregnancy in women suffering from migraine. Postgrad Med J 1978;54:98–102.
13. Peeden JN Jr, Wilroy RS Jr, Soper RG. Prune perineum. Teratology 1979;20:233–6.
14. Spranger JW, Schinzel A, Myers T, Ryan J, Giedion A, Opitz JM. Cerebroarthrodigital syndrome: a newly recognized formal genesis syndrome in three patients with apparent arthromyodysplasia and sacral agenesis, brain malformation and digital hypoplasia. Am J Med Genet 1980;5:13–24.
15. Graham JM Jr, Marin-Padilla M, Hoefnagel D. Jejunal atresia associated with Cafergot ingestion during pregnancy. Clin Pediatr 1983;22:226–8.
16. Au KL, Woo JSK, Wong VCW. Intrauterine death from ergotamine overdosage. Eur J Obstet Gynecol Reprod Biol 1985;19:313–5.
17. Hughes HE, Goldstein DA. Birth defects following maternal exposure to ergotamine, beta blockers, and caffeine. J Med Genet 1988;25:396–9.
18. Czeizel A. Teratogenicity of ergotamine. J Med Genet 1989;26:69–70.
19. Verloes A, Emonts P, Dubois M, Rigo J, Senterre J. Paraplegia and arthrogryposis multiplex of the lower extremities after intrauterine exposure to ergotamine. J Med Genet 1990;27:213–4.
20. de Groot ANJA, van Dongen PWJ, van Roosmalen J, Eskes TKAB. Ergotamine-induced fetal stress: review of side effects of ergot alkaloids during pregnancy. Eur J Obstet Gynecol Reprod Biol 1993;51:73–7.
21. Raymond GV. Teratogen update: ergot and ergotamine. Teratology 1995;51:344–7.
22. Fomina PI. Untersuchungen uber den Ubergang des aktiven Agens des Mutterkorns in die milch stillender Mutter. Arch Gynaek 1934;157:275. As cited by Knowles JA. Excretion of drugs in milk—a review. J Pediatr 1965;66:1068–82.
23. Committee on Drugs, American Academy of Pediatrics. The transfer of drugs and other chemicals into human milk. Pediatrics 2001;108:776–89.
24. Vorherr H. Contraindications to breast-feeding. JAMA 1974;227:676.

Name:	**ERTAPENEM**	Risk Factor:	B_M
Class:	**Antibiotic**		

FETAL RISK SUMMARY

RECOMMENDATION: No Human Data - Probably Compatible

Ertapenem is a broad-spectrum carbapenem antibiotic that is administered by either IM injection or IV infusion. It is structurally related to the beta-lactam antibiotics and belongs to the same class as imipenem (available as imipenem-cilastatin) and meropenem.

Reproduction studies have been conducted in mice and rats. No evidence of structural teratogenicity was observed at IV doses up to three times the recommended human dose of 1 g based on body surface area (mice) and 1.2 times the human exposure at the recommended dose of 1 g based on AUC (rats) (1). However, the maximum dose in mice resulted in decreased fetal weight and decreases in the average number of ossified sacrocaudal vertebrae. The antibiotic had no effect on mating performance, fecundity, fertility, or embryonic survival in either species (1).

Ertapenem crosses the placenta in rats, but this has not been studied in humans. The molecular weight (about 498) is low enough that passage to the fetus should be expected.

No reports describing the use of ertapenem in human pregnancy have been located. No teratogenicity was observed in two animal species, although mild fetal toxicity was observed in one at a dose very close to that used in humans. Moreover, there is no evidence that any beta-lactam antibiotic (e.g., penicillins and cephalosporins) causes developmental toxicity in humans at therapeutic doses. Therefore, if the maternal condition requires the use of ertapenem, the antibiotic probably is safe at anytime during gestation.

BREAST FEEDING SUMMARY

RECOMMENDATION: Limited Human Data - Probably Compatible

Ertapenem is excreted into breast milk (1). Five women 5 to 14 days postpartum were treated with 1 g IV daily for 3 to 10 days. Milk concentrations of the antibiotic were measured at random times for 5 consecutive days after the last dose. Samples obtained within 24 hours of the last dose ranged from <0.13 (lower limit of quantitation) to 0.38 μg/mL. By day 5, ertapenem could not be detected in the milk of four women and was <0.13 μg/mL in one woman (1).

The effects on a nursing infant from exposure to ertapenem via milk are unknown but are of doubtful clinical significance. Most antibiotics are excreted into breast milk in low concentrations, and adverse effects are rare. Potential problems for the nursing infant are modification of bowel flora, direct effects on the infant (e.g., allergic response), and interference with the interpretation of culture results if a fever workup is required.

Reference

1. Product information. Invanz. Merck & Company, 2003.

Name:	**ERYTHRITYL TETRANITRATE**	Risk Factor:	**C_M**
Class:	**Vasodilator**		

See Nitroglycerin or Amyl Nitrite.

Name:	**ERYTHROMYCIN**	Risk Factor:	**B_M**
Class:	**Antibiotic**		

FETAL RISK SUMMARY

RECOMMENDATION: Compatible (Excludes Estolate Salt)

Erythromycin is a macrolide antibiotic. The drug was not teratogenic in female rats fed erythromycin (up to 0.25% of the diet) before and during mating, and throughout gestation and weaning (1).

Erythromycin crosses the placenta but in concentrations too low to treat most pathogens (2–4). Fetal tissue levels increase after multiple doses (4). However, a case has been described in which erythromycin was used successfully to treat maternal syphilis but failed to treat the fetus adequately (5). During pregnancy, erythromycin serum concentrations vary greatly as compared to those in normal men and nonpregnant women, which might account for the low levels observed in the fetus (6).

The estolate salt of erythromycin has been observed to induce hepatotoxicity in pregnant patients (7). Approximately 10% of 161 women treated with the estolate form in the 2nd trimester had abnormally elevated levels of serum glutamic-oxaloacetic transaminase, which returned to normal after therapy was discontinued.

The use of erythromycin in the 1st trimester was reported in a mother who delivered an infant with left absence-of-tibia syndrome (8). The mother was also exposed to other drugs, which makes a relationship to the antibiotic unlikely.

The Collaborative Perinatal Project monitored 50,282 mother-child pairs, 79 of whom had 1st trimester exposure to erythromycin (9, pp. 297–313). For use anytime during pregnancy, 230 exposures were recorded (9, p. 435). No evidence was found to suggest a relationship to large categories of major and minor malformations or to individual defects. Erythromycin, like many other antibiotics, lowers urine estriol concentrations (see also Ampicillin for mechanism and significance) (10). The antibiotic has been used during the 3rd trimester to reduce maternal and infant colonization with group B β-hemolytic streptococcus (11,12). Erythromycin has also been used during pregnancy for the treatment of genital mycoplasmas (13,14). A reduction in the rates of pregnancy loss and low-birth-weight infants was seen in patients with mycoplasma infection after treatment with erythromycin.

In a surveillance study of Michigan Medicaid recipients conducted between 1985 and 1992 involving 229,101 completed pregnancies, 6972 newborns had been exposed to erythromycin during the 1st trimester (F. Rosa, personal communication, FDA, 1993). A total of 320 (4.6%) major birth defects were observed (297 expected). Specific data were available for six defect categories, including (observed/expected) 77/70 cardiovascular defects, 14/11 oral clefts, 1/3 spina bifida, 22/20 polydactyly, 14/12 limb reduction defects, and 11/17 hypospadias. These data do not support an association between the drug and congenital malformations.

A 2003 case-control study, using data from three Swedish health registers, was conducted to identify drug use in early pregnancy that was associated with cardiac defects (15). Cases (cardiovascular defects without known chromosome anomalies) ($N = 5015$) were compared to controls consisting of all infants born in Sweden (1995–2001) ($N = 577{,}730$). Associations were identified for several drugs, some of which were probably due to confounding from the underlying disease or complaint or multiple testing, but some were thought to be true drug effects (15). For erythromycin, there were 27 cases in 1588 exposures (odds ratio 1.91, 95% confidence interval 1.30–2.80) (3).

BREAST FEEDING SUMMARY

RECOMMENDATION: Compatible

Erythromycin is excreted into breast milk (16). Following oral doses of 400 mg every 8 hours, milk levels ranged from 0.4 to 1.6 μg/mL. Oral doses of 2 g/day produced milk concentrations of 1.6-3.2 μg/mL. The milk:plasma ratio in both groups was 0.5. No reports of adverse effects in infants exposed to erythromycin in breast milk have been located. However, three potential problems exist for the nursing infant: modification of bowel flora, direct effects on the infant, and interference with the interpretation of culture results if a fever workup is required. The American Academy of Pediatrics classifies erythromycin as compatible with breast-feeding (17).

References

1. Product information. Ery-Tab. Abbott Laboratories, 2000.
2. Heilman FR, Herrell WE, Wellman WE, Geraci JE. Some laboratory and clinical observations on a new antibiotic, erythromycin (Ilotycin). Proc Staff Meet Mayo Clin 1952;27:285–304.
3. Kiefer L, Rubin A, McCoy JB, Foltz EL. The placental transfer of erythromycin. Am J Obstet Gynecol 1955;69:174–7.
4. Philipson A, Sabath LD, Charles D. Transplacental passage of erythromycin and clindamycin. N Engl J Med 1973;288:1219–20.
5. Fenton LJ, Light LJ. Congenital syphilis after maternal treatment with erythromycin. Obstet Gynecol 1976;47:492–4.
6. Philipson A, Sabath LD, Charles D. Erythromycin and clindamycin absorption and elimination in pregnant women. Clin Pharmacol Ther 1976;19:68–77.
7. McCormack WM, George H, Donner A, Kodgis LF, Albert S, Lowe EW, Kass EH. Hepatotoxicity of erythromycin estolate during pregnancy. Antimicrob Agents Chemother 1977;12:630–5.
8. Jaffe P, Liberman MM, McFadyen I, Valman HB. Incidence of congenital limb-reduction deformities. Lancet 1975;1:526–7.
9. Heinonen OP, Slone D, Shapiro S. *Birth Defects and Drugs in Pregnancy*. Littleton, MA: Publishing Sciences Group, 1977.
10. Gallagher JC, Ismail MA, Aladjem S. Reduced urinary estriol levels with erythromycin therapy. Obstet Gynecol 1980;56:381–2.
11. Merenstein GB, Todd WA, Brown G, Yost CC, Luzier T. Group B β-hemolytic streptococcus: randomized controlled treatment study at term. Obstet Gynecol 1980;55:315–8.
12. Easmon CSF, Hastings MJG, Deeley J, Bloxham B, Rivers RPA, Marwood R. The effect of intrapartum chemoprophylaxis on the vertical transmission of group B streptococci. Br J Obstet Gynaecol 1983;90:633–5.
13. Quinn PA, Shewchuk AB, Shuber J, Lie KI, Ryan E, Chipman ML, Nocilla DM. Efficacy of antibiotic therapy in preventing spontaneous pregnancy loss among couples colonized with genital mycoplasmas. Am J Obstet Gynecol 1983;145:239–44.
14. Kass EH, McCormack WM. Genital mycoplasma infection and perinatal morbidity. N Engl J Med 1984;311:258.
15. Kallen BAJ, Olausson PO. Maternal drug use in early pregnancy and infant cardiovascular defect. Reprod Toxicol 2003;17:255–61.
16. Knowles JA. Drugs in milk. Pediatr Curr 1972;21:28–32.
17. Committee on Drugs, American Academy of Pediatrics. The transfer of drugs and other chemicals into human milk. Pediatrics 2001;108:776–89.

Name:	**ESCITALOPRAM**	Risk Factor:	**C_M**
Class:	**Antidepressant**		

FETAL RISK SUMMARY

RECOMMENDATION: Human Data Suggest Risk in 3rd Trimester

Escitalopram is the S-enantiomer of racemic citalopram. It is a selective serotonin reuptake inhibitor (SSRI) that is indicated for the treatment of depression. The metabolites of escitalopram apparently do not contribute to the antidepressant activity. Plasma protein binding is moderate (56%), but the plasma elimination half-life is long (27–32 hours) (1).

All the antidepressant agents in this class (citalopram, escitalopram, fluoxetine, fluvoxamine, paroxetine, and sertraline) share a similar mechanism of action, although only citalopram and escitalopram have similar chemical structures. These differences could be construed as evidence against any conclusion that they share similar effects on the embryo, fetus, or newborn. In the mouse embryo, however, craniofacial morphogenesis appears to be regulated, at least in part, by serotonin. Interference with serotonin regulation by chemically different inhibitors produces similar craniofacial defects (2). Regardless of the structural differences, therefore, some of the potential adverse effects on the pregnancy also may be similar.

Reproduction studies have been conducted in rats. In rats, doses up to ≥56 times the maximum recommended human dose of 20 mg/day based on body surface area (MRHD) resulted in decreased fetal body weight and delayed ossification. Mild maternal toxicity (clinical signs and decreased body weight gain and food consumption) was evident at the developmental no-effect dose (28 times the MRHD). No teratogenicity was evident at any dose up to 75 times the MRHD. In rats treated throughout pregnancy and through weaning with doses up to 24 times the MRHD, slightly increased offspring mortality and growth retardation were observed at the highest dose. Mild maternal toxicity (same as noted above) was evident at the highest dose. The no-effect dose was 6 times the MRHD (1). (See also Citalopram for fertility studies in rats and teratology studies in rats and rabbits.)

It is not known if escitalopram crosses the human placenta. The molecular weight (about 324 for the free base), moderate plasma protein binding, and prolonged elimination half-life suggest the escitalopram will cross to the embryo and/or fetus.

No reports describing the use of escitalopram in human pregnancy have been located. The animal data suggest that the risk to an embryo/fetus is low. Importantly, no increase in defects or patterns of major defects has been observed with other agents in this class (see also Citalopram, Fluoxetine, Fluvoxamine, Paroxetine, and Sertraline). However, minor malformations and severe perinatal complications were observed with fluoxetine (see Fluoxetine). A 1999 review of SSRI antidepressants concluded that if therapy was required during pregnancy, the SSRIs were a good choice because of their side-effect profile and safety in overdose (3). Because fluoxetine had been studied the most during pregnancy, the reviewers recommended it as their first choice. Additional research, however, is needed on all SSRIs, including escitalopram, to better define their relationship to minor malformations and perinatal morbidity. In addition, investigations are needed on the potential of SSRIs for neurobehavior teratogenicity that might not become evident for years after birth.

BREAST FEEDING SUMMARY

RECOMMENDATION: No Human Data - Potential Toxicity

No reports describing the use of escitalopram during human lactation have been located.

The molecular weight (about 324 for the free base), moderate plasma protein binding (56%), and prolonged elimination half-life (27–32 hours) suggest the escitalopram will be excreted into breast milk. The effects of this exposure on a nursing infant are unknown. However, adverse effects have been observed in infants exposed to citalopram (see Citalopram). Therefore, similar effects should be expected with escitalopram and nursing infants should be closely monitored for evidence of toxicity. The American Academy of Pediatrics classifies other SSRI antidepressants as drugs for which the effect on nursing infants is unknown but may be of concern (e.g., see Fluoxetine).

References

1. Product information. Lexapro. Forest Pharmaceuticals, 2004.
2. Shuey DL, Sadler TW, Lauder JM. Serotonin as a regulator of craniofacial morphogenesis: site specific malformations following exposure to serotonin uptake inhibitors. Teratology 1992;46:367–78.
3. Masand PS, Gupta S. Selective serotonin-reuptake inhibitors: an update. Harv Rev Psychiatry 1999;7:69–84.

Name:	**ESMOLOL**	Risk Factor:	C_M
Class:	**Sympatholytic**		

FETAL RISK SUMMARY

RECOMMENDATION: Compatible - Maternal Benefit >> Embryo/Fetal Risk

Esmolol is a short-acting cardioselective β_1-adrenergic blocking agent that is structurally related to atenolol and metoprolol. The drug is used for the rapid, temporary treatment of supraventricular tachyarrhythmias (e.g., atrial flutter or fibrillation, sinus tachycardia) and for hypertension occurring during surgery. Because hypotension may occur with its use—up to 50% of patients in some trials—the potential for decreased uterine blood flow and resulting fetal hypoxia should be considered.

Reproduction studies in rats with IV doses up to 10 times the maximum human maintenance dose (MHMD) for 30 minutes daily revealed no evidence of embryo or fetal harm (1). Maternal toxicity and lethality were evident at 33 times the MHMD. Studies in pregnant rabbits with non-maternal toxic doses also failed to demonstrate embryo or fetal harm (1).

In pregnant sheep, the mean fetal:maternal serum ratio at the end of an infusion of esmolol was 0.08 (2). The drug was not detectable in the fetus 10 minutes after the end of the infusion. However, the hemodynamic effects in the fetal sheep, in terms of decreases in mean arterial pressure and heart rate, were similar to those in the mothers.

A 31-year-old woman at 22 weeks' gestation complicated by a subarachnoid hemorrhage was treated with esmolol prior to induction of anesthesia (3). The estimated weight of her fetus, by ultrasound, was 350 g. She was administered bolus doses of esmolol of up to 2 mg/kg with a continuous infusion of 200 μg/kg/minute. Fetal heart rate (FHR) decreased from 139–144 beats/minute to 131–137 beats/minute during esmolol treatment. No loss in FHR variability was observed. Administration of the drug was continued during surgery. A healthy, 2880-g boy was delivered at 37 weeks' gestation who was alive and well at 9 months of age.

A 29-year-old woman at 38 weeks' gestation presented with supraventricular tachycardia thought to be due to thyrotoxicosis (4). The FHR was 150–160 beats/minute. A bolus dose of esmolol, 0.5 mg/kg, followed by a continuous infusion of 50 μg/kg/minute was given to the mother. Approximately 20 minutes later, the FHR increased to 170–175 beats/minute; 4 minutes later it fell to 70–80 beats/minute. The severe bradycardia persisted despite stopping the esmolol and an emergency cesarean section was performed to deliver a 2660-g male infant. The infant's initial pulse was 60 beats/minute, but increased to 140 beats/minute within 60 seconds in response to oxygen therapy. The umbilical vein blood pH was 7.09. The mother's arrhythmia was successfully converted after delivery with verapamil. Both mother and infant recovered uneventfully. The authors speculated that the cause of the fetal bradycardia was an esmolol-induced decrease in placental blood flow or interference with fetal compensation for a marginal placental perfusion (4).

A laboring mother at 39 weeks' gestation had a recurrence of tachyarrhythmia (225–235 beats/minute) that resulted in symptomatic hypotension and fetal bradycardia (5). She was treated with esmolol by IV bolus and continuous infusion (total dose 1060 mg) until delivery of a 3390-g female infant with Apgar scores of 7 and 9. Symptoms of β-blockade in the infant included hypotonicity, weak cry, dusky appearance, and apnea with feeding, but except for mild jaundice, other evaluations (calcium, magnesium, and glucose serum levels) were normal. The feeding difficulties had resolved by 48 hours of age and the other symptoms by 60 hours of age.

β-Blockade in the fetus and newborn were described in a case in which the mother was treated with esmolol, 25 μg/kg/minute, for hypertrophic obstructive cardiomyopathy during labor (6). Within 10 minutes of starting esmolol and receiving IV fentanyl, the fetal heart declined from 160 beats/minute to 100 beats/minute with loss of beat-to-beat variability. The newborn had Apgar scores of 8 and 9 at 1 and 5 minutes, respectively, but was hypotensive (mean arterial pressure 34–39 mmHg), mildly hypotonic, hypoglycemic, and fed poorly. All of the symptoms had resolved by 36 hours of age.

A 1994 report described a woman who suffered a myocardial infarction at 26 weeks' gestation who was treated with an infusion of esmolol and other agents (7). She eventually delivered a healthy female infant at 39 weeks.

BREAST FEEDING SUMMARY

RECOMMENDATION: No Human Data - Probably Compatible

No reports describing the use of esmolol during lactation have been located. Because of the indications for this drug and the fact that it must be given by injection, the opportunities for use of esmolol while nursing are probably nil.

References

1. Product information. Brevibloc. Baxter Pharmaceutical, 2000.
2. Ostman PL, Chestnut DH, Robillard JE, Weiner CP, Hdez MJ. Transplacental passage and hemodynamic effects of esmolol in the gravid ewe. Anesthesiology 1988;69:738–41.
3. Losasso TJ, Muzzi DA, Cucchiara RF. Response of fetal heart rate to maternal administration of esmolol. Anesthesiology 1991;74:782–4.
4. Ducey JP, Knape KG. Maternal esmolol administration resulting in fetal distress and cesarean section in a term pregnancy. Anesthesiology 1992;77:829–32.
5. Gilson GJ, Knieriem KJ, Smith JF, Izquierdo L, Chatterjee MS, Curet LB. Short-acting beta-adrenergic blockade and the fetus. A case report. J Reprod Med 1992;37:277–9.
6. Fairley CJ, Clarke JT. Use of esmolol in a parturient with hypertrophic obstructive cardiomyopathy. Br J Anaesthesia 1995;75:801–4.
7. Sanchez-Ramos L, Chami YG, Bass TA, DelValle GO, Adair CD. Myocardial infarction during pregnancy: management with transluminal coronary angioplasty and metallic intracoronary stents.

Name:	**ESTAZOLAM**	Risk Factor:	**X_M**
Class:	**Hypnotic**		

FETAL RISK SUMMARY

RECOMMENDATION: Contraindicated

Estazolam is a benzodiazepine hypnotic agent in the same general class as flurazepam, quazepam, temazepam, and triazolam. It is indicated for the short-term management of insomnia. The metabolites have low potencies and concentrations and are not significant contributors to the hypnotic activity of estazolam. Plasma protein binding of estazolam is high (93%) and the range of estimated elimination half-life varies from 10 to 24 hours (1).

Animal reproduction studies have apparently not been conducted with estazolam. The manufacturer considers the drug contraindicated in pregnancy (1).

It is not known if estazolam crosses the human placenta. The molecular weight (about 295) and moderately long elimination half-life suggest that the drug will be transferred to the embryo/fetus. Of note, the benzodiazepine, diazepam, freely crosses the placenta and accumulates in the fetal circulation (see Diazepam).

No reports describing the use of estazolam in human pregnancy have been located. The effects of this drug on the fetus should be similar to other benzodiazepines (see Diazepam). Maternal use near delivery may potentially cause neonatal motor depression and withdrawal.

BREAST FEEDING SUMMARY

RECOMMENDATION: No Human Data - Potential Toxicity

No reports describing the use of estazolam during human lactation have been located. The molecular weight (about 295) and moderately long elimination half-life (in the range of 10–24 hours) suggest that the drug will be excreted into breast milk. Estazolam and/or its metabolites are excreted in the milk of lactating rats (1). Other agents in this class are excreted into milk in low concentrations (e.g., see Quazepam and Temazepam). No toxicity was observed in the nursing infants exposed to these two agents. However, the effects, if any, on an infant's central nervous system function are unknown. In recognition of this, the American Academy of Pediatrics classified quazepam and temazepam, especially when taken by nursing mothers for long periods, as agents whose effects on an infant are unknown, but may be of concern. Estazolam should be classified similarly.

Reference

1. Product information. ProSom. Abbott Laboratories, 2004.

Name:	**ESTRADIOL**	Risk Factor:	X_M
Class:	**Estrogenic Hormone**		

FETAL RISK SUMMARY

RECOMMENDATION: Contraindicated

Estradiol and its salts (cypionate, valerate) are used for treatment of menopausal symptoms, female hypogonadism, and primary ovarian failure. The more potent synthetic derivative, ethinyl estradiol, has similar indications and is also used in oral contraceptives (see also Oral Contraceptives).

The Collaborative Perinatal Project monitored 614 mother-child pairs with 1st trimester exposure to estrogenic agents (including 48 with exposure to estradiol) (1, pp. 389, 391). An increase in the expected frequency of cardiovascular defects, eye and ear anomalies, and Down's syndrome was found for estrogens as a group but not for estradiol (1, pp. 389, 391, 395). Re-evaluation of these data in terms of timing of exposure, vaginal bleeding in early pregnancy, and previous maternal obstetric history, however, failed to support an association between estrogens and cardiac malformations (2). An earlier study also failed to find any relationship with nongenital malformations (3).

In a surveillance study of Michigan Medicaid recipients conducted between 1985 and 1992 involving 229,101 completed pregnancies, 29 newborns had been exposed to ethinyl estradiol during the 1st trimester (F. Rosa, personal communication, FDA, 1993). Four (13.8%) major birth defects were observed (one expected), including (observed/expected)

1/0.3 cardiovascular defects, and 1/0 hypospadias. No anomalies were observed in four other categories of defects (oral clefts, spina bifida, polydactyly, and limb reduction defects) for which specific data were available. The number of exposures is too small for any conclusion.

Developmental changes in the psychosexual performance of boys have been attributed to *in utero* exposure to estradiol and progesterone (4). The mothers received an estrogen/progestogen regimen for their diabetes. Hormone-exposed males demonstrated a trend to have less heterosexual experience and fewer masculine interests than controls. Estradiol has been administered to women in labor in an attempt to potentiate the cervical ripening effects of prostaglandins (5). No detectable effect was observed. Use of estrogenic hormones during pregnancy is contraindicated.

BREAST FEEDING SUMMARY

RECOMMENDATION: Compatible

Estradiol is used to suppress postpartum breast engorgement in patients who do not desire to breast-feed. Following the administration of vaginal suppositories containing 50 or 100 mg of estradiol to six lactating women who wished to stop breast-feeding, less than 10% of the dose appeared in breast milk (6). The American Academy of Pediatrics classifies estradiol as compatible with breast-feeding (7).

References

1. Heinonen OP, Slone D, Shapiro S. *Birth Defects and Drugs in Pregnancy*. Littleton, MA: Publishing Sciences Group, 1977.
2. Wiseman RA, Dodds-Smith IC. Cardiovascular birth defects and antenatal exposure to female sex hormones: a reevaluation of some base data. Teratology 1984;30:359–70.
3. Wilson JG, Brent RL. Are female sex hormones teratogenic? Am J Obstet Gynecol 1981;141:567–80.
4. Yalom ID, Green R, Fisk N. Prenatal exposure to female hormones. Effect of psychosexual development in boys. Arch Gen Psychiatry 1973;28:554–61.
5. Luther ER, Roux J, Popat R, Gardner A, Gray J, Soubiran E, Korcaz Y. The effect of estrogen priming on induction of labor with prostaglandins. Am J Obstet Gynecol 1980;137:351–7.
6. Nilsson S, Nygren KG, Johansson EDB. Transfer of estradiol to human milk. Am J Obstet Gynecol 1978;132:653–7.
7. Committee on Drugs, American Academy of Pediatrics. The transfer of drugs and other chemicals into human milk. Pediatrics 2001;108:776–89.

Name:	**ESTROGENS, CONJUGATED**	Risk Factor:	X_M
Class:	**Estrogenic Hormone**		

FETAL RISK SUMMARY

RECOMMENDATION: Contraindicated

Conjugated estrogens are a mixture of estrogenic substances (primarily estrone). The Collaborative Perinatal Project monitored 13 mother-child pairs who were exposed to conjugated estrogens during the 1st trimester (1, pp. 389, 391). An increased risk for malformations was found, although identification of the malformations was not provided. Estrogenic agents as a group were monitored in 614 mother-child pairs. An increase in the expected frequency of cardiovascular defects, eye and ear anomalies, and Down's syndrome was reported (1, p. 395). Reevaluation of these data in terms of timing of exposure, vaginal bleeding in early pregnancy, and previous maternal obstetric history, however, failed to support an association between estrogens and cardiac malformations (2).

An earlier study also failed to find any relationship with nongenital malformations (3). No adverse effects were observed in one infant exposed during the 1st trimester to conjugated estrogens (4). However, in an infant exposed during the 4th–7th weeks of gestation to conjugated estrogens, multiple anomalies were found: cleft palate, micrognathia, wormian bones, heart defect, dislocated hips, absent tibiae, bowed fibulae, polydactyly, and abnormal dermal patterns (5). Multiple other agents were also taken during this pregnancy, but only conjugated estrogens and prochlorperazine (see also Prochlorperazine) appeared to have been taken during the critical period for the malformations.

Conjugated estrogens have been used to induce ovulation in anovulatory women (6). They have also been used as partially successful contraceptives when given within 72 hours of unprotected, midcycle coitus (7). No fetal adverse effects were mentioned in either of these reports.

BREAST FEEDING SUMMARY

RECOMMENDATION: No Human Data - Probably Compatible

No reports of adverse effects from conjugated estrogens in the nursing infant have been located. It is possible that decreased milk volume and decreased nitrogen and protein content could occur (see Mestranol, Ethinyl Estradiol).

References

1. Heinonen OP, Slone D, Shapiro S. *Birth Defects and Drugs in Pregnancy*. Littleton, MA: Publishing Sciences Group, 1977.
2. Wiseman RA, Dodds-Smith IC. Cardiovascular birth defects and antenatal exposure to female sex hormones: a reevaluation of some base data. Teratology 1984;30:359–70.
3. Wilson JG, Brent RL. Are female sex hormones teratogenic? Am J Obstet Gynecol 1981;141:567–80.
4. Hagler S, Schultz A, Hankin H, Kunstadter RH. Fetal effects of steroid therapy during pregnancy. Am J Dis Child 1963;106:586–90.
5. Ho CK, Kaufman RL, McAlister WH. Congenital malformations. Cleft palate, congenital heart disease, absent tibiae, and polydactyly. Am J Dis Child 1975;129:714–6.
6. Price R. Pregnancies using conjugated oestrogen therapy. Med J Aust 1980;2:341–2.
7. Dixon GW, Schlesselman JJ, Ory HW, Blye RP. Ethinyl estradiol and conjugated estrogens as postcoital contraceptives. JAMA 1980;244:1336–9.

Name: **ESTRONE** Risk Factor: **X**
Class: **Estrogenic Hormone**

See Estrogens, Conjugated.

Name: **ETANERCEPT** Risk Factor: **B_M**
Class: **Immunologic Agent (Immunomodulator)**

FETAL RISK SUMMARY

RECOMMENDATION: Limited Human Data - Animal Data Suggest Low Risk

Etanercept is a dimeric fusion protein, produced by recombinant DNA technology (Chinese hamster ovary mammalian cell expression system), consisting of the extracellular ligand-binding portion of the human kilodalton (p75) tumor necrosis factor receptor (TNFR) linked to the Fc portion of human IgG1. The protein binds specifically to tumor necrosis factor (TNF), a cytokine involved in inflammatory and immune responses, to block its interaction with cell surface TNFRs (1,2). Etanercept is indicated for reducing the signs and symptoms and delaying structural damage in moderate to severe rheumatoid arthritis, including juvenile arthritis. The drug is administered by SC injection.

Reproduction studies in rats and rabbits at doses 60 to 100 times the human dose revealed no fetal harm (1,2). Animal fertility and carcinogenic studies have not been conducted with etanercept, but it was not mutagenic in *in vitro* and *in vivo* tests.

A 32-year-old woman with a 1-year history of rheumatoid arthritis and infertility was treated with SC etanercept (25 mg twice weekly), oral methotrexate (2.5 mg/week), and rofecoxib (25 mg/day) (3). Three months after stopping methotrexate and rofecoxib, and 4 weeks after the last dose of etanercept (total dose 3300 mg over 64 months), she underwent ovulation induction and intrauterine insemination. A successful pregnancy occurred and she delivered a healthy, 2659-g female infant at term. The baby was doing well at 3 months of age (3).

A 37-year-old woman with infertility secondary to antiphospholipid antibodies and elevated natural killer (NK) cells was treated with etanercept (25 mg SC twice weekly), low-dose aspirin (81 mg/day), and low molecular weight heparin (enoxaparin 30 mg SC daily) (4). The woman also had a history of chronic leukopenia that was attributed to Epstein-Barr virus. She became pregnant 1 month after the start of therapy. All three agents were discontinued at gestational week 32. At about 38 weeks' gestation, she delivered a healthy male (about 2486-g) infant that was doing well at 21 months of age. Although it could not be proven, the authors speculated that etanercept might have played a role in the pregnancy by inhibiting TNF produced by the NK cells in the lining of the woman's uterus (4).

A survey of 600 members of the American College of Rheumatology, partially conducted to determine the outcomes of pregnancies exposed to disease modifying antirheumatic drugs (DMARDs) (etanercept, infliximab, leflunomide, and methotrexate), was published in 2003 (5). From the 175 responders, the outcomes of 15 pregnancies exposed to etanercept were six full term healthy infants, one spontaneous abortion (also taking methotrexate), one elective abortion, three unknown outcomes, and four women still pregnant (5).

In summary, etanercept was not toxic or teratogenic in animal reproduction tests at doses much higher than those used clinically. Although the human pregnancy experience is very limited, there is currently no evidence of embryo/fetal harm. However, the human data are too limited for a full assessment of the risk. An early review recommended that pregnancy should be excluded before etanercept was administered to women of childbearing age and that effective contraception should be used during treatment (6). Another review speculated that etanercept could disrupt pregnancy because of its anti-cytokine activity (7). However, this theoretical concern has not been shown clinically (8). If etanercept is used in pregnancy for the treatment of rheumatoid arthritis, healthcare professionals are encouraged to call the toll free number (877-311-8972) for information about patient enrollment in the OTIS Rheumatoid Arthritis Study.

BREAST FEEDING SUMMARY

RECOMMENDATION: No Human Data - Probably Compatible

No reports describing the use of etanercept during human lactation have been located. The effects of exposure to this protein on a nursing infant are unknown (7). Because etanercept is a protein, it most likely would be digested in the infants' stomach and not absorbed systemically.

References

1. Product information. Enbrel. Immunex, 2001.
2. Product information. Enbrel. Wyeth-Ayerst Pharmaceuticals, 2001.
3. Sills ES, Perloe M, Tucker MJ, Kaplan CR, Palermo GD. Successful ovulation induction, conception, and normal delivery after chronic therapy with etanercept: a recombinant fusion anti-cytokine treatment for rheumatoid arthritis. Am J Reprod Immunol 2001;46:366–8.
4. Wallace DJ, Weisman MH. The use of etanercept and other tumor necrosis factor-α blockers in infertility: it's time to get serious. J Rheumatol 2003;30:1897–9.
5. Chakravarty EF, Sanchez-Yamamoto D, Bush TM. The use of disease modifying antirheumatic drugs in women with rheumatoid arthritis of childbearing age: a survey of practice patterns and pregnancy outcomes. J Rheumatol 2003;30:241–6.
6. Janssen NM, Genta MS. The effects of immunosuppressive and anti-inflammatory medications on fertility, pregnancy, and lactation. Arch Intern Med 2000;160: 610–9.
7. Jarvis B, Faulds D. Etanercept. A review of its use in rheumatoid arthritis. Drugs 1999;57: 945–66.
8. Khanna D, McMahon M, Furst DE. Safety of tumour necrosis factor-α antagonists. Drug Saf 2004;27: 307–24.

Name:	**ETHACRYNIC ACID**	Risk Factor:	B_M*
Class:	**Diuretic**		

FETAL RISK SUMMARY

RECOMMENDATION: Limited Human Data - Animal Data Suggest Low Risk

Ethacrynic acid is a potent diuretic. It has been used for toxemia, pulmonary edema, and diabetes insipidus during pregnancy (1–10).

Reproduction studies in mice and rabbits at doses up to 50 times the human dose showed no evidence of external malformations (11). Doses of 10 or 2.5 times the human dose in rats and dogs, respectively, did not impair fertility or growth and development of pups (11). Intrauterine growth retardation was observed in the offspring of rats at a dose 50 times the human dose, but there was no effect on survival or postnatal development (11).

Although limited 1st trimester human experience has not shown an increased incidence of malformations, ethacrynic acid is not recommended for use in pregnant women (12). Diuretics do not prevent or alter the course of toxemia, but they may decrease placental perfusion (see also Chlorothiazide) (13–15). In general, diuretics are not recommended for the treatment of gestational hypertension because of the maternal hypovolemia characteristic of this disease.

Ototoxicity has been observed in a mother and her newborn following the use of ethacrynic acid and kanamycin during the 3rd trimester (see also Kanamycin) (16).

[*Risk Factor D if used in gestational hypertension.*]

BREAST FEEDING SUMMARY

RECOMMENDATION: No Human Data - Probably Compatible

No reports describing the use of ethacrynic acid during lactation have been located (see also Chlorothiazide). The manufacturer recommends that ethacrynic acid not be used in nursing mothers (11).

References

1. Delgado Urdapilleta J, Dominguez Robles H, Villalobos Roman M, Perez Diaz A. Ethacrynic acid in the treatment of toxemia of pregnancy. Ginecol Obstet Mex 1968;23:271–80.
2. Felman D, Theoleyre J, Dupoizat H. Investigation of ethacrynic acid in the treatment of excessive gain in weight and pregnancy arterial hypertension. Lyon Med 1967;217:1421–8.
3. Sands RX, Vita F. Ethacrynic acid (a new diuretic), pregnancy, and excessive fluid retention. Am J Obstet Gynecol 1968;101:603–9.
4. Kittaka S, Aizawa M, Tokue I, Shimizu M. Clinical results in Edecril tablet in the treatment of toxemia of late pregnancy. Obstet Gynecol (Jpn) 1968;36: 934–7.
5. Mahon R, Dubecq JP, Baudet E, Coqueran J. Use of Edecrin in obstetrics. Bull Fed Soc Gynecol Obstet Lang Fr 1968;20:440–2.
6. Imaizumi S, Suzuoki Y, Torri M, et al. Clinical trial of ethacrynic acid (Edecril) for toxemia of pregnancy. Jpn J Med Consult New Remedies 1969;6: 2364–8.
7. Young BK, Haft JI. Treatment of pulmonary edema with ethacrynic acid during labor. Am J Obstet Gynecol 1970;107:330–1.
8. Harrison KA, Ajabor LN, Lawson JB. Ethacrynic acid and packed-blood-cell transfusion in treatment of severe anaemia in pregnancy. Lancet 1971;1: 11–4.
9. Fort AT, Morrison JC, Fisk SA. Iatrogenic hypokalemia of pregnancy by furosemide and ethacrynic acid: two case reports. J Reprod Med 1971;6:21–2.
10. Pico I, Greenblatt RB. Endocrinopathies and infertility. IV. Diabetes insipidus and pregnancy. Fertil Steril 1969;20:384–92.
11. Product information. Edecrin. Merck, 2000.
12. Wilson AL, Matzke GR. The treatment of hypertension in pregnancy. Drug Intell Clin Pharm 1981;15: 21–6.
13. Pitkin RM, Kaminetzky HA, Newton M, Pritchard JA. Maternal nutrition: a selective review of clinical topics. Obstet Gynecol 1972;40:773–85.
14. Lindheimer MD, Katz AI. Sodium and diuretics in pregnancy. N Engl J Med 1973;288:891–4.
15. Christianson R, Page EW. Diuretic drugs and pregnancy. Obstet Gynecol 1976;48:647–52.
16. Jones HC. Intrauterine ototoxicity: a case report and review of literature. J Natl Med Assoc 1973;65: 201–3.

Name:	**ETHAMBUTOL**	Risk Factor:	**B**
Class:	**Antituberculosis Agent**		

FETAL RISK SUMMARY

RECOMMENDATION: Compatible

No reports linking the use of ethambutol with congenital defects have been located. The drug crosses the placenta to the fetus (1,2). In a woman who delivered at 38 weeks' gestation, ethambutol concentrations in the cord and maternal blood 30 hours after an 800-mg (15 mg/kg) dose were 4.1 and 5.5 ng/mL, respectively, a cord:maternal serum ratio of 0.75 (1). The amniotic fluid ethambutol level was 9.5 ng/mL (1). These levels were within the range (1–5 ng/mL) required to inhibit the growth of *Mycobacterium tuberculosis* (1).

The literature supports the safety of ethambutol in combination with isoniazid and rifampin during pregnancy (3–7). One investigator studied 38 patients (42 pregnancies) receiving antitubercular therapy (3). The minor abnormalities noted were within the expected frequency of occurrence. Another researcher observed six aborted fetuses at 5–12 weeks of age (4). Embryonic optic systems were specifically examined and were found to be normal. Most reviewers consider ethambutol, along with isoniazid and rifampin, to be the safest antituberculosis therapy (8,9). However, long-term follow-up examinations for ocular damage have not been reported, causing concern among some clinicians (10).

BREAST FEEDING SUMMARY

RECOMMENDATION: Limited Human Data - Probably Compatible

Ethambutol is excreted into human milk. Milk concentrations in two women (unpublished data) were 1.4 μg/mL (after an oral dose of 15 mg/kg) and 4.60 μg/mL (dosage not given)

(11). Corresponding maternal serum levels were 1.5 μg/mL and 4.62 μg/mL, respectively, indicating milk:serum ratios of approximately 1:1. The American Academy of Pediatrics classifies ethambutol as compatible with breast-feeding (12).

References

1. Shneerson JM, Francis RS. Ethambutol in pregnancy-foetal exposure. Tubercle 1979;60:167–9.
2. Holdiness MR. Transplacental pharmacokinetics of the antituberculosis drugs. Clin Pharmacokinet 1987;13:125–9.
3. Bobrowitz ID. Ethambutol in pregnancy. Chest 1974;66:20–4.
4. Lewit T, Nebel L, Terracina S, Karman S. Ethambutol in pregnancy: observations on embryogenesis. Chest 1974;66:25–6.
5. Snider DE, Layde PM, Johnson MW, Lyle MA. Treatment of tuberculosis during pregnancy. Am Rev Respir Dis 1980;122:65–79.
6. Brock PG, Roach M. Antituberculous drugs in pregnancy. Lancet 1981;1:43.
7. Kingdom JCP, Kennedy DH. Tuberculous meningitis in pregnancy. Br J Obstet Gynaecol 1989;96:233–5.
8. American Thoracic Society. Treatment of tuberculosis and tuberculosis infection in adults and children. Am Rev Respir Dis 1986;134:355–63.
9. Medchill MT, Gillum M. Diagnosis and management of tuberculosis during pregnancy. Obstet Gynecol Surv 1989;44:81–4.
10. Wall MA. Treatment of tuberculosis during pregnancy. Am Rev Respir Dis 1980;122:989.
11. Snider DE Jr, Powell KE. Should women taking antituberculosis drugs breast-feed? Arch Intern Med 1984;144:589–90.
12. Committee on Drugs, American Academy of Pediatrics. The transfer of drugs and other chemicals into human milk. Pediatrics 2001;108:776–89.

Name: **ETHANOL** Risk Factor: **D***

Class: **Sedative**

FETAL RISK SUMMARY

RECOMMENDATION: Contraindicated

The teratogenic effects of ethanol (alcohol) have been recognized since antiquity, but this knowledge gradually fell into disfavor and was actually dismissed as superstition in the 1940s (1). Approximately three decades later, the characteristic pattern of anomalies that came to be known as the fetal alcohol syndrome (FAS) were rediscovered, first in France and then in the United States (2–5). By 1981, more than 800 clinical and research papers on the FAS had been published (6).

Mild FAS (low birth weight) has been induced by the daily consumption of as little as two drinks (1 ounce of absolute alcohol or about 30 mL) in early pregnancy, but the complete syndrome is usually seen when maternal consumption is four to five drinks (60–75 mL of absolute alcohol) per day or more. The Council on Scientific Affairs of the American Medical Association and the American Council on Science and Health have each published reports on the consequences of maternal alcohol ingestion during pregnancy (7,8). The incidence of the FAS, depending upon the population studied, is estimated to be between 1/300 and 1/2,000 live births with 30%–40% of the offspring of alcoholic mothers expected to show the complete syndrome (7). The true incidence may be even higher because the diagnosis of FAS can be delayed for many years (9) (e.g., see reference 25 below). In addition, the incidence of alcohol abuse seems to be rising. A 1989 report found that alcohol abuse during 1987 in 1,032 pregnant women was 1.4%, compared to 0.7% of 5,602 pregnant women during 1977–1980 (10). The difference in frequency was significant ($p < 0.05$).

Heavy alcohol intake by the father prior to conception has been suspected of producing the FAS (11,12), although this association has been challenged (13). The report by the AMA

Council states that growth retardation and some adverse aspects of fetal development may be a result of paternal influence but conclusive evidence for the complete FAS is lacking (7).

Evidence supporting an association between "regular drinking" by the father in the month before conception and the infant's birth weight was published in two reports, both by the same authors (14,15). "Regular drinking" was defined as "an average of at least 30 ml of ethanol daily or of 75 mL or more on a single occasion at least once a month" (14) "Occasional drinking" was defined as anything less than this. The mean birth weight, 3465 g, of 174 infants of "regular drinking" fathers was 181 g less than the mean birth weight, 3646 g, of 203 infants of "occasional drinking" fathers, a significant difference ($p < 0.001$). Using regression analysis, a 137-g decrease in birth weight was predicted (15). Statistical significance was also present when the data were categorized by sex (males 3561 g vs. 3733 g ($p < 0.05$), females 3364 g vs. 3538 g ($p < 0.05$)), percentage of infants weighing less than 3000 g (15% vs. 9% ($p < 0.05$)), and percentage of infants weighing 4000 g or more (12% vs. 23% ($p < 0.01$)). Infant characteristics unrelated to the father's drinking were length, head circumference, gestational age, and Apgar scores (15). Consideration of the mother's drinking, smoking, and marijuana use did not change the statistical significance of the data. Nor could the differences be attributed to any of 20 reproductive and socioeconomic variables that were examined, including paternal smoking and marijuana use. No increases in structural defects were detected in the infants of the "regular drinking" fathers, but the sample size may have been too small to detect such an increase (14). In contrast to these data, other researchers have been unable to find an association between paternal drinking and infant birth weight (16). Thus, additional research is required, especially because the biologic mechanisms for the proposed association have not been determined (15).

The mechanism of ethanol's teratogenic effect is unknown but may be related to acetaldehyde, a metabolic byproduct of ethanol (7). One researcher reported higher blood levels of acetaldehyde in mothers of children with FAS than in alcoholics who delivered normal children (17). However, the analysis techniques used in that study have been questioned, and the high concentrations may have been a result of artifactual formation of acetaldehyde (18). At the cellular level, alcohol or one of its metabolites may disrupt protein synthesis, resulting in cellular growth retardation with serious consequences for fetal brain development (19). Other proposed mechanisms that may contribute, as reviewed by Shepard (20), include poor protein intake, vitamin B deficiency, lead contamination of alcohol, and genetic predisposition. Of interest, metronidazole, a commonly used anti-infective agent, has been shown to markedly potentiate the fetotoxicity and teratogenicity of alcohol in mice (21). Human studies of this possible interaction have not been reported.

Complete FAS consists of abnormalities in three areas, with a fourth area often involved: (a) craniofacial dysmorphology, (b) prenatal and antenatal growth deficiencies, (c) central nervous system dysfunction, and (d) various other abnormalities (7,8). Problems occurring in the latter area include cardiac and renogenital defects and hemangiomas in about one-half of the cases (3–5,22). Cardiac malformations were described in 43 patients (57%) in a series of 76 children with the FAS evaluated for 0–6 years (age: birth to 18 years) (23). Functional murmurs (12 cases, 16%) and ventricular septal defects (VSD) (20 patients, 26%) accounted for the majority of anomalies. Other cardiac lesions present, in descending order of frequency, were: double-outlet right ventricle and pulmonary atresia; dextrocardia (with VSD); patent ductus arteriosus with secondary pulmonary hypertension; and cor pulmonale. Liver abnormalities have also been reported (24,25). Behavioral problems, including minimal brain dysfunction, are long-term effects of the FAS (1).

Ten-year follow-up of the original 11 children who were first diagnosed as having the FAS was reported in 1985 (25). Of the 11 children, two were dead, one was lost to follow-up, four had borderline intelligence with continued growth deficiency and were dysmorphic, and four had severe intelligence deficiency as well as growth deficiency and dysmorphic appearance. Moreover, the degree of growth deficiency and intellectual impairment was directly related to the degree of craniofacial abnormalities (25). In the eight children examined, height, weight, and head circumference were deficient, especially the latter two parameters. The authors concluded that the slow head growth after birth may explain why, in some cases, the FAS is not diagnosed until 9–12 months of age (25). Cardiac malformations originally observed in the infants, atrial septal defect (one), patent ductus arteriosus (one), and ventricular septal defect (six), had either resolved spontaneously or were no longer clinically significant. Three new features of the FAS were observed: dental malalignment, malocclusion, and eustachian tube dysfunction (associated with maxillary hypoplasia and leading to chronic serous otitis media) (25).

Fetal Alcohol Syndrome (2–9,11–13,22–38)

Craniofacial

- Eyes: short palpebral fissures, ptosis, strabismus, epicanthal folds, myopia, microphthalmia, blepharophimosis
- Ears: poorly formed concha, posterior rotation, eustachian tube dysfunction
- Nose: short, upturned hypoplastic philtrum
- Mouth: prominent lateral palatine ridges, thinned upper vermilion, retrognathia in infancy, micrognathia or relative prognathia in adolescence, cleft lip or palate, small teeth with faulty enamel, Class III malocclusion, poor dental alignment
- Maxilla: hypoplastic

Central nervous system

- Dysfunction demonstrated by mild to moderate retardation, microcephaly, poor coordination, hypotonia, irritability in infancy and hyperactivity in childhood

Growth

- Prenatal (affecting body length more than weight) and postnatal deficiency (length, weight, and head circumference)

Cardiac

- Murmurs, atrial septal defect, ventricular septal defect, great vessel anomalies, tetralogy of Fallot

Renogenital

- Labial hypoplasia, hypospadias, renal defects

Cutaneous

- Hemangiomas, hirsutism in infancy

Skeletal

- Abnormal palmar creases, pectus excavatum, restriction of joint movement, nail hypoplasia, radioulnar synostosis, pectus carinatum, bifid xiphoid, Klippel-Feil anomaly, scoliosis

Muscular

- Hernias of diaphragm, umbilicus or groin, diastasis recti

A study published in 1987 found that craniofacial abnormalities were closely related to alcohol consumption in a dose-response manner (39). Although a distinct threshold was not defined, the data indicated that the consumption of more than six drinks (90 mL of ethanol) per day was clearly related to structural defects, with the critical period for alcohol-induced teratogenicity around the time of conception (39). A 1989 study that examined 595 live singleton births found a significant correlation between alcohol use in the first 2 months of pregnancy and intrauterine growth retardation and structural abnormalities (40). Analysis of alcohol use during the other periods of pregnancy did not show a significant association with these outcomes.

A prospective study conducted between 1974 and 1977 at the Kaiser-Permanente health maintenance organization in Northern California was conducted to determine whether light to moderate drinking during pregnancy was associated with congenital abnormalities (41). A total of 32,870 women met all of the criteria for enrollment in the study. Of the total study population, 15,460 (47%) used alcohol during pregnancy, 17,114 (52%) denied use, and 296 (1%) provided incomplete information on their drinking. Of those drinking, 14,502 (94%) averaged less than one drink/day, 793 (5%) drank one to two drinks/day, 127 (0.8%) consumed three to five drinks/day, and 38 (0.2%) drank six or more drinks/day. The total (major and minor) malformation rates were similar between nondrinkers and light (less than one drink/day) or moderate (one to two drinks/day) drinkers; 78.1/1000, 77.3/1000, and 83.2/1000, respectively. A significant trend ($p = 0.034$) was found with increasing alcohol use and congenital malformations of the sex organs (e.g., absence or hypertrophy of the labia, clitoris, and vagina; defects of the ovaries, fallopian tubes, and uterus; hypoplastic or absent penis or scrotum; intersex and unspecified genital anomalies) (41). Rates per 1000 for defects of the sex organs in nondrinkers and the four drinking groups were 2.8, 2.6, 6.3, 7.9, and 26.3, respectively. Genitourinary malformations (i.e., cryptorchidism, hypospadias, and epispadias) also followed an increasing trend with rates per 1000 women of 27.2, 27.5, 31.5, 47.2, and 78.9 (p value for trend $= 0.04$), respectively. At the levels of alcohol consumption observed in the study, no increase in the other malformations commonly associated with the FAS was found with increasing alcohol use.

A strong association between moderate drinking (>30 mL of absolute alcohol twice per week) and 2nd trimester (15–27 weeks) spontaneous abortions has been found (27,28). Alcohol consumption at this level may increase the risk of miscarriage by 2–4-fold, apparently by acting as an acute fetal toxin. Consumption of smaller amounts of alcohol, such as one drink (approximately 15 mL of absolute alcohol) per week, was not associated with an increased risk of miscarriage in a 1989 report (42).

Ethanol was once used to treat premature uterine contractions. In a retrospective analysis of women treated for premature labor between 1968 and 1973, 239 singleton pregnancies were identified (43). In 136, the women had received oral and/or IV ethanol, in addition to bed rest and oral β-mimetics. The remaining 103 women had been treated only with bed rest and oral β-mimetics. The alcohol group received an average of 38 g of ethanol/day for 2–34 days. In addition, 73 of these women continued to use oral alcohol at home as needed to arrest uterine contractions. Treatment with ethanol was begun at 12 weeks' gestation or less in 82 (60.3%) of the treated women. The mean birth weights of the alcohol-exposed and nonexposed infants were similar, 3385 g vs. 3283 g, respectively. No significant differences were found between the groups in the number of infants who were small for gestational age (weight or length <10th percentile), birth length, fetal and neonatal deaths, and infants with anomalies. No relationship was found between ethanol dose and birth weight, length, or neonatal outcome. None of the exposed infants had features of the typical fetal alcohol syndrome. Psychomotor development (age to sit, walk, speak sentences of a few words, and read) and growth velocity were similar between the two groups. One of the infants whose mother had been treated with IV alcohol was growth retarded from birth to 14 years of age. Eight (6.1%) of 131 alcohol-exposed infants were considered to have problems in school (hyperactivity, carelessness) compared with 2 (2.0%) of 99 controls, but the difference was not significant. Other complications observed were aphasia and impaired hearing in 2 infants of the treated group and a third infant with blindness in the right eye (this infant was delivered at 27 weeks' gestation and the condition was thought to be a consequence of oxygen therapy). The authors concluded that the alcohol treatment for threatened 1st or 2nd trimester abortions did not cause fetal damage (43). However, an earlier study concluded that adverse effects occurred after even short-term exposure (44). This conclusion was reached in an evaluation of 25 children 4–7 years of age whose mothers had been treated with alcohol infusions to prevent preterm labor (44). In comparison with matched controls, seven children born during or within 15 hours of termination of the infusion had significant pathology in developmental and personality evaluations.

Two reports have described neural tube defects in six infants exposed to heavy amounts of alcohol during early gestation (45,46). Lumbosacral meningomyelocele was observed in five of the newborns and anencephaly in one. One of the infants also had a dislocated hip and clubfeet (45).

A possible association between maternal drinking and clubfoot was proposed in a short 1985 report (47). Three of 43 infants, delivered from maternal alcoholics, had fetal talipes equinovarus (clubfoot), an incidence significantly greater than expected ($p < 0.00001$).

Gastroschisis has been observed in dizygotic twins delivered from a mother who consumed 150–180 mL of absolute ethanol/day during the first 10 weeks of gestation (48). Although an association could not be proven, the authors speculated that the defects resulted from the heavy alcohol ingestion.

A 1982 report described four offspring of alcoholic mothers with clinical and laboratory features of combined FAS and DiGeorge syndrome (49). Several characteristics of the two syndromes are similar, including craniofacial, cardiac, central nervous system, renal, and immune defects (49). Features not shared are hypoparathyroidism (part of DiGeorge syndrome) and skeletal anomalies (part of FAS). A possible causative relationship was suggested between maternal alcoholism and the DiGeorge syndrome.

An unusual chromosomal anomaly was discovered in a 2-year-old girl whose mother drank heavily during early gestation (50). The infant's karyotype revealed an isochromosome for the long arm of number 9: 46,XX,−9,+i(9q). The infant had several characteristics of the FAS, including growth retardation. The relationship between the chromosomal defect and alcohol is unknown.

Prospective analysis of 31,604 pregnancies found that the percentage of newborns below the 10th percentile of weight for gestational age increased sharply as maternal alcohol intake increased (51). In comparison to nondrinkers, mean birth weight was reduced 14 g in those newborns whose mothers drank less than one drink/day and 165 g in those newborns whose mothers drank three to five drinks/day. The risk for growth retardation was markedly increased by the ingestion of one to two drinks each day. Other investigators discovered that women who drank more than 100 g of absolute alcohol/week at the time of conception had an increased risk of delivering a growth-retarded infant (52). The risk was twice that of women ingesting less than 50 g/week. Of special significance, the risk for growth retardation was not reduced if drinking was reduced later in pregnancy. However, a 1983 report found that if heavy drinkers reduced their consumption in midpregnancy, growth impairment was also reduced, although an increased incidence of congenital defects was still evident (53). Significantly smaller head circumferences have been measured in offspring of mothers who drank more than an average of 20 mL of alcohol/day compared to nondrinkers (54). In this same study, the incidence of major congenital anomalies in drinkers and nondrinkers was 1.2% vs none (54). These authors concluded that there was no safe level of alcohol consumption in pregnancy.

Alcohol ingestion has been shown to abolish fetal breathing (55). Eleven women, at 37–40 weeks' gestation, were given 0.25 g/kg of ethanol. Within 30 minutes, fetal breathing movements were almost abolished and remained so for 3 hours. No effect on gross fetal body movements or fetal heart rate was observed. However, a 1986 report described four women admitted to a hospital because of marked alcohol intoxication (56). In each case, fetal heart rate tracings revealed no or poor variability and no reactivity to fetal movements or external stimuli. Because of suspected fetal distress, an emergency cesarean section was performed in one patient, but no signs of hypoxia were present in the healthy infant. In the remaining three women, normalization of the fetal heart rate patterns occurred within 11–14 hours when the mothers became sober.

A study of the relationship between maternal alcohol ingestion and the risk of respiratory distress syndrome (RDS) in their infants was published in 1987 (57). Of the 531 infants in the study, 134 were delivered at a gestational age of 28–36 weeks. The 134 mothers of these preterm infants were classified by the amount of alcohol they consumed per occasion into abstainers ($N = 58$) (none), occasional ($N = 21$) (less than 15 mL), social ($N = 15$) (15–30 mL), binge ($N = 12$) (greater than 75 mL), and alcoholic ($N = 28$). The incidence of RDS in the infants from the five groups was 44.8%, 38.1%, 26.7%, 16.7%, and 21.4%, respectively. The difference between abstainers and those frankly alcoholic was significant ($p < 0.05$). Moreover, assuming equal intervals of alcohol intake among the five groups, the decrease in incidence of RDS with increasing alcohol intake was significant ($p < 0.02$). Adjustment of the data for smoking, gestational age, birth weight, Apgar score, and sex of the infant did not change the findings. The authors concluded that chronic alcohol ingestion may have enhanced fetal lung maturation (57).

Neonatal alcohol withdrawal has been demonstrated in offspring of mothers ingesting a mean of 21 ounces (630 mL) of alcohol/week during pregnancy (58). In comparison to infants exposed to an equivalent amount of ethanol only during early gestation or to infants whose mothers never drank, the heavily exposed infants had significantly more withdrawal symptoms. No differences were found between the infants exposed only during early gestation and those never exposed. Electroencephalogram (EEG) testing of infants at 4–6 weeks of age indicated that the irritability and tremors may be due to a specific effect of ethanol on the fetal brain and not to withdrawal or prematurity (59). Persistent EEG hypersynchrony was observed in those infants delivered from mothers who drank more than 60 mL of alcohol/day during pregnancy. The EEG findings were found in the absence of dysmorphology and as a result, the authors suggested that this symptom should be added to the definition of the FAS (59).

Combined fetal alcohol and hydantoin syndromes have been described in several reports (60–63). The infants exhibited numerous similar features from exposure to alcohol and phenytoin. The possibility that the agents are also carcinogenic *in utero* has been suggested by the finding of ganglioneuroblastoma in a 35-month-old boy and Hodgkin's disease in a 45-month-old girl, both with the combined syndromes (see also Phenytoin) (61–63). Adrenal carcinoma in a 13-year-old girl with FAS has also been reported (64). These findings may be fortuitous, but long-term follow-up of children with the FAS is needed.

An unusual cause of FAS was described in 1981 (65). A woman consumed, throughout pregnancy, 480–840 mL/day of an over-the-counter cough preparation. Because the cough syrup contained 9.5% alcohol, the woman was ingesting 45.6–79.8 mL of ethanol/day. The infant had the typical facial features of the FAS, plus an umbilical hernia and hypoplastic labia. Irritability, tremors, and hypertonicity were also evident.

In summary, ethanol is a teratogen and its use during pregnancy, especially during the first 2 months after conception, is associated with significant risk to the fetus and newborn. Heavy maternal use is related to a spectrum of defects collectively termed the fetal alcohol syndrome. Even moderate use may be related to spontaneous abortions and to developmental and behavioral dysfunction in the infant. A safe level of maternal alcohol consumption has not been established (7,8,66). Based on practical considerations, the American Council on Science and Health recommends that pregnant women limit their alcohol consumption to no more than two drinks daily (1 ounce or 30 mL of absolute alcohol) (8). However, the safest course for women who are pregnant, or who are planning to become pregnant, is abstinence (7,66).

[*Risk Factor X if used in large amounts or for prolonged periods.*]

BREAST FEEDING SUMMARY

RECOMMENDATION: Hold Breast Feeding

Although alcohol passes freely into breast milk, reaching concentrations approximating maternal serum levels, the effect on the infant has been considered insignificant except in rare cases or at very high concentrations (67). Recent research on the effects of chronic exposure of the nursing infant to alcohol in breast milk, however, should cause a reassessment of this position.

Chronic exposure to alcohol in breast milk was found to have an adverse effect on psychomotor development of breast-feeding infants in a 1989 report (68). In this study, "breast-fed" was defined as a breast-feeding child who received no more than 473 mL (16 ounces) of its nourishment in the form of supplemental feedings/day. Statistical methods were used to control for alcohol exposure during gestation. Of the 400 infants studied, 153 were breast-fed by mothers who were classified as "heavier" drinkers (i.e., an average daily consumption of 1 ounce of ethanol or about two drinks, or binge drinkers who consumed 2.5 ounces or more of ethanol on a single occasion). The population sampled was primarily white, well-educated, middle-class women who belonged to a health maintenance organization. The investigators measured the mental and psychomotor development of the infants at 1 year of age using the Bayley Scales of Infant Development. Mental development was unrelated to maternal drinking during breast-feeding. In contrast, psychomotor development was adversely affected in a dose-response relation (p for linear trend, 0.006). The mean Psychomotor Development Index (PDI) of infants of mothers who had at least one drink daily was 98, compared to 103 for infants of mothers consuming less alcohol ($p < 0.01$). The decrease in PDI was even greater if only those women not supplementing breast-feeding were considered. Regression analysis predicted that the PDI of totally breast-fed infants of mothers who consumed an average of two drinks daily would decrease by 7.5 points. These associations persisted even after more than 100 potentially confounding variables, including maternal tobacco, marijuana, and heavy caffeine exposures, were controlled for during pregnancy and the first 3 months after delivery. The authors cautioned that their findings were only suggestive and should not be extrapolated to other patient populations because of the relative homogeneity of their sample (68). Although the conclusions of this study have been criticized and defended

(69,70), judgment on the risks to the nursing infant from alcohol in milk must be withheld until additional research has been completed.

The toxic metabolite of ethanol, acetaldehyde, apparently does not pass into milk even though considerable levels can be measured in the mother's blood (71). One report calculated the amount of alcohol received in a single feeding from a mother with a blood concentration of 100 mg/dL (equivalent to a heavy, habitual drinker) as 164 mg, an insignificant amount (72). Maternal blood alcohol levels have to reach 300 mg/dL before mild sedation might be seen in the baby. However, a 1937 report described a case of alcohol poisoning in an 8-day-old breast-fed infant whose mother drank an entire bottle (750 mL) of port wine (73). Symptoms in the child included deep sleep, no response to painful stimuli, abnormal reflexes, and weakly reactive pupils. Alcohol was detected in the infant's blood. The child made an apparently uneventful recovery. Potentiation of severe hypoprothrombic bleeding, a pseudo-Cushing's syndrome, and an effect on the milk-ejecting reflex have been reported in nursing infants of alcoholic mothers (74–76).

Because of the risk of toxicity in a nursing infant, the safest course would be to hold nursing for 1–2 hours for each ounce of alcohol consumed, thereby allowing the alcohol level in milk to decrease. The American Academy of Pediatrics classifies ethanol as compatible with breast-feeding, although it is recognized that adverse effects may occur (77). The Institute of Medicine recommends a maximum daily consumption of 0.5 g/kg ethanol (78).

References

1. Shaywitz BA. Fetal alcohol syndrome: an ancient problem rediscovered. Drug Ther 1978;8:95–108.
2. Lemoine P, Harroussean H, Borteyrn JP. Les enfants de parents alcooliques: anomalies observees. A propos de 127 cas. Quest Med 1968;25:477–82.
3. Ulleland CN. The offspring of alcoholic mothers. Ann N Y Acad Sci 1972;197:167–9.
4. Jones KL, Smith DW, Ulleland CN, Streissguth AP. Pattern of malformation in offspring of chronic alcoholic mothers. Lancet 1973;1:1267–71.
5. Jones KL, Smith DW. Recognition of the fetal alcohol syndrome in early infancy. Lancet 1973;2: 999–1001.
6. Abel EL. *Fetal Alcohol Syndrome, Volume 1: An Annotated and Comprehensive Bibliography*. Boca Raton, FL: CRC Press, 1981. As cited in Anonymous. Alcohol and the fetus—is zero the only option? Lancet 1983;1: 682–3.
7. Council on Scientific Affairs, American Medical Association. Fetal effects of maternal alcohol use. JAMA 1983;249:2517–21.
8. Alcohol use during pregnancy. A report by the American Council on Science and Health. As reprinted in Nutr Today 1982;17:29–32.
9. Lipson AH, Walsh DA, Webster WS. Fetal alcohol syndrome. A great paediatric imitator. Med J Aust 1983;1:266–9.
10. Little BB, Snell LM, Gilstrap LC III, Gant NF, Rosenfeld CR. Alcohol abuse during pregnancy: changes in frequency in a large urban hospital. Obstet Gynecol 1989;74:547–50.
11. Scheiner AP, Donovan CM, Burtoshesky LE. Fetal alcohol syndrome in child whose parents had stopped drinking. Lancet 1979;1:1077–8.
12. Scheiner AP. Fetal alcohol syndrome in a child whose parents had stopped drinking. Lancet 1979;2:858.
13. Smith DW, Graham JM Jr. Fetal alcohol syndrome in child whose parents had stopped drinking. Lancet 1979;2:527.
14. Little RE, Sing CF. Association of father's drinking and infant's birth weight. N Engl J Med 1986;314:1644–5.
15. Little RE, Sing CF. Father's drinking and infant birth weight; report of an association. Teratology 1987;36: 59–65.
16. Rubin DH, Leventhal JM, Krasilnikoff PA, Weile B, Berget A. Fathers' drinking (and smoking) and infants' birth weight. N Engl J Med 1986;315:1551.
17. Veghelyi PV. Fetal abnormality and maternal ethanol metabolism. Lancet 1983;2:53–4.
18. Ryle PR, Thomson AD. Acetaldehyde and the fetal alcohol syndrome. Lancet 1983;2:219–20.
19. Kennedy LA. The pathogenesis of brain abnormalities in the fetal alcohol syndrome: an integrating hypothesis. Teratology 1984;29:363–8.
20. Shepard TH. *Catalog of Teratogenic Agents*. 6th ed. Baltimore, MD: Johns Hopkins University Press, 1989: 54.
21. Damjanov I. Metronidazole and alcohol in pregnancy. JAMA 1986;256:472.
22. FDA Drug Bulletin, *Fetal Alcohol Syndrome*. Volume 7. National Institute on Alcohol Abuse and Alcoholism, 1977:4.
23. Sandor GGS, Smith DF, MacLeod PM. Cardiac malformations in the fetal alcohol syndrome. J Pediatr 1981;98:771–3.
24. Habbick BF, Casey R, Zaleski WA, Murphy F. Liver abnormalities in three patients with fetal alcohol syndrome. Lancet 1979;1:580–1.

E

25. Streissguth AP, Clarren SK, Jones KL. Natural history of the fetal alcohol syndrome: a 10-year follow-up of eleven patients. Lancet 1985;2:85–91.
26. Khan A, Bader JL, Hoy GR, Sinks LF. Hepatoblastoma in child with fetal alcohol syndrome. Lancet 1979;1:1403–4.
27. Harlap S, Shiono PH. Alcohol, smoking and incidence of spontaneous abortions in the first and second trimester. Lancet 1980;2:173–6.
28. Kline J, Shrout P, Stein Z, Susser M, Warburton D. Drinking during pregnancy and spontaneous abortion. Lancet 1980;2:176–80.
29. Hanson JW, Jones KL, Smith DW. Fetal alcohol syndrome experience with 41 patients. JAMA 1976;235:1458–60.
30. Goetzman BW, Kagan J, Blankenship WJ. Expansion of the fetal alcohol syndrome. Clin Res 1975;23:100A.
31. DeBeukelaer MM, Randall CL, Stroud DR. Renal anomalies in the fetal alcohol syndrome. J Pediatr 1977;91:759–60.
32. Qazi Q, Masakawa A, Milman D, McGann B, Chua A, Haller J. Renal anomalies in fetal alcohol syndrome. Pediatrics 1979;63:886–9.
33. Steeg CN, Woolf P. Cardiovascular malformations in the fetal alcohol syndrome. Am Heart J 1979;98:636–7.
34. Halliday HL, Reid MM, McClure G. Results of heavy drinking in pregnancy. Br J Obstet Gynaecol 1982;89:892–5.
35. Beattie JO, Day RE, Cockburn F, Garg RA. Alcohol and the fetus in the west of Scotland. Br Med J 1983;287:17–20.
36. Tsukahara M, Kajii T. Severe skeletal dysplasias following intrauterine exposure to ethanol. Teratology 1988;37:79–80.
37. Charness ME, Simon RP, Greenberg DA. Ethanol and the nervous system. N Engl J Med 1989;321:442–54.
38. Golden NL, Sokol RJ, Kuhnert BR, Bottoms S. Maternal alcohol use and infant development. Pediatrics 1982;70:931–4.
39. Ernhart CB, Sokol RJ, Martier S, Moron P, Nadler D, Ager JW, Wolf A. Alcohol teratogenicity in the human: a detailed assessment of specificity, critical period, and threshold. Am J Obstet Gynecol 1987;156:33–9.
40. Day NL, Jasperse D, Richardson G, Robles N, Sambamoorthi U, Taylor P, Scher M, Stoffer D, Cornelius M. Prenatal exposure to alcohol: effect on infant growth and morphologic characteristics. Pediatrics 1989;84:536–41.
41. Mills JL, Graubard BI. Is moderate drinking during pregnancy associated with an increased risk for malformations? Pediatrics 1987;80:309–14.
42. Halmesmaki E, Valimaki M, Roine R, Ylikahri R, Ylikorkala O. Maternal and paternal alcohol consumption and miscarriage. Br J Obstet Gynaecol 1989;96:188–91.
43. Halmesmaki E, Ylikorkala O. A retrospective study on the safety of prenatal ethanol treatment. Obstet Gynecol 1988;72:545–9.
44. Sisenwin FE, Tejani NA, Boxer HS, DiGiuseppe R. Effects of maternal ethanol infusion during pregnancy on the growth and development of children at four to seven years of age. Am J Obstet Gynecol 1983;147:52–6.
45. Friedman JM. Can maternal alcohol ingestion cause neural tube defects? J Pediatr 1982;101:232–4.
46. Castro-Gago M, Rodriguez-Cervilla J, Ugarte J, Novo I, Pombo M. Maternal alcohol ingestion and neural tube defects. J Pediatr 1984;104:796–7.
47. Halmesmaki E, Raivio K, Ylikorkala O. A possible association between maternal drinking and fetal clubfoot. N Engl J Med 1985;312:790.
48. Sarda P, Bard H. Gastroschisis in a case of dizygotic twins: the possible role of maternal alcohol consumption. Pediatrics 1984;74:94–6.
49. Ammann AJ, Wara DW, Cowan MJ, Barrett DJ, Stiehm ER. The DiGeorge syndrome and the fetal alcohol syndrome. Am J Dis Child 1982;136:906–8.
50. Gardner LI, Mitter N, Coplan J, Kalinowski DP, Sanders KJ. Isochromosome 9q in an infant exposed to ethanol prenatally. N Engl J Med 1985;312:1521.
51. Mills JL, Graubard BI, Harley EE, Rhoads GG, Berendes HW. Maternal alcohol consumption and birth weight. How much drinking during pregnancy is safe? JAMA 1984;252:1875–9.
52. Wright JT, Waterson EJ, Barrison IG, Toplis PJ, Lewis IG, Gordon MG, MacRae KD, Morris NF, Murray-Lyon IM. Alcohol consumption, pregnancy, and low birthweight. Lancet 1983;1:663–5.
53. Rosett HL, Weiner L, Lee A, Zuckerman B, Dooling E, Oppenheimer E. Patterns of alcohol consumption and fetal development. Obstet Gynecol 1983;61:539–46.
54. Davis PJM, Partridge JW, Storrs CN. Alcohol consumption in pregnancy. How much is safe? Arch Dis Child 1982;57:940–3.
55. McLeod W, Brien J, Loomis C, Carmichael L, Probert C, Patrick J. Effect of maternal ethanol ingestion on fetal breathing movements, gross body movements, and heart rate at 37 to 40 weeks' gestational age. Am J Obstet Gynecol 1983;145:251–7.
56. Halmesmaki E, Ylikorkala O. The effect of maternal ethanol intoxication on fetal cardiotocography: a report of four cases. Br J Obstet Gynaecol 1986;93:203–5.
57. Ioffe S, Chernick V. Maternal alcohol ingestion and the incidence of respiratory distress syndrome. Am J Obstet Gynecol 1987;156:1231–5.
58. Coles CD, Smith IE, Fernhoff PM, Falek A. Neonatal ethanol withdrawal: characteristics in clinically normal, nondysmorphic neonates. J Pediatr 1984;105:445–51.
59. Ioffe S, Childiaeva R, Chernick V. Prolonged effects of maternal alcohol ingestion on the neonatal electroencephalogram. Pediatrics 1984;74:330–5.
60. Wilker R, Nathenson G. Combined fetal alcohol and hydantoin syndromes. Clin Pediatr 1982;21:331–4.
61. Seeler RA, Israel JN, Royal JE, Kaye CI, Rao S, Abulaban M. Ganglioneuroblastoma and fetal hydantoin-alcohol syndromes. Pediatrics 1979;63:524–7.
62. Ramilo J, Harris VJ. Neuroblastoma in a child with the hydantoin and fetal alcohol syndrome. The radiographic features. Br J Radiol 1979;52:993–5.
63. Bostrom B, Nesbit ME Jr. Hodgkin disease in a child with fetal alcohol-hydantoin syndrome. J Pediatr 1983;103:760–2.
64. Hornstein L, Crowe C, Gruppo R. Adrenal carcinoma in child with history of fetal alcohol syndrome. Lancet 1977;2:1292–3.
65. Chasnoff IJ, Diggs G, Schnoll SH. Fetal alcohol

effects and maternal cough syrup abuse. Am J Dis Child 1981;135:968.
66. Anonymous. Alcohol and the fetus—is zero the only option? Lancet 1983;1:682–3.
67. Anonymous. Update: drugs in breast milk. Med Lett Drugs Ther 1979;21:21.
68. Little RE, Anderson KW, Ervin CH, Worthington-Roberts B, Clarren SK. Maternal alcohol use during breast-feeding and infant mental and motor development at one year. N Engl J Med 1989;321:425–30.
69. Lindmark B. Maternal use of alcohol and breast-fed infants. N Engl J Med 1990;322:338–9.
70. Little RE. Maternal use of alcohol and breast-fed infants. N Engl J Med 1990;322:339.
71. Kesaniemi YA. Ethanol and acetaldehyde in the milk and peripheral blood of lactating women after ethanol administration. J Obstet Gynaecol Br Commonw 1974;81:84–6.
72. Wilson JT, Brown RD, Cherek DR, Dailey JW, Hilman B, Jobe PC, Manno BR, Manno JE, Redetzki HM, Stewart JJ. Drug excretion in human breast milk. Principles, pharmacokinetics and projected consequences. Clin Pharmacol 1980;5:1–66.
73. Bisdom CJW. Alcohol and nicotine poisoning in nurslings. Maandschrift voor Kindergeneeskunde, Leyden 1937;6:332. As cited in Anonymous. References. JAMA 1937;109:178.
74. Hoh TK. Severe hypoprothrombinaemic bleeding in the breast-fed young infant. Singapore Med J 1969;10:43–9.
75. Binkiewicz A, Robinson MJ, Senior B. Pseudo-Cushing syndrome caused by alcohol in breast milk. J Pediatr 1978;93:965.
76. Cobo E. Effect of different doses of ethanol on the milk-ejecting reflex in lactating women. Am J Obstet Gynecol 1973;115:817–21.
77. Committee on Drugs, American Academy of Pediatrics. The transfer of drugs and other chemicals into human milk. Pediatrics 2001;108:776–89.
78. Howard CR, Lawrence RA. Breast-feeding and drug exposure. Obstet Gynecol Clin North Am 1998;25:195–217.

Name: **ETHCHLORVYNOL** Risk Factor: **C_M**
Class: **Hypnotic**

FETAL RISK SUMMARY

RECOMMENDATION: Limited Human Data - Animal Data Suggest Moderate Risk

No reports linking the use of ethchlorvynol with congenital defects have been located. In pregnant rats, a dose of 40 mg/kg/day was associated with an increase in the number of stillbirths and a lower survival rate among the offspring (1).

The Collaborative Perinatal Project reported 68 patients with 1st trimester exposure to miscellaneous tranquilizers and nonbarbiturate sedatives, 12 of whom had been exposed to ethchlorvynol (2). For the group as a whole, six infants with malformations were delivered, but details on individual exposures were not given.

Animal data indicate that rapid equilibrium occurs between maternal and fetal blood with maximum fetal blood levels measured within 2 hours of maternal ingestion (3). The authors concluded that following maternal ingestion of a toxic or lethal dose, delivery should be accomplished before equilibrium occurs. Neonatal withdrawal symptoms consisting of mild hypotonia, poor suck, absent rooting, poor grasp, and delayed-onset jitteriness, have been reported (B. H. Rumack, P. A. Walravens, personal communication, Dept. of Pediatrics, Univ. of Colorado Medical Center, 1981). The mother had been taking 500 mg daily during the 3rd trimester.

BREAST FEEDING SUMMARY

RECOMMENDATION: No Human Data - Potential Toxicity

No reports describing the use of ethchlorvynol during human lactation have been located. Because the drug rapidly crosses the placenta to the fetus, excretion into milk should be expected. Sedation of the nursing infant is a possible consequence.

References

1. Product information. Placidyl. Abbott Laboratories, 2000.
2. Heinonen OP, Slone D, Shapiro S. *Birth Defects and Drugs in Pregnancy*. Littleton, MA: Publishing Sciences Group, 1977:336–7.
3. Hume AS, Williams JM, Douglas BH. Disposition of ethchlorvynol in maternal blood, fetal blood, amniotic fluid, and chorionic fluid. J Reprod Med 1971;6: 54–6.

E

Name:	**ETHINAMATE**	Risk Factor:	C_M
Class:	**Hypnotic**		

FETAL RISK SUMMARY

RECOMMENDATION: Limited Human Data - No Relevant Animal Data

Ethinamate is a hypnotic used for insomnia. Animal reproduction studies have not been conducted with this drug. The Collaborative Perinatal Project monitored 50,282 mother-child pairs, 68 of whom had 1st trimester exposure to miscellaneous tranquilizers and nonbarbiturate sedatives (1). Three of these exposures were to ethinamate. From the total group of 68, six infants with malformations were delivered, but details on individual exposures were not given.

BREAST FEEDING SUMMARY

RECOMMENDATION: No Human Data - Potential Toxicity

No data are available.

Reference

1. Heinonen OP, Slone D, Shapiro S. *Birth Defects and Drugs in Pregnancy*. Littleton, MA: Publishing Sciences Group, 1977:336.

Name:	**ETHINYL ESTRADIOL**	Risk Factor:	X_M
Class:	**Estrogenic Hormone**		

FETAL RISK SUMMARY

RECOMMENDATION: Contraindicated

Ethinyl estradiol is used frequently in combination with progestins for oral contraception (see Oral Contraceptives). The Collaborative Perinatal Project monitored 89 mother-child pairs who were exposed to ethinyl estradiol during the 1st trimester (1, pp. 389, 391). An increased risk for malformations was found, although identification of the malformations was not provided. Estrogenic agents as a group were monitored in 614 mother-child pairs. An increase in the expected frequency of cardiovascular defects, eye and ear anomalies, and Down's syndrome was reported (1, p. 395).

Reevaluation of these data in terms of timing of exposure, vaginal bleeding in early pregnancy, and previous maternal obstetric history, however, failed to support an association between estrogens and cardiac malformations (2). An earlier study also failed to find any relationship with nongenital malformations (3). In a smaller study, 12 mothers were exposed to ethinyl estradiol during the 1st trimester (4). No fetal abnormalities were observed. Ethinyl estradiol has also been used as a contraceptive when given within 72 hours of unprotected midcycle coitus (5). Use of estrogenic hormones during pregnancy is contraindicated.

BREAST FEEDING SUMMARY

RECOMMENDATION: No Human Data - Probably Compatible

Estrogens are frequently used for suppression of postpartum lactation (6,7). Very small amounts are excreted in milk (7). When used in oral contraceptives, ethinyl estradiol has been associated with decreased milk production and decreased composition of nitrogen and protein content in human milk (8). Although the magnitude of these changes is low, the differences in milk production and composition may be of nutritional importance to nursing infants of malnourished mothers. If breast-feeding is desired, the lowest dose of oral contraceptives should be chosen. Monitoring of infant weight gain and the possible need for nutritional supplementation should be considered (see Oral Contraceptives).

References

1. Heinonen OP, Slone D, Shapiro S. *Birth Defects and Drugs in Pregnancy*. Littleton, MA: Publishing Sciences Group, 1977.
2. Wiseman RA, Dodds-Smith IC. Cardiovascular birth defects and antenatal exposure to female sex hormones: a reevaluation of some base data. Teratology 1984;30:359–70.
3. Wilson JG, Brent RL. Are female sex hormones teratogenic? Am J Obstet Gynecol 1981;141:567–80.
4. Hagler S, Schultz A, Hankin H, Kunstadler RH. Fetal effects of steroid therapy during pregnancy. Am J Dis Child 1963;106:586–90.
5. Dixon GW, Schlesselman JJ, Ory HW, Blye RP. Ethinyl estradiol and conjugated estrogens as postcoital contraceptives. JAMA 1980;244:1336–9.
6. Gilman AG, Goodman LS, Gilman A, eds. *The Pharmacological Basis of Therapeutics*. 6th ed. New York, NY: MacMillan Publishing Co, 1980:1431.
7. Klinger G, Claussen C, Schroder S. Excretion of ethinyloestradiol sulfonate in the human milk. Zentralbl Gynaekol 1981;103:91–5.
8. Lonnerdal B, Forsum E, Hambraeus L. Effect of oral contraceptives on composition and volume of breast milk. Am J Clin Nutr 1980;33:816–24.

Name: **ETHIODIZED OIL** Risk Factor: **D***
Class: **Diagnostic**

FETAL RISK SUMMARY

RECOMMENDATION: Human Data Suggest Risk in 2nd and 3rd Trimesters

Ethiodized oil contains a high concentration of organically bound iodine. Use of this agent close to term has been associated with neonatal hypothyroidism (see Diatrizoate).

[*Risk Factor C according to one manufacturer.*]

BREAST FEEDING SUMMARY

RECOMMENDATION: No Human Data - Probably Compatible

See Potassium Iodide.

Name:	**ETHIONAMIDE**	Risk Factor:	C_M
Class:	**Anti-infective (Antituberculosis)**		

FETAL RISK SUMMARY

RECOMMENDATION: Human Data Suggest Low Risk

The oral anti-infective agent, ethionamide, is indicated for the treatment of tuberculosis when *Mycobacterium tuberculosis* is resistant to isoniazid or rifampin, or when the patient is intolerant to other drugs. Although it apparently has not been studied, the relatively low molecular weight (about 166) suggests that it is transferred to the fetus.

Ethionamide was teratogenic in rats and rabbits at doses higher than those used in humans (1). Nishimura and Tanimura (2), Shepard (3), and Schardein (4) have reviewed nine animal studies involving pregnant mice, rats, and rabbits. All of the studies, except one, showed various developmental anomalies.

Five human studies describing the outcome of pregnancies exposed to ethionamide have been briefly reviewed in three sources (2–4). Only one of the studies found an increased incidence of birth defects, reporting seven cases, two of which were Down's syndrome, from 23 exposed infants (2–4). The other reports found no association with congenital malformations (4).

BREAST FEEDING SUMMARY

RECOMMENDATION: No Human Data - Probably Compatible

No reports describing the use of ethionamide in human lactation have been located. The relatively low molecular weight (about 166) suggests that ethionamide will be excreted into breast milk. The effects of this exposure on a nursing infant are unknown.

References

1. Product information. Trecator. Wyeth-Ayerst Pharmaceuticals, 2001.
2. Nishimura H, Tanimura T. *Clinical Aspects of The Teratogenicity of Drugs*. Amsterdam: Excerpta Medica, 1976:139–41.
3. Shepard TH. *Catalog of Teratogenic Agents*. 9th ed. Baltimore, MD: The Johns Hopkins University Press, 1998:188.
4. Schardein JL. *Chemically Induced Birth Defects*. 3rd ed. New York, NY: Marcel Dekker, 2000:393–4.

Name:	**ETHISTERONE**	Risk Factor:	**D**
Class:	**Progestogenic Hormone**		

FETAL RISK SUMMARY

RECOMMENDATION: Contraindicated

The FDA mandated deletion of pregnancy-related indications for all progestins because of a possible association with congenital anomalies. No reports linking the use of ethisterone alone with congenital defects have been located. The Collaborative Perinatal Project monitored 866 mother-child pairs with 1st trimester exposure to progestational agents (including 2 with exposure to ethisterone) (1, pp. 389, 391). An increase in the expected frequency of cardiovascular defects and hypospadias was observed for the progestational agents as a group, but not for ethisterone as a single agent (1, p. 394). In a subsequent report from the Collaborative Study, a single case of tricuspid atresia and ventricular septal defect was identified with 3rd trimester exposure to ethisterone and ethinyl estradiol (2). Reevaluation of these data in terms of timing of exposure, vaginal bleeding in early pregnancy, and previous maternal obstetric history, however, failed to support an association between female sex hormones and cardiac malformations (3). An earlier study also failed to find any relationship with nongenital malformations (4). (See also Hydroxyprogesterone and Medroxyprogesterone.)

E

BREAST FEEDING SUMMARY

RECOMMENDATION: No Human Data - Probably Compatible

See Oral Contraceptives.

References

1. Heinonen OP, Slone D, Shapiro S. *Birth Defects and Drugs in Pregnancy*. Littleton, MA: Publishing Sciences Group, 1977.
2. Heinonen OP, Slone D, Monson RR, Hook EB, Shapiro S. Cardiovascular birth defects and antenatal exposure to female sex hormones. N Engl J Med 1977;296:67–70.
3. Wiseman RA, Dodds-Smith IC. Cardiovascular birth defects and antenatal exposure to female sex hormones: a reevaluation of some base data. Teratology 1984;30:359–70.
4. Wilson JG, Brent RL. Are female sex hormones teratogenic? Am J Obstet Gynecol 1981;141:567–80.

Name:	**ETHOHEPTAZINE**	Risk Factor:	**C**
Class:	**Analgesic**		

FETAL RISK SUMMARY

RECOMMENDATION: Limited Human Data - No Relevant Animal Data

The Collaborative Perinatal Project monitored 50,282 mother-child pairs, 60 of whom had 1st trimester exposure to ethoheptazine (1, pp. 287–295). For use anytime during pregnancy, 300 exposures were recorded (1, p. 434). Although the numbers were small, a possible relationship may exist between this drug and major or minor malformations. Further, a possible association with individual defects was observed (1, p. 485): congenital dislocation of the hip (three cases); umbilical hernia (three cases); and inguinal hernia (eight cases). Independent confirmation of these associations is required.

BREAST FEEDING SUMMARY

RECOMMENDATION: No Human Data - Probably Compatible

No data are available.

Reference

1. Heinonen OP, Slone D, Shapiro S. *Birth Defects and Drugs in Pregnancy*. Littleton, MA: Publishing Sciences Group, 1977.

Name:	**ETHOPROPAZINE**	Risk Factor:	**C**
Class:	**Parasympatholytic (Anticholinergic)**		

FETAL RISK SUMMARY

RECOMMENDATION: No Human Data - No Relevant Animal Data

Ethopropazine is a phenothiazine compound with anticholinergic activity that is used in the treatment of parkinsonism (see also Atropine and Promethazine). No reports of its use in pregnancy have been located.

BREAST FEEDING SUMMARY

RECOMMENDATION: No Human Data - Probably Compatible

No data are available (see also Atropine and Promethazine).

Name:	**ETHOSUXIMIDE**	Risk Factor:	**C**
Class:	**Anticonvulsant**		

FETAL RISK SUMMARY

RECOMMENDATION: Human Data Suggest Low Risk

Ethosuximide is a succinimide anticonvulsant used in the treatment of petit mal epilepsy. The use of ethosuximide has been reported in 163 pregnancies (1–11). Because of the lack of specific information on the observed malformations, multiple drug therapies, and differences in study methodology, conclusions linking the use of ethosuximide with congenital defects are difficult. Spontaneous hemorrhage in the neonate following *in utero* exposure to ethosuximide has been reported (see also Phenytoin and Phenobarbital) (6). Abnormalities identified with ethosuximide use in 10 pregnancies include patent ductus arteriosus (8 cases); cleft lip and/or palate (7 cases); mongoloid facies, short neck, altered palmar crease and an accessory nipple (1 case); and hydrocephalus (1 case).

Ethosuximide has a much lower teratogenic potential than the oxazolidinedione class of anticonvulsants (see also Trimethadione and Paramethadione) (11,12). The succinimide anticonvulsants should be considered the anticonvulsants of choice for the treatment of petit mal epilepsy during the 1st trimester.

In a surveillance study of Michigan Medicaid recipients conducted between 1985 and 1992 involving 229,101 completed pregnancies, 18 newborns had been exposed to ethosuximide during the 1st trimester (F. Rosa, personal communication, FDA, 1993). No major birth defects were observed (one expected).

BREAST FEEDING SUMMARY

RECOMMENDATION: Limited Human Data - Probably Compatible

Ethosuximide freely enters the breast milk in concentrations similar to the maternal serum (13–15). Two reports measured similar milk:plasma ratios of 1.0 and 0.78 (13,14). No adverse effects on the nursing infant have been reported. The American Academy of Pediatrics classifies ethosuximide as compatible with breast-feeding (16).

References

1. Speidel BD, Meadow SR. Maternal epilepsy and abnormalities of the fetus and newborn. Lancet 1972;2:839–43.
2. Fedrick J. Epilepsy and pregnancy: a report from the Oxford Record Linkage Study. Br Med J 1973;2:442–8.
3. Lowe CR. Congenital malformations among infants born to epileptic women. Lancet 1973;1:9–10.
4. Starreveld-Zimmerman AAE, van der Kolk WJ, Meinardi H, Elshve J. Are anticonvulsants teratogenic? Lancet 1973;2:48–9.
5. Kuenssberg EV, Knox JDE. Teratogenic effect of anticonvulsants. Lancet 1973;2:198.
6. Speidel BD, Meadow SR. Epilepsy, anticonvulsants and congenital malformations. Drugs 1974;8:354–65.
7. Janz D. The teratogenic risk of antiepileptic drugs. Epilepsia 1975;16:159–69.
8. Nakane Y, Okuma T, Takahashi R. Multi-institutional study on the teratogenicity and fetal toxicity of antiepileptic drugs: a report of a collaborative study group in Japan. Epilepsia 1980;21:663–80.
9. Heinonen OP, Slone D, Shapiro S. *Birth Defects and Drugs in Pregnancy*. Littleton, MA: Publishing Sciences Group, 1977:358–9.
10. Dansky L, Andermann E, Andermann F. Major congenital malformations on the offspring of epileptic patients: genetic and environment risk factors. In *Epilepsy, Pregnancy and the Child*. Proceedings of a workshop held in Berlin, September 1980. New York: Raven Press, 1981.
11. Fabro S, Brown NA. Teratogenic potential of anticonvulsants. N Engl J Med 1979;300:1280–1.
12. The National Institute of Health. Anticonvulsants found to have teratogenic potential. JAMA 1981;241:36.
13. Koup JR, Rose JQ, Cohen ME. Ethosuximide pharmacokinetics in pregnant patient and her newborn. Epilepsia 1978;19:535.
14. Kaneko S, Sato T, Suzuki K. The levels of anticonvulsants in breast milk. Br J Clin Pharmacol 1979;7:624–6.
15. Horning MG, Stillwell WG, Nowlin J, Lertratanangkoon K, Stillwill RN, Hill RM. Identification and quantification of drugs and drug metabolites in human breast milk using GC-MS-COM methods. Mod Probl Paediatr 1975;15:73–9.
16. Committee on Drugs, American Academy of Pediatrics. The transfer of drugs and other chemicals into human milk. Pediatrics 2001;108:776–89.

Name: **ETHOTOIN** Risk Factor: **D**

Class: **Anticonvulsant**

FETAL RISK SUMMARY

RECOMMENDATION: Compatible - Maternal Benefit >> Embryo/Fetal Risk

Ethotoin is a low-potency hydantoin anticonvulsant (1). The fetal hydantoin syndrome has been associated with the use of the more potent phenytoin (see Phenytoin). Only six reports describing the use of ethotoin during the 1st trimester have been located (2–4). Congenital malformations observed in two of these cases included cleft lip/palate and patent ductus arteriosus (3,4). No cause-and-effect relationship was established. Although the toxicity of ethotoin appears to be lower than the more potent phenytoin, the occurrence of congenital defects in two fetuses exposed to ethotoin suggests that a teratogenic potential may exist.

BREAST FEEDING SUMMARY

RECOMMENDATION: No Human Data - Probably Compatible

No data are available.

References

1. Schmidt RP, Wilder BJ. Epilepsy. In *Contemporary Neurology Services*. Volume 2. Philadelphia, PA: FA Davis Co, 1968:154.
2. Heinonen OP, Slone D, Shapiro S. *Birth Defects and Drugs in Pregnancy*. Littleton, MA: Publishing Sciences Group, 1977:358–9.

3. Zablen M, Brand N. Cleft lip and palate with the anticonvulsant ethotoin. N Engl J Med 1978;298:285.
4. Nakane Y, Okuma T, Takahashi R, et al. Multi-institutional study on the teratogenicity and fetal toxicity of antiepileptic drugs: a report of a collaborative study group in Japan. Epilepsia 1980;21:663–80.

E

Name:	**ETHYL BISCOUMACETATE**	Risk Factor: **D**
Class:	**Anticoagulant**	

See Coumarin Derivatives.

Name:	**ETHYNODIOL**	Risk Factor: **D**
Class:	**Progestogenic Hormone**	

FETAL RISK SUMMARY

RECOMMENDATION: Contraindicated

Ethynodiol is used primarily in oral contraceptive products (see Oral Contraceptives).

BREAST FEEDING SUMMARY

RECOMMENDATION: No Human Data - Probably Compatible

See Oral Contraceptives.

Name:	**ETODOLAC**	Risk Factor: **C_M***
Class:	**Nonsteroidal Anti-inflammatory**	

FETAL RISK SUMMARY

RECOMMENDATION: Human Data Suggest Risk in 1st and 3rd Trimesters

The nonsteroidal anti-inflammatory drug (NSAID) etodolac is used in the treatment of arthritis, and acute and chronic pain. Etodolac is in a NSAID subclass (pyranocarboxylic acid) that contains no other members.

In reproduction studies with rats the drug produced isolated occurrences of alterations in limb development (polydactyly, oligodactyly, syndactyly, and unossified phalanges) at doses close to human clinical doses (2 to 14 mg/kg/day) (1). These same doses produced oligodactyly and synostosis of metatarsals in rabbits. However, a clear drug or dose-response relationship was not established (1). Similar to other agents in this class, etodolac increased the incidence of dystocia, prolonged gestation, and decreased pup survival in rats (1).

It is not known if etodolac crosses the human placenta. The molecular weight (about 287) is low enough, however, that passage to the fetus should be expected.

A combined 2001 population-based observational cohort study and a case-control study estimated the risk of adverse pregnancy outcome from the use of NSAIDs (2). The use of NSAIDs during pregnancy was not associated with congenital malformations, preterm delivery, or low birth weight, but a positive association was discovered with spontaneous abortions (SABs). A similar study, also published in 2001, failed to find a relationship, in general, between NSAIDs and congenital malformations, but did find a significant association with cardiac defects and orofacial clefts (3). In addition, a 2003 study found a significant association between exposure to NSAIDs in early pregnancy and SABs (4). (See Ibuprofen for details on these three studies.)

In summary, no reports describing the use of etodolac in human pregnancy have been located. The animal data are suggestive of a low risk for congenital malformations. A brief 2003 editorial on the potential for NSAID-induced developmental toxicity concluded that NSAIDs, and specifically those with greater COX-2 affinity, had a lower risk of this toxicity in humans than aspirin (5).

Constriction of the ductus arteriosus *in utero* is a pharmacologic consequence arising from the use of prostaglandin synthesis inhibitors during late pregnancy, as is inhibition of labor, prolongation of pregnancy, and suppression of fetal renal function (see also Indomethacin) (6). Persistent pulmonary hypertension of the newborn may occur if these agents are used in the 3rd trimester close to delivery (6,7). Women attempting to conceive should not use any prostaglandin synthesis inhibitor, including etodolac, because of the findings in a variety of animal models that indicate these agents block blastocyst implantation (8,9). Moreover, as noted above, NSAIDs have been associated with SABs and congenital malformations.

[*Risk Factor D if used in 3rd trimester or near delivery.*]

BREAST FEEDING SUMMARY

RECOMMENDATION: No Human Data - Potential Toxicity

No reports describing the use of etodolac during lactation have been located. Because of the relatively low molecular weight (about 287), the excretion of etodolac into breast milk should be expected. Moreover, because of its long termination adult plasma half-life (7.3 hours), other agents may be preferred during lactation. One reviewer listed several low-risk alternatives (diclofenac, fenoprofen, flurbiprofen, ibuprofen, ketoprofen, ketorolac, and tolmetin) if a NSAID is required while nursing (10).

References

1. Product information. Lodine. Wyeth-Ayerst Laboratories, 2000.
2. Nielsen GL, Sorensen HT, Larsen H, Pedersen L. Risk of adverse birth outcome and miscarriage in pregnant users of non-steroidal anti-inflammatory drugs: population based observational study and case-control study. BMJ 2001;322:266–70.
3. Ericson A, Kallen BAJ. Nonsteroidal anti-inflammatory drugs in early pregnancy. Reprod Toxicol 2001;15:371–5.
4. Li DK, Liu L, Odouli R. Exposure to non-steroidal anti-inflammatory drugs during pregnancy and risk of miscarriage: population based cohort study. BMJ 2003;327:368–71.
5. Tassinari MS, Cook JC, Hurtt ME. NSAIDs and developmental toxicity. Birth Defects Res Part B Dev Reprod Toxicol 2003;68:3–4.
6. Levin DL. Effects of inhibition of prostaglandin synthesis on fetal development, oxygenation, and the fetal circulation. Semin Perinatol 1980;4:35–44.
7. Van Marter LJ, Leviton A, Allred EN, Pagano M, Sullivan KF, Cohen A, Epstein MF. Persistent pulmonary hypertension of the newborn and smoking and aspirin and nonsteroidal antiinflammatory drug consumption during pregnancy. Pediatrics 1996;97:658–63.
8. Matt DW, Borzelleca JF. Toxic effects on the female reproductive system during pregnancy, parturition, and lactation. In Witorsch RJ, editor. *Reproductive Toxicology*. 2nd ed. New York, NY: Raven Press, 1995:175–93.
9. Dawood MY. Nonsteroidal antiinflammatory drugs and reproduction. Am J Obstet Gynecol 1993;169:1255–65.
10. Anderson PO. Medication use while breast feeding a neonate. Neonatal Pharmacol Q 1993;2:3–14.

Name:	**ETOPOSIDE**	Risk Factor:	D_M
Class:	**Antineoplastic**		

FETAL RISK SUMMARY

RECOMMENDATION: Human and Animal Data Suggest Risk

E

Etoposide (VP-16, VP-16-213) is a semisynthetic derivative of podophyllotoxin used as an antineoplastic agent. Low doses of the drug, 1/20th to 1/2 of the recommended clinical dose based on body surface area, are teratogenic and embryocidal in rats and mice (1). A dose-related increase in the occurrence of embryotoxicity and congenital malformations was observed in these animals. Defects included decreased weight, skeletal anomalies, retarded ossification, exencephaly, encephalocele, and anophthalmia. The drug is also mutagenic in mammalian cells and, although not tested in animals, should be considered a potential carcinogen in humans (1).

When etoposide was administered intraperitoneally to pregnant mice during organogenesis, various anomalies were observed, including exencephaly, encephalocele, hydrocephalus, gastroschisis (including abnormal stomach or liver), microphthalmia or anophthalmia, dextrocardia (including missing lung lobe), and axial skeleton defects (2). In whole-embryo rat culture, a concentration of 2 μmol/L (no-observed-adverse-effect-level 1.0 μM; embryotoxic range 2–5 μM) produced growth retardation and brain anomalies (hypoplasia of prosencephalon and edema of rhombencephalon) and microphthalmia (3).

Reported use of etoposide during human pregnancy is limited to five cases (4–8). A 21-year-old woman with a dysgerminoma was treated surgically at 26 weeks' gestation, followed 6 days later with etoposide 100 mg/m^2 and cisplatin 20 mg/m^2, daily for 5 days at 3 - to 4-week intervals (4). Four cycles of chemotherapy were given. Because of oligohydramnios and probable intrauterine growth retardation, labor was induced and she delivered a healthy, 2320-g female infant at 38 weeks. The hematologic profile of the newborn was normal, as was her development at 9 months of age.

A 36-year-old woman at 25 weeks' gestation was treated for acute myeloid leukemia with combination chemotherapy consisting of two courses of etoposide (400 mg/m^2/day, days 8–10), cytarabine (1 g/m^2/day, days 1–3), and daunorubicin (45 mg/m^2/day, days 1–3) (5). No fetal growth was observed during serial ultrasound examinations from 30 to 32 weeks. An emergency cesarean section was performed because of fetal distress at 32 weeks' gestation, 11 days after the second course of chemotherapy. The pale, 1460-g (10th percentile) female infant required resuscitation at birth. Analysis of the cord blood revealed anemia and leukopenia, and profound neutropenia and thrombocytopenia were discovered at 30 hours of age. Following successful therapy, the child, at 1 year of age, was no longer receiving any treatment, had normal peripheral blood counts, and was apparently progressing normally.

A 32-year-old woman at 26 weeks' gestation presented with an unknown primary, poorly differentiated adenocarcinoma of the liver and with a mass in the posterior chamber of the right eye (6). She was treated with daily doses of etoposide 165 mg, bleomycin 30 mg, and cisplatin 55 mg, for 3 days. The patient became profoundly neutropenic, developed septicemia, and went into premature labor. A 1190-g female infant was born with Apgar scores of 3 and 8 at 1 and 5 minutes, respectively. Severe respiratory distress was successful treated over the next 10 days. Although the antineoplastics were chosen because they are highly protein bound (etoposide, 97%; cisplatin, 90% of plasma platinum; bleomycin, no data) and less likely to cross the placenta, marked leukopenia with neutropenia developed in the infant on day 3 (10 days after *in utero* exposure to the chemotherapy). Scalp hair loss and a rapid loss of lanugo were observed at 10 days of age. By 12 weeks of age, substantial hair regrowth had occurred, and at 1 year follow-up, the child was developing normally, except for moderate bilateral sensorineural hearing loss. The investigators could not determine if the deafness was due to the *in utero* exposure to cisplatin or to the maternal and/or neonatal aminoglycoside therapy. The alopecia and bone marrow depression in the infant were attributed to etoposide.

The treatment of nonlymphoblastic acute leukemia, diagnosed at 18 weeks' gestation, was described in a brief 1993 report (7). Therapy consisted of two courses of etoposide 100 mg/m^2/day and daunorubicin 60 mg/m^2/day on days 1–3, and cytarabine 100 mg/m^2/day on days 1–7. Follow-up therapy consisted of mitoxantrone, cytarabine, and amsacrine. The patient eventually delivered a term, 2930-g, healthy male infant who was developing normally.

Non-Hodgkin's lymphoma, diagnosed in a 36-year-old woman at 22 weeks' gestation, was treated with a 12-week chemotherapy course consisting of etoposide (125 mg/m^2), vincristine (1.4 mg/m^2), and bleomycin (9 mg/m^2) in weeks 2, 4, 6, 8, 10, and 12, and cyclophosphamide (375 mg/m^2) and doxorubicin (50 mg/m^2) in weeks 1, 3, 5, 7, 9, and 11 (8). Prednisolone was given during the entire 12-week period. A healthy, 3200-g male infant, delivered 3 weeks after the completion of therapy, was alive and well at 21 months of age. At this time also, the mother delivered another healthy male infant.

Seven reports, including the one above, have described women who became pregnant following treatment with etoposide (8–14) and one report described the return of normal menstrual function after etoposide therapy (15). One woman delivered a normal term infant following treatment with nine courses of etoposide (100mg/m^2/day), cisplatin, dactinomycin, and intrathecal methotrexate 2 years prior to conception for choriocarcinoma (9). Pregnancies occurred about 6–7 years after treatment in three women from a group of 128 women who had been previously treated with high dose chemotherapy for refractory or relapsed Hodgkin's disease (10). The current chemotherapy regimen consisted of etoposide (600–900 mg/m^2), cyclophosphamide and carmustine, followed by either autologous bone marrow or peripheral progenitor cell transplantation. One of the women conceived after receiving a donated ovum and delivered a healthy child. A second woman became pregnant with twins after receiving ovulatory stimulating agents, but aborted both at 5 1/2 months gestation. The third woman spontaneously conceived and delivered a healthy child.

Two women had normal pregnancies and babies after treatment with high dose chemotherapy for relapsed Hodgkin's disease and non-Hodgkin's lymphoma, respectively (11). The first patient was treated with etoposide (800 mg/m^2), carmustine, and melphalan, followed by autologous stem cell transplantation (ASCT). She conceived 19 months after completion of treatment. The second woman received etoposide (1000 mg/m^2), cyclophosphamide, and carmustine, followed by ASCT. She became pregnant 33 months later.

Of 33 women (>18 years old) treated with multiple courses of chemotherapy for ovarian germ cell tumors and fertility conserving surgery, 14 (42%) had successful pregnancies (12). No congenital abnormalities in their offspring were observed. The chemotherapy consisted of etoposide (100 mg/m^2 × 3 days/course), bleomycin, cisplatin, cyclophosphamide, dactinomycin, methotrexate, vincristine, and folinic acid.

A 1993 report described return of ovulation in 25 women younger than 40 years of age from a group of 34 patients treated with etoposide for gestational trophoblastic disease (13). Nine apparently healthy infants were delivered from the group. In another study, 12 women with methotrexate resistant gestational trophoblastic disease were treated with etoposide (100 mg/m^2/day × 5 days every 10 days) (14). Two of the women had successful pregnancies, 3 and 4 years, respectively, after treatment.

E

Etoposide (200 mg/m^2/day × 5 days) was successfully used to treat a cervical pregnancy in one woman (15). Her baseline menstrual function returned 60 days after completion of therapy, but it was not stated if she attempted to conceive. A man who had received etoposide for acute nonlymphoblastic leukemia in a cumulative dose of 3193 mg/m^2, fathered two children, one of whom had a unspecified birthmark (16). There is no evidence that the treatment, that also included irradiation to the brain and lumbar spine, vincristine, thioguanine, doxorubicin, cyclophosphamide, and cytarabine, resulted in the birth defect.

Occupational exposure of the mother to antineoplastic agents during pregnancy may present a risk to the fetus. A position statement from the National Study Commission on Cytotoxic Exposure and a research article involving some antineoplastic agents are presented in the monograph for cyclophosphamide (see Cyclophosphamide).

In summary, etoposide is a potent animal teratogen and potentially, may be a teratogen in humans, but exposure during organogenesis has not been reported. Five cases of maternal exposure to this agent and other antineoplastics during the 2nd and 3rd trimesters resulted in growth retardation and/or severe myelosuppression in three fetuses/newborns, two of whom were delivered prematurely, and reversible alopecia in one. Successful pregnancies, commencing after etoposide treatment, have also been reported.

BREAST FEEDING SUMMARY

RECOMMENDATION: Contraindicated

Etoposide is excreted into breast milk (17). After delivery of a healthy, 2960-g female at 34 weeks' gestation, a 28-year-old woman with acute promyelocytic leukemia in remission (see Mitoxantrone for details of treatment during gestation) was treated with a second consolidation course of cytarabine and mitoxantrone followed by a third consolidation course consisting of etoposide (80 mg/m^2, days 1–5), mitoxantrone (6 mg/m^2, days 1–3), and cytarabine (170 mg/m^2, days 1–5). She maintained milk secretion by pumping her breasts during the chemotherapy courses. The peak milk concentrations of etoposide measured on days 3, 4, and 5 of therapy were approximately (exact concentrations or times of sample collections were not specified) 0.6, 0.6, and 0.8 μg/mL, respectively. Milk concentrations of etoposide were undetectable within 24 hours of drug administration on each day. The rapid disappearance of etoposide from the milk is compatible with the lack of plasma accumulation and an elimination half-life of 4–11 hours in adults (1). Against medical advice, the mother began breast-feeding 21 days after drug administration (see Mitoxantrone).

Because of the potential for severe toxicity in a nursing infant, such as bone marrow depression, alopecia, and carcinogenicity, breast-feeding should be stopped for at least 55 hours after the last dose of etoposide to account for the elimination half-life range noted above. However, if other antineoplastic agents have also been administered, breast-feeding should be withheld until all of the agents have been eliminated from the mother's system.

References

1. Product information. VePesid. Bristol-Myers Squibb Oncology, 2000.
2. Sieber SM, Whang-Peng J, Botkin C, Knutsen T. Teratogenic and cytogenic effects of some plant-derived antitumor agents (vincristine, colchicine, maytansine, VP-16-213 and VM-26) in mice. Teratology 1978;18:31–47.
3. Mirkes PE, Zwelling LA. Embryotoxicity of the intercalating agents in m-AMSA and o-AMSA and the epipodophyllotoxin VP-16 in postimplantation rat embryos in vitro. Teratology 1990;41:679–88.
4. Buller RE, Darrow V, Manetta A, Porto M, DiSaia PJ. Conservative surgical management of dysgerminoma concomitant with pregnancy. Obstet Gynecol 1992;79:887–90.
5. Murray NA, Acolet D, Deane M, Price J, Roberts IAG. Fetal marrow suppression after maternal chemotherapy for leukaemia. Arch Dis Child 1994;71:F209–10.
6. Raffles A, Williams J, Costeloe K, Clark P. Transplacental effects of maternal cancer chemotherapy. Case report. Br J Obstet Gynaecol 1989;96:1099–1100.
7. Brunet S, Sureda A, Mateu R, Domingo-Albos A. Full-term pregnancy in a patient diagnosed with acute leukemia treated with a protocol including VP-16. Med Clin (Barc) 1993;100:757–8.
8. Rodriguez JM, Haggag M. VACOP-B chemotherapy for high grade non-Hodgkin's lymphoma in pregnancy. Clin Oncol (R Coll Radiol) 1995;7:319–20.
9. Bakri YN, Pedersen P, Nassar M. Normal pregnancy after curative multiagent chemotherapy for choriocarcinoma with brain metastases. Acta Obstet Gynecol Scand 1991;70:611–3.
10. Bierman PJ, Bagin RG, Jagannath S, Vose JM, Spitzer G, Kessinger A, Dicke KA, Armitage JO. High dose chemotherapy followed by autologous hematopoietic rescue in Hodgkin's disease: long term follow-up in 128 patients. Ann Oncol 1993;4:767–73.
11. Brice P, Pautier P, Marolleau JP, Castaigne S, Gisselbrecht C. Pregnancy after autologous bone marrow transplantation for malignant lymphomas. Nouv Rev Fr Hematol 1994;36:387–8.
12. Bower M, Fife K, Holden L, Paradinas FJ, Rustin GJS, Newlands ES. Chemotherapy for ovarian germ cell tumours. Eur J Cancer 1996;32A:593–7.
13. Matsui H, Eguchi O, Kimura H, Inaba N, Takamizawa H. The effect of etoposide on ovarian function in patients with gestational trophoblastic disease. Acta Obstet Gynaecol Jpn 1993;45:437–43.
14. Mangili G, Garavaglia E, Frigerio L, Candotti G, Ferrari A. Management of low-risk gestational trophoblastic tumors with etoposide (VP-16) in patients resistant to methotrexate. Gynecol Oncol 1996;61: 218–20.
15. Segna RA, Mitchell DR, Misas JE. Successful treatment of cervical pregnancy with oral etoposide. Obstet Gynecol 1990;76:945–7.
16. Green DM, Zevon MA, Lowrie G, Seigelstein N, Hall B. Congenital anomalies in children of patients who received chemotherapy for cancer in childhood and adolescence. N Engl J Med 1991;325: 141–6.
17. Azuno Y, Kaku K, Fujita N, Okubo M, Kaneko T. Mitoxantrone and etoposide in breast milk. Am J Hematol 1995;48:131–2.

Name: **ETRETINATE** Risk Factor: X_M

Class: **Vitamin/Psoralen**

FETAL RISK SUMMARY

RECOMMENDATION: Contraindicated

Etretinate, an orally active synthetic retinoid and vitamin A derivative, is used for the treatment of severe recalcitrant psoriasis. It is contraindicated in pregnant women and in those likely to become pregnant. Following oral administration, etretinate is stored in subcutaneous fat and is slowly released over a prolonged interval (1,2). In some patients after chronic therapy, detectable serum drug levels may occur up to 2.9 years after treatment has been stopped (2,3). Because of this variable excretion pattern, the exact length of time that pregnancy must be avoided after discontinuing treatment is unknown (2,3).

Like other retinoids (see also Isotretinoin and Vitamin A), etretinate is a potent animal teratogen (4). Data accumulated since release of this drug now indicate that it must be considered a human teratogen as well (1–3,5,6).

As of June 1986, a total of 51 pregnancies had occurred during treatment with etretinate (1,7,8). Of these pregnancies, 23 were still ongoing at the time of the reports and were unable to be evaluated (1). In the remaining 28 cases, 17 resulted in normal infants and three were normal fetuses after induced abortion. Skeletal anomalies were evident in eight cases: three liveborns, one stillbirth at 5 months, and four induced abortions. In addition, marked cerebral abnormalities, including meningomyeloceles, were observed in the stillborn and in three of the aborted fetuses.

A 1988 correspondence listed 22 documented etretinate exposures during pregnancy in West Germany as of September 1988 (9). The outcomes of these pregnancies were six induced abortions (no anomalies observed), four spontaneous abortions (no anomalies observed), six normal infants, and six infants with malformations (9).

Fifty-three pregnancies are known to have occurred following discontinuance of etretinate therapy (1,10). Malformations were observed in a fetus and an infant among the 38 pregnancies with known outcomes. In one case, a 22-year-old woman, treated intermittently over 5 years, became pregnant 4 months after etretinate therapy had been stopped (1,11,12). Serum concentrations of etretinate and the metabolite, etretin, were 7 ng/mL and 8 ng/mL, respectively, during the 8th week of gestation (6 months after the last dose). Following induced abortion at 10 weeks' gestation, the fetus was found to have unilateral skeletal defects of the lower limb consisting of a rudimentary left leg with one toe, missing tibia and fibula, and a hypoplastic femur (11,12). Evaluation of the face, skull, and brain was not possible. The defect was attributed to etretinate.

The second case also involved a 22-year-old woman who conceived 51 weeks after her last dose of etretinate (10). Other than the use of metoclopramide at 8 weeks' gestation for nausea and vomiting, no other drug history was mentioned. A growth-retarded (2850 g, 46 cm long, 3rd percentile) female infant was delivered by cesarean section at 38 weeks' gestation. Multiple congenital anomalies were noted involving the central nervous system, head, face, and heart, which included tetralogy of Fallot, microcephaly, hair whorls, small mandible, asymmetrical nares, protruding ears with malformed antihelices, absent lobules, and enlarged, keyhole-shaped entrances to the external ear canals, strabismus, left peripheral facial nerve paresis, and poor head control. Etretinate was detected in the mother's serum 3.5 months after delivery, but the concentration was below the test's lower limit of accuracy (2 ng/mL). No etretinate was detected in the infant's serum. Etretinate was considered responsible for the defects based partially on the presence of the drug in the mother's serum, and the fact that the pattern of malformation was identical to that observed with isotretinoin, another synthetic retinoid. The author also concluded that women treated with etretinate should avoid conception indefinitely (10).

Some of the defects noted in the above infant are also components of the CHARGE (coloboma, heart defects, choanal atresia, retardation, genital [males only], and ear anomalies) association (13), but in a response, the author of the case immediately above noted that such a relationship does not exclude etretinate as the etiology of the defects (14). Others have questioned whether an indefinite recommendation to avoid pregnancy is practical or necessary (15,16). In West Germany, 2 years of conception avoidance are recommended followed by determination of serum levels of etretinate and its metabolites (16). In six women treated with etretinate from 4–78 months, plasma concentrations of the drug were detected after 12 months in three patients (4, 8, and 8 ng/mL) and after

18 months in one patient (10 ng/mL) (16). Two women had no measurable etretinate 12 and 14 months after stopping therapy. The metabolites, acitretin and cis-acitretin, were detectable in two women (at 8 and 18 months) and five women (at 8–18 months).

The range of malformations, as listed by the manufacturer, includes meningomyelocele; meningoencephalocele; multiple synostoses; facial dysmorphia; syndactylies; absence of terminal phalanges; malformations of hip, ankle, and forearm; low-set ears; high palate; decreased cranial volume; and alterations of the skull and cervical vertebrae (2).

Pronounced jaundice with elevations of the transaminase enzymes, glutamic-oxaloacetic transaminase and glutamic-pyruvic transaminase, was observed in an otherwise normal male newborn following *in utero* exposure to etretinate (17). The cause of the liver pathology was unknown. No other abnormalities were observed, and the infant was normal at 5 months of age.

One source has suggested that male patients treated with etretinate should avoid fathering children during treatment; if this does occur, ultrasound of the fetus is indicated (18). Although there is no evidence that etretinate adversely affects sperm, and even if it did, that this could result in birth defects, the authors defended their comment as practicing "defensive" medicine (19,20).

BREAST FEEDING SUMMARY

RECOMMENDATION: No Human Data - Potential Toxicity

It is not known if etretinate is excreted into human milk (2). The closely related retinoid, vitamin A, is excreted (see Vitamin A) and the presence of etretinate in breast milk should be expected. The manufacturer considers use of the drug during lactation to be contraindicated because of the potential for adverse effects (2).

References

1. Orfanos CE, Ehlert R, Gollnick H. The retinoids: a review of their clinical pharmacology and therapeutic use. Drugs 1987;34:459–503.
2. Roche Scientific Summary. The clinical evaluation of Tegison. Roche Laboratories, Division of Hoffmann-La Roche, Inc., 1986.
3. Anonymous. Etretinate approved. FDA Drug Bull 1986;16:16–7.
4. Kamm JJ. Toxicology, carcinogenicity, and teratogenicity of some orally administered retinoids. J Am Acad Dermatol 1982;6:652–9.
5. Anonymous. Etretinate (Tegison) for skin disease. Drug Ther Bull 1983;21:9–11.
6. Anonymous. Etretinate for psoriasis. Med Lett Drugs Ther 1987;29:9–10.
7. Happle R, Traupe H, Bounameaux Y, Fisch T. Teratogenicity of etretinate in humans. Dtsch Med Wochenschr 1984;109:1476–80.
8. Rosa FW, Wilk AL, Kelsey FO. Teratogen update: vitamin A congeners. Teratology 1986;33:355–64.
9. Hopf G, Mathias B. Teratogenicity of isotretinoin and etretinate. Lancet 1988;2:1143.
10. Lammer EJ. Embryopathy in infant conceived one year after termination of maternal etretinate. Lancet 1988;2:1080–1.
11. Grote W, Harms D, Janig U, Kietzmann H, Ravens U, Schwarze I. Malformation of fetus conceived 4 months after termination of maternal etretinate treatment. Lancet 1985;1:1276.
12. Kietzmann H, Schwarze I, Grote W, Ravens U, Janig U, Harms D. Fetal malformation after maternal etretinate treatment of Darier's disease. Dtsch Med Wochenschr 1986;111:60–2.
13. Blake KD, Wyse RKH. Embryopathy in infant conceived one year after termination of maternal etretinate: a reappraisal. Lancet 1988;2:1254.
14. Lammer E. Etretinate and pregnancy. Lancet 1989;1:109.
15. Greaves MW. Embryopathy in infant conceived one year after termination of maternal etretinate: a reappraisal. Lancet 1988;2:1254.
16. Rinck G, Gollnick H, Orfanos CE. Duration of contraception after etretinate. Lancet 1989;1:845–6.
17. Jager K, Schiller F, Stech P. Congenital ichthyosiforme erythroderma, pregnancy under aromatic retinoid treatment. Hautarzt 1985;36:150–3.
18. Ellis CN, Voorhees JJ. Etretinate therapy. J Am Acad Dermatol 1987;16:267–91.
19. Katz R. Etretinate and paternity. J Am Acad Dermatol 1987;17:509.
20. Ellis CN, Voorhees JJ. Etretinate and paternity (reply). J Am Acad Dermatol 1987;17:509.

E

Name:	**EVANS BLUE**	Risk Factor:	**C**
Class:	**Dye (Diagnostic)**		

FETAL RISK SUMMARY

RECOMMENDATION: Limited Human Data - Probably Compatible

No reports linking the use of Evans blue with congenital defects have been located. The dye is teratogenic in some animal species (1). Evans blue has been injected intra-amniotically for diagnosis of ruptured membranes without apparent effect on the fetus except for temporary staining of the skin (2,3). The use of Evans blue during pregnancy for plasma volume determinations is routine (4–8). No problems in the fetus or newborn have been attributed to this use.

BREAST FEEDING SUMMARY

RECOMMENDATION: No Human Data - Probably Compatible

No data are available.

References

1. Wilson JG. Teratogenic activity of several azo dyes chemically related to trypan blue. Anat Rec 1955;123: 313–34.
2. Atley RD, Sutherst JR. Premature rupture of the fetal membranes confirmed by intraamniotic injection of dye (Evans blue T-1824). Am J Obstet Gynecol 1970;108:993–4.
3. Morrison L, Wiseman HJ. Intra-amniotic injection of Evans blue dye. Am J Obstet Gynecol 1972;113:1147.
4. Quinlivan WLG, Brock JA, Sullivan H. Blood volume changes and blood loss associated with labor. I. Correlation of changes in blood volume measured by I^{131}-albumin and Evans blue dye, with measured blood loss. Am J Obstet Gynecol 1970;106:843–9.
5. Sibai BM, Abdella TN, Anderson GD, Dilts PV Jr. Plasma volume findings in pregnant women with mild hypertension: therapeutic considerations. Am J Obstet Gynecol 1983;145:539–44.
6. Goodlin RC, Anderson JC, Gallagher TF. Relationship between amniotic fluid volume and maternal plasma volume expansion. Am J Obstet Gynecol 1983;146:505–11.
7. Hays PM, Cruikshank DP, Dunn LJ. Plasma volume determination in normal and preeclamptic pregnancies. Am J Obstet Gynecol 1985;151:958–66.
8. Brown MA, Mitar DA, Whitworth JA. Measurement of plasma volume in pregnancy. Clin Sci 1992;83: 29–34.

Name:	**EZETIMIBE**	Risk Factor:	**C_M**
Class:	**Antilipemic Agent**		

FETAL RISK SUMMARY

RECOMMENDATION: No Human Data - Animal Data Suggest Moderate Risk

Ezetimibe selectively inhibits the intestinal absorption of cholesterol and related phytosterols. It is indicated, either alone or in combination with HMG-CoA reductase inhibitors, as adjunctive therapy to diet for the reduction of cholesterol and triglycerides in patients with primary hypercholesterolemia. Ezetimibe is extensively metabolized in the small intestine and liver and both the parent compound and the metabolite are pharmacologically active. In addition, both are highly bound (>90%) to plasma proteins and have an elimination half-life of about 22 hours (1,2).

Reproduction studies have been conducted in rats and rabbits. In rats, there was no evidence of impaired fertility or embryolethal effects at doses up to about 10 times the human exposure at 10 mg/day based on $AUC_{0-24\,hours}$ for total ezetimibe (HDAUC). At the highest dose, increased incidences of skeletal abnormalities (extra pair of thoracic ribs, unossified cervical vertebral centra, shortened ribs). In rabbits, doses up to about 150 times the HDAUC did not cause embryolethal effects but an increased incidence of extra thoracic ribs was observed (1,2).

No evidence of carcinogenicity was observed in mice and rats administered high doses over a 2-year period. There was also no evidence of mutagenic, clastogenic, or genotoxic effects with various other assays (1,2).

It is not known if ezetimibe or its active metabolite crosses the human placenta. The parent compound does cross the rat and rabbit placentas (1,2). The molecular weight (about 409 for the parent compound) and prolonged elimination half-life suggest that passage to the human embryo and/or fetus will occur, but the high plasma protein binding should limit the transfer.

No reports describing the use of ezetimibe in human pregnancy have been located. Although the animal data are suggestive of low risk, the lack of human pregnancy experience prevents an assessment of the risk this agent presents to the embryo and fetus. Generally, discontinuing treatment of hypercholesterolemia during pregnancy is not thought to put the mother at risk. If treatment during pregnancy is mandated, ezetimibe appears to be a better choice than treatment with HMG-CoA reductase inhibitors (i.e., "statins" are contraindicated) and the fibric acid derivative fenofibrate.

BREAST FEEDING SUMMARY

RECOMMENDATION: No Human Data - Potential Toxicity

No reports describing the use of ezetimibe during human lactation have been located. In lactating rats, the milk:plasma ratio for total ezetimibe was approximately 0.5 (1,2). The molecular weight (about 409 for the parent compound) and the prolonged elimination half-life (about 22 hours) for both ezetimibe and its active metabolite suggest that the drug and/or its metabolite will be excreted into breast milk. However, the high plasma protein binding (>90%) should limit the amount excreted. The effects, if any, on a nursing infant from this exposure are unknown. If ezetimibe is taken during lactation, the nursing infant should be closely observed for adverse effects that are commonly seen in adults (such as headache, diarrhea, pharyngitis, sinusitis, arthralgia, etc.).

References

1. Product information. Zetia. Merck/Schering-Plough Pharmaceuticals, 2004.
2. Product information. Zetia. Schering, 2004.

F

Name:	**FAMCICLOVIR**	Risk Factor:	B_M
Class:	**Antiviral**		

FETAL RISK SUMMARY

RECOMMENDATION: Limited Human Data - Animal Data Suggest Low Risk

Famciclovir is a prodrug administered orally for the treatment of infections involving herpes simplex virus types 1 and 2, or varicella zoster virus. After administration, the drug undergoes rapid biotransformation to penciclovir, the active antiviral compound. Specific indications are the treatment of recurrent episodes of genital herpes and the management of acute herpes zoster (shingles) (1).

Carcinogenic, but not embryotoxic or teratogenic, effects were observed in animal studies with famciclovir (1). A significant increase in the incidence of mammary adenocarcinoma was seen in female rats administered famciclovir 600 mg/kg/day, 1.5–9.0 times the levels achieved with the recommended human doses, based on area under the plasma concentration curve (AUC) comparisons for penciclovir. At this dose in female rats, and at doses up to 2.4 times the human dose (AUC comparison) in male mice, marginal increases in the incidence of subcutaneous tissue fibrosarcomas and squamous cell carcinomas of the skin were observed. The tumors, however, were not observed in male rats and female mice. The reason for these interesting gender differences is apparently unknown.

Both famciclovir and the active metabolite, penciclovir, were tested for teratogenicity in pregnant rats and rabbits (1). Based on the penciclovir levels achieved with the recommended human doses (AUC comparison), oral doses of famciclovir up to 21.6 times (rats) and 10.8 times (rabbits) those concentrations had no effect on embryo and fetal development. Intravenous famciclovir also had no effect on embryo and fetal development in either the rat or the rabbit at doses up to 12 and 9 times, respectively, the human dose, based on body surface area (BSA) comparisons. A similar lack of toxicity was observed with intravenous penciclovir at doses in pregnant rats and rabbits up to 2.6 and 4.2 times, respectively, the human dose (BSA).

It is not known whether famciclovir, or its active metabolite penciclovir, crosses the placenta to the fetus. Because of the low molecular weight of famciclovir (about 321), passage to the fetus should be expected.

A 1998 non-interventional observational cohort study described the outcomes of pregnancies in women who had been prescribed one or more of 34 newly marketed drugs by general practitioners in England (2). Data were obtained by questionnaires sent to the prescribing physicians one month after the expected or possible date of delivery. Of 1067 exposed pregnancies, famciclovir was taken during the 1st trimester in seven pregnancies. The outcomes of these pregnancies included one ectopic pregnancy, two missed abortions, and four normal, full-term infants.

The manufacturer (SmithKline Beecham) maintains a pregnancy registry to monitor the maternal-fetal outcomes of women exposed to famciclovir during pregnancy (1). Patients can be registered by calling (800) 366-8900, extension 5231.

BREAST FEEDING SUMMARY

RECOMMENDATION: No Human Data - Potential Toxicity

No studies describing the use of famciclovir during breast-feeding have been located. The drug is concentrated in the milk of lactating rats, achieving milk concentrations higher than those measured in the plasma (1). Because the drug is probably also excreted into human milk, and because of its tumorigenicity observed in rats and mice (see above) and its potential for other toxicity, women taking famciclovir should probably not breast-feed.

References

1. Product information. Famvir. SmithKline Beecham Pharmaceuticals, 2001.
2. Wilton LV, Pearce GL, Martin RM, Mackay FJ, Mann RD. The outcomes of pregnancy in women exposed to newly marketed drugs in general practice in England. Br J Obstet Gynaecol 1998;105:882–9.

Name:	**FAMOTIDINE**	Risk Factor:	B_M
Class:	**Gastrointestinal Agent (Antisecretory)**		

FETAL RISK SUMMARY

RECOMMENDATION: Limited Human Data - Animal Data Suggest Low Risk

Famotidine, a reversible histamine H_2-receptor antagonist that is more potent than either cimetidine or ranitidine, is used in the treatment of gastric and duodenal ulcers and in the therapy of pathologic hypersecretory conditions, such as Zollinger-Ellison syndrome.

Studies in rats and rabbits, using oral doses up to 2000 mg/kg/day and IV doses of 100–200 mg/kg/day, found no evidence of impaired fertility, fetotoxic effects, teratogenicity, or changes in postnatal behavior attributable to famotidine (1,2).

The drug is known to cross the term human placenta based on *in vitro* studies (3). No published reports on the use of famotidine in human pregnancy have appeared in the medical literature.

In a surveillance study of Michigan Medicaid recipients conducted between 1985 and 1992 involving 229,101 completed pregnancies, 33 newborns had been exposed to famotidine during the 1st trimester (F. Rosa, personal communication, FDA, 1993). Two (6.1%) major birth defects were observed (one expected). No anomalies were observed in six defect categories (cardiovascular defects, oral clefts, spina bifida, polydactyly, limb reduction defects, and hypospadias) for which specific data were available. The number of exposures is too small to draw any conclusions.

BREAST FEEDING SUMMARY

RECOMMENDATION: Limited Human Data - Probably Compatible

Famotidine is concentrated in breast milk, but to a lesser degree than either cimetidine or ranitidine (4). Following a single 40-mg dose administered to eight postpartum women who were not breast-feeding, the mean milk:plasma ratios at 2, 6, and 24 hours were 0.41, 1.78, and 1.33, respectively (4). The mean peak milk concentration, 72 ng/mL, occurred at 6 hours compared to 2 hours for plasma (mean 75 ng/mL). Exposure of the nursing infant to famotidine via milk has not been reported. Although a potential risk may exist for adverse effects, the American Academy of Pediatrics classifies a similar drug as compatible with breast-feeding (see Cimetidine). A 1991 reference source suggested that because famotidine and two other similar histamine H_2-receptor antagonists (i.e., nizatidine and roxatidine) are less concentrated in milk, they might be preferred in the nursing woman in place of cimetidine or ranitidine (5).

References

1. Burek JD, Majka JA, Bokelman DL. Famotidine: summary of preclinical safety assessment. Digestion 1985;32(Suppl 1):7–14.
2. Shibata M, Kawano K, Shiobara Y, Yoshinaga T, Fujiwara M, Uchida T, Odani Y. Reproductive studies on famotidine (YM 11170) in rats and rabbits. Oyo Yakuri 1983;26:489–97, 543–78, 831–40. As cited in Shepard TH. *Catalog of Teratogenic Agents*. 6th ed. Baltimore, MD: Johns Hopkins University Press, 1989:273.
3. Dicke JM, Johnson RF, Henderson GI, Kuehl TJ, Schenker S. A comparative evaluation of the transport of H2-receptor antagonists by the human and baboon placenta. Am J Med Sci 1988;295:198–206.
4. Courtney TP, Shaw RW, Cedar E, Mann SG, Kelly JG. Excretion of famotidine in breast milk. Br J Clin Pharmacol 1988;26:639P.
5. Anderson PO. Drug use during breast-feeding. Clin Pharm 1991;10:594–624.

Name: **FELBAMATE** Risk Factor: **C_M**

Class: **Anticonvulsant**

FETAL RISK SUMMARY

RECOMMENDATION: Limited Human Data - Animal Data Suggest Moderate Risk

Little information on the effects in human pregnancy of the antiepileptic agent felbamate is available. The drug is structurally similar to meprobamate. Serious adult toxicity, including fatal cases of aplastic anemia and acute liver failure, was reported by the manufacturer. One adverse pregnancy outcome, an infant with mental retardation whose mother was on monotherapy, has been reported to the Food and Drug Administration (F. Rosa, personal communication, FDA, 1994), but the relationship to the drug is unknown.

Citing information obtained from the manufacturer, one review stated that 10 women had become pregnant while enrolled in clinical trials of the drug and were subsequently dropped from the studies (1). Two of these women underwent elective termination of their pregnancies. A third patient was changed to phenytoin at 4 weeks' gestation and had a spontaneous abortion at 9.5 weeks. The remaining seven women eventually gave birth without any problems, but details on these pregnancies, whether felbamate or other anticonvulsants were continued throughout gestation, and the status of the newborns were not provided.

Felbamate was not teratogenic in rats and rabbits at doses up to 13.9 times and 4.2 times, respectively, the human daily dose on a mg/kg basis, or 3 times and <2 times, respectively, the human dose based on body surface area (2). In rats, however, there was a decrease in pup weight and an increase in pup deaths during lactation. The cause of the deaths was not known. The no-effect dose in rats was 6.9 times the human dose based on a mg/kg basis (1.5 times based on surface area) (2).

The drug crosses the placenta without accumulation in pregnant rats (2,3). Transplacental passage apparently has not been described in humans but should occur because of the low molecular weight (about 238).

BREAST FEEDING SUMMARY

RECOMMENDATION: Limited Human Data - Potential Toxicity

Felbamate is excreted into human milk (2). Although no reports have been located that describe the effects, if any, of exposure to this anticonvulsant via breast milk on human infants, both decreased weight and increased mortality were observed in rat pups of treated dams during lactation (2). The cause of the deaths was not known. Because of the potential for serious toxicity (e.g., aplastic anemia and acute liver failure) in a nursing infant, felbamate should be used cautiously, if at all, during lactation.

F

References

1. Wagner ML. Felbamate: a new antiepileptic drug. Am J Hosp Pharm 1994;51:1657–66.
2. Product information. Felbatol. Wallace Laboratories, 2000.
3. Adusumalli VE, Yang JT, Wong KK, Kucharczyk N, Sofia RD. Felbamate pharmacokinetics in the rat, rabbit, and dog. Drug Metab Dispos 1991;19:1116–25.

Name:	**FELODIPINE**	Risk Factor:	**C_M**
Class:	**Calcium Channel Blocker**		

FETAL RISK SUMMARY

RECOMMENDATION: Limited Human Data - Animal Data Suggest Risk

Felodipine is a calcium channel blocking agent used in the treatment of hypertension. The drug is teratogenic in rabbits, producing digital anomalies consisting of a reduction in size and degree of ossification of the terminal phalanges (1). The frequency and severity of the defects appeared to be dose-related over a range of 0.4 to 4 times the maximum recommended human dose based on body surface area (MRHD). The defects may have been related to reduced uterine blood flow (1). Similar effects were not observed in rats or monkeys. In the latter species, however, an abnormal position of the distal phalanges was observed in about 40% of the fetuses. At doses 4 times the MRHD, delayed parturition with difficult labor, an increased incidence of stillbirths, and a decreased incidence of postnatal survival were noted in rats (1).

A prospective, multicenter cohort study of 78 women (81 outcomes, 3 sets of twins) who had 1st trimester exposure to calcium channel blockers, including 1% to felodipine, was reported in 1996 (2). Compared to controls, no increase in the risk of major congenital malformations was found. A 1997 report described three pregnant women treated with felodipine for chronic essential hypertension (3). Therapy was started before or during the 1st trimester in each case. One woman, treated with felodipine and atenolol throughout gestation, delivered a growth retarded, 2020-g (<5th percentile) female infant at 37 weeks, with Apgar scores of 8 and 9 at 1 and 5 minutes, respectively. The intrauterine growth retardation was most likely a result of atenolol and hypertension. The birth weights of the other two infants were in the 10th and 15th percentile. Although a contribution from felodipine cannot be excluded, the low weights were probably secondary to maternal hypertension.

If felodipine is used in pregnancy, healthcare professionals are encouraged to call the toll free number (800-670-6126) for information about patient enrollment in the Motherisk study.

BREAST FEEDING SUMMARY

RECOMMENDATION: No Human Data - Probably Compatible

F

No reports describing the use of felodipine during human lactation have been located. Because of its relatively low molecular weight (about 384), however, excretion into human milk should be expected. In pregnant rabbits given doses equal to or greater than the MRHD, a significant enlargement of the mammary glands occurred that eventually resolved during lactation (1). Similar changes in rats and monkeys were not observed.

References

1. Product information. Plendil. Merck Sharp & Dohme, 2000.
2. Magee LA, Schick B, Donnenfeld AE, Sage SR, Conover B, Cook L, McElhatton PR, Schmidt MA, Koren G. The safety of calcium channel blockers in human pregnancy: a prospective, multicenter cohort study. Am J Obstet Gynecol 1996;174:823–8.
3. Casele HL, Windley KC, Prieto JA, Gratton R, Laifer SA. Felodipine use in pregnancy. Report of three cases. J Reprod Med 1997;42:378–81.

Name:	**FENFLURAMINE**	Risk Factor:	C_M
Class:	**Anorexiant**		

FETAL RISK SUMMARY

RECOMMENDATION: Contraindicated

Fenfluramine is a sympathomimetic amine used as a anorectic agent in the treatment of obesity. Although its mechanism of action is unknown, it may be related to brain levels of serotonin or to increased glucose utilization (1). The mechanism of action of its dextrorotatory isomer, dexfenfluramine, is thought to be related to serotonin reuptake inhibition and release (see Dexfenfluramine).

A 1971 report described reproductive studies of fenfluramine, conducted in mice, rats, rabbits, and monkeys (*Macaca mulatta*), that found no evidence of structural teratogenicity but observed a dose-related reduction in the birth weight of rat pups (2). A decrease in birth weight was not seen in the other animals. Mice received 10 mg/kg/day; rats, 2, 10, or 20 mg/kg/day; rabbits, 10 or 40 mg/kg/day; and monkeys, 2 mg/kg/day. An unexplained increase in stillbirths of rat pups was observed in the group receiving 2 mg/kg/day. In pregnant monkeys, both fenfluramine and its deethylated metabolite readily crossed the placenta and were measured in amniotic fluid, 1.1 μg/10 mL and 0.36 μg/10 mL, respectively (maternal serum levels not specified) (2).

A significant increase in mortality, as well as a significant reduction in body weight, were observed during the preweaning period in offspring of rats given fenfluramine 20 mg/kg/day orally on days 7–20 of gestation (3). Moreover, although the body weight of fenfluramine-exposed offspring was no different from that of controls by 70 days of age, there was a significant reduction (4.7%) in brain weight. The amount of DNA in the brain and the neuronal cell count density in the cerebellum and hippocampus, however, were similar to those of controls. Behavioral teratogenicity was observed during several tests conducted during the preweaning period, with locomotor development (pivoting) being the most altered. The abnormal behavioral results were also described in a second, similar publication by some of these authors (4).

Two commercial formulations of fenfluramine (Pondimin and Redux) were given to adult female mice before mating and through gestational day 14 (5). Pregnancy outcomes in the two treated groups were compared to a placebo group (5). The doses used (10 mg/kg/day Pondimin and 5 mg/kg/day Redux) were equivalent to the human daily dose based on body surface area. No differences were observed between the three groups in conception rates, maternal food consumption and weight gain, duration of gestation, number of live births, and pup sex ratio. Body weight, length, and head circumference at birth through postnatal day 60 were also similar, as was the time to reach sexual maturation and development milestones (5).

A possible mechanism by which fenfluramine inhibits cortical serotonin fiber outgrowth in newborn rat pups was described in a 1994 paper (6). Using an *in vitro* preparation, the investigators demonstrated that fenfluramine invoked a large increase in serotonin release in fetal tissues, but not in the mother. They postulated that the increased extraneuronal concentration of serotonin in the fetus may be a mechanism by which fenfluramine has produced neurobehavior teratogenicity in animals (6). In an earlier study, however, researchers concluded that the serotonin-releasing action of fenfluramine had no effect on the development of descending spinal serotonergic pathways in rats (7).

A total of 40 women, 30 during the 3rd trimester and 10 during the first 3 days after delivery, were treated with fenfluramine 20 mg 3 times daily for obesity in a study published in 1969 (8). No adverse effects in the fetus or newborn were mentioned, but follow-up of the infants did not appear to have been conducted.

Six congenital malformations from pregnancies exposed to fenfluramine have been reported by the WHO International Drug Monitoring System (F. Rosa, personal communication, FDA, 1997). The anomalies were a urinary tract malformation, a fatal multiple defect involving the limbs and the gastrointestinal tract, ectromelia of one limb, a clubfoot, an atrial septal defect, and multiple nonspecified malformations. The FDA has received two reports involving the use of the combination of fenfluramine and phentermine in early pregnancy (F. Rosa, personal communication, FDA, 1997). A spontaneous abortion occurred in one of the pregnancies. In the other, an infant with bilateral valvular abnormalities, both aortic and pulmonary, with moderate stenosis and displacement was delivered. Because valvular toxicity has been reported in adults taking the combination, a causal relationship in the pregnancy case is potentially possible. No other details of these cases were available.

In summary, fenfluramine is a behavioral teratogen in at least one animal species. It is not known if this occurs in humans, but, except for the cases above, only one study has described the use of fenfluramine during human pregnancy. Both fenfluramine and its metabolite readily cross the placenta in monkeys and presumably, because of the drug's low molecular weight (about 268), in humans. Because the benefits from use of this agent during gestation seem small and the potential risks seem large, the use of fenfluramine during pregnancy should be considered contraindicated. If weight loss is needed during pregnancy, then nonpharmacologic methods such as diet control combined with professional assistance should be used.

BREAST FEEDING SUMMARY

RECOMMENDATION: Contraindicated

No reports describing the use of fenfluramine during human lactation have been located. Its relatively low molecular weight (about 268) probably ensures its excretion into milk. Fenfluramine has demonstrated behavioral toxicity in animals exposed during pregnancy through a mechanism thought to involve the release of serotonin from neurons. Because fenfluramine is readily absorbed from the gastrointestinal tract and has a long plasma half-life (about 20 hours), the nursing infant could be exposed to a potentially neurotoxic agent during a period of rapid brain development. Therefore, the use of fenfluramine during breast-feeding should be considered contraindicated.

References

1. Product information. Pondimin. A. H. Robins, 1997.
2. Gilbert DL, Franko BV, Ward JW, Woodard G, Courtney KD. Toxicologic studies of fenfluramine. Toxicol Appl Pharmacol 1971;19:705–11.
3. Vorhees CV, Brunner RL, Butcher RE. Psychotropic drugs as behavioral teratogens. Science 1979;205:1220–5.
4. Butcher RE, Vorhees CV. A preliminary test battery for the investigation of the behavioral teratology of selected psychotropic drugs. Neurobehav Toxicol 1979;1(Suppl 1):207–12.
5. Rayburn WF, Stewart JD, Gonzalez CL, Christensen HD. Effect of the antiobesity drug fenfluramine given prenatally on growth and development of mice offspring (abstract). Am J Obstet Gynecol 1998;178:S138.
6. Kramer K, Azmitia EC, Whitaker-Azmitia PM. In vitro release of [^{3}H]5-hydroxytryptamine from fetal and maternal brain by drugs of abuse. Brain Res Dev Brain Res 1994;78:142–6.
7. Bell J III, Zhang X, Whitaker-Azmitia PM. 5-HT$_3$ receptor-active drugs alter development of spinal serotonergic innervation: lack of effect of other serotonergic agents. Brain Res 1992;571:293–7.
8. Soto ER, Urdapilleta JD. Fenfluoramina. Droga anorexigenica en la practica obstetrica. Ginecol Obstet Mex 1969;25:425–32.

Name:	**FENOFIBRATE**	Risk Factor:	**C_M**
Class:	**Antilipemic**		

FETAL RISK SUMMARY

RECOMMENDATION: No Human Data - Animal Data Suggest Risk

Fenofibrate is a prodrug that is rapidly hydrolyzed by esterases after oral administration to the active metabolite, fenofibric acid. The active metabolite is further metabolized to inactive metabolites. Fenofibric acid is indicated as adjunctive therapy to diet for the treatment of primary hypercholesterolemia or mixed dyslipidemia, and for hypertriglyceridemia. Fenofibric acid is extensively bound to serum protein (about 99%) and has an elimination half-life of 20 hours (1,2).

Reproduction studies have been conducted in pregnant rats and rabbits (1,2). The drug was embryocidal and teratogenic in pregnant rats given 7 to 10 times the maximum recommended human dose based on body surface area (MRHD). At 9 times the MRHD given before and throughout gestation to rats, reproductive toxicity included delayed parturition in 100% of the dams, a 60% increase in post-implantation loss with a decrease in litter size, reduced birth weight, an increase in spina bifida, and decreased pup survival (40% at birth, 4% during neonatal period, and 0% to weaning). Similar findings were observed at 7 times the MRHD given from day 15 of gestation through weaning. When pregnant rats were dosed at 10 times the MRHD during organogenesis, an increased incidence of congenital malformations was observed, including domed head/hunched shoulders/rounded body/abnormal chest, kyphosis, stunted fetuses, elongated sternal ribs, malformed sternebrae, extra foramen in palatine, misshapen vertebrae, and supernumerary ribs (1). Embryocidal effects were also observed in rabbits. Doses 9 and 18 times the MRHD caused abortions in 10% and 25% of the dams, respectively. At 18 times the MRHD, 7% of the fetuses died (1,2).

Fenofibrate had no mutagenic potential in four different tests, but the drug was carcinogenic in rats, significantly increasing the incidence of liver carcinoma, pancreatic carcinoma and adenomas, and benign testicular interstitial cell tumors in a dose-related manner (1,2). Some of these tumors (pancreatic acinar adenomas and testicular interstitial cell tumors) were also seen in a second strain of rats at lower doses (1,2).

It is not known if fenofibrate or fenofibric acid cross the human placenta. Fenofibrate is rapidly metabolized and is not detected in the plasma (1,2). The molecular weight of the metabolite, fenofibric acid (about 319), and the prolonged elimination half-life suggest that the drug will cross, but the high serum protein binding should limit the amount available for transfer to the embryo or fetus.

No reports describing the use of fenofibrate in human pregnancy have been located. Although the lack of human pregnancy experience prevents an assessment of the risk, the combined animal data are reason for concern if this drug is used for prolong periods in pregnancy. In addition, as with other antilipemic agents, there is apparently no maternal benefit to the use of fenofibrate during gestation. Therefore, fenofibrate should be avoided during pregnancy.

BREAST FEEDING SUMMARY

RECOMMENDATION. No Human Data - Potential Toxicity

No reports describing the use of fenofibrate in human lactation have been located. The relative low molecular weight of the active metabolite (about 319) suggests that it is excreted into breast milk. Although the effect of this exposure on a nursing infant is unknown, women taking fenofibrate should probably not breast-feed because of the carcinogenicity observed in rats.

References

1. Product information. TriCor. Abbott Laboratories, 2001.
2. Product information. Lofibra. GATE Pharmaceuticals, 2004.

Name: **FENOLDOPAM**	Risk Factor: **B_M**
Class: **Antihypertensive**	

FETAL RISK SUMMARY

RECOMMENDATION: No Human Data - Animal Data Suggest Low Risk

An IV infusion of fenoldopam mesylate, a dopamine D_1-like receptor agonist, is indicated for the short-term (up to 48 hours), rapid onset, management of severe hypertension. It is a vasodilator, affecting coronary, renal, mesenteric, and peripheral arteries in animals.

Reproduction studies have been conducted in rats and rabbits with oral doses up to 200 mg/kg/day and 25 mg/kg/day, respectively (1). Although maternal toxicity was evident at the highest doses, no evidence of impaired fertility or fetal harm were observed.

It is not known if fenoldopam mesylate crosses the human placenta. The molecular weight (about 402) is low enough, however, that transfer to the fetus should be expected.

The absence of human pregnancy experience prevents an assessment of the fetal risk from exposure to fenoldopam mesylate, but the animal data is reassuring. Because it is used for the emergency reduction of severe hypertension, the maternal benefit probably outweighs the unknown fetal risk. However, rapid reduction of maternal blood pressure may compromise the placental perfusion resulting in fetal hypoxia and subsequent bradycardia. Fetal death is a potential consequence of this effect. Fetal heart rate monitoring, therefore, is recommended during IV infusions of fenoldopam.

BREAST FEEDING SUMMARY

RECOMMENDATION: No Human Data - Probably Compatible

No reports describing the use of fenoldopam mesylate in human lactation have been located. The molecular weight (about 402), however, suggests that excretion into breast milk probably occurs. The effect of this exposure on a nursing infant are unknown. Fenoldopam mesylate is excreted into the milk of lactating rats (1). Because of the nature of the indication, opportunities for use of this drug during breast-feeding are probably very rare.

Reference

1. Product information. Corlopam. Abbott Laboratories, 2001.

Name:	**FENOPROFEN**	Risk Factor:	**B***
Class:	**Nonsteroidal Anti-inflammatory**		

FETAL RISK SUMMARY

RECOMMENDATION: Human Data Suggest Risk in 1st and 3rd Trimesters

Fenoprofen is a nonsteroidal anti-inflammatory drug (NSAID) in the same subclass (propionic acids) as five other agents (flurbiprofen, ibuprofen, ketoprofen, naproxen, and oxaprozin). It is indicated for the relief of the signs and symptoms of rheumatoid arthritis and osteoarthritis (1). Fenoprofen given to rats during pregnancy and continued until labor resulted in prolonged parturition (1).

It is not known if fenoprofen crosses the human placenta. The molecular weight (about 559) is low enough that passage to the fetus should be expected. However, in one study the drug was used during labor (2). No data were given except that the drug could not be detected in cord blood or amniotic fluid.

In a surveillance study of Michigan Medicaid recipients conducted between 1985 and 1992 involving 229,101 completed pregnancies, 191 newborns had been exposed to fenoprofen during the 1st trimester (F. Rosa, personal communication, FDA, 1993). A total of six (3.1%) major birth defects were observed (eight expected), including (observed/expected) 1/2 cardiovascular defects and 1/1 polydactyly. No anomalies were observed in four other categories of defects (oral clefts, spina bifida, limb reduction defects, and hypospadias) for which specific data were available. These data do not support an association between the drug and congenital defects.

A combined 2001 population-based observational cohort study and a case-control study estimated the risk of adverse pregnancy outcome from the use of NSAIDs (3). The use of NSAIDs during pregnancy was not associated with congenital malformations, preterm delivery, or low birth weight, but a positive association was discovered with spontaneous abortions (SABs). A similar study, also published in 2001, failed to find a relationship, in general between NSAIDs and congenital malformations, but did find a significant association with cardiac defects and orofacial clefts (4). In addition, a 2003 study found a significant association between exposure to NSAIDs in early pregnancy and SABs (5). (See Ibuprofen for details on these three studies.)

A brief 2003 editorial on the potential for NSAID-induced developmental toxicity concluded that NSAIDs, and specifically those with greater COX-2 affinity, had a lower risk of this toxicity in humans than aspirin (6).

Prostaglandin synthesis inhibitors can theoretically cause constriction of the ductus arteriosus *in utero* (see also Indomethacin) (7). Persistent pulmonary hypertension of the newborn may occur if these agents are used in the 3rd trimester close to delivery (7,8). These drugs also have been shown to inhibit labor and prolong pregnancy, both in humans (9) (see also Indomethacin) and in animals (10). Women attempting to conceive should not use any prostaglandin synthesis inhibitor, including fenoprofen, because of the findings in a variety of animal models that indicate these agents block blastocyst implantation (11,12). Moreover, as noted above, NSAIDs have been associated with SABs and congenital malformations.

[*Risk Factor D if used in the 3rd trimester or near delivery.*]

BREAST FEEDING SUMMARY

RECOMMENDATION: Limited Human Data - Probably Compatible

Fenoprofen passes into breast milk in very small quantities. The milk:plasma ratio in nursing mothers given 600 mg every 6 hours for 4 days was approximately 0.017 (2). Although the clinical significance of this amount is unknown, another NSAID in the same subclass is classified as compatible with breast-feeding by the American Academy of Pediatrics (see Ibuprofen).

References

1. Product information. Nalfon. Dista Products, 2001.
2. Rubin A, Chernish SM, Crabtree R, et al. A profile of the physiological disposition and gastro-intestinal effects of fenoprofen in man. Curr Med Res Opin 1974;2:529–44.
3. Nielsen GL, Sorensen HT, Larsen H, Pedersen L. Risk of adverse birth outcome and miscarriage in pregnant users of non-steroidal anti-inflammatory drugs: population based observational study and case-control study. BMJ 2001;322:266–70.
4. Ericson A, Kallen BAJ. Nonsteroidal anti-inflammatory drugs in early pregnancy. Reprod Toxicol 2001; 15:371–5.
5. Li DK, Liu L, Odouli R. Exposure to non-steroidal anti-inflammatory drugs during pregnancy and risk of miscarriage: population based cohort study. BMJ 2003;327:368–71.
6. Tassinari MS, Cook JC, Hurtt ME. NSAIDs and developmental toxicity. Birth Defects Res Part B Dev Reprod Toxicol 2003;68:3–4.
7. Levin DL. Effects of inhibition of prostaglandin synthesis on fetal development, oxygenation, and the fetal circulation. Semin Perinatol 1980;4:35–44.
8. Van Marter LJ, Leviton A, Allred EN, Pagano M, Sullivan KF, Cohen A, Epstein MF. Persistent pulmonary hypertension of the newborn and smoking and aspirin and nonsteroidal antiinflammatory drug consumption during pregnancy. Pediatrics 1996;97:658–63.
9. Fuchs F. Prevention of prematurity. Am J Obstet Gynecol 1976;126:809–20.
10. Powell JG, Cochrane RL. The effects of a number of non-steroidal anti-inflammatory compounds on parturition in the rat. Prostaglandins 1982;23:469–88.
11. Matt DW, Borzelleca JF. Toxic effects on the female

reproductive system during pregnancy, parturition, and lactation. In Witorsch RJ, editor. *Reproductive Toxicology*. 2nd ed. New York, NY: Raven Press, 1995:175–93.

12. Dawood MY. Nonsteroidal antiinflammatory drugs and reproduction. Am J Obstet Gynecol 1993;169:1255–65.

Name: **FENOTEROL** Risk Factor: **B**
Class: **Sympathomimetic (Adrenergic)**

F

FETAL RISK SUMMARY

RECOMMENDATION: Limited Human Data - No Relevant Animal Data

No reports linking the use of fenoterol with congenital defects have been located. Fenoterol, a β-sympathomimetic, has been used to prevent premature labor (1,2). The effects in the mother, fetus, and newborn are similar to those produced by the parent compound (see Metaproterenol). Fenoterol has been shown to inhibit prostaglandin-induced uterine activity at term (3).

Fenoterol was administered to 11 patients 30 minutes before cesarean section under general anesthesia at an infusion rate of 3 μg/minute (4). No adverse effects were seen in the mother, fetus, or newborn after this short exposure. Infusion in hypertensive pregnant patients caused a greater drop in diastolic blood pressure than did the same dose in normotensive pregnant women (5). Other cardiovascular parameters in the mothers and fetuses were comparable between the two groups.

BREAST FEEDING SUMMARY

RECOMMENDATION: No Human Data - Probably Compatible

No data are available.

References

1. Lipshitz J, Baillie P, Davey DA. A comparison of the uterine beta-2-adrenoreceptor selectivity of fenoterol, hexoprenaline, ritodrine and salbutamol. S Afr Med J 1976;50:1969–72.
2. Lipshitz J. The uterine and cardiovascular effects of oral fenoterol hydrochloride. Br J Obstet Gynaecol 1977;84:737–9.
3. Lipshitz J, Lipshitz EM. Uterine and cardiovascular effects of fenoterol and hexoprenaline in prostaglandin $F_{2\alpha}$-induced labor in humans. Obstet Gynecol 1984;63:396–400.
4. Jouppila R, Kauppila A, Tuimala R, Pakarinen A, Moilanen K. Maternal, fetal and neonatal effects of beta-adrenergic stimulation in connection with cesarean section. Acta Obstet Gynecol Scand 1980;59:489–93.
5. Oddoy UA, Joschko K. Effects of fenoterol on blood pressure, heart rate, and cardiotocogram of hypertensive and normotensive women in advanced pregnancy. Zentralbl Gynakol 1982;104:415–21.

Name: **FENTANYL** Risk Factor: **C_M***
Class: **Narcotic Agonist Analgesic**

FETAL RISK SUMMARY

RECOMMENDATION: Human Data Suggest Risk in 3rd Trimester

No reports linking the use of fentanyl with congenital defects have been located. Although not teratogenic in rats, fentanyl impaired fertility and was embryotoxic at IV doses 0.3 times the human dose given for a period of 12 days (1).

The placental transfer of fentanyl has been documented in the 1st and 2nd trimesters (2) and at term (3,11,13,14,16). A study published in 1998 measured fentanyl concentrations in fetal fluids (amniotic and/or chorionic cavities), fetal blood (after 12 weeks' gestation), and maternal serum 5–22 minutes after an IV bolus (1.5 μg/kg) in 42 healthy women scheduled for pregnancy termination (between 6 and 16 weeks' gestation) under general anesthesia (2). Fentanyl was detected in amniotic fluid at less than 12 weeks' gestation, but not later, and in fetal blood. None of the samples of chorionic fluid, however, contained detectable fentanyl (2).

In a study comparing women in labor who received 50 μg or 100 μg of fentanyl IV every hour as needed ($N = 137$) (mean dose 140 μg, range 50–600 μg) to those not requiring analgesia (epidural or narcotic) ($N = 112$), no statistical differences were found in newborn outcome in terms of the incidence of depressed respirations, Apgar scores, and the need for naloxone (3). In blinded measurements taken at 2–4 and 24 hours, no differences were observed between the two groups of infants in respiratory rate, heart rate, blood pressure, adaptive capacity, neurologic evaluation, and overall assessment. The last dose of fentanyl was given a mean of 112 minutes before delivery. Cord blood levels of the narcotic were always significantly lower than maternal serum levels (cord:maternal ratios approximately 0.5 but exact data not given) ($p < 0.03$). Doses used were considered equianalgesic to 5–10 mg of morphine or 37.5–75 mg of meperidine (3).

Respiratory depression has been observed in one infant whose mother received epidural fentanyl during labor (4). Fentanyl may produce loss of fetal heart rate (FHR) variability without causing fetal hypoxia (3,5). However, no effect on FHR variability or accelerations were observed when epidural fentanyl was given to women receiving adequate epidural lidocaine analgesia (6). The narcotic has been combined with bupivacaine for spinal anesthesia during labor (7,8). In four studies, the addition of fentanyl to bupivacaine had no effect on neonatal respiration (9–12) and, in two, did not adversely affect neurobehavioral scores (11,12). Placental transfer of fentanyl was documented in one study with cord:maternal venous plasma ratios of 1.12 for total drug and 1.20 for free drug (11). A study of a continuous epidural infusion of fentanyl and bupivacaine found no accumulation of either drug over a 1–15 hour interval in 21 laboring women and observed no adverse fetal effects (13). The mean cord:maternal venous fentanyl concentration was 0.94.

In 15 women undergoing elective cesarean section, fentanyl 1 μg/kg given IV within 10 minutes of delivery produced an average cord blood:maternal blood ratio over 10 minutes of 0.31 (range 0.06–0.43) (14). No respiratory depression was observed, and all neurobehavioral scores were normal at 4 and 24 hours.

A 1998 case report described respiratory muscle rigidity in a newborn that was attributed to fentanyl (15). Because of severe maternal disease (pulmonary valve stenosis with congestive heart failure and pregnancy-induced hypertension) and Doppler measurements showing periodically absent diastolic flow in the umbilical cord, a cesarean section under general anesthesia was performed at 31 weeks' gestation to deliver a 1440-g male infant. Betamethasone had been given to the mother for fetal lung maturation before delivery. The mother was premedicated with morphine (7.5 mg) and scopolamine (0.3 mg) followed by fentanyl (300 μg; *note: reference states "mg" but assumed to be "μg"*), diazepam (7.5 mg), ketamine (300 mg), and vecuronium (7 mg). The newborn had no respiratory movements and a heart rate of about 100 beats/minute (Apgar score 3 at 1 minute). Attempts to ventilate the infant by mask and then by intubation with positive pressure produced no chest movements until 8 minutes after delivery. A chest x-ray showed normal lungs with no sign of hyaline membrane disease. After treatment of severe respiratory alkalosis at 1 hour of age, the infant made an uneventful recovery and was developing

F

normally at 1 year of age. The author attributed the chest wall rigidity to fentanyl because this is a common adverse effects in adults administered the agent during anesthesia (15).

A 31-year-old woman was treated with transdermal fentanyl patches (125 μg/hour) throughout gestation for severe cervical and lumbar spinal injuries sustained in a road traffic accident before conception (16). An elective cesarean section was performed at 38 weeks' gestation to deliver a healthy, 3.13-kg female infant with Apgar scores of 9 at 1 and 5 minutes, respectively. The infant's head circumference was 35.4 cm (50th percentile). Blood concentrations of fentanyl were mother (pre-delivery) 3.56 ng/mL and infant 1.23 ng/mL (at birth), 0.31 ng/mL (day 1), and <0.25 ng/mL) (day 2). At 24 hours of age, the bottle-fed baby was noted to be jittery, fisting and irritable with a high-pitched cry (16). The mean Finnegan scores (an assessment of acute opioid withdrawal in newborns based on nursing observations) on day 1 and 2 were 4.5 ("mild" is 0–7) with a single peak of 11 ("abstinence" is 8–11) at 72 hours of age (16). Finnegan scores were consistently less than 4 by day 4 and, at 96 hours of age the infant had no signs of opioid withdrawal. No drug therapy of the withdrawal was required at any time. The infant was developing normally at follow-up (16).

[*Risk Factor D if used for prolonged periods or in high doses at term.*]

BREAST FEEDING SUMMARY

RECOMMENDATION: Compatible

Fentanyl is excreted into milk. A study published in 1992 measured fentanyl colostrum concentrations in 13 healthy women who had received fentanyl (2 μg/kg) during cesarean section or postpartum tubal ligation (17). Serum and colostrum samples were collected at six intervals up to 10 hours after drug administration. The peak serum and colostrum fentanyl levels occurred at 0.75 hours, with mean values of 0.19 and 0.40 ng/mL, respectively, falling to undetectable and 0.05 ng/mL, respectively, at 10 hours. Colostrum fentanyl concentrations were always greater than serum levels at every measurement. It was concluded that breast-feeding was safe because of the low colostrum concentrations and the low oral bioavailability of fentanyl (17). The American Academy of Pediatrics classifies fentanyl as compatible with breast-feeding (18).

References

1. Product information. Duragesic. Janssen Pharmaceutica, 2000.
2. Shannon C, Jauniaux E, Gulbis B, Thiry P, Sitham M, Bromley L. Placental transfer of fentanyl in early human pregnancy. Hum Reprod 1998;13:2317–20.
3. Rayburn W, Rathke A, Leuschen MP, Chleborad J, Weidner W. Fentanyl citrate analgesia during labor. Am J Obstet Gynecol 1989;161:202–6.
4. Carrie LES, O'Sullivan GM, Seegobin R. Epidural fentanyl in labour. Anaesthesia 1981;36:965–9.
5. Johnson ES, Colley PS. Effects of nitrous oxide and fentanyl anesthesia on fetal heart-rate variability intra- and postoperatively. Anesthesiology 1980;52:429–30.
6. Viscomi CM, Hood DD, Melone PJ, Eisenach JC. Fetal heart rate variability after epidural fentanyl during labor. Anesth Analg 1990;71:679–83.
7. Justins DM, Francis D, Houlton PG, Reynolds F. A controlled trial of extradural fentanyl in labour. Br J Anaesth 1982;54:409–13.
8. Milon D, Bentue-Ferrer D, Noury D, Reymann JM, Sauvage J, Allain H, Saint-Marc C, van den Driessche J. Peridural anesthesia for cesarean section employing a bupivacaine-fentanyl combination. Ann Fr Anesth Reanim 1983;2:273–9.
9. Benlabed M, Dreizzen E, Ecoffey C, Escourrou P, Migdal M, Gaultier C. Neonatal patterns of breathing after cesarean section with or without epidural fentanyl. Anesthesiology 1990;73:1110–3.
10. Halonen PM, Paatero H, Hovorka J, Haasio J, Korttila K. Comparison of two fentanyl doses to improve epidural anaesthesia with 0.5% bupivacaine for caesarean section. Acta Anaesthesiol Scand 1993;37:774–9.
11. Fernando R, Bonello E, Gill P, Urquhart J, Reynolds F, Morgan B. Neonatal welfare and placental transfer of fentanyl and bupivacaine during ambulatory combined spinal epidural analgesia for labour. Anaesthesia 1997;52:517–24.
12. Porter J, Bonello E, Reynolds F. Effect of epidural

fentanyl on neonatal respiration. Anesthesiology 1998;89:79–85.
13. Bader AM, Fragneto R, Terui K, Arthur GR, Loferski B, Datta S. Maternal and neonatal fentanyl and bupivacaine concentrations after epidural infusion during labor. Anesth Analg 1995;81:829–32.
14. Eisele JH, Wright R, Rogge P. Newborn and maternal fentanyl levels at cesarean section (abstract). Anesth Anal 1982;61:179–80.
15. Lindemann R. Respiratory muscle rigidity in a preterm infant after use of fentanyl during Caesarean section. Eur J Pediatr 1998;157:1012–3.
16. Regan J, Chambers F, Gorman W, MacSullivan R. Neonatal abstinence syndrome due to prolonged administration of fentanyl in pregnancy. Br J Obstet Gynaecol 2000;107:570–2.
17. Steer PL, Biddle CJ, Marley WS, Lantz RK, Sulik PL. Concentration of fentanyl in colostrum after an analgesic dose. Can J Anaesth 1992;39:231–5.
18. Committee on Drugs, American Academy of Pediatrics. The transfer of drugs and other chemicals into human milk. Pediatrics 2001;108:776–89.

Name: **FEXOFENADINE** Risk Factor: C_M

Class: **Antihistamine**

FETAL RISK SUMMARY

RECOMMENDATION: No Human Data - Animal Data Suggest Moderate Risk

Fexofenadine is a second generation (peripherally selective), histamine H_1-receptor antagonist that is used for the relief of symptoms associated with seasonal allergic rhinitis. It is a metabolite of another second generation antihistamine, terfenadine (no longer available). As a group, second generation antihistamines are less sedating than first generation agents.

Fertility studies in rats and reproduction studies in rats and rabbits have been conducted with fexofenadine (1). In rats, doses producing systemic exposures (AUC) that were equal to or greater than 3 times the human exposure (AUC) obtained with a 60-mg twice daily dose (HTD) were associated with dose-related decrease in the number of implantations and an increase in the number of postimplantation losses. No evidence of teratogenicity was noted in pregnant rats and rabbits at oral doses up to 4 and 47 times the HTD, respectively. However, dose-related decreases in pup weight gain and survival were observed in rats at 3 times the HTD (1).

It is not known if fexofenadine crosses the human placenta to the fetus. The molecular weight (about 538 for the free base hydrochloride salt) is low enough, however, that transfer to the fetus should be expected.

No reports describing the use of fexofenadine during human pregnancy have been located. However, studies in rats found dose-related embryo and fetal toxicity, but the risk to a human fetus cannot be assessed at this time. Because of the extensive human data available, several reviews have recommended that oral first generation antihistamines (e.g., chlorpheniramine or tripelennamine) should be considered if antihistamine therapy during pregnancy (especially in the 1st trimester) is required (2–4). The second generation agents cetirizine or loratadine were considered acceptable alternatives, except during the 1st trimester, if a first generation antihistamine was not tolerated.

BREAST FEEDING SUMMARY

RECOMMENDATION: Limited Human Data - Probably Compatible

Consistent with the molecular weight (about 502 for the free base), fexofenadine is excreted into breast milk. Four lactating women were given terfenadine (60 mg every

12 hours for 4 doses), and then milk and plasma samples were collected after the last dose at various times for 30 hours (5). None of the parent compound was detected in the milk or plasma. The maximum concentrations of the active metabolite (i.e., fexofenadine) were 309 and 41 ng/mL, respectively, both occurring approximately 4 hours after the last dose. Based on the 12-hour excretion, the mean milk:plasma ratio was 0.21. The maximum estimated exposure of a nursing infant was 0.45% of the recommended maternal weight-corrected dose (5).

The above estimated exposure of a nursing infant may not be applicable when the mother is actually taking fexofenadine. Moreover, the effect of this exposure on a nursing infant is unknown because the four women did not nurse their infants during the study. However, the American Academy of Pediatrics classifies fexofenadine as compatible with breast-feeding (6).

F

References

1. Product information. Allegra. Hoechst Marion Roussel, 2000.
2. Mazzotta P, Loebstein R, Koren G. Treating allergic rhinitis in pregnancy. Safety considerations. Drug Saf 1999;20:361–75.
3. Horak F, Stubner UP. Comparative tolerability of second generation antihistamines. Drug Saf 1999;20:385–401.
4. Position statement of a joint committee of the American College of Obstetricians and Gynecologists and the American College of Allergy, Asthma and Immunology. The use of newer asthma and allergy medications during pregnancy. Ann Allergy Asthma Immunol 2000;84:475–80.
5. Lucas BD, Purdy CY, Scarim SK, Benjamin S, Abel SR, Hilleman DE. Terfenadine pharmacokinetics in breast milk in lactating women. Clin Pharmacol Ther 1995;57:398–402.
6. Committee on Drugs, American Academy of Pediatrics. The transfer of drugs and other chemicals into human milk. Pediatrics 2001;108:776–89.

Name: **FILGRASTIM** Risk Factor: **C_M**

Class: **Hematopoietic**

FETAL RISK SUMMARY

RECOMMENDATION: Compatible - Maternal Benefit >> Embryo/Fetal Risk

The human granulocyte colony-stimulating factor (G-CSF) filgrastim is a 175-amino acid glycoprotein produced by recombinant DNA technology. Filgrastim is indicated to decrease the incidence of infection, as manifested by febrile neutropenia, in patients with nonmyeloid malignancies receiving myelosuppressive chemotherapy associated with a significant incidence of severe neutropenia with fever. The agent is administered either SC or IV. The elimination half-life is approximately 3.5 hours (1).

Reproduction studies with filgrastim have been conducted in rats and rabbits. No effects on fertility were observed in male and female rats at doses up to 500 μg/kg. (*Note: The human dose is 5–10 μg/kg/day.*) In pregnant rats treated during organogenesis, IV injections up to 575 μg/kg/day were not associated with fetal death, teratogenicity, or behavioral effects. In offspring of pregnant rats treated with doses >20 μg/kg/day, a delay of external differentiation (detachment of auricles and descent of testes) and slight growth retardation were observed. These effects may have been a result of lower maternal body weight during rearing and nursing. At 100 μg/kg/day, newborn pups had decreased body weights and a slightly decreased 4-day survival rate. Treating pregnant rabbits during organogenesis with doses of 80 μg/kg/day resulted in increased resorptions and embryo lethality but not external defects. This dose, however, was maternally toxic (genitourinary bleeding and decreased body weight and food consumption) (1).

Filgrastim crosses the rat placenta late in gestation (2). In a rat study, filgrastim (50 μg/kg) was given twice daily for 2, 4, and 6 days before delivery. Filgrastim crossed the placenta within 30 minutes, reaching peak fetal serum levels 4 hours after the dose. Peak serum levels in the fetuses were 1000-fold lower than levels measured in the dams, but the agent still induced bone marrow and spleen myelopoiesis in the fetus and neonate (2). In a continuation of this study, the investigators demonstrated that the 6-day course of filgrastim administered before delivery significantly increased the survival of pups that were infected at birth with Group B β-hemolytic *Streptococcus* (3).

F

Although it has a very high molecular weight (18,800), filgrastim also crosses the human placenta, at least in the 2nd and 3rd trimesters. A single IV dose of filgrastim (25 μg/kg) was given to 11 women (1 set of twins) with an imminent delivery at $\leq$30 weeks' gestation (4). Ten infants were delivered within 30 hours of the dose (mean 10.8 $\pm$ 8.9 hours) ("early delivery"), and two infants were delivered at 54 and 108 hours ("late delivery"). Three of 10 cord blood samples in the "early delivery" group had G-CSF levels higher than those of 10 untreated controls, but there was no difference in cord blood neutrophil concentrations. Cord blood from the two infants in the "late delivery" group had G-CSF levels similar to those of controls but much higher neutrophil levels that remained elevated for 1 week. The investigators concluded that filgrastim crossed the placenta in amounts sufficient to produce a biologic effect in the fetus, and that this effect was most noticeable in cases where delivery was delayed at least 30 hours after a dose (4).

A 1998 study by the same investigators as above evaluated the effects of filgrastim therapy in women in preterm labor (5). Of the 26 women enrolled in the study, 16 (eight G-CSF subjects and eight controls) delivered within 3 weeks of the dose and were eligible for evaluation. G-CSF cases received a single 25 μg/kg dose administered as an IV infusion over 4 hours, whereas controls received an IV infusion without the drug. No adverse effects on pregnancy duration or maternal discomfort were noted. Neutrophil production was assessed by bone marrow aspiration in neonates 24 hours after delivery. The mean time between G-CSF or placebo administration and delivery was 3.9 and 6.3 days, respectively. Compared with controls, the neonates of case mothers had a significantly greater marrow proliferative pool and a significant improvement in Scores for Neonatal Acute Physiologic State (5).

A 27-year-old patient at 26 weeks' gestation was diagnosed with acute myeloid leukemia (6). Because she was otherwise well, she decided to hold chemotherapy to allow the fetus to mature. The woman became neutropenic and, at 27 weeks' gestation, developed fever secondary to a systemic infection. In addition to antibiotics, a 12-day course of filgrastim (dose not specified) was given to allow further time for fetal maturation. A cesarean section was performed at 32 weeks' gestation to deliver a healthy baby boy (weight and other details not provided). The infant was doing well at 5 months of age (6).

A brief 1996 report described the use of filgrastim in a pregnant woman with acute promyelocytic leukemia (7). In addition to other treatment, filgrastim (75 μg/day SC) was given for 7 days early in the 2nd trimester. She eventually delivered a healthy female infant at term (7).

A number of other studies have reported the use of filgrastim in human pregnancy (8–12). In four of them, the outcomes of 15 pregnancies were (period of exposure shown in parentheses): one normal infant (3rd trimester) (8); two normal infants (throughout), one bilateral hydronephrosis (throughout); one cyclic neutropenia (throughout;

mother also had the disorder); one normal infant (1st trimester); three elective abortions (EABs) (1st trimester; one fetus with "abnormal embryogenesis"); one cyclic neutropenia (3rd trimester; mother also had the disorder); and one infant with cardiac septal defects (3rd trimester) (9); one normal infant (2–3 weeks' gestation); one normal infant and one spontaneous abortion (SAB) (treatment before pregnancy) (10); and one normal infant (3rd trimester) (11).

Two reports from the Severe Chronic Neutropenia International Registry (SCNIR), one in 2002 (12) and the other in 2003 (13), discussed the outcomes of 23 pregnancies in women who were treated with filgrastim. Three women became pregnant during clinical trials and, although they were excluded from the study, continued to receive commercially available filgrastim (12). Two of the women with cyclic neutropenia had normal infants (one with cyclic neutropenia; one electively aborted her first pregnancy, then carried a second pregnancy to term). The third woman had idiopathic neutropenia and she had an EAB because of abnormal bleeding but subsequently died (12). The Registry also collected data on 20 pregnancies in women who had been exposed to filgrastim and 105 pregnancies in women who were not exposed to the agent (historical controls) (13). The outcomes of the exposed group, treated for an average of two trimesters (range one to three), were 13 normal infants, 3 SABs, and 4 EABs (non-medical). Among the 105 historical controls, there were 75 live births (includes two sets of twins and five infants with medical conditions, primarily respiratory), 24 SABs, and 8 EABs (12,13).

The SCNIR also reported the outcomes of nine pregnancies based on information submitted to the manufacturer (12). Of the nine cases, there were four normal infants, one SAB, and four infants with congenital renal and/or cardiac malformations (12).

In summary, neither the animal nor the human pregnancy data suggest a major risk for the human embryo or fetus from maternal filgrastim therapy. Although the human pregnancy experience is limited, no congenital malformations or other toxicities attributable to filgrastim have been observed. The cases submitted to the manufacturer suggest selective reporting (i.e., preferentially reporting of abnormal outcomes). Amounts sufficient to produce a biological effect in the fetus apparently cross the human placenta, at least in the 2nd and 3rd trimesters. Additional study is warranted, but filgrastim treatment should not be withheld because of pregnancy.

BREAST FEEDING SUMMARY

RECOMMENDATION: No Human Data - Probably Compatible

No reports describing the use of filgrastim during human lactation have been located. Filgrastim is a glycoprotein and, although it may be excreted into breast milk, it would probably be digested in a nursing infant's stomach. The risk to a nursing infant is unknown but appears to be low to nonexistent. Therefore, treatment with filgrastim should not be held because of breast-feeding.

References

1. Product information. Neupogen. Amgen, 2004.
2. Medlock ES, Kaplan DL, Cecchini M, Ulich TR, del Castillo J, Andresen J. Granulocyte colony-stimulating factor crosses the placenta and stimulates fetal rat granulopoiesis. Blood 1993;81:916–22.
3. Novales JS, Salva AM, Mondanlou HD, Kaplan DL, del Castillo J, Andresen J, Medlock ES. Maternal administration of granulocyte colony-stimulating factor improves neonatal rat survival after a lethal group B streptococcal infection. Blood 1993;81:923–7.
4. Calhoun DA, Ross C, Christensen RD. Transplacental passage of recombinant human granulocyte colony-stimulating factor in women with an imminent preterm delivery. Am J Obstet Gynecol 1996; 174:1306–11.
5. Calhoun DA, Christensen RD. A randomized pilot trial

of administration of granulocyte colony-stimulating factor to women before preterm delivery. Am J Obstet Gynecol 1998;179:766–71.
6. Cavenagh JD, Richardson DS, Cahill MR, Bernard T, Kelsey SM, Newland AC. Treatment of acute myeloid leukaemia in pregnancy. Lancet 1995;346:441–2.
7. Lin C-P, Huang M-J, Liu H-J, Chang IY, Tsai C-H. Successful treatment of acute promyelocytic leukemia in a pregnant Jehovah's Witness with all-trans retinoic acid, rhG-CSF, and erythropoietin. Am J Hematol 1996;51:251–2.
8. Arango HA, Kalter CS, Decesare SL, Fiorica JV, Lyman GH, Spellacy WN. Management of chemotherapy in a pregnancy complicated by a large neuroblastoma. Obstet Gynecol 1994;84:665–8.
9. Welte K, Boxer LA. Severe chronic neutropenia: pathophysiology and therapy. Semin Hematol 1997; 34:267–78.
10. Cavallaro AM, Lilleby K, Majolino I, Storb R, Appelbaum FR, Rowley SD, Bensinger WI. Three to six year follow-up of normal donors who received recombinant human granulocyte colony-stimulating factor. Bone Marrow Transplant 2000;25:85–9.
11. Sangalli MR, Peek M, McDonald A. Prophylactic granulocyte colony-stimulating factor treatment for acquired chronic severe neutropenia in pregnancy. Aust N Z J Obstet Gynaecol 2001;41:470–1.
12. Cottle TE, Fier CJ, Donadieu J, Kinsey SE. Risk and benefit of treatment of severe chronic neutropenia with granulocyte colony-stimulating factor. Semin Hematol 2002;39:134–40.
13. Dale DC, Cottle TE, Fier CJ, Bolyard AA, Bonilla MA, Boxer LA, Cham B, Freedman MH, Kannourakis G, Kinsey SE, Davis R, Scarlata D, Schwinzer B, Zeidler C, Welte K. Severe chronic neutropenia: treatment and follow-up of patients in the Severe Chronic Neutropenia International Registry. Am J Hematol 2003;72:82–93.

F

Name:	FLAVOXATE	Risk Factor:	B_M
Class:	Urinary Tract Agent (Antispasmodic)		

FETAL RISK SUMMARY

RECOMMENDATION: Limited Human Data - Animal Data Suggest Low Risk

Flavoxate is a tertiary amine that is a direct inhibitor of smooth muscle spasm of the urinary tract. The drug also possesses some antimuscarinic (i.e., atropine-like) activity. It is used for the symptomatic relief of urinary tract discomfort resulting from inflammatory conditions.

Reproduction studies in mice, rats, and rabbits at doses up to 34 times the human therapeutic dose found no evidence of impaired fertility or fetal harm (1–3). At doses approximately 40 times the therapeutic dose, cleft palate (not thought to be drug-induced) and fetal resorption occurred in mice, and intrauterine growth retardation was observed in fetal mice and rabbits (3).

No reports on the placental transfer of flavoxate have been located. The molecular weight (about 392 for the free base) is low enough, however, that passage to the fetus should be expected.

One presentation at a 1975 conference in Yugoslavia described the use of flavoxate during human pregnancy (4). Although specific obstetric data were not provided, IV flavoxate, often as a single dose in combination with antibiotics, was routinely used in pregnant women for the treatment of pyelonephritis. In addition, the effect of flavoxate on uterine contractions, using total IV doses ranging from 100 to 600 mg, was studied in 30 women at term and in 5 women with premature labor at 7–8 months. Uterine contractions were not modified in any of these patients and no fetal or newborn adverse effects were observed.

A 1984 source cited a 1972 study in which IM flavoxate, 100 mg 3 times daily followed by 400 mg/day by suppository, was used as a tocolytic in 66 women with premature labor (3). The 1984 source cited a second study that involved a reduction in the duration of labor in 120 women with a 100-mg IV dose of flavoxate (3). In neither of the cited studies were adverse effects noted in the mothers or fetuses.

In summary, the available human pregnancy data available for flavoxate are very limited and are completely lacking for 1st trimester exposure. Moreover, most of the treated women apparently received short-term therapy (i.e., no more than a few doses), and none involved the oral route with tablets, the only available form of the drug in the United States. The limitations also include a lack of information on the growth and development of the exposed infants. Although these uncertainties markedly limit the validity of any fetal safety assessment, the absence of reported toxicity in the fetus and newborn coupled with the lack of fetal toxicity in animals appear to indicate that the use of flavoxate during the second half of pregnancy presents a small, if any, risk to the fetus. The potential fetal effects of flavoxate exposure in the first half of pregnancy are unknown.

F

BREAST FEEDING SUMMARY

RECOMMENDATION: No Human Data - Probably Compatible

No reports describing the use of flavoxate during lactation have been located. The molecular weight of the drug (about 392 for the free base) is low enough, however, that excretion into milk should be expected. The effect of this exposure on a nursing infant is unknown.

References

1. Product information. Urispas. SmithKline Beecham Pharmaceuticals, 1998.
2. Schardein JL. *Chemically Induced Birth Defects*. 2nd ed. New York, NY: Marcel Dekker, 1993:447.
3. Onnis A, Grella P. *The Biochemical Effects of Drugs in Pregnancy*. Volume 1. West Sussex, England: Ellis Norwood Limited, 1984:221–2.
4. Esposito A. Preliminary studies on the use of flavoxate in obstetrics and gynaecology. International Round Table Discussion on Flavoxate, Opatija, Yugoslavia, March 30, 1975:66–73 (translation provided by BA Wallin, Smith Kline & French Laboratories, 1987).

Name: **FLECAINIDE** Risk Factor: **C_M**

Class: **Antiarrhythmic**

FETAL RISK SUMMARY

RECOMMENDATION: Limited Human Data - Animal Data Suggest Moderate Risk

Flecainide is an antiarrhythmic agent that is structurally related to encainide and procainamide. In one breed of rabbits, flecainide produced dose-related teratogenicity and embryotoxicity at approximately 4 times the usual human dose (1). Structural defects observed were club paws, sternebrae and vertebrae abnormalities, and pale hearts with contracted ventricular septum. Similar toxic effects and malformations were not observed in a second breed of rabbits, or in mice and rats, but dose-related delayed sternebral and vertebral ossification was observed in rat fetuses (1).

Two 1988 reports of human use of flecainide during pregnancy may have described a single incidence of exposure to the drug (2,3). Intravenous flecainide was given to a pregnant woman at 30 weeks' gestation for persistent fetal supraventricular tachycardia resistant to digoxin (2,3). The fetal heart rate pattern quickly converted to a sinus rhythm and the mother was maintained on oral flecainide, 100 mg 3 times daily, until delivery was induced at 38 weeks' gestation. The 3450-g female infant had no cardiac problems during the 10 days of observation. Flecainide concentrations in the cord blood and maternal serum at delivery 5 hours after the last dose were 533 and 833 ng/mL, respectively, a ratio of 0.63 (2).

Flecainide 100 mg twice daily, combined with the β-blocker sotalol, was used throughout gestation in one woman for the treatment of ventricular tachycardia and polymorphous ventricular premature complexes associated with an aneurysm of the left ventricle (4). A cesarean section was performed at approximately 37 weeks' gestation. Flecainide concentrations in umbilical cord and plasma samples at delivery, 11 hours after the last dose, were 0.394 and 0.455 μg/mL, respectively, a ratio of 0.86. No adverse effects, including bradycardia, were observed in the fetus or newborn, who was growing normally at 1 year of age.

A 22-year-old woman at approximately 31 weeks' gestation was treated with flecainide, 100 mg every 8 hours, for fetal arrhythmia associated with fetal hydrops unresponsive to therapeutic levels of digoxin (5). Therapeutic levels of flecainide were measured in the mother over the next 4 days, during which time the fetal heart rate (FHR) converted to a normal sinus rhythm of 120 beats/minute. Approximately 2 days later, a nonreactive nonstress test was documented and flecainide and digoxin were discontinued, but the FHR returned to pretreatment levels within 36 hours. Flecainide was restarted at 150 mg every 12 hours, and within 30 minutes of the first dose, the FHR converted to normal. This dose was continued for 4 days, during which time the FHR remained normal at 120 beats/minute, but with a nonreactive nonstress test. Gradual reduction of the dose to 50 mg every 12 hours maintained a normal FHR with return of a reactive nonstress test and normal beat-to-beat variability. Fetal ascites was completely resolved after 10 days of therapy. A normal 3480-g infant, Apgar scores of 9 and 10 at 1 and 5 minutes, respectively, was delivered vaginally at 41 weeks' gestation. Maternal and fetal serum trough levels at delivery were 0.2 and 0.1 μg/mL, respectively (5). A postnatal echocardiogram performed on the newborn was normal.

A 1991 report described the experimental use of flecainide, 300–400 mg/day orally, in 14 women at a mean gestational age of 31 weeks (range 23–36 weeks) to treat fetal hydrops and ascites secondary to supraventricular tachycardias or atrial flutter (6). The duration of treatment ranged from 2 days to 5 weeks. Although specific data were not given, the cord:maternal plasma ratio at birth was approximately 0.80, and all fetuses had flecainide concentrations within the usual therapeutic range (400–800 μg/L). Twelve of the 14 newborns were alive and well at the time of the report, and one infant, not under treatment at the time, died of sudden infant death syndrome at 4.5 months of age. One intrauterine death occurred after 3 days of therapy and may have been caused by either a flecainide-induced arrhythmia or fetal blood sampling (6).

A woman in the 3rd trimester was initially treated with flecainide 100 mg orally twice daily, then decreased to 50 mg twice daily, for fetal tachycardia that resolved within 4 days (7). The fetal ascites and polyhydramnios also resolved around this time. Approximately 6 weeks after treatment was begun, she gave birth to a 3320-g, male infant. The cord blood:maternal serum ratio of the drug was 0.97 (235.4/241.2 ng/mL), but the flecainide concentration in the amniotic fluid was 6426.5 ng/mL, about 27 times the level in the fetus.

Other publications have described the successful use of flecainide for the treatment of fetal tachycardia (8–14), and in one of these, flecainide and digoxin were considered the drugs of choice for this condition (8). However, flecainide is superior to digoxin for the treatment of tachycardia in hydropic fetuses (9,10).

The loss of fetal heart rate variability and accelerations was described in a case of supraventricular tachycardia treated with 300 mg/day of flecainide during the 3rd trimester (11). The heart rate of the 3690-g male infant returned to a reactive pattern 5 days after delivery. One day later, the infant's serum concentration of flecainide was below the detection level. A general review of drug therapy used for the treatment of fetal arrhythmias was published in 1994 (12). Flecainide has also been used to treat new onset maternal ventricular tachycardia presenting during the 3rd trimester (15).

Conjugated hyperbilirubinemia thought to be caused by flecainide was described in a 1995 reference (16). Flecainide, 150 mg twice daily, was started at about 28 weeks' gestation for the treatment of fetal supraventricular tachycardia after a trial of digoxin and adenosine had failed to halt the arrhythmia. Other fetal complications, in addition to the arrhythmia, were polyhydramnios, ascites, pericardial effusion, cardiomegaly, and tricuspid and mitral valve regurgitation. Successful conversion to a sinus rhythm occurred within 24 hours. The mother discontinued the therapy 1 week later, and a second course of flecainide was started when the fetal tachycardia and ascites reoccurred. The 2843-g, male infant, delivered vaginally at 36 weeks, developed transient conjugated hyperbilirubinemia within a few days of birth. The authors attributed the hyperbilirubinemia to flecainide because no other cause of the toxicity could be found and the drug is known to produce a similar condition in adults. Follow-up of the infant at 2 months of age revealed that the liver toxicity had resolved and at 28 months of age, the child was continuing to do well (16).

BREAST FEEDING SUMMARY

RECOMMENDATION: Limited Human Data - Probably Compatible

Flecainide is concentrated in breast milk (4,17), but no reports of infant exposure to the drug from nursing have been located. A woman was treated throughout gestation and in the postpartum period with flecainide, 100 mg twice daily, and sotalol (see Sotalol) (4). Simultaneous samples of milk and plasma were drawn 3 hours after the second daily dose on the 5th and 7th days postpartum. Flecainide concentrations on day 5 were 0.891 and 0.567 μg/mL, respectively, and 1.093 and 0.500 μg/mL, respectively, on day 7. Milk:plasma ratios were 1.57 and 2.18, respectively. The infant was not breast-fed (4).

Eleven healthy women volunteers who did not intend to breast-feed were given flecainide 100 mg orally every 12 hours for 5.5 days starting on postpartum day 1 (17). The breasts were emptied by a mechanical breast suction pump every 3–4 hours during the study. Peak milk levels of the drug occurred at 3–6 hours after a dose with a mean half-life of elimination of 14.7 hours. The highest daily average concentration of the drug ranged from 270 to 1529 ng/mL, with milk:plasma ratios on days 2, 3, 4, and 5 of 3.7, 3.2, 3.5, and 2.6, respectively. An estimated maximum steady state concentration of flecainide in an infant consuming approximately 700 mL of milk per day (assumed to be the total milk production) was 62 ng/mL, an apparently nontoxic level. Based on this, the investigators concluded that the risk of adverse effects in a nursing infant whose mother was consuming flecainide was minimal (17). The American Academy of Pediatrics classifies flecainide as compatible with breast-feeding (18).

References

1. Product information, Tambocor. 3M Pharmaceuticals, 1993.
2. Wren C, Hunter S. Maternal administration of flecainide to terminate and suppress fetal tachycardia. BMJ 1988;296:249.
3. Macphail S, Walkinshaw SA. Fetal supraventricular tachycardia: detection by routine auscultation and successful *in-utero* management: case report. Br J Obstet Gynaecol 1988;95:1073–6.
4. Wagner X, Jouglard J, Moulin M, Miller AM, Petitjean J, Pisapia A. Coadministration of flecainide acetate and sotalol during pregnancy: lack of teratogenic effects, passage across the placenta, and excretion in human breast milk. Am Heart J 1990;119:700–2.
5. Kofinas AD, Simon NV, Sagel H, Lyttle E, Smith N, King K. Treatment of fetal supraventricular tachycardia with flecainide acetate after digoxin failure. Am J Obstet Gynecol 1991;165:630–1.
6. Allan LD, Chita SK, Sharland GK, Maxwell D, Priestley K. Flecainide in the treatment of fetal tachycardias. Br Heart J 1991;65:46–8.
7. Bourget P, Pons J-C, Delouis C, Fermont L, Frydman R. Flecainide distribution, transplacental passage, and accumulation in the amniotic fluid during the third trimester of pregnancy. Ann Pharmacother 1994;28:1031–4.
8. van Engelen AD, Weijtens O, Brenner JI, Kleinman CS, Copel JA, Stoutenbeek P, Meijboom EJ. Management outcome and follow-up of fetal tachycardia. J Am Coll Cardiol 1994;24:1371–5.
9. Simpson JM, Sharland GK. Fetal tachycardias: management and outcome of 127 consecutive cases. Heart 1998;79:576–81.
10. Wren C. Mechanisms of fetal tachycardia. Heart 1998;79:536–7.
11. van Gelder-Hasker MR, de Jong CLD, de Vries JIP, van Geijn HP. The effect of flecainide acetate on fetal heart rate variability: a case report. Obstet Gynecol 1995;86:667–9.
12. Ito S, Magee L, Smallhorn J. Drug therapy for fetal arrhythmias. Clin Perinatol 1994;21:543–72.
13. Amano K, Harada Y, Shoda T, Nishijima M, Hiraishi S. Successful treatment of supraventricular tachycardia with flecainide acetate: a case report. Fetal Diagn Ther 1997;12:328–31.
14. Jaeggi E, Fouron JC, Drblik SP. Fetal atrial flutter: diagnosis, clinical features, treatment, and outcome. J Pediatr 1998;132:335–9.
15. Connaughton M, Jenkins BS. Successful use of flecainide to treat new onset maternal ventricular tachycardia in pregnancy. Br Heart J 1994;72:297.
16. Vanderhal AL, Cocjin J, Santulli TV, Carlson DE, Rosenthal P. Conjugated hyperbilirubinemia in a newborn infant after maternal (transplacental) treatment with flecainide acetate for fetal tachycardia and fetal hydrops. J Pediatr 1995;126:988–90.
17. McQuinn RL, Pisani A, Wafa S, Chang SF, Miller AM, Frappell JM, Chamberlain GVP, Camm AJ. Flecainide excretion in human breast milk. Clin Pharmacol Ther 1990;48:262–7.
18. Committee on Drugs, American Academy of Pediatrics. The transfer of drugs and other chemicals into human milk. Pediatrics 2001;108:776–89.

Name: **FLOSEQUINAN** Risk Factor: **C_M**

Class: **Vasodilator**

FETAL RISK SUMMARY

RECOMMENDATION: No Human Data - No Relevant Animal Data

Flosequinan is a systemic vasodilator used in the treatment of congestive heart failure. In rats and rabbits, the drug crosses the placenta to the fetus and has been measured in amniotic fluid (1). Fetotoxicity, including delayed calcification, intrauterine deaths, and low fetal viability have been observed in the two animal species. No reports describing the use of this agent in human pregnancy have been located.

BREAST FEEDING SUMMARY

RECOMMENDATION: No Human Data - Probably Compatible

No data are available.

Reference

1. Product information. Manoplax. Boots Pharmaceuticals, Inc., 1993.

Name:	**FLUCONAZOLE**	Risk Factor:	C_M
Class:	**Antifungal**		

F

FETAL RISK SUMMARY

RECOMMENDATION: Human Data Suggest Risk (≥400 mg/day)

Fluconazole is a synthetic triazole antifungal agent. In studies with pregnant rabbits, abortions were noted at a dose 20–60 times the recommended human dose (RHD) but no fetal anomalies (1). In pregnant rats, doses below 20–60 times the RHD produced increases in fetal anatomical variants (supernumerary ribs, renal pelvis dilation, and delays in ossification). At doses of 20–60 times the RHD and higher, embryo deaths were observed as well as structural abnormalities consisting of wavy ribs, cleft palate, and abnormal craniofacial ossification (1). These effects were thought to be consistent with inhibition of estrogen synthesis (1).

One hypothesis for the teratogenic effects of phenytoin involves the production of toxic intermediates, such as an epoxide (arene oxide) (2). Because fluconazole inhibits the cytochrome P450 pathway responsible for phenytoin metabolism, authors of a 1999 study reasoned that the drug combination could provide a test of the hypothesis. The theory was not supported, however, when pretreatment with a nonembryotoxic fluconazole dose doubled (from 6.2% to 13.3%) the incidence of phenytoin-induced cleft palate in mice. Administering both drugs closely together significantly increased the incidence of resorptions ($p < 0.05$) but not malformations. This lack of effect on malformations may have been related to the increased embryo lethality of the combination (2). The mechanism for the teratological interaction between the drugs was unknown.

It is not known if fluconazole crosses the human placenta. The molecular weight (about 306) is low enough, however, that passage to the fetus should be expected.

A case published in 1992 described the pregnancy outcome in a 22-year-old black woman who was treated before and throughout gestation with fluconazole, 400 mg/day orally, for disseminated coccidioidomycosis (3). Premature rupture of the membranes occurred at 27 weeks' gestation; 1 week later, a cesarean section was performed because of chorioamnionitis. A 1145-g female infant with grossly dysmorphic features and with Apgar scores of 0 and 6 at 1 and 5 minutes, respectively, was delivered. The infant died shortly after birth. Anatomic abnormalities included cranioschisis of the frontal bones; craniostenosis of the sagittal suture; hypoplasia of the nasal bones; cleft palate; humeral-radial fusion; bowed tibia and femur; bilateral femoral fractures; contractures of both upper and lower extremities; an incompletely formed right thumb; medial deviation of both feet with a short left first toe; and short right first, fourth, and fifth toes (3). No evidence of coccidioidomycosis was found on microscopic examination.

A 1996 publication described three infants (one of whom is described above) with congenital malformations who had been exposed to fluconazole *in utero* during the 1st trimester or beyond (4). One woman with *Coccidioides immitis* meningitis took 800 mg/day of fluconazole through the first 7 weeks of pregnancy, then resumed therapy during the 9th week of gestation and continued until delivery by cesarean section at 38 weeks' gestation. The male infant was small for gestational age (1878 g), cyanotic, and had poor tone. He suffered a femur fracture when his limbs were straightened for measurement shortly after birth. Multiple malformations were observed involving the *head and face:* brachycephaly, maxillary hypoplasia, small ear helices, exotropia, craniofacial disproportion, large anterior fontanelle, trigonocephaly, supraorbital ridge hypoplasia, and micrognathia; *the skeleton:* femoral bowing, femoral fracture, thin clavicles, ribs, and long bones, and diffuse osteopenia; and *the heart:* tetralogy of Fallot, pulmonary artery hypoplasia, patent foramen ovale, and patent ductus arteriosus.

The pregnancy outcome of a woman (her second pregnancy), first described by Lee et al. in 1992 (3), was also reviewed in the above 1996 reference. In her next pregnancy (her third), she delivered a healthy male infant (4). Although she had been told to take fluconazole 400 mg/day, nontherapeutic serum levels documented that the patient was not compliant with these instructions. After this, the woman conceived a fourth time, and therapeutic serum fluconazole concentrations were documented while she was taking 400 mg/day. Therapy was discontinued when her pregnancy was diagnosed at 4 months' gestation. The full-term female infant (weight not specified) had multiple malformations involving the *head and face:* cleft palate, low-set ears, tracheomalacia, rudimentary epiglottis, and proptosis; *the skeleton:* femoral bowing, clavicular fracture, thin wavy ribs, absent distal phalanx (toe), and arachnodactyly; and *the heart:* ventricular septal defect and pulmonary artery hypoplasia. The infant died at age 3 months from complications related to her tracheomalacia.

The anomalies noted in the 1992 case report were at first thought to be consistent with an autosomal recessive genetic disorder known as the Antley-Bixler syndrome (3). However, because of the second case in the same mother and the third infant, the defects were now thought to represent the teratogenic effect of fluconazole (4). Moreover, several of the defects observed were similar to those described in fetal rats exposed to fluconazole.

In January 1996, the FDA received a report of congenital defects in an infant exposed to 800 mg/day of fluconazole during the 1st trimester (F. Rosa, personal communication, FDA, 1996). Similar to the case described by Lee et al. (3), the infant had craniostenosis of the sagittal suture and a rare bilateral humeral-radial fusion anomaly. Other malformations were rocker-bottom feet and orbital hypoplasia. Additional individual adverse reports involving fluconazole received by the FDA included three cases of cleft palate, one case each of miscarriage with severe shortening of all limbs and of syndactyly, both after a single 150-mg dose in the 1st trimester, and single cases of hydrocephalus, omphalocele, and deafness.

A 1997 case report described a 27-year-old woman with chronic *C. immitis* meningitis who was treated with fluconazole (400 mg/day through the fourth or fifth week, then 800 mg/day) during the first 9 weeks of an unknown pregnancy (5). Fluconazole was stopped when the pregnancy was diagnosed and amphotericin B therapy was initiated. At 22 weeks' gestation, amphotericin B was discontinued and fluconazole was restarted at 1200 mg/day. Spontaneous rupture of the membranes occurred at 31 weeks' gestation and a 1300-g male infant was delivered by cesarean section. Craniofacial anomalies noted in the newborn included a soft calvaria, widely separated sutures, prominent forehead, mild exorbitism, a large, pear-shaped nose, and small ears with overfolded helices (5). Other malformations included immobile elbows, hypoplastic nails, subluxed hips, rocker-bottom feet, and bilateral radiohumeral synostosis. Because of the similarity to the other reported cases, the authors concluded that fluconazole produces a Antley-Bixler-like syndrome (5). [*Note: The malformations observed in this infant are very similar to those described by Rosa above, and may be the same case.*]

In contrast to the above adverse outcomes, a retrospective review of 289 pregnancies was reported in which the mothers received either a single 150-mg dose ($N = 275$), multiple 50-mg doses ($N = 3$), or multiple 150-mg doses ($N = 11$) of fluconazole (6). All of the women were treated during (gestational age of exposure not specified) or shortly before pregnancy for vaginal candidiasis, even though the authors noted that fluconazole was contraindicated for the treatment of this condition in pregnancy. The outcomes of the 289 pregnancies included 178 infants (5 sets of twins), 39 (13.5%) spontaneous abortions, 38 elective abortions, 2 ectopic pregnancies, and 37 unknown outcomes. Four infants with anomalies were observed, but in each case the mother had taken fluconazole before conception (1 week to >26 weeks before the last monthly menstrual period).

A prospective study published in 1996 compared the pregnancy outcomes of 226 women exposed to fluconazole during the 1st trimester with 452 women exposed to nonteratogenic agents (7). The dosage taken by the exposed group consisted of a single, 150 mg dose ($N=105$, 47%), multiple doses of 150 mg ($N=81$, 36%), a 50 mg single dose ($N=3$, 1%), 50 mg multiple doses ($N=23$, 10%), a 100 mg single dose ($N=5$, 2%), or 100 mg multiple doses ($N=9$, 4%). Most women (90.7%) were treated for vaginal candidiasis. There were no differences between the two groups in the number of miscarriages, stillbirths, congenital malformations, prematurity, low birth weight, cesarean section, or prolonged hospital stay. Seven (4.0% of live births) of the exposed women delivered infants with anomalies compared to 17 (4.2% of live births) of controls. There was no pattern among the congenital anomalies in the exposed group except for two cases of trisomy 21.

A brief 1996 case report described a normal pregnancy outcome in a 24-year-old woman treated with 21 days of fluconazole (600 mg/day) (because of intolerance to amphotericin B) for *Torulopsis glabrata* fungemia beginning at 14 weeks' gestation (8). Although the patient's course was complicated by shock and intracerebral hemorrhage, she eventually delivered at term a healthy 2.95-kg infant (sex not specified) who was doing well at 18 months of age.

In another 1996 case report, a 24-year-old woman at about 19 weeks' gestation had chorioretinitis, candidiasis, fever, pneumonia, and low body weight attributed to *Candida albicans* sepsis (9). Because of massive nausea and vomiting after a test dose of amphotericin B, she was treated with IV fluconazole (10 mg/kg/day or about 400 mg/day) for 16 days and then the same dosage orally for another 34 days. She responded well to the antifungal therapy and gave birth at 39 weeks' to a healthy 2834-kg female infant with Apgar scores of 8 and 9 at 1 and 5 minutes, respectively. The infant had normal growth and mental development at 2 years of age (9).

A regional drug information center reported the pregnancy outcomes of 16 women (17 outcomes, 1 set of twins) who had called to inquire about the effect of fluconazole on their pregnancies (10). The median fluconazole dose was 300 mg (range 150–1000 mg) starting at 4 $\pm$ 6 weeks' gestation (range 1–26 weeks). The twins were stillborn (no malformations) but the other 15 newborns were normal.

A 1998 non-interventional observational cohort study described the outcomes of pregnancies in women who had been prescribed one or more of 34 newly marketed drugs by general practitioners in England (11). Data were obtained by questionnaires sent to the prescribing physicians one month after the expected or possible date of delivery. In 831 (78%) of the pregnancies, a newly marketed drug was thought to had been taken during the 1st trimester with birth defects noted in 14 (2.5%) singleton births of the 557 newborns (10 sets of twins). In addition, two birth defects were observed in aborted fetuses. However, few of the aborted fetuses were examined. Fluconazole was taken during the 1st trimester in 48 pregnancies, but the dose and duration of therapy were not specified. The outcomes of these pregnancies included 4 spontaneous abortions, 5 elective abortions, 4 pregnancies lost to follow-up, and 37 normal newborns (3 premature; 2 sets of full-term twins) (11). Although no congenital malformations were observed, the study lacked the sensitivity to identify minor anomalies because of the absence of standardized examinations. Late-appearing major defects may also have been missed because of the timing of the questionnaires.

A short 1998 report described the pregnancy outcome of a 38-year-old woman who had been treated with a single 150-mg oral dose of fluconazole about the date of conception (12). Chorionic villus sampling was conducted at 12 weeks' gestation finding a normal karyotype (46,XY). The male infant, delivered by cesarean section at 39 weeks, had an encephalocele. Echocardiography revealed dextrocardia and that both the pulmonary artery and the aorta emerged from the right ventricle (12). He died at 7 days of age. The cause of the anomalies was unknown, but it could not have been secondary to fluconazole because of the timing of the exposure.

A 42-year-old woman with achalasia at 31 weeks' gestation was diagnosed with *Candida* esophagitis (13). IV fluconazole, 150 mg/day, was given for 14 days with resolution of the vomiting and lessening of her nausea. She was treated before and after fluconazole with parenteral hyperalimentation. An apparently healthy 2438-kg female infant, Apgar scores of 9 and 9 at 1 and 5 minutes, respectively, was delivered at 38 weeks' gestation.

In a 1999 report, fluconazole exposures and pregnancy outcomes were examined using the Danish Jutland Pharmaco-Epidemiological Prescription Database (14). A total of 165 women who had received a single, oral 150-mg dose of fluconazole for vaginal candidiasis just before or during pregnancy from 1991 to 1996 were identified. Of these, 121 had been exposed during the 1st trimester. The outcomes of exposed women were compared to the outcomes of 13,327 women who had not received any prescription medication during their pregnancies (controls). In the comparison of exposed newborns to controls, no elevated risk for preterm delivery (odds ratio [OR] 1.17, 95% confidence interval [CI] 0.63–2.17) or low birth weight (OR 1.19, 95% CI 0.37–3.79) was discovered. Similarly, the prevalence of congenital malformations was 3.3% (4 of 121) in exposed compared to 5.2% (697 of 13,327) in controls (OR 0.65, 95% CI 0.24–1.77) (14).

In summary, although the data are very limited, the use of fluconazole during the 1st trimester appears to be teratogenic with continuous daily doses of 400 mg/day or more. The malformations may be resemble those observed in the Antley-Bixler syndrome. The published experience with the use of smaller doses, such as those prescribed for vaginal fungal infections, suggests that the risk for adverse outcomes is low, if it exists at all. A 1998 review concurred with this assessment (15). In those instances in which continuous, high-dose fluconazole is the only therapeutic choice during the 1st trimester, the patient should be informed of the potential risk to her fetus.

BREAST FEEDING SUMMARY

RECOMMENDATION: Compatible

Fluconazole is excreted into human milk (16,17). A 42-year-old lactating 54.5-kg woman was taking fluconazole 200 mg once daily (16). On her 18th day of therapy (8 days postpartum), milk samples were obtained at 0.5 hour before a dose and at 2, 4, and 10 hours after a dose. Serum samples were drawn 0.5 hour before the dose and 4 hours after the dose. On her last day of therapy (20 days postpartum), milk samples were again collected at 12, 24, 36, and 48 hours after the dose. Peak milk concentrations of fluconazole, up to 4.1 μg/mL, were measured 2 hours after the mother's dose. The milk:plasma ratios at

0.5 hour before dose and 4 hours after dose were both 0.90. The elimination half-lives in the milk and serum were 26.9 hours and 18.6 hours, respectively. No mention was made of the nursing infant.

A 29-year-old woman who was nursing her 12-week-old infant developed a vaginal fungal infection (17). Breast-feeding was halted at the patient's request and she was given 150 mg of fluconazole orally. Fluconazole concentrations were determined in milk (pooled from both breasts) and plasma samples obtained at 2, 5, 24, and 48 hours after the dose. Milk concentrations were 2.93, 2.66, 1.76, and 0.98 μg/mL, respectively, while plasma concentrations were 6.42, 2.79, 2.52, and 1.19 μg/mL, respectively. The milk:plasma ratios were 0.46, 0.85, 0.85, and 0.83, respectively, with half-lives of 30 and 35 hours, respectively, in the milk and plasma. The author estimated that after three plasma half-lives, 87.5% of the dose would have been eliminated from a woman with normal renal function, thereby greatly reducing the amount of drug a nursing infant would ingest (17).

Although the risk to a nursing infant from exposure to fluconazole in breast milk is unknown, the safe use of this antifungal agent in neonates has been reported (18–20). A brief 1989 report described a 48-day-old infant, born at 36 weeks' gestation, who was treated with IV fluconazole, 6 mg/kg/day, for disseminated *Candida albicans* (18). The dosage was reduced to 3 mg/kg/day when a slight, transient increase in serum transaminase values was measured. The infant was discharged home at 80 days of age in good condition. In the second case, IV fluconazole 6 mg/kg/day was administered for 20 days to an approximately 6-week-old, premature infant (born at 28 weeks' gestation) with a disseminated *Candida albicans* infection (19). Results of follow-up studies of the infant during the next 4 months were apparently normal. In a similar case, a 1-month-old premature infant was treated with IV fluconazole (5 mg/kg for 1 hour daily) for 21 days and orally for 8 days for meningitis caused by a *Candida* species (20). He was doing well at 9 months of age.

The safety of fluconazole during breast-feeding cannot be completely extrapolated from these cases, but the dose administered to these infants far exceeds the amount they would have received via breast milk. Because no drug-induced toxicity was encountered in the infants, fluconazole is probably safe to use during breast-feeding. The American Academy of Pediatrics classifies fluconazole as compatible with breast-feeding (21).

References

1. Product information. Diflucan. Pfizer, 2001.
2. Tiboni GM, Iammarrone E, Giampietro F, Lamonaca D, Bellati U, Di Ilio C. Teratological interaction between the bis-triazole antifungal agent fluconazole and the anticonvulsant drug phenytoin. Teratology 1999; 59:81–7.
3. Lee BE, Feinberg M, Abraham JJ, Murthy AR. Congenital malformations in an infant born to a woman treated with fluconazole. Pediatr Infect Dis J 1992; 11:1062–4.
4. Pursley TJ, Blomquist IK, Abraham J, Andersen HF, Bartley JA. Fluconazole-induced congenital anomalies in three infants. Clin Infect Dis 1996;22:336–40.
5. Aleck KA, Bartley DL. Multiple malformation syndrome following fluconazole use in pregnancy: report of an additional patient. Am J Med Genet 1997; 72:253–6.
6. Inman W, Pearce G, Wilton L. Safety of fluconazole in the treatment of vaginal candidiasis. A prescription-event monitoring study, with special reference to the outcome of pregnancy. Eur J Clin Pharmacol 1994;46:115–8.
7. Mastroiacovo P, Mazzone T, Botto LD, Serafini MA, Finardi A, Caramelli L, Fusco D. Prospective assessment of pregnancy outcomes after first-trimester exposure to fluconazole. Am J Obstet Gynecol 1996;175: 1645–50.
8. Kremery V Jr, Huttova M, Masar O. Teratogenicity of fluconazole. Pediatr Infect Dis 1996;15:841.
9. Wiesinger EC, Mayerhofer S, Wenisch C, Breyer S, Graninger W. Fluconazole in *Candida albicans* sepsis during pregnancy: case report and review of the literature. Infection 1996;24:263–6.
10. Campomori A, Bonati M. Fluconazole treatment for vulvovaginal candidiasis during pregnancy. Ann Pharmacother 1997;118–9.
11. Wilton LV, Pearce GL, Martin RM, Mackay FJ, Mann RD. The outcomes of pregnancy in women exposed to newly marketed drugs in general practice in England. Br J Obstet Gynaecol 1998;105:882–9.

12. Sanchez JM, Moya G. Fluconazole teratogenicity. Prenat Diagn 1998;18:862–3.
13. Kalish RB, Garry D, Figueroa R. Achalasia with Candida esophagitis during pregnancy. Obstet Gynecol 1999;94:850.
14. Sorensen HT, Nielsen GL, Olesen C, Larsen H, Steffensen FH, Schonheyder HC, Olsen J, Czeizel AE. Risk of malformations and other outcomes in children exposed to fluconazole *in utero*. Br J Clin Pharmacol 1999;48:234–8.
15. King CT, Rogers PD, Cleary JD, Chapman SW. Antifungal therapy during pregnancy. Clin Infect Dis 1998;27:1151–60.
16. Schilling CG, Seay RE, Larson TA, Meier KR. Excretion of fluconazole in human breast milk (abstract no. 130). Pharmacotherapy 1993;13:287.
17. Force RW. Fluconazole concentrations in breast milk. Pediatr Infect Dis J 1995;14:235–6.
18. Viscoli C, Castagnola E, Corsini M, Gastaldi R, Soliani M, Terragna A. Fluconazole therapy in an underweight infant. Eur J Clin Microbiol Infect Dis 1989;8:925–6.
19. Wiest DB, Fowler SL, Garner SS, Simons DR. Fluconazole in neonatal disseminated candidiasis. Arch Dis Child 1991;66:1002.
20. Gurses N, Kalayci AG. Fluconazole monotherapy for Candidal meningitis in a premature infant. Clin Infect Dis 1996;23:645–6.
21. Committee on Drugs, American Academy of Pediatrics. The transfer of drugs and other chemical into human milk. Pediatrics 2001;108:776–89.

Name: **FLUCYTOSINE** Risk Factor: **C_M**
Class: **Antifungal**

FETAL RISK SUMMARY

RECOMMENDATION: Contraindicated - 1st Trimester

The antifungal agent, flucytosine, was teratogenic in rats at doses 0.27 to 4.7 times the maximum recommended human dose (MRHD), producing vertebral fusions, cleft lip and palate, and micrognathia (1). In mice, a dose 2.7 times the MRHD was associated with a low, nonsignificant, incidence of cleft palate. Flucytosine was not teratogenic in rabbits at 0.68 times the MRHD (1).

Following oral administration, about 4% of the drug is metabolized within the fungal organisms to 5-fluorouracil, an antineoplastic agent (1, 2). Fluorouracil is suspected of producing congenital defects in humans (see Fluorouracil).

Three case reports of pregnant patients treated in the 2nd and 3rd trimesters with flucytosine have been located (3–5). No defects were observed in the newborns.

BREAST FEEDING SUMMARY

RECOMMENDATION: No Human Data - Potential Toxicity

No reports describing the use of flucytosine during lactation have been located. Because of the potential for serious adverse effects in a nursing infant, breast-feeding is not recommended when taking flucytosine.

References

1. Product information. Ancobon. ICN Pharmaceuticals, 2000.
2. Diasio RB, Lakings DE, Bennett JE. Evidence for conversion of 5-fluorocytosine to 5-fluorouracil in humans: possible factor in 5-fluorocytosine clinical toxicity. Antimicrob Agents Chemother 1978;14:903–8.
3. Philpot CR, Lo D. Cryptococcal meningitis in pregnancy. Med J Aust 1972;2:1005–7.
4. Schonebeck J, Segerbrand E. *Candida albicans* septicaemia during first half of pregnancy successfully treated with 5-fluorocytosine. Br Med J 1973;4:337–8.
5. Curole DN. Cryptococcal meningitis in pregnancy. J Reprod Med 1981;26:317–9.

Name:	**FLUMAZENIL**	Risk Factor:	C_M
Class:	**Antidote**		

F

FETAL RISK SUMMARY

RECOMMENDATION: Compatible - Maternal Benefit >> Embryo/Fetal Risk

Flumazenil, a benzodiazepine receptor antagonist, rapidly inhibits the actions of benzodiazepines on the central nervous system. It is indicated for the complete or partial reversal of the sedative effects of benzodiazepines following therapeutic use or for the management of benzodiazepine overdose. Although it has weak partial agonist activity in some animals, flumazenil has little or no agonist action in humans. After IV administration, flumazenil has a mean terminal half-life of 54 minutes (range 41–79 minutes). Approximately 50% of the agent is protein bound in the plasma and the metabolites are inactive (1).

Reproduction studies have been conducted in rats and rabbits. No evidence of impaired fertility was observed in male and female rats at oral doses up to 120 times the human exposure based on AUC obtained with the maximum recommended IV dose of 5 mg (HEMRD). In rats and rabbits, no teratogenicity was observed when flumazenil was given during organogenesis at oral doses up to 120–600 times the HEMRD. However, embryocidal effects (increased pre- and post-implantation losses) were noted in rabbits at 200 times the HEMRD. The no-effect dose was 60 times the HEMRD. In rats, oral doses 120 times the HEMRD during lactation resulted in decreased pup survival and increased pup liver weight at weaning. Other adverse effects noted were delayed incisor eruption and ear opening. The no-effect level was 24 times the HEMRD (1).

It is not known if flumazenil crosses the human placenta to the embryo/fetus. The molecular weight (about 303) and moderate plasma protein binding suggest that transfer may occur, but the very short elimination half-life will mitigate this transfer.

A 1993 case report described the use of flumazenil in a 22-year-old woman at 36 weeks' gestation (2). The woman was somnolent but was able to respond appropriately to questions. She had taken 50–60 5-mg tablets of diazepam. After initial emergency treatment, serum levels approximately 7 hours after ingestion of diazepam and two metabolites (oxazepam and N-desmethyldiazepam) were 1.9, 0.8, and 0.9 μmol/L, respectively. The fetal heart rate was 130–160 beats/minute with decreased variability, absence of accelerations, and occasional decelerations. Flumazenil, 0.3 mg IV, was given to distinguish between fetal asphyxia and an influence of benzodiazepines. Shortly afterwards, the patient awakened and the fetal heart rate was noted to have accelerations and increased variability. Approximately 24 hours later, the maternal and fetal symptoms recurred and a second 0.3 mg dose of IV flumazenil was given. Both the mother and the fetus responded as before and no further doses were required. Two weeks later, she delivered a 3620-g (head circumference 33 cm) healthy, male infant with Apgar scores of 7, 10, and 10 at 1, 5, and 10 minutes, respectively. No adverse effects of the overdose were observed in the infant who was discharged home with his mother at 5 days of age (2).

No reports describing the use of flumazenil during the 1st trimester in humans have been located. Two cases, however, have reported use of the agent in the 3rd trimester. In addition to the above case, a second case report (3) was cited in a 2003 review (4). Although an assessment of the teratogenic risk in humans cannot be made, the animal data suggest the risk is low. Moreover, the indication for flumazenil is such that the maternal benefit should far outweigh the unknown embryo/fetal risk. Therefore, if indicated, flumazenil should not be withheld during pregnancy (5).

BREAST FEEDING SUMMARY

RECOMMENDATION: No Human Data - Probably Compatible

No reports describing the use of flumazenil during human lactation have been located. The molecular weight (about 303) and moderate plasma protein binding suggest that transfer into breast milk may occur, but the very short elimination half-life (mean 54 minutes) will mitigate this transfer. IV flumazenil has been given directly to neonates to reverse the sedative effects of diazepam administered to the mother immediately before delivery (6,7). If indicated, flumazenil should not be withheld during lactation. However, because of the potential for adverse effects in a nursing infant that may be similar to those observed in treated adults (such as fatigue, nausea/vomiting, agitation, and cutaneous vasodilation), holding breast-feeding for a few hours after the last dose to allow drug elimination from the mother should be considered.

References

1. Product information. Romazicon. Roche Pharmaceuticals, 2004.
2. Stahl MMS, Saldeen P, Vinge E. Reversal of fetal benzodiazepine intoxication using flumazenil. Br J Obstet Gynaecol 1993;100:185–8.
3. Shibata T, Kubota N, Yokoyama H. A pregnant woman with convulsion treated with diazepam, which was reversed with flumazenil just prior to cesarean section. [Japanese]. Masui 1994;43:572–4. As cited by Bailey B. Are there teratogenic risks associated with antidotes used in the acute management of poisoned pregnant women? Birth Defects Res Part A Clin Mol Teratol 2003;67:133–40.
4. Bailey B. Are there teratogenic risks associated with antidotes used in the acute management of poisoned pregnant women? Birth Defects Res Part A Clin Mol Teratol 2003;67:133–40.
5. Weinbroum AA, Flaishon R, Sorkine P, Szold O, Rudick V. A risk-benefit assessment of flumazenil in the management of benzodiazepine overdose. Drug Saf 1997;17:181–96.
6. Richard P, Autret E, Bardol J, Soyez C, Barbier P, Jonville AP, Ramponi N. The use of flumazenil in a neonate. J Toxicol Clin Toxicol 1991;29:137–40.
7. Dixon JC, Speidel BD, Dixon JJ. Neonatal flumazenil therapy reverses maternal diazepam. Acta Paediatr 1998;87:225–6.

Name:	FLUNITRAZEPAM	Risk Factor:	D
Class:	Hypnotic		

FETAL RISK SUMMARY

RECOMMENDATION: Human Data Suggest Risk

Flunitrazepam is a benzodiazepine (see also Diazepam). No reports linking the use of flunitrazepam with congenital defects have been located, but other drugs in this group have been suspected of causing fetal malformations (see also Diazepam or Chlordiazepoxide). In contrast to other benzodiazepines, flunitrazepam crosses the placenta slowly (1,2). About 12 hours after a 1-mg oral dose, cord:maternal blood ratios in early and late pregnancy were about 0.5 and 0.22, respectively. Amniotic fluid:maternal serum ratios were in the 0.02–0.07 range in both cases. Accumulation in the fetus may occur after repeated doses (1).

BREAST FEEDING SUMMARY

RECOMMENDATION: Limited Human Data - Potential Toxicity

Flunitrazepam is excreted into breast milk. Following a single 2-mg oral dose in five patients, mean milk:plasma ratios at 11, 15, 27, and 39 hours were 0.61, 0.68, 0.9, and 0.75, respectively (1,2). The effects of these levels on the nursing infant are unknown.

References

1. Kanto J, Aaltonen L, Kangas L, Erkkola R, Pitkanen Y. Placental transfer and breast milk levels of flunitrazepam. Curr Ther Res 1979;26:539–45.
2. Kanto JH. Use of benzodiazepines during pregnancy, labour and lactation, with special reference to pharmacokinetic considerations. Drugs 1982;23:354–80.

F

Name:	**FLUORESCEIN SODIUM**	Risk Factor:	**B**
Class:	**Diagnostic Agent**		

FETAL RISK SUMMARY

RECOMMENDATION: No Human Data - Animal Data Suggest Low Risk

The diagnostic agent, fluorescein sodium (Dye and Coloring Yellow No. 8), is available as a topical solution, dye-impregnated paper strips, and as a solution for IV injection.

No adverse fetal effects were observed in the offspring of pregnant albino rats administered IV sodium fluorescein (10%) at a dose of 5 mL/kg (1). The agent crossed the placenta and distributed throughout the fetuses within 15 minutes. Using phenobarbital in mature rats exposed *in utero* to multiple maternal IV doses of 10% sodium fluorescein, the investigators determined that *in utero* exposure to the dye had no effect on their drug detoxification systems later in life (1). No adverse effects on fetal development were observed when pregnant rats and rabbits were treated by gavage with multiple high doses (up to 1500 mg/kg in rats and up to 250 mg/kg in rabbits) of sodium fluorescein during organogenesis (2). Similarly, no adverse fetal outcomes occurred when pregnant rabbits were administered multiple 1.4-mL IV doses of 10% sodium fluorescein during the first two-thirds of gestation (3).

No reports describing the use of fluorescein sodium during human pregnancy have been located. Use of the topical solution in the eye (as well as IV injection) produces measurable concentrations of the dye in the systemic circulation (see reference #6) and passage to the fetus should be expected.

BREAST FEEDING SUMMARY

RECOMMENDATION: Limited Human Data - Potential Toxicity (IV)
No Human Data - Probably Compatible (Topical)

Fluorescein sodium is excreted into breast milk (4,6). A 29-year-old woman, who suffered acute central vision loss shortly after prematurely delivery of twins, was administered a 5-mL IV dose of 10% fluorescein sodium for diagnostic angiography (4). Her hospitalized infants were not fed her milk because of concern that the fluorescein in the milk could cause a phototoxic reaction if consumed (a severe bullous skin eruption was observed in a premature infant receiving phototherapy for hyperbilirubinemia shortly after administration of IV fluorescein angiography [5]). Milk concentrations of the dye were measured in seven samples collected between 6 and 76 hours after fluorescein administration. The highest and lowest concentrations, 372 ng/mL and 170 ng/mL, were measured at 6 and 76 hours, respectively. The elimination half-life of fluorescein in the woman's milk was approximately 62 hours (4).

In a second case, a 28-year-old woman, 3 months postpartum, was administered a topical 2% solution in both eyes (6). Her infant was not allowed to breast-feed on the day of instillation. Absorption into the systemic circulation was documented with plasma fluorescein concentrations of 36 and 40 ng/mL at 45 and 75 minutes, respectively, after the dose. Milk concentrations at 30, 60, and 90 minutes were 20, 22, and 15 ng/mL, respectively. Because of these data, the authors recommended that mothers should not breast-feed for 8–12 hours after fluorescein topical administration.

The two mothers in the above cases either did not breast-feed or temporarily withheld nursing to allow the dye to clear from their milk because of concerns for a fluorescein-induced phototoxic reaction in their infants. Although the American Academy of Pediatrics classifies fluorescein as compatible with breast-feeding (7), the much higher milk concentrations obtained following IV fluorescein indicate that a risk may exist, especially in those infants undergoing phototherapy, and feeding should be temporarily withheld (8).

References

1. Salem H, Loux JJ, Smith S, Nichols CW. Evaluation of the toxicologic and teratogenic potentials of sodium fluorescein in the rat. Toxicology 1979;12:143 50.
2. Burnett CM, Goldenthal EI. The teratogenic potential in rats and rabbits of D and C Yellow no. 8. Food Chem Toxicol 1986;24:819–23.
3. McEnerney JK, Wong WP, Peyman GA. Evaluation of the teratogenicity of fluorescein sodium. Am J Ophthalmol 1977;84:847–50.
4. Maguire AM, Bennett J. Fluorescein elimination in human breast milk. Arch Ophthalmol 1986;106:718–9.
5. Kearns GL, Williams BJ, Timmons OD. Fluorescein phototoxicity in a premature infant. J Pediatr 1985;107:796–8.
6. Mattern J, Mayer PR. Excretion of fluorescein into breast milk. Am J Ophthalmol 1990;109:598–9.
7. Committee on Drugs, American Academy of Pediatrics. The transfer of drugs and other chemicals into human milk. Pediatrics 2001;108:776–89.
8. Anderson PO. Medication use while breast feeding a neonate. Neonatal Pharmacol Q 1993;2:3–14.

Name:	**FLUOROURACIL**	Risk Factor:	**D***
Class:	**Antineoplastic**		

FETAL RISK SUMMARY

RECOMMENDATION: Contraindicated - 1st Trimester

Fluorouracil was embryotoxic and teratogenic in mice, rats, and hamsters given parenteral doses equivalent to the human dose (1). Although not teratogenic in monkeys, divided doses above 40 mg/kg resulted in abortions. Animal reproduction studies with topical fluorouracil have not been conducted (1).

When applied topically in patients with actinic keratoses, the amount of fluorouracil absorbed systemically is approximately 6% (1). The amount absorbed from mucous membranes is unknown. One manufacturer reported an infant with cleft lip and palate from a woman who appropriately used topical fluorouracil and a second infant with a ventricular septal defect from a woman who used the drug topically on mucous membranes (1). In addition, spontaneous abortions (SABs) have been reported following use on mucous membrane areas (1). It is not known if there is a causative relationship between the topically applied drug and these outcomes.

Following systemic therapy in the 1st trimester (also with exposure to 5 rads of irradiation), multiple defects were observed in an aborted fetus: radial aplasia; absent thumbs and three fingers; hypoplasia of lungs, aorta, thymus, and bile duct; aplasia of esophagus, duodenum, and ureters; single umbilical artery; absent appendix; imperforate anus; and a cloaca (2).

A 33-year-old woman with metastatic breast cancer was treated with a modified radical mastectomy during her 3rd month of pregnancy followed by oophorectomy at 13 weeks' gestation (3). Chemotherapy, consisting of 5-fluorouracil, cyclophosphamide, and doxorubicin, was started at approximately 11 weeks' gestation and continued for six 3-week cyclic courses. Methotrexate was substituted for doxorubicin at this time and the new three-drug regimen was continued until delivery by cesarean section at 35 weeks of a 2260-g female infant. No abnormalities were noted at birth, and continued follow-up at 24 months of age revealed normal growth and development. Toxicity consisting of cyanosis and jerking extremities has been reported in a newborn exposed to fluorouracil in the 3rd trimester (4).

In a surveillance study of Michigan Medicaid recipients conducted between 1985 and 1992 involving 229,101 completed pregnancies, 14 newborns had been exposed to fluorouracil (includes nonsystemic administration) during the 1st trimester (F. Rosa, personal communication, FDA, 1993). One (7.1%) major birth defect was observed (one expected). No anomalies were observed in six defect categories (cardiovascular defects, oral clefts, spina bifida, polydactyly, limb reduction defects, and hypospadias) for which specific data were available.

In a brief 1997 report, three pregnant women with breast cancer were successfully treated with two or three courses of vinorelbine (20–30 mg/m^2) and fluorouracil (500–750 mg/m^2) at 24, 28, and 29 weeks' gestation, respectively (5). Delivery occurred at 34, 41, and 37 weeks' gestation, respectively. One patient also required six courses of epidoxorubicin and cyclophosphamide. Her infant developed transient anemia at 21 days of age that resolved spontaneously. No adverse effects were observed in the other two newborns. All three infants were developing normally at about 2–3 years of age (5).

A 1999 report from France described the outcomes of pregnancies in 20 women with breast cancer who were treated with antineoplastic agents (6). The first cycle of chemotherapy occurred at a mean gestational age of 26 weeks with delivery occurring at a mean 34.7 weeks. A total of 38 cycles were administered during pregnancy with a median of two cycles per woman. None of the women received radiation therapy during pregnancy. The pregnancy outcomes included two SAB (both exposed in the 1st trimester), one intrauterine death (exposed in the 2nd trimester), and 17 live births, one of whom died at 8 days of age without apparent cause. The 16 surviving children were developing normally at a mean follow-up of 42.3 months (6). Fluorouracil (F), in combination with various other agents (cyclophosphamide [C], doxorubicin [D], epirubicin [E], mitoxantrone [M], or vinorelbine [V]) was administered to 16 of the women at a mean dose of 535 mg/m^2 (range 300–750 mg/m^2). The outcomes were one SAB (FCE; 1st trimester), one neonatal death (one cycle of FCE 32 days before birth), and 14 surviving liveborn infants (five FEC, four FV, two FAC, two FCM, and one FD in the 2nd or 3rd trimesters). One of the infants, exposed to two cycles of FCE with the last at 25 days before birth, had transient leukopenia and another was growth retarded (1460-g, born at 33 weeks' gestation after two cycles of FCM) (6).

Amenorrhea has been observed in women treated with fluorouracil for breast cancer, but this was probably caused by concurrent administration of melphalan (see also Melphalan) (7,8). The long-term effects of combination chemotherapy on menstrual and reproductive function have been described in two 1988 reports (9,10). In one report, only 2 of the 40 women treated for malignant ovarian germ cell tumors received fluorouracil (9). The results of this study are discussed in the monograph for cyclophosphamide (see Cyclophosphamide). The other report described the reproductive results of 265 women who had been treated from 1959–1980 for gestational trophoblastic disease (10). Single-agent chemotherapy was administered to 91 women, including 54 cases in which fluorouracil was the only agent used; sequential (single agent) and combination therapies were administered to 67 and 107 women, respectively. Of the total group, 241 were exposed to pregnancy and 205 (85%) of these women conceived, with a total of 355 pregnancies. The time interval between recovery and pregnancy was 1 year or less (8.5%), 1–2 years (32.1%), 2–4 years (32.4%), 4–6 years (15.5%), 6–8 years (7.3%), 8–10 years (1.4%), and more than 10 years (2.8%). A total of 303 (4 sets of twins) liveborn infants resulted from the 355 pregnancies, 3 of whom had congenital malformations: anencephaly, hydrocephalus, and congenital heart disease (one in each case). No gross developmental abnormalities were observed in the dead fetuses. Cytogenetic studies were conducted on the peripheral lymphocytes of 94 children, and no significant chromosomal abnormalities were noted. Moreover, follow-up of the children, more than 80% of the group older than 5 years of age (the oldest was 25 years old), revealed normal development. The reproductive histories and pregnancy outcomes of the treated women were comparable to those of the normal population (10).

Occupational exposure of the mother to antineoplastic agents during pregnancy may present a risk to the fetus. A position statement from the National Study Commission on Cytotoxic Exposure and a research article involving some antineoplastic agents are presented in the monograph for cyclophosphamide (see Cyclophosphamide).

[**Risk Factor X according to manufacturers Allergan and ICN Pharmaceuticals, 2000.*]

BREAST FEEDING SUMMARY

RECOMMENDATION: Contraindicated

No reports describing the use of fluorouracil during lactation have been located. The low molecular weight (about 130) probably indicates that the drug is excreted into milk. Because of the potential for severe toxicity in a nursing infant, women should not nurse while receiving fluorouracil.

References

1. Product information. Efudex. ICN Pharmaceuticals, 2000.
2. Stephens JD, Golbus MS, Miller TR, Wilber RR, Epstein CJ. Multiple congenital anomalies in a fetus exposed to 5-fluorouracil during the first trimester. Am J Obstet Gynecol 1980;137:747–9.
3. Turchi JJ, Villasis C. Anthracyclines in the treatment of malignancy in pregnancy. Cancer 1988;61:435–40.
4. Stadler HE, Knowles J. Fluorouracil in pregnancy: effect on the neonate. JAMA 1971;217:214–5.
5. Cuvier C, Espie M, Extra JM, Marty M. Vinorelbine in pregnancy. Eur J Cancer 1997;33:168–9.
6. Giacalone PL, Laffargue F, Benos P. Chemotherapy for breast carcinoma during pregnancy. Cancer 1999;86:2266–72.
7. Fisher B, Sherman B, Rockette H, Redmond C, Margolese K, Fisher ER. L-Phenylalanine (L-PAM) in the management of premenopausal patients with primary breast cancer. Cancer 1979;44:847–57.
8. Schilsky RL, Lewis BJ, Sherins RJ, Young RC. Gonadal dysfunction in patients receiving chemotherapy for cancer. Ann Intern Med 1980;93:109–14.
9. Gershenson DM. Menstrual and reproductive function after treatment with combination chemotherapy

for malignant ovarian germ cell tumors. J Clin Oncol 1988;6:270–5.
10. Song H, Wu P, Wang Y, Yang X, Dong S. Pregnancy outcomes after successful chemotherapy for choriocarcinoma and invasive mole: long-term follow-up. Am J Obstet Gynecol 1988;158:538–45.

Name: **FLUOXETINE** Risk Factor: **C_M**
Class: **Antidepressant**

FETAL RISK SUMMARY

RECOMMENDATION: Human Data Suggest Risk in 3rd Trimester

Fluoxetine, a selective serotonin reuptake inhibitor (SSRI), is used for the treatment of depression. The chemical structure of fluoxetine is unrelated to other antidepressant agents.

All of the antidepressant agents in the SSRI class (citalopram, escitalopram, fluoxetine, fluvoxamine, paroxetine, and sertraline) share a similar mechanism of action although they have different chemical structures. These differences could be construed as evidence against any conclusion that they share similar effects on the embryo, fetus, or newborn. In the mouse embryo, however, craniofacial morphogenesis appears to be regulated, at least in part, by serotonin. Interference with serotonin regulation by chemically different inhibitors produces similar craniofacial defects (1). Regardless of the structural differences, therefore, some of the potential adverse effects on pregnancy outcome may also be similar.

Reproduction studies in rats and rabbits revealed no evidence of teratogenicity using up to 1.5 and 3.6 times the maximum recommend human daily dose on a body surface area basis [MRHD], respectively, throughout organogenesis (2,3). In rats, however, doses of 1.5 times the MRHD during gestation or 0.9 times the MRHD during gestation and lactation were associated with an increase in stillbirths, a decrease in pup weight, and a decrease in pup survival during the first 7 days postpartum (2). The no-effect dose for pup mortality was 0.6 times the MRHD (2). There was no evidence of developmental neurotoxicity in the surviving pups exposed to 1.5 times the MRHD during gestation (2).

Using uterine rings from midterm (gestation day 14) and term pregnant rats, fluoxetine, and two other antidepressants (imipramine and nortriptyline), were shown to attenuate the activity of serotonin-induced spontaneous uterine contractions (4). Although a direct myometrial role could not be demonstrated for these monoamine reuptake inhibitors, the investigators discussed several other possible pathways that fluoxetine could induce preterm delivery (4).

Administration of fluoxetine to pregnant rats produced a down-regulation of fetal cortical ^{3}H-imipramine binding sites that was still evident 90 days after birth (5). The clinical significance of this finding to the development of the human fetal brain is unknown.

In a study to determine if fluoxetine increased the bleeding risk in neonates, pregnant rats were administered fluoxetine (5.62 mg/kg/day) from day 7 of gestation until the delivery (6). The dose was approximately 5 times the maximum recommended human dose. Compared to controls, fluoxetine-exposed pups had a significantly higher frequency of skin hematomas. The mechanism was thought to be related to the inhibition of serotonin uptake by platelets (6).

Both fluoxetine and the active metabolite norfluoxetine cross the placenta and distribute within the embryo or fetus in rats (7). Consistent with the relatively low molecular weight (about 310 for the free base), fluoxetine and the metabolite desmethylfluoxetine (norfluoxetine) cross the human term placenta. In an *in vitro* experiment using a single placental cotyledon, the mean steady state placental transfer for the two compounds was 8.7% and 9.1%, respectively (8). A 2003 study of the placental transfer of antidepressants found cord blood:maternal serum ratios for fluoxetine and its metabolite that ranged from 0.32–1.36 and 0.12–1.58, respectively (9). The dose-to-delivery interval was 9–37 hours with the highest ratio for the parent drug and metabolite occurring at 26 hours. Moreover, two studies (cited below as references #19 and #20), have documented the human placental transfer of the antidepressant and its active metabolite at term.

During clinical trials with fluoxetine, a total of 17 pregnancies occurred during treatment, even though the women were required to use birth control, suggesting lack of compliance (3). No pregnancy complications or adverse fetal outcomes were observed.

A prospective evaluation of 128 women treated with a mean daily dose of 25.8 mg of fluoxetine during the 1st trimester was reported in 1993 (10). Two matched control groups were selected; one with exposure to tricyclic antidepressants (TCAs) and the other with exposure only to nonteratogens. No differences were found in the rates of major birth defects (2, 0, and 2, respectively) among the groups. An increased risk was observed, although not statistically significant, in the rate of spontaneous abortion when the fluoxetine group was compared to those in the nonteratogen group, 14.8% vs. 7.8% (relative risk 1.9; 95% confidence interval [CI] 0.92–3.92). Because only 74 TCA 1st trimester exposures were available for matching, comparisons between the three groups were based on 74 women in each group. The rates of miscarriage from this analysis were 13.5% (fluoxetine), 12.2% (TCAs), and 6.8% (nonteratogens), again without reaching statistical significance. Because of the increase in the number of spontaneous abortions observed in both antidepressant groups, additional studies are needed to separate the effects of the psychiatric condition from that of the drug therapy. The authors also concluded that exposure to fluoxetine during the 1st trimester was not associated with an increased risk of congenital defects, but that long-term studies were warranted to evaluate the potential neurodevelopmental toxicity of the antidepressant (10).

A 1992 prospective multicenter study evaluated the effects of lithium exposure during the 1st trimester in 148 women (11). One of the pregnancies was terminated at 16 weeks' gestation because of a fetus with Ebstein's anomaly, a rare congenital heart defect. The fetus had been exposed to lithium, fluoxetine, trazodone, and L-thyroxine during the 1st trimester. The defect was probably caused by lithium exposure.

In a surveillance study of Michigan Medicaid recipients conducted between 1985 and 1992 involving 229,101 completed pregnancies, 142 newborns had been exposed to fluoxetine, 109 during the 1st trimester (F. Rosa, personal communication, FDA, 1994). Two (1.8%) major birth defects were observed (five expected), but details of the abnormalities were not available. No anomalies were observed in eight defect categories (cardiovascular defects, oral clefts, spina bifida, polydactyly, limb reduction defects, hypospadias, brain defects, and eye defects) for which specific data were available. These data do not support an association between the drug and congenital defects.

A 1993 letter to the editor from representatives of the manufacturer summarized the postmarketing database for the antidepressant (12). Of the 1103 prospectively reported exposed pregnancies, 761 of which had potentially reached term, data were available for 544 (71%) outcomes, including 91 elective terminations. Among the remaining 453 pregnancies, there were 72 (15.9%) spontaneous abortions, 2 (0.4%) stillbirths, and 20 (4.4%) infants with major malformations, 7 of whom were identified in the post-perinatal period. Details of the aborted fetuses and stillbirths were not given. The malformations observed in the perinatal period were abdominal wall defect (in one twin), atrial septal defect, constricted band syndrome, hepatoblastoma, bilateral hydroceles, gastrointestinal anomaly, intestinal blockage, macrostomia, stubbed and missing digits, trisomy 18, trisomy 21, and ureteral disorder (2 cases). The post-perinatal cases included an arrhythmia, pyloric stenosis (2 cases), tracheal malacia (3 cases), and volvulus. An additional 28 cases of major malformations reported retrospectively to the manufacturer were mentioned, but no details were given other than the fact that the malformations lacked similarity and, thus, were not indicative of a pattern of anomalies (12).

A review that appeared in 1996 (before reference #14) examined the published data relating to the safety of fluoxetine use during gestation and lactation in both experimental animals and humans (13). Using previously published criteria for identifying human teratogens, the authors concluded that the use of fluoxetine during pregnancy did not result in an increased frequency of birth defects or effects on neurobehavior (13).

A prospective study published in 1996 compared the pregnancy outcomes of 228 women who took fluoxetine with 254 nonexposed controls (14). The rates of spontaneous abortion in the two groups were 10% (exposed) and 8.5% (controls), but 13.6% (23 of 169) among those who were enrolled in the study during the 1st trimester and who had 1st trimester exposure. Major structural anomalies were observed in 5.5% (9 of 164) of live-born infants exposed to fluoxetine during the 1st trimester compared to 4.0% (9 of 226) of live-born infants among the controls ($p = 0.63$). No patterns were evident in either group. A total of 250 infants (97 study, 153 controls) were examined (by a physician who was unaware of the infant's drug exposure [15]) for minor anomalies and among those with three or more, 15 (15.5%) were exposed and 10 (6.5%) were not exposed ($p = 0.03$). In comparison to those infants who were exposed during the 1st trimester to fluoxetine or not exposed at all, infants who were exposed late to the drug had a significant increase in perinatal complications, including prematurity (after excluding twins), rate of admission to special-care nurseries (after excluding preterm infants), poor neonatal adaptation, lower mean birth weight and shorter length in full-term infants, and a higher proportion of full-term infants with birth weights at or below the 10th percentile (14). Moreover, two (2.7%) of the full-term infants who were exposed late had persistent pulmonary hypertension, a complication that is estimated to occur in the general population at a rate of 0.07%–0.10%. Although the authors concluded that the number of major structural anomalies and the rate of spontaneous abortions were not significantly increased by fluoxetine exposure in this study, the increased rate of three or more minor anomalies, an unusual finding, is indicative that the drug does affect embryonic development and raises the concern of occult malformations, such as those involving brain development (14). Moreover, the use of fluoxetine late in pregnancy was related to an increase in perinatal complications. In an accompanying editorial (16) and subsequent letters (17,18), various investigators cited perceived problems with the above study, which were addressed in a reply (15).

A 1993 case report described possible fluoxetine-induced toxicity in a term 3580-g male newborn (19). The infant's 17-year-old mother had taken the antidepressant (20 mg/day) throughout most of her pregnancy for severe depression and suicidal ideation. The infant was initially alert and active with mild hypoglycemia (33 mg/dL). Oral 5% dextrose was given and hourly blood glucose samples over the next 4 hours were within normal limits. At 4 hours of age, marked acrocyanosis was noted and the infant became jittery. Tachypnea developed with a respiratory rate of 70 breaths/minute. His condition continued to worsen with symptoms peaking at 36 hours. The symptoms included continuous crying, irritability, moderate to marked tremors, increased muscle tone, a hyperactive Moro reflex, and emesis. An extensive diagnostic work-up, including a drug screen, was negative. The cord blood fluoxetine and norfluoxetine levels were 26 ng/mL and 54 ng/mL, respectively, both within a nontoxic range for adults. The infant was asymptomatic at 96 hours of age, at which time the serum levels of the parent drug and metabolite were <25 ng/mL and 55 ng/mL, respectively. The author attributed the toxic symptoms to fluoxetine (19).

A case report in 1997 described a 3020-g male newborn who was delivered at term from a 34-year-old woman with obsessive-compulsive disorder treated with fluoxetine 60 mg/day (20). Apgar scores were 7 and 8 at 1 and 5 minutes, respectively. After birth, the infant was jittery and hypertonic with mild grunting, flaring, and retracting. Scattered petechiae on the face and trunk and a cephalohematoma were noted. A right, nondisplaced clavicular fracture was noted on chest x-ray. The remainder of the examination and diagnostic work-up was non-revealing. On the second day of life, the serum fluoxetine and norfluoxetine concentrations were 129 ng/mL and 227 ng/mL, respectively, both in the normal adult range (20). The mother did not breast-feed the infant. Marked improvement in the jitteriness was observed by 2 weeks of age, and by 5 months of age, the infant was considered normal. Because of similar symptoms observed in newborns (see references #13 and #15 above) and in adults, the authors attributed the baby's symptoms to fluoxetine. Moreover, the bruising and bleeding were also thought to have been caused by the antidepressant (20).

In a 1996 descriptive case series, the European Network of the Teratology Information Services (ENTIS) prospectively examined the outcomes of 689 pregnancies exposed to antidepressants (21). Multiple-drug therapy occurred in about two-thirds of the mothers. Fluoxetine was used in 96 pregnancies. The outcomes of these pregnancies were 15 elective abortions, 13 spontaneous abortions, 1 stillbirth, 60 normal newborns (includes 6 premature infants), 3 normal infants with neonatal disorder (asphyxia and bradycardia, periventricular bleeding; gastroesophageal regurgitation and bradycardia; and withdrawal symptoms), 2 infants with minor defects (angioma right eyebrow and pilonidal sinus), and 2 infants with congenital defects. The defects (all exposed in the 1st trimester or longer) were ventricular septal defect and hypospadia (exposed to multiple other agents) (21).

Using data from the manufacturer's prospective pregnancy registry, postnatal complications that had been reported in 112 pregnancies (115 infants) exposed to fluoxetine during the 3rd trimester were tabulated in a 1995 reference (22). Maternal doses ranged from 10 to 80 mg/day, but were not reported in 20 pregnancies. Postnatal complications, unrelated to congenital malformations, were noted in 15 singleton term infants, including two infants with jitteriness and three with irritability. Irritability was also observed in one premature infant (gestational age not given). Except in one infant, the complications were considered mild and transitory. No relationship to the maternal dose was observed, but plasma drug levels were not measured in any of the infants (22).

A study published in 1997 described the outcomes among 796 pregnancies with confirmed 1st trimester exposure to fluoxetine that had been reported prospectively to the manufacturer's worldwide fluoxetine pregnancy registry (23) (this is an update of the data presented in reference #12). Of the total number, 37 pregnancies were identified during clinical trials and 759 from spontaneous reports. Spontaneous abortions occurred in 110 (13.8%) cases, and for the remaining 686 pregnancies, malformations, deformations, and disruptions occurred in 34 (5.0%). No consistent pattern of defects were observed, and only one minor malformation was reported. Moreover, no recurring patterns of malformations, increase in unusual defects, or adverse outcomes were observed in 89 infants from 426 retrospectively reported pregnancies. Based on these data, the authors concluded that it was unlikely that the drug was related to an increased risk of malformations (23). Others, however, have previously pointed out that underreporting and documentation of outcomes are problems with these types of surveillance (15).

The neurodevelopment of children between the ages of 16 and 86 months who had been exposed *in utero* for varying lengths of duration to fluoxetine ($N = 55$) or tricyclic antidepressants ($N = 80$), were described in 1997 (24). A control group ($N = 84$) of children not exposed to any agent known to adversely affect the fetus was used for comparison. Assessments of neurodevelopment were based on tests for global IQ and language development and were conducted in a blinded manner. No statistically significant differences were found between the three groups in terms of gestational age at birth, birth weight, and weight, height or head circumference at testing. The mean global IQ scores in the fluoxetine, tricyclic, and control groups were 117, 118, and 115, respectively (*ns*). Moreover, there were no significant differences in the language scores, or assessment of temperament, mood, arousability, activity level, distractibility, or behavior problems (24). In addition, no significant differences between the three groups were found with analysis of the data by comparing those exposed only during the 1st trimester to those exposed throughout pregnancy.

A 1998 non-interventional observational cohort study described the outcomes of pregnancies in women who had been prescribed one or more of 34 newly marketed drugs by general practitioners in England (25). Data were obtained by questionnaires sent to the prescribing physicians one month after the expected or possible date of delivery. In 831 (78%) of the pregnancies, a newly marketed drug was thought to have been taken during the 1st trimester, with birth defects noted in 14 (2.5%) singleton births of the 557 newborns (10 sets of twins). In addition, two birth defects were observed in aborted fetuses. However, few of the aborted fetuses were examined. Fluoxetine was taken during the 1st trimester in 52 pregnancies. The outcomes of these pregnancies included 2 ectopic pregnancies, 6 spontaneous and 6 elective abortions, 11 cases lost to follow-up, 25 normal newborns (1 premature), and 2 infants with major malformations. The birth defects were spina bifida with hydrocephalus (mother also took dothiepin, sodium valproate, and carbamazepine) and congenital hypothyroidism. In addition, one newborn with a normal chromosome pattern had a minor congenital anomaly (single palmar creases) (25).

In a 1998 case report, a 32-year-old woman with bipolar disorder took fluoxetine, buspirone, and carbamazepine (see Breast Feeding Summary for doses and further details) throughout gestation (26). At 42 weeks' gestation she gave birth to a healthy, 3940-g, normally developed, female infant. The mother continued her medications for 3 weeks while exclusively breast-feeding the infant. She reported seizure-like activity in her infant at 3 weeks, 4 months, and 5.5 months of age.

In 1999, the Swedish Medical Birth Registry published the results of a study on the use of antidepressants in early pregnancy and delivery outcome for the years 1995–1997 (27). During the period, 281,728 infants were registered, 531 of whom had been exposed *in utero* to SSRI antidepressants, 15 to SSRIs plus a non-SSRI antidepressant, and 423 to non-SSRI antidepressants. Of the 16 women who used fluoxetine, 15 used it alone and 1 used it in combination with clomipramine. There was no significant differences in relative risk (RR = observed/expected) for birth defects between those exposed to any depressant (total 39; RR 1.13), SSRIs only (total 21; RR 1.12), and non-SSRIs only (total 18; RR 1.15). Similarly, no significant differences in infant survival were observed among the groups. A shorter gestational duration (<37 weeks) was observed for any antidepressant exposure (OR 1.43, 95% CI 1.14–1.80), but no difference between SSRI and non-SSRI antidepressants. Moreover, antidepressant exposure was not associated with an increased risk of low birth weight (defined as <2500 g) among singletons as the crude OR 1.32, 95% CI 0.96–1.80, decreased to 1.03 after adjustment for confounders (27).

The use of fluoxetine in two women was associated with the induction of ovulation that had previously been resistant to clomiphene (28). Although no pregnancies occurred, ovulation continued after fluoxetine was discontinued.

Five male infants exposed to citalopram (30 mg/day), paroxetine (10–40 mg/day), or fluoxetine (20 mg/day) during gestation exhibited withdrawal symptoms at or within a few days of birth and lasting up to 1 month (29). Symptoms included irritability, constant crying, shivering, increased tonus, eating and sleeping problems and convulsions. The four infants exposed to paroxetine and fluoxetine required treatment with chlorpromazine.

A 2002 prospective study compared two groups of mother-child pairs exposed to antidepressants throughout gestation (40 exposed to fluoxetine; 46 to tricyclics) to 36 nonexposed, not depressed controls (30). Offspring were studied between the ages 15 and 71 months for effects of antidepressant exposure in terms of IQ, language, behavior, and temperament. Exposure to antidepressants did not adversely affect the measured parameters, but IQ was significantly and negatively associated with the duration of depression, and language was negatively associated with the number of depression episodes after delivery (30).

The effect of SSRIs on birth outcomes and postnatal neurodevelopment of children exposed prenatally was reported in 2003 (31). Thirty-one children (mean age 12.9 months) exposed during pregnancy to SSRIs (15 sertraline, 8 paroxetine, 7 fluoxetine, and 1 fluvoxamine) were compared to 13 children (mean age 17.7 months) of mothers with depression who elected not to take medications during pregnancy. All of the mothers had healthy lifestyles (i.e., took prenatal vitamins, no smoking, little alcohol use, and regular exercise). The timing of the exposures was 71% in the 1st trimester, 74% in the 3rd trimester, and 45% throughout. The average duration of breast-feeding in the subjects and controls was 6.4 and 8.5 months. Twenty-eight (90%) subjects nursed their infants, 17 of who took SSRIs (10 sertraline, 4 paroxetine, and 3 fluoxetine) compared to 11 (85%) controls, three of whom took sertraline. There were no significant differences between the groups in terms of gestational age at birth, premature births, birth weight and length or, at follow-up, in sex distribution or gain in weight and length (expressed at percentage). Seven (23%) of the exposed infants were admitted to a neonatal intensive care unit (six respiratory distress, four meconium aspiration, and one cardiac murmur) compared to none of the controls ($p = 0.06$). Follow-up examinations were conducted by a pediatric neurologist, psychologist, and a dysmorphologist who were blinded as to the mothers' medications status. The mean Apgar scores at 1 and 5 minutes were lower in the exposed group than in controls, 7.0 vs. 8.2, and 8.4 vs. 9.0, respectively. There was one major defect in each group: small asymptomatic ventricular septal defect (exposed); bilateral lacrimal duct stenosis that required surgery (control). The test outcomes for mental development were similar in the groups, but significant differences in the subjects included a slight delay in psychomotor development and lower behavior motor quality (tremulousness and fine motor movements).

A 2004 prospective study examined the effect of four SSRIs (citalopram, fluoxetine, paroxetine, and sertraline) on newborn neurobehavior, including behavioral state, sleep organization, motor activity, heart rate variability, tremulousness, and startles (32). Seventeen SSRI-exposed, healthy, full-birth-weight newborns and 17 nonexposed, full-birth-weight newborns were matched for maternal cigarette use, social class, and maternal age. A wide range of disrupted neurobehavioral outcomes were shown in the infants exposed *in utero* to SSRIs. After adjustment for gestational age, the exposed infants were found to differ significantly from controls in terms of tremulousness, behavioral states, and sleep organization. Although the effects observed on motor activity, startles, and heart rate variability were not significant after adjustment, the investigators thought they might be mediated through the effects of SSRI exposure on gestational age (32).

In summary, the available animal and human experience indicates fluoxetine is not related to major congenital malformations (33–35). However, one animal study has shown that fluoxetine can produce changes, perhaps permanently, in the fetal brain. Moreover, the increased rate of three or minor anomalies found in one investigation may be evidence that the drug does adversely affect embryonic development. The other studies cited above lacked the sensitivity to identify minor anomalies because of the absence of standardized examinations. Fluoxetine exposure in the 3rd trimester may be related to perinatal complications, neurobehavior disruptions, and a withdrawal syndrome. These potential toxic complications must be weighed against the potential maternal risks of discontinuing antidepressant therapy. The increased incidence of spontaneous abortions in exposed pregnancies needs further investigation. In addition, further investigations of central nervous system development after SSRI exposure are required (36).

BREAST FEEDING SUMMARY

RECOMMENDATION: Limited Human Data - Potential Toxicity

Fluoxetine is excreted into breast milk. A 1990 case report described a woman, 3 months postpartum, who was started on fluoxetine, 20 mg every morning, for depression (37). No drug-related adverse effects were noted in the infant by the mother or the infant's pediatrician. However, the woman's husband, also a pediatrician, thought the nursing infant showed increased irritability during the first 2 weeks of therapy. Two months after treatment had begun, plasma and milk samples were obtained from the mother (time in relationship to the dose was not specified). Plasma concentrations of the antidepressant and its active metabolite, norfluoxetine, were 100.5 and 194.5 ng/mL, respectively. Similar measurements in the milk were 28.8 and 41.6 ng/mL, respectively. The milk:plasma ratios for the parent compound and the metabolite were 0.29 and 0.21, respectively (37).

A 1992 report described a woman treated for postpartum depression with fluoxetine, 20 mg at bedtime, 10 weeks after delivery (38). The dosing time was chosen just before the infant's longest period of sleep to lessen his exposure to the drug. After 53 days of therapy, milk and serum samples were collected 8 hours after the usual dose and 4 hours after a subsequent dose administered to approximate peak concentrations of fluoxetine. Serum concentrations of fluoxetine and the active metabolite at 4 hours were 135 and 149 ng/mL, respectively, and at 8 hours 124 and 141 ng/mL, respectively. The variation in the milk samples was greater, with values at 4 hours of 67 and 52 ng/mL (hand-expressed foremilk), respectively, and at 8 hours of 17 and 13 ng/mL (hand-expressed hindmilk obtained after nursing), respectively. The authors speculated that the variation in milk levels was more likely because of differences in milk composition (foremilk being high in protein and low in fat; hindmilk having a higher fat content) rather than a reflection of maternal serum concentrations. Assuming that the milk contained a steady concentration of 120 ng/mL of fluoxetine and norfluoxetine, and the infant was ingesting 150 mL/kg/day of milk, the authors calculated that the maximum theoretical dose that the infant had received was 15 to 20 μg/kg/day. No adverse effects were observed in the nursing infant's behavior, feeding patterns, or growth during the treatment period (38).

A case study that appeared in 1993 described colicky symptoms consisting of increased crying, irritability, decreased sleep, vomiting, and watery stools in a breast-fed infant whose mother was taking fluoxetine, 20 mg/day (39). The mother had begun breast-feeding the infant immediately after birth and began taking fluoxetine 3 days later. The baby began to show the symptoms noted above at 6 days of age. The mother was enrolled in a study of infant crying at 3 weeks postpartum and at 6 weeks, the infant was switched to a commercial formula for 3 weeks. The mother continued to pump her breasts during this time. She noted a marked change in the infant's behavior shortly after the change to formula feeding. Under an approved study protocol, the mother's breast milk concentrations of fluoxetine and norfluoxetine were measured (by a commercial laboratory), revealing levels of 69 ng/mL and 90 ng/mL, respectively. After 3 weeks of bottle-feeding, feeding with the mother's milk from a bottle was resumed, and within 24 hours the colic returned and she restarted feeding with the commercial formula. Drugs levels of fluoxetine and metabolite, determined by a commercial laboratory, in the infant's serum on the second day after the return to mother's milk were 340 ng/mL and 208 ng/mL, respectively. The authors associated the symptoms of colic with the presence of fluoxetine in the mother's milk (39).

The very high infant serum levels of fluoxetine and metabolite, similar to therapeutic range in adults, are difficult to explain based on the mother's low dose. A 1996 review suggested that one possible explanation was laboratory error (40).

The presence of fluoxetine and its active metabolite, norfluoxetine, were measured in the breast milk of 10 women and in serum or urine of some of the 11 (one set of twins) nursing infants (median age, 185 days) (41). The women had been taking fluoxetine at an unchanged dose for at least 7 days (9 women for at least 14 days, 1 for 7 days) before the study. The mean maternal dose of fluoxetine was 0.39 mg/kg/day (range 0.17–0.85 mg/kg/day). Milk concentrations of fluoxetine, determined from milk samples collected at 2, 5, 8, 12, and 24 hours after a dose (separate samples collected from both breasts of a woman with twins) ranged from 17.4 to 293 ng/mL, whereas those for norfluoxetine ranged from 23.4 to 379.1 ng/mL. In 3 women, the mean milk:plasma ratios for the two agents were 0.88 (range 0.52–1.51) and 0.82 (range 0.60–1.15), respectively. Peak milk concentrations of fluoxetine occurred within 6 hours in 8 women, more than 12 hours in 2 women, and undetermined (because of insufficient samples) in 1 woman. A plasma sample obtained from 1 infant contained no measurable drug or metabolite (limit of detection for both <1 ng/mL). Fluoxetine was detected in 4 of 5 infant urine samples (1.7 to 17.4 ng/mL) and norfluoxetine was measured in two of the five samples (10.5 and 13.3 ng/mL). Based on an ingestion of 1000 mL of milk per day, the authors calculated that the mean infant doses of fluoxetine and norfluoxetine were 0.077 mg/day and 0.084 mg/day, respectively. When these values were converted to fluoxetine equivalents, the mean daily dose from breast milk was 0.165 mg, or about 10.8% of the weight-adjusted maternal dose. No adverse effects in the nursing infants, including alterations in sleeping, eating, or behavior patterns, were reported by the mothers (41).

In a 1998 case report, a 32-year-old woman with bipolar disorder took fluoxetine (20 mg/day), buspirone (45 mg/day), and carbamazepine (600 mg/day) throughout pregnancy and during the first 3 weeks postpartum (26). She reported seizure-like activity in the infant at 3 weeks, 4 months, and 5.5 months of age. Breast milk and infant serum were evaluated for the presence of fluoxetine and metabolite on postpartum days 13 and 21. On day 13, fluoxetine concentrations in breast milk were 45 ng/mL and 68 ng/mL (right and left breasts), whereas norfluoxetine levels were 68 and 57 ng/mL (right and left breasts). On day 21, the milk concentrations of the drug and metabolite were 38 and 28 ng/mL (mixed milk), respectively. The infant's serum had no detectable (test sensitivity not reported) fluoxetine on day 13 but the level was 61 ng/mL on day 21. Norfluoxetine concentrations in infant serum on day 13 and 21 were 58 and 57 ng/mL, respectively. Maternal serum samples were not obtained for fluoxetine analysis. Similar analyses were conducted for buspirone and carbamazepine (see Buspirone and Carbamazepine for results). A neurologic examination of the infant, that included electroencephalography, was within normal limits. The authors were unable to determine the cause of the seizure-like activity, if, indeed, it had occurred (none of the episodes had been observed by medical personnel) (26).

F

Serum and milk concentrations of fluoxetine (maternal dose 20–40 mg/day) and norfluoxetine in four breast-feeding women were reported in a 1998 study (42). Maternal fluoxetine serum concentrations ranged from 71 to 250 ng/mL, whereas the levels for the metabolite were 67 to 177 ng/mL. Hindmilk levels of fluoxetine and norfluoxetine (always higher than foremilk) ranged from 37 to 132 ng/mL and 11 to 74 ng/mL, respectively. Neither the parent drug or metabolite could be detected in the serum or urine samples from the nursing infants. No neurological abnormalities were detected in the infants and all had normal mental and psychomotor performance development up to 12 to 13 months of age as assessed by the Bayley Scales of Infant Development (42).

In 14 breast-feeding women receiving a mean fluoxetine dose of 0.51 mg/kg/day, the mean milk:plasma ratios for the parent drug and metabolite were 0.68 and 0.56, respectively (43). The mean total infant dose (fluoxetine plus active metabolite) was estimated to be 6.81% (range 2.15%–12%) of the weight-adjusted maternal dose. In nine infants for which plasma samples were obtained, fluoxetine was detected in five (range 20–252 ng/mL) and norfluoxetine in seven (range 17–187 ng/mL). In eight cases, the antidepressant had also been taken during pregnancy and three of these infants had the highest plasma concentrations of fluoxetine. Two infants had colic which had resolved in one infant before the study. Two other infants, with the highest plasma levels of fluoxetine, norfluoxetine, or both, exhibited symptoms of withdrawal consisting of uncontrollable crying, irritability, and poor feeding. In one case, however, maternal methadone use may have contributed to the symptoms (43).

An abstract of a study published in 1999 examined the effect of maternal fluoxetine therapy on the weight gain of nursing infants (44). A total of 64 women took the antidepressant during pregnancy and 26 continued the drug during breast feeding. The other 38 women, who also breast-fed their infants but who had discontinued the drug, were used as controls. Fluoxetine exposed nursing infants had a growth curve significantly below the controls, averaging a deficit in weight gain of 392 g (95% Confidence Interval, −5, −780) in measurements taken between 2 weeks and 6 months of age. Although no adverse effects in the exposed nursing infants were reported by the mothers, the reduced growth was thought to be of possible clinical significance if infant weight gain was already of concern (44).

A 2001 case report described a woman who had been taking fluoxetine (40 mg/day) for 8 years, including throughout pregnancy (45). The infant was delivered at 37 weeks' gestation with a birth weight of about 2.76 kg. Apgar scores were 7 and 8 at 1 and 5 minutes, respectively. The infant was drowsy in the immediate postpartum period but was able to nurse. On day 3 of life, the infant was difficult to arouse, stopped rooting, closed her mouth, nursed only for a few minutes, and began to moan and grunt. On day 11, signs and symptoms included fever (102°F), continuous moaning with an expiratory grunt, drowsy and difficult to arouse, and was hypotonic. An examination for sepsis was negative. Breast-feeding was stopped. The mother's serum fluoxetine and norfluoxetine levels were 453 and 422 ng/mL, respectively, whereas her milk levels were 114 and 124 ng/mL, respectively. The infant's serum levels of fluoxetine and metabolite were

<40 ng/mL and 142 ng/mL, respectively. Eight days after nursing was stopped, the infant's serum levels were <40 ng/mL and 86 ng/mL, respectively. The infant recovered over the next 3 weeks (45).

Although some of the above reports described toxicity, the long-term effects on neurobehavior and development from exposure to this potent serotonin reuptake blocker during a period of rapid central nervous system development have not been adequately studied. Furthermore, the reduced weight gain identified in one study may have clinical significance in some situations. As reported by the FDA, the manufacturer was advised to revise the labeling of fluoxetine to contain a recommendation against its use by nursing mothers (46). The current labeling contains this revision (2). In contrast, the authors of a 1996 review stated that they encouraged women to continue breast-feeding while taking the drug (13). Similarly, a recent review of SSRI agents concluded that if there were compelling reasons to treat a mother for postpartum depression, a condition in which a rapid antidepressant effect is important, the benefits of therapy with SSRIs would most likely outweigh the risks (47). The American Academy of Pediatrics classifies the effects of fluoxetine on the nursing infant to be unknown but may be of concern (48).

F

References

1. Shuey DL, Sadler TW, Lauder JM. Serotonin as a regulator of craniofacial morphogenesis: site-specific malformations following exposure to serotonin uptake inhibitors. Teratology 1992;46:367–78.
2. Product information. Prozac. Dista Products, 2000.
3. Cooper GL. The safety of fluoxetine—an update. Br J Psychiatry 1988;153(Suppl 3):77–86.
4. Vedernikov Y, Bolanos S, Bytautiene E, Fulep E, Saade GR, Garfield RE. Effect of fluoxetine on contractile activity of pregnant rat uterine rings. Am J Obstet Gynecol 2000;182:296–9.
5. Montero D, de Ceballos ML, Del Rio J. Down-regulation of ^{3}H-imipramine binding sites in rat cerebral cortex after prenatal exposure to antidepressants. Life Sci 1990;46:1619–26.
6. Stanford MS, Patton JH. In utero exposure to fluoxetine HCl increases hematoma frequency at birth. Pharmacol Biochem Behav 1993;45:959–62.
7. Pohland RC, Byrd TK, Hamilton M, Koons JR. Placental transfer and fetal distribution of fluoxetine in the rat. Toxicol Appl Pharmacol 1989;98:198–205.
8. Heikkinen T, Ekblad U, Laine K. Transplacental transfer of citalopram, fluoxetine, and their primary demethylated metabolites in isolated perfused human placenta. BJOG 2002;109:1003–8.
9. Hendrick V, Stowe ZN, Altshuler LL, Hwang S, Lee E, Haynes D. Placental passage of antidepressant medications. Am J Psychiatry 2003;160:993–6.
10. Pastuszak A, Schick-Boschetto B, Zuber C, Feldkamp M, Pinelli M, Sihn S, Donnenfeld A, McCormack M, Leen-Mitchell M, Woodland C, Gardner A, Hom M, Koren G. Pregnancy outcome following first-trimester exposure to fluoxetine (Prozac). JAMA 1993;269:2246–8.
11. Jacobson SJ, Jones K, Johnson K, Ceolin L, Kaur P, Sahn D, Donnenfeld AE, Rieder M, Santelli R, Smythe J, Pastuszak A, Einarson T, Koren G. Prospective multicentre study of pregnancy outcome after lithium exposure during first trimester. Lancet 1992;339:530–3.
12. Goldstein DJ, Marvel DE. Psychotropic medications during pregnancy: risk to the fetus. JAMA 1993;270:2177.
13. Nulman I, Koren G. The safety of fluoxetine during pregnancy and lactation. Teratology 1996;53:304–8.
14. Chambers CD, Johnson KA, Dick LM, Felix RJ, Jones KL. Birth outcomes in pregnant women taking fluoxetine. N Engl J Med 1996;335:1010–5.
15. Jones KL, Johnson KA, Chambers CD. Birth outcomes in pregnant women taking fluoxetine. N Engl J Med 1997;336:873.
16. Robert E. Treating depression in pregnancy. N Engl J Med 1996;335:1056–8.
17. Cohen LS, Rosenbaum JF. Birth outcomes in pregnant women taking fluoxetine. N Engl J Med 1997;336:872.
18. Goldstein DJ, Sundell KL, Corbin LA. Birth outcomes in pregnant women taking fluoxetine. N Engl J Med 1997;336:872–3.
19. Spencer MJ. Fluoxetine hydrochloride (Prozac) toxicity in a neonate. Pediatrics 1993;92:721–2.
20. Mhanna MJ, Bennet JB II, Izatt SD. Potential fluoxetine chloride (Prozac) toxicity in a newborn. Pediatrics 1997;100:158–9.
21. McElhatton PR, Garbis HM, Elefant E, Vial T, Bellemin B, Mastroiacovo P, Arnon J, Rodriguez-Pinilla E, Schaefer C, Pexieder T, Merlob P, Dal Verme S. The outcome of pregnancy in 689 women exposed to therapeutic doses of antidepressants. A collaborative study of the European Network of Teratology Information Services (ENTIS). Reprod Toxicol 1996;10:285–94.
22. Goldstein DJ. Effects of third trimester fluoxetine exposure on the newborn. J Clin Psychopharmacol 1995;15:417–20.
23. Goldstein DJ, Corbin LA, Sundell KL. Effects of first-trimester fluoxetine exposure on the newborn. Obstet Gynecol 1997;89:713–8.
24. Nulman I, Rovet J, Stewart DE, Wolpin J, Gardner HA, Theis JGW, Kulin N, Koren G. Neurodevelopment of children exposed in utero to antidepressant drugs. N Engl J Med 1997;336:258–62.

25. Wilton LV, Pearce GL, Martin RM, Mackay FJ, Mann RD. The outcomes of pregnancy in women exposed to newly marketed drugs in general practice in England. Br J Obstet Gynaecol 1998;105:882–9.
26. Brent NB, Wisner KL. Fluoxetine and carbamazepine concentrations in a nursing mother/infant pair. Clin Pediatr 1998;37:41–4.
27. Ericson A, Kallen B, Wiholm BE. Delivery outcome after the use of antidepressants in early pregnancy. Eur J Clin Pharmacol 1999;55:503–8.
28. Strain SL. Fluoxetine-initiated ovulatory cycles in two clomiphene-resistant women. Am J Psychiatry 1994;151:620.
29. Nordeng H, Lindemann R, Perminov KV, Reikvam A. Neonatal withdrawal syndrome after in utero exposure to selective serotonin reuptake inhibitors. Acta Paediatr 2001;90:288–91.
30. Nulman I, Rovet J, Stewart DE, Wolpin J, Pace-Asciak P, Shuhaiber S, Koren G. Child development following exposure to tricyclic antidepressants or fluoxetine throughout fetal life: a prospective, controlled study. Am J Psychiatry 2002;159:1889–95.
31. Casper RC, Fleisher BE, Lee-Ancajas JC, Gilles A, Gaylor E, DeBattista A, Hoyme HE. Follow-up of children of depressed mothers exposed or not exposed to antidepressant drugs during pregnancy. J Pediatr 2003;142:402–8.
32. Zeskind PS, Stephens LE. Maternal selective serotonin reuptake inhibitor use during pregnancy and newborn neurobehavior. Pediatrics 2004;113:368–75.
33. Gupta S, Masand PS, Rangwani S. Selective serotonin reuptake inhibitors in pregnancy and lactation. Obstet Gynecol Surv 1998;53:733–6.
34. Austin MPV, Mitchell PB. Psychotropic medications in pregnant women: treatment dilemmas. Med J Aust 1998;169:428–31.
35. Addis A, Koren G. Safety of fluoxetine during the first trimester of pregnancy: a meta-analytical review of epidemiological studies. Psychol Med 2000;30:89–94.
36. Koren G, Pastuszak A. Psychotropic medications during pregnancy: risk to the fetus (reply). JAMA 1993;270:2178.
37. Isenberg KE. Excretion of fluoxetine in human breast milk. J Clin Psychiatry 1990;51:169.
38. Burch KJ, Wells BG. Fluoxetine/norfluoxetine concentrations in human milk. Pediatrics 1992;89: 676–7.
39. Lester BM, Cucca J, Andreozzi L, Flanagan P, Oh W. Possible association between fluoxetine hydrochloride and colic in an infant. J Am Acad Child Adolesc Psychiatry 1993;32:1253–5.
40. Wisner KL, Perel JM, Findling RL. Antidepressant treatment during breast feeding. Am J Psychiatry 1996;153:1132–7.
41. Taddio A, Ito S, Koren G. Excretion of fluoxetine and its metabolite, norfluoxetine, in human breast milk. J Clin Pharmacol 1996;36:42–7.
42. Yoshida K, Smith B, Craggs M, Channi Kumar R. Fluoxetine in breast-milk and developmental outcome of breast-fed infants. Br J Psychiatry 1998;172: 175–9.
43. Kristensen JH, Ilett KF, Hackett LP, Yapp P, Paech M, Begg EJ. Distribution and excretion of fluoxetine and norfluoxetine in human milk. Br J Clin Pharmacol 1999;48:521–7.
44. Chambers CD, Anderson PO, Thomas RG, Dick LM, Felix RJ, Johnson KA, Jones KL. Weight gain in infants breastfed by mothers who take fluoxetine (abstract). Pediatrics 1999;104:1120–1.
45. Hale TW, Shum S, Grossberg M. Fluoxetine toxicity in a breastfed infant. Clin Pediatr 2001;40:681–4.
46. Nightingale SL. Fluoxetine labeling revised to identify phenytoin interaction and to recommend against use in nursing mothers. JAMA 1994;271:1067.
47. Edwards JG, Anerson I. Systematic review and guide to selection of selective serotonin reuptake inhibitors. Drugs 1999;57:507–33.
48. Committee on Drugs, American Academy of Pediatrics. The transfer of drugs and other chemicals into human milk. Pediatrics 2001;108:776–89.

Name: **FLUOXYMESTERONE** Risk Factor: X_M

Class: **Androgenic Hormone**

FETAL RISK SUMMARY

RECOMMENDATION: Contraindicated

The androgenic hormone fluoxymesterone is indicated as replacement therapy in conditions associated with symptoms of deficiency or absence of endogenous testosterone. It is also indicated for the palliation of androgen-responsive recurrent mammary cancer. Fluoxymesterone inhibits the release of testosterone by inhibition of pituitary luteinizing hormone. Large doses may also suppress spermatogenesis by inhibiting follicle-stimulating hormone (1). The relatively low molecular weight (about 336) suggests that the drug will cross the placenta.

Fluoxymesterone (10 mg/day) was given to a 31-year-old woman in the third month of pregnancy for gigantomastia (2). "Several weeks" of therapy had no effect on the size of the breasts nor did diuretic therapy with chlorothiazide (6000 mg/day). The woman was eventually hospitalized at 6 months' gestation because of breast tissue necrosis and hemorrhage. A single IM dose of testosterone and estradiol (Deladumone) had no effect and both breasts continued to enlarge. An 8-day course of combination oral contraceptives was discontinued because of superficial thrombophlebitis in the right thigh. When the breast ulcer became infected, a bilateral simple mastectomy was performed. She eventually delivered a normal healthy, 3.8-kg male infant (2).

No other reports describing the use of fluoxymesterone in human pregnancy have been located. Fluoxymesterone is contraindicated in pregnancy because of the risk for nonadrenal female pseudohermaphroditism (see Testosterone).

F

BREAST FEEDING SUMMARY

RECOMMENDATION: Contraindicated

No reports describing the use of fluoxymesterone during human lactation have been located. Because testosterone and its derivatives inhibit lactation (see Testosterone), fluoxymesterone is contraindicated in women who are breast-feeding.

References

1. Product information. Halotestin. Upjohn, 1995.
2. Moss WH. Gigantomastia with pregnancy. A case report with review of the literature. Arch Surg 1968;96:27–37.

Name:	**FLUPENTHIXOL**	Risk Factor:	**C**
Class:	**Tranquilizer**		

FETAL RISK SUMMARY

RECOMMENDATION: Limited Human Data - No Relevant Animal Data

Flupenthixol crosses the placenta with cord blood levels averaging 24% of maternal serum levels (1). Amniotic fluid concentrations are similar to those in cord blood. Flupenthixol 1 mg daily was used throughout the 2nd and 3rd trimesters in one patient with borderline psychotic depression (2). None of the infants in the above studies was apparently affected by the exposure to flupenthixol.

BREAST FEEDING SUMMARY

RECOMMENDATION: Limited Human Data - Potential Toxicity

Flupenthixol is excreted into breast milk (1,2). In one study, concentrations were about 30% higher than those in maternal serum (1). In a second study, a mother received flupenthixol 1 mg daily throughout the 2nd and 3rd trimesters (2). The dose was increased to 4 mg daily on the 1st postpartum day, then tapered to 2 mg daily over the next 7 weeks. The mother was also receiving nortriptyline. While receiving the 4-mg daily dose, milk concentrations, measured 2–4.5 hours after a dose on postpartum days 6 (four samples) and 20 (two samples), ranged from 2.0–6.8 ng/mL, with a mean of 3.2 ng/mL. The milk:serum ratios for these samples ranged from 0.50–1.62, with a mean of 0.85. No effects of the drug exposure were observed in the nursing infant, who had normal motor development for the first 4 months (2). The significance of chronic exposure of the nursing infant to this drug is unknown, but concern has been expressed about the effects of long-term exposure on the infant's neurobehavioral mechanisms (2).

References

1. Kirk L, Jorgensen A. Concentrations of cis(z)-flupenthixol in maternal serum, amniotic fluid, umbilical cord serum, and milk. Psychopharmacology (Berl) 1980;72:107–8.
2. Matheson I, Skjaeraasen J. Milk concentrations of flupenthixol, nortriptyline and zuclopenthixol and between-breast differences in two patients. Eur J Clin Pharmacol 1988;35:217–20.

Name:	**FLUPHENAZINE**	Risk Factor:	**C**
Class:	**Tranquilizer**		

FETAL RISK SUMMARY

RECOMMENDATION: Human Data Suggest Risk in 3rd Trimester

Fluphenazine is a piperazine phenothiazine in the same group as prochlorperazine. Phenothiazines readily cross the placenta (1).

Shepard reviewed two studies in which fluphenazine was given to pregnant rats at doses up to 100 mg/kg orally without producing adverse fetal effects (2). Pregnant mice were given fluphenazine (1 mg/kg) or diphenylhydantoin (50 mg/kg), or both, by gavage during organogenesis (3). As compared with controls, a significant reduction in fetal weight and length was observed in all treatment groups. The combination produced a significant increase in the incidence of skeletal defects (incomplete ossification of sternebrae and skull bones) and in the incidence of dilated cerebral ventricles (already increased in the fluphenazine-alone group) (3).

An apparently normal pregnancy outcome was described in a woman receiving psychotherapy and being treated with fluphenazine decanoate (2 mL IM every 3 weeks) (4). In addition, she also smoked cigarettes (up to 4 packs/day) and drank four or five cocktails each evening. She eventually delivered a 1-week postterm 3.38-kg, male infant, who developed minor extrapyramidal symptoms (or withdrawal) 4 weeks after delivery. The symptoms readily responded to oral diphenhydramine. At 2 months of age, the infant was healthy and weighed 4.66 kg. The infant boy was reported by the mother to be doing well at 20 months of age.

A 22-year-old woman with schizophrenia was treated with chlorpromazine (up to 1200 mg/day) throughout gestation, fluphenazine decanoate (50 mg IM every 2 weeks) from the 14th week of gestation, and electroconvulsive therapy at 18 weeks' gestation (5). The fluphenazine dose was increased to 100 mg IM every 2 weeks at 24 weeks' gestation. In addition, she smoked 3 to 4 packs of cigarettes per day. An apparently normal, 3.53-kg male infant was delivered by cesarean section at 39 weeks who did well during the first 3 weeks. At that time (6 weeks after the mother's last fluphenazine dose), the infant developed excessive irritability, choreiform and dystonic movements mostly in the upper limbs, jittery behavior, and hypertonicity. Two doses of diphenhydramine given on the 24th and 25th days failed to resolve the condition. Over the next few weeks, the symptoms subsided only to return on the 58th day with the same intensity as earlier (5).

Diphenhydramine (62.5 mg) was restarted every 6 hours with slow improvement in his condition. At 15 weeks of age, the infant's progress appeared normal and at 6 months of age, the diphenhydramine was gradually withdrawn. Follow-up at 15 months of age was normal. The authors attributed the infant's condition to fluphenazine withdrawal (5).

An infant with multiple anomalies was born to a mother treated with fluphenazine enanthate injections throughout pregnancy (6). The mother also took Debendox (see Doxylamine) during the 1st trimester. Anomalies included: ocular hypertelorism with telecanthus, cleft lip and palate, imperforate anus, hypospadias of penoscrotal type, jerky, roving eye movements, episodic rapid nystagmoid movements, rectourethral fistula, and poor ossification of frontal skull bone. Other reports have indicated that the phenothiazines are relatively safe during pregnancy (see also Prochlorperazine).

In a surveillance study of Michigan Medicaid recipients conducted between 1985 and 1992 involving 229,101 completed pregnancies, 13 newborns had been exposed to fluphenazine during the 1st trimester (F. Rosa, personal communication, FDA, 1993). One (7.7%) major birth defect was observed (0.6 expected), a cardiovascular defect (0 expected). The number of exposures is too small for comment.

A 35-year-old woman with schizophrenia was treated throughout gestation with fluphenazine, 10 mg orally twice daily, then decreased to 5 mg orally twice daily during the 3rd trimester (7). The fluphenazine concentration in cord blood was <1.0 ng/mL. She delivered a normal, 2855-g, female infant at 39 weeks' gestation who developed severe rhinorrhea and upper respiratory distress at 8 hours of age. Oral feedings were poor and complicated by periodic episodes of vomiting, course choreoathetoid movements of the arms and legs, and intermittent arching of the body (7). Marked improvement in her symptoms occurred following a single dose of pseudoephedrine solution (0.75 mg) that was repeated once the next day. Although the infant had no further extrapyramidal symptoms, the rhinorrhea and nasal congestion persisted for 3 months.

BREAST FEEDING SUMMARY

RECOMMENDATION: No Human Data - Potential Toxicity

No reports describing the use of fluphenazine during human lactation have been located. Because other phenothiazines cross the placenta and are excreted into milk (see also Prochlorperazine), passage of fluphenazine into milk should be expected. The American Academy of Pediatrics classifies the effects of other antipsychotic phenothiazine agents (e.g., see Chlorpromazine) on the nursing infant to be unknown but may be of concern.

References

1. Moya F, Thorndike V. Passage of drugs across the placenta. Am J Obstet Gynecol 1962;84:1778–98.
2. Shepard TH. *Catalog of Teratogenic Effects*. 8th ed. Baltimore, MD: Johns Hopkins University Press, 1995:190–1.
3. Abdel-Hamid HA, Abdel-Rahman MS, Abdel-Rahman SA. Teratogenic effect of diphenylhydantoin and/or fluphenazine in mice. J Appl Toxicol 1996;16:221–5.
4. Cleary MF. Fluphenazine decanoate during pregnancy. Am J Psychiatry 1977;134:815–6.
5. O'Connor M, Johnson GH, James DI. Intrauterine effect of phenothiazines. Med J Aust 1981;1:416–7.
6. Donaldson GL, Bury RG. Multiple congenital abnormalities in a newborn boy associated with maternal use of fluphenazine enanthate and other drugs during pregnancy. Acta Paediatr Scand 1982;71:335–8.
7. Nath SP, Miller DA, Muraskas JK. Severe rhinorrhea and respiratory distress in a neonate exposed to fluphenazine hydrochloride prenatally. Ann Pharmacother 1996;30:35–7.

Name:	**FLURAZEPAM**	Risk Factor:	X_M
Class:	**Hypnotic**		

F

FETAL RISK SUMMARY

RECOMMENDATION: Limited Human Data - Animal Data Suggest Low Risk

Flurazepam is a benzodiazepine used to induce sleep. No teratogenic or other adverse fetal or postnatal effects were observed in studies using rats and rabbits administered 80 mg/kg and 20 mg/kg, respectively, during various stages of gestation (1). Similarly, no reports of congenital abnormalities attributable to human exposure with flurazepam have been located. One group of investigators classified the risk to the fetus from exposure to flurazepam as "none-minimal," but the quality of the data was judged to be "poor" (2). Studies involving other members of this class, however, have found evidence that some of these agents may cause fetal abnormalities (see Chlordiazepoxide and Diazepam).

Although published data are lacking, the low molecular weight of flurazepam (about 461) suggest it is transferred to the fetus. Data from the manufacturer indicate that an active metabolite of flurazepam crosses the human placenta and may adversely affect the newborn (3). In a case cited in their product information, a woman ingested flurazepam, 30 mg nightly, for 10 days immediately preceding delivery. The newborn appeared sleepy and lethargic during the first 4 days of life. The effect was thought to be a result of a long-acting metabolite, N_1-desalkylflurazepam, found in the newborn's serum.

In a surveillance study of Michigan Medicaid recipients conducted between 1985 and 1992 involving 229,101 completed pregnancies, 73 newborns had been exposed to flurazepam during the 1st trimester (F. Rosa, personal communication, FDA, 1993). Four (5.5%) (three expected) major birth defects were observed, including (observed/expected) 2/1 cardiovascular defects, 1/0 oral clefts, and 1/0 polydactyly. These data do not support an association between the drug and congenital defects.

A brief 1982 case report described convulsions attributable to clomipramine in a newborn who was exposed to that drug and flurazepam throughout gestation (4). The 2360-g male infant was delivered vaginally at 33 weeks' gestation (the reason for the premature delivery was not stated) and had Apgar scores of 9 and 9 at 1 and 5 minutes, respectively. Convulsions, consisting of myoclonic jerks that were unresponsive to phenobarbital, started at 7 hours of age and were eventually successfully treated with IV and oral clomipramine, although the infant remained jittery. The contribution of flurazepam, which is known to cause convulsions after abrupt withdrawal following prolonged use in adults, to the seizures observed in the newborn is unknown. However, a correlation between declining serum levels of clomipramine and its active metabolite and the condition of the infant probably indicates that the seizures were not caused by flurazepam.

BREAST FEEDING SUMMARY

RECOMMENDATION: No Human Data - Potential Toxicity

Studies examining the excretion of flurazepam into breast milk have not been located. However, the passage of this agent and its active, long-acting metabolite into milk should be expected (see also Diazepam). The American Academy of Pediatrics classifies other benzodiazepines as agents whose effects on the nursing infant are unknown but may be of concern (e.g., see Diazepam).

References

1. Hoffmann-LaRoche Company, personal communication, 1979. As cited by Shepard TH. *Catalog of Teratogenic Agents*. 6th ed. Baltimore, MD: Johns Hopkins University Press, 1989:285.
2. Friedman JM, Little BB, Brent RL, Cordero JF, Hanson JW, Shepard TH. Potential human teratogenicity of frequently prescribed drugs. Obstet Gynecol 1990;75:594–9.
3. Product information. Dalmane. Roche Laboratories, 1993.
4. Cowe L, Lloyd DJ, Dawling S. Neonatal convulsions caused by withdrawal from maternal clomipramine. Br Med J 1982;284:1837–8.

F

Name: **FLURBIPROFEN** Risk Factor: B_M*
Class: **Nonsteroidal Anti-inflammatory**

FETAL RISK SUMMARY

RECOMMENDATION: Human Data Suggest Risk in 1st and 3rd Trimesters

Flurbiprofen is a nonsteroidal anti-inflammatory drug (NSAID) that shares the same precautions for human pregnancy use as other NSAIDs. It is in the same subclass (propionic acids) as five other agents (fenoprofen, ibuprofen, ketoprofen, naproxen, and oxaprozin). Flurbiprofen is used in the treatment of arthritis and is available in an ocular formulation for inhibition of intraoperative miosis. No teratogenic effects were observed in mice, rats, and rabbits administered this drug during gestation (1).

Like other NSAIDs, systemic use of flurbiprofen in rats has been associated with prolonged gestation, fetal growth retardation, and decreased fetal survival (2). In one study of pregnant rats, flurbiprofen inhibition of parturition appeared to be dose-related (3).

A combined 2001 population-based observational cohort study and a case-control study estimated the risk of adverse pregnancy outcome from the use of NSAIDs (4). The use of NSAIDs during pregnancy was not associated with congenital malformations, preterm delivery, or low birth weight, but a positive association was discovered with spontaneous abortions (SABs). (A similar study, also published in 2001, failed to find a relationship, in general, between NSAIDs and congenital malformations, but did find a significant association with cardiac defects and orofacial clefts (5). In addition, a 2003 study found a significant association between exposure to NSAIDs in early pregnancy and SABs (6). (See Ibuprofen for details on these three studies.)

In summary, no reports describing the use of flurbiprofen during human pregnancy have been located. A brief 2003 editorial on the potential for NSAID-induced developmental toxicity concluded that NSAIDs, and specifically those with greater COX-2 affinity, had a lower risk of this toxicity in humans than aspirin (7). Two reviews, both on antirheumatic drug therapy in pregnancy, recommended that if a NSAID was needed, agents with short elimination adult half-lives should be used at the maximum tolerated dosage interval, using the smallest effective dose, and that therapy should be stopped within 8 weeks of the expected delivery date (8,9). Flurbiprofen has a short plasma elimination half-life (5.7 hours), but other factors, such as its toxicity profile need to be considered.

Constriction of the ductus arteriosus *in utero* is a pharmacologic consequence arising from the use of prostaglandin synthesis inhibitors during pregnancy, as is inhibition of labor, prolongation of pregnancy, and suppression of fetal renal function (see also Indomethacin) (10). Persistent pulmonary hypertension of the newborn may occur if these agents are used in the 3rd trimester close to delivery (10,11). Women attempting to conceive should not use any prostaglandin synthetase inhibitor, including flurbiprofen, because of the findings in a variety of animal models that indicate these agents block blastocyst implantation (12,13). Moreover, as noted above, NSAIDs have been associated with SABs and congenital malformations.

[*Risk Factor D if used in 3rd trimester or near delivery.*]

BREAST FEEDING SUMMARY

RECOMMENDATION: Compatible

Very small amounts of flurbiprofen are excreted into breast milk (14,15). In 10 nursing mothers, at least 1 month postpartum, a single 100-mg oral dose of flurbiprofen was administered and milk and blood samples were obtained over a 48-hour period (14). The average peak plasma concentration (14.7 μg/mL) occurred at 1.5 hours with a mean half-life of 5.8 hours. The average peak milk concentration was 0.09 μg/mL with an average of 0.05% (range 0.03%–0.07%) of the maternal dose recovered in breast milk. Breast-feeding was discontinued during and after the study.

In a multiple dosing study, 12 lactating women, 3–5 days after delivery, were administered nine doses of flurbiprofen over a 3-day period (50 mg 4 times daily) (15). Paired milk and plasma samples were obtained at several times during the period and after the last dose. The mean maternal plasma half-life of the drug was 4.8 hours. Flurbiprofen milk concentrations were less than 0.05 μg/mL in 10 of the mothers. In the remaining two mothers, only three of their milk samples contained flurbiprofen: 0.06, 0.07, and 0.08 μg/mL. The authors concluded that these small amounts were safe for a nursing infant (15). None of the mothers breast-fed their infants.

The small amounts of flurbiprofen recovered from transitional and mature breast milk seem to indicate that the risk posed by flurbiprofen to a nursing infant is slight, if it exists at all. One reviewer classified flurbiprofen as one of several low-risk alternatives, because of its short adult serum half-life and toxicity profile compared with other similar agents, if a NSAID was required while nursing (16). Other reviewers have also stated that flurbiprofen can be safely used during breast-feeding (17,18). Another NSAID in the same subclass as flurbiprofen is considered compatible with breast-feeding by the American Academy of Pediatrics (see Ibuprofen).

References

1. Product information. Ansaid. The Upjohn Company, 1995.
2. Product information. Ocufen. Allergan America, 1987.
3. Powell JG Jr, Cochrane RL. The effects of a number of non-steroidal anti-inflammatory compounds on parturition in the rat. Prostaglandins 1982;23:469–88.
4. Nielsen GL, Sorensen HT, Larsen H, Pedersen L. Risk of adverse birth outcome and miscarriage in pregnant users of non-steroidal anti-inflammatory drugs: population based observational study and case-control study. BMJ 2001;322:266–70.
5. Ericson A, Kallen BAJ. Nonsteroidal anti-inflammatory drugs in early pregnancy. Reprod Toxicol 2001;15:371–5.
6. Li DK, Liu L, Odouli R. Exposure to non-steroidal anti-inflammatory drugs during pregnancy and risk of miscarriage: population based cohort study. BMJ 2003;327:368–71.
7. Tassinari MS, Cook JC, Hurtt ME. NSAIDs and developmental toxicity. Birth Defects Res Part B Dev Reprod Toxicol 2003;68:3–4.
8. Needs CJ, Brooks PM. Antirheumatic medication in pregnancy. Br J Rheumatol 1985;24:282–90.
9. Ostesen M. Optimisation of antirheumatic drug treatment in pregnancy. Clin Pharmacokinet 1994;27: 486–503.
10. Levin DL. Effects of inhibition of prostaglandin synthesis on fetal development, oxygenation, and the fetal circulation. Semin Perinatol 1980;4:35–44.

11. Van Marter LJ, Leviton A, Allred EN, Pagano M, Sullivan KF, Cohen A, Epstein MF. Persistent pulmonary hypertension of the newborn and smoking and aspirin and nonsteroidal antiinflammatory drug consumption during pregnancy. Pediatrics 1996;97:658–63.
12. Matt DW, Borzelleca JF. Toxic effects on the female reproductive system during pregnancy, parturition, and lactation. In Witorsch RJ, editor. *Reproductive Toxicology*. 2nd ed. New York, NY: Raven Press, 1995: 175–93.
13. Dawood MY. Nonsteroidal antiinflammatory drugs and reproduction. Am J Obstet Gynecol 1993;169: 1255–65.
14. Cox SR, Forbes KK. Excretion of flurbiprofen into breast milk. Pharmacotherapy 1987;7:211–5.
15. Smith IJ, Hinson JL, Johnson VA, Brown RD, Cook SM, Whitt RT, Wilson JT. Flurbiprofen in post-partum women: plasma and breast milk disposition. J Clin Pharmacol 1989;29:174–84.
16. Anderson PO. Medication use while breast feeding a neonate. Neonatal Pharmacol Q 1993;2: 3–14.
17. Goldsmith DP. Neonatal rheumatic disorders. View of the pediatrician. Rheum Dis Clin North Am 1989;15: 287–305.
18. Needs CJ, Brooks PM. Antirheumatic medication during lactation. Br J Rheumatol 1985;24:291–7.

Name:	**FLUVASTATIN**	Risk Factor:	X_M
Class:	**Antilipemic Agent**		

FETAL RISK SUMMARY

RECOMMENDATION: Contraindicated

The cholesterol-lowering, hydrophilic agent fluvastatin (a "statin"), has the same mechanism of action (i.e., inhibition of hepatic 3-hydroxy-3-methylglutaryl-coenzyme A [HMG-CoA] reductase) as other agents in this class (atorvastatin, cerivastatin, lovastatin, pravastatin, and simvastatin). It differs from these other agents in that it is entirely synthetic and is not derived from fungal sources.

Fluvastatin was not teratogenic in rats and rabbits at doses up to 36 and 10 mg/kg/day, respectively (1,2). Moreover, at the highest doses tested in rats for effects on fertility and reproductive performance, 20 mg/kg/day in males and 6 mg/kg/day in females, no adverse effects were observed (2). Significant maternal body weight loss and an increase in stillborns, neonatal morbidity, and maternal morbidity, however, were observed with fluvastatin doses of either 12 or 24 mg/kg/day administered to pregnant rats from the 15th day after coitus through weaning (2). The maternal morbidity was attributed to the occurrence of cardiomyopathy in the affected animals. The adverse effects of fluvastatin were lessened or prevented by the co-administration of mevalonic acid, a product produced by the enzyme HMG-CoA reductase, indicating that the toxicity was a result of inhibition of this enzyme.

Rosa reported finding no recipients of this drug in his 1994 presentation on the outcome of pregnancies following exposure to anticholesterol agents (3). However, a 1999 case report described the pregnancy outcome of a 28-year-old woman who had taken fluvastatin (20 mg/day) for 18 months before conception and during the first 9 weeks of pregnancy (4). The patient, who had a kidney transplantation 6 years before pregnancy, took prednisone, cyclosporine, azathioprine, cephalexin, and ranitidine throughout gestation. She delivered a healthy, 2901-g female infant at term with Apgar scores of 4 and 9 at 1 and 5 minutes, respectively. Except for transient tachypnea, no other complications were noted. At age 19 months, the infant's growth (weight, height, and head circumference all at the 50th percentile or higher) and development were normal (4).

A 2004 report described the outcomes of pregnancy that had been exposed to statins and reported to the FDA (see Lovastatin).

Because the interruption of cholesterol-lowering therapy during pregnancy should have no effect on the long-term treatment of hyperlipidemia, and because cholesterol and other products synthesized from cholesterol are required for fetal development, the use of fluvastatin is contraindicated during pregnancy. If fluvastatin is used in pregnancy, healthcare professionals are encouraged to call the toll free number (800-670-6126) for information about patient enrollment in the Motherisk study.

BREAST FEEDING SUMMARY

F

RECOMMENDATION: Contraindicated

No published reports describing the use of fluvastatin during lactation have been located. The manufacturer reports that fluvastatin is present in breast milk at a milk:plasma ratio of 2 (1). Because of the potential for adverse effects in the nursing infant, the drug should not be used during lactation.

References

1. Product information. Lescol. Sandoz Pharmaceuticals, 1995.
2. Hrab RV, Hartman HA, Cox RH Jr. Prevention of fluvastatin-induced toxicity, mortality, and cardiac myopathy in pregnant rats by mevalonic acid supplementation. Teratology 1994;50:19–26.
3. Rosa F. Anti-cholesterol agent pregnancy exposure outcomes. Presented at the 7th International Organization for Teratogen Information Services, Woods Hole, MA, April 1994.
4. Seguin J, Samuels P. Fluvastatin exposure during pregnancy. Obstet Gynecol 1999;93:847.

Name: **FLUVOXAMINE** Risk Factor: **C_M**

Class: **Antidepressant**

FETAL RISK SUMMARY

RECOMMENDATION: Human Data Suggest Risk in 3rd Trimester

Fluvoxamine is an antidepressant used in the treatment of obsessive-compulsive disorder. Its mechanism of action is unknown, but the drug is a selective serotonin reuptake inhibitor (SSRI) resulting in the potentiation of serotonin activity in the brain. The chemical structure of fluvoxamine is unrelated to other antidepressants.

All the antidepressant agents in the SSRI class (citalopram, escitalopram, fluoxetine, fluvoxamine, paroxetine, and sertraline) share a similar mechanism of action although they have different chemical structures. These differences could be construed as evidence against any conclusion that they share similar effects on the embryo, fetus, or newborn. In the mouse embryo, however, craniofacial morphogenesis appears to be regulated, at least in part, by serotonin. Interference with serotonin regulation by chemically different inhibitors produces similar craniofacial defects (1). Regardless of the structural differences, therefore, some of the potential adverse effects on pregnancy outcome may also be similar.

No evidence of teratogenicity was observed in reproductive studies with rats and rabbits administered oral doses approximately twice the maximum human daily dose on a mg/m^2 basis (MHDD) (2). Increased pup mortality at birth and decreased postnatal pup weight were seen, however, when rats were dosed at 2 and 4 times the MHDD, respectively, throughout pregnancy and weaning. These effects may have been partially a result of maternal toxicity, but a direct toxic effect on the fetuses and pups could not be excluded (2).

No reports describing the transfer across the human placenta have been located. The molecular weight (about 434 for the maleate salt) is low enough, however, that passage to the fetus should be expected.

In a 1996 descriptive case series, the European Network of the Teratology Information Services (ENTIS) prospectively examined the outcomes of 689 pregnancies exposed to antidepressants (3). Multiple drug therapy occurred in about two-thirds of the mothers. Fluvoxamine was used in 67 pregnancies. The outcomes of these pregnancies were 9 elective abortions (1 with defect; see below), 6 spontaneous abortions, 2 stillbirths, 47 normal newborns (includes 2 premature infants), 2 infants with neonatal disorders (withdrawal, cyanosis), and 2 infants with congenital defects. The defects (all exposed in the 1st trimester or longer and to multiple agents) were multicystic left kidney, right megaureter with neonatal renal insufficiency; and hydrocephaly, right diaphragmatic hernia, and agenesis of the corpus callosum (elective abortion) (3).

A 1998 non-interventional observational cohort study described the outcomes of pregnancies in women who had been prescribed one or more of 34 newly marketed drugs by general practitioners in England (4). Data were obtained by questionnaires sent to the prescribing physicians one month after the expected or possible date of delivery. In 831 (78%) of the pregnancies, a newly marketed drug was thought to have been taken during the 1st trimester with birth defects noted in 14 (2.5%) singleton births of the 557 newborns (10 sets of twins). In addition, two birth defects were observed in aborted fetuses. However, few of the aborted fetuses were examined. Fluvoxamine was taken during the 1st trimester in 21 pregnancies. The outcomes of these pregnancies included one ectopic pregnancy, five spontaneous abortions, two elective abortions, nine normal full term newborns, one premature delivery (twins), and three lost to follow-up. One of the elective abortions was for a genetic abnormality (47,XXX) (4).

A prospective, multicenter, controlled cohort study published in 1998 evaluated the pregnancy outcomes of 267 women exposed to one or more of three SSRI antidepressants during the 1st trimester: fluvoxamine ($N = 26$); paroxetine ($N = 97$); and sertraline ($N = 147$) (5). The women were combined into a study group without differentiation as to the drug they had consumed. All of the women had contacted a teratogen information service about their use of the drugs during pregnancy. A randomly selected control group ($N = 267$) was formed from women who had contacted one service after exposure to nonteratogenic agents. The pregnancy outcomes were determined, in most cases, 6 to 9 months after delivery. The study group was significantly more likely to smoke cigarettes and to have had a previous elective abortion but less likely to be a primigravid. Other characteristics, such as a previous spontaneous abortion, alcohol consumption, and maternal age at conception did not differ between the groups. As for pregnancy outcomes, no significant differences were measured in the number of live births, spontaneous or elective abortions, stillbirths, major malformations, birth weight, or gestational age at birth. Nine major malformations were observed in each group. The relative risk for major anomalies was 1.06 (95% confidence interval 0.43–2.62). No clustering of defects was apparent. In the study group, no differences were found in the pregnancy outcomes of smokers compared to nonsmokers. In addition, the outcomes of women who took an antidepressant throughout gestation were similar to those who took an antidepressant only during the 1st trimester (5). One investigator, in response to subsequent correspondence regarding the study (6,7), clarified that all of the 267 women in the study group had taken an antidepressant during embryogenesis (8). Other concerns relating to the outcomes and sample size were also addressed.

The effect of SSRIs on birth outcomes and postnatal neurodevelopment of children exposed prenatally was reported in 2003 (9). Thirty-one children (mean age 12.9 months) exposed during pregnancy to SSRIs (15 sertraline, 8 paroxetine, 7 fluoxetine, and 1 fluvoxamine) were compared to 13 children (mean age 17.7 months) of mothers with depression who elected not to take medications during pregnancy. All of the mothers had healthy lifestyles (i.e., took prenatal vitamins, no smoking, little alcohol use, and regular exercise). The timing of the exposures was 71% in the 1st trimester, 74% in the 3rd trimester, and 45% throughout the pregnancy. The average duration of breast-feeding in the subjects and controls was 6.4 and 8.5 months. Twenty-eight (90%) subjects, 17 of whom took SSRIs (10 sertraline, 4 paroxetine, and 3 fluoxetine), nursed their infants, compared to 11 (85%) controls, three of whom took sertraline. There were no significant differences between the groups in terms of gestational age at birth, premature births, birth weight and length or, at follow-up, in sex distribution or gain in weight and length (expressed at percentage). Seven (23%) of the exposed infants were admitted to a neonatal intensive care unit (six respiratory distress, four meconium aspiration, and one cardiac murmur) compared to none of the controls ($p = 0.06$). Follow-up examinations were conducted by a pediatric neurologist, psychologist, and a dysmorphologist who were blinded as to the mothers' medications status. The mean Apgar scores at 1 and 5 minutes were lower in the exposed group than in controls, 7.0 vs. 8.2, and 8.4 vs. 9.0, respectively. There was one major defect in each group: small asymptomatic ventricular septal defect (exposed); bilateral lacrimal duct stenosis that required surgery (control). The test outcomes for mental development were similar in the groups, but significant differences in the subjects included a slight delay in psychomotor development and lower behavior motor quality (tremulousness and fine motor movements) (9).

In summary, the limited animal and human data do not demonstrate a major teratogenic risk from the use of fluvoxamine during pregnancy. However, the above studies lack the sensitivity to identify minor anomalies because of the absence of standardized examinations. Late-appearing major defects may also have been missed because of the timing of the questionnaires (i.e., 1 month after delivery). Moreover, one study demonstrated that at least one of these drugs (see Fluoxetine) can induce long-term, perhaps permanent, changes in the brain of *in utero* exposed rats. Therefore, even though the clinical significance of this is unknown, the potential for behavioral teratogenicity cannot be excluded and long-term studies of exposed infants are warranted.

BREAST FEEDING SUMMARY

RECOMMENDATION: Limited Human Data - Potential Toxicity

Fluvoxamine is excreted into human milk. A 23-year-old, 70-kg woman in her 12th postpartum week was treated for postnatal depression with fluvoxamine, 100 mg twice daily (2.86 mg/kg/day) (10). Two weeks after the start of therapy, single milk and plasma samples were obtained 5 hours after a dose, and concentrations of 0.09 and 0.31 μg/mL, respectively, were measured. It was estimated that the infant was ingesting about 0.5% of the mother's daily dose (10).

In a brief 1997 communication, plasma and breast milk samples were obtained from a breast-feeding mother 3 hours after her morning fluvoxamine dose (100 mg/day; 1.43 mg/kg/day) (11). The concentrations in the plasma and milk were 0.17 and 0.05 μg/mL, respectively, a milk:plasma ratio of 0.29. The estimated infant dose was slightly less than 0.0075 mg/kg/day (0.5% of the mother's daily dose). The nursing infant had been exposed to the drug in milk for about 3 to 4 weeks when breast-feeding was discontinued. No adverse effects from the exposure were noted on infant assessments conducted up to 21 months of age (11).

Another communication, published in 2000, described a 31-year-old breast-feeding woman, 3 months postpartum, on a stable dose (100 mg twice daily) of fluvoxamine (12). Serum and foremilk samples were collected every hour for 12 hours after a dose. The mean milk:serum ratio was 1.32. The estimated dose ingested by the nursing infant was 48 μg/kg/day or 1.58% of the weight-adjusted maternal dose. Foremilk samples in women ingesting SSRI agents have been shown to contain much less drug than hindmilk because of the higher fat content of hindmilk and the lipid solubility of these drugs (see Paroxetine and Sertraline). Therefore, because only foremilk was collected from each breast, the milk:serum ratio and the actual dose ingested by the infant were probably higher. No adverse effects or unusual behavior was noted in the nursing infant (12).

In a second 2000 communication, a 26-year-old woman was started on fluvoxamine for severe obsessive-compulsive disorder symptoms at 19 days postpartum (13). Approximately 8 weeks later, while on a dose of 25 mg three times daily, six breast milk (2 to 4 ounces) samples were collected (before each dose and before each feeding) over a 24-hour period. Blood samples were obtained from the mother and infant at the same time—10 hours after a dose and 2–3 hours after the last feeding, respectively. Milk concentrations of fluvoxamine varied from 24 to 40 ng/mL over the collection period. Maternal and infant serum concentrations were 20 ng/mL and 9 ng/mL, respectively. The authors speculated that the atypically high infant serum concentration (45% of the mother's level) may have been related to the infant's hepatic function. The estimated maximum dose ingested by the nursing infant was 6 μg/kg/day, or about 0.62% of the weight-adjusted maternal dose. No adverse effects or interference with normal developmental milestones up to 4 months of age was observed in the nursing infant (13).

A 1999 review of SSRI agents concluded that if there were compelling reasons to treat a mother for postpartum depression, a condition in which a rapid antidepressant effect is important, the benefits of therapy with SSRIs would most likely outweigh the risks (14). However, because the long-term effects of exposure to SSRI antidepressants in breast milk on the infant's neurobehavioral development are unknown (no such adverse effects have been identified to date but research is needed), stopping or reducing the frequency of breast-feeding should be considered if therapy with these agents is required. Avoiding nursing around the time of peak maternal concentration (about 4 hours after a dose) may limit infant exposure. The American Academy of Pediatrics classifies fluvoxamine as a drug whose effect on a nursing infant is unknown but may be of concern (15).

References

1. Shuey DL, Sadler TW, Lauder JM. Serotonin as a regulator of craniofacial morphogenesis: site-specific malformations following exposure to serotonin uptake inhibitors. Teratology 1992;46:367–78.
2. Product information. Luvox. Solvay Pharmaceuticals, 1996.
3. McElhatton PR, Garbis HM, Elefant E, Vial T, Bellemin B, Mastroiacovo P, Arnon J, Rodriguez-Pinilla E, Schaefer C, Pexieder T, Merlob P, Dal Verme S. The outcome of pregnancy in 689 women exposed to therapeutic doses of antidepressants. A collaborative study of the European Network of Teratology Information Services (ENTIS). Reprod Toxicol 1996;10:285–94.
4. Wilton LV, Pearce GL, Martin RM, Mackay FJ, Mann RD. The outcomes of pregnancy in women exposed to newly marketed drugs in general practice in England. Br J Obstet Gynaecol 1998;105:882–9.
5. Kulin NA, Pastuszak A, Sage SR, Schick-Boschetto B, Spivey G, Feldkamp M, Ormond K, Matsui D, Stein-Schechman AK, Cook L, Brochu J, Rieder M, Koren G. Pregnancy outcome following maternal use of the new selective serotonin reuptake inhibitors. A

prospective controlled multicenter study. JAMA 1998; 279:609–10.
6. Grush LR. Risk of fetal anomalies with exposure to selective serotonin reuptake inhibitors. JAMA 1998; 279:1873.
7. Witlin AG. Risk of fetal anomalies with exposure to selective serotonin reuptake inhibitors. JAMA 1998; 279:1873.
8. Koren G. In reply. Risk of fetal anomalies with exposure to selective serotonin reuptake inhibitors. JAMA 1998;279:1873–4.
9. Casper RC, Fleisher BE, Lee-Ancajas JC, Gilles A, Gaylor E, DeBattista A, Hoyme HE. Follow-up of children of depressed mothers exposed or not exposed to antidepressant drugs during pregnancy. J Pediatr 2003;142:402–8.
10. Wright S, Dawling S, Ashford JJ. Excretion of fluvoxamine in breast milk. Br J Clin Pharmacol 1991;31:209.
11. Yoshida K, Smith B, Channi Kumar R. Fluvoxamine in breast-milk and infant development. Br J Clin Pharmacol 1997;44:209–13.
12. Hagg S, Granberg K, Carleborg L. Excretion of fluvoxamine into breast milk. Br J Clin Pharmacol 2000; 49:286–8.
13. Arnold LM, Suckow RF, Lichtenstein PK. Fluvoxamine concentrations in breast milk and in maternal and infant sera. J Clin Psychopharmacol 2000;20:491–3.
14. Edwards JG, Anerson I. Systematic review and guide to selection of selective serotonin reuptake inhibitors. Drugs 1999;57:507–33.
15. Committee on Drugs, American Academy of Pediatrics. The transfer of drugs and other chemicals into human milk. Pediatrics 2001;108:776–89.

Name:	**FOLIC ACID**	Risk Factor:	**A***
Class:	**Vitamin**		

FETAL RISK SUMMARY

RECOMMENDATION: Compatible

Folic acid, a water-soluble B complex vitamin, is essential for nucleoprotein synthesis and the maintenance of normal erythropoiesis (1). The National Academy of Sciences' recommended dietary allowance (RDA) for folic acid in pregnancy is 0.4 mg (1). However, a recommended dietary intake of 0.5 mg/day has been proposed that would meet the needs of women with poor folate stores, those with essentially no other dietary folate, and those with multiple pregnancies (2).

Rapid transfer of folic acid to the fetus occurs in pregnancy (3–5). One investigation found that the placenta stores folic acid and transfer occurs only after placental tissue vitamin receptors are saturated (6). Results compatible with this hypothesis were measured in a 1975 study using radiolabeled folate in women undergoing 2nd trimester abortions (7).

Folic acid deficiency is common during pregnancy (8–11). If not supplemented, maternal serum and red blood cell (RBC) folate values decline during pregnancy (8,12–16). Even with vitamin supplements, however, maternal folate hypovitaminemia may result (8). This depletion is thought to result from preferential uptake of folic acid by the fetal circulation such that at birth, newborn levels are significantly higher than maternal levels (8,15–18). At term, mean serum folate in 174 mothers was 5.6 ng/mL (range 1.5–7.6 ng/mL), whereas in their newborns it was 18 ng/mL (range 5.5–66.0 ng/mL) (8). In an earlier study, similar serum values were measured with RBC folate decreasing from 157 ng/mL at 15 weeks' gestation to 118 ng/mL at 38 weeks (12). Folic acid supplementation prevented the decrease in both serum and RBC folate. Although supplementation is common during pregnancy in some countries, not all authorities believe this is necessary for the entire population (19,20). The main controversy is whether all women should receive supplements because of the cost involved in identifying those at risk (19), or whether supplements should be given only to those in whom a clear indication has been established (20).

The most common complication of maternal folic acid deficiency is megaloblastic anemia (9,21–30). Pancytopenia secondary to folate deficiency has also been reported during pregnancy (31). The three main factors involved in the pathogenesis of megaloblastic anemia of pregnancy are depletion of maternal folic acid stores by the fetus, inadequate maternal intake of the vitamin, and faulty absorption (27). Multiple pregnancy, hemorrhage, and hemolytic anemia hasten the decline of maternal levels (13,27). A 1969 study used 1-mg daily supplements to produce a uniformly satisfactory hematologic response in these conditions (29). In anemia associated with β-thalassemia minor, 5 mg/day of folic acid were significantly better than 0.25 mg/day in increasing predelivery hemoglobin concentrations in both nulliparous and multiparous Chinese women (32). Patients with iron deficiency, chronic blood loss, and parasitic infestation were excluded.

The proposed effects on the mother and fetus resulting from folate deficiency, not all of which appear to be related to the vitamin, can be summarized as follows:

Fetal anomalies (neural tube defects; other defects)
Placental abruption
Gestational hypertension (GHTN)
Abortions
Placenta previa
Low birth weight
Premature delivery

Fetal Anomalies (Neural Tube Defects; Other Defects)

Several investigations have suggested a relationship between folic acid deficiency and neural tube defects (NTDs). (Studies conducted with multiple-vitamin products and not specifically with folic acid are described under Vitamins, Multiple.) In a randomized, double blind trial to prevent recurrences of NTDs, 44 women took 4 mg/day of folic acid from before conception through early pregnancy (33). There were no recurrences in this group. A placebo group of 51 women plus 16 noncompliant patients from the treated group had four and two recurrences, respectively. The difference between the supplemented and nonsupplemented patients was significant ($p = 0.04$). Other researchers reported significantly lower RBC folate levels in mothers of infants with NTDs than in mothers of normal infants, but not all of the affected group had low serum folate (34). In a subsequent report by these investigators, very low vitamin B_{12} concentrations were found, suggesting that the primary deficiency may have been a result of this latter vitamin with resulting depletion of RBC and tissue folate (35). A large retrospective study found a protective effect with folate administration during pregnancy, leading to a conclusion that deficiency of this vitamin may be teratogenic (36).

Evidence was published in 1989 that low dietary intake of folic acid is related to the occurrence of NTDs (37). In this Australian population-based case-control study, 77 mothers whose pregnancies involved an isolated NTD were compared to 77 mothers of infants with other defects (control group 1) and 154 mothers of normal infants (control group 2). Free folate intake was classified into four levels (in μg/day): 8.0–79.8, 79.9–115.4, 115.5–180.5, and 180.6–1678.0. After adjustment for potential confounding variables, a statistically significant trend for protection against an NTD outcome was observed with increasing free folate intake in comparison to both control groups: $p = 0.02$ for control group 1, and $p < 0.001$ for control group 2. The odds ratios for the highest intake compared to the control groups were 0.31 and 0.16, respectively. When total folate intake was examined, the trends were less: $p = 0.10$ for control group 1 and $p = 0.03$ for control group 2. In an accompanying editorial comment, criticism of the above study focused on the authors' estimation of dietary folate intake (38). The commentary cited evidence that nutrition tables are unreliable for the estimation of folate content, and that the only conclusion the study could claim was that dietary factors, but not necessarily folate, had a role in the etiology of NTDs.

A 1989 study conducted in California and Illinois examined three groups of patients to determine whether multivitamins had a protective effect against NTDs (39). The groups were composed of women who had a conceptus with an NTD ($N = 571$) and two control groups: those who had a stillbirth or an infant with another defect ($N = 546$), and women who had delivered a normal child ($N = 573$). In this study, NTDs included anencephaly, meningocele, myelomeningocele, encephalocele, rachischisis, iniencephaly, and lipomeningocele. The periconceptional use of multivitamins, both in terms of vitamin supplements only and when combined with fortified cereals, was then evaluated for each of the groups. The outcome of this study, after appropriate adjustment for potential confounding factors, revealed an odds ratio (OR) of 0.95 for NTD-supplemented mothers (i.e., those who received the RDA of vitamins or more) compared to unsupplemented mothers of abnormal infants, and an OR of 1.00 when the NTD group was compared to unsupplemented mothers of normal infants. Only slight differences from these values occurred when the data were evaluated by considering vitamin supplements only (no fortified cereals) or vitamin supplements of any amount (i.e., less than the RDA). Similarly, examination of the data for an effect of folate supplementation on the occurrence of NTDs did not change the results. Thus, this study could not show that the use of either multivitamin or folate supplements reduced the frequency of NTDs. However, the investigators cautioned that their results could not exclude the possibility that vitamins might be of benefit in a high-risk population. Several reasons were proposed by the authors to explain why their results differed from those obtained in other studies: (a) recall bias; (b) a declining incidence of NTDs; (c) geographic differences such that a subset of vitamin-preventable NTDs did not occur in the areas of the current study; and (d) others had not considered the vitamins contained in fortified cereals (39). However, other researchers concluded that this study lead to a null result because (a) the vitamin consumption history was obtained after delivery; (b) the history was obtained after the defect was identified; or (c) the study excluded those women taking vitamins after they knew they were pregnant (40).

In contrast to the above report, a Boston study published in 1989 found a significant effect of folic acid-containing multivitamins on the occurrence of NTDs (40). The study population comprised 22,715 women for whom complete information on vitamin consumption and pregnancy outcomes was available. Women were interviewed at the time of a maternal serum α-fetoprotein screen or an amniocentesis. Thus, in most cases, the interview was conducted before the results of the tests were known to either the patient or the interviewer. A total of 49 women had an NTD outcome (2.2/1000). Among these, three cases occurred in 107 women with a history of previous NTDs (28.0/1000), and two were in 489 women with a family history of NTDs in someone other than an offspring (4.1/1000). After excluding the 87 women whose family history of NTDs was unknown, the incidence of NTDs in the remaining women was 44 cases in 22,093 (2.0/1000). Among the 3157 women who did not use a folic acid-containing multivitamin, 11 cases of NTDs occurred, a prevalence of 3.5/1000. For those using the preparation during the first 6 weeks of pregnancy, 10 cases occurred from a total of 10,713 women (prevalence 0.9/1000). Among mothers who used vitamins during the first 6 weeks that did not contain folic acid, the prevalence was three cases in 926, a ratio of 3.2/1000. When vitamin use was started in the 7th week of gestation, there were 25 cases of NTD from 7795 mothers using the folic acid-multivitamin supplements (3.2/1000; prevalence ratio 0.92) and no cases in the

66 women who started consuming multivitamins without folate. This study, then, observed a markedly reduced risk of NTDs when folic acid-containing multivitamin preparations were consumed in the first 6 weeks of gestation.

A 1989 preliminary report of a Hungarian controlled, double-blind study evaluated the effect on congenital defects and first occurrence of NTDs of periconceptional supplementation with a multivitamin combination containing 0.8 mg folic acid compared to a trace-element supplement (controls) (41). Women were randomized to the vitamin formulation or control 1 month before through 3 months after the last menstrual period. The differences in outcome between the groups (number of subjects 1,302) were not significant. Statistical significance was obtained, however, in the final report, published in 1992 (42) with an accompanying editorial (43), where pregnancy outcome was known in 2104 vitamin-supplemented cases and 2052 controls. Significantly more congenital malformations occurred in the control group (22.9 per 1000 vs. 13.3 per 1000, $p = 0.02$), including six cases of NTDs in controls compared to none in those taking vitamins ($p = 0.029$) (42). The rate of NTD occurrence in the control group corresponded to the expected rate in Hungary (41).

In 1991, the results of an 8-year study to examine the effects of folic acid supplementation, with or without other vitamins, on the recurrence rate of NTDs was published (44). This randomized, double-blind study conducted by the British Medical Research Council (MRC) was carried out at 33 medical centers in the United Kingdom, Australia, Canada, France, Hungary, Israel, and Russia. A total of 1817 women, all of whom had a previous pregnancy affected by an NTD (anencephaly, spina bifida cystica, or encephalocele), were enrolled in the study prior to conception and randomized to one of four treatment groups: folic acid (4 mg/day) ($N = 449$), folic acid (4 mg/day) plus other vitamins ($N = 461$), other vitamins (A, D, B_1, B_2, B_6, C, and nicotinamide) ($N = 453$), and no vitamins (placebo capsules containing ferrous sulfate and dicalcium phosphate) ($N = 454$). Women with epilepsy were excluded, as were those with infants whose NTD was associated with genetic factors. Women who conceived were continued in the study until the 12th week of gestation. The study was terminated after 1195 women had a completed pregnancy where the outcome could be classified as to either NTD or no NTD, because the preventive effect of folic acid was clear. Six NTDs were observed in the two folic acid groups (6/593; 10/1000) and 21 were observed in the nonfolic acid groups (21/602; 35/1000). Analysis of the data indicated that folic acid had prevented 72% of the NTD recurrences compared to other vitamins, which gave no protective effect. The benefit of folic acid was the same for anencephaly as for spina bifida and encephalocele. The study found no evidence that any other vitamin had a protective effect, nor did other vitamins enhance the effect of folic acid. Based on the results of the study, the MRC recommended that all women who have had a previous pregnancy outcome with an NTD should take folic acid supplements. The study could not determine, however, whether 4 mg/day of folic acid was required or whether a smaller dose, such as 0.36 mg, would have been equally efficacious. They speculated, however, that even small doses should have some preventive effect.

The Centers for Disease Control and Prevention (CDC) published interim recommendations for folic acid supplementation based on the MRC study, pending further research to determine the required dose, for women who have had an infant or fetus with an NTD (spina bifida, anencephaly, or encephalocele) (45): 4 mg/day of folic acid at least 4 weeks before conception through the first 3 months of pregnancy. This supplementation was not recommended for (a) women who have never had an infant or fetus with an NTD, (b) relatives of women who have had an infant or fetus with an NTD, (c) women who themselves have spina bifida, and (d) women who take valproic acid (45). Approximately

1 year later, the CDC, in conjunction with other American health agencies, published the recommendation that all women of childbearing age should consume 0.4 mg of folic acid per day either from the diet or from supplements (46). This recommendation included women who had an NTD-affected pregnancy, unless they were planning to become pregnant. In that case, the CDC suggested that the 4-mg/day dose was still appropriate. Although the 0.4-mg dose may be as effective, the higher dose was based on a study designed to prevent NTDs, and the risks of an NTD-affected infant may be greater than the maternal risks from 4 mg/day of folic acid.

Several unanswered questions have been raised by the findings of the MRC trial, in addition to the one involving dosage, including: (a) How long before conception is supplementation needed (47)? (b) What are the risks from supplementation (47–49)? (c) If there are risks, are they the same for 4 mg and 0.4 mg (47–49)? (d) Will the benefits of supplementation be the same for all ethnic groups, even in those with much lower prevalence rates of NTDs (47)? (e) Will the benefits be as great for women who are not at an increased risk for producing a child with an NTD (47)? (f) Can the required folic acid be obtained from food (47)? (g) Is one mechanism of folic acid's action in preventing NTDs related to the correction of genetic defects, such as inborn errors of homocysteine metabolism (50)? and (h) Is folic acid itself or its metabolite, 5-methyltetrahydrofolate (MTHF), the active form of the vitamin (48,49)?

Two uncontrolled trials conducted in the United Kingdom during the MRC study described above provided additional evidence that folic acid supplementation is beneficial in preventing recurrences of NTDs (51,52). Women at high-risk for recurrence, but who refused to be enrolled in the MRC trial, primarily out of fear of being placed in the placebo group, were treated with 4 mg/day of folic acid at least 1 month prior to conception through the 12th week of gestation (51). Of the 255 women supplemented, 234 achieved a pregnancy with 235 fetuses/infants (one set of twins). Two cases of NTDs were observed (spina bifida; encephalocele), a recurrence risk of 8.5/1000, approximately one-third the expected incidence of 30/1000 and nearly identical to the results in the MRC study. In the second trial, 208 high-risk women were treated similarly, but with a multivitamin preparation containing 0.36 mg of folic acid (52). Of the 194 who had delivered (14 were still pregnant), only one NTD was observed (an incidence of 5.2/1000), and that mother admitted poor compliance in taking the vitamins.

The results of three other studies, one conducted in 12 Irish hospitals beginning in 1981 (53), one in Spain between 1974 and 1990 (54), and one in the United States and Canada from 1988 through 1991 (55,56), indicated that folic acid may be protective at a much lower dosage (e.g., 0.3 mg/day or more) than used in the MRC trial. In the American/Canadian study, folic acid (the most commonly used daily dose was 0.4 mg) consumed 28 days before through 28 days after the last menstrual period decreased the risk for first occurrence of NTDs by approximately 60% (55). The investigators also found evidence that a relatively high dietary intake of folate reduced the risk of NTDs (55).

In a search for a possible mechanism of folic acid prevention of NTDs, several studies have compared the concentrations of folic acid in mothers who have produced a child with an NTD with control mothers with no history of NTDs in their infants (57–60). A brief 1991 report found no relation between NTDs and low folate levels in fetal blood, fetal red cells, or maternal blood, thus eliminating poor placental transfer of folic acid as a possible mechanism (57).

A study conducted in Dublin found no difference in serum folate or vitamin B_{12} levels in mothers whose pregnancies ended with an NTD infant or fetus when compared to 395 normal controls (58). The serum samples were obtained during a routine screening program for rubella antibody conducted in three Dublin hospitals. After testing, the samples were frozen and then later used for this study. One hundred sixteen cases of NTDs were identified during the study period, but serum was available for only 32 of the cases: 16 with anencephalus, 15 with spina bifida, and 1 with encephalocele. In half of the cases, serum was obtained between 9 and 13 weeks' gestation. The mean serum folate concentrations in the cases and controls were both 3.4 ng/mL, and levels of vitamin B_{12} were 297 and 277 pg/mL, respectively.

Another trial found significantly lower RBC folate levels in pregnancies ending with an NTD (59). This Scottish study measured vitamin levels in 20 women younger than age 35 years who had a history of two or more NTD pregnancies. A control group of 20 women with no pregnancies ending in NTDs, but matched for age, obstetric history, and social class, was used for comparison. No significant differences between the two groups were found in assays for plasma or serum vitamin A, thiamine, riboflavin, pyridoxine, vitamin B_{12}, folate, vitamin C, vitamin E, total protein, albumin, transferrin, copper, magnesium, zinc, and white cell vitamin C. RBC folate, however, was significantly lower in the case mothers than in controls, 178 vs. 268 ng/mL ($p = 0.005$), respectively, although both were within the normal range (106–614 ng/mL). Moreover, a linear relationship was found between RBC folate and the number of NTD pregnancies. Women who had three or four such pregnancies also had the lowest concentrations of RBC folate (59). The dietary intake of folic acid was lower in the case mothers than in controls, but the difference was not statistically significant. Because the lower RBC folate levels could not be attributed entirely to dietary intake of folic acid, the authors speculated that one factor predisposing to the occurrence of NTDs may be an inherited disorder of folate metabolism (59).

A study conducted in Finland, and published in 1992, was similar in design and findings to the Dublin study described above (60). Serum samples from women who had delivered an infant with an NTD were analyzed and compared to samples from 178 matched controls. Cases of NTDs with known or suspected causes unrelated to vitamins were excluded. Maternal serum had been drawn during the first or second prenatal care appointment for reasons not related to the study, all within 8 weeks of neural tube closure, and kept frozen in a central laboratory. No statistical differences were found between case mothers and controls in serum levels of folate, vitamin B_{12}, and retinol. After adjustment, the odds ratios for being a case mother were 1.00 for folate, 1.05 for vitamin B_{12}, 0.99 for retinol. Several possible explanations have been offered as to why this study was unable to find differences between case and control mothers (61): (a) serum samples may not have been obtained early enough in pregnancy; (b) maternal serum vitamin concentrations may not be a good test of the folic acid deficiency necessary to cause NTDs; and, most likely, (c) the group tested may not have been at risk to have a vitamin-sensitive NTD since the normal incidence of NTDs in the studied population is very low.

At least three publications have commented on the potential risks of high-dose folic acid supplementation (45,62,63). Megaloblastic anemia resulting from vitamin B_{12} deficiency may be masked by folic acid doses of 4 mg/day but still allow the neurologic damage of the deficiency to progress (45,62). Responding to this, a Canadian editorial recommended that a woman's vitamin B_{12} status be checked prior to commencing high-dose folic acid supplementation (62). A second risk identified concerned the inhibition of dihydropteridine reductase (DHPR), a key enzyme in the maintenance of tetrahydrobiopterin levels, by folic acid but not by 5-methyltetrahydrofolate (63). Children with an inherited deficiency of this enzyme have lowered levels of dopamine, noradrenaline, serotonin, and folates in the central nervous system, which results in gross neurologic damage and death if untreated, thus raising the potential that high-dose folic acid could cause damage to embryonic neural tissue.

Folic acid deficiency is a known experimental animal teratogen (64). In humans, the relationship between fetal defects other than NTDs and folate deficiency is less clear. Several reports have claimed an increase in congenital malformations associated with low levels of this vitamin (9,24–26,33,36,65,66), and one study observed a significant decrease in birth defects when a multivitamin-folic acid preparation was used before and during early gestation (see details above) (42). Other investigators have stated that maternal deficiency does not result in fetal anomalies (22,23,67–73). One study found the folate status of mothers giving birth to severely malformed fetuses to be no different from that of the general obstetric population and much better than that of mothers with overt megaloblastic anemia (67). Similar results were found in other series (71–73).

The strongest evidence for an association between folic acid and fetal defects comes from cases treated with drugs that either are folic acid antagonists or induce folic acid deficiency, although agreement with the latter is not universal (70,74,75). The folic acid antagonists, aminopterin and methotrexate, are known teratogens (see Aminopterin and Methotrexate). A very high incidence of defects resulted when aminopterin was used as an unsuccessful abortifacient in the 1st trimester. These antineoplastic agents may cause fetal injury by blocking the conversion of folic acid to tetrahydrofolic acid in both the fetus and the mother.

In contrast, certain anticonvulsants, such as phenytoin and phenobarbital, induce maternal folic acid deficiency, possibly by impairing gastrointestinal absorption or increasing hepatic metabolism of the vitamin (70,74,75). Whether these agents also induce folic acid deficiency in the fetus is less certain, because the fetus seems to be efficient in drawing on available maternal stores of folic acid. Low maternal folate levels, however, have been proposed as a mechanism for the increased incidence of defects observed in infants exposed *in utero* to some anticonvulsants. In a 1984 article, investigators reported research on the relationship between folic acid, anticonvulsants, and fetal defects (74). In the retrospective part of this study, a group of 24 women who were treated with phenytoin and other anticonvulsants produced 66 infants, of whom 10 (15%) had major anomalies. Two of the mothers with affected infants had markedly low RBC folate concentrations. A second group of 22 epileptic women was then given supplements of daily folic acid, 2.5–5.0 mg, starting before conception in 26 pregnancies and within the first 40 days in 6 pregnancies. This group produced 33 newborns (32 pregnancies, 1 set of twins) with no defects, a significant difference from the group not receiving supplementation. Negative associations between anticonvulsant-induced folate deficiency and birth defects have also been reported (70,75). Investigators studied a group of epileptic women taking anticonvulsants and observed only two defects (2.9%) in pregnancies producing a live baby, a rate similar to that expected in a healthy population (70). Although folate levels were not measured in this retrospective survey, maternal folate deficiency was predicted by the authors, based on their current research with folic acid in patients taking anticonvulsants. Another group of researchers observed 20 infants (15%) with defects from 133 women taking anticonvulsants (75). No NTDs were found, but this defect is rare in Finland and an increase in the anomaly could have been missed (75). All of the women were given folate supplements of 0.1–1.0 mg/day (average 0.5 mg/day) from the 6th to 16th weeks of gestation until delivery. Folate levels were usually within the normal range (normal considered to be serum >1.8 ng/mL, RBC >203 ng/mL).

Whole-embryo cultures of rats have been tested with valproic acid and folinic acid, a folic acid derivative (76). The anticonvulsant produced a dose-related increase in the incidence of NTDs that was not prevented by the addition of the vitamin. Experiments in embryonic mice, however, indicated that valproic acid-induced NTDs were related to interference with embryonic folate metabolism (77). Teratogenic doses of valproic acid caused a significant reduction in embryonic levels of formylated tetrahydrofolates and increased the levels of tetrahydrofolate by inhibition of the enzyme glutamate formyltransferase. The result of this inhibition would have serious consequences on embryonic development, including neural tube closure (77).

A review of teratogenic mechanisms involving folic acid and antiepileptic therapy was published in 1992 (78). Several studies conducted by the authors and others demonstrated that phenytoin, phenobarbital, and primidone, but not carbamazepine or valproic acid, significantly reduced serum and RBC levels of folate, and that polytherapy decreased these levels significantly more than monotherapy. Animal studies cited indicated that valproic acid disrupts folic acid metabolism, possibly by inhibiting key enzymes, rather than by lowering concentrations of the vitamin, whereas phenytoin may act on folic acid by both mechanisms (78). Data from a study conducted by the authors indicated that a significant association existed between low serum and RBC folate levels, especially <4 ng/mL, before or early in pregnancy in epileptic women and spontaneous abortions and the occurrence of congenital malformations (78). The reviewers concluded that folic acid supplementation may be effective in preventing some poor pregnancy outcomes in epileptic women.

Another 1992 report, based on the results of a 1990 workshop addressing the use of antiepileptic drugs during pregnancy, offered guidelines to counsel women with epilepsy who plan pregnancy or who are pregnant (79). Included among the guidelines was the recommendation that adequate folic acid be consumed daily, either from the diet or from supplements, to maintain normal serum and RBC levels of folate before and during the first months of pregnancy (i.e., during organogenesis). A specific folic acid dose was not recommended.

Placental Abruption

Several articles have proposed that maternal folic acid status is associated with placental abruption (25,26,28,66,80). In a review and analysis of 506 consecutive cases of abruptio placentae, defective folate metabolism was found as a predisposing factor in 97.5%. The authors theorized that folic acid deficiency early in pregnancy caused irreversible damage to the fetus, chorion, and decidua, leading to abruption, abortion, premature delivery, low birth weight, and fetal malformations. Other studies have discovered that 60% of their patients with abruption were folate deficient, but their numbers were too small for statistical analysis (81). In other series, no correlation was found between low levels of folic acid and this complication (16,69,82).

Gestation Hypertension

A relationship between folate deficiency and GHTN is doubtful. In a study of women with megaloblastic anemia, 14% had GHTN compared with the predicted incidence of 6% for that population (22). In another report, 22 (61%) of 36 GHTN patients had folate deficiency, but the authors were unable to conclude that the association was causative (66,81). Other investigators have also failed to find a relationship between low levels of the vitamin and GHTN (23,27). In one of these studies, the incidence of GHTN in megaloblastic anemia was 12.2%, compared with 14.0% in normoblastic anemia (27). A second group of investigators studied folate levels in 101 preeclamptic and 17 eclamptic women and compared them with 52 normal controls and 29 women with overt megaloblastic anemia (83). No correlation was found between levels of folic acid and the complications.

Abortions and Placenta Previa

Several papers have associated folic acid deficiency with abortion (25,26,66,78,80, 84–86). The cause of some abortions, as proposed by some, is faulty folate metabolism in early pregnancy, producing irreversible injury to the fetus and placenta (80). Others have been unable to detect any significant relationship between serum and RBC folate levels and abortion (12,68,87). In a series of 66 patients with early spontaneous abortions, the incidence of folate deficiency was the same as in those with uncomplicated pregnancies (87). These researchers did find a relationship between low folic acid levels and placenta previa. However, others found no evidence of an association between folate deficiency and either abortion or antepartum hemorrhage (12).

Low Birth Weight and Prematurity

The relationship between prematurity, low birth weight, and folic acid levels has been investigated. In one study, significantly lower folate levels were measured in the blood of low-birth-weight neonates as compared with normal-weight infants (18). In a 1960 report, the incidences of both premature delivery and infants with a birth weight less than 2500 g were increased in folate-deficient mothers (22). These patients all had severe megaloblastic anemia and a poor standard of nutrition. In a later study of 510 infants from folate-deficient mothers, 276 (56%) weighed 2500 g or less, compared with a predicted incidence of 8.6% (80). A study of women with uterine bleeding during pregnancy found a significant association between serum folate and low birth weight (85). Similarly, another study reported a significant relationship between folate levels at the end of the 2nd trimester and newborn birth weight (88). A 1992 report described the effects of supplementation with ferrous sulfate (325 mg/day) and folic acid (1 mg/day), beginning at the first prenatal visit, on infant birth weight (89). A significant association between low serum folate levels at 30 weeks' gestation and fetal growth retardation (defined as below the 15th percentile for gestational age) was discovered. Adjustment for psychosocial status, maternal race, body mass index, smoking history, history of a low-birth-weight infant, and infant gender did not change the results. In contrast, others have found no association between folic acid deficiency and prematurity (27,69,90,91) or between serum folate and birth weight (12,69,92,93).

Two reports have alluded to problems with high folic acid levels in the mother during pregnancy (94,95). An isolated case report described an anencephalic fetus whose mother was under psychiatric care (94). She had been treated with very high doses of folic acid and vitamins B_1, B_6, and C. The relationship between the vitamins and the defect is questionable. A 1984 study examined the effect of folic acid, zinc, and other nutrients on pregnancy outcome (95). Total complications of pregnancy (infection, bleeding, fetal distress, prematurity or death, pregnancy-induced hypertension, and tissue fragility) were associated with high serum folate and low serum zinc levels. The explanation offered for these surprising findings was that folate inhibits intestinal absorption of zinc, which, they proposed, was responsible for the complications. This study also found an association between low folate and abortion.

Summary

Folic acid deficiency during pregnancy is a common problem in undernourished women and in women not receiving supplements. The relationship between folic acid levels and various maternal or fetal complications is complex. Evidence has accumulated that interference with folic acid metabolism or folate deficiency induced by drugs such as anticonvulsants and some antineoplastics that occurs early in pregnancy results in congenital anomalies. Moreover, a substantial body of evidence is now available that non-drug-induced folic acid deficiency, or abnormal folate metabolism, is related to the occurrence of birth defects and some NTDs. Lack of the vitamin or its metabolites may also be responsible for some cases of spontaneous abortion and intrauterine growth retardation. For other complications, it is probable that a number of factors, of which folic acid deficiency may be one, contribute to poor pregnancy outcome. Thus, to ensure good maternal and fetal health, all pregnant women should receive sufficient dietary or supplementary folic acid to maintain normal maternal folate levels. The CDC and other U.S. health agencies recommend a daily consumption of 0.4 mg of folic acid, from either the diet or supplements or both, for all women of childbearing age before the onset of pregnancy (46,96).

An increased risk of adverse fetal outcome can be lowered by folic acid supplementation in at least two groups of women: (a) Women with a history of a fetus or infant with an NTD should receive supplementation with 4 mg/day of folic acid beginning 1 month (3 months have been recommended in England [97]) before conception and continuing through the 12th week of gestation (45,97,98). (b) Women receiving antiepileptic medications should receive sufficient folic acid from either the diet or supplementation or both to maintain normal serum and RBC levels of the vitamin beginning before conception through the period of organogenesis. (A specific dosage recommendation has not been located for women receiving anticonvulsants.)

[*Risk Factor C if used in doses above the RDA.*]

BREAST FEEDING SUMMARY

RECOMMENDATION: Compatible

Folic acid is actively excreted into breast milk (99–108). Accumulation of folate in milk takes precedence over maternal folate needs (99). Levels of folic acid are relatively low in colostrum but as lactation proceeds, concentrations of the vitamin rise (100–102). Folate levels in newborns and breast-fed infants are consistently higher than those in mothers and normal adults (103,104). In Japanese mothers, mean breast milk folate concentrations were 141.4 ng/mL, resulting in a total intake by the infant of 14–25 μg/kg/day (104). Much lower mean levels were measured in pooled human milk in an English study examining preterm (26 mothers, 29–34 weeks) and term (35 mothers, 39 weeks or longer) patients (102). Preterm milk folate concentrations rose from 10.6 ng/mL (colostrum) to 30.5 ng/mL (16–196 days), whereas term milk folate concentrations increased during the same period from 17.6 to 42.3 ng/mL.

Supplementation with folic acid is apparently not needed in mothers with good nutritional habits (102–106). Folic acid deficiency and megaloblastic anemia did not develop in women not receiving supplements even when lactation exceeded I year (102,103). In another study, maternal serum and red blood cell folate levels increased significantly after 1 mg of folic acid/day for 4 weeks, but milk folate levels remained unchanged (104). Investigators gave well-nourished lactating women a multivitamin preparation containing 0.8 mg of folic acid (105). At 6 months postpartum, milk concentrations of folate did not differ significantly from those of controls who were not receiving supplements. Other investigators measured more than adequate blood folate levels in American breast-fed infants during the 1st year of life (106). The mean milk concentration of folate consumed by these infants was 85 ng/mL.

In patients with poor nutrition, lactation may lead to severe maternal folic acid deficiency and megaloblastic anemia (99). For these patients, there is evidence that low folate levels, as part of the total nutritional status of the mother, are related to the length of the lactation period (102). In one study, lactating mothers with megaloblastic anemia were treated with 5 mg/day of folic acid for 3 days (101). Breast milk folate rose from 7–9 ng/mL to 15–40 ng/mL 1 day after treatment began. The elevated levels were maintained for 3 weeks without further treatment. Nine lower-socioeconomic-status women were treated with multivitamins containing 0.8 mg of folic acid and were compared with seven untreated controls (107). Breast milk folate was significantly higher in the treated women. In another study of lactating women with low nutritional status, supplementation with folic acid, 0.2–10.0 mg/day, resulted in mean milk concentrations of 2.3–5.6 ng/mL (108). Milk concentrations were directly proportional to dietary intake.

Folic acid concentrations were determined in preterm and term milk in a study to determine the effect of storage time and temperature (109). Storage of milk in a freezer resulted in progressive decreases over 3 months such that the RDA of folate for infants could not be provided from milk stored for this length of time. Storage in a refrigerator for 24 hours did not affect folate levels.

The National Academy of Sciences' RDA for folic acid during lactation is 0.280 mg (1). If the lactating woman's diet adequately supplies this amount, maternal supplementation with folic acid is not needed. Maternal supplementation with the RDA for folic acid is recommended for those patients with inadequate nutritional intake. The American Academy of Pediatrics considers maternal consumption of folic acid to be compatible with breast-feeding (110).

References

1. American Hospital Formulary Service. *Drug Information 1997*. Bethesda, MD: American Society of Health-System Pharmacists, 1997:2809–11.
2. Herbert V. Recommended dietary intakes (RDI) of folate in humans. Am J Clin Nutr 1987;45:661–70.
3. Frank O, Walbroehl G, Thomson A, Kaminetzky H, Kubes Z, Baker H. Placental transfer: fetal retention of some vitamins. Am J Clin Nutr 1970;23:662–3.
4. Kaminetzky HA, Baker H, Frank O, Langer A. The effects of intravenously administered water-soluble vitamins during labor in normovitaminemic and hypovitaminemic gravidas on maternal and neonatal blood vitamin levels at delivery. Am J Obstet Gynecol 1974;120:697–703.
5. Hill EP, Longo LD. Dynamics of maternal-fetal nutrient transfer. Fed Proc 1980;39:239–44.
6. Baker H, Frank O, Deangelis B, Feingold S, Kaminetzky HA. Role of placenta in maternal-fetal vitamin transfer in humans. Am J Obstet Gynecol 1981;141:792–6.
7. Landon MJ, Eyre DH, Hytten FE. Transfer of folate to the fetus. Br J Obstet Gynaecol 1975;82:12–9.
8. Baker H, Frank O, Thomason AD, Langer A, Munves ED, De Angelis B, Kaminetzky HA. Vitamin profile of 174 mothers and newborns at parturition. Am J Clin Nutr 1975;28:59–65.
9. Kaminetzky HA, Baker H. Micronutrients in pregnancy. Clin Obstet Gynecol 1977;20:263–80.
10. Dostalova L. Correlation of the vitamin status between mother and newborn during delivery. *Dev Pharmacol Ther* 1982;4(Suppl 1):45–57.
11. Bruinse HW, Berg HVD, Haspels AA. Maternal serum folacin levels during and after normal pregnancy. Eur J Obstet Gynecol Reprod Biol 1985;20:153–8.
12. Chanarin I, Rothman D, Ward A, Perry J. Folate status and requirement in pregnancy. Br Med J 1968;2:390–4.
13. Ball EW, Giles C. Folic acid and vitamin B_{12} levels in pregnancy and their relation to megaloblastic anemia. J Clin Pathol 1964;17:165–74.
14. Ek J, Magnus EM. Plasma and red blood cell folate during normal pregnancies. Acta Obstet Gynecol Scand 1981;60:247–51.
15. Baker H, Ziffer H, Pasher I, Sobotka H. A Comparison of maternal and foetal folic acid and vitamin B_{12} at parturition. Br Med J 1958;1:978–9.
16. Avery B, Ledger WJ. Folic acid metabolism in well-nourished pregnant women. Obstet Gynecol 1970;35:616–24.
17. Ek J. Plasma and red cell folate values in newborn infants and their mothers in relation to gestational age. J Pediatr 1980;97:288–92.
18. Baker H, Thind IS, Frank O, DeAngelis B, Caterini H, Liquria DB. Vitamin levels in low-birth-weight newborn infants and their mothers. Am J Obstet Gynecol 1977;129:521–4.
19. Horn E. Iron and folate supplements during pregnancy: supplementing everyone treats those at risk and is cost effective. BMJ 1988;297:1325, 1327.
20. Hibbard BM. Iron and folate supplements during pregnancy: supplementation is valuable only in selected patients. BMJ 1988;297:1324, 1326.
21. Chanarin I, MacGibbon BM, O'Sullivan WJ, Mollin DL. Folic-acid deficiency in pregnancy: the pathogenesis of megaloblastic anaemia of pregnancy. Lancet 1959;2:634–9.
22. Gatenby PBB, Lillie EW. Clinical analysis of 100 cases of severe megaloblastic anaemia of pregnancy. Br Med J 1960;2:1111–4.
23. Pritchard JA, Mason RA, Wright MR. Megaloblastic anemia during pregnancy and the puerperium. Am J Obstet Gynecol 1962;83:1004–20.
24. Fraser JL, Watt HJ. Megaloblastic anemia in

pregnancy and the puerperium. Am J Obstet Gynecol 1964;89:532–4.
25. Hibbard BM. The role of folic acid in pregnancy: with particular reference to anaemia, abruption and abortion. J Obstet Gynaecol Br Commonw 1964;71: 529–42.
26. Hibbard BM, Hibbard ED, Jeffcoate TNA. Folic acid and reproduction. Acta Obstet Gynecol Scand 1965;44:375–400.
27. Giles C. An account of 335 cases of megaloblastic anaemia of pregnancy and the puerperium. J Clin Pathol 1966;19:1–11.
28. Streiff RR, Little AB. Folic acid deficiency in pregnancy. N Engl J Med 1967;276:776–9.
29. Pritchard JA, Scott DE, Whalley PJ. Folic acid requirements in pregnancy-induced megaloblastic anemia. JAMA 1969;208:1163–7.
30. Rothman D. Folic acid in pregnancy. Am J Obstet Gynecol 1970;108:149–75.
31. Solano FX Jr, Councell RB. Folate deficiency presenting as pancytopenia in pregnancy. Am J Obstet Gynecol 1986;154:1117–8.
32. Leung CF, Lao TT, Chang AMZ. Effect of folate supplement on pregnant women with beta-thalassaemia minor. Eur J Obstet Gynecol Reprod Biol 1989;33:209–13.
33. Laurence KM, James N, Miller MH, Tennant GB, Campbell H. Double-blind randomised controlled trial of folate treatment before conception to prevent recurrence of neural tube defects. Br Med J 1981;282:1509–11.
34. Smithells RW, Sheppard S, Schorah CJ. Vitamin deficiencies and neural tube defects. Arch Dis Child 1976;51:944–50.
35. Schorah CJ, Smithells RW, Scott J. Vitamin B_{12} and anencephaly. Lancet 1980;1:880.
36. Nelson MM, Forfar JO. Associations between drugs administered during pregnancy and congenital abnormalities of the fetus. Br Med J 1971;1:523–7.
37. Bower C, Stanley FJ. Dietary folate as a risk factor for neural-tube defects: evidence from a case-control study in Western Australia. Med J Aust 1989; 150:613–9.
38. Mann J. Dietary folate and neural-tube defects. Med J Aust 1989;150:609.
39. Mills JL, Rhoads GG, Simpson JL, Cunningham GC, Conley MR, Lassman MR, Walden ME, Depp OR, Hoffman HJ. The absence of a relation between the periconceptional use of vitamins and neural-tube defects. N Engl J Med 1989;321:430–5.
40. Milunsky A, Jick H, Jick SS, Bruell CL, MacLaughlin DS, Rothman KJ, Willett W. Multivitamin/folic acid supplementation in early pregnancy reduces the prevalence of neural tube defects. JAMA 1989; 262:2847–2852.
41. Czeizel A, Fritz G. Letter to the editor. JAMA 1989;262:1634.
42. Czeizel AE, Dudás I. Prevention of the first occurrence of neural-tube defects by periconceptional vitamin supplementation. N Engl J Med 1992;327:1832–5.
43. Rosenberg IH. Editorial. Folic acid and neural-tube defects—time for action? N Engl J Med 1992;327:1875–7.
44. MRC Vitamin Study Research Group. Prevention of neural tube defects: results of the Medical Research Council vitamin study. Lancet 1991;338: 131–7.
45. CDC. Use of folic acid for prevention of spina bifida and other neural tube defects—1983–1991. MMWR 1991;40:513–6.
46. CDC. Recommendations for the use of folic acid to reduce the number of cases of spina bifida and other neural tube defects. MMWR 1992;41(RR-14):1–7.
47. Anonymous. Folic acid and neural tube defects. Lancet 1991;338:153–4.
48. Scott JM, Kirke P, O'Broin S, Weir DG. Folic acid to prevent neural tube defects. Lancet 1991;338:505.
49. Lucock MD, Wild J, Hartley R, Levene MI, Schorah CJ. Vitamins to prevent neural tube defects. Lancet 1991;338:894–5.
50. Steegers-Theunissen RPM, Boers GHJ, Trijbels FJM, Eskes TKAB. Neural-tube defects and derangement of homocysteine metabolism. N Engl J Med 1991; 324:199–200.
51. Laurence KM. Folic acid to prevent neural tube defects. Lancet 1991;338:379.
52. Super M, Summers EM, Meylan B. Preventing neural tube defects. Lancet 1991;338:755–6.
53. Kirke PN, Daly LE, Elwood JH for the Irish Vitamin Study Group. A randomised trial of low dose folic acid to prevent neural tube defects. Arch Dis Child 1992;67:1442–6.
54. Martinez-Frias M-L, Rodriguez-Pinilla E. Folic acid supplementation and neural tube defects. Lancet 1992;340:620.
55. Werler MM, Shapiro S, Mitchell AA. Periconceptional folic acid exposure and risk of occurrent neural tube defects. JAMA 1993;269:1257–61.
56. Oakley GP Jr. Folic acid - preventable spina bifida and anencephaly (editorial). JAMA 1993;269:1292–3.
57. Holzgreve W, Tercanli S, Pietrzik K. Vitamins to prevent neural tube defects. Lancet 1991;338:639–40.
58. Molloy AM, Kirke P, Hillary I, Weir DG, Scott JM. Maternal serum folate and vitamin B_{12} concentrations in pregnancies associated with neural tube defects. Arch Dis Child 1985;60:660–5.
59. Yates JRW, Ferguson-Smith MA, Shenkin A, Guzman-Rodriguez R, White M, Clark BJ. Is disordered folate metabolism the basis for the genetic predisposition to neural tube defects? Clin Genet 1987;31:279–87.
60. Mills JL, Tuomilehto J, Yu KF, Colman N, Blaner WS, Koskela P, Rundle WE, Forman M, Tolvanen L, Rhoads GG. Maternal vitamin levels during pregnancies producing infants with neural tube defects. J Pediatr 1992;120:863–71.
61. Holmes LB. Prevention of neural tube defects (editorial). J Pediatr 1992;120:918–9.
62. Glanville NT, Cook HW. Folic acid and prevention of neural tube defects. CMAJ 1992;146:39.
63. Leeming RJ, Blair JA, Brown SE. Vitamins to prevent neural tube defects. Lancet 1991;338:895.
64. Shepard TH. *Catalog of Teratogenic Agents*. 6th ed. Baltimore, MD: Johns Hopkins University Press, 1989:285–8.
65. Hibbard ED, Smithells RW. Folic acid metabolism and human embryopathy. Lancet 1965;1:1254.
66. Stone ML. Effects on the fetus of folic acid deficiency in pregnancy. Clin Obstet Gynecol 1968;11: 1143–53.

F

67. Scott DE, Whalley PJ, Pritchard JA. Maternal folate deficiency and pregnancy wastage. II. Fetal malformation. Obstet Gynecol 1970;36:26–8.
68. Pritchard JA, Scott DE, Whalley PJ, Haling RF Jr. Infants of mothers with megaloblastic anemia due to folate deficiency. JAMA 1970;211:1982–4.
69. Kitay DZ, Hogan WJ, Eberle B, Mynt T. Neutrophil hypersegmentation and folic acid deficiency in pregnancy. Am J Obstet Gynecol 1969;104:1163–73.
70. Pritchard JA, Scott DE, Whalley PJ. Maternal folate deficiency and pregnancy wastage. IV. Effects of folic acid supplements, anticonvulsants, and oral contraceptives. Am J Obstet Gynecol 1971;109:341–6.
71. Emery AEH, Timson J, Watson-Williams EJ. Pathogenesis of spina bifida. Lancet 1969;2:909–10.
72. Hall MH. Folates and the fetus. Lancet 1977;1:648–9.
73. Emery AEH. Folates and fetal central-nervous-system malformations. Lancet 1977;1:703.
74. Biale Y, Lewenthal H. Effect of folic acid supplementation on congenital malformations due to anticonvulsive drugs. Eur J Obstet Gynecol Reprod Biol 1984;18:211–6.
75. Hiilesmaa VK, Teramo K, Granstrom M-L, Bardy AH. Serum folate concentrations during pregnancy in women with epilepsy: relation to antiepileptic drug concentrations, number of seizures, and fetal outcome. Br Med J 1983;287:577–9.
76. Hansen DK, Grafton TF. Lack of attenuation of valproic acid-induced effects by folinic acid in rat embryos in vitro. Teratology 1991;43:575–82.
77. Wegner C, Nau H. Alteration of embryonic folate metabolism by valproic acid during organogenesis: implications for mechanism of teratogenesis. Neurology 1992;42(Suppl 5):17–24.
78. Dansky LV, Rosenblatt DS, Andermann E. Mechanisms of teratogenesis: folic acid and antiepileptic therapy. Neurology 1992;42(Suppl 5):32–42.
79. Delgado-Escueta AV, Janz D. Consensus guidelines: preconception counseling, management, and care of the pregnant woman with epilepsy. Neurology 1992;42(Suppl 5):149–60.
80. Hibbard BM, Jeffcoate TNA. Abruptioplacentae. Obstet Gynecol 1966;27:155–67.
81. Stone ML, Luhby AL, Feldman R, Gordon M, Cooperman JM. Folic acid metabolism in pregnancy. Am J Obstet Gynecol 1967;99:638–48.
82. Whalley PJ, Scott DE, Pritchard JA. Maternal folate deficiency and pregnancy wastage. I. Placental abruption. Am J Obstet Gynecol 1969;105:670–8.
83. Whalley PJ, Scott DE, Pritchard JA. Maternal folate deficiency and pregnancy wastage. III. Pregnancy-induced hypertension. Obstet Gynecol 1970;36:29–31.
84. Martin JD, Davis RE. Serum folic acid activity and vaginal bleeding in early pregnancy. J Obstet Gynaecol Br Commonw 1964;71:400–3.
85. Martin RH, Harper TA, Kelso W. Serum-folic-acid in recurrent abortions. Lancet 1965;1:670–2.
86. Martin JD, Davis RE, Stenhouse N. Serum folate and vitamin B12 levels in pregnancy with particular reference to uterine bleeding and bacteriuria. J Obstet Gynaecol Br Commonw 1967;74:697–701.
87. Streiff RR, Little B. Folic acid deficiency as a cause of uterine hemorrhage in pregnancy. J Clin Invest 1965;44:1102.
88. Whiteside MG, Ungar B, Cowling DC. Iron, folic acid and vitamin B_{12} levels in normal pregnancy, and their influence on birth-weight and the duration of pregnancy. Med J Aust 1968;1:338–42.
89. Goldenberg RL, Tamura T, Cliver SP, Cutter GR, Hoffman HJ, Copper RL. Serum folate and fetal growth retardation: a matter of compliance? Obstet Gynecol 1992;79:719–22.
90. Husain OAN, Rothman D, Ellis L. Folic acid deficiency in pregnancy. J Obstet Gynaecol Br Commonw 1963;70:821–7.
91. Abramowicz M, Kass EH. Pathogenesis and prognosis of prematurity (continued). N Engl J Med 1966;275:938–43.
92. Scott KE, Usher R. Fetal malnutrition: its incidence, causes, and effects. Am J Obstet Gynecol 1966;94:951–63.
93. Varadi S, Abbott D, Elwis A. Correlation of peripheral white cell and bone marrow changes with folate levels in pregnancy and their clinical significance. J Clin Pathol 1966;19:33–6.
94. Averback P. Anencephaly associated with megavitamin therapy. Can Med Assoc J 1976;114:995.
95. Mukherjee MD, Sandstead HH, Ratnaparkhi MV, Johnson LK, Milne DB, Stelling HP. Maternal zinc, iron, folic acid, and protein nutriture and outcome of human pregnancy. Am J Clin Nutr 1984;40:496–507.
96. CDC. Recommendations for use of folic acid to reduce number of spina bifida cases and other neural tube defects. MMWR 1992;41(RR-14):1–7. As cited in Anonymous. From the Centers for Disease Control and Prevention. JAMA 1993;269:1233, 1236, 1238.
97. Hibbard BM. Folates and fetal development. Br J Obstet Gynaecol 1993;100:307–9.
98. Committee on Obstetrics: Maternal and Fetal Medicine. American College of Obstetrics and Gynecology. Folic acid for the prevention of recurrent neural tube defects. No. 120. March 1993.
99. Metz J. Folate deficiency conditioned by lactation. Am J Clin Nutr 1970;23:843–7.
100. Cooperman JM, Dweck HS, Newman LJ, Garbarino C, Lopez R. The folate in human milk. Am J Clin Nutr 1982;36:576–80.
101. Ford JE, Zechalko A, Murphy J, Brooke OG. Comparison of the B vitamin composition of milk from mothers of preterm and term babies. Arch Dis Child 1983;58:367–72.
102. Ek J. Plasma, red cell, and breast milk folacin concentrations in lactating women. Am J Clin Nutr 1983;38:929–35.
103. Ek J, Magnus EM. Plasma and red blood cell folate in breastfed infants. Acta Paediatr Scand 1979;68:239–43.
104. Tamura T, Yoshimura Y, Arakawa T. Human milk folate and folate status in lactating mothers and their infants. Am J Clin Nutr 1980;33:193–7.
105. Thomas MR, Sneed SM, Wei C, Nail PA, Wilson M, Sprinkle EE III. The effects of vitamin C, vitamin B_6, vitamin B_{12}, folic acid, riboflavin, and thiamine on the breast milk and maternal status of well-nourished

women at 6 months postpartum. Am J Clin Nutr 1980;33:2151–6.
106. Smith AM, Picciano MF, Deering RH. Folate intake and blood concentrations of term infants. Am J Clin Nutr 1985;41:590–8.
107. Sneed SM, Zane C, Thomas MR. The effects of ascorbic acid, vitamin B_6, vitamin B_{12}, and folic acid supplementation on the breast milk and maternal nutritional status of low socioeconomic lactating women. Am J Clin Nutr 1981;34:1338–46.
108. Deodhar AD, Rajalakshmi R, Ramakrishnan CV. Studies on human lactation. Part III. Effect of dietary vitamin supplementation on vitamin contents of breast milk. Acta Paediatr 1964;53:42–8.
109. Bank MR, Kirksey A, West K, Giacoia G. Effect of storage time and temperature on folacin and vitamin C levels in term and preterm human milk. Am J Clin Nutr 1985;41:235–42.
110. Committee on Drugs, American Academy of Pediatrics. The transfer of drugs and other chemicals into human milk. Pediatrics 2001;108:776–89.

Name: **FOMEPIZOLE** Risk Factor: C_M
Class: **Antidote**

FETAL RISK SUMMARY

RECOMMENDATION: Compatible - Maternal Benefit >> Embryo/Fetal Risk

Fomepizole, given IV every 12 hours for 48 hours or longer, is a competitive inhibitor of alcohol dehydrogenase, an enzyme that catalyzes the oxidation of alcohol to acetaldehyde. The enzyme also catalyzes the initial steps in the metabolism of ethylene glycol and methanol to their toxic metabolites. Fomepizole is indicated as an antidote for ethylene glycol (such as antifreeze or coolants) or methanol ingestion. It undergoes extensive metabolism to inactive metabolites. The elimination half-life has not been determined (1).

According to the manufacturer, animal reproduction studies have not been conducted with fomepizole. One source cited a 1982 abstract, however, that reported that the drug was not teratogenic in mice (2).

It is not known if fomepizole crosses the human placenta to the embryo or fetus. The very low molecular weight (about 82), however, suggests that the drug will cross the placenta.

Only one report describing the use of fomepizole in human pregnancy has been located. A 21-year-old woman at 11 weeks' gestation in her second pregnancy was treated with fomepizole (two doses of 15 mg IV over 30 minutes, approximately 8 hours apart) for inhalation of carburetor cleaner (3). The cleaner contained a mixture of methanol, toluene, methylene chloride, and carbon dioxide. Her history included chronic abuse of toluene and inhalants. After release from the hospital, she was again admitted for the same problem about 6 weeks later and was treated with one dose of fomepizole. Attempts to contact the patient after discharge were unsuccessful and the eventual outcome of the pregnancy was unknown (3).

Other than the above case, no other human pregnancy experience is available. Although an assessment of the risk this agent presents to a human embryo or fetus cannot be made, the maternal benefits should far outweigh the unknown fetal risks. Therefore, the drug should not be withheld because of pregnancy (4).

BREAST FEEDING SUMMARY

RECOMMENDATION: Hold Breast Feeding

No reports describing the use of fomepizole during human lactation have been located. The very low molecular weight (about 82), however, suggests that the drug will be excreted into breast milk. The effects of this exposure on a nursing infant are unknown (the most common adverse effects in patients and normal volunteers were headache, nausea, dizziness, and bad taste/metallic taste [1]). Because the maternal benefits of therapy are great, breast-feeding should be temporarily discontinued, at least until the therapy is completed and the drug eliminated from the maternal system. The time required to eliminate the drug is unknown, but waiting for 24 hours would allow for nearly complete elimination if the half-life were 5 hours or less. Moreover, fomepizole is extensively metabolized to inactive metabolites and this will serve to lessen infant exposure.

F

References

1. Product information. Antizol. Orphan Medical, 2000.
2. Giknis MLA, Damjanov I. The effects of pyrazole and its derivatives on the transplacental embryotoxicity of ethanol. Teratology 1982;25:43A–4A. As cited by Schardein JL. *Chemically Induced Birth Defects*. 3rd Ed. New York, NY: Marcel Dekker, 2000:633.
3. Velez LI, Kulstad E, Shepherd G, Roth B. Inhalational methanol toxicity in pregnancy treated twice with fomepizole. Vet Hum Toxicol 2003;45:28–30.
4. Bailey B. Are there teratogenic risks associated with antidotes used in the acute management of poisoned pregnant women? Birth Defects Res Part A Clin Mol Teratol 2003;67:133–40.

Name:	**FONDAPARINUX**	Risk Factor:	$\mathbf{B_M}$
Class:	**Anticoagulant**		

FETAL RISK SUMMARY

RECOMMENDATION: No Human Data - Animal Data Suggest Low Risk

Fondaparinux is a synthetic selective inhibitor of activated factor X (Xa) that is administered by SC injection. The drug is indicated for the prophylaxis of deep vein thrombosis in patients undergoing hip fracture, hip replacement, or knee replacement surgery. Distribution to extravascular fluid is characterized as minor. The drug is extensively (at least 94%) and specifically bound to antithrombin III but not to other plasma proteins or red blood cells. The binding to antithrombin III significantly potentiates the neutralization of factor Xa by antithrombin III. Fondaparinux has no effect on thrombin or platelet function. The metabolism of fondaparinux has not been investigated, but most of a dose is excreted unchanged in the urine. The drug is contraindicated in patients who weigh less than 50 kg because total clearance in this group is reduced by approximately 30% (1).

Reproduction studies in pregnant rats and rabbits at SC doses up to 32 and 65 times the recommended human dose based on body surface area, respectively, revealed no evidence of impaired fertility or fetal harm (1).

Fondaparinux did not cross the placenta in an *in vitro* human dually perfused cotyledon model using placentas from six healthy white women approximately 31 years of age (2,3). The dose tested corresponded to the therapeutic plasma concentrations observed with the recommended human dose. The result is consistent with the high molecular weight (about 1728) and minimal extravascular distribution of fondaparinux.

No reports describing the use of fondaparinux in human pregnancy have been located. However, based on the evidence that the drug does not cross the human placenta and the absence of fetal harm in animal experiments, the embryo/fetal risk in human pregnancy appears to very low, if it exists at all. Therefore, if the maternal condition requires the drug, it should not be withheld because of pregnancy.

BREAST FEEDING SUMMARY

RECOMMENDATION: No Human Data - Probably Compatible

The use of fondaparinux during human lactation has not been described. In spite of the high molecular weight (about 1728), however, the drug is excreted in the milk of lactating rats (1). Consequently, excretion into human milk should be expected. The potential effects of this exposure on a nursing infant are unknown, but appear to be clinically insignificant.

References

1. Product information. Arixtra. Sanofi-Synthelabo, 2003.
2. Lagrange F, Brun J-L, Vergnes MC, Paolucci F, Nadal T, Lenq J-J, Saux MC, Bannwarth B. Fondaparinux sodium does not cross the placental barrier. Study using the *in-vitro* human dually perfused cotyledon model. Clin Pharmacokinet 2002;41(Suppl 2):47–9.
3. Lagrange F, Vergnes C, Brun JL, Paolucci F, Nadal T, Leng JJ, Saux MC, Banwarth B. Absence of placental transfer of pentasaccharide (Fondaparinux, Arixtra) in the dually perfused human cotyledon in vitro. Thromb Haemost 2002;87:831–5.

Name: **FOSAMPRENAVIR** Risk Factor: C_M
Class: **Antiviral**

FETAL RISK SUMMARY

RECOMMENDATION: Compatible - Maternal Benefit >> Embryo/Fetal Risk

Fosamprenavir is a prodrug of amprenavir, an inhibitor of human immunodeficiency virus (HIV) protease. After *in vivo* conversion in the gut during absorption, amprenavir binds to the active site of HIV-1 protease to prevent the processing of viral Gag and Gag-Pol polyprotein precursors, resulting in the formation of immature, non-infectious viral particles. Fosamprenavir is indicated, in combination with other antiretroviral agents, for the treatment of HIV infection (1). Fosamprenavir/amprenavir is in the same class of protease inhibitors as atazanavir, indinavir, lopinavir, nelfinavir, ritonavir, and saquinavir.

Fosamprenavir was not mutagenic or genotoxic in assays conducted *in vitro* and *in vivo*. The agent did not impair fertility or general reproductive performance in male and female rats treated with doses producing systemic exposures of 3 (males) or 4 (females) times the systemic exposure ($AUC_{0-24\,hours}$) obtained with the maximum recommended human dose when given alone (AUC-MRHD), or similar to the systemic exposure obtained with the maximum recommended human dose when given in combination with ritonavir (AUC-MRHD-RIT) (1).

Reproduction studies have been conducted in pregnant rats and rabbits. In rats given fosamprenavir from gestational days 6 to 17, no major effects on embryo-fetal development were observed at doses 0.7 and 2 times the AUC-MRHD-RIT and AUC-MRHD, respectively. Dosing of female rats before and during mating, throughout gestation and during the first six postpartum days was associated with a reduction in pup survival and body weights. An increased incidence of abortion was observed in pregnant rabbits given fosamprenavir from gestational days 7 to 20 at doses 0.3 and 0.8 times the AUC-MRHD-RIT and AUC-MRHD, respectively. In contrast, amprenavir was associated with abortions and an increase in the incidence of minor skeletal variations (deficient ossification of the femur, humerus, and trochlea) in rabbits at a dose about 1/20th the human exposure obtained from the recommended dose (1).

Consistent with its molecular weight (about 506), amprenavir crosses the rat and rabbit placentas to the fetus. Amprenavir also has been shown to readily cross the *ex vivo* human placenta (see Amprenavir).

The Antiretroviral Pregnancy Registry reported, for the period January 1989 through January 2004, prospective data (reported to the Registry before the outcomes were known) involving 1537 live births that had been exposed during the 1st trimester to one or more antiretroviral agents (2). Forty-seven of the newborns had congenital defects (3.1%, 95% confidence interval [CI] 2.3–4.1). In the 2407 live births with earliest exposure in the 2nd/3rd trimesters, there were 56 infants with defects (2.3%, 95% CI 1.8–3.0). The prevalence rates for the two periods did not differ significantly. There were 103 infants with birth defects among 3944 live births with exposure anytime during pregnancy (2.6%, 95% CI 2.1–3.2). The prevalence rate did not differ significantly from the rate expected in a non-exposed population (2). There were four outcomes exposed to fosamprenavir (four in the 1st trimester and none in the 2nd/3rd trimesters) in combination with other antiretroviral agents. There were no birth defects in the exposed group. In reviewing the birth defects of prospective and retrospective (pregnancies reported after the outcomes were known) registered cases, and clinical reports, the Registry concluded that there was no pattern of anomalies to suggest a common cause (2). (See Lamivudine for required statement.)

The Food and Drug Administration (FDA) issued a public health advisory on the association between protease inhibitors and diabetes mellitus (3). Because pregnancy is a risk factor for hyperglycemia, there was concern that these antiviral agents would exacerbate this risk. An abstract published in 2000 described the results of a study involving 34 pregnant women treated with protease inhibitors (none with fosamprenavir or amprenavir) compared to 41 controls that evaluated the association with diabetes (4). No association between protease inhibitors and an increased incidence of gestational diabetes was found.

Although the limited human data does not allow a prediction as to the safety of fosamprenavir during pregnancy, the animal data indicates that the drug may represent a low risk to the developing fetus. Two reviews, one in 1996 and the other in 1997, concluded that all women currently receiving antiretroviral therapy should continue to receive therapy during pregnancy and that treatment of the mother with monotherapy should be considered inadequate therapy (5,6). In 1998, the Centers for Disease Control and Prevention (CDC) made a similar recommendation that antiretroviral therapy should be continued during pregnancy, but discontinuation of all therapy during the 1st trimester was a consideration (3). If indicated, therefore, protease inhibitors, including fosamprenavir, should not be withheld in pregnancy because the expected benefit to the HIV-positive mother probably outweighs the unknown risk to the fetus. However, one review suggested that during pregnancy ritonavir (see Ritonavir) was the drug of choice among the protease inhibitors (6). Pregnant women taking protease inhibitors should be monitored for hyperglycemia. The efficacy and safety of combined therapy in preventing vertical transmission of HIV to the newborn, however, are unknown, and zidovudine remains the only antiretroviral agent recommended for this purpose (5,6).

BREAST FEEDING SUMMARY

RECOMMENDATION: Contraindicated

No reports describing the use of fosamprenavir during lactation have been located. Amprenavir is excreted into the milk of lactating rats. In addition, the molecular weight of amprenavir (about 506) is low enough that excretion into breast milk should be expected (see Amprenavir).

Reports on the use of fosamprenavir during human lactation are unlikely because the antiviral agent is used in the treatment of human immunodeficiency virus (HIV) infections. HIV-1 is transmitted in milk, and in developed countries, breast-feeding is not recommended (5–9). In developing countries, breast-feeding is undertaken, despite the risk, because there are no affordable milk substitutes available. Until 1999, no studies had been published that examined the effect of any antiretroviral therapy on HIV-1 transmission in milk. In 1999, a study involving zidovudine was published that measured a 38% reduction in vertical transmission of HIV-1 infection in spite of breast-feeding when compared to controls (see Zidovudine).

F

References

1. Product information. Lexiva. GlaxoSmithKline, 2003.
2. Antiretroviral Pregnancy Registry Steering Committee. *Antiretroviral Pregnancy Registry International Interim Report for 1 January 1989 through 31 January 2004.* Wilmington, NC: Registry Coordinating Center, 2004.
3. CDC. Public Health Service Task Force recommendations for the use of antiretroviral drugs in pregnant women infected with HIV-1 for maternal health and for reducing perinatal HIV-1 transmission in the United States. MMWR 1998;47:No. RR-2.
4. Fassett M, Kramer F, Stek A. Treatment with protease inhibitors in pregnancy is not associated with an increased incidence of gestational diabetes (abstract). Am J Obstet Gynecol 2000;182:S97.
5. Carpenter CCJ, Fischi MA, Hammer SM, Hirsch MS, Jacobsen DM, Katzenstein DA, Montaner JSG, Richman DD, Saag MS, Schooley RT, Thompson MA, Vella S, Yeni PG, Volberding PA. Antiretroviral therapy for HIV infection in 1996. JAMA 1996;276:146–54.
6. Minkoff H, Augenbraun M. Antiretroviral therapy for pregnant women. Am J Obstet Gynecol 1997;176:478–89.
7. Brown ZA, Watts DH. Antiviral therapy in pregnancy. Clin Obstet Gynecol 1990;33:276–89.
8. de Martino M, Tovo P-A, Pezzotti P, Galli L, Massironi E, Ruga E, Floreea F, Plebani A, Gabiano C, Zuccotti GV. HIV-1 transmission through breast-milk: appraisal of risk according to duration of feeding. AIDS 1992;6:991–7.
9. Van de Perre P. Postnatal transmission of human immunodeficiency virus type 1: the breast-feeding dilemma. Am J Obstet Gynecol 1995;173:483–7.

Name:	**FOSCARNET**	Risk Factor:	**C_M**
Class:	**Antiviral**		

FETAL RISK SUMMARY

RECOMMENDATION: Compatible - Maternal Benefit >> Embryo/Fetal Risk

Foscarnet has antiviral *in vitro* activity against all known herpesviruses, including cytomegalovirus (CMV), herpes simplex virus (HSV) types 1 and 2, human herpesvirus 6, Epstein-Barr virus, and varicella-zoster virus (1). The drug is also active *in vitro* against the human immunodeficiency virus (HIV) (2). It is used in patients with acquired immunodeficiency syndrome (AIDS) who have CMV retinitis or in immunocompromised patients with mucocutaneous acyclovir-resistant HSV infections.

Reproductive studies in pregnant rats with SC doses of 150 mg/kg/day, approximately one-eighth the estimated maximum daily human exposure based on area under the plasma concentration curve (AUC) comparison, caused an increase in the frequency of skeletal malformations or variations (1). Administration to pregnant rabbits with 75 mg/kg/day, approximately one-third the human dose (AUC comparison), produced similar skeletal defects or variations. In addition, dose-related genotoxic effects were seen in two *in vitro* tests and in one *in vivo* test in mice (1).

It is not known if foscarnet crosses the human placenta. The molecular weight (about 300 for the sodium salt) is low enough, however, that passage to the fetus should be expected.

Only one report describing the use of foscarnet during human pregnancy has been located. A 21-year-old woman at 18 weeks' gestation was treated with an 8-day course of IV foscarnet (total dose 43.8 g) for severe, genital acyclovir-resistant HSV type 2 (2). The patient also had a 3-year history of HIV disease that was being treated with saquinavir, lamivudine, and zidovudine. After discharge from the hospital, repeat cultures yielded HSV type 2 sensitive to acyclovir and she was treated with oral doses of this antiviral agent for the remainder of her pregnancy. She underwent a cesarean section at term to deliver a healthy, HIV-negative, female infant who was developing normally at 1 year of age. The authors, citing information received from the manufacturer, briefly reviewed two other cases of IV foscarnet therapy (2). In one case, a HIV-negative woman with acyclovir-resistant HSV encephalitis and retinitis had been treated with foscarnet (60 mg/kg IV every 8 hours) for 17 days starting at 32 weeks' gestation. She eventually delivered a healthy infant at term. The second case involved a HIV-positive patient who was treated with foscarnet (40 mg/kg IV every 8 hours) for genital HSV type 2 beginning at 29 weeks' gestation. No further information was available on this case (2).

One 1992 review suggested that the antiviral drug would be a first-line agent for pregnant HIV-positive patients with sight-threatening CMV retinitis (3). Because of the frequent occurrence of renal toxicity experienced with foscarnet in adults, however, the reviewer recommended frequent antepartum testing of the fetus and close monitoring of the amniotic fluid volume to observe for fetal renal toxicity.

BREAST FEEDING SUMMARY

RECOMMENDATION: Contraindicated

No reports describing the use of foscarnet during human lactation have been located. Foscarnet was concentrated in the milk of lactating rats given 75 mg/kg/day SC, with milk levels 3 times higher than the peak maternal blood concentrations (1). Because excretion into human milk most likely occurs, and because of the potentially severe toxicity that might occur in a nursing infant, women receiving foscarnet should not breast-feed.

References

1. Product information. Foscavir. AstraZeneca, 2001.
2. Alvarez-McLeod A, Havlik J, Drew KE. Foscarnet treatment of genital infection due to acyclovir-resistant herpes simplex virus type 2 in a pregnant patient with AIDS: case report. Clin Infect Dis 1999;29:937–8.
3. Watts DH. Antiviral agents. Obstet Gynecol Clin North Am 1992;19:563–85.

Name:	**FOSFOMYCIN**	Risk Factor:	**B_M**
Class:	**Antibiotic**		

FETAL RISK SUMMARY

RECOMMENDATION: Compatible

Fosfomycin is a synthetic, broad-spectrum, bactericidal phosphonic acid antibiotic given as a single 3-g oral dose of the trometamol salt for the treatment of uncomplicated urinary tract infections (acute cystitis) in women (1). Outside of the United States, other salt forms (calcium salt for oral administration, disodium salt for IM or IV dosing) are also available. Following absorption, fosfomycin tromethamine is rapidly converted to the free acid, fosfomycin.

Studies in male and female rats found no effect on fertility or impairment of reproductive performance (1). No teratogenic effects were observed in pregnant rats administered doses up to 1000 mg/kg/day, about 9 and 1.4 times the human dose based on body weight and mg/m^2 (HD), respectively (1). In pregnant rabbits, fetotoxicity was observed at doses up to 1000 mg/kg/day, about 9 and 2.7 times the HD, respectively, a maternally toxic dose in the rabbit.

The placental transfer of fosfomycin, following a single 1-g IM dose (14–20 mg/kg), was studied in a group of women at term in active labor (2). Samples of maternal and fetal blood were obtained before delivery at 30, 90, and 120–210 minutes after the dose in 7, 8, and 7 women, respectively. Mean maternal blood concentrations of fosfomycin at the three time intervals were 14.24, 23.32, and 15.86 μg/mL, respectively, while those in the fetal blood were 1.58, 5.35, and 11.5 μg/mL, respectively.

Although the above study was conducted with IM dosing, the results appear to be comparable to those expected after oral dosing. The mean maximum maternal serum concentration of fosfomycin, after a single 3-g oral dose of fosfomycin tromethamine under fasting conditions, was 26.1 μg/mL within 2 hours (1). As should be expected because of the normal physiologic changes that occur during gestation, pregnant women will have lower peak levels. In four pregnant women at 28–32 weeks' gestation after a single 3-g oral dose, the mean peak serum level at 2 hours was 20.5 μg/mL (3).

A number of reports have described the use of fosfomycin during human pregnancy. Although appropriate precautions had been taken to exclude and prevent pregnancies during clinical trials, three women conceived shortly after enrolling and all received a single 3-g oral dose of fosfomycin (H. A. Schneier, personal communication, Forest Laboratories, 1997). The dose was apparently consumed about 3 days before conception in one case, 8 days after the last menstrual period (i.e., probably before conception) in a second, and 14 days after the last menstrual period (i.e., assumed to be around the time of conception) in a third. The first woman was lost to follow-up and the other two delivered healthy male newborns who were developing normally at 3 years of age.

In a case of stillbirth reported by the manufacturer to the FDA, the mother was hospitalized following a car accident and approximately 10 days later received a single 3-g oral dose of fosfomycin for a urinary tract infection (H. A. Schneier, personal communication, Forest Laboratories, 1997). About 5 days later ultrasound demonstrated no fetal heartbeat and an induced abortion was performed. The cause of death was thought to be caused by progressive multiple placental infarctions and fetal hypotrophy.

Several published reports have studied the efficacy and safety of oral fosfomycin during pregnancy (3–14). The drug has been used in all trimesters of pregnancy without apparent harm to the fetus or newborn.

A 1998 non-interventional observational cohort study described the outcomes of pregnancies in women who had been prescribed one or more of 34 newly marketed drugs by general practitioners in England (15). Of 1067 exposed pregnancies, fosfomycin was taken during the 1st trimester in two, both concluding with normal, full-term infants.

In summary, the lack of teratogenicity in animals and the apparently safe use of fosfomycin during human pregnancy appears to indicate that the drug presents a low risk, if any, to the fetus.

BREAST FEEDING SUMMARY

RECOMMENDATION: No Human Data - Probably Compatible

No reports describing the use of fosfomycin during human lactation have been located. Because of its relatively low molecular weight (about 259) and its transfer across the placenta, passage into milk should be anticipated. The risk to a nursing infant from this exposure is unknown, but modification of the infant's bowel flora may occur.

F

References

1. Product information. Monurol. Forest Laboratories, 2001.
2. Ferreres L, Paz M, Martin G, Gobernado M. New studies on placental transfer of fosfomycin. Chemotherapy 1977;23(Suppl 1):175–9.
3. De Cecco L, Ragni N. Urinary tract infections in pregnancy: Monuril single-dose treatment versus traditional therapy. Eur Urol 1987;13(Suppl 1): 108–13.
4. Ragni N. Fosfomycin trometamol single dose versus pipemidic acid 7 days in the treatment of bacteriuria in pregnancy. Clinical report, 29 November 1990. Data on file, Forest Laboratories.
5. Reeves DS. Treatment of bacteriuria in pregnancy with single dose fosfomycin trometamol: a review. Infection 1992;20(Suppl 4):S313–6.
6. Moroni M. Monuril effectiveness and tolerability in the treatment and prevention of urinary tract infections. Clinical report. Data on file, Forest Laboratories.
7. Paladini A, Paladini AA, Balbi C, Carati L. Efficacy and safety of fosfomycin trometamol in the treatment of bacteriuria in pregnancy. Clinical report. Data on file, Forest Laboratories.
8. Ragni N, Pivetta C, Paccagnella F, Foglia G, Del Bono GP, Fontana P. Urinary tract infections in pregnancy. In Neu HC, Williams JD, eds. *New Trends in Urinary Tract Infections. International Symposium Rome 1987*. Basel: Karger, 1988:197–206.
9. Zinner S. Fosfomycin trometamol versus pipemidic acid in the treatment of bacteriuria in pregnancy. Chemotherapy 1990;36(Suppl 1):50–2.
10. Marone P, Concia E, Catinella M, Andreoni M, Guaschino S, Marino L, Grossi F, Cellani F. Fosfomycin trometamol in the treatment of urinary tract infections during pregnancy. A multicenter study. *3rd International Congress, Infections in Obstetrics and Gynecology*, Pavia, Italy, 1988.
11. Thoumsin H, Aghayan M, Lambotte R. Fosfomycin trometamol versus nitrofurantoin in multiple dose in pregnant women. Preliminary results. Infection 1990;18(Suppl 2):S94–7.
12. Moroni M. Monurol in lower uncomplicated urinary tract infections in adults. Eur Urol 1987;13(Suppl 1): 101–4.
13. De Andrade J, Mendes Carvalho Lopes C, Carneiro daSilva D, Champi Ribeiro MG, Souza JEMR. Fosfomycin trometamol single-dose in the treatment of uncomplicated urinary tract infections in cardiac pregnant or non pregnant women. A controlled study. J Bras Ginec 1994;104:345–51.
14. Gobernado M, Perez de Leon A, Santos M, Mateo C, Ferreres L. Fosfomycin in the treatment of gynecological infections. Chemotherapy 1977;23(Suppl 1): 287–92.
15. Wilton LV, Pearce GL, Martin RM, Mackay FJ, Mann RD. The outcomes of pregnancy in women exposed to newly marketed drugs in general practice in England. Br J Obstet Gynaecol 1998;105:882–9.

Name: **FOSINOPRIL** Risk Factor: C_M*

Class: **Antihypertensive**

FETAL RISK SUMMARY

RECOMMENDATION: Human Data Suggest Risk in 2nd and 3rd Trimesters

Fosinopril is an angiotensin-converting enzyme inhibitor. In reproduction studies in rats at doses about 80 to 250 times the maximum recommended human dose on a mg/kg basis [MRHD], three similar orofacial malformations and one fetus with situs inversus were observed (1). No teratogenic effects were observed in rabbits at a dose up to 25 times the MRHD (1).

No reports of the use of this agent in human pregnancy have been located, but this class of drugs should be used with caution, if at all, during gestation. Use of angiotensin-converting enzyme inhibitors limited to the 1st trimester does not appear to present a significant risk to the fetus, but fetal exposure after this time has been associated with teratogenicity and severe toxicity in the fetus and newborn, including death. See Captopril or Enalapril for a summary of fetal and neonatal effects from these agents. If fosinopril is used in pregnancy, healthcare professionals are encouraged to call the toll free number (800-670-6126) for information about patient enrollment in the Motherisk study.

[*Risk Factor D_M if used in 2nd or 3rd trimesters.*]

BREAST FEEDING SUMMARY

RECOMMENDATION: No Human Data - Probably Compatible

No published reports describing the use of fosinopril during lactation have been located. The manufacturer states that the drug can be detected in milk after a daily dose of 20 mg given for 3 days (1). Although the effects of this exposure on a nursing infant are unknown, the American Academy of Pediatrics classifies two other similar agents (see Captopril and Enalapril) as compatible with breast-feeding.

Reference

1. Product information. Monopril. Bristol-Myers Squibb, 2000.

Name:	**FROVATRIPTAN**	Risk Factor:	C_M
Class:	**Antimigraine**		

FETAL RISK SUMMARY

RECOMMENDATION: No Human Data - Animal Data Suggest Low Risk

Frovatriptan is an oral selective serotonin (5-hydroxytryptamine; 5-HT) receptor agonist that has high affinity for 5-HT_{1B} and 5-HT_{1D} receptors. The drug is closely related to almotriptan, eletriptan, rizatriptan, and zolmitriptan. (See also Almotriptan, Eletriptan, Rizatriptan, and Zolmitriptan.) It is indicated for the acute treatment of migraine with or without aura in adults. Protein binding is minimal (about 15%). Several metabolites have been identified, but only one has affinity, lower than frovatriptan, for the $5\text{-HT}_{1B/1D}$ receptors. The mean terminal elimination half-life of frovatriptan is about 26 hours (1).

Reproduction studies have been conducted in rats and rabbits. In rats, frovatriptan was given during organogenesis at oral doses ranging from 130 to 1300 times the maximum recommended human dose based on body surface area (MRHD). Dose-related increases in the incidences of dilated ureters, unilateral and bilateral pelvic cavitation, hydronephrosis, and hydroureters. The renal effects were thought to be consistent with a slight delay in fetal maturation. A no-effect dose for this toxicity was not established. Skeletal variations (incomplete ossification of the sternebrae, skull and nasal bones) were observed at all doses. In pregnant rabbits, oral doses up to 210 times the MRHD during organogenesis revealed no effects on fetal development (1).

It is not known if frovatriptan or its less active metabolite crosses the human placenta to the fetus. The molecular weight of the parent compound (about 243 for the free base), however, is low enough that passage to the fetus should be expected. In addition, the minimal protein binding and prolonged elimination half-life suggest that the drug will be available for transfer at the maternal-fetal interface.

No reports describing the use of frovatriptan in human pregnancy have been located. The animal data are suggestive of low risk, but an assessment of the actual risk cannot be determined until human pregnancy experience is available.

BREAST FEEDING SUMMARY

RECOMMENDATION: No Human Data - Probably Compatible

No reports describing the use of frovatriptan during human lactation have been located. In lactating rats, the agent is concentrated in milk with the maximum concentration about four times higher than that measured in the blood (1). The molecular weight (about 243 for the free base), low plasma protein binding, and prolonged elimination half-life suggest that the drug will be excreted into breast milk. The effects of this exposure on a nursing infant are unknown.

Reference

1. Product information. Frova. Elan Biopharmaceuticals, 2004.

Name:	**FURAZOLIDONE**	Risk Factor:	**C**
Class:	**Anti-infective**		

FETAL RISK SUMMARY

RECOMMENDATION: Limited Human Data - No Relevant Animal Data

No reports linking the use of furazolidone with congenital defects have been located. The Collaborative Perinatal Project monitored 50,282 mother-child pairs, 132 of whom had 1st trimester exposure to furazolidone (1). No association with malformations was found. Theoretically, furazolidone could produce hemolytic anemia in a glucose-6-phosphate dehydrogenase-deficient newborn if given at term. Placental passage of the drug has not been reported.

BREAST FEEDING SUMMARY

RECOMMENDATION: No Human Data - Potential Toxicity

No data are available.

Reference

1. Heinonen OP, Slone D, Shapiro S. *Birth Defects and Drugs in Pregnancy*. Littleton, MA: Publishing Sciences Group, 1977:299–302.

Name:	**FUROSEMIDE**	Risk Factor:	C_M*
Class:	**Diuretic**		

FETAL RISK SUMMARY

RECOMMENDATION: Human Data Suggest Low Risk

Furosemide is a potent diuretic. The drug has caused maternal deaths and abortions in rabbits at doses 2, 4, and 8 times the maximum recommended human dose of 600 mg/day (1). An increase in the incidence and severity of hydronephrosis (distention of the renal pelvis and in some cases of the ureters) has also been observed in the offspring of mice and rabbits (1). Wavy ribs and some skeletal defects have been observed in the offspring of rats given furosemide during organogenesis (2). These effects appeared to be caused directly or indirectly by the diuretic action of the drug (2).

Cardiovascular disorders, such as pulmonary edema, severe hypertension, or congestive heart failure, are probably the only valid indications for this drug in pregnancy. Furosemide crosses the placenta (3). Following oral doses of 25–40 mg, peak concentrations in cord serum of 330 ng/mL were recorded at 9 hours. Maternal and cord levels were equal at 8 hours. Increased fetal urine production after maternal furosemide therapy has been observed (4,5). Administration of furosemide to the mother has been used to assess fetal kidney function by provoking urine production, which is then visualized by ultrasonic techniques (6,7). Diuresis was found more often in newborns exposed to furosemide shortly before birth than in controls (8). Urinary sodium and potassium levels in the treated newborns were significantly greater than in the nonexposed controls.

In a surveillance study of Michigan Medicaid recipients conducted between 1985 and 1992 involving 229,101 completed pregnancies, 350 newborns had been exposed to furosemide during the 1st trimester (F. Rosa, personal communication, FDA, 1993). A total of 18 (5.1%) major birth defects were observed (15 expected). Specific data were available for six defect categories, including (observed/expected) 2/4 cardiovascular defects, 1/1 oral clefts, 0/0 spina bifida, 1/1 polydactyly, 1/1 limb reduction defects, and 3/1 hypospadias. Only with the latter defect is there a suggestion of an association, but other factors, including the mother's disease, concurrent drug use, and chance, may be involved.

After the 1st trimester, furosemide has been used for edema, hypertension, and toxemia of pregnancy without causing fetal or newborn adverse effects (9–31). Many investigators now consider diuretics contraindicated in pregnancy, except for patients with cardiovascular disorders, because they do not prevent or alter the course of toxemia and might decrease placental perfusion (32–35). A 1984 study determined that the use of diuretics for hypertension in pregnancy prevented normal plasma volume expansion and did not change perinatal outcome (36). Thus, diuretics are not recommended for the treatment of gestational hypertension because of the maternal hypovolemia characteristic of this disease.

Administration of the drug during pregnancy does not significantly alter amniotic fluid volume (30). Serum uric acid levels, which are increased in toxemia, are further elevated by furosemide (37). No association was found in a 1973 study between furosemide and low platelet counts in the neonate (38). Unlike the thiazide diuretics, neonatal thrombocytopenia has not been reported for furosemide.

[*Risk Factor D if used in gestational hypertension.*]

BREAST FEEDING SUMMARY

RECOMMENDATION: Limited Human Data - Probably Compatible

Furosemide is excreted into breast milk (1,39). No reports of adverse effects in nursing infants have been found. Thiazide diuretics have been used to suppress lactation (see Chlorothiazide).

F

References

1. Product information. Furosemide. Mylan Pharmaceuticals, 2000.
2. Shepard TH. *Catalog of Teratogen Agents*. 9th ed. Baltimore, MD: The Johns Hopkins University Press, 1998:215.
3. Beermann B, Groschinsky-Grind M, Fahraeus L, Lindstroem B. Placental transfer of furosemide. Clin Pharmacol Ther 1978;24:560–2.
4. Wladimiroff JW. Effect of furosemide on fetal urine production. Br J Obstet Gynaecol 1975;82: 221–4.
5. Stein WW, Halberstadt E, Gerner R, Roemer E. Effect of furosemide on fetal kidney function. Arch Gynakol 1977;224:114–5.
6. Barrett RJ, Rayburn WF, Barr M Jr. Furosemide (Lasix) challenge test in assessing bilateral fetal hydronephrosis. Am J Obstet Gynecol 1983;147:846–7.
7. Harman CR. Maternal furosemide may not provoke urine production in the compromised fetus. Am J Obstet Gynecol 1984;150:322–3.
8. Pecorari D, Ragni N, Autera C. Administration of furosemide to women during confinement, and its action on newborn infants. Acta Biomed (Italy) 1969;40:2–11.
9. Pulle C. Diuretic therapy in monosymptomatic edema of pregnancy. Minerva Med 1965;56:1622–3.
10. DeCecco L. Furosemide in the treatment of edema in pregnancy. Minerva Med 1965;56:1586–91.
11. Bocci A, Pupita F, Revelli E, Bartoli E, Molaschi M, Massobrio A. The water-salt metabolism in obstetrics and gynecology. Minerva Ginecol 1965;17: 103–10.
12. Sideri L. Furosemide in the treatment of oedema in gynaecology and obstetrics. Clin Ter 1966;39: 339–46.
13. Wu CC, Lee TT, Kao SC. Evaluation of new diuretic (furosemide) on pregnant women. A pilot study. J Obstet Gynecol Republ China 1966;5:318–20.
14. Loch EG. Treatment of gestosis with diuretics. Med Klin 1966;61:1512–5.
15. Buchheit H, Nicolai KH. Influence of furosemide (Lasix) on gestational edemas. Med Klin 1966;61: 1515–8.
16. Tanaka T. Studies on the clinical effect of Lasix in edema of pregnancy and toxemia of pregnancy. Sanka To Fujinka 1966;41:914–20.
17. Merger R, Cohen J, Sadut R. Study of the therapeutic effects of furosemide in obstetrics. Rev Fr Gynecol 1967;62:259–65.
18. Nascimento R, Fernandes R, Cunha A. Furosemide as an accessory in the therapy of the toxemia of pregnancy. Hospital (Portugal) 1967;71:137–40.
19. Finnerty FA Jr. Advantages and disadvantages of furosemide in the edematous states of pregnancy. Am J Obstet Gynecol 1969;105:1022–7.
20. Das Gupta S. Frusemide in blood transfusion for severe anemia in pregnancy. J Obstet Gynaecol India 1970;20:521–5.
21. Kawathekar P, Anusuya SR, Sriniwas P, Lagali S. Diazepam (Calmpose) in eclampsia: a preliminary report of 16 cases. Curr Ther Res 1973;15:845–55.
22. Pianetti F. Our results in the treatment of parturient patients with oedema during the five years 1966–1970. Atti Accad Med Lomb 1973;27:137–40.
23. Azcarte Sanchez S, Quesada Rocha T, Rosas Arced J. Evaluation of a plan of treatment in eclampsia (first report). Ginecol Obstet Mex 1973;34:171–86.
24. Bravo Sandoval J. Management of pre-eclampsia-eclampsia in the third gyneco-obstetrical hospital. Cir Cirjjands 1973;41:487–94.
25. Franck H, Gruhl M. Therapeutic experience with nortensin in the treatment of toxemia of pregnancy. Munch Med Wochenschr 1974;116:521–4.
26. Cornu P, Laffay J, Ertel M, Lemiere J. Resuscitation in eclampsia. Rev Prat 1975;25:809–30.
27. Finnerty FA Jr. Management of hypertension in toxemia of pregnancy. Hosp Med 1975;11:52–65.
28. Saldana-Garcia RH. Eclampsia: maternal and fetal mortality. Comparative study of 80 cases. In VIII World Congress of Gynecology and Obstetrics. Int Cong Ser 1976;396:58–9.
29. Palot M, Jakob L, Decaux J, Brundis JP, Quereux C, Wahl P. Arterial hypertensions of labor and the postpartum period. Rev Fr Gynecol Obstet 1979;74:173–6.
30. Votta RA, Parada OH, Windgrad RH, Alvarez OH, Tomassinni TL, Patori AA. Furosemide action on the creatinine concentration of amniotic fluid. Am J Obstet Gynecol 1975;123:621–4.
31. Clark AD, Sevitt LH, Hawkins DF. Use of furosemide in severe toxaemia of pregnancy. Lancet 1972;1:35–6.
32. Pitkin RM, Kaminetzky HA, Newton M, Pritchard JA. Maternal nutrition: a selective review of clinical topics. Obstet Gynecol 1972;40:773–85.
33. Lindheimer MD, Katz AI. Sodium and diuretics in pregnancy. N Engl J Med 1973;288:891–4.
34. Christianson R, Page EW. Diuretic drugs and pregnancy. Obstet Gynecol 1976;48:647–52.
35. Gant NF, Madden JD, Shteri PK, MacDonald PC. The metabolic clearance rate of dehydroisoandrosterone sulfate. IV. Acute effects of induced hypertension, hypotension, and natriuresis in normal and hypertensive pregnancies. Am J Obstet Gynecol 1976;124:143–8.
36. Sibai BM, Grossman RA, Grossman HG. Effects of diuretics on plasma volume in pregnancies with long-term hypertension. Am J Obstet Gynecol 1984; 150:831–5.

37. Carswell W, Semple PF. The effect of furosemide on uric acid levels in maternal blood, fetal blood and amniotic fluid. J Obstet Gynaecol Br Commonw 1974;81:472–4.
38. Jerkner K, Kutti J, Victorin L. Platelet counts in mothers and their newborn infants with respect to antepartum administration of oral diuretics. Acta Med Scand 1973;194:473–5.
39. Product information. Lasix. Hoechst-Roussel Pharmaceuticals, 1990.

F

G

Name:	**GABAPENTIN**	Risk Factor:	**C_M**
Class:	**Anticonvulsant**		

FETAL RISK SUMMARY

RECOMMENDATION: Limited Human Data - Animal Data Suggest Risk

Gabapentin is an anticonvulsant used as adjunctive therapy for the treatment of partial seizures in patients with epilepsy (1,2). It is not known whether gabapentin crosses the human placenta to the fetus. Because of its lack of protein binding and low molecular weight (about 171), however, transfer to the fetus should be expected.

Fetotoxicity in mice exposed during organogenesis to maternal oral doses of about 1 to 4 times the maximum recommended human dose based on body surface area (MRHD) was characterized by delayed ossification of bones in the skull, vertebrae, forelimbs, and hindlimbs (2). The no-effect dose in mice was about one-half of the MRHD. Delayed ossification was also observed in rats exposed *in utero* to less than 1 to 5 times the MRHD. Hydroureter or hydronephrosis was observed in rat pups exposed *in utero* during organogenesis and during the perinatal and postnatal periods after similar doses. The causes of the urinary tract anomalies were unclear (2). The no-effect dose in rats during organogenesis was approximately equal to the MRHD in the teratogenicity study. When compared with controls, exposure to gabapentin during organogenesis did not increase congenital malformations, other than hydroureter or hydronephrosis in rats, in mice, rats, and rabbits at 4, 5, or 8 times, respectively, the MRHD. In rabbits, doses less than about one-quarter to 8 times the MRHD caused an increased incidence of postimplantation fetal loss (2).

Only four published reports have been located that describe the human use of gabapentin during gestation. In addition, no cases of fetal or newborn adverse outcomes had been reported to the FDA through 1996 (F. Rosa, personal communication, FDA, 1996).

In a brief 1995 communication, a newborn exposed to gabapentin and carbamazepine during pregnancy had a cyclops holoprosencephaly (no nose and one eye) (3). Of the seven suspected cases of holoprosencephaly described in this report, five involved the use of carbamazepine (two cases of monotherapy and three of combined therapy). Because of the lack of family histories, an association with familial holoprosencephaly or maternal neurologic problems could not be excluded (3).

The Lamotrigine Pregnancy Registry, an ongoing project conducted by the manufacturer, was first published in January 1997, followed by interim reports with the latest release in July 2004 (see Lamotrigine for consensus statement required for the use of these data) (4). One of the cases prospectively identified following 1st trimester exposure to lamotrigine (400–800 mg/day during gestation) involved a 29-year-old woman who also received gabapentin (dose not specified) before and throughout pregnancy. She gave birth at 37 weeks' gestation to a male infant with skin tags on the left ear, no opening to the ear canal on the right ear, jaundice, and intermittent tremors that occurred for about 5 days after birth. No defects were observed in 13 other live births in which the combination of gabapentin and lamotrigine was used during pregnancy with or without other anticonvulsants (4).

A 1998 non-interventional observational cohort study described the outcomes of pregnancies in women who had been prescribed one or more of 34 newly marketed drugs by general practitioners in England (5). Data were obtained by questionnaires sent to the prescribing physicians one month after the expected or possible date of delivery. In 831 (78%) of the pregnancies, a newly marketed drug was thought to have been taken during the 1st trimester with birth defects noted in 14 (2.5%) singleton births of the 557 newborns (10 sets of twins). In addition, two birth defects were observed in aborted fetuses. However, few of the aborted fetuses were examined. Gabapentin was taken during the 1st trimester in 17 pregnancies. The outcomes of these pregnancies included 2 spontaneous abortions, 4 elective abortions, and 11 normal newborns (1 premature) (5). Although no congenital malformations were observed, the study lacked the sensitivity to identify minor anomalies. Late-appearing major defects may also have been missed as a consequence of the timing of the questionnaires.

A 1996 review reported 16 pregnancies exposed to gabapentin from preclinical trials and postmarketing surveillance (6). The outcomes of these pregnancies included five elective abortions, one ongoing pregnancy, seven normal infants, and three infants with birth defects. No specific information was provided on the defects other than the fact that there was no pattern of malformation and all were receiving polytherapy for epilepsy (6).

In summary, the limited human data do not allow an assessment as to the safety of gabapentin in pregnancy. Because the agent is often combined with other anticonvulsants, the actual cause of a defect may be obscured. Of note, no distinguishable pattern of malformations has been reported. Based on this limited evidence, if a woman's condition requires gabapentin, the benefits of therapy to her appear to outweigh the potential risks to her fetus.

BREAST FEEDING SUMMARY

RECOMMENDATION: No Human Data - Probably Compatible

No reports describing the use of gabapentin during human lactation have been located. Because of its low molecular weight (about 171), transfer into milk should be expected. The effects of this exposure on a nursing infant are unknown.

References

1. Dichter MA, Brodie MJ. New antiepileptic drugs. N Engl J Med 1996;334:1583–90.
2. Product information. Neurontin. Parke-Davis, 2001.
3. Rosa F. Holoprosencephaly and antiepileptic exposures. Teratology 1995;51:230.
4. Lamotrigine Pregnancy Registry. Interim Report. 1 September 1992 through 31 March 2004. Glaxo Wellcome, July 2004.
5. Wilton LV, Pearce GL, Martin RM, Mackay FJ, Mann RD. The outcomes of pregnancy in women exposed to newly marketed drugs in general practice in England. Br J Obstet Gynaecol 1998;105:882–9.
6. Morrell MJ. The new antiepileptic drugs and women: efficacy, reproductive health, pregnancy, and fetal outcome. Epilepsia 1996;37(Suppl 6):S34–S44.

Name:	**GADOPENTETATE DIMEGLUMINE**	Risk Factor:	C_M
Class:	**Diagnostic Agent**		

FETAL RISK SUMMARY

RECOMMENDATION: Limited Human Data - Animal Data Suggest Risk

Gadopentetate dimeglumine is an IV paramagnetic contrast agent used for magnetic resonance imaging. Although no congenital malformations were observed, doses 2.5 times the human dose in rats and 7.5–12.5 times the human dose in rabbits resulted in slight retardation of development (1).

G

Gadopentetate dimeglumine crosses the placenta to the fetus in rabbits (2). Pregnant rabbits were given 0.1 mmol/kg IV in the 3rd trimester. Drug concentrations (μg/g) in fetal tissues at 5 and 60 minutes were placenta (16.6 and 6.1), liver (2.8 and 1.6), brain (0.4 and 0.6), muscle (3.2 and 3.9), heart (2.2 and 3.1), and kidneys (4.3 and 6.8). The amounts in the placenta and kidneys were sufficient for imaging and possibly for fetal toxicity (2).

A 1992 case report described the inadvertent IV bolus administration of gadopentetate dimeglumine (0.2 mmol/kg) to a woman with multiple sclerosis shortly after conception (3). Her last menstrual period had occurred 23 days before the magnetic resonance imaging procedure, thus giving her an estimated gestational length of 9 days. Because this was before the period of organogenesis, the authors of the report concluded that the most likely adverse effect would have been an early spontaneous abortion, rather than congenital malformations. A normal pregnancy occurred, however, terminating in the delivery of a healthy baby girl at 39 weeks' gestation. The infant was developing normally at 3 months of age (3).

BREAST FEEDING SUMMARY

RECOMMENDATION: Compatible

Gadopentetate dimeglumine is excreted in small amounts in the milk of lactating rats given a dose of 5 mmol/kg (1). The manufacturer reported that less than 0.2% of the total dose was transferred to the nursing pups during a 24-hour period (1).

A 2000 study described the excretion of gadopentetate dimeglumine into the breast milk of 19 women (4). One woman who was undergoing magnetic resonance imaging received 0.2 mmol/kg IV (15 mmol), but the other 18 subjects received 0.1 mmol/kg (mean 5.9 mmol). Breast-feeding was stopped for at least 24 hours. A mean of four (range one to seven) samples of breast milk were collected over 24 hours. The cumulative amount of drug excreted into milk over 24 hours was 0.57 μmol (range 0.05–3.0 μmol). This amount was a mean 0.009% (range 0.001%–0.04%) of the mother's dose. Because the amount excreted into milk would be far less than the recommended IV dose for neonates (200 μmol/kg) combined with the fact that very little of orally administered gadopentetate dimeglumine is absorbed systemically, the authors concluded that waiting 24 hours to resume breast feeding was not warranted (4). The American Academy of Pediatrics classifies gadopentetate dimeglumine as compatible with breast-feeding (5).

References

1. Product information. Magnevist. Berlex Laboratories, 1993.
2. Novak Z, Thurmond AS, Ross PL, Jones MK, Thornburg KL, Katzberg RW. Gadolinium-DTPA transplacental transfer and distribution in fetal tissue in rabbits. Invest Radiol 1993;28:828–30.
3. Barkhof F, Heijboer RJJ, Algra PR. Inadvertent IV administration of gadopentetate dimeglumine during early pregnancy. AJR Am J Roentgenol 1992;158:1171.
4. Kubik-Huch RA, Gottstein-Aalame NM, Frenzel T, Seifert B, Puchert E, Wittek S, Debatin JF. Gadopentetate dimeglumine excretion into human breast milk during lactation. Radiology 2000;216:555–8.
5. Committee on Drugs, American Academy of Pediatrics. The transfer of drugs and other chemicals into human milk. Pediatrics 2001;106:776–89.

Name: **GALANTAMINE** Risk Factor: B_M

Class: **Cholinesterase Inhibitor (CNS Agent)**

FETAL RISK SUMMARY

RECOMMENDATION: No Human Data - Animal Data Suggest Low Risk

Galantamine is a reversible cholinesterase inhibitor that is indicated for the treatment of mild to moderate dementia of the Alzheimer's type. The metabolites are apparently inactive. Plasma protein binding is low (18%) and the plasma elimination half-life is about 7 hours (1).

Reproduction studies have been conducted in rats and rabbits. In rats, a dose three times the maximum recommended human dose based on body surface area (MRHD) given for 14 days before mating through organogenesis caused a slight increase in skeletal variations. No major malformations were observed with a dose seven times the MRHD. When rats were given doses three and seven times the MRHD from the beginning of organogenesis through postpartum day 21, pup weights were decreased. However, no other adverse effects on postnatal development were observed. The above doses also caused slight maternal toxicity. No impairment of fertility was observed in female rats given doses up to seven times the MRHD for 14 days or in male rats for 60 days before mating. In rabbits, doses up to 32 times the MRHD during organogenesis revealed no evidence of teratogenicity (1).

It is not known if galantamine crosses the human placenta. The molecular weight (about 287 for the free base), low plasma protein binding, and the moderately long plasma elimination half-life suggest that the drug will cross to the embryo and/or fetus.

No reports describing the use of galantamine in human pregnancy have been located. Because of its indication, such reports should be rare. Moreover, the animal data suggest that the risk to the embryo and/or fetus is low. Therefore, inadvertent exposure to galantamine during pregnancy should not be a reason for pregnancy termination.

BREAST FEEDING SUMMARY

RECOMMENDATION: No Human Data - Potential Toxicity

No reports describing the use of galantamine during human lactation have been located. Because of its indication, such reports should be rare. The molecular weight (about 287 for the free base), its low plasma protein binding (18%) and moderately long plasma elimination half-life (about 7 hours) suggest that galantamine will be excreted into breast milk. The effects of this exposure on a nursing infant are unknown.

Reference

1. Product information. Reminyl. Janssen Pharmaceutica Products, 2004.

Name:	**GANCICLOVIR**	Risk Factor:	C_M
Class:	**Antiviral**		

FETAL RISK SUMMARY

RECOMMENDATION: Compatible - Maternal Benefit >> Embryo/Fetal Risk

Ganciclovir, a synthetic nucleoside analogue that inhibits replication of herpes viruses, is used in the treatment of cytomegalovirus (CMV) retinitis and other viral infections.

The drug is embryotoxic in mice and rabbits, causing fetal resorption in at least 85% of animals exposed to 2 times the human dose based on AUC (HD) (1). One month old male offspring of female mice administered 1.7 times HD before and during gestation and during lactation had hypoplastic testes and seminal vesicles and pathologic changes in the nonglandular region of the stomach (1). In pregnant rabbits given doses 2 times the HD, fetal effects included growth retardation and teratogenicity (cleft palate, anophthalmia/microphthalmia, aplastic kidneys and pancreas, hydrocephaly, and brachygnathia).

Ganciclovir is both carcinogenic and mutagenic in mice (1). Moreover, inhibition of spermatogenesis has been observed in mice and dogs. One study using cultured fetal rat hepatocytes, however, found little or no toxic effects, in terms of cell growth and cell membrane permeability, of high concentrations (0.5–30 μg/mL) of ganciclovir (2).

Passage of ganciclovir across the perfused human placenta has been reported (2,3). In a 1993 report, ganciclovir was found initially to concentrate at the maternal placental surface and then to cross passively, without metabolism, to the fetus (2). In a second study, ganciclovir and acyclovir were discovered to cross the placenta in approximately similar amounts by simple diffusion (3).

Only two reports have been located that describe the use of ganciclovir during human pregnancy (4,5). In the first case, a 31-year-old woman received a renal transplant approximately 3 weeks after her last menstrual period (LMP) (8 and 10 days after unprotected intercourse) (4). Medications related to maintaining the transplant included methylprednisolone tapered to prednisone, azathioprine, and cyclosporine. Other drugs added shortly after surgery were trimethoprim, nifedipine and acyclovir. Her worsening hypertension was controlled with nifedipine. Six weeks after surgery (9 weeks after her LMP), she developed CMV infection that was treated with IV ganciclovir (2.5 mg/kg twice daily) for 2 weeks and a single dose of IV CMV hyperimmune globulin. CMV cultures were negative after treatment and remained so throughout the reminder of the pregnancy. A normal 2640-g male infant was born at 38 weeks' gestation with Apgar scores of 9 and 9 at 1 and 5 minutes, respectively. Placental villitis consistent with CMV was noted and the infant had a positive CMV urine culture, but he remained healthy and was developing normally at 18 months of age (4).

The second case involved a 29-year-old CMV negative woman who had received a CMV positive liver transplant. She became pregnant 5 months after the transplant (5). She received ganciclovir (1-g orally three times daily), tacrolimus, and prednisone before conception and throughout the 1st trimester. Ganciclovir was discontinued when pregnancy was diagnosed at 3 months gestation. Steroid-induced hyperglycemia was not observed, but worsening preeclampsia and fetal distress resulted in delivery at 30 weeks' gestation of a 790-g female infant with Apgar scores of 4 and 7 at 1 and 5 minutes, respectively. No malformations were observed and, except for her small size and mild respiratory problems, she did well and was discharged home on day 50 of life. The author also mentioned three other, unpublished, ganciclovir-treated pregnancies that had been reported to the manufacturer. One patient had been lost to follow-up, one had been treated with IV ganciclovir during the last 4 weeks of pregnancy, and one had been treated with oral ganciclovir from 14 to 18 weeks' gestation. The two pregnancies with known outcomes resulted in normal infants (5).

CMV is the most common cause of congenital viral infection in the United States, infecting 0.2%–2.2% of all liveborn infants (6). Approximately 40% of primary CMV infections occurring during pregnancy will result in transplacental passage of the virus to the fetus (6). A relatively small percentage of these infants, however, will exhibit structural damage, such as symmetric growth retardation, hepatosplenomegaly, chorioretinitis, microphthalmia, cerebral calcification, hydrocephaly, and microcephaly. Some infants who have been infected *in utero* will develop later toxicity as evidenced by deafness (CMV is the leading cause of congenital hearing loss), mental retardation, and impaired psychomotor development (6). The effectiveness of ganciclovir in preventing or ameliorating these effects is unknown. Only five cases of its use in human pregnancy are known, but no adverse effects attributable to ganciclovir were apparent in the four cases with outcome details, although one infant had a positive CMV urine culture without signs or symptoms of infection. Long-term evaluation of the four exposed infants for late-appearing toxicity, however, has not been reported. Because of the potential for fetal toxicity and the known toxic effects in animals, some investigators have recommended that ganciclovir should only be used during pregnancy for life-threatening disease or in immunocompromised patients with major cytomegalovirus infections, such as retinitis (1,3,7). Currently, the only approved indications for ganciclovir are for the treatment of CMV retinitis or prevention of CMV disease in immunocompromised patients or in solid-organ transplant recipients (1).

BREAST FEEDING SUMMARY

RECOMMENDATION: No Human Data - Potential Toxicity

No reports describing the use of ganciclovir during lactation have been located. Because of the potential for serious toxicity in a nursing infant, mothers taking ganciclovir should probably not breast-feed. The pharmacokinetics of ganciclovir in newborns with congenital cytomegalovirus infections has been reported (8).

References

1. Product information. Cytovene. Roche Laboratories, 2001.
2. Henderson GI, Hu ZQ, Yang Y, Perez TB, Devi BG, Frosto TA, Schenker S. Ganciclovir transfer by human placenta and its effects on rat fetal cells. Am J Med Sci 1993;306:151–6.
3. Gilstrap LC, Bawdon RE, Roberts SW, Sobhi S. The transfer of the nucleoside analog ganciclovir across the perfused human placenta. Am J Obstet Gynecol 1994;170:967–73.
4. Miller BW, Howard TK, Goss JA, Mostello DJ, Holcomb WL Jr, Brennan DC. Renal transplantation one week after conception. Transplantation 1995;60:1353–4.
5. Pescovitz MD. Absence of teratogenicity of oral

ganciclovir used during early pregnancy in a liver transplant recipient. Transplantation 1999;67:758–9.
6. American College of Obstetricians and Gynecologists. Perinatal viral and parasitic infections. *ACOG Practice Bulletin*. No. 20, September 2000.
7. DeArmond B. Safety considerations in the use of ganciclovir in immunocompromised patients. Transplant Proc 1991;23(Suppl 1):26–9.
8. Trang JM, Kidd L, Gruber W, Storch G, Demmler G, Jacobs R, Dankner W, Starr S, Pass R, Stagno S, Alford C, Soong S-J, Whitley RJ, Sommadossi J-P, and the NIAID Collaborative Antiviral Study Group. Linear single-dose pharmacokinetics of ganciclovir in newborns with congenital cytomegalovirus infections. Clin Pharmacol Ther 1993;53:15–21.

G

Name: **GARLIC**
Class: **Herb**
Risk Factor: **C**

FETAL RISK SUMMARY

RECOMMENDATION: Compatible

Allium sativum L. (family, Alliaceae), better known as garlic, is a perennial bulb used as a food flavoring. In much higher doses, the herb has been used for medicinal purposes since ancient times. The medicinal parts of garlic are the whole fresh bulb, the dried bulb, and the oil. Studies have demonstrated antibacterial, antimycotic, lipid-lowering, and platelet aggregation inhibition properties. Garlic may prolong bleeding and clotting time and enhance fibrinolytic activity. The average daily doses for medicinal indications are 4 g of fresh garlic, 8 mg of essential oil, or one or two fresh garlic cloves (1–5).

The primary chemical constituents of garlic are the alliins (alkylcysteine sulfoxides), in particular the odorless, colorless amino acid, allylliin (S-allyl-L-cysteine sulfoxide). This amino acid, which has no pharmacologic activity, is converted by the enzyme, allinase (released from neighboring vascular bundle sheath cells by cutting or crushing the bulb) to allicin (diallyl-disulfide-mono-S-oxide but also known as diallyl thiosulfinate responsible for the pungent characteristic garlic odor), a sulfur-containing volatile oil. The unstable allicin then undergoes further changes to two major products, diallyldisulfide (a predominant compound in garlic breath) and diallytrisulfide, and several minor products, cycloalliin, vinyl dithiins, ajoene (4,5,9, trithiadodeca-1,6,11-triene 9-oxide), and methylallyltrisulfide (1–4).

Depending on the method of preparation, commercial garlic products may vary widely in their content of allicin, especially those in oil (3). In some cases, no detectable levels of allicin were found. A 1992 study that evaluated 18 garlic preparations of the approximate 70 that were commercially available in Germany found that only five had an allicin content equivalent to 4 g of fresh garlic, the average daily dose required for therapeutic effects (3). The other 13 products were considered "expensive placebos" because they had no pharmacologic activity (3).

Korean garlic juice was administered to rats to investigate whether it would protect against embryotoxicity induced by maternal ingestion of methylmercuric chloride (6). Analysis of Korean garlic juice indicated that it contained several types of free amino acids, including (numbers in parentheses are the number of amino acids for each type) neutral ($N = 7$), sulfur-containing ($N = 3$), acidic ($N = 2$), basic ($N = 2$), imino acid ($N = 1$), and aromatic acid ($N = 3$) with a total content of approximately 55 mg/mL. The pregnant rats were given 20 mg of methylmercuric chloride on gestational day 7 and then treated with either 0.5 or 1.0 g/kg Korean garlic juice or saline. A fourth group of rats was not treated with mercury or garlic juice. Korean garlic juice was effective, in a dose-related manner, in preventing or reversing the toxicity of organic mercury in terms of increasing maternal and fetal body weights, increasing fetal survival, and decreasing mercury levels in the organs and blood of dams and fetuses (6). The investigators concluded that the effects of Korean garlic juice were most likely a result of the thiol groups found on several of the amino acids that resulted in chelation of the mercury, thereby protecting essential maternal and fetal enzyme systems (6).

Some of the chemical components apparently cross the placenta of animals and humans. In fetal sheep, the taste system develops between 50 and 100 days after conception (8). To determine if garlic crosses the sheep placenta, sheep were administered 6 mL of Egyptian garlic oil by gavage on approximately day 110 of gestation (7). A sensory panel of 16 judges, selected because of demonstrated ability to detect dilute concentrations of garlic in water, were used to determine if the odor was present in allantoic and amniotic fluid, fetal blood, and maternal blood. Samples were drawn at 0, 50, 100, and 150 minutes after the maternal dose. Paired samples (treated and untreated) were presented to each judge. Garlic odor was detected in amniotic fluid at 100 and 150 minutes, and in allantoic fluid, fetal blood, and maternal blood at 50, 100, and 150 minutes. In a brief letter, one correspondent said the odor of garlic had been noted on the breath of some human newborns (8). In a 1995 study, a sensory panel of 13 judges, screened for normal olfactory function, smelled paired samples of amniotic fluid from 10 women (9). Forty-eight minutes before amniocentesis in the 2nd trimester, five of the women received capsules containing the essential oil of garlic and five received placebo capsules containing lactose. The odor of garlic was judged stronger in four of the five women who had ingested the capsules with garlic. Therefore, this study demonstrated that components of garlic were transferred across the placenta and altered the odor of amniotic fluid (9). Although the specific components of garlic in the amniotic fluid were not identified, allicin (diallyl thiosulfinate) and at least one of its degradation products (diallyldisulfide) were most likely present, because these are responsible for the characteristic odor of garlic (see above).

Two brief reports by a group of investigators in London stated that garlic might have benefits in preventing preeclampsia and intrauterine growth retardation (IUGR) (10,11). In an *in vitro* experiment, the investigators added increasing concentrations of garlic extract to a homogenate of human placental villous tissue to demonstrate a dose-related increase in nitric oxide synthase (enzyme that produces nitric oxide) activity (10). Because both calcium-dependent and calcium-independent nitric oxide synthase activities are decreased in preeclampsia and IUGR, the researchers speculated that garlic might be beneficial in these vascular conditions. In the second study, also using human placental villous tissue, both garlic extract and perchloric acid-treated garlic extract (allicin-negative) were shown to have cyclooxygenase inhibitor activity similar that of aspirin (11).

In summary, ingestion of garlic as a food flavoring appears to be safe during pregnancy. The herb has been used since ancient times and its use is so common that it is doubtful it presents any risk to the embryo or fetus. Some components of garlic do cross the placenta to the fetus, as shown by detection of a garlic odor in the amniotic fluid and on the newborn's breath. The use of high-dose garlic during gestation is not common and apparently has not been reported. Moreover, the lack of standardization of therapeutic garlic preparations would make any such study suspect unless analysis of the chemical constituents of the actual product used in the study was also reported. The complete lack of data on the outcome of animal or human pregnancies after high-dose garlic does not allow any assessment of its fetal risk. At least one source considers the use of large amounts of garlic during pregnancy to be contraindicated because of the potential for inducing menstruation or uterine contractions (5).

BREAST FEEDING SUMMARY

RECOMMENDATION: Compatible

At least some garlic constituents are excreted into breast milk. A 1994 study in lactating mice evaluated the effects on xenobiotic metabolizing enzymes in mouse pups from garlic administered to the mother (12). The lactating mice received either 200 or 400 mg/kg of crushed fresh garlic diluted in a volume of 0.1 mL of water for 14 or 21 days postpartum. Significant hepatic enzyme changes were measured in both the dams and pups, but the clinical significance of the changes is unknown.

Eight women, all exclusively breast-feeding their 3- to 4-month old infants, were the subject of a study published in 1991 examining the effect of garlic on the odor of breast milk and the nursling's behavior (13). None of the women was a regular user of garlic and their consumption of other sulfur-containing foods was limited before and during the study. In addition to breast-feeding, milk samples were also collected from the women every hour for 4 hours. They were given either placebo or garlic (1.5 g of garlic extract) capsules on alternate days. A sensory panel of 11 judges, all screened for normal olfactory function, were able to consistently detect the odor of garlic from paired samples of expressed milk (treated and untreated) with a peak effect at 2 hours. It also appeared that the nursing infants detected the garlic odor because when the mother had ingested garlic capsules, the infants attached to the breast for significantly longer periods and sucked more. Although not significant, the infants also tended to consume more milk, but consumption may have been limited by the amount of milk available to the infant (13). A subsequent study confirmed that infants attached to the breast longer than usual when their mothers started taking garlic but that this effect disappeared with continued garlic ingestion (14).

The clinical significance of the above investigations is unknown. A review on the effect of various flavors in milk concluded that it was not known whether flavors such as garlic in milk had any effect on the subsequent development of food habits or willingness to accept new foods at weaning or later in life (15).

In summary, garlic ingestion by a lactating woman may impart garlic odor to her milk. The clinical significance of occasional garlic odor in milk appears to relate only to the amount of time the infant will be attached to the breast and this effect will disappear if the mother ingests the herb frequently.

References

1. Allium Sativum. Garlic. *PDR for Herbal Medicines*, Montvale, NJ: Medical Economics, 1998:626–8.
2. Garlic. Blumenthal M, Senior Editor. *The Complete German Commission E Monographs. Therapeutic Guide to Herbal Medicines*. Austin, TX: American Botanical Council, 1998:134.
3. Robbers JE, Tyler VE. *Tyler's Herbs of Choice. The Therapeutic Use of Phytomedicinals*. Binghamton, NY: Haworth Press, 2000:132–7.
4. Garlic. *The Lawrence Review of Natural Products*. St. Louis, MO: Facts and Comparisons, April, 1994.
5. Garlic. *Natural Medicines Comprehensive Database*. Stockton, CA: Therapeutic Research Faculty, 1999: 366–8.
6. Lee JH, Kang HS, Roh J. Protective effects of garlic juice against embryotoxicity of methylmercuric chloride administered to pregnant Fischer 344 rats. Yonsei Med J 1999;40:483–9.
7. Nolte DL, Provenza FD, Callan R, Panter KE. Garlic in the ovine fetal environment. Physiol Behav 1992;52:1091–3.
8. Snell SB. Garlic on the baby's breath. Lancet 1973; 2:43.
9. Mennella JA, Johnson A, Beauchamp GK. Garlic ingestion by pregnant women alters the odor of amniotic fluid. Chem Senses 1995;20:207–9.
10. Das I, Khan NS, Sooranna SR. Nitric oxide synthase activation is a unique mechanism of garlic action. Biochem Soc Trans 1995;23:136S.
11. Das I, Patel S, Sooranna SR. Effects of aspirin and garlic on cyclooxygenase-induced chemiluminescence in human term placenta. Biochem Soc Trans 1997;25:99S.
12. Chhabra SK, Rao AR. Transmammary exposure of mouse pups to allium sativum (garlic) and its effect on the neonatal hepatic xenobiotic metabolizing enzymes of mice. Nutr Res 1994;14:195–210.

13. Mennella JA, Beauchamp GK. Maternal diet alters the sensory qualities of human milk and the nursling's behavior. Pediatrics 1991;88:737–44.
14. Mennella JA, Beauchamp GK. The effects of repeated exposure to garlic-flavored milk on the nursling's behavior. Pediatr Res 1993;34:805–8.
15. Mennella JA. Mother's milk: a medium for early flavor experiences. J Hum Lact 1995;11:39–45.

Name:	**GATIFLOXACIN**	Risk Factor:	C_M
Class:	**Anti-infective (Quinolone)**		

FETAL RISK SUMMARY

RECOMMENDATION: Human Data Suggest Low Risk

Gatifloxacin is a synthetic, broad-spectrum, fluoroquinolone antibacterial agent. It is in the same anti-infective class as ciprofloxacin, enoxacin, gemifloxacin, levofloxacin, lomefloxacin, moxifloxacin, norfloxacin, ofloxacin, sparfloxacin, and trovafloxacin. Gatifloxacin is available in both oral and injectable formulations (1).

In reproduction studies with rats and rabbits, oral doses up to 0.7 and 1.9 times the human exposure obtained from the maximum dose (AUC-MHD), respectively, were not teratogenic (1). Rat fetal toxicity (delayed skeletal ossification, including wavy ribs) was noted at doses ≥0.7 times the AUC-MHD, and skeletal malformations occurred at about 1.0 times the AUC-MHD. Additional evidence of rat fetal toxicity, at doses 1.0 times the AUC-MHD given late in pregnancy and continuing during lactation, included increases in postimplantation loss and neonatal and perinatal death. No adverse fetal effects were seen at doses of 0.2 and 1.9 times the AUC-MHD, respectively, in rats or rabbits. No adverse effects on fertility or reproduction were observed in rats at oral doses up to about 1.0 times the AUC-MHD (1).

It is not known if gatifloxacin crosses the human placenta. The molecular weight of the hydrate (about 402) is low enough that transfer to the fetus should be expected.

No reports describing the use of either the IV or oral forms of gatifloxacin during human pregnancy have been located. The animal toxicity observed at doses equivalent to the maximum human exposure should be considered before this anti-infective is used in pregnant women. Moreover, some reviewers have concluded that all fluoroquinolones should be considered contraindicated in pregnancy (see Ciprofloxacin and Norfloxacin) because safer alternatives are usually available.

BREAST FEEDING SUMMARY

RECOMMENDATION: No Human Data - Probably Compatible

No reports describing the use of gatifloxacin in human lactation have been located. The molecular weight (about 402 for the hydrated form) suggests that the agent will be excreted into breast milk. Gatifloxacin is excreted in the milk of lactating rats (1). The effects of this exposure on a nursing infant are unknown. However, the American Academy of Pediatrics classifies another fluoroquinolone (ciprofloxacin) as compatible with breast-feeding (see Ciprofloxacin).

Reference

1. Product information. Tequin. Bristol-Myers-Squibb, 2001.

Name:	**GEMFIBROZIL**	Risk Factor:	C_M
Class:	**Antilipemic Agent**		

G

FETAL RISK SUMMARY

RECOMMENDATION: Limited Human Data - Animal Data Suggest Risk

The reproductive effects of the serum lipid-lowering agent, gemfibrozil, have been studied in rats and rabbits. In male and female rats, gemfibrozil was tumorigenic (benign liver nodules, liver carcinoma, and benign Leydig cell tumors) at 0.2 and 1.3 times the human exposure (based on AUC) (1). Treatment of female rats before and during gestation with 0.6 and 2 times the human dose (based on body surface area) produced dose-related decreases in the conception rate, birth weight, and pup growth during lactation, and increased skeletal variations (1). Anophthalmia was observed rarely. The highest dose also resulted in an increased rate of stillbirths. Pregnant rabbits given 1 and 3 times the human dose during organogenesis had a decreased litter size and, at the highest dose, an increased incidence of parietal bone variations (1). Two other studies have found no evidence of reproductive or teratogenic effects in rats and rabbits (2,3).

A 1992 report described the use of gemfibrozil starting at 20 weeks' gestation in a 33-year-old woman with eruptive xanthomas (4). The patient had a similar condition in her first pregnancy that included hypertriglyceridemia, fulminant pancreatitis, and acute respiratory distress syndrome (4). A dose of 600 mg 4 times daily for 2 months lowered the triglyceride level from 7530 to 4575 mg/dL, and the total cholesterol level from 1515 to 1325 mg/dL, but the xanthomas persisted throughout her pregnancy. A healthy, term infant (birth weight and sex not specified) was eventually delivered.

In a surveillance study of Michigan Medicaid recipients conducted between 1985 and 1992 involving 229,101 completed pregnancies, 8 newborns had been exposed to gemfibrozil during the 1st trimester and 7 in the 2nd or 3rd trimesters (5). One defect, a structural brain anomaly, was observed in an infant delivered from a mother who took the agent after the 1st trimester. In a separate case included in this report, an infant with Pierre Robin syndrome, suspected of being associated with 1st trimester exposure to gemfibrozil, was reported retrospectively to the FDA (5).

BREAST FEEDING SUMMARY

RECOMMENDATION: No Human Data - Potential Toxicity

No reports describing the use of gemfibrozil during lactation have been located. The relatively low molecular weight (about 250) probably indicates that the drug will be excreted into milk. Gemfibrozil should probably not be used in breast-feeding women because of the potential for severe toxicity, including tumors, in the nursing infant.

References

1. Product information. Lopid. Parke-Davis, 2000.
2. Kurtz SM, Fitzgerald JE, Fisken RA, Schardein JL, Reutner TF, Lucas JA. Toxicological studies on gemfibrozil. Proc R Soc Med 1976;69(Suppl 2):15–23. As cited in Schardein JL. *Chemically Induced Birth Defects*. 2nd ed. New York, NY: Marcel Dekker, 1993:81.
3. Fitzgerald JE, Petrere JA, De La Iglesia FA. Experimental studies on reproduction with the lipid-regulating agent gemfibrozil. Fund Appl Toxicol 1987;8:454–64. As cited in Shepard TH. *Catalog of Teratogenic Agents*. 7th ed. Baltimore, MD: Johns Hopkins University Press, 1992:188.

4. Jaber PW, Wilson BB, Johns DW, Cooper PH, Ferguson JE II. Eruptive xanthomas during pregnancy. J Am Acad Dermatol 1992;27:300–2.
5. Rosa F. Anti-cholesterol agent pregnancy exposure outcomes. Presented at the 7th International Organization for Teratogen Information Services, Woods Hole, MA, April 1994.

Name:	**GEMIFLOXACIN**	Risk Factor:	C_M
Class:	**Anti-infective (Quinolone)**		

FETAL RISK SUMMARY

RECOMMENDATION: Human Data Suggest Low Risk

Gemifloxacin is a synthetic, broad-spectrum, fluoroquinolone antibacterial agent. It is in the same anti-infective class as ciprofloxacin, enoxacin, gatifloxacin, levofloxacin, lomefloxacin, moxifloxacin, norfloxacin, ofloxacin, sparfloxacin, and trovafloxcin. Gemifloxacin is available in an oral formulation. Gemifloxacin and its metabolites are primarily eliminated in the feces (about 61%) with the remainder excreted in the urine (about 36%). Plasma protein binding ranges from 55% to 73% and the elimination half-life is about 7 hours (range 4–12 hours) (1).

Reproduction studies have been conducted with gemifloxacin in mice, rats and rabbits. Fetal growth retardation was observed in all three species given doses resulting in exposures, based on AUC, that were 2-, 4-, and 3-fold greater, respectively, than those obtained in women given oral doses of 325 mg HDAUC. The growth retardation appeared to be reversible in rats, but this was not studied in mice and rabbits. In rats, a dose 8 times the HDAUC caused fetal brain and ocular malformations but also caused maternal toxicity. The no-observed-effect level (i.e., NOEL) in pregnant animals was about 0.8–3 times the HDAUC (1).

It is not known if gemifloxacin crosses the human placenta. The molecular weight of the mesylate salt (about 485), plasma protein binding (55%–73%), and elimination half-life (about 7 hours), however, suggest that passage to the fetus should be expected.

No reports describing the use of gemifloxacin during human pregnancy have been located. The animal toxicity (fetal growth retardation) observed at exposures close to those obtained in humans should be considered before this agent is used in pregnant women. Moreover, some reviewers have concluded that all fluoroquinolones should be considered contraindicated in pregnancy (e.g., see Ciprofloxacin and Norfloxacin) because safer alternatives are usually available.

BREAST FEEDING SUMMARY

RECOMMENDATION: No Human Data - Probably Compatible

No reports describing the use of gemifloxacin in lactating humans have been located. The anti-infective is excreted into the milk of lactating rats (1). This is consistent with its molecular weight (about 485), plasma protein binding (55%–73%), and elimination half-life (about 7 hours). The effects of this exposure on a nursing infant are unknown. However, other fluoroquinolones are classified by the American Academy of Pediatrics as compatible with breast-feeding (see Ciprofloxacin).

Reference

1. Product information. Factive. GeneSoft Pharmaceuticals, 2004.

Name: **GENTAMICIN** Risk Factor: **C**

Class: **Antibiotic (Aminoglycoside)**

FETAL RISK SUMMARY

RECOMMENDATION: Human Data Suggest Low Risk

Gentamicin is an aminoglycoside antibiotic. The antibiotic did not impair fertility or cause fetal harm in rats and rabbits (1). Not surprisingly, gentamicin produces dose-related nephrotoxicity in fetal rats (2–4). High doses (110 mg/kg/day SC) of gentamicin during gestation have also been shown to produce significant and persistent increases in the blood pressure, as well as nephrotoxicity, in exposed rat offspring (5).

G

Gentamicin rapidly crosses the placenta into the fetal circulation and amniotic fluid (6–15). Following 40–80-mg IM doses given to patients in labor, peak cord serum levels averaging 34%–44% of maternal levels were obtained at 1–2 hours (6,9,13,14). Following a single 80-mg IM injection before delivery, mean peak amniotic fluid concentrations (5.17 μg/mL) occurred at 8 hours (14). No toxicity attributable to gentamicin was seen in any of the newborns. Patients undergoing 1st and 2nd trimester abortions were given 1 mg/kg IM (10). Gentamicin could not be detected in their cord serum before 2 hours. Amniotic fluid levels were undetectable at this dosage up to 9 hours after injection. Doubling the dose to 2 mg/kg allowed detectable levels in the fluid in one of two samples 5 hours after injection.

The pharmacokinetics of gentamicin in 23 women with pyelonephritis at a mean gestational age of 21.8 weeks were described in 1994 (16). Similar to that observed in postpartum women, standard weight-adjusted doses of gentamicin produced low, subtherapeutic serum levels in most of the women.

A brief study published in 2000 compared gentamicin serum levels in infants of women who had received the antibiotic IV (240-mg single daily dose vs. 80 mg 3 times daily) during labor (17). In the single daily dose group ($N = 11$), all of the mothers had received one dose a mean 5.12 hours before delivery, whereas in the divided dose group ($N = 10$), 9 of 10 mothers received one dose a mean 4.72 hours before delivery. The mean serum levels in the newborn infants were 1.94 $\pm$ 0.63 and 0.98 $\pm$ 0.45 μg/mL, respectively ($p = 0.01$). There was no correlation between the infant's serum level and the time interval from the mother's dose (17). Based on their analysis, the authors concluded that the divided dose regimen was best for women in labor (17).

In an abstract published in 1997, women undergoing mid-trimester terminations received gentamicin either as a 10-mg intra-amniotic infusion ($N = 16$) or a single 80-mg IV dose (18). Low median gentamicin plasma levels were measured in the mothers and fetuses after the intra-amniotic dose; 0.28 μg/mL (mothers) and 0.4 μg/mL (fetuses). In contrast, the median amniotic fluid concentration, 46 μg/mL, was sustained for greater than 24 hours. After IV dosing, amniotic fluid concentrations were low throughout the study (median 0.35 μg/mL). The authors concluded that intra-amniotic infusions of gentamicin was a safe method to administer the antibiotic without reaching toxic levels in the mother or the fetus (18).

Intra-amniotic instillations of gentamicin were given to 11 patients with premature rupture of the membranes (19). Ten patients received 25 mg every 12 hours and one received 25 mg every 8 hours, for a total of 1–19 doses per patient. Maternal gentamicin serum levels ranged from 0.063 to 6 μg/mL (all but one were less than 0.6 μg/mL and that one was believed to be caused by error). Cord serum levels varied from 0.063 to 2 μg/mL (all but two were less than 0.6 μg/mL). No harmful effects were seen in the newborns after prolonged exposure to high local concentrations of gentamicin.

Only one report linking the use of gentamicin to congenital defects has been located. A 34-year-old woman, who was not known to be pregnant at the time, received a 10-day course of gentamicin (300 mg/day) in gestational week 7 (20). The appropriateness of this dose cannot be determined because the mother's height and weight and renal function were not given. The mother was also treated with prednisolone (50 mg/day for 5 days) for an "allergic reaction" to the antibiotic. She delivered an apparently healthy 2950-g (6 pounds 8 ounces) male infant at 37 weeks' gestation. His growth after birth was less than the 5th percentile and at 4.5 years of age, the child was evaluated for short stature (<5th percentile). At this time, he was noted to have impaired renal function. Ultrasound examination revealed small kidneys, both <5th centile for age, with increased echotexture, markedly decreased corticomedullary differentiation, and small bilateral cysts. Although the exact cause of the renal cystic dysplasia was unknown, and a potential genetic defect could not be excluded, the authors speculated, on the basis of animal studies, that the combination of gentamicin and prednisolone had induced the abnormal nephrogenesis.

G

Gentamicin, in combination with ampicillin ($N = 62$), was compared to two groups of women treated with cefazolin ($N = 58$) or ceftriaxone ($N = 59$) in a randomized trial of the treatment of acute pyelonephritis in pregnancy (21). The mean gestational age at the start of therapy was 14 to 15 weeks. There were no significant differences between the three groups in clinical or pregnancy outcomes. The pregnancy outcomes included gestational age at delivery, preterm delivery, birth weight, neonatal intensive care admission, and length of stay in the neonatal intensive care if admitted (21).

The population-based dataset of the Hungarian Case-Control Surveillance of Congenital Abnormalities, covering the period of 1980–1996, was used to evaluate the teratogenicity of aminoglycoside antibiotics (parenteral gentamicin, streptomycin, tobramycin, and oral neomycin) in a study published in 2000 (22). A case group of 22,865 women who had fetuses or newborns with congenital malformations were compared to 38,151 women who had no newborns with structural defects. A total of 38 cases and 42 controls were treated with aminoglycosides. There were 19 women in the case and control groups, 0.08% and 0.05%, respectively, treated with gentamicin (odds ratio 1.7, 95% confidence interval 0.9–3.2). A case-control pair analysis for the 2nd and 3rd months of gestation also failed to show a risk for teratogenicity. The investigators concluded that there was no detectable teratogenic risk for structural defects for any of the aminoglycoside antibiotics (22). They also concluded, although it was not investigated in this study, that the risk of deafness after *in utero* aminoglycoside exposure was small.

Ototoxicity, which is known to occur after gentamicin therapy, has not been reported as an effect of *in utero* exposure. However, eighth cranial nerve toxicity in the fetus is well known following exposure to other aminoglycosides (see Kanamycin and Streptomycin) and may potentially occur with gentamicin. Gentamicin and vancomycin, both of which can cause ototoxicity and nephrotoxicity, have been used together during pregnancy without apparent harm to the fetus or newborn (see Vancomycin).

Potentiation of $MgSO_4$-induced neuromuscular weakness has been reported in a neonate exposed during the last 32 hours of pregnancy to 24 g of $MgSO_4$ (23). The depressed infant was treated with gentamicin for sepsis at 12 hours of age. After the second dose, the infant's condition worsened with rapid onset of respiratory arrest. Emergency treatment was successful, and no lasting effects of the toxic interaction were noted.

BREAST FEEDING SUMMARY

RECOMMENDATION: Compatible

Small amounts of gentamicin are excreted into breast milk and absorbed by the nursing infant. In a reference published in 1994, 10 women, who had just delivered term infants, were administered antibiotic prophylaxis with gentamicin, 80 mg IM 3 times daily (24). On the 4th day of a 5-day therapy course, milk and serum samples were obtained. The mean maternal serum levels of gentamicin at 1 and 7 hours after a dose were 3.94 and 1.02 μg/mL, respectively. Mean milk levels at 1, 3, 5, and 7 hours after a dose were 0.42, 0.48, 0.49, and 0.41 μg/mL, respectively, providing mean milk:plasma ratios at 1 and 7 hours of 0.11 and 0.44, respectively. The infants were allowed to breast-feed 1 hour after a dose and serum samples were collected 1 hour later. Five of the 10 infants had detectable (above 0.27 μg/mL) gentamicin serum levels with a mean level of 0.41 μg/mL.

G

In a case report, a nursing infant developed two grossly bloody stools while his mother was receiving gentamicin and clindamycin (25). The condition cleared rapidly when breast feeding was discontinued. Although both antibiotics are known to be excreted into milk, the cause of the infant's diarrhea cannot be determined with certainty. The American Academy of Pediatrics classifies gentamicin as compatible with breast-feeding (26).

References

1. Product information. Garamycin. Schering, 1997.
2. Mallie J-P, Coulon G, Billerey C, Faucourt A, Morin J-P. In utero aminoglycosides-induced nephrotoxicity in rat neonates. Kidney Int 1988;33:36–44.
3. Smaoui H, Mallie J-P, Schaeverbeke M, Robert A, Schaeverbeke J. Gentamicin administered during gestation alters glomerular basement membrane development. Antimicrob Agents Chemother 1993;37:1510–7.
4. Lelievre-Pegorier M, Euzet S, Merlet-Benichou C. Effect of fetal exposure to gentamicin on phosphate transport in young rat kidney. Am J Physiol 1993;265:F807–12.
5. Stahlmann R, Chahoud I, Thiel R, Klug S, Forster C. The developmental toxicity of three antimicrobial agents observed only in nonroutine animal studies. Reprod Toxicol 1997;11:1–7.
6. Percetto G, Baratta A, Menozzi M. Observations on the use of gentamicin in gynecology and obstetrics. Minerva Ginecol 1969;21:1–10.
7. von Kobyletzki D. Experimental studies on the transplacental passage of gentamicin. Presented at Fifth International Congress on Chemotherapy, Vienna, 1967.
8. von Koblyetzki D, Wahlig H, Gebhardt F. Pharmacokinetics of gentamicin during delivery. Antimicrobial Anticancer Chemotherapy—Proceedings of the Sixth International Congress on Chemotherapy, Tokyo, 1969;1:650–2.
9. Yoshioka H, Monma T, Matsuda S. Placental transfer of gentamicin. J Pediatr 1972;80:121–3.
10. Garcia S, Ballard C, Martin C, Ivler D, Mathies A, Bernard B. Perinatal pharmacology of gentamicin. Clin Res 1972;20:252.
11. Daubenfeld O, Modde H, Hirsch H. Transfer of gentamicin to the foetus and the amniotic fluid during a steady state in the mother. Arch Gynecol 1974;217:233–40.
12. Kauffman R, Morris J, Azarnoff D. Placental transfer and fetal urinary excretion of gentamicin during constant rate maternal infusion. Pediatr Res 1975;9:104–7.
13. Weinstein A, Gibbs R, Gallagher M. Placental transfer of clindamycin and gentamicin in term pregnancy. Am J Obstet Gynecol 1976;124:688–91.
14. Creatsas G, Pavlatos M, Lolis D, Kaskarelis D. Ampicillin and gentamicin in the treatment of fetal intrauterine infections. J Perinat Med 1980;8:13–8.
15. Gilstrap LC III, Bawdon RE, Burris J. Antibiotic concentration in maternal blood, cord blood, and placental membranes in chorioamnionitis. Obstet Gynecol 1988;72:124–5.
16. Graham JM, Blanco JD, Oshiro BT, Magee KP. Gentamicin levels in pregnant women with pyelonephritis. Am J Perinatol 1994;11:40–41.
17. Regev RH, Litmanowitz I, Arnon S, Shiff J, Dolfin T. Gentamicin serum concentrations in neonates born to gentamicin-treated mothers. Pediatr Infect Dis J 2000;19:890–1.
18. Barak J, Mankuta D, Pak I, Glezerman M, Katz M, Danon A. Transabdominal amnioinfusion of gentamicin: a pharmacokinetic study of maternal plasma and intraamniotic levels (abstract). Am J Obstet Gynecol 1997;176:S59.
19. Freeman D, Matsen J, Arnold N. Amniotic fluid and maternal and cord serum levels of gentamicin after intra-amniotic instillation in patients with premature rupture of the membranes. Am J Obstet Gynecol 1972;113:1138–41.
20. Hulton S-A, Kaplan BS. Renal dysplasia associated with in utero exposure to gentamicin and corticosteroids. Am J Med Genet 1995;58:91–3.

21. Wing DA, Hendershott CM, Debuque L, Millar LK. A randomized trial of three antibiotic regimens for the treatment of pyelonephritis in pregnancy. Obstet Gynecol 1998;92:249–53.
22. Czeizel AE, Rockenbauer M, Olsen J, Sorensen HT. A teratological study of aminoglycoside antibiotic treatment during pregnancy. Scand J Infect Dis 2000; 32:309–13.
23. L'Hommedieu CS, Nicholas D, Armes DA, Jones P, Nelson T, Pickering LK. Potentiation of magnesium sulfate-induced neuromuscular weakness by gentamicin, tobramycin, and amikacin. J Pediatr 1983; 102:629–31.
24. Celiloglu M, Celiker S, Guven H, Tuncok Y, Demir N, Erten O. Gentamicin excretion and uptake from breast milk by nursing infants. Obstet Gynecol 1994;84: 263–5.
25. Mann CF. Clindamycin and breast-feeding. Pediatrics 1980;66:1030–1.
26. Committee on Drugs, American Academy of Pediatrics. The transfer of drugs and other chemicals into human milk. Pediatrics 2001;108:776–89.

Name:	**GENTIAN VIOLET**	Risk Factor:	**C**
Class:	**Disinfectant/Anthelmintic**		

FETAL RISK SUMMARY

RECOMMENDATION: Limited Human Data - No Relevant Animal Data

The Collaborative Perinatal Project monitored 50,282 mother-child pairs, 40 of whom had 1st trimester exposure to gentian violet (1). Evidence was found to suggest a relationship to malformations based on defects in 4 patients. Independent confirmation is required to determine the actual risk.

BREAST FEEDING SUMMARY

RECOMMENDATION: No Human Data - Potential Toxicity

No data are available.

Reference

1. Heinonen OP, Slone D, Shapiro S. *Birth Defects and Drugs in Pregnancy*. Littleton, MA: Publishing Sciences Group, 1977:302.

Name:	**GINGER**	Risk Factor:	**C**
Class:	**Herb**		

FETAL RISK SUMMARY

RECOMMENDATION: Compatible

The rhizome of the perennial plant, ginger (*Zingiber officinale*) is used as a dried powdered spice in foods and as a natural medicine for its alleged carminative, cardiotonic, antithrombotic, antibacterial, antioxidant, antitussive, antiemetic, stimulant, antihepatotoxic, anti-inflammatory, antimutagenic, diaphoretic, diuretic, spasmolytic, immunostimulant, and cholagogue actions (1). The active ingredients in ginger are thought to be primarily a class of structurally cardiotonic compounds called gingerols. Other pharmacologically active compounds that have been identified in ginger include shogaol, dehydrogingerdiones, gingerdiones, and zingerone. Some of these ingredients inhibit prostaglandin synthetase (cyclooxygenase) but, in some cases, this activity may be confined only to fresh ginger (1).

In a reproduction study in rats, ginger tea (20 g/L or 50 g/L) was given to rats during organogenesis (days 6 through 15) via their drinking water (2). The lower concentration (20 g/L) was equivalent to the ginger tea consumed by humans (2). No maternal toxicity or teratogenicity were seen, but early embryonic loss was double that of the controls ($p < 0.05$) at both doses. In addition, surviving fetuses, especially females, were significantly heavier than controls and had more advanced skeletal growth (2). Another rat study used a patented standardized ethanol extract of *Zingiber officinale* (EV.EXT 33) to administer doses up to 1000 mg/kg/day during organogenesis (3). Compared to a control group, no embryo toxicity, teratogenicity, or treatment-related adverse effects were observed in the pregnant rats or their offspring.

G

Several authors have commented on or reported, with mixed results, studies examining the antiemetic properties of ginger in nonpregnant patients (4–10), and a review of this topic was published in 2000 (11). The oral dosage in the studies varied from 1 to 2 g/day of the powdered root or rhizome. Although the exact mechanism of action is unknown, it appears to be a local effect in the gastrointestinal tract rather than a central action (7,10). The effect may be mediated by antagonism of gastrointestinal 5-hydroxytryptamine (serotonin) to prevent stimulation of the vagus nerve and, thus, the vomiting center (8,10). One author commented that ginger has been long used in Chinese herbal or folk medicine for the treatment of pregnancy-induced nausea and vomiting (5).

The efficacy of ginger as an antiemetic in pregnancy was studied in a double-blind, randomized, cross-over trial involving women with hyperemesis gravidarum (12). All the subjects had been admitted to a hospital with hyperemesis and if their symptoms persisted for more than 2 days, they were enrolled in the study after giving informed consent. A total of 27 women at a mean gestational age of about 11 weeks completed the study. The women were administered either powdered root of ginger (1 g/day) or placebo for 4 days, then nothing for 2 days, then given the alternate agent for 4 days. More patients stated a preference for ($p = 0.003$), and had greater relief from their symptoms ($p = 0.035$), with ginger than with placebo. No maternal adverse effects were observed. The pregnancy outcomes were one spontaneous abortion in the 12th week of gestation, one elective abortion for reasons other than nausea and vomiting, and 25 normal living infants. The mean gestational age at delivery was 39.9 weeks (range 36–41 weeks) with a mean birth weight of 3585 g (range 2450–5150 g). All had Apgar scores of 9–10 at 5 minutes, and none had a congenital abnormality (12).

In a comment relating to the above study, one author urged caution in the use of ginger during pregnancy, citing ginger's action as a thromboxane synthetase inhibitor, which, theoretically, could affect testosterone receptor binding and result in adverse sex steroid differentiation of the fetal brain (13). Although the author's research failed to find evidence of toxicity caused by ginger, he recommended that it not be used in pregnancy until this effect was studied. No published reports to refute or support this alleged effect, however, have been located.

A 2001 randomized, double-masked study also evaluated the effect on ginger on nausea and vomiting of pregnancy (14). Ginger 1 g/day was compared to placebo for 4 days starting at a mean gestational age of about 10 weeks. Ginger resulted in a significant decrease in the severity of nausea and vomiting. No adverse effects on pregnancy outcome were detected (14).

The result of a prospective study of women consuming ginger in the 1st trimester for nausea and vomiting was reported in 2003 (15). The pregnancy outcomes of the exposed women were compared to a control group who were exposed to nonteratogenic drugs that were not antiemetics. The outcomes in the 187 ginger-exposed subjects were

3 spontaneous abortions, 1 elective abortion (Down's syndrome), 2 stillbirths, and 181 live births. Three liveborn infants had birth defects: ventricular septal defect; right lung abnormality; and a kidney abnormality (pelviectasis). In addition, a female child was later diagnosed with idiopathic central precocious puberty at 2 years of age. The mean birth weight was 3542 g and the mean gestational age at birth was 39 weeks. Except that more control infants weighed <2500 g, the outcomes between the groups did not differ significantly. Sixty-six women rated the effectiveness of the ginger in controlling nausea and vomiting. On a 10-point scale (0 being no effect and 10 the best effect), the mean score was 3.3 (within the "mild effect" range) (15).

A 2004 randomized, controlled trial was conducted in women at less than 16 weeks' gestation (16). Women were treated for 3 weeks with either ginger ($N = 146$) (1.05 g/day) or vitamin B6 ($N = 145$) (75 mg/day) and the efficacy of the treatments were measured at 7, 14, and 21 days. The median gestational age at the start of the study in the two groups was 8.5 and 8.6 weeks', respectively. There was no difference between the groups, averaged over time, in reducing nausea, retching, or vomiting. There also was no difference in the pregnancy outcomes, except that the ginger group had slightly more live births (16).

BREAST FEEDING SUMMARY

RECOMMENDATION: No Human Data - Probably Compatible

No studies describing the use of ginger during lactation have been located. It is unlikely, however, that small doses of ginger, such as those used as a spice, would affect a nursing infant. The effects, if any, of the higher doses used as an antiemetic are also unknown, but probably of little consequence to the infant. The oral bioavailability of ginger and its active ingredients, however, has not been studied in animals or humans.

References

1. Ginger. *The Review of Natural Products*. St. Louis, MO: Facts and Comparisons, May 2000.
2. Wilkinson JM. Effect of ginger tea on the fetal development of Sprague-Dawley rats. Reprod Toxicol 2000;14:507–12.
3. Weidner MS, Sigwart K. Investigation of the teratogenic potential of a Zingiber officinale extract in the rat. Reprod Toxicol 2001;15:75–80.
4. Mowrey DB, Clayson DE. Motion sickness, ginger, and psychophysics. Lancet 1982;1:655–7.
5. Liu WHD. Ginger root, a new antiemetic. Anaesthesia 1990;45:1085.
6. Bone ME, Wilkinson DJ, Young JR, McNeil J, Charlton S. Ginger root—a new antiemetic. The effect of ginger root on postoperative nausea and vomiting after major gynaecological surgery. Anaesthesia 1990;45:669–71.
7. Phillips S, Ruggier R, Hutchinson SE. *Zingiber officinale* (Ginger)—an antiemetic for day case surgery. Anaesthesia 1993;48:715–7.
8. Lumb AB. Mechanism of antiemetic effect of ginger. Anaesthesia 1993;48:1118.
9. Arfeen Z, Owen H, Plummer JL, Ilsley AH, Sorby-Adams RAC, Doecke CJ. A double-blind randomized controlled trial of ginger for the prevention of postoperative nausea and vomiting. Anaesth Intensive Care 1995;23:449–52.
10. Visalyaputra S, Petchpaisit N, Somcharoen K, Choavaratana R. The efficacy of ginger root in the prevention of postoperative nausea and vomiting after outpatient gynaecological laparoscopy. Anaesthesia 1998;53:486–510.
11. Ernst E, Pittler MH. Efficacy of ginger for nausea and vomiting: a systematic review of randomized clinical trials. Br J Anaesth 2000;84:367–71.
12. Fischer-Rasmussen W, Kjaer SK, Dahl C, Asping U. Ginger treatment of hyperemesis gravidarum. Eur J Obstet Gynecol Reprod Biol 1990;38:19–24.
13. Backon J. Ginger in preventing nausea and vomiting of pregnancy: a caveat due to its thromboxane synthetase activity and effect on testosterone binding. Eur J Obstet Gynecol Reprod Biol 1991;42:163.
14. Vutyavanich T, Kraisarin T, Ruangsri RA. Ginger for nausea and vomiting in pregnancy: randomized, double-masked, placebo-controlled trial. Obstet Gynecol 2001;97:577–82.
15. Portnoi G, Chng LA, Karimi-Tabesh L, Koren G, Tan MP, Einarson A. Prospective comparative study of the safety and effectiveness of ginger for the treatment of nausea and vomiting in pregnancy. Am J Obstet Gynecol 2003;189:1374–7.
16. Smith C, Crowther C, Willson K, Hotham N, McMillian V. A randomized controlled trial of ginger to treat nausea and vomiting of pregnancy. Obstet Gynecol 2004;103:639–45.

Name:	GINKGO BILOBA	Risk Factor:	C
Class:	Herb		

G

FETAL RISK SUMMARY

RECOMMENDATION: No Human Data - Animal Data Suggest Low Risk

Ginkgo biloba (scientific name) is a popular herbal preparation. The dioecious ginkgo tree may live as long as several hundred to a thousand years. It is the sole survivor of the family *Ginkgoaceae* that dates back more than 200 million years. The tree, which may grow to a height of 30 to 40 meters (approximately 98 to 131 feet), has fan-shaped leaves and is indigenous to China, Japan, and Korea (1–3). Commercial plantations of ginkgo trees in the United States, however, are pruned to shrub height to allow mechanical picking of the leaves (4).

The medicinal parts of ginkgo are the fresh and dried leaves, and the seeds separated from their fleshy outer layer (2). Ginkgo leaf extract, however, is the most commonly used form of this herb (3). Numerous uses have been recommended for the various IV (not available in United States) and oral preparations of ginkgo leaf extract, such as for symptomatic relief of organic brain syndrome (e.g., cerebral insufficiency, anxiety and stress, memory impairment, headache, dementias, etc.), intermittent claudication and other circulatory disorders, asthma, and vertigo, and tinnitus of vascular origin (1–5).

Ginkgo seed, although not commercially available in the United States, is used orally as an antitussive and expectorant, as an aid for digestion, to prevent drunkenness, in asthma and bronchitis, and for genitourinary complaints (3). Topical uses include scabies and skin sores. Roasted seeds with the pulp removed are eaten for food in Japan and China (3).

The content of active compounds in ginkgo leaves may vary widely depending upon the season (1,6). Seasonal and other factors, such as location and method of harvest, may result in a variance as much as 300% in the concentrations of active compounds (6). Ginkgo leaf extract is prepared using an acetone-water extraction process and subsequent purification steps without adding concentrates or isolated ingredients (2–5). A number of chemical constituents have been identified in the extract (percentages refer to German Commission E standards): 22%–27% flavanone glycosides (flavonoids consisting of monosides, biosides, and triosides of quercetin, kaempferol, isorhamnetins, and 3′-*O*-methylmyristicins); 5%–7% terpene lactones (terpenoids) (2.8%–3.4% ginkgolides A, B, C, and M [trilactonic diterpenes], 2.6%–3.2% bilobalide [trilactone sesquiterpene]); and less than 5 ppm of ginkgolic acids (1–5). Other chemical constituents found in the leaf before processing, in addition to those identified in the extract, include amino acid 6-hydroxykynurenic acid, bioflavonoids (dimeric bioflavones: amentoflavone, bilobetin, ginkgetin, isoginkgetin, 5-methoxybilobetin, sciadopitysin) (about 40 different bioflavonoids have been identified), terpene lactone (ginkgolide J), steroids (sitosterol, stigmasterol), polyprenols, organic acids (shikimic, vanillic, ascorbic, p-coumaric), benzoic acid derivatives, carbohydrates, straight chain hydrocarbons, alcohol, ketones, and 2-hexenol (1). A 1993 reference detailed the chemical structures of the active ingredients (flavonoids and terpene lactones) (7).

The seed contains 38% carbohydrate, 4% protein, and less than 2% fat (1). This part of the tree is not marketed in the United States, but may contaminate other ginkgo products (8). Chemicals found in the seed are alkaloids (e.g., ginkgotoxin), amino acids, cyanogenetic glycosides, and long-chain phenols (e.g., anacardic acid, bilobol, and cardanol) (1).

Reproduction studies in animals have revealed no mutagenic or teratogenic effects (1). No teratogenicity was observed in pregnant rats given oral doses up to 1600 mg/kg/day (1).

In a sperm penetration assay, zona-free hamster oocytes were incubated for 1 hour with two concentrations of ginkgo biloba, 0.1 mg/mL and 1.0 mg/mL, dissolved in HEPES-buffered synthetic human tubal fluid (modified HTF) (9). Fresh human donor sperm was suspended in the modified HTF and then mixed with the oocytes for 3 hours. Modified HTF served as the control. At the 0.1 mg/mL concentration, three of nine oocytes were penetrated, whereas at 1.0 mg/mL, zero (0 of 8) penetration occurred. The decrease in penetration was not associated with a decrease in sperm motility (9). In the second part of the study, sperm were incubated with the herbal solutions for 7 days (9). Neither concentration caused significant sperm DNA denaturation or mutation of a selected sperm sentinel gene (BRCA1 exon 11 gene), but the higher concentration reduced sperm viability compared with controls. Extrapolation of these data to the reproductive risk of ginkgo biloba in males is difficult, in part because the concentration of the herb in semen or sperm has not been studied (9). Moreover, although the doses used in this study are small fractions of the actual recommended human dose, usually expressed in milligrams of ginkgo, there is no published evidence that the adverse effects observed have occurred *in vivo*.

Although some ginkgo preparations may be standardized, the standardization of any herbal product as to its constituents, concentrations, and the presence of contaminants is generally lacking. Consumption of these products during pregnancy may result in fetal exposure to unintended chemicals and doses.

In summary, no reports describing the use of ginkgo biloba during human pregnancy have been located. No mutagenicity in animals or human sperm was observed and no teratogenicity occurred in one animal species, but the data and details of the animal studies are very limited. Moreover, a large number of chemicals have been identified from this herb and none have undergone rigorous reproductive testing. However, because ginkgo is an ancient herb and its use is widespread, it is doubtful that a major teratogenic effect or other significant reproductive toxicity would have escaped notice. More subtle or low-incidence effects, however, including structural and behavioral teratogenicity, the induction of abortions, and infertility may have escaped detection, and further study is required before human reproductive risk or safety can be assessed.

Because of the uncertainties described above, various sources can be found that either state there are no restrictions against it use in pregnancy (5) or that the herb is contraindicated during gestation (1,3,10). The safest course is to avoid ginkgo products during pregnancy.

BREAST FEEDING SUMMARY

RECOMMENDATION: No Human Data - Potential Toxicity

No reports describing the use of ginkgo biloba during lactation have been located. Although one source states that there are no restrictions to its use during lactation (5), other sources consider the use of the herb during lactation to be contraindicated (1,3,10). The latter course is the safest because of the large number of chemical compounds in the herb and the complete lack of information on the effects of exposure to these substances in a nursing infant.

References

1. Ginkgo. *The Review of Natural Products*. St. Louis, MO: Facts and Comparisons. March, 1998.
2. Ginkgo Biloba. *PDR for Herbal Medicines*. Montvale, NJ: Medical Economics. 1998:871–3.
3. Ginkgo Leaf, Ginkgo Leaf Extract, Ginkgo Seed. *Natural Medicines Comprehensive Database*. Stockton, CA: Therapeutic Research Faculty. 1999:377–81.
4. Robbers JE, Tyler VE. *Tyler's Herbs of Choice. The Therapeutic Use of Phytomedicinals*. Binghamton, NY: Haworth Press. 2000:141–6.
5. Ginkgo biloba leaf extract. Blumenthal M, senior editor. *The Complete German Commission E Monographs. Therapeutic Guide to Herbal Medicines*. Austin, TX: American Botanical Council. 1998:136–8.
6. Product information. BioGinkgo 27/7. Pharmanex, 1998.
7. Sticher O. Quality of Ginkgo preparations. Planta Medica 1993;59:2–11.
8. Boullata JI, Nace AM. Safety issues with herbal medicine. Pharmacotherapy 2000;20:257–69.
9. Ondrizek RR, Chan PJ, Patton WC, King A. An alternative medicine study of herbal effects on the penetration of zona-free hamster oocytes and the integrity of sperm deoxyribonucleic acid. Fertil Steril 1999;71:517–22.
10. Wong AHC, Smith M, Boon HS. Herbal remedies in psychiatric practice. Arch Gen Psychiatry 1998;55:1033–44.

Name:	**GINSENG**	Risk Factor:	**B**
Class:	**Herb**		

FETAL RISK SUMMARY

RECOMMENDATION: Limited Human Data - Animal Data Suggest Low Risk

Ginseng is a plant that is found throughout the world. The root is considered the most important part of plant as it contains the pharmacologically active ginsenosides. Ginseng has been used in medicine for more than 2000 years. The herb is promoted as having multiple pharmacologic effects, including adaptogenic, CNS, cardiovascular, endocrine, ergogenic, antineoplastic, and immunomodulatory effects. It is available as fresh or dried roots, extracts, solutions, tablets, sodas, teas, chewing gum, cigarettes, and candy (1–3).

Although the name ginseng (common names, if given, shown in parentheses) commonly refers to *Panax quinquefollus* L. (American or Canadian ginseng) or *P. ginseng* C.A. Meyer (Asian, Chinese, Korean, or Oriental ginseng; red ginseng [steamed]), one source listed seven other recognized medicinal ginsengs (1). They are *P. japonicus* var *bipinnatifidus*, *P. japonicus* C. A. Meyer (Japanese, Chikusetsu, or zhu je ginseng), *P. japonicus* var *major*, *P. notoginseng* (Western or Five-fingers ginseng; Sang; San-chi; Tien-chan or tienqi ginseng), *P. pseudoginseng* subsp. *himalaicus* (Himalayan ginseng), *P. pseudoginseng* var *major* (Zhuzishen), and *P. vietnamensis* Ha et Grushv. (Vietnamese ginseng) (1).

A 1994 letter stated that there were eight species and three varieties of genus *Panax* in the northern hemisphere (4). The eight species were *ginseng*, *quinquefolium*, *notoginseng*, *pseudoginseng*, *zingigerensis*, *trifolus*, *stipuleanatus*, and *japonicus*. The varieties of *P. japonicus* were identified as var *major*, var *angustifolius*, and var *bipinnatifidus*.

Ginseng products are commercially available as food flavorings and herbal medicines. Although the minor constituents of ginseng listed below might have some role, the principal pharmacologically active ingredients of ginseng appear to be a group of steroid-like compounds linked to sugars, called saponins (ginsenosides) (1). At least 13 major saponins, as well as numerous minor glycosides, have been identified. Minor constituents include volatile oils, beta-elemene, sterols, acetylenes, polysaccharides, starch, flavonoids, peptides, various B-complex vitamins, minerals, enzymes, and choline (1). Xanthines (e.g., caffeine, theophylline, and theobromine), produced by the plant, may also be present in various concentrations and may contribute to the pharmacologic action of the product (1).

The actual amount of ginsenosides in commercial preparations varies widely. This variance partially reflects poor quality control, but may also depend upon the species, age of the root, location, season of harvest, and preservation or curing method (1). In addition, products sold as ginseng may actually contain no ginsenosides (2,5). For example, other herbal species that do not contain ginsenosides are also called "ginseng," such as Siberian ginseng (*Eleutherococcus senticosus*; active constituents are eleutherosides) and Brazilian ginseng (*Pfaffia paniculata*) (6). In addition, Chinese silk vine (*Periploca sepium*), an herb that contains cardiac glycosides but no ginsenosides, is a common substitute for Siberian ginseng (7).

A reproduction study with rats was conducted with an extract (G115) of Oriental ginseng (*P. ginseng*) (8). Two generations of rats, male and female, were fed a diet supplemented with ginseng extract at doses of 1.5, 5, or 15 mg/kg/day or a control diet. No differences in treatment-related effects were observed between the groups in terms of body weights, food consumption, and hematological and clinical chemical data. In addition, no differences were noted in ophthalmic, gross and histopathological examinations, or in autopsies (8).

Ginseng (*P. ginseng*) was used as a fetal protectant in a study involving rats given hexavalent chromium throughout gestation (9). Hexavalent chromium, the most toxic form of chromium for the embryo and fetus, was fed to two groups of female rats in their drinking water. In one of the groups, ginseng (20 mg/kg/day) was also given. A third group received ginseng only, whereas a control group received neither agent. The rats receiving chromium plus ginseng had significantly better pregnancy outcomes than those receiving only chromium in terms of increased maternal weight gain, fewer pre- and post-implantation losses, resorptions, and stillbirths, and lower rates of visceral and skeletal anomalies (9).

The effects of American ginseng (*P. quinquefolium*) on male copulatory behavior have been studied in rats (10). Doses of 10–100 mg/kg/day given for 28 days significantly stimulated copulatory behavior. In comparison to controls, no effects were noted on plasma luteinizing hormone or testosterone levels, or on sex organs, but plasma prolactin concentrations were significantly decreased in ginseng-treated animals (10).

Three brief reports have described an estrogen-like effect (11) and vaginal bleeding (12,13) in three postmenopausal women taking ginseng (*P. ginseng* in two; unknown source in one).

A 30-year-old woman took an herbal preparation alleged to be pure Siberian ginseng (1300 mg/day - twice the manufacturer's recommended dose) throughout pregnancy and during the first 2 weeks of breast-feeding (14). In late pregnancy, she had repeated occurrences of premature uterine contractions. She also thought that the hair growth on her head, face, and pubic region had increased and was thicker. The term, 3.3-kg male infant had thick black hair in the pubic region and over the entire forehead, and swollen, red nipples (14). The mother stopped breast-feeding 2 weeks postpartum on medical advice because she did not want to stop taking the herb. At 7.5 weeks of age, the infant's weight (5.8 kg) and length (60.6 cm) were above the 97th percentile, but the pubic and forehead hair, which had begun to fallout at 2 weeks, was scant. A physical examination revealed enlarged testes (volume = 3 mL) that were otherwise normal. In addition, there was no evidence of adrenogenital syndrome as the serum concentrations of 17-hydroxyprogesterone, testosterone, and cortisol were within normal ranges. The investigators noted that ginseng increases testosterone levels in male rats and testes growth in rabbits, and could significantly increase corticotropin and corticosteroid levels. Therefore, they concluded that the product she was taking might have caused the hirsutism in the mother and infant and the infant's excessive weight gain (14).

In response to the above case, a representative for a government agency argued that the cited animal studies involving ginseng had no relevance because the active constituents of Siberian ginseng were eleutherosides that are completely different from ginsenosides (15). In reply, one of the investigators stated that they had recently given the woman doses either of her Siberian ginseng or placebo in a double-blind manner. Her testosterone levels were undetectable when she was taking the herb and normal when she received placebo. The investigator hypothesized that the product she was taking contained a compound that suppressed, but acted like, endogenous testosterone (16). In the last correspondence on this case, three bulk lots of powder supposedly containing Siberian ginseng were obtained from the manufacturer of the product taken by the woman. The lot dates overlapped the period of her pregnancy. Chemical analysis revealed that the powder was actually Chinese silk vine (*P. sepium*), the bark of which contains cardioactive glycosides (17). Inadvertent substitution of Chinese silk vine for Siberian ginseng had occurred previously and may have resulted because of confusion surrounding the Chinese names of the herbs (17).

A brief 1991 correspondence compared the outcomes of 88 Asian women who had taken ginseng during pregnancy with 88 matched controls who had not taken the herb (18). No statistically significant differences were found in the mode of delivery, birth weight, low birth weight (<2500 g), preterm delivery (<37 weeks), low Apgar scores (<7), and stillbirths or neonatal deaths. Regarding pregnancy complications, there were no differences in the incidence of gestational diabetes, or antepartum or postpartum hemorrhage, but significantly more controls than subjects had preeclampsia (1 vs. 8; $p < 0.02$). No mention was made of congenital malformations in either group (18).

In summary, ginseng is an ancient popular herb that is used extensively throughout the world. The reproductive effects of the herb in pregnant animals, except in one case, have not been studied. Similarly, only one small study has investigated its effect in human pregnancy, but the study did not mention if birth defects were observed. Like most herbal preparations, there appears to be little or no quality control in the production of commercial products, and mislabeling of these products is probably common. Ginseng is known to act on multiple organ systems. Depending on the product ingested and the dose and duration of use, the herb can produce clinically significant adverse reactions in nonpregnant patients. Hypertension and hypoglycemia have been reported with ginseng (1). These effects could complicate pregnancies with hypertensive disorders or diabetes. However, because ginseng has been used in medicine for more than 2000 years and its current use is widespread, it is doubtful if it causes major birth defects or other clinically significant developmental toxicity. More subtle or low-incidence effects, however, including structural and behavioral teratogenicity, the induction of abortions, and infertility may have escaped detection. Further study using products identified by chemical analysis is required before human reproductive risk or safety can be assessed.

BREAST FEEDING SUMMARY

RECOMMENDATION: No Human Data - Potential Toxicity

No studies describing the use of ginseng during human lactation have been located. Confusion has arisen in the past over the actually identity of commercial products (see above), so without chemical analysis the actual herb ingested is uncertain. Ginseng can affect multiple organ systems in users and, potentially, could adversely affect a nursing infant if the ginsenosides (active constituents) were excreted into breast milk. However, it is doubtful if ginseng has caused clinically significant effects in nursing infants because of its ancient and widespread use. Although more subtle affects on a nursing infant could have been missed, the proven benefits of breast-feeding may outweigh the unknown risk from exposure to the active and inactive constituents of ginseng. Women taking this herb and nursing should be informed of this uncertainty.

References

1. Ginseng, Panax. *The Review of Natural Products*. St. Louis, MO: Facts and Comparisons, February 2001.
2. Robbers JE, Tyler VE. *Tyler's Herbs of Choice*. Binghamton, NY: Haworth Herbal Press, 1999:238.
3. Attele AS, Wu JA, Yuan CS. Ginseng pharmacology. Multiple constituents and multiple actions. Biochem Pharmacol 1999;58:1685–93.
4. Vigano C, Ceppi E. What is in ginseng? Lancet 1994;344:619.
5. Cui J, Garle M, Eneroth P, Björkem I. What do commercial ginseng preparations contain? Lancet 1994; 344:134.
6. Walker AF. What is in ginseng? Lancet 1994;344:619.
7. Wong HCG. Probable false authentication of herbal plants: ginseng. Arch Intern Med 1999;159:1142.
8. Hess FG Jr, Parent RA, Cox GE, Stevens KR, Becci PJ. Reproduction study in rats of ginseng extract G115. Food Chem Toxicol 1982;20:189–92.
9. Elsaleed EM, Nada SA. Teratogenicity of hexavalent chromium in rats and the beneficial role of ginseng. Bull Environ Contam Toxicol 2002;68:361–8.
10. Murphy LL, Cadena RS, Chavez D, Ferraro JS. Effect of American ginseng (*Panax quinquefolium*) on male copulatory behavior in the rat. Physiol Behavior 1998;64:445–50.
11. Punnonen R, Lukola A. Oestrogen-like effect of ginseng. Br Med J 1980;281:1110.
12. Greenspan EM. Ginseng and vaginal bleeding. JAMA 1983;249:2018.
13. Palop-Larrea V, Gonzálvez-Perales JL, Catalán-Oliver C, Belenguer-Varea A, Martínez-Mir I. Metrorrhagia and ginseng. Ann Pharmacother 2000;34:1347–8.
14. Koren G, Randor S, Martin S, Danneman D. Maternal ginseng use associated with neonatal androgenization. JAMA 1990;264:2866.
15. Awang DVC. Maternal use of ginseng and neonatal androgenization. JAMA 1991;265:1828.
16. Koren G. Maternal use of ginseng and neonatal androgenization. JAMA 1991;265:1828.
17. Awang DVC. Maternal use of ginseng and neonatal androgenization. JAMA 1991;266:363.
18. Chin RKH. Ginseng and common pregnancy disorders. Asia Oceania J Obstet Gynaecol 1991;17: 379–80.

Name:	**GITALIN**	Risk Factor:	**C**
Class:	**Cardiac Glycoside**		

See Digitalis.

Name:	**GLATIRAMER**	Risk Factor:	$\mathbf{B_M}$
Class:	**Immunologic Agent (Immunosuppressive)**		

FETAL RISK SUMMARY

RECOMMENDATION: Compatible - Maternal Benefit >> Embryo/Fetal Risk

Glatiramer (copolymer-1) is an immunosuppressant agent given by SC injection to reduce the frequency of relapses in patients with relapsing-remitting multiple sclerosis. It is the acetate salts of synthetic polypeptides containing four naturally occurring amino acids: L-glutamic acid, L-alanine, L-lysine, and L-tyrosine (1). Chemically, glatiramer is designated glutamic acid polymer with L-alanine, L-lysine, and L-tyrosine (1).

Reproduction studies during organogenesis have been conducted in rats and rabbits at SC doses up to 18 and 36 times the human dose of 20 mg on a body surface area basis (HD), respectively (1). No adverse fetal effects were observed in either species. Pregnant rats were also given glatiramer at doses up to approximately 18 times the HD from gestational day 15 and throughout lactation. No significant effects were observed on delivery or pup growth or development (1). Multigeneration fertility and reproductive performance studies conducted in rats at SC doses up to 18 times the HD revealed no adverse effects on reproductive parameters (1).

It is not known if glatiramer crosses the human placenta to the fetus. The molecular weights of the polypeptides average 4700 to 11,000, suggesting that they do not cross by simple diffusion.

No published reports on the use of glatiramer during human pregnancy have been found. Based solely on animal data, the drug does not appear to present a significant risk to the fetus. Among 979 patients treated during premarketing clinical trials or in the postmarketing period, vaginal hemorrhage occurred with a frequency of at least 1/100 and abortions with a frequency between 1/100 and 1/1000 (1). Although the cause of these outcomes is unknown, they may have occurred by chance or from the disease and may not be specifically related to glatiramer.

In spite of the uncertainty surrounding the use of glatiramer during pregnancy, the benefits of the drug in reducing the number of relapses of multiple sclerosis appears to outweigh the potential risks to the fetus. The patient should be advised of the lack of human data and the potential risk of abortion. If she consents, starting therapy after the 1st trimester, if possible, and after confirming that she has a viable pregnancy is probably the safest course.

BREAST FEEDING SUMMARY

RECOMMENDATION: No Human Data - Probably Compatible

No reports describing the use of glatiramer during lactation have been located. Because of the high molecular weight (4700–11,000), it is doubtful that the unmetabolized agent is excreted into breast milk.

Reference

1. Product information. Copaxone. TevaMarion Partners, 2000.

Name:	**GLIMEPIRIDE**	Risk Factor:	**C_M**
Class:	**Oral Hypoglycemic**		

FETAL RISK SUMMARY

RECOMMENDATION: No Human Data - Animal Data Suggest Low Risk

Glimepiride is a second-generation sulfonylurea in the same class as glipizide and glyburide (see also Glipizide and Glyburide). It is used as an adjunct to diet and exercise, either alone or in combination with other oral agents, in the treatment of type II diabetes (non-insulin-dependent diabetes mellitus). It has also been used in combination with insulin when diet, exercise, and an oral hypoglycemic have not controlled hyperglycemia.

Reproduction studies in animals have been conducted with glimepiride (1). No teratogenic effects were observed in rats and rabbits given doses up to approximately 4,000 and 60 times, respectively, the maximum recommended human dose based on body surface area (MRHD). However, in some studies, rat pups, nursing from mothers given high doses of glimepiride during pregnancy and lactation, developed skeletal deformities consisting of shortening, thickening, and bending of the humerus during the postnatal period (1). Moreover, fetotoxicity (intrauterine death) occurred in both rats and rabbits at 50 and 0.1 times, respectively, the MRHD. The fetotoxicity, that had also been observed with other sulfonylureas, occurred only at doses that produced maternal hypoglycemia and was thought to be due to that affect (1). No effect on the fertility of male and female rats was noted at doses up to 4,000 times the MRHD (1).

It is not known if glimepiride crosses the placenta, but the molecular weight (about 491) is low enough that transfer to the fetus should be expected. Hypoglycemia in the newborn may occur if glimepiride is taken close to delivery.

No reports describing the use of glimepiride during human pregnancy have been located. Insulin is the treatment of choice for pregnant diabetic patients because, in general, other hypoglycemic agents do not provide adequate glycemic control. Moreover, insulin, unlike most oral agents, does not cross the placenta to the fetus, thus eliminating the additional concern that the drug therapy itself will adversely effect the fetus. Carefully prescribed insulin therapy provides better control of the mother's glucose, thereby preventing the fetal and neonatal complications that occur with this disease. High maternal glucose levels, as may occur in diabetes mellitus, are closely associated with a number of maternal and fetal adverse effects, including fetal structural anomalies if the hyperglycemia occurs early in gestation. To prevent this toxicity, most experts, including the American College of Obstetricians and Gynecologists, recommend that insulin be used for types I and II diabetes occurring during pregnancy and, if diet therapy alone is not successful, for gestational diabetes (2,3).

BREAST FEEDING SUMMARY

RECOMMENDATION: No Human Data - Probably Compatible

No reports describing the use of glimepiride during human lactation have been located. Consistent with its relatively low molecular weight (about 491), significant concentrations of glimepiride have been found in rat milk and in the serum of rat pups (1). Because neonatal hypoglycemia is a potential effect, women taking glimepiride should consider changing to insulin therapy during the nursing period (1).

References

1. Product information. Amaryl. Hoechst Marion Roussel, 2000.
2. American College of Obstetricians and Gynecologists. Diabetes and pregnancy. *Technical Bulletin*. No. 200, December 1994.
3. Coustan DR. Management of gestational diabetes. Clin Obstet Gynecol 1991;34:558–64.

Name:	**GLIPIZIDE**	Risk Factor:	**C_M**
Class:	**Oral Hypoglycemic**		

FETAL RISK SUMMARY

RECOMMENDATION: Limited Human Data - Animal Data Suggest Low Risk

Glipizide is an oral sulfonylurea agent, structurally similar to glyburide, that is used for the treatment of adult-onset diabetes mellitus. It is not the treatment of choice for the pregnant diabetic patient.

Reproductive studies in male and female rats showed no effect on fertility (1). Mild fetotoxicity (type not specified), observed at all doses tested in rats, was thought to be caused by the hypoglycemic action of glipizide. No teratogenic effects were observed in rats or rabbits (1).

In an abstract (2) and later in a full report (3), the *in vitro* placental transfer, using a single cotyledon human placenta, of four oral hypoglycemic agents was described. As expected, molecular weight was the most significant factor for drug transfer, with dissociation constant (pKa) and lipid solubility providing significant additive effect. The cumulative percent placental transfer at 3 hours of the four agents and their approximate molecular weights (shown in parenthesis) were tolbutamide (270) 21.5%, chlorpropamide (277) 11.0%, glipizide (446) 6.6%, and glyburide (494) 3.9%.

A 1984 source cited a study that described the use of glipizide in four diabetic patients from the 32nd week of gestation through delivery (4). No adverse effects in the fetuses were observed.

A study published in 1995 assessed the risk of congenital malformations in infants of mothers with non-insulin-dependent diabetes (NIDDM) during a 6-year period (5). Women were included in the study if, during the first 8 weeks of pregnancy, they had not participated in a preconception care program and then had been treated either with diet alone (Group 1), diet and oral hypoglycemic agents (predominantly chlorpropamide, glyburide, or glipizide) (Group 2), or diet and exogenous insulin (Group 3). The 302 women eligible for analysis gave birth to 332 infants (5 sets of twins and 16 with two or three separate singleton pregnancies during the study period). A total of 56 (16.9%) infants had one or more congenital malformations, 39 (11.7%) of which were classified as major anomalies (defined as those that were either lethal, caused significant morbidity, or required surgical repair). The major anomalies were divided among those involving the central nervous system, face, heart and great vessels, gastrointestinal, genitourinary, and skeletal (includes caudal regression syndrome) systems. Minor anomalies included all of these, except those of the central nervous system, and a miscellaneous group composed of sacral skin tags, cutis aplasia of the scalp, and hydroceles. The number of infants in each group and the number of major and minor anomalies observed were Group 1: 125 infants, 18 (14.4%) major, 6 (4.8%) minor; Group 2: 147 infants, 14 (9.5%) major, 9 (6.1%) minor; and Group 3: 60 infants, 7 (11.7%) major, 2 (3.3%) minor. There were no statistical differences among the groups. Six (4.1%) of the infants exposed *in utero* to oral hypoglycemic agents and 4 other infants in the other two groups had ear anomalies (included among those with face defects). Other than the incidence of major anomalies, two other important findings of this study were (a) the independent associations between the risk of major anomalies (but not minor defects) and poor glycemic control in early pregnancy and (b) a younger maternal age at the onset of diabetes (5). Moreover, the study did not find an association between the use of oral hypoglycemics during organogenesis and congenital malformations, in that the observed anomalies appeared to be related to poor maternal glycemic control (5).

In summary, although the use of glipizide may be beneficial for decreasing the incidence of fetal and newborn morbidity and mortality in developing countries where the proper use of insulin is problematic, insulin is still the treatment of choice for this disease during pregnancy. Oral hypoglycemic agents are not indicated for the pregnant diabetic, because they will not provide good control in patients who cannot be controlled by diet alone (6). Moreover, insulin, unlike glipizide, does not cross the placenta and, thus, eliminates the additional concern that the drug therapy itself is adversely affecting the fetus. Carefully prescribed insulin therapy will provide better control of the mother's blood glucose, thereby preventing the fetal and neonatal complications that occur with this disease. High maternal glucose levels, as may occur in diabetes mellitus, are closely associated with a number of maternal and fetal adverse effects, including fetal structural anomalies if the hyperglycemia occurs early in gestation. To prevent this toxicity, most experts, including the American College of Obstetricians and Gynecologists, recommend that insulin be used for types I and II diabetes occurring during pregnancy and, if diet therapy alone is not successful, for gestational diabetes (7,8). If glipizide is used during pregnancy, therapy should be changed to insulin, and glipizide should be discontinued before delivery (the exact time before delivery is unknown) to lessen the possibility of prolonged hypoglycemia in the newborn.

BREAST FEEDING SUMMARY

RECOMMENDATION: No Human Data - Probably Compatible

No reports have been located that describe the use of glipizide during lactation. Other antidiabetic sulfonylurea agents are excreted into milk (e.g., see Chlorpropamide and Tolbutamide) and excretion of glipizide should be expected. The effect on the nursing infant from this exposure is unknown but hypoglycemia is a potential toxicity.

References

1. Product information. Glucotrol. Pfizer Inc., 1997.
2. Elliott B, Schenker S, Langer O, Johnson R, Prihoda T. Oral hypoglycemic agents: profound variation exists in their rate of human placental transfer (abstract). Am J Obstet Gynecol 1992;166:368.
3. Elliott BD, Schenker S, Langer O, Johnson R, Prihoda T. Comparative placental transport of oral hypoglycemic agents in humans: a model of human placental drug transfer. Am J Obstet Gynecol 1994;171:653–60.
4. Onnis A, Grella P. *The Biochemical Effects of Drugs in Pregnancy*. Vol. 2. West Sussex, England: Ellis Horwood Limited, 1984:174–5.
5. Towner D, Kjos SL, Leung B, Montoro MM, Xiang A, Mestman JH, Buchanan TA. Congenital malformations in pregnancies complicated by NIDDM. Diabetes Care 1995;18:1446–51.
6. Friend JR. Diabetes. Clin Obstet Gynecol 1981;8: 353–82.
7. American College of Obstetricians and Gynecologists. Diabetes and pregnancy. *Technical Bulletin* No. 200, December 1994.
8. Coustan DR. Management of gestational diabetes. Clin Obstet Gynecol 1991;34:558–64.

Name: **GLYBURIDE** Risk Factor: **C_M**

Class: **Oral Hypoglycemic**

FETAL RISK SUMMARY

RECOMMENDATION: Human Data Suggest Low Risk

Glyburide is a second-generation, oral sulfonylurea agent, structurally similar to acetohexamide and glipizide, that is used for the treatment of adult-onset diabetes mellitus. It is not the treatment of choice for the pregnant diabetic patient. Glyburide is metabolized to inactive metabolites. The decrease in glyburide serum levels is biphasic with a terminal half-life of about 10 hours (1).

No fetotoxicity or teratogenicity was observed in pregnant mice, rats, and rabbits fed large doses of the agent (2). In pregnant rats, glyburide crossed the placenta to the fetus (fetal:maternal ratio 0.541) in amounts similar to diazepam (fetal:maternal ratio 0.641) (3).

In studies using *in vitro* techniques with human placentas, only relatively small amounts of glyburide were observed to transfer from the maternal to the fetal circulation (4–9), and the use of placentas from diabetic patients (5) or with high glucose concentrations (6) did not change the amounts transferred. Concentrations used on the maternal side of the perfused placenta model were approximately 800 ng/mL, much higher than the average peak serum level of 140–350 ng/mL obtained after a single 5-mg oral dose (7). Transport of the drug to the fetal side of the placenta was 0.62% at 2 hours.

In an abstract (8), and later in a full report (9), the *in vitro* placental transfer, using a single cotyledon human placenta, of four oral hypoglycemic agents was described. As expected, molecular weight was the most significant factor for drug transfer, with the dissociation constant (pKa) and lipid solubility providing a significant additive effect. The cumulative percent placental transfer at 3 hours of the four agents and their approximate molecular weights (shown in parenthesis) were tolbutamide (270) 21.5%, chlorpropamide (277) 11.0%, glipizide (446) 6.6%, and glyburide (494) 3.9%. In another abstract, this same group of investigators, using similar *in vitro* techniques with human placentas, demonstrated that glyburide did not increase glucose transfer to the fetus or affect the placental uptake of glucose (10). *In vivo* studies of glyburide human placental transport have not been located.

A commentary in 2001 considered several factors (pKa, molecular weight, lipid solubility, elimination half-life, and protein binding) that could limit glyburide from crossing the placenta (11). The author concluded that the short elimination half-life (4 hours) and extensive protein binding (99.8%) were the major determinants limiting transplacental transfer (11).

A 1991 report described the outcomes of pregnancies in 21 non-insulin-dependent diabetic women who were treated with oral hypoglycemic agents (17 sulfonylureas, 3 biguanides, and 1 unknown type) during the 1st trimester (12). The duration of exposure ranged from 3 to 28 weeks, but all patients were changed to insulin therapy at the first prenatal visit. Forty non-insulin-dependent diabetic women matched for age, race, parity, and glycemic control served as a control group. Eleven (52%) of the exposed infants had major or minor congenital malformations compared with 6 (15%) of the controls. Moreover, ear defects, a malformation that is observed, but uncommonly, in diabetic embryopathy, occurred in six of the exposed infants and in none of the controls. Two of the infants with defects (anencephaly; ventricular septal defect) were exposed *in utero* to glyburide during the first 10 and 23 weeks of gestation, respectively, but these and the other malformations observed, with the possible exception of the ear defects, were thought to be related to poor blood glucose control during organogenesis. The cluster of ear defects, however, suggested a drug effect or synergism between the drug and lack of metabolic control in the mother (12). Sixteen livebirths occurred in the exposed group compared to 36 in controls. The groups did not differ in the incidence of hypoglycemia at birth (53% vs. 53%), but 3 of the exposed newborns (not exposed to glyburide) had severe hypoglycemia lasting 2, 4, and 7 days, even though the mothers had not used oral hypoglycemics close to delivery. This was attributed to irreversible β-cell hyperplasia that may have been increased by exposure to oral hypoglycemics. Hyperbilirubinemia was noted in 10 (67%) of 15 exposed newborns compared to 13 (36%) of controls ($p < 0.04$), and polycythemia and hyperviscosity requiring partial exchange transfusions were observed in 4 (27%) of 15 exposed vs. 1 (3.0%) control ($p < 0.03$) (1 exposed infant was not included in these data because of delivery after completion of study) (12).

The use of glyburide in all phases of human gestation has been reported in other studies (13–17). In these studies, glyburide (glibenclamide) was either used alone or combined with the oral antihyperglycemic agent, metformin (see Metformin). Neonatal hypoglycemia (blood glucose <25 mg/dL) was present in 4 of 15 (27%) newborns who were exposed to glyburide during gestation (14,15). This adverse effect was 3.5 times that observed in a group of newborns whose mothers were treated with insulin. Moreover, in one newborn, the hypoglycemia persisted for more than 48 hours (14).

A study published in 1995 assessed the risk of congenital malformations in infants of mothers with non-insulin-dependent diabetes (NIDDM) over a 6-year period (18). Women were included in the study if, during the first 8 weeks of pregnancy, they had not participated in a preconception care program and then had been treated either with diet alone (Group 1), diet and oral hypoglycemic agents (predominantly chlorpropamide, glyburide, or glipizide) (Group 2), or diet and exogenous insulin (Group 3). The 302 women eligible for analysis gave birth to 332 infants (5 sets of twins and 16 with two or three separate singleton pregnancies during the study period). A total of 56 (16.9%) of the infants had one or more congenital malformations, 39 (11.7%) of which were classified as major anomalies (defined as those that were either lethal, caused significant morbidity, or required surgical repair). The major anomalies were divided among those involving the central nervous system, face, heart and great vessels, gastrointestinal, genitourinary, and skeletal (includes caudal regression syndrome) systems. Minor anomalies included all of these, except those of the central nervous system, and a miscellaneous group composed of sacral skin tags, cutis aplasia of the scalp, and hydroceles. The number of infants in each group and the number of major and minor anomalies observed were Group 1: 125 infants, 18 (14.4%) major, 6 (4.8%) minor; Group 2: 147 infants, 14 (9.5%) major, 9 (6.1%) minor; and Group 3: 60 infants, 7 (11.7%) major, 2 (3.3%) minor. There were no statistical differences among the groups. Six (4.1%) of the infants exposed *in utero* to oral hypoglycemic agents and four other infants in the other two groups had ear anomalies (included among those with face defects). Another important finding of this study was the independent association between the risk of major anomalies and poor glycemic control in early pregnancy. The study did not find an association between the use of oral hypoglycemics during organogenesis and congenital malformations because the observed anomalies appeared to be related to poor maternal glycemic control (18).

In a surveillance study of Michigan Medicaid recipients conducted between 1985 and 1992 involving 229,101 completed pregnancies, 37 newborns had been exposed to glyburide during the 1st trimester (F. Rosa, personal communication, FDA, 1993). One (2.7%) major birth defect was observed (two expected), which was a cardiovascular defect (0.4 expected). No anomalies were observed in five other categories of defects (oral clefts, spina bifida, polydactyly, limb reduction defects, and hypospadias) for which specific data were available.

A study published in 2000 compared the pregnancy outcomes in gestational diabetic women with singleton pregnancies who were randomly assigned to treatment with glyburide or insulin (19). A majority of the women (83%) were Hispanic, mostly Mexican American. The study was not blinded. The goals of treatment were the achievement of a mean glucose concentration of 90–105 mg% and fasting, preprandial, and postprandial glucose levels of 60–90 mg%, 80–95 mg%, and <120 mg%, respectively. A total of 404 women were enrolled, 201 in the glyburide group and 203 in the insulin group. The mean pretreatment glucose concentrations, fasting, preprandial, and postprandial concentrations, and the glycosylated hemoglobins in the glyburide and insulin groups were 114 mg% vs. 116 mg%, 104 mg% vs. 108 mg%, 104 mg% vs. 107 mg%, 130 mg% vs. 129 mg%, and 5.7% vs. 5.6%, respectively. These results are indicative of mild hyperglycemia. There were no significant differences between the groups in terms of any characteristic, including the gestational age at start of therapy and at delivery. The mean doses of glyburide and insulin were 9 ± 6 mg/day and 85 ± 48 units/day, respectively.

Eight (4%) of the women randomized to glyburide failed to achieve good glycemic control and were changed to insulin. During treatment, the mean blood glucose concentrations and the mean fasting, preprandial, and postprandial values did not differ significantly between the glyburide and insulin groups. Nor was there a difference in the mean glycosylated hemoglobin values, 5.5% vs. 5.4%, respectively, measured late in the 3rd trimester. In 12 randomly selected women, the glyburide maternal serum concentrations ranged from 50 to 150 ng/mL, whereas glyburide was undetectable in cord serum, at a mean 8 ± 4 hours after the last dose. No significant differences were measured between the groups in terms of neonatal features, metabolic outcomes, or perinatal mortality (19).

Two reports described their experience with the use of glyburide for the treatment of gestational diabetes not controlled by diet (20,21). Both reported favorable control of glucose levels with relatively few patients requiring a change to insulin therapy.

In summary, although the use of glyburide may be beneficial for decreasing the incidence of fetal and newborn morbidity and mortality in developing countries and in some populations where the proper use of insulin is problematic, insulin is still the treatment of choice for this disease. However, the available evidence suggests that glyburide may be an acceptable alternative in gestational diabetes. Moreover, the agent does not appear to cross the placenta in detectable amounts. Insulin is the treatment of choice for diabetic types I and II. For non-insulin-dependent diabetics (type II), close control of the mother's blood glucose with insulin, preferably starting before conception, will help to prevent the fetal and neonatal complications that occur with this disease. High maternal glucose levels, as may occur in diabetes mellitus, are closely associated with a number of maternal and fetal adverse effects, including fetal structural anomalies if the hyperglycemia occurs early in gestation. To prevent this toxicity, most experts, including the American College of Obstetricians and Gynecologists, recommend that insulin be used for types I and II diabetes occurring during pregnancy and, if diet therapy alone is not successful, for gestational diabetes (22,23).

BREAST FEEDING SUMMARY

RECOMMENDATION: No Human Data - Probably Compatible

No reports have been located that describe the use of glyburide during lactation. Other antidiabetic sulfonylurea agents are excreted into milk (e.g., see Chlorpropamide and Tolbutamide) and excretion of glyburide should be expected. The effect on the nursing infant from this exposure is unknown but hypoglycemia is a potential toxicity.

References

1. Product information. Diaβeta. Aventis Pharmaceuticals, 2004.
2. Shepard TH. *Catalog of Teratogenic Agents*. 8th ed. Baltimore, MD: Johns Hopkins University Press, 1995:202.
3. Sivan E, Feldman B, Dolitzki M, Nevo N, Dekel N, Karasik A. Glyburide crosses the placenta *in vivo* in pregnant rats. Diabetologia 1995;38:753–6.
4. Elliott BD, Langer O, Schenker S, Johnson RF. Insignificant transfer of glyburide occurs across the human placenta. Am J Obstet Gynecol 1991;165:807–12.
5. Elliott BD, Bynum D, Langer O. Glyburide does not cross the diabetic placenta in significant amounts. Society of Perinatal Obstetricians Abstracts. Am J Obstet Gynecol 1993;168:360.
6. Elliott BD, Bynum D, Langer O. Maternal hyperglycemia does not alter in-vitro placental transfer of the oral hypoglycemic agent glyburide. Society of Perinatal Obstetricians Abstracts. Am J Obstet Gynecol 1993;168:360.
7. Elliott B, Langer O, Schenker S, Johnson R. Glyburide is insignificantly transported to the fetal circulation by the human placenta *in vitro* (abstract). Am J Obstet Gynecol 1991;164:247.
8. Elliott B, Schenker S, Langer O, Johnson R, Prihoda T. Oral hypoglycemic agents: profound variation exists in their rate of human placental transfer. Society of Perinatal Obstetricians Abstracts. Am J Obstet Gynecol 1992;166:368.
9. Elliott BD, Schenker S, Langer O, Johnson R, Prihoda T.

Comparative placental transport of oral hypoglycemic agents in humans: a model of human placental drug transfer. Am J Obstet Gynecol 1994;171:653–60.
10. Elliott BD, Crosby-Schmidt C, Langer O. Human placental glucose uptake and transport are not altered by pharmacologic levels of the oral hypoglycemic agent, glyburide. Society of Perinatal Obstetricians Abstracts. Am J Obstet Gynecol 1994;170:321.
11. Koren G. Glyburide and fetal safety; transplacental pharmacokinetic considerations. Reprod Toxicol 2001;15:227–9.
12. Piacquadio K, Hollingsworth DR, Murphy H. Effects of in-utero exposure to oral hypoglycaemic drugs. Lancet 1991;338:866–9.
13. Coetzee EJ, Jackson WPU. Diabetes newly diagnosed during pregnancy. A 4-year study at Groote Schuur Hospital. S Afr Med J 1979;56:467–75.
14. Coetzee EJ, Jackson WPU. Pregnancy in established non-insulin- dependent diabetics; a five-and-a-half year study at Groote Schuur Hospital. S Afr Med J 1980;58:795–802.
15. Coetzee EJ, Jackson WPU. Oral hypoglycaemics in the first trimester and fetal outcome. S Afr Med J 1984;65:635–7.
16. Coetzee EJ, Jackson WPU. The management of non-insulin-dependent diabetes during pregnancy. Diabetes Res Clin Pract 1986;5:281–7.
17. Ravina A. Insulin-dependent diabetes of pregnancy treated with the combination of sulfonylurea and insulin. Isr J Med Sci 1995;31:623–5.
18. Towner D, Kjos SL, Leung B, Montoro MM, Xiang A, Mestman JH, Buchanan TA. Congenital malformations in pregnancies complicated by NIDDM. Diabetes Care 1995;18:1446–51.
19. Langer O, Conway DL, Berkus MD, Xenakis EMJ, Gonzales O. A comparison of glyburide and insulin in women with gestational diabetes mellitus. N Engl J Med 2000;343:1134–8.
20. Velazquez MD, Bolnick J, Cloakey D, Gonzalez JL, Curet LB. The use of glyburide in the management of gestational diabetes. Obstet Gynecol 2003; 101(Suppl):88S.
21. Kremer CJ, Duff P. Glyburide for the treatment of gestational diabetes. Am J Obstet Gynecol 2004;190:1438–9.
22. American College of Obstetricians and Gynecologists. Diabetes and pregnancy. *Technical Bulletin*. No. 200. December 1994.
23. Coustan DR. Management of gestational diabetes. Clin Obstet Gynecol 1991;34:558–64.

Name: **GLYCERIN** Risk Factor: **C**
Class: **Diuretic**

FETAL RISK SUMMARY

RECOMMENDATION: No Human Data - Probably Compatible

No data are available.

BREAST FEEDING SUMMARY

RECOMMENDATION: No Human Data - Probably Compatible

No data are available.

Name: **GLYCOPYRROLATE** Risk Factor: **B_M**
Class: **Parasympatholytic (Anticholinergic)**

FETAL RISK SUMMARY

RECOMMENDATION: Limited Human Data - No Relevant Animal Data

Glycopyrrolate is an anticholinergic agent.

In pregnant sheep, the transfer of glycopyrrolate (0.025 mg/kg) across the placenta was significantly less than that of atropine (0.05 mg/kg) (1). No change in maternal or fetal arterial pressure, fetal heart rate, or beat-to-beat variability was observed. In pregnant dogs, the placental passage of glycopyrrolate was again significantly less than that of atropine (2).

In a large prospective study, 2,323 patients were exposed to this class of drugs during the 1st trimester, only 4 of whom took glycopyrrolate (3). A possible association was found between the total group and minor malformations. Glycopyrrolate has been used before cesarean section to decrease gastric secretions (4–7). Maternal heart rate, but not blood pressure, was increased. Uterine activity increased as expected for normal labor. Fetal heart rate and variability were not changed significantly, confirming the limited placental transfer of this quaternary ammonium compound. No effects in the newborns were observed.

Glycopyrrolate has been recommended as the anticholinergic of choice during anesthesia for electroconvulsive therapy in pregnant patients (8).

BREAST FEEDING SUMMARY

RECOMMENDATION: No Human Data - Probably Compatible

No data are available (see also Atropine).

References

1. Murad SHN, Conklin KA, Tabsh KMA, Brinkman CR III, Erkkola R, Nuwayhid B. Atropine and glycopyrrolate: hemodynamic effects and placental transfer in the pregnant ewe. Anesth Analg 1981;60:710–4.
2. Proakis AG, Harris GB. Comparative penetration of glycopyrrolate and atropine across the blood-brain and placental barriers in anesthetized dogs. Anesthesiology 1978;48:339–44.
3. Heinonen OP, Slone D, Shapiro S. *Birth Defects and Drugs in Pregnancy*. Littleton, MA: Publishing Sciences Group, 1977:346–53.
4. Diaz DM, Diaz SF, Marx GF. Cardiovascular effects of glycopyrrolate and belladonna derivatives in obstetric patients. Bull N Y Acad Med 1980;56:245–8.
5. Abboud TK, Read J, Miller F, Chen T, Valle R, Henriksen EH. Use of glycopyrrolate in the parturient: effect on the maternal and fetal heart and uterine activity. Obstet Gynecol 1981;57:224–7.
6. Roper RE, Salem MG. Effects of glycopyrrolate and atropine combined with antacid on gastric acidity. Br J Anaesth 1981;53:1277–80.
7. Abboud T, Raya J, Sadri S, Grobler N, Stine L, Miller F. Fetal and maternal cardiovascular effects of atropine and glycopyrrolate. Anesth Analg 1983;62:426–30.
8. Wise MG, Ward SC, Townsend-Parchman W, Gilstrap LC III, Hauth JC. Case report of ECT during high-risk pregnancy. Am J Psychiatry 1984;141:99–101.

Name:	**GOLD SODIUM THIOMALATE**	Risk Factor:	C_M
Class:	**Immunologic Agent (Antirheumatic)**		

FETAL RISK SUMMARY

RECOMMENDATION: Limited Human Data - Animal Data Suggest Low Risk

Gold sodium thiomalate is indicated in the treatment of active rheumatoid arthritis.

Teratogenic effects were observed in rats and rabbits given SC doses 140 and 175 times the usual human dose, respectively, during organogenesis (1). In rats, the defects were hydrocephaly and microphthalmia, whereas those in rabbits were limb malformations and gastroschisis.

Gold compounds have been used for the treatment of maternal rheumatoid arthritis and other conditions in a small number of pregnancies (2–7). One review noted that several pregnant patients had been treated with gold salts without harmful effects observed in the newborns (2). In a Japanese report, 119 patients were treated during the 1st trimester with gold, 26 of whom received the drug throughout pregnancy (3). Two anomalies were observed in the newborns—a dislocated hip in one infant and a flattened acetabulum in another infant—but the association with the therapy is unknown. A German case history involved a woman who received her last injection of gold for chronic polyarthritis in the 3rd week of pregnancy (4). A growth-retarded, 1750-g female infant was delivered at 40 weeks' gestation. Other than the low birth weight, no other abnormalities were noted in the infant, whose development during the next 2 years was normal. In another case, a woman had been treated with gold sodium thiomalate (sodium aurothiomalate) for 2 years immediately prior to pregnancy, receiving her last dose when several weeks pregnant (5). No adverse effects in the newborn were mentioned.

Gold compounds cross the placenta. A patient who had received a total dose of 570 mg of gold sodium thiomalate from before conception through the 20th week of gestation elected to terminate her pregnancy (6). No obvious fetal abnormalities were observed, but gold deposits were found in the fetal liver and kidneys. A second patient received monthly 100-mg injections of gold throughout pregnancy (7). The last dose, given 3 days prior to delivery, produced a cord serum concentration of 2.25 μg/mL, 57% of the simultaneous maternal serum level. No anomalies were observed in the infant.

Although gold compounds apparently do not pose a major risk to the fetus, the clinical experience is limited and long-term follow-up studies of exposed fetuses have not been reported. If gold compounds are used in pregnancy for the treatment of rheumatoid arthritis, healthcare professionals are encouraged to call the toll free number (877-311-8972) for information about patient enrollment in the OTIS Rheumatoid Arthritis study.

BREAST FEEDING SUMMARY

RECOMMENDATION: Limited Human Data - Probably Compatible

Gold is excreted in milk (5,8–10). A woman received a total aurothioglucose dose of 135 mg in the postpartum period (8). Gold levels in two milk samples collected a week apart were 8.64 and 9.97 μg/mL. The validity of these figures has been challenged on a mathematical basis, so the exact amount excreted is open to question (9). In addition, the timing of the samples in relation to the dose was not given. Of interest, however, was the demonstration of gold levels in the infant's red blood cells (0.354 μg/mL) and serum (0.712 μg/mL) obtained on the same date as the second milk sample. The author speculated that this unexpected oral absorption may have been the cause of various unexplained adverse reactions noted in nursing infants of mothers receiving gold injections, such as rashes, nephritis, hepatitis, and hematologic abnormalities (8).

Another report described a lactating woman who was treated with 50 mg of gold sodium thiomalate weekly for 7 weeks after an initial 20-mg dose (total dose 370 mg) (10). Milk and infant urine samples collected 66 hours after the last dose yielded gold levels of 22 and 0.4 ng/mL, respectively. Repeat samples collected 7 days after an additional 25-mg dose produced milk and urine levels of 40 and <0.4 ng/mL, respectively. Three months after cessation of therapy, transient facial edema was observed in the nursing infant, but it was not known whether this was related to the maternal gold administration.

In a 1986 report, two women were given IM injections of gold sodium thiomalate (5). One patient received 20 mg on day 1 followed by 50 mg on day 3. Milk concentrations rose from a low of 17 ng/mL (1.4% of simultaneous maternal serum) 10 hours after the first dose to a peak of 153 ng/mL (approximately 4.6% of maternal serum) 22 hours after the second dose. The second patient received three doses of the gold salt: 10 mg on day 1, 20 mg on day 8, and 20 mg on day 12. The peak milk concentration, 185 ng/mL (10.4% of maternal serum), occurred 3 hours after the third dose. The levels of gold in the milk of both patients increased steadily over the sampling periods. The investigators estimated that the nursing infant would receive about 20% of the maternal dose (5).

In summary, three studies have described the excretion of gold into breast milk, with milk concentrations in two of the studies being similar in magnitude. Gold absorption by the nursing infant has been documented. Although adverse effects have been suggested, a direct cause-and-effect relationship has not been proven. At least one set of investigators cautioned that nursing should be avoided because of the prolonged maternal elimination time after gold administration and the potential for toxicity in the infant (5). However, the American Academy of Pediatrics classifies gold salts as compatible with breast-feeding (11).

References

1. Product information. Myochrysine. Merck, 2000.
2. Freyberg RH, Ziff M, Baum J. Gold therapy for rheumatoid arthritis. In Hollander JL, McCarty DJ Jr, eds. *Arthritis and Allied Conditions*. 8th ed. Philadelphia, PA: Lea & Febiger, 1972:479.
3. Miyamoto T, Miyaji S, Horiuchi Y, Hara M, Ishihara K. Gold therapy in bronchial asthma-special emphasis upon blood level of gold and its teratogenicity. J Jpn Soc Intern Med 1974;63:1190–7.
4. Fuchs U, Lippert TH. Gold therapy and pregnancy. Dtsch Med Wochenschr 1986;111:31–4.
5. Ostensen M, Skavdal K, Myklebust G, Tomassen Y, Aarbakke J. Excretion of gold into human breast milk. Eur J Clin Pharmacol 1986;31:251–2.
6. Rocker I, Henderson WJ. Transfer of gold from mother to fetus. Lancet 1976;2:1246.
7. Cohen DL, Orzel J, Taylor A. Infants of mothers receiving gold therapy. Arthritis Rheum 1981;24:104–5.
8. Blau SP. Metabolism of gold during lactation. Arthritis Rheum 1973;16:777–8.
9. Gottlieb NL. Suggested errata. Arthritis Rheum 1974; 17:1057.
10. Bell RAF, Dale IM. Gold secretion in maternal milk. Arthritis Rheum 1976;19:1374.
11. Committee on Drugs, American Academy of Pediatrics. The transfer of drugs and other chemicals into human milk. Pediatrics 2001;108:776–89.

Name:	**GRANISETRON**	Risk Factor:	B_M
Class:	**Antiemetic**		

FETAL RISK SUMMARY

RECOMMENDATION: No Human Data - Animal Data Suggest Low Risk

Granisetron is an antiemetic used for the prevention of nausea and vomiting in patients receiving cancer chemotherapy. The drug is a selective 5-hydroxytryptamine$_3$ (5-HT_3) receptor antagonist with little or no affinity for other serotonin receptors (1). No evidence of an effect on plasma prolactin concentrations has been found in clinical studies.

Reproductive studies at doses up to 146 and 96 times, respectively, the recommended human dose (based on body surface area) in pregnant rats and rabbits found no evidence of impaired fertility or harm to the fetus (1). Shepard reviewed three studies conducted in rats and rabbits before and after conception or in the perinatal and postnatal periods that found no adverse fetal effects or drug-related effects on behavior (2).

It is not known whether granisetron crosses the placenta to the fetus. The molecular weight (about 349) is low enough, however, that passage to the fetus should be expected.

No reports describing the use of granisetron during human gestation have been located. Because of the indication for this drug, the opportunity for fetal exposure appears to be minimal.

BREAST FEEDING SUMMARY

RECOMMENDATION: No Human Data - Probably Compatible

No reports describing the use of granisetron during lactation have been located. The indication for granisetron therapy, however, suggests that the opportunities for use of the drug during lactation are minimal. Because of its low molecular weight (about 349), transfer into breast milk should be expected.

References

1. Product information. Kytril. SmithKline Beecham Pharmaceuticals, 1997.
2. Shepard TH. *Catalog of Teratogenic Agents*. 8th ed. Baltimore, MD: Johns Hopkins University Press, 1995:204–5.

Name: **GRISEOFULVIN** Risk Factor: **C**

Class: **Antifungal**

FETAL RISK SUMMARY

RECOMMENDATION: Limited Human Data - Animal Data Suggest Risk

Griseofulvin is a fungistatic antibiotic derived from a species of *Penicillium*. The drug is tumorigenic, embryotoxic, and teratogenic in some species of animals. Chronic oral exposure to griseofulvin in several strains of mice has induced hepatic and thyroid tumors (1). Hepatic tumors were also induced by relatively low weekly SC doses in mice during the first 3 weeks of life (1). Multiple malformations, including defects of the eye, skeleton, urogenital tract, and the central nervous system, were observed in fetuses of pregnant rats injected with 50–500 mg/kg on days 11 to 14 of gestation (2). Daily doses of 1250–1500 mg/kg (about 60 to 75 times the usual human dose) on days 6 through 15 of gestation in rats produced tail defects and occasional exencephaly (2). Because of the animal toxicity, at least one publication suggested that it not be given during pregnancy (3).

Human placental transfer of griseofulvin has been demonstrated at term (4). The reported use of the antifungal agent in human pregnancy, described below, is limited.

In a surveillance study of Michigan Medicaid recipients conducted between 1985 and 1992 involving 229,101 completed pregnancies, 34 newborns had been exposed to griseofulvin during the 1st trimester (F. Rosa, personal communication, FDA, 1993). One (2.9%) major birth defect was observed (one expected). No anomalies were observed in six defect categories (cardiovascular defects, oral clefts, spina bifida, polydactyly, limb reduction defects, and hypospadias) for which specific data were available. The number of exposures is too small to draw any conclusions.

A possible interaction between oral contraceptives and griseofulvin has been reported in 22 women (5). Transient intermenstrual bleeding in 15, amenorrhea in 5, and unintended pregnancies in 2 were described.

In a report from investigators at the U.S. Food and Drug Administration, two sets of conjoined twins were observed in a sample of more than 20,000 birth defect cases with 1st trimester drug exposure (6). The first case involved female twins conjoined at the head and chest (craniothoracopagus syncephalus), and the second case involved male dicephalic twins joined in the thorax and lumbar areas with a single seven-chamber heart. In both cases the mothers had taken griseofulvin during early pregnancy. Fission with twinning is normally completed by the 20th day after ovulation, and thus, the cause of conjoined twinning would have to be present prior to this time (6). In both cases, maternal griseofulvin use was the only drug exposure (of those drugs under surveillance by the FDA). Because the incidence of conjoined twins is rare (approximately 1 in 50,000 births) and thoracopagus is even less common (1 in 250,000), the authors concluded that the cases provided evidence for an association with griseofulvin (6). The FDA investigators also examined other data on 1st trimester griseofulvin exposure involving 55,736 deliveries from one geographical area between 1980 and 1983 (6). Of these cases, griseofulvin was taken during the first 3 months by 37 mothers, two of whom delivered infants with birth defects—one with a congenital heart defect and one with an unknown defect. The incidence of 5.4% (2 of 37) was approximately the incidence in the total sample. However, in 4264 women with spontaneous or threatened abortion diagnoses, 7 had been prescribed the drug during the preceding 3 months, a relative risk of 2.5 (95% Confidence Interval 1.01–6.1) (6).

Prompted by the above report, investigators in two other countries reported data from their respective congenital anomaly registries (7,8). The report from Hungary found 39 sets of conjoined twins in a sample of more than 100,000 cases of congenital anomalies observed between 1970 and 1986 (griseofulvin was marketed in Hungary in 1970) (7). None of the mothers of the 39 conjoined twins took griseofulvin. The prevalence of conjoined twins in Hungary is approximately 1 in 60,000 births (7). The investigators also reported data from their case-control surveillance system for the period 1980–1984 (7). Of 6,786 congenital anomaly cases, 2 were exposed to griseofulvin-one infant with a heart defect was exposed during the 2nd and 3rd months, and one infant with pyloric stenosis was exposed during the 1st month. Three exposures occurred in the 10,962 matched controls, all in the late 2nd and 3rd trimesters.

The second report involved data from the International Clearinghouse for Birth Defects Monitoring Systems (8). None of the 47 sets of conjoined twins in more than 3 million births had been exposed to griseofulvin. Thus, neither of these reports was able to support the FDA report of an association between griseofulvin and the rare defect. However, because the use of an antifungal agent is seldom essential during pregnancy, griseofulvin should be avoided during this time (6).

BREAST FEEDING SUMMARY

RECOMMENDATION: No Human Data - Potential Toxicity

No reports describing the use of griseofulvin during lactation have been located. Because of the tumorigenicity demonstrated in one animal species and the potential for other toxicities in a nursing infant, the use of griseofulvin during breast-feeding does not appear to be warranted.

References

1. Product information. Fulvicin. Schering, 2000.
2. Shepard TH. *Catalog of Teratogenic Agents*. 9th ed. Baltimore, MD: Johns Hopkins University Press, 1998: 224–5.
3. Anonymous. Griseofulvin: a new formulation and some old concerns. Med Lett Drugs Ther 1976;18:17.
4. Rubin A, Dvornik D. Placental transfer of griseofulvin. Am J Obstet Gynecol 1965;92:882–3.
5. van Dijke CPH, Weber JCP. Interaction between oral contraceptives and griseofulvin. Br Med J 1984;288: 1125–6.
6. Rosa FW, Hernandez C, Carlo WA. Griseofulvin teratology, including two thoracopagus conjoined twins. Lancet 1987;1:171.
7. Metneki J, Czeizel A. Griseofulvin teratology. Lancet 1987;1:1042.
8. Knudsen LB. No association between griseofulvin and conjoined twinning. Lancet 1987;2:1097.

Name:	**GUAIFENESIN**	Risk Factor:	**C**
Class:	**Respiratory Drug (Expectorant)**		

FETAL RISK SUMMARY

RECOMMENDATION: Compatible

The Collaborative Perinatal Project monitored 197 mother-child pairs with 1st trimester exposure to guaifenesin (1, p. 478). An increase in the expected frequency of inguinal hernias was found. For use anytime during pregnancy, 1336 exposures were recorded (1, p. 442). In this latter case, no evidence for an association with malformations was found. In another large study in which 241 women were exposed to the drug during pregnancy, no strong association was found between guaifenesin and congenital defects (2).

A 1981 report described a woman who consumed, throughout pregnancy, 480–840 mL/day of a cough syrup (3). The potential maximum daily doses based on 840 mL of syrup were 16.8 g of guaifenesin, 5.0 g of pseudoephedrine, 1.68 g of dextromethorphan, and 79.8 mL of ethanol. The infant had features of the fetal alcohol syndrome (see Ethanol) and displayed irritability, tremors, and hypertonicity. It is not known whether guaifenesin or the other drugs, other than ethanol, were associated with the adverse effects observed in the infant.

In a surveillance study of Michigan Medicaid recipients conducted between 1985 and 1992 involving 229,101 completed pregnancies, 141 newborns had been exposed to guaifenesin during the 1st trimester (F. Rosa, personal communication, FDA, 1993). A total of nine (6.4%) major birth defects were observed (six expected), including two cardiovascular defects (1.4 expected). No anomalies were observed in five other categories of defects (oral clefts, spina bifida, polydactyly, limb reduction defects, and hypospadias) for which specific data were available. An additional 1338 newborns were exposed to the general class of expectorants during the 1st trimester with 63 (4.7%) major birth defects observed (57 expected). Specific malformations were (observed/expected) 9/13 cardiovascular defects, 0/2 oral clefts, 1/1 spina bifida, 7/4 polydactyly, 1/2 limb reduction defects, and 3/3 hypospadias. These data do not support an association between either guaifenesin or the general class of expectorants and congenital defects.

BREAST FEEDING SUMMARY

RECOMMENDATION: No Human Data - Probably Compatible

No reports describing the use of guaifenesin during lactation have been located.

References

1. Heinonen OP, Slone D, Shapiro S. *Birth Defects and Drugs in Pregnancy*. Littleton, MA: Publishing Sciences Group, 1977.
2. Aselton P, Jick H, Milunsky A, Hunter JR, Stergachis A. First-trimester drug use and congenital disorders. Obstet Gynecol 1985;65:451–5.
3. Chasnoff IJ, Diggs G, Schnoll SH. Fetal alcohol effects and maternal cough syrup abuse. Am J Dis Child 1981;135:968.

Name: GUANABENZ	Risk Factor: C_M
Class: Sympatholytic (Antihypertensive)	

G

FETAL RISK SUMMARY

RECOMMENDATION: No Human Data - Animal Data Suggest Moderate Risk

Guanabenz is a centrally acting, α_2-adrenergic agonist that acts as an antihypertensive agent by decreasing sympathetic outflow from the brain. In one study, no increase in fetal malformations was observed in rats and rabbits treated with the drug during organogenesis (1). However, an increase in perinatal mortality was observed with doses that produced sedation in the mothers. In mice, oral doses of guanabenz 3–6 times the maximum recommended human dose resulted in a possible increase in skeletal malformations, primarily costal and vertebral (2). No reports describing the use of guanabenz in human pregnancy have been located.

BREAST FEEDING SUMMARY

RECOMMENDATION: No Human Data - Potential Toxicity

No reports describing the use of guanabenz during lactation have been located. The relatively low molecular weight (about 291), however, probably indicates that the drug is excreted into breast milk. The potential effects on a nursing infant from this exposure are unknown.

References

1. Akatsuka K, Hashimoto T, Takeuchi K, Yanagisawa Y, Kogure M. Reproduction studies of guanabenz in the rat and rabbit. J Toxicol Sci 1982;11:93–151. As cited in Shepard TH. *Catalog of Teratogenic Agents*. 6th ed. Baltimore, MD: Johns Hopkins University Press, 1989: 305.
2. Product information. Wytensin. Wyeth-Ayerst Laboratories, 1993.

Name: GUANADREL	Risk Factor: B_M
Class: Sympatholytic (Antihypertensive)	

FETAL RISK SUMMARY

RECOMMENDATION: No Human Data - Animal Data Suggest Low Risk

Guanadrel is a peripherally acting antiadrenergic agent used in the treatment of hypertension. In pregnant rats and rabbits, doses of 30 and 100 mg/kg/day had no effect on the length of gestation (1). At the higher dose, a low incidence, apparently not statistically significant (about 6%), of congenital malformations involving the viscera, soft tissue, and skeleton were observed (1). No fetal harm was observed in either species treated with up to 12 times the maximum recommended human dose (2). No reports describing the use of guanadrel in human pregnancy have been located.

BREAST FEEDING SUMMARY

RECOMMENDATION: No Human Data - Potential Toxicity

No reports describing the use of guanadrel during lactation have been located. The molecular weight (about 525), however, probably indicates that some excretion into breast milk will occur. The potential effects on a nursing infant from this exposure are unknown.

References

1. Palmer JD, Nugent CA. Guanadrel sulfate: a postganglionic sympathetic inhibitor for the treatment of mild to moderate hypertension. Pharmacotherapy 1983;3:220–9.
2. Product information. Hylorel. Medeva Pharmaceuticals, 2000.

G

Name:	**GUANETHIDINE**	Risk Factor:	**C_M**
Class:	**Sympatholytic (Antihypertensive)**		

FETAL RISK SUMMARY

RECOMMENDATION: Limited Human Data - Animal Data Suggest Low Risk

Guanethidine is a peripherally acting, antiadrenergic agent used in the treatment of hypertension. In nonpregnant adults, the drug is often combined with diuretics. Because orthostatic hypotension resulting from adrenergic inhibition and unopposed parasympathetic function is a common problem with this agent, its usefulness in the pregnant patient is markedly reduced (1–4).

In a reproduction study in pregnant rats, guanethidine 10 mg/kg/day (average human dose <1.0 mg/kg/day) produced no adverse effects in the offspring (5). Guanethidine was listed in a later reference as a drug that causes maternal death before any effect on the fetus is observed (6). Without citing details, another publication cited guanethidine as a drug capable of producing embryopathy (i.e., death or malformation or both) in laboratory animals (7).

Guanethidine neurotoxicity has been observed in newborn rats and mice who were given the drug early in postnatal life (8,9). In one study, newborn rats were given guanethidine (50 mg/kg SC) once daily for 5 days starting on postnatal day 2 (8). In contrast to adult rats, a possible drug-induced delay in cellular proliferation resulting in initially low brain weights occurred that was thought to be related to passage of guanethidine into the brain because of immature function of the neonatal blood-brain barrier (8). An earlier study found a dysfunctional blood-brain barrier in newborn mice, but not in adult mice, when administration of guanethidine caused a long-lasting reduction in brain catecholamine (norepinephrine and dopamine) levels (9). It is not known if these neurotoxicities would have occurred in the animal fetuses from exposure to the much smaller amounts of drug that would have presumably resulted after placental transfer.

No studies relating to the placental transfer of guanethidine in animals or humans have been located. The commercially available form of the drug, guanethidine monosulfate, has a molecular weight of about 296 that is low enough that passage to the fetus in measurable amounts should occur.

Several reports have described the use of guanethidine during all phases of human pregnancy (10–16). The Collaborative Perinatal Project monitored 50,282 mother-child pairs, 13 of whom had 1st trimester exposure to a miscellaneous group of antihypertensives, 2 of which were exposed to guanethidine (10). There was 1 infant with a malformation from the total group of 13.

Three references described the use of guanethidine during the 3rd trimester for the treatment of preeclampsia (11–13). Although the outcomes of many of these pregnancies were poor, including fetal death, they appeared to be related to the severity of the mother's disease rather than to the drug therapy. In a fourth reference, the use of guanethidine, tolazoline, phentolamine, and methyldopa for severe hypertension of pregnancy were curtailed over a 3-year period in favor of reserpine and phenoxybenzamine because the authors concluded that the latter two agents gave better control of hypertension, improvement of renal function, and greater predictability of results (14). No fetal or newborn adverse effects were mentioned. A fifth reference also concluded that guanethidine was not an effective antihypertensive, in comparison to other available agents, for the treatment of severe hypertension presenting late in pregnancy (15).

A 1977 report described a 29-year-old woman who was treated with guanethidine (10 mg/day) and hydrochlorothiazide (50 mg twice daily) for hypertension during the first 12 weeks of pregnancy (16). This therapy was stopped, and she was eventually diagnosed with pheochromocytoma that was resected during delivery of a healthy, full-term, 5400-g female infant. The infant was alive and well at 8 years of age.

In summary, although most reports of guanethidine have not been associated with drug-induced adverse fetal or newborn outcome, only three cases of 1st trimester exposure have been described. Two of these were reported in a surveillance study in which one malformed infant was delivered from a group of 13 women who took miscellaneous antihypertensives. Thus, the available data are too limited to assess its safety during early human pregnancy. Moreover, the use of this potent antihypertensive has been supplanted by safer, more effective agents for pregnant women. Because of this, it probably should be considered as a drug of last choice during pregnancy (1).

BREAST FEEDING SUMMARY

RECOMMENDATION: Limited Human Data - Potential Toxicity

The manufacturer states that very small amounts of guanethidine are excreted into milk (17), but published reports describing the use of guanethidine during lactation have not been located. The relatively low molecular weight (about 296) of the commercially available form, guanethidine monosulfate, is consistent with the passage of the drug into milk. Because neurotoxicity has been observed in newborn mice and rats given the drug directly (see above) and because of the potential adverse effects on an infant's blood pressure, use during human lactation is not recommended.

References

1. Sullivan JM. Blood pressure elevation in pregnancy. Prog Cardiovasc Dis 1974;16:375–94.
2. Finnerty FA Jr. Hypertension in pregnancy. Clin Obstet Gynecol 1975;18:145–54.
3. Kelly JV. Drugs used in the management of toxemia of pregnancy. Clin Obstet Gynecol 1977;20:395–409.
4. Berkowitz RL. Anti-hypertensive drugs in the pregnant patient. Obstet Gynecol Surv 1980;35:191–204.
5. West GB. Drugs and rat pregnancy. J Pharm Pharmacol 1962;14:828–30.
6. West GB. Pregnancy tests using new drugs (abstract). Biochem Pharmacol 1963;12(Suppl):246–7.
7. Woollam DHM. Principles of teratogenesis: mode of

action of thalidomide. Proc R Soc Med 1965;58: 497–501.
8. Bartolome J, Bartolome M, Seidler FJ, Anderson TR, Slotkin TA. Effects of early postnatal guanethidine administration on adrenal medulla and brain of developing rats. Biochem Pharmacol 1976;25: 2387–90.
9. Liuzzi A, Foppen FH, Angeletti PU. Adrenaline, noradrenaline and dopamine levels in brain and heart after administration of 6-hydroxydopamine and guanethidine to newborn mice. Biochem Pharmacol 1974;23:1041–4.
10. Heinonen OP, Sloan D, Shapiro S. *Birth Defects and Drugs in Pregnancy*. Littleton, MA: Publishing Sciences Group, 1977:372–3.
11. Coyle MG, Greig M, Walker J. Blood-progesterone and urinary pregnanediol and oestrogens in foetal death from severe pre-eclampsia. Lancet 1962;2: 275–7.
12. Daftary SN, Desa Souza JM, Kumar A, Mandrekar SS, Lotlikar KD, Sheth UK. A controlled clinical trial of guanethidine in toxemia of pregnancy. Indian J Med Sci 1963;17:812–8.
13. Wallace SJ, Michie EA. A follow-up study of infants born to mothers with low oestriol excretion during pregnancy. Lancet 1966;2:560–3.
14. Maughan GB, Shabanah EH, Toth A. Experiments with pharmacologic sympatholysis in the gravid. Am J Obstet Gynecol 1967;97:764–76.
15. Ratnam SS, Lean TH, Sivasamboo R. A comparison of hypotensive drugs in patients with hypertensive disorders in late pregnancy. Aust N Z J Obstet Gynaecol 1971;11:78–84.
16. Leak D, Carroll JJ, Robinson DC, Ashworth EJ. Management of pheochromocytoma during pregnancy. Can Med Assoc J 1977;116:371–5.
17. Product information. Ismelin. Ciba Pharmaceutical, 1995.

G

Name: **GUANFACINE**	Risk Factor: B_M
Class: **Sympatholytic (Antihypertensive)**	

FETAL RISK SUMMARY

RECOMMENDATION: Limited Human Data - Animal Data Suggest Low Risk

Guanfacine is a centrally acting antihypertensive agent. The drug did not produce reproductive dysfunction or adverse fetal effects in rats and rabbits given doses 70 and 20 times the maximum recommended human dose (MRHD) (1). At doses 200 and 100 times the MRHD, respectively, increased fetal mortality and maternal toxicity were observed. Although guanfacine crosses the placenta in animals (1,2), this has not been studied in humans.

The manufacturer is aware of two unreported cases of exposure during pregnancy that resulted in the birth of healthy infants (personal communication, A. H. Robins Company, 1987). A third patient, who was participating in a clinical trial of the drug for the treatment of hypertension, became pregnant during treatment (3). Guanfacine therapy was discontinued at approximately 8 weeks of gestation. She subsequently delivered a healthy male infant.

Guanfacine is not approved for the treatment of preeclampsia, but one study has been located that describes the use of the agent for this purpose. A 1980 German report summarized the use of guanfacine for the treatment of hypertension secondary to preeclampsia in 30 women (4). The gestational ages of the women at the time of treatment were not specified. Therapy was administered for 16–68 days with doses ranging from 1–4 mg/day (mean dose approximately 2 mg/day). Mean systolic blood pressures (supine/standing) before treatment were about 160/164 mm Hg compared with 136/139 mm Hg just before parturition. Mean diastolic pressures (supine/standing) before treatment and just before delivery were 105/106 and 88/92 mm Hg, respectively. No significant changes in fetal heart rate were observed during the trial. Six infants were growth retarded, but this was probably secondary to the maternal hypertension. No drug-induced adverse effects were observed in any of the infants, and all were developing normally on follow-up (duration of follow-up not specified).

BREAST FEEDING SUMMARY

RECOMMENDATION: No Human Data - Potential Toxicity

Guanfacine is excreted into the milk of animals, but human studies have not been located. In rats, milk concentrations of guanfacine were 75% of the level in the plasma (1). The molecular weight (about 283 for the hydrochloride salt) is low enough that excretion into human milk should be expected. The potential effects on a nursing infant from this exposure are unknown. Guanfacine reduces serum prolactin concentrations in some patients and, theoretically, could cause inhibition of milk secretion.

References

1. Product information. Tenex. A. H. Robins Company, 2000.
2. Sorkin EM, Heel RC. Guanfacine. A review of its pharmacodynamic and pharmacokinetic properties, and therapeutic efficacy in the treatment of hypertension. Drugs 1986;31:301–36.
3. Karesoja M, Takkunen H. Guanfacine, a new centrally acting antihypertensive agent in long-term therapy. Curr Ther Res 1981;29:60–5.
4. Philipp E. Guanfacine in the treatment of hypertension due to pre-eclamptic toxaemia in thirty women. Br J Clin Pharmacol 1980;10(Suppl 1):137S–40S.

H

Name: **HALOPERIDOL** Risk Factor: C_M

Class: **Tranquilizer**

FETAL RISK SUMMARY

RECOMMENDATION: Limited Human Data - Animal Data Suggest Low Risk

Animal reproductive studies with haloperidol in mice, rats, rabbits, and dogs have not revealed a teratogenic effect attributable to this tranquilizer (1,2). In rodents, doses 2 to 8 times the usual maximum human dose (oral or parenteral) were associated with an increased incidence of resorption, reduced fertility, delayed delivery, and pup mortality (1,2). With single injections up to maternal toxic levels in hamsters, haloperidol was associated with fetal mortality and dose-related anomalies (3). Exposure of male rats *in utero* to haloperidol throughout most of gestation had no effect on typical parameters of adult sexual activity other than subtle changes involving ultrasonic vocalization (4).

Two reports describing limb reduction malformations in two infants after 1st trimester use of haloperidol have been located (5,6). In one of these cases, high doses (15 mg/day) were used (6). Defects observed in the two infants were ectromelia (phocomelia) (5); and multiple upper- and lower-limb defects, and an aortic valve defect (6). The infant in the latter case died. Other investigations have not observed these defects in haloperidol-exposed pregnancies (7–11).

In 98 of 100 patients treated with haloperidol for hyperemesis gravidarum in the 1st trimester, no effects were produced on birth weight, duration of pregnancy, sex ratio, or fetal or neonatal mortality, and no malformations were found in abortuses, stillborn, or liveborn infants (7). Two of the patients were lost to follow-up. In 31 infants with severe reduction deformities born over a 4-year period, none of the mothers remembered taking haloperidol (8). Haloperidol has been used for the control of chorea gravidarum and manic-depressive illness during the 2nd and 3rd trimesters (12,13). During labor, the drug has been administered to the mother without causing neonatal depression or other effects in the newborn (9).

In a surveillance study of Michigan Medicaid recipients conducted between 1985 and 1992 involving 229,101 completed pregnancies, 56 newborns had been exposed to haloperidol during the 1st trimester (F. Rosa, personal communication, FDA, 1993). Three (5.4%) (two expected) major birth defects were observed, two of which were cardiovascular defects (0.6 expected). No anomalies were observed in five other defect categories (oral clefts, spina bifida, polydactyly, limb reduction defects, and hypospadias) for which specific data were available.

A 1989 report described a case of withdrawal emergent syndrome, a subtype of tardive dyskinesia, in a newborn infant that had been exposed to oral haloperidol (2–6 mg/day) throughout gestation (14). The mother had been treated with haloperidol for schizophrenia, but she stopped the drug 2 weeks before delivery at 38 weeks' gestation. The male infant (weight not given except as "appropriate for gestational age") had Apgar scores of 8 and 9 at 1 and 5 minutes, respectively. One hour after delivery he became irritable and developed continuous tongue thrust. In addition, poor suck resulting in difficult feeding, vomiting, abdominal posturing of the hands, and tremors of the trunk and extremities were noted. By 8 days of age, all of the signs had resolved except for the tongue thrusting. This symptom continued to persist at 6 months of age, but otherwise, his development and examination were normal (14). A second, similar case of tardive dyskinesia was described in a 2003 case report (15). The mother had been treated for schizophrenia with haloperidol 200 mg IM every 2 weeks throughout gestation. She received her last dose 3 weeks before delivery of an infant (sex and weight not given) with Apgar scores of 9 and 9 at 1 and 5 minutes, respectively. The newborn was noted to be jittery and developed diarrhea and metabolic acidosis. Irritability increased over the next 8 days when tonic-clonic movements in all extremities were noted (seizures were excluded by an electroencephalogram) as well as tongue thrusting and torticollis. Treatment with clonazepam resolved the condition and the infant was discharged home at 21 days of age (15).

Premature labor, loss of fetal cardiac variability and acceleration, an unusual fetal heart rate pattern (double phase baseline), and depression at birth (Apgar scores of 4 and 7 at 1 and 5 minutes, respectively), were observed in a comatose mother and her infant after an acute overdose of an unknown amount of haloperidol and lithium at 31 weeks' gestation (16). Because of progressive premature labor, the 1526-g female infant was delivered about 3 days after the overdose. The lithium concentrations of the maternal plasma, amniotic fluid, and cord vein plasma were all greater than 4 mmol/L (severe toxic effect >2.5 mmol/L) whereas the maternal level of haloperidol at delivery was about 1.6 ng/mL. The effects observed in the fetus and newborn were attributed to cardiac and cerebral manifestations of lithium intoxication. No follow-up on the infant was reported (16).

BREAST FEEDING SUMMARY

RECOMMENDATION: Limited Human Data - Potential Toxicity

Haloperidol is excreted into breast milk. In one patient receiving an average of 29.2 mg/day, a milk level of 5 ng/mL was detected (17). When the dose was decreased to 12 mg, a level of 2 ng/mL was measured. In a second patient taking 10 mg daily, milk levels up to 23.5 ng/mL were found (18). A milk:plasma ratio of 0.6–0.7 was calculated. No adverse effects were noted in the nursing infant.

A 1992 reference measured haloperidol in the breast milk of three women receiving chronic therapy (19). The maternal doses were 3, 4, and 6 mg/day, and the corresponding haloperidol concentrations in their milk were 32, 17, and 4.7 ng/mL, respectively. The patient receiving 6 mg/day, but with the lowest milk concentration, was thought to be noncompliant with her therapy. No mention of nursing infants was made (19).

A study published in 1998 described 12 mothers who breast-fed their infants while taking haloperidol, chlorpromazine or trifluoperazine for bipolar depression (3 cases), manic disorder (1 case), schizoaffective disorder (5 cases), or schizophrenia (3 cases) (20). Haloperidol was given in a dose ranging from 1 to 40 mg/day. The age of the nursing infants at the start of therapy ranged from 1 to 18 weeks. Using an enzyme immunoassay technique, the range of concentrations in foremilk and hindmilk were <10–988 ng/mL and 23–140 ng/mL, respectively, whereas the range of ratios of foremilk and hindmilk to maternal plasma were 0.8–5.2 and 1.7–8.0, respectively. Plasma concentrations of haloperidol in the four nursing infants that were tested were 0.8, 1.2 and 2.1, 6.8, and 8.0 ng/mL, respectively. Two of the samples (6.8 and 8.0 ng/mL) were in the adult range. In addition, the urine of all seven infants tested contained haloperidol in concentrations ranging from 1.6 to 7.9 ng/mL. The maximum infant dose ingested was 3% of the weight-adjusted maternal dose. As assessed using the Bayley Scales of Infant Development, all three of the infants whose mothers were taking both haloperidol (20–40 mg/day) and chlorpromazine (200–600 mg/day) showed a decline in mental and psychomotor development from the first (at 1–4 months of age) to the second assessment (at 12–18 months of age). Because of this decline, the investigators concluded that breast-feeding might not be best if a breast-feeding mother is taking neuroleptics, either alone or in combination, at the upper end of their recommended dose ranges (20).

The American Academy of Pediatrics classifies haloperidol as an agent whose effect on the nursing infant is unknown but may be of concern (21).

References

1. Tuchmann-Duplessis H, Mercier-Parot L. Influence of neuroleptics on prenatal development in mammals. In: *Malformations, Tumors and Mental Defects, Pathogenetic Correlations*. H Tuchmann-Duplessis, G Fanconi and GR Burgio, eds. Milan: Carlo Erba Foundation, 1971. As cited in Shepard TH. *Catalog of Teratogenic Agents*. 6th ed. Baltimore, MD: Johns Hopkins University Press, 1989:308–9.
2. Product information. Haldol. Ortho-McNeil Pharmaceutical, 2000.
3. Gill TS, Guram MS, Geber WF. Haloperidol teratogenicity in the fetal hamster. Dev Pharmacol Ther 1982;4:1–5. As cited in Elia J, Katz IR, Simpson GM. Teratogenicity of psychotherapeutic medications. Psychopharmacol Bull 1987;23:531–86.
4. Bignami G, Laviola G, Alleva E, Cagiano R, Lacomba C, Cuomo V. Developmental aspects of neurobehavioural toxicity. Toxicol Lett 1992;64/65:231–7.
5. Dieulangard P, Coignet J, Vidal JC. Sur un cas d'ectrophocomelie peut-etre d'origine medicamenteuse. Bull Fed Gynecol Obstet 1966;18:85–7.
6. Kopelman AE, McCullar FW, Heggeness L. Limb malformations following maternal use of haloperidol. JAMA 1975;231:62–4.
7. Van Waes A, Van de Velde E. Safety evaluation of haloperidol in the treatment of hyperemesis gravidarum. J Clin Pharmacol 1969;9:224–7.
8. Hanson JW, Oakley GP. Haloperidol and limb deformity. JAMA 1975;231:26.
9. Ayd FJ Jr. Haloperidol: fifteen years of clinical experience. Dis Nerv Syst 1972;33:459–69.
10. Magnier P. On hyperemesis gravidarum; a therapeutical study of R 1625. Gynecol Prat 1964;15:17–23.
11. Loke KH, Salleh R. Electroconvulsive therapy for the acutely psychotic pregnant patient: a review of 3 cases. Med J Malaysia 1983;38:131–3.
12. Donaldson JO. Control of chorea gravidarum with haloperidol. Obstet Gynecol 1982;59:381–2.
13. Nurnberg HG. Treatment of mania in the last six months of pregnancy. Hosp Community Psychiatry 1980;31:122–6.
14. Sexon WR, Barak Y. Withdrawal emergent syndrome in an infant associated with maternal haloperidol therapy. J Perinatol 1989;9:170–2.
15. Collins KO, Comer JB. Maternal haloperidol therapy associated with dyskinesia in a newborn. Am J Health Syst Pharm 2003;60:2253–5.
16. Nishiwaki T, Tanaka K, Sekiya S. Acute lithium intoxication in pregnancy. Int J Gynecol Obstet 1996;52:191–2.
17. Stewart RB, Karas B, Springer PK. Haloperidol excretion in human milk. Am J Psychiatry 1980;137:849–50.
18. Whalley LJ, Blain PG, Prime JK. Haloperidol secreted in breast milk. Br Med J 1981;282:1746–7.
19. Ohkubo T, Shimoyama R, Sugawara K. Measurement of haloperidol in human breast milk by high-performance liquid chromatography. J Pharm Sci 1992;81:947–9.
20. Yoshida K, Smith B, Craggs M, Kumar R. Neuroleptic drugs in breast milk: a study of pharmacokinetics and of possible adverse effects in breast-fed infants. Psychol Med 1998;28:81–91.
21. Committee on Drugs, American Academy of Pediatrics. The transfer of drugs and other chemicals into human milk. Pediatrics 2001;108:776–89.

Name:	**HALOTHANE**	Risk Factor:	**B**
Class:	**General Anesthetic**		

FETAL RISK SUMMARY

RECOMMENDATION: Limited Human Data - Animal Data Suggest Low Risk

Halothane, a nonflammable, volatile liquid administered via vaporizer, is indicated for the induction and/or maintenance of anesthesia during surgery. It is a fluorinated inhalation anesthetic agent that was the first such agent in a class that now includes desflurane, enflurane, isoflurane, methoxyflurane, and sevoflurane. Halothane has a high blood-gas partition coefficient (2.5) compared with other anesthetics in this class (1). The agent has been used in obstetric anesthesia since the 1950s.

In a 1968 reproduction study, pregnant rats were administered a subanesthetic mixture of 0.8% halothane in 25% oxygen-nitrogen for 12 hours at different stages of gestation (2). Higher incidences of lumbar ribs, vertebral anomalies, and fetal resorptions were observed. An abstract published the same year described the effects on pregnant mice exposed to either 1% or 1.5% halothane for 3 hours during organogenesis (3). An increased incidence of cleft palate, limb hematomas, and ossification defects in the limbs was observed.

An increased incidence of resorptions, as well as decreased fetal weight and length, was observed in pregnant hamsters exposed on the ninth, tenth, or eleventh day of gestation to a mixture of 0.6% halothane and 60% nitrous oxide (4). In contrast, subanesthetic concentrations of halothane (50 to 3200 parts per million [ppm]) administered to rats on days 8–12 of pregnancy did not increase fetal death and resorptions rates, growth retardation, or frequency of skeletal anomalies (5). Skeletal variations and ossification defects were observed in all groups but were not dose related.

In a 1978 study, male and female mice were exposed to subanesthetic and anesthetic concentrations of halothane before mating (5–7 days/week for 9 weeks), then the females were exposed daily throughout gestation (6). Halothane exposures ranged from 0.025 to 4.0 MAC hours/day. (*Note: The minimum alveolar anesthetic concentration [MAC] is the concentration that causes immobility in 50% of patients exposed to a noxious stimulus such as a surgical incision; it represents the* ED_{50} *[7].*) Maternal (decreased weight gain), fetal (decreased weight and length), and neonatal (decreased early postnatal weight gain) toxicity were observed at 0.4 MAC hour/day or more. At 1.2 MAC hours/day, the pregnancy rate, implantation rate, and number of live fetuses per litter were all significantly decreased, but the percentage of resorptions and postnatal offspring survival were not altered. The smallest dose at which toxicity was observed was estimated to be 40 times greater than the level of occupational exposure in unscavenged operating rooms (6). Two studies of similar design using subanesthetic mixtures of halothane and nitrous oxide found a decrease in ovulation and implantation and a slight decrease in fetal growth (8,9). No increase in resorptions or major defects was observed in either study. However, cytogenetic damage to bone marrow and spermatogonial cells were noted after prolonged exposure (8,9).

High subanesthetic concentrations of halothane or halothane plus nitrous oxide resulted in fetal growth retardation in pregnant rats, but did not increase fetal death or congenital malformations (10). Another study in rats also found no minor or major congenital defects using 0.75 MAC of halothane (0.8%) for 6 hours/day for 3 consecutive days at different intervals during gestation (11).

A 1999 study examined the effects on mice exposed to 1.2 MAC of halothane (1.5%) before and during gestation (12). The dose was equivalent to that used clinically. Treatment before gestation had no effect on fertility or the number of live young delivered. Compared with controls, there were an increased number of offspring deaths before weaning, and the immune response of the offspring was impaired. The clinical significance of the impairment was unknown (12).

The effects of halothane on growing neural tips (growth cones) in the forebrains of neonatal rat pups were described in a 1993 report (13). The pups were exposed to three concentrations of halothane (0.5%, 0.75%, and 1.0%) over a 6-hour period on postnatal day 1. A dose-response on the activity of a growth cone enzyme (protein kinase C, PKC) was found, with the lowest concentration having no effect on the enzyme. The 1.0%

concentration, however, reduced the activity to about 71%. The 0.75% dose also reduced the PKC activity but to a lesser degree. The authors thought that the reduced enzyme activity could be related to long-term morphologic or behavioral neuroabnormalities in the pups (13).

The low molecular weight (about 197) suggests that halothane will cross the placenta to the fetus. In agreement, research has demonstrated the rapid uptake of halothane by the fetus (14). Two reviews have concluded that, in general, inhalational anesthetic agents are freely transferred to fetal tissues (15,16), and in most cases, the maternal and fetal blood concentrations are approximately equivalent (16). Lower levels were reported in a 1977 study in which 15 women undergoing cesarean section received 0.65% halothane combined with 50% nitrous oxide in oxygen (17). The umbilical vein:maternal artery ratio at delivery was 0.35. The ratio in a second group of 15 women who received the anesthetic mixture with 0.2% halothane was 0.51. The time from start of halothane to delivery was about 10.5 minutes in both groups.

Pregnant women, at least in early gestation, require less halothane for anesthesia than nonpregnant women. A 1996 study compared eight women scheduled for pregnancy termination at 8–13 weeks gestation with eight nonpregnant women undergoing laparoscopic sterilization (18). In pregnant women the median MAC of 0.58 volume% (range 0.53–0.58) was less than that in nonpregnant women, 0.75 volume% (range 0.70–0.78) ($p = 0.0005$). The percentage decrease (95% confidence interval) for pregnant women was 27% (20% to 27%). Similar results were found with enflurane (18).

Halothane and similar anesthetic agents (e.g., isoflurane and enflurane) have a relaxant effect on the pregnant uterus (1,19–24). This effect has been known since the 1950s and was considered one reason to avoid using halothane during routine, uncomplicated obstetric procedures (1,19). A 1970 study using low concentrations (0.5% or 0.8%) found no increase in blood loss at cesarean section (23). However, it was recognized that decreasing uterine tone could result in increased postpartum hemorrhage. Indeed, a 1989 review concluded that halothane, isoflurane, and enflurane all increased blood loss through a dose-related depression of uterine activity (24). In agreement with the dose-related uterine effects, a 1991 reviewer thought that low halothane concentrations (0.5% or less) were not associated with an increased risk of uterine hemorrhage (25). In the 1970 study cited above, the 0.8% concentration of halothane was associated with an increased incidence of maternal hypotension, most likely secondary to compression of the inferior vena cava by the uterus and vasodilatation (23). However, uterine blood flow is maintained during maternal hypotension because of uterine artery dilation (24). In addition, low concentrations of halothane (0.25%–0.5%) did not depress the neonatal cardiac or respiratory systems (24).

Halothane was once frequently prescribed for both vaginal and cesarean deliveries (17,20,26,27). For example, one hospital conducted 2500 vaginal deliveries over a 6-year period with a combination of halothane, nitrous oxide, and oxygen (20). The decline in obstetric use was probably a result of the availability of agents with reduced solubility in blood (e.g., see Desflurane and Isoflurane) and the recognition that general anesthesia can cause depression of the newborn.

Several studies have documented decreased initial Apgar scores in newborns following cesarean section under general anesthesia (17,23,26–28). Because the halothane concentrations often were subanesthetic and combined with nitrous oxide, it was not always clear whether the depression was secondary to a specific agent or the combination. In one study, reducing the amount of nitrous oxide from 75% to 50% and adding 0.5% halothane substantially improved the Apgar scores at 2 minutes (23). In an earlier study

H

that combined halothane anesthesia with succinylcholine, reducing the halothane dose markedly improved the condition of the newborns as measured by Apgar scores (26). Another study found no difference in Apgar scores between groups given 0.3%–0.5% halothane combined with either 40% or 25% nitrous oxide (27). In a direct comparison between 0.5% halothane and 0.75% isoflurane, both combined with 50% nitrous oxide, the isoflurane group required significantly less succinylcholine, recovered faster from anesthesia, and had less uterine relaxation and bleeding (28). The mean Apgar scores were significantly higher at 1 minute in the isoflurane group (7.4 vs. 6.7), but were similar at 5 minutes (8.9 vs. 8.8).

A 1989 study compared 0.5% halothane, 0.5% isoflurane, and 1.0% isoflurane ($N = 20$ in each group) during cesarean section delivery (29). No differences among the groups were observed in the incidence of low 1-minute Apgar scores or in the Neurologic and Adaptive Capacity Scores (NACS) at 15 minutes, 2 hours, and 24 hours. The percentage of infants who scored 35–40 on the NACS was similar in the three groups (29). A small 1983 study compared the neonatal outcomes in four groups (10 patients each) of women receiving general anesthesia for cesarean section: 50% nitrous oxide and 50% oxygen either alone or combined with 0.5% halothane, 1.0% enflurane, or 0.75% isoflurane (30). There were no differences among the groups in low Apgar scores at 1 minute and 5 minutes, neonatal neurobehavioral assessment 2–4 hours after delivery, or maternal or umbilical blood gas analysis at delivery. A randomized study examined the effects of halothane ($N = 32$) and isoflurane ($N = 34$) (both at 0.7 MAC) on newborn Apgar scores and acid-base status after anesthesia for emergency cesarean section (31). There were no statistically significant differences in the percentage of infants with low Apgar scores (<7) at 1 minute and 5 minutes. Similarly, there were no significant differences in the hydrogen ion concentration, partial pressure of carbon dioxide, partial pressure of oxygen, or base deficit in blood samples from umbilical arteries and veins (31).

The Collaborative Perinatal Project monitored 50,282 mother-child pairs, 25 of whom had 1st trimester exposure to halothane (32). Two children had unspecified malformations, but there was no evidence of an association between halothane and the defects (32). A 1965 report on fetal hazards of surgery during pregnancy described the outcomes of 20 women who were administered general anesthesia (halothane plus nitrous oxide) during pregnancy (7, 9, and 4 women in the 1st, 2nd, and 3rd trimesters, respectively) (33). One unspecified birth defect was observed (timing of exposure not specified).

A possible association between surgery in the 1st trimester and neural tube defects (NTDs) was published in 1990 (34). Using data from Swedish health care registries, investigators studied 2252 infants whose mothers had surgery during the 1st trimester. Six of the infants had NTD (expected 2.5), one of whom was thought to have Meckel's syndrome. An additional infant had a diagnosis of hydranencephaly, but the autopsy report indicated the diagnosis was uncertain and it may have been a very large encephalocele. In the total group, 572 had operations during the period of neural tube closure (gestational weeks 4 and 5). Mothers of five of the six infants with NTD (expected 0.6) had surgery during this period, but only one had been exposed to halothane (in combination with nitrous oxide). The mother of the hydranencephaly case had surgery in gestational week 8 and was exposed to halothane in combination with thiopental and succinylcholine. The authors could not determine whether the findings represented a causal association with surgery or just a random occurrence (34).

Chronic occupational exposure to anesthetic gases in operating rooms during pregnancy has raised concerns that such exposure could cause spontaneous abortions (35,36). The principal concern relates to unscavenged environments in which high concentrations of halothane (0.001% or 10 ppm) and nitrous oxide (0.03% or 300 ppm) had been measured (35). Lower concentrations of halothane also have been reported near the anesthesiologist (1–26 ppm) and the surgeon (1–2 ppm) (37). A 1988 review cited a number of studies investigating the possible association between occupational exposure to anesthetic gases and adverse pregnancy outcomes (15). The reviewer concluded that serious methodological weaknesses in these studies precluded arriving at a firm conclusion, but a slightly increased risk of miscarriage was a possibility. However, there was no evidence of an association between occupational exposure and congenital anomalies (15).

A review published in 1991 briefly evaluated the possibility that some drugs and environmental agents could cause behavioral teratogenicity (38). Anesthetics (e.g., halothane) were listed as "suspected" human behavioral teratogens apparently based solely on animal studies. However, specific data for any anesthetic agent, including halothane, were not cited.

A 2004 study, however, found a significant association between maternal occupational exposure to waste anesthetic gases during pregnancy and developmental deficits in their children, including gross and fine motor ability, inattention/hyperactivity, and IQ performance (see Nitrous Oxide).

A 1993 study evaluated the effect of halothane anesthesia for fetal surgery in pregnant ewes (39). Compared with ketamine, halothane decreased fetal cardiac output and placental blood flow. An increase in total vascular resistance, highest in the placenta, resulted in the shunting of blood away from the placenta (39). The combination of these effects resulted in depressed respiratory gas exchange. The investigators concluded that halothane was a poor anesthetic for fetal surgery (39).

In summary, halothane has demonstrated teratogenicity and toxicity in some animal studies, but this may have occurred at maternally toxic doses. The potential for long-term behavioral teratogenicity in animals or humans has not been adequately studied but such studies are needed. The anesthetic does not appear to cause human structural anomalies nor does it appear to be related to embryotoxicity (e.g., abortions), but this is based on limited 1st-trimester experience. Others also have reached this same conclusion (15). In addition, general anesthesia usually involves the use of multiple pharmacologic agents which complicates attempts at fetal risk assessment. In the past, halothane frequently was used during delivery for analgesia and anesthesia. This use does not appear to affect the newborn any differently than use of other general anesthetic agents does. The uterine effects of halothane (relaxation and increased blood loss) also appear to be similar to those of other agents in this class. All anesthetic agents can cause depression in the newborn that may last for 24 hours or more. The potential reproductive toxicity (spontaneous abortion and infertility) of occupational exposure to halothane has not been adequately studied.

BREAST FEEDING SUMMARY

RECOMMENDATION: Limited Human Data - Probably Compatible

Halothane is excreted into breast milk (40–42). Breast milk samples were collected on 2 days from a lactating anesthesiologist while she was working (40). The milk concentrations of 2 ppm were consistent with the concentrations at the anesthesiologist's face in the operating room. Because respiratory excretion of halothane by operating room personnel continues for up to 72 hours, the authors thought that the trace milk concentrations would be detectable for a similar period of time (40).

No reports measuring the amount of halothane excreted in milk of patients who have received halothane anesthesia have been located. Of interest, a 1993 reference stated that respiratory excretion of halothane in patients may occur for up to 20 days after exposure and that trace amounts of halothane should be expected in milk during that interval (41). One review considered the potential amounts in milk after halothane anesthesia, when nursing was feasible, to be negligible (42). The American Academy of Pediatrics classifies halothane as a drug that usually is compatible with breast-feeding (43).

References

1. Product information. Halothane. Abbott Laboratories, 1975.
2. Basford AB, Fink BR. The teratogenicity of halothane in the rat. Anesthesiology 1968;29:1167–73.
3. Smith BE, Usubliaga LE, Lehrer SB. Cleft palate induced by halothane anesthesia in C-57 black mice (abstract). Teratology 1971;4:242.
4. Bussard DA, Stoelting RK, Peterson C, Ishaq M. Fetal changes in hamsters anesthetized with nitrous oxide and halothane. Anesthesiology 1974;41:275–8.
5. Lansdown ABG, Pope WDB, Halsey MJ, Bateman PE. Analysis of fetal development in rats following maternal exposure to subanesthetic concentrations of halothane. Teratology 1976;13:299–304.
6. Wharton RS, Mazze RI, Baden JM, Hitt BA, Dooley JR. Fertility, reproduction and postnatal survival in mice chronically exposed to halothane. Anesthesiology 1978;48:167–74.
7. Trevor AJ, Miller RD. General anesthetics. In Katzung BG, ed. *Basic and Clinical Pharmacology*. 8th ed. New York: McGraw-Hill, 2001:426.
8. Coate WB, Kapp RW Jr, Lewis TR. Chronic exposure to low concentrations of halothane – nitrous oxide: reproductive and cytogenetic effects in the rat. Anesthesiology 1979;50:310–8.
9. Coate WB, Kapp RW Jr, Ulland BM. Toxicity of low concentration long-term exposure to an airborne mixture of nitrous oxide and halothane. J Environ Pathol Toxicol 1979;2:209–31.
10. Pope WDB, Halsey MJ, Lansdown ABG, Simmonds A, Bateman PE. Fetotoxicity in rats following chronic exposure to halothane, nitrous oxide, or methoxyflurane. Anesthesiology 1978;48:11–6.
11. Mazze RI, Fujinaga M, Rice SA, Harris SB, Baden JM. Reproductive and teratogenic effects of nitrous oxide, halothane, isoflurane, and enflurane in Sprague-Dawley rats. Anesthesiology 1986;64:339–44.
12. Puig NR, Amerio N, Piaggio E, Barragan J, Comba JO, Elena GA. Effects of halothane reexposure in female mice and their offspring. Reprod Toxicol 1999;13:361–7.
13. Saito S, Fujita T, Igarashi M. Effects of inhalational anesthetics on biochemical events in growing neuronal tips. Anesthesiology 1993;79:1338–47.
14. Dwyer R, Fee JPH, Moore J. Uptake of halothane and isoflurane by mother and baby during caesarean section. Br J Anaesth 1995;74:379–83.
15. Friedman JM. Teratogen update: anesthetic agents. Teratology 1988;37:69–77.
16. Kanto J. Risk-benefit assessment of anaesthetic agents in the puerperium. Drug Saf 1991;6:285–301.
17. Latto IP, Waldron BA. Anaesthesia for caesarean section. Br J Anaesth 1977;49:371–8.
18. Chan MTV, Mainland P, Gin T. Minimum alveolar concentration of halothane and enflurane are decreased in early pregnancy. Anesthesiology 1996;85:782–6.
19. Crawford JS. The place of halothane in obstetrics. Br J Anaesth 1962;34:386–90.
20. Stoelting VK. Fluothane in obstetric anesthesia. Anesth Analg 1964;43:243–6.
21. Munson ES, Embro WJ. Enflurane, isoflurane, and halothane and isolated human uterine muscle. Anesthesiology 1977;46:11–4.
22. Naftalin NJ, McKay DM, Phear WPC, Goldberg AH. The effects of halothane on pregnant and nonpregnant human myometrium. Anesthesiology 1977;46:15–9.
23. Moir DD. Anaesthesia for caesarean section. Br J Anaesth 1970;42:136–42.
24. Quail AW. Modern inhalational anaesthetic agents. A review of halothane, isoflurane and enflurane. Med J Aust 1989;150:95–102.
25. Nandi PR, Morrison PF, Morgan BM. Effects of general anaesthesia on the fetus during caesarean section. Anaesth Rev 1991;8:103–22.
26. Johnstone M, Breen PJ. Halothane in obstetrics: elective caesarean section. Br J Anaesth 1966;38:386–93.
27. Galbert MW, Gardner AE. Use of halothane in a balanced technic for cesarean section. Anesth Analg 1972;51:701–4.
28. Ghaly RG, Flynn RJ, Moore J. Isoflurane as an alternative to halothane for caesarean section. Anaesthesia 1988;43:5–7.
29. Abboud TK, D'Onofrio I, Reyes A, Mosaad P, Zhu J, Mantilla M, Gangolly J, Crowell D, Cheung M, Afrasiabi A, Khoo N, Davidson J, Steffens Z, Zaki N. Isoflurane or halothane for cesarean section: comparative maternal and neonatal effects. Acta Anaesthesiol Scand 1989;33:578–81.
30. Warren TM, Datta S, Ostheimer GW, Naulty JS, Weiss JB, Morrison JA. Comparison of the maternal and neonatal effects of halothane, enflurane, and isoflurane for cesarean delivery. Anesth Analg 1983;62:516–20.
31. Mokriski BK, Malinow AM. Neonatal acid-base status following general anesthesia for emergency abdominal delivery with halothane or isoflurane. J Clin Anesth 1992;4:97–100.
32. Heinonen OP, Slone D, Shapiro S. *Birth Defects and Drugs in Pregnancy*. Littleton, MA: Publishing Sciences Group, 1977:358–60.
33. Shnider SM, Webster GM. Am J Obstet Gynecol 1965;92:891–900.
34. Kallen B, Mazze RI. Neural tube defects and first trimester operations. Teratology 1990;41:717–20.
35. Corbett TH. Anesthetics as a cause of abortion. Fertil Steril 1972;23:866–9.

36. Brodsky JB. Anesthesia and surgery during early pregnancy and fetal outcome. Clin Obstet Gynecol 1983;26:449–57.
37. Corbett TH. Cancer and congenital anomalies associated with anesthetics. Ann N Y Acad Sci 1976;271: 58–66.
38. Nelson BK. Evidence for behavioral teratogenicity in humans. J Appl Toxicol 1991;11:33–7.
39. Sabik JF, Assad RS, Hanley FL. Halothane as an anesthetic for fetal surgery. J Pediatr Surg 1993;28:542–7.
40. Cote CJ, Kenepp NB, Reed SB, Strobel GE. Trace concentrations of halothane in human breast milk. Br J Anaesth 1976;48:541–3.
41. Lee JJ, Rubin AP. Breast feeding and anaesthesia. Anaesthesia 1993;48:616–25.
42. Spigset O. Anaesthetic agents and excretion in breast milk. Acta Anaesthesiol Scand 1994;38:94–103.
43. Committee on Drugs, American Academy of Pediatrics. The transfer of drugs and other chemicals into human milk. Pediatrics 2001;108:776–89.

Name: **HEMIN** Risk Factor: **C_M**

Class: **Hematopoietic**

FETAL RISK SUMMARY

RECOMMENDATION: No Human Data - No Relevant Animal Data

The enzyme inhibitor hemin (previously known as hematin) limits the hepatic and/or marrow synthesis of porphyrin. It is indicated for the amelioration of recurrent attacks of acute intermittent porphyria that are temporally related to the menstrual cycle (1). Hemin is an iron molecule derived from human red blood cells. Although multiple steps have been taken to lessen the chance of blood-borne infection, a risk still exists for the transmission of infectious agents, such as viruses, and for the agent that causes Creutzfeldt-Jacob disease (1).

Reproduction studies in animals have not been conducted. It is not known if hemin can cross the human placenta to the fetus. As a natural constituent of human blood, it is unlikely that clinically significant amounts would cross to the fetal compartment.

A 1989 review summarized the prevalence, genetics, biochemistry, classification and the treatment of acute intermittent porphyria (2). The authors also cited evidence that female hormones affect the onset and expression of the disease. Before an understanding of the disease and improved prenatal care was achieved, porphyria was associated with significant maternal mortality and poor pregnancy outcome (2). Although they did not specifically state that hemin treatment was indicated during pregnancy, they did state that patients with acute attacks should be hospitalized for symptomatic treatment. They also noted that treatment with hematin (*now known as hemin*) could shorten the duration of the attack and reduce its severity (2).

Earlier, a brief response to a question concerning porphyria and pregnancy hinted to the potential severity of this disease. The author, although noting the lack of information relating to the potential to cause adverse pregnancy outcomes, still recommended hematin therapy for an acute porphyric attack "before considering termination of pregnancy" (3). Responding to this recommendation, another author suggested that glucose infusions were safer and expressed concern that the anticoagulant effect of hemin could jeopardize a pregnancy (4). However, hemin was not thought to have a clinically significant anticoagulant effect at low doses and was indicated in pregnancy if glucose infusions were not effective in reversing the disease process (5).

A 34-year-old woman, in the first or second month of pregnancy, was treated with hematin, 3 mg/kg/day administered as an IV infusion for 5 days, for an exacerbation of acute intermittent porphyria (6). A second IV infusion course, 1.5 mg/kg/day for 2 weeks, was started 41 days after the first course. No adverse fetal effects of the exposure were noted and the woman eventually delivered a healthy, 2570-g male infant at 39 weeks' gestation. At follow-up, no evidence of porphyria was noted in the 5-year-old child (6).

A 1984 study investigated the effect of hematin on bilirubin binding (7). Cord blood of newborn infants with ABO hemolytic disease was thought to contain endogenous hematin, which could increase the risk of kernicterus. In an *in vitro* experiment, hematin was added to bilirubin-enriched cord blood and was found to have a significant adverse effect on bilirubin binding. However, the high concentrations required were not physiologic and, thus, were not thought to have clinical significance for infants with ABO-isoimmune hemolysis (7).

In summary, animal reproduction studies have not been conducted with hemin and there is only one report on its use in human pregnancy. The citations above, however, suggest that hemin has been used more frequently in pregnant women. The primary embryo or fetal risk from hemin appears to be from the transmission of viruses or other agents from a hemin-induced maternal infection or from a hemin-induced maternal adverse reaction (e.g., thrombocytopenia or coagulopathy). Therefore, the drug should not be withheld because of pregnancy.

BREAST FEEDING SUMMARY

RECOMMENDATION: No Human Data - Probably Compatible

No reports describing the use of hemin during lactation have been located. Hemin is an enzyme inhibitor that is derived from human red blood cells. It is doubtful if hemin is excreted in milk, but even if small amounts were excreted, they would be digested in the infant's gut.

References

1. Product information. Panhematin. Ovation Pharmaceuticals, 2004.
2. Kanaan C, Veille JC, Lakin M. Pregnancy and acute intermittent porphyria. Obstet Gynecol Surv 1989;44:244–9.
3. Bissell DM. Acute intermittent porphyria and pregnancy. JAMA 1985;252:1457.
4. Loftin EB III. Hematin therapy in acute porphyria. JAMA 1985;254:613.
5. Bissell DM. In reply: Hematin therapy in acute porphyria. JAMA 1985;254:1457.
6. Wenger S, Meisinger V, Brücke T, Deecke L. Acute porphyric neuropathy during pregnancy—effect of haematin therapy. Eur Neurol 1998;39:187–8.
7. Kirk JJ, Ritter DA, Kenny JD. The effect of hematin on bilirubin binding in bilirubin-enriched neonatal cord serum. Biol Neonate 1984;45:53–7.

Name:	**HEPARIN**	Risk Factor:	**C_M**
Class:	**Anticoagulant**		

FETAL RISK SUMMARY

RECOMMENDATION: Compatible

No reports linking the use of heparin during gestation with congenital defects have been located. Other problems, at times lethal to the fetus or neonate, may be related to heparin or to the severe maternal disease necessitating anticoagulant therapy. Hall and co-workers (1) reviewed the use of heparin and other anticoagulants during pregnancy (167 references) (see also Coumarin Derivatives). They concluded from the published cases in which heparin was used without other anticoagulants that significant risks existed for the mother and fetus and that heparin was not a clearly superior form of anticoagulation during pregnancy. Nageotte and co-workers (2) analyzed the same data to arrive at a different conclusion.

	Hall	*Nageotte*
Total number of cases	135	120
Term liveborn—no complications	86	86
Premature—survived without complications	19	19
Liveborn—complications (not specified)	1	1
Premature—expired		
Heparin therapy appropriate*	10	5
Heparin therapy not appropriate*	4[a]	
Severe maternal disease making successful outcome of pregnancy unlikely	1[b]	
Spontaneous abortions		
Unknown cause	2	1
Maternal death due to pulmonary embolism	1	
Stillbirths		
Heparin therapy appropriate*	17	8
Heparin therapy not appropriate*	7[c]	
Heparin and Coumadin used	2	

*Appropriateness as determined by current standards
[a]Hypertension of pregnancy (4)
[b]Tricuspid atresia (1)
[c]Hypertension of pregnancy (6); proliferative glomerulonephritis (1)

By eliminating the 15 cases in which maternal disease or other drugs were the most likely cause of the fetal problem, the analysis of Nageotte and co-workers results in a 13% (15 of 120) unfavorable outcome vs. the 22% (30 of 135) of Hall and associates. This new value appears to be significantly better than the 31% (133 of 426) abnormal outcome reported for coumarin derivatives (see Coumarin Derivatives). Furthermore, in contrast to coumarin derivatives in which a definite drug-induced pattern of malformations has been observed (fetal warfarin syndrome), heparin has not been related to congenital defects nor does it cross the placenta (3–5). Consequently, the mechanism of heparin's adverse effect on the fetus, if it exists, must be indirect. Hall and co-workers theorized that fetal effects may be caused by calcium (or other cation) chelation resulting in the deficiency of that ion(s) in the fetus. A more likely explanation, in light of the report of the Nageotte group, is severe maternal disease that could be relatively independent of heparin. Thus, heparin appears to have major advantages over oral anticoagulants as the treatment of choice during pregnancy (6–13).

A retrospective study, published in 1989, lends support to the argument that heparin therapy is safe for the mother and fetus (14). A total of 77 women were treated with heparin during 100 pregnancies. In 98 pregnancies, therapy was administered for the prevention or treatment of venous thromboembolism, and in 2, treatment was because of prosthetic heart valves. In comparison with normal pregnancies, no difference was seen in the treated mothers in terms of prematurity, spontaneous abortions, stillbirths, neonatal deaths, or congenital malformations (6). Two bleeding episodes occurred, but there were no symptomatic thrombolic events.

In a surveillance study of Michigan Medicaid recipients conducted between 1985 and 1992 involving 229,101 completed pregnancies, 65 newborns had been exposed to heparin during the 1st trimester (F. Rosa, personal communication, FDA, 1993). Seven (10.8%) major birth defects were observed (three expected). Specific data were available for six defect categories, including (observed/expected) 4/0.6 cardiovascular defects, 0/0 oral clefts, 0/0 spina bifida, 1/0 polydactyly, 0/0 limb reduction defects, and 1/0 hypospadias. The data for total malformations and for cardiovascular defects are suggestive of possible associations, but other factors, most likely the mother's disease, but also possibly concurrent drug therapy and chance, are probably involved.

Long-term heparin therapy during pregnancy has been associated with maternal osteopenia (15–19). Both low-dose (10,000 units/day) and high-dose heparin have been implicated, but the latter is more often related to this complication. One study found bone demineralization to be dose related, with more severe changes occurring after long-term therapy (>25 weeks) and in patients who had also received heparin in a previous pregnancy (18). The significant decrease in 1,25-dihydroxyvitamin D levels measured in heparin-treated pregnant patients may be related to the pathogenesis of this adverse effect (16,17). Similar problems have not been reported in newborns.

H

BREAST FEEDING SUMMARY

RECOMMENDATION: Compatible

Heparin is not excreted into breast milk because of its high molecular weight (15,000) (20).

References

1. Hall JG, Pauli RM, Wilson KM. Maternal and fetal sequelae of anticoagulation during pregnancy. Am J Med 1980;68:122–40.
2. Nageotte MP, Freeman RK, Garite TJ, Block RA. Anticoagulation in pregnancy. Am J Obstet Gynecol 1981; 141:472.
3. Flessa HC, Kapstrom AB, Glueck HI, Will JJ, Miller MA, Brinker B. Placental transport of heparin. Am J Obstet Gynecol 1965;93:570–3.
4. Russo R, Bortolotti U, Schivazappa L, Girolami A. Warfarin treatment during pregnancy: a clinical note. Haemostasis 1979;8:96–8.
5. Moe N. Anticoagulant-therapy in the prevention of placental infarction and perinatal death. Obstet Gynecol 1982;59:481–3.
6. Hellgren M, Nygards EB. Long-term therapy with subcutaneous heparin during pregnancy. Gynecol Obstet Invest 1982;13:76–89.
7. Cohen AW, Gabbe SG, Mennuti MT. Adjusted-dose heparin therapy by continuous intravenous infusion for recurrent pulmonary embolism during pregnancy. Am J Obstet Gynecol 1983;146:463–4.
8. Howell R, Fidler J, Letsky E. The risks of antenatal subcutaneous heparin prophylaxis: a controlled trial. Br J Obstet Gynaecol 1983;90:1124–8.
9. Vellenga E, van Imhoff GW, Aarnoudse JG. Effective prophylaxis with oral anticoagulants and low-dose heparin during pregnancy in an antithrombin III deficient woman. Lancet 1983;2:224.
10. Bergqvist A, Bergqvist D, Hallbook T. Deep vein thrombosis during pregnancy. Acta Obstet Gynecol Scand 1983;62:443–8.
11. Michiels JJ, Stibbe J, Vellenga E, van Vliet HHDM. Prophylaxis of thrombosis in antithrombin III-deficient women during pregnancy and delivery. Eur J Obstet Gynecol Reprod Biol 1984;18:149–53.
12. Nelson DM, Stempel LE, Fabri PJ, Talbert M. Hickman catheter use in a pregnant patient requiring therapeutic heparin anticoagulation. Am J Obstet Gynecol 1984;149:461–2.
13. Romero R, Duffy TP, Berkowitz RL, Chang E, Hobbins JC. Prolongation of a preterm pregnancy complicated by death of a single twin *in utero* and disseminated intravascular coagulation: effects of treatment with heparin. N Engl J Med 1984;310:772–4.
14. Ginsberg JS, Kowalchuk G, Hirsh J, Brill-Edwards P, Burrows R. Heparin therapy during pregnancy: risks to the fetus and mother. Arch Intern Med 1989;149:2233–6.
15. Wise PH, Hall AJ. Heparin-induced osteopenia in pregnancy. Br Med J 1980;281:110–1.
16. Aarskog D, Aksnes L, Lehmann V. Low 1,25-dihydroxyvitamin D in heparin-induced osteopenia. Lancet 1980;2:650–1.
17. Aarskog D, Aksnes L, Markestad T, Ulstein M, Sagen N. Heparin-induced inhibition of 1,25-dihydroxyvitamin D formation. Am J Obstet Gynecol 1984;148: 1141–2.
18. De Swiet M, Dorrington Ward P, Fidler J, Horsman A, Katz D, Letsky E, Peacock M, Wise PH. Prolonged

heparin therapy in pregnancy causes bone demineralization. Br J Obstet Gynaecol 1983;90:1129–34.
19. Griffiths HT, Liu DTY. Severe heparin osteoporosis in pregnancy. Postgrad Med J 1984;60:424–5.
20. O'Reilly RA. Anticoagulant, antithrombotic, and thrombolytic drugs. In Gilman AG, Goodman LS, Gilman A, eds. *The Pharmacological Basis of Therapeutics*. 6th ed. New York, NY: MacMillan, 1980:1350.

Name:	**HEROIN**	Risk Factor:	**B***
Class:	**Narcotic Agonist Analgesic**		

FETAL RISK SUMMARY

RECOMMENDATION: Human Data Suggest Risk in 3rd Trimester

In the United States, heroin exposure during pregnancy is confined to illicit use as opposed to other countries, such as Great Britain, where the drug is commercially available. The documented fetal toxicity of heroin derives from the illicit use and resulting maternal-fetal addiction. In the form available to the addict, heroin is adulterated with various substances (such as lactose, glucose, mannitol, starch, quinine, amphetamines, strychnine, procaine, or lidocaine) or contaminated with bacteria, viruses, or fungi (1,2). Maternal use of other drugs, abused and nonabused, is likely. It is, therefore, difficult to separate entirely the effects of heroin on the fetus from the possible effects of other chemical agents, multiple diseases with addiction, and lifestyle.

Heroin rapidly crosses the placenta, entering fetal tissues within 1 hour of administration. Withdrawal of the drug from the mother causes the fetus to undergo simultaneous withdrawal. Intrauterine death may occur from meconium aspiration (3,4).

Assessment of fetal maturity and status is often difficult because of uncertain dates and an accelerated appearance of mature lecithin : sphingomyelin ratios (5).

Until recently, the incidence of congenital anomalies was not thought to be increased (6–8). Current data, however, suggest that a significant increase in major anomalies can occur (9). In a group of 830 heroin-addicted mothers, the incidence of infants with congenital abnormalities was significantly greater than in a group of 400 controls (9). Higher rates of jaundice, respiratory distress syndrome, and low Apgar scores were also found. Malformations reported with heroin are multiple and varied with no discernible patterns of defects (6–13). In addition, all of the mothers in the studies reporting malformed infants were consuming numerous other drugs, including drugs of abuse.

Characteristics of infants delivered from a heroin-addicted mother may be (14):

Accelerated liver maturity with a lower incidence of jaundice (8,15)
Lower incidence of hyaline membrane disease after 32 weeks' gestation (5,16)
Normal Apgar scores (6)
(*Note:* The findings of Ostrea and Chavez (9) are in disagreement with the above statements.)
Low birth weight; up to 50% weigh less than 2500 g
Small size for gestational age
Narcotic withdrawal in about 85% (58%–91%): symptoms apparent usually within the first 48 hours with some delaying up to 6 days; incidence is directly related to daily dose and length of maternal addiction; hyperactivity, respiratory distress, fever, diarrhea, mucus secretion, sweating, convulsions, yawning, and face scratching (7,8)
Meconium staining of amniotic fluid

Elevated serum magnesium levels when withdrawal signs are present (up to twice normal)
Increased perinatal mortality; rates up to 37% in some series (13)

Random chromosomal damage was significantly higher when Apgar scores were 6 or less (12,17). However, only one case has appeared relating chromosomal abnormalities to congenital anomalies (12). The clinical significance of this is doubtful. The lower incidence of hyaline membrane disease may be caused by elevated prolactin blood levels in fetuses of addicted mothers (18).

Long-term effects on growth and behavior have been reported (19). As compared with controls, children ages 3–6 years who were delivered from addicted mothers were found to have lower weights, lower heights, and impaired behavioral, perceptual, and organizational abilities.

[*Risk Factor D if used for prolonged periods or in high doses at term.*]

BREAST FEEDING SUMMARY

RECOMMENDATION: Contraindicated

Heroin crosses into breast milk in sufficient quantities to cause addiction in the infant (20). A milk:plasma ratio has not been reported. Previous investigators have considered nursing as one method for treating the addicted newborn (21). The American Academy of Pediatrics classifies heroin abuse as a contraindication to breast-feeding (22).

References

1. Anonymous. Diagnosis and management of reactions to drug abuse. Med Lett Drugs Ther 1980;22:74.
2. Thomas L. Notes of a biology-watcher. N Engl J Med 1972;286:531–3.
3. Chappel JN. Treatment of morphine-type dependence. JAMA 1972;221:1516.
4. Rementeria JL, Nunag NN. Narcotic withdrawal in pregnancy: stillbirth incidence with a case report. Am J Obstet Gynecol 1973;116:1152–6.
5. Gluck L, Kulovich MV. Lecithin/sphingomyelin ratios in amniotic fluid in normal and abnormal pregnancy. Am J Obstet Gynecol 1973;115:539–46.
6. Reddy AM, Harper RG, Stern G. Observations on heroin and methadone withdrawal in the newborn. Pediatrics 1971;48:353–8.
7. Stone ML, Salerno LJ, Green M, Zelson C. Narcotic addiction in pregnancy. Am J Obstet Gynecol 1971;109:716–23.
8. Zelson C, Rubio E, Wasserman E. Neonatal narcotic addiction: 10 year observation. Pediatrics 1971;48: 178–89.
9. Ostrea EM, Chavez CJ. Perinatal problems (excluding neonatal withdrawal) in maternal drug addiction: a study of 830 cases. J Pediatr 1979;94:292–5.
10. Perlmutter JF. Drug addiction in pregnant women. Am J Obstet Gynecol 1967;99:569–72.
11. Krause SO, Murray PM, Holmes JB, Burch RE. Heroin addiction among pregnant women and their newborn babies. Am J Obstet Gynecol 1958;75:754–8.
12. Kushnick T, Robinson M, Tsao C. 45,X chromosome abnormality in the offspring of a narcotic addict. Am J Dis Child 1972;124:772–3.
13. Naeye RL, Blanc W, Leblanc W, Khatamee MA. Fetal complications of maternal heroin addiction: abnormal growth, infections and episodes of stress. J Pediatr 1973;83:1055–61.
14. Perlmutter JF. Heroin addiction and pregnancy. Obstet Gynecol Surv 1974;29:439–46.
15. Nathenson G, Cohen MI, Liff IF, McNamara H. The effect of maternal heroin addiction on neonatal jaundice. J Pediatr 1972;81:899–903.
16. Glass L, Rajegowda BK, Evans HE. Absence of respiratory distress syndrome in premature infants of heroin-addicted mothers. Lancet 1971;2:685–6.
17. Amarose AP, Norusis MJ. Cytogenetics of methadone-managed and heroin-addicted pregnant women and their newborn infants. Am J Obstet Gynecol 1976;124:635–40.
18. Parekh A, Mukherjee TK, Jhaveri R, Rosenfeld W, Glass L. Intrauterine exposure to narcotics and cord blood prolactin concentrations. Obstet Gynecol 1981;57:447–9.
19. Wilson GS, McCreary R, Kean J, Baxter JC. The development of preschool children of heroin-addicted mothers: a controlled study. Pediatrics 1979;63: 135–41.
20. Lichtenstein PM. Infant drug addiction. N Y Med J 1915;102:905. As reported by Cobrinik RW, Hood RT Jr, Chusid E. The effect of maternal narcotic addiction on the newborn infant. Pediatrics 1959;24:288–304.
21. Cobrinik RW, Hood RT Jr, Chusid E. The effect of maternal narcotic addiction on the newborn infant. Pediatrics 1959;24:288–304.
22. Committee on Drugs, American Academy of Pediatrics. The transfer of drugs and other chemicals into human milk. Pediatrics 2001;108;776–89.

Name:	**HETACILLIN**	Risk Factor:	**B**
Class:	**Antibiotic (Penicillin)**		

Hetacillin breaks down in aqueous solution to ampicillin and acetone (see Ampicillin).

Name:	**HEXACHLOROPHENE**	Risk Factor:	**C_M**
Class:	**Anti-infective**		

FETAL RISK SUMMARY

RECOMMENDATION: Compatible (Topical; Excludes Mucous Membranes)

H

Hexachlorophene, a polychlorinated biphenol compound, is a topical antiseptic used primarily as a surgical hand scrub and as a bacteriostatic skin cleanser. Although no longer recommended, hexachlorophene has also been used as a douching agent and in feminine hygiene sprays. The drug is rapidly absorbed systemically following topical administration to injured skin, but percutaneous absorption also occurs across intact skin (1–3). Because of very rapid absorption, hexachlorophene should not be used on mucous membranes or injured skin (1,2).

Blood concentrations of the anti-infective have been documented in premature and full-term newborns who were bathed with hexachlorophene and in adults after chronic handwashing (3). Central nervous system toxicity has been observed following the topical use of hexachlorophene in burn patients and after intravaginal application (3).

Hexachlorophene crosses the human placenta (4,5). In one study, newborn whole cord blood concentrations ranged from 0.003 to 0.182 μg/g with a mean of 0.022 μg/g (1 μg/g = 1 ppm) (4). The source of the drug was thought to be from vaginal sprays used by the mothers and from preparation of the skin immediately before delivery. In a second study, a commercially available 3% emulsion of hexachlorophene was used as antiseptic lubricant for vaginal examinations during labor (5). At delivery, detectable maternal serum concentrations of the drug occurred in 12 of 28 women (range 0.142–0.942 μg/mL) and in the whole cord blood of 9 of 28 newborns (range 0.177–0.617 μg/mL). Because of the potential for toxicity, the authors recommended the use of alternative lubricants.

A number of studies have examined the reproductive toxicity of hexachlorophene in various animal species (6–14). A marked reduction in the sperm count was observed in male rats administered a single oral dose of 125 mg/kg (6). In pregnant rats, dose-related teratogenicity was demonstrated following acute and chronic oral dosing (6–9). No malformations resulted with relatively low doses (6–8), but high maternal doses were associated with cleft palate (8) and with microphthalmia, anophthalmia, and rib anomalies (9). Intravaginal administration of hexachlorophene in pregnant rats resulted in frequent microphthalmia, anophthalmia, wavy ribs, and less frequently, cleft palate in the offspring (10,11). Blood concentrations were 6–10 times higher after vaginal or oral administration than after dermal application (11). Oral doses of 6 mg/kg/day in pregnant rabbits produced defects of the ribs in a small percentage of exposed fetuses, indicating a minimal teratogenic response (9).

Three studies have described the distribution of hexachlorophene in the fetuses of pregnant mice, rats, and monkeys (12–14). In fetal mice, the drug selectively accumulated in the brain, optic vesicles, and neural tube in early gestation (12). During late gestation, high fetal concentrations were measured in the blood, liver, and intestine. A similar pattern of distribution during gestation was described in fetal monkeys (13). In both mice and monkeys, a partial blood-brain barrier was demonstrated to hexachlorophene in term fetuses (12,13). Hexachlorophene crossed the placenta in pregnant rats after both oral and dermal administration with concentrations detected in the placenta, amniotic fluid, and fetus (14).

Only one study has associated the routine use of hexachlorophene with human teratogenicity (15). The results of the investigation were summarized as a news item in a medical journal approximately a year before publication of the original study (16). In a retrospective analysis of the pregnancy outcomes among nurses who had washed their hands with hexachlorophene during the 1st trimester, 25 severe malformations were observed in 460 neonates (15). No major congenital defects were observed among 233 newborns delivered from similarly employed mothers who did not use hexachlorophene. The exposed nurses had worked at one of six Swedish hospitals between 1969 and 1975, and had washed their hands 10 to 60 times/day with either a 0.5% or 3% hexachlorophene liquid soap. Three of the hospitals also used a 0.3% or 0.5% hexachlorophene hand cream. Among the exposed group, 46 newborns, in addition to the 25 with major defects, had minor malformations for a total of 71 affected infants (15.4%). The major malformations included cleft lip and/or palate, microphthalmia, anal atresia and hypospadias, cystic kidneys, esophageal atresia and kidney defects, limb reductions, diaphragmatic hernia, neural tube defects, pulmonary stenosis, and cardiac defects. Minor malformations included dislocations of the hip, undescended testes, polydactyly, various foot anomalies, and mild cardiac defects. Eight (3.4%) minor malformations were observed in the control group.

Criticisms of this study on methodological grounds have been published (17,18). Most of the hexachlorophene-exposed nurses were selected because of an infant malformation, not on the basis of exposure to the drug, thus leading to a higher rate of malformations in the exposed group. The selection of the control group was also criticized and was considered, at least on statistical grounds, not to be representative of random selection (17). Concern was expressed over the identification of the minor defects and how diligently these defects were searched for at the various hospitals (18). Furthermore, another study evaluated delivery data on women working in Swedish hospitals from 1973–1975 and compared them with births in the general Swedish population during the same period (19). A cluster of malformed infants was found in 1973–1974 that was similar to that observed in the report associating defects with hexachlorophene. However, the rates of perinatal deaths and congenital malformations did not differ between 3007 infants born to women heavily exposed to hexachlorophene in 31 hospitals and 1653 infants born to women working in 18 hospitals where the antiseptic was not used at all or was used only sporadically (19).

In summary, one report has suggested that heavy use of hexachlorophene during the 1st trimester may cause birth defects in exposed offspring, but several criticisms have been directed at this study on methodological grounds. Moreover, in nonprimate animal species, only very high levels (i.e., those approaching maternal toxicity) of hexachlorophene are teratogenic. These considerations, coupled with the absence of confirming reports in humans, suggest a lack of an association between routine handwashing with hexachlorophene and human congenital malformations. Because of other toxicities, use of the antiseptic on mucous membranes, such as in the vagina, or on injured skin should be avoided.

BREAST FEEDING SUMMARY

RECOMMENDATION: Compatible

Hexachlorophene has been detected in the milk of lactating rats following a single oral dose of 10 mg/kg on the 2nd postpartum day (14). Detectable milk concentrations of hexachlorophene were found 1 hour after the dose.

In humans, hexachlorophene has been measured in milk following the presumed use of the antiseptic as a nipple wash between nursings (20). The specific history of hexachlorophene use by the women was not available. Six samples of milk were found to have a range of hexachlorophene levels from trace (<2 ppb) to 9.0 ppb (1 ng/g = 1 ppb). The authors concluded that the milk concentrations of hexachlorophene found in their study were too low to present a risk to a nursing infant. The American Academy of Pediatrics has not found any reports describing signs or symptoms in a nursing infant or effect on lactation after use of the drug, but notes that nipple washing with hexachlorophene may contaminate the milk (21).

H

References

1. American Hospital Formulary Service. *Drug Information 1997*. Bethesda, MD: American Society of Health-System Pharmacists, 1997:2716 8.
2. Product information. pHisoHex. Sanofi Winthrop Pharmaceuticals, 1993.
3. Lockhart JD. How toxic is hexachlorophene? Pediatrics 1972;50:220–35.
4. Curley A, Hawk RE, Kimbrough RD, Nathenson G, Finberg L. Dermal absorption of hexachlorophene in infants. Lancet 1971;2:296–7.
5. Strickland DM, Leonard RG, Stavchansky S, Benoit T, Wilson RT. Vaginal absorption of hexachlorophene during labor. Am J Obstet Gynecol 1983;147: 769–72.
6. Thorpe E. Some pathological effects of hexachlorophene in the rat. J Comp Pathol 1967;77: 137–42.
7. Gaines TB, Kimbrough RD. The oral and dermal toxicity of hexachlorophene in rats. Toxicol Appl Pharmacol 1971;19:375–6.
8. Oakley GP, Shepard TH. Possible teratogenicity of hexachlorophene in rats (abstract). Teratology 1972;5:264.
9. Kennedy GL Jr, Smith SH, Keplinger ML, Calandra JC. Evaluation of the teratological potential of hexachlorophene in rabbits and rats. Teratology 1975;12:83–8.
10. Kimmel CA, Moore W Jr, Stara JF. Hexachlorophene teratogenicity in rats. Lancet 1972;2:765.
11. Kimmel CA, Moore W Jr, Hysell DK, Stara JF. Teratogenicity of hexachlorophene in rats. Comparison of uptake following various routes of administration. Arch Environ Health 1974;28:43–8.
12. Brandt I, Dencker L, Larsson Y. Transplacental passage and embryonic-fetal accumulation of hexachlorophene in mice. Toxicol Appl Pharmacol 1979;49:393–401.
13. Brandt I, Dencker L, Larsson KS, Siddall RA. Placental transfer of hexachlorophene (HCP) in the marmoset monkey (*Callithrix jacchus*). Acta Pharmacol Toxicol 1983;52:310–3.
14. Kennedy GL Jr, Dressler IA, Keplinger ML, Calandra JC. Placental and milk transfer of hexachlorophene in the rat. Toxicol Appl Pharmacol 1977;40: 571–6.
15. Halling H. Suspected link between exposure to hexachlorophene and malformed infants. Ann N Y Acad Sci 1979;320:426–35.
16. Check W. New study shows hexachlorophene is teratogenic in humans. JAMA 1978;240:513–4.
17. Källen B. Hexachlorophene teratogenicity in humans disputed. JAMA 1978;240:1585–6.
18. Janerich DT. Environmental causes of birth defects: the hexachlorophene issue. JAMA 1979;241: 830–1.
19. Baltzar B, Ericson A, Källen B. Pregnancy outcome among women working in Swedish hospitals. N Engl J Med 1979;300:627–8.
20. West RW, Wilson DJ, Schaffner W. Hexachlorophene concentrations in human milk. Bull Environ Contam Toxicol 1975;13:167–9.
21. Committee on Drugs, American Academy of Pediatrics. The transfer of drugs and other chemicals into human milk. Pediatrics 2001;108:776–89.

Name: **HEXAMETHONIUM** Risk Factor: **C**
Class: **Antihypertensive**

FETAL RISK SUMMARY

RECOMMENDATION: Limited Human Data - No Relevant Animal Data

No reports linking the use of hexamethonium with congenital defects have been located. Hexamethonium crosses the placenta and accumulates in the amniotic fluid. The drug has been used in the treatment of preeclampsia and essential hypertension. Its use in these conditions is no longer recommended. Three cases of paralytic ileus and one case of delayed passage of meconium have been reported (1,2).

BREAST FEEDING SUMMARY

RECOMMENDATION: No Human Data - Potential Toxicity

No data are available.

References

1. Morris N. Hexamethonium in the treatment of pre-eclampsia and essential hypertension during pregnancy. Lancet 1953;1:322–4.
2. Hallum JL, Hatchuel WLF. Congenital paralytic ileus in a premature baby as a complication of hexamethonium bromide therapy for toxemia of pregnancy. Arch Dis Child 1954;29:354–6.

Name: **HEXOCYCLIUM** Risk Factor: **C**
Class: **Parasympatholytic (Anticholinergic)**

FETAL RISK SUMMARY

RECOMMENDATION: No Human Data - No Relevant Animal Data

Hexocyclium is an anticholinergic agent. No reports of its use in pregnancy have been located (see also Atropine).

BREAST FEEDING SUMMARY

RECOMMENDATION: No Human Data - Probably Compatible

No data are available (see also Atropine).

Name: **HEXOPRENALINE** Risk Factor: **C**
Class: **Sympathomimetic (Adrenergic)**

FETAL RISK SUMMARY

RECOMMENDATION: Limited Human Data - Animal Data Suggest Low Risk

Hexoprenaline is a β_2-sympathomimetic used as an IV tocolytic agent and as an oral or inhaled bronchodilator in the symptomatic treatment of bronchial asthma and chronic obstructive pulmonary disease. It is structurally similar to several other sympathomimetics, including epinephrine, norepinephrine, and isoproterenol. Although available in other countries, it is not yet available in the United States.

Unpublished reproductive data involving hexoprenaline in rats and rabbits were cited in a 1977 review (1). No embryotoxic or teratogenic effects were noted in pregnant rats administered hexoprenaline 5 mg/kg/day between days 6 and 15. However, a slight decrease in the fertility index did occur. An increase in the number of stillborn and a decrease in fetal weight were observed in pregnant rabbits dosed with 0.5 mg/kg/day between days 16 and 18 of pregnancy (1). For comparison, the human oral dose for bronchodilation is approximately 0.04 mg/kg/day, based on 3 mg/day in a 70-kg human, whereas the usual tocolytic dose is approximately 0.1 μg/minute (about 0.002 mg/kg/day for a 70-kg human).

In a study with pregnant rats at day 14 of gestation, a bolus injection of hexoprenaline 0.5 μg/kg followed immediately by a 30-minute infusion of 0.1 μg/kg/minute, increased blood flow to the placenta by 198% (2). This dose also increased the percentage of cardiac output distributed to the placenta by 229%. Renal blood flow was reduced by 24% (2).

H

Because of its relatively low molecular weight (about 519 for the sulfate salt), hexoprenaline should cross the placenta to the fetus. However, no measurable levels of radioactivity were found in fetal blood following administration of carbon-14-labeled hexoprenaline to pregnant sheep (3). Pregnant rabbits were given a 0.015-mg/kg dose of carbon-14-labeled hexoprenaline and the amounts of labeled drug were determined in the maternal and fetal compartments over a 60-minute interval (4). Very small amounts of radioactivity were measured in the fetal compartment, which the authors considered "insignificant." In an *in vitro* perfused human placenta module, the transfer of ^{14}C-labeled hexoprenaline to the fetal side was approximately 1.1%, significantly less than the transfer of three other β-sympathomimetics labeled with tritium (^{3}H-fenoterol 2.3%, ^{3}H-ritodrine 2.4%, and ^{3}H-albuterol 2.8%) (5). The doses used for each drug were considered similar to those used in clinical practice and had equivalent tocolytic effects. The low placental transfer of these agents may have resulted from the use of only about 5% of the exchange area of the total placenta and a short measurement interval (5).

At least four studies have described the human use of hexoprenaline as a tocolytic (6–9). A 1976 study compared the uterine selectivity of four tocolytic agents (equivalent IV bolus doses are shown in parentheses), hexoprenaline (7.5 μg), albuterol (200 μg), fenoterol (50 μg), and ritodrine (6 mg) (6). The study drugs were administered in a predetermined sequence to 10 women at term with oxytocin-induced labor. Hexoprenaline had the least effect on the maternal heart as measured by an increase in pulse rate. All of the drugs caused transient hypotension with the most pronounced effect on the diastolic blood pressure. Although the difference was not significant, hexoprenaline stopped uterine contractions for the longest average time (12.94 minutes) and ritodrine stopped uterine contractions for the shortest average time (8.63 minutes). The average time for the other two agents was about 10.3 minutes. All of the agents produced a transient rise in the fetal heart rate of about 10 beats/minute and an increase in beat-to-beat variation.

A second report by the same investigators compared the uterine and cardiovascular effects of a 20-minute IV infusion of the four tocolytics used in the study above (7). The dose infused per minute was 1/20th of the IV bolus dose. All of the drugs significantly reduced the activity of the uterus to less than 30% of the initial level, but the tocolytic effect of ritodrine lasted nearly twice as long as the effects of the other three agents. As in their first study, hexoprenaline produced the smallest rise in maternal pulse rate and the smallest increase in systolic blood pressure. The decrease in diastolic blood pressure was similar among the four drugs. No adverse fetal or neonatal effects were observed other than a slight rise in the fetal heart rate and an increase in beat-to-beat variability prior to birth. A 1981 study of 20 women in labor reported that 30 minutes of a hexoprenaline infusion, at doses up to 0.3 μg/minute, decreased the uterine activity by nearly 74% while increasing the maternal pulse rate by 25% (8). No significant change was observed in the fetal heart rate.

IV infusions of hexoprenaline (0.38 μg/minute) and fenoterol (2.5 μg/minute) as tocolytics in prostaglandin $F_{2\alpha}$-induced labor were compared in a 1984 study (9). Both drugs were alternatively infused for 20 minutes in each of 12 women at term. Uterine activity (pressure, intensity, and frequency) was reduced to less than 29% of the initial activity by both drugs. As in the above two studies, hexoprenaline produced the least effect on maternal pulse rate. The effects on systolic and diastolic pressure were similar. Other than the fetal heart rate changes noted above, no adverse effects on the fetuses or newborns were observed.

H

Like other β-sympathomimetic tocolytic agents, hexoprenaline has been used in the emergency treatment of fetal distress resulting from various causes during labor (10–12). A 1977 study described the successful treatment of six women in labor with a single, 10-μg IV bolus dose of hexoprenaline for acute, severe fetal bradycardia (10). Fetal acidosis was documented in three of the cases. The Apgar scores were 7–9 in five infants (4 in one infant) at 1 minute, and 7–10 in six infants at 5 minutes. In a 1986 study, 12 women with severe fetal distress from various causes in labor were treated with a 7.5–10-μg IV bolus of hexoprenaline followed by an IV infusion of the drug titrated to inhibit uterine contractions (11). According to protocol, all were delivered by cesarean section approximately 40 minutes after the IV bolus dose. Nine of the newborns had Apgar scores of 7 or greater at 1 minute (2 in one infant, 6 in two), and 12 had Apgar scores of 8 or greater at 5 minutes. The mean fetal scalp pH before treatment was 7.17, and the mean cord blood pH was 7.31. A randomized, controlled study published in 1997 studied the benefits and disadvantages of therapy with a β-sympathomimetic in 37 women in labor at 35 weeks' gestation or more who were scheduled for cesarean section because of fetal distress (12). Comparisons were made between the maternal, fetal, and newborn outcomes for the study group (hexoprenaline; $N = 17$) and the controls (no therapy; $N = 20$). The mean time to cesarean section was 60 minutes in the study group and 54 minutes for the controls. The study group received a 10-μg IV bolus of hexoprenaline ($N = 17$) administered over 5 minutes. There were no statistical differences between the groups in the main outcomes measured: cord blood gas values, Apgar scores at 1 and 5 minutes, need for resuscitation, and admission to the neonatal intensive care unit (12). Significantly more fetuses, however, had an improvement in their heart rate patterns after hexoprenaline. Two infants in the control group were stillborn; one had hydrocephalus, and the other was delivered vaginally 55 minutes after the onset of fetal distress.

Fetal and maternal cardiac toxicities have been reported with the use of hexoprenaline tocolysis (13–16). A 1991 case report described severe fetal tachycardia in a woman at 32 weeks' gestation given a 10-μg IV bolus dose of hexoprenaline for fetal distress (13). The patient had been treated 3 days earlier with glucocorticoids for fetal lung maturity and with indomethacin and hexoprenaline (for 4 hours) followed by oral fenoterol for tocolysis. Because of the suspected occurrence of intrauterine infection 3 days later, fenoterol was stopped and oxytocin was initiated for labor induction. Shortly thereafter, with the fetal heart rate at 160–175 beats/minute, a sudden deceleration to 80 beats/minute occurred without evidence of a hypertonic uterine contraction. Oxytocin was discontinued, and an IV bolus of hexoprenaline was administered. The fetal heart rate increased to at least 210 beats/minute. A 1440-g, male infant was delivered by emergency cesarean section with

Apgar scores of 2, 3, and 5 at 1, 5, and 10 minutes, respectively. The infant survived after ventilation for 24 hours. No evidence of infection or cardiac defect was found.

A healthy, 20-year-old woman at 33 weeks' gestation was treated with an IV infusion of hexoprenaline 0.15 μg/minute, increased to 0.3 μg/minute over 20 minutes, for preterm labor (14). Her pulse rate increased from 80 beats/minute to 112–124 beats/minute. After 1.5 hours, her pulse suddenly increased to 160 beats/minute and became irregular. Her blood pressure remained unchanged at 90/60 mm Hg. An electrocardiogram (ECG) revealed atrial fibrillation that reverted spontaneously to a normal sinus rhythm 8 hours later. She had no further symptoms of cardiac dysfunction or preterm labor and eventually delivered, at term, a 3220-g female infant with Apgar scores of 6 and 9 at 1 and 5 minutes, respectively. In the absence of other known causes, the atrial fibrillation was attributed to hexoprenaline.

Hexoprenaline 9 μg/hour was used for tocolysis in a healthy 29-year-old patient with preterm labor at 32 weeks' gestation (15). Her baseline pulse rate was 95 beats/minute. An IV infusion of verapamil was added to prevent maternal tachycardia, but after 24 hours the patient developed retrosternal pain, dyspnea, palpitations, and nausea. An ECG revealed supraventricular tachycardia with a rate of 180 beats/minute. Her blood pressure fell from 95/60 mm Hg to 70/45 mm Hg. The hexoprenaline dose was reduced to 6 μg/hour and then discontinued 5 hours later. Other measures, including digoxin, continuous verapamil, carotid sinus massage, and Valsalva maneuvers, failed to stop the arrhythmia. Metoprolol (5 mg IV), a cardioselective β-adrenergic blocking agent, was administered 52 hours after the onset of the tachycardia, and 4 hours later the heart rate fell to 100 beats/minute. The fetal heart rate remained in the 130–140-beats/minute range throughout and did not appear to be affected by any of the above events. In the absence of labor, the patient was treated with oral metoprolol (100 mg/day) until the recurrence of tachycardia (130 beats/minute) with signs of cardiac decompensation at 39 weeks' gestation. A cesarean section was performed to deliver a 3850-g female infant with Apgar scores of 9, 10, and 10 at 1, 5, and 10 minutes, respectively. In the absence of cardiac disease, the authors thought the tachycardia was most likely induced by hexoprenaline (15).

Two studies have reported follow-up examinations of 72 children exposed *in utero* to hexoprenaline during the 3rd trimester (16,17). Examinations were conducted during the first week of life in 28 (16), at a mean age of 15 months (range 2–40 months) in 23 (17), and at 3 years of age in 21 (16). The mean maternal hexoprenaline dose in one group was 51.103 mg over an average period of 13.8 days (17). The examinations included general health, neurological development, ECG, blood analyses, and ultrasonography (not all of the examinations were conducted in each group). Except for an incidental systolic murmur in two children and borderline cardiomegaly in a third, all of the children appeared to be developing within normal limits.

Like all β-sympathomimetics, hexoprenaline may cause transient maternal hyperglycemia with an increase in serum insulin levels (18). Sustained neonatal hypoglycemia may be observed if maternal hyperglycemia occurs close to delivery.

In summary, no reports describing the use of hexoprenaline during early human pregnancy have been located. Although several studies have investigated the use of the drug as a tocolytic agent, the amount of published research is less than that available for other similar agents (e.g., see Terbutaline and Ritodrine). Hexoprenaline does not appear to offer any advantage over these tocolytic agents. As with any β-sympathomimetic, including hexoprenaline, avoiding continuous IV infusions will lessen the chance of serious maternal cardiac toxicity. The administration of the drug as a bronchodilator during pregnancy has not been reported.

BREAST FEEDING SUMMARY

RECOMMENDATION: No Human Data - Probably Compatible

No reports describing the use of hexoprenaline during lactation have been located. The molecular weight of the sulfate salt of hexoprenaline (about 519) is low enough, however, that passage into milk should be expected. The effects of this exposure on a nursing infant are unknown, but other β-sympathomimetics (e.g., see Terbutaline) are considered compatible with breast-feeding.

References

1. Pinder RM, Brogden RN, Speight TM, Avery GS. Hexoprenaline: A review of its pharmacological properties and therapeutic efficacy with particular reference to asthma. Drugs 1977;14:1–28.
2. Lipshitz J, Ahokas RA, Broyles K, Anderson GD. Effect of hexoprenaline on uteroplacental blood flow in the pregnant rat. Am J Obstet Gynecol 1986;154:310–4.
3. Lipshitz J, Yau MK, Meyer MC, Ahokas RA, Maduska AL, Whybrew WD, Anderson GD, Morrison JC, Schneider J. Hexoprenaline pharmacokinetics in pregnant and nonpregnant sheep. Res Commun Chem Pathol Pharmacol 1981;34:3–16.
4. Lipshitz J, Broyles K, Whybrew WD, Ahokas RA, Anderson GD. Placental transfer of ^{14}C-hexoprenaline. Am J Obstet Gynecol 1982;142:313–5.
5. Sodha RJ, Schneider H. Transplacental transfer of beta-adrenergic drugs studied by an *in vitro* perfusion method of an isolated human placental lobule. Am J Obstet Gynecol 1983;147:303–10.
6. Lipshitz J, Baillie P, Davey DA. A comparison of the uterine beta$_2$ -adrenoreceptor selectivity of fenoterol, hexoprenaline, ritodrine and salbutamol. S Afr Med J 1976;50:1969–72.
7. Lipshitz J, Baillie P. Uterine and cardiovascular effects of beta$_2$ -selective sympathomimetic drugs administered as an intravenous infusion. S Afr Med J 1976;50:1973–7.
8. Bernaschek G, Hondros K, Schaller A. Intrauterine pressure and fetal and maternal heart rate on administration of the beta-mimetic agent, hexoprenaline during labour. Wien Klin Wochenschr 1981;93:541–7.
9. Lipshitz J, Lipshitz EM. Uterine and cardiovascular effects of fenoterol and hexoprenaline in prostaglandin $F_{2\alpha}$-induced labor in humans. Obstet Gynecol 1984;63:396–400.
10. Lipshitz J. Use of a β_2-sympathomimetic drug as a temporizing measure in the treatment of acute fetal distress. Am J Obstet Gynecol 1977;129:31–6.
11. Lipshitz J, Shaver DC, Anderson GD. Hexoprenaline tocolysis for intrapartum fetal distress and acidosis. J Reprod Med 1986;31:1023–6.
12. Kulier R, Gulmezogul AM, Hofmeyr GJ, Van Gelderen CJ. Beta-mimetics in fetal distress: a randomised controlled trial. J Perinat Med 1997;25:97–100.
13. D'Hooghe TM, Odendaal HJ. Severe fetal tachycardia after administration of hexoprenaline to the mother. S Afr Med J 1991;80:594–5.
14. Frederiksen MC, Toig RM, Depp R III. Atrial fibrillation during hexoprenaline therapy for premature labor. Am J Obstet Gynecol 1983;145:108–9.
15. Frigo P, Eppel W, Frank A, Ulm M, Golaszewski T, Gruber W. Management of supraventricular tachycardia during hexoprenaline therapy for preterm labour: benefit of cardioselective beta blockade? Gynecol Obstet Invest 1995;39:212–4.
16. Wilk F. Hexoprenaline tocolysis - side effects in the child? Z Geburtshilfe Perinatol 1985;189:232–4.
17. Trittenwein G, Rosegger H, Beitzke H, Lichtenegger W, Rosanelli K, Zeichen HL. Heart function in infants and small children, whose mothers required tocolysis with hexoprenaline sulfate (Gynipral). Wien Klin Wochenschr 1986;98:613–7.
18. Lipshitz F, Vinik AI. The effects of hexoprenaline, a β_2-sympathomimetic drug, on maternal glucose, insulin, glucagon, and free fatty acid levels. Am J Obstet Gynecol 1978;130:761–4.

Name:	**HOMATROPINE**	Risk Factor:	**C**
Class:	**Parasympatholytic (Anticholinergic)**		

FETAL RISK SUMMARY

RECOMMENDATION: Limited Human Data - No Relevant Animal Data

Homatropine is an anticholinergic agent. The Collaborative Perinatal Project monitored 50,282 mother-child pairs, 26 of whom used homatropine in the 1st trimester (1, pp. 346–353). For use anytime during pregnancy, 86 exposures were recorded (1, p. 439). Only for anytime use was a possible association with congenital defects discovered. In addition, when the group of parasympatholytics was taken as a whole (2,323 exposures), a possible association with minor malformations was found (1, pp. 346–353).

BREAST FEEDING SUMMARY

RECOMMENDATION: No Human Data - Probably Compatible

See Atropine.

Reference

1. Heinonen OP, Slone D, Shapiro S. *Birth Defects and Drugs in Pregnancy*. Littleton, MA: Publishing Sciences Group, 1977.

H

Name:	**HORMONAL PREGNANCY TEST TABLETS**	Risk Factor:	**X**
Class:	**Estrogenic/Progestogenic Hormones**		

See Oral Contraceptives.

Name:	**HYDRALAZINE**	Risk Factor:	**C_M**
Class:	**Antihypertensive**		

FETAL RISK SUMMARY

RECOMMENDATION: Human Data Suggest Risk in 3rd Trimester

No reports linking the use of hydralazine with congenital defects have been located. In England, hydralazine is the most commonly used antihypertensive agent in pregnant women (1). Neonatal thrombocytopenia and bleeding secondary to maternal ingestion of hydralazine have been reported in three infants (2). In each case, the mother had consumed the drug daily throughout the 3rd trimester. This complication has also been reported in series examining severe maternal hypertension and may be related to the disease rather than to the drug (3,4).

Hydralazine readily crosses the placenta to the fetus (5). Serum concentrations in the fetus are equal to or greater than those in the mother.

The Collaborative Perinatal Project monitored 50,282 mother-child pairs, 8 of whom had 1st trimester exposure to hydralazine (6, p. 372). For use anytime during pregnancy, 136 cases were recorded (6, p. 441). No defects were observed with 1st trimester use. There were 8 infants born with defects who were exposed in the 2nd or 3rd trimesters. This incidence (5.8%) is greater than the expected frequency of occurrence, but the severe maternal disease necessitating the use of hydralazine is probably responsible. Patients with preeclampsia are at risk for a marked increase in fetal mortality (7–10).

In a surveillance study of Michigan Medicaid recipients conducted between 1985 and 1992 involving 229,101 completed pregnancies, 40 newborns had been exposed to hydralazine during the 1st trimester (F. Rosa, personal communication, FDA, 1993). One (2.5%) major birth defect was observed (two expected), a hypospadias (none expected).

A number of studies involving the use of hydralazine either alone or in combination with other antihypertensives have found the drug to be relatively safe for the fetus (4,7–17). Fatal maternal hypotension has been reported in one patient after combined therapy with hydralazine and diazoxide (18).

In a woman with chronic hypertension maintained on methyldopa, an increase in blood pressure at about 35 weeks' gestation prompted the addition of hydralazine, 25 mg twice daily, to the treatment regimen (19). Fetal premature atrial contractions were diagnosed 1 week later, but tachyarrhythmias, which can be initiated by premature atrial contractions, were not observed (19). Hospitalization with bed rest allowed the patient's blood pressure to decline enough to discontinue hydralazine therapy. Within 24 hours of stopping hydralazine, the fetal arrhythmia resolved. The infant was delivered at 38 weeks and cardiac evaluation after discharge at 3 days indicated a regular heart rate.

A syndrome resembling lupus erythematosus was diagnosed in a 29-year-old woman treated with IV hydralazine during the 28th week of pregnancy (20). The patient received 425 mg during a 6-day period for the treatment of hypertension. IV methyldopa was administered on the 6th day of therapy. Labor was induced for fetal distress and a 780-g, growth-retarded male infant was delivered vaginally. The infant expired at 36 hours of age secondary to cardiac tamponade induced by 7 mL of clear sterile transudate in the pericardial space. Lupus-like symptoms consisting of macular rash, arthralgia, and bilateral pleural effusion developed in the mother on the 5th day of hydralazine therapy and gradually resolved after discontinuance of the drug and delivery. The findings of pericardial effusion and cardiac tamponade in the infant were also thought to represent clinical evidence of a lupus-like syndrome (20). The symptoms in both the mother and fetus were attributed to hydralazine sensitivity resulting in the induction of a lupus-like syndrome.

BREAST FEEDING SUMMARY

RECOMMENDATION: Limited Human Data - Probably Compatible

Hydralazine is excreted into breast milk (5). In one patient treated with 50 mg 3 times daily, the milk:plasma ratio 2 hours after a dose was 1.4. This value is in close agreement with the predicted ratio calculated from the pK_a (21). The available dose of hydralazine in 75 mL of milk was estimated to be 13 μg (5). No adverse effects were noted in the nursing infant from this small concentration. The American Academy of Pediatrics classifies hydralazine as compatible with breast-feeding (22).

References

1. de Swiet M. Antihypertensive drugs in pregnancy. Br Med J 1985;291:365–6.
2. Widerlov E, Karlman I. Storsater J. Hydralazine-induced neonatal thrombocytopenia. N Engl J Med 1980;303:1235.
3. Brazy JE, Grimm JK, Little VA. Neonatal manifestations of severe maternal hypertension occurring before the thirty-sixth week of pregnancy. J Pediatr 1982;100:265–71.
4. Sibai BM, Anderson GD. Pregnancy outcome of intensive therapy in severe hypertension in first trimester. Obstet Gynecol 1986;67:517–22.
5. Liedholm H, Wahlin-Boll E, Ingemarsson I, Melander A. Transplacental passage and breast milk concentrations of hydralazine. Eur J Clin Pharmacol 1982;21:417–9.
6. Heinonen OP, Slone D, Shapiro S. *Birth Defects and Drugs in Pregnancy*. Littleton, MA: Publishing Sciences Group, 1977.
7. Bott-Kanner G, Schweitzer A, Schoenfeld A, Joel-Cohen J, Rosenfeld JB. Treatment with propranolol and hydralazine throughout pregnancy in a hypertensive patient. Isr J Med Sci 1978;14:466–8.
8. Pritchard JA, Pritchard SA. Standardized treatment of 154 consecutive cases of eclampsia. Am J Obstet Gynecol 1975;123:543–52.
9. Chapman ER, Strozier WE, Magee RA. The clinical use of Apresoline in the toxemias of pregnancy. Am J Obstet Gynecol 1954;68:1109–17.
10. Johnson GT, Thompson RB. A clinical trial of intravenous Apresoline in the management of toxemia of late pregnancy. J Obstet Gynecol 1958;65:360–6.
11. Kuzniar J, Skret A, Piela A, Szmigiel Z, Zaczek T.

Hemodynamic effects of intravenous hydralazine in pregnant women with severe hypertension. Obstet Gynecol 1985;66:453–8.
12. Hogstedt S, Lindeberg S, Axelsson O, Lindmark G, Rane A, Sandstrom B, Lindberg BS. A prospective controlled trial of metoprolol-hydralazine treatment in hypertension during pregnancy. Acta Obstet Scand 1985;64:505–10.
13. Gallery EDM, Ross MR, Gyory AZ. Antihypertensive treatment in pregnancy: analysis of different responses to oxprenolol and methyldopa. Br Med J 1985;291:563–6.
14. Horvath JS, Korda A, Child A, Henderson-Smart D, Phippard A, Duggin GG, Hall BM, Tiller DJ. Hypertension in pregnancy: a study of 142 women presenting before 32 weeks' gestation. Med J Aust 1985;143:19–21.
15. Rosenfeld J, Bott-Kanner G, Boner G, Nissenkorn A, Friedman S, Ovadia J, Merlob P, Reisner S, Paran E, Zmora E, Biale Y, Insler V. Treatment of hypertension during pregnancy with hydralazine monotherapy or with combined therapy with hydralazine and pindolol. Eur J Obstet Gynecol Reprod Biol 1986;22:197–204.
16. Mabie WC, Gonzalez AR, Sibai BM, Amon E. A comparative trial of labetalol and hydralazine in the acute management of severe hypertension complicating pregnancy. Obstet Gynecol 1987;70:328–33.
17. Owen J, Hauth JC. Polyarteritis nodosa in pregnancy: a case report and brief literature review. Am J Obstet Gynecol 1989;160:606–7.
18. Henrich WL, Cronin R, Miller PD, Anderson RJ. Hypotensive sequelae of diazoxide and hydralazine therapy. JAMA 1977;237:264–5.
19. Lodeiro JG, Feinstein SJ, Lodeiro SB. Fetal premature atrial contractions associated with hydralazine. Am J Obstet Gynecol 1989;160:105–7.
20. Yemini M, Shoham(Schwartz) Z, Dgani R, Lancet M, Mogilner BM, Nissim F, Bar-Khayim Y. Lupus-like syndrome in a mother and newborn following administration of hydralazine: a case report. Eur J Obstet Gynecol Reprod Biol 1989;30:193–7.
21. Daily JW. Anticoagulant and cardiovascular drugs. In Wilson JT, ed. *Drugs in Breast Milk*. Balgowlah, Australia: ADIS Press, 1981:61–4.
22. Committee on Drugs, American Academy of Pediatrics. The transfer of drugs and other chemicals into human milk. Pediatrics 2001;108:776–89.

Name:	**HYDRIODIC ACID**	Risk Factor:	**D**
Class:	**Respiratory Drug (Expectorant)**		

The active ingredient of hydriodic acid is iodide (see Potassium Iodide).

Name:	**HYDROCHLOROTHIAZIDE**	Risk Factor:	$\mathbf{B_M}$
Class:	**Diuretic**		

See Chlorothiazide.

Name:	**HYDROCODONE**	Risk Factor:	**C***
Class:	**Narcotic Agonist Analgesic/ Respiratory Drug (Antitussive)**		

FETAL RISK SUMMARY

RECOMMENDATION: Human Data Suggest Risk in 3rd Trimester

Hydrocodone is a centrally acting narcotic agent that is related to codeine. It is combined with other drugs for use an analgesic or as an antitussive. In a reproductive study in hamsters, a single SC injection (102 mg/kg) during the critical period of central nervous system organogenesis produced malformations (cranioschisis and various other lesions) in 3.4% of the offspring (1). Because of its narcotic properties, withdrawal could theoretically occur in infants exposed *in utero* to prolonged maternal ingestion of hydrocodone.

In a surveillance study of Michigan Medicaid recipients conducted between 1985 and 1992 involving 229,101 completed pregnancies, 332 newborns had been exposed to

hydrocodone during the 1st trimester (F. Rosa, personal communication, FDA, 1993). A total of 24 (7.2%) major birth defects were observed (14 expected), five of which were cardiovascular defects (three expected). No anomalies were observed in five other defect categories (oral clefts, spina bifida, polydactyly, limb reduction defects, and hypospadias) for which specific data were available. The total number of malformations is suggestive of a possible association, but other factors, including the mother's disease, concurrent drug use, and chance, may be involved.

At a 1996 meeting, data on 118 women using hydrocodone ($N = 40$) or oxycodone ($N = 78$) during the 1st trimester for postoperative pain, general pain, or upper respiratory infection were matched with a similar group using codeine for these purposes (2). Six (5.1%) of the infants exposed to hydrocodone or oxycodone had malformations, an odds ratio of 2.61 (95% confidence interval 0.6–11.5) ($p = 0.13$). There was no pattern evident among the six malformations.

H

[**Risk Factor D if used for prolonged periods or in high doses at term.*]

BREAST FEEDING SUMMARY

RECOMMENDATION: No Human Data - Probably Compatible

No reports describing the use of hydrocodone during human lactation have been located. Because of the relatively low molecular weight (about 381), passage into milk should be expected. Although occasional maternal doses of hydrocodone probably present a minimal risk for adverse effects during nursing, infants should be monitored for gastrointestinal effects, sedation, and changes in feeding patterns.

References

1. Geber WF, Schramm LC. Congenital malformations of the central nervous system produced by narcotic analgesics in the hamster. Am J Obstet Gynecol 1975;123:705–13.
2. Schick B, Hom M, Tolosa J, Librizzi R, Donnfeld A. Preliminary analysis of first trimester exposure to oxycodone and hydrocodone (abstract). Presented at the Ninth International Conference of the Organization of Teratology Information Services, Salt Lake City, Utah, May 2–4, 1996. Reprod Toxicol 1996;10:162.

Name:	**HYDROCORTISONE**	Risk Factor:	**C***
Class:	**Corticosteroid**		

FETAL RISK SUMMARY

RECOMMENDATION: Human Data Suggest Risk

Hydrocortisone (Cortisol; Compound F) is a corticosteroid secreted by the adrenal cortex. An inactive precursor, cortisone (Compound E), is also secreted by the adrenal cortex and is converted by reduction, primarily by the liver, to hydrocortisone (1). Hydrocortisone is used for a variety of indications. Physiologic doses are used to treat adrenal hormone deficiency, and higher, pharmacologic amounts for the anti-inflammatory and immunosuppressant properties and other effects.

A number of studies have described the effects of hydrocortisone or cortisone on the pregnancy outcomes of experimental animals (2–11,13–15). In five different strains of pregnant mice administered a daily IM dose of cortisone ranging from 0.625 to 10.0 mg for 4 to 5 days, a dose-related and strain-related incidence of cleft palate and resorption were observed (2). Depending on the day of gestation that treatment started, the percentage of young with cleft palate ranged from 2.9% to 79.1%. (Pups with cleft lip and palate similar to the spontaneous defects that sometimes occur in untreated pups were excluded [2].) In contrast, no cases of cleft palate were observed in the young from control mice injected with an inert cortisone-free vehicle. Other anomalies observed in the offspring of treated groups included marked intrauterine growth retardation (IUGR), shortening of the head and mandible, and spina bifida.

In a continuation of the above work, this same research group studied the effects on pregnant mice of a daily, 2.5-mg IM cortisone dose given for 4 consecutive days beginning on gestational days 7 through 18 (3). The maximum percentage of litters resorbed occurred on day 7 (88%) and declined thereafter as the gestational age increased at the first dose. Depending on the mother's genotype, the 4-day cortisone treatment beginning on gestational day 11 resulted in an incidence of cleft palate in the offspring varying from 4% to 100%. Much of this and earlier experiments was reviewed by these investigators in a 1957 paper (4).

Hydrocortisone was shown to produce an incidence of cleft palate in mice offspring similar to cortisone (95%) in genetically susceptible pregnant mice treated with 2.5 mg/day IM for 4 days starting on the 10th or 11th gestational day (5). No other gross external malformations were observed in the offspring.

The effect of cortisone treatment in mice on litter size, birth weight, cleft palate, gestation length, and spontaneous cleft lip (with or without palate) has been investigated (6). Litter size was reduced only if treatment was begun before the 12th gestational day, whereas birth weight was primarily reduced (mean reduction 31.2%) by treatment after this time. Cortisone administration had no effect on mean gestation length or on the frequency of spontaneous cleft lip but did induce cleft palate in some offspring. A 1998 correspondence reiterated the negative effect of cortisone on intrauterine growth that was found in this study (7).

The teratogenic potency of three corticosteroids to produce cleft palate in mice was the subject of a study published in 1965 (8). Therapeutically equivalent IM doses of hydrocortisone (4 mg), prednisolone (1 mg), or dexamethasone (0.15 mg) were administered to pregnant mice (weight 20 to 25 g) on gestational days 11 through 14. After exclusion of offspring with spontaneous cleft lip and palate, the frequency of cleft palate with the three agents was 18%, 77%, and 100%, respectively (8). In another study, cleft palate (palatoschisis) and cataract were frequently observed in the offspring of pregnant mice (weight 20 g) administered 1 mg of hydrocortisone SC for 2 to 4 days between gestational days 9 and 16 (9). Resorption of part or all of the litters was common.

One study investigated the effect on reproduction in rabbits of IM cortisone, 1 to 5.7 mg/kg/day administered for 1 to 33 days (10). Gross congenital anomalies were not seen in offspring that survived, but IUGR was evident in some. Further, a marked increase in fetal and neonatal death was observed. In a later study, pregnant rabbits received IM cortisone, 25 or 30 mg (approximately 7 to 8 mg/kg/day), for 4 days beginning on gestational day 14 or 15 (11). (Total gestation time in rabbits is 31–34 days [12].) Seventeen of the 35 embryos had a cleft palate, including 9 of the 12 born dead. Embryos with cleft palate, living or stillborn, usually weighed less than their siblings. In addition, two of the seven exposed litters were completely resorbed. All 36 offspring from nonexposed controls were born alive without cleft palate.

Reduced lung and body weights were observed in rabbit fetuses given a 2-mg IM injection of hydrocortisone on gestational day 24 (13). Treated fetuses also had fewer lung cells as indicated by decreased DNA per lung. The deficiencies in the number of lung cells and the weights of lung and body recovered within 30 days of birth. In a 1979 study, hydrocortisone, 57 mg/kg/day intraperitoneal on day 12 or 15 of gestation, had no effect on the development of brain monoamine cell bodies or the arrival of axon terminals in the regions where the synapses form (14).

A study published in 1991 demonstrated that a single, 250 mg/kg SC dose of hydrocortisone in pregnant mice on gestational days 11 through 17 could induce polycystic kidney disease in the fetus (15). (Total gestation time in mice is 18–20 days [12].) The highest incidence of the defect occurred after exposure on gestational day 12, corresponding to the expected onset of metanephric renal differentiation in the fetal mouse (15).

Hydrocortisone and cortisone cross the human placenta to the fetus (16–19). Six pregnant women, immediately before an elective cesarean section at term, received a continuous IV infusion of a mixture of radioactive-labeled hydrocortisone and cortisone (16). By measurement of the hormones in the mothers and newborns, the investigators demonstrated that most (about 75%) of the hydrocortisone in the fetus was endogenous, whereas most of the cortisone was from the mother. Two other studies described low transfer of hydrocortisone to the fetus because of placental metabolism (17,18). The placenta is a rich source of the enzyme, 11β-ol-dehydrogenase, which can convert hydrocortisone to cortisone, the biologically inactive 11-ketosteroid (17,18). In an *in vivo* experiment, radioactive-labeled IV hydrocortisone was administered to five women immediately before an elective abortion at 13 to 18 weeks' gestation (17). The concentrations of hydrocortisone and cortisone in umbilical cord serum and the placenta exhibited similar patterns: about 15% for hydrocortisone and 85% for cortisone, indicating that most of hydrocortisone crossing the placenta had been converted to cortisone (17). Using a perfused human placenta, one investigation discovered that the percentage of hydrocortisone converted to cortisone in three different perfusion mediums was 73% (buffer), 85% (1% human serum albumin), and 78% (washed calf red blood cells) (18).

In a 1982 report, researchers measured the concentration of hydrocortisone in the cord blood of 71 premature infants (mean gestational age 32.5 weeks) after administration of the drug in an attempt to prevent respiratory distress syndrome (RDS) (19). The mothers received an IV dose of 100 mg, followed by 100 mg IM every 8 hours up to a total of 400 mg. The infants were delivered between 6 minutes and 85 hours after the first dose. The peak cord blood concentration (32 μg/100 mL) occurred approximately 1 hour after a dose, representing a 3.8-fold increase over endogenous levels (8.5 μg/100 mL). Nearly all of the exogenous hydrocortisone was cleared between doses as indicated by the elimination half-life of about 2 hours (19).

Hydrocortisone is frequently prescribed during human pregnancy and case reports and other references have described the use of this agent or its precursor, cortisone, during pregnancies that produced an infant with a congenital malformation. In most cases, however, a relationship between the drug and the outcome cannot be determined.

The Collaborative Perinatal Project monitored 50,282 mother-child pairs, of whom 21 and 34 infants, respectively, were exposed in the 1st trimester to hydrocortisone and cortisone (20, pp. 388–400). Three of the infants exposed *in utero* to hydrocortisone had a major malformation (relative risk [RR] 2.79), whereas one infant had a defect following exposure to cortisone (RR 0.46) (types of defect not specified). There were 74 exposures to hydrocortisone anytime during pregnancy with three malformed infants (RR 1.70) (20, pp. 443). Although the number of exposures is limited, no evidence of an association with congenital malformations was found with these data (20, pp. 398).

Several case reports have described congenital anomalies in newborns exposed to corticosteroids with and without other drug exposures (21–25). Some of these cases are included in the review discussed below (26). A brief 1953 correspondence describes four infants with defects (club foot, coarctation of the aorta, cataract, and hypospadias) who were delivered to mothers treated during the 1st trimester with cortisone for nausea and vomiting (21). Microcephaly was noted in a newborn whose mother was treated with two 100-mg IV doses of hydrocortisone and a single IM dose of procaine penicillin at about the 8th week of gestation (22). A male cyclops with a single orbit containing one eyeball with two corneas and two irides was described in a 1973 publication (23). The mother had been treated with "high doses" (specifics not given) of cortisone, procaine penicillin, and sodium salicylate at about 4 weeks fetal age for symptoms of diarrhea, fever, and a maculopapular rash. The infant died 5 minutes after birth. In addition to the cyclops, the nose was absent and the ears were low set, and at autopsy, the brain was found to be small and severely malformed. Although the mother had a positive rubella titer, a definite diagnosis of rubella could not be made (23). Moreover, the defects noted in the infant were not consistent with those required for a diagnosis of congenital rubella syndrome (see Vaccine, Rubella). Two malformed infants, one with gastroschisis and the other with hydrocephalus, were briefly noted in a 1965 reference (24). The mothers had used cortisone (doses not specified) throughout their pregnancies for ulcerative colitis and severe asthma, respectively. Bilateral nuclear cataract was diagnosed in a male infant who had been exposed to prednisone (15–60 mg/day) throughout gestation for maternal Crohn's disease (25). In addition, "high dose" (amount not specified) cortisone had been given during the 6th month of gestation.

A brief 1995 article reviewed the available literature to assess whether the use of corticosteroids (hydrocortisone, cortisone, prednisone, prednisolone, or dexamethasone) during the first 70 days after human conception was teratogenic (26). The disorders treated were mainly systemic lupus erythematosus, asthma, and infertility. From 18 case reports, the researchers identified 26 exposed pregnancies of which 7 (27%) ended with malformed offspring (26). Four (57%) of the anomalies were cleft palate (three of these cases are described below in references 27–29); the other three anomalies were bilateral nuclear cataract, gastroschisis, and hydrocephalus. Although the number of infants with congenital defects is much higher than expected, the authors thought it likely that they represented reporting bias (26). In addition, they reviewed 17 reported series of 457 mothers exposed to the corticosteroids during the 1st trimester. In this group, 16 (3.5%) of the offspring, an incidence close to that expected, had malformations. Of these, two had cleft palate (0.2 expected based on population frequency) (26). The other defects were anencephaly ($N = 2$), clubfoot ($N = 3$), dislocated hip ($N = 1$), coarctation of the aorta ($N = 2$; 1 with a positive family history), transposition of the great vessels ($N = 1$; with a positive family history), cataract ($N = 2$; 1 with a positive family history), hypospadias ($N = 2$), and undescended testis ($N = 1$) (26). Other adverse effects, including stillbirth, neonatal death, prematurity, and low birth weight, accounted for 21% of the outcomes, but the authors were unable to separate the effect of the drug treatment from the disease process itself. They concluded that there was little teratogenic risk, if any, from the use of corticosteroids in human pregnancy (26).

The first reported case of cleft palate in an infant delivered from a woman treated with cortisone was published in 1956 (27). A 30-year-old woman with idiopathic steatorrhea was administered oral cortisone, 100 mg three times daily, beginning on the 38th day of pregnancy. Therapy was gradually tapered and then discontinued about 9 weeks later when pregnancy was diagnosed. The woman eventually delivered a term stillborn male child with a cleft palate. The cause of death was thought to be intrauterine anoxia. A second case was also reported in 1956 (28). A woman with disseminated lupus erythematosus was treated throughout her pregnancy with oral cortisone (100 mg/day) and tolazoline (400 mg/day). She delivered a premature, growth-retarded, 2 pound 11 ounce (about 1.22 kg) male infant at between 35 and 36 weeks' gestation. The infant, who died of pneumonia 14 days after birth, had a cleft palate but no other malformations were observed at autopsy. A 1962 paper mentioned an infant with a cleft palate whose mother had taken 62.5 mg/day of cortisone during the first 6 months of pregnancy (29).

A 1960 reference cited pregnancy outcome data from 31 reports totaling 260 pregnancies exposed to pharmacologic doses of cortisone or its analogues (30). The outcomes included 8 stillborn, 1 abortion, 15 premature infants, and 7 newborns with various disorders, one of which involved transient adrenocortical failure. (Disorders in the other six were not specified.) The authors did not attempt to list the type or frequency of congenital defects, stating only that most "showed no malformations." They did, however, mention four cases of cleft palate (two from their series and two from unpublished data) in infants exposed to large doses of corticosteroids during the 1st trimester (30).

Data from the MADRE (an acronym for MAlformation DRug Exposure surveillance) project was published in 1994 (31). This large surveillance study, a part of the International Clearinghouse for Birth Defects Monitoring Systems, compared congenital malformations with 1st trimester drug exposures from six different countries (Australia, France, Israel, Italy, Japan, and South America) during a 2-year period (1990–1991) (31). A total of 1448 infants with birth defects were studied. Most of the programs, however, did not report abortions. Moreover, individual drugs were not identified but were grouped into 45 pharmacologic classes. The maternal drug exposure history was determined by interview in the postpartum period. Of interest, seven infants with facial clefts (cleft lip $N = 5$, cleft lip and palate $N = 2$) were exposed to systemic corticosteroids (OR 3.16; 95% CI 1.08–7.91; $p = 0.04$). The authors noted that the association may have occurred by chance (31).

The MADRE database again was used in a 2003 case-control study (32). The time interval for data collection was now 13 years (1990–2002) and included 11,150 reported congenital malformations (including live births, stillbirths, and induced abortion) with 1st trimester drug exposure. For the present study, cases were defined as infants with cleft lip and/or palate and exposure to systemic corticosteroids during the 1st trimester. Controls were defined as infants with any other birth defect. There were nine cases of cleft lip or cleft palate (OR 2.10, 95% CI 1.03–4.26). Two of the cases were cleft palate only (OR 1.17, 95% CI 0.28–4.92) and seven were cleft lip $\pm$ palate (OR 2.59, 95% CI 1.18–5.67). Because of a decreasing trend of the number of cases per year and animal data, the results were thought to suggest a possible interaction with environmental pesticides (32).

The case-control study Spanish Collaborative Study of Congenital Malformations, surveying more than 1.2 million infants born live from 1976 to 1995, was published in 1995 (33). The study's purpose was to determine if the occurrence of nonsyndromic cleft lip (with or without cleft palate) was related to 1st trimester exposure to systemic corticosteroids. Three control groups were used: (a) paired controls; (b) controls born at the same hospital $\pm$ 45 days of the case's birth date; and (c) malformed infants without oral clefts. Statistical analysis was employed to control for four potential confounding factors: (a) maternal smoking; (b) maternal hyperthermia; (c) first-degree malformed relatives with cleft lip with or without cleft palate; and (d) 1st trimester drug exposure to anticonvulsants, benzodiazepines, metronidazole, or sex hormones. A total of 1184 case infants were identified with nonsyndromic oral clefts, five (0.42%) of whom were exposed during the 1st trimester to corticosteroids. Among the 31,752 control infants, 36 (0.11%) had been exposed to corticosteroids during the 1st trimester. None of the five case infants had been exposed to known teratogens or known risk factors for oral clefts during the 1st trimester. Based on four cases (a case of cleft soft palate was excluded), there was an increased risk of cleft lip (with or without cleft palate) following 1st trimester exposure to systemic corticosteroids (OR 6.55, 95% CI 1.44–29.76, $p = 0.015$) (32). Control of the four confounding factors made the association slightly stronger (OR 6.64, 95% CI 1.46–30.18, $p = 0.014$). The corticosteroids identified in these four cases were hydrocortisone ($N = 1$; 40 mg/day throughout pregnancy), prednisone ($N = 2$; 15–30 mg/day during 1st trimester), and triamcinolone ($N = 1$; 8 mg/day during 2nd month) (33).

Another large case-control study of the teratogenic potential of oral and topical corticosteroids involving 1,923,413 total births from 1980 to 1994 was conducted with the Hungarian Case-Control Surveillance of Congenital Abnormalities and published in 1997 (34). Among the 20,830 malformed case infants, 322 (1.55%) were exposed to systemic corticosteroids (all oral except for four that received parenteral doses) during the 1st trimester compared with 503 (1.41%) (all oral except for three that received parenteral doses) of the 35,727 normal control infants ($p = 0.19$). A corticosteroid ointment was used in 73 (0.35%) of the cases and in 118 (0.33%) of the controls ($p = 0.69$). A corticosteroid spray was used by eight case mothers (0.04%) and 11 controls (0.03%) ($p = 0.63$), but the offspring from those mothers were excluded from the detailed analysis because of the small numbers. The indications for systemic corticosteroids during the 1st trimester were primarily for asthma, hay fever, rheumatoid disorders, and subfertility, whereas the ointments were used for skin diseases. Most of the systemic exposures in both cases and controls were to dexamethasone and prednisolone. None of the patients in either group received systemic hydrocortisone and only 15 cases and 22 controls received systemic cortisone. Hydrocortisone ointment was used by 24 case mothers and 32 controls. No association between the rate of different abnormalities and the use of corticosteroids (oral and ointment) in the 2nd and 3rd months of gestation or during the 1st trimester was found based on the analysis of the case-control pairs. In the 1st gestational month, three cases with cleft lip (with or without cleft palate) (OR 5.88, 95% CI 1.70–20.32) and multiple defects (OR 4.88, 95% CI 1.41–16.88) were observed. However, exposures that occurred only during the 1st gestational month (the 1st half of this month is before conception and the other half involves the processes of pre-implantation and implantation) cannot cause defects because this time is before the critical period for induction of congenital malformations (34).

In a case-control study published in 1999, the California Birth Defects Monitoring Program evaluated the association between selected congenital anomalies and the use of corticosteroids 1 month before to 3 months after conception (periconceptional period) (35). Case infants or fetal deaths diagnosed with orofacial clefts, conotruncal defects, neural tubal defects (NTDs), and limb anomalies were identified from a total of 552,601 births that occurred from 1987 through the end of 1989. Controls, without birth defects, were selected from the same data base. Following exclusion of known genetic syndromes, mothers of case and control infants were interviewed by telephone, an average of 3.7 years (cases) or 3.8 years (controls) after delivery, to determine various exposures during the periconceptional period. The number of interviews completed were orofacial cleft case mothers ($N = 662$, 85% of eligible), conotruncal case mothers ($N = 207$, 87%), NTD case mothers ($N = 265$, 84%), limb anomaly case mothers ($N = 165$, 82%), and control mothers ($N = 734$, 78%) (34). Orofacial clefts were classified into four phenotypic groups: isolated cleft lip with or without cleft palate (ICLP, $N = 348$), isolated cleft palate (ICP, $N = 141$), multiple cleft lip with or without cleft palate (MCLP, $N = 99$), and multiple cleft palate (MCP, $N = 74$). A total of 13 mothers reported using corticosteroids during the periconceptional period for a wide variety of indications. Six case mothers of ICLP and 3 of ICP used corticosteroids (unspecified corticosteroid $N = 1$, prednisone $N = 2$, cortisone $N = 3$, triamcinolone acetonide $N = 1$, dexamethasone $N = 1$, and cortisone plus prednisone $N = 1$). One case mother of an infant with NTD used cortisone and an injectable unspecified corticosteroid, and three controls used corticosteroids (hydrocortisone $N = 1$ and prednisone $N = 2$). The odds ratio for corticosteroid use and ICLP was 4.3 (95% CI 1.1–17.2), whereas the odds ratio for ICP and corticosteroid use was 5.3 (95% CI 1.1–26.5). No increased risks were observed for the other anomaly groups. Commenting on their results, the investigators thought that recall bias was unlikely because they did not observe increased risks for other malformations, and it was unlikely that the mothers would have known of the suspected association between corticosteroids and orofacial clefts (35).

H

A 2002 study, using data from a Danish prescription database and a birth registry, examined the relationship between topical corticosteroids and low birth weight, malformations, and preterm delivery (36). The pregnancy outcomes of 363 women, who had received prescriptions for the drugs 30 days before conception and/or during pregnancy, were compared to 9263 controls, who had received no prescriptions at all. The incidence of birth defects in 170 pregnancies with 1st trimester exposure was 1.8% (3 of 170) and in controls 3.6%. The defects in the exposed group were clubfoot, flat foot, and metatarsus varus. For use anytime in pregnancy, no associations were found with low birth weight and preterm delivery. Stratification by corticosteroid strength (weak to very strong) did not change any of the results (36).

In a 2004 report, the Israeli Teratogen Information Service prospectively collected and followed 311 pregnancies exposed to systemic corticosteroids (37). The pregnancy outcomes, in terms of major congenital defects, of exposed and 790 controls did not differ significantly (4.6% vs. 2.6%). There were no cases of oral clefts in the exposed group. However, significant differences were observed in the rates of spontaneous abortion (11.5% vs. 7.0%) and preterm births (22.7% vs. 10.8%). Moreover, exposed infants had a lower median birth weight (3080 vs. 3290 g) and were born at an earlier median gestational age (39 vs. 40 weeks). The study had a power to find a 2.5-fold increase in the overall rate of major congenital defects (37).

Hydrocortisone was only partly successful in an attempt to prevent *in utero* virilization by adrenal suppression of a female fetus with congenital adrenal hyperplasia (21-hydroxylase deficiency) (38). A daily oral dose of 40 mg was started at 9.4 weeks' gestation and increased to 50 mg/day during mid-pregnancy. At delivery, low amniotic fluids of estriol suggested only partial suppression of the fetal adrenal glands. The infant had moderate virilization as indicated by clitoral hypertrophy and slight posterior fusion. In contrast, dexamethasone was used successfully in a second mother (see Dexamethasone). The failure of hydrocortisone to prevent virilization was probably a result of the lower placental transfer and adrenal suppression potency compared with dexamethasone (38).

Hydrocortisone has been used in attempts to enhance fetal lung maturation and, thus, prevent RDS (18,39–48). This therapy is relatively nontoxic to the fetus. However, hydrocortisone is no longer used for this purpose because very large doses are required to overcome placental metabolism and relatively short half-life of the corticosteroid in the fetus. Compared with a corticosteroid frequently used to prevent RDS (betamethasone

24 mg/treatment course), at least a 2000 mg/treatment course of hydrocortisone would have to be administered to achieve therapeutically equivalent results (48).

Both hydrocortisone and cortisone have been used to treat pregnancy-induced severe nausea and vomiting (i.e., hyperemesis gravidarum) (21,49,50). Although this therapy appears to be successful, its risks, especially in the 1st trimester (e.g., see reference 21), indicate that corticosteroids should not be used as primary therapy.

Hydrocortisone and other systemic and inhaled corticosteroids are frequently prescribed to control the symptoms of severe asthma during pregnancy (51–57). Most authorities believe that these agents are relatively safe in pregnancy and that their benefit to both the mother and her pregnancy clearly outweigh the potential risks to the fetus (51–56). One author, however, suggested caution in their use around the time of palate closure and in women with a family history of cleft lip (with or without cleft palate) (51). A recent study of 824 pregnant asthmatic patients matched with 678 controls (all singleton pregnancies in both groups) found no significant relationship between major congenital malformations and 1st trimester exposure to corticosteroids (oral, inhaled, or intranasal) (53). However, significant associations were found between corticosteroid use and preeclampsia (exposed 11.4% vs controls 7.1%, $p = 0.014$), preterm birth (exposed 6.4% vs. controls 3.8%, $p = 0.048$), and low birth weight (exposed 6.0% vs. controls 3.3%, $p = 0.032$) (53). Other references have reported IUGR as a complication of systemic corticosteroids (54–56). The latter reference quantified the impaired fetal growth as about a 300- to 400-g decrease in birth weight (56).

In summary, hydrocortisone and its inactive precursor, cortisone, appear to present a small risk to the human fetus. These corticosteroids produce dose-related teratogenic and toxic effects in genetically susceptible experimental animals consisting of cleft palate, cataracts, spontaneous abortion, IUGR, and polycystic kidney disease. Although the large number of data do not support these effects in the great majority of human pregnancies, adverse outcomes have been observed and may have been caused by corticosteroids. Moreover, the decrease in birth weight and a small increase in the incidence of cleft lip with or without cleft palate is supported by large epidemiologic studies. In addition, cataracts, resulting from a toxicity observed in humans administered the drug directly, have been reported in human offspring exposed *in utero*, but a causal relationship to maternal corticosteroid use is less certain. Because the benefits of corticosteroids appear to far outweigh the fetal risks, these agents should not be withheld if the mother's condition requires their use. The mother, however, should be informed of the risks so that she can actively participate in the decision on whether to use these agents during her pregnancy.

[**Risk Factor D if used in 1st trimester.*]

BREAST FEEDING SUMMARY

RECOMMENDATION: Limited Human Data - Probably Compatible

Trace amounts of endogenous hydrocortisone (cortisol) are excreted into breast milk (57,58). The amount of the corticosteroid in milk varies from 0.2 to 32 ng/mL with the highest mean concentrations (25.5 ng/mL) measured in colostrum during late pregnancy (58). The concentration of hydrocortisone in colostrum averages 7.5% of the plasma level.

No reports describing the excretion of exogenous hydrocortisone or cortisone into human milk have been located. It is unlikely, however, that these agents pose a risk to a nursing infant. Prednisone, a corticosteroid more potent than hydrocortisone, is excreted in trace amounts into milk and is classified as compatible with breast-feeding (see Prednisone). Moreover, a 1997 review stated that corticosteroids have been used safely during lactation (54).

References

1. American Hospital Formulary Service. *Drug Information 1999*. Bethesda, MD: American Society of Health-System Pharmacists, 1999:2637.
2. Fraser FC, Fainstat TD. Production of congenital defects in the offspring of pregnant mice treated with cortisone. Progress report. Pediatrics 1951;8:527–33.
3. Fraser FC, Kalter H, Walker BE, Fainstat TD. The experimental production of cleft palate with cortisone and other hormones. J Cell Comp Physiol 1954;43(Suppl 1):235–59.
4. Fraser FC, Walker BE, Trasler DG. Experimental production of congenital cleft palate: genetic and environmental factors. Pediatrics 1957;19:782–7.
5. Kalter H, Fraser FC. Production of congenital defects in the offspring of pregnant mice treated with compound F. Nature 1952;169:665.
6. Kalter H. Factors influencing the frequency of cortisone-induced cleft palate in mice. J Exp Zool 1957;134:449–67.
7. Kalter H. Fetal growth restriction induced by cortisone 40 years ago. Am J Obstet Gynecol 1998;179:835.
8. Pinsky L, DiGeorge AM. Cleft palate in the mouse: a teratogenic index of glucocorticoid potency. Science 1965;147:402–3.
9. Rogoyski A, Trzcinska-Dabrowska Z. Corticosteroid-induced cataract and palatoschisis in the mouse fetus. Am J Ophthalmol 1969;68:128–33.
10. DeCosta EJ, Abelman MA. Cortisone and pregnancy. An experimental and clinical study of the effects of cortisone on gestation. Am J Obstet Gynecol 1952;64:746–67.
11. Fainstat T. Cortisone-induced congenital cleft palate in rabbits. Endocrinology 1954;55:502–8.
12. Shepard TH. *Catalog of Teratogenic Agents*. 8th ed. Baltimore, MD: The Johns Hopkins University Press, 1995.
13. Kotas RV, Mims LC, Hart LK. Reversible inhibition of lung cell number after glucocorticoid injection into fetal rabbits to enhance surfactant appearance. Pediatrics 1974;53:358–61.
14. Van Geijn HP, Zuspan FP, Copeland SJ, Vorys AS, Zuspan MF, Scott GD. The effects of hydrocortisone on the development of the amine system in the fetal brain. Am J Obstet Gynecol 1979;135:743–50.
15. Crocker JFS, Ogborn MR. Glucocorticoid teratogenesis in the developing nephron. Teratology 1991;43:571–4.
16. Beitins IZ, Bayard F, Ances IG, Kowarski A, Migeon CJ. The metabolic clearance rate, blood production, interconversion and transplacental passage of cortisol and cortisone in pregnancy near term. Pediatr Res 1973;7:509–19.
17. Pearson Murphy BE, Clark SJ, Donald IR, Pinsky M, Vedady D. Conversion of maternal cortisol to cortisone during placental transfer to the human fetus. Am J Obstet Gynecol 1974;118:538–41.
18. Levitz M, Jansen V, Dancis J. The transfer and metabolism of corticosteroids in the perfused human placenta. Am J Obstet Gynecol 1978;132:363–6.
19. Ballard PL, Liggins GC. Glucocorticoid activity in cord serum: comparison of hydrocortisone and betamethasone regimens. J Pediatr 1982;101:468–70.
20. Heinonen OP, Slone D, Shapiro S. *Birth Defects and Drugs in Pregnancy*. Littleton, MA: Publishing Sciences Group, 1977.
21. Guilbeau JA Jr. Effects of cortisone on fetus. Am J Obstet Gynecol 1953;64:227.
22. Reisman LE, Matheny A. Corticosteroids in pregnancy. Lancet 1968;1:592–3.
23. Khudr G, Olding L. Cyclopia. Am J Dis Child 1973;125;120–2.
24. Malpas P. Foetal malformation and cortisone therapy. Br Med J 1965;1:795.
25. Kraus AM. Congenital cataract and maternal steroid ingestion. J Pediatr Ophthalmol 1975;12:107–8.
26. Fraser FC, Sajoo A. Teratogenic potential of corticosteroids in humans. Teratology 1995;51:45–6.
27. Harris JWS, Ross IP. Cortisone therapy in early pregnancy: relation to cleft palate. Lancet 1956;1:1045–7.
28. Doig RK, Coltman OM. Cleft palate following cortisone therapy in early pregnancy. Lancet 1956;2:730.
29. Popert AJ. Pregnancy and adrenocortical hormones. Some aspects of the interaction in rheumatic diseases. Br Med J 1962;1:967–72.
30. Bongiovanni AM, McPadden AJ. Steroids during pregnancy and possible fetal consequences. Fertil Steril 1960;11:181–6.
31. Robert E, Vollset SE, Botto L, Lancaster PAL, Merlob P, Mastroiacovo P, Cocchi G, Ashizawa M, Sakamoto S, Orioli I. Malformation surveillance and maternal drug exposure: the MADRE project. Int J Risk Safety Med 1994;6:75–118.
32. Pradat P, Robert-Gnansia E, Di Tanna GL, Rosano A, Lisi A, Mastroiacovo, and all contributors to the MADRE database. First trimester exposure to corticosteroids and oral clefts. Birth Defects Res Part A Clin Mol Teratol 2003;67:968–70.
33. Rodriguez-Pinilla E, Martinez-Frias ML. Corticosteroids during pregnancy and oral clefts: a case-control study. Teratology 1998;58:2–5.
34. Czeizel AE, Rockenbauer M. Population-based case-control study of teratogenic potential of corticosteroids. Teratology 1997;56:335–40.
35. Carmichael SL, Shaw GM. Maternal corticosteroid use and risk of selected congenital anomalies. Am J Med Genet 1999;86:242–4.
36. Mygind H, Thulstrup AM, Pedersen L, Larsen H. Risk of intrauterine growth retardation, malformations and other birth outcomes in children after topical use of corticosteroids in pregnancy. Acta Obstet Gynecol Scand 2002;81:234–9.
37. Gur C, Diav-Citrin O, Shechtman S, Arnon J, Ornoy A. Pregnancy outcome after first trimester exposure

H

to corticosteroids: a prospective controlled study. Reprod Toxicol 2004;18:93–101.
38. David M, Forest MG. Prenatal treatment of congenital adrenal hyperplasia resulting from 21-hydroxylase deficiency. J Pediatr 1984;105:799–803.
39. Taeusch HW Jr. Glucocorticoid prophylaxis for respiratory distress syndrome: a review of potential toxicity. J Pediatr 1975;87:617–23.
40. Dluholucky S, Babic J, Taufer I. Reduction of incidence and mortality of respiratory distress syndrome by administration of hydrocortisone to mother. Arch Dis Child 1976;51:420–3.
41. Zuspan FP, Cordero L, Semchyshyn S. Effects of hydrocortisone on lecithin-sphingomyelin ratio. Am J Obstet Gynecol 1977;128:571–4.
42. Morrison JC, Whybrew WD, Bucovaz ET, Schneider JM. Injection of corticosteroids into mother to prevent neonatal respiratory distress syndrome. Am J Obstet Gynecol 1978;131:358–66.
43. Beck JC, Johnson JWC. Maternal administration of glucocorticoids. Clin Obstet Gynecol 1980;23:93–113.
44. Semchyshyn S, Zuspan FP, Cordero L. Cardiovascular response and complications of glucocorticoid therapy in hypertensive pregnancies. Am J Obstet Gynecol 1983;145:530–3.
45. Schmidt PL, Sims ME, Strassner HT, Paul RH, Mueller E, McCart D. Effect of antepartum glucocorticoid administration upon neonatal respiratory distress syndrome and perinatal infection. Am J Obstet Gynecol 1984;148:178–86.
46. Iams JD, Barrows H. Management of preterm prematurely ruptured membranes: a retrospective comparison of observation versus use of steroids and timed delivery. Am J Obstet Gynecol 1984;150:977–81.
47. Iams JD, Talbert ML, Barrows H, Sachs L. Management of preterm prematurely ruptured membranes: a prospective randomized comparison of observation versus use of steroids and timed delivery. Am J Obstet Gynecol 1985;151:32–8.
48. Ward RM. Pharmacologic enhancement of fetal lung maturation. Clin Perinatol 1994;21:523–42.
49. Wells CN. Treatment of hyperemesis gravidarum with cortisone. I. Fetal results. Am J Obstet Gynecol 1953;66:598–601.
50. Taylor R. Successful management of hyperemesis gravidarum using steroid therapy. QJM 1996;89:103–7.
51. Greenberg F. The potential teratogenicity of allergy and asthma treatment in pregnancy. Immunol Aller Prac 1985;7:15–20.
52. D'Alonzo GE. The pregnant asthmatic patient. Semin Perinatol 1990;14:119–29.
53. Schatz M, Zeiger RS, Harden K, Hoffman CC, Chilingar L, Petitti D. The safety of asthma and allergy medications during pregnancy. J Allergy Clin Immunol 1997;100:301–6.
54. Venkataraman MT, Shanies HM. Pregnancy and asthma. J Asthma 1997;34:265–71.
55. Schatz M, Zeiger RS. Asthma and allergy in pregnancy. Clin Perinatol 1997;24:407–32.
56. Report of the Working Group on Asthma and Pregnancy. Management of asthma during pregnancy. National Institutes of Health. NIH Publication No. 93–3279. 1993:18–9.
57. Rosner W, Beers PC, Awan T, Khan MS. Identification of corticosteroid-binding globulin in human milk: measurement with a filter disk assay. J Clin Endocrinol Metab 1976;42:1064–73.
58. Kulski JK, Hartmann PE. Changes in the concentration of cortisol in milk during different stages of human lactation. Aust J Exp Biol Med Sci 1981;59:769–78.

Name:	**HYDROFLUMETHIAZIDE**	Risk Factor:	C_M
Class:	**Diuretic**		

See Chlorothiazide.

Name:	**HYDROMORPHONE**	Risk Factor:	**B***
Class:	**Narcotic Agonist Analgesic**		

FETAL RISK SUMMARY

RECOMMENDATION: Human Data Suggest Risk in 3rd Trimester

No reports linking the use of hydromorphone with congenital defects have been located. Withdrawal could occur in infants exposed *in utero* to prolonged maternal ingestion of hydromorphone. Use of the drug in pregnancy is primarily confined to labor. Respiratory depression in the neonate similar to that produced by meperidine or morphine should be expected (1).

[**Risk Factor D if used for prolonged periods or in high doses at term.*]

BREAST FEEDING SUMMARY

RECOMMENDATION: Limited Human Data - Probably Compatible

Hydromorphone is excreted into breast milk (2). Eight healthy, lactating women were given a single dose of 2 mg hydromorphone by nasal spray and serial blood and milk samples were collected over 24 hours. Infants were not allowed to nurse during the study. Little of the drug was found in milk fat (skim milk:whole milk ratio 0.98). The milk:plasma ratio was about 2.6 and the estimated infant dose (based on 150 mL/kg/day) was 0.67% of the mother's weight adjusted dose (2). The effect of these amounts, if any, on a nursing infant are unknown but appear to be clinically insignificant. However, further study, especially with multiple dosing, is warranted.

References

1. Bonica J. *Principles and Practice of Obstetric Analgesia and Anesthesia*. Philadelphia, PA: FA Davis, 1967:251.
2. Edwards JE, Rudy AC, Wermeling DP, Desai N, McNamara PJ. Hydromorphone transfer into breast milk after intranasal administration. Pharmacotherapy 2003;23:153–8.

Name:	**HYDROXYCHLOROQUINE**	Risk Factor:	**C**
Class:	**Antimalarial/Immunologic Agent (Antirheumatic)**		

FETAL RISK SUMMARY

RECOMMENDATION: Limited Human Data - Probably Compatible

Hydroxychloroquine is used for the treatment of malaria, discoid and systemic lupus erythematosus (SLE), and rheumatoid arthritis. A 1988 review described several references relating to animal studies with the closely related agent, chloroquine (1). In pregnant mice, rats, rabbits, and monkeys, chloroquine crosses the placenta to the fetus (1). In fetal mice and monkeys, the drug accumulates for long intervals, up to 5 months in mice, in the melanin structures of the eyes and inner ears (1,2). Teratogenicity studies with chloroquine using monkeys have not been published. However, in rats, only high doses were teratogenic, producing skeletal and ocular defects (1). In pregnant mice, chloroquine alone was not teratogenic, but in combination with radiation, a significant increase in cleft palates and tail anomalies was observed (1). No similar data are available for hydroxychloroquine.

Published data relating to the use of hydroxychloroquine during human pregnancy are scarce but do not indicate that the drug poses a significant risk to the fetus. The Collaborative Perinatal Project monitored 50,282 mother-child pairs, 2 of whom had 1st trimester exposure to hydroxychloroquine (3). Neither child had a congenital malformation. A 1974 reference reported no abnormalities in a fetus after a therapeutic abortion at 14 weeks' gestation (4). The fetus had been exposed to the antimalarial agent, 200 mg twice daily, since the time of conception. Examination of the temporal bones, the embryonal precartilage, the anlages of the auditory ossicles, and the membranous labyrinth demonstrated a normal 14-week stage of development, indicating an apparent lack of drug-induced ototoxicity in this fetus (4). A short 1983 communication described the use of 200 mg/day of hydroxychloroquine during the first 16 weeks of gestation for the treatment of maternal discoid lupus erythematosus (5). A male infant was eventually delivered who was alive and well at 2 years of age.

The use of hydroxychloroquine during 27 pregnancies in 23 women with mild to moderate SLE was described in a 1995 abstract (6). In 17 of the pregnancies, the drug was used at a dose of 200–400 mg daily throughout gestation. The outcomes of these cases included 2 miscarriages, 2 perinatal deaths, 1 infant with congenital heart block (in a Ro-positive mother), and 12 normal newborns. In six other pregnancies, hydroxychloroquine was started after conception, three during the 1st trimester. In the remaining four cases, therapy was stopped after diagnosis of pregnancy, resulting in a worsening of the disease and higher doses of prednisolone, and pregnancy termination in one because of severe renal lupus. No fetal or newborn adverse effects related to hydroxychloroquine were observed. A follow-up of 20 newborns for at least 3 years found that all were healthy. The authors concluded that hydroxychloroquine was safe in pregnancy, and because of the risk of lupus flare, discontinuing therapy during pregnancy represented a greater danger to the fetus (6).

Other investigators have reached similar conclusions as to the safety of hydroxychloroquine in the treatment of SLE during pregnancy (7,8). These authors described nine pregnancies (plus seven from an earlier paper) in which hydroxychloroquine (200 mg/day) was used throughout gestation without producing congenital malformations. In the present series of nine pregnancies, five newborns were delivered preterm and four at term. Long-term follow-up of the children exposed *in utero* has been normal. Because of the very long elimination half-life of the drug from maternal tissues (weeks to months), the authors concluded that discontinuing the drug when pregnancy was known would not eliminate fetal exposure, but could jeopardize the pregnancy from a lupus flare (7,8).

The use of hydroxychloroquine as an antimalarial, instead of chloroquine, has been recommended because of the belief that hydroxychloroquine is less toxic (1). However, little data are available to substantiate this practice, either in terms of congenital malformations or in optic or otic toxicity. From published reports of fetal exposure to either chloroquine or hydroxychloroquine, one source cited an incidence of 7 infants with congenital anomalies from 188 live births, a rate of 4.5% (1). This value is within the expected 3%–6% incidence of congenital malformations in a nonexposed population.

In summary, hydroxychloroquine does not seem to pose a significant risk to the fetus, especially with lower doses. No reports of retinal or ototoxicity after *in utero* exposure have been located. The Centers for Disease Control and Prevention (CDC) stated that hydroxychloroquine may be used during pregnancy for antimalarial prophylaxis because the agent has not been shown to be harmful to the fetus in prophylactic doses (9,10). The adult antimalarial prophylactic dose is 400 mg/week (2). The use of higher doses for prolonged periods, such as those used for SLE, acute attacks of malaria, and rheumatoid arthritis, probably represents an increased fetal risk, but the magnitude of this increase is unknown. At least one source has recommended that the use of hydroxychloroquine for rheumatoid arthritis or SLE be avoided during pregnancy (1), but recent reports (6–8) do not support this conclusion. Moreover, stopping therapy when a pregnancy became known would not, as discussed above, stop exposure of the embryo and fetus to the drug, but could increase the risk because of a lupus flare. If hydroxychloroquine is used in pregnancy for the treatment of rheumatoid arthritis, healthcare professionals are encouraged to call the toll free number (877-311-8972) for information about patient enrollment in the OTIS Rheumatoid Arthritis study.

BREAST FEEDING SUMMARY

RECOMMENDATION: Limited Human Data - Probably Compatible

Two reports have described the excretion of small amounts of hydroxychloroquine into breast milk. A 27-year-old woman was treated with hydroxychloroquine, 400 mg (310 mg base) each night, for an exacerbation of lupus erythematosus (11). She had been breast-feeding her infant for 9 months. No mention of the infant's condition or of the presence of toxic effects was made by the authors of this report. Milk samples were collected 2.0, 9.5, and 14.0 hours after one dose and 17.7 hours after a second dose. Milk concentrations of hydroxychloroquine base at the four times were 1.46, 1.09, 1.09, and 0.85 μg/mL, respectively. A maternal blood sample was collected 15.5 hours after the first dose. Hydroxychloroquine base concentrations in whole blood and plasma were 1.76 and 0.20 μg/mL, respectively. The authors estimated that the infant was consuming, based on 1000 mL of milk, a daily dose of 1.1 mg hydroxychloroquine base, or approximately 0.35% of the mother's daily dose (11).

H

Much lower milk concentrations of drug were obtained from a 28-year-old woman who was being treated with hydroxychloroquine, 200 mg twice daily, for rheumatoid arthritis (12). Treatment had been stopped for 6 months during pregnancy and then restarted 2 months later because of arthritis relapse. A total of 3.2 μg of the drug was recovered from her milk over a 48-hour interval, representing 0.0005% of the mother's dose. The highest milk concentration of the agent, 10.6 ng/mL, was found in the 39–48 hour sample. It was not stated whether the infant was allowed to breast-feed.

Because of the slow elimination rate and the potential for accumulation of a toxic amount in the infant, breast-feeding during daily therapy with hydroxychloroquine should be undertaken cautiously (11–13). The administration of once-weekly doses, such as those used for malaria prophylaxis, would markedly reduce the amount of drug available to the nursing infant and, consequently, produce a much lower risk of accumulation and toxicity. Although breast-feeding during maternal malarial prophylaxis is not thought to be harmful, the amount of hydroxychloroquine in milk is insufficient to provide protection against malaria in the infant (10). The American Academy of Pediatrics classifies the drug as compatible with breast-feeding (14).

References

1. Roubenoff R, Hoyt J, Petri M, Hochberg MC, Hellmann DB. Effects of antiinflammatory and immunosuppressive drugs on pregnancy and fertility. Semin Arthritis Rheum 1988;18:88–110.
2. Product information. Plaquenil. Sanofi Winthrop Pharmaceuticals, 1997.
3. Heinonen OP, Slone D, Shapiro S. *Birth Defects and Drugs in Pregnancy*. Littleton, MA: Publishing Sciences Group, 1977:299.
4. Ross JB, Garatsos S. Absence of chloroquine-induced ototoxicity in a fetus. Arch Dermatol 1974;109:573.
5. Suhonen R. Hydroxychloroquine administration in pregnancy. Arch Dermatol 1983;119:185–6.
6. Buchanan NMM, Toubi E, Khamashta MA, Lima F, Kerslake S, Hughes GRV. The safety of hydroxychloroquine in lupus pregnancy: experience in 27 pregnancies (abstract). Br J Rheumatol 1995;34(Suppl 1):14.
7. Parke AL, Rothfield NF. Antimalarial drugs in pregnancy—the North American experience. Lupus 1996;5(Suppl 1):567–9.
8. Parke A, West B. Hydroxychloroquine in pregnant patients with systemic lupus erythematosus. J Rheumatol 1996;23:1715–8.
9. CDC. Adverse reactions and contraindications to antimalarials. MMWR 1988;37:282–3.
10. CDC. Recommendations for the prevention of malaria among travelers. MMWR 1990;39:1–10.
11. Nation RL, Hackett LP, Dusci LJ, Ilett KF. Excretion of hydroxychloroquine in human milk. Br J Clin Pharmacol 1984;17:368–9.
12. Ostensen M, Brown ND, Chiang PK, Aarbakke J. Hydroxychloroquine in human breast milk. Eur J Clin Pharmacol 1985;28:357.
13. Anderson PO. Drug use during breast-feeding. Clin Pharm 1991;10:594–624.
14. Committee on Drugs, American Academy of Pediatrics. The transfer of drugs and other chemicals into human milk. Pediatrics 2001;108:776–89.

Name:	**HYDROXYPROGESTERONE**	Risk Factor:	**D**
Class:	**Progestogenic Hormone**		

FETAL RISK SUMMARY

RECOMMENDATION: Contraindicated - 1st Trimester

The FDA mandated deletion of pregnancy-related indications from all progestins because of a possible association with congenital anomalies. Ambiguous genitalia of both male and female fetuses have been reported with hydroxyprogesterone (see also Norethindrone, Norethynodrel) (1–4).

The Collaborative Perinatal Project monitored 866 mother-child pairs with 1st trimester exposure to progestational agents (including 162 with exposure to hydroxyprogesterone) (5, pp. 389, 391). An increase in the expected frequency of cardiovascular defects and hypospadias was observed for both estrogens and progestogens (5, p. 394; 6). Re-evaluation of these data in terms of timing of exposure, vaginal bleeding in early pregnancy, and previous maternal obstetric history, however, failed to support an association between female sex hormones and cardiac malformations (7).

Dillon (8,9) reported six infants with malformations exposed to hydroxyprogesterone during various stages of gestation. The congenital defects included spina bifida, anencephalus, hydrocephalus, tetralogy of Fallot, common truncus arteriosus, cataract, and ventricular septal defect. Complete absence of both thumbs and dislocated head of the right radius in a child have been associated with hydroxyprogesterone (9). Use of diazepam in early pregnancy and the lack of similar reports make an association doubtful.

A 1985 study described 2,754 offspring born to mothers who had vaginal bleeding during the 1st trimester (10). Of the total group, 1,608 of the newborns were delivered from mothers treated during the 1st trimester with either oral medroxyprogesterone (20–30 mg/day), 17-hydroxyprogesterone (500 mg/week by injection), or a combination of the two. Medroxyprogesterone was used exclusively in 1274 (79.2%) of the study group. The control group consisted of 1146 infants delivered from mothers who bled during the 1st trimester but who were not treated. There were no differences between the study and control groups in the overall rate of malformations (120 vs. 123.9/1000, respectively) or in the rate of major malformations (63.4 vs. 71.5/1000, respectively). Another 1985 study compared 988 infants, exposed *in utero* to various progesterones, to a matched cohort of 1976 unexposed controls (11). No association between the use of progestins, primarily progesterone and 17-hydroxyprogesterone, and fetal malformations was discovered.

Developmental changes in the psychosexual performance of boys has been attributed to *in utero* exposure to hydroxyprogesterone (12). The mothers received an estrogen-progestogen regimen for their diabetes. Hormone-exposed males demonstrated a trend to have less heterosexual experience and fewer masculine interests than controls.

Although additional studies are required, the administration of hydroxyprogesterone during pregnancy might prevent premature labor (13–21), but it was not effective in twin pregnancies (22). No increase in the incidence of fetal adverse effects was observed. The progesterone also has been used in early gestation to prevent spontaneous abortion, but the results have been mixed (23,24).

Because several issues still exist, including the long-term safety, the American College of Obstetricians and Gynecologists (ACOG) recommends that the use of hydroxyprogesterone should be restricted to only women with a documented history of spontaneous birth before 37 weeks' gestation (25).

BREAST FEEDING SUMMARY

RECOMMENDATION: No Human Data - Probably Compatible

No data are available.

References

1. Dayan E, Rosa FW. Fetal ambiguous genitalia associated with sex hormone use early in pregnancy. ADR Highlights 1981:1–14. Food and Drug Administration, Division of Drug Experience.
2. Wilkins L. Masculinization of female fetus due to use of orally given progestins. JAMA 1960;172;1028–32.
3. Wilkins L, Jones HW, Holman GH, Stempfel RS Jr. Masculinization of the female fetus associated with administration of oral and intramuscular progestins during gestation: non-adrenal female pseudohermaphrodism. J Clin Endocrinol Metab 1958;68: 559–85.
4. Evans ANW, Brooke OG, West RJ. The ingestion by pregnancy women of substances toxic to the fetus. Practitioner 1980;224:315–9.
5. Heinonen OP, Slone D, Shapiro S. *Birth Defects and Drugs in Pregnancy*. Littleton, MA: Publishing Sciences Group, 1977.
6. Heinonen OP, Slone D, Monson RR, Hook EB, Shapiro S. Cardiovascular birth defects and antenatal exposure to female sex hormones. N Engl J Med 1977;296: 67–70.
7. Wiseman RA, Dodds-Smith IC. Cardiovascular birth defects and antenatal exposure to female sex hormones: a reevaluation of some base data. Teratology 1984;30:359–70.
8. Dillon S. Congenital malformations and hormones in pregnancy. Br Med J 1976;2:1446.
9. Dillon S. Progestogen therapy in early pregnancy and associated congenital defects. Practitioner 1970; 205:80–4.
10. Katz Z, Lancet M, Skornik J, Chemke J, Mogilner BM, Klinberg M. Teratogenicity of progestogens given during the first trimester of pregnancy. Obstet Gynecol 1985;65:775–80.
11. Resseguie LJ, Hick JF, Bruen JA, Noller KL, O'Fallon WM, Kurland LT. Congenital malformations among offspring exposed in utero to progestins, Olmsted County, Minnesota, 1936–1974. Fertil Steril 1985;43:514–9.
12. Yalom ID, Green R, Fisk N. Prenatal exposure to female hormones. Effect on psychosexual development in boys. Arch Gen Psychiatry 1973;28:554–61.
13. Johnson JWC, Austin KL, Jones GS, Davis GH, King TM. Efficacy of 17-hydroxyprogesterone caproate in the prevention of premature labor. N Engl J Med 1975;293:675–80.
14. Johnson JWC, Lee PA, Zachary AS, Calhoun S, Migeon CJ. High-risk prematurity-progestin treatment and steroid studies. Obstet Gynecol 1979;54:412–8.
15. Kauppila A, Hartikainen-Sorri AL, Janne O, Tuimala R, Jarvinen PA. Suppression of threatened premature labor by administration of cortisol and 17α-hydroxyprogesterone caproate: a comparison with ritodrine. Am J Obstet Gynecol 1980;138: 404–8.
16. Varma TR, Morsman J. Evaluation of the use of Proluton-depot (hydroxyprogesterone hexanoate) in early pregnancy. Int J Gynecol Obstet 1982;20: 13–7.
17. Hauth JC, Gilstrap LC III, Brekken AL, Hauth JM. The effect of 17α-hydroxyprogesterone caproate on pregnancy outcome in an active-duty military population. Am J Obstet Gynecol 1983;146:187–90.
18. Yemini M, Borenstein R, Dreazen E, Apelman Z, Mogilner BM, Kessler I, Lancet M. Prevention of premature labor by 17α-hydroxyprogesterone caproate. Am J Obstet Gynecol 1985;151:574–7.
19. Keirse MJNC. Progesterone administration in pregnancy may prevent preterm delivery. Br J Obstet Gynecol 1990;97:149–54.
20. Meis PJ, Klebanoff M, Thom E, Dombrowski MP, Sibai B, Moawad AH, Spong CY, Hauth JC, Miodovnik M, Varner MW, Leveno KJ, Caritis SN, Iams JD, Wapner RJ, Conway D, O'Sullivan MJ, Carpenter M, Mercer B, Ramin SM, Thorp JM, Peaceman AM, for the National Institute of Child Health and Human Development Maternal-Fetal Medicine Units Network. Prevention of recurrent preterm delivery by 17 alpha-hydroxyprogesterone caproate. N Engl J Med 2003;348:2379–85.
21. Greene MF. Progesterone and preterm delivery—déjà vu all over again. N Engl J Med 2003;348:2453–5.
22. Hartikainen-Sorri AL, Kauppila A, Tuimala R. Inefficacy of 17-hydroxyprogesterone caproate in the prevention of prematurity in twin pregnancy. Obstet Gynecol 1980;56:692–5.
23. Reijnders FJL, Thomas GMG, Doesburg WH, Rolland R, Eskes TKAB. Endocrine effects of 17 alpha-hydroxyprogesterone caproate during early pregnancy: a double-blind clinical trial. Br J Obstet Gynecol 1988;95:462–8.
24. Prietl G, Diedrich K, van der Ven HH, Luckhaus J, Krebs D. The effect of 17α-hydroxyprogesterone caproate/oestradiol valerate on the development and outcome of early pregnancies following in vitro fertilization and embryo transfer: a prospective and randomized controlled trial. Hum Reprod 1992;7:1–5.
25. Committee on Obstetric Practice, American College of Obstetricians and Gynecologists. Use of progesterone to reduce preterm birth. *ACOG Committee Opinion*. Number 291, November 2003.

Name:	**HYDROXYUREA**	Risk Factor:	**D**
Class:	**Antineoplastic**		

FETAL RISK SUMMARY

RECOMMENDATION: Limited Human Data - Animal Data Suggest Risk

Hydroxyurea, an antineoplastic agent, is teratogenic in animals. Shepard reviewed nine studies describing the effects of this agent on the embryos and fetuses of a variety of animal species (1). Anomalies observed included defects of the central nervous system, palate, and skeleton, depressed DNA synthesis, extensive cell death in limb buds and central nervous system, impaired postnatal learning, and decreased body and brain growth (rats), beak defects (chick embryos), and neural tube and cardiac defects (hamsters) (1). A 1999 report, evaluating the combined prenatal toxicity of hydroxyurea and 6-mercaptopurine riboside in mice, determined that the NOAEL (no-observed-adverse-effect level) of a single, intraperitoneal dose of hydroxyurea administered on day 11 of gestation was 250 mg/kg (2). An increase in gross structural abnormalities was observed at the 300- and 350-mg/kg dose levels.

Published human pregnancy experience with hydroxyurea is limited to 19 cases, 5 of which were electively terminated and 1 ended in a stillbirth (3–16). Two women, both with acute myelocytic leukemia, were treated with five-drug chemotherapy regimens at 17 and 27 weeks' gestation, respectively (3). In both cases, hydroxyurea (8 mg) was given as an initial, single IV dose. One woman underwent an elective abortion of a grossly normal fetus 4 weeks after the start of chemotherapy. The second patient delivered a premature infant at 31 weeks with no evidence of birth defects, again 4 weeks after the start of therapy. Follow-up at 13.5 months revealed normal growth and development.

A 1991 report described the use of oral hydroxyurea, 0.5–1.0 g/day, throughout gestation in a woman with chronic myelocytic leukemia (CML) (4). A spontaneous vaginal delivery at 36 weeks' gestation resulted in the birth of a normal, healthy 2670-g male infant with normal blood counts. The infant's growth and development have been normal through 26 months of age. A subsequent brief report described a similar patient treated with 1–3 g/day orally before and throughout gestation (5). Hydroxyurea therapy was stopped (to prevent a potential cytopenia in the fetus) 1 week before a planned cesarean section at 38 weeks' gestation. A healthy 3100-g male infant was delivered, without evidence of hematologic abnormalities, whose growth and development remain normal at 32 months of age. A 1992 report listed a pregnant woman with CML who was treated in the 1st trimester with hydroxyurea and three other agents (6). She elected to terminate her pregnancy.

Four other studies have reported on the use of hydroxyurea for CML during pregnancy (7–10). A 1992 publication described two women who were treated before and throughout gestation with oral doses of 1.5 g/day (7). Eclampsia developed at 26 weeks' gestation in one woman resulting in the delivery of a stillborn male fetus without gross abnormalities who had a normal phenotype. The second patient had a vaginal delivery at 40 weeks of a healthy 3.2-kg male infant with normal phenotype. No follow-up evaluation of the infant was mentioned. The clinical course of a pregnant woman with CML was discussed in a 1993 report (8). She required 1.5–3 g/day during pregnancy for her disease. At 37 weeks' gestation, she delivered a healthy baby girl who had normal blood counts and no evidence of congenital defects. A second 1993 report described a woman with CML treated unsuccessfully with interferon alfa before pregnancy and then with hydroxyurea (9).

At the patient's request, all therapy was stopped before conception. Hydroxyurea therapy (dose not specified) was reinstituted during the 2nd trimester and continued until 1 month before the delivery of a normal, term, 3.4-kg, male infant. The infant was developing normally at approximately 11 months of age. In another case, a woman received hydroxyurea, 1.5–2.5 g/day, throughout gestation and delivered a term, 3.44-kg female infant who was normal at age 6 weeks (10).

A 1994 report described a woman with primary thrombocythemia who had lost two previous pregnancies from stillbirths (11). She was treated with hydroxyurea (1–2 g/day) prior to and during the first 6 weeks of her third pregnancy. She delivered a healthy male infant at 35 weeks' gestation. Two other publications have also reported the use of hydroxyurea in pregnant women with essential thrombocythemia (12,13). In one case, the dose and exposure time was not specified but the pregnancy was elective terminated because of maternal complications (12). In the other case, 0.5–1.0 g/day was used from 18 to 28 weeks' gestation and a healthy male infant was delivered at 37 weeks' gestation (13).

Three reports have described the use of hydroxyurea for the management of sickle cell disease in pregnant women (14–16). In a study published in 1995, three women conceived while receiving the drug (14). All stopped the therapy when pregnancy was diagnosed. One delivered a normal, full-term infant, and two had elective pregnancy terminations. A 1999 report described one woman with sickle cell disease who had received hydroxyurea (1 g/day) and folic acid (5 mg/day) for 3 years before pregnancy (15). She discontinued hydroxyurea when pregnancy was confirmed at 9 weeks' gestation and delivered a normal male baby at 39 weeks' with Apgar scores of 8 and 10 at 1 and 5 minutes, respectively. The 3.24-kg newborn, length 55 cm and head circumference 31 cm, was developing normally at 15 months. Another 1999 publication reported two pregnancies that were exposed to hydroxyurea very early in gestation (16). Both women were being treated for sickle cell disease with the drug (1g/day and 0.5 g/day), in addition to folic acid and other drugs, and both discontinued hydroxyurea when pregnancy was confirmed at approximately 5 and 4 weeks, respectively. One woman delivered a 2750-g, male infant at 37 weeks' gestation with Apgar scores of 8 and 9 at 1 and 5 minutes, respectively. The infant was developing normally at age 17 months. The second woman delivered a premature, 1365-g, male baby at 32.5 weeks' gestation with Apgar scores of 8 and 9 at 1 and 5 minutes, respectively. Because of his prematurity, the infant required treatment for respiratory distress syndrome, hyperbilirubinemia, patent ductus arteriosus, and sepsis during the first 6 weeks, but was developing normally at age 21 months (16).

The outcomes of pregnancies exposed to chemotherapy gestational trophoblastic disease before conception were evaluated two reports, one in 1984 and the other in 1998 (17,18). In 436 long-term survivors treated with chemotherapy between 1958 and 1978, 69 (16%) received hydroxyurea as part of their treatment regimens (17). Of the 69 women, 14 (20%) had at least one live birth (numbers in parentheses refer to mean/maximum hydroxyurea dose in grams) (3.6/8.0), 3 (4%) had no live births (6.3/16.0), 3 (4%) failed to conceive (3.0/6.0), and 49 (71%) did not try to conceive (9.4/47.0). Additional details, including congenital anomalies observed, are described in the monograph for methotrexate (see Methotrexate) (17). In the 1998 report, 336 women, who had tried to conceive, had previously received various combinations of chemotherapeutic agents, some of which included hydroxyurea (18). In comparison to a group receiving single-agent therapy ($N = 392$; methotrexate), no differences in pregnancy outcome were observed in the number of live births, unsuccessful pregnancies, and an inability to become pregnant. Only 18 major or minor congenital abnormalities (affecting 1.7% of the births) were reported.

However, the stillbirth rate in all women treated for gestational trophoblastic disease was significantly higher than that of the general population (odds ratio 2.87; 95% confidence interval 2.44–3.03; $p < 0.001$) (18). One woman treated for acute lymphoid leukemia with a combination of nine antineoplastic agents, one of which was hydroxyurea, conceived two pregnancies, 2 and 4 years after chemotherapy was stopped (19). Apparently normal-term infants, a 3850-g male and a 3550-g female, resulted and both were doing well at 7 and 4.5 years, respectively.

Occupational exposure of the mother to antineoplastic agents during pregnancy may present a risk to the fetus. A position statement from the National Study Commission on Cytotoxic Exposure and a research article involving some antineoplastic agents are presented in the monograph for cyclophosphamide (see Cyclophosphamide).

In summary, although hydroxyurea is teratogenic in animals, no fetal anomalies have been observed in 13 human pregnancies that resulted in live infants in which the drug was used to treat maternal disease. In some of these cases, however, hydroxyurea was discontinued very early in gestation. Therefore, the data are too limited to draw conclusions about the safety of this agent during pregnancy or about the long-term growth and development of children exposed *in utero*.

BREAST FEEDING SUMMARY

RECOMMENDATION: Contraindicated

Hydroxyurea is excreted into human milk. A 29-year-old breast-feeding woman with recently diagnosed chronic myelogenous leukemia was treated with hydroxyurea, 500 mg orally 3 times daily (20). Breast-feeding was halted before initiation of the chemotherapy. Milk samples were collected 2 hours after the last dose for 7 days. Because of technical difficulties with the analysis, milk concentrations of hydroxyurea could only be determined on days 1, 3, and 4. The mean level of hydroxyurea was 6.1 μg/mL (range 3.8–8.4 μg/mL). Serum concentrations were not measured. Although these concentrations are low, the potential for adverse effects in the infant suggests that nursing should be considered contraindicated during hydroxyurea therapy.

References

1. Shepard TH. *Catalog of Teratogenic Agents*. 7th ed. Baltimore, MD: Johns Hopkins University Press, 1992:206–7.
2. Platzek T, Schwabe R. Combined prenatal toxicity of 6-mercaptopurine riboside and hydroxyurea in mice. Teratog Carcinog Mutagen 1999;19:223–32.
3. Doney KC, Kraemer KG, Shepard TH. Combination chemotherapy for acute myelocytic leukemia during pregnancy: three case reports. Cancer Treat Rep 1979;63:369–71.
4. Patel M, Dukes IAF, Hull JC. Use of hydroxyurea in chronic myeloid leukemia during pregnancy: a case report. Am J Obstet Gynecol 1991;165:565–6.
5. Tertian G, Tchernia G, Papiernik E, Elefant E. Hydroxyurea and pregnancy. Am J Obstet Gynecol 1992;166:1868.
6. Zemlickis D, Lishner M, Degendorfer P, Panzarella T, Sutcliffe SB, Koren G. Fetal outcome after in utero exposure to cancer chemotherapy. Arch Intern Med 1992;152:573–6.
7. Delmer A, Rio B, Bauduer F, Ajchenbaum F, Marie J-P, Zittoun R. Pregnancy during myelosuppressive treatment for chronic myelogenous leukaemia. Br J Haematol 1992;82:783–4.
8. Jackson N, Shukri A, Ali K. Hydroxyurea treatment for chronic myeloid leukaemia during pregnancy. Br J Haematol 1993;85:203–4.
9. Fitzgerald JM, McCann SR. The combination of hydroxyurea and leucapheresis in the treatment of chronic myeloid leukaemia in pregnancy. Clin Lab Haematol 1993;15:63–5.
10. Szanto F, Kovacs L. Successful delivery following continuous cytostatic therapy of a leukemic pregnant woman. Ovr Hetil 1994;134:527–9. (Hungarian). As cited by Diav-Citrin O, Hunnisett L, Sher GD, Koren G. Hydroxyurea use during pregnancy: a case report in sickle cell disease and review of the literature. Am J Hematol 1999;60:148–50.
11. Cinkotai KI, Wood P, Donnai P, Kendra J. Pregnancy after treatment with hydroxyurea in a patient with primary thrombocythaemia and a history of recurrent abortion. J Clin Pathol 1994;47:769–70.

12. Fernandez H. Essential thrombocythemia and pregnancy. J Gynecol Obstet Biol Reprod 1994;23:103–4. (French). As cited by Diav-Citrin O, Hunniset L, Sher GD, Koren G. Hydroxyurea use during pregnancy: a case report in sickle cell disease and review of the literature. Am J Hematol 1999;60:148–50.
13. Dell'Isola A, De Rosa G, Catalano D. Essential thrombocythemia in pregnancy. A case report and general considerations. Minerva Ginecol 1997;49: 165–72. (Italian). As cited by Diav-Citrin O, Hunnisett L, Sher GD, Koren G. Hydroxyurea use during pregnancy: a case report in sickle cell disease and review of the literature. Am J Hematol 1999;60:148–50.
14. Charache S, Terrin ML, Moore RD, Dover GJ, Barton FB, Eckert SV, McMahon RP, Bonds DR, and the Investigators of the Multicenter Study of Hydroxyurea in Sickle Cell Anemia. Effect of hydroxyurea on the frequency of painful crises in sickle cell anemia. N Engl J Med 1995;332:1317–22.
15. Diav-Citrin O, Hunnisett L, Sher GD, Koren G. Hydroxyurea use during pregnancy: a case report in sickle cell disease and review of the literature. Am J Hematol 1999;60:148–50.
16. Byrd DC, Pitts SR, Alexander CK. Hydroxyurea in two pregnant women with sickle cell anemia. Pharmacotherapy 1999;19:1459–62.
17. Rustin GJS, Booth M, Dent J, Salt S, Rustin F, Bagshawe KD. Pregnancy after cytotoxic chemotherapy for gestational trophoblastic tumours. Br Med J 1984;288:103–6.
18. Woolas RP, Bower M, Newlands ES, Seckl M, Short D, Holden L. Influence of chemotherapy for gestational trophoblastic disease on subsequent pregnancy outcome. Br J Obstet Gynaecol 1998;105:1032–5.
19. Pajor A, Zimonyi I, Koos R, Lehoczky D, Ambrus C. Pregnancies and offspring in survivors of acute lymphoid leukemia and lymphoma. Eur J Obstet Gynecol Reprod Biol 1991;40:1–5.
20. Sylvester RK, Lobell M, Teresi ME, Brundage D, Dubowy R. Excretion of hydroxyurea into milk. Cancer 1987;60:2177–8.

Name: **HYDROXYZINE** Risk Factor: **C**

Class: **Antihistamine**

FETAL RISK SUMMARY

RECOMMENDATION: Human Data Suggest Low Risk

Hydroxyzine belongs to the same class of compounds as buclizine, cyclizine, and meclizine. The drug is teratogenic in mice and rats, but not in rabbits, at high doses (1–5). One report suggested that hydroxyzine teratogenicity was mediated by a metabolite (norchlorcyclizine) that was common to four antihistamines (hydroxyzine, buclizine, meclizine, and chlorcyclizine) (3). High-dose hydroxyzine (6–12 mg/kg/day) resulted in abortions in rhesus monkeys (6). The manufacturer considers hydroxyzine to be contraindicated in early pregnancy because of the lack of clinical data (1,2).

In 100 patients treated in the 1st trimester with oral hydroxyzine (50 mg daily) for nausea and vomiting, no significant difference from nontreated controls was found in fetal wastage or anomalies (7). A woman treated with 60 mg/day of hydroxyzine during the 3rd trimester gave birth to a normal infant (8).

The Collaborative Perinatal Project monitored 50,282 mother-child pairs, 50 of whom had 1st trimester exposure to hydroxyzine (9, pp. 335–337, 341). For use anytime during pregnancy, 187 exposures were recorded (9, p. 438). Based on 5 malformed children, a possible relationship was found between 1st trimester use and congenital defects.

In a surveillance study of Michigan Medicaid recipients conducted between 1985 and 1992 involving 229,101 completed pregnancies, 828 newborns had been exposed to hydroxyzine during the 1st trimester (F. Rosa, personal communication, FDA, 1993). A total of 48 (5.8%) major birth defects were observed (42 expected). Specific data were available for six defect categories, including (observed/expected) 9/8 cardiovascular defects, 1/0.4 spina bifida, 0/2 polydactyly, 2/1 limb reduction defects, 0/2 hypospadias, and 3/1 oral clefts. Only with the latter defect is there a suggestion of a possible association, but other factors, including the mother's disease, concurrent drug use, and chance, may be involved.

Withdrawal in a newborn exposed to hydroxyzine 600 mg/day throughout gestation has been reported (10). The mother, who was being treated for severe eczema and asthma, was also treated with phenobarbital, 240 mg/day for 4 days then 60 mg/day, for mild preeclampsia during the 3-week period before delivery. Symptoms in the newborn, some beginning 15 minutes after birth, consisted of a shrill cry, jitteriness with clonic movements of the upper extremities, irritability, and poor feeding. The presumed drug-induced withdrawal persisted for approximately 4 weeks and finally resolved completely after 2 weeks of therapy with phenobarbital and methscopolamine. The infant was apparently doing well at 9 months of age. Although phenobarbital withdrawal could not be excluded, and neonatal withdrawal is a well-known complication of phenobarbital pregnancy use, the author concluded the symptoms in the infant were primarily caused by hydroxyzine (10).

A 1996 report described the use of hydroxyzine, droperidol, diphenhydramine, and metoclopramide in 80 women with hyperemesis gravidarum (11). The mean gestational age at the start of treatment was 10.9 weeks. All women received approximately 200 mg/day of hydroxyzine in divided dosage for up to a week after discharge from the hospital, and 12 (15%) required a second course of therapy for recurrence of their symptoms. Three of the mothers (all treated in the 2nd trimester) delivered offspring with congenital defects: Poland's syndrome, fetal alcohol syndrome, and hydrocephalus and hypoplasia of the right cerebral hemisphere. Only the latter anomaly is a potential drug effect, but the most likely cause was thought to be the result of an *in utero* fetal vascular accident or infection (11).

A 2001 study, using a treatment method similar to the above study, described the use of droperidol and diphenhydramine in 28 women hospitalized for hyperemesis gravidarum (12). Pregnancy outcomes in the study group were compared to a historical control of 54 women who had received conventional anti-emetic therapy. Oral metoclopramide and hydroxyzine were used after discharge from the hospital. Therapy was started in the study and control groups at mean gestational ages of 9.9 and 11.1 weeks, respectively. The study group appeared to have more severe disease then controls as suggested by a greater mean loss from the pre-pregnancy weight, 2.07 kg vs. 0.81 kg (*n.s.*), and a slightly lower serum potassium level, 3.4 vs. 3.5 mmol/L (*n.s.*). Compared to controls, the droperidol group had a shorter duration of hospitalization (3.53 vs. 2.82 days, $p = 0.023$), fewer readmissions (38.9% vs. 14.3%, $p = 0.025$), and lower average daily nausea and vomiting scores (both $p < 0.001$). There were no statistical differences in outcomes (study vs. controls) in terms of spontaneous abortions ($N = 0$ vs. $N = 2$ [4.3%]), elective abortions ($N = 3$ [12.0%] vs. $N = 3$ [6.5%]), Apgar scores at 1, 5, and 10 minutes, age at birth (37.3 vs. 37.9 weeks), and birth weight (3114 vs. 3347 g) (12). In controls, there was one (2.4%) major malformation of unknown cause, an acardiac fetus in a set of triplets, and one newborn with a genetic defect (Turner's syndrome). There was also one unexplained major birth defect (4.4%) in the droperidol group (bilateral hydronephrosis), and two genetic defects (translocation of chromosomes 3 and 7; tyrosinemia) (12).

A prospective controlled study published in 1997 evaluated the teratogenic risk of hydroxyzine and cetirizine (see also Cetirizine) in human pregnancy (13). A total of 120 pregnancies (2 sets of twins) exposed to either hydroxyzine ($N = 81$) or cetirizine ($N = 39$) during pregnancy were identified and compared to 110 controls. The control group was matched for maternal age, smoking, and alcohol use. The drugs were taken during the 1st trimester in 53 (65%) of the hydroxyzine cases and in 37 (95%) of the cetirizine exposures for a variety of indications (e.g., rhinitis, urticaria, pruritic urticarial papules and plaques of pregnancy, sedation, and other nonspecified reasons). Fourteen spontaneous abortions (hydroxyzine 3, cetirizine 6, controls 5) and 11 induced abortions (hydroxyzine 6, controls 5) occurred in the three groups. Among the live births, there were no statistical differences between the groups in birth weight, gestational age at delivery, rate of cesarean section, or neonatal distress. In the hydroxyzine group, two of the live births had major malformations; one with a ventricular septal defect and one with a complex congenital heart defect (also exposed to carbamazepine). A third infant, exposed after organogenesis, also had a ventricular septal defect. Minor abnormalities were observed in four hydroxyzine-exposed infants: one case each of hydrocele, inguinal hernia, hypothyroidism (mother also taking propylthiouracil), and strabismus. Two minor anomalies were observed in liveborn infants exposed to cetirizine during organogenesis; one with an ectopic kidney and one with undescended testes. No major abnormalities were seen in this group. In the control group, no major malformations were observed, but five infants had minor defects (dislocated hip, growth hormone deficiency, short lingual frenulum, and two unspecified defects). Statistically, there were no differences between the groups in outcome (13).

H

A 1997 article compared the published pregnancy outcomes, in terms of congenital malformations, of various first and second generation antihistamines (14). Based on 995 hydroxyzine-exposed liveborn infants, the authors calculated a relative risk for any congenital malformation that ranged from 1.2 to 3.4 (95% confidence interval 0.4 to 0.9, 1.6 to 17.9). Based on their analysis of published reports, the authors concluded that, in pregnancy, chlorpheniramine is the oral antihistamine of choice and that diphenhydramine should be used if a parenteral antihistamine is required (14).

During labor, hydroxyzine has been shown to be safe and effective for the relief of anxiety (15,16). No effect on the progress of labor or on neonatal Apgar scores was observed. In a study published in 1978, however, a 75-mg IM dose administered during labor caused a statistically significant decrease in fetal heart rate (FHR) variability in 10 of 16 cases (17). Maximal effects on the FHR were observed within 25 minutes after which they returned to normal values. Administration of hydroxyzine close to delivery reduces newborn platelet aggregation, but the clinical significance of this is unknown (18).

BREAST FEEDING SUMMARY

RECOMMENDATION: No Human Data - Probably Compatible

No reports describing the use of hydroxyzine during lactation have been located. The molecular weight (about 448) is low enough that excretion into breast milk should be expected. The effects, if any, on the nursing infant are unknown.

References

1. Product information. Vistaril. Pfizer, 1997.
2. Product information. Atarax. Pfizer, 1997.
3. King CTG, Howell J. Teratogenic effect of buclizine and hydroxyzine in the rat and chlorcyclizine in the mouse. Am J Obstet Gynecol 1966;95:109–11.
4. Posner HS, Darr A. Fetal edema from benzhydrylpiperazines as a possible cause of oral-facial malformations in rats. Toxicol Appl Pharmacol 1970;17:67–75.
5. Walker BE, Patterson A. Induction of cleft palate in mice by tranquilizers and barbiturates. Teratology 1974;10:159–64.
6. Steffek AJ, King CTG, Wilk AL. Abortive effects and comparative metabolism of chlorcyclizine in various mammalian species. Teratology 1968;1:399–406.
7. Erez S, Schifrin BS, Dirim O. Double-blind evaluation of hydroxyzine as an antiemetic in pregnancy. J Reprod Med 1971;7:57–9.
8. Romero R, Olsen TG, Chervenak FA, Hobbins JC. Pruritic urticarial papules and plaques of pregnancy. A case report. J Reprod Med 1983;28:615–9.
9. Heinonen OP, Slone D, Shapiro S. *Birth Defects and*

Drugs in Pregnancy. Littleton, MA: Publishing Sciences Group, 1977.
10. Prenner BM. Neonatal withdrawal syndrome associated with hydroxyzine hydrochloride. Am J Dis Child 1977;131:529–30.
11. Nageotte MP, Briggs GG, Towers CV, Asrat T. Droperidol and diphenhydramine in the management of hyperemesis gravidarum. Am J Obstet Gynecol 1996;174:1801–6.
12. Turcotte V, Ferreira E, Duperron L. Utilité du dropéridol et de la diphenhydramine dans l'hyperemesis gravidarum. J Soc Obstet Gynaecol Can 2001;23:133–9.
13. Einarson A, Bailey B, Jung G, Spizzirri D, Baillie M, Koren G. Prospective controlled study of hydroxyzine and cetirizine in pregnancy. Ann Allergy Asthma Immunol 1997;78:183–6.
14. Schatz M, Petitti D. Antihistamines and pregnancy. Ann Allergy Asthma Immunol 1997;78:157–9.
15. Zsigmond EK, Patterson RL. Double-blind evaluation of hydroxyzine hydrochloride in obstetric anesthesia. Anesth Analg (Cleve) 1967;46:275–80.
16. Amato G, Corsini D, Pelliccia E. Personal experience with a combination of Althesin and Atarax in caesarean section. Minerva Anestesiol 1980;46:671–4.
17. Petrie RH, Yeh S-Y, Murata Y, Paul RH, Hon EH, Barron BA, Johnson RJ. The effects of drugs on fetal heart rate variability. Am J Obstet Gynecol 1978;130:294–9.
18. Whaun JM, Smith GR, Sochor VA. Effect of prenatal drug administration on maternal and neonatal platelet aggregation and PF_4 release. Haemostasis 1980;9:226–37.

H

Name:	***l*-HYOSCYAMINE**	Risk Factor:	C_M
Class:	**Parasympatholytic (Anticholinergic)**		

FETAL RISK SUMMARY

RECOMMENDATION: Limited Human Data - No Relevant Animal Data

l-Hyoscyamine is an anticholinergic agent. No published reports of its use in pregnancy have been located (see also Belladonna or Atropine).

In a surveillance study of Michigan Medicaid recipients conducted between 1985 and 1992 involving 229,101 completed pregnancies, 281 newborns had been exposed to *l*-hyoscyamine during the 1st trimester (F. Rosa, personal communication, FDA, 1993). A total of 12 (4.3%) major birth defects were observed (11 expected). Specific data were available for six defect categories, including (observed/expected) 1/3 cardiovascular defects, 0/0.5 oral clefts, 0/0 spina bifida, 0/1 hypospadias, 2/1 polydactyly, and 2/0.5 limb reduction defects. Only with the latter two defects is there a suggestion of a possible association, but other factors, including the mother's disease, concurrent drug use, and chance, may be involved.

BREAST FEEDING SUMMARY

RECOMMENDATION: No Human Data - Probably Compatible

See Atropine.

Name:	**HYPERALIMENTATION, PARENTERAL**	Risk Factor:	C
Class:	**Nutrient**		

FETAL RISK SUMMARY

RECOMMENDATION: Compatible

Parenteral hyperalimentation (TPN) is the administration of an IV solution designed to provide complete nutritional support for a patient unable to maintain adequate nutritional intake. The solution is normally composed of dextrose (5%–35%), amino acids (3.5%–5%), vitamins, electrolytes, and trace elements. Lipids (IV fat emulsions) are often given with TPN to supply essential fatty acids and calories (see Lipids). A number of studies describing the use of TPN in pregnant women have been published (1–26). A report of four additional cases with a review of the literature appeared in 1986 (27), followed by another review in 1990 (28). This latter review also included an in depth discussion of indications, fluid, caloric (including lipids), electrolyte, and vitamin requirements for gestation and lactation, and monitoring techniques (28).

Maternal indications for TPN have been varied, with duration of therapy ranging from a few days to the entire pregnancy. Eleven patients were treated during the 1st trimester (1–5). No fetal complications attributable to TPN, including newborn hypoglycemia, have been identified in any of the reports. Intrauterine growth retardation occurred in five infants, and one of whom died, but the retarded growth and neonatal death were most likely caused by the underlying maternal disease (2–4,6–9,22). In a group of eight women treated with TPN for severe hyperemesis gravidarum who delivered live babies, the ratio of birth weight to standard mean weight for gestational age was greater than 1.0 in each case (5).

Obstetric complications included the worsening of one mother's renal hypertension after TPN was initiated, but the relationship between the effect and the therapy is not known (8). In a second case, resistance to oxytocin-induced labor was observed; but, again, the relationship to TPN is not clear (9).

Maternal and fetal death secondary to cardiac tamponade during central hyperalimentation has been reported (29). A 22-year-old woman in the 3rd trimester of pregnancy was treated with TPN for severe hyperemesis gravidarum. Seven days after commencing central TPN therapy, the patient experienced acute sharp retrosternal pain and dyspnea (29). Cardiac tamponade was subsequently diagnosed, but the mother and the fetus expired before the condition could be corrected. Percutaneous pericardiocentesis yielded 70 mL of fluid that was a mixture of the TPN and lipid solutions that the patient had been receiving.

A stillborn male fetus was delivered at 22 weeks' gestation from a 31-year-old woman with hyperemesis gravidarum following 8 weeks of parenteral hyperalimentation with lipid emulsion (fat composed 24% of total calories) (30). The tan-yellow placenta showed vacuolated syncytial cells and Hofbauer cells that stained for fat (30).

In summary, the use of total parenteral hyperalimentation does not seem to pose a significant risk to the fetus or newborn provided that normal procedures, as with nonpregnant patients, are followed to prevent maternal complications.

BREAST FEEDING SUMMARY

RECOMMENDATION: No Human Data - Probably Compatible

No problems should be expected in nursing infants whose mothers are receiving total parenteral hyperalimentation.

References

1. Hew LR, Deitel M. Total parenteral nutrition in gynecology and obstetrics. Obstet Gynecol 1980;55:464–8.
2. Tresadern JC, Falconer GF, Turnberg LA, Irving MH. Successful completed pregnancy in a patient maintained on home parenteral nutrition. Br Med J 1983;286:602–3.
3. Tresadern JC, Falconer GF, Turnberg LA, Irving MH. Maintenance of pregnancy in a home parenteral nutrition patient. JPEN J Parenter Enteral Nutr 1984;8:199–202.
4. Breen KJ, McDonald IA, Panelli D, Ihle B. Planned pregnancy in a patient who was receiving home parenteral nutrition. Med J Aust 1987;146:215–7.
5. Levine MG, Esser D. Total parenteral nutrition for the treatment of severe hyperemesis gravidarum: maternal nutritional effects and fetal outcome. Obstet Gynecol 1988;72:102–7.

6. Gineston JL, Capron JP, Delcenserie R, Delamarre J, Blot M, Boulanger JC. Prolonged total parenteral nutrition in a pregnant woman with acute pancreatitis. J Clin Gastroenterol 1984;6:249–52.
7. Lakoff KM, Feldman JD. Anorexia nervosa associated with pregnancy. Obstet Gynecol 1972;39:699–701.
8. Lavin JP Jr, Gimmon Z, Miodovnik M, von Meyenfeldt M, Fischer JE. Total parenteral nutrition in a pregnant insulin-requiring diabetic. Obstet Gynecol 1982;59:660–4.
9. Weinberg RB, Sitrin MD, Adkins GM, Lin CC. Treatment of hyperlipidemic pancreatitis in pregnancy with total parenteral nutrition. Gastroenterology 1982;83:1300–5.
10. Di Costanzo J, Martin J, Cano N, Mas JC, Noirclerc M. Total parenteral nutrition with fat emulsions during pregnancy—nutritional requirements: a case report. JPEN J Parenter Enteral Nutr 1982;6:534–8.
11. Young KR. Acute pancreatitis in pregnancy: two case reports. Obstet Gynecol 1982;60:653–7.
12. Rivera-Alsina ME, Saldana LR, Stringer CA. Fetal growth sustained by parenteral nutrition in pregnancy. Obstet Gynecol 1984;64:138–41.
13. Seifer DB, Silberman H, Catanzarite VA, Conteas CN, Wood R, Ueland K. Total parenteral nutrition in obstetrics. JAMA 1985;253:2073–5.
14. Benny PS, Legge M, Aickin DR. The biochemical effects of maternal hyperalimentation during pregnancy. N Z Med J 1978;88:283–5.
15. Cox KL, Byrne WJ, Ament ME. Home total parenteral nutrition during pregnancy: a case report. JPEN J Parenter Enteral Nutr 1981;5:246–9.
16. Gamberdella FR. Pancreatic carcinoma in pregnancy: a case report. Am J Obstet Gynecol 1984;149: 15–7.
17. Loludice TA, Chandrakaar C. Pregnancy and jejunoileal bypass: treatment complications with total parenteral nutrition. South Med J 1980;73:256–8.
18. Main ANH, Shenkin A, Black WP, Russell RI. Intravenous feeding to sustain pregnancy in patient with Crohn's disease. Br Med J 1981;283:1221–2.
19. Webb GA. The use of hyperalimentation and chemotherapy in pregnancy: a case report. Am J Obstet Gynecol 1980;137:263–6.
20. Stowell JC, Bottsford JE Jr, Rubel HR. Pancreatitis with pseudocyst and cholelithiasis in third trimester of pregnancy: management with total parenteral nutrition. South Med J 1984;77:502–4.
21. Martin R, Trubow M, Bistrian BR, Benotti P, Blackburn GL. Hyperalimentation during pregnancy: a case report. JPEN J Parenter Enteral Nutr 1985;9:212–5.
22. Herbert WNP, Seeds JW, Bowes WA, Sweeney CA. Fetal growth response to total parenteral nutrition in pregnancy: a case report. J Reprod Med 1986;31: 263–6.
23. Hatjis CG, Meis PJ. Total parenteral nutrition in pregnancy. Obstet Gynecol 1985;66:585–9.
24. Adami GF, Friedman D, Cuneo S, Marinari G, Gandolfo P, Scopinaro N. Intravenous nutritional support in pregnancy. Experience following biliopancreatic diversion. Clin Nutr 1992;11:106–9.
25. Satin AJ, Twickler D, Gilstrap LC III. Esophageal achalasia in late pregnancy. Obstet Gynecol 1992;79:812–4.
26. Teuscher AU, Sutherland DER, Robertson RP. Successful pregnancy after pancreatic islet autotransplantation. Transplant Proc 1994;26:3520.
27. Lee RV, Rodgers BD, Young C, Eddy E, Cardinal J. Total parenteral nutrition during pregnancy. Obstet Gynecol 1986;68:563–71.
28. Wolk RA, Rayburn WF. Parenteral nutrition in obstetric patients. Nutr Clin Pract 1990;5:139–52.
29. Greenspoon JS, Masaki DI, Kurz CR. Cardiac tamponade in pregnancy during central hyperalimentation. Obstet Gynecol 1989;73:465–6.
30. Jasnosz KM, Pickeral JJ, Graner S. Fat deposits in the placenta following maternal total parenteral nutrition with intravenous lipid emulsion. Arch Pathol Lab Med 1995;119:555–7.

I

Name:	**IBUPROFEN**	Risk Factor:	**B_M***
Class:	**Nonsteroidal Anti-inflammatory**		

FETAL RISK SUMMARY

RECOMMENDATION: Human Data Suggest Risk in 1st and 3rd Trimesters

Ibuprofen is a nonsteroidal anti-inflammatory drug (NSAID) indicated for the reduction of fever and mild to moderate pain. It is the same subclass (propionic acids) as five other NSAIDs (fenoprofen, flurbiprofen, ketoprofen, naproxen, and oxaprozin). No evidence of developmental abnormalities was observed in reproduction studies in rats and rabbits at doses slightly less then the maximum human clinical dose (1).

No published reports linking the use of ibuprofen with congenital defects have been located. The manufacturer has received information by a voluntary reporting system on the use of ibuprofen in 50 pregnancies (2). Seven of these cases were reported retrospectively and 43 prospectively. The results of the retrospective cases included one fetal death (cause of death unknown, no abnormalities observed) after 3rd trimester exposure, and one spontaneous abortion (SAB) without abnormality. Five infants with defects were observed, including an anencephalic infant exposed during the 1st trimester to ibuprofen and Bendectin (doxylamine succinate and pyridoxine hydrochloride), petit mal seizures progressing to grand mal convulsions, cerebral palsy (the fetus had also been exposed to other drugs), a hearsay report of microphthalmia with nasal cleft and mildly rotated palate, and tooth staining (2) (M. M. Westland, personal communication, The Upjohn Company, 1981). A cause-and-effect relationship between the drug and these defects is doubtful.

Prospectively, 23 of the exposed pregnancies ended in normal outcomes, 1 infant was stillborn, and 1 ended in SAB, both without apparent abnormality (2). Seven of the pregnancies were electively terminated, three had unknown outcomes, and eight of the pregnancies were still progressing at the time of the report.

In a surveillance study of Michigan Medicaid recipients conducted between 1985 and 1992 involving 229,101 completed pregnancies, 3,178 newborns had been exposed to ibuprofen during the 1st trimester (F. Rosa, personal communication, FDA, 1993). A total of 143 (4.5%) major birth defects were observed (129 expected). Specific data were available for six defect categories, including (observed/expected) 33/30 cardiovascular defects, 7/5 oral clefts, 3/2 spina bifida, 11/9 polydactyly, 5/5 limb reduction defects, and 4/8 hypospadias. These data do not support an association between the drug and congenital defects.

A combined 2001 population-based observational cohort study and a case-control study estimated the risk of adverse pregnancy outcome from the use of NSAIDs (3). The studies were based on data from the Danish birth registry and the North Jutland County's hospital discharge registry collected between 1991 and 1998. Only those women who had received a prescription for a NSAID at doses equivalent to 400 mg or 600 mg of ibuprofen were classified as exposed (NSAID doses equivalent to 200 mg of ibuprofen are over-the-counter in Denmark). The cohort involved 1462 pregnant women who had received a NSAID prescription in the interval from 30 days before conception to birth and a reference group of 17,259 pregnant women who had not been prescribed any drugs during pregnancy. In both groups, only pregnancies lasting longer than 28 weeks were included. There were 1106 women (76%) who had received a NSAID prescription between 30 days before conception and the end of the 1st trimester. The prevalences of congenital malformations in infants of these women and the reference group were ($N = 46$, 4.2%, 95% confidence interval [CI] 3.0%–5.3% vs. $N = 564$, 3.3%, 95% CI 3.0%–3.5%), respectively; adjusted odds ratio (OR) 1.27 (95% CI 0.93–1.75). A total of 997 women received a NSAID prescription in the 2nd and/or 3rd trimesters. In this group, the OR for preterm delivery was 1.05 (95% CI 0.80–1.39) and for low birth weight (excluding preterm infants) 0.79 (95% CI 0.45–1.38). Adjusting the data for the use of indomethacin (the tocolytic of choice in Denmark) did not affect the results. There was no evidence of a specific grouping of defects or of a dose-response relationship for adverse birth outcome. Based on the analysis, the authors concluded that NSAIDs were not associated with adverse birth outcome (3).

In the case-control portion of the above study, cases were defined as first recorded SAB in women who had received a prescription for NSAIDs in the 12 weeks before the date of discharge from the hospital after the SAB (63 of 4,268 women who had SAB) (3). The controls were 29,750 primiparous women who had live births, 318 of whom had received a prescription for NSAIDs in the 1st trimester. The data was analyzed for the time from receiving a NSAID prescription in the weeks before the SAB (or missed abortion), adjusted for maternal age. The OR (95% CI) for 1 week, 2–3 weeks, 4–6 weeks, 7–9 weeks, and 10–12 weeks before the SAB were 6.99 (2.75–17.74), 3.00 (1.21–7.44), 4.38 (2.66–7.20), 2.69 (1.81–4.00), and 1.26 (0.85–1.87), respectively. The results indicated that NSAIDs were associated with SAB because the OR decreased as the interval from assumed NSAID exposure to SAB increased (3).

A 2003 population-based cohort study involving 1055 pregnant women investigated the prenatal use of aspirin, NSAIDs, and acetaminophen (4). Fifty-three women (5%) reported use of NSAIDs around the time of conception or during pregnancy, 13 of whom had a SAB. After adjustment, an 80% increased risk of SAB was found for NSAIDs (adjusted hazard ratio 1.8, 95% CI 1.0–3.2). Moreover, the association was stronger if the initial use of drugs was around conception of if they were used longer than 1 week (4). A similar association was found with aspirin, but it was weaker because there were only 22 exposures (5 SAB). No association was observed with acetaminophen (4).

A prospective study of drug use in the 1st trimester examined the relationship between NSAIDs ($N = 2557$ infants born to exposed women) and congenital malformations (5). After adjustment, the OR for any birth defect was 1.04 (95% CI 0.84–1.29). However, the OR for cardiac defects ($N = 36$) and orofacial clefts ($N = 6$) were 1.86 (95% CI 1.32–2.62) and 2.61 (95% 1.01–6.78), respectively. There was no drug specificity for cardiac malformations, but five of the six cases of orofacial clefts had been exposed to naproxen (5).

A 2003 case-control study was conducted to identify drug use in early pregnancy that was associated with cardiac defects (6). Cases (cardiovascular defects without known chromosome anomalies) were drawn from three Swedish health registers ($N = 5015$) and controls consisting of all infants born in Sweden (1995–2001) ($N = 577,730$). Among the NSAIDs, only naproxen had a positive association with the defects (see Naproxen). For ibuprofen, there were 4124 pregnant women exposed and 37 cases of cardiac defects (OR 1.08, 95% CI 0.78–1.50) (6).

A 1996 case-control study of gastroschisis found a significantly elevated risk for ibuprofen ($N = 6$; OR 4.0, 95% CI 1.0–16.0) and other medications and exposures. A significant association was also found for aspirin ($N = 7$; OR 4.67, 95% CI 1.21–18.05). The data supported a vascular hypothesis for the pathogenesis of gastroschisis (7).

The use of ibuprofen as a tocolytic agent has been associated with reduced amniotic fluid volume (8–10). Fourteen (82.3%) of 17 women treated with a NSAID had decreased amniotic fluid volume (8). Of the 17 women, ibuprofen, 1200–2400 mg/day, was used alone in 3 pregnancies and was combined with ritodrine in one. The other 13 women were treated with indomethacin (see also Indomethacin). One woman who was treated with ibuprofen for 44 days had a return to a normal amniotic fluid volume after the drug was stopped (time for reversal not specified).

Ibuprofen, 600 mg every 6 hours, was used as a tocolytic in a woman with a triplet pregnancy at approximately 26 weeks' gestation (9). Terbutaline and magnesium sulfate were combined with ibuprofen at various times for tocolysis. Oligohydramnios in each sac (pockets <1 cm) was documented by ultrasonogram on the 20th day of therapy and ibuprofen therapy was stopped. Therapy was restarted 5 days later when normal fluid volume for the three fetuses was observed but oligohydramnios was again evident after 4 days and ibuprofen was discontinued. Tocolysis was then maintained with terbutaline and normal fluid volumes were observed 5 days after the second course of ibuprofen. The triplets were eventually delivered by elective cesarean section at 35 weeks' gestation, but no details on the infants were given (9).

A brief 1992 abstract described the results of using ibuprofen, 1200–2400 mg/day, as a tocolytic agent in 52 pregnancies (61 fetuses) up to 32 weeks' gestation (10). Amniotic fluid volumes were evaluated every 1–2 weeks. No cases of true oligohydramnios were observed, although 3 cases of low-normal fluid occurred that resolved after discontinuation of ibuprofen. Periodic Doppler echocardiography during therapy revealed a non-dose-related mild constriction of the ductus arteriosus in 4 (6.6%) of the fetuses. Ductal constriction was observed in three of the fetuses within 1 week of starting ibuprofen. Normal echocardiograms were obtained in all four cases within 1 week of discontinuing therapy (10).

Ibuprofen is commonly used by pregnant women according to a 2003 study that identified the medications taken by a rural population (11). Among 578 participants, 86 (15%) took ibuprofen during pregnancy, including 20 during the 3rd trimester. Ibuprofen was the fourth most commonly used over-the-counter medication (after acetaminophen, calcium carbonate, and cough drops) (11).

Constriction of the ductus arteriosus *in utero* is a pharmacologic consequence arising from the use of prostaglandin synthesis inhibitors during pregnancy (see also Indomethacin) (12). Persistent pulmonary hypertension of the newborn may occur if these agents are used in the 3rd trimester close to delivery (12,13). These drugs also have been shown to inhibit labor and prolong pregnancy, both in humans (14) and in animals (15). Women attempting to conceive should not use any prostaglandin synthesis inhibitor, including ibuprofen, because of the findings in a variety of animal models that indicate these agents block blastocyst implantation (16,17). Moreover, as noted above, NSAIDs have also been associated with SAB and possibly with congenital malformations.

[*Risk Factor D if used in 3rd trimester or near delivery.*]

BREAST FEEDING SUMMARY

RECOMMENDATION: Compatible

Ibuprofen is excreted into human milk. Two studies were unable to detect the drug (18–20), but a third study using a more sensitive assay (lower limit 2.5 ng/mL) was able to quantify ibuprofen in milk (21). In 12 patients taking 400 mg every 6 hours for 24 hours, an assay capable of detecting 1 μg/mL failed to demonstrate ibuprofen in the milk (18,19). In a second report, a woman was treated with 400 mg twice daily for 3 weeks (20). Milk levels shortly before and up to 8 hours after drug administration were all less than 0.5 μg/mL.

The third study involved a lactating woman who underwent maxillary surgery (21). After surgery, she took ibuprofen 400 mg six times over a 42.5-hour interval for postoperative pain. Ten breast milk samples were collected during this same period. Ibuprofen was detected (13 ng/mL) 30 minutes after the first dose. The maximum milk concentration, 181 ng/mL, was found 20.5 hours after the first dose (about 5 hours after the third dose). Although the infant was not nursing, the infant's weight adjusted dose would have been an estimated 0.0008% of the mother's dose (21).

The American Academy of Pediatrics classifies ibuprofen as compatible with breastfeeding (22).

References

1. Product information. Motrin. McNeil Consumer, 2000.
2. Barry WS, Meinzinger MM, Howse CR. Ibuprofen overdose and exposure *in utero:* results from a postmarketing voluntary reporting system. Am J Med 1984; 77(1A):35–9.
3. Nielsen GL, Sorensen HT, Larsen H, Pedersen L. Risk of adverse birth outcome and miscarriage in pregnant users of non-steroidal anti-inflammatory drugs: population based observational study and case-control study. BMJ 2001;322:266–70.
4. Li DK, Liu L, Odouli R. Exposure to non-steroidal anti-inflammatory drugs during pregnancy and risk of miscarriage: population based cohort study. BMJ 2003;327:368–71.
5. Ericson A, Kallen BAJ. Nonsteroidal anti-inflammatory drugs in early pregnancy. Reprod Toxicol 2001; 15:371–5.
6. Kallen BAJ, Olausson PO. Maternal drug use in early pregnancy and infant cardiovascular defect. Reprod Toxicol 2003;17:255–61.
7. Torfs CP, Katz EA, Bateson TF, Lam PK, Curry CJR. Maternal medications and environmental exposures as risk factors for gastroschisis. Teratology 1996;54: 84–92.
8. Hickok DE, Hollenbach KA, Reilley SF, Nyberg DA. The association between decreased amniotic fluid volume and treatment with nonsteroidal anti-inflammatory agents for preterm labor. Am J Obstet Gynecol 1989;160:1525–31.
9. Wiggins DA, Elliott JP. Oligohydramnios in each sac of a triplet gestation caused by Motrin—fulfilling Kock's postulates. Am J Obstet Gynecol 1990;162: 460–1.
10. Hennessy MD, Livingston EC, Papagianos J, Killam AP. The incidence of ductal constriction and oligohydramnios during tocolytic therapy with ibuprofen (abstract). Am J Obstet Gynecol 1992;166:324.
11. Glover DD, Amonkar M, Rybeck BF, Tracy TS. Prescription, over-the-counter, and herbal medicine use in a rural, obstetric population. Am J Obstet Gynecol 2003;188:1039–45.
12. Levin DL. Effects of inhibition of prostaglandin synthesis on fetal development, oxygenation, and the fetal circulation. Semin Perinatol 1980;4: 35–44.
13. Van Marter LJ, Leviton A, Allred EN, Pagano M, Sullivan KF, Cohen A, Epstein MF. Persistent pulmonary hypertension of the newborn and smoking and aspirin and nonsteroidal antiinflammatory drug consumption during pregnancy. Pediatrics 1996;97:658–63.
14. Fuchs F. Prevention of prematurity. Am J Obstet Gynecol 1976;126:809–20.
15. Powell JG, Cochrane RL. The effects of a number of non-steroidal anti-inflammatory compounds on parturition in the rat. Prostaglandins 1982;23: 469–88.
16. Matt DW, Borzelleca JF. Toxic effects on the female reproductive system during pregnancy, parturition, and lactation. In Witorsch RJ, ed. *Reproductive Toxicology*. 2nd ed. New York, NY: Raven Press, 1995: 175–93.
17. Dawood MY. Nonsteroidal antiinflammatory drugs and reproduction. Am J Obstet Gynecol 1993;169: 1255–65.
18. Townsend RJ, Benedetti T, Erickson S, Gillespie WR, Albert KS. A study to evaluate the passage of ibuprofen into breast milk (abstract). Drug Intell Clin Pharm 1982;16:482–3.
19. Townsend RJ, Benedetti TJ, Erickson S, Cengiz C, Gillespie WR, Gschwend J, Albert KS. Excretion of ibuprofen into breast milk. Am J Obstet Gynecol 1984; 149:184–6.
20. Weibert RT, Townsend RJ, Kaiser DG, Naylor AJ. Lack

of ibuprofen secretion into human milk. Clin Pharm 1982;1:457–8.
21. Walter K, Dilger C. Ibuprofen in human milk. Br J Clin Pharmacol 1997;44:209–13.
22. Committee on Drugs, American Academy of Pediatrics. The transfer of drugs and other chemicals into human milk. Pediatrics 2001;108:776–89.

Name: **IBUTILIDE** Risk Factor: **C_M**
Class: **Antiarrhythmic**

FETAL RISK SUMMARY

RECOMMENDATION: No Human Data - Animal Data Suggest Moderate Risk

Ibutilide is a cardiac antiarrhythmic agent with predominantly class III (cardiac action potential prolongation) properties (1). Other available class III antiarrhythmic agents are amiodarone, sotalol, and bretylium (2). Ibutilide is administered by IV injection only. It undergoes rapid and extensive hepatic metabolism to eight metabolites, only one of which is active. Ibutilide has an average elimination half-life of about 6 hours (range 2–12 hours) (1).

Dose-related teratogenic, embryocidal effects, and fetal toxicity were observed in rats given ibutilide orally on days 6–15 of gestation (1,3,4). The no-observed-adverse-effect level (NOAEL), corrected for the 3% oral bioavailability, was 5 mg/kg/day, approximately the same as the maximum recommended human dose on a mg/m^2 basis (MRHD). Scoliosis was observed at a dose double the MRHD, but the incidence was not significantly different from controls (4). At four and eight times the MRHD, a significant dose-response effect was observed for adactyly, interventricular septal defects, scoliosis, and pharynx and palate malformations (4). A significant increase in embryo resorptions and fetal toxicity occurred at eight times the MRHD (4).

No reports describing the use of ibutilide in human pregnancy have been located. Similarly, human placental transfer of ibutilide has apparently not been studied. The molecular weight (about 443 for the fumarate salt), however, is low enough that passage to the fetus should be expected.

In summary, animal data in the one species tested suggest a moderate risk to the human embryo/fetus. The lack of human reports, however, prevents an assessment of the risk, but the benefits of therapy might outweigh the fetal risk, especially after the 1st trimester. This conclusion is based on two considerations. First, the indication for ibutilide (i.e., rapid conversion of atrial fibrillation or atrial flutter of recent onset to sinus rhythm) is indicative of severe maternal disease that would be, in itself, harmful to the fetus if not treated. Second, treatment with ibutilide would most likely be short-term and occur in a hospital with the fetus under surveillance.

BREAST FEEDING SUMMARY

RECOMMENDATION: No Human Data - Probably Compatible

No reports describing the use of ibutilide during lactation have been located. It is doubtful if such reports will occur because of the indication for this drug. In addition, its low oral bioavailability (about 3% in rats) suggests a nursing infant would absorb minimal amounts.

References

1. Product information. Corvert, Pharmacia & Upjohn, 2000.
2. Granberry MC. Ibutilide: A new class III antiarrhythmic agent. Am J Health Syst Pharm 1998;55:255–60.
3. Marks TA, Terry RD. Developmental toxicity of ibutilide fumarate in rats (abstract). Teratology 1995;49:406.
4. Marks TA, Terry RD. Developmental toxicity of ibutilide fumarate in rats after oral administration. Teratology 1996;54:157–64.

Name: **IDARUBICIN** Risk Factor: **D_M**

Class: **Antineoplastic**

FETAL RISK SUMMARY

RECOMMENDATION: Limited Human Data - Animal Data Suggest Risk

Idarubicin, an anthracycline antineoplastic antibiotic agent, is a DNA-intercalating analogue of daunorubicin. It is used in the treatment of acute myeloid leukemia.

In pregnant rats, a dose 10% of the human dose (HD) produced embryotoxicity and teratogenicity without causing maternal toxicity. Embryotoxicity, but not teratogenicity, occurred in rabbits treated with doses up to about 20% of the HD. However, this dose caused maternal toxicity (1).

Shepard reviewed three reproductive studies in which IV doses up to 0.2 mg/kg were given to rats (2). When treatment occurred early in pregnancy, fetal loss, intrauterine growth retardation (IUGR), decreased ossification, and skeletal defects such as fused ribs were observed at the highest dose. These effects were not seen when treatment occurred perinatally. Infertility may have occurred in the second generation.

A 26-year-old woman at 20 weeks' gestation presented with acute myeloblastic leukemia and was treated with an induction course of cytarabine and daunorubicin that failed to halt the disease progression (3). At approximately 23 weeks' gestation, a second induction course was started with mitoxantrone and cytarabine. Complete remission was achieved 60 days from the start of therapy. Weekly ultrasound examinations documented normal fetal growth. Because of the long interval required for remission, treatment was changed to idarubicin (10 mg/m^2, days 1 and 2) and cytarabine. She tolerated this therapy and was discharged home, but returned 2 days later complaining of abdominal pain and the loss of fetal movements. A stillborn, 2200-g fetus (gestational age not specified) without evidence of congenital malformations was delivered after induction. Permission for an autopsy was denied. Although the authors did not specify a mechanism, they concluded that the cause of the fetal death was caused by idarubicin.

A 1998 case report described a woman with acute myeloid leukemia who was treated with idarubicin and cytarabine during the 2nd trimester (4). Treatment was begun at 21 weeks' gestation with IV idarubicin 10 mg/m^2 on days 1, 3, and 5, and IV cytarabine 100 mg/m^2 on days 1 through 10. A 6-day consolidation course of IV cytarabine, 1000 mg/m^2 every 12 hours, was given 6 weeks later. Complete remission was documented after recovery from this course. IUGR and decreased fetal movements were diagnosed at 32 weeks' gestation and a week and half later, a 1408-g female infant was delivered by cesarean section. Apgar scores were 4, 7, and 10 at 1, 5, and 10 minutes, respectively. Except for hyperbilirubinemia, the infant was healthy and was doing well on discharge. An echocardiographic examination revealed no evidence of cardiac anomalies or signs of cardiomyopathy (4).

A 22-year-old woman at 22 weeks' gestation with acute lymphoblastic leukemia type T was treated with idarubicin (9 mg/m^2 on days 1, 2, 3, and 8), cyclophosphamide (750 mg/m^2 on days 1 and 8), vincristine (2 mg/day on days 1, 8, 15, and 22), and prednisone (60 mg/m^2 on days 1–7 and 15–21) (5). The patient tolerated the therapy except for agranulocytosis with fever that was treated with antibiotics. A complete remission was documented by 27 weeks' gestation. Before consolidation chemotherapy, a 1024-g male infant was delivered by cesarean section 1 week later. Apgar scores were 6, 8, and 8 at 1, 5, and 10 minutes, respectively. Neonatal complications, related to prematurity, were respiratory distress syndrome, necrotizing enterocolitis, and grade II ventricular hemorrhage (5). In addition, acute heart failure occurred during the first 3 days after birth (5). Diffuse cardiomyopathy involving both ventricles and the interventricular septum without anomalies was revealed by echocardiography. The condition was thought to be related to the chemotherapy, especially, idarubicin (5). With supportive care, the cardiac function returned to normal within 3 days. Except for slight delay in the acquisition of language, the infant was progressing normally at 18 months of age.

Occupational exposure of the mother to antineoplastic agents during pregnancy may present a risk to the fetus. A position statement from the National Study Commission on Cytotoxic Exposure and a research article involving some antineoplastic agents are presented in the monograph for cyclophosphamide (see Cyclophosphamide).

BREAST FEEDING SUMMARY

RECOMMENDATION: Contraindicated

No reports describing the use of idarubicin during lactation have been located. The molecular weight (about 498 for the free base) is low enough, however, that excretion into breast milk should be expected. Because of the potential toxicity, a woman treated with this drug should not breast-feed until idarubicin and its cytoxic and presumed active metabolite, idarubicinol, have been eliminated from her system. Idarubicin has a mean terminal half-life of 20–22 hours (range 4–46 hours), but the estimated mean terminal half-life of idarubicinol exceeds 45 hours (1). Thus, elimination of the two agents may require 10 days or longer. The American Academy of Pediatrics classifies other similar antineoplastic agents (e.g., doxorubicin) as contraindicated during breast-feeding because of the potential for immune suppression and an unknown effect on growth or association with carcinogenesis (6).

References

1. Product information. Idamycin. Pharmacia, 1996.
2. Shepard TH. *Catalog of Teratogenic Agents*. 8th ed. Baltimore, MD: Johns Hopkins University Press, 1995: 1290.
3. Reynoso EE, Huerta F. Acute leukemia and pregnancy - fatal fetal outcome after exposure to idarubicin during the second trimester. Acta Oncol 1994;33: 703–16.
4. Claahsen HL, Semmekrot BA, van Dongen PWJ, Mattijssen V. Successful fetal outcome after exposure to idarubicin and cytosine-arabinoside during the second trimester of pregnancy—a case report. Am J Perinatol 1998;15:295–7.
5. Achtari C, Hohlfeld P. Cardiotoxic transplacental effect of idarubicin administered during the second trimester of pregnancy. Am J Obstet Gynecol 2000;183: 511–2.
6. Committee on Drugs, American Academy of Pediatrics. The transfer of drugs and other chemicals into human milk. Pediatrics 2001;108:776–89.

Name:	**IDOXURIDINE**	Risk Factor:	**C**
Class:	**Antiviral**		

FETAL RISK SUMMARY

RECOMMENDATION: No Human Data - Animal Data Suggest Risk

Idoxuridine has not been studied in human pregnancy. The drug is teratogenic in some species of animals after injection and ophthalmic use (1,2).

BREAST FEEDING SUMMARY

RECOMMENDATION: No Human Data - Potential Toxicity

No data are available.

References

1. Nishimura H, Tanimura T. *Clinical Aspects of The Teratogenicity of Drugs*. New York, NY: American Elsevier, 1976:148, 258–9.
2. Itoi M, Gefter JW, Kaneko N, Ishii Y, Ramer RM, Gasset AR. Teratogenicities of ophthalmic drugs. I. Antiviral ophthalmic drugs. Arch Ophthalmol 1975;93:46–51.

Name:	**IFOSFAMIDE**	Risk Factor:	**D_M**
Class:	**Antineoplastic**		

FETAL RISK SUMMARY

RECOMMENDATION: Contraindicated - 1st Trimester

Ifosfamide is chemically related to the nitrogen mustards and is a synthetic analog of cyclophosphamide. (See also Cyclophosphamide.) Ifosfamide is a prodrug that requires metabolic activation by microsomal liver enzymes to produce biologically active metabolites. It is indicated for the treatment of germ cell testicular cancer. Combination with a prophylactic agent such as mesna is recommended to prevent hemorrhagic cystitis (1).

Ifosfamide was carcinogenic in rats (including a significant incidence of leiomyosarcomas and mammary fibroadenomas in female rats) and mutagenic in several assays (1). Reproduction studies have been conducted in pregnant mice, rats, and rabbits. In mice, a single dose of 30 mg/m^2 (1/40th the daily recommended human dose of 1200 mg/m^2) administered on gestational day 11 caused an increase in the incidence of resorptions and anomalies (not specified). Evidence of embryo lethality was observed in rats given 54-mg/m^2 doses on gestational days 6–15. Embryotoxic effects (not specified) were observed when a smaller dose (18 mg/m^2) was administered over the same period. Embryotoxicity and teratogenicity were observed in rabbits given 88 mg/m^2/day on gestational days 6–18 (1). Maternal toxicity was not mentioned in any of the above studies.

A 1973 study described the teratogenic and embryotoxic effects of various single intraperitoneal doses (5, 10, and 20 mg/kg) of ifosfamide given to mice on gestational day 11 (2). Only the 20-mg/kg dose was embryolethal (significantly increased resorption rates), but significant fetal toxicity (decreased body weight and/or crown-rump length) was observed with the 10- and 20-mg/kg doses. A number of anomalies were observed in the highest dose group: open eyes, internal and external hydrocephalus, microphakia, micromelia, adactyly, syndactyly, microcaudate, kinky tails, kidney ectopia, and hydronephrosis. Both 10- and 20-mg/kg doses increased the number of skeletal defects and the 5-mg/kg dose was associated with a significant increase in supernumerary ribs. Finally, a single SC dose of 45 mg/kg administered to 1-day-old mice resulted in reduced body weight and altered development (2).

In sexually mature male rabbits, single IV doses of ifosfamide (0, 60, 90, 120, or 240 mg/kg) caused transient and dose-dependent depression of spermatocytogenesis, spermiogenesis, and sperm maturation in comparison to controls (3). In the second part of this study, using the same methods, the investigators combined ifosfamide with mesna (a uroprotectant agent) (4). Three groups of male rabbits were given different doses of the combination (ifosfamide 30, 45 or 60 mg/kg plus mesna 6, 9 or 12 mg/kg, followed by a second equal dose of mesna 4 hours later). Each group received 10 weekly treatments. Controls were given either mesna alone (three groups) or saline (one group). Dose-related ifosfamide-mesna suppression of spermatogenesis and epididymal sperm maturation was observed. In addition, the investigators noted incomplete recovery of the germinal epithelium (4).

A 1997 review stated that ifosfamide is less toxic for stem cell spermatogonia (type A spermatogonia) than is cyclophosphamide (5). In 15 of 16 patients who received 15–30 g/m^2 of ifosfamide, the median follicle-stimulating hormone levels returned to normal. In addition, there was no evidence of an increased risk of malformations or malignancies in offspring fathered by patients with germ cell cancer after chemotherapy (5). However, a 2003 study confirmed that ifosfamide exposure is a potential cause of male infertility (6). A significant ($p = 0.005$) dose-dependent relationship was observed between increasing doses of ifosfamide and infertility in patients treated for osteosarcoma.

It is not known if ifosfamide or its active metabolites cross the placenta to the fetus. The low molecular weight of the parent prodrug (about 261), however, suggests that it reaches the fetal circulation.

Only two reports describing the use of ifosfamide in human pregnancy have been located. A 20-year-old woman at 23 weeks' gestation was treated with ifosfamide (5 g/day on days 1 and 2), vincristine (2 mg/day on days 1 and 14), and dactinomycin (1 mg/day on days 1 and 2) for advanced rhabdomyosarcoma of the face (7). In addition to the antineoplastics, the patient also received mesna and urate oxidase (used for the treatment of hyperuricemia). A second course of therapy was given 4 weeks later. At initiation of the chemotherapy, the fetal weight was estimated to be at the 20th percentile with normal amniotic fluid volume and active movements. At the time of the second course of chemotherapy, ultrasound revealed a complete absence of amniotic fluid, an empty fetal bladder, cessation of fetal growth, and absence of fetal movements. An emergency cesarean section was performed 2 weeks later after evidence of continued anhydramnios, intrauterine growth arrest, and acute fetal hypoxia. A 720-g female was delivered with Apgar scores of 3, 7, and 7 at 1, 5, and 10 minutes, respectively. An ultrasound of the neonate revealed bilateral intraventricular hemorrhage and left occipital meningeal hematomas. Anuria persisted, and the girl died at age 7 days. Autopsy noted extensive cerebral lesions associated with prematurity but no renal lesions or chromosome abnormalities. The placenta had large areas of ischemic necrosis without evidence of chorioamnionitis. No cancer cells were found in the fetus or placenta. The authors speculated that the lack of renal lesions suggested that causes in addition to ifosfamide-induced toxicity should be considered to explain the anuria in the fetus and newborn (7).

In contrast to the above study, a 21-year-old woman was treated with three courses of ifosfamide/mesna (each 5 g/m^2 three times weekly) and doxorubicin (50 mg/m^2 three times weekly) for Ewing's sarcoma of the pelvis (8). The three courses were given in the 27th, 30th, and 33rd week of pregnancy. Mild intrauterine growth retardation was detected by ultrasound. A cesarean section at the beginning of the 36th gestational week delivered a 42-cm-long, 1300-g female infant. No adverse effects were noted in the infant who was doing well at 2 years of age (8).

In summary, ifosfamide is carcinogenic and mutagenic in experimental studies. In addition, it is teratogenic and embryotoxic in three animal species at doses far less than the recommended human dose. One of the infants in the two published cases of fetal exposure to ifosfamide did well after exposure in the 3rd trimester. However, in the other case, treatment was begun in the 2nd trimester and resulted in severe fetal toxicity and eventual death of the neonate. Although the exact cause of the severe renal toxicity was unknown, ifosfamide-induced toxicity could not be excluded. Because of the above findings and the close relationship of ifosfamide to cyclophosphamide, a known human teratogen, ifosfamide should be considered an agent with a high potential for human teratogenicity and embryo/fetal toxicity.

BREAST FEEDING SUMMARY

RECOMMENDATION: Contraindicated

No studies describing the use of ifosfamide during lactation have been located. Ifosfamide is excreted into breast milk (1). This is consistent with its low molecular weight (about 261). Although the amount of ifosfamide in milk was not stated, severe toxicity in a nursing infant is a potential concern (e.g., bone marrow depression, urinary and central nervous systems toxicity). Therefore, women receiving ifosfamide should not breast-feed.

References

1. Product information. Ifex. Bristol-Myers Squibb, 2000.
2. Bus JS, Gibson JE. Teratogenicity and neonatal toxicity of Ifosfamide in mice. Proc Soc Exp Biol Med 1973; 143:965–70.
3. Ypsilantis P, Papaioannou N, Psalla D, Politou M, Simopoulos C. Effects of single dose administration of ifosfamide on testes and semen characteristics in the rabbit. Reprod Toxicol 2003;17:237–45.
4. Ypsilantis P, Papaioannou N, Psalla D, Politou M, Pitiakoudis M, Simopoulos C. Effects of subchronic ifosfamide-mesna treatment on testes and semen characteristics in the rabbit. Reprod Toxicol 2003;17: 699–708.
5. Pont J, Albrecht W. Fertility after chemotherapy for testicular germ cell cancer. Fertil Steril 1997;68:1–5.
6. Longhi A, Macchiagodena M, Vitali G, Bacci G. Fertility in male patients treated with neoadjuvant chemotherapy for osteosarcoma. J Pediatr Hematol Oncol 2003;25:292–6.
7. Fernandez H, Diallo A, Baume D, Papiernik E. Anhydramnios and cessation of fetal growth in a pregnant mother with polychemotherapy during the second trimester. Prenat Diag 1989;9:681–2.
8. Merimsky O, Chevalier TL, Missenard G, Lepechoux C, Cojean-Zelek I, Mesurolle B, Le Cesne A. Management of cancer in pregnancy: a case of Ewing's sarcoma of the pelvis in the third trimester. Ann Oncol 1999;10:345–50.

Name:	**IMIPENEM-CILASTATIN SODIUM**	Risk Factor:	C_M
Class:	**Antibiotic**		

FETAL RISK SUMMARY

RECOMMENDATION: Limited Human Data - Animal Data Suggest Low Risk

Imipenem, a semisynthetic carbapenem related to the β-lactam antibiotics, is only available in the United States in a 1:1 combination with the enzyme inhibitor cilastatin sodium. The latter agent is a specific, reversible inhibitor of dehydropeptidase I, an enzyme that is present in the proximal renal tubular cells and inactivates imipenem. By inhibiting this enzyme, cilastatin results in higher urinary concentrations of imipenem.

Reproductive studies in pregnant rabbits and rats with imipenem at doses up to 2 and 30 times, respectively, and with cilastatin sodium at 10 and 33 times, respectively, the maximum recommended human dose showed no evidence of adverse fetal effects (1). Similar negative findings were found with imipenem-cilastatin sodium in pregnant mice and rats treated with doses up to 11 times the maximum human dose (1).

Adverse effects observed in pregnant cynomolgus monkeys given either 40 mg/kg/day (bolus IV) or 160 mg/kg/day (SC injection) included loss of appetite, weight loss, emesis, diarrhea, abortion, and death in some animals (1). No significant toxicity was observed in nonpregnant monkeys given 180 mg/kg/day SC. An IV infusion of 100 mg/kg/day (approximately 3 times the maximum daily recommended human IM dose) in pregnant monkeys did not produce significant maternal toxicity or teratogenic effects, but it did result in an increase in embryonic loss.

Imipenem-cilastatin crosses the placenta to the fetus (2,3). Seven women at a mean gestational age of 8.6 weeks' gestation (immediately before pregnancy termination) and seven at a mean gestational age of 38.7 weeks' were given a single 20-minute IV infusion of 500 mg of imipenem-cilastatin (2). A third, nonpregnant group was also studied. Maternal plasma and amniotic fluid samples were collected at frequent intervals for 8 hours. In comparison with nonpregnant women, imipenem concentrations in maternal plasma were significantly lower in both early and late pregnancy. The mean concentrations in the amniotic fluid in early and late pregnancy were 0.07 and 0.72 μg/mL, respectively. At delivery, the mean cord venous and arterial blood concentrations were 1.72 and 1.64 μg/mL, respectively, representing a fetal:maternal mean ratio of 0.33 (venous) and 0.31 (arterial). Transfer of both imipenem and cilastatin across the placenta at term was observed in two Japanese studies (3,4). Peak concentrations of both agents were about 30% of those measured in the maternal blood (4). Both drugs were also transferred to the amniotic fluid, with the highest concentrations occurring, after a single dose, at about 5–6 hours. Peak amniotic fluid:maternal blood ratios for imipenem and cilastatin were approximately 0.30 and 0.45, respectively (4).

No reports describing the use of this antibiotic-enzyme inhibitor combination in the 1st trimester of nonterminated human pregnancies have been located. Three references, however, consider imipenem-cilastatin to be a safe and effective agent during the perinatal period (3–5).

BREAST FEEDING SUMMARY

RECOMMENDATION: Limited Human Data - Probably Compatible

Small amounts of imipenem-cilastatin are excreted into breast milk (3). These amounts are comparable to other β-lactam antibiotics (3). The effects, if any, on a nursing infant are unknown.

References

1. Product information. Primaxin. Merck & Co., 1994.
2. Heikkila A, Renkonen O-V, Erkkola R. Pharmacokinetics and transplacental passage of imipenem during pregnancy. Antimicrob Agents Chemother 1992;36:2652–5.
3. Matsuda S, Suzuki M, Oh K, Ishikawa M, Soma A, Takada H, Shimizu T, Makinoda S, Fujimoto S, Chimura T, Morisaki N, Matsuo M, Cho N, Fukunaga K, Kunii K, Tamaya T, Hayasaki M, Ito K, Izumi K, Takagi H, Ninomiya K, Tateno M, Okada H, Yamamoto T,

Yasuda J, Kanao M, Hirabayashi K, Okada E. Pharmacokinetic and clinical studies on imipenem/cilastatin sodium in the perinatal period. Jpn J Antibiot 1988;11:1731–41.
4. Hirabayashi K, Okada E. Pharmacokinetic and clinical studies of imipenem/cilastatin sodium in the perinatal period. Jpn J Antibiot 1988;11:1797–1804.
5. Cho N, Fukunaga K, Kunii K, Kobayashi I, Tezuka K. Studies on imipenem/cilastatin sodium in the perinatal period. Jpn J Antibiot 1988;11:1758–73.

Name: **IMIPRAMINE** Risk Factor: **C**

Class: **Antidepressant**

FETAL RISK SUMMARY

RECOMMENDATION: Human Data Suggest Low Risk

Shepard reviewed six animal reproductive studies involving imipramine in 1989 (1). Some defects were observed in one investigation using rabbits, but other studies with mice, rats, rabbits, and monkeys revealed no evidence of drug-induced teratogenicity.

Bilateral amelia was reported in one child whose mother had ingested imipramine during pregnancy (2). An analysis of 546,505 births, 161 with 1st trimester exposure to imipramine, however, failed to find an association with limb reduction defects (3–15). Reported malformations other than limb reduction were defective abdominal muscles (1 case); diaphragmatic hernia (2 cases); exencephaly, cleft palate, adrenal hypoplasia (1 case); cleft palate (2 cases); and renal cystic degeneration (1 case) (4–6). These reports indicate that imipramine is not a major cause of congenital limb deformities.

In a surveillance study of Michigan Medicaid recipients conducted between 1985 and 1992 involving 229,101 completed pregnancies, 75 newborns had been exposed to imipramine during the 1st trimester (F. Rosa, personal communication, FDA, 1993). Six (8.0%) major birth defects were observed (three expected), including (observed/expected) 3/0.8 cardiovascular defects, 1/0.2 spina bifida, and 1/0.2 hypospadias. No anomalies were observed in three other defect categories (oral clefts, polydactyly, and limb reduction defects) for which specific data were available. Only with cardiovascular defects is there a suggestion of an association, but other factors, including the mother's disease, concurrent drug use, and chance, may be involved.

In a 1996 descriptive case series, the European Network of the Teratology Information Services (ENTIS) prospectively examined the outcomes of 689 pregnancies exposed to antidepressants (16). Multiple drug therapy occurred in about two-thirds of the mothers. Imipramine exposure occurred in 30 pregnancies (1 set of twins). The outcomes of these pregnancies were 1 elective abortion, 3 spontaneous abortions, 25 normal newborns, and 2 infants with congenital defects. The defects (all exposed in the 1st trimester or longer) were six fingers on right hand, and an omphalocele (16).

Neonatal withdrawal symptoms have been reported with the use of imipramine during pregnancy (17–19). Symptoms observed in the infants during the 1st month after birth were colic, cyanosis, rapid breathing, and irritability. Urinary retention in the neonate has been associated with maternal use of nortriptyline (chemically related to imipramine) (20).

A 2002 prospective study compared two groups of mother-child pairs exposed to antidepressants throughout gestation (46 exposed to tricyclics: 12 to imipramine, 40 to fluoxetine) to 36 nonexposed, not depressed controls (21). Offspring were studied between the ages of 15 and 71 months for effects of antidepressant exposure in terms of IQ, language, behavior, and temperament. Exposure to antidepressants did not adversely affect the measured parameters, but IQ was significantly and negatively associated with the duration of depression, and language was negatively associated with the number of depression episodes after delivery (21).

BREAST FEEDING SUMMARY

RECOMMENDATION: Limited Human Data - Potential Toxicity

Imipramine and its metabolite, desipramine, enter breast milk in low concentrations (22–24). A milk:plasma ratio of 1 has been suggested (22). Assuming a therapeutic serum level of 200 ng/mL, an infant consuming 1000 mL of breast milk would ingest a daily dose of about 0.2 mg. Ten nursing infants of mothers taking antidepressants (four with imipramine 75–150 mg/day) were compared to 15 bottle-fed infants of mothers with depression who did not breast-feed (24). Concentrations of imipramine in fore- and hindmilk ranged from 34–408 ng/mL and 48–622 ng/mL, respectively. The milk:maternal plasma ratios were 0.7–1.7 and 1.2–2.3, respectively. Two infants had plasma levels: 0.6 ng/mL (mother's dose 75 mg/day) and 3.3–7.4 ng/mL (mother's dose 75–100 mg/day). No toxic effects or delays in development were observed in the infants. The estimated daily dose consumed by the infants was about 1% of the mother's weight-adjusted dose (24).

The clinical significance of these amounts is unknown. The American Academy of Pediatrics classifies imipramine as an agent whose effect on the nursing infant is unknown but may be of concern (25).

References

1. Shepard TH. *Catalog of Teratogenic Agents*. 6th ed. Baltimore, MD: Johns Hopkins University Press, 1989: 345–6.
2. McBride WG. Limb deformities associated with iminodibenzyl hydrochloride. Med J Aust 1972;1:492.
3. Heinonen OP, Slone D, Shapiro S. *Birth Defects and Drugs in Pregnancy*. Littleton, MA: Publishing Sciences Group, 1977:336–7.
4. Kuenssberg EV, Knox JDE. Imipramine in pregnancy. Br Med J 1972;2:29.
5. Barson AJ. Malformed infant. Br Med J 1972;2:45.
6. Idanpaan-Heikkila J, Saxen L. Possible teratogenicity of imipramine/chloropyramine. Lancet 1973;2:282–3.
7. Crombie DL, Pinsent R, Fleming D. Imipramine in pregnancy. Br Med J 1972;1:745.
8. Sim M. Imipramine and pregnancy. Br Med J 1972; 2:45.
9. Scanlon FJ. Use of antidepressant drugs during the first trimester. Med J Aust 1969;2:1077.
10. Rachelefsky GS, Flynt JW, Eggin AJ, Wilson MG. Possible teratogenicity of tricyclic antidepressants. Lancet 1972;1:838.
11. Banister P, Dafoe C, Smith ESO, Miller J. Possible teratogenicity of tricyclic antidepressants. Lancet 1972;1:838–9.
12. Jacobs D. Imipramine (Tofranil). S Afr Med J 1972;46: 1023.
13. Australian Drug Evaluation Committee. Tricyclic antidepressant and limb reduction deformities. Med J Aust 1973;1:766–9.
14. Morrow AW. Imipramine and congenital abnormalities. N Z Med J 1972;75:228–9.
15. Wilson JG. Present status of drugs as teratogens in man. Teratology 1973;7:3–15.
16. McElhatton PR, Garbis HM, Elefant E, Vial T, Bellemin B, Mastroiacovo P, Arnon J, Rodriguez-Pinilla E, Schaefer C, Pexieder T, Merlob P, Dal Verme S. The outcome of pregnancy in 689 women exposed to therapeutic doses of antidepressants. A collaborative study of the European Network of Teratology Information Services (ENTIS). Reprod Toxicol 1996;10:285–94.
17. Hill RM. Will this drug harm the unborn infant? South Med J 1977;67:1476–80.
18. Eggermont E. Withdrawal symptoms in neonate associated with maternal imipramine therapy. Lancet 1973;2:680.
19. Shrand H. Agoraphobia and imipramine withdrawal? Pediatrics 1982;70:825.
20. Shearer WT, Schreiner RL, Marshall RE. Urinary retention in a neonate secondary to maternal ingestion of nortriptyline. J Pediatr 1972;81:570–2.
21. Nulman I, Rovet J, Stewart DE, Wolpin J, Pace-Asciak P, Shuhaiber S, Koren G. Child development following exposure to tricyclic antidepressants or fluoxetine throughout fetal life: a prospective, controlled study. Am J Psychiatry 2002;159:1889–95.
22. Sovner R, Orsulak PJ. Excretion of imipramine and desipramine in human breast milk. Am J Psychiatry 1979;136:451–2.
23. Erickson SH, Smith GH, Heidrich F. Tricyclics and breast-feeding. Am J Psychiatry 1979;136:1483.
24. Yoshida K, Smith B, Craggs M, Kumar RC. Investigation of pharmacokinetics and of possible adverse effects in infants exposed to tricyclic antidepressants in breast-milk. J Affect Disord 1997;43:225–37.
25. Committee on Drugs, American Academy of Pediatrics. The transfer of drugs and other chemicals into human milk. Pediatrics 2001;108:776–89.

Name:	**IMMUNE GLOBULIN, HEPATITIS B**	Risk Factor:	**C_M**
Class:	**Serum**		

FETAL RISK SUMMARY

RECOMMENDATION: Compatible

Hepatitis B immune globulin is used to provide passive immunity following exposure to hepatitis B. When hepatitis B occurs during pregnancy, an increased rate of abortion and prematurity may be observed (1). No risk to the fetus from the immune globulin has been reported (1,2). The American College of Obstetricians and Gynecologists *Technical Bulletin* No. 160 recommends use of hepatitis B immune globulin in pregnancy for postexposure prophylaxis (1).

BREAST FEEDING SUMMARY

RECOMMENDATION: No Human Data - Probably Compatible

No data are available.

References

1. American College of Obstetricians and Gynecologists. Immunization during pregnancy. *Technical Bulletin*. No. 160, October 1991.
2. Amstey MS. Vaccination in pregnancy. Clin Obstet Gynaecol 1983;10:13–22.

Name:	**IMMUNE GLOBULIN INTRAMUSCULAR**	Risk Factor:	**C_M**
Class:	**Serum**		

FETAL RISK SUMMARY

RECOMMENDATION: Compatible

Immune globulin IM (IGIM) is a solution of immunoglobulin, primarily immunoglobulin G, prepared from pooled plasma that takes 2–5 days to obtain adequate serum levels (1). It is indicated for postexposure prophylaxis of hepatitis A and measles (rubeola), and in the prevention of serious infections in patients with immunoglobulin deficiencies. In cases of rubella exposure of the pregnant woman, IGIM, 0.55 mL/kg, administered as soon as possible after exposure may prevent or modify maternal infection, but there is no evidence that it will prevent fetal infection (2). However, its use in such cases may be of benefit in women who will not consider therapeutic abortion (2).

The American College of Obstetricians and Gynecologists *Technical Bulletin* No. 160 recommends the use of IGIM for postexposure prophylaxis of hepatitis A and measles (rubeola) (3). No risk to the fetus from this therapy has been reported (3).

BREAST FEEDING SUMMARY

RECOMMENDATION: No Human Data - Probably Compatible

No data are available.

References

1. Product information. Gammar. Armour Pharmaceutical Co., 1993.
2. American Academy of Pediatrics and the American College of Obstetricians and Gynecologists. *Guidelines for Perinatal Care*. 3rd Ed. Elk Grove Village, IL: American Academy of Pediatrics, and Washington, DC: American College of Obstetricians and Gynecologists, 1992:129.
3. American College of Obstetricians and Gynecologists. Immunization during pregnancy. *Technical Bulletin*. No. 160, October 1991.

Name:	**IMMUNE GLOBULIN INTRAVENOUS**	Risk Factor:	**C_M**
Class:	**Serum**		

FETAL RISK SUMMARY

RECOMMENDATION: Compatible

I

Immune globulin IV (IGIV) is a solution of immunoglobulin, primarily immunoglobulin G (IgG), prepared from pooled plasma that, in contrast to the IM preparation, provides immediate serum concentrations of antibodies (1).

IgG administered IV was shown to cross the human placenta in significant amounts only if the gestational age was greater than 32 weeks (2). Placental transfer was also a function of dose, as well as gestational age. Four subclasses of IgG and two different antibodies in the preparation also crossed to the fetus in a similar manner (2). Others have found that the placental transfer of exogenous IgG is dependent on the dose and duration of treatment and, possibly, on the method of IgG preparation (3).

A 1988 review of IGIV summarized the clinical indications for the product in pregnancy (4). The indications included hypogammaglobulinemia such as common variable immunodeficiency, autoimmune diseases such as chronic immune thrombocytopenic purpura, and alloimmune disorders such as severe Rh-immunization disease and alloimmune thrombocytopenia. Recent reports have described the use of IGIV for the prevention of intracranial hemorrhage in fetal alloimmune thrombocytopenia (5,6), recurrent abortions caused by antiphospholipid antibodies (7,8), neonatal congenital heart block caused by maternal antibodies to Ro (SS-A) and La (SS-B) autoantigens (9), and severe isoimmunization with either Rh or Kell antibodies (10). No adverse effects were observed in the fetus or newborns in any of the above reports, but caution has been advised in its use to prevent spontaneous abortion (11).

BREAST FEEDING SUMMARY

RECOMMENDATION: No Human Data - Probably Compatible

No data are available.

References

1. Product information. Gamimune N. Miles, Inc., 1993.
2. Sidiropoulos D, Herrmann U Jr, Morell A, von Muralt G, Barandun S. Transplacental passage of intravenous immunoglobulin in the last trimester of pregnancy. J Pediatr 1986;109:505–8.
3. Smith CIE, Hammarström SL. Intravenous immunoglobulin in pregnancy. Obstet Gynecol 1985; 66(Suppl):39S–40S.
4. Sacher RA, King JC. Intravenous gamma-globulin in pregnancy: a review. Obstet Gynecol Surv 1988; 44:25–34.
5. Lynch L, Bussel JB, McFarland JG, Chitkara U, Berkowitz RL. Antenatal treatment of alloimmune thrombocytopenia. Obstet Gynecol 1992;80: 67–71.
6. Wenstrom KD, Weiner CP, Williamson RA. Antenatal

treatment of fetal alloimmune thrombocytopenia. Obstet Gynecol 1992;80:433–5.
7. Scott JR, Branch DW, Kochenour NK, Ward K. Intravenous immunoglobulin treatment of pregnant patients with recurrent pregnancy loss caused by antiphospholipid antibodies and Rh immunization. Am J Obstet Gynecol 1988;159:1055–6.
8. Orvieto R, Achiron A, Ben-Rafael Z, Achiron R. Intravenous immunoglobulin treatment for recurrent abortions caused by antiphospholipid antibodies. Fertil Steril 1991;56:1013–20.
9. Kaaja R, Julkunen H, Ämmälä P, Teppo A-M, Kurki P. Congenital heart block: successful prophylactic treatment with intravenous gamma globulin and corticosteroid therapy. Am J Obstet Gynecol 1991;165:1333–4.
10. Chitkara U, Bussel J, Alvarez M, Lynch L, Meisel RL, Berkowitz RL. High-dose intravenous gamma globulin: does it have a role in the treatment of severe erythroblastosis fetalis? Obstet Gynecol 1990;76:703–8.
11. Marzusch K, Tinneberg H, Mueller-Eckhardt G, Kaveri SV, Hinney B, Redman C. Is immunotherapy justified for recurrent spontaneous abortion? Lancet 1992, 339:1543.

Name:	**IMMUNE GLOBULIN, RABIES**	Risk Factor:	C_M
Class:	**Serum**		

FETAL RISK SUMMARY

RECOMMENDATION: Compatible

Rabies immune globulin is used to provide passive immunity following exposure to rabies combined with active immunization with rabies vaccine (1). Because rabies is nearly 100% fatal if contracted, both the immune globulin and the vaccine should be given for postexposure prophylaxis (1). No risk to the fetus from the immune globulin has been reported (see also Vaccine, Rabies (Human)) (1,2). The American College of Obstetricians and Gynecologists *Technical Bulletin* No. 160 recommends use of rabies immune globulin in pregnancy for postexposure prophylaxis (1).

BREAST FEEDING SUMMARY

RECOMMENDATION: No Human Data - Probably Compatible

No data are available.

References

1. American College of Obstetricians and Gynecologists. Immunization during pregnancy. *Technical Bulletin*. No. 160, October 1991.
2. Amstey MS. Vaccination in pregnancy. Clin Obstet Gynaecol 1983;10:13–22.

Name:	**IMMUNE GLOBULIN, TETANUS**	Risk Factor:	C_M
Class:	**Serum**		

FETAL RISK SUMMARY

RECOMMENDATION: Compatible

Tetanus immune globulin is used to provide passive immunity following exposure to tetanus combined with active immunization with tetanus toxoid (1). Tetanus produces severe morbidity and mortality in both the mother and newborn. No risk to the fetus from the immune globulin has been reported (1,2). The American College of Obstetricians and Gynecologists

Technical Bulletin No. 160 recommends the use of tetanus immune globulin in pregnancy for postexposure prophylaxis (1).

BREAST FEEDING SUMMARY

RECOMMENDATION: No Human Data - Probably Compatible

No data are available.

References

1. American College of Obstetricians and Gynecologists. Immunization during pregnancy. *Technical Bulletin*. No. 160, October 1991.
2. Amstey MS. Vaccination in pregnancy. Clin Obstet Gynaecol 1983;10:13–22.

Name:	**IMMUNE GLOBULIN, VARICELLA-ZOSTER (HUMAN)**	Risk Factor:	**C**
Class:	**Serum**		

FETAL RISK SUMMARY

RECOMMENDATION: Compatible

Varicella-Zoster (human) immune globulin (VZIG) is obtained from the plasma of normal volunteer blood donors. In most of United States, it is available from the American Red Cross Blood Services.

Varicella-zoster immune globulin is indicated for susceptible (seronegative) pregnant women exposed to chickenpox because of the increased severity of maternal chickenpox, including death, in adults compared with children (1–13). One reference cited the increased risk of complications in adults as 9–25-fold greater than in children (4). It is not known whether administration of VZIG to the mother will protect the fetus from infection or the low risk of defects associated with the congenital varicella syndrome (1,9,11,12). Moreover, VZIG may modify the mother's infection such that she has a subclinical, asymptomatic infection, but not prevent fetal infection or disease (1,9,10,12).

Congenital malformations following intrauterine varicella in pregnancy are relatively uncommon, but case reports have periodically appeared since 1947 (5–7,9,10,14–18). In addition to cicatricial skin lesions, defects associated with this syndrome involve the brain, eyes, skeleton, and gastrointestinal and genitourinary tracts, with the highest risk occurring if the mother has varicella between the 8th and 21st weeks of gestation (5,7,9,18), although one case occurred when the mother had varicella at 25.5 weeks' gestation (19). One review (9) found that the incidence of congenital malformations after 1st trimester chickenpox infection was 2.3% (3/131; 95% confidence intervals 0.5%–6.5%), but a second review (5) found a lower rate of 1.3% (4/308) if all cases of intrauterine varicella infection were included.

There is no known fetal risk from passive immunization of pregnant women with varicella-zoster immune globulin (1,13). Administration of VZIG to newborns of mothers who develop varicella within a 5-day interval before or 48 hours after delivery is recommended (1,5,9,11–13).

The American College of Obstetricians and Gynecologists *Technical Bulletin* No. 160 recommends one IM dose of the immune globulin be given to healthy pregnant women within 96 hours of exposure to varicella to protect against maternal, but not congenital, infection (13).

BREAST FEEDING SUMMARY

RECOMMENDATION: No Human Data - Probably Compatible

No data are available.

References

1. Centers for Disease Control. Immunization Practices Advisory Committee. Varicella-zoster immune globulin for the prevention of chickenpox. MMWR 1984;33:84–100.
2. Enders G. Management of varicella-zoster contact and infection in pregnancy using a standardized varicella-zoster ELISA test. Postgrad Med J 1985;61(Suppl 4):23–30.
3. McGregor JA, Mark S, Crawford GP, Levin MJ. Varicella zoster antibody testing in the care of pregnant women exposed to varicella. Am J Obstet Gynecol 1987;157:281–4.
4. Greenspoon JS, Masaki DI. Screening for varicella-zoster immunity and the use of varicella zoster immune globulin in pregnancy. Am J Obstet Gynecol 1989,160.1020–1.
5. Sterner G, Forsgren M, Enocksson E, Grandien M, Granstrom G. Varicella-zoster infections in late pregnancy. Scand J Infect Dis 1990;Suppl 71:30–5.
6. Prober CG, Gershon AA, Grose C, McCracken GH Jr, Nelson JD. Consensus: varicella-zoster infections in pregnancy and the perinatal period. Pediatr Infect Dis J 1990;9:865–9.
7. Brunell PA. Varicella in pregnancy, the fetus, and the newborn: problems in management. J Infect Dis 1992;166(Suppl 1):S42–7.
8. Wallace MR, Hooper DG. Varicella in pregnancy, the fetus, and the newborn: problems in management. J Infect Dis 1993;167:254.
9. McIntosh D, Isaacs D. Varicella zoster virus infection in pregnancy. Arch Dis Child Fetal Neonatal 1993;68:1–2.
10. Faix RG. Maternal immunization to prevent fetal and neonatal infection. Clin Obstet Gynecol 1991;34:277–87.
11. Committee on Infectious Diseases, American Academy of Pediatrics. Varicella-zoster infections. In *Report of the Committee on Infectious Diseases*. 22nd ed. Elk Grove Village, IL: American Academy of Pediatrics, 1991:521–2.
12. Brown ZA, Watts DH. Antiviral therapy in pregnancy. Clin Obstet Gynecol 1990;33:276–89.
13. American College of Obstetricians and Gynecologists. Immunization during pregnancy. *Technical Bulletin*. No. 160, October 1991.
14. Laforet EG, Lynch CL Jr. Multiple congenital defects following maternal varicella: report of a case. N Engl J Med 1947;236:534–7.
15. Brice JEH. Congenital varicella resulting from infection during second trimester of pregnancy. Arch Dis Child 1976;51:474–6.
16. Bai APV, John TJ. Congenital skin ulcers following varicella in late pregnancy. J Pediatr 1979;94:65–7.
17. Preblud SR, Cochi SL, Orenstein WA. Varicella-zoster infection in pregnancy. N Engl J Med 1986;315:1416–7.
18. Alkalay AL, Pomerance JJ, Rimoin DL. Fetal varicella syndrome. J Pediatr 1987;111:320–3.
19. Salzman MB, Sood SK. Congenital anomalies resulting from maternal varicella at $25^1/_2$ weeks of gestation. Pediatr Infect Dis J 1992;11:504–5.

Name:	**INDAPAMIDE**	Risk Factor:	B_M*
Class:	**Diuretic**		

FETAL RISK SUMMARY

RECOMMENDATION: Limited Human Data - Animal Data Suggest Low Risk

Indapamide is an oral active antihypertensive-diuretic of the indoline class that is closely related to the thiazide diuretics (see also Chlorothiazide for a discussion of this class of diuretics). No evidence of impaired fertility, fetal harm, or effect on postnatal development was observed in mice, rats, or rabbits given doses up to 6,250 times the therapeutic human dose during pregnancy (1). However, fetal growth retardation has been reported in rats dosed at 1000 mg/kg/day (2).

In a surveillance study of Michigan Medicaid recipients conducted between 1985 and 1992 involving 229,101 completed pregnancies, 46 newborns had been exposed to indapamide during the 1st trimester (F. Rosa, personal communication, FDA, 1993). Three (6.5%) major birth defects were observed (two expected). Details on the malformations were not available, but no anomalies were observed in six defect categories (cardiovascular defects, oral clefts, spina bifida, polydactyly, limb reduction defects, and hypospadias) for which specific data were available.

In general, diuretics are not recommended for the treatment of gestational hypertension because of the maternal hypovolemia characteristic of this disease.

[*Risk Factor D if used in gestational hypertension.*]

BREAST FEEDING SUMMARY

RECOMMENDATION: No Human Data - Probably Compatible

No reports describing the use of indapamide during lactation have been located. The closely related thiazide diuretics have been used to suppress lactation (see Chlorothiazide).

I

References

1. Product information. Indapamide Tablets, USP. Mylan Pharmaceuticals, 2000.
2. Seki T, Fujitani M, Osumi S, Yamamoto T, Eguchi K, Inoue N, Sakka N, Suzuki MR. Reproductive studies of indapamide. Yakuri to Chiryo 1982;10:1325–35, 1337–53, 1355–414. As cited in Shepard TH. *Catalog of Teratogenic Agents*. 6th ed. Baltimore, MD: Johns Hopkins University Press, 1989:347.

Name:	**INDIGO CARMINE**	Risk Factor:	**B**
Class:	**Dye (Diagnostic)**		

FETAL RISK SUMMARY

RECOMMENDATION: Limited Human Data - No Relevant Animal Data

Indigo carmine is used as a diagnostic dye. No reports linking its use with congenital defects have been located. Intra-amniotic injection has been conducted without apparent effect on the fetus (1–3). Because of its known toxicities after IV administration, however, the dye should not be considered totally safe (4).

A report of jejunal atresia, possibly secondary to the use of methylene blue (see Methylene Blue) during genetic amniocentesis in pregnancies with twins was published in 1992 (5). A portion of this report described 67 newborns treated for the defect, 20 of whom were one of a set of twins. Of these latter cases, 2nd-trimester amniocentesis had been performed with indigo carmine in 1 case and with methylene blue in 18 cases. An accompanying commentary noted that indigo carmine, like methylene blue, is a vasoconstrictor and may also induce small-bowel atresia (6).

A brief 1993 report described the use of indigo carmine in women with twins who underwent amniocentesis between 1977 and 1991 in the United States (7). A total of 195 women were included, 78 (40%) of whom were administered indigo carmine during the procedure. Of the 156 fetuses (total data included live births, stillbirths, intrauterine deaths, and fetuses that were electively terminated; specific data for indigo carmine was not given), 7 (4.5%) had a major birth defect. Included in this number were two infants from the same set of twins who had syndactyly, clubfoot (one), hydrocephaly (one), urethral obstruction sequence (one), and multiple congenital defects (two) (7). None of the exposed infants had small intestinal atresia.

BREAST FEEDING SUMMARY

RECOMMENDATION: No Human Data - Probably Compatible

No data are available.

References

1. Elias S, Gerbie AB, Simpson JL, Nadler HL, Sabbagha RE, Shkolnik A. Genetic amniocentesis in twin gestations. Am J Obstet Gynecol 1980;138:169–74.
2. Horger EO III, Moody LO. Use of indigo carmine for twin amniocentesis and its effect on bilirubin analysis. Am J Obstet Gynecol 1984;150:858–60.
3. Pijpers L, Jahoda MGJ, Vosters RPL, Niermeijer MF, Sachs ES. Genetic amniocentesis in twin pregnancies. Br J Obstet Gynaecol 1988;95:323–6.
4. Fribourg S. Safety of intraamniotic injection of indigo carmine. Am J Obstet Gynecol 1981;140:350–1.
5. Van Der Pol JG, Wolf H, Boer K, Treffers PE, Leschot NJ, Hey HA, Vos A. Jejunal atresia related to the use of methylene blue in genetic amniocentesis in twins. Br J Obstet Gynaecol 1992;99:141–3.
6. McFadyen I. The dangers of intra amniotic methylene blue. Br J Obstet Gynaecol 1992;99:89–90.
7. Cragan JD, Martin ML, Khoury MJ, Fernhoff PM. Dye use during amniocentesis and birth defects. Lancet 1993;341:1352.

Name: **INDINAVIR** Risk Factor: **C_M**

Class: **Antiviral**

FETAL RISK SUMMARY

RECOMMENDATION: Compatible - Maternal Benefit >> Embryo/Fetal Risk

The antiretroviral agent, indinavir, is an inhibitor of the human immunodeficiency virus (HIV) protease, an enzyme that is required for the cleavage of viral polyprotein precursors into active functional proteins found in infectious HIV. Other drugs in this class are amprenavir, nelfinavir, ritonavir, and saquinavir.

Indinavir was not teratogenic in rats and rabbits at doses comparable to or slightly higher than those used in humans (1). In rats, however, an increase in the incidence of supernumerary ribs (at exposures at or less than those in humans) and cervical ribs (at exposures at or slightly greater than those in humans) were observed. These changes were not observed in rabbits and no effects were noted on embryonic and/or fetal survival or on fetal weight in either rats or rabbits. A study in dogs (because fetal exposure was about 2% of maternal levels in rabbits) observed no indinavir-related effects on embryo or fetal survival, fetal weight, or teratogenicity. At the highest dose tested in dogs, 80 mg/kg/day, fetal drug levels were about 50% of the maternal levels (1).

A study of the developmental toxicity of indinavir in rats was reported in 2000 (2). Pregnant rats were given an oral dose of 500 mg/kg once daily during day 6 to 15 of gestation or twice daily from day 9 to 11 of gestation (a dose of 640 mg/kg/day produces systemic exposure in the rat that is comparable to or slightly greater than human exposure). In both groups, an increased incidence of supernumerary ribs and variations of the vertebral ossification centers occurred, but no effects on litter sizes, fetal weight, or viability were observed (2). Unilateral anophthalmia was observed in 7 pups (3%) from 2 of the 19 litters

(2). On examination, the ocular bulbs were noted to be absent and the bulbar cavity was filled with an enlarged lacrimal gland. No such cases were noted in controls. Other postnatal abnormalities included delayed fur development, eye opening, and slightly earlier descent of the testis. In addition, some liver changes were noted in dams (hepatocellular inclusions of lipids and myelin figure-like structures) and in offspring (infiltration with granulocytes) (2).

It is not known if indinavir crosses the human placenta. The molecular weight (about 712 for the sulfate salt) is low enough that transfer to the fetus should be expected. The drug has been found in fetal plasma of rats, rabbits, dogs, and Rhesus monkeys (1). In Rhesus monkeys, fetal plasma drug levels were 1% to 2% of maternal plasma levels about 1 hour after a dose given in the 3rd trimester (1).

The pharmacokinetics of indinavir during pregnancy have been reported in two women (800 mg every 8 hours) (3). A marked decrease in maternal drug concentrations occurred around 33–34 weeks' gestation, suggesting that women may be exposed to subtherapeutic levels late in pregnancy (3).

The Antiretroviral Pregnancy Registry reported, for the period January 1989 through January 2004, prospective data (reported to the Registry before the outcomes were known) involving 1537 live births that had been exposed during the 1st trimester to one or more antiretroviral agents (4). Forty-seven of the newborns had congenital defects (3.1%, 95% confidence interval [CI] 2.3–4.1). In the 2407 live births with earliest exposure in the 2nd/3rd trimesters, there were 56 infants with defects (2.3%, 95% CI 1.8–3.0). The prevalence rates for the two periods did not differ significantly. There were 103 infants with birth defects among 3944 live births with exposure anytime during pregnancy (2.6%, 95% CI 2.1–3.2). The prevalence rate did not differ significantly from the rate expected in a nonexposed population (4). There were 281 outcomes exposed to indinavir (179 in the 1st trimester and 102 in the 2nd/3rd trimesters) in combination with other antiretroviral agents. There were five birth defects among the 1st trimester exposures and one in those exposed in the 2nd/3rd trimesters. In reviewing the birth defects of prospective and retrospective (pregnancies reported after the outcomes were known) registered cases, and clinical reports, the Registry concluded that there was no pattern of anomalies to suggest a common cause (4). (See Lamivudine for required statement.)

In an unusual case, a woman was exposed to HIV through self-insemination with fresh semen obtained from a man with a high HIV ribonucleic acid viral load (>750,000 copies/mL plasma) (5). Ten days later, she was started on a prophylactic regimen of indinavir (2400 mg/day), zidovudine (600 mg/day), and lamivudine (300 mg/day). Pregnancy was confirmed 14 days after insemination. The indinavir dose was reduced to 1800 mg/day, 4 weeks after the start of therapy because of the development of renal calculi. All antiretroviral therapy was stopped after 9 weeks because of negative tests for HIV. She gave birth at 40 weeks' gestation to a healthy 3490-g male infant, without evidence of HIV disease, who was developing normally at 2 years of age (5).

The experience of one perinatal center with the treatment of HIV-infected pregnant women was summarized in a 1999 abstract (6). Of 55 women receiving ≥3 antiviral drugs, 39 were treated with a protease inhibitor (5 with indinavir). The outcomes included 2 spontaneous abortions, 5 elective abortions, 27 newborns, and 5 ongoing pregnancies. One woman was taken off of indinavir because of ureteral obstruction and another (drug therapy not specified) developed gestational diabetes. None of the newborns tested positive for HIV or had major congenital anomalies or complications (6).

A study published in 1999 evaluated the safety, efficacy, and perinatal transmission rates of HIV in 30 pregnant women receiving various combinations of antiretroviral agents

(7). Many of the women were substance abusers. Protease inhibitors (indinavir [*N* = 6], nelfinavir [*N* = 7], and saquinavir [*N* = 1] in combination with nelfinavir) were used in 13 of the women. Antiretroviral therapy was initiated at a median of 14 weeks' gestation (range preconception to 32 weeks). In spite of previous histories of extensive antiretroviral experience and of vertical transmission of HIV, combination therapy was effective in treating maternal disease and in preventing transmission to the current newborns. The outcomes of the pregnancies treated with protease inhibitors appeared to be similar to the 17 cases that did not receive these agents, except that the birth weights were lower (7).

Indinavir has frequently produced hyperbilirubinemia in adults, but it is not known whether treatment of the mother prior to delivery will exacerbate physiologic hyperbilirubinemia in the neonate (1). No such effects have been observed in Rhesus monkey neonates exposed *in utero* to indinavir during the 3rd trimester (1).

A public health advisory has been issued by the Food and Drug Administration (FDA) on the association between protease inhibitors and diabetes mellitus (8). Because pregnancy is a risk factor for hyperglycemia, there was concern that these antiviral agents would exacerbate this risk. An abstract published in 2000 described the results of a study involving 34 pregnant women treated with protease inhibitors (4 with indinavir) compared to 41 controls that evaluated the association with diabetes (9). No relationship between protease inhibitors and an increased incidence of gestational diabetes was found.

A multicenter, retrospective survey of pregnancies exposed to protease inhibitors was published in 2000 (10). There were 92 liveborn infants delivered from 89 women (3 sets of twins) at six health care centers. One nonviable infant, born at 22 weeks' gestation, died. The surviving 91 infants were evaluated in terms of adverse effects, prematurity rate, and frequency of HIV-1 transmission. Most of the infants were exposed *in utero* to a single protease inhibitor, but a few were exposed to more than one because of sequential or double combined therapy. The number of newborns exposed to each protease inhibitor was indinavir (*N* = 23), nelfinavir (*N* = 39), ritonavir (*N* = 5), and saquinavir (*N* = 34). Protease inhibitors were started before conception in 18, during the 1st, 2nd, or 3rd trimesters in 12, 44, and 14, respectively, and not reported in one. Other antiretrovirals used with the protease inhibitors included four nucleoside reverse transcriptase inhibitors (NRTI) (didanosine, lamivudine, stavudine, and zidovudine). The most common NRTI regimen was a combination of zidovudine and lamivudine (65% of women). In addition, seven women were enrolled in the AIDS Clinical Trials Group Protocol 316 and, at the start of labor, received either a single dose of the non-nucleoside reverse transcriptase inhibitor, nevirapine, or placebo. Maternal conditions, thought possibly or likely to be related to therapy, were mild anemia in eight, severe anemia in one (probably secondary to zidovudine), and thrombocytopenia in one. Gestational diabetes mellitus was observed in three women (3.3%), a rate similar to the expected prevalence of 2.6% in a nonexposed population (10). One mother developed postpartum cardiomyopathy and died 2 months after birth of twins, but the cause death was not known. For the surviving newborns, there was no increase in adverse effects over that observed in previous clinical trials of HIV-positive women, including the prevalence of anemia (12%), hyperbilirubinemia (6%; none exposed to indinavir), and low birth weight (20.6%). Premature delivery occurred in 19.1% of the pregnancies (close to the expected rate). The percentage of infants infected with HIV was 0 (95% CI 0%–3%) (10).

In summary, the limited human data do not suggest a major embryo/fetal risk, but the animal data involving birth defects is a concern. The finding of anophthalmia in rat pups at a systemic exposure approximately equivalent to human exposure needs further investigation. The authors of that study also observed anophthalmia in a rat experiment with ritonavir (1 of 113 offspring, unpublished data), another protease inhibitor (2). An editorial, accompanying this study, reviewed how the changes in the treatment of HIV disease (e.g., multiple combinations of drugs; use of agents throughout gestation) were altering the risk:benefit ratio of antiretroviral therapy during pregnancy (11).

Two reviews, one in 1996 and the other in 1997, concluded that all women currently receiving antiretroviral therapy should continue to receive therapy during pregnancy and that treatment of the mother with monotherapy should be considered inadequate therapy (12,13). In 1998, the Centers for Disease Control and Prevention (CDC) made a similar recommendation that antiretroviral therapy should be continued during pregnancy, but discontinuation of all therapy during the 1st trimester was a consideration (8). If indicated, therefore, protease inhibitors, including indinavir, should not be withheld in pregnancy (with the possible exception of the 1st trimester) because the expected benefit to the HIV-positive mother probably outweighs the unknown risks to the fetus. For indinavir, these theoretical risks include birth defects, hyperbilirubinemia, complications of maternal diabetes, and renal stones. Pregnant women taking protease inhibitors should be monitored for hyperglycemia. Because of the potential for hyperbilirubinemia with indinavir, one review suggested that ritonavir (see Ritonavir) may be a more appropriate first-choice drug (13). Moreover, indinavir has been associated with the development of renal stones in adults and, if significant human placental transfer occurs, maternal usage near delivery may, theoretically, cause development of renal toxicity in the newborn. The combination of immature neonatal renal function and the potential for suboptimal hydration may allow for high or prolonged concentrations of the drug leading to crystallization and renal stones. Finally, the efficacy and safety of combined therapy in preventing vertical transmission of HIV to the newborn are unknown, and zidovudine remains the only antiretroviral agent currently recommended for this purpose (12,13).

BREAST FEEDING SUMMARY

RECOMMENDATION: Contraindicated

No reports describing the use of indinavir during lactation have been located. The antiviral agent is excreted into the milk of lactating rats (1). The molecular weight (about 712 for the sulfate salt) is low enough that excretion into breast milk should be expected.

Reports on the use of indinavir during lactation are unlikely because of the potential toxicity in the nursing infant, especially hyperbilirubinemia, and because the drug is indicated in the treatment of patient's with HIV. HIV type 1 (HIV-1) is transmitted in milk, and in developed countries, breast-feeding is not recommended (12–16). In developing countries, breast-feeding is undertaken, despite the risk, because there are no affordable milk substitutes available. Until 1999, no studies have been published that examined the effect of any antiretroviral therapy on HIV-1 transmission in milk. In that year, a study involving zidovudine was published that measured a 38% reduction in vertical transmission of HIV-1 infection in spite of breast-feeding when compared to controls (see Zidovudine).

References

1. Product information. Crixivan. Merck, 2001.
2. Riecke K, Schultz TG, Shakibaei M, Krause B, Chahoud I, Stahlmann R. Developmental toxicity of the HIV-protease inhibitor indinavir in rats. Teratology 2000;62:291–300.
3. Hayashi S, Beckerman K, Homma M, Kosel BW, Aweeka FT. Pharmacokinetics of indinavir in HIV-positive pregnant women. AIDS 2000;14:1061–2.
4. Antiretroviral Pregnancy Registry Steering Committee. *Antiretroviral Pregnancy Registry International Interim Report for 1 January 1989 through 31 January 2004.* Wilmington, NC: Registry Coordinating Center, 2004.

5. Bloch M, Carr A, Vasak E, Cunningham P, Smith D. The use of human immunodeficiency virus postexposure prophylaxis after successful artificial insemination. Am J Obstet Gynecol 1999;181:760–1.
6. Stek A, Kramer F, Fassen M, Khoury M. The safety and efficacy of protease inhibitor therapy for HIV infection during pregnancy (abstract). Am J Obstet Gynecol 1999;180:S7.
7. McGowan JP, Crane M, Wiznia AA, Blum S. Combination antiretroviral therapy in human immunodeficiency virus-infected pregnant women. Obstet Gynecol 1999;94:641–6.
8. CDC. Public Health Service Task Force recommendations for the use of antiretroviral drugs in pregnant women infected with HIV-1 for maternal health and for reducing perinatal HIV-1 transmission in the United States. MMWR 1998:47:No. RR-2.
9. Fassett M, Kramer F, Stek A. Treatment with protease inhibitors in pregnancy is not associated with an increased incidence of gestational diabetes (abstract). Am J Obstet Gynecol 2000;182:S97.
10. Morris AB, Cu-Uvin S, Harwell JI, Garb J, Zorrilla C, Vajaranant M, Dobles AR, Jones TB, Carlan S, Allen DY. Multicenter review of protease inhibitors in 89 pregnancies. J Acquir Immune Defic Syndr 2000;25: 306–11.
11. Miller RK. Anti-HIV therapy during pregnancy: risk-benefit ratio. Teratology 2000;62:288–90.
12. Carpenter CCJ, Fischi MA, Hammer SM, Hirsch MS, Jacobsen DM, Katzenstein DA, Montaner JSG, Richman DD, Saag MS, Schooley RT, Thompson MA, Vella S, Yeni PG, Volberding PA. Antiretroviral therapy for HIV infection in 1996. JAMA 1996;276:146–54.
13. Minkoff H, Augenbraun M. Antiretroviral therapy for pregnant women. Am J Obstet Gynecol 1997; 176:478–89.
14. Brown ZA, Watts DH. Antiviral therapy in pregnancy. Clin Obstet Gynecol 1990;33:276–89.
15. de Martino M, Tovo P-A, Pezzotti P, Galli L, Massironi E, Ruga E, Floreea F, Plebani A, Gabiano C, Zuccotti GV. HIV-1 transmission through breast-milk: appraisal of risk according to duration of feeding. AIDS 1992;6:991–7.
16. Van de Perre P. Postnatal transmission of human immunodeficiency virus type 1: the breast feeding dilemma. Am J Obstet Gynecol 1995;173:483–7.

I

Name:	**INDOMETHACIN**	Risk Factor:	**B**[M]
Class:	**Nonsteroidal Anti-inflammatory**		

FETAL RISK SUMMARY

RECOMMENDATION: Human Data Suggest Risk in 1st and 3rd Trimesters

Indomethacin is a nonsteroidal anti-inflammatory drug (NSAID). It is indicated for the relief of the signs and symptoms of moderate-to-severe rheumatoid arthritis, osteoarthritis, gouty arthritis, ankylosing spondylitis, and acute painful shoulder (bursitis and/or tendinitis). Indomethacin is in the same subclass (acetic acids) as three other NSAIDs (diclofenac, sulindac, and tolmetin).

Shepard reviewed four reproduction studies on the use of indomethacin in mice and rats (1). Fused ribs, vertebral abnormalities, and other skeletal defects were seen in mouse fetuses, but no malformations were observed in rats except for premature closure of the ductus arteriosus in some fetuses. A 1990 report described an investigation on the effects of several nonsteroidal anti-inflammatory agents on mouse palatal fusion both *in vivo* and *in vitro* (2). All of the compounds were found to induce some degree of cleft palate, although indomethacin was associated with the lowest frequency of cleft palate of the five agents tested (diclofenac, indomethacin, mefenamic acid, naproxen, and sulindac).

Indomethacin crosses the placenta to the fetus with concentrations in the fetus equal to those in the mother (3). Twenty-six women, between 23 and 37 weeks' gestation, who were undergoing cordocentesis for varying indications, were given a single 50-mg oral dose approximately 6 hours before the procedure. Mean maternal and fetal indomethacin levels were 218 and 219 ng/mL, respectively, producing a mean ratio of 0.97. The mean amniotic fluid level, 21 ng/mL, collected during cordocentesis, was significantly lower than the maternal and fetal concentrations. Neither fetal nor amniotic fluid concentrations varied with gestational age.

In a surveillance study of Michigan Medicaid recipients conducted between 1985 and 1992 involving 229,101 completed pregnancies, 114 newborns had been exposed to indomethacin during the 1st trimester (F. Rosa, personal communication, FDA, 1993). Seven (6.1%) major birth defects were observed (five expected), two of which were cardiovascular defects (one expected). No anomalies were observed in five other defect categories (oral clefts, spina bifida, polydactyly, limb reduction defects, and hypospadias) for which specific data were available.

A combined 2001 population-based observational cohort study and a case-control study estimated the risk of adverse pregnancy outcome from the use of NSAIDs (4). The use of NSAIDs during pregnancy was not associated with congenital malformations, preterm delivery, or low birth weight, but a positive association was discovered with spontaneous abortions (SABs). A similar study, also published in 2001, failed to find a relationship, in general, between NSAIDs and congenital malformations, but did find a significant association with cardiac defects and orofacial clefts (5). In addition, a 2003 study found a significant association between exposure to NSAIDs in early pregnancy and SABs (6). (See Ibuprofen for details on these three studies.)

A brief 2003 editorial on the potential for NSAID-induced developmental toxicity concluded that NSAIDs, and specifically those with greater COX-2 affinity, had a lower risk of this toxicity in humans than aspirin (7).

Indomethacin is occasionally used in the treatment of premature labor (8–40). The drug acts as a prostaglandin synthesis inhibitor and is an effective tocolytic agent, including in those cases resistant to β-mimetics. Niebyl (33) reviewed this topic in 1981. Daily doses ranged from 100 to 200 mg usually by the oral route, but rectal administration was used as well. In most cases, indomethacin, either alone or in combination with other tocolytics, was successful in postponing delivery until fetal lung maturation had occurred. More recent reviews on the use of indomethacin as a tocolytic agent appeared in 1992 (37) and 1993 (38). The latter review concluded that the prostaglandin synthesis inhibitors, such as indomethacin, might be the only effective tocolytic drugs (38).

In a 1986 report, 46 infants exposed *in utero* to indomethacin for maternal tocolysis were compared with two control groups: (a) 43 infants exposed to other tocolytics and (b) 46 infants whose mothers were not treated with tocolytics (34). Indomethacin-treated women received one or two courses of 150 mg orally over 24 hours, all before 34 weeks' gestation. No significant differences were observed between the groups in Apgar scores, birth weight, or gestational age at birth. Similarly, no differences were found in the number of neonatal complications such as hypocalcemia, hypoglycemia, respiratory distress syndrome, need for continuous positive airway pressure, pneumothorax, patent ductus arteriosus, sepsis, exchange transfusion for hyperbilirubinemia, congenital anomalies, or mortality (34).

A 1989 study compared indomethacin, 100-mg rectal suppository followed by 25 mg orally every 4 hours for 48 hours, with IV ritodrine in 106 women in preterm labor with intact membranes who were at a gestational age of 32 weeks or less (39). Fifty-two women received indomethacin and 54 received ritodrine. Thirteen (24%) of the ritodrine group developed adverse drug reactions severe enough to require discontinuance of the drug and a change to magnesium sulfate: cardiac arrhythmia ($N = 1$), chest pain ($N = 2$), tachycardia ($N = 3$), and hypotension ($N = 7$). None of the indomethacin-treated women developed drug intolerance ($p < 0.01$). The outcomes of the pregnancies were similar, regardless of whether delivery occurred close to the time of therapy or not. Of those delivered within 48 hours of initiation of therapy, the mean glucose level in the ritodrine-exposed newborns ($N = 9$) was significantly higher than the level in those exposed to indomethacin

($N = 8$), 198 vs. 80 mg/dL ($p < 0.05$), respectively. No cases of premature closure of the ductus arteriosus or pulmonary hypertension were observed. A reduction in amniotic fluid volume was noted in 3 (5.6%) of the ritodrine group and in 6 (11.5%) of those treated with indomethacin. On a cost basis, tocolysis with indomethacin was 17 times less costly than tocolysis with ritodrine (39).

The tocolytic effects of indomethacin and magnesium sulfate ($MgSO_4$) were compared in a study of women in labor at less than 32 weeks' gestation (40). A total of 49 women were treated with indomethacin, 100 mg per rectum followed by 25 mg orally every 4 hours for 48 hours, whereas 52 women were administered IV $MgSO_4$. Women who had responded to the initial treatment were then changed to oral terbutaline. All women received betamethasone and vitamin K and some received IV phenobarbital as prophylaxis against hyaline membrane disease and neonatal intracranial hemorrhage. Both indomethacin and $MgSO_4$ were effective in delaying delivery more than 48 hours, 90% vs. 85%, respectively, and combined with terbutaline, in extending the gestation, 22.9 vs. 22.7 days, respectively (40). Renal function of the newborns delivering at ≤48 hours (indomethacin, $N = 5$; $MgSO_4$, $N = 8$) as measured by blood urea nitrogen, creatinine, and urine output during the first 2 days after birth were statistically similar between the groups. Other neonatal outcomes, including the incidence of respiratory distress syndrome, intraventricular hemorrhage (all grades), and intraventricular hemorrhage (grades 3 and 4), were also similar. Tocolytic therapy was discontinued in eight (15%) of the women treated with $MgSO_4$ because of maternal adverse reactions compared with none in the indomethacin group ($p < 0.05$) (40).

Complications associated with the use of indomethacin during pregnancy may include premature closure of the ductus arteriosus, which may result in primary pulmonary hypertension of the newborn and, in severe cases, neonatal death (8–12,37,38,41–48). Ductal constriction is dependent on the gestational age of the fetus, starting as early as 27 weeks (49,50), and increasing markedly at 27–32 weeks (50,51), and occurs with similar frequency in singleton and multiple gestations (51). Furthermore, constriction is independent of fetal serum indomethacin levels (49,50). Primary pulmonary hypertension of the newborn is caused by the shunting of the right ventricular outflow into the pulmonary vessels when the fetal ductus arteriosus narrows. This results in pulmonary arterial hypertrophy (48). Persistent fetal circulation occurs after birth secondary to pulmonary hypertension shunting blood through the foramen ovale, bypassing the lungs and still patent ductus arteriosus, with resultant difficulty in adequate oxygenation of the neonate (48).

Using fetal echocardiography, researchers described the above effects in a study of 13 women (14 fetuses, 1 set of twins) between the gestational ages of 26.5 and 31.0 weeks (48). The patients were treated with 100–150 mg of indomethacin orally per day. Fetal ductal constriction occurred in 7 of 14 fetus's 9.5–25.5 hours after the first dose and was not correlated with either gestational age or maternal indomethacin serum levels. In two other cases not included in the present series, ductal constriction did not occur until several weeks after the start of therapy. Tricuspid regurgitation was observed in three of the fetuses with ductal constriction. This defect was caused by the constriction-induced elevated pressure in the right ventricular outflow tract producing mild endocardial ischemia with papillary muscle dysfunction (48). All cases of constriction, including two of the three with tricuspid regurgitation, resolved within 24 hours after indomethacin was discontinued. The third tricuspid case returned to normal 40 hours after resolution of the ductal constriction. No cases of persistent fetal circulation were observed in the 11 newborns studied. Some have questioned the methods used in the above study and whether the results actually reflected fetal ductal constriction (52). In response, the authors of the original paper defended their techniques based on both animal and human experimental findings (53).

A 1987 report described a patient with premature labor who was treated for 29 days between 27 and 32 weeks' gestation with a total indomethacin dose of 6.2 g (54). The woman delivered a female infant who had patent ductus arteriosus that persisted for 4 weeks. A macerated twin fetus, delivered at the same time as the surviving infant, was thought to have died before the initiation of treatment.

Administration of indomethacin to the mother results in reduced fetal urine output. Severe oligohydramnios, meconium staining, constriction of the ductus arteriosus, and death were reported in the offspring of three women treated for preterm labor at 32–33 weeks' gestation (55). Indomethacin doses were 100 mg (one case) and 400 mg (two cases) during the first 24 hours followed by 100 mg/day for 2–5 days. Two of the fetuses were stillborn, and the third died within 3 hours of birth. A second report described a woman with preterm labor at 24 weeks' gestation that was treated with IV ritodrine and indomethacin, 300 mg/day, for 8 weeks (56). A reduction in the amount of amniotic fluid was noted at 28 weeks' gestation (after 4 weeks of therapy), and severe oligohydramnios was present 4 weeks later. Filling of the fetal bladder could not be visualized at this time. The infant, who expired 47 hours after birth, had the characteristic facies of Potter's syndrome (i.e., oligohydramnios sequence), but autopsy revealed a normal urinary tract with normal kidneys. Both cardiac ventricles were hypertrophic and the lungs showed no evidence of pulmonary hypertension (56).

In a 1987 study involving eight patients with polyhydramnios and premature uterine contractions, indomethacin, administered by oral tablets or vaginal suppositories in a dose of 2.2–3.0 mg/kg/day, resolved the condition in each case (57). Four of the patients had diabetes mellitus. The gestational age of the patients at the start of treatment ranged between 21.5 and 34 weeks. The duration of therapy, which was stopped between 34.5 and 38 weeks' gestation, ranged from 2 to 11 weeks. The average gestational age at birth was 38.6 weeks and none was premature. All infants were normal at birth and at follow-up for 2–6 months. In addition to the reduced urine output, indomethacin was thought to have minimized the amount of fluid produced by the amnion and chorion (57).

A case report described a 33-year-old woman with a low serum α-fetoprotein level at 16 weeks' gestation and symptomatic polyhydramnios and preterm labor at 26 weeks' gestation that was treated with indomethacin, 25 mg orally every 4 hours, after therapeutic decompression had removed 3000 mL of amniotic fluid (58). During the 9 weeks of therapy, periodic fetal echocardiography was conducted to ensure that the fetal ductus arteriosus remained patent. Fetal urine output declined significantly (<50%) as determined by ultrasound examinations during therapy. Therapy was stopped at 35 weeks' gestation, and a 2280-g female infant was delivered vaginally a week later. Chromosomal analysis of the amniotic fluid at 26 weeks and of the infant after birth revealed 46 chromosomes with an additional marker or ring chromosome. No structural defects were noted in the infant, who was developing normally at 3 months of age (58).

In two women treated for premature labor, indomethacin-induced oligohydramnios was observed 1 week and 3.5 weeks after starting therapy (59). Treatment was continued for 3 weeks in one patient and for 8 weeks in the other, with therapy discontinued at 31 and 32 weeks' gestation, respectively. Within a week of stopping indomethacin, amniotic fluid volume had returned to normal in both patients. Ultrasonography revealed that both fetuses had regular filling of their bladders. The newborns, delivered 3–4 weeks after indomethacin treatment was halted, had normal urine output. Neither premature closure of the ductus arteriosus nor pulmonary hypertension was observed (59). Another case of reversible indomethacin-induced oligohydramnios was reported in 1989 (60). The woman was treated from 20–28 weeks' gestation with indomethacin, 100–200 mg/day, plus various other tocolytic agents for premature labor. Ten days after indomethacin therapy was stopped, the volume of amniotic fluid was normal. She was eventually delivered of a 2905-g female infant at 36 weeks' gestation. Development was normal at 1 year of age (60).

The effects of tocolytic therapy on amniotic fluid volume were the subject of a 1989 study (61). Of 27 women meeting the criteria for the study, 13 were treated either with indomethacin alone ($N = 9$) or indomethacin combined with ritodrine ($N = 2$), terbutaline ($N = 1$), or magnesium sulfate ($N = 1$). Indomethacin dosage varied from 100 to 200 mg/day with a mean duration of treatment of 15.3 days (range 5–44 days). Four other patients were treated with ibuprofen, another nonsteroidal anti-inflammatory agent. Fourteen of the 17 patients (82.3%) either had a decrease in amniotic fluid volume to low-normal levels or had oligohydramnios compared with none of the 10 women treated only with terbutaline, ritodrine, or magnesium sulfate ($p < 0.001$). The mean time required to reaccumulate amniotic fluid in 7 women after stopping nonsteroidal anti-inflammatory therapy was 4.4 days. In one other woman who had an ultrasound examination after therapy was discontinued, amniotic fluid volume remained in the low-normal range (61).

A study published in 1988 described the treatment with indomethacin, 100–150 mg/day, for premature labor in eight women at 27–32 weeks' gestation (62). Fetal urine output fell from a mean pretreatment value of 11.2 to 2.2 mL/hour at 5 hours, then stabilized at 1.8 mL/hour at 12 and 24 hours. Mean output 24 hours after stopping indomethacin was 13.5 mL/hour. No correlation was found between maternal indomethacin serum levels and hourly fetal urine output. Three of the four fetuses treated with indomethacin every 4 hours had ductal constriction at 24 hours that apparently resolved after therapy was halted. All newborns had normal renal function in the neonatal period.

Fetal adverse effects described during treatment of premature labor with indomethacin in recent studies include primary pulmonary hypertension (four cases) (35,63), ductal constriction with or without tricuspid regurgitation (36,64–67), and, in infants younger than 30 weeks' gestational age, a significantly increased incidence compared with controls of intracranial hemorrhage, necrotizing enterocolitis, and patent ductus arteriosus requiring ligation (68,69). A possible interaction between cocaine abuse and indomethacin resulting in fetal anuria, generalized massive edema, and neonatal gastrointestinal hemorrhage has been reported (70).

A number of reports have described the use of indomethacin for the treatment of symptomatic polyhydramnios in singleton and multiple pregnancies (71–82), including a 1991 review of this indication (83). Indomethacin-induced constriction of the ductus arteriosus and tricuspid regurgitation were observed in some of the studies (70,72,74,80). In one report, indomethacin was used to treat polyhydramnios because of feto-fetal transfusion syndrome in two sets of twins (80). One twin survived from each pregnancy, but one was oliguric (urine output 0.5 mL/kg/hour) and the other was anuric requiring peritoneal dialysis. The authors speculated that the renal failure in both infants was secondary to indomethacin. A unilateral pleural effusion developed in one twin fetus after 28 days of indomethacin therapy for polyhydramnios, possibly because of ductus arteriosus constriction (82). The condition resolved completely within 48 hours of stopping the drug.

A probable drug interaction between indomethacin and β-blockers resulting in severe maternal hypertension was reported in two women in 1989 (84). One woman, with a history of labile hypertension of 6 years' duration, was admitted at 30 weeks' gestation for control of her blood pressure. She was treated with propranolol 80 mg/day with good response. Indomethacin was started because of premature uterine contractions occurring at 32 weeks' gestation. An initial 200-mg rectal dose was followed by 25 mg orally/day. On the 4th day of therapy, the patient suffered a marked change in blood pressure, which rose from 135/85 mm Hg to 240/140 mm Hg, with cardiotocographic signs of fetal distress. A cesarean section was performed, but the severely growth-retarded newborn died 72 hours later. The second patient developed signs and symptoms of preeclampsia at 31 weeks' gestation. She was treated with pindolol 15 mg/day with good blood pressure response. Two weeks later, indomethacin was started, as in the first case, for preterm labor. On the 5th day of therapy, blood pressure rose to 230/130 mm Hg. Signs of fetal distress were evident and a cesarean section was performed. The low-weight infant survived (84). In a brief letter referring to the above study, one author proposed that the mechanism of nonsteroidal anti-inflammatory-induced hypertension may be related to the inhibition of prostaglandin synthesis in the renal vasculature (85). On the basis of this theory, the author recommended that all similar agents should be avoided in women with preeclampsia. Although the mechanism is unknown, one source has reviewed several cases of the interaction with the observation that indomethacin may inhibit the effects of β-blockers, as well as antihypertensives in general (86).

Severe complications after *in utero* exposure to indomethacin were reported in three preterm infants (87). The three mothers had been treated with indomethacin, 200–300 mg/day, for 4 weeks, 3 days, and 2 days immediately before delivery. Complications in the newborns included edema or hydrops, oliguric renal failure (<0.5 mL/kg/hour) lasting for 1–2 days, gastrointestinal bleeding occurring on the 4th and 6th days (2 infants), subcutaneous bruising, intraventricular hemorrhage (1 infant), absent platelet aggregation (2 infants; not determined in the third infant), and perforation of the terminal ileum. The authors attributed the problems to maternal indomethacin therapy because of (a) the absence of predisposing factors, and the lack of diagnostic evidence, for necrotizing enterocolitis, and (b) the close similarity and sequential pattern of the signs and symptoms in the three newborns (87).

A single case of phocomelia with agenesis of the penis has been described, but the relationship between indomethacin and this defect is unknown (88). Inhibition of platelet aggregation may have contributed to postpartum hemorrhage in 3 of 16 women given a 100-mg indomethacin suppository during term labor (19).

In summary, the use of indomethacin as a tocolytic agent during the latter half of pregnancy may cause constriction of the fetal ductus arteriosus, with or without tricuspid regurgitation. These effects are usually transient and reversible if therapy is stopped an adequate time before delivery. Premature closure of the ductus arteriosus can result in primary pulmonary hypertension of the newborn that, in severe cases, may be fatal (89). Reduced fetal urine output should be expected when indomethacin is administered to the mother. This may be therapeutic in cases of symptomatic polyhydramnios, but the complications of this therapy may be severe. Oliguric renal failure, hemorrhage, and intestinal perforation have been reported in premature infants exposed immediately before delivery. Use of indomethacin with antihypertensive agents, particularly the β-blockers, has been associated with severe maternal hypertension and resulting fetal distress. Short courses of indomethacin, such as 24–48 hours with allowance of at least 24 hours or more between the last dose and delivery, should prevent complications of this therapy in the newborn. Use of the smallest effective dose is essential, although maternal serum levels of indomethacin that are effective for tocolysis have not yet been defined (48) and, at least one complication, ductal constriction, is independent of fetal drug serum levels (49,50). Restriction of indomethacin tocolysis to gestational ages between 24 and 32 completed weeks, when therapy for premature labor is most appropriate, will also lessen the incidence of complications (38), although a higher rate of newborn complications has been observed when delivery occurred before 30 weeks' gestation (68,69). Other uses of indomethacin, such as for analgesia or inflammation, have not been studied in pregnancy but should be approached with caution because of the effects described above. Moreover, women attempting to conceive should not use any prostaglandin synthesis inhibitor, including indomethacin, because of the findings in a variety of animal models that indicate these agents block blastocyst implantation (90,91). In addition, as noted above, NSAIDs have been associated with SABs and congenital malformations.

[*Risk Factor D if used for longer than 48 hours or after 34 weeks' gestation or close to delivery.*]

BREAST FEEDING SUMMARY

RECOMMENDATION: Limited Human Data - Probably Compatible

Indomethacin is excreted in breast milk. Although an earlier reference speculated that milk levels were similar to maternal plasma levels (92), a study published in 1991 reported a median milk:plasma ratio of 0.37 in 7 of 16 women taking 75–300 mg/day (93). The other nine women did not have measurable drug levels in both milk and plasma. The investigators calculated that the total infant dose ingested (assuming 100% absorption) ranged from 0.07% to 0.98% (median 0.18%) of the weight-adjusted maternal dose (93).

A case report of possible indomethacin-induced seizures in a breast-fed infant has been published (92), although the causal link between the two events has been questioned (94). The mother was taking 200 mg/day (3 mg/kg/day). The American Academy of Pediatrics noted the above possible adverse reaction but classified indomethacin as compatible with breast-feeding (95).

References

1. Shepard TH. *Catalog of Teratogenic Agents*. 6th ed. Baltimore, MD: Johns Hopkins University Press, 1989: 348–9.
2. Montenegro MA, Palomino H. Induction of cleft palate in mice by inhibitors of prostaglandin synthesis. J Craniofac Genet Dev Biol 1990;10:83–94.
3. Moise KJ Jr, Ou C-N, Kirshon B, Cano LE, Rognerud C, Carpenter RJ Jr. Placental transfer of indomethacin in the human pregnancy. Am J Obstet Gynecol 1990;162:549–54.
4. Nielsen GL, Sorensen HT, Larsen H, Pedersen L. Risk of adverse birth outcome and miscarriage in pregnant users of non-steroidal anti-inflammatory drugs: population based observational study and case-control study. BMJ 2001;322:266–70.
5. Ericson A, Kallen BAJ. Nonsteroidal anti-inflammatory drugs in early pregnancy. Reprod Toxicol 2001;15:371–5.
6. Li DK, Liu L, Odouli R. Exposure to non-steroidal anti-inflammatory drugs during pregnancy and risk of miscarriage: population based cohort study. BMJ 2003;327:368–71.
7. Tassinari MS, Cook JC, Hurtt ME. NSAIDs and developmental toxicity. Birth Defects Res Part B Dev Reprod Toxicol 2003;68:3–4.
8. Atad J, David A, Moise J, Abramovici H. Classification of threatened premature labor related to treatment with a prostaglandin inhibitor: indomethacin. Biol Neonate 1980;37:291–6.
9. Gonzalez CHL, Jimenez PG, Pezzotti y R MA, Favela EL. Hipertension pulmonar persistente en el recien nacido por uso prenatal de inhibidores de las prostaglandinas (indometacina). Informe de un caso. Ginecol Obstet Mex 1980;48:103–10.
10. Sureau C, Piovani P. Clinical study of indomethacin for prevention of prematurity. Eur J Obstet Gynecol Reprod Biol 1983;46:400–2.
11. Van Kets H, Thiery M, Derom R, Van Egmond H, Baele G. Perinatal hazards of chronic antenatal tocolysis with indomethacin. Prostaglandins 1979;18:893–907.
12. Van Kets H, Thiery M, Derom R, Van Egmond H, Baele G. Prostaglandin synthase inhibitors in preterm labor. Lancet 1980;2:693.
13. Blake DA, Niebyl JR, White RD, Kumor KM, Dubin NH,

Robinson JC, Egner PG. Treatment of premature labor with indomethacin. Adv Prostaglandin Thromboxane Res 1980;8:1465–7.
14. Grella P, Zanor P. Premature labor and indomethacin. Prostaglandins 1978;16:1007–17.
15. Karim SMM. On the use of blockers of prostaglandin synthesis in the control of labor. Adv Prostaglandin Thromboxane Res 1978;4:301–6.
16. Katz Z, Lancet M, Yemini M, Mogilner BM, Feigl A, Ben Hur H. Treatment of premature labor contractions with combined ritodrine and indomethacine. Int J Gynaecol Obstet 1983;21:337–42.
17. Niebyl JR, Blake DA, White RD, Kumor KM, Dubin NH, Robinson JC, Egner PG. The inhibition of premature labor with indomethacin. Am J Obstet Gynecol 1980;136:1014–9.
18. Peteja J. Indometacyna w zapobieganiu porodom przedwczesnym. Ginekol Pol 1980;51:347–53.
19. Reiss U, Atad J, Rubinstein I, Zuckerman H. The effect of indomethacin in labour at term. Int J Gynaecol Obstet 1976;14:369–74.
20. Souka AR, Osman N, Sibaie F, Einen MA. Therapeutic value of indomethacin in threatened abortion. Prostaglandins 1980;19:457–60.
21. Spearing G. Alcohol, indomethacin, and salbutamol. Obstet Gynecol 1979;53:171–4.
22. Chimura T. The treatment of threatened premature labor by drugs. Acta Obstet Gynaecol Jpn 1980;32:1620–4.
23. Suzanne F, Fresne JJ, Portal B, Baudon J. Essai therapeutique de l'indometacine dans les menaces d'accouchement premature: a propos de 30 observations. Therapie 1980;35:751–60.
24. Tinga DJ, Aranoudse JG. Post-partum pulmonary oedema associated with preventive therapy for premature labor. Lancet 1979;1:1026.
25. Dudley DKL, Hardie MJ. Fetal and neonatal effects of indomethacin used as a tocolytic agent. Am J Obstet Gynecol 1985;151:181–4.
26. Gamissans O, Canas E, Cararach V, Ribas J, Puerto B, Edo A. A study of indomethacin combined with ritodrine in threatened preterm labor. Eur J Obstet Gynecol Reprod Biol 1978;8:123–8.
27. Wiqvist N, Lundstrom V, Green K. Premature labor and indomethacin. Prostaglandins 1975;10:515–26.
28. Wiqvist N, Kjellmer I, Thiringer K, Ivarsson E, Karlsson K. Treatment of premature labor by prostaglandin synthetase inhibitors. Acta Biol Med Germ 1978;37:923–30.
29. Zuckerman H, Reiss U, Rubinstein I. Inhibition of human premature labor by indomethacin. Obstet Gynecol 1974;44:787–92.
30. Zuckerman H, Reiss U, Atad J, Lampert I, Ben Ezra S, Sklan D. The effect of indomethacin on plasma levels of prostaglandin $F_{2\alpha}$ in women in labour. Br J Obstet Gynaecol 1977;84:339–43.
31. Zuckerman H, Shalev E, Gilad G, Katzuni E. Further study of the inhibition of premature labor by indomethacin. Part I. J Perinat Med 1984;12:19–23.
32. Zuckerman H, Shalev E, Gilad G, Katzuni E. Further study of the inhibition of premature labor by indomethacin. Part II. Double-blind study. J Perinat Med 1984;12:25–9.
33. Niebyl JR. Prostaglandin synthetase inhibitors. Semin Perinatol 1981;5:274–87.
34. Niebyl JR, Witter FR. Neonatal outcome after indomethacin treatment for preterm labor. Am J Obstet Gynecol 1986;155:747–9.
35. Besinger RE, Niebyl JR, Keyes WG, Johnson TRB. Randomized comparative trial of indomethacin and ritodrine for the long-term treatment of preterm labor. Am J Obstet Gynecol 1991;164:981–8.
36. Evans DJ, Kofinas AD, King K. Intraoperative amniocentesis and indomethacin treatment in the management of an immature pregnancy with completely dilated cervix. Obstet Gynecol 1992;79:881–2.
37. Leonardi MR, Hankins GDV. What's new in tocolytics. Clin Perinatol 1992;19:367–84.
38. Higby K, Xenakis EM-J, Pauerstein CJ. Do tocolytic agents stop preterm labor? A critical and comprehensive review of efficacy and safety. Am J Obstet Gynecol 1993;168:1247–59.
39. Morales WJ, Smith SG, Angel JL, O'Brien WF, Knuppel RA. Efficacy and safety of indomethacin versus ritodrine in the management of preterm labor: a randomized study. Obstet Gynecol 1989;74:567–72.
40. Morales WJ, Madhav H. Efficacy and safety of indomethacin compared with magnesium sulfate in the management of preterm labor: A randomized study. Am J Obstet Gynecol 1993;169:97–102.
41. Levin DL. Effects of inhibition of prostaglandin synthesis on fetal development, oxygenation, and the fetal circulation. Semin Perinatol 1980;4:35–44.
42. Csaba IF, Sulyok E, Ertl T. Relationship of maternal treatment with indomethacin to persistence of fetal circulation syndrome. J Pediatr 1978;92:484.
43. Levin DL, Fixler DE, Morriss FC, Tyson J. Morphologic analysis of the pulmonary vascular bed in infants exposed in utero to prostaglandin synthetase inhibitors. J Pediatr 1978;92:478–83.
44. Rubaltelli FF, Chiozza ML, Zanardo V, Cantarutti F. Effect on neonate of maternal treatment with indomethacin. J Pediatr 1979;94:161.
45. Manchester D, Margolis HS, Sheldon RE. Possible association between maternal indomethacin therapy and primary pulmonary hypertension of the newborn. Am J Obstet Gynecol 1976;126:467–9.
46. Goudie BM, Dossetor JFB. Effect on the fetus of indomethacin given to suppress labour. Lancet 1979;2:1187–8.
47. Mogilner BM, Ashkenazy M, Borenstein R, Lancet M. Hydrops fetalis caused by maternal indomethacin treatment. Acta Obstet Gynecol Scand 1982;61:183–5.
48. Moise KJ Jr, Huhta JC, Sharif DS, Ou CN, Kirshon B, Wasserstrum N, Cano L. Indomethacin in the treatment of premature labor: effects on the fetal ductus arteriosus. N Engl J Med 1988;319:327–31.
49. Van Den Veyver I, Moise K Jr, Ou C-N, Carpenter R Jr. The effect of gestational age and fetal indomethacin levels on the incidence of constriction of the fetal ductus arteriosus (abstract). Am J Obstet Gynecol 1993;168:373.
50. Van Den Veyver IB, Moise KJ Jr, Ou C-N, Carpenter RJ Jr. The effect of gestational age and fetal indomethacin levels on the incidence of constriction of the fetal ductus arteriosus. Obstet Gynecol 1993;82:500–3.
51. Moise KJ Jr. Effect of advancing gestational age on the frequency of fetal ductal constriction in association

with maternal indomethacin use. Am J Obstet Gynecol 1993;168:1350–3.
52. Ovadia M. Effects of indomethacin on the fetus. N Engl J Med 1988;319:1484.
53. Moise KJ Jr, Huhta JC, Mari G. Effects of indomethacin on the fetus. N Engl J Med 1988;319:1485.
54. Atad J, Lissak A, Rofe A, Abramovici H. Patent ductus arteriosus after prolonged treatment with indomethacin during pregnancy: case report. Int J Gynaecol Obstet 1987;25:73–6.
55. Itskovitz J, Abramovici H, Brandes JM. Oligohydramnion, meconium and perinatal death concurrent with indomethacin treatment in human pregnancy. J Reprod Med 1980;24:137–40.
56. Veersema D, de Jong PA, van Wijck JAM. Indomethacin and the fetal renal nonfunction syndrome. Eur J Obstet Gynecol Reprod Biol 1983; 16:113–21.
57. Cabrol D, Landesman R, Muller J, Uzan M, Sureau C, Saxena BB. Treatment of polyhydramnios with prostaglandin synthetase inhibitor (indomethacin). Am J Obstet Gynecol 1987;157:422–6.
58. Kirshon B, Cotton DB. Polyhydramnios associated with a ring chromosome and low maternal serum α-fetoprotein levels managed with indomethacin. Am J Obstet Gynecol 1988;158:1063–4.
59. De Wit W, Van Mourik I, Wiesenhaan PF. Prolonged maternal indomethacin therapy associated with oligohydramnios. Case reports. Br J Obstet Gynecol 1988;95:303–5.
60. Goldenberg RL, Davis RO, Baker RC. Indomethacin-induced oligohydramnios. Am J Obstet Gynecol 1989;160:1196–7.
61. Hickok DE, Hollenbach KA, Reilley SF, Nyberg DA. The association between decreased amniotic fluid volume and treatment with nonsteroidal anti-inflammatory agents for preterm labor. Am J Obstet Gynecol 1989;160:1525–31.
62. Kirshon B, Moise KJ Jr, Wasserstrum N, Ou CN, Huhta JC. Influence of short-term indomethacin therapy on fetal urine output. Obstet Gynecol 1988;72:51–3.
63. Demandt E, Legius E, Devlieger H, Lemmens F, Proesmans W, Eggermont E. Prenatal indomethacin toxicity in one member of monozygous twins; a case report. Eur J Obstet Gynecol Reprod Biol 1990;35:267–9.
64. Eronen M, Pesonen E, Kurki T, Ylikorkala O, Hallman M. The effects of indomethacin and a β-sympathomimetic agent on the fetal ductus arteriosus during treatment of premature labor: a randomized double-blind study. Am J Obstet Gynecol 1991;164: 141–6.
65. Hallak M, Reiter AA, Ayres NA, Moise KJ Jr. Indomethacin for preterm labor: fetal toxicity in a dizygotic twin gestation. Obstet Gynecol 1991;78:911–3.
66. Rosemond RL, Boehm FH, Moreau G, Karmo H. Tricuspid regurgitation: a method of monitoring patients treated with indomethacin (abstract). Am J Obstet Gynecol 1992;166:336.
67. Bivins HA Jr, Newman RB, Fyfe DA, Campbell BA, Stramm SL. Randomized comparative trial of indomethacin and terbutaline for the long term treatment of preterm labor (abstract). Am J Obstet Gynecol 1993;168:375.
68. Norton M, Merril J, Kuller J, Clyman R. Neonatal complications after antenatal indomethacin for preterm labor (abstract). Am J Obstet Gynecol 1993;168: 303.
69. Norton ME, Merrill J, Cooper BAB, Kuller JA, Clyman RI. Neonatal complications after the administration of indomethacin for preterm labor. N Engl J Med 1993;329:1602–7.
70. Carlan SJ, Stromquist C, Angel JL, Harris M, O'Brien WF. Cocaine and indomethacin: fetal anuria, neonatal edema, and gastrointestinal bleeding. Obstet Gynecol 1991;78:501–3.
71. Kirshon B, Mari G, Moise KJ Jr. Indomethacin therapy in the treatment of symptomatic polyhydramnios. Obstet Gynecol 1990;75:202–5.
72. Mari G, Moise KJ Jr, Deter RL, Kirshon B, Carpenter RJ. Doppler assessment of the renal blood flow velocity waveform during indomethacin therapy for preterm labor and polyhydramnios. Obstet Gynecol 1990;75:199–201.
73. Mamopoulos M, Assimakopoulos E, Reece EA, Andreou A, Zheng X-Z, Mantalenakis S. Maternal indomethacin therapy in the treatment of polyhydramnios. Am J Obstet Gynecol 1990;162:1225–9.
74. Kirshon B, Mari G, Moise KJ Jr, Wasserstrum N. Effect of indomethacin on the fetal ductus arteriosus during treatment of symptomatic polyhydramnios. J Reprod Med 1990;35:529–32.
75. Smith LG Jr, Kirshon B, Cotton DB. Indomethacin treatment of polyhydramnios and subsequent infantile nephrogenic diabetes insipidus. Am J Obstet Gynecol 1990;163:98–9.
76. Ash K, Harman CR, Gritter H. TRAP sequence - successful outcome with indomethacin treatment. Obstet Gynecol 1990;76:960–2.
77. Malas HZ, Hamlett JD. Acute recurrent polyhydramnios - management with indomethacin. Br J Obstet Gynaecol 1991;98:583–7.
78. Nordstrom L, Westgren M. Indomethacin treatment for polyhydramnios. Effective but potentially dangerous? Acta Obstet Gynecol Scand 1992;71:239–41.
79. Dolkart LA, Eshwar KP, Reimers FT. Indomethacin therapy and chronic hemodialysis during pregnancy. A case report. J Reprod Med 1992;37:181–3.
80. Buderus S, Thomas B, Fahnenstich H, Kowalewski S. Renal failure in two preterm infants: toxic effect of prenatal maternal indomethacin treatment? Br J Obstet Gynaecol 1993;100:97–8.
81. Deeny M, Haxton MJ. Indomethacin use to control gross polyhydramnios complicating triplet pregnancy. Br J Obstet Gynaecol 1993;100:281–2.
82. Murray HG, Stone PR, Strand L, Flower J. Fetal pleural effusion following maternal indomethacin therapy. Br J Obstet Gynaecol 1993;100:277–82.
83. Moise KJ Jr. Indomethacin therapy in the treatment of symptomatic polyhydramnios. Clin Obstet Gynecol 1991;34:310–8.
84. Schoenfeld A, Freedman S, Hod M, Ovadia Y. Antagonism of antihypertensive drug therapy in pregnancy by indomethacin? Am J Obstet Gynecol 1989;161: 1204–5.
85. Mousavy SM. Indomethacin induces hypertensive crisis in preeclampsia irrespective of prior antihypertensive drug therapy. Am J Obstet Gynecol 1991; 165:1577.
86. Hansen PD. *Drug Interactions*. 5th ed. Philadelphia, PA: Lea & Febiger, 1985:36.

87. Vanhaesebrouck P, Thiery M, Leroy JG, Govaert P, de Praeter C, Coppens M, Cuvelier C, Dhont M. Oligohydramnios, renal insufficiency, and ileal perforation in preterm infants after intrauterine exposure to indomethacin. J Pediatr 1988;113:738–43.
88. Di Battista C, Landizi L, Tamborino G. Focomelia ed agenesia del pene in neonato. Minerva Pediatr 1975;27:675. As cited in Dukes MNG, ed. *Side Effects of Drugs Annual 1*. Amsterdam: Excerpta Medica, 1977:89.
89. Van Marter LJ, Leviton A, Allred EN, Pagano M, Sullivan KF, Cohen A, Epstein MF. Persistent pulmonary hypertension of the newborn and smoking and aspirin and nonsteroidal antiinflammatory drug consumption during pregnancy. Pediatrics 1996;97:658–63.
90. Matt DW, Borzelleca JF. Toxic effects on the female reproductive system during pregnancy, parturition, and lactation. In Witorsch RJ, ed. *Reproductive Toxicology*. 2nd ed. New York, NY: Raven Press, 1995:175–93.
91. Dawood MY. Nonsteroidal antiinflammatory drugs and reproduction. Am J Obstet Gynecol 1993;169:1255–65.
92. Eeg-Olofsson O, Malmros I, Elwin CE, Steen B. Convulsions in a breast-fed infant after maternal indomethacin. Lancet 1978;2:215.
93. Lebedevs TH, Wojnar-Horton RE, Yapp P, Roberts MJ, Dusci LJ, Hackett LP, Ilett KF. Excretion of indomethacin in breast milk. Br J Clin Pharmacol 1991;32:751–4.
94. Fairhead FW. Convulsions in a breast-fed infant after maternal indomethacin. Lancet 1978;2:576.
95. Committee on Drugs, American Academy of Pediatrics. The transfer of drugs and other chemicals into human milk. Pediatrics 2001;108:776–89.

Name: **INFLIXIMAB** Risk Factor: **C_M**

Class: **Antirheumatic Agent/ Gastrointestinal Agent**

FETAL RISK SUMMARY

RECOMMENDATION: Limited Human Data - No Relevant Animal Data

Infliximab, a chimeric (mouse/human) IgG1 monoclonal antibody, is indicated for the treatment of rheumatoid arthritis (in combination with methotrexate) and for severe Crohn's disease, including fistulizing Crohn's disease. Infliximab binds specifically to human tumor necrosis factor alpha (TNFα) to inhibit its activity. The agent has an elimination half-life of 8.0–9.5 days (1).

Animal reproduction studies have not been conducted with infliximab because it does not cross-react with TNFα in species other than humans and chimpanzees (1). However, when a reproduction study was conducted in mice with an analogous antibody that binds specifically to mouse TNFα, no evidence of maternal toxicity, embryo toxicity, or teratogenicity was observed (1,2).

It is not known if infliximab crosses the human placenta to the fetus. Although the molecular weight is very high (about 149,100), another antibody, immune globulin G, has been shown to cross the human placenta if the gestational age was greater than 32 weeks (see Immune Globulin, Intravenous). The amount transferred was also a function of dose. Moreover, the long elimination half-life indicates that the drug will be at the maternal:fetal interface for a prolonged interval.

A 2001 case report described the pregnancy outcome of a 26-year-old woman with Crohn's disease who had received infliximab early in gestation (3). The woman had a 6-year history of Crohn's disease and was symptomatic with a rectovaginal fistula while receiving azathioprine, metronidazole, and mesalamine. She was given two infusions of infliximab (dose not specified); the first occurred at about 1–2 weeks' gestation and the second at about 2–3 weeks. A planned third infusion was canceled when her pregnancy was diagnosed. She eventually delivered a premature 681-g infant at 24 weeks of conception who died 3 days later (3).

The author of the above report also cited data received from the manufacturer on 27 women who had been treated with infliximab immediately before or during the

1st trimester (3). Of the 27 women, 3 aborted spontaneously, 1 had an elective abortion (for personal reasons), and 6 delivered term infants. (No information was given on the condition of the infants.) Another woman had received infliximab during the 1st trimester and delivered an infant with tetralogy of Fallot. No data were provided on the remaining 16 pregnancies. The author noted the close relationship between infliximab's mechanism of action and that of thalidomide, a known human teratogen that decreases the production of TNFα (3). This relationship has been noted by others (4).

In an extension of the above report (some of the same data are reported), a 2001 abstract evaluated data from 59 women who had received infliximab before or during pregnancy for the treatment of Crohn's disease ($N = 45$), rheumatoid arthritis ($N = 5$; not specified if these cases also received methotrexate), or unknown disease ($N = 9$) (5). The cases were retrieved from the infliximab postmarketing safety database. Treating physicians were contacted to document pregnancy outcomes. The timing of exposures were before pregnancy ($N = 27$), before pregnancy and during 1st trimester ($N = 11$), and during the 1st trimester ($N = 5$), and unknown ($N = 16$). Pregnancy outcomes were known for 36 cases (time of exposure not specified): live births ($N = 26$), spontaneous abortion ($N = 5$), and elective abortion ($N = 5$). Among the live births, two had complications: 681-g infant delivered at 23 weeks' and died at age 3 weeks; and an infant with tetralogy of Fallot (corrected surgically) that is otherwise currently healthy. The investigators concluded the outcomes were consistent with those expected in healthy women (5).

In a 2003 case report, a 29-year-old woman with chronic, severe Crohn's disease received three infusions of infliximab (600 mg/dose) over a 6-week period (6). Three months later, she received a fourth infusion of 500 mg. This dose was given approximately 3 days after conception. She eventually delivered a healthy infant at 36 weeks' gestation (birth weight and other details not specified). The child has normal growth and development at 20 months of age (6).

A survey of 600 members of the American College of Rheumatology, partially conducted to determine the outcomes of pregnancies exposed to disease modifying antirheumatic drugs (DMARD) (etanercept, infliximab, leflunomide, and methotrexate), was published in 2003 (7). From the 175 responders, the outcomes of two pregnancies exposed to infliximab were one full term healthy infant and one unknown outcome (7).

In summary, animal reproduction studies were not conducted with infliximab because the mechanism of action is different from that in humans. In addition, the limited human pregnancy data are inadequate to assess the embryo/fetal risk. Moreover, the agent may be used with methotrexate, a potential teratogen, for the treatment of rheumatoid arthritis. It is not known if the antibody can cross the placenta early in gestation when all of the known exposures to infliximab have occurred. If it is similar to immune globulin G, clinically significant amounts would cross only late in gestation and thus would present no direct risk to the embryo or fetus during early development. An indirect risk during any stage of gestation may exist because of the potential for severe maternal toxicity in some patient populations. This includes increased incidence of mortality in patients with moderate to severe congestive heart failure and an increased risk of severe infections. The similarity between the mechanism of action of infliximab and thalidomide is of interest. However, decreased production of TNFα may not be a primary cause of the teratogenicity of thalidomide (see Thalidomide). Theoretically, TNFα antagonists could interfere with implantation and ovulation, but this has not been shown clinically (8). If infliximab is used in pregnancy for the treatment of rheumatoid arthritis, healthcare professionals are encouraged to call the toll free number (877-311-8972) for information about patient enrollment in the OTIS Rheumatoid Arthritis study.

BREAST FEEDING SUMMARY

RECOMMENDATION: No Human Data - Probably Compatible

No reports describing the use of infliximab during human lactation have been located. Even if it were excreted into breast milk, the antibody would probably be digested in the gastrointestinal tract. Therefore, the risk of toxicity in a nursing infant from exposure via milk would most likely be nil. The manufacturer states that infants should not breast-feed from women receiving the antibody (1).

References

1. Product information. Remicade. Centocor, 2001.
2. Treacy G. Using an analogous monoclonal antibody to evaluate the reproductive and chronic toxicity potential for a humanized anti-TNFα monoclonal antibody. Hum Exp Toxicol 2000;19:226–8.
3. Srinivasan R. Infliximab treatment and pregnancy outcome in active Crohn's disease. Am J Gastroenterol 2001;96:2274–5.
4. Stein RB, Hanauer SB. Comparative tolerability of treatments for inflammatory bowel disease. Drug Safety 2000;23:429–48.
5. Antoni CE, Furst D, Manger B, Lichtenstein GR, Keenan GF, Healy DE, Jacobs SJ, Katz Erlangen JA. Outcome of pregnancy in women receiving Remicade (infliximab) for the treatment of Crohn's disease or rheumatoid arthritis (abstract). Arthritis Rheum 2001;44(Suppl 9):S152.
6. Burt MJ, Frizelle FA, Barbezar GO. Pregnancy and exposure to infliximab (anti-tumor necrosis factor-alpha monoclonal antibody. J Gastroenterol Hepatol 2003;18:465–6.
7. Chakravarty EF, Sanchez-Yamamoto D, Bush TM. The use of disease modifying antirheumatic drugs in women with rheumatoid arthritis of childbearing age: a survey of practice patterns and pregnancy outcomes. J Rheumatol 2003;30:241–6.
8. Khanna D, McMahon M, Furst DE. Safety of tumour necrosis factor-α antagonists. Drug Saf 2004;27:307–24.

Name:	INSULIN	Risk Factor:	B
Class:	Antidiabetic		

FETAL RISK SUMMARY

RECOMMENDATION: Compatible

Insulin, a naturally occurring hormone, is the drug of choice for the control of diabetes mellitus in pregnancy. Because it is a very large molecule, it was thought that insulin does not cross the human placenta. Research published in 1990, however, found that animal (bovine or porcine) insulin does cross the human placenta as an insulin-antibody complex, and that the amount of transfer directly correlated with the amount of anti-insulin antibody in the mother (1). Moreover, high concentrations of animal insulin in cord blood were significantly associated with the development of fetal macrosomia, suggesting that the transferred insulin had biologic activity and that the fetal condition was determined by factors other than the mother's glycemic control (1). This latter conclusion has been challenged (2,3) and defended (4) and, at present, requires additional study. The results of the study do underscore the argument that immunogenic insulin should not be used in women who may become pregnant (1,2).

Infants of diabetic mothers are at risk for an increased incidence of congenital anomalies, 3 to 5 times that of normal controls (5–12). The rate of malformations appears to be related to maternal glycemic control in the 1st trimester of pregnancy, but the exact mechanisms causing structural defects are unknown. A 1996 review examined this issue and concluded that uncontrolled diabetes, occurring very early in gestation (i.e., before

8 weeks of gestation), causes an abnormal metabolic fuel state and that this condition leads to a number of processes, operating via a common pathway, that results in cell injury (11).

Congenital malformations are now the most common cause of perinatal death in infants of diabetic mothers (5,6). Not only is the frequency of major defects increased but also the frequency of multiple malformations (affecting more than one organ system) (5). Malformations observed in infants of diabetic mothers include the following (9,10,12–14):

Caudal regression syndrome (includes anomalies of lower neural tube resulting in sacral agenesis and defects of lumbar vertebrae; defects of lower extremities, gastrointestinal and genitourinary tracts [15])
Femoral hypoplasia and unusual facies syndrome
Spina bifida, hydrocephalus, other central nervous system defects
Anencephalus
Cardiovascular: transposition of great vessels; ventricular septal defect; atrial septal defect
Anal and rectal atresia
Renal: agenesis, multicystic dysplasia, ureter duplex
Gastrointestinal: situs inversus, tracheoesophageal fistula, bowel atresias, imperforate anus, small left colon

Infants of diabetic mothers may have significant perinatal morbidity, even when the mothers have been under close diabetic control (12). Perinatal morbidity in one series affected 65% (169/260) of the infants and included hypoglycemia, hyperbilirubinemia, hypocalcemia, and polycythemia (16).

In contrast to the data relating to the adverse fetal effects of poor maternal hyperglycemia control, animal studies have documented that short periods of hypoglycemia during early organogenesis are associated with malformations of the skeleton and heart (17–19), and reduced growth, including some major organs (20). Although hypoglycemia in humans has not been shown to be teratogenic (21,22), at least one author has concluded that this has not been adequately studied (23).

BREAST FEEDING SUMMARY

RECOMMENDATION: Compatible

Insulin is a naturally occurring constituent of the blood. It does not pass into breast milk.

References

1. Menon RK, Cohen RM, Sperling MA, Cutfield WS, Mimouni F, Khoury JC. Transplacental passage of insulin in pregnant women with insulin-dependent diabetes mellitus. N Engl J Med 1990;323:309–15.
2. Kimmerle R, Chantelau EA. Transplacental passage of insulin. N Engl J Med 1991;324:198.
3. Ben-Shlomo I, Dor J, Zohar S, Mashiach S. Transplacental passage of insulin. N Engl J Med 1991;324:198.
4. Menon RK, Sperling MA, Cohen RM. Transplacental passage of insulin. N Engl J Med 1991;324:199.
5. Dignan PSJ. Teratogenic risk and counseling in diabetes. Clin Obstet Gynecol 1981;24:149–59.
6. Friend JR. Diabetes. Clin Obstet Gynaecol 1981; 8:353–82.
7. Miller E, Hare JW, Cloherty JP, Dunn PJ, Gleason RE, Soeldner JS, Kitzmiller JL. Elevated maternal hemoglobin A_{1c} in early pregnancy and major congenital anomalies in infants of diabetic mothers. N Engl J Med 1981;304:1331–4.
8. Soler NG, Walsh CH, Malins JM. Congenital malformations in infants of diabetic mothers. Q J Med 1976;45:303–13.
9. American College of Obstetricians and Gynecologists. Diabetes and pregnancy. *Technical Bulletin*. No. 200, December 1994.
10. Towner D, Kjos SL, Leung B, Montoro MM, Xiang A, Mestman JH, Buchanan TA. Congenital malformations in pregnancies complicated by NIDDM. Diabetes Care 1995;18:1446–51.
11. Reece EA, Homko CJ, Wu Y-K. Multifactorial basis of the syndrome of diabetic embryopathy. Teratology 1996;54:171–82.

12. Steel JM, Johnstone FD. Guidelines for the management of insulin-dependent diabetes mellitus in pregnancy. Drugs 1996;52:60–70.
13. Cousins L. Etiology and prevention of congenital anomalies among infants of overt diabetic women. Clin Obstet Gynecol 1991;34:481–93.
14. Hinson RM, Miller RC, Macri CJ. Femoral hypoplasia and maternal diabetes: consider femoral hypoplasia/unusual facies syndrome. Am J Perinatol 1996;13:433–6.
15. Escobar LF, Weaver DD. Caudal regression syndrome. In Buyse ML, Editor-in-Chief. *Birth Defects Encyclopedia*. Volume 1. Dover, MA: Center for Birth Defects Information Services, 1990:296–7.
16. Gabbe SG, Mestman JH, Freeman RK, Goebelsmann UT, Lowensohn RI, Nochimson D, Cetrulo C, Quilligan EJ. Management and outcome of pregnancy in diabetes mellitus, classes B to R. Am J Obstet Gynecol 1977;129:723–32.
17. Tanigawa K, Kawaguchi M, Tanaka O, Kato Y. Skeletal malformations in rat offspring. Long-term effect of maternal insulin-induced hypoglycemia during organogenesis. Diabetes 1991;40:1115–21.
18. Peet JH, Sadler TW. Mouse embryonic cardiac metabolism under euglycemic and hypoglycemic conditions. Teratology 1996;54:20–26.
19. Smoak IW. Brief hypoglycemia alters morphology, function, and metabolism of the embryonic mouse heart. Reprod Toxicol 1997;11:495–502.
20. Lueder FL, Buroker CA, Kim S-B, Flozak AS, Ogata ES. Differential effects of short and long durations of insulin-induced maternal hypoglycemia upon fetal rat tissue growth and glucose utilization. Pediatr Res 1992;32:436–40.
21. Kimmerle R, Heinemann L, Delecki A, Berger M. Severe hypoglycemia incidence and predisposing factors in 85 pregnancies of type I diabetic women. Diabetes Care 1992;15:1034–7.
22. Kalter H. Letter to the editor. Teratology 1996;54:266.
23. Sadler TW. Letter from the editor. Teratology 1996; 54:266.

Name:	**INTERFERON, ALFA**	Risk Factor:	C_M
Class:	**Antineoplastic/Immunologic Agent (Immunomodulator)**		

FETAL RISK SUMMARY

RECOMMENDATION: Limited Human Data - Probably Compatible

Interferon alfa is a family of at least 23 structurally similar subtypes of human proteins and glycoproteins that have antiviral, antineoplastic, and immunomodulating properties (1). Five preparations are available in the United States: interferon alfa-n3, interferon alfa-N1 (orphan drug status), interferon alfa-2a, interferon alfa-2b, and peginterferon alfa-2B. Interferon alfa-2c has been used in pregnancy, but this product is not available in the United States. No reports describing the placental transfer of interferon alfa have been located.

Shepard reviewed four studies in which human interferon alfa (subtype not specified) was administered by various parenteral routes to rats and rabbits during pregnancy (2–5). No teratogenicity or adverse developmental changes were observed in the offspring.

Interferon alfa-2a produced a statistically significant increase in abortions in rhesus monkeys given 20–500 times the human dose (6). No teratogenic effects, however, were observed in this species when doses of 1–25 million IU/kg/day were administered during the early to mid fetal period (day 22 to day 70 of gestation) (6). Interferon alfa-2b also had abortifacient effects in rhesus monkeys treated with 7.5–30 million IU/kg (90–360 times the human dose) (7). Reproduction studies have not been conducted with interferon alfa-n3 (8).

Administration of interferon alfa to female sheep before conception resulted in an increased number of pregnant ewes and embryonic survival (9). This effect may have been the result of enhanced biochemical communication between the mother and conceptus (9). A study published in 1986 demonstrated that human fetal blood and organs, placenta, membranes, amniotic fluid, and decidua contain significant concentrations of interferon alfa (10). In contrast, maternal blood and blood and tissues from nonpregnant adults contained little or none of these proteins. The investigators concluded that one of the effects of interferon alfa may involve the preservation of the fetus as a homograft (10). Other effects and actions of endogenous interferons (alfa, beta, and gamma) in relation to animal and human pregnancies and the presence of these proteins in various maternal and fetal tissues have been summarized in two reviews (11,12).

A number of reports have described the use of interferon alfa in all phases of pregnancy for the treatment of leukemia (13–20). The first reported case involved a woman with chronic myelogenous leukemia (CML) who was treated before conception and throughout a normal pregnancy with 4 million units/m^2 (6.4 million units) of interferon alfa-2a every other day (13). She delivered a term, healthy, 3487-g female infant whose growth and development continued to be normal at 15 months of age. The newborn had an elevated white blood cell count (40,000/mm^3) that normalized at 48 hours of age with no signs or symptoms of infection. Since this report, 10 other pregnancies have been described in which interferon alfa was used for CML or hairy cell leukemia (14–20).

In one case, a woman was treated with interferon alfa-2c (not available in the United States) (16). In two of the pregnancies, the concentrations of interferon alfa in the newborns were <0.6 and <1 U/mL, respectively, while those in the mothers were 20.8 and 58 U/mL, respectively (18). Normal pregnancy outcomes were observed in all of the above cases and there were no fetal or newborn toxic effects attributable to interferon alfa (13–20). In addition, four infants have been followed for periods ranging from 6 to 44 months and all had normal growth and development (14).

A 1995 reference reported the use of interferon alfa-2a for the treatment of multiple myeloma before and during approximately the first 6 weeks of pregnancy (21). The woman delivered a normal male infant at 38 weeks' gestation.

As noted above, interferon alfa does not appear to cross the placenta to the fetus. A study published in 1995 specifically evaluated this in two HIV-seropositive women who were undergoing abortions at 19 and 24 weeks (22). Both women were given a single IM injection of 5 million U interferon alfa-2a. Peak blood concentrations of the drug were reached at 3 hours in both women, 100 U and 400 U, respectively. Fetal blood and amniotic fluid samples were drawn at 1 hour from one fetus and at 4 hours from the other. Concentrations in the four samples were all below the detection limit of the assay (<2 U).

A number of pregnant women have been treated with interferon alfa (usually interferon alfa-2a) for essential thrombocythemia (23–34), although not without controversy (35–37). In some of these cases, the women were receiving interferon therapy at the time of conception (23,24,26,28,29) and, in most, the treatment was continued throughout pregnancy (26,28,29). No adverse effects in the fetuses or in the newborns attributable to the drug therapy were reported.

An HIV-infected pregnant woman was treated with IM interferon alfa, 2 million units twice weekly, and oral and IV glycyrrhizin during the 3rd trimester (38). Two weeks after interferon alfa was started, an elective cesarean section was performed at 37 weeks' gestation. The healthy, 2320-g female was alive and well at 4 years of age without evidence of HIV infection.

Two reports have described the use of interferon alfa for the treatment of chronic hepatitis C (39,40). In both cases treatment was started before conception and continued into the 2nd trimester. Interferon alfa treatment throughout the 1st trimester also occurred in a woman with advanced Hodgkin's disease (41). Normal newborns resulted in all three of these pregnancies.

In summary, based on a limited number of human cases, the maternal administration of interferon alfa does not appear to pose a significant risk to the developing embryo and fetus. There does not seem to be a difference in risk among the subtypes but, in many cases, the actual product used was not specified. Although very high doses are abortifacient in rhesus monkeys, doses used clinically apparently do not have this effect. No teratogenic or other reproductive toxicity, other than that noted above, has been observed in animals, and no toxicity of any type attributable to interferon alfa has been observed in humans. However, because of the antiproliferative activity of these agents, they should be used cautiously during gestation until more data are available to assess their risk.

BREAST FEEDING SUMMARY

RECOMMENDATION: Limited Human Data - Probably Compatible

Interferon alfa is excreted into breast milk. A study published in 1996 measured interferon alfa milk concentrations in two women who had been treated with the drug throughout the 2nd and 3rd trimesters for CML (18). Both women were receiving 8 million units SC 3 times a week at the time of delivery. Immediately postpartum, milk concentrations in the two patients were 1.4 and 6 U/mL (time of the last dose in relationship to milk sampling not specified), while the serum levels in the mothers were 20.8 and 58 U/mL, respectively. The authors did not specify if the infants were allowed to breast-feed.

Breast-feeding was allowed in a second reference (25). The woman was being treated with interferon alfa-2a, 3 million units SC 3 times weekly, for essential thrombocythemia. Nursing was halted 2 weeks postpartum because of the onset of bilateral mastitis. In a 2000 case report, a woman with malignant melanoma received 30 million IU IV over 30 minutes (42). Breast milk samples were collected before (to measure endogenous interferon alfa) and after the infusion. Only small amounts of interferon alfa were transferred into milk (peak level 1551 IU/mL vs. 1249 IU/mL before infusion). The infant did not breast-feed during the therapy.

The American Academy of Pediatrics classifies interferon alfa as compatible with breast-feeding (43).

References

1. American Hospital Formulary Service. *Drug Information 1997*. Bethesda, MD: American Society of Health-System Pharmacists, 1997:775–804.
2. Matsumoto T, Nakamura K, Imai M, Aoki H, Okugi M, Shimoi H, Hagita K. Reproduction studies of human interferon α (interferon alpha). (I) Teratological study in rabbits. Iyakuhin Kenkyu 1986;17:397–404. As cited by Shepard TH. *Catalog of Teratogenic Agents*. 7th ed. Baltimore, MD: Johns Hopkins University Press, 1992:220–1.
3. Matsumoto T, Nakamura K, Imai M, Aoki H, Okugi M, Shimoi H, Hagita K. Reproduction studies of human interferon α (interferon alpha). (III) Teratological study in rats. Iyakuhin Kenkyu 1986;17:417–38. As cited by Shepard TH. *Catalog of Teratogenic Agents*. 7th ed. Baltimore, MD: Johns Hopkins University Press, 1992:220–1.
4. Matsumoto T, Nakamura K, Imai M, Aoki H, Okugi M, Shimoi H, Hagita K. Perinatal studies of human interferon α (interferon alpha). (IV) Teratological study in rats. Iyakuhin Kenkyu 1986;17:439–57. As cited by Shepard TH. *Catalog of Teratogenic Agents*. 7th ed. Baltimore, MD: Johns Hopkins University Press, 1992: 220–1.
5. Shibutani Y, Hamada Y, Kurokawa M, Inoue K, Shichi S. Toxicity studies of human lymphoblastoid interferon α. Teratogenicity study in rats. Iyakuhin Kenkyu 1987;18:60–78. As cited by Shepard TH. *Catalog of Teratogenic Agents*. 7th ed. Baltimore, MD: Johns Hopkins University Press, 1992:220–1.

6. Product information. Roferon-A. Roche Laboratories, 2001.
7. Product information. Intron A. Schering, 2001.
8. Product information. Alferon N. Interferon Sciences, 2001.
9. Nephew KP, McClure KE, Day ML, Xie S, Roberts RM, Pope WF. Effects of intramuscular administration of recombinant bovine interferon-alpha$_I$1 during the period of maternal recognition of pregnancy. J Anim Sci 1990;68:2766–70.
10. Chard T, Craig PH, Menabawey M, Lee C. Alpha interferon in human pregnancy. Br J Obstet Gynaecol 1986;93:1145–9.
11. Chard T. Interferon in pregnancy. J Develop Physiol 1989;11:271–6.
12. Roberts RM, Cross JC, Leaman DW. Interferons as hormones of pregnancy. Endocr Rev 1992;13:432–52.
13. Baer MR. Normal full-term pregnancy in a patient with chronic myelogenous leukemia treated with α-interferon. Am J Hematol 1991;37:66.
14. Baer MR, Ozer H, Foon KA. Interferon-α therapy during pregnancy in chronic myelogenous leukaemia and hairy cell leukaemia. Br J Haematol 1992,81:167–9.
15. Crump M, Wang X-H, Sermer M, Keating A. Successful pregnancy and delivery during α-interferon therapy for chronic myeloid leukemia. Am J Hematol 1992;40:238–43.
16. Reichel RP, Linkesch W, Schetitska D. Therapy with recombinant interferon alpha-2c during unexpected pregnancy in a patient with chronic myeloid leukaemia. Br J Haematol 1992;82:472–3.
17. Delmer A, Rio B, Bauduer F, Ajchenbaum F, Marie J-P, Zittoun R. Pregnancy during myelosuppressive treatment for chronic myelogenous leukaemia. Br J Haematol 1992;82:783–4.
18. Haggstrom J, Adriansson M, Hybbinette T, Harnby E, Thorbert G. Two cases of CML treated with alpha-interferon during second and third trimester of pregnancy with analysis of the drug in the new-born immediately postpartum. Eur J Haematol 1996;57:101–2.
19. Lipton JH, Derzko CM, Curtis J. Alpha-interferon and pregnancy in a patient with CML. Hematol Oncol 1996;14:119–22.
20. Kuroiwa M, Gondo H, Ashida K, Kamimura T, Miyamoto T, Niho Y, Tsukimori K, Nakano H, Ohga S. Interferon-alpha therapy for chronic myelogenous leukemia during pregnancy. Am J Hematology 1998;59:101–2.
21. Sakata H, Karamitsos J, Kundaria B, DiSaia PJ. Case report of interferon alfa therapy for multiple myeloma during pregnancy. Am J Obstet Gynecol 1995;172:217–9.
22. Pons J-C, Lebon P, Frydman R, Delfraissy J-F. Pharmacokinetics of interferon-alpha in pregnant women and fetoplacental passage. Fetal Diagn Ther 1995;10:7–10.
23. Pardini S, Dore F, Murineddu M, Bontigli S, Longinotti M, Grigliotti B, Spano B. α2b-Interferon therapy and pregnancy—report of a case of essential thrombocythemia. Am J Hematol 1993;43:78–9.
24. Petit JJ, Callis M, Fernandez de Sevilla A. Normal pregnancy in a patient with essential thrombocythemia treated with interferon-α_{2b}. Am J Hematol 1992;40:80.
25. Thornley S, Manoharan A. Successful treatment of essential thrombocythemia with alpha interferon during pregnancy. Eur J Haematol 1994;52:63–4.
26. Williams JM, Schlesinger PE, Gray AG. Successful treatment of essential thrombocythaemia and recurrent abortion with alpha interferon. Br J Haematol 1994;88:647–8.
27. Vianelli N, Gugliotta L, Tura S, Bovicelli L, Rizzo N, Gabrielli A. Interferon-α2a treatment in a pregnant woman with essential thrombocythemia. Blood 1994;83:874–5.
28. Shpilberg O, Shimon I, Sofer O, Dolitski M, Ben-Bassat I. Transient normal platelet counts and decreased requirement for interferon during pregnancy in essential thrombocythaemia. Br J Haematol 1996;92:491–3.
29. Pulik M, Lionnet F, Genet P, Petitdidier C, Jary L. Platelet counts during pregnancy in essential thrombocythaemia treated with recombinant α-interferon. Br J Haematol 1996;93:495.
30. Delage R, Demers C, Cantin G, Roy J. Treatment of essential thrombocythemia during pregnancy with interferon-α. Obstet Gynecol 1996;87:814–7.
31. Schmidt HH, Neumeister P, Kainer F, Karpf EF, Linkesch W, Sill H. Treatment of essential thrombocythemia during pregnancy: antiabortive effect of interferon-α? Ann Hematol 1998;77:291–2.
32. Diez-Martin JL, Banas MH, Fernandez MN. Childbearing age patients with essential thrombocythemia: should they be placed on interferon? Am J Hematol 1996;52:331–2.
33. Cincotta R, Higgins JR, Tippett C, Gallery E, North R, McMahon LP, Brennecke SP. Management of essential thrombocythaemia during pregnancy. Aust N Z J Obstet Gynaecol 2000;40:33–7.
34. Vantroyen B, Vanstraelen D. Management of essential thrombocythemia during pregnancy with aspirin, interferon alpha-2a and no treatment. Acta Haematol 2002;107:158–69.
35. Randi ML, Barbone E, Girolami A. Normal pregnancy and delivery in essential thrombocythemia even without interferon therapy. Am J Hematol 1994;45:270–1.
36. Petit J. Normal pregnancy and delivery in essential thrombocythemia even without interferon therapy. In reply. Am J Hematol 1994;45:271.
37. Frezzato M, Rodeghiero F. Pregnancy in women with essential thrombocythaemia. Br J Haematol 1996;93:977.
38. Sagara Y. Management of pregnancy of HIV infected woman. Early Hum Dev 1992;29:231–2.
39. Ruggiero G, Andreana A, Zampino R. Normal pregnancy under inadvertent alpha-interferon therapy for chronic hepatitis C. J Hepatol 1996;24:646.
40. Trotter JF, Zygmunt AJ. Conception and pregnancy during interferon-alpha therapy for chronic hepatitis C. J Clin Gastroenterol 2001;32:76–8.
41. Ferrari VD, Jirillo A, Lonardi F, Pavanato G, Bonciarelli G. Pregnancy during alpha-interferon therapy in patients with advanced Hodgkin's disease. Eur J Cancer 1995;31A;2121–2.
42. Kimar AR, Hale TW, Mock RE. Transfer of interferon alfa into human breast milk. J Hum Lact 2000;16:226–8.
43. Committee on Drugs, American Academy of Pediatrics. The transfer of drugs and other chemicals into human milk. Pediatrics 2001;108:776–89.

Name: **INTERFERON BETA-1B** Risk Factor: C_M

Class: **Immunologic Agent (Immunomodulator)**

FETAL RISK SUMMARY

RECOMMENDATION: Limited Human Data - Animal Data Suggest Moderate Risk

Interferon beta-1b, prepared by recombinant DNA technology, is used for the symptomatic treatment of multiple sclerosis and investigationally in the therapy of AIDS, some neoplasms, and acute non-A/non-B hepatitis. No teratogenic effects were observed in rhesus monkeys given doses up to 0.42 mg/kg/day (13.3 million IU, 40 times the recommended human dose based on body surface area [RHD]) on gestation days 20–70 (1). However, dose-related abortifacient activity occurred in these monkeys with doses of 0.028–0.42 mg/kg/day (2.8–40 times the RHD).

Although no published reports of its use in human pregnancy have been located, the manufacturer states that spontaneous abortions occurred in four patients who were participating in the Betaseron Multiple Sclerosis clinical trial (1). The relationship between interferon beta-1b and the abortions cannot be determined, at least partially because of the lack of details involving this clinical trial, such as the timing of abortion to drug administration, the dose used, the clinical condition of the women, and the number of pregnant women in the trial. Also unknown is the effect of multiple sclerosis on early pregnancy, although it appears that the physiologic immunomodulation that occurs in pregnancy offers some protection from relapses of the disease during gestation (2,3).

BREAST FEEDING SUMMARY

RECOMMENDATION: No Human Data - Probably Compatible

No data are available.

References

1. Product information. Betaseron. Berlex Laboratories, 1994.
2. Hutchinson M. Pregnancy in multiple sclerosis. J Neurol Neurosurg Psychiatry 1993;56:1043–5.
3. Roullet E, Verdier-Taillefer M-H, Armarenco P, Gharbi G, Alperovitch A, Marteau R. Pregnancy and multiple sclerosis: a longitudinal study of 125 remittent patients. J Neurol Neurosurg Psychiatry 1993;56:1062–5.

Name: **INTERFERON GAMMA-1B** Risk Factor: C_M

Class: **Immunologic Agent (Immunomodulator)**

FETAL RISK SUMMARY

RECOMMENDATION: No Human Data - Animal Data Suggest Low Risk

No reports describing the use of interferon gamma-1b in human pregnancy have been located. Interferon gamma-1b, produced by recombinant DNA technology, is used to reduce the frequency and severity of serious infections in patients who have chronic granulomatous disease (1). Because of this indication, the opportunities for its use in human pregnancy should be rare.

Interferon gamma-1b has abortifacient activity in nonhuman primates treated with a dose approximately 100 times the human dose (1). Similar activity was observed in mice treated with maternally toxic doses. Other effects noted in mice were an increased incidence of uterine bleeding and decreased neonatal viability (1). However, no evidence of teratogenicity was found in primates with doses of 2–100 times the human dose (1).

Treatment of pregnant mice with 5000 units/day for 6 days produced maternal and fetal hematologic toxicity (2). In addition to an increase in aborted fetuses and decreased fetal weight, severe anomalies, consisting of inhibition or retardation of eye formation and brain hematomas, were observed in surviving fetuses (2).

Two reviews have summarized the effects and actions of endogenous interferons (alfa, beta, and gamma) in animal and human pregnancies and the presence of these proteins in various maternal and fetal tissues (3,4).

BREAST FEEDING SUMMARY

RECOMMENDATION: No Human Data - Probably Compatible

No data are available.

I

References

1. Product information. Actimmune. Genentech, Inc., 1994.
2. Vassiliadis S, Athanassakis I. Type II interferon may be a potential hazardous therapeutic agent during pregnancy. Br J Haematol 1992;82:782–3.
3. Chard T. Interferon in pregnancy. J Develop Physiol 1989;11:271–6.
4. Roberts RM, Cross JC, Leaman DW. Interferons as hormones of pregnancy. Endocr Rev 1992;13:432–52.

Name:	**IOCETAMIC ACID**	Risk Factor: **D**
Class:	**Diagnostic**	

FETAL RISK SUMMARY

RECOMMENDATION: Human Data Suggest Risk in 2nd and 3rd Trimesters

Iocetamic acid contains a high concentration of organically bound iodine. See Diatrizoate for possible effects on the fetus and neonate.

BREAST FEEDING SUMMARY

RECOMMENDATION: No Human Data - Probably Compatible

See Potassium Iodide.

Name:	**IODAMIDE**	Risk Factor: **D**
Class:	**Diagnostic**	

FETAL RISK SUMMARY

RECOMMENDATION: Human Data Suggest Risk in 2nd and 3rd Trimesters

The various preparations of iodamide contain a high concentration of organically bound iodine. See Diatrizoate for possible effects on the fetus and newborn.

BREAST FEEDING SUMMARY

RECOMMENDATION: Limited Human Data - Probably Compatible

Iodamide is excreted into breast milk. A woman, 7 weeks postpartum, received the contrast medium for urography (1). Nine hours after the dose, no measurable drug was identified by spectrophotometer. (See Potassium Iodide.)

Reference

1. FitzJohn TP, Williams DG, Laker MF, Owen JP. Intravenous urography during lactation. Br J Radiol 1982; 55:603–5.

I

Name:	**IODINATED GLYCEROL**	Risk Factor:	X_M
Class:	**Respiratory Drug (Expectorant)**		

FETAL RISK SUMMARY

RECOMMENDATION: Human Data Suggest Risk in 2nd and 3rd Trimesters

Iodinated glycerol is a stable complex containing 50% organically bound iodine (see Potassium Iodide). In a surveillance study of Michigan Medicaid recipients conducted between 1985 and 1992 involving 229,101 completed pregnancies, 1453 newborns had been exposed to iodinated glycerol during the 1st trimester (F. Rosa, personal communication, FDA, 1993). A total of 65 (4.5%) major birth defects were observed (61 expected). Specific data were available for six defect categories, including (observed/expected) 11/15 cardiovascular defects, 0/2 oral clefts, 1/1 spina bifida, 8/4 polydactyly, 1/2 limb reduction defects, and 1/3 hypospadias. An additional 1338 newborns were exposed to the general class of expectorants during the 1st trimester with 63 (4.7%) major birth defects observed (57 expected). Specific malformations were (observed/expected) 9/13 cardiovascular defects, 0/2 oral clefts, 1/1 spina bifida, 7/4 polydactyly, 1/2 limb reduction defects, and 3/3 hypospadias. These data do not support an association between 1st trimester use of either iodinated glycerol or the general class of expectorants and congenital defects.

BREAST FEEDING SUMMARY

RECOMMENDATION: No Human Data - Probably Compatible

See Potassium Iodide.

Name:	**IODINE**	Risk Factor:	**D**
Class:	**Anti-infective**		

See Potassium Iodide.

Name:	**IODIPAMIDE**	Risk Factor:	**D**
Class:	**Diagnostic**		

FETAL RISK SUMMARY

RECOMMENDATION: Human Data Suggest Risk in 2nd and 3rd Trimesters

The various preparations of iodipamide contain a high concentration of organically bound iodine. See Diatrizoate for possible effects on the fetus and newborn.

BREAST FEEDING SUMMARY

RECOMMENDATION: No Human Data - Probably Compatible

See Potassium Iodide.

I

Name:	**IODOQUINOL**	Risk Factor:	**C**
Class:	**Amebicide**		

FETAL RISK SUMMARY

RECOMMENDATION: Limited Human Data - No Relevant Animal Data

Iodoquinol (diiodohydroxyquinoline; diiodohydroxyquin) is used in the treatment of intestinal amebiasis. It has been used in pregnancy apparently without causing fetal harm.

Two case reports described the use of iodoquinol in pregnancy for the treatment of a rare skin disease. The first case involved a woman with chronic acrodermatitis enteropathica who was treated with the amebicide in the 2nd and 3rd trimesters of her first pregnancy (1). She delivered a typical achondroplastic dwarf who died in 30 minutes. The second case also involved a woman with the same disorder who took iodoquinol throughout gestation (2). Dosage during the 1st trimester, 1.3 g/day, was systematically increased during pregnancy in an attempt to control the cutaneous lesions, eventually reaching 6.5 g/day during the last 4 weeks. A normal male infant was delivered at term. Physical examinations of the infant, including ophthalmic examinations, were normal at birth and at 6 weeks follow-up.

The Collaborative Perinatal Project monitored 50,282 mother-child pairs, 169 of whom had 1st trimester exposure to iodoquinol (3, pp. 299, 302). Ten of the infants were born with a congenital malformation, corresponding to a hospital standardized relative risk (SRR) of 0.88. Based on three infants, an SRR of 6.6 for congenital dislocation of the hip was calculated, but this association is not interpretable without confirming evidence (3, pp. 467, 473). For use anytime during pregnancy, 172 exposures were recorded (3, pp. 434, 435). With the same caution as noted above, an SRR of 1.68 (95% confidence interval 0.62–3.58) was estimated based on malformations in 6 infants. The SRR for congenital dislocation of the hip after use anytime during pregnancy was 6.5 (3, p. 486).

BREAST FEEDING SUMMARY

RECOMMENDATION: Limited Human Data - Probably Compatible

No reports describing the use of iodoquinol during lactation have been located. Although the oral bioavailability is low, the molecular weight (397) should allow transfer of some drug from the plasma into the milk. In addition, protein-bound serum iodine levels may be increased with the administration of iodoquinol and persist for as long as 6 months after discontinuation of therapy (4). The effects on a nursing infant from this exposure are unknown, but because iodide is concentrated in breast milk, serum and urinary iodide levels in the infant may be elevated (see Potassium Iodide).

References

1. Vedder JS, Griem S. Acrodermatitis enteropathica (Danbolt-Closs) in five siblings: efficacy of diodoquin in its management. J Pediatr 1956;48:212–9.
2. Verburg DJ, Burd LI, Hoxtell EO, Merrill LK. Acrodermatitis enteropathica and pregnancy. Obstet Gynecol 1974;44:233–7.
3. Heinonen OP, Slone D, Shapiro S. *Birth Defects and Drugs in Pregnancy*. Littleton, MA: Publishing Sciences Group, 1977.
4. Product information. Yodoxin. Glenwood, 2000.

I

Name:	**IODOTHYRIN**	Risk Factor:	**A**
Class:	**Thyroid**		

FETAL RISK SUMMARY

RECOMMENDATION: Compatible

Iodothyrin is a combination product containing thyroid, iodized calcium, and peptone. See Thyroid.

BREAST FEEDING SUMMARY

RECOMMENDATION: Compatible

See Levothyroxine and Liothyronine.

Name:	**IODOXAMATE**	Risk Factor:	**D**
Class:	**Diagnostic**		

FETAL RISK SUMMARY

RECOMMENDATION: Human Data Suggest Risk in 2nd and 3rd Trimesters

The various preparations of iodoxamate contain a high concentration of organically bound iodine. See Diatrizoate for possible effects on the fetus and newborn.

BREAST FEEDING SUMMARY

RECOMMENDATION: No Human Data - Probably Compatible

See Potassium Iodide.

Name:	**IOHEXOL**	Risk Factor:	**D**
Class:	**Diagnostic**		

FETAL RISK SUMMARY

RECOMMENDATION: Human Data Suggest Risk in 2nd and 3rd Trimesters

Iohexol, a nonionic radiopaque agent, contains a high concentration of organically bound iodine (140–350 mg iodine/mL). Iohexol was not detected in the fetuses or amniotic fluid of mid-term rabbits (1).

Use of organically bound iodine preparations near term has resulted in hypothyroidism in some newborns (see Diatrizoate). Appropriate measures should be taken to treat neonatal hypothyroidism if diagnostic tests with iohexol are required close to delivery.

BREAST FEEDING SUMMARY

RECOMMENDATION: Limited Human Data - Probably Compatible

Iohexol is excreted into the milk of rabbits (1) and humans (2). In rabbits, the amount measured in milk was 1.6% of the administered dose (1). Four lactating women received the IV contrast media (1 mL/kg–350 mg iodine/mL) in the postpartum period (1 week to 14 months) (2). Breast-feeding was stopped for 48 hours. The amount excreted over a 24-hour period was 0.5% of the maternal weight-adjusted dose. This amount does not appear to be clinically significant (2). The American Academy of Pediatrics classifies iohexol as compatible with breast-feeding (3).

References

1. Bourrinet P, Dencausse A, Havard P, Violas X, Bonnemain B. Transplacental passage and milk excretion of iobitridol. Invest Radiol 1995;30:156–8.
2. Nielsen ST, Matheson I, Rasmussen JN, Skinnemoen K, Andrew E, Hafsahl G. Excretion of iohexol and metrizoate in human breast milk. Acta Radiol 1987;28:523–6.
3. Committee on Drugs, American Academy of Pediatrics. The transfer of drugs and other chemicals into human milk. Pediatrics 2001;108:776–89.

Name:	**IOPANOIC ACID**	Risk Factor:	**D**
Class:	**Diagnostic**		

FETAL RISK SUMMARY

RECOMMENDATION: Human Data Suggest Risk in 2nd and 3rd Trimesters

Iopanoic acid contains a high concentration of organically bound iodine. See Diatrizoate for possible effects on the fetus and newborn.

BREAST FEEDING SUMMARY

RECOMMENDATION: Limited Human Data - Probably Compatible

Iopanoic acid is excreted in breast milk. Cholecystography was performed in 11 lactating patients with iopanoic acid (1). The mean amount of iodine administered to five patients was 2.77 g (range 1.98–3.96 g) and the mean amount excreted in breast milk during the next 19–29 hours was 20.8 mg (0.08%) (range 6.72–29.9 mg). The nursing infants showed no reaction to the contrast media. The American Academy of Pediatrics classifies iopanoic acid as compatible with breast-feeding (2).

References

1. Holmdahl KH. Cholecystography during lactation. Acta Radiol 1956;45:305–7.
2. Committee on Drugs, American Academy of Pediatrics. The transfer of drugs and other chemicals into human milk. Pediatrics 2001;108:776–89.

Name: **IOTHALAMATE**
Class: **Diagnostic**
Risk Factor: **D**

FETAL RISK SUMMARY

RECOMMENDATION: Human Data Suggest Risk in 2nd and 3rd Trimesters

Iothalamate has been used for diagnostic procedures during pregnancy. Amniography was performed in one patient to diagnose monoamniotic twinning shortly before an elective cesarean section (1). No effect on the two newborns was mentioned. In a second study, 17 women were given either iothalamate or metrizoate for ascending phlebography during various stages of pregnancy (2). Two patients, one exposed in the 1st trimester and one in the 2nd trimester, were diagnosed as having deep vein thrombosis and were treated with heparin. The baby from the 2nd trimester patient was normal, but the other newborn had hyperbilirubinemia and undescended testis. The relationship between the diagnostic agents (or other drugs) and the defects is not known.

Use of other organically bound iodine preparations near term has resulted in hypothyroidism in some newborns (see Diatrizoate). Thus, appropriate measures should be taken to treat neonatal hypothyroidism if diagnostic tests with iothalamate are required close to delivery.

BREAST FEEDING SUMMARY

RECOMMENDATION: No Human Data - Probably Compatible

See Potassium Iodide.

References

1. Dunnihoo DR, Harris RE. The diagnosis of monoamniotic twinning by amniography. Am J Obstet Gynecol 1966;96:894–5.
2. Kierkegaard A. Incidence and diagnosis of deep vein thrombosis associated with pregnancy. Acta Obstet Gynecol Scand 1983;62:239–43.

Name: **IPODATE**
Class: **Diagnostic**
Risk Factor: **D**

FETAL RISK SUMMARY

RECOMMENDATION: Human Data Suggest Risk in 2nd and 3rd Trimesters

Ipodate contains a high concentration of organically bound iodine. See Diatrizoate for possible effects on the fetus and newborn.

BREAST FEEDING SUMMARY

RECOMMENDATION: No Human Data - Probably Compatible

See Potassium Iodide.

Name:	**IPRATROPIUM**	Risk Factor:	**B_M**
Class:	**Parasympatholytic**		

FETAL RISK SUMMARY

RECOMMENDATION: Human Data Suggest Low Risk

Ipratropium, an anticholinergic compound chemically related to atropine, is a quaternary ammonium bromide used as a bronchodilator for the treatment of bronchospasm. Its use during pregnancy is primarily confined to patients with severe asthma (1).

Ipratropium was not teratogenic in mice, rats, and rabbits when administered either orally or by inhalation (2). Oral doses used in the reproductive toxicity studies were 2000, 200,000, and 26,000 times the maximum recommended human daily dose (MRHDD), respectively. Doses used by inhalation in rats and rabbits were, respectively, 312 and 375 times the MRHDD. Schardein cited a German study that found no evidence of teratogenicity in mice, rats, and rabbits (3). A Japanese study involving rats and rabbits that found no adverse fetal effects except a slight weight reduction was described by Shepard (4).

Data from a surveillance study of Medicaid patients between 1982 and 1994 indicated that 37 women took this drug during the 1st trimester (F. Rosa, personal communication, FDA, 1996). One malformation, a renal obstruction, was observed. Preliminary analysis found no brain defects among 80 recipients following exposure anytime during pregnancy.

A 1991 brief report described the use of nebulized ipratropium, among other drugs, in the treatment of life-threatening status asthmaticus in a pregnant patient at 12.5 weeks' gestation (5). She eventually delivered a term 3440-g male infant (information on the condition of the newborn was not provided).

A number of sources recommend the use of inhaled ipratropium for severe asthma, especially in those not responding adequately to other therapy (1,6–8). The consensus appears to be that although human data are rare, there is no evidence that the drug is hazardous to the fetus. Moreover, it produces less systemic effects than atropine (1), and may have an additive bronchodilatory effect to β_2 agonists (6).

BREAST FEEDING SUMMARY

RECOMMENDATION: No Human Data - Probably Compatible

No reports describing the excretion of ipratropium into human milk have been located. A chemically related drug, atropine, is considered compatible with breast-feeding by the American Academy of Pediatrics (9), although definitive data on the appearance of atropine in milk has not been published. Ipratropium is lipid-insoluble and, similar to other quaternary ammonium bases, may appear in milk. The amounts, although unknown, are probably clinically insignificant, however, especially after inhalation.

References

1. Report of the Working Group on Asthma and Pregnancy. *Management of Asthma During Pregnancy.* Washington, DC: National Institutes of Health Publication No. 93–3279, Public Health Service, US Department of Health and Human Services, 1993:20.
2. Product information. Atrovent. Boehringer Ingelheim Pharmaceuticals, 1996.
3. Schardein JL. *Chemically Induced Birth Defects.* 2nd ed. New York, NY: Marcel Dekker, 1993:343.
4. Shepard TH. *Catalog of Teratogenic Agents.* 8th ed. Baltimore, MD: Johns Hopkins University Press, 1995:238.
5. Gilchrist DM, Friedman JM, Werker D. Life-threatening status asthmaticus at 12.5 weeks' gestation. Chest 1991;100:285–6.
6. D'Alonzo GE. The pregnant asthmatic patient. Semin Perinatol 1990;14:119–29.
7. Schatz M. Asthma during pregnancy: interrelationships and management. Ann Allergy 1992;68:123–33.
8. Moore-Gillon J. Asthma in pregnancy. Br J Obstet Gynaecol 1994;101:658–60.
9. Committee on Drugs, American Academy of Pediatrics. The transfer of drugs and other chemicals into human milk. Pediatrics 1994;93:137–50.

Name:	**IPRINDOLE**	Risk Factor:	**C**
Class:	**Antidepressant**		

No data are available (see Imipramine).

Name:	**IPRONIAZID**	Risk Factor:	**C**
Class:	**Antidepressant**		

No data are available (see Phenelzine).

Name:	**IRBESARTAN**	Risk Factor:	C_M*
Class:	**Antihypertensive**		

FETAL RISK SUMMARY

RECOMMENDATION: Human Data Suggest Risk in 2nd and 3rd Trimesters

Irbesartan is a selective angiotensin II receptor antagonist that is used either alone, or in combination with other antihypertensive agents, for the treatment of hypertension. Irbesartan blocks the vasoconstrictor and aldosterone-secreting effects of angiotensin II by preventing angiotensin II from binding to AT_1 receptors.

Reproduction studies have been conducted in rats and rabbits during pregnancy (1). In the pregnant rat, doses approximately equal to or higher than the maximum recommended human dose of 300 mg/day on a body surface area basis (MRHD) were associated with increased incidences of renal pelvic cavitation, hydroureter and/or absence of renal papilla. At 4 times the MRHD, subcutaneous edema was observed in the fetuses. The anomalies appeared to be related to late, rather than early, gestational exposure (1). Doses approximately 1.5 times the MRHD in pregnant rabbits produced maternal mortality and abortion. Surviving rabbits had a slight increase in early resorptions (1). No adverse effects on fertility or reproductive performance were seen in male and female rats at an oral dose about 5 times the MRHD (1).

It is not known if irbesartan crosses the human placenta to the fetus. The molecular weight (about 429) is low enough, however, that transfer to the fetus should be expected. The drug does cross the placentas of rats and rabbits in late gestation (1).

No reports describing the use of irbesartan during human pregnancy have been located. The antihypertensive mechanisms of action of irbesartan and angiotensin-converting enzyme (ACE) inhibitors are very close. That is, the former selectively blocks the binding of angiotensin II to AT1 receptors, whereas the latter prevents the formation of angiotensin II itself. Therefore, use of this drug during the 2nd and 3rd trimesters may cause teratogenicity and severe fetal and neonatal toxicity that is identical to that seen with ACE inhibitors (e.g., see Captopril or Enalapril). Fetal toxic effects may include anuria, oligohydramnios, fetal hypocalvaria, intrauterine growth retardation, prematurity, and patent ductus arteriosus. Anuria-associated oligohydramnios may produce fetal limb contractures, craniofacial deformation, and pulmonary hypoplasia. Severe anuria and hypotension, that is resistant to both pressor agents and volume expansion, may occur in the newborn following *in utero* exposure to irbesartan. Newborn renal function and blood pressure should be closely monitored. If irbesartan is used in pregnancy, healthcare professionals are encouraged to call the toll free number (800-670-6126) for information about patient enrollment in the Motherisk study.

[**Risk factor D_M if used in 2nd or 3rd trimesters.*]

I

BREAST FEEDING SUMMARY

RECOMMENDATION: No Human Data - Probably Compatible

No reports describing the use irbesartan during human lactation have been located. The agent is found in the milk of lactating rats (1). Because of the relatively low molecular weight (about 429), excretion into human breast milk should also be expected. The effects of this exposure on a nursing infant are unknown. The American Academy of Pediatrics, however, classifies ACE inhibitors, a closely related group of antihypertensive agents, as compatible with breast-feeding (see Captopril or Enalapril).

Reference

1. Product information. Avapro. Bristol-Myers Squibb, 2000.

Name:	**ISOCARBOXAZID**	Risk Factor:	**C**
Class:	**Antidepressant**		

FETAL RISK SUMMARY

RECOMMENDATION: Limited Human Data - No Relevant Animal Data

Isocarboxazid is a monoamine oxidase inhibitor. The Collaborative Perinatal Project monitored 21 mother-child pairs exposed to these drugs during the 1st trimester, 1 of which was exposed to isocarboxazid (1). An increased risk of malformations was found. Details of the single case with exposure to isocarboxazid were not given.

BREAST FEEDING SUMMARY

RECOMMENDATION: No Human Data - Potential Toxicity

No data are available.

Reference

1. Heinonen OP, Slone D, Shapiro S. *Birth Defects and Drugs in Pregnancy*. Littleton, MA: Publishing Sciences Group, 1977:336–7.

Name: **ISOETHARINE** Risk Factor: **C**

Class: **Sympathomimetic (Adrenergic)**

FETAL RISK SUMMARY

RECOMMENDATION: Limited Human Data - No Relevant Animal Data

No reports linking the use of isoetharine with congenital defects have been located. Isoetharine-like drugs are teratogenic in some animal species, but human teratogenicity has not been suspected (1,2).

The Collaborative Perinatal Project monitored 50,282 mother-child pairs, 3082 of whom had 1st trimester exposure to sympathomimetic drugs (3, pp. 345–356). For use anytime during pregnancy, 9719 exposures were recorded (3, p. 439). An association in the 1st trimester was found between the sympathomimetic class of drugs as a whole and minor malformations (not life-threatening or major cosmetic defects), inguinal hernia, and clubfoot (3, pp. 345–356). Sympathomimetics are often administered in combination with other drugs to alleviate the symptoms of upper respiratory infections. Thus, the fetal effects of sympathomimetics, other drugs, and viruses cannot be totally separated. However, indiscriminate use of this class of drugs, especially in the 1st trimester, is not without risk.

In a surveillance study of Michigan Medicaid recipients conducted between 1985 and 1992 involving 229,101 completed pregnancies, 22 newborns had been exposed to isoetharine during the 1st trimester (F. Rosa, personal communication, FDA, 1993). No major birth defects were observed (one expected).

BREAST FEEDING SUMMARY

RECOMMENDATION: No Human Data - Probably Compatible

No data are available.

References

1. Nishimura H, Tanimura T. *Clinical Aspects of The Teratogenicity of Drugs*. New York, NY: American Elsevier, 1976:231.
2. Shepard TH. *Catalog of Teratogenic Agents*. 3rd ed. Baltimore, MD: Johns Hopkins University Press, 1980:134–5.
3. Heinonen OP, Slone D, Shapiro S. *Birth Defects and Drugs in Pregnancy*. Littleton, MA: Publishing Sciences Group, 1977.

Name: **ISOFLURANE** Risk Factor: **B**

Class: **General Anesthetic**

FETAL RISK SUMMARY

RECOMMENDATION: Limited Human Data - Animal Data Suggest Low Risk

The nonflammable general anesthetic isoflurane is in the same class of volatile liquid halogenated agents as desflurane, enflurane, halothane, methoxyflurane, and sevoflurane.

It is closely related to desflurane and enflurane. The only difference between isoflurane and desflurane is the presence of a chlorine atom in isoflurane instead of a fluorine atom. This small difference, however, produces marked pharmacokinetic and clinical effects. The potency of isoflurane is five times that of desflurane, the blood-gas partition coefficient is increased (i.e., increased solubility in blood) (1.46 vs. 0.42), as is tissue solubility (brain-blood partition coefficient 1.6 vs. 1.3), and recovery from anesthesia is slower (1).

In an animal reproductive study, mean anesthetic concentrations (about 1.6%) of isoflurane were administered to male and female rats for 5-day intervals up to 15 days before pairing (2). No adverse effects on mating and fertility indices were observed. Studies for structural anomalies were conducted in pregnant rats and rabbits in the same way. Three groups of rats received mean anesthetic doses of 1.6%–1.7% for 5-day intervals between day 1 and day 15 of gestation, whereas three groups of rabbits received mean doses of 2.3% for 4- or 5-day intervals between day 6 and day 18 of gestation. No congenital malformations related to the exposures were found in either animal species (2). In the third segment of this study, pregnant rats were exposed to isoflurane 1.74% for 1 hour/day on gestation days 15–20. Maternal weight gain was significantly less in the exposed group, and fetal survival was also decreased (2).

Three dose-levels of isoflurane were administered in a reproduction study with pregnant mice: trace (0.006%), subanesthetic (0.06%), and light anesthetic (0.6%) (3). No adverse maternal or fetal effects were observed when the two smaller concentrations were administered for 4 hours daily on days 6–15 of pregnancy. When given the same way, the light anesthetic dose, however, resulted in significantly lower maternal weight gain. Fetal toxicity included a significant decrease in fetal weight, decreased skeletal ossification, minor hydronephrosis, and increased pelvic cavitation (3). In addition, an increased incidence of cleft palate was observed (12.1% vs. 0.75% for controls). The incidence of cleft palate also was higher than that observed in previous experiments with halothane (1.2%) or enflurane (1.9%) (3).

In a second study by the authors of the above report, the effects of four general anesthetic agents were compared in pregnant rats (4). The doses and agents used were nitrous oxide (75%; 0.55 MAC), enflurane (1.65%; 0.75 MAC), halothane (0.8%; 0.75 MAC), and isoflurane (1.05%; 0.75 MAC). (*Note: the minimum alveolar anesthetic concentration [MAC] is the concentration that causes immobility in 50% of patients exposed to a noxious stimulus such as a surgical incision; it represents the* ED_{50} *[5].*) Each agent was administered for 6 hours on each of three consecutive days in one of three gestational periods: pregnancy days 8–10, 11–13, or 14–16. Compared with controls, significantly decreased maternal weight gain was observed in three of the groups (nitrous oxide, isoflurane, and enflurane) after exposure on days 14–16. Exposure on those days resulted in significantly decreased fetal weight in all four groups and, when exposure occurred on days 8–10, in three groups (all except nitrous oxide). Nitrous oxide exposure during days 14–16 resulted in significant increases in total fetal wastage and resorptions (3-fold increases). However, no major or minor teratogenic effects were observed in any of the groups (4).

The teratogenic potential of isoflurane, enflurane, and sevoflurane was studied by evaluating the effect of each agent on the proliferation and differentiation of cells exiting from the G1-phase of the cell cycle (6). The theory behind the study was that normal development during embryogenesis, organogenesis, and histogenesis depended upon the proliferation and differentiative processes of cell migration (6). For example, valproate, a known human teratogen, is a potent G1-phase inhibitor of the *in vitro* proliferation rate at concentrations less than two times the therapeutic plasma concentration. At anesthetic concentrations less than two times the MAC, the antiproliferative potency of the three agents was isoflurane = enflurane >> sevoflurane. However, in the growth-arrested cell population, there was no specific accumulation of any cell cycle phase and no specific effect on the G1 phase. The investigators concluded that the three agents lacked the specific *in vitro* characteristics of valproate (6).

Three anesthetic agents, isoflurane, halothane, and methoxyflurane, were administered to pregnant (near term) and nonpregnant ewes in a study designed to determine the requirement for inhaled anesthetic agents (7). The MAC was decreased in the pregnant animals in each case—40%, 25%, and 32% less, respectively. In a 1994 study, women at 8–12 weeks' gestation (all undergoing termination of pregnancy) were matched with women undergoing gynecologic surgery (8). The MAC was reduced by 28% in comparison to the nonpregnant controls (median end-tidal concentration 0.775% vs. 1.075%, respectively).

Two reviews have concluded that, in general, inhalational anesthetics are freely transferred to fetal tissues (9,10) and, in most cases, the maternal and fetal concentrations are equivalent (10). The low molecular weight (about 185) and the presence of isoflurane in the maternal brain support this assertion. In agreement, research has demonstrated the rapid uptake of isoflurane by the fetus (11).

A 1991 case report described two liver transplant procedures, 3 days apart, in a pregnant woman at approximately 21 weeks' gestation (12). Isoflurane was the only inhaled anesthetic agent used, although a number of other drugs were administered during the combined 24.4 hours of anesthesia. The woman eventually delivered a healthy infant by cesarean section (12).

Subanesthetic doses of isoflurane have been used for labor analgesia (13–15). A study published in 1985 compared the self-administration of isoflurane (0.75% in oxygen) or 50% nitrous oxide in oxygen given in a random sequence in 32 women (13). Isoflurane use resulted in better analgesia but increased drowsiness. The condition of the newborns was not mentioned. A 1989 study used isoflurane (0.2%–0.7%) or 30%–60% nitrous oxide (30 in each group) for labor analgesia (14). Seven percent of the newborns in both groups were depressed (1 minute Apgar scores 5–7), but all had Apgar scores of 8–10 at 5 minutes. There was also no difference in neonatal neurobehavior as measured by the Neurologic and Adaptive Capacity Scores (NACS) at 15 minutes, 2 hours, and 24 hours of age. Although specific percentages were not given, it was stated that there was no significant difference between the groups in the percentage of infants who scored 35–40 on the NACS. Mothers in the isoflurane group had higher concentrations of fluoride in their urine at 12–24 hours postpartum than those who had received nitrous oxide (36.5 vs. 23.6 μmol/L), but the fluoride blood levels were similar (<5.6 μmol/L). The fluoride urine levels in the newborns (first void) also were similar (<5.6 μmol/L) (14). In a 1993 report, 17 laboring women received alternating doses of 0.2% isoflurane plus 50% nitrous oxide/oxygen or nitrous oxide/oxygen alone, each over 1-hour intervals, for a total of 3 hours (15). Analgesia was significantly better when the women were receiving isoflurane. Progressive drowsiness was noted over the 3-hour period, but it was not considered clinically significant. The newborns were delivered vaginally and all had 1-and 5-minute Apgar scores of 8 to 10. Neurobehavior assessment was not conducted (15).

Isoflurane has been used for anesthesia during cesarean section (11,16–19). As with vaginal delivery, some degree of neonatal depression may occur as indicated by Apgar scores less than 7 at 1 minute (11,16–18) or a NACS less than 35 at 2 and 24 hours of age (16). A small 1983 study compared the neonatal outcomes in four groups (10 patients each) of women receiving general anesthesia for cesarean section: 50% nitrous oxide and

50% oxygen either alone, or combined with 0.5% halothane, 1.0% enflurane, or 0.75% isoflurane (19). One newborn had an Apgar score less than 7 at 1 minute (enflurane group), but all newborns in all groups had scores of 7 or greater at 5 minutes. There were no significant differences between the groups in neonatal neurobehavior assessment 2–4 hours after delivery or in maternal or umbilical blood gas analysis at delivery.

In a 1977 *in vitro* study, isoflurane was shown to have a statistically significant depressive effect on myometrial strips from non-gravid and gravid uteri (20). Three anesthetic agents, isoflurane, enflurane, and halothane, were studied at three concentrations (0.5, 1.0, and 1.5 MAC). The amount of depression was dose-related for each agent and was similar with all agents (20). Another study also demonstrated a dose-related relaxing effect of isoflurane (0.5%, 1.0%, and 1.5%) on isolated gravid human uterine muscle (21). All doses caused a significant decrease in uterine activity, but oxytocin, in a dose similar to that used clinically, reversed the effects of the anesthetic (21). In another study, the subjective assessment of maternal blood loss and uterine relaxation was less for isoflurane than for halothane (16).

A study published in 1998 evaluated the exposure of nine nurses in a post-anesthesia care unit (PACU) to exhaled isoflurane and desflurane and compared these exposures to the National Institute of Occupational Safety and Health (NIOSH) recommended exposure limits (22). The NIOSH recommendation for volatile anesthetics (without concomitant nitrous oxide exposure) is a maximum of 2 parts per million, but has not been adopted by the Occupational Safety and Health Administration. Moreover, the recommended limit is controversial and is thought by some to be inappropriately low (22). However, a potential for reproductive risk (spontaneous abortion and infertility) is thought to exist for some anesthetic agents. The study involved exposure in the PACU to exhaled anesthetic gases from 50 adult patients (isoflurane $N - 19$, desflurane $N - 31$) over an approximately 1-hour recovery time. About one-half of the patients were extubated in the PACU. Exposure was continuously measured from the shoulders (i.e., breathing zone) of the nurses. Breathing-zone anesthetic concentrations of isoflurane and desflurane exceeded the NIOSH limits in 37% and 87% of the cases, respectively. These exposures were above the limit 12% of the time for isoflurane and 49% of the time for desflurane. The investigators listed several limitations to their study and concluded that the results might represent a "worst-case analysis" (22).

A 2004 study found a significant association between maternal occupational exposure to waste anesthetic gases during pregnancy and developmental deficits in their children, including gross and fine motor ability, inattention/hyperactivity, and IQ performance (see Nitrous Oxide).

In summary, isoflurane was not teratogenic in mice, rats, and rabbits at doses that did not cause maternal toxicity. No reports of its use early in human gestation have been located. The absence of human experience during organogenesis prevents an assessment of the risk for structural anomalies. In addition, general anesthesia usually involves the use of multiple pharmacological agents. Although no teratogenicity has been observed with two other halogenated general anesthetic agents (halothane and methoxyflurane), only halothane has 1st trimester human exposure data (9). Isoflurane has been used immediately prior to delivery for analgesia and anesthesia. This use does not appear to affect the newborn any differently than other general anesthetic agents. The uterine effects of isoflurane (relaxation and increased blood loss) also appear to be similar to other agents in this class (23). All anesthetic agents can cause depression in the newborn that may last for 24 hours or more. The potential reproductive toxicity (spontaneous abortion and infertility) of occupational exposure to isoflurane has not been studied but is a concern based on the exposure concentration found in one study. Furthermore, occupational exposure to nitrous oxide was also measured in that study, and indicated that the nurses were exposed to both nitrous oxide and volatile anesthetic agents at the same time.

BREAST FEEDING SUMMARY

RECOMMENDATION: No Human Data - Probably Compatible

Although isoflurane has been administered during labor and delivery, the effects of this exposure on the infant that begins nursing immediately after birth have not been described. Isoflurane is probably excreted into colostrum and milk as suggested by its presence in the maternal blood and its low molecular weight (about 185), but the toxic potential of this exposure for the infant is unknown. However, the risk to a nursing infant from exposure to isoflurane via milk is probably very low (24,25). Another halogenated inhalation anesthetic, halothane, is classified as compatible with breast-feeding by the American Academy of Pediatrics (see Halothane).

References

1. Eger EI II. Desflurane animal and human pharmacology: aspects of kinetics, safety, and MAC. Anesth Analg 1992;75:S3–9.
2. Kennedy GL Jr, Smith SH, Keplinger ML, Calandra JG, Reproductive and teratologic studies with isoflurane. Drug Chem Toxicol 1977–78;1:75–88.
3. Mazze RI, Wilson AI, Rice SA, Baden JM. Fetal development in mice exposed to isoflurane. Teratology 1985;32:339–45.
4. Mazze RI, Fujinaga M, Rice SA, Harris SB, Baden JM. Reproductive and teratogenic effects of nitrous oxide, halothane, isoflurane, and enflurane in Sprague-Dawley rats. Anesthesiology 1986;64:339–44.
5. Trevor AJ, Miller RD. General anesthetics. In Katzung BG, ed. *Basic and Clinical Pharmacology*. 8th ed. New York: McGraw-Hill, 2001:426.
6. O'Leary G, Bacon CL, Odumeru O, Fagan C, Fitzpatrick T, Gallagher HC, Moriarty DC, Regan CM. Antiproliferative actions of inhalational anesthetics: comparisons to the valproate teratogen. Int J Dev Neurosci 2000;18:39–45.
7. Palahniuk RJ, Shnider SM, Eger EI II. Pregnancy decreases the requirement for inhaled anesthetic agents. Anesthesiology 1974;41:82–3.
8. Gin T, Chan MTV. Decrease minimum alveolar concentration of isoflurane in pregnant humans. Anesthesiology 1994;81:829–32.
9. Friedman JM. Teratogen update: anesthetic agents. Teratology 1988;37:69–77.
10. Kanto J. Risk-benefit assessment of anaesthetic agents in the puerperium. Drug Saf 1991;6:285–301.
11. Dwyer R, Fee JPH, Moore J. Uptake of halothane and isoflurane by mother and baby during caesarean section. Br J Anaesthesia 1995;74:379–83.
12. Merritt WT, Dickstein R, Beattie C, Burdick J, Klein A. Liver transplantation during pregnancy: anesthesia for two procedures in the same patient with successful outcome of pregnancy. Transplant Proc 1991;23:1996–7.
13. McLeod DD, Ramayya GP, Tunstall ME. Self-administered isoflurane in labour. A comparative study with Entonox. Anaesthesia 1985;40:424–6.
14. Abboud TK, Gangolly J, Mosaad P, Crowell D. Isoflurane in obstetrics. Anesth Analg 1989;68:388–91.
15. Wee MYK, Hasan MA, Thomas TA. Isoflurane in labour. Anaesthesia 1993;48:369–72.
16. Ghaly RG, Flynn RJ, Moore J. Isoflurane as an alternative to halothane for caesarean section. Anaesthesia 1988;43:5–7.
17. Abboud TK, Zhu J, Richardson M, Peres Da Silva E, Donovan M. Intravenous propofol vs. thiamylal-isoflurane for caesarean section, comparative maternal and neonatal effects. Acta Anaesthesiol Scand 1995;39:205–9.
18. Stuart JC, Kan AF, Rowbottom SJ, Yau G, Gin T. Acid aspiration prophylaxis for emergency caesarean section. Anaesthesia 1996;51:415–21.
19. Warren TM, Datta S, Ostheimer GW, Naulty JS, Weiss JB, Morrison JA. Comparison of the maternal and neonatal effects of halothane, enflurane, and isoflurane for cesarean section. Anesth Analg 1983;62:516–20.
20. Munson ES, Embro WJ. Enflurane, isoflurane, and halothane and isolated human uterine muscle. Anesthesiology 1977;46:11–4.
21. Abadir AR, Humayun SG, Calvello D, Gintautas J. Effects of isoflurane and oxytocin on gravid human uterus in vitro (abstract). Anesth Analg 1987;66:S1.
22. Sessler DI, Badgwell JM. Exposure of postoperative nurses to exhaled anesthetic gases. Anesth Analg 1998;87:1083–8.
23. Quail AW. Modern inhalational anaesthetic agents. A review of halothane, isoflurane and enflurane. Med J Aust 1989;150:95–102.
24. Lee JJ, Rubin AP. Breast feeding and anaesthesia. Anaesthesia 1993;48:616–25.
25. Spigset O. Anaesthetic agents and excretion in breast milk. Acta Anaesthesiol Scand 1994;38:94–103.

Name: **ISOFLUROPHATE** Risk Factor: **C**
Class: **Parasympathomimetic (Cholinergic)**

FETAL RISK SUMMARY

RECOMMENDATION: No Human Data - Probably Compatible

Isoflurophate is used in the eye. No reports of its use in pregnancy have been located. As a quaternary ammonium compound, it is ionized at physiologic pH and transplacental passage in significant amounts would not be expected (see also Neostigmine).

BREAST FEEDING SUMMARY

RECOMMENDATION: No Human Data - Probably Compatible

No data are available.

Name: **ISOMETHEPTENE** Risk Factor: **C**
Class: **Sympathomimetic (Adrenergic)**

FETAL RISK SUMMARY

RECOMMENDATION: Limited Human Data - No Relevant Animal Data

The sympathomimetic drug, isometheptene, is commercially available in combination with dichloralphenazone and acetaminophen (e.g., Isocom, Isopap, Midchlor, Midrin, and Migratine) for the treatment of tension and vascular (migraine) headaches (see also Dichloralphenazone and Acetaminophen). No animal reproductive studies of isometheptene have been located.

The Collaborative Perinatal Project, conducted between 1958 and 1965, recorded eight 1st trimester exposures to isometheptene among 96 mothers who had consumed a miscellaneous group of sympathomimetics (1). From these 96 mothers, 7 children had congenital malformations producing a standardized relative risk (SRR) of 0.96. When only malformations showing uniform rates by hospital were analyzed, the number of children with defects decreased to 4 (SRR 0.81). The authors of this study concluded there was no association between these agents and congenital anomalies.

A 1984 source briefly reviewed isometheptene (2). Although citing no primary references, the authors concluded that the agent was not contraindicated in pregnancy because of the lack of reports of harmful effects on the fetus, the mother, and the pregnancy (2).

BREAST FEEDING SUMMARY

RECOMMENDATION: No Human Data - Probably Compatible

No data are available.

References

1. Heinonen OP, Slone D, Shapiro S. *Birth Defects and Drugs in Pregnancy*. Littleton, MA: Publishing Sciences Group, 1977:346.
2. Onnis A, Grella P. *The Biochemical Effects of Drugs in Pregnancy*. Volume 1. West Sussex, England: Ellis Horwood Limited, 1984:179.

Name:	**ISONIAZID**	Risk Factor:	**C**
Class:	**Antituberculosis Agent**		

I

FETAL RISK SUMMARY

RECOMMENDATION: Compatible - Maternal Benefit >> Embryo/Fetal Risk

Isoniazid is used in the prevention and treatment of pulmonary tuberculosis. Reproduction studies in mice, rats, and rabbits have not revealed teratogenic effects, but embryocidal effects were observed in rats and rabbits (1).

An official statement of the American Thoracic Society, published in 1986, recommends isoniazid as part of the treatment regimen for women who have tuberculosis during pregnancy (2). Other reviewers also consider isoniazid as part of the treatment of choice for tuberculosis occurring during pregnancy (3).

Isoniazid crosses the placenta to the fetus (4–6). In a 1955 study, 19 women in labor were given a single 100-mg dose of isoniazid 0.25–4.25 hours before delivery (4). The mean maternal serum concentration at birth was 0.32 μg/mL compared with a cord blood level of 0.22 μg/mL. The mean cord:maternal ratio was 0.73, but in seven of the patients, cord blood concentrations exceeded those in the maternal plasma. Another study examined the placental transfer of isoniazid in two women who had been treated with 300 mg/day during the 3rd trimester (5). One hour before delivery, the women were given a single 300-mg IM dose. Mean cord blood and maternal serum concentrations were 4 and 6.5 μg/mL, respectively, a ratio of 0.62. These studies and the elimination kinetics of intrauterine acquired isoniazid in the newborn were reviewed in 1987 (6).

Reports discussing fetal effects of isoniazid during pregnancy reflect multiple drug therapies. Early reports identified retarded psychomotor activity, psychic retardation, convulsions, myoclonia, myelomeningocele with spina bifida and talipes, and hypospadias as possible effects related to isoniazid therapy during pregnancy (7,8). The Collaborative Perinatal Project monitored 85 patients who received isoniazid during the 1st trimester (9, pp. 299, 313). They observed 10 malformations, an incidence almost twice the expected rate, but they cautioned that their findings required independent confirmation. For use anytime during pregnancy, 146 mother-child pairs were exposed to isoniazid, with malformations that may have been produced after the 1st trimester observed in 4 infants (9, p. 435). This was close to the expected frequency. Adverse outcomes in the fetus and newborn after intrauterine exposure to isoniazid have not been confirmed by other studies (10–15). Retrospective analysis of more than 4900 pregnancies in which isoniazid was administered demonstrated rates of malformations similar to those in control populations (0.7%–2.3%). A 1980 review also found no association between isoniazid and fetal anomalies (16).

In a surveillance study of Michigan Medicaid recipients conducted between 1985 and 1992 involving 229,101 completed pregnancies, 11 newborns had been exposed to

isoniazid during the 1st trimester (F. Rosa, personal communication, FDA, 1993). One (9.1%) major birth defect was observed (0.5 expected), a case of polydactyly.

A case report of a malignant mesothelioma in a 9-year-old child who was exposed to isoniazid *in utero* was published in 1980 (17). The authors suggested a possible carcinogenic effect of isoniazid because of the rarity of malignant mesotheliomas during the first decade and supportive animal data. However, an earlier study examined 660 children up to 16 years of age and found no association with carcinogenic effects (18).

An association between isoniazid and hemorrhagic disease of the newborn has been suspected in two infants (19). The mothers were also treated with rifampin and ethambutol and in a third case, only with these latter two drugs. Although other reports of this potentially serious reaction have not been found, prophylactic vitamin K_1 is recommended at birth (see Phytonadione).

In summary, isoniazid does not appear to be a human teratogen. The American Thoracic Society recommends use of the drug for tuberculosis occurring during pregnancy because, "Untreated tuberculosis represents a far greater hazard to a pregnant woman and her fetus than does treatment of the disease" (2).

I

BREAST FEEDING SUMMARY

RECOMMENDATION: Limited Human Data - Probably Compatible

No reports of isoniazid-induced effects in the nursing infant have been located, but the potential for interference with nucleic acid function and for hepatotoxicity may exist (20,21). Both isoniazid and its metabolite, acetylisoniazid, are excreted in breast milk (21–23). A woman was given a single oral dose of 300 mg after complete weaning of her infant (21). Both isoniazid and the metabolite were present in her milk within 1 hour with peak levels of isoniazid (16.6 μg/mL) occurring at 3 hours and those of the metabolite (3.76 μg/mL) at 5 hours. At 5 and 12 hours after the dose, isoniazid levels in the milk were twice the levels in simultaneously obtained plasma. Levels of acetylisoniazid were similar in plasma and milk at 5 and 12 hours. The elimination half-life for milk isoniazid was calculated to be 5.9 hours, whereas that of the metabolite was 13.5 hours. Both were detectable in milk 24 hours after the dose. The 24-hour excretion of isoniazid was estimated to be 7 mg. Two other studies also reported substantial excretion of isoniazid into human milk (22,23). A milk:plasma ratio of 1.0 was reported in one of these studies (22). In another, milk levels 3 hours after a maternal dose of 5 mg/kg were 6 μg/mL (23). Doubling the maternal dose doubled the milk concentration.

Based on the above information, at least one review concluded that women can safely breast-feed their infants while taking isoniazid if, among other precautions, the infant is periodically examined for signs and symptoms of peripheral neuritis or hepatitis (20). Moreover, the American Academy of Pediatrics classifies isoniazid as compatible with breast-feeding (24).

References

1. Product information. Rifamate. Hoechst Marion Roussel, 2000.
2. American Thoracic Society. Treatment of tuberculosis and tuberculosis infection in adults and children. Am Rev Respir Dis 1986;134:355–63.
3. Medchill MT, Gillum M. Diagnosis and management of tuberculosis during pregnancy. Obstet Gynecol Surv 1989;44:81–4.
4. Bromberg YM, Salzberger M, Bruderman I. Placental transmission of isonicotinic acid hydrazide. Gynaecologia 1955;140:141–4.
5. Miceli JN, Olson WA, Cohen SN. Elimination kinetics of

isoniazid in the newborn infant. Dev Pharmacol Ther 1981;2:235–9.
6. Holdiness MR. Transplacental pharmacokinetics of the antituberculosis drugs. Clin Pharmacokinet 1987;13:125–9.
7. Weinstein L, Dalton AC. Host determinants of response to antimicrobial agents. N Engl J Med 1968; 279:524–31.
8. Lowe CR. Congenital defects among children born to women under supervision or treatment for pulmonary tuberculosis. Br J Prev Soc Med 1964;18:14–6.
9. Heinonen OP, Slone D, Shapiro S. *Birth Defects and Drugs in Pregnancy*. Littleton, MA: Publishing Sciences Group, 1977.
10. Marynowski A, Sianozecka E. Comparison of the incidence of congenital malformations in neonates from healthy mothers and from patients treated because of tuberculosis. Ginekol Pol 1972;43:713.
11. Jentgens H. Antituberkulose Chimotherapie und Schwangerschaft sabbruch. Prax Klin Pneumol 1973; 27:479.
12. Ludford J, Doster B, Woolpert SF. Effect of isoniazid on reproduction. Am Rev Respir Dis 1973;108: 1170–4.
13. Scheinhorn DJ, Angelillo VA. Antituberculosis therapy in pregnancy; risks to the fetus. West J Med 1977;127:195–8.
14. Good JT, Iseman MD, Davidson PT, Lakshminarayan S, Sahn SA. Tuberculosis in association with pregnancy. Am J Obstet Gynecol 1981;140:492–8.
15. Kingdom JCP, Kennedy DH. Tuberculous meningitis in pregnancy. Br J Obstet Gynaecol 1989;96:233–5.
16. Snider DE Jr, Layde PM, Johnson MW, Lyle MA. Treatment of tuberculosis during pregnancy. Am Rev Respir Dis 1980;122:65–79.
17. Tuman KJ, Chilcote RR, Gerkow RI, Moohr JW. Mesothelioma in child with prenatal exposure to isoniazid. Lancet 1980;2:362.
18. Hammond DC, Silidoff IJ, Robitzek EH. Isoniazid therapy in relation to later occurrence of cancer in adults and in infants. Br Med J 1967;2:792–5.
19. Eggermont E, Logghe N, Van De Casseye W, Casteels-Van Daele M, Jaeken J, Cosemans J, Verstraete M, Renaer M. Haemorrhagic disease of the newborn in the offspring of rifampicin and isoniazid treated mothers. Acta Paediatr Belg 1976;29:87–90.
20. Snider DE Jr, Powell KE. Should women taking antituberculosis drugs breast-feed? Arch Intern Med 1984;144:589–90.
21. Berlin CM Jr, Lee C. Isoniazid and acetylisoniazid disposition in human milk, saliva and plasma. Fed Proc 1979;38:426.
22. Vorherr H. Drugs excretion in breast milk. Postgrad Med 1974;56:97–104.
23. Ricci G, Copaitich T. Modalta di eliminazione dili'isoniazide somministrata per via orale attraverso il latte di donna. Rass Clin Ter 1954–5;209:53–4.
24. Committee on Drugs, American Academy of Pediatrics. The transfer of drugs and other chemicals into human milk. Pediatrics 2001;108:776–89.

Name: **ISOPROPAMIDE** Risk Factor: **C**

Class: **Parasympatholytic**

FETAL RISK SUMMARY

RECOMMENDATION: Limited Human Data - No Relevant Animal Data

Isopropamide is an anticholinergic quaternary ammonium iodide. The Collaborative Perinatal Project monitored 50,282 mother-child pairs, 180 of whom used isopropamide in the 1st trimester (1, pp. 346–353). For use anytime during pregnancy, 1071 exposures were recorded (1, p. 439). In neither case was evidence found for an association with malformations. However, when the group of parasympatholytics was taken as a whole (2,323 exposures), a possible association with minor malformations was found (1, pp. 346–353).

BREAST FEEDING SUMMARY

RECOMMENDATION: No Human Data - Probably Compatible

No data are available (see also Atropine).

Reference

1. Heinonen OP, Slone D, Shapiro S. *Birth Defects and Drugs in Pregnancy*. Littleton, MA: Publishing Sciences Group, 1977.

Name:	**ISOPROTERENOL**	Risk Factor:	**C**
Class:	**Sympathomimetic**		

FETAL RISK SUMMARY

RECOMMENDATION: Limited Human Data - Animal Data Suggest Moderate Risk

No reports linking the human use of isoproterenol with congenital defects have been located. Isoproterenol was not teratogenic in rats and rabbits, but was in hamsters (1,2).

The Collaborative Perinatal Project monitored 50,282 mother-child pairs, 31 of whom had 1st trimester exposure to isoproterenol (3, pp. 346–347). No evidence was found to suggest a relationship between large categories of major or minor malformations or to individual defects. However, an association in the 1st trimester was found between the sympathomimetic class of drugs as a whole and minor malformations (not life-threatening or major cosmetic defects), inguinal hernia, and clubfoot (3, pp. 345–356).

In a surveillance study of Michigan Medicaid recipients conducted between 1985 and 1992 involving 229,101 completed pregnancies, 16 newborns had been exposed to isoproterenol during the 1st trimester (F. Rosa, personal communication, FDA, 1993). One (6.3%) major birth defect was observed (0.7 expected), an oral cleft.

Sympathomimetics are often administered in combination with other drugs to alleviate the symptoms of upper respiratory infections. Thus, the fetal effects of sympathomimetics, other drugs, and viruses cannot be totally separated.

Isoproterenol has been used during pregnancy to accelerate heart rhythm when high-grade atrioventricular block is present and to treat ventricular arrhythmias associated with prolonged QT intervals (4). Because of its β-adrenergic effect, the agent will inhibit contractions of the pregnant uterus (4). Of incidental interest, five-term, nonlaboring pregnant women were discovered to have an increased resistance to the chronotropic effect of isoproterenol in comparison to nonpregnant women (5). One fetus had an isolated 5-beats/minute late deceleration 2 minutes after the mother received 0.25 μg of the drug (5).

BREAST FEEDING SUMMARY

RECOMMENDATION: No Human Data - Probably Compatible

No data are available.

References

1. Nishimura H, Tanimura T. *Clinical Aspects of The Teratogenicity of Drugs*. New York, NY: American Elsevier, 1976;231–2.
2. Shepard TH. *Catalog of Teratogenic Agents*. 3rd ed. Baltimore, MD: Johns Hopkins University Press, 1980;191.
3. Heinonen OP, Slone D, Shapiro S. *Birth Defects and Drugs in Pregnancy*. Littleton, MA: Publishing Sciences Group, 1977.
4. Tamari I, Eldar M, Rabinowitz B, Neufeld HN. Medical treatment of cardiovascular disorders during pregnancy. Am Heart J 1982;104:1357–63.
5. DeSimone CA, Leighton BL, Norris MC, Chayen B, Menduke H. The chronotropic effect of isoproterenol is reduced in term pregnant women. Anesthesiology 1988;69:626–8.

Name:	**ISOSORBIDE**	Risk Factor:	**C**
Class:	**Diuretic**		

FETAL RISK SUMMARY

RECOMMENDATION: Limited Human Data - Probably Compatible

Isosorbide is an osmotic diuretic used for the short-term reduction of intraocular pressure in acute glaucoma before and after intraocular surgery.

No published reports describing the use of isosorbide in pregnancy have been located. In a surveillance study of Michigan Medicaid recipients conducted between 1985 and 1992 involving 229,101 completed pregnancies,, 13 newborns had been exposed to isosorbide during the 1st trimester (F. Rosa, personal communication, FDA, 1993). No major birth defects were observed (0.6 expected).

I

BREAST FEEDING SUMMARY

RECOMMENDATION: No Human Data - Probably Compatible

No data are available.

Name:	**ISOSORBIDE DINITRATE**	Risk Factor:	**C_M**
Class:	**Vasodilator**		

FETAL RISK SUMMARY

RECOMMENDATION: Limited Human Data - Animal Data Suggest Moderate Risk

Isosorbide is a nitric oxide donor, similar to nitroglycerin that is used in the management of angina pectoris and of heart failure. It is administered sublingually, as chewable tablets, and as oral tablets. An oral spray is also available outside of the United States. The molecular weight (about 236) is low enough that passage to the fetus should be expected.

The drug produces dose-related embryotoxicity in rabbits at doses 35 and 150 times the maximum recommended human dose (1). (See also Nitroglycerin or Amyl Nitrite.)

Two full reports and one abstract have described the use of isosorbide dinitrate during human pregnancy (2–4). However, all of the pregnancies in these reports had pre-scheduled elective terminations for nonmedical reasons shortly after the drug exposure. In a 1996 study (first published as an abstract in 1995), 18 women in the 2nd trimester received a single 5-mg sublingual dose of isosorbide dinitrate (2,3). Statistically significant decreases in the maternal systolic and diastolic blood pressures were observed 6 minutes after the dose. The blood pressures gradually returned to control levels over the ensuing 30 minutes. The mean maternal heart rate significantly increased from about 85 beats/minute to 96 beats/minute at 6 minutes, but declined to near control levels at 8 minutes. The mean systolic-diastolic flow velocity ratios in the umbilical and uterine arteries declined significantly, reaching nadirs at 6 and 10 minutes, respectively, before gradually returning to pre-dose levels. These findings suggested that isosorbide dinitrate may be beneficial in reversing the effects of endothelial cell dysfunction-induced generalized vasoconstriction and increased vascular resistance to flow in the uteroplacental circulation, such as occurs in preeclampsia (2,3).

In a similar investigation by these same researchers, 11 women at a mean gestational age of 10.0 weeks (range 8.2–11.6 weeks) were given a single 5-mg sublingual dose of the drug (4). The results of this study were comparable to the researchers previous work and led them to a similar conclusion that isosorbide dinitrate may be effective in reversing the effects of the endothelial cell dysfunction that is observed in preeclampsia (4).

BREAST FEEDING SUMMARY

RECOMMENDATION: No Human Data - Probably Compatible

No reports describing the use of isosorbide dinitrate during lactation have been located. The molecular weight (about 236) is low enough that excretion into breast milk should be expected. The effects of this exposure on a nursing infant are unknown.

References

1. Product information. Isordil. Wyeth-Ayerst Laboratories, 1993.
2. Thaler I, Amit A, Itskovitz J. The effect of isosorbide dinitrate, a nitric oxide donor, on human uterine and placental vascular resistance in patients with preeclampsia (abstract). Am J Obstet Gynecol 1995;172:387.
3. Thaler I, Amit A, Jakobi P, Itskovitz-Eldor J. The effect of isosorbide dinitrate on uterine artery and umbilical artery flow velocity waveforms at mid-pregnancy. Obstet Gynecol 1996;88:838–43.
4. Amit A, Thaler I, Paz Y, Itskovity-Eldor J. The effect of a nitric oxide donor on Doppler flow velocity waveforms in the uterine artery during the first trimester of pregnancy. Ultrasound Obstet Gynecol 1998;11:94–8.

Name:	**ISOSORBIDE MONONITRATE**	Risk Factor:	**C_M**
Class:	**Vasodilator**		

FETAL RISK SUMMARY

RECOMMENDATION: No Human Data - Animal Data Suggest Moderate Risk

The vasodilator isosorbide mononitrate is the major active metabolite of isosorbide dinitrate. In rats and rabbits administered doses up to 250 mg/kg/day, no adverse effects on reproduction and development were observed, but doses of 500 mg/kg/day in rats caused significant increases in prolonged gestation, prolonged parturition, stillbirth, and neonatal death (1). No reports on the use of isosorbide mononitrate in human pregnancy have been located (see also Isosorbide Dinitrate).

BREAST FEEDING SUMMARY

RECOMMENDATION: No Human Data - Probably Compatible

No data are available.

Reference

1. Product information. Ismo. Wyeth-Ayerst Laboratories, 1993.

Name: **ISOTRETINOIN**

Class: **Vitamin**

Risk Factor: **X_M**

FETAL RISK SUMMARY

RECOMMENDATION: Contraindicated

Isotretinoin (Accutane) is a vitamin A isomer used for the treatment of severe, recalcitrant cystic acne. The animal teratogenicity of this drug was well documented before its approval for human use in 1982 (1,2). The mechanism of isotretinoin teratogenicity in animals may involve cytotoxic peroxyl free radical generation by metabolism with prostaglandin synthase (3). Newborn mice exposed *in utero* to isotretinoin at a critical point in gestation had characteristic craniofacial and limb malformations, but concurrent treatment with aspirin, a prostaglandin synthase inhibitor, resulted in a dose-dependent decrease in the overall incidence of abnormalities, the number of anomalies per fetus, and the incidence of specific craniofacial and limb defects (3).

I

Shortly after its approval, several publications appeared warning of the human teratogenic potential if isotretinoin were administered to women who were pregnant or who may become pregnant (4–9). In the 22 months following its introduction (September 1982–July 5, 1984), the manufacturer, the U.S. Food and Drug Administration (FDA), and the Centers for Disease Control and Prevention (CDC) received reports on 154 isotretinoin-exposed pregnancies (10). Some of these cases had been described in earlier reports (11–20). Of the 154 pregnancies, 95 were electively aborted, 12 aborted spontaneously, 26 infants were born without major defects (some may not have been exposed during the critical gestational period), and 21 had major malformations (10). Three of the 21 infants were stillborn and 9 died after birth. A characteristic pattern of defects was observed in the 21 infants that closely resembled that seen in animal experiments (10). The syndrome of defects observed in these infants and in other reported cases (21–34) consists of all or part of the following:

Central nervous system:
Hydrocephalus
Facial (VII nerve) palsy
Posterior fossa structure defects
Cortical and cerebellar defects
Cortical blindness
Optic nerve hypoplasia
Retinal defects
Microphthalmia

Craniofacial:
Microtia or anotia
Low-set ears
Agenesis or marked stenosis of external ear canals
Micrognathia
Small mouth
Microcephaly
Triangular skull

Facial dysmorphism
Depressed nasal bridge
Cleft palate
Hypertelorism

Cardiovascular:
Conotruncal malformations:
Transposition of great vessels
Tetralogy of Fallot
Double-outlet right ventricle
Truncus arteriosus communis
Ventricular septal defect
Atrial septal defect

Branchial-arch mesenchymal-tissue defects:
Interrupted or hypoplastic aortic arch
Retroesophageal right subclavian artery

Thymic defects:
Ectopia, hypoplasia, or aplasia

Miscellaneous defects (sporadic occurrence):
Spina bifida
Nystagmus
Hepatic abnormality
Hydroureter
Decreased muscle tone
Large scrotal sac
Simian crease
Limb reduction

Other defects have been reported with isotretinoin, but in these cases exposure had either been terminated before conception or was outside the critical period for the defect (33). These defects are thought to be nonteratogenic or have occurred by chance (33). Similarly, three reports of anomalies in children in which only the father was exposed (biliary atresia and ventricular septal defect; four-limb ectromelia and hydrocephalus; anencephaly) also probably occurred by chance (33).

A 1985 case report proposed that reduction deformities observed in all four limbs of a male infant were induced by isotretinoin (35,36). Other evidence suggested that these defects may have been secondary to amniotic bands (37). However, a 1991 reference described an infant and a fetus with limb reduction deformities after 1st trimester exposure to isotretinoin (38). A 17-year-old mother took 50 mg/day of isotretinoin for 10 days during the 2nd month of gestation. Abnormalities present in the infant were absence of the right clavicle and nearly absent right scapula, a short humerus, and a short, broad, completely synostotic right radius and ulna (38). Other defects present were asymmetrical ventriculomegaly, minor dysmorphic facial features, a short sternum with a sterno-umbilical raphe, and developmental delay (38). The second case involved an 18-year-old woman who took 60 mg/day of isotretinoin during the first 62 days of gestation (38). The pregnancy was terminated at 22 weeks' gestation because of fetal hydrocephalus and cystic kidney. Multiple defects were noted in the fetus, including an absent left thumb but with normal proximal bony structures, a single umbilical artery, anal and vaginal atresia, urethral agenesis with dysplastic, multicystic kidneys, and other malformations consistent with isotretinoin exposure (38).

Because isotretinoin causes central nervous system abnormalities, concern has been raised over the potential for adverse behavioral effects in infants who seemingly are normal at birth (39). Long-term studies are in progress to evaluate behavioral toxicities, such as mental retardation and learning disabilities, but have not been concluded because the exposed children are still too young for tests to produce meaningful results (40).

The teratogenic mechanism of isotretinoin and its main metabolite, 4-oxo-isotretinoin, is thought to result from an adverse effect on the initial differentiation and migration of cephalic neural crest cells (10,41). Daily doses in the range of 0.5–1.5 mg/kg were usually ingested in cases with adverse outcome (10), but doses as low as 0.2 mg/kg or lower may also have caused teratogenicity (34,42). The critical period of exposure is believed to be 2–5 weeks after conception, but clinically it is difficult to establish the exact dating in many cases (33). Because of the high proportion of spontaneous abortions in prospectively identified exposed women, the CDC commented that fetotoxicity may be a more common adverse outcome than liveborn infants with abnormalities (11).

The lack of reports of isotretinoin-induced abnormalities from areas other than the United States and Canada caused speculation that this was caused by the use of lower doses, more restricted use in women, or later marketing of the drug (43). Several groups of investigators have responded to this, and although under diagnosis and underreporting may contribute, the reasons are still unclear (42,45–47).

An autosomal or X-linked recessive syndrome with features of isotretinoin-induced defects has been described in three male siblings (48). Although the mother had no history of isotretinoin or vitamin A use, the authors did not rule out a defect in vitamin A metabolism.

In a follow-up to a previous report involving 36 pregnancies, investigators noted the outcome of an additional 21 pregnancies exposed in the 1st trimester to isotretinoin (49). The outcomes of the 57 pregnancies were 9 spontaneous abortions, 1 malformed stillborn, 10 malformed live births, and 37 normal live births. In this population, the absolute risk for a major defect in pregnancies extending to 20 weeks' gestation or longer was 23% (11 of 48) (49).

In a surveillance study of Michigan Medicaid recipients conducted between 1985 and 1992 involving 229,101 completed pregnancies, 6 newborns had been exposed to isotretinoin during the 1st trimester (F. Rosa, personal communication, FDA, 1993). One (16.7%) major birth defect was observed (0.3 expected). Specific data was not available for the anomaly, but it was not one of six defect categories (cardiovascular defects, oral clefts, spina bifida, polydactyly, limb-reduction defects, and hypospadias) for which specific data were available.

The outcome of pregnancies occurring after the discontinuation of isotretinoin was described in a 1989 article (50). Of 88 prospectively ascertained pregnancies, conception occurred in 77 within 60 days of the last dose of the drug. In 10 cases, the date of conception (defined as 14 days after the last menstrual period) occurred within 2–5 days after the last dose of isotretinoin. These 10 pregnancies ended in 2 spontaneous abortions and 8 normal infants. Three women who had taken their last dose within 2 days of the estimated date of conception delivered normal infants. The outcomes of all 88 pregnancies were as follows: 8 (9.1%) spontaneous abortions, 1 abnormal birth (details not provided), 75 (85.3%) normal infants, and 4 (4.5%) infants with congenital malformations. The defects observed were small anterior fontanelle (1 case), congenital cataract with premature hypertrophic vitreous membrane (1 case), congenital cataract (1 case), and hypospadias (1 case). The mothers had taken their last dose of isotretinoin 33, 22, 17, and 55 days before conception, respectively. These anomalies are not characteristic of those reported with *in utero* exposure to isotretinoin. In an additional 13 cases obtained retrospectively, 5 ended in spontaneous abortions, 4 normal infants were delivered, and 4 infants had congenital defects: syndactyly (1 case), Down's syndrome (1 case), hypoplasia of left side of heart (1 case), and unknown defects (1 case). In the cases of known defects, the mothers had stopped isotretinoin at least 9 months before conception. As with the prospective cases, the defects described in the three infants were not those typical of isotretinoin-induced anomalies. Moreover, retrospective reports are probably more likely to report abnormal outcomes and to underreport normal infants (50).

In summary, isotretinoin is a potent human teratogen. Critically important is the fact that a high percentage of the recipients of this drug are women in their childbearing years. Estimates have appeared indicating that 38% of isotretinoin users are women aged 13–19 years (14). Pregnancy must be excluded and prevented in these and other female patients before isotretinoin is prescribed.

Fortunately, in one study the drug did not interfere with the action of oral contraceptive steroids (51). Initially, recommendations included stopping therapy at least 1 month before conception (14), but others indicated that shorter intervals between the last dose of isotretinoin and conception were apparently safe (50). Labeling by the manufacturer currently states that a negative serum pregnancy 2 weeks before beginning therapy is required (52,53). A recent statement by the Teratology Society supplemented the manufacturer's recommendations, for treatment of women of childbearing potential with isotretinoin, with additional recommendations and reviewed the animal and human teratogenicity of this agent (53).

BREAST FEEDING SUMMARY

RECOMMENDATION: No Human Data - Potential Toxicity

It is not known whether isotretinoin or its metabolite, 4-oxo-isotretinoin, is excreted into human milk. The closely related retinoid, vitamin A, is excreted (see Vitamin A), and the presence of isotretinoin in breast milk should be expected.

References

1. Voorhees JJ, Orfanos CE. Oral retinoids. Arch Dermatol 1981;117:418–21.
2. Kamm JJ. Toxicology, carcinogenicity, and teratogenicity of some orally administered retinoids. J Am Acad Dermatol 1982;6:652–9.
3. Kubow S. Inhibition of isotretinoin teratogenicity by acetylsalicylic acid pretreatment in mice. Teratology 1992;45:55–63.
4. Perry MD, McEvoy GK. Isotretinoin: new therapy for severe acne. Clin Pharm 1983;2:12–9.
5. Henderson IWD, Rice WB. Accutane. Can Med Assoc J 1983;129:682.
6. Shalita AR, Cunningham WJ, Leyden JJ, Pochi PE, Strauss JS. Isotretinoin treatment of acne and related disorders: an update. J Am Acad Dermatol 1983;9:629–38.
7. Anonymous. Update on isotretinoin (Accutane) for acne. Med Lett Drugs Ther 1983;25:105–6.
8. Conner CS. Isotretinoin: a reappraisal. Drug Intell Clin Pharm 1984;18:308–9.
9. Ward A, Brogden RN, Heel RC, Speight TM, Avery GS. Isotretinoin. A review of its pharmacological properties and therapeutic efficacy in acne and other skin disorders. Drugs 1984;28:6–37.
10. Lammer EJ, Chen DT, Hoar RM, Agnish ND, Benke PJ, Braun JT, Curry CJ, Fernhoff PM, Grix AW Jr, Lott IT, Richard JM, Sun SC. Retinoic acid embryopathy. N Engl J Med 1985;313:837–41.
11. Anonymous. Isotretinoin—a newly recognized human teratogen. MMWR 1984;33:171–3.
12. Anonymous. Update on birth defects with isotretinoin. FDA Drug Bull 1984;14:15–6.
13. Rosa FW. Teratogenicity of isotretinoin. Lancet 1983; 2:513.
14. Anonymous. Adverse effects with isotretinoin. FDA Drug Bull 1983;13:21–3.

15. Braun JT, Franciosi RA, Mastri AR, Drake RM, O'Neil BL. Isotretinoin dysmorphic syndrome. Lancet 1984;1:506–7.
16. Hill RM. Isotretinoin teratogenicity. Lancet 1984; 1:1465.
17. Benke PJ. The isotretinoin teratogen syndrome. JAMA 1984;251:3267–9.
18. Fernhoff PM, Lammer EJ. Craniofacial features of isotretinoin embryopathy. J Pediatr 1984;105:595–7.
19. Lott IT, Bocian M, Pribram HW, Leitner M. Fetal hydrocephalus and ear anomalies associated with maternal use of isotretinoin. J Pediatr 1984;105:597–600.
20. De La Cruz E, Sun S, Vangvanichyakorn K, Desposito F. Multiple congenital malformations associated with maternal isotretinoin therapy. Pediatrics 1984;74:428–30.
21. Stern RS, Rosa F, Baum C. Isotretinoin and pregnancy. J Am Acad Dermatol 1984;10:851–4.
22. Marwick C. More cautionary labeling appears on isotretinoin. JAMA 1984;251:3208–9.
23. Zarowny DP. Accutane Roche: risk of teratogenic effects. Can Med Assoc J 1984;131:273.
24. Hall JG. Vitamin A: a newly recognized human teratogen. Harbinger of things to come? J Pediatr 1984; 105:583–4.
25. Robertson R, MacLeod PM. Accutane-induced teratogenesis. CMAJ 1985;133:1147–8.
26. Willhite CC, Hill RM, Irving DW. Isotretinoin-induced craniofacial malformations in humans and hamsters. J Craniofac Genet Dev Biol 1986;2(Suppl):193–209.
27. Cohen M, Rubinstein A, Li JK, Nathenson G. Thymic hypoplasia associated with isotretinoin embryopathy. Am J Dis Child 1987;141:263–6.
28. Millan SB, Flowers FP, Sherertz EF. Isotretinoin. South Med J 1987;80:494–9.
29. Jahn AF, Ganti K. Major auricular malformations due to Accutane (isotretinoin). Laryngoscope 1987;97:832–5.
30. Bigby M, Stern RS. Adverse reactions to isotretinoin: a report from the adverse drug reaction reporting system. J Am Acad Dermatol 1988;18:543–52.
31. Anonymous. Birth defects caused by isotretinoin—New Jersey. MMWR 1988;37:171–2, 177.
32. Orfanos CE, Ehlert R, Gollnick H. The retinoids: a review of their clinical pharmacology and therapeutic use. Drugs 1987;34:459–503.
33. Rosa FW, Wilk AL, Kelsey FO. Teratogen update: vitamin A congeners. Teratology 1986;33:355–64.
34. Rosa FW. Retinoic acid embryopathy. N Engl J Med 1986;315:262.
35. McBride WG. Limb reduction deformities in child exposed to isotretinoin in utero on gestation days 26–40 only. Lancet 1985;1:1276.
36. McBride WG. Isotretinoin and reduction deformities. Lancet 1985;2:503.
37. Lammer EJ, Flannery DB, Barr M. Does isotretinoin cause limb reduction defects? Lancet 1985;2:328.
38. Rizzo R, Lammer EJ, Parano E, Pavone L, Argyle JC. Limb reduction defects in humans associated with prenatal isotretinoin exposure. Teratology 1991;44: 599–604.
39. Vorhees CV. Retinoic acid embryopathy. N Engl J Med 1986;315:262–3.
40. Lammer EJ. Retinoic acid embryopathy (in reply). N Engl J Med 1986;315:263.
41. Webster WS, Johnston MC, Lammer EJ, Sulik KK. Isotretinoin embryopathy and the cranial neural crest: an in vivo and in vitro study. J Craniofac Genet Dev Biol 1986;6:211–22.
42. Ayme S, Julian C, Gambarelli D, Mariotti B, Maurin N. Isotretinoin dose and teratogenicity. Lancet 1988;1:655.
43. Rosa F. Isotretinoin dose and teratogenicity. Lancet 1987;2:1154.
44. Robert E. Isotretinoin dose and teratogenicity. Lancet 1988;1:236.
45. Lammer EJ, Schunior A, Hayes AM, Holmes LB. Isotretinoin dose and teratogenicity. Lancet 1988;2:503–4.
46. Hope G, Mathias B. Teratogenicity of isotretinoin and etretinate. Lancet 1988;2:1143.
47. Lancaster PAL. Teratogenicity of isotretinoin. Lancet 1988;2:1254.
48. Kawashima H, Ohno I, Ueno Y, Nakaya S, Kato E, Taniguchi N. Syndrome of microtia and aortic arch anomalies resembling isotretinoin embryopathy. J Pediatr 1987;111:738–40.
49. Lammer EJ, Hayes AM, Schunior A, Holmes LB. Risk for major malformation among human fetuses exposed to isotretinoin (13-cis-retinoic acid). Teratology 1987;35:68A.
50. Dai WS, Hsu M-A, Itri LM. Safety of pregnancy after discontinuation of isotretinoin. Arch Dermatol 1989;125:363–5.
51. Orme M, Back DJ, Shaw MA, Allen WL, Tjia J, Cunliffe WJ, Jones DH. Isotretinoin and contraception. Lancet 1984;2:752–3.
52. Product information. Accutane. Roche Dermatologics, 1993.
53. Public Affairs Committee, The Teratology Society. Recommendations for isotretinoin use in women of childbearing potential. Teratology 1991;44:1–6.

Name:	**ISOXSUPRINE**	Risk Factor:	**C**
Class:	**Sympathomimetic (Vasodilator)**		

FETAL RISK SUMMARY

RECOMMENDATION: Limited Human Data - No Relevant Animal Data

No reports linking the use of isoxsuprine with congenital defects have been located. Isoxsuprine, a β-sympathomimetic, is indicated for vasodilation, but it has been used to prevent premature labor (1–6). Uterine inhibitory effects usually require high IV doses, which increase the risk for serious adverse effects (7,8). Maternal heart rate increases and blood pressure decreases are usually mild at lower doses (2,4,6). A decrease in the incidence of neonatal respiratory distress syndrome has been observed (9). However, in one study, neonatal respiratory depression was increased if cord serum levels exceeded 10 ng/mL (10). The depression was always associated with hypotension, so the mechanism of the defect may have been related to pulmonary hypoperfusion.

Neonatal toxicity is generally rare if cord levels of isoxsuprine are less than 2 ng/mL (corresponding to a drug-free interval of more than 5 hours), but levels greater than 10 ng/mL (drug-free interval of 2 hours of less) were associated with severe neonatal problems (10). These problems include hypocalcemia, hypoglycemia, ileus, hypotension, and death (10–12). Hypotension and neonatal death occurred primarily in infants of 26–31 weeks' gestation, especially if cord levels exceeded 10 ng/mL, and in infants whose mothers developed hypotension or tachycardia during isoxsuprine infusion (10,11). Neonatal ileus, up to 33% in some series, was not related to cord isoxsuprine concentrations, but hypotension and hypocalcemia were directly related, reaching 89% and 100%, respectively, when cord levels exceeded 10 ng/mL (10,12). Fetal tachycardia is a common side effect. As compared with controls, no increase in late or variable decelerations was seen (10). In contrast to the above, infusion of isoxsuprine 30 minutes before cesarean section under general anesthesia was not observed to produce adverse effects in the mother, fetus, or newborn (13). Cord concentrations were not measured.

Long-term evaluation of infants exposed to β-mimetics *in utero* has been reported but not specifically for isoxsuprine (14). No harmful effects in the infants resulting from this exposure were observed.

The Collaborative Perinatal Project monitored 50,282 mother-child pairs, 54 of whom were exposed to isoxsuprine during the 1st trimester (15, pp. 346–347). For use anytime during pregnancy, 858 exposures were recorded (15, p. 439). In neither case was evidence found for an association with malformations.

BREAST FEEDING SUMMARY

RECOMMENDATION: No Human Data - Probably Compatible

No data are available.

References

1. Bishop EH, Woutersz TB. Isoxsuprine, a myometrial relaxant. A preliminary report. Obstet Gynecol 1961;17:442–6.
2. Hendricks CH, Cibils LA, Pose SV, Eskes TKAB. The pharmacological control of excessive uterine activity with isoxsuprine. Am J Obstet Gynecol 1961;82:1064–78.
3. Bishop EH, Woutersz TB. Arrest of premature labor. JAMA 1961;178:812–4.
4. Stander RW, Barden TP, Thompson JF, Pugh WR, Werts CE. Fetal cardiac effects of maternal isoxsuprine infusion. Am J Obstet Gynecol 1964;89:792–800.
5. Hendricks CH. The use of isoxsuprine for the arrest of premature labor. Clin Obstet Gynecol 1964;7:687–94.
6. Allen HH, Short H, Fraleigh DM. The use of isoxsuprine in the management of premature labor. Appl Ther 1965;7:544–7.
7. Anonymous. Drugs acting on the uterus. Br Med J 1964;1:1234–6.
8. Briscoe CC. Failure of oral isoxsuprine to prevent prematurity. Am J Obstet Gynecol 1966;95:885–6.
9. Kero P, Hirvonen T, Valimaki I. Perinatal isoxsuprine and respiratory distress syndrome. Lancet 1973;2:198.
10. Brazy JE, Little V, Grimm J, Pupkin M. Risk:benefit considerations for the use of isoxsuprine in the treatment of premature labor. Obstet Gynecol 1981;58:297–303.
11. Brazy JE, Pupkin MJ. Effects of maternal isoxsuprine administration on preterm infants. J Pediatr 1979;94:444–8.
12. Brazy JE, Little V, Grimm J. Isoxsuprine in the perinatal period. II. Relationships between neonatal symptoms, drug exposure, and drug concentration at the time of birth. J Pediatr 1981;98:146–51.

13. Jouppila R, Kauppila A, Tuimala R, Pakarinen A, Moilanen K. Maternal, fetal and neonatal effects of beta-adrenergic stimulation in connection with cesarean section. Acta Obstet Gynecol Scand 1980;59:489–93.
14. Freysz H, Willard D, Lehr A, Messer J. Boog G. A long term evaluation of infants who received a beta-mimetic drug while in utero. J Perinat Med 1977;5:94–9.
15. Heinonen OP, Slone D, Shapiro S. *Birth Defects and Drugs in Pregnancy*. Littleton, MA: Publishing Sciences Group, 1977.

Name: **ISRADIPINE** Risk Factor: **C_M**

Class: **Calcium Channel Blocker**

FETAL RISK SUMMARY

RECOMMENDATION: Limited Human Data - Animal Data Suggest Low Risk

Isradipine is a calcium channel blocking agent used in the treatment of hypertension. The drug is not teratogenic in rats or rabbits at doses 150 and 25 times the maximum recommended human dose, respectively (1). Embryotoxicity was not observed in either species at doses that were not maternally toxic (1).

In a study to determine the effects of isradipine on maternal and fetal hemodynamics, 27 women with pregnancy-induced hypertension in the 3rd trimester were treated with the drug, 2.5 mg twice daily for 4 days then 5 mg twice daily (2). Hemodynamic measurements, conducted before and after 1 week of therapy, demonstrated a significant reduction in mean arterial pressure without a significant change in uteroplacental or fetal blood flows. The lack of change in uteroplacental blood flow suggested that there was uterine vasodilatation with decreased uterine vascular resistance (2). No fetal adverse effects were observed.

A 1992 study examined the effect of isradipine on three standardized physical stress tests in 14 women under treatment for hypertension (3 with essential hypertension, 11 with preeclampsia) (3). Treatment with isradipine, 5 mg once daily for 4 days then 5 mg twice daily, was begun at a mean 33 weeks' gestation with delivery occurring at a mean of 38 weeks. The pregnancy outcomes were normal except for one newborn whose birth weight was below the 10th percentile and transient hyperbilirubinemia in two neonates.

Several other studies have described the use of isradipine in pregnant women (4–8). No adverse fetal effects attributable to the drug were observed. Isradipine crosses the placenta to the fetus at term (4).

BREAST FEEDING SUMMARY

RECOMMENDATION: No Human Data - Probably Compatible

No reports describing the use of isradipine during human lactation have been located. The relatively low molecular weight (about 371), however, suggests that the drug is excreted into breast milk. The potential effects of this exposure on a nursing infant are unknown.

References

1. Product information. DynaCirc. Sandoz Pharmaceuticals, 1993.
2. Lunell N-O, Garoff L, Grunewald C, Nisell H, Nylund L, Sarby B, Thornstrom S. Isradipine, a new calcium antagonist: effects on maternal and fetal hemodynamics. J Cardiovasc Pharmacol 1991;18(Suppl 3):S37–40.
3. Lunell NO, Grunewald C, Nisell H. Effect of isradipine on responses to standardized physical stress tests in hypertension of pregnancy. J Cardiovasc Pharmacol 1992;19(Suppl 3):S99–101.
4. Lunnell NO, Bondesson U, Grunewald C, Ingemarsson I, Nisell H, Wide-Swensson D. Transplacental passage of

isradipine in the treatment of pregnancy-induced hypertension. Am J Hypertens 1993;6:110S–1S.
5. Wide-Swensson DH, Ingemarsson I, Lunell NO, Forman A, Skajaa K, Lindberg B, Lindeberg S, Marsal K, Andersson KE. Calcium channel blockade (isradipine) in treatment of hypertension in pregnancy: a randomized placebo-controlled study. Am J Obstet Gynecol 1995;173:872–8.
6. Maharaj B, Khedun SM, Moodley J, Madhanpall N, van der Byl K. Intravenous isradipine in the management of severe hypertension in pregnant and nonpregnant patients. A pilot study. Am J Hypertens 1994;7:61S–3S.
7. Kublickas M, Lunell NO, Grunewald C, Nisell H. Effect of isradipine on maternal renal artery pulsatility index in hypertensive pregnancy. Hypertens Pregn 1995;14:277–85.
8. Resch B, Mache CJ, Windhager T, Holzer H, Leitner G, Muller W. FK 506 and successful pregnancy in a patient after renal transplantation. Transplant Proc 1998;30:163–4.

Name:	**ITRACONAZOLE**	Risk Factor:	C_M
Class:	**Antifungal**		

FETAL RISK SUMMARY

RECOMMENDATION: Human Data Suggest Low Risk

Itraconazole is a triazole antifungal agent that is structurally related to a number of other antifungal agents, including the imidazole-derivatives butoconazole, clotrimazole, and ketoconazole, and to the triazoles, fluconazole and terconazole (1).

A dose-related increase in toxicity and teratogenicity was found in both rats and mice (2). In pregnant rats treated with a dosage range 5 to 20 times the maximum recommended human dose (MRHD), maternal and embryo toxicity were observed, as were major skeletal malformations. In mice given 10 times the MRHD, maternal toxicity, embryo toxicity, and malformations consisting of encephaloceles or macroglossia occurred.

It is not known if itraconazole crosses the human placenta. The molecular weight (about 706) is low enough that passage to the fetus should be expected.

Cohort data presented at a 1996 meeting on single-dose fluconazole or itraconazole exposures during organogenesis did not demonstrate adverse outcomes in approximately 70 exposed pregnancies (3). However, the FDA has received 14 case reports of malformations following use of itraconazole, 4 of which involved limb defects (includes 1 case of agenesis of the fingers and toes (3).

A 1998 non-interventional observational cohort study described the outcomes of pregnancies in women who had been prescribed one or more of 34 newly marketed drugs by general practitioners in England (4). Data were obtained by questionnaires sent to the prescribing physicians one month after the expected or possible date of delivery. In 831 (78%) of the pregnancies, a newly marketed drug was thought to have been taken during the 1st trimester with birth defects noted in 14 (2.5%) singleton births of the 557 newborns (10 sets of twins). In addition, two birth defects were observed in aborted fetuses. However, few of the aborted fetuses were examined. Itraconazole was taken during the 1st trimester in 41 pregnancies. The outcomes of these pregnancies included 1 ectopic pregnancy, 2 spontaneous abortions, 6 elective abortions, 2 cases lost to follow-up, and 30 normal newborns (1 premature) (4). One of the normal, full-term newborns, however, had a minor congenital anomaly consisting of a thin, prominent and protruding left ear. Although no major congenital malformations were observed, the study lacked the sensitivity to identify minor anomalies because of the absence of standardized examinations. Late-appearing major defects may also have been missed as a consequence of the timing of the questionnaires.

A prospective cohort study published in 2000 evaluated the pregnancy outcomes of 198 women exposed to itraconazole in the 1st trimester (5). The pregnancy exposures had been reported to the manufacturer, before the outcomes were known, between April 1989 and June 1998. The median itraconazole dose was 200 mg (range 50–800 mg) with mean therapy duration of 8.5 days (range 1–90 days). A matched control group ($N = 198$) was formed from pregnant women who had contacted the Motherisk Program, a teratogen information service in Toronto, Canada. The control group had not been exposed to any known teratogens (acceptable exposures were acetaminophen, penicillins, prenatal vitamins, dental radiography, or no exposures). There were no statistical differences between the groups in gravidity, parity, alcohol use, or cigarette smoking, but the maternal age in the study group was significantly less than controls (30.1 vs. 31.0 years). Among pregnancy outcomes, there were no statistical differences between the groups in delivery method, rates of term, preterm, and postterm deliveries, 1- and 5-minute Apgar scores, sex ratios, and rates of neonatal complications. Significantly more pregnancy losses occurred in the exposed group than in controls (relative risk 1.75, 95% confidence interval 1.47–2.09), including spontaneous abortions (12.6% vs. 4.0%), elective abortions (7.5% vs. 0.5%), and fetal deaths (1.5% vs. 1.0%). The authors attributed these differences to group differences, rather than to effects of itraconazole exposure (5). In addition, the birth weight of exposed newborns was significantly lower than controls (3.33 vs. 3.46 kg), but this finding was probably not clinically significant (5). There was no statistical difference between the groups in major congenital malformations. Among the 156 live births in the study group there were five infants (3.2%) with major anomalies (microphthalmia, dysplasia of the right hand, pyloric stenosis, hip joint dysplasia, and congenital heart disease [type not specified]). There were nine newborns (4.8%) with major defects among the 187 controls with live births (congenital heart disease [three cases—two with ventricular septal defect and one not specified], hypospadias requiring surgery [two cases], and one each of oversized tongue, congenital hip dislocation, cleft palate, and Down's syndrome with atrioventricular canal). The study had 80% power to detect a 3-fold increased risk of major defects (5), but no evaluation was conducted for minor defects.

In summary, the available human data do not show that itraconazole poses a significant risk for major anomalies in humans. None of the above studies, however, adequately looked for minor malformations. Moreover, another azole antifungal agent, fluconazole, has demonstrated a possible dose-related relationship with major malformations (see Fluconazole). Therefore, the safest course is to avoid itraconazole, if possible, during organogenesis. If inadvertent exposure does occur during the 1st trimester, or if itraconazole must be used during early pregnancy, the woman can be reassured that the risk to her embryo or fetus, if it exists at all, is most likely low.

BREAST FEEDING SUMMARY

RECOMMENDATION: Limited Human Data - Potential Toxicity

Itraconazole is excreted into breast milk. Two healthy, lactating women each took two oral doses of 200 mg 12 hours apart (total dose 400 mg) (E. K. Cazzaniga and A. Chanlam, personal communication, Janssen Pharmaceuticals, 1996). Neither infant was allowed to nurse during the study. At 4, 24, and 48 hours after the second dose, the average milk concentrations of itraconazole were 70, 28, and 16 ng/mL, respectively. At 72 hours, the milk level was 20 ng/mL in one woman and not detectable (<5 ng/mL) in the other. The average milk:plasma ratios at 4, 24, and 48 hours were 0.51, 1.61, and 1.77, respectively. Using the 4-hour concentration (the approximate time of the peak plasma level), and assuming the infants consumed 500 mL of milk/day, the maximum 24-hour average dose the infants would have received was 35 μg.

Although the above amount seems small, peak plasma concentrations in healthy male volunteers taking itraconazole 200 mg twice daily were not reached until about 15 days (2). The mean peak concentration of the parent compound in these volunteers was 2282 ng/mL, or about 15 times the average peak concentration measured in the two women above. Moreover, the mean plasma concentration of one of the metabolites (hydroxyitraconazole) exceeded that of the parent compound. Additionally, in animal studies, itraconazole accumulated in fatty tissues, omentum, liver, kidney, and skin tissues at levels 2–20 times the corresponding plasma concentration (2). Thus, continuous daily dosing, even with lower doses, should result in milk levels of the drug much higher than those found above and could result in widespread tissue accumulation in nursing infants. Because the potential effects of this exposure have not been studied, women taking itraconazole should probably not breast-feed.

I

References

1. American Hospital Formulary Service. *Drug Information 1997*. Bethesda, MD: American Society of Health-System Pharmacists, 1997:93–5.
2. Product information. Sporanox. Janssen Pharmaceutica, 2001.
3. Rosa F. Azole fungicide pregnancy risks. Presented at the Ninth International Conference of the Organization of Teratology Information Services, May 2–4, 1996, Salt Lake City, Utah.
4. Wilton LV, Pearce GL, Martin RM, Mackay FJ, Mann RD. The outcomes of pregnancy in women exposed to newly marketed drugs in general practice in England. Br J Obstet Gynaecol 1998;105:882–9.
5. Bar-Oz B, Moretti ME, Bishai R, Mareels G, Van Tittelboom T, Verspeelt J, Koren G. Pregnancy outcome after in utero exposure to itraconazole: a prospective cohort study. Am J Obstet Gynecol 2000;183:617–20.

Name: **IVERMECTIN** Risk Factor: C_M

Class: **Anthelmintic**

FETAL RISK SUMMARY

RECOMMENDATION: Human Data Suggest Low Risk

Ivermectin is a semisynthetic anthelmintic. It is a mixture of two components derived from the avermectins, a class of antiparasitic agents isolated from the fermentation of *Streptomyces avermitilis*. Ivermectin is indicated for the treatment of intestinal strongyloidiasis infections caused by the nematode *Strongyloides stercoralis* and onchocerciasis caused by the nematode *Onchocerca volvulus* (1).

In reproduction studies with mice, rats, and rabbits, ivermectin was teratogenic when given in repeated doses of 0.2, 8.1, and 4.5 times, respectively, the maximum recommended human dose based on body surface area. The malformations observed, cleft palate (in all three species) and clubbed forepaws in rabbits, however, were only observed at or near doses producing maternal toxicity. The results were thought to indicate that ivermectin was not selectively fetal toxic to the developing fetus (1).

It is not known if ivermectin crosses the human placenta. The molecular weights of the two components in the product, approximately 875 and 861, are low enough that some exposure of the embryo or fetus probably occurs.

A well-conducted study published in 1990 described the pregnancy outcomes of women who were inadvertently exposed to ivermectin during (1987–1989) community-based ivermectin distribution programs for onchocerciasis on a Liberian rubber plantation (14,000 people) (2). The average oral ivermectin dose was 150 μg/kg as a single dose. Because the women did not recall the date of their last menstrual period before delivery, pregnancy exposure was defined as a delivery occurring within 40 weeks of treatment. During the distribution programs, 2884 women received treatment, including 200 (7%) that were inadvertently treated during pregnancy. Of those treated during pregnancy, 85% were treated in the first 12 weeks of pregnancy and 36% occurred within the first 4 weeks (2). The outcomes of all pregnancies were followed up by a field census team, systematic examination of all babies born at the hospital, and a year-round plantation-wide surveillance system of all births and deaths (2). All children under 12 months of age were examined by a physician and children aged 12–24 months were examined by a pediatrician. Among the 203 pregnancy outcomes from exposed pregnancies, there were 10 (4.9%) abnormal events—5 stillbirths and 5 congenital malformations (single-dose exposure in weeks before delivery shown in parentheses): anal atresia (34 weeks); cleft palate and lip (33 weeks); Pierre-Robin syndrome, micrognathia, glossoptosis, low-slung ears, and shortening of limbs in a stillborn infant (32 weeks); Turner's syndrome (24 weeks); and deafness plus probable ventricular septal defect (VSD) (33 weeks). Among the 1,767 pregnancy outcomes not exposed to ivermectin, there were 76 (4.3%) abnormal events: 55 stillbirths or miscarriages and 21 congenital anomalies. The congenital anomalies were: polydactyly ($N = 6$), convergent strabismus ($N = 3$), talipes equinovarus ($N = 2$), unspecified ($N = 2$), and 1 each deafness, facial malformations, hypopigmented skin, hypospadias, microcephaly, Down's syndrome, syndactyly, and VSD. There were no significant differences between the treated and untreated groups in the rates of congenital malformations, stillbirths, or all abnormalities (congenital malformations, stillbirths, and miscarriages). There also was no statistical differences in terms of health status and malformations between infants (ages 2–7 months) and children (ages 12–24 months) whose mothers had been treated in comparison to untreated controls, matched for age, sex, and distance from the hospital (2).

A brief 1993 communication from Cameroon described the outcomes of pregnancies in 110 women who had inadvertently received ivermectin treatment during a mass treatment campaign for onchocerciasis (3). During the 2-year campaign, 401 of 2,710 women were excluded from treatment because of pregnancy. Of the remaining 2,389 women who were treated, 110 were discovered to be pregnant during regularly scheduled follow-up. Treatment was considered to have been given during pregnancy if delivery occurred within 40 weeks of ivermectin distribution. A comparison of the 110 women treated during gestation to the 401 pregnant women who did not receive treatment revealed no statistical differences in early abortion (<4 months) (3.6% vs. 2.2%), late abnormal events (abortion, miscarriage, stillbirth) (15.5% vs. 11%), children lost to follow-up (7.3% vs. 11.2%), infants with malformations (0 vs. 0.5%), or normal infants (74.5% vs. 75.8%). The prevalence of all abnormal obstetric events of treated women was similar to that of those not treated ($p > 0.37$). Only two newborns with congenital malformations were observed, both in the untreated group. In a second analysis, pregnancy outcomes of 97 women treated in the 1st trimester were compared with the outcomes of 142 untreated women. As before, no statistical differences were observed. The authors concluded that ivermectin did not present a major risk to the fetus (3).

In summary, ivermectin was teratogenic in three animal species, but only at doses at or near those producing maternal toxicity. No teratogenicity or toxicity attributable to ivermectin has been observed in limited human pregnancy experience. A 1997 review, citing a World Health Organization reference, stated that because of the high risk of blindness from onchocerciasis, and the lack of reported adverse outcomes, the use of ivermectin after the 1st trimester was probably acceptable (4).

BREAST FEEDING SUMMARY

RECOMMENDATION: Limited Human Data - Probably Compatible

Ivermectin is excreted into breast milk, but its use during breast-feeding has not been reported. Four healthy women, who had lost their babies at birth, were given a single 150-μg/kg oral ivermectin dose after an overnight fast (5). Ivermectin was detected in the plasma and breast milk within 1 hour. The mean peak concentration in plasma was 37.9 ng/mL and in milk was 14.1 ng/mL. The mean milk:plasma ratio was 0.51 (range 0.39–0.57). The steady-state ivermectin concentration in milk over a 24-hour period was approximately 10 ng/mL. The investigators estimated that the dose a 1-month old African infant would receive from breast milk was 2.75 μg/kg. This dose is much lower than an estimated dose of 21.8 μg/kg they calculated for a 1-month-old infant (5). (*Note*: In the United States, because the safety and effectiveness has not been established, ivermectin is not recommended for children who weigh less than 15 kg [1].) In Nigeria, where the study was conducted, lactating women within the first week of breast-feeding were excluded from community wide ivermectin distribution because of the concerns for infant safety (5). The investigators concluded, however, that the benefits of treatment for the lactating woman, combined with the impracticality of withholding nursing for a week, the low drug levels in milk, and the lack of reported adverse effects in nursing infants in their population, suggested that the drug should be given to the mother regardless of her lactation status (5). The American Academy of Pediatrics classifies ivermectin as compatible with breast-feeding (6).

I

References

1. Product information. Stromectol. Merck, 2002.
2. Pacque M, Munoz B, Poetschke G, Foose J, Greene BM, Taylor HR. Pregnancy outcome after inadvertent ivermectin treatment during community-based distribution. Lancet 1990;336:1486–9.
3. Chippaux JP, Gardon-Wendel N, Gardon J, Ernould JC. Absence of any adverse effect of inadvertent ivermectin treatment during pregnancy. Tran R Soc Trop Med Hyg 1993;87:318.
4. de Silva N, Guyatt H, Bundy D. Anthelmintics. A comparative review of their clinical pharmacology. Drugs 1997;53:769–88.
5. Ogbuokiri JE, Ozumba BC, Okonkwo PO. Ivermectin levels in human breastmilk. Eur J Clin Pharmacol 1993;45:389–90.
6. Committee on Drugs, American Academy of Pediatrics. The transfer of drugs and other chemicals into human milk. Pediatrics 2001;108:776–89.

K

Name: **KANAMYCIN** Risk Factor: **D**

Class: **Antibiotic (Aminoglycoside)**

FETAL RISK SUMMARY

RECOMMENDATION: Human Data Suggest Risk

Kanamycin is an aminoglycoside antibiotic. At term, the drug was detectable in cord serum 15 minutes after a 500-mg IM maternal dose (1). Mean cord serum levels at 3–6 hours were 6 μg/mL. Amniotic fluid levels were undetectable during the first hour, then rose during the next 6 hours to a mean value of 5.5 μg/mL. No effects on the infants were mentioned.

Eighth cranial nerve damage has been reported following *in utero* exposure to kanamycin (2,3). In a retrospective survey of 391 mothers who had received kanamycin, 50 mg/kg, for prolonged periods during pregnancy, 9 (2.3%) children were found to have hearing loss (2). Complete hearing loss in a mother and her infant was reported after the mother had been treated during pregnancy with kanamycin, 1 g/day IM for 4.5 days (3). Ethacrynic acid, an ototoxic diuretic, was also given to the mother during pregnancy.

Except for ototoxicity, no reports of congenital defects caused by kanamycin have been located. Embryos were examined from five patients who aborted during the 11th–12th week of pregnancy and who had been treated with kanamycin during the 6th and 8th weeks (2). No abnormalities in the embryos were found.

BREAST FEEDING SUMMARY

RECOMMENDATION: Limited Human Data - Probably Compatible

Kanamycin is excreted into breast milk. Milk:plasma ratios of 0.05–0.40 have been reported (4). A 1-g IM dose produced peak milk levels of 18.4 μg/mL (5). No effects were reported in the nursing infants. Because oral absorption of kanamycin is poor, ototoxicity would not be expected. However, three potential problems exist for the nursing infant: modification of bowel flora, direct effects on the infant, and interference with the interpretation of culture results if a fever workup is required. The American Academy of Pediatrics classifies kanamycin as compatible with breast-feeding (6).

References

1. Good R, Johnson G. The placental transfer of kanamycin during late pregnancy. Obstet Gynecol 1971;38:60–2.
2. Nishimura H, Tanimura T. *Clinical Aspects of The Teratogenicity of Drugs*. New York, NY: American Elsevier, 1976:131.
3. Jones HC. Intrauterine ototoxicity. A case report and review of literature. J Natl Med Assoc 1973;65:201–3.
4. Wilson JT. Milk/plasma ratios and contraindicated drugs. In Wilson JT, ed. *Drugs in Breast Milk*. Balgowlah, Australia: ADIS Press, 1981:79.
5. O'Brien T. Excretion of drugs in human milk. Am J Hosp Pharm 1974;31:844–54.
6. Committee on Drugs, American Academy of Pediatrics. The transfer of drugs and other chemicals into human milk. Pediatrics 2001;108:776–89.

Name:	**KAOLIN/PECTIN**	Risk Factor:	**C**
Class:	**Antidiarrheal**		

FETAL RISK SUMMARY

RECOMMENDATION: No Human Data - Probably Compatible

Kaolin is a hydrated aluminum silicate clay used for its adsorbent properties in diarrhea, and pectin is a polysaccharide obtained from plant tissues that is used as a solidifying agent. Neither agent is absorbed into the systemic circulation.

No reports have related the use of the kaolin/pectin mixture in pregnancy with adverse fetal outcome. There have been reports of iron-deficiency anemia and hypokalemia secondary to the eating of clays (i.e., geophagia) containing kaolin (1–3). The mechanism for this is thought to be either a reduction in the intake of foods containing absorbable iron or an interference with the absorption of iron. In humans, iron-deficiency anemia may significantly enhance the chance for a low-birth-weight infant and preterm delivery (4,5).

Female rats fed a diet containing 20% kaolin became anemic and delivered pups with a significant decrease in birth weight (6). When an iron supplement was added to the kaolin-fortified diet, no anemia or reduced birth weight was observed.

K

BREAST FEEDING SUMMARY

RECOMMENDATION: No Human Data - Probably Compatible

Other than producing anemia in the mother after prolonged, chronic use, the kaolin/pectin mixture should have no effect on lactation or the nursing infant.

References

1. Mengel CE, Carter WA, Horton ES. Geophagia with iron deficiency and hypokalemia: cachexia africana. Arch Intern Med 1964;114:470–4.
2. Talington KM, Gant NF Jr, Scott DE, Pritchard JA. Effect of ingestion of starch and some clays on iron absorption. Am J Obstet Gynecol 1970;108:262–7.
3. Roselle HA. Association of laundry starch and clay ingestion with anemia in New York City. Arch Intern Med 1970;125:57–61.
4. Scholl TO, Hediger ML, Fischer RL, Shearer JW. Anemia vs iron deficiency: increased risk of preterm delivery in a prospective study. Am J Clin Nutr 1992;55:985–8.
5. Macgregor MW. Maternal anaemia as a factor in prematurity and perinatal mortality. Scott Med J 1963;8:134–40.
6. Patterson EC, Staszak DJ. Effects of geophagia (kaolin ingestion) on the maternal blood and embryonic development in the pregnant rat. J Nutr 1977;107:2020–5.

Name:	**KETAMINE**	Risk Factor:	**B**
Class:	**General Anesthetic**		

FETAL RISK SUMMARY

RECOMMENDATION: Limited Human Data - Animal Data Suggest Low Risk

Ketamine is a rapid-acting IV general anesthetic agent related in structure and action to phencyclidine. No teratogenic or other adverse fetal effects have been observed in reproduction studies during organogenesis and near delivery with rats, mice, rabbits, and dogs (1–5). In one study with pregnant rats, a dose of 120 mg/kg/day for 5 days during organogenesis resulted in no malformations or effect on fetal weight (4).

Ketamine rapidly crosses the placenta to the fetus in animals and humans (6,7). Pregnant ewes were given 0.7 mg/kg IV, and 1 minute later the maternal and fetal concentrations of ketamine were 1230 ng/mL and 470 ng/mL (ratio 0.38), respectively (6). Maternal effects were slight, transitory increases in maternal mean arterial pressure and cardiac output, respiratory acidosis, and an increase in uterine tone without changes in uterine blood flow. In humans, the placental transfer of ketamine was documented in a study in which a dose of 250 mg IM was administered when the fetal head reached the perineum (7). The ketamine concentration in cord venous plasma at the 0- to 10-minute dose-to-delivery interval was 0.61 μg/mL, compared with 1.03 μg/mL at the 10- to 30-minute interval, reflecting absorption following the IM route.

Pregnant monkeys (*Macaca nemistrina*) were administered ketamine in a dose of 2 mg/kg IV ($N = 3$) or 1 mg/kg IV ($N = 2$) in an investigation of the anesthetic's effects on the fetus and newborn (8). No fetal effects were observed from either dose. The newborns from the mothers given 2 mg/kg, but not those exposed to lower doses, however, had profound respiratory depression.

The use of ketamine (CI-581) for obstetric anesthesia was first described in 1966 (9). Since then, a large number of references have documented its use for this purpose (10–38). Among the maternal and newborn complications reported with ketamine are oxytocic properties, an increase in maternal blood pressure, newborn depression, and an increased tone of newborn skeletal musculature. These adverse effects were usually related to higher doses (1.5–2.2 mg/kg IV) administered during early studies rather than to the lower doses (0.2–0.5 mg/kg IV) now commonly used.

Ketamine usually demonstrates a dose-related oxytocic effect with an increase in uterine tone, and in frequency and intensity of uterine contractions (9–12,22,37), but one investigator reported weakened uterine contractions following a 250-mg dose administered IM when the fetal head reached the perineum (7). Uterine tetany was observed in one case (12). Low doses (0.275–1.1 mg/kg IV) of ketamine increased only uterine contractions, whereas a higher dose (2.2 mg/kg IV) resulted in a marked increase in uterine tone (22). Maximum effects were observed within 2–4 minutes of the dose. In one study, however, the effect on uterine contractions from an IV dose of 1 mg/kg, followed by succinylcholine 1 mg/kg, was no different from thiopental (14). No effect on intra-uterine pressure was measured in 12 term patients treated with ketamine 2 mg/kg IV, in contrast to a marked uterine pressure increase in patients in early pregnancy undergoing termination (39). Similarly, in 12 women given ketamine 2.2 mg/kg IV for termination of pregnancy at 8–19 weeks, uterine pressure and the intensity and frequency of contractions were increased (40).

Several investigators have noted a marked increase in maternal blood pressure, up to 30%–40% in systolic and diastolic in some series, during ketamine induction (7,10,12,13,15,23,24). An increased maternal heart rate is usually observed. These effects are dose-related with the greatest increases occurring when 2–2.2 mg/kg IV was administered, but smaller elevations of pressure and pulse have been noted with lower IV doses.

Maternal ketamine anesthesia may cause depression of the newborn (7,12, 15–18,21,23,26,32). As with the other complications, the use of higher doses (1.5–2.2 mg/kg IV) resulted in the highest incidence of low neonatal Apgar scores and requirements for newborn resuscitation. The induction-to-delivery (ID) interval is an important determinant for neonatal depression (7,21,32,34). In two studies, neonatal depression was markedly lower or absent if the ID interval was less than 10 minutes (7,32). In a third report, significant depression occurred with an ID interval of 9.2 minutes, but a dose of 2.1 mg/kg IV had been used (21).

The use of ketamine in low doses apparently has little effect on fetal cardiovascular status or acid-base balance as evidenced by neonatal blood gases (7,24,26,29,31–33). In one study, a ketamine dose of 25 mg IV administered with nitrous oxide and oxygen within 4 minutes of delivery did not adversely affect neonatal blood pressure (38).

Ketamine doses of 2 mg/kg IV have been associated with excessive neonatal muscle tone, sometimes with apnea (10,11,17). In some cases, the increased muscle tone made endotracheal intubation difficult. In contrast, lower doses (e.g., 0.25–1 mg/kg) have not been associated with this complication (24).

Neonatal neurobehavior, as measured by the Scanlon Group of Early Neonatal Neurobehavioral Tests during the first 2 days, is depressed following maternal ketamine (1 mg/kg IV) anesthesia but less than the effect measured after thiopental anesthesia (4 mg/kg IV) (41,42). In these studies, spinal anesthesia with 6–8 mg of tetracaine was associated with the best performance, general anesthesia with ketamine was intermediate, and that with thiopental was the poorest in performance.

In summary, although ketamine anesthesia close to delivery may induce dose-related, transient toxicity in the newborn, these effects are usually avoided with the use of lower maternal doses. No reports of malformations in humans (43) or in animals attributable to ketamine have been located, although experience with the anesthetic agent during human organogenesis apparently has not been published.

K

BREAST FEEDING SUMMARY

RECOMMENDATION: No Human Data - Probably Compatible

Because ketamine is a general anesthetic agent, breast-feeding would not be possible while using the drug, and no reports have been located that measured the amount of the agent in milk. The elimination half-life of ketamine has been reported to be 2.17 hours in unpremedicated patients (31). Thus, the drug should be undetectable in the mother's plasma approximately 11 hours after a dose. Nursing after this time should not expose the infant to pharmacologically significant amounts of ketamine.

References

1. Nishimura H, Tanimura T. *Clinical Aspects of The Teratogenicity of Drugs*. New York, NY: American Elsevier, 1976:178.
2. Schardein JL. *Chemically Induced Birth Defects*. 2nd ed. New York, NY: Marcel Dekker, 1993:148.
3. Onnis A, Grella P. *The Biochemical Effects of Drugs in Pregnancy*. Volume 1. West Sussex, England: Ellis Norwood, 1984:18–9.
4. El-Karum AHA, Benny R. Embryotoxic and teratogenic action of ketamine. Ain Shams Med J 1976;27: 459–63.
5. Product information. Ketalar. Parke-Davis, 1993.
6. Craft JB Jr, Coaldrake LA, Yonekura ML, Dao SD, Co EG, Roizen MF, Mazel P, Gilman R, Shokes L, Trevor AJ. Ketamine, catecholamines, and uterine tone in pregnant ewes. Am J Obstet Gynecol 1983;146:429–34.
7. Nishijima M. Ketamine in obstetric anesthesia: special reference to placental transfer and its concentration in blood plasma. Acta Obstet Gynaecol Jpn 1972;19: 80–93. Cited in Anonymous. Operative obstetrics and anesthesia. Obstet Gynecol Surv 1975;30:605–6.
8. Eng M, Bonica JJ, Akamatsu TJ, Berges PU, Ueland K. Respiratory depression in newborn monkeys at caesarean section following ketamine administration. Br J Anaesth 1975;47:917–21.
9. Chodoff P, Stella JG. Use of CI-581 a phencyclidine derivative for obstetric anesthesia. Anesth Analg 1966;45:527–30.
10. Bovill JG, Coppel DL, Dundee JW, Moore J. Current status of ketamine anaesthesia. Lancet 1971;1: 1285–8.
11. Moore J, McNabb TG, Dundee JW. Preliminary report on ketamine in obstetrics. Br J Anaesth 1971;43: 779–82.
12. Little B, Chang T, Chucot L, Dill WA, Enrile LL, Glazko AJ, Jassani M, Kretchmer H, Sweet AY. Study of ketamine as an obstetric anesthetic agent. Am J Obstet Gynecol 1972;113:247–60.
13. McDonald JS, Mateo CV, Reed EC. Modified nitrous oxide or ketamine hydrochloride for cesarean section. Anesth Analg 1972;51:975–83.
14. Peltz B, Sinclair DM. Induction agents for caesarean

section. A comparison of thiopentone and ketamine. Anaesthesia 1973;28:37–42.
15. Meer FM, Downing JW, Coleman AJ. An intravenous method of anaesthesia for caesarean section. Part II: ketamine. Br J Anaesth 1973;45:191–6.
16. Galbert MW, Gardner AE. Ketamine for obstetrical anesthesia. Anesth Analg 1973;52:926–30.
17. Corssen G. Ketamine in obstetric anesthesia. Clin Obstet Gynecol 1974;17:249–58.
18. Janeczko GF, El-Etr AA, Younes S. Low-dose ketamine anesthesia for obstetrical delivery. Anesth Analg 1974;53:828–31.
19. Akamatsu TJ, Bonica JJ, Rehmet R, Eng M, Ueland K. Experiences with the use of ketamine for parturition. I. Primary anesthetic for vaginal delivery. Anesth Analg 1974;53:284–7.
20. Krantz ML. Ketamine in obstetrics: comparison with methoxyflurane. Anesth Analg 1974;53:890–3.
21. Downing JW, Mahomedy MC, Jeal DE, Allen PJ. Anaesthesia for caesarean section with ketamine. Anaesthesia 1976;31:883–92.
22. Galloon S. Ketamine for obstetric delivery. Anesthesiology 1976;44:522–4.
23. Ellingson A, Haram K, Sagen N. Ketamine and diazepam as anaesthesia for forceps delivery. A comparative study. Acta Anaesth Scand 1977;21:37–40.
24. Maduska AL, Hajghassemali M. Arterial blood gases in mothers and infants during ketamine anesthesia for vaginal delivery. Anesth Analg 1978;57:121–3.
25. Dich-Nielsen J, Holasek J. Ketamine as induction agent for caesarean section. Acta Anaesth Scand 1982;26:139–42.
26. White PF, Way WL, Trevor AJ. Ketamine—its pharmacology and therapeutic uses. Anesthesiology 1982; 56:119–36.
27. Hill CR, Schultetus RR, Dharamraj CM, Banner TE, Berman LS. Wakefulness during cesarean section with thiopental, ketamine, or thiopental-ketamine combination (abstract). Anesthesiology 1993;59:A419.
28. Schultetus RR, Paulus DA, Spohr GL. Haemodynamic effects of ketamine and thiopentone during anaesthetic induction for caesarean section. Can Anaesth Soc J 1985;32:592–6.
29. Bernstein K, Gisselsson L, Jacobsson L, Ohrlander S. Influence of two different anaesthetic agents on the newborn and the correlation between foetal oxygenation and induction-delivery time in elective caesarean section. Acta Anaesthesiol Scand 1985;29:157–60.
30. Schultetus RR, Hill CR, Dharamraj CM, Banner TE, Berman LS. Wakefulness during cesarean section after anesthetic induction with ketamine, thiopental, or ketamine and thiopental combined. Anesth Analg 1986;65:723–8.
31. Reich DL, Silvay G. Ketamine: an update on the first twenty-five years of clinical experience. Can J Anaesth 1989;36:186–97.
32. Baraka A, Louis F, Dalleh R. Maternal awareness and neonatal outcome after ketamine induction of anaesthesia for caesarean section. Can J Anaesth 1990;37:641–4.
33. Rowbottom SJ, Gin T, Cheung LP. General anaesthesia for caesarean section in a patient with uncorrected complex cyanotic heart disease. Anaesth Intensive Care 1994;22:74–8.
34. Krissel J, Dick WF, Leyser KH, Gervais H, Brockerhoff P, Schranz D. Thiopentone, thiopentone/ketamine, and ketamine for induction of anaesthesia in caesarean section. Eur J Anaesthesiol 1994;11:115–22.
35. Conway JB, Posner M. Anaesthesia for caesarean section in a patient with Watson's syndrome. Can J Anaesth 1994;41:1113–6.
36. Maleck W. Ketamine and thiopentone in caesarean section. Eur J Anaesthesiol 1995;12:533.
37. Marx GF, Hwang HS, Chandra P. Postpartum uterine pressures with different doses of ketamine. Anesthesiology 1979;50:163–6.
38. Marx GF, Cabe CM, Kim YI, Eidelman AI. Neonatal blood pressures. Anaesthesist 1976;25:318–22.
39. Oats JN, Vasey DP, Waldron BA. Effects of ketamine on the pregnant uterus. Br J Anaesth 1979;51:1163–6.
40. Galloon S. Ketamine and the pregnant uterus. Can Anaesth Soc J 1973;20:141–5.
41. Hodgkinson R, Marx GF, Kim SS, Miclat NM. Neonatal neurobehavioral tests following vaginal delivery under ketamine, thiopental, and extradural anesthesia. Anesth Analg 1977;56:548–53.
42. Hodgkinson R, Bhatt M, Kim SS, Grewal G, Marx GF. Neonatal neurobehavioral tests following cesarean section under general and spinal anesthesia. Am J Obstet Gynecol 1978;132:670–4.
43. Friedman JM. Teratogen update: anesthetic agents. Teratology 1988;37:69–77.

Name:	**KETOCONAZOLE**	Risk Factor:	**C_M**
Class:	**Antifungal**		

FETAL RISK SUMMARY

RECOMMENDATION: **Limited Human Data - Animal Data Suggest Risk (Oral)**
No Human Data - Probably Compatible (Topical)

Ketoconazole is a synthetic, broad-spectrum antifungal agent. The antimycotic agent is embryotoxic and teratogenic in rats, producing syndactyly and oligodactyly at a dose

10 times the maximum recommended human dose (weight basis) (1,2). However, the dose caused maternal toxicity. Ketoconazole has been used, apparently without fetal harm, for the treatment of vaginal candidiasis occurring during pregnancy (3).

In a surveillance study of Michigan Medicaid recipients conducted between 1985 and 1992 involving 229,101 completed pregnancies, 20 newborns had been exposed to oral ketoconazole during the 1st trimester (F. Rosa, personal communication, FDA, 1993). No major birth defects were observed (one expected). Between 1992 and 1996, the FDA has received six reports of limb defects (F. Rosa, personal communication, FDA, 1996).

Limb malformations were reported in a 1985 abstract (4). A Turkish woman had used ketoconazole, 200 mg daily, during the first 7 weeks of gestation. Hydrops fetalis was diagnosed at 29 weeks' gestation and she delivered a female infant at 30.5 weeks' gestation. The infant, with a normal karyotype (46,XX), had multiple anomalies of the limbs (further details not specified).

Women infected with human immunodeficiency virus frequently have vaginal candidiasis. Maternal symptoms, such as pruritus, may require treatment; in these cases, therapeutic and prophylactic ketoconazole regimens are recommended, even though the fungal infection has little perinatal significance (5).

Ketoconazole inhibits steroidogenesis in fungal cells. In humans, high doses, such as those above 400 mg/day, impair testosterone and cortisol synthesis (6–9). Because of this effect, ketoconazole has been used in the treatment of hypercortisolism (10). A review summarizing the treatment of 67 cases of Cushing's syndrome occurring during pregnancy did not find any cases treated with ketoconazole (10). A 1990 report, however, described a ketoconazole-treated 36-year-old pregnant woman with Cushing's syndrome (11). The pregnancy, in addition to Cushing's syndrome, was complicated by hypertension, the diagnosis of diabetes mellitus at 9 weeks' gestation, and intrauterine growth retardation. Ketoconazole, 200 mg every 8 hours, was started at 32 weeks' gestation and continued for 5 weeks because of maternal clinical deterioration resulting from the sustained hypercortisolism. Rapid clinical improvement was noted in the mother after therapy was begun. A growth-retarded, 2080-g, but otherwise normal, female infant was delivered by elective cesarean section at 37 weeks. The Apgar scores were 9 and 9 at 1 and 5 minutes, respectively. No clinical or biochemical evidence of adrenal insufficiency was found in the newborn. The infant's basal cortisol and adrenocorticotropic hormone levels, 306 nmol/L and 8.1 pmol/L, respectively, were normal. The child was growing normally at 18 months of age.

K

BREAST FEEDING SUMMARY

RECOMMENDATION: No Human Data - Probably Compatible

Ketoconazole is excreted into breast milk (12). A 41-year-old, 82-kg woman took 200 mg/day for 10 days while nursing her 1-month-old infant. Five manually expressed milk samples were collected over a 24-hour interval (1.75–24 hours post-dose) on day 10. The maximum milk concentration (0.22 μg/mL) was measured at 3.25 hours post-dose. Ketoconazole was undetectable (detection limit 0.005 μg/mL) at 24 hours post-dose. The mean milk concentration, based on AUC for 0–24 hours, was 0.068 μg/mL. The level corresponded to an estimated infant dose (based on 150 mL/kg/day) of 0.01 mg/kg/day (maximum estimated dose 0.033 mg/kg/day). The dose was about 0.4% of the mother's weight-adjusted dose. No adverse effects were observed in the infant (12).

The effects on the nursing infant from exposure to drug in the milk are unknown, but the exposure in the above case does not appear to be clinically significant. The American Academy of Pediatrics classifies ketoconazole as compatible with breast-feeding (13).

References

1. Product information. Nizoral. Janssen Pharmaceutics, 1997.
2. Nishikawa S, Hara T, Miyazaki H, Ohguro Y. Reproduction studies of KW-1414 in rats and rabbits. Clin Report 1984;18:1433–88.
   As cited in Shepard TH. *Catalog of Teratogenic Agents*. 6th ed. Baltimore, MD: Johns Hopkins University Press, 1989:1075.
3. Luscher KP, Schneitter J, Vogt HP. Frequency of candidiasis during pregnancy and therapy with ketokonazol ovula. Schweiz Rundsch Med Prax 1987;76:1285–7.
4. Lind J. Limb malformations in a case of hydrops fetalis with ketoconazole use during pregnancy (abstract). Arch Gynecol 1985;237(Suppl):398.
5. Minkoff HL. Care of pregnant women infected with human immunodeficiency virus. JAMA 1987;258:2714–7.
6. Hobbs ER. Coccidioidomycosis. Dermatol Clin 1989;7:227–39.
7. Pont A, Williams PL, Loose DS, Feldman D, Reitz RE, Bochra C, Stevens DA. Ketoconazole blocks adrenal steroid synthesis. Ann Intern Med 1982;97:370–2.
8. Engelhardt D, Mann K, Hormann R, Braun S, Karl HJ. Ketoconazole inhibits cortisol secretion of an adrenal adenoma *in vivo* and *in vitro*. Klin Wochenschr 1983;61:373–5.
9. Divers MJ. Ketoconazole treatment of Cushing's syndrome in pregnancy. Am J Obstet Gynecol 1990;163:1101.
10. Aron DC, Schnall AM, Sheeler LR. Cushing's syndrome and pregnancy. Am J Obstet Gynecol 1990;162:244–52.
11. Amado JA, Pesquera C, Gonzalez EM, Otero M, Freijanes J, Alvarez A. Successful treatment with ketoconazole of Cushing's syndrome in pregnancy. Postgrad Med J 1990;66:221–3.
12. Moretti ME, Ito S, Koren G. Disposition of maternal ketoconazole in breast milk. Am J Obstet Gynecol 1995;173:1625–8.
13. Committee on Drugs, American Academy of Pediatrics. The transfer of drugs and other chemicals into human milk. Pediatrics 2001;108:776–89.

Name:	**KETOPROFEN**	Risk Factor:	**B_M***
Class:	**Nonsteroidal Anti-inflammatory**		

FETAL RISK SUMMARY

RECOMMENDATION: Human Data Suggest Risk in 1st and 3rd Trimesters

Ketoprofen is a nonsteroidal anti-inflammatory drug (NSAID) that is indicated for the management of the signs and symptoms of rheumatoid arthritis and osteoarthritis. It is in the same subclass (propionic acids) as five other NSAIDs (fenoprofen, flurbiprofen, ibuprofen, naproxen, and oxaprozin).

Reproductive studies in mice and rats at about 0.2 times the maximum recommended human dose based on body surface area revealed no teratogenic or embryotoxic effects (1). In rabbits, maternally toxic doses were embryotoxic but not teratogenic (1). Shepard reviewed four animal studies using mice, rats, and monkeys and found no adverse fetal effects or congenital malformations (2).

Consistent with the low molecular weight (about 254), ketoprofen crosses the human placenta. A 1998 study, using a human isolated perfused placenta, demonstrated transfer of the drug (3). The investigators had previously shown that the drug crosses to the fetus and is detectable in the newborn (4).

In a surveillance study of Michigan Medicaid recipients conducted between 1985 and 1992 involving 229,101 completed pregnancies, 112 newborns had been exposed to ketoprofen during the 1st trimester (F. Rosa, personal communication, FDA, 1993). Three (2.7%) major birth defects were observed (five expected), including (expected/observed)

1/1 cardiovascular defect and 1/0.3 polydactyly. No anomalies were observed in four other categories of defects (oral clefts, spina bifida, limb reduction defects, and hypospadias) for which specific data were available.

A combined 2001 population-based observational cohort study and a case-control study estimated the risk of adverse pregnancy outcome from the use of NSAIDs (5). The use of NSAIDs during pregnancy was not associated with congenital malformations, preterm delivery, or low birth weight, but a positive association was discovered with spontaneous abortions (SABs). A similar study, also published in 2001, failed to find a relationship, in general, between NSAIDs and congenital malformations, but did find a significant association with cardiac defects and orofacial clefts (6), In addition, a 2003 study found a significant association between exposure to NSAIDs in early pregnancy and SABs (7). (See Ibuprofen for details on these three studies.)

A brief 2003 editorial on the potential for NSAID-induced developmental toxicity concluded that NSAIDs, and specifically those with greater COX-2 affinity, had a lower risk of this toxicity in humans than aspirin (8).

Constriction of the ductus arteriosus *in utero* is a pharmacologic consequence arising from the use of prostaglandin synthesis inhibitors during pregnancy (see also Indomethacin) (9). Persistent pulmonary hypertension of the newborn may occur if these agents are used in the 3rd trimester close to delivery (9,10). These drugs also have been shown to inhibit labor and prolong pregnancy, both in humans (11) (see also Indomethacin) and in animals (12). Women attempting to conceive should not use any prostaglandin synthesis inhibitor, including ketoprofen, because of the findings in a variety of animal models that indicate these agents block blastocyst implantation (13,14). Moreover, as noted above, NSAIDs have been associated with SABs and congenital malformations.

[*Risk Factor D if used in 3rd trimester or near delivery*]

K

BREAST FEEDING SUMMARY

RECOMMENDATION: No Human Data - Probably Compatible

No reports on the use of ketoprofen in lactating humans have been located. The low molecular weight (about 254) suggests that the drug will be excreted into breast milk. The effects of this exposure on a nursing infant are unknown. Ketoprofen is excreted into the milk of lactating dogs, with milk concentrations about 4%–5% of plasma levels (1). Another NSAID in the same subclass is classified as compatible with breast-feeding by the American Academy of Pediatrics (see Ibuprofen).

References

1. Product information. Orudis, Oruvail. Wyeth-Ayerst Pharmaceuticals, 2000.
2. Shepard TH. *Catalog of Teratogenic Agents*. 6th ed. Baltimore, MD: Johns Hopkins University Press, 1989: 364.
3. Lagrange F, Pehourcq F, Bannwarth B, Leng JJ, Saux MC. Passage of S-(+)- and R-(−)-ketoprofen across the human isolated perfused placenta. Fundam Clin Pharmacol 1998;12:286–91.
4. Labat L, Llanas B, Demotes-Mainard F, Lagrange F, Demarquez JL, Bannwarth B. Accumulation of S-ketoprofen in neonates after maternal administration of the racemate. Fundam Clin Pharmacol 1995;9:62. As cited in Lagrange F, Pehourcq F, Bannwarth B, Leng JJ, Saux MC. Passage of S-(+)- and R-(−)-ketoprofen across the human isolated perfused placenta. Fundam Clin Pharmacol 1998;12:286–91.
5. Nielsen GL, Sorensen HT, Larsen H, Pedersen L. Risk of adverse birth outcome and miscarriage in pregnant users of non-steroidal anti-inflammatory drugs: population based observational study and case-control study. BMJ 2001;322:266–70.
6. Ericson A, Kallen BAJ. Nonsteroidal anti-inflammatory drugs in early pregnancy. Reprod Toxicol 2001;15:371–5.
7. Li DK, Liu L, Odouli R. Exposure to non-steroidal anti-inflammatory drugs during pregnancy and risk of miscarriage: population based cohort study. BMJ 2003;327:368–71.
8. Tassinari MS, Cook JC, Hurtt ME. NSAIDs and

developmental toxicity. Birth Defects Res Part B Dev Reprod Toxicol 2003;68:3–4.
9. Levin DL. Effects of inhibition of prostaglandin synthesis on fetal development, oxygenation, and the fetal circulation. Semin Perinatol 1980;4:35–44.
10. Van Marter LJ, Leviton A, Allred EN, Pagano M, Sullivan KF, Cohen A, Epstein MF. Persistent pulmonary hypertension of the newborn and smoking and aspirin and nonsteroidal antiinflammatory drug consumption during pregnancy. Pediatrics 1996;97:658–63.
11. Fuchs F. Prevention of prematurity. Am J Obstet Gynecol 1976;126:809–20.
12. Powell JG, Cochrane RL. The effects of a number of non-steroidal anti-inflammatory compounds on parturition in the rat. Prostaglandins 1982;23:469–88.
13. Matt DW, Borzelleca JF. Toxic effects on the female reproductive system during pregnancy, parturition, and lactation. In Witorsch RJ, editor. *Reproductive Toxicology*. 2nd ed. New York, NY: Raven Press, 1995:175–93.
14. Dawood MY. Nonsteroidal antiinflammatory drugs and reproduction. Am J Obstet Gynecol 1993;169:1255–65.

Name: **KETOROLAC** Risk Factor: **C_M***
Class: **Nonsteroidal Anti-inflammatory**

FETAL RISK SUMMARY

RECOMMENDATION: Human Data Suggest Risk in 1st and 3rd Trimesters

K

Ketorolac is a nonsteroidal anti-inflammatory drug (NSAID) indicated for the short-term (≤5 days) treatment of pain. The drug is also available as a solution for ocular pain. Ketorolac is in a NSAID subclass (pyrrolizine carboxylic acid) with no other members.

Ketorolac was not teratogenic in rats (1.0 times the human area under the plasma concentration curve [AUC]) and rabbits (0.37 times the human AUC) treated with daily oral doses of the drug during organogenesis (1). Oral dosing in rats at 0.14 times the human AUC after day 17 of gestation caused dystocia and decreased pup survivability (1).

In a study using chronically catheterized pregnant sheep, an infusion of ketorolac completely blocked the ritodrine-induced increase of prostaglandin $F_{2\alpha}$, a potent uterine stimulant, in the uterine venous plasma (2,3). The researchers speculated that ritodrine stimulation of prostaglandin synthesis in pregnant uterine tissue might contribute to the tachyphylaxis sometimes observed with the tocolytic agent.

It is not known if ketorolac crosses the human placenta. The molecular weight (about 376) is low enough, however, that passage to the fetus should be expected.

A combined 2001 population-based observational cohort study and a case-control study estimated the risk of adverse pregnancy outcome from the use of NSAIDs (4). The use of NSAIDs during pregnancy was not associated with congenital malformations, preterm delivery, or low birth weight, but a positive association was discovered with spontaneous abortions (SABs). A similar study, also published in 2001, failed to find a relationship, in general, between NSAIDs and congenital malformations, but did find a significant association with cardiac defects and orofacial clefts (5). In addition, a 2003 study found a significant association between exposure to NSAIDs in early pregnancy and SABs (6). (See Ibuprofen for details on these three studies.)

A brief 2003 editorial on the potential for NSAID-induced developmental toxicity concluded that NSAIDs, and specifically those with greater COX-2 affinity, had a lower risk of this toxicity in humans than aspirin (7).

A randomized, double-blind study published in 1992 compared single doses of ketorolac 10 mg IM, meperidine 50 mg IM, and meperidine 100 mg IM in multiparous women in labor (8). All patients also received a single dose of prochlorperazine (for nausea and vomiting) and ranitidine for acid reflux. Ineffective pain relief was observed in all three treatment groups, but both doses of meperidine were superior to ketorolac. Duration of labor was similar between the three groups, as was the occurrence of adverse effects, including maternal blood loss. One-minute Apgar scores were significantly greater in the ketorolac group compared with the meperidine groups, most likely because of the lack of respiratory depressant effects of ketorolac, but this difference was not observed at 5 minutes (8).

A 1997 abstract and later full report described the use of ketorolac for acute tocolysis in preterm labor (9,10). Women, at ≤32 weeks' gestation, were randomized to receive either ketorolac ($N = 45$), 60 mg IM followed by 30 mg IM every 4–6 hours, or magnesium sulfate ($N = 43$), 6 g IV followed by 3–6 g/hour IV. Therapy was stopped if 48 hours lapsed, labor progressed (>4 cm), severe side effects occurred, or uterine quiescence was achieved (9,10). Ketorolac was significantly better than magnesium sulfate in the time required to stop uterine contractions (2.7 vs. 6.2 hours), but no difference was found between the two regimens for the other parameters (failed tocolysis, birth weight, gestational age at delivery, and neonatal morbidity). There was no difference in the incidence of maternal and neonatal adverse effects between the groups (9,10).

Because ketorolac is a prostaglandin synthesis inhibitor, constriction of the ductus arteriosus *in utero* and fetal renal impairment are potential complications when multiple doses of the drug are administered during the latter half of pregnancy (11) (see also Indomethacin). Premature closure of the ductus can result in primary pulmonary hypertension of the newborn that, in severe cases, may be fatal (11,12). Other complications that have been associated with NSAIDs are inhibition of labor and prolongation of pregnancy (see above). Women attempting to conceive should not use any prostaglandin synthesis inhibitor, including ketorolac, because of the findings in a variety of animal models that indicate these agents block blastocyst implantation (13,14). Moreover, as noted above, NSAIDs have been associated with SABs and congenital malformations.

[**Risk Factor D if used in the 3rd trimester or near delivery.*]

K

BREAST FEEDING SUMMARY

RECOMMENDATION: Limited Human Data - Probably Compatible

Ketorolac is excreted into breast milk (15). Ten women, 2 to 6 days postpartum, were given oral ketorolac, 10 mg 4 times daily for 2 days. Their infants were not allowed to breast-feed during the study. Four of the women had milk concentrations of the drug below the detection limit of the assay (<5 ng/mL) and were excluded from analysis. In the remaining six women, the mean milk:plasma ratios 2 hours after doses 1, 3, 5, and 7 ranged from 0.016 to 0.027, corresponding to mean milk concentrations ranging from 5.2 to 7.9 ng/mL. Based on a milk production of 400 to 1000 mL/day, the investigators estimated that the maximum amount of drug available to a nursing infant would range from 3.16 to 7.9 μg/day (note: the cited reference indicated 3.16 to 7.9 *mg/day*, but this appears to be an error), equivalent to 0.16% to 0.40% of the mother's dose on a weight-adjusted basis. These amounts were considered clinically insignificant (15). The American Academy of Pediatrics classifies ketorolac as compatible with breast-feeding (16).

References

1. Product information. Toradol. Roche Laboratories, 2000.
2. Rauk PN, Laifer SA. Ketorolac blocks ritodrine-stimulated production of $PGF_{2\alpha}$ in pregnant sheep (abstract). Am J Obstet Gynecol 1992;166:274.
3. Rauk PN, Laifer SA. The prostaglandin synthesis inhibitor ketorolac blocks ritodrine-stimulated production of prostaglandin $F_{2\alpha}$ in pregnant sheep. Obstet Gynecol 1993;81:323–6.
4. Nielsen GL, Sorensen HT, Larsen H, Pedersen L. Risk

of adverse birth outcome and miscarriage in pregnant users of non-steroidal anti-inflammatory drugs: population based observational study and case-control study. BMJ 2001;322:266–70.
5. Ericson A, Kallen BAJ. Nonsteroidal anti-inflammatory drugs in early pregnancy. Reprod Toxicol 2001;15:371–5.
6. Li DK, Liu L, Odouli R. Exposure to non-steroidal anti-inflammatory drugs during pregnancy and risk of miscarriage: population based cohort study. BMJ 2003;327:368–71.
7. Tassinari MS, Cook JC, Hurtt ME. NSAIDs and developmental toxicity. Birth Defects Res Part B Dev Reprod Toxicol 2003;68:3–4.
8. Walker JJ, Johnston J, Fairlie FM, Lloyd J, Bullingham R. A comparative study of intramuscular ketorolac and pethidine in labour pain. Eur J Obstet Gynecol Reprod Biol 1992;46:87–94.
9. Schorr SJ, Ascarelli MH, Rust OA, Ross EL, Calfee EF, Perry KG Jr, Morrison JC. Ketorolac is a safe and effective drug for acute tocolysis (abstract). Am J Obstet Gynecol 1997;176:S7.
10. Schorr SJ, Ascarelli MH, Rust OA, Ross EL, Calfee EL, Perry KG Jr, Morrison JC. A comparative study of ketorolac (Toradol) and magnesium sulfate for arrest of preterm labor. South Med J 1998;91:1028–32.
11. Levin DL. Effects of inhibition of prostaglandin synthesis on fetal development, oxygenation, and the fetal circulation. Semin Perinatol 1980;4:35–44.
12. Van Marter LJ, Leviton A, Allred EN, Pagano M, Sullivan KF, Cohen A, Epstein MF. Persistent pulmonary hypertension of the newborn and smoking and aspirin and nonsteroidal antiinflammatory drug consumption during pregnancy. Pediatrics 1996;97:658–63.
13. Matt DW, Borzelleca JF. Toxic effects on the female reproductive system during pregnancy, parturition, and lactation. In Witorsch RJ, editor. *Reproductive Toxicology*. 2nd ed. New York, NY: Raven Press, 1995:175–93.
14. Dawood MY. Nonsteroidal antiinflammatory drugs and reproduction. Am J Obstet Gynecol 1993;169:1255–65.
15. Wischnik A, Manth SM, Lloyd J, Bullingham R, Thompson JS. The excretion of ketorolac tromethamine into breast milk after multiple oral dosing. Eur J Clin Pharmacol 1989;36:521–4.
16. Committee on Drugs, American Academy of Pediatrics. The transfer of drugs and other chemicals into human milk. Pediatrics 2001;108:776–89.

L

Name:	**LABETALOL**	Risk Factor:	C_M
Class:	**Sympatholytic (Antihypertensive)**		

FETAL RISK SUMMARY

RECOMMENDATION: Human Data Suggest Low Risk

Labetalol, a combined α/β-adrenergic blocking agent, has been used for the treatment of hypertension occurring during pregnancy (1–29). No teratogenicity was observed in rats and rabbits at oral doses 6 and 4 times the maximum recommended human dose (MRHD), respectively (30). However, increased fetal resorptions occurred in both species at doses approximately equivalent to the MRHD. In rabbits, IV doses up to 1.7 times the MRHD revealed no drug-related fetal harm (30).

Labetalol crosses the human placenta to produce cord serum concentrations averaging 40%–80% of peak maternal levels (1–5). Maternal serum and amniotic fluid concentrations are approximately equivalent 1–3 hours after a single IV dose (4). After oral dosing (1–42 days) in eight women, amniotic fluid concentrations of labetalol were in the same range as, but lower than, the plasma concentrations in six of the women (6). The pharmacokinetics of labetalol in pregnant patients has been reported (7,8). A 1988 article briefly reviewed some of the experience with labetalol in pregnancy (31).

In a surveillance study of Michigan Medicaid recipients conducted between 1985 and 1992 involving 229,101 completed pregnancies, 29 newborns had been exposed to labetalol during the 1st trimester (F. Rosa, personal communication, FDA, 1993). Four (13.8%) major birth defects were observed (one expected). Details on the malformations were not available, but no anomalies were observed in six defect categories (cardiovascular defects, oral clefts, spina bifida, polydactyly, limb reduction defects, and hypospadias) for which specific data were available. Although the number of exposures is small, the incidence of malformations is suggestive of an association, but other factors, including the mother's disease, concurrent drug use, and chance, may be involved.

No published reports of fetal malformations attributable to labetalol have been located, but experience during the 1st trimester, except for the surveillance study described above, is lacking. Most reports have found no adverse effects on birth weight, head circumference, Apgar scores, or blood glucose control after *in utero* exposure to labetalol (9–13). One case of neonatal hypoglycemia has been mentioned, but the mother was also taking a thiazide diuretic (2). Offspring of mothers treated with labetalol had a significantly higher birth weight than infants of atenolol-treated mothers, 3280 g vs. 2750 g, respectively (14). However, in a study comparing labetalol plus hospitalization with hospitalization alone for the treatment of mild preeclampsia presenting at 26–35 weeks' gestation, labetalol treatment did not improve perinatal outcome, and a significantly higher number of labetalol-exposed infants were growth retarded, 19.1% (18 of 94) vs. 9.3% (9 of 97), respectively (15).

Fetal heart rate is apparently unaffected by labetalol treatment of hypertensive pregnant women. However, two studies have observed newborn bradycardia in five infants (16,17). In one infant, bradycardia was marked (<100 beats/minute) and persistent (17). All five infants survived. Hypotension was noted in another infant delivered by cesarean section at 28 weeks' gestation (1). In a study examining the effects of labetalol exposure on term (37 weeks or greater) newborns, mild transient hypotension, which resolved within 24 hours, was observed in 11 infants, as compared with 11 matched controls (18). Maternal dosage varied from 100 to 300 mg 3 times daily with the last dose given within 12 hours of birth. The mean systolic blood pressures at 2 hours of age in exposed and nonexposed infants were 58.8 and 63.3 mm Hg ($p < 0.05$), respectively. Other measures of β-blockade, such as heart and respiratory rates, palmar sweating, blood glucose control, and metabolic and vasomotor responses to cold stress, did not differ between the groups. The investigators concluded that labetalol did not cause clinically significant β-blockade in mature newborn infants (18).

Several investigations have shown a lack of effect of labetalol treatment on uterine contractions (1–3,16,19–21). One study did report a higher incidence of spontaneous labor in labetalol-treated mothers (6 of 10) than in a similar group treated with methyldopa (2 of 9) (22). In another report, 3 of 31 patients treated with labetalol experienced spontaneous labor, one of whom delivered prematurely (23). The authors attributed the uterine activity to the drug because no other causes were found. However, because most trials with labetalol in hypertensive women have not shown this effect, it is questionable whether the drug has any direct effect on uterine contractility.

L

Labetalol does not change uteroplacental blood flow despite a drop in blood pressure (2,4,5,24,25). The lack of effect on blood flow was probably caused by reduced peripheral resistance.

Labetalol apparently reduces the incidence of hyaline membrane disease in premature infants by increasing the production of pulmonary surfactant (1,2,4,16,26). The mechanism for this effect may be mediated through β_2-adrenoceptor agonist activity that the drug partially possesses (1,2,4,16,26).

Follow-up studies have been completed at 6 months of age on 10 infants exposed *in utero* to labetalol (27). All infants demonstrated normal growth and development. In addition, no ocular toxicity has been observed in newborns, even though labetalol has an affinity for ocular melanin (1,2,26).

In summary, the use of labetalol for the treatment of maternal hypertension does not seem to pose a risk to the fetus, except possibly in the 1st trimester, and may offer advantages over the use of agents with only β-blocker activity. A 2000 meta-analysis concluded that IV labetalol for late-onset hypertension in pregnancy was safer than IV hydralazine or diazoxide in terms of drug-induced maternal hypotension and fewer cesarean sections (32). However, one study has demonstrated growth retardation when used for the treatment of mild preeclampsia. Some β-blockers may cause intrauterine growth retardation (IUGR) and reduced placental weight, especially those lacking intrinsic sympathomimetic activity (ISA) (i.e., partial agonist). Treatment beginning early in the 2nd trimester results in the greatest weight reductions, whereas treatment restricted to the 3rd trimester primarily affects only placental weight. Labetalol does not possess ISA. However, IUGR and reduced placental weight may potential occur with all agents within this class. Although growth retardation is a serious concern, the benefits of maternal therapy with labetalol (or β-blockers) in some cases, might outweigh the risks to the fetus and must be judged on a case-by-case basis. If used near delivery, the newborn infant should be closely observed for 24–48 hours for signs and symptoms of

β-blockade. Long-term effects of *in utero* to labetalol have not been studied but warrant evaluation.

BREAST FEEDING SUMMARY

RECOMMENDATION: Limited Human Data - Probably Compatible

Labetalol is excreted into breast milk (1,6). In 24 lactating women, 3 days postpartum, administration of 330–800 mg/day produced a mean milk level of 33 ng/mL. No adverse effects were observed in the nursing infants. One patient, consuming 1200 mg/day, had a mean milk concentration of 600 ng/mL, but this woman did not breast-feed. Three women, 6–9 days postpartum, consumed daily doses of labetalol of 600, 600, and 1200 mg, and produced peak milk concentrations of the drug of 129, 223, and 662 ng/mL, respectively (6). Peak concentrations of labetalol in the milk occurred between 2 and 3 hours after a dose. Measurable plasma concentrations of labetalol were found in only one infant: 18 ng/mL at 4 hours and 21 ng/mL at 8 hours. Although no adverse effects have been reported, nursing infants should be closely observed for bradycardia, hypotension, and other symptoms of α/β-blockade. Long-term effects of exposure to labetalol from milk have not been studied but warrant evaluation. The American Academy of Pediatrics classifies labetalol as compatible with breast-feeding (33).

L

References

1. Michael CA. Use of labetalol in the treatment of severe hypertension during pregnancy. Br J Clin Pharmacol 1979;8(Suppl 2):211S–5S.
2. Riley AJ. Clinical pharmacology of labetalol in pregnancy. J Cardiovasc Pharmacol 1981;3(Suppl 1):S53–S9.
3. Andrejak M, Coevoet B, Fievet P, Gheerbrant JD, Comoy E, Leuillet P, Verhoest P, Boulanger JC, Vitse M, Fournier A. Effect of labetalol on hypertension and the renin-angiotensin-aldosterone and adrenergic systems in pregnancy. In Riley A, Symonds EM, eds. *The Investigation of Labetalol in The Management of Hypertension in Pregnancy*. Amsterdam: Excerpta Medica, 1982:77–87.
4. Lunell NO, Hjemdahl P, Fredholm BB, Lewander R, Nisell H, Nylund L, Persson B, Sarby J, Wager J, Thornstrom S. Acute effects of labetalol on maternal metabolism and uteroplacental circulation in hypertension of pregnancy. In Riley A, Symonds EM, eds. *The Investigation of Labetalol in The Management of Hypertension in Pregnancy*. Amsterdam: Excerpta Medica, 1982:34–45.
5. Nylund L, Lunell NO, Lewander R, Sarby B, Thornstrom S. Labetalol for the treatment of hypertension in pregnancy. Acta Obstet Gynecol Scand 1984; 118(Suppl):71–3.
6. Lunell NO, Kulas J, Rane A. Transfer of labetalol into amniotic fluid and breast milk in lactating women. Eur J Clin Pharmacol 1985;28:597–9.
7. Rubin PC. Drugs in pregnancy. In Riley A, Symonds EM. eds. *The Investigation of Labetalol in The Management of Hypertension in Pregnancy*. Amsterdam: Excerpta Medica, 1982:28–33.
8. Rubin PC, Butters L, Kelman AW, Fitzsimons C, Reid JL. Labetalol disposition and concentration-effect relationships during pregnancy. Br J Clin Pharmacol 1983;15:465–70.
9. Lamming GD, Broughton Pipkin F, Symonds EM. Comparison of the alpha and beta blocking drug, labetalol, and methyl dopa in the treatment of moderate and severe pregnancy-induced hypertension. Clin Exp Hypertens 1980;2:865–95.
10. Lotgering FK, Derkx FMH, Wallenburg HCS. Primary hyperaldosteronism in pregnancy. Am J Obstet Gynecol 1986;155:986–8.
11. Mabie WC, Gonzalez AR, Sibai BM, Amon E. A comparative trial of labetalol and hydralazine in the acute management of severe hypertension complicating pregnancy. Obstet Gynecol 1987;70:328–33.
12. Plouin P-F, Breart G, Maillard F, Papiernik E, Relier J-P. Comparison of antihypertensive efficacy and perinatal safety of labetalol and methyldopa in the treatment of hypertension in pregnancy: a randomized controlled trial. Br J Obstet Gynaecol 1988;95:868–76.
13. Pickles CJ, Symonds EM, Broughton Pipkin F. The fetal outcome in a randomized trial of labetalol versus placebo in pregnancy-induced hypertension. Br J Obstet Gynaecol 1989;96:38–43.
14. Lardoux H, Gerard J, Blazquez G, Chouty F, Flouvat B. Hypertension in pregnancy: evaluation of two beta blockers atenolol and labetalol. Eur Heart J 1983;4(Suppl G):35–40.
15. Sibai BM, Gonzalez AR, Mabie WC, Moretti M. A comparison of labetalol plus hospitalization versus hospitalization alone in the management of preeclampsia remote from term. Obstet Gynecol 1987;70:323–7.
16. Michael CA, Potter JM. A comparison of labetalol with other antihypertensive drugs in the treatment of hypertensive disease of pregnancy. In Riley A, Symonds, EM. eds. *The Investigation of Labetalol in*

The Management of Hypertension in Pregnancy. Amsterdam: Excerpta Medica, 1982:111–22.
17. Davey DA, Dommisse J, Garden A. Intravenous labetalol and intravenous dihydralazine in severe hypertension in pregnancy. In Riley A, Symonds EM, eds. *The Investigation of Labetalol in The Management of Hypertension in Pregnancy*. Amsterdam: Excerpta Medica, 1982:52–61.
18. MacPherson M, Broughton Pipkin F, Rutter N. The effect of maternal labetalol on the newborn infant. Br J Obstet Gynaecol 1986;93:539–42.
19. Redman CWG. A controlled trial of the treatment of hypertension in pregnancy: labetalol compared with methyldopa. In Riley A, Symonds EM, eds. *The Investigation of Labetalol in The Management of Hypertension in Pregnancy*. Amsterdam: Excerpta Medica, 1982:101–10.
20. Walker JJ, Crooks A, Erwin L, Calder AA. Labetalol in pregnancy-induced hypertension: fetal and maternal effects. In Riley A, Symonds EM, eds. *The Investigation of Labetalol in The Management of Hypertension of Pregnancy*. Amsterdam: Excerpta Medica, 1982: 148–60.
21. Thulesius O, Lunell NO, Ibrahim M, Moberger B, Angilivilayil C. The effect of labetalol on contractility of human myometrial preparations. Acta Obstet Gynecol 1987;66:237–40.
22. Lamming GD, Symonds EM. Use of labetalol and methyldopa in pregnancy-induced hypertension. Br J Clin Pharmacol 1979;8(Suppl 2):217S–22S.
23. Jorge CS, Fernandes L, Cunha S. Labetalol in the hypertensive states of pregnancy. In Riley A, Symonds EM, eds. *The Investigation of Labetalol in The Management of Hypertension of Pregnancy*. Amsterdam: Excerpta Medica, 1982:124–30.
24. Lunell NO, Nylund L, Lewander R, Sarby B. Acute effect of an antihypertensive drug, labetalol, on uteroplacental blood flow. Br J Obstet Gynaecol 1982;89:640–4.
25. Jouppila P, Kirkinen P, Koivula A, Ylikorkala O. Labetalol does not alter the placental and fetal blood flow or maternal prostanoids in pre-eclampsia. Br J Obstet Gynaecol 1986;93:543–7.
26. Michael CA. The evaluation of labetalol in the treatment of hypertension complicating pregnancy. Br J Clin Pharmacol 1982;13(Suppl):127S–31S.
27. Symonds EM, Lamming GD, Jadoul F, Broughton Pipkin F. Clinical and biochemical aspects of the use of labetalol in the treatment of hypertension in pregnancy: comparison with methyldopa. In Riley A, Symonds EM, eds. *The Investigation of Labetalol in The Management of Hypertension in Pregnancy*. Amsterdam: Excerpta Medica, 1982:62–76.
28. Smith AM. Beta-blockers for pregnancy hypertension. Lancet 1983;1:708–9.
29. Walker JJ, Bonduelle M, Greer I, Calder AA. Antihypertensive therapy in pregnancy. Lancet 1983;1:932–3.
30. Product information. Normodyne. Schering, 2000.
31. Frishman WH, Chesner M. Beta-adrenergic blockers in pregnancy. Am Heart J 1988;115:147–52.
32. Magee LA, Elran E, Bull SB, Logan A, Koren G. Risks and benefits of β-receptor blockers for pregnancy hypertension: overview of the randomized trials. Eur J Obstet Gynecol Reprod Biol 2000;88:15–26.
33. Committee on Drugs, American Academy of Pediatrics. The transfer of drugs and other chemicals into human milk. Pediatrics 2001;108:776–89.

L

Name:	**LACTULOSE**	Risk Factor:	$\mathbf{B_M}$
Class:	**Laxative**		

FETAL RISK SUMMARY

RECOMMENDATION: No Human Data - Probably Compatible

Lactulose is a synthetic disaccharide that is biodegraded only by bacteria in the colon to the low molecular weight acids, lactic acid, formic acid, and acetic acid. Small amounts of lactulose, about 3% of a dose, are absorbed following oral administration (1).

No impairment of fertility or fetal harm have been observed in pregnant mice, rats, and rabbits at doses up to 3 or 6 times the usual human oral dose (2). No reports on the use of this product in human pregnancy or lactation have been located, but the risk to the fetus and the newborn appears to be negligible.

BREAST FEEDING SUMMARY

RECOMMENDATION: No Human Data - Probably Compatible

No data are available.

References

1. Product information. Cephulac. Marion Merrell Dow, 1992.
2. Product information. Duphalac. Solvay Pharmaceuticals, 2000.

Name:	**LAETRILE**	Risk Factor:	**C**
Class:	**Unclassified/Antineoplastic**		

FETAL RISK SUMMARY

RECOMMENDATION: No Human Data - No Relevant Animal Data

Laetrile is a nonapproved agent used for the treatment of cancer. There are no studies of laetrile in pregnancy. A concern for possible gestational cyanide poisoning has been reported (1). Because of an increased amount of β-glycosidase present in the intestinal flora, the oral route would theoretically be more toxic than the parenteral route in liberation of hydrogen cyanide, which is present in various sources of laetrile (1). Long-term follow-up has been recommended because neurologic evidence of chronic cyanide exposure may not be recognizable in the infant.

BREAST FEEDING SUMMARY

RECOMMENDATION: No Human Data - Potential Toxicity

No data are available.

Reference

1. Peterson RG, Ruman BH. Laetrile and pregnancy. Clin Toxicol 1979;15:181–4.

Name:	**LAMIVUDINE**	Risk Factor:	**C_M**
Class:	**Antiviral**		

FETAL RISK SUMMARY

RECOMMENDATION: Compatible - Maternal Benefit >> Embryo/Fetal Risk

Lamivudine (2′,3′-dideoxy-3′-thiacytidine, 3TC), an antiviral agent structurally similar to zalcitabine, inhibits viral reverse transcription via viral DNA chain termination (1). It is classified as a nucleoside analog reverse transcriptase inhibitor (NRTI) that is used for the treatment of human immunodeficiency virus (HIV) infection. Other drugs in this class are abacavir, didanosine, stavudine, zalcitabine, and zidovudine. Lamivudine is believed to be converted by intracellular enzymes to the active metabolite, lamivudine-5′-triphosphate (3TC-TP).

No teratogenic effects were observed in rats and rabbits administered lamivudine up to approximately 130 and 60 times, respectively, the usual human adult dose (1). Early embryo lethality was observed in rabbits at doses close to those used in humans and above. This effect was not observed in rats given up to 130 times the usual human dose. Lamivudine crossed the placenta to the fetus in both animal types.

Adverse effects on neurobehavior development in mice offspring resulting from a combination of lamivudine and zidovudine were described in a 2001 study (2). Pregnant mice received both drugs from day 10 of gestation to delivery. The effects on somatic and sensorimotor development were minor but more marked in exposed offspring then when either drug was given alone (2). Both developmental endpoints were delayed with respect to control animals. Further, alterations of social behavior were observed in both sexes of exposed offspring (2).

The low molecular weight (about 229) of lamivudine is predictive of placental transfer. A study published in 1997 described the human placental transfer of lamivudine using an *ex vivo* single cotyledon perfusion system (3). Lamivudine crossed the placenta to the fetal side by simple diffusion. Transfer did not appear to be affected by the presence of zidovudine. Confirming this, a 1998 study found that combination therapy with zidovudine did not affect the pharmacokinetics of lamivudine (4). Lamivudine freely crossed the placenta when given near term with nearly equivalent drug levels in the mother, cord blood, and newborn.

The Antiretroviral Pregnancy Registry reported, for the period January 1989 through January 2004, prospective data (reported to the Registry before the outcomes were known) involving 1537 live births that had been exposed to one or more antiretroviral agents during the 1st trimester (5). Forty-seven of the newborns had congenital defects (3.1%, 95% confidence interval [CI] 2.3–4.1). In the 2407 live births with earliest exposure in the 2nd/3rd trimesters, there were 56 infants with defects (2.3%, 95% CI 1.8–3.0). The prevalence rates for the two periods did not differ significantly. There were 103 infants with birth defects among 3944 live births with exposure anytime during pregnancy (2.6%, 95% CI 2.1–3.2). The prevalence rate did not differ significantly from the rate expected in a nonexposed population (5). There were 3185 outcomes exposed to lamivudine (1185 in the 1st trimester and 2000 in the 2nd/3rd trimesters) in combination with other antiretroviral agents. There were 34 (2.9%, 95% CI 2.0–4.0) birth defects among the 1st trimester exposures and 47 (2.4%, 95% CI 1.7–3.1) in those exposed in the 2nd/3rd trimesters. In reviewing the birth defects of prospective and retrospective (pregnancies reported after the outcomes were known) registered cases, and clinical reports, the Registry concluded that there was no pattern of anomalies to suggest a common cause (5). (See required statement below.)

A study published in 1999 evaluated the safety, efficacy, and perinatal transmission rates of HIV in 30 pregnant women receiving various combinations of antiretroviral agents (6). Many of the women were substance abusers. Lamivudine was taken by 29 women in various combinations that included zidovudine, nelfinavir, indinavir, stavudine, nevirapine, and saquinavir. Antiretroviral therapy was initiated at a median of 14 weeks' gestation (range preconception to 32 weeks). In spite of previous histories of extensive antiretroviral experience and of vertical transmission of HIV, combination therapy was effective in treating maternal disease and in preventing transmission to the current newborns. The outcomes of the pregnancies included one stillbirth, one case of microcephaly, and five infants with birth weights less than 2500 g, two of which were premature (6).

In an unusual case, a woman was exposed to HIV through self-insemination with fresh semen obtained from a man with a high HIV ribonucleic acid viral load (>750,000 copies/mL plasma) (7). Ten days later, she was started on a prophylactic regimen of lamivudine (300 mg/day), zidovudine (600 mg/day), and indinavir (2400 mg/day). Pregnancy was confirmed 14 days after insemination. The indinavir dose was reduced to 1800 mg/day, 4 weeks after the start of therapy because of the development of renal calculi. All antiretroviral therapy was stopped after 9 weeks because of negative tests for HIV. She gave birth at 40 weeks' gestation to a healthy 3490-g male infant, without evidence of HIV disease, who was developing normally at 2 years of age (7).

Several reports have described the apparent safe use of lamivudine, usually in combination with other agents, during human pregnancy (8–11). Occasional mild adverse effects were observed in the newborns (e.g., anemia), but no birth defects attributable to drug therapy. In one report, lamivudine concentrations in the newborn were similar to those in the mother (10).

A 1999 report from France described the possible association of zidovudine and lamivudine (NRTIs) use in pregnancy with mitochondrial dysfunction in the offspring (12). Mitochondrial disease is relatively rare in France (estimated prevalence 1 in 5,000–20,000 children) (12). From an ongoing epidemiological survey of 1,754 mother-child pairs exposed to zidovudine and other agents during pregnancy, however, 8 children with possible mitochondrial dysfunction were identified. None of the eight infants were infected with HIV, but all received prophylaxis for up to 6 weeks after birth with the same antiretroviral regimen as given during pregnancy. Four of the cases were exposed to zidovudine alone and four to a combination of zidovudine and lamivudine. Two from the combination group died at about 1 year of age. All eight cases had abnormally low respiratory-chain enzyme activities. The authors concluded that their results supported the hypothesis of a causative association between mitochondrial respiratory-chain dysfunction and NRTIs. Moreover, the toxicity may have been potentiated by combination of these agents (12).

In a paper following the above study, investigators noted that NRTIs inhibit DNA polymerase γ, the enzyme responsible for mitochondrial DNA replication (13). They then hypothesized that this inhibition would induce depletion of mitochondrial DNA and mitochondrial DNA-encoded mitochondrial enzymes, thus resulting in mitochondrial dysfunction (13). Moreover, they stated that support for their hypothesis was suggested by the closeness of the clinical manifestations of inherited mitochondrial diseases with the adverse effects attributed to NRTIs. These adverse effects included polyneuropathy, myopathy, cardiomyopathy, pancreatitis, bone marrow suppression, and lactic acidosis. They also postulated this mechanism was involved in the development of a lipodystrophy syndrome of peripheral fat wasting and central adiposity, a condition that has been thought to be related to protease inhibitors (13).

A commentary on the above two studies concluded that the evidence for NRTI-induced mitochondrial dysfunction was equivocal (14). First, the clinical presentations in the infants were varied and not suggestive of a single cause; indeed, three of infants were symptom-free and one had Leigh's syndrome, a classic mitochondrial disease (14). Second, the clinical features, in some cases, were not suggestive of mitochondrial dysfunction. Although three had neurological symptoms, none had raised levels of lactate in the cerebrospinal fluid. Moreover, histological or histochemical features of mitochondrial disease were only found in two cases. Finally, low mitochondrial DNA, that would have been direct evidence of NRTI toxicity, was not found in the three cases in which it was measured (14).

A case of combined transient mitochondrial and peroxisomal β-oxidation dysfunction after exposure to NRTIs (lamivudine and zidovudine) combined with protease inhibitors (ritonavir and saquinavir) throughout gestation was reported in 2000 (15). A male infant was delivered at 38 weeks' gestation. He received postnatal prophylaxis with lamivudine and zidovudine for 4 weeks until the agents were discontinued because of anemia. Other adverse effects that were observed in the infant (age at onset) were hypocalcemia (shortly after birth), Group B streptococcal sepsis, ventricular extrasystoles, prolonged metabolic acidosis, and lactic acidemia (8 weeks), a mild elevation of long chain fatty acids (9 weeks), and neutropenia (3 months). The metabolic acidosis required treatment until 7 months of age, whereas the elevated plasma lactate resolved over 4 weeks. Cerebrospinal fluid lactate was not determined nor was a muscle biopsy conducted. Both the neutropenia and the cardiac dysfunction had resolved by 1 year of age. The elevated plasma fatty acid level was confirmed in cultured fibroblasts, but other peroxisomal functions (plasmalogen biosynthesis and catalase staining) were normal. Although mitochondrial dysfunction has been linked to NRTIs, the authors were unable to identify the cause of the combined abnormalities in the infant (15). The child was reported to be healthy and developing normally at 26 months of age.

A case of life-threatening anemia following *in utero* exposure to antiretroviral agents was described in 1998 (16). A 30-year-old woman with HIV infection was treated with zidovudine, didanosine, and trimethoprim/sulfamethoxazole (three times weekly) during the 1st trimester. Vitamin supplementation was also given. Because of an inadequate response, didanosine was discontinued and lamivudine and zalcitabine were started in the 3rd trimester. Two weeks before delivery the HIV viral load was undetectable. At term, a pale, male infant was delivered who developed respiratory distress shortly after birth. Examination revealed a hyperactive precordium and hepatomegaly without evidence of hydrops. The hematocrit was 11% with a reticulocyte count of zero. An extensive work-up of the mother and infant failed to determine the cause of the anemia. Bacterial and viral infections, including HIV, parvovirus B19, cytomegalovirus, and others, were excluded. The infant received a transfusion and was apparently doing well at 10 weeks of age. Because no other cause of the anemia could be found, the authors attributed the condition to bone morrow suppression, most likely to zidovudine (16). A contribution of the other agents to the condition, however, could not be excluded.

In summary, the animal and human data suggest that lamivudine presents a low risk to the developing fetus for structural malformations. Theoretically, exposure to agents in this class at the time of implantation could result in impaired fertility as a result of embryonic cytotoxicity (see, e.g., Didanosine, Stavudine, Zidovudine, or Zalcitabine), but this has not been studied in humans. The risk of mitochondrial dysfunction with NRTIs needs confirmation. However, even if an association is proven, the risk of mortality and morbidity from HIV infection appears to far outweigh the risk of mitochondrial dysfunction (14).

Two reviews, one in 1996 and the other in 1997, concluded that all women currently receiving antiretroviral therapy should continue to receive therapy during pregnancy and that treatment of the mother with monotherapy should be considered inadequate therapy (17,18). In 1998, the Centers for Disease Control and Prevention (CDC) made a similar recommendation that antiretroviral therapy should be continued during pregnancy, but discontinuation of all therapy during the 1st trimester was a consideration (19). If indicated, therefore, lamivudine should not be withheld in pregnancy (with the possible exception of the 1st trimester) because the expected benefit to the HIV-positive mother probably outweighs the unknown risk to the fetus.

A review published in 2000 described seven clinical trials that have been effective in reducing perinatal transmission, five with zidovudine alone, one with zidovudine plus lamivudine, and one with nevirapine (20). Six of the trials were in less-developed countries. Prolonged use of zidovudine in the mother and infant was the most effective for preventing vertical transmission, but also the most expensive. The combination of lamivudine and zidovudine, consisting of antepartum, intrapartum, and postpartum maternal therapy with continued therapy in the infant for 1 week, may have been as effective as prolonged zidovudine (20). More data are needed, however, before the efficacy and safety of combined therapy in preventing vertical transmission of HIV to the newborn can be assessed. Currently, zidovudine remains the only antiretroviral agent recommended for this purpose in developed countries (17,18).

Required statement: "The Registry's analytic approach is to evaluate specific classes of antiretroviral drugs (NRTIs [nucleoside analog reverse transcriptase inhibitor(s)], nnRTIs [non-nucleoside reverse transcriptase inhibitor(s)], NtRTIs [nucleotide reverse transcriptase inhibitors], and PIs [protease inhibitor(s)]). Currently there are six specific drugs with large enough groups of exposed women to warrant a separate analysis. These drugs are abacavir, lamivudine, nelfinavir, nevirapine, stavudine, and zidovudine.

For lamivudine and zidovudine sufficient numbers of first trimester exposures have been monitored to detect at least a 1.5-fold increase in risk of overall birth defects and a 2-fold increase in risk of birth defects in the more common classes, cardiovascular and genitourinary systems. No such increases have been detected to date. For abacavir, nelfinavir, nevirapine, and stavudine sufficient numbers of first trimester exposures have been monitored to detect at least a two-fold increase in risk of overall birth defects. No such increases have detected to date.

To date, the Registry has not demonstrated an increased prevalence of birth defects overall, or in the specific classes studied, or among women exposed to abacavir, lamivudine, nelfinavir, nevirapine, stavudine, or zidovudine individually or in combination during the first trimester when compared with observed rates for 'early diagnoses' in population-based birth defects surveillance systems. While the Registry to date has not detected a major teratogenic signal overall or within classes of drugs or the six individual drugs analyzed separately, the population exposed and monitored to date is not sufficient to detect an increase in the risk of relatively rare defects. These findings should provide some assurance when counseling patients." (*Note:* "early diagnoses" *is defined as "birth defects identified in live births either prior to birth or during the first day of life."*)

BREAST FEEDING SUMMARY

RECOMMENDATION: Contraindicated

Lamivudine is excreted into breast milk. In 10 women on lamivudine monotherapy (300 mg/day), the mean drug concentrations in maternal serum and breast milk were 0.55 and 1.22 μg/mL, respectively (4). The infants were not allowed to breast-feed. The agent is also excreted into the milk of lactating rats at concentrations slightly greater than those in the maternal plasma (1). Both of these findings are supported by the low molecular weight (about 229) of lamivudine.

Reports on the use of lamivudine during breast-feeding are unlikely because the antiviral agent is used in the treatment of human immunodeficiency virus (HIV) infections. HIV-1 is transmitted in milk, and in developed countries, breast-feeding is not recommended (17,18,21–23). In developing countries, breast-feeding is undertaken, despite the risk, because there are no affordable milk substitutes available. Until 1999, no studies had been published that examined the effect of any antiretroviral therapy on HIV-1 transmission in milk. In that year, a study involving zidovudine was published that measured a 38% reduction in vertical transmission of HIV-1 infection despite breast-feeding when compared to controls (see Zidovudine).

References

1. Product information. Epivir. Glaxo Wellcome, 2001.
2. Venerosi A, Valanzano A, Alleva E, Calamandrei G. Prenatal exposure to anti-HIV drugs: neurobehavioral effects of zidovudine (AZT) + lamivudine (3TC) treatment in mice. Teratology 2001;63:26–37.
3. Bloom SL, Dias KM, Bawdon RE, Gilstrap LC III. The maternal-fetal transfer of lamivudine in the ex vivo human placenta. Am J Obstet Gynecol 1997;176:291–3.
4. Moodley J, Moodley D, Pillay K, Coovadia H, Saba J, van Leeuwen R, Goodwin C, Harrigan PR, Moore KHP, Stone C, Plumb R, Johnson MA. Pharmacokinetics and antiretroviral activity of lamivudine alone or when coadministered with zidovudine in human immunodeficiency virus type 1-infected pregnant women and their offspring. J Infect Dis 1998;178:1327–33.
5. Antiretroviral Pregnancy Registry Steering Committee. *Antiretroviral Pregnancy Registry International Interim Report for 1 January 1989 through 31 January 2004*. Wilmington, NC: Registry Coordinating Center, 2004.
6. McGowan JP, Crane M, Wiznia AA, Blum S. Combination antiretroviral therapy in human immunodeficiency virus-infected pregnant women. Obstet Gynecol 1999;94:641–6.
7. Bloch M, Carr A, Vasak E, Cunningham P, Smith D. The use of human immunodeficiency virus postexposure prophylaxis after successful artificial insemination. Am J Obstet Gynecol 1999;181:760–1.
8. Scott GB, Tuomala R. Combination antiretroviral therapy during pregnancy. AIDS 1998;12:2495–7.
9. Lorenzi P, Spicher VM, Laubereau B, Hirschel B, Kind C, Rudin C, Irion O, Kaiser L. Antiretroviral therapies in pregnancy: maternal, fetal and neonatal effects. Swiss HIV Cohort Study, the Swiss Collaborative HIV and Pregnancy Study, and the Swiss Neonatal HIV Study. AIDS 1998;12:F241–7.
10. Grubert TA, Wintergerst U, Lutz-Friedrich R, Belohradsky BH, Rolinski B. Long-term antiretroviral combination therapy including lamivudine in HIV-1 infected women during pregnancy. AIDS 1999;13:1430–1.
11. Ristola M, Salo E, Ammala P, Suni J. Combined stavudine and lamivudine during pregnancy. AIDS 1999;13:285.
12. Blanche S, Tardieu M, Rustin P, Slama A, Barret B, Firtion G, Ciraru-Vigneron N, Lacroix C, Rouzioux C, Mandelbrot L, Desguerre I, Rotig A, Mayaux MJ, Delfraissy JF. Persistent mitochondrial dysfunction and perinatal exposure to antiretroviral nucleoside analogues. Lancet 1999;354:1084–9.
13. Brinkman K, Smeitink JA, Romijn JA, Reiss P. Mitochondrial toxicity induced by nucleoside-analogue reverse-transcriptase inhibitors is a key factor in the pathogenesis of antiretroviral-therapy-related lipodystrophy. Lancet 1999;354:1112–15.
14. Morris AAM, Carr A. HIV nucleoside analogues: new adverse effects on mitochondria? Lancet 1999;354:1046–7.
15. Stojanov S, Wintergerst U, Belohradsky BH. Mitochondrial and peroxisomal dysfunction following perinatal exposure to antiretroviral drugs. AIDS 2000;14:1669.
16. Watson WJ, Stevens TP, Weinberg GA. Profound anemia in a newborn infant of a mother receiving antiretroviral therapy. Pediatr Infect Dis J 1998;17:435–6.
17. Carpenter CCJ, Fischi MA, Hammer SM, Hirsch MS, Jacobsen DM, Katzenstein DA, Montaner JSG, Richman DD, Saag MS, Schooley RT, Thompson MA, Vella S, Yeni PG, Volberding PA. Antiretroviral therapy for HIV infection in 1996. JAMA 1996;276;146–54.
18. Minkoff H, Augenbraun M. Antiretroviral therapy for pregnant women. Am J Obstet Gynecol 1997;176:478–89.
19. CDC. Public Health Service Task Force recommendations for the use of antiretroviral drugs in pregnant women infected with HIV-1 for maternal health and for reducing perinatal HIV-1 transmission in the United States. MMWR 1998;47:No. RR-2.
20. Mofenson LM, McIntrye JA. Advances and research directions in the prevention of mother-to-child HIV-1 transmission. Lancet 2000;355:2237–44.
21. Brown ZA, Watts DH. Antiviral therapy in pregnancy. Clin Obstet Gynecol 1990;33:276–89.
22. de Martino M, Tovo P-A, Tozzi AE, Pezzotti P, Galli L, Livadiotti S, Caselli D, Massironi E, Ruga E, Fioredda F, Plebani A, Gabiano C, Zuccotti GV. HIV-1 transmission through breast-milk: appraisal of risk according to duration of feeding. AIDS 1992;6:991–7.
23. Van de Perre P. Postnatal transmission of human immunodeficiency virus type 1: the breast feeding dilemma. Am J Obstet Gynecol 1995;173:483–7.

Name:	**LAMOTRIGINE**	Risk Factor:	C_M
Class:	**Anticonvulsant**		

FETAL RISK SUMMARY

RECOMMENDATION: Human Data Suggest Low Risk

Lamotrigine is an anticonvulsant, chemically unrelated to existing antiepileptic drugs, that is used as adjunctive therapy for the treatment of partial seizures in patients with epilepsy (1).

Lamotrigine was not teratogenic in animal reproductive studies involving mice, rats, and rabbits using oral doses that were 1.2, 0.5, and 1.1 times, respectively, the highest usual human maintenance dose (500 mg/day) based on body surface area (HUHMD) (1). Secondary fetal toxicity consisting of reduced fetal weight or delayed ossification, however, was observed at these doses in mice and rats, but not in rabbits. Behavioral teratogenicity was observed in the offspring of rats dosed with 0.1 and 0.5 times the HUHMD during organogenesis. No teratogenic effects were observed after IV bolus doses in the above animals, but an increased incidence of intrauterine fetal death occurred in rats dosed at 0.6 times the HUHMD (1). Similarly, an increase in fetal deaths occurred in rats dosed orally at 0.1, 0.14, or 0.3 times the HUHMD during the latter part of gestation. Postnatal deaths were also observed with the two highest doses.

Lamotrigine reduces fetal folate levels in rats, an effect known to be associated with malformations in animals and humans (1). Human fetal folate levels have apparently not been investigated, but in studies with nonpregnant humans, the drug's weak inhibitory action of dihydrofolate reductase did not produce a significant reduction in folate levels (2). Serum folate and red blood cell folate concentrations were within the 95% confidence interval (CI) of the baseline values.

Lamotrigine crosses the human placenta (3–5). A 24-year-old woman had been treated before and throughout gestation with the anticonvulsant (300 mg/day) in combination with valproic acid (3). The latter drug was discontinued during the 3rd week of pregnancy. Her lamotrigine serum levels decreased from 17.8 μg/mL (2 weeks after her last dose of valproic acid) to 2.52 μg/mL at week 34, but she remained seizure-free throughout pregnancy. She delivered a healthy, 3620-g male infant at 39 weeks' gestation. The umbilical cord blood lamotrigine concentration was 3.26 μg/mL, indicating a probable cord:maternal serum ratio of 1 (maternal serum level at delivery not reported). On the second day after delivery and a few hours after commencing suckling, the serum concentrations in the infant and mother were 2.79 and 3.88 μg/mL, respectively, a ratio of 0.7. A 1997 case report found that maternal lamotrigine plasma levels decreased during pregnancy (4). She delivered a healthy infant (weight and sex not given) at term. At delivery, the umbilical cord:maternal plasma ratio was 1.2 (4).

In a 2000 report, maternal and cord plasma concentrations of lamotrigine were determined at term delivery in nine women (10 pregnancies; 1 woman with 2 pregnancies also reported in reference #3) (5). Maternal and cord plasma levels were similar. At 72 hours postpartum, median lamotrigine levels in the infants were 75% of the cord plasma levels (range 50%–100%). The placental transfer is consistent with the low molecular weight (about 256). Moreover, during the first 2 weeks after delivery, the median increase in maternal plasma concentration/dose ratio was 170%, a significant increase (5).

A 2004 report described 12 pregnancies treated with lamotrigine monotherapy for epilepsy (6). An increase in seizure frequency and/or severity occurred in nine pregnancies that were attributed to a gradual decrease in the serum-to-dose ratio to 40% of baseline. Consequently, the doses were increased in seven pregnancies. Three to 10 days after delivery, toxic symptoms (dizziness, diplopia, or ataxia) occurred in three of the women with dose increases (lamotrigine serum levels were 12–14 μg/mL, a high normal range). The symptoms resolved when the dose was decreased (6).

An interim report of the Lamotrigine Pregnancy Registry, an ongoing project conducted by the manufacturer, was issued in 2004 (7). The data covered reported pregnancy exposures from September 1992 through March 2004. The outcomes of 785 prospectively enrolled pregnancies (reported to the registry before the pregnancy outcome was known) are summarized in the latest report. There were 794 outcomes (7 sets of twins and 1 set of triplets). Lamotrigine monotherapy occurred in 482 outcomes. The earliest exposure by trimester was 455 (1st), 18 (2nd), 4 (3rd), and 5 (unspecified). The outcomes with 1st trimester exposure were 22 spontaneous abortions (SABs), 17 elective abortions (EABs) (no birth defects), 2 fetal deaths, 402 live births without major birth defects, 1 EAB (with major defect), and 11 live births with major birth defects. The 27 outcomes with earliest exposure in the 2nd, 3rd or unspecified trimesters all involved live births without birth defects. The frequency of major defects among the 1st trimester monotherapy exposures was 2.9% (12 of 414; includes only live births and EAB with birth defect). In the pregnancies reported prospectively, there was no consistent pattern among the outcomes with major birth defects (7).

Lamotrigine polytherapy (lamotrigine plus other antiepileptic agents) occurred in 312 outcomes (includes 88 outcomes of polytherapy with valproate) (7). The earliest exposure by trimester was 298 (1st), 9 (2nd), 4 (3rd), and 1 (unspecified). The outcomes with 1st trimester exposure were 14 SABs, 13 EABs (no birth defects), 1 fetal death, 254 live births without major birth defects, 3 EABs (with major defects), and 13 live births with major birth defects. The 14 outcomes with earliest exposure in the 2nd, 3rd, or unspecified trimesters all involved live births without birth defects. The frequency of major defects among the 1st trimester polytherapy exposures was 5.9% (16 of 270; includes only live births and EABs with birth defects). When the polytherapy outcomes with earliest exposure in the 1st trimester included valproate, the frequency of major defects was 12.5% (11 of 88). In the pregnancies reported prospectively, there was no consistent pattern among the outcomes with major birth defects (7).

L

Retrospective cases (reported after the pregnancy outcome was known) are often biased (only adverse outcomes are reported), but they are useful in identifying specific patterns of anomalies suggestive of a common cause (7). There were 70 pregnancy outcomes reported retrospectively (reported after the outcomes were known) to the Registry, 64 involving earliest exposure to lamotrigine in the 1st trimester and 6 with an unspecified trimester of exposure. Thirty-two involved monotherapy and 38 were antiepileptic drug polytherapy. In the pregnancy outcomes reported retrospectively, there was no consistent pattern in the birth defects (7). (See required statement below.)

As of 1996, the FDA had received three disparate reports of birth defects in which lamotrigine, in combination with other anticonvulsants, was used during the affected pregnancy (F. Rosa, personal communication, FDA, 1996).

A 1998 non-interventional observational cohort study described the outcomes of pregnancies in women who had been prescribed one or more of 34 newly marketed drugs by general practitioners in England (8). Data were obtained by questionnaires sent to the prescribing physicians one month after the expected or possible date of delivery. In 831 (78%) of the pregnancies, a newly marketed drug was thought to have taken during the 1st trimester with birth defects noted in 14 (2.5%) singleton births of the 557 newborns (10 sets of twins). In addition, two birth defects were observed in aborted fetuses. However, few of the aborted fetuses were examined. Lamotrigine was taken during the 1st trimester in 59 pregnancies. The outcomes of these pregnancies included 10 spontaneous abortions, 1 missed abortion, 9 elective abortions, 35 normal newborns (4 premature), and 4 newborns with congenital malformations. The malformations observed were: ventricular septal defect; congenital respiratory stridor; palatal cleft (soft palate only), hypospadiasis, undescended testes (mother had convulsions early in gestation); abdominal distension with possible congenital intestinal obstruction. In three of these cases, lamotrigine was given in various combinations with other anticonvulsants (e.g., carbamazepine, phenytoin, phenobarbital, and/or sodium valproate). In addition, the study lacked the sensitivity to identify minor anomalies because of the absence of standardized examinations. Late-appearing major defects may also have been missed due to the timing of the questionnaires (8).

In summary, the animal and human data do not appear to indicate a major risk for congenital malformations or fetal loss following 1st trimester exposure to lamotrigine. At least two reviews have concluded that this anticonvulsant may be associated with a lower risk of teratogenicity (9,10). In general, women with epilepsy have a higher risk of delivering an infant with a malformation than those who do not have this condition. In some cases, the cause of a defect is most likely the anticonvulsant, but based on the small number of diverse anomalies described above, there does not appear to be a pattern suggesting that lamotrigine is a significant human teratogen (7). More data are needed, however, to confirm or refute this initial assessment.

Required statement: "If the baseline frequency of total birth defects is 3 in 100 live births, a sample size of 414 first trimester lamotrigine monotherapy exposures has an 80 percent chance (80% power) of correctly detecting at least a 1.79-fold increase from baseline in the frequency of birth defects. Currently, the frequency of major birth defects in the Registry is 2.9%. While this frequency is encouraging, the lamotrigine monotherapy sample size to date remains too small for formal comparisons of the frequency of specific birth defects.

The Lamotrigine Pregnancy Registry Advisory Committee notes the higher frequency of major malformations within the groups exposed to AED combinations that include both lamotrigine and valproate. Because the number of AEDs used may be inextricably tied to the frequency and severity of seizures, it is difficult to assess the contribution of each of these factors to the risk of major malformations. The Committee will continue to monitor the frequency and pattern of birth defects exposed to the combination of lamotrigine and valproate." (See reference #7 for full Committee Consensus statement.)

BREAST FEEDING SUMMARY

RECOMMENDATION: Limited Human Data - Potential Toxicity

Lamotrigine is excreted into breast milk (1,3–5). A 24-year-old mother had been treated throughout gestation with lamotrigine (see details above) and on the second day following delivery, she began nursing her infant (3). At this time she was taking 300 mg/day, decreased to 200 mg/day approximately 6 weeks postpartum to lessen the drug exposure of the infant. From day 2 to day 145 after delivery, 11 maternal serum and 9 milk samples (about 2–3 hours after the morning dose) were drawn, with lamotrigine serum concentrations ranging from 3.59 to 9.61 μg/mL and milk levels ranging from 1.26 to 6.51 μg/mL. The mean milk:serum ratio was 0.56 with a high correlation ($r = 0.959$, $p < 0.01$) between the serum and milk. The infant's serum levels (about 1–2 hours after breast feeding), determined at the same times as the mother's, ranged from <0.2 μg/mL (during weaning) to 2.79 μg/mL. No adverse effects were observed in the nursing infant either during breast-feeding or during weaning (3).

A 60-kg woman took lamotrigine 200 mg/day throughout gestation and during nursing (4). Two weeks after delivery, the milk:maternal plasma ratio was 0.6. The infant's plasma level, which had been similar to the mother's plasma level at birth, was now 25% of the maternal levels. No adverse effects were observed in the nursing infant (4).

L

In a 2000 report, nine women (10 pregnancies, one woman with two pregnancies also reported in reference #3) received lamotrigine throughout gestation (see Fetal Risk Summary above) and continued the drug during breast-feeding (5). The median milk:maternal plasma ratio 2–3 weeks after delivery was 0.61 (range 0.47–0.77). The lamotrigine plasma concentrations in the infants were approximately 30% (range 23%–50%) of the corresponding maternal plasma levels. The estimated infant lamotrigine dose was ≥0.2–1 mg/kg/day, assuming a milk intake of 150 mL/kg/day, about 9% of the weight-adjusted maternal daily dose. Because of the slow elimination in the infant (most likely due to reduced hepatic glucuronidation capacity), the marked increase in maternal plasma lamotrigine concentrations that occurred after birth (see Fetal Risk Summary above), and the fact that infant drug levels may not have reached steady-state concentrations, the infant exposure could eventually result in therapeutic plasma lamotrigine levels. No adverse effect in the nursing infants was observed (5).

As with any drug, a mother who must take lamotrigine to control her disease and who chooses to nurse her infant should carefully monitor the infant for adverse effects. Some anticonvulsants have produced adverse effects in nursing infants (see Phenobarbital and Primidone); whereas others are considered compatible with breast-feeding (see Carbamazepine, Phenytoin, and Valproic Acid). Although no adverse effects have been seen in nursing infants of mothers taking lamotrigine, the number of known cases are too small adequately assess the safety of this drug during lactation. Monitoring infant serum levels of lamotrigine may be required.

Because of the potential for therapeutic serum concentrations in the infant, the American Academy of Pediatrics classifies lamotrigine as a drug for which the effect on a nursing infant is unknown but may be of concern (11).

References

1. Product information. Lamictal. Glaxo Wellcome, 1997.
2. Betts T, Goodwin G, Withers RM, Yuen AWC. Human safety of lamotrigine. Epilepsia 1991;32(Suppl 2): S17–21.
3. Rambeck B, Kurlemann G, Stodieck SRG, May TW, Jurgens U. Concentrations of lamotrigine in a mother on lamotrigine treatment and her newborn child. Eur J Clin Pharmacol 1997;51:481–4.
4. Tomson T, Ohman I, Sigurd V. Lamotrigine in pregnancy and lactation: a case report. Epilepsia 1997; 38:1039–41.
5. Ohman I, Vitols S, Tomson T. Lamotrigine in pregnancy: pharmacokinetics during delivery, in the neonate, and during lactation. Epilepsia 2000;41: 709–13.
6. de Haan GJ, Edelbroek P, Segers J, Engelsman M, Lindhout D, Devile-Notschaele M, Augustijn P. Gestation-induced changes in lamotrigine pharmacokinetics: a monotherapy study. Neurology 2004;63:571–3.
7. Lamotrigine Pregnancy Registry. Interim Report. 1 September 1992 through 31 March 2004. Glaxo Wellcome, July 2004.
8. Wilton LV, Pearce GL, Martin RM, Mackay FJ, Mann RD. The outcomes of pregnancy in women exposed to newly marketed drugs in general practice in England. Br J Obstet Gynaecol 1998;105:882–9.
9. Dichter MA, Brodie MJ. New antiepileptic drugs. N Engl J Med 1996;334:1583–90.
10. Morrell MJ. The new antiepileptic drugs and women: efficacy, reproductive health, pregnancy, and fetal outcome. Epilepsia 1996;37(Suppl 6):S34–S44.
11. Committee on Drugs, American Academy of Pediatrics. The transfer of drugs and other chemicals into human milk. Pediatrics 2001;108:776–89.

Name:	**LANATOSIDE C**	Risk Factor:	**C**
Class:	**Cardiac Glycoside**		

See Digitalis.

Name:	**LANSOPRAZOLE**	Risk Factor:	B_M
Class:	**Gastrointestinal Agent (Antisecretory)**		

FETAL RISK SUMMARY

RECOMMENDATION: Limited Human Data - Animal Data Suggest Low Risk

Lansoprazole is a proton pump inhibitor that blocks gastric acid secretion by a direct inhibitory effect on the gastric parietal cell (1). It is used for the treatment of gastric and duodenal ulcer, erosive esophagitis, gastroesophageal reflux disease (GERD), and pathologic hypersecretory conditions, such as Zollinger-Ellison syndrome. It is also used in combination with amoxicillin and/or clarithromycin for *Helicobacter pylori* eradication to reduce the risk of duodenal ulcer recurrence.

Reproductive studies have been conducted in pregnant rats and rabbits at oral doses up to 40 and 16 times, respectively, the recommended human dose based on body surface area (1). No evidence was found that these doses impaired fertility or caused fetal harm. Similar to other proton pump inhibitors, lansoprazole is carcinogenic in mice and rats producing dose-related gastric, testicular, and liver tumors (1). In addition, positive results were seen with lansoprazole in the *in vitro* human lymphocyte chromosomal aberration assays, but the Ames mutation assay and other genotoxic animal tests were negative (1).

In a study published in 1990, lansoprazole at a dose of 50 or 300 mg/kg was not teratogenic in pregnant rats, but a decrease in fetal weight occurred (2). Schardein also cited a 1990 study, which appears to be similar to the one cited above, that found no evidence of teratogenicity in rats and rabbits (3).

It is not known if lansoprazole crosses the human placenta. The molecular weight (about 369) is low enough, however, that passage to the fetus should be expected. Another proton pump inhibitor, omeprazole, has a molecular weight (about 345) and chemical structure that is very similar to lansoprazole, and it is known to cross the human placenta (see Omeprazole).

A 1998 non-interventional observational cohort study described the outcomes of pregnancies in women who had been prescribed one or more of 34 newly marketed drugs by general practitioners in England (4). Data were obtained by questionnaires sent to the prescribing physicians one month after the expected or possible date of delivery. In 831 (78%) of the pregnancies, a newly marketed drug was thought to had been taken during the 1st trimester with birth defects noted in 14 (2.5%) singleton births of the 557 live newborns (10 sets of twins). In addition, two birth defects were observed in aborted fetuses. However, few of the aborted fetuses were examined. Lansoprazole was taken during the 1st trimester in six pregnancies. Seven healthy newborns (one premature; one set of twins) were delivered (4).

Data from the Swedish Medical Birth Registry were presented in 1998 (5). A total of 553 infants (6 sets of twins) were delivered from 547 women who had used acid-suppressing drugs early in pregnancy. A number of other pharmaceutical agents, identified only by drug category, were also used by these women. Seventeen infants with birth defects were identified (3.1%; 95% Confidence Interval [CI] 1.8–4.9) compared with the crude malformation rate of 3.9% in the Registry. The odds ratio (OR) for a congenital malformation, stratified for birth year, maternal age, parity, and smoking was 0.72 (95% CI 0.41–1.24) (5). The OR for malformations after proton pump blocker exposure was 0.91

(95% CI 0.45–1.84) compared to 0.46 (95% CI 0.17–1.20) for H_2-receptor antagonists (OR 0.86, 95% CI 0.33–2.23; $p = 0.13$). Of the 17 infants with birth defects, 10 had been exposed to proton pump blockers, 6 to H_2 antagonists, and 1 to both classes of drug. Six of the defects in the proton pump inhibitor group were cardiovascular defects (see also Omeprazole), whereas only one such defect occurred in those exposed to H_2 antagonists. Lansoprazole was the only acid-suppressing drug exposure in 13 infants. Two birth defects were observed in this group: atrial septum defect and an undescended testicle (5).

In a study published in 1999, investigators linked data from a Danish prescription database to a birth registry to evaluate the risks of proton pump inhibitors for congenital malformations, low birth weight, and preterm delivery (<37 weeks' gestation) (6). From a total of 51 women who had filled a prescription for these drugs sometime during pregnancy, 38 (omeprazole $N = 35$, lansoprazole $N = 3$) had done so during the interval of 30 days before conception to the end of the 1st trimester. A control group, consisting of 13,327 pregnancies in which the mother had not obtained a prescription for reimbursed medication from 30 days before conception to the end of her pregnancy, was used for comparison. The prevalence of major congenital anomalies in controls was 5.2%. Three major birth defects (7.9%), two of which were cardiovascular anomalies, were observed from the 38 pregnancies possibly exposed in the 1st trimester (specific drug exposure not given): ventricular septum defect; pyloric stenosis; and one case of patent ductus arteriosus, atrial septum defect, hydronephrosis, and agenesis of the iris. In comparison to controls, the adjusted (for maternal age, birth order, gestational age, and smoking, but not for alcohol abuse) relative risks for the three outcomes were congenital malformations 1.6 (95% CI 0.5–5.2), low birth weight 1.8 (95% CI 0.2–13.1), and preterm delivery (not adjusted for gestational age) 2.3 (95% CI 0.9–6.0). Although the study found no elevated risks for the three outcomes, the investigators cautioned that more data were needed to assess the possible association between proton pump inhibitors and cardiac malformations or preterm delivery (6).

In summary, the lack of teratogenicity in animals is reassuring, but the limited human pregnancy experience prevents an assessment of the risk from this drug. Birth defects, including cardiac defects, have been reported in pregnancies exposed to a proton pump inhibitor (see also Omeprazole), but there is no evidence of a causal association. Most likely, the observed defects were the result of many factors, including possibly the severity of the disease and concurrent use of other drugs. The data do warrant continued investigation. In addition, the studies lacked the sensitivity to detect minor anomalies because of the absence of standardized examinations. Late-appearing major defects may also have been missed as a consequence of the timing of some data collection. The carcinogenicity data are a potential concern, but the dose-related nature of the tumors and the presumable limited *in utero* exposure to the drug during human gestation probably indicates a negligible risk. However, as with all drug therapy, avoidance of lansoprazole during pregnancy, especially during the 1st trimester, is the safest course. If lansoprazole is required or if inadvertent exposure does occur early in gestation, the known risk to the embryo/fetus appears to be low. Long-term follow-up of offspring exposed during gestation is warranted.

BREAST FEEDING SUMMARY

RECOMMENDATION: No Human Data - Potential Toxicity

No reports describing the use of lansoprazole during human lactation have been located. Both lansoprazole and its metabolites are excreted in the milk of lactating rats (1), and their excretion in human milk should be expected. Because of the carcinogenicity observed in animals, and the potential for suppression of gastric acid secretion in the nursing infant, the use of lansoprazole during lactation should probably be avoided.

References

1. Product information. Prevacid. Tap Pharmaceuticals, 2001.
2. Schardein JL, Furuhashi T, Ooshima Y. Reproductive and developmental toxicity studies of lansoprazole (ag-1749) in rats and rabbits. Yakuri to Rinsho 1990;18:S2773–83. As cited by Shepard TH. *Catalog of Teratogenic Agents*. 8th ed. Baltimore, MD: Johns Hopkins University Press, 1995:245.
3. Schardein JL, Furuhashi T, Ooshima Y. Reproductive and developmental toxicity studies of lansoprazole (AG-1749) in rats and rabbits. Jpn Pharmacol Ther 1990;18(Suppl 10):119–29. As cited by Schardein JL. *Chemically Induced Birth Defects*. 2nd ed. New York, NY: Marcel Dekker, 1993:447.
4. Wilton LV, Pearce GL, Martin RM, Mackay FJ, Mann RD. The outcomes of pregnancy in women exposed to newly marketed drugs in general practice in England. Br J Obstet Gynaecol 1998;105:882–9.
5. Kallen B. Delivery outcome after the use of acid-suppressing drugs in early pregnancy with special reference to omeprazole. Br J Obstet Gynaecol 1998;105: 877–81.
6. Nielsen GL, Sorensen HT, Thulstrup, Tage-Jensen U, Olesen C, Ekbom A. The safety of proton pump inhibitors in pregnancy. Aliment Pharmacol Ther 1999;13: 1085–9.

Name: **LEFLUNOMIDE** Risk Factor: X_M

Class: **Immunologic Agent (Antirheumatic)**

FETAL RISK SUMMARY

RECOMMENDATION: Contraindicated

Leflunomide, a pyrimidine synthesis inhibitor, is indicated for the treatment of active rheumatoid arthritis to reduce signs and symptoms and retard structural damage. The drug is metabolized to an active metabolite that has an elimination half-life of about 2 weeks (1).

Leflunomide is contraindicated in pregnancy because it has exhibited dose related teratogenicity and embryo/fetal toxicity in animals at doses that resulted in systemic exposures at or below those obtained in humans. Therefore, in women of childbearing age, leflunomide should not be started until pregnancy has been excluded and the use of reliable contraception has been confirmed (1).

In reproduction studies with pregnant rats during organogenesis, an oral dose that produced systemic exposure approximately 10% of the human exposure level based on area under the plasma concentration curve (HE) was teratogenic (anophthalmia or microphthalmia and internal hydrocephalus) (1). This dose also resulted in an increase in embryo death and a decrease in maternal and surviving fetuses' body weight. In rabbits, an oral dose equivalent to the maximum HE during organogenesis resulted in fused, dysplastic sternebrae (1). No teratogenic effects were noted at lower doses in either species. In rats treated with doses 1% of the HE for 14 days before mating and continued until the end of lactation, more than 90% of the offspring failed to survive the postnatal period (1).

Leflunomide was not carcinogenic in rats, but mice exhibited dose-related increases in lymphoma (males) and bronchoalveolar adenomas and carcinomas combined (females). The incidence of the lung tumors, however, was within the spontaneous range for the mouse strain (2). The drug was not mutagenic or clastogenic in various assays although a minor metabolite (4-trifluoromethylaniline; TFMA) was in some tests (1). Because of the very low amounts of this metabolite, the results were not thought to be clinically significant (2).

It is not known if leflunomide crosses the human placenta. The molecular weight (about 270) is low enough that passage to the fetus should be expected. It is also not known if the active metabolite can cross the placenta or if the fetus can metabolize the parent compound to the active metabolite.

Because it may take up to 2 years to reach non-detectable plasma levels (<0.02 μg/mL) of the active metabolite, the manufacturer has developed a drug elimination procedure in the event that a woman taking leflunomide becomes pregnant: (a) administer cholestyramine 8 g 3 times daily for 11 days (not necessarily consecutive unless there is a need to lower the plasma level rapidly); and (b) verify plasma levels less than 0.02 μg/mL by two tests at least 14 days apart. If plasma levels are higher than 0.02 μg/mL, additional cholestyramine treatment should be considered (1).

Information relating to the risks of leflunomide use in human pregnancy has been published (2,3). A 2000 review on the treatment of rheumatic diseases briefly mentioned the agent, stating that it was contraindicated in pregnancy (3). It also reviewed the drug elimination procedure in the manufacturer's product literature. A 2001 reference thoroughly reviewed the reproductive risks of leflunomide and provided detailed information on counseling of men and women who might have been exposed to the agent and were either contemplating fathering a child, were pregnant, or were planning a pregnancy (2). The drug blood level considered safe was 0.03 μg/mL, which was 123 and 136 times lower than the no-effect blood levels in rats and rabbits, respectively. The safe concentration was about 0.1% of the average steady-state plasma level of the active metabolite. The author mentioned that approximately 30 women had become pregnant on leflunomide, 29 of whom were exposed to therapeutic levels of the drug during early organogenesis in spite of initiating the drug elimination protocol as soon as pregnancy was diagnosed. Only 3 pregnancies were continuing (no outcome data available), however, as 27 women had elected to undergo termination (2).

A survey of 600 members of the American College of Rheumatology, partially conducted to determine the outcomes of pregnancies exposed to disease modifying antirheumatic drugs (DMARD) (etanercept, infliximab, leflunomide, and methotrexate), was published in 2003 (4). From the 175 responders, the outcomes of 10 pregnancies exposed to leflunomide were two full term healthy infants, one preterm delivery, one spontaneous abortion, two elective abortions, two unknown outcomes, and two women still pregnant. Cholestyramine was definitely used in two pregnancies and may have been used in all (4).

In summary, leflunomide is an animal teratogen but, except for the data above, no human pregnancy experience has been published and the risk for congenital malformations cannot be determined. The drug and its active metabolite are eliminated from the body very slowly and may take up to 2 years to reach non-detectable plasma metabolite levels. The drug is contraindicated in pregnancy. In women of childbearing age, pregnancy should be excluded and the woman should be on a reliable contraceptive before starting therapy. In the event of inadvertent conceptions, a drug elimination procedure has been developed and is included in the product information. However, the procedure for preventing embryo exposure to therapeutic levels in unplanned pregnancies, based on the above report, appears to be clinically ineffective. In inadvertent pregnancies, the procedure, to be at least partially effective, should be initiated no later then the time of the first missed menstrual period (2). Pregnancy loss and anomalies occurring early in organogenesis would still be a risk, but drug-induced microcephaly and mental retardation would be prevented (2). A pregnancy registry and cohort study has been established to monitor fetal outcomes of pregnant women exposed to leflunomide for the treatment of rheumatoid arthritis (5). Healthcare providers are encouraged to register such patients by calling the toll free number (877-311-8972) (1,2).

BREAST FEEDING SUMMARY

RECOMMENDATION: No Human Data - Potential Toxicity

No reports describing the use of leflunomide during lactation have been located. The molecular weight (about 270) is low enough that excretion into breast milk should be expected. The effects of this exposure on a nursing infant are unknown. Because of the potential for serious adverse effects and without information on the amount of drug in milk, nursing mothers receiving this drug should probably not breast-feed (2).

References

1. Product information. Arava. Aventis Pharmaceuticals, 2001.
2. Brent RL. Teratogen update: reproductive risks of leflunomide (Arava); a pyrimidine synthesis inhibitor: counseling women taking leflunomide before or during pregnancy and men taking leflunomide who are contemplating fathering a child. Teratology 2001;63:106–12.
3. Janssen NM, Genta MS. The effects of immunosuppressive and anti-inflammatory medications on fertility, pregnancy, and lactation. Arch Intern Med 2000;160:610–9.
4. Chakravarty EF, Sanchez-Yamamoto D, Bush TM. The use of disease modifying antirheumatic drugs in women with rheumatoid arthritis of childbearing age: a survey of practice patterns and pregnancy outcomes. J Rheumatol 2003;30:241–6.
5. Jones KL, Johnson DL, Chambers CD. Monitoring leflunomide (Arava) as a new potential teratogen. Teratology 2002;65:200–2.

L

Name:	**LEPIRUDIN**	Risk Factor:	**B_M**
Class:	**Hematologic Agent (Thrombin Inhibitor)**		

FETAL RISK SUMMARY

RECOMMENDATION: No Human Data - Animal Data Suggest Low Risk

The polypeptide lepirudin (rDNA) is a recombinant hirudin derived from yeast cells that is indicated for anticoagulation in patients with heparin-induced thrombocytopenia and associated thromboembolic disease. It is composed of 65 amino acids and is administered as a continuous IV infusion. Lepirudin binds to thrombin to directly block the thrombogenic activity of thrombin (1).

Reproduction studies with lepirudin have been conducted in rats and rabbits. In pregnant rats, IV doses up to 1.2 times the maximum recommended daily human dose based on body surface area (MRHD) during organogenesis and the perinatal-postnatal period revealed no evidence of fetal harm. However, increased rat maternal mortality from undetermined causes was noted. Studies with pregnant rabbits at IV doses up to 2.4 times the MRHD also found no evidence of embryo or fetal harm (1).

In spite of the high molecular weight of lepirudin (about 6970), the drug crosses the placenta of pregnant rats (1). Because of the similarities between rat and human placentas, exposure of the human embryo/fetus may occur.

No reports describing the use of lepirudin during human pregnancy have been located. Although no fetal harm was observed in two animal species, the passage of lepirudin across the rat placenta suggests that the agent may also cross the human placenta. The effects of this potential exposure on a human embryo or fetus, including hemorrhage, are unknown. However, if a pregnant woman requires lepirudin therapy, the benefits to her appear to outweigh the theoretical risks to her embryo/fetus.

BREAST FEEDING SUMMARY

RECOMMENDATION: No Human Data - Probably Compatible

No studies describing the use of lepirudin during lactation have been located. The high molecular weight (about 6970) suggests that excretion into milk does not occur. However, lepirudin may cross the placenta and may also be present in breast milk. Although the effects of lepirudin exposure of a nursing infant via breast milk are unknown, the polypeptide would probably be digested in the stomach.

Reference

1. Product information. Refludan. Aventis Pharmaceuticals, 2002.

Name:	**LEUCOVORIN**	Risk Factor:	C_M
Class:	**Vitamin**		

L

FETAL RISK SUMMARY

RECOMMENDATION: Compatible

Leucovorin (folinic acid) is an active metabolite of folic acid (1). It has been used for the treatment of megaloblastic anemia during pregnancy (2). See Folic Acid.

BREAST FEEDING SUMMARY

RECOMMENDATION: Compatible

Leucovorin (folinic acid) is an active metabolite of folic acid (1). See Folic Acid.

References

1. American Hospital Formulary Service. *Drug Information 1997*. Bethesda, MD: American Society of Health-System Pharmacists, 1997:2890–93.
2. Scott JM. Folinic acid in megaloblastic anaemia of pregnancy. Br Med J 1957;2:270–2.

Name:	**LEUPROLIDE**	Risk Factor:	X_M
Class:	**Antineoplastic/Hormone**		

FETAL RISK SUMMARY

RECOMMENDATION: Contraindicated

Leuprolide is a synthetic nonapeptide analogue of naturally occurring gonadotropin-releasing hormone that inhibits the secretion of gonadotropin when given continuously and in therapeutic doses.

Leuprolide causes a dose-related increase in the incidence of major malformations in pregnant rabbits, but not in rats (1). The most frequently observed malformations in rabbits were vertebral anomalies and hydrocephalus (J. D. Miller, personal communication, Tap Pharmaceuticals, Inc., 1992). The doses tested were 1/300–1/3 of the typical human dose. Increased fetal mortality and decreased fetal weights were observed in both animal species with the higher test doses.

In humans, spontaneous abortions or intrauterine growth retardation are theoretically possible because leuprolide suppresses endometrial proliferation. The risk of these adverse outcomes is considered greater than the risk of congenital malformations because the affected organs in animal studies do not depend on the presence of gonadal steroids for normal development (J. D. Miller, personal communication, Tap Pharmaceuticals, Inc., 1992).

The manufacturer is maintaining a registry of inadvertent human exposures during pregnancy to leuprolide and currently has more than 100 such cases (J. D. Miller, personal communication, Tap Pharmaceuticals, Inc., 1992). No cases of congenital defects attributable to the drug have been reported, although the numbers are too small to draw conclusions as to the risk for perinatal mortality, low birth weight, or teratogenicity.

BREAST FEEDING SUMMARY

RECOMMENDATION: Contraindicated

No data are available.

Reference

1. Product information. Lupron. Tap Pharmaceuticals, Inc., 1990.

Name:	**LEVALLORPHAN**	Risk Factor:	**D**
Class:	**Narcotic Antagonist**		

FETAL RISK SUMMARY

RECOMMENDATION: Limited Human Data - No Relevant Animal Data

Levallorphan is a narcotic antagonist that is used to reverse respiratory depression from narcotic overdose. It has been used in combination with alphaprodine or meperidine during labor to reduce neonatal depression (1–6). Although some benefits were initially claimed, caution in the use of levallorphan during labor has been advised for the following reasons (7): (a) a statistically significant reduction in neonatal depression has not been demonstrated; (b) the antagonist also reduces analgesia; and (c) the antagonist may increase neonatal depression if an improper narcotic-narcotic antagonist ratio is used.

As indicated above, levallorphan may cause respiratory depression in the absence of narcotics or if a critical ratio is exceeded (7). Because of these considerations, the use in pregnancy of levallorphan either alone or in combination therapy should be discouraged. If a narcotic antagonist is indicated, other agents that do not cause respiratory depression, such as naloxone, are preferred.

BREAST FEEDING SUMMARY

RECOMMENDATION: No Human Data - Potential Toxicity

No data are available.

References

1. Backner DD, Foldes FF, Gordon EH. The combined use of alphaprodine (Nisentil) hydrochloride and levallorphan tartrate for analgesia in obstetrics. Am J Obstet Gynecol 1957;74:271–82.
2. Roberts H, Kuck MAC. Use of alphaprodine and levallorphan during labour. Can Med Assoc J 1960;83:1088–93.
3. Roberts H, Kane KM, Percival N, Snow P, Please NW. Effects of some analgesic drugs used in childbirth. Lancet 1957;1:128–32.
4. Bullough J. Use of premixed pethidine and antagonists in obstetrical analgesia with special reference to cases in which levallorphan was used. Br Med J 1959;2:859–62.
5. Posner AC. Combined pethidine and antagonists in obstetrics. Br Med J 1960;1:124–5.
6. Bullough J. Combined pethidine and antagonists in obstetrics. Br Med J 1960;1:125.
7. Bonica JJ. *Principles and Practice of Obstetric Analgesia and Anesthesia*. Philadelphia, PA: FA Davis, 1967:254–9.

Name: **LEVETIRACETAM** Risk Factor: C_M

Class: **Anticonvulsant**

L

FETAL RISK SUMMARY

RECOMMENDATION: No Human Data - Animal Data Suggest Risk

Levetiracetam is an anticonvulsant used as adjunctive therapy in the treatment of partial-onset seizures in epilepsy. It is chemically unrelated to other anticonvulsant agents. Levetiracetam is minimally protein bound (<10%) and it is not metabolized by the liver (1,2). Major metabolism occurs by enzymatic hydrolysis of the acetamide group to produce the carboxylic acid metabolite (1). Levetiracetam does not inhibit and is not a high affinity substrate for epoxide hydrolase (1). Reports describing the effects (if any) of levetiracetam on folic acid have not been located.

In reproduction studies with pregnant rats, maternal doses approximately equivalent to the maximum recommended human dose (3000 mg) on a body surface area basis (MRHD) administered throughout pregnancy and lactation were associated with an increased incidence of minor fetal skeletal abnormalities and retarded growth pre- and postnatally (1). When doses six times the MRHD were used, increased pup mortality and behavioral alterations were observed. The developmental no-effect dose administered throughout pregnancy and lactation was 0.2 times the MRHD. Dosing at 12 times the MRHD given only during organogenesis resulted in reduced fetal weights and an increased incidence of fetal skeletal variations. The developmental no-effect dose during organogenesis was four times the MRHD. No evidence of fetal or neonatal harm was observed with doses up to six times the MRHD during the last third of pregnancy and throughout lactation. None of the studied doses produced maternal toxicity (1).

In pregnant rabbits, increased embryo/fetal mortality and an increased incidence of minor skeletal abnormalities were observed at maternal doses 4 times the MRHD administered during organogenesis. When a dose 12 times the MRHD was used, decreased fetal weight and increased incidences of fetal malformations were noted, but maternal toxicity was also evident at this dose. The developmental no-effect dose was 1.3 times the MRHD (1).

It is not known if levetiracetam crosses the human placenta. The low molecular weight (about 170) and the lack of protein binding, however, suggest that exposure of the embryo and fetus should be expected.

An estimated 20% to 30% of epileptic patients have seizures not well controlled by monotherapy and require anticonvulsant polytherapy (2). Clinical studies of levetiracetam have demonstrated efficacy in partial-onset seizures with a good tolerability profile. In addition, its lack of hepatic metabolism and low protein binding result in a low risk of interaction with other drugs, including other anticonvulsants and oral contraceptives. Although comparison studies with other adjunctive anticonvulsants (e.g. felbamate, gabapentin, lamotrigine, tiagabine, topiramate, and vigabatrin) have not been conducted, it should be added to the list of agents to consider in cases of treatment-refractory partial-onset seizures (2).

In summary, experimental animal data indicate that levetiracetam causes embryo and fetal toxicity at or near the human dose. Teratogenicity was demonstrated in one species but only at maternal toxic doses. No reports describing the use of levetiracetam during human pregnancy have been located. However, its low molecular weight and complete oral bioavailability suggest that significant amounts will cross the placenta. The risk of this anticonvulsant to the human embryo/fetus is unknown (3). It is not known if levetiracetam causes folic acid deficiency, but it will usually be combined with other anticonvulsants, some of which may cause folic acid deficiency. Therefore, daily supplementation with 4–5 mg of folic acid, combined with multivitamins that include adequate amounts of other B vitamins, may be indicated. Because levetiracetam use in human pregnancy is likely, physicians are encouraged to register pregnant subjects receiving the anticonvulsant, before pregnancy outcome is known, in the Antiepileptic Drug Pregnancy Registry by calling (888) 233-2334 (toll free) (1).

BREAST FEEDING SUMMARY

RECOMMENDATION: No Human Data - Probably Compatible

No reports describing the use of levetiracetam during lactation have been located. The low molecular weight (about 170) and low protein binding (<10%) suggest that levetiracetam will be excreted into breast milk. The effects of this exposure on a nursing infant are unknown. Of note, however, other anticonvulsants are classified as compatible with breast-feeding by the American Academy of Pediatrics (see Carbamazepine, Phenytoin, and Valproic Acid).

References

1. Product information. Keppra. UCB Pharma, 2002.
2. Dooley M, Plosker GL. Levetiracetam. A review of its adjunctive use in the management of partial onset seizures. Drugs 2000;60:871–93.
3. Anonymous. Two new drugs for epilepsy. Med Lett Drugs Ther 2000;42:33–5.

Name:	**LEVODOPA**	Risk Factor:	C_M
Class:	**Antiparkinsonian Agent**		

FETAL RISK SUMMARY

RECOMMENDATION: Limited Human Data - Animal Data Suggest Moderate Risk

Levodopa, a metabolic precursor to dopamine, is primarily used for the treatment and prevention of symptoms related to Parkinson's disease. The active agent for this purpose is thought to be dopamine, which is formed in the brain after metabolism of levodopa. Levodopa crosses the blood-brain barrier, but dopamine does not. Combination with carbidopa (see also Carbidopa), an agent that inhibits the decarboxylation of extracerebral levodopa, allows for lower doses of levodopa, fewer adverse drug effects related to peripheral dopamine, and higher amounts of levodopa available for passage to the brain and eventual conversion to dopamine.

Levodopa, either alone or in combination with carbidopa, has caused visceral and skeletal malformations in rabbits (1). Doses of 125 or 250 mg/kg/day in pregnant rabbits produced malformations of the fetal circulatory system (2). This teratogenicity was not observed at 75 mg/kg/day, but all three doses produced fetal toxicity manifested by decreased litter weight and an increased incidence of stunted and resorbed fetuses. In mice, no teratogenicity was observed with doses of 125, 250, and 500 mg/kg/day, but at the highest dose, fetuses were significantly smaller than controls (2). A similar, significant decrease in the weights of newborn mice was observed in a study in which pregnant mice were fed levodopa 40 mg/g of food, but not at lower doses (3). The number of pregnancies and the number of newborns were also significantly decreased in those treated at 40 mg/g compared with those treated with 0, 10, or 20 mg/g of food.

Levodopa, in oral doses of 1–1000 mg/kg/day, administered to pregnant rats during the 1st week of gestation, produced a dose-related occurrence in brown fat (interscapular brown adipose tissue) hemorrhage and vasodilation in the newborns (4). A similar response was observed with dopamine. The addition of carbidopa (MK-486) to levodopa resulted in a significant decrease in this toxicity, implying that the causative agent was dopamine.

A study published in 1978 examined the effect of carbidopa (20 mg/kg SC every 12 hours × 7 days) and levodopa plus carbidopa (200/20 mg/kg SC every 12 hours × 7 days) on the length of gestation in pregnant rats (5). Only the combination had a statistically significant effect on pregnancy duration, causing a delay in parturition of 12 hours. The results were thought to be consistent with dopamine inhibition of oxytocin release.

Because Parkinson's disease is relatively uncommon in women of childbearing age, only a few reports, some involving uses other than for parkinsonism, have been located that describe the use of levodopa, with or without carbidopa, in human pregnancy (6–21).

Placental transfer of levodopa at term was documented in a 1989 report (6). A 34-year-old multiparous woman, with a 6-year history of Parkinson's disease, was treated with a proprietary combination of levodopa and benserazide (Madopar, not available in the United States), three 250-mg tablets/day. When pregnancy was diagnosed (15th day post-conception), the combination therapy was discontinued and treatment with levodopa (up to 5000 mg/day) alone was started. After 5 months, because of worsening parkinsonism, she was again treated with levodopa/benserazide (six 250-mg tablets/day). She eventually gave birth to a normal, 3070-g female infant who had no signs or symptoms of toxicity from the drug therapy during the first 8 days of life. Her 1-minute Apgar score was 2; then improved to 7 and 10 at 3 and 5 minutes, respectively. The cord plasma level of levodopa was 0.38 μg/mL compared with 2.7 μg/mL in the mother's plasma, a ratio of 0.14.

A 1995 reference described the placental transfer of levodopa and the possible fetal metabolism of the drug to dopamine, its active metabolite (7). A 34-year-old woman with juvenile Parkinson's disease was treated with carbidopa/levodopa (200/800 mg/day) during two pregnancies (see also Carbidopa). Both pregnancies were electively terminated, one at 8 weeks' gestation and the other at 10 weeks' gestation. Mean concentrations of levodopa (expressed as ng/mg protein) in the maternal serum, placental tissue (including umbilical cord), fetal peripheral organs (heart, kidney, muscle), and fetal neural tissue (brain and spinal cord) were 8.5, 33.6, 7.4, and 7.7, respectively. Corresponding mean concentrations of dopamine at these sites were 0.10, <0.03, 0.29, and 1.01, respectively. The levels in the placentas and fetuses for both levodopa and dopamine were much higher than those measured in control tissue. Moreover, the relatively high concentrations of dopamine in fetal peripheral organs and neural tissue implied that the fetuses had metabolized levodopa. The investigators cautioned that, because neurotransmitters were known to alter early neural development in animals and in cultured cells, the increased amounts of dopamine found in their study suggested that chronic use of levodopa during gestation could induce long-term damage (7).

The pregnancy outcomes of two women who were treated with levodopa or carbidopa/levodopa during three pregnancies were described in a 1985 paper (8). The first woman, with at least a 7-year history of parkinsonism, conceived while being treated with carbidopa/levodopa (five 25/250-mg tablets/day) and amantadine (100 mg twice daily). She had delivered a normal male infant approximately 6 years earlier, but no medical treatment had been given during that pregnancy. Amantadine was immediately discontinued when the current pregnancy was diagnosed. Other than slight vaginal bleeding in the 1st trimester, there were no maternal or fetal complications. She gave birth to a normal term infant (sex and weight not specified) who was doing well at 1.5 years of age. The second patient, a 32-year-old woman with parkinsonism first diagnosed at age 23, was being treated with levodopa (4 g/day) when a pregnancy of about 6 months' duration was diagnosed. Attempts to lower her levodopa dose were unsuccessful. She delivered a term, male, 7-lb 2-oz (about 3235-g) infant. Two years later, while still undergoing treatment with levodopa, she delivered a term, female, 6-lb 8-oz (about 2951-g) infant. Both children were alive and well at 7 and 5 years, respectively.

L

A 1987 retrospective report described the use of carbidopa/levodopa, starting before conception, in five women during seven pregnancies, one of which was electively terminated during the 1st trimester (9). A sixth woman, taking levodopa plus amantadine, had a miscarriage at 4 months. All of the other pregnancies went to term (newborn weights and sexes not specified). Maternal complications in three pregnancies included slight 1st trimester vaginal bleeding, nausea and vomiting during the 8th and 9th months (the only patient who reported nausea and vomiting after the 1st trimester) and depression that resolved postpartum, and preeclampsia. One infant, whose mother took amantadine and carbidopa/levodopa and whose pregnancy was complicated by preeclampsia, had an inguinal hernia. No adverse effects or congenital anomalies were noted in the other five newborns and all remained healthy at follow-up (approximately 1–5 years of age).

A 27-year-old woman, with a history of chemotherapy and radiotherapy for non-Hodgkin's lymphoma occurring approximately 4 years earlier had developed a progressive parkinsonism syndrome that was treated with a proprietary preparation of carbidopa/levodopa (co-careldopa, Sinemet Plus; 375 mg/day) (10). She conceived 5 months after treatment began and eventually delivered a healthy, 3540-g male infant at term. Apgar scores were both 9 at 1 and 10 minutes. Co-careldopa had been continued throughout her pregnancy.

A brief case report, published in 1997, described a normal outcome in the 3rd pregnancy of a woman with levodopa-responsive dystonia (Segawa's type) who was treated throughout gestation with 500 mg/day of levodopa alone (11). The male infant weighed 2350 g at birth and was developing normally at the time of the report. Two previous pregnancies had occurred while the woman was being treated with daily doses of levodopa 100 mg and carbidopa 10 mg. Spontaneous abortions had occurred in both pregnancies; one at 6 weeks and the other at 12 weeks. An investigation failed to find any cause for the miscarriages.

Two 1998 case reports described the use of levodopa, in combination with selegiline and benserazide, during human pregnancy (see Selegiline for details) (12,13). In another 1998 case report, a woman took levodopa/carbidopa (Sinemet CR 50/200) four times daily throughout gestation (14). Healthy male infants were delivered in all three pregnancies.

A brief 1996 communication included data obtained from a manufacturer (the Roche Drug Safety database) on the effects of levodopa on the fetus during human pregnancy (15). This database, current up to March 31, 1995, had six reports involving the use of levodopa/benserazide during gestation. The outcomes of these pregnancies included two elective terminations, one spontaneous abortion, two normal outcomes, and one lost to follow-up. No information was available on the condition of the fetuses in the three abortions. Another normal pregnancy outcome, without further details, from a mother who used levodopa/benserazide during gestation, was also cited (16). To the knowledge of these authors, two of whom were representatives of the manufacturer, no reports of human birth defects resulting from use of levodopa had been discovered.

A study designed to investigate the inhibitory effect of levodopa on prolactin levels in late pregnancy was reported in 1973 (17). Four women in the 3rd trimester of pregnancy were given a single oral dose of levodopa, 1000 mg. A statistically significant decrease in serum prolactin occurred, with the lowest levels measured 4 hours after the dose, but 2 hours later the levels had returned to pretreatment values, similar to nontreated controls. No further decreases in prolactin were measured during the next 3 days. All of the treated women eventually delivered normal infants at or near term.

L

Levodopa has been used in the treatment of coma resulting from fulminant hepatic failure occurring during pregnancy (18,19). A 22-year-old woman, in her 6th month of pregnancy, had severe viral hepatitis with a grade IV coma (18). She was successfully treated with levodopa, 1 g orally every 6 hours, neomycin, vitamins, and parenteral hydrocortisone (1000 mg/day). Recovery from the coma occurred 24–48 hours after the start of levodopa. Approximately 3 months later, she delivered a full-term infant (details of the infant and its condition were not included). In the second case, a 30-year-old woman in her 5th month of gestation was treated for 1 week with levodopa, 1 g orally every 6 hours (19). This patient, who also had viral hepatitis, began to recover consciousness 1 hour after the first dose of levodopa and was fully awake within 24–48 hours. She delivered a term, healthy infant (sex and weight not specified).

Angiotensin pressor responsiveness (vascular sensitivity) was decreased by the administration of levodopa in pregnancy (mean 29–30 weeks, range 24–36 weeks' gestation) (20). Five patients were treated with a single 500-mg oral dose and 16 received 1000 mg. Only the higher dose produced a significant decrease in angiotensin sensitivity. The authors hypothesized that chronic treatment with levodopa might not only decrease angiotensin sensitivity but also decrease pregnancy-induced hypertension. No data were provided on the outcome of these pregnancies following the study. The effect of levodopa on plasma prolactin secretion and inhibition of the renin-aldosterone axis was reported in a subsequent paper by this same group of investigators (21). Using methods and a patient population nearly identical with those of their previous study, the investigators found that a 1000-mg oral dose of levodopa produced a significant decrease in serum prolactin, plasma renin activity, and plasm aldosterone.

In summary, levodopa-induced teratogenicity and dose-related toxicity have been observed in animals, but no adverse outcomes associated with this drug have been observed in a limited number of human pregnancies. Although conditions requiring the use of levodopa during the childbearing years are relatively uncommon, exposure to this agent during gestation does not appear to present a major risk to the fetus. However, evaluation of the effect of chronic *in utero* exposure to dopamine, the active metabolite of levodopa, on neurodevelopment is warranted.

BREAST FEEDING SUMMARY

RECOMMENDATION: Limited Human Data - Probably Compatible

Levodopa is excreted into breast milk. A 1998 case report described a woman who took levodopa/carbidopa (Sinemet CR 50/200) four times daily throughout gestation (14). She continued the therapy after delivery and during breast-feeding. At about 5 months postpartum, the peak concentration of levodopa in milk (based on 5 mL milk samples) was 1.6 nmol/mL, 3 hours after a dose. The milk:plasma ratio, based on area under the concentration curves (6 hours for plasma and milk) was 0.28. When the dose was changed to two tablets of Sinemet 25/100 four times daily, the peak milk concentration (3 hours after a dose) was 3.47 nmol/mL and the milk:plasma ratio was 0.32. With both tablet strengths, the milk concentrations returned to baseline in 6 hours. The authors estimated that the nursing infant was ingesting 0.127–0.181 mg/day (0.016–0.023 mg/kg/day) of levodopa. No adverse effects were observed in the infant and he was developing normally at 2 years of age (14).

Levodopa inhibits prolactin release in both animals (22) and humans (17,21). In lactating rats, levodopa injected IP in doses of 1.25, 2.5, 5, and 10 mg/100 g body weight produced a dose-related inhibition of milk ejection (22). Doses of 5 and 10 mg/100 g body weight, but not lower doses, prevented the release of prolactin induced by suckling. Small doses of oxytocin given immediately before suckling produced a normal milk-ejection response, indicating that the mechanism of inhibition by levodopa was not caused by mammary gland response but to an increase in catecholamines at the hypothalamic-hypophysial axis (22).

In one study, four women in the 3rd trimester of pregnancy received a single 1000-mg oral dose of levodopa (17). A significant decrease in serum prolactin occurred with the lowest concentration at 4 hours. Two hours later, the level had returned to pretreatment values. After delivery at or near term, all of the women had completely normal lactation. A second study also found that a single 1000-mg oral dose of levodopa produced a significant decrease in serum prolactin (21).

Clinical evidence of lactation inhibition was provided in a 1974 study (23). Ten female patients with a history of inappropriate galactorrhea were treated orally with levodopa, 500–3500 mg/day. Partial to complete suppression of lactation was observed in the women, but when treatment was stopped, lactation returned to normal levels.

References

1. Product information. Sinemet. DuPont Pharmaceuticals, 1997.
2. Staples RE, Mattis PA. Teratology of L-dopa (abstract). Teratology 1973;8:238.
3. Cotzia GC, Miller ST, Tang LC, Papavila PS. Levodopa, fertility, and longevity. Science 1977;196:549–50.
4. Kitchin KT, DiStefano V. L-Dopa and brown fat hemorrhage in the rat pup. Toxicol Appl Pharmacol 1976;38:251–63.
5. Seybold VS, Miller JW, Lewis PR. Investigation of a dopaminergic mechanism for regulating oxytocin release. J Pharmacol Exp Ther 1978;207:605–10.
6. Allain H, Bentue-Ferrer D, Milon D, Moran P, Jacquemard F, Defawe G. Pregnancy and parkinsonism. A case report without problem. Clin Neuropharmacol 1989;12:217–9.
7. Merchant CA, Cohen G, Mytilineou C, DiRocco A, Moros D, Molinari S, Yahr MD. Human transplacental transfer of carbidopa/levodopa. J Neural Transm Park Dis Dement Sect 1995;9:239–42.
8. Cook DG, Klawans HL. Levodopa during pregnancy. Clin Neuropharmacol 1985;8:93–5.
9. Golbe LI. Parkinson's disease and pregnancy. Neurology 1987;37:1245–9.
10. Ball MC, Sagar HJ. Levodopa in pregnancy. Mov Disord 1995;10:115.

11. Nomoto M, Kaseda S, Iwata S, Osame M, Fukuda T. Levodopa in pregnancy. Mov Disord 1997;12: 261.
12. Hagell P, Odin P, Vinge E. Pregnancy in Parkinson' disease: a review of the literature and a case report. Mov Disord 1998;13:34–8.
13. Kupsch A, Oertel WH. Selegiline, pregnancy, and Parkinson' disease. Mov Disord 1998;13:175–94.
14. Thulin PC, Woodward WR, Carter JH, Nutt JG. Levodopa in human breast milk: clinical implications. Neurology 1998;50:1920–1.
15. von Graeventiz KS, Shulman LM, Revell SP. Levodopa in pregnancy. Mov Disord 1996;11:115–6.
16. Bauherz G. Pregnancy and Parkinson's disease. A case report. N Trends Clin Neuropharmacol 1994;8:142. As cited by von Graeventiz KS, Shulman LM, Revell SP. Levodopa in pregnancy. Mov Disord 1996;11: 115–6.
17. Pujol-Amat P, Gamissans O, Calaf J, Benito E, Perez-Lopez FR, L'Hermite M, Robyn C. Influence of L-dopa on serum prolactin, human chorionic somatomammotropin (HCS) and human chorionic gonadotrophin (HCG) during the last trimester of pregnancy. In: Human Prolactin. Proceedings of the International Symposium on Human Prolactin, Brussels, June 12–14, 1973:316–20.
18. Datta DV, Maheshwari YK, Aggarwal ML. Levodopa in fulminant hepatic failure: preliminary report. Am J Med Sci 1976;272:95–9.
19. Chajek T, Friedman G, Berry EM, Abramsky O. Treatment of acute hepatic encephalopathy with L-dopa. Postgrad Med J 1977;53:262–5.
20. Kaulhausen H, Oney T, Feldmann R, Leyendecker G. Decrease of vascular angiotensin sensitivity by L-dopa during human pregnancy. Am J Obstet Gynecol 1981;140:671–5.
21. Kaulhausen H, Oney T, Leyendecker G. Inhibition of the renin-aldosterone axis and of prolactin secretion during pregnancy by L-dopa. Br J Obstet Gynaecol 1982;89:483–88.
22. Prilusky J, Deis RP. Effect of L-dopa on milk ejection and prolactin release in lactating rats. J Endocrinol 1975;67:397–401.
23. Ayalon D, Peyser MR, Toaff R, Cordova T, Harell A, Franchimont P, Lindner HR. Effect of L-dopa on galactopoiesis and gonadotropin levels in the inappropriate lactation syndrome. Am J Obstet Gynecol 1974;44:159–70.

Name: **LEVOFLOXACIN** Risk Factor: C_M

Class: **Anti-infective (Quinolone)**

FETAL RISK SUMMARY

RECOMMENDATION: Human Data Suggest Low Risk

Levofloxacin is a synthetic, broad-spectrum antibacterial agent that is the optical isomer of ofloxacin. As a fluoroquinolone, it is in the same class as ciprofloxacin, enoxacin, lomefloxacin, norfloxacin, ofloxacin, and sparfloxacin. Nalidixic acid is also a quinolone drug.

Reproduction studies of levofloxacin in rats with oral doses up to 3 or 18 times the maximum recommended human dose (MRHD) based on body surface area or body weight, respectively, and with IV doses up to 1 or 5 times the MRHD (in surface area or body weight, respectively) found no evidence of impaired fertility or reproductive performance (1). No teratogenicity was observed in pregnant rats at oral doses of 14 or 82 times the MRHD, respectively, or with IV doses of 2.7 or 16 times the MRHD, respectively (1). However, decreased fetal weight and increased fetal loss were observed at high doses. In pregnant rabbits, oral doses at 1.6 or 5 times the MRHD, respectively, and IV doses at 0.8 or 2.5 times the MRHD, respectively, did not cause teratogenicity (1).

No studies describing the placental transfer of levofloxacin have been located. Because of its relatively low molecular weight (about 370), transfer to the fetus should be expected. In addition, ofloxacin crosses the placenta (see Ofloxacin), and levofloxacin would be expected to possess similar properties.

In a prospective follow-up study conducted by the European Network of Teratology Information Services (ENTIS), data on 549 pregnancies exposed to fluoroquinolones (none to levofloxacin; 93 to ofloxacin) (see also Ofloxacin) were described in a 1996 reference (2). Data on another 116 prospective and 25 retrospective pregnancy exposures to the antibacterials were also included. Of the 666 cases with known outcome, 32 (4.8%) of the embryos, fetuses, or newborns had congenital malformations. From previous epidemiologic data, the authors concluded that the 4.8% frequency of malformations did not exceed the background rate (2). Finally, 25 retrospective reports of infants with anomalies, who had been exposed *in utero* to fluoroquinolones, were described, but no specific patterns of major congenital malformations were detected.

The authors of the above study concluded that pregnancy exposure to quinolones was not an indication for termination, but that this class of antibacterials should still be considered contraindicated in pregnant women. Moreover, this study did not address the issue of cartilage damage from quinolone exposure and the authors recognized the need for follow-up studies of this potential toxicity in children exposed *in utero*. Because of their own and previously published findings, they further recommended that the focus of future studies should be on malformations involving the abdominal wall and urogenital system and on limb reduction defects (2).

In summary, although no reports describing the use of levofloxacin during human gestation have been located, the available evidence for other members of this class, including the optical isomer, ofloxacin, indicates that a causal relationship with birth defects cannot be excluded (see Ofloxacin), although the lack of a pattern among the anomalies is reassuring (see Ciprofloxacin). Because of these concerns and the available animal data, the use of levofloxacin during pregnancy, especially during the 1st trimester, should be considered contraindicated. A 1993 review on the safety of fluoroquinolones concluded that these antibacterials should be avoided during pregnancy because of the difficulty in extrapolating animal mutagenicity results to humans and because interpretation of this toxicity is still controversial (3). The authors of this review were not convinced that fluoroquinolone-induced fetal cartilage damage and subsequent arthropathies were a major concern, even though this effect had been demonstrated in several animal species after administration to both pregnant and immature animals and in occasional human case reports involving children (3). Others have also concluded that fluoroquinolones should be considered contraindicated in pregnancy, because safer alternatives are usually available (2).

BREAST FEEDING SUMMARY

RECOMMENDATION: No Human Data - Probably Compatible

When first marketed, the administration of levofloxacin during breast-feeding was not recommended because of the potential for arthropathy (based on animal data) and other serious toxicity in the nursing infant (1). Phototoxicity has been observed with quinolones when exposure to excessive sunlight (i.e., ultraviolet light) has occurred (1). Well-differentiated squamous cell carcinomas of the skin has been produced in mice who were exposed chronically to some fluoroquinolones and periodic ultraviolet light (e.g., see Lomefloxacin), but studies to evaluate the carcinogenicity of levofloxacin in this manner have not been conducted.

No reports describing the use of levofloxacin in lactation have been located. Because levofloxacin is the optical isomer of ofloxacin, its passage into milk should be similar, and the milk concentrations of ofloxacin are about the same as those in the maternal serum (see Ofloxacin). Both ofloxacin and another fluoroquinolone, ciprofloxacin, are classified as compatible with breast-feeding by the American Academy of Pediatrics (see Ofloxacin and Ciprofloxacin).

References

1. Product information. Levaquin. Ortho-McNeil Pharmaceutical, 1997.
2. Schaefer C, Amoura-Elefant E, Vial T, Ornoy A, Garbis H, Robert E, Rodriguez-Pinilla E, Pexieder T, Prapas N, Merlob P. Pregnancy outcome after prenatal quinolone exposure. Evaluation of a case registry of the European Network of Teratology Information Services (ENTIS). Eur J Obstet Gynecol Reprod Biol 1996;69:83–9.
3. Norrby SR, Lietman PS. Safety and tolerability of fluoroquinolones. Drugs 1993;45(Suppl 3):59–64.

Name:	**LEVORPHANOL**	Risk Factor:	C_M*
Class:	**Narcotic Agonist Analgesic**		

FETAL RISK SUMMARY

RECOMMENDATION: Human Data Suggest Risk in 3rd Trimester

No reports linking the use of levorphanol with human congenital defects have been located. A single oral dose of 25 mg/kg was teratogenic in mice (1). At this dose, nearly 50% of the mouse embryos died.

Use of the drug during labor should be expected to produce neonatal depression to the same degree as other narcotic analgesics (2).

[**Risk Factor D if used for prolonged periods or in high doses at term.*]

L

BREAST FEEDING SUMMARY

RECOMMENDATION: No Human Data - Probably Compatible

No reports describing the use of levorphanol during lactation have been located. The molecular weight (about 444) is low enough, however, that passage into breast milk should be expected. Moreover, the drug is structurally similar to morphine, which is excreted into milk (see Morphine). The potential for long-term effects on neurobehavior and development in a nursing infant from exposure to levorphanol in milk are unknown but warrant study.

References

1. Product information. Levo-Dromoran. ICN Pharmaceuticals, 2000.
2. Bonica JJ. *Principles and Practice of Obstetric Analgesia and Anesthesia*. Philadelphia, PA: FA Davis, 1967:251.

Name:	**LEVOTHYROXINE**	Risk Factor:	A_M
Class:	**Thyroid**		

FETAL RISK SUMMARY

RECOMMENDATION: Compatible

Levothyroxine (T_4) is a naturally occurring thyroid hormone produced by the mother and the fetus. It is used during pregnancy for the treatment of hypothyroidism (see also Liothyronine and Thyroid). Most investigators have concluded that there is negligible transplacental passage of the drug at physiologic serum concentrations (1–6). However, maternal-fetal transfer of sufficient amounts of T_4 to protect the congenital hypothyroid fetus and newborn has been demonstrated (7).

In a surveillance study of Michigan Medicaid recipients conducted between 1985 and 1992 involving 229,101 completed pregnancies, 554 newborns had been exposed to levothyroxine during the 1st trimester (F. Rosa, personal communication, FDA, 1993). A total of 25 (4.5%) major birth defects were observed (24 expected). Specific data were available for six defect categories, including (observed/expected) 5/6 cardiovascular defects, 0/1 oral clefts, 0/0.3 spina bifida, 1/2 polydactyly, 1/1 limb reduction defects, and 1/1 hypospadias. These data do not support an association between the drug and congenital defects.

In a study of 25 neonates born with an autosomal recessive disorder that completely prevents iodination of thyroid proteins and, thus, the synthesis of T_4, the thyroid hormone was measured in their cord serum in concentrations ranging from 35 to 70 nmol/L. Because the newborns were unable to synthesize the hormone, the T_4 must have come from the mothers (7). The investigators then studied 15 newborns with thyroid agenesis and measured similar cord levels of T_4. The mean serum half-life of T_4 in the neonates was only 3.6 days, indicating that T_4 would be below the level of detection between 8 and 19 days after birth (7). Although the amounts measured were below normal values of T_4 (80–170 nmol/L), the amounts were sufficient to protect the infants initially from impaired mental development. A possible mechanism for this protection may involve increased conversion of T_4 to T_3 in the cerebral cortex in hypothyroid fetuses, and when combined with a decreased rate of T_3 degradation, the net effect is to normalize intracellular levels of the active thyroid hormone in the brain (7).

Several reports have described the direct administration of T_4 to the fetus and amniotic fluid (5,7–13). In almost identical cases, two fetuses were treated in the 3rd trimester with IM injections of T_4, 120 μg, every 2 weeks for four doses in an attempt to prevent congenital hypothyroidism (5,9). Their mothers had been treated with radioactive iodine (I^{131}) at 13 and 13.5 weeks' gestation. Both newborns were hypothyroid at birth and developed respiratory stridor, but neither had physical signs of cretinism. At the time of the reports, one child had mild developmental retardation at 3 years of age (5). The second infant was stable with a tracheostomy tube in place at 6 months of age (9). In a third mother who inadvertently received I^{131} at 10–11 weeks' gestation, intra-amniotic T_4, 500 μg, was given weekly during the last 7 weeks of pregnancy (10). Evidence was found that the T_4 was absorbed by the fetus. A male infant who developed normally was delivered. In a study to determine the metabolic fate of T_4 *in utero*, 700 μg of T_4 were injected intra-amniotically 24 hours before delivery in five full-term healthy patients (11). Serum T_4 levels were increased in all infants. Intra-amniotic T_4, 200 μg, was given to eight women in whom premature delivery was inevitable or was indicated to enhance fetal lung maturity (12). The patients ranged in gestational age between 29 and 32 weeks. No respiratory distress syndrome was found in the eight newborn infants. Delivery occurred 1–49 days after the injection. The dimensions of a large fetal goiter, secondary to propylthiouracil, were decreased but not eliminated within 5 days of an intra-amniotic 200-μg dose of T_4 administered at 34.5 weeks' gestation (13). Serial lecithin:sphingomyelin (L:S) ratios before and after the injection demonstrated no effect of T_4 on fetal lung maturity.

In a large prospective study, 537 mother-child pairs were exposed to levothyroxine and thyroid (desiccated) during the 1st trimester (14, pp. 388–400). For use anytime during pregnancy, 780 exposures were reported (14, p. 443). After 1st trimester exposure, possible associations were found with cardiovascular anomalies (9 cases), Down's syndrome (3 cases), and polydactyly in blacks (3 cases). Because of the small numbers involved, the statistical significance of these findings is unknown and independent confirmation is required. Maternal hypothyroidism itself has been reported to be responsible for poor pregnancy outcome (15–17). Others have not found this association, claiming that fetal development is not directly affected by maternal thyroid function (18).

Combination therapy with thyroid-antithyroid drugs was advocated at one time for the treatment of hyperthyroidism but is now considered inappropriate (see Propylthiouracil).

BREAST FEEDING SUMMARY

RECOMMENDATION: Compatible

Levothyroxine (T_4) is excreted into breast milk in low concentrations. The effect of this hormone on the nursing infant is controversial (see also Liothyronine and Thyrotropin). Two reports have claimed that sufficient quantities are present to partially treat neonatal hypothyroidism (19,20). A third study measured high T_4 levels in breast-fed infants but was unsure of its significance (21). In contrast, four competing studies have found that breast-feeding does not alter either T_4 levels or thyroid function in the infant (22–25). Although all of the investigators, on both sides of the issue, used sophisticated available methods to arrive at their conclusions, the balance of evidence weighs in on the side of those claiming lack of effect because they have relied on increasingly refined means to measure the hormone (26–28). The reports are briefly summarized below.

L

In 19 healthy euthyroid mothers not taking thyroid replacement therapy, mean milk T_4 concentrations in the 1st postpartum week were 3.8 ng/mL (19). Between 8 and 48 days, the levels rose to 42.7 ng/mL and then decreased to 11.1 ng/mL after 50 days postpartum. The daily excretion of T_4 at the higher levels is about the recommended daily dose for hypothyroid infants. An infant was diagnosed as athyrotic shortly after breast-feeding was stopped at age 10 months (19). Growth was at the 97th percentile during breast-feeding, but the bone age remained that of a newborn. In this study, mean levels of T_4 in breast milk during the last trimester (12 patients) and within 48 hours of delivery (22 patients) were 14 and 7 ng/mL, respectively. A 1983 report measured significantly greater serum levels of T_4 in 22 breast-fed infants than those in 25 formula-fed babies, 131.1 vs. 118.4 ng/mL, respectively (22). The overlap between the two groups, however, casts doubt on the physiologic significance of the differences.

In 77 euthyroid mothers, measurable amounts of T_4 were found in only 5 of 88 milk specimens collected over 43 months of lactation with 4 of the positive samples occurring within 4 days of delivery (22). Concentrations ranged from 8 to 13 ng/mL. A 1980 report described four exclusively breast-fed infants with congenital hypothyroidism that were diagnosed between the ages of 2 and 79 days (23). Breast-feeding did not hinder making the diagnosis. Another 1980 research report evaluated clinical and biochemical thyroid parameters in 45 hypothyroid infants, 12 of whom were breast-fed (24). No difference was detected between the breast-fed and bottle-fed babies, leading to the conclusion that breast milk did not offer protection against the effects of congenital hypothyroidism. In a 1985 study, serum concentrations of T_4 were similar in breast-fed and bottle-fed infants at 5, 10, and 15 days postpartum (25).

The discrepancies described above can be partially explained by the various techniques used to measure milk T_4 concentrations. Japanese researchers failed to detect milk T_4 using four different methods of radioimmunoassay (RIA) (26). Using three competitive protein-binding assays, highly variable T_4 levels were recovered from milk and a standard solution. Although the RIA methods were not completely reliable, because recovery from a standardized solution exceeded 100% with one method, the researchers concluded that milk T_4 concentrations must be very low and had no influence on the pituitary-thyroid axis of normal babies. No difficulty was encountered with measuring serum T_4 levels, which were not significantly different between breast-fed and bottle-fed infants (26). Swedish investigators using RIA methods also failed to find T_4 in milk (27). A second group of Swedish researchers used a gas chromatography-mass spectrometry technique to determine that the concentration of T_4 in milk was less than 4 ng/mL (28).

In summary, levothyroxine breast milk levels, as determined by modern laboratory techniques, are apparently too low to protect a hypothyroid infant completely from the effects of the disease. The levels are also too low to interfere with neonatal thyroid screening programs (25). Breast-feeding, however, probably offers better protection to infants with congenital hypothyroidism than does formula feeding. The American Academy of Pediatrics classifies levothyroxine as compatible with breast-feeding (29).

References

1. Grumbach MM, Werner SC. Transfer of thyroid hormone across the human placenta at term. J Clin Endocrinol Metab 1956,16:1392–5.
2. Kearns JE, Hutson W. Tagged isomers and analogues of thyroxine (their transmission across the human placenta and other studies). J Nucl Med 1963;4:453–61.
3. Fisher DA, Lehman H, Lackey C. Placental transport of thyroxine. J Clin Endocrinol Metab 1964;24:393–400.
4. Fisher DA, Klein AH. Thyroid development and disorders of thyroid function in the newborn. N Engl J Med 1981;304:702–12.
5. Van Herle AJ, Young RT, Fisher DA, Uller RP, Brinkman CR III. Intrauterine treatment of a hypothyroid fetus. J Clin Endocrinol Metab 1975;40:474–7.
6. Bachrach LK, Burrow GN. Maternal-fetal transfer of thyroxine. N Engl J Med 1989;321:1549.
7. Vulsma T, Gons MH, de Vijlder JJM. Maternal-fetal transfer of thyroxine in congenital hypothyroidism due to a total organification defect or thyroid agenesis. N Engl J Med 1989;321:13–6.
8. Larsen PR. Maternal thyroxine and congenital hypothyroidism. N Engl J Med 1989;321:44–6.
9. Jafek BW, Small R, Lillian DL. Congenital radioactive-iodine induced stridor and hypothyroidism. Arch Otolaryngol 1974;99:369–71.
10. Lightner ES, Fisher DA, Giles H, Woolfenden J. Intra-amniotic injection of thyroxine (T_4) to a human fetus. Am J Obstet Gynecol 1977;127:487–90.
11. Klein AH, Hobel CJ, Sack J, Fisher DA. Effect of intraamniotic fluid thyroxine injection on fetal serum and amniotic fluid iodothyronine concentrations. J Clin Endocrinol Metab 1978;47:1034–7.
12. Mashiach S, Barkai G, Sach J, Stern E, Goldman B, Brish M, Serr DM. Enhancement of fetal lung maturity by intra-amniotic administration of thyroid hormone. Am J Obstet Gynecol 1978;130:289–93.
13. Weiner S, Scharf JI, Bolognese RJ, Librizzi RJ. Antenatal diagnosis and treatment of fetal goiter. J Reprod Med 1980;24:39–42.
14. Heinonen OP, Slone D, Shapiro S. *Birth Defects and Drugs in Pregnancy*. Littleton, MA: Publishing Sciences Group, 1977.
15. Potter JD. Hypothyroidism and reproductive failure. Surg Gynecol Obstet 1980;150:251–5.
16. Pekonen F, Teramo K, Ikonen E, Osterlund K, Makinen T, Lamberg BA. Women on thyroid hormone therapy: pregnancy course, fetal outcome, and amniotic fluid thyroid hormone level. Obstet Gynecol 1984;63:635–8.
17. Man EB, Shaver BA Jr, Cooke RE. Studies of children born to women with thyroid disease. Am J Obstet Gynecol 1958;75:728–41.
18. Montoro M, Collea JV, Frasier SD, Mestman JH. Successful outcome of pregnancy in women with hypothyroidism. Ann Intern Med 1981;94:31–4.
19. Sack J, Amado O, Lunenfeld. Thyroxine concentration in human milk. J Clin Endocrinol Metab 1977;45:171–3.
20. Bode HH, Vanjonack WJ, Crawford JD. Mitigation of cretinism by breast-feeding. Pediatrics 1978;62:13–6.
21. Hahn HB Jr, Spiekerman AM, Otto WR, Hossalla DE. Thyroid function tests in neonates fed human milk. Am J Dis Child 1983;137:220–2.
22. Varma SK, Collins M, Row A, Haller WS, Varma K. Thyroxine, triiodothyronine, and reverse triiodothyronine concentrations in human milk. J Pediatr 1978;93:803–6.
23. Abbassi V, Steinour TA. Successful diagnosis of congenital hypothyroidism in four breast-fed neonates. J Pediatr 1980;97:259–61.
24. Letarte J, Guyda H, Dussault JH, Glorieux J. Lack of protective effect of breast-feeding in congenital hypothyroidism: report of 12 cases. Pediatrics 1980;65:703–5.
25. Franklin R, O'Grady C, Carpenter L. Neonatal thyroid function: comparison between breast-fed and bottle-fed infants. J Pediatr 1985;106:124–6.
26. Mizuta H, Amino N, Ichihara K, Harada T, Nose O, Tanizawa O, Miyai K. Thyroid hormones in human milk and their influence on thyroid function of breast-fed babies. Pediatr Res 1983;17:468–71.
27. Jansson L, Ivarsson S, Larsson I, Ekman R. Tri-iodothyronine and thyroxine in human milk. Acta Paediatr Scand 1983;72:703–5.
28. Moller B, Bjorkhem I, Falk O, Lantto O, Larsson A. Identification of thyroxine in human breast milk by gas chromatography-mass spectrometry. J Clin Endocrinol Metab 1983;56:30–4.
29. Committee on Drugs, American Academy of Pediatrics. The transfer of drugs and other chemicals into human milk. Pediatrics 2001;108:776–89.

Name:	**LIDOCAINE**	Risk Factor:	B_M
Class:	**Local Anesthetic/Cardiac Drug**		

FETAL RISK SUMMARY

RECOMMENDATION: Compatible

Lidocaine is a local anesthetic that is also used for the treatment of cardiac ventricular arrhythmias. The majority of the information on the drug in pregnancy derives from its use as a local anesthetic during labor and delivery. Reproduction studies have revealed no evidence of fetal harm in pregnant rats at doses up to 6.6 times the human dose (1).

The drug rapidly crosses the placenta to the fetus, appearing in the fetal circulation within a few minutes after administration to the mother. Cord:maternal serum ratios range between 0.50 and 0.70 after IV and epidural anesthesia (2–12). In 25 women just before delivery, a dose of 2–3 mg/kg was given by IV infusion at a rate of 100 mg/minute (2). The mean cord:maternal serum ratio in 9 patients who received 3 mg/kg was 0.55. A mean ratio of 1.32 was observed in nonacidotic newborns following local infiltration of the perineum for episiotomy (13). A similarly elevated ratio was measured in an acidotic newborn (14). The infant had umbilical venous/arterial pH values of 7.23/7.08 and a lidocaine cord:maternal serum ratio of 1.32 following epidural anesthesia. Because lidocaine is a weak base, the high ratio may have been caused by ion trapping (14).

Both the fetus and the newborn are capable of metabolizing lidocaine (8,9). The elimination half-life of lidocaine in the newborn following maternal epidural anesthesia averaged 3 hours (8). After local perineal infiltration for episiotomy, lidocaine was found in neonatal urine for at least 48 hours after delivery (13).

A number of studies have examined the effect of lidocaine on the newborn. In one report, offspring of mothers receiving continuous lumbar epidural blocks had significantly lower scores on tests of muscle strength and tone than did controls (15). Results of other tests of neurobehavior did not differ from those of controls. In contrast, four other studies failed to find adverse effects on neonatal neurobehavior following lidocaine epidural administration (10–12,16). Continuous infusion epidural analgesia with lidocaine has been used without effect on the fetus or newborn (17).

Lidocaine may produce central nervous system depression in the newborn with high serum levels. Of eight infants with lidocaine levels greater than 2.5 μg/mL, four had Apgar scores of 6 or less (3). Three infants with levels above 3.0 μg/mL were mildly depressed at birth (3). A 1973 study observed fetal tachycardia (3 cases) and bradycardia (3 cases) after paracervical block with lidocaine in 12 laboring women (18). The authors were unable to determine whether these effects were a direct effect of the drug. Accidental direct injection into the fetal scalp during local infiltration for episiotomy led to apnea, hypotonia, and fixed, dilated pupils 15 minutes after birth in one infant (19). Lidocaine-induced seizures occurred at 1 hour. The lidocaine concentration in the infant's serum at 2 hours was 14 μg/mL. The heart rate was 180 beats/minute. Following successful treatment, physical and neurologic examinations at 3 days and again at 7 months were normal.

Lidocaine is the treatment of choice for ventricular arrhythmias (20,21). A 1984 report described the use of therapeutic lidocaine doses (100 mg IV injection followed by 4 mg/minute infusion) in a woman who was successfully resuscitated after a cardiac arrest at 18 weeks' gestation (22). A normal infant was delivered at 38 weeks' gestation.

Neurologic development was normal at 17 months of age, but growth was below the 10th percentile.

The Collaborative Perinatal Project monitored 50,282 mother-child pairs, 293 of whom had exposure to lidocaine during the 1st trimester (23, pp. 358–363). No evidence of an association with large classes of malformations was found. Greater than expected risks were found for anomalies of the respiratory tract (three cases), tumors (two cases), and inguinal hernias (eight cases), but the statistical significance is unknown and independent confirmation is required (23, pp. 358–363, 477). For use anytime during pregnancy, 947 exposures were recorded (23, pp. 440, 493). From these data, no evidence of an association with large categories of major or minor malformations or to individual defects was found.

BREAST FEEDING SUMMARY

RECOMMENDATION: Limited Human Data - Probably Compatible

Small amounts of lidocaine are excreted into breast milk (24). A 37-year-old, lactating woman was treated with intravenous lidocaine for acute onset ventricular arrhythmia secondary to chronic mitral valve prolapse. The woman had been nursing her 10-month-old infant up to the time of treatment. She was treated with lidocaine, 75 mg over 1 minute, followed by a continuous infusion of 2 mg/minute (23 μg/kg/minute). A second 50-mg dose was given 5 minutes after the first bolus dose. The woman's serum lidocaine level 5 hours after initiation of therapy was 2 μg/mL. The drug concentration in a milk sample, obtained 2 hours later when therapy was stopped, was 0.8 μg/mL (40% of maternal serum). Although the infant was not allowed to nurse during and immediately following the mother's therapy, the potential for harm of the infant from exposure to lidocaine in breast milk is probably very low. The American Academy of Pediatrics classifies lidocaine as compatible with breast-feeding (25).

L

References

1. Product information. Xylocaine. AstraZeneca, 2000.
2. Shnider SM, Way EL. The kinetics of transfer of lidocaine (Xylocaine) across the human placenta. Anesthesiology 1968;29:944–50.
3. Shnider SM, Way EL. Plasma levels of lidocaine (Xylocaine) in mother and newborn following obstetrical conduction anesthesia: clinical applications. Anesthesiology 1968;29:951–8.
4. Lurie AO, Weiss JB. Blood concentrations of mepivacaine and lidocaine in mother and baby after epidural anesthesia. Am J Obstet Gynecol 1970;106:850–6.
5. Petrie RH, Paul WL, Miller FC, Arce JJ, Paul RH, Nakamura RM, Hon EH. Placental transfer of lidocaine following paracervical block. Am J Obstet Gynecol 1974;120:791–801.
6. Zador G, Lindmark G, Nilsson BA. Pudendal block in normal vaginal deliveries. Acta Obstet Gynecol Scand 1974;Suppl 34:51–64.
7. Blankenbaker WL, DiFazio CA, Berry FA Jr. Lidocaine and its metabolites in the newborn. Anesthesiology 1975;42:325–30.
8. Brown WU Jr, Bell GC, Lurie AO, Weiss JB, Scanlon JW, Alper MH. Newborn blood levels of lidocaine and mepivacaine in the first postnatal day following maternal epidural anesthesia. Anesthesiology 1975; 42:698–707.
9. Kuhnert BR, Knapp DR, Kuhnert PM, Prochaska AL. Maternal, fetal, and neonatal metabolism of lidocaine. Clin Pharmacol Ther 1979;26:213–20.
10. Abboud TK, Sarkis F, Blikian A, Varakian L. Lack of adverse neurobehavioral effects of lidocaine. Anesthesiology 1982;57(Suppl):A404.
11. Kileff M, James FM III, Dewan D, Floyd H, DiFazio C. Neonatal neurobehavioral responses after epidural anesthesia for cesarean section with lidocaine and bupivacaine. Anesthesiology 1982;57(Suppl):A403.
12. Abboud TK, David S, Costandi J, Nagappala S, Haroutunian S, Yeh SY. Comparative maternal, fetal and neonatal effects of lidocaine versus lidocaine with epinephrine in the parturient. Anesthesiology 1984;61(Suppl):A405.
13. Philipson EH, Kuhnert BR, Syracuse CD. Maternal, fetal, and neonatal lidocaine levels following local perineal infiltration. Am J Obstet Gynecol 1984;149: 403–7.
14. Brown WU Jr, Bell GC, Alper MH. Acidosis, local anesthetics, and the newborn. Obstet Gynecol 1976; 48:27–30.
15. Scanlon JW, Brown WU Jr, Weiss JB, Alper MH. Neurobehavioral responses of newborn infants after maternal epidural anesthesia. Anesthesiology 1974; 40:121–8.
16. Abboud TK, Williams V, Miller F, Henriksen EH, Doan T, Van Dorsen JP, Earl S. Comparative fetal, maternal,

and neonatal responses following epidural analgesia with bupivacaine, chloroprocaine, and lidocaine. Anesthesiology 1981;55(Suppl):A315.
17. Chestnut DH, Bates JN, Choi WW. Continuous infusion epidural analgesia with lidocaine: efficacy and influence during the second stage of labor. Obstet Gynecol 1987;69:323–7.
18. Liston WA, Adjepon-Yamoah KK, Scott DB. Foetal and maternal lignocaine levels after paracervical block. Br J Anaesth 1973;45:750–4.
19. Kim WY, Pomerance JJ, Miller AA. Lidocaine intoxication in a newborn following local anesthesia for episiotomy. Pediatrics 1979;64:643–5.
20. Tamari I, Eldar M, Rabinowitz B, Neufeld HN. Medical treatment of cardiovascular disorders during pregnancy. Am Heart J 1982;104:1357–63.
21. Rotmensch HH, Elkayam U, Frishman W. Antiarrhythmic drug therapy during pregnancy. Ann Intern Med 1983;98:487–97.
22. Stokes IM, Evans J, Stone M. Myocardial infarction and cardiac arrest in the second trimester followed by assisted vaginal delivery under epidural analgesia at 38 weeks gestation. Case report. Br J Obstet Gynaecol 1984;91:197–8.
23. Heinonen OP, Slone D, Shapiro S. *Birth Defects and Drugs in Pregnancy*. Littleton, MA: Publishing Sciences Group, 1977.
24. Zeisler JA, Gaarder TD, De Mesquita SA. Lidocaine excretion in breast milk. Drug Intell Clin Pharm 1986; 20:691–3.
25. Committee on Drugs, American Academy of Pediatrics. The transfer of drugs and other chemicals into human milk. Pediatrics 2001;108:776–89.

Name: **LINCOMYCIN** Risk Factor: **B**

Class: **Antibiotic**

FETAL RISK SUMMARY

RECOMMENDATION: Compatible

No reports linking the use of lincomycin with congenital defects have been located. The antibiotic crosses the placenta, achieving cord serum levels about 25% of the maternal serum level (1,2). Multiple IM injections of 600 mg did not result in accumulation in the amniotic fluid (2). No effects on the newborn were observed.

The progeny of 302 patients treated at various stages of pregnancy with oral lincomycin, 2 g/day for 7 days, were evaluated at various intervals up to 7 years after birth (3). As compared with a control group, no increases in malformations or in delayed developmental defects were observed.

BREAST FEEDING SUMMARY

RECOMMENDATION: Compatible

Lincomycin is excreted into breast milk. Six hours following oral dosing of 500 mg every 6 hours for 3 days, serum and milk levels in nine patients averaged 1.37 and 1.28 μg/mL, respectively, a milk:plasma ratio of 0.9 (1). Much lower milk:plasma ratios of 0.13–0.17 have also been reported (4). Although no adverse effects have been reported, three potential problems exist for the nursing infant: modification of bowel flora, direct effects on the infant, and interference with the interpretation of culture results if a fever workup is required.

References

1. Medina A, Fiske N, Hjelt-Harvey I, Brown CD, Prigot A. Absorption, diffusion, and excretion of a new antibiotic, lincomycin. Antimicrob Agents Chemother 1963; 189–96.
2. Duignan NM, Andrews J, Williams JD. Pharmacological studies with lincomycin in late pregnancy. Br Med J 1973;3:75–8.
3. Mickal A, Panzer JD. The safety of lincomycin in pregnancy. Am J Obstet Gynecol 1975;121:1071–4.
4. Wilson JT. Milk/plasma ratios and contraindicated drugs. In Wilson JT, ed. *Drugs in Breast Milk*. Balgowlah, Australia: ADIS Press, 1981:78–9.

Name:	**LINDANE**	Risk Factor:	**B_M**
Class:	**Scabicide/Pediculicide**		

FETAL RISK SUMMARY

RECOMMENDATION: Limited Human Data - Animal Data Suggest Low Risk

Lindane (γ-benzene hexachloride) is used topically for the treatment of lice and scabies. Small amounts are absorbed through the intact skin and mucous membranes (1).

No published reports linking the use of this drug with toxic or congenital defects have been located, but one reference suggested that it should be used with caution because of its potential to produce neurotoxicity, convulsions, and aplastic anemia (2). Animal studies have not shown a teratogenic effect (3,4) and in one, lindane seemed to have a protective effect when given with known teratogens (5). Multigeneration reproduction studies in mice, rats, rabbits, pigs, and dogs at oral doses up to 10 times the human dose have revealed no evidence of impaired fertility or fetal harm (6).

In a surveillance study of Michigan Medicaid recipients conducted between 1985 and 1992 involving 229,101 completed pregnancies, 1417 newborns had been exposed to topical lindane during the 1st trimester (F. Rosa, personal communication, FDA, 1993). A total of 64 (4.5%) major birth defects were observed (60 expected). Specific data were available for six defect categories, including (observed/expected) 17/14 cardiovascular defects, 4/2 oral clefts, 0/0.7 spina bifida, 1/4 polydactyly, 2/2 limb reduction defects, and 7/3 hypospadias. Only with the latter defect is there a suggestion of a possible association, but other factors, including concurrent drug use and chance, may be involved.

If maternal treatment is required, the manufacturers recommend using lindane no more than twice during a pregnancy (6,7). However, because of lindane's potentially serious toxicity, the Centers for Disease Control and Prevention (CDC) recommends, in pregnant women, permethrin or pyrethrins with piperonyl butoxide for the treatment of lice infestations and permethrin for the treatment of scabies (see Permethrin and Pyrethrins with Piperonyl Butoxide) (8).

BREAST FEEDING SUMMARY

RECOMMENDATION: Limited Human Data - Probably Compatible

Lindane is excreted into breast milk after ingestion of the agent from treated foods (6). Concentrations in milk ranged from 0 to 113 ppb.

No reports describing the use of lindane in lactating women have been located. Based on theoretical considerations, a manufacturer estimated the upper limit of lindane levels in breast milk to be approximately 30 ng/mL after maternal application (E. D. Rickard, personal communication, Reed & Carnrick Pharmaceuticals, 1983). A nursing infant consuming 1000 mL of milk/day would thus ingest about 30 μg/day of lindane. This is in the same general range that the infant would absorb after direct topical application (E. D. Rickard, personal communication, 1983). These amounts are probably clinically insignificant. Waiting 4 days after discontinuing lindane lotion, however, should prevent exposure of a nursing infant to any drug in the milk (6).

References

1. American Hospital Formulary Service. *Drug Information 1997*. Bethesda, MD: American Society of Health-System Pharmacists, 1997:2711–3.
2. Sanmiguel GS, Ferrer AP, Alberich MT, Genaoui BM. Consideraciones sobre el tratamiento de la infancia y en el embarazo. Actas Dermosifilogr 1980;71:105–8.
3. Palmer AK, Cozens DD, Spicer EJF, Worden AN. Effects of lindane upon reproduction function in a 3-generation study of rats. Toxicology 1978;10:45–54.
4. Palmer AK, Bottomley AM, Worden AN, Frohberg H, Bauer A. Effect of lindane on pregnancy in the rabbit and rat. Toxicology 1978;10:239–47.
5. Shtenberg AI, Torchinski I. Adaptation to the action of several teratogens as a consequence of preliminary administration of pesticides to females. Biull Eksp Biol Med 1977;83:227–8.
6. Product information. Lindane Lotion USP 1%. Alpharma, 2001.
7. Product information. Kwell. Reed & Carnrick Pharmaceuticals, 1990.
8. CDC. 1998 guidelines for treatment of sexually transmitted diseases. MMWR 1998;47(RR-1):106–8.

Name:	**LINEZOLID**	Risk Factor:	C_M
Class:	**Anti-infective**		

FETAL RISK SUMMARY

RECOMMENDATION: Compatible - Maternal Benefit >> Embryo/Fetal Risk

Linezolid, is a synthetic, oxazolidinone class, antibacterial agent that is indicated for the treatment of gram positive bacteria, including vancomycin-resistant enterococcus (VRE). It is available in both oral and IV formulations.

Reproduction studies have been conducted in pregnant mice and rats (1). No evidence of teratogenicity was seen in mice and rats at doses that were 4 and 1 times the expected human exposure based on area under the plasma concentration curve (EHE), respectively. However, in mice, embryo and fetal toxicity (embryo death, including total litter loss, decreased fetal weight, and an increased incidence of costal cartilage fusion) and maternal toxicity (clinical signs and reduced weight gain) were seen at this dose. In pregnant rats, doses 0.13 and 0.64 times the EHE resulted in slight fetal toxicity (reduced fetal weight and ossification of sternebrae). The higher dose (0.64 times the EHE) caused slight maternal toxicity consisting of reduced body weight gain. When this dose was given during pregnancy and lactation, pup survival was decreased on postnatal days 1 to 4. In addition, when surviving pups reached maturity and were mated, they had decreased fertility as evidenced by an increase in pre-implantation loss (1).

It is not known if linezolid crosses the human placenta. The molecular weight (about 337) is low enough that transfer to the fetus should be expected.

No reports describing the use of linezolid during human pregnancy have been located. Because of the lack of human pregnancy data, other antibiotics with this experience should be used if possible. If no other alternatives are available and linezolid must be used, the maternal benefit appears to outweigh the unknown fetal risk.

BREAST FEEDING SUMMARY

RECOMMENDATION: No Human Data - Potential Toxicity

Linezolid and the inactive metabolites are excreted in the milk of lactating rats at concentrations similar to those in the plasma. The molecular weight (about 337) is low enough that excretion into breast milk should also be expected. The effects of this exposure on a nursing infant are unknown. Because myelosuppression has occurred in animals (dogs and rats) exposed to doses at or below the EHE (1), and reversible thrombocytopenia (duration dependent) in adult humans, women taking linezolid should probably not breast-feed.

Reference

1. Product information. Zyvox. Pharmacia & Upjohn, 2001.

Name:	**LIOTHYRONINE**	Risk Factor:	A_M
Class:	**Thyroid**		

FETAL RISK SUMMARY

RECOMMENDATION: Compatible

Liothyronine (T_3) is a naturally occurring thyroid hormone produced by the mother and the fetus. It is used during pregnancy for the treatment of hypothyroidism (see also Levothyroxine and Thyroid). There is little or no transplacental passage of the hormone at physiologic serum concentrations (1–3). Limited placental passage of T_3 to the fetus has been demonstrated following very large doses (4,5).

In a large prospective study, 34 mother-child pairs were exposed to liothyronine during the 1st trimester (6). No association between the drug and fetal defects was found. Maternal hypothyroidism itself has been reported to be responsible for poor pregnancy outcome (7). Others have not found this association, claiming that fetal development is not directly affected by maternal thyroid function (8).

Combination therapy with thyroid-antithyroid drugs was advocated at one time for the treatment of hyperthyroidism but is now considered inappropriate (see Propylthiouracil).

BREAST FEEDING SUMMARY

RECOMMENDATION: Compatible

T_3 is excreted into breast milk in low concentrations. The effect on the nursing infant is not thought to be physiologically significant, although at least one report concluded otherwise (9). An infant was diagnosed as athyrotic shortly after breast-feeding was stopped at age 10 months (9). Growth was at the 97th percentile during breast-feeding, but the bone age remained that of a newborn. Mean levels of T_3 in breast milk during the last trimester (12 patients) and within 48 hours of delivery (22 patients) were 1.36 and 2.86 ng/mL, respectively. A 1978 study reported milk concentrations varying between 0.4 and 2.38 ng/mL (range 0.1–5 ng/mL) from the day of delivery to 148 days postpartum (10). No liothyronine was detected in a number of the samples. Levels in three instances, collected 16, 20, and 43 months postpartum, ranged from 0.68 to 4.5 ng/mL with the highest concentration measured at 20 months. From the 1st week through 148 days post-delivery, the calculated maximum amount of T_3 that a nursing infant would have ingested was 2.1–2.6 μg/day, far less than the dose required to treat congenital hypothyroidism (10). However, it was concluded that this was enough to mask the symptoms of the disease without halting its progression. In a study comparing serum T_3 levels between 22 breast-fed and 29 formula-fed infants, significantly higher levels were found in the breast-feeding group (11). The levels, 2.24 and 1.79 ng/mL, were comparable to previous reports and probably were of doubtful clinical significance. A 1980 report described four exclusively breast-fed infants with congenital hypothyroidism that were diagnosed between the ages of 2 and 79 days (12). Breast-feeding did not hinder making the diagnosis. Another 1980 research report evaluated clinical and biochemical thyroid parameters in 45 hypothyroid infants, 12 of whom were breast-fed (13). No difference was detected between the breast-fed and bottle-fed babies, leading to the conclusion that breast milk does not offer protection against the effects of congenital hypothyroidism. As reported in a 1985 paper, serum concentrations of T_3 were similar in breast-fed and bottle-fed infants at 5, 10, and 15 days postpartum (14).

Japanese researchers found a T_3 milk:plasma ratio of 0.36 (15). No correlation was discovered between serum T_3 and milk T_3 or total daily T_3 excretion. Neither was there a correlation between milk T_3 levels and milk protein concentration or daily volume of milk. They concluded that breast-feeding has no influence on the pituitary-thyroid axis of normal babies. A Swedish investigation measured higher levels of T_3 in milk 1–3 months after delivery as compared with T_3 levels in early colostrum (16). The concentrations were comparable to the studies cited above.

In summary, liothyronine breast milk concentrations are too low to protect a hypothyroid infant completely from the effects of the disease. The levels are also too low to interfere with neonatal thyroid screening programs (14).

References

1. Grumbach MM, Werner SC. Transfer of thyroid hormone across the human placenta at term. J Clin Endocrinol Metab 1956;16:1392–5.
2. Kearns JE, Hutson W. Tagged isomers and analogues of thyroxine (their transmission across the human placenta and other studies). J Nucl Med 1963;4:453–61.
3. Fisher DA, Lehman H, Lackey C. Placental transport of thyroxine. J Clin Endocrinol Metab 1964;24:393–400.
4. Raiti S, Holzman GB, Scott RI, Blizzard RM. Evidence for the placental transfer of tri-iodothyronine in human beings. N Engl J Med 1967;277:456–9.
5. Dussault J, Row VV, Lickrish G, Volpe R. Studies of serum triiodothyronine concentration in maternal and cord blood: transfer of triiodothyronine across the human placenta. J Clin Endocrinol Metab 1969;29:595–606.
6. Heinonen OP, Slone D, Shapiro S. *Birth Defects and Drugs in Pregnancy*. Littleton, MA: Publishing Sciences Group, 1977:388–400.
7. Potter JD. Hypothyroidism and reproductive failure. Surg Gynecol Obstet 1980;150:251–5.
8. Montoro M, Collea JV, Frasier SD, Mestman JH. Successful outcome of pregnancy in women with hypothyroidism. Ann Intern Med 1981;94:31–4.
9. Bode HH, Vanjonack WJ, Crawford JD. Mitigation of cretinism by breast-feeding. Pediatrics 1978;62:13–6.
10. Varma SK, Collins M, Row A, Haller WS, Varma K. Thyroxine, triiodothyronine, and reverse triiodothyronine concentrations in human milk. J Pediatr 1978;93:803–6.
11. Hahn HB Jr, Spiekerman AM, Otto WR, Hossalla DE. Thyroid function tests in neonates fed human milk. Am J Dis Child 1983;137:220–2.
12. Abbassi V, Steinour TA. Successful diagnosis of congenital hypothyroidism in four breast-fed neonates. J Pediatr 1980;97:259–61.
13. Letarte J, Guyda H, Dussault JH, Glorieux J. Lack of protective effect of breast-feeding in congenital hypothyroidism: report of 12 cases. Pediatrics 1980;65:703–5.
14. Franklin R, O'Grady C, Carpenter L. Neonatal thyroid function: comparison between breast-fed and bottle-fed infants. J Pediatr 1985;106:124–6.
15. Mizuta H, Amino N, Ichihara K, Harade T, Nose O, Tanizawa O, Miyai K. Thyroid hormones in human milk and influence on thyroid function of breast-fed babies. Pediatr Res 1983;17:468–71.
16. Jansson L, Ivarsson S, Larsson I, Ekman R. Triiodothyronine and thyroxine in human milk. Acta Paediatr Scand 1983;72:703–5.

Name:	**LIOTRIX**	Risk Factor:	**A**
Class:	**Thyroid**		

Liotrix is a synthetic combination of levothyroxine and liothyronine (see Levothyroxine and Liothyronine).

Name:	**LIPIDS**	Risk Factor:	**C**
Class:	**Nutrient**		

FETAL RISK SUMMARY

RECOMMENDATION: Compatible

Lipids (IV fat emulsions) are a mixture of neutral triglycerides, primarily unsaturated fatty acids, prepared from either soybean or safflower oil. Egg yolk phospholipids are used as an emulsifier. Most fatty acids readily cross the placenta to the fetus (1,2).

A number of reports have described the use of lipids during pregnancy in conjunction with dextrose/amino acid solutions (see Hyperalimentation, Parenteral) (3–14). However, one investigator concluded in 1977 that lipid infusions were contraindicated during pregnancy because (a) an excessive increase in serum triglycerides, often with ketonemia, would result because of the physiologic hyperlipemia present during pregnancy; (b) premature labor would occur; and (c) placental infarctions would occur from fat deposits and cause placental insufficiency (15). A brief 1986 correspondence also stated that lipids were contraindicated because of the danger of inducing premature uterine contractions with the potential for abortion or premature delivery (16). This conclusion was based on the observation that lipids contain arachidonic acid, a precursor to prostaglandins E_2 and $F_{2\alpha}$ (16). However, another investigator concluded that concentrations of arachidonic acid must arise from decidual membranes or amniotic fluid (i.e., must be very close to the myometrium) to produce this effect (17).

A 1986 report described four women in whom parenteral hyperalimentation was used during pregnancy, two of whom also received lipids, and, in addition, reviewed the literature for both total parenteral nutrition and lipid use during gestation (18). These authors concluded that there was no evidence that lipid emulsions had an adverse effect on pregnancy (18).

The effect of oral administration of a triglyceride emulsion on the fetal breathing index was described in a 1982 publication (19). Six women, at 32 weeks' gestation, ingested 100 mL of the emulsion containing 67 g of triglycerides and were compared with six women, also at 32 weeks' gestation, which drank mineral water. No correlation was noted between the fetal breathing index and plasma free fatty acids, glucose, insulin, glucagon, total cortisol, free cortisol, or triglyceride levels (19).

Cardiac tamponade, resulting in maternal and fetal death, has been reported in a woman receiving central hyperalimentation with lipids for severe hyperemesis gravidarum (see Hyperalimentation, Parenteral, for details of this case) (20).

A stillborn male fetus was delivered at 22 weeks' gestation from a 31-year-old woman with hyperemesis gravidarum who had been treated with total IV hyperalimentation and lipid emulsion for 8 weeks (21). The tan-yellow placenta showed vacuolated syncytial cells and Hofbauer cells that stained for fat (21). The placental fat deposits, the first to be described with parenteral lipids, were thought to be the cause of the fetal demise (21).

Based on limited clinical experience, intravenous lipids apparently do not pose a significant risk to the mother or fetus, although the case above is indicative that the therapy is not without danger. Standard precautions, as taken with nonpregnant patients, should be followed when administering these solutions during pregnancy.

BREAST FEEDING SUMMARY

RECOMMENDATION: No Human Data - Probably Compatible

No reports describing the use of IV lipids during lactation have been located.

References

1. Elphick MC, Filshie GM, Hull D. The passage of fat emulsion across the human placenta. Br J Obstet Gynaecol 1978;85:610–8.
2. Hendrickse W, Stammers JP, Hull D. The transfer of free fatty acids across the human placenta. Br J Obstet Gynaecol 1985;92:945–52.
3. Hew LR, Deitel M. Total parenteral nutrition in gynecology and obstetrics. Obstet Gynecol 1980;55:464–8.
4. Tresadern JC, Falconer GF, Turnberg LA, Irving MH. Successful completed pregnancy in a patient maintained on home parenteral nutrition. Br Med J 1983; 286:602–3.
5. Tresadern JC, Falconer GF, Turnberg LA, Irving MH. Maintenance of pregnancy in a home parenteral nutrition patient. JPEN J Parenter Enteral Nutr 1984;8: 199–202.
6. Seifer DB, Silberman H, Catanzarite VA, Conteas CN, Wood R, Ueland K. Total parenteral nutrition in obstetrics. JAMA 1985;253;2073–5.
7. Lavin JP Jr, Gimmon Z, Miodovnik M, von Meyenfeldt M, Fischer JE. Total parenteral nutrition in a pregnant insulin-requiring diabetic. Obstet Gynecol 1982;59:660–4.
8. Rivera-Alsina ME, Saldana LR, Stringer CA. Fetal growth sustained by parenteral nutrition in pregnancy. Obstet Gynecol 1984;64:138–41.
9. Di Costanzo J, Martin J, Cano N, Mas JC, Noirclerc M. Total parenteral nutrition with fat emulsions during pregnancy—nutritional requirements: a case report. JPEN J Parenter Enteral Nutr 1982;6: 534–8.
10. Young KR. Acute pancreatitis in pregnancy: two case reports. Obstet Gynecol 1982;60:653–7.
11. Breen KJ, McDonald IA, Panelli D, Ihle B. Planned pregnancy in a patient who was receiving home parenteral nutrition. Med J Aust 1987;146:215–7.
12. Levine MG, Esser D. Total parenteral nutrition for the treatment of severe hyperemesis gravidarum: maternal nutritional effects and fetal outcome. Obstet Gynecol 1988;72:102–7.
13. Herbert WNP, Seeds JW, Bowes WA, Sweeney CA. Fetal growth response to total parenteral nutrition in pregnancy: a case report. J Reprod Med 1986;31: 263–6.
14. Hatjis CG, Meis PJ. Total parenteral nutrition in pregnancy. Obstet Gynecol 1985;66:585–9.
15. Heller L. Parenteral nutrition in obstetrics and gynecology. In Greep JM, Soeters PB, Wesdorp RIC, et al, eds. *Current Concepts in Parenteral Nutrition*. The Hague: Martinus Nijhoff Medical Division, 1977:179–86.
16. Neri A. Fetal growth sustained by parenteral nutrition in pregnancy. Obstet Gynecol 1986;67:753.
17. Saldana LR. Fetal growth sustained by parenteral nutrition in pregnancy (in reply). Obstet Gynecol 1986;67:753.
18. Lee RV, Rodgers BD, Young C, Eddy E, Cardinal J. Total parenteral nutrition during pregnancy. Obstet Gynecol 1986;68:563–71.
19. Neldam S, Hornnes PJ, Kuhl C. Effect of maternal triglyceride ingestion on fetal respiratory movements. Obstet Gynecol 1982;59:640–2.
20. Greenspoon JS, Masaki DI, Kurz CR. Cardiac tamponade in pregnancy during central hyperalimentation. Obstet Gynecol 1989;73:465–6.
21. Jasnosz KM, Pickeral JJ, Graner S. Fat deposits in the placenta following maternal total parenteral nutrition with intravenous lipid emulsion. Arch Pathol Lab Med 1995;119:555–7.

Name: **LISINOPRIL** Risk Factor: **C_M***

Class: **Antihypertensive**

FETAL RISK SUMMARY

RECOMMENDATION: Human Data Suggest Risk in 2nd and 3rd Trimesters

Lisinopril is a long-acting angiotensin I-converting enzyme (ACE) inhibitor used for the treatment of hypertension (see also Captopril and Enalapril). The drug is not teratogenic in mice, rats, and rabbits treated with doses up to 55, 33, and 0.15 times, respectively, the maximum recommended human daily dose based on body surface area (1).

Use of lisinopril limited to the 1st trimester does not appear to present a significant risk to the fetus, but fetal exposure after this time has been associated with teratogenicity and severe toxicity in the fetus and newborn, including death. The pattern of fetal toxicity, including teratogenicity, appears to be similar to that experienced with captopril and enalapril.

In a surveillance study of Michigan Medicaid recipients conducted between 1985 and 1992 involving 229,101 completed pregnancies, 15 newborns had been exposed to lisinopril during the 1st trimester (F. Rosa, personal communication, FDA, 1993). Two (13.3%) major birth defects were observed (0.6 expected), one of which was polydactyly (none expected). No anomalies were observed in five other categories of defects (cardiovascular defects, oral clefts, spina bifida, limb reduction defects, and hypospadias) for which specific data were available.

Two cases of lisinopril-induced perinatal renal failure in newborns were published in a 1991 abstract (2). Additional details were not provided other than that both infants had been exposed *in utero* to the agent. The authors noted, however, that the effects of angiotensin-converting enzyme inhibitors in the newborn are prolonged unless removed by dialysis, because 95% of the active metabolites are eliminated by renal excretion (2).

In a 2000 report, a woman with normal amniotic fluid volume and fetal measurements by ultrasound consistent with 18 weeks' gestation presented with severe chronic hypertension (3). She had been treated before conception and during the first 16 weeks with lisinopril but had self-stopped therapy 2 weeks before presentation. Because a combination of methyldopa, nifedipine, and labetalol failed to control her blood pressure, lisinopril was re-added to her regimen. At 22 weeks' gestation, the amniotic fluid index was 8 but declined to 0 at 24 weeks' gestation. A cesarean section was performed at about 27 weeks' gestation because of deteriorating maternal and fetal condition. The growth retarded, 680-g (3rd percentile) female infant had minimal respiratory distress syndrome. Severe renal impairment (maximum urine output 0.3 mL/kg/hour) was present during the first 6 days before improving after corrective surgery for bowel perforations secondary to necrotizing enterocolitis. She was discharged home on day 102 (3).

An 18-year-old woman received lisinopril, 10 mg/day, throughout gestation for the treatment of essential hypertension (4). No mention of amniotic fluid levels during pregnancy was made in this brief report. She delivered a premature, 1.48-kg, anuric infant at 33 weeks' gestation. Fetal calvarial hypoplasia was present. The normal sized kidneys showed no evidence of perfusion on renal ultrasonography. An open biopsy at 11 weeks of age showed extensive atrophy and loss of tubules with interstitial fibrosis. The findings were compatible with exposure to a nephrotoxic agent. Peritoneal dialysis was instituted on day 8. Measurements of the drug in the dialysate indicated that removal of lisinopril was occurring. At 12 months of age, the infant continued to require dialysis (4).

Three cases of *in utero* exposure to ACE inhibitors, one of which was lisinopril, were reported in a 1992 abstract (5). The infant, delivered at 32 weeks' gestation because of severe oligohydramnios and fetal distress, suffered from intrauterine growth retardation, hypocalvaria, renal tubular dysplasia, and persistent renal insufficiency. The profound neonatal hypotension and anuria observed at birth improved only after dialysis. At the time of the report, the 15-month-old infant was maintained on dialysis.

A 1992 reference described the effects of ACE inhibitors on pregnancy outcome (6). Among 106,813 women enrolled in the Tennessee Medicaid program who delivered either a liveborn or stillborn infant, 19 had taken either lisinopril, captopril, or enalapril during gestation. Two of the infants had adverse outcomes (see Enalapril and Captopril for details).

Six pregnancies treated with lisinopril were reported in a 1997 study of 19 pregnancies exposed to ACE inhibitors (7). Lisinopril therapy was stopped in the 1st trimester in four pregnancies and at 20 and 25 weeks' gestation, respectively, in the others. No congenital anomalies or renal dysfunction were noted in the six neonates (7).

A case of lisinopril-induced fetopathy and hypocalvaria was included in a study examining the causes of fetal skull hypoplasia (8). Among 14 known cases of hypocalvaria or acalvaria, 5 were caused by ACE inhibitors. The authors speculated that the underlying pathogenetic mechanism in these cases is fetal hypotension (8).

A 1991 article examining the teratogenesis of ACE inhibitors cited evidence linking fetal calvarial hypoplasia with the use of these agents after the 1st trimester (9). The proposed mechanism was drug-induced oligohydramnios that allowed the uterine musculature to exert direct pressure on the fetal skull. This mechanical insult, combined with drug-induced fetal hypotension, could inhibit peripheral perfusion and ossification of the calvaria (9).

In summary, ACE inhibitors present a major risk to the fetus in terms of toxicity, including fetal and neonatal renal failure, intrauterine growth retardation, prematurity, severe neonatal hypotension, and fetal and neonatal death. Oligohydramnios may occur resulting in pulmonary hypoplasia, limb contractures, persistent patent ductus arteriosus, craniofacial deformation, and neonatal death (10,11). These agents appear to be teratogenic when used in the 2nd and 3rd trimesters, causing fetal calvarial hypoplasia and renal anomalies (see also Captopril and Enalapril). The cause of these defects is probably related to fetal hypotension and decreased renal blood flow. Because of these reports, some investigators contend that drugs in this class should not be used in pregnancy (10–13). In those cases in which lisinopril must be used to treat the mother's disease, close monitoring of amniotic fluid levels and fetal well-being are required. Newborn renal function and blood pressure should also be monitored. If oligohydramnios occurs, stopping the drug may resolve the problem but may not improve infant outcome because of irreversible fetal damage (10). Guidelines for counseling exposed pregnant patients have been published and should be of benefit to health professionals faced with this task (9,10). If lisinopril is used in pregnancy, healthcare professionals are encouraged to call the toll free number (800-670-6126) for information about patient enrollment in the Motherisk study.

[**Risk Factor* D_M *if used in 2nd or 3rd trimesters.*]

BREAST FEEDING SUMMARY

RECOMMENDATION: No Human Data - Probably Compatible

No reports describing the use of lisinopril during human lactation have been located. The drug is excreted in the milk of lactating rats (1). The molecular weight (about 442) is low enough that excretion into breast milk should be expected. Two similar agents are present in milk in low concentrations and are classified by the American Academy of Pediatrics as compatible with breast-feeding (see Captopril and Enalapril).

References

1. Product information. Prinivil. Merck, 2001.
2. Rosa F, Bosco L. Infant renal failure with maternal ACE inhibition (abstract). Am J Obstet Gynecol 1991;164:273.
3. Tomlinson AJ, Campbell J, Walker JJ, Morgan C. Malignant primary hypertension in pregnancy treated with lisinopril. Ann Pharmacother 2000;34:180–2.
4. Bhatt-Mehta V, Deluga KS. Chronic renal failure (CRF) in a neonate due to in-utero exposure to lisinopril. Presented at the 12th Annual Meeting of the American College of Clinical Pharmacy, Minneapolis, MN, August 20, 1991, Abstract No. 43.
5. Pryde PG, Nugent CE, Sedman AB, Barr M Jr. ACE inhibitor fetopathy (abstract). Am J Obstet Gynecol 1992;166:348.
6. Piper JM, Ray WA, Rosa FW. Pregnancy outcome following exposure to angiotensin-converting enzyme inhibitors. Obstet Gynecol 1992;80:429–32.
7. Lip GYH, Churchill D, Beevers M, Auckett A, Beevers DG. Angiotensin-converting-enzyme inhibitors in early pregnancy. Lancet 1997;350:1446–7.
8. Barr M Jr, Cohen MM Jr. ACE inhibitor fetopathy and hypocalvaria: the kidney-skull connection. Teratology 1991;44:485–95.
9. Brent RL, Beckman DA. Angiotensin-converting enzyme inhibitors, an embryopathic class of drugs with

unique properties: information for clinical teratology counselors. Teratology 1991;43:543–6.
10. Barr M Jr. Teratogen update: angiotensin-converting enzyme inhibitors. 1994;50:399–409.
11. Shotan A, Widerhorn J, Hurst A, Elkayam U. Risks of angiotensin-converting enzyme inhibition during pregnancy: experimental and clinical evidence, potential mechanisms, and recommendations for use. Am J Med 1994;96:451–6.
12. Lindheimer MD, Katz AI. Hypertension in pregnancy. N Engl J Med 1985;313:675–80.
13. Lindheimer MD, Barron WM. Enalapril and pregnancy-induced hypertension. Ann Intern Med 1988;108:91.

Name: **LITHIUM** Risk Factor: **D**
Class: **Tranquilizer**

FETAL RISK SUMMARY

RECOMMENDATION: Human Data Suggest Risk

Lithium is used for the treatment of manic episodes of manic-depressive illness. The drug is available as either lithium carbonate or lithium citrate.

The use of lithium during the 1st trimester may be related to an increased incidence of congenital defects, particularly of the cardiovascular system. A 1987 review of psychotherapeutic drugs in pregnancy evaluated several reproduction studies of lithium in animals, including mice, rats, rabbits, and monkeys, and observed no teratogenicity except in rats (1).

Lithium freely crosses the placenta, equilibrating between maternal and cord serum (1–6). Amniotic fluid concentrations exceed cord serum levels (3).

Frequent reports have described the fetal effects of lithium, the majority from data accumulated by the Lithium Baby Register (1,2,7–15). The Register, founded in Denmark in 1968 and later expanded internationally, collects data on known cases of 1st trimester exposure to lithium. By 1977, the Register included 183 infants, 20 (11%) with major congenital anomalies (13). Of the 20 malformed infants, 15 involved cardiovascular defects, including 5 with the rare Ebstein's anomaly. Others have also noted the increased incidence of Ebstein's anomaly in lithium-exposed babies (16). Two new case reports bring the total number of infants with cardiovascular defects to 17, or 77% (17 of 22) of the known malformed children (17,18). Ebstein's anomaly has been diagnosed in the fetus during the 2nd trimester by echocardiography (19). Details on 16 of the malformed infants are given below.

AUTHOR	CASE NO.	DEFECT
Weinstein and Goldfield (12)	1	Coarctation of aorta
	2	High intraventricular septal defect
	3	Stenosis of aqueduct with hydrocephalus, spina bifida with sacral meningomyelocele, bilateral talipes equinovarus with paralysis; atonic bladder, patulous rectal sphincter and rectal prolapse (see also reference 7)
	4	Unilateral microtia
	5	Mitral atresia, rudimentary left ventricle without inlet or outlet, aorta and pulmonary artery arising from right ventricle, patent ductus arteriosus, left superior vena cava

(continued)

AUTHOR	CASE NO.	DEFECT
Weinstein and Goldfield (12) *(contd.)*	6	Mitral atresia
	7	Ebstein's anomaly
	8	Single umbilical artery, bilateral hypoplasia of maxilla
	9	Ebstein's anomaly
	10	Atresia of tricuspid valve
	11	Ebstein's anomaly
	12	Patent ductus arteriosus, ventricular septal defect
	13	Ebstein's anomaly
Rane et al. (17)	14	Dextrocardia and situs solitus, patent ductus arteriosus, juxtaductal aortic coarctation
Weinstein (13)	15	Ebstein's anomaly
Arnon et al. (18)	16	Massive tricuspid regurgitation, atrial flutter, congestive heart failure

In 60 of the children born without malformations, follow-up comparisons with nonexposed siblings did not show an increased frequency of physical or mental anomalies (20).

The fetal toxicity of lithium, particularly in regards to cardiac abnormalities and Ebstein's anomaly, was discussed in two 1988 references (21,22). As an indication of the rarity of Ebstein's anomaly, only approximately 300 cases of the defect have been recorded in the literature since Ebstein first described it approximately 100 years ago (21). One author concluded that the majority of tricuspid valve malformations, such as Ebstein's anomaly, are not related to drug therapy and, thus, the association between lithium and Ebstein's anomaly is weak (22).

A 1996 case report described multiple anomalies in an aborted male fetus of a woman treated with lithium carbonate monotherapy for a schizodepressive disorder (23). Maternal plasma levels before pregnancy varied between 0.58 and 0.73 mmol/L, but were not determined during gestation. Following diagnosis of multiple defects, the pregnancy was terminated at 22 weeks. The findings in the fetus were deep-seated ears, clubfeet, bilateral agenesis of the kidneys (Potter's syndrome), and a septal defect with transposition of the great vessels (23). In addition, the placenta had portions that were poorly vascularized and villi of different sizes. A causal association in this case between lithium and the defects cannot be determined. Moreover, Potter's syndrome is thought to be a genetic defect (24).

A prospective study published in 1992 gathered data from four teratogen information centers in Canada and the United States on lithium exposure in pregnancy (25). A total of 148 pregnant women using lithium (mean daily dose 927 mg) during the 1st trimester were matched by age with 148 controls. Ten women using lithium were lost to postnatal follow-up, but information was available on the fetal echocardiograms performed. The number of live births in the two groups were 76% (105/138) and 83% (123/148), respectively. One stillbirth, in the exposed group, was observed. Other outcomes (figures based on 148 women in each group) included spontaneous abortion (9% vs. 8%), therapeutic abortion (10% vs. 6%), and ectopic pregnancy (1 case vs. 0 case). None of these differences were statistically significant. However, the birthweight of lithium-exposed infants was significantly higher than that of controls, 3475 g vs. 3383 g, $p = 0.02$), even though significantly more of their mothers smoked cigarettes than did controls (31.8% vs. 15.5%, $p = 0.002$). Three exposed infants and three controls had congenital malformations. The defects observed after lithium exposure were two infants with neural tube defects (hydrocephalus and meningomyelocele—also exposed to carbamazepine during the 1st trimester; spina bifida and tethered cord) and one with meromelia who was delivered at 23 weeks' gestation and died shortly after birth. Defects in the offspring of control mothers were a ventricular septal defect (one), congenital hip dislocation (one), and cerebral palsy and torticollis (one). In addition to the above cases, one of the therapeutic abortions in the lithium group was a pregnancy terminated at 16 weeks' gestation for a severe form of Ebstein's anomaly. The mother had also taken fluoxetine, trazodone, and L-thyroxine in the 1st trimester. Ebstein's anomaly has an incidence of 1 in 20,000 in the general population (25); thus, the appearance of this case is consistent with an increased risk for the heart defect among infants of women using lithium. However, a larger sample size is still needed to define the actual magnitude of the risk. The investigators concluded that lithium is not an important human teratogen and that, because it is beneficial in the therapy of major affective disorders, women may continue the drug during pregnancy. They cautioned, however, that adequate screening tests, including level II ultrasound and fetal echocardiography, were required when lithium is used during gestation (25).

A 1994 reference evaluated the teratogenic risk of 1st trimester exposure to lithium and summarized the treatment recommendations for lithium use in women with bipolar disorder (26). Included in their assessment were four case-controlled studies in which no cases of Ebstein's anomaly occurred among 207 lithium-exposed pregnancies as compared with 2 cases of the defects among 398 nonexposed controls. These data led them to the conclusion that the risk of teratogenicity after 1st trimester exposure to lithium was lower than previously reported (26). Reaching a similar conclusion, another review, published in 1995, concluded that the risk of teratogenicity with lithium was low in women with carefully controlled therapy, but that therapy should probably be avoided during the period of cardiac organogenesis (2nd–4th month of pregnancy) (27).

Concerning nonteratogenic effects, lithium toxicity in the fetus and newborn has been reported frequently:

Cyanosis (3,17,28–32,38)
Hypotonia (3,11,28–35,38)
Bradycardia (17,29,32,34,36,38)
Thyroid depression with goiter (3,11,35)
Atrial flutter (37)
Hepatomegaly (32,38)
Electrocardiogram abnormalities (T-wave inversion) (29,36)
Cardiomegaly (30,32,37,38)
Gastrointestinal bleeding (36)
Diabetes insipidus (3,32,38,39)
Polyhydramnios (38,39)
Seizures (38)
Shock (32)

Most of these toxic effects are self-limiting, returning to normal in 1–2 weeks. This corresponds with the renal elimination of lithium from the infant. The serum half-life of lithium in newborns is prolonged, averaging 68–96 hours, as compared with the adult value of 10–20 hours (4,17). Two of the reported cases of nephrogenic diabetes insipidus persisted for 2 months or longer (3,32).

Premature labor, loss of fetal cardiac variability and acceleration, an unusual fetal heart rate pattern (double phase baseline), and depression at birth (Apgar scores of 4 and 7 at 1 and 5 minutes, respectively) were observed in a comatose mother and her infant after an acute overdose of an unknown amount of lithium and haloperidol at 31 weeks' gestation (40). Because of progressive premature labor, the female, 1526-g infant was delivered about 3 days after the overdose. The lithium concentrations of the maternal plasma, amniotic fluid, and cord vein plasma were all greater than 4 mmol/L (severe toxic effect >2.5 mmol/L), whereas the maternal level of haloperidol at delivery was about 1.6 ng/mL (40). The effects observed in the fetus and newborn were attributed to cardiac and cerebral manifestations of lithium intoxication. No follow-up on the infant was reported.

In a surveillance study of Michigan Medicaid recipients conducted between 1985 and 1992 involving 229,101 completed pregnancies, 62 newborns had been exposed to lithium during the 1st trimester (F. Rosa, personal communication, FDA, 1993). Two (3.2%) major birth defects were observed (three expected), one of which was a polydactyly (0.2 expected). No anomalies were observed in five other categories of defects (cardiovascular defects, oral clefts, spina bifida, limb reduction defects, and hypospadias) for which specific data were available.

Fetal red blood cell choline levels are elevated during maternal therapy with lithium (41). The clinical significance of this effect on choline, the metabolic precursor to acetylcholine, is unknown but may be related to the teratogenicity of lithium because of its effect on cellular lithium transport (41). In an *in vitro* study, lithium had no effect on human sperm motility (42).

A review published in 1995 used a unique system to assess the reproductive toxicity of lithium in animals and humans (43). Following an extensive evaluation of the available literature, for both experimental animals and humans, up through the early 1990s, a committee concluded that lithium, at concentrations within the human therapeutic range, could induce major malformations (particularly cardiac) and may be associated with neonatal toxicity. The evaluation included an assessment of human reproductive toxicity from lithium exposure in food, mineral supplements, swimming pools and spas, and drinking water, as well as from other environmental or occupational exposures. Because a linear relationship between lithium and toxicity was assumed, these exposures, which produce concentrations of lithium well below therapeutic levels, were not thought to produce human toxicity (43).

In the mother, renal lithium clearance rises during pregnancy, returning to pre-pregnancy levels shortly after delivery (44). In four patients, the mean clearance before delivery was 29 mL/minute, declining to 15 mL/minute 6–7 weeks after delivery, a statistically significant difference ($p < 0.01$). These data emphasize the need to monitor lithium levels closely before and after pregnancy (44).

In summary, lithium should be avoided during pregnancy if possible, especially during the period of organogenesis. In those cases in which 1st trimester use is unavoidable, adequate screening tests, including level II ultrasound and fetal echocardiography (e.g., at 18–20 weeks' gestation [45]), should be performed (25,26,45). Serum levels should also be monitored. Use of the drug near term may produce severe toxicity in the newborn, which is usually reversible. The long-term effects of *in utero* lithium exposure on postnatal development are unknown but warrant investigation.

BREAST FEEDING SUMMARY

RECOMMENDATION: Limited Human Data - Potential Toxicity

Lithium is excreted into breast milk (6,29,46–49). Milk levels are approximately 40%–50% of the maternal serum concentration (29,47,48). Infant serum and milk levels are approximately equal. In a 2003 study, milk lithium levels were determined in 11 lactating women (daily dose 600–1500 mg) that were taking the drug for the management of bipolar disorder (49). No adverse effects were observed in the infants. The estimated infant dose from milk ranged from 0% to 30% of the mother's weight-adjusted dose. These data suggested that monitoring lithium levels in milk and/or the infant's blood, combined with close observation of the nursing infant for adverse effects, was a rational approach (49).

Although no toxic effects in the nursing infant have been reported, long-term effects from this exposure have not been studied. Because of the near therapeutic blood concentrations in infants, the American Academy of Pediatrics classifies lithium as a drug that should be given to nursing mothers with caution (50).

References

1. Elia J, Katz IR, Simpson GM. Teratogenicity of psychotherapeutic medications. Psychopharmacol Bull 1987;23:531–86.
2. Weinstein MR, Goldfield M. Lithium carbonate treatment during pregnancy: report of a case. Dis Nerv Syst 1969;30:828–32.
3. Mizrahi EM, Hobbs JF, Goldsmith DI. Nephrogenic diabetes insipidus in transplacental lithium intoxication. J Pediatr 1979;94:493–5.
4. Mackay AVP, Loose R, Glen AIM. Labour on lithium. Br Med J 1976;1:878.
5. Schou M, Amdisen A. Lithium and placenta. Am J Obstet Gynecol 1975;122:541.
6. Sykes PA, Quarrie J, Alexander FW. Lithium carbonate and breast-feeding. Br Med J 1976;2:1299.
7. Schou M, Amdisen A. Lithium in pregnancy. Lancet 1970;1:1391.
8. Aoki FY, Ruedy J. Severe lithium intoxication: management without dialysis and report of a possible teratogenic effect of lithium. Can Med Assoc J 1971;105:847–8.
9. Goldfield M, Weinstein MR. Lithium in pregnancy: a review with recommendations. Am J Psychiatry 1971;127:888–93.
10. Goldfield MD, Weinstein MR. Lithium carbonate in obstetrics: guidelines for clinical use. Am J Obstet Gynecol 1973;116:15–22.
11. Schou M, Goldfield MD, Weinstein MR, Villeneuve A. Lithium and pregnancy. I. Report from the register of lithium babies. Br Med J 1973;2:135–6.
12. Weinstein MR, Goldfield MD. Cardiovascular malformations with lithium use during pregnancy. Am J Psychiatry 1975;132:529–31.
13. Weinstein MR. Recent advances in clinical psychopharmacology. I. Lithium carbonate. Hosp Form 1977;12:759–62.
14. Linden S, Rich CL. The use of lithium during pregnancy and lactation. J Clin Psychiatry 1983;44:358–61.
15. Pitts FN. Lithium and pregnancy (editorial). J Clin Psychiatry 1983;44:357.
16. Nora JJ, Nora AH, Toews WH. Lithium, Ebstein's anomaly, and other congenital heart defects. Lancet 1974;2:594–5.
17. Rane A, Tomson G, Bjarke B. Effects of maternal lithium therapy in a newborn infant. J Pediatr 1978;93:296–7.
18. Arnon RG, Marin-Garcia J, Peeden JN. Tricuspid valve regurgitation and lithium carbonate toxicity in a newborn infant. Am J Dis Child 1981;135:941–3.
19. Allan LD, Desai G, Tynan MJ. Prenatal echocardiographic screening for Ebstein's anomaly for mothers on lithium therapy. Lancet 1982;2:875–6.
20. Schou M. What happened later to the lithium babies? A follow-up study of children born without malformations. Acta Psychiatr Scand 1976;54:193–7.
21. Warkany J. Teratogen update: lithium. Teratology 1988;38:593–6.
22. Källén B. Comments on teratogen update: lithium. Teratology 1988;38:597.
23. Eikmeier G. Fetal malformations under lithium treatment. Eur Psychiatry 1996;11:376–7.
24. Moel DI. Renal agenesis, bilateral. In Buyse ML, Editor-in-Chief. *Birth Defects Encyclopedia*. Volume II. Dover, MA: Center for Birth Defects Information Service, 1990:1460–1.
25. Jacobson SJ, Jones K, Johnson K, Ceolin L, Kaur P, Sahn D, Donnenfeld AE, Rieder M, Santelli R, Smythe J, Pastuszak A, Einarson T, Koren G. Prospective multicentre study of pregnancy outcome after lithium exposure during first trimester. Lancet 1992;339:530–3.
26. Cohen LS, Friedman JM, Jefferson JW, Johnson EM, Weiner ML. A reevaluation of risk of *in utero* exposure to lithium. JAMA 1994;271:146–50.
27. Leonard A, Hantson Ph, Gerber GB. Mutagenicity, carcinogenicity and teratogenicity of lithium compounds. Mutat Res 1995;339:131–7.
28. Woody JN, London WL, Wilbanks GD Jr. Lithium toxicity in a newborn. Pediatrics 1971;47:94–6.
29. Tunnessen WW Jr, Hertz CG. Toxic effects of lithium in newborn infants: a commentary. J Pediatr 1972; 81:804–7.
30. Piton M, Barthe ML, Laloum D, Davy J, Poilpre E,

L

Venezia R. Acute lithium intoxication. Report of two cases: mother and her newborn. Therapie 1973;28:1123–44.
31. Wilbanks GD, Bressler B, Peete CH Jr, Cherny WB, London WL. Toxic effects of lithium carbonate in a mother and newborn infant. JAMA 1970;213:865–7.
32. Morrell P, Sutherland GR, Buamah PK, Oo M, Bain HH. Lithium toxicity in a neonate. Arch Dis Child 1983;58:539–41.
33. Silverman JA, Winters RW, Strande C. Lithium carbonate therapy during pregnancy: apparent lack of effect upon the fetus. Am J Obstet Gynecol 1971;109:934–6.
34. Strothers JK, Wilson DW, Royston N. Lithium toxicity in the newborn. Br Med J 1973;3:233–4.
35. Karlsson K, Lindstedt G, Lundberg PA, Selstam U. Transplacental lithium poisoning: reversible inhibition of fetal thyroid. Lancet 1975;1:1295.
36. Stevens D, Burman D, Midwinter A. Transplacental lithium poisoning. Lancet 1974;2:595.
37. Wilson N, Forfar JC, Godman MJ. Atrial flutter in the newborn resulting from maternal lithium ingestion. Arch Dis Child 1983;58:538–9.
38. Krause S, Ebbesen F, Lange AP. Polyhydramnios with maternal lithium treatment. Obstet Gynecol 1990;75:504–6.
39. Ang MS, Thorp JA, Parisi VM. Maternal lithium therapy and polyhydramnios. Obstet Gynecol 1990;76:517–9.
40. Nishiwaki T, Tanaka K, Sekiya S. Acute lithium intoxication in pregnancy. Int J Gynecol Obstet 1996;52:191–2.
41. Mallinger AG, Hanin I, Stumpf RL, Mallinger J, Kopp U, Erstling C. Lithium treatment during pregnancy: a case study of erythrocyte choline content and lithium transport. J Clin Psychiatry 1983;44:381–4.
42. Levin RM, Amsterdam JD, Winokur A, Wein AJ. Effects of psychotropic drugs on human sperm motility. Fertil Steril 1981;36:503–6.
43. Moore JA, and an IEHR Expert Scientific Committee. An assessment of lithium using the IEHR evaluative process for assessing human developmental and reproductive toxicity of agents. Reprod Toxicol 1995;9:175–210.
44. Schou M, Amdisen A, Steenstrup OR. Lithium and pregnancy. II. Hazards to women given lithium during pregnancy and delivery. Br Med J 1973;2:137–8.
45. Committee on Drugs. American Academy of Pediatrics. Use of psychoactive medication during pregnancy and possible effects on the fetus and newborn. Pediatrics 2000;105:880–7.
46. Fries H. Lithium in pregnancy. Lancet 1970;1:1233.
47. Schou M, Amdisen A. Lithium and pregnancy. III. Lithium ingestion by children breast-fed by women on lithium treatment. Br Med J 1973;2:138.
48. Kirksey A, Groziak SM. Maternal drug use: evaluation of risks to breast-fed infants. World Rev Nutr Diet 1984;43:60–79.
49. Moretti ME, Koren G, Verjee Z, Ito S. Monitoring lithium in breast milk: an individualized approach for breast-feeding mothers. Ther Drug Monit 2003;25:364–6.
50. Committee on Drugs, American Academy of Pediatrics. The transfer of drugs and other chemicals into human milk. Pediatrics 2001;108:776–89.

Name:	**LOMEFLOXACIN**	Risk Factor:	C_M
Class:	**Anti-infective (Quinolone)**		

FETAL RISK SUMMARY

RECOMMENDATION: Human Data Suggest Low Risk

Lomefloxacin is an oral, synthetic, broad-spectrum antibacterial agent. As a fluoroquinolone, it is the same class of agents as ciprofloxacin, enoxacin, levofloxacin, norfloxacin, ofloxacin, and sparfloxacin. Nalidixic acid is also a quinolone drug.

Reproductive studies have been conducted in rats, rabbits, and monkeys (1). No evidence of impaired fertility, in male or female rats, or fetal harm in pregnant rats was observed at doses up to 8 times the recommended human dose (RHD) based on body surface area. In rabbits, maternal and fetal toxicity was evident at a dose 2 times the RHD (RHD-BSA) (34 times the RHD based on body weight [RHD-BW]) consisting of reduced placental weight and variations of the coccygeal vertebrae. Pregnant monkeys dosed at 3–6 times the RHD-BSA, (6–12 times the RHD-BW) had an increased incidence of fetal loss, but no teratogenic effects were observed. As with other quinolones, multiple doses of lomefloxacin produced permanent lesions and erosion of cartilage in weight-bearing joints leading to lameness in immature rats and dogs (1).

It is not known whether lomefloxacin crosses the placenta to the human fetus, but the molecular weight (about 388) is low enough that transfer to the fetus should be expected. No reports describing the use of the antibacterial in human gestation have been located.

In a prospective follow-up study conducted by the European Network of Teratology Information Services (ENTIS), data on 549 pregnancies exposed to fluoroquinolones (none to lomefloxacin) were described in a 1996 reference (2). Data on another 116 prospective and 25 retrospective pregnancy exposures to the antibacterials were also included. Of the 666 cases with known outcome, 32 (4.8%) of the embryos, fetuses, or newborns had congenital malformations. From previous epidemiologic data, the authors concluded that the 4.8% frequency of malformations did not exceed the background rate (2). Finally, 25 retrospective reports of infants with anomalies, who had been exposed *in utero* to fluoroquinolones, were analyzed, but no specific patterns of major congenital malformations were detected.

The authors of the above study concluded that pregnancy exposure to quinolones was not an indication for termination, but that this class of antibacterial agents should still be considered contraindicated in pregnant women. Moreover, this study did not address the issue of cartilage damage from quinolone exposure and the authors recognized the need for follow-up studies of this potential toxicity in children exposed *in utero*. Because of their own and previously published findings, they further recommended that the focus of future studies should be on malformations involving the abdominal wall and urogenital system and on limb-reduction defects (2).

In summary, although no reports describing the use of lomefloxacin during human gestation have been located, the available evidence for other members of this class indicates that a causal relationship with birth defects cannot be excluded (see Ciprofloxacin, Norfloxacin, or Ofloxacin), although the lack of a pattern among the anomalies is reassuring. Because of these concerns and the available animal data, the use of lomefloxacin during pregnancy, especially during the 1st trimester, should be considered contraindicated. A 1993 review on the safety of fluoroquinolones concluded that these antibacterials should be avoided during pregnancy because of the difficulty in extrapolating animal mutagenicity results to humans and because interpretation of this toxicity is still controversial (3). The authors of this review were not convinced that fluoroquinolone-induced fetal cartilage damage and subsequent arthropathies were a major concern, even though this effect had been demonstrated in several animal species after administration to both pregnant and immature animals and in occasional human case reports involving children (3). Others have also concluded that fluoroquinolones should be contraindicated in pregnancy, because safer alternatives are usually available (2).

BREAST FEEDING SUMMARY

RECOMMENDATION: No Human Data - Probably Compatible

When first marketed, the administration of lomefloxacin during breast-feeding was not recommended because of the potential for arthropathy and other serious toxicity in the nursing infant (1). Phototoxicity has been observed when lomefloxacin was given chronically to mice, who were also exposed periodically to ultraviolet light (1). Moreover, most of the mice exposed to the combination of drug and ultraviolet light eventually developed well-differentiated squamous cell carcinoma of the skin (1). The tumors were not observed in mice exposed only to the drug.

No reports describing the use of lomefloxacin in human lactation have been located. Other quinolones are excreted into milk and, because of its relatively low molecular weight (about 388), the passage of lomefloxacin into milk should be expected. The American

Academy of Pediatrics classifies ciprofloxacin and ofloxacin as compatible with breast-feeding (see Ciprofloxacin and Ofloxacin).

References

1. Product information. Maxaquin. G. D. Searle, 1997.
2. Schaefer C, Amoura-Elefant E, Vial T, Ornoy A, Garbis H, Robert E, Rodriguez-Pinilla E, Pexieder T, Prapas N, Merlob P. Pregnancy outcome after prenatal quinolone exposure. Evaluation of a case registry of the European Network of Teratology Information Services (ENTIS). Eur J Obstet Gynecol Reprod Biol 1996;69:83–9.
3. Norrby SR, Lietman PS. Safety and tolerability of fluoroquinolones. Drugs 1993;45(Suppl 3):59–64.

Name: **LOPERAMIDE** Risk Factor: **B_M**
Class: **Antidiarrheal**

FETAL RISK SUMMARY

RECOMMENDATION: Limited Human Data - Animal Data Suggest Low Risk

No published reports linking the use of loperamide with congenital defects have been located. Reproduction studies with rats and rabbits at doses up to 30 times the human dose have revealed no evidence of impaired fertility, teratogenicity, or other fetal harm (1).

In a surveillance study of Michigan Medicaid recipients conducted between 1985 and 1992 involving 229,101 completed pregnancies, 108 newborns had been exposed to loperamide during the 1st trimester (F. Rosa, personal communication, FDA, 1993). Six (5.6%) major birth defects were observed (five expected), three of which were cardiovascular defects (one expected). No anomalies were observed in five other defect categories (oral clefts, spina bifida, polydactyly, limb reduction defects, and hypospadias) for which specific data were available. The number of cardiovascular defects suggests a possible association, but other factors, including the mother's disease, concurrent drug use, and chance, may be involved.

BREAST FEEDING SUMMARY

RECOMMENDATION: Limited Human Data - Probably Compatible

No reports describing the use of loperamide during lactation have been located. However, one study investigated loperamide oxide, a pharmacologically inactive prodrug that is reduced to loperamide as it progresses through the intestinal tract, during lactation (2). Six women in the immediate postpartum period, who were not nursing, were given two 4-mg oral doses of loperamide oxide 12 hours apart. Simultaneous plasma and milk samples were collected 12 hours after the first dose, and 6 and 24 hours after the second dose. Small amounts of loperamide oxide were measured in some of the plasma samples, but the mean loperamide oxide milk concentrations were less than 0.10 ng/mL (detection limit) at each sampling time. Mean loperamide milk concentrations for the three samples were 0.18, 0.27, and 0.19 ng/mL, respectively, corresponding to milk:plasma ratios of 0.50, 0.37, and 0.35, respectively. Although these amounts are very small, an earlier source recommended that loperamide should not be used in the lactating mother because of the potential for adverse effects in the nursing infant (3). However, because of the absence of these effects, the American Academy of Pediatrics classifies loperamide as compatible with breast-feeding (4).

References

1. Product information. Imodium. McNeil Consumer, 2000.
2. Nikodem VC, Hofmeyr GJ. Secretion of the antidiarrhoeal agent loperamide oxide in breast milk. Eur J Clin Pharmacol 1992;42:695–6.
3. Stewart JJ. Gastrointestinal drugs. In Wilson JT, ed. *Drugs in Breast Milk*. Balgowlah, Australia: ADIS Press, 1981:71.
4. Committee on Drugs, American Academy of Pediatrics. The transfer of drugs and other chemicals into human milk. Pediatrics 2001;108:776–89.

Name:	**LOPINAVIR**	Risk Factor:	**C_M**
Class:	**Antiviral**		

FETAL RISK SUMMARY

RECOMMENDATION: Compatible - Maternal Benefit >> Embryo/Fetal Risk

Lopinavir, an inhibitor of human immunodeficiency virus protease, prevents cleavage of the Gag-Pol polyproteins resulting in the production of immature, non-infectious viral particles. The agent is only available in a fixed combination (133.3 mg lopinavir/33.3 mg ritonavir per capsule). Ritonavir is a potent inhibitor of CYP3A isozyme from the hepatic cytochrome P450 system that is responsible for the metabolism of lopinavir, thereby increasing the plasma levels of lopinavir. The plasma levels of ritonavir are very low; therefore, the antiviral activity of the combination is due to lopinavir. Plasma protein binding of lopinavir is high (98%–99%), primarily by α_1-acid glycoprotein, but some is bound to albumin. The average half-life of lopinavir over a 12-hour dosing interval is 5–6 hours (1).

Reproduction studies have been conducted in rats and rabbits. In rats, doses producing systemic exposures that were approximately 0.7 (lopinavir)/1.8 (ritonavir) times the human exposure obtained with the recommended dose of 400/100 mg twice daily based on AUC (HE) resulted in embryonic and fetal toxicity (early resorption, decreased fetal viability and body weight, increased incidences of skeletal variations and skeletal ossification delays). This dose was maternal toxic. Developmental toxicity (decreased pup survival) also was observed in a peri- and postnatal rat study at doses producing exposures equal to or greater than about 0.3 (lopinavir)/0.7 (ritonavir) times the HE. In rabbits, maternal toxic doses (0.6 [lopinavir]/1.0 [ritonavir]) did not result in embryonic or fetal development toxicity (1).

It is not known if lopinavir crosses the human placenta. Small amounts of ritonavir are thought to cross the human placenta (see Ritonavir). The molecular weight (about 629) and lipid solubility of lopinavir are similar enough to ritonavir that some placental transfer of lopinavir should be expected. The extensive protein binding, however, should limit the amount crossing to the embryo or fetus. In a 2002 study, the cord:maternal blood ratio 12.25 hours after lopinavir (533 mg twice daily in combination with lamivudine and abacavir) in a woman delivering at term (38 ± 1 week) was <0.1 (<250 ng/mL/3105 ng/mL) (2,3).

The Antiretroviral Pregnancy Registry reported, for the period January 1989 through January 2004, prospective data (reported to the Registry before the outcomes were known) involving 1537 live births that had been exposed during the 1st trimester to one or more antiretroviral agents (4). Forty-seven of the newborns had congenital defects (3.1%, 95% confidence interval [CI] 2.3–4.1). In the 2407 live births with earliest exposure in the 2nd/3rd trimesters, there were 56 infants with defects (2.3%, 95% CI 1.8–3.0). The prevalence rates for the two periods did not differ significantly. There were 103 infants with birth defects among 3944 live births with exposure anytime during pregnancy (2.6%, 95% CI 2.1–3.2). The prevalence rate did not differ significantly from the rate expected in a nonexposed population (4). There were 207 outcomes exposed to lopinavir (68 in the 1st trimester and 139 in the 2nd/3rd trimesters) in combination with other antiretroviral agents. There were two birth defects in infants exposed in the 1st trimester and two exposed in the 2nd/3rd trimesters. In reviewing the birth defects of prospective and retrospective (pregnancies reported after the outcomes were known) registered cases, and clinical reports, the Registry concluded that there was no pattern of anomalies to suggest a common cause (4). (See Lamivudine for required statement.)

No reports, other than the data above, describing the use of the lopinavir/ritonavir combination with other antiretroviral agents in human pregnancy have been located. The animal data are suggestive of moderate risk because the exposure for lopinavir was less than the human therapeutic exposure. Higher doses could not be used because of the maternal toxicity. Similar animal toxicity has been observed with ritonavir (see Ritonavir). The limited human experience suggests that the embryo/fetal risk is low, at least for structural anomalies. Past reviewers have concluded that all women currently receiving antiretroviral therapy should continue to receive therapy during pregnancy (5–7). Discontinuing all therapy, however, until after 10–12 weeks' gestation is an option (7,8). If indicated, therefore, lopinavir/ritonavir should not be withheld in pregnancy, except possibly in the 1st trimester, because the expected benefit for the HIV-positive mother appears to outweigh the unknown risks to the fetus. The efficacy and safety of combined therapy in preventing vertical transmission of HIV to the newborn, however, are unknown, and zidovudine remains the only antiretroviral agent recommended for this purpose (8).

L

BREAST FEEDING SUMMARY

RECOMMENDATION: Contraindicated

No reports have been located that describe the use of the combination product lopinavir/ritonavir during human lactation. The molecular weights of lopinavir (about 629) and ritonavir (about 721), combined with their lipid solubility suggest that the drugs will be excreted into human breast milk, though the extensive plasma protein binding (98%–99%) should limit this excretion. The effects of this exposure on a nursing infant are unknown. However, reports on the use of lopinavir/ritonavir during lactation are unlikely because the combination is indicated in the treatment of patient's with HIV. HIV type 1 (HIV-1) is transmitted in milk, and in developed countries, breast-feeding is not recommended (5,6,9–12). In developing countries, breast-feeding is undertaken, despite the risk, because there are no affordable milk substitutes available.

References

1. Product information. Kaletra. Abbott Laboratories, 2004.
2. Marzolini C, Rudin C, Decosterd LA, Telenti A, Schreyer A, Biollaz J, Buclin T, and the Swiss Mother + Child HIV Cohort Study. Transplacental passage of protease inhibitors at delivery. AIDS 2002;16:889–93.
3. Marzolini C, Beguin A, Telenti A, Schreyer A, Buclin T, Biollaz J, Decosterd LA. Determination of lopinavir and nevirapine by high-performance liquid chromatography after solid-phase extraction: application for the assessment of their transplacental passage at delivery. J Chromatogr B Analyt Technol Biomed Life Sci 2002;774:127–40.
4. Antiretroviral Pregnancy Registry Steering Committee. *Antiretroviral Pregnancy Registry International Interim Report for 1 January 1989 through 31 January*

2004. Wilmington, NC: Registry Coordinating Center, 2004.
5. Carpenter CCJ, Fischi MA, Hammer SM, Hirsch MS, Jacobsen DM, Katzenstein DA, Montaner JSG, Richman DD, Saag MS, Schooley RT, Thompson MA, Vella S, Yeni PG, Volberding PA. Antiretroviral therapy for HIV infection in 1996. JAMA 1996;276:146–54.
6. Minkoff H, Augenbraun M. Antiretroviral therapy for pregnant women. Am J Obstet Gynecol 1997; 176:478–89.
7. Centers for Disease Control and Prevention. Public Health Service Task Force recommendations for the use of antiretroviral drugs in pregnant women infected with HIV-1 for maternal health and for reducing perinatal HIV-1 transmission in the United States. MMWR 1998;47:No. RR-2.
8. Public Health Service Task Force Perinatal HIV Guidelines Working Group. Summary of the updated recommendations from the Public Health Service Task Force to reduce perinatal human immunodeficiency virus-1 transmission in the United States. Obstet Gynecol 2002;99:1117–26.
9. Brown ZA, Watts DH. Antiviral therapy in pregnancy. Clin Obstet Gynecol 1990;33:276–89.
10. de Martino M, Tovo P-A, Pezzotti P, Galli L, Massironi E, Ruga E, Floreea F, Plebani A, Gabiano C, Zuccotti GV. HIV-1 transmission through breast-milk: appraisal of risk according to duration of feeding. AIDS 1992;6:991–7.
11. Van de Perre P. Postnatal transmission of human immunodeficiency virus type 1: the breast-feeding dilemma. Am J Obstet Gynecol 1995;173:483–7.
12. American College of Obstetricians and Gynecologists. Breastfeeding: maternal and infant aspects. *Educational Bulletin*. No. 258, July 2000.

Name:	**LORACARBEF**	Risk Factor:	**B_M**
Class:	**Antibiotic (Cephalosporin)**		

FETAL RISK SUMMARY

RECOMMENDATION: Compatible

Loracarbef is an oral, synthetic, β-lactam antibiotic that is closely related to the cephalosporin class of antibiotics. Reproduction studies in mice, rats, and rabbits found no evidence of impaired fertility, or reproductive performance, or fetal harm at doses up to 4, 10, and 4 times, respectively, the maximum human dose based on body surface area (1).

No reports describing the use of loracarbef in human pregnancy have been located. The closely related cephalosporins are usually considered safe to use during pregnancy (see various cephalosporins for published human experience).

BREAST FEEDING SUMMARY

RECOMMENDATION: Compatible

No reports describing the use of loracarbef during human lactation have been located. Low concentrations of the closely related cephalosporins have been measured, however, and the presence of loracarbef in milk should be expected. Three potential problems exist for the nursing infant exposed to loracarbef in milk: modification of bowel flora, direct effects on the infant, and interference with the interpretation of culture results if a fever workup is required. Although not specifically listing loracarbef, the American Academy of Pediatrics classifies other cephalosporin antibiotics as compatible with breast-feeding (2).

References

1. Product information. Lorabid. Eli Lilly and Company, 1997.
2. Committee on Drugs, American Academy of Pediatrics. The transfer of drugs and other chemicals into human milk. Pediatrics 2001;108:776–89.

Name:	**LORATADINE**	Risk Factor:	B_M
Class:	**Antihistamine**		

FETAL RISK SUMMARY

RECOMMENDATION: Limited Human Data - Animal Data Suggest Low Risk

Loratadine, a second-generation histamine H_1-receptor antagonist, is used for the treatment of symptoms related to seasonal allergic rhinitis. Studies with rats and rabbits with oral doses up to 75 and 150 times, respectively, the maximum recommended human daily oral dose based on body surface area found no evidence of teratogenicity (1). Treatment of pregnant rats from gestational day 7 through postpartum day 4 with doses up to 26 times the human clinical exposure revealed no evidence of antiandrogenic activity, as demonstrated by a lack of effect on androgen-dependent development in male offspring (2).

It is not known if loratadine crosses the human placenta. The molecular weight (about 383) is low enough, however, that passage to the fetus should be expected.

The FDA has received six reports of adverse outcomes following exposure during pregnancy, including two cases of cleft palate, and one case each of microtia and microphthalmia, deafness, tricuspid dysplasia, and diaphragmatic hernia (F. Rosa, personal communication, FDA, 1996). A relationship, if any, between loratadine and the outcomes cannot be determined from these data.

L

A 1998 non-interventional observational cohort study described the outcomes of pregnancies in women who had been prescribed one or more of 34 newly marketed drugs by general practitioners in England (3). Data were obtained by questionnaires sent to the prescribing physicians one month after the expected or possible date of delivery. In 831 (78%) of the pregnancies, a newly marketed drug was thought to have been taken during the 1st trimester with birth defects noted in 14 (2.5%) singleton births of the 557 newborns (10 sets of twins). In addition, two birth defects were observed in aborted fetuses. However, few of the aborted fetuses were examined. Loratadine was taken during the 1st trimester in 18 pregnancies. The outcomes of these pregnancies included 2 elective abortions and 16 normal, term infants (3).

A 2002 study found no increased risk of teratogenicity or other pregnancy or newborn complications for antihistamines when used in early pregnancy for the treatment of nausea and vomiting (N = 12,394) and allergy (N = 5,041) (4). In the study, 1,769 women used loratadine.

A collaborative 2003 report gathered data from four teratology information services (Canada, Israel, Italy, and Brazil) pertaining to 1st trimester loratadine exposures in 161 pregnancies (5). The outcomes of these pregnancies were compared to 161 nonexposed controls. The average daily dose of loratadine was 11.3 mg. The live birth rate, gestational age at delivery, and birth weight in the two groups were similar. There were five congenital malformations (kidney defect, aortic valve stenosis, unspecified chromosomal abnormalities, bilateral inguinal hernia, and congenital hip dislocation) in the loratadine group and six in the controls. The sample size had an 80% power to detect a 3.5-fold increase in the overall rate of defects (5).

In 2004, the Centers for Disease Control and Prevention (CDC) summarized their analysis of data from The National Birth Defects Prevention Study that examined the association between loratadine and hypospadias (6). The study population consisted of 563 male infants with hypospadias and 1444 male infants with no major birth defects. Cases and controls were born between October 1997 and June 2001. In the cases, 46 (8.2%) had multiple congenital malformations that were not recognized as phenotypes, and in 517 (91.8%) hypospadias was an isolated defect. Exposure to loratadine occurred in 11 cases and 22 controls (adjusted odds ratio [OR] 0.96, 95% confidence interval [CI] 0.41–2.22). For nonsedating (including loratadine) and sedating antihistamines, the OR (and 95% CI) were 0.95 (0.48–1.89) and 1.02 (0.68–1.53), respectively. Thus, neither type of antihistamine was associated with hypospadias (6).

In summary, no evidence of increased teratogenicity has been found in animals or humans. The human pregnancy experience is adequate to show that the drug is not a major human teratogen. Moreover, a significant increase in loratadine-induced congenital malformations would be unusual, as no other antihistamine has been shown to be a major human teratogen. If an oral antihistamine agent is required during pregnancy, first generation agents such as chlorpheniramine or tripelennamine should be considered. Previous reviews published before the availability of the above studies, concluded that loratadine and cetirizine were acceptable alternatives, except during the 1st trimester, if a first generation drug was not tolerated (7–9).

BREAST FEEDING SUMMARY

RECOMMENDATION: Limited Human Data - Probably Compatible

Loratadine and its metabolite, descarboethoxyloratadine, are excreted into human milk (1,10). Six lactating women were given a single 40-mg dose (10). The peak milk concentration, 29.2 ng/mL, occurred within 2 hours of the dose, whereas the peak plasma level, 30.5 ng/mL, was measured 1 hour after the dose. The mean milk:plasma area under the concentration curve (AUC) ratios for the parent compound and the active metabolite, measured during 48 hours, were 1.17 and 0.85, respectively (1,10). During 48 hours, the mean amounts of loratadine and metabolite recovered from the milk were 4.2 μg (0.010% of the dose) and 6.0 μg (equivalent to 7.5 μg of loratadine; 0.019% of the dose), respectively. A 4-kg infant ingesting this milk would have received a dose equivalent to 0.46% of the mother's dose on a mg/kg basis (10). Based on this estimate, and the fact that the dose used in the study was 4 times the current recommended dose, there is probably little clinical risk to a nursing infant whose mother was taking 10 mg of loratadine per day. The American Academy of Pediatrics classifies loratadine as compatible with breast-feeding (11).

References

1. Product information. Claritin. Schering Corporation, 2001.
2. McIntyre BS, Vancutsem PM, Treinen KA, Morrissey RE. Effects of perinatal loratadine exposure on male rat reproductive organ development. Reprod Toxicol 2003;17:691–7.
3. Wilton LV, Pearce GL, Martin RM, Mackay FJ, Mann RD. The outcomes of pregnancy in women exposed to newly marketed drugs in general practice in England. Br J Obstet Gynaecol 1998;105:882–9.
4. Kallen B. Use of antihistamine drugs in early pregnancy and delivery outcome. J Matern Fetal Neonatal Med 2002;11:146–52.
5. Moretti ME, Caprara D, Coutinho CJ, Bar-Oz B, Berkovitch M, Addis A, Jovanovski E, Schuler-Faccini L, Koren G. Fetal safety of loratadine use in the first trimester of pregnancy: a multicenter study. J Allergy Clin Immunol 2003;111:479–83.
6. Werler M, McCloskey C, Edmonds LD, Olney R, Honein MA, Reefhuis J. Evaluation of an association between loratadine and hypospadias—United States, 1997–2001. MMWR 2004;53:219–21.
7. Mazzotta P, Loebstein R, Koren G. Treating allergic rhinitis in pregnancy. Safety considerations. Drug Saf 1999;20:361–75.
8. Horak F, Stubner UP. Comparative tolerability of second generation antihistamines. Drug Saf 1999;20: 385–401.
9. Position statement of a joint committee of the American College of Obstetricians and Gynecologists and

the American College of Allergy, Asthma and Immunology. The use of newer asthma and allergy medications during pregnancy. Ann Allergy Asthma Immunol 2000;84:475–80.
10. Hilbert J, Radwanski E, Affrime MB, Perentesis G, Symchowicz S, Zampaglione N. Excretion of loratadine in human breast milk. J Clin Pharmacol 1988;28:234–9.
11. Committee on Drugs, American Academy of Pediatrics. The transfer of drugs and other chemicals into human milk. Pediatrics 2001;108:776–89.

Name:	**LORAZEPAM**	Risk Factor:	**D_M**
Class:	**Sedative**		

FETAL RISK SUMMARY

RECOMMENDATION: Human Data Suggest Risk in 1st and 3rd Trimesters

Lorazepam is a benzodiazepine indicated for the treatment of status epilepticus and as a preanesthetic sedative. Reproduction studies have been conducted in mice, rats, and two strains of rabbits (1). Occasional, non-dose-related malformations (reduction of tarsals, tibia, metatarsals, malrotated limbs, gastroschisis, malformed skull, and microphthalmia) were observed in rabbits, but these defects have also randomly occurred in controls. Fetal resorptions and increased fetal loss occurred in rabbits at oral (40 mg/kg) and IV (4 mg/kg) doses and higher (1).

Lorazepam crosses the placenta, achieving cord levels similar to maternal serum concentrations (2–5). Placental transfer is slower than that of diazepam, but high IV doses may produce the "floppy infant" syndrome (3). (See Diazepam for a description of this syndrome.)

A case reported in 1996 described an otherwise healthy male infant, who had been exposed throughout gestation to lorazepam (7.5–12.5 mg/day) and clozapine (200–300 mg/day), who developed transient, mild floppy infant syndrome after delivery at 37 weeks' gestation (6). The mother had taken the combination therapy for the treatment of schizophrenia. The hypotonia, attributed to lorazepam because of the absence of such reports in pregnancies exposed to clozapine alone, resolved 5 days after birth.

An abstract published in 1999 found an association between lorazepam and anal atresia (7). Using data from a French pregnancy registry, the investigators reported that among infants exposed to benzodiazepines 5 of 6 cases of anal atresia were exposed to lorazepam ($p = 0.01$) (7).

Lorazepam has been used in labor to potentiate the effects of narcotic analgesics (8). Although not statistically significant, a higher incidence of respiratory depression occurred in the exposed newborn infants.

BREAST FEEDING SUMMARY

RECOMMENDATION: Limited Human Data - Potential Toxicity

Lorazepam is excreted into breast milk in low concentrations (9,10). In one study, no effects on the nursing infant were reported (9), but the slight delay in establishing feeding was a cause for concern (11). Milk:plasma ratios in four women who had received 3.5 mg orally of lorazepam 4 hours earlier ranged from 0.15 to 0.26 (9). The mean milk concentration was 8.5 ng/mL. In another study, 5 mg of oral lorazepam was given 1 hour before labor induction and the effects on feeding behavior were measured in the newborn infants (12). During the first 48 hours, no significant effect was observed on volume of milk consumed or duration of feeding. The American Academy of Pediatrics classifies the effects of lorazepam on the nursing infant as unknown but may be of concern if exposure is prolonged (13).

References

1. Product information. Ativan. Wyeth-Ayerst Pharmaceuticals, 2000.
2. de Groot G, Maes RAA, Defoort P, Thiery M. Placental transfer of lorazepam. IRCS J Med Sci 1975;3:290.
3. McBride RJ, Dundee JW, Moore J, Toner W, Howard PJ. A study of the plasma concentrations of lorazepam in mother and neonate. Br J Anaesth 1979;51:971–8.
4. Kanto J, Aaltonen L, Liukko P, Maenpaa K. Transfer of lorazepam and its conjugate across the human placenta. Acta Pharmacol Toxicol (Copenh) 1980; 47:130–4.
5. Kanto JH. Use of benzodiazepines during pregnancy, labour and lactation, with particular reference to pharmacokinetic considerations. Drugs 1982;23:354–80.
6. Di Michele V, Ramenghi LA, Sabatino G. Clozapine and lorazepam administration in pregnancy. Eur Psychiatry 1996;11:214.
7. Bonnot O, Vollset SE, Godet PF, Robert E. Maternal exposure to lorazepam and anal atresia in newborns? Results from a hypothesis generating study of benzodiazepines and malformations (abstract). Teratology 1999;59:439–40.
8. McAuley DM, O'Neill MP, Moore J, Dundee JW. Lorazepam premedication for labour. Br J Obstet Gynaecol 1982;89:149–54.
9. Whitelaw AGL, Cummings AJ, McFadyen IR. Effect of maternal lorazepam on the neonate. Br Med J 1981;282:1106–8.
10. Summerfield RJ, Nielsen MS. Excretion of lorazepam into breast milk. Br J Anaesth 1985;57:1042–3.
11. Johnstone M. Effect of maternal lorazepam on the neonate. Br Med J 1981;282:1973.
12. Johnstone MJ. The effect of lorazepam on neonatal feeding behaviour at term. Pharmatherapeutica 1982;3:259–62.
13. Committee on Drugs, American Academy of Pediatrics. The transfer of drugs and other chemicals into human milk. Pediatrics 2001;108:776–89.

Name: **LOSARTAN** Risk Factor: **C_M***

Class: **Antihypertensive**

FETAL RISK SUMMARY

RECOMMENDATION: Human Data Suggest Risk in 2nd and 3rd Trimesters

Losartan is a selective angiotensin II receptor antagonist that is used, either alone or in combination with other antihypertensive agents, for the treatment of hypertension. Losartan, and its active metabolite, block the vasoconstrictor and aldosterone-secreting effects of angiotensin II by preventing angiotensin II from binding to AT_1 receptors.

Reproduction studies have been conducted in pregnant rats (1–3). At oral doses greater than 3 times the maximum recommended human dose of 100 mg on a body surface area basis (MRHD), reduced body weight, delayed physical and behavioral development, mortality, and renal toxicity were observed in rat fetuses and neonates (1–3). These adverse effects were attributed to exposure during late pregnancy (gestational days 15–20) and/or during lactation (1,2). A later study, however, found that the amounts of losartan and its active metabolite crossing to the rat fetus were much higher than those excreted in milk, suggesting that the renal toxicity was a result of transplacental exposure (4). The irreversible renal abnormalities in the newborn pups included dilatation of the renal pelvis, edema of the renal papilla, medial hypertrophy of intracortical arterioles, chronic renal inflammation, and irregular scarring of the renal parenchyma (2).

In fertility and reproductive performance studies, a significant decrease in fetal implants in rats was noted at a maternally toxic oral dose, approximately 24 times the MRHD. No effects on implants/pregnant female, percent post-implantation loss, or live pups/litter at parturition were observed at an oral dose approximately 12 times the MRHD (1–3).

A study published in 1999 compared the effects of losartan (an AT_1 receptor blocker) to an investigational agent, PD123319 (an AT_2 receptor inhibitor), on the developing fetal rat heart (5). Both agents markedly decreased newborn cardiac collagen content, suggesting that angiotensin II receptors are involved in the development of cardiac tissue during gestation. The hearts, however, appeared normal in size, shape, and structure. Compared to controls, PD123319 had no effect on birth weight, whereas losartan caused intrauterine growth retardation (5).

It is not known if losartan or its active metabolite crosses the human placenta to the fetus. Both the drug and its active metabolite cross the rat placenta in significant amounts only during late gestation (1,4). Moreover, the amounts in the rat fetal plasma were significantly higher than those found in maternal milk during lactation (4). In sheep at 125–132 days' gestation (mean 130 days), a bioassay indicated that losartan (10 mg/kg IV) did not cross the placenta (6). The significance of this finding for humans is unknown because the sheep placenta is epitheliochorial whereas the human placenta is hemomonochorial (6). However, because the molecular weight of losartan potassium (about 461) is low enough, passage to the human fetus should be expected.

A post-marketing safety surveillance study of losartan, published in 1999, described the outcomes of four human pregnancies (7). Three of the pregnancies were exposed to the drug in the 1st trimester and the fourth pregnancy was diagnosed about 2 months after stopping the drug. In the first case, the woman became pregnant while taking losartan and the drug was discontinued at approximately 8 weeks' gestation. Because of worsening renal failure, dialysis was required during pregnancy. She delivered a growth-retarded infant at 29 weeks who died at 9 days of age. In the second case, losartan was stopped 6 weeks after the last menstrual period. The woman delivered prematurely at 30 weeks because of preeclampsia. The infant was reported to be doing well. The third pregnancy ended with a spontaneous abortion (no specific embryo data) at 6 to 8 weeks' gestation while the woman was receiving losartan. Finally, a spontaneous abortion (no specific embryo data) occurred at 6 weeks' gestation in a woman who had stopped losartan about 2 months before the pregnancy was diagnosed. Because of the timing of the exposures, none of the outcomes appears to be related to the use of losartan. They are probably a consequence of the women's severe hypertension.

In a 2001 case report, anhydramnios was diagnosed at 31 weeks' gestation in a 31-year-old woman with periarteritis nodosa (8). Hypertension had developed at 17 weeks' gestation and losartan, 50 mg/day, had been started. Therapy was changed to methyldopa (750 mg/day), but 2 days later the woman noticed no fetal movements. Ultrasound confirmed intrauterine fetal death and she delivered a stillborn 1592-g male infant the next day. The infant had facial and limb deformities characteristic of oligohydramnios. At autopsy, pulmonary hypoplasia and hypoplastic skull bones with wide sutures were observed, but no other apparent abnormalities, including the kidneys and urinary tract, were noted. The anhydramnios and resulting fatal fetal abnormalities were attributed to losartan (8).

Two additional case reports followed the above report (9,10). A 42-year-old woman was treated with losartan (dose not specified), hydrochlorothiazide, felodipine, and metoprolol throughout gestation (9). Oligohydramnios was diagnosed at 33 weeks' gestation. A 2180-g female infant was born at 36 weeks' with limb deformities (varus of left foot, right clubfoot, and fixed external rotation of the right knee). Potter's facies, pulmonary hypertension and anuria were present and the infant died of respiratory distress on day 4. Autopsy revealed a patent ductus arteriosus and abnormal kidneys (9). In the second case, a 35-year-old woman with hypertension was treated with losartan (50 mg/day) throughout gestation (10). An examination at 22 weeks' gestation was normal but oligohydramnios was noted 34 weeks' gestation. Losartan was stopped and an amnioinfusion was given, but the woman developed signs of infection and a hypotonic male infant (weight not given) was delivered. Apgar scores were 1, 4, and 4 at 1, 5, and 10 minutes, respectively. The infant had persistent hypotension, anuria, and multivisceral failure and died on day 4 (10).

The antihypertensive mechanisms of action of losartan and angiotensin-converting enzyme (ACE) inhibitors are very close. That is, the former selectively blocks the binding of angiotensin II to AT_1 receptors, whereas the latter prevents the formation of angiotensin II itself. Therefore, use of this drug during the 2nd and 3rd trimesters may cause teratogenicity and severe fetal and neonatal toxicity that is identical to that seen with ACE inhibitors (e.g., see Captopril or Enalapril). Fetal toxic effects may include anuria, oligohydramnios, fetal hypocalvaria, intrauterine growth retardation, prematurity, and patent ductus arteriosus. Anuria-associated oligohydramnios may produce fetal limb contractures, craniofacial deformation, and pulmonary hypoplasia. Severe anuria and hypotension, that is resistant to both pressor agents and volume expansion, may occur in the newborn following *in utero* exposure to losartan. Newborn renal function and blood pressure should be closely monitored. If losartan is used in pregnancy, healthcare professionals are encouraged to call the toll free number (800-670-6126) for information about patient enrollment in the Motherisk study.

[*Risk factor D_M if used in 2nd or 3rd trimesters.*]

L

BREAST FEEDING SUMMARY

RECOMMENDATION: No Human Data - Probably Compatible

No reports describing the use of losartan during human lactation have been located. The drug and its active metabolite are found in the milk of lactating rats (1). Because the molecular weight (about 461) of losartan potassium is low enough, excretion into human breast milk should also be expected. The effects of this exposure on a nursing infant are unknown. The American Academy of Pediatrics, however, classifies ACE inhibitors, a closely related group of antihypertensive agents, as compatible with breast-feeding (see Captopril or Enalapril).

References

1. Product information. Cozaar. Merck, 2001.
2. Spence SG, Allen HL, Cukierski MA, Manson JM, Robertson RT, Eydelloth RS. Defining the susceptible period of developmental toxicity for the AT_1-selective angiotensin II receptor antagonist losartan in rats. Teratology 1995;51:367–82.
3. Spence SG, Cukierski MA, Manson JM, Robertson RT, Eydelloth RS. Evaluation of the reproductive and developmental toxicity of the AT_1-selective angiotensin II receptor antagonist losartan in rats. Teratology 1995;51:383–97.
4. Spence SG, Zacchei AG, Lee LL, Baldwin CL, Berna RA, Mattson BA, Eydelloth RS. Toxicokinetic analysis of losartan during gestation and lactation in the rat. Teratology 1996;53:245–52.
5. Lamparter S, Sun Y, Weber KT. Angiotensin II receptor blockade during gestation attenuates collagen formation in the developing rat heart. Cardiovascular Res 1999;43:165–72.
6. Stevenson KM, Gibson KJ, Lumbers ER. Comparison of the transplacental transfer of enalapril, captopril and losartan in sheep. Br J Pharmacol 1995;114: 1495–1501.
7. Mann RD, Mackay F, Pearce G, Freemantle S, Wilton LV. Losartan: a study of pharmacovigilance data on 14 522 patients. J Hum Hypertens 1999;13:551–7.
8. Saji H, Yamanaka M, Hagiwara, Ijiri R. Losartan and fetal toxic effects. Lancet 2001;357:363.
9. Lambot MA, Vermeylen D, Noel JC. Angiotensin-II-receptor inhibitors in pregnancy. Lancet 2001;357: 1619–20.
10. Martinovic J, Benachi A, Laurent N, Daikha-Dahmane F, Gubler MC. Fetal toxic effects and angiotensin-II-receptor antagonists. Lancet 2001;358:241–2.

Name:	**LOVASTATIN**	Risk Factor:	X_M
Class:	**Antilipemic Agent**		

FETAL RISK SUMMARY

RECOMMENDATION: Contraindicated

Lovastatin, a 3-hydroxy-3-methylglutaryl-coenzyme A (HMG-CoA) reductase inhibitor ("statins") that is lipophilic, is used to lower elevated levels of cholesterol. The drug is teratogenic in mice and rats, producing decreased fetal weight and skeletal malformations in exposed fetuses, at doses of 800 mg/kg/day (40 and 80 times the recommended maximum human dose based on body surface area [MRHD], respectively) (1,2). No teratogenic effects were observed in rabbits administered doses up to 15 mg/kg/day (3 times the MRHD), the maximum tolerated dose (1,2).

A surveillance study of lovastatin exposures during pregnancy, conducted by the manufacturer, was reported in 1996 (2). Among 76 women, most taking the drug before conception and then discontinuing it sometime during the 1st trimester when pregnancy was diagnosed, 19 (25%) outcomes were unknown, 1 (1.3%) outcome was pending, and 8 (11%) were electively aborted. None of the products of conception from the elective abortions underwent morphologic and/or chromosomal evaluations (3). Of the 48 pregnancies with known outcomes, there were 3 (6.3%) spontaneous abortions, 1 (2.1%) stillbirth (cord wrapped around newborn's neck; mother took unknown dose throughout gestation), 1 (2.1%) case of foot edema (probably because of labor arrest requiring cesarean section; mother took 20 mg/day during first 5 weeks), 4 (8.3%) infants with congenital defects, and 39 (81.3%) normal outcomes (all exposed during all or a portion of the 1st trimester). The details of the infants with defects (all reported retrospectively) were (dose and exposure in weeks from last menstrual period): atrial, ventricular septal defect, cerebral dysfunction, infant died at 1 month of age (40 mg/day, 0–5 weeks); vertebral defect, anal atresia, tracheoesophageal fistula with esophageal atresia (VATER association), mother also took dextroamphetamine at same time (10 mg/day, 6–11 weeks); and spina bifida, elective abortion at 18 weeks (20 mg/day, 0–3 weeks); holoprosencephaly (dose unknown, 0–6 weeks). The case involving the VATER association is also described below. Based on the timing of exposure, only the case of spina bifida can be excluded as being lovastatin-induced because the critical period for neural tube defects does not begin until the 5th week (3rd week postconception) and the mother took the drug only during the 1st week postconception (conception was estimated to have occurred in all cases 2 weeks after the last menstrual period) (2). Although the remaining three defects may have occurred by chance, an association with lovastatin cannot be excluded.

In a surveillance study of Michigan Medicaid recipients conducted between 1985 and 1992 involving 229,101 completed pregnancies, 3 newborns had been exposed to lovastatin during the 1st trimester (F. Rosa, personal communication, FDA, 1993). One (33.3%) major birth defect was observed (none expected), a cardiovascular defect. Eight other exposures to lovastatin occurred after the 1st trimester without apparent fetal harm (4).

Three retrospective spontaneous reports of birth defects suspected of being associated with 1st-trimester use of lovastatin have been received by the FDA (4). The anomalies described were aortic hypoplasia, ventricular septal defect with cerebral dysfunction, and death (one case); anal atresia and renal dysplasia (one case); and short forearm, absent thumb, and thoracic scoliosis (one case).

A case report describing the use of lovastatin in a human pregnancy was published in 1992 (5). A woman was treated for 5 weeks with lovastatin and dextroamphetamine, starting approximately 6 weeks from her last menstrual period, for progressive weight gain and hypercholesterolemia. Therapy was discontinued when her pregnancy was diagnosed at 11 weeks' gestation. A female infant was delivered by cesarean section at 39 weeks' gestation. Gestational age was confirmed by an ultrasound examination at 21 weeks' gestation and the Dubowitz score at birth. The infant had a constellation of malformations termed the VATER association (vertebral anomalies, anal atresia, tracheoesophageal fistula with esophageal atresia, renal and radial dysplasias) (5). Specific anomalies included an asymmetric chest, thoracic scoliosis, absent left thumb, foreshortened left forearm, left elbow contracture, fusion of the ribs on the left, butterfly vertebrae in the thoracic and lumbar spine, left radial aplasia, and a lower esophageal stricture (5). Chromosomal analysis was normal, and the family history was noncontributory. This case is also described above (see reference 2).

The cause of the defects in the above infant is unknown. Experiments with mice and rabbits indicate that amphetamines are teratogenic, but the anomalies primarily involve the heart and central nervous system (6). Moreover, the use of amphetamines during human pregnancy for medical indications has not been found to present a significant risk to the fetus in terms of fetotoxicity or teratogenicity (see Amphetamines). Although the cause of the infant's defects cannot be determined, drug-induced teratogenicity cannot be excluded because *in utero* exposure occurred during a critical period (i.e., 4th–9th weeks of embryogenesis) and in light of the skeletal defects observed in rats with lovastatin (6).

A 2004 report evaluated 20 cases of adverse pregnancy outcomes reported to the FDA after exposures to statins (7). The cases were among 178 cases of 1st trimester pregnancy exposure to cholesterol-lowering statin drugs reported to the FDA. There were 52 cases suitable for evaluation after exclusion for spontaneous abortions, elective abortions, pregnancy loss due to maternal diseases, fetal genetic disorders, transient neonatal disorders, or those loss to follow-up. In the 52 cases, there were 20 reports of malformation. *Central Nervous System (drug, dose, and exposure time in weeks after last menstrual period shown in parentheses)*: (1) holoprosencephaly (cerivastatin, 0.25 mg/day, 0–8 weeks); (2) holoprosencephaly (defective septum separating lateral cerebral ventricles), atrial septal defect, aortic hypoplasia, death at 1 month of age (lovastatin, 40 mg/day, 0–7 weeks); (3) aqueductal stenosis with hydrocephalus, limb deficiency (right banded, atretic thumb) (lovastatin, 40 mg/day, 0–4.5 weeks); (4) neural tube defect, myelocele, duplication of spinal cord, cerebellar herniation with hydrocephalus, apparent agenesis of palate (lovastatin, 20 mg/day, 1st trimester); (5) spina bifida, right arm abnormality (mother also type 1 diabetic) (atorvastatin, unknown dose, until pregnancy recognized). *Limb-Deficiency*: (1) same as #3 above; (2) right leg fibula and tibia 9% shorter than left side, agenesis of one tarsal bone, right foot 16% shorter than left (reported at 4 years of age) (simvastatin, 20 mg/day, 0–6 weeks); (3) left leg femur 16% shorter than right, foot with aplasia of metatarsals and phalanges 3, 4, and 5, additional VACTERL defects—left renal dysplasia, reversed laterality of aorta, disorganized lumbosacral vertebrae, single umbilical artery, additional findings—clitoral hypertrophy, vaginal and uterine agenesis (mother also took drug similar to progesterone 10 days/month, 0–13 weeks) (simvastatin, 10 mg/day, 0–13 weeks); (4) left arm aplasia of radius and thumb, shortened ulna, additional VACTERL defects—left arthrogryposis, thoracic scoliosis, fusion of ribs on left, butterfly vertebrae in thoracic and lumbar region, esophageal stricture, anal atresia, renal dysplasia, additional findings—hemihypertrophy of entire left side, craniofacial anomalies (including asymmetric ears, ptosis of eyelids, high arched palate), torticollis (mother also took dextroamphetamine, 6–11 weeks) (lovastatin, 10 mg/day, 6–11 weeks); (5) limb-reduction deficiency, transverse deficiency of otherwise normal radius and ulna superior to wrist structures, with aplasia of all distal structures (atorvastatin, 10 mg/day, 0–9 weeks) (7).

The other 11 cases of malformations were simvastatin: cleft lip with intrauterine growth retardation, cleft lip, polydactyly, duodenal atresia, hypospadias, clubfoot, and unspecified major abnormalities; atorvastatin: cleft palate and esophageal atresia; lovastatin: microtia with absent auditory canal and severe unspecified deformity (7). All of the 20 defects involved a lipophilic statin (i.e., atorvastatin, cerivastatin, lovastatin, and simvastatin). There were no malformations in the 14 cases of exposure to pravastatin, a hydrophilic agent with low tissue penetration that is not related to reproductive toxicity in animals (see Pravastatin). Because of the voluntary nature of the reports to the FDA, the authors thought that the reports were likely to be biased toward severe outcomes. However, the nature of some of the CNS and limb-deficiency malformations (i.e., primarily the cases of holoprosencephaly and VACTERL association) might be consistent with the inhibition of cholesterol biosynthesis (7).

In summary, infants with malformations following *in utero* exposure to lovastatin have been described in published and unpublished reports. A causal relationship between the drug and some of the defects is possible, but additional data are needed. Until such data are available, inadvertent exposure to any of the drugs in this class (atorvastatin, cerivastatin, fluvastatin, lovastatin, pravastatin, rosuvastatin, and simvastatin) should not be a reason for pregnancy termination. Because there is apparently no maternal benefit for the use of lovastatin during gestation and because of the human cases and the teratogenicity observed in one animal species, the drug should be avoided during pregnancy. If lovastatin is used in pregnancy, healthcare professionals are encouraged to call the toll free number (800-670-6126) for information about patient enrollment in the Motherisk study.

BREAST FEEDING SUMMARY

RECOMMENDATION: Contraindicated

Lovastatin is excreted in the milk of lactating rats (8), but no studies involving humans have been published. Because there is potential for adverse effects in the infant, the drug should not be used by women who are nursing.

References

1. Product information. Mevacor. Merck, 2000.
2. Manson JM, Freyssinges C, Ducrocq MB, Stephenson WP. Postmarketing surveillance of lovastatin and simvastatin exposure during pregnancy. Reprod Toxicol 1996;10:439–46.
3. Manson JM. Postmarketing surveillance of lovastatin and simvastatin exposure during pregnancy (Reply). Reprod Toxicol 1997;11:641–2.
4. Rosa F. Anti-cholesterol agent pregnancy exposure outcomes. Presented at the 7th International Organization for Teratogen Information Services, Woods Hole, MA, April 1994.
5. Ghidini A, Sicherer S, Willner J. Congenital abnormalities (VATER) in baby born to mother using lovastatin. Lancet 1992;339:1416–7.
6. Shepard TH. *Catalog of Teratogenic Agents*. 6th ed. Baltimore, MD: Johns Hopkins University Press, 1989: 197–8.
7. Edison RJ, Muenke M. Central nervous system and limb anomalies in case reports of first-trimester statin exposure. N Engl J Med 2004;350:1579–82.
8. Product information. Mevacor. Merck Sharp & Dohme, 1993.

Name:	**LOXAPINE**	Risk Factor:	**C**
Class:	**Tranquilizer**		

FETAL RISK SUMMARY

RECOMMENDATION: No Human Data - Animal Data Suggest Risk

No reports on the use of loxapine in human pregnancy have been located. In reproductive studies with mice, rats, rabbits, and dogs, a low incidence of exencephaly was observed in mouse fetuses, but no embryotoxicity or teratogenicity was found in the other species (1,2). The highest dose in rats and dogs was 2 times the maximum recommended human dose (2). Renal papillary abnormalities were found in offspring of rats treated from midgestation with doses approximately equivalent to the usual human dose (2).

BREAST FEEDING SUMMARY

RECOMMENDATION: No Human Data - Potential Toxicity

No reports describing the use of loxapine during human lactation have been located. The drug is excreted into the milk of lactating dogs (2). The relatively low molecular weight of loxapine (about 328) suggests that the drug would also be excreted into human milk. The potential effects of this exposure on a nursing infant are unknown.

L

References

1. Mineshita T, Hasewaga Y, Inoue Y, Kozen T, Yamamoto A. Teratological studies on fetuses and suckling young mice and rats of S-805. Oyo Yakuri 1970;4:305–16. As cited in Shepard TH. *Catalog of Teratogenic Agents.* 6th ed. Baltimore, MD: Johns Hopkins University Press, 1989:378.
2. Product information. Loxitane. Watson Laboratories, 2000.

Name:	**LYNESTRENOL**	Risk Factor:	**D**
Class:	**Progestogenic Hormone**		

FETAL RISK SUMMARY

RECOMMENDATION: Contraindicated - 1st Trimester

The Food and Drug Administration mandated deletion of pregnancy-related indications from all progestins because of a possible association with congenital anomalies. No reports linking the use of lynestrenol with congenital defects have been located (see Hydroxyprogesterone, Norethynodrel, Norethindrone, Medroxyprogesterone, Ethisterone). One reference cited 16 women who had used lynestrenol for contraception and gave birth to normal infants following cessation of treatment (1). No conclusions can be made from this report. Use of progestogens during pregnancy is not recommended.

BREAST FEEDING SUMMARY

RECOMMENDATION: No Human Data - Probably Compatible

See Oral Contraceptives.

Reference

1. Ravn J. Pregnancy and progeny after long-term contraceptive treatment with low-dose progestogens. Curr Med Res Opin 1975;2:616–9.

Name:	**LYPRESSIN**	Risk Factor:	C_M
Class:	**Pituitary Hormone, Synthetic**		

FETAL RISK SUMMARY

RECOMMENDATION: Compatible

Lypressin is a synthetic polypeptide structurally identical to the major active component of vasopressin. See Vasopressin.

BREAST FEEDING SUMMARY

RECOMMENDATION: Compatible

See Vasopressin.

Name:	**LYSERGIC ACID DIETHYLAMIDE**	Risk Factor:	C
Class:	**Hallucinogen**		

FETAL RISK SUMMARY

RECOMMENDATION: Contraindicated

Lysergic acid diethylamide (LSD, lysergide) is a chemical used for its hallucinogenic properties. The drug does not have a legal indication in the United States. Illicitly obtained LSD is commonly adulterated with a variety of other chemicals (e.g., amphetamines) (1,2). In some cases, doses sold illicitly as LSD may contain little or none of the chemical; as a result, the actual amount of LSD ingested cannot be determined (1). In addition, persons consuming the hallucinogen often consume multiple abuse drugs simultaneously, such as marijuana, opiates, alcohol, amphetamines, STP (dimethyloxyamphetamine, or DOM, a synthetic hallucinogen), barbiturates, cocaine, and other prescription and nonprescription substances. Further complicating the situation are the lifestyles that some of these persons live, which are often not conducive to good fetal health. As a consequence, the effects of pure LSD on the human fetus can only be evaluated by examining those cases in which the chemical was administered under strict medical supervision. These cases, however, are few in number. Most data are composed of sample populations who ingested the chemical in an unsupervised environment. Correct interpretation of this latter material is extremely difficult and, although cited in this monograph, must be viewed cautiously.

The passage of LSD across the human placenta has not been studied. The molecular weight of the chemical (about 323) is low enough, however, that rapid passage to the fetus should be expected. LSD has been shown to cross the placenta in mice with early 1st trimester fetal levels averaging 5 times the levels measured in late gestation (3).

Concerns with fetal exposure to LSD have primarily focused on chromosomal damage (both chromatid-type and chromosome-type abnormalities), an increased risk of spontaneous abortions, and congenital malformations. These topics are discussed in the sections below.

A 1967 report was the first to claim that the use of LSD could cause chromosomal abnormalities in human leukocytes (4). Because these abnormalities could potentially result in carcinogenic, mutagenic, and teratogenic effects in current or future generations, at least 25 studies were published in the next 7 years. These studies were the subject of three reviews published in the 1970s with all three arriving at similar conclusions (2,5,6). First, in the majority of studies, the addition of LSD to cells *in vitro* caused chromosomal breakage, but a dose-response relationship was not always apparent. The clinical relevance of the *in vitro* studies was questionable because pure LSD was used, usually with much higher levels than could be achieved in humans, and the *in vitro* systems lacked the normal protective mechanisms of metabolism and excretion that are present in the body. Second, only a slight transitory increase in chromosomal breaks was seen in a small percentage (14%) of the subjects administered pure LSD. A much higher percentage of persons (49%) consuming illicit LSD was observed to have chromosomal damage. The abnormalities in this latter group were probably related to the effects of multiple drug abuse and not to LSD alone. Four prospective studies found no definitive evidence that LSD damages lymphocyte chromosomes *in vitro* (2). Third, there was no evidence that the chromosomal defects observed in illicit LSD users were expressed as an increased incidence of leukemias or other neoplasia. Fourth, mutagenic changes were only observed in experimental organisms (e.g., *Drosophila*) when massive doses (2,000–10,000 μg/mL) were used. Because of this, LSD was believed to be a weak mutagen, but mutagenicity was thought to be unlikely after exposure to any concentration used by humans (5). Finally, the reviewers found no compelling evidence for a teratogenic effect of LSD, either in animals or humans.

A 1974 investigation involving 50 psychiatric patients, who had been treated for varying intervals under controlled conditions with pure LSD, provided further confirmation that the chemical does not cause chromosomal damage (7). Chromosomal analyses of these patients were compared with those of 50 nonexposed controls matched for age, sex, and marital status. The analysis was blinded so that the investigators did not know the origin of the samples. No significant difference between the groups in chromosomal abnormalities was observed. In another 1974 reference (not included in the previously cited reviews), involving only two subjects, no evidence of chromosomal damage was found in their normal offspring (8). The two women had been treated medically with pure LSD before pregnancy. Thus, the predominance of evidence indicates that LSD does not induce chromosomal aberrations, and even if it did, it has no clinical significance to the fetus.

The question of whether fetal wastage could be induced by LSD exposure was investigated in a study published in 1970 (9). This investigation involved 148 pregnancies (81 patients) in which either the father ($N = 60$) or the mother ($N = 21$) had ingested LSD. In 12 pregnancies, exposure occurred both before and during pregnancy. In the 136 pregnancies in which the exposure occurred only before conception, 118 involved the administration of pure LSD (the medical group) and 18 involved both medical and illicit LSD exposure (the combined group). The spontaneous abortion rates for these two populations were 14% (17 of 118) and 28% (5 of 18), respectively. In 83 of the pregnancies, only the father had been exposed to LSD. Excluding these, the incidences of fetal loss for the medical and combined groups are 26% (11 of 43) and 40% (4 of 10), respectively. In the 12 pregnancies in which LSD was consumed both before and during gestation, 3 were in the medical group and 9 were in the combined group. The frequency of spontaneous abortions in these cases was 33% (1 of 3) and 56% (5 of 9). In the combined sample, however, one woman accounted for five abortions and one liveborn infant. If she is excluded, the incidence of fetal wastage in the combined group is zero.

In the medical group, the number of women (12 of 46; 26%) with fetal wastage is high. However, 25 of these pregnancies occurred in women undergoing psychotherapy, and 21 occurred in an experimental setting (9). The number of spontaneous abortions in the psychotherapy group ($N = 9$) (36%) was more than twice the incidence in the experimental sample ($N = 3$) (14%). The authors speculated that the greater frequency of fetal wastage in the women undergoing psychotherapy may have been caused by the greater emotional stress that often accompanies such therapy. The increased rate in the combined sample (9 of 19; 47%) was probably caused by the use of multiple abuse drugs, other nondrug factors, and the inclusion of one woman with five abortions and one live birth. Exclusion of this latter patient decreases the combined sample incidence to 31% (4 of 13). Thus, although other studies examining the incidence of spontaneous abortions in LSD-exposed women have not been located, it appears unlikely that pure LSD administered in a controlled condition is an abortifacient. The increased rate of fetal wastage that was observed in the 1970 study was probably caused by a combination of factors, rather than only to the ingestion of LSD.

A number of case reports have described LSD use in pregnancies ending with poor outcomes since the first report in 1967 of an exposed infant with major malformations (10–25). All of these reports, however, are biased in the respect that malformed infants exposed *in utero* to LSD are much more likely to be reported than exposed normal infants and are also more frequently reported than nonexposed malformed infants (2). Most of the reports either involved multiple drug exposures, including abuse drugs, or other drug exposures could probably be deduced because of the illicit nature of LSD. With these cautions, the reports are briefly described below.

The first mention of an anomaly observed in an infant exposed *in utero* to LSD appeared in a 1967 editorial (10). The editorial, citing a report in a lay publication, briefly described a case of LSD exposure in a pregnancy that ended in a malformed infant with megacolon. Apparently, details of this case have never been published in the medical literature.

The first case report in the medical literature also appeared in 1967 and involved a female infant with unilateral fibular aplastic syndrome (11,12). The mother had taken LSD 4 times between the 25th and 98th days of gestation with one dose occurring during the time of most active lower limb differentiation (11). Defects in the infant, which were characteristic of the syndrome, included absence of the fibula and lateral rays of the foot, anterior bowing of the shortened tibia, shortening of the femur, and dislocated hip. A second case involving limb defects and LSD exposure was published in 1968 (13). The infant, with a right terminal transverse acheiria defect (absence of the hand), was the offspring of a woman who had taken LSD both before and during early gestation. She had also smoked marijuana throughout the pregnancy and had taken a combination product containing dicyclomine, doxylamine, and pyridoxine for 1st trimester nausea. Another infant with a terminal transverse deficit, also exposed to LSD and marijuana, was described in 1969 (14). The defect involved portions of the fingers on the left hand, syndactyly of the right hand with shortened fingers, and talipes equinovarus of the left foot. Two of these same authors described another exposed infant with amputation deformities of the third finger of the right hand and the third toe of the left foot (15). A critique of these latter three case histories concluded that the defects in the infants could have been caused by amniotic band syndrome (26). Limb defects and intrauterine growth retardation were observed in an offspring of a malnourished mother who had used LSD, marijuana, methadone, and cigarettes during gestation (16). The anomalies consisted of partial adactyly of the hands and feet, syndactyly of the remaining fingers, and defective formation of the legs and forearms. In a study of 140 women using LSD and marijuana followed up through 148 pregnancies, 8 of 83 liveborn infants had major defects as did 4 of 14 embryos examined after induced abortion (17). The incidence of defects in this sample was 8.1% (12 of 148) and may have been higher if the other abortuses had been examined. Only one of the liveborn infants had a limb defect (absence of both feet) combined with spina bifida occulta and hemangiomas. Defects in the other 7 infants were: myelomeningocele with hydrocephalus in 3 babies (1 with clubfoot); tetralogy of Fallot; hydrocephalus; right kidney neuroblastoma; and hydrocephalus and congestive heart failure. A limb defect was one of several anomalies found in a male infant whose mother ingested LSD both before and during gestation (18). The abnormalities included absent left arm, syndactyly, anencephaly with ectopic placenta, cleft lip and palate, coloboma of the iris, cataract, and corneal opacity with vascularization. At least one author thought the limb and cranial defects in this latter case may have been caused by amniotic band syndrome (27). This opinion was contested by the original authors, who stated that the limb defects were true aplasia and not an amputation deformity (28). Similarly, they claimed that the cranial anomaly was not a form of encephalocele, which an amniotic band could have caused, but a true anencephaly (28). Congenital anomalies were observed in 11 of 120 liveborn infants in a previously cited study that examined the effects of LSD on spontaneous abortions and other pregnancy outcomes (9). Nine of the 11 infants had limb defects that were, in most cases, easily correctable with either special shoes or casts. None of the 11 cases appears to be related to LSD exposure. The defects were (the number of cases and possible causes are shown in parentheses): turned-in feet (6 cases, 4 familial, 2 unknown); "crimped" ureter (1 case, familial); tibial rotation (2 cases, 2 familial); pyloric stenosis (1 case, possibly genetic); bone deformity of legs and deafness (1 case, postrubella syndrome) (9).

Other infants with ocular defects, in addition to the case mentioned immediately above, have been described. A mother who ingested LSD, marijuana, meprobamate, amphetamines, and hydrochlorothiazide throughout pregnancy delivered an infant with generalized hypotonia, a high-pitched cry, brachycephaly with widely separated sutures, bilateral cephalohematomas, a right eye smaller than the left and with a cataract, and overlapping second and third toes (19). Two other cases of ocular defects were published in 1978 and 1980 (20,21). In one case, a premature female infant was delivered from a 16-year-old mother who had consumed LSD, cocaine, and heroin during the 1st trimester (20). The infant, who died 1 hour after birth, had microphthalmos, intraocular cartilage, cataract, persistent hyperplastic primary vitreous, and retinal dysplasia. A hypoplastic left lung and a defect in the diaphragm were also noted. The second case involved another premature female infant born to a mother enrolled in a methadone program who also used LSD (21). The infant had left anophthalmia but no other defects.

Various other malformations have been reported after *in utero* LSD exposure (22–25). Complete exstrophy of the bladder, epispadias, widely separated pubic rami, and bilateral inguinal hernias were observed in a newborn exposed to LSD, marijuana, and mephentermine (22). The mother had consumed LSD 12–15 times during an interval extending from 2 months before conception to 2.5 months into pregnancy. A mother, who ingested LSD at the time of conception, produced a female infant with multiple defects including a short neck, left hemithorax smaller than the right, protuberant abdomen because of a

L

severe thoracolumbar lordosis, a thoracolumbar rachischisis, craniolacunia, long fingers, clubfeet, and defects of the urinary tract and brain (23). The infant died at 41 days of age. Other drug exposures consisted of cigarettes, an estrogen preparation (type not specified) that was used unsuccessfully to induce menstruation, and medroxyprogesterone for 1st trimester bleeding. Because the case resembled a previously described cluster of unusual defects (i.e., spondylothoracic dysplasia, Jarcho-Levin syndrome), which is caused by an autosomal recessive mode of inheritance, the authors could not exclude this mechanism. In a case of a female infant with multiple anomalies compatible with trisomy 13 with D/D translocation, the mother had last used LSD 9 months before conception (24). She had also used marijuana, barbiturates, and amphetamines throughout gestation and, presumably, before conception. The authors theorized that the defect may have been caused by LSD-induced damage to maternal germ cells before fertilization. A 1971 study evaluated 47 infants born to parents who had used LSD (25). Maternal use of the drug could be documented in only 30 of the cases and multiple other abuse drugs were consumed. Abnormalities observed in 8 (17%) of the infants were transient hearing loss and ventricular septal defect, cortical blindness, tracheoesophageal fistula, congenital heart disease (type not specified), congenital neuroblastoma, spastic diplegia, and seizure disorders in 2 infants.

Two other case reports involving the combined use of LSD and marijuana with resulting adverse fetal outcomes do not appear to have any relationship to either drug (29,30). One of these involved a report of six infants with persistent ductus arteriosus, one of whom was exposed to LSD and marijuana during early gestation (29). The history of maternal drug use was coincidental. The second case described an infant who died at 2.5 months of age of a bilateral *in utero* cerebral vascular accident and resulting porencephaly (30). The mother had used LSD, marijuana, alcohol, and other abuse drugs, including cocaine. This latter drug was thought to be the causative agent.

In contrast to the above reports, a large body of research has been published describing the maternal (and paternal) ingestion of LSD without apparent fetal consequences (1,7–9,31–36). A number of reviews have also examined the teratogenic potential of the chemical and have concluded that a causal relationship between congenital malformations and LSD does not exist (2,5,6,37–45). (See reference 6 for an excellent critique of the early investigations in laboratory animals.)

In summary, the available data indicate that pure LSD does not cause chromosomal abnormalities, spontaneous abortions, or congenital malformations. There are no published cases of fetal anomalies when only pure LSD was administered under medical supervision. Early descriptions of congenital abnormalities involved patients who had used or were using illicit LSD and are believed to be examples of reporting bias, the effects of multiple drugs, or other nondrug factors. However, long-term follow-up of exposed infants has never been reported. This is an area that warrants additional research.

BREAST FEEDING SUMMARY

RECOMMENDATION: Contraindicated

No reports have been located concerning the passage of lysergic acid diethylamide into breast milk. Because the drug has a relatively low molecular weight (about 323), which should allow its transfer into milk, and because its psychotomimetic effects are produced at extremely low concentrations, the use of LSD during lactation is contraindicated.

References

1. Warren RJ, Rimoin DL, Sly WS. LSD exposure in utero. Pediatrics 1970;45:466–9.
2. Matsuyama SS, Jarvik LF. Cytogenetic effects of psychoactive drugs. Mod Probl Pharmacopsychiatry 1975;10:99–132.
3. Idanpaan-Heikkila JE, Schoolar JC. LSD: Autoradiographic study on the placental transfer and tissue distribution in mice. Science 1969;164:1295–7.
4. Cohen MM, Marinello MJ, Back N. Chromosomal damage in human leukocytes induced by lysergic acid diethylamide. Science 1967;155:1417–9.
5. Dishotsky NI, Loughman WD, Mogar RE, Lipscomb WR. LSD and genetic damage: Is LSD chromosome damaging, carcinogenic, mutagenic, or teratogenic? Science 1971;172:431–40.
6. Long SY. Does LSD induce chromosomal damage and malformations? A review of the literature. Teratology 1972;6:75–90.
7. Robinson JT, Chitham RG, Greenwood RM, Taylor JW. Chromosome aberrations and LSD: a controlled study in 50 psychiatric patients. Br J Psychiatry 1974;125:238–44.
8. Fernandez J, Brennan T, Masterson J, Power M. Cytogenetic studies in the offspring of LSD users. Br J Psychiatry 1974;124:296–8.
9. McGlothlin WH, Sparkes RS, Arnold DO. Effect of LSD on human pregnancy. JAMA 1970;212:1483–7.
10. Anonymous. Hallucinogen and teratogen? Lancet 1967;2:504–5.
11. Zellweger H, McDonald JS, Abbo G. Is lysergic-acid diethylamide a teratogen? Lancet 1967;2:1066–8.
12. Zellweger H, McDonald JS, Abbo G. Is lysergide a teratogen? Lancet 1967;2:1306.
13. Hecht F, Beals RK, Lees MH, Jolly H, Roberts P. Lysergic-acid-diethylamide and cannabis as possible teratogens in man. Lancet 1968;2:1087.
14. Carakushansky G, Neu RL, Gardner LI. Lysergide and cannabis as possible teratogens in man. Lancet 1969;1:150–1.
15. Assemany SR, Neu RL, Gardner LI. Deformities in a child whose mother took L.S.D. Lancet 1970;1:1290.
16. Jeanbart P, Berard MJ. A propos d'un cas personnel de malformations congenitales possiblement dues au LSD-25: revue de la litterature. Union Med Can 1971;100:919–29.
17. Jacobson CB, Berlin CM. Possible reproductive detriment in LSD users. JAMA 1972;222:1367–73.
18. Apple DJ, Bennett TO. Multiple systemic and ocular malformations associated with maternal LSD usage. Arch Ophthalmol 1974;92:301–3.
19. Bogdanoff B, Rorke LB, Yanoff M, Warren WS. Brain and eye abnormalities: possible sequelae to prenatal use of multiple drugs including LSD. Am J Dis Child 1972;123:145–8.
20. Chan CC, Fishman M, Egbert PR. Multiple ocular anomalies associated with maternal LSD ingestion. Arch Ophthalmol 1978;96:282–4.
21. Margolis S, Martin L. Anophthalmia in an infant of parents using LSD. Ann Ophthalmol 1980;12:1378–81.
22. Gelehrter TD. Lysergic acid diethylamide (LSD) and exstrophy of the bladder. J Pediatr 1970;77:1065–6.
23. Eller JL, Morton JM. Bizarre deformities in offspring of user of lysergic acid diethylamide. N Engl J Med 1970;283:395–7.
24. Hsu LY, Strauss L, Hirschhorn K. Chromosome abnormality in offspring of LSD user: D trisomy with D/D translocation. JAMA 1970;211:987–90.
25. Dumars KW Jr. Parental drug usage: effect upon chromosomes of progeny. Pediatrics 1971;47:1037–41.
26. Blanc WA, Mattison DR, Kane R, Chauhan P. L.S.D., intrauterine amputations, and amniotic-band syndrome. Lancet 1971;2:158–9.
27. Holmes LB. Ocular malformations associated with maternal LSD usage. Arch Ophthalmol 1975;93:1061.
28. Apple DJ. Ocular malformations associated with maternal LSD usage (in reply). Arch Ophthalmol 1975;93:1061.
29. Brown R, Pickering D. Persistent transitional circulation. Arch Dis Child 1974;49:883–5.
30. Tenorio GM, Nazvi M, Bickers GH, Hubbird RH. Intrauterine stroke and maternal polydrug abuse. Clin Pediatr 1988;27:565–7.
31. Cohen MM, Hirschhorn K, Frosch WA. In vivo and in vitro chromosomal damage induced by LSD-25. N Engl J Med 1967;277:1043–9.
32. Sato H, Pergament E. Is lysergide a teratogen? Lancet 1968;1:639–40.
33. Egozcue J, Irwin S, Maruffo CA. Chromosomal damage in LSD users. JAMA 1968;204:214–8.
34. Cohen MM, Hirschhorn K, Verbo S, Frosch WA, Groeschel MM. The effect of LSD-25 on the chromosomes of children exposed in utero. Pediatr Res 1968;2:486–92.
35. Hulten M, Lindsten J, Lidberg L, Ekelund H. Studies on mitotic and meiotic chromosomes in subjects exposed to LSD. Ann Genet (Paris) 1968;11:201–10.
36. Aase JM, Laestadius N, Smith DW. Children of mothers who took L.S.D. in pregnancy. Lancet 1970;2:100–1.
37. Hoffer A. Effect of LSD on chromosomes. Can Med Assoc J 1968;98:466.
38. Smart RG, Bateman K. The chromosomal and teratogenic effects of lysergic acid diethylamide: a review of the current literature. Can Med Assoc J 1968;99:805–10.
39. Rennert OM. Drug-induced somatic alterations. Clin Obstet Gynecol 1975;18:185–98.
40. Glass L, Evans HE. Perinatal drug abuse. Pediatr Ann 1979;8:84–92.
41. VanBlerk GA, Majerus TC, Myers RAM. Teratogenic potential of some psychopharmacologic drugs: a brief review. Int J Gynaecol Obstet 1980;17:399–402.
42. Chernoff GF, Jones KL. Fetal preventive medicine: teratogens and the unborn baby. Pediatr Ann 1981;10:210–7.
43. Stern L. In vivo assessment of the teratogenic potential of drugs in humans. Obstet Gynecol 1981;58:3S–8S.
44. Lee CC, Chiang CN. Maternal-fetal transfer of abused substances: pharmacokinetic and pharmacodynamic data. NIDA Res Monogr 1985;60:110–47.
45. McLane NJ, Carroll DM. Ocular manifestations of drug abuse. Surv Ophthalmol 1986;30:298–313.

L

Name:	L-LYSINE	Risk Factor:	C
Class:	**Nutrient (Amino Acid)**		

FETAL RISK SUMMARY

RECOMMENDATION: No Human Data - Probably Compatible

L-Lysine is an essential amino acid that has been occasionally used for the treatment and prophylaxis of herpes simplex infections (the effectiveness of this indication is questionable). No reports on the use of the commercial formulation in human pregnancy have been located.

L-Lysine is actively transported across the human placenta to the fetus with a steady-state fetal:maternal ratio of approximately 1.6:1 (1,2). Fetal tissues retain most of the essential amino acids, including L-lysine, in preference to the nonessential amino acids (3).

One published case has been located that described a woman with familial hyperlysinemia because of deficiency of the enzymes lysine ketoglutarate reductase and saccharopine dehydrogenase (4). The woman gave birth to a normal child. No details of the pregnancy or the child were provided other than that the child was normal. Serum lysine levels, which were regularly above 10 mg/dL and may have been as high as 20 mg/dL or more when the disorder was detected, were not measured during the pregnancy or in the baby.

L

BREAST FEEDING SUMMARY

RECOMMENDATION: No Human Data - Probably Compatible

No data are available.

References

1. Schneider H, Mohlen KH, Dancis J. Transfer of amino acids across the in vitro perfused human placenta. Pediatr Res 1979;13:236–40.
2. Schneider H, Mohlen KH, Challier JC, Dancis J. Transfer of glutamic acid across the human placenta perfused in vitro. Br J Obstet Gynaecol 1979;86:299–306.
3. Velazquez A, Rosado A, Bernal A, Noriega L, Arevalo N. Amino acid pools in the feto-maternal system. Biol Neonate 1976;29:28–40.
4. Dancis J, Hutzler J, Ampola MG, Shih VE, van Gelderen HH, Kirby LT, Woody NC. The prognosis of hyperlysinemia: an interim report. Am J Hum Genet 1983;35:438–42.

M

Name:	**MAGNESIUM SULFATE**	Risk Factor:	**B**
Class:	**Anticonvulsant/Laxative**		

FETAL RISK SUMMARY

RECOMMENDATION: Compatible

Magnesium sulfate ($MgSO_4$) is commonly used as an anticonvulsant for toxemia and as a tocolytic agent for premature labor during the last half of pregnancy. Concentrations of magnesium, a natural constituent of human serum, are readily increased in both the mother and fetus following maternal therapy, with cord serum levels ranging from 70% to 100% of maternal concentrations (1–6). Elevated levels in the newborn may persist for up to 7 days, with an elimination half-life of 43.2 hours (2). The elimination rate is the same in premature and full-term infants (2). Intravenous magnesium sulfate did not cause lower Apgar scores in a study of women treated for pregnancy-induced hypertension, although the magnesium levels in the newborns reflected hypermagnesemia (6). The mean cord magnesium level, 5.3 mEq/dL, was equal to the mean maternal serum level.

No reports linking the use of magnesium sulfate to congenital defects have been located. The Collaborative Perinatal Project (CPP) monitored 50,282 mother-child pairs, 141 of which had exposure to magnesium sulfate during pregnancy (7). No evidence was found to suggest a relationship to congenital malformations.

In a 1987 report, 17 women who had been successfully treated with IV magnesium sulfate for preterm labor, were given 1 g of magnesium gluconate every 4 hours after the IV magnesium had been discontinued (8). A mean serum magnesium level before any therapy was 1.44 mg/dL. Two hours after an oral dose (12–24 hours after discontinuation of IV magnesium), the mean magnesium serum level was 2.16 mg/dL, a significant increase ($p < 0.05$). A group of 568 women was randomly assigned to receive either 15 mmol of magnesium-aspartate hydrochloride ($N = 278$) or 13.5 mmol of aspartic acid ($N = 290$) per day (9). Therapy was started as early as possible in the pregnancies, but not later than 16 weeks' gestation. Women receiving the magnesium tablets had fewer hospitalizations ($p < 0.05$), fewer preterm deliveries, and less frequent referral of the newborn to the neonatal intensive care unit ($p < 0.01$) (9). In a double-blind randomized, controlled clinical study, 374 young women (mean age approximately 18 years) were treated with either 365 mg of elemental magnesium/day (provided by six tablets of magnesium-aspartate hydrochloride, each containing 60.8 mg of elemental magnesium) ($N = 185$) or placebo tablets containing aspartic acid only ($N = 189$) (10). Treatment began at approximately a mean gestational age of 18 weeks (range 13–24 weeks). In addition, both groups received prenatal vitamins containing 100 mg of elemental magnesium. In contrast to the reference cited above, the magnesium therapy did not improve the outcome of the pregnancies, as judged by the nonsignificant differences between the groups in incidences of preeclampsia, fetal growth retardation, preterm labor, birth weight, gestational age at delivery, and number of infants admitted to the special care unit (10).

Most studies have been unable to find a correlation between cord serum magnesium levels and newborn condition (2,5,11–15). In a study of 7,000 offspring of mothers treated with $MgSO_4$ for toxemia, no adverse effects from the therapy were noted in fetuses or newborns (5). Other studies have also observed a lack of toxicity (16,17). A 1983 investigation of women at term with pregnancy-induced hypertension compared newborns of magnesium-treated mothers with newborns of untreated mothers (15). No differences in neurologic behavior were observed between the two groups except that exposed infants had decreased active tone of the neck extensors on the 1st day after birth.

Newborn depression and hypotonia have been reported as effects of maternal magnesium therapy in some series, but intrauterine hypoxia could not always be eliminated as a potential cause or contributing factor (2,11,12,18–20). In a study reporting on the effects of IV magnesium on Apgar scores, the most common negative score was assigned for color rather than for muscle tone (6).

A 1971 report described two infants with magnesium levels greater than 8 mg/dL who were severely depressed at birth (13). Spontaneous remission of toxic symptoms occurred after 12 hours in one infant, but the second had residual effects of anoxic encephalopathy. In a 1982 study, activities requiring sustained muscle contraction, such as head lag, ventral suspension, suck reflex, and cry response, were impaired up to 48 hours after birth in infants exposed *in utero* to magnesium (14). A hypertensive woman treated with 11 g of magnesium sulfate within 3.5 hours of delivery gave birth to a depressed infant without spontaneous respirations, movement, or reflexes (21). An exchange transfusion at 24 hours reversed the condition. In another study, decreased gastrointestinal motility, ileus, hypotonia, and patent ductus arteriosus occurring in the offspring of mothers with severe hypertension were thought to be caused by maternal drug therapy, including magnesium sulfate (22). However, the authors could not relate their findings to any particular drug or drugs and could not completely eliminate the possibility that the effects were caused by the severe maternal disease.

M

A mild decrease in cord calcium concentrations has been reported in mothers treated with magnesium (3,13,15). In contrast, a 1980 study reported elevated calcium levels in cord blood following magnesium therapy (4). No newborn symptoms were associated with either change in serum calcium concentrations. However, long-term maternal tocolysis with IV magnesium sulfate may cause injury to the newborn as described below.

In an investigation of five newborn infants whose mothers had been treated with IV magnesium sulfate for periods ranging from 5 to 14 weeks, radiographic bony abnormalities were noted in two of the infants (18). One of the mothers, a class C diabetic who had been insulin-dependent for 12 years, was treated with IV magnesium for 14 weeks, beginning at 21 weeks' gestation. A 2030-g female infant was delivered vaginally at 35 weeks' gestation following spontaneous rupture of the mother's membranes. The maternal histories of this and another case treated for 6 weeks were described in 1986 (19). The infant had frank rachitic changes of the long bones and the calvaria. Serum calcium at 6 hours of age was normal. She was treated with IV calcium gluconate for 3 days, and then given bottle feedings without additional calcium or vitamin D. Scout films for an IV pyelogram taken at 4 months of age because of a urinary tract infection showed no bony abnormalities. Growth over the first 3 years has been consistently at the 3rd percentile for height, weight, and head circumference. Dental enamel hypoplasia, especially of the central upper incisors, was the only physical abnormality noted at 3 years of age. The second infant's mother had been treated with IV magnesium for 9 weeks beginning at

25 weeks' gestation. The 2190-g female infant was delivered vaginally at 34 weeks because of spontaneous rupture of the mother's membranes. Hypocalcemia (5.8 mg/dL, normal 6.0–10.0 mg/dL) was measured at 6 hours of age. A chest radiograph taken on the 1st day revealed lucent bands at the distal ends of the metaphyses (18). She was treated with IV calcium for 5 days and then given bottle feedings without additional calcium or vitamin D. A scout film for an IV pyelogram at 5 months of age showed no bony abnormalities. In the remaining three cases, the mothers had been treated with IV magnesium for 4–6 weeks, and their infants were normal on examination. The authors hypothesized that the fetal hypermagnesemia produced by the long-term maternal administration of magnesium caused a depression of parathyroid hormone release that resulted in fetal hypocalcemia (18).

In another study of long-term IV magnesium tocolysis, 22 women were treated for an average of 26.3 ± 19.2 days (maximum duration in any patient was 75 days) (20). Two infants delivered from this group were noted to have wide-spaced fontanelles and parietal bone thinning. These effects returned to normal with time. A third newborn, delivered from a mother belonging to an intermediate group treated with IV magnesium for an average of 6.3 ± 1.9 days, sustained a parietal bone fracture during an instrumental delivery and developed spastic quadriplegia (20).

More recent studies have also described the adverse effects of prolonged magnesium therapy on fetal bone mineralization (23–27). The mechanism of this reaction appears to be increased, persistent urinary calcium losses in the mother and her fetus (26,27). In one investigation, increases in 1,25-dihydroxyvitamin D and parathyroid hormone in both the mother and the fetus may have prevented more severe hypocalcemia (27).

Clinically significant drug interactions have been reported, one in a newborn and three in mothers, after maternal administration of $MgSO_4$. In one case, an interaction between *in utero* acquired magnesium and gentamicin was reported in a newborn 24 hours after birth (28,29). The mother had received 24 g of $MgSO_4$ during the 32 hours preceding birth of a neurologically depressed female infant. Gentamicin, 2.5 mg/kg IM every 12 hours, was begun at 12 hours of age for presumed sepsis. The infant developed respiratory arrest following the second dose of gentamicin, which resolved after the antibiotic was stopped. Animal experiments confirmed the interaction. The maternal cases involved an interaction between magnesium and nifedipine (30,31). One report described two women who were hospitalized at 30 and 32 weeks' gestation, respectively, for hypertension (30). In both cases, oral methyldopa, 2 g, and IV $MgSO_4$, 20 g, daily were ineffective in lowering the mother's blood pressure. Oral nifedipine, 10 mg, was given, and a marked hypotensive response occurred 45 minutes later. The blood pressures before nifedipine in the women were 150/110 and 140/105 mm Hg, and decreased to 80/50 and 90/60 mm Hg, respectively, after administration of the calcium channel blocker. Blood pressure returned to previous levels 25–30 minutes later. Both infants were delivered following the hypotensive episodes, but only one survived. In the third maternal case, a woman in premature labor at 32 weeks' gestation, was treated with oral nifedipine, 60 mg over 3 hours, then 20 mg every 8 hours (31). Because uterine contractions returned, intravenous $MgSO_4$ was begun 12 hours later followed by the onset of pronounced muscle weakness after 500 mg had been administered. Her symptoms included jerky movements of the extremities, difficulty in swallowing, paradoxical respirations, and an inability to lift her head from the pillow. The magnesium was stopped and the symptoms resolved during the next 25 minutes. The reaction was attributed to nifedipine potentiation of the neuromuscular blocking action of magnesium.

Maternal hypothermia with maternal and fetal bradycardia apparently caused by IV magnesium sulfate has been reported (32). The 30-year-old woman, at about 31 weeks' gestation, was being treated for premature labor. She had received a single, 12-mg IM dose of betamethasone at the same time that magnesium therapy was started. Her oral temperature fell from 99.8°F to 97°F, 2 hours after the infusion had been increased from 2 g/hour to 3 g/hour. Twelve hours after admission to the hospital, her heart rate fell to 64 beats/minute (baseline 80 beats/minute), while the fetal heart rate decreased to 110 beats/minute (baseline 140–150 beats/minute). A rectal temperature at this time was 95.8°F, and the patient complained of lethargy and diplopia. Her serum magnesium level was 6.6 mg/dL. Magnesium therapy was discontinued and all signs and symptoms returned to baseline values within 6 hours. Neither the mother nor the fetus suffered adversely from the effects attributed to magnesium.

In summary, the administration of magnesium sulfate to the mother for anticonvulsant or tocolytic effects does not usually pose a risk to the fetus or newborn. Long-term infusions of magnesium may be associated with sustained hypocalcemia in the fetus resulting in congenital rickets. Neonatal neurologic depression may occur with respiratory depression, muscle weakness, and loss of reflexes. The toxicity is not usually correlated with cord serum magnesium levels. Offspring of mothers treated with this drug close to delivery should be closely observed for signs of toxicity during the first 24–48 hours after birth. Caution is also advocated with the use of aminoglycoside antibiotics during this period.

BREAST FEEDING SUMMARY

RECOMMENDATION: Compatible

Magnesium salts may be encountered by nursing mothers who are using over-the-counter laxatives. A study in which 50 mothers received an emulsion of magnesium and liquid petrolatum or mineral oil found no evidence of changes or frequency of stools in nursing infants (33). In 10 preeclamptic patients receiving magnesium sulfate, 1 g/hour IV during the first 24 hours after delivery, magnesium levels in breast milk were 64 μg/mL, as compared with 48 μg/mL in nontreated controls (34). Twenty-four hours after stopping the drug, milk levels in treated and nontreated patients were 38 and 32 μg/mL, respectively. By 48 hours, the levels were identical in the two groups. Milk:plasma ratios were 1.9 and 2.1 in treated and nontreated patients, respectively. The American Academy of Pediatrics classifies magnesium sulfate as compatible with breast-feeding (35).

References

1. Chesley LC, Tepper I. Plasma levels of magnesium attained in magnesium sulfate therapy for preeclampsia and eclampsia. Surg Clin North Am 1957;37:353–67.
2. Dangman BC, Rosen TS. Magnesium levels in infants of mothers treated with $MgSO_4$. Pediatr Res 1977;11:415 (Abstract #262).
3. Cruikshank DP, Pitkin RM, Reynolds WA, Williams GA, Hargis GK. Effects of magnesium sulfate treatment on perinatal calcium metabolism. I. Maternal and fetal responses. Am J Obstet Gynecol 1979;134:243–9.
4. Donovan EF, Tsang RC, Steichen JJ, Strub RJ, Chen IW, Chen M. Neonatal hypermagnesemia: effect on parathyroid hormone and calcium homeostasis. J Pediatr 1980;96:305–10.
5. Stone SR, Pritchard JA. Effect of maternally administered magnesium sulfate on the neonate. Obstet Gynecol 1970;35:574–57.
6. Pruett KM, Kirshon B, Cotton DB, Adam K, Doody KJ. The effects of magnesium sulfate therapy on Apgar scores. Am J Obstet Gynecol 1988;159:1047–18.
7. Heinonen OP, Slone D, Shapiro S. *Birth Defects and Drugs in Pregnancy*. Littleton, MA: Publishing Sciences Group, 1977:440.
8. Martin RW, Gaddy DK, Martin JN Jr, Lucas JA, Wiser WL, Morrison JC. Tocolysis with oral magnesium. Am J Obstet Gynecol 1987;156:433–44.
9. Spatling L, Spatling G. Magnesium supplementation in pregnancy: a double-blind study. Br J Obstet Gynaecol 1988;95:120–15.
10. Sibai BM, Villar L. MA, Bray E. Magnesium supplementation during pregnancy: a double-blind

randomized controlled clinical trial. Am J Obstet Gynecol 1989;161:115–19.
11. Lipsitz PJ, English IC. Hypermagnesemia in the newborn infant. Pediatrics 1967;40:856–62.
12. Lipsitz PJ. The clinical and biochemical effects of excess magnesium in the newborn. Pediatrics 1971;47: 501–59.
13. Savory J, Monif GRG. Serum calcium levels in cord sera of the progeny of mothers treated with magnesium sulfate for toxemia of pregnancy. Am J Obstet Gynecol 1971;110:556–59.
14. Rasch DK, Huber PA, Richardson CJ, L'Hommedieu CS, Nelson TE, Reddi R. Neurobehavioral effects of neonatal hypermagnesemia. J Pediatr 1982;100:272–26.
15. Green KW, Key TC, Coen R, Resnik R. The effects of maternally administered magnesium sulfate on the neonate. Am J Obstet Gynecol 1983;146:29–33.
16. Sibai BM, Lipshitz J, Anderson GD, Dilts PV Jr. Reassessment of intravenous $MgSO_4$ therapy in preeclampsia-eclampsia. Obstet Gynecol 1981;57:199–202.
17. Hutchinson HT, Nichols MM, Kuhn CR, Vasicka A. Effects of magnesium sulfate on uterine contractility, intrauterine fetus, and infant. Am J Obstet Gynecol 1964;88:747–58.
18. Lamm CI, Norton KI, Murphy RJC, Wilkins IA, Rabinowitz JG. Congenital rickets associated with magnesium sulfate infusion for tocolysis. J Pediatr 1988;113:1078–82.
19. Wilkins IA, Goldberg JD, Phillips RN, Bacall CJ, Chervenak FA, Berkowitz RL. Long-term use of magnesium sulfate as a tocolytic agent. Obstet Gynecol 1986;67:38S–40S.
20. Dudley D, Gagnon D, Varner M. Long-term tocolysis with intravenous magnesium sulfate. Obstet Gynecol 1989;73:373–8.
21. Brady JP, Williams HC. Magnesium intoxication in a premature infant. Pediatrics 1967;40:100–13.
22. Brazy JE, Grimm JK, Little VA. Neonatal manifestations of severe maternal hypertension occurring before the thirty-sixth week of pregnancy. J Pediatr 1982;100:265–71.
23. Holcomb WL Jr, Shackelford GD, Petrie RH. Prolonged magnesium therapy affects fetal bone (abstract). Am J Obstet Gynecol 1991;164:386.
24. Smith LG Jr, Schanler RJ, Burns P, Moise KJ Jr. Effect of magnesium sulfate therapy ($MgSO_4$) on the bone mineral content of women and their newborns (abstract). Am J Obstet Gynecol 1991;164:427.
25. Holcomb WL Jr, Shackelford GD, Petrie RH. Magnesium tocolysis and neonatal bone abnormalities: a controlled study. Obstet Gynecol 1991;78:611–4.
26. Smith LG Jr, Burns PA, Schanler RJ. Calcium homeostasis in pregnant women receiving long-term magnesium sulfate therapy for preterm labor. Am J Obstet Gynecol 1992;167:45–51.
27. Cruikshank DP, Chan GM, Doerrfeld D. Alterations in vitamin D and calcium metabolism with magnesium sulfate treatment of preeclampsia. Am J Obstet Gynecol 1993;168:1170–7.
28. L'Hommedieu CS, Nicholas D, Armes DA, Jones P, Nelson T, Pickering LK. Potentiation of magnesium sulfate-induced neuromuscular weakness by gentamicin, tobramycin, and amikacin. J Pediatr 1983;102: 629–31.
29. L'Hommedieu CS, Huber PA, Rasch DK. Potentiation of magnesium-induced neuromuscular weakness by gentamicin. Crit Care Med 1983;11:55–6.
30. Waisman GD, Mayorga LM, Camera MI, Vignolo CA, Martinotti A. Magnesium plus nifedipine: potentiation of hypotensive effect in preeclampsia? Am J Obstet Gynecol 1988;159:308–9.
31. Snyder SW, Cardwell MS. Neuromuscular blockade with magnesium sulfate and nifedipine. Am J Obstet Gynecol 1989;161:35–6.
32. Rodis JF, Vintzileos AM, Campbell WA, Deaton JL, Nochimson DJ. Maternal hypothermia: an unusual complication of magnesium sulfate therapy. Am J Obstet Gynecol 1987;156:435–6.
33. Baldwin WF. Clinical study of senna administration to nursing mothers: assessment of effects on infant bowel habits. Can Med Assoc J 1963;89:566–8.
34. Cruikshank DP, Varner MW, Pitkin RM. Breast milk magnesium and calcium concentrations following magnesium sulfate treatment. Am J Obstet Gynecol 1982;143:685–8.
35. Committee on Drugs, American Academy of Pediatrics. The transfer of drugs and other chemicals into human milk. Pediatrics 2001;108:776–9.

Name:	**MANDELIC ACID**	Risk Factor:	**C**
Class:	**Urinary Germicide**		

FETAL RISK SUMMARY

RECOMMENDATION: Limited Human Data - No Relevant Animal Data

Mandelic acid is available as a single agent and in combination with methenamine (see also Methenamine). The Collaborative Perinatal Project reported 30 1st trimester exposures for this drug (1, pp. 299, 302). For use anytime in pregnancy, 224 exposures were recorded (1, p. 435). Only in the latter group was a possible association with malformations found, but independent confirmation is required.

BREAST FEEDING SUMMARY

RECOMMENDATION: Limited Human Data - Probably Compatible

Mandelic acid is excreted into breast milk. In six mothers given 12 g/day, milk levels averaged 550 μg/mL (2). The drug was found in the urine of all infants. It was estimated that an infant would receive an average dose of 86 mg/kg/day by this route. The effect of this exposure on a nursing infant is unknown.

References

1. Heinonen OP, Slone D, Shapiro S. Birth Defects and Drugs in Pregnancy. Littleton, MA: Publishing Sciences Group, 1977.
2. Berger H. Excretion of mandelic acid in breast milk. Am J Dis Child 1941;61:256–61.

Name:	**MANNITOL**	Risk Factor:	**C**
Class:	**Diuretic**		

FETAL RISK SUMMARY

RECOMMENDATION: No Human Data - Probably Compatible

Mannitol is an osmotic diuretic. No reports of its use in pregnancy following IV administration have been located. Mannitol, given by intra-amniotic injection, has been used for the induction of abortion (1).

M

BREAST FEEDING SUMMARY

RECOMMENDATION: No Human Data - Probably Compatible

No data are available.

Reference

1. Craft IL, Mus BD. Hypertonic solutions to induce abortions. Br Med J 1971;2:49.

Name:	**MAPROTILINE**	Risk Factor:	**B_M**
Class:	**Antidepressant**		

FETAL RISK SUMMARY

RECOMMENDATION: Limited Human Data - Animal Data Suggest Low Risk

Maprotiline is a tetracyclic antidepressant. No published reports linking the use of maprotiline to congenital defects have been located. Animal studies have failed to demonstrate teratogenicity, carcinogenicity, mutagenicity, or impairment of fertility (1,2).

In a surveillance study of Michigan Medicaid recipients, involving 229,101 completed pregnancies, conducted between 1985 and 1992, 13 newborns had been exposed to maprotiline during the 1st trimester (F. Rosa, personal communication, FDA, 1993). Two (15.4%) major birth defects were observed (0.6 expected), one of which was an oral cleft (none expected). No anomalies were observed in five other defect categories (cardiovascular defects, spina bifida, polydactyly, limb reduction defects, and hypospadias) for which specific data were available. The number of exposures is too small for an assessment of the embryo/fetal risk.

In a 1996 descriptive case series, the European Network of the Teratology Information Services (ENTIS) prospectively examined the outcomes of 689 pregnancies exposed to antidepressants (3). Multiple drug therapy occurred in about two thirds of the mothers. Maprotiline was used in 107 pregnancies. The outcomes of these pregnancies were 17 elective abortions, 11 spontaneous abortions, 2 stillbirths, 72 normal newborns (includes 7 premature infants), 3 normal infants with neonatal disorder (hypotonia in 2; diabetes associated disorder in 1), and 2 infants with congenital defects. The defects (all exposed in the 1st trimester or longer; both exposed to multiple other agents) were facial dysmorphology, nasal hypoplasia, bone immaturity, and bilateral talipes.

A 2002 prospective study compared two groups of mother-child pairs exposed to antidepressants throughout gestation (46 exposed to tricyclics or tetracyclics—1 to maprotiline; 40 to fluoxetine) to 36 nonexposed, not depressed controls (4). Offspring were studied between the ages 15 and 71 months for effects of antidepressant exposure in terms of IQ, language, behavior, and temperament. Exposure to antidepressants did not adversely affect the measured parameters, but IQ was significantly and negatively associated with the duration of depression, and language was negatively associated with the number of depression episodes after delivery (4).

BREAST FEEDING SUMMARY

RECOMMENDATION: Limited Human Data - Potential Toxicity

Maprotiline is excreted into breast milk (5). Milk:plasma ratios of 1.5 and 1.3 have been reported following a 100-mg single dose and 150 mg in divided doses for 120 hours. Multiple dosing resulted in milk concentrations of unchanged maprotiline of 0.2 μg/mL. Although this amount is low, the significance to the nursing infant is not known.

References

1. Product information. Ludiomil. CIBA, 1993.
2. Esaki K, Tanioka Y, Tsukada M, Izumiyama K. Teratogenicity of maprotiline tested by oral administration to mice and rats (Japanese). CIEA Preclinical Report 1976;2:69–77. As cited in Shepard TH. Catalog of Teratogenic Agents. 6th ed. Baltimore, MD: Johns Hopkins University Press, 1989:384.
3. McElhatton PR, Garbis HM, Elefant E, Vial T, Bellemin B, Mastroiacovo P, Arnon J, Rodriguez-Pinilla E, Schaefer C, Pexieder T, Merlob P, Dal Verme S. The outcome of pregnancy in 689 women exposed to therapeutic doses of antidepressants. A collaborative study of the European Network of Teratology Information Services (ENTIS). Reprod Toxicol 1996;10:285–94.
4. Nulman I, Rovet J, Stewart DE, Wolpin J, Pace-Asciak P, Shuhaiber S, Koren G. Child development following exposure to tricyclic antidepressants or fluoxetine throughout fetal life: a prospective, controlled study. Am J Psychiatry 2002;159:1889–95.
5. Reiss W. The relevance of blood level determinations during the evaluation of maprotiline in man. In Murphy JE, ed. *Research and Clinical Investigation in Depression*. Northampton, England: Cambridge Medical Publications, 1980:19–38.

Name:	**MARIJUANA**	Risk Factor:	**X**
Class:	**Hallucinogen**		

FETAL RISK SUMMARY

RECOMMENDATION: Contraindicated

Marijuana (cannabis; hashish) is a natural substance that is smoked for its hallucinogenic properties. (One marijuana cigarette is commonly referred to as a "joint.") Hashish is a potent concentrated form of marijuana. The main psychoactive ingredient, delta-9-tetrahydrocannabinol (Δ-9-THC, THC), is also available in a commercial oral formulation (dronabinol) for use as an antiemetic agent. Natural preparations of marijuana may vary widely in their potency and, except for the commercial preparation, no standardization exists either for the THC content or for the presence of contaminants. Only the commercially available oral formulation can be legally used in the United States.

The use of marijuana by pregnant women is common. Most investigators have reported incidences of 3%–16% (1–17). Other researchers have proposed that even these figures represent underreporting, especially in the 1st month when pregnancy may not be suspected (18–20). Because of the illicit nature of marijuana, many women will simply not admit to its use (4,8). Data from the Ottawa Prenatal Prospective Study in Canada indicated that 20% of their patients used marijuana during the year before pregnancy, with the incidence declining to about one half after the women knew they were pregnant (13). In addition, heavy marijuana use (more than five joints/week or the use of hashish), when compared with alcohol or nicotine usage, was the least reduced of the three agents during pregnancy (21).

Although the use of marijuana by pregnant women is common, the effects of this use on the pregnancies and the fetuses are still unclear. Part of this problem is attributable to the close association between marijuana, alcohol, cigarette smoking, other abuse drugs, and lifestyles that may increase perinatal risk (1–3,6,7). Moreover, studies have relied on maternal self-reporting of the amount and timing of exposures to marijuana and the other substances. Controlling for these confounders becomes a daunting task of almost all studies. However, sufficient data appear to be available to allow classification of the major concerns surrounding exposure to marijuana during pregnancy. These concerns are:

Placental passage of Δ-9-THC
Pregnancy complications
  Length of gestation
  Quality and duration of labor
  Effect on maternal hormone levels
Fetal or newborn complications
  Intrauterine growth
  Structural defects
  Neurobehavioral defects
Leukemia
Miscellaneous effects

Placental Passage

Δ-9-THC and a metabolite, 9-carboxy-THC, cross the placenta to the fetus at term (4,22). Data for other periods of gestation and for other metabolites are not available. A 1982 study found measurable amounts of 9-carboxy-THC, but not THC, in two cord blood samples but did not quantify the concentrations (4). In a study of 10 women who daily smoked up to five marijuana cigarettes, maternal serum samples were drawn 10–20 minutes before corresponding cord blood samples (22). The time interval between last exposure and sampling ranged from 5–26 hours. This is well beyond the time of peak THC levels that occur 3–8 minutes after beginning to smoke (23). Maternal levels of THC were below the limit of sensitivity (0.2 ng/mL) in five samples and ranged from 0.4 to 6 ng/mL in the others. Measurable cord blood concentrations of THC were found in three samples and varied between 0.3 and 1.0 ng/mL. The maternal plasma:cord blood ratios for these three samples were 2.7, 4, and 6. The metabolite, 9-carboxy-THC, was measured in all maternal and cord blood samples, ranging between 2.3 and 125 ng/mL and 0.4 and 18 ng/mL, respectively. Plasma:cord blood ratios for the metabolite varied from 1.7 to 7.8.

Pregnancy Complications

Length of Gestation

Marijuana-induced complications of pregnancy are controversial, with different studies producing conflicting results. One of these areas of controversy involves the effect of marijuana on length of gestation. A 1980 prospective study of 291 women found no relationship between maternal use of marijuana and gestational length (3). Similar results were reported from two studies: one in 1982 involving 1690 women (24) and one in 1989 with 1226 women (25). Of interest, marijuana use by the women in the latter study was confirmed with urine assays (25). A significantly shorter gestational period was found in 1246 users in a retrospective study of 12,424 pregnancies, but this difference disappeared when the data were controlled for nicotine exposure, demographic characteristics, and medical and obstetric histories (9).

In contrast to the above reports, three groups of investigators have associated regular marijuana use with shorter gestations (1,10,14) and one group with longer gestations (26). In 36 women using marijuana two or more times/week, 9 (25%) delivered prematurely, a rate much higher than the 5.1% for users of marijuana one time or less/week and the 5.6% for nonusers (1). Investigation of 583 women who delivered single live births, a continuation of the 1980 study mentioned above, now revealed that heavy use of marijuana (more than five marijuana cigarettes/week) was significantly associated with a reduction of 0.8 week's gestational length after adjustment for the mother's prepregnancy weight (10). A total of 84 women (14.4%) used marijuana in this population, 18 of whom were classified as heavy users. A large prospective study of 3857 pregnancies ending in singleton live births found that regular marijuana use (two to three times/month or more) was associated with an increased risk of preterm (<37 weeks) delivery for white women but not for nonwhite women (14). For the 122 regular white users, 8.2% delivered prematurely compared with 3.8% of 105 occasional users (one marijuana cigarette or less/month) and 4.0% of 2778 nonusers. In the nonwhite groups, the incidences of shortened gestation for the 86 regular, 53 occasional, and 706 nonusers were 10.5%, 11.3%, and 8.8%, respectively. In a population of lower socioeconomic status women, the total amount of marijuana used during pregnancy was positively correlated with an average 2 days' prolongation of gestation (26). However, the authors of this study noted that their evidence for a longer gestational period was weak in terms of magnitude.

Quality and Duration of Labor

A second pregnancy complication examined frequently is the effect of marijuana on the quality and duration of labor. No association between marijuana and duration of labor, including precipitate labor and the type of presentation at birth, was found in the Ottawa Prenatal Prospective Study (3,5,8) or in another study (26). In contrast, other investigators found a significant difference in precipitate labor (<3 hours total) between users (29%) and nonusers (3%) (4,27). Although not significant, 31% of users (11 of 35) had prolonged, protracted, or arrested labor as compared with 19% (7 of 36) nonusers (4,27). Because of the dysfunctional labor, 57% of the newborn infants in the user group had meconium staining vs. 25% among nonusers, a situation that probably resulted in the observation that 41% of newborn infants of users required resuscitation compared with 21% of infants of nonusers. Adjustment of the data for race, income, smoking, alcohol use, and first physician visit did not change the findings. A second study by these latter investigators using a different group of patients produced similar results in the incidence of dysfunctional labor, precipitate labor, and meconium staining, but the differences between users and nonusers were not significant (7).

Maternal Hormone Levels

In nonhuman primates, marijuana disrupts the menstrual cycle by inhibiting ovulation through its effects on the pituitary trophic hormones (luteinizing hormone and follicle-stimulating hormone), prolactin, and resulting decreases in estrogen and progesterone levels (16). Tolerance to these effects has been reported (16). Similar effects have been observed in human clinical studies (16).

Thirteen pregnant women who were regular users of marijuana (once/month to four times/day), were matched with controls (28). No effect of this exposure was measured on the levels of human chorionic gonadotropin (hCG), pregnancy-specific β-1-glycoprotein, placental lactogen, progesterone, 17-hydroxyprogesterone, estradiol, and estriol.

Fetal or Newborn Complications

Concerns with the fetal complications arising from maternal marijuana use center around the effects on intrauterine growth, structural anomalies, and neurobehavioral complications in the newborn infant. A recent report has now indicated that induction of leukemia in childhood must also be considered. As with pregnancy complications, conflicting reports are common.

M

Intrauterine Growth

Data of the Ottawa Prenatal Prospective Study indicated no significant reduction in birth weight or head circumference (after adjustment for other factors) in babies of marijuana users (3,5,8,10,13). Compared with infants of nonusers, birth weight actually increased by an average of 67 g in irregular users (one marijuana cigarette or less/week) and 117 g in moderate users (two to five/week), whereas heavy use (more than five marijuana cigarettes/week) was associated with a nonsignificant reduction of 52 g (10). Other studies have observed no effect on growth after adjustment of their data (1,7,9,26,29–33). However, in one study, a reduction of 0.55 cm in infant length, but not in head circumference, was correlated with maternal use of three marijuana cigarettes/day in the 1st trimester (26). Use during the remainder of pregnancy or the total amount smoked during pregnancy did not significantly affect the infant's length or head circumference. One study, however, did find a significantly smaller head size in offspring of mothers who were heavy marijuana users (32). In addition, one group of investigators found no association between marijuana and preterm delivery or abruptio placentae (30).

A number of researchers have reported positive correlations with reduced intrauterine growth (after adjustment). In one study, use of less than three joints/week was associated with a significant decrease in birth weight of 95 g compared with that of controls, and use of three or more cigarettes/week was associated with a significant reduction of 139 g (24,34). A related 1989 study found that marijuana use during pregnancy, when confirmed by positive urine assays, was independently associated with impaired fetal growth, and that the effects of cocaine abuse were additive but not synergistic (25). However, they could not demonstrate a cause-and-effect relationship with marijuana because of other factors, such as the markedly elevated blood levels of carbon monoxide that occur with marijuana use (blood carboxyhemoglobin levels after smoking marijuana are about

5 times those observed after smoking tobacco) (25). Of 1,226 mothers who were studied, 331 (27%) used marijuana during gestation as determined by history and positive urine assay. Only 278 (84%) of these would have been detected by history alone. After controlling for potential confounding variables, infants of marijuana users with positive urine assays ($N = 202$), compared to infants of nonusers ($N = 895$), had significantly lower birth weight (79 g) and length (0.52 cm), but not head circumference. The birth weight and length measurements did not differ statistically if only self-reported marijuana use was considered, demonstrating the importance of a biologic marker in studies involving this drug (25).

A study, conducted from 1975 to 1983 in two phases, found decreased birth weight only in the second phase (17). The two phases, involving 1434 and 1381 patients, respectively, differed primarily in their assessment of marijuana use early in pregnancy. In the first phase, 9.3% used marijuana, with consumption of two to four joints/month associated with a significant increase in birth weight. No trend was observed with more- or less-frequent use. In the second phase, with 10.3% users, weight reductions were found in all classifications of marijuana exposure: 127 g for two to three joints/week, 143 g for four to six joints/week, and 230 g for daily use (17). The authors speculated that the difference between the groups may have been related to the use of other abuse drugs (e.g., cocaine) or changes in the composition or contaminants of marijuana. In a 1986 study, regular marijuana use (two to three times or more/month) was correlated with an increased risk of low-birth-weight (<2500 g) and small-for-gestational-age (SGA) infants in whites only (14). The rates of low-birth-weight and SGA infants in users ($N = 122$) and nonusers ($N = 3490$) were 8.2% vs. 2.7%, and 12.5% vs. 4.9%, respectively. In 845 nonwhites, no differences between users and nonusers were observed. In a 1984 report, examination of 462 infants, 16% of whom were exposed to marijuana and alcohol during early gestation, found a significant correlation between maternal marijuana use and decreased body length at 8 months of age (11). Body weight and head circumference were not significantly affected.

In three case reports on the same five infants, low birth weight (all <2500 g) with reduced head circumference and length were observed (35–37). Two of the infants were premature (<37 weeks). The mothers of these infants smoked 2–14 marijuana cigarettes/day during pregnancy with one also using alcohol, cocaine, and nicotine, and two mothers using nicotine. In a 1999 study, positive pregnancy test urine samples were screened for several drugs, including marijuana (38). Those testing positive for marijuana had significantly lower birth weight, an increased risk of prematurity, and a lower gestational age at delivery.

A 1997 meta-analysis on the effect of marijuana on birth weight identified 10 studies in which the results were adjusted for cigarette smoking, and five of these met their criteria for analysis (39). The pooled odds ratio for any use of marijuana and low birth weight was 1.09 (95% confidence interval 0.94–1.27). They concluded that, in the amounts typically used by pregnant women, there was insufficient evidence that marijuana caused low birth weight (39). In a 2001 study, exposure to marijuana during pregnancy was not associated with any growth measurement or timing of pubertal milestones in a group of 152 adolescents (13- to 16-year-olds) that had been followed longitudinally since birth (40).

Structural Defects

Animal research in the 1960s and 1970s yielded inconclusive evidence on the teratogenicity of marijuana and its active ingredients unless high doses were used in certain species (41–44). In humans, most investigators and reviewers have concluded either that marijuana does not produce structural defects or that insufficient data exist to reach any conclusion (1,13,25,26,29,45–56). However, one reviewer cautioned that marijuana-induced birth defects could be rare and easily missed (55), and another observed that marijuana could potentiate known teratogens by lowering the threshold for their effects (49). A previously mentioned study that used urine assays to document marijuana exposure found that the drug was not associated with minor (either singly or as a constellation of three) or major congenital anomalies (25).

Because marijuana use is so common in women during pregnancy, and because of its frequent association with alcohol and other abuse drugs, it is not surprising that a number of studies and case reports have described congenital malformations in infants whose mothers were smoking marijuana. With some exceptions, the majority of these investigators did not attribute the observed defects to marijuana, but they are chronicled here mainly for a complete record.

Several reports have described the combined maternal use of marijuana and lysergic acid diethylamide (LSD) in cases ending with poor fetal outcome (57–65). A 1968 report described an infant with right terminal transverse acheiria (absence of hand) (57). The mother had taken LSD early in the gestation before she knew she was pregnant. She had also smoked marijuana throughout the pregnancy and had taken a combination product containing dicyclomine, doxylamine, and pyridoxine for 1st trimester nausea. A second infant with a terminal transverse deficit, who was also exposed to the two hallucinogens, was described in 1969 (58). The defect involved portions of fingers of the left hand. Syndactyly of the right hand with shortened fingers and talipes equinovarus of the left foot were also present. A critique of these case reports and others concluded that the defects in the two infants might have been caused by amniotic band syndrome (59). Complete exstrophy of the bladder, epispadias, widely separated pubic rami, and bilateral inguinal hernias were observed in a newborn exposed to LSD, marijuana, and mephentermine (60). Marijuana was allegedly used only twice by the mother. In another case, a female infant with multiple anomalies compatible with trisomy 13 with D/D translocation was delivered from a 22-year-old mother who had last used LSD 9 months before conception (61). The mother used marijuana, barbiturates, and amphetamines throughout gestation and, presumably, before conception. The authors speculated that the defect may have been caused by LSD-induced damage of maternal germ cells before fertilization. A 1972 case report described an infant with multiple eye and central nervous system defects consisting of brachycephaly with widely separated sutures, bilateral cephalohematomas, a right eye smaller than the left, a possible cataract, and multiple brain anomalies (62). The mother had taken marijuana, LSD, and other drugs throughout pregnancy. In a study of 140 women using LSD and marijuana followed through 148 pregnancies, 8 of 83 liveborn infants had major defects as did 4 of 14 embryos examined after induced abortion (63). The incidence of defects in this sample is high (8.1%), but many of the women were using multiple other abuse drugs and had lifestyles that probably were not conducive to good fetal health. Two other reports involving the combined use of marijuana and LSD with resulting adverse fetal outcomes do not appear to have any relationship to either drug (64,65). One of these involved a report of six cases of persistent ductus arteriosus, one of which was exposed to marijuana *in utero* (64). The history of maternal marijuana use was coincidental. The second case described an infant who died at 2.5 months of age of a bilateral *in utero* cerebrovascular accident and resulting porencephaly (65). The mother had used marijuana, LSD, alcohol, and other abuse drugs, including cocaine. This latter drug was thought to be the causative agent.

In one of two fatal cases of congenital hypothalamic hamartoblastoma tumor, an infant exposed to marijuana also had congenital heart disease and skeletal anomalies suggestive of the Ellis-von Creveld syndrome (i.e., chondroectodermal dysplasia syndrome) (66). In addition to marijuana, the mother had used cocaine and methaqualone during early pregnancy, but the authors did not attribute the defects to a particular agent. In a report of an infant with a random pattern of amputations and constrictions consistent with the amniotic band sequence, the mother's occasional use of marijuana was coincidental (67).

In contrast to the above case reports, in which marijuana use was apparently not related to structural defects, studies have reported possible associations with the drug (9,24, 35–37,68,69). In a large study involving 12,424 women of whom 1246 (10%) used marijuana during pregnancy, a crude association between one or more major malformations and marijuana was discovered; no association was found with minor malformations (9). Logistic regression was used to control confounding variables, and although the odds ratio (1.36) was suggestive, the association between marijuana and the defects was not significant. In 1690 mother-child pairs, women who smoked marijuana, but who only drank small amounts of alcohol, were 5 times more likely than nonusers to deliver an infant with features compatible with the fetal alcohol syndrome (see Ethanol) (24). The relative risk for this defect in marijuana users was 12.7 compared with 2.0 in nonusers. In a series of case reports, five infants were described with congenital defects suggestive of the fetal alcohol syndrome (35–37). In addition to daily marijuana use by the mothers, one used alcohol, cocaine, and nicotine; two used nicotine only; and two denied the use of other drugs (35). One study compared 25 marijuana users with 25 closely matched nonusing controls in a search for minor anomalies (68). Infants were examined at a mean age of 28.8 months. No relationship between the drug and minor malformations was found, but the authors could not exclude the existence of a possible relationship at birth, since some minor anomalies disappear with age. Of interest, three infants had severe epicanthal folds, three had true ocular hypertelorism, and all were the offspring of heavy users (more than five joints/week) (68).

A 2004 report from the Atlanta Birth Defects Case-Control Study identified an association between maternal marijuana use and ventricular septal defects (VSD) in the offspring (69). The cases, 122 infants with isolated simple VSD, were compared to 3029 control infants. Maternal marijuana use was determined by self-report combined with paternal proxy-reports of the mother's exposure. The odds ratio (OR) for maternal use of marijuana and VSD, after adjustment, was 1.90, 95% confidence interval (CI) 1.29–2.81. The risk of VSD increased with regular (3 or more days/week) marijuana use. A similar analysis for heavy (10 or more drinks/week) maternal alcohol consumption produced an OR of 2.10, 95% CI 0.75–5.87 (69).

Strabismus was diagnosed in 24% (7 of 29) of the infants delivered from mothers maintained on methadone throughout pregnancy in a 1987 report (70). This percentage was approximately 4–8 times the expected incidence of the eye defect in the general population. Two (29%) of the seven infants were also exposed *in utero* to marijuana vs. three (14%) of the nonaffected infants. Although use of other abuse drugs was common, the authors attributed the eye condition to low birth weight and, possibly, an unknown contribution from methadone (70). However, in the Ottawa Prenatal Prospective Study, 35% of the marijuana-exposed infants compared to 6% of the controls had significantly more than one of the following eye problems: myopia, strabismus, abnormal oculomotor functioning, or unusual discs (13). The examiner was blinded to the prenatal histories of the infants.

Neurobehavioral Defects

Significant alterations in neurobehavior in offspring of regular marijuana users were noted in the Ottawa Prenatal Prospective Study (3,5,13,15,71–80). After adjustment for nicotine and alcohol use, *in utero* exposure to marijuana was associated with increased tremors and exaggerated startles, both spontaneous and in response to minimal stimuli (13,15). Decreased visual responses, including poorer visual habituation to light, were also observed in these infants. In addition, a slight increase in irritability was noted. In early data from the Ottawa group, a distinctive shrill, high-pitched, cat-like cry, reminiscent of the cry considered to be symptomatic of drug withdrawal, was heard from a large number of the offspring of regular users (3). No differences were noted between exposed and nonexposed infants in terms of lateralization, muscle tone, hand-to-mouth behavior, general activity, alertness, or lability of states (3). On follow-up examinations, the abnormalities in neonatal neurobehavior apparently did not result in poorer performance on cognitive and motor tests at 18 and 24 months (13). The investigators cautioned that they were unable to determine whether the follow-up results were truly indicative of a return to normal or were related to insensitivity of the available tests (13).

In a longitudinal analysis of exposed offspring, a series of additional reports from the Ottawa Prenatal Prospective Study appeared covering the period of 1989 to 2001 (71–80). Offspring exposed prenatally to marijuana were evaluated at 9 and 30 days of age (71). Exposure was associated with symptoms similar to mild narcotic withdrawal (tremors associated with Moro reflex, increased fine tremor, and startles). Children exposed *in utero* were evaluated by a series of tests at 12 and 24 months of age (72). A positive association was found between maternal use of marijuana and the cognitive composite score at 12 months but not at 24 months. At 36- and 48-month follow up, significantly lower scores in verbal and memory were associated with maternal use of the drug during pregnancy (73). However, no association was found with lower verbal or cognitive scores at 60- and 72-month evaluation (74); however in the latter evaluation, a dose-response association was found with a possible deficit in sustained attention and a higher rating by the mothers on the impulsive/hyperactive scale (75). In children who were 6–9 years of age, parental ratings of behavior problems, visual-perceptual tasks, language comprehension, and distractibility, after adjustment for the home environment condition, were not associated with marijuana exposure (76). No association was found between marijuana and reading or language outcomes in children 9–12 years of age (77). Although subsequent analysis found no association between exposure and global intelligence or verbal, it did find a negative association with executive function tasks that require impulse control and visual analysis/hypothesis testing (78). Prenatal marijuana exposure did not adversely affect basic visuoperceptual tasks in 9- to 12-year-olds, but a negative association was found with performance in visual problem-solving situations (79). This latter finding could be explained by marijuana's negative impact on problem-solving situations requiring integration, analysis, and synthesis (i.e., executive functions) (79). In 13- to 16-year-olds, prenatal marijuana exposure was associated with the stability of attention over time (increased errors of omissions) (80). This finding was similar to what was found in 6 year olds (see reference 75 above). Several reviews by the above investigators have summarized their findings (81–86).

A 1984 report examining maternal drinking and neonatal withdrawal found that marijuana use had no effect on the signs of withdrawal in their patients (87). In another study, no increase in startles, tremors, or other neurobehavioral measures at birth was noted in exposed infants (26). Marijuana exposure also had no effect on muscle tone. Evaluation at 1 year of age found no significant differences in growth or in mental and motor development between infants exposed *in utero* to either none or varying amounts of the drug (26).

A 1994 study of children exposed to marijuana during the 1st and 2nd trimesters found significant negative effects on the performance of 3-year-old children on the Stanford-Binet Intelligence Scale (88). Although the effects were small, they indicated that, on average, exposed children would have a lower IQ compared to nonexposed children. In another study, infants were assessed at 9 and 19 months of age (88). At 9 months, 3rd trimester marijuana use (>1 joint/day) was associated with delayed mental development, but not on infants at 19 months of age (89). In a third study from this group, children exposed prenatally were evaluated at 10 years of age (90). A significant relationship between prenatal exposure to marijuana and increased hyperactivity, impulsivity, inattention, increased delinquency, and externalizing problems was found.

Leukemia

The development of leukemia in children exposed to marijuana during gestation has been suggested in a 1989 report (91). In a multicenter study conducted between 1980 and 1984 by the Children's Cancer Study Group, *in utero* marijuana exposure was significantly related to the development of acute nonlymphoblastic leukemia (ANLL). Of the 204 cases that were analyzed, marijuana use was found in 10 mothers, only one of whom used other (LSD) mind-altering drugs. An 11th case mother used methadone. Only 1 of the 203 closely matched healthy controls was exposed to abuse drugs. The 10-fold risk induced by marijuana exposure was statistically significant. The mean age of ANLL diagnosis was significantly younger in the exposed children than in nonexposed children: 37.7 months vs. 96.1 months, respectively. Based on the French-American-British system of classification, the morphology of the leukemias also differed significantly, with 70% of the exposed cases presenting with monocytic (M5) or myelomonocytic (M4) morphology compared with 31% of the nonexposed cases. Additionally, only 10% of the exposed children had M1 or M2 (myelocytic) morphology vs. 58% of the nonexposed children. The authors were able to exclude reporting bias but could not exclude the possibility that the association was related to other factors, such as the presence of herbicides or pesticides on the marijuana (91).

Miscellaneous Effects. Early concerns (92,93) that marijuana-induced chromosomal damage could eventually lead to congenital defects have been largely laid to rest (46,55,56). The clinical significance of any drug-induced chromosomal abnormality is doubtful (55). Finally, heavy marijuana use in males has been associated with decreased sperm production (16,93). However, the clinical significance of this finding has been questioned, since there is no evidence that the reduction in sperm counts is related to infertility (16,93).

Summary

The use of marijuana in pregnancy has produced conflicting reports on the length of gestation, the quality and duration of labor, fetal growth, congenital defects, and neurobehavior in the newborn. These effects have been the subject of a number of reviews (16,42,43,45–49,52–56,81–86,94–96). A meta-analysis and a longitudinal study could not find associations between marijuana and low birth weight or growth in adolescents, but an association with lower birth weight and length was found when biomarkers were used to document maternal exposure. The possible association of *in utero* marijuana exposure with leukemia in children should be a major concern of any woman who chooses to use this drug during pregnancy. No pattern of malformations has been observed that could be considered characteristic of *in utero* marijuana exposure. However, there is evidence that marijuana might potentiate the fetal effects of alcohol and may be associated with an increased risk of ventricular septal defects. Two research centers have concluded that prenatal marijuana use adversely effects neurobehavior in infants and adolescents. In the neonatal period, exposed infants may have symptoms similar to mild narcotic withdrawal. In older children, the negative effects included decreased problem solving ability, inattention, increased hyperactivity, impulsivity and delinquency, and externalization of problems. Some of these results were found even after controlling for the home environment. In most studies, the use of marijuana is closely associated with the use of nicotine and alcohol, and the abuse of other drugs, both prescription and illicit, occurs frequently. Moreover, maternal self-reporting of the amounts and timing of the exposures to marijuana and other abuse substances is common. Separating the effects of these confounding exposures from the effects of marijuana is a daunting task. In addition, failure to account for the varying concentrations of Δ-9-THC contained in the natural product, the presence of contaminants, and the underreporting of maternal marijuana use could very well have changed the findings of many studies. Therefore, the associations with structural and neurobehavior defects require continued study.

BREAST FEEDING SUMMARY

RECOMMENDATION: Contraindicated

Δ-9-Tetrahydrocannabinol (Δ-9-THC; THC), the main active ingredient of marijuana (cannabis, hashish), is excreted into breast milk (26,49,97,98). Analysis of THC and two metabolites, 11-hydroxy-THC and 9-carboxy-THC, were conducted on the milk of two women who had been nursing for 7 and 8 months and who smoked marijuana frequently (97). A THC concentration of 105 ng/mL, but no metabolites, was found in the milk of the woman smoking one pipe of marijuana daily. In the second woman, who smoked seven pipes/day, concentrations of THC, 11-hydroxy-THC, and 9-carboxy-THC were 340 ng/mL, 4 ng/mL, and none, respectively. The analysis was repeated in the second mother, approximately 1 hour after the last use of marijuana, by using simultaneously obtained samples of milk and plasma. Concentrations (in ng/mL) of the active ingredient and metabolites in milk and plasma (ratios shown in parenthesis) were 60.3 and 7.2 (8.4), 1.1 and 2.5 (0.4), and 1.6 and 19 (0.08), respectively. The marked differences in THC found between the milk samples was thought to be related to the amount of marijuana smoked and the interval between smoking and sample collection. A total fecal sample from the infant yielded levels of 347 ng of THC, 67 ng of 11-hydroxy-THC, and 611 ng of 9-carboxy-THC. Because of the large concentration of metabolites, the authors interpreted this as evidence that the nursing infant was absorbing and metabolizing the THC from the milk. Despite the evidence that the fat-soluble THC was concentrated in breast milk, both nursing infants were developing normally (97).

In animals, THC decreases the amount of milk produced by suppressing the production of prolactin and, possibly, by a direct action on the mammary glands (49). Although data on this effect are not available in humans, maternal marijuana use does not seem grossly to affect the nursing infant (26). In 27 infants evaluated at 1 year of age who were exposed to marijuana via the milk, compared with 35 nonexposed infants, no significant differences were found in terms of age at weaning, growth, and mental or motor development (26).

Although no adverse effects of marijuana exposure from breast milk have been reported, follow up of these infants is inadequate. At the present time, the long-term effects of this exposure are unknown and additional research to determine these effects, if any, is warranted (98). The American Academy of Pediatrics classifies marijuana as a drug that should not be used by nursing mothers (99).

References

1. Gibson GT, Baghurst PA, Colley DP. Maternal alcohol, tobacco and cannabis consumption and the outcome of pregnancy. Aust N Z J Obstet Gynaecol 1983;23: 15–9.
2. Fried PA, Watkinson B, Grant A, Knights RM. Changing patterns of soft drug use prior to and during pregnancy: a prospective study. Drug Alcohol Depend 1980;6:323–43.
3. Fried PA. Marihuana use by pregnant women: neurobehavioral effects in neonates. Drug Alcohol Depend 1980;6:415–24.
4. Greenland S, Staisch KJ, Brown N, Gross SJ. The effects of marijuana use during pregnancy. I. A preliminary epidemiologic study. Am J Obstet Gynecol 1982;143:408–13.
5. Fried PA. Marihuana use by pregnant women and effects on offspring: an update. Neurobehav Toxicol Teratol 1982;4:451–4.
6. Rayburn W, Wible-Kant J, Bledsoe P. Changing trends in drug use during pregnancy. J Reprod Med 1982; 27:569–75.
7. Greenland S, Richwald GA, Honda GD. The effects of marijuana use during pregnancy. II. A study in a low-risk home-delivery population. Drug Alcohol Depend 1983;11:359–66.
8. Fried PA, Buckingham M, Von Kulmiz P. Marijuana use during pregnancy and perinatal risk factors. Am J Obstet Gynecol 1983;146:992–4.
9. Linn S, Schoenbaum SC, Monson RR, Rosner R, Stubblefield PC, Ryan KJ. The association of marijuana use with outcome of pregnancy. Am J Public Health 1983;73:1161–4.
10. Fried PA, Watkinson B, Willan A. Marijuana use during pregnancy and decreased length of gestation. Am J Obstet Gynecol 1984;150:23–7.
11. Barr HM, Streissguth AP, Martin DC, Herman CS. Infant size at 8 months of age: relationship to maternal use of alcohol, nicotine, and caffeine during pregnancy. Pediatrics 1984;74:336–41.
12. Zuckerman BS, Hingson RW, Morelock S, Amaro H, Frank D, Sorenson JR, Kayne HL, Timperi R. A pilot study assessing maternal marijuana use by urine assay during pregnancy. Natl Inst Drug Abuse Res Monogr Ser 1985;57:84–93.
13. Fried PA. Postnatal consequences of maternal marijuana use. Natl Inst Drug Abuse Res Monogr Ser 1985; 59:61–72.
14. Hatch EE, Bracken MB. Effect of marijuana use in pregnancy on fetal growth. Am J Epidemiol 1986; 124:986–93.
15. Fried PA, Makin JE. Neonatal behavioural correlates of prenatal exposure to marihuana, cigarettes and alcohol in a low risk population. Neurotoxicol Teratol 1987;9:1–7.
16. Smith CG, Asch RH. Drug abuse and reproduction. Fertil Steril 1987;48:355–73.
17. Kline J, Stein Z, Hutzler M. Cigarettes, alcohol and marijuana: varying associations with birthweight. Int J Epidemiol 1987;16:44–51.
18. Day NL, Wagener DK, Taylor PM. Measurement of substance use during pregnancy: methodologic issues. Natl Inst Drug Abuse Res Monogr Ser 1985;59: 36–47.
19. Hingson R, Zuckerman B, Amaro H, Frank DA, Kayne H, Sorenson JR, Mitchell J, Parker S, Morelock S, Timperi R. Maternal marijuana use and neonatal outcome: uncertainty posed by self-reports. Am J Public Health 1986;76:667–9.
20. Little RE, Uhl CN, Labbe RF, Abkowitz JL, Phillips ELR. Agreement between laboratory tests and self-reports of alcohol, tobacco, caffeine, marijuana and other drug use in post-partum women. Soc Sci Med 1986;22:91–8.
21. Fried PA, Barnes MV, Drake ER. Soft drug use after pregnancy compared to use before and during pregnancy. Am J Obstet Gynecol 1985;151:787–92.
22. Blackard C, Tennes K. Human placental transfer of cannabinoids. N Engl J Med 1984;311:797.
23. Busto U, Bendayan R, Sellers EM. Clinical pharmacokinetics of non-opiate abused drugs. Clin Pharmacokinet 1989;16:1–26.
24. Hingson R, Alpert JJ, Day N, Dooling E, Kayne H, Morelock S, Oppenheimer E, Zuckerman B. Effects of maternal drinking and marijuana use on fetal growth and development. Pediatrics 1982;70:539–46.
25. Zuckerman B, Frank DA, Hingson R, Amaro H, Levenson SM, Kayne H, Parker S, Vinci R, Aboagye K, Fried LE, Cabral H, Timperi R, Bauchner H. Effects of maternal marijuana and cocaine use on fetal growth. N Engl J Med 1989;320:762–78.
26. Tennes K, Avitable N, Blackard C, Boyles C, Hassoun B, Holmes L, Kreye M. Marijuana: prenatal and postnatal exposure in the human. Natl Inst Drug Abuse Res Monogr Ser 1985;59:48–60.
27. Greenland S, Staisch KJ, Brown N, Gross SJ. Effects of marijuana on human pregnancy, labor, and delivery. Neurobehav Toxicol Teratol 1982;4:447–50.
28. Braunstein GD, Buster JE, Soares JR, Gross SJ. Pregnancy hormone concentrations in marijuana users. Life Sci 1983;33:195–9.
29. Rosett HL, Weiner L, Lee A, Zuckerman B, Dooling E, Oppenheimer E. Patterns of alcohol consumption and fetal development. Obstet Gynecol 1983;61: 539–546.
30. Shiono PM, Klebanoff MA, Nugent RP, Cotch MF, Wilkins DG, Rollins DE, Carey JC, Behrman RE. The impact of cocaine and marijuana use on low birth weight and preterm birth. A multicenter study. Am J Obstet Gynecol 1995;172:19–27.
31. Cornelius MD, Taylor PM, Geva D, Day NL. Prenatal tobacco and marijuana use among adolescents: effect on offspring gestational age, growth, and morphology. Pediatrics 1995;95:738–43.
32. Fried PA, Watkinson B, Gray R. Growth from birth to early adolescence in offspring prenatally exposed to cigarettes and marijuana. Neurotoxicol Teratol 1999;21:513–25.
33. Fergusson DM, Horwood LJ, Northstone K, ALSPAC

M

Team. Maternal use of cannabis and pregnancy outcome. BJOG 2002;109:21–7.
34. Zuckerman B, Alpert JJ, Dooling E, Oppenheimer E, Hingson R, Day N, Rosett H. Substance abuse during pregnancy and newborn size. Pediatr Res 1980;15:524.
35. Qazi QH, Mariano E, Milman DH, Beller E, Crombleholme W. Abnormalities in offspring associated with prenatal marihuana exposure. Dev Pharmacol Ther 1985;8:141–8.
36. Qazi QH, Mariano E, Beller E, Milman DH, Crombleholme W. Abnormalities in offspring associated with prenatal marihuana exposure. Pediatr Res 1983;17:153A.
37. Qazi QH, Milman DH. Nontherapeutic use of psychoactive drugs. N Engl J Med 1983;309:797–8.
38. Sherwood RA, Keating J, Kavvadia V, Greenough A, Peters TJ. Substance misuse in early pregnancy and relationship to fetal outcome. Eur J Pediatr 1999;158:488–92.
39. English DR, Hulse GK, Milne E, Holman CDJ, Bower CI. Maternal cannabis use and birth weight: a meta-analysis. Addiction 1997;92:1553–60.
40. Fried PA, James DS, Watkinson B. Growth and pubertal milestones during adolescence in offspring prenatally exposed to cigarettes and marihuana. Neurotoxicol Teratol 2001;23:431–6.
41. Abel EL. Prenatal exposure to cannabis: a critical review of effects on growth, development, and behavior. Behav Neural Biol 1980;29:137–56.
42. VanBlerk GA, Majerus TC, Myers RAM. Teratogenic potential of some psychopharmacologic drugs: a brief review. Int J Gynaecol Obstet 1980;17:399–402.
43. Lee CC, Chiang CN. Maternal-fetal transfer of abused substances: pharmacokinetic and pharmacodynamic data. Natl Inst Drug Abuse Res Monogr Ser 1985;60:110–47.
44. Shepard TH. *Catalog of Teratogenic Agents*. 5th ed. Baltimore, MD: Johns Hopkins University Press, 1986: 353–6.
45. Rennert OM. Drug-induced somatic alterations. Clin Obstet Gynecol 1975;18:185–98.
46. Matsuyama S, Jarvik L. Effects of marihuana on the genetic and immune systems. Natl Inst Drug Abuse Res Monogr Ser 1977;14:179–93.
47. Nahas GG. Current status of marijuana research: symposium on marijuana held July 1978 in Reims, France. JAMA 1979;242:2775–8.
48. Glass L, Evans HE. Perinatal drug abuse. Pediatr Ann 1979;8:84–92.
49. Harclerode J. The effect of marijuana on reproduction and development. Natl Inst Drug Abuse Res Monogr Ser 1980;31:137–66.
50. Chernoff GF, Jones KL. Fetal preventive medicine: teratogens and the unborn baby. Pediatr Ann 1981; 10:210–7.
51. Stern L. In vivo assessment of the teratogenic potential of drugs in humans. Obstet Gynecol 1981;58: 3S–8S.
52. Shy KK, Brown ZA. Maternal and fetal well-being. West J Med 1984;141:807–15.
53. Tennes K. Effects of marijuana on pregnancy and fetal development in the human. Natl Inst Drug Abuse Res Monogr Ser 1984;44:115–23.
54. Mullins CL, Gazaway PM III. Alcohol and drug use in pregnancy: a case for management. Md Med J 1985;34:991–6.
55. Hollister LE. Health aspects of cannabis. Pharmacol Rev 1986;38:1–20.
56. O'Connor MC. Drugs of abuse in pregnancy—an overview. Med J Aust 1987;147:180–3.
57. Hecht F, Beals RK, Lees MH, Jolly H, Roberts P. Lysergic-acid-diethylamide and cannabis as possible teratogens in man. Lancet 1968;2:1087.
58. Carakushansky G, Neu RL, Gardner LI. Lysergide and cannabis as possible teratogens in man. Lancet 1969;1:150–1.
59. Blanc WA, Mattison DR, Kane R, Chauhan P. L.S.D., intrauterine amputations, and amniotic-band syndrome. Lancet 1971;2:158–9.
60. Gelehrter TD. Lysergic acid diethylamide (LSD) and exstrophy of the bladder. J Pediatr 1970;77:1065–6.
61. Hsu LY, Strauss L, Hirschorn K. Chromosome abnormality in offspring of LSD user. JAMA 1970;211: 987–90.
62. Bogdanoff B, Rorke LB, Yanoff M, Warren WS. Brain and eye abnormalities. Am J Dis Child 1972;123: 145–8.
63. Jacobson CB, Berlin CM. Possible reproductive detriment in LSD users. JAMA 1972;222:1367–73.
64. Brown R, Pickering D. Persistent transitional circulation. Arch Dis Child 1974;49:883–5.
65. Tenorio GM, Nazvi M, Bickers GH, Hubbird RH. Intrauterine stroke and maternal polydrug abuse. Clin Pediatr 1988;27:565–7.
66. Huff DS, Fernandes M. Two cases of congenital hypothalamic hamartoblastoma, polydactyly, and other congenital anomalies (Pallister-Hall syndrome). N Engl J Med 1982;306:430–1.
67. Lage JM, VanMarter LJ, Bieber FR. Questionable role of amniocentesis in the etiology of amniotic band formation. A case report. J Reprod Med 1988;33:71–3.
68. O'Connell CM, Fried PA. An investigation of prenatal cannabis exposure and minor physical anomalies in a low risk population. Neurobehav Toxicol Teratol 1984;6:345–50.
69. Williams LJ, Correa A, Rasmussen S. Maternal lifestyle factors and risk for ventricular septal defects. Birth Defects Res Part A Clin Mol Teratol 2004;70:59–64.
70. Nelson LB, Ehrlich S, Calhoun JH, Matteucci T, Finnegan LP. Occurrence of strabismus in infants born to drug-dependent women. Am J Dis Child 1987;141:175–8.
71. Fried PA, Watkinson B, Dillon RF, Dulberg CS. Neonatal neurological status in a low-risk population after prenatal exposure to cigarettes, marijuana, and alcohol. J Dev Behav Pediatr 1987;8:318–26.
72. Fried PA, Watkinson B. 12- and 24-month neurobehavioural follow-up of children prenatally exposed to marihuana, cigarettes and alcohol. Neurotoxicol Teratol 1988;10:305–13.
73. Fried PA, Watkinson B. 36- and 48-month neurobehavioral follow-up of children prenatally exposed to marijuana, cigarettes, and alcohol. J Dev Behav Pediatr 1990;11:49–58.
74. Fried PA, O'Connell CM, Watkinson B. 60- and 72-month follow-up of children prenatally exposed to marijuana, cigarettes, and alcohol: cognitive and language assessment. J Dev Behav Pediatr 1992;13: 383–91.

75. Fried PA, Watkinson B, Gray R. A follow-up study of attentional behavior in 6-year-old children exposed prenatally to marihuana, cigarettes, and alcohol. Neurotoxicol Teratol 1992;14:299–311.
76. O'Connell CM, Fried PA. Prenatal exposure to cannabis: a preliminary report of postnatal consequences in school-age children. Neurotoxicol Teratol 1991;13:631–9.
77. Fried PA, Watkinson B, Siegel LS. Reading and language in 9- to 12-year olds prenatally exposed to cigarettes and marijuana. Neurotoxicol Teratol 1997;19:171–83.
78. Fried PA, Watkinson B, Gray R. Differential effects on cognitive functioning in 9- to 12-year-olds prenatally exposed to cigarettes and marihuana. Neurotoxicol Teratol 1998;20:293–306.
79. Fried PA, Watkinson B. Visuoperceptual functioning differs in 9- to 12-year-olds prenatally exposed to cigarettes and marihuana. Neurotoxicol Teratol 2000;22:11–20.
80. Fried PA, Watkinson B. Differential effects on facets of attention in adolescents prenatally exposed to cigarettes and marihuana. Neurotoxicol Teratol 2001;23:421–30.
81. Fried PA. Cigarettes and marijuana: are there measurable long-term neurobehavioral teratogenic effects? Neurotoxicol 1989;10:577–83.
82. Fried PA. Postnatal consequences of maternal marijuana use in humans. Ann N Y Acad Sci 1989;562:123–32.
83. Fried PA. Marijuana use during pregnancy: consequences for the offspring. Semin Perinatol 1991;15:280–7.
84. Fried PA. Behavioral outcomes in preschool and school-age children exposed prenatally to marijuana: a review and speculative interpretation. Natl Inst Drug Abuse Res Monogr 1996;164:242–60.
85. Fried PA, Smith AM. A literature review of the consequences of prenatal marihuana exposure. An emerging theme of a deficiency in aspects of executive function. Neurotoxicol Teratol 2001;23:1–11.
86. Fried PA. Conceptual issues in behavioral teratology and their application in determining long-term sequelae of prenatal marihuana exposure. J Child Psychol Psychiatry 2002;43:81–102.
87. Coles CD, Smith IE, Fernhoff PM, Falek A. Neonatal ethanol withdrawal: characteristics in clinically normal, nondysmorphic neonates. J Pediatr 1984;105:445–51.
88. Day NL, Richardson GA, Goldschmidt L, Robles N, Taylor PM, Stoffer DS, Cornelius MD, Geva D. Effect of prenatal marijuana exposure on the cognitive development of offspring at age three. Neurotoxicol Teratol 1994;16:169–75.
89. Richardson GA, Day NL, Goldschmidt L. Prenatal alcohol, marijuana, and tobacco use: infant mental and motor development. Neurotoxicol Teratol 1995;17:479–87.
90. Goldschmidt L, Day NL, Richardson GA. Effects of prenatal marijuana exposure on child behavior problems at age 10. Neurotoxicol Teratol 2000;22:325–36.
91. Robison LL, Buckley JD, Daigle AE, Wells R, Benjamin D, Arthur DC, Hammond GD. Maternal drug use and risk of childhood nonlymphoblastic leukemia among offspring: an epidemiologic investigation implicating marijuana (a report from the Children's Cancer Study Group). Cancer 1989;63:1904–11.
92. Stenchever MA, Kunysz TJ, Allen MA. Chromosome breakage in users of marihuana. Am J Obstet Gynecol 1974;118:106–13.
93. Matsuyama SS, Jarvik LF. Cytogenetic effects of psychoactive drugs. Mod Probl Pharmacopsychiatry 1975;10:99–132.
94. Abel EL. Marihuana and sex: a critical survey. Drug Alcohol Depend 1981;8:1–22.
95. Nahas GG. Cannabis: toxicological properties and epidemiological aspects. Med J Aust 1986;145:82–7.
96. Walker A, Rosenberg M, Balaban-Gil K. Neurodevelopmental and neurobehavioral sequelae of selected substances of abuse and psychiatric medications in utero. Child Adolesc Psychiatr Clin N Am 1999;8:845–67.
97. Perez-Reyes M, Wall ME. Presence of delta-9-tetrahydrocannabinol in human milk. N Engl J Med 1982;307:819–20.
98. Arena JM. Drugs and chemicals excreted in breast milk. Pediatr Ann 1980;9:452–7.
99. Committee on Drugs, American Academy of Pediatrics. The transfer of drugs and other chemicals into human milk. Pediatrics 2001;108:776–89.

M

Name:	**MAZINDOL**	Risk Factor:	**C**
Class:	**Central Stimulant/Anorexiant**		

FETAL RISK SUMMARY

RECOMMENDATION: No Human Data - No Relevant Animal Data

No data are available.

BREAST FEEDING SUMMARY

RECOMMENDATION: No Human Data - Potential Toxicity

No data are available.

Name:	**MEBANAZINE**	Risk Factor:	**C**
Class:	**Antidepressant**		

No data are available (see Phenelzine).

Name:	**MEBENDAZOLE**	Risk Factor:	**C_M**
Class:	**Anthelmintic**		

FETAL RISK SUMMARY

RECOMMENDATION: Human Data Suggest Low Risk

Mebendazole is a synthetic anthelminthic agent. Although embryotoxic and teratogenic in rats at single oral doses approximately equal to the human dose based on body surface area (1), this effect has not been observed in multiple other animal species (2).

One manufacturer has reports of first trimester mebendazole exposure in 170 pregnancies going to term without an identifiable teratogenic risk (1). There was also no increased risk of spontaneous abortion following 1st trimester exposure. An earlier manufacturer knew of only one malformation, a digital reduction of one hand, in 112 infants exposed *in utero* to the drug (3).

In a surveillance study of Michigan Medicaid recipients conducted between 1985 and 1992 involving 229,101 completed pregnancies, 64 newborns had been exposed to mebendazole during the 1st trimester (F. Rosa, personal communication, FDA, 1993). Four (6.3%) major birth defects were observed (three expected), one of which was a limb reduction defect (none expected). No anomalies were observed in five other defect categories (cardiovascular defects, oral clefts, spina bifida, polydactyly, and hypospadias) for which specific data were available.

During a 1984 outbreak of trichinosis (*Trichinella spiralis*) in Lebanon, four pregnant patients were treated with mebendazole and corticosteroids (4). Two women, both in the 1st trimester, had miscarriages. The authors did not mention if this was caused by the disease or the drug. Neither fetus was examined. The remaining two patients, both in the 3rd trimester, delivered healthy infants. In a separate case, a pregnant patient, also with trichinosis, was treated with mebendazole and delivered a normal infant (5). The period of pregnancy when the infection and treatment occurred was not specified.

In Sri Lanka, *Necator americanus*, one of the two known causes of hookworm, is endemic and it is an important contributor to iron-deficiency anemia in pregnancy (6). Consequently, the routine use of mebendazole is recommended in the 2nd trimester of pregnancy. A study published in 1999 compared the pregnancy outcomes of women treated with mebendazole ($N = 5275$) to a control group ($N = 1737$) that was not treated (6). There was no significant difference in the rate of major congenital malformations for exposures anytime during pregnancy, 1.8% (97 of 5275) vs. 1.5% (26 of 1737), odds ratio (OR) 1.24, 95% confidence interval (CI) 0.8–1.91. For 1st trimester exposure, the incidence was 2.5% (10 of 407), OR 1.66, 95% CI 0.81–3.56, $p = 0.23$ (6). In other comparisons between the two groups, significant decreases occurred in the exposed group in the incidence of stillbirths and perinatal deaths (1.9% vs. 3.3%, $p = 0.0004$), and low ($\leq$1500 g) birth weights (1.1% vs. 2.3%, $p = 0.0003$) (6). The researchers concluded that although there was no significant increase in the number of major defects associated with mebendazole, the agent should not be used during the 1st trimester, and a small increased risk of defects could not be excluded (6).

A 2003 prospective controlled cohort study reported the outcomes of 192 pregnancies exposed to mebendazole, most of which (71.5%) involved 1st trimester exposure (7). The rate of major birth defects, spontaneous abortions, and median birth weight did not differ significantly between the exposed and matched control groups, 3.3% vs. 1.7%, 11.5% vs. 9.4%, and 3222 g vs 3258 g, respectively. However, more pregnancies were electively terminated in the study group than in controls, 11.5% vs. 1.6%. There was no pattern in the defects to suggest a single cause. Moreover, the timing of the exposures made a causative association with the malformations implausible (7).

A 1985 review of intestinal parasites and pregnancy concluded that treatment of the pregnant patient should only be considered if the "parasite is causing clinical disease or may cause public health problems" (8). When indicated, mebendazole was recommended for the treatment of *Trichuris trichiura* (whipworm) occurring during pregnancy. A 1986 review recommended mebendazole therapy, when indicated, for the treatment of *Ascaris lumbricoides* (roundworm) and *Enterobius vermicularis* (threadworm, seatworm, or pinworm) (9), although another review recommended piperazine for this purpose, despite the known poor absorption of mebendazole (10).

BREAST FEEDING SUMMARY

RECOMMENDATION: Limited Human Data - Probably Compatible

One nursing woman, in her 10th week of lactation, was treated with mebendazole (100 mg twice daily for 3 days) for a roundworm infection (11). Immediately before this she had been treated for 7 days with metronidazole for genital *Trichomonas vaginalis*. Milk production decreased markedly on the 2nd day of mebendazole therapy and stopped completely within 1 week. Although no mechanism was suggested, the author concluded that the halt in lactation was mebendazole-induced.

In contrast to the above report, a 1994 reference described no effect on lactation or breast-feeding in four postpartum women treated with mebendazole, 100 mg twice daily for 3 days, for various intestinal parasites (12). In one of the patients, the maternal plasma concentration of mebendazole at the end of therapy was less than 20 ng/mL, and milk levels were undetectable. The decreased milk production in the above case was attributed to maternal anxiety from having passed a roundworm per rectum (12).

On the basis of more recent data, breast-feeding should not be withheld during mebendazole therapy. Only about 2%–10% of an oral dose is absorbed (13) and, as expected, the amounts of the drug excreted into milk are below the level of detection and appear to be clinically insignificant.

References

1. Product information. Vermox. McNeil Consumer, 2000.
2. Beard TC, Rickard MD, Goodman HT. Medical treatment for hydatids. Med J Aust 1978;1:6335–5.
3. Shepard TH. *Catalog of Teratogenic Agents*, 8th ed. Baltimore, MD: Johns Hopkins University Press, 1995: 261.
4. Blondheim DS, Klein R, Ben-Dror G, Schick G. Trichinosis in southern Lebanon. Isr J Med Sci 1984;20: 141–4.
5. Draghici O, Vasadi T, Draghici G, Codrea A, Mihuta A, Dragan S, Biro S, Mocuja D, Mihuja S. Comments with reference to a trichinellosis focus. Rev Ig (Bacteriol) 1976;21:99–104.
6. de Silva NR, Sirisena JLGJ, Gunasekera DPS, Ismail MM, de Silva HJ. Effect of mebendazole therapy during pregnancy on birth outcome. Lancet 1999;353: 1145–9.
7. Diav-Citrin O, Shechtman S, Arnon J, Lubart I, Ornoy A. Pregnancy outcome after gestational exposure to

mebendazole: a prospective controlled cohort study. Am J Obstet Gynecol 2003;188:282–5.
8. D'Alauro F, Lee RV, Pao-In K, Khairallah M. Intestinal parasites and pregnancy. Obstet Gynecol 1985;66:639–43.
9. Ellis CJ. Antiparasitic agents in pregnancy. Clin Obstet Gynecol 1986;13:269–75.
10. Leach FN. Management of threadworm infestation during pregnancy. Arch Dis Child 1990;65:399–400.
11. Rao TS. Does mebendazole inhibit lactation? N Z Med J 1983;96:589–90.
12. Kurzel RB, Toot PJ, Lambert LV, Mihelcic AS. Mebendazole and postpartum lactation. N Z Med J 1994;107:439.
13. American Hospital Formulary Service. Drug Information 1997. Bethesda, MD: American Society of Health-System Pharmacists, 1997:44–6.

Name:	**MECAMYLAMINE**	Risk Factor:	C_M
Class:	**Antihypertensive**		

FETAL RISK SUMMARY

RECOMMENDATION: No Human Data - Animal Data Suggest Low Risk

Mecamylamine, a secondary amine, is a potent antihypertensive and ganglionic blocker that is indicated for the management of moderately severe to severe essential hypertension and uncomplicated cases of malignant hypertension (1,2). The antihypertensive effect is predominantly orthostatic, but supine blood pressure is also significantly reduced.

Although the manufacturers state that animal reproduction studies have not been conducted (1,2), a 1998 study observed no teratogenicity in pregnant rat and rabbit experiments (3).

Mecamylamine crosses the human placenta to the fetus (1,2). This is consistent with its relatively low molecular weight (about 168 for the free base).

Except for a single case included with other antihypertensives in the data of the Collaborative Perinatal Project (4), no reports on the use of mecamylamine during human pregnancy have been located. The near absence of human and animal reproduction data prevents an assessment of the fetal risk. However, lowering of maternal hypertension may compromise the placental perfusion, resulting in fetal hypoxia (as indicated by bradycardia) and death.

BREAST FEEDING SUMMARY

RECOMMENDATION: No Human Data - Probably Compatible

No reports describing the use of mecamylamine in human lactation have been located. The low molecular weight (about 168 for the free base) suggests that the drug is excreted into breast milk. The effect of this exposure on a nursing infant is unknown.

References

1. Product information. Inversine. Layton Bioscience, 2001.
2. Product information. Inversine. Merck, 2001.
3. Schroeder RE, Betlach CJ. Subcutaneous developmental toxicity studies in rats and rabbits with nicotine and mecamylamine in combination. Toxicologist 1998;42:257. As cited by Schardein JL. *Chemically Induced Birth Defects*. 3rd ed. New York, NY: Marcel Dekker, 2000:527.
4. Heinonen OP, Slone D, Shapiro S. Birth Defects and Drugs in Pregnancy. Littleton, MA: Publishing Sciences Group, 1977:372.

Name:	**MECHLORETHAMINE**	Risk Factor:	**D_M**
Class:	**Antineoplastic**		

FETAL RISK SUMMARY

RECOMMENDATION: Contraindicated - 1st Trimester

Mechlorethamine is an alkylating antineoplastic agent. The drug produced congenital malformations in rats and ferrets when given as a single SC injection of 1 mg/kg (2–3 times the maximum recommended human dose) (1).

Mechlorethamine has been used in pregnancy, usually in combination with other antineoplastic drugs. Most reports have not shown an adverse effect in the fetus, even when mechlorethamine was given during the 1st trimester (2–6). Two malformed infants have resulted following 1st trimester use of mechlorethamine:

Oligodactyly of both feet with webbing of third and fourth toes, four metatarsals on left, three on right, bowing of right tibia, cerebral hemorrhage (7)
Malformed kidneys-markedly reduced size and malpositioned (8)

Data from one review indicated that 40% of the infants exposed to anticancer drugs were of low birth weight (4). Long-term studies of growth and mental development in offspring exposed to mechlorethamine during the 2nd trimester, the period of neuroblast multiplication, have not been conducted (9).

Ovarian function has been evaluated in 27 women previously treated with mechlorethamine and other antineoplastic drugs (10). Excluding three patients who received pelvic radiation, 13 (54%) maintained regular cyclic menses and, overall, 13 normal children were born after therapy. Other successful pregnancies have been reported following combination chemotherapy with mechlorethamine (11–17). Ovarian failure is apparently often gradual in onset and is age related (10). Mechlorethamine therapy in males has been observed to produce testicular germinal cell depletion and azoospermia (15,16,18,19).

Occupational exposure of the mother to antineoplastic agents during pregnancy may present a risk to the fetus. A position statement from the National Study Commission on Cytotoxic Exposure and a research article involving some antineoplastic agents are presented in the monograph for cyclophosphamide (see Cyclophosphamide).

BREAST FEEDING SUMMARY

RECOMMENDATION: Contraindicated

No reports describing the use of mechlorethamine during lactation have been located. The low molecular weight (about 157 for the free base) suggests that the drug passes into milk. Although it undergoes rapid chemical transformation in water and body fluids, it is not known if exposure to this biologic alkylating agent in breast milk poses a significant risk to a nursing infant. Because of the potential for serious adverse reactions, however, breast-feeding should be discontinued while the mother is receiving therapy.

References

1. Product information. Mustargen. Merck, 2000.
2. Hennessy JP, Rottino A. Hodgkin's disease in pregnancy with a report of twelve cases. Am J Obstet Gynecol 1952;63:756–64.
3. Riva HL, Andreson PS, O'Grady JW. Pregnancy and Hodgkin's disease: a report of eight cases. Am J Obstet Gynecol 1953;66:866–70.
4. Nicholson HO. Cytotoxic drugs in pregnancy: review of reported cases. J Obstet Gynaecol Br Commonw 1968;75:307–312.
5. Jones RT, Weinerman ER. MOPP (nitrogen mustard, vincristine, procarbazine, and prednisone) given during pregnancy. Obstet Gynecol 1979;54:477–8.
6. Johnson IR, Filshie GM. Hodgkin's disease diagnosed in pregnancy: case report. Br J Obstet Gynaecol 1977;84:791–2.
7. Garrett MJ. Teratogenic effects of combination chemotherapy. Ann Intern Med 1974;80:667.
8. Mennuti MT, Shepard TH, Mellman WJ. Fetal renal malformation following treatment of Hodgkin's disease during pregnancy. Obstet Gynecol 1975;46: 194–6.
9. Dobbing J. Pregnancy and leukaemia. Lancet 1977; 1:1155.
10. Schilsky RL, Sherins RJ, Hubbard SM, Wesley MN, Young RC, DeVita VT Jr. Long-term follow-up of ovarian function in women treated with MOPP chemotherapy for Hodgkin's disease. Am J Med 1981;71: 552–6.
11. Ross GT. Congenital anomalies among children born of mothers receiving chemotherapy for gestational trophoblastic neoplasms. Cancer 1976;37:1043–7.
12. Johnson SA, Goldman JM, Hawkins DF. Pregnancy after chemotherapy for Hodgkin's disease. Lancet 1979;2:93.
13. Whitehead E, Shalet SM, Blackledge G, Todd I, Crowther D, Beardwell CG. The effect of combination chemotherapy on ovarian function in women treated for Hodgkin's disease. Cancer 1983;52:988–93.
14. Andrieu JM, Ochoa-Molina ME. Menstrual cycle, pregnancies and offspring before and after MOPP therapy for Hodgkin's disease. Cancer 1983;52:435–8.
15. Dein RA, Mennuti MT, Kovach P, Gabbe SG. The reproductive potential of young men and women with Hodgkin's disease. Obstet Gynecol Surv 1984;39: 474–82.
16. Schilsky RL, Lewis BJ, Sherins RJ, Young RC. Gonadal dysfunction in patients receiving chemotherapy for cancer. Ann Intern Med 1980;93:109–14.
17. Shalet SM, Vaughan Williams CA, Whitehead E. Pregnancy after chemotherapy induced ovarian failure. Br Med J 1985;290:898.
18. Sherins RJ, Olweny CLM, Ziegler JL. Gynecomastia and gonadal dysfunction in adolescent boys treated with combination chemotherapy for Hodgkin's disease. N Engl J Med 1978;299:12–6.
19. Sherins RJ, DeVita VT Jr. Effect of drug treatment for lymphoma on male reproductive capacity: studies of men in remission after therapy. Ann Intern Med 1973;79:216–20.

M

Name: **MECLIZINE** Risk Factor: **B_M**

Class: **Antihistamine/Antiemetic**

FETAL RISK SUMMARY

RECOMMENDATION: Compatible

Meclizine is a piperazine antihistamine that is frequently used as an antiemetic (see also Buclizine and Cyclizine). The drug is teratogenic in animals, causing cleft palates in rats at 25–50 times the human dose, but apparently not in humans (1). Since late 1962, the question of meclizine's effect on the fetus has been argued in numerous citations, the bulk of which are case reports and letters (2–28). Three studies involving large numbers of patients have concluded that meclizine is not a human teratogen (29–31).

The Collaborative Perinatal Project (CPP) monitored 50,282 mother-child pairs, 1014 of whom had exposure to meclizine in the 1st trimester (29, p. 328). For use anytime during pregnancy, 1463 exposures were recorded (29, p. 437). In neither group was evidence found to suggest a relationship to large categories of major or minor malformations. Several possible associations with individual malformations were found, but their statistical significance is unknown (29, pp. 328, 437, 475). Independent confirmation is required to determine the actual risk.

Respiratory defects (7 cases)
Eye and ear defects (7 cases)

Inguinal hernia (18 cases)
Hypoplasia cordis (3 cases)
Hypoplastic left heart syndrome (3 cases)

The CPP study indicated a possible relationship to ocular malformations, but the authors warned that the results must be interpreted with extreme caution (32). The FDA's Over-the-Counter Laxative Panel, acting on the data from the CPP study, concluded that meclizine was not teratogenic (33). A second large prospective study covering 613 1st trimester exposures supported these negative findings (30). No harmful effects were found in the exposed offspring as compared with the total sample. Finally, in a 1971 report, significantly fewer infants with malformations were exposed to antiemetics in the 1st trimester as compared with controls (31). Meclizine was the third most commonly used antiemetic.

An association between exposure during the last 2 weeks of pregnancy to antihistamines in general and retrolental fibroplasia in premature infants has been reported. See Brompheniramine for details.

BREAST FEEDING SUMMARY

RECOMMENDATION: No Human Data - Probably Compatible

No reports describing the use of meclizine during lactation have been located. The molecular weight (about 464), however, is low enough that passage into milk should be anticipated. The potential effects of this exposure on a nursing infant are unknown. Some agents in this class (e.g., see Brompheniramine and Diphenhydramine) have been classified by their manufacturers as contraindicated during nursing because of the increased sensitivity of newborn or premature infants to antihistamines.

M

References

1. Product information. Antivert. Pfizer, 2000.
2. Watson GI. Meclozine ("Ancoloxin") and foetal abnormalities. Br Med J 1962;2:1446.
3. Smithells RW. "Ancoloxin" and foetal abnormalities. Br Med J 1962;2:1539.
4. Diggorg PLC, Tomkinson JS. Meclozine and foetal abnormalities. Lancet 1962;2:1222.
5. Carter MP, Wilson FW. "Ancoloxin" and foetal abnormalities. Br Med J 1962;2:1609.
6. Macleod M. "Ancoloxin" and foetal abnormalities. Br Med J 1962;2:1609.
7. Lask S. "Ancoloxin" and foetal abnormalities. Br Med J 1962;2:1609.
8. Leck IM. "Ancoloxin" and foetal abnormalities. Br Med J 1962;2:1610.
9. McBride WG. Drugs and foetal abnormalities. Br Med J 1962;2:1681.
10. Fagg CG. "Ancoloxin" and foetal abnormalities. Br Med J 1962;2:1681.
11. Barwell TE. "Ancoloxin" and foetal abnormalities. Br Med J 1962;2:1681–2.
12. Woodall J. "Ancoloxin" and foetal abnormalities. Br Med J 1962;2:1682.
13. McBride WG. Drugs and congenital abnormalities. Lancet 1962;2:1332.
14. Lenz W. Drugs and congenital abnormalities. Lancet 1962;2:1332–3.
15. David A, Goodspeed AH. "Ancoloxin" and foetal abnormalities. Br Med J 1963;1:121.
16. Gallagher C. "Ancoloxin" and foetal abnormalities. Br Med J 1963;1:121–12.
17. Watson GI. "Ancoloxin" and foetal abnormalities. Br Med J 1963;1:122.
18. Mellin GW, Katzenstein M. Meclozine and foetal abnormalities. Lancet 1963;1:222–3.
19. Salzmann KD. "Ancoloxin" and foetal abnormalities. Br Med J 1963;1:471.
20. Burry AF. Meclozine and foetal abnormalities. Br Med J 1963;1:1476.
21. Smithells RW, Chinn ER. Meclozine and foetal abnormalities. Br Med J 1963;1:1678.
22. O'Leary JL, O'Leary JA. Nonthalidomide ectromelia. Report of a case. Obstet Gynecol 1964;23:17–20.
23. Smithells RW, Chinn ER. Meclozine and foetal malformations: a prospective study. Br Med J 1964;1:217–8.
24. Pettersson F. Meclozine and congenital malformations. Lancet 1964;1:675.
25. Yerushalmy J, Milkovich L. Evaluation of the teratogenic effect of meclizine in man. Am J Obstet Gynecol 1965;93:553–62.
26. Sadusk JF Jr, Palmisano PA. Teratogenic effect of meclizine, cyclizine, and chlorcyclizine. JAMA 1965;194:987–9.

27. Lenz W. Malformations caused by drugs in pregnancy. Am J Dis Child 1966;112:99–106.
28. Lenz W. How can the teratogenic action of a factor be established in man? South Med J 1971;64(Suppl 1): 41–7.
29. Heinonen OP, Slone D, Shapiro S. *Birth Defects and Drugs in Pregnancy*. Littleton, MA: Publishing Sciences Group, 1977.
30. Milkovich L, Van den Berg BJ. An evaluation of the teratogenicity of certain antinauseant drugs. Am J Obstet Gynecol 1976;125:244–8.
31. Nelson MM, Forfar JO. Associations between drugs administered during pregnancy and congenital abnormalities of the fetus. Br Med J 1971;1: 523–7.
32. Shapiro S, Kaufman DW, Rosenberg L, Slone D, Monson RR, Siskind V, Heinonen OP. Meclizine in pregnancy in relation to congenital malformations. Br Med J 1978;1:483.
33. Anonymous. Pink Sheets. Meclizine, cyclizine not teratogenic. FDC Rep 1974:2.

Name: **MECLOFENAMATE** Risk Factor: **B***

Class: **Nonsteroidal Anti-inflammatory**

FETAL RISK SUMMARY

RECOMMENDATION: Human Data Suggest Risk in 1st and 3rd Trimesters

The nonsteroidal anti-inflammatory drug (NSAID), meclofenamate sodium, is used in the treatment of acute and chronic pain, arthritis, and primary dysmenorrhea. It is in the same NSAID subclass (fenamates) as mefenamic acid.

Reproduction studies in mice, rats, and rabbits during organogenesis found no teratogenic effects (1–3), but postimplantation losses were observed in rats (3). Although apparently not reported, animal reproductive toxicities observed with other agents in the class, such as prolonged gestation, dystocia, intrauterine growth retardation, and decreased fetal and neonatal survival, should also be expected with meclofenamate.

It is not known if meclofenamate crosses the human placenta. The molecular weight of the free acid (about 313) is low enough, however, that passage to the fetus should be expected.

In a surveillance study of Michigan Medicaid recipients conducted between 1985 and 1992 involving 229,101 completed pregnancies, 166 newborns had been exposed to meclofenamate during the 1st trimester (F. Rosa, personal communication, FDA, 1993). Six (3.6%) major birth defects were observed (seven expected), including one cardiovascular defect (two expected) and one oral cleft (three expected). No anomalies were observed in four other categories of defects (spina bifida, polydactyly, limb reduction defects, and hypospadias) for which specific data were available. These data do not support an association between the drug and congenital defects.

A combined 2001 population-based observational cohort study and a case-control study estimated the risk of adverse pregnancy outcome from the use of NSAIDs (4). The use of NSAIDs during pregnancy was not associated with congenital malformations, preterm delivery, or low birth weight, but a positive association was discovered with spontaneous abortions (SABs). A similar study, also published in 2001, failed to find a relationship, in general, between NSAIDs and congenital malformations, but did find a significant association with cardiac defects and orofacial clefts (5). In addition, a 2003 study found a significant association between exposure to NSAIDs in early pregnancy and SABs (6). (See Ibuprofen for details on these three studies.)

A brief 2003 editorial on the potential for NSAID-induced developmental toxicity concluded that NSAIDs, and specifically those with greater COX-2 affinity, had a lower risk of this toxicity in humans than aspirin (7).

Two reviews, both on antirheumatic drug therapy in pregnancy, recommended that if an NSAID was needed, agents with short elimination adult half-lives should be used at the maximum tolerated dosage interval, using the lowest effective dose, and that therapy should be stopped within 8 weeks of the expected delivery date (8,9). Meclofenamate has a short plasma elimination half-life (2 hours), but other factors, such as its toxicity profile, need to be considered.

Constriction of the ductus arteriosus *in utero* is a pharmacologic consequence arising from the use of prostaglandin synthesis inhibitors during pregnancy, as is inhibition of labor, prolongation of pregnancy, and suppression of fetal renal function (see also Indomethacin) (10). Persistent pulmonary hypertension of the newborn may occur if these agents are used in the 3rd trimester close to delivery (10,11). Women attempting to conceive should not use any prostaglandin synthesis inhibitor, including meclofenamate, because of the findings in a variety of animal models that indicate these agents block blastocyst implantation (12,13). Moreover, as noted above, NSAIDs have been associated with SABs and congenital malformations.

[**Risk Factor D if used in 3rd trimester or near delivery.*]

BREAST FEEDING SUMMARY

RECOMMENDATION: No Human Data - Probably Compatible

No reports describing the use of meclofenamate sodium during lactation have been located. The molecular weight of the free acid (about 313) suggests that the drug will be excreted into breast milk. The effects of this exposure on a nursing infant are unknown, but other NSAIDs are classified as compatible with breast-feeding by the American Academy of Pediatrics (see Ibuprofen and Indomethacin).

References

1. Product information. Meclomen. Parke-Davis, 1993.
2. Schardein JL, Blatz AT, Woosley ET, Kaump DH. Reproduction studies on sodium meclofenamate in comparison to aspirin and phenylbutazone. Toxicol Appl Pharmacol 1969;15:46–55. As cited in Schardein JL. *Chemically Induced Birth Defects*. 2nd ed. New York, NY: Marcel Dekker, Inc., 1993:131.
3. Petrere JA, Humphrey RR, Anderson JA, Fitzgerald JE, De La Iglesia FA. Studies on reproduction in rats with meclofenamate sodium, a nonsteroidal antiinflammatory agent. Fund Appl Toxicol 1985;5:665–71. As cited in Shepard TH. *Catalog of Teratogenic Agents*. 7th ed. Baltimore, MD: Johns Hopkins University Press, 1992:2444–5.
4. Nielsen GL, Sorensen HT, Larsen H, Pedersen L. Risk of adverse birth outcome and miscarriage in pregnant users of non-steroidal anti-inflammatory drugs: population based observational study and case-control study. BMJ 2001;322:266–70.
5. Ericson A, Kallen BAJ. Nonsteroidal anti-inflammatory drugs in early pregnancy. Reprod Toxicol 2001;15:371–5.
6. Li DK, Liu L, Odouli R. Exposure to non-steroidal anti-inflammatory drugs during pregnancy and risk of miscarriage: population based cohort study. BMJ 2003;327:368–71.
7. Tassinari MS, Cook JC, Hurtt ME. NSAIDs and developmental toxicity. Birth Defects Res Part B Dev Reprod Toxicol 2003;68:3–4.
8. Needs CJ, Brooks PM. Antirheumatic medication in pregnancy. Br J Rheumatol 1985;24:282–90.
9. Ostensen M. Optimisation of antirheumatic drug treatment in pregnancy. Clin Pharmacokinet 1994; 27:486–503.
10. Levin DL. Effects of inhibition of prostaglandin synthesis on fetal development, oxygenation, and the fetal circulation. Semin Perinatol 1980;4: 35–44.
11. Van Marter LJ, Leviton A, Allred EN, Pagano M, Sullivan KF, Cohen A, Epstein MF. Persistent pulmonary hypertension of the newborn and smoking and aspirin and nonsteroidal antiinflammatory drug consumption during pregnancy. Pediatrics 1996;97:658–63.
12. Matt DW, Borzelleca JF. Toxic effects on the female reproductive system during pregnancy, parturition, and lactation. In Witorsch RJ, ed. *Reproductive Toxicology*. 2nd ed. New York, NY: Raven Press, 1995: 175–93.
13. Dawood MY. Nonsteroidal antiinflammatory drugs and reproduction. Am J Obstet Gynecol 1993;169: 1255–65.

Name: **MEDROXYPROGESTERONE** Risk Factor: X_M

Class: **Progestogenic Hormone**

FETAL RISK SUMMARY

RECOMMENDATION: Contraindicated

Medroxyprogesterone acetate (MPA) is a derivative of progesterone that is available in both parenteral and oral formulations. The indications for this hormone include contraception (either alone or in combination with an estrogen), secondary amenorrhea and abnormal uterine bleeding caused by hormonal imbalance in the absence of organic pathology, and in combination with estrogens for the treatment of vasomotor symptoms associated with menopause, vulvar and vaginal atrophy, and the prevention of osteoporosis. There are currently no pregnancy-related indications for this hormone.

A 1977 report described reproduction tests conducted with MPA in mice, rats, and rabbits (1). In each species, once daily subcutaneous doses of 0.1–3000 mg/kg/day were given during organogenesis for 3, 6, or 9 consecutive days. Untreated controls were used for each species. No congenital defects attributable to the hormone were observed in mice and rats. In two breeds of rabbits, however, a dose-related increase in cleft palate was observed at 3, 10, and 30 mg/kg/day. The absence of a significant dose-response at doses >30 mg/kg/day was thought to result from the mortality caused by the higher doses (1).

In an attempt to explain the teratogenic effects observed in rabbits, the same investigative group examined the binding of MPA to glucocorticoid receptors in appropriate rat and rabbit target tissues (2). Their results indicated that, in rabbits but not in rats, MPA was as effective as natural glucocorticoids in competing for selected binding sites. They theorized that the MPA-induced cleft palates in their original experiment might have been caused by the hormone binding to specific glucocorticoid receptors and not due to its progestational activity (2).

An experiment to determine a possible mechanism for progestogen-induced hypospadias was reported in 1982 (3). Pregnant rats were given MPA at doses of 1, 10, and 100 times, respectively, the human contraceptive dose equivalent based on body weight (HCDE) on days 13–20 of gestation. Norethisterone, alone or in combination with ethinylestradiol, was also given to other pregnant rats at similar doses. Compared to untreated controls, no effect was observed from these agents on dehydroepiandrosterone metabolism by fetal Wolffian ducts. Inhibition of this testosterone precursor had been shown previously to cause severe hypospadias in male rats and was thought to be a possible mechanism for similar defects in human males (3).

Mice given SC MPA (5–900 mg/kg) before implantation (day 2 of pregnancy) had sporadic increases in dead and resorbed fetuses, decreased fetal weight, and an increase in the incidence of cleft palate and malformed fetuses (4). These effects were not dose-related. Treatment with 30 mg/kg on gestational day 9 was associated with increased rates of respiratory and urinary tract defects. In addition, increased incidences of cleft palate were observed with this dose on several days between gestational days 1 and 12 (4). The methods used in this animal study have been criticized and its findings considered to have questionable relevancy (5) and defended (6).

The fetal effects of IM MPA were studied in pregnant baboons administered during organogenesis that were 1, 10, and 40 times, respectively, the HCDE (7). Only the two highest doses were teratogenic, causing anomalies only in the target organs: male external genitalia (short penis, hypospadias, underdeveloped glans and prepuce, and bilateral cryptorchidism), female external genitalia (clitoral hypertrophy, labial fusion, and female pseudohermaphroditism), and adrenal gland hypoplasia (only at 40 times the HCDE) (7).

Pregnant mice were treated during organogenesis with subdermal pellets that delivered MPA at daily doses 25, 250, and 2,500 times, respectively, the human dose equivalent (HDE) (8). No increase in nongenital malformations was noted at any dose, but the two highest doses caused embryotoxicity (resorptions and decreased weight). In addition, no evidence was found for limb reduction defects even when endochondral bone growth was inhibited (8).

An *in vivo* model in pregnant mice of intrauterine inflammation was developed using lipopolysaccharide (LPS) from *Escherichia coli* (9). At a gestational length corresponding to about 28 to 29 weeks in humans, the animals were pretreated with either MPA or progesterone before LPS was infused into the uterus. The preterm delivery rates were 91% (LPS alone), 63% (LPS + progesterone), and 0% (LPS + MPA). All of the undelivered fetuses in the first two groups died within 48 hours, whereas most fetuses survived in the LPS + MPA group. The investigators concluded that the progestational and anti-inflammatory properties of MPA prevented inflammation-induced preterm parturition and preserved fetal viability (9).

Although the Food and Drug Administration (FDA) mandated deletion of pregnancy-related indications from all progestins years ago because of concerns for congenital anomalies, MPA was once used to prevent early abortions. A 1964 report described the use of the hormone for that purpose in 239 women (10). Of the 203 women who went to term, 172 were treated with MPA (oral or IM) before the 12th week of gestation. The average daily dose was 5 to 50 mg orally with a total dose ranging from less than 50 mg to more than 7,000 mg. In six cases, MPA (IM) was the only agent used. Among the 174 infants (2 sets of twins), there were 92 males and 82 females. The outcomes included one stillborn, one newborn with congenital heart disease (no details provided), and one case of mild, transient clitoral enlargement. The infant's mother had received oral MPA 25 mg/day for 7 days during the 6th week of gestation. At 6 months of age, the clitoral hypertrophy had resolved (10).

An unusual cluster of multiple anomalies was observed in a newborn female exposed *in utero* during the 1st trimester to MPA (for first-trimester bleeding), lysergic acid diethylamide (LSD), and cigarette smoking (11). The authors of the report could not exclude an autosomal recessive mode of inheritance as a cause of the defects (see Lysergic Acid Diethylamide).

A total of 259 1st trimester exposures to MPA were reported in a 1975 letter (12). Pregnancies exposed to estrogens or progesterones were identified prospectively over a 3-year period (1966–1968). Women were interviewed during pregnancy about early drug use and their outcomes compared to women who were not exposed to sex hormones. Of those exposed to MPA, 30 infants had congenital malformations, some of which were minor anomalies. Among major defects, there were eight cases involving male genitalia (undescended testis [$N = 4$], hypospadias [$N = 2$], and hydrocele [$N = 2$]), four infants with talipes, two heart defects, and three infants with defects of blood-vessel development (hemangioma, telangiectasia [$N = 2$]). No causal association could be determined because of the nature of indications for the hormones (e.g., threatened or previous abortions) (12).

M

As of 1981, 14 cases of ambiguous genitalia of the fetus had been reported to the FDA, although the literature is more supportive of the 19-nortestosterone derivatives (see Norethindrone, Norethynodrel) (13). Moreover, a 1979 review proposed that the use of progestins during the 1st trimester was a possible cause of hypospadias (14).

A brief 1982 correspondence described the use of oral MPA (40 mg/day) to support an *in vitro* fertilization procedure (15). The drug was given for 10 days after fertilization was confirmed and restarted about 3 weeks later for threatened abortion (vaginal bleeding and a fall in basal temperature). The second course was continued until 16 weeks' gestation by menstrual dates. A 2340-g male infant was delivered at term that, except for growth retardation, was otherwise healthy (15). The potential adverse consequences of the drug therapy on female (virilization) and male (hypospadias) fetuses were the subject of later correspondence on this report (16).

The Collaborative Perinatal Project monitored 866 mother-child pairs with 1st trimester exposure to progestational agents, including 130 with exposure to MPA (17, p. 389). An increase in the expected frequency of cardiovascular defects (also see FDA data below) and hypospadias was observed for the progestational agents as a group (17, p. 394). The cardiovascular defects included a ventricular septal defect and tricuspid atresia (18). Re-evaluation of these data in terms of timing of exposure, vaginal bleeding in early pregnancy, and previous maternal obstetric history, however, failed to support an association between female sex hormones and cardiac malformations (19). Other studies have also failed to find any relationship with nongenital malformations (20,21).

In a surveillance study of Michigan Medicaid recipients conducted between 1985 and 1992 involving 229,101 completed pregnancies, 407 newborns had been exposed to MPA during the 1st trimester (F. Rosa, personal communication, FDA, 1993). A total of 15 (3.7%) major birth defects were observed (13 expected), including (observed/expected) 7/4 cardiovascular defects and 1/1 oral clefts. No malformations were observed in four other defect categories (spina bifida, polydactyly, limb reduction defects, and hypospadias) for which specific data were available. Only the number of cardiovascular defects is suggestive of an association, but other factors, including the mother's disease, concurrent drug use, and chance, may be involved.

One infant of a set of triplets was found to have an additional lumbar rib and hemivertebrae at two levels of the spinal column (22). In addition, the infant had a small, deformed right ear. The pregnancy had resulted from *in vitro* fertilization following ovulation induction with clomiphene citrate. Because of threatened abortion, the mother had been treated with oral MPA (80 mg/d) from the fourth week after embryo transfer throughout the 30-week gestation. The authors thought the combination of ear, spinal, and rib malformations was probably consistent with the Goldenhar syndrome (oculoauriculovertebral anomaly) (22).

A 1985 study described 2754 infants born to mothers who had vaginal bleeding during the 1st trimester (23). Of the total group, 1608 of the newborns were delivered from mothers treated during the 1st trimester with either oral MPA (20–30 mg/d), 17-hydroxyprogesterone (500 mg/week by injection), or a combination of the two. MPA was used exclusively in 1274 (79.2%) of the study group. The control group consisted of 1146 infants delivered from mothers who bled during the 1st trimester but who were not treated. There were no differences between the study and control groups in the overall rate of malformations (120 vs. 123.9/1,000, respectively) or in the rate of major malformations (63.4 vs. 71.5/1,000, respectively) (23). Another 1985 study compared 988 infants exposed *in utero* to various progesterones with a matched cohort of 1,976 unexposed controls (24). Only 60 infants were exposed to MPA. No association between progestins, primarily progesterone and 17-hydroxyprogesterone, and fetal malformations was discovered.

A 1988 report from Thailand described the outcomes of pregnancies of 1229 women who had used MPA before the index pregnancy compared with 4023 women who had used no contraception (controls) and 3038 who had used oral contraceptives (pill) (25). No differences were observed between the groups in terms of stillbirths, multiple pregnancies, or birth weight. Women who had used MPA had a similar incidence of major and minor malformations and deformations as controls, but both groups had significantly increased incidences of these outcomes compared with pill users. There was a significantly increased association of polysyndactyly in the MPA group compared to the other two groups (rate per 1000: 8.1 vs. 1.7 and 1.2). However, only 3 of the 10 cases had exposure to MPA during gestation and in 5 cases; the last injection of the hormone had occurred more than 9 months before conception. Thus, a causal association between MPA and syndactyly was thought to be unlikely. Another unexpected finding was an increase in the number of chromosomal anomalies ($N = 5$) found in the MPA group relative to the controls ($N = 3$) and pill users ($N = 2$). Adjustment by maternal age did not affect these results. Because of the unrelated nature of the defects, the lack of confirming studies, and the distant timing of the exposure in some cases, the authors concluded that the association had occurred by chance (25).

Using the same population base as above, the same investigators studied the effects of *in utero* exposure to steroid contraceptives on birth weight (26). A total of 1573 pregnancies were exposed to injectable MPA (830 accidental pregnancies and 743 infants conceived before the use of the steroid), 601 to oral contraceptives, and 2578 planned pregnancies (controls). Both the injectable and oral contraceptive groups had increased risks for low birth weight infants (<2500 g), but this result was thought to be partial the result of confounders. However, the risk of low birth weight infants was significantly increased in accidental pregnancies when MPA was given within 4 weeks of conception (odds ratio [OR] 1.9, 95% confidence interval [CI] 1.4–3.2) (26). The researchers then investigated the effect of steroid contraceptives on neonatal and infant survival (27). As above, three groups were formed consisting of 1431 children of women who had received injectable MPA during pregnancy, 565 children exposed *in utero* to oral contraceptives, and 2307 control infants with no exposure to hormonal contraceptives. After adjustment (including adjustment for birth weight), the neonatal and infant death rates in those exposed to MPA were nonsignificant. However, there was a relation between shorter injection-to-conception intervals and an increased risk of death: OR 2.5 (95% CI 1.1–5.7) interval ≤4 weeks, OR 2.1 (95% CI 1.0–4.6) interval 5–8 weeks, and OR 0.9 (95% CI 0.4–2.4) interval ≥9 weeks (27). The investigators concluded that infants of pregnancies that occur 1–2 months after an injection of MPA might be at increased risk of low birth weight and death (26,27).

A commentary on the methodology used in the above two studies raised concerns about the validity of the results (28). In particular, criticism involved the comparison groups, establishing the timing of conception, and the biologic plausibility of the effects on birth weight. The authors, however, defended the methods used in the studies and their findings (29).

In the fourth study from the research group in Thailand, no increased risk of impaired growth in height, after adjustment for socioeconomic factors, was found in

M

children (up to the age of 17 years) exposed to MPA during pregnancy ($N = 1207$) and/or during breast-feeding ($N = 1215$) (30). However, there was a delay in the onset of reported pubic hair growth among girls exposed to MPA during pregnancy. No other effects on attainment of puberty (i.e., menarche and breast development) were observed (30).

Another 1988 report focused on the potential teratogenicity of MPA (31). Three groups of women were formed: subfertile women with a history of recurrent spontaneous abortion ($N = 180$) or threatened abortion ($N = 269$), and matched subfertile controls ($N = 464$). The women in the first groups were treated with oral MPA (80–120 mg/d) from the 5th or 7th week of pregnancy until the 18th week. The number of pregnancies in each group was 199, 309, and 508, respectively, and the total number of infants was 161, 205, and 428, respectively. Early pregnancy wastage was high in all groups. Congenital malformations were noted in 15/366 (4.1%) in the treated groups and 15/428 (3.5%) in the controls (difference not significant). Of note, there were two cases of hypospadias: one in the treated group and one in controls. The investigators concluded that MPA was not teratogenic (31).

A possible association between MPA and epispadias, with or without bladder exstrophy, was reported in 1991 (32). Among 20,650 infants delivered at one hospital over a 5-year period, four male infants had epispadias and two of the four also had bladder exstrophy. In each case, MPA had been given to the mother to prevent 1st trimester threatened abortion. The infants were delivered at term, with a mean birth weight of 2980 g. The cluster of these rare defects suggested to the authors that a relationship to the drug was possible (32).

In summary, MPA demonstrates dose-related teratogenicity and toxicity in animals. Although the hormone is contraindicated in human pregnancy, inadvertent exposure to therapeutic doses does not appear to represent a significant risk of structural defects. Fetal growth retardation might be a low-risk complication if MPA is administered within 4 weeks of conception. However, confirmation of this finding is needed.

BREAST FEEDING SUMMARY

RECOMMENDATION: Compatible

Medroxyprogesterone (MPA) has not been shown to affect lactation adversely (33,34). A 1981 review concluded that use of the drug by the mother would not have a significant effect on the nursing infant (35). Milk production and duration of lactation may be increased if the drug is given in the puerperium. This effect might be secondary to the increase in basal serum prolactin levels that has been shown to occur with depot-MPA (34). If breast-feeding is desired, MPA may be used safely (37,38). A 1996 study found no effect on the urine hormonal profiles of male infants nursing from mothers receiving a depot injection of MPA (38). The American Academy of Pediatrics classifies MPA as compatible with breast-feeding (39).

References

1. Andrew FD, Staples RE. Prenatal toxicity of medroxyprogesterone acetate in rabbits, rats, and mice. Teratology 1977;15:25–32.
2. Kimmel GL, Hartwell BS, Andrew FD. A potential mechanism in medroxyprogesterone acetate teratogenesis. Teratology 1979;19:171–6.
3. Briggs MH. Hypospadias, androgen biosynthesis, and synthetic progestogens during pregnancy. Int J Fertil 1982;27:70–2.
4. Eibs HG, Spielmann H, Hagele M. Teratogenic effects of cyproterone acetate and medroxyprogesterone treatment during the pre- and postimplantation

period of mouse embryos. I. Teratology 1982;25:27–36.
5. Marks TA. Comments on two recent papers dealing with the teratogenicity of medroxyprogesterone acetate. Teratology 1984;31:313–5.
6. Spielmann H. Reply to comments on two articles dealing with the teratogenicity of cyproterone acetate (CA) and medroxyprogesterone acetate (MPA). Teratology 1985;32:319–20.
7. Prahalada S, Carroad E, Hendrickx AG. Embryotoxicity and maternal serum concentrations of medroxyprogesterone acetate (MPA) in baboons (*Papio cynocephalus*). Contraception 1985;32:497–515.
8. Carbone JP, Figurska K, Buck S, Brent RL. Effect of gestational sex steroid exposure on limb development and endochondral ossification in the pregnant C57Bl/6J mouse: I. Medroxyprogesterone acetate. Teratology 1990;42:121–30.
9. Elovitz M, Wang Z. Medroxyprogesterone acetate, but not progesterone, protects against inflammation-induced parturition and intrauterine fetal demise. Am J Obstet Gynecol 2004;190:693–701.
10. Burstein R, Wasserman HC. The effect of Provera on the fetus. Obstet Gynecol 1964;23:931–4.
11. Eller JL, Morton JM. Bizarre deformities in offspring of user of lysergic acid diethylamide. N Engl J Med 1970;283:395–7.
12. Harlap S, Prywes R, Davies AM. Birth defects and oestrogens and progesterones in pregnancy. Lancet 1975;1:682–3.
13. Dayan E, Rosa FW. Fetal ambiguous genitalia associated with sex hormones use early in pregnancy. Food and Drug Administration, Division of Drug Experience. ADR Highlights 1981:1–14.
14. Aarskog D. Maternal progestins as a possible cause of hypospadias. N Engl J Med 1979;300:75–8.
15. Yovich J, Puzey A, De'Atta R, Roberts R, Reid S, Grauaug A. In-vitro fertilisation pregnancy with early progestogen support. Lancet 1982;2:378–9.
16. Barlow SM. Medroxyprogesterone in in-vitro fertilisation. Lancet 1982;2:1408.
17. Heinonen OP, Slone D, Shapiro S. *Birth Defects and Drugs in Pregnancy*. Littleton, MA: Publishing Sciences Group, 1977.
18. Heinonen OP, Slone D, Monson RR, Hook EB, Shapiro S. Cardiovascular birth defects and antenatal exposure to female sex hormones. N Engl J Med 1977;296:67–70.
19. Wiseman RA, Dodds-Smith IC. Cardiovascular birth defects and antenatal exposure to female sex hormones: a reevaluation of some base data. Teratology 1984;30:359–70.
20. Wilson JG, Brent RL. Are female sex hormones teratogenic? Am J Obstet Gynecol 1981;141:567–80.
21. Dahlberg K. Some effects of depo-medroxyprogesterone acetate (DMPA): observations in the nursing infant and in the long-term user. Int J Gynaecol Obstet 1982;20:43–8.
22. Yovich JL, Stanger JD, Grauaug AA, Lunay GG, Hollingsworth P, Mulcahy MT. Fetal abnormality (Goldenhar syndrome) occurring in one of triplet infants derived from in vitro fertilization with possible monozygotic twinning. J In Vitro Fert Embryo Transf 1985;2:27–32.
23. Katz Z, Lancet M, Skornik J, Chemke J, Mogilner BM, Klinberg M. Teratogenicity of progestogens given during the first trimester of pregnancy. Obstet Gynecol 1985;65:775–80.
24. Resseguie LJ, Hick JF, Bruen JA, Noller KL, O'Fallon WM, Kurland LT. Congenital malformations among offspring exposed *in utero* to progestins, Olmsted County, Minnesota, 1936–74. Fertil Steril 1985;43:514–9.
25. Pardthaisong T, Gray RH, McDaniel EB, Chandacham A. Steroid contraceptive use and pregnancy outcome. Teratology 1988;38:51–8.
26. Pardthaisong T, Gray RH. *In utero* exposure to steroid contraceptives and outcome of pregnancy. Am J Epidemiol 1991;134:795–803.
27. Gray RH, Pardthaisong T. In utero exposure to steroid contraceptives and survival during infancy. Am J Epidemiol 1991;134:804–11.
28. Hogue CJR. Invited commentary: The contraceptive technology tightrope. Am J Epidemiol 1991;134:812–5.
29. Gray RH, Pardthaisong T. The author's response to Hogue. Am J Epidemiol 1991;134:816–7.
30. Pardthaisong T, Yenchit C, Gray R. The long-term growth and development of children exposed to Depo-Provera during pregnancy and lactation. Contraception 1992;45:313–24.
31. Yovich JL, Turner SR, Draper R. Medroxyprogesterone acetate therapy in early pregnancy has no apparent fetal effects. Teratology 1988;38:135–44.
32. Blickstein I, Katz Z. Possible relationship of bladder exstrophy and epispadias with progestins taken during early pregnancy. Br J Urol 1991;68:105–6.
33. Guiloff E, Ibarra-Polo A, Zanartu J, Toscanini C, Mischler TW, Gomez-Rogers C. Effect of contraception on lactation. Am J Obstet Gynecol 1974;118:42–5.
34. Karim M, Ammar R, El Mahgoub S, El Ganzoury B, Fikri F, Abdou Z. Injected progesterone and lactation. Br Med J 1971;1:200–3.
35. Schwallie PC. The effect of depot-medroxyprogesterone acetate on the fetus and nursing infant: a review. Contraception 1981;23:375–86.
36. Ratchanon S, Taneepanichskul S. Depot medroxyprogesterone acetate and basal serum prolactin levels in lactating women. Obstet Gynecol 2000;96:926–8.
37. Sapire KE, Dommisse J. Injectable contraception and lactation. S Afr Med J 1995;85:1302–3.
38. Virutamasen P, Leepipatpaiboon S, Kriengsinyot R, Vichaidith P, Ndavi Muia P, Sekadde-Kigondu CB, Mati JKG, Forest MG, Dikkeschei LD, Wolthers BG, d'Arcangues C. Pharmacodynamic effects of depot-medroxyprogesterone acetate (DMPA) administered to lactating women on their male infants. Contraception 1996;54:153–7.
39. Committee on Drugs, American Academy of Pediatrics. The transfer of drugs and other chemicals into human milk. Pediatrics 2001;108:776–89.

Name:	**MEFENAMIC ACID**	Risk Factor:	C_M*
Class:	**Nonsteroidal Anti-inflammatory**		

FETAL RISK SUMMARY

RECOMMENDATION: Human Data Suggest Risk in 1st and 3rd Trimesters

Mefenamic acid, a nonsteroidal anti-inflammatory drug (NSAID), is used for the short-term treatment of pain and for primary dysmenorrhea. It is in the same NSAID subclass (fenamates) as meclofenamate.

Although mefenamic acid causes toxic effects in pregnant animals similar to those produced by other agents in this class (decreased fertility, delayed parturition, increase in the number of resorptions, and decreased pup survival), no congenital malformations were observed in studies involving rats, rabbits, and dogs at doses up to 10 times those used in humans (1). In one study of pregnant rats, inhibition of parturition by mefenamic acid appeared to be dose-related (2).

Consistent with its low molecular weight (about 241), mefenamic acid crosses the human placenta to the fetus. Fetal concentrations of the drug, 40–180 minutes after a 500-mg dose administered to 13 women at 15–22 weeks' gestation, were 32%–54% of the maternal plasma concentrations (3).

A combined 2001 population-based observational cohort study and a case-control study estimated the risk of adverse pregnancy outcome from the use of NSAIDs (4). The use of NSAIDs during pregnancy was not associated with congenital malformations, preterm delivery, or low birth weight, but a positive association was discovered with spontaneous abortions (SABs). A similar study, also published in 2001, failed to find a relationship, in general, between NSAIDs and congenital malformations, but did find a significant association with cardiac defects and orofacial clefts (5). In addition, a 2003 study found a significant association between exposure to NSAIDs in early pregnancy and SABs (6). (See Ibuprofen for details on these three studies.)

A brief 2003 editorial on the potential for NSAID-induced developmental toxicity concluded that NSAIDs, and specifically those with greater COX-2 affinity, had a lower risk of this toxicity in humans than aspirin (7).

Mefenamic acid, 500 mg 3 times a day, was used as a tocolytic in a double-blind, randomized human study (8). Compared with controls, preterm delivery occurred less in the mefenamic acid group (15% vs. 40%, $p < 0.005$), and birth weights were higher. No adverse effects were observed in the newborns exposed *in utero* to mefenamic acid.

An infant, delivered by urgent cesarean section at 34 weeks' gestation, had marked cyanosis after *in utero* exposure to mefenamic acid used to prevent premature delivery (9). Echocardiography of the infant demonstrated a small (1- to 2-mm) patent ductus arteriosus. The authors concluded that the maternal drug therapy was responsible for the premature closure of the ductus.

Constriction of the ductus arteriosus *in utero* is a pharmacologic consequence arising from the use of prostaglandin synthesis inhibitors during pregnancy, as is inhibition of labor, prolongation of pregnancy, and suppression of fetal renal function (see also Indomethacin) (10). Persistent pulmonary hypertension of the newborn may occur if these agents are used in the 3rd trimester close to delivery (10,11). Women attempting to conceive should not use any prostaglandin synthesis inhibitor, including mefenamic acid, because of the findings in a variety of animal models that indicate these agents block blastocyst implantation (12,13). Moreover, as noted above, NSAIDs have been associated with SABs and congenital malformations.

[**Risk Factor D if used in 3rd trimester or near delivery.*]

BREAST FEEDING SUMMARY

RECOMMENDATION: Limited Human Data - Probably Compatible

Small amounts of mefenamic acid are excreted into breast milk and absorbed by the nursing infant (14). Ten nursing mothers in the immediate postpartum period were given a 500-mg oral loading dose followed by 250 mg 3 times daily for 3 days. Blood and milk samples were obtained 2 hours after the first daily dose on postpartum days 2–4. Blood and urine samples were obtained from the infants 1 hour after nursing on postpartum day 4. The averages of the mean daily concentrations of mefenamic acid in maternal plasma and milk were 0.94 and 0.17 μg/mL, respectively, corresponding to a milk:plasma ratio of 0.18. In 3 of the mothers, breast milk concentrations of mefenamic acid plus metabolites ranged from 0.62 to 1.99 μg/mL. The mean infant blood concentration of mefenamic acid was 0.08 μg/mL, whereas the mean urine concentration of mefenamic acid plus metabolites was 9.8 μg/mL (14).

One reviewer concluded that because of the potential toxicity of mefenamic acid, other agents (diclofenac, fenoprofen, flurbiprofen, ibuprofen, ketoprofen, ketorolac, and tolmetin) were safer alternatives if a NSAID was required during nursing (15). However, the American Academy of Pediatrics classifies mefenamic acid as usually compatible with breast-feeding (16).

M

References

1. Product information. Ponstel. Parke-Davis, 1995.
2. Powell JG Jr, Cochrane RL. The effects of a number of non-steroidal anti-inflammatory compounds on parturition in the rat. Prostaglandins 1982;23:469–88.
3. MacKenzie IZ, Graf AK, Mitchell MD. Prostaglandins in the fetal circulation following maternal ingestion of a prostaglandin synthetase inhibitor during mid-pregnancy. Int J Gynaecol Obstet 1985;23:455–8.
4. Nielsen GL, Sorensen HT, Larsen H, Pedersen L. Risk of adverse birth outcome and miscarriage in pregnant users of non-steroidal anti-inflammatory drugs: population based observational study and case-control study. BMJ 2001;322:266–70.
5. Ericson A, Kallen BAJ. Nonsteroidal anti-inflammatory drugs in early pregnancy. Reprod Toxicol 2001;15:371–5.
6. Li DK, Liu L, Odouli R. Exposure to non-steroidal anti-inflammatory drugs during pregnancy and risk of miscarriage: population based cohort study. BMJ 2003;327:368–71.
7. Tassinari MS, Cook JC, Hurtt ME. NSAIDs and developmental toxicity. Birth Defects Res Part B Dev Reprod Toxicol 2003;68:3–4.
8. Mital P, Garg S, Khuteta RP, Khuteta S, Mital P. Mefenamic acid in prevention of premature labor. J R Soc Health 1992;112:214–6.
9. Menahem S. Administration of prostaglandin inhibitors to the mother; the potential risk to the fetus and neonate with duct-dependent circulation. Reprod Fertil Dev 1991;3:489–94.
10. Levin DL. Effects of inhibition of prostaglandin synthesis on fetal development, oxygenation, and the fetal circulation. Semin Perinatol 1980;4:35–44.
11. Van Marter LJ, Leviton A, Allred EN, Pagano M, Sullivan KF, Cohen A, Epstein MF. Persistent pulmonary hypertension of the newborn and smoking and aspirin and nonsteroidal antiinflammatory drug consumption during pregnancy. Pediatrics 1996;97:658–63.
12. Matt DW, Borzelleca JF. Toxic effects on the female reproductive system during pregnancy, parturition, and lactation. In Witorsch RJ, ed. *Reproductive Toxicology*. 2nd ed. New York, NY: Raven Press, 1995:175–93.
13. Dawood MY. Nonsteroidal antiinflammatory drugs and reproduction. Am J Obstet Gynecol 1993;169:1255–65.
14. Buchanan RA, Eaton CJ, Koeff ST, Kinkel AW. The breast milk excretion of mefenamic acid. Curr Ther Res Clin Exp 1968;10:592–6.
15. Anderson PO. Medication use while breast feeding a neonate. Neonatal Pharmacol Q 1993;2:3–14.
16. Committee on Drugs, American Academy of Pediatrics. The transfer of drugs and other chemicals into human milk. Pediatrics 2001;108:776–89.

Name:	**MEFLOQUINE**	Risk Factor:	C_M
Class:	**Antimalarial**		

FETAL RISK SUMMARY

RECOMMENDATION: Compatible

Mefloquine is a quinoline-methanol antimalarial agent used in the prevention and treatment of malaria caused by *Plasmodium falciparum*, including chloroquine-resistant strains, or by *Plasmodium vivax*. At high doses (80–160 mg/kg/day), mefloquine is teratogenic in mice, rats, and rabbits, and, at one dose (160 mg/kg/day), it is embryotoxic in rabbits (1). Smaller doses (20–50 mg/kg/day) impaired fertility in rats, but no adverse effect was observed on spermatozoa in humans taking 250 mg/week for 22 weeks (1).

A study published in 1990 examined the pharmacokinetics of mefloquine during the 3rd trimester of pregnancy (2). Twenty women were treated with either 250 mg of mefloquine base ($N = 10$) or 125 mg of base ($N = 10$) weekly until delivery at term. Peak and trough concentrations of mefloquine were lower than those measured in nonpregnant adults, and the terminal elimination half-life was 11.6 ± 7.9 days. The half-life reported in nonpregnant adults is 15–33 days (1). No obstetric complications were observed at either dosage level, including during labor, and no toxicity was observed in the exposed infants. Normal infant development was observed during a 2-year follow-up.

The risks of complications from malarial infection occurring during pregnancy are increased, especially in women not living in endemic areas (i.e., nonimmune women) (3–6). Infection is associated with a number of severe maternal and fetal outcomes: maternal death, anemia, abortion, stillbirth, prematurity, low birth weight, fetal distress, and congenital malaria (3–7). However, one of these outcomes, low birth weight with the resulting increased risk of infant mortality, may have other causes inasmuch as it has not been established that antimalarial chemoprophylaxis can prevent this complication (4). Increased maternal morbidity and mortality includes adult respiratory distress syndrome, pulmonary edema, massive hemolysis, disseminated intravascular coagulation, acute renal failure, and hypoglycemia (5–7). Severe *P. falciparum* malaria in pregnant nonimmune women has a poor prognosis and may be associated with asymptomatic uterine contractions, intrauterine growth retardation, fetal tachycardia, fetal distress, placental insufficiency because of intense parasitization, and hypoglycemia (4,7). The exacerbation of this latter adverse effect has not been reported with mefloquine (7), but it occurs frequently with quinine (7–9). Because of the severity of this disease in pregnancy, chemoprophylaxis is recommended for women of childbearing age who are traveling in areas where malaria is present (3–5). However, some authors state that mefloquine should not be used for prophylaxis during pregnancy, especially during the 1st trimester, because of the potential for fetotoxicity (3–5,7,10–14), except in areas where chloroquine-resistant *P. falciparum* is present (11). An editorial comment to one reference stated that recent data indicated the use of mefloquine during early pregnancy could result in congenital defects, but no other information was provided (15).

Two reports have described the therapeutic use of mefloquine during pregnancy without causing adverse fetal effects (4,16). A 24-year-old woman presented at 33 weeks' gestation with fever, scleral icterus, and tender splenomegaly secondary to *P. falciparum* infection involving 3% of her erythrocytes (16). After two attempts to administer doses of mefloquine (750 and 500 mg), both of which were vomited, predosing with

IV metoclopramide allowed the woman to tolerate three 250-mg doses spaced 4 hours apart and two 250-mg doses the following day (total dose 1250 mg). Maternal fever resolved the day after therapy and, at 5 days, no parasites were observed in the mother's blood. Two months later, a 3405-g infant (sex not specified) was delivered by cesarean section for pelvic disproportion and poor beat-to-beat fetal heart rate variability. Apgar scores at 1 and 5 minutes were 6 and 9, respectively. The child was developing normally at 2 months.

An unpublished double-blind, randomized controlled study from Thailand conducted between 1983 and 1989 was briefly described in a World Health Organization (WHO) publication (4) and a 1993 review (13). A total of 178 pregnant women were randomized to two groups; one group received mefloquine 500 mg every 8 hours for two doses ($N = 87$), and the other group received quinine 600 mg every 8 hours for 7 days ($N = 91$). Although the exact stages of pregnancy at the time of treatment were not specified, a small number of the women in the mefloquine group were in the 1st trimester (4,13). All of the women were followed to term. The incidence of uterine contractions, premature labor, and fetal distress in the mefloquine and quinine groups were 18% vs. 25%, 1% vs. 5%, and 2% vs. 4%, respectively (4). None of the differences was statistically significant. No stillbirths occurred, but one spontaneous abortion was observed in each group, 21 days after mefloquine and 37 days after quinine; neither was thought to be related to drug treatment (4). The 21-day cure rate was 97% among those treated with mefloquine compared with 86% of those treated with quinine. Three newborns had congenital malformations, but these were believed to be unrelated to the drug therapy (13). The study investigators concluded that the therapeutic use of mefloquine during pregnancy was safe and effective. The WHO Scientific Group concluded, however, that because of the small number of patients, treatment with mefloquine should be undertaken cautiously during the first 12–14 weeks of gestation (4).

Two trials of mefloquine prophylaxis in pregnancy were reviewed in a 1993 reference (13). An unpublished study compared weekly prophylaxis with either mefloquine ($N = 468$) or chloroquine ($N = 1312$) in asymptomatic pregnant women (13). Mefloquine was more effective than chloroquine in preventing fetal growth retardation and was also effective in reducing placental *P. falciparum* infections. In another double-blind, placebo-controlled trial, prophylaxis during the second half of pregnancy with 250 mg/week for 1 month followed by 125 mg/week until delivery in 360 Karen women (living on the Thailand-Burma border) was 95% effective in preventing malaria (13). The incidence of stillbirths was similar between mefloquine ($N = 4$) and placebo ($N = 5$).

A presentation made at a 1991 conference described the follow-up of 98 prospectively recorded pregnancy exposures to mefloquine (17). Five diverse congenital malformations were observed, an incidence that does not support mefloquine-induced teratogenicity.

BREAST FEEDING SUMMARY

RECOMMENDATION: Limited Human Data - Probably Compatible

Mefloquine is excreted into human milk (1,18). Two women, who were not breast-feeding, were given a single 250-mg dose, 2–3 days after delivery (18). Milk samples were collected from both women during the first 4 days after dosing, and from one woman at various intervals up to 56 days. The milk:plasma ratios in the two women during the first 4 days were 0.13 and 0.16, respectively. In one woman, the ratio was 0.27 calculated over 56 days. The investigators estimated that a 4-kg infant consuming 1000 mL of milk daily would ingest 0.08 mg/day of the mother's dose (18), or approximately 4% of the dose would be recovered from the milk (1,18). Although these amounts are not thought to be harmful to the nursing infant, they are insufficient to provide adequate protection against malaria (3).

Long-term effects of mefloquine exposure via breast milk have not been studied. Because the antimalarial agent has a long plasma half-life, averaging nearly 12 days during pregnancy (2) and 14.4–18.0 days during and after lactation (18), weekly prophylactic doses of mefloquine will result in continuous exposure of a nursing infant. Moreover, higher milk concentrations of mefloquine than those reported should be expected after therapeutic or weekly prophylactic doses (18).

References

1. Product information. Lariam. Roche Laboratories, 1993.
2. Nosten F, Karbwang J, White NJ, Honeymoon, Na Bangchang K, Bunnag D, Harinasuta T. Mefloquine antimalarial prophylaxis in pregnancy: dose finding and pharmacokinetic study. Br J Clin Pharmacol 1990; 30:79–85.
3. Centers for Disease Control. Recommendations for the prevention of malaria among travelers. MMWR 1990;39:1–10.
4. World Health Organization. Practical chemotherapy of malaria. WHO Tech Rep Ser 1990;805:1–141.
5. Subramanian D, Moise KJ Jr, White AC Jr. Imported malaria in pregnancy: report of four cases and review of management. Clin Infect Dis 1992;15:408–13.
6. World Health Organization. Severe and complicated malaria. Trans R Soc Trop Med Hyg 1990;84(Suppl 2):1–65.
7. Nathwani D, Currie PF, Douglas JG, Green ST, Smith NC. *Plasmodium falciparum* malaria in pregnancy: a review. Br J Obstet Gynaecol 1992;99:118–21.
8. Phillips RE, Looareesuwan S, White NJ, Silamut K, Kietinun S, Warrell DA. Quinine pharmacokinetics and toxicity in pregnant and lactating women with falciparum malaria. Br J Clin Pharmacol 1986;21:677–83.
9. White NJ, Warrell DA, Chanthavanich P, Looareesuwan S, Warrell MJ, Krishna S, Williamson DH, Turner RC. Severe hypoglycemia and hyperinsulinemia in falciparum malaria. N Engl J Med 1983;309:61–6.
10. Bradley D. Prophylaxis against malaria for travelers from the United Kingdom. BMJ 1993;306:1247–52.
11. Barry M, Bia F. Pregnancy and travel. JAMA 1989; 261:728–31.
12. Lackritz EM, Lobel HO, Howell BJ, Bloland P, Campbell CC. Imported *Plasmodium falciparum* malaria in American travelers to Africa. JAMA 1991;265:383–5.
13. Palmer KJ, Holliday SM, Brogden RN. Mefloquine. A review of its antimalarial activity, pharmacokinetic properties and therapeutic efficacy. Drugs 1993;45:430–75.
14. Baker L, Van Schoor JD, Bartlett GA, Lombard JH. Malaria prophylaxis—the South African viewpoint. S Afr Med J 1993;83:126–9.
15. Raccurt CP, Le Bras M, Ripert C, Cuisinier-Raynal JC, Carteron B, Buestel ML. Paludisme d'importation à Bordeaux: évaluation du risque d'infectation par Plasmodium falciparum en fonction de la destination. Bull WHO 1991;69:85–91.
16. Collignon P, Hehir J, Mitchell D. Successful treatment of falciparum malaria in pregnancy with mefloquine. Lancet 1989;1:967.
17. Elefant E, Boyer M, Roux C. Presentation at the 4th International Conference of Teratogen Information Services, Chicago, IL, April 18–20, 1991 (F. Rosa, personal communication, 1993).
18. Edstein MD, Veenendaal JR, Hyslop R. Excretion of mefloquine in human breast milk. Chemotherapy 1988;34:165–9.

Name: **MELOXICAM** Risk Factor: C_M*

Class: **Nonsteroidal Anti-inflammatory**

FETAL RISK SUMMARY

RECOMMENDATION: Human Data Suggest Risk in 1st and 3rd Trimesters

The nonsteroidal anti-inflammatory drug (NSAID), meloxicam, shares the same mechanism of action and uses as other agents in this class. It is an oxicam derivative in the same subclass as piroxicam. No published reports linking meloxicam to human congenital malformations have been located.

Reproduction studies have been conducted in the rat and rabbit. In rabbits, oral doses 64.5 times the human dose at 15 mg/day for a 50-kg adult based on body surface area (HD) given throughout organogenesis resulted in an increased incidence of cardiac septal defects

(1). Embryo lethality was observed at ≥5.4 times the HD. In pregnant rats, no teratogenicity was noted at doses up to 2.2 times the HD. An increase in stillbirths, however, occurred at oral doses about ≥0.5 times the HD and a decrease in pup survival at 2.1 times the HD, when these doses were administered throughout organogenesis (1). At ≥0.5 times the HD in late gestation, meloxicam was associated with stillbirths, an increased length of delivery time, and delayed parturition. At doses ≥0.07 times the HD during late gestation and lactation, reductions in birth index, live births, and neonatal survival were seen in rats.

It is not known if meloxicam crosses the human placenta. The molecular weight (about 351), however, is low enough that transfer to the fetus should be expected. Meloxicam does cross the rat placenta (1).

A combined 2001 population-based observational cohort study and a case-control study estimated the risk of adverse pregnancy outcome from the use of NSAIDs (2). The use of NSAIDs during pregnancy was not associated with congenital malformations, preterm delivery, or low birth weight, but a positive association was discovered with spontaneous abortions (SABs). A similar study, also published in 2001, failed to find a relationship, in general, between NSAIDs and congenital malformations, but did find a significant association with cardiac defects and orofacial clefts (3). In addition, a 2003 study found a significant association between exposure to NSAIDs in early pregnancy and SABs (4). (See Ibuprofen for details on these three studies.)

A brief 2003 editorial on the potential for NSAID-induced developmental toxicity concluded that NSAIDs, and specifically those with greater COX-2 affinity, had a lower risk of this toxicity in humans than aspirin (5).

Constriction of the ductus arteriosus *in utero* is a pharmacologic consequence arising from the use of prostaglandin synthesis inhibitors during pregnancy (see also Indomethacin) (6). Persistent pulmonary hypertension of the newborn may occur if these agents are used in the 3rd trimester close to delivery (6,7). These drugs have also been shown to inhibit labor and prolong gestation, both in humans (8) (see also Indomethacin) and in animals (1,9). Women attempting to conceive should not use any prostaglandin synthesis inhibitor, including meloxicam, because of the findings in a variety of animal models that indicate these agents block blastocyst implantation (10,11). Moreover, as noted above, NSAIDs have been associated with SABs and congenital malformations.

[*Risk Factor D if used in 3rd trimester or near term.*]

BREAST FEEDING SUMMARY

RECOMMENDATION: No Human Data - Probably Compatible

No reports describing the use of meloxicam during lactation have been located. The drug is excreted into the milk of lactating rats at concentrations higher than those in the plasma (1). The molecular weight (about 351) is low enough that excretion into breast milk should be expected. The effects of this exposure on a nursing infant are unknown, but a similar agent, piroxicam, is classified as compatible with breast-feeding by the American Academy of Pediatrics (see Piroxicam).

References

1. Product information. Mobic. Boehringer Ingelheim Pharmaceuticals, 2001.
2. Nielsen GL, Sorensen HT, Larsen H, Pedersen L. Risk of adverse birth outcome and miscarriage in pregnant users of non-steroidal anti-inflammatory drugs: population based observational study and case-control study. BMJ 2001;322:266–70.
3. Ericson A, Kallen BAJ. Nonsteroidal anti-inflammatory drugs in early pregnancy. Reprod Toxicol 2001;15:371–5.

4. Li DK, Liu L, Odouli R. Exposure to non-steroidal anti-inflammatory drugs during pregnancy and risk of miscarriage: population based cohort study. BMJ 2003;327:368–71.
5. Tassinari MS, Cook JC, Hurtt ME. NSAIDs and developmental toxicity. Birth Defects Res Part B Dev Reprod Toxicol 2003;68:3–4.
6. Levin DL. Effects of inhibition of prostaglandin synthesis on fetal development, oxygenation, and the fetal circulation. Semin Perinatol 1980;4:35–44.
7. Van Marter LJ, Leviton A, Allred EN, Pagano M, Sullivan KF, Cohen A, Epstein MF. Persistent pulmonary hypertension of the newborn and smoking and aspirin and nonsteroidal antiinflammatory drug consumption during pregnancy. Pediatrics 1996;97:658–63.
8. Fuchs F. Prevention of prematurity. Am J Obstet Gynecol 1976;126:809–20.
9. Powell JG, Cochrane RL. The effects of a number of non-steroidal anti-inflammatory compounds on parturition in the rat. Prostaglandins 1982;23:469–88.
10. Matt DW, Borzelleca JF. Toxic effects on the female reproductive system during pregnancy, parturition, and lactation. In Wilorsch RJ, ed. *Reproductive Toxicology*. 2nd ed. New York, NY: Raven Press, 1995:175–93.
11. Dawood MY. Nonsteroidal antiinflammatory drugs and reproduction. Am J Obstet Gynecol 1993; 169:1255–65.

Name:	**MELPHALAN**	Risk Factor:	**D_M**
Class:	**Antineoplastic**		

FETAL RISK SUMMARY

RECOMMENDATION: Contraindicated - 1st Trimester

Melphalan, a phenylalanine derivative of nitrogen mustard, is a bifunctional alkylating agent. No reports linking the use of melphalan with congenital defects have been located. The drug is mutagenic as well as carcinogenic (1–8). These effects have not been described in infants following *in utero* exposure. Although there are no supportive data of a teratogenic effect in humans, melphalan is structurally similar to other alkylating agents that have produced defects (see Chlorambucil, Mechlorethamine, Cyclophosphamide).

Reproduction studies in rats with oral doses of 6 to 18 mg/m^2/day for 10 days, or with a single intraperitoneal dose of 18 mg/m^2 revealed embryolethal and teratogenic effects (9). Congenital anomalies included the brain (underdevelopment, deformation, meningocele, and encephalocele), eye (anophthalmia and microphthalmos), reduction of the mandible and tail, and hepatocele.

Studies examining the placental transfer of melphalan have not been found. The molecular weight (about 305) is low enough, however, that transfer across the placenta to the fetus should be expected.

Data from one review indicated that 40% of the infants exposed to anticancer drugs were of low birth weight (10). Long-term studies of growth and mental development in offspring exposed to melphalan and other antineoplastic drugs during the 2nd trimester, the period of neuroblast multiplication, have not been conducted (11).

Melphalan has caused suppression of ovarian function resulting in amenorrhea (11–14). These effects should be considered before administering the drug to patients in their reproductive years. However, in 436 long-term survivors treated with chemotherapy between 1958 and 1978 for gestational trophoblastic tumors, 15 received melphalan as part of their treatment regimens (15). Three of these women had at least one live birth (mean melphalan dose 18 mg; maximum dose 24 mg), and the remaining 12 did not attempt to conceive. Complete details of this study are discussed in the monograph for methotrexate (see Methotrexate).

Occupational exposure of the mother to antineoplastic agents during pregnancy may present a risk to the fetus. A position statement from the National Study Commission on

Cytotoxic Exposure and a research article on some antineoplastic agents are presented in the monograph for cyclophosphamide (see Cyclophosphamide).

BREAST FEEDING SUMMARY

RECOMMENDATION: Contraindicated

No reports describing the use of melphalan during lactation have been located. Excretion into breast milk, however, should be expected because of the relatively low (about 305) molecular weight. Because of the potential for severe toxicity in the nursing infant, women receiving this antineoplastic agent should not nurse.

References

1. Sharpe HB. Observations on the effect of therapy with nitrogen mustard or a derivative on chromosomes of human peripheral blood lymphocytes. Cell Tissue Kinet 1971;4:501–4.
2. Kyle RA, Pierre RV, Bayrd ED. Multiple myeloma and acute myelomonocytic leukemia. N Engl J Med 1970;283:1121–5.
3. Kyle RA. Primary amyloidosis in acute leukemia associated with melphalan. Blood 1974;44:333–7.
4. Burton IE, Abbott CR, Roberts BE, Antonis AH. Acute leukemia after four years of melphalan treatment for melanoma. Br Med J 1976;1:20.
5. Peterson HS. Erythroleukemia in a melphalan treated patient with primary macroglobulinaemia. Scand J Haematol 1973;10:5–11.
6. Stavem P, Harboe M. Acute erythroleukaemia in a patient treated with melphalan for the cold agglutinin syndrome. Scand J Haematol 1971;8: 375–9.
7. Einhorn N. Acute leukemia after chemotherapy (melphalan). Cancer 1978;41:444–7.
8. Reimer RR, Hover R, Fraumen JF, Young RC. Acute leukemia after alkylating agent therapy of ovarian cancer. N Engl J Med 1977,297:177–81.
9. Product information. Alkeran. Glaxo Wellcome, 2000.
10. Nicholson HO. Cytotoxic drugs in pregnancy: review of reported cases. J Obstet Gynaecol Br Commonw 1968;75:307–12.
11. Dobbing J. Pregnancy and leukaemia. Lancet 1977; 1:11–5.
12. Rose DP, David PE. Ovarian function in patients receiving adjuvant chemotherapy for breast cancer. Lancet 1977;1:1174–6.
13. Ahmann DL. Repeated adjuvant chemotherapy with phenylalanine mustard or 5-fluorouracil, cyclophosphamide and prednisone with or without radiation. Lancet 1978;1:893–6.
14. Schilsky RL, Lewis DJ, Sherins RJ, Young RC. Gonadal dysfunction in patients receiving chemotherapy for cancer. Ann Intern Med 1980;93:109–14.
15. Rustin GJS, Booth M, Dent J, Salt S, Rustin F, Bagshawe KD. Pregnancy after cytotoxic chemotherapy for gestational trophoblastic tumours. Br Med J 1984;288:103–6.

Name:	**MENADIONE**	Risk Factor:	C_M
Class:	**Vitamin**		

FETAL RISK SUMMARY

RECOMMENDATION: Human Data Suggest Risk in 3rd Trimester

Menadione (vitamin K_3) is a synthetic, fat-soluble form of vitamin K used to prevent hypoprothrombinemia resulting from vitamin K deficiency. The water-soluble derivative of menadione, menadiol sodium phosphate, also known as vitamin K_3, is available for parenteral use.

Vitamin K_1 occurs naturally in a variety of foods and is synthesized by the normal intestinal flora (see Phytonadione). Administration of vitamin K during pregnancy is usually not required unless the mother develops hypoprothrombinemia or is taking certain drugs that may produce severe vitamin K deficiency in the fetus, resulting in hemorrhagic disease of the newborn (e.g., anticonvulsants, warfarin, rifampin, isoniazid). Early attempts to prevent maternal-induced hemorrhagic disease of the newborn by administering vitamin K_3

to the mother shortly before delivery often resulted in marked hyperbilirubinemia and kernicterus in the newborn, especially in premature infants (1–4). Several large reviews have described the relationship between vitamin K and bilirubin and have discussed the toxicity of the vitamin K analogues (1–4). Because menadione and menadiol may produce newborn toxicity, phytonadione is considered the drug of choice for administration during pregnancy or to the newborn (5,6).

BREAST FEEDING SUMMARY

RECOMMENDATION: No Human Data - Probably Compatible

See Phytonadione.

References

1. Lane PA, Hathaway WE. Vitamin K in infancy. J Pediatr 1985;106:351–9.
2. Payne NR, Hasegawa DK. Vitamin K deficiency in newborns: a case report in á-1-antitrypsin deficiency and a review of factors predisposing to hemorrhage. Pediatrics 1984;73:712–6.
3. Wynn RM. The obstetric significance of factors affecting the metabolism of bilirubin, with particular reference to the role of vitamin K. Obstet Gynecol Surv 1963;18:333–54.
4. Finkel MJ. Vitamin K1 and the vitamin K analogues. Clin Pharmacol Ther 1961;2:795–814.
5. Committee on Nutrition, American Academy of Pediatrics. Vitamin K compounds and the water-soluble analogues. Pediatrics 1961;28:501–7.
6. Committee on Nutrition, American Academy of Pediatrics. Vitamin and mineral supplement needs in normal children in the United States. Pediatrics 1980;66:1015–21.

Name:	**MEPENZOLATE**	Risk Factor:	**C**
Class:	**Parasympatholytic (Anticholinergic)**		

FETAL RISK SUMMARY

RECOMMENDATION: Limited Human Data - No Relevant Animal Data

Mepenzolate is an anticholinergic quaternary ammonium bromide. In a large prospective study, 2,323 patients were exposed to this class of drugs during the 1st trimester, 1 of whom took mepenzolate (1). A possible association was found between the total group and minor malformations.

BREAST FEEDING SUMMARY

RECOMMENDATION: No Human Data - Probably Compatible

No data are available (see Atropine).

Reference

1. Heinonen OP, Slone D, Shapiro S. *Birth Defects and Drugs in Pregnancy*. Littleton, MA: Publishing Sciences Group, 1977:346–53.

Name:	**MEPERIDINE**	Risk Factor:	**B***
Class:	**Narcotic Agonist Analgesic**		

FETAL RISK SUMMARY

RECOMMENDATION: Human Data Suggest Risk in 3rd Trimester

Fetal problems have not been reported from the therapeutic use of meperidine in pregnancy except when it has been given during labor. Like all narcotics, maternal and neonatal addiction are possible from inappropriate use. Neonatal depression, at times fatal, has historically been the primary concern following obstetric meperidine analgesia. Controversy has now arisen over the potential long-term adverse effects resulting from this use.

The placental transfer of meperidine is very rapid, appearing in cord blood within 2 minutes following IV administration (1). It is detectable in amniotic fluid 30 minutes after IM injection (2). Cord blood concentrations average 70%–77% (range 45%–106%) of maternal plasma levels (3,4). The drug has been detected in the saliva of newborns for 48 hours following maternal administration during labor (5). Concentrations in pharyngeal aspirates were higher than in either arterial or venous cord blood.

In a surveillance study of Michigan Medicaid recipients conducted between 1985 and 1992 involving 229,101 completed pregnancies, 62 newborns had been exposed to meperidine during the 1st trimester (F. Rosa, personal communication, FDA, 1993). Three (4.8%) major birth defects were observed (three expected), including (observed/expected) 1/0 polydactyly and 1/0 hypospadias. No malformations were observed in four other defect categories (cardiovascular defects, oral clefts, spina bifida, and limb reduction defects) for which specific data were available.

Respiratory depression in the newborn following use of the drug in labor is time- and dose-dependent. The incidence of depression increases markedly if delivery occurs 60 minutes or longer after injection, reaching a peak at around 2–3 hours after injection (6,7). Whether this depression is caused by metabolites of meperidine (e.g., normeperidine) or the drug itself is currently not known (2,8–10). However, recent work suggests that these effects are related to unmetabolized meperidine and not to normeperidine (7).

Impaired behavioral response and electroencephalographic changes persisting for several days have been observed (11,12). These persistent effects may be partially explained by the slow elimination of meperidine and normeperidine from the neonate over several days (13,14). One group of investigators related depressed attention and social responsiveness during the first 6 weeks of life to high cord-blood levels of meperidine (15). An earlier study reported long-term follow up of 70 healthy neonates born to mothers who had received meperidine within 2 hours of birth (16,17). Psychologic and physical parameters at 5 years of age were similar in both exposed and control groups. Academic progress and behavior during the 3rd and 4th years in school were also similar.

The Collaborative Perinatal Project monitored 50,282 mother-child pairs, 268 of whom had 1st trimester exposure to meperidine (18, pp. 287–295). For use anytime during pregnancy, 1,100 exposures were recorded (18, p. 434). No evidence was found to suggest a relationship to large categories of major or minor malformations. A possible association between the use of meperidine in the 1st trimester and inguinal hernia was found based on six cases (18, p. 471). The statistical significance of this association is unknown and independent confirmation is required.

[*Risk Factor D if used for prolonged periods or in high doses at term.*]

BREAST FEEDING SUMMARY

RECOMMENDATION: Compatible

Meperidine is excreted into breast milk (19,20). In a group of mothers who had received meperidine during labor, the breast-fed infants had higher saliva levels of the drug for up to 48 hours after birth than a similar group that was bottle-fed (5). In nine nursing mothers, a single 50-mg IM dose produced peak levels of 0.13 μg/mL at 2 hours (20). After 24 hours, the concentrations decreased to 0.02 μg/mL. Average milk:plasma ratios for the nine patients were greater than 1.0. No adverse effects in nursing infants were reported in any of the above studies. The American Academy of Pediatrics classifies meperidine as compatible with breast-feeding (21).

References

1. Crawford JS, Rudofsky S. The placental transmission of pethidine. Br J Anaesth 1965;37: 929–33.
2. Szeto HH, Zervoudakis IA, Cederquist LL, Inturrise CE. Amniotic fluid transfer of meperidine from maternal plasma in early pregnancy. Obstet Gynecol 1978;52:59–62.
3. Apgar V, Burns JJ, Brodie BB, Papper EM. The transmission of meperidine across the human placenta. Am J Obstet Gynecol 1952;64:1368–70.
4. Shnider SM, Way EL, Lord MJ. Rate of appearance and disappearance of meperidine in fetal blood after administration of narcotic to the mother. Anesthesiology 1966;27:227–8.
5. Freeborn SF, Calvert RT, Black P, MacFarlane T, D'Souza SW. Saliva and blood pethidine concentrations in the mother and the newborn baby. Br J Obstet Gynaecol 1980;87:966–9.
6. Morrison JC, Wiser WL, Rosser SI, Gayden JO, Bucovaz ET, Whybrew WD, Fish SA. Metabolites of meperidine related to fetal depression. Am J Obstet Gynecol 1973;115:1132–7.
7. Belfrage P, Boreus LO, Hartvig P, Irestedt L, Raabe N. Neonatal depression after obstetrical analgesia with pethidine. The role of the injection-delivery time interval and the plasma concentrations of pethidine and norpethidine. Acta Obstet Gynecol Scand 1981;60:43–9.
8. Morrison JC, Whybrew WD, Rosser SI, Bucovaz ET, Wiser WL, Fish SA. Metabolites of meperidine in the fetal and maternal serum. Am J Obstet Gynecol 1976;126:997–1002.
9. Clark RB, Lattin DL. Metabolites of meperidine in serum. Am J Obstet Gynecol 1978;130:113–5.
10. Morrison JC. Reply to Drs. Clark and Lattin. Am J Obstet Gynecol 1978;130:115–7.
11. Borgstedt AD, Rosen MG. Medication during labor correlated with behavior and EEG of the newborn. Am J Dis Child 1968;115:21–4.
12. Hodgkinson R, Bhatt M, Wang CN. Double-blind comparison of the neurobehaviour of neonates following the administration of different doses of meperidine to the mother. Can Anaesth Soc J 1978;25: 405–11.
13. Cooper LV, Stephen GW, Aggett PJA. Elimination of pethidine and bupivacaine in the newborn. Arch Dis Child 1977;52:638–41.
14. Kuhnert BR, Kuhnert PM, Prochaska AL, Sokol RJ. Meperidine disposition in mother, neonate and nonpregnant females. Clin Pharmacol Ther 1980;27: 486–91.
15. Belsey EM, Rosenblatt DB, Lieberman BA, Redshaw M, Caldwell J, Notarianni L, Smith RL, Beard RW. The influence of maternal analgesia on neonatal behaviour. I. Pethidine. Br J Obstet Gynaecol 1981;88: 398–406.
16. Buck C, Gregg R, Stavraky K, Subrahmaniam K, Brown J. The effect of single prenatal and natal complications upon the development of children of mature birthweight. Pediatrics 1969;43:942–55.
17. Buck C. Drugs in pregnancy. Can Med Assoc J 1975; 112:1285.
18. Heinonen O, Slone D, Shapiro S. *Birth Defects and Drugs in Pregnancy*. Littleton, MA: Publishing Sciences Group, 1977.
19. Vorherr H. Drug excretion in breast milk. Postgrad Med 1974;56:97–104.
20. Peiker G, Muller B, Ihn W, Noschel H. Excretion of pethidine in mother's milk. Zentralbl Gynaekol 1980; 102:537–41.
21. Committee on Drugs, American Academy of Pediatrics. The transfer of drugs and other chemicals into human breast milk. Pediatrics 2001;108: 776–89.

M

Name: **MEPHENTERMINE** Risk Factor: **C**
Class: **Sympathomimetic (Adrenergic)**

FETAL RISK SUMMARY

RECOMMENDATION: Limited Human Data - No Relevant Animal Data

Mephentermine is a sympathomimetic used in emergencies to treat hypotension. Because of the nature of its indication, experience in pregnancy with mephentermine is limited. Mephentermine's primary action is to increase cardiac output as a result of enhanced cardiac contraction and, to a lesser extent, from peripheral vasoconstriction (1). Its effect on uterine blood flow should be minimal (1).

A newborn infant with complete exstrophy of the bladder, epispadias, widely separated pubic rami, and bilateral inguinal hernias was described in a 1970 publication (2). The infant's mother, a 19-year-old woman, had used lysergic acid diethylamide (LSD) on at least 12–15 occasions during the 2 months before conception and during the first 2.5 months of pregnancy. In addition, she had smoked marijuana twice and had ingested mephentermine sulfate once during the above interval. The cause of the defects observed in the infant is unknown.

BREAST FEEDING SUMMARY

RECOMMENDATION: No Human Data - Probably Compatible

No data are available.

M

References

1. Smith NT, Corbascio AN. The use and misuse of pressor agents. Anesthesiology 1970;33:58–101.
2. Gelehrter TD. Lysergic acid diethylamide (LSD) and exstrophy of the bladder. J Pediatr 1970;77:1065–6.

Name: **MEPHENYTOIN** Risk Factor: **C**
Class: **Anticonvulsant**

FETAL RISK SUMMARY

RECOMMENDATION: Compatible - Maternal Benefit >> Embryo/Fetal Risk

Mephenytoin is a hydantoin anticonvulsant similar to phenytoin (see Phenytoin). The drug is infrequently prescribed because of the greater incidence of serious side effects as compared with phenytoin (1). There have been reports of 12 infants with 1st trimester exposure to mephenytoin (2–5). No evidence of adverse fetal effects was found.

BREAST FEEDING SUMMARY

RECOMMENDATION: No Human Data - Probably Compatible

No data are available.

References

1. Rall TW, Shleifer LS. Drugs effective in the treatment of the epilepsies. In Goodman AG, Goodman LS, Gilman A, eds. *The Pharmacological Basis of Therapeutics.* 6th ed. New York, NY: Macmillan Publishing, 1980: 456.
2. Fedrick J. Epilepsy and pregnancy: a report from the Oxford Linkage Study. Br Med J 1973;2:442–8.
3. Heinonen O, Slone D, Shapiro S. *Birth Defects and Drugs in Pregnancy.* Littleton, MA: Publishing Sciences Group, 1977:358–9.
4. Annegers JF, Elveback LR, Hauser WA, Kurland LT. Do anticonvulsants have a teratogenic effect? Arch Neurol 1974;31:364–73.
5. Speidel BD, Meadow SR. Maternal epilepsy and abnormalities of the fetus and newborn. Lancet 1972;2: 839–43.

Name: **MEPHOBARBITAL** Risk Factor: **D_M**
Class: **Anticonvulsant/Sedative**

M

FETAL RISK SUMMARY

RECOMMENDATION: Compatible - Maternal Benefit >> Embryo/Fetal Risk

Mephobarbital (methylphenobarbital; methylphenobarbitone) is a barbiturate with sedative, hypnotic, and anticonvulsant properties. Although specific information is not available, barbiturates readily cross the placenta with highest concentrations in the placenta, fetal liver and brain (1). The drug is demethylated by the liver to phenobarbital (see Phenobarbital).

The Collaborative Perinatal Project monitored 50,282 mother-child pairs, 8 of whom had 1st trimester exposure to mephobarbital (2). No evidence was found to suggest a relationship to large categories of major or minor malformations or to individual defects. Hemorrhagic disease and barbiturate withdrawal in the newborn are theoretically possible, although they have not been reported in humans with mephobarbital.

A 2000 study, using data from the MADRE (an acronym for MAlformation and DRug Exposure) surveillance project, assessed the human teratogenicity of anticonvulsants (3). Among 8005 malformed infants, cases were defined as infants with a specific malformation, whereas controls were infants with other anomalies. Of the total group, 299 were exposed in the 1st trimester to anticonvulsants. Among these, exposure to monotherapy occurred in the following: phenobarbital ($N = 65$), mephobarbital ($N = 10$), carbamazepine ($N = 46$), valproic acid ($N = 80$), phenytoin ($N = 24$), and other agents ($N = 16$). Statistically significant associations (CI not overlapping 1 and $p \leq 0.05$) were found between mephobarbital monotherapy and cardiac defects ($N = 4$) and cleft lip/palate ($N = 4$). When all 1st trimester exposures (mono- and polytherapy) were evaluated, a significant association was found with cleft lip/palate ($N = 4$). Although the study confirmed some previously known associations, several new associations with anticonvulsants were discovered and require independent confirmation (see also Carbamazepine, Phenobarbital, Phenytoin, and Valproic Acid) (3).

BREAST FEEDING SUMMARY

RECOMMENDATION: No Human Data - Potential Toxicity

See Phenobarbital.

References

1. Product information. Mebaral. Sanofi-Synthelabo, 2001.
2. Heinonen O, Slone D, Shapiro S. *Birth Defects and Drugs in Pregnancy*. Littleton, MA: Publishing Sciences Group, 1977:336.
3. Arpino C, Brescianini S, Robert E, Castilla EE, Cocchi G, Cornel MC, de Vigan C, Lancaster PAL, Merlob P, Sumiyoshi Y, Zampino G, Renzi C, Rosano A, Mastroiacovo P. Teratogenic effects of antiepileptic drugs: use of an international database on malformations and drug exposure (MADRE). Epilepsia 2000;41:1436–43.

Name:	**MEPINDOLOL**	Risk Factor:	**C***
Class:	**Sympatholytic (Antihypertensive)**		

FETAL RISK SUMMARY

RECOMMENDATION: Human Data Suggest Risk in 2nd and 3rd Trimesters

Mepindolol is a nonselective β-adrenergic blocking agent. No reports of its use in pregnancy have been located.

The use near delivery of some agents in this class has resulted in persistent β-blockade in the newborn (see Acebutolol, Atenolol, and Nadolol). Thus, newborns exposed *in utero* to mepindolol should be closely observed during the first 24–48 hours after birth for bradycardia and other symptoms. The long-term effects of *in utero* exposure to β-blockers have not been studied but warrant evaluation.

Some β-blockers may cause intrauterine growth retardation (IUGR) and reduced placental weight, especially those lacking intrinsic sympathomimetic activity (ISA) (i.e., partial agonist). Treatment beginning early in the 2nd trimester results in the greatest weight reductions, whereas treatment restricted to the 3rd trimester primarily affects only placental weight. It is not known if mepindolol possesses ISA. However, IUGR and reduced placental weight may potentially occur with all agents within this class. Although growth retardation is a serious concern, the benefits of maternal therapy with β-blockers, in some cases, might outweigh the risks to the fetus and must be judged on a case-by-case basis.

[**Risk Factor D if used in 2nd or 3rd trimesters.*]

BREAST FEEDING SUMMARY

RECOMMENDATION: Limited Human Data - Potential Toxicity

Mepindolol is excreted into breast milk (1). Following a 20-mg dose, mean milk concentrations in five mothers at 2 and 6 hours were 18 and 16 ng/mL, respectively, with a milk:plasma ratio at 2 hours of 0.35. Continuous dosing of 20 mg daily for 5 days produced milk levels at 2 and 6 hours of 22 and 33 ng/mL. The milk:plasma ratio at 6 hours was 0.61. At a detection limit of 1 ng/mL, mepindolol could be found in the serum of only one of the five breast-fed infants. Although no adverse effects were observed, nursing infants should be closely watched for bradycardia and other signs and symptoms of β-blockade. Long-term effects of exposure to β-blockers from milk have not been studied but warrant evaluation.

Reference

1. Krause W, Stoppelli I, Milia S, Rainer E. Transfer of mepindolol to newborns by breast-feeding mothers after single and repeated daily doses. Eur J Clin Pharmacol 1982;22:53–5.

Name:	**MEPROBAMATE**	Risk Factor:	**D**
Class:	**Sedative**		

FETAL RISK SUMMARY

RECOMMENDATION: Contraindicated - 1st Trimester

Meprobamate is used in the treatment of anxiety disorders or for the short-term treatment of the symptoms of anxiety. The drug crosses the placenta to the fetus and has been measured in umbilical cord blood at or near maternal plasma levels (1).

Schardein reviewed seven reproduction studies in mice, rats, and rabbits (2). Meprobamate caused digital defects in mice and neurobehavior toxicity in rats. However, because most of the studies involved parenteral administration, the findings cannot be used to assess the degree of human risk (2).

Meprobamate use in pregnancy has been associated with an increased risk of congenital anomalies (1.9%–12.1%) (3,4). In one study of 395 patients, 8 defects were observed: congenital heart disease (2 with multiple other defects) (5 cases), Down's syndrome (1 case), deafness (partial) (1 case), and deformed elbows and joints (1 case) (3). Another report described multiple anomalies, including congenital heart defects, in a newborn exposed to meprobamate (5). The mother of this patient was treated very early in the 1st trimester with meprobamate and propoxyphene. Malformations observed were omphalocele, defective anterior abdominal wall, defect in diaphragm, congenital heart disease with partial ectopic cordis secondary to sternal cleft, and dysplastic hips. Multiple defects of the eye and central nervous system were observed in a newborn exposed to multiple drugs, including meprobamate and LSD (6).

M

The Collaborative Perinatal Project monitored 50,282 mother-child pairs, 356 of whom were exposed in the 1st trimester to meprobamate (7,8). No association of meprobamate with large classes of malformations or with individual defects was found. Others also have failed to find a relationship between the use of meprobamate and congenital malformations (9).

In a surveillance study of Michigan Medicaid recipients conducted between 1985 and 1992 involving 229,101 completed pregnancies, 75 newborns had been exposed to meprobamate during the 1st trimester (F. Rosa, personal communication, FDA, 1993). Three (4.0%) major birth defects were observed (three expected), including (observed/expected) 1/0 oral clefts and 2/0 polydactyly. No anomalies were observed in four other defect categories (cardiovascular defects, spina bifida, limb reduction defects, and hypospadias) for which specific data were available. Only with the cases of polydactyly is there a suggestion of a possible association, but other factors, such as the mother's disease, concurrent drug use, and chance, may be involved.

In summary, few indications exist for meprobamate in the pregnant woman. If therapy is required, avoiding the 1st trimester is the safest course, but inadvertent exposure does not appear to represent a major risk.

BREAST FEEDING SUMMARY

RECOMMENDATION: Limited Human Data - Potential Toxicity

Meprobamate is excreted into breast milk (1,10). Milk concentrations are 2–4 times that of maternal plasma. The effect on the nursing infant is unknown.

References

1. Product information. Miltown. Wallace Laboratories, 2000.
2. Schardein JL. *Chemically Induced Birth Defects*. 3rd ed. New York: Marcel Dekker, 2000:243.
3. Milkovich L, van den Berg BJ. Effects of prenatal meprobamate and chlordiazepoxide hydrochloride on human embryonic and fetal development. N Engl J Med 1974;291:1268–71.
4. Crombie DL, Pinsent RJ, Fleming DM, Rumeau-Rouguette C, Goujard J, Huel G. Fetal effects of tranquilizers in pregnancy. N Engl J Med 1975;293:198–9.
5. Ringrose CAD. The hazard of neurotropic drugs in the fertile years. Can Med Assoc J 1972;106:1058.
6. Bogdanoff B, Rorke LB, Yanoff M, Warren WS. Brain and eye abnormalities: possible sequelae to prenatal use of multiple drugs including LSD. Am J Dis Child 1972;123:145–8.
7. Heinonen OP, Slone D, Shapiro S. *Birth Defects and Drugs in Pregnancy*. Littleton, MA: Publishing Sciences Group, 1977:336–37.
8. Hartz SC, Heinonen OP, Shapiro S, Siskind V, Slone D. Antenatal exposure to meprobamate and chlordiazepoxide in relation to malformations, mental development, and childhood mortality. N Engl J Med 1975;292:726–8.
9. Belafsky HA, Breslow S, Hirsch LM, Shangold JE, Stahl MB. Meprobamate during pregnancy. Obstet Gynecol 1969;34:378–86.
10. Wilson JT, Brown RD, Cherek DR, Dailey JW, Hilman B, Jobe PC, Manno BR, Manno JE, Redetzki HM, Stewart JJ. Drug excretion in human breast milk: principles, pharmacokinetics and projected consequences. Clin Pharmacokinet 1980;5:1–66.

Name: **MERCAPTOPURINE** Risk Factor: **D_M**

Class: **Antineoplastic**

FETAL RISK SUMMARY

RECOMMENDATION: Human Data Suggest Risk in 3rd Trimester

Mercaptopurine (6-MP) is an antimetabolite antineoplastic agent. References citing the use of mercaptopurine in 79 human pregnancies have been located, including 34 cases in which the drug was used in the 1st trimester (1–21). Excluding those pregnancies that ended in abortion or stillbirths, congenital abnormalities were observed in only one infant (10). Defects noted in the infant were cleft palate, microphthalmia, hypoplasia of the ovaries and thyroid gland, corneal opacity, cytomegaly, and intrauterine growth retardation. The anomalies were attributed to busulfan.

Neonatal toxicity as a result of combination chemotherapy has been observed in three infants: pancytopenia (6), microangiopathic hemolytic anemia (9), and transient severe bone marrow hypoplasia (12). In the latter case, administration of mercaptopurine was stopped 3.5 weeks before delivery because of severe maternal myelosuppression. No chemotherapy was given during this period and her peripheral blood counts were normal during the final 2 weeks of her pregnancy (12).

In another case, a 34-year-old woman with acute lymphoblastic leukemia was treated with multiple antineoplastic agents from 22 weeks' gestation until delivery of a healthy female infant 18 weeks later (14). Mercaptopurine was administered throughout the 3rd trimester. Chromosomal analysis of the newborn revealed a normal karyotype (46,XX) but with gaps and a ring chromosome. The clinical significance of these findings is unknown, but since these abnormalities may persist for several years, the potential existed for an increased risk of cancer, as well as for a risk of genetic damage in the next generation (14).

Data from one review indicated that 40% of the infants exposed to anticancer drugs were of low birth weight (2). This finding was not related to the timing of exposure. In addition, except in a few cases, long-term studies of growth and mental development in infants exposed to mercaptopurine during the 2nd trimester, the period of neuroblast multiplication, have not been conducted (22). However, growth and development were normal in 13 infants (one set of twins) examined for 6 months to 10 years (12,15,16, 18–21).

Severe oligospermia has been described in a 22-year-old male receiving sequential chemotherapy of cyclophosphamide, methotrexate, and mercaptopurine for leukemia (23). After treatment was stopped, the sperm count returned to normal and the patient fathered a healthy female child. Others have also observed reversible testicular dysfunction (24).

Ovarian function in females exposed to mercaptopurine does not seem to be affected adversely (25–29). An investigator noted in 1980 that long-term analysis of human reproduction following mercaptopurine therapy had not been reported (30). However, a brief 1979 correspondence described the reproductive performance of 314 women after treatment of gestational trophoblastic tumors, 159 of whom had conceived with a total of 218 pregnancies (28). Excluding the 17 women still pregnant at the time of the report, 38 (79%) of 48 women, exposed to mercaptopurine as part of their therapy, delivered live, term infants. A more detailed report of these and additional patients was published in 1984 (31). This latter study, and another published in 1988 (32), both involving women treated for gestational trophoblastic neoplasms, are discussed below.

In 436 long-term survivors treated with chemotherapy between 1958 and 1978, 95 (22%) received mercaptopurine as part of their treatment regimens (31). Of the 95 women, 33 (35%) had at least one live birth (numbers given in parentheses refer to mean/maximum mercaptopurine dose in grams) (5.9/30.0), 3 (3%) conceived but had no live births (5.3/14.0), 3 (3%) failed to conceive (1.3/2.0), and 56 (59%) did not try to conceive (5.4/30.0). Additional details, including congenital anomalies observed, are described in the monograph for methotrexate (see Methotrexate).

M

A 1988 report described the reproductive results of 265 women who had been treated from 1959 to 1980 for gestational trophoblastic disease (32). Single-agent chemotherapy was administered to 91 women, including 26 cases in which mercaptopurine was the only agent used, whereas sequential (single agent) and combination therapy was administered to 67 and 107 women, respectively. Of the total group, 241 were exposed to pregnancy and 205 (85%) of these women conceived, with a total of 355 pregnancies. The time interval between recovery and pregnancy was 1 year or less (8.5%), 1–2 years (32.1%), 2–4 years (32.4%), 4–6 years (15.5%), 6–8 years (7.3%), 8–10 years (1.4%), and more than 10 years (2.8%). A total of 303 (4 sets of twins) liveborn infants resulted from the 355 pregnancies, 3 of whom had congenital malformations: anencephaly, hydrocephalus, and congenital heart disease (1 in each case). No gross developmental abnormalities were observed in the dead fetuses. Cytogenetic studies were conducted on the peripheral lymphocytes of 94 children and no significant chromosomal abnormalities were noted. Moreover, follow-up of the children, with more than 80% of the group older than 5 years of age (the oldest was 25 years), revealed normal development. The reproductive histories and pregnancy outcomes of the treated women were comparable to those of the normal population (32).

Occupational exposure of the mother to antineoplastic agents during pregnancy may present a risk to the fetus. A position statement from the National Study Commission on Cytotoxic Exposure and a research article involving some antineoplastic agents are presented in the monograph for cyclophosphamide (see Cyclophosphamide).

BREAST FEEDING SUMMARY

RECOMMENDATION: No Human Data - Potential Toxicity

No reports describing the use of mercaptopurine during lactation have been located. Because of the relatively low molecular weight (about 170), transfer into milk should be expected. Because of the potential for severe toxicity in the nursing infant, women receiving this antineoplastic agent should not nurse.

References

1. Moloney WC. Management of leukemia in pregnancy. Ann N Y Acad Sci 1964;114:857–67.
2. Nicholson HO. Cytotoxic drugs in pregnancy: review of reported cases. J Obstet Gynaecol Br Commonw 1968;75:307–12.
3. Gililland J, Weinstein L. The effects of cancer chemotherapeutic agents on the developing fetus. Obstet Gynecol Surv 1983;38:6–13.
4. Wegelius R. Successful pregnancy in acute leukaemia. Lancet 1975;2:1301.
5. Nicholson HO. Leukaemia and pregnancy: a report of five cases and discussion of management. J Obstet Gynaecol Br Commonw 1968;75:517–20.
6. Pizzuto J, Aviles A, Noriega L, Niz J, Morales M, Romero F. Treatment of acute leukemia during pregnancy: presentation of nine cases. Cancer Treat Rep 1980;64:679–83.
7. Burnier AM. Discussion. In Plows CW. Acute myelomonocytic leukemia in pregnancy: report of a case. Am J Obstet Gynecol 1982;143:41–3.
8. Dara P, Slater LM, Armentrout SA. Successful pregnancy during chemotherapy for acute leukemia. Cancer 1981;47:845–6.
9. McConnell JF, Bhoola R. A neonatal complication of maternal leukemia treated with 6-mercaptopurine. Postgrad Med J 1973;49:211–3.
10. Diamond J, Anderson MM, McCreadie SR. Transplacental transmission of busulfan (Myleran) in a mother with leukemia: production of fetal malformation and cytomegaly. Pediatrics 1960;25:85–90.
11. Khurshid M, Saleem M. Acute leukaemia in pregnancy. Lancet 1978;2:534–5.
12. Okun DB, Groncy PK, Sieger L, Tanaka KR. Acute leukemia in pregnancy: transient neonatal myelosuppression after combination chemotherapy in the mother. Med Pediatr Oncol 1979;7:315–9.
13. Doney KC, Kraemer KG, Shepard TH. Combination chemotherapy for acute myelocytic leukemia during pregnancy: three case reports. Cancer Treat Rep 1979;63:369–71.
14. Schleuning M, Clemm C. Chromosomal aberrations in a newborn whose mother received cytotoxic treatment during pregnancy. N Engl J Med 1987;317:1666–7.
15. Turchi JJ, Villasis C. Anthracyclines in the treatment of malignancy in pregnancy. Cancer 1988;61:435–40.
16. Feliu J, Juarez S, Ordonez A, Garcia-Paredes ML, Gonzalez-Baron M, Montero JM. Acute leukemia and pregnancy. Cancer 1988;61:580–4.
17. Haerr RW, Pratt AT. Multiagent chemotherapy for sarcoma diagnosed during pregnancy. Cancer 1985;56:1028–33.
18. Frenkel EP, Meyers MC. Acute leukemia and pregnancy. Ann Intern Med 1960;53:656–71.
19. Loyd HO. Acute leukemia complicated by pregnancy. JAMA 1961;178:1140–3.
20. Lee RA, Johnson CE, Hanlon DG. Leukemia during pregnancy. Am J Obstet Gynecol 1962;84:455–8.
21. Coopland AT, Friesen WJ, Galbraith PA. Acute leukemia in pregnancy. Am J Obstet Gynecol 1969;105:1288–9.
22. Dobbing J. Pregnancy and leukaemia. Lancet 1977;1:1155.
23. Hinkes E, Plotkin D. Reversible drug-induced sterility in a patient with acute leukemia. JAMA 1973;223:1490–1.
24. Lendon M, Palmer MK, Hann IM, Shalet SM, Jones PHM. Testicular histology after combination chemotherapy in childhood for acute lymphoblastic leukaemia. Lancet 1978;2:439–41.
25. Schilsky RL, Lewis BJ, Sherins RJ, Young RC. Gonadal dysfunction in patients receiving chemotherapy for cancer. Ann Intern Med 1980;93:109–14.
26. Gasser C. Long-term survival (cures) in childhood acute leukemia. Paediatrician 1980;9:344–57.
27. Bacon C, Kernahan J. Successful pregnancy in acute leukaemia. Lancet 1975;2:515.
28. Walden PAM, Bagshawe KD. Pregnancies after chemotherapy for gestational trophoblastic tumours. Lancet 1979;2:1241.
29. Sanz MH, Rafecas FJ. Successful pregnancy during chemotherapy for acute promyelocytic leukemia. N Engl J Med 1982;306:939.
30. Steckman ML. Treatment of Crohn's disease with 6-mercaptopurine: what effects on fertility? N Engl J Med 1980;303:817.
31. Rustin GJS, Booth M, Dent J, Salt S, Rustin F, Bagshawe KD. Pregnancy after cytotoxic chemotherapy for gestational trophoblastic tumours. Br Med J 1984;288:103–6.
32. Song H, Wu P, Wang Y, Yang X, Dong S. Pregnancy outcomes after successful chemotherapy for choriocarcinoma and invasive mole: long-term follow-up. Am J Obstet Gynecol 1988;158:538–45.

Name:	**MEROPENEM**	Risk Factor:	B_M
Class:	**Antibiotic**		

FETAL RISK SUMMARY

RECOMMENDATION: No Human Data - Animal Data Suggest Low Risk

Meropenem is an intravenous broad-spectrum, carbapenem antibiotic. The drug belongs to the same class of antibiotics as imipenem.

Reproduction studies in rats and cynomolgus monkeys at doses up to 1.8 and 3.7 times, respectively, the usual human dose (1 g every 8 hours), found no evidence of impaired fertility or fetal harm, except for slight changes in fetal weight in rats at doses of 0.4 times the usual human dose or greater (1).

Placental passage in animals or humans has apparently not been studied, but the low molecular weight (about 438) suggests that placental transfer to the fetus occurs. Moreover, the drug is distributed into a large number of human tissues, including the endometrium, fallopian tubes, and ovaries (1).

No reports have been located that described the use of meropenem in human pregnancy. Although the lack of published human pregnancy experience does not allow an assessment of the fetal risk, another carbapenem antibiotic is considered safe to use during the perinatal period (i.e., 28 weeks' gestation or later) and, most likely, meropenem can be classified similarly. The fetal risk of use before this period is unknown.

BREAST FEEDING SUMMARY

RECOMMENDATION: No Human Data - Probably Compatible

No reports describing the use of meropenem during lactation have been located. Because of its relatively low molecular weight (about 438), excretion into milk should be expected. The potential effects of the antibiotic on a nursing infant are unknown.

Reference

1. Product information. Merrem. Zeneca Pharmaceuticals, 1997.

Name:	**MESALAMINE**	Risk Factor:	B_M
Class:	**Anti-inflammatory Bowel Disease Agent**		

FETAL RISK SUMMARY

RECOMMENDATION: Compatible

Mesalamine (5-aminosalicylic acid, 5-ASA) is administered by either rectal suspension or suppository for the treatment of distal ulcerative colitis, proctosigmoiditis, and proctitis. It also results from metabolism in the large intestine of the oral preparation sulfasalazine, which is split to mesalamine and sulfapyridine, and from balsalazide and olsalazine, oral formulations that are metabolized in the colon to mesalamine. The history, pharmacology, and pharmacokinetics of mesalamine and olsalazine were extensively reviewed in a 1992 reference (1).

Reproduction studies in rats and rabbits at oral doses of 480 mg/kg/day observed no fetal toxicity or teratogenicity (2).

Sulfasalazine and one of the metabolites, sulfapyridine, readily cross the placenta and could displace bilirubin from albumin if the concentrations were great enough. Mesalamine, however, is bound to different sites on albumin than bilirubin and, thus, has no bilirubin-displacing ability (3). Moreover, only small amounts of mesalamine are absorbed from the cecum and colon into the systemic circulation, and most of this is rapidly excreted in the urine (4).

A 1987 reference reported the concentrations of mesalamine and its metabolite, acetyl-5-aminosalicylic acid, in amniotic fluid at 16 weeks' gestation and in maternal and cord plasma at term in women treated prophylactically with sulfasalazine 3 g/day (5). The drug and metabolite levels and the number of patients were as follows: amniotic fluid ($N = 4$), 0.02–0.08 μg/mL and 0.07–0.77 μg/mL, respectively; maternal plasma ($N = 5$), 0.08–0.29 μg/mL and 0.31–1.27 μg/mL, respectively; and cord plasma ($N = 5$), <0.02–0.10 μg/mL and 0.29–1.80 μg/mL, respectively. No effects on the fetus or newborn from the maternal drug therapy were mentioned. At delivery in a woman taking 1 g of mesalamine 3 times daily, the concentrations of the drug and its metabolite, 3.3 hours after the last dose, in the mother's serum were 1.2 and 2.8 μg/mL, respectively, and in the umbilical cord serum, 0.4 and 5.7 μg/mL, respectively (6). The cord:maternal serum ratios were 0.33 and 2.0, respectively.

A review of drug therapy for ulcerative colitis recommended that women taking mesalamine to maintain remission of the disease should continue the drug when trying to conceive or when pregnant (7). A study published in 1993 described the course of 19 pregnancies in 17 women (ulcerative colitis $N = 10$; Crohn's disease $N = 7$) who received mesalamine (mean dose 1.7 g/d; range 0.8–2.4 g/d) throughout gestation (8). Full-term deliveries occurred in 18 and one patient, with a history of four previous miscarriages, suffered a spontaneous abortion. No congenital malformations were observed.

Only one report has described possible *in utero* mesalamine-induced toxicity that may have occurred during 2nd trimester exposure to the drug (9). The 24-year-old mother was treated, between the 13th and 24th week of gestation, for Crohn's disease with 4 g/day of mesalamine for 5 weeks, then tapered to 2 g/day for 6 weeks, and then stopped. A fetal ultrasound at 17 weeks' gestation was normal, but a second examination at 21 weeks showed bilateral renal hyperechogenicity (9). The term male infant had a serum creatinine at birth of 115 μmol/L (normal 18–35 μmol/L). Renal hyperechogenicity was confirmed at various times up to 6 months of age. At this age, the serum creatinine was 62 μmol/L with a creatinine clearance of 52 mL/min (normal 80–90 mL/min). A renal biopsy at 6 months of age showed focal tubulointerstitial lesions with interstitial fibrosis and tubular atrophy in the absence of cell infiltration (9). Because no other cause of the renal lesions could be found and there was some resemblance to lesions induced by the prostaglandin synthesis inhibitor, indomethacin, the authors attributed the defect to mesalamine (9). A letter published in response to this study, however, questioned the association between the drug and observed renal defect because of the lack of toxicity in an unpublished series of 60 exposed pregnancies and the lack of evidence that mesalamine causes renal prostaglandin synthesis inhibition *in utero* (10).

A 1997 report described the successful outcomes of 19 pregnancies followed prospectively in 16 women with proven distal colitis (11). The women received either 4-g mesalamine enemas three times weekly or a 500-mg mesalamine suppository every night throughout gestation. No fetal abnormalities were observed during pregnancy and all of the full-term offspring were normal at birth and at a median follow-up of 2 years (range 2 months–5 years) (11).

A 1998 prospective study reported the pregnancy outcomes of 165 women exposed to mesalamine (146 during the 1st trimester) who had contacted a teratogen information service (TIS) (12). The study patients were compared to 165 matched controls who had called the TIS concerning nonteratogenic exposures. There were no significant differences between the two groups in spontaneous abortions (6.7% vs. 8.5%), ectopic pregnancies (0.6% vs. 0%), or elective abortions (none were associated with malformed fetuses) (4.2% vs. 1.8%). There was one major defect (an extra right thumb) in the study group compared

M

to five major anomalies in controls (*n.s.*). Eight subjects had minor malformations compared to five controls (*n.s.*). However, compared to controls, significantly more preterm deliveries occurred in subjects (13.0% vs. 4.7%), the mean birth weight was lower (3253 g vs. 3461 g), and the mean maternal weight gain was lower (13.1 kg vs. 15.6 kg) (12).

A 2004 report described the pregnancy outcomes of 113 women who were being treated for inflammatory bowel disease (39 ulcerative colitis; 73 Crohn's disease; and 1 indeterminate colitis) (13). In the group, there were 207 pregnancies, 100 during treatment with a 5-ASA agent (mesalamine, sulfasalazine, balsalazide, or olsalazine) at some time during pregnancy. Other agents used included 49 cases with prednisone, 101 with azathioprine or mercaptopurine, 27 with metronidazole, 18 with ciprofloxacin, and 2 with cyclosporine. The pregnancy outcomes of the first eligible pregnancy in the 113 women were 2 ectopic pregnancies, 2 elective abortions, 16 spontaneous abortions, 6 premature infants, 85 full-term infants (1 set of twins), and 3 major defects (2.7%). However, one of the "defects" was a case of immature lungs, which is not considered a congenital defect. The other two defects were imperforate anus and an unspecified heart defect. In addition, the two elective abortions were for unspecified fetal defects. The study concluded that there was no evidence that any of the drugs used either alone or in combination was associated with poor pregnancy outcomes (13).

In contrast to sulfasalazine, mesalamine apparently has no adverse effect on spermatogenesis. Treatment of males with sulfasalazine may adversely affect spermatogenesis (14–18), but either stopping therapy or changing to mesalamine allows recovery of sperm production, usually within 3 months (15–18).

In summary, the maternal benefits of therapy with mesalamine appear to outweigh the potential risks to the fetus. No teratogenic effects caused by mesalamine have been described and, although toxicity in the fetus has been reported in one case, a causal relationship between the drug and that outcome is controversial.

BREAST FEEDING SUMMARY

RECOMMENDATION: Limited Human Data - Potential Toxicity

Small amounts of mesalamine are excreted into human milk. A 1990 report described the excretion of mesalamine and its metabolite, acetyl-5-aminosalicylic acid, into breast milk (19). The woman was receiving 500 mg 3 times daily for ulcerative colitis. In a single plasma and milk sample obtained 5.25 hours after a dose, milk and plasma levels of mesalamine were 0.11 and 0.41 μg/mL, respectively, a milk:plasma ratio of 0.27. Milk and plasma levels of acetyl-5-aminosalicylic acid were 12.4 and 2.44 μg/mL, respectively, a ratio of 5.1. In another study, women treated prophylactically with 3 g/day of sulfasalazine had milk levels of mesalamine and acetyl-5-aminosalicylic acid of 0.02 and 1.13–3.44 μg/mL, respectively (5). No adverse effects on the nursing infants were mentioned.

Low concentrations of mesalamine and its metabolite were also found in a woman taking 1 g, 3 times daily (6). Maternal serum levels of the drug and metabolite, determined at 7 and 11 days postpartum, were 0.6 and 1.1 μg/mL (day 7) and 1.1 and 1.8 μg/mL (day 11), respectively. Milk concentrations of the drug and metabolite at these times were 0.1 and 18.1 μg/mL (day 7) and 0.1 and 12.3 μg/mL (day 11), respectively, representing milk:plasma ratios for mesalamine of 0.17 and 0.09 (day 7 and 11), respectively, and for the metabolite of 16.5 and 6.8 (day 7 and 11), respectively. The estimated daily intake by the infant of mesalamine and metabolite was 0.065 mg (0.015 mg/kg) and 10 mg (2.3 mg/kg), respectively, considered to be negligible amounts (6).

A study published in 1993 described the excretion of olsalazine, a prodrug that is partially (2.4%) absorbed into the systemic circulation before conversion of the remainder by colonic bacteria into two molecules of mesalamine (see Olsalazine), in the breast milk of a woman 4 months' postpartum (20). Following a 500-mg oral dose, olsalazine, olsalazine sulfate, and mesalamine were undetectable in breast milk up to 48 hours (detection limits 0.5 μmol/L, 0.2 μmol/L, and 1.0 μmol/L, respectively). Acetyl-5-aminosalicylic concentrations at 10, 14, and 24 hours, were 0.8, 0.86, and 1.24 μmol/L, respectively, but undetectable (detection limit 1.0 μmol/L) during the first 6 hours and after 24 hours. The quantities detected were considered clinically insignificant (20).

Diarrhea in a nursing infant, apparently because of the rectal administration of mesalamine to the mother, has been reported (21). The mother had relapsing ulcerative proctitis. Six weeks after childbirth, treatment was begun with 500-mg mesalamine suppositories twice daily. Her exclusively breast-fed infant developed watery diarrhea 12 hours after the mother's first dose. After 2 days of therapy, the mother stopped the suppositories and the infant's diarrhea stopped 10 hours later. Therapy was reinstituted on four occasions with diarrhea developing each time in the infant 8–12 hours after the mother's first dose and stopping 8–12 hours after therapy was halted. Because of the severity of the mother's disease, breast-feeding was discontinued and no further episodes of diarrhea were observed in the infant (21).

Because of the adverse effect described above, a possible allergic reaction, nursing infants of women being treated with mesalamine or olsalazine should be closely observed for changes in stool consistency. The American Academy of Pediatrics classifies 5-aminosalicylic acid (i.e., mesalamine) as a drug that has produced adverse effects in a nursing infant and should be used with caution during breast-feeding (22).

M

References

1. Segars LW, Gales BJ. Mesalamine and olsalazine: 5-aminosalicylic acid agents for the treatment of inflammatory bowel disease. Clin Pharm 1992;11: 514–28.
2. Product information. Asacol. Procter & Gamble Pharmaceuticals, 2000.
3. Jarnerot G, Andersen S, Esbjorner E, Sandstrom B, Brodersen R. Albumin reserve for binding of bilirubin in maternal and cord serum under treatment with sulphasalazine. Scand J Gastroenterol 1981;16: 1049–55.
4. Berlin CM Jr, Yaffe SJ. Disposition of salicylazosulfapyridine (Azulfidine) and metabolites in human breast milk. Dev Pharmacol Ther 1980;1:313–9.
5. Christensen LA, Rasmussen SN, Hansen SH, Bondesen S, Hvidberg EF. Salazosulfapyridine and metabolites in fetal and maternal body fluids with special reference to 5-aminosalicylic acid. Acta Obstet Gynecol Scand 1987;66:433–5.
6. Klotz U, Harings-Kaim A. Negligible excretion of 5-aminosalicylic acid in breast milk. Lancet 1993;342: 618–9.
7. Kamm MA, Senapati A. Drug management of ulcerative colitis. BMJ 1992;305:35–8.
8. Habal FM, Hui G, Greenberg GR. Oral 5-aminosalicylic acid for inflammatory bowel disease in pregnancy: safety and clinical course. Gastroenterology 1993;105:1057–60.
9. Colombel J-F, Brabant G, Gubler M-C, Locquet A, Comes M-C, Dehennault M, Delcroix M. Renal insufficiency in infant: side-effect of prenatal exposure to mesalazine? Lancet 1994;344:620–1.
10. Marteau P, Devaux CB. Mesalazine during pregnancy. Lancet 1994;344:1708–9.
11. Bell CM, Habal FM. Safety of topical 5-aminosalicylic acid in pregnancy. Am J Gastroenterol 1997;92: 2201–2.
12. Diav-Citrin O, Park Y-H, Veerasuntharam G, Polachek H, Bologa M, Pastuszak A, Koren G. The safety of mesalamine in human pregnancy: a prospective controlled cohort study. Gastroenterology 1998;114:23–8.
13. Moskovitz DN, Bodian C, Chapman ML, Marion JF, Rubin PH, Scherl E, Present DH. The effect on the fetus of medications used to treat pregnant inflammatory bowel-disease patients. Am J Gastroenterol 2004;99:656–61.
14. Freeman JG, Reece VAC, Venables CW. Sulphasalazine and spermatogenesis. Digestion 1982;23:68–71.
15. Toovey S, Hudson E, Hendry WF, Levi AJ. Sulphasalazine and male infertility: reversibility and possible mechanism. Gut 1981;22:445–51.
16. O'Morain C, Smethurst P, Dore CJ, Levi AJ. Reversible male infertility due to sulphasalazine: studies in man and rat. Gut 1984;25:1078–84.
17. Chatzinoff M, Guarino JM, Corson SL, Batzer FR, Friedman LS. Sulfasalazine-induced abnormal sperm penetration assay reversed on changing to 5-aminosalicylic acid enemas. Dig Dis Sci 1988;33:108–10.

18. Delaere KP, Strijbos WE, Meuleman EJ. Sulphasalazine-induced reversible male infertility. Acta Urol Belg 1989;57:29–33.
19. Jenss H, Weber P, Hartmann F. 5-Aminosalicylic acid and its metabolite in breast milk during lactation. Am J Gastroenterol 1990;85:331.
20. Miller LG, Hopkinson JM, Motil KJ, Corboy JE, Andersson S. Disposition of olsalazine and metabolites in breast milk. J Clin Pharmacol 1993;33:703–6.
21. Nelis GF. Diarrhoea due to 5-aminosalicylic acid in breast milk. Lancet 1989;1:383.
22. Committee on Drugs, American Academy of Pediatrics. The transfer of drugs and other chemicals into human milk. Pediatrics 2001;108:776–89.

Name: **MESNA** Risk Factor: **B_M**

Class: **Cytoprotective Agent (Antineoplastic)**

FETAL RISK SUMMARY

RECOMMENDATION: Compatible - Maternal Benefit >> Embryo/Fetal Risk

Mesna (sodium 2-mercaptoethane sulfonate) is a cytoprotective agent that is used to prevent hemorrhagic cystitis caused by ifosfamide (approved indication) and cyclophosphamide (off label indication). Upon administration, the agent is rapidly oxidized to its only metabolite, mesna disulfide (dimesna). Dimesna remains in the intravascular compartment and is rapidly eliminated by the kidneys where it is changed back to mesna. The elimination half-lives of mesna and dimesna in the blood are 0.36 and 1.17 hours, respectively (1).

Reproduction studies have been conducted in rats and rabbits. Both species were given doses up to 1000 mg/kg during pregnancy without evidence of fetal harm (1). Two published studies studied the reproductive effects of mesna in pregnant rats and rabbits (2,3). In rats, IV doses up to 800 mg/kg on days 7–17 were associated with lumbar ribs at 400 mg/kg and decreased fetal weight at 800 mg/kg (2). Increased open field activity was observed in rat pups exposed *in utero* to doses of 400 mg/kg or higher. In pregnant rabbits treated similarly, decreased fetal weights and lumbar ribs were observed with doses of 600 mg/kg or higher (3).

In a 1986 study with rats, two doses of mesna were evaluated to determine if they were protective against cyclophosphamide-induced teratogenicity (4). The low dose (5 mg/kg) offered no protection, but the high dose (30 mg/kg) significantly decreased the number of fetuses with external and skeletal malformations. However, the protection was not sufficiently extensive to be considered effective in protecting pregnant women exposed to cyclophosphamide (4).

In a 2003 study, mesna was combined with ifosfamide to determine if the cytoprotective agent could decrease the toxic effects of ifosfamide on the testes and semen characteristics of rabbits (5). Three groups of male rabbits were given different doses of the combination (ifosfamide 30, 45, or 60 mg/kg plus mesna 6, 9, or 12 mg/kg, followed by a second equal dose of mesna 4 hours later, respectively). Each group received 10 weekly treatments. Controls were given either mesna alone (three groups) or saline (one group). Dose-related ifosfamide-mesna suppression of spermatogenesis and epididymal sperm maturation was observed. In addition, the investigators noted incomplete recovery of the germinal epithelium (5).

It is not known if mesna crosses the human placenta. The molecular weight (about 164) is low enough to cross the placenta, but the short elimination half-life of the parent compound and its rapid metabolism to a metabolite that is restricted to the intravascular compartment suggest that little, if any, exposure of embryo or fetus occurs.

Two reports have described the use of mesna in human pregnancy. In both cases, mesna was combined with ifosfamide in the 2nd and/or 3rd trimesters (see Ifosfamide).

In summary, the limited animal and human data and the pharmacokinetic properties of mesna suggest that the drug poses little, if any, risk to a human fetus. There is no experience, however, in the 1st trimester. Moreover, mesna is probably not protective against ifosfamide- or cyclophosphamide-induced birth defects if these chemotherapy agents are used in the 1st trimester. However, the maternal benefits from use of the agent with ifosfamide or cyclophosphamide to lessen or prevent hemorrhagic cystitis appear to outweigh the unknown fetal risks.

BREAST FEEDING SUMMARY

RECOMMENDATION: No Human Data - Probably Compatible

No reports describing the use of mesna during lactation have been located. The molecular weight (about 164) is low enough for excretion into breast milk, but the short elimination half-life of the parent compound (0.36 hours) and its rapid metabolism to a metabolite that is restricted to the intravascular compartment suggest that little, if any, of the drug will appear in milk. However, mesna is always combined with ifosfamide or cyclophosphamide and women receiving these antineoplastic agents should not breast-feed.

References

1. Product information. Mesna. Gensia Sicor Pharmaceuticals, 2000.
2. Komai Y, Itoh I, Iriyam K, Ishimura K, Fuchigami K, Kobayashi F. Reproduction study of mesna - teratogenicity study in rats by intravenous administration. Kiso to Rinsho 1990;24:6553–94. As cited by Shepard TH. *Catalog of Teratogenic Agents.* 10 th ed. Baltimore, MD: The Johns Hopkins University Press, 2001:323.
3. Komai Y, Itoh I, Ishimura K, Fuchigami K, Kobayashi F. Reproduction study of mesna - teratogenicity study in rabbits by intravenous administration. Kiso to Rinsho 1990;24:6596–602. As cited by Shepard TH. *Catalog of Teratogenic Agents.* 10 th ed. Baltimore, MD: The Johns Hopkins University Press, 2001:323.
4. Slott VL, Hales BF. Sodium 2-mercaptoethane sulfonate protection against cyclophosphamide-induced teratogenicity in rats. Toxicol Appl Pharmacol 1986;82:80–6.
5. Ypsilantis P, Papaioannou N, Psalla D, Politou M, Pitiakoudis M, Simopoulos C. Effects of subchronic ifosfamide-mesna treatment on testes and semen characteristics in the rabbit. Reprod Toxicol 2003;17: 699–708.

M

Name:	**MESORIDAZINE**	Risk Factor:	**C**
Class:	**Tranquilizer**		

FETAL RISK SUMMARY

RECOMMENDATION: No Human Data - No Relevant Animal Data

Mesoridazine is a piperidyl phenothiazine. Phenothiazines readily cross the placenta (1). No specific information on its use in pregnancy has been located. Although occasional reports have attempted to link various phenothiazine compounds with congenital malformations, the bulk of the evidence indicates that these drugs are safe for the mother and fetus (see Chlorpromazine).

BREAST FEEDING SUMMARY

RECOMMENDATION: No Human Data - Potential Toxicity

A 1978 review stated that mesoridazine is excreted into breast milk (2). Specific data for mesoridazine were not provided, but the review did state that no significant neonatal effects had been observed with phenothiazines. The American Academy of Pediatrics classifies mesoridazine as an agent whose effect on the nursing infant is unknown but may be of concern (3).

References

1. Moya F, Thorndike V. Passage of drugs across the placenta. Am J Obstet Gynecol 1962;84:1778–98.
2. Ananth J. Side effects in the neonate from psychotropic agents excreted through breast-feeding. Am J Psychiatry 1978;135:801–5.
3. Committee on Drugs, American Academy of Pediatrics. The transfer of drugs and other chemicals into human milk. Pediatrics 2001;108:776–89.

Name: **MESTRANOL** Risk Factor: X_M

Class: **Estrogenic Hormone**

FETAL RISK SUMMARY

RECOMMENDATION: Contraindicated

Mestranol is the 3-methyl ester of ethinyl estradiol. Mestranol is used frequently in combination with progestins for oral contraception (see Oral Contraceptives). Congenital malformations attributed to the use of mestranol alone have not been reported.

M

The Collaborative Perinatal Project monitored 614 mother-child pairs with 1st trimester exposure to estrogenic agents (including 179 with exposure to mestranol) (1, pp. 389, 391). An increase in the expected frequency of cardiovascular defects, eye and ear anomalies, and Down's syndrome was found for estrogens as a group but not for mestranol (1, pp. 389, 391, 395). Re-evaluation of these data in terms of timing of exposure, vaginal bleeding in early pregnancy, and previous maternal obstetric history, however, failed to support an association between estrogens and cardiac malformations (2). An earlier study also failed to find any relationship with nongenital malformations (3). The use of estrogenic hormones during pregnancy is contraindicated.

In a surveillance study of Michigan Medicaid recipients conducted between 1985 and 1992 involving 229,101 completed pregnancies, 190 newborns had been exposed to mestranol during the 1st trimester (F. Rosa, personal communication, FDA, 1993). A total of 13 (6.8%) major birth defects were observed (8 expected). Specific data were available for six defect categories, including (observed/expected) 1/2 cardiovascular defects, 1/0.5 oral clefts, 0/0 spina bifida, 0/0.5 polydactyly, 1/0.5 limb reduction defects, and 0/0.5 hypospadias.

BREAST FEEDING SUMMARY

RECOMMENDATION: Limited Human Data - Probably Compatible

Estrogens are frequently used for suppression of postpartum lactation (4). Doses of 100–150 μg of ethinyl estradiol (equivalent to 160–240 μg of mestranol) for 5–7 days are used (4). Mestranol, when used in oral contraceptives with doses of 30-80 μg, has been associated with decreased milk production, lower infant weight gain, and decreased composition of nitrogen and protein content of human milk (5–7). The magnitude of these changes is low. However, the changes in milk production and composition may be of nutritional importance in malnourished mothers. If breast-feeding is desired, the lowest dose of oral contraceptives should be chosen. Monitoring of infant weight gain and the possible need for nutritional supplementation should be considered (see Oral Contraceptives).

References

1. Heinonen OP, Slone D, Shapiro S. *Birth Defects and Drugs in Pregnancy*. Littleton, MA: Publishing Sciences Group, 1977.
2. Wiseman RA, Dodds-Smith IC. Cardiovascular birth defects and antenatal exposure to female sex hormones: a reevaluation of some base data. Teratology 1984;30:359–70.
3. Wilson JG, Brent RL. Are female sex hormones teratogenic? Am J Obstet Gynecol 1981,141:567–80.
4. Gilman AG, Goodman LS, Gilman A. *The Pharmacological Basis of Therapeutics*. New York, NY: Macmillan, 1980:1431.
5. Kora SJ. Effect of oral contraceptives on lactation. Fertil Steril 1969;20:419–23.
6. Miller GH, Hughs LR. Lactation and genital involution effects of a new low-dose oral contraceptive on breast-feeding mothers and their infants. Obstet Gynecol 1970;35:44–50.
7. Lonnerdal B, Forsum E, Hambraeus L. Effect of oral contraceptives on composition and volume of breast milk. Am J Clin Nutr 1980;33:816–24.

Name: **METAPROTERENOL** Risk Factor: **C_M**

Class: **Sympathomimetic (Adrenergic)**

FETAL RISK SUMMARY

RECOMMENDATION: Compatible

Metaproterenol, a selective β_2 adrenergic agonist, is used as a bronchodilator for bronchial asthma and for reversible bronchospasm occurring in bronchitis and emphysema.

Reproduction studies in mice, rats, and rabbits have been conducted (1). No embryotoxic or fetotoxic effects, or teratogenicity was observed in rats at 40 mg/kg (approximately 25 times the maximum recommended human oral dose [MRHOD]), but embryo toxicity was observed in mice at 31 times the MRHOD. In rabbits, oral doses 620 times the human inhalation dose and 62 times the MRHOD caused both embryotoxic and teratogenic (skeletal anomalies, hydrocephalus, and skull bone separation) effects.

No published reports linking the use of metaproterenol with congenital defects have been located. In a surveillance study of Michigan Medicaid recipients conducted between 1985 and 1992 involving 229,101 completed pregnancies, 361 newborns had been exposed to metaproterenol during the 1st trimester (F. Rosa, personal communication, FDA, 1993). A total of 17 (4.7%) major birth defects were observed (15 expected). Specific data were available for six defect categories, including (observed/expected) 3/4 cardiovascular defects, 1/1 oral clefts, 0/0 spina bifida, 1/1 limb reduction defects, 0/1 hypospadias, and 3/1 polydactyly. Only with the latter defect is there a suggestion of a possible association, but other factors, including the mother's disease, concurrent drug use, and chance, may be involved.

Metaproterenol has been used to prevent premature labor (2–4). Its use for this purpose has been largely assumed by ritodrine, albuterol, or terbutaline. Like all β-mimetics, metaproterenol causes maternal and, to a lesser degree, fetal tachycardia. Maternal hypotension and hyperglycemia and neonatal hypoglycemia should be expected (see also Ritodrine, Albuterol, and Terbutaline). Long-term evaluation of infants exposed *in utero* to β-mimetics has been reported, but not specifically for metaproterenol (5). No harmful effects in the infants were observed.

In summary, selective β_2-agonists, including metaproterenol, are commonly used during gestation for the treatment of asthma (6). Fetal tachycardia may occur, but because there is no evidence of fetal injury, there is no contraindication to their use in pregnancy (6).

BREAST FEEDING SUMMARY

RECOMMENDATION: No Human Data - Probably Compatible

No reports describing the use of metaproterenol during lactation have been located. However, agents in this class, including metaproterenol, are commonly used in the treatment of asthma and there is no contraindication to their use during breast-feeding (6). Neonatal tachycardia, hypoglycemia, or tremor are potential adverse effects (6).

References

1. Product information. Alupent. Boehringer Ingelheim, 2000.
2. Baillie P, Meehan FP, Tyack AJ. Treatment of premature labour with orciprenaline. Br Med J 1970;4:154–5.
3. Tyack AJ, Baillie P, Meehan FP. In-vivo response of the human uterus to orciprenaline in early labour. Br Med J 1971;2:741–3.
4. Zilianti M, Aller J. Action of orciprenaline on uterine contractility during labor, maternal cardiovascular system, fetal heart rate, and acid-base balance. Am J Obstet Gynecol 1971;109:1073–9.
5. Freysz H, Willard D, Lehr A, Messer J, Boog G. A long term evaluation of infants who received a β-mimetic drug while in utero. J Perinat Med 1977;5:94–9.
6. Report of the Working Group on Asthma and Pregnancy. *Management of Asthma During Pregnancy*. U.S. Department of Health and Human Services, NIH Publication No. 93–3279, September 1993:19.

M

Name: **METARAMINOL** Risk Factor: **C_M**

Class: **Sympathomimetic (Adrenergic)**

FETAL RISK SUMMARY

RECOMMENDATION: Human Data Suggest Risk in 2nd and 3rd Trimesters

Metaraminol is a sympathomimetic used in emergencies to treat hypotension. Animal reproduction studies have not been conducted with this drug.

Because of the nature of its indications, experience in pregnancy with metaraminol is limited. Normally, uterine vessels are maximally dilated and have only α-adrenergic receptors (1). Use of the predominantly α-adrenergic stimulant, metaraminol, could cause constriction of these vessels and reduce uterine blood flow, thereby producing fetal hypoxia (bradycardia). Metaraminol may also interact with oxytocics or ergot derivatives to produce severe persistent maternal hypertension (1). Rupture of a cerebral vessel is possible. If a pressor agent is indicated, other drugs such as ephedrine should be considered.

BREAST FEEDING SUMMARY

RECOMMENDATION: No Human Data - Probably Compatible

No data are available.

Reference

1. Smith NT, Corbascio AN. The use and misuse of pressor agents. Anesthesiology 1970;33:58–101.

Name: **METAXALONE** Risk Factor: **B**
Class: **Skeletal Muscle Relaxant**

FETAL RISK SUMMARY

RECOMMENDATION: No Human Data - No Relevant Animal Data

Metaxalone is a skeletal muscle relaxant that is indicated as an adjunct to rest and physical therapy and other measures for the relief of discomforts associated with acute, painful musculoskeletal conditions. The agent has no direct effect on muscles. It is thought to act centrally as a sedative. Metaxalone is metabolized by the liver and the unidentified metabolites are excreted in the urine. The mean terminal elimination half-life is approximately 2.4 hours (1).

Reproduction studies in rats revealed no evidence of impaired fertility or fetal harm (1). Further details of these studies have apparently not been published.

It is not known if metaxalone crosses the human placenta. The relatively low molecular weight (about 221) suggests, however, that transfer to the fetal compartment should be expected.

No reports describing the use of metaxalone in human pregnancy have been located. The manufacturer states that postmarketing experience has not revealed evidence of fetal harm (1), but additional details are not provided. The very limited, incomplete animal data and absence of reported human pregnancy experience prevents an assessment of human embryo/fetal risk. Therefore, avoid the 1st trimester, if possible if metaxalone is required in pregnancy.

M

BREAST FEEDING SUMMARY

RECOMMENDATION: No Human Data - Potential Toxicity

No reports describing the use of metaxalone during lactation have been located. The relatively low molecular weight (about 221) suggests the drug will be excreted into breast milk. The effects of this exposure on a nursing infant are unknown. Because the drug is thought to be a central acting sedative, nursing infants should be closely observed for sedation.

Reference

1. Product information. Skelaxin. Monarch Pharmaceuticals, 2004.

Name: **METFORMIN** Risk Factor: **B_M**
Class: **Oral Antihyperglycemic**

FETAL RISK SUMMARY

RECOMMENDATION: Human Suggest Low Risk

Metformin is an oral, biguanide, antihyperglycemic agent that is chemically and pharmacologically unrelated to the sulfonylureas. Its mechanism of action is thought to include decreased hepatic glucose production, decreased intestinal absorption of glucose, and increased peripheral uptake and utilization of glucose (1,2). The latter two mechanisms result in improved insulin sensitivity (i.e., decreased insulin requirements) (1,2).

Reproduction studies found no evidence of impaired fertility in male and female rats and no evidence of teratogenicity in rats and rabbits at doses up to 600 mg/kg/day, approximately 2 times the maximum recommended human dose on a mg/m^2 basis (1). A partial placental barrier to metformin was observed, however, based on fetal concentrations (1).

Shepard (3) and Schardein (4) cited a study in rats that observed teratogenesis (neural tube closure defects and edema) in rat fetuses exposed to metformin. The drug did not appear to be a major teratogen because less than 0.5% of the rat fetuses in mothers fed 500–1000 mg/kg developed anophthalmia and anencephaly (3). Higher doses in this study were embryotoxic (5).

A 1994 abstract described the teratogenic effects of high metformin concentrations on early somite mouse embryos exposed *in vitro* (6). At levels much higher than those obtained clinically, metformin produced neural tube defects and malformations of the heart and eye. In contrast, a study that also appeared in 1994 observed no major malformations in mouse embryos exposed in culture to similar concentrations of metformin (7). About 10% of the embryos, however, demonstrated a transient delay in closure of cranial neuropores.

In an experiment using the human single-cotyledon model with placentas obtained from diabetic patients and normal controls, researchers measured the effect of metformin on the uptake and transport of glucose in both the maternal-to-fetal and fetal-to-maternal directions (8). A second publication described only the results of the experiments studying the effect of metformin on the maternal-to-fetal direction of glucose (9). Compared with controls, metformin had no effect on the movement of glucose in either direction (8,9).

Among 26 women undergoing treatment for polycystic ovary syndrome (PCOS) with metformin, 1.5 g/day for 8 weeks, 3 became pregnant during treatment (10). The women were involved in a study to determine whether metformin was effective in normalizing the condition that is characterized by insulin resistance and hyperandrogenism. One of the pregnancies aborted after 2 months, but the outcomes of the other two were not mentioned. In three reports from the same center, women who had successfully conceived while taking metformin for PCOS were continued on the agent during pregnancy (11–13). Metformin reduced the incidences of 1st trimester spontaneous abortion and gestational diabetes without causing birth defects or neonatal or maternal complications. The therapy had no adverse effect on birth weight or height, or growth and development at 3 and 6 months of age (12).

A number of references have described the use of metformin during all stages of gestation for the control of maternal diabetes (14–22). A 1979 reference described the therapy of gestational diabetes that included the use of metformin alone ($N = 15$), glyburide alone ($N = 9$), or metformin plus glyburide ($N = 6$) in women who were not controlled on diet alone and did not require insulin (16). None of the newborns developed symptomatic hypoglycemia, and only one infant had a congenital defect (ventricular septal defect). Although the treatment group was not specified, ventricular septal defects are commonly associated with poorly controlled diabetes occurring early in gestation (22).

A 1979 reference described the pregnancy outcomes of 60 obese women who received metformin in the 2nd and the 3rd trimester for diabetes (preexisting [$N = 39$] or gestational [$N = 21$]) that was not controlled by diet alone (17). The drug was not effective in 21 (54%) and 6 (29%) of the patients, respectively. The pregnancy outcomes, in terms of hyperbilirubinemia, polycythemia, necrotizing enterocolitis, and major congenital abnormalities, were not better than those observed in another group of insulin-dependent and non-insulin-dependent diabetic women treated by the investigators, except for perinatal mortality. None of the newborns had symptoms of hypoglycemia. The three infants with congenital malformations had defects (two heart defects and one sacral agenesis) that were most likely caused by poorly controlled diabetes occurring early in gestation (17).

In another report, metformin in combination with diet ($N = 22$) and glyburide ($N = 45$) was used during pregnancy for the treatment of preexisting diabetes (18). No cases of lactic acidosis or neonatal hypoglycemia were observed with metformin and diet alone, but the latter complication did occur when glyburide was added. Neonatal hypoglycemia is a well-known complication of sulfonylurea agents ingested too close to delivery (e.g., see Chlorpropamide). In an earlier reference, 56 patients received metformin up to 24 hours of delivery without adverse effects in the newborns (15).

Metformin was used during the 1st trimester in 21 pregnancies described in a 1984 report (19). A minor abnormality (polydactyly) was observed in a newborn whose mother had taken metformin and glyburide. Based on this and previous experience, these investigators proposed a treatment regimen for the management of women with non-insulin-dependent diabetes mellitus (NIDDM) (i.e., type II diabetes mellitus) who become pregnant consisting of diet and treatment with metformin and glyburide as necessary (20). If this regimen did not provide control of the blood glucose, a change to insulin therapy was recommended (20). These investigators concluded that the drug therapy was not teratogenic and did not cause ketosis and that neonatal hypoglycemia was preventable if the therapy was changed to insulin before delivery.

A 1990 reference addressed the problem of treating diabetes in tropical countries where the availability of medical support and facilities is poor (21). The author recommended that gestational diabetes, not responding to diet alone, be treated with sulfonylurea agents or metformin or both because the initiation of insulin therapy in developing countries was difficult.

The fetal effects of oral hypoglycemic agents on the fetuses of women attending a diabetes and pregnancy clinic were reported in 1991 (22). All of the women ($N = 21$) had NIDDM and were treated during organogenesis with oral agents (1 with metformin, 2 with phenformin, 17 with sulfonylureas, and 1 with an unknown agent), with a duration of exposure of 3–28 weeks. A control group ($N = 40$) of similar women with NIDDM who were also attending the clinic, matched for age, race, parity, and glycemic control, was used for comparison. Both groups of patients were changed to insulin therapy at the first prenatal visit. From the study group, 11 infants (52%) had congenital malformations, compared with 6 (15%) from the controls ($p < 0.002$). Moreover, six of the newborns from the study group (none in the control group) had ear defects, a malformation that is observed, albeit uncommonly, in diabetic embryopathy (22). No defects were seen in the one infant exposed to metformin. Sixteen live births occurred in the exposed group, compared with 36 in controls. The groups did not differ in the incidence of hypoglycemia at birth (53% vs. 53%), but three of the exposed newborns had severe hypoglycemia lasting 2, 4, and 7 days, respectively, even though the mothers had not used the oral agents close to delivery. In one of these cases, the mother had been taking metformin 1500 mg daily for 28 weeks. Hyperbilirubinemia was noted in 10 (67%) of 15 exposed liveborn infants, compared with 13 (36%) of the controls, and polycythemia and hyperviscosity requiring partial-exchange transfusions were observed in 4 (27%) of 15 exposed vs. 1 (3.0%) control (one exposed infant was not included in these data because the child presented after completion of the study) (22).

In summary, although the use of metformin may be beneficial for decreasing the incidence of fetal and/or newborn morbidity and mortality in developing countries where the proper use of insulin is problematic, insulin is still the treatment of choice for this disease. Moreover, insulin, unlike metformin, does not cross the placenta and, thus, eliminates the additional concern that the drug therapy itself is adversely affecting the fetus. Carefully prescribed insulin therapy will provide better control of the mother's blood glucose, thereby preventing the fetal and neonatal complications that occur with this disease. High maternal glucose levels, as may occur in diabetes mellitus, are closely associated with a number of maternal and fetal adverse effects, including fetal structural anomalies if the hyperglycemia occurs early in gestation. To prevent this toxicity, most experts, including the American College of Obstetricians and Gynecologists, recommend that insulin be used for types I and II diabetes occurring during pregnancy and, if diet therapy alone is not successful, for gestational diabetes (23,24).

BREAST FEEDING SUMMARY

RECOMMENDATION: Compatible

Metformin is excreted in the milk of lactating rats, obtaining levels comparable to those in the plasma (1). Consistent with its low molecular weight (about 166), metformin is also excreted into human milk. In seven women taking metformin (500 mg three times daily), the mean milk:plasma ratio was 0.35 and the average metformin concentration over the dosing interval was 0.27 μg/mL (25). The average infant dose received from the milk was 0.04 mg/kg/day, or about 0.28% of the maternal weight adjusted dose. A second study involving eight women (three at steady state and five after a single 500-mg dose) estimated that nursing infants would ingest about 0.11%–0.21% of the maternal weight adjusted dose (26). For the women at steady state, the milk:plasma ratios (based on AUC) were 0.37–0.71. Of interest, the concentration-time profile of the drug was relatively flat in all subjects (26). Both of these studies concluded that metformin use during nursing was safe (25,26).

M

References

1. Product information. Glucophage. Bristol-Myers Squibb, 1997.
2. Klepser TB, Kelly MW. Metformin hydrochloride: an antihyperglycemic agent. Am J Health-Syst Pharm 1997;54:893–903.
3. Shepard TH. *Catalog of Teratogenic Agents*. 8th ed. Baltimore, MD: Johns Hopkins University Press, 1995:270.
4. Schardein JL. *Chemically Induced Birth Defects*. 2nd ed. New York, NY: Marcel Dekker, 1993:417–8.
5. Onnis A, Grella P. *The Biochemical Effects of Drugs in Pregnancy*. Volume 2. West Sussex, England: Ellis Horwood Limited, 1984:179.
6. Miao J, Smoak IW. In vitro effects of the biguanide, metformin, on early-somite mouse embryos (abstract). Teratology 1994;49:389.
7. Denno KM, Sadler TW. Effects of the biguanide class of oral hypoglycemic agents on mouse embryogenesis. Teratology 1994;49:260–6.
8. Elliott B, Schuessling F, Langer O. The oral antihyperglycemic agent metformin does not affect glucose uptake and transport in the human diabetic placenta (abstract). Am J Obstet Gynecol 1997;176: S182.
9. Elliott B, Langer O, Schuessling F. Human placental glucose uptake and transport are not altered by the oral antihyperglycemic agent metformin. Am J Obstet Gynecol 1997;176:527–30.
10. Velazquez EM, Mendoza S, Hamer T, Sosa F, Glueck CJ. Metformin therapy in polycystic ovary syndrome reduces hyperinsulinemia, insulin resistance, hyperandrogenemia, and systolic blood pressure, while facilitating normal menses and pregnancy. Metabolism 1994;43:647–54.
11. Glueck CJ, Phillips H, Cameron D, Sieve-Smith L, Wang P. Continuing metformin throughout pregnancy in women with polycystic ovary syndrome appears to safely reduce first-trimester spontaneous abortion: a pilot study. Fertil Steril 2001;75:46–52.
12. Glueck CJ, Wang P, Goldenberg, Sieve-Smith L. Pregnancy outcomes among women with polycystic ovary syndrome treated with metformin. Hum Reprod 2002;17:2858–64.
13. Glueck CJ, Wang P, Kobayashi S, Phillips H, Sieve-Smith L. Metformin therapy throughout pregnancy reduces the development of gestational diabetes in women with polycystic ovary syndrome. Fertil Steril 2002;77:520–5.
14. Brearley BF. The management of pregnancy in diabetes mellitus. Practitioner 1975;215:644–52.
15. Jackson WPU, Coetzee EJ. Side-effects of metformin. S Afr Med J 1979;56:1113–4.

16. Coetzee EJ, Jackson WPU. Diabetes newly diagnosed during pregnancy. A 4-year study at Groote Schuur Hospital. S Afr Med J 1979;56:467–75.
17. Coetzee RJ, Jackson WPU. Metformin in management of pregnant insulin-independent diabetics. Diabetologia 1979;16:241–5.
18. Coetzee EJ, Jackson WPU. Pregnancy in established non-insulin-dependent diabetics. A five-and-a-half year study at Groote Schuur Hospital. S Afr Med J 1980;58:795–802.
19. Coetzee EJ, Jackson WPU. Oral hypoglycaemics in the first trimester and fetal outcome. S Afr Med J 1984;65:635–7.
20. Coetzee EJ, Jackson WPU. The management of non-insulin-dependent diabetes during pregnancy. Diabetes Res Clin Pract 1986;5:281–7.
21. Gill G. Practical management of diabetes in the tropics. Trop Doct 1990;20:4–10.
22. Piacquadio K, Hollingsworth DR, Murphy H. Effects of in-utero exposure to oral hypoglycaemic drugs. Lancet 1991;338:866–9.
23. American College of Obstetricians and Gynecologists. Diabetes and pregnancy. Technical Bulletin No. 200, December 1994.
24. Coustan DR. Management of gestational diabetes. Clin Obstet Gynecol 1991;34:558–64.
25. Hale TW, Kristensen JH, Hackett LP, Kohan R, Ilett KF. Transfer of metformin into human milk. Diabetologia 2002;45:1509–14.
26. Gardiner SJ, Kirkpatrick CMJ, Begg EJ, Zhang M, Moore MP, Saville DJ. Transfer of metformin into human milk. Clin Pharmacol Ther 2003;73:71–7.

Name: **METHACYCLINE** Risk Factor: **D**

Class: **Antibiotic (Tetracycline)**

See Tetracycline.

Name: **METHADONE** Risk Factor: **B***

Class: **Narcotic Agonist Analgesic**

M

FETAL RISK SUMMARY

RECOMMENDATION: Human Data Suggest Risk in 3rd Trimester

Methadone use in pregnancy is almost exclusively related to the treatment of heroin addiction. No increase in congenital defects has been observed. However, since these patients normally consume a wide variety of drugs, it is not possible to separate completely the effects of methadone from the effects of other agents. Neonatal narcotic withdrawal and low birth weight seem to be the primary problems.

Withdrawal symptoms occur in approximately 60%–90% of the infants (1–6). One study concluded that the intensity of withdrawal was increased if the daily maternal dosage exceeded 20 mg (5). When withdrawal symptoms do occur, they normally start within 48 hours after delivery, but a small percentage may be delayed up to 7–14 days (1). One report observed initial withdrawal symptoms appearing up to 28 days after birth, but the authors do not mention if mothers of these infants were breast feeding (6). Methadone concentrations in breast milk are reported to be sufficient to prevent withdrawal in addicted infants (see Breast Feeding Summary below). Some authors believe methadone withdrawal is more intense than that occurring with heroin (1). Less than one-third of symptomatic infants, require therapy (1–5). A lower incidence of hyaline membrane disease is seen in infants exposed *in utero* to chronic methadone and may be due to elevated blood levels of prolactin (7).

Infants of drug-addicted mothers are often small for gestational age. In some series, one-third or more of the infants weigh less than 2500 g (1,2,4). The newborns of methadone addicts may have a higher birth weights than comparable offspring of heroin addicts for reasons that remain unclear (4).

Other problems occurring in the offspring of methadone addicts are increased mortality, sudden infant death syndrome (SIDS), jaundice, and thrombocytosis. A correlation between drug addiction and SIDS has been suggested with 20 cases (2.8%) in a group of 702 infants, but the data could not attribute the increase to a single drug (8,9). Another study of 313 infants of methadone-addicted mothers reported 2 cases (0.6%) of SIDS, an incidence similar to the overall experience of that location (4). In one study, a positive correlation was found between severity of neonatal withdrawal and the incidence of SIDS (9). Maternal withdrawal during pregnancy has been observed to produce a marked response of the fetal adrenal glands and sympathetic nervous system (10). An increased stillborn and neonatal mortality rate has also been reported (11). Both reports recommend against detoxification of the mother during gestation. Jaundice is comparatively infrequent in both heroin- and methadone-exposed newborns. However, a higher rate of severe hyperbilirubinemia in methadone-exposed infants than in a comparable group of heroin-exposed infants has been observed (1). Thrombocytosis developing in the 2nd week of life, with some platelet counts exceeding 1,000,000/mm^3 and persisting for more than 16 weeks, has been reported (12). The condition was not related to withdrawal symptoms or neonatal treatment. Some of these infants also had increased circulating platelet aggregates.

Respiratory depression is not a significant problem, and Apgar scores are comparable to those of a nonaddicted population (1–5). Long-term effects on the behavior and gross motor development skills are not known.

[*Risk Factor D if used for prolonged period or in high doses at term.*]

M

BREAST FEEDING SUMMARY

RECOMMENDATION: Limited Human Data - Probably Compatible

Methadone is excreted into breast milk and claims have been made that it could prevent withdrawal in addicted infants. One study reported an average milk concentration in 10 patients of 0.27 μg/mL, representing an average milk:plasma ratio of 0.83 (13). The same investigators earlier reported levels ranging from 0.17 to 5.6 μg/mL in the milk of mothers on methadone maintenance (2). At least one infant death has been attributed to methadone obtained through breast milk (14). However, a recent report claimed that methadone enters breast milk in very low quantities that are clinically insignificant (15).

A 1997 report described two cases where the mothers were taking high maintenance doses of methadone (73 and 60 mg/day) (16). Both mothers breast-fed their infants. The average milk:plasma ratios were 0.66 and 1.22, respectively. The amounts of methadone in milk were considered to negligible (16). A 2000 study evaluated eight lactating women who were taking methadone (25–180 mg/day) (17). The mean amount of methadone in milk was 95 ng/mL (range 27–260 ng/mL). Based on an estimated newborn milk intake of 475 mL/day, the estimated mean daily methadone dose was 0.05 mg/day. No adverse effects of the exposure were observed during the duration of breast-feeding (2.5–21 months) or during weaning (17). The American Academy of Pediatrics classifies methadone as compatible with breast-feeding (18).

References

1. Zelson C, Lee SJ, Casalino M. Neonatal narcotic addiction. N Engl J Med 1973;289:1216–20.
2. Blinick G, Jerez E, Wallach RC. Methadone maintenance, pregnancy and progeny. JAMA 1973; 225:477–9.
3. Strauss ME, Andresko M, Stryker JC, Wardell JN, Dunkel LD. Methadone maintenance during pregnancy: pregnancy, birth and neonate characteristics. Am J Obstet Gynecol 1974;120:895–900.
4. Newman RG, Bashkow S, Calko D. Results of 313

consecutive live births of infants delivered to patients in the New York City methadone maintenance program. Am J Obstet Gynecol 1975;121:233–7.
5. Ostrea EM, Chavez CJ, Strauss ME. A study of factors that influence the severity of neonatal narcotic withdrawal. J Pediatr 1976;88:642–5.
6. Kandall SR, Gartner LM. Delayed presentation of neonatal methadone withdrawal. Pediatr Res 1973; 7:320.
7. Parekh A, Mukherjee TK, Jhaveri R, Rosenfeld W, Glass L. Intrauterine exposure to narcotics and cord blood prolactin concentrations. Obstet Gynecol 1981;57:447–9.
8. Pierson PS, Howard P, Kleber HD. Sudden deaths in infants born to methadone maintained addicts. JAMA 1972;220:1733–4.
9. Chavez CJ, Ostrea EM, Stryker JC, Smialek Z. Sudden infant death syndrome among infants of drug-dependent mothers. J Pediatr 1979;95: 407–9.
10. Zuspan FP, Gumpel JA, Mejia-Zelaya A, Madden J, David R. Fetal stress from methadone withdrawal. Am J Obstet Gynecol 1975;122:43–6.
11. Rementeria JL, Nunag NN. Narcotic withdrawal in pregnancy: stillbirth incidence with a case report. Am J Obstet Gynecol 1973;116:1152–6.
12. Burstein Y, Giardina PJV, Rausen AR, Kandall SR, Siljestrom K, Peterson CM. Thrombocytosis and increased circulating platelet aggregates in newborn infants of polydrug users. J Pediatr 1979;94:895–9.
13. Blinick G, Inturrisi CE, Jerez E, Wallach RC. Methadone assays in pregnant women and progeny. Am J Obstet Gynecol 1975;121:617–21.
14. Smialek JE, Monforte JR, Aronow R, Spitz WU. Methadone deaths in children-a continuing problem. JAMA 1977;238:2516–7.
15. Anonymous. Methadone in breast milk. Med Lett Drugs Ther 1979;21:52.
16. Geraghty B, Graham EA, Logan B, Weiss EL. Methadone levels in breast milk. J Hum Lact 1997; 13:227–30.
17. McCarthy JJ, Posey BL. Methadone levels in human milk. J Hum Lact 2000;16:115–20.
18. Committee on Drugs, American Academy of Pediatrics. The transfer of drugs and other chemicals into human milk. Pediatrics 2001;108:776–89.

Name: **METHAMPHETAMINE** Risk Factor: C_M
Class: **Central Stimulant**

M

See Amphetamine.

Name: **METHANTHELINE** Risk Factor: **C**
Class: **Parasympatholytic (Anticholinergic)**

FETAL RISK SUMMARY

RECOMMENDATION: Limited Human Data - No Relevant Animal Data

Methantheline is an anticholinergic quaternary ammonium bromide. In a large prospective study, 2323 patients were exposed to this class of drugs during the 1st trimester, 2 of whom took methantheline (1). A possible association was found between the total group and minor malformations.

BREAST FEEDING SUMMARY

RECOMMENDATION: No Human Data - Probably Compatible

No data are available (see also Atropine).

Reference

1. Heinonen OP, Slone D, Shapiro S. *Birth Defects and Drugs in Pregnancy*. Littleton, MA: Publishing Sciences Group, 1977:346–53.

Name:	**METHAQUALONE**	Risk Factor:	**D**
Class:	**Hypnotic**		

FETAL RISK SUMMARY

RECOMMENDATION: Limited Human Data - No Relevant Animal Data

No reports linking the use of methaqualone with congenital defects have been located. One manufacturer was not aware of any adverse effects following 1st trimester use (R.R. Smith, personal communication, William H. Rorer, Inc., 1972). The autopsy of a 6-day-old infant found a congenital hypothalamic hamartoblastoma and multiple malformations (1). The baby had been exposed to methaqualone, marijuana, and cocaine early in gestation but the correlation to any of these agents is unknown. Methaqualone is often used as an illicit abuse drug. Separating fetal effects from adulterants or other drugs is not possible. Because of the abuse potential, methaqualone is not recommended during pregnancy.

BREAST FEEDING SUMMARY

RECOMMENDATION: No Human Data - Potential Toxicity

No data are available.

M

Reference

1. Huff DS, Fernandes M. Two cases of congenital hypothalamic hamartoblastoma, polydactyly, and other congenital anomalies (Pallister-Hall syndrome). N Engl J Med 1982;306:430–1.

Name:	**METHARBITAL**	Risk Factor:	**D**
Class:	**Anticonvulsant/Sedative**		

FETAL RISK SUMMARY

RECOMMENDATION: No Human Data - No Relevant Animal Data

No reports linking the use of metharbital with congenital defects have been located. Metharbital is demethylated to barbital by the liver (see also Phenobarbital).

BREAST FEEDING SUMMARY

RECOMMENDATION: Limited Human Data - Potential Toxicity

Metharbital's metabolite, barbital, has been demonstrated in breast milk in trace amounts (1). No reports linking the use of metharbital with adverse effects in the nursing infant have been located.

Reference

1. Kwit NT, Hatcher RA. Excretion of drugs in milk. Am J Dis Child 1935;40:900–4.

Name: **METHAZOLAMIDE** | Risk Factor: **C**
Class: **Diuretic (Carbonic Anhydrase Inhibitor)**

FETAL RISK SUMMARY

RECOMMENDATION: No Human Data - Probably Compatible

Methazolamide is a carbonic anhydrase inhibitor used in glaucoma to lower intraocular pressure. No reports describing the use of methazolamide in human pregnancy have been located. The drug is teratogenic in some animal species (1). (See also Acetazolamide.)

BREAST FEEDING SUMMARY

RECOMMENDATION: No Human Data - Probably Compatible

No data are available.

Reference

1. Product information. Neptazane. Lederle Laboratories, 1988.

Name: **METHDILAZINE** | Risk Factor: **C**
Class: **Antihistamine**

No data are available. See Promethazine for representative agent in this class.

Name: **METHENAMINE** | Risk Factor: **C_M**
Class: **Urinary Germicide**

FETAL RISK SUMMARY

RECOMMENDATION: Compatible

Methenamine, in either the mandelate or the hippurate salt form, is used for chronic suppressive treatment of bacteriuria. In two studies, the mandelate form was given to 120 patients and the hippurate to 70 patients (1,2). No increases in congenital defects or other problems as compared with controls were observed.

The Collaborative Perinatal Project reported 49 1st trimester exposures to methenamine (3, pp. 299, 302). For use anytime in pregnancy, 299 exposures were recorded (3, p. 435). Only in the latter group was a possible association with malformations found. Independent confirmation is required.

In a surveillance study of Michigan Medicaid recipients conducted between 1985 and 1992 involving 229,101 completed pregnancies, 209 newborns had been exposed to methenamine during the 1st trimester (F. Rosa, personal communication, FDA, 1993). Eight (3.8%) major birth defects were observed (nine expected). Specific data were available for six defect categories, including (observed/expected) 1/2 cardiovascular defects, 1/0.5 oral clefts, 0/0 spina bifida, 1/1 polydactyly, 1/0.5 limb reduction defects, and 0/0.5 hypospadias. These data do not support an association between the drug and congenital defects.

Methenamine interferes with the determination of urinary estrogen (4). Urinary estrogen was formerly used to assess the condition of the fetoplacental unit, depressed levels being associated with fetal distress. This assessment is now made by measuring unconjugated estriol, which is not affected by methenamine.

BREAST FEEDING SUMMARY

RECOMMENDATION: Limited Human Data - Probably Compatible

Methenamine is excreted into breast milk. Peak levels occur at 1 hour (5). No adverse effects on the nursing infant have been reported.

References

1. Gordon SF. Asymptomatic bacteriuria of pregnancy. Clin Med 1972;79:22–4.
2. Furness ET, McDonald PJ, Beasley NV. Urinary antiseptics in asymptomatic bacteriuria of pregnancy. N Z Med J 1975;81:417–9.
3. Heinonen OP, Slone D, Shapiro S. *Birth Defects and Drugs in Pregnancy*. Littleton, MA: Publishing Sciences Group, 1977.
4. Kivinen S, Tuimala R. Decreased urinary oestriol concentrations in pregnant women during hexamine hippurate treatment. Br Med J 1977;2:682.
5. Sapeika N. The excretion of drugs in human milk-a review. J Obstet Gynaecol Br Emp 1947;54:426–31.

Name: **METHICILLIN** Risk Factor: B_M

Class: **Antibiotic (Penicillin)**

FETAL RISK SUMMARY

RECOMMENDATION: Compatible

Methicillin is a penicillin antibiotic (see also Penicillin G). The drug rapidly crosses the placenta into the fetal circulation and amniotic fluid (1,2). Following a 500-mg IV dose over 10–15 minutes, peak levels of 13.0 and 10.5 μg/mL were measured in maternal and fetal serums, respectively, at 30 minutes (1). Equilibration occurred between the two serums within 1 hour. No effects were reported in the infants.

No reports linking the use of methicillin with congenital defects have been located. The Collaborative Perinatal Project monitored 50,282 mother-child pairs, 3546 of whom had 1st trimester exposure to penicillin derivatives (3, pp. 297–313). For use anytime during pregnancy, 7171 exposures were recorded (3, p. 435). In neither group was evidence found to suggest a relationship to large categories of major or minor malformations or to individual defects.

BREAST FEEDING SUMMARY

RECOMMENDATION: Compatible

No data are available (see Penicillin G).

References

1. Depp R, Kind A, Kirby W, Johnson W. Transplacental passage of methicillin and dicloxacillin into the fetus and amniotic fluid. Am J Obstet Gynecol 1970;107:1054–7.
2. MacAulay M, Molloy W, Charles D. Placental transfer of methicillin. Am J Obstet Gynecol 1973;115:58–65.
3. Heinonen OP, Slone D, Shapiro S. *Birth Defects and Drugs in Pregnancy*. Littleton, MA: Publishing Sciences Group, 1977.

Name:	**METHIMAZOLE**	Risk Factor:	**D**
Class:	**Antithyroid**		

FETAL RISK SUMMARY

RECOMMENDATION: Human Data Suggest Risk

Methimazole, a thiourea antithyroid agent, is used for the treatment of hyperthyroidism. Methimazole readily crosses the placenta to the fetus. Two patients undergoing 2nd trimester therapeutic abortions were given a single 10-mg ^{35}S-labeled oral dose 2 hours before pregnancy termination (1). Fetal:maternal serum ratios were 0.72 and 0.81, representing 0.22% and 0.24% of the administered dose. In the same study, three patients at 14, 14, and 20 weeks' gestation were given an equimolar dose of carbimazole (16.6 mg). Fetal:maternal serum ratios were 0.80–1.09 with 0.17%–0.87% of the total radioactivity in the fetus. The highest serum and tissue levels were found in the 20-week-old fetus (1).

A comparison of the placental transfer of methimazole and propylthiouracil (PTU) in the perfused human term placental lobule was reported in 1997 (2). There were no significant differences between the drugs and the investigators concluded that the drugs have similar placental transfer kinetics (2).

Early references reported 11 cases of scalp defects (aplasia cutis congenita) in newborns exposed *in utero* to methimazole or carbimazole (converted *in vivo* to methimazole) (3–7). In two of the 11 infants, umbilical defects (patent urachus in one; patent vitelline duct in another) were also observed, suggesting to one investigator, because of the rarity of these defects, that the combination of anomalies represented a possible malformation syndrome (5). In one of the above cases, the α-fetoprotein level was elevated in both the maternal serum (3–18 standard deviations [SD] above normal) and the amniotic fluid (2.4–4 SD above normal) (7). The 6-cm scalp defect was the only defect found in the newborn that had been exposed during the 1st trimester to methimazole (10 mg/day).

In contrast, a 1987 study examined the records of 49,091 live births for cases of congenital skin defects (8). Twenty-five (0.05%) such cases were identified, 13 (0.03%) of which were confined to the scalp. In the sample of 48,057 women, 24 were treated with methimazole or carbimazole during the 1st trimester, but none of these mothers produced children with the skin defects. The authors concluded that they could not exclude an association between the therapy and scalp defects, but if it existed, it was a weak association (8).

Defects observed in two infants exposed to the antithyroid agents in two other reports were imperforate anus (4) and transposition of the great arteries (died at 3 days of age) (9). In a large prospective study, 25 patients were exposed to one or more noniodide thyroid suppressants during the 1st trimester, 9 of whom took methimazole (10). From the total

M

group, 4 children with nonspecified malformations were found, suggesting that the drugs may be teratogenic. However, because 16 of the group took other antithyroid drugs, the relationship between methimazole and the anomalies cannot be determined. In a study of 25 infants exposed to carbimazole, 2 were found to have defects: bilateral congenital cataracts and partial adactyly of the right foot (11). Because no pattern of malformations has emerged from these reports, it appears that these malformations were not associated with the drug therapy. In addition, other reports have described the use of methimazole and carbimazole during pregnancy without fetal anomalies (12–26).

In a surveillance study of Michigan Medicaid recipients conducted between 1985 and 1992 involving 229,101 completed pregnancies, 5 newborns had been exposed to methimazole during the 1st trimester (F. Rosa, personal communication, FDA, 1993). One (20.0%) major birth defect was observed (none expected), a hypospadias.

A 1984 report described the relationship between maternal Graves' disease and major structural malformations of external organs, including the oral cavity, in 643 newborns (27). Of 167 newborns delivered from mothers who were hyperthyroid during gestation, 117 were exposed *in utero* to methimazole. In 50 newborns, the mothers received no treatment, other than subtotal thyroidectomy before or during pregnancy. The incidences of anomalies in these two groups were 1.7% (2 of 117) and 6.0% (3 of 50), respectively. For 476 neonates the mothers were euthyroid during gestation, with 126 receiving treatment with methimazole and 350 receiving no treatment (other than surgery). No malformations were observed in the methimazole-exposed infants and only 1 (0.3%) occurred in the patients not receiving drug therapy. The difference in malformation rates between the nonexposed neonates in the hyperthyroid and euthyroid groups was significant (6% vs. 0.3%, $p < 0.01$). Similarly, the difference between the two groups in total malformations, 3% (5 of 167) vs. 0.2% (1 of 476) was also significant ($p < 0.01$). The defects observed were malformation of the earlobe (methimazole-exposed, hyperthyroid), omphalocele (methimazole-exposed, hyperthyroid), imperforate anus (hyperthyroid), anencephaly (hyperthyroid), harelip (hyperthyroid), and polydactyly (euthyroid). The authors concluded that the disease itself causes congenital malformations and that the use of methimazole lessened the risk for adverse outcome (27).

A 1987 case report described a female infant (46,XX) who had been exposed throughout gestation to methimazole and propranolol given for maternal hyperthyroidism (28). Choanal atresia was noted at birth and treated surgically. At 6 months of age, she was noted to be developmentally delayed, especially in gross motor development, and had mild neurosensory hearing loss bilaterally and recurrent dacryocystitis. By 3.5 years, her development continued to be markedly delayed. Her height and weight were below the 3rd percentile, and a small area of alopecia was noted in the parietal region close to the midline on the otherwise normal scalp. Although the chest was symmetrical, both nipples were absent (athelia). Other abnormalities noted at this time were upper slanting palpebral fissures and epicanthal folds, a broad nasal bridge with slightly anteverted nostrils, and a tented upper lip with a short philtrum (28).

Two cases of esophageal atresia and tracheoesophageal fistula in newborn infants exposed throughout gestation to methimazole (30 mg/day) were reported in 1992 (29). The mothers were euthyroid during pregnancy. Both newborns were small for gestational age and had palpable goiters with laboratory evidence of hypothyroidism. Surgical correction of the defects was attempted but the infants died of post-operative sepsis and renal failure. At autopsy, in addition to the defects noted above, one infant had a ventricular septal defect and a Meckel's diverticulum, and both had diffuse goiters. Because of the relatively low frequency of esophageal atresia and tracheoesophageal fistula (1:3000–1:4500), the authors attributed the defects to use of methimazole (29).

A 1992 study reported no difference in the intellectual capacity of offspring of 31 mothers with Graves disease who were treated during gestation with either methimazole ($N = 15$) or propylthiouracil (PTU) ($N = 16$) when compared with nonexposed controls (30). The ages of the subjects ranged from 4 to 23 years. None was hypothyroid or had goiter at birth. There were no differences between the antithyroid drugs, and there was no correlation between dosage used and intelligence (30).

Two reports, one in 1994 and the other in 1995, described aplasia cutis in two newborns exposed during pregnancy to methimazole (31,32). In reviewing their case and previously published cases, the authors of the 1994 publication were uncertain of a causal association between the drug and the scalp defect (31). The other group of authors concluded that the evidence indicated a strong association between the drug and aplasia cutis (32). Both groups concluded, because no such cases had been reported with PTU, that this drug was preferred for the treatment of hyperthyroidism during pregnancy (31,32).

A female infant exposed *in utero* to methimazole during the first 2 months of pregnancy and then to PTU until term was described in a 1997 abstract (33). Birth weight and length were normal as was the chromosomal analysis (46,XX). Malformations observed in the infant were choanal atresia, right iris/retinal coloboma, right renal pelvis ectasia, and minor facial anomalies.

A brief 1996 report described multiple malformations in a newborn of a woman who was treated with methimazole (34). Metoprolol (150 mg/day) and methimazole (30 mg/day) were taken throughout most of the 1st trimester. Levothyroxine was also administered during most of the pregnancy. Metoprolol was discontinued at about 9 weeks' gestation and the methimazole dose was gradually tapered until a subtotal thyroidectomy was performed at 18 weeks. Premature labor could not be arrested and a 750-g, male infant was delivered at 27 weeks with Apgar scores of 1, 0, and 3 at 1, 5, and 10 minutes, respectively. Major malformations evident were choanal atresia, esophageal atresia with tracheoesophageal fistula, omphaloenteric connection, and multiple ventricular septal defects. The infant died at 6 weeks of age secondary to complications arising from corrective surgery (34).

A 1998 case report described a 3-year-old boy with choanal atresia (surgically corrected shortly after birth), hypoplastic nipples (hypothelia; see also reference #28 above for a case of athelia), and developmental delay (35). He had been exposed throughout a 34-week gestation to carbimazole, but was euthyroid at birth. He was hypotonic at birth and remained so at 3 years of age. He had mild global but predominantly motor, developmental delay. His height and weight were at the 10th percentile or less. Other features noted were short upslanting palpebral fissures (length <3rd percentile), small nose and mouth, and a short philtrum. The nipples were hypoplastic and inverted. The mother had a normal, healthy child before and after the subject case. The authors suggested that the combination of malformations represented a rare but distinct syndrome of methimazole teratogenicity (35).

A case of multiple defects in an newborn infant exposed *in utero* to methimazole (20 mg/day) was reported in 1999 (36). The mother, who was euthyroid on therapy, had taken methimazole for 9 years prior to conception and was continued on the drug during the first 7 gestational weeks (i.e., 9 weeks after the first day of the last menstrual period [LMP]). At that time, she was changed to PTU for the remainder of her pregnancy. A

1475-g (25th–50th percentile) male preterm infant was delivered at 31 gestational weeks because of premature rupture of the membranes. The Apgar scores, length, and head circumference were not recorded, but severe respiratory distress required assisted ventilation. Anomalies observed in the infant were bilateral choanal atresia, esophageal atresia and tracheoesophageal fistula, patent ductus arteriosus (closed spontaneously at 2 months), and periventricular leukomalacia with bilateral parieto-occipital cavitations. The latter defect was confirmed by magnetic resonance imaging (MRI) at age 2 years and was thought to be of possible hypoxic-ischemic origin and related to prematurity. At 7 months of age, abdominal sonography, chromosomal analysis, and brain-stem auditory evoked responses were normal. An eye examination revealed bilateral convergent strabismus, mildly pale papillae, and diffuse depigmentation of the fundi. Severe psychomotor retardation with mixed tetraparesis was evident. At 4.25 years, the weight and height were both below the 3rd percentile for age, he was unable to walk or sit without support, and language was absent. Physical examination noted dolichocephaly, bilateral ptosis of the eyelid with inner epicanthal fold, convergent squint, mild malar hypoplasia, small nose with moderately anteverted nostrils, long and flat philtrum, a highly arched palate, bilateral bridged palmar creases, axial hypotonia and limb hypertonia, poor head control, Moro-like reflexes, and bilateral talipes varus. A localized (6 × 6 cm) patchy defect consisting of short, sparse, kinky, and hypopigmented hair in the occipital region was also noted. On the basis of previously reported cases, the defects suggested to the authors that they represented a specific teratogenic malformation syndrome (36).

A 2000 report described various congenital abnormalities observed in a term, female infant of a woman who was kept euthyroid throughout pregnancy with methimazole 30 mg/day (37). Aplasia cutis congenita was noted at birth. Seizures were noted at 18 months of age. At 3 years of age, her height, weight, and head circumference were normal (75th–80th percentile) as was her psychomotor development. Minor facial abnormalities consisted of hypertrichosis of the eyelashes and synophrys. There were areas of hyperpigmented skin on the back, two supernumerary nipples, bilateral syndactylies between the third and fourth fingers and between the second and third toes, dystrophic, small and shortened fingernails, and longitudinal ridges on a finger of each hand. A brain MRI, electroencephalogram, and karyotyping were normal. The authors considered this case to represent a new combination of signs, including abnormalities of various tissues of ectodermal origin (fingernails and skin anomalies) and epilepsy that were associated with *in utero* exposure to methimazole (37).

Several reports have studied pregnancies complicated by hyperthyroidism and the effects of methimazole and carbimazole on maternal and fetal thyroid indexes (23,38–41). In separate pregnancies in a mother with Graves disease, fetal thyrotoxicosis was treated with 20–40 mg/day of carbimazole with successful resolution of fetal tachycardia in both cases and disappearance of fetal goiter in the first infant (23). A woman with hyperthyroidism was treated with a partial thyroidectomy before pregnancy (39). She subsequently had four pregnancies, all of which were complicated by fetal hyperthyroidism. No antithyroid therapy was administered during her first two pregnancies. The first ended in a late stillbirth, and the second resulted in a child with skull deformities. Both adverse outcomes were compatible with fetal hyperthyroidism. Carbimazole was administered in the next two pregnancies and both resulted in normal infants (39).

A 1992 abstract and a later full report described a retrospective evaluation of hyperthyroid pregnancy outcomes treated with either methimazole ($N = 36$) or PTU ($N = 99$) (42,43). One newborn (2.8%) in the methimazole group had a birth defect (inguinal hernia) whereas three (3.0%) defects were observed in those exposed to PTU (ventricular septal defect; pulmonary stenosis; patent ductus arteriosus in a term infant). No scalp defects were observed.

A 2001 report described the pregnancy outcomes of 241 women counseled by Teratology Information Services (TIS) associated with the European Network of Teratology Information Services because of exposure to carbimazole (20–40 mg/day) or methimazole (8–50 mg/day) during the 1st trimester (44). The control group consisted of 1089 pregnant women who had contacted the TIS concerning exposures to nonteratogenic agents. There was no increase in the rate of major birth defects in the exposed pregnancies compared to controls. However, two newborns had defects (choanal atresia; esophageal atresia) that were consistent with the anomalies postulated for methimazole embryopathy (44)

A 2003 case report described the outcomes of two pregnancies with hyperthyroidism (45). Diagnosis of the disease was made in the 2nd trimester and methimazole was started at 14 and 16 weeks' gestation, respectively. In the first case, discordant female twins (2000 g and 1200 g) were delivered at 33.5 weeks. Twin A was normal but twin B had esophageal atresia and tracheoesophageal fistula. After corrective surgery, she was growing adequately at 9 months of age. In the second case, intrauterine growth retardation occurred and a 1400-g female infant was delivered at 33 weeks. Apgar scores were 6 and 10 at 1 and 5 minutes, respectively. The infant developed jaundice and examination revealed a complete absence of the biliary ducts and tree. At age 18 months the infant old was awaiting a liver transplantation. Both affected infants were euthyroid at birth. Because the observed defects have been associated with 1st trimester methimazole exposure, the authors raised the question whether the actual teratogen was untreated hyperthyroidism (45).

Two cases of major congenital defects were described in another 2003 report (46). Both pregnancies (one with twins) were treated with methimazole in the 1st trimester. In one case, methimazole (10 mg/day) was replaced with propylthiouracil at 8 weeks. A 2550-g, euthyroid female infant was delivered at 36 weeks with Apgar scores of 5, 7, and 7 at 1, 5, and 10 minutes, respectively. Defects recognized in the infant included choanal atresia, aplasia cutis, umbilical hernia, sacral pilonidal sinus, limb hypertonia, and downslanting palpebral fissures. Additional follow up could not be obtained. In the second case (twins), the mother received methimazole 40 mg/day until the 18th week, when the dose was decreased to 20 mg/day. The male twins were euthyroid with birth weights of 1850 g and 1900 g with Apgar scores of 9 and 9 at 1 and 5 minutes, respectively. No malformations were detected in the larger twin. However, the smaller twin had a full-thickness defect of the parietal scalp and a small omphalocele. At 12 months of age, the small twin had mild global (mostly motor) developmental delay, whereas development in the larger twin was normal (46).

Treatment of maternal hyperthyroidism may result in mild fetal hypothyroidism because of increased levels of fetal pituitary thyrotropin (17,20,40,47). This usually resolves within a few days without treatment (20). An exception to this occurred in one newborn exposed to 30 mg of carbimazole daily to term who appeared normal at birth but who developed hypothyroidism evident at 2 months of age with subsequent mental retardation (12).

A brief 1992 report from Spain examined the relationship between the illicit and uncontrolled use of methimazole in cattle feed as a weight enhancer and the appearance of congenital scalp aplasia cutis in humans (48). Seven cases of the rare malformation were observed in 1990–1991 in regions thought to have used methimazole in cattle food. The investigators speculated that pregnant women eating the meat of methimazole-exposed cattle would expose their fetuses to the drug (48).

Small, usually nonobstructing goiters in the newborn have been reported frequently with PTU (see Propylthiouracil). Only two goiters have been reported in carbimazole-exposed newborns and none with methimazole (9). Long-term follow-up of 25 children exposed *in utero* to carbimazole has shown normal growth and development (11).

Combination therapy with thyroid-antithyroid drugs was advocated at one time but is now considered inappropriate (see also Propylthiouracil) (18,22,47,49,50). Two reasons contributed to this change: (a) use of thyroid hormones may require higher doses of the antithyroid drug to be used, and (b) placental transfer of levothyroxine and liothyronine is minimal and not sufficient to reverse fetal hypothyroidism (see also Levothyroxine and Liothyronine) (20).

A 2002 review of the fetal effects of antithyroid drugs concluded that the evidence for a specific methimazole syndrome is inadequate (51). However, the cluster of case of case reports of aplasia cutis congenita cases suggests a weak association but additional studies are required (51).

In summary, because of the possible association with aplasia cutis and other malformations, and the passage of methimazole into breast milk, many investigators, including two in 1984 (52), consider PTU to be the drug of choice for the medical treatment of hyperthyroidism during pregnancy. However, this opinion is not universal (50). A specific pattern of rare congenital malformations secondary to exposure to methimazole during the first 7 weeks of gestation (9 weeks after the LMP) has been suggested that consists of some or all of the following: scalp or patchy hair defects, choanal atresia, esophageal atresia with tracheoesophageal fistula, minor facial anomalies, hypoplastic or absent nipples, and psychomotor delay. These defects may indicate a phenotype for methimazole embryopathy (35,36), but the complete spectrum of anomalies may still need further definition (37). Some of these defects have also been seen in untreated hyperthyroidism. If methimazole or carbimazole is used, the lowest possible dose to control the maternal disease should be given (9,47). One review recommended that the dosage should be adjusted to maintain the maternal free thyroxine levels in a mildly thyrotoxic range (41).

BREAST FEEDING SUMMARY

RECOMMENDATION: Compatible

Methimazole is excreted into breast milk (53–57). In a patient given 10 mg of radiolabeled carbimazole (converted *in vivo* to methimazole), the milk:plasma ratio was a fairly constant 1.05 over 24 hours (38). This represented about 0.47% of the given radioactive dose. In a second study, a patient was administered 2.5 mg of methimazole every 12 hours (54). The mean milk:plasma ratio was 1.16, representing 16–39 μg of methimazole in the daily milk supply. Extrapolation of these results to a daily dose of 20 mg indicated that approximately 3 mg/day would be excreted into the milk (54). Five lactating women were given 40 mg of carbimazole, producing a mean milk:plasma ratio at 1 hour of 0.72 (55). For the 8-hour period after dosing, the milk:plasma ratio was 0.98. A new radioimmunoassay was used to measure methimazole milk levels after a single 40-mg oral dose in four lactating women. The mean milk:plasma ratio during the first 8 hours was 0.97, with 70 μg excreted in the milk (55).

A 1987 publication described the results of carbimazole therapy in a woman breast-feeding twins (57). Two months after delivery, the mother was started on carbimazole, 30 mg/day. The dose was decreased as she became euthyroid. Three paired milk:plasma levels revealed ratios of 0.30–0.70. The mean free methimazole concentration in milk, determined between 2–16 weeks of therapy, was 43 ng/mL (range 0–92 ng/mL). Peak milk levels occurred 2–4 hours after a dose. Mean plasma levels in the twins were 45 ng/mL (range 0–105 ng/mL) and 52 ng/mL (range 0–156 ng/mL), with the highest concentrations occurring while the mother was taking 30 mg/day. No evidence of thyroid suppression was found clinically or after thyroid function tests in the nursing twins (57).

Two other studies also found no effect on clinical status or thyroid function in nursing infants of mothers taking carbimazole or methimazole (58,59). In one report, no adverse effects were observed during a 3-week study of 11 infants whose mothers were taking carbimazole 5–15 mg/day (58). In the other study, normal thyroid function in 35 nursing infants, whose mothers were taking methimazole, was documented over periods ranging from 1 to 6 months (59). Most mothers were taking 5–10 mg/day, but six received 20 mg/day for 1 month and then tapered to 5 mg/day.

Because the amounts found in some studies may cause thyroid dysfunction in the nursing infant, methimazole and carbimazole have, in the past, been considered contraindicated during lactation. If antithyroid drug therapy was required, PTU was considered the treatment of choice, partially because PTU is ionized at physiologic pH and because 80% of the drug is protein bound (60). Methimazole is neither ionized nor protein bound, but small doses of methimazole (e.g., 10–20 mg/day or less) do not appear to pose a major risk to the nursing infant if thyroid function is monitored at frequent (e.g., weekly or biweekly) intervals (58–60).

In 2000, a long-term study confirmed the lack of toxicity in infants of mothers being treated with methimazole (61). A total of 139 thyrotoxic lactating mothers and their nursing infants were studied, 51 of whom were treated with methimazole during pregnancy and continued their treatment during lactation. The other 88 women started methimazole therapy during lactation with 10–20 mg/day for 1 month, 10 mg/day during the second month, and then 5–10 mg/day thereafter. Methimazole serum levels in six infants whose mothers were taking 20 mg/day were <0.03 μg/mL, 2 hours after breast-feeding. No effects on infant thyroid function were detected at various times up to 12 months. In a blinded assessment, the total IQ scores, including verbal and performance IQ, of 14 children (age 48–74 months) exposed to methimazole in milk did not differ from those of 17 nonexposed controls (61).

The American Academy of Pediatrics classifies methimazole and carbimazole as compatible with breast-feeding (62).

References

1. Marchant B, Brownlie EW, Hart DM, Horton PW, Alexander WD. The placental transfer of propylthiouracil, methimazole and carbimazole. J Clin Endocrinol Metab 1977;45:1187–93.
2. Mortimer RH, Cannell GR, Addison RS, Johnson LP, Roberts MS, Bernus I. Methimazole and propylthiouracil equally cross the perfused human term placental lobule. J Clin Endocrinol Metab 1997;82:3099–102.
3. Milham S Jr, Elledge W. Maternal methimazole and congenital defects in children. Teratology 1972;5:125.
4. Mujtaba Q, Burrow GN. Treatment of hyperthyroidism in pregnancy with propylthiouracil and methimazole. Obstet Gynecol 1975;46:282–6.
5. Milham S Jr. Scalp defects in infants of mothers treated for hyperthyroidism with methimazole or carbimazole during pregnancy. Teratology 1985;32:321.
6. Kalb RE, Grossman ME. The association of aplasia cutis congenita with therapy of maternal thyroid disease. Pediatr Dermatol 1986;3:327–30.
7. Farine D, Maidman J, Rubin S, Chao S. Elevated alpha-fetoprotein in pregnancy complicated by aplasia cutis after exposure to methimazole. Obstet Gynecol 1988;71:996–7.
8. Van Dijke CP, Heydendael RJ, De Kleine MJ. Methimazole, carbimazole, and congenital skin defects. Ann Intern Med 1987;106:60–1.
9. Sugrue D, Drury MI. Hyperthyroidism complicating pregnancy: results of treatment by antithyroid drugs in 77 pregnancies. Br J Obstet Gynaecol 1980;87:970–5.
10. Heinonen OP, Slone D, Shapiro S. *Birth Defects and Drugs in Pregnancy*. Littleton, MA: Publishing Sciences Group, 1977:388–400.
11. McCarroll AM, Hutchinson M, McAuley R, Montgomery DAD. Long-term assessment of children

exposed in utero to carbimazole. Arch Dis Child 1976;51:532–6.
12. Hawe P, Francis HH. Pregnancy and thyrotoxicosis. Br Med J 1962;2:817–22.
13. Herbst AL, Selenkow HA. Combined antithyroid-thyroid therapy of hyperthyroidism in pregnancy. Obstet Gynecol 1963;21:543–50.
14. Reveno WS, Rosenbaum H. Observation on the use of antithyroid drugs. Ann Intern Med 1964;60:982–9.
15. Herbst AL, Selenkow HA. Hyperthyroidism during pregnancy. N Engl J Med 1965;273:627–33.
16. Talbert LM, Thomas CG Jr, Holt WA, Rankin P. Hyperthyroidism during pregnancy. Obstet Gynecol 1970;36:779–85.
17. Refetoff S, Ochi Y, Selenkow HA, Rosenfield RL. Neonatal hypothyroidism and goiter in one infant of each of two sets of twins due to maternal therapy with antithyroid drugs. J Pediatr 1974;85:240–4.
18. Mestman JH, Manning PR, Hodgman J. Hyperthyroidism and pregnancy. Ann Intern Med 1974;134: 434–9.
19. Ramsay I. Attempted prevention of neonatal thyrotoxicosis. Br Med J 1976;2:1110.
20. Low L, Ratcliffe W, Alexander W. Intrauterine hypothyroidism due to antithyroid-drug therapy for thyrotoxicosis during pregnancy. Lancet 1978;2:370–1.
21. Robinson PL, O'Mullane NH, Alderman B. Prenatal treatment of fetal thyrotoxicosis. Br Med J 1979;1: 383–4.
22. Kock HCLV, Merkus JMWM. Graves' disease during pregnancy. Eur J Obstet Gynecol Reprod Biol 1983;14:323–30.
23. Pekonen F, Teramo K, Makinen T, Ikonen E, Osterlund K, Lamberg BA. Prenatal diagnosis and treatment of fetal thyrotoxicosis. Am J Obstet Gynecol 1984;150:893–4.
24. Jeffcoate WJ, Bain C. Recurrent pregnancy-induced thyrotoxicosis presenting as hyperemesis gravidarum. Case report. Br J Obstet Gynaecol 1985;92:413–5.
25. Johnson IR, Filshie GM. Hodgkin's disease diagnosed in pregnancy: case report. Br J Obstet Gynaecol 1977;84:791–2.
26. Ramsay I, Kaur S, Krassas G. Thyrotoxicosis in pregnancy: results of treatment by antithyroid drugs combined with T_4. Clin Endocrinol (Oxf) 1983;18: 73–85.
27. Momotani N, Ito K, Hamada N, Ban Y, Nishikawa Y, Mimura T. Maternal hyperthyroidism and congenital malformation in the offspring. Clin Endocrinol (Oxf) 1984;20:695–700.
28. Greenberg, F. Choanal atresia and athelia: methimazole teratogenicity or a new syndrome? Am J Med Genet 1987;28:931–4.
29. Ramirez A, Espinosa de los Monteros A, Parra A, De Leon B. Esophageal atresia and tracheoesophageal fistula in two infants born to hyperthyroid women receiving methimazole (Tapazol) during pregnancy. Am J Med Genet 1992;44:200–2.
30. Eisenstein Z, Weiss M, Katz Y, Bank H. Intellectual capacity of subjects exposed to methimazole or propylthiouracil in utero. Eur J Pediatr 1992;151:558–9.
31. Mandel SJ, Brent GA, Larsen PR. Review of antithyroid drug use during pregnancy and report of a case of aplasia cutis. Thyroid 1994;4:129–33.
32. Vogt T, Stolz W, Landthaler M. Aplasia cutis congenita after exposure to methimazole: a causal relationship? Br J Dermatol 1995;133:994–6.
33. Hall BD. Methimazole as a teratogenic etiology of choanal atresia/multiple congenital anomaly syndrome (abstract). Am J Hum Genet 1997;61(Suppl):A100. As cited in Clementi M, Di Gianantonio E, Pelo E, Mammi I, Basile RT, Tenconi R. Methimazole embryopathy: delineation of the phenotype. Am J Med Genet 1999;83:43–6.
34. Johnsson E, Larsson G, Ljunggren M. Severe malformations in infant born to hyperthyroid woman on methimazole. Lancet 1997;350:1520.
35. Wilson LC, Kerr BA, Wilkinson R, Fossard C, Donnai D. Choanal atresia and hypothelia following methimazole exposure in utero: a second report. Am J Med Genet 1998;75:220–2.
36. Clementi M, Di Gianantonio E, Pelo E, Mammi I, Basile RT, Tenconi R. Methimazole embryopathy: delineation of the phenotype. Am J Med Genet 1999;83: 43–6.
37. Martin-Danavit T, Edery P, Plauchu H, Attia-Sobol J, Raudrant D, Aurand JM, Thomas L. Ectodermal abnormalities associated with methimazole intrauterine exposure. Am J Med Genet 2000;94:338–40.
38. Hardisty CA, Munro DS. Serum long acting thyroid stimulator protector in pregnancy complicated by Graves' disease. Br Med J 1983;286:934–5.
39. Cove DH, Johnston P. Fetal hyperthyroidism: experience of treatment in four siblings. Lancet 1985;1: 430–2.
40. Burrow GN. The management of thyrotoxicosis in pregnancy. N Engl J Med 1985;313:562–5.
41. Momotani N, Noh J, Oyanagi H, Ishikawa N, Ito K. Antithyroid drug therapy for Graves' disease during pregnancy: optimal regimen for fetal thyroid status. N Engl J Med 1986;315:24–8.
42. Wing D, Millar L, Koonings P, Montoro M, Mestman J. A comparison of PTU versus Tapazole in the treatment of hyperthyroidism (abstract). Am J Obstet Gynecol 1992;166:308.
43. Wing DA, Millar LK, Koonings PP, Montoro MN, Mestman JH. A comparison of propylthiouracil versus methimazole in the treatment of hyperthyroidism in pregnancy. Am J Obstet Gynecol 1994;170:90–5.
44. Di Gianantonio E, Schaefer C, Mastroiacovo PP, Cournot MP, Benedicenti F, Reuvers M, Occupati B, Robert E, Bellemin B, Addis A, Arnon J, Clementi M. Adverse effects of prenatal methimazole exposure. Teratology 2001;64:262–6.
45. Seoud M, Nassar A, Usta I, Mansour M, Salti I, Younes K. Gastrointestinal malformations in two infants born to women with hyperthyroidism untreated in the first trimester. Am J Perinatol 2003;20:59–62.
46. Ferraris S, Valenzise M, Lerone M, Divizia MT, Rosaia L, Blaid D, Nemelka O, Ferrero GB, Silengo M. Malformations following methimazole exposure in utero: an open issue. Birth Defects Res Part A Clin Mol Teratol 2003;67:989–92.
47. Burr WA. Thyroid disease. Clin Obstet Gynecol 1981;8:341–51.
48. Martinez-Frias ML, Cereijo A, Rodriguez-Pinilla E, Urioste M. Methimazole in animal feed and congenital aplasia cutis. Lancet 1992;339:7424–3.
49. Anonymous. Transplacental passage of thyroid hormones. N Engl J Med 1967;277:486–7.

M

50. Mestman JH. Hyperthyroidism in pregnancy. Clin Obstet Gynecol 1997;40:45–64.
51. Diav-Citrin O, Ornoy A. Teratogen update: antithyroid drugs—methimazole, carbimazole, and propylthiouracil. Teratology 2002;65:38–44.
52. Bachrach LK, Burrow GN. Aplasia cutis congenita and methimazole. Can Med Assoc J 1984;130:1264.
53. Low LCK, Lang J, Alexander WD. Excretion of carbimazole and propylthiouracil in breast milk. Lancet 1979;2:1011.
54. Tegler L, Lindstrom B. Antithyroid drugs in milk. Lancet 1980;2:591.
55. Johansen K, Andersen AN, Kampmann JP, Hansen JM, Mortensen HB. Excretion of methimazole in human milk. Eur J Clin Pharmacol 1982;23:339–41.
56. Cooper DS, Bode HH, Nath B, Saxe V, Malcof F, Ridgway EC. Methimazole in man: studies using a newly developed radioimmunoassay for methimazole. J Clin Endocrinol Metab 1984;58:473–9.
57. Rylance GW, Woods CG, Donnelly MC, Oliver JS, Alexander WD. Carbimazole and breastfeeding. Lancet 1987;1:928.
58. Lamberg BA, Ikonen E, Osterlund K, Teramo K, Pekonen F, Peltola J, Valimaki M. Antithyroid treatment of maternal hyperthyroidism during lactation. Clin Endocrinol (Oxf) 1984;21:81–7.
59. Azizi F. Effect of methimazole treatment of maternal thyrotoxicosis on thyroid function in breast-feeding infants. J Pediatr 1996;128:855–8.
60. Cooper DS. Antithyroid drugs: to breast-feed or not to breast-feed. Am J Obstet Gynecol 1987;157:234–5.
61. Azizi F, Khoshniat M, Bahrainian M, Hedayati M. Thyroid function and intellectual development of infants nursed by mothers taking methimazole. J Clin Endocrinol Metab 2000;85:3233–8.
62. Committee on Drugs, American Academy of Pediatrics. The transfer of drugs and other chemicals into human milk. Pediatrics 2001;108:776–89.

Name: **METHIXENE** Risk Factor: **C**
Class: **Parasympatholytic (Anticholinergic)**

FETAL RISK SUMMARY

RECOMMENDATION: No Human Data - No Relevant Animal Data

Methixene is an anticholinergic agent. No reports of its use in pregnancy have been located (see also Atropine).

BREAST FEEDING SUMMARY

RECOMMENDATION: No Human Data - Probably Compatible

No data are available (see also Atropine).

Name: **METHOCARBAMOL** Risk Factor: **C**
Class: **Muscle Relaxant**

FETAL RISK SUMMARY

RECOMMENDATION: Human Data Suggest Low Risk

The centrally acting muscle relaxant, methocarbamol, is not teratogenic in animals (personal communication, A.H. Robins Company, 1987). The agent crosses the placenta to the fetus in dogs, (1) but apparently placental transfer in humans has not been studied.

One manufacturer has an unpublished case on file relating to a mother who consumed methocarbamol, 1 g 4 times/day, throughout gestation (personal communication, A. H. Robins Company, 1987). The mother also used marijuana, and possibly other illicit substances, during her pregnancy. No physical or developmental abnormalities were noted at birth, but the infant did exhibit withdrawal symptoms consisting of prolonged crying, restlessness, easy irritability, and seizures. The infant was hospitalized for 2 months following birth to treat these symptoms. No further withdrawal symptoms or seizures were observed following discharge from the hospital. Follow-up neurologic examination indicated that developmental patterns were normal.

The above manufacturer also has informal data on file obtained from the Boston Collaborative Drug Surveillance Program (personal communication, A. H. Robins Company, 1987). These data, compiled between 1977 and 1981, relate to the use of methocarbamol by pregnant patients of the Puget Sound Group Health Cooperative in Seattle, Washington. During the data collection interval, 27 1st trimester exposures to the muscle relaxant were documented. None of the exposed infants had a congenital malformation.

The Collaborative Perinatal Project monitored 50,282 mother-child pairs, 22 of whom were exposed to methocarbamol during the 1st trimester (2, pp. 358, 360). One of these infants had an inguinal hernia. For use anytime during pregnancy, 119 exposures were recorded (2, p. 493). In this latter group, 6 infants had an inguinal hernia. An association between the drug and the defect cannot be determined from these data.

In a surveillance study of Michigan Medicaid recipients conducted between 1985 and 1992 involving 229,101 completed pregnancies, 340 newborns had been exposed to methocarbamol during the 1st trimester (F. Rosa, personal communication, FDA, 1993). A total of 13 (3.8%) major birth defects were observed (14 expected), including (observed/expected) 1/1 polydactyly and 1/1 limb reduction defect. No anomalies were observed in four other defect categories (cardiovascular defects, oral clefts, spina bifida, and hypospadias) for which specific data were available. These data do not support an association between the drug and congenital defects.

The authors of a 1982 study of 350 patients with congenital contractures of the joints (arthrogryposis) concluded that only 15 had been exposed to a possible teratogen (3). One of the 15 cases involved a 24-year-old woman who had consumed, at 2 months of gestation, methocarbamol and propoxyphene, 750 mg and 65 mg, respectively, 2–3 times/day for 3 days to treat severe back pain. The term female infant was noted at birth to have multiple joint contractures involving the thumbs, wrists, elbows, knees, and feet. The latter was described as a bilateral equinovarus deformity. There were practically no foot creases. Other abnormalities present were frontal bosselation, a midline hemangioma, and weak abdominal musculature. Development was normal at 3 years of age except for the joint contractures, which had improved with time, and a grade I/VI systolic murmur.

Because of the muscle-relaxant properties of methocarbamol, the authors of the above study attributed the defect to this drug. Their review of the literature and of the records of the Centers for Disease Control and Prevention failed to find any other cases of arthrogryposis with maternal methocarbamol ingestion. Moreover, no reports have appeared since then relating the defect to maternal use of the drug. A case of arthrogryposis, however, had been previously described with propoxyphene ingestion (see Propoxyphene for details) (4). Therefore, based on the present information, it is unlikely that a relationship exists between maternal use of methocarbamol and congenital contractures in the newborn.

BREAST FEEDING SUMMARY

RECOMMENDATION: No Human Data - Probably Compatible

Methocarbamol is excreted in the milk of dogs (1), but human studies have not been located. Because newborns have been directly treated for tetanus with methocarbamol, any amounts excreted in milk are probably not clinically significant.

References

1. Campbell AD, Coles FK, Eubank LL, Huf EG. Distribution and metabolism of methocarbamol. J Pharmacol Exp Ther 1961;131:18–25.
2. Heinonen OP, Slone D, Shapiro S. *Birth Defects and Drugs in Pregnancy*. Littleton, MA: Publishing Sciences Group, 1977.
3. Hall JG, Reed SD. Teratogens associated with congenital contractures in humans and in animals. Teratology 1982;25:173–91.
4. Barrow MV, Souder DE. Propoxyphene and congenital malformations. JAMA 1971;217:1551–2.

Name: **METHOTREXATE** Risk Factor: X_M

Class: **Antineoplastic/Immunologic Agent (Antirheumatic)**

FETAL RISK SUMMARY

RECOMMENDATION: Contraindicated

Methotrexate is a folic acid antagonist. A number of references describing the use of this antineoplastic agent in pregnancy have been located (1–28). Methotrexate-induced congenital defects (also known as the aminopterin-methotrexate syndrome) are similar to those produced by another folic acid antagonist, aminopterin (see also Aminopterin) (6). Anomalies in two infants were absence of lambdoid and coronal sutures, oxycephaly, absence of frontal bone, low-set ears, hypertelorism, dextroposition of heart, absence of digits on feet, growth retardation, very wide posterior fontanelle, hypoplastic mandible, and multiple anomalous ribs (2); and oxycephaly caused by absent coronal sutures, large anterior fontanelle, depressed and wide nasal bridge, low-set ears, long webbed fingers, and wide-set eyes (3).

A 1990 report described the pregnancy outcomes of eight women who were treated with low-dose oral methotrexate for rheumatic disease during 10 pregnancies (17). The outcomes included two elective abortions (no details given for these cases), three SABs and five normal full-term live births. In the eight pregnancies (six women) with details, the methotrexate weekly dose (usually given as a single dose) was 7.5 mg in seven and 10 mg in one. In the live birth group, the mean methotrexate exposure was 6.8 weeks postconception (range 2–15 weeks), whereas in the spontaneous abortion (SAB) group the mean exposure was 7 weeks (range 4–9 weeks). The mean cumulative methotrexate dose prior to conception was 1384 mg (range 165–3545 mg) (live births) and 333 mg (range 45–775 mg) (SAB). Other drugs taken by the women included aspirin, nonsteroidal anti-inflammatory agents, prednisone (<10 mg/day), and hydroxychloroquine. Folate supplements had been taken in three of the five pregnancies ending in live births and in all three of the SAB cases. No obvious differences were apparent between the live birth and SAB groups in terms of smoking, use of alcohol, or the use of other drugs. Information on the long-term development of the five live births was obtained by telephone interview at a mean age of 11.5 years (range 3.7–16.7 years). All of the children were healthy and had experienced normal physical and mental development (one child had a minor speech impediment that had resolved with speech therapy) (17).

A 1993 case report and review described the pregnancy outcome of a 39-year-old woman with severe rheumatoid arthritis who was exposed to methotrexate and other drugs shortly after conception (18). For about 6 months before conception she had been taking methotrexate (7.5 mg once weekly), ibuprofen (6.4 g/day), misoprostol (0.4 mg/day), and cimetidine (600 mg) or sucralfate (3 g) per day. All medications were stopped within

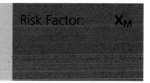

10 days of the last menstrual period (as determined by ultrasound at 5–6 weeks' gestation). A healthy full-term, 3962-g male infant was delivered by cesarean section (breech presentation) with Apgar scores of 8 and 9 at 1 and 5 minutes, respectively. Examination by a dysmorphologist when the infant was 12 weeks of age revealed a healthy, normal infant with no evidence of embryopathy (18).

A 25-year-old woman at 30 weeks' gestation was diagnosed with metastatic choriocarcinoma of the vagina and lungs (19). The woman was treated with IV methotrexate 20 mg/day for 5 days. Five days later, she delivered a preterm male infant with an Apgar of 10 (no other details were given). The mother and infant were alive and well at 12 months' follow-up (19).

In a 1994 reference, data relating to methotrexate use before or during pregnancy were gathered from programs participating in the Organization of Teratology Information Services (OTIS) and the European Network of Teratology Information Services (ENTIS) (20). The survey resulted in data for 21 prospectively ascertained cases. Seven exposures occurred more than 1 year before conception and they were excluded from the analysis. In the remaining 14 cases, 9 were exposed within 1 year of conception and 5 were exposed during pregnancy. Four of the five pregnancy exposures occurred within the first 6 weeks of gestation with a duration of exposure of 1–3 weeks and one single dose exposure occurred at 37–38 weeks' gestation. Doses ranged from 7.5 mg/week (one woman had been taking this dose for 3 years) to a single 42 mg IV dose. All of these outcomes resulted in healthy infants without birth defects (one delivered at 36 weeks). In the women exposed within 1 year of pregnancy, the duration of exposures ranged from a few weeks to 6 years. The doses were known in four cases (7.5 mg/week in three, 12.5 mg/wk in one). The outcomes of these nine cases were four SABs, four healthy infants, and one infant born at term with a cavernous hemangioma. The authors concluded that the limited data confirmed that the critical time for methotrexate-induced defects was 6–8 weeks postconception and the critical dose was ≥10 mg/week (20).

A 1997 case report described an adverse pregnancy outcome in a 20-year-old woman with polyarticular rheumatoid arthritis who had been treated with oral doses of methotrexate (10–12.5 mg/week) for about 5–6 years (21). Folic acid (1 mg/day) was also prescribed, but her compliance with therapy was unclear. The woman discontinued treatment at about 8 weeks' gestation (estimated dose during gestation about 100 mg). At 35 weeks' she gave birth to a 1.79-kg female (normal 46,XX karyotype) infant with intrauterine growth retardation (IUGR) and multiple congenital anomalies. The defects included brachycephaly, a 0.5-cm anterior fontanelle, coronal ridging, shallow orbits with hypertelorism, retrognathia, malformed ears, palate with a posterior groove and a bifid uvula, umbilical hernia, spinal defects (dorsal kyphosis with L5 and S1 hemivertebrae), deformed thumb, bilateral simian creases, hypoplastic nails, reduction of radial ray on right side, syndactyly of fourth and fifth toes, absent fifth metatarsal bone, and cardiovascular defects (double-outlet right ventricle, doubly committed ventricular septal defect, transposed great vessels, restrictive atrial septal defect, pulmonary stenosis, and an aberrant right subclavian artery (21). The infant died at 6 months of age. The authors concluded that the anomalies were consistent with methotrexate-induced embryopathy (21).

A 26-year-old man with fetal methotrexate syndrome and two children with mild manifestations of the syndrome were described in 1998 (22). In the adult's case, his mother (who gave him up for adoption) had attempted to terminate the pregnancy at 6–8 weeks' gestation with an unknown amount of methotrexate. His malformations included hypertelorism, ptosis of the eyelids, short palpebral fissures, sparse eyebrows, prominent nose, low-set ears, a widow's peak at the frontal hairline, flexion contractures of the metacarpophalangeal joints of both thumbs and syndactyly of all fingers (all repaired surgically), four metacarpals, and a single fused hypoplastic nub of tissue at the forefoot (corrected surgically with reconstruction of all toes). His physical growth was retarded, but his psychomotor development was normal, as is his intelligence. The first child, a 9-year-old male, was exposed to 80 mg/week of methotrexate for 6 doses at 7.5–28.5 weeks' gestation. His mother, with an undetected pregnancy, had been treated for breast cancer with methotrexate, fluorouracil (1200 mg/week times 10 doses), and radiation (total dose estimated to be 14 rads). He was born at 29 weeks with a birth weight of 820 g (small for gestational age) and he remains growth retarded. Malformations included hypertelorism, a frontal hair whorl, upsweep of the frontal hairline, microcephaly, low-set ears, micrognathia, right palmar simian crease, and borderline mental retardation (composite IQ of 70) (22). The second child is a 3.5-year-old male infant who was born at 29 weeks' gestation with a normal weight (1160 g; 50th percentile). His mother had undergone a failed elective abortion (dilatation, suction, and curettage; 11 weeks after the last menstrual period [LMP]) and then, because of large uterine myomas, had chosen to have a medical abortion with methotrexate. She received 100 mg bi-weekly from about 13 to 19 weeks' and 200 mg bi-weekly from 19 to 25 weeks', but this abortion attempt also failed. Birth defects noted were a bulging forehead, bi-temporal narrowing, upward slanting palpebral fissures, sparse hair on the temporal areas, low-set ears, broad nasal tip, and a high arched palate (22). He has had chronic diarrhea since 9 months of age. An intestinal biopsy revealed villous atrophy. His psychomotor development has been normal. At 34 months, his weight and length were retarded, but his head circumference was normal (75th percentile) (22).

A 1999 report described the outcomes of pregnancies in 20 women with breast cancer who were treated with antineoplastic agents (23). (See also Fluorouracil.) Methotrexate (25 mg/m^2), in combination with epirubicin and vincristine, was administered to one woman at 6 weeks' gestation. The pregnancy ended in a SAB (23).

Another 1999 reference reported the outcome of a male infant (normal karyotype 46, XY) whose mother had been treated for chronic severe psoriasis with 12.5 mg methotrexate three times weekly during the first 8 weeks postconception (24). He was delivered at 40 weeks' gestation with Apgar scores of 2, 5, and 6 at 1, 5, and 10 minutes, respectively. Birth weight, length, and head circumference were severely retarded (<3rd percentile). Malformations included widely separated sutures and large fontanelles, bilateral epicanthal folds and sparse eyebrows laterally with hypoplastic supraorbital ridges, broad nasal bridge, anteverted nares, smooth long philtrum, hypoplastic nipples, small umbilical hernia, diastasis recti, a shawl scrotum, decreased extension of the elbows, short bilateral proximal phalanges of the third, fourth, and fifth fingers, and mildly hypoplastic fingernails (24). The only neurologic abnormality noted was mild hypotonia. At 20 months, he was still growth retarded. He had a triangular face (trigonocephaly) with a prominent metopic suture and the open anterior fontanelle finally closed at age 30 months. Generalized tonic-clonic seizures associated with fever were noted at 1 and 2 years (both of his older sisters had a similar episode during the first 2 years of life). Developmental testing revealed mental retardation with significant early motor and cognitive delays (24).

A 23-year-old woman underwent an attempted abortion at 8 weeks' gestation with IM methotrexate 100 mg followed by misoprostol 800 μg 4 days later (25). Four weeks later she still had a viable pregnancy but could not afford hospitalization for surgical termination. She eventually delivered a 2050-g female infant at term with Apgar scores of 4 and 8 at 1 and 5 minutes, respectively. The infant was hypotonic. All growth parameters (weight, height, and head circumference) were severely growth retarded. Multiple malformations were noted including a disproportionately long head (dolichocephaly), a prominent broad nose, hypertelorism, short palpebral fissure, small mouth, micrognathia, fifth-finger clinodactyly, extra flexion creases on the thumbs, mild syndactyly of the second and third toes with fourth and fifth toe clinodactyly, and hypoplastic toenails. Severe growth retardation was evident at the 12 and 18 month examinations. The mother declined developmental testing of the child, but stated that the usual developmental milestones were normal (25).

A 2002 case report described the pregnancy outcome of a woman who was treated for psoriasis with two doses of methotrexate 7.5 mg/day at 3.5 weeks postconception (26). She also was taking sertraline and smoked cigarettes. An ultrasound examination at 18 weeks' gestation revealed multiple anomalies and the pregnancy was terminated 2 weeks later. The male fetus (normal 46,XY karyotype) had a wide anterior fontanelle, sloping forehead, undermineralization of the skull, low-set and poorly formed ears, absent auditory canals, flat nose, micrognathia, multiple skeletal abnormalities (absent and slender ribs, a hemivertebrae, and fusion of the third through fifth lumbar vertebral bodies), limb defects (absent left radius, hypoplastic right radius, bilaterally short forearms, hypoplastic left thumb, and clinodactyly of the fifth digit bilaterally), tracheal atresia, markedly hypoplastic lungs, cardiovascular defects (left ventricle mildly hypoplastic, ventricular septal defect, persistent right subclavian artery with an arterial ring, and absent left and right pulmonary arteries), malrotated intestines, duodenal atresia, a Meckel's diverticulum, multiple accessory spleens, enlarged left liver lobe, and a two-vessel umbilical cord (26).

M

A 2003 case reported a failed pregnancy termination attempt at 6 weeks' gestation with IM methotrexate 75 mg and oral misoprostol 400 μg (27). The pregnancy was terminated at 27 weeks secondary to ultrasound diagnosis of methotrexate embryopathy. Autopsy revealed a 918-g female (normal karyotype) fetus with upper extremities that were asymmetric in length, bilateral shortening of the radii and ulnae, asymmetric in length lower extremities with bilateral absent fibulae, polydactyly of the right foot, small head, prominent eyes, low-set ears, micrognathia, and a two-vessel umbilical cord (27).

A survey of 600 members of the American College of Rheumatology, partially conducted to determine the outcomes of pregnancies exposed to disease modifying antirheumatic drugs (DMARDs) (etanercept, infliximab, leflunomide, and methotrexate), was published in 2003 (28). From the 175 responders, the outcomes of 39 pregnancies exposed to methotrexate were 21 full-term healthy infants, 7 spontaneous abortions (1 with a congenital malformation), 8 elective abortions, 1 woman still pregnant, and 2 live-born infants with birth defects. No information was available on the three cases with malformations and whether these were believed to have resulted from methotrexate exposure (28).

Possible retention of methotrexate in maternal tissues before conception was suggested as the cause of a rare pulmonary disorder in a newborn, desquamating fibrosing alveolitis (29). The infant's mother had conceived within 6 months of completing treatment with the antineoplastic. (Note: A later publication from these investigators, which included this case, noted that the newborn was conceived within 2 months of treatment termination [see reference 41]. In addition, a sister of the infant born 3 years later developed the same disorder, although a third child born from the mother 1 year later developed normally.) Previous studies have shown that methotrexate may persist for prolonged periods in human tissues (30). However, conception occurred 3 months after discontinuance of therapy in one case (31), after 6 months in a second (13), and after 7 months in a third (32). Four (one set of twins) normal infants resulted from these latter pregnancies. Therefore, the association between methotrexate and the pulmonary disorder is unknown.

Two cases of severe newborn myelosuppression have been reported after methotrexate use in pregnancy. In one case, pancytopenia was discovered in a 1000-g male newborn after exposure to six different antineoplastic agents, including methotrexate, in the 3rd trimester (4). The second infant, delivered at 31 weeks' gestation, was exposed to methotrexate only during the 12th week of pregnancy (9). The severe bone marrow hypoplasia was most likely caused by the use of mercaptopurine near delivery.

Data from one review indicated that 40% of the infants exposed to cytotoxic drugs were of low birth weight (1). This finding was not related to the timing of the exposure. Long-term studies of growth and mental development in offspring exposed to antineoplastic agents during the 2nd trimester, the period of neuroblast multiplication, have not been conducted (32,34). Several studies, however, have followed individual infants for periods ranging from 2 to 84 months and have not discovered any problems (9–13,15,16).

Methotrexate crosses the placenta to the fetus (14). A 34-year-old mother was treated with multiple antineoplastic agents for acute lymphoblastic leukemia beginning in her 22nd week of pregnancy. Weekly intrathecal methotrexate (10 mg/m^2) was administered from approximately 26 to 29 weeks' gestation, after which the dose was increased to 20 mg/m^2 weekly until delivery at 40 weeks' gestation. Methotrexate levels in cord serum and red cells were 1.86×10^{-9} mol/L, and 2.6×10^{-9} mol/g of hemoglobin, respectively, with 29% as the polyglutamate metabolite (14).

In the case described above, chromosomal analysis of the newborn revealed a normal karyotype (46,XX), but with gaps and a ring chromosome (14). The clinical significance of these findings is unknown, but because these abnormalities may persist for several years, the potential existed for an increased risk of cancer as well as for a risk of genetic damage in the next generation (14).

M

Successful pregnancies have followed the use of methotrexate before conception (13,29,31,32,35–41). Apparently, ovarian and testicular dysfunction is reversible (34, 42–45). Two studies, one in 1984 and one in 1988, both involving women treated for gestational trophoblastic neoplasms, have analyzed reproductive function after methotrexate therapy and are described below (41,46).

In 438 long-term survivors treated with chemotherapy between 1958 and 1978, 436 received methotrexate either alone or in combination with other antineoplastic agents (41). This report was a continuation of a brief 1979 correspondence that discussed some of the same patients (29). The mean duration of chemotherapy was 4 months, with a mean interval from completion of therapy to the first pregnancy of 2.7 years. Conception occurred within 1 year of therapy completion in 45 women, resulting in 31 live births, 1 anencephalic stillbirth, 7 spontaneous abortions, and 6 elective abortions. Of the 436 women, 187 (43%) had at least one live birth (numbers given in parentheses refer to mean/maximum methotrexate dose in grams when used alone; mean/maximum dose in grams when used in combination) (1.26/6.0; 1.22/6.8), 23 (5%) had no live births (1.56/2.6; 1.33/6.5), 7 (2%) failed to conceive (1.30/1.6; 1.95/4.5), and 219 (50%) did not try to conceive (1.10/2.0; 2.20/34.5). The average ages at the end of treatment in the four groups were 24.9, 24.4, 24.4, and 31.5 years, respectively. Congenital abnormalities noted were anencephaly (2), spina bifida (1), tetralogy of Fallot (1), talipes equinovarus (1), collapsed lung (1), umbilical hernia (1), desquamative fibrosing alveolitis (1; same case as described above), asymptomatic heart murmur (1), and mental retardation (1). An 11th child had tachycardia but developed normally after treatment. One case of sudden infant death syndrome occurred in a female infant at 4 weeks of age. None of these outcomes differed statistically from that expected in a normal population (41).

The 1988 report described the reproductive results of 265 women who had been treated from 1959 to 1980 for gestational trophoblastic disease (46). Single-agent chemotherapy was administered to 91 women, only 2 of whom received methotrexate. Sequential (single agent) and combination therapy were administered to 67 and 107 women, respectively, but the individual agents used were not specified. Further details of this study are provided in the monograph for mercaptopurine (see Mercaptopurine).

The long-term effects of combination chemotherapy on menstrual and reproductive function have also been described in women treated for malignant ovarian germ cell tumors (47). Only 2 of the 40 women treated received methotrexate. The results of this study are discussed in the monograph for cyclophosphamide (see Cyclophosphamide).

A 34-year-old man, being treated with oral methotrexate for Reiter's syndrome, fathered a normal full-term female infant (48). The man had been receiving treatment with the drug intermittently for approximately 5 years and continuously for 5 months before conception.

Occupational exposure of the mother to antineoplastic agents during pregnancy may present a risk to the fetus. A position statement from the National Study Commission on Cytotoxic Exposure and a research article involving some antineoplastic agents are presented in the monograph for cyclophosphamide (see Cyclophosphamide).

In summary, the use of methotrexate during organogenesis is associated with a spectrum of congenital defects collectively called methotrexate embryopathy or the fetal aminopterin-methotrexate syndrome. The critical period of exposure is 6–8 weeks post-conception (8–10 weeks after the first day of the LMP) and the critical dose is thought to be 10 mg or more/week (18,20). Typical characteristics of the syndrome are IUGR, a marked decrease in ossification of the calvarium, hypoplastic supraorbital ridges, small, low-set ears, micrognathia, limb abnormalities, and occasional mental retardation (24). Exposure in the 2nd and 3rd trimesters may be associated with fetal toxicity and mortality. Although methotrexate may persist in tissues for long periods, pregnancies occurring after treatment with methotrexate do not appear to be at a risk any different from that of an unexposed population. If methotrexate is used in pregnancy for the treatment of rheumatoid arthritis, healthcare professionals are encouraged to call the toll free number (877-311-8972) for information about patient enrollment in the OTIS Rheumatoid Arthritis study.

BREAST FEEDING SUMMARY

RECOMMENDATION: Contraindicated

Methotrexate is excreted into breast milk in low concentrations (49). After a dose of 22.5 mg/day, milk concentrations of 0.26 μg/dL have been measured with a milk:plasma ratio of 0.08. The significance of this small amount is not known. However, because the drug may accumulate in neonatal tissues, breast-feeding is contraindicated. The American Academy of Pediatrics classifies methotrexate as a cytotoxic drug that may interfere with cellular metabolism of the nursing infant (50).

References

1. Nicholson HO. Cytotoxic drugs in pregnancy: review of reported cases. J Obstet Gynaecol Br Commonw 1968;75:307–12.
2. Milunsky A, Graef JW, Gaynor MF. Methotrexate-induced congenital malformations. J Pediatr 1968; 72:790–5.
3. Powell HR, Ekert H. Methotrexate-induced congenital malformations. Med J Aust 1971;2:1076–7.
4. Pizzuto J, Aviles A, Noriega L, Niz J, Morales M, Romero F. Treatment of acute leukemia during pregnancy: presentation of nine cases. Cancer Treat Rep 1980;64:679–83.

5. Dara P, Slater LM, Armentrout SA. Successful pregnancy during chemotherapy for acute leukemia. Cancer 1981;47:845–6.
6. Warkany J. Teratogenicity of folic acid antagonists. Cancer Bull 1981;33:76–7.
7. Burnier AM. Discussion. In Plows CW. Acute myelomonocytic leukemia in pregnancy: report of a case. Am J Obstet Gynecol 1982;143:41–3.
8. Khurshid M, Saleem M. Acute leukaemia in pregnancy. Lancet 1978;2:534–5.
9. Okun DB, Groncy PK, Sieger L, Tanaka KR. Acute leukemia in pregnancy: transient neonatal myelosuppression after combination chemotherapy in the mother. Med Pediatr Oncol 1979;7:315–9.
10. Doney KC, Kraemer KG, Shepard TH. Combination chemotherapy for acute myelocytic leukemia during pregnancy: three case reports. Cancer Treat Rep 1979;63:369–71.
11. Karp GI, von Oeyen P, Valone F, Khetarpal VK, Israel M, Mayer RJ, Frigoletto FD, Garnick MB. Doxorubicin in pregnancy; possible transplacental passage. Cancer Treat Rep 1983;67:773–7.
12. Feliu J, Juarez S, Ordonez A, Garcia-Paredes ML, Gonzalez-Baron M, Montero JM. Acute leukemia and pregnancy. Cancer 1988;61:580–4.
13. Turchi JJ, Villasis C. Anthracyclines in the treatment of malignancy in pregnancy. Cancer 1988;61:435–40.
14. Schleuning M, Clemm C. Chromosomal aberrations in a newborn whose mother received cytotoxic treatment during pregnancy. N Engl J Med 1987;317:1666–7.
15. Frenkel EP, Meyers MC. Acute leukemia and pregnancy. Ann Intern Med 1960;53:656–71.
16. Coopland AT, Friesen WJ, Galbraith PA. Acute leukemia in pregnancy. Am J Obstet Gynecol 1969;105:1288–9.
17. Kozlowski RD, Steinbrunner JV, MacKenzie AH, Clough JD, Wilke WS, Segal AM. Outcome of first-trimester exposure to low-dose methotrexate in eight patients with rheumatic disease. Am J Med 1990;88:589–92.
18. Feldkamp M, Carey JC. Clinical teratology counseling and consultation case report: low dose methotrexate exposure in the early weeks of pregnancy. Teratology 1993;47:533–9.
19. Gangadharan VP, Chitrathara K, Satishkumar K, Rajan B, Nair MK. Successful management of choriocarcinoma with pregnancy. Acta Oncol 1994;33:76–7.
20. Donnenfeld AE, Pastuszak A, Noah JS, Schick B, Rose NC, Koren G. Methotrexate exposure prior to and during pregnancy. Teratology 1994;49:79–81.
21. Buckley LM, Bullaboy CA, Leichtman L, Marquez M. Multiple congenital anomalies associated with weekly low-dose methotrexate treatment of the mother. Arthritis Rheum 1997;40:971–3.
22. Bawle EV, Conard JV, Weiss L. Adult and two children with fetal methotrexate syndrome. Teratology 1998;57:51–5.
23. Giacalone PL, Laffargue F, Benos P. Chemotherapy for breast carcinoma during pregnancy. Cancer 1999;86:2266–72.
24. Del Campo M, Kosaki K, Bennett FC, Jones KL. Developmental delay in fetal aminopterin/methotrexate syndrome. Teratology 1999;60:10–12.
25. Wheeler M, O'Meara P, Stanford M. Fetal methotrexate and misoprostol exposure: the past revisited. Teratology 2002;66:73–6.
26. Nguyen C, Duhl AJ, Escallon CS, Blakemore KJ. Multiple anomalies in a fetus exposed to low-dose methotrexate in the first trimester. Obstet Gynecol 2002;99:599–602.
27. Chapa JB, Hibbard JU, Weber EM, Abramowicz JS, Verp MS. Prenatal diagnosis of methotrexate embryopathy. Obstet Gynecol 2003;101:1104–7.
28. Chakravarty EF, Sanchez-Yamamoto D, Bush TM. The use of disease modifying antirheumatic drugs in women with rheumatoid arthritis of childbearing age: a survey of practice patterns and pregnancy outcomes. J Rheumatol 2003;30:241–6.
29. Walden PAM, Bagshawe KD. Pregnancies after chemotherapy for gestational trophoblastic tumours. Lancet 1979;2:1241.
30. Charache S, Condit PT, Humphreys SR. Studies on the folic acid vitamins. IV. The persistence of amethopterin in mammalian tissues. Cancer 1960;13:236–40.
31. Barnes AB, Link DA. Childhood dermatomyositis and pregnancy. Am J Obstet Gynecol 1983;146:335–6.
32. Sivanesaratnam V, Sen DK. Normal pregnancy after successful treatment of choriocarcinoma with cerebral metastases: a case report. J Reprod Med 1988;33:402–3.
33. Dobbing J. Pregnancy and leukaemia. Lancet 1977;1:1155.
34. Schilsky RL, Lewis BJ, Sherins RJ, Young RC. Gonadal dysfunction in patients receiving chemotherapy for cancer. Ann Intern Med 1980;93:109–14.
35. Bacon C, Kernahan J. Successful pregnancy in acute leukaemia. Lancet 1975;2:515.
36. Wegelius R. Successful pregnancy in acute leukaemia. Lancet 1975;2:1301.
37. Ross GT. Congenital anomalies among children born of mothers receiving chemotherapy for gestational trophoblastic neoplasms. Cancer 1976;37:1043–7.
38. Gasser C. Long-term survival (cures) in childhood acute leukemia. Paediatrician 1980;9:344–57.
39. Sanz MA, Rafecas FJ. Successful pregnancy during chemotherapy for acute promyelocytic leukemia. N Engl J Med 1982;306:939.
40. Deeg HJ, Kennedy MS, Sanders JE, Thomas ED, Storb R. Successful pregnancy after marrow transplantation for severe aplastic anemia and immunosuppression with cyclosporine. JAMA 1983;250:647.
41. Rustin GJS, Booth M, Dent J, Salt S, Rustin F, Bagshawe KD. Pregnancy after cytotoxic chemotherapy for gestational trophoblastic tumours. Br Med J 1984;288:103–6.
42. Hinkes E, Plotkin D. Reversible drug-induced sterility in a patient with acute leukemia. JAMA 1973;223:1490–1.
43. Sherins RJ, DeVita VT Jr. Effect of drug treatment for lymphoma on male reproductive capacity. Ann Intern Med 1973;79:216–20.
44. Lendon M, Palmer MK, Hann IM, Shalet SM, Jones PHM. Testicular histology after combination chemotherapy in childhood for acute lymphoblastic leukaemia. Lancet 1978;2:439–41.
45. Evenson DP, Arlin Z, Welt S, Claps ML, Melamed MR. Male reproductive capacity may recover following drug treatment with the L-10 protocol for acute lymphocytic leukemia. Cancer 1984;53:30–6.

46. Song H, Wu P, Wang Y, Yang X, Dong S. Pregnancy outcomes after successful chemotherapy for choriocarcinoma and invasive mole: long-term follow-up. Am J Obstet Gynecol 1988;158:538–45.
47. Gershenson DM. Menstrual and reproductive function after treatment with combination chemotherapy for malignant ovarian germ cell tumors. J Clin Oncol 1988;6:270–5.
48. Perry WH. Methotrexate and teratogenesis. Arch Dermatol 1983;119:874.
49. Johns DG, Rutherford LD, Keighton PC, Vogel CL. Secretion of methotrexate into human milk. Am J Obstet Gynecol 1972;112:978–80.
50. Committee on Drugs, American Academy of Pediatrics. The transfer of drugs and other chemicals into human milk. Pediatrics 2001;108:776–89.

Name:	**METHOTRIMEPRAZINE**	Risk Factor:	**C**
Class:	**Sedative/Analgesic**		

FETAL RISK SUMMARY

RECOMMENDATION: Limited Human Data - No Relevant Animal Data

Methotrimeprazine, a propylamino phenothiazine in the same class as chlorpromazine, is used primarily as a sedative and analgesic. Although specific data are not available, other phenothiazines readily cross the placenta and methotrimeprazine should be expected to enter the fetus.

Methotrimeprazine has been used for obstetric analgesia (1,2). The drug does not affect the force, duration, and frequency of uterine contractions, nor does it affect fetal heart tones (1,2). The manufacturer, however, has unsubstantiated data on file that methotrimeprazine may increase the rate of cervical dilation (2). No adverse effects were observed in more than 800 newborns exposed to the drug during labor (2).

In a prospective study that compared 315 women consuming phenothiazines during the 1st trimester with 11,099 non-exposed controls, malformations were observed in 11 exposed infants (3.5%) vs. 178 controls (1.6%) (3). In the phenothiazine group, methotrimeprazine was taken by 18 women, 2 of whom delivered children with defects: 1 with hydrocephalus and 1 with a cardiac malformation (type not specified).

A cause-and-effect relationship between methotrimeprazine and the defects cannot be determined from this study. However, other phenothiazines are generally considered safe for both mother and fetus if used occasionally in low doses (e.g., see Chlorpromazine) and methotrimeprazine can probably be classified similarly. Other reviewers have also concluded that the phenothiazines are not teratogenic (4,5).

BREAST FEEDING SUMMARY

RECOMMENDATION: No Human Data - Potential Toxicity

No data are available (see also Chlorpromazine).

References

1. DeKornfeld TJ, Pearson JW, Lasagna L. Methotrimeprazine in the treatment of labor pain. N Engl J Med 1964;270:391–4.
2. Levoprome: methotrimeprazine parenteral. Lederle Laboratories, December 1966:15.
3. Rumeau-Rouquette C, Goujard J, Huel G. Possible teratogenic effect of phenothiazines in human beings. Teratology 1976;15:57–64.
4. Ayd FJ Jr. Children born of mothers treated with chlorpromazine during pregnancy. Clin Med 1964;71:1758–63.
5. Ananth J. Congenital malformations with psychopharmacologic agents. Compr Psychiatry 1975;16:437–45.

Name: **METHOXAMINE** Risk Factor: C_M
Class: **Sympathomimetic (Adrenergic)**

FETAL RISK SUMMARY

RECOMMENDATION: Human Data Suggest Risk

Methoxamine is a sympathomimetic used in emergencies to treat hypotension. Because of the nature of its indications, experience with methoxamine in pregnancy is limited. Uterine vessels are normally maximally dilated and they have only α-adrenergic receptors (1). Use of the predominantly α-adrenergic stimulant, methoxamine, could cause constriction of these vessels and reduce uterine blood flow, thereby producing fetal hypoxia and bradycardia. These effects, including adverse effects on the fetal acid-base status, have been observed in pregnant ewes and monkeys at doses comparable to those used in humans (2).

Methoxamine may interact with oxytocics or ergot derivatives to produce severe persistent maternal hypertension (1). Rupture of a cerebral vessel is possible. If a pressor agent is indicated, other drugs, such as ephedrine, should be considered.

BREAST FEEDING SUMMARY

RECOMMENDATION: No Human Data - Probably Compatible

No data are available.

References

1. Smith NT, Corbascio AN. The use and misuse of pressor agents. Anesthesiology 1970;33:58–101.
2. Product information. Vasoxyl. Glaxo Wellcome, 2000.

Name: **METHOXSALEN** Risk Factor: C_M
Class: **Psoralen**

FETAL RISK SUMMARY

RECOMMENDATION: Compatible

Methoxsalen (8-methoxypsoralen), available in oral capsules and as a topical lotion, is used as a photosensitizer in conjunction with long-wave UVA radiation (PUVA) for the symptomatic control of severe psoriasis. Reproductive toxicity testing of the agent in animals has not been conducted (1). Shepard reviewed a closely related compound, 5-methoxypsoralen (5-MOP), that was not teratogenic in pregnant mice given up to 500 mg/kg/day, but was teratogenic in rabbits (type of malformations not specified) fed 70 or 560 mg/kg/day (2).

Because PUVA treatments are mutagenic, investigators, in a 1991 report, described the pregnancy outcomes among 1380 patients (892 men and 488 women) who had received the therapy (3). Of the men, 99 (11.1%) reported 167 pregnancies in their partners, whereas 94 (19.3%) of the women reported 159 pregnancies. Among the men, 34% (55 of 163; data missing for 4 pregnancies) received PUVA therapy near the time of conception. In the women, 20% (31 of 158; data missing for 1 pregnancy) received treatment at the time of conception or during pregnancy. The difference in the incidence of spontaneous abortions among those exposed (men 3.6% vs. women 12.9%) was thought to be related to reporting bias, but the total rate of abortions is no different from that expected in a nonexposed population. No congenital malformations were reported in the offspring of the exposed patients.

A 1993 publication described the outcome of 689 infants born before maternal PUVA treatment, 502 infants conceived and born after treatment, and 14 infants whose mothers had received the therapy during pregnancy (4). No difference among the three groups was noted in sex ratio, twinning, and mortality rate after birth. A significant increase in low-birth-weight infants was observed in those conceived and born after maternal treatment, an effect, the authors concluded, that may have resulted from the mother's disease. No congenital abnormalities were observed in the 14 infants exposed *in utero* to PUVA therapy. In the other two groups, 3.6% (25 of 689) and 3.2% (16 of 502) of the infants had congenital defects.

PUVA treatment occurred around the time of conception or during the 1st trimester of pregnancy (none treated after the 1st trimester) in 41 women identified by the European Network of Teratology Information Services (5). Of these cases, 32 were treated before conception and during the 1st trimester, 8 were treated only during the 1st trimester, and 1 stopped treatment 2 weeks before conception. The number of treatments was described as normal (two to three per week) in 27 cases, less than normal in 6 cases, greater than normal in 2, and unknown in 6 women. The maximum daily dose of methoxsalen was 40 mg. Four (10%) of the pregnancies terminated with a spontaneous abortion (a normal incidence), 6 were voluntarily terminated, 1 woman was lost to follow up, and 31 infants (1 set of twins) were live born. Two of the infants had low birth weights (2120 g and 2460 g), but neither was attributable to the mother's therapy or to psoriasis. No malformations were observed at birth or in the neonatal period. The sample size in this study allowed the authors to exclude a 6-fold increase in the risk for all malformations (5).

In summary, although methoxsalen combined with UVA is mutagenic, carcinogenic, and cataractogenic in humans, it does not appear to be a significant human teratogen. However, the long-term effects of *in utero* exposure to methoxsalen, such as cancer, have not been studied but warrant investigation.

BREAST FEEDING SUMMARY

RECOMMENDATION: Hold Breast Feeding

No reports describing the use of methoxsalen during breast-feeding have been located, nor is it known whether the drug is excreted into breast milk. Because the drug acts as a photosensitizer, breast feeding should be stopped and the milk discarded, probably for at least 24 hours (approximately 95% of a dose is excreted in the urine as metabolites within 24 hours [1]), if the drug is administered.

References

1. Product information. Oxsoralen. ICN Pharmaceuticals, 1995.
2. Shepard TH. *Catalog of Teratogenic Agents*. 7th ed. Baltimore, MD: Johns Hopkins University Press, 1992: 257.
3. Stern RS, Lange R. Members of The Photochemotherapy Follow-up Study. Outcomes of pregnancies among women and partners of men with a history of exposure to methoxsalen photochemotherapy (PUVA) for the treatment of psoriasis. Arch Dermatol 1991;127: 347–50.
4. Gunnarskog JG, Källén AJB, Lindelöf BG, Sigurgeirsson B. Psoralen photochemotherapy (PUVA) and pregnancy. Arch Dermatol 1993;129:320–3.
5. Garbis H, Eléfant E, Bertolotti E, Robert E, Serafini MA, Prapas N. Pregnancy outcome after periconceptional and first-trimester exposure to methoxsalen photochemotherapy. Arch Dermatol 1995;131:492–3.

Name: **METHSCOPOLAMINE** Risk Factor: **C**
Class: **Parasympatholytic (Anticholinergic)**

FETAL RISK SUMMARY

RECOMMENDATION: Limited Human Data - No Relevant Animal Data

Methscopolamine is an anticholinergic quaternary ammonium bromide derivative of scopolamine (see also Scopolamine). In a large prospective study, 2323 patients were exposed to this class of drugs during the 1st trimester, 2 of whom took methscopolamine (1). A possible association was found in the total group between this class of drugs and minor malformations.

BREAST FEEDING SUMMARY

RECOMMENDATION: No Human Data - Probably Compatible

No data are available (see also Atropine).

Reference

1. Heinonen OP, Slone D, Shapiro S. *Birth Defects and Drugs in Pregnancy*. Littleton, MA: Publishing Sciences Group, 1977:346–53.

M

Name: **METHSUXIMIDE** Risk Factor: **C**
Class: **Anticonvulsant**

FETAL RISK SUMMARY

RECOMMENDATION: Limited Human Data - No Relevant Animal Data

Methsuximide is a succinimide anticonvulsant used in the treatment of petit mal epilepsy. The use of methsuximide during the 1st trimester has been reported in only five pregnancies (1,2). No evidence of adverse fetal effects was found. Methsuximide has a much lower teratogenic potential than the oxazolidinedione class of anticonvulsants (see Trimethadione) (3,4). The succinimide anticonvulsants should be considered the anticonvulsants of choice for the treatment of petit mal epilepsy during the 1st trimester (see Ethosuximide).

BREAST FEEDING SUMMARY

RECOMMENDATION: No Human Data - Probably Compatible

No data are available.

References

1. Annegers JF, Elveback LR, Hauser WA, Kurland LT. Do anticonvulsants have a teratogenic effect? Arch Neurol 1974;31:364–73.
2. Heinonen OP, Slone D, Shapiro S. *Birth Defects and Drugs in Pregnancy*. Littleton, MA: Publishing Sciences Group, 1977:358–9.
3. Fabro S, Brown NA. Teratogenic potential of anticonvulsants. N Engl J Med 1979;300:1280–1.
4. The National Institutes of Health. Anticonvulsants found to have teratogenic potential. JAMA 1981;241:36.

Name:	**METHYCLOTHIAZIDE**	Risk Factor:	**B_M***
Class:	**Diuretic**		

FETAL RISK SUMMARY

RECOMMENDATION: Limited Human Data - Probably Compatible

Methyclothiazide is a member of the thiazide class of diuretics (see Chlorothiazide).

Reproduction studies in rats and rabbits at doses up to 4 mg/kg/day (about 20 times the maximum recommended human dose) did not observe any evidence of impaired fertility or fetal harm (1).

In general, diuretics are not recommended for the treatment of gestational hypertension because of the maternal hypovolemia characteristic of this disease.

[**Risk Factor D if used in gestational hypertension.*]

BREAST FEEDING SUMMARY

RECOMMENDATION: Limited Human Data - Probably Compatible

See Chlorothiazide.

Reference

1. Product information. Enduron. Abbott Laboratories, 2000.

M

Name:	**METHYLDOPA**	Risk Factor:	**B_M**
Class:	**Antihypertensive**		

FETAL RISK SUMMARY

RECOMMENDATION: Compatible

Methyldopa is a central acting, antiadrenergic agent used in the treatment of hypertension. It has been used frequently in pregnancy for this indication.

Reproduction studies in mice, rats, and rabbits at doses 1.4, 0.2, and 1.1 times, respectively, the maximum recommended human dose on a body surface area basis (MRHD), revealed no fetal harm (1). No impairment of fertility was noted in male or female rats at 0.2 times the MRHD. At higher doses (0.5 and 1 times the MRHD) in male rats, however, methyldopa decreased sperm count, sperm motility, the number of late spermatids, and the male fertility index (1).

Methyldopa crosses the placenta and achieves fetal concentrations similar to the maternal serum concentration (2–4). The Collaborative Perinatal Project monitored only one mother-child pair in which 1st trimester exposure to methyldopa was recorded (5). No abnormalities were found.

In a surveillance study of Michigan Medicaid recipients conducted between 1985 and 1992 involving 229,101 completed pregnancies, 242 newborns had been exposed to methyldopa during the 1st trimester (F. Rosa, personal communication, FDA, 1993). A total of 11 (4.5%) major birth defects were observed (10 expected). Specific data were available for six defect categories, including (observed/expected) 1/2 cardiovascular defects, 1/0 oral clefts, 0/0 spina bifida, 1/1 polydactyly, 0/0 limb reduction defects, and 0/1 hypospadias. These data do not support an association between the drug and congenital defects.

A decrease in intracranial volume has been reported after 1st trimester exposure to methyldopa (6,7). Children evaluated at 4 years of age showed no association between small head size and retarded mental development (8). Review of 1157 hypertensive pregnancies demonstrated no adverse effects from methyldopa administration (9–21). A reduced systolic blood pressure of 4–5 mm Hg in 24 infants for the first 2 days after delivery has been reported (22). This mild reduction in blood pressure was not considered significant. An infant born with esophageal atresia with fistula, congenital heart disease, absent left kidney, and hypospadias was exposed to methyldopa throughout gestation (23). The mother also took clomiphene early in the 1st trimester.

BREAST FEEDING SUMMARY

RECOMMENDATION: Limited Human Data - Probably Compatible

Methyldopa is excreted into breast milk in small amounts. In four lactating women taking 750–2000 mg/day, milk levels of free and conjugated methyldopa ranged from 0.1 to 0.9 μg/mL (2). A milk:plasma ratio could not be determined because simultaneous plasma levels were not obtained. The American Academy of Pediatrics classifies methyldopa as compatible with breast-feeding (24).

M

References

1. Product information. Aldomet. Merck, 2000.
2. Jones HMR, Cummings AJ. A study of the transfer of á-methyldopa to the human foetus and newborn infant. Br J Clin Pharmacol 1978;6:432–4.
3. Jones HMR, Cummings AJ, Setchell KDR, Lawson AM. Pharmacokinetics of methyldopa in neonates. Br J Clin Pharmacol 1979;8:433–40.
4. Cummings AJ, Whitelaw AGL. A study of conjugation and drug elimination in the human neonate. Br J Clin Pharmacol 1981;12:511–5.
5. Heinonen OP, Slone D, Shapiro S. *Birth Defects and Drugs in Pregnancy*. Littleton, MA: Publishing Sciences Group, 1977:372.
6. Myerscough PR. Infant growth and development after treatment of maternal hypertension. Lancet 1980;1:883.
7. Moar VA, Jefferies MA, Mutch LMM, Dunsted MK, Redman CWG. Neonatal head circumference and the treatment of maternal hypertension. Br J Obstet Gynaecol 1978;85:933–7.
8. Dunsted M, Moar VA, Redman CWG. Infant growth and development following treatment of maternal hypertension. Lancet 1980;1:705.
9. Redman CWG, Beilin LJ, Bonnar J, Ounsted MK. Fetal outcome in trial of antihypertensive treatment in pregnancy. Lancet 1976;2:753–6.
10. Hamilton M, Kopelman H. Treatment of severe hypertension with methyldopa. Br Med J 1963;1:151–5.
11. Abramowsky CR, Vegas ME, Swinehart G, Gyves MT. Decidual vasculopathy of the placenta in lupus erythematosus. N Engl J Med 1980;303:668–72.
12. Gallery EDM, Sounders DM, Hunyor SN, Gyory AZ. Randomised comparison of methyldopa and oxprenolol for treatment of hypertension in pregnancy. Br Med J 1979;1:1591–4.
13. Gyory AZ, Gallery ED, Hunyor SN. Effect of treatment of maternal hypertension with oxprenolol and α-methyldopa on plasma volume, placental and birth weights. Eighth World Congress of Cardiology, Tokyo, 1978; abstract No. 1098.
14. Arias F, Zamora J. Antihypertensive treatment and pregnancy outcome in patients with mild chronic hypertension. Obstet Gynecol 1979;53:489–94.
15. Redman CWG, Beilin LJ, Bonnar J. A trial of hypotensive treatment in pregnancy. Clin Sci Mol Med 1975;49:3–4.
16. Tcherdakoff P, Milliez P. Traitement de l'hypertension arterielle par alphamethyldopa au cours de la grossesse. Proc Premier Symposium National, Hypertension Arterielle, Cannes, 1970:207–9.
17. Lselve A, Berger R, Vial JY, Gaillard MF. Alphamethyldopa/Aldomet and reserpine/Serpasil: treatment of pregnancy hypertensions. J Med Lyon 1968; 1369–75.
18. Leather HM, Humphreys DM, Baker P, Chadd MA. A controlled trial of hypotensive agents in hypertension in pregnancy. Lancet 1968;2:488–90.
19. Hamilton H. Some aspects of the long-term treatment of severe hypertension with methyldopa. Postgrad Med J 1968;44:66–9.
20. Skacel K, Sklendvsky A, Gazarek F, Matlocha Z, Mohapl M. Therapeutic use of alpha-methyldopa in cases of late toxemia of pregnancy. Cesk Gynekol 1967;32:78–80.

21. Kincaid-Smith P, Bullen M. Prolonged use of methyldopa in severe hypertension in pregnancy. Br Med J 1966;1:274–6.
22. Whitelaw A. Maternal methyldopa treatment and neonatal blood pressure. Br Med J 1981;283:471.
23. Ylikorkala O. Congenital anomalies and clomiphene. Lancet 1975;2:1262–3.
24. Committee on Drugs, American Academy of Pediatrics. The transfer of drugs and other chemicals into human milk. Pediatrics 2001;108:776–89.

Name:	**METHYLENE BLUE**	Risk Factor:	C_M*
Class:	**Urinary Germicide/Diagnostic Dye**		

FETAL RISK SUMMARY

RECOMMENDATION: Human Data Suggest Risk in 2nd and 3rd Trimesters

Methylene blue has been administered orally for its weak urinary germicide properties or injected into the amniotic fluid to diagnose premature rupture of the membranes. For oral dosing, nine exposures in the 1st trimester have been reported (1, p. 299). No congenital abnormalities were observed. For use anytime during pregnancy, 46 exposures were reported (1, pp. 434–435). Based on three malformed infants, a possible association with malformations (type not specified) was found.

Diagnostic intra-amniotic injection of methylene blue has resulted in hemolytic anemia, hyperbilirubinemia, and methemoglobinemia in the newborn (2–11). Doses of the dye in most reports ranged from 10 to 70 mg, but in one case, 200 mg was injected into the amniotic cavity (7). Deep-blue staining of the newborn may occur after injection of the agent into the amniotic fluid (7–9,11). One author suggested that smaller doses, such as 1.6 mg, would be adequate to confirm the presence of ruptured membranes without causing hemolysis (2).

In a 1989 report, 1 mL of a 1% solution (10 mg) was used to diagnose suspected membrane rupture in a woman with premature labor at 26 weeks' gestation (12). A 920-g girl was born 18 hours later who was stained a deep blue. The clinical assessment of hypoxia was impaired by the skin color as was pulse oximetry. A transcutaneous oxygen monitor was eventually used to measure arterial blood gas so that ventilator therapy could be regulated. No evidence of hemolysis was observed. The bluish tinge persisted for more than 2 weeks despite frequent baths.

Inadvertent intrauterine injection in the 1st trimester has been reported (13). No adverse effects were reported in the full-term neonate.

Multiple ileal occlusions were found in seven newborns born to mothers with twin pregnancies, at three different medical centers, who had received diagnostic intra-amniotic methylene blue into one of the amniotic sacs at 15–17 weeks' gestation (14). The doses in these cases ranged from 10 to 30 mg. Four of the infants required surgery for intestinal obstruction, but no information was given on the other three. The authors speculated that the mechanism of the adverse effect was related either to hemolysis or to acute intestinal hypoxia secondary to methylene blue-induced release of norepinephrine and subsequent vasoconstriction (14).

In an abstract published in 1992, data on jejunal and ileal atresia in twins were reported from Australia (15). Higher risks of atresia were found in twins, compared to singletons, and in twins delivered from older mothers. When undiluted 1% methylene blue was used in one group, one twin in nine of 40 (22.5%) twin pregnancies had atresia, compared to three cases among 53 (5.7%) in those exposed to a 0.25% solution.

A third report of the above complication appeared in 1992 (16). Intra-amniotic methylene blue, 10–20 mg, was used in 86 of 89 consecutive twin pregnancies for prenatal diagnosis. No dye was used in three pregnancies for technical reasons. Jejunal atresia occurred in 17 (19%) of the pregnancies; in 15 of the affected cases, it was possible to determine that the affected fetus had been the one exposed to the dye. All of the infants required surgery to relieve the intestinal obstruction. A portion of this report also described 67 newborns that were treated for jejunal atresia, 20 of whom were one of a set of twins (16). Of the 20 newborns from twins, 18 had been exposed to methylene blue during 2nd-trimester amniocentesis. Because the incidence of jejunal atresia was much higher than expected and because the dye appears to cause the defect, the authors of the study (16) and an accompanying commentary (17) recommended avoidance of methylene blue for this purpose. The commentary also alluded to the vasoconstrictor properties of methylene blue as a possible mechanism (17).

A brief 1993 report described the use of methylene blue dye in women with twins who underwent amniocentesis in the Atlanta, Georgia, area between 1977 and 1991 (18). A total of 195 women were included, 4 (2%) of whom were administered methylene blue during the procedure. Of the eight fetuses, one had anencephaly (no association with the dye), but no cases of small intestinal atresia were observed.

A 1993 article reviewed the teratogenicity and newborn adverse effects resulting from intraamniotic injection of methylene blue (19). The most frequent adverse effects in newborns were hyperbilirubinemia, hemolytic anemia with or without Heinz body formation, blue staining of the skin, and occasionally methemoglobinemia and fetal death. Respiratory distress was also frequently observed but may have been related to other causes. The structural defects observed were jejunal-ileal atresias, but the mechanism of the bowel injury is unknown. Based on the pharmacologic properties of the dye, the most likely mechanism was thought to be vascular disruption caused by methylene blue-induced arterial constriction. However, methemoglobinemia- and hemolytic anemia-induced hypoxia causing a shunting of blood away from the intestine with resulting ischemia and atresia, or a direct toxic effect from the dye when swallowed with amniotic fluid were other possible mechanisms (19).

In summary, the intraamniotic injection of methylene blue to detect ruptured membranes should be discouraged. If indicated, other dyes, such as indigo carmine or Evans blue appear to be safer alternatives, although both have limited pregnancy data (see Indigo Carmine and Evans Blue) (19).

[*Risk Factor D if injected intraamniotically.*]

BREAST FEEDING SUMMARY

RECOMMENDATION: No Human Data - Probably Compatible

No data are available.

References

1. Heinonen OP, Slone D, Shapiro S. *Birth Defects and Drugs in Pregnancy*. Littleton, MA: Publishing Sciences Group, 1977.
2. Plunkett GD. Neonatal complications. Obstet Gynecol 1973;41:476–7.
3. Cowett RM, Hakanson DO, Kocon RW, Oh W. Untoward neonatal effect of intraamniotic administration of methylene blue. Obstet Gynecol 1976;48:74S–5S.
4. Kirsch IR, Cohen HJ. Heinz body hemolytic anemia from the use of methylene blue in neonates. J Pediatr 1980;96:276–8.
5. Crooks J. Haemolytic jaundice in a neonate after intra-amniotic injection of methylene blue. Arch Dis Child 1982;57:872–3.
6. McEnerney JK. McEnerney LN. Unfavorable neonatal outcome after intraamniotic injection of methylene blue. Obstet Gynecol 1983;61:35S–6S.

7. Serota FT, Bernbaum JC, Schwartz E. The methylene-blue baby. Lancet 1979;2:1142–3.
8. Vincer MJ, Allen AC, Evans JR, Nwaesei C, Stinson DA. Methylene-blue-induced hemolytic anemia in a neonate. CMAJ 1987;136:503–4.
9. Spahr RC, Salsburey DJ, Krissberg A, Prin W. Intraamniotic injection of methylene blue leading to methemoglobinemia in one of twins. Int J Gynaecol Obstet 1980;17:477–8.
10. Poinsot J, Guillois B, Margis D, Carlhant D, Boog G, Alix D. Neonatal hemolytic anemia after intra-amniotic injection of methylene blue. Arch Fr Pediatr 1988;45:657–60.
11. Fish WH, Chazen EM. Toxic effects of methylene blue on the fetus. Am J Dis Child 1992;146:1412–3.
12. Troche BI. The methylene-blue baby. N Engl J Med 1989;320:1756–7.
13. Katz Z, Lancet M. Inadvertent intrauterine injection of methylene blue in early pregnancy. N Engl J Med 1981;304:1427.
14. Nicolini U, Monni G. Intestinal obstruction in babies exposed in utero to methylene blue. Lancet 1990;336:1258–9.
15. Lancaster PAL, Pedisich EL, Fisher CC, Robertson RD. Intra-amniotic methylene blue and intestinal atresia in twins (abstract). J Perinat Med 1992;20(Suppl 1):262.
16. Van Der Pol JG, Wolf H, Boer K, Treffers PE, Leschot NJ, Hey HA, Vos A. Jejunal atresia related to the use of methylene blue in genetic amniocentesis in twins. Br J Obstet Gynaecol 1992;99:141–3.
17. McFadyen I. The dangers of intra-amniotic methylene blue. Br J Obstet Gynaecol 1992;99:89–90.
18. Cragan JD, Martin ML, Khoury MJ, Fernhoff PM. Dye use during amniocentesis and birth defects. Lancet 1993;341:1352.
19. Cragan JD. Teratogen update: methylene blue. Teratology 1999;60:42–48.

Name:	**METHYLERGONOVINE MALEATE**	Risk Factor:	**C**
Class:	**Oxytocic**		

FETAL RISK SUMMARY

RECOMMENDATION: Contraindicated

Methylergonovine maleate (methylergometrine maleate; methylergobasine maleate) is an ergot alkaloid derivative used in the treatment of postpartum and postabortion hemorrhage. It is contraindicated during pregnancy because it may cause sustained, tetanic uterine contractions and resulting fetal compromise.

Only one animal reproductive study has been located that has investigated the effect of methylergonovine on the fetus (1). Thirteen albino rats were administered 0.5 mg/kg intraperitoneally twice daily from the 12th through the 21st day (second half of gestation) after sperm were found in the vaginal smears of the animals (1). Three other groups received different ergot alkaloids and another group acted as controls. Three (23%) of the methylergonovine group failed to conceive or resorbed their concepti compared with an average of 17% (10 of 58) in the other three treated groups and 17% (2 of 12) in the controls. The surviving pups were not examined for congenital malformations (drug-induced anomalies not expected) but their birth weights were similar to those of pups in the control group.

The Collaborative Perinatal Project monitored 50,282 mother-child pairs, 32 of whom were exposed to ergot derivatives other than ergotamine during the 1st trimester (2). Five of this group were exposed to methylergonovine maleate; 18, to ergonovine; 5, to ergot; 3, to dihydroergotamine; and 1, to methysergide. Three children with any malformation were observed in the total group, but only one had a malformation considered easily recognizable among the 12 medical centers participating in the study. The authors concluded that, although the numbers were small, there was no evidence that these agents were teratogenic (2).

A 1979 report described the effects of methylergonovine on a woman in the first stage of labor (i.e., from onset of labor to full dilation of the cervix) at 43 weeks' gestation (3). The woman was accidentally given 0.2 mg methylergonovine IM that had been ordered for a postpartum patient. Within 20 minutes, uterine hypertonus was evident, and the fetal heart rate (FHR) decreased to 80 to 90 beats/minute with increased variability. IV epinephrine (0.5 mL of 1:1000) was administered with a rapid decline in excessive uterine activity but the FHR fell to 40 to 50 beats/minute (most likely because of epinephrine-induced vasoconstriction) before slowly returning to baseline. When uterine tetany returned, a second dose of epinephrine (1/6 mL) was required, producing similar effects on uterine activity and the FHR, but of shorter duration. A 6-pound 0.25-ounce (about 2731-g) male infant was delivered 6 hours later with Apgar scores of 5 and 7 at 1 and 5 minutes, respectively. Examinations of the infant over the next 9 months were normal.

A similar case of accidental (i.e., a dose intended for another patient) methylergonovine administration resulting in uterine hypertonus was reported in 1988 (4). The 18-year-old woman at 37 weeks' gestation in the first stage of labor with uterine contractions every 2 to 3 minutes and a partially dilated and effaced cervix received 0.2 mg methylergonovine IM. Six minutes later, the FHR fell from 150 to 70 beats/minute and uterine hypertonus was detected on palpation. Terbutaline, 0.25 mg IV reversed the fetal bradycardia but did not relax the uterus. Magnesium sulfate, 4-g IV loading dose followed by 2 g/hour, also failed to reverse the hypertonus. Adverse changes in the fetus, including loss of FHR beat-to-beat variability, late decelerations, development of tachycardia (170 beats/minute), and acidosis (scalp pH 7.12), impelled the authors to perform a cesarean section, under general anesthesia, to deliver the 7-pound 15-ounce (about 3604-g) male infant. Apgar scores were 8 and 9 at 1 and 5 minutes, respectively. At delivery, the umbilical artery blood had a pH of 7.13, confirming the diagnosis of metabolic acidosis (4). The infant did well after delivery and was discharged home at 4 days of age.

In summary, methylergonovine does not appear to be a major teratogen in either animals or humans, but the data are too limited for any conclusion. The drug is contraindicated during pregnancy because of its propensity to cause sustained, tetanic uterine contractions that result in fetal hypoxia. Because of this, it is used as an alternate drug to oxytocin for management of the third stage of labor (i.e., from delivery of the infant to delivery of the placenta) and for the treatment of postpartum or postabortion hemorrhage. Care must be taken before administering this agent to confirm that the intended recipient has delivered her fetus.

BREAST FEEDING SUMMARY

RECOMMENDATION: Compatible

Small amounts of methylergonovine are excreted into breast milk. During the first 4 days postpartum, eight lactating women (not stated whether the women were nursing) were treated with the drug, 0.125 mg orally 3 times daily, because of incomplete uterine involution (5). On the 5th postpartum day, a 0.25-mg oral dose was administered, and milk and plasma samples were collected 1 and 8 hours later. Methylergonovine concentrations in the milk were determined by radioimmunoassay. Measurable (test sensitivity 0.5 ng/mL) amounts were found in four of the eight milk samples at 1 hour (average 0.8 ng/mL; range 0.6–1.3 ng/mL) and in one sample at 8 hours (1.2 ng/mL). Seven other milk samples had detectable amounts of the drug, but the concentrations were <0.5 ng/mL. In contrast, all eight of the plasma samples had measurable drug (average 2.5 ng/mL; range 0.6–4.4 ng/mL). At 8 hours after the dose, two plasma samples had measurable drug (0.5 and 0.6 ng/mL), and one had detectable drug (<0.5 ng/mL). In the four cases at 1 hour that had measurable drug in both the plasma and milk, the milk:plasma ratio was about 0.3. Because of the lack of accumulation of methylergonovine in the plasma or milk, the authors concluded that the use of the drug during breast-feeding would not affect the infant (5).

Higher plasma, and presumably, milk–drug levels may have occurred at 3 hours after a dose based on other research conducted by these investigators (6). In this study, conducted in the same manner as the study described above but with drug levels determined on the 3rd and 6th postpartum days, maternal plasma levels of methylergonovine at 1 and 3 hours after a 0.25-mg oral dose were about 1.7 ng/mL and 2 ng/mL, respectively (5,6). The authors, however, did not believe that measurement of the higher drug levels would have changed their conclusion (5).

The effect of methylergonovine, which is structurally related to bromocriptine, a known inhibitor of prolactin secretion and human lactation, on suckling-induced release of prolactin and subsequent milk production is controversial. In a study published in 1975, 14 women received a 0.2 mg IM dose of the drug after delivery of the placenta and 15 other women acted as controls (7). Serum prolactin levels before drug administration in the two groups were 90.1 and 93.6 ng/mL, respectively. At 80 to 90 minutes after delivery, the mean serum prolactin concentration in the treated group was 141 ng/mL (difference not significant from baseline). In contrast, the level in the controls was 266 ng/mL, significantly higher than baseline and the methylergonovine group.

Similar effects of methylergonovine on prolactin release were published in a 1975 reference (8). A 0.2-mg IM dose administered on the 3rd postpartum day produced a statistically significant decrease in serum prolactin between 45 and 60 minutes after injection. At 180 minutes after the dose, the prolactin levels began to rise, but they still had not returned to baseline by 240 minutes.

In another 1975 report, 10 breast-feeding mothers in the immediate postpartum period were treated with methylergonovine, 0.2 mg orally 3 times daily for 7 days (9). A similar group of 10 breast-feeding women received no medication. Plasma prolactin concentrations in both groups were measured each morning. No significant difference between the groups in prolactin concentrations was measured with plasma levels of prolactin decreasing from a mean of 144 ng/mL (both groups) to 41 ng/mL (methylergonovine) and 37 ng/mL (controls) at 7 days. Milk let-down occurred between the 2nd and 4th postpartum day in both groups. Moreover, the mean milk volume production (estimated by infant weight gain and residual milk obtained by electric breast pump) on the 7th postpartum day was 386 mL in the treated group and 367 mL in the controls.

Contrary to the above study, two reports, one in 1976 (10) and one in 1979 (11), described the inhibitory effects of ergot derivatives on prolactin secretion and lactation. In the 1976 paper, ergonovine, an agent closely related to methylergonovine, was given to 10 women in a dose of 0.2 mg orally, 3 times daily from the 1st through the 7th postpartum day (10). None of the women nursed their infants. Six other women who were not breast feeding acted as controls. Blood samples for serum prolactin measurement were drawn each morning in both groups. Before-treatment mean serum prolactin concentrations in the ergonovine and control groups were 537 and 562 ng/mL, respectively, and on postpartum day 7 they were 89.7 and 218.0 ng/mL, respectively. Moreover, the serum prolactin concentrations were significantly lower each day than the levels in the ergonovine group. Three of the ergonovine-treated women showed progressive lactation inhibition, whereas the other seven women had painful breast engorgement and spontaneous milk let-down.

Two other women in the above study received ergonovine 0.2 mg IV before nursing on the 5th postpartum day (10). One of these women also received ergonovine, 0.2 mg orally 3 times daily, before and after the IV dose. In the woman who received both IV and oral doses, the normal rise in serum prolactin induced by suckling was abolished.

The 1979 report described the effects of methylergonovine, 0.2 mg orally 3 times daily, in 30 breast-feeding women compared with 30 nonmedicated, breast-feeding control women (11). Plasma prolactin concentrations were determined in both groups on postpartum days 1, 3, and 7. Milk yields, estimated by weighing the nursing baby before and after suckling, were determined on postpartum days 3 and 7. In the control group, mean plasma prolactin levels on days 1, 3, and 7 were 374.1, 226.2, and 166.3 ng/mL, respectively. Mean plasma prolactin levels in the treated group on these days were 352.9, 219.6, and 88.7 ng/mL, respectively. Only the levels on day 7 were statistically different (11). Milk production (in g/day) was significantly less in the treated group compared with the controls on days 3 and 7 (specific weights of milk not stated).

In summary, methylergonovine is excreted into breast milk in very small quantities. No accumulation of the drug in breast milk has been measured. This ergot derivative appears to inhibit release of prolactin, including that induced by suckling, resulting in a decreased milk production, but not to the same degree as the structurally related drug bromocriptine. The clinical significance of the lactation suppression and the exposure of the nursing infant to the drug, however, is most likely nil. This may be a result of its usual short-term use after delivery and its lower potency (on a mg-to-mg basis) as a prolactin-release inhibitor. No adverse effects attributable to methylergonovine in a nursing infant have been reported. Moreover, methylergonovine is one of the most commonly prescribed drugs during the first postpartum week.

References

1. Sommer AF, Buchanan AR. Effects of ergot alkaloids on pregnancy and lactation in the albino rat. Am J Physiol 1955;180:296–300.
2. Heinonen OP, Slone D, Shapiro S. *Birth Defects and Drugs in Pregnancy*. Littleton, MA: Publishing Sciences Group, 1977:357–65.
3. Wong R, Paul RH. Methergine-induced uterine tetany treated with epinephrine: case report. Am J Obstet Gynecol 1979;134:602–3.
4. Moise KJ Jr, Carpenter RJ Jr. Methylergonovine-induced hypertonus in term pregnancy. A case report. J Reprod Med 1988;33:771–3.
5. Erkkola R, Kanto J, Allonen H, Kleimola T, Mantyla R. Excretion of methylergometrine (methylergonovine) into the human breast milk. Int J Clin Pharmacol Biopharm 1978;16:579–80.
6. Allonen H, Juvakoski R, Kanto J, Laitinen S, Mantyla R, Kleimola T. Methylergometrine: comparison of plasma concentrations and clinical response of two brands. Int J Clin Pharmacol Biopharm 1978;16:340–2.
7. Weiss G, Klein S, Shenkman L, Kataoka K, Hollander CS. Effect of methylergonovine on puerperal prolactin secretion. Obstet Gynecol 1975;46:209–10.
8. Perez-Lopez FR, Delvoye P, Denayer P, L'Hermite M, Roncero MC, Robyn C. Effect of methylergobasine maleate on serum gonadotrophin and prolactin in humans. Acta Endocrinol 1975;79:644–57.
9. Del Pozo E, Brun Del Re R, Hinselmann M. Lack of effect of methyl-ergonovine on postpartum lactation. Am J Obstet Gynecol 1975;123:845–6.
10. Canales ES, Garrido JT, Zarate A, Mason M, Soria J. Effect of ergonovine on prolactin secretion and milk let-down. Obstet Gynecol 1976;48:228–9.
11. Peters F, Lummerich M, Breckwoldt M. Inhibition of prolactin and lactation by methylergometrine hydrogen maleate. Acta Endocrinol 1979;91:213–6.

Name:	**METHYLPHENIDATE**	Risk Factor:	**C_M**
Class:	**Central Stimulant**		

FETAL RISK SUMMARY

RECOMMENDATION: Limited Human Data - Animal Data Suggest Moderate Risk

Methylphenidate is a mild central nervous system stimulant used in the treatment of attention deficit disorders and in narcolepsy.

Reproductive testing with methylphenidate in mice found no teratogenicity (1). In rabbits, doses about 40 times the maximum recommended human dose based on body surface area (MRHD) were teratogenic (increased incidence of spina bifida) (2). The no-effect dose for embryo-fetal development was about 11 times the MRHD. No teratogenic effects were observed in rats, but a dose seven times the MRHD caused maternal toxicity and fetal skeletal variations. The no-effect dose in rats was two times the MRHD. Dosing in rats throughout gestation and lactation at four times the MRHD resulted in decreased body weight gain in the offspring. In this case, the no-effect dose was equal to the MRHD (2).

The Collaborative Perinatal Project monitored 3,082 mother-child pairs with exposure to sympathomimetic drugs, 11 of which were exposed to methylphenidate (3). No evidence for an increased malformation rate was found.

In a surveillance study of Michigan Medicaid recipients conducted between 1985 and 1992 involving 229,101 completed pregnancies, 13 newborns had been exposed to methylphenidate during the 1st trimester (F. Rosa, personal communication, FDA, 1993). One (7.7%) major birth defect was observed (one expected), a cardiovascular defect (none expected).

A report of an infant with microtia following *in utero* exposure to methylphenidate from the 3rd to the 6th week of pregnancy appeared in a 1962 publication (4). No other details of the case were provided, other than the fact that the mother did not take antinausea medication and she had no virus infection during gestation.

A 1975 report described a male infant, delivered at 30 weeks' gestation, with multiple congenital limb malformations that had been exposed during the first 7 weeks of pregnancy to haloperidol (15 mg/day), methylphenidate (30 mg/day), and phenytoin (300 mg/day) (5). The mother had also taken tetracycline and a decongestant for a cold during the 1st trimester. The infant died at 2 hours of age of a subdural hemorrhage. Limb malformations included a thumb and two fingers on each hand, syndactyly of the two fingers on the right hand, deformed radius and missing ulna in the left forearm, four toes on the right foot, shortened right tibia, and incomplete development of the right midfoot ossification centers (5). A defect of the aortic valve (bicuspid with a notch in one of the valve leaflets) was also found. The chromosomal analysis was normal and the mother had no family history of limb malformations (5).

A study published in 1993 examined the effects on the fetus and newborn of IV pentazocine and methylphenidate abuse during pregnancy (6). During a 2-year (1987–1988) period, 39 infants (38 pregnancies, 1 set of twins) were identified in the study population as being subjected to the drug abuse during gestation, a minimum incidence of 5 cases per 1000 live births. Many of the mothers had used cigarettes (34%), alcohol (71%), or abused other drugs (26%). The median duration of IV pentazocine and methylphenidate abuse was 3 years (range 1–9 years), with a median frequency of 14 injections/week (range 1–70 injections/week). Among the infants, 8 were delivered prematurely, 12 were growth retarded, and 11 had withdrawal symptoms after birth. Four of the infants had birth defects including twins with fetal alcohol syndrome, one with a ventricular septal defect, and one case of polydactyly. Of the 21 infants that had formal developmental testing, 17 had normal development and 4 had low-normal developmental quotients (6).

BREAST FEEDING SUMMARY

RECOMMENDATION: No Human Data - Potential Toxicity

No reports describing the use of methylphenidate during lactation have been located. Because of its relatively low molecular weight (about 270), passage into milk should be expected. The effects of this predicted exposure on a nursing infant are unknown.

References

1. Takano K, Tanimura T, Nishimura H. Effects of some psychoactive drugs administered to pregnant mice upon the development of their offspring. Congenital Anom 1963;3:2. As cited in Schardein JL. *Chemically Induced Birth Defects*. 2nd ed. New York, NY: Marcel Dekker, 1993:223.
2. Product information. Ritalin LA. Novartis Pharmaceuticals, 2004.
3. Heinonen OP, Slone D, Shapiro S. *Birth Defects and Drugs in Pregnancy*. Littleton, MA: Publishing Sciences Group, 1977:346–7.
4. Smithells RW. Thalidomide and malformations in Liverpool. Lancet 1962;1:1270–3.
5. Kopelman AE, McCullar FW, Heggeness L. Limb malformations following maternal use of haloperidol. JAMA 1975;231:62–4.
6. Debooy VD, Seshia MMK, Tenenbein M, Casiro OG. Intravenous pentazocine and methylphenidate abuse during pregnancy. Maternal lifestyle and infant outcome. Am J Dis Child 1993;147:1062–5.

Name:	**METHYLTESTOSTERONE**	Risk Factor:	X_M
Class:	**Androgenic Hormone Risk**		

See Testosterone.

Name:	**METOCLOPRAMIDE**	Risk Factor:	B_M
Class:	**Antiemetic/Gastrointestinal Stimulant**		

FETAL RISK SUMMARY

RECOMMENDATION: Compatible

Metoclopramide has been used during pregnancy as an antiemetic and to decrease gastric emptying time (1–24). Reproductive studies in mice, rats, and rabbits at doses up to 250 times the human dose have revealed no evidence of impaired fertility or fetal harm as a result of the drug (25). Metoclopramide (10 mg IV) in pregnant sheep increased maternal heart rate, but had no effect on maternal blood pressure, uterine blood flow, or fetal hemodynamic variables (26).

No congenital malformations or other fetal or newborn adverse effects attributable to the drug have been observed. Except for the one study noted below (7), long-term evaluation of infants exposed *in utero* to metoclopramide has not been reported.

Metoclopramide crosses the placenta at term (1–3). Cord:maternal plasma ratios were 0.57–0.84 after administration of IV doses just before cesarean section. Placental transfer during other stages of pregnancy has not been studied.

Nine reports have described the use of metoclopramide for the treatment of nausea and vomiting occurring in early pregnancy (4–7, 20–24). Administration of the drug in two of these studies was begun at 7–8 weeks' gestation (4,5) and at 6 weeks in another (6). The exact timing of pregnancy was not specified in one report (7). Daily doses ranged between 10 and 60 mg. Metoclopramide was as effective as other antiemetics for this indication and superior to placebo (8,9). Normal infant development for up to 4 years was mentioned in one study, but no details were provided (7).

In another case of metoclopramide use for nausea and vomiting, the drug was started at 10 weeks' gestation (20). Dosage was not specified. At 18 weeks, after 8 weeks of therapy, the patient developed a neuropsychiatric syndrome with acute asymmetrical axonal motor-sensory polyneuropathy and marked anxiety, depression, irritability, and memory and concentration difficulties (20). Acute porphyria was diagnosed based on the presence of increased porphyrin precursors in the patient's urine. Metoclopramide was discontinued and the patient was treated with a high-carbohydrate diet. Eventually, a normal, 3500-g infant was delivered at term. The woman recovered except for slight residual weakness in the lower extremities. The investigators speculated that the pregnancy itself, the starvation, the drug, or a combination of these may have precipitated the acute attack (20).

A 1996 report described the use of metoclopramide, droperidol, diphenhydramine, and hydroxyzine in 80 women with hyperemesis gravidarum (21). The mean gestational age at the start of treatment was 10.9. All of the women received metoclopramide 40 mg/day orally for approximately 7 days, and 12 (15%) required a second course because of the recurrence of their symptoms of nausea and vomiting. Three of the mothers (all treated in the 2nd trimester) delivered offspring with congenital defects: Poland's syndrome, fetal alcohol syndrome, and hydrocephalus and hypoplasia of the right cerebral hemisphere. Only the latter anomaly is a potential drug effect, but the most likely cause was thought to be the result of an *in utero* fetal vascular accident or infection (21).

A 2001 study, using a treatment method similar to that in the above study, described the use of droperidol and diphenhydramine in 28 women hospitalized for hyperemesis gravidarum (22). Pregnancy outcomes in the study group were compared to a historical control of 54 women who had received conventional antiemetic therapy. Oral metoclopramide and hydroxyzine were used after discharge from the hospital. Therapy was started in the study and control groups at mean gestational ages of 9.9 and 11.1 weeks', respectively. The study group appeared to have more severe disease then controls as suggested by a greater mean loss from the pre-pregnancy weight, 2.07 kg vs. 0.81 kg (*n.s.*), and a slightly lower serum potassium level, 3.4 vs. 3.5 mmol/L (*n.s.*). Compared to controls, the droperidol group had a shorter duration of hospitalization (3.53 vs. 2.82 days, $p = 0.023$), fewer readmissions (38.9% vs. 14.3%, $p = 0.025$), and lower average daily nausea and vomiting scores (both $p < 0.001$). There were no statistical differences ($p > 0.05$) in outcomes (study vs. controls) in terms of spontaneous abortions ($N = 0$ vs. $N = 2$ [4.3%]), elective abortions ($N = 3$ [12.0%] vs. $N = 3$ [6.5%]), Apgar scores at 1, 5, and 10 minutes, age at birth (37.3 vs. 37.9 weeks'), and birth weight (3114 vs. 3347 g) (22). In controls, there was one (2.4%) major malformation of unknown cause, an acardiac fetus in a set of triplets, and one newborn with a genetic defect (Turner syndrome). There was also one unexplained major birth defect (4.4%) in the droperidol group (bilateral hydronephrosis), and two genetic defects (translocation of chromosomes 3 and 7; tyrosinemia) (22).

The Pharmaco-Epidemiological Prescription Database of North Jutland County (Denmark) identified 309 women with singleton pregnancies who filled prescriptions for metoclopramide during a 6-year period (1991–1996) (23). The pregnancy outcomes of this group were compared to 13,327 women who did not receive prescriptions of any kind during pregnancy. The mean birth weights of the metoclopramide and control groups were nearly identical, 3480 g vs. 3470 g, respectively. No significant differences were found between the groups in terms of congenital malformations (odds ratio [OR] 1.11, 95% confidence interval [CI] 0.6–2.1), low birth weight (OR 1.79, 95% CI 0.8–3.9), or preterm delivery (OR 1.02, 95% CI 0.6–1.7) (23).

A brief 2000 communication examined the outcome of 126 women who had received metoclopramide for nausea and vomiting of pregnancy during the 1st trimester (24). The pregnancy outcomes of these women, who had called one of five teratogen information centers (one each in Italy and Brazil and three in Israel), were compared with a control group of 126 women who had contacted the centers for information on nonteratogenic and nonembryotoxic drug exposures, matched for age, smoking status, and alcohol use. The pregnancy outcomes were similar between the groups in terms of live births, spontaneous abortions, gestational age at delivery, rate of prematurity, birth weight, fetal distress, and major malformations. Both groups had five infants with major birth defects. In the metoclopramide group, two infants had patent ductus arteriosus, two had ventricular septal defects (VSD), and one had hypospadias. The birth defects in the infants born to the control group were two cases of VSD and one each of bilateral syndactyly of the foot, hypospadias, and an inguinal hernia. The gross motor development (as measured by the Denver Development Scale) of the infants in the two groups at ages 4 to 15 months were also similar (24).

In a surveillance study of Michigan Medicaid recipients conducted between 1985 and 1992 involving 229,101 completed pregnancies, 192 newborns had been exposed to metoclopramide during the 1st trimester (F. Rosa, personal communication, FDA, 1993). Ten (5.2%) major birth defects were observed (eight expected), including (observed/expected) 1/2 cardiovascular defects and 1/1 polydactyly. No anomalies were observed in four other defect categories (oral clefts, spina bifida, limb reduction defects, and hypospadias) for which specific data were available. These data do not support an association between the drug and congenital defects.

A 1997 case report described the signs and symptoms of acute intermittent porphyria in a 29-year-old woman at 13 weeks' gestation (27). The patient presented with abdominal pain, constipation, and vomiting and was treated with IV metoclopramide. Her symptoms worsened with treatment and included weakness of the lower extremities and a severe neuropsychiatric syndrome consisting of both autonomic and neurologic functions. Metoclopramide was stopped and she was treated with high-dose IV glucose and a high carbohydrate diet. Evaluation of urine and stool porphyrin precursors confirmed the diagnosis. She eventually delivered a normal, 2760-g infant at term. The authors concluded that the severe maternal symptoms were brought on by metoclopramide, a porphyrinogenic agent, and starvation resulting from hyperemesis (27).

Several studies have examined the effect of metoclopramide on gastric emptying time during labor for the prevention of Mendelson's syndrome (i.e., pulmonary aspiration of acid gastric contents and resulting chemical pneumonitis and pulmonary edema) (1,3, 10–16,28,29). Gastroesophageal reflux was decreased as was the gastric emptying time. The drug was effective in preventing vomiting during anesthesia. No effects were noted on the course of labor or the fetus. Apgar scores and results of neurobehavioral tests did not differ from those of controls (1,3,10,16), nor did newborn heart rates or blood pressures (1).

The effect of metoclopramide on maternal and fetal prolactin secretion during pregnancy and labor has been studied (2,17,18). The drug is a potent stimulator of prolactin release from the anterior pituitary by antagonism of hypothalamic dopaminergic receptors. However, transplacentally acquired metoclopramide did not cause an increased prolactin release from the fetal pituitary and maternal prolactin did not cross the placenta to the fetus (2,17). In two other studies, 10 mg of intravenous metoclopramide administered during labor did not affect the levels of maternal or fetal thyroid-stimulating hormone or thyroid hormones (19), or maternal growth hormone concentrations (30).

BREAST FEEDING SUMMARY

RECOMMENDATION: Limited Human Data - Potential Toxicity

Metoclopramide is excreted into breast milk. Because of ion trapping of the drug in the more acidic (as compared with plasma) milk, accumulation occurs with milk:plasma ratios of 1.8–1.9 after steady-state conditions are reached (31–33).

Several studies have examined the effect of metoclopramide as a lactation stimulant in women with inadequate or decreased milk production (31–43). One study involved 23 women who had delivered prematurely (mean gestational length, 30.4 weeks) (41). The drug, by stimulating the release of prolactin from the anterior pituitary, was effective in increasing milk production with doses of 20–45 mg/day (9,32–42). Doses of 15 mg/day were not effective (37). In one study, metoclopramide caused a shift in the amino acid composition of milk, suggesting an enhanced rate of transition from colostrum to mature milk (38). No effect on the serum levels of prolactin, thyroid-stimulating hormone, or free thyroxin was observed in nursing infants in a 1985 study of 11 women with lactational insufficiency (39). A 1994 investigation found a positive response in 78% (25 of 32) of treated women, but the increase in daily milk production was inversely correlated with maternal age (43).

The total daily dose that would be consumed by a nursing infant during the maternal use of 30 mg/day has been estimated to be 1–45 μg/kg/day (31–33). This is much less than the maximum daily dose of 500 μg/kg recommended in infants (9) or the 100 μg/kg/day dosage that has been given to premature infants (44). Metoclopramide was detected in the plasma of one of five infants whose mothers were taking 10 mg, 3 times daily (32,33). Adverse effects have been observed in only two infants, both with mild intestinal discomfort (36,37). In one case the mother was consuming 30 mg/day (36), and in the other, 45 mg/day (37).

In summary, metoclopramide apparently represents a small risk to the nursing infant with maternal doses of 45 mg or less/day. Mild adverse effects have been reported in only two nursing infants. One review has stated that the drug should not be used during breast-feeding because of the potential risks to the neonate (45), but there are no published studies to substantiate this caution. The American Academy of Pediatrics classifies metoclopramide as a drug for which the effect on a nursing infant is unknown but may be of concern because it is a dopaminergic blocking agent (46).

M

References

1. Bylsma-Howell M, Riggs KW, McMorland GH, Rurak DW, Ongley R, McErlane B, Price JDE, Axelson JE. Placental transport of metoclopramide: assessment of maternal and neonatal effects. Can Anaesth Soc J 1983;30:487–92.
2. Arvela P, Jouppila R, Kauppila A, Pakarinen A, Pelkonen O, Tuimala R. Placental transfer and hormonal effects of metoclopramide. Eur J Clin Pharmacol 1983;24:345–8.
3. Cohen SE, Jasson J, Talafre M-L, Chauvelot-Moachon L, Barrier G. Does metoclopramide decrease the volume of gastric contents in patients undergoing cesarean section? Anesthesiology 1984;61:604–7.
4. Lyonnet R, Lucchini G. Metoclopramide in obstetrics. J Med Chir Prat 1967;138:352–5.
5. Sidhu MS, Lean TH. The use of metoclopramide (Maxolon) in hyperemesis gravidarum. Proc Obstet Gynaecol Soc Singapore 1970;1:1–4.
6. Guikontes E, Spantideas A, Diakakis J. Ondansetron and hyperemesis gravidarum. Lancet 1992;340:1223.
7. Martynshin MYA, Arkhengel'skii AE. Experience in treating early toxicoses of pregnancy with metoclopramide. Akush Ginekol 1981;57:44–5.
8. Pinder RM, Brogden RN, Sawyer PR, Speight TM, Avery GS. Metoclopramide: a review of its pharmacological properties and clinical use. Drugs 1976;12:81–131.
9. Harrington RA, Hamilton CW, Brogden RN, Linkewich JA, Romankiewicz JA, Heel RC. Metoclopramide: an update review of its pharmacological properties and clinical use. Drugs 1983;25:451–94.

10. McGarry JM. A double-blind comparison of the anti-emetic effect during labour of metoclopramide and perphenazine. Br J Anaesth 1971;43: 613–5.
11. Howard FA, Sharp DS. Effect of metoclopramide on gastric emptying during labour. Br Med J 1973;1: 446–8.
12. Brock-Utne JG, Dow TGB, Welman S, Dimopoulos GE, Moshal MG. The effect of metoclopramide on the lower oesophageal sphincter in late pregnancy. Anaesth Intens Care 1978;6:26–9.
13. Hey VMF, Ostick DG. Metoclopramide and the gastro-oesophageal sphincter. Anaesthesia 1978;33: 462–5.
14. Feeney JG. Heartburn in pregnancy. Br Med J 1982; 284:1138–9.
15. Murphy DF, Nally B, Gardiner J, Unwin A. Effect of metoclopramide on gastric emptying before elective and emergency caesarean section. Br J Anaesth 1984;56:1113–6.
16. Vella L, Francis D, Houlton P, Reynolds F. Comparison of the antiemetics metoclopramide and promethazine in labour. Br Med J 1985;290: 1173–5.
17. Messinis IE, Lolis DE, Dalkalitsis N, Kanaris C, Souvatzoglou A. Effect of metoclopramide on maternal and fetal prolactin secretion during labor. Obstet Gynecol 1982;60:686–8.
18. Bohnet HG, Kato K. Prolactin secretion during pregnancy and puerperium: response to metoclopramide and interactions with placental hormones. Obstet Gynecol 1985;65:789–92.
19. Roti E, Robuschi G, Emanuele R, d'Amato L, Gnudi A, Fatone M, Benassi L, Foscolo MS, Gualerzi C, Braverman LE. Failure of metoclopramide to affect thyrotropin concentration in the term human fetus. J Clin Endocrinol Metab 1983;56:1071–5.
20. Milo R, Neuman M, Klein C, Caspi E, Arlazoroff A. Acute intermittent porphyria in pregnancy. Obstet Gynecol 1989;73:450–2.
21. Nageotte MP, Briggs GG, Towers CV, Asrat T. Droperidol and diphenhydramine in the management of hyperemesis gravidarum. Am J Obstet Gynecol 1996;174:1801–6.
22. Turcotte V, Ferreira E, Duperron L. Metoclopramide in breast milk and newborn (abstract). J Soc Obstet Gynaecol Can 2001;23:133–9.
23. Sorensen HT, Nielsen GL, Christensen K, Tage-Jensen U, Ekborn A, Baron J, and the Euromap study group. Birth outcome following maternal use of metoclopramide. Br J Clin Pharmacol 2000;49: 264–8.
24. Berkovitch M, Elbirt D, Addis A, Schuler-Faccini L, Ornoy A. Fetal effects of metoclopramide therapy for nausea and vomiting of pregnancy. N Engl J Med 2000;343:445–6.
25. Product information. Reglan. A.H. Robins, 1997.
26. Eisenach JC, Dewan DM. Metoclopramide exaggerates stress-induced tachycardia in pregnant sheep. Anesth Analg 1996;82:607–11.
27. Shenhav S, Gemer O, Sassoon E, Segal S. Acute intermittent porphyria precipitated by hyperemesis and metoclopramide treatment in pregnancy. Acta Obstet Gynecol Scand 1997;76:484–5.
28. Orr DA, Bill KM, Gillon KRW, Wilson CM, Fogarty DJ, Moore J. Effects of omeprazole, with and without metoclopramide, in elective obstetric anaesthesia. Anaesthesia 1993;48:114–9.
29. Stuart JC, Kan AF, Rowbottom SJ, Yau G, Gin T. Acid aspiration prophylaxis for emergency caesarean section. Anaesthesia 1996;51:415–21.
30. Robuschi G, Emanuele R, d'Amato L, Salvi M, Montermini M, Gnudi A, Roti E. Failure of metoclopramide to release GH in pregnant women. Horm Metab Res 1983;15:460–1.
31. Lewis PJ, Devenish C, Kahn C. Controlled trial of metoclopramide in the initiation of breast feeding. Br J Clin Pharmacol 1980;9:217, 219.
32. Pelkonen O, Arvela P, Kauppila A, Koivisto M, Kivinen S, Ylikorkala O. Metoclopramide in breast milk and newborn. Acta Physiol Scand 1982;(Suppl 502):62 (Abstract).
33. Kauppila A, Arvela P, Koivisto M, Kivinen S, Ylikorkala O, Pelkonen O. Metoclopramide and breast feeding: transfer into milk and the newborn. Eur J Clin Pharmacol 1983;25:819–23.
34. Sousa PLR. Metoclopramide and breast-feeding. Br Med J 1975;1:512.
35. Guzman V, Toscano G, Canales ES, Zarate A. Improvement of defective lactation by using oral metoclopramide. Acta Obstet Gynecol Scand 1979;58: 53–5.
36. Kauppila A, Kivinen S, Ylikorkala O. Metoclopramide increases prolactin release and milk secretion in puerperium without stimulating the secretion of thyrotropin and thyroid hormones. J Clin Endocrinol Metab 1981;52:436–9.
37. Kauppila A, Kivinen S, Ylikorkala O. A dose response relation between improved lactation and metoclopramide. Lancet 1981;1:1175–7.
38. de Gezelle H, Ooghe W, Thiery M, Dhont M. Metoclopramide and breast milk. Eur J Obstet Gynecol Reprod Biol 1983;15:31–6.
39. Kauppila A, Anunti P, Kivinen S, Koivisto M, Ruokonen A. Metoclopramide and breast feeding: efficacy and anterior pituitary responses of the mother and the child. Eur J Obstet Gynecol Reprod Biol 1985;19: 19–22.
40. Gupta AP, Gupta PK. Metoclopramide as a lactogogue. Clin Pediatr 1985;24:269–72.
41. Ehrenkranz RA, Ackerman BA. Metoclopramide effect on faltering milk production by mothers of premature infants. Pediatrics 1986;78:614–20.
42. Budd SC, Erdman SH, Long DM, Trombley SK, Udall JN Jr. Improved lactation with metoclopramide. Clin Pediatr 1993;32:53–7.
43. Toppare MF, Laleli Y, Senses DA, Kitaper F, Kaya IS, Dilmen U. Metoclopramide for breast milk production. Nutrition Res 1994;14:1019–29.
44. Sankaran K, Yeboah E, Bingham WT, Ninan A. Use of metoclopramide in preterm infants. Dev Pharmacol Ther 1982;5:114–9.
45. Lewis JH, Weingold AB. The Committee on FDA-Related Matters, American College of Gastroenterology. The use of gastrointestinal drugs during pregnancy and lactation. Am J Gastroenterol 1985;80:912–23.
46. Committee on Drugs, American Academy of Pediatrics. The transfer of drugs and other chemicals into human milk. Pediatrics 2001;108:776–89.

M

Name: **METOLAZONE** Risk Factor: **B_M***
Class: **Diuretic**

FETAL RISK SUMMARY

RECOMMENDATION: Limited Human Data - Probably Compatible

Metolazone is structurally related to the thiazide diuretics. See Chlorothiazide.

Reproduction studies in mice, rats, and rabbits at doses up to 50 mg/kg/day revealed no evidence of fetal harm (1).

In general, diuretics are not recommended for the treatment of gestational hypertension because of the maternal hypovolemia characteristic of this disease.

[*Risk Factor D is used in gestational hypertension.*]

BREAST FEEDING SUMMARY

RECOMMENDATION: Limited Human Data - Probably Compatible

See Chlorothiazide.

Reference

1. Product information. Mykrox. Medeva Pharmaceuticals, 2000.

Name: **METOPROLOL** Risk Factor: **C_M***
Class: **Sympatholytic (Antihypertensive)**

FETAL RISK SUMMARY

RECOMMENDATION: Human Data Suggest Risk in 2nd and 3rd Trimesters

Metoprolol, a cardioselective β_1-adrenergic blocking agent, has been used during pregnancy for the treatment of maternal hypertension and tachycardia (1–10). Reproductive studies in mice and rats have found no evidence of impaired fertility or teratogenicity (11). In rats, however, increases in fetal loss and decreases in neonatal survival were observed at doses up to 55.5 times the maximum daily human dose (11).

The drug readily crosses the placenta, producing approximately equal concentrations of metoprolol in maternal and fetal serum at delivery (1–3). The serum half-lives of metoprolol determined in five women during the 3rd trimester and repeated 3–5 months after delivery were similar (1.3 vs. 1.7 hours, respectively), but peak levels during pregnancy were only 20%–40% of those measured later (4). Neonatal serum levels of metoprolol increase up to 4-fold in the first 2–5 hours after birth, then decline rapidly during the next 15 hours (2,3).

No fetal malformations attributable to metoprolol have been reported, but experience during the 1st trimester is limited. Twins, exposed throughout gestation to metoprolol 200 mg/day plus other antihypertensive agents for severe maternal hypertension, were reported to be doing well at 10 months of age (7).

In a surveillance study of Michigan Medicaid recipients conducted between 1985 and 1992 involving 229,101 completed pregnancies, 52 newborns had been exposed to metoprolol during the 1st trimester (F. Rosa, personal communication, FDA, 1993). Three (5.8%) major birth defects were observed (two expected). No anomalies were observed in six defect categories (cardiovascular defects, oral clefts, spina bifida, polydactyly, limb reduction defects, and hypospadias) for which specific data were available.

A 1978 study described 101 hypertensive pregnant patients treated with metoprolol alone (57 patients) or combined with hydralazine (44 patients) compared with 97 patients treated with hydralazine alone (1). The duration of pregnancy at the start of antihypertensive treatment was 34.1 weeks (range 13–41 weeks) for the metoprolol group and 32.5 weeks (range 12–40 weeks) for the hydralazine group. The metoprolol group experienced a lower rate of perinatal mortality (2% vs. 8%) and a lower incidence of intrauterine growth retardation (11.7% vs. 16.3%). No signs or symptoms of β-blockade were noted in the fetuses or newborns in this or other studies (1,2,5).

The use of metoprolol in a pregnant patient with pheochromocytoma has been reported (5). High blood pressure had been controlled with prazosin, an α-adrenergic blocking agent, but the onset of maternal tachycardia required the addition of metoprolol during the last few weeks of pregnancy. No adverse effects were observed in the newborn.

The acute effects of metoprolol on maternal hemodynamics have been studied (12). Nine women at a mean gestational age of 36.7 ± 3.0 weeks with a diagnosis of gestational hypertension were given a single oral dose of 100 mg of metoprolol. Statistically significant ($p < 0.01$) decreases were observed in maternal heart rate, systolic and diastolic blood pressure, and cardiac output. No significant change was noted in mean blood volume or intervillous blood flow. An improvement was observed in four women for the latter parameter, but a reduction occurred in another four. The intervillous blood flow did not change in the ninth patient.

Cardiac palpitations, accompanied by lightheadedness and dyspnea but without syncope, developed in a previously healthy 33-year-old woman at 10 weeks' gestation (13). A diagnosis of ventricular tachycardia and mitral valve prolapse with mild mitral regurgitation was diagnosed at 22 weeks and treatment with metoprolol, 50 mg twice daily, was begun. Four weeks later, quinidine was added to the regimen because of recurrent palpitations. Intrauterine growth retardation (IUGR) was noted during her obstetric care and she eventually gave birth at term to a healthy, 4-pound 15-ounce (about 2242-g) newborn. Follow-up of the infant was not mentioned.

New-onset ventricular tachycardia was diagnosed in seven pregnant women among whom four were treated with metoprolol (250–450 mg/d) throughout the remainder of their pregnancy (14). Metoprolol therapy in a fifth patient did not resolve the arrhythmia and it was discontinued. Treatment was started in the 1st trimester in one, during the 2nd trimester in one, and in the 3rd trimester in two. All four were delivered at term of healthy newborns with birth weights (in grams) (daily metoprolol dose shown in parenthesis) of 3380 (250 mg), 3462 (350 mg), 3560 (250 mg), and 2535 (450 mg).

A retrospective study published in 1992 reported the follow-up of 35 very low-birth-weight (≤1500 g) infants who had been exposed *in utero* to maternal antihypertensive therapy (15). Nineteen of the infants (mean birth weight 1113 g) had been exposed to β-blockers (metoprolol $N = 15$, propranolol $N = 4$; combination with hydralazine or clonidine in 17 cases) whereas in 16 cases (mean birth weight 1102 g), other antihypertensives (hydralazine alone $N = 11$, hydralazine plus clonidine $N = 3$, hydralazine plus methyldopa $N = 1$, and diuretics $N = 1$) had been used. The metoprolol dose ranged from 100 to 200 mg/day, whereas that of hydralazine varied from 30 to 150 mg/day. The mean duration of therapy was similar in both groups (12 vs. 11 days). Among the 19 β-blocker-exposed infants, 7 died, 4 within 15 days of birth, compared with no deaths in the other group ($p = 0.006$). The authors speculated that the β-blockade might have impaired the infant's adaptation to the postnatal environment by inhibition of the sympathoadrenal system (15).

Although the use of metoprolol for maternal disease does not seem to pose a major risk to the fetus, the long-term effects of *in utero* exposure to β-blockers have not been studied. Persistent β-blockade has been observed in newborns exposed near delivery to other members of this class (see Acebutolol, Atenolol, and Nadolol). Thus, newborns exposed *in utero* to metoprolol should be closely observed during the first 24–48 hours after birth for bradycardia and other symptoms.

Some β-blockers may cause IUGR (as may have occurred in some of the cases above) and reduced placental weight, especially those lacking intrinsic sympathomimetic activity (ISA) (i.e., partial agonist). Treatment beginning early in the 2nd trimester results in the greatest weight reductions, whereas treatment restricted to the 3rd trimester primarily affects only placental weight. Metoprolol does not possess ISA. Although growth retardation is a serious concern, the benefits of maternal therapy, in some cases, might outweigh the risks to the fetus and must be judged on a case-by-case basis.

[*Risk Factor D if used in 2nd or 3rd trimesters.*]

BREAST FEEDING SUMMARY

RECOMMENDATION: Limited Human Data - Potential Toxicity

M

Metoprolol is concentrated in breast milk (1,3,16–18). Milk concentrations are approximately 3 times (range 2.0–3.7) those found simultaneously in the maternal serum (reported range 2.0–3.7). No adverse effects have been observed in nursing infants exposed to metoprolol in milk. On the basis of calculations from a 1984 study, a mother ingesting 200 mg/day of metoprolol would provide only about 225 μg in 1000 mL of her milk (3). To minimize this exposure even further, one reference suggested waiting 3–4 hours after a dose to breast-feed (18). Although these levels are probably clinically insignificant, nursing infants should be closely observed for signs or symptoms of β-blockade. The long-term effects of exposure to β-blockers from milk have not been studied but warrant evaluation. The American Academy of Pediatrics classifies metoprolol as compatible with breast-feeding (19).

References

1. Sandstrom B. Antihypertensive treatment with the adrenergic beta-receptor blocker metoprolol during pregnancy. Gynecol Invest 1978;9:195–204.
2. Lundborg P, Agren G, Ervik M, Lindeberg S, Sandstrom B. Disposition of metoprolol in the newborn. Br J Clin Pharmacol 1981;12:598–600.
3. Lindeberg S, Sandstrom B, Lundborg P, Regardh CG. Disposition of the adrenergic blocker metoprolol in the late-pregnant woman, the amniotic fluid, the cord blood and the neonate. Acta Obstet Gynecol Scand 1984;118(Suppl):61–4.
4. Hogstedt S, Lindberg B, Rane A. Increased oral clearance of metoprolol in pregnancy. Eur J Clin Pharmacol 1983;24:217–20.
5. Venuto R, Burstein P, Schneider R. Pheochromocytoma: antepartum diagnosis and management with tumor resection in the puerperium. Am J Obstet Gynecol 1984;150:431–2.
6. Robson DJ, Jeeva Ray MV, Storey GAC, Holt DW. Use of amiodarone during pregnancy. Postgrad Med J 1985;61:75–7.
7. Coen G, Cugini P, Gerlini G, Finistauri D, Cinotti GA. Successful treatment of long-lasting severe hypertension with captopril during a twin pregnancy. Nephron 1985;40:498–500.
8. Gallery EDM. Hypertension in pregnant women. Med J Aust 1985;143:23–7.
9. Hogstedt S, Lindeberg S, Axelsson O, Lindmark G, Rane A, Sandstrom B, Lindberg BS. A prospective controlled trial of metoprolol–hydralazine treatment in hypertension during pregnancy. Acta Obstet Gynecol Scand 1985;64:505–10.
10. Frishman WH, Chesner M. Beta-adrenergic blockers in pregnancy. Am Heart J 1988;115:147–52.
11. Product information. Lopressor. CibaGeneva Pharmaceuticals, 1997.

12. Suonio S, Saarikoski S, Tahvanainen K, Paakkonen A, Olkkonen H. Acute effects of dihydralazine mesylate, furosemide, and metoprolol on maternal hemodynamics in pregnancy-induced hypertension. Am J Obstet Gynecol 1985;155:122–5.
13. Braverman AC, Bromley BS, Rutherford JD. New onset ventricular tachycardia during pregnancy. Int J Cardiol 1991;33:409–12.
14. Brodsky M, Doria R, Allen B, Sato D, Thomas G, Sada M. New-onset ventricular tachycardia during pregnancy. Am Heart J 1992;123:933–41.
15. Kaaja R, Hiilesmaa V, Holma K, Jarvenpaa A-L. Maternal antihypertensive therapy with beta-blockers associated with poor outcome in very-low birthweight infants. Int J Gynecol Obstet 1992;38:195–9.
16. Sandstrom B, Regardh CG. Metoprolol excretion into breast milk. Br J Clin Pharmacol 1980;9:518–9.
17. Liedholm H, Melander A, Bitzen PO, Helm G, Lonnerholm G, Mattiasson I, Nilsson B. Accumulation of atenolol and metoprolol in human breast milk. Eur J Clin Pharmacol 1981;20:229–31.
18. Kulas J, Lunell NO, Rosing U, Steen B, Rane A. Atenolol and metoprolol. A comparison of their excretion into human breast milk. Acta Obstet Scand 1984;118(Suppl):65–9.
19. Committee on Drugs, American Academy of Pediatrics. The transfer of drugs and other chemicals into human milk. Pediatrics 2001;108:776–89.

Name: **METRIZAMIDE** Risk Factor: **D**

Class: **Diagnostic**

FETAL RISK SUMMARY

RECOMMENDATION: Human Data Suggests Risk in 2nd and 3rd Trimesters

Metrizamide contains a high concentration of organically bound iodine. See Diatrizoate for possible effects on the fetus and newborn.

BREAST FEEDING SUMMARY

RECOMMENDATION: Limited Human Data - Probably Compatible

Metrizamide is excreted into milk in small quantities (1). A woman was injected with 5.06 g of metrizamide into the subarachnoid space. Milk levels increased linearly with time, but only 1.1 mg (0.02%) of the dose was recovered in 44.3 hours. This amount of contrast media probably does not pose a risk to the nursing infant. The American Academy of Pediatrics classifies metrizamide as compatible with breast-feeding (2).

References

1. Ilett KF, Hackett LP, Paterson JW, McCormick CC. Excretion of metrizamide in milk. Br J Radiol 1981;54:537–8.
2. Committee on Drugs, American Academy of Pediatrics. The transfer of drugs and other chemicals into human milk. Pediatrics 2001;108:776–89.

Name: **METRIZOATE** Risk Factor: **D**

Class: **Diagnostic**

FETAL RISK SUMMARY

RECOMMENDATION: Human Data Suggest Risk in 2nd and 3rd Trimesters

Metrizoate has been used for phlebography during pregnancy for the diagnosis of deep vein thrombosis (1). Seventeen pregnant women were given either metrizoate or iothalamate at various stages of gestation. Two patients, one exposed in the 1st trimester and one in the 2nd trimester, were diagnosed as having a thrombosis and were treated with heparin. Although the baby of the mother exposed in the 2nd trimester was normal, the other newborn had hyperbilirubinemia and undescended testis. The relationship between the diagnostic agents and the defect is unknown.

Use of organically bound iodine preparations near term has resulted in hypothyroidism in some newborns (see Diatrizoate). Appropriate measures should be taken to treat neonatal hypothyroidism if diagnostic tests with metrizoate are required close to delivery.

BREAST FEEDING SUMMARY

RECOMMENDATION: Limited Human Data - Probably Compatible

Metrizoate is excreted into breast milk. Two lactating women received the IV contrast media (1 mL/kg, 350 mg iodine/mL) in the postpartum period (1 week; 4 weeks) (2). Breast-feeding was suspended for 48 hours. The amount excreted over a 24-hour period was 0.3% of the maternal weight adjusted dose. This amount does not appear to be clinically significant (2). The American Academy of Pediatrics classifies metrizoate as compatible with breast-feeding (3).

References

1. Kierkegaard A. Incidence and diagnosis of deep vein thrombosis associated with pregnancy. Acta Obstet Gynecol Scand 1983;62:239–43.
2. Nielsen ST, Matheson I, Rasmussen JN, Skinnemoen K, Andrew E, Hafsahl G. Excretion of iohexol and metrizoate in human breast milk. Acta Radiol 1987;28:523–6.
3. Committee on Drugs, American Academy of Pediatrics. The transfer of drugs and other chemicals into human milk. Pediatrics 2001;108:776–89.

M

Name: **METRONIDAZOLE**	Risk Factor:	$\mathbf{B_M}$
Class: **Anti-infective/Amebicide/Trichomonacide**		

FETAL RISK SUMMARY

RECOMMENDATION: Human Data Suggest Low Risk

Metronidazole possesses trichomonacidal and amebicidal activity as well as effectiveness against certain bacteria. The drug crosses the placenta to the fetus throughout gestation with a cord:maternal plasma ratio at term of approximately 1.0 (1–3). The pharmacokinetics of metronidazole in pregnant women have been reported (4,5).

Reproduction studies have been conducted in mice (at oral doses about 0.1 times the human dose) and in rats (at doses up to 5 times the human dose) have revealed no fetal harm (6). After intraperitoneal administration in mice, however, some fetal deaths were noted (6).

The use of metronidazole in pregnancy is controversial. The drug is mutagenic in bacteria and carcinogenic in rodents, and although these properties have never been shown in humans, concern for these toxicities have led some to advise against the use of metronidazole in pregnancy (7,8). However, no association with human cancer has been proven (8,9).

A 1995 case report described a 32-year-old woman who was treated with metronidazole during the 12th and 13th weeks of pregnancy with 500 mg/day orally plus 500 mg/day intravaginally for 10 days (10). She eventually delivered an apparently normal, 3640-g male infant at term. Fifteen days later, the infant was diagnosed with adrenal neuroblastoma with hepatic metastasis (eventual outcome not mentioned). The authors acknowledged that neuroblastoma was the second most common malignant solid tumor in childhood and that a causal relationship between the tumor and metronidazole in this case could not be established (10).

A retrospective cohort study of childhood cancer and *in utero* exposure to metronidazole was reported in 1998 (11). The cohort included 328,846 children younger than 5 years of age who had been born to women (ages 15 to 44 years) enrolled from 1975 through 1992 in Tennessee Medicaid at any time between the last menstrual period and the date of delivery. Exposure to metronidazole was based on Medicaid pharmacy prescription records. A statewide childhood cancer database was developed to identify study cases. In the cohort, 8.1% were exposed *in utero* to metronidazole and 91.9% were not exposed. From 952 children younger than 5 years of age in the cancer database, 175 met the criteria for the study (first primary cancer before age 5 years, a Tennessee resident, and seen at a Tennessee hospital at the time of diagnosis) (11). The study was limited to children under the age of 5 years to minimize the loss to out-of-state migration (expected to be no more than 6% [12]). None of the study cases had a history of therapeutic radiation or exposure to chemotherapy before their cancer diagnosis. The cancer type, number of cases, adjusted relative risk (RR), and 95% confidence interval (95% CI) were, for all cancers: $N = 175$, RR 0.81, 95% CI 0.41–1.59; for leukemia: $N = 42$, no exposed cases; for central nervous system tumors: $N = 30$, RR 1.23, 95% CI 0.29–5.21; for neuroblastoma: $N = 28$, RR 2.60, 95% CI 0.89–7.59; and other cancers: $N = 75$, RR 0.57, 95% CI 0.18–1.82. Although none of the observed relative risks were statistically significant, the authors stated that the increased risk for neuroblastoma needed further evaluation (11).

M

In a brief comment, other investigators agreed with the conclusions of the above study but expressed concern that the frequent use of medications during pregnancy combined with the rarity of childhood cancer made it difficult to establish a carcinogenic effect (12). In addition, limiting the study to children younger than 5 years of age prevented the identification of potential effects on later developing cancers such as Hodgkin's disease, Ewing's sarcoma, and osteosarcoma (12).

Several studies, individual case reports, and reviews have described the safe use of metronidazole during pregnancy (13–27). Included among these is a 1972 review summarizing 20 years of experience with the drug and involving 1469 pregnant women, 206 of whom were treated during the 1st trimester (27). No association with congenital malformations, abortions, or stillbirths was found. Some investigations, however, have found an increased risk when the agent was used early in pregnancy (9,28–30).

In a 1979 report, metronidazole was used in 57 pregnancies including 23 during the 1st trimester (9). Three of the 1st trimester exposures ended in spontaneous abortion (a normal incidence), and in the remaining 20 births, there were five congenital anomalies: hydrocele (two), congenital dislocated hip (female twin), metatarsus varus, and mental retardation (both parents mentally retarded). Analysis of the data is not possible because of the small numbers and possible involvement of genetic factors (9).

The Collaborative Perinatal Project monitored 50,282 mother-child pairs, 31 of whom had 1st trimester exposure to metronidazole (28). A possible association with malformations was found (RR 2.02) based on defects in four children, but independent confirmation is required.

Two mothers, treated with metronidazole during the 5th–7th weeks of gestation for amebiasis, gave birth to infants with midline facial defects (29). Diiodohydroxyquinoline was also used in one of the pregnancies. One of the infants had holotelencephaly and one had unilateral cleft lip and palate.

A mother treated for trichomoniasis between the 6th and 7th weeks of gestation gave birth to a male infant with a cleft of the hard and soft palate, optic atrophy, a hypoplastic, short philtrum, and a Sydney crease on the left hand (30). The mother was also taking an antiemetic medication (Bendectin) on an "as needed" basis. Chromosomal analysis of the infant was normal. The relationship between metronidazole and the defects is unknown.

As of May 1987, the FDA had received reports of 27 adverse outcomes associated with use of metronidazole: spontaneous abortions ($N = 3$), brain defects ($N = 6$), limb defects ($N = 5$), genital defects ($N = 3$), unspecified defects ($N = 3$), and 1 each of craniostenosis, peripheral neuropathy, ventricular septal defect, retinoblastoma, obstructive uropathy, and a chromosomal defect (31). In this same report, the authors, from data obtained from the Michigan Medicaid program between 1980 and 1983, cited 1,020 other cases in which metronidazole use in the 1st trimester for treatment of vaginitis was not linked with birth defects. In an additional 63 cases, use of the agent for this indication was linked to a birth defect diagnosis. On the basis of these data, the estimated RR of a birth defect was 0.92 (95% CI 0.7–1.2) (31). Of the 122 infants with oral clefts, none was exposed to metronidazole. An estimated RR for spontaneous abortion of 1.67 (95% CI 1.4–2.0) was determined from 135 exposures among 4,264 spontaneous abortions compared to 1020 exposures among 55,736 deliveries.

In a continuation of the study cited immediately above, 229,101 completed pregnancies of Michigan Medicaid recipients were evaluated between 1985 and 1992 (F. Rosa, personal communication, FDA, 1993). Of this group, 2,445 newborns had been exposed to metronidazole during the 1st trimester. A total of 100 (4.1%) major birth defects were observed (97 expected). Specific data were available for six defect categories, including (observed/expected) 23/24 cardiovascular defects, 1/1 spina bifida, 4/7 polydactyly, 2/4 limb reduction defects, 7/6 hypospadias, and 8/4 oral clefts. Only with oral clefts is there a suggestion of a possible association, but in view of the outcomes observed between 1980 and 1983, other factors, such as the mother's disease, concurrent drug use, and chance, are probably involved.

Using data from the Tennessee Medicaid program, pregnancy outcomes of women ($N = 1,307$) who had filled a prescription for metronidazole between 30 days before and 120 days after the onset of their last normal menstrual period were compared with those of women who had not filled such a prescription (32). The groups were matched for age, race, year of delivery, and hospital. Data were available for 1322 exposed (1318 livebirths; 4 stillbirths) and 1328 nonexposed (1320 livebirths; 8 stillbirths) infants. The occurrence of birth defects was similar in the two groups; 96 in the exposed group and 80 in the nonexposed group (adjusted odds ratio [OR] 1.2; 95% CI 0.9–1.6). Similar results were obtained when congenital malformations were analyzed by specific types, including those of the central nervous system, heart, gastrointestinal tract, musculoskeletal system, urogenital system, respiratory tract, chromosomal, and by multiple organ systems. The investigators concluded that the use of metronidazole was not associated with an increased risk for birth defects (32).

A study published in 1995 conducted a meta-analysis of seven studies (from a total of 32 references identified in their search) that met their criteria for assessing the safety of metronidazole use in human pregnancy (33). The criteria required exposure during the 1st trimester and comparison of these outcomes to the outcomes of pregnancies that were not exposed or only exposed during the 3rd trimester. Six of the studies were prospective and one was retrospective. The OR (exposure vs. no exposure during the 1st trimester) for the seven studies was 0.93 (95% CI 0.73–1.18) and, for the six prospective studies, 1.02 (95% CI 0.48–2.18). Based on these findings, the investigators concluded that the use of metronidazole during the 1st trimester was not associated with an increase risk of congenital defects (33).

A second meta-analysis, similar in design to that of the study described above, evaluated the risk for birth defects after the use of metronidazole early in pregnancy (34). Five studies, one unpublished case-control and four published cohort studies, met the inclusion criteria. As in the study immediately above, the OR 1.08 (95% CI 0.90–1.29) indicated that exposure to metronidazole during the 1st trimester was not associated with birth defects (34).

A large ethnically homogeneous population-based dataset (Hungarian Case-Control Surveillance of Congenital Abnormalities, 1980–1991) was used in a study published in 1998 to evaluate whether the use of metronidazole in the 1st trimester was associated with congenital anomalies (35). The background rate of congenital malformations in the dataset was 4.0%–4.7% (liveborn, stillborn, and selectively terminated fetuses). Minor abnormalities and congenital abnormality syndromes of known origin were excluded. Among 17,300 cases with birth defects, 665 (3.8%) were treated with metronidazole (oral and IV) in the 2nd to 3rd months of gestation (dating from last menstrual period). In comparison, among 30,663 matched controls, 1,041 (3.4%) were treated with metronidazole (oral and IV) during this period of gestation. Using the McNemar analysis of case-control pairs, the only defect with a positive association was cleft lip ± palate (nine cases) (adjusted OR 8.54, 95% CI 1.06–68.86). The investigators concluded that the most likely reasons for the association were recall bias or chance alone, but that a true association could not be ruled out. However, because of the prevalence of isolated cleft lip (with or without cleft palate) in their population and the prevalence of exposure to metronidazole during the 2nd and 3rd months of pregnancy, their analysis suggested that even a true association would increase the prevalence of the defect from 100 cases/100,000 births to only 103 cases/100,000 births. Moreover, the finding was not confirmed when the comparison was made with the total control group (35).

A population-based cohort study on the use of metronidazole during pregnancy from 1991 to 1996 was conducted in Denmark and reported in 1999 (36). An estimated 35,000 pregnancies were used in the risk analysis for the specific outcomes of congenital abnormalities, low birth weight (<2500 g) and preterm birth (<37 weeks). Data on the use of metronidazole were determined from a prescription data base and classified as either exposure from 30 days before conception to the end of the 1st trimester (group 1) or during the 2nd and 3rd trimesters (group 2). A total of 138 prescriptions to the agent were obtained by 124 women during the study period. A control group of 13,327 pregnancies was used for comparison. Outcome data were determined independently from exposure information. On the basis of the prevalence rates of congenital anomalies in the exposed (group 1) and control groups of 2.4% and 5.2%, respectively, no increased risk for malformations was found (OR 0.44, 95% CI 0.11–1.81). The two birth defects in group 1 were transpositio vasorum with ventricular septum defect and hypertelorism. Preterm birth occurred in 6 of the 124 exposed women (4.8%) and in 793 of 13,327 controls (6.0%) (adjusted OR 0.80, 95% CI 0.35–1.83). After adjustment for maternal age, birth order, gestational age, and smoking, there was no difference in mean birth weight between those exposed and the controls (36). The investigators acknowledged the major limitations of their study: low statistical power owing to the small number of exposed subjects; the inability to control

M

for potentially confounding factors; and the lack of information on spontaneous abortions and fetuses aborted for prenatal diagnosis of malformations. They concluded, however, that their results showed no evidence of major teratogenicity and no indication for the termination of pregnancies because of exposure to metronidazole (36).

Metronidazole has been shown to markedly potentiate the fetotoxicity and teratogenicity of alcohol in mice (37). Human studies of this possibly clinically significant interaction have not been reported.

A 2001 prospective, controlled cohort study evaluated the pregnancy outcomes of 217 women exposed to metronidazole (86.2% exposed in 1st trimester) (38). The women had consulted a Teratogen Information Service concerning their exposure to the drug. A matched control group consisted of 612 women who had called about nonteratogenic exposures. There were no statistical differences between the groups in terms of spontaneous abortions (7.8% vs. 7.2%), stillbirths (0.0% vs. 0.2%), preterm delivery (6.8% vs. 5.7%), or rate of major birth defects (2.6% vs. 2.1%). However, exposed cases had a lower birth weight than controls (3253 g vs. 3375 g, $p = 0.004$) (38).

A number of reports have described the use of metronidazole in pregnant women with bacterial vaginosis in attempts to reduce the incidence of preterm births (39–49). A 1994 randomized, double-blind, placebo-controlled study found that two courses of oral metronidazole (400 mg twice daily for 2 days) administered at 24 and 29 weeks' gestation, respectively, were effective in suppressing *Gardnerella vaginalis* for 2–3 months in the majority of women with bacterial vaginosis (39).

M

A prospective, randomized, double-blind, placebo-controlled study first published in abstract form in 1993 (40) and then in full in 1994 (41) compared a 7-day course of oral metronidazole (750 mg/d) to a 7-day course of placebo in women with bacterial vaginosis and a history of preterm birth (<37 weeks' gestation) in the preceding pregnancy from either idiopathic preterm labor or premature rupture of membranes. The women were enrolled between 13 and 20 weeks' gestation. Compared to the placebo group ($N = 36$), the pregnancy outcomes of the active drug group ($N = 44$) included significantly fewer admissions for preterm labor (27% vs. 78%, $p < 0.05$), fewer preterm births (18% vs. 39%, $p < 0.05$), fewer newborns with birth weight <2500 g (14% vs. 33%, $p < 0.05$), and fewer cases of premature rupture of membranes (5% vs. 33%, $p < 0.05$) (41).

Another prospective randomized, double-blind, placebo-controlled study first published in abstract form in 1993 (42) and then in full in 1995 (43) described the effect of a 7-day course of oral metronidazole (750 mg/d) combined with a 14-day course of oral erythromycin base (999 mg/d) in pregnant women at increased risk for preterm delivery (based on a history of spontaneous preterm delivery or pre-pregnancy body weight less than 50 kg) (43). At enrollment (at a mean 23 weeks' gestation for both groups), 41% of the 433 women in the active drug group had bacterial vaginosis compared to 46% of the 191 women receiving placebo. If a second examination (at a mean 27.6 weeks' gestation for both groups) revealed bacterial vaginosis, a second course of active drugs or placebo were administered. Eight women were lost to follow-up. A total of 110 women (26%) in the active group delivered preterm (<37 weeks) compared to 68 women (36%) in the placebo group ($p = 0.01$). However, the rates of preterm delivery in those without bacterial vaginosis were nearly identical (22% in the active drug group vs. 25% in the placebo group, $p = 0.55$). In contrast, in those with bacterial vaginosis, the rates of preterm delivery were 31% for the active drug group compared to 49% in those receiving placebo $p = 0.006$. The positive association with anti-infective treatment existed both for women with a history of preterm birth (39% vs. 57%, $p = 0.02$) and pre-pregnancy body weight of less than 50 kg (14% vs. 33%, $p = 0.04$) (43).

A 1997 randomized, placebo-controlled also found that the beneficial effect of a 2-day course of oral metronidazole (400 mg twice daily) on prolonging pregnancy was restricted to those women with bacterial vaginosis and a previous history of spontaneous preterm birth (44). Metronidazole therapy was started at 24 weeks' gestation and repeated at 29 weeks if *G. vaginalis* was still present.

Another 1997 randomized, double-blind, placebo-controlled study administered a combination of metronidazole and ampicillin to 59 women and placebo to 51 women (45). The subjects in both groups had threatened idiopathic preterm labor and intact membranes. The anti-infective regimen was an 8-day course of metronidazole (500 mg IV every 8 hours for 24 hours, then 400 mg orally every 8 hours for 7 days) and ampicillin (2 g IV every 6 hours for 24 hours, then pivampicillin 500 mg orally every 8 hours for 7 days). The women were enrolled in the study at 26 to 34 weeks' gestation from six clinics in the Copenhagen area. Treatment with the anti-infectives was associated with prolongation of gestation (47.5 days vs. 27 days, $p < 0.05$), higher gestational age at birth (37 weeks vs. 34 weeks, $p < 0.05$), reduced preterm birth rate (40% vs. 63%, $p < 0.05$), and a lower rate of admission to neonatal intensive care unit (40% vs. 63%, $p < 0.05$) (44). The incidences of maternal (5% vs. 0%, $p = 0.30$) and neonatal (10% vs. 22%, $p = 0.18$) infectious morbidity, however, were statistically similar between the groups. In four other reports, all from the same source, gestational metronidazole treatment of women with asymptomatic bacterial vaginosis, but without a history of previous preterm birth, either did not reduce the risk of preterm birth (46–48), or increased the risk for that outcome (49).

Metronidazole was not effective in preventing preterm delivery among pregnant women with asymptomatic *Trichomonas vaginalis* infection in a 2001 report (50). Women were screened for the infection at 16–23 weeks' gestation and then randomized to either metronidazole ($N = 320$) or placebo ($N = 297$). The metronidazole group received two 2-g doses 48 hours apart at randomization and then again at 24–29 weeks' gestation. Preterm delivery (<37 weeks') occurred in 19% of the treated group and about 11% of the controls (50).

In summary, although some of the available reports have arrived at conflicting conclusions as to the safety of metronidazole in pregnancy, the majority of the published evidence suggests that the anti-infective does not represent a significant risk of structural defects to the fetus. At present, it is not possible to assess the risk to the fetus from the carcinogenic potential of metronidazole. The answer to the question of transplacental carcinogenic potential of metronidazole has major public health implications, but may never be answered because of the rarity of childhood cancers and the inability to identify potentially confounding environmental factors in older children and adults. The manufacturer considers metronidazole to be contraindicated during the 1st trimester in patients with trichomoniasis or bacterial vaginosis (6). The use of metronidazole for trichomoniasis or vaginosis during the 2nd and 3rd trimesters is acceptable. For other indications, metronidazole can be used during pregnancy if there are no other alternatives with established safety profiles.

BREAST FEEDING SUMMARY

RECOMMENDATION: **Hold Breast Feeding (Single Dose)**
Limited Human Data - Potential Toxicity (Divided Dose)

Metronidazole is excreted into breast milk. Following a single 2-g oral dose in three patients, peak milk concentrations in the 50–60 μg/mL range were measured at

2–4 hours (51). With normal breast-feeding, infants would have received about 25 mg of metronidazole during the next 48 hours. By interrupting feedings for 12 hours, infant exposure to the drug would have been reduced to 9.8 mg, or 3.5 mg if feeding had been stopped for 24 hours (51).

In women treated with divided oral doses of either 600 or 1200 mg/day, the mean milk levels were 5.7 and 14.4 μg/mL, respectively (52). The milk:plasma ratios in both groups were approximately 1.0. The mean plasma concentrations in the exposed infants were about 20% of the maternal plasma drug level. Eight women treated with metronidazole rectal suppositories, 1 g every 8 hours, produced a mean milk drug level of 10 μg/mL with maximum concentrations of 25 μg/mL (53).

One report described diarrhea and secondary lactose intolerance in a breast-fed infant whose mother was receiving metronidazole (54). The relationship between the drug and the events is unknown. Except for this one case, no reports of adverse effects in metronidazole-exposed nursing infants have been located. However, because the drug is mutagenic and carcinogenic in some test species (see Fetal Risk Summary), unnecessary exposure to metronidazole should be avoided.

If a single, 2-g oral dose of metronidazole is used for treating trichomoniasis, the American Academy of Pediatrics recommends discontinuing breast-feeding for 12–24 hours to allow excretion of the drug (55).

References

1. Amon K, Amon I, Huller H. Maternal-fetal passage of metronidazole. In *Advances in Antimicrobial and Antineoplastic Chemotherapy*. Proceedings of the VII International Congress of Chemotherapy, Prague, 1971:113–5.
2. Heisterberg L. Placental transfer of metronidazole in the first trimester of pregnancy. J Perinat Med 1984;12:43–5.
3. Karhunen M. Placental transfer of metronidazole and tinidazole in early human pregnancy after a single infusion. Br J Clin Pharmacol 1984;18:254–7.
4. Amon I, Amon K, Franke G, Mohr C. Pharmacokinetics of metronidazole in pregnant women. Chemotherapy 1981;27:73–9.
5. Visser AA, Hundt HKL. The pharmacokinetics of a single intravenous dose of metronidazole in pregnant patients. J Antimicrob Chemother 1984;13: 279–83.
6. Product information. Flagyl. G.D. Searle, 2000.
7. Anonymous. Is Flagyl dangerous? Med Lett Drugs Ther 1975;17:53–4.
8. Finegold SM. Metronidazole. Ann Intern Med 1980; 93:585–7.
9. Beard CM, Noller KL, O'Fallon WM, Kurland LT, Dockerty MB. Lack of evidence for cancer due to use of metronidazole. N Engl J Med 1979;301:519–22.
10. Carvajal A, Sanchez A, Hurtarte G. Metronidazole during pregnancy. Int J Gynecol Obstet 1995;48: 323–4.
11. Thapa PB, Whitlock JA, Brockman Worrell KG, Gideon P, Mitchel EF Jr, Roberson P, Pais R, Ray WA. Prenatal exposure to metronidazole and risk of childhood cancer. A retrospective cohort study of children younger than 5 years. Cancer 1998;83:1461–8.
12. Berbel-Tornero O, Lopez-Andreu JA, Ferris-Tortajada J. Prenatal exposure to metronidazole and risk of childhood cancer. A retrospective cohort study of children younger than 5 years. Cancer 1999;85:2494–5.
13. Gray MS. Trichomonas vaginalis in pregnancy: the results of metronidazole therapy on the mother and child. J Obstet Gynaecol Br Commonw 1961;68: 723–9.
14. Robinson SC, Johnston DW. Observations on vaginal trichomoniasis. II. Treatment with metronidazole. Can Med Assoc J 1961;85:1094–6.
15. Luthra R, Boyd JR. The treatment of trichomoniasis with metronidazole. Am J Obstet Gynecol 1962;83:1288–93.
16. Schram M, Kleinman H. Use of metronidazole in the treatment of trichomoniasis. Am J Obstet Gynecol 1962;83:1284–7.
17. Andrews MC, Andrews WC. Systemic treatment of trichomonas vaginitis. South Med J 1963;56: 1214–8.
18. Zacharias LF, Salzer RB, Gunn JC, Dierksheide EB. Trichomoniasis and metronidazole. Am J Obstet Gynecol 1963;86:748–52.
19. Kotcher E, Frick CA, Giesel LO, Jr. The effect of metronidazole on vaginal microbiology and maternal and neonatal hematology. Am J Obstet Gynecol 1964;88:184–9.
20. Scott-Gray M. Metronidazole in obstetric practice. J Obstet Gynaecol Br Commonw 1964;71:82–5.
21. Perl G. Metronidazole treatment of trichomoniasis in pregnancy. Obstet Gynecol 1965;25:273–6.
22. Peterson WF, Stauch JE, Ryder CD. Metronidazole in pregnancy. Am J Obstet Gynecol 1966;94:343–9.
23. Robinson SC, Mirchandani G. Trichomonas vaginalis. V. Further observations on metronidazole (Flagyl) (including infant follow-up). Am J Obstet Gynecol 1965;93:502–5.
24. Mitchell RW, Teare AJ. Amoebic liver abscess in

pregnancy. Case reports. Br J Obstet Gynaecol 1984;91:393–5.
25. Morgan I. Metronidazole treatment in pregnancy. Int J Gynaecol Obstet 1978;15:501–2.
26. Sands RX. Pregnancy, trichomoniasis, and metronidazole. Am J Obstet Gynecol 1966;94:350–3.
27. Berget A, Weber T. Metronidazole and pregnancy. Ugeskr Laeger 1972;134:2085–9. As cited in Shepard TH. *Catalog of Teratogenic Agents*. 6th ed. Baltimore, MD: Johns Hopkins University Press, 1989: 426.
28. Heinonen OP, Slone D, Shapiro S. *Birth Defects and Drugs in Pregnancy*. Littleton, MA: Publishing Sciences Group, 1977:298, 299, 302.
29. Cantu JM, Garcia-Cruz D. Midline facial defect as a teratogenic effect of metronidazole. Birth Defects 1982;18:85–8.
30. Greenberg F. Possible metronidazole teratogenicity and clefting. Am J Med Genet 1985;22:825.
31. Rosa FW, Baum C, Shaw M. Pregnancy outcomes after first-trimester vaginitis drug therapy. Obstet Gynecol 1987;69:751–5.
32. Piper JM, Mitchel EF, Ray WA. Prenatal use of metronidazole and birth defects: no association. Obstet Gynecol 1993;82:348–52.
33. Burtin P, Taddio A, Ariburnu O, Einarson TR, Koren G. Safety of metronidazole in pregnancy: a meta-analysis. Am J Obstet Gynecol 1995;172: 525–9.
34. Caro-Paton T, Carvajal A, Martin de Diego I, Martin-Arias LH, Alvarez Requejo A, Rodriguez Pinilla E. Is metronidazole teratogenic? A meta-analysis. Br J Clin Pharmacol 1997;44:179–82.
35. Czeizel AE, Rockenbauer M. A population based case-control teratologic study of oral metronidazole treatment during pregnancy. Br J Obstet Gynaecol 1998;105:322–7.
36. Sorensen HT, Larsen H, Jensen ES, Thulstrup AM, Schonheyder HC, Nielsen GL, Czeizel A, and the EUROMAP Study Group. Safety of metronidazole during pregnancy: a cohort study of risk of congenital abnormalities, preterm delivery and low birth weight in 124 women. J Antimicrob Chemother 1999;44: 854–5.
37. Damjanov I. Metronidazole and alcohol in pregnancy. JAMA 1986;256:472.
38. Diav-Citrin O, Shechtman S, Gotteiner T, Arnon J, Ornoy A. Pregnancy outcome after gestational exposure to metronidazole: a prospective controlled cohort study. Teratology 2001;63:186–92.
39. McDonald HM, O'Loughlin JA, Vigneswaran R, Jolley PT, McDonald PJ. Bacterial vaginosis in pregnancy and efficacy of short-course oral metronidazole treatment: a randomized controlled trial. Obstet Gynecol 1994;84:343–8.
40. Morales WJ, Schorr S, Albritton J. Effect of metronidazole in patients with history of preterm birth and bacterial vaginosis: a placebo control double blind study (abstract). Am J Obstet Gynecol 1993;168: 377.
41. Morales WJ, Schorr S, Albritton J. Effect of metronidazole in patients with preterm birth in preceding pregnancy and bacterial vaginosis: a placebo-controlled, double-blind study. Am J Obstet Gynecol 1994;171:345–9.
42. Hauth J, Goldenberg R, Andrews W, Copper R, Schmid T. Efficacy of metronidazole plus erythromycin to decrease bacterial vaginosis and other markers of altered vaginal flora (abstract). Am J Obstet Gynecol 1993;168:421.
43. Hauth JC, Goldenberg RL, Andrews WW, DuBard MB, Copper RL. Reduced incidence of preterm delivery with metronidazole and erythromycin in women with bacterial vaginosis. N Engl J Med 1995;333: 1732–6.
44. McDonald HM, O'Loughlin JA, Vigneswaran R, Jolley PT, Harvey JA, Bof A, McDonald PJ. Impact of metronidazole therapy on preterm birth in women with bacterial vaginosis flora (*Gardnerella vaginalis*): a randomized, placebo controlled trial. Br J Obstet Gynaecol 1997;104:1391–7.
45. Svare J, Langhoff-Roos J, Andersen LF, Kryger-Baggesen N, Borch-Christensen H, Heisterberg L, Kristensen J. Ampicillin-metronidazole treatment in idiopathic preterm labour: a randomized controlled multicentre trial. Br J Obstet Gynaecol 1997;104: 892–7.
46. Klebanoff M, Carey JC, for the NICHD MFMU Network, Bethesda, MD. Metronidazole did not prevent preterm birth in asymptomatic women with bacterial vaginosis (abstract). Am J Obstet Gynecol 1999;180:S2.
47. Hauth JC, for the NICHD MFMU Network, Bethesda, MD. Response of the three components of a vaginal gram stain score to metronidazole treatment and in relation to preterm birth (abstract). Am J Obstet Gynecol 2000;182:S56.
48. Carey J, Klebanoff MA, Hauth JC, Hillier SL, Thom EA, Ernest JM, Heine RP, Nugent RP, Fischer ML, Leveno KJ, Wapner R, Varner M, and the National Institute of Child Health and Human Development Network of Maternal-Fetal Medicine Units. Metronidazole to prevent preterm delivery in pregnant women with asymptomatic bacterial vaginosis. N Engl J Med 2000;342:534–40.
49. Carey JC, Klebanoff M, for the NICHD MFMU Network, Bethesda MD. Metronidazole treatment increased the risk of preterm birth in asymptomatic women with trichomonas (abstract). Am J Obstet Gynecol 2000;182:Ss13.
50. Klebanoff MA, Carey JC, Hauth JC, Hillier SL, Nugent RP, Thom EA, Ernest JM, Heine RP, Wapner RJ, Trout W, Moawad A, Leveno KJ, and the National Institute of Child Health and Human Development Network of Maternal-Fetal Medicine Units. Failure of metronidazole to prevent preterm delivery among pregnant women with asymptomatic *Trichomonas vaginalis* infection. N Engl J Med 2001;345:487–93.
51. Erickson SH, Oppenheim GL, Smith GH. Metronidazole in breast milk. Obstet Gynecol 1981;57:48–50.
52. Heisterberg L, Branebjerg PE. Blood and milk concentrations of metronidazole in mothers and infants. J Perinat Med 1983;11:114–20.
53. Moore B, Collier J. Drugs and breast-feeding. Br Med J 1979;2:211.
54. Clements CJ. Metronidazole and breast feeding. N Z Med J 1980;92:329.
55. Committee on Drugs, American Academy of Pediatrics. The transfer of drugs and other chemicals into human milk. Pediatrics 2001;108:776–89.

Name:	**METYROSINE**	Risk Factor:	C_M
Class:	**Antihypertensive**		

FETAL RISK SUMMARY

RECOMMENDATION: Limited Human Data - No Relevant Animal Data

Metyrosine, an enzyme inhibitor, is used in patients with pheochromocytoma for preoperative preparation, management when surgery is contraindicated, or as chronic treatment of malignant pheochromocytoma. The drug inhibits tyrosine hydroxylase, the enzyme that catalyzes the conversion of tyrosine to dihydroxyphenylalanine, the first transformation in catecholamine biosynthesis (1).

No reproduction studies in animals have been located. The molecular weight of the compound (195) is low enough that transfer to the fetus should be expected.

A case report published in 1986 described the pregnancy of a 24-year-old woman at 30 weeks' gestation who was managed for recurrent pheochromocytoma with a combination of metyrosine, prazosin (α_1-adrenergic blocker), and timolol (β-adrenergic blocker) (2). Hypertension had been noted at her first prenatal visit at 12 weeks' gestation. Because of declines in fetal breathing, body movements, and amniotic fluid volume that began 2 weeks after the start of therapy, a cesarean section was conducted at 33 weeks. The 1450-g female infant had Apgar scores of 3 and 5 at 1 and 5 minutes, respectively. Mild metabolic acidosis was found on analysis of umbilical cord blood gases. Multiple infarcts were noted in the placenta but no evidence of metastatic tumor. The growth-retarded infant did well and was discharged home on day 53 of life (2).

BREAST FEEDING SUMMARY

RECOMMENDATION: No Human Data - Potential Toxicity

No reports describing the use of metyrosine during human lactation have been located. The molecular weight (195) is low enough that excretion into breast milk probably occurs. The effects of this exposure on a nursing infant are unknown.

References

1. Product information. Demser. Merck, 2001.
2. Devoe LD, O'Dell BE, Castillo RA, Hadi HA, Searle N. Metastatic pheochromocytoma in pregnancy and fetal biophysical assessment after maternal administration of alpha-adrenergic, beta-adrenergic, and dopamine antagonists. Obstet Gynecol 1986;68:15S–8S.

Name:	**MEXILETINE**	Risk Factor:	C_M
Class:	**Antiarrhythmic**		

FETAL RISK SUMMARY

RECOMMENDATION: Limited Human Data - Animal Data Suggest Low Risk

Mexiletine is a local anesthetic, orally active, antiarrhythmic agent structurally similar to lidocaine. The drug is not teratogenic in pregnant mice, rats, and rabbits given doses up to and including maternal toxicity (1–3). Human pregnancy experience with mexiletine is limited to three women, one treated throughout gestation, one starting during the 14th week, and one at 32 weeks (4–6). No adverse effects attributable to mexiletine were mentioned in these reports.

A healthy 2600-g male infant was delivered at 39 weeks' gestation (Apgar scores 9 and 10 at 1 and 5 minutes, respectively) to a 26-year-old primigravida woman who had been treated throughout her pregnancy with mexiletine (200 mg 3 times daily) and atenolol (50 mg/d) for ventricular tachycardia with multifocal ectopic beats (4). A serum mexiletine level obtained from the infant 9 hours after birth was 0.4 μg/mL (normal therapeutic range 0.75–2.0 μg/mL) (4). Heart rates during a normal newborn course were 120–160 beats/minute. Postpartum, the mother continued both mexiletine and atenolol. The infant was fed breast milk only, and by 17 days of age, his weight had decreased to 2155 g. The weight loss was attributed to failure to feed and was corrected with maternal education and formula supplementation. Breast feeding was halted at 3 months of age. Gastroesophageal reflux, presenting with seizure-like episodes but with a normal neurologic examination and electroencephalogram, was diagnosed at 8 months of age. The condition responded to corrective measures, and growth and development were appropriate at 10 months of age (4).

A 1981 report described the treatment of a 30-year-old woman with cardiac palpitations with 600 mg/day of mexiletine and 60 mg/day of propranolol starting at approximately 14 weeks' gestation (5). A healthy infant (birth weight and sex not specified) was delivered 5 months later.

A 34-year-old woman was treated at 32 weeks' gestation with a combination of mexiletine 200 mg 3 times daily and propranolol 40 mg 3 times daily for paroxysmal ventricular tachycardia (6). A normal male infant (birth weight not given) was delivered by spontaneous vaginal birth at 39 weeks' gestation. Bradycardia, most likely as a result of propranolol, was noted in the infant during the first 6 hours after birth. The heart rate was 90 beats/minute, before increasing to a normal rate of 120 beats/minute. An electrocardiogram was normal. The cord blood and maternal serum mexiletine concentrations at birth were both 0.3 μg/mL.

On the basis of the very limited published information in animals and humans, mexiletine does not appear to present a significant risk to the fetus. However, three reviews on the use of cardiovascular drugs during pregnancy caution that too few data are available to assess the safety of this agent during pregnancy (7–9).

M

BREAST FEEDING SUMMARY

RECOMMENDATION: Limited Human Data - Probably Compatible

Mexiletine is excreted into breast milk in concentrations exceeding those in the maternal serum (5,6). Three cases have been reported in which a nursing infant was exposed to the drug via the milk with drug levels determined in two of these cases. All three infants had been exposed to mexiletine *in utero*, and no adverse effects attributable to the drug were noted. The American Academy of Pediatrics classifies mexiletine as compatible with breast-feeding (10).

Milk and serum mexiletine concentrations in a woman described above, who was taking 600 mg/day in divided doses, were 0.6 and 0.3 μg/mL, respectively, 2 days postpartum, and 0.8 and 0.7 μg/mL, respectively, 6 weeks after delivery (6). These levels represented milk:plasma ratios of 2.0 and 1.1, respectively. Mexiletine was not detected in serum samples from the breast-fed infant at either sampling time, and there were no adverse effects observed in the infant. A second report, appearing 1 year later, described the excretion of the antiarrhythmic agent into breast milk of a woman also taking 600 mg/day in divided doses (5). Again, no adverse effects were noted in the breast-fed infant. Twelve paired milk and serum levels, collected from the mother between the 2nd and 5th postpartum days, yielded peak concentrations of 0.959 μg/mL in the milk compared with 0.724 μg/mL in the serum, a ratio of 1.32 (mean ratio 1.45, range 0.78–1.89).

Failure to feed was observed in a wholly breast-fed infant whose mother was taking mexiletine (600 mg/d) and atenolol (50 mg/d) (4). The infant's weight dropped from 2600 g at birth to 2155 g at 17 days of age. An acceptable growth curve was obtained with maternal education and formula supplementation for the next 2.5 months, after which breast-feeding was stopped (4).

References

1. Matsuo A, Kast A, Tsunenari Y. Reproduction studies of mexiletine hydrochloride by oral administration. Iyakuhin Kenkyu 1983;14:527–49. As cited in Shepard TH. *Catalog of Teratogenic Agents*. 6th ed. Baltimore, MD: Johns Hopkins University Press, 1989:427.
2. Nishimura M, Kast A, Tsunenari Y. Reproduction studies of mexiletine hydrochloride by intravenous administration. Ikakuhin Kenkyu 1983;14:550–70. As cited in Shepard TH. *Catalog of Teratogenic Agents*. 6th ed. Baltimore, MD: Johns Hopkins University Press, 1989:427.
3. Product information. Mexitil. Boehringer Ingelheim, 1992.
4. Lownes HE, Ives TJ. Mexiletine use in pregnancy and lactation. Am J Obstet Gynecol 1987;157: 446–7.
5. Lewis AM, Patel L, Johnston A, Turner P. Mexiletine in human blood and breast milk. Postgrad Med J 1981;57:546–7.
6. Timmis AD, Jackson G, Holt DW. Mexiletine for control of ventricular dysrhythmias in pregnancy. Lancet 1980;2:647–8.
7. Tamari I, Eldar M, Rabinowitz B, Neufeld HN. Medical treatment of cardiovascular disorders during pregnancy. Am Heart J 1982;104:1357–63.
8. Rotmensch HH, Rotmensch S, Elkayam U. Management of cardiac arrhythmias during pregnancy. Current concepts. Drugs 1987;33:623–33.
9. Brodsky M, Doria R, Allen B, Sato D, Thomas G, Sada M. New-onset ventricular tachycardia during pregnancy. Am Heart J 1992;123:933–41.
10. Committee on Drugs, American Academy of Pediatrics. The transfer of drugs and other chemicals into human milk. Pediatrics 2001;108:776–89.

Name: **MICONAZOLE** Risk Factor: C_M

Class: **Antifungal Antibiotic**

FETAL RISK SUMMARY

RECOMMENDATION: Compatible (Topical)

Miconazole is normally used as a topical antifungal agent. Small amounts are absorbed from the vagina (1). Use in pregnant patients with vulvovaginal candidiasis (moniliasis) has not been associated with an increase in congenital malformations (1–7). Effects following IV use are unknown.

In data obtained from the Michigan Medicaid program between 1980 and 1983, a total of 2092 women were exposed to miconazole during the 1st trimester from a total sample of 97,775 deliveries not linked to a birth defect diagnosis (8). Of 6564 deliveries linked to such a diagnosis, miconazole was used in 144 cases. The estimated relative risk for birth defects from these data was 1.02 (95% confidence limits [CI] 0.9–1.2). An estimated relative risk for spontaneous abortions of 1.38 (95% CI 1.2–1.5) was calculated based on 250 miconazole exposures among 4264 abortions compared with 2236 1st trimester exposures among 55,736 deliveries (8). Moreover, no association was found between miconazole use and oral clefts, spina bifida, or cardiovascular defects. Although the relative risks for total birth defects or the three specific defects were not increased, the authors could not exclude the possibility of an association with other specific defects (8).

In an extension of the above investigation, data were obtained for 229,101 completed pregnancies between 1985 and 1992, in which 7266 newborns had been exposed to miconazole administered vaginally during the 1st trimester (F. Rosa, personal communication, FDA, 1993). A total of 304 (4.2%) major birth defects were observed (273 expected). Specific data were available for six defect categories, including (observed/expected) 77/73 cardiovascular defects, 14/12 oral clefts, 3/4 spina bifida, 22/21 polydactyly, 12/12 limb reduction defects, and 20/17 hypospadias. These data do not support an association between the drug and congenital defects.

BREAST FEEDING SUMMARY

RECOMMENDATION: No Human Data - Probably Compatible

No data are available.

References

1. Product information. Monistat. Ortho Pharmaceutical, 1990.
2. Culbertson C. Monistat: a new fungicide for treatment of vulvovaginal candidiasis. Am J Obstet Gynecol 1974;120:973–6.
3. Wade A, ed. *Martindate. The Extra Pharmacopoeia*. 27th ed. London: Pharmaceutical Press, 1977:648.
4. Davis JE, Frudenfeld JH, Goddard JL. Comparative evaluation of Monistat and Mycostatin in the treatment of vulvovaginal candidiasis. Obstet Gynecol 1974;44:403–6.
5. Wallenburg HCS, Wladimiroff JW. Recurrence of vulvovaginal candidosis during pregnancy. Comparison of miconazole vs nystatin treatment. Obstet Gynecol 1976;48:491–4.
6. McNellis D, McLeod M, Lawson J, Pasquale SA. Treatment of vulvovaginal candidiasis in pregnancy: a comparative study. Obstet Gynecol 1977;50:674–8.
7. Weisberg M. Treatment of vaginal candidiasis in pregnant women. Clin Therap 1986;8:563–7.
8. Rosa FW, Baum C, Shaw M. Pregnancy outcomes after first-trimester vaginitis drug therapy. Obstet Gynecol 1987;69:751–5.

M

Name: **MIDAZOLAM** Risk Factor: **D_M**

Class: **Sedative**

FETAL RISK SUMMARY

RECOMMENDATION: Limited Human Data - Animal Data Suggest Low Risk

Midazolam is a short-acting benzodiazepine used for anesthetic induction. Reproduction studies in rats and rabbits at 10 and 5 times the human dose, respectively, found no evidence of teratogenicity in either species or impairment of fertility in rats (1). No reports have been located that describe the use of midazolam in humans during the 1st or 2nd trimesters.

Midazolam crosses the human placenta, but this transfer, at least after oral and IM use, appears to be slower than that experienced with other benzodiazepines, such as diazepam, oxazepam, or lorazepam (2). In 13 patients given 15 mg of midazolam orally a mean of 11.4 hours (range 10.5–12.4 hours) before cesarean section, only 1 had measurable levels of the drug at the time of surgery: maternal venous level was 12 ng/mL and cord venous level was 7 ng/mL. No patient had detectable levels of the drug in the amniotic fluid. A second group of patients ($N = 11$) were administered 15 mg of midazolam orally a mean of 34.3 minutes (15–60 minutes) before cesarean section. The mean serum concentrations in maternal venous, umbilical venous, and umbilical arterial blood were 12.7, 8.4, and 5.7 ng/mL, respectively. The cord venous:maternal venous and cord arterial:maternal venous ratios were 0.74 and 0.45, respectively. Six patients in a third group were administered midazolam, 0.05 mg/kg IM, 18–45 minutes (mean 30.5 minutes) before cesarean section. Drug levels from the same sampling sites and ratios obtained in the second group were measured in this group, with results of 40.0, 21.7, and 12.8 ng/mL, respectively, and 0.56 and 0.32, respectively. None of the 1- and 5-minute Apgar scores of the 30 infants was less than 7, and no adverse effects attributable to midazolam were observed in the newborns (2).

The placental transfer of midazolam and its metabolite, α-hydroxymidazolam, was described in a 1989 reference (3). (See reference 7 for the clinical and physiologic condition of the newborns.) Twenty women were given 0.03 mg/kg of midazolam IV for anesthesia induction before cesarean section. The mean concentrations of midazolam in the mothers' serum and cord blood were 339 and 318 ng/mL (ratio 0.66), respectively. Similar measurements of the metabolite produced values of 22 and 5 (ratio 0.28), respectively. The elimination half-life of midazolam in the newborn infants was 6.3 hours (3).

Plasma levels of midazolam were measured at frequent intervals up to 2 hours after a 5-mg IV dose administered to two groups of pregnant patients in a study published in 1985 (4). Levels were significantly higher in 12 patients in early labor than in 8 women undergoing elective cesarean section. No reason was given for the significant difference. Data on the exposed newborns were not given.

Midazolam, 0.2 mg/kg ($N = 26$), or thiopental, 3.5 mg/kg ($N = 26$), was combined with succinylcholine for rapid-sequence IV induction before cesarean section in a study examining the effects of these agents on the newborn (5). Five of the newborns exposed to midazolam required tracheal intubation compared to one in the thiopental group, a significant difference ($p < 0.05$). The authors concluded that thiopental was superior to midazolam for this procedure.

A 1989 study compared the effects of midazolam 0.3 mg/kg ($N = 20$) with thiopental 4 mg/kg ($N = 20$) in mothers undergoing induction of anesthesia before cesarean section (6). The only difference found between the groups was a significantly higher (mean 7.9 mm Hg) diastolic blood pressure in the midazolam group during, but not after, induction. Characteristics of the newborns from the midazolam and thiopental groups (both $N = 19$) were compared in the second part of this study (7). Oxygen via face mask was required in five midazolam-exposed newborns compared to three in the thiopental group. Respiratory depression on day 1 and hypoglycemia and jaundice on day 3 were also observed in the midazolam group. Moreover, three statistically significant ($p < 0.05$) neurobehavioral adverse effects, from the 19 tested, consisting of body temperature, general body tone, and arm recoil, were noted after midazolam exposure during the first 2 hours after birth. Other parameters that were inferior in the midazolam group, but that did not reach statistical significance, were palmar grasp, resistance against pull, and startle reaction (7). Although these differences do not meet all of the criteria for "floppy infant syndrome" (see Diazepam), they do indicate that the use of midazolam before cesarean section has a depressant effect on the newborn that is greater than that observed with thiopental.

BREAST FEEDING SUMMARY

RECOMMENDATION: Limited Human Data - Potential Toxicity

Midazolam is excreted into breast milk. In a study published in 1990, 12 women in the immediate postpartum period took 15 mg orally at night for 5 nights (8). No measurable concentrations of midazolam or the metabolite, hydroxy-midazolam, were detected (<10 nmol/L) in milk samples collected a mean 7 hours (range 6–8 hours) after drug intake during the 5-day period. One mother, however, who was accidentally given a second dose (total dose 30 mg) did have a milk concentration of 30 nmol/L (milk:plasma ratio 0.20) at 7 hours. The authors estimated that the exposure of the infant would be nil in early breast milk if nursing was held for 4 hours after a 15-mg dose. In addition, two women were studied at 2–3 months postpartum. In six paired milk and serum samples collected up to 6 hours after a 15-mg dose, the mean milk:plasma ratio was 0.15. On the basis of an average milk concentration of 10 nmol/L, a nursing infant would ingest an estimated 0.33 μg of midazolam and 0.34 μg of metabolite per 100 mL of milk if nursed within 4–6 hours of the maternal dose (8).

The American Academy of Pediatrics classifies midazolam as a drug for which the effect on a nursing infant is unknown but may be of concern (9).

References

1. Product information. Versed. Roche Laboratories, 1997.
2. Kanto J, Sjovall S, Erkkola R, Himberg J-J, Kangas L. Placental transfer and maternal midazolam kinetics. Clin Pharmacol Ther 1983;33:786–91.
3. Bach V, Carl P, Ravlo O, Crawford ME, Jensen AG, Mikkelsen BO, Crevoisier C, Heizmann P, Fattinger K. A randomized comparison between midazolam and thiopental for elective cesarean section anesthesia. III. Placental transfer and elimination in neonates. Anesth Analg 1989;68:238–42.
4. Wilson CM, Dundee JW, Moore J, Collier PS, Mathews HLM, Thompson EM. A comparison of plasma midazolam levels in non-pregnant and pregnant women at parturition. Br J Clin Pharmacol 1985;20:256P–7P.
5. Bland BAR, Lawes EG, Duncan PW, Warnell I, Downing JW. Comparison of midazolam and thiopental for rapid sequence anesthetic induction for elective cesarean section. Anesth Analg 1987;66:1165–8.
6. Crawford ME, Carl P, Bach V, Ravlo O, Mikkelsen BO, Werner M. A randomized comparison between midazolam and thiopental for elective cesarean section anesthesia. I. Mothers. Anesth Analg 1989;68:229–33.
7. Ravlo O, Carl P, Crawford ME, Bach V, Mikkelsen BO, Nielsen HK. A randomized comparison between midazolam and thiopental for elective cesarean section anesthesia: II. Neonates. Anesth Analg 1989;68:234–7.
8. Matheson I, Lunde PKM, Bredesen JE. Midazolam and nitrazepam in the maternity ward: milk concentrations and clinical effects. Br J Clin Pharmacol 1990;30:787–93.
9. Committee on Drugs, American Academy of Pediatrics. The transfer of drugs and other chemicals into human milk. Pediatrics 2001;108:776–89.

Name:	**MIDODRINE**	Risk Factor:	C_M
Class:	**Sympathomimetic (Adrenergic)**		

FETAL RISK SUMMARY

RECOMMENDATION: No Human Data - Animal Data Suggest Risk

The active metabolite of midodrine, desglymidrodrine, is a α_1-adrenergic receptor agonist that increases the vascular tone to raise blood pressure. It is indicated for the treatment of symptomatic orthostatic hypotension. Marked increases in systolic blood pressure greater than 200 mm Hg may occur, which in itself could jeopardize the fetus. No reports describing the use of midodrine during human pregnancy have been located.

Reproduction studies have been conducted in pregnant rats and rabbits (1). At doses 13 and 7 times, respectively, the maximum human dose based on body surface area, embryo toxicity (resorptions) and reduced fetal weights occurred in both species, and decreased fetal survival was noted in rabbits. No teratogenicity was observed in either species.

It is not known if midodrine or its metabolite cross the human placenta. The molecular weight (about 255 for the free base) is low enough that transfer to the fetus should be expected.

BREAST FEEDING SUMMARY

RECOMMENDATION: No Human Data - Potential Toxicity

No reports describing the use of midodrine in human lactation have been located. The molecular weight (about 255 for the free base) suggests that the drug will be excreted into breast milk. The effect of this exposure on a nursing infant is unknown. Because severe systolic hypertension is a potential effect in an infant, women who are taking midodrine should probably not breast-feed.

Reference

1. Product information. ProAmatine. Shire US, 2001.

Name:	**MIFEPRISTONE**	Risk Factor:	**X**
Class:	**Antiprogestogen**		

FETAL RISK SUMMARY

RECOMMENDATION: Contraindicated

Mifepristone (RU 38486; RU 486) is an orally active, synthetic antiprogestogen that has been used primarily for the termination of pregnancy. At higher doses, the drug also has antiglucocorticoid effects. The mechanism of action of mifepristone, which exerts its antiprogestogen effect at the level of the receptor, and the physiologic effects it produces in both animals and humans have been studied and reviewed in a number of references (1–16). A 1993 review summarized the drug's antiprogestin and other pharmacologic effects in humans (17).

Mifepristone rapidly crosses the placenta to the fetus in both monkeys (18) and humans (19,20). The fetal:maternal ratio decreased from 0.31 to 0.18 in monkeys between the 2nd and 3rd trimesters (18). In 13 women undergoing 2nd-trimester abortions, a single 100-mg oral dose produced fetal cord blood concentrations of mifepristone ranging from 20 ng/mL (30 minutes) to 400 ng/mL (18 hours) (19). The peak maternal concentration (1500 ng/mL) was attained in 1–2 hours, and the average fetal:maternal ratio was approximately 0.33. In contrast to a simple diffusion process observed in monkeys (18), an active transport mechanism was suggested because the fetal concentration increased exponentially (19). In the second human study, a lower mean fetal:maternal ratio (0.11) was measured at 17.2 ± 8.6 hours in six women treated with 600 mg of mifepristone for 2nd-trimester abortion (20). Maternal plasma concentrations of aldosterone, progesterone, estradiol, or cortisol did not change significantly 4 hours after mifepristone, but a significant increase in fetal aldosterone occurred at this time, rising from 999 pmol/L to 1699 pmol/L. Mean changes in the fetal levels of the other three steroids were not significant.

A large number of studies have investigated the use of mifepristone as an abortive agent, either when given alone (21–36), or when combined with a prostaglandin analog

(24,30,37–51). The drug has also been studied for labor induction after 2nd trimester intrauterine death (52,53), as a cervical ripening agent in the 1st trimester (54–59), in the 2nd trimester (60), and at term (61–63). Although mifepristone, especially when combined with a prostaglandin analogue, is an effective abortive agent, it has not been effective when used for the termination of ectopic pregnancies (64,65). The use of mifepristone as a postcoital contraceptive or for routine administration during the mid to late luteal phase to prevent a potential early pregnancy by induction of menses (i.e., contragestation) has also been frequently investigated (22,66–79).

Mifepristone is teratogenic in rabbits and the effect is both dose and duration dependent (80). Abnormalities observed included growth retardation, nonfused eyelids and large fontanelle, opened cranial vault with exposure of the meninges and hemorrhagic or necrotic nervous tissue, necrotic destruction of the upper part of the head and brain, and absence of closure of the vertebral canal (80). At doses approximating those used in clinical practice, no evidence of teratogenicity was observed in postimplantation rat embryos exposed to mifepristone in culture (81). Similarly, no teratogenicity was observed after *in vitro* exposure of monkey embryos to mifepristone (82,83).

In humans, only six cases have been reported of exposure to mifepristone that was not followed by subsequent abortion. Although specific details were not provided, in the United Kingdom Multicenter Trial (gestational age ≤36–69 days from last menstrual period), one woman changed her mind after taking mifepristone and her pregnancy continued until a normal infant was delivered at term (41). In 1989, brief mention was made of fetal malformations discovered after pregnancy termination at 18 weeks' gestation (84). Additional information on this and one other case was published in 1991 (85–87). A 25-year-old primigravida was treated with 600 mg of mifepristone at 5 weeks' gestation, but then decided not to proceed with termination (85,86). Severe malformations were observed by ultrasound examination at 17 weeks' gestation, consisting of an absence of amniotic sac, stomach, gallbladder, and urinary tract, and the pregnancy was stopped with prostaglandin at 18 weeks (85). The 190-g fetus had typical features of the sirenomelia sequence (sympodia; caudal regression syndrome): fused lower limbs with a single flexed foot containing seven toes, no external genitalia or anal or urethral openings, and absence of internal reproductive organs, lower urinary tract, and kidneys. Other anomalies were hypoplastic lungs, a cleft palate, and a cleft lip. Sirenomelia is thought to date back to the primitive streak stage during the 3rd week of gestation, and, thus, in this case, before exposure to mifepristone (85). However, induction of cleft palate and cleft lip occurs at approximately 36 days of gestation (85) and may have been a consequence of drug exposure.

A normal outcome was achieved in the second case in which a 30-year-old woman was treated with 400 mg of mifepristone 6 weeks after her last menstrual period, but then decided to continue her pregnancy (85). She eventually delivered a healthy, 3030-g male baby at 41 weeks' gestation. Three other normal infants have been described after *in utero* exposure to mifepristone (59,88). All three were participants in clinical trials who decided to continue their pregnancies after treatment with mifepristone at 8, 8, and 9 weeks' gestation (88). The latter patient vomited 1.5 hours after taking the drug and reported seeing at least one partially digested tablet in the vomit. Delivery occurred at 40 weeks (4150-g male), 39 weeks (3930-g male), and 41 weeks (3585 g-female), respectively. Follow-ups of the infants at 15, 9, and 6 months, respectively, were completely normal.

In summary, mifepristone (RU 486) is a potent antiprogestogen compound that is mainly used for the termination of pregnancy, usually in combination with a prostaglandin agent. It has also been used for cervical ripening before abortion and is currently being studied as an aid in the induction of labor at term. It is teratogenic in one animal species, but not in two others, one of which is a primate species. Data are too limited to determine whether the drug is a human teratogen. Because the incidence of successful abortion after mifepristone is high, but not total, women should be informed of the risk for embryotoxicity if their pregnancy continues after use of this drug.

BREAST FEEDING SUMMARY

RECOMMENDATION: Contraindicated

No data have been located on the excretion of mifepristone in breast milk. Because the drug is well absorbed after oral administration, it should not be used during breast-feeding because of its potent antihormonal effects. However, as a result of the limited indications for this agent, the opportunities for its use during lactation should be infrequent.

References

1. Garfield RE, Gasc JM, Baulieu EE. Effects of the antiprogesterone RU 486 on preterm birth in the rat. Am J Obstet Gynecol 1987;157:1281–5.
2. Roblero LS, Fernandez O, Croxatto HB. The effects of RU486 on transport, development and implantation of mouse embryos. Contraception 1987;36:549–55.
3. Burgess KM, Jenkin G, Ralph MM, Thorburn GD. Effect of the antiprogestin RU486 on uterine sensitivity to oxytocin in ewes in late pregnancy. J Endocrinol 1992;134:353–60.
4. Haluska GJ, Stanczyk FZ, Cook MJ, Novy MJ. Temporal changes in uterine activity and prostaglandin response to RU486 in rhesus macaques in late gestation. Am J Obstet Gynecol 1987;157:1487–95.
5. Cullingford TE, Pollard JW. RU 486 completely inhibits the action of progesterone on cell proliferation in the mouse uterus. J Reprod Fertil 1988;83:909–14.
6. Haluska GJ, West NB, Novy MJ, Brenner RM. Uterine estrogen receptors are increased by RU486 in late pregnant rhesus macaques but not after spontaneous labor. J Clin Endocrinol Metab 1990;70:181–6.
7. Haluska GJ, Mitchell MD, Novy MJ. Amniotic fluid lipoxygenase metabolites during spontaneous labor and after RU486 treatment during late pregnancy in rhesus macaques. Prostaglandins 1990;40:99–105.
8. Juneja SC, Dodson MG. In vitro effect of RU 486 on sperm-egg interaction in mice. Am J Obstet Gynecol 1990;163:216–21.
9. Cabrol D, Carbonne B, Bienkiewicz A, Dallot E, Alj AE, Cedard L. Induction of labor and cervical maturation using mifepristone (RU 486) in the late pregnant rat. Influence of a cyclooxygenase inhibitor (diclofenac). Prostaglandins 1991;42:71–9.
10. Smith SK, Kelly RW. The effect of the antiprogestins RU 486 and ZK 98734 on the synthesis and metabolism of prostaglandins $F_{2\alpha}$ and E_2 in separated cells from early human decidua. J Clin Endocrinol Metab 1987;65:527–34.
11. Das C, Catt KJ. Antifertility actions of the progesterone antagonist RU 486 include direct inhibition of placental hormone secretion. Lancet 1987;2:599–601.
12. Anonymous. Mifepristone—contragestive agent or medical abortifacient. Lancet 1987;2:1308–10.
13. Hill NCW, Selinger M, Ferguson J, Lopez Bernal A, Mackenzie IZ. The physiological and clinical effects of progesterone inhibition with mifepristone (RU 486) in the second trimester. Br J Obstet Gynaecol 1990;97:487–92.
14. Baulieu EE. RU-486 as an antiprogesterone steroid. From receptor to contragestion and beyond. JAMA 1989;262:1808–14.
15. Guillebaud J. Medical termination of pregnancy. Combined with prostaglandin RU 486 is effective. Br Med J 1990;301:352–4.
16. Brogden RN, Goa KL, Faulds D. Mifepristone. A review of its pharmacodynamic and pharmacokinetic properties, and therapeutic potential. Drugs 1993;45:384–409.
17. Spitz IM, Bardin CW. Mifepristone (RU 486)—a modulator of progestin and glucocorticoid action. N Engl J Med 1993;329:404–12.
18. Wolf JP, Chillik CF, Itskovitz J, Weyman D, Anderson TL, Ulmann A, Baulieu EE, Hodgen GD. Transplacental passage of a progesterone antagonist in monkeys. Am J Obstet Gynecol 1988;159:238–42.
19. Frydman R, Taylor S, Ulmann A. Transplacental passage of mifepristone. Lancet 1985;2:1252.
20. Hill NCW, Selinger M, Ferguson J, MacKenzie IZ. The placental transfer of mifepristone (RU 486) during the second trimester and its influence upon maternal and fetal steroid concentrations. Br J Obstet Gynaecol 1990;97:406–11.
21. Kovacs L, Sas M, Resch BA, Ugocsai G, Swahn ML, Bygdeman M, Rowe PJ. Termination of very early pregnancy by RU 486—an antiprogestational compound. Contraception 1984;29:399–410.
22. Haspels AA. Interruption of early pregnancy by an antiprogestational compound, RU 486. Eur J Obstet Gynecol Reprod Biol 1985;20:169–75.
23. Vervest HAM, Haspels AA. Preliminary results with the antiprogestational compound RU-486 (mifepristone) for interruption of early pregnancy. Fertil Steril 1985;44:627–32.
24. Bygdeman M, Swahn ML. Progesterone receptor blockage. Effect on uterine contractility and early pregnancy. Contraception 1985;32:45–51.
25. Couzinet B, Strat NL, Ulmann A, Baulieu EE, Schaison G. Termination of early pregnancy by the

M

progesterone antagonist RU 486 (mifepristone). N Engl J Med 1986;315:1565–70.

26. Shoupe D, Mishell DR Jr, Brenner PF, Spitz IM. Pregnancy termination with a high and medium dosage regimen of RU 486. Contraception 1986;33:455–61.
27. Mishell DR Jr, Shouupe D, Brenner PF, Lacarra M, Horenstein J, Lahteenmaki P, Spitz IM. Termination of early gestation with the anti-progestin steroid RU 486: medium versus low dose. Contraception 1987;35:307–21.
28. Urquhart DR, Templeton AA. Mifepristone (RU 486) and second-trimester termination. Lancet 1987; 2:1405.
29. Birgerson L, Odlind V. Early pregnancy termination with antiprogestins: a comparative clinical study of RU 486 given in two dose regimens and epostane. Fertil Steril 1987,48:565–70.
30. Cameron IT, Michie AF, Baird DT. Therapeutic abortion in early pregnancy with antiprogestogen RU486 alone or in combination with prostaglandin analogue (Gemeprost). Contraception 1986;34:459–68.
31. Grimes DA, Mishell DR Jr, Shoupe D, Lacarra M. Early abortion with a single dose of the antiprogestin RU-486. Am J Obstet Gynecol 1988;158:1307–12.
32. Cameron IT, Baird DT. Early pregnancy termination: a comparison between vacuum aspiration and medical abortion using prostaglandin (16,16 dimethyl-trans-δ_2-PGE_1 methyl ester) or the antiprogestogen RU 486. Br J Obstet Gynaecol 1988;95:271–6.
33. Maria B, Stampf F, Goepp A, Ulmann A. Termination of early pregnancy by a single dose of mifepristone (RU 486), a progesterone antagonist. Eur J Obstet Gynecol Reprod Biol 1988;28:249–55.
34. Frydman R, Fernandez H, Pons JC, Ulmann A. Mifepristone (RU486) and therapeutic late pregnancy termination: a double-blind study of two different doses. Hum Reprod 1988;3:803–6.
35. Ylikorkala O, Alfthan H, Kaariainen M, Rapeli T, Lahteenmaki P. Outpatient therapeutic abortion with mifepristone. Obstet Gynecol 1989;74:653–7.
36. Gottlieb C, Bygdeman M. The use of antiprogestin (RU 486) for termination of second trimester pregnancy. Acta Obstet Gynecol Scand 1991;70:199–203.
37. Rodger MW, Baird DT. Induction of therapeutic abortion in early pregnancy with mifepristone in combination with prostaglandin pessary. Lancet 1987;2: 1415–8.
38. Swahn ML, Bygdeman M. The effect of the antiprogestin RU 486 on uterine contractility and sensitivity to prostaglandin and oxytocin. Br J Obstet Gynaecol 1988;95:126–34.
39. Hill NCW, Ferguson J, MacKenzie IZ. The efficacy of oral mifepristone (RU 38,486) with a prostaglandin E_1 analog vaginal pessary for the termination of early pregnancy: complications and patient acceptability. Am J Obstet Gynecol 1990;162:414–7.
40. Silvestre L, Dubois C, Renault M, Rezvani Y, Baulieu EE, Ulmann A. Voluntary interruption of pregnancy with mifepristone (RU 486) and a prostaglandin analogue. N Engl J Med 1990;322:645–8.
41. UK Multicentre Trial. The efficacy and tolerance of mifepristone and prostaglandin in first trimester termination of pregnancy. Br J Obstet Gynaecol 1990;97:480–6.
42. Norman JE, Thong KJ, Baird DT. Uterine contractility and induction of abortion in early pregnancy by misoprostol and mifepristone. Lancet 1991;338:1233–6.
43. Anonymous. Misoprostol and legal medical abortion. Lancet 1991;338:1241–2.
44. World Health Organization. Pregnancy termination with mifepristone and gemeprost: a multicenter comparison between repeated doses and a single dose of mifepristone. Fertil Steril 1991;56:32–40.
45. Norman JE, Thong KJ, Rodger MW, Baird DT. Medical abortion in women of ≤56 days amenorrhoea: a comparison between gemeprost (a PGE_1 analogue) alone and mifepristone and gemeprost. Br J Obstet Gynaecol 1992;99:601–6.
46. Ulmann A, Silvestre L, Chemama L, Rezvani Y, Renault M, Aguillaume CJ, Baulieu EE. Medical termination of early pregnancy with mifepristone (RU 486) followed by a prostaglandin analogue; study in 16,369 women. Acta Obstet Gynecol Scand 1992;71:278–283.
47. Baird DT, Norman JE, Thong KJ, Glasier AF. Misoprostol, mifepristone, and abortion. Lancet 1992;339:313.
48. Thong KJ, Baird DT. A study of gemeprost alone, dilapan or mifepristone in combination with gemeprost for the termination of second trimester pregnancy. Contraception 1992;46:11–7.
49. Thong KJ, Baird DT. Induction of abortion with mifepristone and misoprostol in early pregnancy. Br J Obstet Gynaecol 1992;99:1004–7.
50. Heard M, Guillebaud J. Medical abortion. Safe, effective, and legal in Britain. BMJ 1992;304:195–6.
51. Peyron R, Aubeny E, Targosz V, Silvestre L, Renault M, Elkik F, Leclerc P, Ulmann A, Baulieu E-E. Early termination of pregnancy with mifepristone (RU 486) and the orally active prostaglandin misoprostol. N Engl J Med 1993;328:1509–13.
52. Cabrol D, Bouvier D'Yvoire M, Mermet E, Cedard L, Sureau C, Baulieu EE. Induction of labour with mifepristone after intrauterine fetal death. Lancet 1985;2:1019.
53. Cabrol D, Dubois C, Cronje H, Gonnet JM, Guillot M, Maria B, Moodley J, Oury JF, Thoulon JM, Treisser A, Ulmann D, Correl S, Ulmann A. Induction of labor with mifepristone (RU 486) in intrauterine fetal death. Am J Obstet Gynecol 1990;163:540–2.
54. Radestad A, Christensen NJ, Stromberg L. Induced cervical ripening with mifepristone in first trimester abortion; a double-blind randomized biomechanical study. Contraception 1988;38:301–12.
55. Durlot F, Dubois C, Brunerie J, Frydman R. Efficacy of progesterone antagonist RU486 (mifepristone) for pre-operative cervical dilatation during first trimester abortion. Hum Reprod 1988;3:583–4.
56. Lefebvre Y, Proulx L, Elie R, Poulin O, Lanza E. The effects of RU-38486 on cervical ripening. Clinical studies. Am J Obstet Gynecol 1990;162:61–5.
57. Johnson N, Bryce FC. Could antiprogesterones be used as alternative cervical ripening agents? Am J Obstet Gynecol 1990;162:688–90.
58. World Health Organization. The use of mifepristone (RU 486) for cervical preparation in first trimester pregnancy termination by vacuum aspiration. Br J Obstet Gynaecol 1990;97:260–6.
59. Cohn M, Stewart P. Pretreatment of the primigravid uterine cervix with mifepristone 30 h prior to termination of pregnancy: a double blind study. Br J Obstet Gynaecol 1991;98:778–82.

60. Frydman R, Taylor S, Pons JC, Forman RG, Ulmann A. Obstetrical indications for mifepristone. Adv Contracept 1986;2:269–70.
61. Li Y, Perezgrovas R, Gazal OS, Schwabe C, Anderson LL. Antiprogesterone, RU 486, facilitates parturition in cattle. Endocrinology 1991;129:765–70.
62. Wolf JP, Sinosich M, Anderson TL, Ulmann A, Baulieu EE, Hodgen GD. Progesterone antagonist (RU 486) for cervical dilation, labor induction, and delivery in monkeys; effectiveness in combination with oxytocin. Am J Obstet Gynecol 1989;160:45–7.
63. Frydman R, Lelaidier C, Baton-Saint-Mleux C, Fernandez H, Vial M, Bourget P. Labor induction in women at term with mifepristone (RU 486): a double-blind randomized, placebo-controlled study. Obstet Gynecol 1992;80:972–5.
64. Levin JH, Lacarra M, d'Ablain G, Grimes DA, Vermesh M. Mifepristone (RU 486) failure in an ovarian heterotopic pregnancy. Am J Obstet Gynecol 1990;163:543–4.
65. Pansky M, Golan A, Bukovsky I, Caspi E. Nonsurgical management of tubal pregnancy. Necessity in view of the changing clinical appearance. Am J Obstet Gynecol 1991;164:888–95.
66. Ulmann A. Uses of RU 486 for contragestion: an update. Contraception 1987;36(Suppl):27–31.
67. Nieman LK, Choate TM, Chrousos GP, Healy DL, Morin M, Renquist D, Merriam GR, Spitz IM, Bardin CW, Baulieu EE, Loriaux DL. The progesterone antagonist RU 486; a potential new contraceptive agent. N Engl J Med 1987;316:187–91.
68. Psychoyos A, Prapas I. Inhibition of egg development and implantation in rats after post-coital administration of the progesterone antagonist RU 486. J Reprod Fertil 1987;80:487–91.
69. Baulieu EE, Ulmann A, Philibert D. Contragestion by antiprogestin RU 486: a review. Arch Gynecol Obstet 1987;241:73–85.
70. Lahteenmaki P, Rapeli T, Kaariainen M, Alfthan H, Ylikorkala O. Late postcoital treatment against pregnancy with antiprogesterone RU 486. Fertil Steril 1988;50:36–8.
71. Dubois C, Ulmann A, Baulieu EE. Contragestion with late luteal administration of RU 486 (mifepristone). Fertil Steril 1988;50:593–6.
72. Couzinet B, Le Strat N, Silvestre L, Schaison G. Late luteal administration of the antiprogesterone RU486 in normal women: effects on the menstrual cycle events and fertility control in a long-term study. Fertil Steril 1990;54:1039–44.
73. Swahn ML, Gemzell K, Bygdeman M. Contraception with mifepristone. Lancet 1991;338:942–3.
74. Glasier A, Thong KJ, Dewar M, Mackie M, Baird DT. Postcoital contraception with mifepristone. Lancet 1991;337:1414–5.
75. Batista MC, Bristow TL, Mathews J, Stokes WS, Loriaux DL, Nieman LK. Daily administration of the progesterone antagonist RU 486 prevents implantation in the cycling guinea pig. Am J Obstet Gynecol 1991;165:82–6.
76. Glasier A, Thong KJ, Dewar M, Mackie M, Baird DT. Mifepristone (RU 486) compared with high-dose estrogen and progestogen for emergency postcoital contraception. N Engl J Med 1992;327:1041–4.
77. Grimes DA, Cook RJ. Mifepristone (RU 486)—an abortifacient to prevent abortion? N Engl J Med 1992;327:1088–9.
78. Hamel RP, Lysaught MT. Mifepristone (RU 486)—an abortifacient to prevent abortion? N Engl J Med 1993;328:354.
79. Grimes DA, Cook RJ. Mifepristone (RU 486)—an abortifacient to prevent abortion? Reply. N Engl J Med 1993;328:355.
80. Jost A. New data on the hormonal requirement of the pregnant rabbit; partial pregnancies and fetal anomalies resulting from treatment with a hormonal antagonist, given at a sub-abortive dosage. C R Acad Sci III 1986;303:281–4.
81. Hardy RP, New DAT. Effects of the anti-progestin RU 38486 on rat embryos growing in culture. Food Chem Toxicol 1991;29:361–2.
82. Avrech OM, Golan A, Weinraub Z, Bukovsky I, Caspi E. New tools for the trade. Reply. Fertil Steril 1992;57:1139–40.
83. Wolf JP, Chillik CF, Dubois C, Ulmann A, Baulieu EE, Hodgen GD. Tolerance of perinidatory primate embryos to RU486 exposure in vitro and in vivo. Contraception 1990;41:85–92.
84. Henrion R. RU 486 abortions. Nature 1989;338:110.
85. Pons JC, Imbert MC, Elefant E, Roux C, Herschkorn P, Papiernik E. Development after exposure to mifepristone in early pregnancy. Lancet 1991;338:763.
86. Ulmann A, Rubin I, Barnard J. Development after in-utero exposure to mifepristone. Lancet 1991;338:1270.
87. Pons JC, Papiernik E. Mifepristone teratogenicity. Lancet 1991;338:1332–3.
88. Lim BH, Lees DAR, Bjornsson S, Lunan CB, Cohn MR, Stewart P, Davey A. Normal development after exposure to mifepristone in early pregnancy. Lancet 1990;336:257–8.

Name:	**MIGLITOL**	Risk Factor:	**B_M**
Class:	**Oral Hypoglycemic**		

FETAL RISK SUMMARY

RECOMMENDATION: No Human Data - Probably Compatible

Miglitol is an oral α-glucosidase inhibitor, in the same class as acarbose (see Acarbose), that delays the digestion of ingested carbohydrates within the gastrointestinal tract, thereby reducing the rise in blood glucose following meals (1). It is used either alone or in combination with a sulfonylurea as an adjunct to diet in the management of type II diabetes (non-insulin-dependent diabetes mellitus). In contrast to acarbose, miglitol is readily absorbed into the systemic circulation, but the absorption is saturable at high doses. In addition, miglitol is not metabolized and is excreted unchanged in the urine with a elimination half-life of approximately 2 hours (1).

Reproduction studies have been conducted in animals with miglitol. In rats and rabbits at doses up to 12 and 10 times, respectively, the maximum recommended human exposure based on body surface area (MRHE), no evidence of teratogenicity was observed. In addition, no evidence of impaired fertility or fetal harm were noted at doses up to 4 and 3 times the MRHE, respectively, in these species. At 12 and 10 times the MRHE in rats and rabbits, respectively, maternal and/or fetal toxicity was noted. In rats, fetotoxicity was characterized by a slight but significant reduction in fetal weight. In rabbits, a slight reduction in fetal weight, an increased number of non-viable fetuses, and delayed ossification of the fetal skeleton were evident. In the rat peri-postnatal study, an increase in stillborns occurred at 4 times the MRHE (1).

Placental transfer of miglitol has been documented in pregnant rats after oral administration (2). It is not known if miglitol crosses the human placenta, but the molecular weight (about 207) is low enough that transfer to the fetus should be expected.

No reports describing the use of miglitol during human pregnancy have been located. Miglitol is normally used either alone or in combination with oral hypoglycemic agents, and these hypoglycemic drugs are not indicated for the pregnant diabetic as they may not provide good control in patients who cannot be controlled by diet alone. Carefully prescribed insulin therapy provides better control of the mother's glucose, thereby preventing the fetal and neonatal complications that occur with this disease. Moreover, insulin, unlike most oral agents, does not cross the placenta to the fetus, thereby eliminating the additional concern that the drug therapy itself will adversely affect the fetus. High maternal glucose levels, as may occur in diabetes mellitus, are closely associated with a number of maternal and fetal adverse effects, including fetal structural anomalies if the hyperglycemia occurs early in gestation. To prevent this toxicity, most experts, including the American College of Obstetricians and Gynecologists, recommend that insulin be used for types I and II diabetes in pregnancy and, if diet therapy alone is not successful, for gestational diabetes (3,4).

BREAST FEEDING SUMMARY

RECOMMENDATION: Limited Human Data - Probably Compatible

Miglitol is excreted into the milk of lactating rats. The mean milk:plasma ratio, based on area under the concentration curve, was 1.3 (2). Consistent with its relatively low molecular weight (about 207), miglitol is also excreted into human milk (1). The total amount excreted, however, is very small, accounting only for 0.02% of a 100-mg dose (only 50%–70% of a 100–mg dose is bioavailable) (1). The estimated exposure of a nursing infant was about 0.4% of the mother's dose. The effects of this exposure on a nursing infant are unknown, but the manufacturer recommends that miglitol not be used during lactation (1). A 2000 review also stated that miglitol should not be used during breast-feeding (5).

References

1. Product information. Glyset. Pharmacia & Upjohn, 2000.
2. Ahr H-J, Boberg M, Brendel E, Krause HP, Steinke W. Pharmacokinetics of miglitol. Absorption, distribution, metabolism, and excretion following administration to rats, dogs, and man. Arzneim-Forsch/Drug Res 1997;47:734–45.
3. American College of Obstetricians and Gynecologists. Diabetes and pregnancy. *Technical Bulletin*. No. 200, December 1994.
4. Coustan DR. Management of gestational diabetes. Clin Obstet Gynecol 1991;34:558–64.
5. Campbell LK, Baker DE, Campbell RK. Miglitol: assessment of its role in the treatment of patients with diabetes mellitus. Ann Pharmacother 2000;34:1291–301.

Name: **MILRINONE** Risk Factor: C_M

Class: **Cardiac Agent**

FETAL RISK SUMMARY

RECOMMENDATION: No Human Data - Animal Data Suggest Risk

Milrinone is used IV for the treatment of congestive heart disease. Reproductive studies in rats (dosages up to 40 mg/kg/day) and rabbits (dosages up to 12 mg/kg/day) have revealed an increased resorption rate, but no teratogenic effects (1). No reports describing the use of this drug in human pregnancy have been located.

In an experiment with four pregnant baboons at 155–165 days' gestation (term 175 days), milrinone was given as an IV bolus of 75 μg/kg followed by a continuous infusion of 1 μg/kg/minute for 180 minutes (loading and maintenance doses considered maximal in humans) (2). Placental transfer was demonstrated as early as 5 minutes after beginning. At steady state (60 minutes), the maternal:fetal concentration ratio was 4:1. Although a significant increase in maternal heart rate was measured during the experiment, no significant changes were observed in the maternal mean arterial pressure or in the fetal heart rate and arterial blood gasses or pH values. All four fetuses appeared normal at birth.

BREAST FEEDING SUMMARY

RECOMMENDATION: No Human Data - Probably Compatible

No data are available.

References

1. Product information. Primacor. Sanofi Pharmaceuticals, 2000.
2. Atkinson BD, Fishburne JI Jr, Hales KA, Levy GH, Rayburn WF. Placental transfer of milrinone in the nonhuman primate (baboon). Am J Obstet Gynecol 1996;174:895–6.

Name: **MINERAL OIL** Risk Factor: **C**

Class: **Laxative**

FETAL RISK SUMMARY

RECOMMENDATION: Compatible

Mineral oil is an emollient laxative. The drug is generally considered nonabsorbable. Chronic use may lead to decreased absorption of fat-soluble vitamins.

BREAST FEEDING SUMMARY

RECOMMENDATION: Compatible

No data are available.

Name:	**MINOCYCLINE**	Risk Factor:	**D**
Class:	**Antibiotic (Tetracycline)**		

See Tetracycline.

Name:	**MINOXIDIL**	Risk Factor:	**C_M**
Class:	**Antihypertensive**		

FETAL RISK SUMMARY

RECOMMENDATION: Limited Human Data - Animal Data Suggest Moderate Risk

Minoxidil is a potent antihypertensive peripheral vasodilator. It is indicated for the treatment of hypertension that is symptomatic or associated with target organ damage. Minoxidil is considered a second-line antihypertensive therapy because of the potential for severe adverse effects. After oral dosing, minoxidil is nearly completely (90%) metabolized to metabolites that have much less antihypertensive effects. The average plasma elimination half-life of the parent compound is 4.2 hours (1).

Minoxidil is also used topically for the treatment of androgenetic alopecia (male baldness) and alopecia areata. After topical application, it is poorly absorbed from normal intact skin, with an average of 1.4% (range 0.3–4.5%) entering the systemic circulation. Steady state concentrations in the plasma are reached at the end of the third dosing interval (36 hours) (2).

Reproduction studies have been conducted in rats and rabbits (1–3). In rats, no evidence of teratogenicity or fetotoxicity was observed after an oral dose that was five times the human dose (1,2). Similarly, no teratogenicity was observed with a SC dose (80 mg/kg/day) that produced maternal toxicity (1). The oral dose, however, reduced the conception rate (2). There also was no teratogenicity in the offspring of pregnant rabbits given an oral dose that was five times the human dose, but an increased incidence of fetal resorptions was noted (1,2).

Pregnant rats were administered minoxidil at doses of 3 and 10 mg/kg/day on gestational days 6–15 (3). No evidence of teratogenicity or acute toxicity was observed. However, in the 10 mg/kg/day group, there was a higher than expected incidence of retinal folds in the eyes of offspring. Additional studies did not confirm this finding. In pregnant rabbits, similar doses administered on gestational days 6–18 resulted in fewer live pups per litter. At the highest dose, there was a higher incidence of resorptions (3).

It is not known if minoxidil crosses the human placenta. The molecular weight (about 209) is low enough, however, that fetal exposure should be expected. Moreover, the moderately long elimination half-life (4.2 hours) should increase the opportunity for drug transfer to the fetal compartment. In addition, the two cases of hypertrichosis described below suggest that minoxidil crosses the placenta.

Information on the use of oral minoxidil in human pregnancy is very limited, and only four cases of fetal exposure have been located (4–6). In one report, minoxidil was used throughout gestation with no effect seen in the healthy newborn (4). A second report involved a mother with a history of renal artery stenosis and malignant hypertension who was treated throughout gestation with minoxidil, captopril, and propranolol (5). Three of her four previous pregnancies had ended in midgestation stillbirths. The most recent stillbirth, her fourth pregnancy, involved a 500-g male infant with low-set ears but no gross anomalies. The mother had been treated with the above regimen plus furosemide. In her second pregnancy, she was treated with only hydrochlorothiazide and delivered a normal term infant. No information was available on the first and third pregnancies, both of which ended in stillbirths.

In her current pregnancy, daily doses of the three drugs were 10 mg, 50 mg, and 160 mg, respectively. The infant, delivered by cesarean section at 38 weeks' gestation, had multiple abnormalities, including an omphalocele (repaired on the 2nd day), pronounced hypertrichosis of the back and extremities, depressed nasal bridge, low-set ears, micrognathia, bilateral fifth finger clinodactyly, undescended testes, a circumferential midphallic constriction, a large ventriculoseptal defect, and a brain defect consisting of slightly prominent sulci, especially the basal cisterns and interhemispheric fissure. Growth retardation was not evident, but the weight (3170 g, 60th percentile), length (46 cm, 15th percentile), and head circumference (32.5 cm, 25th percentile) were disproportionate. Neurologic, skeletal, and kidney examinations were normal. Marked hypotension (30–50 mm Hg systolic) was present, which resolved after 24 hours. Heart rate, blood glucose, and renal function were normal.

M

The infant's hospital course was marked by failure to thrive, congestive heart failure, prolonged physiologic jaundice, and eight episodes of hyperthermia (>38.5°C without apparent cause) at 2–6 weeks of age. The hypertrichosis, which was much less prominent at 2 months of age, is a known side effect of minoxidil therapy in both children and adults, and the condition in this infant was thought to be caused by that drug. The cause of the other defects could not be determined, but a chromosomal abnormality was excluded based on a normal male karyotype (46,XY) determined after a midgestation amniocentesis (5).

Interestingly, captopril (see Captopril) is known to cause structural defects (hypocalvaria or acalvaria) and severe renal toxicity (anuria), but none of the anomalies observed in the above infant have been reported with captopril. The relatively low dose of 50 mg/day (recommended dose 50–150 mg/day) may have protected the fetus from the characteristic renal toxicity observed with angiotensin 1-converting enzyme inhibitors.

Two additional cases of *in utero* exposure to oral minoxidil were reported to the FDA and published in 1987 (6). The first infant was the product of a 32-week gestation in a 22-year-old woman with severe uncontrolled renal hypertension who was treated during pregnancy with minoxidil, methyldopa, hydralazine, furosemide, and phenobarbital. The 1770-g infant died of congenital heart disease the day after delivery. Defects noted at autopsy were transposition of the great vessels and pulmonic bicuspid valvular stenosis. Hypertrichosis was not observed. No conclusions can be drawn on the cause of the cardiac defects. The second infant, delivered near term and weighing 3220 g, was exposed throughout gestation to minoxidil (5 mg/day) plus metoprolol (100 mg/day) and prazosin (20 mg/day). The mother had severe hypertension secondary to chronic nephritis. Hypertrichosis was evident in both the mother and the newborn, but no other abnormalities were noted in the infant. The excessive hair growth, which was longest in the sacral area, gradually disappeared during the following 2–3 months. Normal development was noted at 2 years of age (6).

Two reports have described the outcomes of pregnancies exposed to topical minoxidil (7,8). A 14-week gestation was diagnosed in a nondiabetic 28-year-old, primigravid, woman who had used minoxidil 2% topical solution to treat hair loss during the 1st trimester (7). Her pregnancy was terminated at 17 weeks' gestation because an ultrasound examination had revealed oligohydramnios, a single umbilical artery, and multiple, severe anomalies. The woman also had experienced a flu-like upper respiratory disease during the 7th to 9th weeks of gestation, which had been treated with trimethoprim-sulfamethoxazole (2 tablets twice daily for 2 weeks) and erythromycin (500 mg four times daily for 1 week). At termination, no evidence of infection was found with a negative TORCH (toxoplasmosis, other infections, rubella, cytomegalovirus, and herpes simplex) test. Malformations in the male fetus included a transverse reduction deformity of the lower limbs and pelvis, agenesis of the cloacal membrane, imperforate anus, absence of external genitalia and bladder, renal agenesis, esophageal atresia, tracheoesophageal fistula, hypoplastic left thumb and thenar eminence, 11 ribs, and absence of L5, sacrum, and pelvis (7). There was no evidence of an amniotic band, and the cause of the malformations remained unknown. Trimethoprim is a folate antagonist and is believed to cause congenital anomalies but not of the type observed in this infant. (See Trimethoprim.) The constellation of defects was thought to represent a severe form of caudal regression syndrome, although the most severe form of this syndrome, the sirenomelia complex, could not be completely excluded (7).

A 28-year-old woman applied a 2% solution of minoxidil on her whole scalp to treat a diffuse bristly-hair condition for at least 1 year and throughout her current pregnancy (8). She experienced a brief flu-like syndrome at the 9th week of gestation (maximum temperature 38.5°C). The woman elected to terminate her pregnancy at about 22 weeks' gestation after an ultrasound examination revealed a fetus with multiple anomalies. The 450-g female fetus had extradural occipital hematomas, funnel-like posterior cranial base, hypoplastic middle cranial base, underdeveloped cerebellar lobes, fourth ventricle dilation, and diffuse intracerebral hemorrhages. Other defects included a globose heart, partial subaortic stenosis, mesentery commune, and a significantly increased length of the sigmoid colon Histologic examination of the brain revealed multiple areas of necrosis, diffuse areas of white matter demyelinization with reactive gliosis, with capillary agglomerates. There also was dilation and congestion of cerebral small vessels and capillaries. The woman stopped the minoxidil and gave birth to a normal infant 2 years later. The cause of the malformations could not be determined, but the authors thought they were secondary to minoxidil (8).

In summary, minoxidil is not teratogenic in rats and rabbits, but some fetotoxicity was observed in rabbits. The human pregnancy experience is too limited, after both oral dosing and topical application, to determine the risk of teratogenicity. A possible exception involves the two infants exposed *in utero* to oral minoxidil who had hypertrichosis. This is a known adverse effect in adults and, indeed, one of the mothers had hypertrichosis. However, the causes of the multiple congenital malformations observed in one of these infants and the heart defects in the other are unknown. Similarly, the causes of the multiple anomalies observed in two fetuses after minoxidil topical application also are unknown. Although the doses applied in these two cases were not specified, only small amounts of topically applied minoxidil are absorbed into the systemic circulation. Of interest, both mothers had a flu-like illness in the 1st trimester. Even if these malformations are not related to drug exposure, the potential toxicity of oral minoxidil is severe enough to preclude its use in pregnancy. One of these toxicities includes large orthostatic decreases in blood pressure that could severely jeopardize placental perfusion. Although the possibility of a causal relationship to malformations after topical application appears to be remote, the safest course is to avoid applying the agent during the 1st trimester.

BREAST FEEDING SUMMARY

RECOMMENDATION: Limited Human Data - Probably Compatible

Minoxidil is excreted into breast milk (4). Levels in the milk ranged from 41.7 ng/mL (1 hour) to 0.3 ng/mL (12 hours), with milk:plasma ratios during this interval varying from 0.67 to 1.0. No adverse effects were observed in the infant. The American Academy of Pediatrics classifies minoxidil as compatible with breast-feeding (9).

References

1. Product information. Loniten. Pharmacia & Upjohn, 2002.
2. Product information. Rogaine. RxMed: Pharmaceutical Information, 2004.
3. Carlson RG, Feenstra ES. Toxicologic studies with the hypotensive agent minoxidil. Toxicol Appl Pharmacol 1977;39:1–11.
4. Valdivieso A, Valdes G, Spiro TE, Westerman RL. Minoxidil in breast milk. Ann Intern Med 1985;102:135.
5. Kaler SG, Patrinos ME, Lambert GH, Myers TF, Karlman R, Anderson CL. Hypertrichosis and congenital anomalies associated with maternal use of minoxidil. Pediatrics 1987;79:434–6.
6. Rosa FW, Idanpaan-Heikkila J, Asanti R. Fetal minoxidil exposure. Pediatrics 1987;80:120.
7. Rojansky N, Fasouliotis SJ, Ariel H, Nadjari M. Extreme caudal agenesis. Possible drug-related etiology? J Reprod Med 2002;47:241–5.
8. Smorlesi C, Caldarella A, Caramelli L, Di Lollo S, Moroni F. Topically applied minoxidil may cause fetal malformation: a case report. Birth Defects Res Part A Clin Mol Teratol 2003;67:997–1001.
9. Committee on Drugs, American Academy of Pediatrics. The transfer of drugs and other chemicals into human milk. Pediatrics 2001;108:776–89.

Name: **MIRTAZAPINE** Risk Factor: C_M

Class: **Antidepressant**

FETAL RISK SUMMARY

RECOMMENDATION: No Human Data - Animal Data Suggest Low Risk

Mirtazapine is a tetracyclic antidepressant that is chemically unrelated to selective serotonin reuptake inhibitors, tricyclic antidepressants, and monoamine oxidase inhibitors. Although the exact mechanism of action is unknown, the antidepressant effect is thought to result from an increase in central noradrenergic and serotonergic activity (1). Mirtazapine is also a potent inhibitor of histamine (H_1) inhibitors, a property that probably explains the marked sedation often seen with this agent.

No teratogenic effects were observed in rats given doses up to 100 mg/kg or in rabbits given doses up to 40 mg/kg, 20 and 17 times the maximum recommended human dose based on body surface area, respectively (1). Toxicity observed in rats at the maximum dose (but not at 15 mg/kg) included an increase in postimplantation losses, increased pup deaths during the first 3 days of lactation, and lower pup birth weights.

It is not known whether mirtazapine crosses the placenta to the fetus. Because of its low molecular weight (about 265), however, transfer to the fetus in measurable amounts should be anticipated.

Mirtazapine was approved by the FDA for use in the United States in June 1996. No published reports describing the use of this drug in human pregnancy have been located. Moreover, no reports of adverse pregnancy outcomes related to mirtazapine have been reported to the FDA (F. Rosa, personal communication, FDA, 1996). If mirtazapine is used in pregnancy, healthcare professionals are encouraged to call the toll free number (800-670-6126) for information about patient enrollment in the Motherisk study.

BREAST FEEDING SUMMARY

RECOMMENDATION: No Human Data - Potential Toxicity

No reports describing the use of mirtazapine during lactation have been located. Because other antidepressants are excreted into milk (see Maprotiline, another tetracyclic antidepressant) and because of its relatively low molecular weight (about 265), the passage of mirtazapine into milk should be expected. Moreover, the long-term effects on neurobehavior and development from exposure to this class of agents during a period of rapid central nervous system development have not been studied. The American Academy of Pediatrics classifies other antidepressants as drugs for which the effect on nursing infants is unknown but may be of concern (2).

References

1. Product information. Remeron. Organon, 1997.
2. Committee of Drugs, American Academy of Pediatrics. The transfer of drugs and other chemicals into human milk. Pediatrics 2001;108:776–89.

M

Name:	**MISOPROSTOL**	Risk Factor:	**X_M**
Class:	**Gastrointestinal Agent (Antisecretory)**		

FETAL RISK SUMMARY

RECOMMENDATION: Contraindicated (Oral)
Human Data Suggest Low Risk (Term Cervical Ripening)

Misoprostol, a synthetic prostaglandin E_1 analogue is used to prevent gastric ulcers induced by nonsteroidal anti-inflammatory agents. It is contraindicated in pregnancy because of the risk of uterine bleeding and contractions that may result in abortion. Although not indicated for such, misoprostol is routinely used for cervical ripening in term pregnancies and for 2nd trimester pregnancy termination.

In reproduction studies reported by the manufacturer, misoprostol was not teratogenic in rats and rabbits at doses 625 and 63 times the maximum recommended human dose (MRHD), respectively (1). At 6.25–625 times the MRHD, however, dose-related pre- and post-implantation losses and a significant decrease in the number of live pups were seen in rats (1). In another study, however, teratogenicity observed in pregnant rabbits given doses of 300–1500 μg/kg on days 7–19 included spinal bifida, caudal vertebral defects, umbilical hernia, and gastroschisis (2).

In a surveillance study of Michigan Medicaid recipients conducted between 1985 and 1992 involving 229,101 completed pregnancies, 5 newborns had been exposed to misoprostol during the 1st trimester (F. Rosa, personal communication, FDA, 1993). One (20.0%) major birth defect was observed (none expected), a cardiovascular defect.

During the initial clinical trials, menstrual complaints were higher among nonpregnant women treated with misoprostol (3.7%) than with placebo (1.7%) (3). In a clinical study designed to assess the effect of misoprostol on the pregnant uterus, 111 women, who had consented to an elective 1st-trimester abortion, were treated with either placebo or one or two 400-μg doses of the prostaglandin. All 6 of the women who aborted spontaneously the day following treatment had received misoprostol. Uterine bleeding occurred in 45% (25 of 56) of the women treated with misoprostol compared with 4% (2 of 55) of the placebo-treated women (3).

Misoprostol has been combined with the antiprogestogen mifepristone (RU 486) to induce legal abortion (see also Mifepristone) (4–7). Some of the advantages of this prostaglandin analogue over similar agents are that it is effective, active by the oral route, inexpensive, and stable at room temperature (4,5). In one study, 40 women were treated with 400 μg of the drug 7 days before surgical termination of pregnancy (6). Only two of the women from this group had a complete abortion. In a second part of the study, 21 women were given 200–1000 μg of misoprostol 48 hours after a 200-mg dose of mifepristone, resulting in a complete abortion in 18 women (6). Similar effectiveness was found in a large study published in 1993 involving 895 women who received misoprostol, either 4 or 48 hours after a dose of mifepristone (7).

A 1991 reference cited the use of misoprostol as an illegal abortifacient in Brazil (8). The drug is freely available as an over-the-counter product in that country, where abortions are illegal. At one university hospital maternity unit, 20 women sought emergency treatment for uterine bleeding in 1988 after an unsuccessful attempt to induce abortion with misoprostol. In 1990, the number rose to 525. The usual dose consumed was 800 μg (two 200-μg tablets orally plus two tablets vaginally), but some women may have taken as much as 9200 μg (46 tablets) (8).

M

Five infants with congenital malformations who had been exposed during the 1st trimester to misoprostol in unsuccessful attempts at abortion were described in a 1991 case report (9). The total dose was 1200 μg in two of the mothers and 400–600 μg in the other three cases. The five infants had an unusual defect of the frontotemporal region of the skull consisting of an asymmetric, well-circumscribed anomaly of the cranium and overlying scalp, exposing the dura mater and underlying cerebrum. Surgical correction of the defect was attempted within 4 days of birth in each of the cases, but one infant died of severe infection. Although the authors conceded that a later-acting agent was suggested by the nature of the defect, three of the mothers denied any further attempts to terminate their pregnancies after the use of misoprostol (9). In a later publication, two of the authors described more fully the defects of the scalp and cranium in three of the newborns (10).

Two additional reports describing the use of misoprostol as an abortifacient by Brazilian women appeared in 1993 (11,12). In Rio de Janeiro during a 9-month period of 1991, of 803 women admitted to hospitals with abortion complications, 458 (57%) had self-administered misoprostol to induce abortion (11). Most (80%) of these women had used the drug alone. The median dose used was 800 μg (range 200–16,800 μg) with 65% taking it orally, 29% orally and vaginally, and 6% vaginally only. The most frequently cited reasons by the women for seeking medical care were vaginal bleeding (80%) and uterine cramps (78%). Only 8% of the women reported vomiting and diarrhea. Morbidity among the 458 women included heavy bleeding (19%) (1% required blood transfusion), infection (17%), curettage required (85%), uterine perforation after curettage (1%), and systemic collapse (1%). In Fortaleza, Brazil, misoprostol use accounted for 444 (75%) of 593 incomplete abortions treated in a hospital by uterine evacuation during 1991 (12).

Complications observed in the 444 women included 144 (32%) with infection, 1 with septic shock, 3 with hypovolemic shock, and 1 with uterine perforation.

A 1992 report from Brazil questioned the teratogenicity of misoprostol (13). Since 1990, 29 women had contacted a teratogen information counseling service after unsuccessful attempts at inducing abortion with misoprostol during the 1st trimester. The mean dose used by these women was 4000 μg (20 tablets), with a range of 200 μg (one tablet) to 11,200 μg (56 tablets). The women were monitored with ultrasonography during the remainder of their pregnancies. The results of the pregnancies were: spontaneous abortions (2nd trimester), 3; still pregnant, 3; lost to follow-up, 6; and normal infants, 17 (one with preauricular tag). Of the 17 normal infants, 8 were examined by the authors, 4 were examined by pediatricians not associated with the authors, and in 5 cases verbal information was received from the mothers (13). The absence of data for the 9 (31%) cases, however, lessens the ability to interpret this report.

Seven cases of limb defects involving the hands and feet following 1st-trimester use of misoprostol (dose range 600–1800 μg) as an unsuccessful abortifacient were described in a 1993 report (14). Four of the infants demonstrated bilateral palsy of cranial nerves, leading to a diagnosis of Möbius sequence (6th and 7th nerve palsies). An additional five cases (one with limb deficiency, one with limb deficiency and Möbius sequence, and three with Möbius sequence) following failed abortion attempts with misoprostol were appended to the report, but specific details were not given. In the seven pregnancies with sufficient detail, misoprostol exposure was thought to have occurred between 30 and 60 days following conception. The investigators attributed the anomalies to misoprostol-induced vascular disruption (14). In a 1993 invited editorial on the strengths and weaknesses of case reports, the publication of the above research was thought to be valid because the association with birth defects was biologically plausible and there were other reports supporting a causal association (15).

A brief report (16) and abstract (17) suggested that a possible mechanism for Möbius syndrome was flexion of the embryo in the area of cranial nuclei 6 and 7 that resulted in vascular disruption of the region bent. The cranial nuclei 6 and 7 are located in a region of the embryo that would be bent if there was pressure in a cephalocaudal direction. The hypothesis proposed that flexing of the region would result in decreased blood flow and hemorrhage and/or cell death of the cranial nuclei. It was hypothesized that misoprostol-induced uterine contractions early in gestation, before there was sufficient amniotic fluid to cushion the embryo, would cause the flexing if the embryo was correctly positioned. Experiments in rat embryos confirmed that hemorrhage would occur in this region after mechanical flexion in the proposed direction. Although limb reduction defects are often associated with Möbius syndrome and may also be a result of mechanical factors, the author's hypothesis could not reasonably explain these defects (16,17).

A 1998 study (18) and earlier abstract (19) compared the frequency of 1st trimester misoprostol use in 96 infants with Möbius syndrome with 96 infants with neural tube defects (NTDs). In the 96 infants with Möbius syndrome, there were no differences in the clinical appearance between those exposed to misoprostol (N = 47; 46 for attempted abortion) and those not exposed (N = 49): bilateral facial-nerve (cranial nerve 7) paralysis, 34 vs. 36; unilateral facial-nerve paralysis, 13 vs. 13; abducens-nerve (cranial nerve 6) paralysis, 39 vs. 37; other cranial nerve palsy, 10 vs. 8; all limb defects, 31 vs. 28; club feet only, 25 vs. 18; limb reduction, 6 vs. 10; orofacial anomalies, 18 vs. 11; mental retardation, 26 vs. 26; other defects, 15 vs. 14 (all *n.s.*). Misoprostol was used in 47 cases of Möbius syndrome and 3 cases of NTD (odds ratio 29.7, 95% confidence interval [CI] 11.6–76.0). Among the 47 cases of misoprostol use, 20 took the drug orally, 20 took it both orally and vaginally, 3 took it vaginally only, and 4 could not recall how they took the drug. The authors concluded that attempted abortion with misoprostol was associated with an increased risk of Möbius syndrome (18,19).

A 1994 abstract reported a case of a woman who took misoprostol 600 μg/day for 2 days at 7 weeks' gestation in an unsuccessful attempt to induce abortion (20). An elective abortion at 17 weeks' gestation revealed a male fetus with an omphalocele, left leg below-the-knee amputation, absence of the middle and distal phalanges of four fingers of the right hand with distal fusion by amniotic band, and evidence of early amniotic rupture. Although the mother had had chicken pox at 12 weeks, there was no evidence in the placenta or fetus of viral infection.

The Latin-America Collaborative Study of Congenital Malformations found 12 misoprostol-exposed newborns among 5708 malformed and 5708 nonmalformed matched controls (21). Each of the exposures involved unsuccessful attempts by the women to induce abortion. Four of the infants were in the control group, but the maternal dose (1000 μg) was known in only one case. Of the eight exposed infants, two had Down's syndrome (doses 1400 μg and 4000 μg) and two had minor anomalies (café-au-lait spot on right leg, dose 600 μg; extranumerary nipple on left, dose 400 μg). These cases do not appear to be related to misoprostol. In the remaining four infants, the authors characterized the defects as suggestive of misoprostol-induced *in utero* vascular disruption (maternal dose shown in parenthesis) (21):

Missing metacarpals and phalanges; hypoplasia of thumbs and two fingers; partial syndactyly of two fingers; peculiar face with prominent nasal bridge and ocular hypertelorism; weak cry (400 μg)

Complete bilateral cleft lip and palate; ocular hypertelorism; short limbs; absence of thumbs and 5th fingers; skin tags on one finger; stiff knees; bilateral talipes equinovarus (dose unknown)

Skin scar over T2-T3; no evidence of spina bifida by x-ray (dose unknown)

Gastroschisis (1400 μg)

In a second report from the above group, they found 57 newborn infants exposed to misoprostol among 9653 newborns: 34 in 4673 malformed infants and 23 in 4980 control infants (*n.s.*) (22). In comparing exposed vs. nonexposed malformed infants, significant differences were measured for four vascular disruption malformations that had been reported by others: arthrogryposis (5.88% vs. 0.73%), hydrocephalus (11.76% vs. 3.04%), terminal transverse limb reduction (8.82% vs. 0.67%), and limb constriction ring or skin scars (8.82% vs. 0.24%). No cases of cranial nerve palsies (e.g., Möbius sequence) were in the registry because these types of defects would not be obvious at birth. Significant associations with two other malformations that had not been reported previously were holoprosencephaly (5.88% vs. 0.34%) and bladder exstrophy (2.94% vs. 0.06%). However, the authors recommended caution in interpreting these latter defects as causal associations. They concluded that there was a causal association between the four vascular disruption defects and the use of misoprostol as an abortifacient (22).

Of note, a 1996 report provided detailed descriptions of three cases of arthrogryposis (i.e., arthrogryposis multiplex congenita; the use of the shorter term, arthrogryposis, implies multiple, nonprogressive congenital joint contractures) after failed mechanical attempts at pregnancy termination (23). The cause of the defect was thought to be vascular disruption resulting in nerve damage that led to fetal akinesia and subsequent contractures (23).

A relative risk of >7.0 for congenital malformations, particularly Möbius sequence, was found among 732 children born after 1990 who were attending five outpatient genetic clinics in Brazil (24). About 10% of the children had been exposed *in utero* to misoprostol. There were 25 cases of Möbius syndrome, 24 cases of reduction of phalanges, and 227 cases with isolated malformations. Associations with misoprostol occurred in 17 (68%), 7 (29%), and 15 (6.6%), respectively, of the cases (24).

A below-the-knee amputation was observed in a female newborn delivered at 29 weeks' gestation because of fetal distress (25). An abortion had been attempted at about 13 weeks' under medical supervision. A single misoprostol tablet (strength not specified) had been inserted vaginally for 4 days, but only some vaginal bleeding had occurred on day 4. Spontaneous rupture of the membranes was documented at about 26 weeks' gestation (25).

A 1998 study proposed that the abnormalities observed in children exposed *in utero* during the 1st trimester to misoprostol were induced by uterine contractions that caused vascular disruption in the fetuses, including ischemia of the brainstem (26). Of the 42 infants with congenital malformations, 17 had equinovarus with cranial nerve defects (usually of nerves 5, 6, and 7), 10 had equinovarus as part of a more extensive arthrogryposis, and 9 had terminal transverse-limb defects. Five children had a distinctive arthrogryposis, without cranial nerve injury, that was confined to the legs. Severe amyoplasia of the legs was confirmed in five children by electromyography, and two of the cases had deficient anterior horn cell activity. Eight had hydrocephalus associated with increased pressure that required shunt placement to relieve. One child had an omphalocele but no evidence of cranial nerve defects of arthrogryposis (26).

A 1997 abstract and 1999 full report described a prospective, observational cohort study of 86 misoprostol-exposed pregnancies compared with 86 pair-matched controls (27,28). All of the women had called a teratogen information service regarding pregnancy exposure to either misoprostol or nonteratogenic agents. There were no statistical differences between the groups in the rates of major (2/67 vs. 2/81) or minor (7/67 vs. 3/81) malformations, gestational age at birth, prematurity, birth weight, low birth weight, sex ratio, or rates of cesarean section. However, there were more abortions in the exposed group, 17.1% vs. 5.8%, relative risk 2.97, 95% CI 1.12–7.88. The sample size had limited power as it was only able to detect an eight-fold increase in the risk of major malformations (28).

A study published in 2000 reported the clinical evaluations of 15 children (8 males, 7 females; average age 2 years) from Salvador and Brazil with misoprostol-induced arthrogryposis (29). Their mothers had taken 400–4800 μg of misoprostol, orally or vaginally, from 8 to 12 weeks' gestation for attempted abortions. Common pathologic features in the children were growth retardation, underdeveloped bones, short feet with equinovarus, rigidity of joints with skin dimples and webs, neurologic impaired leg movement, bilateral symmetrical hypoplasia or atrophy of limb muscles, and absent tendon reflexes. Twelve had normal intelligence (information not available for the other three). Other abnormalities included neurogenic bladder/bowel ($N = 9$), hip dislocation ($N = 6$), upper and lower limb deformity ($N = 5$), cryptorchidism ($N = 2$), inguinal hernia ($N = 2$), and single cases of medullar stenosis/syringomyelia, spina bifida, abdominal muscle hypoplasia, and nail hypoplasia. Neurogenic patterns suggestive of anterior horn cell defects were observed on electromyogram in five children (29).

In another 2000 report, a multicenter, case-control study compared the frequency of misoprostol exposure in 93 children with vascular disruption anomalies (subjects) and 279 children with other types of defects (controls) (30). All of the children were born after 1992. Congenital malformations classified as vascular disruptions in the subject cases were Möbius syndrome ($N = 29$), transverse limb reduction ($N = 27$), hemifacial microsomia ($N = 16$), arthrogryposis ($N = 9$), microtia ($N = 9$), porencephalic cyst ($N = 2$), and hypoglossia hypodactyly ($N = 1$). Misoprostol exposure (all for attempted abortion) occurred in 32 subject cases (34.4%) compared to 12 controls (4.3%), $p < 0.0000001$. In 16 subjects, misoprostol was used between the 5th and 8th week after the last menstrual period, and in two the exposure occurred after the 1st trimester. There was no difference between the two groups in the misoprostol dose taken. Based on their data, the investigators concluded that misoprostol was associated with vascular disruption defects (30).

A case of maternal misoprostol overdosage resulting in fetal death was reported in 1994 (31). In a suicide attempt, a 19-year-old woman at 31 weeks' gestation ingested 6000 μg (thirty 200-μg tablets) and 8 mg of trifluoperazine. She was seen 2 hours later at a hospital complaining of feeling hot, chills, shortness of breath, restlessness, and discomfort. A tetanic uterus was observed, and physical examination revealed her cervix to be dilated to 5 cm with 80% effacement. Fetal movements and heart motion (by sonogram) were absent 1 hour after admission (3 hours after ingestion), and 1 hour later she delivered a stillborn 1,800-g fetus that was diffusely ecchymotic. Postmortem examination was remarkable only for diffuse head and upper body bruising (31).

Misoprostol has been used for the induction of labor in cases involving intrauterine fetal death (IUFD) or when medical or genetic reasons existed for pregnancy termination (32–34). In 20 cases of IUFD, pregnancy termination occurred a mean 9.2 hours after the start of oral misoprostol, 400 μg every 4 hours (mean total dose 1,000 μg) (32). Maternal adverse effects were common. A second study, involving 72 women with IUFD at 18–40 weeks' gestation, used a lower dose (100 μg; one-half of an oral 200-μg tablet) introduced into the vaginal posterior fornix every 12 hours (up to 48 hours) until effective contractions and cervical dilatation were obtained (33). Only 6 women (8%) required treatment between 24 and 48 hours and all had delivered within 48 hours (mean 12.6 hours; range 2–48 hours). None of the women required surgical intervention. Other than one case of abruptio placentae, no complications were observed. A dose of 200 μg, also administered vaginally, was used in a third study with a comparison group receiving a 20-mg prostaglandin E_2 (PGE_2) vaginal suppository every 3 hours (34). Successful abortions were obtained within 24 hours in 89% (25 of 28) of women treated with misoprostol and in 81% (22 of 27) of women administered PGE_2 (*n.s.*). The remaining three misoprostol-treated women had successful abortions within 38 hours (similar data for PGE2 were not given). Complete abortions (passage of the fetus and the placenta simultaneously) occurred in 43% and 32% of the misoprostol- and PGE_2-treated groups, respectively. Significantly more women experienced adverse effects (pyrexia, uterine pain, vomiting, and diarrhea) with PGE_2 than with misoprostol, and the difference in average cost between the treatments was large ($315.30 for PGE2 versus $0.97 for misoprostol). Two other studies have described the use of intravaginal misoprostol (200–800 μg) to successfully induce legal abortion at gestational ages ranging from 11 to 23 weeks (35,36).

Several reports and communications have described the use of misoprostol for cervical ripening and labor induction in the 3rd trimester (37–43). The doses used were 50–100 μg administered either as a single dose or at 4-hour intervals, but one group of investigators was studying a 25-μg dose (42). Tachysystole was observed in some cases, but the uterine hyperstimulation was not associated with an increased incidence of fetal distress or a higher rate of operative deliveries. The American College of Obstetricians and Gynecologists considers low dose (e.g., 25 μg) intravaginal misoprostol to be effective for inducing labor in pregnant women who have unfavorable cervices (44,45).

In summary, the prostaglandin E_1 analogue, misoprostol, is a potent uterine stimulant that induces abortion after either oral or vaginal administration early in pregnancy. The drug has been used as an illicit abortifacient and most cases of birth defects have been associated with abortion attempts. However, congenital malformations have also been associated with the therapeutic use of the drug. The teratogenic mechanism appears to be related to the induction of uterine contractions that deform the embryo, resulting in vascular disruption, hemorrhage, and cell death. Some authors consider the potential teratogenicity of misoprostol following an unsuccessful abortion attempt a reason to proceed cautiously with the use of the drug for this purpose, particularly in countries with limited medical services (46). Investigational and clinical use during the 2nd and 3rd trimesters have demonstrated the utility of misoprostol for labor induction and cervical ripening. Misoprostol appears to be superior, in terms of maternal morbidity and cost, to PGE_2 when used for 2nd-trimester pregnancy terminations and for cervical ripening.

BREAST FEEDING SUMMARY

RECOMMENDATION: No Human Data - Potential Toxicity

No studies describing the use of misoprostol during human lactation have been located. The manufacturer considers the drug to be contraindicated during nursing because of the potential for severe, drug-induced diarrhea in the nursing infant (1). Natural occurring PGE_1, however, is excreted into milk in concentrations similar to that in maternal plasma and may have an important function (e.g., cytoprotection) in the gastrointestinal tract of the nursing infant (47).

References

1. Product information. Cytotec. G.D. Searle, 2001.
2. Clemens GR, Hilbish KG, Hartnagel RE Jr, Schluter G, Reynolds JA. Developmental toxicity including teratogenicity of E_1 prostaglandins in rabbits. The Toxicologist 1997;36.260. As cited in Gonzalez CH, Marques-Dias MJ, Kim CA, Sugayama SMM, Da Paz JA, Huson SM, Holmes LB. Congenital abnormalities in Brazilian children associated with misoprostol misuse in first trimester of pregnancy. Lancet 1998;351:1624–7.
3. Lewis JH. Summary of the 29th meeting of the Gastrointestinal Drugs Advisory committee, Food and Drug Administration—June 10, 1985. Am J Gastroenterol 1985;80:743–5.
4. Anonymous. Misoprostol and legal medical abortion. Lancet 1991;338:1241–2.
5. Baird DT, Norman JE, Thong KJ, Glasier AF. Misoprostol, mifepristone, and abortion. Lancet 1992;339:313.
6. Norman JE, Thong KJ, Baird DT. Uterine contractility and induction of abortion in early pregnancy by misoprostol and mifepristone. Lancet 1991;338:1233–6.
7. Peyron R, Aubeny E, Targosz V, Silvestre L, Renault M, Elkik F, Leclerc P, Ulmann A, Baulieu E-E. Early termination of pregnancy with mifepristone (RU 486) and the orally active prostaglandin misoprostol. N Engl J Med 1993;328:1509–13.
8. Schonhofer PS. Brazil: misuse of misoprostol as an abortifacient may induce malformations. Lancet 1991;337:1534–5.
9. Fonseca W, Alencar AJC, Mota FSB, Coelho HLL. Misoprostol and congenital malformations. Lancet 1991;338:56.
10. Fonseca W, Alencar AJC, Pereira RMM, Misago C. Congenital malformation of the scalp and cranium after failed first trimester abortion attempt with misoprostol. Clin Dysmorphol 1993;2:76–80.
11. Costa SH, Vessey MP. Misoprostol and illegal abortion in Rio de Janeiro, Brazil. Lancet 1993;341:1258–61.
12. Coêlho HLL, Teixeira AC, Santos AP, Forte FB, Morais SM, Vecchia CL, Tognoni G, Herxheimer A. Misoprostol and illegal abortion in Fortaleza, Brazil. Lancet 1993;341:1261–3.
13. Schuler L, Ashton PW, Sanseverino MT. Teratogenicity of misoprostol. Lancet 1992;339:437.
14. Gonzalez CH, Vargas FR, Perez ABA, Kim CA, Brunoni D, Marques-Dias MJ, Leone CR, Neto JC, Llerena JC Jr, Cabral de Almeida JC. Limb deficiency with or without Möbius sequence in seven Brazilian children associated with misoprostol use in the first trimester of pregnancy. Am J Med Genet 1993;47:59–64.
15. Brent RL. Congenital malformation case reports: the editor's and reviewer's dilemma. Am J Med Genet 1993;47:872–4.
16. Shepard TH. Möbius syndrome after misoprostol: a possible teratogenic mechanism. Lancet 1995;346:780.
17. Shepard TH, Lemire RJ. Möbius syndrome: a possible teratogenic mechanism (abstract). Teratology 1996;53:86.
18. Pastuszak AL, Schuler L, Speck-Martins CE, Coelho KEFA, Cordello SM, Vargas F, Brunoni D, Schwarz IVD, Larrandaburu M, Safattle H, Meloni VFA, Koren G. Use of misoprostol during pregnancy and Möbius' syndrome in infants. N Engl J Med 1998;338:1881–5.
19. Pastuszak AL, Schuler L, Coelho KA, Vargas F, Brunoni D, Speck-Martin C, Larrandaburu M. Misoprostol use during pregnancy is associated with an increased risk for Möbius sequence (abstract). Teratology 1997;55:36.
20. Genest DR, Richardson A, Rosenblatt M, Holmes L. Limb defects and omphalocele in a 17 week fetus

M

following first trimester misoprostol exposure (abstract). Teratology 1994;49:418.
21. Castilla EE, Orioli IM. Teratogenicity of misoprostol: data from the Latin-American Collaborative Study of Congenital Malformations (ECLAMC). Am J Med Genet 1994;51:161–2.
22. Orioli IM, Castilla EE. Epidemiological assessment of misoprostol teratogenicity. Br J Obstet Gynaecol 2000;107:519–23.
23. Hall JG. Arthrogryposis associated with unsuccessful attempts at termination of pregnancy. Am J Med Genet 1996;63:293–300.
24. Vargas FR, Brunoni D, Gonzalez C, Kim C, Meloni V, Conte A, Bortolotto E, Almeida JCC, Llerena JC, Duarte A, Albano L, Oliveira S, Cavalcanti D, Castilla EE. Investigation of the teratogenic potential of misoprostol (abstract). Teratology 1997;55:104.
25. Hofmeyr GJ, Milos D, Nikodem VC, de Jager M. Limb reduction anomaly after failed misoprostol abortion. S Afr Med J 1998;88:566–7.
26. Gonzalez CH, Marques-Dias MJ, Kim CA, Sugayama SMM, Da Paz JA, Huson SM, Holmes LB. Congenital abnormalities in Brazilian children associated with misoprostol misuse in first trimester of pregnancy. Lancet 1998;351:1624–7.
27. Schuler L, Pastuszak A, Sanseverino MT, Orioli IM, Brunoni D, Koren G. Pregnancy outcome after abortion attempt with misoprostol (abstract). Teratology 1997;55:36.
28. Schuler L, Pastuszak A, Sanseverino MTV, Orioli IM, Brunoni D, Ashton-Prolla P, Da Costa FS, Giugliani R, Couto AM, Brandao SB, Koren G. Pregnancy outcome after exposure to misoprostol in Brazil: a prospective, controlled study. Reprod Toxicol 1999;13:147–51.
29. Coelho KEFA, Sarmento MVF, Veiga CM, Speck-Martins CE, Safatle HPN, Castro CV, Niikawa N. Misoprostol embryotoxicity: clinical evaluation of fifteen patients with arthrogryposis. Am J Med Genet 2000;95:297–301.
30. Vargas FR, Schuler-Faccini L, Brunoni D, Kim C, Meloni VFA, Sugayama SMM, Albano L, Llerena JC Jr, Almeida JCC, Duarte A, Cavalcanti DP, Goloni-Bertollo E, Conte A, Koren G, Addis A. Prenatal exposure to misoprostol and vascular disruption defects: a case-control study. Am J Med Genet 2000;95:302–6.
31. Bond GR, Zee AV. Overdosage of misoprostol in pregnancy. Am J Obstet Gynecol 1994;171:561–2.
32. Mariani-Neto C, Leao EJ, Barreto EMCP, Kenj G, Aquino MMA, Tuffi VHB. Use of misoprostol for labor induction in stillbirth. Rev Paul Med 1987;105:325–8.
33. Bugalho A, Bique C, Machungo F, Fandes A. Induction of labor with intravaginal misoprostol in intrauterine fetal death. Am J Obstet Gynecol 1994;171:538–41.
34. Jain JK, Mishell DR Jr. A comparison of intravaginal misoprostol with prostaglandin E_2 for termination of second-trimester pregnancy. N Engl J Med 1994;331:290–3.
35. Bugalho A, Bique C, Almeida L, Bergström S. Pregnancy interruption by vaginal misoprostol. Gynecol Obstet Invest 1993;36:226–9.
36. Bugalho A, Bique C, Almeida L, Faúndes A. The effectiveness of intravaginal misoprostol (Cytotec) in inducting abortion after eleven weeks of pregnancy. Stud Fam Plann 1993;24:319–23.
37. Margulies M, Perez GC, Voto LS. Misoprostol to induce labour. Lancet 1992;339:64.
38. Sanchez-Ramos L, Kaunitz AM, Del Valle GO, Delke I, Schroeder A, Briones DK. Labor induction with the prostaglandin E_1 methyl analogue misoprostol versus oxytocin: a randomized trial. Obstet Gynecol 1993;81:332–6.
39. Fletcher HM, Mitchell S, Frederick J, Brown D. Intravaginal misoprostol as a cervical ripening agent. Br J Obstet Gynaecol 1993;100:641–44.
40. Sanchez-Ramos L, Chen A, Briones D, Del Valle GO, Gaudier FL, Delke I. Premature rupture of membranes at term: induction of labor with intravaginal misoprostol tablets (PGE_1) or intravenous oxytocin (abstract). Am J Obstet Gynecol 1994;170:380.
41. Fletcher H, Mitchell S, Frederick J, Simeon D, Brown D. Intravaginal misoprostol versus dinoprostone as cervical ripening and labor-inducing agents. Obstet Gynecol 1994;83:244–7.
42. Sanchez-Ramos L, Kaunitz A. Intravaginal misoprostol versus dinoprostone as cervical ripening and labor-inducing agents. Obstet Gynecol 1994;83:799–800.
43. Fletcher H. Intravaginal misoprostol versus dinoprostone as cervical ripening and labor-inducing agents (reply). Obstet Gynecol 1994;83:800–1.
44. Committee on Obstetric Practice, American College of Obstetricians and Gynecologists. Induction of labor with misoprostol. *Committee Opinion*. No. 228, November 1999.
45. Committee on Obstetric Practice, American College of Obstetricians and Gynecologists. Response to Searle's drug warning on misoprostol. *Committee Opinion*. No. 248, December 2000.
46. Fonseca W, Misago C, Kanji N. Misoprostol plus mifepristone. Lancet 1991;338:1594.
47. Shimizu T, Yamashiro Y, Yabuta K. Prostaglandins E_1, E_2, and $F_{2\alpha}$ in human milk and plasma. Biol Neonate 1992;61:222–5.

M

Name: **MITOXANTRONE**		Risk Factor: **D_M**
Class: **Antineoplastic**		

FETAL RISK SUMMARY

RECOMMENDATION: Contraindicated - 1st Trimester

This synthetic anthracenedione, structurally related to doxorubicin, is an antineoplastic antibiotic used in the treatment of acute nonlymphocytic leukemia. Other uses of this agent include cancers of the breast, ovary, and liver, and refractory lymphomas. Mitoxantrone is toxic to DNA and has a cytocidal effect on both proliferating and nonproliferating human cells (1). The mean half-life of mitoxantrone is 5.8 days (range 2.3–13.0 days) and may be longer in tissue. Moreover, the drug accumulates after multiple dosing in plasma and tissue.

Mitoxantrone administration to pregnant rats at a dose 0.05 times the recommended human dose on a mg/m^2 basis (RHD) caused decreased fetal weight and retarded development of the fetal kidney (1). Although not teratogenic in rabbits, a dose 0.01 times the RHD was associated with an increased incidence of premature delivery (1).

Two case reports, both during the 2nd trimester, have described the use of mitoxantrone in human pregnancy (2,3). A 26-year-old woman at 20 weeks' gestation presented with acute myeloblastic leukemia and was treated with an induction course of cytarabine and daunorubicin that failed to halt the disease progression (2). At approximately 23 weeks' gestation, a second induction course was started with mitoxantrone (12 mg/m^2, days 1–3) and cytarabine (days 1–4). Complete remission was achieved 60 days from the start of therapy. Weekly ultrasound examinations documented normal fetal growth. Because of the long interval required for remission, treatment was changed to idarubicin and cytarabine for the consolidation phase. Shortly after the start of this therapy, the woman delivered a 2200-g stillborn infant (gestational age not specified). No apparent congenital malformations were observed but permission for an autopsy was refused. The authors speculated that the fetal death was secondary to the use of idarubicin.

In the second case, a 28-year-old woman at 24 week's gestation with acute promyelocytic leukemia was treated with an induction course of behenoyl-cytosine arabinoside (enocytabine; converted *in vivo* to cytarabine), daunorubicin, and 6-mercaptopurine (3). Following a rapid, complete remission and her first consolidation therapy with cytarabine and mitoxantrone (dose not specified), a cesarean section was performed at 34 weeks' gestation to deliver a healthy 2960-g female infant who was alive and well at 16 months of age.

A 1999 report from France described the outcomes of pregnancies in 20 women with breast cancer who were treated with antineoplastic agents (4). The first cycle of chemotherapy occurred at a mean gestational age of 26 weeks with delivery occurring at a mean 34.7 weeks. A total of 38 cycles were administered during pregnancy with a median of two cycles per woman. None of the women received radiation therapy during pregnancy. The pregnancy outcomes included two spontaneous abortions (both exposed in the 1st trimester), one intrauterine death (exposed in the 2nd trimester), and 17 live births, one of whom died at 8 days of age without apparent cause. The 16 surviving children were developing normally at a mean follow-up of 42.3 months (4). Mitoxantrone, in combination with cyclophosphamide and fluorouracil, was administered to two of the women at a mean dose of 12 mg/m^2. The outcomes were two surviving liveborn infants, both exposed in the 2nd trimester. One of the infants was growth retarded (1460 g, born at 33 weeks' gestation after two cycles of chemotherapy) (4).

Occupational exposure of the mother to antineoplastic agents during pregnancy may present a risk to the fetus. A position statement from the National Study Commission on Cytotoxic Exposure and a research article involving some antineoplastic agents are presented in the monograph for cyclophosphamide (see Cyclophosphamide).

BREAST FEEDING SUMMARY

RECOMMENDATION: Contraindicated

Mitoxantrone is excreted in breast milk (3). After delivery at 34 weeks' gestation, a 28-year-old woman with acute promyelocytic leukemia in remission (case described above) was treated with a second consolidation therapy course of cytarabine and mitoxantrone. She maintained milk secretion by pumping her breasts during this and a third consolidation course consisting of mitoxantrone (6 mg/m^2, days 1–3), etoposide, and behenoyl-cytosine arabinoside (enocytabine; converted *in vivo* to cytarabine). The milk concentration of mitoxantrone on the 3rd day of this last course of therapy was 120 ng/mL and was still high (18 ng/mL) 28 days later. Although data on the drug concentration in milk were not yet available and against the authors' advisement, the patient voluntarily began to breast-feed her infant 21 days after drug administration. Her infant, exposed to mitoxantrone *in utero* and during nursing, was doing well at 16 months of age.

Although no adverse effects were observed in the above infant, the long-term consequences of such exposure are unknown. Mitoxantrone accumulates in the plasma and tissue after multiple doses and is slowly eliminated from the body (1). Because of its long elimination time and the uncertainty over the potential toxicity, women who have been treated with this agent should not breast-feed. The American Academy of Pediatrics classifies doxorubicin, an antineoplastic agent structurally related to mitoxantrone, as contraindicated during breast-feeding (see Doxorubicin).

M

References

1. Product information. Novantrone. Immunex, 2000.
2. Reynoso EE, Huerta F. Acute leukemia and pregnancy—fatal fetal outcome after exposure to idarubicin during the second trimester. Acta Oncologica 1994;33:703–16.
3. Azuno Y, Kaku K, Fujita N, Okubo M, Kaneko T, Matsumoto N. Mitoxantrone and etoposide in breast milk. Am J Hematol 1995;48:131–2.
4. Giacalone PL, Laffargue F, Benos P. Chemotherapy for breast carcinoma during pregnancy. Cancer 1999;86:2266–72.

Name:	**MODAFINIL**	Risk Factor:	**C_M**
Class:	**Central Stimulant**		

FETAL RISK SUMMARY

RECOMMENDATION: Limited Human Data - Animal Data Suggest Low Risk

Modafinil is indicated to improve wakefulness in patients with excessive daytime sleepiness associated with narcolepsy. Its mechanism of action is unknown, but its pharmacologic profile is not identical to that of sympathomimetic agents. Plasma protein binding, primarily to albumin, is moderate (about 60%). Modafinil is extensively (>90%) metabolized by the liver. After chronic dosing, the elimination half-life is about 15 hours (1).

Reproduction studies have been conducted in rats and rabbits. In rats, doses 10 times the maximum recommended human daily dose of 200 mg based on body surface area (MRHDD) given throughout organogenesis were associated with increased resorptions, hydronephrosis, and skeletal variations. No maternal toxicity was observed at this dose. The no-effect dose for these effects was 5 times the MRHDD. Doses up to 4.8 times the MRHDD given to male and female rats before and during gestation had no effect on fertility. In rabbits, no embryotoxicity was observed at doses up to 10 times the MRHDD during organogenesis. However, the sample sizes and doses were inadequate to assess the toxic effects on fertility or reproduction (1).

It is not known if modafinil crosses the human placenta. The molecular weight (about 273), moderate plasma protein binding, and long elimination half-life suggest that the drug will cross to the embryo/fetus.

The manufacturer cited the outcomes of nine pregnancies that were exposed to modafinil, but few details were given. There were seven normal births, one birth of a healthy male infant that occurred 3 weeks before the expected range of delivery dates (based on ultrasound), and one woman had a spontaneous abortion (also had history of previous spontaneous abortions).

In summary, no other human pregnancy data, except for the above nine cases, are available. The animal data are suggestive of low risk, but the absence of adequate human pregnancy experience prevents an assessment of the risk to the embryo/fetus. Therefore, avoiding modafinil in the 1st trimester is the safest course, but inadvertent exposure during this period does not appear to represent a major risk of embryo/fetal harm.

BREAST FEEDING SUMMARY

RECOMMENDATION: No Human Data - Potential Toxicity

No reports describing the use of modafinil during human lactation have been located. The relatively low molecular weight (about 273), moderate plasma protein binding (about 60%), and the long elimination half-life (about 15 hours) suggest that the drug will be excreted in breast milk. The effects of this exposure on a nursing infant are unknown. However, if a lactating woman uses modafinil, her infant should be closely observed for adverse effects that are commonly seen in adults (i.e., headache, infection, nausea, nervousness, anxiety, and insomnia).

M

Reference

1. Product information. Provigil. Cephalon, 2004.

Name:	**MOEXIPRIL**	Risk Factor:	C_M*
Class:	**Antihypertensive**		

FETAL RISK SUMMARY

RECOMMENDATION: Human Data Suggest Risk in 2nd and 3rd Trimesters

The prodrug, moexipril, is rapidly metabolized to the active drug, moexiprilat. It is indicated in the management of hypertension either alone, or in combination with thiazide diuretics. The active metabolite, moexiprilat, is a competitive inhibitor of angiotensin I–converting enzyme (ACE inhibitor), thereby preventing the conversion of angiotensin I to angiotensin II.

Reproduction studies have been conducted in pregnant rats and rabbits (1). Doses up to 90.9 and 0.7 times, respectively, the maximum recommended human dose on a body surface area basis revealed no embryotoxic, fetotoxic, or teratogenic effects.

It is not known if moexipril or moexiprilat cross the human placenta. The molecular weight (about 535 for the hydrochloride salt forms) is low enough, however, that transfer to the fetus should be expected.

No reports describing the use of moexipril during human pregnancy have been located. Based on the human pregnancy experience with other ACE inhibitors, moexipril exposure during the 1st trimester would not be expected to represent a risk to the fetus. However, use of moexipril during the 2nd and 3rd trimesters may cause teratogenicity and severe fetal and neonatal toxicity (see Captopril or Enalapril). Fetal toxic effects may include anuria, oligohydramnios, fetal hypocalvaria, intrauterine growth retardation, prematurity, and patent ductus arteriosus. Anuria-associated oligohydramnios may produce fetal limb contractures, craniofacial deformation, and pulmonary hypoplasia. Severe anuria and hypotension that is resistant to both pressor agents and volume expansion may occur in the newborn following *in utero* exposure to ACE inhibitors.

In cases in which the mother's disease requires moexipril (or another ACE inhibitor), the lowest possible dose should be used. Close monitoring of amniotic fluid levels and fetal well-being should be conducted during gestation followed by close observation of renal function and blood pressure in the newborn. If moexipril is used in pregnancy, healthcare professionals are encouraged to call the toll free number (800-670-6126) for information about patient enrollment in the Motherisk study.

[*Risk Factor D if used in the 2nd and/or 3rd trimesters according to the manufacturer.*]

BREAST FEEDING SUMMARY

M

RECOMMENDATION: No Human Data - Probably Compatible

No reports describing the use of moexipril in human lactation have been located. The molecular weight (about 535 for the salt forms of the parent drug and metabolite) suggests that excretion into breast milk should be expected. The effect of this exposure on a nursing infant are unknown. However, other ACE inhibitors are excreted into breast milk and are considered compatible with breast-feeding by the American Academy of Pediatrics (see Captopril and Enalapril).

Reference

1. Product information. Univasc. Schwarz Pharma, 2001.

Name:	**MOLINDONE**	Risk Factor:	**C**
Class:	**Tranquilizer**		

FETAL RISK SUMMARY

RECOMMENDATION: Limited Human Data - Animal Data Suggest Low Risk

Molindone is an antipsychotic drug. Reproduction studies in mice, rats, and rabbits at doses of 20–40 mg/kg/day, 20–40 mg/kg/day, and 5–20 mg/kg/day, respectively, revealed no evidence of teratogenicity, but a slight increase in fetal resorptions occurred in mice at the tested doses (1).

The only reported use of molindone in human pregnancy was in a woman who gave birth at term to normal twin boys (2). The mother had ingested 9800 mg of molindone during her 9-month pregnancy. No abnormalities in physical or mental development were noted in their first 20 years of life.

BREAST FEEDING SUMMARY

RECOMMENDATION: No Human Data - Potential Toxicity

No reports describing the use of molindone during lactation have been located. The molecular weight (about 313) is low enough, however, that excretion into breast milk should be expected. The effect of exposure of the nursing infant to the drug from milk is unknown.

References

1. Product information. Moban. Endo Pharmaceuticals, 2000.
2. Ayd FJ Jr. Moban: the first of a new class of neuroleptics. In Ayd FJ Jr., ed. *Rational Psychopharmacotherapy and the Right to Treatment*. Baltimore, MD: Ayd Medical Communications, 1975:91–106.

Name: **MONTELUKAST** Risk Factor: **B_M**
Class: **Respiratory (Leukotriene Receptor Antagonist)**

FETAL RISK SUMMARY

RECOMMENDATION: Limited Human Data - Probably Compatible

Montelukast, an oral inhibitor of the cysteinyl leukotriene $CysLT_1$ receptor, is indicated for the prophylaxis and chronic treatment of asthma. Reproduction studies in rats and rabbits at doses up to 320 and 490 times the maximum recommended human daily oral dose based on body surface area (MRHD), respectively, found no evidence of teratogenicity (1). The drug impaired the fertility of female rats at 160 times, but not at 80 times, the MRHD. Fertility in male rats was not affected by oral doses up to 650 times the MRHD (1).

It is not known if montelukast crosses the human placenta. The molecular weight (about 608) is low enough, however, that transfer to the fetus should be expected. The drug crosses the placenta in rats and rabbits (1).

The manufacturer maintains a pregnancy registry for montelukast (2). As of July 2003, there were 243 prospective (reported before outcome of pregnancy known) reports of exposure during gestation. The outcomes of these pregnancies were: 35 pending, 71 lost to follow-up, 2 spontaneous abortions, 2 elective abortions, and 134 live births (1 set of twins). In the live births, 116 were known to have been exposed in the 1st trimester. Congenital anomalies were observed in four live births exposed in the 1st trimester: absent left hand (amniotic band deformity); hypospadias; slight valgus foot deviation; and triploidy 69XXY (elective abortion). There were 24 retrospective (reported after the outcome of pregnancy known) reports of exposure, two of which had defects (both exposed in 1st trimester): bilateral sensorineural hearing loss; and trisomy 18 (spontaneous abortion) (2).

During clinical trials, 38 women received montelukast with or without standard asthma therapy (beta-adrenergic agents, corticosteroids, theophylline, and/or cromolyn sodium) (2). In all cases, montelukast treatment was limited to the 1st trimester. The outcome of three pregnancies was pending or lost to follow-up. The pregnancy of one woman, who was also receiving loratadine, an antihistamine, terminated in a 1st trimester spontaneous abortion. In another, the report could not determine if her abortion was spontaneous or elective. Seven other women had spontaneous abortions in the 1st trimester, and nine pregnancies were electively terminated (none for identified medical indications). One fetal death at 28–30 weeks' gestation was attributed to preeclampsia, intraventricular cranial hemorrhage, immaturity, and placental infarcts (2). No congenital malformations were observed in the fetus by macroscopic analysis. Healthy, full-term infants were delivered from the remaining 16 pregnancies. No differences in the pregnancy outcomes were observed between the montelukast group and those who received placebo or beclomethasone (2).

In summary, montelukast is not teratogenic in animals, and the few adverse outcomes in humans do not demonstrate a pattern that suggests a common etiology. However, the human data are very limited and lack sufficient power to detect an increased risk of congenital malformations or other adverse outcomes. One source states that montelukast may be safe to use during pregnancy, but this conclusion was based solely on animal studies (3). A 2000 position statement of the American College of Obstetricians and Gynecologists (ACOG) and the American College of Allergy, Asthma and Immunology (ACAAI) recommended that montelukast could be considered in patients with recalcitrant asthma who had shown a uniquely favorable response to the drug prior to becoming pregnant (4). If montelukast is used in pregnancy, healthcare professionals are encouraged to call the toll free number (800-670-6126) for information about patient enrollment in the Motherisk study.

BREAST FEEDING SUMMARY

M

RECOMMENDATION: No Human Data - Probably Compatible

No reports describing the use of montelukast during human lactation have been located. The molecular weight (about 608) is sufficiently low, however, that excretion into breast milk should be expected. The drug is excreted into the milk of lactating rats (1). The potential effects on a nursing infant from exposure to the drug in milk are unknown.

References

1. Product information. Singulair. Merck, 2000.
2. Merck Pregnancy Registry for Singulair (montelukast sodium). Fifth annual report on exposure during pregnancy. February 1998 through July 2003.
3. Anonymous. Drugs for asthma. Med Lett Drugs Ther 2000;42:19–24.
4. Joint Committee of the American College of Obstetricians and Gynecologists (ACOG) and the American College of Allergy, Asthma and Immunology (ACAAI). The use of newer asthma and allergy medications during pregnancy. Ann Allergy Asthma Immunol 2000;84:475–80.

Name:	**MORICIZINE**	Risk Factor:	B_M
Class:	**Antiarrhythmic**		

FETAL RISK SUMMARY

RECOMMENDATION: No Human Data - Animal Data Suggest Low Risk

Moricizine is an orally active agent used in the treatment of ventricular tachycardia. The drug is neither teratogenic nor fetotoxic in rats and rabbits at doses up to 6.7 and 4.7 times the maximum recommended human dose (1). No reports of the use of moricizine in human pregnancy have been located.

BREAST FEEDING SUMMARY

RECOMMENDATION: Limited Human Data - Probably Compatible

The excretion of moricizine in human milk has been documented in one patient (data on file, Roberts Pharmaceutical Corporation, 1993), but no details on the amount in milk or its relationship to maternal levels are available. The clinical significance to the nursing infant is unknown.

Reference

1. Product information. Ethmozine. Roberts Pharmaceutical, 2000.

Name:	**MORPHINE**	Risk Factor:	$\mathbf{C_M}$*
Class:	**Narcotic Agonist Analgesic**		

FETAL RISK SUMMARY

RECOMMENDATION: Human Data Suggest Risk in 3rd Trimester

No reports linking the therapeutic use of morphine with major congenital defects have been located. The narcotic is not teratogenic in rats at a dose 35 times the usual human dose (1).

Bilateral horizontal nystagmus persisting for 1 year was reported in one addicted newborn (2). Like all narcotics, placental transfer of morphine is very rapid (3,4). Maternal addiction with subsequent neonatal withdrawal is well known following illicit use (see also Heroin) (2,5,6). Morphine was widely used in labor until the 1940s, when it was largely displaced by meperidine. Clinical impressions that meperidine caused less respiratory depression in the newborn were apparently confirmed (7,8). Other clinicians reported no difference between narcotics in the degree of neonatal depression when equianalgesic IV doses were used (4). Epidural use of morphine has been reported in women in labor but with unsatisfactory analgesic effects (9). The intrathecal route, however, has provided safe and effective analgesia without fetal or newborn toxicity (10–12).

The Collaborative Perinatal Project monitored 50,282 mother–child pairs, 70 of whom had 1st trimester exposure to morphine (13, pp. 287–295). For use anytime during pregnancy, 448 exposures were recorded (13, p. 434). No evidence was found to suggest a relationship to large categories of major or minor malformations. A possible association with inguinal hernia (10 cases) after anytime use was observed (13, p. 484). The statistical significance of this association is unknown and independent confirmation is required.

[**Risk Factor D if used for prolonged periods or in high doses at term.*]

BREAST FEEDING SUMMARY

RECOMMENDATION: Limited Human Data - Probably Compatible

Past reports have indicated that only trace amounts of morphine enter breast milk and the clinical significance of this was unknown (14–16). In a 1990 report, however, much higher concentrations of morphine were measured in the breast milk of one woman and in her infant's serum (17). A 30-year-old, 75-kg woman with systemic lupus erythematosus and severe arthritic back pain was treated with morphine, 50 mg every 6 hours, during the 3rd trimester and then with tapering doses during breast feeding. At the time of the study, the normal, healthy 3.5-kg infant was 21 days of age. One day before the study, the dose was 10 mg every 6 hours and then was tapered to 5 mg every 6 hours on the study day. Milk sampling times and morphine concentrations were: 4.5 hours after a dose (before feeding), 100 ng/mL; 4.75 hours after a dose (at end of feeding), 10 ng/mL; and 0.5 hours after a dose, 12 ng/mL (reported as 12 ng/L). A blood sample drawn from the infant 1 hour after a feeding (4 hours after a dose) had a morphine concentration of 4 ng/mL, a close approximation to the estimated therapeutic level. It was presumed that the infant had been exposed to much higher morphine concentrations from the milk before dose tapering and, thus, had higher therapeutic serum concentrations. Using pharmacokinetic calculations, the authors estimated that the infant was receiving between 0.8% and 12% of the maternal dose (17). No adverse effects of the exposure were observed in the infant.

The American Academy of Pediatrics classifies morphine as compatible with breast-feeding (18). However, the long-term effects on neurobehavior and development are unknown but warrant study.

References

1. Product information. Duramorph. Elkins-Sinn, 2000.
2. Perlstein MA. Congenital morphinism. A rare cause of convulsions in the newborn. JAMA 1947;135:633.
3. Fisher DE, Paton JB. The effect of maternal anesthetic and analgesic drugs on the fetus and newborn. Clin Obstet Gynaecol 1974;17:275–87.
4. Bonica JJ. Principles and Practice of Obstetric Analgesia and Anesthesia. Philadelphia, PA: FA Davis, 1967:247.
5. McMullin GP, Mobarak AN. Congenital narcotic addiction. Arch Dis Child 1970;45:140–1.
6. Cobrinik RW, Hodd RT Jr, Chusid E. The effect of maternal narcotic addiction on the newborn infant. Pediatrics 1959;24:288–304.
7. Gilbert G, Dixon AB. Observations on Demerol as an obstetric analgesic. Am J Obstet Gynecol 1943;45:320–6.
8. Way WL, Costley EC, Way EL. Respiratory sensitivity of the newborn infant to meperidine and morphine. Clin Pharmacol Ther 1965;6:454–61.
9. Nybell-Lindahl G, Carlsson C, Ingemarsson I, Westgren M, Paalzow L. Maternal and fetal concentrations of morphine after epidural administration during labor. Am J Obstet Gynecol 1981;139:20–1.
10. Baraka A, Noueihid R, Hajj S. Intrathecal injection of morphine for obstetric analgesia. Anesthesiology 1981;54:136–40.
11. Bonnardot JP, Maillet M, Colau JC, Millot F, Deligne P. Maternal and fetal concentration of morphine after intrathecal administration during labour. Br J Anaesth 1982;54:487–9.
12. Brizgys RV, Shnider SM. Hyperbaric intrathecal morphine analgesia during labor in a patient with Wolff-Parkinson-White syndrome. Obstet Gynecol 1984;64:44S–6S.
13. Heinonen OP, Slone D, Shapiro S. *Birth Defects and Drugs in Pregnancy*. Littleton, MA: Publishing Sciences Group, 1977.
14. Terwilliger WG, Hatcher RA. The elimination of morphine and quinine in human milk. Surg Gynecol Obstet 1934;58:823–6.
15. Kwit NT, Hatcher RA. Excretion of drugs in milk. Am J Dis Child 1935;49:900–4.
16. Anonymous. Drugs in breast milk. Med Lett Drugs Ther 1979;21:21–4.
17. Robieux I, Koren G, Vandenbergh H, Schneiderman J. Morphine excretion in breast milk and resultant exposure of a nursing infant. J Toxicol Clin Toxicol 1990;28:365–70.
18. Committee on Drugs, American Academy of Pediatrics. The transfer of drugs and other chemicals into human milk. Pediatrics 2001;108:776–89.

Name: **MOXALACTAM** Risk Factor: C_M

Class: **Antibiotic (Cephalosporin)**

FETAL RISK SUMMARY

RECOMMENDATION: Compatible

Moxalactam is a cephalosporin antibiotic. No controlled studies on its use in pregnancy have been located. The drug crosses the placenta to the fetus, producing a mean peak level at 1 hour in the cord blood of 38.4 μg/mL following a 1-g IV dose (R. Kammer, personal communication, Eli Lilly and Company, 1985). Peak amniotic fluid levels of 10.3 μg/mL occurred at 7.5 hours.

BREAST FEEDING SUMMARY

RECOMMENDATION: Compatible

Moxalactam is excreted into breast milk (1). In eight women receiving 2 g every 8 hours, mean daily concentrations of the antibiotic varied from 1.56 to 3.66 μg/mL, representing a daily dose of 0.86–2.01 mg. Because moxalactam is acid stable, the authors cautioned that colonization of the infant's bowel with gram-positive organisms could occur, resulting in a risk for enterocolitis (1). Because of this theoretical risk, they advised against breast-feeding if the mother was being treated with moxalactam. The American Academy of Pediatrics classifies moxalactam as compatible with breast-feeding (2).

References

1. Miller RD, Keegan KA, Thrupp LD, Brann J. Human breast milk concentration of moxalactam. Am J Obstet Gynecol 1984;148:348–9.
2. Committee on Drugs, American Academy of Pediatrics. The transfer of drugs and other chemicals into human milk. Pediatrics 2001;108:776–89.

Name: **MOXIFLOXACIN** Risk Factor: **C_M**

Class: **Anti-infective (Quinolone)**

M

FETAL RISK SUMMARY

RECOMMENDATION: Human Data Suggest Low Risk

Moxifloxacin is an oral synthetic, broad-spectrum, fluoroquinolone anti-infective agent. It is in the same anti-infective class as ciprofloxacin, enoxacin, gatifloxacin, lomefloxacin, levofloxacin, norfloxacin, ofloxacin, sparfloxacin, and trovafloxacin.

In reproduction studies with pregnant rats, doses up to 0.24 times the maximum recommended human dose based on systemic exposure determined by area under the plasma concentration curve (MRHD) were not teratogenic (1). At this dose, fetal toxicity was observed, as indicated by decreased fetal body weight and slightly delayed fetal skeletal development. Moreover, in a pre- and postnatal development study, the highest dose (0.24 times the MRHD) was associated with increases in pregnancy duration and prenatal loss, reduced pup birth weight, decreased neonatal survival, and treatment related maternal death during gestation. In pregnant rabbits given an IV dose during organogenesis that was approximately equal to the MRHD (a maternal toxic dose), decreased fetal body weights and delayed fetal skeletal ossification were observed. In addition, there was an increased fetal and litter incidence of rib and vertebral malformations when these effects were combined. No evidence of teratogenicity was seen when cynomolgus monkeys were given oral doses up to 2.5 times the MRHD, but fetal growth retardation did occur at the highest dose.

It is not known if moxifloxacin crosses the human placenta. The molecular weight (about 402 for the free base) is low enough that transfer to the fetus should be expected.

No reports describing the use of moxifloxacin during human pregnancy have been located. Animal toxicity was observed at doses at or less than the maximum human exposure, but these doses also resulted in maternal toxicity. Some reviewers, however, have concluded that all fluoroquinolones should be considered contraindicated in pregnancy (e.g., see Ciprofloxacin and Norfloxacin), because safer alternatives are usually available.

BREAST FEEDING SUMMARY

RECOMMENDATION: No Human Data - Probably Compatible

No reports describing the use of moxifloxacin in human lactation have been located. The molecular weight (about 402 for the free base) suggests that the agent will be excreted into breast milk. Moxifloxacin is excreted in the milk of lactating rats (1). The effects of this exposure on a nursing infant are unknown. However, two other fluoroquinolones are classified as compatible with breast-feeding by the American Academy of Pediatrics (see Ciprofloxacin and Ofloxacin).

Reference

1. Product information. Avelox. Bayer, 2001.

Name: **MYCOPHENOLATE MOFETIL** Risk Factor: **C_M**

Class: **Immunologic Agent (Immunosuppressive)**

M

FETAL RISK SUMMARY

RECOMMENDATION: No Human Data - Animal Data Suggest Risk

Mycophenolate mofetil is a purine synthesis inhibitor that is used as an immunosuppressant agent in the prophylaxis of organ rejection in patients receiving allogeneic renal and liver transplants (1,2). Following oral administration, the drug undergoes rapid and complete hydrolysis to mycophenolic acid, the active moiety (2).

Reproductive studies have been conducted in rats and rabbits (2). In both species, in the absence of maternal toxicity, fetal resorptions and malformations (type not specified) were observed at doses of 6 mg/kg/day (0.03 times the recommended human dose based on body surface area basis [RHD]) in rats and 90 mg/kg/day (0.92 times the RHD) in rabbits. In rats, a dose of 4.5 mg/kg/day (0.02 times the RHD) produced malformations, principally of the head and eyes (2).

It is not known if mycophenolate mofetil or the active metabolite, mycophenolic acid, crosses the human placenta to the fetus. The molecular weight of the prodrug (about 434), however, is low enough that transfer to the fetus probably occurs. The animal data cited above support this assessment.

A 2001 case report described the use of mycophenolate mofetil during pregnancy (3). The 33-year-old woman, with an unknown pregnancy at the time of surgery, had received a renal transplant at about 6–7 weeks' gestation. Postoperatively, she had been treated with mycophenolate, tacrolimus, corticosteroids, cefepime, and vancomycin. After discharge from the hospital, she was maintained on acyclovir, nifedipine, trimethoprim/sulfamethoxazole, tacrolimus (14 mg/d), mycophenolate (2 g/d), and prednisone

(25 mg/d). The pregnancy was diagnosed on posttransplantation day 100, at which time the two anti-infectives were discontinued and the mycophenolate dose reduced to 1 g/day. The woman delivered a 2,250-g female infant at about 34 weeks' with Apgar scores of 5 and 8 at 1 and 5 minutes, respectively. The birth weight, length, and head circumference were at the 75th percentile, 75th–90th percentile, and 10th–25th percentile, respectively. The infant had hypoplastic finger and toenails and shortened fifth fingers bilaterally. An aberrant blood vessel between the trachea and esophagus was found later. The infant was hospitalized three times during her first year with pneumonia (thought to have been caused in part by aspiration of stomach contents). Since then, the child has been healthy and was growing and developing normally at 3 years of age (3).

Severe congenital malformations were detailed in a 2004 case report (4). A 27-year-old woman had received a renal transplant 2 years before her pregnancy and had been maintained on mycophenolate (500 mg/d), tacrolimus (9 mg/d), and prednisone (15 mg/d). Her pregnancy was diagnosed at 13 weeks' gestation. At this time, azathioprine (50 mg/d) was substituted for mycophenolate. Multiple malformations were detected at 22 weeks' and the pregnancy was terminated. Defects included complete agenesis of the corpus callosum, cleft lip/palate, micrognathia, ocular hypertelorism, microtia and external auditory duct atresia, and a left pelvic ectopic kidney. The fetus had a normal male karyotype. One year later, the woman had another pregnancy and delivered a normal 2640-g male infant who was growing and developing normally at follow-up. During this pregnancy, the woman had been maintained on azathioprine, tacrolimus, and prednisone (4).

In summary, the animal data suggest risk for structural defects, but the human data are too limited to assess. However, use of the drug during pregnancy may represent a risk to the fetus. Women of childbearing potential who are prescribed this agent should be informed of this risk. The manufacturer recommends these women use effective contraception before and during therapy and for 6 weeks after therapy is stopped (2).

M

BREAST FEEDING SUMMARY

RECOMMENDATION: Contraindicated

Mycophenolate mofetil is excreted into the milk of lactating rats (2). Reports of human use during lactation have not been found. The molecular weight of the drug (about 434) is low enough, however, that passage into human milk should be expected. Mycophenolate mofetil is rapidly and completely hydrolyzed to mycophenolic acid upon absorption. Because of the potential for serious adverse effects in a nursing infant, including an increased frequency of certain infections and the possible development of lymphoma observed in adults (2), mycophenolate mofetil should be considered contraindicated during breastfeeding.

References

1. Casele HL, Laifer SA. Pregnancy after liver transplantation. Semin Perinatol 1998;22:149–55.
2. Product information. CellCept. Roche Pharmaceuticals, 1998.
3. Pergola PE, Kancharla A, Riley DJ. Kidney transplantation during the first trimester of pregnancy: immunosuppression with mycophenolate mofetil, tacrolimus, and prednisone. Transplantation 2001;71:994–7.
4. Le Ray C, Coulomb A, Elefant E, Frydman R, Audibert F. Mycophenolate mofetil in pregnancy after renal transplantation: a case of major fetal malformations. Obstet Gynecol 2004;103:1091–4.

N

Name:	**NABUMETONE**	Risk Factor:	**C_M***
Class:	**Nonsteroidal Anti-inflammatory**		

FETAL RISK SUMMARY

RECOMMENDATION: Human Data Suggest Risk in 1st and 3rd Trimesters

The nonsteroidal anti-inflammatory drug (NSAID), nabumetone, is used in the acute and chronic treatment of arthritis. Nabumetone is a prodrug that partially undergoes hepatic conversion to an active metabolite. It is in an NSAID subclass (naphthylalkanones) that contains no other agents.

The drug was not teratogenic in rats and rabbits but did produce toxicity similar to other agents in this class, including delayed parturition, dystocia, decreased fetal growth, and decreased fetal survival (1,2). Increased postimplantation loss in rats was observed at a dose equal to the average human exposure at the maximum recommended dose (1).

It is not known if nabumetone crosses the human placenta. The molecular weight (about 228) is low enough, however, that passage to the fetus should be expected.

A combined 2001 population-based observational cohort study and a case–control study estimated the risk of adverse pregnancy outcome from the use of NSAIDs (3). The use of NSAIDs during pregnancy was not associated with congenital malformations, preterm delivery, or low birth weight, but a positive association was discovered with spontaneous abortions (SABs). A similar study, also published in 2001, failed to find a relationship, in general, between NSAIDs and congenital malformations, but did find a significant association with cardiac defects and orofacial clefts (4). In addition, a 2003 study found a significant association between exposure to NSAIDs in early pregnancy and SABs (5). (See Ibuprofen for details on these three studies.)

A brief 2003 editorial on the potential for NSAID-induced developmental toxicity concluded that NSAIDs, and specifically those with greater COX-2 affinity, had a lower risk of this toxicity in humans than aspirin (6).

Constriction of the ductus arteriosus *in utero* is a pharmacologic consequence arising from the use of prostaglandin-synthesis inhibitors during pregnancy, as is inhibition of labor, prolongation of pregnancy, and suppression of fetal renal function (see also Indomethacin) (7). Persistent pulmonary hypertension of the newborn may occur if these agents are used in the 3rd trimester close to delivery (7,8). Women who are attempting to conceive should not use any prostaglandin synthesis inhibitor, including nabumetone, because of the findings in a variety of animal models that indicate these agents block blastocyst implantation (9,10). Moreover, as noted above, NSAIDs have been associated with SABs and congenital malformations.

[**Risk Factor D if used in 3rd trimester or near delivery.*]

BREAST FEEDING SUMMARY

RECOMMENDATION: No Human Data - Potential Toxicity

No reports describing the use of nabumetone during human lactation have been located. The molecular weight (about 228) is low enough that excretion into breast milk should be expected. The active metabolite is excreted into the milk of lactating rats (1).

One reviewer listed several NSAIDs (diclofenac, fenoprofen, flurbiprofen, ibuprofen, ketoprofen, ketorolac, and tolmetin) that were considered safer alternatives to other agents (nabumetone not mentioned) if these drugs were required during nursing (11). Because of the long serum elimination half-life (≥22.5 hours) of the active metabolite in adults and the unknown amounts of the drug that are excreted into milk, any of these choices are probably preferable.

References

1. Product information. Relafen. SmithKline Beecham Pharmaceuticals, 2001.
2. Toshiyaki F, Kadoh Y, Fujimoto Y, Tenshio A, Fuchigami K, Ohtsuka T. Toxicity study of nabumetone (iii)—teratological studies. Kiso to Rinsho 1988;22:2975–85. As cited in Shepard TH. *Catalog of Teratogenic Agents*. 7th ed. Baltimore, MD: Johns Hopkins University Press, 1992:275–6.
3. Nielsen GL, Sorensen HT, Larsen H, Pedersen L. Risk of adverse birth outcome and miscarriage in pregnant users of non-steroidal anti-inflammatory drugs: population based observational study and case-control study. BMJ 2001;322:266–70.
4. Ericson A, Kallen BAJ. Nonsteroidal anti-inflammatory drugs in early pregnancy. Reprod Toxicol 2001;15:371–5.
5. Li DK, Liu L, Odouli R. Exposure to non-steroidal anti-inflammatory drugs during pregnancy and risk of miscarriage: population based cohort study. BMJ 2003;327:368–71.
6. Tassinari MS, Cook JC, Hurtt ME. NSAIDs and developmental toxicity. Birth Defects Res (Part B) 2003;68:3–4.
7. Levin DL. Effects of inhibition of prostaglandin synthesis on fetal development, oxygenation, and the fetal circulation. Semin Perinatol 1980;4:35–44.
8. Van Marter LJ, Leviton A, Allred EN, Pagano M, Sullivan KF, Cohen A, Epstein MF. Persistent pulmonary hypertension of the newborn and smoking and aspirin and nonsteroidal antiinflammatory drug consumption during pregnancy. Pediatrics 1996;97:658–63.
9. Matt DW, Borzelleca JF. Toxic effects on the female reproductive system during pregnancy, parturition, and lactation. In Witorsch RJ, editor. *Reproductive Toxicology*. 2nd ed. New York, NY: Raven Press, 1995:175–93.
10. Dawood MY. Nonsteroidal antiinflammatory drugs and reproduction. Am J Obstet Gynecol 1993;169:1255–65.
11. Anderson PO. Medication use while breast feeding a neonate. Neonatal Pharmacol Q 1993;2:3–14.

N

Name:	**NADOLOL**	Risk Factor:	**C_M***
Class:	**Sympatholytic (Antihypertensive)**		

FETAL RISK SUMMARY

RECOMMENDATION: Human Data Suggest Risk in 2nd and 3rd Trimesters

Nadolol is a nonselective β_1, β_2-adrenergic blocking agent used for hypertension and angina pectoris. The drug is not teratogenic in rats, hamsters, and rabbits, but embryotoxicity and fetotoxicity were observed in the latter species (1,2).

In a surveillance study of Michigan Medicaid recipients conducted between 1985 and 1992 involving 229,101 completed pregnancies, 71 newborns had been exposed to nadolol during the 1st trimester (F. Rosa, personal communication, FDA, 1993). One

(1.4%) major birth defect was observed (three expected), a cardiovascular defect (one expected).

Only one published case of the use of nadolol in pregnancy has been located (3). A mother with immunoglobulin A nephropathy and hypertension was treated throughout pregnancy with nadolol, 20 mg/day, plus a diuretic (triamterene/hydrochlorothiazide) and thyroid. The infant, delivered by emergency cesarean section at 35 weeks' gestation, was growth retarded and exhibited tachypnea (68 breaths/minute) and mild hypoglycemia (20 mg/dL). Depressed respirations (23 breaths/minute), slowed heart rate (112 beats/minute), and hypothermia (96.5 °F) occurred at 4.5 hours of age. The lowered body temperature responded to warming, but the cardiorespiratory depression, with brief episodes of bradycardia, persisted for 72 hours. Nadolol serum concentrations in cord blood and in the infant at 12 and 38 hours after delivery were 43, 145, and 80 ng/mL, respectively. The cause of some or all of the effects observed in this infant may have been β-blockade (3). However, maternal disease could not be excluded as the sole or contributing factor behind the intrauterine growth retardation (IUGR) and hypoglycemia (3). In addition, hydrochlorothiazide may have contributed to the low blood glucose (see Chlorothiazide).

The authors identified several characteristics of nadolol in the adult that could potentially increase its toxicity in the fetus and newborn, including a long serum half-life (17–24 hours), lack of metabolism (excreted unchanged by the kidneys), and low protein binding (30%) (3). Because of these factors, other β-blockers may be safer for use during pregnancy, although persistent β-blockade has also been observed with acebutolol and atenolol. As with other agents in this class, long-term effects of *in utero* β-blockade have not been studied but warrant evaluation.

Some β-blockers may cause IUGR (as may have occurred in the case above) and reduced placental weight, especially those lacking intrinsic sympathomimetic activity (ISA) (i.e., partial agonist). Treatment beginning early in the 2nd trimester results in the greatest weight reductions, whereas treatment restricted to the 3rd trimester primarily affects only placental weight. Nadolol does not possess ISA. However, IUGR and reduced placental weight may potentially occur with all agents within this class. Although growth retardation is a serious concern, the benefits of maternal therapy with β-blockers, in some cases, might outweigh the risks to the fetus and this must be judged on a case-by-case basis.

[**Risk Factor D if used in 2nd or 3rd trimester.*]

BREAST FEEDING SUMMARY

RECOMMENDATION: Limited Human Data - Potential Toxicity

Nadolol is excreted into breast milk (3,4). A mother taking 20 mg of nadolol/day had a concentration in her milk of 146 ng/mL 38 hours after delivery (3). In 12 lactating women ingesting 80 mg once daily for 5 days, mean steady-state levels of nadolol, approximately 357 ng/mL, were attained at 3 days. This level was approximately 4.6 times higher than simultaneously measured maternal serum levels (4). By calculation, a 5-kg infant would have received 2%–7% of the adult therapeutic dose, but the infants were not allowed to breast-feed (4).

Because experience is lacking, nursing infants of mothers consuming nadolol should be closely observed for symptoms of β-blockade. Long-term effects of exposure to β-blockers from milk have not been studied but warrant evaluation. The

American Academy of Pediatrics classifies nadolol as compatible with breast-feeding (5).

References

1. Product information. Corgard. Bristol Laboratories, 1993.
2. Saegusa T, Suzuki T, Narama I. Reproduction studies of nadolol: a new α-adrenergic blocking agent. Yakuri to Chiryo 1983;11:5119–38. As cited in Shepard TH. *Catalog of Teratogenic Agents*. 6th ed. Baltimore, MD: Johns Hopkins University Press, 1989:440.
3. Fox RE, Marx C, Stark AR. Neonatal effects of maternal nadolol therapy. Am J Obstet Gynecol 1985;152:1045–6.
4. Devlin RG, Duchin KL, Fleiss PM. Nadolol in human serum and breast milk. Br J Clin Pharmacol 1981;12:393–6.
5. Committee on Drugs, American Academy of Pediatrics. The transfer of drugs and other chemicals into human milk. Pediatrics 2001;108:776–89.

Name: **NADROPARIN** Risk Factor: **B**

Class: **Anticoagulant**

FETAL RISK SUMMARY

RECOMMENDATION: Limited Human Data - Probably Compatible

Nadroparin is a low molecular weight heparin prepared by depolymerization of heparin obtained from porcine intestinal mucosa (1). It is not available in the United States (see also Dalteparin and Enoxaparin).

One report described the prophylactic use of nadroparin throughout pregnancy in seven women, all with a history of deep vein thrombosis of a lower limb, with familial thrombophilia (2). The pregnancies resulted in normal, healthy newborns. No maternal thromboembolic or hemorrhagic complications were observed, and thrombocytopenia did not occur. Osteoporosis was not studied (2).

Nadroparin has an average molecular weight of about 4500 (1). Because this is a relatively large molecule, it probably does not cross the placenta and, thus, presents a low risk to the fetus.

BREAST FEEDING SUMMARY

RECOMMENDATION: No Human Data - Probably Compatible

No reports describing the use of nadroparin during lactation have been located. Nadroparin, a low molecular weight heparin, still has a relatively high molecular weight (average 4500) and, as such, should not be expected to be excreted into human milk. Because nadroparin would be inactivated in the gastrointestinal tract, the risk to a nursing infant from ingesting the drug from milk appears to be negligible.

References

1. Reynold JEF, ed. *Martindale. The Extra Pharmacopoeia*. 30th ed. London: The Pharmaceutical Press, 1993:231–2.
2. Boda Z, Laszlo P, Rejto L, Tornai I, Pfliegler G, Blasko G, Rak K. Low molecular weight heparin as thromboprophylaxis in familial thrombophilia during the whole of pregnancy. Thromb Haemost 1996;76:128.

N

Name: **NAFCILLIN** Risk Factor: **B**
Class: **Antibiotic (Penicillin)**

FETAL RISK SUMMARY

RECOMMENDATION: Compatible

Nafcillin is a penicillin antibiotic (see also Penicillin G). No reports linking its use with congenital defects have been located. The Collaborative Perinatal Project monitored 50,282 mother-child pairs, 3546 of whom had 1st trimester exposure to penicillin derivatives (1, pp. 297–313). For use any time during pregnancy, 7171 exposures were recorded (1, p. 435). In neither group was evidence found to suggest a relationship to large categories of major or minor malformations or to individual defects.

BREAST FEEDING SUMMARY

RECOMMENDATION: Compatible

No data are available (see Penicillin G).

Reference

1. Heinonen OP, Slone D, Shapiro S. *Birth Defects and Drugs in Pregnancy*. Littleton, MA: Publishing Sciences Group, 1977.

Name: **NALBUPHINE** Risk Factor: **B_M***
Class: **Narcotic Agonist–Antagonist Analgesic**

FETAL RISK SUMMARY

RECOMMENDATION: Human Data Suggest Risk in 3rd Trimester

No congenital defects have been reported in humans or in experimental animals following the use of nalbuphine in pregnancy (1). Reproduction studies in rats and rabbits at doses up to 14 and 31 times, respectively, the maximum recommended human dose (MRHD) revealed no evidence of impaired fertility or fetal harm (2). Administration to rats at doses 8–17 times the MRHD during at least the last third of gestation and during lactation reduced both neonatal body weight and survival (2).

Nalbuphine has both narcotic agonist and antagonist effects. Prolonged use during pregnancy could theoretically result in fetal addiction with subsequent withdrawal in the newborn (see also Pentazocine). Use of the drug in labor may produce fetal distress and neonatal respiratory depression comparable to that produced by meperidine (1–6).

Nalbuphine crosses the placenta to the fetus (6,7). The cord:maternal serum ratio in five women in active labor given 20 mg as an IV bolus ranged from 0.37 to 6.03 (7). A sixth patient given 15 mg had a ratio of 1.24. Umbilical cord concentrations of nalbuphine obtained 3–10 hours after a dose varied from "not detectable" to 46 ng/mL. The terminal half-life of the drug in the mothers was 2.4 $\pm$ 0.4 hours.

A sinusoidal fetal heart rate pattern was observed after a 10-mg IV dose administered to a woman in labor at 42 weeks' gestation (8). The sinusoidal pattern persisted for at least 2.25 hours, and periodic late decelerations became evident. A cesarean section was performed to deliver a healthy baby girl with Apgar scores of 8 and 9 at 1 and 5 minutes, respectively. The infant did well following delivery. The authors attributed the persistent sinusoidal pattern to the prolonged plasma half-life in adults (8).

A 1987 reference compared the use of nalbuphine administered during labor via either a patient-controlled analgesia (PCA) IV pump or by direct IV-push doses (9). No differences were observed between the groups in terms of fetal distress, as evidenced by late decelerations or abnormal scalp blood pH, or in Apgar scores, but specific details on the newborns were not given. However, the fetuses of women receiving nalbuphine by the PCA system had a higher incidence of variable heart rate decelerations.

[**Risk Factor D if used for prolonged periods or in high doses at term.*]

BREAST FEEDING SUMMARY

RECOMMENDATION: No Human Data - Probably Compatible

No reports describing the use of nalbuphine during lactation have been located. Because of the rapid transfer across the placenta, excretion into breast milk should also be expected. The manufacturer states that small amounts (less than 1% of the mother's dose) are excreted into breast milk but that these amounts are clinically insignificant (2).

References

1. Miller RR. Evaluation of nalbuphine hydrochloride. Am J Hosp Pharm 1980;37:942–9.
2. Product information. Nubain. Endo Pharmaceuticals, 2000.
3. Guillonneau M, Jacqz-Aigrain E, De Crepy A, Zeggout H. Perinatal adverse effects of nalbuphine given during parturition. Lancet 1990;335:1588.
4. Sgro C, Escousse A, Tennenbaum D, Gouyon JB. Perinatal adverse effects of nalbuphine given during labour. Lancet 1990;336:1070.
5. Wilson CM, McClean E, Moore J, Dundee JW. A double-blind comparison of intramuscular pethidine and nalbuphine in labour. Anaesthesia 1986;41:1207–13.
6. Frank M, McAteer EJ, Cattermole R, Loughnan B, Stafford LB, Hitchcock AM. Nalbuphine for obstetric analgesia. Anaesthesia 1987;42:697–703.
7. Wilson SJ, Errick JK, Balkon J. Pharmacokinetics of nalbuphine during parturition. Am J Obstet Gynecol 1986;155:340–4.
8. Feinstein SJ, Lodeiro JG, Vintzileos AM, Campbell WA, Montgomery JT, Nochimson DJ. Sinusoidal fetal heart rate pattern after administration of nalbuphine hydrochloride: a case report. Am J Obstet Gynecol 1986;154:159–60.
9. Podlas J, Breland BD. Patient-controlled analgesia with nalbuphine during labor. Obstet Gynecol 1987;70:202–4.

Name:	**NALIDIXIC ACID**	Risk Factor:	C_M
Class:	**Urinary Germicide**		

FETAL RISK SUMMARY

RECOMMENDATION: Limited Human Data - Animal Data Suggest Moderate Risk

No reports linking the use of nalidixic acid, a quinolone antibacterial agent, with congenital defects have been located. At oral doses 6 times the human dose, nalidixic acid was embryocidal and teratogenic in rats (1). Prolongation of pregnancy was also noted, especially at 4 times the human dose. Similar to other agents in this class, nalidixic acid causes arthropathy in immature animals (1).

N

Chromosomal damage was not observed in human leukocytes cultured with varying concentrations of the drug (2). One author cautioned that the drug should be avoided in late pregnancy because it may produce hydrocephalus (3). However, a subsequent report examined the newborns of 63 patients treated with nalidixic acid at various stages of gestation (4). No defects attributable to the drug or intracranial hypertension were observed.

BREAST FEEDING SUMMARY

RECOMMENDATION: Compatible

Nalidixic acid is excreted into breast milk in low concentrations (5–7). Hemolytic anemia was reported in one infant with glucose-6-phosphate dehydrogenase deficiency whose mother was taking 1 g 4 times a day (5). Milk levels were not measured in this case, but the author noted data from the manufacturer in which milk levels from four women taking a similar dose were found to be 4 μg/mL. The milk:plasma ratio has been reported as 0.08–0.13 (6).

A 1980 report described the excretion of unmetabolized nalidixic acid into the breast milk of 13 women, 3–8 days postpartum, following a 2-g oral dose (7). Nursing was suspended on the day of the test. Milk was collected from each woman for a 24-hour period and serum samples were taken 7 hours after the dose. The highest milk concentration of the drug occurred in the sample collected from 0 to 4 hours, 0.64 μg/mL, but the total unchanged drug excreted over 24 hours was only 0.003% of the mother's dose. The milk:serum ratio at 7 hours was 0.061, and the minimal inhibitory concentration of about 3 μg/mL was never reached (7).

N

The quantities measured above are normally considered insignificant (8). Although noting the single case of hemolytic anemia described above, the American Academy of Pediatrics classifies nalidixic acid as compatible with breast-feeding (9).

References

1. Product information. NegGram. Sanofi Winthrop Pharmaceuticals, 1997.
2. Stenchever MA, Powell W, Jarvis JA. Effect of nalidixic acid on human chromosome integrity. Am J Obstet Gynecol 1970;107:329–30.
3. Asscher AW. Diseases of the urinary system. Urinary tract infections. Br Med J 1977;1:1332.
4. Murray EDS. Nalidixic acid in pregnancy. Br Med J 1981;282:224.
5. Belton EM, Jones RV. Hemolytic anemia due to nalidixic acid. Lancet 1965;2:691.
6. Wilson JT. Milk/plasma ratios and contraindicated drugs. In Wilson JT, ed. *Drugs in Breast Milk*. Balgowlah, Australia: ADIS Press, 1981:78–9.
7. Traeger A, Peiker G. Excretion of nalidixic acid via mother's milk. Arch Toxicol 1980;Suppl 4:388–90.
8. Takyi BE. Excretion of drugs in human milk. J Hosp Pharm 1970;28:317–25.
9. Committee on Drugs, American Academy of Pediatrics. The transfer of drugs and other chemicals into human milk. Pediatrics 2001;108:776–89.

Name:	**NALORPHINE**	Risk Factor:	**D**
Class:	**Narcotic Antagonist**		

FETAL RISK SUMMARY

RECOMMENDATION: Human Data Suggest Risk

Nalorphine is a narcotic antagonist that is used to reverse respiratory depression from narcotic overdose. It has been used either alone or in combination with meperidine or morphine during labor to reduce neonatal depression (1–6). Nalorphine has also been given to the newborn to prevent neonatal asphyxia (3,7). Although some benefits were initially claimed, caution in the use of nalorphine during labor has been advised for the following reasons: (a) a statistically significant reduction in neonatal depression has not been demonstrated; (b) the antagonist reduces analgesia; and (c) the antagonist may increase neonatal depression if an improper narcotic-to-narcotic antagonist ratio is used (8).

An adverse effect on fetal cord blood pH, pCO_2, and base deficit was shown when nalorphine was given in combination with meperidine during labor (9). As indicated above, nalorphine may cause respiratory depression in the absence of narcotics or if the critical ratio is exceeded (8). Because of these considerations, the use of nalorphine either alone or in combination therapy in pregnancy should be discouraged. If a narcotic antagonist is indicated, other agents that do not cause respiratory depression, such as naloxone, are preferred.

BREAST FEEDING SUMMARY

RECOMMENDATION: No Human Data - Probably Compatible

No data are available.

References

1. Cappe BE, Himel SZ, Grossman F. Use of a mixture of morphine and N-allylnormorphine as an analgesic. Am J Obstet Gynecol 1953;66:1231–4.
2. Echenhoff JE, Hoffman GL, Funderburg LW. N-Allylnormorphine: an antagonist to neonatal narcosis produced by sedation of the parturient. Am J Obstet Gynecol 1953;65:1269–75.
3. Echenhoff JE, Funderburg LW. Observations in the use of the opiate antagonists nalorphine and levallorphan. Am J Med Sci 1954;228:546–53.
4. Baker FJ. Pethidine and nalorphine in labor. Anaesthesia 1957;12:282–92.
5. Gordon DWS, Pinker GD. Increased pethidine dosage in obstetrics associated with the use of nalorphine. J Obstet Gynaecol Br Commonw 1958;65:606–11.
6. Bullough J. Use of premixed pethidine and antagonists in obstetrical analgesia with special reference to cases in which levallorphan was used. Br Med J 1959,2:859–62.
7. Paterson S, Prescott F. Nalorphine in prevention of neonatal asphyxia due to maternal sedation with pethidine. Lancet 1954;1:490–3.
8. Bonica JJ. *Principles and Practice of Obstetric Analgesia and Anesthesia*. Philadelphia, PA: FA Davis, 1967:254–9.
9. Hounslow D, Wood C, Humphrey M, Chang A. Intrapartum drugs and fetal blood pH and gas status. J Obstet Gynaecol Br Commonw 1973;80:1007–12.

Name:	**NALOXONE**	Risk Factor:	B_M
Class:	**Narcotic Antagonist**		

FETAL RISK SUMMARY

RECOMMENDATION: Compatible

Naloxone is a narcotic antagonist that is used to reverse the effects of narcotic overdose. The drug has no intrinsic respiratory depressive actions or other narcotic effects of its own (1). Naloxone has been shown to cross the placenta, appearing in fetal blood 2 minutes after a maternal dose and gradually increasing over 10–30 minutes (2).

Reproduction studies in mice and rats at doses up to 50 times the usual human dose revealed no evidence of impaired fertility or fetal harm (3).

In three reports, naloxone was given to mothers in labor after the administration of meperidine (4–6). One study found that 18–40 μg/kg (maternal weight) given IV provided the best results in comparison with controls who did not receive meperidine or naloxone (5). In measurements of newborn neurobehavior, groups treated in labor with either meperidine or meperidine plus naloxone (0.4 mg) were compared with a nontreated control group (6). The control group scored better in the first 24 hours than either of the treated groups and, after 2 hours, no difference was found between meperidine and meperidine plus naloxone-treated patients. Women in active labor received 1.0 mg of morphine intrathecal followed in 1 hour by a 0.4-mg IV bolus of naloxone plus 0.6 mg/hour or placebo as constant infusion for 23 hours (7). A reduction in some morphine-induced maternal side effects was seen with naloxone, but no significant differences with placebo were found for fetal heart rate or variability, Apgar scores, umbilical venous and arterial gases, neonatal respirations, or neurobehavioral examination scores. Cord:maternal serum ratio for naloxone was 0.50. Naloxone has also been safely given to newborns within a few minutes of delivery (8–13).

Naloxone has been used at term to treat fetal heart rate baselines with low beat-to-beat variability not caused by maternally administered narcotics (14). This use was based on the assumption that the heart-rate patterns were caused by elevated fetal endorphins. In one case, however, naloxone may have enhanced fetal asphyxia, leading to fatal respiratory failure in the newborn (14). Based on the above data, naloxone should not be given to the mother just before delivery to reverse the effects of narcotics in the fetus or newborn unless narcotic toxicity is evident. Information on its fetal effects during pregnancy, other than labor, is not available.

In a study of the effects of naloxone on fetal behavior, 54 pregnant women with gestational ages between 37 and 39 weeks were evenly divided into two groups (15). One group received 0.4 mg of naloxone and the other received an equal volume of saline placebo. In the group receiving naloxone, significant increases were observed in the number, duration, and amplitude of fetal heart rate accelerations. Significant increases were also observed in the number of fetal body movements and the percentage of time spent breathing. Moreover, significantly more fetuses exposed to naloxone were actively awake than those not exposed. The investigators attributed their findings to reversal of the effects of fetal endorphins.

BREAST FEEDING SUMMARY

RECOMMENDATION: No Human Data - Probably Compatible

No data are available.

References

1. Jaffe JH, Martin WR. Opioid analgesics and antagonists. In Gilman AG, Goodman LS, Gilman A, eds. *The Pharmacological Basis of Therapeutics*. 6th ed. New York, NY: Macmillan, 1980:522–5.
2. Finster M, Gibbs C, Dawes GS, et al. Placental transfer of meperidine (Demerol) and naloxone (Narcan). Presented at the Annual Meeting of the American Society of Anesthesiologists, Boston, October 4, 1972. In Clark RB, Beard AG, Greifenstein FE, Barclay DL. Naloxone in the parturient and her infant. South Med J 1976;69:570–5.
3. Product information. Narcan. Endo Pharmaceuticals, 2000.
4. Clark RB. Transplacental reversal of meperidine depression in the fetus by naloxone. J Arkansas Med Soc 1971;68:128–30.
5. Clark RB, Beard AG, Greifenstein FE, Barclay DL. Naloxone in the parturient and her infant. South Med J 1976;69:570–5.
6. Hodgkinson R, Bhatt M, Grewal G, Marx GF. Neonatal neurobehavior in the first 48 hours of life: effect of the administration of meperidine with and without naloxone in the mother. Pediatrics 1978;62:294–8.
7. Brookshire GL, Shnider SM, Abboud TK, Kotelko DM, Nouiehed R, Thigpen JW, Khoo SS, Raya JA, Foutz SE, Brizgys RV. Effects of naloxone on the mother and

neonate after intrathecal morphine for labor analgesia. Anesthesiology 1983;59:A417.
8. Evans JM, Hogg MIJ, Rosen M. Reversal of narcotic depression in the neonate by naloxone. Br Med J 1976;2:1098–1100.
9. Wiener PC, Hogg MIJ, Rosen M. Effects of naloxone on pethidine-induced neonatal depression. II. Intramuscular naloxone. Br Med J 1977;2:229–31.
10. Wiener PC, Hogg MIJ, Rosen M. Effects of naloxone on pethidine-induced neonatal depression. I. Intravenous naloxone. Br Med J 1977;2:228–9.
11. Gerhardt T, Bancalari E, Cohen H, Rocha LF. Use of naloxone to reverse narcotic respiratory depression in the newborn infant. J Pediatr 1977;90:1009–12.
12. Bonta BW, Gagliardi JV, Williams V, Warshaw JB. Naloxone reversal of mild neurobehavioral depression in normal newborn infants after routine obstetric analgesia. J Pediatr 1979;94:102–5.
13. Welles B, Belfrage P, de Chateau P. Effects of naloxone on newborn infant behavior after maternal analgesia with pethidine during labor. Acta Obstet Gynecol Scand 1984;63:617–9.
14. Goodlin RC. Naloxone and its possible relationship to fetal endorphin levels and fetal distress. Am J Obstet Gynecol 1981;139:16–9.
15. Arduini D, Rizzo G, Dell'Acqua S, Mancuso S, Romanini C. Effect of naloxone on fetal behavior near term. Am J Obstet Gynecol 1987;156:474–8.

Name: **NALTREXONE** Risk Factor: C_M
Class: **Narcotic Antagonist**

FETAL RISK SUMMARY

RECOMMENDATION: Limited Human Data - Animal Data Suggest Moderate Risk

Naltrexone is an opioid antagonist that is used in the treatment of alcohol dependence and to block the effects of exogenously administered opioids. The agent is a synthetic congener of oxymorphone and is also related to another opioid antagonist, naloxone.

In fertility studies, a significant increase in pseudopregnancy and a decrease in the pregnancy rate after mating was observed in rats administered 100 mg/kg/day orally (16 times the recommended human therapeutic dose based on body surface area [RHTD]) (1). No adverse effects on male rat fertility were seen at this dose. A significant increase in early fetal loss was observed in rats and rabbits at 5 and 18 times the RHTD, respectively (1). No evidence of teratogenicity was found in either species at doses up to 32 and 65 times the RHTD, respectively, administered during organogenesis. Because rats do not form appreciable amounts of the major metabolite found in humans (6-β-naltrexol), the potential reproductive toxicity of the metabolite is unknown (1).

An animal study published in 1984 evaluated the reproductive effects of naltrexone in rats and rabbits (2). In rats, prolonged administration of naltrexone at doses that did not affect body weight produced excitatory signs in both sexes, increased production of seminal plugs in males, and decreases in estrus cycling and fertility in females. No adverse effect on mating activity was observed, but there was an increase in pseudopregnancy in those receiving 100 mg/kg/day. Fertility was also reduced (i.e., fewer females became pregnant) when both sexes received this dose. No evidence of teratogenicity or embryo toxicity was noted in either pregnant rats or rabbits (2). When administered to rats near term (20 days' gestation), naltrexone crossed the placenta and was measured in all fetal tissues (3). Apparently, the human placental transfer of naltrexone has not been studied, but the relatively low molecular weight of the drug (about 378) indicates that transfer to the fetus should be expected.

In an experiment with stressed (noise and light at unpredictable frequency) pregnant rats, a continuous infusion of naltrexone (10 mg/kg/day) was administered by implanted minipumps from day 17 of gestation (4). Compared to controls receiving an infusion of vehicle only, naltrexone prevented the reduction in anogenital distance in male pups and restored the growth rate in both sexes. Other adverse fetal effects of prenatal stress were also prevented by naltrexone, leading the authors to conclude that some of the morphologic and behavioral changes induced by prenatal stress may result from excess opioid activity (4).

The effects of daily injections of naltrexone (50 mg/kg) administered to rats throughout gestation on fetal growth were described in a 1997 publication (5). Compared to controls given daily injections of saline, naltrexone-exposed pups had greater body weights, crown-rump lengths, and organ and skeletal muscle weights. Naltrexone had no effect on the length of gestation, course of pregnancy, litter size, or viability of the mother or offspring (5). The effects on growth were attributed to the blocking of endogenous opioids.

Decreased sensitivity to morphine has been observed in rat offspring exposed *in utero* to naltrexone (6,7). The appreciation of pain was not affected. However, insensitivity was not observed to butorphanol (7). These results raise the possibility that, later in life, morphine would provide less effective analgesia in human offspring who were exposed during gestation to naltrexone.

Other rat studies have also demonstrated that naltrexone can modify behavior of both the mother and the offspring (8–10). Naltrexone was administered at parturition to ewes lambing for the first time (8). Compared to controls, naltrexone significantly delayed the onset of maternal behavior (licking and bleating) toward the newborn. The drug facilitated sexual behavior in adult male rats who had been exposed *in utero* (9). Another study found that naltrexone exposure throughout gestation modified postnatal behavioral development of rat offspring (10). The investigators concluded that blocking the endogenous opioid systems during embryogenesis altered the somatic, physical, and behavioral development after birth. Of interest, a 1998 study found that naltrexone was present in the brains and hearts of newborn rats after maternal administration during gestation, but it was not present on postnatal days 2 and 10 (11). The investigators concluded that the somatic and neurobiological acceleration observed in previous studies was not due to opioid receptor blockade during the postnatal period (11).

Two 1993 reports, from the same research group, described the use of naltrexone (25–150 mg/day for 4–100 weeks) in 138 women with various grades of hypothalamic or hyperandrogenic ovarian failure (12,13). A total of 24 pregnancies in 22 women were achieved. Naltrexone was discontinued as soon as pregnancy had been diagnosed. Four pregnancies ended in an early spontaneous abortion, six women had delivered (no data provided on newborn condition), eight pregnancies were ongoing, and no information was given for six cases. A 1995 study of women with functional hypothalamic amenorrhea, however, found that even after priming with exogenous estradiol and progesterone or pulsatile gonadotropin-releasing hormone, the continued use of naltrexone alone did not maintain gonadotropin secretion and eventual ovulation (14).

Continuous naltrexone (50 mg/day), either alone or with intermittent clomiphene, has been used successfully in women with clomiphene resistant normogonadotrophic anovulation (15). In this study, 19 of 22 women achieved ovulation and 12 singleton pregnancies were documented. Naltrexone was discontinued when pregnancy was diagnosed. The outcomes of the pregnancies included two spontaneous abortions and eight ongoing pregnancies (15).

Except for the reports above in which the naltrexone was discontinued very early in gestation, no other references describing the use of the agent during human pregnancy have been located. Although naltrexone did not produce gross structural abnormalities in any of the animal studies, it did alter some opioid receptors in the brain that appeared to have long-lasting consequences. This potential for behavioral alteration in humans cannot be assessed because of the lack of data, but concern is warranted.

BREAST FEEDING SUMMARY

RECOMMENDATION: No Human Data - Potential Toxicity

No reports describing the use of naltrexone during human lactation have been located. Naltrexone and its metabolite, 6-β-naltrexol, are excreted into the milk of lactating rats (1). Because the molecular weight (about 378) is low enough, excretion into human breast milk should be expected. The effects of this exposure on a nursing infant are unknown, but there appears to be the potential for altering opioid receptors in the brain. In addition, based on studies in adults, baseline levels of some hormones of hypothalamic, pituitary, adrenal, and gonadal origin may also be altered (1).

References

1. Product information. Revia. DuPont Pharma, 2000.
2. Christian MS. Reproductive toxicity and teratology evaluations of naltrexone. J Clin Psychiatry 1984;45:7–10.
3. Zagon IS, Hurst WJ, McLaughlin PJ. Transplacental transfer of naltrexone in rats. Life Sci 1997;61:1261–7.
4. Keshet GI, Weinstock M. Maternal naltrexone prevents morphological and behavioral alterations induced in rats by prenatal stress. Pharmacol Biochem Behav 1995;50:413–9.
5. McLaughlin PJ, Tobias SW, Lang CM, Zagon IS. Chronic exposure to the opioid antagonist naltrexone during pregnancy: maternal and offspring effects. Physiol Behav 1997;62:501–8.
6. Harry GJ, Rosecrans JA. Behavioral effects of perinatal naltrexone exposure: a preliminary investigation. Pharmacol Biochem Behav 1979;11(Suppl):19–22.
7. Zagon IS, Tobias SW, Hytrek SD, McLaughlin PJ. Opioid receptor blockade throughout prenatal life confers long-term insensitivity to morphine and alters μ opioid receptors. Pharmacol Biochem Behav 1998;59:201–7.
8. Caba M, Poindron P, Krehbiel D, Levy F, Romeyer A, Venier G. Naltrexone delays the onset of maternal behavior in primiparous parturient ewes. Pharmacol Biochem Behav 1995;52:743–8.
9. Cohen E, Keshet G, Shavit Y, Weinstock M. Prenatal naltrexone facilitates male sexual behavior in the rat. Pharmacol Biochem Behav 1996;54:183–8.
10. McLaughlin PJ, Tobias SW, Lang CM, Zagon IS. Opioid receptor blockade during prenatal life modifies postnatal behavioral development. Pharmacol Biochem Behav 1997;58:1075–82.
11. Zagon IS, Hurst WJ, McLaughlin PJ. Naltrexone is not detected in preweaning rats following transplacental exposure: implications for growth modulation. Life Sci 1998;62:221–8.
12. Wildt L, Leyendecker G, Sir-Petermann T, Waibel-Treber S. Treatment with naltrexone in hypothalamic ovarian failure: induction of ovulation and pregnancy. Hum Reprod 1993;8;350–8.
13. Wildt L, Sir-Petermann T, Leyendecker G, Waibel-Treber S, Rabenbauer B. Opiate antagonist treatment of ovarian failure. Hum Reprod 1993;8(Suppl 2):168–74.
14. Couzinet B, Young J, Brailly S, Chanson P, Schaison G. Even after priming with ovarian steroids or pulsatile gonadotropin-releasing hormone administration, naltrexone is unable to induce ovulation in women with functional hypothalamic amenorrhea. J Clin Endocrinol Metab 1995;80:2102–7.
15. Roozenburg BJ, van Dessel HJHM, Evers JLH, Bots RSGM. Successful induction of ovulation in normogonadotrophic clomiphene resistant anovulatory women by combined naltrexone and clomiphene citrate treatment. Hum Reprod 1997;12:1720–2.

Name:	**NAPROXEN**	Risk Factor:	B_M*
Class:	**Nonsteroidal Anti-inflammatory**		

FETAL RISK SUMMARY

RECOMMENDATION: Human Data Suggest Risk in 1st and 3rd Trimesters

Naproxen is a nonsteroidal anti-inflammatory drug (NSAID) used in the management of the signs and symptoms of rheumatoid arthritis, osteoarthritis, ankylosing spondylitis, and juvenile arthritis. It is in same subclass (propionic acids) as five other NSAIDs (fenoprofen, flurbiprofen, ibuprofen, ketoprofen, and oxaprozin). Drugs in this class have been shown to inhibit labor and to prolong the length of pregnancy (1).

At 0.23–0.28 times the human systemic exposure at the recommended dose, no evidence of impaired fertility or fetal harm was seen in mice, rats, and rabbits (2). A 1990 report described an investigation on the effects of several nonsteroidal anti-inflammatory agents on mouse palatal fusion both *in vivo* and *in vitro* (3). The compounds, including naproxen, were found to induce cleft palate.

Consistent with the relatively low molecular weight (about 230), naproxen readily crosses the placenta to the fetal circulation. Twenty-eight women received two 500-mg naproxen doses, the first within 10.5 to 15 hours and the second within 4 hours of an elective 1st trimester pregnancy termination (4). Mean naproxen levels in maternal serum, fetal tissue, coelomic fluid, and amniotic fluid were 69.5, 6.4, 1.85, and 0.14 μg/mL. The mean fetal:maternal drug ratio was 0.092 (4). In a woman at 30 weeks' gestation treated with 250 mg of naproxen every 8 hours for four doses, plasma levels in twins 5 hours after the last dose were 59.5 and 68 μg/mL (5).

In a surveillance study of Michigan Medicaid recipients conducted between 1985 and 1992 involving 229,101 completed pregnancies, 1448 newborns had been exposed to naproxen during the 1st trimester (F. Rosa, personal communication, FDA, 1993). A total of 70 (4.8%) major birth defects were observed (62 expected). Specific data were available for six defect categories, including (observed/expected) 14/14 cardiovascular defects, 2/2 oral clefts, 0/1 spina bifida, 3/4 polydactyly, 2/2 limb reduction defects, and 3/3 hypospadias. These data do not support an association between the drug and congenital defects.

A combined 2001 population-based observational cohort study and a case-control study estimated the risk of adverse pregnancy outcome from the use of NSAIDs (6). The use of NSAIDs during pregnancy was not associated with congenital malformations, preterm delivery, or low birth weight, but a positive association was discovered with spontaneous abortions (SABs). A similar study, also published in 2001, failed to find a relationship, in general, between NSAIDs and congenital malformations, but did find a significant association with cardiac defects and orofacial clefts (7). In addition, a 2003 study found a significant association between exposure to NSAIDs in early pregnancy and SABs (8). (See Ibuprofen for details on these three studies.)

A brief 2003 editorial on the potential for NSAID-induced developmental toxicity concluded that NSAIDs, and specifically those with greater COX-2 affinity, had a lower risk of this toxicity in humans than aspirin (9).

A 2003 study using data from three Swedish health registers (1995–2001) that included maternal drug history collected prospectively, identified 1142 infants with orofacial clefts (isolated or with other malformations, excluding chromosome anomalies) (10). Compared to the expected number ($N = 2.9$) of orofacial clefts, there were eight naproxen-exposed cases, a relative risk of 2.72 (95% confidence interval [CI] 1.17–5.36).

A 2003 case-control study, using data from the same Swedish registers as in the above study, was conducted to identify drug use in early pregnancy that was associated with cardiac defects (11). Cases (cardiovascular defects without known chromosome anomalies) ($N = 5015$) were compared to controls consisting of all infants born in Sweden (1995–2001) ($N = 577,730$). Associations were identified for several drugs, some of which were probably due to confounding from the underlying disease or complaint or multiple testing, but some were thought to be true drug effects (11). For NSAIDs, the total exposed, number of cases, and odds ratios with 95%CI for NSAIDs were NSAIDs (all) (7698; 80 cases; 1.24, 0.99–1.55), naproxen (1679; 24 cases; 1.70, 1.14–2.54), diclofenac (1362; 15 cases; 1.30, 0.78–2.16), ibuprofen (4124; 37 cases; 1.08, 0.78–1.50), and aspirin (5920; 52 cases; 1.01, 0.76–1.33). Five of the defects observed with naproxen were two infants with transposition of the great vessels and three with endocardial cushion defects (one infant had both defects). The authors noted that further studies were needed to verify or reject the hypothesis (11).

A 2004 case report described a 24-year-old woman who took naproxen (550 mg about twice a week), bisoprolol (5 mg/day), and sumatriptan (100 mg about once a week) for migraine headaches during the first 5 weeks of pregnancy (12). An elective cesarean section was performed at 37 weeks' gestation for breech presentation to deliver a 3125-g male infant. The infant had a wide bilateral cleft lip/palate, marked hypertelorism, a broad nose, and bilateral but asymmetric toe abnormalities (missing and hypoplastic phalanges) (12).

Prostaglandin synthesis inhibitors may cause constriction of the ductus arteriosus *in utero*, which may result in primary pulmonary hypertension of the newborn (13–15). The dose, duration, and period of gestation are important determinants of these effects. Most studies of NSAIDs used as tocolytics have indicated that the fetus is relatively resistant to premature closure of the ductus before the 34th or 35th week of gestation (see Indomethacin). However, three fetuses (one set of twins) exposed to naproxen at 30 weeks for 2–6 days in an unsuccessful attempt to halt premature labor had markedly decreased plasma concentrations of prostaglandin E (6,15). Primary pulmonary hypertension of the newborn with severe hypoxemia, increased blood clotting times, hyperbilirubinemia, and impaired renal function were observed in the newborns. One infant died 4 days after birth, probably because of subarachnoid hemorrhage. Autopsy revealed a short and constricted ductus arteriosus. Use in other patients for premature labor at 34 weeks or earlier has not result in neonatal problems (17,18).

In a case report published in 2000, a mother took an over-the-counter preparation of naproxen 220 mg twice a day over the 4 days immediately preceding birth of a term 3790-g male infant (19). Within 2 hours of birth, the infant developed typical signs and symptoms of primary pulmonary hypertension with a closed ductus arteriosus. Conservative management was initiated and the infant was improving by the sixth postnatal day. At 6 weeks of age, the infant was doing well clinically without cyanosis.

Because of the potential newborn toxicity, naproxen should not be used late in the 3rd trimester (2,6,20). Moreover, women attempting to conceive should not use any prostaglandin synthesis inhibitor, including naproxen, because of the findings in a variety of animal models that indicate these agents block blastocyst implantation (21,22). In addition, as noted above, NSAIDs have been associated with SABs and congenital malformations.

[**Risk Factor D if used in 3rd trimester or near delivery.*]

BREAST FEEDING SUMMARY

RECOMMENDATION: Limited Human Data - Probably Compatible

Naproxen passes into breast milk in very small quantities. The milk:plasma ratio is approximately 0.01 (2). Following 250 or 375 mg twice daily, maximum milk levels were found 4 hours after a dose and ranged from 0.7 to 1.25 μg/mL and 1.76 to 2.37 μg/mL, respectively (23,24). The total amount of naproxen excreted in the infant's urine was 0.26% of the mother's dose. The effect on the infant from these amounts is unknown. The American Academy of Pediatrics classifies naproxen as compatible with breast-feeding (25).

References

1. Fuchs F. Prevention of prematurity. Am J Obstet Gynecol 1976;126:809–20.
2. Product information. Naprosyn. Roche Laboratories, 2000.
3. Montenegro MA, Palomino H. Induction of cleft palate in mice by inhibitors of prostaglandin synthesis. J Craniofac Genet Dev Biol 1990;10:83–94.
4. Siu SSN, Yeung JHK, Lau TK. An in-vivo study on placental transfer of naproxen in early human pregnancy. Hum Reprod 2002;17:1056–9.
5. Wilkinson AR. Naproxen levels in preterm infants after maternal treatment. Lancet 1980;2:591–2.
6. Nielsen GL, Sorensen HT, Larsen H, Pedersen L. Risk of adverse birth outcome and miscarriage in pregnant users of non-steroidal anti-inflammatory drugs: population based observational study and case-control study. BMJ 2001;322:266–70.
7. Ericson A, Kallen BAJ. Nonsteroidal anti-inflammatory drugs in early pregnancy. Reprod Toxicol 2001;15:371–5.
8. Li DK, Liu L, Odouli R. Exposure to non-steroidal anti-inflammatory drugs during pregnancy and risk of miscarriage: population based cohort study. BMJ 2003;327:368–71.
9. Tassinari MS, Cook JC, Hurtt ME. NSAIDs and developmental toxicity. Birth Defects Res (Part B) 2003;68:3–4.
10. Kallen B. Maternal drug use and infant cleft lip/palate with special reference to corticoids. Cleft Palate Craniofac J 2003;40:624–8.
11. Kallen BAJ, Olausson PO. Maternal drug use in early pregnancy and infant cardiovascular defect. Reprod Toxicol 2003;17:255–61.
12. Kajantie E, Somer M. Bilateral cleft lip and palate, hypertelorism and hypoplastic toes. Clin Dysmorphol 2004;13:195–6.
13. Levin DL. Effects of inhibition of prostaglandin synthesis on fetal development, oxygenation, and the fetal circulation. Semin Perinatol 1980;4:35–44.
14. Rudolph AM. The effects of nonsteroidal antiinflammatory compounds on fetal circulation and pulmonary function. Obstet Gynecol 1981;58(Suppl):63s–7s.
15. Van Marter LJ, Leviton A, Allred EN, Pagano M, Sullivan KF, Cohen A, Epstein MF. Persistent pulmonary hypertension of the newborn and smoking and aspirin and nonsteroidal antiinflammatory drug consumption during pregnancy. Pediatrics 1996;97:658–63.
16. Wilkinson AR, Aynsley-Green A, Mitchell MD. Persistent pulmonary hypertension and abnormal prostaglandin E levels in preterm infants after maternal treatment with naproxen. Arch Dis Child 1979;54:942–5.
17. Gerris J, Jonckheer M, Sacre-Smits L. Acute hyperthyroidism during pregnancy: a case report and critical analysis. Eur J Obstet Gynecol Reprod Biol 1981;12:271–80.
18. Wiqvist N, Kjellmer I, Thiringer K, Ivarsson E, Karlsson K. Treatment of premature labor by prostaglandin synthetase inhibitors. Acta Biol Med Germ 1978;37:923–30.
19. Talati AJ, Salim MA, Korones SB. Persistent pulmonary hypertension after maternal naproxen ingestion in a term newborn: a case report. Am J Perinatol 2000;17:69–71.
20. Anonymous. PG-synthetase inhibitors in obstetrics and after. Lancet 1980;2:185–6.
21. Matt DW, Borzelleca JF. Toxic effects on the female reproductive system during pregnancy, parturition, and lactation. In Witorsch RJ, ed. *Reproductive Toxicology*. 2nd editor New York, NY: Raven Press, 1995:175–93.
22. Dawood MY. Nonsteroidal antiinflammatory drugs and reproduction. Am J Obstet Gynecol 1993; 169:1255–65.
23. Jamali F, Tam YK, Stevens RD. Naproxen excretion in breast milk and its uptake by suckling infant (abstract). Drug Intell Clin Pharm 1982;16:475.
24. Jamali F, Stevens DRS. Naproxen excretion in milk and its uptake by the infant. Drug Intell Clin Pharm 1983;17:910–11.
25. Committee on Drugs, American Academy of Pediatrics. The transfer of drugs and other chemicals into human milk. Pediatrics 2001;108:776–89.

N

Name: **NARATRIPTAN** Risk Factor: C_M

Class: **Antimigraine**

FETAL RISK SUMMARY

RECOMMENDATION: Limited Human Data - Animal Data Suggest Moderate Risk

Naratriptan is an oral selective serotonin (5-hydroxytryptamine; 5-HT) receptor subtype agonist used for the acute treatment of migraine headaches. The safety and effectiveness of naratriptan have not been established for cluster headaches (1).

Developmental toxicity was observed in pregnant rats and rabbits at oral doses producing maternal plasma drug levels as low as 11 and 2.5 times, respectively, the plasma levels in humans receiving the maximum recommended daily dose (MRDD) of 5 mg (1). Toxicity consisted of embryo lethality, minor fetal structural variations, pup mortality, and offspring growth retardation. In pregnant rats during the period of organogenesis, daily oral doses of 10, 60, and 340 mg/kg/day that resulted in maternal plasma levels 11, 70, and 470 times the human plasma levels obtained with the MRDD, respectively, were associated with dose-related increases in embryonic death and in the incidence of fetal structural variations: incomplete, irregular ossification of skull bones, sternebrae, and ribs (1). A no-effect dose for these toxicities was not established. The highest dose was associated with maternal toxicity as evidenced by decreased body weight gain. When naratriptan was administered before and throughout the mating period at 60 mg/kg/day or greater, there was an increase in pre-implantation loss. Impairment of fertility in both male (testicular effects) and female (anestrus) rats occurred at higher doses. Exposure to the two highest doses—60 and 340 mg/kg/day—late in gestation and during lactation resulted in offspring behavioral impairment (tremors) and decreased viability and growth (1).

Pregnant rabbits received daily oral doses during organogenesis that produced maternal plasma levels ranging from 2.5 to 140 times the human levels produced by the MRDD on a body surface area basis (1). Developmental toxicity, observed at all doses, consisted of embryonic death and fetal variations (major blood vessel variations, supernumerary ribs, and incomplete skeletal ossification). Fetal skeletal malformation (fused sternebrae) was observed in one rabbit subspecies at the highest dose. A no-effect dose for these toxicities was not established (1).

No reports describing the placental transfer of naratriptan in humans have been located. However, the relatively low molecular weight of the compound, about 372 for the hydrochloride salt, suggests that the drug will cross to the fetus.

A manufacturer's pregnancy registry, covering 1 January 1996 through 30 April 2004, has outcome data for 40 prospectively enrolled (reported before pregnancy outcome was known) pregnancies exposed to naratriptan (some also exposed to sumatriptan) (2). There were 35 exposures in the 1st trimester and 5 in the 2nd trimester. The outcomes included 35 live births, 3 spontaneous abortions, 1 elective abortion, and 1 infant (exposed to naratriptan and sumatriptan in the 1st trimester) with a small ventricular septal defect that was expected to close spontaneously. Retrospective reports (reported after the outcome was known) are often biased (only adverse outcomes are reported). There were two retrospective reports of adverse outcomes exposed in the 1st trimester (2). (See Sumatriptan for required statement).

In summary, naratriptan is not an animal teratogen but does produce dose-related embryo and fetal developmental toxicity. Human pregnancy experience, however, is too limited to assess the safety of the drug or its teratogenic potential. A 1998 review on the safety of migraine treatment in pregnancy recommended that naratriptan and other similar agents (see Sumatriptan) be avoided during pregnancy (3).

BREAST FEEDING SUMMARY

RECOMMENDATION: No Human Data - Probably Compatible

Naratriptan is excreted in the milk of nursing rats (1), but no reports describing the use of naratriptan during human lactation have been located. The molecular weight of the hydrochloride salt (about 372) is low enough, however, that passage into the milk should be expected. The effects of this exposure, if any, on a nursing infant are unknown.

References

1. Product information. Amerge. Glaxo Wellcome, 1999.
2. Sumatriptan and Naratriptan Pregnancy Registry. Interim Report. 1 January 1996 through 30 April 2004. Glaxo Wellcome, July 2004.
3. Pfaffenrath V, Rehm M. Migraine in pregnancy. What are the safest treatment options? Drug Saf 1998; 19:383–8.

Name: **NATEGLINIDE** Risk Factor: **C_M**

Class: **Oral Hypoglycemic**

FETAL RISK SUMMARY

RECOMMENDATION: Limited Human Data - Animal Data Suggest Low Risk

Nateglinide is an amino-acid derivative that is used as an oral insulin secretagogue. It is structurally unrelated to the oral sulfonylurea agents. Nateglinide is indicated for the management of type 2 diabetes mellitus (non-insulin dependent) as monotherapy to lower blood glucose when hyperglycemia cannot be adequately controlled by diet and exercise. The drug is rapidly cleared from the plasma with an elimination half-life of approximately 1.5 hours. It is protein bound (98%) primarily by serum albumin and to a lesser degree by α_1 acid glycoprotein. Although the major metabolites are less potent antidiabetic agents, a minor metabolite has antidiabetic potency similar to that of the parent compound (1).

Reproduction studies with nateglinide have been conducted in rats and rabbits. In rats, no evidence of teratogenicity was observed at doses up to approximately 60 times the human therapeutic exposure from the recommended dose of 120 mg three times daily before meals (HTE). Decreased body weights in offspring were observed when these doses were administered in the perinatal and postnatal periods. In rabbits, a dose approximately 40 times the HTE adversely affected embryonic development and increased the incidence of gallbladder agenesis or small gallbladder (1).

It is not known if nateglinide crosses the human placenta. The relatively low molecular weight (about 317) suggests that exposure of the embryo and/or fetus is possible, but the short plasma elimination half-life and extensive protein binding should limit the amount of drug available to cross to the fetal compartment.

In a 2004 case report, a 39-year-old woman took pravastatin (80 mg/day), metformin (2 g/day), and nateglinide (360 mg/day) during the first 24 weeks of gestation (2). All therapy was discontinued and insulin was started for her diabetes. At term, the woman delivered a healthy 2.4-kg male infant (head circumference 34 cm, length 46 cm) with Apgar scores of 8 and 9 at 1 and 5 minutes, respectively. The infant's growth and development were normal at follow-up examinations during the first 6 months of life (2).

In summary, the animal data suggest a low risk for developmental toxicity, but only one report of human pregnancy experience has been located. Insulin is the treatment of choice for pregnant diabetics if diet and exercise cannot control the maternal hyperglycemia. Insulin does not cross the placenta to the fetus and, thus, eliminates the additional concern that the drug therapy itself may adversely affect the fetus. Although a potential role in gestational diabetes may exist for some oral hypoglycemics (e.g., see Glyburide), carefully prescribed insulin therapy will provide better control of the mother's blood glucose, thereby preventing the fetal and neonatal complications that occur with this disease. In general, if oral hypoglycemics are used during pregnancy, consideration should be given to changing the therapy to insulin to lessen the possibility of prolonged hypoglycemia in the newborn. The rapid elimination and extensive protein binding of nateglinide, however, may lessen the potential for this adverse effect.

BREAST FEEDING SUMMARY

RECOMMENDATION: No Human Data - Probably Compatible.

No reports describing the use of nateglinide during human lactation have been located. The relatively low molecular weight (about 317) suggests that excretion into milk may occur, but the short elimination half-life (1.5 hours) and extensive protein binding (98%) should limit the amount of drug and active metabolites available for excretion into milk. In lactating rats given doses approximately 60 times the human exposure from the recommended dose of 120 mg three times daily before meals, the milk:plasma ratio, based on area under the concentration versus time curve, was 1:4 (1).

References

1. Product information. Starlix. Novartis Pharmaceuticals, 2004.
2. Teelucksingh S, Youssef JE, Sohan K, Ramsewak S. Prolonged inadvertent pravastatin use in pregnancy. Reprod Toxicol 2004;18:299–300.

Name: **NEDOCROMIL SODIUM** Risk Factor: **B_M**

Class: **Respiratory Anti-inflammatory (Inhaled)**

N

FETAL RISK SUMMARY

RECOMMENDATION: Limited Human Data - Animal Data Suggest Low Risk

Nedocromil sodium is an inhaled anti-inflammatory agent used in the prevention of asthma. Because of its mast cell-stabilizing properties, it is also available as a 2% ophthalmic solution for the treatment of itching associated with allergic conjunctivitis. Its respiratory action appears to be similar to that of cromolyn sodium. Each activation of the meter delivers 1.75 mg nedocromil from the mouthpiece. In asthmatic patients, the absolute bioavailability after chronic dosing (2 activations four times/day for 1 month) was approximately 5% of the administered dose (1). No accumulation was observed after chronic use. With chronic administration in the eye, less than 4% of the total dose is absorbed systemically (2).

No effects on fertility in male and female mice and rats were observed with a SC dose of nedocromil sodium 100 mg/kg/day, about 30 and 60 times the maximum recommended human daily inhalation dose on a body surface basis (MRHID), respectively (1). In reproduction studies, no evidence of teratogenicity or fetal harm was revealed when 100 mg/kg/day SC was given to pregnant mice, rats, and rabbits (30, 60, and 116 times the MRHID, respectively) (1). The SC dose was more than 1600 times the maximum recommended human daily ocular dose on a mg/kg basis (2).

It is not known if nedocromil sodium crosses the human placenta. The molecular weight of the drug (about 415) is low enough that transfer to the fetus should be expected. The low systemic bioavailability (e.g., mean peak plasma concentrations in the 1.6–2.8-ng/mL range [1]), however, suggests that the amounts reaching the embryo or fetus are clinically insignificant.

A report published in 1988 described three women who became pregnant while enrolled in a trial of nedocromil (3). All three were withdrawn from the study because of their pregnancy. One woman stopped the therapy 5 weeks after her last menstrual period. She and another woman (gestational age when therapy stopped not specified) had normal pregnancies. The third woman stopped nedocromil therapy at 8 weeks' gestation and had a spontaneous abortion 5 days later. The abortion was thought to be unrelated to treatment (3).

A 1998 noninterventional observational cohort study described the outcomes of pregnancies in women who had been prescribed one or more of 34 newly marketed drugs by general practitioners in England (4). Data were obtained by questionnaires sent to the prescribing physicians 1 month after the expected or possible date of delivery. In 831 (78%) of the pregnancies, a newly marketed drug was thought to have been taken during the 1st trimester with birth defects noted in 14 (2.5%) singleton births of the 557 newborns (10 sets of twins). In addition, two birth defects were observed in aborted fetuses. However, few of the aborted fetuses were examined. Nedocromil was taken during the 1st trimester in 35 pregnancies. The outcomes of these pregnancies included 1 spontaneous abortion; 8 elective abortions; 3 cases lost to follow-up; 22 normal, term infants; and 1 newborn with a birth defect (4). The birth defect, in an infant born to a 22-year-old woman, was categorized as congenital heart disease (no details given). Other maternal drug exposures in this case included aminophylline, corticosteroids, and salbutamol. Although the cause of the one major congenital malformation observed is unknown, the study lacks the sensitivity to identify minor anomalies because of the absence of standardized examinations. Late-appearing major defects may also have been missed because of the timing of the questionnaires.

N

In summary, the absence of animal embryo/fetal toxicity, the limited human systemic bioavailability, and the outcomes of the exposed human pregnancies appear to indicate that nedocromil sodium is not a major teratogenic risk. Although this assessment is based on limited pregnancy experience, the benefits in preventing maternal asthma probably outweigh any potential fetal harm. Because of the greater pregnancy experience, cromolyn sodium may be the preferred choice (see Cromolyn Sodium).

BREAST FEEDING SUMMARY

RECOMMENDATION: No Human Data - Probably Compatible

No reports describing the use of nedocromil sodium during human lactation have been located. After IV administration, the drug is excreted into the milk of lactating rats (2). Although the molecular weight of the drug (about 415) is low enough to allow excretion into breast milk, the very small amounts in the systemic circulation (see above) suggests that the potential for harm in a nursing infant is nil.

References

1. Product information. Tilade. Rhone-Poulenc Rorer Pharmaceuticals, 2000.
2. Product information. Alocril. Allergan, 2001.
3. Carrasco E, Sepulveda R. The acceptability, safety and efficacy of nedocromil sodium in long-term clinical use in patients with perennial asthma. J Int Med Res 1988;16:394–401.
4. Wilton LV, Pearce GL, Martin RM, Mackay FJ, Mann RD. The outcomes of pregnancy in women exposed to newly marketed drugs in general practice in England. Br J Obstet Gynaecol 1998;105:882–9.

Name: **NEFAZODONE** Risk Factor: **C_M**
Class: **Antidepressant**

FETAL RISK SUMMARY

RECOMMENDATION: No Human Data - Animal Data Suggest Moderate Risk

Nefazodone is structurally unrelated to other antidepressants. Although its exact mechanism of action is unknown, it inhibits neuronal reuptake of serotonin and norepinephrine.

No teratogenic effects were observed in reproductive toxicity studies involving rats and rabbits dosed, respectively, at 5 and 6 times the maximum human daily dose based on body surface area (MHDD) (1). Increased early pup mortality was observed, however, when dosing at 5 times the MHDD in rats began during gestation and continued until weaning. Moreover, decreased pup weights were seen at this and lower doses. The no-effect dose for pup mortality was 1.3 times the MHDD (1).

A 2003 prospective controlled study described the outcomes of 147 pregnancies exposed in the 1st trimester (52 exposed throughout gestation) to either nefazodone or trazodone, a closely related antidepressant (2). The data were collected from five teratology information services in Canada (two sites), the United States (two sites), and Italy. The outcomes were compared to two control groups (one exposed to other antidepressants and one exposed to nonteratogens). There were no significant differences between the three groups in terms of spontaneous abortions, elective abortions, stillbirths, major malformations, gestational age at birth, or birth weights. In the study group, there were two (1.6%) major malformations: neural tube defect and Hirschsprung disease (2).

N

BREAST FEEDING SUMMARY

RECOMMENDATION: Limited Human Data - Potential Toxicity

Nefazodone is excreted into breast milk. A 1999 report described an analytical method for determining the concentrations of nefazodone and its metabolites in human plasma and milk (3). In addition, in one woman taking 200 mg twice daily, the paired concentrations of nefazodone in milk and plasma (trough) were 57 and 617 ng/mL, respectively; the milk:plasma ratio was 0.09. In two other subjects, one taking 50 mg twice daily and the other 50 mg in the morning and 100 mg in the evening, the trough plasma levels were <50 ng/mL, whereas the paired milk concentrations were 687 and 213 ng/mL, respectively (3).

A 35-year-old woman gave birth to a premature female infant at 27 weeks' gestation (4). The infant was fed the mother's breast milk from a bottle while in the hospital. The mother was started on nefazodone, 200 mg in the morning and 100 mg at night, because of depression 7 weeks after delivery. One week later, the mother began breast-feeding. At 9 weeks of age, the 2.1-kg infant was readmitted to the hospital because of drowsiness, lethargy, failure to maintain body temperature, and poor feeding. Breast-feeding was stopped 1 week later and the infant's symptoms resolved gradually over 72 hours. Maternal blood and breast milk were collected immediately before the 200 mg morning dose and at intervals up to 6 hours (for milk) or 12 hours (for blood). The milk:plasma ratio (based on area under the concentration curve over 12 hours) for nefazodone was 0.27, and 0.02–0.19 for three metabolites that were identified. The maximum concentrations in milk and plasma were 358 ng/mL (at 3 hours) and 1270 ng/mL (at 1 hour), respectively.

The estimated infant dose, relative to the weight-adjusted total daily maternal dose, was 0.3% for nefazodone and 0.45% for the parent drug plus metabolites. The investigators speculated that the sedative effects might have resulted from reduced clearance of the drug secondary to the infant's prematurity (4).

The long-term effects on neurobehavior and development from exposure to antidepressants during a period of rapid central nervous system development have not been studied. The American Academy of Pediatrics classifies the effects of other antidepressants on nursing infants as unknown but may be of concern (5).

References

1. Product information. Serzone. Bristol-Myers Squibb, 1996.
2. Einarson A, Bonari L, Voyer-Lavigne S, Addis A, Matsui D, Johnson Y, Koren G. A multicentre prospective controlled study to determine the safety of trazodone and nefazodone use during pregnancy. Can J Psychiatry 2003;48:106–9.
3. Dodd S, Buist A, Burrows GD, Maguire KP, Norman TR. Determination of nefazodone and its pharmacologically active metabolites in human blood plasma and breast milk by high-performance liquid chromatography. J Chromatogr B Biomed Sci Appl 1999;730:249–55.
4. Yapp P, Ilett KF, Kristensen JH, Hackett LP, Paech MJ, Rampono J. Drowsiness and poor feeding in a breast-fed infant: association with nefazodone and its metabolites. Ann Pharmacother 2000;34:1269–72.
5. Committee on Drugs, American Academy of Pediatrics. The transfer of drugs and other chemicals into human milk. Pediatrics 2001;108:776–89.

Name: **NELFINAVIR** Risk Factor: B_M

Class: **Antiviral**

FETAL RISK SUMMARY

RECOMMENDATION: Compatible - Maternal Benefit >> Embryo/Fetal Risk

Nelfinavir is an inhibitor of human immunodeficiency virus (HIV) protease (PI). In *in vitro* tests, the agent was found to be active against both type 1 and type 2 (HIV-1 and HIV-2) (1). Other drugs in this class are amprenavir, indinavir, ritonavir, and saquinavir. Protease is an enzyme that is required for the cleavage of viral polyprotein precursors into active functional proteins found in infectious HIV. Nelfinavir, usually in combination with other antiretroviral agents, is indicated for the treatment of HIV infections.

Reproduction studies with nelfinavir have been conducted in rats and rabbits (1). No effects on fertility, mating, embryo survival, or fetal development were observed in rats given doses that produced plasma concentrations comparable to those measured in humans with therapeutic doses. Exposure of pregnant rats from mid-gestation through lactation had no effect on survival, growth, development to weaning, or subsequent fertility of the offspring (1). In rabbits, doses up to a maternal toxic dose (decreased maternal body weight) had no effect on fetal development. However, even at the highest dose, the systemic exposure in rabbits was significantly less than that observed in humans (1).

It is not known if nelfinavir crosses the human placenta to the fetus. The molecular weight of the free base (about 568) is low enough that transfer to the fetus should be expected.

A 2004 study, using data (through July 2002) from the Antiretroviral Pregnancy Registry (see below), reported 301, 1st trimester exposures to nelfinavir (2). The prevalence rate of birth defects, based on nine cases, was 3.0% (95% confidence interval [CI] 1.4–5.6).

This rate was similar to the expected rate of 3.1% in the Centers for Disease Control and Prevention's (CDC) population-based surveillance system (2).

The Antiretroviral Pregnancy Registry reported for the period from January 1989 through January 2004, prospective data (reported to the Registry before the outcomes were known) involving 1537 live births that had been exposed during the 1st trimester to one or more antiretroviral agents (3). Forty-seven of the newborns had congenital defects (3.1%, 95% CI 2.3–4.1). In the 2407 live births with earliest exposure in the 2nd/3rd trimesters, there were 56 infants with defects (2.3%, 95% CI 1.8–3.0). The prevalence rates for the two periods did not differ significantly. There were 103 infants with birth defects among 3944 live births with exposure any time during pregnancy (2.6%, 95% CI 2.1–3.2). The prevalence rate did not differ significantly from the expected rate in the CDC's system. There were 1286 outcomes exposed to nelfinavir (416 in the 1st trimester and 870 in the 2nd/3rd trimesters) in combination with other antiretroviral agents. There were 15 (3.6%, 95% CI 2.0–5.9) birth defects among the 1st trimester exposures and 19 (2.2%, 95% CI 1.3–3.4) in those exposed in the 2nd/3rd trimesters. In reviewing the birth defects of prospective and retrospective (pregnancies reported after the outcomes were known) registered cases, and clinical reports, the Registry concluded that there was no pattern of anomalies to suggest a common cause (3). (See Lamivudine for required statement.)

A study published in 1999 evaluated the safety, efficacy, and perinatal transmission rates of HIV in 30 pregnant women receiving various combinations of antiretroviral agents (4). Many of the women were substance abusers. Protease inhibitors (nelfinavir $N = 7$, indinavir $N = 6$, and saquinavir $N = 1$ in combination with nelfinavir) were used in 13 of the women. Antiretroviral therapy was initiated at a median of 14 weeks' gestation (range preconception to 32 weeks). Despite previous histories of extensive antiretroviral experience and of vertical transmission of HIV, combination therapy was effective in treating maternal disease and in preventing transmission to the current newborns. The outcomes of the pregnancies treated with protease inhibitors appeared to be similar to the 17 cases that did not receive these agents, except that the birth weights were lower (4).

The Food and Drug Administration (FDA) issued a public health advisory in 1998 on the association between protease inhibitors and diabetes mellitus (5). Because pregnancy is a risk factor for hyperglycemia, there was concern that these antiviral agents would exacerbate this risk. An abstract published in 2000 described the results of a study involving 34 pregnant women treated with protease inhibitors (30 with nelfinavir) compared to 41 controls that evaluated the association with diabetes (6). No association between protease inhibitors and an increased incidence of gestational diabetes was found.

A 1999 abstract reported the effect of protease inhibitors (nelfinavir, indinavir, ritonavir, or saquinavir) in combination with two or more other antiretroviral agents in 39 pregnant women (7). Nelfinavir was the most commonly used protease inhibitor. The mean gestational age at the start of protease inhibitor therapy was 31 weeks (range 8–39 weeks). All of the newborns tested HIV-negative. Based on these outcomes, and the lack of congenital anomalies and serious neonatal complications, and the mother's response to therapy, the authors concluded that protease inhibitor therapy during pregnancy was effective for maternal HIV disease and contributed to the very low rate of perinatal HIV transmission (7).

A multicenter, retrospective survey of pregnancies exposed to protease inhibitors was published in 2000 (8). There were 92 live born infants delivered from 89 women (3 sets of twins) at six health care centers. One nonviable infant, born at 22 weeks' gestation, died. The surviving 91 infants were evaluated in terms of adverse effects, prematurity rate, and frequency of HIV-1 transmission. Most of the infants were exposed *in utero* to a single protease inhibitor, but a few were exposed to more than one because of sequential or double combined therapy. The number of newborns exposed to each protease inhibitor was indinavir ($N = 23$), nelfinavir ($N = 39$), ritonavir ($N = 5$), and saquinavir ($N = 34$). Protease inhibitors were started before conception in 18, and during the 1st, 2nd, or 3rd trimesters in 12, 44, and 14, respectively, and not reported in 1. Other antiretrovirals used with the protease inhibitors included four nucleoside reverse-transcriptase inhibitors (NRTIs) (didanosine, lamivudine, stavudine, and zidovudine). The most common NRTI regimen was a combination of zidovudine and lamivudine (65% of women). In addition, seven women were enrolled in the AIDS Clinical Trials Group Protocol 316 and, at the start of labor, received either a single dose of the non-nucleoside reverse transcriptase inhibitor nevirapine, or placebo. Maternal conditions thought possibly or likely to be related to therapy were mild anemia in eight, severe anemia in one (probably secondary to zidovudine), and thrombocytopenia in one. Gestational diabetes mellitus was observed in three women (3.3%), a rate similar to the expected prevalence of 2.6% in a nonexposed population. One mother developed postpartum cardiomyopathy and died 2 months after birth of twins, but the cause death was not known. For the surviving newborns, there was no increase in adverse effects over that observed in previous clinical trials of HIV-positive women, including the prevalence of anemia (12%), hyperbilirubinemia (6%; none exposed to indinavir), and low birth weight (20.6%). Premature delivery occurred in 19.1% of the pregnancies (close to the expected rate). The percentage of infants infected with HIV was 0 (95% CI 0%–3%) (8).

In summary, the lack of animal toxicity and the human pregnancy data suggest that nelfinavir is not a major teratogen. Two reviews, one in 1996 and the other in 1997, concluded that all women currently receiving antiretroviral therapy should continue to receive therapy during pregnancy and that treatment of the mother with monotherapy should be considered inadequate therapy (9,10). In 1998, the Centers for Disease Control and Prevention (CDC) made a similar recommendation that antiretroviral therapy should be continued during pregnancy, but discontinuation of all therapy during the 1st trimester was a consideration (5). If indicated, therefore, protease inhibitors, including nelfinavir, should not be withheld in pregnancy (with the possible exception of the 1st trimester) because the expected benefit to the HIV-positive mother probably outweighs the known risk to the fetus. Pregnant women taking protease inhibitors should be monitored for hyperglycemia. The efficacy and safety of combined therapy in preventing vertical transmission of HIV to the newborn, however, are unknown, and zidovudine remains the only antiretroviral agent recommended for this purpose (9,10).

BREAST FEEDING SUMMARY

RECOMMENDATION: Contraindicated

No reports describing the use of nelfinavir during human lactation have been located. The molecular weight of the free base (about 568) is low enough that excretion into breast milk should be expected. The agent is excreted in the milk of lactating rats (1).

Reports on the use of nelfinavir during human lactation are unlikely because the antiviral agent is used in the treatment of human immunodeficiency virus (HIV) infections. HIV-1 is transmitted in milk, and, in developed countries, breast-feeding is not recommended (9–13). In developing countries, breast-feeding is undertaken, despite the risk, because there are no affordable milk substitutes available. Until 1999, no studies had been published that examined the effect of any antiretroviral therapy on HIV-1 transmission in milk. In that year, a study of zidovudine measured a 38% reduction in vertical transmission of HIV-1 infection when compared to controls despite breast-feeding (see Zidovudine).

References

1. Product information. Agouron Pharmaceuticals, 2001.
2. Covington DL, Conner SD, Doi PA, Sinson J, Daniels EM. Risk of birth defects associated with nelfinavir exposure during pregnancy. Obstet Gynecol 2004;103:1181–9.
3. Antiretroviral Pregnancy Registry Steering Committee, Antiretroviral Pregnancy Registry International Interim Report for 1 January 1989 through 31 January 2004. Wilmington, NC: Registry Coordinating Center; 2004.
4. McGowan JP, Crane M, Wiznia AA, Blum S. Combination antiretroviral therapy in human immunodeficiency virus-infected pregnant women. Obstet Gynecol 1999;94:641–6.
5. CDC. Public Health Service Task Force recommendations for the use of antiretroviral drugs in pregnant women infected with HIV-1 for maternal health and for reducing perinatal HIV-1 transmission in the United States. MMWR 1998;47:No. RR 2.
6. Fassett M, Kramer F, Stek A. Treatment with protease inhibitors in pregnancy is not associated with an increased incidence of gestational diabetes (abstract). Am J Obstet Gynecol 2000;182:S97.
7. Stek A, Kramer F, Fassett M, Khoury M. The safety and efficacy of protease inhibitor therapy for HIV infection during pregnancy (abstract). Am J Obstet Gynecol 1999;180:S7.
8. Morris AB, Cu-Uvin S, Harwell JI, Garb J, Zorrilla C, Vajaranant M, Dobles AR, Jones TB, Carlan S, Allen DY. Multicenter review of protease inhibitors in 89 pregnancies. J Acquir Immune Defic Syndr 2000;25:306–11.
9. Carpenter CCJ, Fischi MA, Hammer SM, Hirsch MS, Jacobsen DM, Katzenstein DA, Montaner JSG, Richman DD, Saag MS, Schooley RT, Thompson MA, Vella S, Yeni PG, Volberding PA. Antiretroviral therapy for HIV infection in 1996. JAMA 1996;276:146–54.
10. Minkoff H, Augenbraun M. Antiretroviral therapy for pregnant women. Am J Obstet Gynecol 1997;176:478–89.
11. Brown ZA, Watts DH. Antiviral therapy in pregnancy. Clin Obstet Gynecol 1990;33:276–89.
12. de Martino M, Tovo P-A, Pezzotti P, Galli L, Massironi E, Ruga E, Floreea F, Plebani A, Gabiano C, Zuccotti GV. HIV-1 transmission through breast-milk: appraisal of risk according to duration of feeding. AIDS 1992;6:991–7.
13. Van de Perre P. Postnatal transmission of human immunodeficiency virus type 1: the breast-feeding dilemma. Am J Obstet Gynecol 1995;173:483–7.

N

Name:	**NEOMYCIN**	Risk Factor:	**C**
Class:	**Antibiotic (Aminoglycoside)**		

FETAL RISK SUMMARY

RECOMMENDATION: Human Data Suggest Low Risk

Neomycin is an aminoglycoside antibiotic. Small amounts of neomycin (about 3%) are absorbed from the normal gastrointestinal tract (GI) after oral and rectal administration (1). Larger systemic amounts may be obtained if GI motility is impaired. A single 4-g oral dose has produced peak plasma concentrations of 2.5–6.1 μg/mL, 1–4 hours after the dose (1).

No reports describing the passage of neomycin across the placenta to the fetus have been located, but this should be expected (see other aminoglycosides Amikacin, Gentamicin, Kanamycin, Streptomycin, and Tobramycin).

Ototoxicity, which is known to occur after oral, topical, and parenteral neomycin therapy, has not been reported as an effect of *in utero* exposure. However, eighth cranial nerve toxicity in the fetus is well known following exposure to kanamycin and streptomycin and may potentially occur with neomycin.

Oral neomycin therapy, 2 g daily, depresses urinary estrogen excretion, apparently by inhibiting steroid conjugate hydrolysis in the gut (2). The fall in estrogen excretion resembles the effect produced by ampicillin but occurs about 2 days later. Urinary estriol was formerly used to assess the condition of the fetoplacental unit, depressed levels being associated with fetal distress. This assessment is now made by measuring plasma conjugated estriol, which is not usually affected by neomycin.

The Collaborative Perinatal Project monitored 50,282 mother-child pairs, 30 of whom had 1st trimester exposure to neomycin (3). No evidence was found to suggest a relationship to large categories of major or minor malformations or to individual defects.

The population-based dataset of the Hungarian Case-Control Surveillance of Congenital Abnormalities, covering the period of 1980–1996, was used to evaluate the teratogenicity of aminoglycoside antibiotics (parenteral gentamicin, streptomycin, tobramycin, and oral neomycin) in a study published in 2000 (4). A case group of 22,865 women who had fetuses or newborns with congenital malformations were compared to 38,151 women who had no newborns with structural defects. A total of 38 cases and 42 controls were treated with aminoglycosides. There were 12 cases (0.05%) and 14 controls (0.04%) treated with oral neomycin (odds ratio 1.4, 95% confidence interval 0.7–3.1). A case-control pair analysis for the 2nd and 3rd months of gestation also failed to show a risk for teratogenicity. The investigators concluded that there was no detectable teratogenic risk for structural defects for any of the aminoglycoside antibiotics (4). They also concluded, although it was not investigated in this study, that the risk of deafness after *in utero* aminoglycoside exposure was small.

BREAST FEEDING SUMMARY

RECOMMENDATION: No Human Data - Probably Compatible

No reports describing the use of neomycin during human lactation have been located. Small amounts of other aminoglycosides (e.g., see Gentamicin) are excreted into breast milk and absorbed by the nursing infant. Neomycin was excreted into the milk of lactating cows and ewes after a single 10 mg/kg IM dose that produced peak concentrations of approximately 35 μg/mL at 1–2 hours (5). The very limited systemic bioavailability of oral neomycin in humans (about 3% for a normal GI tract), however, suggests that clinically insignificant amounts of neomycin would appear in breast milk.

N

References

1. American Hospital Formulary Service. *Drug Information 2000*. Bethesda, MD: American Society of Health-System Pharmacists, 2000:73–4.
2. Pulkkinen M, Willman K. Reduction of maternal estrogen excretion by neomycin. Am J Obstet Gynecol 1973;115:1153.
3. Heinonen OP, Slone D, Shapiro S. *Birth Defects and Drugs in Pregnancy*. Littleton, MA: Publishing Sciences Group, 1977:297–301.
4. Czeizel AE, Rockenbauer M, Olsen J, Sorensen HT. A teratological study of aminoglycoside antibiotic treatment during pregnancy. Scand J Infect Dis 2000;32:309–13.
5. Ziv G, Sulman FG. Distribution of aminoglycoside antibiotics in blood and milk. Res Vet Sci 1974;17:68–74.

Name: **NEOSTIGMINE** Risk Factor: **C_M**
Class: **Parasympathomimetic (Cholinergic)**

FETAL RISK SUMMARY

RECOMMENDATION: Limited Human Data - No Relevant Animal Data

Neostigmine is a quaternary ammonium compound with anticholinesterase activity used in the diagnosis and treatment of myasthenia gravis and to reverse muscle relaxation from competitive (nondepolarizing) muscle relaxants.

Although neostigmine is ionized at physiologic pH, the molecular weight (about 223) is low enough that transfer of the nonionized fraction to the fetus should be expected. Circumstantial evidence for neostigmine placental transfer was presented in a 1996 case report (1). A woman with a pregnancy of 31 weeks' gestation, undergoing surgery for a fractured elbow, was given IV neostigmine (5 mg) and glycopyrrolate (1 mg) to reverse muscle paralysis at the end of the procedure. The fetal heart rate immediately decreased from 115–130 beats/minute to 90–110 beats/minute and then gradually returned to 130 beats/minute within 1 hour. Four days later, surgical repair of the elbow was again required. At the end of this surgery, neostigmine (5 mg) and atropine (0.4 mg) were given IV and no change in the fetal heart rate was observed. The authors attributed the different effects on the fetal heart rate to the greater placental transfer of atropine in comparison to glycopyrrolate (see also Glycopyrrolate), that resulted in blocking the transplacental muscarinic effects of neostigmine (1).

The safe use of neostigmine in the treatment of maternal myasthenia gravis or other conditions has been reported (2–12). One study described 22 exposures to neostigmine in the 1st trimester (2). No relationship to congenital defects was found. A 1973 study reported the use of IM neostigmine (0.5 mg/day) for 3 days as a pregnancy test in 27 women with "uncertain pregnancies" at 5–14 weeks' gestation (3). Although vaginal bleeding occurred in seven (26%) patients, only one aborted and the remaining 26 pregnancies went to term without complications. In a 1983 report, two women with myasthenia gravis were treated throughout gestation with neostigmine, 105 mg/day (combined with pyridostigmine and ambenonium) and 300 mg/day (combined with pyridostigmine), respectively, without apparent fetal harm (12).

One investigator considers neostigmine to be one of the drugs of choice for pregnant patients with myasthenia gravis (4). This author also cautioned that IV anticholinesterases should not be used in pregnancy because of the potential for inducing premature labor and suggested that IM neostigmine be used in place of IV edrophonium for diagnostic purposes (4). This recommendation, however, should be approached with caution in view of the high rate of vaginal bleeding following IM neostigmine described above.

Transient muscular weakness has been observed in about 20% of newborns of mothers with myasthenia gravis (10). The neonatal myasthenia is caused by transplacental passage of anti-acetylcholine receptor immunoglobulin G antibodies (10).

BREAST FEEDING SUMMARY

RECOMMENDATION: Limited Human Data - Probably Compatible

No reports describing the use of neostigmine, a quaternary ammonium compound, during lactation have been located. Two publications have stated that the drug is not excreted into breast milk (11,13). However, pyridostigmine, another quaternary ammonium compound, is found in breast milk (see Pyridostigmine). Thus, although neostigmine is ionized at physiologic pH, the molecular weight (about 223) is low enough that the nonionized fraction should be excreted into milk. The effects, if any, on a nursing infant from exposure to neostigmine in milk are unknown.

References

1. Clark RB, Brown MA, Lattin DL. Neostigmine, atropine, and glycopyrrolate: does neostigmine cross the placenta? Anesthesiology 1996;84:450–2.
2. Heinonen OP, Slone D, Shapiro S. *Birth Defects and Drugs in Pregnancy*. Littleton, MA: Publishing Sciences Group, 1977:345–56.
3. Brunclik V, Hauser GA. Short-term therapy in secondary amenorrhea. Ther Umsch 1973;30:496–502.

4. McNall PG, Jafarnia MR. Management of myasthenia gravis in the obstetrical patient. Am J Obstet Gynecol 1965;92:518–25.
5. Foldes FF, McNall PG. Myasthenia gravis: a guide for anesthesiologists. Anesthesiology 1962;23: 837–72.
6. Chambers DC, Hall JE, Boyce J. Myasthenia gravis and pregnancy. Obstet Gynecol 1967;29:597–603.
7. Hay DM. Myasthenia gravis and pregnancy. J Obstet Gynaecol Br Commonw 1969;76:323–9.
8. Blackhall MI, Buckley GA, Roberts DV, Roberts JB, Thomas BH, Wilson A. Drug-induced neonatal myasthenia. J Obstet Gynaecol Br Commonw 1969; 76:157–62.
9. Eden RD, Gall SA. Myasthenia gravis and pregnancy: a reappraisal of thymectomy. Obstet Gynecol 1983;62:328–33.
10. Plauche WC. Myasthenia gravis in pregnancy: an update. Am J Obstet Gynecol 1979;135:691–7.
11. Fraser D, Turner JWA. Myasthenia gravis and pregnancy. Proc R Soc Med 1963;56:379–81.
12. Lefvert AK, Osterman PO. Newborn infants to myasthenic mothers: a clinical study and an investigation of acetylcholine receptor antibodies in 17 children. Neurology 1983;33:133–8.
13. Wilson JT. Pharmacokinetics of drug excretion. In Wilson JT, ed. *Drugs in Breast Milk*. Balgowlah, Australia: ADIS Press, 1981:17.

Name: **NEVIRAPINE** Risk Factor: C_M
Class: **Antiviral**

FETAL RISK SUMMARY

RECOMMENDATION: Compatible - Maternal Benefit >> Embryo/Fetal Risk

Nevirapine is used in combination with other antiviral agents in the treatment of human immunodeficiency virus (HIV) infections. It is a non-nucleoside reverse transcriptase inhibitor (nNRTI). Other agents in this class include delavirdine and efavirenz.

No teratogenic effects were observed in reproductive studies with rats and rabbits (1). In rats, however, a significant decrease in fetal weight occurred at doses producing systemic levels approximately 50% higher (based on AUC) than those seen with the recommended human dose. Moreover, impaired fertility was noted in female rats at doses producing levels approximately equal to those seen with the recommended human dose (1).

Nevirapine readily crosses the human placenta to the fetus (1). In a study reported by the manufacturer, nevirapine crossed the placentas of 10 HIV type 1 (HIV-1)-infected women given a single oral dose of 100 or 200 mg a mean 5.8 hours before delivery (1). The placental transfer is consistent with the low molecular weight of about 266.

A study published in 1998 described the pharmacokinetics of nevirapine in 18 HIV-1-infected women who received the drug in active labor (2). In the first cohort, 10 women were treated with 100 mg or 200 mg of nevirapine, but no drug was given to their infants. Based on the pharmacokinetic data in the first cohort, eight additional women were given a 200-mg dose of nevirapine during active labor and their infants received a 2-mg/kg dose 48–72 hours after birth. In this latter cohort, delivery occurred a median 5.4 hours after dosing. The median cord blood nevirapine concentration was 1106 ng/mL, resulting in a median ratio of cord blood:maternal plasma of 82.9% (range 71.9%–120.2%) (2). The median calculated nevirapine concentration 7 days after birth was 215 ng/mL (range 112–275 ng/mL) (2). Maintaining the concentration above 100 ng/mL (10 times the *in vitro* 50% inhibitory concentration [IC_{50}] against HIV) during labor and in the neonate during the 7 days of life was a specific goal of the study (2). No adverse effects due to nevirapine or HIV-infected infants were observed.

A 1999 study also described the pharmacokinetics of a single 200 mg dose of nevirapine given to 20 HIV-infected women during labor and to 13 of the neonates at 72 hours

(3). The median cord:maternal blood ratio was 0.75. The target drug level (>100 ng/mL; 10 times the IC_{50}) in the neonates was maintained in all infants at 7 days of age, irrespective of whether they received nevirapine at 72 hours. No serious adverse effects attributable to nevirapine were observed (3).

The Antiretroviral Pregnancy Registry reported, for the period January 1989 through January 2004, prospective data (reported to the Registry before the outcomes were known) involving 1537 live births that had been exposed during the 1st trimester to one or more antiretroviral agents (4). Forty-seven of the newborns had congenital defects (3.1%, 95% confidence interval [CI] 2.3–4.1). In the 2407 live births with earliest exposure in the 2nd/3rd trimesters, there were 56 infants with defects (2.3%, 95% CI 1.8–3.0). The prevalence rates for the two periods did not differ significantly. There were 103 infants with birth defects among 3944 live births with exposure any time during pregnancy (2.6%, 95% CI 2.1–3.2). The prevalence did not differ significantly from that expected in a nonexposed population (4). There were 1193 outcomes exposed to nevirapine (332 in the 1st trimester and 861 in the 2nd/3rd trimesters) in combination with other antiretroviral agents. There were 7 (2.1%, 95% CI 0.9–4.3) birth defects among the 1st trimester exposures and 19 (2.2%, 95% CI 1.3–3.4) in those exposed in the 2nd/3rd trimesters. In reviewing the birth defects of prospective and retrospective (pregnancies reported after the outcomes were known) registered cases, and clinical reports, the Registry concluded that there was no pattern of anomalies to suggest a common cause (4). (See Lamivudine for required statement.)

A 2000 case report described the pregnancy outcomes of two pregnant women with HIV infection who were treated with the anti-infective combination, trimethoprim/sulfamethoxazole, for prophylaxis against *Pneumocystis carinii*, concurrently with antiretroviral agents (5). One of the cases involved a 31-year-old woman who presented at 15 weeks' gestation. She was receiving trimethoprim/sulfamethoxazole, didanosine, stavudine, nevirapine, and vitamin B supplements (specific vitamins and dosage not given) that had been started before conception. A fetal ultrasound at 19 weeks' gestation revealed spina bifida and ventriculomegaly. The patient elected to terminate her pregnancy. The fetus did not have HIV infection. Defects observed at autopsy included ventriculomegaly, an Arnold-Chiari malformation, sacral spina bifida, and a lumbosacral meningomyelocele. The authors attributed the neural tube defects to the antifolate activity of trimethoprim (5).

A study published in 1999 evaluated the safety, efficacy, and perinatal transmission rates of HIV in 30 pregnant women receiving various combinations of antiretroviral agents (6). Many of the women were substance abusers. Nevirapine was used in combination with zidovudine, didanosine, and/or lamivudine in two of the women. Antiretroviral therapy was initiated at a median of 14 weeks' gestation (range preconception to 32 weeks). Despite previous histories of extensive antiretroviral experience and of vertical transmission of HIV, combination therapy was effective in treating maternal disease and in preventing transmission to the current newborns. No adverse outcomes were noted in the two nevirapine-exposed cases (6).

A 1999 study compared the safety and efficacy of a short-course of nevirapine to zidovudine for the prevention of mother-to-child transmission of HIV-1 (7). At the onset of labor, women were randomly assigned to receive either a single dose of nevirapine (200 mg) plus a single dose (2 mg/kg) to their infants 24–72 hours after birth (N = 310) or zidovudine (600 mg then 300 mg every 3 hours until delivery) plus 4 mg/kg twice daily for 7 days to their infants (N = 308). Nearly all (98.8%) of the women breast-fed their infants immediately after birth. Up to age 14–16 weeks, significantly fewer infants in the

N

nevirapine group were HIV-1 infected, lowering the risk of infection or death, compared with zidovudine, by 48% (95% CI, 24–65) (7). The prevalence of maternal and infant adverse effects was similar in the two groups. In an accompanying study, the nevirapine regimen was shown to be cost-effective in various seroprevalence settings (8).

In summary, no teratogenicity was observed in two animal species but toxicity was noted in one. Although there might be a risk for toxicity in the embryo/fetus, the human data suggest that the risk is low. Exposure of the human embryo/fetus is likely to occur because the agent, at least at term, readily crosses the human placenta. Two reviews, one in 1996 and the other in 1997, concluded that all women currently receiving antiretroviral therapy should continue to receive therapy during pregnancy and that treatment of the mother with monotherapy should be considered inadequate therapy (9,10). In 1998, the Centers for Disease Control and Prevention (CDC) made a similar recommendation that antiretroviral therapy should be continued during pregnancy, but discontinuation of all therapy during the 1st trimester was a consideration (11).

Although the study cited above (7) has shown that single doses of nevirapine administered to mothers and their infants were more effective in lowering the risk of HIV infection and death than a short course of maternal and newborn zidovudine, confirmation of these findings is required before nevirapine can be recommended for this purpose. Moreover, *in utero* exposure to nevirapine during the 2nd and 3rd trimesters may induce hepatic cytochrome P450 CYP3A metabolism, thereby increasing the drug's clearance in the newborn (12). Therefore, offspring of pregnant women chronically treated with nevirapine may not receive protection from HIV infection for the full 7 days observed in those not exposed to chronic dosing (12). Because the efficacy and safety of combined therapy in preventing vertical transmission of HIV to the newborn are unknown, zidovudine remains the only antiretroviral agent recommended for this purpose in developed countries (9,10). A review published in 2000 reviewed seven clinical trials that have been effective in reducing perinatal transmission, five with zidovudine alone, one with zidovudine plus lamivudine, and one with nevirapine (13). Six of the trials were in developing countries. Prolonged use of zidovudine in the mother and infant was the most effective for preventing vertical transmission, but also the most expensive. Single-dose nevirapine (in the mother and infant) was the least expensive and the simplest regimen to administer (13).

BREAST FEEDING SUMMARY

RECOMMENDATION: Contraindicated

Nevirapine is excreted into breast milk. In a study reported by the manufacturer, nevirapine was found in the breast milk of 10 women with HIV-1 infection given a single oral dose of 100 or 200 mg a mean 5.8 hours before delivery (1). In 21 HIV-infected women who had received a single 200-mg dose of nevirapine during labor, the median milk:maternal plasma ratio was 60.5% (range 25.3%–122.2%) (3). At 48 hours after birth, the median breast milk concentration was 454 ng/mL (range 219–972 ng/mL), declining to 103 ng/mL (range 50–309 ng/mL) 7 days after birth (3).

HIV-1 is transmitted in milk, and in developed countries, breast-feeding is not recommended (9,10,14–16). In developing countries, breast-feeding is undertaken, despite the risk, because there are no affordable milk substitutes available. Zidovudine, zidovudine plus lamivudine, and nevirapine have all been shown to reduce, but not eliminate, the risk of HIV-1 transmission during breast-feeding (see also Lamivudine and Zidovudine) (13).

References

1. Product information. Viramune. Roxane Laboratories, 2001.
2. Mirochnick M, Fenton T, Gagnier P, Pav J, Gwynne M, Siminski S, Sperling RS, Beckerman K, Jimenez E, Yogev R, Spector SA, Sullivan JL, for the Pediatric AIDS Clinical Trials Group Protocol 250 team. Pharmacokinetics of nevirapine in human immunodeficiency virus type 1-infected pregnant women and their neonates. J Infect Dis 1998;178:368–74.
3. Musoke P, Guay LA, Bagenda D, Mirochnick M, Nakabiito C, Fleming T, Elliott T, Horton S, Dransfield K, Pav JW, Murarka A, Allen M, Fowler MG, Mofenson L, Hom D, Mmiro F, Jackson JB. A phase I/II study of the safety and pharmacokinetics of nevirapine in HIV-1-infected pregnant Ugandan women and their neonates (HIVNET 006). AIDS 1999;13:479–86.
4. Antiretroviral Pregnancy Registry Steering Committee, Antiretroviral Pregnancy Registry International Interim Report for 1 January 1989 through 31 January 2004. Wilmington, NC: Registry Coordinating Center; 2004.
5. Richardson MP, Osrin D, Donaghy S, Brown NA, Hay, Sharland M. Spinal malformations in the fetuses of HIV infected women receiving combination antiretroviral therapy and co-trimoxazole. Eur J Obstet Gynecol Reprod Biol 2000;93:215–7.
6. McGowan JP, Crane M, Wiznia AA, Blum S. Combination antiretroviral therapy in human immunodeficiency virus-infected pregnant women. Obstet Gynecol 1999;94:641–6.
7. Guay LA, Musoke P, Fleming T, Bagenda D, Allen M, Nakabiito C, Sherman J, Bakaki P, Ducar C, Deseyve M, Emel L, Mirochnick M, Fowler MG, Mofenson L, Miotti P, Dransfield K, Bray D, Mmiro F, Jackson JB. Intrapartum and neonatal single-dose nevirapine compared with zidovudine for prevention of mother-to-child transmission of HIV-1 in Kampala, Uganda: HIVNET 012 randomised trial. Lancet 1999;354:795–802.
8. Marseille E, Kahn JG, Mmiro F, Guay L, Musoke P, Fowler MG, Jackson JB. Cost effectiveness of single-dose nevirapine regimen for mothers and babies to decrease vertical HIV-1 transmission in sub-Saharan Africa. Lancet 1999;354:803–9.
9. Carpenter CCJ, Fischi MA, Hammer SM, Hirsch MS, Jacobsen DM, Katzenstein DA, Montaner JSG, Richman DD, Saag MS, Schooley RT, Thompson MA, Vella S, Yeni PG, Volberding PA. Antiretroviral therapy for HIV infection in 1996. JAMA 1996;276:146–54.
10. Minkoff H, Augenbraun M. Antiretroviral therapy for pregnant women. Am J Obstet Gynecol 1997;176:478–89.
11. CDC. Public Health Service Task Force recommendations for the use of antiretroviral drugs in pregnant women infected with HIV-1 for maternal health and for reducing perinatal HIV-1 transmission in the United States. MMWR 1998;47:No. RR-2.
12. Taylor GP, Lyall EGH, Back D, Ward C, Tudor-Williams G. Pharmacological implications of lengthened in-utero exposure to nevirapine. Lancet 2000;355:2134–5.
13. Mofenson LM, McIntyre JA. Advances and research directions in the prevention of mother-to-child HIV-1 transmission. Lancet 2000;355:2237–44.
14. Brown ZA, Watts DH. Antiviral therapy in pregnancy. Clin Obstet Gynecol 1990;33:276–89.
15. de Martino M, Tovo P-A, Pezzotti P, Galli L, Massironi E, Ruga E, Floreea F, Plebani A, Gabiano C, Zuccotti GV. HIV-1 transmission through breast-milk: appraisal of risk according to duration of feeding. AIDS 1992;6:991–7.
16. Van de Perre P. Postnatal transmission of human immunodeficiency virus type 1: the breast feeding dilemma. Am J Obstet Gynecol 1995;173:483–7.

Name:	**NIACIN**	Risk Factor:	**A***
Class:	**Vitamin/Antilipemic Agent**		

FETAL RISK SUMMARY

RECOMMENDATION: Compatible

Niacin, a B complex vitamin, is converted in humans to niacinamide, the active form of vitamin B_3. See Niacinamide.

[**Risk Factor C if used in doses above the RDA or C_M for doses typically used for lipid disorders.*]

BREAST FEEDING SUMMARY

RECOMMENDATION: Compatible

See Niacinamide.

Name:	**NIACINAMIDE**	Risk Factor:	**A***
Class:	**Vitamin**		

FETAL RISK SUMMARY

RECOMMENDATION: Compatible

Niacinamide, a water-soluble B complex vitamin, is an essential nutrient required for lipid metabolism, tissue respiration, and glycogenolysis (1). Both niacin, which is converted to niacinamide *in vivo*, and niacinamide are available commercially and are collectively known as vitamin B_3. The recommended dietary allowance of the National Academy of Sciences for niacin in pregnancy is 17 mg (1).

Only two reports have been located that link niacinamide with maternal or fetal complications. A 1948 study observed an association between niacinamide deficiency and pregnancy-induced hypertension (PIH) (2). Other B complex vitamins have also been associated with this disease, but any relationship between vitamins and PIH is controversial (see other B complex vitamins). One patient with hyperemesis gravidarum presented with neuritis, reddened tongue, and psychosis (3). She was treated with 100 mg of niacin plus other B complex vitamins, resulting in the rapid disappearance of her symptoms. The authors attributed her response to the niacin.

Niacinamide is actively transported to the fetus (4,5). Higher concentrations are found in the fetus and newborn, rather than in the mother (5–8). Deficiency of niacinamide in pregnancy is uncommon except in women with poor nutrition (6,7). At term, mean niacinamide values in 174 mothers were 3.9 μg/mL (range 2.0–7.2 μg/mL) and in their newborns 5.8 μg/mL (range 3.0–10.5 μg/mL) (6). Conversion of the amino acid, tryptophan, to niacin and then to niacinamide is enhanced in pregnancy (9).

[**Risk Factor C if used in doses above the RDA.*]

N

BREAST FEEDING SUMMARY

RECOMMENDATION: Compatible

Niacin, the precursor to niacinamide, is actively excreted into breast milk (10). Reports on the excretion of niacinamide in milk have not been located, but it is probable that it also is actively transferred. In a study of lactating women with low nutritional status, supplementation with niacin in doses of 2.0–60.0 mg/day resulted in mean milk concentrations of 1.17–2.75 μg/mL (10). Milk concentrations were directly proportional to dietary intake. A 1983 English study measured niacin levels in pooled human milk obtained from mothers of preterm (26 mothers, 29–34 weeks) and term (35 mothers, 39 weeks or longer) infants (11). Niacin in milk from preterm mothers rose from 0.65 μg/mL (colostrum) to 2.05 μg/mL (16–196 days), whereas that in milk from term mothers increased during the same period from 0.50 to 1.82 μg/mL.

The recommended dietary allowance (RDA) of the National Academy of Sciences for niacin during lactation is 20 mg (1). If the diet of the lactating woman adequately supplies this amount, supplementation with niacinamide is not needed. Maternal supplementation with the RDA for niacinamide is recommended for those patients with inadequate nutritional intake.

References

1. American Hospital Formulary Service. *Drug Information 1997*. Bethesda, MD: American Society of Health-System Pharmacists, 1997: 2811–13.
2. Hobson W. A dietary and clinical survey of pregnant women with particular reference to toxaemia of pregnancy. J Hyg 1948;46:198–216.
3. Hart BF, McConnell WT. Vitamin B factors in toxic psychosis of pregnancy and the puerperium. Am J Obstet Gynecol 1943;46:283.
4. Hill EP, Longo LD. Dynamics of maternal-fetal nutrient transfer. Fed Proc 1980;39:239–44.
5. Kaminetzky HA, Baker H, Frank O, Langer A. The effects of intravenously administered water-soluble vitamins during labor in normovitaminemic and hypovitaminemic gravidas on maternal and neonatal blood vitamin levels at delivery. Am J Obstet Gynecol 1974;120:697–703.
6. Baker H, Frank O, Thomson AD, Langer A, Munves ED, De Angelis B, Kaminetzky HA. Vitamin profile of 174 mothers and newborns at parturition. Am J Clin Nutr 1975;28:59–65.
7. Baker H, Frank O, Deangelis B, Feingold S, Kaminetzky HA. Role of placenta in maternal-fetal vitamin transfer in humans. Am J Obstet Gynecol 1981;141:792–6.
8. Baker H, Thind IS, Frank O, DeAngelis B, Caterini H, Lquria DB. Vitamin levels in low-birth-weight newborn infants and their mothers. Am J Obstet Gynecol 1977;129:521–4.
9. Wertz AW, Lojkin ME, Bouchard BS, Derby MB. Tryptophan-niacin relationships in pregnancy. Am J Nutr 1958;64:339–53.
10. Deodhar AD, Rajalakshmi R, Ramakrishnan CV. Studies on human lactation. Part III. Effect of dietary vitamin supplementation on vitamin contents of breast milk. Acta Paediatr Scand 1964;53:42–8.
11. Ford JE, Zechalko A, Murphy J, Brooke OG. Comparison of the B vitamin composition of milk from mothers of preterm and term babies. Arch Dis Child 1983;58:367–72.

Name: **NIALAMIDE** Risk Factor: **C**
Class: **Antidepressant**

FETAL RISK SUMMARY

RECOMMENDATION: No Human Data - Animal Data Suggest Low Risk

No reports describing the use of this monoamine oxidase inhibitor in human pregnancy have been located. No teratogenic effects were observed in the offspring of female rats administered this drug before and during gestation, and to the pups after weaning (1). However, decreased fertility and neurobehavioral changes were observed in the young rats (1).

BREAST FEEDING SUMMARY

RECOMMENDATION: No Human Data - Potential Toxicity

No data are available.

Reference

1. Tuchmann-Duplessis H, Mercier-Parot L. Modifications du comportement sexual chez des descendants de rats traites par un inhibiteur des monoamine-oxydases. C R Acad Sci (Paris) 1963;256:2235–7. As cited in Shepard TH. *Catalog of Teratogenic Agents*. 6th ed. Baltimore, MD: Johns Hopkins University Press, 1989:447.

Name: **NICARDIPINE** Risk Factor: **C_M**
Class: **Calcium Channel Blocker**

FETAL RISK SUMMARY

RECOMMENDATION: Limited Human Data - Animal Data Suggest Risk

Nicardipine is a calcium channel blocking agent used in the treatment of angina and hypertension. The drug has also been used as a tocolytic in premature labor.

Dose-related embryotoxicity, but not teratogenicity, was observed in reproduction studies using IV nicardipine in rats and rabbits (1). Embryotoxic doses were about 2.5 and 0.5 times, respectively, the maximum recommended human dose (MRHD). At 50 times the MRHD in rats, dystocia, reduced birth weights, reduced neonatal survival, and reduced neonatal weight gain were noted (1). In one type of rabbit, but not in another, high doses (about 75 times the MRHD) were embryocidal (1). Two studies with rats reported that *in utero* exposure had no effect on postnatal function or subsequent fertility (2,3).

Nicardipine 20 μg/kg/minute was infused for 2 minutes in 15 near-term ewes given angiotensin II 5 μg/minute (4). Transient bradycardia was observed in the fetuses, followed by hypercapnia and acidemia. These changes were associated with a decrease in fetal placental blood flow and an increase in fetal vascular resistance, and five fetuses died 65 minutes after nicardipine was given. In the second part of this study in the pregnant ewe, nicardipine was found to reverse maternal angiotensin II-induced systemic vasoconstriction, including that of the renal and endomyometrial vascular beds, but it caused a significant increase in placental vascular resistance (5).

The use of nicardipine as a tocolytic agent was first investigated in an experiment by using excised rabbit uterus and in laboring (either spontaneous or induced) rats (6). In both species, the calcium channel blocker was effective in abolishing uterine contractions. A 1983 study investigated the effect of nicardipine and nifedipine on isolated human pregnant-term and nonpregnant myometrium (7). Nicardipine was a more potent tocolytic than nifedipine in pregnant myometrium, but its onset of action was slower.

Because the cardiovascular and myometrial responses of pregnant rabbits are similar to those observed in human pregnancies (8), a series of studies was conducted in the rabbit with nicardipine to determine its effectiveness as a tocolytic agent and its safety for the mother and the fetus (8–10). A statistically significant inhibition of uterine contractions was recorded in each study, but this effect was accompanied by maternal tachycardia, an increase in cardiac output, a drop in both diastolic and systolic blood pressure and mean arterial pressure, and a decrease in uteroplacental blood flow. The authors of these studies cautioned that further trials were necessary because the decrease in uteroplacental blood flow would seriously jeopardize the fetus (9,10).

In a study to determine the tocolytic effects of nicardipine in a primate species, pregnant rhesus monkeys with spontaneous uterine contractions were treated with an IV bolus of 500 μg, followed by a continuous infusion of 6 μg/kg/minute for 1 hour (11). Placental transfer of nicardipine was demonstrated with peak fetal concentrations ranging from 7 to 35 ng/mL compared with maternal peak levels of 175–865 ng/mL. Although a marked tocolytic effect was observed, significant acidemia and hypoxemia developed in the fetuses.

The tocolytic effects of nicardipine have been reported (12–14). The agent compared favorably to albuterol (12) and magnesium sulfate (13,14). No adverse effects in the newborns attributable to nicardipine were observed.

The direct effects of nicardipine on the fetus were investigated in a study using fetal sheep (15). Infusions of nicardipine, either 50 μg or 100 μg, had minimal, nonsignificant effects on mean arterial and diastolic blood pressure and no effect on fetal heart rate, fetal arterial blood gas values, and maternal cardiovascular variables. The authors concluded that the fetal hypoxia observed in other animal studies, when nicardipine was administered to the mother, was not due to changes in umbilical or ductal blood flow but to a decrease in maternal uterine blood flow (15).

A single 10-mg dose of nicardipine was given to eight women with acute hypertension (diastolic blood pressure >105 mm Hg) in the 3rd trimester of pregnancy (16). A significant decrease in maternal diastolic, but not in systolic, pressure was observed during the next 60 minutes with an onset at 15 minutes.

Nicardipine has been used in human pregnancy for the treatment of hypertension (17,18). Forty women with mild or moderate hypertension (25 with gestational hypertension, 3 with preeclampsia, and 12 with chronic hypertension) were treated with oral nicardipine 20 mg 3 times a day, beginning at 28 weeks' gestation through the 7th postpartum day, a mean duration of 9 weeks (17). An additional 20 women were treated with IV nicardipine for severe preeclampsia, 5 of whom also had chronic hypertension, beginning at a mean 33 weeks' gestation (range 27–40 weeks). The IV dose used was based on body weight: 2 mg/hour ($N = 9$; <80 kg), 4 mg/hour ($N = 8$; 80–90 kg), and 6 mg/hour ($N = 3$; >90 kg). The mean duration of IV therapy was 5.3 days (range 2–15 days). Low placental passage of nicardipine was demonstrated in 10 women, 7 on oral therapy and 3 receiving IV therapy, but no accumulation of the drug was observed in the fetus. No perinatal deaths, fetal adverse effects, or adverse neonatal outcomes attributable to nicardipine were observed during treatment. Both umbilical and cerebral Doppler velocimetry remained stable throughout the study (17).

A study published in 1994 compared nicardipine and metoprolol in the treatment of hypertension (gestational, preeclampsia, and chronic) during pregnancy (18). Fifty patients were treated in each group starting at a gestational age of about 29 weeks. Nicardipine decreased maternal systolic and diastolic blood pressure and umbilical artery resistance significantly more than metoprolol and significantly fewer patients required a cesarean section for fetal distress (6% vs. 28%). The difference in birth weights in the two groups was 201 g (2952 vs. 2751 g) (*n.s.*) (18).

A prospective multicenter cohort study of 78 women (81 outcomes; 3 sets of twins) who had 1st trimester exposure to calcium channel blockers (none of whom took nicardipine) was reported in 1996 (19). Compared with controls, no increased risk of congenital malformations was found.

N

BREAST FEEDING SUMMARY

RECOMMENDATION: No Human Data - Probably Compatible

The manufacturer states that significant amounts of nicardipine appear in milk of lactating rats (1). No reports on the use of nicardipine during human lactation have been located.

References

1. Product information. Cardene. Wyeth-Ayerst Pharmaceuticals, 2000.
2. Sejima Y, Sado T. Teratological study of 2-(N-benzyl-N-methylamino) ethyl methyl 2,6-dimethyl-4-m-nitrophenyl)-1,4-dihydropyridine-3,5-dicarboxylate hydrochloride (YC-93) in rats. Kiso to Rinsho 1979;13:1149–59. As cited in Shepard TH. *Catalog of Teratogenic Agents.* 6th ed. Baltimore, MD: Johns Hopkins University Press, 1989:447.
3. Sato T, Nagaoka T, Fuchigami K, Ohsuga F, Hatano M. Reproductive studies of 2-(N-benzyl-N-methylamino) ethyl methyl 2,6-dimethyl-4-m-nitrophenyl)-1,4-dihydropyridine-3,5-dicarboxylate hydrochloride (YC-93) in rats and rabbits. Kiso to Rinsho 1979;13:1160–76. As cited in Shepard TH. *Catalog of Teratogenic Agents.* 6th ed. Baltimore, MD: Johns Hopkins University Press, 1989:447.
4. Parisi VM, Salinas J, Stockmar EJ. Fetal vascular responses to maternal nicardipine administration in the hypertensive ewe. Am J Obstet Gynecol 1989;161:1035–9.
5. Parisi VM, Salinas J, Stockmar EJ. Placental vascular responses to nicardipine in the hypertensive ewe. Am J Obstet Gynecol 1989;161:1039–43.
6. Csapo AI, Puri CP, Tarro S, Henzel MR. Deactivation of the uterus during normal and premature labor by the calcium antagonist nicardipine. Am J Obstet Gynecol 1982;142:483–91.
7. Maigaard S, Forman A, Andersson KE, Ulmsten U. Comparison of the effects of nicardipine and nifedipine on isolated human myometrium. Gynecol Obstet Invest 1983;16:354–66.
8. Lirette M, Holbrook RH, Katz M. Effect of nicardipine HCl on prematurely induced uterine activity in the pregnant rabbit. Obstet Gynecol 1985;65:31–6.

9. Litette M, Holbrook RH, Katz M. Cardiovascular and uterine blood flow changes during nicardipine HCl tocolysis in the rabbit. Obstet Gynecol 1987;69: 79–82.
10. Holbrook RH Jr, Lirette M, Katz M. Cardiovascular and tocolytic effects of nicardipine HCl in the pregnant rabbit: comparison with ritodrine HCl. Obstet Gynecol 1987;69:83–7.
11. Ducsay CA, Thompson JS, Wu AT, Novy MJ. Effects of calcium entry blocker (nicardipine) tocolysis in rhesus macaques: fetal plasma concentrations and cardiorespiratory changes. Am J Obstet Gynecol 1987;157:1482–6.
12. Jannet D, Abankwa A, Guyard B, Carbonne B, Marpeau L, Milliez J. Nicardipine versus salbutamol in the treatment of premature labor. A prospective randomized study. Eur J Obstet Gynaecol Reprod Med 1997;73:11–6.
13. Ross EL, Ross BS, Dickerson GA, Fischer RG, Morrison JC. Oral nicardipine versus intravenous magnesium sulfate for the treatment of preterm labor (abstract). Am J Obstet Gynecol 1998;178: S181.
14. Larmon JE, Ross BS, May WL, Dickerson GA, Fischer RG, Morrison JC. Oral nicardipine versus intravenous magnesium sulfate for the treatment of preterm labor. Am J Obstet Gynecol 1999;181:1432–7.
15. Holbrook RH, Voss EM, Gibson RN. Ovine fetal cardiorespiratory response to nicardipine. Am J Obstet Gynecol 1989;161:718–21.
16. Walker JJ, Mathers A, Bjornsson S, Cameron AD, Fairlie FM. The effect of acute and chronic antihypertensive therapy on maternal and fetoplacental Doppler velocimetry. Eur J Obstet Gynecol Reprod Biol 1992;43:193–9.
17. Carbonne B, Jannet D, Touboul C, Khelifati Y, Milliez J. Nicardipine treatment of hypertension during pregnancy. Obstet Gynecol 1993;81:908–14.
18. Jannet D, Carbonne B, Sebban E, Milliez J. Nicardipine versus metoprolol in the treatment of hypertension during pregnancy: a randomized comparative trial. Obstet Gynecol 1994;84:354–9.
19. Magee LA, Schick B, Donnenfeld AE, Sage SR, Conover B, Cook L, McElhatton PR, Schmidt MA, Koren G. The safety of calcium channel blockers in human pregnancy: a prospective, multicenter cohort study. Am J Obstet Gynecol 1996;174: 823–8.

Name: **NICOTINYL ALCOHOL** Risk Factor: **C**

Class: **Vasodilator**

N

FETAL RISK SUMMARY

RECOMMENDATION: Limited Human Data - No Relevant Animal Data

Nicotinyl alcohol is converted in the body to niacin, the active form. Only one report of its use in pregnancy has been located. The Collaborative Perinatal Project recorded one 1st trimester exposure to nicotinyl alcohol and 14 other patients exposed to other vasodilators (1). From this small group of 15 patients, 4 malformed children were produced, a statistically significant incidence ($p < 0.02$). It was not stated whether nicotinyl alcohol was taken by the mother of one of the affected infants. Although the data serve as a warning, the number of patients is so small that conclusions as to the relative safety of this drug in pregnancy cannot be made.

BREAST FEEDING SUMMARY

RECOMMENDATION: No Human Data - Probably Compatible

No data are available.

Reference

1. Heinonen OP, Slone D, Shapiro S. *Birth Defects and Drugs in Pregnancy*. Littleton, MA: Publishing Sciences Group, 1977:371–3.

Name:	**NICOUMALONE**	Risk Factor:	**D**
Class:	**Anticoagulant**		

See Coumarin Derivatives.

Name:	**NIFEDIPINE**	Risk Factor:	C_M
Class:	**Calcium Channel Blocker**		

FETAL RISK SUMMARY

RECOMMENDATION: Human Data Suggest Low Risk

The use of nifedipine, a calcium channel-blocking agent, during pregnancy is controversial. Studies in pregnant sheep with IV infusions of the drug indicate that a progressive decrease in mean maternal arterial blood pressure occurs without a significant alteration of uterine vascular resistance (1). The hypotensive effect of nifedipine resulted in a decrease in uterine blood flow and fetal arterial oxygen content. Other investigators have reported similar results in animals with other calcium channel blockers (2). Although these studies indicated the potential problems with nifedipine, the investigators cautioned that their findings were preliminary and needed to be confirmed in humans (1,3).

Reproduction studies with nifedipine have been conducted in mice, rats, and rabbits (4). The drug was teratogenic (digital anomalies similar to those reported with phenytoin) in rats and rabbits, an effect that might have resulted from compromised uterine blood flow. Other toxicities were noted in the embryos and fetuses of mice, rats, and rabbits at doses 3.5 to 42 times the maximum recommended human dose (MRHD) on a weight basis, or doses higher or lower than the MRHD based on body surface area (4). These toxicities included stunted fetuses (mice, rats, rabbits), rib deformities (mice), cleft palate (mice), embryo and fetal deaths (mice, rats, rabbits), and prolonged pregnancy and decreased neonatal survival (rats; not evaluated in other species) (4). Small placentas and underdeveloped chorionic villi were observed in monkeys at doses equivalent to or less than the MRHD based on body surface area (4).

In a surveillance study of Michigan Medicaid recipients conducted between 1985 and 1992 involving 229,101 completed pregnancies, 37 newborns had been exposed to nifedipine during the 1st trimester (F. Rosa, personal communication, FDA, 1993). Two (5.4%) major birth defects were observed (two expected), one of which was a cardiovascular defect (0.5 expected). No anomalies were observed in five other categories of defects (oral clefts, spina bifida, polydactyly, limb reduction defects, and hypospadias) for which specific data were available.

A human study was reported in 1988 in which nine hypertensive pregnant women in the 3rd trimester were treated with 5 mg of nifedipine sublingually and compared with nine hypertensive women treated with placebo (5). The women were randomly assigned to the two groups but treatment was not blinded. Both maternal arterial blood pressure and uterine artery perfusion pressure were significantly lowered by nifedipine, but no apparent reduction in uteroplacental blood flow was detected. The investigators interpreted their findings as suggestive of a relative uterine vasodilation and a relative decrease in uterine vascular resistance that was proportional to the decrease in blood pressure.

Nifedipine has been used during the 2nd and 3rd trimesters for the treatment of severe hypertension (6). No fetal heart rate changes were observed after reduction of maternal blood pressure, nor were other adverse effects noted in the fetus or newborn. In a 1987 study, 23 women with severe hypertension of various causes (4 gestational, 17 essential, 1 renal, and 1 systemic lupus erythematosus) who either failed to respond to first-line therapy (atenolol, methyldopa, or hydralazine) and had slow-release nifedipine, 40–120 mg/day, added to their regimens ($N = 22$), or nifedipine, 40 mg/day, was used as initial therapy ($N = 1$) (7). Good blood pressure control was obtained in 20 women. The mean duration of therapy was 8.75 weeks (range 1–24 weeks). There were three perinatal deaths (rate 130/1000), but none could be attributed to drug therapy. The mean gestational age at delivery was 35 weeks (range 29–39 weeks), and 15 (71%) of the 21 liveborn infants were delivered by cesarean section. A high percentage of the 22 infants with accessible data were growth retarded, 9 (41%) had birth weights at or below the 3rd percentile, and 20 (91%) were at or below the 10th percentile for body weight. The investigators could not determine whether this outcome was caused by the severe maternal disease, drug therapy, or a combination of both (7).

Nifedipine has been used as a tocolytic agent. An *in vitro* study using pregnant human myometrium found that nifedipine caused a dose-related decrease in contraction strength and lengthened the period of contraction in a non-dose-related manner (8). In three studies totaling 31 women, nifedipine was used for this purpose (9–11). In one patient, nifedipine, 20 mg 3 times daily combined with terbutaline, was given for a total of 55 days (10). A study involving 60 women in presumed early labor was reported in 1986 (11). Women were included in this open trial if they had a singleton pregnancy and intact membranes, were between 20 and 35 weeks' gestation, and were contracting at least once every 10 minutes, and if their cervix was less than 4 cm dilated. Included among the various exclusions were a history of midtrimester abortion or previous preterm delivery. The women were equally divided into three groups: nifedipine, ritodrine, and no treatment. Nifedipine dosage was 30 mg orally followed by 20 mg every 8 hours for 3 days. Ritodrine was initially administered as a standard IV infusion followed by 48 hours of oral therapy. The days from presentation to delivery in the nifedipine, ritodrine, and no treatment groups were 36.3, 25.1, and 19.3 days ($p < 0.001$ nifedipine compared with the other two groups), respectively (11). No complications of the therapy were found in any of the infants from the three studies. Two of the studies (9,10) conducted follow-up examinations of the infants at 5–12 months of age and all were alive and well.

Two apparently clinically significant drug interactions when nifedipine and magnesium were used concurrently have been reported (12,13). A woman, at 32 weeks' gestation in premature labor, was treated with 60 mg of nifedipine orally for 3 hours followed by 20 mg every 8 hours. Uterine contractions returned 12 hours later and IV magnesium sulfate was started followed by the onset of pronounced muscle weakness after 500 mg had been administered. Her symptoms consisted of jerky movements of the extremities, difficulty in swallowing, paradoxical respirations, and an inability to raise her head from the pillow (12). The muscle weakness resolved 25 minutes after the magnesium was stopped. The effects were attributed to nifedipine potentiation of the neuromuscular blocking action of magnesium. In a second report, two women were hospitalized for hypertension at 30 and 32 weeks' gestation (13). In both cases, oral methyldopa 2 g and IV magnesium sulfate 20 g daily were ineffective in lowering the mother's blood pressure. Oral nifedipine 10 mg was given, and a marked hypotensive response occurred 45 minutes later. The blood pressures before nifedipine were 150/110 and 140/105 mm Hg, respectively, then decreased to 80/50 and 90/60 mm Hg, respectively, after administration of the calcium channel blocker. The blood pressures returned to the previous levels 25–30 minutes later. Both infants were delivered following the hypotensive episodes, but only one survived.

The pharmacokinetics of nifedipine in pregnant women have been studied (14).

A prospective, multicenter cohort study of 78 women (81 outcomes; 3 sets of twins) who had 1st-trimester exposure to calcium channel blockers, including 44% to nifedipine, was reported in 1996 (15). Compared with controls, no increase in the risk of major congenital malformations was found.

In summary, the experience with nifedipine in human pregnancy is limited, although the agent has been used for tocolysis and as an antihypertensive agent in pregnant women. The agent does not appear to be a major human teratogen based on the results of two studies. Severe adverse reactions, however, have occurred when the drug was combined with IV magnesium sulfate. Moreover, IV nifedipine in pregnant rhesus monkeys has been associated with fetal hypoxemia and acidosis (16). Because of this and other animal studies, nifedipine should probably be reserved for women with severe hypertension who are unresponsive to standard therapy or in controlled trials until this toxicity has been studied more carefully. If nifedipine is used in pregnancy, healthcare professionals are encouraged to call the toll free number (800-670-6126) for information about patient enrollment in the Motherisk study.

BREAST FEEDING SUMMARY

RECOMMENDATION: Limited Human Data - Probably Compatible

Nifedipine is excreted into breast milk (17). A woman with persistent hypertension after premature delivery at 26 weeks' gestation was treated with nifedipine 30 mg every 8 hours for 48 hours, then 20 mg every 8 hours for 48 hours, then 10 mg every 8 hours for 36 hours. Concentrations of the drug in milk were related to dosage and the time interval between the dose and milk collection. Peak concentrations and time of occurrence were 53.35 ng/mL 30 minutes after 30 mg, 16.35 ng/mL 1 hour after 20 mg, and 12.89 ng/mL 30 minutes after 10 mg. The estimated milk half-lives after the three doses were 2.4 hours (30 mg), 3.1 hours (20 mg), and 1.4 hours (10 mg). In comparison with controls, nifedipine had no effect on milk composition. The authors concluded that these amounts, representing less than 5% of a therapeutic dose, posed little risk to a nursing infant. If desired, delaying breast feeding by 3–4 hours after a dose would significantly decrease the amount of drug ingested by the infant (17). The American Academy of Pediatrics classifies nifedipine as compatible with breast-feeding (18).

References

1. Harake B, Gilbert RD, Ashwal S, Power GG. Nifedipine: effects on fetal and maternal hemodynamics in pregnant sheep. Am J Obstet Gynecol 1987;157:1003–8.
2. Holbrook RH Jr. Effects of calcium antagonists during pregnancy. Am J Obstet Gynecol 1989;160:1018.
3. Gilbert RD. Effects of calcium antagonists during pregnancy (reply). Am J Obstet Gynecol 1989;160:1018–9.
4. Product information. Procardia. Pfizer, 2000.
5. Lindow SW, Davies N, Davey DA, Smith JA. The effect of sublingual nifedipine on uteroplacental blood flow in hypertensive pregnancy. Br J Obstet Gynaecol 1988;95:1276–81.
6. Walters BNJ, Redman CWG. Treatment of severe pregnancy-associated hypertension with the calcium antagonist nifedipine. Br J Obstet Gynaecol 1984;91:330–6.
7. Constantine G, Beevers DG, Reynolds AL, Luesley DM. Nifedipine as a second line antihypertensive drug in pregnancy. Br J Obstet Gynaecol 1987;94;1136–42.
8. Bird LM, Anderson NC Jr, Chandler ML, Young RC. The effects of aminophylline and nifedipine on contractility of isolated pregnant human myometrium. Am J Obstet Gynecol 1987;157:171–7.
9. Ulmsten U, Andersson K-E, Wingerup L. Treatment of premature labor with the calcium antagonist nifedipine. Arch Gynecol 1980;229:1–5.

N

10. Kaul AF, Osathanondh R, Safon LE, Frigoletto FD Jr, Friedman PA. The management of preterm labor with the calcium channel-blocking agent nifedipine combined with the â-mimetic terbutaline. Drug Intell Clin Pharm 1985;19:369–71.
11. Read MD, Wellby DE. The use of a calcium antagonist (nifedipine) to suppress preterm labour. Br J Obstet Gynaecol 1986;93:933–7.
12. Snyder SW, Cardwell MS. Neuromuscular blockade with magnesium sulfate and nifedipine. Am J Obstet Gynecol 1989;161:35–6.
13. Waisman GD, Mayorga LM, Camera MI, Vignolo CA, Martinotti A. Magnesium plus nifedipine: potentiation of hypotensive effect in preeclampsia? Am J Obstet Gynecol 1988;159:308–9.
14. O'Neill S, Osathanondh R, Kaul AF, Scavone JM, Bromley BS, Malin MA. The pharmacokinetics of nifedipine in pregnant women (abstract). Drug Intell Clin Pharm 1986;20:460–1.
15. Magee LA, Schick B, Donnenfeld AE, Sage SR, Conover B, Cook L, McElhatton PR, Schmidt MA, Koren G. The safety of calcium channel blockers in human pregnancy: a prospective, multicenter cohort study. Am J Obstet Gynecol 1996;174:823–8.
16. Ducsay CA, Cook MJ, Veille JC, Novy MJ. Nifedipine tocolysis in pregnant rhesus monkeys: maternal and fetal cardiorespiratory effects. Abstract No. 79, Society of Perinatal Obstetricians Annual Meeting, Las Vegas, Nevada, February, 1985.
17. Ehrenkranz RA, Ackerman BA, Hulse JD. Nifedipine transfer into human milk. J Pediatr 1989;114:478–80.
18. Committee on Drugs, American Academy of Pediatrics. The transfer of drugs and other chemicals into human milk. Pediatrics 2001;108:776–89.

Name:	**NIMODIPINE**	Risk Factor:	C_M
Class:	**Calcium Channel Blocker**		

FETAL RISK SUMMARY

RECOMMENDATION: Limited Human Data - Animal Data Suggest Risk

Nimodipine is a dihydropyridine calcium channel blocker used to reduce the incidence and severity of ischemic deficits in patients with subarachnoid hemorrhage after rupture of congenital aneurysms. Nimodipine shares similar hemodynamic effects with other calcium channel blockers, but does not usually produce a marked lowering of blood pressure. In clinical studies involving nonpregnant patients, only about 5% of the subjects experienced a marked lowering of blood pressure (1).

In studies with male and female rats, nimodipine had no effect on fertility or reproductive performance at doses up to about four times the equivalent human dose of 60 mg every 4 hours in a 50-kg patient (EHD) (1). Reproduction studies have been conducted in rats and rabbits. Nimodipine was teratogenic in rabbits, producing an increase in the incidence of malformations and stunted fetuses at oral doses of 1 to 10 mg/kg/day (1). In rats, nimodipine dosing during organogenesis was embryotoxic, causing resorptions and stunted fetal growth, but except for skeletal variations, caused no malformations (1). The dose used in rats was about 12 times the EHD. Oral doses about four times the EHD administered late in organogenesis and continued to nearly the end of gestation or for 21 days after delivery were associated with an increase in skeletal variations, stunted fetuses and stillbirths but no malformations (1).

The placental transfer of nimodipine early in human gestation has apparently not been studied. However, consistent with its relatively low molecular weight (about 418), nimodipine crosses the human placenta at term. An abstract and later full report described the use of nimodipine for the management of preeclampsia (2,3). Ten women at 38 ± 2 weeks' gestation with preeclampsia were treated with nimodipine, 30 mg orally every 4 hours. Delivery occurred within 24 hours of starting nimodipine and continued for 24 hours after delivery. Both systolic and diastolic blood pressure were significantly reduced after nimodipine administration without evidence of fetal distress. At delivery, the median nimodipine concentrations in the maternal and umbilical cord serum were 7.32 and 2.6 ng/mL, respectively (fetal:maternal ratio 0.36). In four patients who were delivered by cesarean section within 2 hours of the first dose, the maternal and cord serum levels were 9.68 and 3.46 ng/mL, respectively (fetal:maternal ratio 0.36). The median Apgar scores were 8 (range 6–10) and 9 (range 8–10) at 1 and 5 minutes, respectively. No adverse effects of the drug treatment were observed in the newborns and all were doing well at 6-week follow-up (3). One newborn was excluded from the above data because the mother suffered a ruptured uterus. Although severely depressed at birth (Apgar scores 1 and 5 at 1 and 5 minutes, respectively), the infant was successfully resuscitated and was developing normally at 6 weeks of age (3).

A prospective, multicenter cohort study of 78 women (81 outcomes; 3 sets of twins) who had 1st trimester exposure to calcium channel blockers, including 11% to nimodipine, was reported in 1996 (4). Compared with controls, the women experienced no increase in major congenital malformations.

Nimodipine also has been used for its cerebral vasodilator characteristics in the treatment of eclampsia complicated by cerebral vasospasm and edema (5–7). In the first two cases, delivery of the fetus had occurred before initiation of therapy (5,6). The use of nimodipine in combination with magnesium sulfate was not recommended because of the risk for maternal heart block (6). In the third report, seizures in four pregnant patients were halted with IV clonazepam (average dose 3 mg, range 1–5 mg), followed by IV nimodipine (1 mg/hr for 20 minutes, then 2 mg/hr) to control blood pressure (mean dose 1.83 mg) (7). The four live-born infants were delivered by cesarean section once maternal blood pressure was controlled. The mean birth weight was 1822 g (range 1460–2800 g). Individual Apgar scores were not provided, but two infants had 5-minute Apgar scores of less than 7. One mother died of severe postpartum complications, and another developed multiorgan disease secondary to severe preeclampsia/eclampsia (7).

A 1998 abstract described an ongoing international, multicenter, randomized, controlled trial comparing the effects of nimodipine and magnesium sulfate in the prevention of eclampsia (8). Another study involving 21 women with severe preeclampsia compared oral nimodipine with IV magnesium sulfate for the prevention of seizures (9). Neither report provided data on newborns.

In summary, nimodipine is teratogenic and toxic in experimental animals. However, human data early in gestation are insufficient to assess the risk to the embryo or fetus. Only a few calcium channel blockers have any human data on exposure during early gestation. Based on this very limited information, these agents do not appear to be major human teratogens. However, more information is required before any conclusion can be reached as to the potential teratogenic risk of these agents. In addition, maternal hypotension caused by nimodipine is a potential, but yet unreported, complication that could jeopardize the fetus. An *in vitro* study has examined the potential use of nimodipine as a tocolytic agent (10). Thus, additional data on the potential for nimodipine-induced maternal hypotension may be forthcoming.

BREAST FEEDING SUMMARY

RECOMMENDATION: Limited Human Data - Probably Compatible

Nimodipine and its metabolites are concentrated in the milk of lactating rats (1). The drug is also excreted into the milk of humans. In a 1996 case report, a 36-year-old woman, 3 weeks postpartum, experienced a transient clinical syndrome of paresthesias (arm and face) associated with motor dysphasia (11). The symptoms resolved but perioral dysesthesia and motor dysphasia recurred after cerebral angiography. Because the symptoms were thought possibly to be vascular spasm secondary to angiographic examination, the woman was treated with IV nimodipine (formulation not available in the United States). Over a 24-hour interval, she received a total dose of 46 mg (1 mg/hr for 2 hours, then 2 mg/hr). Milk samples were collected (50–60 mL/collection) by the patient every 3–4 hours during nimodipine therapy and blood samples were drawn about every 6 hours. The infant was not allowed to nurse during this period. Nimodipine milk concentrations ranged from 0.42 ng/mL (0.5 hours) to 4.70 ng/mL (26 hours; 2 hours after the infusion ended), whereas the maternal serum concentrations ranged from 3.54 to 10.83 ng/mL. The milk:serum ratios at 0.5, 7.5, and 13.5 hours were 0.12, 0.06, and 0.15, respectively. Assuming a milk intake of 150 mL/kg/day, the authors estimated that the infant would have received 0.008% to 0.092% of the mother's weight-adjusted dose. This exposure was thought to be clinically insignificant (11).

References

1. Product information. Nimotop. Bayer, 2002.
2. Belfort M, Saade G, Cruz A, Adam K, Kirshon B, Kramer W, Moise K Jr. Nimodipine as an alternative to magnesium sulfate in the management of severe preeclampsia: maternal and fetal effects (abstract). Am J Obstet Gynecol 1994;170:412.
3. Belfort MA, Saade GR, Moise KJ Jr, Cruz A, Adam K, Kramer W, Kirshon B. Nimodipine in the management of preeclampsia: maternal and fetal effects. Am J Obstet Gynecol 1994;171:417–24.
4. Magee LA, Schick B, Donnenfeld AE, Sage SR, Conover B, Cook L, McElhatton PR, Schmidt MA, Koren G. The safety of calcium channel blockers in human pregnancy: a prospective, multicenter cohort study. Am J Obstet Gynecol 1996;174:823–8.
5. Horn EH, Filshie M, Kerslake RW, Jaspan T, Worthington BS, Rubin PC. Widespread cerebral ischaemia treated with nimodipine in a patient with eclampsia. BMJ 1990;301:794.
6. Belfort MA, Carpenter RJ Jr, Kirshon B, Saade GR, Moise KJ Jr. The use of nimodipine in a patient with eclampsia: color flow Doppler demonstration of retinal artery relaxation. Am J Obstet Gynecol 1993;169:204–6.
7. Anthony J, Mantel G, Johanson R, Dommisse J. The haemodynamic and respiratory effects of intravenous nimodipine used in the treatment of eclampsia. Br J Obstet Gynaecol 1996;103:518–22.
8. Belfort M, Anthony J, Saade G and the Nimodipine Study Group. Interim report of the nimodipine vs. magnesium sulfate for seizure prophylaxis in severe preeclampsia study: an international, randomized, controlled trial (abstract). Am J Obstet Gynecol 1998;178:S7.
9. Belfort MA, Saade GR, Yared M, Grunewald C, Herd JA, Varner MA, Nisell H. Change in estimated cerebral perfusion pressure after treatment with nimodipine or magnesium sulfate in patients with preeclampsia. Am J Obstet Gynecol 1999;181:402–7.
10. Kaya T, Cetin A, Cetin M, Sarioglu Y. Effects of endothelin-1 and calcium channel blockers on contractions in human myometrium. A study on myometrial strips from normal and diabetic pregnant women. J Reprod Med 1999;44:115–21.
11. Carcas AJ, Abad-Santos F, de Rosendo JM, Frias J. Nimodipine transfer into human breast milk and cerebrospinal fluid. Ann Pharmacother 1996;30:148–50.

Name: **NISOLDIPINE** Risk Factor: C_M

Class: **Calcium Channel Blocker**

FETAL RISK SUMMARY

RECOMMENDATION: No Human Data - Animal Data Suggest Risk

Nisoldipine is a calcium channel blocker indicated for the treatment of hypertension, either alone or in combination with other antihypertensive agents. The elimination half-life (about 7–12 hours) of this agent allows for once daily dosing.

Animal reproduction studies have been conducted in three different species (1). No teratogenicity was observed in rats and rabbits, but fetotoxicity, most likely due to maternal toxicity, did occur in both species. Decreased fetal weight was observed in pregnant rats given doses about 5 and 16 times the maximum recommended human dose based on body surface area (MRHD). At the higher dose, increased postimplantation loss (resorption) was also noted. In pregnant rabbits, decreased fetal and placental weights occurred at doses approximately 10 times the MRHD. At a dose 30 times the MRHD in pregnant monkeys, the only surviving fetus had forelimb and vertebral abnormalities not previously seen in control monkeys of the same strain (1). In this particular study, control monkeys also had increased rates of abortion and mortality (1).

It is not known if nisoldipine crosses the human placenta. The molecular weight (about 388) is low enough, however, that placental transfer should be expected.

No reports describing the use of nisoldipine during human pregnancy have been located. A 1992 abstract did report the successful use of the agent in 12 women for the treatment of severe postpartum pregnancy-induced hypertension (2). Other calcium channel blockers (e.g., see Nicardipine, Nifedipine, and Verapamil) have been used for maternal hypertension and as tocolytic agents.

Although the lack of human pregnancy data prevents an assessment of the fetal risk, the absence of teratogenicity and the observance of fetotoxicity only at maternal toxic doses is reassuring. Other calcium channel blockers have been extensively used in human pregnancy as antihypertensives and tocolytics without evidence of major congenital defects or fetal toxicity (see Nicardipine, Nifedipine, and Verapamil).

BREAST FEEDING SUMMARY

RECOMMENDATION: No Human Data - Probably Compatible

No reports describing the use of nisoldipine in human lactation have been reported. The molecular weight (about 388) is low enough that excretion into breast milk should be expected. The effects of this exposure on a nursing infant are unknown. Other calcium channel blockers are excreted in milk and are classified as compatible with breast-feeding by the American Academy of Pediatrics (see Diltiazem, Nifedipine, and Verapamil).

N

References

1. Product information. Sular. AstraZeneca Pharmaceuticals, 2001.
2. Belfort M. Nisoldipine: preliminary results using a new orally administered calcium antagonist in the treatment of severe postpartum pregnancy induced hypertension(PIH) (abstract). Am J Obstet Gynecol 1992;166:440.

Name:	**NITAZOXANIDE**	Risk Factor:	B_M
Class:	**Anti-Infective (Antiprotozoal)**		

FETAL RISK SUMMARY

RECOMMENDATION: No Human Data - Animal Data Suggest Low Risk

Nitazoxanide is an oral synthetic antiprotozoal agent approved for the treatment of diarrhea caused by *Cryptosporidium parvum* and *Giardia lamblia* in pediatric patients between the ages of 1 and 11 years (1). However, the drug has been used in children and adults for a wide variety of gastrointestinal and hepatic infections, including those associated with acquired immunodeficiency syndrome (AIDS) (2–10). Nitazoxanide is a prodrug that is rapidly hydrolyzed during absorption to the active metabolites, tizoxanide and tizoxanide glucuronide (1). The parent compound, nitazoxanide, is not detected in plasma. Tizoxanide is extensively bound to plasma proteins (>99.9%) (1). The terminal elimination half-life of tizoxanide is 7.3 hours (11).

Reproduction studies have been conducted in rats and rabbits. In rats, doses up to 48 times the human clinical dose based on body surface area (HCD) revealed no evidence of fetal harm. Higher doses (up to 66 times the HCD) had no effect on fertility in male and female rats. In rabbits, doses up to three times the HCD revealed no evidence of impaired fertility or fetal harm (1).

It is not known if the active metabolites of nitazoxanide cross the human placenta (nitazoxanide itself is not detected in the plasma). The molecular weight of one of the active metabolites, tizoxanide (about 265), is low enough for placental passage, but the extensive plasma protein binding will limit the amount of drug transferred to the embryo or fetus.

No reports describing the use of nitazoxanide in human pregnancy have been located. Although the animal data are suggestive of low risk, the absence of human pregnancy experience prevents an assessment of risk the drug represents to an embryo or fetus. If indicated, nitazoxanide should not be withheld during pregnancy. However, until human pregnancy data are available, exposure to the agent should be avoided in the 1st trimester, if possible.

BREAST FEEDING SUMMARY

RECOMMENDATION: No Human Data - Probably Compatible

No reports describing the use of nitazoxanide during human lactation have been located. It is not known if the active metabolites of nitazoxanide are excreted into breast milk (nitazoxanide itself is not detected in the plasma). The molecular weight of one of the active metabolites, tizoxanide (about 265), is low enough to pass into milk, but the extensive plasma protein binding (>99.9%) will limit the amount of drug in milk. The effects of this exposure on a nursing infant are unknown, but are probably not clinically significant. However, the nursing infant should be monitored for gastrointestinal symptoms.

References

1. Product information. Alinia. Romark Pharmaceuticals, 2004.
2. Rossignol JF, Maisonneuve H. Nitazoxanide in the treatment of *Taenia saginata* and *Hymenolepis nana* infections. Am J Trop Med Hyg 1984;33:511–2.
3. Murphy JR, Friedman JC. Pre-clinical toxicology of nitazoxanide—a new antiparasitic compound. J Appl Toxicol 1985;5:49–52.
4. Dubreuil L, Houcke I, Mouton Y, Rossignol JF. In vitro evaluation of activities of nitazoxanide and tizoxanide against anaerobes and aerobic organisms. Antimicrob Agents Chemother 1996;40:2266–70.
5. Romero Cabello R, Guerrero LR, Munoz Garcia MDR, Geyne Cruz A. Nitazoxanide for the treatment of intestinal protozoan and helminthic infections in Mexico. Trans R Soc Trop Med Hyg 1997;91:701–3.
6. Doumbo O, Rossignol JF, Pichard E, Traore HA, Dembele M, Diakite M, Traore F, Diallo DA. Nitazoxanide in the treatment of cryptosporidial diarrhea and other intestinal parasitic infections associated with acquired immunodeficiency syndrome in tropical Africa. Am J Trop Med Hyg 1997;56:637–9.
7. Megraud F, Occhialini A, Rossignol JF. Nitazoxanide, a potential drug for eradication of *Helicobacter pylori* with no cross-resistance to metronidazole. Antimicrob Agents Chemother 1998;42:2836–40.
8. Rossignol JF, Abaza H, Friedman H. Successful treatment of human fascioliasis with nitazoxanide. Trans R Soc Trop Med Hyg 1998;92:103–4.
9. Yamamoto Y, Hakki A, Friedman H, Okubo S, Shimamura T, Hoffman PS, Rossignol JF. Nitazoxanide, a nitrothiazolide antiparasitic agent with anti-vacuolating toxin activity. Chemotherapy 1999;45:303–12.
10. Bicart-See A, Massip P, Linas MD, Datry A. Successful treatment with nitazoxanide of *Enterocytozoon bieneusi* microsporidiosis in a patient with AIDS. Antimicrob Agents Chemother 2000;44:167–8.
11. Stockis A, Deroubaix X, Lins R, Jeanbaptiste B, Calderon P, Rossignol JF. Pharmacokinetics of nitazoxanide after single oral dose administration in 6 healthy volunteers. Int J Clin Pharmacol Ther 1996;34:349–51.

Name:	**NITROFURANTOIN**	Risk Factor:	B_M
Class:	**Urinary Germicide**		

FETAL RISK SUMMARY

RECOMMENDATION: Human Data Suggest Risk in 3rd Trimester

The anti-infective agent nitrofurantoin is commonly used in pregnancy for the treatment and prophylaxis of urinary tract infections. No reports linking the use of nitrofurantoin with congenital defects have been located.

Impaired fertility, teratogenicity, and other fetal adverse effects were not observed in rats and rabbits treated with nitrofurantoin before and during gestation (1,2). Doses used were up to 6 times the human dose (1). In mice, a dose 68 times the human dose (on a mg/kg basis) was associated with fetal growth retardation and a low incidence of minor and common malformations (1). When a dose 25 times the human dose was administered, fetal malformations were not observed (1). A dose 19 times the human dose (on a mg/kg basis) induced lung papillary adenomas in mice offspring, but the relationship of this to potential human carcinogenesis is unknown (1).

In a surveillance study of Michigan Medicaid recipients conducted between 1985 and 1992 involving 229,101 completed pregnancies, 1292 newborns had been exposed to nitrofurantoin during the 1st trimester (F. Rosa, personal communication, FDA, 1993). A total of 52 (4.0%) major birth defects were observed (55 expected). Specific data were available for six defect categories, including (observed/expected) 15/12 cardiovascular defects, 1/2 oral clefts, 0/2 spina bifida, 4/4 polydactyly, 3/2 limb reduction defects, and 5/3 hypospadias. These data do not support an association between the drug and congenital defects.

One manufacturer (Norwich-Eaton Laboratories) has collected more than 1,700 case histories describing the use of this drug during various stages of pregnancy (95 references) (personal communication, 1981). None of the reports observed deleterious effects on the fetus. In a published study, a retrospective analysis of 91 pregnancies in which nitrofurantoin was used yielded no evidence of fetal toxicity (3). Other studies have also supported the safety of this drug in pregnancy (4).

Nitrofurantoin is capable of inducing hemolytic anemia in glucose-6-phosphate dehydrogenase (G-6-PD)-deficient patients and in patients whose red blood cells are deficient in reduced glutathione (5). One manufacturer considers nitrofurantoin to be contraindicated in pregnant women at term (38–42 weeks' gestation), when the onset of labor is imminent, or during labor and delivery, because of the risk of hemolytic anemia in the newborn secondary to immature erythrocyte enzyme systems (glutathione instability) (1). A 1990 reference, citing data from a manufacturer's database, mentioned nine cases of hemolytic anemia in newborns whose mothers had taken the drug late in pregnancy (6). None of the mothers or infants were tested for G-6-PD deficiency and there was no information available as to whether the mothers were also affected. A 2000 case report published in France described hemolytic anemia in a full-term newborn whose mother had taken nitrofurantoin during the last month of pregnancy (7). The authors attributed the toxicity to the drug.

Nitrofurantoin has been reported to cause discoloration of the primary teeth when given to an infant; by implication, this could occur from *in utero* exposure (8). However, the fact that the baby was also given a 14-day course of tetracycline, an antibiotic known to cause this adverse effect, and the lack of other confirming reports make the likelihood of a causal relationship remote (9).

In a 1995 report, 22 studies of nitrofurantoin use in pregnancy were evaluated for a meta-analysis (10). Only four of the studies met the inclusion criteria of the investigators. The pooled odds ratio (OR) for malformations after use of the drug in the 1st trimester was 1.29 (95% confidence interval [CI] 0.25–6.57). These results demonstrated no significant correlation between nitrofurantoin use in early gestation and congenital malformations (10).

A 2003 case–control study, using data from three Swedish health registers, was conducted to identify drug use in early pregnancy that was associated with cardiac defects (11). Cases (cardiovascular defects without known chromosome anomalies) (N = 5015) were compared to controls consisting of all infants born in Sweden (1995–2001) (N = 577,730). Associations were identified for several drugs, some of which were probably due to confounding from the underlying disease or complaint or multiple testing, but some were thought to be true drug effects. For nitrofurantoin, there were 30 cases in 2060 exposures (OR 1.68, 95% CI 1.17–2.40) (11).

When given orally in high doses of 10 mg/kg/day to young males, nitrofurantoin may produce slight-to-moderate transient spermatogenic arrest (12). The lower doses used clinically do not seem to have this effect.

In summary, nitrofurantoin is not an animal teratogen with doses close to those used in humans, and there are no data suggesting that it is a human teratogen. However, there appears to be risk of hemolytic anemia in newborns, including those who are not G-6-PD deficient, which are exposed *in utero* to nitrofurantoin close to delivery. Although the incidence is unknown, the rare reports of this toxicity combined with the popularity of the drug for urinary tract infections in pregnant women suggests that the risk is rare. The safest course, however, would be to avoid nitrofurantoin close to delivery.

BREAST FEEDING SUMMARY

RECOMMENDATION: Limited Human Data - Probably Compatible

Nitrofurantoin is excreted into breast milk. In one study, the drug could not be detected in 20 samples from mothers receiving 100 mg 4 times daily (13). In a second study, nine mothers were given 100 mg every 6 hours for 1 day, then either 100 mg or 200 mg the next morning (14). Only two of the four patients receiving the 200-mg dose excreted measurable amounts of nitrofurantoin, 0.3–0.5 μg/mL. Although these amounts are negligible, the authors cautioned that infants with G-6-PD deficiency may develop hemolytic anemia from this exposure (14).

A 2001 study concluded that nitrofurantoin is actively transported into milk, by an unknown mechanism, resulting in a milk:plasma (M–P) ratio of 6.21 (15). The observed M–P ratio was about 22-fold greater then the predicted ratio (0.28) that was determined in the study. Four lactating women, who did not breast-feed during the study, were given a single 100-mg capsule of nitrofurantoin macrocrystals with a standardized high-fat breakfast. Nine serum and milk samples were drawn after the dose over a 12-hour interval. The mean milk drug concentration in each patient during the 12-hour interval was approximately 1.3 μg/mL. Based on this, the investigators estimated that if a 60-kg woman was taking 100 mg twice daily, the infant dose would be 0.2 mg/kg, or about 6% of the mother's weight-adjusted dose. Although this exposure was thought to be low, the authors concluded that nursing infants younger than 1 month of age and those with a high frequency of G-6-PD deficiency or sensitivity to nitrofurantoin may be at risk for toxicity (15).

The above studies suggest that there is a potential for nitrofurantoin-induced toxicity from exposure to the drug in breast milk. Determining the magnitude of the risk is not possible because of the absence of published reports describing toxicity in breast-fed infants, but the risk appears to be rare. The American Academy of Pediatrics classifies nitrofurantoin as compatible with breast-feeding (16).

References

1. Product information. Macrodantin. Procter & Gamble Pharmaceuticals, 2001.
2. Prytherch JP, Sutton ML, Denine EP. General reproduction, perinatal–postnatal and teratology studies of nitrofurantoin macrocrystals in rats and rabbits. J Toxicol Environ Health 1984;13:811–23. As cited in Shepard TH. *Catalog of Teratogenic Agents*. 6th ed. Baltimore, MD: Johns Hopkins University Press, 1989:454.
3. Hailey FJ, Fort H, Williams JC, Hammers B. Foetal safety of nitrofurantoin macrocrystals therapy during pregnancy: a retrospective analysis. J Int Med Res 1983;11:364–9.
4. Lenke RR, VanDorsten JP, Schifrin BS. Pyelonephritis in pregnancy: a prospective randomized trial to prevent recurrent disease evaluating suppressive therapy with nitrofurantoin and close surveillance. Am J Obstet Gynecol 1983;146:953–7.
5. Powell RD, DeGowin RL, Alving AS. Nitrofurantoin-induced hemolysis. J Lab Clin Med 1963;62:1002–3.
6. Gait JE. Hemolytic reactions to nitrofurantoin in patients with glucose-6-phosphate dehydrogenase deficiency: theory and practice. DICP 1990;24:1210–3.
7. Bruel H, Guillemant V, Saladin-Thiron C, Chabrolle JP, Lahary A, Poinsot J. Hemolytic anemia in a newborn after maternal treatment with nitrofurantoin at the end of pregnancy. Arch Pediatr 2000;7:745–7.
8. Ball JS, Ferguson AN. Permanent discoloration of primary dentition by nitrofurantoin. Br Med J 1962;2:1103.
9. Duckworth R, Swallow JN. Nitrofurantoin and teeth. Br Med J 1962;2:1617.
10. Ben David S, Einarson T, Ben David Y, Nulman I, Pastuszak A, Koren G. The safety of nitrofurantoin during the first trimester of pregnancy: meta analysis. Fundam Clin Pharmacol 1995;9:503–7.
11. Kallen BAJ, Olausson PO. Maternal drug use in early pregnancy and infant cardiovascular defect. Reprod Toxicol 2003;17:255–61.
12. Nelson WO, Bunge RG. The effect of therapeutic dosages of nitrofurantoin (Furadantin) upon spermatogenesis in man. J Urol 1957;77:275–81.
13. Hosbach RE, Foster RB. Absence of nitrofurantoin from human milk. JAMA 1967;202:1057.
14. Varsano I, Fischl J, Shochet SB. The excretion of orally ingested nitrofurantoin in human milk. J Pediatr 1973;82:886–7.
15. Gerk PM, Kuhn RJ, Desai NS, McNamara PJ. Active transport of nitrofurantoin into human milk. Pharmacotherapy 2001;21:669–75.
16. Committee on Drugs, American Academy of Pediatrics. The transfer of drugs and other chemicals into human milk. Pediatrics 2001;108:776–89.

N

Name: **NITROGLYCERIN** Risk Factor: **B***

Class: **Vasodilator**

FETAL RISK SUMMARY

RECOMMENDATION: Human Data Suggest Low Risk

Nitroglycerin (glyceryl trinitrate) is primarily indicated for the treatment or prevention of angina pectoris. Because of the nature of this use, experience in pregnancy is limited. The drug, a rapid-onset, short-acting vasodilator, has been used to control severe hypertension during cesarean section (1,2). Use of nitroglycerin sublingually for angina during pregnancy without fetal harm has also been reported (3). Recent investigations, discussed below, have explored the use of nitroglycerin as both an emergency and routine tocolytic agent.

Reproductive studies in rats and rabbits have been conducted with nitroglycerin (4–6). No adverse fetal effects or postnatal changes were observed in these experiments.

The Collaborative Perinatal Project recorded seven 1st trimester exposures to nitroglycerin and amyl nitrite plus eight other patients exposed to other vasodilators (7). From this small group of 15 patients, 4 malformed children were produced, a statistically significant incidence ($p < 0.02$). The data did not indicate whether nitroglycerin was taken by any of the mothers of the affected infants. Because of the lack of specific information and the small number of patients, no conclusions as to the relative safety of nitroglycerin in the 1st trimester can be made from this study. Moreover, the authors of this study emphasized that statistical significance could not be used to infer causal relationships and that independent confirmation from other studies was required.

The use of nitroglycerin in gestational hypertension has been described (8–11). In three patients, IV infusions of nitroglycerin were effective in rapidly correcting the hemodynamic disturbances of gestational hypertension complicated by hydrostatic pulmonary edema, but a rapid improvement in arterial oxygenation did not occur (8). In another study by the same investigators, the effectiveness of IV nitroglycerin to decrease blood pressure in six women with gestational hypertension was dependent on the patient's volume status (9). When volume expansion was combined with nitroglycerin therapy, a marked resistance to the hypotensive effect of the drug was observed. In two of the women treated with IV nitroglycerin alone, significant reductions in blood pressure occurred, resulting in fetal heart rate changes that included late decelerations and bradycardia. Recovery occurred after nitroglycerin therapy was terminated and then restarted at a lower dose. In three other fetuses, a loss of beat-to-beat variability (average variability <5 beats/minute) was noted. Therapy was continued and no abnormalities were observed in the umbilical blood gases or Apgar scores.

An abstract published in 1996 described the use of transdermal nitroglycerin patches (releasing 10 mg in 24 hours) in the treatment of gestational hypertension (10). The 24-hour mean systemic and diastolic blood pressures were significantly decreased (5% and 7%, respectively). In a 1995 study, 12 women with severe preeclampsia received an infusion of nitroglycerin starting at 0.25 μg/kg/minute with stepwise dosage increases until a diastolic blood pressure of 100 mm Hg was achieved (11). The mean systolic blood pressure decreased from 161 to 138 mm Hg, whereas diastolic pressure decreased from a mean of 116 to 103 mm Hg. The umbilical artery pulsatility index changed significantly but not the uterine pulsatility index, implying vasodilation in the umbilical circulation and avoidance of adverse impairment of fetoplacental perfusion (11).

Lowering of maternal blood pressure and a lessening of the hemodynamic responses to endotracheal intubation were beneficial effects obtained from IV nitroglycerin in six women with severe preeclampsia (12). A progressive flattening of fetal heart rate beat-to-beat variability was observed in all six patients. Prevention of an increase in mean arterial pressure of greater than 20% was achieved in only two of the women, and all had nausea, retching, and vomiting that was apparently non-dose-related.

Myocardial infarction, secondary to development of a thrombus on an artificial aortic valve, occurred in a 25-year-old woman at 26 weeks' gestation (13). A portion of her initial treatment consisted of both oral and IV nitroglycerin, with the latter being continued for an unspecified interval. Maternal diastolic blood pressure was maintained above 50 mm Hg while on nitroglycerin and, apparently, no fetal distress was observed. A viable 2608-g male infant was eventually delivered at 35 weeks' gestation, but specific details were not provided on his condition.

A 1993 reference described two women, one with triplets, who sustained myocardial infarctions during pregnancy, at 16 and 28 weeks' gestation, and who were treated with

IV nitroglycerin and other agents (14). In addition, mild chest pain occurring during labor was successfully treated with sublingual nitroglycerin in one of the women. Both patients survived and eventually delivered infants apparently unaffected by the treatment. Another report described a woman at 26 weeks' gestation that was treated with IV nitroglycerin and other agents for a myocardial infarction (15). She eventually delivered a healthy female infant by cesarean section at 39 weeks.

In gravid ewes, IV nitroglycerin was effective in counteracting norepinephrine-induced uterine vasoconstriction (16). The antihypertensive effect resulted in a significantly decreased mean aortic pressure but did not significantly change uterine blood flow or uterine vascular conductance. A 1994 abstract reported no adverse effects on fetal cardiorespiratory function in sheep from a 2-hour IV infusion of nitroglycerin at 3 times the minimum effective tocolytic dose (17).

The use of nitroglycerin during cesarean section to allow delivery of babies entrapped by a contracted uterus has been described in two case reports (18,19). In the first case, the head of a baby presenting as a double footling breech was trapped in the hypertonic upper segment (18). Uterine relaxation was achieved with a 1000-μg (1-mg) IV bolus of nitroglycerin. The mother's blood pressure fell to 70/30 mm Hg but responded to ephedrine. The Apgar scores of the 3090-g, term infant were 5 and 9 at 1 and 5 minutes, respectively. In the second case, a woman received a 100-μg bolus of nitroglycerin to quickly relax a contracted uterus and to allow the successful delivery of her twins (19). Other than a systolic blood pressure decrease (preoperative pressure 120 mm Hg; after nitroglycerin 85 mm Hg) that responded rapidly to ephedrine, no other adverse effects from nitroglycerin were encountered in the mother or her newborns.

Two references have discussed the use of IV nitroglycerin as a short-acting tocolytic agent during intrapartum external cephalic version (20,21) and one involving internal podalic version (22). A woman in premature labor (uterine contractions every 2 minutes with the cervix dilated to 9 cm) at 30 weeks 5 days was given a 50-μg IV bolus of nitroglycerin (20). The uterus relaxed palpably within 20 seconds and the fetus was repositioned to allow for vaginal delivery. A decrease in the maternal blood pressure was noted (145/100 to 130/75 mm Hg, then stabilizing at 130/85 mm Hg within 2 minutes), but the heart rate and oxygen saturation remained unchanged. The premature infant was delivered vaginally shortly after rupture of the membranes and start of an oxytocin infusion. A second mother at 39 weeks 4 days of gestation received a 100-μg IV bolus dose before external cephalic version (blood pressure decreased from 120/60 to 112/60 mm Hg within 1 minute) and subsequently underwent a vaginal delivery of a healthy infant.

In the second report, a woman delivered one twin vaginally and then received a 50-μg IV nitroglycerin bolus to allow external version of the second transverse-lie twin (21). No significant maternal adverse effects (e.g., headache or dizziness) or changes in blood pressure or heart rate were observed. The healthy twin was delivered vaginally 45 minutes after the version.

Internal podalic version and total breech extraction of the second twin was accomplished in a third case with sublingual nitroglycerin by aerosol after the uterus had contracted down upon the operator's forearm (22). Two 400-μg boluses were given resulting in uterine relaxation within 30 seconds. No adverse effects on the newborn were observed.

Three cases of total breech extraction, with internal podalic version in two, of the second twin were aided by the use of nitroglycerin spray (0.4 mg) administered sublingually after either contraction of the uterine corpus and lower segment or uterine or cervical contractions with failure of the fetal head to engage (23). Minimal changes were observed in the maternal blood pressures and pulses. All three newborns were doing well.

A 1996 report described nine cases of internal podalic version of a second nonvertex twin with the assistance of an IV bolus of nitroglycerin (1 mg in eight, 1.5 mg in one) (24). One of the women had a panic attack that required general anesthesia for sedation, although the version was successful. In another case, nitroglycerin failed to induce uterine relaxation, and an emergency cesarean section was required for fetal distress. Postpartum hemorrhage (2000 mL) occurred in a third woman. A significant fall in maternal blood pressure was observed in all cases, but no adverse effects from the decrease occurred in the mothers or newborns (24).

Transdermal patches of nitroglycerin have been tested as tocolytics in 13 women in preterm labor (23–33 weeks' gestation) (25). Most of the women received a single patch that delivered 10 mg of nitroglycerin for 24 hours, but some patients were given a second patch if uterine contractions had not subsided within 1 hour. Patches were changed every 24 hours. The mean prolongation of pregnancy, as of the date of a subsequent report (one woman was still pregnant), was 59 days (26). The babies who had been delivered were all doing well.

Small IV bolus doses of nitroglycerin (60 or 90 μg × 1 or 2 doses) were used in 24 laboring women for severe fetal distress, related to uterine hyperactivity that was unresponsive to standard measures (27). Six of the patients developed hypotension with a mean nadir of 93.2 mm Hg (minimum 85 mm Hg) that was reversed with a single dose of ephedrine (4.5–6 mg). Four newborns had low 1-minute Apgar scores (3, 4, 5, and 6), but all newborns had Apgar scores of 9 or 10 and were vigorous at 5 minutes.

Nitroglycerin has also been used to relax the uterus in postpartum cases with retained placenta (28–31), two of which occurred in patients with an inverted uterus (30,31). The IV bolus dose was 500 μg in 15 women (28), 50 μg (some patients required two doses) in 23 cases (29,30), and 100 μg in 1 woman (31). No significant changes in blood pressure or heart rate were recorded, and no adverse effects, such as headache, palpitations, or prolonged uterine relaxation, were observed.

In summary, the use of nitroglycerin during pregnancy does not seem to present a risk to the fetus. However, the number of women treated during pregnancy is limited, especially during the 1st trimester. With the smaller doses reported, transient decreases in the mother's blood pressure may occur, but these do not appear to be sufficient to jeopardize placental perfusion. Nitroglycerin appears to be a safe, effective, rapid-onset, short-acting tocolytic agent. The use of transdermal nitroglycerin patches may also prove to be effective when longer periods of tocolysis are required. With any route of administration, however, additional studies are required to determine the safest effective dose.

[**Several manufacturers state that animal studies have not been conducted with nitroglycerin and, thus, assign the Risk Factor C. As noted above, however, animal studies have been conducted.*]

BREAST FEEDING SUMMARY

RECOMMENDATION: No Human Data - Probably Compatible

No data are available.

References

1. Snyder SW, Wheeler AS, James FM III. The use of nitroglycerin to control severe hypertension of pregnancy during cesarean section. Anesthesiology 1979;51:563–4.
2. Hood DD, Dewan DM, James FM III, Bogard TD, Floyd HM. The use of nitroglycerin in preventing the hypertensive response to tracheal intubation in severe preeclamptics. Anesthesiology 1983;59:A423.
3. Diro M, Beydown SN, Jaramillo B, O'Sullivan MJ, Kieval J. Successful pregnancy in a woman with a left ventricular cardiac aneurysm: a case report. J Reprod Med 1983;28:559–63.
4. Oketani Y, Mitsuzono T, Ichikawa K, Itono Y, Gojo T, Gofuku M, Konoha N. Toxicological studies on nitroglycerin (NK-843). 6. Teratological studies in rabbits. Oyo Yakuri 1981;22:633–38. As cited in Schardein JL. *Chemically Induced Birth Defects*. 2nd ed. New York, NY: Marcel Dekker, 1993:91.
5. Oketani Y, Mitsuzono T, Ichikawa K, Itono Y, Gojo T, Gofuku M, Konoha N. Toxicological studies on nitroglycerin (NK-843). 8. Teratological study in rats. Oyo Yakuri 1981;22:737–51. As cited in Schardein JL. *Chemically Induced Birth Defects*. 2nd ed. New York, NY: Marcel Dekker, 1993:91.
6. Sato K, Taniguchi H, Ohtsuka T, Himeno Y, Uchiyama K, Koide M, Hoshino K. Reproductive studies of nitroglycerin applied dermally to pregnant rats and rabbits. Clin Report 1984;18:3511–86. As cited in Shepard TH. *Catalog of Teratogenic Agents*. 7th ed. Baltimore, MD: Johns Hopkins University Press, 1992:285.
7. Heinonen OP, Slone D, Shapiro S. *Birth Defects and Drugs in Pregnancy*. Littleton, MA: Publishing Sciences Group, 1977:371–3.
8. Cotton DB, Jones MM, Longmire S, Dorman KF, Tessem J, Joyce TH III. Role of intravenous nitroglycerin in the treatment of severe pregnancy-induced hypertension complicated by pulmonary edema. Am J Obstet Gynecol 1986;154:91–3.
9. Cotton DB, Longmire S, Jones MM, Dorman KF, Tessem J, Joyce TH III. Cardiovascular alterations in severe pregnancy-induced hypertension: effects of intravenous nitroglycerin coupled with blood volume expansion. Am J Obstet Gynecol 1986;154:1053–9.
10. Facchinetti F, Neri I, Volpe A. Glyceryl trinitrate lowers blood pressure in patients with gestational hypertension (abstract). Am J Obstet Gynecol 1996;174:455.
11. Grunewald C, Kublickas M, Carlstrom K, Lunell N-O, Nisell H. Effects of nitroglycerin on the uterine and umbilical circulation in severe preeclampsia. Obstet Gynecol 1995;86:600–4.
12. Longmire S, Leduc L, Jones MM, Hawkins JL, Joyce TH III, Cotton DB. The hemodynamic effects of intubation during nitroglycerin infusion in severe preeclampsia. Am J Obstet Gynecol 1991;164:551–6.
13. Ottman EH, Gall SA. Myocardial infarction in the third trimester of pregnancy secondary to an aortic valve thrombus. Obstet Gynecol 1993;81:804–5.
14. Sheikh AU, Harper MA. Myocardial infarction during pregnancy: management and outcome of two pregnancies. Am J Obstet Gynecol 1993;169:279–84.
15. Sanchez-Ramos L, Chami YG, Bass TA, DelValle GO, Adair CD. Myocardial infarction during pregnancy: management with transluminal coronary angioplasty and metallic intracoronary stents. Am J Obstet Gynecol 1994;171:1392–3.
16. Wheeler AS, James FM III, Meis PJ, Rose JC, Fishburne JI, Dewan DM, Urban RB, Greiss FC Jr. Effects of nitroglycerin and nitroprusside on the uterine vasculature of gravid ewes. Anesthesiology 1980;52:390–4.
17. Bootstaylor B, Roman C, Heymann MA, Parer JT. Fetal cardiorespiratory effects of nitroglycerin in the near term pregnant sheep (abstract). Am J Obstet Gynecol 1994;170:281.
18. Roblin SH, Hew EM, Bernstein A. Uterine relaxation can be life saving. Can J Anaesth 1991;38:939–40.
19. Mayer DC, Weeks SK. Antepartum uterine relaxation with nitroglycerin at caesarean delivery. Can J Anaesth 1992;39:166–9.
20. Belfort MA. Intravenous nitroglycerin as a tocolytic agent for intrapartum external cephalic version. S Afr Med J 1993;83:656.
21. Abouleish AE, Corn SB. Intravenous nitroglycerin for intrapartum external version of the second twin. Anesth Analg 1994;78:808–9.
22. Greenspoon JS, Kovacic A. Breech extraction facilitated by glyceryl trinitrate sublingual spray. Lancet 1991;338:124–5.
23. Rosen DJD, Velez J, Greenspoon JS. Total breech extraction of the second twin with uterine relaxation induced by nitroglycerin sublingual spray. Israel J Obstet Gynecol 1994;5:18–21.
24. Dufour Ph, Vinatier D, Vanderstichele S, Subtil D, Ducloy JC, Puech F, Codaccionni X, Monnier JC. Intravenous nitroglycerin for intrapartum internal podalic version of the second non-vertex twin. Eur J Obstet Gynecol Reprod Biol 1996;70:29–32.
25. Lees C, Campbell S, Jauniaux E, Brown R, Ramsay B, Gibb D, Moncada S, Martin JF. Arrest of preterm labour and prolongation of gestation with glyceryl trinitrate, a nitric oxide donor. Lancet 1994;343:1325–6.
26. Lees C, Campbell S, Martin J, Moncada S, Brown R, Jauniaux E, Ramsay B, Gibb D. Glyceryl trinitrate in management of preterm labour. Authors' reply. Lancet 1994;344:553–4.
27. Mercier FJ, Dounas M, Bouaziz H, Lhuissier C, Benhamou D. Intravenous nitroglycerin to relieve intrapartum fetal distress related to uterine hyperactivity: a prospective observational study. Anesth Analg 1997;84:1117–20.
28. Peng ATC, Gorman RS, Shulman SM, DeMarchis E, Nyunt K, Blancato LS. Intravenous nitroglycerin for uterine relaxation in the postpartum patient with retained placenta. Anesthesiology 1989;71:172–3.
29. DeSimone CA, Norris MC, Leighton BL. Intravenous nitroglycerin aids manual extraction of a retained placenta. Anesthesiology 1990;73:787.
30. Altabef KM, Spencer JT, Zinberg S. Intravenous nitroglycerin for uterine relaxation of an inverted uterus. Am J Obstet Gynecol 1992;166:1237–8.
31. Dayan SS, Schwalbe SS. The use of small-dose intravenous nitroglycerin in a case of uterine inversion. Anesth Analg 1996;82:1091–3.

N

Name: **NITROPRUSSIDE** Risk Factor: **C**
Class: **Antihypertensive**

FETAL RISK SUMMARY

RECOMMENDATION: Human and Animal Data Suggest Risk

No reports linking the use of sodium nitroprusside with congenital defects have been located. Nitroprusside has been used in pregnancy to produce deliberate hypotension during aneurysm surgery or to treat severe hypertension (1–8). Transient fetal bradycardia was the only adverse effect noted (1). One advantage of nitroprusside is the very rapid onset of action and the return to pretreatment blood pressure levels when the drug is stopped (8). Balanced against this is the potential accumulation of cyanide in the fetus.

Nitroprusside crosses the placenta and produces fetal cyanide concentrations higher than maternal levels in animals (9). This effect has not been studied in humans. A 1984 article reviewed the potential fetal toxicity of nitroprusside (6). Avoidance of prolonged use and the monitoring of serum pH, plasma cyanide, red blood cell cyanide, and methemoglobin levels in the mother were recommended. Standard doses of nitroprusside apparently do not pose a major risk of excessive accumulation of cyanide in the fetal liver (6).

BREAST FEEDING SUMMARY

RECOMMENDATION: No Human Data - Potential Toxicity

No data are available.

N

References

1. Donchin Y, Amirav B, Sahar A, Yarkoni S. Sodium nitroprusside for aneurysm surgery in pregnancy. Br J Anaesth 1978;50:849–51.
2. Paull J. Clinical report of the use of sodium nitroprusside in severe pre-eclampsia. Anaesth Intensive Care 1975;3:72.
3. Rigg D, McDonogh A. Use of sodium nitroprusside for deliberate hypotension during pregnancy. Br J Anaesth 1981;53:985–7.
4. Willoughby JS. Case reports: Sodium nitroprusside, pregnancy and multiple intracranial aneurysms. Anaesth Intensive Care 1984;12:358–60.
5. Stempel JE, O'Grady JP, Morton MJ, Johnson KA. Use of sodium nitroprusside in complications of gestational hypertension. Obstet Gynecol 1982;60: 533–8.
6. Shoemaker CT, Meyers M. Sodium nitroprusside for control of severe hypertensive disease of pregnancy: a case report and discussion of potential toxicity. Am J Obstet Gynecol 1984;149:171–3.
7. Willoughby JS. Review article: sodium nitroprusside, pregnancy and multiple intracranial aneurysms. Anaesth Intensive Care 1984;12:351–7.
8. de Swiet M. Antihypertensive drugs in pregnancy. Br Med J 1985;291:365–6.
9. Lewis PE, Cefalo RC, Naulty JS, Rodkey RL. Placental transfer and fetal toxicity of sodium nitroprusside. Gynecol Invest 1977;8:46.

Name: **NITROUS OXIDE** Risk Factor: **C**
Class: **General Anesthetic**

FETAL RISK SUMMARY

RECOMMENDATION: Human and Animal Data Suggest Risk

Nitrous oxide (N_2O; Laughing Gas) is a nonflammable, nonexplosive gas that is widely used as an analgesic and general anesthetic. It is always administered with at least 20% oxygen to prevent hypoxia. The blood-gas coefficient is relatively low (0.47) as is tissue solubility (brain-gas coefficient 0.50) (1).

Animal Studies

In a 1967 study, pregnant rats were exposed to 45%–50% nitrous oxide for 2, 4, or 6 days starting on gestational day 8 (2). Compared to nonexposed controls, there was a dose-related increase in embryonic death and resorptions, growth retardation, and skeletal malformations (vertebrae and ribs), and the male–female sex ratio of surviving fetuses was lower (2). Resorptions and fetal deaths were significantly increased in rats exposed to nitrous oxide (0.1% or 1.5%) mixed with oxygen for 8 or 24 hours per day for several days during midgestation (3). A lower concentration (0.01%) had no effect on the incidence of resorptions but did increase the number of fetal deaths.

A 1978 study did not observe teratogenic effects, changes in surviving fetal sex ratio, or increased fetal loss in pregnant rats exposed 8 hours per day throughout gestation to nitrous oxide (1%, 10%, or 50%) or nitrous oxide (10%) plus halothane (0.16%) (4). However, fetal growth retardation was observed in all four groups exposed to nitrous oxide. Exposure of pregnant rats to 50% nitrous oxide for 25 minutes per day for 3 consecutive days in mid-gestation resulted in an increase in fetal death rate, but no effects on fetal growth were observed (5). In another study, pregnant rats were exposed to nitrous oxide either alone (0.005% or 0.05%) or a mixture of nitrous oxide (0.05%) and halothane (0.001%) for 7 hours per day during the first 15 days of gestation (6,7). No adverse embryo or fetal effects were observed.

Continuous exposure of gravid rats to nitrous oxide (0.5%) from gestational day 1 to day 19 resulted in a significant increase in the incidence of resorptions, growth retardation, and skeletal anomalies, and a lower male female sex ratio of surviving fetuses (8). In a follow-up to this study, the threshold dose required to produce some of these effects was determined using exposures of 0.0, 0.1%, 0.05%, and 0.025% (9). Only the group exposed to 0.1% had an increased incidence of resorptions and growth retardation. The same group of investigators reported a third study in which gravid rats were intermittently exposed (6 hours per day, 5 days per week) to nitrous oxide 0.0, 0.025%, 0.05%, 0.1%, and 0.5% throughout gestation (10). A significant reduction in litter size was noted only in the highest exposure group, but no signs of fetal resorption or skeletal malformations were found in any group.

Pregnant hamsters were exposed to nitrous oxide (70%–95%) mixed with oxygen for 24 hours during organogenesis (11). An increased incidence of fetal death was only observed at concentrations of 90%–95%, but hypoxia-induced mortality could not be excluded. A small but significant number of fetuses had malformations (cleft palate, limb defects, gut herniation, and fetal edema), but a dose-effect relationship was not observed (11). The effects on pregnant hamsters from exposure to a combination of nitrous oxide (60%) and halothane (0.6%) for 3 hours per day on gestational days 9, 10, or 11 was reported in 1974 (12). No effects were noted on the sex ratio of surviving fetuses. Compared to controls, resorptions were increased on day 11, and decreased fetal weight was noted in the groups exposed on days 10 and 11 (12).

In a 1980 study, pregnant rats were exposed to nitrous oxide (70%–75%) or xenon (70%–75%) for 24 hours on gestational day 9 (13). Compared to controls and the xenon-exposed group, the nitrous oxide group had a significant increase in the incidence of resorptions and congenital malformations (delayed maturation of the skeletal system, fused ribs, encephalocele, hydrocephalus, anophthalmia, microphthalmia, gastroschisis, and gonadal agenesis) (13). The above experiment was repeated by another group with four different concentrations of nitrous oxide: 0.75%, 7.5%, 25%, and 75% (14). The threshold for toxicity was determined to be greater than 25% because only those animals exposed to the 75% concentration had increased incidences of resorptions and both major and minor congenital malformations. However, all exposures caused a significant increase in minor variants involving the ribs and sternum (14).

In another study by the above investigators, the effect of nitrous oxide in pregnant rats was compared to three other general anesthetic agents (see also Enflurane, Halothane, and Isoflurane) (15). The nitrous oxide dose was 75% (0.55 MAC). (*Note: the minimum alveolar anesthetic concentration [MAC] is the concentration that causes immobility in 50% of patients exposed to a noxious stimulus such as a surgical incision; it represents the* ED_{50} *[16].*) Each agent was administered for 6 hours on each of three consecutive days in one of three periods: gestational days 8–10, 11–13, or 14–16. Compared with controls, significantly decreased maternal weight gain was observed in three of the groups (nitrous oxide, isoflurane, and enflurane) after exposure on days 14–16. Exposure on those days resulted in significantly decreased fetal weight in all four groups, and when exposure occurred on days 8–10, in three groups (all except nitrous oxide). Nitrous oxide exposure during days 14–16 resulted in significant increases in total fetal wastage and resorptions (3-fold increases). However, no major or minor congenital defects were observed in any of the groups (15).

No evidence of reproductive toxicity was observed in mice exposed to nitrous oxide (0.5%, 5%, or 50%) for 4 hours per day on days 6–15 of gestation (17). In the same experiment, the fertility of male mice exposed in the same way for 9 weeks was not affected. Based on their previous work, they concluded that the order of reproductive toxicity was halothane > enflurane > methoxyflurane > nitrous oxide (17). Of interest, a 1990 study found that brief exposure of 2-cell mouse preimplantation embryos to nitrous oxide/oxygen (60%/40%) caused disruption to subsequent embryo cleavage and blastocyst development (18).

A 1989 study determined the susceptible period for nitrous oxide teratogenicity in rats (19). Pregnant rats were exposed to 60% nitrous oxide for 24 hours on each of gestational days 6–12. There were no differences among the seven groups in the number of live fetuses, fetal weight, and sex ratio. However, compared to controls, there was a significant increase in the mean percentage of resorptions/litter and number of litters with resorptions on days 8 and 11. Major skeletal anomalies (ribs and vertebrae) were increased only on day 9, but minor skeletal defects were increased on days 8 and 9. Right sided aortic arch and left sided umbilical artery, defects indicative of altered laterality, were increased on day 8 and hydrocephalus was increased on gestational day 9 (19).

A 1986 mouse study tested the hypothesis that prenatal nitrous oxide exposure (75% with 25% oxygen for 6 hours on gestational day 14) or postnatal exposure (same mixture for 4 hours on postnatal day 2) would cause permanent damage to the developing brain and behavioral effects (20). Compared to controls, offspring (postnatal day 6 to 6 months of age) exposed prenatally or postnatally were noted to have several abnormal behavioral effects that included preweaning motor development and general activity. When they reached adulthood, their brains were also noted to have significant morphologic changes (20). A 1986 rat study also found that *in utero* exposure caused permanent alterations in the spontaneous motor output of the brain that affected females more than males (21). By using a slightly different exposure protocol during rat pregnancy, these same investigators did observe subtle differences from controls in growth rates at 14 and 21 days and reduced reflex suspension, indicating that normal development had been interrupted (22). In a fourth study, mouse offspring exposed *in utero* to nitrous oxide during organogenesis had hyporeactivity of the startle reflex at 60 and 95 days of age (23).

The effects of nitrous oxide on growing neural tips (growth cones) in the forebrains of neonatal rat pups were described in a 1993 report (24). The pups were exposed to three concentrations of nitrous oxide (25%, 50%, and 75%) over a 6-hour period on postnatal day 1. A dose-response on the activity of a growth cone enzyme (protein kinase C, PKC) was found, with the lowest concentration having no effect on the enzyme. The 75% concentration, however, reduced the activity to about 63%. The 50% dose also reduced the PKC activity but to a lesser degree. The authors thought that the reduced enzyme activity could be related to long-term morphologic or behavioral neuroabnormalities in the pups (24).

The effect of nitrous oxide on rat fertility was described in a 1990 study (25). Adult virgin female rats were exposed to the gas during their 4-day ovulatory cycles. Nitrous oxide disrupted luteinizing hormone releasing hormone (LHRH) (now known as *gonadotropin-releasing hormone*) cells in the hypothalamus. This disruption resulted in the inhibition of LHRH release and, thus, ovulation (25).

Human

Placental Passage

Nitrous oxide rapidly crosses the human placenta to the fetus, thereby obtaining amounts in the fetal circulation nearly equivalent to those in the mother (26–31). In a 1970 study, umbilical vein and artery nitrous oxide concentrations ranged up to 91% of maternal levels and increased progressively with increasing duration of anesthesia (27).

Spontaneous Abortion

A number of reports have described the association between spontaneous abortions (SABs) and exposure to anesthetic gasses in the operating room, dental office, or during surgery (32–46). In addition, several reviews have examined this topic (47–55).

The principal concern for chronic exposure to anesthetic gasses relates to unscavenged environments in which high concentrations of gases, such as nitrous oxide, have been measured. A 1972 reference cited studies that measured levels of nitrous oxide in the operating room averaging 130 ppm (0.013%) but with peak concentrations as high as 428 ppm (0.048%) (32). Even higher levels (e.g., 9700 ppm or 0.97%) were measured in the anesthesiologist's inhalational zone. A 1970 report described the results of a survey from a group of nurses (67 operating room/92 general duty) and physicians (50 anesthetists/81 specialists other than anesthesia) that were routinely exposed to anesthetics in the operating room (33). In the first group, 29.7% of the pregnancies of operating room nurses ended in SAB, compared to 8.8% in the controls. In the second group, the SAB incidence was 37.8% and 10.3%, respectively. In both exposed groups, the SAB occurred earlier than the controls (8th vs. 10th week). However, the study could not identify a specific anesthetic agent, nor could it establish a cause-effect relationship (33).

The results of a national survey of operating room personnel was reported in 1974 (34). The survey included the memberships of four organizations, essentially covering all personnel in the United States who were continuously exposed to low levels of anesthetic gasses: American Society of Anesthesiologists (ASA), American Association of Nurse Anesthetists (AANA), Association of Operating Room Nurses (AORN), and Association of Operating Room Technicians (AORT). Two control groups were surveyed: American Academy of Pediatrics (AAP) and American Nurses Association (ANA). At the time of the survey, about 21% of the operating rooms were ventilated and anesthetic-scavenged. The rates of SAB among the respondents (organization and total number of pregnancies shown in parentheses) were 17.1% (ASA; 468), 17.0% (AANA; 1826), and 19.5% (AORN/AORT; 2781). The results were statistically significant when compared to women working outside of the operating room. However, no difference was found with the controls for the time (in gestational weeks) of the abortions or for a decrease in the sex ratio of exposed pregnancies (34).

A survey of women physicians in England and Wales to determine the outcome of pregnancies was reported in 1977 (35). The analysis involved 9044 pregnancies that were classified into three groups: working anesthetists ($N = 670$), other medical specialties (includes medical students but excludes radiologists) ($N = 6377$), and physicians not currently working ($N = 1997$). The adjusted SAB rates were 13.8%, 13.8%, and 12.0%, respectively. For stillbirths, the rates were 17.3%, 8.3%, and 10.3% (*n.s.*), respectively (35). Another survey in England of anesthetists exposed to anesthetics, male and female, appeared in 1979 (36). The SAB rates (percentage of known conceptions) for exposed fathers, mothers, both parents, and nonexposed controls were 15.7%, 34.4%*, 23.1%*, and 9.8%, respectively (*significant compared to controls).

Because dentist and their assistants may be exposed to even higher concentrations of anesthetic gases than personnel in hospital operating rooms, a survey of this population was undertaken and reported in 1980 (37). The responding sample size involved more than 22,000 dentists (98.5% male) and more than 21,000 chairside assistants (99.1% female). Only about 19% of the individuals were exposed to halogenated anesthetic gases in addition to nitrous oxide. The two groups were further classified by the amount of exposure in the year before conception (nonusers, light [1–2999 hours in past decade], and heavy [more than 3,000 hours in past decade]). After adjustment for smoking, age, and pregnancy history, a significant association was found between use of anesthetics and the rate of SAB in chairside assistants (8.1% nonusers, 14.2% light, and 19.1% heavy). The association also was significant for wives of dentists but the rates of SAB were about half of those for the assistants (37). In a brief 1986 report, six SABs were observed in four female personnel over a 17-month interval (38). These persons worked in an oral surgery department that used 35% nitrous oxide in oxygen as a sedative during procedures. In the operating rooms, the range of nitrous oxide concentrations were 0.01–0.04% but were as high as 0.07% when the patient talked (38). A 1995 study found a significant increase in SAB among female dental assistants who worked for 3 or more hours per week in offices not using scavenging equipment (39). After adjustment for age, smoking, and number of amalgams prepared, the relative risk (RR) was 2.6 (95% confidence interval [CI] 1.3–5.0).

In contrast to the above reports, two studies found no association between chronic exposure to nitrous oxide and SAB, and a third found only a partial association (40–42). In comparison to unexposed controls, the adjusted odds ratios (ORs) for SAB in dental assistants working in unscavenged clinics or dental school services in Denmark were 0.9 (95% CI 0.4–2.1) and 0.3 (0.0–1.8), respectively (40). In a Swedish study of 1711 midwives, the use of nitrous oxide (>50% of deliveries) was not associated with an increased risk of SAB (OR 0.95, 95% CI 0.62–1.47) (41). The study could not determine if scavenging equipment for waste gas was used. The investigators concluded that night work and high workload increased the risk of SAB (41). In an earlier study, the rates of SAB were compared for 563 married female anesthetists, working and not working, to 828 female physician controls (42). The rates were 18.3%, 13.7%, and 14.7%, respectively.

A 1980 report described the outcomes of 187 women who had been exposed to inhalational anesthetics (mostly nitrous oxide) during work or by their husbands, and who had surgery during pregnancy (43). The study was an extension of the study involving occupational exposure to inhalational anesthetics and SAB in wives of dentists and dental assistants ($N = 12{,}929$) (see reference #37). The rates of 1st trimester SAB in four groups classified as controls ($N = 8654$; no exposure or surgery), exposure/no surgery ($N = 4088$), no exposure/surgery ($N = 122$), and exposure/surgery ($N = 65$) were 5.1%, 8.6%, 8.0%, and 14.8%, respectively. The rates for 2nd trimester SAB were 1.4%, 2.6%, 6.9%, and 0, respectively (43). A Canadian study compared pregnant women who where undergoing incidental surgery with pregnant women not undergoing surgery (44). Surgery (usually gynecologic) under general anesthesia in the 1st or 2nd trimesters was associated with an increased risk of SAB (estimated risk ratio [ERR] 2.0, 95% CI 1.10–3.64). The risk was also increased following procedures under general anesthesia that were remote from the conceptus (ERR 1.54, 95% CI 1.03–2.30) (44). A 1986 study in 433 women (9 sets of twins) of general anesthesia with nitrous oxide given in the 1st and 2nd trimesters was unable to find an association between the anesthetic and SAB (45).

Finally, a 1985 study combined the data from six studies to determine the risk of SAB in operating room personnel (46). The low RR was 1.3 (95% CI 1.2–1.4) for pregnant physicians and nurses.

Infertility - Female

An increased rate of infertility in anesthetists was noted in a 1972 study (42). In this survey of women anesthetists in the United Kingdom, 65 (12%) of the 563 married anesthetists reported infertility of unknown cause compared to 6% of controls. However, 36 (44%) eventually conceived, even though 92% of them continued to work (42). A 1979 survey reported that 30% of anesthetists (includes both sexes) had difficulty in conceiving, but unexpected infertility occurred in only 3% (37).

A 1992 study examined the effect of environmental nitrous oxide on the fertility of dental assistants (56). A group of 7000 female dental assistants was surveyed, and 459 were determined to be eligible for the study because they had met all inclusion criteria, including conception, within the previous 4 years. Of those eligible, 418 (91%) completed the telephone interview. Data were collected over 13 menstrual cycles (about 1 year). The primary statistical analysis involved a comparison of the adjusted fecundability ratio (an estimate of the conception rate for exposed women relative to that for unexposed women in each menstrual cycle of unprotected intercourse) (56). No difference in the ratio was observed in the 121 assistants who worked <5 hours/week ($N = 85$; ratio 1.05) or ≥ 5 hours/week ($N = 36$; ratio 1.15) in scavenged offices. In contrast, among the 60 assistants who worked in unscavenged offices, the 41 working <5 hours/week had a significantly higher adjusted ratio (1.01) than the 19 working ≥ 5 hours/week (0.41). Thus, the latter group was only 41% as likely as unexposed women to conceive during each menstrual cycle. In addition, the study examined the occurrence of SAB. Among the 325 pregnancies (93 excluded because they were pregnant at the time of data collection), 10 were in the "high exposure" unscavenged group. Their SAB rate was 50% (5/10), whereas 25 (8%) of the remaining 315 pregnancies aborted (56). An accompanying editorial and later correspondence discussed the implications of the study (57–61).

A 1996 study involving Swedish midwives obtained results similar to those above (62). As in the above study, data were collected over 13 menstrual cycles. In 84% of the responders ($N = 3985$) to a mailed questionnaire, the adjusted fecundability ratios of three groups, compared to those working in the day time, were two-shift rotations 0.78, three-shift rotations 0.77, night-shift only 0.82, respectively. The effect of nitrous oxide was noted only for midwives exposed to more than 30 deliveries/month where the gas was used (ratio 0.64) (62).

The effects of general anesthesia on pregnancy rates in patients who were undergoing embryo transfer after *in vitro* fertilization were described in a 1995 study (63). Analgesia for ovum retrieval and embryo transfer was sedation (opiates, diazepam, promethazine)/local anesthesia (120 cycles; 88 patients), epidural block (139 cycles; 111 patients), and general anesthesia (nitrous oxide, halothane, opiates, and barbiturates) (173 cycles; 112 patients). The groups did not differ in embryo yield or number or quality of embryos transferred. However, the clinical pregnancy rates for the general anesthesia group were significantly lower than that for the other two groups: 25.8%, 23.7%, and 14.5%, respectively. The delivery rate also was significantly lower for the general anesthesia group: 19.2%, 20.1%, and 8.7%, respectively. The authors concluded that the adverse effect of general anesthesia occurred after embryo transfer and was probably related to nitrous oxide exposure (63). However, a 1999 study with data from seven fertility programs involving gamete intrafallopian transfer found no significant difference in the clinical pregnancy or delivery rates between women who had received nitrous oxide (or other anesthetic agents) and those who did not (64).

Infertility - Male

A survey of 5507 male anesthetists in the United Kingdom found no association between paternal work in operating rooms and SAB, infertility, or the frequency of congenital anomalies (65). However, if the mother was also exposed, the risk of SAB may be increased by 158% to 271%. A 1987 review suggested that male fertility could be affected by direct nitrous oxide inactivation of vitamin B_{12} (cyanocobalamin) (66). The inactivation of this vitamin could result in a reduction of methionine synthetase that is essential for normal cell division (66). A later review discussed the effect of nitrous oxide on cyanocobalamin-dependent methionine synthetase and other factors that eventually impair DNA synthesis and could cause infertility (67).

N

Congenital Malformations

Several studies have examined the relationship between 1st trimester exposure to nitrous oxide and congenital malformations (34–36,42–46,68–74). Two early studies did not find such a relationship, but the number of exposed cases was small (68,69). A larger study also found no relationship between surgical anesthesia and congenital malformations (44). In another previously cited study, the overall rate of birth defects in live-births was no different in 583 anesthetists (5.2%) and 828 controls (4.9%) (42). However, when analyzed separately, working anesthetists had a significantly higher rate of offspring with defects (6.5%) than those who were not working (2.5%), but not significantly higher than controls.

A 1974 survey of 621 female nurse-anesthetists, with a response rate of 84.5%, found an incidence of birth defects (major and minor) in offspring of working mothers of 16.4%, compared to 5.7% when the mother was not working (70). Nearly one half of the defects in the exposed group were cutaneous anomalies. In the 1974 national survey cited above, the congenital abnormality rates (all skin anomalies were excluded) in the groups (unexposed vs. exposed) were ASA (3.4% vs. 5.9%), AANA (5.9% vs. 9.6%), and AORN/AORT (7.0% vs 7.7%) (34). The first two comparisons were statistically significant. The survey also provided the congenital malformation rates (excluding skin anomalies) for wives of the male survey respondents in the three groups: 5.4%, 8.2%, and 6.4%, respectively (34). A 1977 survey found a significant rate of heart/great vessel defects in working anesthetists (13.8%), in comparison to a combined group of other physicians (3.6%), or an earlier population-based study (6.6%) (35). However, no differences were found for other congenital anomalies (neural tube defects [NTD], oral clefts, talipes, congenital hip dislocation, hydrocele, hypospadias, and epispadias, and genitourinary). The rates of development or congenital abnormalities (percentage of live births) in a 1979 survey of anesthetists exposed to anesthetics were 9.3% ($N = 22$) for exposed fathers, 4.8% ($N = 1$) for exposed mothers, and 15.0% (N = 3) when both parents were exposed (36). These rates did not differ significantly from nonexposed controls.

No significant increase in the incidence of birth defects was found in a 1980 study of surgery during early pregnancy (43). Anesthetics for surgery were used in 187 women during the 1st trimester and in 100 women during the 2nd trimester. The rates of defects in the offspring of mothers who had surgery in the 1st and 2nd trimesters, but no occupational exposure to inhalational anesthetics, were 3.1% and 5.8%, respectively. For surgery plus occupational exposure, the rates were 7.2% and 2.3%, respectively. The differences were not significant (43). A 1986 study analyzed the outcomes of 375 cases (8 sets of twins) of cervical cerclage and 58 other surgeries (1 set of twins) conducted under general anesthesia with nitrous oxide (45). Cases were further stratified by the gestational week when surgery was conducted (>16 weeks or ≤16 weeks). None of the observed birth defects could be attributed to anesthetic exposure (45). A 1985 study combined the results from six studies to derive an RR for congenital abnormalities of 1.2 (95% CI 1.0–1.4) for pregnant physicians and nurses working in operating rooms (46).

Using data from three Swedish health care registries for the years 1973 to 1981, a 1989 study analyzed 5405 cases of nonobstetric surgical operations that occurred during pregnancy (71). The types of anesthesia were general (about 54%; 99% using combinations with nitrous oxide), regional (about 14%), and unknown (32%). The rates of congenital malformations, stillbirths, infant death within 7 days of birth, and decreased birth weights were determined by the trimester in which the operation was performed. For congenital malformations, the RR and 95% CI for the 1st, 2nd, and 3rd trimesters and the total group were 1.0 (0.8–1.4), 0.9 (0.6–1.2), 1.5 (1.1–2.2) and 1.1 (0.9–1.3), respectively. The rate for all defects was about 5%; about 1.9% for major anomalies. Both rates were similar to those in the total Swedish population. The risk for stillbirths also was not significantly different from the general population (RR 1.4, 95% CI 1.0–1.8), but the risk of infant death within 7 days of birth was increased (RR 2.1, 95% CI 1.6–2.7). Most of the infant deaths (70%) occurred in infants of very-low birth-weight. The rates of low-birth-weight (<2500 g) and very-low-birth-weight (<1500 g) infants were increased in all trimesters and for the total the RR (95% CI) were 2.0 (1.8–2.2) and 2.2 (1.8–2.8). The reduced weights were due to prematurity and intrauterine growth retardation. For all mothers who were operated on, the prematurity rate was 7.47% vs. 5.13% in controls ($p < 0.001$) (71).

Using the same data as in the above study, study investigators found a possible association between surgery in the 1st trimester and NTD, and these findings were published in 1990 (72). The investigators studied 2252 infants whose mothers had surgery during the 1st trimester. Six of the infants had NTD (expected 2.5), one of whom was thought to have Meckel's syndrome. An additional infant had a diagnosis of hydranencephaly, but the autopsy report indicated the diagnosis was uncertain and it may have been a very large encephalocele. In the total group, 572 had operations during the period of neural tube closure (gestational weeks 4 and 5). Mothers of five of the six infants with NTD (expected 0.6) had surgery during this period, but only three had been exposed to nitrous oxide. The mother of the hydranencephaly case had surgery in gestational week 8 and was not exposed to nitrous oxide. The authors could not determine whether the findings represented a causal association with surgery or just a random occurrence (72).

In a 1994 population-based, case-control study, 12 (1.7%) of 694 mothers of infants with central nervous system (CNS) defects had surgery under general anesthesia in the 1st trimester, compared to 34 (1.1%) of 2984 controls (73). Analysis of total CNS defects

N

and 1st trimester exposure to general anesthesia revealed the following: NTD (345 cases; 3 exposed), OR 0.7, 95% CI 0.2, 2.4; microcephaly (91 cases; 1 exposed), OR 1.7, 95% CI 0.2, 13.5; hydrocephalus (198 cases; 7 exposed), OR 3.8, 95% CI 1.6, 9.1. When isolated CNS defects were analyzed, the OR and 95% CI for the three defects were 1.1 (0.3, 4.9), 3.8 (0.4, 33.0), and 0.0 (0.00, 4.1) (all nonsignificant). However, when the analysis included multiple CNS defects, there were 70 cases (7 exposed) of hydrocephalus (OR 9.6, 95% CI 3.8, 24.6), 8 cases (3 exposed) of hydrocephalus and eye defects (OR 39.6, 95% CI 7.5, 209.2), and 2 cases (2 exposed) of hydrocephalus and cataracts (OR infinity, 95% CI 1329, infinity). Although the investigators identified several limitations of their study, including the inability to identify the specific medications used for general anesthesia, the findings do warrant additional study (73).

The Collaborative Perinatal Project monitored 50,282 mother-child pairs, 76 of whom were exposed to nitrous oxide during the 1st trimester (74). Four malformed infants were observed, a hospital standardized relative risk of 0.75. There was no evidence of an association between the gas and the defects (74).

Neurotoxicity

The mechanism of action of nitrous oxide, at anesthetic concentrations, is thought to involve blockade of *N*-methyl-D-aspartate (NMDA) glutamate receptors (75–79). This action also produces neurotoxic effects, which can be prevented by drugs (e.g., benzodiazepines, barbiturates, halothane, isoflurane, propofol, scopolamine, and atropine) that enhance GABAergic (γ-amino-n-butyric acid) inhibition (75,77). However, the addition of ketamine, another NMDA antagonist, to nitrous oxide without concomitant use of a GABA agonist has been shown in animals to potentiate the neurotoxicity of nitrous oxide (80). Recent evidence has shown that the neurotoxicity of ethanol, a NMDA antagonist and a potentiator of GABA transmission, is different in immature brains than in adult brains (81). Therefore, the potential exists that the common use of nitrous oxide and GABAergic agents together during general anesthesia in obstetrics and pediatrics could cause neuroteratogenicity during human brain growth spurts (synaptogenesis; 3rd trimester to several years after birth) (81–83). Animal studies in 7-day-old rats have demonstrated this teratogenicity, as evidenced by widespread apoptotic neurodegeneration, deficits in hippocampal synaptic function, and persistent impairment of memory and learning (84).

A 2004 study examined the association between exposure of mothers to waste anesthetic gases during pregnancy and development of their offspring (85). Although the specific gases were not identified, the timing of the exposures (1983–1996) and practice patterns suggested that nitrous oxide, halothane, and isoflurane were the most likely agents. Forty children (age 5–13 years) born to female anesthesiologists and operating room nurses who were exposed to waste anesthetic gases were compared to 40 female physicians and nurses (matched for children's age, gender, and maternal occupation) who worked in hospitals during their pregnancies but who did not work in operating rooms (unexposed controls). All children underwent standardized developmental tests to evaluate their medical and neurodevelopmental state and the mothers were interviewed. The developmental milestones in the two groups were similar, but the exposed children had a significantly lower gross motor ability and more evidence of inattention/hyperactivity. Moreover, the level of exposure was significantly and negatively correlated with fine motor ability and IQ performance. The investigators concluded that the results supported the hypothesis that occupational exposure to waste anesthetic gases during pregnancy might be a risk factor for minor neurological deficits in the offspring (85).

Miscellaneous Effects

Subanesthetic doses of nitrous oxide have been used for analgesia in laboring patients (86–93). The effects on the fetus do not appear to be any different from those of other general anesthetics (92). When used as an analgesic, nitrous oxide has no direct effect on uterine activity (87,94). In contrast, prolonged general anesthesia with nitrous oxide may cause neonatal acidosis and an increased incidence of low Apgar scores (95). A 1988 study concluded that the use of high intermittent doses of nitrous oxide used for obstetric analgesia was associated with a risk of developing amphetamine addiction in later life (96). The mechanism was thought to be an effect of imprinting. However, this study has been criticized for several design flaws and conclusions (88).

A 2-minute inhalation dose of 30% nitrous oxide with oxygen for analgesia at term resulted in a decrease in both maternal and fetal central vascular resistance (97). Although this dose is usually safe for the mother or fetus, the cerebral hyperemia induced by nitrous oxide might increase the risk of intracranial hemorrhage in preterm infants (97).

Decreased birth weight, but not preterm birth, was associated with occupational exposure to nitrous oxide in a 1999 study based on a survey of the Swedish Midwifes Association (98). Chronic nitrous oxide exposure during the 2nd trimester was associated with 77 g decrease in birth weight (95% CI 129, 24) and an increase in the odds of infants being small-for-gestational-age (OR 1,8, 95% CI 1.1, 2.8) (99). In a 1977 survey, the offspring of working anesthetists had significantly lower birth weights and a higher proportion of infants weighing 2500 g or less than did two other physician groups (35). Lower birth weights also were observed in offspring of female anesthetists in a 1979 survey (36). Female infants were particularly under weight. Moreover, there was a lower male:female sex ratio in the offspring of female anesthetists (36). The author, however, has had to defend his research (99).

A 1991 population-based case-control study conducted in Sweden found an association between childhood leukemia and nitrous oxide anesthesia during delivery (100). Mothers of the 411 cases were more likely than controls to have received the anesthetic (OR 1.3, 95% CI 1.0, 1.6).

Summary

A large amount of data has been published concerning the reproductive toxicity of nitrous oxide. Abortions and growth retardation have been consistently observed in animal studies, but the exposures to the gas were usually much higher and of greater duration than the exposures that occur in humans. Structural anomalies, usually involving the skeleton, were inconsistently found. Neuroteratogenicity also has been noted in animal studies and, in some cases, permanent changes in the brains of animals exposed *in utero* have been found. Thus, in animals, nitrous oxide is an embryo and fetal toxin that may have long-lasting consequences.

The evidence for human reproductive toxicity is not as clear. Much of the data relating to SAB, infertility, and decreased birth weight is based on voluntary responses to surveys that involved self-reported outcomes. These retrospective reports are subject to self-selection and/or recall bias. Moreover, many studies have evaluated exposure to nitrous oxide in operating rooms or dental offices, rather than to individuals, and have not quantified the amount and type of anesthetic gas exposure (46,101). In addition, the studies have not always accounted for confounding variables, such as the introduction of scavenging equipment and ventilation, maternal age, smoking, and other drug exposures, and have characterized nitrous oxide exposure based only on job title (102). Nevertheless, there does appear to be an increase in the incidence of SAB and infertility related to chronic exposure to nitrous oxide, but the dose and magnitude of these effects need further study. Moreover, general anesthesia in the 1st and 2nd trimesters has been associated with reduced birth weight, but the causative agents have not been identified.

The information for nitrous oxide and congenital malformations is less confusing, but many of the limitations identified above also apply to this patient population. However, the available data do not appear to suggest that acute or chronic exposure to nitrous oxide at any time in pregnancy represents a major risk for congenital anomalies. Although nitrous oxide is the most commonly used general anesthetic agent, it is never administered alone, being combined with a number of other agents. Therefore, the safest course is to postpone elective surgical procedures until after pregnancy or, at the minimum, until after the period of organogenesis. Moreover, because even operating rooms that are scavenged and ventilated are not entirely free of waste anesthetic gases, women who might become pregnant and are working in these areas should be counseled as to the potential risks and offered positions in areas free of nitrous oxide contamination. Recent data have shown that offspring of mothers with occupational exposure could have long-term neurodevelopmental deficits. Finally, long-term neurotoxicity studies of infants exposed *in utero* to nitrous oxide during the 3rd trimester or during the first few years after birth are warranted.

BREAST FEEDING SUMMARY

RECOMMENDATION: Compatible

No reports describing the use of nitrous oxide during lactation have been located. The solubility in blood and tissue is low. Moreover, the plasma half-life is very short (<3 minutes) and, thus, it is unlikely that a nursing infant would be exposed to the agent in milk or that it would be orally bioavailable to the infant (103).

N

References

1. Steward A, Allott PR, Cowles AL, Mapleson WW. Solubility coefficients for inhaled anaesthetics for water, oil and biological media. Br J Anaesth 1973;45: 282–93.
2. Fink BR, Shepard TH, Blandau RJ. Teratogenic activity of nitrous oxide. Nature 1967;214:146–8.
3. Corbett TH, Cornell RG, Endres JL, Millard RI. Effect of low concentrations of nitrous oxide on rat pregnancy. Anesthesiology 1973;39:299–301.
4. Pope WDB, Halsey MJ, Phil D, Lansdown ABG, Simmonds A, Bateman PE. Fetotoxicity in rats following chronic exposure to halothane, nitrous oxide, or methoxyflurane. Anesthesiology 1978;48: 11–6.
5. Ramazzotto LJ, Carlin RD, Warchalowski GA. Effects of nitrous oxide during organogenesis in the rat. J Dent Res 1979;58:1940–3.
6. Coate WB, Kapp RW Jr, Lewis TR. Chronic exposure to low concentrations of halothane-nitrous oxide. Anesthesiology 1979;50:310–8.
7. Coate WB, Kapp RW Jr, Ulland BM, Lewis TR. Toxicity of low concentration long-term exposure to an airborne mixture of nitrous oxide and halothane. J Environ Pathol Toxicol 1979;2:209–31.
8. Vieira E. Effect of the chronic administration of nitrous oxide 0.5% to gravid rats. Br J Anaesth 1979;51:283–7.
9. Vieira E, Cleaton-Jones P, Austin JC, Moyes DG, Shaw R. Effects of low concentrations of nitrous oxide on rat fetuses. Anesth Analg 1980;59:175–7.
10. Vieira E, Cleaton-Jones P, Moyes D. Effects of low intermittent concentrations of nitrous oxide on the developing rat fetus. Br J Anaesth 1983;55:67–9.
11. Shah RM, Burdett DN, Donaldson D. The effects of nitrous oxide on the developing hamster embryos. Can J Physiol Pharmacol 1979;57:1229–32.
12. Bussard DA, Stoelting RK, Peterson C, Ishaq M. Fetal changes in hamsters anesthetized with nitrous oxide and halothane. Anesthesiology 1974;41:275–8.
13. Lane GA, Nahrwold ML, Tait AR, Taylor-Busch M, Cohen PJ, Beaudoin AR. Anesthetics as teratogens: nitrous oxide is fetotoxic, xenon is not. Science 1980;210:899–901.
14. Mazze RI, Wilson AI, Rice SA, Baden JM. Reproduction and fetal development in rats exposed to nitrous oxide. Teratology 1984;30:259–65.
15. Mazze RI, Fujinaga M, Rice SA, Harris SB, Baden JM. Reproductive and teratogenic effects of nitrous oxide, halothane, isoflurane, and enflurane in Sprague-Dawley rats. Anesthesiology 1986;64:339–44.
16. Trevor AJ, Miller RD. General anesthetics. In Katzung BG, ed. *Basic and Clinical Pharmacology*. 8th ed. New York: McGraw-Hill, 2001:426.
17. Mazze RI, Wilson AI, Rice SA, Baden JM. Reproduction and fetal development in mice chronically exposed to nitrous oxide. Teratology 1982;26:11–6.

18. Warren JR, Shaw B, Steinkampf MP. Effects of nitrous oxide on preimplantation mouse embryo cleavage and development. Biol Reprod 1990;43:158–61.
19. Fujinaga M, Baden JM, Mazze RI. Susceptible period of nitrous oxide teratogenicity in Sprague-Dawley rats. Teratology 1989;40:439–44.
20. Rodier PM. Inhalant anesthetics as neuroteratogens. Ann N Y Acad Sci 1986;477:42–8.
21. Mullenix PJ, Moore PA, Tassinari MS. Behavioral toxicity of nitrous oxide in rats following prenatal exposure. Toxicol Ind Health 1986;2:273–87.
22. Tassinari MS, Mullenix PJ, Moore PA. The effects of nitrous oxide after exposure during middle and late gestation. Toxicol Ind Health 1986;2:261–71.
23. Rice SA. Effect of prenatal N_2O exposure on startle reflex reactivity. Teratology 1990;42:373–81.
24. Saito S, Fujita T, Igarashi M. Effects of inhalational anesthetics on biochemical events in growing neuronal tips. Anesthesiology 1993;79:1338–47.
25. Kugel G, Letelier C, Zive MA, King JC. Nitrous oxide and infertility. Anesth Prog 1990;37:176–80.
26. Cohen EN, Paulson WJ, Wall J, Elert B. Thiopental, curare, and nitrous oxide anesthesia for cesarean section with studies on placental transmission. Surg Gynecol Obstet 1953;97:456–62.
27. Marx GF, Joshi CW, Orkin LR. Placental transmission of nitrous oxide. Anesthesiology 1970;32:429–32.
28. Morgan CA, Paull J. Drugs in obstetric anaesthesia. Anaesth Intens Care 1980;8:278–88.
29. Nandi PR, Morrison PF, Morgan BM. Effects of general anaesthesia on the fetus during caesarean section. Anaesth Rev 1991;8:103–22.
30. Friedman JM. Teratogen update: anesthetic agents. Teratology 1988;37:69–77.
31. Kanto J. Risk-benefit assessment of anaesthetic agents in the puerperium. Drug Saf 1991;6:285–301.
32. Corbett TH. Anesthetics as a cause of abortion. Fertil Steril 1972;23:866–9.
33. Cohen EN, Bellville JW, Brown BW Jr. Anesthesia, pregnancy, and miscarriage: a study of operating room nurses and anesthetists. Anesthesiology 1971;35:343–7.
34. Ad Hoc Committee on the Effect of Trace Anesthetics on the Health of Operating Room Personnel, American Society of Anesthesiologists. Occupational disease among operating room personnel: a national study. Anesthesiology 1974;41:321–40.
35. Pharoah POD, Alberman E, Doyle P. Outcome of pregnancy among women in anaesthetic practice. Lancet 1977;1:34–6.
36. Tomlin PJ. Health problems of anaesthetists and their families in the West Midlands. Br Med J 1979;1:779–84.
37. Cohen EN, Brown BW, Wu ML, Whitcher CE, Brodsky JB, Gift HC, Greenfield W, Jones TW, Driscoll EJ. Occupational disease in dentistry and chronic exposure to trace anesthetic gases. J Am Dent Assoc 1980;101:21–31.
38. Schuyt HC, Brakel K, Oostendorp SGLM, Schiphorst BJM. Abortion among dental personnel exposed to nitrous oxide. Anaesthesia 1986;41:82–3.
39. Rowland AS, Baird DD, Shore DL, Weinberg CR, Savitz DA, Wilcox AJ. Nitrous oxide and spontaneous abortion in female dental assistants. Am J Epidemiol 1995;141:531–8.
40. Heidam LZ. Spontaneous abortions among dental assistants, factory workers, painters, and gardening workers: a follow up study. J Epidemiol Comm Health 1984;38:149–55.
41. Axelsson G, Ahlborg G Jr, Bodin L. Shift work, nitrous oxide exposure, and spontaneous abortion among Swedish midwives. Occup Environ Med 1996;53:374–8.
42. Knill-Jones RP, Rodrigues LV, Moir DD, Spence AA. Anaesthetic practice and pregnancy - controlled survey of women anaesthetists in the United Kingdom. Lancet 1972;1:1326–8.
43. Brodsky JB, Cohen EN, Brown BW Jr, Wu ML, Whitcher C. Surgery during pregnancy and fetal outcome. Am J Obstet Gynecol 1980;138:1165–7.
44. Duncan PG, Pope WDB, Cohen MM, Greer N. Fetal risk of anesthesia and surgery during pregnancy. Anesthesiology 1986;64:790–4.
45. Crawford JS, Lewis M. Nitrous oxide in early human pregnancy. Anaesthesia 1986;41:900–5.
46. Buring JE, Hennekens CH, Mayrent SL, Rosner B, Greenberg ER, Colton T. Health experience of operating room personnel. Anesthesiology 1985;62:325–30.
47. Spence AA, Knill-Jones RP. Is there a health hazard in anaesthetic practice? Br J Anaesth 1978;50:713–9.
48. Brodsky JB. Anesthesia and surgery during early pregnancy and fetal outcome. Clin Obstet Gynecol 1983;26:449–57.
49. Aldridge LM, Tunstall ME. Nitrous oxide and the fetus. Br J Anaesth 1986;58:1348–56.
50. Eger EI II. Fetal injury and abortion associated with occupational exposure to inhaled anesthetics. AANA J 1991;59:309–12.
51. Shortridge-McCauley LA. Reproductive hazards: an overview of exposures to health care workers. AAOHN J 1995;43:614–21.
52. Donaldson D, Meechan JG. The hazards of chronic exposure to nitrous oxide: an update. Br Dent J 1995;178:95–100.
53. Sessler DI. Risks of occupational exposure to waste-anesthetic gases. Acta Anaesthesiol Scand 1997;41(Suppl 111):237–9.
54. Wasylko L, Matsui D, Dykxhoorn SM, Rieder MJ, Weinberg S. A review of common dental treatments during pregnancy: implications for patients and dental personnel. J Can Dent Assoc 1998;64:434–9.
55. Smith DA. Hazards of nitrous oxide exposure in healthcare personnel. AANA J 1998;66:390–3.
56. Rowland AS, Baird DD, Weinberg CR, Shore DL, Shy CM, Wilcox AJ. Reduced fertility among women employed as dental assistants exposed to high levels of nitrous oxide. N Engl J Med 1992;327:993–7.
57. Baird PA. Occupational exposure to nitrous oxide—not a laughing matter. N Engl J Med 1992;327:1026–7.
58. Gray RH. Nitrous oxide and fertility. N Engl J Med 1993;328:284.
59. Rowland AS, Baird DD, Weinberg CR. Nitrous oxide and fertility (reply). N Engl J Med 1993;328:284.
60. Brodsky JB. Nitrous oxide and fertility. N Engl J Med 1993;328:284–5.

61. Baird PA. Nitrous oxide and fertility (reply). N Engl J Med 1993;328:285.
62. Ahlborg G Jr, Axelsson G, Bodin L. Shift work, nitrous oxide exposure and subfertility among Swedish midwifes. Int J Epidemiol 1996;25:783–90.
63. Gonen O, Shulman A, Ghetler Y, Shapiro A, Judeiken R, Beyth Y, Ben-Nun I. The impact of different types of anesthesia on in vitro fertilization-embryo transfer treatment outcome. J Assist Reprod Genet 1995;12:678–82.
64. Beilin Y, Bodian CA, Mukherjee T, Andres LA, Vincent RD Jr, Hock DL, Sparks AET, Munson AK, Minnich ME, Steinkampf MP, Christman GM, McKay RSF, Eisenkraft JB. The use of propofol, nitrous oxide, or isoflurane does not affect the reproductive success rate following gamete intrafallopian transfer (GIFT). Anesthesiology 1999;90:36–41.
65. Knill-Jones RP, Newman BJ, Spence AA. Anaesthetic practice and pregnancy. Lancet 1975;2:807–9.
66. Buckley DN, Brodsky JB. Nitrous oxide and male fertility. Reprod Toxicol 1987;1:93–7.
67. Louis-Ferdinand RT. Myelotoxic, neurotoxic and reproductive adverse effects of nitrous oxide. Adverse Drug React Toxicol Rev 1994;13:193–206.
68. Shnider SM, Webster GM. Maternal and fetal hazards of surgery during pregnancy. Am J Obstet Gynecol 1965;92:891–900.
69. Mellin GW. Comparative teratology. Anesthesiology 1968;29:1–4.
70. Corbett TH, Cornell RG, Endres JL, Lieding K. Birth defects among children of nurse-anesthetists. Anesthesiology 1974;41:341–4.
71. Mazze RI, Kallen B. Reproductive outcome after anesthesia and operation during pregnancy: a registry study of 5405 cases. Am J Obstet Gynecol 1989;161:1178–85.
72. Kallen B, Mazze RI. Neural tube defects and first trimester operations. Teratology 1990;41:717–20.
73. Sylvester GC, Khoury MJ, Lu X, Erickson JD. First-trimester anesthesia exposure and the risk of central nervous system defects: a population-based case-control study. Am J Public Health 1994;84:1757–60.
74. Heinonen OP, Sloan D, Shapiro S. *Birth Defects and Drugs in Pregnancy*. Littleton, MA: Publishing Sciences Group, 1977:358–60.
75. Jevtovic-Todorovic V, Todorovic SM, Mennerick S, Powell S, Dikranian K, Benshoff N, Zorumski CF, Olney JW. Nitrous oxide (laughing gas) is an NMDA antagonist, neuroprotectant and neurotoxin. Nat Med 1998;4:460–3.
76. Mennerick S, Jevtovic-Todorovic V, Todorovic SM, Shen W, Olney JW, Zorumski CF. Effect of nitrous oxide on excitatory and inhibitory synaptic transmission in hippocampal cultures. J Neurosci 1998;18:9716–26.
77. Jevtovic-Todorovic V, Beals J, Benshoff N, Olney JW. Prolonged exposure to inhalational anesthetic nitrous oxide kills neurons in adult rat brain. Neuroscience 2003;122:609–16.
78. Jevtovic-Todorovic V, Wozniak DF, Benshoff ND, Olney JW. A comparative evaluation of the neurotoxic properties of ketamine and nitrous oxide. Brain Res 2001;895:264–7.
79. Olney JW, Wozniak DF, Farber NB, Jevtovic-Todorovic V, Bittigau P, Ikonomidou C. The enigma of fetal alcohol neurotoxicity. Ann Med 2002;34:109–19.
80. Jevtovic-Todorovic V, Benshoff N, Olney JW. Ketamine potentiates cerebrocortical damage induced by the common anaesthetic agent nitrous oxide in adult rats. Br J Pharmacol 2000;130:1692–8.
81. Olney JW, Farber NB, Wozniak DF, Jevtovic-Todorovic V, Ikonomidou C. Environmental agents that have the potential to trigger massive apoptotic neurodegeneration in the developing brain. Environ Health Perspect 2000;108(Suppl 3):383–8.
82. Olney JW, Wozniak DF, Jevtovic-Todorovic V, Farber NB, Bittigau P, Ikonomidou C. Drug-induced apoptotic neurodegeneration in the developing brain. Brain Pathol 2002;12:488–98.
83. Ikonomidou C, Bittigau P, Koch C, Genz K, Hoerster F, Felderhoff-Mueser U, Tenkova T, Dikranian K, Olney JW. Neurotransmitters and apoptosis in the developing brain. Biochem Pharmacol 2001;62:401–5.
84. Jevtovic-Todorovic V, Hartman RE, Izumi Y, Benshoff ND, Dikranian K, Zorumski CF, Olney JW, Wozniak DF. Early exposure to common anesthetic agents causes widespread neurodegeneration in the developing rat brain and persistent learning deficits. J Neurosci 2003;23:876–82.
85. Ratzon NZ, Ornoy A, Pardo A, Rachel M, Hatch M. Development evaluation of children born to mothers occupationally exposed to waste anesthetic gases. Birth Defects Res Part A Clin Mol Teratol 2004;70:476–82.
86. Harrison RF, Shore M, Woods T, Mathews G, Gardiner J, Unwin A. A comparison study of transcutaneous electrical nerve stimulation (TENS), Entonox, pethidine + promazine and lumbar epidural for pain relief in labor. Acta Obstet Gynecol Scand 1987;66:914.
87. Marx GF, Katsnelson T. The introduction of nitrous oxide analgesia into obstetrics. Obstet Gynecol 1992;80:715–8.
88. Irestedt L. Current status of nitrous oxide for obstetric pain relief. Acta Anaesthesiol Scand 1994;38:771–2.
89. Ross JAS, Tunstall ME, Campbell DM, Lemon JS. The use of 0.25% isoflurane premixed in 50% nitrous oxide and oxygen for pain relief in labour. Anaesthesia 1999;54:1166–72.
90. King R, Hepp M. Isoflurane Entonox mixtures for pain relief during labour. Anaesthesia 2000;55:711.
91. Ross JAS. Isoflurane Entonox mixtures for pain relief during labour (reply). Anaesthesia 2000;55:711–2.
92. Stefani SJ, Hughes SC, Shnider SM, Levinson G, Abboud TK, Henriksen EH, Williams V, Johnson J. Neonatal neurobehavioral effects of inhalation analgesia for vaginal delivery. Anesthesiology 1982;56:351–5.
93. Abboud TK, Swart F, Zhu J, Donovan MM, Peres Da Silva E, Yakal K. Desflurane analgesia for vaginal delivery. Acta Anaesthesiol Scand 1995;39:259–61.
94. Baxi LV, Petrie RH. Pharmacologic effects on labor: effects of drugs on dystocia, labor, and uterine activity. Clin Obstet Gynecol 1987;30:19–32.
95. Datta S, Ostheimer GW, Weiss JB, Brown WU Jr, Alper MH. Neonatal effect of prolonged anesthetic induction for cesarean section. Obstet Gynecol 1981;58:331–5.

96. Jacobson B, Nyberg K, Eklund G, Bygdeman M, Rydberg U. Obstetric pain medication and eventual adult amphetamine addiction in offspring. Acta Obstet Gynecol Scand 1988;67:677–82.
97. Polvi HJ, Pirhonen JP, Erkkola RU. Nitrous oxide inhalation: effects on maternal and fetal circulations at term. Obstet Gynecol 1996;87:1045–8.
98. Bodin L, Axelsson G, Ahlborg G Jr. The association of shift work and nitrous oxide exposure in pregnancy with birth weight and gestational age. Epidemiology 1999;10:429–36.
99. Tomlin PJ. Health problems of anaesthetists and their families. Br Med J 1979;1:1280–1.
100. Zack M, Adam HO, Ericson A. Maternal and perinatal risk factors for childhood leukemia. Cancer Res 1991;51:3696–701.
101. Dale O, Husum B. Nitrous oxide: at threat to personnel and global environment? Acta Anaesthesiol Scand 1994;38:777–9.
102. Jones HE, Balster RL. Inhalant abuse in pregnancy. Obstet Gynecol Clin North Am 1998;25:153–67.
103. Hale TW. Anesthetic medications in breastfeeding mothers. J Hum Lact 1999;15:185–94.

Name: **NIZATIDINE** Risk Factor: **B_M**
Class: **Gastrointestinal Agent (Antisecretory)**

FETAL RISK SUMMARY

RECOMMENDATION: Limited Human Data - Animal Data Suggest Low Risk

Nizatidine is an H_2-receptor antagonist that inhibits gastric acid secretion. In pregnant rats and rabbits given oral doses up to 506 mg/kg/day, no adverse effects were observed on fertility, and no teratogenic effects occurred with doses up to 1500 mg/kg/day, although some abortions occurred in rabbits, but not rats, at the highest dose (1). In reproduction studies reported by the manufacturer, no evidence of impaired fertility or fetal harm was observed in rats given oral doses up to 1500 mg/kg/day (40.5 times the recommended human dose based on body surface area [RHD]) or rabbits at doses up to 275 mg/kg/day (14.6 times the RHD) (2).

A single cotyledon perfusion model was used to determine the placental transfer of nizatidine in both term human and preterm baboon placentas (3). In both systems, nizatidine was transferred at about 40% of the freely diffusible reference compound. Nizatidine transfer across the placentas was the same in both directions (i.e., mother-to-fetus and fetus-to-mother).

Based on studies in male humans (4) and animals (5,6), nizatidine does not appear to have antiandrogenic effects like those observed with cimetidine (see Cimetidine). Reversible impotence, however, has been described in men treated with nizatidine for therapeutic indications (7).

A genetic counselor was consulted about a woman who had taken nizatidine during the 14th through the 16th post-conception weeks (TM Gardner, personal communication, Jefferson Medical College, 1996). The woman delivered a healthy, 7 pound 13 ounce male infant at 37 weeks' gestation who was doing well at 1 month of age.

BREAST FEEDING SUMMARY

RECOMMENDATION: Limited Human Data - Probably Compatible

Small amounts of nizatidine are excreted into breast milk (8). Three women, who had been breast-feeding for 3–8 months, were administered nizatidine (150 mg) as a single dose and as multiple doses given every 12 hours for five doses. Serum and milk samples from both breasts were collected at intervals up to 12 hours after a dose. The mean total amount of drug measured in the milk from both breasts during a 12-hour interval was 96.1 μg. This amount represented 0.064% of the maternal dose. Peak concentrations of the drug in milk occurred between 1 and 2 hours after a dose.

Although the infants were not allowed to breast-feed during the above study, the small amounts excreted into the milk are probably not significant. Other drugs in this class are excreted into milk (see Cimetidine and Ranitidine). The American Academy of Pediatrics classifies one of these agents as compatible with breast-feeding (see Cimetidine).

References

1. Morton DM. Pharmacology and toxicology of nizatidine. Scand J Gastroenterol 1987;22(Suppl 136):1–8.
2. Product information. Axid. Eli Lilly, 2000.
3. Dicke JM, Johnson RF, Henderson GI, Kuehl TJ, Schenker S. A comparative evaluation of the transport of H_2-receptor antagonists by the human and baboon placenta. Am J Med Sci 1988;295:198–206.
4. Van Thiel DH, Gavaler JS, Heyl A, Susen B. An evaluation of the anti-androgen effects associated with H_2 antagonist therapy. Scand J Gastroenterol 1987;22(Suppl 136):24–8.
5. Neubauer BL, Goode RL, Best KL, Hirsch KS, Lin T-M, Pioch RP, Probst KS, Tinsley FC, Shaar CJ. Endocrine effects of new histamine H_2-receptor antagonist, nizatidine (LY139037), in the male rat. Toxicol Appl Pharmacol 1990;102:219–32.
6. Probst KS, Higdon GL, Fisher LF, McGrath JP, Adams ER, Emmerson JL. Preclinical toxicology studies with nizatidine, a new H_2-receptor antagonist: acute, subchronic, and chronic toxicity evaluations. Fundam Appl Toxicol 1989;13:778–92.
7. Kassianos GC. Impotence and nizatidine. Lancet 1989;1:963.
8. Obermeyer BD, Bergstrom RF, Callaghan JT, Knadler MP, Golichowski A, Rubin A. Secretion of nizatidine into human breast milk after single and multiple doses. Clin Pharmacol Ther 1990;47:724–30.

Name:	**NONOXYNOL-9/OCTOXYNOL-9**	Risk Factor:	**C**
Class:	**Vaginal Spermicides**		

FETAL RISK SUMMARY

RECOMMENDATION: Contraindicated

Nonoxynol-9 and octoxynol-9 are vaginal spermicides used to prevent conception. These agents, applied intravaginally, act by inactivating sperm after direct contact. Although human data are lacking, in animals, nonoxynol-9 rapidly crosses the vaginal wall into the systemic circulation (1). Octoxynol should also be expected to act in a similar manner. The use of vaginal spermicides just before conception or inadvertently during the early stages of pregnancy has led to investigations of their effects on the fetus. The effects studied include congenital malformations, spontaneous abortions (SABs), low birth weight, stillbirth, sex ratio at birth, frequency of multiple births, and premature delivery.

A causal relationship between vaginal spermicides and congenital abnormalities was first tentatively proposed in a 1981 study comparing 763 spermicide users and 3902 nonuser controls (2). The total number of infants with malformations was low: 17 (2.2%) in the exposed group and 39 (1.0%) in the nonexposed group. Malformations thought to be associated with spermicide use were limb reduction deformities (3 cases), neoplasms (2 cases), chromosomal abnormalities (Down's syndrome) (3 cases), and hypospadias (2 cases). An earlier investigation, published in 1977, had concluded there was no causal relationship between spermicides and congenital defects, although there was an increased incidence of limb-reduction defects in infants of users (11 of 93) as compared with nonusers (8 of 186) (3). Three reports appeared in 1982 that suggested a possible relationship between spermicide use and congenital malformations (4–6). In a case–control study conducted by one of the co-authors of the 1981 investigation, a positive association with Down's syndrome was proposed when in a group of 16 affected infants, 4 were from users of spermicides (4). In another case-control study, increased risk ratios after spermicide use, although not statistically significant, were reported for limb-reduction defects (relative risk 2.00; six infants) and hypospadias (relative risk 4.00; eight infants) (5). Finally, an English study observed, among other defects, 2 cases each of hypospadias, limb reduction deformity, and Down's syndrome among infants of 1103 spermicide users (6). The authors stated that their data were not conclusive, but the occurrence rates of these particular defects were higher than those observed in a comparative nonuser group.

Several criticisms have been directed at the original 1981 study (7–10). First, an infant was presumed exposed if the mother had a prescription filled at a designated pharmacy within 600 days of delivery. No attempt was made to ascertain actual use of the product or whether the mothers, either users or nonusers, had purchased a spermicide without a prescription (7–9). In a subsequent correspondence, all of the study's exposed cases of limb reduction deformity (three cases), Down's syndrome (three cases), and neoplasm (two cases) were re-examined in terms of the exact timing of spermicide use (10). The data suggested that spermicides were not used near the time of conception in these cases. However, this does not eliminate the possibility that spermicides may act directly on the ovum before conception (11). Second, the four types of malformations lack a common cause and time of occurrence (9). Even a single type of defect, such as limb-reduction deformity, has a varied origin (9). Third, the total number of infants with malformations was low (2.2% vs. 1.0%). Because these values are comparable to the 2%–5% reported incidence of major malformations in hospital-based studies, the apparent association may have been caused by a lower than expected rate of defects in the nonexposed group rather than an increase in the exposed infants (7,9). Fourth, no confounding variables other than maternal age were adjusted (9).

A number of investigators have been unable to reproduce the results published in 1981 (8,12–19). In a study examining 188 infants with chromosomal abnormalities or limb-reduction defects, no relationship between periconceptional use of spermicides and these defects was observed (8). No association between spermicide use at conception and any congenital malformation was observed in a study comparing 1427 cases with 3001 controls (12). In a prospective study of 34,660 women controlled for age, time in pregnancy, concentration of spermicide used, and other confounding variables, the malformation rate of spermicide users was no greater than in users of other contraceptive methods (13–15). A cohort study, the Collaborative Perinatal Project involving 50,282 mother-child pairs, found no greater risk for limb reduction deformities, neoplasm, Down's syndrome, or hypospadias in children exposed *in utero* to spermicides (16). One group of investigators interviewed 12,440 women during delivery and found no relationship between the last contraceptive method used and congenital malformations (17). Spermicides were the last contraceptive method used by 3,891 (31%) of the women. A 1987 case-control study of infants with Down's syndrome ($N = 265$), hypospadias ($N = 396$), limb reduction defects ($N = 146$), neoplasms ($N = 116$), or neural tube defects ($N = 215$) compared with 3,442 control infants with a wide variety of other defects was unable to establish any causal relationship to maternal spermicide use (18). The authors investigated spermicide usage at three different time intervals: preconceptional (1 month before to 1 month after the last menstrual period), first trimester (first 4 lunar months), and any use during lifetime without producing a positive association. A similar study, involving 13,729 women who had produced 154 fetuses with trisomy, 98 with trisomy 21 (i.e., Down's syndrome), also failed to find any association with spermicides (19). In addition, a letter from one researcher argued that an association between vaginal spermicides, or any environmental risk factor for that matter, and trisomies was implausible based on an understanding of the origin of these defects (20).

An association between vaginal spermicides and SABs was found in five studies (21–25). A strong association was found among subjects who had obtained a spermicide within 12 weeks of conception (21). Another study demonstrated approximately twice the rate of SABs in women who continued to use spermicides after conception compared with users before or close to the time of conception (22). However, a 1985 critique concluded that both sets of investigators had seriously biased their results by failing to adjust for potentially confounding variables (9). In a study involving women aborting spontaneously before the 28th week of gestation and controls delivering after the 28th week, women who used spermicides at the time of conception demonstrated a 5-fold increase in chromosomal anomalies on karyotype examinations in 929 cases (23). Although no association between spermicide use and chromosomally normal abortion was found in a study involving 6339 women, spermicide use of longer than 1 year was more common in cases of aborting trisomic conception than in controls (24). In an earlier report, the same authors observed an odds ratio of 4.8 for the association between abortuses with anomalies and unexposed controls (25). Two of these latter studies (23,25) did not adjust for confounding variables.

Three studies have found no association with SABs (6,14,26). No significant risk for SAB was observed in a large cohort study involving 17,032 subjects (6) or in another study examining periconceptional spermicide use (14). In a well-designed, large prospective study involving 32,123 subjects, spermicide use before conception was associated with a significant reduction in SAB during the 2nd trimester (26).

Three studies found no association between spermicide use and birth weight (6,14,22), but one study did find such an association (5). In this latter investigation, spermicide use after the last menstrual period was significantly associated with a lower mean birth weight among female infants of both smoking and nonsmoking mothers. For male births, an association with lower birth weight was found only when the mothers smoked. The authors were unable to determine whether these relationships were causal. Spermicide use before the last menstrual period had no effect on birth weight.

Under miscellaneous effects, a case-control study of 73 nontraumatic stillbirths found no relationship with the use of vaginal spermicides (27). No association between sex ratio at birth or frequency of multiple births and spermicides was found in one study (6). However, in a 1976 national survey, female births were approximately 25% higher among women using spermicides near the time of conception compared with nonusers, a statistically significant difference (22). Finally, a 1985 study found no evidence of a relationship between spermicide use and preterm delivery (14).

A 1990 reference reported the meta-analysis of previous studies to determine whether maternal spermicide use is detrimental to the developing fetus (28). Negative associations were found between the periconceptual and postconceptual maternal use of spermicides and teratogenicity, SAB, stillbirth, reduced fetal weight, prematurity, or an increased incidence of female births.

In summary, the available evidence indicates that the use of vaginal spermicides, either before or during early pregnancy, does not pose a risk of congenital malformations to the fetus. Three authors of the original 1981 paper reporting a relationship between spermicides and congenital defects have commented that available data now argue against a causal association (29). In addition, the FDA has issued a statement that spermicides do not cause birth defects (30). There is also controversy about whether the 1981 study should have been published (31,32). The data for SABs, low birth weight, stillbirths, sex ratios at birth, frequency of multiple births, and premature delivery also indicate it is unlikely that these factors are influenced by spermicide use.

BREAST FEEDING SUMMARY

RECOMMENDATION: No Human Data - Possible Toxicity

Although human data are lacking, nonoxynol-9 is rapidly excreted into the milk of lactating rats (1). Similar excretion in humans should be expected for both nonoxynol-9 and octoxynol-9. If excretion does occur, the effect on the nursing infant is unknown.

References

1. Chvapil M, Eskelson CD, Stiffel V, Owen JA, Droegemueller W. Studies on nonoxynol-9. II. Intravaginal absorption, distribution, metabolism and excretion in rats and rabbits. Contraception 1980;22:325–39.
2. Jick H, Walker AM, Rothman KJ, Hunter JR, Holmes LB, Watkins RN, D'Ewart DC, Danford A, Madsen S. Vaginal spermicides and congenital disorders. JAMA 1981;245:1329–32.
3. Smith ESO, Dafoe CS, Miller JR, Banister P. An epidemiological study of congenital reduction deformities of the limbs. Br J Prev Soc Med 1977;31:39–41.
4. Rothman KJ. Spermicide use and Down's syndrome. Am J Public Health 1982;72:399–401.
5. Polednak AP, Janerich DT, Glebatis DM. Birth weight and birth defects in relation to maternal spermicide use. Teratology 1982;26:27–38.
6. Huggins G, Vessey M, Flavel R, Yeates D, McPherson K. Vaginal spermicides and outcome of pregnancy: findings in a large cohort study. Contraception 1982;25:219–30.
7. Oakley GP Jr. Spermicides and birth defects. JAMA 1982;247:2405.
8. Cordero JF, Layde PM. Vaginal spermicides, chromosomal abnormalities and limb reduction defects. Fam Plann Perspect 1983;15:16–8.
9. Bracken MB. Spermicidal contraceptives and poor reproductive outcomes: the epidemiologic evidence against an association. Am J Obstet Gynecol 1985;151:552–6.
10. Watkins RN. Vaginal spermicides and congenital disorders: the validity of a study. JAMA 1986;256:3095.
11. Jick H, Walker A, Rothman KJ. Vaginal spermicides and congenital disorders: the validity of a study—in reply. JAMA 1986;256:3095–6.
12. Bracken MB, Vita K. Frequency of non-hormonal contraception around conception and association with congenital malformations in offspring. Am J Epidemiol 1983;117:281–91.
13. Mills JL, Harley EE, Reed GF, Berendes HW. Are spermicides teratogenic? JAMA 1982;248:2148–51.
14. Mills JL, Reed GF, Nugent RP, Harley EE, Berendes HW. Are there adverse effects of periconceptional spermicide use? Fertil Steril 1985;43:442–6.
15. Harlap S, Shiono PH, Ramcharan S. Congenital abnormalities in the offspring of women who used oral and other contraceptives around the time of conception. Int J Fertil 1985;30:39–47.
16. Shapiro S, Slone D, Heinonen OP, Kaufman DW, Rosenberg L, Mitchell AA, Helmrich SP. Birth defects and vaginal spermicides. JAMA 1982;247:2381–4.
17. Linn S, Schoenbaum SC, Monson RR, Rosner B, Stubblefield PG, Ryan KJ. Lack of association between contraceptive usage and congenital malformations in offspring. Am J Obstet Gynecol 1983;147:923–8.
18. Louik C, Mitchell AA, Werler MM, Hanson JW, Shapiro S. Maternal exposure to spermicides in relation to certain birth defects. N Engl J Med 1987;317:474–8.
19. Warburton D, Neugut RH, Lustenberger A, Nicholas AG, Kline J. Lack of association between spermicide use and trisomy. N Engl J Med 1987;317:478–82.
20. Bracken MB. Vaginal spermicides and congenital disorders: study reassessed, not retracted. JAMA 1987;257:2919.
21. Jick H, Shiota K, Shepard TH, Hunter JR, Stergachis A, Madsen S, Porter JB. Vaginal spermicides and miscarriage seen primarily in the emergency room. Teratog Carcinog Mutagen 1982;2:205–10.
22. Scholl TO, Sobel E, Tanfer K, Soefer EF, Saidman B. Effects of vaginal spermicides on pregnancy outcome. Fam Plann Perspect 1983;15:244, 249–50.
23. Warburton D, Stein Z, Kline J, Strobino B. Environmental influences on rates of chromosome anomalies in spontaneous abortions (abstract). Am J Hum Genet 1980;32:92A.
24. Strobino B, Kline J, Lai A, Stein Z, Susser M, Warburton D. Vaginal spermicides and spontaneous abortion of known karyotype. Am J Epidemiol 1986;123:431–43.
25. Strobino B, Kline J, Stein Z, Susser M, Warburton D. Exposure to contraceptive creams, jellies and douches and their effect on the zygote (abstract). Am J Epidemiol 1980;112:434.
26. Harlap S, Shiono PH, Ramcharan S. Spontaneous foetal losses in women using different contraceptives around the time of conception. Int J Epidemiol 1980;9:49–56.
27. Porter JB, Hunter-Mitchell J, Jick H, Walker AM. Drugs and stillbirth. Am J Public Health 1986;76:1428–31.
28. Einarson TR, Koren G, Mattice D, Schechter-Tsafriri O. Maternal spermicide use and adverse reproductive outcome: a meta-analysis. Am J Obstet Gynecol 1990;162:655–60.
29. Jick H, Walker AM, Rothman KJ. The relation between vaginal spermicides and congenital disorders—in reply. JAMA 1987;258:2066.
30. Anonymous. Data do not support association between spermicides, birth defects. FDA Drug Bull 1986;16:21.

N

31. Mills JL. Reporting provocative results; can we publish "hot" papers without getting burned? JAMA 1987;258:3428–9.
32. Holmes LB. Vaginal spermicides and congenital disorders: the validity of a study—in reply. JAMA 1986; 256:3096.

Name: **NOREPINEPHRINE** Risk Factor: **C**

Class: **Sympathomimetic (Adrenergic)**

FETAL RISK SUMMARY

RECOMMENDATION: Human and Animal Data Suggest Risk

Norepinephrine (noradrenaline; levarterenol) is a direct-acting adrenergic agent that is used for acute hypotension and as an adjunct in the treatment of cardiac arrest. It is a mixture of the racemic stereoisomer and is given by IV infusion. Norepinephrine readily crosses the placenta (1), consistent with its relatively low molecular weight (about 169).

In animal reproduction studies, norepinephrine has caused situs inversus (rat embryos) (*l*-isomer only; no effect from *d*-form) (2); cataract (rat embryos) (3); hemorrhages of cephalic, skin, and extremity structures (chick embryo) (4); and microscopic liver abnormalities and delayed skeletal ossification (hamsters) (5).

In a 1995 study in pregnant ewes (123–137 days' gestation), a high maternal dose (40 μg/minute) of norepinephrine given by IV infusion caused a significant decrease in maternal placental blood flow (6). Although fetal arterial pressure did not change, transient ($\leq$2.5 hours) but statistically significant decreases in fetal oxygenation, fetal urine flow, and lung liquid flow were observed. Because the average human maintenance dose is much less (about 2–4 μg/minute), the clinical significance of these changes to a human fetus is unknown.

Uterine vessels are normally maximally dilated, and they have only α-adrenergic receptors (7). Use of the α- and β-adrenergic stimulant, norepinephrine, could cause constriction of these vessels and reduce uterine blood flow, thereby producing fetal hypoxia (bradycardia). Norepinephrine may also interact with oxytocics or ergot derivatives to produce severe persistent maternal hypertension (7). Rupture of a cerebral vessel is possible. If a pressor agent is indicated, other drugs, such as ephedrine, should be considered.

N

BREAST FEEDING SUMMARY

RECOMMENDATION: No Human Data - Potential Toxicity

No reports describing the use of norepinephrine in lactation have been located. Use of the agent during breast-feeding would not be expected because of the indications for use.

References

1. Morgan CD, Sandler M, Panigel M. Placental transfer of catecholamines in vitro and in vivo. Am J Obstet Gynecol 1972;112:1068–75.
2. Fujinaga M, Maze M, Hoffman BB, Baden JM. Activation of á-1 adrenergic receptors modulates the control of left/right sidedness in rat embryos. Dev Biol 1992;150:419–21. As cited in Shepard TH. *Catalog of Teratogenic Agents*. 9th ed. Baltimore, MD: The Johns Hopkins University Press, 1998:340.
3. Pitel M, Lerman S. Studies on the fetal rat lens. Effects of intrauterine adrenalin and noradrenalin. Invest Ophthalmol 1962;1:406–12. As cited in Shepard TH. *Catalog of Teratogenic Agents*. 9th ed. Baltimore, MD: The Johns Hopkins University Press, 1998:340.
4. Gatling RR. The effect of sympathomimetic agents on the chick embryo. Am J Pathol 1962;40:113–27.
5. Hirsch KS, Fritz HI. A comparison of mescaline with epinephrine and norepinephrine in the hamster.

Teratology 1974;9:A19–A20. As cited in Schardein TH. *Chemically Induced Birth Defects*. 3rd ed. New York, NY: Marcel Dekker, 2000:360, 364.
6. Stevens AD, Lumbers ER. Effects of intravenous infusions of noradrenaline into the pregnant ewe on uterine blood flow, fetal renal function, and lung liquid flow. Can J Physiol Pharmacol 1995;73:202–8.
7. Smith NT, Corbascio AN. The use and misuse of pressor agents. Anesthesiology 1970;33:58–101.

Name: **NORETHINDRONE**	Risk Factor: X_M
Class: **Progestogenic Hormone**	

FETAL RISK SUMMARY

RECOMMENDATION: Contraindicated

Norethindrone is a progestogen derived from 19-nortestosterone. It is used in oral contraceptives and hormonal pregnancy tests (no longer available in the United States). Masculinization of the female fetus has been associated with norethindrone (1–3). One researcher observed an 18% incidence of masculinization of female infants born to mothers given norethindrone (2). A more conservative estimate for the incidence of masculinization caused by synthetic progestogens has been reported as 0.3% (4).

The Collaborative Perinatal Project monitored 866 mother–child pairs with 1st trimester exposure to progestational agents (including 132 with exposure to norethindrone) (5, pp. 389, 391). Evidence of an increased risk of malformation was found for norethindrone. An increase in the expected frequency of cardiovascular defects and hypospadias was also observed for progestational agents as a group (5, p. 394; 6). Re-evaluation of these data in terms of timing of exposure, vaginal bleeding in early pregnancy, and previous maternal obstetric history, however, failed to support an association between female sex hormones and cardiac malformations (7). An earlier study also failed to find any relationship with nongenital malformations (3). One investigator observed two infants with malformations who were exposed to norethindrone (8). The congenital defects included spina bifida and hydrocephalus. The relationship between norethindrone and the anomalies is unknown.

In a surveillance study of Michigan Medicaid recipients conducted between 1985 and 1992 involving 229,101 completed pregnancies, 238 newborns had been exposed to norethindrone (see also Oral Contraceptives) shortly before or after conception (F. Rosa, personal communication, FDA, 1993). A total of 20 (8.4%) major birth defects were observed (10 expected). Specific data were available for six defect categories, including (observed/expected) 2/2 cardiovascular defects, 1/0.5 oral clefts, 0/0 spina bifida, 0/1 polydactyly, 0/0.5 limb reduction defects, and 1/1 hypospadias. The total number of congenital malformations suggests a moderate association between the drug and the incidence of congenital defects, but the study could not determine the percentage of women who presumably stopped the hormone before conception or the number of anomalies as a result of prematurity (F. Rosa, personal communication, FDA, 1993).

BREAST FEEDING SUMMARY

RECOMMENDATION: Limited Human Data - Probably Compatible

Norethindrone exhibits a dose-dependent suppression of lactation (9). Lower infant weight gain, decreased milk production, and decreased composition of nitrogen and protein

N

content of human milk have been associated with norethindrone and estrogenic agents (10–13). The magnitude of these changes is low. However, the changes in milk production and composition may be of nutritional importance in malnourished mothers. If breast-feeding is desired, the lowest dose of oral contraceptives should be chosen. Monitoring of infant weight gain and the possible need for nutritional supplementation should be considered. The American Academy of Pediatrics classifies norethindrone as compatible with breast-feeding (14).

References

1. Hagler S, Schultz A, Hankin H, Kunstadter RN. Fetal effects of steroid therapy during pregnancy. Am J Dis Child 1963;106:586–90.
2. Jacobson BD. Hazards of norethindrone therapy during pregnancy. Am J Obstet Gynecol 1962;84:962–8.
3. Wilson JG, Brent RL. Are female sex hormones teratogenic? Am J Obstet Gynecol 1981;141:567–80.
4. Bongiovanni AM, McFadden AJ. Steroids during pregnancy and possible fetal consequences. Fertil Steril 1960;11:181–4.
5. Heinonen OP, Slone D, Shapiro S. *Birth Defects and Drugs in Pregnancy*. Littleton, MA: Publishing Sciences Group, 1977.
6. Heinonen OP, Slone D, Monson RR, Hook EB, Shapiro S. Cardiovascular birth defects and antenatal exposure to female sex hormones. N Engl J Med 1977;296:67–70.
7. Wiseman RA, Dodds-Smith IC. Cardiovascular birth defects and antenatal exposure to female sex hormones: a reevaluation of some base data. Teratology 1984;30:359–70.
8. Dillon S. Congenital malformations and hormones in pregnancy. Br Med J 1976;2:1446.
9. Guiloff E, Ibarra-Polo A, Zanartu J, Toscanini C, Mischler TW, Gomez-Rogers C. Effect of contraception on lactation. Am J Obstet Gynecol 1974;118:42–5.
10. Karim M, Ammarr R, El-Mahgoubh S, El-Ganzoury B, Fikri F, Abdou I. Injected progestogen and lactation. Br Med J 1971;1:200–3.
11. Kora SJ. Effect of oral contraceptives on lactation. Fertil Steril 1969;20:419–23.
12. Miller GH, Hughes LR. Lactation and genital involution effects of a new low-dose oral contraceptive on breast-feeding mothers and their infants. Obstet Gynecol 1970;35:44–50.
13. Lonnerdal B, Forsum E, Hambraeus L. Effect of oral contraceptives on composition and volume of breast milk. Am J Clin Nutr 1980;33:816–24.
14. Committee on Drugs, American Academy of Pediatrics. Transfer of drugs and other chemicals into human milk. Pediatrics 2001;108:776–89.

Name: **NORETHYNODREL** Risk Factor: X_M

Class: **Progestogenic Hormone**

FETAL RISK SUMMARY

RECOMMENDATION: Contraindicated

Norethynodrel is a progestogen derived from 19-nortestosterone. It is used in oral contraceptive agents and hormonal pregnancy tests (no longer available in the United States). Masculinization of the female infant has been associated with norethynodrel (1,2). The Collaborative Perinatal Project monitored 866 mother-child pairs with 1st trimester exposure to progestational agents (including 154 with exposure to norethynodrel) (3, pp. 389, 391). Fetuses exposed to norethynodrel were not at an increased risk for malformation. However, an increase in the expected frequency of cardiovascular defects and hypospadias was observed for progestational agents as a group (3, p. 394; 4). Re-evaluation of these data in terms of timing of exposure, vaginal bleeding in early pregnancy, and previous maternal obstetric history, however, failed to support an association between female sex hormones and cardiac malformations (5). An earlier study also failed to find any relationship with nongenital malformations (1). One investigator observed three infants exposed to norethynodrel and mestranol during the 1st trimester, who had congenital defects, including atrial and ventricular septal defects (one infant), hypospadias (one infant), and inguinal hernias (two infants) (6). The relationship between the anomalies and the exposure to the hormones is unknown.

BREAST FEEDING SUMMARY

RECOMMENDATION: Limited Human Data - Probably Compatible

Norethynodrel exhibits a dose-dependent suppression of lactation (7). Lower infant weight gain, decreased milk production, and decreased composition of nitrogen and protein content of human milk have been associated with similar synthetic progestogens and estrogen products (see Norethindrone, Mestranol, Ethinyl Estradiol, Oral Contraceptives) (8–10). The magnitude of these changes is low. However, the changes in milk production and composition may be of nutritional importance in malnourished mothers. If breast-feeding is desired, the lowest dose of oral contraceptives should be chosen. Monitoring of infant weight gain and the possible need for nutritional supplementation should be considered. The American Academy of Pediatrics classifies norethynodrel as compatible with breast-feeding (11).

References

1. Wilson JG, Brent RL. Are female sex hormones teratogenic? Am J Obstet Gynecol 1981;141:567–80.
2. Hagler S, Schultz A, Hankin H, Kunstadter RN. Fetal effects of steroid therapy during pregnancy. Am J Dis Child 1963;106:586–90.
3. Heinonen OP, Slone D, Shapiro S. *Birth Defects and Drugs in Pregnancy*. Littleton, MA: Publishing Sciences Group, 1977.
4. Heinonen OP, Slone D, Monson RR, Hook EB, Shapiro S. Cardiovascular birth defects and antenatal exposure to female hormones. N Engl J Med 1977;296:67–70.
5. Wiseman RA, Dodds-Smith IC. Cardiovascular birth defects and antenatal exposure to female sex hormones: a reevaluation of some base data. Teratology 1984;30:359–70.
6. Dillon S. Congenital malformations and hormones in pregnancy. Br Med J 1976;2:1446.
7. Guiloff E, Ibarra-Polo A, Zanartu J, Toscanini C, Mischler TW, Gomez-Rogers C. Effect of contraception on lactation. Am J Obstet Gynecol 1974;118:42–5.
8. Kora SJ. Effect of oral contraceptives on lactation. Fertil Steril 1969;20:419–23.
9. Miller GH, Hughes LR. Lactation and genital involution effects of a new low-dose oral contraceptive on breast-feeding mothers and their infants. Obstet Gynecol 1970;35:44–50.
10. Lonnerdal B, Forsum E, Hambraeus L. Effect of oral contraceptives on composition and volume of breast milk. Am J Clin Nutr 1980;33:816–24.
11. Committee on Drugs, American Academy of Pediatrics. The transfer of drugs and other chemicals into human milk. Pediatrics 2001;108:776–89.

Name: **NORFLOXACIN** Risk Factor: **C_M**
Class: **Anti-infective (Quinolone)**

FETAL RISK SUMMARY

RECOMMENDATION: Human Data Suggest Low Risk

Norfloxacin is an oral, synthetic, broad-spectrum antibacterial agent. As a fluoroquinolone, it is in the same class as ciprofloxacin, enoxacin, levofloxacin, lomefloxacin, ofloxacin, and sparfloxacin. Nalidixic acid is also a quinolone drug.

In rats, high doses of norfloxacin administered before and at various intervals during gestation, including during organogenesis, did not produce an increase in congenital abnormalities, adverse effects on fertility, fetotoxicity, or changes in postnatal function in the offspring (1,2). Embryo lethality, but not teratogenicity, was observed in rabbits given 100 mg/kg (1), and in cynomolgus monkeys given 200 or 300 mg/day ($\geq$200 mg/kg/day) (3). In the monkeys, plasma concentrations (about 3 times human therapeutic levels) were high enough to produce maternal toxicity (3). In the second part of this study, the cause of the embryotoxicity was found to be directly related to a decrease in placental-derived progesterone production (4).

In reproductive studies reported by the manufacturer, no evidence of teratogenicity was found in mice, rats, rabbits, or monkeys at 6–50 times the maximum daily human dose on a body weight basis (MDHD) (5). Embryonic loss was observed in monkeys with doses 10 times the MDHD (peak plasma levels about 2 times those obtained in humans).

A 1991 reference evaluated the toxic effects of norfloxacin on rat liver and kidney DNA in mothers and their fetuses (6). Single oral doses of the antibiotic, ranging from 1 to 8 mmol/kg (319–2552 weight), about 30 times the human dose, were administered to pregnant rats on the 17th day of gestation. No DNA damage was observed in the female rats at any dose, but at 4 and 8 mmol/kg, a statistically significant decrease in the percentage of double-stranded DNA (i.e., an increase in DNA damage) was observed in fetal tissues. Because a dose-response relationship with the DNA fragmentation was lacking, and because of the very high doses administered, the investigators concluded that the results did not indicate genotoxicity, but most likely a nonspecific consequence of fetal toxicity. Thus, the potential for mutagenic and carcinogenic risk in humans was probably nil (6).

The effects of norfloxacin on spermatogenesis and sperm abnormalities were studied using a mouse sperm morphology test following either single or five consecutive daily doses of 2 and 4 mmol/kg (7). Norfloxacin stimulated spermatogenesis, presumably through a hormonal action, and may have had a mutagenic effect that resulted in an increase in abnormal sperm morphology. However, because a significant dose-response relationship for adverse morphology was not observed, the investigators could not conclude with certainty that the antibiotic induced abnormal sperm (7).

In humans, norfloxacin crosses the placenta, appearing in cord blood and in amniotic fluid (T.P. Dowling, personal communication, Merck & Co, Inc., 1987). Following a single oral 200-mg dose given to nine patients, cord blood and amniotic fluid levels varied from undetectable to 0.18 μg/mL and undetectable to 0.19 μg/mL, respectively. Cord blood levels were about one half of maternal serum levels. In another 14 women administered a single 200-mg dose, the peak maternal serum, cord blood, and amniotic fluid levels were 1.1, 0.38, and 0.92 μg/mL, respectively.

No congenital malformations were observed in the infants of 38 women who received either norfloxacin (N = 28) or ciprofloxacin (N = 10) during pregnancy (35 in the 1st trimester) (8). Most (N = 35) received the drugs for the treatment of urinary tract infections. Matched to a control group, the fluoroquinolone-exposed pregnancies had a significantly higher rate of cesarean section for fetal distress and their infants were significantly heavier. No differences were found between the groups in infant development or in the musculoskeletal system.

A surveillance study on the use of fluoroquinolones during pregnancy was conducted by the Toronto Motherisk Program among members of the Organization of Teratology Information Services and briefly reported in 1995 (9). Pregnancy outcome data were available for 134 cases, of which 61 were exposed to norfloxacin, 68 to ciprofloxacin, and 5 to both drugs. Most (90%) were exposed during the first 13 weeks postconception. Fluoroquinolone-exposed pregnancies were compared with matched controls and there were no differences in live births (87% vs. 86%), terminations (3% vs. 5%), miscarriages (10% vs. 9%), abnormal outcomes (7% vs. 4%), cesarean section rate (12% vs. 22%), fetal distress (15% vs. 15%), and pregnancy weight gain (15 kg vs. 16 kg). The birth weights of exposed infants was a mean 162 g higher than those in the control group and their gestations were a mean 1 week longer.

In a prospective follow-up study conducted by the European Network of Teratology Information Services (ENTIS), data on 549 pregnancies exposed to fluoroquinolones (318 to norfloxacin) were described in a 1996 reference (10). Data on another 116 prospective and 25 retrospective pregnancy exposures to the antibacterials were also included. From the 549 follow-up cases, 509 were treated during the 1st trimester, 22 after the 1st trimester, and in 18 cases the exposure occurred at an unknown gestational time. The live-born infants were delivered at a mean gestational age of 39.4 ± 1.5 weeks and had a mean birth weight of 3302 ± 495 g, length of 50.3 ± 2.3 cm, and head circumference of 34.9 ± 1.5 cm. Of the 549 pregnancies, there were 415 live-born infants (390 exposed during the 1st trimester), 356 of which were normal term deliveries (including 1 set of twins), 15 were premature, 6 were small-for-gestational age (intrauterine growth retardation [IUGR], <10th percentile), 20 had congenital anomalies (19 from mothers exposed during the 1st trimester; 4.9%), and 18 had postnatal disorders unrelated to either prematurity, low birth weight, or malformations (10). Of the remaining 135 pregnancies, there were 56 spontaneous abortions or fetal deaths (none late) (1 malformed fetus), and 79 elective abortions (4 malformed fetuses). A total of 116 (all involving ciprofloxacin) prospective cases were obtained from a manufacturer's registry (8). Among these, there were 91 live-born infants, 6 of whom had malformations. Of the remaining 25 pregnancies, 15 were terminated (no malformations reported), and 10 aborted spontaneously (1 embryo with acardia, no data available on a possible twin). Thus, of the 666 cases with known outcomes, 32 (4.8%) of the embryos, fetuses, or newborns had congenital malformations. From previous epidemiologic data, the authors concluded that the 4.8% frequency of malformations did not exceed the background rate (10). Finally, 25 retrospective reports of infants with anomalies, who had been exposed *in utero* to fluoroquinolones, were analyzed, but no specific patterns of major congenital malformations were detected.

The defects observed in 12 infants followed up prospectively and in 16 infants reported retrospectively who were exposed to norfloxacin were (10):

Source: Prospective ENTIS

Trisomy 18, heart defect
Diastasis recti, mild hypospadias
Patient ductus arteriosus (term)
Central nervous system calcification, cataract
Urogenital malformation (no uterus and gonad)
Fossa posterior hypoplasia
Bilateral uretero-vesical reflux, hydronephrosis
Herniation of abdominal viscera, rudimentary umbilical cord, severe kyphoscoliosis, absent diaphragma and pericardium, ectopia cordis, imperforated anus, ambiguous genitalia, urinary bladder not identifiable (pregnancy terminated)
Anencephaly (pregnancy terminated)
Trisomy 21
Unilateral cryptorchidism
Macroglossia (2nd trimester exposure) (pregnancy terminated)

Source: Retrospective Reports

1st Trimester Exposure:

Abdominal and thoracic wall defects, lungs outside of thoracic cavity, pericardium visible (pregnancy terminated)

Achondroplastic dwarfism, (pregnancy terminated)
Renal and ureteral agenesis, pulmonary hypoplasia
Supraumbilical hernia
Intestinal cystic duplication
Ventricular septal defect
Penoscrotal hypospadias

2nd Trimester Exposure:
Dysplastic hips
Hypertelorism, cryptorchism, small penis, short thorax, heart valves dysplasia
Urachal abnormality

3rd trimester exposure:
Microretrognathia
Two nevi, 4 × 2 and 2 × 2 cm
Talipes valgus
Hands and feet syndactyly
Trisomy 21
Short limbs (possibly familial)

The authors of the above study concluded that pregnancy exposure to quinolones was not an indication for termination, but that this class of antibacterials should still be considered contraindicated in pregnant women (10). Moreover, this study did not address the issue of cartilage damage from quinolone exposure and the authors recognized the need for follow-up studies of this potential toxicity in children exposed *in utero*. Because of their own and previously published findings, they further recommended that the focus of future studies should be on malformations involving the abdominal wall and urogenital system, and on limb reduction defects.

In a surveillance study of Michigan Medicaid recipients conducted between 1985 and 1992 involving 229,101 completed pregnancies, 139 newborns had been exposed to norfloxacin, 79 during the 1st trimester (F. Rosa, personal communication, FDA, 1994). Five (6.3%) major birth defects were observed (three expected), one of which was a brain defect that occurred in an infant whose mother consumed the drug after the 1st trimester. Details of the remaining cases were not available, but none of the abnormalities was included in seven other categories of defects (cardiovascular defects, oral clefts, spina bifida, polydactyly, limb-reduction defects, hypospadias, and eye defects) for which specific data were available.

A 1998 prospective multi-center study reported the pregnancy outcomes of 200 women exposed to fluoroquinolones compared to 200 matched controls (11). Subjects were pregnant women who had called one of four teratogen information services concerning their exposure to fluoroquinolones. The agents, number of subjects, and daily doses were ciprofloxacin ($N = 105$; 500–1000 mg), norfloxacin ($N = 93$; 400–800 mg), and ofloxacin ($N = 2$; 200–400 mg). The most common infections involved the urinary tract (69.4%) or the respiratory tract (24%). The fewer live births in the fluoroquinolone group (173 vs. 188, $p = 0.02$) were attributable to the greater number of spontaneous abortions (18 vs. 10, $p = 0.17$) and induced abortions (9 vs. 2, $p = 0.06$). There were no differences between the groups in terms of premature birth, fetal distress, method of delivery, low birth weight (<2500 g), or birth weight. Among the live-born infants exposed during organogenesis, major malformations were observed in 3 infants of 133 subjects and 5 of 188 controls ($p = 0.54$). The defects in subject infants were two cases of ventricular septal defect and one case of patent ductus arteriosus, whereas those in controls were two cases of ventricular septal defect, one case of atrial septal defect with pulmonic valve stenosis, one case of hypospadias, and one case of displaced hip. There were also no differences between the children of the groups in gross motor development milestone achievements (musculoskeletal functions: lifting, sitting, crawling, standing, or walking) as measured by the Denver Developmental Scale (11).

In summary, the use of norfloxacin during human gestation does not appear to be associated with an increased risk of major congenital malformations. Although a number of birth defects have occurred in the offspring of women who had taken this drug during pregnancy, the lack of a pattern among the anomalies is reassuring. However, a causal relationship with some of the birth defects cannot be excluded. Because of this and the available animal data, the use of norfloxacin during pregnancy, especially during the 1st trimester, should be approached with caution. A 1993 review on the safety of fluoroquinolones concluded that these antibacterials should be avoided during pregnancy because of the difficulty in extrapolating animal mutagenicity results to humans and because interpretation of this toxicity is still controversial (12). The authors of this review were not convinced that fluoroquinolone-induced fetal cartilage damage and subsequent arthropathies were a major concern, even though this effect had been demonstrated in several animal species after administration to both pregnant and immature animals and in occasional human case reports involving children (12). Others have also concluded that fluoroquinolones should be considered contraindicated in pregnancy, because safer alternatives are usually available (10).

BREAST FEEDING SUMMARY

RECOMMENDATION: No Human Data - Probably Compatible

The administration of norfloxacin during breast-feeding is not recommended because of the potential for arthropathy and other serious toxicity in the nursing infant (5). Phototoxicity has been observed with some members of the quinolone class of drugs when exposure to excessive sunlight (i.e., ultraviolet [UV] light) has occurred (5). Well-differentiated squamous cell carcinomas of the skin have been produced in mice who were exposed chronically to some quinolones and periodic UV light (e.g., see Lomefloxacin), but studies to evaluate the carcinogenicity of norfloxacin in this manner have not been conducted.

The manufacturer reports that the drug was not detected in milk following a single 200-mg oral dose administered to nursing mothers (5). However, this dose is one fourth of the normal recommended daily dose and, thus, may not be indicative of excretion after normal use. Similarly, a 1991 review cited a study that the antibacterial was undetectable in milk, but no details on dosage were given (13).

In a study published in 1994, lactating ewes were administered a single IV dose of norfloxacin (25 mg/kg) during nursing (14). Milk concentrations of the antibacterial agent were up to 40 times higher than corresponding serum levels, and therapeutic levels were measured in the serum of suckling lambs.

Although it is not known whether norfloxacin is excreted into human milk, the high concentrations of the drug found in the milk of ewes, the relatively low molecular weight (about 319), and the excretion of other quinolones are evidence that the passage of norfloxacin most likely occurs. Both ciprofloxacin and ofloxacin are classified by the American Academy of Pediatrics as compatible with breast-feeding (see individual agents).

References

1. Irikura T, Imada O, Suzuki H, Abe Y. Teratological study of 1-ethyl-6-fluoro-1, 4-dihydro-4-oxo-7-(1-piperazinyl)-3-quinolinecarboxilic acid (AM-715). Kiso to Rinsho 1981;15:5251–63. As cited in Shepard TH. *Catalog of Teratogenic Agents*. 7th ed. Baltimore, MD: Johns Hopkins University Press, 1992:290.
2. Irikura T, Suzuki H, Sugimoto T. Reproductive studies of AM-715. Chemotherapy 1981:29:886–94, 895–914, 915–31. As cited in Shepard TH. *Catalog of Teratogenic Agents*. 7th ed. Baltimore, MD: Johns Hopkins University Press, 1992:290.
3. Cukierski MA, Prahalada S, Zacchei AG, Peter CP, Rodgers JD, Hess DL, Cukierski MJ, Tarantal AF, Nyland T, Robertson RT, Hendrickx AG. Embryotoxicity studies of norfloxacin in cynomolgus monkeys. I. Teratology studies and norfloxacin plasma concentrations in pregnant and nonpregnant monkeys. Teratology 1989;39:39–52. As cited in Shepard TH. *Catalog of Teratogenic Agents*. 7th ed. Baltimore, MD: Johns Hopkins University Press, 1992:290.
4. Cukierski MA, Hendrickx AG, Prahalada S, Tarantal AF, Hess DL, Lasley BL, Peter CP, Tarara R, Robertson RT. Embryotoxicity studies of norfloxacin in cynomolgus monkeys. II. Role of progesterone. Teratology 1992;46:429–38.
5. Product information. Noroxin. Merck & Company, 1997.
6. Pino A, Maura A, Villa F, Masciangelo L. Evaluation of DNA damage induced by norfloxacin in liver and kidney of adult rats and in fetal tissues after transplacental exposure. Mutat Res Lett 1991;264:81–5.
7. Maura A, Pino A. Induction of sperm abnormalities in mice by norfloxacin. Mutat Res Lett 1991;264: 197–200.
8. Berkovitch M, Pastuszak A, Gazarian M, Lewis M, Koren G. Safety of the new quinolones in pregnancy. Obstet Gynecol 1994;84:535–8.
9. Pastuszak A, Andreou R, Schick B, Sage S, Cook L, Donnenfeld A, Koren G. New postmarketing surveillance data supports a lack of association between quinolone use in pregnancy and fetal and neonatal complications. Reprod Toxicol 1995;9:584.
10. Schaefer C, Amoura-Elefant E, Vial T, Ornoy A, Garbis H, Robert E, Rodriguez-Pinilla E, Pexieder T, Prapas N, Merlob P. Pregnancy outcome after prenatal quinolone exposure. Evaluation of a case registry of the European Network of Teratology Information Services (ENTIS). Eur J Obstet Gynecol Reprod Biol 1996;69:83–9.
11. Loebstein R, Addis A, Ho E, Andreou R, Sage S, Donnenfeld AE, Schick B, Bonati M, Mortetti M, Lalkin A, Pastuszak A, Koren G. Pregnancy outcome following gestational exposure to fluoroquinolones: a multicenter prospective controlled study. Antimicrob Agents Chemother 1998;42:1336–9.
12. Norrby SR, Lietman PS. Safety and tolerability of fluoroquinolones. Drugs 1993;45(Suppl 3): 59–64.
13. Takase Z, Shirafuji H, Uchida M. Basic and clinical studies of AM-715 in the field of obstetrics and gynecology. Chemotherapy (Tokyo) 1981;29(Suppl 4): 697–704. As cited by Anderson PO. Drug use during breast-feeding. Clin Pharmacol 1991;10:594–624.
14. Soback S, Gips M, Bialer M, Bor A. Effect of lactation on single-dose pharmacokinetics of norfloxacin nicotinate in ewes. Antimicrob Agents Chemother 1994;38:2336–9.

Name:	NORGESTREL	Risk Factor:	X_M
Class:	**Progestogenic Hormone**		

Norgestrel is commonly used as an oral contraceptive either alone or in combination with estrogens (see Oral Contraceptives).

Name:	NORTRIPTYLINE	Risk Factor:	C
Class:	**Antidepressant**		

FETAL RISK SUMMARY

RECOMMENDATION: Human Data Suggest Low Risk

Nortriptyline is a tricyclic antidepressant. Limb reduction anomalies have been reported with nortriptyline (1,2). However, one of these children was not exposed until after the critical period for limb development (3). The second infant was also exposed to sulfamethizole and heavy cigarette smoking (1). Evaluation of data from 86 patients with 1st trimester exposure to amitriptyline, the active precursor of nortriptyline, does not support the drug as a major cause of congenital limb deformities (see Amitriptyline). Urinary retention in the neonate has been associated with maternal use of nortriptyline (4).

In a surveillance study of Michigan Medicaid recipients conducted between 1985 and 1992 involving 229,101 completed pregnancies, 61 newborns had been exposed to nortriptyline during the 1st trimester (F. Rosa, personal communication, FDA, 1993). Two (3.3%) major birth defects were observed (two expected), both cardiovascular anomalies (0.5 expected).

In a 1996 descriptive case series, the European Network of the Teratology Information Services (ENTIS) prospectively examined the outcomes of 689 pregnancies exposed to antidepressants (5). Multiple drug therapy occurred in about two-thirds of the mothers. There were four exposures to nortriptyline. The outcomes of these pregnancies were four normal newborns (one premature) without birth defects (5).

A 2002 prospective study compared two groups of mother–child pairs exposed to antidepressants throughout gestation (46 exposed to tricyclics: 3 to nortriptyline; 40 to fluoxetine) to 36 nonexposed, not depressed controls (6). Offspring were studied between the ages 15 and 71 months for effects of antidepressant exposure in terms of IQ, language, behavior, and temperament. Exposure to antidepressants did not adversely affect the measured parameters, but IQ was significantly and negatively associated with the duration of depression, and language was negatively associated with the number of depression episodes after delivery (6).

BREAST FEEDING SUMMARY

RECOMMENDATION: Limited Human Data - Potential Toxicity

Nortriptyline is excreted into breast milk in low concentrations (7–11). A milk level in one patient was 59 ng/mL, representing a milk:serum ratio of 0.7 (8). A second patient was treated with nortriptyline, 100 mg daily, during the 2nd and 3rd trimesters, then stopped 2 weeks before an elective cesarean section (10). Treatment was restarted at 125 mg every night on the 1st postpartum day, then decreased to 75 mg nightly over the next 7 weeks. The mother was also receiving flupenthixol. Milk concentrations of nortriptyline, measured 11–13.5 hours after a dose on postpartum days 6 (four samples), 20 (two samples), and 48 (two samples), ranged from 90 to 404 ng/mL, mean 230 ng/mL. The milk:serum ratios for these samples ranged from 0.87 to 3.71 (mean 1.62). No effects of the drug exposure were observed in the nursing infant, who had normal motor development for the first 4 months. Infant serum concentrations were not determined (10).

Nortriptyline was not detected in the serum of other breast-fed infants when their mothers were taking the drug (8,9,11); however, low levels (5–11 ng/mL) of the metabolite, 10-hydroxynortriptyline, were measured in the serum of two infants in one study (11). In this latter study, no evidence of accumulation in nursing infants after long-term (e.g., >50 days) maternal use of the antidepressant was observed (11). A 1996 review of antidepressant treatment during breast-feeding found no information that nortriptyline exposure during nursing resulted in quantifiable amounts of the parent compound in an infant or that the exposure caused adverse effects (12).

The significance of chronic exposure of the nursing infant to the antidepressant is unknown, but concern has been expressed about the effects of long-term exposure on the infant's neurobehavioral mechanisms (10). The American Academy of Pediatrics classifies nortriptyline as a drug for which the effect on nursing infants is unknown but may be of concern (13).

References

1. Bourke GM. Antidepressant teratogenicity? Lancet 1974;1:98.
2. McBride WG. Limb deformities associated with iminobenzyl hydrochloride. Med J Aust 1972;1:492.
3. Australian Drug Evaluation Committee. Tricyclic antidepressants and limb reduction deformities. Med J Aust 1973;1:768–9.
4. Shearer WT, Schreiner RL, Marshall RE. Urinary retention in a neonate secondary to maternal ingestion of nortriptyline. J Pediatr 1972;81:570–2.
5. McElhatton PR, Garbis HM, Elefant E, Vial T, Bellemin B, Mastroiacovo P, Arnon J, Rodriguez-Pinilla E, Schaefer C, Pexieder T, Merlob P, Dal Verme S. The outcome of pregnancy in 689 women exposed to therapeutic doses of antidepressants. A collaborative study of the European Network of Teratology Information Services (ENTIS). Reprod Toxicol 1996;10:285–94.
6. Nulman I, Rovet J, Stewart DE, Wolpin J, Pace-Asciak P, Shuhaiber S, Koren G. Child development following exposure to tricyclic antidepressants or fluoxetine throughout fetal life: a prospective, controlled study. Am J Psychiatry 2002;159:1889–95.
7. Bader TF, Newman K. Amitriptyline in human breast milk and the nursing infant's serum. Am J Psychiatry 1980;137:855–6.
8. Erickson SH, Smith GH, Heidrich F. Tricyclics and breast feeding. Am J Psychiatry 1979;136:1483.
9. Brixen-Rasmussen L, Halgrener J, Jorgensen A. Amitriptyline and nortriptyline excretion in human breast milk. Psychopharmacology (Berlin) 1982;76:94–5.
10. Matheson I, Skjaeraasen J. Milk concentrations of flupenthixol, nortriptyline and zuclopenthixol and between-breast differences in two patients. Eur J Clin Pharmacol 1988;35;217–20.
11. Wisner KL, Perel JM. Serum nortriptyline levels in nursing mothers and their infants. Am J Psychiatry 1991;148:1234–6.
12. Wisner KL, Perel JM, Findling RL. Antidepressant treatment during breast-feeding. Am J Psychiatry 1996;153:1132–7.
13. Committee on Drugs, American Academy of Pediatrics. The transfer of drugs and other chemicals into human milk. Pediatrics 2001;108:776–89.

Name:	**NOVOBIOCIN**	Risk Factor:	**C**
Class:	**Antibiotic**		

N

FETAL RISK SUMMARY

RECOMMENDATION: Limited Human Data - No Relevant Animal Data

No reports linking the use of novobiocin with congenital defects have been located. One study listed 21 patients exposed to the drug in the 1st trimester (1). No association with malformations was found. Because novobiocin may cause jaundice due to inhibition of glucuronyl transferase, its use near term is not recommended (2).

BREAST FEEDING SUMMARY

RECOMMENDATION: Limited Human Data - Probably Compatible

Novobiocin is excreted into breast milk. Concentrations up to 7 μg/ml have been reported with milk:plasma ratios of 0.10.25 (3,4). Although adverse effects have not been reported, three potential problems exist for the nursing infant: modification of bowel flora, direct effects on the infant, and interference with the interpretation of culture results if a fever workup is required.

References

1. Heinonen OP, Slone D, Shapiro S. *Birth Defects and Drugs in Pregnancy*. Littleton, MA: Publishing Sciences Group, 1977:297, 301.
2. Weistein L. Antibiotics. IV. Miscellaneous antimicrobial, antifungal, and antiviral agents. In Goodman LS, Gilman A, eds. *The Pharmacological Basis of Therapeutics*. 4th ed. New York, NY: Macmillan, 1970: 1292.
3. Knowles JA. Excretion of drugs in milk—a review. J Pediatr 1965;66:1068–82.
4. Anderson PO. Drugs and breast feeding—a review. Drug Intell Clin Pharm 1977;11:208–23.

Name: **NUTMEG** Risk Factor: **C**
Class: **Herb**

FETAL RISK SUMMARY

RECOMMENDATION: Compatible

Nutmeg, the dried aromatic seeds of the tree *Myristica fragrans*, is used as a common spice. The seeds contain a toxic chemical, myristicium that has anticholinergic properties. A 1987 case report described an accidental overdose of grated nutmeg in a pregnant woman at 30 weeks' gestation (1). The woman used 1 tablespoon of the spice (equivalent to approximately 7 g, or one whole grated nutmeg) instead of the suggested amount of 1/8 teaspoon in a recipe for cookies (1). After ingesting some of the cookies, she developed a sinus tachycardia (170 beats/minute), hypertension (170/80 mm Hg), and a sensation of impending doom, but no mydriasis. The fetal heart rate was 160–170 beats/minute with loss of long-term variability. It returned to its normal baseline of 120–140 beats/minute within 12 hours. A diagnosis of atropine-like poisoning was made based on the history and physical findings (1). Following nonspecific treatment for poisoning, the mother made an uneventful recovery and was discharged home after 24 hours. Approximately 10 weeks later, she delivered a healthy infant.

BREAST FEEDING SUMMARY

RECOMMENDATION: No Human Data - Probably Compatible

No data are available.

N

Reference

1. Lavy G. Nutmeg intoxication in pregnancy; a case report. J Reprod Med 1987;32:63–4.

Name: **NYLIDRIN** Risk Factor: **C_M**
Class: **Vasodilator**

FETAL RISK SUMMARY

RECOMMENDATION: Limited Human Data - No Relevant Animal Data

Nylidrin is a β-adrenergic receptor stimulant used as a vasodilator in the United States. The drug has been studied in Europe as a tocolytic agent for premature labor and for the treatment of hypertension in pregnancy (1–7). Systolic blood pressure is usually unchanged, with a fall in total peripheral resistance greater than the decrease in diastolic pressure (8,9). Although maternal hyperglycemia has been observed, especially in diabetic patients, this or other serious adverse effects were not reported in the above studies in mothers or in newborns.

BREAST FEEDING SUMMARY

RECOMMENDATION: No Human Data - Probably Compatible

No data are available.

References

1. Neubuser D. Comparative investigation of two inhibitors of labour (TV 399 and buphenin). Geburtshilfe Fraunheilkd 1972;32:781–6.
2. Castren O, Gummerus M, Saarikoski S. Treatment of imminent premature labour. Acta Obstet Gynecol Scand 1975;54:95–100.
3. Gummerus M. Prevention of premature birth with nylidrin and verapamil. Z Geburtshilfe Perinatol 1975; 179:261–6.
4. Wolff F, Bolte A, Berg R. Does an additional administration of acetylsalicylic acid reduce the requirement of beta mimetics in tocolytic treatment? Geburtshilfe Fraunheilkd 1981;41:293–6.
5. Hofer U, Ammann K. The oral tocolytic longtime therapy and its effects on the child. Ther Umsch 1978;35:417–21.
6. Retzke VU, Schwarz R, Lanckner W, During R. Dilatol for hypertension therapy in pregnancy. Zentralbl Gynaekol 1979;101:1034–8.
7. During VR, Mauch I. Effects of nylidrin (Dilatol) on blood pressure of hypertensive patients in advanced pregnancy. Zentralbl Gynaekol 1980;102:193–8.
8. Retzke VU, Schwarz R, Barten G. Cardiovascular effects of nylidrin (Dilatol) in pregnancy. Zentralbl Gynaekol 1976;98:1059–65.
9. During VR, Reincke R. Action of nylidrin (Dilatol) on utero-placental blood supply. Zentralbl Gynaekol 1981;103:214–9.

Name:	**NYSTATIN**	Risk Factor:	C_M
Class:	**Antifungal Antibiotic**		

N

FETAL RISK SUMMARY

RECOMMENDATION: Compatible

Nystatin is poorly absorbed after oral administration and from intact skin and mucous membranes. Animal studies have not been conducted with this antifungal agent.

The Collaborative Perinatal Project found a possible association with congenital malformations after 142 1st trimester exposures, but this was probably related to its use as an adjunct to tetracycline therapy (1, p. 313). No association was found following 230 exposures anytime in pregnancy (1, p. 435). Other investigators have reported its safe use in pregnancy (2–5).

In a surveillance study of Michigan Medicaid recipients conducted between 1985 and 1992 involving 229,101 completed pregnancies, 489 newborns had been exposed to nystatin during the 1st trimester (F. Rosa, personal communication, FDA, 1993). A total of 20 (4.1%) major birth defects were observed (21 expected). Specific data were available for six defect categories, including (observed/expected) 3/5 cardiovascular defects, 1/1 oral clefts, 0/0 spina bifida, 1/1 polydactyly, 1/1 limb reduction defects, and 2/1 hypospadias. These data do not support an association between the drug and congenital defects.

BREAST FEEDING SUMMARY

RECOMMENDATION: Compatible

Because nystatin is poorly absorbed, if at all, serum and milk levels would not occur.

References

1. Heinonen OP, Slone D, Shapiro S. *Birth Defects and Drugs in Pregnancy*. Littleton, MA: Publishing Sciences Group, 1977.
2. Culbertson C. Monistat: a new fungicide for treatment of vulvovaginal candidiasis. Am J Obstet Gynecol 1974;120:973–6.
3. David JE, Frudenfeld JH, Goddard JL. Comparative evaluation of Monistat and Mycostatin in the treatment of vulvovaginal candidiasis. Obstet Gynecol 1974;44: 403–6.
4. Wallenburg HCS, Wladimiroff JW. Recurrence of vulvovaginal candidosis during pregnancy. Comparison of miconazole vs nystatin treatment. Obstet Gynecol 1976;48:491–4.
5. Rosa FW, Baum C, Shaw M. Pregnancy outcomes after first-trimester vaginitis drug therapy. Obstet Gynecol 1987;69:751–5.

N

O

Name: **OCTREOTIDE**
Class: **Miscellaneous**

Risk Factor: B_M

FETAL RISK SUMMARY

RECOMMENDATION: Limited Human Data - Animal Data Suggest Low Risk

This cyclic octapeptide (Octreotide; SMS-201-995), an analogue of the natural hormone, somatostatin, is used to reduce blood levels of growth hormone and somatomedin C in patients with acromegaly, and for the symptomatic treatment of patients with profuse watery diarrhea as a result of metastatic carcinoid tumors or vasoactive intestinal peptide-secreting tumors. It has also been used to reduce insulin requirements for patients with diabetes mellitus; to reduce output from gastrointestinal, enteric, and pancreatic fistulas; in the treatment of variceal bleeding; and for various other indications.

No evidence of impaired fertility, teratogenicity, or fetal harm was observed in pregnant rats and rabbits given up to 16 times the highest human dose based on body surface area (1).

Octreotide crosses the human placenta to the fetus (2,3). A 31-year-old infertile woman was treated with octreotide 300 μg/day for hyperthyroidism induced by a thyroid stimulating hormone (TSH)-secreting macroadenoma (2,3). The patient became euthyroid, with return of normal menstruation, after 3 months of therapy. She was found to be pregnant 1 month later and octreotide treatment was stopped. Because her symptoms recurred, therapy was reinstated at 6 months' gestation and continued until an elective cesarean section at 8 months' gestation delivered a normal infant (weight 3300 g, length 51 cm, sex not specified). The concentration of octreotide in umbilical cord serum at delivery was 359 pg/mL compared with the mean maternal level (measured on two different occasions 1 month earlier) of 890 pg/mL (range 764–1191 pg/mL) (2). Although the amount of drug in the newborn was only about 40% that in the mother, the authors concluded that octreotide crossed the placenta by passive diffusion for two reasons (3). First, only the unbound fraction of octreotide is available for placental transfer and, second, the drug is 60%–65% bound to maternal lipoprotein. Thus, assuming that the mother's concentration had not changed significantly, the unbound maternal fraction and the infant's serum level were close to unity. Subsequently, the concentration of octreotide in the infant's serum decreased to 251 pg/mL at 3 hours of age and was undetectable (<20 pg/mL) when next measured (at 40 days).

The cord serum concentrations of TSH, thyroid hormones, prolactin, and growth hormone were normal at birth, at 3 hours, and at 40 and 104 days of age (3). Because the infant's pituitary–thyroid function was not affected by exposure to octreotide at these concentrations, the authors speculated that the somatostatin receptors on thyrotroph cells, as suggested by studies in animals, are not completely functional at birth (3).

The pregnancy of a previously infertile 37-year-old woman who was treated with octreotide for acromegaly during the first 8 weeks of gestation was described in a 1989 reference (4). Treatment, 100 μg SC 3 times daily, was started within approximately 4 days of conception and discontinued when pregnancy was diagnosed at 8 weeks. A healthy male infant (weight 2530 g, length 46.0 cm) was delivered by cesarean section 2 weeks before term because of the mother's age and imminent fetal asphyxia. No malformations were apparent and his subsequent development at the time of report (age not specified but estimated to be about 9 months) was normal.

A 37-year-old woman with primary amenorrhea was discovered to have acromegaly as a result of pituitary macroadenoma (5). She was treated with octreotide and bromocriptine with reappearance of her menses occurring 7 months later. Treatment with octreotide (300 μg 3 times daily) and bromocriptine (20 mg/day) was continued until a 1-month pregnancy was diagnosed approximately 7 months later. She eventually delivered, by emergency cesarean section for fetal distress, a term 3540 g, 50-cm male infant with no evidence of congenital defects. Except for requiring mechanical ventilation for 3 days because of neonatal asphyxia, his subsequent development was satisfactory.

A 1999 case report described the pregnancy of a 36-year-old woman who was treated with octreotide (240 μg/day) for a pituitary adenoma (6). The woman had clinical and laboratory signs of acromegaly. Treatment was started at 13 weeks' gestation and continued until delivery at 40 weeks' gestation of a 3288-g, normal female infant with Apgar scores of 8 and 9 at 1 and 5 minutes, respectively, who was developing normally. Cord concentrations of growth hormone, thyrotropin, and prolactin were within normal limits.

In another 1999 case report, a 27-year-old woman with acromegaly was treated throughout the 1st trimester of an unknown pregnancy with SC octreotide (7). At 4 months of pregnancy, she received a continuous infusion of octreotide immediately before surgical resection of the tumor. Postoperative treatment consisted of hydrocortisone, thyroxine, and bromocriptine. Pregnancy was diagnosed at 6 months and at 39 weeks, she delivered a 3780-g healthy, female infant who was doing well (7).

In summary, octreotide is not teratogenic or toxic in two animal species, but published reports have described only five women who were treated during portions of their pregnancies. Although all of the outcomes were normal, the data are too limited to assess the human embryo/fetal risk. The drug crosses the placenta to the fetus and has been measured in the newborn.

O

BREAST FEEDING SUMMARY

RECOMMENDATION: No Human Data - Probably Compatible

It is not known whether octreotide is transferred to breast milk, but this should be expected because of the documented placental passage. No reports have been located that described the use of this agent during lactation. However, because of probable digestion following oral therapy, the risk to the nursing infant appears to be nonexistent.

References

1. Product information. Sandostatin. Novartis Pharmaceuticals, 2000.
2. Caron P, Gerbeau C, Pradayrol L. Maternal-fetal transfer of octreotide. N Engl J Med 1995;333:601–2.
3. Caron P, Gerbeau C, Pradayrol L, Cimonetta C, Bayard F. Successful pregnancy in an infertile woman with a thyrotropin-secreting macroadenoma treated with somatostatin analog (octreotide). J Clin Endocrinol Metab 1996;81:1164–8.
4. Landolt AM, Schmid J, Karlsson ERC, Boerlin V. Successful pregnancy in a previously infertile woman treated with SMS-201-995 for acromegaly. N Engl J Med 1989;320:621–2.
5. Montini M, Pagani G, Gianola D, Pagani MD, Piolini R,

Camboni MG. Acromegaly and primary amenorrhea: ovulation and pregnancy induced by SMS 201-995 and bromocriptine. J Endocrinol Invest 1990;13:193.
6. Takeuchi K, Funakoshi T, Oomori S, Maruo T. Successful pregnancy in an acromegalic woman treated with octreotide. Obstet Gynecol 1999;93:848.
7. Mozas J, Ocon E, Lopez de la Torre M, Suarez AM, Miranda JA, Herruzo AJ. Successful pregnancy in a woman with acromegaly treated with somatostatin analog (octreotide) prior to surgical resection. Int J Gynecol Obstet 1999;65:71–3.

Name:	**OFLOXACIN**	Risk Factor:	C_M
Class:	**Anti-infective (Quinolone)**		

FETAL RISK SUMMARY

RECOMMENDATION: Human Data Suggest Low Risk

Ofloxacin is a synthetic, broad-spectrum antibacterial agent available in oral and parenteral formulations. As a fluoroquinolone, it is in the same class as ciprofloxacin, enoxacin, lomefloxacin, norfloxacin, and sparfloxacin.

A study published in 1986 observed no ofloxacin-induced malformations with high doses in pregnant rats and rabbits (1). Similarly, no evidence of teratogenicity was observed in pregnant rats and rabbits at doses 11 times the recommended maximum human dose based on body surface area (RMHD) or 4 times the RMHD, respectively (2). These doses were fetotoxic, however, causing reduced birth weight, increased mortality, and, in rats only, minor skeletal variations. In rats dosed at 5 times the RMHD, no adverse effects were seen on late fetal development, labor, delivery, lactation, neonatal viability, or subsequent growth of the newborn (2).

In a study investigating the pharmacokinetics of ofloxacin, 20 pregnant women, between 19 and 25 weeks' gestation (mean 22.2 weeks), were scheduled for pregnancy termination because the fetuses were affected with β-thalassemia major (3). Two doses of ofloxacin, 400 mg IV every 12 hours, were given before abortion. Serum and amniotic fluid concentrations were determined concomitantly at 6, 10, and 12 hours after dosing. Mean maternal serum concentrations at these times were 0.68, 0.21, and 0.07 μg/mL, respectively, compared with mean amniotic fluid levels of 0.25, 0.15, and 0.13 μg/mL, respectively. The amniotic fluid:maternal serum ratios were 0.37, 0.71, and 1.86, respectively.

In a prospective follow-up study conducted by the European Network of Teratology Information Services (ENTIS), data on 549 pregnancies exposed to fluoroquinolones (93 to ofloxacin) were described in a 1996 reference (4). Data on another 116 prospective and 25 retrospective pregnancy exposures to the antibacterials were also included. From the 549 follow-up cases, 509 were treated during the 1st trimester, 22 after the 1st trimester, and in 18 cases, the exposure occurred at an unknown gestational time. The live-born infants were delivered at a mean gestational age of 39.4 $\pm$ 1.5 weeks and had a mean birth weight of 3302 $\pm$ 495 g, length of 50.3 $\pm$ 2.3 cm, and head circumference of 34.9 $\pm$ 1.5 cm. Of the 549 pregnancies, there were 415 live-born infants (390 exposed during the 1st trimester), 356 of which were normal-term deliveries (including one set of twins), 15 were premature, 6 were small-for-gestational age (intrauterine growth retardation [IUGR], <10th percentile), 20 had congenital anomalies (19 from mothers exposed during the 1st trimester; 4.9%), and 18 had postnatal disorders unrelated to either prematurity, low birth weight, or malformations (4). Of the remaining 135 pregnancies, there were 56 spontaneous abortions or fetal deaths (none late) (1 malformed fetus), and 79 elective abortions (4 malformed fetuses). A total of 116 (all involving ciprofloxacin) prospective cases were obtained from the manufacturer's registry (4). Among these, there were 91 live-born infants, 6 of whom had malformations. Of the remaining 25 pregnancies, 15 were terminated (no malformations reported), and 10 aborted spontaneously (1 embryo with acardia, no data available on a possible twin). Thus, of the 666 cases with known outcome, 32 (4.8%) of the embryos, fetuses, or newborns had congenital malformations. From previous epidemiologic data, the authors concluded that the 4.8% frequency of malformations did not exceed the background rate (4). Finally, 25 retrospective reports of infants with anomalies who had been exposed *in utero* to fluoroquinolones were analyzed, but no specific patterns of major congenital malformations were detected.

The defects observed in seven infants followed up prospectively (no ofloxacin-exposed cases among the retrospective reports), all exposed to ofloxacin during the 1st trimester, were as follows (4):

Source: Prospective ENTIS
Myelomeningocele, hydrocephaly
Ureterostenosis
Mal descensus testis
Hypospadias
Hernia inguinalis left side
Bilateral hip dysplasia
Small atrial septal defect

The authors of the above study concluded that pregnancy exposure to quinolones was not an indication for termination, but that this class of antibacterials should still be considered contraindicated in pregnant women (4). Moreover, this study did not address the issue of cartilage damage from quinolone exposure and the authors recognized the need for follow-up studies of this potential toxicity in children exposed *in utero*. Because of their own and previously published findings, they further recommended that the focus of future studies should be on malformations involving the abdominal wall and urogenital system, and on limb reduction defects.

A 1998 prospective multi-center study reported the pregnancy outcomes of 200 women exposed to fluoroquinolones compared to 200 matched controls (5). Subjects were pregnant women who had called one of four teratogen information services concerning their exposure to fluoroquinolones. The agents, number of subjects, and daily doses were ciprofloxacin, ($N = 105$; 500–1000 mg), norfloxacin ($N = 93$; 400–800 mg), and ofloxacin ($N = 2$; 200–400 mg). The most common infections involved the urinary tract (69.4%) or the respiratory tract (24%). The fewer live births in the fluoroquinolone group (173 vs. 188, $p = 0.02$) was attributable to the greater number of spontaneous abortions (18 vs. 10, $p = 0.17$) and induced abortions (9 vs. 2, $p = 0.06$). There were no differences between the groups in terms of premature birth, fetal distress, method of delivery, low birth weight (<2500 g), or birth weight. Among the live-born infants exposed during organogenesis, major malformations were observed in 3 infants of 133 subjects and 5 of 188 controls ($p = 0.54$). The defects in subject infants were two cases of ventricular septal defect and one case of patent ductus arteriosus, whereas those in controls were two cases of ventricular septal defect, one case of atrial septal defect with pulmonic valve stenosis, one case of hypospadias, and one case of displaced hip. There were also no differences between the children of the groups in gross motor development milestone achievements (musculoskeletal functions: lifting, sitting, crawling, standing, or walking) as measured by the Denver Developmental Scale (5).

In summary, the use of ofloxacin during human gestation does not appear to be associated with an increased risk of major congenital malformations. Although a number of birth defects have occurred in the offspring of women who had taken this drug during pregnancy, the lack of a pattern among the anomalies is reassuring. However, a causal relationship with some of the birth defects cannot be excluded. Because of this and the available animal data, the use of ofloxacin during pregnancy, especially during the 1st trimester, should be approached with caution. A 1993 review on the safety of fluoroquinolones concluded that these antibacterials should be avoided during pregnancy because of the difficulty in extrapolating animal mutagenicity results to humans and because interpretation of this toxicity is still controversial (6). The authors of this review were not convinced that fluoroquinolone-induced fetal cartilage damage and subsequent arthropathies were a major concern, even though this effect had been demonstrated in several animal species after administration to both pregnant and immature animals and in occasional human case reports involving children (6). Others have also concluded that fluoroquinolones should be considered contraindicated in pregnancy, because safer alternatives are usually available (4).

BREAST FEEDING SUMMARY

RECOMMENDATION: Limited Human Data - Probably Compatible

When ofloxacin was first marketed, its use during lactation was not recommended because of the potential for arthropathy and other serious toxicity in the nursing infant (2). Phototoxicity has been observed with quinolones when exposure to excessive sunlight (i.e., ultraviolet [UV] light) has occurred (2). Well-differentiated squamous cell carcinomas of the skin has been produced in mice who were exposed chronically to some fluoroquinolones and periodic UV light (e.g., see Lomefloxacin), but studies to evaluate the carcinogenicity of ofloxacin in this manner have not been conducted.

O

Ofloxacin is excreted into breast milk in concentrations approximately equal to those in maternal serum (2,3). Ten lactating women were given three oral doses of ofloxacin, 400 mg each (3). Six simultaneous serum and milk samples were drawn between 2 and 24 hours after the third dose of the antibiotic. The mean peak serum level occurred at 2 hours (2.45 μg/mL), then steadily fell to 0.03 μg/mL at 24 hours. Milk concentrations exhibited a similar pattern, with a mean peak level measured at 2 hours (2.41 μg/mL), and the lowest amount at 24 hours (0.05 μg/mL). The mean milk:serum ratio varied from 0.98 to 1.66, with the highest ratio occurring 24 hours after the last dose. The manufacturer reports that following a single 200-mg dose, milk and serum concentrations of ofloxacin were similar (2).

The American Academy of Pediatrics classifies ofloxacin as compatible with breastfeeding (7).

References

1. Takayama S, Watanabe T, Akiyama Y, Ohura K, Harada S, Matsuhashi K, Mochida K, Yamashita N. Reproductive toxicity of ofloxacin. Arzneim Forsch 1986;36:1244–8. As cited in Shepard TH. *Catalog of Teratogenic Agents*. 7th ed. Baltimore, MD: Johns Hopkins University Press, 1992:296.
2. Product information. Floxin. Ortho-McNeil Pharmaceutical, 2000.
3. Giamarellou H, Kolokythas E, Petrikkos G, Gazis J, Aravantinos D, Sfikakis P. Pharmacokinetics of three newer quinolones in pregnant and lactating women. Am J Med 1989;87(Suppl 5A):49S–51S.
4. Schaefer C, Amoura-Elefant E, Vial T, Ornoy A, Garbis H, Robert E, Rodriguez-Pinilla E, Pexieder T, Prapas N, Merlob P. Pregnancy outcome after prenatal quinolone exposure. Evaluation of a case registry of the European Network of Teratology Information Services (ENTIS). Eur J Obstet Gynecol Reprod Biol 1996;69:83–9.

5. Loebstein R, Addis A, Ho E, Andreou R, Sage S, Donnenfeld AE, Schick B, Bonati M, Mortetti M, Lalkin A, Pastuszak A, Koren G. Pregnancy outcome following gestational exposure to fluoroquinolones: a multicenter prospective controlled study. Antimicrob Ag Chemother 1998;42:1336–9.
6. Norrby SR, Lietman PS. Safety and tolerability of fluoroquinolones. Drugs 1993;45(Suppl 3):59–64.
7. Committee on Drugs, American Academy of Pediatrics. The transfer of drugs and other chemicals into human milk. Pediatrics 2001;108:776–89.

Name: **OLANZAPINE**		Risk Factor: C_M
Class: **Antipsychotic**		

FETAL RISK SUMMARY

RECOMMENDATION: Human Data Suggest Low Risk

Olanzapine, a thienobenzodiazepine-class psychotropic agent, is indicated for the management of schizophrenia and bipolar mania. The mechanism of action for either indication is unknown but may involve a combination of dopamine and serotonin type 2 ($5HT_2$) antagonism in the management of schizophrenia. The drug has a relatively long elimination half-life (mean 30 hours, range 21–54 hours) (1). The long half-life is partially a result of extensive protein binding to albumin (90%) and to α_1-acid glycoprotein (77%) (2).

In reproductive studies in rats and rabbits, no evidence of teratogenicity was observed at doses up to 9 and 30 times the maximum recommended human dose based on body surface area (MRHD), respectively (1). In rats, early resorption and increased numbers of nonviable fetuses were observed at 9 times the MRHD. In addition, prolonged gestations were noted at 5 times the MRHD. In rabbits administered a maternal toxic dose (30 times the MRHD), increased resorptions and decreased fetal weight were indications of fetotoxicity (1).

Olanzapine and/or its metabolites cross the rat placenta (1,3). Consistent with the low molecular weight (about 312), an *in vitro* experiment demonstrated that olanzapine also crosses the human placenta. In a 1999 study that used a near-term human placenta-perfused single cotyledon system, up to 14% of [^{14}C]-olanzapine crossed from the maternal to the fetal compartment over 4 hours (2). The initial concentration (10 ng/mL) was equal to the peak human plasma concentration observed after a 10-mg dose. Although no placental oxidative metabolites were found, the glucuronide metabolite did cross the placenta, but at a slightly slower rate than that of the parent drug (2).

In its product information, the manufacturer reported seven pregnancies exposed to olanzapine during clinical trials (1). The outcomes of these pregnancies were one spontaneous abortion, three elective abortions, one neonatal death due to a cardiovascular defect (no specific data given), and two normal births.

A 2000 report expanded the above database, describing the outcomes of 37 prospectively identified pregnancies that had been exposed to olanzapine during clinical trials (4). The mean daily maternal dose, in 30 of these pregnancies, was 12.9 mg (range 5–25 mg/day; median dose 10 mg/day). There were 3 spontaneous abortions (SABs), 13 elective abortions, and 1 ectopic pregnancy that was aborted. There was one stillbirth at 37 weeks' gestation after premature rupture of the membranes. This pregnancy, exposed to an unknown dose in the 2nd and 3rd trimesters, had been complicated by gestational diabetes, thrombocytopenia, hepatitis, and polydrug abuse. In 19 pregnancies, there were 16 normal newborns without complications (exposure times: 8 in 1st trimester, 1 in 1st and 2nd trimesters, 6 throughout gestation, and 1 unknown exposure time). Among the remaining three outcomes, one infant exposed *in utero* to 20 mg/day was delivered by cesarean section at 30 weeks. The birth weight and length were 2.13 kg and 40 cm. The pregnancy had been complicated by gestational diabetes, hypothyroidism, preeclampsia, and abnormal liver enzymes. The infant recovered from respiratory distress and hypoglycemia after 2 weeks of therapy. A second infant, whose mother had taken 10 mg/day throughout gestation, was delivered 10 days after term because of fetal distress (birth weight 3.66 kg). The neonatal examination was normal. Finally, one infant, exposed only during the 1st trimester to an unknown dose, had meconium aspiration after a cesarean section for postmaturity. The eventually neonatal outcome of this case was not given. No congenital malformations were observed in the 19 newborns (4).

In addition to the prospective cases, the above report also described the outcomes of 11 retrospectively identified olanzapine-exposed pregnancies (4). Although retrospective reports are considered to be biased, they are useful as early indicators of fetal risks if a cluster of defects or abnormalities is observed. The results of these pregnancies were as follows: SABs (2 cases; 1st trimester, dose unknown); fetal death (olanzapine and risperidone overdose, timing and doses unknown); unilateral dysplastic kidney (1st trimester, dose unknown); and Down's syndrome (timing and dose unknown). The case of unilateral dysplastic kidney does not appear to be related to the drug exposure. Most likely, a chemical insult during development would have produced bilateral kidney damage (4). Three infant complications also are worth noting, but their relationship to olanzapine is unknown: (a) cardiomegaly, jaundice, somnolence, heart murmur (1st and 3rd trimesters, 5 mg/day); (b) convulsion at 12 days of age (1st and 3rd trimesters, 20 mg/day; electroencephalogram and laboratory tests were normal); and (c) heart murmur, sudden infant death at 2 months of age (throughout gestation, 10 mg/day) (4).

In a 2002 reference, the authors briefly reported the outcomes of 96 olanzapine-exposed pregnancies in a further expansion of the above prospective case registry (5). The new material was based on a 2001 written communication with the manufacturer. The outcomes included 69 normal births, 12 SABs, 3 stillbirths, 2 premature births, 7 perinatal complications, and 1 major malformation. Neither the perinatal complications nor the malformation was detailed (5).

Another report of olanzapine use in human pregnancy appeared in 2000 (6). A 40-year-old obese woman with a 24-year complicated history of schizophrenia and chronic hypertension was treated throughout pregnancy with olanzapine. During the first month she received 20 mg/day and then, because of sedation, 15 mg/day for the remainder of gestation. Her mental disease was stable throughout, but pregnancy was complicated by excessive weight gain (79 lb; 35.9 kg), gestational diabetes, and severe preeclampsia (hypertension, proteinuria, and elevated liver function tests). Because of worsening preeclampsia, a cesarean section was performed at 30 weeks' gestation to deliver a 4 lb, 11 oz (about 2128 g) viable female infant. Apgar scores were 7 and 9 at 1 and 5 minutes, respectively. No other information on the infant was provided (6).

A 31-year-old woman with paranoid schizophrenia was treated with olanzapine (10 mg/day) from the 2nd trimester until delivery and then continued during breast-feeding (7). The patient was hospitalized for treatment of a psychotic episode in the 18th gestational week, and olanzapine was started at this time. Hospitalization was continued for over 3 months. A normal 3190-g female infant was born at term with Apgar scores of 9, 10, and 10 at 1, 5, and 10 minutes, respectively. Olanzapine plasma levels in the mother and infant on the first day after delivery were 33.4 and 11.3 ng/mL. The infant was breast-fed (see Breast Feeding Summary). At 7 months of age, the infant was not able to roll from the back to the ventral position, possibly suggesting impaired motor development.

No impairment, however, was noted at 11 months. At this age, head circumference was approximately at the 50th percentile, whereas height and weight were around the 97th percentile (7).

A 2001 case report described the pregnancy of a 38-year-old woman who was treated with olanzapine, 7.5 mg/day, for maintenance treatment of schizoaffective disorder (8). She took the drug throughout a 38-week pregnancy, eventually delivering a 3883-g female infant by cesarean section. Apgar scores were 9 and 9 at 1 and 5 minutes, respectively. The infant's length and head circumference were 21.75 and 14.75 inches, respectively. No abnormalities were noted. The mother, who was advised not to breast-feed, required a dose increase to 12.5 mg/day after delivery. The infant's growth was described as normal with weights at 6, 18, and 24 months of age of 6.8 kg (25th percentile), 10.4 kg (50th percentile), and 12.2 kg (75th percentile), respectively. No other measurements were available. She was doing well at age 26 months (8).

A post-marketing surveillance study of olanzapine that was conducted in England identified 18 pregnancies; 11 of these pregnant women took the drug in the 1st trimester and 3 during the 2nd/3rd trimesters (9). The outcomes were 11 live births, 2 SABs, 3 elective abortions, and 1 unknown outcome. In another case, exposure to the drug was uncertain. One of the elective abortions was for a fetus with a lumbar myelomeningocele (9).

A 37-year-old woman with paranoid schizophrenia was started on olanzapine in the 8th week of gestation (10). She had not received antipsychotics for 3 months prior to this time. Her daily dose was titrated to 25 mg over the next 3 months. She discontinued therapy against medical advice at 32 weeks' because she felt well. She remained well and eventually delivered a healthy 3-kg male infant by cesarean section at 39 weeks' gestation. The Apgar scores were 9 and 10 at 1 and 5 minutes, respectively (10).

Concern that switching a patient from typical neuroleptics (e.g., fluphenazine) to an atypical agent, such as olanzapine, may result in pregnancy was expressed in a brief 1998 communication (11). An unmarried 41-year-old woman with a 22-year history of schizophrenia, paranoid type, and bipolar disorder had been unsuccessfully treated with multiple agents. Her regimen, immediately prior to olanzapine, was depot fluphenazine decanoate (75 mg IM every 2 weeks) and carbamazepine (400 mg/day). Because she remained chronically delusional and thought disordered, her regimen was changed to olanzapine, eventually reaching a maintenance dose of 12.5 mg/day. An 8-week pregnancy was diagnosed 14 weeks after the start of olanzapine. An elective abortion was performed at the patient's request. The authors attributed the pregnancy to a normalization of prolactin levels, such as that observed with clozapine, another atypical neuroleptic (11). However, the manufacturer states that hyperprolactinemia does occur with olanzapine and that a modest elevation of prolactin levels persists during chronic therapy (1).

A 27-year-old woman at 24 weeks' gestation was started on olanzapine when she developed a recurrence of her psychosis (12). The initial dose of 2.5 mg/day had to be gradually increased to 20 mg/day to control her symptoms. After 1 month at 20 mg/day, her dose was tapered over a period of 8 weeks and then discontinued 10 days before delivery. At term, she delivered a 2.9-kg male infant with Apgar scores of 8 and 9 at 1 and 5 minutes, respectively. The infant was growing and developing normally at 3 months of age (12).

In summary, olanzapine is not an animal teratogen in two species, but dose-related embryo and fetal toxicity were observed. Although no structural congenital malformations attributable to olanzapine have been reported in humans, the number of exposures is too low to assess the fetal risk. One inadvertent pregnancy was attributed to olanzapine-induced normalization of prolactin levels, but the opposite effect (i.e., hyperprolactinemia) is reported by the manufacturer. More study of this potential concern is warranted. Because olanzapine is indicated for severe debilitating mental disease, the benefits to the mother probably outweigh the potential risks to the fetus. A 1996 review on the management of psychiatric illness concluded that patients with histories of chronic psychosis or severe bipolar illness represent a high-risk group (for both the mother and the fetus) and should be maintained on pharmacologic therapy before and during pregnancy (13). However, a 2000 review stated that the human pregnancy data were too limited to recommend olanzapine (14).

BREAST FEEDING SUMMARY

RECOMMENDATION: Limited Human Data - Potential Toxicity

Consistent with the molecular weight (about 312) and the prolonged elimination half-life (mean 30 hours, range 21–54 hours), olanzapine is excreted into breast milk (15-17) and the milk of lactating rats (1,3). Several reports have described the use of olanzapine in lactating women.

One mother took 5 mg/day in the 1st and 3rd trimesters and continued the drug during breast-feeding (4). The infant had cardiomegaly, jaundice, somnolence, and a heart murmur. At 7 days of age, the infant was changed to bottle-feeding, but sedation and jaundice continued. No other details were provided, but the authors stated that the continued sedation and jaundice suggested that they were not drug-induced (4). However, the elimination half-life of olanzapine in adults is prolonged and, although the neonatal half-life is unknown, it may be longer because of immature hepatic and renal function. If comparable, it would take about 4–11 days for the infant to eliminate from its system approximately 97% of the drug that was obtained during pregnancy and/or nursing. Thus, a causal relationship cannot be excluded without knowing additional information. In a second case, the mother started olanzapine 10 mg/day for paranoid schizophrenia 2 months after delivery (4). She was also taking paroxetine, trifluoperazine, and procyclidine. No adverse effects were reported in the infant.

The third case involved a woman who took olanzapine 10 mg/day throughout the second half of pregnancy and during 2 months of lactation (7). Plasma levels in the mother and infant 1 day after delivery were 33.4 and 11.3 ng/mL, respectively. The infant's level is attributable to drug acquired while *in utero*. During nursing, the mother's and infant's plasma levels were determined at 2 and 6 weeks postpartum. Maternal levels were 39.5 and 32.8 ng/mL, respectively, whereas those in the infant were <2 and <2 ng/mL, respectively. No adverse effects of this exposure were noted in the infant (see Fetal Risk Summary for development and growth measures at 11 months of age) (7).

In a 2002 study, five lactating women were started on olanzapine for postpartum psychosis (15). After 5 days of therapy, one to three paired samples per patient (nine samples) of maternal plasma and milk were drawn 11 to 23 hours after a dose. The mean milk:plasma ratio was 0.46 (range 0.2–0.84). The median infant dose was 1.6% (range 0–2.5%) of the weight-adjusted maternal dose (15). The highest milk concentrations (21 mg/L at 11 hours post-dose and 16 mg/mL at 23 hours post-dose) occurred in the woman taking the highest dose (10 mg/day). The other women were taking 2.5 mg/day, and their milk levels ranged from <1 to 8 mg/L. The olanzapine plasma level in one infant 15 hours after the mother's 2.5 mg dose was <1 μg/L. No adverse effects in the infants were observed (15).

A 2003 study reported the milk concentrations of olanzapine in seven women, two of whom started treatment during pregnancy (16). The women had been taking olanzapine a mean 114 days (range 19–395) and the mean age of the infants was 2.4 months (range 0.1–4.3). Multiple maternal plasma and milk samples were collected over 12- or 24-hour intervals. In six women, the median maternal dose was 7.5 mg/day (range 5–20) or 131.5 μg/kg (range 75–286) and the median peak plasma concentration and time post-dose were 29 μg/L (range 15–73) and 2.5 hours (1.5–4.5), respectively. The median peak drug concentration in milk occurred 5.2 hours (range 0.7–13.2) after the dose and the median concentration was 8.8 μg/L (range 1.2–22.7). The median milk-to-plasma area-under-the-curve ratio was 0.38. Olanzapine plasma levels in the infants were below the detection limit (1–5 μg/L). No adverse effects were observed or measured in the nursing infants. For the seventh woman, the milk:plasma ratio was 0.75 at 6 hours post-dose based on a single sample collection. Sedation had been noted in her infant 3 weeks before the study and her dose had been halved to 5 mg/day. Sedation was not observed in infant at the time of the study (16).

Olanzapine 20 mg/day was given to a 32-year-old woman hospitalized 9 days after delivery for a postpartum psychotic disorder (17). Although she had been breast-feeding her infant, she decided to stop nursing on admission. Serial milk samples were drawn for 10 days with olanzapine concentrations ranging from 7.6 (day 2) to 27.5 ng/mL. The milk:plasma ratio ranged from 0.35 to 0.42. If nursing had been continued, the infant would have consumed a dose that was approximately 4% of the maternal weight-adjusted dose, or about 0.011 mg/kg/day (17). Therefore, the infant exposure would have been very low.

In summary, sedation is a frequent adverse effect in adults treated with olanzapine and has occurred in nursing infants whose mothers were taking the drug. Reducing the maternal dose may eliminate this problem, but the potential effect on control of the mother's disease must be considered. The prolonged adult elimination half-life and the potential for long-term neurodevelopment toxicity in a nursing infant should be considered before olanzapine is prescribed during lactation.

References

1. Product information. Zyprexa. Eli Lilly, 2001.
2. Schenker S, Yang Y, Mattiuz E, Tatum D, Lee M. Olanzapine transfer by human placenta. Clin Exp Pharmacol Physiol 1999;26:691–7.
3. Chay SH, Herman JL. Disposition of the novel antischizophrenic drug [^{14}C] Olanzapine in male Fischer 344 and female CD rats following single oral dose administration. Arzneimittel-Forschung 1998;48:446–54.
4. Goldstein DJ, Corbin LA, Fung MC. Olanzapine-exposed pregnancies and lactation: early experience. J Clin Psychopharmacol 2000;20:399–403.
5. Ernst CL, Goldberg JF. The reproductive safety profile of mood stabilizers, atypical antipsychotics, and broad-spectrum psychotropics. J Clin Psychiatry 2002;63(Suppl 4):42–55.
6. Littrell KH, Johnson CG, Peabody CD, Hilligoss N. Antipsychotics during pregnancy. Am J Psychiatry 2000;157:1342.
7. Kirchheiner J, Berghofer A, Bolk-Weischedel D. Healthy outcome under olanzapine treatment in a pregnant woman. Pharmacopsychiatry 2000;33:78–80.
8. Malek-Ahmadi P. Olanzapine in pregnancy. Ann Pharmacother 2001;35:1294–5.
9. Biwsas PN, Wilton LV, Pearce GL, Freemantle S, Shakir SAW. The pharmacovigilance of olanzapine: results of a post-marketing surveillance study on 8858 patients in England. J Psychopharmacol 2001;15:265–71.
10. Lim LM. Olanzapine and pregnancy. Aust N Z J Psychiatry 2001;35:856–7.
11. Dickson RA, Dawson DT. Olanzapine and pregnancy. Can J Psychiatry 1998;43:196–7.
12. Mendhekar DN, War L, Sharma JB, Jiloha RC. Olanzapine and pregnancy. Pharmacopsychiatry 2002;35:122–3.
13. Altshuler LL, Cohen L, Szuba MP, Burt VK, Gitlin M, Mintz J. Pharmacologic management of psychiatric illness during pregnancy: dilemmas and guidelines. Am J Psychiatry 1996;153:592–606.
14. Committee on Drugs, American Academy of Pediatrics. Use of psychoactive medication during pregnancy and possible effects on the fetus and newborn. Pediatrics 2000;105:880–7.
15. Croke S, Buist A, Hackett LP, Ilett KF, Norman TR, Burrows GD. Olanzapine excretion in human breast milk: estimation of infant exposure. Int J Neuropsychopharmacol 2002;5:243–7.
16. Gardiner SJ, Kristensen JH, Begg EJ, Hackett LP, Wilson DA, Ilett KF, Kohan R, Rampono J. Transfer of

olanzapine into breast milk, calculation of infant drug dose, and effect on breast-fed infants. Am J Psychiatry 2003;160:1428–31.

17. Ambresin G, Berney P, Schulz P, Bryois C. Olanzapine excretion into breast milk: a case report. J Clin Psychopharmacol 2004;24:93–5.

Name: **OLEANDOMYCIN** Risk Factor: **C**
Class: **Antibiotic**

FETAL RISK SUMMARY

RECOMMENDATION: Limited Human Data - No Relevant Animal Data

No reports linking the use of oleandomycin or its triacetyl ester, troleandomycin, with congenital defects have been located. One study listed nine patients exposed to the drugs in the 1st trimester (1). No association with malformations was found.

BREAST FEEDING SUMMARY

RECOMMENDATION: No Human Data - Probably Compatible

No data are available.

Reference

1. Heinonen OP, Slone D, Shapiro S. *Birth Defects and Drugs in Pregnancy*. Littleton, MA: Publishing Sciences Group, 1977:297,301.

Name: **OLMESARTAN** Risk Factor: **C_M***
Class: **Antihypertensive**

FETAL RISK SUMMARY

RECOMMENDATION: Human Data Suggest Risk in 2nd and 3rd Trimesters

The prodrug olmesartan medoxomil is hydrolyzed to olmesartan during absorption from the gastrointestinal tract. No additional metabolism occurs. Olmesartan is a selective angiotensin II receptor antagonist that is indicated, either alone or in combination with other antihypertensive agents, for the treatment of hypertension. Olmesartan blocks the vasoconstrictor and aldosterone-secreting effects of angiotensin II by preventing angiotensin II from binding to the AT_1 receptors. Other drugs in this class include candesartan, eprosartan, irbesartan, telmisartan, and valsartan. The terminal elimination half-life is about 13 hours.

Reproductive studies with olmesartan have been conducted in rats and rabbits. No evidence of teratogenicity was observed in either species at doses up 240 and 0.5 times, respectively, the maximum recommended human dose based on body surface area (MRHD). Higher doses in rabbits could not be administered because they caused maternal death. In rats, doses equal to or greater than about 0.4 times the MRHD caused fetal toxicity (decreases in pup birth weight and weight gain). Higher doses (equal to or greater than about 2 times the MRHD) resulted in delays in developmental milestones and dose-related increases in the incidence of dilation of the renal pelvis. The no-observed effect dose for developmental toxicity was about 0.1 times the MRHD.

It is not known if olmesartan crosses the human placenta. The molecular weight (about 559) is low enough that passage to the fetus should be expected. In addition, the relatively long terminal elimination half-life will increase the time that the drug remains at the maternal-fetal placental interface.

No reports describing the use of olmesartan during human pregnancy have been located. The antihypertensive mechanisms of action of olmesartan and angiotensin converting enzyme (ACE) inhibitors are very close. That is, the former selectively blocks the binding of angiotensin II to AT_1 receptors, whereas the latter prevents the formation of angiotensin II itself. Therefore, use of this drug during the 2nd and 3rd trimesters may cause teratogenicity and severe fetal and neonatal toxicity identical to that seen with ACE inhibitors (see Captopril or Enalapril). Fetal toxic effects may include anuria, oligohydramnios, fetal hypocalvaria, intrauterine growth retardation, prematurity, and patent ductus arteriosus. Anuria-associated oligohydramnios may produce fetal limb contractures, craniofacial deformation, and pulmonary hypoplasia. Severe anuria and hypotension, resistant to both pressor agents and volume expansion, may occur in the newborn following *in utero* exposure to olmesartan. Newborn renal function and blood pressure should be closely monitored. If olmesartan is used in pregnancy, healthcare professionals are encouraged to call the toll free number (800-670-6126) for information about patient enrollment in the Motherisk study.

[**Risk Factor* D_M *if used in 2nd or 3rd trimesters.*]

BREAST FEEDING SUMMARY

RECOMMENDATION: No Human Data - Probably Compatible

No reports describing the use of olmesartan during human lactation have been located. The drug is excreted in low concentration into the milk of lactating rats (1). The molecular weight (about 559) is low enough that excretion into breast milk should be expected. The effects of this exposure on a nursing infant are unknown. The American Academy of Pediatrics, however, classifies ACE inhibitors, a closely related group of antihypertensive agents, as compatible with breast-feeding (see Captopril or Enalapril).

Reference

1. Product information. Benicar. Sankyo Pharma, 2004.

Name: **OLSALAZINE** Risk Factor: C_M
Class: **Anti-inflammatory Bowel Disease Agent**

FETAL RISK SUMMARY

RECOMMENDATION: Compatible

Olsalazine is used for the maintenance of remission of ulcerative colitis in patients who cannot tolerate sulfasalazine. It is poorly absorbed, approximately 2.4% after oral administration, with the remainder reaching the colon intact where it is converted into two molecules of 5-aminosalicylic acid (mesalamine) by colonic bacteria (1). The history, pharmacology, and pharmacokinetics of mesalamine and olsalazine were reviewed extensively in a 1992 reference (2).

Reproductive studies with olsalazine in rats have revealed reduced fetal weights, retarded ossifications, and immaturity of the fetal visceral organs with doses 5–20 times the recommended human dose on a weight basis (1). No reports describing adverse fetal effects following the use of olsalazine in human pregnancy have been located.

The use of 5-aminosalicylic acid, the active metabolite of olsalazine, in human pregnancy is discussed under Mesalamine (see Mesalamine).

BREAST FEEDING SUMMARY

RECOMMENDATION: Limited Human Data - Potential Toxicity

The active metabolite of olsalazine, 5-aminosalicylic acid (mesalamine), is excreted into human milk (see Mesalamine). In one study, however, only a metabolite of mesalamine, acetyl-5-aminosalicylic acid, was detected in breast milk after the ingestion of olsalazine (see Mesalamine) (3). Because diarrhea has occurred in a nursing infant of a mother receiving mesalamine (see Mesalamine), nursing infants of women being treated with olsalazine should be closely observed for changes in stool consistency.

References

1. Product information. Dipentum. Pharmacia & Upjohn, 2000.
2. Segars LW, Gales BJ. Mesalamine and olsalazine: 5-aminosalicylic acid agents for the treatment of inflammatory bowel disease. Clin Pharm 1992;11:514–28.
3. Miller LG, Hopkinson JM, Motil KJ, Corboy JE, Andersson S. Disposition of olsalazine and metabolites in breast milk. J Clin Pharmacol 1993;33:703–6.

Name:	**OMEPRAZOLE**	Risk Factor:	**C_M**
Class:	**Gastrointestinal Agent (Antisecretory)**		

FETAL RISK SUMMARY

RECOMMENDATION: Human Data Suggest Low Risk

The antisecretory agent, omeprazole, a proton pump inhibitor, suppresses gastric acid secretion by a direct inhibitory effect on the gastric parietal cell (1). It is used for the treatment of duodenal and gastric ulcers, erosive esophagitis, and pathologic hypersecretory conditions, such as Zollinger-Ellison syndrome.

In reproductive studies in pregnant rats and rabbits, doses up to approximately 345 and 172 times, respectively, the normal human dose produced no evidence of teratogenicity, but dose-related embryo and fetal mortality was observed (1). A dose-dependent increase in gastric cell carcinoid tumors has been observed in rats (1). The *in vitro* Ames mutagen assay was negative. Other tests for genotoxicity in mice and rats were either borderline or negative (1).

Omeprazole crosses the placenta to the fetus in sheep (2) and in humans (3). In sheep, the fetal:maternal ratio of total omeprazole, after both low and high dosage, was 0.2, but the ratio of unbound drug was 0.5 (2). Urinary clearance of the drug was low in both the mother and the fetus.

Placental passage of omeprazole in humans was demonstrated in a study published in 1989 (3). Twenty women were administered a single 80-mg oral dose of omeprazole the night before scheduled cesarean sections with a mean dosing-to-general anesthesia induction time interval of 853 minutes (range of 765–977 minutes) (3). At the time of surgery, maternal omeprazole levels ranged from 0 to 271 nmol/L. The drug concentration in 13 of the 20 infants (both arterial and venous umbilical samples were drawn in most cases) either was 0 or below the minimum detection limit (20 nmol/L). In the remaining 7 infants, omeprazole cord blood concentrations ranged from 21 to 109 nmol/L. No adverse effects attributable to the drug were observed either at birth or at follow-up in 7 days.

The FDA has received reports following pregnancy exposure to omeprazole, of 11 specified birth defects, 4 of which were anencephaly and 1 of which was a hydranencephaly that developed de novo after starting omeprazole in the 13th gestational week (F. Rosa, personal communication, FDA, 1996).

A paper published in 1995 described the use of omeprazole, 20 mg daily for esophageal reflux, by a woman in two consecutive pregnancies that were terminated because of severe congenital anomalies—anencephaly in one and severe talipes in the other (4). The first pregnancy was the result of a gamete intrafallopian transfer (GIFT) procedure, and the second occurred after a natural conception. Both aborted fetuses had normal chromosomal patterns.

A woman with Zollinger-Ellison syndrome was treated in two of her three pregnancies with omeprazole (5). In her first pregnancy, she had been treated with ranitidine (300 mg/day) and other therapy during the 2nd and 3rd trimesters and delivered a healthy, 2560-g boy at 37 weeks' gestation. She then presented at 11 weeks' gestation in her second pregnancy, complaining of abdominal pain and vomiting. Her symptoms were controlled with omeprazole (120 mg/day), which was continued until delivery of a healthy, 2610-g girl. During the third pregnancy, she was treated throughout gestation with omeprazole (180 mg/day) and cimetidine (450 mg/day), delivering a healthy term 2550-g male infant.

Data from the Swedish Medical Birth Registry were presented in 1998 (6). A total of 553 infants (6 sets of twins) were delivered from 547 women who had used acid-suppressing drugs early in pregnancy. A number of other pharmaceutical agents, identified only by drug category, were also used by these women. Seventeen infants with birth defects were identified (3.1%; 95% confidence interval [CI] 1.8–4.9) compared with the crude malformation rate of 3.9% in the Registry. The odds ration (OR) for a congenital malformation, stratified for birth year, maternal age, parity, and smoking was 0.72 (95% CI 0.41–1.24 (6). The OR for malformations after proton pump blocker exposure was 0.91 (95% CI 0.45–1.84) compared with 0.46 (95% CI 0.17–1.20) for H_2-receptor antagonists (OR 0.86, 95% CI 0.33–2.23; $p = 0.13$). Of the 17 infants with birth defects, 10 had been exposed to proton pump blockers, 6 to H_2 antagonists, and 1 to both classes of drug. Six of the defects in the proton pump inhibitor group were cardiovascular defects (see also Lansoprazole), whereas only one such defect occurred in those exposed to H_2 antagonists. Omeprazole was the only acid-suppressing drug exposure in 262 infants. Twenty other offspring were exposed *in utero* to omeprazole combined either with cimetidine (2 infants) or ranitidine (18 infants). Eight birth defects (3.1%) were observed in the group where omeprazole was the only acid-suppressing agent used. The defects were ventricular septum defect ($N = 3$), and one each of patent ductus arteriosus, unspecified cardiac defect, urethral valve (detected at 1 month of age), facial anomaly (type not specified), and

Down's syndrome. In addition, one infant with hypospadias was observed in a newborn exposed to a combination of omeprazole and ranitidine (6).

A prospective cohort study published in 1998 described the pregnancy outcomes of 113 women exposed to omeprazole (101 during organogenesis) matched to 113 disease-paired controls (exposed to H_2-receptor antihistamines) and 113 controls who were exposed to nonteratogenic agents (e.g., dental radiation, acetaminophen) (7). All of the subjects and controls had contacted a teratogen information service to inquire about drug exposures during their pregnancy. Omeprazole-exposed women were from Canada ($N = 59$), Italy ($N = 41$), and France ($N = 13$), whereas all of the 226 controls were from Canada (Motherisk Program in Toronto). There were no significant differences between the groups in alcohol use and smoking. However, omeprazole-exposed women used significantly more antipeptic and prokinetic agents (histamine blockers, antacids, sucralfate, bismuth subsalicylate, calcium carbonate, and cisapride) than women in the two control groups. Pregnancy outcomes were determined from information supplied by the women shortly after delivery. No significant differences between the three groups in terms of live births, spontaneous abortions, elective abortions, gestational age at delivery, preterm delivery, cesarean section, and birth weight were observed (7). The incidence of major anomalies in live births exposed during the 1st trimester in the three groups were 4 of 78 (5.1%), 3 of 98 (3.1%), and 2 of 66 (3.0%), respectively. The four malformations in omeprazole-exposed infants were ventricular septal defect, polycystic kidneys, ureteropelvic junction stenosis, and patent ductus arteriosus. In disease-paired controls, the three defects were atrial septal defect and two cases of ventricular septal defect, whereas in nonteratogenic controls the two malformations were atrial septal defect with pulmonary stenosis and developmental delay. Although the study lacked the statistical power to detect a small increase in major malformations, the authors concluded that it was unlikely that omeprazole was a major teratogen (7).

A 1998 non-interventional observational cohort study described the outcomes of pregnancies in women who had been prescribed one or more of 34 newly marketed drugs by general practitioners in England (8). Data were obtained by questionnaires sent to the prescribing physicians one month after the expected or possible date of delivery. In 831 (78%) of the pregnancies, a newly marketed drug was thought to have been taken during the 1st trimester with birth defects noted in 14 (2.5%) singleton births of the 557 newborns (10 sets of twins). In addition, two birth defects were observed in aborted fetuses. However, few of the aborted fetuses were examined. Omeprazole was taken during the 1st trimester in five pregnancies. The outcomes of these pregnancies included one elective abortion and four normal, full-term infants (8).

The pregnancy outcomes of nine women who had taken omeprazole (20–60 mg/day) during gestation were described in 1998 publication (9). Four of the women took omeprazole during the 1st trimester and five started treatment in the 2nd or 3rd trimesters. No complications or congenital malformations were observed in the offspring or during subsequent follow-up periods ranging from 2 to 12 years (9).

In a study published in 1999, investigators linked data from a Danish prescription database to a birth registry to evaluate the risks of proton pump inhibitors for congenital malformations, low birth weight, and preterm delivery (<37 weeks') (10). From a total of 51 women who had filled a prescription for these drugs sometime during pregnancy, 38 (omeprazole $N = 35$, lansoprazole $N = 3$) had done so during the interval of 30 days before conception to the end of the 1st trimester. A control group, consisting of 13,327 pregnancies in which the mother had not obtained a prescription for reimbursed medication from 30 days before conception to the end of her pregnancy, was used for comparison. The prevalence of major congenital anomalies in the controls was 5.2%. Three major birth defects (7.9%), two of which were cardiovascular anomalies, were observed from the 38 pregnancies possibly exposed in the 1st trimester (specific drug exposure not given): ventricular septum defect; pyloric stenosis; and one case of patent ductus arteriosus, atrial septum defect, hydronephrosis, and agenesis of the iris. Compared with controls, the adjusted (for maternal age, birth order, gestational age, and smoking, but not for alcohol abuse) relative risks for the three outcomes were congenital malformations 1.6 (95% CI 0.5–5.2), low birth weight 1.8 (95% CI 0.2–13.1), and preterm delivery (not adjusted for gestational age) 2.3 (95% CI 0.9–6.0). Although the study found no elevated risks for the three outcomes, the investigators cautioned that more data were needed to assess the possible association between proton pump inhibitors and cardiac malformations or preterm delivery (10).

Two databases, one from England and the other from Italy, were combined in a study published in 1999 that was designed to assess the incidence of congenital malformations in women who had received a prescription for an acid-suppressing drug (omeprazole, cimetidine, or ranitidine) during the 1st trimester (11). Nonexposed women were selected from the same databases to form a control group. Spontaneous abortions and elective abortions (except two cases of prenatally diagnosed congenital anomalies that were grouped with stillbirths) were excluded from the analysis. Stillbirths were defined as any pregnancy loss occurring at 28 weeks' gestation or later. Omeprazole was taken in 134 pregnancies, resulting in 139 live births (11 [7.9%] premature), 5 (3.7%) of whom had a congenital malformation. There were no stillbirths or neonatal deaths. The malformations were (shown by system) head/face (tongue tie), heart (septal defects $N = 2$), muscle/skeleton (dysplastic hip/dislocation/clicking hip), and genital/urinary (congenital hydrocele/inguinal hernia). In addition, three newborns had a small head circumference for gestational age. In comparison, the outcomes of 1547 nonexposed pregnancies included 1560 live births (115 [7.4%] premature), 15 stillbirths (includes 2 elective abortions for anomalies), and 10 neonatal deaths. Sixty-four (4.1%) of the newborns had malformations, including defects of the central nervous system ($N = 2$), head/face ($N = 13$), eye ($N = 2$), heart ($N = 7$), muscle/skeleton ($N = 13$), genital/urinary ($N = 18$), gastrointestinal ($N = 2$), and those that were polyformation ($N = 3$) or known genetic anomalies ($N = 4$). There were 21 newborns who were small for gestational age, and 78 had a small head circumference for gestational age. The relative risk of malformation (adjusted for mother's age and prematurity) associated with omeprazole was 0.9 (95% CI 0.4–2.4), with cimetidine 1.3 (95% CI 0.7–2.6), and with ranitidine 1.5 (95% CI 0.9–2.6) (11).

A 1998 case report described a 41-year-old woman with refractory gastroesophageal reflux disease (GERD) who was treated with omeprazole (20 mg/day) starting at 29 weeks' gestation (12). Previous treatment with ranitidine (late 1st trimester), cisapride (2nd trimester), or a combination of the two had been unsuccessful. A slightly premature male child (birth weight not given) with fetal bradycardia was delivered in the 36th week with Apgar scores of 6 and 9 at 1 and 5 minutes, respectively. He was doing well at 1 year of age (12).

Several investigations have studied the effect of omeprazole for prophylaxis against aspiration pneumonitis in emergency cesarean section (13–18). No adverse effects were noted in the newborns.

In summary, the lack of teratogenicity in animals and the bulk of the human 1st trimester exposure data indicate that omeprazole is not a major human teratogen. None of the cohort studies measured a significant increase in the rates of major birth defects, but they lacked the power to detect small increases in birth defects or rare malformations. The small cluster of cardiac defects observed in one study after omeprazole exposure appears to be an errant signal as it was not confirmed in other studies. Most likely, cardiac and other defects observed in all studies were the result of many factors, including possibly the severity of the disease and concurrent use of other drugs. The data, however, do warrant continued investigation. In addition, the studies lacked the sensitivity to detect minor anomalies because of the absence of standardized examinations. Late appearing major defects may also have been missed because of the timing of some of the data collection. The gastric tumors observed in rats are a potential concern for human offspring, but the dose-related nature of the tumors and the limited *in utero* exposure during gestation probably indicate a negligible risk. However, as with all drug therapy, avoidance of omeprazole during pregnancy, especially during the 1st trimester, is the safest course. If omeprazole is required or if inadvertent exposure does occur early in gestation, the known risk to the embryo/fetus appears to be low. Long-term follow-up of offspring exposed during gestation is warranted.

BREAST FEEDING SUMMARY

RECOMMENDATION: Limited Human Data - Potential Toxicity

Only one report describing the use of omeprazole during human lactation has been located. A woman with refractory GERD was treated with omeprazole (20 mg/day) for 7–8 weeks before delivering a premature male infant (birth weight not given) at 36 weeks' gestation (see above) (12). Treatment was continued during breast-feeding. During this time, the woman fed her infant son just before taking her dose at 8 AM, refrained from nursing for 4 hours, and then expressed and discarded her milk at 12 noon. At 3 weeks postpartum, blood and milk samples were obtained at 8 AM and then every 30 minutes for 4 hours (i.e., until 12 noon). The milk was obtained by expressing but the volume of the samples was not specified. Maternal serum concentrations began to rise 90 minutes after the dose, reached 950 nM at 12 noon, and appeared to be still rising. Breast milk levels also began to rise at 90 minutes and peaked at 180 minutes at 58 nM. The infant was doing well at 1 year of age.

The above case report estimated a maximum daily omeprazole exposure of 4 μg, but the calculation was based on a consumption of only 200 mL of milk/day for a 5-kg infant (40 mL/kg/day). A more acceptable value is 150 mL/kg/day (19). Moreover, the milk samples were obtained by expression and the volumes expressed were not given. This is clinically relevant because hindmilk obtained at the end of a feeding is 4–5 times higher in fat than in foremilk (20). For lipid soluble drugs, such as omeprazole, hindmilk would be expected to contain most of the drug in milk.

In concurrence with the above case report, the relatively low molecular weight of omeprazole (about 345) predicts that it will be excreted into human milk. In rats, administration of omeprazole at a dose 35–345 times the human dose during late gestation and lactation resulted in decreased pup weight gain (1). The clinical significance of this for nursing human infants is unknown.

One source has stated that the safety of a drug during breast-feeding can be arbitrarily defined as no more than 10% of the adult dose standardized by weight if a therapeutic dose for infants is not known (13). Until additional studies show that omeprazole meets this criterion, the use of omeprazole during breast-feeding should probably be avoided. Other concerns, such as the carcinogenicity observed in animals and the potential for suppression of gastric acid secretion in the nursing infant, also warrant further study.

References

1. Product information. Prilosec. AstraZeneca, 2001.
2. Ching MS, Morgan DJ, Mihaly GW, Hardy KF, Smallwood RA. Placental transfer of omeprazole in maternal and fetal sheep. Dev Pharmacol Ther 1986;9:323–31.
3. Moore J, Flynn RJ, Sampaio M, Wilson CM, Gillon KRW. Effect of single-dose omeprazole on intragastric acidity and volume during obstetric anaesthesia. Anaesthesia 1989;44:559–62.
4. Tsirigotis M, Yazdani N, Craft I. Potential effects of omeprazole in pregnancy. Hum Reprod 1995;10:2177–8.
5. Harper MA, McVeigh JE, Thompson W, Ardill JES, Buchanan KD. Successful pregnancy in association with Zollinger-Ellison syndrome. Am J Obstet Gynecol 1995;173:863–4.
6. Kallen B. Delivery outcome after the use of acid-suppressing drugs in early pregnancy with special reference to omeprazole. Br J Obstet Gynaecol 1998;105:877–81.
7. Lalkin A, Loebstein R, Addis A, Ramezani-Namin F, Mastroiacovo P, Mazzone T, Vial T, Bonati M, Koren G. The safety of omeprazole during pregnancy: a multicenter prospective controlled study. Am J Obstet Gynecol 1998;179:727–30.
8. Wilton LV, Pearce GL, Martin RM, Mackay FJ, Mann RD. The outcomes of pregnancy in women exposed to newly marketed drugs in general practice in England. Br J Obstet Gynaecol 1998;105:882–9.
9. Brunner G, Meyer H, Athmann C. Omeprazole for peptic ulcer disease in pregnancy. Digestion 1998;59:651–4.
10. Nielsen GL, Sorensen HT, Thulstrup, Tage-Jensen U, Olesen C, Ekbom A. The safety of proton pump inhibitors in pregnancy. Aliment Pharmacol Ther 1999;13:1085–9.
11. Ruigomez A, Rodriguez LAG, Cattaruzzi C, Troncon MG, Agostinis L, Wallander MA, Johansson S. Use of cimetidine, omeprazole, and ranitidine in pregnant women and pregnancy outcomes. Am J Epidemiol 1999;150:476–81.
12. Marshall JK, Thomson ABR, Armstrong D. Omeprazole for refractory gastroesophageal reflux disease during pregnancy and lactation. Can J Gastroenterol 1998;12:225–7.
13. Yau G, Kan AF, Gin T, Oh TE. A comparison of omeprazole and ranitidine for prophylaxis against aspiration pneumonitis in emergency caesarean section. Anaesthesia 1992;47:101–4.
14. Orr DA, Bill KM, Gillon KRW, Wilson CM, Fogarty DJ, Moore J. Effects of omeprazole, with and without metoclopramide, in elective obstetric anaesthesia. Anaesthesia 1993;48:114–9.
15. Rocke DA, Rout CC, Gouws E. Intravenous administration of the proton pump inhibitor omeprazole reduces the risk of acid aspiration at emergency cesarean section. Anesth Analg 1994;78:1093–8.
16. Gin T. Intravenous omeprazole before emergency cesarean section. Anesth Analg 1995;80:848.
17. Rocke DA, Rout CC. Intravenous omeprazole before emergency cesarean section. Anesth Analg 1995;80:848–9.
18. Stuart JC, Kan AF, Rowbottom SJ, Gin T. Acid aspiration prophylaxis for emergency caesarean section. Anaesthesia 1996;51:415–21.
19. Ito S. Drug therapy for breast-feeding women. N Engl J Med 2000;343:118–26.
20. Lawrence RA, Lawrence RM. *Breastfeeding. A Guide for The Medical Profession*. 5th ed. St. Louis, MO: Mosby, 1999:360.

Name:	**ONDANSETRON**	Risk Factor:	**B_M**
Class:	**Antiemetic**		

FETAL RISK SUMMARY

RECOMMENDATION: Limited Human Data - Animal Data Suggest Low Risk

Ondansetron is a potent antiemetic indicated for the prevention and treatment of chemotherapy-induced nausea and vomiting. No adverse effects on fertility or on the fetus were observed in reproduction studies in rats and rabbits at IV doses up to 4 mg/kg/day (1).

Ondansetron has been used in the treatment of hyperemesis gravidarum (2–6). A 21-year-old primigravida with severe nausea and vomiting was treated unsuccessfully for approximately 4 weeks, beginning at 6 weeks' gestation, with IV metoclopramide, 10 mg 3 times daily, rectal dimenhydrinate, 100 mg twice daily, and IV fluids (2). Because her condition was considered life-threatening for both her and her fetus, ondansetron 8 mg IV 3 times daily was instituted at 11 weeks' gestation and continued for 14 days. Significant improvement was noted in the patient's condition from the 2nd day of therapy. The woman eventually gave birth at term to a healthy 3.2-kg girl.

A second report on the use of ondansetron for severe nausea and vomiting in pregnancy involved a 22-year-old woman with renal impairment and nephrotic syndrome (3). Treatment with the antiemetic was begun at 30 weeks' gestation with 8 mg IV 3 times daily for 1 day, then orally (dose not specified) until 33 weeks' gestation. A healthy 2052-g female infant was delivered at 36 weeks by elective cesarean section. The infant remained in good health at an unspecified follow-up period.

A randomized, double-blind study, first published as an abstract (4) and then as a full report (5), compared IV ondansetron (10 mg) (N = 15) with IV promethazine (50 mg) (N = 15) for the treatment of hyperemesis gravidarum. Both drugs were given as an initial dose followed by as-needed doses every 8 hours. The mean gestational ages of the two groups at the start of therapy were 11.0 and 10.2 weeks, respectively. No differences were observed between the two groups in terms of duration of hospitalization, nausea score, number of doses received, treatment failures, and daily weight gain. The only adverse effect observed was sedation in eight women who received promethazine compared with none in the ondansetron group. No mention was made of the pregnancy outcomes in either group.

Ondansetron, 8 mg IV twice daily, was administered to a woman at 14 weeks' gestation after 6 weeks of unsuccessful therapy with intermittent use of promethazine, prochlorperazine, metoclopramide, and IV hydration (6). IV ondansetron was able to control her vomiting, but not her nausea, and 2 days later she was converted to oral therapy (4 mg) that was taken intermittently (1–2 times daily) until 33 weeks' gestation. Nausea occurred throughout her pregnancy, with occasional episodes of vomiting. She eventually delivered a healthy, 2.7-kg male infant at 39 weeks' who was doing well at early follow-up.

BREAST FEEDING SUMMARY

RECOMMENDATION: No Human Data - Probably Compatible

No reports describing the use of ondansetron during human lactation have been located. The drug has been found in the milk of lactating rats (1). Because of this and its relatively low molecular weight (about 366), excretion into breast milk should be expected. The effects of exposure to the drug on a nursing infant are unknown.

References

1. Product information. Zofran. Glaxo Wellcome, 1997.
2. Guikontes E, Spantideas A, Diakakis J. Ondansetron and hyperemesis gravidarum. Lancet 1992;340:1223.
3. World MJ. Ondansetron and hyperemesis gravidarum. Lancet 1993;341:185.
4. Sullivan CA, Johnson CA, Roach H, Martin RW, Stewart DK, Morrison JC. A prospective, randomized, double-blind comparison of the serotonin antagonist ondansetron to a standardized regimen of promethazine for hyperemesis gravidarum. A preliminary investigation (abstract). Am J Obstet Gynecol 1995;172:299.
5. Sullivan CA, Johnson CA, Roach H, Martin RW, Stewart DK, Morrison JC. A pilot study of intravenous ondansetron for hyperemesis gravidarum. Am J Obstet Gynecol 1996;174:1565–8.
6. Tincello DG, Johnstone MJ. Treatment of hyperemesis gravidarum with the 5-HT_3 antagonist ondansetron (Zofran). Postgrad Med J 1996;72:688–9.

Name:	OPIPRAMOL	Risk Factor:	C
Class:	Antidepressant		

No data are available (see Imipramine).

Name:	OPIUM	Risk Factor:	B*
Class:	Narcotic Antidiarrheal		

FETAL RISK SUMMARY

RECOMMENDATION: Human Data Suggest Risk in 3rd Trimester

The effects of opium are caused by morphine (see Morphine). The Collaborative Perinatal Project monitored 50,282 mother-child pairs, 36 of whom had 1st trimester exposure to opium (1, pp. 287–295). For use anytime during pregnancy, 181 exposures were recorded (1, p. 434). Four of the 1st-trimester exposed infants had congenital defects, but these numbers are too small to draw any conclusion about a relationship between the drug and major or minor malformations. A possible association with inguinal hernia based on seven cases after anytime exposure was suggested (1, p. 485) (see also Morphine for similar findings). The statistical significance of these associations is unknown and independent confirmation is required.

Narcotic withdrawal was observed in a newborn whose mother was treated for regional ileitis with deodorized tincture of opium during the 2nd and 3rd trimesters (2). Symptoms of withdrawal in the infant began at 48 hours of age.

[**Risk Factor D if used for prolonged periods or in high doses at term.*]

O

BREAST FEEDING SUMMARY

RECOMMENDATION: No Human Data - Probably Compatible

See Morphine.

References

1. Heinonen OP, Slone D, Shapiro S. *Birth Defects and Drugs in Pregnancy*. Littleton, MA: Publishing Sciences Group, 1977.
2. Fisch GR, Henley WL. Symptoms of narcotic withdrawal in a newborn infant secondary to medical therapy of the mother. Pediatrics 1961;28:852–3.

Name:	OPRELVEKIN	Risk Factor:	C_M
Class:	Hematopoietic		

FETAL RISK SUMMARY

RECOMMENDATION: No Human Data - Animal Data Suggest Risk

Oprelvekin is a protein produced by recombinant DNA technology from *Escherichia coli* that differs from natural interleukin-11 (IL-11) by one terminal amino acid. This difference does not affect its bioactivity as a thrombopoietic growth factor that indirectly stimulates increased platelet production. It is indicated for the prevention of severe thrombocytopenia and the reduction in the need for platelet transfusions following myelosuppressive chemotherapy. The terminal half-life is about 6.9 hours (1).

Reproductive studies have been conducted in rats and rabbits. Oprelvekin was embryocidal in rats at doses 2 to 20 times the human dose based on body weight (HD). Maternal toxicity (transient hypoactivity and dyspnea) and prolonged estrus cycle were evident at these doses. Embryo/fetal effects included increased early embryonic deaths and decreased numbers of live fetuses. At 20 times the HD, retarded fetal development occurred, as evidenced by low fetal weight, and reduced number of ossified sacral and caudal vertebrae. Doses ≥2 times the HD used throughout gestation and lactation resulted in increased newborn mortality, decreased viability index on day 4 of lactation, and decreased pup body weights. In pregnant rabbits, doses 0.02 to 2 times the HD were maternal toxic (decreased fecal/urine eliminations, decreased food consumption and body weight loss). These doses caused abortion, increased embryonic and fetal deaths, and decreased numbers of live fetuses. No teratogenicity was observed in rabbits at doses up to 0.6 times HD (1).

It is not known if oprelvekin crosses the human placenta. Oprelvekin is a 177-amino acid protein with a molecular weight of about 19,000, but proteins can cross to the embryo and fetus.

No reports describing the use of oprelvekin in human pregnancy have been located. The animal data suggest a risk of toxicity but not teratogenicity. However, the absence of human pregnancy experience prevents an assessment the drug represents to the embryo and fetus.

BREAST FEEDING SUMMARY

RECOMMENDATION: No Human Data - Probably Compatible

No reports describing the use of oprelvekin during lactation have been located. Oprelvekin is a 177-amino acid protein with a molecular weight of about 19,000. Although it may be excreted into breast milk, it would most likely be digested in the infant's gastrointestinal tract. Therefore, the risk to a nursing infant from exposure to the drug in milk appears to be very low or nonexistent.

Reference

1. Product information. Neumega. Wyeth Pharmaceuticals, 2004.

Name:	**ORAL CONTRACEPTIVES**	Risk Factor:	X_M
Class:	**Estrogenic/Progestogenic Hormones**		

FETAL RISK SUMMARY

RECOMMENDATION: Contraindicated

Oral contraceptives contain a 19–nortestosterone progestin and a synthetic estrogen (see Mestranol, Norethindrone, Norethynodrel, Ethinyl Estradiol, Progesterone, Hydroxyprogesterone, and Ethisterone). Because oral contraceptives are primarily combination products, it is difficult to separate entirely the fetal effects of progestogens and estrogens. Two groups of investigators have reviewed the effects of these hormones on the fetus (133 references) (1,2). Several potential problems were discussed: congenital heart defects, central nervous system defects, limb reduction malformations, general malformations, and modified development of sexual organs. Except for the latter category, no firm evidence has appeared that establishes a causal relationship between oral contraceptives and various congenital anomalies. The acronym VACTERL (Vertebral, Anal, Cardiac, Tracheal, Esophageal, Renal or Radial, and Limb) has been used to describe the fetal malformations produced by oral contraceptives or the related hormonal pregnancy test preparations (no longer available in the United States) (2,3). The use of this acronym should probably be abandoned in favor of more conventional terminology as a large variety of malformations have been reported with estrogen–progestogen–containing products (1–11). The Population Council estimates that even if the study findings for VACTERL malformations are accurate, such abnormalities would occur in only 0.07% of the pregnancies exposed to oral contraceptives (12). Some reviewers have concluded that the risk to the fetus for nongenital malformations after *in utero* exposure to these agents is small, if indeed it exists at all (2).

In contrast to the above, the effect of estrogens and some synthetic progestogens on the development of the sexual organs is well established (2). Masculinization of the female infant has been associated with norethindrone, norethynodrel, hydroxyprogesterone, medroxyprogesterone, and diethylstilbestrol (2,13,14). The incidence of masculinization of female infants exposed to synthetic progestogens is reported to be approximately 0.3% (15). Pseudohermaphroditism in the male infant is not a problem, because of the low doses of estrogen employed in oral contraceptives (14).

Increased serum bilirubin in neonates of mothers taking oral contraceptives or progestogens before and after conception has been observed (16). Icterus occasionally reached clinically significant levels in infants whose mothers were exposed to the progestogens.

Concern that oral contraceptives may be a risk factor for preeclampsia has been suggested based on the known effects of oral contraceptives on blood pressure (17). However, a retrospective controlled review of 341 patients found no association between this effect and the drugs (17).

Possible interactions between oral contraceptives and tetracycline, rifampin, ampicillin, or chloramphenicol resulting in pregnancy have been reported (18–25). The mechanism for this interaction may involve the interruption of the enterohepatic circulation of contraceptive steroids by inhibiting gut hydrolysis of steroid conjugates, resulting in lower concentrations of circulating steroids.

BREAST FEEDING SUMMARY

RECOMMENDATION: Compatible

Use of oral contraceptives during lactation has been associated with shortened duration of lactation, decreased infant weight gain, decreased milk production, and decreased composition of nitrogen and protein content of milk (26–29). The American Academy of Pediatrics has reviewed this subject (30) (37 references). Although the magnitude of these changes is low, the changes in milk production and composition may be of nutritional importance in malnourished mothers.

In general, progestin-only contraceptives demonstrate no consistent alteration of breast milk composition, volume, or duration of lactation (30). The composition and volume of breast milk will vary considerably even in the absence of steroidal contraceptives (29). Both estrogens and progestins cross into milk. An infant consuming 600 mL of breast milk daily from a mother using contraceptives containing 50 μg of ethinyl estradiol will probably receive a daily dose in the range of 10 ng (30). This is in the same range as the amount of natural estradiol received by infants of mothers not using oral contraceptives. Progestins also pass into breast milk, although naturally occurring progestins have not been identified. One study estimated 0.03, 0.15, and 0.3 μg of *d*-norgestrel/600 mL of milk from mothers receiving 30, 150, and 250 μg of the drug, respectively (31). A milk:plasma ratio of 0.15 for norgestrel was calculated by the authors (31). A ratio of 0.16 has been calculated for lynestrenol (31,32).

Reports of adverse effects are lacking except for one child with mild breast tenderness and hypertrophy who was exposed to large doses of estrogen (30). If breast-feeding is desired, the lowest effective dose of oral contraceptives should be chosen. Infant weight gain should be monitored, and the possible need for nutritional supplements should be considered. The American Academy of Pediatrics classifies combination oral contraceptives as compatible with breast-feeding (33).

References

1. Ambani LM, Joshi NJ, Vaidya RA, Devi PK. Are hormonal contraceptives teratogenic? Fertil Steril 1977;28:791–7.
2. Wilson JG, Brent RL. Are female sex hormones teratogenic? Am J Obstet Gynecol 1981;141:567–80.
3. Corcoran R, Entwistle GC. VACTERL congenital malformations and the male fetus. Lancet 1975;2:981–2.
4. Nora JJ, Nora AH. Can the pill cause birth defects? N Engl J Med 1974;294:731–2.
5. Kasan PN, Andrews J. Oral contraceptives and congenital abnormalities. Br J Obstet Gynaecol 1980;87:545–51.
6. Kullander S, Kallen B. A prospective study of drugs and pregnancy. Acta Obstet Gynecol Scand 1976;55:221–4.
7. Oakley GP, Flynt JW. Hormonal pregnancy test and congenital malformations. Lancet 1973;2:256–7.
8. Savolainen E, Saksela E, Saxen L. Teratogenic hazards of oral contraceptives analyzed in a national malformation register. Am J Obstet Gynecol 1981;140:521–4.
9. Frost O. Tracheo-oesophageal fistula associated with hormonal contraception during pregnancy. Br Med J 1976;3:978.
10. Redline RW, Abramowsky CR. Transposition of the great vessels in an infant exposed to massive doses of oral contraceptives. Am J Obstet Gynecol 1981;141:468–9.
11. Farb HF, Thomason J, Carandang FS, Sampson MB, Spellacy WH. Anencephaly twins and HLA-B27. J Reprod Med 1980;25:166–9.
12. Department of Medical and Public Affairs. *Population Reports*. Washington, D.C.: George Washington University Medical Center, 1975;2:A29–51.
13. Bongiovanni AM, DiGeorge AM, Grumbach MM. Masculinization of the female infant associated with estrogenic therapy alone during gestation: four cases. J Clin Endocrinol Metab 1959;19:1004–11.
14. Hagler S, Schultz A, Hankin H, Kunstadter RH. Fetal effects of steroid therapy during pregnancy. Am J Dis Child 1963;106:586–90.
15. Bongiovanni AM, McFadden AJ. Steroids during pregnancy and possible fetal consequences. Fertil Steril 1960;11:181–4.
16. McConnell JB, Glasgow JF, McNair R. Effect on neonatal jaundice of oestrogens and progestogens taken before and after conception. Br Med J 1973;3:605–7.
17. Bracken MB, Srisuphan W. Oral contraception as a risk factor for preeclampsia. Am J Obstet Gynecol 1982;142:191–6.
18. Bacon JF, Shenfield GM. Pregnancy attributable to interaction between tetracycline and oral contraceptives. Br Med J 1980;1:283.
19. Stockley I. Interactions with oral contraceptives. Pharm J 1976;216:140.
20. Reiners D, Nockefinck L, Breurer H. Rifampin and the "pill" do not go well together. JAMA 1974;227:608.
21. Dosseter EJ. Drug interactions with oral contraceptives. Br Med J 1975;1:1967.
22. Pullskinnen MO, Williams K. Reduced maternal plasma and urinary estriol during ampicillin treatment. Am J Obstet Gynecol 1971;109:895–6.
23. Friedman GI, Huneke AL, Kim MH, Powell J. The effect of ampicillin on oral contraceptive effectiveness. Obstet Gynecol 1980;55:33–7.
24. Back DJ, Breckenridge AM. Drug interactions with oral contraceptives. IPFF Med Bull 1978;12:1–2.
25. Orme ML, Back DJ. Therapy with oral contraceptive steroids and antibiotics. J Antimicrob Chemother 1979;5:124–6.
26. Miller GH, Hughes LR. Lactation and genital involution effects of a new low-dose oral contraceptive on breast-feeding mothers and their infants. Obstet Gynecol 1970;35:44–50.
27. Kora SJ. Effect of oral contraceptives on lactation. Fertil Steril 1969;20:419–23.
28. Guiloff E, Ibarra-Polo A, Zanartu J, Tuscanini C, Mischler TW, Gomez-Rodgers C. Effect of contraception on lactation. Am J Obstet Gynecol 1974;118:42–5.
29. Lonnerdal B, Forsum E, Hambraeus L. Effect of oral contraceptives on consumption and volume of breast milk. Am J Clin Nutr 1980;33:816–24.
30. Committee on Drugs, American Academy of

O

Pediatrics. Breast-feeding and contraception. Pediatrics 1981;68:138–40.
31. Nilsson S, Nygren KC, Johansson EDB. D-Norgestrel concentrations in maternal plasma, milk, and child plasma during administration of oral contraceptives to nursing women. Am J Obstet Gynecol 1977;129:178–83.
32. van der Molen HJ, Hart PG, Wijmenga HG. Studies with 4-^{14}C-lynestrol in normal and lactating women. Acta Endocrinol 1969;61:255–74.
33. Committee on Drugs, American Academy of Pediatrics. The transfer of drugs and other chemicals into human milk. Pediatrics 2001;108:776–89.

Name: **ORLISTAT** Risk Factor: **B_M**

Class: **Gastrointestinal Agent (Lipase Inhibitor)**

FETAL RISK SUMMARY

RECOMMENDATION: No Human Data - Animal Data Suggest Low Risk

Orlistat is a lipase inhibitor used in the management of obesity. The agent inhibits the absorption of dietary fats. The mechanism of action of orlistat involves bonding to gastric and pancreatic lipases, thereby inactivating these enzymes. The inactive enzymes are unable to hydrolyze dietary fat to absorbable free fatty acids and monoglycerides (1). The systemic bioavailability of orlistat is minimal (1).

Reproductive studies in rats and rabbits at doses up to 23 and 47 times the recommended human daily dose on a body surface area basis (RHD) revealed no evidence of embryotoxicity or teratogenicity (1). In two rat studies, but not in two others, doses of 6 and 23 times the RHD were associated with an increased incidence of dilated cerebral ventricles. At 12 times the RHD in rats, no evidence of impaired fertility was observed (1).

It is not known if orlistat crosses the placenta. Although the molecular weight (about 496) is low enough for passage to the fetus, the minimal systemic bioavailability of the agent following oral administration suggests that little, if any, of the agent would be available for transfer from the maternal circulation.

No reports describing the use of orlistat during human pregnancy have been located. Because of its minimal systemic bioavailability, orlistat appears to present a very low risk, if any, to the embryo or fetus. Orlistat may cause a deficiency of fat soluble vitamins (vitamins A [both retinol and beta-carotene], D, and E) if a daily multiple vitamin supplement is not taken. The vitamin should be taken either 2 hours before or after an orlistat dose (1). Maternal deficiency of these vitamins may result in fetal adverse effects (see also Vitamin A, Vitamin D, and Vitamin E). If orlistat is used in pregnancy, healthcare professionals are encouraged to call the toll free number (800-670-6126) for information about patient enrollment in the Motherisk study.

BREAST FEEDING SUMMARY

RECOMMENDATION: No Human Data - Probably Compatible

No reports describing the use of orlistat during human lactation have been located. The minimal systemic bioavailability suggests that the drug would not be found in breast milk, but maternal hypovitaminosis A, D, and E may occur (see above).

Reference

1. Product information. Xenical. Roche Laboratories, 2000.

Name:	**ORPHENADRINE**	Risk Factor:	**C**
Class:	**Skeletal Muscle Relaxant**		

FETAL RISK SUMMARY

RECOMMENDATION: Limited Human Data - No Relevant Animal Data

Orphenadrine is an anticholinergic agent used in the treatment of painful skeletal muscle conditions. In a study using pregnant rats, large oral doses (15 and 30 mg) produced enlarged bladders containing blood, but no other anomalies, in 8 of 159 fetuses (1). No published reports of its use in pregnancy have been located (see also Atropine).

In a surveillance study of Michigan Medicaid recipients involving 229,101 completed pregnancies conducted between 1985 and 1992, 411 newborns had been exposed to orphenadrine during the 1st trimester (F. Rosa, personal communication, FDA, 1993). A total of 11 (2.7%) major birth defects were observed (16 expected), including (observed/expected) 2/4 cardiovascular defects and 1/1 polydactyly. No anomalies were observed in four other defect categories (oral clefts, spina bifida, limb reduction defects, and hypospadias) for which specific data were available. These data do not support an association between the drug and congenital defects.

BREAST FEEDING SUMMARY

RECOMMENDATION: No Human Data - Probably Compatible

No data are available (see also Atropine).

Reference

1. Beall JR. A teratogenic study of chlorpromazine, orphenadrine, perphenazine, and LSD-25 in rats. Toxicol Appl Pharmacol 1972;21:230–6. As cited in Shepard TH. *Catalog of Teratogenic Agents*. 6th ed. Baltimore, MD: Johns Hopkins University Press, 1989:476–7.

O

Name:	**OSELTAMIVIR**	Risk Factor:	**C_M**
Class:	**Antiviral**		

FETAL RISK SUMMARY

RECOMMENDATION: No Human Data - Animal Data Suggest Low Risk

Oseltamivir is an ethyl ester prodrug that is metabolized primarily in the liver by esterases to oseltamivir carboxylate, the active agent. The drug is active against influenza viruses, Types A and B, and is given orally for the treatment of uncomplicated acute illness due to influenza infection.

In reproduction studies, doses up to approximately 100 times the human systemic exposure based on AUC (0 to 24 hours) of oseltamivir carboxylate (HSE) had no effects on fertility or mating performance in male and female rats, or on embryo-fetal development (1). Similarly, doses in rabbits up to 50 times the HSE also had no effect on embryo-fetal development (1). In both species, fetal exposure to the antiviral agent was documented. Although a dose-dependent increase in the incidence rates of skeletal abnormalities and variants were observed in both species, the individual incidence rate of each defect remained within the expected background rates of occurrence (1).

It is not known if oseltamivir or oseltamivir carboxylate cross the placenta to the human fetus. The molecular weight (about 312 for the free base of oseltamivir) is low enough that transfer to the fetus should be expected.

No reports describing the use of oseltamivir during human pregnancy have been located. The lack of embryo and fetal toxicity in two animal species is reassuring, but an assessment of the risk this antiviral agent presents to a human embryo or fetus cannot be determined.

BREAST FEEDING SUMMARY

RECOMMENDATION: No Human Data - Probably Compatible

No reports describing the use of oseltamivir during human lactation have been located. In lactating rats, both oseltamivir and oseltamivir carboxylate are excreted into milk (1). Because the molecular weight of oseltamivir (about 312 for the free base) is low enough, excretion into breast milk should be expected. The effects of this exposure on a nursing infant are unknown.

Reference

1. Product information. Tamiflu. Roche Laboratories, 2000.

Name:	**OUABAIN**	Risk Factor:	**B**
Class:	**Cardiac Glycoside**		

See Digitalis.

Name:	**OXACILLIN**	Risk Factor:	B_M
Class:	**Antibiotic (Penicillin)**		

FETAL RISK SUMMARY

RECOMMENDATION: Compatible

Oxacillin is a penicillin antibiotic (see also Penicillin G). The drug crosses the placenta in low concentrations. Cord serum and amniotic fluid levels were less than 0.3 μg/mL in 15 of 18 patients given 500 mg orally 0.5–4 hours before cesarean section (1). No effects were seen in the infants.

The Collaborative Perinatal Project monitored 50,282 mother-child pairs, 3546 of whom had 1st trimester exposure to penicillin derivatives (2, pp. 297–313). For use anytime during pregnancy, 7171 exposures were recorded (2, p. 435). In neither group was evidence found to suggest a relationship to large categories of major or minor malformations or to individual defects.

A 1999 study used the population-based data-set of the Hungarian Case-Control Surveillance of Congenital Abnormalities (1980–1996) to evaluate the teratogenicity of oxacillin (3). The data base contained 22,865 fetuses or newborns with congenital malformations and 38,151 matched control newborns without birth defects. The mothers of 14 cases (4 in the 1st trimester) and 19 controls (8 in the 1st trimester) were treated with oxacillin during pregnancy. No associations were discovered based on a comparison with the expected rates in 24 congenital anomaly groups (3).

An interaction between oxacillin and oral contraceptives resulting in pregnancy has been reported (4). Other penicillins (e.g., see Ampicillin) have been suspected of this interaction, but not all investigators believe it occurs. Although controversial, an alternate means of contraception may be a practical solution if both drugs are consumed at the same time.

BREAST FEEDING SUMMARY

RECOMMENDATION: Compatible

Oxacillin is excreted in breast milk in low concentrations (1). Although no adverse effects have been reported, three potential problems exist for the nursing infant: modification of bowel flora, direct effects on the infant (e.g., allergic response), and interference with the interpretation of culture results if a fever workup is required.

References

1. Prigot A, Froix C, Rubin E. Absorption, diffusion, and excretion of new penicillin, oxacillin. Antimicrob Agents Chemother 1962:402–10.
2. Heinonen OP, Slone D, Shapiro S. *Birth Defects and Drugs in Pregnancy*. Littleton, MA: Publishing Sciences Group, 1977.
3. Czeizel AE, Rockenbauer M, Sorensen HT, Olsen J. Teratogenic evaluation of oxacillin. Scand J Infect Dis 1999;31:311–2.
4. Silber TJ. Apparent oral contraceptive failure associated with antibiotic administration. J Adolesc Health Care 1983;4:287–9.

O

Name: **OXAPROZIN** Risk Factor: **C_M***

Class: **Nonsteroidal Anti-inflammatory**

FETAL RISK SUMMARY

RECOMMENDATION: Human Data Suggest Risk in 1st and 3rd Trimesters

Oxaprozin is a nonsteroidal anti-inflammatory drug (NSAID) used in the treatment of acute and chronic arthritis. It is in the same subclass (propionic acids) as five other NSAIDs (fenoprofen, flurbiprofen, ibuprofen, ketoprofen, and naproxen).

The drug produced infrequent congenital malformations in rabbits treated with doses in the usual human range, but not in mice and rats (1). No teratogenic effects were observed in two other studies of pregnant rats and rabbits (2–5). A dose-dependent constriction of the ductus arteriosus, similar to that produced by other nonsteroidal anti-inflammatory agents, was observed in fetal rats (5).

It is not known if oxaprozin crosses the human placenta. The molecular weight (about 293) is low enough, however, that passage to the fetus should be expected.

A combined 2001 population-based observational cohort study and a case-control study estimated the risk of adverse pregnancy outcome from the use of NSAIDs (6). The use of NSAIDs during pregnancy was not associated with congenital malformations, preterm delivery, or low birth weight, but a positive association was discovered with spontaneous abortions (SABs). A similar study, also published in 2001, failed to find a relationship, in general, between NSAIDs and congenital malformations, but did find a significant association with cardiac defects and orofacial clefts (7). In addition, a 2003 study found a significant association between exposure to NSAIDs in early pregnancy and SABs (8). (See Ibuprofen for details on these three studies.)

A brief 2003 editorial on the potential for NSAID-induced developmental toxicity concluded that NSAIDs, and specifically those with greater COX-2 affinity, had a lower risk of this toxicity in humans than aspirin (9).

Constriction of the ductus arteriosus *in utero* is a pharmacologic consequence arising from the use of prostaglandin synthesis inhibitors during pregnancy, as is inhibition of labor, prolongation of pregnancy, and suppression of fetal renal function (see also Indomethacin) (10). Persistent pulmonary hypertension of the newborn may occur if these agents are used in the 3rd trimester close to delivery (10,11). Women attempting to conceive should not use any prostaglandin synthesis inhibitor, including oxaprozin, because of the findings in a variety of animal models that indicate these agents block blastocyst implantation (12,13). Moreover, as noted above, NSAIDs have been associated with SABs and congenital malformations.

[**Risk Factor D if used in 3rd trimester or near delivery.*]

BREAST FEEDING SUMMARY

RECOMMENDATION: No Human Data - Potential Toxicity

No reports describing the use of oxaprozin during human lactation have been located. The drug has been found in the milk of lactating rats (1). The molecular weight (about 293) is low enough that excretion into breast milk should be expected. One reviewer listed several NSAIDs (diclofenac, fenoprofen, flurbiprofen, ibuprofen, ketoprofen, ketorolac, and tolmetin) that were considered safer alternatives to other agents (oxaprozin not mentioned) if a NSAID was required while nursing (14). Because of the long terminal elimination half-life (approximately 42 hours or longer) in adults and the unknown amount of oxaprozin that is excreted into milk, any of these choices are probably preferable.

O

References

1. Product information. Daypro. G.D. Searle, 2001.
2. Yamada T, Nishiyama T, Sasajima M, Nakane S. Reproduction studies of oxaprozin in the rat and rabbit. Iyakuhin Kenkyu 1984;15:207–92. As cited in Shepard TH. *Catalog of Teratogenic Agents*. 7th ed. Baltimore, MD: Johns Hopkins University Press, 1992:299–300.
3. Yamada T, Norariya T, Sasajima M, Nakane S. Reproduction studies of oxaprozin. II. Teratology study in rats. Iyakuhin Kenkyu 1984;15:225–49. As cited in Schardein JL. *Chemically Induced Birth Defects*. 2nd ed. New York, NY: Marcel Dekker, 1993:132–3.
4. Yamada T, Uchida H, Sasajima M, Nakane S. Reproduction studies of oxaprozin. III. Teratogenicity study in rabbits. Iyakuhin Kenkyu 1984;15:250–64. As cited in Schardein JL. *Chemically Induced Birth Defects*. 2nd ed. New York, NY: Marcel Dekker, 1993:132–3.
5. Yamada T, Inoue T, Hara M, Ohba Y, Nakame S, Uchida H. Reproductive studies of oxaprozin and studies on the fetal ductus arteriosus. Clin Report 1984;18:514–25, 528–36. As cited in Shepard TH. *Catalog of Teratogenic Agents*. 7th ed. Baltimore, MD: Johns Hopkins University Press, 1992:299–300.
6. Nielsen GL, Sorensen HT, Larsen H, Pedersen L. Risk of adverse birth outcome and miscarriage in pregnant users of non-steroidal anti-inflammatory drugs: population based observational study and case-control study. BMJ 2001;322:266–70.
7. Ericson A, Kallen BAJ. Nonsteroidal anti-inflammatory drugs in early pregnancy. Reprod Toxicol 2001; 15:371–5.
8. Li DK, Liu L, Odouli R. Exposure to non-steroidal anti-inflammatory drugs during pregnancy and risk of miscarriage: population based cohort study. BMJ 2003;327:368–71.
9. Tassinari MS, Cook JC, Hurtt ME. NSAIDs and developmental toxicity. Birth Defects Res Part B Dev Reprod Toxicol 2003;68:3–4.
10. Levin DL. Effects of inhibition of prostaglandin synthesis on fetal development, oxygenation, and the fetal circulation. Semin Perinatol 1980;4:35–44.
11. Van Marter LJ, Leviton A, Allred EN, Pagano M, Sullivan KF, Cohen A, Epstein MF. Persistent pulmonary hypertension of the newborn and smoking and aspirin and nonsteroidal antiinflammatory drug consumption during pregnancy. Pediatrics 1996;97:658–63.
12. Matt DW, Borzelleca JF. Toxic effects on the female reproductive system during pregnancy, parturition,

and lactation. In Witorsch RJ, ed. *Reproductive Toxicology*. 2nd ed. New York, NY: Raven Press, 1995: 175–93.
13. Dawood MY. Nonsteroidal antiinflammatory drugs and reproduction. Am J Obstet Gynecol 1993;169: 1255–65.
14. Anderson PO. Medication use while breast feeding a neonate. Neonatal Pharmacol Q 1993;2:3–14.

Name:	**OXAZEPAM**	Risk Factor:	**D**
Class:	**Sedative**		

FETAL RISK SUMMARY

RECOMMENDATION: Human Data Suggest in 1st and 3rd Trimesters

Oxazepam is an active metabolite of diazepam (see also Diazepam). It is a member of the benzodiazepine group. The drug, both free and conjugated forms, crosses the placenta achieving average cord:maternal serum ratios of 0.6 during the 2nd trimester and 1.1 at term (1). Large variations between patients for placental transfer have been observed (1–3). Passage of oxazepam is slower than diazepam, but the clinical significance of this is unknown (4). Two reports have suggested that the use of oxazepam in preeclampsia would be safer for the newborn infant than diazepam (5,6). However, it is doubtful whether either drug is indicated for this condition.

A 1989 report described characteristic dysmorphic features, growth retardation, and central nervous system defects in eight infants exposed either to oxazepam, 75 mg/day or more, or diazepam, 30 mg/day or more (7). See Diazepam for a detailed description of the infants. The authors concluded that the clinical characteristics observed in the infants probably represented a teratogenic syndrome related to benzodiazepines (7).

O

BREAST FEEDING SUMMARY

RECOMMENDATION: No Human Data - Potential Toxicity

Specific data relating to oxazepam usage in lactating women have not been located. Oxazepam, an active metabolite of diazepam, was detected in the urine of an infant exposed to high doses of diazepam during lactation (8). The infant was lethargic and demonstrated an electroencephalographic pattern compatible with sedative medication (see Diazepam).

References

1. Kangas L, Erkkola R, Kanto J, Eronen M. Transfer of free and conjugated oxazepam across the human placenta. Eur J Clin Pharmacol 1980;17:301–4.
2. Kanto J, Erkkola R, Sellman R. Perinatal metabolism of diazepam. Br Med J 1974;1:641–2.
3. Mandelli M, Morselli PL, Nordio S, Pardi G, Principi N, Seveni F, Tognoni G. Placental transfer of diazepam and its disposition in the newborn. Clin Pharmacol Ther 1975;17:564–72.
4. Kanto JH. Use of benzodiazepines during pregnancy, labour and lactation, with particular reference to pharmacokinetic considerations. Drugs 1982;23:354–80.
5. Gillberg C. "Floppy infant syndrome" and maternal diazepam. Lancet 1977;2:612–3.
6. Drury KAD, Spalding E, Donaldson D, Rutherford D. Floppy-infant syndrome: Is oxazepam the answer? Lancet 1977;2:1126–7.
7. Laegreid L, Olegard R, Walstrom J, Conradi N. Teratogenic effects of benzodiazepine use during pregnancy. J Pediatr 1989;114:126–31.
8. Patrick MJ, Tilstone WJ, Reavey P. Diazepam and breastfeeding. Br Med J 1972;1:542–3.

Name:	**OXCARBAZEPINE**	Risk Factor:	C_M
Class:	**Anticonvulsant**		

FETAL RISK SUMMARY

RECOMMENDATION: Limited Human Data - Animal Data Suggest Risk

Oxcarbazepine is an orally active anticonvulsant agent used as either monotherapy or adjunctive therapy in the treatment of partial seizures. The chemical structure of oxcarbazepine is closely related to that of another anticonvulsant, carbamazepine. Oxcarbazepine is rapidly metabolized to an active 10-monohydroxy metabolite (10-hydroxy-10,11-dihydrocarbamazepine; MHD) that is primarily responsible for the anticonvulsant activity.

In fertility studies with the active metabolite (MHD), an oral dose, 2 times the maximum recommended human dose based on body surface area (MRHD) administered to rats before and during mating and during early gestation caused disruption of the estrous cyclicity and a reduction in the numbers of corpora lutea, implantations, and live embryos (1). In pregnant rats, the administration of oral oxcarbazepine during organogenesis, at doses approximately 1.2 and 4 times the MRHD, caused increased incidences of fetal malformations (craniofacial, cardiovascular, and skeletal) and variations (1). Developmental toxicity (embryo/fetal death and growth retardation) was observed with oxcarbazepine at 4 times the MRHD. Oxcarbazepine (0.6 times the MRHD) or its active metabolite (1 times the MRHD) given during the latter part of gestation and throughout lactation were associated with persistent reductions in offspring body weights and, in the case of oxcarbazepine, altered behavior (decreased activity). Embryo and fetal death but no birth defects were observed in rabbits given oral doses of the active metabolite (1.5 times the MRHD) during organogenesis (1).

In a strain of mice susceptible to the teratogenic effects of carbamazepine, the highest tolerable oral dose of oxcarbazepine (1100 mg/kg/day) produced a lower incidence of teratogenicity (8% vs. 5% in controls; *n.s.*) than the epoxide metabolite of carbamazepine (14%–27% vs. 6% in controls; $p < 0.05$) (2). Concurrent treatment with phenobarbital did not increase the incidence of congenital malformations over that observed with oxcarbazepine alone.

In agreement with the relatively low molecular weight (about 252) of the parent drug, oxcarbazepine and its metabolite have been found in the fetus (3,4). In a woman who was taking oxcarbazepine monotherapy (300 mg 3 times daily) throughout gestation, maternal and term newborn plasma concentrations of the drug and its metabolite (MHD) were approximately equal (3). The healthy, 3700-g female infant had mild facial dysmorphism with a discrete epicanthus and a broad nasal bridge. Her development at 13 months of age was normal without signs of mental retardation or neurologic deficit.

In three women taking oxcarbazepine (600–1800 mg/day; time of last dose not specified), maternal and cord blood were obtained at delivery and analyzed for parent drug, active metabolite (MHD), and the inactive metabolite of MHD (4). The three agents were detected in all samples. In another part of the study, oxcarbazepine was metabolized to MHD in a dual recirculating human placental perfusion system, suggesting that the same metabolic process occurs *in vivo* (4). MHD, however, was not metabolized to the inactive metabolite by the placenta. No placental metabolism of carbamazepine was observed in the perfusion system.

The author of a 1994 report very briefly reviewed the pregnancy outcomes of 27 women treated with oxcarbazepine (5). The outcomes included 1 infant born with "some dysmorphic features" (which disappeared later in life), 3 spontaneous abortions, 1 infant with spina bifida (whose mother also received valproate), 1 newborn with "amniotic bands," and 22 normal infants (including 1 set of twins).

A 1996 review discussed the effects of oxcarbazepine and other anticonvulsants (6). Compared with carbamazepine, oxcarbazepine causes less induction of the cytochrome P450 enzyme system. However, oxcarbazepine may compromise the efficacy of hormonal contraception (6). The outcomes of 12 pregnancies treated with oxcarbazepine (3 spontaneous abortions and 9 normal newborns) were listed without further details.

In summary, oxcarbazepine is embryo and fetal toxic and teratogenic in some animal species. Although no major congenital malformations have been reported, with the possible exception of one case, mild facial defects have been observed. Of note, carbamazepine has also been associated with neural tube defects and minor craniofacial malformations (see Carbamazepine). The combined human data, however, are too limited to assess the absolute risk to the fetus. The effect of oxcarbazepine on folic acid levels or metabolism is unknown (6). Until this information is available, the safest course is to give folic acid supplementation with oxcarbazepine, as is done with other antiepileptic agents. In addition, metabolism of oxcarbazepine does not result in epoxide metabolites (4,6,7). Because these intermediate arene oxide metabolites have been associated with teratogenicity (see Carbamazepine, Phenytoin, and Valproic Acid), this may indicate a lower risk of teratogenicity with oxcarbazepine compared to the other agents.

BREAST FEEDING SUMMARY

RECOMMENDATION: Limited Human Data - Probably Compatible

Only one published report describing the use of oxcarbazepine during human lactation has been located. In a woman who took oxcarbazepine (900 mg/day) throughout gestation and during lactation (see case discussion above), the milk:plasma ratios of the drug and its active metabolite (MHD) were 0.5 (3). No adverse effects in the nursing infant from the exposure were mentioned. The manufacturer also states that the milk:plasma ratio for both agents is 0.5 (1). Because the American Academy of Pediatrics classifies carbamazepine as compatible with breast-feeding (see Carbamazepine), oxcarbazepine can probably be similarly classified.

References

1. Product information. Trileptal. Novartis Pharmaceuticals, 2001.
2. Bennett GD, Amore BM, Finnell RH, Wlodarczyk B, Kalhorn TF, Skiles GL, Nelson SD, Slattery JT. Teratogenicity of carbamazepine-10,11-epoxide and oxcarbazepine in the SWV mouse. J Pharmacol Exp Ther 1996;279:1237–42.
3. Bulau P, Paar WD, von Unruh GE. Pharmacokinetics of oxcarbazepine and 10-hydroxy-carbazepine in the newborn child of an oxcarbazepine-treated mother. Eur J Clin Pharmacol 1988;34:311–3.
4. Pienimaki P, Lampela E, Hakkola J, Arvela P, Raunio H, Vahakangas K. Pharmacokinetics of oxcarbazepine and carbamazepine in human placenta. Epilepsia 1997;38:309–16.
5. Andermann E. Pregnancy and oxcarbazepine. Epilepsia 1994;35(Suppl 3):S26.
6. Morrell MJ. The new antiepileptic drugs and women: efficacy, reproductive health, pregnancy, and fetal outcome. Epilepsia 1996;37(Suppl 6):S34–S44.
7. Grant SM, Faulds D. Oxcarbazepine. A review of its pharmacology and therapeutic potential in epilepsy, trigeminal neuralgia and affective disorders. Drugs 1992;43:873–88.

Name:	**OXPRENOLOL**	Risk Factor:	**C***
Class:	**Sympatholytic (Antihypertensive)**		

FETAL RISK SUMMARY

RECOMMENDATION: Human Data Suggest Risk in 2nd and 3rd Trimesters

Oxprenolol, a nonselective β-adrenergic blocking agent, has been used for the treatment of hypertension occurring during pregnancy (1–4). Oxprenolol and other β-blockers are generally considered safe and effective for this purpose by some reviewers (5,6). However, one reviewer recommended that agents with either cardioselectivity or α-blocking activity may be preferred to the nonselective blockers because these agents would be less likely to interfere with uterine perfusion (5). Other suggested guidelines governing the use of β-blockers in pregnancy were (a) if possible, avoid use in the 1st trimester; (b) use the lowest possible dose; and (c) if possible, discontinue the drugs 2–3 days before delivery (5). Oxprenolol crosses the placenta, but mean fetal serum levels at term are only about 25%–37% of maternal concentrations (4,6).

No fetal malformations or other fetal adverse effects attributable to oxprenolol have been reported, but experience during the 1st trimester is lacking. The drug has been compared with methyldopa in two studies of pregnant hypertensive women (1,2). In one of these studies, oxprenolol-exposed infants were significantly larger, 3051 g vs. 2654 g, than offspring of methyldopa-treated mothers (1). The difference was thought to be caused by the greater maternal plasma volume expansion and placental growth observed in the β-blocker group (1). In a follow-up report, the investigators noted that the differences between the two groups disappeared after 10 weeks of treatment (7). A 1983 study found no difference between oxprenolol- and methyldopa-treated groups in birth weight, placental weight, head circumference, and Apgar scores (2). In a third study, the combination of oxprenolol and prazosin (an α-adrenergic blocking agent) was effective for the control of severe essential hypertension in 25 pregnant women but not effective in 19 patients with gestational hypertension (3).

Although β-blockade of the newborn has not been reported in the offspring of oxprenolol-treated mothers, this complication has occurred with other members of this class (see Acebutolol, Atenolol, and Nadolol). Thus, close observation of the newborn for bradycardia and other symptoms of β-blockade are recommended during the first 24–48 hours after birth. Long-term effects of *in utero* exposure to β-blockers have not been studied but warrant evaluation.

Some β-blockers may cause intrauterine growth retardation (IUGR) and reduced placental weight, especially those lacking intrinsic sympathomimetic activity (ISA) (i.e., partial agonist). Treatment beginning early in the 2nd trimester results in the greatest weight reductions, whereas treatment restricted to the 3rd trimester primarily affects only placental weight. It is not known if oxprenolol possesses ISA. However, IUGR and reduced placental weight may potentially occur with all agents within this class. Although growth retardation is a serious concern, the benefits of maternal therapy with β-blockers, in some cases, might outweigh the risks to the fetus and must be judged on a case-by-case basis.

[**Risk Factor D if used in 2nd or 3rd trimesters.*]

O

BREAST FEEDING SUMMARY

RECOMMENDATION: Limited Human Data - Potential Toxicity

Oxprenolol is excreted into breast milk. In nine lactating women given 80 mg twice daily, the mean milk concentration of oxprenolol 105–135 minutes after a dose was 118 ng/mL (9). When a dose of 160 mg twice daily was given to three women, mean milk levels were 160 ng/mL. Finally, one woman was treated with 320 mg twice daily, producing a milk level of 470 ng/mL. The milk:plasma ratios for the three regimens were 0.14, 0.16, and 0.43, respectively. The mean milk:plasma ratio in another study was 0.45 (8). These low ratios, relative to other β-blockers, may be caused by the high maternal serum protein binding (80%) that negates trapping of the weakly basic drug in the relatively acidic milk (8). Based on calculations, a mother ingesting 240 mg/day would provide a 3-kg infant with a dose of 0.07 mg/kg in 500 mL of milk (8). This amount is probably clinically insignificant.

Although no adverse reactions have been noted in nursing infants of mothers treated with oxprenolol, infants should be closely observed for bradycardia and other symptoms of β-blockade. Long-term effects of exposure to β-blockers from milk have not been studied but warrant evaluation. The American Academy of Pediatrics classifies oxprenolol as compatible with breast-feeding (10).

References

1. Gallery EDM, Saunders DM, Hunyor SN, Gyory AZ. Randomized comparison of methyldopa and oxprenolol for treatment of hypertension in pregnancy. Br Med J 1979;1:1591–4.
2. Fidler J, Smith V, Fayers P, DeSwiet M. Randomized controlled comparative study of methyldopa and oxprenolol in treatment of hypertension in pregnancy. Br Med J 1983;286:1927–30.
3. Lubbe WF, Hodge JV. Combined α- and α-adrenoceptor antagonism with prazosin and oxprenolol in control of severe hypertension in pregnancy. N Z Med J 1981;94:169–72.
4. Lubbe WF. More on beta-blockers in pregnancy. N Engl J Med 1982;307:753.
5. Frishman WH, Chesner M. Beta-adrenergic blockers in pregnancy. Am Heart J 1988;115:147–52.
6. Gallery EDM. Hypertension in pregnant women. Med J Aust 1985;143:23–7.
7. Gallery EDM, Ross MR, Gyory AZ. Antihypertensive treatment in pregnancy: analysis of different responses to oxprenolol and methyldopa. Br Med J 1985;291:563–6.
8. Sioufi A, Hillion D, Lumbroso P, Wainer R, Olivier-Martin M, Schoeller JP, Colussi D, Leroux F, Mangoni P. Oxprenolol placental transfer, plasma concentrations in newborns and passage into breast milk. Br J Clin Pharmacol 1984;18:453–6.
9. Fidler J, Smith V, DeSwiet M. Excretion of oxprenolol and timolol in breast milk. Br J Obstet Gynaecol 1983;90:961–5.
10. Committee on Drugs, American Academy of Pediatrics. The transfer of drugs and other chemicals into human milk. Pediatrics 2001;108:776–89.

Name:	OXTRIPHYLLINE	Risk Factor:	C
Class:	Respiratory Drug (Bronchodilator)		

FETAL RISK SUMMARY

RECOMMENDATION: Compatible

Oxtriphylline is a methylxanthine that is metabolized to theophylline. Theophylline has been found in cord blood but not in the serum of an infant whose mother had taken oxtriphylline during pregnancy (1). No adverse effects in the infant were observed (see also Theophylline).

In a surveillance study of Michigan Medicaid recipients conducted between 1985 and 1992 involving 229,101 completed pregnancies, 63 newborns had been exposed to oxtriphylline during the 1st trimester (F. Rosa, personal communication, FDA, 1993). One (1.6%) major birth defect was observed (three expected). No anomalies were observed in six defect categories (cardiovascular defects, oral clefts, spina bifida, polydactyly, limb reduction defects, and hypospadias) for which specific data were available.

BREAST FEEDING SUMMARY

RECOMMENDATION: Compatible

No data are available. See also Theophylline.

Reference

1. Labovitz E, Spector S. Placental theophylline transfer in pregnant asthmatics. JAMA 1982;247:786–8.

Name:	**OXYBUTYNIN**	Risk Factor:	**B_M**
Class:	**Urinary Tract Agent (Antispasmodic)**		

FETAL RISK SUMMARY

RECOMMENDATION: No Human Data - Animal Data Suggest Low Risk

Oxybutynin is a tertiary amine that is a direct inhibitor of smooth muscle spasm of the urinary tract. The drug also possesses some antimuscarinic activity (about one-fifth of the anticholinergic activity of atropine). It is used for the relief of symptoms associated with bladder instability and nocturnal enuresis.

Reproduction studies in the hamster, mouse, rat, and rabbit have not demonstrated definite evidence of impaired fertility or fetal harm (1–3). No fetal harm was noted in female rats dosed orally with oxybutynin, 20–160 mg/kg/day (maximum recommended human dose is 20 mg/day or less than 0.5 mg/kg/day for an average adult) (4).

Reports describing the use of oxybutynin during human pregnancy have not been located. It is not known if the drug crosses the placenta to the fetus. The molecular weight (about 394 for the hydrochloride salt) is low enough, however, that passage to the fetus should be expected.

BREAST FEEDING SUMMARY

RECOMMENDATION: No Human Data - Probably Compatible

No reports describing the use of oxybutynin during human lactation have been located. The molecular weight (about 358 for the free base) is low enough, however, that

O

excretion into milk should be expected. The effect of this exposure on a nursing infant is unknown.

References

1. Product information. Ditropan. ALZA Pharmaceuticals, 2000.
2. Schardein JL. *Chemically Induced Birth Defects*. 2nd ed. New York, NY: Marcel Dekker, 1993:645.
3. Edwards JA, Reid YJ, Cozens DD. Reproductive toxicity studies with oxybutynin hydrochloride. Toxicology 1986;40:31–44.
4. Department of Research and Development, Marion Laboratories. *A Compendium. Ditropan. A New Urinary Tract Antispasmodic*. Kansas City, MO: Marian Laboratories, 1975:16.

Name:	**OXYCODONE**	Risk Factor:	$\mathbf{B_M}$*
Class:	**Narcotic Agonist Analgesic**		

FETAL RISK SUMMARY

RECOMMENDATION: Human Data Suggest Risk in 3rd Trimester

Oxycodone is a narcotic analgesic available as a single agent or in combination with nonnarcotic analgesics, such as acetaminophen or aspirin. Reproduction studies in rats and rabbits at doses up to 4 and 60 times the human dose of 120 mg/day in a 60 kg adult (0.7 and 19 times the human dose based on mg/m^2), respectively, found no evidence of fetal harm (1).

O

The Collaborative Perinatal Project monitored 50,282 mother-child pairs, 8 of whom had 1st trimester exposure to oxycodone (2). No evidence was found to suggest a relationship to large categories of major or minor malformations or to individual defects.

In a surveillance study of Michigan Medicaid recipients conducted between 1985 and 1992 involving 229,101 completed pregnancies, 281 newborns had been exposed to oxycodone during the 1st trimester (F. Rosa, personal communication, FDA, 1993). A total of 13 (4.6%) major birth defects were observed (12 expected), including (observed/expected) 3/3 cardiovascular defects and 1/1 hypospadias. No anomalies were observed in four other defect categories (oral clefts, spina bifida, polydactyly, and limb reduction defects) for which specific data were available. These data do not support an association between the drug and congenital defects.

At a 1996 meeting, data were presented on 118 women using oxycodone ($N = 78$) or hydrocodone ($N = 40$) during the 1st trimester for postoperative pain, general pain, or upper respiratory infection who were matched with a similar group using codeine for these purposes (3). Six (5.1%) of the infants exposed to oxycodone or hydrocodone had malformations, an odds ratio of 2.61 (95% confidence interval 0.6–11.5) ($p = 0.13$). There was no pattern evident among the six malformations.

[**Risk Factor D if used for prolonged periods or in high doses at term.*]

BREAST FEEDING SUMMARY

RECOMMENDATION: Limited Human Data - Probably Compatible

Oxycodone is excreted into breast milk. Six healthy postpartum women received a combination product of oxycodone and acetaminophen, one or two capsules every 4–7 hours, while breast-feeding their newborn infants (4). Maternal plasma levels were in the expected range of 14 to 35 ng/mL, and milk concentrations ranged from <5 to 226 ng/mL. Peak milk concentrations occurred 1.5–2.0 hours after the first dose, then at variable times after multiple doses. Although a large degree of variability was present, the mean milk:plasma ratio was 3.4:1. No mention was made of any effects observed in the nursing infants.

Although occasional maternal doses of oxycodone for analgesia probably present a minimal risk for adverse effects during nursing, infants should be monitored for gastrointestinal effects, sedation, and changes in feeding patterns.

References

1. Product information. Oxycontin. Purdue Frederick, 1997.
2. Heinonen OP, Slone D, Shapiro S. *Birth Defects and Drugs in Pregnancy*. Littleton, MA: Publishing Sciences Group, 1977:287.
3. Schick B, Horn M, Tolosa J, Librizzi R, Donnfeld A. Preliminary analysis of first trimester exposure to oxycodone and hydrocodone (abstract). Presented at the Ninth International Conference of the Organization of Teratology Information Services, Salt Lake City, Utah, May 2–4, 1996. Reprod Toxicol 1996;10:162.
4. Marx CM, Pucino F, Carlson JD, Driscoll JW, Ruddock V. Oxycodone excretion in human milk in the puerperium (abstract). Drug Intell Clin Pharm 1986;20:474.

Name: **OXYMETAZOLINE** Risk Factor: **C**

Class: **Sympathomimetic (Adrenergic)**

FETAL RISK SUMMARY

RECOMMENDATION: Limited Human Data - No Relevant Animal Data

Oxymetazoline, an α-adrenergic agent, is a long-acting vasoconstrictor used topically in nasal decongestant sprays. No reports associating oxymetazoline with congenital abnormalities have been located. The Collaborative Perinatal Project recorded only 2 cases of exposure from 50,282 mother-child pairs (1). Although there was no indication of risk for malformations, the number of women exposed is too small for any conclusion.

Uterine vessels are normally maximally dilated and have only α-adrenergic receptors (2). Use of the α-adrenergic agent, oxymetazoline, could cause constriction of these vessels and reduce uterine blood flow, thereby producing fetal hypoxia and bradycardia. A 1985 case report illustrated this toxicity when a nonreactive nonstress test and a positive contraction stress test were discovered in a 20-year-old woman at 41 weeks' gestation (3). Persistent late fetal heart rate decelerations were observed, and blood obtained from the fetal scalp revealed a pH of 7.23. The mother had self-administered a nasal spray containing 0.05% oxymetazoline, two sprays in each nostril, 6 times in a 15.5-hour interval before the nonstress test with the last dose administered 0.5 hour before testing. The recommended dosage interval for the preparation was every 12 hours. Approximately 6 hours after the last dose the late decelerations disappeared and the normal beat-to-beat variability returned about 0.5 hour later. A normal male infant with Apgar scores of 9 and 9 at 1 and 5 minutes, respectively, was delivered spontaneously 14 hours after the last dose.

In contrast to the above case, a 1990 report described the results of a single dose (two full squirts) of 0.05% oxymetazoline (4). The drug was self-administered by 12 women with allergic rhinitis, sinusitis, or an upper respiratory tract infection. The otherwise healthy women were between 27 and 39 weeks' gestation. The effects of this dose on the maternal and fetal circulations were measured at 15-minute intervals for 2 hours after the dose. No significant changes were observed for maternal blood pressures or pulse rates, fetal aortic blood flow velocity, and fetal heart rate, or for the systolic to diastolic ratios in the uterine arcuate artery and umbilical artery. The investigators concluded that oxymetazoline, when administered at the recommended frequency, did not pose a risk for the healthy patient. Women with borderline placental reserve, however, should use the agent cautiously (4).

BREAST FEEDING SUMMARY

RECOMMENDATION: No Human Data - Probably Compatible

No data are available.

References

1. Heinonen OP, Slone D, Shapiro S. *Birth Defects and Drugs in Pregnancy*. Littleton, MA: Publishing Sciences Group, 1977:346.
2. Smith NT, Corbascio AN. The use and misuse of pressor agents. Anesthesiology 1970;33:58–101.
3. Baxi LV, Gindoff PR, Pregenzer GJ, Parras MK. Fetal heart rate changes following maternal administration of a nasal decongestant. Am J Obstet Gynecol 1985;153:799–800.
4. Rayburn WF, Anderson JC, Smith CV, Appel LL, Davis SA. Uterine and fetal doppler flow changes from a single dose of a long-acting intranasal decongestant. Obstet Gynecol 1990;76:180–2.

Name:	**OXYMORPHONE**	Risk Factor:	**B***
Class:	**Narcotic Agonist Analgesic**		

FETAL RISK SUMMARY

RECOMMENDATION: Human Data Suggest Risk in 3rd Trimester

No reports linking the use of oxymorphone with congenital defects have been located. Use of this drug during labor produces neonatal respiratory depression to the same degree as other narcotic analgesics (1–4).

[**Risk Factor D if used for prolonged periods or in high doses at term.*]

BREAST FEEDING SUMMARY

RECOMMENDATION: No Human Data - Probably Compatible

No data are available.

References

1. Simeckova M, Shaw W, Pool E, Nichols EE. Numorphan in labor—a preliminary report. Obstet Gynecol 1960;16:119–23.
2. Sentnor MH, Solomons E, Kohl SG. An evaluation of oxymorphone in labor. Am J Obstet Gynecol 1962;84:956–61.
3. Eames GM, Pool KRS. Clinical trial of oxymorphone in labor. Br Med J 1964;2:353–5.
4. Ransom S. Oxymorphone as an obstetric analgesic—a clinical trial. Anesthesia 1966;21:464–71.

Name: **OXYPHENBUTAZONE** Risk Factor: **C**
Class: **Nonsteroidal Anti-inflammatory**

See Phenylbutazone.

Name: **OXYPHENCYCLIMINE** Risk Factor: **C**
Class: **Parasympatholytic (Anticholinergic)**

FETAL RISK SUMMARY

RECOMMENDATION: Limited Human Data - No Relevant Animal Data

Oxyphencyclimine is an anticholinergic agent. In a large prospective study, 2323 patients were exposed to this class of drugs during the 1st trimester, 1 of whom took oxyphencyclimine (1). A possible association was found between the total group and minor malformations.

BREAST FEEDING SUMMARY

RECOMMENDATION: No Human Data - Probably Compatible

No data are available (see also Atropine).

Reference

1. Heinonen OP, Slone D, Shapiro S. *Birth Defects and Drugs in Pregnancy*. Littleton, MA: Publishing Sciences Group, 1977:346–53.

Name: **OXYPHENONIUM** Risk Factor: **C**
Class: **Parasympatholytic (Anticholinergic)**

FETAL RISK SUMMARY

RECOMMENDATION: No Human Data - No Relevant Animal Data

Oxyphenonium is an anticholinergic quaternary ammonium bromide. No reports of its use in pregnancy have been located (see also Atropine).

BREAST FEEDING SUMMARY

RECOMMENDATION: No Human Data - Probably Compatible

No data are available (see also Atropine).

Name:	**OXYTETRACYCLINE**	Risk Factor:	**D**
Class:	**Antibiotic (Tetracycline)**		

See Tetracycline.

P

Name:	**PACLITAXEL**	Risk Factor:	D_M
Class:	**Antineoplastic**		

FETAL RISK SUMMARY

RECOMMENDATION: Limited Human Data - Animal Data Suggest Risk

Paclitaxel, a novel antineoplastic agent, is indicated for the treatment of advanced ovarian cancer but also is used in other malignancies. The drug is a natural product obtained by extraction from *Taxus brevifolia* (Pacific yew tree) (1,2). Paclitaxel is an antimicrotubule agent, an action that results in the inhibition of the normal reorganization of the microtubule network that is essential for vital interphase and mitotic cellular functions (1). The pharmacokinetics of paclitaxel is markedly affected by the dose and infusion rate with elimination half-lives varying from approximately 13 to 53 hours. Approximately 89%–98% of the agent is protein bound (1). The free commercial form of paclitaxel contains the vehicle polyoxyethylated castor oil (also known as polyoxyl 35 castor oil) (1,2).

Reproduction studies in pregnant rabbits at doses about 0.2 times the maximum recommended human daily dose based on body surface area (MRHDD) caused embryo and fetal toxicity (increased resorptions and intrauterine deaths). However, maternal toxicity was observed at this dose. No teratogenic effects were noted at a dose about 0.07 times the MRHDD, but the teratogenic potential of higher doses could not be assessed because of extensive fetal mortality (1).

The carcinogenic potential of paclitaxel has not been studied. The drug was not mutagenic in one test but was clastogenic *in vitro* (human lymphocytes) and *in vivo* (micronucleus test in mice). Fertility in male and female rats was impaired at doses about 0.04 times the MRHHD, and, at this dose, increased embryo and fetal toxicity was observed (1).

Interestingly, a 1995 research report concluded that some, paclitaxel-induced, embryotoxicity in animals might be a result of the polyoxyethylated castor oil vehicle (2). In an experiment with chick embryos, the researchers compared free paclitaxel containing the vehicle with liposome-encapsulated paclitaxel. At a dose of 1.5 μg/egg, 60% of the embryos either died or were malformed. A 20-fold higher dose was required to produce the same degree of toxicity with the liposome-encapsulated product (2).

In a follow-up to the above study, the same group of researchers compared the developmental toxicity in rats of free and encapsulated paclitaxel (3). Free paclitaxel, at a dose of 10 mg/kg (approximately 0.4 times the MRHHD) given IV once on gestation day 8 (determined to be the most sensitive day for the production of paclitaxel-induced malformations), produced maternal toxicity and resorption of all embryos in surviving dams. At 2 mg/kg (about 0.08 times the MRHHD) of free paclitaxel, embryo/fetal toxicity (increased resorptions and reduced fetal weight) and anomalies (exencephaly, anencephaly, ventral wall defects, facial clefts, anophthalmia, diaphragmatic hernia, and malformations of the kidney, cardiovascular system, and tail) were observed (3). In contrast, no toxicity or anomalies were observed with a 2 mg/kg IV dose of encapsulated paclitaxel. At 10 mg/kg, toxicity and malformations were noted that were similar to those observed with the free drug at 2 mg/kg. Thus, encapsulation appeared to increase the dose needed to produce toxicity and malformations (3).

It is not known if paclitaxel crosses the placenta to the human fetus. The molecular weight (about 854) and extensive protein binding suggest that transfer to the fetal compartment is limited. Encapsulation of paclitaxel, however, could markedly increase or decrease the amount of drug crossing the placenta to the fetus (3). The authors of the above study cited examples in perfused *in vitro* human placentas in which liposome encapsulation reduced placental transfer. In contrast, they also cited studies in intact rats and rabbits that showed that encapsulation could enhance placental transfer, possibly by a process involving placental intracellular sequestration and degradation of liposomes (3).

Only two cases of exposure to paclitaxel during human pregnancy, both in the 2nd and 3rd trimesters, have been located (4,5). A 33-year-old woman was diagnosed with ovarian carcinoma at 27 weeks' gestation (4). Six days after debulking surgery that preserved the pregnancy, she received the first cycle of paclitaxel (135 mg/m^2) over 24 hours and cisplatin (75 mg/m^2) over 4 hours. She received two more cycles of chemotherapy at 3-week intervals. Appropriate fetal growth was documented by ultrasound. Fetal lung maturity was demonstrated at 37 weeks' gestation and a cesarean section was performed to deliver a 2800-g female with Apgar scores of 9 and 10 at 1 and 5 minutes, respectively, and normal blood counts. The infant had normal growth and development to 30 months of age (4).

A 2003 report described the pregnancy outcome of a 30-year-old woman treated with carboplatin and paclitaxel during the 2nd and 3rd trimesters (5). She was diagnosed with an advanced stage of serous papillary adenocarcinoma of the ovary in the 1st trimester. The woman underwent an exploratory laparotomy at 7.5 weeks' gestation and consented to chemotherapy beginning at 16–17 weeks. She received six cycles of carboplatin (dose specified as AUC 5) and paclitaxel (175 mg/m^2) and was delivered by cesarean hysterectomy 3 weeks after the last cycle, at 35.5 weeks. The newborn (sex not specified) had Apgar scores of 9, 9, and 9 at 1, 5, and 10 minutes, respectively. Birth weight was 2500 g (44th percentile), and the physical examination and laboratory tests were normal. In addition, the placenta appeared grossly normal. The infant was doing well at 15 months of age with no evidence of neurologic, renal, growth, or hematologic effects from the exposure (5).

In a novel case report, a 21-year-old woman was diagnosed with metastatic ovarian cancer that was initially treated with surgery that left her uterus, right fallopian tube and ovary *in situ* (6). She was then enrolled into a phase I transplant protocol and received three cycles of paclitaxel (225 mg/m^2) and carboplatin (dose specified as AUC 6). Subsequent high-dose chemotherapy was then given (paclitaxel, carboplatin, and/or cyclophosphamide). After her chemotherapy, the woman received a successful transplant of autologous peripheral blood stem cells. Approximately 16 months after the transplant she conceived but had a 1st trimester miscarriage. She conceived again several months later and eventually delivered a healthy full-term, 3000-g female infant. The child was developing normally at 17 months of age (6).

A 30-year-old woman became pregnant approximately 2 years after treatment of stage IIB fallopian tube carcinoma with paclitaxel and cisplatin (7). She was diagnosed with an asymptomatic intra-abdominal recurrence at 16 weeks' gestation but refused additional therapy. A 2888-g male infant was delivered by cesarean section at 37 weeks. No additional information about the infant was given.

In summary, paclitaxel produces embryo and fetal toxicity and is teratogenic in animals. In addition, the drug was clastogenic in *in vitro* and *in vivo* tests. In animals, compared with the free drug, liposome-encapsulation of paclitaxel appears to markedly increase the dose at which toxicity and teratogenicity are observed. Whether this also would occur in human pregnancy is not known. The human pregnancy experience is too limited to assess the potential for embryo/fetal toxicity. However, the animal data suggest there is a risk of congenital malformations from exposure during organogenesis. Use after this period appears to be relatively safe, but the fetus should be monitored appropriately.

BREAST FEEDING SUMMARY

RECOMMENDATION: Contraindicated

No reports describing the use of paclitaxel during human lactation have been located. In rats, milk concentrations appeared to be higher than maternal plasma levels and declined in parallel with the maternal levels (1). Because of the potential for serious toxicity in a nursing infant, women receiving this agent should not breast-feed (8).

References

1. Product information. Paclitaxel Injection. Faulding Pharmaceutical, 2003.
2. Scialli AR, DeSesso JM, Rahman A, Husain SR, Goeringer GC. Embryotoxicity of free and liposome-encapsulated Taxol in the chick. Pharmacology 1995;51:145–51.
3. Scialli AR, Waterhouse TB, DeSesso JM, Rahman A, Goeringer GC. Protective effect of liposome encapsulation on paclitaxel developmental toxicity in the rat. Teratology 1997;56:305–10.
4. Sood AK, Shahin MS, Sorosky JI. Paclitaxel and platinum chemotherapy for ovarian carcinoma during pregnancy. Gynecol Oncol 2001;83:599–600.
5. Méndez LE, Mueller A, Salom E, González-Quintero VH. Paclitaxel and carboplatin chemotherapy administered during pregnancy for advanced epithelial ovarian cancer. Obstet Gynecol 2003;102:1200–2.
6. Seiden MV, Spitzer TR, McAfee S, Fuller AF. Successful pregnancy after high-dose cyclophosphamide, carboplatinum, and Taxol with peripheral blood stem cell transplant in a young woman with ovarian cancer. Gynecol Oncol 2001;83:412–4.
7. Adolph A, Le T, Khan K, Biem S. Recurrent metastatic fallopian tube carcinoma in pregnancy. Gynecol Oncol 2001;81:110–2.
8. Leslie KK. Chemotherapy and pregnancy. Clin Obstet Gynecol 2002;45:153–64.

Name:	**PANCURONIUM**	Risk Factor:	C_M
Class:	**Skeletal Muscle Relaxant**		

FETAL RISK SUMMARY

RECOMMENDATION: Limited Human Data - Animal Data Suggest Low Risk

Pancuronium (pancuronium bromide) is a competitive (non-depolarizing) neuromuscular blocking agent. Structurally, it is a bisquaternary ammonium compound (i.e., contains two quaternary ammonium groups) and is commercially available as the dibromide. Pancuronium is used to induce skeletal muscle relaxation during anesthesia and other procedures, and has been used to produce fetal muscle paralysis during intrauterine procedures.

Unpublished reproduction studies in rats and rabbits with pancuronium did not reveal any effect on the number of resorptions, litter size, birth weight and vitality, or the frequency of malformations (gross, skeletal, and internal organs) (1). Pregnant rats (average gestational length 21–22 days [2]) received intraperitoneal doses of 0.16 mg/kg/day either from the 7th to the 14th day or from the 1st to the 20th day of gestation, whereas pregnant rabbits (average gestational length 31–34 days [2]) were given IV doses of 0.02 mg/kg/day from day 8 to day 16 of gestation.

Theoretically, the combination of relatively high molecular weight (about 733 for the dibromide) and the presence of two quaternary ammonium groups that are ionized at physiologic pH should limit the placental transfer of pancuronium. An animal study, published in 1973, appeared to confirm the lack of significant transfer when cumulative IV doses up to 16.3 mg/kg administered to pregnant ferrets (neuromuscular block in the mother complete at 0.015 mg/kg) did not cause neuromuscular blockade in the fetus during a 1-hour observation period (3). The fetus was responsive to pancuronium-induced blockade by direct administration. Furthermore, the lack of adverse effects in newborns after mean doses of 0.0875 mg/kg at cesarean section led some authors to conclude that the drug did not cross the placenta (4). However, several human studies have demonstrated placental transfer, at least near term, when pancuronium was used during cesarean section (5–11).

Maternal IV bolus doses between 0.04 mg/kg and 0.12 mg/kg (approximately 2.8–8.6 times the maternal ED_{50}, the dose producing a 50% depression of evoked twitch tension [12]), resulted in mean umbilical vein:maternal vein ratios ranging from 0.19 to 0.26. These ratios were higher than those measured with atracurium, fazadinium, pipecuronium, rocuronium, *d*-tubocurarine, and vecuronium (13). No clinical evidence of neuromuscular blockade was observed in five studies in which the neonatal condition was noted (5–9), but in one of the studies (9), the Neurologic and Adaptive Capacity Scores (NACS) system indicated that neonatal depression was present. The NACS evaluates adaptive capacity, passive and active muscular tone, primary reflexes, and general assessment (13). The maximum score possible is 40 with a score of 35–40 denoting a normal, vigorous baby.

The NACS was measured at 15 minutes, 2 hours, and 24 hours in seven newborns whose mothers had been given IV doses of *d*-tubocurarine (3 mg), thiopental (4mg/kg), succinylcholine (1.5 mg/kg), and pancuronium (0.04 mg/kg) immediately prior to cesarean section (9). Five newborns (71%) had a NACS value <35 at 15 minutes, three were <35 at 2 hours, and none were <35 at 24 hours (9). Although the NACS indicated depression, no neonatal adverse effects were actually observed (9). A 1998 review, commenting on this and other studies of neuromuscular relaxants in pregnancy, thought the low NACS values might have been caused by a contribution from the other anesthetic agents (13).

The direct administration of pancuronium has been reported in animals and humans (14–38). A 1989 report compared the effects of pancuronium (0.5 mg/kg IV over 5 minutes) and *d*-tubocurarine (3.0 mg/kg IV over 5 minutes) on the heart rate and mean arterial pressure of fetal lambs (14). Whereas pancuronium significantly increased both rate and pressure, both measures were significantly decreased by *d*-tubocurarine. Only pancuronium effected fetal pH and PCO_2, increasing the former and decreasing the latter. The human studies, discussed below, all involve pancuronium administration during the second half of gestation.

In a study published in 1988, the baseline fetal heart rate (FHR), number of accelerations, and beat-to-beat variability were assessed before and after an IV bolus dose of pancuronium (0.05–0.10 mg/kg) was given to 17 fetuses before transfusion (15). Twenty minutes after transfusion, no changes were noted in the baseline FHR, although some heart rate patterns appeared "sinusoidal-like," but significant decreases in accelerations ($p = 0.003$) and variability ($p = 0.0003$) were observed (15). The transient FHR changes were not indicative of fetal compromise and returned to normal when the fetus "awakened" (15). A 1991 abstract reported significantly less bradycardia with the use of pancuronium

P

(0.3 mg/kg) compared with no muscle relaxant after cordocentesis (3.6% [8/224] vs. 8.2% [27/329], $p = 0.04$) and a near-significant difference after intravascular transfusion (7.9% [9/114] vs. 40% [2/5], $p = 0.06$) (16).

Pancuronium (0.1 mg/kg IV) was administered to 20 fetuses immediately before blood transfusion at 28 to 34 weeks' gestation (17). A control group of 20 fetuses matched for gestational age and hematocrit who did not receive pancuronium was used for comparison. After transfusion, compared with controls, fetuses that received pancuronium had significantly fewer FHR accelerations (mean 0 vs 3.0, $p < 0.0005$), less change in the baseline FHR (increase 1.5 beats/minute vs. decrease 4 beats/minute, $p < 0.0005$), lower mean minute range in FHR variation (17.3 vs. 34.7, $p < 0.0001$), and less short-term variation (3.4 vs. 7.35, $p = 0.0001$). Another study compared FHR changes after the use of pancuronium or vecuronium for intravascular transfusion, fetal thoracentesis, or paracentesis (18). Specific details were not provided for the pancuronium group, but the authors concluded that the pancuronium-induced increase in FHR and decrease in variability made it less desirable than vecuronium, which caused no FHR changes.

Fetal death at 25.5 weeks' gestation, that was apparently the result of a cord hematoma, occurred 2 hours after an intravascular intrauterine transfusion (19). The authors thought that the accident was related to the injection of pancuronium before confirmation of needle placement by aspiration of fetal blood. The results of an autopsy confirmed that the cause of death was compression of the umbilical vein by the hematoma with subsequent umbilical venous thrombosis.

Fetal administration of pancuronium immediately preceding magnetic resonance imaging (MRI) has been described in a number of publications (20–28). Most doses varied from 0.08 to 0.3 mg/kg (IV into the umbilical vein or IM) (20–25), two used 0.5 mg IM (26,27), and one reported 100 mg (*sic*) into the intrahepatic vein of each twin (28).

Direct fetal administration of pancuronium for intrauterine procedures, such as cordocentesis and intravascular transfusion, has been reported (29–38). The fetal dose ranged from 0.1 to 0.3 mg/kg IV or IM, but in one report, a single 0.5-mg IM dose was administered (29). In another study, pancuronium (0.15 mg/kg of the estimated total fetal body weights of twins) was administered in two cases to the smaller of a set of twins (38). The procedure was undertaken in an attempt to diagnose twin-twin transfusion syndrome. In the first case, the FHR patterns of both twins showed lack of accelerations and decreased variability and, in addition, the larger twin had a "sinusoidal-like" pattern. In the second case, absent accelerations and decreased variability occurred only in the smaller twin (38).

A continuous infusion of morphine, midazolam, and pancuronium was administered for 10 hours to allow mechanical ventilation in a seriously ill, pregnant (about 35 weeks) woman with pneumonia caused by *Legionella pneumophila* (39). No evidence of fetal harm was observed during the infusion, but the fetus was noted to have a consistent pattern of "sleeping." Approximately 3 to 4 weeks later, at 40 weeks' gestation, the mother gave birth to a healthy female infant.

In summary, pancuronium has been administered directly to the fetus during the last half of pregnancy and to the mother at cesarean section without causing fetal harm. Although no teratogenicity was observed in two animal species, the use of pancuronium in early human pregnancy has not been reported. The drug is known to cross the human placenta to the fetus, at least near term. Placental transfer early in pregnancy has not been reported. Large or repetitive doses and/or prolonged dose-to-delivery intervals may potentially result in newborn depression, but the clinical significance of this appears to be low. Moreover, other anesthetic agents may contribute to the condition. In addition, transient FHR changes, such as decreased accelerations and beat-to-beat variability, and an occasional sinusoidal-like pattern, have been observed after direct fetal administration, but apparently this does not indicate fetal compromise.

BREAST FEEDING SUMMARY

RECOMMENDATION: No Human Data - Probably Compatible

No reports describing the use of pancuronium in a lactating woman have been located. Because of the nature of the drug and its indications, such reports are unlikely to occur. Moreover, because pancuronium is a bisquaternary ammonium compound, it is ionized at physiologic pH. Only the nonionized form would be available for excretion into milk, and this would probably be only trace amounts (40). In addition, compounds of this type are poorly absorbed from the gastrointestinal tract (40).

References

1. Speight TM, Avery GS. Pancuronium bromide: A review of its pharmacological properties and clinical application. Drugs 1972;4:163–226.
2. Shepard TH. *Catalog of Teratogenic Agents*. 9th ed. Baltimore, MD: Johns Hopkins University Press, 1998.
3. Evans CA, Waud DR. Do maternally administered neuromuscular blocking agents interfere with fetal neuromuscular transmission? Anesth Analg 1973;52:548–52.
4. Neeld JB Jr, Seabrook PD Jr, Chastain GM, Frederickson EL. A clinical comparison of pancuronium and tubocurarine for cesarean section anesthesia. Anesth Analg 1974;53:7–11.
5. Speirs I, Sim AW. The placental transfer of pancuronium bromide. Br J Anaesth 1972;44:370–3.
6. Booth PN, Watson MJ, McLeod K. Pancuronium and the placental barrier. Anaesthesia 1977;32:320–3.
7. Duvaldestin P, Demetriou M, Henzel D, Desmonts JM. The placental transfer of pancuronium and its pharmacokinetics during caesarian section. Acta Anaesthiol Scand 1978;22:327–33.
8. Abouleish E, Wingard LB Jr, De La Vega S, Uy N. Pancuronium in caesarean section and its placental transfer. Br J Anaesth 1980;52:531–6.
9. Dailey PA, Fisher DM, Shnider SM, Baysinger CL, Shinohara Y, Miller RD, Abboud TK, Kim KC. Pharmacokinetics, placental transfer, and neonatal effects of vecuronium and pancuronium administered during cesarean section. Anesthesiology 1984;60:569–74.
10. Heaney GAH. Pancuronium in maternal and foetal serum. Br J Anaesth 1974;46:282–7.
11. Wingard LB Jr, Abouleish E, West DC, Goehl TJ. Modified fluorometric quantitation of pancuronium bromide and metabolites in human maternal and umbilical serums. J Pharm Sci 1979;68:914–5.
12. Agoston S, Crul JF, Kersten UW, Scaf AHJ. Relationship of the serum concentration of pancuronium to its neuromuscular activity in man. Anesthesiology 1977;47:509–12.
13. Guay J, Grenier Y, Varin F. Clinical pharmacokinetics of neuromuscular relaxants in pregnancy. Clin Pharmacokinet 1998;34:483–96.
14. Chestnut DH, Weiner CP, Thompson CS, McLaughlin GL. Intravenous administration of *d*-tubocurarine and pancuronium in fetal lambs. Am J Obstet Gynecol 1989;160:510–3.
15. Pielet BW, Socol ML, MacGregor SN, Dooley SL, Minogue J. Fetal heart rate changes after fetal intravascular treatment with pancuronium bromide. Am J Obstet Gynecol 1988;159:640–3.
16. Weiner C. Pancuronium protects against fetal bradycardia following umbilical cord puncture (abstract). Am J Obstet Gynecol 1991;164:335.
17. Spencer JAD, Ronderos-Dumit D, Rodeck CH. The effect of neuromuscular blockade on human fetal heart rate and its variation. Br J Obstet Gynaecol 1994;101:121–4.
18. Watson WJ, Atchison SR, Harlass FE. Comparison of pancuronium and vecuronium for fetal neuromuscular blockade during invasive procedures. J Matern Fetal Med 1996;5:151–4.
19. Seeds JW, Chescheir NC, Bowes WA Jr, Owl-Smith FA. Fetal death as a complication of intrauterine intravascular transfusion. Obstet Gynecol 1989;74:461–3.
20. Williamson RA, Weiner CP, Yuh WTC, Abu-Yousef MM. Magnetic resonance imaging of anomalous fetuses. Obstet Gynecol 1989;73:952–6.
21. Lituania M, Passamonti U, Cordone MS, Magnano GM, Toma P. Schizencephaly: prenatal diagnosis by computed sonography and magnetic resonance imaging. Prenat Diagn 1989;9:649–55.
22. Toma P, Lucigrai G, Dodero P, Lituania M. Prenatal detection of an abdominal mass by MR imaging performed while the fetus is immobilized with pancuronium bromide. AJR Am J Roentgenol 1990;154:1049–50.
23. Toma P, Costa A, Magnano GM, Cariati M, Lituania M. Holoprosencephaly: prenatal diagnosis by sonography and magnetic resonance imaging. Prenat Diagn 1990;10:429–36.
24. Wenstrom KD, Williamson RA, Weiner CP, Sipes SL,

P

Yuh WTC. Magnetic resonance imaging of fetuses with intracranial defects. Obstet Gynecol 1991;77: 529–32.
25. Okamura K, Murotsuki J, Sakai T, Matsumoto K, Shirane R, Yajima A. Prenatal diagnosis of lissencephaly by magnetic resonance image. Fetal Diagn Ther 1993;8:56–9.
26. Lenke RR, Persutte WH, Nemes JM. Use of pancuronium bromide to inhibit fetal movement during magnetic resonance imaging. A case report. J Reprod Med 1989;34:315–7.
27. Horvath L, Seeds JW. Temporary arrest of fetal movement with pancuronium bromide to enable antenatal magnetic resonance imaging of holoprosencephaly. Am J Perinatol 1989;6:418–20.
28. Zoppini C, Vanzulli A, Kustermann A, Rizzuti T, Selicorni A, Nicolini U. Prenatal diagnosis of anatomical connections in conjoined twins by use of contrast magnetic resonance imaging. Prenat Diagn 1993; 13:995–9.
29. Seeds JW, Corke BC, Spielman FJ. Prevention of fetal movement during invasive procedures with pancuronium bromide. Am J Obstet Gynecol 1986;155:818–9.
30. Moise KJ Jr, Carpenter RJ Jr, Deter RL, Kirshon B, Diaz SF. The use of neuromuscular blockade during intrauterine procedures. Am J Obstet Gynecol 1987;157:874–9.
31. Copel JA, Grannum PA, Harrison D, Hobbins JC. The use of intravenous pancuronium bromide to produce fetal paralysis during intravascular transfusion. Am J Obstet Gynecol 1988;158:170–1.
32. Moise KJ Jr, Deter RL, Kirshon B, Adam K, Patton DE, Carpenter RJ Jr. Intravenous pancuronium bromide for fetal neuromuscular blockade during intrauterine transfusion for red-cell alloimmunization. Obstet Gynecol 1989;74:905–8.
33. Fan SZ, Huang FY, Lin SY, Wang YP, Hsieh FJ. Intrauterine neuromuscular blockade in fetus. Anaesth Sinica 1990;28:31–4.
34. Weiner CP, Wenstrom KD, Sipes SL, Williamson RA. Risk factors for cordocentesis and fetal intravascular transfusion. Am J Obstet Gynecol 1991;165:1020–5.
35. Fan SZ, Susetio L, Tsai MC. Neuromuscular blockade of the fetus with pancuronium or pipecuronium for intra-uterine procedures. Anaesthesia 1994;49: 284–6.
36. Mouw RJC, Hermans J, Brandenburg HCR, Kanhai HHH. Effects of pancuronium or atracurium on the anemic fetus during and directly after intrauterine transfusion (IUT): a double blind randomized study (abstract). Am J Obstet Gynecol 1997;176:S18.
37. Mouw RJC, Klumper F, Hermans J, Brandenburg HCR, Kanhai HHH. Effect of atracurium or pancuronium on the anemic fetus during and directly after intravascular intrauterine transfusion. A double blind randomized study. Acta Obstet Gynecol Scand 1999;78:763–7.
38. Tanaka M, Natori M, Ishimoto H, Kohno H, Kobayashi T, Nozawa S. Intravascular pancuronium bromide infusion for prenatal diagnosis of twin-twin transfusion syndrome. Fetal Diagn Ther 1992;7:36–40.
39. Eisenberg VH, Eidelman LA, Arbel R, Ezra Y. Legionnaire's disease during pregnancy: a case presentation and review of the literature. Eur J Obstet Gynecol Reprod Biol 1997;72:15–8.
40. Spigset O. Anaesthetic agents and excretion in breast milk. Acta Anaesthesiol Scand 1994;38:94–103.

Name:	**PANTOPRAZOLE**	Risk Factor:	**B_M**
Class:	**Gastrointestinal Agent (Antisecretory)**		

FETAL RISK SUMMARY

RECOMMENDATION: No Human Data - Animal Data Suggest Low Risk

Pantoprazole is a proton pump inhibitor that blocks gastric acid secretion by a direct inhibitory effect on the gastric parietal cell (1). It is used in the short-term treatment of erosive esophagitis associated with gastroesophageal reflux disease (GERD).

Reproductive studies have been conducted in pregnant rats and rabbits at doses up to 88 and 16 times, respectively, the recommended human dose based on body surface area (1). No evidence was found at these doses of impaired fertility or fetal harm.

Similar to other proton pump inhibitors, pantoprazole is carcinogenic in mice and rats (gastrointestinal, liver, and thyroid) (1). The dose-related nature of the tumors and the presumable limited *in utero* exposure to the drug during human gestation probably indicates a negligible risk. In addition, positive results were seen with pantoprazole in the *in vitro* human lymphocyte chromosomal aberration assays, and in some mutagenic tests with mice, rats, and hamsters. However, negative results were obtained in the *in vitro* Ames mutation assay and in the mammalian cell-forward gene mutation assay, and in several other tests of mutagenicity (1).

It is not known if pantoprazole crosses the human placenta. The molecular weight (about 432 for the hydrated form) is low enough, however, that passage to the fetus should be expected. Another proton pump inhibitor, omeprazole, has a similar molecular weight (about 345) and chemical structure and it is known to cross the human placenta (see Omeprazole).

No reports describing the use of pantoprazole during human pregnancy have been located. Human pregnancy experience with two other proton pump inhibitors (see Lansoprazole and Omeprazole) have not shown a causal relationship with congenital malformations. In some cases, for both agents, malformations may have been missed because of the design and size of the studies. The animal and cell toxicity data are a potential concern, but the absence of follow-up studies prevents a risk assessment for exposed offspring. As with all drug therapy, avoidance of pantoprazole during pregnancy, especially during the 1st trimester, is the safest course. If pantoprazole is required or if inadvertent exposure does occur early in gestation, the known risk to the embryo/fetus for congenital defects, based on animal data for pantoprazole and the published experience for other proton pump inhibitors, appears to be low. Long-term follow-up of offspring exposed during gestation is warranted.

BREAST FEEDING SUMMARY

RECOMMENDATION: No Human Data - Potential Toxicity

No reports describing the use of pantoprazole during human lactation have been located. Both pantoprazole and the inactive metabolites are excreted into the milk of lactating rats (1). The animal data and the relatively low molecular weight (about 432 for the hydrated form) suggest that pantoprazole excretion into human milk should be expected. Because of the carcinogenicity and mutagenicity in animals, the chromosomal aberrations in human lymphocytes, and the potential for suppression of gastric acid secretion in the nursing infant, the use of pantoprazole during lactation should probably be avoided until clinical data are available.

Reference

1. Product information. Protonix. Wyeth-Ayerst Pharmaceuticals, 2001.

Name:	**PANTOTHENIC ACID**	Risk Factor:	**A***
Class:	**Vitamin**		

FETAL RISK SUMMARY

RECOMMENDATION: Compatible

Pantothenic acid, a water-soluble B complex vitamin, acts as a coenzyme in the metabolism or synthesis of a number of carbohydrates, proteins, lipids, and steroid hormones (1). The U.S. recommended daily allowance (RDA) for pantothenic acid or its derivatives (dexpanthenol and calcium pantothenate) in pregnancy is 10.0 mg (2).

No reports of maternal or fetal complications associated with pantothenic acid have been located. Deficiency of this vitamin was not found in two studies evaluating maternal vitamin levels during pregnancy (3,4). Like other B complex vitamins, newborn pantothenic acid levels are significantly greater than maternal levels (3–6). At term, mean pantothenate levels in 174 mothers were 430 ng/mL (range 250–710 ng/mL) and in their newborns 780 ng/mL (range 400–1480 ng/mL) (3). Placental transfer of pantothenate to the fetus is by active transport, but it is slower than transfer of other B complex vitamins (7,8). In one report, low-birth-weight infants had significantly lower levels of pantothenic acid than did normal weight infants (6).

[**Risk Factor C if used in doses above the RDA.*]

BREAST FEEDING SUMMARY

RECOMMENDATION: Compatible

Pantothenic acid is excreted in breast milk with concentrations directly proportional to intake (9,10). With a dietary intake of 8–15 mg/day, mean milk concentrations average 1.93–2.35 μg/mL (9). In a group of mothers who had delivered premature babies (28–34 weeks' gestational age), pantothenic acid milk levels were significantly greater than a comparable group with term babies (39–41 weeks) (10). Milk levels in the preterm group averaged 3.91 μg/mL up to 40 weeks' gestational age and then fell to 3.16 μg/mL. For the term group, levels at 2 and 12 weeks postpartum were 2.57 and 2.55 μg/mL, respectively. A 1983 English study measured pantothenic acid levels in pooled human milk obtained from preterm (26 mothers: 29–34 weeks) and term (35 mothers: 39 weeks or longer) patients (11). Milk from mothers of preterm infants rose from 1.29 μg/mL (colostrum) to 2.27 μg/mL (16–196 days), whereas milk from mothers of term infants increased during the same period from 1.26 μg/mL to 2.61 μg/mL.

An RDA for pantothenic acid during lactation has not been established. However, because this vitamin is required for good health, amounts at least equal to the RDA for pregnancy are recommended. If the diet of the lactating woman adequately supplies this amount, maternal supplementation with pantothenic acid is probably not required. Supplementation with the pregnancy RDA for pantothenic acid is recommended for those women with inadequate nutritional intake.

P

References

1. American Hospital Formulary Service. *Drug Information 1997*. Bethesda, MD: American Society of Health-System Pharmacists, 1997:2813–5.
2. *Recommended Dietary Allowances*. 9th ed. Washington, DC: National Academy of Sciences, 1980:122–4.
3. Baker H, Frank O, Thomson AD, Langer A, Munves ED, De Angelis B, Kaminetzky HA. Vitamin profile of 174 mothers and newborns at parturition. Am J Clin Nutr 1975;28:59–65.
4. Baker H, Frank O, Deangelis B, Feingold S, Kaminetzky HA. Role of placenta in maternal-fetal vitamin transfer in humans. Am J Obstet Gynecol 1981;141:792–6.
5. Cohenour SH, Calloway DH. Blood, urine, and dietary pantothenic acid levels of pregnant teenagers. Am J Clin Nutr 1972;25:512–7.
6. Baker H, Thind IS, Frank O, DeAngelis B, Caterini H, Louria DB. Vitamin levels in low-birth-weight newborn infants and their mothers. Am J Obstet Gynecol 1977;129:521–4.
7. Hill EP, Longo LD. Dynamics of maternal-fetal nutrient transfer. Fed Proc 1980;39:239–44.
8. Kaminetsky HA, Baker H, Frank O, Langer A. The effects of intravenously administered water-soluble vitamins during labor in normovitaminemic and hypovitaminemic gravidas on maternal and neonatal blood vitamin levels at delivery. Am J Obstet Gynecol 1974;120:697–703.
9. Deodhar AD, Rajalakshmi R, Ramakrishnan CV. Studies on human lactation. Part III. Effect of dietary vitamin supplementation on vitamin contents of breast milk. Acta Paediatr Scand 1964;53:42–8.
10. Song WO, Chan GM, Wyse BW, Hansen RG. Effect of pantothenic acid status on the content of the vitamin in human milk. Am J Clin Nutr 1984;40:317–24.
11. Ford JE, Zechalko A, Murphy J, Brooke OG. Comparison of the B vitamin composition of milk from mothers of preterm and term babies. Arch Dis Child 1983;58:367–72.

Name: **PARAMETHADIONE** Risk Factor: **D_M**
Class: **Anticonvulsant**

FETAL RISK SUMMARY

RECOMMENDATION: Contraindicated - 1st Trimester

Paramethadione is an oxazolidinedione anticonvulsant used in the treatment of petit mal epilepsy. There have been three families (10 pregnancies) in which an increase in spontaneous abortion or abnormalities has been reported (1,2). Paramethadione is considered equivalent to trimethadione in regard to its fetal effects. In fact, one of the families described by German and colleagues (3) was included in the fetal trimethadione syndrome (see Trimethadione). This patient had one normal infant after anticonvulsant medications were withdrawn. Malformations reported in two additional families by Rutman (2) are consistent with fetal paramethadione-trimethadione syndrome. The malformations included tetralogy of Fallot, mental retardation, failure to thrive, and increased incidence of spontaneous abortions (2). Because paramethadione has demonstrated both clinical and experimental fetal risk greater than other anticonvulsants, its use should be abandoned in favor of other anticonvulsants for the treatment of petit mal epilepsy (see also Ethosuximide, Phensuximide, and Methsuximide) (4–6).

BREAST FEEDING SUMMARY

RECOMMENDATION: No Human Data - Probably Compatible

No data are available.

References

1. German J, Ehlers KH, Kowal A, DeGeorge PU, Engle MA, Passarge E. Possible teratogenicity of trimethadione and paramethadione. Lancet 1970;2:261–2.
2. Rutman JT. Anticonvulsants and fetal damage. N Engl J Med 1973;189:696–7.
3. German J, Kowal A, Ehlers KH. Trimethadione and human teratogenesis. Teratology 1970;3:349–62.
4. National Institute of Health. Anticonvulsants found to have teratogenic potential. JAMA 1981;245:36.
5. Fabro S, Brown NA. Teratogenic potential of anticonvulsants. N Engl J Med 1979;300:1280–1.
6. Hill RM. Managing the epileptic patient during pregnancy. Drug Ther 1976:204–5.

Name: **PAREGORIC** Risk Factor: **B***
Class: **Antidiarrheal**

FETAL RISK SUMMARY

RECOMMENDATION: Human Data Suggest Risk in 3rd Trimester

Paregoric is a mixture of opium powder, anise oil, benzoic acid, camphor, glycerin, and ethanol. Its action is mainly caused by morphine (see also Morphine). The Collaborative Perinatal Project monitored 50,282 mother-child pairs, 90 of whom had 1st trimester exposure to paregoric (1, pp. 287–295). For use anytime during pregnancy, 562 exposures were recorded (1, p. 434). No evidence was found to suggest a relationship to large categories of major or minor malformations or to individual defects.

[**Risk Factor D if used for prolonged periods or in high doses at term.*]

BREAST FEEDING SUMMARY

RECOMMENDATION: Limited Human Data - Probably Compatible

See Morphine.

Reference

1. Heinonen OP, Slone D, Shapiro S. *Birth Defects and Drugs in Pregnancy*. Littleton, MA: Publishing Sciences Group, 1977.

Name:	**PARGYLINE**	Risk Factor:	**C_M**
Class:	**Antihypertensive**		

FETAL RISK SUMMARY

RECOMMENDATION: No Human Data - No Relevant Animal Data

No data are available.

BREAST FEEDING SUMMARY

RECOMMENDATION: No Human Data - Potential Toxicity

No data are available.

Name:	**PARNAPARIN**	Risk Factor:	**B**
Class:	**Anticoagulant**		

P

FETAL RISK SUMMARY

RECOMMENDATION: No Human Data - Probably Compatible

Parnaparin is a low-molecular-weight heparin prepared by depolymerization of heparin obtained from porcine intestinal mucosa (1). It is not available in the United States (see also Dalteparin and Enoxaparin). Parnaparin has a molecular weight in the range of 4000–5000 (1). Because this is relatively large molecule, it probably does not cross the placenta and, thus, presents a low risk to the fetus.

BREAST FEEDING SUMMARY

RECOMMENDATION: No Human Data - Probably Compatible

No reports describing the use of Parnaparin during lactation have been located. Parnaparin, a low molecular-weight-heparin, still has a relatively high molecular weight (4000–5000) and, as such, should not be expected to be excreted into human milk. Because Parnaparin would be inactivated in the gastrointestinal tract, the risk to a nursing infant from ingestion of the drug from milk appears to be negligible.

Reference

1. Reynold JEF, ed. *Martindale. The Extra Pharmacopoeia*. 30th ed. London, UK: The Pharmaceutical Press, 1993:232.

Name: **PAROMOMYCIN** Risk Factor: **C**

Class: **Antibiotic (Aminoglycoside)/Amebicide**

FETAL RISK SUMMARY

RECOMMENDATION: Limited Human Data - Probably Compatible

Paromomycin is an aminoglycoside antibiotic used for intestinal amebiasis. No reports linking this agent with congenital malformations have been located. Because it is poorly absorbed, with almost 100% of an oral dose excreted unchanged in the feces, little if any of the drug will reach the fetus.

Two women, one at 13 weeks' and the other at 23 weeks' gestation, were treated for a symptomatic intestinal infection caused by *Giardia lamblia* (1). Both delivered normal female infants at term. A 1985 review of intestinal parasites and pregnancy concluded that treatment of the pregnant patient should only be considered if the "parasite is causing clinical disease or may cause public health problems" (2). When indicated, paromomycin was recommended for the treatment of protozoan infections caused by *G. lamblia* and *Entamoeba histolytica*, and for tapeworm infestations occurring during pregnancy (2).

BREAST FEEDING SUMMARY

RECOMMENDATION: No Human Data - Probably Compatible

P

Paromomycin excretion in human milk is not expected because the drug is not absorbed into the systemic circulation after oral dosing. Following parenteral administration to lactating ewes, only 0.018% of the dose was recovered from the milk during a 12-hour period (3). The poor lipid solubility of the antibiotic limited its passage into milk (3).

References

1. Kreutner AK, Del Bene VE, Amstey MS. Giardiasis in pregnancy. Am J Obstet Gynecol 1981;140:895–901.
2. D'Alauro F, Lee RV, Pao-In K, Khairallah M. Intestinal parasites and pregnancy. Obstet Gynecol 1985;66:639–43.
3. Ziv G, Sulman FG. Distribution of aminoglycoside antibiotics in blood and milk. Res Vet Sci 1974;17:68–74.

Name: **PAROXETINE** Risk Factor: **C_M**

Class: **Antidepressant**

FETAL RISK SUMMARY

RECOMMENDATION: Human Data Suggest Risk in 3rd Trimester

Paroxetine is thought to manifest its antidepressant activity as a selective serotonin reuptake inhibitor (SSRI), thereby potentiating the activity of serotonin in the brain. Its chemical structure is unrelated to other antidepressants, including those classified as SSRI agents. Paroxetine is metabolized to inactive metabolites.

All the antidepressant agents in the SSRI class (citalopram, escitalopram, fluoxetine, fluvoxamine, paroxetine, and sertraline) share a similar mechanism of action although they have different chemical structures. These differences could be construed as evidence against any conclusion that they share similar effects on the embryo, fetus, or newborn. In the mouse embryo, however, craniofacial morphogenesis appears to be regulated, at least in part, by serotonin. Interference with serotonin regulation by chemically different inhibitors produces similar craniofacial defects (1). Regardless of the structural differences, therefore, some of the potential adverse effects on pregnancy outcome may also be similar.

In reproduction studies with rats and rabbits, paroxetine was not teratogenic at doses up to 50 mg/kg/day and 6 mg/kg/day, respectively (2). These doses were equivalent to 9.7 and 2.2 times, respectively, the maximum recommended human dose based on body surface area (MRHD) for depression and social anxiety (DSAD) disorder, and 8.1 and 1.9 times, respectively, the MRHD for obsessive compulsive disorder (OCD). In rats dosed at 0.19 times the MRHD for DSAD and 0.16 times the MRHD for OCD, there was an increase in pup deaths when paroxetine was used during the last trimester and continued during lactation. The cause of the deaths was not known (2). In another study, no embryotoxic or teratogenic effects were observed in either of these species at doses up to 43.0 mg/kg and 5.1 mg/kg, respectively (3).

In a 1999 abstract and a full report in the same year, the effects of paroxetine on behavioral changes in developing mice was studied (4,5). The drug was administered for 2 weeks before conception and throughout gestation. A similar group of mice were administered placebo for comparison. The daily dose (30 mg/kg/day) was known to achieve levels in the mouse serum equivalent to the upper human therapeutic level and to obtain levels in the fetal mouse brain equivalent to those in the adult mouse (5). No drug-induced facial abnormalities were seen nor were any differences between the exposed and control groups in terms of pregnancy duration, litter size, and sex ratio. Body weights, however, were significantly lower for the exposed pups (both male and female) at least through postnatal day 5. Most of the behavioral tests showed no differences between the groups but subtle differences in anxiety testing and adult male aggressiveness were noted. Although stating that these findings require confirmation, the investigators speculated that these effects may have resulted from the effect of paroxetine on the development of the postsynaptic serotonin (1A) receptors (5).

Consistent with the low molecular weight (about 329 for the free base), paroxetine crosses the human placenta. A 2003 study of the placental transfer of SSRI antidepressants found cord blood:maternal serum ratios ranging from 0.05–0.91 (6). The dose-to-delivery interval was 6–40 hours with the highest ratio occurring at 21 hours.

The FDA has received 10 reports of birth defects, including 4 involving clubfoot and 2 cases of cutaneous hemangioma (F. Rosa, personal communication, FDA, 1995).

The results of a postmarketing survey of paroxetine, conducted in England between March 1991 and March 1992, were published in 1993 (7). A total of 137 pregnancies were identified, including 66 in which the drug was stopped before the last menstrual period. In this group, there were 12 deliveries, 9 spontaneous abortions, 5 elective terminations, and 40 unknown outcomes. Among the remaining 71 pregnancies, 63 were known to be exposed during the 1st trimester, but the dates of exposure were uncertain in 8. The outcomes in the combined exposed group were 44 newborns (3 sets of twins; 1 twin stillborn, cause not specified), 9 spontaneous abortions, 12 elective terminations, and

9 unknown outcomes. There were no congenital anomalies in the liveborn infants (data not provided for the abortions or stillborn) (7).

A 1998 non-interventional observational cohort study described the outcomes of pregnancies in women who had been prescribed one or more of 34 newly marketed drugs by general practitioners in England (8). Data were obtained by questionnaires sent to the prescribing physicians one month after the expected or possible date of delivery. In 831 (78%) of the pregnancies, a newly marketed drug was thought to had been taken during the 1st trimester with birth defects noted in 14 (2.5%) singleton births of the 557 newborns (10 sets of twins). In addition, two birth defects were observed in aborted fetuses. However, few of the aborted fetuses were examined. Paroxetine was taken during the 1st trimester in 63 pregnancies. The outcomes of these pregnancies included 8 spontaneous abortions, 11 elective abortions, 1 intrauterine death, 2 stillborns (twins), 3 cases lost to follow-up, 41 normal infants (3 premature plus 2 sets of full term twins). No birth defects were noted in any of the outcomes (8).

In a 1996 descriptive case series, the European Network of the Teratology Information Services (ENTIS) prospectively examined the outcomes of 689 pregnancies exposed to antidepressants (9). Multiple drug therapy occurred in about two-thirds of the mothers. Paroxetine was used in three pregnancies, all with normal outcomes.

A prospective, multicenter, controlled cohort study published in 1998 evaluated the pregnancy outcomes of 267 women exposed to one or more of three SSRI antidepressants during the 1st trimester: fluvoxamine ($N = 26$), paroxetine ($N = 97$), and sertraline ($N = 147$) (10). The women were combined into a study group without differentiation as to the drug they had consumed. All of the women had contacted a teratogen information service about their use of the drugs during pregnancy. A randomly selected control group ($N = 267$) was formed from women who had contacted one service after exposure to nonteratogenic agents. The pregnancy outcomes were determined, in most cases, 6 to 9 months after delivery. The study group was significantly more likely to smoke cigarettes and to have had a previous elective abortion but less likely to be primigravid. Other characteristics, such as a previous spontaneous abortion, alcohol consumption, and maternal age at conception, did not differ between the groups. As for pregnancy outcomes, no significant differences were measured in the number of live births, spontaneous or elective abortions, stillbirths, major malformations, birth weight, or gestational age at birth. Nine major malformations were observed in each group. The relative risk for major anomalies was 1.06 (95% confidence interval [CI] 0.43–2.62). No clustering of defects was apparent. In the study group, no differences were found in the pregnancy outcomes of smokers compared to nonsmokers. In addition, the outcomes of women who took an antidepressant throughout gestation were similar to those who took an antidepressant only during the 1st trimester (10). One of the investigators, in response to subsequent correspondence regarding the study (11,12), clarified that all of the 267 women in the study group had taken an antidepressant during embryogenesis (13). Other concerns relating to the outcomes and sample size were also addressed.

In 1999, the Swedish Medical Birth Registry published the results of a study on the use of antidepressants in early pregnancy and delivery outcome for the years 1995–1997 (14). During the period, 281,728 infants were registered, 531 of whom had been exposed *in utero* to SSRI antidepressants, 15 to SSRIs plus a non-SSRI antidepressant, and 423 to non-SSRI antidepressants. Of the 122 women who used paroxetine, 118 used it alone, 1 used it in combination with sertraline, and 3 used it in combination with non-SSRI antidepressants (clomipramine, amitriptyline, or nortriptyline). There was no significant differences in relative risk (RR = observed/expected) for birth defects between those exposed to any depressant (total 39; RR 1.13), SSRIs only (total 21; RR 1.12), and non-SSRIs only (total 18; RR 1.15). Similarly, no significant differences in infant survival were observed among the groups. A shorter gestational duration (<37 weeks) was observed for any antidepressant exposure (odds ratio [OR] 1.43, 95% CI 1.14–1.80), but no difference between SSRI and non-SSRI antidepressants. Moreover, antidepressant exposure was not associated with an increased risk of low birth weight (defined as <2500 g) among singletons as the crude OR 1.32, 95% CI 0.96–1.80, decreased to 1.03 after adjustment for confounders (14).

A 2001 case report described complications consistent with neonatal withdrawal in four neonates exposed during pregnancy to paroxetine (15). The infants were delivered at 37–38 weeks' gestation and one mother breast fed her infant. The maternal medications were paroxetine (10 mg/day); paroxetine (60 mg/day from early pregnancy to 35 weeks, then 120 mg/day to delivery as a result of a dispensing error, then decreased to 60 mg/day during breast-feeding) plus desipramine (150 mg/day); paroxetine (20 mg/day) plus buspirone (30 mg/day); and paroxetine (20 mg/day) plus trazodone (50 mg/day) and diphenhydramine (25 mg each night). Neonatal withdrawal has also been reported with diphenhydramine (see Diphenhydramine). The symptoms in the four infants included jitteriness, irritability, lethargy, myoclonus, vomiting, and hypothermia. In one infant, serum levels of paroxetine and desipramine on days 5 and 15 of age were 48 and 70 ng/mL, respectively, and <10 and <10 ng/mL, respectively. In a second infant, the serum paroxetine concentration on day 2 was 66 ng/mL, whereas trazodone was undetectable. Two infants were hypoglycemic (one shortly after birth and one at 40 hours of age), but both mothers had gestational diabetes mellitus. Necrotizing enterocolitis was also observed in two infants. The authors speculated that this condition might have been related to rebound activation of platelets after discontinuance of paroxetine exposure resulting in a hypercoagulable state. The withdrawal symptoms in one infant resolved over a few days, but some symptoms in the other three were still apparent at discharge on days 5, 22, and 24 of age, respectively (15).

Another 2001 report described withdrawal symptoms in newborn infants exposed in utero to SSRIs (16). Male infants exposed to paroxetine ($N = 3$; 10–40 mg/day), citalopram ($N = 1$; 30 mg/day), or fluoxetine ($N = 1$; 20 mg/day) during gestation exhibited withdrawal symptoms at or within a few days of birth and lasting up to 1 month. Symptoms included irritability, constant crying, shivering, increased tonus, eating and sleeping problems and convulsions. The four infants exposed to paroxetine and fluoxetine required treatment with chlorpromazine (16).

Paroxetine withdrawal was suspected in a third 2001 case report (17). The mother had taken paroxetine (40 mg/day) throughout pregnancy and delivered a 2690-g female infant at 35 weeks' gestation. Apgar scores were 9, 10, and 10 at 1, 5, and 10 minutes, respectively. The premature infant was bottle-fed and did well during the first few days, but then became irritable, lethargic, hypertonic, apathetic, and jittery. Tube feeding was required. A complete physical examination did not reveal a cause for the symptoms. The infant improved without therapy and was discharged home at 18 days of age. After delivery, the mother's serum paroxetine concentration was 126 μg/L (therapeutic levels 10–150 μg/L). Because of previous reports, the authors attributed the premature birth and the infant's symptoms to paroxetine (17).

In a 2002 study, the pregnancy outcomes of 55 women taking paroxetine (median dose 20 mg/day) in the 3rd trimester were reported (18). Twelve neonates had complications requiring short-term intensive treatment and prolonged hospitalization. The complications, all resolving within 1–2 weeks, included respiratory distress ($N = 9$; 3 preterm infants), hypoglycemia ($N = 2$), and jaundice ($N = 1$). Compared to controls, significantly more infants were premature. In contrast, only three complications were observed in 54 matched controls. Twenty-seven women in the comparison group had used paroxetine (median dose 20 mg/day) in the 1st and 2nd trimesters, but not in the 3rd trimester. Only 3rd trimester exposure was associated with respiratory distress (odds ratio 9.53, 95% confidence interval 1.14–79.30) (18).

The effect of SSRIs on birth outcomes and postnatal neurodevelopment of children exposed prenatally was reported in 2003 (19). Thirty-one children (mean age 12.9 months) exposed during pregnancy to SSRIs (15 sertraline, 8 paroxetine, 7 fluoxetine, and 1 fluvoxamine) were compared to 13 children (mean age 17.7 months) of mothers with depression who elected not to take medications during pregnancy. All of the mothers had healthy lifestyles (i.e., took prenatal vitamins, no smoking, little alcohol use, and regular exercise). The timing of the exposures was 71% in the 1st trimester, 74% in the 3rd trimester, and 45% throughout. The average duration of breast-feeding in the subjects and controls was 6.4 and 8.5 months. Twenty-eight (90%) subjects nursed their infants, 17 of who took SSRIs (10 sertraline, 4 paroxetine, and 3 fluoxetine) compared to 11 (85%) controls, three of whom took sertraline. There were no significant differences between the groups in terms of gestational age at birth, premature births, birth weight and length or, at follow-up, in sex distribution or gain in weight and length (expressed at percentage). Seven (23%) of the exposed infants were admitted to a neonatal intensive care unit (six respiratory distress, four meconium aspiration, and one cardiac murmur) compared to none of the controls ($p = 0.06$). Follow-up examinations were conducted by a pediatric neurologist, psychologist, and a dysmorphologist who were blinded as to the mother's mediations status. The mean Apgar scores at 1 and 5 minutes were lower in the exposed group than in controls, 7.0 vs. 8.2, and 8.4 vs. 9.0, respectively. There was one major defect in each group: small asymptomatic ventricular septal defect (exposed); bilateral lacrimal duct stenosis that required surgery (control). The test outcomes for mental development were similar in the groups, but significant differences in the subjects included a slight delay in psychomotor development and lower behavior motor quality (tremulousness and fine motor movements) (19).

A 2004 case report described a term 3750-g male newborn who had a normal examination at birth except that he did not cry in the delivery room or afterward (20). The mother had taken paroxetine 20 mg/day throughout the pregnancy. The infant was bottle-fed and had a normal appetite. He was discharged home at 48 hours of age, but was readmitted 2 days later because of lethargy and the absence of cry. The only abnormality detected on examination was the lack of reaction to pain stimulation. On the day 6 of life, an electroencephalogram (EEG) was abnormal (". . . depressed background activity with trace alternance and independent spike and wave activity; somatosensory-evoked potentials on the posterior tibial were impossible to elicit."). The infant began crying and responded to pain stimulation on day 13 of life and an EEG on day 14 showed marked improvement. Physical examination at 6 weeks of age was normal (20).

A 2004 prospective study examined the effect of four SSRIs (citalopram, fluoxetine, paroxetine, and sertraline) on newborn neurobehavior, including behavioral state, sleep organization, motor activity, heart rate variability, tremulousness, and startles (21). Seventeen SSRI-exposed, healthy, full-birth-weight newborns and 17 nonexposed, full-birth-weight newborns were matched for maternal cigarette use, social class, and maternal age. A wide range of disrupted neurobehavioral outcomes were shown in the infants exposed *in utero* to SSRIs. After adjustment for gestational age, the exposed infants were found to differ significantly from controls in terms of tremulousness, behavioral states, and sleep organization. Although the effects observed on motor activity, startles, and heart rate variability were not significant after adjustment, the investigators thought they might be mediated through the effects of SSRI exposure on gestational age (21).

In summary, the animal data and limited human pregnancy experience suggests that paroxetine does not pose a major teratogenic risk. Disruptions in neurobehavior and a withdrawal syndrome have been observed after exposure to paroxetine in the 3rd trimester. Moreover, at least one study has demonstrated that a SSRI (see Fluoxetine) can induce long-term, perhaps permanent, changes in the brain of *in utero* exposed rats. Studies of the long-term neurobehavior effects of SSRI agents on gestational exposed offspring are needed.

BREAST FEEDING SUMMARY

RECOMMENDATION: Limited Human Data - Potential Toxicity

Paroxetine is excreted into breast milk. A brief 1996 correspondence described a 39-year-old, 60-kg woman with a recurrent depressive and obsessive disorder who was started on paroxetine 20 mg/day (333 μg/kg/day) 3 days after delivery (22). One week later, analysis of a milk sample for paroxetine revealed a concentration of 7.6 ng/mL. Assuming that the infant ingested 0.15 L/kg of milk per day, the authors estimated that the daily weight-adjusted dose was 0.34% of the mother's dose. The minimum milk:plasma ratio (obtained 4 hours after a dose) was estimated to be 0.09. No data were available on the effects of this exposure on the nursing infant (22).

Breast milk concentrations of paroxetine in seven lactating women were reported in a 1999 publication (23). In six women receiving a paroxetine dose of 10–40 mg/day, milk and maternal serum samples were obtained 4–7 hours and 24 hours after a dose. The samples corresponded to either close to peak milk concentrations or trough levels. Based on area under the curve (AUC) calculations, the mean estimated daily infant dose was 1.4% (range 0.7%–2.9%) of the weight-adjusted maternal dose. The mean milk:serum ratio was 0.69 (range 0.39–1.11). In a seventh woman, frequent sampling during two 24-hour periods (one at 20 mg/day and one at 40 mg/day, 7 weeks apart) resulted in estimated daily infant doses of 1.0% and 2.0%, respectively, of the weight-adjusted maternal dose. The milk:serum ratios were 0.69 and 0.72, respectively. The study also measured paroxetine concentrations in foremilk and hindmilk at two steady-state doses (20 and 40 mg/day) in one subject. Drug levels in hindmilk were a mean 78% (range 16%–169%) higher than those in foremilk. The increase paralleled the increase in milk triglycerides and was thought to be consistent with the lipophilic properties of the drug. No adverse effects of the exposure were observed in the seven nursing infants (23).

In a two-phase study published in 1999, the dose of paroxetine received by 10 nursing infants from breast milk was estimated (24). In six subjects sampled over 24 hours, the mean daily estimated infant dose was 1.13% (range 0.5%–1.7%) of the weight-adjusted maternal dose (based on AUC). The mean milk:plasma ratio was 0.39 (range 0.32–0.51). In the second phase, milk and serum samples were obtained from four subjects around a normal infant feeding time. In this case, the mean infant dose was 1.25% (range 0.38%–2.24%) of the maternal dose and the mean milk:plasma ratio was 0.96 (range 0.31–3.33). The milk:plasma ratio was similar for fore and hind milk. Paroxetine was detected (limit 2 ng/mL) in the plasma of one of the eight infants tested, but the concentration was below the level of quantification for the assay (4 ng/mL). No adverse effects were noted in any of the infants (24).

A 2000 study described the excretion of paroxetine into breast milk (25). Sixteen women on a stable paroxetine dose (mean 23.1 mg/day; range 10–50 mg/day) were studied during the postpartum period (range 4–55.2 weeks). Seven of the women had continued their prenatal paroxetine, four had started the antidepressant postpartum, and data were not available for five subjects. Milk samples were collected after a dose at 4- to 6-hour intervals over a 24-hour period. The mean milk concentration was 41.6 ng/mL (range 2–101 ng/mL). Paroxetine concentrations were higher in hindmilk than in foremilk. No detectable levels of paroxetine (all <2 ng/mL) were found in the infants serum, including the 10 infants who were exclusively breast-fed. No adverse effects in the nursing infants were reported by the mothers upon direct interview (25).

In another 2000 report, maternal serum, breast milk, and infant serum samples were obtained from 24 mother-infant pairs (mean infant age 4.5 months) 6 hours after a paroxetine dose (26). In 13 of the pairs, the infants were exclusively breast-fed. All of the mothers were on a stable dose of paroxetine (10–40 mg/day for at least 30 days). One mother-infant pair was tested twice; once at 10 mg/day and again at 40 mg/day. The mean maternal serum, breast milk, and infant serum concentrations (ng/mL) were 45.2, 19.2, and not detectable (<0.1 ng/mL), respectively. The mean milk:plasma ratio, infant dose, and percent of maternal dose were 0.53, 2.88 μg/kg/day, and 1.1%, respectively. No adverse effects of the drug exposure were noted in the nursing infants, but the investigators recognized the need for follow-up studies to evaluate the potential for long-term effects (26).

In a 2002 report, the pregnancy outcomes of 55 women who had taken paroxetine during the 3rd trimester were reported (see Fetal Risk Summary) (18). Thirty-six of the women breast-fed their infants. Eight of the women reported adverse symptoms in their infants: alertness ($N = 6$), constipation ($N = 3$), sleepiness ($N = 1$), and irritability ($N = 1$). No adverse events were reported in 44 breast-fed infants in the comparison group (18).

A 1999 review of SSRI agents concluded that if there were compelling reasons to treat a mother for postpartum depression, a condition in which a rapid antidepressant effect is important, the benefits of therapy with SSRIs would most likely outweigh the risks (27). However, because the long-term effects of exposure to SSRI antidepressants in breast milk on the infant's neurobehavioral development are unknown (no such adverse effects have been identified to date but research is needed), stopping or reducing the frequency of breast-feeding should be considered if therapy with these agents is required. Avoiding nursing around the time of peak maternal concentration (about 4 hours after a dose) may limit infant exposure. The American Academy of Pediatrics classifies paroxetine as a drug for which the effect on nursing infants is unknown but may be of concern (28).

P

References

1. Shuey DL, Sadler TW, Lauder JM. Serotonin as a regulator of craniofacial morphogenesis: site-specific malformations following exposure to serotonin uptake inhibitors. Teratology 1992;46:367–78.
2. Product information. Paxil. SmithKline Beecham Pharmaceuticals, 2000.
3. Baldwin JA, Davidson EJ, Pritchard AL, Ridings JE. The reproductive toxicology of paroxetine. Acta Psychiatr Scand Suppl 1989;350:37–9.
4. Coleman F, Christensen D, Gonzalez C, Rayburn W. Behavioral changes in developing mice after prenatal exposure to paroxetine (Paxil) (abstract). Am J Obstet Gynecol 1999;180:S61.
5. Coleman FH, Christensen HD, Gonzalez CL, Rayburn WF. Behavioral changes in developing mice after prenatal exposure to paroxetine (Paxil). Am J Obstet Gynecol 1999;181:1166–71.
6. Hendrick V, Stowe ZN, Altshuler LL, Hwang S, Lee E, Haynes D. Placental passage of antidepressant medications. Am J Psychiatry 2003;160:993–6.
7. Inman W, Kubota K, Pearce G, Wilton L. PEM report number 6. Paroxetine. Pharmacoepidemiol Drug Saf 1993;2:393–422.
8. Wilton LV, Pearce GL, Martin RM, Mackay FJ, Mann RD. The outcomes of pregnancy in women exposed to newly marketed drugs in general practice in England. Br J Obstet Gynaecol 1998;105:882–9.
9. McElhatton PR, Garbis HM, Elefant E, Vial T,

Bellemin B, Mastroiacovo P, Arnon J, Rodriguez-Pinilla E, Schaefer C, Pexieder T, Merlob P, Dal Verme S. The outcome of pregnancy in 689 women exposed to therapeutic doses of antidepressants. A collaborative study of the European Network of Teratology Information Services (ENTIS). Reprod Toxicol 1996;10:285–94.
10. Kulin NA, Pastuszak A, Sage SR, Schick-Boschetto B, Spivey G, Feldkamp M, Ormond K, Matsui D, Stein-Schechman AK, Cook L, Brochu J, Rieder M, Koren G. Pregnancy outcome following maternal use of the new selective serotonin reuptake inhibitors. A prospective controlled multicenter study. JAMA 1998; 279:609–10.
11. Grush LR. Risk of fetal anomalies with exposure to selective serotonin reuptake inhibitors. JAMA 1998; 279:1873.
12. Witlin AG. Risk of fetal anomalies with exposure to selective serotonin reuptake inhibitors. JAMA 1998;279:1873.
13. Koren G. In reply. Risk of fetal anomalies with exposure to selective serotonin reuptake inhibitors. JAMA 1998;279:1873–4.
14. Ericson A, Kallen B, Wiholm BE. Delivery outcome after the use of antidepressants in early pregnancy. Eur J Clin Pharmacol 1999;55:503–8.
15. Stiskal JA, Kulin N, Koren G, Ho T, Ito S. Neonatal paroxetine withdrawal syndrome. Arch Dis Child Fetal Neonatal Ed 2001;84:F134–5.
16. Nordeng H, Lindemann R, Perminov KV, Reikvam A. Neonatal withdrawal syndrome after in utero exposure to selective serotonin reuptake inhibitors. Acta Paediatr 2001;90:288–91.
17. Nijhuis IJM, Kok-Van Rooij GWM, Bosschaart AN. Withdrawal reactions of a premature neonate after maternal use of paroxetine. Arch Dis Child Neonatal Ed 2001;84:F77.
18. Costei AM, Kozer E, Ho T, Ito S, Koren G. Perinatal outcome following third trimester exposure to paroxetine. Arch Pediatr Adolesc Med 2002;156:1129–32.
19. Casper RC, Fleisher BE, Lee-Ancajas JC, Gilles A, Gaylor E, DeBattista A, Hoyme HE. Follow-up of children of depressed mothers exposed or not exposed to antidepressant drugs during pregnancy. J Pediatr 2003;142:402–8.
20. Morag I, Batash D, Keidar R, Bulkowstein M, Heyman E. Paroxetine use throughout pregnancy: does it pose any risk to the neonate? J Toxicol Clin Toxicol 2004;42:97–100.
21. Zeskind PS, Stephens LE. Maternal selective serotonin reuptake inhibitor use during pregnancy and newborn neurobehavior. Pediatrics 2004;113:368–75.
22. Spigset O, Carleborg L, Norstrom A, Sandlund M. Paroxetine level in breast milk. J Clin Psychiatry 1996;57:39.
23. Ohman R, Hagg S, Carleborg L, Spigset O. Excretion of paroxetine into breast milk. J Clin Psychiatry 1999;60:519–23.
24. Begg EJ, Duffull SB, Saunders DA, Buttimore RC, Ilett KF, Hackett LP, Yapp P, Wilson DA. Paroxetine in human milk. Br J Clin Pharmacol 1999;48:142–7.
25. Stowe ZN, Cohen LS, Hostetter A, Ritchie JC, Owens MJ, Nemeroff CB. Paroxetine in human breast milk and nursing infants. Am J Psychiatry 2000;157:185–9.
26. Misri S, Kim J, Riggs KW, Kostaras X. Paroxetine levels in postpartum depressed women, breast milk, and infant serum. J Clin Psychiatry 2000;61:828–32.
27. Edwards JG, Anerson I. Systematic review and guide to selection of selective serotonin reuptake inhibitors. Drugs 1999;57:507–33.
28. Committee on Drugs, American Academy of Pediatrics. The transfer of drugs and other chemicals into human milk. Pediatrics 2001;108:776–89.

Name:	**PASSION FLOWER**	Risk Factor:	**C**
Class:	**Herb**		

FETAL RISK SUMMARY

RECOMMENDATION: No Human Data - No Relevant Animal Data

The herbal product used for medicinal purposes usually refers to the plant, *Passiflora incarnata*, but the common name, passion flower, may refer to many of the approximately 400 species of the genus *Passiflora* (1,2). Some species are grown for their flowers. In addition, some species produce edible fruit, such as *P. incarnata*, *P. edulis*, and *P. quadrangularis*. The plant is a perennial vine that may reach 10 meters in length. It is indigenous to the southeastern United States to South America. The medicinal parts include the whole or cut dried herb and the fresh aerial parts (1,2). In this review, the term passion flower will only refer to *P. incarnata*, the product used in herbal medicine.

Commercial products of passion flower are available for both oral and topical administration. A number of indications have been claimed for passion flower, including nervousness (e.g., hysteria, nervous exhaustion, pediatric nervousness and excitability), neuralgia, insomnia, pain, asthma and other bronchial disorders, generalized seizures, compresses for burns, hemorrhoids (externally), and for menopausal complaints (1–4).

As with most herbs, a relatively large number of chemical compounds are contained in the commercial product: Flavonoids (content 2.5%; includes flavone di-C-glycosides shaftoside, isoshaftoside, isovitexin, iso-orientin, vicenin, lucenin, saponarin, and passiflorine), maltol (0.05%), cyanogenic glycosides (gynocardine [less than 0.1%]), and indole alkaloids (harman, harmine, harmaline, harmalol, and harmin) are the primary constituents (1–4). The alkaloids, however, are reportedly present in subtherapeutic amounts (5). Other constituents include free flavonoids (apigenin, luteolin, quercetin, and campherol), several acid compounds (phenolic, linoleic, linolenic, palmitic, oleic, myristic, formic, and butyric acids), coumarins, phytosterols, and essential oil (1).

The pharmacologic activity of passion flower apparently derives from the flavonoids and alkaloids (1,3). A few studies have apparently documented the sedative action of passion flower in animals and humans. The FDA prohibited the use of passion flower in over-the-counter (OTC) products in 1978 because it had not been proven to be safe and effective (5), but the product is apparently available as a herbal remedy.

No reports have been located describing the use of passion flower in human pregnancy. However, two sources have cited reports that the herb is contraindicated during pregnancy because of the uterine stimulant action of the harman (harmala) alkaloids (harman, harmaline) shown in animals and because of the presence of cyanogenic glycoside gynocardine (1,3). In contrast, the German Commission E monographs state that there are no contraindications (4).

In summary, the use of passion flower has apparently not been reported during human pregnancy. Typically, with herbal products, a large number of chemicals have been identified from this herb and none has undergone reproductive testing. Because passion flower has been in use for hundreds of years or longer, it is doubtful that a major teratogenic effect or other significant reproductive toxicity would have escaped notice. More subtle or low-incidence effects, however, including structural and behavioral teratogenicity, the induction of abortions because of its uterine stimulant properties, and infertility, may have escaped detection, and further study is required before human reproductive risk or safety can be assessed.

In addition to the above concerns, standardization of any herbal product is often questionable (6). As such, the presence of therapeutic or subtherapeutic amounts of active ingredients, or their complete absence, in a given preparation cannot be predicted. Commercial herbal products may also be adulterated with unlabeled ingredients (6). Because of these uncertainties, the consumption of passion flower during gestation should be avoided.

BREAST FEEDING SUMMARY

RECOMMENDATION: No Human Data - Potential Toxicity

No reports describing the use of passion flower during lactation have been located. Because of the large number of chemical compounds in the herb, the lack of standardization of commercial products, and the complete lack of information on the effects of exposure to these substances in a nursing infant, the use of passion flower during breast-feeding should be avoided.

References

1. Passion Flower. *The Review of Natural Products*. St. Louis, MO: Facts and Comparisons, March, 1999.
2. Passiflora Incarnata. *PDR for Herbal Medicines*. Montvale, NJ: Medical Economics, 1998:1015–6.
3. Passion Flower. *Natural Medicines Comprehensive Database*. Stockton, CA: Therapeutic Research Faculty, 1999:645–6.
4. Passionflower Herb. Blumenthal M, Senior Editor. *The Complete German Commission E Monographs. Therapeutic Guide to Herbal Medicines*. Austin, TX: American Botanical Council. 1998:179–80.
5. Robbers JE, Tyler VE. *Tyler's Herbs of Choice. The Therapeutic Use of Phytomedicinals*. Binghamton, NY: Haworth Press, 2000:159–60.
6. Miller LG, Hume A, Harris IM, Jackson EA, Kanmaz TJ, Cauffield JS, Chin TWF, Knell M. White paper on herbal products. American College of Clinical Pharmacy. Pharmacotherapy 2000;20:877–91.

Name: **PEGFILGRASTIM** Risk Factor: **C_M**
Class: **Hematopoietic**

FETAL RISK SUMMARY

RECOMMENDATION: No Human Data - Animal Data Suggest Low Risk

Pegfilgrastim is a covalent conjugate of monomethoxypolyethylene glycol and filgrastim that results in reduced renal elimination and prolonged persistence in the serum. (See also Filgrastim.) Pegfilgrastim is indicated to decrease the incidence of infection, as manifested by febrile neutropenia, in patients with non-myeloid malignancies receiving myelosuppressive chemotherapy associated with a clinically significant incidence of febrile neutropenia. The serum half-life depends on the dose and the number of neutrophils, ranging from 15–80 hours after SC injection (1).

Reproduction studies have been conducted in rats and rabbits. In rats, pegfilgrastim given SC in doses up to 1000 μg/kg/dose every other day during organogenesis caused no embryotoxic or fetotoxic outcome. However, an increased incidence of wavy ribs was observed at the maximum dose. When doses up to 1000 μg/kg/dose were given once weekly from gestation day 6 through lactation day 18, no maternal toxicity or adverse effects on the growth or development of offspring were observed. The highest dose was about 23 times the recommended human dose (RHD). In addition, the once-weekly dose in male and nonpregnant female rats had no effect on reproductive performance, fertility, or sperm parameters. In rabbits, SC doses as low as four times the RHD given every other day were maternally toxic (decreased food consumption and maternal weight gain) and fetotoxic (decreased body weights). At about 16 times the RHD or higher, there was an increased incidence of resorptions and abortions with a corresponding decrease in the number of live fetuses (1).

Pegfilgrastim crosses the rat placenta in very low levels (<0.5%) (1). It is not known if the drug crosses the human placenta, but filgrastim apparently reaches the fetus late in gestation in amounts sufficient to produce a biologic effect. (See Filgrastim.) The molecular weight of pegfilgrastim (about 39,000) is twice that of filgrastim (about 19,000) because of the polyethylene glycol. The addition of this non-amino acid moiety may prevent the transfer of pegfilgrastim in amounts sufficient to produce a biologic effect in the fetus.

No reports describing the use of pegfilgrastim in human pregnancy have been located. Although the animal data do not suggest fetal risk, the absence of human pregnancy experience prevents an assessment of the embryo/fetal risk. Filgrastim has been used in

P

the pregnancy without apparent fetal harm. (See Filgrastim.) Therefore, until human data are available, filgrastim would be preferred over pegfilgrastim in pregnancy.

BREAST FEEDING SUMMARY

RECOMMENDATION: No Human Data - Probably Compatible

No reports describing the use of pegfilgrastim during human lactation have been located. Pegfilgrastim is composed of monomethoxypolyethylene glycol and filgrastim that are chemically bound together. This produces a compound with a very long half-life (15–80 hours) and a very high molecular weight (about 39,000). Excretion into breast milk is doubtful, but even if the drug were excreted, it probably would be digested in a nursing infant's stomach. The risk to a nursing infant is unknown but appears to be low to nonexistent. Therefore, treatment with pegfilgrastim should not be withheld because of breast-feeding.

Reference

1. Product information. Neulasta. Amgen, 2004.

Name: **PEMOLINE** Risk Factor: **B_M**
Class: **Central Stimulant**

FETAL RISK SUMMARY

RECOMMENDATION: No Human Data - Animal Data Suggest Low Risk

Pemoline, used for the treatment of attention deficit disorder, is a central nervous system stimulant that is chemically unrelated to amphetamines and methylphenidate. Reproduction studies in mice, rats, and rabbits showed no evidence of impaired fertility or adverse effects in the fetus (1,2). Doses used in the studies with pregnant rats and rabbits were 18.75 and 37.5 mg/kg/day, respectively (1). In rats, however, a dose of 37.5 mg/kg/day, much higher than the recommended starting dose in humans (37.5 mg/day), was associated with an increased incidence of stillbirths and cannibalization. Moreover, in rats dosed with 18.75 and 37.5 mg/kg/day, decreased postnatal survival of offspring was observed (1).

No published reports describing the use of pemoline during human pregnancy have been located. Because of its relatively low molecular weight (about 176), moderate plasma protein binding (about 50%), and long serum half-life (about 12 hours), embryo/fetal exposure should be expected. A 1984 source stated that no harmful effects had been reported in the human fetus and that the agent was not contraindicated in pregnancy (3).

BREAST FEEDING SUMMARY

RECOMMENDATION: No Human Data - Potential Toxicity

It is not known whether pemoline is excreted into human breast milk. No reports describing the use of this drug during lactation have been located. The relatively low molecular weight (about 176), moderate plasma protein binding (about 50%), and long serum half-life (about 12 hours), suggest that pemoline will be excreted into milk. The effects of exposure on a nursing infant, if any, are unknown.

References

1. Product information. Cylert. Abbott Laboratories, 2005.
2. Schardein JL. *Chemically Induced Birth Defects*. 2nd ed. New York, NY: Marcel Dekker, 1993:223.
3. Onnis A, Grella P. *The Biochemical Effects of Drugs in Pregnancy. Volume 1: Drugs Active on The Nervous, Cardiovascular and Haemopoietic Systems*. West Sussex, England: Ellis Horwood Limited, 1984:161.

Name: **PENBUTOLOL** Risk Factor: **C_M***

Class: **Sympatholytic (Antihypertensive)**

FETAL RISK SUMMARY

RECOMMENDATION: Human Data Suggest Risk in 2nd and 3rd Trimesters

Penbutolol is a nonselective β_1, β_2-adrenergic blocking agent used in the treatment of hypertension. No teratogenic effects were noted in mice, rats, and rabbits treated with doses up to 250 times the maximum recommended human dose (MRHD) (1,2). A slight increase in fetal and newborn mortality was observed in rabbits given 156 times the MRHD (2). In rats dosed at 200 times the MRHD, decreased pup body weight and survival were observed (2). In mice, the drug produced no behavioral changes in the exposed offspring (1).

No reports describing the use of penbutolol in human pregnancy have been located. If used near delivery, the newborn infant should be closely observed for 24–48 hours for signs and symptoms of β-blockade. Long-term effects of *in utero* exposure to β-blockers have not been studied but warrant evaluation.

Some β-blockers may cause intrauterine growth retardation (IUGR) and reduced placental weight, especially those lacking intrinsic sympathomimetic activity (ISA) (i.e., partial agonist). Treatment beginning early in the 2nd trimester results in the greatest weight reductions, whereas treatment restricted to the 3rd trimester primarily affects only placental weight. Penbutolol does possess ISA. However, IUGR and reduced placental weight may potentially occur with all agents within this class. Although growth retardation is a serious concern, the benefits of maternal therapy with β-blockers, in some cases, might outweigh the risks to the fetus and must be judged on a case-by-case basis.

[**Risk Factor D if used in 2nd or 3rd trimesters.*]

BREAST FEEDING SUMMARY

RECOMMENDATION: No Human Data - Potential Toxicity

No reports describing the use of penbutolol during human lactation have been located. If penbutolol is used during nursing, the infant should be closely monitored for hypotension, bradycardia, and other signs or symptoms of β-blockade. Long-term effects of exposure to β-blockers from milk have not been studied but warrant evaluation.

References

1. Sugisaki T, Takagi S, Seshimo M, Hayashi S, Miyamoto M. Reproductive studies of penbutolol sulfate given orally to mice. Oyo Yakuri 1981;22:289–305. As cited in Shepard TH. *Catalog of Teratogenic Agents*. 6th ed. Baltimore, MD: Johns Hopkins University Press, 1989:487.
2. Product information. Levatol. Schwarz Pharma, 1997.

Name:	PENICILLAMINE	Risk Factor:	D
Class:	Chelating Agent		

FETAL RISK SUMMARY

RECOMMENDATION: Human Data Suggest Risk

Penicillamine is a chelating agent used in the treatment of Wilson's disease, cystinuria, and severe rheumatoid arthritis. Reproductive studies in rats at doses 6 times higher than the maximum recommended human dose revealed fetal anomalies consisting of skeletal defects, cleft palates, and fetal resorptions (1).

The use of penicillamine during pregnancy has been observed in more than 100 pregnancies (2–20). The mothers were treated for rheumatoid arthritis, cystinuria, or Wilson's disease. Most of the pregnancies resulted in healthy newborns that developed normally, but anomalies were observed in 8 infants:

Cutis laxa, hypotonia, hyperflexion of hips and shoulders, pyloric stenosis, vein fragility, varicosities, impaired wound healing, death (3)
Cutis laxa, growth retardation, inguinal hernia, simian crease, perforated bowel, death (7)
Cutis laxa (4)
Cutis laxa, mild micrognathia, low-set ears, inguinal hernia (12)
Cutis laxa, inguinal hernia (13)
Marked flexion deformities of extremities, dislocated hips, hydrocephalus, intraventricular hemorrhage, death (14)
Cerebral palsy, blindness, bilateral talipes, sudden infant death at 3 months (14)
Hydrocephalus (14)
Ventricular septal defect (small) (9)
Bilateral cleft lip with totally cleft palate (19)

The relationship of the last five cases listed above to penicillamine is controversial because they did not include connective tissue anomalies. The drug may be partially responsible, but other factors, such as maternal infections and surgery, may have a stronger association with the defects (14).

A 2000 review cited data from the literature involving 111 women with Wilson's disease who had 153 pregnancies (20). The outcomes included 144 normal neonates (1 premature), 4 elective abortions, 1 spontaneous abortion, and 4 cases of birth defects (mannosidosis; cleft lip and palate; 2 transient cutis laxa).

Penicillamine crosses the placenta to the fetus. A mother was treated for cystinuria throughout gestation with penicillamine hydrochloride 1050 mg/day (843 mg of penicillamine base) (2). The drug was found in the urine of her newborn infant. The baby's physical and mental development was normal at 3 months.

A 1993 report described the effects of untreated Wilson's disease on a fetus (21). A 23-year-old woman, diagnosed with Wilson's disease at 12 years of age, had been treated with penicillamine but she had stopped the therapy when she was 15 years old. Liver cirrhosis, thrombocytopenia, and low serum proteins developed during the 2nd trimester and, when the diagnosis of Wilson's disease was remade (the patient had withheld information about her past history), an elective cesarean section was performed at 36 weeks' gestation. The 2380-g male infant had hepatomegaly, elevated liver enzymes, slightly low serum ceruloplasmin, and high excretion of urinary copper. His development during the first year has been normal, as is his current serum ceruloplasmin concentration, but his liver enzymes have remained elevated, possibly because of copper accumulation in the fetal liver (21).

Several conflicting recommendations have appeared in the literature concerning the use of penicillamine during pregnancy. The authors of one review believe the drug should be avoided during pregnancy (22). Another suggested that therapy with penicillamine should be continued during pregnancy in women with Wilson's disease, but stopped in those with rheumatoid arthritis (23). Still others have recommended continuing therapy during the treatment of Wilson's disease, except during the 1st trimester (24).

Although the evidence is incomplete, maintaining the daily dose at 500 mg or less may reduce the incidence of penicillamine-induced toxicity in the newborn (6,11). The manufacturer recommends, however, that the dose be limited to 1 g/day and, if cesarean section is planned, to 250 mg/day for 6 weeks before delivery and postoperatively until wound healing is complete (1). If penicillamine is used in pregnancy for the treatment of rheumatoid arthritis, healthcare professionals are encouraged to call the toll free number (877-311-8972) for information about patient enrollment in the OTIS Rheumatoid Arthritis study.

BREAST FEEDING SUMMARY

RECOMMENDATION: No Human Data - Potential Toxicity

No reports describing the use of penicillamine during lactation have been located. Authors of one review recommend avoiding penicillamine during lactation (21). However, a 2000 review stated that no adverse effects in nursing infants have been reported by nursing mothers who were taking penicillamine, even though one study found lower amounts of zinc and copper in milk (20).

References

1. Product information. Cuprimine. Merck & Co, 1997.
2. Crawhall JC, Scowen EF, Thompson CJ, Watts RWE. Dissolution of cystine stones during d-penicillamine treatment of a pregnant patient with cystinuria. Br Med J 1967;2:216–8.
3. Mjolnerod OK, Rasmussen K, Dommerud SA, Gjeruldsen ST. Congenital connective-tissue defect probably due to D-penicillamine treatment in pregnancy. Lancet 1971;1:673–5.
4. Laver M, Fairley KF. D-Penicillamine treatment in pregnancy. Lancet 1971;1:1019–20.
5. Scheinberg IH, Sternlieb I. Pregnancy in penicillamine-treated patients with Wilson's disease. N Engl J Med 1975;293:1300–3.
6. Marecek Z, Graf M. Pregnancy in penicillamine-treated patients with Wilson's disease. N Engl J Med 1976;295:841–2.
7. Solomon L, Abrams G, Dinner M, Berman L. Neonatal abnormalities associated with d-penicillamine treatment during pregnancy. N Engl J Med 1977;296:54–5.
8. Walshe JM. Pregnancy in Wilson's disease. Q J Med 1977;46:73–83.
9. Lyle WH. Penicillamine in pregnancy. Lancet 1978;1:606–7.
10. Linares A, Zarranz JJ, Rodriguez-Alarcon J, Diaz-Perez JL. Reversible cutis laxa due to maternal d penicillamine treatment. Lancet 1979;2:43.
11. Endres W. D-penicillamine in pregnancy—to ban or not to ban? Klin Wochenschr 1981;59:535–7.
12. Harpey JP, Jaudon MC, Clavel JP, Galli A, Darbois Y. Cutis laxa and low serum zinc after antenatal exposure to penicillamine. Lancet 1983;2:858.
13. Beck RB, Rosenbaum KN, Byers PH, Holbrook KA, Perry LW. Ultrastructural findings in the fetal penicillamine syndrome (abstract). Presented at the 13th Annual Birth Defects Conference, March of Dimes and University of California, San Diego, June 1980.
14. Gal P, Ravenel SD. Contractures and hydrocephalus with penicillamine and maternal hypotension. J Clin Dysmorphol 1984;2:9–12.
15. Gregory MC, Mansell MA. Pregnancy and cystinuria. Lancet 1983;2:1158–60.
16. Dupont P, Irion O, Béguin F. Pregnancy in a patient with treated Wilson's disease: a case report. Am J Obstet Gynecol 1990;163:1527–8.
17. Hartard C, Kunze K. Pregnancy in a patient with Wilson's disease treated with D-penicillamine and zinc sulfate. Eur Neurol 1994;34:337–40.
18. Berghella V, Steele D, Spector T, Cambi F, Johnson A. Successful pregnancy in a neurologically impaired

P

woman with Wilson's disease. Am J Obstet Gynecol 1997;176:712–4.
19. Martinez-Frias ML, Rodriguez-Pinilla E, Bermejo E, Blanco M. Prenatal exposure to penicillamine and oral clefts: case report. Am J Med Genet 1998;76:274–5.
20. Sternlieb I. Wilson's disease and pregnancy. Hepatology 2000;31:531–2.
21. Oga M, Matsui N, Anai T, Yoshimatsu J, Inoue I, Miyakawa I. Copper disposition of the fetus and placenta in a patient with untreated Wilson's disease. Am J Obstet Gynecol 1993;169:196–8.
22. Ostensen M, Husby G. Antirheumatic drug treatment during pregnancy and lactation. Scand J Rheumatol 1985;14:1–7.
23. Miehle W. Current aspects of D-penicillamine and pregnancy. Z Rheumatol 1988;47(Suppl 1):20–3.
24. Woods SE, Colón VF. Wilson's disease. Am Fam Physician 1989;40:171–8.

Name:	**PENICILLIN G**	Risk Factor:	**B_M**
Class:	**Antibiotic (Penicillin)**		

FETAL RISK SUMMARY

RECOMMENDATION: Compatible

Penicillin G is used routinely for maternal infections during pregnancy. Reproduction studies in mice, rats, and rabbits revealed no evidence of impaired fertility or fetal harm (1).

Several investigators have documented its rapid passage into the fetal circulation and amniotic fluid (2–6). Therapeutic levels are reached in both sites except for the amniotic fluid during the 1st trimester (6). At term, maternal serum and amniotic fluid concentrations are equal 60–90 minutes after IV administration (3). Continuous IV infusions (10,000 U/hour) produced equal concentrations of penicillin G at 20 hours in maternal serum, cord serum, and amniotic fluid (3).

The early use of penicillin G was linked to increased uterine activity and abortion (7–11). It is not known whether this was related to impurities in the drug or to penicillin itself. No reports of this effect have appeared since a report published in 1950 (11). An anaphylactic reaction in a pregnant patient reportedly led to the death of her fetus *in utero* (12).

Only one reference has linked the use of penicillin G with congenital abnormalities (13). An examination of hospital records indicated that in three of four cases the administration of penicillin G had been followed by the birth of a malformed baby. A retrospective review of additional patients exposed to antibiotics in the 1st trimester indicated an increase in congenital defects. Unfortunately, the authors did not analyze their data for each antibiotic, so no causal relationship to penicillin G could be shown (13,14). In another case, a patient was treated in early pregnancy with high doses of penicillin G procaine IV*, cortisone, and sodium salicylate (15). A cyclopic male was delivered at term but died 5 minutes later. The defect was attributed to salicylates, cortisone, or maternal viremia.

In a controlled study, 110 patients received one to three antibiotics during the 1st trimester for a total of 589 weeks (16). Penicillin G was given for a total of 107 weeks. The incidence of birth defects was no different than in a nontreated control group.

The Collaborative Perinatal Project monitored 50,282 mother-child pairs, 3546 of whom had 1st trimester exposure to penicillin derivatives (17, pp. 297–313). For use anytime during pregnancy, 7171 exposures were recorded (17, p. 435). In neither group was evidence found to suggest a relationship to large categories of major or minor malformations or to individual defects. From these data, it is unlikely that penicillin G is teratogenic.

[**Penicillin G procaine should not be given IV. The Editors are assuming the drug was either given IM or the procaine form was not used. We have not been able to contact the authors to clarify these assumptions.*]

P

BREAST FEEDING SUMMARY

RECOMMENDATION: Compatible

Penicillin G is excreted into breast milk in low concentrations. Milk:plasma ratios following IM doses of 100,000 U in 11 patients varied between 0.02 and 0.13 (18). The maximum concentration measured in milk was 0.6 U/mL after this dose. Although no adverse effects were reported, three potential problems exist for the nursing infant: modification of bowel flora, direct effects on the infant (e.g., allergic response), and interference with the interpretation of culture results if a fever workup is required.

References

1. Product information. Pfizerpen. Pfizer, 2000.
2. Herrel W, Nichols D, Heilman D. Penicillin. Its usefulness, limitations, diffusion and detection, with analysis of 150 cases in which it was employed. JAMA 1944;125:1003–11.
3. Woltz J, Zintel H. The transmission of penicillin to amniotic fluid and fetal blood in the human. Am J Obstet Gynecol 1945;50:338–40.
4. Hutter A, Parks J. The transmission of penicillin through the placenta. A preliminary report. Am J Obstet Gynecol 1945;49:663–5.
5. Woltz J, Wiley M. The transmission of penicillin to the previable fetus. JAMA 1946;131:969–70.
6. Wasz-Hockert O, Nummi S, Vuopala S, Jarvinen P. Transplacental passage of azidocillin, ampicillin and penicillin G during early and late pregnancy. Acta Paediatr Scand (Suppl) 1970;206:109–10.
7. Lentz J, Ingraham N Jr, Beerman H, Stokes J. Penicillin in the prevention and treatment of congenital syphilis. JAMA 1944;126:408–13.
8. Leavitt H. Clinical action of penicillin on the uterus. J Vener Dis Inf 1945;26:150–3.
9. McLachlan A, Brown D. The effects of penicillin administration on menstrual and other sexual functions. Br J Vener Dis 1947;23:1–10.
10. Mazingarbe A. Le pencilline possede-t-elle une action abortive? Gynecol Obstet 1946;45:487.
11. Perin L, Sissmann R, Detre F, Chertier A. La pencilline a-t-elle une action abortive? Bull Soc Fr Dermatol 1950;57:534–8.
12. Kosim H. Intrauterine fetal death as a result of anaphylactic reaction to penicillin in a pregnant woman. Dapim Refuiim 1959;18:136–7.
13. Carter M, Wilson F. Antibiotics and congenital malformations. Lancet 1963;1:1267–8.
14. Carter M, Wilson F. Antibiotics in early pregnancy and congenital malformations. Dev Med Child Neurol 1965;7:353–9.
15. Khudr G, Olding L. Cyclopia. Am J Dis Child 1973;125:120–2.
16. Ravid R, Toaff R. On the possible teratogenicity of antibiotic drugs administered during pregnancy-a prospective study. In Klingberg M, Abramovici A, Chemki J, eds. *Drugs and Fetal Development*. New York, NY: Plenum Press, 1972:505–10.
17. Heinonen OP, Slone D, Shapiro S. *Birth Defects and Drugs in Pregnancy*. Littleton, MA: Publishing Sciences Group, 1977.
18. Greene H, Burkhart B, Hobby G. Excretion of penicillin in human milk following parturition. Am J Obstet Gynecol 1946;51:732–3.

P

Name: **PENICILLIN G, BENZATHINE** Risk Factor: **B_M**

Class: **Antibiotic (Penicillin)**

FETAL RISK SUMMARY

RECOMMENDATION: Compatible

Benzathine penicillin G is a combination of an ammonium base and penicillin G suspended in water (see also Penicillin G). Reproduction studies in mice, rats, and rabbits have revealed no evidence of impaired fertility or fetal harm (1).

The pharmacokinetics of benzathine penicillin G in healthy women at 38–39 weeks' gestation, 1–7 days before delivery, have been described (2). Penicillin concentrations were measured in maternal serum, maternal cerebrospinal fluid, cord serum, and amniotic fluid. Because of the wide range of concentrations measured, the authors concluded that the altered pharmacokinetics occurring at this time may adversely affect the efficacy of the drug to prevent congenital syphilis.

BREAST FEEDING SUMMARY

RECOMMENDATION: Compatible

See Penicillin G.

References

1. Product information. Bicillin L-A. Wyeth-Ayerst Pharmaceuticals, 2000.
2. Nathan L, Bawdon RE, Sidawi JE, Stettler RW, McIntire DM, Wendel GD Jr. Penicillin levels following the administration of benzathine penicillin G in pregnancy. Obstet Gynecol 1993;82:338–42.

Name:	**PENICILLIN G, PROCAINE**	Risk Factor:	B_M
Class:	**Antibiotic (Penicillin)**		

FETAL RISK SUMMARY

RECOMMENDATION: Compatible

Procaine penicillin G is an equimolar combination of procaine and penicillin G suspended in water (1). The combination is broken down *in vivo* into the two components. Reproduction studies in mice, rats, and rabbits have revealed no evidence of impaired fertility or fetal harm (2) (see also Penicillin G).

A case report described the use of high doses of penicillin G procaine IV*, cortisone, and sodium salicylate in early pregnancy followed by the delivery at term of a cyclopic male infant (3). The lethal defect was attributed to salicylates, cortisone, or maternal viremia.

[**Penicillin G procaine should not be given IV. The Editors are assuming the drug was either given IM or the procaine form was not used. We have been unable to contact the authors of the paper to clarify these assumptions.*]

P

BREAST FEEDING SUMMARY

RECOMMENDATION: Compatible

See Penicillin G.

References

1. Mandel G, Sande M. Antimicrobial agents (continued). Penicillins and cephalosporins. In Gilman AG, Goodman LS, Gilman A, eds. *The Pharmacological Basis of Therapeutics*. 6th ed. New York, NY: Macmillan, 1980:1137.
2. Product information. Bicillin C-R. Wyeth-Ayerst Pharmaceuticals, 2000.
3. Khudr G, Olding L. Cyclopia. Am J Dis Child 1973; 125:120–2.

Name:	**PENICILLIN V**	Risk Factor:	**B**
Class:	**Antibiotic (Penicillin)**		

FETAL RISK SUMMARY

RECOMMENDATION: Compatible

No reports linking the use of penicillin V with congenital defects have been located. The Collaborative Perinatal Project monitored 50,282 mother-child pairs, 3,546 of whom had

1st trimester exposure to penicillin derivatives (1, pp. 297–313). For use anytime during pregnancy, 7171 exposures were recorded (1, p. 435). In neither group was evidence found to suggest a relationship to large categories of major or minor malformations or to individual defects.

In a surveillance study of Michigan Medicaid recipients conducted between 1985 and 1992 involving 229,101 completed pregnancies, 4597 newborns had been exposed to penicillin V during the 1st trimester (F. Rosa, personal communication, FDA, 1993). A total of 202 (4.4%) major birth defects were observed (195 expected). Specific data were available for six defect categories, including (observed/expected) 46/56 cardiovascular defects, 5/7 oral clefts, 3/2 spina bifida, 17/13 polydactyly, 7/8 limb reduction defects, and 8/11 hypospadias. These data do not support an association between the drug and congenital defects.

Penicillin V depresses both plasma-bound and urinary excreted estriol (2). Urinary estriol was formerly used to assess the condition of the fetoplacental unit, depressed levels being associated with fetal distress. This assessment is now made by measuring plasma-unconjugated estriol, which is not usually affected by penicillin V.

The pharmacokinetics of penicillin V during the 2nd and 3rd trimesters have been reported (3). Elimination of the drug is enhanced at these stages of pregnancy.

BREAST FEEDING SUMMARY

RECOMMENDATION: Compatible

No data are available (see Penicillin G).

References

1. Heinonen OP, Slone D, Shapiro S. *Birth Defects and Drugs in Pregnancy*. Littleton, MA: Publishing Sciences Group, 1977.
2. Pulkkinen M, Willman K. Maternal oestrogen levels during penicillin treatment. Br Med J 1971,4:48.
3. Heikkilä AM, Erkkola RU. The need for adjustment of dosage regimen of penicillin V during pregnancy. Obstet Gynecol 1993;81:919–21.

P

Name:	**PENTAERYTHRITOL TETRANITRATE**	Risk Factor:	**C**
Class:	**Vasodilator**		

FETAL RISK SUMMARY

RECOMMENDATION: Limited Human Data - No Relevant Animal Data

Pentaerythritol tetranitrate is a long-acting agent used for the prevention of angina pectoris. Because of the nature of its indication, experience in pregnancy is limited.

The Collaborative Perinatal Project recorded 3 1st trimester exposures to pentaerythritol tetranitrate and 12 other patients exposed to other vasodilators (1). From this small sample, four malformed children were produced, a statistically significant incidence ($p < 0.02$). It was not reported whether pentaerythritol tetranitrate was taken by any of the mothers of the affected infants. Although these data serve as a warning, the number of patients is so small that conclusions as to the relative safety of this drug cannot be made.

BREAST FEEDING SUMMARY

RECOMMENDATION: No Human Data - Probably Compatible

No data are available.

Reference

1. Heinonen OP, Slone D, Shapiro S. *Birth Defects and Drugs in Pregnancy*. Littleton, MA: Publishing Sciences Group, 1977.

Name: **PENTAMIDINE** Risk Factor: C_M

Class: **Antiprotozoal**

FETAL RISK SUMMARY

RECOMMENDATION: Compatible - Maternal Benefit >> Embryo/Fetal Risk

Pentamidine is an antiprotozoal agent indicated for the treatment of pneumonia caused by *Pneumocystis carinii,* a common opportunistic infection in patients suffering from human immunodeficiency virus (HIV) disease. The mechanism of action of this agent is not fully known. *In vitro* tests have indicated that pentamidine inhibits the synthesis of DNA, RNA, phospholipids, and proteins, and it may be a folic acid antagonist by inhibiting dihydrofolate reductase (1,2).

Pentamidine was not teratogenic in pregnant rats treated with doses similar to those used in humans (3). However, these doses were embryocidal when administered during embryogenesis (3). Significant placental transfer was observed in rats administered pentamidine in late pregnancy (4). By the 12th hour, fetal brain tissue concentrations of pentamidine were statistically similar to the maternal serum levels achieved 2 hours after the dose.

In an experiment using *in vitro* perfused human placentas, the placental transfer of pentamidine in humans was undetectable with therapeutic maternal concentrations of approximately 2 μg/mL (5). The level of sensitivity of the high-performance liquid chromatography method was 0.05 μg/mL. When peak concentrations of pentamidine on the maternal side were increased to approximately 14 μg/mL, fetal levels were consistently 0.2 μg/mL at 30 minutes. Pentamidine did concentrate in placental tissue at all drug levels studied, but the clinical significance of this to placental function is unknown (5).

In contrast to the above, a study published in 1995 used a more sensitive test to document the placental transfer of pentamidine at about 33 weeks' gestation (6). A 21-year-old HIV-infected woman received pentamidine, 200 mg (3.4 mg/kg) IV daily, for 7 days before a cesarean section. A maternal serum sample, drawn 8 hours after her seventh dose, was 0.0813 μg/mL (free base). The pentamidine concentration in the cord blood sample, obtained 16.5 hours after the dose, was 0.0132 μg/mL.

The U.S. Centers for Disease Control and Prevention (CDC) recommends aerosolized pentamidine as one of two treatment regimens for prophylaxis against *P. carinii* in persons infected with HIV (7,8). However, because the safety of this treatment has not been established in human pregnancies, the CDC advises against this use in pregnant women

(7,8). Others have cited information from the manufacturer that the use of aerosolized pentamidine is contraindicated in pregnancy (9).

A 1988 reference cited a concern that pregnant health care workers involved in the care of patients treated with aerosolized pentamidine might be at risk for fetal harm (10). An estimation of this risk, based on a pharmacokinetic model, was published in 1994 (11). The maximum exposure of health care workers, at two different hospitals, to aerosolized pentamidine was estimated to be 1.7 and 9.8 μg/kg/day (IV equivalent). The authors then calculated the embryolethal and teratogenic IV-equivalent reference doses, based on pregnant rat data, to be 0.08 and 4 μg/kg/day, respectively. Comparison of the estimated actual exposures to the predicted toxic levels led to the conclusion that improvement was needed in the methods used to reduce pentamidine exposure of health care workers (11).

An argument favoring the use of pentamidine in the pregnant patient with active *P. carinii* pneumonia, when other treatment regimens had failed, was put forth in a 1987 article (12). Moreover, this same source, in a 1990 reference, argued that the availability of aerosolized pentamidine for prophylaxis should be disclosed to the pregnant HIV-seropositive patient "as part of the informed consent process" (13). This latter position is strengthened by the *in vitro* data cited above relating to the placental transfer of the agent. Because aerosolized pentamidine results in very low systemic concentrations, fetal exposure to the drug by this route is probably minimal and below the level of detection.

The use of aerosolized and IV pentamidine during gestation in women with HIV infection has been described (14–17). A 1992 abstract described the use of aerosolized pentamidine, 300 mg/month, in 15 women during the 2nd and 3rd trimesters (14). No significant effects on the course of pregnancy or on the fetus or newborn were observed. The second reference reported five pregnancies (six fetuses, one set of twins) that were treated with aerosolized pentamidine, zidovudine, and other drugs (15). One woman was treated throughout her 39-week gestation, one from 10 to 39 weeks' gestation, and three during the 2nd and 3rd trimesters. The outcomes of the exposed pregnancies included one growth-retarded infant, one with albinism, one with congenital cytomegalovirus infection, and three normal infants. The latter two references described IV pentamidine in five women (16) and aerosolized drug in nine (16,17). No adverse fetal effects of the drug were reported.

BREAST FEEDING SUMMARY

RECOMMENDATION: Contraindicated

Because systemic concentrations achieved with aerosolized pentamidine are very low, breast milk levels of the drug after administration via this route are probably nil. However, no reports of lactating women administered pentamidine by any route (IM, IV, or by inhalation) have been located.

References

1. Product information. Pentam. Lyphomed, Inc., 1991.
2. Drake S, Lampasona V, Nicks HL, Schwarzmann SW. Pentamidine isethionate in the treatment of *Pneumocystis carinii* pneumonia. Clin Pharm 1985;4:507–16.
3. Harstad TW, Little BB, Bawdon RE, Knoll K, Roe D, Gilstrap LC III. Embryofetal effects of pentamidine isethionate administered to pregnant Sprague-Dawley rats. Am J Obstet Gynecol 1990;163:912–6.
4. Little BB, Harstad TH, Bawdon RE, Sobhi S, Roe DA, Knoll KA, Ghali FE. Pharmacokinetics of pentamidine in Sprague-Dawley rats in late pregnancy. Am J Obstet Gynecol 1991;164:927–30.

5. Fortunato SJ, Bawdon RE. Determination of pentamidine transfer in the *in vitro* perfused human cotyledon with high-performance liquid chromatography. Am J Obstet Gynecol 1989;160:759–61.
6. Schwebke K, Fletcher CV, Acosta EP, Henry K. Pentamidine concentrations in a mother with AIDS and in her neonate. Clin Infect Dis 1995;20:1569–70.
7. CDC. Guidelines for prophylaxis against *Pneumocystis carinii* pneumonia for persons infected with human immunodeficiency virus. MMWR 1989;38(Suppl 5): 1–9.
8. CDC. Guidelines for prophylaxis against *Pneumocystis carinii* pneumonia for persons infected with human immunodeficiency virus. JAMA 1989;262:335–9.
9. Sarti GM. Aerosolized pentamidine in HIV; promising new treatment for *Pneumocystis carinii* pneumonia. Postgrad Med 1989;86:54–69.
10. Conover B, Goldsmith JC, Buehler BA, Maloley BA, Windle ML. Aerosolized pentamidine and pregnancy. Ann Intern Med 1988;109:927.
11. Ito S, Koren G. Estimation of fetal risk from aerosolized pentamidine in pregnant healthcare workers. Chest 1994;106:1460–2.
12. Minkoff HL. Care of pregnant women infected with human immunodeficiency virus. JAMA 1987;258: 2714–7.
13. Minkoff HL, Moreno JD. Drug prophylaxis for human immunodeficiency virus-infected pregnant women; ethical considerations. Am J Obstet Gynecol 1990;163:1111–4.
14. Nana D, Tannenbaum I, Landesman S, Mendez H, Moroso G, Minkoff H. Pentamidine prophylaxis in pregnancy (abstract). Am J Obstet Gynecol 1992;166:387.
15. Sperling RS, Stratton P, O'Sullivan MJ, Boyer P, Watts DH, Lambert JS, Hammill H, Livingston EG, Gloeb DJ, Minkoff H, Fox HE. A survey of zidovudine use in pregnant women with human immunodeficiency virus infection. N Engl J Med 1992;326:857–61.
16. Stratton P, Mofenson LM, Willoughby AD. Human immunodeficiency virus infection in pregnant women under care at AIDS clinical trials centers in the United States. Obstet Gynecol 1992;79:364–8.
17. Gates HS Jr, Barker CD. Pneumocystis carinii pneumonia in pregnancy. A case report. J Reprod Med 1993;38:483–6.

Name: **PENTAZOCINE** Risk Factor: **C***
Class: **Narcotic Agonist-Antagonist Analgesic**

FETAL RISK SUMMARY

RECOMMENDATION: Human Data Suggest Risk in 3rd Trimester

No reports linking the use of pentazocine with congenital defects have been located. As reported by the manufacturer, reproductive studies in animals did not found embryotoxic or teratogenic effects (1). In a 1975 reference, however, increasing single SC doses of pentazocine (98–570 mg/kg) administered to hamsters during the critical period of central nervous system (CNS) organogenesis resulted in a significant increase in the number of offspring with malformations (exencephaly, cranioschisis, and various other CNS lesions) (2). Maternal death was observed in 10% of the mothers at the highest dose, but not with the lower doses.

The drug rapidly crosses the placenta, resulting in cord blood levels of 40%–70% of maternal serum (3). Withdrawal has been reported in infants exposed *in utero* to chronic maternal ingestion of pentazocine (4–8). Symptoms, presenting within 24–48 hours of birth, consist of trembling and jitteriness, marked hyperirritability, hyperactivity with hypertonia, high-pitched cry, diaphoresis, diarrhea, vomiting, and opisthotonic posturing.

During labor, increased overall uterine activity has been observed after pentazocine, but without changes in fetal heart rate (9). In equianalgesic doses, most studies report no significant differences between meperidine and pentazocine in pain relief, length of labor, or Apgar scores (10–15). However, meperidine in one study was observed to produce significantly lower Apgar scores than pentazocine, especially in repeated doses (16). Severe neonatal respiratory depression may also occur with pentazocine (10,16).

A 1982 report from New Orleans described 24 infants born of mothers using the IV combination of pentazocine/tripelennamine (T's and blue's) (17). Doses were unknown but probably ranged from 200 to 600 mg of pentazocine and 100 to 250 mg of tripelennamine. Six of the newborns were exposed early in pregnancy. Birth weights for 11 of the infants were less than 2500 g; 9 of these were premature (<37 weeks) and 2 were small for gestational age. Daily or weekly exposure throughout pregnancy produced withdrawal symptoms, occurring within 7 days of birth, in 15 of 16 infants. Withdrawal was thought to be related to pentazocine, but antihistamine withdrawal has been reported (see Diphenhydramine). Thirteen of 15 infants became asymptomatic 3–11 days following onset of withdrawal, but symptoms persisted for up to 6 months in 2.

Three cases of maternal bacterial endocarditis were observed following IV drug abuse, one of which involved the injection of pentazocine/tripelennamine intermittently throughout pregnancy (18). Following satisfactory antibiotic treatment for the infection, the mother gave birth at term to a healthy, male infant.

In a study published in 1983, three groups of pregnant women were evaluated in a perinatal addiction program in the Chicago area (19). One group ($N = 13$) was composed of women addicted to pentazocine/tripelennamine. A second group consisted of women who conceived while self-administering heroin, and who were then converted to low-dose (5–40 mg/day) methadone ($N = 46$). The third group consisted of drug-free controls ($N = 27$). The three groups were statistically similar as to mean maternal age, educational level, gravidity, cigarette smoking, and mean weight gain during pregnancy. Heavy alcohol users were excluded. All infants were delivered at term. Apgar scores were similar among the three groups of newborns, and no significant perinatal complications were observed. Mean birth weight, length, and head circumference were similar between the two drug groups. Compared with the drug-free controls, the pentazocine/tripelennamine-exposed infants weighed less (2799 vs. 3479 g, $p < 0.0001$), were shorter (48.1 vs. 51.1 cm, $p < 0.002$), and had smaller heads (32.9 vs. 34.7 cm, $p < 0.003$). Neonatal withdrawal was observed in both drug-exposed infant groups. Withdrawal characteristics observed in the pentazocine/tripelennamine infants were similar to those seen in the methadone group, consisting of irritability, voracious sucking, and feeding difficulties (19). However, none of these infants required therapy for their symptoms. Neonatal behavior was evaluated using the Brazelton Neonatal Behavioral Assessment Scale. Results of these tests indicated that the infants exposed to the drug combination had interactive deficits and withdrawal similar to the methadone-addicted babies (19).

P

In 1986, nearly the same data as above were published but with the addition of a group exposed to mixed sedative/stimulant ($N = 22$) and a group exposed to phencyclidine ($N = 9$) (20). The outcome of the pentazocine/tripelennamine group was the same as above.

Another study described the effects of pentazocine/tripelennamine abuse in 50 pregnancies identified retrospectively from 23,779 deliveries occurring between January 1, 1981, and June 30, 1983 (21). Compared with matched controls, users of the combination were more likely to have no prenatal care ($p < 0.005$), to be anemic ($p < 0.001$), and to have syphilis ($p < 0.001$), gonorrhea ($p < 0.01$), or hepatitis ($p < 0.005$). Moreover, their infants were more likely to be small for gestational age ($p < 0.01$), to have lower birth weights (3260 g vs. 2592 g, $p < 0.01$), to have a 1-minute Apgar score less than 7 ($p < 0.025$), and to have neonatal withdrawal ($p < 0.001$). No congenital abnormalities were observed in the infants exposed to the drug combination.

A study published in 1993 examined the effects on the fetus and newborn of IV pentazocine and methylphenidate abuse during pregnancy (22). During a 2-year (1987–1988) period, 39 infants (38 pregnancies, 1 set of twins) were identified in the study population as being subjected to the drug abuse during gestation, a minimum incidence of 5 cases per 1000 live births. Many of the mothers had used cigarettes (34%) or alcohol (71%) or abused other drugs (26%). The median duration of IV pentazocine and methylphenidate abuse was 3 years (range 1–9 years) with a median frequency of 14 injections/week (range 1–70 injections/week). Among the infants, 8 were delivered prematurely, 12 were growth-retarded, and 11 had withdrawal symptoms after birth. Four of the infants had birth defects, including twins with fetal alcohol syndrome, one with a ventricular septal defect, and one case of polydactyly. Of the 21 infants that had formal developmental testing, 17 had normal development and 4 had low-normal developmental quotients (22).

In summary, pentazocine does not appear to cause structural malformations in humans, but behavioral teratogenicity, either from the drug itself, the mother's lifestyle, other drug abuse, or a combination of these factors, is a common finding. Moreover, its abuse during pregnancy is associated with intrauterine growth retardation and withdrawal in the newborn.

[**Risk Factor D if used for prolonged periods or in high doses at term.*]

BREAST FEEDING SUMMARY

RECOMMENDATION: No Human Data - Probably Compatible

No reports describing the use of pentazocine during lactation have been located. The relatively low molecular weight (about 285), however, probably indicates that the drug is excreted into milk. The effects of this predicted exposure on a nursing infant are unknown, but small, infrequent doses most likely present a minimal risk.

References

1. Product information. Talwin. Sanofi Winthrop Pharmaceuticals, 1997.
2. Geber WF, Schramm LC. Congenital malformations of the central nervous system produced by narcotic analgesics in the hamster. Am J Obstet Gynecol 1975;123:705–13.
3. Beckett AH, Taylor JF. Blood concentrations of pethidine and pentazocine in mother and infant at time of birth. J Pharm Pharmacol 1967;19(Suppl):50s–2s.
4. Goetz RL, Bain RV. Neonatal withdrawal symptoms associated with maternal use of pentazocine. J Pediatr 1974;84:887–8.
5. Scanlon JW. Pentazocine and neonatal withdrawal symptoms. J Pediatr 1974;85:735–6.
6. Kopelman AE. Fetal addiction to pentazocine. Pediatrics 1975;55:888–9.
7. Reeds TO. Withdrawal symptoms in a neonate associated with maternal pentazocine abuse. J Pediatr 1975;87:324.
8. Preis O, Choi SJ, Rudolph N. Pentazocine withdrawal syndrome in the newborn infant. Am J Obstet Gynecol 1977;127:205–6.
9. Filler WW, Filler NW. Effect of a potent non-narcotic analgesic agent (pentazocine) on uterine contractility and fetal heart rate. Obstet Gynecol 1966;28:224–32.
10. Freedman H, Tafeen CH, Harris H. Parenteral Win 20,228 as analgesic in labor. N Y State J Med 1967;67:2849–51.
11. Duncan SLB, Ginsburg J, Morris NF. Comparison of pentazocine and pethidine in normal labor. Am J Obstet Gynecol 1969;105:197–202.
12. Moore J, Hunter RJ. A comparison of the effects of pentazocine and pethidine administered during labor. J Obstet Gynaecol Br Commonw 1970;77:830–6.
13. Mowat J, Garrey MM. Comparison of pentazocine and pethidine in labour. Br Med J 1970;2:757–9.
14. Levy DL. Obstetric analgesia. Pentazocine and meperidine in normal primiparous labor. Obstet Gynecol 1971;38:907–11.
15. Moore J, Ball HG. A sequential study of intravenous analgesic treatment during labour. Br J Anaesth 1974;46:365–72.
16. Refstad SO, Lindbaek E. Ventilatory depression of the newborn of women receiving pethidine or pentazocine. Br J Anaesth 1980;52:265–70.
17. Dunn DW, Reynolds J. Neonatal withdrawal symptoms associated with "T's and blue's" (pentazocine and tripelennamine). Am J Dis Child 1982;136:644–5.
18. Pastorek JG, Plauche WC, Faro S. Acute bacterial endocarditis in pregnancy: a report of three cases. J Reprod Med 1983;28:611–4.
19. Chasnoff IJ, Hatcher R, Burns WJ, Schnoll SH. Pentazocine and tripelennamine ("T's and blue's"): effects on the fetus and neonate. Dev Pharmacol Ther 1983;6:162–9.
20. Chasnoff IJ, Burns KA, Burns WJ, Schnoll SH. Prenatal drug exposure: effects on neonatal and infant growth and development. Neurobehavior Toxicol Teratol 1986;8:357–62.
21. von Almen WF II, Miller JM Jr. "Ts and blues" in pregnancy. J Reprod Med 1986;31:236–9.
22. Debooy VD, Seshia MMK, Tenenbein M, Casiiro OG. Intravenous pentazocine and methylphenidate abuse during pregnancy. Maternal lifestyle and infant outcome. Am J Dis Child 1993;147:1062–5.

Name: **PENTOBARBITAL** Risk Factor: **D_M**
Class: **Sedative/Hypnotic**

FETAL RISK SUMMARY

RECOMMENDATION: Limited Human Data - Probably Compatible

No reports linking the use of pentobarbital with congenital defects have been located. The Collaborative Perinatal Project monitored 50,282 mother-child pairs, 250 of whom had 1st trimester exposure to pentobarbital (1). No evidence was found to suggest a relationship to large categories of major or minor malformations or to individual defects. Hemorrhagic disease and barbiturate withdrawal in the newborn are theoretical possibilities (see also Phenobarbital).

BREAST FEEDING SUMMARY

RECOMMENDATION: Limited Human Data - Potential Toxicity

Pentobarbital is excreted into breast milk (2). Breast milk levels of 0.17 μg/mL have been detected 19 hours after a dose of 100 mg daily for 32 days. The effect on the nursing infant is not known.

References

1. Heinonen OP, Slone D, Shapiro S. *Birth Defects and Drugs in Pregnancy*. Littleton, MA: Publishing Sciences Group, 1977:336–7.
2. Wilson JT, Brown RD, Cherek DR, Dailey JW, Hilman B, Jobe PC, Manno BR, Manno JE, Redetzki HM, Stewart JJ. Drug excretion in human breast milk: principles, pharmacokinetics and projected consequences. Clin Pharmacokinet 1980;5:1–66.

Name: **PENTOXIFYLLINE** Risk Factor: **C_M**
Class: **Hemorheologic Agent**

P

FETAL RISK SUMMARY

RECOMMENDATION: Limited Human Data - Animal Data Suggest Moderate Risk

Pentoxifylline is a synthetic xanthine derivative used to lower blood viscosity in peripheral vascular and cerebrovascular diseases. No published reports of its use in human pregnancy have been located.

Reproduction studies in rats and rabbits at oral doses up to 4.2 and 3.5 times the maximum recommended human dose on a surface area basis revealed no evidence of teratogenicity (1). In rats, however, an increased incidence of resorptions was seen at the maximum dose (1).

In a surveillance study of Michigan Medicaid recipients conducted between 1985 and 1992 involving 229,101 completed pregnancies, 34 newborns had been exposed to pentoxifylline during the 1st trimester (F. Rosa, personal communication, FDA, 1993). Five (14.7%) major birth defects were observed (one expected), including (observed/expected) 2/0 cardiovascular defects and 1/0 spina bifida. No anomalies were observed in four other defect categories (oral clefts, polydactyly, limb reduction defects, and hypospadias) for which specific data were available. Although the number of exposures is small, the total number of defects and both specific defects are suggestive of possible associations, but other factors, including the mother's disease, concurrent drug use, and chance, may be involved.

Pentoxifylline causes a significant increase in sperm motility, but not concentration, and may be useful in patients with normogonadotrophic asthenozoospermia (2).

BREAST FEEDING SUMMARY

RECOMMENDATION: Limited Human Data - Probably Compatible

Pentoxifylline is excreted into human milk. Five healthy women, who had been breast-feeding for at least 6 weeks, were given a single 400-mg sustained-release tablet of pentoxifylline (commercially available formulation) after a 4-hour fast (3). The mean milk:plasma ratio of unmetabolized pentoxifylline at 4 hours was 0.87. Mean milk:plasma ratios for the three major metabolites at 4 hours were 0.76, 0.54, and 1.13. Mean milk concentration of pentoxifylline at 2 hours (73.9 ng/mL) was approximately twice as much as that occurring at 4 hours (35.7 ng/mL) (3). Pentoxifylline and its metabolites are stable in breast milk for 3 weeks when stored at −15°C (4).

References

1. Product information. Trental. Hoechst Roussel, 2000.
2. Shen M-R, Chiang P-H, Yang R-C, Hong C-Y, Chen S-S. Pentoxifylline stimulates human sperm motility both *in vitro* and after oral therapy. Br J Clin Pharmacol 1991;31:711–4.
3. Witter FR, Smith RV. The excretion of pentoxifylline and its metabolites into human breast milk. Am J Obstet Gynecol 1985;151:1094–7.
4. Bauza MT, Smith RV, Knutson DE, Witter FR. Gas chromatographic determination of pentoxifylline and its major metabolites in human breast milk. J Chromatogr 1984;310:61–9.

Name: **PERGOLIDE** Risk Factor: **B_M**

Class: **Antiparkinsonian Agent**

FETAL RISK SUMMARY

RECOMMENDATION: Limited Human Data - Animal Data Suggest Low Risk

Pergolide is an ergot derivative, dopamine receptor agonist (D1 and D2 receptor sites) that is indicated as an adjunct in the treatment of the signs and symptoms of Parkinson disease (1). As a dopamine receptor agonist, pergolide is 10 to 1000 times more potent, on a milligram-to-milligram basis, than bromocriptine. Pergolide inhibits the secretion of prolactin in humans and has been used for the treatment of prolactinomas (2,3). However, this use has decreased because of the high incidence of adverse effects (similar to bromocriptine) and the observation of uterine neoplasms in rodents (4). Some pergolide metabolites have been shown to be dopamine agonists in animals (1). No information is available on the pharmacokinetics of pergolide, but approximately 90% is bound to plasma proteins (1).

Reproduction studies have been conducted in mice and rabbits (1,5,6). In male and female mice, no effect on fertility was observed with oral doses up to 14 times the maximum human dose (based on 6 mg/day equivalent to 0.12 mg/kg/day) (MHD), but a dose

47 times the MHD caused a decrease in fertility (1). No evidence of fetal harm was observed in pregnant mice and rabbits treated with oral doses up to 375 and 133 times the MHD, respectively (1). In mice, reduced fetal weight was observed at 500 times the MHD (5). This high dose also decreased startle amplitudes in postnatal male mice (5).

In another reproductive and developmental toxicity study, male and female mice were administered pergolide (0–50 parts per million [ppm]) in the diet (6). Fewer pregnancies occurred with the highest dose (equivalent to approximately 5 mg/kg/day [*42 times the MHD*]) (6). Pergolide was administered to female mice throughout gestation and during lactation. Doses of 15 or 50 ppm (about 1.5–5 mg/kg/day [*12.5–42 times the MHD*]) during pregnancy caused fetal growth retardation. During lactation, the 50 ppm dose was associated with maternal and pup toxicity (decreased body weight). The no adverse-effect-level was 0.5 mg/kg/day (*about 4 times the MHD*) (6).

Prolonged (2-year) exposure in mice and rats with dietary doses up to 340 and 12 times the MHD, respectively, was associated with uterine neoplasms in both species (1). A low incidence of endometrial sarcomas was observed in mice and of endometrial adenomas and carcinomas in rats. The neoplasms were attributed to the high estrogen/progesterone ratios that resulted from the prolactin-inhibiting action of pergolide. It was not thought to be a risk for women treated with the drug because these endocrine mechanisms are not present in humans, but no human data confirm this conclusion (1).

It is not known if pergolide can cross the placenta to the embryo or fetus. The molecular weight (about 315), however, is low enough that distribution to the fetal compartment should be expected.

In premarketing studies, 39 pregnancies were exposed to pergolide (dose, timing, and other details not provided) (1). The outcomes of these cases were 33 healthy infants, 3 newborns with major anomalies, and 3 with minor defects (no details provided on the malformations).

A 2002 case report described the use of pergolide in a 35-year-old woman throughout gestation (7). The woman was started on pergolide (3 mg/day) and levodopa (200 mg/day) about 3 years before conception. She continued these doses until delivery of a normal term infant (sex and weight not specified), with Apgar scores of 9 (assumed to mean 9 and 9 at 1 and 5 minutes, respectively). The healthy child was developing normally at 13 months of age (7).

In summary, pergolide is not teratogenic in two animal species, but dose-related fetal toxicity was evident in one species. The animal reproduction tests, however, only involved pergolide alone, not in combination with levodopa/carbidopa as it often is used clinically. Human pregnancy experience is limited to the one case report and the premarketing studies that involved 39 pregnancies. Except for the number of major and minor defects, no other information was provided. Based only on the small number of cases, the incidence of major anomalies (7.7%) in the newborns is higher than the expected background incidence of approximately 3%. Of interest, another dopamine agonist with extensive human pregnancy data (see Bromocriptine) does not appear to be related to congenital malformations. In treatment of Parkinson's disease, pergolide is used concomitantly with levodopa/carbidopa. Although the data are very limited, these latter agents do not appear to present a major risk to the fetus. (See Levodopa and Carbidopa.) Because Parkinson disease is relatively uncommon during the childbearing years, the use of pergolide during pregnancy also will be uncommon. Moreover, pergolide is not the drug of choice for the treatment of hyperprolactinemic disorders. Therefore, even though additional data are required before the risk to a human pregnancy, if any, can be better assessed, it appears doubtful that such data will be forthcoming soon. Until additional pregnancy experience has been obtained, the safest course is to avoid pergolide, if possible, during the 1st trimester. However, inadvertent exposure during this period should not be a basis for termination.

BREAST FEEDING SUMMARY

RECOMMENDATION: Contraindicated

No reports describing the use of pergolide during human lactation have been located. The relatively low molecular weight (about 315), however, is low enough that excretion into breast milk should be expected. The effects, if any, of this exposure on a nursing infant are unknown. Infants should be closely monitored for adverse events that are common in adults, such as digestive complaints (e.g., nausea and constipation). Pergolide inhibits prolactin secretion and may inhibit lactation. Until data to the contrary are available, pergolide should not be used during lactation.

References

1. Product information. Permax. Amarin Pharmaceuticals, 2003.
2. Ferrari C, Crosignani PG. Medical treatment of hyperprolactinaemic disorders. Hum Reprod 1986;1:507–14.
3. Orrego JJ, Chandler WF, Barkan AL. Pergolide as primary therapy for macroprolactinomas. Pituitary 2000; 3:251–6.
4. Colao A, di Sarno A, Pivonello R, di Somma C, Lombardi G. Dopamine receptor agonists for treating prolactinomas. Exper Opin Investig Drugs 2002;11:787–800.
5. Shepard TH. *Catalog of Teratogenic Agents*. 10th ed. Baltimore, MD: The Johns Hopkins University Press, 2001:398.
6. Hoyt JA, Byrd RA, Owen NV. Reproductive and developmental toxicity of the dopamine agonist pergolide mesylate in mice. Arzneimittelforschung 1994;44: 1177–83.
7. De Mari M, Zenzola A, Lamberti P. Antiparkinsonian treatment in pregnancy. Mov Disord 2002;17:428–32.

Name: **PERINDOPRIL** Risk Factor: C_M*
Class: **Antihypertensive**

FETAL RISK SUMMARY

RECOMMENDATION: Human Data Suggest Risk in 2nd and 3rd Trimesters

Perindopril, a competitive inhibitor of angiotensin I-converting enzyme (ACE), is a prodrug that is hydrolyzed *in vivo* to the active agent, perindoprilat. The agent is used in the management of essential hypertension.

Reproduction studies have been conducted with perindopril in mice, rats, rabbits, and cynomolgus monkeys (1). No evidence of teratogenicity was observed in these species at doses 6, 670, 50, and 17 times, respectively, the maximum recommended human dose on a body surface area basis for a 50-kg adult (MRHD). At 6 times the MRHD in rats, no adverse effects on reproductive performance or fertility were observed in male and female rats (1).

It is not known if either perindopril or its metabolite, perindoprilat, crosses the human placenta to the fetus. The relatively low molecular weights of perindopril (about 368 for the free acid or 442 for the salt form) and perindoprilat (less than the prodrug) suggest that transfer to the fetus will occur.

No reports describing the use of perindopril during human pregnancy have been located. Although ACE inhibitors do not appear to cause embryo or fetal harm when used only during the 1st trimester, their use during the 2nd and 3rd trimesters may cause teratogenicity and severe fetal and neonatal toxicity. The mechanism of these adverse effects are thought to be related to fetal hypotension and decreased renal blood flow. Fetal toxic effects may include anuria, oligohydramnios, fetal hypocalvaria, intrauterine growth retardation, prematurity, and patent ductus arteriosus. Anuria-associated oligohydramnios may produce fetal limb contractures, craniofacial deformation, and pulmonary hypoplasia. Severe anuria and hypotension, that is resistant to both pressor agents and volume expansion, may occur in the newborn following *in utero* exposure to ACE inhibitors, including perindopril (see also Captopril and Enalapril). Newborn renal function and blood pressure should be closely monitored. If perindopril is used in pregnancy, healthcare professionals are encouraged to call the toll free number (800-670-6126) for information about patient enrollment in the Motherisk study.

[**Risk Factor* D_M *if used in the 2nd and 3rd trimesters.*]

BREAST FEEDING SUMMARY

RECOMMENDATION: No Human Data - Probably Compatible

No reports describing the use of the prodrug perindopril during human lactation have been located. Perindopril excreted into the milk of lactating rats (1). The relatively low molecular weights of perindopril (about 368 for the free acid or 442 for the salt form) and its active metabolite, perindoprilat (molecular weight less than perindopril), are suggestive that both would be excreted into breast milk if present in the maternal circulation. The effects on a nursing infant from exposure to perindopril or perindoprilat in milk are unknown. However, other agents in this class are excreted into milk and, because the amounts are low and no adverse effects have been observed in nursing infants, are classified as compatible with breast feeding by the American Academy of Pediatrics (see also Captopril and Enalapril).

Reference

1. Product information. Aceon. Solvay Pharmaceuticals, 2000.

Name:	**PERMETHRIN**	Risk Factor:	B_M
Class:	**Scabicide**		

FETAL RISK SUMMARY

RECOMMENDATION: Compatible

Permethrin, a pyrethroid, is indicated for the topical treatment of *Sarcoptes scabiei* (scabies) infestations. The drug is also active against lice, ticks, fleas, mites, and other arthropods. In patients with moderate to severe scabies, systemic absorption was estimated to be 2% or less of the dose (1,2).

Oral reproduction studies with permethrin have been conducted in mice, rats, and rabbits at doses of 200–400 mg/kg/day (1,2). No adverse effects on fertility or evidence of fetal harm were observed in these studies. Species-specific carcinogenesis was observed in mouse studies but negative results were seen in rats. Genetic toxic studies revealed no evidence of mutagenicity (1,2). Only the highest oral concentrations (2500–4000 ppm) of permethrin administered after implantation were found to lower significantly the protein and glycogen contents of rat placentas, but this had no statistical effect on the number of live fetuses (3).

Although no studies of permethrin placental transfer have been located, the molecular weight (about 391) is low enough that transfer should occur. However, because only small amounts are absorbed systemically and these are rapidly metabolized by ester hydrolysis to inactive metabolites, the opportunity for fetal exposure to permethrin appears to be minimal, if it occurs at all.

A 1995 case report described the use of multiple courses of permethrin and other agents in a pregnant woman who had developed crusted scabies (4). She was initially treated at 2 months' gestation with monosulfiram (a pesticide not available in the United States). Relapse occurred at 5 months' gestation and she was treated with two total-body (24-hour) applications of malathion 0.5% liquid and one total-body (24-hour) application of monosulfiram 25% solution. Three weeks later another relapse occurred and she was treated with permethrin 5% cream to the whole body for 12 hours. Because live mites were found the next day, a sulfur/tar/coconut oil soak to the scalp three times daily followed by two total body benzyl benzoate 25% treatments within 24 hours. Then permethrin cream was used weekly for 3 weeks. A healthy male infant was delivered at term (4).

The Centers for Disease Control and Prevention (CDC) considers permethrin or pyrethrins with piperonyl butoxide to be the treatments of choice for pubic lice in pregnant women (5). Although not specifically mentioned, permethrin or pyrethrins with piperonyl butoxide should also be used if other body areas of a pregnant woman, such as the head, are infested with lice. For pregnant women with scabies, permethrin is considered the treatment of choice in the United States and the United Kingdom (5,6).

BREAST FEEDING SUMMARY

RECOMMENDATION: Compatible

No reports describing the use of topical permethrin during lactation have been located. Although the molecular weight (about 391) is low enough for excretion into breast milk, the minimal systemic absorption and rapid metabolism suggests that little, if any, of the drug will be found in milk. The CDC considers permethrin or pyrethrins with piperonyl butoxide to be the treatment of choice for pubic lice during lactation (5). For lactating women with scabies, permethrin is considered the treatment of choice in the United States and the United Kingdom (5,6).

References

1. Product information. Elimite. Allergan, 2001.
2. Product information. Acticin. Bertek Pharmaceuticals, 2001.
3. Spencer F, Berhane Z. Uterine and fetal characteristics in rats following a post-implantational exposure to permethrin. Bull Environ Contam Toxicol 1982;29:84–8.
4. Judge MR, Kobza-Black A. Crusted scabies in pregnancy. Br J Dermatol 1995;132:116–9.
5. CDC. 1998 Guidelines for treatment of sexually transmitted diseases. MMWR 1998;47:1–116.
6. Clinical Effectiveness Group (Association of Genitourinary Medicine and the Medical Society for the Study of Venereal Diseases). National guideline for the management of scabies. Sex Transm Inf 1999;75(Suppl):S76–7.

Name: **PERPHENAZINE** Risk Factor: **C**
Class: **Tranquilizer**

FETAL RISK SUMMARY

RECOMMENDATION: Limited Human Data - No Relevant Animal Data

Perphenazine is a piperazine phenothiazine in the same group as prochlorperazine (see Prochlorperazine). The phenothiazines readily cross the placenta to the fetus (1).

The Collaborative Perinatal Project monitored 50,282 mother-child pairs, 63 of whom had 1st trimester exposure to perphenazine (2). For use anytime during pregnancy, 166 exposures were recorded. No evidence was found in either group to suggest neither a relationship to malformations, nor an effect on perinatal mortality rates, birth weight, or intelligence quotient scores at 4 years of age.

In a surveillance study of Michigan Medicaid recipients conducted between 1985 and 1992 involving 229,101 completed pregnancies, 140 newborns had been exposed to perphenazine during the 1st trimester (F. Rosa, personal communication, FDA, 1993). Five (3.6%) major birth defects were observed (six expected), four of which were cardiovascular defects (one expected). No anomalies were observed in five other defect categories (oral clefts, spina bifida, polydactyly, limb reduction defects, and hypospadias) for which specific data were available. The number of cardiovascular defects is suggestive of a possible association, but other factors, including the mother's disease, concurrent drug use, and chance, may be involved.

A case of maternal suicide attempt with a combination of amitriptyline (725 mq) and perphenazine (58 mg) at 8 days' gestation was described in a 1980 abstract (3). An infant was eventually delivered with multiple congenital defects. The abnormalities included microcephaly, "cotton-like" hair with pronounced shedding, cleft palate, micrognathia, ambiguous genitalia, foot deformities, and undetectable dermal ridges (3).

Perphenazine has been used as an antiemetic during normal labor without producing any observable effect on the newborn (4).

Although occasional published reports have attempted to link various phenothiazine compounds with congenital defects, the bulk of the evidence suggests that the therapeutic use of these drugs are safe for the mother and fetus (see also Chlorpromazine). A possible association between perphenazine, amitriptyline, or both and congenital defects is suggested by a single case, but without confirming evidence no conclusions can be reached.

BREAST FEEDING SUMMARY

RECOMMENDATION: Limited Human Data - Potential Toxicity

Perphenazine is excreted into human milk (5). A 50-kg, lactating 22-year-old woman was taking perphenazine 12 mg twice daily (480 μg/kg) for postpartum psychosis. She had a 1-month-old child. During a 24-hour interval, she produced 510 mL of milk that contained 3.2 ng/mL (7.8 nmol/L) of perphenazine. Because of toxicity, her dose was decreased to 8 mg twice daily, with a proportionate decrease in the concentration in milk to 2.1 ng/mL. The mean milk:plasma ratio from samples drawn at various times during the day was approximately 1. Calculated on the infant's weight of 3.5 kg, the authors estimated that the infant would consume about 0.1% of the mother's dose, based on a μg/kg/day basis. Because they did not consider this exposure to be clinically significant, breast-feeding was started. For the next 3.5 months, while the mother was on perphenazine, the infant's growth and development were normal. Although no adverse effects were observed in this single case, the American Academy of Pediatrics classifies perphenazine as a drug for which the effect on nursing infants is unknown but may be of concern (6).

References

1. Moya F, Thorndike V. Passage of drugs across the placenta. Am J Obstet Gynecol 1962;84:1778–98.
2. Slone D, Siskind V, Heinonen OP, Monson RR, Kaufman DW, Shapiro S. Antenatal exposure to the phenothiazines in relation to congenital malformations, perinatal mortality rate, birth weight, and intelligence quotient score. Am J Obstet Gynecol 1977;128:486–8.
3. Wertelecki W, Purvis-Smith SG, Blackburn WR. Amitriptyline/perphenazine maternal overdose and birth defects (abstract). Teratology 1980;21:74A.
4. McGarry JM. A double-blind comparison of the anti-emetic effect during labour of metoclopramide and perphenazine. Br J Anaesth 1971;43:613–5.
5. Olesen OV, Bartels U, Poulsen JH. Perphenazine in breast milk and serum. Am J Psychiatry 1990;147:1378–9.
6. Committee on Drugs, American Academy of Pediatrics. The transfer of drugs and other chemicals into human milk. Pediatrics 2001;108:776–89.

Name:	**PHENACETIN**	Risk Factor:	**B**
Class:	**Analgesic/Antipyretic**		

FETAL RISK SUMMARY

RECOMMENDATION: Compatible

Phenacetin, in combination products, is routinely used during pregnancy. It is metabolized mainly to acetaminophen (see also Acetaminophen).

The Collaborative Perinatal Project monitored 50,282 mother-child pairs, 5546 of whom had 1st trimester exposure to phenacetin (1, pp. 286–295). Although no evidence was found to suggest a relationship to large categories of major or minor malformations, possible associations were found with several individual defects (1, p. 471): craniosynostosis (6 cases); adrenal syndromes (5 cases); anal atresia (7 cases); and accessory spleen (5 cases). The statistical significance of these associations is unknown and independent confirmation is required. Further, phenacetin is rarely used alone, being consumed usually in combination with aspirin and caffeine. For use anytime during pregnancy, 13,031 exposures were recorded (1, p. 434). With the same qualifications, possible associations with individual defects were found (1, p. 483): musculoskeletal (6 cases); hydronephrosis (8 cases); and adrenal anomalies (8 cases).

In a surveillance study of Michigan Medicaid recipients conducted between 1985 and 1992 involving 229,101 completed pregnancies, 368 newborns had been exposed to phenacetin during the 1st trimester (F. Rosa, personal communication, FDA, 1993). A total of 24 (6.5%) major birth defects were observed (16 expected), including (observed/expected) 6/4 cardiovascular defects, 1/1 polydactyly, and 2/1 hypospadias. No anomalies were observed in three other defect categories (oral clefts, spina bifida, and limb reduction defects) for which specific data were available. These data do not support an association between the drug and congenital defects.

BREAST FEEDING SUMMARY

RECOMMENDATION: Compatible

Phenacetin is excreted into breast milk, appearing along with its major metabolite, acetaminophen (2). A patient who consumed two tablets of Empirin Compound with

Codeine No. 3 (aspirin-phenacetin-caffeine-codeine) produced an average phenacetin milk concentration of 71 ng/mL (2). Milk:plasma ratios in this and a second patient varied from 0.16 to 0.90 (2).

References

1. Heinonen OP, Slone D, Shapiro S. *Birth Defects and Drugs in Pregnancy*. Littleton, MA: Publishing Sciences Group, 1977.
2. Findlay JWA, DeAngelis RL, Kearney MF, Welch RM, Findlay JM. Analgesic drugs in breast milk and plasma. Clin Pharmacol Ther 1981;29:625–33.

Name:	**PHENAZOCINE**	Risk Factor:	**C***
Class:	**Narcotic Agonist Analgesic**		

FETAL RISK SUMMARY

RECOMMENDATION: Human Data Suggest Risk in 3rd Trimester

No reports linking the use of phenazocine with congenital defects in humans have been located. In a reproductive study with hamsters, increasing doses (100–240 mg/kg) administered as single SC injections during the critical period of central nervous system organogenesis resulted in a significant increase in malformations (exencephaly and cranioschisis) in the offspring (1). Maternal mortality was not observed at the doses tested.

Phenazocine is not commercially available in the United States. Withdrawal could theoretically occur in infants exposed *in utero* to prolonged maternal ingestion of phenazocine. Phenazocine may cause neonatal respiratory depression when used in labor (2,3).

[**Risk Factor D if used for prolonged period or in high doses at term.*]

BREAST FEEDING SUMMARY

RECOMMENDATION: No Human Data - Probably Compatible

No data are available.

References

1. Geber WF, Schramm LC. Congenital malformations of the central nervous system produced by narcotic analgesics in the hamster. Am J Obstet Gynecol 1975;123:705–13.
2. Sadove M, Balagot R, Branion J Jr, Kobak A. Report on the use of a new agent, phenazocine, in obstetric analgesia. Obstet Gynecol 1960;16:448–53.
3. Corbit J, First S. Clinical comparison of phenazocine and meperidine in obstetric analgesia. Obstet Gynecol 1961;18:488–91.

Name:	**PHENAZOPYRIDINE**	Risk Factor:	**B_M**
Class:	**Urinary Tract Agent (Analgesic)**		

FETAL RISK SUMMARY

RECOMMENDATION: Limited Human Data - Probably Compatible

No reports linking the use of phenazopyridine with congenital defects have been located. The Collaborative Perinatal Project monitored 50,282 mother-child pairs, 219 of whom had 1st trimester exposure to phenazopyridine (1, pp. 299–308). For use anytime during pregnancy, 1,109 exposures were recorded (1, p. 435). In neither group was evidence found to suggest a relationship to large categories of major or minor malformations or to individual defects.

In a surveillance study of Michigan Medicaid recipients conducted between 1985 and 1992 involving 229,101 completed pregnancies, 496 newborns had been exposed to phenazopyridine during the 1st trimester (F. Rosa, personal communication, FDA, 1993). A total of 27 (5.4%) major birth defects were observed (21 expected), including (observed/expected) 7/5 cardiovascular defects and 1/1 oral cleft. No anomalies were observed in four other defect categories (spina bifida, polydactyly, limb reduction defects, and hypospadias) for which specific data were available. These data do not support an association between the drug and congenital defects.

BREAST FEEDING SUMMARY

RECOMMENDATION: No Human Data - Probably Compatible

No data are available.

Reference

1. Heinonen OP, Slone D, Shapiro S. *Birth Defects and Drugs in Pregnancy*. Littleton, MA: Publishing Sciences Group, 1977.

Name:	**PHENCYCLIDINE**	Risk Factor:	**X**
Class:	**Hallucinogen**		

P

FETAL RISK SUMMARY

RECOMMENDATION: Contraindicated

Phencyclidine (PCP) is an illicit drug used for its hallucinogenic effects. Transfer to the fetus has been demonstrated in humans with placental metabolism of the drug (1–7). Qualitative analysis of the urine from two newborns revealed phencyclidine levels of 75 ng/mL or greater up to 3 days after birth (2). In 24 (12%) of 200 women evaluated at a Los Angeles hospital, cord blood PCP levels ranged from 0.10 to 5.80 ng/mL (3). Cord blood concentrations were twice as high as maternal serum—1215 vs. 514 pg/mL in one woman who allegedly consumed her last dose approximately 53 days before delivery (4). PCP in the newborn's urine was found to be 5841 pg/mL (4).

Relatively few studies have appeared on the use of phencyclidine during pregnancy, but fetal exposure may be more common than this lack of reporting indicates. During a 9-month period of 1980–1981 in a Cleveland hospital, 30 of 519 (5.8%) consecutively screened pregnant patients were discovered to have PCP exposure (8). In a subsequent report from this same hospital, 2,327 pregnant patients were screened for PCP exposure between 1981 and 1982 (6). Only 19 patients (0.8%) had positive urine samples, but up to 256 (11%) or more may have tested positive with more frequent checking (6). In the Los Angeles study cited above, 12% were exposed (3). However, the specificity of the chemical screening methods used in this latter report have been questioned (7).

Most pregnancies in which the mother used phencyclidine apparently end with healthy newborns (3,4,9). However, case reports involving four newborns indicate that the use of this agent may result in long-term damage (2,9,10):

Depressed at birth, jittery, hypertonic, poor feeding (2) (2 infants)
Irritable, poor feeding and sucking reflex (9) (1 infant)
Triangular-shaped face with pointed chin, narrow mandibular angle, antimongoloid slanted eyes, poor head control, nystagmus, inability to track visually, respiratory distress, hypertonic, jitteriness (10) (1 infant)

Irritability, jitteriness, hypertonicity, and poor feeding were common features in the affected infants. In three of the neonates, most of the symptoms had persisted at the time of the report. In the case with the malformed child, no causal relationship with PCP could be established. Marijuana was also taken, and it is a known teratogen in some animal species (11). However, marijuana is not considered to be a human teratogen (see Marijuana).

A study published in 1992 described the effects of PCP on human fetal cerebral cortical neurons in culture (12). High levels of the drug caused progressive degeneration and death of the neurons whereas sublethal concentrations inhibited axonal outgrowth. Because the fetal central nervous system can concentrate and retain PCP, these results suggested that PCP exposure during pregnancy could produce profound functional impairments (12).

Abnormal neurobehavior in the newborn period was observed in nine infants delivered from mothers who had used PCP during pregnancy (13). The abnormality was significantly more than that observed in control infants and those exposed *in utero* to opiates, sedative/stimulants, or the combination of pentazocine and tripelennamine (i.e., T's and blue's). However, by 2 years of age, the mental and psychomotor development of all of the drug-exposed infants, including those exposed to PCP, were similar to controls.

BREAST FEEDING SUMMARY

RECOMMENDATION: Contraindicated

Phencyclidine (PCP) is excreted into breast milk (14). One lactating mother, who took her last dose 40 days previously, excreted 3.90 ng/mL in her milk. In animal studies, milk concentrations of PCP were 10 times those of plasma (1). Women consuming PCP should not breast-feed. The American Academy of Pediatrics considers the drug to be contraindicated during breast-feeding (15).

P

References

1. Nicholas JM, Lipshitz J, Schreiber EC. Phencyclidine: its transfer across the placenta as well as into breast milk. Am J Obstet Gynecol 1982;143:143–6.
2. Strauss AA, Modanlou HD, Bosu SK. Neonatal manifestations of maternal phencyclidine (PCP) abuse. Pediatrics 1981;68:550–2.
3. Kaufman KR, Petrucha RA, Pitts FN Jr, Kaufman ER. Phencyclidine in umbilical cord blood: preliminary data. Am J Psychiatry 1983;140:450–2.
4. Petrucha RA, Kaufman KR, Pitts FN. Phencyclidine in pregnancy: a case report. J Reprod Med 1982;27: 301–3.
5. Rayburn WF, Holsztynska EF, Domino EF. Phencyclidine: biotransformation by the human placenta. Am J Obstet Gynecol 1984;148:111–2.
6. Golden NL, Kuhnert BR, Sokol RJ, Martier S, Bagby BS. Phencyclidine use during pregnancy. Am J Obstet Gynecol 1984;148:254–9.
7. Lipton MA. Phencyclidine in umbilical cord blood: some cautions. Am J Psychiatry 1983;140:449.
8. Golden NL, Sokol RJ, Martier S, Miller SI. A practical method for identifying angel dust abuse during pregnancy. Am J Obstet Gynecol 1982;142: 359–61.
9. Lerner SE, Burns RS. Phencyclidine use among youth: history, epidemiology, and acute and chronic intoxication. In Petersen R, Stillman R, eds. *Phencyclidine (PCP) Abuse: An Appraisal*. National Institute on Drug Abuse Research Monograph No. 21, US Government Printing Office, 1978.
10. Golden NL, Sokol RJ, Rubin IL. Angel dust: possible effects on the fetus. Pediatrics 1980;65:18–20.

11. Persaud TVN, Ellington AC. Teratogenic activity of cannabis resin. Lancet 1968;2:406–7.
12. Mattson MP, Rychlik B, Cheng B. Degenerative and axon outgrowth-altering effects of phencyclidine in human fetal cerebral cortical cells. Neuropharmacology 1992;31:279–91.
13. Chasnoff IJ, Burns KA, Burns WJ, Schnoll SH. Prenatal drug exposure: effects on neonatal and infant growth and development. Neurobehavior Toxicol Teratol 1986;8:357–62.
14. Kaufman KR, Petrucha RA, Pitts FN Jr, Weekes ME. PCP in amniotic fluid and breast milk: case report. J Clin Psychiatry 1983;44:269–70.
15. Committee on Drugs, American Academy of Pediatrics. The transfer of drugs and other chemicals into human milk. Pediatrics 2001;108:776–89.

Name:	**PHENDIMETRAZINE**	Risk Factor:	**C**
Class:	**Central Stimulant/Anorexiant**		

FETAL RISK SUMMARY

RECOMMENDATION: No Human Data - No Relevant Animal Data

Phendimetrazine is a sympathomimetic amine that has pharmacologic activity similar to the amphetamines. It is used for the management of obesity. No animal or human reproductive data are available (see also Phentermine or Amphetamine).

BREAST FEEDING SUMMARY

RECOMMENDATION: No Human Data - Potential Toxicity

No reports describing the use phendimetrazine during lactation have been located. The molecular weight (341 for the tartrate salt) is low enough, however, that excretion into breast milk should be expected.

Name:	**PHENELZINE**	Risk Factor:	**C**
Class:	**Antidepressant**		

P

FETAL RISK SUMMARY

RECOMMENDATION: Limited Human Data - Animal Data Suggest Moderate Risk

Phenelzine is a monoamine oxidase (MOA) inhibitor used in the treatment of depression. In reproduction studies with mice at doses above the maximum recommended human dose, a significant decrease in the number of viable offspring per mouse was observed (1).

The Collaborative Perinatal Project monitored 21 mother-child pairs exposed to MOA inhibitors during the 1st trimester, 3 of which were exposed to phenelzine (2). An increased risk of malformations was found (standardized relative risk 2.62). Details of the 3 cases with phenelzine exposure are not available.

BREAST FEEDING SUMMARY

RECOMMENDATION: No Human Data - Potential Toxicity

No reports describing the use of phenelzine during lactation have been located. The molecular weight (about 234 for the sulfate salt) is low enough, however, that excretion into breast milk should be expected.

References

1. Product information. Nardil. Parke-Davis, 2000.
2. Heinonen OP, Slone D, Shapiro S. *Birth Defects and Drugs in Pregnancy*. Littleton, MA: Publishing Sciences Group, 1977:336–7.

Name:	**PHENINDIONE**	Risk Factor:	**D**
Class:	**Anticoagulant**		

See Coumarin Derivatives.

Name:	**PHENIRAMINE**	Risk Factor:	**C**
Class:	**Antihistamine**		

FETAL RISK SUMMARY

RECOMMENDATION: Limited Human Data - Probably Compatible

The Collaborative Perinatal Project monitored 50,282 mother-child pairs, 831 of whom were exposed to pheniramine during the 1st trimester (1, pp. 322–334). A possible relationship between this use and respiratory malformations and eye/ear defects was found, but independent confirmation is required. For use anytime during pregnancy, 2442 exposures were recorded (1, pp. 436–437). No evidence was found in this group to suggest a relationship to congenital anomalies.

An association between exposure during the last 2 weeks of pregnancy to antihistamines in general and retrolental fibroplasia in premature infants has been reported. See Brompheniramine for details.

BREAST FEEDING SUMMARY

RECOMMENDATION: No Human Data - Probably Compatible

No data are available.

Reference

1. Heinonen OP, Slone D, Shapiro S. *Birth Defects and Drugs in Pregnancy*. Littleton, MA: Publishing Sciences Group, 1977.

Name:	**PHENOBARBITAL**	Risk Factor:	**D**
Class:	**Sedative/Anticonvulsant**		

FETAL RISK SUMMARY

RECOMMENDATION: Human Data Suggest Risk

Phenobarbital has been used widely in clinical practice as a sedative and anticonvulsant since 1912 (1). The drug crosses the placenta to the fetus at birth (2). Factors significantly influencing placental transfer were duration of maternal treatment, gestational age, and arterial cord pH (2).

The potential teratogenic effects of phenobarbital were recognized in 1964 along with phenytoin (3). Since this report, there have been numerous reviews and studies on the teratogenic effects of phenobarbital either alone or in combination with phenytoin and other anticonvulsants. Based on this literature, the epileptic pregnant woman taking phenobarbital in combination with other antiepileptics has a 2–3 times greater risk for delivering a child with congenital defects over the general population (4–11).

It has not always been known if the increased risk of congenital anomalies was caused by antiepileptic drugs, the disease itself, genetic factors, or a combination of these factors. A 1991 study of epileptic mothers who had been treated with either phenobarbital or carbamazepine, or the two agents in combination during pregnancy concluded that major and minor anomalies appeared to be more related to the mother's disease than to the drugs (11). An exception to this was the smaller head circumference observed in infants exposed *in utero* to either phenobarbital alone or in combination with carbamazepine. However, an earlier publication thought there was evidence that drugs were the causative factor (12).

A prospective study published in 1999 described the outcomes of 517 pregnancies of epileptic mothers identified at one Italian center from 1977 (13). Excluding genetic and chromosomal defects, malformations were classified as severe structural defects, mild structural defects, and deformations. Minor anomalies were not considered. Spontaneous ($N = 38$) and early ($N = 20$) voluntary abortions were excluded from the analysis, as were 7 pregnancies that delivered at other hospitals. Of the remaining 452 outcomes, 427 were exposed to anticonvulsants of which 313 involved monotherapy: phenobarbital ($N = 83$), carbamazepine ($N = 113$), valproate ($N = 44$), primidone ($N = 35$), phenytoin ($N = 31$), clonazepam ($N = 6$), and other ($N = 1$). There were no defects in the 25 pregnancies not exposed to anticonvulsants. Of the 42 (9.3%) outcomes with malformations, 24 (5.3%) were severe, 10 (2.2%) were mild, and 8 (1.8%) were deformities. There were four malformations with phenobarbital monotherapy: two (2.4%) were severe (Fallot's tetralogy, hydronephrosis), one (1.2%) was mild (umbilical and inguinal hernia), and one (1.2%) deformation (hip dislocation). The investigators concluded that the anticonvulsants were the primary risk factor for an increased incidence of congenital malformations (see also Carbamazepine, Clonazepam, Phenytoin, Primidone, and Valproic Acid) (13).

P

A 2001 prospective study provides further evidence that the congenital defects observed in the offspring of epileptic mothers treated with anticonvulsants are caused by drugs (14). The prospective cohort study, conducted from 1986 to 1993 at five maternity hospitals, was designed to determine if anticonvulsant agents or other factors (e.g., genetic) were responsible for the constellation of abnormalities seen in infants of mothers treated with anticonvulsants during pregnancy. A total of 128,049 pregnant women were screened at delivery for exposure to anticonvulsant drugs. Three groups of singleton infants were identified: (a) exposed to anticonvulsant drugs, (b) not exposed to anticonvulsant drugs but with a maternal history of seizures, and (c) not exposed to anticonvulsant drugs and with no maternal history of seizures (control group). For a variety of reasons, including exposure to other teratogens, many identified infants were excluded, leaving 316, 98, and 508 infants, respectively, in the three groups for analysis. Anticonvulsant monotherapy occurred in 223 women: phenytoin ($N = 87$), phenobarbital ($N = 64$), carbamazepine ($N = 58$), and too few cases for analysis with valproic acid, clonazepam, diazepam, and lorazepam. Ninety-three infants were exposed to two or more anticonvulsant drugs. All infants were examined systematically (blinded as to group in 93% of the cases) for embryopathy associated with anticonvulsant exposure (major malformations, hypoplasia of the midface and fingers, microcephaly, and intrauterine growth retardation). Compared to controls, significant ($p \leq 0.05$, confidence limits not overlapping 1) associations between anticonvulsants and anticonvulsant embryopathy were: phenobarbital monotherapy 26.6% (17/64), phenytoin monotherapy 20.7% (18/87), all infants exposed to anticonvulsant monotherapy 20.6% (46/223), exposed to two or more anticonvulsants 28.0% (26/93), and all infants exposed to anticonvulsants (mono- and poly-therapy) 22.8% (72/316). Nonsignificant associations were found for carbamazepine monotherapy (13.8% (8/58), nonexposed infants with a maternal history of seizures 6.1% (6/98), and controls 8.5% (43/508). The investigators concluded that the distinctive pattern of physical abnormalities observed in infants exposed to anticonvulsants during gestation was caused by the drugs, rather than by epilepsy itself (14).

A phenotype, as described for phenytoin in the fetal hydantoin syndrome (FHS), apparently does not occur with phenobarbital (see Phenytoin for details of FHS). However, as summarized by Janz (15), some of the minor malformations composing the FHS have been occasionally observed in infants of epileptic mothers treated only with phenobarbital.

The effects of prenatal exposure to phenobarbital on central nervous system development of offspring have been studied in both animals (16–18) and humans (11,19–22). The neural development in 90-day-old offspring of female rats given phenobarbital in doses of 0, 20, 40, or 60 mg/kg/day before and throughout gestation were described in a 1992 study (16). The drug produced dose- and sex-dependent changes in the electroencephalograms of the offspring. Lower doses resulted in adverse changes in learning and attentional focus, whereas higher doses also adversely affected neural function related to slow-wave sleep and receptor homeostasis. An earlier study measured the long-term effects on the offspring of rats from exposure to 40 mg/kg/day of phenobarbital from day 12 to day 19 of gestation (17). The effects included delays in the onset of puberty, disorders in the estrous cycle, infertility, and altered concentrations of sex steroids, gonadotropic hormones, and estrogen receptors. The changes represented permanent alterations in sexual maturation. A similar study measured decreases in the concentration of testosterone in the plasma and brain of exposed fetal rats (18). These changes persisted into adult life, indicating that phenobarbital may lead to sexual dysfunction in mature animals.

In a 1991 human study, the cognitive development (as measured by school career, reading, spelling, and arithmetic skills) of children who had been exposed *in utero* to either phenobarbital alone or in combination with carbamazepine was significantly impaired in comparison with children of nonepileptic mothers (11). A similar finding, but not significant, was suggested when the phenobarbital-exposed children were compared with children exposed only to carbamazepine.

In a 1988 study designed to evaluate the effect of *in utero* exposure to anticonvulsants on intelligence, 148 Finnish children of epileptic mothers were compared with 105 controls (19). Previous studies had either shown intellectual impairment from this exposure or no effect. Of the 148 children of epileptic mothers, 129 were exposed to anticonvulsant therapy during the first 20 weeks of pregnancy, 2 were only exposed after 20 weeks, and 17 were not exposed. In those mothers treated during pregnancy, 22 received phenobarbital in combination with other anticonvulsants, all during the first 20 weeks. The children were evaluated at 5.5 years of age for both verbal and nonverbal measures of intelligence. A child was considered mentally deficient if the results of both tests were less than 71. Two of the 148 children of epileptic mothers were diagnosed as mentally deficient and 2 others had borderline intelligence (the mother of one of these latter children had not been treated with anticonvulsant medication). None of the controls was considered

P

mentally deficient. Both verbal (110.2 vs. 114.5, $p < 0.05$) and nonverbal (108.7 vs. 113.2, $p < 0.05$) intelligence scores were significantly lower in the study group children than in controls. In both groups, intelligence scores were significantly lower when seven or more minor anomalies were present ($p = 0.03$). However, the presence of hypertelorism and digital hypoplasia, two minor anomalies considered typical of exposure to phenytoin, was not predictive of low intelligence (19).

A 1996 study also described the effects of *in utero* phenobarbital exposure on cognitive performance (20). Intelligence scores of Danish adult men, born between 1959 and 1961, who had been exposed to prenatal phenobarbital were measured. Their mothers had no history of central nervous system disorder and there was no exposure to other psychopharmacological drugs. Two double-blind studies using different measures of general intelligence were conducted on subjects (total = 114) and controls (total = 153). The test scores of matched controls were used to predict scores for each exposed subject. The exposure effects were then estimated by comparing the predicted to the observed scores. Phenobarbital exposure was associated with significantly lower verbal intelligence scores (about 0.5 SD). Exposure in the 3rd trimester was the most detrimental. The magnitude of the intelligence deficit was increased by lower socioeconomic status and being the offspring of an unwanted pregnancy (20).

A two-part 2000 study evaluated the effects of prenatal phenobarbital and phenytoin exposure on brain development and cognitive functioning in adults (21). Subjects and matched controls, delivered at a mean 40 weeks' gestation, were retrospectively identified from birth records covering the years between 1957 and 1972. Maternal diseases of the subjects included epilepsy (treated with anticonvulsants) and other conditions in which anticonvulsants were used as sedatives (nausea, vomiting, or emotional problems), whereas the control group had no maternal pathologies. Only those exposed prenatally to phenobarbital alone or phenobarbital plus phenytoin had sufficient subjects to analyze. The mean occipitofrontal circumference for phenobarbital-exposed neonates was not different from controls (34.49 vs. 34.50 cm), but it was significantly smaller for phenobarbital plus phenytoin subjects compared to phenobarbital alone or controls (33.82 cm, $p = 0.003$). In the follow-up part of the study, no differences in adult cognitive functioning (intelligence, attention, and memory) were found between the exposed and control groups. More subjects than controls, however, were mentally retarded (4 vs. 2; causes of retardation not known except for one case of autism in controls) and more had persistent learning problems (12% vs. 1%). The investigators concluded that phenobarbital plus phenytoin reduced occipitofrontal circumference but may only affect cognitive capacity in susceptible offspring (21).

The relationship between maternal anticonvulsant therapy, neonatal behavior, and neurological function in children was reported in a 1996 study (22). Among newborns exposed to maternal monotherapy, 18 were exposed to phenobarbital (including primidone), 13 to phenytoin, and 8 to valproic acid. Compared to controls, neonates exposed to phenobarbital had significantly higher mean apathy and optimality scores. Phenytoin-exposed neonates also had a significantly higher mean apathy score. However, the neonatal optimality and apathy scores did not correlate with neurological outcome of the children at 6 years of age. In contrast, those exposed to valproic acid had optimality and apathy scores statistically similar to controls but a significantly higher hyperexcitability score. Moreover, the hyperexcitability score correlated with later minor and major neurological dysfunction at age 6 years (22).

The Collaborative Perinatal Project monitored 50,282 mother-child pairs, 1415 of whom had 1st trimester exposure to phenobarbital (23, pp. 336–339). For use anytime during pregnancy, 8037 exposures were recorded (23, p. 438). In neither group was evidence found to suggest a relationship to large categories of major or minor malformations, although a possible association with Down's syndrome was shown statistically. However, a relationship between phenobarbital and Down's syndrome is unlikely.

In a surveillance study of Michigan Medicaid recipients conducted between 1985 and 1992 involving 229,101 completed pregnancies, 334 newborns had been exposed to phenobarbital during the 1st trimester (F. Rosa, personal communication, FDA, 1993). A total of 20 (6.0%) major birth defects were observed (14 expected). Specific data were available for six defect categories, including (observed/expected) 8/3 cardiovascular defects, 1/1 oral clefts, 1/0 spina bifida, 1/1 polydactyly, 0/1 limb reduction defects, and 1/1 hypospadias. Only the data for cardiovascular defects is suggestive of a possible association.

The effects of exposure (at any time during the 2nd or 3rd month after the last menstrual period) to folic acid antagonists on embryo/fetal development were evaluated in a large, multicenter, case-control surveillance study published in 2000 (24). The report was based on data collected between 1976 and 1998 from 80 maternity or tertiary care hospitals. Mothers were interviewed within 6 months of delivery about their use of drugs during pregnancy. Folic acid antagonists were categorized into two groups: group I—dihydrofolate reductase inhibitors (aminopterin, methotrexate, sulfasalazine, pyrimethamine, triamterene, and trimethoprim); group II—agents that affect other enzymes in folate metabolism, impair the absorption of folate, or increase the metabolic breakdown of folate (carbamazepine, phenytoin, primidone, and phenobarbital). The case subjects were 3870 infants with cardiovascular defects, 1962 with oral clefts, and 1100 with urinary tract malformations. Infants with defects associated with a syndrome were excluded as were infants with coexisting neural tube defects (NTDs; known to be reduced by maternal folic acid supplementation). Too few infants with limb-reduction defects were identified to be analyzed. Controls (N = 8,387) were infants with malformations other than oral clefts and cardiovascular, urinary tract, limb-reduction, and NTDs, but included infants with chromosomal and genetic defects. The risk of malformations in control infants would not have been reduced by vitamin supplementation, and none of the controls used folic acid antagonists. For group I cases, the relative risks (RRs) of cardiovascular defects and oral clefts were 3.4 (95% confidence interval [CI] 1.8–6.4) and 2.6 (95% CI 1.1–6.1), respectively. For group II cases, the RRs of cardiovascular and urinary tract defects, and oral clefts were 2.2 (95% CI 1.4–3.5), 2.5 (95% CI 1.2–5.0), and 2.5 (95% CI 1.5–4.2), respectively. Maternal use of multivitamin supplements with folic acid (typically 0.4 mg) reduced the risks in group I cases, but not in group II cases (24).

Thanatophoric dwarfism was found in a stillborn infant exposed throughout gestation to phenobarbital (300 mg/day), phenytoin (200 mg/day), and amitriptyline (>150 mg/day) (25). The cause of the malformation could not be determined, but both drug and genetic causes were considered.

A 2000 study, using data from the MADRE (an acronym for MAlformation and DRug Exposure) surveillance project, assessed the human teratogenicity of anticonvulsants (26). Among 8,005 malformed infants, cases were defined as infants with a specific malformation, whereas controls were infants with other anomalies. Of the total group, 299 were exposed in the 1st trimester to anticonvulsants. Among these, exposure to monotherapy occurred in the following: phenobarbital (N = 65), mephobarbital (N = 10), carbamazepine (N = 46), valproic acid (N = 80), phenytoin (N = 24), and other agents (N = 16). Statistically significant associations (CI do not overlap 1 and $p \leq 0.05$) were found with phenobarbital monotherapy and cardiac defects (N = 12), and cleft lip/palate (N = 11). When all

1st trimester exposures (mono- and polytherapy) were evaluated, significant associations were found between phenobarbital and cardiac defects ($N = 20$), cleft lip/palate ($N = 19$), and persistent left superior vena cava/other anomalies of the circulatory system ($N = 3$). Although the study confirmed some previously known associations, several new associations with anticonvulsants were discovered and require independent confirmation (see also Carbamazepine, Mephobarbital, Phenytoin, and Valproic Acid) (26).

Phenobarbital and other anticonvulsants (e.g., phenytoin) may cause early hemorrhagic disease of the newborn (27–36). Hemorrhage occurs during the first 24 hours after birth and may be severe or even fatal. The exact mechanism of the defect is unknown but may involve phenobarbital induction of fetal liver microsomal enzymes that deplete the already low reserves of fetal vitamin K (36). This results in suppression of the vitamin K-dependent coagulation factors II, VII, IX, and X. A 1985 review summarized the various prophylactic treatment regimens that have been proposed (see Phenytoin for details) (36).

Barbiturate withdrawal has been observed in newborns exposed to phenobarbital *in utero* (37). The average onset of symptoms in 15 addicted infants was 6 days (range 3–14 days). These infants had been exposed during gestation to doses varying from 64 to 300 mg/day with unknown amounts in four patients.

Phenobarbital may induce folic acid deficiency in the pregnant woman (38–40). A discussion of this effect and the possible consequences for the fetus are presented under Phenytoin (see also reference 24 above).

High-dose phenobarbital, contained in an anti-asthmatic preparation, was reported in a mother giving birth to a stillborn full-term female infant with complete triploidy (41). The authors speculated on the potential for phenobarbital-induced chromosomal damage. However, an earlier *in vitro* study found no effect of phenobarbital on the incidence of chromosome gaps, breaks, or abnormal forms (42). Any relationship between the drug and the infant's condition is probably coincidental.

Phenobarbital and cholestyramine have been used to treat cholestasis of pregnancy (43,44). Although no drug-induced fetal complications were noted, the therapy was ineffective for this condition. An earlier study, however, reported the successful treatment of intrahepatic cholestasis of pregnancy with phenobarbital, resulting in the normalization of serum bilirubin concentrations (45). The drug has also been used in the last few weeks of pregnancy to reduce the incidence and severity of neonatal hyperbilirubinemia (46).

Antenatal phenobarbital, either alone or in combination with vitamin K, has been used to reduce the incidence and severity of intraventricular hemorrhage in very-low-birth-weight infants (47–54). The therapy seemed to consistently reduce the frequency of grade 3 and grade 4 hemorrhage, and infant mortality from this condition. A 1991 review of this therapy summarized several proposed mechanisms by which phenobarbital might produce this beneficial effect (55). However, three studies (50,52,54), one involving 668 infants (treated and controls) (54), have concluded that the risk of intraventricular hemorrhage or early death in preterm infants is not decreased by antenatal phenobarbital.

In a study using the same subjects and controls as in reference 53 above, antenatal phenobarbital (10 mg/kg IV, then 100 mg orally every 24 hours until delivery or until completion of 34 weeks' gestation) had no effect, compared to nonexposed controls, on neurodevelopment as measured serially up to age 3 years (56). In contrast, another study using the same subjects and controls as a previous study (reference 52) found that antenatal phenobarbital (720–780 mg IV, then 60 mg IV every 6 hours until delivery or 34 weeks' gestation) significantly impaired developmental outcome as measured at age 2 years (57,58).

In summary, phenobarbital therapy in the epileptic pregnant woman presents a risk to the fetus in terms of major and minor congenital defects, hemorrhage at birth, and addiction. Adverse effects on neurobehavioral development have also been reported. The risk to the mother, however, is greater if the drug is withheld and seizure control is lost. The risk:benefit ratio, in this case, favors continued use of the drug during pregnancy at the lowest possible level to control seizures. Use of the drug in nonepileptic patients does not seem to pose a significant risk for structural defects, but neurodevelopment, hemorrhage, and addiction in the newborn are still concerns.

BREAST FEEDING SUMMARY

RECOMMENDATION: Limited Human Data - Potential Toxicity

Phenobarbital is excreted into breast milk (59–64). In two reports, the milk:plasma ratio varied between 0.4 and 0.6 (60,61). The amount of phenobarbital ingested by the nursing infant has been estimated to reach 2–4 mg/day (62). The pharmacokinetics of phenobarbital during lactation have been reviewed (61). Because of slower elimination in the nursing infant, accumulation may occur to the point that blood levels in the infant may actually exceed those of the mother (61). Phenobarbital-induced sedation has been observed in three nursing infants probably caused by this accumulation (59).

A case of withdrawal in a 7-month-old nursing infant after abrupt weaning from a mother taking phenobarbital, primidone, and carbamazepine has been reported (64). The mother had taken the anticonvulsant agents throughout gestation and during lactation. The baby's serum phenobarbital level at approximately 8 weeks of age was 14.8 μmol/L, near the lower level of the therapeutic range. At 7 months of age, the mother abruptly stopped nursing her infant, and shortly thereafter withdrawal symptoms were observed in the infant consisting of episodes of "startle" responses and infantile spasms confirmed by electroencephalography. The infant was treated with phenobarbital with prompt resolution of her symptoms and she was gradually weaned from the drug during a 6-month interval. Her neurologic and mental development were normal during the subsequent 5-year follow-up period (64).

Women consuming phenobarbital during breast-feeding, especially those on high doses, should be instructed to observe their infants for sedation. Phenobarbital levels in the infant should also be monitored to avoid toxic concentrations (61,65). The American Academy of Pediatrics classifies phenobarbital as a drug that has caused major adverse effects in some nursing infants, and it should be given to nursing women with caution (65).

References

1. Hauptmann A. Luminal bei epilepsie. Munchen Med Wochenschr 1912;59:1907–8.
2. De Carolis MP, Romagnoli C, Frezza S, D'Urzo E, Muzil U, Mezza A, Ferrazzani S, De Carolis S. Placental transfer of phenobarbital: what is new? Dev Pharmacol Ther 1992;19:19–26.
3. Janz D, Fuchs V. Are anti-epileptic drugs harmful when given during pregnancy? German Med Monogr 1964;9:20–3.
4. Hill RB. Teratogenesis and anti-epileptic drugs. N Engl J Med 1973;289:1089–90.
5. Bodendorfer TW. Fetal effects of anticonvulsant drugs and seizure disorders. Drug Intell Clin Pharm 1978;12:14–21.
6. Committee on Drugs, American Academy of Pediatrics. Anticonvulsants and pregnancy. Pediatrics 1977;63:331–3.
7. Nakane Y, Okoma T, Takahashi R, Sato Y, Wada T, Sato T, Fukushima Y, Kumashiro H, Ono T, Takahashi T, Aoki Y, Kazamatsuri H, Inami M, Komai S, Seino M, Miyakoshi M, Tanimura T, Hazama H, Kawahara R, Otuski S, Hosokawa K, Inanaga K, Nakazawa Y, Yamamoto K. Multi-institutional study of the teratogenicity and fetal toxicity of anti-epileptic drugs: a

report of a collaborative study group in Japan. Epilepsia 1980;21:633–80.
8. Andermann E, Dansky L, Andermann F, Loughnan PM, Gibbons J. Minor congenital malformations and dermatoglyphic alterations in the offspring of epileptic women; a clinical investigation of the teratogenic effects of anticonvulsant medication. In *Epilepsy, Pregnancy and the Child*. Proceedings of a Workshop in Berlin, September 1980. New York, NY: Raven Press, 1981.
9. Dansky L, Andermann E, Andermann F. Major congenital malformations in the offspring of epileptic patients. In *Epilepsy, Pregnancy and the Child*. Proceedings of a Workshop in Berlin, September 1980. New York, NY: Raven Press, 1981.
10. Janz D. The teratogenic risks of antiepileptic drugs. Epilepsia 1975;16:159–69.
11. van der Pol MC, Hadders-Algra M, Huisjes HJ, Touwen BCL. Antiepileptic medication in pregnancy: late effects on the children's central nervous system development. Am J Obstet Gynecol 1991;164:121–8.
12. Hanson JW, Buehler BA. Fetal hydantoin syndrome: current status. J Pediatr 1982;101:816–8.
13. Canger R, Battino D, Canevini MP, Fumarola C, Guidolin L, Vignoli A, Mamoli D, Palmieri C, Molteni F, Granata T, Hassibi P, Zamperini P, Pardi G, Avanzini G. Malformations in offspring of women with epilepsy: a prospective study. Epilepsia 1999;40:1231–6.
14. Holmes LB, Harvey EA, Coull BA, Huntington KB, Khoshbin S, Hayes AM, Ryan LM. The teratogenicity of anticonvulsant drugs. N Engl J Med 2001;344: 1132–8.
15. Janz D. Antiepileptic drugs and pregnancy: altered utilization patterns and teratogenesis. Epilepsia 1982;23(Suppl 1):S53–S63.
16. Livezey GT, Rayburn WF, Smith CV. Prenatal exposure to phenobarbital and quantifiable alterations in the electroencephalogram of adult rat offspring. Am J Obstet Gynecol 1992;167:1611–5.
17. Gupta C, Sonawane BR, Yaffe SJ, Shapiro BH. Phenobarbital exposure in utero: alterations in female reproductive function in rats. Science 1980;208:508–10.
18. Gupta C, Yaffe SJ, Shapiro BH. Prenatal exposure to phenobarbital permanently decreases testosterone and causes reproductive dysfunction. Science 1982;216:640–2.
19. Gaily E, Kantola-Sorsa E, Granstrom ML. Intelligence of children of epileptic mothers. J Pediatr 1988;113:677–84.
20. Reinisch JM, Sanders SA, Mortensen EL, Rubin DB. In utero exposure to phenobarbital and intelligence deficits in adult men. JAMA 1995;274:1518–25.
21. Dessens AB, Cohen-Kettenis PT, Mellenbergh GJ, Koppe JG, van de Poll NE, Boer K. Association of prenatal phenobarbital and phenytoin exposure with small head size at birth and with learning problems. Acta Paediatr 2000;89:533–41.
22. Koch S, Jager-Roman E, Losche G, Nau H, Rating D, Helge H. Antiepileptic drug treatment in pregnancy: drug side effects in the neonate and neurological outcome. Acta Paediatr 1996;84:739–46.
23. Heinonen OP, Slone D, Shapiro S. *Birth Defects and Drugs in Pregnancy*. Littleton, MA: Publishing Sciences Group, 1977.
24. Hernandez-Diaz S, Werler MM, Walker AM, Mitchell AA. Folic acid antagonists during pregnancy and the risk of birth defects. N Engl J Med 2000;343:1608–14.
25. Rafla NM, Meehan FP. Thanatophoric dwarfism; drugs and antenatal diagnosis; a case report. Eur J Obstet Gynecol Reprod Biol 1990;38:161–5.
26. Arpino C, Brescianini S, Robert E, Castilla EE, Cocchi G, Cornel MC, de Vigan C, Lancaster PAL, Merlob P, Sumiyoshi Y, Zampino G, Renzi C, Rosano A, Mastroiacovo P. Teratogenic effects of antiepileptic drugs: use of an international database on malformations and drug exposure (MADRE). Epilepsia 2000;41:1436–43.
27. Spiedel BD, Meadow SR. Maternal epilepsy and abnormalities of the fetus and the newborn. Lancet 1972;2:839–43.
28. Bleyer WA, Skinner AL. Fatal neonatal hemorrhage after maternal anticonvulsant therapy. JAMA 1976;235:826–7.
29. Lawrence A. Anti-epileptic drugs and the foetus. Br Med J 1963;2:1267.
30. Kohler HG. Haemorrhage in the newborn of epileptic mothers. Lancet 1966;1:267.
31. Mountain KR, Hirsh J, Gallus AS. Neonatal coagulation defect due to anticonvulsant drug treatment in pregnancy. Lancet 1970;1:265–8.
32. Evans AR, Forrester RM, Discombe C. Neonatal haemorrhage during anticonvulsant therapy. Lancet 1970;1:517–8.
33. Margolin FG, Kantor NM. Hemorrhagic disease of the newborn. An unusual case related to maternal ingestion of an anti-epileptic drug. Clin Pediatr (Phila) 1972;11:59–60.
34. Srinivasan G, Seeler RA, Tiruvury A, Pildes RS. Maternal anticonvulsant therapy and hemorrhagic disease of the newborn. Obstet Gynecol 1982;59:250–2.
35. Payne NR, Hasegawa DK. Vitamin K deficiency in newborns: a case report in α-1-antitrypsin deficiency and a review of factors predisposing to hemorrhage. Pediatrics 1984;73:712–6.
36. Lane PA, Hathaway WE. Vitamin K in infancy. J Pediatr 1985;106:351–9.
37. Desmond MM, Schwanecke RP, Wilson GS, Yasunaga S, Burgdorff I. Maternal barbiturate utilization and neonatal withdrawal symptomatology. J Pediatr 1972; 80:190–7.
38. Pritchard JA, Scott DE, Whalley PJ. Maternal folate deficiency and pregnancy wastage. IV. Effects of folic acid supplements, anticonvulsants, and oral contraceptives. Am J Obstet Gynecol 1971;109:341–6.
39. Hiilesmaa VK, Teramo K, Granstrom ML, Bardy AH. Serum folate concentrations during pregnancy in women with epilepsy: relation to antiepileptic drug concentrations, number of seizures, and fetal outcome. Br Med J 1983;287:577–9.
40. Biale Y, Lewenthal H. Effect of folic acid supplementation on congenital malformations due to anticonvulsive drugs. Eur J Obstet Reprod Biol 1984;18: 211–6.
41. Halbrecht I, Komlos L, Shabtay F, Solomon M, Book JA. Triploidy 69,XXX in a stillborn girl. Clin Genet 1973;4:210–2.
42. Stenchever MA, Jarvis JA. Effect of barbiturates on the chromosomes of human cells in vitro—a negative report. J Reprod Med 1970;5:69–71.
43. Heikkinen J, Maentausta O, Ylostalo P, Janne O. Serum bile acid levels in intrahepatic cholestasis of pregnancy

during treatment with phenobarbital or cholestyramine. Eur J Obstet Reprod Biol 1982;14:153–62.
44. Shaw D, Frohlich J, Wittmann BAK, Willms M. A prospective study of 18 patients with cholestasis of pregnancy. Am J Obstet Gynecol 1982;142:621–5.
45. Espinoza J, Barnafi L, Schnaidt E. The effect of phenobarbital on intrahepatic cholestasis of pregnancy. Am J Obstet Gynecol 1974;119:234–8.
46. Valaes T, Kipouros K, Petmezaki S, Solman M, Doxiadis SA. Effectiveness and safety of prenatal phenobarbital for the prevention of neonatal jaundice. Pediatr Res 1980;14:947–52.
47. Morales WJ, Koerten J. Prevention of intraventricular hemorrhage in very low birth weight infants by maternally administered phenobarbital. Obstet Gynecol 1986;68:295–9.
48. Shankaran S, Cepeda EE, Ilagan N, Mariona F, Hassan M, Bhatia R, Ostrea E, Bedard MP, Poland RL. Antenatal phenobarbital for the prevention of neonatal intracerebral hemorrhage. Am J Obstet Gynecol 1986;154:53–7.
49. De Carolis S, De Carolis MP, Caruso A, Oliva GC, Romagnoli C, Ferrazzani S, Umberto M, Luciano R, Mancuso S. Antenatal phenobarbital in preventing intraventricular hemorrhage in premature newborns. Fetal Ther 1988;3:224–9.
50. Kaempf JW, Porreco R, Molina R, Hale K, Pantoja AF, Rosenberg AA. Antenatal phenobarbital for the prevention of periventricular and intraventricular hemorrhage: a double-blind, randomized, placebo-controlled, multihospital trial. J Pediatr 1990;117:933–8.
51. Thorp JA, Parriott J, Ferrette-Smith D, Holst V, Meyer BA, Cohen GR, Yeast JD, Johnson J, Anderson J. Antepartum vitamin K (VK) and phenobarbital (PB) for preventing intraventricular hemorrhage (IVH) in the premature newborn: a randomized double blind placebo controlled trial (abstract). Am J Obstet Gynecol 1993;168:367.
52. Thorp JA, Parriott J, Ferrette-Smith D, Meyer BA, Cohen GR, Johnson J. Antepartum vitamin K and phenobarbital for preventing intraventricular hemorrhage in the premature newborn: a randomized, double-blind, placebo-controlled trial. Obstet Gynecol 1994;83:70–6.
53. Shankaran S, Cepeda E, Muran G, Mariona F, Johnson S, Kazzi SN, Poland R, Bedard MP. Antenatal phenobarbital therapy and neonatal outcome I: effect on intracranial hemorrhage. Pediatrics 1996;97:644–8.
54. Shankaran S, Papile LA, Wright LL, Ehrenkranz RA, Mele L, Lemons JA, Korones SB, Stevenson DK, Donovan EF, Stoll BJ, Fanaroff AA, Oh W. The effect of antenatal phenobarbital therapy on neonatal intracranial hemorrhage in preterm infants. N Engl J Med 1997;337:466–71.
55. Morales WJ. Antenatal therapy to minimize neonatal intraventricular hemorrhage. Clin Obstet Gynecol 1991;34:328–35.
56. Shankaran S, Woldt E, Nelson J, Bedard M, Delaney-Black V. Antenatal phenobarbital therapy and neonatal outcome II: neurodevelopmental outcome at 36 months. Pediatrics 1996;97:649–52.
57. Thorpe JA, Yeast JD, Cohen GR, Poskin M, Peng V, Hoffman E. Does in-utero phenobarbital lower IQ: follow up of the intracranial hemorrhage prevention trial (abstract). Am J Obstet Gynecol 1997;176:S117.
58. Thorp JA, O'Connor M, Jones AMH, Hoffman EL, Belden B. Does perinatal phenobarbital exposure affect developmental outcome at age 2? Am J Perinatol 1999;16:51–60.
59. Tyson RM, Shrader EA, Perlman HN. Drugs transmitted through breast-milk. II. Barbiturates. J Pediatr 1938;13:86–90.
60. Kaneko S, Sata T, Suzuki K. The levels of anticonvulsants in breast milk. Br J Clin Pharmacol 1979;7:624–7.
61. Nau H, Kuhnz W, Egger HJ, Rating D, Helge H. Anticonvulsants during pregnancy and lactation: transplacental, maternal and neonatal pharmacokinetics. Clin Pharmacokinet 1982;7:508–43.
62. Horning MG, Stillwell WG, Nowlin J, Lertratanangkoon K, Stillwell RN, Hill RM. Identification and quantification of drugs and drug metabolites in human breast milk using GC-MS-COM methods. Mod Probl Paediatr 1975;15:73–9.
63. Reith H, Schafer H. Antiepileptic drugs during pregnancy and the lactation period. Pharmacokinetic data. Dtsch Med Wochenschr 1979;104:818–23.
64. Knott C, Reynolds F, Clayden G. Infantile spasms on weaning from breast milk containing anticonvulsants. Lancet 1987;2:272–3.
65. Committee on Drugs, American Academy of Pediatrics. The transfer of drugs and other chemicals into human breast milk. Pediatrics 2001;108:776–89.

Name: **PHENOLPHTHALEIN** Risk Factor: **C**
Class: **Laxative**

FETAL RISK SUMMARY

RECOMMENDATION: Limited Human Data - Probably Compatible

The mechanism of action of the laxative phenolphthalein is similar to that of the anthraquinone purgatives (i.e., cascara sagrada, casanthranol, danthron, and senna). Small amounts of the laxative are absorbed into the systemic circulation. It is not known if the drug crosses the placenta, although the molecular weight is low enough (approximately 318) for placental transfer to occur. No studies describing the use of phenolphthalein in experimental animals have been located.

Phenolphthalein was used by 236 mother-child pairs during the 1st trimester (1, pp. 384–387) and 806 anytime during pregnancy (1, pp. 442,497) in the Collaborative Perinatal Project. No evidence was found to associate the use of this drug with major or minor malformations.

BREAST FEEDING SUMMARY

RECOMMENDATION: Limited Human Data - Probably Compatible

Phenolphthalein that had undergone conjugation, but not unmetabolized phenolphthalein, was excreted into breast milk in concentrations up to 1.0 μg/mL after a single 200- to 800-mg dose in 22 lactating women (2). Bowel movements occurred in 16 of the women after the dose, but none of the nursing infants had diarrhea. The possibility that conjugated phenolphthalein may undergo deconjugation in the infant's bowel, and thus by implication, produce diarrhea in the infant, has concerned some investigators (3). However, no reports of adverse effects following use of this produce during nursing have been located.

References

1. Heinenon OP, Slone D, Shapiro S. *Birth Defects and Drugs in Pregnancy*. Littleton, MA: Publishing Sciences Group, 1977.
2. Burgess DE. Constipation in obstetrics. In Jones FA, Godding EW, eds. *Management of Constipation*. Oxford: Blackwell Scientific Publications, 1972:176–88. As cited by Leng-Peschlow E. Risk assessment for senna during pregnancy. Pharmacology 1992;44(Suppl 1):20–2.
3. Odenthal KP, Ziegler D. In vitro effects of anthraquinones on rat intestine and uterus. Pharmacology 1988;36(Suppl 1):57–65.

Name:	**PHENOXYBENZAMINE**	Risk Factor:	**C_M**
Class:	**Antihypertensive**		

FETAL RISK SUMMARY

RECOMMENDATION: Compatible - Maternal Benefit >> Embryo/Fetal Risk

Phenoxybenzamine, a long-acting α-adrenergic blocking agent, is used for the treatment of hypertension caused by pheochromocytoma. Because of the lack of well-controlled studies, the effect of phenoxybenzamine on pregnant animals is not known (B. A. Wallin, personal communication, Smith Kline & French Laboratories, 1987). Animal and *in vitro* experiments conducted by the manufacturer, however, have indicated the drug has carcinogenic and mutagenic activity. Neither of these adverse outcomes, nor other fetal harm, has been reported in the relatively few human studies that have been published.

In a study using pregnant rats, phenoxybenzamine, with or without the β-blocker propranolol, had no effect on implantation of the fertilized ovum, nor was there any interference with the antifertility effect of an intrauterine contraceptive device placed in the uterus of rats (1).

Only one study has evaluated the human transplacental passage of phenoxybenzamine (2). A 22-year-old woman with pheochromocytoma was treated with phenoxybenzamine, 10 mg 3 times daily, and labetalol, 100 mg 3 times daily, for 26 days beginning at 33 weeks' gestation. She received her last dose of phenoxybenzamine 2 hours before delivery. The mean concentrations of the drug (each sample analyzed in triplicate) in the cord and maternal plasma and in the amniotic fluid were 103.3, 66, and 79.3 ng/mL, respectively, representing a cord:maternal plasma ratio of 1.6. Serum samples for phenoxybenzamine obtained from the infant (also determined in triplicate) at 32 and 80 hours of age contained mean concentrations of 22.3 ng/mL and none detected (limit of detection 10 ng/mL), respectively. The 2475-g male infant had depressed respiratory effort and hypotonia at birth, and was hypotensive during the first 2 days of life. The cause of the hypotension could not be determined, but may have been caused by both drugs. He subsequently did well and was discharged home 14 days after delivery.

No reports describing the use of phenoxybenzamine early in the 1st trimester of pregnancy have been located. Early *in vitro* studies of phenoxybenzamine indicated the drug abolished the *l*-norepinephrine–stimulated contractile activity of animal and human myometrium (3,4). However, a phenoxybenzamine infusion for 3 hours had no significant effect on the uterine activity in two pregnant women (4). One study included the use of phenoxybenzamine for the treatment of essential hypertension, toxemia, and cardiovascular renal disease occurring during pregnancy (3). No adverse fetal effects were observed.

Because of the relative rarity of pheochromocytoma, only a small number of cases have been found in which phenoxybenzamine was used during pregnancy. In 23 pregnancies, phenoxybenzamine administration was begun in the 2nd or 3rd trimesters and continued for periods ranging from 1 day to 16 weeks (5–21). Therapy was started at 10 weeks' gestation in a 24th case and continued for approximately 25 weeks when a 2665-g healthy male infant was delivered by cesarean section (22). Seventeen other pregnancies ended with either a cesarean section ($N = 13$) or vaginal delivery ($N = 4$) of a healthy infant before resection of the pheochromocytoma. In some of the cases the infant was growth retarded, probably secondary to uncontrolled maternal hypertension before treatment, but all survived. One fetus apparently survived the initial surgery to remove the mother's tumor, but the outcome of the pregnancy was not discussed (17). In another case, phenoxybenzamine was begun at 17 weeks' gestation and continued for 7 days before surgery (20). Following successful tumor resection, the patient's pregnancy went to term and terminated with the vaginal delivery of a normal healthy female infant.

Fetal mortality occurred in four cases. One involved a therapeutic abortion performed at approximately 12 weeks' gestation during the surgical removal of the mother's tumor (15). A second fetal death occurred when the mother, in her 5th–6th month of pregnancy, died 2 days after extensive surgery to remove a metastatic pheochromocytoma (5). Another fetal loss involved a woman whose pheochromocytoma was diagnosed at 7 months' gestation (15). Therapy with phenoxybenzamine was begun, but the fetus died *in utero* (details of therapy were not given). The fourth case of fetal mortality involved a 15-year-old woman at 25.5 weeks' gestation that was treated for 3 days with oral phenoxybenzamine in preparation for surgery (8). On the 3rd day of therapy, her membranes spontaneously ruptured followed by a hypertensive crisis requiring a phentolamine infusion. A spontaneous abortion occurred shortly thereafter of a severely growth-retarded fetus. Thus, only two of the fetal deaths occurred during pharmacologic therapy of the mother's disease.

The low incidences of maternal (4%; 1 of 24) and fetal (9%; 2 of 22) mortality when α-blockade with phenoxybenzamine is used is much better than the mortality observed in undiagnosed pheochromocytoma complicating pregnancy. A 1971 review of 89 cases of unsuspected tumor found that maternal and fetal mortality rates were 48% and 54.4%, respectively (23). A more recent review cited incidences of maternal and fetal mortality without α-blockade of 9% and 50%, respectively (19). When all cases of α-blockade (i.e., those receiving either phenoxybenzamine, phentolamine, or both) administered during pregnancy were considered, maternal mortality was 3% (1 of 29) and fetal loss was 19% (5 of 27) (2 cases excluded because fetal death *in utero* had occurred at the time of diagnosis) (19).

Long-term follow-up of infants exposed *in utero* to phenoxybenzamine has only been reported in three cases (7,10,13). The follow-up periods ranged from 2 to 8 years, and all three were normal healthy children.

In summary, the use of phenoxybenzamine during pregnancy to treat hypertension secondary to pheochromocytoma is indicated for the reduction of maternal and fetal mortality, especially after 24 weeks' gestation when surgical intervention is associated with high rates of these outcomes (20). Maternal α-blockade may also reduce or eliminate the adverse effect of hypertension on placental perfusion and subsequent poor fetal growth. No adverse fetal effects related to this drug treatment have been observed, but drug-induced hypotension in a newborn may have occurred.

BREAST FEEDING SUMMARY

RECOMMENDATION: No Human Data - Potential Toxicity

P

No reports describing the use of phenoxybenzamine during human lactation have been located. The molecular weight of the drug (about 340) is low enough, however, that passage into milk should be expected. The potential effects of this exposure on a nursing infant, including, but not limited to, hypotension, are unknown.

References

1. Sethi A, Chaudhury RR. Effect of adrenergic receptor-blocking drugs in pregnancy in rats. J Reprod Fertil 1970;21:551–4.
2. Santeiro ML, Stromquist C, Wyble L. Phenoxybenzamine placental transfer during the third trimester. Ann Pharmacother 1996;30:1249–51.
3. Maughan GB, Shabanah EH, Toth A. Experiments with pharmacologic sympatholysis in the gravid. Am J Obstet Gynecol 1967;97:764–76.
4. Wansbrough H, Nakanishi H, Wood C. The effect of adrenergic receptor blocking drugs on the human uterus. J Obstet Gynaecol Br Commonw 1968;75:189–98.
5. Brown RB, Borowsky M. Further observations on intestinal lesions associated with pheochromocytomas. A case of malignant pheochromocytoma in pregnancy. Ann Surg 1960;151:683–92.
6. Lawee D. Pheochromocytoma associated with pregnancy. Can Med Assoc J 1970;103:1185–7.
7. Simanis J, Amerson JR, Hendee AE, Anton AH. Unresectable pheochromocytoma in pregnancy. Pharmacology and biochemistry. Am J Med 1972;53:381–5.
8. Brenner WE, Yen SSC, Dingfelder JR, Anton AH. Pheochromocytoma: Serial studies during pregnancy. Am J Obstet Gynecol 1972;113:779–88.
9. Smith AM. Phaeochromocytoma and pregnancy. J Obstet Gynaecol Br Commonw 1973;80:848–51.
10. Griffith MI, Felts JH, James FM, Meyers RT, Shealy GM, Woodruff LF Jr. Successful control of pheochromocytoma in pregnancy. JAMA 1974;229:437–9.
11. Awitti-Sunga SA, Ursell W. Phaeochromocytoma

in pregnancy. Case report. Br J Obstet Gynaecol 1975;82:426–8.
12. Coombes GB. Phaeochromocytoma presenting in pregnancy. Proc R Soc Med 1976;69:224–5.
13. Leak D, Carroll JJ, Robinson DC, Ashworth EJ. Management of pheochromocytoma during pregnancy. Can Med Assoc J 1977;116:371–5.
14. Burgess GE III. Alpha blockade and surgical intervention of pheochromocytoma in pregnancy. Obstet Gynecol 1979;53:266–70.
15. Modlin IM, Farndon JR, Shepherd A, Johnston IDA, Kennedy TL, Montgomery DAD, Welbourn RB. Phaeochromocytomas in 72 patients: clinical and diagnostic features, treatment and long term results. Br J Surg 1979;66:456–65.
16. Fudge TL, McKinnon WMP, Geary WL. Current surgical management of pheochromocytoma during pregnancy. Arch Surg 1980;115:1224–5.
17. Coetzee A, Hartwig N, Erasmus FR. Feochromositoom tydens swangerskap. Die narkosehantering van 'n pasient. S Afr Med J 1981;59:861–2.
18. Stonham J, Wakefield C. Phaeochromocytoma in pregnancy: caesarean section under epidural analgesia. Anaesthesia 1983;38:654–8.
19. Stenstrom G, Swolin K. Pheochromocytoma in pregnancy. Experience of treatment with phenoxybenzamine in three patients. Acta Obstet Gynecol Scand 1985;64:357–61.
20. Combs CA, Easterling TR, Schmucker BC, Benedetti TJ. Hemodynamic observations during paroxysmal hypertension in a pregnancy with pheochromocytoma. Obstet Gynecol 1989;74:439–41.
21. Bakri YN, Ingemansson SE, Ali A, Parikh S. Pheochromocytoma and pregnancy: report of three cases. Acta Obstet Gynecol Scand 1992;71:301–4.
22. Lyons CW, Colmorgen GHC. Medical management of pheochromocytoma in pregnancy. Obstet Gynecol 1988;72:450–1.
23. Schenker JG, Chowers I. Pheochromocytoma and pregnancy. Review of 89 cases. Obstet Gynecol Surv 1971;26:739–47.

Name:	**PHENPROCOUMON**	Risk Factor:	**D**
Class:	**Anticoagulant**		

See Coumarin Derivatives.

Name:	**PHENSUXIMIDE**	Risk Factor:	**D**
Class:	**Anticonvulsant**		

FETAL RISK SUMMARY

RECOMMENDATION: Human Data Suggest Risk

The use of phensuximide, the first succinimide anticonvulsant used in the treatment of petit mal epilepsy, has been reported in three pregnancies (1,2). Because of multiple drug therapy and difference in study methodology, conclusions linking the use of phensuximide with congenital defects are difficult. Fetal abnormalities identified with the three pregnancies include ambiguous genitalia, inguinal hernia, and pyloric stenosis. Phensuximide has a much lower teratogenic potential than the oxazolidinedione class of anticonvulsants (see Trimethadione) (3,4). Because of a high incidence of toxic effects, the new succinimides should be considered in favor of phensuximide for the treatment of petit mal epilepsy (see Ethosuximide, Methsuximide) (5).

BREAST FEEDING SUMMARY

RECOMMENDATION: No Human Data - Potential Toxicity

No data are available.

References

1. Fedrick J. Epilepsy and pregnancy: A report from the Oxford Record Linkage Study. Br Med J 1973;2:442–8.
2. McMullin GP. Teratogenic effects of anticonvulsants. Br Med J 1971;2:430.
3. Fabro S, Brown NA. Teratogenic potential of anticonvulsants. New Engl J Med 1979;300:1280–1.
4. The National Institutes of Health. Anticonvulsants found to have teratogenic potential. JAMA 1981;241:36.
5. Schmidt RP, Wilder BJ. Epilepsy. In *Contemporary Neurology Series*, No. 2. Philadelphia, PA: FA Davis, 1968:159.

Name: **PHENTERMINE** Risk Factor: C_M

Class: **Anorexiant**

FETAL RISK SUMMARY

RECOMMENDATION: Contraindicated

Phentermine (phenyl-tertiary-butylamine) is a sympathomimetic amine that has activity as a central nervous system stimulant. Similar to other drugs in this class, such as the amphetamines, it is used as an appetite suppressant in the treatment of obesity. In addition to other adverse effects, hypertension has occurred in adults treated with this agent.

Reproduction studies in animals investigating if phentermine is teratogenic have not been conducted. A closely related compound, chlorphentermine (30 mg/kg/day SC), was administered to pregnant rats during the last 5 days of gestation (1). Phospholipidosis was evident in the lungs of the mothers and the newborn rats, and 83% of the latter died within 24 hours of birth. Another group treated with phentermine (30 mg/kg/day SC) in a similar manner did not develop the complication and did not die. A subsequent reference suggested that the chlorphentermine-induced pup mortality was consistent with retardation of fetal pulmonary maturity (2).

No studies have been located that described the placental transfer of phentermine in animals or humans, but because of its low molecular weight (about 186), exposure of the fetus to the drug should be expected.

A study published in 1962 described the use of phentermine in 118 women who were treated for obesity during the 3rd trimester of pregnancy up to delivery (3). Women weighing less than 200 pounds were given 30 mg each morning, while those weighing more than 200 pounds were given with 30 mg twice daily. The weights of the patients before treatment ranged from 180 to 315 pounds. Adverse outcomes occurred in five women with stillborn infants (three females and two males), one of whom was caused by abruptio placentae. The cause of the other stillborns, whose weights ranged from 9 to 10 pounds, was not mentioned, other than the statement that one mother had mild preeclampsia.

The FDA has received two reports involving the use of the combination, fenfluramine and phentermine, in early pregnancy (F. Rosa, personal communication, FDA, 1997). A spontaneous abortion occurred in one of the pregnancies. In the other, an infant with bilateral valvular abnormalities, both aortic and pulmonary, with moderate stenosis and displacement was delivered. Because valvular toxicity has been reported in adults taking the combination, a causal relationship in the pregnancy case is potentially possible. No other details of these cases were available.

That any real benefit is derived from the use of phentermine for weight control during pregnancy is doubtful, and its use during gestation, especially during the 1st trimester, should be considered contraindicated. Moreover, although the causes of the stillbirths in the human study cited above were not fully elucidated and may not have been caused by maternal treatment with phentermine, the high incidence is disturbing and is a reason to withhold use of the drug during pregnancy.

BREAST FEEDING SUMMARY

RECOMMENDATION: Contraindicated

No reports describing the use of phentermine during lactation have been located. Based on its low molecular weight (about 186), however, the excretion of phentermine into breast milk should be expected. Because central nervous system stimulation and other adverse reactions may occur in a nursing infant exposed to this drug in milk, breast-feeding should be considered a contraindication if the mother is taking phentermine.

References

1. Thoma-Laurie D, Walker ER, Reasor MJ. Neonatal toxicity in rats following in utero exposure to chlorphentermine or phentermine. Toxicology 1982;24:85–94.
2. Kacew S, Reasor MJ. Newborn response to cationic amphiphilic drugs. Fed Proc 1985;44:2323–2327.
3. Sands RX. Obesity and pregnancy. Weight control with a resinate. Am J Obstet Gynecol 1962;83:1617–21.

Name: **PHENTOLAMINE** Risk Factor: **C_M**
Class: **Antihypertensive**

FETAL RISK SUMMARY

RECOMMENDATION: Compatible - Maternal Benefit >> Embryo/Fetal Risk

The short-acting α-adrenergic blocker, phentolamine, is used for the treatment of severe hypertension secondary to maternal pheochromocytoma. Animal studies with phentolamine have observed neither teratogenicity nor embryotoxicity (1). No reports of adverse fetal outcome in humans have been located, but 1st trimester experience with this agent has not been documented, nor have studies describing the placental transfer of phentolamine in humans been found. However, although apparently not teratogenic, phentolamine must be used with caution because of the marked decrease in maternal blood pressure that can occur with resulting fetal anoxia.

Early *in vitro* and *in vivo* investigations of phentolamine indicated the drug inhibited the *l*-norepinephrine-stimulated contractile activity of human myometrium (2–4). A 1971 investigation, however, examined the effect of combined α-adrenergic blockade (phentolamine) and β-adrenergic stimulation (isoxsuprine) on oxytocin-stimulated uterine activity in six women just before undergoing therapeutic abortion at 16–20 weeks' gestation (5). The results indicated that phentolamine had no effect on uterine activity, while isoxsuprine inhibited uterine contractions. Moreover, the uterine inhibitory effect of β-stimulation was independent of α-blockade.

In one study, phentolamine was used for approximately 10 weeks for the treatment of toxemia (2). No adverse effects in the fetus were observed and the infant was alive and well at 18 months. However, the authors commented that they had stopped using phentolamine for this purpose because prolonged use in a few cases had resulted in "jitters" in the newborns, especially in premature infants (2).

The most common use of phentolamine in pregnancy is for the diagnosis of pheochromocytoma. Administration of phentolamine to patients with this disease causes a marked drop in blood pressure. Because of the very rapid half-life (19 minutes) of the drug, the return to the pretest blood pressures usually occurs in less than 30 minutes (1). A 1971 review article of pheochromocytoma in pregnancy cited 22 cases of the disease identified between 1955–1966 in which the diagnosis was made during pregnancy with phentolamine (6). Three additional cases were published in 1969 (7) and 1973 (8). Reflecting the high maternal and fetal mortality that can occur with this disease, 21% (3 of 14) of the mothers and 43% (6 of 14) of the fetuses died.

Phentolamine has been used for the short-term management of severe hypertension caused by pheochromocytoma, including those cases occurring during surgery to deliver the fetus or to resect the tumor (9–12). No adverse effects on the fetus or newborn attributable to phentolamine from this use have been reported, but fetal hypoxia is a potential complication.

BREAST FEEDING SUMMARY

RECOMMENDATION: No Human Data - Potential Toxicity

No data are available.

References

1. Product information. Regitine. Ciba-Geigy Corporation, 1991.
2. Maughan GB, Shabanah EH, Toth A. Experiments with pharmacologic sympatholysis in the gravid. Am J Obstet Gynecol 1967;97:764–76.
3. Wansbrough H, Nakanishi H, Wood C. The effect of adrenergic receptor blocking drugs on the human uterus. J Obstet Gynaecol Br Commonw 1968;75:189–98.
4. Althabe O Jr, Schwarcz RL Jr, Sala NL, Fisch L. Effect of phentolamine methanesulfonate upon uterine contractility induced by l-norepinephrine in pregnancy. Am J Obstet Gynecol 1968;101:1083–8.
5. Jenssen H. Inhibition of oxytocin-induced uterine activity in midpregnancy by combined adrenergic α-blockade and β-stimulation. Acta Obstet Gynecol Scand 1971;50:135–9.
6. Schenker JG, Chowers I. Pheochromocytoma and pregnancy. Review of 89 cases. Obstet Gynecol Surv 1971;26:739–47.
7. Hendee AE, Martin RD, Waters WC III. Hypertension in pregnancy: toxemia or pheochromocytoma? Am J Obstet Gynecol 1969;105:64–72.
8. Smith AM. Phaeochromocytoma and pregnancy. J Obstet Gynaecol Br Commonw 1973;80:848–51.
9. Anton AH, Brenner WE, Yen SS, Dingfelder JR. Pheochromocytoma: studies during pregnancy, premature delivery and surgery. Abstract Presented at the 5th International Congress on Pharmacology, July 23–28, 1972, San Francisco, California, p. 8, #43.
10. Simanis J, Amerson JR, Hendee AE, Anton AH. Unresectable pheochromocytoma in pregnancy. Pharmacology and biochemistry. Am J Med 1972;53:381–5.
11. Brenner WE, Yen SSC, Dingfelder JR, Anton AH. Pheochromocytoma: serial studies during pregnancy. Am J Obstet Gynecol 1972;113:779–88.
12. Burgess GE III. Alpha blockade and surgical intervention of pheochromocytoma in pregnancy. Obstet Gynecol 1979;53:266–70.

P

Name: **PHENYLBUTAZONE** Risk Factor: **C_M***
Class: **Nonsteroidal Anti-Inflammatory**

FETAL RISK SUMMARY

RECOMMENDATION: Human Data Suggest Risk in 1st and 3rd Trimesters

Reproductive studies with phenylbutazone in rats and rabbits have not revealed teratogenicity or adverse fetal effects (1,2). However, an increase in stillbirths and decreased survival of newborns have been observed in these species (3).

In a surveillance study of Michigan Medicaid recipients conducted between 1985 and 1992 involving 229,101 completed pregnancies, 27 newborns had been exposed to phenylbutazone during the 1st trimester (F. Rosa, personal communication, FDA, 1993). The total number of major birth defects observed was not available, but at least two (7.4%) occurred (one expected), including (observed/expected) 1/0.3 cardiovascular defects and 1/0 spina bifida. No anomalies were observed in four other defect categories (oral clefts, polydactyly, limb reduction defects, and hypospadias) for which specific data were available.

Two reports have been located that describe congenital defects in the offspring of mothers consuming phenylbutazone during pregnancy (4,5). A causal relationship was not established in either case. One review on the use of antirheumatic drug treatment during pregnancy stated that phenylbutazone is nonteratogenic in humans (6). The drug is known to cross the placenta to the human fetus (7–9).

Constriction of the ductus arteriosus *in utero* is a pharmacologic consequence arising from the use of prostaglandin synthesis inhibitors during pregnancy (see also Indomethacin) (10). Persistent pulmonary hypertension of the newborn may occur if these agents are used in the 3rd trimester close to delivery (10). These drugs also have been shown to inhibit labor and prolong pregnancy, both in humans (11) (see also Indomethacin) and in animals (12). Women attempting to conceive should not use any prostaglandin synthesis inhibitor, including phenylbutazone, because of the findings in a variety of animal models that indicate these agents block blastocyst implantation (13,14). In addition, a possible association between this class of agents and abortions may exist (see Ibuprofen).

[**Risk Factor D if used in 3rd trimester or near delivery.*]

BREAST FEEDING SUMMARY

RECOMMENDATION: Limited Human Data - Probably Compatible

Phenylbutazone is excreted into breast milk in low concentrations, although some investigators failed to detect the drug 3 hours after maternal administration (15). The drug has been measured in infant serum after breast-feeding, but no adverse effects in the nursing infant have been reported. The American Academy of Pediatrics classifies phenylbutazone as compatible with breast-feeding (16).

References

1. Larsen V, Bredahl E. The embryotoxic effects on rabbits of monophenylbutazone (Monazen) compared with phenylbutazone and thalidomide. Acta Pharmacol Toxicol 1966;24:453–5. As cited in Shepard TH. *Catalog of Teratogenic Agents*. 6th ed. Baltimore, MD: Johns Hopkins University Press, 1989:500.
2. Schardein JL, Blatz AT, Woosley ET, Kaup DH. Reproductive studies on sodium meclofenamate in comparison to aspirin and phenylbutazone. Toxicol Appl Pharmacol 1969;15:46–55. As cited in Shepard TH. *Catalog of Teratogenic Agents*. 6th ed. Baltimore, MD: Johns Hopkins University Press, 1989:500.
3. Product information. Butazolidin. Geigy Pharmaceuticals, 1993.
4. Tuchmann-Duplessis H. Medication in the course of pregnancy and teratogenic malformation. Concours Med 1967;89:2119–20.
5. Kullander S, Kallen B. A prospective study of drugs in pregnancy. Acta Obstet Gynecol Scand 1976;55:289–95.
6. Ostensen M, Husby G. Antirheumatic drug treatment during pregnancy and lactation. Scand J Rheumatol 1985;14:1–7.
7. Leuxner E, Pulver R. Verabreichung von irgapryin bei schwangeren und wochnerinnen. Munchen Med Wochenschr 1956;98:84–6.
8. Strobel S, Leuxner E. Uber die zullassigkeit der verabreichung von butazolidin bei schwangeren und wochnerinnen. Med Klin 1957;39:1708–10.
9. Akbaraly R, Leng JJ, Brachet-Liermain A, White P, Laclau-Lacrouts B. Trans-placental transfer of four anti-inflammatory agents. A study carried out by in vitro perfusion. J Gynecol Obstet Biol Reprod (Paris) 1981;10:7–11.

P

10. Levin DL. Effects of inhibition of prostaglandin synthesis on fetal development, oxygenation, and the fetal circulation. Semin Perinatol 1980;4:35–44.
11. Fuchs F. Prevention of prematurity. Am J Obstet Gynecol 1976;126:809–20.
12. Powell JG, Cochrane RL. The effects of a number of non-steroidal anti-inflammatory compounds on parturition in the rat. Prostaglandins 1982;23:469–88.
13. Matt DW, Borzelleca JF. Toxic effects on the female reproductive system during pregnancy, parturition, and lactation. In Witorsch RJ, ed. *Reproductive Toxicology*. 2nd ed. New York, NY: Raven Press, 1995:175–93.
14. Dawood MY. Nonsteroidal antiinflammatory drugs and reproduction. Am J Obstet Gynecol 1993;169:1255–65.
15. Wilson JT. Milk/plasma ratios and contraindicated drugs. In Wilson JT, ed. *Drugs in Breast Milk*. Balgowlah, Australia: ADIS Press, 1981:78–9.
16. Committee on Drugs, American Academy of Pediatrics. The transfer of drugs and other chemicals into human milk. Pediatrics 2001;108:776–89.

Name:	**PHENYLEPHRINE**	Risk Factor:	**C**
Class:	**Sympathomimetic (Adrenergic)**		

FETAL RISK SUMMARY

RECOMMENDATION: Human Data Suggest Risk

Phenylephrine is a sympathomimetic used in emergency situations to treat hypotension and to alleviate allergic symptoms of the eye and ear. Uterine vessels are normally maximally dilated and they have only α-adrenergic receptors (1). Use of the predominantly α-adrenergic stimulant, phenylephrine, could cause constriction of these vessels and reduce uterine blood flow, thereby producing fetal hypoxia (bradycardia). Phenylephrine may also interact with oxytocics or ergot derivatives to produce severe persistent maternal hypertension (1). Rupture of a cerebral vessel is possible. If a pressor agent is indicated, other drugs such as ephedrine should be considered. Sympathomimetic amines are teratogenic in some animal species, but human teratogenicity has not been suspected (2,3).

P

The Collaborative Perinatal Project monitored 50,282 mother-child pairs, 1249 of whom had 1st trimester exposure to phenylephrine (4, pp. 345–356). For use anytime during pregnancy, 4,194 exposures were recorded (4, p. 439). An association was found between 1st trimester use of phenylephrine and malformations; association with minor defects was greater than with major defects (4, pp. 345–356). For individual malformations, several possible associations were found (4, pp. 345–356, 476, 491):

First trimester
Eye and ear (8 cases)
Syndactyly (6 cases)
Preauricular skin tag (4 cases)
Clubfoot (3 cases)

Anytime use
Congenital dislocation of hip (15 cases)
Other musculoskeletal defects (4 cases)
Umbilical hernia (6 cases)

Independent confirmation of these findings is required. For the sympathomimetic class of drugs as a whole, an association was found between 1st trimester use and minor malformations (not life-threatening or major cosmetic defects), inguinal hernia, and clubfoot (4, pp. 345–356).

Sympathomimetics are often administered in combination with other drugs to alleviate the symptoms of upper respiratory infections. Thus, the fetal effects of sympathomimetics, other drugs, and viruses cannot be totally separated. However, indiscriminate use of this class of drugs, especially in the 1st trimester, is not without risk.

Phenylephrine has been used as a stress test to determine fetal status in high-risk pregnancies (5). In the United States, however, this test is normally conducted with oxytocin.

BREAST FEEDING SUMMARY

RECOMMENDATION: No Human Data - Probably Compatible

No reports describing the use of phenylephrine during human lactation have been located. The molecular weight (about 167) of the drug, however, is low enough that passage into breast milk should be expected. The effects of this exposure on a nursing infant are unknown.

References

1. Smith NT, Corbascio AN. The use and misuse of pressor agents. Anesthesiology 1970;33:58–101.
2. Nashimura H, Tanimura T. *Clinical Aspects of the Teratogenicity of Drugs*. Amsterdam: Excerpta Medica, 1976:231.
3. Shepard TH. *Catalog of Teratogenic Agents*. 3rd ed. Baltimore, MD: Johns Hopkins University Press, 1980: 134–5.
4. Heinonen OP, Slone D, Shapiro S. *Birth Defects and Drugs in Pregnancy*. Littleton, MA: Publishing Sciences Group, 1977.
5. Eguchi K, Yonezawa M, Hagegawa T, Lin TT, Ejiri K, Kudo T, Sekiba K, Takeda Y. Fetal activity determination and Neo-Synephrine test for evaluation of fetal well-being in high risk pregnancies. Nippon Sank Fujinka Gakkai Zasshi 1980;32:663–8.

Name: **PHENYLPROPANOLAMINE** Risk Factor: **C**

Class: **Sympathomimetic (Adrenergic)**

FETAL RISK SUMMARY

RECOMMENDATION: Limited Human Data - No Relevant Animal Data

Phenylpropanolamine is a sympathomimetic used for anorexia and to alleviate the symptoms of allergic disorders or upper respiratory infections. Uterine vessels are normally maximally dilated and they have only α-adrenergic receptors (1). Use of the α- and β-adrenergic stimulant, phenylpropanolamine, could cause constriction of these vessels and reduce uterine blood flow, thereby producing fetal hypoxia (bradycardia). This drug is a common component of proprietary mixtures containing antihistamines and other drugs. Thus, it is difficult to separate the effects of phenylpropanolamine on the fetus from other drugs, disease states, and viruses.

Sympathomimetic amines are teratogenic in some animal species, but human teratogenicity has not been suspected (2,3). The Collaborative Perinatal Project monitored 50,282 mother-child pairs, 726 of whom had 1st trimester exposure to phenylpropanolamine (4, pp. 345–356). For use anytime during pregnancy, 2489 exposures were recorded (4, p. 439). An association was found between 1st trimester use of phenylpropanolamine and malformations; association with minor defects was greater than with major defects (4, pp. 345–356). For individual malformations, several possible associations were found (4, pp. 345–356, 477, 491):

First trimester
Hypospadias (4 cases)
Eye and ear (7 cases) (statistically significant)
Polydactyly (6 cases)
Cataract (3 cases)
Pectus excavatum (7 cases)

Anytime use
Congenital dislocation of hip (12 cases)

Independent confirmation of these findings is required. For the sympathomimetic class of drugs as a whole, an association was found between 1st trimester use and minor malformations (not life-threatening or major cosmetic defects), inguinal hernia, and clubfoot (4, pp. 345–356). Indiscriminate use of this class of drugs, especially in the 1st trimester, is not without risk.

A case of infantile malignant osteopetrosis was described in a 4-month-old boy exposed *in utero* on several occasions to Contac (chlorpheniramine, phenylpropanolamine, and belladonna alkaloids), but this is a known genetic defect (5). The infant also had a continual "stuffy" nose.

BREAST FEEDING SUMMARY

RECOMMENDATION: No Human Data - Probably Compatible

No data are available.

References

1. Smith NT, Corbascio AN. The use and misuse of pressor agents. Anesthesiology 1970;33:58–101.
2. Nishimura H, Tanimura T. *Clinical Aspects of the Teratogenicity of Drugs*. Amsterdam: Excerpta Medica, 1976:231.
3. Shepard TH. *Catalog of Teratogenic Drugs*. 3rd ed. Baltimore, MD: Johns Hopkins University Press, 1980: 134–5.
4. Heinonen OP, Slone D, Shapiro S. *Birth Defects and Drugs in Pregnancy*. Littleton, MA: Publishing Sciences Group, 1977.
5. Golbus MS, Koerper MA, Hall BD. Failure to diagnose osteopetrosis in utero. Lancet 1976;2:1246.

Name: **PHENYLTOLOXAMINE** Risk Factor: **C**
Class: **Antihistamine**

FETAL RISK SUMMARY

RECOMMENDATION: No Human Data - No Relevant Animal Data

No data are available.

BREAST FEEDING SUMMARY

RECOMMENDATION: No Human Data - Probably Compatible

No data are available.

Name:	**PHENYTOIN**	Risk Factor:	**D**
Class:	**Anticonvulsant**		

FETAL RISK SUMMARY

RECOMMENDATION: Compatible - Maternal Benefit >> Embryo/Fetal Risk

Phenytoin is a hydantoin anticonvulsant introduced in 1938. The teratogenic effects of phenytoin were recognized in 1964 (1). Since this report there have been numerous reviews and studies on the teratogenic effects of phenytoin and other anticonvulsants. Based on this literature, the epileptic pregnant woman taking phenytoin, either alone or in combination with other anticonvulsants, has a 2–3 times greater risk for delivering a child with congenital defects over the general population (2–9).

It was not always known whether this increased risk was caused by antiepileptic drugs, the disease itself, genetic factors, or a combination of these, although past evidence indicated that drugs were the causative factor. Fifteen epidemiologic studies cited by reviewers in 1982 found an incidence of defects in treated epileptics varying from 2.2% to 26.1% (9). In each case, the rate for treated patients was higher than for untreated epileptics or normal controls. Animal studies have also implicated drugs and have suggested that a dose-related response may occur (9). Two studies cited below provides further evidence that the congenital defects observed in the offspring of epileptic mothers treated with anticonvulsants are caused by drugs.

A prospective study published in 1999 described the outcomes of 517 pregnancies of epileptic mothers identified at one Italian center from 1977 (10). Excluding genetic and chromosomal defects, malformations were classified as severe structural defects, mild structural defects, and deformations. Minor anomalies were not considered. Spontaneous ($N = 38$) and early ($N = 20$) voluntary abortions were excluded from the analysis, as were 7 pregnancies that delivered at other hospitals. Of the remaining 452 outcomes, 427 were exposed to anticonvulsants of which 313 involved monotherapy: phenytoin ($N = 31$), carbamazepine ($N = 113$), phenobarbital ($N = 83$), valproate ($N = 44$), primidone ($N = 35$), clonazepam ($N = 6$), and other ($N = 1$). There were no defects in the 25 pregnancies not exposed to anticonvulsants. Of the 42 (9.3%) outcomes with malformations, 24 (5.3%) were severe, 10 (2.2%) were mild, and 8 (1.8%) were deformities. There were three malformations with phenytoin monotherapy: none were severe, one (3.2%) was mild (umbilical hernia), and two (6.4%) deformations (club foot and hip dislocation). The investigators concluded that the anticonvulsants were the primary risk factor for an increased incidence of congenital malformations (see also Carbamazepine, Clonazepam, Phenobarbital, Primidone, and Valproic Acid) (10).

A prospective cohort study, conducted from 1986 to 1993 at five maternity hospitals, was designed to determine if anticonvulsant agents or other factors (e.g., genetic) were responsible for the constellation of abnormalities seen in infants of mothers treated with anticonvulsants during pregnancy (11). A total of 128,049 pregnant women were screened at delivery for exposure to anticonvulsant drugs. Three groups of singleton infants were identified: (a) exposed to anticonvulsant drugs, (b) not exposed to anticonvulsant drugs but with a maternal history of seizures, and (c) not exposed to anticonvulsant drugs and with no maternal history of seizures (control group). After applying exclusion criteria, including exposure to other teratogens, 316, 98, and 508 infants, respectively, were analyzed. Anticonvulsant monotherapy occurred in 223 women: phenytoin ($N = 87$), phenobarbital

P

($N = 64$), carbamazepine ($N = 58$), and too few cases for analysis with valproic acid, clonazepam, diazepam, and lorazepam. Ninety-three infants were exposed to two or more anticonvulsant drugs. All infants were examined systematically (blinded as to group in 93% of the cases) for embryopathy associated with anticonvulsant exposure (major malformations, hypoplasia of the midface and fingers, microcephaly, and intrauterine growth retardation). Compared to controls, significant ($p \leq 0.05$, confidence limits not overlapping 1) associations between anticonvulsants and anticonvulsant embryopathy were: phenytoin monotherapy 20.7% (18/87), phenobarbital monotherapy 26.6% (17/64), any monotherapy 20.6% (46/223), exposed to two or more anticonvulsants 28.0% (26/93), and all infants exposed to anticonvulsants (mono- and polytherapy) 22.8% (72/316). Nonsignificant associations were found for carbamazepine monotherapy 13.8% (8/58), nonexposed infants with a maternal history of seizures 6.1% (6/98), and controls 8.5% (43/508). The investigators concluded that the distinctive pattern of physical abnormalities observed in infants exposed to anticonvulsants during gestation was due to the drugs, rather than to epilepsy itself (11).

A study published in 1990 provided evidence that, at least in some cases, the teratogenic effects of phenytoin are secondary to elevated levels of oxidative metabolites (epoxides) (12). Epoxides are normally eliminated by the enzyme epoxide hydrolase, but in some individuals, low activity of this enzyme is present. By measuring the enzyme's activity in a number of subjects, the investigators proposed a trimodal distribution that is regulated by a single gene with two allelic forms. The three phenotypes proposed were: low activity (homozygous for the recessive allele), intermediate activity (heterozygous), and high activity (homozygous for the dominant allele). In the prospective portion of the study, 19 pregnant women with epilepsy, who were being treated with phenytoin monotherapy, had an amniocentesis performed and the microsomal epoxide hydrolase activity in amniocytes was determined. Four of the 19 had low activity (<30% of standard), whereas 15 had normal activity (>30% of standard). As predicted, only the four fetuses with low activity had clinical evidence of the fetal hydantoin syndrome (12).

P

In contrast to the above study, a 1999 study with mice involving fluconazole and phenytoin was unable to provide support for the theory that toxic intermediates, such as epoxides, were the cause of phenytoin-induced congenital defects (13). Because fluconazole inhibits the cytochrome P450 pathway responsible for phenytoin metabolism, the authors of this study reasoned that the drug combination could provide a test of the hypothesis. Pretreatment of mice with a nonembryotoxic fluconazole dose, however, doubled (from 6.2% to 13.3%; $p < 0.05$) the incidence of phenytoin-induced cleft palate. Administering both drugs closely together significantly increased the incidence of resorptions ($p < 0.05$) but not malformations. This lack of effect on malformations may have been related to the increased embryo lethality of the combination. The mechanism for the teratological interaction between the drugs was unknown (13).

In a surveillance study of Michigan Medicaid recipients conducted between 1985 and 1992 involving 229,101 completed pregnancies, 332 newborns had been exposed to phenytoin during the 1st trimester (F. Rosa, personal communication, FDA, 1993). A total of 15 (4.5%) major birth defects were observed (13 expected), including (observed/expected) 5/3 cardiovascular defects, 1/0 spina bifida, and 1/1 hypospadias. No anomalies were observed in three other defect categories (oral clefts, polydactyly, and limb reduction defects) for which specific data were available.

A recognizable pattern of malformations, now known as the fetal hydantoin syndrome (FHS), was partially described in 1968 when Meadow (14) observed distinct facial abnormalities in infants exposed to phenytoin and other anticonvulsants. In 1973, two groups of investigators, in independent reports, described unusual anomalies of the fingers and toes in exposed infants (15,16). The basic syndrome consists of variable degrees of hypoplasia and ossification of the distal phalanges and craniofacial abnormalities. Clinical features of the FHS, not all of which are apparent in every infant, are as follows (14–16):

Craniofacial
Broad nasal bridge
Wide fontanelle
Low-set hairline
Broad alveolar ridge
Metopic ridging
Short neck
Ocular hypertelorism
Microcephaly
Cleft lip and/or palate
Abnormal or low-set ears
Epicanthal folds
Ptosis of eyelids
Coloboma
Coarse scalp hair

Limbs
Small or absent nails
Hypoplasia of distal phalanges
Altered palmar crease
Digital thumb
Dislocated hip

Impaired growth, both physical and mental, and congenital heart defects, are often observed in conjunction with the FHS.

Numerous other defects have been reported to occur after phenytoin exposure in pregnancy. Janz, in a 1982 review (17), stated that nearly all possible types of malformations may be observed in the offspring of epileptic mothers. This statement is supported by the large volume of literature describing various anomalies that have been attributed to phenytoin with or without other anticonvulsants (1–9,14–58).

In one of the above cases, the mother took phenytoin (300 mg/day) during the first 7 months of gestation and phenobarbital (90 mg/day) during the last 2 months (54). The full-term female infant had features of FHS (hypoplastic nails and flat nasal bridge), hydrocephalus, a left porencephalic cyst, and an encephalocele. She died at 2.5 months of age of bronchopneumonia. An autopsy of the brain revealed both gross and microscopic abnormalities. The defects were consistent with changes produced early in fetal development and with tissue destruction resulting in the second half of gestation (54).

A possible association between phenytoin and the rare defect, holoprosencephaly, was reported in 1993 (56). Because of psychomotor and petit mal seizures, the mother was treated with phenytoin (350 mg/day) and primidone (500 mg/day) during gestation. Except for microcephaly, fetal sonography detected no pathology. The female infant was born after 36 weeks of gestation with both weight and length above the 50th percentile. The Apgar scores were 3, 9, and 10 at 1, 5, and 10 minutes, respectively. The occipitofrontal head circumference (31 cm) was below the 25th percentile. Malformations evident on examination were microcephaly, narrow forehead, hypertelorism, hypoplastic midface with anteverted nostrils, smooth philtrum, and thin vermillion border lip. Distal phalanges and nails on all fingers and nails were noted to be hypoplastic. A sacral dimple was also noted. Ultrasound examination revealed a right-sided renal duplication, hepatomegaly, a mild ventricular septal defect, and bilateral hip dysplasia. An electroencephalogram revealed significantly delayed visual evoked potentials. A partial lobar holoprosencephaly with ventral fusion of the cerebral hemispheres was noted on magnetic resonance imaging of the brain. Coarse gyri and horizontal cleavage, but no sagittal cleavage, was noted in the frontal lobe. The corpus callosum was absent. Although both parents suffered from epilepsy, there was no consanguinity and the infant's karyotype was normal (46,XX), thus a genetic cause of the holoprosencephaly was thought to be unlikely (56).

Authors of correspondence relating to the above report noted that they had also identified a case of holoprosencephaly in a stillborn infant exposed *in utero* to anticonvulsants (59). Unfortunately, the clinical examination did not record the presence or absence of minor physical features characteristic of the FHS. Based on their experience, however, establishing an association between phenytoin and the defect would be very difficult because of the infrequent *in utero* exposure to anticonvulsants (1:250 births), the even lower frequency of exposure to phenytoin monotherapy (1:844 births), and the rarity of holoprosencephaly (1:10,000) (59).

Thanatophoric dwarfism was found in a stillborn infant exposed throughout gestation to phenytoin (200 mg/day), phenobarbital (300 mg/day), and amitriptyline (>150 mg/day) (60). The cause of the malformation could not be determined, but both drug and genetic causes were considered.

A 2000 study, using data from the MADRE (an acronym for MAlformation and DRug Exposure) surveillance project, assessed the human teratogenicity of anticonvulsants (61). Among 8,005 malformed infants, cases were defined as infants with a specific malformation, whereas controls were infants with other anomalies. Of the total group, 299 were exposed in the 1st trimester to anticonvulsants. Among these, exposure to monotherapy occurred in the following: phenytoin ($N = 24$), phenobarbital ($N = 65$), mephobarbital ($N = 10$), carbamazepine ($N = 46$), valproic acid ($N = 80$), and other agents ($N = 16$). No statistically significant associations (CI not overlapping 1 and $p \leq 0.05$) were found with phenytoin monotherapy or polytherapy. Although the study confirmed some previously known associations, several new associations with anticonvulsants were discovered and require independent confirmation (see also Carbamazepine, Mephobarbital, Phenobarbital, and Valproic Acid) (61).

Twelve case reports have been located that, taken in sum, suggest phenytoin is a human transplacental carcinogen (18–28,62). Tumors reported to occur in infants after *in utero* exposure to phenytoin include:

Neuroblastoma (6 cases) (18–22,62)
Ganglioneuroblastoma (1 case) (23)
Melanotic neuroectodermal tumor (1 case) (24)
Extrarenal Wilms' tumor (1 case) (25)
Mesenchymoma (1 case) (26)
Lymphangioma (1 case) (27)
Ependymoblastoma (1 case) (28)

Children exposed *in utero* to phenytoin should be closely observed for several years because tumor development may take that long to express itself. A 1989 study, however, found no *in utero* exposures to phenytoin among 188 cases of childhood neuroblastoma diagnosed between 1969 and 1988 at their center (63). But the investigators did conclude that an increased risk of the neoplasm in children with FHS was still a possibility.

Phenytoin and other anticonvulsants (e.g., phenobarbital) may cause early hemorrhagic disease of the newborn (18,64–78). Hemorrhage occurs during the first 24 hours after birth and may be severe or even fatal. The exact mechanism of the defect is unknown but may involve phenytoin induction of fetal liver microsomal enzymes that deplete the already low reserves of fetal vitamin K (78). This results in suppression of the vitamin K-dependent coagulation factors II, VII, IX, and X. Phenytoin-induced thrombocytopenia has also been reported as a mechanism for hemorrhage in the newborn (75). A 1985 review summarized the various prophylactic treatment regimens that have been proposed (78):

Administering 10 mg of oral vitamin K daily during the last 2 months of pregnancy
Administering 20 mg of oral vitamin K daily during the last 2 weeks of pregnancy
Avoiding salicylates and administering vitamin K during labor
Caesarean section if a difficult or traumatic delivery is anticipated
Administering intravenous vitamin K to the newborn in the delivery room plus cord blood clotting studies

Although all of the above suggestions are logical, none has been tested in controlled trials. The reviewers recommended immediate IM vitamin K and close observation of the infant (see also Phytonadione) (78).

Of interest, a 1995 study suggested that anticonvulsant-induced vitamin K deficiency may be the mechanism that causes the maxillonasal hypoplasia seen in the FHS (79). They proposed early vitamin K supplementation of at-risk pregnancies to prevent this disfiguring malformation.

Liver damage was observed in an infant exposed during gestation to phenytoin and valproic acid (80). Although they were unable to demonstrate which anticonvulsant caused the injury, the authors concluded that valproic acid was the more likely offending agent.

Phenytoin may induce folic acid deficiency in the epileptic patient by impairing gastrointestinal absorption or by increasing hepatic metabolism of the vitamin (81–83). Whether phenytoin also induces folic acid deficiency in the fetus is less certain because the fetus seems to be efficient in drawing on available maternal stores of folic acid (see Folic Acid). Low maternal folate levels, however, have been proposed as one possible mechanism for the increased incidence of defects observed in infants exposed *in utero* to phenytoin. In a 1984 report, two investigators studied the relationship between folic acid, anticonvulsants, and fetal defects (81). In the retrospective part of this study, a group of 24 women treated with phenytoin and other anticonvulsants produced 66 infants, 10 (15%) with major anomalies. Two of the mothers with affected infants had markedly low red blood cell folate concentrations. A second group of 22 epileptic women was then supplemented with daily folic acid, 2.5–5.0 mg, starting before conception in 26 pregnancies and within the first 40 days in 6. This group produced 33 newborns (32 pregnancies, 1 set of twins) with no defects, a significant difference from the nonsupplemented group. Loss of seizure control caused by folic acid lowering of phenytoin serum levels, which is known to occur, was not a problem in this small series (81).

Negative associations between phenytoin-induced folate deficiency have been reported (82,83). In one study, mothers were given supplements with an average folic acid dose of 0.5 mg/day from the 6th to 16th week of gestation until delivery (83). Defects were observed in 20 infants (15%) from the 133 women taking anticonvulsants, which is similar to the reported frequency in pregnant patients not given supplements. Folate levels were usually within the normal range for pregnancy.

The effects of exposure (at any time during the 2nd or 3rd month after the last menstrual period) to folic acid antagonists on embryo/fetal development were evaluated in a large, multicenter, case-control surveillance study published in 2000 (84). The report was based on data collected between 1976 and 1998 from 80 maternity or tertiary care hospitals. Mothers were interviewed within 6 months of delivery about their use of drugs during pregnancy. Folic acid antagonists were categorized into two groups: group I—dihydrofolate reductase inhibitors (aminopterin, methotrexate, sulfasalazine, pyrimethamine, triamterene, and trimethoprim); group II—agents that affect other enzymes in folate metabolism, impair the absorption of folate, or increase the metabolic breakdown of folate (carbamazepine, phenytoin, primidone, and phenobarbital). The case subjects were 3870 infants with cardiovascular defects, 1962 with oral clefts, and 1100 with urinary tract malformations. Infants with defects associated with a syndrome were excluded as were infants with coexisting neural tube defects (NTDs; known to be reduced by maternal folic acid supplementation). Too few infants with limb-reduction defects were identified to be analyzed. Controls ($N = 8,387$) were infants with malformations other than oral clefts and cardiovascular, urinary tract, and limb-reduction defects and NTDs, but included infants with chromosomal and genetic defects. The risk of malformations in control infants would not have been reduced by vitamin supplementation, and none of the controls used folic acid antagonists. For group I cases, the relative risks (RRs) of cardiovascular defects and oral clefts were 3.4 (95% confidence interval [CI] 1.8–6.4) and 2.6 (95% CI 1.1–6.1), respectively. For group II cases, the RRs of cardiovascular and urinary tract defects, and oral clefts were 2.2 (95% CI 1.4–3.5), 2.5 (95% CI 1.2–5.0), and 2.5 (95% CI 1.5–4.2), respectively. Maternal use of multivitamin supplements with folic acid (typically 0.4 mg) reduced the risks in group I cases, but not in group II cases (84).

P

The pharmacokinetics and placental transport of phenytoin have been extensively studied and reviewed (85–87). Plasma concentrations of phenytoin may fall during pregnancy. Animal studies and recent human reports suggest a dose-related teratogenic effect of phenytoin (88,89). Although these results are based on a small series of patients, it is reasonable to avoid excessively high plasma concentrations of phenytoin. Close monitoring of plasma phenytoin concentrations is recommended to maintain adequate seizure control and prevent potential fetal hypoxia.

Placental function in women taking phenytoin has been evaluated (90). No effect was detected from phenytoin as measured by serum human placental lactogen, 24-hour urinary total estriol excretion, placental weight, and birth weight.

In a study evaluating thyroid function, no differences were found between treated epileptic pregnant women and normal pregnant controls (91). Thyroxine levels in the cord blood of anticonvulsant-exposed infants were significantly lower than in controls, but this was shown to be caused by altered protein binding and not altered thyroid function. Other parameters studied—thyrotropin, free thyroxine, and triiodothyronine—were similar in both groups.

The effect of phenytoin on maternal and fetal vitamin D metabolism was examined in a 1984 study (92). In comparison to normal controls, several significant differences were found in the level of various vitamin D compounds and in serum calcium, but the values were still within normal limits. No alterations were found in alkaline phosphatase and phosphate concentrations. The authors doubted whether the observed differences were of major clinical significance.

Phenytoin may be used for the management of digitalis-induced arrhythmias that are unresponsive to other agents and for refractory ventricular tachyarrhythmias (93–95). This short-term use has not been reported to cause problems in the exposed fetuses. The drug has also been used for anticonvulsant prophylaxis in severe preeclampsia (96).

In a 1988 study designed to evaluate the effect of *in utero* exposure to anticonvulsants on intelligence, 148 Finnish children of epileptic mothers were compared with 105 controls (97). Previous studies had either shown intellectual impairment from this exposure or no effect. Of the 148 children of epileptic mothers, 129 were exposed to anticonvulsant therapy during the first 20 weeks of pregnancy, 2 were only exposed after 20 weeks, and 17 were not exposed. In those mothers treated during pregnancy, 103 received phenytoin (monotherapy in 54 cases), all during the first 20 weeks. The children were evaluated at 5.5 years of age for both verbal and nonverbal measures of intelligence. A child was considered mentally deficient if the results of both tests were less than 71. Two of the 148 children of epileptic mothers were diagnosed as mentally deficient and 2 others had borderline intelligence (the mother of one of these latter children had not been treated with anticonvulsant medication). None of the controls was considered mentally deficient. Both verbal (110.2 vs. 114.5, $p < 0.05$) and nonverbal (108.7 vs. 113.2, $p < 0.05$) intelligence scores were significantly lower in the study group children than in controls. In both groups, intelligence scores were significantly lower when seven or more minor anomalies were present ($p = 0.03$). However, the presence of hypertelorism and digital hypoplasia, two minor anomalies considered typical of exposure to phenytoin, was not predictive of low intelligence (97).

A prospective, controlled, blinded observational 1994 study compared the global IQ and language development of children exposed *in utero* to either phenytoin ($N = 36$) or carbamazepine ($N = 34$) monotherapy to their respective matched controls (98). The cognitive tests were administered to the children between the ages of 18 and 36 months. The maternal IQ scores and socioeconomic status in the phenytoin subjects and their controls were similar, 90 vs. 93.9, and 40.8 vs. 40.9, respectively, as they were in the carbamazepine subjects and controls, 96.5 vs. 96.0, and 44.7 vs. 46.1, respectively. Compared to controls, phenytoin-exposed children had a lower mean global IQ than their matched controls (113.4 vs. 103.1; 95% CI 4.9 to 15.8 points; $p = 0.038$). The verbal comprehension and expressive language scores were also significantly ($p < 0.05$) lower, 0.2 vs. 1.1, and −0.47 vs. 0.2, respectively. In contrast, no significant differences were measured either in IQ or language development scores between carbamazepine-exposed children and their matched controls. No correlation between the daily dose (mg/kg) of either anticonvulsant and global IQ was found. Major malformations were observed in two phenytoin-exposed children (cleft palate and hypospadias; meningomyelocele and hydrocephalus), none of the phenytoin controls, two carbamazepine-exposed children (missing last joint of right index finger and nail hypoplasia; hypospadias), and one carbamazepine control (pulmonary atresia). The study results suggested that phenytoin had a clinically important negative effect on neurobehavioral development that was independent of maternal or environmental factors (98). In subsequent correspondence relating to the above study (99,100), various perceived problems were cited and were addressed in a reply (101).

The relationship between maternal anticonvulsant therapy, neonatal behavior, and neurological function in children was reported in a 1996 study (102). Among newborns exposed to maternal monotherapy, 18 were exposed to phenobarbital (including primidone), 13 to phenytoin, and 8 to valproic acid. Compared to controls, neonates exposed to phenobarbital had significantly higher mean apathy and optimality scores. Phenytoin-exposed neonates also had a significantly higher mean apathy score. However, the neonatal optimality and apathy scores did not correlate with neurological outcome of the children at 6 years of age. In contrast, those exposed to valproic acid had optimality and apathy scores statistically similar to controls but a significantly higher hyperexcitability score. Moreover, the hyperexcitability score correlated with later minor and major neurological dysfunction at age 6 years (102).

A two-part 2000 study evaluated the effects of prenatal phenobarbital and phenytoin exposure on brain development and cognitive functioning in adults (103). Subjects and controls, delivered at a mean 40 weeks' gestation, were retrospectively identified from birth records covering the years between 1957 and 1972. Maternal diseases of the subjects included epilepsy (treated with anticonvulsants) and other conditions in which anticonvulsants were used as sedatives (nausea, vomiting, or emotional problems), whereas the matched control group had no maternal pathologies. Only those exposed prenatally to phenobarbital alone or phenobarbital plus phenytoin had sufficient subjects to analyze. The mean occipitofrontal circumference for phenobarbital-exposed neonates was not different from controls (34.49 vs. 34.50 cm), but it was significantly smaller for phenobarbital plus phenytoin subjects compared to phenobarbital alone or controls (33.82 cm, $p = 0.003$). In the follow-up part of the study, no difference in adult cognitive functioning (intelligence, attention, and memory) were found between the exposed and control groups. More subjects than controls, however, were mentally retarded (4 vs. 2; one control had autism) and more had persistent learning problems (12% vs. 1%). The investigators concluded that phenobarbital plus phenytoin reduced occipitofrontal circumference but may only affect cognitive capacity in susceptible offspring (103).

In summary, the use of phenytoin during pregnancy involves significant risk to the fetus in terms of major and minor congenital abnormalities and hemorrhage at birth. Adverse effects on neurodevelopment have also been reported. The risk to the mother, however, is also great if the drug is not used to control her seizures. The risk:benefit ratio, in this case, favors continued use of the drug during pregnancy. Frequent determinations of phenytoin levels are recommended to maintain the lowest level required to prevent seizures and possibly to lessen the likelihood of fetal anomalies. Based on recent research, consideration should also be given to monitoring folic acid levels simultaneously with phenytoin determinations and administering folic acid very early in pregnancy or before conception to those women shown to have low folate concentrations.

BREAST FEEDING SUMMARY

RECOMMENDATION: Compatible

Phenytoin is excreted into breast milk. Milk:plasma ratios range from 0.18 to 0.54 (85,103–107). The pharmacokinetics of phenytoin during lactation have been reviewed (85). The reviewers concluded that little risk to the nursing infant was present if maternal levels were kept in the therapeutic range. However, methemoglobinemia, drowsiness, and decreased sucking activity have been reported in one infant (108). Except for this one case, no other reports of adverse effects with the use of phenytoin during lactation have been located. The American Academy of Pediatrics classifies phenytoin as compatible with breast-feeding (109).

References

1. Janz D, Fuchs V. Are anti-epileptic drugs harmful when given during pregnancy? German Med Monogr 1964;9:20–3.
2. Hill RB. Teratogenesis and antiepileptic drugs. N Engl J Med 1973;289:1089–90.
3. Janz D. The teratogenic risk of antiepileptic drugs. Epilepsia 1975;16:159–69.
4. Bodendorfer TW. Fetal effects of anticonvulsant drugs and seizure disorders. Drug Intell Clin Pharm 1978;12:14–21.
5. Committee on Drugs, American Academy of Pediatrics. Anticonvulsants and pregnancy. Pediatrics 1977;60:331–3.
6. Nakane Y, Okuma T, Takahashi R, Sato Y, Wada T, Sato T, Fukushima Y, Kumashiro H, Ono T, Takahashi T, Aoki Y, Kazamatsuri H, Inami M, Komai S, Seino M, Miyakoshi M, Tanimura T, Hazama H, Kawahara R, Otuski S, Hosokawa K, Inanaga K, Nakazawa Y, Yamamoto K. Multi-institutional study of the teratogenicity and fetal toxicity of antiepileptic drugs: A report of a collaborative study group in Japan. Epilepsia 1980;21:663–80.
7. Andermann E, Dansky L, Andermann F, Loughnan PM, Gibbons J. Minor congenital malformations and dermatoglyphic alterations in the offspring of epileptic women: a clinical investigation of the teratogenic effects of anticonvulsant medication. In *Epilepsy, Pregnancy and the Child*. Proceedings of a Workshop in Berlin, September 1980. New York, NY: Raven Press, 1981.
8. Dansky L, Andermann E, Andermann F. Major congenital malformations in the offspring of epileptic patients. In *Epilepsy, Pregnancy and the Child*. Proceedings of a Workshop in Berlin, September 1980. New York, NY: Raven Press, 1981.
9. Hanson JW, Buehler BA. Fetal hydantoin syndrome: Current status. J Pediatr 1982;101:816–8.
10. Canger R, Battino D, Canevini MP, Fumarola C, Guidolin L, Vignoli A, Mamoli D, Palmieri C, Molteni F, Granata T, Hassibi P, Zamperini P, Pardi G, Avanzini G. Malformations in offspring of women with epilepsy: a prospective study. Epilepsia 1999;40:1231–6.
11. Holmes LB, Harvey EA, Coull BA, Huntington KB, Khoshbin S, Hayes AM, Ryan LM. The teratogenicity of anticonvulsant drugs. N Engl J Med 2001;344:1132–8.
12. Buehler BA, Delimont D, Van Waes M, Finnell RH. Prenatal prediction of risk of the fetal hydantoin syndrome. N Engl J Med 1990;322:1567–72.
13. Tiboni GM, Iammarrone E, Giampietro F, Lamonaca D, Bellati U, Di Ilio C. Teratological interaction between the bis-triazole antifungal agent fluconazole and the anticonvulsant drug phenytoin. Teratology 1999;59:81–7.
14. Meadow SR. Anticonvulsant drugs and congenital abnormalities. Lancet 1968;2:1296.
15. Loughnan PM, Gold H, Vance JC. Phenytoin teratogenicity in man. Lancet 1973;1:70–2.
16. Hill RM, Horning MG, Horning EC. Antiepileptic drugs and fetal well-being. In Boreus L, ed. *Fetal Pharmacology*. New York, NY: Raven Press, 1973: 375–9.
17. Janz D. Antiepileptic drugs and pregnancy: altered utilization patterns and teratogenesis. Epilepsia 1982;23(Suppl 1):S53–S63.
18. Allen RW Jr, Ogden B, Bentley FL, Jung AL. Fetal hydantoin syndrome, neuroblastoma, and hemorrhagic disease in a neonate. JAMA 1980;244:1464–5.
19. Ramilo J, Harris VJ. Neuroblastoma in a child with the hydantoin and fetal alcohol syndrome. The radiographic features. Br J Radiol 1979;52: 993–5.
20. Pendergrass TW, Hanson JW. Fetal hydantoin syndrome and neuroblastoma. Lancet 1976;2:150.
21. Sherman S, Roizen N. Fetal hydantoin syndrome and neuroblastoma. Lancet 1976;2:517.
22. Ehrenbard LT, Chaganti RSK. Cancer in the fetal hydantoin syndrome. Lancet 1981;2:97.
23. Seeler RA, Israel JN, Royal JE, Kaye CI, Rao S, Abulaban M. Ganglioneuroblastoma and fetal hydantoin-alcohol syndromes. Pediatrics 1979;63:524–7.
24. Jimenez JF, Seibert RW, Char F, Brown RE, Seibert JJ. Melanotic neuroectodermal tumor of infancy and fetal hydantoin syndrome. Am J Pediatr Hematol Oncol 1981;3:9–15.
25. Taylor WF, Myers M, Taylor WR. Extrarenal Wilms' tumour in an infant exposed to intrauterine phenytoin. Lancet 1980;2:481–2.
26. Blattner WA, Hanson DE, Young EC, Fraumeni JF. Malignant mesenchymoma and birth defects. JAMA 1977;238:334–5.
27. Kousseff BG. Subcutaneous vascular abnormalities in fetal hydantoin syndrome. Birth Defects Orig Artic Ser 1982;18:51–4.
28. Lipson A, Bale P. Ependymoblastoma associated with prenatal exposure to diphenylhydantoin and methylphenobarbitone. Cancer 1985;55:1859–62.
29. Corcoran R, Rizk MW. VACTERL congenital malformation and phenytoin therapy? Lancet 1976;2:960.
30. Pinto W Jr, Gardner LI, Rosenbaum P. Abnormal genitalia as a presenting sign in two male infants with hydantoin embryopathy syndrome. Am J Dis Child 1977;131:452–5.
31. Hoyt CS, Billson FA. Maternal anticonvulsants and optic nerve hypoplasia. Br J Ophthalmol 1978;62: 3–6.
32. Wilson RS, Smead W, Char F. Diphenylhydantoin teratogenicity: ocular manifestations and related deformities. J Pediatr Ophthalmol Strabismus 1970;15:137–40.
33. Dabee V, Hart AG, Hurley RM. Teratogenic effects of diphenylhydantoin. Can Med Assoc J 1975;112: 75–7.
34. Anderson RC. Cardiac defects in children of mothers receiving anticonvulsant therapy during pregnancy. J Pediatr 1976;89:318–9.
35. Hill RM, Verniaud WM, Horning MG, McCulley LB, Morgan NF. Infants exposed in utero to antiepileptic drugs. A prospective study. Am J Dis Child 1974;127:645–53.

36. Stankler L, Campbell AGM. Neonatal acne vulgaris: a possible feature of the fetal hydantoin syndrome. Br J Dermatol 1980;103:453–5.
37. Ringrose CAD. The hazard of neurotropic drugs in the fertile years. Can Med Assoc J 1972;106:1058.
38. Pettifor JM, Benson R. Congenital malformations associated with the administration of oral anticoagulants during pregnancy. J Pediatr 1975;86:459–61.
39. Biale Y, Lewenthal H, Aderet NB. Congenital malformations due to anticonvulsant drugs and congenital abnormalities. Obstet Gynecol 1975;45:439–42.
40. Aase JM. Anticonvulsant drugs and congenital abnormalities. Am J Dis Child 1974;127:758.
41. Lewin PK. Phenytoin associated congenital defects with Y-chromosome variant. Lancet 1973;I:559.
42. Yang TS, Chi CC, Tsai CJ, Chang MJ. Diphenylhydantoin teratogenicity in man. Obstet Gynecol 1978;52:682–4.
43. Mallow DW, Herrick MK, Gathman G. Fetal exposure to anticonvulsant drugs. Arch Pathol Lab Med 1980;104:215–8.
44. Hirschberger M, Kleinberg F. Maternal phenytoin ingestion and congenital abnormalities: Report of a case. Am J Dis Child 1975;129:984.
45. Hanson JW, Myrianthopoulos NC, Sedgwick Harvey MA, Smith DW. Risks to the offspring of women treated with hydantoin anticonvulsants, with emphasis on the fetal hydantoin syndrome. J Pediatr 1976;89:662–8.
46. Shakir RA, Johnson RH, Lambie DG, Melville ID, Nanda RN. Comparison of sodium valproate and phenytoin as single drug treatment in epilepsy. Epilepsia 1981;22:27–33.
47. Michalodimitrakis M, Parchas S, Coutselinis A. Fetal hydantoin syndrome: Congenital malformation of the urinary tract—a case report. Clin Toxicol 1981;18:1095–7.
48. Phelan MC, Pellock JM, Nance WE. Discordant expression of fetal hydantoin syndrome in heteropaternal dizygotic twins. N Engl J Med 1982;307:99–101.
49. Kousseff BG, Root ER. Expanding phenotype of fetal hydantoin syndrome. Pediatrics 1982;70:328–9.
50. Wilker R, Nathenson G. Combined fetal alcohol and hydantoin syndromes. Clin Pediatr 1982;21:331–4.
51. Kogutt MS. Fetal hydantoin syndrome. South Med J 1984;77:657–8.
52. Krauss CM, Holmes LB, VanLang QN, Keith DA. Four siblings with similar malformations after exposure to phenytoin and primidone. J Pediatr 1984;105: 750–5.
53. Pearl KN, Dickens S, Latham P. Functional palatal incompetence in the fetal anticonvulsant syndrome. Arch Dis Child 1984;59:989–90.
54. Trice JE, Ambler M. Multiple cerebral defects in an infant exposed in utero to anticonvulsants. Arch Pathol Lab Med 1985;109:521–3.
55. D'Souza SW, Robertson IG, Donnai D, Mawer G. Fetal phenytoin exposure, hypoplastic nails, and jitteriness. Arch Dis Child 1990;65:320–4.
56. Kotzot D, Weigl J, Huk W, Rott HD. Hydantoin syndrome with holoprosencephaly: a possible rate teratogenic effect. Teratology 1993;48:15–19.
57. Shaw GM, Wasserman CR, O'Malley CD, Lammer EJ, Finnell RH. Orofacial clefts and maternal anticonvulsant use. Reprod Toxicol 1995;9:97–8.
58. Sabry MA, Farag TI. Hand anomalies in fetal-hydantoin syndrome: from nail/phalangeal hypoplasia to unilateral acheiria. Am J Med Genet 1996;62:410–2.
59. Holmes LB, Harvey EA. Holoprosencephaly and the teratogenicity of anticonvulsants. Teratology 1994;49:82.
60. Rafla NM, Meehan FP. Thanatophoric dwarfism; drugs and antenatal diagnosis: A case report. Eur J Obstet Gynecol Reprod Biol 1990;38:161–5.
61. Arpino C, Brescianini S, Robert E, Castilla EE, Cocchi G, Cornel MC, de Vigan C, Lancaster PAL, Merlob P, Sumiyoshi Y, Zampino G, Renzi C, Rosano A, Mastroiacovo P. Teratogenic effects of antiepileptic drugs: use of an international database on malformations and drug exposure (MADRE). Epilepsia 2000; 41:1436–43.
62. Al-Shammri S, Guberman A, Hsu E. Neuroblastoma and fetal exposure to phenytoin in a child without dysmorphic features. Can J Neurol Sci 1992;19: 243–5.
63. Koren G, Demitrakoudis D, Weksberg R, Reider M, Shear NH, Sonely M, Shandling B, Spielberg SP. Neuroblastoma after prenatal exposure to phenytoin: cause and effect? Teratology 1989;40:157–62.
64. Lawrence A. Antiepileptic drugs and the foetus. Br Med J 1963;2:1267.
65. Kohler HG. Haemorrhage in newborn of epileptic mothers. Lancet 1966;1:267.
66. Douglas H. Haemorrhage in the newborn. Lancet 1966;1:816–7.
67. Monnet P, Rosenberg D, Bovier-Lapierre M. Terapeutique anticomitale administree pendant la grosses et maladie hemorragique du nouveau-ne. As cited in Bleyer WA, Skinner AL. Fetal neonatal hemorrhage after maternal anticonvulsant therapy. JAMA 1976;235:626–7.
68. Davis PP. Coagulation defect due to anticonvulsant drug treatment in pregnancy. Lancet 1970;1:413.
69. Evans AR, Forrester RM, Discombe C. Neonatal haemorrhage following maternal anticonvulsant therapy. Lancet 1970;1:517–8.
70. Stevensom MM, Bilbert EF. Anticonvulsants and hemorrhagic diseases of the newborn infant. J Pediatr 1970;77:516.
71. Speidel BD, Meadow SR. Maternal epilepsy and abnormalities of the foetus and newborn. Lancet 1972;2:839–40.
72. Truog WE, Feusner JH, Baker DL. Association of hemorrhagic disease and the syndrome of persistent fetal circulation with the fetal hydantoin syndrome. J Pediatr 1980;96:112–4.
73. Solomon GE, Hilgartner MW, Kutt H. Coagulation defects caused by diphenylhydantoin. Neurology 1972;22:1165–71.
74. Griffiths AD. Neonatal haemorrhage associated with maternal anticonvulsant therapy. Lancet 1981;2:1296–7.
75. Page TE, Hoyme HE, Markarian M, Jones KL. Neonatal hemorrhage secondary to thrombocytopenia: an occasional effect of prenatal hydantoin exposure. Birth Defects Orig Artic Ser 1982;18:47–50.
76. Srinivasan G, Seeler RA, Tiruvury A, Pildes RS. Maternal anticonvulsant therapy and hemorrhagic disease of the newborn. Obstet Gynecol 1982;59:250–2.

77. Payne NR, Hasegawa DK. Vitamin K deficiency in newborns: a case report in α-1-antitrypsin deficiency and a review of factors predisposing to hemorrhage. Pediatrics 1984;73:712–6.
78. Lane PA, Hathaway WE. Vitamin K in infancy. J Pediatr 1985;106:351–9.
79. Howe AM, Lipson AH, Sheffield LJ, Haan EA, Halliday JL, Jenson F, David DJ, Webster WS. Prenatal exposure to phenytoin, facial development, and a possible role for vitamin K. Am J Med Genet 1995;58: 238–44.
80. Felding I, Rane A. Congenital liver damage after treatment of mother with valproic acid and phenytoin? Acta Paediatr Scand 1984;73: 565–8.
81. Biale Y, Lewenthal H. Effect of folic acid supplementation on congenital malformations due to anticonvulsive drugs. Eur J Obstet Reprod Biol 1984;18: 211–6.
82. Pritchard JA, Scott DE, Whalley PJ. Maternal folate deficiency and pregnancy wastage. IV. Effects of folic acid supplements, anticonvulsants, and oral contraceptives. Am J Obstet Gynecol 1971;109: 341–6.
83. Hiilesmaa VK, Teramo K, Granstrom ML, Bardy AH. Serum folate concentrations during pregnancy in women with epilepsy: relation to antiepileptic drug concentrations, number of seizures, and fetal outcome. Br Med J 1983;287:577–9.
84. Hernandez-Diaz S, Werler MM, Walker AM, Mitchell AA. Folic acid antagonists during pregnancy and the risk of birth defects. N Engl J Med 2000;343: 1608–14.
85. Nau H, Kuhnz W, Egger HJ, Rating D, Helge H. Anticonvulsants during pregnancy and lactation: transplacental, maternal and neonatal pharmacokinetics. Clin Pharmacokinet 1982;7: 508–43.
86. Chen SS, Perucca E, Lee JN, Richens A. Serum protein binding and free concentrations of phenytoin and phenobarbitone in pregnancy. Br J Clin Pharmacol 1982;13:547–52.
87. van der Klign E, Schobben F, Bree TB. Clinical pharmacokinetics of antiepileptic drugs. Drug Intell Clin Pharm 1980;14:674–85.
88. Dansky L, Andermann E, Sherwin AL, Andermann F. Plasma levels of phenytoin during pregnancy and the puerperium. In *Epilepsy, Pregnancy and the Child*. Proceedings of a Workshop held in Berlin, September 1980. New York, NY: Raven Press, 1981.
89. Dansky L, Andermann E, Andermann F, Sherwin AL, Kinch RA. Maternal epilepsy and congenital malformation: correlation with maternal plasma anticonvulsant levels during pregnancy. In *Epilepsy, Pregnancy and the Child*. Proceedings of a Workshop held in Berlin, September 1980. New York, NY: Raven Press, 1981.
90. Hiilesmaa VK. Evaluation of placental function in women on antiepileptic drugs. J Perinat Med 1983;11:187–92.
91. Carriero R, Andermann E, Chen MF, Eeg-Oloffson O, Kinch RAH, Klein G, Pearson Murphy BE. Thyroid function in epileptic mothers and their infants at birth. Am J Obstet Gynecol 1985;151: 641–4.
92. Markestad T, Ulstein M, Strandjord RE, Aksnes L, Aarskog D. Anticonvulsant drug therapy in human pregnancy: effects on serum concentrations of vitamin D metabolites in maternal and cord blood. Am J Obstet Gynecol 1984;150:254–8.
93. Tamari I, Eldar M, Rabinowitz B, Neufeld HN. Medical treatment of cardiovascular disorders during pregnancy. Am Heart J 1982;104:1357–63.
94. Rotmensch HH, Elkayam U, Frishman W. Antiarrhythmic drug therapy during pregnancy. Ann Intern Med 1983;98:487–497.
95. Rotmensch HH, Rotmensch S, Elkayam U. Management of cardiac arrhythmias during pregnancy: Current concepts. Drugs 1987;33:623–33.
96. Ryan G, Lange IR, Naugler MA. Clinical experience with phenytoin prophylaxis in severe preeclampsia. Am J Obstet Gynecol 1989;161:1297–304.
97. Gaily E, Kantola-Sorsa E, Granstrom M-L. Intelligence of children of epileptic mothers. J Pediatr 1988,113.677–84.
98. Scolnik D, Nulman I, Rovet J, Gladstone D, Czuchta D, Gardner HA, Gladstone R, Ashby P, Weksberg R, Einarson T, Koren G. Neurodevelopment of children exposed in utero to phenytoin and carbamazepine monotherapy. JAMA 1994;271:767–770.
99. Jeret JS. Neurodevelopment after in utero exposure to phenytoin and carbamazepine. JAMA 1994;272:850.
100. Loring DW, Meador KJ, Thompson WO. Neurodevelopment of children exposed *in utero* to phenytoin and carbamazepine. JAMA 1994;272:850–1.
101. Koren G. Neurodevelopment of children exposed in utero to phenytoin and carbamazepine. JAMA 1994;272:851.
102. Koch S, Jager-Roman E, Losche G, Nau H, Rating D, Helge H. Antiepileptic drug treatment in pregnancy: drug side effects in the neonate and neurological outcome. Acta Paediatr 1996;84:739–46.
103. Dessens AB, Cohen-Kettenis PT, Mellenbergh GJ, Koppe JG, van de Poll NE, Boer K. Association of prenatal phenobarbital and phenytoin exposure with small head size at birth and with learning problems. Acta Paediatr 2000;89:533–41.
104. Horning MG, Stillwell WG, Nowling J, Lertratanangkoon K, Stillwell RN, Hill RM. Identification and quantification of drugs and drug metabolites in human breast milk using GC-MS-COM methods. Mod Probl Pediatr 1975;15:73–9.
105. Svensmark O, Schiller PJ. 5-5-Diphenylhydantoin (Dilantin) blood level after oral or intravenous dosage in man. Acta Pharmacol Toxicol 1960;16: 331–46.
106. Kok THHG, Taitz LS, Bennett MJ, Holt DW. Drowsiness due to clemastine transmitted in breast milk. Lancet 1982;1:914–5.
107. Steen B, Rane A, Lonnerholm G, Falk O, Elwin CE, Sjoqvist F. Phenytoin excretion in human breast milk and plasma levels in nursed infants. Ther Drug Monit 1982;4:331–4.
108. Finch E, Lorber J. Methaemoglobinaemia in the newborn: Probably due to phenytoin excreted in human milk. J Obstet Gynaecol Br Emp 1954;61:833.
109. Committee on Drugs, American Academy of Pediatrics. The transfer of drugs and other chemicals into human milk. Pediatrics 2001;108:776–89.

Name:	**PHYSOSTIGMINE**	Risk Factor:	**C**
Class:	**Parasympathomimetic (Cholinergic)**		

FETAL RISK SUMMARY

RECOMMENDATION: Limited Human Data - No Relevant Animal Data

Physostigmine is rarely used in pregnancy. No reports linking its use with congenital defects have appeared. One report described its use in 15 women at term to reverse scopolamine-induced twilight sleep (1). Apgar scores of 14 of the newborns ranged from 7 to 9 at 1 minute and 8 to 10 at 5 minutes. One infant was depressed at birth and required resuscitation, but the mother had also received meperidine and diazepam. No other effects in the infants were mentioned.

Physostigmine is an anticholinesterase agent, but it does not contain a quaternary ammonium element. It crosses the blood-brain barrier and should be expected to cross the placenta (2).

Transient muscular weakness has been observed in about 20% of newborns of mothers with myasthenia gravis (3–5). The neonatal myasthenia is caused by transplacental passage of anti-acetylcholine receptor immunoglobulin G antibodies (5).

BREAST FEEDING SUMMARY

RECOMMENDATION: No Human Data - Probably Compatible

No data are available.

References

1. Smiller BG, Bartholomew EG, Sivak BJ, Alexander GD, Brown EM. Physostigmine reversal of scopolamine delirium in obstetric patients. Am J Obstet Gynecol 1973;116:326–9.
2. Taylor P. Anticholinesterase agents. In Gilman AG, Goodman LS, Gilman A, eds. *The Pharmacological Basis of Therapeutics*. 6th ed. New York, NY: Macmillan, 1980:100–19.
3. McNall PG, Jafarnia MR. Management of myasthenia gravis in the obstetrical patient. Am J Obstet Gynecol 1965;92:518–25.
4. Blackhall MI, Buckley GA, Roberts DV, Roberts JB, Thomas BH, Wilson A. Drug-induced neonatal myasthenia. J Obstet Gynaecol Br Commonw 1969;76:157–62.
5. Plauche WG. Myasthenia gravis in pregnancy: An update. Am J Obstet Gynecol 1979;135:691–7.

Name:	**PHYTONADIONE**	Risk Factor:	**C_M**
Class:	**Vitamin**		

FETAL RISK SUMMARY

RECOMMENDATION: Compatible

Phytonadione is a synthetic, fat-soluble substance identical to vitamin K_1, the natural vitamin found in a variety of foods (1). It is used for the prevention and treatment of hypoprothrombinemia caused by to vitamin K deficiency (1). Animal reproduction studies have not been conducted with phytonadione.

In a surveillance study of Michigan Medicaid recipients conducted between 1985 and 1992 involving 229,101 completed pregnancies, 5 newborns had been exposed to

phytonadione during the 1st trimester (F. Rosa, personal communication, FDA, 1993). Four (80.0%) major birth defects were observed (none expected), including 2/0 cardiovascular defects and 1/0 spina bifida. No anomalies were observed in four other defect categories (oral clefts, polydactyly, limb reduction defects, and hypospadias) for which specific data were available.

The use of phytonadione (vitamin K_1) during pregnancy and in the newborn has been the subject of several large reviews (2–5). Administration of vitamin K during pregnancy is usually not required because of the abundance of natural sources in food and the synthesis of the vitamin by the normal intestinal flora. Vitamin K_1 is indicated for maternal hypoprothrombinemia and for the prevention of hemorrhagic disease of the newborn (HDN) induced by maternal drugs, such as anticonvulsants, warfarin, rifampin, and isoniazid (2–5).

The placental transfer of vitamin K_1 is poor (6,7). A 1982 study found no detectable vitamin K (<0.10 ng/mL) in the cord blood of nine term infants, although adequate levels (mean 0.20 ng/mL) were present in eight of the nine mothers (6). Vitamin K_1, 1 mg IV, was then given to six additional mothers shortly before delivery (11–47 minutes), resulting in plasma vitamin K_1 values of 45–93 ng/mL. Vitamin K_1 was detected in only four of the six cord blood samples (ranging from 0.10–0.14 ng/mL), and its appearance did not seem to be time dependent. In a 1990 study, women were administered one or two doses of vitamin K_1 10 mg IM at 4-day intervals, and if not delivered, followed by daily oral 20-mg doses until the end of the 34th week or delivery (7). Treated subjects had significantly higher vitamin K_1 maternal and cord plasma levels than controls (11.592 vs. 0.102 ng/mL and 0.024 vs. 0.010 ng/mL, respectively). Although the median plasma vitamin K_1 levels in the mothers treated only with IM doses were similar to those treated with IM and oral doses, cord plasma levels in the latter group were significantly higher (0.42 vs. 0.017 ng/mL). No correlation was found between cord plasma levels of vitamin K_1 and gestational age or duration of therapy (7).

Vitamin K_1 is nontoxic in doses less than 20 mg (3). In a double- blind trial, 933 women at term were given 20 mg of either K_1 or K_2, the naturally occurring vitamins (8). No toxicity from either vitamin was found, including any association with low birth weight, asphyxia, neonatal jaundice, or perinatal mortality.

Oral vitamin K_1 has been suggested during the last 2 weeks of pregnancy for women taking anticonvulsants to prevent hypoprothrombinemia and hemorrhage in their newborns, but the effectiveness of this therapy has not been proven (2,3). In a group of mothers receiving phenindione, an oral anticoagulant, 10–30 mg of vitamin K_1 was given either IV or intra-amniotically 2–4 days before delivery (9). In a separate group, 2.5–3.0 mg of vitamin K_1 was injected IM into the fetuses at the same interval before delivery. Only in this latter group were coagulation factors significantly improved.

In summary, phytonadione (vitamin K_1) is the treatment of choice for maternal hypoprothrombinemia and for the prevention of HDN. Maternal supplements are not needed except for those patients deemed at risk for vitamin K deficiency. A recommended dietary intake from food of vitamin K_1 during pregnancy of 45 μg (100 nmol) has been proposed (10).

P

BREAST FEEDING SUMMARY

RECOMMENDATION: Compatible

Levels of phytonadione (vitamin K_1) in breast milk are naturally low with most samples having less than 20 ng/mL and many less than 5 ng/mL (2,3). In 20 lactating women, colostrum and mature milk concentrations were 2.3 and 2.1 ng/mL, less than half that found in cow's milk (11). Administration of a single 20-mg oral dose of phytonadione to one mother produced a concentration of 140 ng/mL at 12 hours with levels at 48 hours still about double normal values (11). In another study, 40 mg orally of vitamin K_1 or K_3 (menadione) were given to mothers within 2 hours after delivery (12). Effects from either vitamin on the prothrombin time of the breast-fed newborns were nil to slight during the first 3 days.

Natural levels of vitamin K_1 or K_2 in milk will not provide adequate supplies of the vitamin for the breast-fed infant (2,3). The vitamin K_1-dependent coagulation factors II, VII, IX, and X, are dependent on gestational age (2). In the newborn, these factors are approximately 30%–60% of normal and do not reach adult levels until about 6 weeks (2). Although not all newborns are vitamin K_1 deficient, many are deficient because of poor placental transfer of the vitamin. Exclusive breast-feeding will not prevent further decline of these already low stores and the possible development of deficiency in 48–72 hours (2,3). In addition, the intestinal flora of breast-fed infants may produce less vitamin K than the flora of formula-fed infants (2). The potential consequence of this deficiency is hemorrhagic disease of the newborn.

The American Academy of Pediatrics has suggested that HDN be defined as "a hemorrhagic disorder of the first days of life caused by a deficiency of vitamin K and characterized by deficiency of prothrombin and proconvertin (stable factor, factor VII), and probably of other factors" (13). The hemorrhage is frequently life threatening with intracranial bleeds common. A 1985 review (2) identified three types of HDN:

Early HDN (onset 0–24 hours)
Classic HDN (onset 2–5 days)
Late HDN (onset 1–12 months)

The maternal ingestion of certain drugs, such as anticonvulsants, warfarin, or antituberculous agents, is one of the known causes of early and classic HDN, whereas breast-feeding has been shown to be a cause of classic and late HDN (2). The administration of phytonadione to the newborn prevents HDN by preventing further decline of factors II, VII, IX, and X (2).

The use of prophylactic vitamin K_1 in all newborns is common in the United States but is controversial in other countries (2). The Committee on Nutrition, American Academy of Pediatrics, recommended in 1961, and again in 1980, that all newborns receive 0.5–1.0 mg of parenteral vitamin K_1 (13,14). The Committee recommended that administration to the mother prenatally should not be substituted for newborn prophylaxis (13). The bleeding risk in breast-fed infants who did not receive prophylactic vitamin K_1 is 15–20 times greater than in infants fed cow's milk, given vitamin K_1, or both (2). In spite of this evidence, new cases of HDN are still reported (3,15). In a recent report, 10 breast-fed infants with intracranial hemorrhage as a result of vitamin K deficiency were described (15). Onset of the bleeding was between 27 and 47 days of age with three infants dying and three having permanent brain injury. Milk levels of total vitamin K ($K_1 + K_2$) varied between 1.36 and 9.17 ng/mL. None of the infants had been given prophylactic therapy at birth.

In summary, the natural vitamin K content of breast milk is too low to protect the newborn from vitamin K deficiency and resulting hemorrhagic disease. The administration of vitamin K to the mother to increase milk concentrations may be possible but needs further study. All newborns should receive parenteral prophylactic therapy at birth consisting of 0.5–1.0 mg of phytonadione. Larger or repeat doses may be required for infants whose mothers are consuming anticonvulsants or oral anticoagulants (2,13). The American Academy of Pediatrics classifies vitamin K_1 as compatible with breast-feeding (16).

References

1. American Hospital Formulary Service. *Drug Information 1997*. Bethesda, MD: American Society of Health-System Pharmacists, 1997:2834–36.
2. Lane PA, Hathaway WE. Vitamin K in infancy. J Pediatr 1985;106:351–9.
3. Payne NR, Hasegawa DK. Vitamin K deficiency in newborns: a case report in α-1-antitrypsin deficiency and a review of factors predisposing to hemorrhage. Pediatrics 1984;73:712–6.
4. Wynn RM. The obstetric significance of factors affecting the metabolism of bilirubin, with particular reference to the role of vitamin K. Obstet Gynecol Surv 1963;18:333–54.
5. Finkel MJ. Vitamin K_1 and the vitamin K analogues. J Clin Pharmacol Ther 1961;2:795–814.
6. Shearer MJ, Rahim S, Barkhan P, Stimmler L. Plasma vitamin K_1 in mothers and their newborn babies. Lancet 1982;2:460–3.
7. Kazzi NJ, Ilagan NB, Liang K-C, Kazzi GM, Grietsell LA, Brans YW. Placental transfer of vitamin K_1 in preterm pregnancy. Obstet Gynecol 1990;75:334–7.
8. Blood Study Group of Gynecologists. Effect of vitamins K_2 and K_1 on the bleeding volume during parturition and the blood coagulation disturbance of newborns by a double blind controlled study. Igaku no Ayumi 1971;76:818. As cited in Nishimura H, Tanimura T. *Clinical Aspects of the Teratogenicity of Drugs*. New York, NY: American Elsevier, 1976:253.
9. Larsen JF, Jacobsen B, Holm HH, Pedersen JF, Mantoni M. Intrauterine injection of vitamin K before delivery during anticoagulant therapy of the mother. Acta Obstet Gynecol Scand 1978;57:227–30.
10. Olson JA. Recommended dietary intakes (RDI) of vitamin K in humans. Am J Clin Nutr 1987;45:687–92.
11. Haroon Y, Shearer MJ, Rahim S, Gunn WG, McEnery G, Barkhan P. The content of phylloquinone (vitamin K_1) in human milk, cows' milk and infant formula foods determined by high-performance liquid chromatography. J Nutr 1982;112:1105–17.
12. Dyggve HV, Dam H, Sondergaard E. Influence on the prothrombin time of breast-fed newborn babies of one single dose of vitamin K_1 or Synkavit given to the mother within 2 hours after birth. Acta Obstet Gynecol Scand 1956;35:440–4.
13. Committee on Nutrition, American Academy of Pediatrics. Vitamin K compounds and the water soluble analogues. Pediatrics 1961;28:501–7.
14. Committee on Nutrition, American Academy of Pediatrics. Vitamin and mineral supplement needs in normal children in the United States. Pediatrics 1980;66:1015–21.
15. Motohara K, Matsukura M, Matsuda I, Iribe K, Ikeda T, Kondo Y, Yonekubo A, Yamamoto Y, Tsuchiya F. Severe vitamin K deficiency in breast-fed infants. J Pediatr 1984;105:943–5.
16. Committee on Drugs, American Academy of Pediatrics. The transfer of drugs and other chemicals into human milk. Pediatrics 2001;108:776–89.

Name: **PILOCARPINE** Risk Factor: **C_M**

Class: **Parasympathomimetic (Cholinergic)**

P

FETAL RISK SUMMARY

RECOMMENDATION: Limited Human Data - Probably Compatible

Pilocarpine is used topically in the eye for glaucoma or as oral tablets in the treatment of dry mouth. In reproduction studies in rats at a dose about 26 times the maximum human oral dose based on body surface area (MRHD), adverse effects consisting of a decrease in fetal weight and an increase in the incidence of skeletal variations were observed (1). These effects may have been secondary to maternal toxicity (1). In another study with rats, doses approximately 10 times the MRHD during gestation and lactation were associated with an increased incidence of stillbirths, whereas doses 5 or more times the MRHD were associated with decreased neonatal survival and reduced pup body weights (1).

A single report of the topical use during pregnancy has been located. A woman with glaucoma was treated throughout gestation with topical pilocarpine, two drops twice daily, timolol, two drops each eye, and oral acetazolamide (2). Within 48 hours of delivery at 36 weeks' gestation, the infant presented with hyperbilirubinemia, hypocalcemia, hypomagnesemia, and metabolic acidosis. The toxic effects, attributed to the carbonic anhydrase inhibitor, acetazolamide (see Acetazolamide), resolved quickly on treatment. Mild hypertonicity requiring physiotherapy was observed at examinations at 1, 3, and 8 months of age.

BREAST FEEDING SUMMARY

RECOMMENDATION: No Human Data - Probably Compatible

No reports describing the use of pilocarpine during lactation have been located. Because of the relatively low molecular weight (about 209 for the free base), excretion into breast milk should be expected.

References

1. Product information. Salagen. MGI Pharma, 2000.
2. Merlob P, Litwin A, Mor N. Possible association between acetazolamide administration during pregnancy and metabolic disorders in the newborn. Eur J Obstet Gynecol Reprod Biol 1990;35:85–8.

Name:	**PIMOZIDE**	Risk Factor:	C_M
Class:	**Antipsychotic**		

FETAL RISK SUMMARY

RECOMMENDATION: No Human Data - Animal Data Suggest Low Risk

Pimozide is an orally active antipsychotic agent that blocks dopaminergic receptors on neurons in the central nervous system. It is indicated for the suppression of motor and phonic tics in patients with Tourette's disorder who have failed to respond satisfactorily to standard treatment. Pimozide is extensively metabolized, primarily in the liver, but the antipsychotic activity of the metabolites has not been determined. In schizophrenic patients, the mean serum elimination half-life was about 55 hours (1).

Reproduction studies have been conducted in rats and rabbits. In rats, oral doses up to eight times the maximum human dose (HD) (*assumed to be based on weight*) were not teratogenic, but decreased pregnancies and retarded fetal development were observed. The decreased pregnancies were thought to be due to an inhibition or delay in implantation, an effect in rodents that has been observed with other antipsychotic drugs. Although rat fertility studies were not adequate to assess all aspects of fertility, pimozide did cause prolonged estrus cycles similar to that observed with other antipsychotics. In the rabbit, dose-related (doses not specified) maternal toxicity, mortality, decreased weight gain, and embryo toxicity, including increased resorptions, were noted (1).

Dose-related increases in pituitary and mammary gland tumors in female mice were observed in long-term studies. The latter tumors may have been related to drug-induced elevated prolactin levels. Doses up to 50 times the HD were not tumorigenic in rats, but the limited number of animals surviving this study makes the findings unclear (1).

It is not known if pimozide crosses the human placenta. The molecular weight (about 462) and prolong elimination half-life suggest that the drug will cross to the embryo/fetus.

No reports describing the use of pimozide in human pregnancy have been located. The animal data do not suggest a risk of teratogenicity, but the lack of a meaningful comparison to the human dose limits the data's usefulness. In addition, the absence of human pregnancy experience prevents an assessment of the risk for the embryo and/or fetus. However, other antipsychotics are not considered major human teratogens. The use of antipsychotics, including pimozide, close to delivery may cause extrapyramidal effects (e.g., Parkinson-like; akinesia) in the newborn (2). Until human pregnancy experience has been reported, the safest course is to avoid pimozide in pregnancy, especially in the 1st trimester and close to delivery. Inadvertent exposure early in gestation, however, does not appear to represent a major risk.

BREAST FEEDING SUMMARY

RECOMMENDATION: No Human Data - Potential Toxicity

No reports describing the use of pimozide during human lactation have been located. The molecular weight (about 462) and prolong elimination half-life suggest that the drug will be excreted into breast milk. The effects, including effects on neurodevelopment, of this exposure on a nursing infant are unknown. If a woman taking this drug decides to breast-feed, her infant should be closely monitored for adverse effects seen in adults, such as extrapyramidal reactions (Parkinson-like; akinesia), sedation, and constipation.

References

1. Product information. Orap. Gate Pharmaceuticals, 2004.
2. Committee on Drugs. American Academy of Pediatrics. Use of psychoactive medication during pregnancy and possible effects on the fetus and newborn. Pediatrics 2000;105:880–7.

Name:	**PINDOLOL**	Risk Factor:	B_M*
Class:	**Sympatholytic (Antihypertensive)**		

FETAL RISK SUMMARY

RECOMMENDATION: Human Data Suggest Risk in 2nd and 3rd Trimesters

Pindolol, a nonselective β-adrenergic blocking agent, has been used for the treatment of hypertension occurring during pregnancy (1–7). Reproductive studies in rats and rabbits at doses exceeding 100 times the maximum recommended human dose (MRHD) found no evidence of embryotoxicity or teratogenicity (8). Impaired mating behavior and increased mortality of offspring were observed in female rats given doses 35 times the MRHD before and through 21 days of lactation (8). At 118 times the MRHD, increased fetal resorptions were noted (8).

A 1988 review compared the effects of β-blockers, including pindolol, in pregnancy and concluded that these agents are relatively safe (9) (see comment below).

Pindolol crosses the placenta to the fetus with maternal serum levels higher than cord concentrations (10). Cord:maternal serum ratios at 2 and 6 hours after the last dose were 0.37 and 0.67, respectively. Elimination half-lives in fetal and maternal serum were 1.6 hours and 2.2 hours, respectively.

The effect of pindolol on uteroplacental blood flow was studied in 10 women with gestational hypertension given a 10-mg oral dose (11). A significant fall in the mean maternal blood pressure and mean arterial blood pressure occurred, but no significant changes were observed in maternal or fetal heart rates, uteroplacental blood flow index, or uteroplacental vascular resistance. In contrast, a 1992 study, comparing the effects of pindolol and propranolol in women with preeclampsia, found a significant reduction in uterine artery vascular resistance, prompting the authors to conclude that pindolol acted, at least in part, through a peripheral vascular mechanism (12).

No fetal malformations attributable to pindolol have been reported, but experience in the 1st trimester is lacking. In a study comparing three β-blockers for the treatment of hypertension during pregnancy, the mean birth weight of pindolol-exposed babies was slightly higher than that of the acebutolol group and much higher than that of the offspring of atenolol-treated mothers (3375 g vs. 3160 g vs. 2745 g) (2). It is not known whether these differences were caused by the degree of maternal hypertension, the potency of the drugs used, or a combination of these and other factors.

The preliminary results of another study found that more than a third of the infants delivered from hypertensive women treated with pindolol were of low birth weight, but the authors thought this did not differ significantly from the expected rate for this population (3). In mothers treated with pindolol or atenolol, a decrease in the basal fetal heart rate was noted only in the atenolol-exposed fetuses (4). Additionally, in a prospective randomized study comparing 27 pindolol-treated women with 24 atenolol-treated women, no differences between the groups were found in gestational length, birth weight, Apgar scores, rates of cesarean section, or umbilical cord blood glucose levels (5). Treatment in both groups started at about 33 weeks' gestation.

A 1986 reference described the comparison of pindolol plus hydralazine with hydralazine alone for the treatment of maternal hypertension (6). Treatment in both groups was started at about 25 weeks' gestation. The newborn outcomes of the two groups, including birth weights, were similar.

A 1992 report described the outcomes of 29 women with gestational hypertension in the 3rd trimester (7). The women were randomized to receive either the cardioselective β-blocker, atenolol ($N = 13$), or the nonselective β-blocker, pindolol ($N = 16$). The mean maternal arterial blood pressure decrease in the two groups was 9 and 7.8 mm Hg, respectively (*n.s.*). In comparing before and after therapy, several significant changes were measured in fetal hemodynamics with atenolol but, except for fetal heart rate, no significant changes were measured with pindolol. The atenolol-induced changes included a decrease in fetal heart rate, increases in the pulsatility indexes (and thus, the peripheral vascular resistance) of the fetal thoracic descending aorta, the abdominal aorta, and the umbilical artery and a decrease in the umbilical venous blood flow. Although no difference was observed in the birth weights in the two groups, the placental weight in atenolol-treated pregnancies was significantly less (529 g vs. 653 g, respectively).

An apparently significant drug interaction occurred when a woman, who was being treated with pindolol for preeclampsia, had indomethacin added for tocolysis to her therapy (13). Two weeks after starting pindolol, 15 mg/day, indomethacin was started with a 200-mg rectal loading dose followed by 25 mg daily for 5 days. A sudden rise in blood pressure (230/130 mm Hg) occurred on the 5th day with cardiotocographic changes in fetal vitality (13). A low-birth-weight newborn infant was delivered by cesarean section and the mother's blood pressure returned to normal (125/85 mm Hg) in the postpartum period. A similar interaction occurred in another patient who was being treated with propranolol (13).

β-Blockade in the newborn has not been reported in the offspring of pindolol-treated mothers. However, because this complication has been observed in infants exposed to other β-blockers (see Acebutolol, Atenolol, and Nadolol), close observation of the newborn is recommended during the first 24–48 hours after birth. Long-term effects of *in utero* exposure to β-blockers have not been studied but warrant evaluation.

Some β-blockers may cause intrauterine growth retardation (IUGR) and reduced placental weight, especially those lacking intrinsic sympathomimetic activity (ISA) (i.e., partial agonist). Treatment beginning early in the 2nd trimester results in the greatest weight reductions, whereas treatment restricted to the 3rd trimester primarily affects only placental weight. Pindolol does possess ISA. However, IUGR and reduced placental weight may potentially occur with all agents within this class. Although growth retardation is a serious concern, the benefits of maternal therapy with β-blockers, in some cases, might outweigh the risks to the fetus and must be judged on a case-by-case basis.

[**Risk Factor D if used in 2nd or 3rd trimesters.*]

BREAST FEEDING SUMMARY

RECOMMENDATION: No Human Data - Potential Toxicity

No reports describing the use of pindolol during human lactation have been located. The manufacturer, however, states that pindolol is excreted in human milk (8). Because β-blockade has been observed in nursing infants exposed to other β-blockers (see Acebutolol and Atenolol), infants should be closely observed for bradycardia and other symptoms of β-blockade. Long-term effects of exposure to β-blockers from milk have not been studied but warrant evaluation.

References

1. Dubois D, Petitcolas J, Temperville B, Klepper A. Beta blockers and high-risk pregnancies. Int J Biol Res Pregnancy 1980;1:141–5.
2. Dubois D, Petitcolas J, Temperville B, Klepper A, Catherine PH. Treatment of hypertension in pregnancy with β-adrenoceptor antagonists. Br J Clin Pharmacol 1982;13(Suppl):375S–8S.
3. Sukerman-Voldman E. Pindolol therapy in pregnant hypertensive patients. Br J Clin Pharmacol 1982;13(Suppl):379S.
4. Ingemarsson I, Liedholm H, Montan S, Westgren M, Melander A. Fetal heart rate during treatment of maternal hypertension with beta-adrenergic antagonists. Acta Obstet Gynecol Scand 1984;118(Suppl):95–7.
5. Tuimala R, Hartikainen-Sorri A-L. Randomized comparison of atenolol and pindolol for treatment of hypertension in pregnancy. Curr Ther Res 1988;44:579–84.
6. Rosenfeld J, Bott-Kanner G, Boner G, Nissenkorn A, Friedman S, Ovadia J, Merlob P, Reisner S, Paran E, Zmora E, Biale Y, Insler V. Treatment of hypertension during pregnancy with hydralazine monotherapy or with combined therapy with hydralazine and pindolol. Eur J Obstet Gynecol Reprod Biol 1986;22:197–204.
7. Montan S, Ingemarsson I, Marsal K, Sjoberg N-O. Randomized controlled trial of atenolol and pindolol in human pregnancy: effects on fetal haemodyndamics. BMJ 1992;304:946–9.
8. Product information. Visken. Sandoz Pharmaceuticals, 1997.
9. Frishman WH, Chesner M. Beta-adrenergic blockers in pregnancy. Am Heart J 1988;115:147–52.
10. Grunstein S, Ellenbogen A, Anderman S, Davidson A, Jaschevatsky O. Transfer of pindolol across the placenta in hypertensive pregnant women. Curr Ther Res 1985;37:587–91.
11. Lunell NO, Nylund L, Lewander R, Sarby B, Wager J. Uteroplacental blood flow in pregnancy hypertension after the administration of a beta-adrenoceptor blocker, pindolol. Gynecol Obstet Invest 1984;18:269–74.
12. Meizner I, Paran E, Katz M, Holcberg G, Insler V. Flow velocity analysis of umbilical and uterine artery flow in pre-eclampsia treated with propranolol or pindolol. J Clin Ultrasound 1992;20:115–9.
13. Schoenfeld A, Freedman S, Hod M, Ovadia Y. Antagonism of antihypertensive drug therapy in pregnancy by indomethacin? Am J Obstet Gynecol 1989;161:1204–5.

P

Name:	**PIOGLITAZONE**	Risk Factor:	C_M
Class:	**Oral Antihyperglycemic**		

FETAL RISK SUMMARY

RECOMMENDATION: No Human Data - Animal Data Suggest Moderate Risk

Pioglitazone, a thiazolidinedione antidiabetic agent, is used as an adjunct to diet and exercise to improve glycemic control in patients with type II diabetes mellitus. It is used either alone or in combination with other antidiabetic agents (insulin, metformin, or sulfonylureas). Pioglitazone is not an insulin secretagogue, but acts to decrease insulin resistance in the periphery and in the liver (i.e., decreases insulin requirements). Thus, it requires the presence of insulin for its action. Pioglitazone undergoes extensive metabolism by hydroxylation and oxidation, and at least three of the metabolites are pharmacologically active (1).

Reproduction studies with pioglitazone have been conducted in rats and rabbits at doses up to 17 and 40 times, respectively, the maximum recommended human dose on a body surface area basis (MRHD) (1). In pregnant rats, at 10 or more times the MRHD, pioglitazone was embryotoxic as evidenced by increased postimplantation losses, delayed development, and reduced fetal weights. At 2 or more times the MRHD during late gestation and in the lactation period, delayed development was observed that was attributed to decreased body weights. Embryotoxicity was observed in rabbits dosed at 40 times the MRHD (1).

It is not known if pioglitazone or its active metabolites cross the placenta to the fetus. The molecular weight of the parent compound (about 393 for the hydrochloride salt) is low enough, however, that transfer to the fetus should be expected.

No reports describing the use of pioglitazone during human pregnancy have been located. Insulin is the treatment of choice for pregnant diabetic patients because, in general, other hypoglycemic agents do not provide adequate glycemic control. Moreover, insulin, unlike most oral agents, does not cross the placenta to the fetus, thus eliminating the additional concern that the drug therapy itself will adversely effect the fetus. Carefully prescribed insulin therapy provides better control of the mother's glucose, thereby preventing the fetal and neonatal complications that occur with this disease. High maternal glucose levels, as may occur in diabetes mellitus, are closely associated with a number of maternal and fetal adverse effects, including fetal structural anomalies if the hyperglycemia occurs early in gestation. To prevent this toxicity, most experts, including the American College of Obstetricians and Gynecologists, recommend that insulin be used for types I and II diabetes occurring during pregnancy and, if diet therapy alone is not successful, for gestational diabetes (2,3).

BREAST FEEDING SUMMARY

RECOMMENDATION: No Human Data - Probably Compatible

No reports describing the use of pioglitazone during human lactation have been located. The molecular weight of pioglitazone (about 393 for the hydrochloride salt) is low enough, however, that secretion into breast milk should be expected. Pioglitazone has been detected in the milk of lactating rats (1). In addition, at least three active metabolites have been identified and these also may be transferred into milk. The effects on a nursing infant from exposure to the drug in milk are unknown.

References

1. Product information. Actos. Takeda Pharmaceuticals America, 2000.
2. American College of Obstetricians and Gynecologists. Diabetes and pregnancy. *Technical Bulletin*. No. 200, December 1994.
3. Coustan DR. Management of gestational diabetes. Clin Obstet Gynecol 1991;34:558–64.

Name:	PIPERACETAZINE	Risk Factor:	C
Class:	Tranquilizer		

FETAL RISK SUMMARY

RECOMMENDATION: No Human Data - No Relevant Animal Data

Piperacetazine is a piperidyl phenothiazine. The phenothiazines readily cross the placenta (1). No specific information on the use of piperacetazine in pregnancy has been located. Although occasional reports have attempted to link various phenothiazine compounds with congenital malformations, the bulk of the evidence indicates that these drugs are safe for the mother and fetus (see also Chlorpromazine).

BREAST FEEDING SUMMARY

RECOMMENDATION: No Human Data - Potential Toxicity

No reports describing the excretion of piperacetazine into breast milk have been located.

Reference

1. Moya F, Thorndike V. Passage of drugs across the placenta. Am J Obstet Gynecol 1962;84:1778–98.

Name:	PIPERACILLIN	Risk Factor:	B_M
Class:	Antibiotic (Penicillin)		

FETAL RISK SUMMARY

RECOMMENDATION: Compatible

Piperacillin, a piperazine derivative of ampicillin, is a broad-spectrum penicillin (see also Ampicillin). Animal reproduction studies in mice and rats at doses up to 4 times the human dose have shown no evidence of impaired fertility or fetal harm (1).

No reports linking the use of piperacillin with congenital defects in humans have been located. Piperacillin has been used between 24 and 35 weeks' gestation in women with premature rupture of the membranes to delay delivery (2). No adverse maternal or fetal effects were observed.

Piperacillin rapidly crosses the placenta to the fetus (3). Three women, between 22 and 33 weeks' gestation, were administered a single 4-g IV dose of the antibiotic immediately before intrauterine exchange transfusion for Rh isoimmunization. The mean concentrations of piperacillin in fetal serum was 20 $\pm$ 12 μg/mL, in maternal serum 121 $\pm$ 50 μg/mL (fetal:maternal ratio 0.17), and in amniotic fluid 0.9 $\pm$ 0.4 μg/mL.

The pharmacokinetics of piperacillin during pregnancy have been reported (4). Women were administered a 4-g IV dose just before cesarean section. The mean venous cord concentration was 9.7 μg/mL, representing a mean fetal:maternal ratio of 0.27. As with other penicillins, an increased clearance of the antibiotic was observed during pregnancy.

BREAST FEEDING SUMMARY

RECOMMENDATION: Compatible

Piperacillin is excreted in small amounts into breast milk (1). Although concentrations are low, three potential problems exist for the nursing infant: modification of bowel flora, direct effects on the infant, and interference with the interpretation of culture results if a fever workup is required.

References

1. Product information. Pipracil. Lederle Laboratories, 2000.
2. Lockwood CJ, Costigan K, Ghidini A, Wein R, Cetrulo C, Alvarez M, Berkowitz RL. Double-blind, placebo-controlled trial of piperacillin sodium in preterm membrane rupture (abstract). Am J Obstet Gynecol 1993;168:378.
3. Brown CEL, Christmas JT, Bawdon RE. Placental transfer of cefazolin and piperacillin in pregnancies remote from term complicated by Rh isoimmunization. Am J Obstet Gynecol 1990;163:938–43.
4. Heikkilä A, Erkkola R. Pharmacokinetics of piperacillin during pregnancy. J Antimicrob Chemother 1991; 28:419–23.

Name:	**PIPERAZINE**	Risk Factor:	**B**
Class:	**Anthelmintic**		

FETAL RISK SUMMARY

RECOMMENDATION: Limited Human Data - No Relevant Animal Data

No published reports linking the use of piperazine with congenital defects have been located. A review of the treatment of threadworm infestation during pregnancy cited a personal communication involving two infants with congenital malformations who were exposed to piperazine (1). One of the infants had bilateral hare lip, cleft palate, and anophthalmia, but exposure to piperazine had occurred at 12 and 14 weeks' gestation. The mother in the second case had taken the anthelmintic at 6 and 8 weeks' gestation and her infant had a defect of the right foot. Based on the scarcity of reports, the possibility of a causal relationship in the latter case is probably remote.

The Collaborative Perinatal Project monitored 50,282 mother-child pairs, 3 of whom had 1st trimester exposure to piperazine. No evidence was found to suggest a relationship to malformations (2).

BREAST FEEDING SUMMARY

RECOMMENDATION: Hold Breast Feeding

Piperazine is excreted in breast milk (2), but specific data have not been located. According to one reviewer, the mother should take her dose of the drug immediately following feeding her infant, and then express and discard her milk during the next 8 hours (2).

References

1. Heinonen OP, Slone D, Shapiro S. *Birth Defects and Drugs in Pregnancy*. Littleton, MA: Publishing Sciences Group, 1977:299.
2. Leach FN. Management of threadworm infestation during pregnancy. Arch Dis Child 1990;65:399–400.

Name: **PIPERIDOLATE** Risk Factor: **C**
Class: **Parasympatholytic (Anticholinergic)**

FETAL RISK SUMMARY

RECOMMENDATION: Limited Human Data - No Relevant Animal Data

Piperidolate is an anticholinergic agent. In a large prospective study, 2323 patients were exposed to this class of drugs during the 1st trimester, 16 of whom took piperidolate (1). A possible association was found between the total group and minor malformations.

BREAST FEEDING SUMMARY

RECOMMENDATION: No Human Data - Probably Compatible

No data are available (see also Atropine).

Reference

1. Heinonen OP, Slone D, Shapiro S. *Birth Defects and Drugs in Pregnancy*. Littleton, MA: Publishing Sciences Group, 1977:346–53.

Name: **PIROXICAM** Risk Factor: **C_M***
Class: **Nonsteroidal Anti-Inflammatory**

FETAL RISK SUMMARY

RECOMMENDATION: Human Data Suggest Risk in 1st and 3rd Trimesters

Piroxicam is a nonsteroidal anti-inflammatory drug (NSAID) used for relief of the signs and symptoms of rheumatoid arthritis and osteoarthritis. It is in the same NSAID subclass (oxicams) as meloxicam.

Animal reproduction studies in rabbits and rats have not shown drug-related embryotoxicity or teratogenicity (1–3). However, decreased fetal growth was observed in some species (2).

In a surveillance study of Michigan Medicaid recipients conducted between 1985 and 1992 involving 229,101 completed pregnancies, 161 newborns had been exposed to piroxicam during the 1st trimester (F. Rosa, personal communication, FDA, 1993). Six (3.7%) major birth defects were observed (seven expected). Specific data were available for six defect categories, including (observed/expected) 1/2 cardiovascular defects, 1/0 oral clefts, 1/0 spina bifida, 1/0.5 polydactyly, 0/0 limb reduction defects, and 0/0 hypospadias. These data do not support an association between the drug and congenital defects.

A combined 2001 population-based observational cohort study and a case-control study estimated the risk of adverse pregnancy outcome from the use of NSAIDs (4). The use of NSAIDs during pregnancy was not associated with congenital malformations, preterm delivery, or low birth weight, but a positive association was discovered with spontaneous abortions (SABs). A similar study, also published in 2001, failed to find a relationship, in general, between NSAIDs and congenital malformations, but did find a significant association with cardiac defects and orofacial clefts (5). In addition, a 2003 study found a significant association between exposure to NSAIDs in early pregnancy and SABs (6). (See Ibuprofen for details on these three studies.)

A brief 2003 editorial on the potential for NSAID-induced developmental toxicity concluded that NSAIDs, and specifically those with greater COX-2 affinity, had a lower risk of this toxicity in humans than aspirin (7).

Constriction of the ductus arteriosus *in utero* is a pharmacologic consequence arising from the use of prostaglandin synthesis inhibitors during pregnancy (see also Indomethacin) (8). Persistent pulmonary hypertension of the newborn may occur if these agents are used in the 3rd trimester close to delivery (8,9). These drugs also have been shown to inhibit labor and prolong pregnancy, both in humans (10) (see also Indomethacin) and in animals (11). Women attempting to conceive should not use any prostaglandin synthesis inhibitor, including piroxicam, because of the findings in a variety of animal models that indicate these agents block blastocyst implantation (12,13). Moreover, as noted above, NSAIDs have been associated with SABs and congenital malformations.

[**Risk Factor D if used in 3rd trimester or near delivery.*]

BREAST FEEDING SUMMARY

RECOMMENDATION: Limited Human Data - Probably Compatible

Piroxicam is excreted into breast milk. A nursing woman, 9 months postpartum, was treated with piroxicam 20 mg/day for 4 months (14). Maternal serum concentrations of the drug 2.5 and 15.0 hours after a dose were 5.85 and 4.79 μg/mL, respectively. Milk levels varied between 0.05 and 0.17 μg/mL. Based on an ingested volume of 600 mL/day, the investigators estimated the infant would have received a daily dose of about 0.05 mg. However, no drug was detectable in the infant's serum. A second woman stopped nursing her 8-month-old infant when she was treated with piroxicam 40 mg/day (14). Milk concentrations of the drug ranged from 0.11 to 0.22 μg/mL, with the highest level measured 2.5 hours after the second dose. In both cases, the concentration of the drug in milk was approximately 1% of the mother's serum levels. These amounts probably do not present a risk to the nursing infant (15). The American Academy of Pediatrics classifies piroxicam as compatible with breast-feeding (16).

References

1. Product information. Feldene. Pfizer, 2001.
2. Sakai T, Ofsuki I, Noguchi F. Reproduction studies on piroxicam. Yakuri to Chiryo 1980;8:4655–71. As cited in Shepard TH. *Catalog of Teratogenic Agents*. 6th ed. Baltimore, MD: Johns Hopkins University Press, 1989:513.
3. Perraud J, Stadler J, Kessedjian MJ, Monro AM. Reproductive studies with the anti-inflammatory agent, piroxicam: modification of classical protocols. Toxicology 1984;30:59–63.
4. Nielsen GL, Sorensen HT, Larsen H, Pedersen L. Risk of adverse birth outcome and miscarriage in pregnant users of non-steroidal anti-inflammatory drugs: population based observational study and case-control study. BMJ 2001;322:266–70.
5. Ericson A, Kallen BAJ. Nonsteroidal anti-inflammatory drugs in early pregnancy. Reprod Toxicol 2001;15:371–5.
6. Li DK, Liu L, Odouli R. Exposure to non-steroidal anti-inflammatory drugs during pregnancy and risk of miscarriage: population based cohort study. BMJ 2003;327:368–71.
7. Tassinari MS, Cook JC, Hurtt ME. NSAIDs and developmental toxicity. Birth Defects Res Part B Dev Reprod Toxicol 2003;68:3–49.
8. Levin DL. Effects of inhibition of prostaglandin synthesis on fetal development, oxygenation, and the fetal circulation. Semin Perinatol 1980;4:35–44.
9. Van Marter LJ, Leviton A, Allred EN, Pagano M, Sullivan KF, Cohen A, Epstein MF. Persistent pulmonary hypertension of the newborn and smoking and aspirin and nonsteroidal antiinflammatory drug consumption during pregnancy. Pediatrics 1996;97:658–63.
10. Fuchs F. Prevention of prematurity. Am J Obstet Gynecol 1976;126:809–20.
11. Powell JG, Cochrane RL. The effects of a number of

non-steroidal anti-inflammatory compounds on parturition in the rat. Prostaglandins 1982;23:469–88.
12. Matt DW, Borzelleca JF. Toxic effects on the female reproductive system during pregnancy, parturition, and lactation. In Witorsch RJ, ed. *Reproductive Toxicology*. 2nd ed. New York, NY: Raven Press, 1995:175–93.
13. Dawood MY. Nonsteroidal antiinflammatory drugs and reproduction. Am J Obstet Gynecol 1993;169:1255–65.
14. Ostensen M. Piroxicam in human breast milk. Eur J Clin Pharmacol 1983;25:829–30.
15. Ostensen M, Husby G. Antirheumatic drug treatment during pregnancy and lactation. Scand J Rheumatol 1985;14:1–7.
16. Committee on Drugs, American Academy of Pediatrics. The transfer of drugs and other chemicals into human milk. Pediatrics 2001;108:776–89.

Name: **PLICAMYCIN** — Risk Factor: X_M
Class: **Antineoplastic**

FETAL RISK SUMMARY

RECOMMENDATION: Contraindicated - 1st Trimester

No reports on the use of plicamycin (formerly named mithramycin) during pregnancy have been located. Occupational exposure of the mother to antineoplastic agents during pregnancy may present a risk to the fetus. A position statement from the National Study Commission on Cytotoxic Exposure and a research article involving some antineoplastic agents are presented in the monograph for cyclophosphamide (see Cyclophosphamide).

BREAST FEEDING SUMMARY

RECOMMENDATION: Contraindicated

No data are available.

Name: **PODOFILOX** — Risk Factor: C_M
Class: **Keratolytic Agent**

FETAL RISK SUMMARY

RECOMMENDATION: Contraindicated

Podofilox (podophyllotoxin) is the active compound in podophyllum resin. No teratogenicity was observed in pregnant rabbits after once daily topical use for 13 days at doses up to five times the maximum human dose (1).

See Podophyllum.

BREAST FEEDING SUMMARY

RECOMMENDATION: No Human Data - Potential Toxicity

No data are available.

Reference

1. Product information. Condylox. Oclassen Pharmaceuticals, 2000.

Name:	**PODOPHYLLUM**	Risk Factor:	**C**
Class:	**Keratolytic Agent**		

FETAL RISK SUMMARY

RECOMMENDATION: Contraindicated

Podophyllum is the dried rhizomes and roots of *Podophyllum peltatum* (American mandrake, May apple) (1). Podophyllum resin is the dried mixture of resins extracted from podophyllum (1). Podophyllotoxin (podofilox), the major active compound in podophyllum resin, and podophyllum are keratolytic agents whose caustic action is thought to be caused by the arrest of mitosis in metaphase. In addition to its antimitotic effect, podophyllum also has cathartic action, but should not be used for this purpose because of the potential for severe drug-induced toxicity (2).

Three reproductive studies in rats and mice with podophyllum or podophyllotoxin found no teratogenic effects, but resorptions occurred when the agents were used early in gestation (3–5). A 1952 study observed no teratogenic changes in mice, rats, and rabbits with podophyllotoxin (6). Two other studies involving podophyllum reported embryotoxicity, but not teratogenicity, in mice (7) and only minor skeletal changes in rats (8). Another agent derived from *P. peltatum* that is present in podophyllum resin, peltatin (α and β forms), was not teratogenic in mice (9).

The first report of human teratogenicity related to podophyllum appeared in 1962 (10). A 24-year-old woman took herbal "slimming tablets," containing podophyllum and other extracts, from the 5th to 9th weeks of gestation, a total of 3.5 weeks. The estimated daily dose of podophyllum was 180 mg. The term, female infant had multiple anomalies, including an absent right thumb and radius, a supernumerary left thumb, a probable septal defect of the heart, a defect of the right external ear, and skin tags. The malformations were attributed to the antimitotic action of podophyllum (10).

In contrast to the above outcome, a woman at 26 weeks' gestation was treated with multiple applications of 20% podophyllum resin in compound benzoin tincture for condylomata acuminata (genital human papillomavirus infection) that covered the entire vulva, the minor and major labia, and a portion of the vagina (11). In addition, the woman was accidentally given 5 mL of the preparation orally, a potentially fatal dose. Toxic symptoms in the mother included persistent, severe coughing, nausea and vomiting, and hypotension, all of which had resolved within 72 hours. Three months later, the mother delivered a normal, 3560-g, male infant who was doing well.

A 1972 report described severe peripheral neuropathy and intrauterine fetal death in a woman at either 32 or 34 weeks' (both dates were used) gestation following the administration of 7.5 mL (1.88 g of podophyllum) of 25% podophyllum resin to florid vulval warts that were friable and bled easily (12). General anesthesia (nitrous oxide and oxygen) was used during application of podophyllum. Fetal heart sounds were lost 2 days after the application of podophyllum, and 10 days later a stillborn female infant was delivered. The woman's symptoms and death of her fetus were attributed to podophyllum poisoning, apparently from systemic absorption of the drug. She eventually recovered, and within a year or two, she had an uneventful pregnancy and normal infant.

Minor congenital malformations consisting of a simian crease on the left hand and a preauricular skin tag were observed in a newborn whose mother had been treated with five applications of 25% podophyllum resin between the 23rd and 29th weeks of pregnancy for condyloma acuminata (13). Although the authors attributed the skin tag to the drug, podophyllum was not related to either anomaly because of the late timing of exposure (14).

The Collaborative Perinatal Project recorded 14 1st trimester exposures to podophyllum (presumably oral) among 50 mothers who had used a group of miscellaneous gastrointestinal drugs (15). From this group, 1 (2%) infant with an unspecified congenital malformation was observed (standardized relative risk 0.27). It was not stated whether podophyllum was taken by the mother of the affected infant.

In summary, although it is uncertain whether podophyllum is a human teratogen, products containing this drug should not be used during pregnancy for the treatment of genital warts (human papillomavirus infections) because of the potential severe myelotoxicity and neurotoxicity in the mother. Although one author believes the topical application of podophyllum resin is safe during pregnancy (16), most other sources consider it a dangerous agent to use during this period, especially because of the availability of alternative, safer treatments. The American College of Obstetricians and Gynecologists (17) and other reviews (18) and reference sources (1) all state that the drug is contraindicated during pregnancy. The contraindication to the use of podophyllum agents includes the use of podophyllotoxin (i.e., podofilox) during pregnancy and on the vagina or cervix at any time (17).

BREAST FEEDING SUMMARY

RECOMMENDATION: No Human Data - Potential Toxicity

No data are available.

References

1. American Hospital Formulary Service. *Drug Information 1997*. Bethesda, MD: American Society of Health-System Pharmacists, 1997:2754–5.
2. Rosenstein G, Rosenstein H, Freeman M, Weston N. Podophyllum—a dangerous laxative. Pediatrics 1976;57:419–21.
3. Wiesner BP, Yudkin J. Control of fertility by antimitotic agents. Nature (London) 1955;176:249–50. As cited in Shepard TH. *Catalog of Teratogenic Agents*. 7th ed. Baltimore, MD: Johns Hopkins University Press, 1992:322.
4. Thiersch JB. Effects of podophyllin (P) and podophyllotoxin (PT) on the rat litter in utero. Proc Soc Exp Biol Med 1963;113:124–7. As cited in Shepard TH. *Catalog of Teratogenic Agents*. 7th ed. Baltimore, MD: Johns Hopkins University Press, 1992:322.
5. Chaube S, Murphy ML. The teratogenic effects of the recent drugs active in cancer chemotherapy. In Woollam DHM, ed. *Advances in Teratology*. New York, NY: Logos and Academic Press, 1968;3:181–237. As cited in Shepard TH. *Catalog of Teratogenic Agents*. 7th ed. Baltimore, MD: Johns Hopkins University Press, 1992:322.
6. Didcock KA, Picard CW, Robson JM. The action of podophyllotoxin on pregnancy. J Physiol (London) 1952;117:65P–6P. As cited in Schardein JL. *Chemically Induced Birth Defects*. 2nd ed. New York, NY: Marcel Dekker, 1993:491.
7. Joneja MG, LeLiever WC. Effects of vinblastine and podophyllin on DBA mouse fetuses. Toxicol Appl Pharmacol 1974;27:408–14. As cited in Schardein JL. *Chemically Induced Birth Defects*. 2nd ed. New York, NY: Marcel Dekker, 1993:446.
8. Dwornik JJ, Moore KL. Congenital anomalies produced in the rat by podophyllin. Anat Rec 1967;157:237. As cited in Schardein JL. *Chemically Induced Birth Defects*. 2nd ed. New York, NY: Marcel Dekker, 1993:446.
9. Wiesner BP, Wolfe M, Yudkin J. The effects of some antimitotic compounds on pregnancy in the mouse. Stud Fertil 1958;9:129–36. As cited in Schardein JL. *Chemically Induced Birth Defects*. 2nd ed. New York, NY: Marcel Dekker, 1993:805.
10. Cullis JE. Congenital deformities and herbal "slimming tablets." Lancet 1962;2:511–2.
11. Balucani M, Zellers DD. Podophyllum resin poisoning with complete recovery. JAMA 1964;189:639–40.
12. Chamberlain MJ, Reynolds AL, Yeoman WB. Toxic effect of podophyllum application in pregnancy. Br Med J 1972;3:391–2.
13. Karol MD, Conner CS, Watanabe AS, Murphrey KJ. Podophyllum: suspected teratogenicity from topical application. Clin Toxicol 1980;16:283–6.
14. Fraser FC. Letter to the editor. Mod Med Canada 1981;36:1508.
15. Heinonen OP, Slone D, Shapiro S. *Birth Defects and Drugs in Pregnancy*. Littleton, MA: Publishing Sciences Group, 1977:385.

P

16. Bargman H. Is podophyllin a safe drug to use and can it be used during pregnancy? Arch Dermatol 1988;124:1718–20.
17. American College of Obstetricians and Gynecologists. Genital human papillomavirus infections. *Technical Bulletin*, No. 193, June 1994.
18. Patsner B, Baker DA, Orr JW Jr. Human papillomavirus genital tract infections during pregnancy. Clin Obstet Gynecol 1990;33:258–67.

Name:	**POLYMYXIN B**	Risk Factor:	**B**
Class:	**Antibiotic**		

FETAL RISK SUMMARY

RECOMMENDATION: Compatible (Topical)

No reports linking the use of polymyxin B with congenital defects have been located. Although available for injection, polymyxin B is used almost exclusively by topical administration. In one study, seven exposures were recorded in the 1st trimester (1). No association with congenital defects was observed.

BREAST FEEDING SUMMARY

RECOMMENDATION: Compatible (Topical)

No data are available.

Reference

1. Heinonen OP, Slone D, Shapiro S. *Birth Defects and Drugs in Pregnancy*. Littleton, MA: Publishing Sciences Group, 1977:297.

Name:	**POLYTHIAZIDE**	Risk Factor:	**C***
Class:	**Diuretic**		

FETAL RISK SUMMARY

RECOMMENDATION: No Human Data - Probably Compatible

Polythiazide is a thiazide diuretic. In general, diuretics are not recommended for the treatment of gestational hypertension because of the maternal hypovolemia characteristic of this disease. See Chlorothiazide.

[**Risk Factor D if used in gestational hypertension.*]

BREAST FEEDING SUMMARY

RECOMMENDATION: No Human Data - Probably Compatible

See Chlorothiazide.

Name:	**POTASSIUM CHLORIDE**	Risk Factor:	**A**
Class:	**Electrolyte**		

FETAL RISK SUMMARY

RECOMMENDATION: Compatible

Potassium chloride is a natural constituent of human tissues and fluids. Exogenous potassium chloride may be indicated as replacement therapy for pregnant women with low serum potassium levels, such as those receiving diuretics. Because high or low levels are detrimental to maternal and fetal cardiac function, serum levels should be closely monitored.

In a surveillance study of Michigan Medicaid recipients conducted between 1985 and 1992 involving 229,101 completed pregnancies, 35 newborns had been exposed to oral potassium salts during the 1st trimester (F. Rosa, personal communication, FDA, 1993). One (2.9%) infant with major birth defects was observed (one expected), a case of limb reduction and hypospadias.

BREAST FEEDING SUMMARY

RECOMMENDATION: Compatible

Human milk is naturally low in potassium (1). If maternal serum levels are maintained in a physiologic range, no harm will result in the nursing infant from the administration of potassium chloride to the mother.

Reference

1. Wilson JT. Production and characteristics of breast milk. In Wilson JT, ed. *Drugs in Breast Milk*. Balgowlah, Australia: ADIS Press, 1981:12.

Name:	**POTASSIUM CITRATE**	Risk Factor:	**A**
Class:	**Electrolyte**		

See Potassium Chloride.

Name:	**POTASSIUM GLUCONATE**	Risk Factor:	**A**
Class:	**Electrolyte**		

See Potassium Chloride.

Name:	**POTASSIUM IODIDE**	Risk Factor:	**D**
Class:	**Respiratory Drug (Expectorant)**		

FETAL RISK SUMMARY

RECOMMENDATION: Human Data Suggest Risk in 2nd and 3rd Trimesters

The primary concern with the use of potassium iodide and the anti-infective, iodine, during pregnancy relates to the effect of iodide on the fetal thyroid gland. Because aqueous solutions of iodine are in equilibrium with the ionized form, all iodide or iodine products are considered as one group.

Iodide readily crosses the placenta to the fetus (1). When used for prolonged periods or close to term, iodide may cause hypothyroidism and goiter in the fetus and newborn. Short-term use, such as a 10-day preparation course for maternal thyroid surgery, does not carry this risk and is apparently safe (2,3). A 1983 review tabulated 49 cases of congenital iodide goiter dating back to 1940 (66 references) (4). In 14 cases, the goiter was large enough to cause tracheal compression resulting in death. Cardiomegaly was present in 3 surviving newborns and in 1 of the fatalities. In a majority of the cases, exposure to the iodide as a result of maternal asthma treatment.

Four studies have shown the potential hazard resulting from the use of povidone-iodine during pregnancy (5–8). In each case, significant absorption of iodine occurred in the mother and fetus following topical, vaginal, or perineal use before delivery. Transient hypothyroidism was demonstrated in some newborns (5,8).

Because a large number of prescription and over-the-counter medications contain iodide or iodine, pregnant patients should consult with their physician before using these products. The American Academy of Pediatrics considers the use of iodides as expectorants during pregnancy to be contraindicated (9).

BREAST FEEDING SUMMARY

RECOMMENDATION: Limited Human Data - Probably Compatible

Iodide is concentrated in breast milk (4,10,11). In one report, a breast-feeding mother used povidone-iodine vaginal gel daily for 6 days without douching (10). Two days after stopping the gel, the mother noted an odor of iodine on the 7 1/2-month-old baby. The free iodide serum:milk ratio 1 day later was approximately 23:1. By day 7, the ratio had fallen to about 4:1 but then rose again on day 8 to 10:1. Serum and urine iodide levels in the infant were grossly elevated. No problems or alterations in thyroid tests were noted in the baby.

In a 2000 case report, a woman delivered a female infant at 29 weeks' gestation by cesarean section (11). An abscess of the abdominal wall 1 week after delivery was treated with IV antibiotics and iodine tampons (each tampon contained about 10.5 mg of iodine). Full breast-feeding of the infant was begun approximately 20 days after birth. At 29 days, neonatal hypothyroidism was diagnosed: thyroid-stimulating hormone (TSH) level 287.9 μU/mL (normal range 0.45–10.0 μU/mL). Iodine levels in the mother's milk and infant urine were 4410 μg/L (normal range 29–490 μg/L) and 3932 μg/L (normal $<$185 μg/L), respectively. At 32 days, iodine tampons and breast-feeding were stopped and the infant was given levothyroxine (25 μg/day). Six days later, thyroid function had normalized and breast-feeding was restarted. The infant's thyroid function remained normal over a 4-month follow-up period (11).

Use of povidone-iodine immediately before delivery as a topical anesthetic for epidural anesthesia or cesarean section produced iodine overload in newborn infants who were breast-fed as evidenced by increased neonatal TSH concentrations (12). Breast-fed infants had a 25- to 30-fold increase in the recall rate at screening for congenital hypothyroidism (TSH >50 mU/L) compared with bottle-fed infants.

The normal iodine content of human milk has been recently assessed (13). Mean iodide levels in 37 lactating women were 178 μg/L. This is approximately 4 times the recommended daily allowance (RDA) for infants. The RDA for iodine was based on the amount of iodine found in breast milk in earlier studies (13). The higher levels now are probably caused by dietary supplements of iodine (e.g., salt, bread, cow's milk). The significance to the nursing infant from the chronic ingestion of higher levels of iodine is not known. The American Academy of Pediatrics, although recognizing that the maternal use of iodides during lactation may affect the infant's thyroid activity by producing elevated iodine levels in breast milk, classifies the agents as compatible with breast-feeding (14).

References

1. Wolff J. Iodide goiter and the pharmacologic effects of excess iodide. Am J Med 1969;47:101–24.
2. Herbst AL, Selenkow HA. Hyperthyroidism during pregnancy. N Engl J Med 1965;273:627–33.
3. Selenkow HA, Herbst AL. Hyperthyroidism during pregnancy. N Engl J Med 1966;274:165–6.
4. Mehta PS, Mehta SJ, Vorherr H. Congenital iodide goiter and hypothyroidism: a review. Obstet Gynecol Surv 1983;38:237–47.
5. l'Allemand D, Gruters A, Heidemann P, Schurnbrand P. Iodine-induced alterations of thyroid function in newborn infants after prenatal and perinatal exposure to povidone iodine. J Pediatr 1983;102: 935–8.
6. Bachrach LK, Burrow GN, Gare DJ. Maternal-fetal absorption of povidone-iodine. J Pediatr 1984;104: 158–9.
7. Jacobson JM, Hankins GV, Young RL, Hauth JC. Changes in thyroid function and serum iodine levels after prepartum use of a povidone-iodine vaginal lubricant. J Reprod Med 1984;29:98–100.
8. Danziger Y, Pertzelan A, Mimouni M. Transient congenital hypothyroidism after topical iodine in pregnancy and lactation. Arch Dis Child 1987;62: 295–6.
9. Committee on Drugs. American Academy of Pediatrics. Adverse reactions to iodide therapy of asthma and other pulmonary diseases. Pediatrics 1976;57:272–4.
10. Postellon DC, Aronow R. Iodine in mother's milk. JAMA 1982;247:463.
11. Casteels K, Punt S, Bramswig J. Transient neonatal hypothyroidism during breast-feeding after postnatal maternal topical iodine treatment. Eur J Pediatr 2000;159:716–7.
12. Chanoine JP, Boulvain M, Bourdoux P, Pardou A, Van Thi HV, Ermans AM, Delange F. Increased recall rate at screening for congenital hypothyroidism in breast-fed infants born to iodine overloaded mothers. Arch Dis Child 1988;63:1207–10.
13. Gushurst CA, Mueller JA, Green JA, Sedor F. Breast milk iodide: reassessment in the 1980s. Pediatrics 1984;73:354–7.
14. Committee on Drugs, American Academy of Pediatrics. The transfer of drugs and other chemicals into human milk. Pediatrics 2001;108:776–89.

P

Name:	**POVIDONE-IODINE**	Risk Factor:	**D**
Class:	**Anti-infective**		

See Potassium Iodide.

Name:	**PRALIDOXIME**	Risk Factor:	**C_M**
Class:	**Antidote**		

FETAL RISK SUMMARY

RECOMMENDATION: Compatible - Maternal Benefit >> Embryo/Fetal Risk

Pralidoxime (2-PAM) reactivates cholinesterase (mainly outside of the central nervous system) that has been inactivated by phosphorylation because of an organophosphate pesticide or related compound. Its most critical effect is relieving the paralysis of the muscles of respiration. Pralidoxime is short-acting (apparent half-life 74–77 minutes) and is not bound to plasma proteins. Pralidoxime is available in an auto-injector that can be used rapidly in cases of exposure to nerve agents possessing anticholinesterase activity (organophosphate poisoning) (1).

Animal reproduction studies have not been conducted with pralidoxime.

It is not known if pralidoxime crosses the human placenta to the embryo or fetus. Pralidoxime chloride is a quaternary ammonium compound, but the molecular weight of the free base (about 137) is low enough for passage across the placenta. The rapid elimination of the drug, however, should mitigate this transfer.

A 1988 report described the pregnancy outcomes of two women who were treated with pralidoxime for self-induced organophosphorus insecticide poisoning (2). In the first case, a 22-year-old primigravida at 36 weeks' gestation was admitted to the hospital 3 hours after ingesting methamidophos. She was treated with pralidoxime and atropine and eventually recovered. Forty-four days after poisoning, she delivered a healthy 2.85-kg male infant with an Apgar score of 8 at 1 minute. The second case involved a 25-year-old woman at 16 weeks' gestation who ingested fenthion. She also was treated with pralidoxime and atropine and made a full recovery. She delivered a healthy 3.83-kg infant (Apgar 10 at 1 minute) 24 weeks after intoxication (2).

In summary, reproduction studies with pralidoxime have not been conducted and the human pregnancy experience is limited to two cases. No other reports describing the use of this drug in human pregnancy have been located. Although the risk this agent represents in pregnancy cannot be assessed, the maternal benefit clearly outweighs any concern regarding embryo or fetal toxicity. Therefore, pralidoxime should not be withheld because of pregnancy.

BREAST FEEDING SUMMARY

RECOMMENDATION: Hold Breast Feeding

No reports describing the use of pralidoxime during lactation have been located. Pralidoxime chloride is a quaternary ammonium compound, but the molecular weight of the free base (about 137) is low enough for excretion into breast milk. The rapid elimination of the drug, however, should mitigate this transfer into milk. Moreover, the emergency nature of its use suggests that nursing is unlikely when it has been used. In any event, the maternal benefit is clear and breast-feeding should be held for at least 6–7 hours (about five half-lives) after a dose is given.

References

1. Product information. Pralidoxime Chloride Injection (Auto-Injector). Meridian Medical Technologies, 2002.
2. Karalliedde L, Senanayake N, Ariaratnam A. Acute organophosphorus insecticide poisoning during pregnancy. Hum Toxicol 1988;7:363–4.

Name:	**PRAMIPEXOLE**	Risk Factor:	C_M
Class:	**Antiparkinsonian Agent**		

FETAL RISK SUMMARY

RECOMMENDATION: No Human Data - Animal Data Suggest Low Risk

Pramipexole is a nonergoline dopamine agonist indicated for the treatment of the signs and symptoms of idiopathic Parkinson disease. The drug has high specificity for the D2 and D3 receptor subtypes. Pramipexole undergoes little if any metabolism, and no metabolites in plasma or urine have been identified. The plasma protein binding of the agent is low (about 15%) and the elimination half-life, in young healthy adults, is about 8 hours. Pramipexole is commonly used in combination with levodopa.

Reproduction studies have been conducted in rats and rabbits. In pregnant rats given pramipexole throughout gestation, a dose 5.4 times the highest recommended human clinical dose (1.5 mg three times daily) based on body surface area (HRHCD) inhibited implantation. A lower dose (3.2 times the HRHCD), administered during organogenesis, caused a high incidence of total resorptions. At this dose, the AUC was 4.3 times the AUC of adults taking 1.5 mg three times daily. These adverse effects were thought to be secondary to the prolactin-lowering effect of the drug and prevented an adequate evaluation of the teratogenic potential of pramipexole (1). Prolactin is required for implantation and pregnancy maintenance in rats but not in rabbits or humans. Offspring postnatal growth was inhibited when pramipexole, at doses approximately equal to the HRHCD or higher, was given to rats during the latter half of pregnancy and throughout lactation. In pregnant rabbits treated during organogenesis with doses 71 times the AUC of adults taking 1.5 mg three times daily, no evidence of adverse effects on embryo or fetal development was observed.

In a 2-year carcinogenicity study in mice, dietary administration of pramipexole, at doses up to 11 times the HRHCD, was not associated with a significant increase in tumors. A similar study in rats, at doses up to 12.5 times the AUC of adults taking 1.5 mg three times daily, also was negative for tumors (1).

It is not known if pramipexole crosses the human placenta. The low molecular weight (about 302; 211 for the free base), low protein binding, and prolonged elimination half-life, however, suggest that the drug will cross to the embryo and fetus.

No reports describing the use of pramipexole during human pregnancy have been located. The limited animal data do not suggest a significant risk for teratogenicity or toxicity. The toxicity observed in rats apparently was caused by mechanisms not present in human pregnancy. However, the complete absence of human pregnancy experience prevents an assessment of the human risk. Since Parkinson disease is relatively uncommon during the childbearing years, the use of pramipexole during pregnancy also will be uncommon. Until data on such use are available, the safest course is to avoid, if possible, the use of pramipexole during the 1st trimester.

BREAST FEEDING SUMMARY

RECOMMENDATION: No Human Data - Potential Toxicity

No reports describing the use of pramipexole during human lactation have been located. Pramipexole is excreted into the milk of lactating rats (1). This is consistent with its low molecular weight (about 211 for the free base) and low protein binding (about 15%). Probably secondary to ion trapping (milk is slightly acidic compared with the plasma), the drug accumulated in rat milk (milk:plasma ratio 3–6:1) (1). Excretion into human breast milk, with possibly accumulation, also should be expected. The effects, if any, of this exposure on a nursing infant are unknown. Infants should be monitored for adverse events commonly observed in adults, such as extrapyramidal disorders (e.g., dyskinesia), hallucinations, somnolence, nausea, and constipation. Pramipexole inhibits prolactin secretion and may inhibit lactation. Until data on its safe use are available, pramipexole should not be used during lactation.

Reference

1. Product information. Mirapex. Pharmacia & Upjohn, 2003.

Name:	**PRAMOXINE**	Risk Factor:	**C_M**
Class:	**Local Anesthetic**		

FETAL RISK SUMMARY

RECOMMENDATION: Compatible

Pramoxine is a local anesthetic used for topical anesthesia. It is administered either alone or combined with hydrocortisone or other ingredients for the temporary relief of pain and itching secondary to minor skin irritations resulting from burns, sunburn, cuts, abrasions, insect bites, and hemorrhoids and other anorectal disorders. Pramoxine is typically formulated in a 1% concentration. Animal reproduction studies with pramoxine have not been conducted.

The molecular weight of pramoxine (about 294 for the free base) is low enough to cross the placenta, but the amount, if any, that is absorbed after topical administration into the systemic circulation is unknown. A 1985 review stated that pramoxine and similar anorectal products were not absorbed (1). However, even if some were absorbed systemically, the maternal plasma concentration would be very low and thus, the amount available for transfer to the embryo or fetus should be negligible.

Even though no studies describing the use of pramoxine during animal or human pregnancy have been located (1,2), because symptomatic hemorrhoids occur frequently in pregnancy, products containing pramoxine probably have been used during gestation. Because there is insignificant systemic absorption, there does not appear to be a risk to the embryo or fetus from pramoxine.

BREAST FEEDING SUMMARY

RECOMMENDATION: No Human Data - Probably Compatible

No studies describing the use of pramoxine during lactation have been located. The molecular weight of the free base (about 294) is low enough for excretion into breast milk, but the drug is not thought to be absorbed (1). Even if some absorption does occur, the amount in the maternal plasma should be very low so that little, if any, drug would appear in milk. The risk to a nursing infant is probably nil.

References

1. Lewis JH, Weingold AB, The Committee on FDA-Related Matters, American College of Gastroenterology. The use of gastrointestinal drugs during pregnancy and lactation. Am J Gastroenterol 1985;80:912–23.
2. Friedman JM. Teratogen update: anesthetic agents. Teratology 1988;37:69–77.

Name: **PRAVASTATIN**
Class: **Antilipemic Agent**
Risk Factor: **X_M**

FETAL RISK SUMMARY

RECOMMENDATION: Contraindicated

Pravastatin is used to lower elevated levels of cholesterol. It is a hepatic 3-hydroxy-3-methylglutaryl-coenzyme A [HMG-CoA] reductase inhibitor ("statin") similar to other agents in this class (atorvastatin, cerivastatin, fluvastatin, lovastatin, and simvastatin). Pravastatin is structurally related to lovastatin and simvastatin but, in contrast to the lipophilic properties of these agents, it is hydrophilic.

Pravastatin was not teratogenic in rats and rabbits administered doses up to 240 times and 20 times, respectively, the human exposure based on surface area (HE) (1). Similarly, no adverse effects on fertility or reproductive performance were observed in rats with doses up to 120 times the HE (1).

The Food and Drug Administration has received a single report of a fetal loss in a mother taking pravastatin, but further details are not available (F. Rosa, personal communication, FDA, 1995).

In a 2004 case report, a 39-year-old woman took pravastatin (80 mg/day), metformin (2 g/day), and nateglinide (360 mg/day) during the first 24 weeks of gestation (2). All therapy was discontinued and insulin was started for her diabetes. At term, the woman delivered a healthy 2.4-kg male infant (head circumference 34 cm, length 46 cm) with Apgar scores of 8 and 9 at 1 and 5 minutes, respectively. The infant's growth and development were normal at follow-up examinations during the first 6 months of life (2).

A 2004 report described the outcomes of pregnancy that had been exposed to statins and reported to the FDA (see Lovastatin).

Because the interruption of cholesterol-lowering therapy during pregnancy should have no effect on the long-term treatment of hyperlipidemia, and because of the human data reported with lovastatin, the use of pravastatin is contraindicated during pregnancy. However, evidence suggesting that pravastatin has a lower risk of developmental toxicity because of its hydrophilic properties has been published (see Lovastatin). If pravastatin is used in pregnancy, healthcare professionals are encouraged to call the toll free number (800-670-6126) for information about patient enrollment in the Motherisk study.

BREAST FEEDING SUMMARY

RECOMMENDATION: Contraindicated

No reports describing the use of pravastatin during lactation have been located. The manufacturer reports that pravastatin is excreted into breast milk in small amounts (1). Because of the potential for adverse effects in the nursing infant, the drug should not be used during lactation.

References

1. Product information. Pravachol. Bristol-Myers Squibb, 2000.
2. Teelucksingh S, Youssef JE, Sohan K, Ramsewak S. Prolonged inadvertent pravastatin use in pregnancy. Reprod Toxicol 2004;18:299–300.

Name:	**PRAZIQUANTEL**	Risk Factor:	B_M
Class:	**Anthelmintic**		

FETAL RISK SUMMARY

RECOMMENDATION: Limited Human Data - Animal Data Suggest Moderate Risk

Praziquantel is a systemic anthelmintic used in the treatment of parasitic infections involving cestodes (tapeworms), including neurocysticercosis, and trematode (flukes) infestations of the liver and other tissues. The drug is rapidly and nearly completely (80%) absorbed following oral administration (1). The various metabolites are excreted primarily by the kidneys.

Praziquantel was not carcinogenic in rats and hamsters but mutagenic effects in Salmonella tests were observed in one laboratory (1). The mutagenicity was not confirmed in the same tested strain by other laboratories (1). Similarly, a study published in 1982 found no mutagenic effects in five strains of Salmonella exposed to praziquantel (2). A 1984 review also described negative mutagenic results in a variety of tests, including those with mice, rats, and humans, and negative carcinogenic results in tests with rats and hamsters (3). A 1997 review, however, cited studies that observed a co-mutagenic effect between praziquantel and several mutagens and carcinogens (4). Praziquantel has also been shown in *in vitro* studies to induce micronuclei in hamster embryonic cells and lymphocytes (4). Moreover, in some pigs and humans, praziquantel was found to induce hyperploid lymphocytes and structural chromosomal aberrations (4).

Reproduction studies in mice, rats, and rabbits at doses up to 40 times the human dose (human dose 60–75 mg/kg over 1 day) showed no evidence of impaired fertility or teratogenicity (1,3). An increase in the abortion rate in rats, however, was observed at doses 3 times the single human therapeutic dose (1). No teratogenicity was observed in other studies in rats and rabbits with doses up to 300 mg/kg (5,6) or in rats with doses up to 450 mg/kg (2). Compared with controls, the administration of praziquantel and ivermectin (another anthelmintic agent) to possums at 8- to 10-week intervals throughout the breeding season to the time of emergence of young from the pouch had no significant effect on the number of births or survival of the young to emergence (7).

Authors of a study published in 1985 concluded that treatment of parasitic disease with potentially teratogenic or toxic drugs might not always be indicated in otherwise healthy pregnant women (8). For example, in their study, they found that treatment of some gastrointestinal parasites, including some tapeworms and liver flukes, could be postponed until after delivery unless the parasite was causing clinical disease or public health problems (8). Similarly, reviews in 1996 and 1997 recommended avoiding praziquantel during pregnancy (9,10).

The authors are aware of two cases of neurocysticercosis treated with praziquantel during gestation, but no outcome information is available in either case. A 1996 case report, however, described the use of praziquantel for the treatment of neurocysticercosis in a 17-year-old pregnant woman (11). She received praziquantel, 1050 mg 3 times daily, for 21 days starting at about 8 weeks' gestation. Seizures, which occurred at the time of presentation and again 4 days after the start of anticysticercus therapy, were successfully controlled with phenytoin and carbamazepine. She eventually delivered a 2.5-kg girl at term. Other than documented anemia, no other abnormalities or malformations were found. The placenta appeared normal on gross examination.

In summary, praziquantel is not an animal teratogen, but human data are limited to one case. The lack of published human data prevents any assessment of a human risk. Recent data have indicated that the agent may be mutagenic and carcinogenic in humans, especially in developing countries where infections of trematodes and cestodes are frequent and multiple treatment courses may be prescribed. Moreover, the presence of other environmental mutagens combined with praziquantel may increase the risk for mutagenicity (4). Because of this potential toxicity, the use of praziquantel during pregnancy should be reserved for those cases in which the parasite is causing clinical illness or public health problems.

BREAST FEEDING SUMMARY

RECOMMENDATION: No Human Data - Potential Toxicity

Because praziquantel is excreted into breast milk at a concentration of about one-fourth that of the maternal serum, the manufacturer advises holding nursing on the day of treatment and during the subsequent 72 hours (1). The drug is excreted primarily in the urine with 80% of the dose being eliminated within 4 days (12). About 90% of this elimination, however, occurs in the first 24 hours (12).

No reports describing the use of praziquantel during nursing have been located, but a 1996 review recommended avoiding praziquantel during lactation (9). The effects, if any, on a healthy, noninfected nursing infant from exposure to the drug via breast milk are unknown. Because adverse reactions induced by the death of an infecting parasite have been observed in treated adults (7), nursing infants with parasitic infections sensitive to praziquantel may be at risk for similar adverse effects. Moreover, the potential for mutagenic and carcinogenic effects of the drug should be considered (see Fetal Risk Summary).

References

1. Product information. Biltricide. Bayer Corporation, 1999.
2. Ni YC, Shao BR, Zhan CQ, Xu YQ, Ha SH, Jiao PY. Mutagenic and teratogenic effects of anti-schistosomal praziquantel. Chin Med J 1982;95:494–8.
3. Frohberg H. Results of toxicological studies on praziquantel. Arzneimittelforschung 1984;34:1137–44.
4. Montero R, Ostrosky P. Genotoxic activity of praziquantel. Mutat Res 1997;387:123–39.
5. Muermann P, Von Eberstein M, Frohberg H. Notes on the tolerance of Droncit. Summary of trial results. Ved Med Rev 1976;2:142–65. As cited by Schardein JL. *Chemical Induced Birth Defects*. 2nd ed. New York, NY: Marcel Dekker, 1993:402–15.
6. Muermann P, Von Eberstein M, Frohberg H. Notes on the tolerance of Droncit. Summary of trial results. Vet Med Rev 1976;2:142–65. As cited by Shepard TH. *Catalog of Teratogenic Agents*. 8th ed. Baltimore, MD: Johns Hopkins University Press, 1995:350.
7. Viggers KL, Lindenmayer DB, Cunningham RB, Donnelly CF. The effects of parasites on a wild population of the Mountain Brushtail possum (*Trichosurus caninus*) in south-eastern Australia. Int J Parasitol 1998;28:747–55.
8. D'Alauro F, Lee RV, Pao-In K, Khairallah M. Intestinal parasites and pregnancy. Obstet Gynecol 1985;66:639–43.
9. Volkheimer G. Intestinal helminthiasis-general practice problem of the gastroenterologist. Z Gastroenterol 1996;34:534–41.
10. de Silva N, Guyatt H, Bundy D. Anthelmintics. A

P

comparative review of their clinical pharmacology. Drugs 1997;53:769–88.
11. Paparone PW, Menghetti RA. Case report: neurocysticercosis in pregnancy. N J Med 1996;93:91–4.
12. Reynolds JEF, editor. *Martindale. The Extra Pharmacopoeia*. 31st ed. London, England: Royal Pharmaceutical Society, 1996:123–5.

Name:	**PRAZOSIN**	Risk Factor:	**C**
Class:	**Sympatholytic (Antihypertensive)**		

FETAL RISK SUMMARY

RECOMMENDATION: Limited Human Data - Animal Data Suggest Low Risk

Prazosin is an α_1-adrenergic blocking agent used for hypertension. No evidence of teratogenicity was observed in reproduction studies with rats, rabbits, and monkeys at doses more than 225, 225, and 12 times, respectively, the usual maximum recommended human dose (1). A decreased litter size at birth in rats, however, was observed at the maximum dose.

The molecular weight of prazosin (about 384 for the free base) is low enough that transfer across the placenta to the fetus is likely. Consistent with this, a 1995 study using a 5-mg delayed release formulation in three women measured umbilical cord blood concentrations at delivery that were 9%–23% of the maternal plasma levels 8–15 hours after the last dose (2).

In two studies, prazosin was combined with oxprenolol or atenolol, β-adrenergic blockers, in the treatment of pregnant women with severe essential hypertension or gestational hypertension (3,4). The combinations were effective in the first group but less so in the patients with gestational hypertension. No adverse effects attributable to the drugs were noted. Prazosin, 20 mg/day, was combined with minoxidil and metoprolol throughout gestation to treat severe maternal hypertension secondary to chronic nephritis (5). The child, normal except for hypertrichosis as a result of minoxidil, was doing well at 2 years of age.

P

Prazosin has been used during the 3rd trimester in patients with pheochromocytoma (6,7). In one case, blood pressure was well controlled, but maternal tachycardia required the addition of a β-blocker. A healthy male infant was delivered by cesarean section (6).

A case report published in 1986 described the pregnancy of a 24-year-old woman at 30 weeks' gestation who was managed for recurrent pheochromocytoma with a combination of prazosin, metyrosine (a tyrosine hydroxylase inhibitor), and timolol (a β-adrenergic blocker) (7). Hypertension had been noted at her first prenatal visit at 12 weeks' gestation. Because of declines in fetal breathing, body movements, and amniotic fluid volume that began 2 weeks after the start of therapy, a cesarean section was conducted at 33 weeks' gestation. The 1450-g female infant had Apgar scores of 3 and 5 at 1 and 5 minutes, respectively. Mild metabolic acidosis was found on analysis of umbilical cord blood gases. Multiple infarcts were noted in the placenta but no evidence of metastatic tumor. The growth-retarded infant did well and was discharged home on day 53 of life (7).

BREAST FEEDING SUMMARY

RECOMMENDATION: Limited Human Data - Potential Toxicity

No reports describing the use of prazosin during lactation have been located. The manufacturer reports that small amounts are excreted into human milk (1). This is consistent with the relatively low molecular weight (about 384 for the free base) of the drug. The effects on a nursing infant from exposure to the drug from breast milk are unknown.

References

1. Product information. Minipress. Pfizer, 2000.
2. Bourget P, Fernandez H, Edouard D, Lesne-Hulin A, Ribou F, Baton-Saint-Mleux C, Lelaidier C. Disposition of a new rate-controlled formulation of prazosin in the treatment of hypertension during pregnancy: transplacental passage of prazosin. Eur J Drug Metab Pharmacokinet 1995;20:233–41.
3. Lubbe WF, Hodge JV. Combined alpha- and beta-adrenoceptor antagonism with prazosin and oxprenolol in control of severe hypertension in pregnancy. N Z Med J 1981;94:169–72.
4. Lubbe WF. More on beta-blockers in pregnancy. N Engl J Med 1982;307:753.
5. Rosa FW, Idanpaan-Heikkila J, Asanti R. Fetal minoxidil exposure. Pediatrics 1987;80:120.
6. Venuto R, Burstein P, Schneider R. Pheochromocytoma: antepartum diagnosis and management with tumor resection in the puerperium. Am J Obstet Gynecol 1984;150:431–2.
7. Devoe LD, O'Dell BE, Castillo RA, Hadi HA, Searle N. Metastatic pheochromocytoma in pregnancy and fetal biophysical assessment after maternal administration of alpha-adrenergic, beta-adrenergic, and dopamine antagonists. Obstet Gynecol 1986;68:15S–8S.

Name:	**PREDNISOLONE**	Risk Factor:	**C***
Class:	**Corticosteroid**		

FETAL RISK SUMMARY

RECOMMENDATION: Human Data Suggest Risk

Prednisolone is the biologically active form of prednisone (see Prednisone). The placenta can oxidize prednisolone to inactive prednisone or less active cortisone (see Cortisone).

[**Risk Factor D if used in 1st trimester.*]

BREAST FEEDING SUMMARY

RECOMMENDATION: Compatible

See Prednisone.

Name:	**PREDNISONE**	Risk Factor:	**C***
Class:	**Corticosteroid**		

FETAL RISK SUMMARY

RECOMMENDATION: Human Data Suggest Risk

Prednisone is metabolized to prednisolone. There are a number of studies in which pregnant patients received either prednisone or prednisolone (see also various antineoplastic agents for additional references) (1–14).

Although most reports describing the use of prednisone or prednisolone during gestation have not observed abnormal outcomes, four large epidemiologic studies have associated the use of corticosteroids in the 1st trimester with nonsyndromic orofacial clefts. Specific agents were not identified in three of these studies (see Hydrocortisone for details), but in one 1999 study, discussed below, the corticosteroids were listed.

In a case-control study, the California Birth Defects Monitoring Program evaluated the association between selected congenital anomalies and the use of corticosteroids 1 month before to 3 months after conception (periconceptional period) (15). Case infants or fetal deaths diagnosed with orofacial clefts, conotruncal defects, neural tubal defects (NTDs), and limb anomalies were identified from a total of 552,601 births that occurred from 1987 through the end of 1989. Controls, without birth defects, were selected from the same data base. Following exclusion of known genetic syndromes, mothers of case and control infants were interviewed by telephone, an average of 3.7 years (cases) or 3.8 years (controls) after delivery, to determine various exposures during the periconceptional period. The number of interviews completed were orofacial cleft case mothers ($N = 662$, 85% of eligible), conotruncal case mothers ($N = 207$, 87%), NTD case mothers ($N = 265$, 84%), limb anomaly case mothers ($N = 165$, 82%), and control mothers ($N = 734$, 78%) (15). Orofacial clefts were classified into four phenotypic groups: isolated cleft lip with or without cleft palate (ICLP, $N = 348$), isolated cleft palate (ICP, $N = 141$), multiple cleft lip with or without cleft palate (MCLP, $N = 99$), and multiple cleft palate (MCP, $N = 74$). A total of 13 mothers reported using corticosteroids during the periconceptional period for a wide variety of indications. Six case mothers of infants with ICLP and three of infants with ICP used corticosteroids (unspecified corticosteroid $N = 1$, prednisone $N = 2$, cortisone $N = 3$, triamcinolone acetonide $N = 1$, dexamethasone $N = 1$, and cortisone plus prednisone $N = 1$). One case mother of an infant with NTD used cortisone and an injectable unspecified corticosteroid, and three controls used corticosteroids (hydrocortisone $N = 1$ and prednisone $N = 2$). The odds ratio (OR) for corticosteroid use and ICLP was 4.3 (95% confidence interval [CI] 1.1–17.2), whereas the OR for ICP and corticosteroid use was 5.3 (95% CI 1.1–26.5). No increased risks were observed for the other anomaly groups. Commenting on their results, the investigators thought that recall bias was unlikely because they did not observe increased risks for other malformations, and it was also unlikely that the mothers would have known of the suspected association between corticosteroids and orofacial clefts (15).

A prospective cohort study and meta-analysis of corticosteroid use in pregnancy was reported in 2000 (16). In the prospective study, 187 outcomes (184 pregnancies, 3 sets of twins) exposed to prednisone were compared to the outcomes in 188 controls. Prednisone-exposed infants were delivered at a lower gestational age (38 vs. 39.5 weeks), had an increased rate of premature delivery (17% vs. 5%), and had a lower birth weight (3112 g vs. 3429 g) (all statistically significant). There was no significant difference in the rate of major birth defects (3.6% vs. 2%) and there was no cluster of malformations suggesting a common cause. The defects in the prednisone-exposed cases were Hirschsprung's disease; double-outlet right ventricle, valvar, and subvalvar pulmonary stenosis, hypothyroidism, hypospadias; undescended testicle; and cleft palate, hypospadias. Two cases were excluded from the analysis because the cause of the defects was known (genetic history and maternal infection) (16). In their meta-analysis, they found a small increase in major malformations (OR 3.03, 95% CI 1.08–8.54) for 1st trimester corticosteroid exposure (16). In addition, case-control studies showed a significant association with oral clefts (OR 3.35, 95% CI 1.97–5.69) (16).

In a surveillance study of Michigan Medicaid recipients conducted between 1985 and 1992 involving 229,101 completed pregnancies, 143, 236, and 222 newborns had been exposed to prednisolone, prednisone, and methylprednisolone, respectively, during the 1st trimester (F. Rosa, personal communication, FDA, 1993). The number of birth defects, the number expected, and the percent for each drug were 11/6 (7.7%), 11/10 (4.7%), and 14/9 (6.3%), respectively. Specific details were available for six defect categories (observed/expected): cardiovascular defects (2/1,2/2,3/2), oral clefts (0/0,0/0,0/0), spina bifida (0/0,0/0,0/0), polydactyly (0/0,0/1,0/1), limb reduction defects (0/0,0/0,1/0), and hypospadias (1/0,0/1,1/1), respectively. These data do not support an association between the drugs and congenital defects, except for a possible association between prednisolone and the total number of defects. In the latter case, other factors, such as the mother's disease, concurrent drug use, and chance may be involved.

Immunosuppression was observed in a newborn exposed to high doses of prednisone with azathioprine throughout gestation (17). The newborn had lymphopenia, decreased survival of lymphocytes in culture, absence of IgM, and reduced levels of IgG. Recovery occurred at 15 weeks of age. However, these effects were not observed in a larger group of similarly exposed newborns (18). A 1968 study reported an increase in the incidence of stillbirths following prednisone therapy during pregnancy (7). Increased fetal mortality has not been confirmed by other investigators.

An infant exposed to prednisone throughout pregnancy was born with congenital cataracts (1). The eye defect was consistent with reports of subcapsular cataracts observed in adults receiving corticosteroids. The relationship in this case between the cataracts and prednisone is unknown, but other reports have also described cataracts after corticosteroid use during gestation (see Hydrocortisone).

In a 1970 case report, a female infant with multiple deformities was described (19). Her father had been treated several years before conception with prednisone, azathioprine, and radiation for a kidney transplant. The authors speculated that the child's defects might have been related to the father's immunosuppressive therapy. A relationship to prednisone seems remote because previous studies have shown that the drug has no effect on chromosome number or morphology (20). High, prolonged doses of prednisolone (30 mg/day for at least 4 weeks) may damage spermatogenesis (21). Recovery may require 6 months after the drug is stopped.

Prednisone has been used successfully to prevent neonatal respiratory distress syndrome when premature delivery occurs between 28 and 36 weeks of gestation (22). Therapy between 16 and 25 weeks of gestation had no effect on lecithin:sphingomyelin ratios (23).

In summary, prednisone and prednisolone apparently pose a small risk to the developing fetus. One of these risks appears to be orofacial clefts. Although the available evidence supports their use to control various maternal diseases, the mother should be informed of this risk so that she can actively participate in the decision on whether to use these agents during her pregnancy. If prednisone (or prednisolone) is used in pregnancy for the treatment of rheumatoid arthritis, healthcare professionals are encouraged to call the toll free number (877-311-8972) for information about patient enrollment in the OTIS Rheumatoid Arthritis study.

[*Risk Factor D if used in 1st trimester.*]

BREAST FEEDING SUMMARY

RECOMMENDATION: Compatible

Trace amounts of prednisone and prednisolone have been measured in breast milk (24–27). Following a 10-mg oral dose of prednisone, milk concentrations of prednisone and prednisolone at 2 hours were 26.7 and 1.6 ng/mL, respectively (24). The authors estimated the infant would ingest approximately 28.3 μg in 1000 mL of milk. In a second study using radioactive-labeled prednisolone in seven patients, a mean of 0.14% of a 5-mg oral dose was recovered per liter of milk during 48–61 hours (25).

In six lactating women, prednisolone doses of 10–80 mg/day resulted in milk concentrations ranging from 5% to 25% of maternal serum levels (26). The milk:plasma ratio increased with increasing serum concentrations. For maternal doses of 20 mg 1–2 times daily, the authors concluded that the nursing infant would be exposed to minimal amounts of steroid. At higher doses, they recommended waiting at least 4 hours after a dose before nursing was performed. However, even at 80 mg/day, the nursing infant would ingest <0.1% of the dose, which corresponds to <10% of the infant's endogenous cortisol production (26).

A 1993 report described the pharmacokinetics of prednisolone in milk (27). Following a 50-mg IV dose, an average of 0.025% (range 0.010%–0.049%) was recovered from the milk. The data suggested a rapid, bidirectional transfer of unbound prednisolone between the milk and serum (27). The investigators concluded that the measured milk concentrations of the steroid did not pose a clinically significant risk to a nursing infant.

Although nursing infants were not involved in the above studies, it is doubtful whether the amounts measured are clinically significant. The American Academy of Pediatrics classifies prednisolone and prednisone as compatible with breast-feeding (28).

References

1. Kraus AM. Congenital cataract and maternal steroid injection. J Pediatr Ophthalmol 1975;12:107–8.
2. Durie BGM, Giles HR. Successful treatment of acute leukemia during pregnancy: Combination therapy in the third trimester. Arch Intern Med 1977;137:90–1.
3. Nolan GH, Sweet RL, Laros RK, Roure CA. Renal cadaver transplantation followed by successful pregnancies. Obstet Gynecol 1974;43:732–9.
4. Grossman JH III, Littner MR. Severe sarcoidosis in pregnancy. Obstet Gynecol 1977;50(Suppl):81s–4s.
5. Cutting HO, Collier TM. Acute lymphocytic leukemia during pregnancy: Report of a case. Obstet Gynecol 1964;24:941–5.
6. Hanson GC, Ghosh S. Systemic lupus erythematosus and pregnancy. Br Med J 1965;2:1227–8.
7. Warrell DW, Taylor R. Outcome for the foetus of mothers receiving prednisolone during pregnancy. Lancet 1968;1:117–8.
8. Walsh SD, Clark FR. Pregnancy in patients on long-term corticosteroid therapy. Scott Med J 1967;12: 302–6.
9. Zulman JI, Talal N, Hoffman GS, Epstein WV. Problems associated with the management of pregnancies in patients with systemic lupus erythematosus. J Rheumatol 1980;7:37–49.
10. Hartikainen-Sorri AL, Kaila J. Systemic lupus erythematosus and habitual abortion: Case report. Br J Obstet Gynaecol 1980;87:729–31.
11. Minchinton RM, Dodd NJ, O'Brien H, Amess JAL, Waters AH. Autoimmune thrombocytopenia in pregnancy. Br J Haematol 1980;44:451–9.
12. Tozman ECS, Urowitz MB, Gladman DD. Systemic lupus erythematosus and pregnancy. J Rheumatol 1980;7:624–32.
13. Karpatkin M, Porges RF, Karpatkin S. Platelet counts in infants of women with autoimmune thrombocytopenia: Effect of steroid administration to the mother. N Engl J Med 1981;305:936–9.
14. Pratt WR. Allergic diseases in pregnancy and breast-feeding. Ann Allergy 1981;47:355–60.
15. Carmichael SL, Shaw GM. Maternal corticosteroid use and risk of selected congenital anomalies. Am J Med Genet 1999;86:242–4.
16. Park-Wyllie L, Mazzotta P, Pastuszak A, Moretti ME, Beique L, Hunnisett L, Friesen MH, Jacobson S, Kasapinovic S, Chang D, Diav-Citrin O, Chitayat D, Nulman I, Einarson TR, Koren G. Birth defects after maternal exposure to corticosteroids: prospective cohort study and meta-analysis of epidemiological studies. Teratology 2000;62:385–82.
17. Cote CJ, Meuwissen HJ, Pickering RJ. Effects on the neonate of prednisone and azathioprine administered to the mother during pregnancy. J Pediatr 1974;85:324–8.
18. Cederqvist LL, Merkatz IR, Litwin SD. Fetal immunoglobulin synthesis following maternal immunosuppression. Am J Obstet Gynecol 1977;129:687–90.
19. Tallent MB, Simmons RL, Najarian JS. Birth defects in child of male recipient of kidney transplant. JAMA 1970;211:1854–5.
20. Jensen MK. Chromosome studies in patients treated with azathioprine and amethopterin. Acta Med Scand 1967;182:445–55.
21. Mancini RE, Larieri JC, Muller F, Andrada JA, Saraceni DJ. Effect of prednisolone upon normal and pathologic human spermatogenesis. Fertil Steril 1966;17:500–13.
22. Szabo I, Csaba I, Novak P, Drozgyik I. Single-dose glucocorticoid for prevention of respiratory-distress syndrome. Lancet 1977;2:243.
23. Szabo I, Csaba I, Bodis J, Novak P, Drozgyik J, Schwartz J. Effect of glucocorticoid on fetal lecithin and sphingomyelin concentrations. Lancet 1980;1:320.
24. Katz FH, Duncan BR. Entry of prednisone into human milk. N Engl J Med 1975;293:1154.
25. McKenzie SA, Selley JA, Agnew JE. Secretion of prednisone into breast milk. Arch Dis Child 1975;50: 894–6.
26. Ost L, Wettrell G, Bjorkhem I, Rane A. Prednisolone excretion in human milk. J Pediatr 1985;106:1008–11.

27. Greenberger PA, Odeh YK, Frederiksen MC, Atkinson AJ Jr. Pharmacokinetics of prednisolone transfer to breast milk. Clin Pharmacol Ther 1993;53:324–8.
28. Committee on Drugs, American Academy of Pediatrics. The transfer of drugs and other chemicals into human milk. Pediatrics 2001;108:776–89.

Name:	**PRIMAQUINE**	Risk Factor:	**C**
Class:	**Antimalarial**		

FETAL RISK SUMMARY

RECOMMENDATION: Limited Human Data - Probably Compatible

No reports linking the use of primaquine with congenital defects have been located. Primaquine may cause hemolytic anemia in patients with glucose-6-phosphate dehydrogenase deficiency. Pregnant patients at risk for this disorder should be tested accordingly (1). If possible, the drug should be withheld until after delivery (2). However, if prophylaxis or treatment is required, primaquine should not be withheld (3).

BREAST FEEDING SUMMARY

RECOMMENDATION: No Human Data - Probably Compatible

No data are available.

References

1. Trenholme GM, Parson PE. Therapy and prophylaxis of malaria. JAMA 1978;240:2293–5.
2. Anonymous. Chemoprophylaxis of malaria. MMWR 1978;27:81–90.
3. Diro M, Beydoun SN. Malaria in pregnancy. South Med J 1982;75:959–62.

P

Name:	**PRIMIDONE**	Risk Factor:	**D**
Class:	**Anticonvulsant**		

FETAL RISK SUMMARY

RECOMMENDATION: Human Data Suggest Risk

Primidone, a structural analogue of phenobarbital (see also Phenobarbital), is effective against generalized convulsive seizures and psychomotor attacks. The epileptic patient on anticonvulsant medication is at a higher risk for having a child with congenital defects than the general population (1–7). A total of 323 infants who were exposed to primidone during the 1st trimester have been noted in various publications (4,8–17). Of the 41 malformed infants described in these reports, only 3 infants were exposed to primidone alone during gestation (8,15,16). The anomalies observed in these 3 infants were similar to those observed in the fetal hydantoin syndrome (see Phenytoin).

Acardia, a rare congenital defect, was described in 1996 case report (18). The 28-year-old mother with two healthy children and a long history of epilepsy had taken primidone (500 mg/day) until the 3rd month of pregnancy. She stopped the drug at this time because of concern for malformations. Her pregnancy history included three epileptic seizures in months 4, 5, and 8. She had no prenatal care during the pregnancy until she presented at term. An ultrasound revealed a twin pregnancy. A cesarean section was performed to deliver a normal 2300-g female infant and a female acardiac acephalic monster. Both were in a single amniotic cavity. The normal female infant did well with no problems in the neonatal period. Genetic studies on the anomalous twin could not be conducted because of delay in receiving permission to study it. At autopsy, the head and upper extremities were totally absent and the major internal organs (heart, lungs, liver, spleen, pancreas, and the upper gastrointestinal tract) could not be identified. Structures that were identified included the small intestine with a blind proximal ending, colon with an anal opening, two adrenal glands, two hypoplastic kidneys and ureters, bladder, uterus and tubes, two ovaries, and a single umbilical artery and vein. The cause of the rare defect could not be determined.

In a surveillance study of Michigan Medicaid recipients conducted between 1985 and 1992 involving 229,101 completed pregnancies, 36 newborns had been exposed to primidone during the 1st trimester (F. Rosa, personal communication, FDA, 1993). One (2.8%) major birth defect was observed (two expected). Details were not available on the single case, but no anomalies were observed in six defect categories (cardiovascular defects, oral clefts, spina bifida, polydactyly, limb reduction defects, and hypospadias) for which specific data were available.

The effects of exposure (at any time during the 2nd or 3rd month after the last menstrual period) to folic acid antagonists on embryo/fetal development were evaluated in a large, multicenter, case-control surveillance study published in 2000 (19). The report was based on data collected between 1976 and 1998 from 80 maternity or tertiary care hospitals. Mothers were interviewed within 6 months of delivery about their use of drugs during pregnancy. Folic acid antagonists were categorized into two groups: group I—dihydrofolate reductase inhibitors (aminopterin, methotrexate, sulfasalazine, pyrimethamine, triamterene, and trimethoprim); group II—agents that affect other enzymes in folate metabolism, impair the absorption of folate, or increase the metabolic breakdown of folate (carbamazepine, phenytoin, primidone, and phenobarbital) (18). The case subjects were 3870 infants with cardiovascular defects, 1962 with oral clefts, and 1100 with urinary tract malformations. Infants with defects associated with a syndrome were excluded, as were infants with coexisting neural tube defects (NTDs; known to be reduced by maternal folic acid supplementation). Too few infants with limb-reduction defects were identified to be analyzed. Controls ($N = 8,387$) were infants with malformations other than oral clefts and cardiovascular, urinary tract, and limb-reduction defects and NTDs, but included infants with chromosomal and genetic defects. The risk of malformations in control infants would not have been reduced by vitamin supplementation, and none of the controls used folic acid antagonists. For group I cases, the relative risks (RRs) of cardiovascular defects and oral clefts were 3.4 (95% confidence interval [CI] 1.8–6.4) and 2.6 (95% CI 1.1–6.1), respectively. For group II cases, the RRs of cardiovascular and urinary tract defects, and oral clefts were 2.2 (95% CI 1.4–3.5), 2.5 (95% CI 1.2–5.0), and 2.5 (95% CI 1.5–4.2), respectively. Maternal use of multivitamin supplements with folic acid (typically 0.4 mg) reduced the risks in group I cases, but not in group II cases (19).

A prospective study published in 1999 described the outcomes of 517 pregnancies of epileptic mothers identified at one Italian center from 1977 (20). Excluding genetic and chromosomal defects, malformations were classified as severe structural defects, mild structural defects, and deformations. Minor anomalies were not considered. Spontaneous

($N = 38$) and early ($N = 20$) voluntary abortions were excluded from the analysis, as were 7 pregnancies that delivered at other hospitals. Of the remaining 452 outcomes, 427 were exposed to anticonvulsants of which 313 involved monotherapy: primidone ($N = 35$), carbamazepine ($N = 113$), phenobarbital ($N = 83$), valproate ($N = 44$), phenytoin ($N = 31$), clonazepam ($N = 6$), and other ($N = 1$). There were no defects in the 25 pregnancies not exposed to anticonvulsants. Of the 42 (9.3%) outcomes with malformations, 24 (5.3%) were severe, 10 (2.2%) were mild, and 8 (1.8%) were deformities. There were three malformations with primidone monotherapy: two (5.7%) were severe (intraventricular defect and hypospadias), and one (2.8%) was mild (undescended testis and inguinal hernia). The investigators concluded that the anticonvulsants were the primary risk factor for an increased incidence of congenital malformations (see also Carbamazepine, Clonazepam, Phenobarbital, Phenytoin, and Valproic Acid) (20).

There are other potential complications associated with the use of primidone during pregnancy. Neurologic manifestations in the newborn, such as overactivity and tumors, have been associated with use of primidone in pregnancy (16,21). Neonatal hemorrhagic disease with primidone alone or in combination with other anticonvulsants has been reported (14,22–26). Suppression of vitamin K_1-dependent clotting factors is the proposed mechanism of the hemorrhagic effect (14,22). Administration of prophylactic vitamin K_1 to the infant immediately after birth is recommended (see Phytonadione, Phenytoin, and Phenobarbital).

BREAST FEEDING SUMMARY

RECOMMENDATION: Limited Human Data - Potential Toxicity

Primidone is excreted into breast milk (27). Because primidone undergoes limited conversion to phenobarbital, breast milk concentrations of phenobarbital should be anticipated (see Phenobarbital). A milk:plasma ratio of 0.8 for primidone has been reported (27). The amount of primidone available to the nursing infant is small, with milk concentrations of 2.3 μg/mL. No reports linking adverse effects to the nursing infant have been located, however, patients that breast-feed should be instructed to watch for potential sedative effects in the infant. The American Academy of Pediatrics classifies primidone as an agent that has been associated with significant effects in some nursing infants and should be used with caution in the lactating woman (28).

References

1. Hill RB. Teratogenesis and antiepileptic drugs. N Engl J Med 1973;289:1089–90.
2. Bodendorfer TW. Fetal effect of anticonvulsant drugs and seizure disorders. Drug Intell Clin Pharm 1978;12:14–21.
3. Committee on Drugs, American Academy of Pediatrics. Anticonvulsants and pregnancy. Pediatrics 1977;63:331–3.
4. Nakane Y, Okuma T, Takahashi R, Sato Y, Wada T, Sato T, Fukushima Y, Kumashiro H, Ono T, Takahashi T, Aoki Y, Kazamatsuri H, Inami M, Komai S, Seino M, Miyakoshi M, Tanimura T, Hazama H, Kawahara R, Otuski S, Hosokawa K, Inanaga K, Nakazawa Y, Yamamoto K. Multi-institutional study on the teratogenicity and fetal toxicity of antiepileptic drugs: a report of a collaborative study group in Japan. Epilepsia 1980;21:663–80.
5. Andermann E, Dansky L, Andermann F, Loughnan PM, Gibbons J. Minor congenital malformations and dermatoglyphic alterations in the offspring of epileptic women: a clinical investigation of the teratogenic effects of anticonvulsant medication. In *Epilepsy, Pregnancy and the Child.* Proceedings of a Workshop held in Berlin, September 1980. New York, NY: Raven Press, 1981.
6. Danksy L, Andermann F. Major congenital malformations in the offspring of epileptic patients. In *Epilepsy, Pregnancy and the Child.* Proceedings of a Workshop held in Berlin, September 1980. New York, NY: Raven Press, 1981.

P

7. Janz D. The teratogenic risks of antiepileptic drugs. Epilepsia 1975;16:159–69.
8. Lowe CR. Congenital malformations among infants born to epileptic women. Lancet 1973;1:9–10.
9. Lander CM, Edwards BE, Eadie MJ, Tyrer JH. Plasma anticonvulsants concentrations during pregnancy. Neurology 1977;27:128–31.
10. Speidel BD, Meadow SR. Maternal epilepsy and abnormalities of the fetus and newborn. Lancet 1972;2: 839–43.
11. McMullin GP. Teratogenic effects of anticonvulsants. Br Med J 1971;4:430.
12. Fedrick J. Epilepsy and pregnancy: a report from the Oxford Record Linkage Study. Br Med J 1973;2:442–8.
13. Biale Y, Lewenthal H, Aderet NB. Congenital malformations due to anticonvulsant drugs. Obstet Gynecol 1975;45:439–42.
14. Thomas P, Buchanan N. Teratogenic effect of anticonvulsants. J Pediatr 1981;99:163.
15. Myhree SA, Williams R. Teratogenic effects associated with maternal primidone therapy. J Pediatr 1981;99: 160–2.
16. Rudd NL, Freedom RM. A possible primidone embryopathy. J Pediatr 1979;94:835–7.
17. Heinonen OP, Slone D, Shapiro S. *Birth Defects and Drugs in Pregnancy*. Littleton, MA: Publishing Sciences Group, 1977:358.
18. Kutlay B, Bayramoglu S, Kutlar AI, Yesildaglar N. An acardiac acephalic monster following in-utero antiepileptic drug exposure. Eur J Obstet Gynecology Reprod Med 1996;65:245–8.
19. Hernandez-Diaz S, Werler MM, Walker AM, Mitchell AA. Folic acid antagonists during pregnancy and the risk of birth defects. N Engl J Med 2000;343:1608–14.
20. Canger R, Battino D, Canevini MP, Fumarola C, Guidolin L, Vignoli A, Mamoli D, Palmieri C, Molteni F, Granata T, Hassibi P, Zamperini P, Pardi G, Avanzini G. Malformations in offspring of women with epilepsy: a prospective study. Epilepsia 1999;40:1231–6.
21. Martinez G, Snyder RD. Transplacental passage of primidone. Neurology 1973;23:381–3.
22. Kohler HG. Haemorrhage in the newborn of epileptic mothers. Lancet 1966;1:267.
23. Bleyer WA, Skinner AL. Fatal neonatal hemorrhage after maternal anticonvulsant therapy. JAMA 1976;235:826–7.
24. Mountain KR, Hirsh J, Gallus AS. Neonatal coagulation defect due to anticonvulsant drug treatment in pregnancy. Lancet 1970;1:265–8.
25. Evans AR, Forrester RM, Discombe C. Neonatal hemorrhage following maternal anticonvulsant therapy. Lancet 1970;1:517–8.
26. Margolin DO, Kantor NM. Hemorrhagic disease of the newborn: an unusual case related to maternal ingestion of antiepileptic drug. Clin Pediatr (Phila) 1972;11:59–60.
27. Kaneko S, Sato T, Suzuki K. The levels of anticonvulsants in breast milk. Br J Clin Pharmacol 1979;7: 624–7.
28. Committee on Drugs, American Academy of Pediatrics. The transfer of drugs and other chemicals into human milk. Pediatrics 2001;108:776–89.

Name: **PROBENECID** Risk Factor: **C**

Class: **Miscellaneous (Uricosuric)**

FETAL RISK SUMMARY

RECOMMENDATION: Limited Human Data - No Relevant Animal Data

No reports linking the use of probenecid with congenital defects have been located. Probenecid has been used during pregnancy without producing adverse effects in the fetus or in the infant (1–3). The manufacturer reports that the drug crosses the placenta and appears in cord blood (4).

In a surveillance study of Michigan Medicaid recipients conducted between 1985 and 1992 involving 229,101 completed pregnancies, 339 newborns had been exposed to probenecid during the 1st trimester (F. Rosa, personal communication, FDA, 1993). A total of 17 (5.0%) major birth defects were observed (14 expected). Specific data were available for six defect categories, including (observed/expected) 5/3 cardiovascular defects, 1/1 oral clefts, 0/0 spina bifida, 1/1 polydactyly, 0/1 limb reduction defects, and 1/1 hypospadias. These data do not support an association between the drug and congenital defects.

BREAST FEEDING SUMMARY

RECOMMENDATION: No Human Data - Potential Toxicity

No reports describing the use of probenecid during lactation have been located. The molecular weight (about 286) is low enough, however, that excretion into breast milk should be expected. The effects on a nursing infant from exposure to the drug in breast milk are unknown.

References

1. Beidleman B. Treatment of chronic hypoparathyroidism with probenecid. Metabolism 1958;7:690–8.
2. Lee FI, Loeffler FE. Gout and pregnancy. J Obstet Gynaecol Br Commonw 1962;69:299.
3. Batt RE, Cirksena WJ, Lebhertz TB. Gout and salt-wasting renal disease during pregnancy. Diagnosis, management and follow-up. JAMA 1963;186:835–8.
4. Product information. Benemid. Merck, 2000.

Name:	**PROBUCOL**	Risk Factor:	**B_M**
Class:	**Antilipemic Agent**		

FETAL RISK SUMMARY

RECOMMENDATION: Limited Human Data - Animal Data Suggest Low Risk

Probucol is used to lower serum cholesterol concentrations. In animal reproductive tests, probucol given during organogenesis to pregnant rats (up to 1000 mg/kg) and rabbits (administered unspecified amounts) produced no adverse fetal effects (1). The manufacturer reports a similar lack of evidence of fertility impairment or fetal harm in pregnant rats and rabbits given up to 50 times the human dose (2).

In a surveillance study of Michigan Medicaid recipients conducted between 1985 and 1992 involving 229,101 completed pregnancies, 11 newborns had been exposed to probucol during the 1st trimester (3). Two other infants were exposed after the 1st trimester. No congenital malformations were observed in the 13 infants.

BREAST FEEDING SUMMARY

RECOMMENDATION: No Human Data - Potential Toxicity

No human data are available. The manufacturer states that probucol is excreted into the milk of lactating animals (2), but specific data were not provided. Because of this, excretion into human milk should be expected.

References

1. Molello JA, Thompson DJ, LeBeau JE. Eight year toxicity study in monkeys and reproduction studies in rats and rabbits with a new hypocholesterolemic agent, probucol (abstract). Toxicol Appl Pharmacol 1979;648:A98. As cited in Shepard TH. *Catalog of Teratogenic Agents*. 7th ed. Baltimore, MD: Johns Hopkins University Press, 1992:327.
2. Product information. Lorelco. Marion Merrell Dow, 1994.
3. Rosa F. Anti-cholesterol agent pregnancy exposure outcomes. Presented at the 7th International Organization for Teratogen Information Services, Woods Hole, MA, April 1994.

P

Name: **PROCAINAMIDE** Risk Factor: **C_M**
Class: **Antiarrhythmic**

FETAL RISK SUMMARY

RECOMMENDATION: Limited Human Data - No Relevant Animal Data

Procainamide is a cardiac drug used for the termination and prophylaxis of atrial and ventricular tachyarrhythmias (1). Animal reproduction studies with procainamide have not been conducted. The use of procainamide during human pregnancy has not been associated with congenital anomalies or other adverse fetal effects (1–9).

Successful cardioversion with procainamide of a fetal supraventricular tachycardia presenting at 30 weeks' gestation has been reported (4). Therapy with digoxin alone and digoxin combined with propranolol failed to halt the arrhythmia. Procainamide was then combined with digoxin, resulting in cardioversion to a sinus rhythm and resolution of fetal ascites and pericardial effusion. During the following 3 weeks, the mother was maintained on oral procainamide, 1 g every 6 hours, and digoxin. Maternal serum levels of procainamide varied from 2.4 to 4.1 μg/mL. The abnormal rhythm returned at 33 weeks' gestation, and control became increasingly difficult. Additional therapy with procainamide increased the maternal serum concentration to 6.8 μg/mL. During the last 24 hours, four IV bolus doses of procainamide (700 mg 3 times, 650 mg once) were administered plus a maintenance dose of 3 mg/minute. Three hours after the last bolus dose, a 2650-g female infant was delivered by cesarean section. Serum procainamide concentrations in the newborn and mother were 4.3 and 15.6 μg/mL, respectively, a ratio of 0.28. During the subsequent neonatal course, the infant was successfully treated for congestive heart failure and persistent supraventricular tachycardia. The electrocardiogram was normal at 6 months of age.

In a case similar to the one described above, therapy with digoxin, verapamil, and procainamide failed to control fetal supraventricular tachycardia presenting at 24 weeks' gestation (5). At cordocentesis, procainamide concentrations in the fetus and mother were 11.7 and 12.8 μg/mL (ratio 0.91), respectively. Levels of the active metabolite, *N*-acetylprocainamide, were 3.0 and 3.5 μg/mL (ratio 0.86), respectively. Cardioversion was eventually accomplished with direct fetal digitalization by periodic IM injection.

Procainamide was prescribed for a woman in her 24th week of gestation for ventricular tachycardia (7). She was treated with doses up to 2000 mg every 6 hours, combined with metoprolol 100 mg every 12 hours, until delivery of a healthy, 3155-g girl at 38 weeks' gestation. Maternal and mixed cord blood concentrations of procainamide were 6.0 and 6.4 μg/mL (fetal:maternal ratio 1.1), respectively. Similar analysis for *N*-acetylprocainamide yielded levels of 9.4 and 8.7 μg/mL (ratio 0.9), respectively. No fetal or newborn adverse effects were observed.

BREAST FEEDING SUMMARY

RECOMMENDATION: Limited Human Data - Probably Compatible

Procainamide and its active metabolite, *N*-acetylprocainamide, are accumulated in breast milk (10). A woman was treated with procainamide, 375 mg 4 times daily, for premature ventricular contractions during the 3rd trimester (10). The dose was increased to 500 mg 4 times daily 1 week before delivery at 39 weeks' gestation. Simultaneous serum and milk samples were obtained in the postpartum period (exact time not specified) every 3 hours for a total of 15 hours. Procainamide (500 mg) was administered orally at hours 0, 6, and 12 immediately after samples were obtained. Mean serum concentrations of procainamide and *N*-acetylprocainamide were 1.1 and 1.6 μg/mL, respectively, while the concentrations in the milk were 5.4 and 3.5 μg/mL, respectively. The mean milk:serum ratios for the parent drug and the metabolite were 4.3 (range 1.0–7.3) and 3.8 (range 1.0–6.2), respectively. The amount of drug available to the nursing infant based on a hypothetical serum level of 8 μg/mL was estimated to be 64.8 μg/mL (procainamide plus metabolite). Assuming the infant could ingest 1000 mL of milk/day (thought to be unlikely), this would only provide about 65 mg of total active drug. This amount was not expected to yield clinically significant serum concentrations (10). The American Academy of Pediatrics classifies procainamide as compatible with breast feeding (11). However, the long-term effects of exposure in the nursing infant to procainamide and its metabolites are unknown, particularly in regard to potential drug toxicity (e.g., development of antinuclear antibodies and lupus-like syndrome).

References

1. Rotmensch HH, Elkayam U, Frishman W. Antiarrhythmic drug therapy during pregnancy. Ann Intern Med 1983;98:487–97.
2. Mendelson CL. Disorders of the heartbeat during pregnancy. Am J Obstet Gynecol 1956;72:1268–301.
3. Tamari I, Eldar M, Rabinowitz B, Neufeld HN. Medical treatment of cardiovascular disorders during pregnancy. Am Heart J 1982;104:1357–63.
4. Dumesic DA, Silverman NH, Tobias S, Golbus MS. Transplacental cardioversion of fetal supraventricular tachycardia with procainamide. N Engl J Med 1982;307:1128–31.
5. Weiner CP, Thompson MIB. Direct treatment of fetal supraventricular tachycardia after failed transplacental therapy. Am J Obstet Gynecol 1988;158:570–3.
6. Little BB, Gilstrap LC III. Cardiovascular drugs during pregnancy. Clin Obstet Gynecol 1989;32:13–20.
7. Allen NM, Page RL. Procainamide administration during pregnancy. Clin Pharm 1993;12:58–60.
8. Kanzaki T, Murakami M, Kobayashi H, Takahashi S, Chiba Y. Hemodynamic changes during cardioversion in utero: A case report of supraventricular tachycardia and atrial flutter. Fetal Diagn Ther 1993;8:37–44.
9. Hallak M, Neerhof MG, Perry R, Nazir M, Huhta JC. Fetal supraventricular tachycardia and hydrops fetalis: Combined intensive, direct, and transplacental therapy. Obstet Gynecol 1991;78:523–5.
10. Pittard WB III, Glazier H. Procainamide excretion in human milk. J Pediatr 1983;102:631–3.
11. Committee on Drugs, American Academy of Pediatrics. The transfer of drugs and other chemicals into human milk. Pediatrics 2001;108:776–89.

Name:	**PROCARBAZINE**	Risk Factor:	**D_M**
Class:	**Antineoplastic**		

FETAL RISK SUMMARY

RECOMMENDATION: Contraindicated - 1st Trimester

The use of procarbazine, in combination with other antineoplastic agents, during pregnancy has been described in nine patients, five during the 1st trimester (1–8). One of the 1st trimester exposures was electively terminated, but no details on the fetus were given (5). Congenital malformations were observed in the remaining four 1st trimester exposures (1–4):

Multiple hemangiomas (1)
Oligodactyly of both feet with webbing of third and fourth toes, four metatarsals on left, three on right, bowing of right tibia, cerebral hemorrhage, spontaneously aborted at 24 weeks' gestation (2)

Malformed kidneys - markedly reduced size and malposition (3)
Small secundum atrial septal defect, intrauterine growth retardation (4)

A patient in her 12th week of pregnancy received procarbazine, 50 mg daily, in error for 30 days when she was given the drug instead of an iron/vitamin supplement (6). A normal 3575-g male infant was delivered at term.

Long-term studies of growth and mental development in offspring exposed to procarbazine during the 2nd trimester, the period of neuroblast multiplication, have not been conducted (9). Data from one review indicated that 40% of the infants exposed to anticancer drugs were of low birth weight (10). This finding was not related to the timing of exposure.

Procarbazine is mutagenic and carcinogenic in animals (11). In combination with other antineoplastic drugs, procarbazine may produce gonadal dysfunction in males and females (12–17). Ovarian and testicular function may return to normal, with successful pregnancies possible, depending on the patient's age at the time of therapy and the total dose of chemotherapy received (16–20).

Occupational exposure of the mother to antineoplastic agents during pregnancy may present a risk to the fetus. A position statement from the National Study Commission on Cytotoxic Exposure and a research article involving some antineoplastic agents are presented in the monograph for cyclophosphamide (see Cyclophosphamide).

BREAST FEEDING SUMMARY

RECOMMENDATION: Contraindicated

No reports describing the use of procarbazine during lactation have been located. The molecular weight (about 222 for the free base) is low enough, however, that excretion into breast milk should be expected. Because of the potential for tumorigenicity, women receiving this drug should not nurse (21).

References

1. Wells JH, Marshall JR, Carbone PP. Procarbazine therapy for Hodgkin's disease in early pregnancy. JAMA 1968;205:935–7.
2. Garrett MJ. Teratogenic effects of combination chemotherapy. Ann Intern Med 1974;80:667.
3. Mennuti MT, Shepard TH, Mellman WJ. Fetal renal malformation following treatment of Hodgkin's disease during pregnancy. Obstet Gynecol 1975;46:194–6.
4. Thomas PRM, Peckham MJ. The investigation and management of Hodgkin's disease in the pregnant patient. Cancer 1976;38:1443–51.
5. Daly H, McCann SR, Hanratty TD, Temperley IJ. Successful pregnancy during combination chemotherapy for Hodgkin's disease. Acta Haematol (Basel) 1980;64:154–6.
6. Daw EG. Procarbazine in pregnancy. Lancet 1970;2:984.
7. Johnson IR, Filshie GM. Hodgkin's disease diagnosed in pregnancy: case report. Br J Obstet Gynaecol 1977;84:791–2.
8. Jones RT, Weinerman ER. MOPP (nitrogen mustard, vincristine, procarbazine, and prednisone) given during pregnancy. Obstet Gynecol 1979;54:477–8.
9. Dobbing J. Pregnancy and leukaemia. Lancet 1977;1:1155.
10. Nicholson HO. Cytotoxic drugs in pregnancy: review of reported cases. J Obstet Gynecol Br Commonw 1968;75:307–12.
11. Lee IP, Dixon RL. Mutagenicity, carcinogenicity and teratogenicity of procarbazine. Mutat Res 1978;55:1–14.
12. Sherins RJ, DeVita VT Jr. Effect of drug treatment for lymphoma on male reproductive capacity: studies of men in remission after therapy. Ann Intern Med 1973;79:216–20.
13. Sherins RJ, Olweny CLM, Ziegler JL. Gynecomastia and gonadal dysfunction in adolescent boys treated with combination chemotherapy for Hodgkin's disease. N Engl J Med 1978;299:12–6.
14. Johnson SA, Goldman JM, Hawkins DF. Pregnancy after chemotherapy for Hodgkin's disease. Lancet 1979;2:93.
15. Card RT, Holmes IH, Sugarman RG, Storb R, Thomas ED. Successful pregnancy after high dose chemotherapy and marrow transplantation for treatment of aplastic anemia. Exp Hematol 1980;8:57–60.
16. Schilsky RL, Sherins RJ, Hubbard SM, Wesley MN, Young RC, DeVita VT Jr. Long-term follow-up of ovarian function in women treated with MOPP chemotherapy for Hodgkin's disease. Am J Med 1981;71:552–6.
17. Shalet SM, Vaughan Williams CA, Whitehead E. Pregnancy after chemotherapy induced ovarian failure. Br Med J 1985;290:898.
18. Whitehead E, Shalet SM, Blackledge G, Todd I,

Crowther D, Beardwell CG. The effect of combination chemotherapy on ovarian function in women treated for Hodgkin's disease. Cancer 1983;52:988–93.
19. Andrieu JM, Ochoa-Molina ME. Menstrual cycle, pregnancies and offspring before and after MOPP therapy for Hodgkin's disease. Cancer 1983;52:435–8.
20. Schapira DV, Chudley AE. Successful pregnancy following continuous treatment with combination chemotherapy before conception and throughout pregnancy. Cancer 1984;54:800–3.
21. Product information. Matulane. Sigma-Tau Pharmaceuticals, 2000.

Name: **PROCHLORPERAZINE** Risk Factor: **C**
Class: **Tranquilizer/Antiemetic**

FETAL RISK SUMMARY

RECOMMENDATION: Compatible

Prochlorperazine is a piperazine phenothiazine. In one rat study, prochlorperazine produced significant postnatal weight decrease, increased fetal mortality, and minor behavioral changes, but no structural defects (1). In a second rat study, an increased incidence of cleft palate, a few anencephalic fetuses, and one double monster was observed (2).

The drug readily crosses the placenta (3). Prochlorperazine has been used to treat nausea and vomiting of pregnancy. Most studies have found the drug to be safe for this indication (see also Chlorpromazine) (4–6).

The Collaborative Perinatal Project (CPP) monitored 50,282 mother-child pairs, 877 of whom had 1st trimester exposure to prochlorperazine (6). For use anytime during pregnancy, 2023 exposures were recorded. No evidence was found in either group to suggest a relationship to malformations or an effect on perinatal mortality rate, birth weight, or intelligence quotient scores at 4 years of age.

In a separate study using data from the CPP, offspring of psychotic or neurotic mothers who had consumed prochlorperazine for 1–2 months during gestation ($N = 30$) were significantly taller than nonexposed controls ($N = 71$) at 4 months and at 1 year of age (7). Those who had been exposed for longer than 2 months ($N = 8$) were also taller than controls at both ages, but not significantly so. Offspring ($N = 21$) of normal women, who had taken the drug for more than 2 months during pregnancy, were significantly taller than nonexposed controls ($N = 68$) at 1 year of age but no difference was measured at 7 years of age. Moreover, the mean weight of exposed children of normal mothers was significantly greater than controls at 1 year of age, but not at 7 years of age. The mechanisms behind these effects were not clear, but may have been related to the dopamine receptor-blocking action of the drug.

Five infants exposed to prochlorperazine, and, in some cases, to multiple other drugs, during the 1st trimester are described below:

Cleft palate, micrognathia, congenital heart defects, skeletal defects (8)
Thanatophoric dwarfism (short limb anomaly) (9)
Hypoplasia of radium and ulnar bones with a vestigial wrist and hand (10)
Below-the-elbow amputation in one arm and small atrophic hand attached to the stump (11)
Below-the-knee amputation in one limb, with rudimentary foot attached to stump (one twin) (11)

The relationship between prochlorperazine and the above defects is unknown. The case of dwarfism was probably caused by genetic factors. No evidence of amniotic bands was observed in the two cases involving amputations, both of whom were exposed during the mothers' treatment for hyperemesis gravidarum (11).

A 1963 report described phocomelia of the upper limbs in a male infant exposed to two phenothiazines during gestation (12). The mother had not taken prochlorperazine until approximately the 13th week of gestation, so no association between the drug and the defect is possible. However, the other agent, trifluoperazine, was taken early in pregnancy (see also Trifluoperazine). In another study, no increase in defects or pattern of malformations were observed in 76 infants (2 sets of twins) exposed *in utero* to the antiemetic (13).

In a surveillance study of Michigan Medicaid recipients conducted between 1985 and 1992 involving 229,101 completed pregnancies, 704 newborns had been exposed to prochlorperazine during the 1st trimester (F. Rosa, personal communication, FDA, 1993). A total of 24 (3.4%) major birth defects were observed (29 expected). Specific data were available for six defect categories, including (observed/expected) 6/7 cardiovascular defects, 1/1 oral clefts, 0/0 spina bifida, 1/2 polydactyly, 1/1 limb reduction defects, and 0/2 hypospadias. These data do not support an association between the drug and congenital defects.

In summary, although there are isolated reports of congenital defects in children exposed to prochlorperazine *in utero*, the majority of the evidence indicates that this drug and the general class of phenothiazines are safe for both mother and fetus if used occasionally in low doses. Other reviewers have also concluded that the phenothiazines are not teratogenic (14,15).

BREAST FEEDING SUMMARY

RECOMMENDATION: No Human Data - Potential Toxicity

No reports describing the excretion of prochlorperazine into breast milk have been located, but the drug has been found in the milk of lactating dogs (16). Because other phenothiazines appear in human milk (e.g., chlorpromazine), excretion of prochlorperazine should be expected. Sedation is a possible effect in the nursing infant.

P

References

1. Vorhees CV, Brunner RL, Butcher RE. Psychotropic drugs as behavioral teratogens. Science 1979;205:1220–5. As cited in Shepard TH. *Catalog of Teratogenic Agents*. 6th ed. Baltimore, MD: Johns Hopkins University Press, 1989:525–6.
2. Roux C. Action teratogene de la prochlorpemazine. Arch Fr Pediatr 1959;16:968–71. As cited in Shepard TH. *Catalog of Teratogenic Agents*. 6th ed. Baltimore, MD: Johns Hopkins University Press, 1989:525–6.
3. Moya F, Thorndike V. Passage of drugs across the placenta. Am J Obstet Gynecol 1962;84:1778–98.
4. Reider RO, Rosenthal D. Wender P, Blumenthal H. The offspring of schizophrenics. Fetal and neonatal deaths. Arch Gen Psychiatry 1975;32:200–11.
5. Milkovich L, Van den Berg BJ. An evaluation of the teratogenicity of certain antinauseant drugs. Am J Obstet Gynecol 1976;125:244–8.
6. Slone D, Siskind V, Heinonen OP, Monson RR, Kaufman DW, Shapiro S. Antenatal exposure to the phenothiazines in relation to congenital malformations, perinatal mortality rate, birth weight, and intelligence quotient score. Am J Obstet Gynecol 1977;128:486–8.
7. Platt JE, Friedhoff AJ, Broman SH, Bond RN, Laska E, Lin SP. Effects of prenatal exposure to neuroleptic drugs on children's growth. Neuropsychopharmacology 1988;1:205–12.
8. Ho CK, Kaufman RL, McAlister WH. Congenital malformations. Cleft palate, congenital heart disease, absent tibiae, and polydactyly. Am J Dis Child 1975;129:714–6.
9. Farag RA, Ananth J. Thanatophoric dwarfism associated with prochlorperazine administration. NY State J Med 1978;78:279–82.
10. Freeman R. Limb deformities: possible association with drugs. Med J Aust 1972;1:606–7.
11. Rafla N. Limb deformities associated with prochlorperazine. Am J Obstet Gynecol 1987;156:1557.
12. Hall G. A case of phocomelia of the upper limbs. Med J Aust 1983;1:449–50.

13. Mellin GW. Report of prochlorperazine during pregnancy from the fetal life study bank (abstract). Teratology 1975;11:28A.
14. Ayd FJ Jr. Children born of mothers treated with chlorpromazine during pregnancy. Clin Med 1964; 71:1758–63.
15. Ananth J. Congenital malformations with psychopharmacologic agents. Compr Psychiatry 1975;16: 437–45.
16. Knowles JA. Excretion of drugs in milk—a review. J Pediatr 1965;66:1068–82.

Name:	**PROCYCLIDINE**	Risk Factor:	**C**
Class:	**Parasympatholytic (Anticholinergic)**		

FETAL RISK SUMMARY

RECOMMENDATION: No Human Data - No Relevant Animal Data

Procyclidine is an anticholinergic agent used in the treatment of parkinsonism. No reports of its use in pregnancy have been located (see also Atropine).

BREAST FEEDING SUMMARY

RECOMMENDATION: No Human Data - Probably Compatible

No data are available (see also Atropine).

Name:	**PROGUANIL**	Risk Factor:	**B**
Class:	**Antimalarial**		

FETAL RISK SUMMARY

RECOMMENDATION: Compatible - Maternal Benefit >> Embryo/Fetal Risk

Proguanil is not available in the United States as a single agent, but is available in combination with atovaquone (see also Atovaquone). Proguanil, a biguanide compound that inhibits plasmodial dihydrofolate reductase, has been frequently used in other parts of the world for causal prophylaxis (defined as absolute prevention) of *Plasmodium falciparum* malaria since 1948. It is now known, however, that no chemoprophylaxis regimen ensures complete protection against infection with malaria (1). Proguanil is also indicated for the suppression of other forms of malaria and reduced transmission of infection, but because of its slow action it is not used for the acute treatment of malaria. Combination with other antimalarial agents such as chloroquine is common because of the rapid development of drug resistance. Proguanil is converted *in vivo* to cycloguanil, the active metabolite. Because it is a folate antagonist, pregnant women taking proguanil should also take folic acid supplements (2–6). One reviewer recommended either 5 mg/day of folic acid or 5 mg/week of folinic acid (leucovorin) at least during the 1st trimester (6). Moreover, because iron deficiency anemia is often present in some regions, a combination of proguanil, iron, and folic acid has been recommended (7).

A reproductive study in pregnant rats given proguanil and the active metabolite, cycloguanil, was summarized by Shepard (8) and also cited by Schardein (9). Proguanil,

30 mg/kg every 4 hours, was given by gavage on days 1, 9, and 13 of gestation. No effects on the embryos or fetuses were observed. In contrast, the same dose of cycloguanil on day 1 of gestation caused death in 90% of the embryos. As with proguanil, no effects were observed from exposure to cycloguanil on days 9 and 13.

Antimalarial agents, including proguanil, are used routinely during pregnancy because the risks from the disease far outweigh the risks to the fetus from drug therapy (3,4). The risks of complications from maternal malarial infection are increased during pregnancy, especially in primigravidas and in women not living in endemic areas (i.e., nonimmune women) (10–13). Infection is associated with a number of severe maternal and fetal outcomes: maternal death, anemia, abortion, stillbirth, prematurity, low birth weight, intrauterine growth retardation, fetal distress, and congenital malaria (10–15). One of these outcomes, low birth weight with the resulting increased risk of infant mortality, may have other causes, however, inasmuch as it has not been established that antimalarial chemoprophylaxis can completely prevent this complication (11). Increased maternal morbidity and mortality includes adult respiratory distress syndrome, pulmonary edema, massive hemolysis, disseminated intravascular coagulation, acute renal failure, and hypoglycemia (12–14). Severe *Plasmodium falciparum* malaria in pregnant nonimmune women has a poor prognosis and may be associated with asymptomatic uterine contractions, intrauterine growth retardation, fetal tachycardia, fetal distress, placental insufficiency because of intense parasitization, and hypoglycemia (11,14). Because of the severity of this disease in pregnancy, chemoprophylaxis is recommended for women of childbearing age traveling in areas where malaria is present (5,10–12).

Of 200 Nigerian women enrolled in a randomized double-blind trial, 160 were given an initial curative chloroquine course (600 mg base once), followed by prophylaxis regimens consisting of proguanil, 100 mg/day, with or without daily iron supplements or 1 mg/day of folic acid (16,17). A control group of 40 women received no treatment. All patients were primigravidas seen before 24 weeks' gestation. In the treated groups, the prevalence of falciparum parasitemia was decreased from 32%–35% to about 2% at gestational weeks 28 and 36. Benefits of the regimens that included iron and/or folic acid were reductions in (a) severe anemia during pregnancy (from 18% to 3%), (b) megaloblastic erythropoiesis at or before delivery (from 56% to 25%), and (c) anemia at 6 weeks postpartum (from 61% to 29%). However, the mean birth weight was increased by only 132 g in treated compared with untreated pregnancies (difference not significant). Other than a single case of talipes and two infants with umbilical hernias, no other birth defects were observed. The authors stated that no association with the maternal treatment groups was evident, but the groups the infants were in was not specified (16).

In the first of a series of four reports, a study published in 1993 described the use of proguanil, either alone ($N = 124$) (200 mg once daily) or in combination with chloroquine ($N = 90$) (300 mg base once weekly), or of chloroquine alone ($N = 113$) (300 mg base once weekly) as malarial chemoprophylaxis during pregnancy in Tanzania (18). Chemoprophylaxis was begun after a single curative dose of pyrimethamine/sulfadoxine (Fansidar) was administered to clear preexisting parasitemia. Both proguanil chemoprophylaxis regimens were superior to chloroquine alone. The proguanil regimens were well tolerated by the mothers, with no cases of mouth ulcers and palmar or plantar skin scaling, although a few of the women complained of nausea. Based on urinary levels of proguanil and cycloguanil, they concluded that better protection from infection would have been achieved if a 12-hour dosing regimen with proguanil had been used (18).

In the second report, the effects of drug therapy on maternal hemoglobin, placental malaria, and birth weight were examined (19). As above, either proguanil alone or proguanil in combination with chloroquine were superior to chloroquine alone, producing higher levels of maternal hemoglobin, higher birth weights, and less placental malaria. The difference in outcomes between the two proguanil groups was not significant, however, leading the investigators to the conclusion that chemoprophylaxis with proguanil alone was suitable for this particular region.

The third and fourth reports in the series related to the effects of the therapy on the maternal malaria immunity and the transfer of maternal antibodies to the fetus and subsequent immunity of the offspring during early infancy (20,21). The data demonstrated that the chemoprophylaxis regimens did not significantly interfere with the maternal-fetal transfer of antisporozoite antibodies but that antibody levels at birth did not alter the first occurrence of malaria parasitemia in the infant (21).

The pharmacokinetics of proguanil in pregnant and postpartum women was described in a 1993 report (22). Ten healthy women in the 3rd trimester were given a single 200-mg oral dose and four of the women were restudied 2 months after delivery. The pharmacokinetics of proguanil during pregnancy and postpartum were similar, but the blood concentrations of the active metabolite, cycloguanil, were markedly decreased during late gestation. The mean maximum concentration (ng/mL) of cycloguanil in plasma and whole blood during pregnancy was 12.5 and 11.9, respectively, compared with postpartum levels of 28.4 and 22.4, respectively. Moreover, the proguanil:cycloguanil ratio based on the area under the plasma concentration curve (AUC) was 16.7 during pregnancy and 7.8 following pregnancy. The decreased conversion to the active antimalarial metabolite may have been caused by estrogen inhibition of the enzyme that metabolizes proguanil (22). Although the antimalarial prophylaxis concentration of cycloguanil is not known with certainty, these data indicate that the currently recommended dose of 200 mg/day may need to be doubled during late pregnancy to achieve the same blood levels as those obtained 2 months postpartum (22).

P

In summary, no adverse fetal or newborn effects attributable to the use of proguanil during gestation have been reported. It is considered by some to be the least toxic prophylactic agent available (23). Moreover, most investigators have concluded that proguanil is safe to use during pregnancy (1–6,10,18,23–25).

BREAST FEEDING SUMMARY

RECOMMENDATION: Limited Human Data - Probably Compatible

No reports quantifying the amount of proguanil excreted in breast milk have been located. At least two reports have stated that agents used for malaria prophylaxis, such as proguanil, are excreted in small amounts in milk (2,10). These amounts, however, are too small for adequate malaria chemoprophylaxis of a nursing infant (2,10). Because proguanil is recommended for malaria protection in infants of any age (2,10,25), the use of the agent by a nursing woman is probably safe. Studies are needed, however, to measure the amount of proguanil and the active metabolite, cycloguanil, in milk and to determine the safety of this exposure in the nursing infant.

References

1. Barry M, Bia F. Pregnancy and travel. JAMA 1989;261:728–31.
2. Luzzi GA, Peto TEA. Adverse effects of antimalarials. An update. Drug Saf 1993;8:295–311.
3. Cook GC. Prevention and treatment of malaria. Lancet 1988;1:32–7.
4. Bradley DJ, Phillips-Howard PA. Prophylaxis against malaria for travelers from the United Kingdom. BMJ 1989;299:1087–9.
5. Ellis CJ. Antiparasitic agents in pregnancy. Clin Obstet Gynaecol 1986;13:269–75.
6. Spracklen FHN. Malaria 1984 Part I. Malaria prophylaxis. S Afr Med J 1984;65:1037–41.
7. Fleming AF. The aetiology of severe anaemia in pregnancy in Ndola, Zambia. Ann Trop Med Parasitol 1989;83:37–49.
8. Shepard TH. *Catalog of Teratogenic Agents*. 8th ed. Baltimore, MD: Johns Hopkins University Press, 1995:118.
9. Schardein JL. *Chemically Induced Birth Defects*. 2nd ed. New York, NY: Marcel Dekker, 1993:403.
10. Centers for Disease Control. Recommendations for the prevention of malaria among travelers. MMWR 1990;39(RR-3):1–10.
11. World Health Organization. Practical chemotherapy of malaria. WHO Tech Rep Ser 1990;805:1–141.
12. Subramanian D, Moise KJ Jr, White AC Jr. Imported malaria in pregnancy: report of four cases and review of management. Clin Infect Dis 1992;15:408–13.
13. World Health Organization. Severe and complicated malaria. Trans R Soc Trop Med Hyg 1990;84(Suppl 2):1–65.
14. Nathwani D, Currie PF, Douglas JG, Green ST, Smith NC. *Plasmodium falciparum* malaria in pregnancy: a review. Br J Obstet Gynaecol 1992;99:118–21.
15. Steketee RW, Wirima JJ, Slutsker L, Heymann DL, Breman JG. The problem of malaria and malaria control in pregnancy in sub-Saharan Africa. Am J Trop Med Hyg 1996;55(Suppl):2–7.
16. Fleming AF, Ghatoura GBS, Harrison KA, Briggs ND, Dunn DT. The prevention of anaemia in pregnancy in primigravidae in the Guinea Savanna of Nigeria. Ann Trop Med Parasitol 1986;80:211–33.
17. Fleming AF. Antimalarial prophylaxis in pregnant Nigerian women. Lancet 1990;335:45.
18. Mutabingwa TK, Malle LN, de Geus A, Oosting J. Malaria chemosuppression in pregnancy. I. The effect of chemosuppressive drugs on maternal parasitaemia. Trop Geogr Med 1993;45:6–14.
19. Mutabingwa TK, Malle LN, de Geus A, Oosting J. Malaria chemosuppression in pregnancy. II. Its effect on maternal haemoglobin levels, placental malaria and birth weight. Trop Geogr Med 1993;45:49–55.
20. Mutabingwa TK, Malle LN, Eling WMC, Verhave JP, Meuwissen JHETh, de Geus A. Malaria chemosuppression in pregnancy. III. Its effects on the maternal malaria immunity. Trop Geogr Med 1993;45:103–9.
21. Mutabingwa TK, Malle LN, Verhave JP, Eling WMC, Meuwissen JHETh, de Geus A. Malaria chemosuppression during pregnancy. IV. Its effects on the newborn's passive malaria immunity. Trop Geogr Med 1993;45:150–6.
22. Wangboonskul J, White NJ, Nosten F, ter Kuile F, Moody RR, Taylor RB. Single dose pharmacokinetics of proguanil and its metabolites in pregnancy. Eur J Clin Pharmacol 1993;44:247–51.
23. Olsen VV. Why not proguanil in malaria prophylaxis? Lancet 1983;1:649.
24. Anonymous. Malaria in pregnancy. Lancet 1983;2:84–5.
25. Anonymous. Prevention of malaria in pregnancy and early childhood. Br Med J 1984;289:1296–7.

Name: **PROMAZINE** Risk Factor: **C**
Class: **Tranquilizer**

FETAL RISK SUMMARY

RECOMMENDATION: Limited Human Data - Probably Compatible

Promazine is a propylamino phenothiazine structurally related to chlorpromazine. The drug readily crosses the placenta (1,2).

The Collaborative Perinatal Project monitored 50,282 mother-child pairs, 50 of whom had 1st trimester exposure to promazine (3). For use anytime during pregnancy, 347 exposures were recorded. No evidence was found in either group to suggest a relationship to malformations or an effect on perinatal mortality rate, birth weight, or intelligence quotient scores at 4 years of age.

A possible relationship between the use of promazine (100 mg or more) in labor and neonatal hyperbilirubinemia was reported in 1975 (4). In addition, a study published in 1980 found that the administration of promazine close to delivery caused a reduction in neonatal platelet aggregation (5). The clinical significance of this effect is unknown.

Although occasional reports have attempted to link various phenothiazine compounds with congenital defects, the bulk of the evidence indicates that these drugs are safe for mother and fetus (see also Chlorpromazine).

BREAST FEEDING SUMMARY

RECOMMENDATION: No Human Data - Potential Toxicity

No reports describing the use of promazine during human lactation have been located. Because the agent readily crosses the placenta, excretion into breast milk should be expected. The effects, if any, on a nursing infant are unknown, but sedation is a possibility.

References

1. Moya F, Thorndike V. Passage of drugs across the placenta. Am J Obstet Gynecol 1962;84:1778–98.
2. O'Donoghue SEF. Distribution of pethidine and chlorpromazine in maternal, foetal and neonatal biological fluids. Nature 1971;229:124–5.
3. Slone D, Siskind V, Heinonen OP, Monson RR, Kaufman DW, Shapiro S. Antenatal exposure to the phenothiazines in relation to congenital malformations, perinatal mortality rate, birth weight, and intelligence quotient score. Am J Obstet Gynecol 1977;128:486–8.
4. John E. Promazine and neonatal hyperbilirubinemia. Med J Aust 1975;2:342–4.
5. Whaun JM, Smith GR, Sochor VA. Effect of prenatal drug administration on maternal and neonatal platelet aggregation and PF4 release. Haemostasis 1980;9:226–37.

Name: **PROMETHAZINE** Risk Factor: **C**

Class: **Antihistamine/Antiemetic**

FETAL RISK SUMMARY

RECOMMENDATION: Compatible

Promethazine is a phenothiazine antihistamine that is sometimes used as an antiemetic in pregnancy and as an adjunct to narcotic analgesics during labor.

The Collaborative Perinatal Project monitored 50,282 mother-child pairs, 114 of whom had promethazine exposure in the 1st trimester (1, pp. 323–324). For use anytime during pregnancy, 746 exposures were recorded (1, p. 437). In neither group was evidence found to suggest a relationship to large categories of major or minor malformations or to individual defects. A 1964 report also failed to show an association between 165 cases of promethazine exposure in the 1st trimester and malformations (2). In a 1971 reference, infants of mothers who had ingested antiemetics during the 1st trimester actually had significantly fewer abnormalities when compared with controls (3). Promethazine was the most commonly used antiemetic in this latter study.

In a surveillance study of Michigan Medicaid recipients conducted between 1985 and 1992 involving 229,101 completed pregnancies, 1,197 newborns had been exposed to promethazine during the 1st trimester (F. Rosa, personal communication, FDA, 1993). A total of 61 (5.1%) major birth defects were observed (51 expected). Specific data were available for six defect categories, including (observed/expected) 1/2 oral clefts, 0/1 spina bifida, 4/3 polydactyly, 1/2 limb reduction defects, 1/3 hypospadias, and 17/12 cardiovascular defects. Only with the latter defect is there a suggestion of a possible association, but other factors, including the mother's disease, concurrent drug use, and chance, may be involved.

At term, the drug rapidly crosses the placenta, appearing in cord blood within 1.5 minutes of an IV dose (4). Fetal and maternal blood concentrations are at equilibrium in 15 minutes, with infant levels persisting for at least 4 hours.

Several investigators have studied the effect of promethazine on labor and the newborn (5–13). Significant neonatal respiratory depression was seen in a small group of patients (5). However, in three large series, no clinical evidence of promethazine-induced respiratory depression was found (6–8). In a series of 33 mothers at term, 28 received either promethazine alone (one patient) or a combination of meperidine with promethazine or phenobarbital (27 patients). Transient behavioral and electroencephalographic changes, persisting for less than 3 days, were seen in all newborns (10). These and other effects prompted one author to recommend that promethazine should not be used during labor (14).

Maternal tachycardia as a result of promethazine (mean increase 30 beats/minute) or promethazine-meperidine (mean increase 42 beats/minute) was observed in one series (9). The maximum effect occurred about 10 minutes after injection. The fetal heart rate did not change significantly.

The antiemetic effects of promethazine 25 mg and metoclopramide 10 mg following the use of meperidine in labor were described in a study involving 477 women (13). Both drugs were superior to placebo as antiemetics, but significantly more of the promethazine-treated mothers had persistent sedation that extended into the immediate postpartum period. Moreover, an antianalgesic effect, as evidenced by pain score, duration of analgesia, and an increased need for meperidine, was observed when promethazine was used.

Fatal shock was reported in a pregnant woman with an undiagnosed pheochromocytoma given promethazine (15). A precipitous drop in blood pressure resulted from administration of the drug, probably secondary to unmasking of hypovolemia (15).

Effects on the uterus have been mixed, with both increases and decreases in uterine activity reported (8,9,11).

Promethazine used during labor has been shown to markedly impair platelet aggregation in the newborn but less so in the mother (12,16). Although the clinical significance of this is unknown, the degree of impairment in the newborn is comparable to those disorders associated with a definite bleeding state.

Promethazine has been used to treat hydrops fetalis in cases of anti-erythrocytic isoimmunization (17). Six patients were treated with 150 mg/day orally between the 26th and 34th weeks of gestation while undergoing intraperitoneal transfusions. No details on the infants' conditions were given except that all were born alive. Other authors have reported similarly successful results in Rh-sensitized pregnancies (18,19). As described by some authors, doses up to 6.5 mg/kg/day may be required (18). However, a 1991 review concluded that the benefits of promethazine in the treatment of Rh immunization were marginal and may be hazardous to the fetus (20).

Two female anencephalic infants were born to mothers after ovulatory stimulation with clomiphene (21). One of the mothers had taken promethazine for morning sickness. No association between promethazine and this defect has been suggested.

BREAST FEEDING SUMMARY

RECOMMENDATION: No Human Data - Probably Compatible

Available laboratory methods for the accurate detection of promethazine in breast milk are not clinically useful because of the rapid metabolism of phenothiazines (M. Lipshutz, personal communication, Wyeth Laboratories, 1981). Because of the low molecular weight (about 284), however, passage of the drug into breast milk, should be expected. The potential effects of this exposure on a nursing infant are unknown.

References

1. Heinonen OP, Slone D, Shapiro S. *Birth Defects and Drugs in Pregnancy*. Littleton, MA: Publishing Sciences Group, 1977.
2. Wheatley D. Drugs and the embryo. Br Med J 1964; 1:630.
3. Nelson MM, Forfar JO. Association between drugs administered during pregnancy and congenital abnormalities of the fetus. Br Med J 1971;1:523–7.
4. Moya F, Thorndike V. The effects of drugs used in labor on the fetus and newborn. Clin Pharmacol Ther 1963;4:628–53.
5. Crawford JS, as quoted by Moya F, Thorndike V. The effects of drugs used in labor on the fetus and newborn. Clin Pharmacol Ther 1963;4:628–53.
6. Powe CE, Kiem IM, Fromhagen C, Cavanagh D. Propiomazine hydrochloride in obstetrical analgesia. JAMA 1962;181:290–4.
7. Potts CR, Ullery JC. Maternal and fetal effects of obstetric analgesia. Am J Obstet Gynecol 1961;81: 1253–9.
8. Carroll JJ, Moir RS. Use of promethazine (Phenergan) hydrochloride in obstetrics. JAMA 1958;168: 2218–24.
9. Riffel HD, Nochimson DJ, Paul RH, Hon EH. Effects of meperidine and promethazine during labor. Obstet Gynecol 1973;42:738–45.
10. Borgstedt AD, Rosen MG. Medication during labor correlated with behavior and EEG of the newborn. Am J Dis Child 1968;115:21–4.
11. Zakut H, Mannor SM, Serr DM. Effect of promethazine on uterine contractions. Harefuah 1970;78:61–2. As cited in Anonymous. References and reviews. JAMA 1970;211:1572.
12. Corby DG, Shulman I. The effects of antenatal drug administration on aggregation of platelets of newborn infants. J Pediatr 1971;79:307–13.
13. Vella L, Francis D, Houlton P, Reynolds F. Comparison of the antiemetics metoclopramide and promethazine in labour. Br Med J 1985;290:1173–5.
14. Hall PF. Use of promethazine (Phenergan) in labour. CMAJ 1987;136:690–1.
15. Montminy M, Teres D. Shock after phenothiazine administration in a pregnant patient with a pheochromocytoma: A case report and literature review. J Reprod Med 1983;28:159–62.
16. Whaun JM, Smith GR, Sochor VA. Effect of prenatal drug administration on maternal and neonatal platelet aggregation and PF4 release. Haemostasis 1980;9:226–37.
17. Bierme S, Bierme R. Antihistamines in hydrops foetalis. Lancet 1967;1:574.
18. Gusdon JP Jr. The treatment of erythroblastosis with promethazine hydrochloride. J Reprod Med 1981;26:454–8.
19. Charles AG, Blumenthal LS. Promethazine hydrochloride therapy in severely Rh-sensitized pregnancies. Obstet Gynecol 1982;60:627–30.
20. Bowman JM. Antenatal suppression of Rh alloimmunization. Clin Obstet Gynecol 1991;34:296–303.
21. Dyson JL, Kohler HC. Anencephaly and ovulation stimulation. Lancet 1973;1:1256–7.

P

Name:	**PROPAFENONE**	Risk Factor:	C_M
Class:	**Antiarrhythmic**		

FETAL RISK SUMMARY

RECOMMENDATION: Limited Human Data - Animal Data Suggest Moderate Risk

Propafenone is an orally active antiarrhythmic used in the treatment of ventricular tachycardia. No teratogenic effects have been observed in studies with rabbits and rats, but propafenone was embryotoxic in both species when given in doses of 10 and 40 times the maximum recommended human dose, respectively (1).

Propafenone, in combination with β-methyldigoxin 400 μg/day, was administered to a 22-year-old woman between 24 and 26 weeks' gestation in an unsuccessful attempt to treat refractory fetal supraventricular tachycardia and hydrops fetalis (2). The daily dose of propafenone was 850 mg. Because transplacental passage of the antiarrhythmics was hindered by the fetal hydrops, successful resolution of the condition eventually required direct umbilical vein injections of amiodarone (see Amiodarone).

BREAST FEEDING SUMMARY

RECOMMENDATION: No Human Data - Probably Compatible

No data are available.

References

1. Product information. Rythmol. Knoll Pharmaceuticals, 2000.
2. Gembruch U, Manz M, Bald R, Rüddel H, Redel DA, Schlebusch H, Nitsch J, Hansmann M. Repeated intravascular treatment with amiodarone in a fetus with refractory supraventricular tachycardia and hydrops fetalis. Am Heart J 1989;118:1335–8.

Name: **PROPANTHELINE** Risk Factor: C_M
Class: **Parasympatholytic (Anticholinergic)**

FETAL RISK SUMMARY

RECOMMENDATION: Limited Human Data - No Relevant Animal Data

Propantheline is an anticholinergic quaternary ammonium bromide. The Collaborative Perinatal Project monitored 50,282 mother-child pairs, 33 of whom used propantheline in the 1st trimester (1). No evidence was found for an association with congenital malformations. However, when the group of parasympatholytics were taken as a whole (2,323 exposures), a possible association with minor malformations was found (1).

BREAST FEEDING SUMMARY

RECOMMENDATION: No Human Data - Probably Compatible

No data are available (see also Atropine).

P

Reference

1. Heinonen OP, Slone D, Shapiro S. *Birth Defects and Drugs in Pregnancy*. Littleton, MA: Publishing Sciences Group, 1977:346–53.

Name: **PROPOFOL** Risk Factor: B_M
Class: **Hypnotic**

FETAL RISK SUMMARY

RECOMMENDATION: Limited Human Data - Animal Data Suggest Low Risk

A number of studies have described the use during cesarean section of propofol, a hypnotic agent used for the IV induction and maintenance of anesthesia (1–20). Apparently, the drug has not been used during the 1st and 2nd trimesters in humans. Reproduction studies in rats and rabbits at doses 6 times the recommended human induction dose revealed no evidence of impaired fertility or fetal harm (21).

The pharmacokinetics of propofol in women undergoing cesarean section was reported in 1990 (1). Propofol rapidly crosses the placenta and distributes in the fetus (2–12). The fetal:maternal (umbilical vein:maternal vein) ratio is approximately 0.7. Doses were administered either by IV bolus, by continuous infusion, or by both methods.

Several studies have examined the effect of maternal propofol anesthesia on infant Apgar scores, time to sustained spontaneous respiration, and Neurologic and Adaptative Capacity Score (NACS) or Early Neonatal Neurobehavioural Scale (ENNS) (1,2,4,5,7,8,11–18). Most investigators reported no difference in the Apgar scores of infants exposed to propofol either alone or when compared with other general anesthesia techniques, such as thiopental with enflurane or isoflurane (2,5,7,8,14–18). Moreover, no correlation was found between the Apgar scores and umbilical arterial or venous concentration of propofol (2,5,8,11,15).

In one study infants ($N = 20$) exposed to a maternal propofol dose of 2.8 mg/kg had significantly lower Apgar scores at 1 and 5 minutes compared with infants ($N = 20$) whose mothers were treated with thiopental 5 mg/kg ($p < 0.05$) (13). The Apgar scores in both groups were significantly lower ($p < 0.002$) when compared with infants born by spontaneous vaginal delivery. The induction-to-delivery and uterine incision-to-delivery intervals in the two treatment groups were nearly identical. Five propofol-exposed infants had profound muscular hypotonus at birth and at 5 minutes, and one newborn was somnolent (13). Propofol-exposed infants were evaluated using the ENNS and found to have a depression in alert state, pinprick and placing reflexes, and mean decremental count in Moro and light reflexes 1 hour after birth, but not at 4 hours (13). Five (25%) of the infants exhibited generalized irritability and continuous crying at 1 hour, but not at 4 hours.

In contrast, most studies found no difference in the NACS or time to sustained spontaneous respiration between various groups with propofol IV bolus doses of 2.5 mg/kg, or when continuous infusion doses were no higher than 6 mg/kg/hour (2,5,8,14–16). Higher doses, such as 9 mg/kg/hour, were correlated with a depressed NACS (8,12, 14–16,18).

BREAST FEEDING SUMMARY

RECOMMENDATION: Limited Human Data - Probably Compatible

Small amounts of propofol are excreted into breast milk and colostrum following use of the agent for the induction and maintenance of maternal anesthesia during cesarean section (3). Two groups of women were studied. The first group consisted of four women who had received a mean IV propofol dose of 2.55 mg/kg, a mean of 25.9 minutes before delivery. The mean total dose received by patients in this group was 155.5 mg. The second group consisted of three women who had received a mean IV dose of 2.51 mg/kg plus a mean infusion of 5.08 mg/kg/hour. The mean total dose in this group was 247.4 mg, and the mean time to delivery was 20.2 minutes. Breast milk or colostrum samples were collected at various intervals from 4 to 24 hours after delivery. Propofol concentrations in the seven patients varied between 0.048 and 0.74 μg/mL, with the highest levels predictably occurring at 4–5 hours in group 2. In one patient from group 2, the milk/colostrum concentration was 0.74 μg/mL at 5 hours and fell to 0.048 μg/mL (6% of the initial sample) at 24 hours. These amounts were considered negligible when compared with the amounts the infants received before birth from placental transfer of the drug (3).

References

1. Gin T, Gregory MA, Chan K, Buckley T, Oh TE. Pharmacokinetics of propofol in women undergoing elective caesarean section. Br J Anaesth 1990;64:148–53.
2. Dailland P, Lirzin JD, Cockshott ID, Jorrot JC, Conseiller C. Placental transfer and neonatal effects of propofol administered during cesarean section (abstract). Anesthesiology 1987;67:A454.
3. Dailland P, Cockshott ID, Lirzin JD, Jacquinot P, Jorrot JC, Devery J, Harmey JL, Conseiller C. Intravenous propofol during cesarean section: Placental transfer, concentrations in breast milk, and neonatal effects. A preliminary study. Anesthesiology 1989;71:827–34.
4. Moore J, Bill KM, Flynn RJ, McKeating KT, Howard PJ. A comparison between propofol and thiopentone as induction agents in obstetric anaesthesia. Anaesthesia 1989;44:753–7.
5. Dailland P, Jacquinot P, Lirzin JD, Jorrot JC. Neonatal effects of propofol administered to the mother in anesthesia in cesarean section. Can Anesthesiol 1989;37:429–33.
6. Dailland P, Jacquinot P, Lirzin JD, Jorrot JC, Conseiller C. Comparative study of propofol with thiopental for general anesthesia in cesarean section. Ann Fr Anesth Reanim 1989;8(Suppl):R65.
7. Valtonen M, Kanto J, Rosenberg P. Comparison of propofol and thiopentone for induction of anaesthesia for elective caesarean section. Anaesthesia 1989;44:758–62.
8. Gin T, Gregory MA. Propofol for caesarean section. Anaesthesia 1990;45:165.
9. Pagnoni B, Casalino S, Monzani R, Lazzarini A, Tiengo M. Placental transfer of propofol in elective cesarean section. Minerva Anestesiol 1990;56:877–9.
10. Maglione F, Guarini MC, Montanari A, Cirillo F, Postiglione M, Pica M, Amorena M, De Liguoro M. Determination of propofol blood levels in mothers and newborns in anesthesia for cesarean section. Minerva Anestesiol 1990;56:881–3.
11. Gin T, Gregory MA, Chan K, Oh TE. Maternal and fetal levels of propofol at caesarean section. Anaesth Intensive Care 1990;18:180–4.
12. Gin T, Yau G, Chan K, Gregory MA, Oh TE. Disposition of propofol infusions for caesarean section. Can J Anaesth 1991;38:31–6.
13. Celleno D, Capogna G, Tomassetti M, Costantino P, Di Feo G, Nisini R. Neurobehavioural effects of propofol on the neonate following elective caesarean section. Br J Anaesth 1989;62:649–54.
14. Gin T, Yau G, Gregory MA. Propofol during cesarean section. Anesthesiology 1990;73:789.
15. Gin T, Yau G, Chan K, Gregory MA, Kotur CF. Recovery from propofol infusion anaesthesia for caesarean section. Neurosci Lett (Suppl) 1990;37:S44.
16. Gregory MA, Gin T, Yau G, Leung RKW, Chan K, Oh TE. Propofol infusion anaesthesia for caesarean section. Can J Anaesth 1990;37:514–20.
17. Gin T, Gregory MA, Oh TE. The haemodynamic effects of propofol and thiopentone for induction of caesarean section. Anaesth Intensive Care 1990;18:175–9.
18. Yau G, Gin T, Ewart MC, Kotur CF, Leung RKW, Oh TE. Propofol for induction and maintenance of anaesthesia at caesarean section. Anaesthesia 1991;46:20–3.
19. Costantino P, Emanuelli M, Muratori F, Sebastiani M. Propofol versus thiopentone as induction agents in cesarean section. Minerva Anestesiol 1990;56:865–70.
20. Alberico FP. Propofol in anesthesia induction for cesarean section. Minerva Anestesiol 1990;56:871.
21. Product information. Diprivan. AstraZeneca, 2000.

Name: **PROPOXYPHENE** Risk Factor: **C***

Class: **Narcotic Agonist Analgesic**

FETAL RISK SUMMARY

RECOMMENDATION: Human Data Suggest Risk in 3rd Trimester

Four case reports, involving five patients, have described the use of propoxyphene during pregnancies that resulted in infants with congenital abnormalities (1–4). However, other drugs were used in each case and any association may be fortuitous:

Pierre Robin syndrome, arthrogryposis, severe mental and growth retardation (1 infant) (1)
Absence of left forearm and radial two digits, syndactyly of ulnar three digits and left fourth and fifth toes, hypoplastic left femur (1 infant) (2)
Omphalocele, defective anterior left wall, diaphragmatic defect, congenital heart disease with partial ectopic cordis because of sternal cleft, dysplastic hips (1 infant) (2)

Micrognathia, widely spaced sutures, beaked nose, bifid uvula, defects of toes, withdrawal seizures (1 infant) (3)
Bilateral anophthalmia (1 infant) (4)

A 1982 study of 350 patients with congenital contractures of the joints (arthrogryposis) concluded that only 15 had been exposed to a possible teratogen (5). One of the 15 cases involved a 24-year-old woman who had consumed, at 2 months gestation, propoxyphene (65 mg) and methocarbamol (750 mg) 2–3 times daily for 3 days to treat severe back pain. The term female infant was noted at birth to have multiple joint contractures involving the thumbs, wrists, elbows, knees, and feet. The latter were described as a bilateral equinovarus deformity. There were practically no foot creases. Other abnormalities present were frontal bosselation, a midline hemangioma, and weak abdominal musculature. Development was normal at 3 years of age except for the joint contractures, which had improved with time, and a grade I/VI systolic murmur. The cause of the malformations was unknown, although the authors speculated that there may have been a link to methocarbamol (5).

The Collaborative Perinatal Project monitored 50,282 mother-child pairs, 686 of whom had 1st trimester exposure to propoxyphene (6, pp. 287–295). For use anytime during pregnancy, 2914 exposures were recorded (6, p. 434). No evidence was found in either group to suggest a relationship to large categories of major or minor malformations or, in the 1st trimester, to individual defects. Five possible associations with individual defects after anytime use were observed, but independent confirmation is required (6, p.484): microcephaly (6 cases); persistent ductus arteriosus (5 cases); cataract (5 cases); benign tumors (12 cases); and clubfoot (18 cases).

In a surveillance study of Michigan Medicaid recipients conducted between 1985 and 1992 involving 229,101 completed pregnancies, 1,029 newborns had been exposed to propoxyphene during the 1st trimester (F. Rosa, personal communication, FDA, 1993). A total of 41 (4.0%) major birth defects were observed (43 expected). Specific data were available for six defect categories, including (observed/expected) 10/10 cardiovascular defects, 2/2 oral clefts, 0/1 spina bifida, 3/3 polydactyly, 0/2 limb reduction defects, and 1/2 hypospadias. These data do not support an association between the drug and congenital defects.

Neonatal withdrawal has been reported in five infants (3,7–10). The relationship between heavy maternal ingestion of this drug and neonatal withdrawal seems clear. The infants were asymptomatic with normal Apgar scores until 3.5–14 hours after delivery. Withdrawal was marked by the onset of irritability, tremors, diarrhea, fever, high-pitched cry, hyperactivity, hypertonicity, diaphoresis, and, in two cases, seizures. Symptoms began to subside by day 4, usually without specific therapy. Examinations after 2–3 months were normal.

Propoxyphene has been used in labor without causing neonatal respiratory depression (11). However, a significant shortening of the first stage of labor occurred without an effect on uterine contractions.

[**Risk Factor D if used for prolonged periods.*]

BREAST FEEDING SUMMARY

RECOMMENDATION: Limited Human Data - Probably Compatible

Propoxyphene passes into breast milk, but the amounts and clinical significance are unknown. In one case, a nursing mother attempted suicide with propoxyphene (12). The

P

concentration of the drug in her breast milk was found to be 50% of her plasma level. By calculation, the authors predicted a mother consuming a maximum daily dose of the drug would provide her infant with 1 mg/day. The American Academy of Pediatrics classifies propoxyphene as compatible with breast-feeding (13).

References

1. Barrow MV, Souder DE. Propoxyphene and congenital malformations. JAMA 1971;217:1551–2.
2. Ringrose CAD. The hazard of neurotrophic drugs in the fertile years. Can Med Assoc J 1972;106:1058.
3. Golden NL, King KC, Sokol RJ. Propoxyphene and acetaminophen: possible effects on the fetus. Clin Pediatr 1982;21:752–4.
4. Golden SM, Perman KI. Bilateral clinical anophthalmia: drugs as potential factors. South Med J 1980; 73:1404–7.
5. Hall JG, Reed SD. Teratogens associated with congenital contractures in humans and in animals. Teratology 1982;25:173–91.
6. Heinonen OP, Slone D, Shapiro S. *Birth Defects and Drugs in Pregnancy*. Littleton, MA: Publishing Sciences Group, 1977.
7. Tyson HK. Neonatal withdrawal symptoms associated with maternal use of propoxyphene hydrochloride (Darvon). J Pediatr 1974;85:684–5.
8. Klein RB, Blatman S, Little GA. Probable neonatal propoxyphene withdrawal: a case report. Pediatrics 1975;55:882–4.
9. Quillan WW, Dunn CA. Neonatal drug withdrawal from propoxyphene. JAMA 1976;235:2128.
10. Ente G, Mehra MC. Neonatal drug withdrawal from propoxyphene hydrochloride. N Y State J Med 1978;78:2084–5.
11. Eddy NB, Friebel H, Hahn KJ, Halbach H. Codeine and its alternatives for pain and cough relief. 2. Alternates for pain relief. Bull WHO 1969;40:1–53.
12. Catz C, Guiacoia G. Drugs and breast milk. Pediatr Clin North Am 1972;19:151–66.
13. Committee on Drugs, American Academy of Pediatrics. The transfer of drugs and other chemicals into human milk. Pediatrics 2001;108:776–89.

Name: **PROPRANOLOL** Risk Factor: **C_M***

Class: **Sympatholytic (Antihypertensive)**

FETAL RISK SUMMARY

RECOMMENDATION: Human Data Suggest Risk in 2nd and 3rd Trimesters

P

Propranolol, a nonselective β-adrenergic blocking agent, has been used for various indications in pregnancy:

Maternal hyperthyroidism (1–7)
Pheochromocytoma (8)
Maternal cardiac disease (6,7,9–20)
Fetal tachycardia or arrhythmia (21,22)
Maternal hypertension (7,20,23–30)
Dysfunctional labor (31)
Termination of pregnancy (32)

Reproduction studies in rats revealed embryotoxicity (increased resorption sites and reduced litter sizes) and reduced neonatal survival at doses up to about 10 times the maximum recommended human dose (MRHD) (33). No embryotoxicity was observed in rabbits at doses up to about 20 times the MRHD. No teratogenicity was noted in either species.

The drug readily crosses the placenta (2,6,12,16,22,29,34,35). Cord serum levels varying between 19% and 127% of maternal serum have been reported (2,16,22,29). Oxytocic effects have been demonstrated following IV, extra-amniotic injections, and high oral dosing (17,31,32,36,37). IV propranolol has been shown to block or decrease the marked increase in maternal plasma progesterone induced by vasopressin or theophylline (38). The pharmacokinetics of propranolol in pregnancy have been described (39). Plasma levels and elimination were not significantly altered by pregnancy.

A number of fetal and neonatal adverse effects have been reported following the use of propranolol in pregnancy. Whether these effects were caused by propranolol, maternal disease, other drugs consumed concurrently, or a combination of these factors is not always clear. Daily doses of 160 mg or higher seem to produce the more serious complications, but lower doses have also resulted in toxicity. Analysis of 23 reports involving 167 liveborn infants exposed to chronic propranolol *in utero* is shown below (1–4,6,7,9,11–14,20,22–24,26–29,40–43):

NO.	CASES	%
Intrauterine growth retardation (IUGR)	23	14
Hypoglycemia	16	10
Bradycardia	12	7
Respiratory depression at birth	6	4
Hyperbilirubinemia	6	4
Small placenta (size not always noted)	4	2
Polycythemia	2	1
Thrombocytopenia (40,000/mm^3)	1	0.6
Hyperirritability	1	0.6
Hypocalcemia with convulsions	1	0.6
Blood coagulation defect	1	0.6

Two infants were reported to have anomalies (pyloric stenosis; crepitus of hip), but the authors did not relate these to propranolol (27,40). In another case, a malformed fetus was spontaneously aborted from a 30-year-old woman with chronic renovascular hypertension (44). The patient had been treated with propranolol, amiloride, and captopril for her severe hypertension. Malformations included absence of the left leg below the midthigh and no obvious skull formation above the brain tissue. The authors attributed the defect either to captopril alone or to a combination effect of the three drugs (44), but recent reports have associated fetal calvarial hypoplasia with captopril (see Captopril).

In a surveillance study of Michigan Medicaid recipients conducted between 1985 and 1992 involving 229,101 completed pregnancies, 274 newborns had been exposed to propranolol during the 1st trimester (F. Rosa, personal communication, FDA, 1993). A total of 11 (4.0%) major birth defects were observed (12 expected), including (observed/expected) 3/3 cardiovascular defects and 2/1 hypospadias. No anomalies were observed in four other defect categories (oral clefts, spina bifida, polydactyly, and limb reduction defects) for which specific data were available.

Respiratory depression was noted in four of five infants whose mothers were given 1 mg of propranolol IV just before cesarean section (45). None of the five controls in the double-blind study was depressed at birth. The author suggested the mechanism may have been β-adrenergic blockade of the cervical sympathetic discharge that occurs at cord clamping.

Fetal bradycardia was observed in 2 of 10 patients treated with propranolol, 1 mg/minute for 4 minutes, for dysfunctional labor (31). No lasting effects were seen in the babies. In a retrospective study, 8 markedly hypertensive patients (9 pregnancies) treated with propranolol were compared with 15 hypertensive controls not treated with propranolol (25). Other antihypertensives were used in both groups. A significant difference was found between the perinatal mortality rates, with 7 deaths in the propranolol group (78%) and only 5 deaths in the controls (33%). However, a possible explanation for the difference may have been the more severe hypertension and renal disease in the propranolol group than in the controls (46).

IUGR may be related to propranolol. Several possible mechanisms for this effect, if indeed it is associated with the drug, have been reviewed (47). Premature labor has been suggested as a possible complication of propranolol therapy in patients with gestational hypertension (42). In nine women treated with propranolol for gestational hypertension, three delivered prematurely. The author speculated that these patients were relatively hypovolemic and when a compensatory increase in cardiac output failed to occur, premature delivery resulted. However, another report on chronic propranolol use in 14 women did not observe premature labor (43).

In a randomized, double-blind trial, 36 patients at term were given either 80 mg of propranolol or placebo (48). Fetal heart rate reaction to a controlled sound stimulus was then measured at 1, 2, and 3 hours. The heart rate reaction in the propranolol group was significantly depressed, compared with placebo, at all three time intervals.

The reactivity of nonstress tests (NSTs) was affected by propranolol in two hypertensive women in the 2nd and 3rd trimesters (49). One woman was taking 20 mg every 6 hours and the other 10 mg 3 times daily. Repeated NSTs were nonreactive in both women, but immediate follow-up contraction stress tests were negative. The NSTs became reactive 2 and 10 days, respectively, after propranolol was discontinued.

In summary, propranolol has been used during pregnancy for maternal and fetal indications. The drug is apparently not a teratogen, but fetal and neonatal toxicity may occur. A 1988 review on the use of β-blockers, including propranolol, during pregnancy concluded that these agents are relatively safe (50), but some β-blockers, including propranolol, may cause IUGR and reduced placental weight, especially those lacking intrinsic sympathomimetic activity (ISA) (i.e., partial agonist). Treatment beginning early in the 2nd trimester results in the greatest weight reductions, whereas treatment restricted to the 3rd trimester primarily affects only placental weight. Propranolol does not possess ISA. However, IUGR and reduced placental weight may potentially occur with all agents within this class. Although growth retardation is a serious concern, the benefits of maternal therapy with β-blockers, in some cases, might outweigh the risks to the fetus and must be judged on a case-by-case basis.

Newborn infants of women consuming the drug near delivery should be closely observed during the first 24–48 hours after birth for bradycardia, hypoglycemia, and other symptoms of β-blockade. Long-term effects of *in utero* exposure to β-blockers have not been studied but warrant evaluation.

[**Risk Factor D if used in 2nd or 3rd trimesters.*]

BREAST FEEDING SUMMARY

RECOMMENDATION: Limited Human Data - Potential Toxicity

Propranolol is excreted into breast milk. Peak concentrations occur 2–3 hours after a dose (12,20,43,51). Milk levels have ranged from 4 to 64 ng/mL, with milk:plasma ratios of

0.2–1.5 (12,20,29,50). Although such adverse effects as respiratory depression, bradycardia, and hypoglycemia have not been reported, nursing infants exposed to propranolol in breast milk should be closely observed for these symptoms of β-blockade. Long-term effects of exposure to β-blockers from milk have not been studied but warrant evaluation. The American Academy of Pediatrics classifies propranolol as compatible with breast-feeding (52).

References

1. Jackson GL. Treatment of hyperthyroidism in pregnancy. Pa Med 1973;76:56–7.
2. Langer A, Hung CT, McA'Nulty JA, Harrigan JT, Washington E. Adrenergic blockade: a new approach to hyperthyroidism during pregnancy. Obstet Gynecol 1974;44:181–6.
3. Bullock JL, Harris RE, Young R. Treatment of thyrotoxicosis during pregnancy with propranolol. Am J Obstet Gynecol 1975;121:242–5.
4. Lightner ES, Allen HD, Loughlin G. Neonatal hyperthyroidism and heart failure: a different approach. Am J Dis Child 1977;131:68–70.
5. Levy CA, Waite JH, Dickey R. Thyrotoxicosis and pregnancy. Use of preoperative propranolol for thyroidectomy. Am J Surg 1977;133:319–21.
6. Habib A, McCarthy JS. Effects on the neonate of propranolol administered during pregnancy. J Pediatr 1977;91:808–11.
7. Pruyn SC, Phelan JP, Buchanan GC. Long-term propranolol therapy in pregnancy: maternal and fetal outcome. Am J Obstet Gynecol 1979;135:485–9.
8. Leak D, Carroll JJ, Robinson DC, Ashworth EJ. Management of pheochromocytoma during pregnancy. Can Med Assoc J 1977;116:371–5.
9. Turner GM, Oakley CM, Dixon HG. Management of pregnancy complicated by hypertrophic obstructive cardiomyopathy. Br Med J 1968;4:281–4.
10. Barnes AB. Chronic propranolol administration during pregnancy: a case report. J Reprod Med 1970;5:79–80.
11. Schroeder JS, Harrison DC. Repeated cardioversion during pregnancy. Am J Cardiol 1971;27:445–6.
12. Levitan AA, Manion JC. Propranolol therapy during pregnancy and lactation. Am J Cardiol 1973;32:247.
13. Reed RL, Cheney CB, Fearon RE, Hook R, Hehre FW. Propranolol therapy throughout pregnancy: a case report. Anesth Analg (Cleve) 1974;53:214–8.
14. Fiddler GI. Propranolol pregnancy. Lancet 1974;2:722–3.
15. Kolibash AE, Ruiz DE, Lewis RP. Idiopathic hypertrophic subaortic stenosis in pregnancy. Ann Intern Med 1975;82:791–4.
16. Cottrill CM, McAllister RG Jr, Gettes L, Noonan JA. Propranolol therapy during pregnancy, labor, and delivery: Evidence for transplacental drug transfer and impaired neonatal drug disposition. J Pediatr 1977;91:812–4.
17. Datta S, Kitzmiller JL, Ostheimer GW, Schoenbaum SC. Propranolol and parturition. Obstet Gynecol 1978;51:577–81.
18. Diaz JH, McDonald JS. Propranolol and induced labor: Anesthetic implications. Anesth Rev 1979;6:29–32.
19. Oakley GDG, McGarry K, Limb DG, Oakley CM. Management of pregnancy in patients with hypertrophic cardiomyopathy. Br Med J 1979;1:1749–50.
20. Bauer JH, Pape B, Zajicek J, Groshong T. Propranolol in human plasma and breast milk. Am J Cardiol 1979;43:860–2.
21. Eibschitz I, Abinader EG, Klein A, Sharf M. Intrauterine diagnosis and control of fetal ventricular arrhythmia during labor. Am J Obstet Gynecol 1975;122:597–600.
22. Teuscher A, Boss E, Imhof P, Erb E, Stocker FP, Weber JW. Effect of propranolol on fetal tachycardia in diabetic pregnancy. Am J Cardiol 1978;42:304–7.
23. Gladstone GR, Hordof A, Gersony WM. Propranolol administration during pregnancy: Effects on the fetus. J Pediatr 1975;86:962–4.
24. Tcherdakoff PH, Colliard M, Berrard E, Kreft C, Dupry A, Bernaille JM. Propranolol in hypertension during pregnancy. Br Med J 1978;2:670.
25. Lieberman BA, Stirrat GM, Cohen SL, Beard RW, Pinker GD, Belsey E. The possible adverse effect of propranolol on the fetus in pregnancies complicated by severe hypertension. Br J Obstet Gynaecol 1978;85:678–83.
26. Eliahou HE, Silverberg DS, Reisin E, Romen I, Mashiach S, Serr DM. Propranolol for the treatment of hypertension in pregnancy. Br J Obstet Gynaecol 1978;85:431–6.
27. Bott-Kanner G, Schweitzer A, Schoenfeld A, Joel-Cohen J, Rosenfeld JB. Treatment with propranolol and hydralazine throughout pregnancy in a hypertensive patient: a case report. Isr J Med Sci 1978;14:466–8.
28. Bott-Kanner G, Reisner SH, Rosenfeld JB. Propranolol and hydralazine in the management of essential hypertension in pregnancy. Br Obstet Gynaecol 1980;87:110–4.
29. Taylor EA, Turner P. Anti-hypertensive therapy with propranolol during pregnancy and lactation. Postgrad Med J 1981;57:427–30.
30. Serup J. Propranolol for the treatment of hypertension in pregnancy. Acta Med Scand 1979;206:333.
31. Mitrani A, Oettinger M, Abinader EG, Sharf M, Klein A. Use of propranolol in dysfunctional labour. Br J Obstet Gynaecol 1975;82:651–5.
32. Amy JJ, Karim SMM. Intrauterine administration of 1-noradrenaline and propranolol during the second trimester of pregnancy. J Obstet Gynaecol Br Commonw 1974;81:75–83.
33. Product information. Inderal. Wyeth-Ayerst Laboratories, 1997.
34. Smith MT, Livingstone I, Eadie MJ, Hooper WD, Triggs EJ. Metabolism of propranolol in the human

P

maternal-placental-foetal unit. Eur J Clin Pharmacol 1983;24:727–32.
35. Erkkola R, Lammintausta R, Liukko P, Anttila M. Transfer of propranolol and sotalol across the human placenta. Acta Obstet Gynecol Scand 1982;61:31–4.
36. Barden TP, Stander RW. Myometrial and cardiovascular effects of an adrenergic blocking drug in human pregnancy. Am J Obstet Gynecol 1968;101:91–9.
37. Wansbrough H, Nakanishi H, Wood C. The effect of adrenergic receptor blocking drugs on the human fetus. J Obstet Gynaecol Br Commonw 1968;75: 189–98.
38. Fylling P. Dexamethasone or propranolol blockade of induced increase in plasma progesterone in early human pregnancy. Acta Endocrinol (Copenh) 1973;72:569–72.
39. Smith MT, Livingstone I, Eadie MJ, Hooper WD, Triggs EJ. Chronic propranolol administration during pregnancy: maternal pharmacokinetics. Eur J Clin Pharmacol 1983;25:481–90.
40. O'Connor PC, Jick H, Hunter JR, Stergachis A, Madsen S. Propranolol and pregnancy outcome. Lancet 1981;2:1168.
41. Caldroney RD. Beta-blockers in pregnancy. N Engl J Med 1982;306:810.
42. Goodlin RC. Beta blocker in pregnancy-induced hypertension. Am J Obstet Gynecol 1982;143:237.
43. Livingstone I, Craswell PW, Bevan EB, Smith MT, Eadie MJ. Propranolol in pregnancy: three year prospective study. Clin Exp Hypertens (B) 1983;2:341–50.
44. Duminy PC, Burger P du T. Fetal abnormality associated with the use of captopril during pregnancy. S Afr Med J 1981;60:805.
45. Tunstall ME. The effect of propranolol on the onset of breathing at birth. Br J Anaesth 1969;41:792.
46. Rubin PC. Beta-blockers in pregnancy. N Engl J Med 1981;305:1323–6.
47. Redmond GP. Propranolol and fetal growth retardation. Semin Perinatol 1982;6:142–7.
48. Jensen OH. Fetal heart rate response to a controlled sound stimulus after propranolol administration to the mother. Acta Obstet Gynecol Scand 1984;63: 199–202.
49. Margulis E, Binder D, Cohen AW. The effect of propranolol on the nonstress test. Am J Obstet Gynecol 1984;148:340–1.
50. Frishman WH, Chesner M. Beta-adrenergic blockers in pregnancy. Am Heart J 1988;115:147–52.
51. Karlberg B, Lundberg O, Aberg H. Excretion of propranolol in human breast milk. Acta Pharmacol Toxicol (Copenh) 1974;34:222–4.
52. Committee on Drugs, American Academy of Pediatrics. The transfer of drugs and other chemicals into human milk. Pediatrics 2001;108:776–89.

Name:	**PROPYLTHIOURACIL**	Risk Factor: **D**
Class:	**Antithyroid**	

FETAL RISK SUMMARY

RECOMMENDATION: Compatible - Maternal Benefit >> Embryo/Fetal Risk

Propylthiouracil (PTU) has been used for the treatment of hyperthyroidism during pregnancy since its introduction in the 1940s (1–39). The drug prevents synthesis of thyroid hormones and inhibits peripheral deiodination of levothyroxine (T_4) to liothyronine (T_3) (40).

PTU crosses the placenta. Four patients undergoing therapeutic abortion were given a single 15-mg ^{35}S-labeled oral dose 2 hours before pregnancy termination (41). Serum could not be obtained from two 8-week-old fetuses, but 0.0016%–0.0042% of the given dose was found in the fetal tissues. In two other fetuses at 12 and 16 weeks of age, the fetal:maternal serum ratios were 0.27 and 0.35, respectively, with 0.020% and 0.025% of the dose in the fetuses. A 1986 report described the pharmacokinetics of PTU in six pregnant, hyperthyroid women (42). Serum concentrations of PTU consistently decreased during the 3rd trimester. At delivery in five patients, 1–9 hours after the last dose of 100–150 mg, the mean maternal serum concentration of PTU was 0.19 μg/mL (range <0.02–0.52 μg/mL) compared with a mean cord blood level of 0.36 μg/mL (range 0.03–0.67 μg/mL). The cord:maternal serum ratio was 1.9 (42).

The primary effect on the fetus from transplacental passage of PTU is the production of a mild hypothyroidism when the drug is used close to term. This usually resolves within a few days without treatment (34). Clinically, the hypothyroid state may be observed as a goiter in the newborn and is the result of increased levels of fetal pituitary thyrotropin (24). The incidence of fetal goiter after PTU treatment in reported cases is approximately 12% (29 goiters/241 patients) (1–37,43). Some of these cases may have been caused by coadministration of iodides (9,11,18,22). Use of PTU early in pregnancy does not produce fetal goiter because the fetal thyroid does not begin hormone production until approximately the 11th or 12th week of gestation (44). Goiters from PTU exposure are usually small and do not obstruct the airway as do iodide-induced goiters (see also Potassium Iodide) (43–45). However, two reports have been located that described PTU-induced goiters in newborns that were sufficiently massive to produce tracheal compression resulting in death in one infant and moderate respiratory distress in the second (7,10). In two other PTU-exposed fetuses, clinical hypothyroidism was evident at birth with subsequent retarded mental and physical development (10–12). One of these infants was also exposed to high doses of iodide during gestation (12). PTU-induced goiters are not predictable or dose dependent, but the smallest possible dose of PTU should be used, especially during the 3rd trimester (19,33,44–46). No effect on intellectual or physical development from PTU-induced hypothyroxinemia was observed in comparison studies between exposed and nonexposed siblings (19,47).

Congenital anomalies have been reported in seven newborns exposed to PTU *in utero* (14,17,21,27,34). This incidence is well within the expected rate of malformations. Maternal hyperthyroidism itself has been shown to be a cause of malformations (48). No association between PTU and defects has been suggested. The reported defects were as follows: congenital dislocation of hip (14); cryptorchidism (17); muscular hypotonicity (17); syndactyly of hand and foot (I^{131} also used) (21); hypospadias (27); aortic atresia (27); and choanal atresia (34).

In a large prospective study, 25 patients were exposed to one or more noniodide thyroid suppressants during the 1st trimester, 16 of whom took PTU (49). From the total group, 4 children with nonspecified malformations were found, suggesting that this group of drugs may be teratogenic. However, because of the maternal disease and the use of other drugs (i.e., methimazole in 9 women and other thiouracil derivatives in 2), the relationship between PTU and the anomalies cannot be determined. This study also noted that independent confirmation of the data was required (49).

In a surveillance study of Michigan Medicaid recipients conducted between 1985 and 1992 involving 229,101 completed pregnancies, 35 newborns had been exposed to PTU during the 1st trimester (F. Rosa, personal communication, FDA, 1993). One (2.9%) major birth defect was observed (one expected), a case of hypospadias (none expected).

A 1992 abstract and a later full report described a retrospective evaluation of hyperthyroid pregnancy outcomes treated with either PTU ($N = 99$) or methimazole ($N = 36$) (50,51). Three (3.0%) defects were observed in those exposed to PTU (ventricular septal defect; pulmonary stenosis; patent ductus arteriosus in a term infant), whereas one newborn (2.8%) had a defect (inguinal hernia) in the methimazole group. No scalp defects were observed.

In comparison with other antithyroid drugs, propylthiouracil is considered the drug of choice for the medical treatment of hyperthyroidism during pregnancy (see also Carbimazole, Methimazole, Potassium Iodide) (34,36,44–46). Combination therapy with thyroid-antithyroid drugs was advocated at one time but is now considered inappropriate

(25,26,34,36,44–46,52). Two reasons for this change are that (a) the use of thyroid hormones may require higher doses of PTU to be used, and (b) placental transfer of T_4 and T_3 is minimal and not sufficient to reverse fetal hypothyroidism (see also Levothyroxine and Liothyronine).

BREAST FEEDING SUMMARY

RECOMMENDATION: Compatible

Propylthiouracil (PTU) is excreted into breast milk in low amounts. In a patient given 100 mg of radiolabeled PTU, the milk:plasma ratio was a constant 0.55 for a 24-hour period, representing about 0.077% of the given radioactive dose (53). In a second study, nine patients were given an oral dose of 400 mg (54). Mean serum and milk levels at 90 minutes were 7.7 μg/mL and 0.7 μg/mL, respectively. The average amount excreted in milk during 4 hours was 99 μg, about 0.025% of the total dose. One mother took 200–300 mg daily while breast-feeding. No changes in any of the infant's thyroid parameters were observed (54).

Based on these two reports, PTU does not seem to pose a significant risk to the breast-fed infant, but periodic evaluation of the infant's thyroid function would be prudent. A 1987 review of antithyroid medication during lactation considered PTU the drug of choice because it is ionized at physiologic pH and protein bound (80%), both limiting its transfer into milk (55).

An interesting study published in 2000 found that the physician's advice was the only significant predictor of a woman's choice to breast-feed during PTU therapy (56). In the postpartum period, a group of 36 hyperthyroid women who required PTU were compared with 30 women who no longer required PTU therapy and 36 healthy women (controls). The breast-feeding initiation rates in the three groups were 44%, 83%, and 83%, respectively. In 15 of the women receiving PTU who breast-fed, advice on breast-feeding was given by 22 physicians (20 in favor, 1 against, and 1 equivocal). In those women taking PTU that formula fed, 11 received advice from 17 physicians (4 in favor, 12 against, and 1 equivocal) (56).

The American Academy of Pediatrics classifies propylthiouracil as compatible with breast-feeding (57).

References

1. Astwood EB, VanderLaan WP. Treatment of hyperthyroidism with propylthiouracil. Ann Intern Med 1946;25:813–21.
2. Bain L. Propylthiouracil in pregnancy: Report of a case. South Med J 1947;40:1020–1.
3. Lahey FH, Bartels EC. The use of thiouracil, thiobarbital and propylthiouracil in patients with hyperthyroidism. Ann Surg 1947;125:572–81.
4. Reveno WS. Propylthiouracil in the treatment of toxic goiter. J Clin Endocrinol Metab 1948;8:866–74.
5. Eisenberg L. Thyrotoxicosis complicating pregnancy. N Y State J Med 1950;50:1618–9.
6. Astwood EB. The use of antithyroid drugs during pregnancy. J Clin Endocrinol Metab 1951;11:1045–56.
7. Aaron HH, Schneierson SJ, Siegel E. Goiter in newborn infant due to mother's ingestion of propylthiouracil. JAMA 1955;159:848–50.
8. Waldinger C, Wermer OS, Sobel EH. Thyroid function in infant with congenital goiter resulting from exposure to propylthiouracil. J Am Med Wom Assoc 1955;10:196–7.
9. Bongiovanni AM, Eberlein WR, Thomas PZ, Anderson WB. Sporadic goiter of the newborn. J Clin Endocrinol Met 1956;16:146–52.
10. Krementz ET, Hooper RG, Kempson RL. The effect on the rabbit fetus of the maternal administration of propylthiouracil. Surgery 1957;41:619–31.
11. Branch LK, Tuthill SW. Goiters in twins resulting from propylthiouracil given during pregnancy. Ann Intern Med 1957;46:145–8.
12. Man EB, Shaver BA Jr, Cooke RE. Studies of children born to women with thyroid disease. Am J Obstet Gynecol 1958;75:728–41.
13. Becker WF, Sudduth PG. Hyperthyroidism and pregnancy. Ann Surg 1959;149:867–74.
14. Greenman GW, Gabrielson MO, Howard-Flanders J,

Wessel MA. Thyroid dysfunction in pregnancy. N Engl J Med 1962;267:426–31.

15. Herbst AL, Selenkow HA. Combined antithyroid-thyroid therapy of hyperthyroidism in pregnancy. Obstet Gynecol 1963;21:543–50.
16. Reveno WS, Rosenbaum H. Observations on the use of antithyroid drugs. Ann Intern Med 1964;60:982–9.
17. Herbst AL, Selenkow HA. Hyperthyroidism during pregnancy. N Engl J Med 1965;273:627–33.
18. Burrow GN. Neonatal goiter after maternal propylthiouracil therapy. J Clin Endocrinol Metab 1965;25:403–8.
19. Burrow GN, Bartsocas C, Klatskin EH, Grunt JA. Children exposed in utero to propylthiouracil. Am J Dis Child 1968;116:161–5.
20. Talbert LM, Thomas CG Jr, Holt WA, Rankin P. Hyperthyroidism during pregnancy. Obstet Gynecol 1970;36:779–85.
21. Hollingsworth DR, Austin E. Thyroxine derivatives in amniotic fluid. J Pediatr 1971;79:923–9.
22. Ayromlooi J. Congenital goiter due to maternal ingestion of iodides. Obstet Gynecol 1972;39:818–22.
23. Worley RJ, Crosby WM. Hyperthyroidism during pregnancy. Am J Obstet Gynecol 1974;119:150–5.
24. Refetoff S, Ochi Y, Selenkow HA, Rosenfield RL. Neonatal hypothyroidism and goiter in one infant of each of two sets of twins due to maternal therapy with antithyroid drugs. J Pediatr 1974;85:240–4.
25. Mestman JH, Manning PR, Hodgman J. Hyperthyroidism and pregnancy. Arch Intern Med 1974;134:434–9.
26. Goluboff LG, Sisson JC, Hamburger JI. Hyperthyroidism associated with pregnancy. Obstet Gynecol 1974;44:107–16.
27. Mujtaba Q, Burrow GN. Treatment of hyperthyroidism in pregnancy with propylthiouracil and methimazole. Obstet Gynecol 1975;46:282–6.
28. Serup J, Petersen S. Hyperthyroidism during pregnancy treated with propylthiouracil. Acta Obstet Gynecol Scand 1977,56.463–6.
29. Petersen S, Serup J. Case report: neonatal thyrotoxicosis. Acta Paediatr Scand 1977;66:639–42.
30. Serup J. Maternal propylthiouracil to manage fetal hyperthyroidism. Lancet 1978;2:896.
31. Wallace EZ, Gandhi VS. Triiodothyronine thyrotoxicosis in pregnancy. Am J Obstet Gynecol 1978;130:106–7.
32. Weiner S, Scharf JI, Bolognese RJ, Librizzi RJ. Antenatal diagnosis and treatment of a fetal goiter. J Reprod Med 1980;24:39–42.
33. Sugrue D, Drury MI. Hyperthyroidism complicating pregnancy: results of treatment by antithyroid drugs in 77 pregnancies. Br J Obstet Gynaecol 1980;87:970–5.
34. Cheron RG, Kaplan MM, Larsen PR, Selenkow HA, Crigler JF Jr. Neonatal thyroid function after propylthiouracil therapy for maternal Graves' disease. N Engl J Med 1981;304:525–8.
35. Check JH, Rezvani I, Goodner D, Hopper B. Prenatal treatment of thyrotoxicosis to prevent intrauterine growth retardation. Obstet Gynecol 1982;60:122–4.
36. Kock HCLV, Merkus JMWM. Graves' disease during pregnancy. Eur J Obstet Gynecol Reprod Biol 1983;14:323–30.
37. Hollingsworth DR, Austin E. Observations following I131 for Graves disease during first trimester of pregnancy. South Med J 1969;62:1555–6.
38. Burrow GN. The management of thyrotoxicosis in pregnancy. N Engl J Med 1985;313:562–5.
39. Momotani N, Noh J, Oyanagi H, Ishikawa N, Ito K. Antithyroid drug therapy for Graves' disease during pregnancy. Optimal regiment for fetal thyroid status. N Engl J Med 1986;315:24–8.
40. American Hospital Formulary Service. *Drug Information 1997*. Bethesda, MD: American Society of Health-System Pharmacists, 1997:2487–8.
41. Marchant B, Brownlie EW, Hart DM, Horton PW, Alexander WD. The placental transfer of propylthiouracil, methimazole and carbimazole. J Clin Endocrinol Metab 1977;45:1187–93.
42. Gardner DF, Cruikshank DP, Hays PM, Cooper DS. Pharmacology of propylthiouracil (PTU) in pregnant hyperthyroid women: Correlation of maternal PTU concentrations with cord serum thyroid function tests. J Clin Endocrinol Metab 1986;62:217–20.
43. Ramsay I, Kaur S, Krassas G. Thyrotoxicosis in pregnancy: Results of treatment by antithyroid drugs combined with T_4. Clin Endocrinol (Oxf) 1983;18:73–85.
44. Burr WA. Thyroid disease. Clin Obstet Gynecol 1981;8:341–51.
45. Burrow GN. Hyperthyroidism during pregnancy. N Engl J Med 1978,298:150–3.
46. Burrow GN. Maternal-fetal considerations in hyperthyroidism. Clin Endocrinol Metab 1978;7:115–25.
47. Burrow GN, Klatskin EH, Genel M. Intellectual development in children whose mothers received propylthiouracil during pregnancy. Yale J Biol Med 1978;51:151–6.
48. Momotani N, Ito K, Hamada N, Ban Y, Nishikawa Y, Mimura T. Maternal hyperthyroidism and congenital malformations in the offspring. Clin Endocrinol (Oxf) 1984;20:695–700.
49. Heinonen OP, Slone D, Shapiro S. *Birth Defects and Drugs in Pregnancy*. Littleton, MA: Publishing Sciences Group, 1977:388–400.
50. Wing D, Millar L, Koonings P, Montoro M, Mestman J. A comparison of PTU versus Tapazole in the treatment of hyperthyroidism (abstract). Am J Obstet Gynecol 1992;166:308.
51. Wing DA, Millar LK, Koonings PP, Montoro MN, Mestman JH. A comparison of propylthiouracil versus methimazole in the treatment of hyperthyroidism in pregnancy. Am J Obstet Gynecol 1994;170:90–5.
52. Anonymous. Transplacental passage of thyroid hormones. N Engl J Med 1967;277:486–7.
53. Low LCK, Lang J, Alexander WD. Excretion of carbimazole and propylthiouracil in breast milk. Lancet 1979;2:1011.
54. Kampmann JP, Johansen K, Hansen JM, Helweg J. Propylthiouracil in human milk. Lancet 1980;1:736–8.
55. Cooper DS. Antithyroid drugs: to breast-feed or not to breast-feed. Am J Obstet Gynecol 1987;157:234–5.
56. Lee A, Moretti ME, Collantes A, Chong D, Mazzotta P, Koren G, Merchant SS, Ito S. Choice of breast-feeding and physicians' advice: a cohort study of women receiving propylthiouracil. Pediatrics 2000;106:27–30.
57. Committee on Drugs, American Academy of Pediatrics. The transfer of drugs and other chemicals into human milk. Pediatrics 2001;108:776–89.

P

Name:	**PROTAMINE**	Risk Factor:	C_M
Class:	**Antiheparin**		

FETAL RISK SUMMARY

RECOMMENDATION: Compatible - Maternal Benefit >> Embryo/Fetal Risk

Protamine is used to neutralize the anticoagulant effect of heparin. No reports of its use in pregnancy have been located. Reproduction studies in animals have not been conducted (1).

BREAST FEEDING SUMMARY

RECOMMENDATION: No Human Data - Probably Compatible

No data are available.

Reference

1. Product information. Protamine sulfate. Eli Lilly, 1993.

Name:	**PROTIRELIN**	Risk Factor:	C_M
Class:	**Thyroid**		

FETAL RISK SUMMARY

RECOMMENDATION: Limited Human Data - Animal Data Suggest Moderate Risk

P

Protirelin is a synthetic tripeptide that is thought to be structurally identical to naturally occurring thyrotropin-releasing hormone (TRH). TRH stimulates the release of thyroid-stimulating hormone (TSH) and prolactin from the pituitary.

Reproduction studies in rats and rabbits at doses 6 and 1.5 times, respectively, the human dose have shown an increased number of resorptions in rabbits, but not in rats (1).

The published experience in human pregnancy for this agent is restricted to studies evaluating its role, in combination with corticosteroids, in the acceleration of fetal lung maturity. No reports describing the use in human pregnancy of only TRH, either for fetal lung maturation or for diagnostic assessment of thyroid function, have been located.

Several research studies have demonstrated that cord blood levels of liothyronine (T_3) and levothyroxine (T_4) are lower, and TSH levels are higher, in infants with respiratory distress syndrome (RDS), when compared with healthy matched controls without clinical evidence of lung immaturity (2–5). Moreover, a 1975 publication reported a higher incidence of RDS in premature infants with congenital hypothyroidism (6). In studies of animals and humans, when T_3 or T_4 was administered directly to the fetus, or in experiments involving fetal lung cultures, significant increases were measured in the synthesis of phosphatidylcholine, a major constituent of lung surfactant (2,7–11). Combining thyroid hormones with corticosteroids, such as dexamethasone, produced an additive effect on phosphatidylcholine synthesis that was greater than that produced by either agent alone

(7–11). These data suggest that the thyroid hormones act at different receptors in the fetal lung than those stimulated by corticosteroids (6–11).

In contrast to T_3, T_4, and TSH, which either do not cross the human placenta or cross in negligible amounts, TRH is rapidly transferred across the animal and human placenta to the fetus and stimulates fetal TSH, T_3, and T_4 (2,12,13). Research published in 1991 indicated that the fetal pituitary is capable of responding to TRH with an increase in TSH by at least the 25th week of gestation (13). Moreover, the fetal response to TRH is much greater than the maternal response, which may be caused by lower concentrations of fetal thyroid hormone and resulting reduced negative feedback on the pituitary (13). It is these characteristics that have stimulated research on the use of TRH for fetal lung maturation.

In fetal rabbits, the maternal administration of TRH enhanced functional and morphologic fetal lung maturation (12). The first human study comparing the use of TRH and corticosteroids with corticosteroids alone was published in 1989 (5). In this study, 248 women who were at risk for delivery before 34 weeks' gestation and who had a lecithin:sphingomyelin (L:S) ratio less than 2.0 (maturity defined as an L:S ratio 2.0 or greater) were randomized into a study group ($N = 119$) or controls ($N = 129$). Mothers in the study group were treated with TRH (400 μg IV every 8 hours for 6 doses) plus betamethasone (12 mg IM every 24 hours for 2 doses). Control patients received the betamethasone doses only. Infants delivered from the study group within 1 week of therapy had a greater increase in L:S ratio, fewer respirator days, and a lower incidence of bronchopulmonary dysplasia, indicating that the combination of TRH with betamethasone was superior to betamethasone alone (5). Adverse effects occurred in 35% of the study group mothers, consisting of nausea, flushing, hot flashes, and palpitations, all resolving within 20 minutes (5). No adverse fetal or newborn effects were observed, a finding similar to other studies (2,12).

BREAST FEEDING SUMMARY

RECOMMENDATION: Limited Human Data - Probably Compatible

Three nursing women, 5–6 weeks postpartum, were treated with 1–300 μg of TRH (14). Doses of 1–2 μg produced no significant change in maternal TSH or prolactin. When the doses were increased to 6–300 μg, significant increases in both TSH and prolactin were measured. Suckling alone produced a much greater effect on serum prolactin than did TRH, but had no effect on serum TSH levels.

Administration of TRH will increase maternal levels of T_3 and T_4, and both hormones are excreted into breast milk in low concentrations (see Liothyronine and Levothyroxine).

References

1. Product information. Thyrel TRH. Ferring Pharmaceuticals, 2000.
2. Moya FR, Gross I. Prevention of respiratory distress syndrome. Semin Perinatol 1988;12:348–58.
3. Cuestas RA, Lindall A, Engel RR. Low thyroid hormones and respiratory-distress syndrome of the newborn. Studies on cord blood. N Engl J Med 1976;295:297–302.
4. Klein AH, Foley B, Foley TP, MacDonald HM, Fisher DA. Thyroid function studies in cord blood from premature infants with and without RDS. J Pediatr 1981;98: 818–20.
5. Morales WJ, O'Brien WF, Angel JL, Knuppel RA, Sawai S. Fetal lung maturation: the combined use of corticosteroids and thyrotropin-releasing hormone. Obstet Gynecol 1989;73:111–6.
6. Smith DW, Klein AM, Henderson JR, Myrianthopoulos NC. Congenital hypothyroidism—signs and symptoms in the newborn period. J Pediatr 1975;87:958–62.
7. Gross I, Wilson CM. Fetal lung in organ culture. IV. Supra-additive hormone interactions. J Appl Physiol 1982;52:1420–5.
8. Gonzales LK, Ballard PL. Glucocorticoid and thyroid hormone stimulation of phosphatidylcholine (PC) synthesis in cultured human fetal lung (abstract). Pediatr Res 1984;18:310A.

9. Gross I, Dynia DW, Wilson CM, Ingleson LD, Gewolb IH, Rooney SA. Glucocorticoid-thyroid hormone interactions in fetal rat lung. Pediatr Res 1984;18:191–6.
10. Ballard PL, Hovey ML, Gonzales LK. Thyroid hormone stimulation of phosphatidylcholine synthesis in cultured fetal rabbit lung. J Clin Invest 1984;74:898–905.
11. Warburton D, Parton L, Buckley S, Cosico L, Enns G, Saluna T. Combined effects of corticosteroid, thyroid hormones, and β-agonist on surfactant, pulmonary mechanics, and β-receptor binding in fetal lamb lung. Pediatr Res 1988;24:166–70.
12. Devaskar U, Nitta K, Szewczyk K, Sadiq HF, deMello D. Transplacental stimulation of functional and morphologic fetal rabbit lung maturation: effect of thyrotropin-releasing hormone. Am J Obstet Gynecol 1987;157:460–4.
13. Thorpe-Beeston JG, Nicolaides KH, Snijders RJM, Butler J, McGregor AM. Fetal thyroid-stimulating hormone response to maternal administration of thyrotropin-releasing hormone. Am J Obstet Gynecol 1991;164:1244–5.
14. Gautvik KM, Weintraub BD, Graeber CT, Maloof F, Zuckerman JE, Tashjian AH Jr. Serum prolactin and TSH: effects of nursing and pyroGlu-His-ProNH$_2$ administration in postpartum women. J Clin Endocrinol Metab 1973;36:135–9.

Name:	**PROTRIPTYLINE**	Risk Factor:	**C**
Class:	**Antidepressant**		

FETAL RISK SUMMARY

RECOMMENDATION: No Human Data - Animal Data Suggest Low Risk

Protriptyline, a dibenzocycloheptene derivative, is a tricyclic antidepressant. Other antidepressants in this class are amitriptyline and its metabolite, nortriptyline.

Reproduction studies in mice, rats, and rabbits at doses about 10 times greater than the recommended human dose had no apparent adverse effects on reproduction (1).

No reports on the use of protriptyline during human pregnancy have been located. See also Amitriptyline and Nortriptyline.

BREAST FEEDING SUMMARY

RECOMMENDATION: No Human Data - Potential Toxicity

P

No reports describing the use of protriptyline during lactation have been located. The molecular weight (about 264 for the free base) is low enough, however, that excretion into breast milk should be expected. The effects on a nursing infant from exposure to the drug in breast milk are unknown. The American Academy of Pediatrics classifies amitriptyline, a similar antidepressant, as a drug whose effect on the nursing infant is unknown but may be of concern (see Amitriptyline).

Reference

1. Product information. Vivactil. Merck, 2000.

Name:	**PSEUDOEPHEDRINE**	Risk Factor:	**C**
Class:	**Sympathomimetic (Adrenergic)**		

FETAL RISK SUMMARY

RECOMMENDATION: Limited Human Data - No Relevant Animal Data

Pseudoephedrine is a sympathomimetic used to alleviate the symptoms of allergic disorders or upper respiratory infections. It is a common component of proprietary mixtures containing antihistamines and other ingredients. Thus, it is difficult to separate the effects of pseudoephedrine on the fetus from those of other drugs, disease states, and viruses.

Sympathomimetic amines are teratogenic in some animal species, but human teratogenicity has not been suspected (1). The Collaborative Perinatal Project monitored 50,282 mother-child pairs, 3,082 of whom had 1st trimester exposure to sympathomimetic drugs (2, pp. 345–356). For use anytime during pregnancy, 9,719 exposures were recorded (2, p. 439). An association in the 1st trimester was found between the sympathomimetic class of drugs as a whole and minor malformations (not life-threatening or major cosmetic defects), inguinal hernia, and clubfoot (2, pp. 345–356). However, independent confirmation of these results is required (2, pp. 345–356).

In a surveillance study of Michigan Medicaid recipients conducted between 1985 and 1992 involving 229,101 completed pregnancies, 940 newborns had been exposed to pseudoephedrine during the 1st trimester (F. Rosa, personal communication, FDA, 1993). A total of 37 (3.9%) major birth defects were observed (40 expected). Specific data were available for six defect categories, including (observed/expected) 3/9 cardiovascular defects, 2/2 oral clefts, 0/0 spina bifida, 3/3 polydactyly, 0/2 limb reduction defects, and 0/2 hypospadias. These data do not support an association between the drug and congenital defects.

A case-controlled surveillance study published in 1992 reported a significantly elevated relative risk of 3.2 (95% confidence interval, 1.3–7.7) for the use of pseudoephedrine during the 1st trimester and 76 exposed cases with gastroschisis (3). A total of 2142 infants with other malformations formed a control group. Relative risks for other drugs were salicylates 1.6, acetaminophen 1.7, ibuprofen 1.3, and phenylpropanolamine 1.5. Because some of these drugs are vasoactive substances, and because the cause of gastroschisis is thought to involve vascular disruption of the omphalomesenteric artery (3), the investigators compared the use of 1st trimester pseudoephedrine and other drugs in relation to a heterogeneous group of malformations, other than gastroschisis, suspected of also having a vascular origin. In this case, however, the relative risk for the drugs approximated unity. These data suggested that the association between pseudoephedrine and the other drugs and gastroschisis may have been caused by an underlying maternal illness (3).

A 1981 report described a woman who consumed, throughout pregnancy, 480–840 mL/day of a cough syrup (4). The potential maximum daily doses based on 840 mL of syrup were 5.0 g of pseudoephedrine, 16.8 g of guaifenesin, 1.68 g of dextromethorphan, and 79.8 mL of ethanol. The infant had features of the fetal alcohol syndrome (see Ethanol) and displayed irritability, tremors, and hypertonicity. It is not known whether the ingredients, other than the ethanol, were associated with the adverse effects observed in the infant.

BREAST FEEDING SUMMARY

RECOMMENDATION: Limited Human Data - Probably Compatible

Pseudoephedrine is excreted into breast milk (5). Three mothers, who were nursing healthy infants, were given an antihistamine-decongestant preparation containing 60 mg of pseudoephedrine and 2.5 mg of triprolidine. Two of the mothers had been nursing for 14 weeks, and one had been nursing for 18 months. Milk concentrations of pseudoephedrine were higher than plasma levels in all three patients, with peak milk concentrations occurring at 1.0–1.5 hours. The milk:plasma ratios at 1, 3, and 12 hours in one subject were 3.3, 3.9, and 2.6, respectively. The investigators calculated that 1000 mL of milk produced during 24 hours would contain 0.25–0.33 mg of pseudoephedrine base, approximately 0.5–0.7%

of the maternal dose (5). The American Academy of Pediatrics classifies pseudoephedrine as compatible with breast-feeding (6).

References

1. Nishimura H, Tanimura T. *Clinical Aspects of the Teratogenicity of Drugs*. Amsterdam: Excerpta Medica, 1976:231.
2. Heinonen OP, Slone D, Shapiro S. *Birth Defects and Drugs in Pregnancy*. Littleton, MA: Publishing Sciences Group, 1977.
3. Werler MM, Mitchell AA, Shapiro S. First trimester maternal medication use in relation to gastroschisis. Teratology 1992;45:361–7.
4. Chasnoff IJ, Diggs G. Fetal alcohol effects and maternal cough syrup abuse. Am J Dis Child 1981;135:968.
5. Findlay JWA, Butz RF, Sailstad JM, Warren JT, Welch RM. Pseudoephedrine and triprolidine in plasma and breast milk of nursing mothers. Br J Clin Pharmacol 1984;18:901–6.
6. Committee on Drugs, American Academy of Pediatrics. The transfer of drugs and other chemicals into human milk. Pediatrics 2001;108:776–89.

Name: **PYRANTEL PAMOATE** Risk Factor: **C**
Class: **Anthelmintic**

FETAL RISK SUMMARY

RECOMMENDATION: No Human Data - Animal Data Suggest Low Risk

No reports on the use of this drug in human pregnancy have been located. Shepard cited two studies in which no congenital defects or postnatal effects were observed in pregnant rats fed doses up to 3000 mg/kg or in pregnant rabbits given 1000 mg/kg (1,2).

BREAST FEEDING SUMMARY

RECOMMENDATION: No Human Data - Probably Compatible

No data are available.

P

References

1. Owaki Y, Sakai T, Momiyama H. Teratological studies on pyrantel pamoate in rats. Oyo Yakuri 1971;5:41–50. As cited in Shepard TH. *Catalog of Teratogenic Agents*. 6th ed. Baltimore, MD: Johns Hopkins University Press, 1989:536.
2. Owaki Y, Sakai T, Momiyama H. Teratological studies on pyrantel pamoate in rabbits. Oyo Yakuri 1971;5:33–39. As cited in Shepard TH. *Catalog of Teratogenic Agents*. 6th ed. Baltimore, MD: Johns Hopkins University Press, 1989:536.

Name: **PYRAZINAMIDE** Risk Factor: **C_M**
Class: **Antituberculosis Agent**

FETAL RISK SUMMARY

RECOMMENDATION: Limited Human Data - No Relevant Animal Data

Pyrazinamide is a synthetic antituberculosis agent derived from niacinamide. Animal reproduction studies have not been conducted with this drug (1).

A single report has been located that describes the use of pyrazinamide in a pregnant woman. She had been treated for cavitary pulmonary tuberculosis with three other agents for 5 months before the addition of pyrazinamide at 26 weeks' gestation for persistent positive sputum cultures (2). No drug-related fetal toxicity was mentioned. However, this and other references caution that pyrazinamide should not be routinely used because of the lack of information pertaining to its fetal effects (2–4).

BREAST FEEDING SUMMARY

RECOMMENDATION: Limited Human Data - Probably Compatible

Pyrazinamide is excreted into human milk. In one non-breast-feeding patient given an oral 1-g dose of pyrazinamide, the peak concentration of the drug, 1.5 μg/mL, was measured in the milk at 3 hours (5). The peak concentration in the maternal plasma, 42.0 μg/mL, occurred at 2 hours.

References

1. Product information. Pyrazinamide. Lederle Laboratories, 2000.
2. Margono F, Mroueh J, Garely A, White D, Duerr A, Minkoff HL. Resurgence of active tuberculosis among pregnant women. Obstet Gynecol 1994;83:911–4.
3. American Thoracic Society. Treatment of tuberculosis and tuberculosis infection in adults and children. Am Rev Respir Dis 1986;134:355–63.
4. Hamadeh MA, Glassroth J. Tuberculosis and pregnancy. Chest 1992;101:1114–20.
5. Holdiness MR. Antituberculosis drugs and breast-feeding. Arch Intern Med 1984;144:1888.

Name:	**PYRETHRINS WITH PIPERONYL BUTOXIDE**	Risk Factor:	**C**
Class:	**Pediculicide**		

FETAL RISK SUMMARY

RECOMMENDATION: No Human Data - Probably Compatible

Pyrethrins with piperonyl butoxide is a synergistic combination product used topically for the treatment of lice infestations. It is not effective for the treatment of scabies (mite infestations). Pyrethrins with piperonyl butoxide is considered the drug of choice for lice (1). Although no reports of its use in pregnancy have been located, topical absorption is poor, so potential toxicity should be less than that of lindane (see also Lindane) (2). For this reason, use of the combination is probably preferred over lindane in the pregnant patient.

BREAST FEEDING SUMMARY

RECOMMENDATION: No Human Data - Probably Compatible

No data are available.

References

1. Anonymous. Drugs for parasitic infections. In *Handbook for Antimicrobial Therapy*. New Rochelle, NY: The Medical Letter, Inc., 1984:100.
2. Robinson DH, Shepherd DA. Control of head lice in schoolchildren. Curr Ther Res 1980;27:1–6.

Name:	**PYRIDOSTIGMINE**	Risk Factor:	**C**
Class:	**Parasympathomimetic (Cholinergic)**		

FETAL RISK SUMMARY

RECOMMENDATION: Limited Human Data - Animal Data Suggest Low Risk

Pyridostigmine is a quaternary ammonium compound with anticholinesterase activity used in the treatment of myasthenia gravis. The agent was not teratogenic in rats at doses up to 30 mg/kg/day, but maternal and fetal toxicity (reduced weight) were observed at the highest dose (1).

Although it is ionized at physiologic pH, the low molecular weight of pyridostigmine (about 261) allows the nonionized fraction to cross to the fetus. Pyridostigmine concentrations have been determined at birth in maternal plasma, cord blood, and amniotic fluid (2). Two women with long-term myasthenia gravis were treated throughout gestation with pyridostigmine, 360 mg and 420 mg per day, respectively. The latter woman was also treated with neostigmine (105 mg/day) and ambenonium (60 mg/day). In the first case, the maternal plasma, cord blood, and amniotic drug concentrations were 77, 65, and 290 ng/mL, respectively, and in the second, 53, 39, and 300 ng/mL, respectively. Thus, the cord blood:maternal plasma ratios were 0.84 and 0.74, respectively, whereas the amniotic fluid:maternal plasma ratios were 3.8 and 5.7 respectively (2).

Caution has been advised against the use in pregnancy of IV anticholinesterases because they may cause premature labor (3,4). This effect on the pregnant uterus increases near term.

A number of reports have described the apparent safe use of pyridostigmine during human gestation (2–16). However, a case report published in 2000 described microcephaly and central nervous system (CNS) injury in a newborn that was attributed to high-dose pyridostigmine (17). The infant's mother was a 24-year-old primigravida with a 14-year history of myasthenia gravis. She required high-dose pyridostigmine (1500–3000 mg/day) throughout gestation to control her diplopia and ptosis. In comparison, the average recommended daily dose is 600 mg, with daily doses up to 1500 mg required in severe cases (18). The mother denied smoking and the use of other drugs during pregnancy. At 36 weeks' gestation, an emergency cesarean section for fetal bradycardia was conducted, delivering a severely growth-retarded (1880-g, <2nd percentile), hypotonic male infant with Apgar scores of 3 and 8 at 1 and 5 minutes, respectively. Shortly after birth, neonatal myasthenia gravis was diagnosed and two exchange transfusions were used to lower his acetylcholine receptor antibody titer and IV immunoglobulin was administered. The infant required immediate intubation because of poor respiratory effort and was continued on the respirator until age 3.5 months. Mild finger and wrist contractures and bilateral cryptorchidism were noted at birth, but he had no abnormal ocular findings (17). The head circumference was 33.5 cm at birth and 37 cm (<5th percentile) at 3 months of age. By about 5 months of age, a number of dysmorphic features were noted, including a broad nasal bridge with a prominent nose, slight downslanting palpebral fissures, high arched palate, short neck, broad chest, campylodactyly, and hammer toes (17). He continued to do poorly, requiring additional hospitalizations and mechanical ventilation. At 4.5 months, he was discharged home but readmitted 1 week later because of prolonged apnea and cyanosis. His weight (5.1 kg, 10th percentile) and head circumference (38 cm, <2nd percentile) were still retarded and he remained hypotonic. A cranial ultrasound, karyotyping,

P

and TORCH titers (i.e., toxoplasmosis, other infections, rubella, cytomegalovirus, and herpes simplex) were normal or negative and there was no evidence of craniosynostosis. A brain magnetic resonance imaging scan at 5 months revealed apparent brachycephaly and mild ventriculomegaly. At 9 months of age, he still required nasal oxygen, tone was normal, and the joint contractures had resolved, but his reflexes were brisk and ankle clonus was evident. Because no other cause could be identified, the authors attributed the microcephaly and CNS injury to pyridostigmine (17).

Both antenatal and neonatal myasthenia gravis have been reported and either may result in perinatal death. Both forms of the disorder are caused by transplacental passage of antiacetylcholine receptor immunoglobulin G antibodies (11,19). The inhibited fetal skeletal muscle movement and development may result in pulmonary hypoplasia, arthrogryposis multiplex, and polyhydramnios (19).

Transient muscular weakness has been observed in about 20% of newborns of mothers with myasthenia gravis (11,19).

BREAST FEEDING SUMMARY

RECOMMENDATION: Limited Human Data - Probably Compatible

Pyridostigmine is excreted into breast milk. Levels in two women receiving 120–300 mg/day were 2–25 ng/mL, representing milk:plasma ratios of 0.36–1.13 (15). Although pyridostigmine is an ionized quaternary ammonium compound, these values indicate that the nonionized fraction crosses easily into breast milk. The drug was not detected in the infants nor were any adverse effects noted. The authors estimated that the two infants were ingesting 0.1% or less of the maternal doses (15). The American Academy of Pediatrics classifies pyridostigmine as compatible with breast feeding (20).

References

1. Levine BS, Parker RM. Reproductive and developmental toxicity studies of pyridostigmine bromide in rats. Toxicology 1991;69:291–300.
2. Lefvert AK, Osterman PO. Newborn infants to myasthenic mothers: a clinical study and an investigation of acetylcholine receptor antibodies in 17 children. Neurology 1983;33:133–8.
3. Foldes FF, McNall PG. Myasthenia gravis: a guide for anesthesiologists. Anesthesiology 1962;23:837–72.
4. McNall PG, Jafarnia MR. Management of myasthenia gravis in the obstetric patient. Am J Obstet Gynecol 1965;92:518–25.
5. Plauche WC. Myasthenia gravis in pregnancy. Am J Obstet Gynecol 1964;88:404–9.
6. Chambers DC, Hall JE, Boyce J. Myasthenia gravis and pregnancy. Obstet Gynecol 1967;29:597–603.
7. Hay DM. Myasthenia gravis and pregnancy. J Obstet Gynaecol Br Commonw 1969;76:323–9.
8. Heinonen OP, Slone D, Shapiro S. *Birth Defects and Drugs in Pregnancy*. Littleton, MA: Publishing Sciences Group, 1977:345–56.
9. Blackhall MI, Buckley GA, Roberts DV, Roberts JB, Thomas BH, Wilson A. Drug-induced neonatal myasthenia. J Obstet Gynaecol Br Commonw 1969;76:157–62.
10. Rolbin SH, Levinson G, Shnider SM, Wright RG. Anesthetic considerations for myasthenia gravis and pregnancy. Anesth Analg (Cleve) 1978;57:441–7.
11. Plauche WC. Myasthenia gravis in pregnancy: An update. Am J Obstet Gynecol 1979;135:691–7.
12. Eden RD, Gall SA. Myasthenia gravis and pregnancy: A reappraisal of thymectomy. Obstet Gynecol 1983;62:328–33.
13. Cohen BA, London RS, Goldstein PJ. Myasthenia gravis and preeclampsia. Obstet Gynecol 1976;48(Suppl):35S–7S.
14. Catanzarite VA, McHargue AM, Sandberg EC, Dyson DC. Respiratory arrest during therapy for premature labor in a patient with myasthenia gravis. Obstet Gynecol 1984;64:819–22.
15. Hardell LI, Lindstrom B, Lonnerholm G, Osterman PO. Pyridostigmine in human breast milk. Br J Clin Pharmacol 1982;14:565–7.
16. Carr SR, Gilchrist JM, Abuelo DN, Clark D. Treatment of antenatal myasthenia gravis. Obstet Gynecol 1991;78:485–9.
17. Niesen CE, Shah NS. Pyridostigmine-induced microcephaly. Neurology 2000;54:1873–4.
18. Product information. Mestinon. ICN Pharmaceuticals, 2000.
19. Gilchrist JM. Muscle disease in the pregnant woman. Adv Neurol 1994;64:193–208.
20. Committee on Drugs, American Academy of Pediatrics. The transfer of drugs and other chemicals into human milk. Pediatrics 2001;108:776–89.

Name:	**PYRIDOXINE**	Risk Factor:	**A**
Class:	**Vitamin**		

FETAL RISK SUMMARY

RECOMMENDATION: Compatible

Pyridoxine (vitamin B_6), a water-soluble B complex vitamin, acts as an essential coenzyme involved in the metabolism of amino acids, carbohydrates, and lipids (1). The National Academy of Sciences' recommended dietary allowance (RDA) for pyridoxine in pregnancy is 2.2 mg (1).

Pyridoxine is actively transported to the fetus (2–4). Like other B complex vitamins, concentrations of pyridoxine in the fetus and newborn are higher than in the mother and are directly proportional to maternal intake (5–16). Actual pyridoxine levels vary from report to report because of the nutritional status of the populations studied and the microbiologic assays used, but usually indicate an approximate newborn:maternal ratio of 2:1 with levels ranging from 22–87 ng/mL for newborns and 13–51 ng/mL for mothers (4,14–16).

Pyridoxine deficiency without clinical symptoms is common during pregnancy (10,16–34). Clinical symptoms consisting of oral lesions have been reported, however, in severe B6 deficiency (35). Supplementation with multivitamin products reduces, but does not always eliminate, the incidence of pyridoxine hypovitaminemia (16).

Severe vitamin B_6 deficiency is teratogenic in experimental animals (36,37). No reports of human malformations linked to B_6 deficiency have been located. A brief report in 1976 described an anencephalic fetus resulting from a woman treated with high doses of pyridoxine and other vitamins and nutrients for psychiatric reasons, but the relationship between the defect and the vitamins is unknown (38).

The effects on the mother and fetus resulting from pyridoxine deficiency or excess are controversial. These effects can be summarized as follows:

P

Gestational hypertension
Gestational diabetes mellitus
Infantile convulsions
Nausea and vomiting of pregnancy
Congenital malformations
Miscellaneous effects

Gestational Hypertension

Several researchers have claimed that pyridoxine deficiency is associated with the development of gestational hypertension (GH) (12,39–41); others have not found this relationship (10,19,42,43). One group of investigators demonstrated that women with GH excreted larger amounts of xanthurenic acid in their urine after a loading dose of *dl*-tryptophan than did normal pregnant women (39). Although the test only was partially specific for GH, they theorized that it could be of value for early detection of the disease and was indicative of abnormal pyridoxine-niacin-protein metabolism. In another study, 410 women treated with 10 mg of pyridoxine daily were compared with 410 controls (40). GH occurred in 18 (4.4%) of the untreated controls and in 7 (1.7%) of the pyridoxine-supplemented patients, a significant difference. In an earlier report, no significant differences were found between women with GH and normal controls in urinary excretion of 4-pyridoxic acid, a pyridoxine metabolite, after a loading dose of the vitamin (19). Some investigators have measured lower levels of pyridoxine in mothers with GH than in mothers without GH (12). The difference in levels between the newborns of GH and normal mothers was more than 2-fold and highly significant. In a 1961 Swedish report, pyridoxine levels in 10 women with GH were compared with those in 26 women with uncomplicated pregnancies (42). The difference between the mean levels of the two groups, 25 and 33 ng/mL, respectively, was not significant. Similarly, others have been unable to find a correlation between pyridoxine levels and GH (10,43).

Gestational Diabetes Mellitus

Pyridoxine levels were studied in 14 pregnant women with an abnormal glucose tolerance test (GTT), and 13 of these patients were shown to be pyridoxine deficient (44). All were placed on a diet and given 100 mg of pyridoxine/day for 14 days, after which only two were diagnosed as having gestational diabetes mellitus. The effect of the diet on the GTT was said to be negligible, although a control group was not used. Other investigators duplicated these results in 13 women using the same dose of pyridoxine but without mentioning any dietary manipulation and without controls (45). However, a third study was unable to demonstrate a beneficial effect in four patients with an abnormal GTT using 100 mg of B_6 for 21 days (46). Moreover, all of the mothers had large-for-gestational-age infants, an expected complication of diabetic pregnancies. In 13 gestational diabetic women treated with the doses of pyridoxine described above, an improvement was observed in the GTT in 2 patients, a worsening was seen in 6, and no significant change occurred in the remaining 5 (47).

Infantile Convulsions

An association between pyridoxine and infantile convulsions was first described in the mid-1950s (48–52). Some infants fed a diet deficient in this vitamin developed intractable seizures that responded only to pyridoxine. A 1967 publication reviewed this complication in infants and differentiated between the states of pyridoxine deficiency and dependency (53). Whether or not these states can be induced *in utero* is open to question. As noted earlier, pyridoxine deficiency is common during pregnancy, even in well-nourished women, but the fetus accumulates the vitamin, although at lower levels, even in the face of maternal hypovitaminemia. Reports of seizures in newborn infants delivered from mothers with pyridoxine deficiency have not been located. On the other hand, high doses of pyridoxine early in gestation in one patient were suspected of altering the normal metabolism of pyridoxine, leading to intractable convulsions in the newborn (54). The woman, in whom two pregnancies were complicated by hyperemesis gravidarum, was treated with frequent injections of pyridoxine and thiamine, 50 mg each (54). The first newborn began convulsing 4 hours after birth and died within 30 hours. The second infant began mild twitching at 3 hours of age and progressed to severe generalized convulsions on the 5th day. Successful treatment was eventually accomplished with pyridoxine but not before marked mental retardation had occurred. The authors of this report postulated that the fetus, exposed to high doses of pyridoxine, developed an adaptive enzyme system that was capable of rapidly metabolizing the vitamin; following delivery, this adaptation was manifested by pyridoxine dependency and convulsions (54). Since this case, more than 50 additional cases of pyridoxine dependency have been reported, and the disease is now thought to be an inherited autosomal recessive disorder (55).

A 1967 report described *in utero* dependency-induced convulsions in three successive pregnancies in one woman (56). The first two newborns died—one during the 7th week and one on day 2—as a result of intractable convulsions. During the third pregnancy, *in utero* convulsions stopped after the mother was treated with 110 mg/day of pyridoxine 4 days before delivery. Following birth, the newborn was treated with pyridoxine. Convulsions occurred on three separate occasions when vitamin therapy was withheld and then abated when therapy was restarted. Late-onset seizures in a female infant were reported in 1999 (57). The mother had taken pyridoxine 80 mg/day throughout pregnancy and intermittently when the nursing infant was between 1 and 10 weeks of age. Four days after birth, the infant had two generalized colonic seizures. Then, at 3.5 months of age, the infant became irritable and fussy and had a cluster of 12 generalized seizures, each lasting 2–5 minutes, over 4 days. Laboratory tests and an electroencephalogram, taken when the infant was not seizing, were normal. A single dose of pyridoxine 100 mg IV was given and she was seizure-free for 3 weeks. Then three more seizures occurred over 4 days. She was given 100 mg oral pyridoxine and then 12.5 mg/day thereafter. The infant is now 7-months-old and has been seizure-free with normal temperament and development since starting oral pyridoxine (57).

Nausea and Vomiting of Pregnancy

The first use of pyridoxine for severe nausea and vomiting of pregnancy (hyperemesis gravidarum) was reported in 1942 (58). Individual injections ranged from 10 to 100 mg, with total doses up to 1500 mg being given. Satisfactory relief was obtained in most cases. In one study, patients were successfully treated with IM doses of 50–100 mg 3 times weekly (59). Another report described a single patient with hyperemesis who responded to an IV mixture of high-dose B complex vitamins, including 50 mg of pyridoxine, each day for 3 days (60). Much smaller doses were used in a study of 17 patients (61). IM doses of 5 mg every 2–4 days were administered to these patients, with an immediate response observed in 12 women and all responding by the second dose. Oral doses of 60–80 mg/day up to a total dose of 2500 mg gave partial or complete relief from nausea and vomiting in 68 patients; an additional 10 patients required oral plus injectable pyridoxine (62). A success rate of 95% was claimed in a study of 62 women treated with a combination of pyridoxine and suprarenal cortex (adrenal cortex extract) (63). None of the preceding six studies was double-blind or controlled. The effect of pyridoxine on blood urea concentrations in hyperemesis has been investigated (64). Blood urea was decreased below normal adult levels in pregnant women and even lower in patients with hyperemesis. Pyridoxine, 40 mg/day orally for 3 days, significantly increased blood urea only in women with hyperemesis. In another measure of the effect of pyridoxine on hyperemesis, elevated serum glutamic acid levels observed with this condition were returned to normal pregnant values after pyridoxine therapy (65). However, another investigator could not demonstrate any value from pyridoxine therapy in 16 patients (66). Placebos were used but the study was not blinded. In addition, only 1 of 16 patients had hyperemesis gravidarum with the remaining 15 presenting with lesser degrees of nausea and vomiting. Based on the above studies, it is impossible to judge the effectiveness of the vitamin in allaying true hyperemesis gravidarum. More than likely, the effect of hydration, possibly improved prenatal care, the attention of health care personnel, the transitory nature of hyperemesis, the lack of strict diagnostic criteria in classifying patients with the disease, and other factors were involved in the reversal of the symptoms of the women involved in these studies. The vitamin, however, does appear to reduce nausea and vomiting of pregnancy as demonstrated in the two investigations described below.

Two studies have demonstrated that oral doses of pyridoxine are effective in alleviating nausea and vomiting of pregnancy (67–69). A randomized, double-blind, placebo-controlled study, found that pyridoxine, 25 mg orally every 8 hours for 72 hours, administered to 31 women at a mean gestational age of 9.3 weeks, significantly reduced severe nausea ($p < 0.01$) and vomiting ($p < 0.05$) of pregnancy (67,68). A second study, using pyridoxine 10 mg orally every 8 hours for 5 days in 167 women at a mean gestational age of 10.9 weeks, produced a significant reduction in nausea ($p = 0.0008$) and nearly a significant decrease in the number of vomiting episodes ($p = 0.0552$) (69).

Congenital Malformations

A recent case report suggested a link between high doses of pyridoxine and phocomelia (70). The mother, who weighed only 47 kg, took 50 mg of pyridoxine daily plus unknown doses of lecithin and vitamin B_{12} through the first 7 months of pregnancy. The full-term female infant was born with a near-total amelia of her left leg at the knee. A relationship between any of the drugs and the defect is doubtful.

The combination of doxylamine and pyridoxine (Bendectin, others) has been the focus of considerable debate in the past. The debate centered on whether the preparation was teratogenic. The combination had been used by millions of women for pregnancy-induced nausea and vomiting but was removed from the market by the manufacturer because of a number of large legal awards against the company. Jury decisions notwithstanding, the available scientific evidence indicates the combination is not teratogenic (see Doxylamine).

Pyridoxine has been shown to protect fetal rats from β-aminopropionitrile–induced palatal clefting when given before and during administration of the chemical (71). The same protection may occur in humans. In a case-control study from two sites in the Philippines, women with offspring with an oral cleft (cleft lip, with or without cleft palate) had worst pyridoxine deficiency than controls (72). The association was strongest if the mother also had lower folate levels. However, folate-oral cleft associations were inconsistent and were thought to be a result of differing pyridoxine status in the two populations studied. In contrast, poor maternal pyridoxine status was consistently associated with an increased risk of oral clefts (72).

Miscellaneous Effects

Among miscellaneous effects, two studies were unable to associate low maternal concentrations of pyridoxine with premature labor (29,43). Similarly, no correlation was found between low levels and stillbirths (10,40). However, 1-minute Apgar scores were significantly related to low maternal and newborn pyridoxine concentrations (14,73). The effects of pyridoxine supplementation in black pregnant women have been studied (74). Lower maternal serum lipid, fetal weight, and placental weight, and the frequency of placental vascular sclerosis were observed. Others have not found a correlation between pyridoxine levels and birth weight (15,43,73). In an unusual report, pregnant women given daily 20-mg supplements of pyridoxine by either lozenges or capsules had less dental disease than untreated controls (75). The best cariostatic effect was seen in patients in the lozenge group.

In summary, pyridoxine deficiency during pregnancy is a common problem in unsupplemented women. Supplementation with oral pyridoxine reduces but does not eliminate the frequency of deficiency. No definitive evidence has appeared that indicates mild to moderate deficiency of this vitamin is a cause of maternal or fetal complications. Most of the studies with this vitamin have been open and uncontrolled. If a relationship does exist with poor pregnancy outcome, it is probable that a number of factors, of which pyridoxine may be one, contribute to the problem. A significant reduction in nausea and vomiting of pregnancy, however, appears to occur with pyridoxine. The available data are sufficient to conclude that the combination of pyridoxine and doxylamine is safe and effective for nausea and vomiting of pregnancy.

P

Severe deficiency or abnormal metabolism is related to fetal and infantile convulsions and possibly to other conditions. However, the association of pyridoxine deficiency, with or without folate deficiency, and oral clefts requires confirmation. High doses apparently pose little risk to the fetus.

Because pyridoxine is required for good maternal and fetal health, and an increased demand for the vitamin occurs during pregnancy, supplementation of the pregnant woman with the RDA for pyridoxine is recommended.

BREAST FEEDING SUMMARY

RECOMMENDATION: Compatible

Pyridoxine (vitamin B_6) is excreted into breast milk (14,76–82). Concentrations in milk are directly proportional to intake (76–82). In well-nourished women, pyridoxine levels varied, depending on intake, from 123 to 314 ng/mL (76–78). Peak pyridoxine milk levels occurred 3–8 hours after ingestion of a vitamin supplement (76,78,79). A 1983 study measured pyridoxine levels in pooled human milk obtained from preterm (26 mothers: 29–34 weeks) and term (35 mothers: 39 weeks or longer) patients (80). Levels in milk obtained from preterm mothers rose from 11.1 ng/mL (colostrum) to 62.2 ng/mL (16–196 days), whereas levels in milk from term mothers increased during the same period from 17.0 to 107.1 ng/mL. In a 1985 study, daily supplements of 0–20 mg resulted in milk concentrations of 93–413 ng/mL, corresponding to an infant intake of 0.06–0.28 mg/day (79). A significant correlation was found between maternal intake and infant intake. Most infants, however, did not receive the RDA for infants (0.3 mg) even when the mother was consuming 8 times the RDA for lactating women (2.5 mg) (79). In lactating women with low nutritional status, supplementation with pyridoxine, 0.4–40 mg/day, resulted in mean milk concentrations of 80–158 ng/mL (81).

Convulsions have been reported in infants fed a pyridoxine-deficient diet (see discussion under Fetal Risk Summary) (49–54). Seizures were described in two breast-fed infants, one of whom was receiving only 67 μg/day in the milk (83). Intake in the second infant was not determined. A similar report involved three infants whose mothers had levels less than 20 ng/mL (at 7 days postpartum) or less than 60 ng/mL (at 4 weeks) of pyridoxine in their milk (84). The convulsions responded promptly to pyridoxine therapy in all five of these infants.

Very large doses of pyridoxine have been reported to have a lactation-inhibiting effect (85). Using oral doses of 600 mg/day, lactation was successfully inhibited in 95% of patients within 1 week as compared with only 17% of placebo-treated controls. Very high IV doses of pyridoxine, 600 mg infused for 1 hour in healthy, nonlactating young adults, successfully suppressed the rise in prolactin induced by exercise (86). However, because use of this dose and method of administration in lactating women would be unusual, the relevance of these data to breast-feeding is limited. With dosage much closer to physiologic levels, such as 20 mg/day, no effect on lactation has been observed (79). In addition, two separate trials, using 450 mg and 600 mg/day in divided oral doses, failed to reproduce the lactation-inhibiting effect observed earlier or to show any suppression of serum prolactin levels (87,88). One writer, however, has suggested that pyridoxine be removed from multivitamin supplements intended for lactating women (89). This proposal has invoked sharp opposition from other correspondents who claimed the available evidence does not support a milk-inhibiting property for pyridoxine (90,91). Moreover, a study published in 1985 examined the effects of pyridoxine supplements, 0.5 or 4.0 mg/day started 24 hours after delivery, on lactation (92). Women receiving the higher dose of pyridoxine had significantly higher concentrations of plasma pyridoxal phosphate ($p < 0.01$) and milk total vitamin B_6 ($p < 0.05$) at 1, 3, 6, and 9 months. Plasma prolactin concentrations were similar between the two groups throughout the study. The American Academy of Pediatrics classifies pyridoxine as compatible with breast-feeding (93).

In summary, the National Academy of Sciences' RDA for pyridoxine during lactation is 2.1 mg (1). If the diet of the lactating woman adequately supplies this amount, maternal supplementation with pyridoxine is not required (82). Supplementation with the RDA for pyridoxine is recommended for those women with inadequate nutritional intake.

References

1. American Hospital Formulary Service. *Drug Information 1997*. Bethesda, MD: American Society of Health-System Pharmacists, 1997:2815–7.
2. Frank O, Walbroehl G, Thomson A, Kaminetzky H, Kubes Z, Baker H. Placental transfer: fetal retention of some vitamins. Am J Clin Nutr 1970;23:662–3.
3. Hill EP, Longo LD. Dynamics of maternal-fetal nutrient transfer. Fed Proc 1980;39:239–44.
4. Baker H, Frank O, Deangelis B, Feingold S, Kaminetzky HA. Role of placenta in maternal-fetal vitamin transfer in humans. Am J Obstet Gynecol 1981;141:792–6.
5. Wachstein M, Moore C, Graffeo LW. Pyridoxal phosphate (B_6-al-PO_4) levels of circulating leukocytes in maternal and cord blood. Proc Soc Exp Biol Med 1957;96:326–8.
6. Wachstein M, Kellner JD, Ortiz JM. Pyridoxal phosphate in plasma and leukocytes of normal and pregnant subjects following B_6 load tests. Proc Soc Exp Biol Med 1960;103:350–3.
7. Brin M. Thiamine and pyridoxine studies of mother and cord blood. Fed Proc 1966;25:245.
8. Contractor SF, Shane B. Blood and urine levels of vitamin B_6 in the mother and fetus before and after loading of the mother with vitamin B_6. Am J Obstet Gynecol 1970;107:635–40.
9. Brin M. Abnormal tryptophan metabolism in pregnancy and with the oral contraceptive pill. II. Relative levels of vitamin B_6-vitamers in cord and maternal blood. Am J Clin Nutr 1971;24:704–8.
10. Heller S, Salkeld RM, Korner WF. Vitamin B_6 status in pregnancy. Am J Clin Nutr 1973;26:1339–48.
11. Kaminetzky HA, Baker H, Frank O, Langer A. The effects of intravenously administered water-soluble vitamins during labor in normovitaminemic and hypovitaminemic gravidas on maternal and neonatal blood vitamin levels at delivery. Am J Obstet Gynecol 1974;120:697–703.
12. Brophy MH, Siiteri PK. Pyridoxal phosphate and hypertensive disorders of pregnancy. Am J Obstet Gynecol 1975;121:1075–9.
13. Bamji MS. Enzymic evaluation of thiamin, riboflavin and pyridoxine status of parturient women and their newborn infants. Br J Nutr 1976;35:259–65.
14. Roepke JLB, Kirksey A. Vitamin B_6 nutriture during pregnancy and lactation. I. Vitamin B_6 intake, levels of the vitamin in biological fluids, and condition of the infant at birth. Am J Clin Nutr 1979;32:2249–56.
15. Baker H, Thind IS, Frank O, DeAngelis B, Caterini H, Lquria DB. Vitamin levels in low-birth-weight newborn infants and their mothers. Am J Obstet Gynecol 1977;129:521–4.
16. Baker H, Frank O, Thomason AD, Langer A, Munves ED, De Angelis B, Kaminetzky HA. Vitamin profile of 174 mothers and newborns at parturition. Am J Clin Nutr 1975;28:59–65.
17. Wachstein M, Gudaitis A. Disturbance of vitamin B_6 metabolism in pregnancy. J Lab Clin Med 1952;40:550–7.
18. Wachstein M, Gudaitis A. Disturbance of vitamin B_6 metabolism in pregnancy. II. The influence of various amounts of pyridoxine hydrochloride upon the abnormal tryptophane load test in pregnant women. J Lab Clin Med 1953;42:98–107.
19. Wachstein M, Gudaitis A. Disturbance of vitamin B_6 metabolism in pregnancy. III. Abnormal vitamin B_6 load test. Am J Obstet Gynecol 1953;66:1207–13.
20. Wachstein M, Lobel S. Abnormal tryptophan metabolites in human pregnancy and their relation to deranged vitamin B_6 metabolism. Proc Soc Exp Biol Med 1954;86:624–7.
21. Zartman ER, Barnes AC, Hicks DJ. Observations on pyridoxine metabolism in pregnancy. Am J Obstet Gynecol 1955;70:645–9.
22. Turner ER, Reynolds MS. Intake and elimination of vitamin B_6 and metabolites by women. J Am Diet Assoc 1955;31:1119–20.
23. Page EW. The vitamin B_6 requirement for normal pregnancy. West J Surg Obstet Gynecol 1956;64:96–103.
24. Coursin DB, Brown VC. Changes in vitamin B_6 during pregnancy. Am J Obstet Gynecol 1961;82:1307–11.
25. Brown RR, Thornton MJ, Price JM. The effect of vitamin supplementation on the urinary excretion of tryptophan metabolites by pregnant women. J Clin Invest 1961;40:617–23.
26. Hamfelt A, Hahn L. Pyridoxal phosphate concentration in plasma and tryptophan load test during pregnancy. Clin Chim Acta 1969;25:91–6.
27. Rose DP, Braidman IP. Excretion of tryptophan metabolites as affected by pregnancy, contraceptive steroids, and steroid hormones. Am J Clin Nutr 1971;24:673–83.
28. Kaminetzky HA, Langer A, Baker H, Frank O, Thomson AD, Munves ED, Opper A, Behrle FC, Glista B. The effect of nutrition in teen-age gravidas on pregnancy and the status of the neonate. I. A nutritional profile. Am J Obstet Gynecol 1973;115:639–46.
29. Shane B, Contractor SF. Assessment of vitamin B_6

P

status. Studies on pregnant women and oral contraceptive users. Am J Clin Nutr 1975;28:739–47.
30. Cleary RE, Lumeng L, Li TK. Maternal and fetal plasma levels of pyridoxal phosphate at term: adequacy of vitamin B_6 supplementation during pregnancy. Am J Obstet Gynecol 1975;121:25–8.
31. Lumeng L, Cleary RE, Wagner R, Yu PL, Li TK. Adequacy of vitamin B_6 supplementation during pregnancy: a prospective study. Am J Clin Nutr 1976;29:1376–83.
32. Anonymous. Requirement of vitamin B_6 during pregnancy. Nutr Rev 1976;34:15–6.
33. Dostalova L. Correlation of the vitamin status between mother and newborn during delivery. Dev Pharmacol Ther 1982;4(Suppl 1):45–57.
34. Hunt IF, Murphy NJ, Martner-Hewes PM, Faraji B, Swendseid ME, Reynolds RD, Sanchez A, Mejia A. Zinc, vitamin B-6, and other nutrients in pregnant women attending prenatal clinics in Mexico. Am J Clin Nutr 1987;46:563–9.
35. Bapurao S, Raman L, Tulpule PG. Biochemical assessment of vitamin B_6 nutritional status in pregnant women with orolingual manifestations. Am J Clin Nutr 1982;36:581–6.
36. Davis SD. Immunodeficiency and runting syndrome in rats from congenital pyridoxine deficiency. Nature 1974;251:548–50. As cited in Shepard TH. *Catalog of Teratogenic Agents*. 6th ed. Baltimore, MD: Johns Hopkins University Press, 1989:537–8.
37. Davis SD, Nelson T, Shepard TH. Teratogenicity of vitamin B_6 deficiency: Omphalocele, skeletal and neural defects, and splenic hypoplasia. Science 1970;169: 1329–30. As cited in Shepard TH. *Catalog of Teratogenic Agents*. 6th ed. Baltimore, MD: Johns Hopkins University Press, 1989:537–8.
38. Averback P. Anencephaly associated with megavitamin therapy. Can Med Assoc J 1976;114:995.
39. Sprince H, Lowy RS, Folsome CE, Behrman J. Studies on the urinary excretion of "xanthurenic acid" during normal and abnormal pregnancy: a survey of the excretion of "xanthurenic acid" in normal nonpregnant, normal pregnant, pre-eclamptic, and eclamptic women. Am J Obstet Gynecol 1951;62:84–92.
40. Wachstein M, Graffeo LW. Influence of vitamin B_6 on the incidence of preeclampsia. Obstet Gynecol 1956;8:177–80.
41. Kaminetzky HA, Baker H. Micronutrients in pregnancy. Clin Obstet Gynecol 1977;20:363–80.
42. Diding NA, Melander SEJ. Serum vitamin B_6 level in normal and toxaemic pregnancy. Acta Obstet Gynecol Scand 1961;40:252–61.
43. Hillman RW, Cabaud PG, Nilsson DE, Arpin PD, Tufano RJ. Pyridoxine supplementation during pregnancy. Clinical and laboratory observations. Am J Clin Nutr 1963;12:427–30.
44. Coelingh Bennink HJT, Schreurs WHP. Improvement of oral glucose tolerance in gestational diabetes by pyridoxine. Br Med J 1975;3:13–5.
45. Spellacy WN, Buhi WC, Birk SA. Vitamin B_6 treatment of gestational diabetes mellitus. Studies of blood glucose and plasma insulin. Am J Obstet Gynecol 1977;127:599–602.
46. Perkins RP. Failure of pyridoxine to improve glucose tolerance in gestational diabetes mellitus. Obstet Gynecol 1977;50:370–2.
47. Gillmer MDG, Mazibuko D. Pyridoxine treatment of chemical diabetes in pregnancy. Am J Obstet Gynecol 1979;133:499–502.
48. Snyderman SE, Holt LE, Carretero R, Jacobs K. Pyridoxine deficiency in the human infant. J Clin Nutr 1953;1:200–7.
49. Molony CJ, Parmalee AH. Convulsions in young infants as a result of pyridoxine (vitamin B_6) deficiency. JAMA 1954;154:405–6.
50. Coursin DB. Vitamin B_6 deficiency in infants. Am J Dis Child 1955;90:344–8.
51. Coursin DB. Effects of vitamin B_6 on the central nervous activity in childhood. Am J Clin Nutr 1956;4:354–63.
52. Molony CJ, Parmelee AH. Convulsions in young infants as a result of pyridoxine (vitamin B_6) deficiency. JAMA 1954;154:405–6.
53. Scriver CR. Vitamin B_6 deficiency and dependency in man. Am J Dis Child 1967;113:109–14.
54. Hunt AD Jr, Stokes J Jr, McCrory WW, Stroud HH. Pyridoxine dependency: report of a case of intractable convulsions in an infant controlled by pyridoxine. Pediatrics 1954;13:140–5.
55. Bankier A, Turner M, Hopkins IJ. Pyridoxine dependent seizures—a wider clinical spectrum. Arch Dis Child 1983;58:415–8.
56. Bejsovec MIR, Kulenda Z, Ponca E. Familial intrauterine convulsions in pyridoxine dependency. Arch Dis Child 1967;42:201–7.
57. South M. Neonatal seizures after use of pyridoxine in pregnancy. Lancet 1999;353:1940.
58. Willis RS, Winn WW, Morris AT, Newsom AA, Massey WE. Clinical observations in treatment of nausea and vomiting in pregnancy with vitamins B_1 and B_6. A preliminary report. Am J Obstet Gynecol 1942;44:265–71.
59. Weinstein BB, Mitchell GJ, Sustendal GF. Clinical experiences with pyridoxine hydrochloride in treatment of nausea and vomiting of pregnancy. Am J Obstet Gynecol 1943;46:283–5.
60. Hart BF, McConnell WT. Vitamin B factors in toxic psychosis of pregnancy and the puerperium. Am J Obstet Gynecol 1943;46:283.
61. Varas O. Treatment of nausea and vomiting of pregnancy with vitamin B_6. Bol Soc Chilena Obstet Ginecol 1943;8:404. As abstracted in Am J Obstet Gynecol 1945;50:347–8.
62. Weinstein BB, Wohl Z, Mitchell GJ, Sustendal GF. Oral administration of pyridoxine hydrochloride in the treatment of nausea and vomiting of pregnancy. Am J Obstet Gynecol 1944;47:389–94.
63. Dorsey CW. The use of pyridoxine and suprarenal cortex combined in the treatment of the nausea and vomiting of pregnancy. Am J Obstet Gynecol 1949;58:1073–8.
64. McGanity WJ, McHenry EW, Van Wyck HB, Watt GL. An effect of pyridoxine on blood urea in human subjects. J Biol Chem 1949;178:511–6.
65. Beaton JR, McHenry EW. Observations on plasma glutamic acid. Fed Proc 1951;10:161.
66. Hesseltine HC. Pyridoxine failure in nausea and vomiting of pregnancy. Am J Obstet Gynecol 1946;51:82–6.
67. Sahakian V, Rouse DJ, Rose NB, Niebyl JR. Vitamin B_6 for nausea and vomiting of pregnancy (abstract). Am J Obstet Gynecol 1991;164:322.

68. Sahakian V, Rouse D, Sipes S, Rose NB, Niebyl J. Vitamin B_6 is effective therapy for nausea and vomiting of pregnancy: a randomized double-blind placebo-controlled study. Obstet Gynecol 1991;78: 33–6.
69. Vutyavanich T, Wongtra-ngan S, Ruangsri R-a. Pyridoxine for nausea and vomiting of pregnancy: a randomized, double-blind, placebo-controlled trial. Am J Obstet Gynecol 1995;173:881–4.
70. Gardner LI, Welsh-Sloan J, Cady RB. Phocomelia in infant whose mother took large doses of pyridoxine during pregnancy. Lancet 1985;1:636.
71. Jacobsson C, Granstrom G. Effects of vitamin B_6 on beta-aminopropionitrile–induced palatal cleft formation in the rat. Cleft Palate Craniofac J 1997;34:95–100.
72. Munger RG, Sauberlich HE, Corcoran C, Nepomuceno B, Daack-Hirsch S, Solon FS. Maternal vitamin B-6 and folate status and risk of oral cleft birth defects in the Philippines. Birth Defects Res (Part A) 2004;70:464–71.
73. Schuster K, Bailey LB, Mahan CS. Vitamin B_6 status of low-income adolescent and adult pregnant women and the condition of their infants at birth. Am J Clin Nutr 1981;34:1731–5.
74. Swartwout JR, Unglaub WG, Smith RC. Vitamin B_6, serum lipids and placental arteriolar lesions in human pregnancy. A preliminary report. Am J Clin Nutr 1960;8:434–44.
75. Hillman RW, Cabaud PG, Schenone RA. The effects of pyridoxine supplements on the dental caries experience of pregnant women. Am J Clin Nutr 1962;10:512–5.
76. West KD, Kirksey A. Influence of vitamin B_6 intake on the content of the vitamin in human milk. Am J Clin Nutr 1976;29:961–9.
77. Thomas MR, Kawamoto J, Sneed SM, Eakin R. The effects of vitamin C, vitamin B_6, and vitamin B_{12} supplementation on the breast milk and maternal status of well nourished women. Am J Clin Nutr 1979;32:1679–85.
78. Sneed SM, Zane C, Thomas MR. The effects of ascorbic acid, vitamin B_6, vitamin B_{12}, and folic acid supplementation on the breast milk and maternal nutritional status of low socioeconomic lactating women. Am J Clin Nutr 1981;34:1338–46.
79. Styslinger L, Kirksey A. Effects of different levels of vitamin B-6 supplementation on vitamin B-6 concentrations in human milk and vitamin B-6 intakes of breastfed infants. Am J Clin Nutr 1985;41:21–31.
80. Ford JE, Zechalko A, Murphy J, Brooke OG. Comparison of the B vitamin composition of milk from mothers of preterm and term babies. Arch Dis Child 1983;58:367–72.
81. Deodhar AD, Rajalakshmi R, Ramakrishnan CV. Studies on human lactation. Part III. Effect of dietary vitamin supplementation vitamin contents of breast milk. Acta Pediatr 1964;53:42–8.
82. Thomas MR, Sneed SM, Wei C, Nail PA, Wilson M, Sprinkle EE III. The effects of vitamin C, vitamin B_6, vitamin B_{12}, folic acid, riboflavin, and thiamine on the breast milk and maternal status of well-nourished women at 6 months postpartum. Am J Clin Nutr 1980;33:2151–6.
83. Bessey OA, Adam DJD, Hansen AE. Intake of vitamin B_6 and infantile convulsions: a first approximation of requirements of pyridoxine in infants. Pediatrics 1957;20:33–44.
84. Kirksey A, Roepke JLB. Vitamin B-6 nutriture of mothers of three breast-fed neonates with central nervous system disorders. Fed Proc 1981;40:864.
85. Foukas MD. An antilactogenic effect of pyridoxine. J Obstet Gynaecol Br Commonw 1973;80:718–20.
86. Moretti C, Fabbri A, Gnessi L, Bonifacio V, Fraioli F, Isidori A. Pyridoxine (B_6) suppresses the rise in prolactin and increases the rise in growth hormone induced by exercise. N Engl J Med 1982;307:444–5.
87. MacDonald HN, Collins YD, Tobin MJW, Wijayaratne, DN. The failure of pyridoxine in suppression of puerperal lactation. Br J Obstet Gynaecol 1976;83:54–5.
88. Canales ES, Soria J, Zarate A, Mason M, Molina M. The influence of pyridoxine on prolactin secretion and milk production in women. Br J Obstet Gynaecol 1976;83:387–8.
89. Greentree LB. Dangers of vitamin B_6 in nursing mothers. N Engl J Med 1979;300:141–2.
90. Lande NI. More on dangers of vitamin B_6 in nursing mothers. N Engl J Med 1979,300.926–7.
91. Rivlin RS. More on dangers of vitamin B_6 in nursing mothers. N Engl J Medi 1979;300:927.
92. Andon MB, Howard MP, Moser PB, Reynolds RD. Nutritionally relevant supplementation of vitamin B_6 in lactating women: Effect on plasma prolactin. Pediatrics 1985;76:769–73.
93. Committee on Drugs, American Academy of Pediatrics. The transfer of drugs and other chemicals into human milk. Pediatrics 2001;108:776–89.

Name: **PYRILAMINE** Risk Factor: **C**
Class: **Antihistamine**

FETAL RISK SUMMARY

RECOMMENDATION: Limited Human Data - Probably Compatible

Pyrilamine is used infrequently during pregnancy. The Collaborative Perinatal Project monitored 50,282 mother-child pairs, 121 of whom had pyrilamine exposure in the 1st trimester

(1, pp. 323–324). No evidence was found to suggest a relationship to large categories of major or minor malformations. For use anytime during pregnancy, 392 exposures were recorded (1, pp. 436–437). A possible association with malformations was found on the basis of 12 defects, 6 of which involved benign tumors (1, p. 489).

An association between exposure during the last 2 weeks of pregnancy to antihistamines in general and retrolental fibroplasia in premature infants has been reported. See Brompheniramine for details.

BREAST FEEDING SUMMARY

RECOMMENDATION: No Human Data - Probably Compatible

No data are available.

Reference

1. Heinonen OP, Slone D, Shapiro S. *Birth Defects and Drugs in Pregnancy*. Littleton, MA: Publishing Sciences Group, 1977.

Name: **PYRIMETHAMINE** Risk Factor: **C_M**
Class: **Antimalarial**

FETAL RISK SUMMARY

RECOMMENDATION: Compatible - Maternal Benefit >> Embryo/Fetal Risk

Pyrimethamine is a folic acid antagonist (inhibitor of dihydrofolate reductase) used in combination with other agents primarily for the treatment and prophylaxis of malaria, but also for toxoplasmosis. Shepard reviewed 15 studies that evaluated the reproductive effects of pyrimethamine in rats, mice, and hamsters (1). Malformations in fetal rats included cleft palate, mandibular hypoplasia, limb defects, and neural tube defects. In some cases, the teratogenic dose was similar to the human dose. At slightly higher doses in rats, pyrimethamine caused chromosomal aberrations such as trisomy or chromosomal mosaicism (1).

A 1993 study found in pregnant rats and mice that oral folic acid potentiated the embryotoxicity of pyrimethamine, but that decreased embryotoxicity was observed when folic acid was given intraperitoneally (2). The mechanism of the increased toxicity appeared to be reduced plasma levels of 5-methyltetrahydrofolic acid in the dams. 5-Methyltetrahydrofolic acid is the principal active folate in plasma and it undergoes a large amount of enterohepatic circulating (2). Folic acid inhibited the absorption of the active folate from the intestine.

Reproduction studies, reported by the manufacturer, revealed teratogenicity in rats, hamsters, and miniature pigs (3). In rats, oral doses 7 times the human dose for chemoprophylaxis of malaria (HDCM) or 2.5 times the human dose for toxoplasmosis (HDT), caused cleft palate, brachygnathia, oligodactyly, and microphthalmia. Meningocele was seen in hamsters, given doses 170 times the HDCM or HDT, and cleft palate occurred in miniature pigs at 5 times the HDCM or HDT (3).

In an *in vitro* study using human perfused placentas, the transfer rate of pyrimethamine was about 30% (4). The results suggested that the placental transfer was independent of maternal concentration and the transfer occurred by passive diffusion (4).

Antimalarial agents, including pyrimethamine, are used routinely during pregnancy because the risks from the disease far outweigh the risks to the fetus from drug therapy (see Proguanil for a discussion on the maternal and fetal risks of malaria during pregnancy).

Although some folic acid antagonists are human teratogens (e.g., see Methotrexate), this does not seem to occur with pyrimethamine (5–11). One case report, however, did describe a severe defect of the abdominal and thoracic wall (exteriorization of the heart, lungs, and most of the abdominal viscera) (possible variant of ectopia cordis) and a missing left arm in an infant exposed to the drug (12). The woman had been treated with chloroquine, 100 mg/day, plus a combination of dapsone (100 mg) and pyrimethamine (12.5 mg) (Maloprim) on post-conception days 10, 20, and 30. However, an association between the drug and the defect has been questioned (13,14). Moreover, most studies describing the use of pyrimethamine in pregnant women for the treatment or prophylaxis of malaria have found the drug to be relatively safe and effective (14–29), although some recommend avoiding the drug during the 1st trimester (25).

Two reviews of toxoplasmosis (*Toxoplasma gondii*) in pregnancy were published in 1994 (30,31). Pyrimethamine, in combination with sulfadiazine, was recommended in both as the most effective treatment after the infection had reached the fetus. No fetal adverse effects of this therapy have been observed.

In spite of the animal study above that described increased embryotoxicity after oral folic acid, if pyrimethamine is used during pregnancy, folic acid (5 mg/day) or folinic acid (leucovorin; 5 mg/day) supplementation is recommended, especially during the 1st trimester, to prevent folate deficiency (5–9,14,25,30).

BREAST FEEDING SUMMARY

RECOMMENDATION: Limited Human Data - Probably Compatible

Pyrimethamine is excreted into breast milk (32,33). Mothers treated with 25–75 mg orally produced peak concentrations of 3.1–3.3 μg/mL at 6 hours (32). The drug was detectable in breast milk up to 48 hours after a dose. Malaria parasites were completely eliminated in infants up to 6 months of age who were entirely breast-fed. In a 1986 study, three women were treated with a combination tablet containing 100 mg of dapsone and 12.5 mg of pyrimethamine at 2–5 days postpartum (33). Blood and milk samples were collected up to 227 hours after the dose. The milk:plasma area under the concentration-time curve ratios ranged from 0.46 to 0.66. Based on an estimated ingestion of 1000 mL of milk/day, the infants would have consumed between 16.8% and 45.6% of the maternal doses during a 9-day period. The American Academy of Pediatrics classifies pyrimethamine as compatible with breast-feeding (34).

References

1. Shepard TH. *Catalog of Teratogenic Agents*. 8th ed. Baltimore, MD: Johns Hopkins University Press, 1995:362–3.
2. Kudo G, Tsunematsu K, Shimoda M, Kokue E. Effects of folic acid on pyrimethamine teratogenesis in rats. Adv Exp Med Biol 1993;338:469–72.
3. Product information. Daraprim. Glaxo Wellcome, 2000.
4. Peytavin G, Leng JJ, Forestier F, Saux MC, Hohlfeld P, Farinotti R. Placental transfer of pyrimethamine studied in an ex vivo placental perfusion model. Biol Neonate 2000;78:83–5.
5. Anonymous. Prevention of malaria in pregnancy and early childhood. Br Med J 1984;1296–7.
6. Spracklen FHN. Malaria 1984 Part I. Malaria prophylaxis. S Afr Med J 1984;65:1037–41.

7. Spracklen FHN, Monteagudo FSE. Therapeutic protocol No. 3. Malaria prophylaxis. S Afr Med J 1986;70:316.
8. Brown GV. Chemoprophylaxis of malaria. Med J Aust 1986;144:696–702.
9. Cook GC. Prevention and treatment of malaria. Lancet 1988;1:32–7.
10. Barry M, Bia F. Pregnancy and travel. JAMA 1989;261:728–31.
11. Stekette RW, Wirima JJ, Slutsker L, Heymann DL, Breman JG. The problem of malaria and malaria control in pregnancy in sub-Saharan Africa. Am J Trop Med Hyg 1996;55:2–7.
12. Harpey J-P, Darbois Y, Lefebvre G. Teratogenicity of pyrimethamine. Lancet 1983;2:399.
13. Smithells RW, Sheppard S. Teratogenicity of Debendox and pyrimethamine. Lancet 1983;2:623–4.
14. Main EK, Main DM, Krogstad DJ. Treatment of chloroquine-resistant malaria during pregnancy. JAMA 1983;249:3207–9.
15. Anonymous. Pyrimethamine combinations in pregnancy. Lancet 1983;2:1005–7.
16. Morley D, Woodland M, Cuthbertson WFJ. Controlled trial of pyrimethamine in pregnant women in an African village. Br Med J 1964;1:667–8.
17. Gilles HM, Lawson JB, Sibelas M, Voller A, Allan N. Malaria, anaemia and pregnancy. Ann Trop Med Parasitol 1969;63:245–63.
18. Heinonen OP, Slone D, Shapiro. *Birth Defects and Drugs in Pregnancy*. Littleton, MA: Publishing Sciences Group, 1977:299,302.
19. Bruce-Chwatt LJ. Malaria and pregnancy. Br Med J 1983;286:1457–8.
20. Anonymous. Malaria in pregnancy. Lancet 1983;2:84–5.
21. Strang A, Lachman E, Pitsoe SB, Marszalek A, Philpott RH. Malaria in pregnancy with fatal complications. Case report. Br J Obstet Gynaecol 1984;91:399–403.
22. Nahlen BL, Akintunde A, Alakija T, Nguyen-Dinh P, Ogunbode O, Edungbola LD, Adetoro O, Breman JG. Lack of efficacy of pyrimethamine prophylaxis in pregnant Nigerian women. Lancet 1989;2:830–4.
23. Keuter M, van Eijk A, Hoogstrate M, Raasveld M, van de Ree M, Ngwawe WA, Watkins WM, Were JBO, Brandling-Bennett AD. Comparison of chloroquine, pyrimethamine and sulfadoxine, and chlorproguanil and dapsone as treatment for falciparum malaria in pregnant and non-pregnant women, Kakamega district, Kenya. BMJ 1990;301:466–70.
24. Greenwood AM, Armstrong JRM, Byass P, Snow RW, Greenwood BM. Malaria chemoprophylaxis, birth weight and child survival. Trans Roy Soc Trop Med Hyg 1992;86:483–5.
25. Luzzi GA, Peto TEA. Adverse effects of antimalarials. An Update. Drug Saf 1993;8:295–311.
26. Greenwood AM, Menendez C, Todd J, Greenwood BM. The distribution of birth weights in Gambian women who received malaria chemoprophylaxis during their first pregnancy and in control women. Trans Roy Soc Trop Med Hyg 1994;88:311–2.
27. Schultz LJ, Steketee RW, Macheso A, Kazembe P, Chitsulo L, Wirima JJ. The efficacy of antimalarial regimens containing sulfadoxine-pyrimethamine and/or chloroquine in preventing peripheral and placental *Plasmodium falciparum* infection among pregnant women in Malawi. Am J Trop Med Hyg 1994;51:515–22.
28. Menendez C, Todd J, Alonso PL, Lulat S, Francis N, Greenwood BM. Malaria chemoprophylaxis, infection of the placenta and birth weight in Gambian primigravidae. J Trop Med Hyg 1994;97:244–8.
29. Sowunmi A, Akindele JA, Omitowoju GO, Omigbodun AO, Oduola AMJ, Salako LA. Intramuscular sulfadoxine-pyrimethamine in uncomplicated chloroquine-resistant falciparum malaria during pregnancy. Trans Roy Soc Trop Med Hyg 1993;87:472.
30. Wong S-Y, Remington JS. Toxoplasmosis in pregnancy. Clin Infect Dis 1994;18:853–62.
31. Matsui D. Prevention, diagnosis, and treatment of fetal toxoplasmosis. Clin Perinatol 1994;21:675–88.
32. Clyde DF, Shute GT, Press J. Transfer of pyrimethamine in human milk. J Trop Med Hyg 1956;59:277–84.
33. Edstein MD. Veerendaal JR, Newman K, Hyslop R. Excretion of chloroquine, dapsone and pyrimethamine in human milk. Br J Clin Pharmacol 1986;22:733–5.
34. Committee on Drugs, American Academy of Pediatrics. The transfer of drugs and other chemicals into human milk. Pediatrics 2001;108:776–89.

Name: **PYRVINIUM PAMOATE** Risk Factor: **C**
Class: **Anthelmintic**

FETAL RISK SUMMARY

RECOMMENDATION: No Human Data - No Relevant Animal Data

No data are available.

BREAST FEEDING SUMMARY

RECOMMENDATION: No Human Data - Probably Compatible

No data are available.

Q

Name:	**QUAZEPAM**	Risk Factor: X_M
Class:	**Hypnotic**	

FETAL RISK SUMMARY

RECOMMENDATION: Human Data Suggest Risk in 1st and 3rd Trimesters

Quazepam is a benzodiazepine that is used as a hypnotic for the short-term management of insomnia. No major abnormalities were observed in mice and rabbits at doses up to 400 and 134 times the human dose, respectively (1). Minor defects observed in mice were delayed ossification of the sternum, vertebrae, distal phalanges, and supraoccipital bones (1). The manufacturer considers the drug to be contraindicated during pregnancy (1).

No reports of human use of quazepam during human pregnancy have been located, but the effects of this agent on the fetus following prolonged use should be similar to those observed with other benzodiazepines (see also Diazepam). Maternal use near delivery may potentially cause neonatal motor depression and withdrawal.

BREAST FEEDING SUMMARY

RECOMMENDATION: Limited Human Data - Potential Toxicity

Quazepam is excreted into breast milk (2). Four healthy, lactating volunteers, who agreed not to breast-feed their infants, were given a single 15-mg dose of the hypnotic, and blood and milk samples were collected at scheduled times during a 48-hour interval. Mean cumulative amounts of quazepam and its two major active metabolites excreted into milk during the 48-hour period were 11.6 μg (range 2.4–32.8 μg) quazepam, 4.0 μg (range 1.3–10.0 μg) 2-oxoquazepam, and 1.0 μg (range 0.4–1.6 μg) *N*-desalky-2-oxoquazepam. These amounts represented 0.08%, 0.02%, and 0.09% of the dose, respectively. Milk concentrations of quazepam and 2-oxoquazepam were always higher than those in the plasma, with milk-to-plasma ratios of 4.18 and 2.02, respectively. Because of the lipophilic properties of quazepam, these ratios are much higher than those observed with diazepam (see Diazepam). The investigators estimated that following a multiple-dose regimen, only 28.7 μg/day of the three compounds combined would be excreted into milk, representing 0.19% of the daily dose. Moreover, they concluded that the pharmacokinetics of quazepam indicated that accumulation would not occur, except for *N*-desalky-2-oxoquazepam, the metabolite excreted in milk in the smallest amounts (2).

Although the amounts measured in the above study are small, the effects, if any, on a nursing infant's central nervous system function are unknown. The American Academy of Pediatrics classifies quazepam, especially when taken by nursing mothers for long periods, as a drug for which the effect on nursing infants is unknown but may be of concern (3).

References

1. Product information. Doral. Wallace Laboratories, 1994.
2. Hilbert JM, Gural RP, Symchowicz S, Zampaglione N. Excretion of quazepam into human breast milk. J Clin Pharmacol 1984;24:457–62.
3. Committee on Drugs, American Academy of Pediatrics. The transfer of drugs and other chemicals into human milk. Pediatrics 2001;108:776–89.

Name:	**QUETIAPINE**	Risk Factor:	**C_M**
Class:	**Antipsychotic**		

FETAL RISK SUMMARY

RECOMMENDATION: Limited Human Data - Animal Data Suggest Risk

Quetiapine is an antipsychotic agent that is a dibenzothiazepine derivative. Other antipsychotic agents in the same class are clozapine, loxapine, and olanzapine. These agents are often referred to as atypical antipsychotics. Quetiapine is indicated for the treatment of schizophrenia. Its mechanism of action is unknown, but it is thought to be related to dopamine type 2 and serotonin type 2 receptor antagonism. The drug also is an antagonist of histamine H_1 and adrenergic α_1 receptors and may cause somnolence and orthostatic hypotension, respectively (1).

Reproduction studies have been conducted in rats and rabbits (1). No evidence of teratogenicity was observed in pregnant rats or rabbits at oral doses up to 2.4 times the maximum human dose on a body surface basis (MHD) during organogenesis. However, minor soft tissue malformations (carpal/tarsal flexure) were noted in rabbit fetuses at 2.4 times the MHD. Embryo/fetal toxicity were observed in both species but the doses used (in rats only with the highest dose and in rabbits with all doses) also caused maternal toxicity (decreased weight gain and/or death). Delays in skeletal ossification were observed in rats at doses equivalent to 0.6 and 2.4 times the MHD. Similar fetal effects were observed in rabbits at doses 1.2 and 2.4 times the MHD. Reduced fetal body weights were noted at the highest doses in both species. No drug-related effects were noted in rat offspring in a perinatal/postnatal study using oral doses that were 0.1–0.24 times the MHD (1).

Q

Quetiapine decreased mating and fertility in male rats given oral doses up to 1.8 times the MHD (1). The adverse effects (increased interval to mate and number of matings required for successful impregnation) continued to be observed in the high-dose group 2 weeks after treatment had been stopped. In male rats, the no-effect dose for impaired mating and fertility was 0.3 times the MHD. Quetiapine also adversely effected mating and fertility in female rats. At an oral dose 0.6 times the MHD, drug effects included decreases in mating and in matings resulting in pregnancy, and increases in the interval to mate and in irregular estrus cycles (also noted at 0.1 times the MHD). The no-effect dose in female rats was 0.01 times the MHD.

It is not known if quetiapine can cross the placenta to the fetus. The molecular weight (about 767 for the base), a protein binding of 86%, and a moderately long elimination half-life (6 hours) suggest that the drug will reach the fetus.

A 38-year-old woman with paranoid-type schizophrenia was started on quetiapine (300 mg/day) after an unsuccessful trial with zuclopenthixol (2). After a marked improvement in her symptoms, she conceived with her pregnancy being diagnosed at 17 weeks' gestation when she reported amenorrhea. At 20 weeks' gestation her dose was lowered to

200 mg/day; 2 weeks later her dose was reduced to 150 mg/day (cited as 200 mg bid then 150 mg bid, but stated to be reductions in her dose). She eventually gave birth to a healthy 3120-g male infant with Apgar scores of 9 and 10 at 1 and 5 minutes, respectively. Birth length was 48 cm. The infant was developing normally at 6 months of age (2).

In summary, quetiapine is a potent atypical antipsychotic that may cause clinically significant improvements in the symptoms experienced by a schizophrenic patient. In certain situations, this improvement may result in an increased opportunity for conception and subsequent pregnancy. Quetiapine is not teratogenic in rats and rabbits, but only low doses ($\leq$2.4 times the MHD) have been evaluated. Administration of higher doses was prevented because of significant maternal, embryo, and fetal toxicity. Human pregnancy experience is limited to a single case and thus, when combined with the animal reproduction data, prevents an assessment of the risk to the fetus. In addition, quetiapine dosing in male and female rats causes mating and fertility problems at doses that are a fraction of those prescribed to humans. However, because quetiapine is indicated for severe, debilitating mental disease, the benefits to the mother appear to outweigh the potential risks to the fetus (3). A 1996 review on the management of psychiatric illness concluded that patients with histories of chronic psychosis or severe bipolar illness represent a high-risk group (for both the mother and the fetus) and should be maintained on pharmacologic therapy before and during pregnancy (4).

BREAST FEEDING SUMMARY

RECOMMENDATION: No Human Data - Potential Toxicity

No studies describing the use of quetiapine during human lactation have been located. The drug is excreted into the milk of experimental animals. Consistent with its molecular weight (about 767 for the base), protein binding of 86%, and the elimination half-life of 6 hours, quetiapine is also probably excreted into breast milk. The effects of this exposure on a nursing infant are unknown. The manufacturer recommends women receiving quetiapine should not breast-feed (1).

References

1. Product information. Seroquel. AstraZeneca Pharmaceuticals, 2003.
2. Tenyi T, Trixler M, Keresztes Z. Quetiapine and pregnancy. Am J Psychiatry 2002;159:674.
3. Cutler AJ, Goldstein JM, Tumas JA. Dosing and switching strategies for quetiapine fumarate. Clin Ther 2002;24:209–22.
4. Althuler LL, Cohen L, Szuba MP, Burt VK, Gitlin M, Mintz J. Pharmacologic management of psychiatric illness during pregnancy: dilemmas and guidelines. Am J Psychiatry 1996;153:592–606.

Name: **QUINACRINE** Risk Factor: **C**

Class: **Antimalarial/Anthelmintic**

FETAL RISK SUMMARY

RECOMMENDATION: Limited Human Data - No Relevant Animal Data

Studies in pregnant rabbits with quinacrine produced increased fetal mortality, but no structural defects were observed (1). In humans, a newborn with renal agenesis, hydronephrosis, spina bifida, megacolon, and hydrocephalus whose mother received quinacrine 0.1 g/day during the 1st trimester has been reported (2). Topical application of solutions containing 125 mg/mL of quinacrine directly into the uterine cavity has resulted in tubal occlusion and infertility (3).

BREAST FEEDING SUMMARY

RECOMMENDATION: No Human Data - Probably Compatible

No data are available.

References

1. Rothschild B, Levy G. Action de la quinacrine sur la gestation chez le rat. C R Soc Biol 1950;144:1350–2. As cited in Shepard TH. *Catalog of Teratogenic Agents*. 6th ed. Baltimore, MD: Johns Hopkins University Press, 1989:542.
2. Vevera J, Zatlovkal F. Pfipad uruzenych malformact zpusobenych pravdepodobne atebrinem-ym uranem tehotenstui. In Nishmura H, Tanimura T, eds. *Clinical Aspects of The Teratogenicity of Drugs*. New York, NY: American Elsevier, 1976:145.
3. Zipper JA, Stachetti E, Medel M. Human fertility control by transvaginal application of quinacrine on the fallopian tube. Fertil Steril 1970;21:581–9.

Name: **QUINAPRIL** Risk Factor: C_M*

Class: **Antihypertensive**

FETAL RISK SUMMARY

RECOMMENDATION: Human Data Suggest Risk in 2nd and 3rd Trimesters

Quinapril is an angiotensin-converting enzyme (ACE) inhibitor. No teratogenic effects were observed in reproduction studies in rats and rabbits with doses 180 and 1 times the maximum recommended human dose, respectively (1).

No reports of the use of this agent in human pregnancy have been located, but this class of drugs should be used with caution, if at all, during gestation. Use of ACE inhibitors limited to the 1st trimester does not appear to present a significant risk to the fetus, but fetal exposure after this time is associated with teratogenicity and severe toxicity in the fetus and newborn, including death. See Captopril or Enalapril for a summary of fetal and neonatal effects from these agents. If quinapril is used in pregnancy, health care professionals are encouraged to call the toll free number (800-670-6126) for information about patient enrollment in the Motherisk study.

[**Risk Factor* D_M *if used in 2nd or 3rd trimesters.*]

BREAST-FEEDING SUMMARY

RECOMMENDATION: Limited Human Data - Probably Compatible

Quinapril is excreted into breast milk. Six healthy mothers who had been breast-feeding for at least 2 weeks were given a single 20 mg oral dose of quinapril (2). Serial blood and milk samples were collected over 24 hours. The mean milk:plasma ratio was 0.12 based on AUC, but no drug was detected in milk after 4 hours. The metabolite (quinaprilat) was not detected in any of the milk samples. The estimated infant dose was 1.6% of the mother's weight-adjusted dose (2).

The amount of quinapril measured in the above study is clinically insignificant. Although data from women receiving daily doses of the drug are needed, quinapril is probably compatible with nursing.

The American Academy of Pediatrics classifies captopril and enalapril as compatible with breast-feeding (see Captopril and Enalapril).

References

1. Product information. Accupril. Parke-Davis, 2000.
2. Begg EJ, Robson RA, Gardiner SJ, Hudson LF, Reece PA, Olson SC, Posvar EL, Sedman AJ. Quinapril and its metabolite quinaprilat in human milk. Br J Clin Pharmacol 2001;51:478–81.

Name:	**QUINETHAZONE**	Risk Factor:	**C***
Class:	**Diuretic**		

FETAL RISK SUMMARY

RECOMMENDATION: No Human Data - No Relevant Animal Data

Quinethazone is structurally related to the thiazide diuretics. In general, diuretics are not recommended for the treatment of gestational hypertension because of the maternal hypovolemia characteristic of this disease. See Chlorothiazide.

[**Risk Factor D if used in gestational hypertension.*]

BREAST FEEDING SUMMARY

RECOMMENDATION: No Human Data - Probably Compatible

See Chlorothiazide.

Name:	**QUINIDINE**	Risk Factor:	C_M
Class:	**Antiarrhythmic/Antimalarial**		

FETAL RISK SUMMARY

RECOMMENDATION: Compatible

No reports linking the use of quinidine with congenital defects have been located. Animal reproduction studies have apparently not been conducted with quinidine.

Quinidine has been in use as an antiarrhythmic drug for more than 100 years (1) and in pregnancy, at least back to the 1920s (2–8). Eighth cranial nerve damage is associated with high doses of the optical isomer, quinine, but not with quinidine (4). Neonatal thrombocytopenia has been reported after maternal use of quinidine (5).

Quinidine crosses the placenta and achieves fetal serum levels similar to maternal levels (1,6–8). In a 1979 case, a woman taking 600 mg every 8 hours plus an additional dose of 300 mg (2100 mg/day) had serum and amniotic fluid levels of 5.8 and 10.6 μg/mL, respectively, 10 days before term (6). Three days later, 10 hours after the last dose, a healthy male infant was delivered by elective cesarean section. Quinidine concentrations in the serum, cord blood, and amniotic fluid were 3.4, 2.8, and 9.3 μg/mL, respectively (6). The cord blood:serum ratio was 0.82. The cord blood levels were greater than those measured in three other reports (1,7,8).

In a 1984 study, three women maintained on quinidine, 300 mg every 6 hours, and digoxin had serum levels of quinidine at delivery ranging from 0.7 to 2.1 μg/mL (7). A quinidine level in one amniotic fluid sample was 0.9 μg/mL, whereas cord blood levels ranged from <0.5 to 1.6 μg/mL. In two of the three cases, cord blood:serum ratios were 0.2 and 0.9.

In a 1985 report, a woman taking quinidine, 400 mg every 6 hours, plus digoxin and propranolol, was electively delivered by cesarean section 18 hours after the last dose (8). The quinidine concentration in the cord blood was 0.8 μg/mL.

One case involved a woman in whom quinidine doses were escalated during a 6-day interval from 300 mg every 6 hours to 1500 mg every 6 hours (1). On day 8, the dosage was reduced to 1500 mg every 8 hours, then to 1200 mg every 8 hours on day 9, and stopped on day 10. Amniotic fluid levels of quinidine and the metabolite, 3-hydroxyquinidine, on day 10 were 2.2 and 9.7 μg/mL, respectively. At delivery 2 days later, cord blood contained 0.5 μg/mL of quinidine and 0.7 μg/mL of the metabolite.

In a surveillance study of Michigan Medicaid recipients involving 229,101 completed pregnancies conducted between 1985 and 1992, 17 newborns had been exposed to quinidine during the 1st trimester (F. Rosa, personal communication, FDA, 1993). One (5.9%) major birth defect was observed (one expected). No anomalies were observed in six defect categories (cardiovascular defects, oral clefts, spina bifida, polydactyly, limb reduction defects, and hypospadias) for which specific data were available.

The drug has been used in combination with digoxin to treat fetal supraventricular and reciprocating atrioventricular tachycardia (7,8). The authors of one of these reports consider quinidine to be the drug of choice after digoxin for the treatment of persistent fetal tachyarrhythmias (8). A 1990 report described an unsuccessful attempt of maternal transplacental cardioversion with quinidine for a rare case of fetal ventricular tachycardia associated with nonimmune hydrops fetalis at 30 weeks' gestation (9). A dose of 200 mg quinidine 4 times daily was given for 3 days before worsening preeclampsia with breech presentation required delivery by cesarean section. The newborn died 5 hours after birth.

A 33-year-old woman with new-onset, sustained ventricular tachycardia was treated with metoprolol, 50 mg twice daily, at 22 weeks' gestation (10). Because of recurrent palpitations, quinidine (dose not specified) was added to the regimen at 26 weeks' gestation; with the attainment of a therapeutic quinidine level, the combination was successful in controlling the ectopic beats. Combination therapy was continued until term when a healthy, growth-retarded, 4-lb 15-oz (approximately 2240-g) infant was delivered. Intrauterine growth retardation apparently developed after maternal combination therapy was initiated, but a discussion of its cause was not included in the reference, nor were maternal blood pressures given.

A mother treated with quinidine for a fetal supraventricular tachycardia developed symptoms of quinidine toxicity consisting of severe nausea and vomiting, diarrhea, lightheadedness, and tinnitus (1). Electrocardiographic changes were consistent with quinidine toxicity. Her dosage had been increased during an interval of 6 days in a manner described above, producing serum quinidine levels of 1.4–3.3 μg/mL (the therapeutic range in the author's laboratory was 1.5–5.0 μg/mL) (1). At the highest dose, her serum level was

2.3 μg/mL. Levels of the metabolite 3-hydroxyquinidine rose from 1.1 to 6.8 μg/mL during the 6-day interval, eventually reaching 9.7 μg/mL 1 day after quinidine was discontinued. The 3-hydroxyquinidine:quinidine ratio varied from 0.8 (on day 2) to 3.7 (on day 10). These ratios were much higher than those observed in previously reported patients (1). Because the fetal heart rate continued to be elevated, with only occasional reductions to 120–130 beats/minute, and fetal lung maturity had been demonstrated, labor was induced, resulting in the delivery of a 3540-g infant with hydrops fetalis. The infant required pharmacologic therapy to control the supraventricular tachycardia. The maternal toxicity was attributed to the elevated levels of 3-hydroxyquinidine, because concentrations of quinidine were in the low to mid-therapeutic range (1).

In an *in vitro* study using plasma from 16 normal pregnant women, quinidine concentrations between 0.5 and 5.0 μg/mL were shown to inhibit plasma pseudocholinesterase activity (11). Inhibition varied from 29% (0.5 μg/mL) to 71% (5.0 μg/mL). Pseudocholinesterase is responsible for the metabolism of succinylcholine and ester-type local anesthetics (e.g., procaine, tetracaine, cocaine, and chloroprocaine) (11). The quinidine-induced inhibition of this enzyme, which is already significantly decreased by pregnancy itself, could potentially result in toxicity if these agents were used in a mother maintained on quinidine.

A 21-year-old woman in premature labor at 31 weeks' gestation was treated with IV quinidine and exchange transfusion for severe, apparently chloroquine-resistant, malaria (12). Parasitemia with *Plasmodium falciparum* greater than 12% was shown on blood smears before treatment and then fell to 1% after treatment. Initial therapy with 1 g oral chloroquine was unsuccessful and approximately 12 hours later, she was given an IV loading dose of quinidine, 10 mg base/kg over 2 hours, followed by a continuous infusion of 0.02 mg/kg/minute and exchange transfusion. No potentiation of labor was observed during quinidine therapy, although the mother was receiving IV magnesium sulfate for tocolysis. Because of fetal distress, thought to be caused by uteroplacental insufficiency as a result of maternal parasitemia or fever, a cesarean section was performed to deliver a 1570-g male infant with Apgar scores of 5 and 7 at 1 and 5 minutes, respectively. Except for respiratory difficulty during the first 6 hours, the infant had an uneventful hospital course, including a negative blood smear for malaria.

The use of quinidine during pregnancy has been classified in reviews of cardiovascular drugs as relatively safe for the fetus (13–16). In therapeutic doses, the oxytocic properties of quinidine have been rarely observed, but high doses can produce this effect and may result in abortion (15,17).

BREAST FEEDING SUMMARY

RECOMMENDATION: Limited Human Data - Probably Compatible

Quinidine is excreted into breast milk (6). A woman taking 600 mg every 8 hours had milk and serum concentrations determined on the 5th postpartum day, 3 hours after a dose (6). Levels in the two samples were 6.4 and 9.0 μg/mL, respectively, a milk:serum ratio of 0.71. A quinidine level of 8.2 μg/mL was noted in a milk sample on the preceding day (time relationship to the dose not specified) but a simultaneous serum concentration was not determined. The infant in this case did not breast-feed. The American Academy of Pediatrics classifies quinidine as compatible with breast-feeding (18).

References

1. Killeen AA, Bowers LD. Fetal supraventricular tachycardia treated with high-dose quinidine: toxicity associated with marked elevation of the metabolite, 3(S)-3-hydroxyquinidine. Obstet Gynecol 1987;70: 445–9.
2. Meyer J, Lackner JE, Schochet SS. Paroxysmal tachycardia in pregnancy. JAMA 1930;94:1901–4.
3. McMillan TM, Bellet S. Ventricular paroxysmal tachycardia: report of a case in a pregnant girl of sixteen years with an apparently normal heart. Am Heart J 1931;7:70–8.
4. Mendelson CL. Disorders of the heartbeat during pregnancy. Am J Obstet Gynecol 1956;72: 1268–1301.
5. Domula VM, Weissach G, Lenk H. Uber die auswirkung medikamentoser Behandlung in der Schwangerschaft auf das Gerennungspotential des Neugeborenen. Zentralbl Gynaekol 1977;99:473.
6. Hill LM, Malkasian GD Jr. The use of quinidine sulfate throughout pregnancy. Obstet Gynecol 1979;54: 366–8.
7. Spinnato JA, Shaver DC, Flinn GS, Sibai BM, Watson DL, Marin-Garcia J. Fetal supraventricular tachycardia: in utero therapy with digoxin and quinidine. Obstet Gynecol 1984;64:730–5.
8. Guntheroth WG, Cyr DR, Mack LA, Benedetti T, Lenke RR, Petty CN. Hydrops from reciprocating atrioventricular tachycardia in a 27-week fetus requiring quinidine for conversion. Obstet Gynecol 1985;66(Suppl): 29S–33S.
9. Sherer DM, Sadovksy E, Menashe M, Mordel N, Rein AJJT. Fetal ventricular tachycardia associated with nonimmunologic hydrops fetalis: a case report. J Reprod Med 1990;35:292–4.
10. Braverman AC, Bromely BS, Rutherford JD. New onset ventricular tachycardia during pregnancy. Int J Cardiol 1991;33:409–12.
11. Kambam JR, Franks JJ, Smith BE. Inhibitory effect of quinidine on plasma pseudocholinesterase activity in pregnant women. Am J Obstet Gynecol 1987;157:897–9.
12. Wong RD, Murthy ARK, Mathisen GE, Glover N, Thornton PJ. Treatment of severe Falciparum malaria during pregnancy with quinidine and exchange transfusion. Am J Med 1992;92:561–2.
13. Rotmensch HH, Elkayam U, Frishman W. Antiarrhythmic drug therapy during pregnancy. Ann Intern Med 1983;98:487–97.
14. Tamari I, Eldar M, Rabinowitz B, Neufeld HN. Medical treatment of cardiovascular disorders during pregnancy. Am Heart J 1982;104:1357–63.
15. Rotmensch HH, Rotmensch S, Elkayam U. Management of cardiac arrhythmias during pregnancy: current concepts. Drugs 1987;33:623–33.
16. Ward RM. Maternal drug therapy for fetal disorders. Semin Perinatol 1992;16:12–20.
17. Bigger JT, Hoffman BF. Antiarrhythmic drugs. In Gilman AG, Goodman LS, Gilman A eds. *The Pharmacological Basis of Therapeutics*. 6th ed. New York, NY: MacMillan, 1980:768.
18. Committee on Drugs, American Academy of Pediatrics. The transfer of drugs and other chemicals into human milk. Pediatrics 2001;108: 776–89.

Name: **QUININE** Risk Factor: **D***
Class: **Antimalarial**

FETAL RISK SUMMARY

RECOMMENDATION: Human Data Suggest Risk

Nishimura and Tanimura (1) summarized the human case reports of teratogenic effects linked with quinine in 21 infants who were exposed during the 1st trimester after unsuccessful abortion attempts (some infants had multiple defects and are listed more than once):

Central nervous system (CNS) anomalies (6 with hydrocephalus) (10 cases)
Limb defects (3 dysmelias) (8 cases)
Facial defects (7 cases)
Heart defects (6 cases)
Digestive organ anomalies (5 cases)
Urogenital anomalies (3 cases)
Hernias (3 cases)
Vertebral anomaly (1 case)

The malformations noted are varied, although CNS anomalies and limb defects were the most frequent. Auditory defects and optic nerve damage have also been reported (1–5). These reports usually concern the use of quinine in toxic doses as an abortifacient. Quinine has also been used for the induction of labor in women with intrauterine fetal death (6). Epidemiologic observations do not support an increased teratogenic risk or increased risk of congenital deafness over non-quinine-exposed patients (1,7). Neonatal and maternal thrombocytopenia purpura and hemolysis in glucose-6-phosphate dehydrogenase-deficient newborns has been reported (8,9).

In a surveillance study of Michigan Medicaid recipients conducted between 1985 and 1992 and involving 229,101 completed pregnancies, 35 newborns had been exposed to quinine during the 1st trimester (F. Rosa, personal communication, FDA, 1993). Two (5.7%) major birth defects were observed (one expected). No anomalies were observed in six defect categories (cardiovascular defects, oral clefts, spina bifida, polydactyly, limb reduction defects, and hypospadias) for which specific data were available.

Quinine has effectively been replaced by newer agents for the treatment of malaria. Although no increased teratogenic risk can be documented for therapeutic doses, its use during pregnancy should be avoided. One manufacturer considers the drug to be contraindicated in pregnancy (10). However, some investigators believe quinine should be used for the treatment of chloroquine-resistant *Plasmodium falciparum* malaria (11).

[**Risk Factor X according to the manufacturer, Merrell Dow, 1993.*]

BREAST FEEDING SUMMARY

RECOMMENDATION: Limited Human Data - Probably Compatible

Quinine is excreted into breast milk. Following 300- and 640-mg oral doses in six patients, the drug was detectable in milk up to 23 hours after a dose with concentrations ranging from trace to 2.2 μg/mL (12). No adverse effects were reported in the nursing infants. Patients at risk for glucose-6-phosphate dehydrogenase deficiency should not be breast-fed until this disease can be ruled out. The American Academy of Pediatrics classifies quinine as compatible with breast-feeding (13).

References

1. Nishimura H, Tanimura T. *Clinical Aspects of The Teratogenicity of Drugs*. New York, NY: American Elsevier, 1976:140–3.
2. Robinson GC, Brummitt JR, Miller JR. Hearing loss in infants and preschool children. II. Etiological considerations. Pediatrics 1963;32:115–24.
3. West RA. Effect of quinine upon auditory nerve. Am J Obstet Gynecol 1938;36:241–8.
4. McKinna AJ. Quinine induced hypoplasia of the optic nerve. Can J Ophthalmol 1966;1:261.
5. Morgon A, Charachon D, Brinquier N. Disorders of the auditory apparatus caused by embryopathy or foetopathy. Prophylaxis and treatment. Acta Otolaryngol (Stockh) 1971;291(Suppl):5.
6. Mukherjee S, Bhose LN. Induction of labor and abortion with quinine infusion in intrauterine fetal deaths. Am J Obstet Gynecol 1968;101:853–4.
7. Heinonen OP, Slone D, Shapiro S. *Birth Defects and Drugs in Pregnancy*. Littleton, MA: Publishing Sciences Group, 1977:299, 302, 333.
8. Mauer MA, DeVaux W, Lahey ME. Neonatal and maternal thrombocytopenic purpura due to quinine. Pediatrics 1957;19:84–7.
9. Glass L, Rajegowda BK, Bowne E, Evans HE. Exposure to quinine and jaundice in a glucose-6-phosphate dehydrogenase-deficient newborn infant. Pediatrics 1973;82:734–5.
10. Product information. Quinamm. Merrell Dow, 1990.
11. Strang A, Lachman E, Pitsoe SB, Marszalek A, Philpott RH. Malaria in pregnancy with fatal complications: case report. Br J Obstet Gynaecol 1984;91: 399–403.
12. Terwilliger WG, Hatcher RA. The elimination of morphine and quinine in human milk. Surg Gynecol Obstet 1934;58:823–6.
13. Committee on Drugs, American Academy of Pediatrics. The transfer of drugs and other chemicals into human milk. Pediatrics 2001;108:776–89.

Name:	QUINUPRISTIN/DALFOPRISTIN	Risk Factor:	B_M
Class:	Antibiotic		

FETAL RISK SUMMARY

RECOMMENDATION: Compatible - Maternal Benefit >> Embryo/Fetal Risk

The semisynthetic pristinamycin derivatives quinupristin/dalfopristin are streptogramin antibacterial agents that are combined in a ratio of 30:70 (weight/weight). The antibacterial combination is indicated for the treatment of vancomycin-resistant *Enterococcus faecium*. It also is active against *Staphylococcus aureus* and *Streptococcus pyogenes*. Depending on the bacterium, the combination exhibits both bacteriostatic and bactericidal action. Although quinupristin and dalfopristin are the main active components circulating in the plasma, both agents are converted to several active metabolites (1).

In reproduction studies with rats, no adverse effects on fertility, or perinatal/postnatal development were observed with the combination at doses up to approximately 0.4 times the human dose based on body surface area (HD). In addition, no evidence of impaired fertility or fetal harm was observed in pregnant mice, rats, and rabbits at approximately 0.5, 2.5, and 0.5 times the HD, respectively (1). In four genetic toxicity assays, the results with the combination and the individual antibacterial agents were negative. In a fifth test (Chinese hamster ovary cell chromosome aberration assay), dalfopristin was associated with structural chromosome aberrations, but the combination and quinupristin were not (1).

It is not known whether quinupristin or dalfopristin cross the human placenta to the fetus. Quinupristin is a combination of three peptide macrolactones in which the main component (>88%) has a molecular weight of about 1022. Dalfopristin has a molecular weight of about 691 (1). It is possible, therefore, that both agents and/or their metabolites could cross to the fetus. However, in a study with rats, the combination did not cross the placenta in significant amounts (2). Other than the fact that the antibiotic was given on gestation day 17, specific data, such as the dosage and amount crossing the placenta, were not given in the study.

No reports describing the use of quinupristin/dalfopristin in human pregnancy have been located. The drug does not cause teratogenicity or embryo/fetal toxicity in experimental animals. However, in pregnant rats the antibiotic combination may not reach the embryo or fetus in significant amounts. Placental passage in humans has not been studied. Because the indication for the combination involves potentially life-threatening infections, the maternal benefit of therapy appears to far outweigh the unknown embryo or fetal risk.

BREAST FEEDING SUMMARY

RECOMMENDATION: No Human Data - Potential Toxicity

The use of quinupristin/dalfopristin during human lactation has not been reported. The combination is excreted in the milk of lactating rats (1,3). The relatively high molecular weights for the two components (about 1022 and 691, respectively), however, suggests that only small amounts, if any, will pass into human milk. A review published in 2000 concluded that quinupristin/dalfopristin was unlikely to pass into breast milk because of its molecular size and weakly acidic nature (4). However, if the antibiotic were present in milk, it could alter the bowel flora of a nursing infant. Because of the special indication for the antibiotic (vancomycin-resistant *E. faecium*) and the potential for the development of strains resistant to quinupristin/dalfopristin, breast-feeding is not recommended.

References

1. Product information. Synercid. Aventis Pharmaceuticals, 2002.
2. Bergeron M, Montay G. The pharmacokinetics of quinupristin/dalfopristin in laboratory animals and in humans. J Antimicrob Chemother 1997;39(Suppl A): 129–38.
3. Rubinstein E, Prokocimer P, Talbot GH. Safety and tolerability of quinupristin/dalfopristin: administration guidelines. J Antimicrob Chemother 1999;44(Topic A):37–46.
4. Chin KG, Mactal-Haaf C, McPherson CE III. Use of anti-infective agents during lactation: Part I – beta-lactam antibiotics, vancomycin, quinupristin-dalfopristin, and linezolid. J Hum Lact 2000;16:351–8.

Q

R

Name: **RABEPRAZOLE** Risk Factor: B_M
Class: **Gastrointestinal Agent (Antisecretory)**

FETAL RISK SUMMARY

RECOMMENDATION: No Human Data - Animal Data Suggest Low Risk

Rabeprazole is a proton pump inhibitor that blocks gastric acid secretion by a direct inhibitory effect on the gastric parietal cell (1). It is used for the treatment of duodenal ulcer, erosive or ulcerative gastroesophageal reflux disease (GERD), and the long-term treatment of pathologic hypersecretory conditions, such as Zollinger-Ellison syndrome.

Reproductive studies have been conducted in rats and rabbits at IV doses up to 13 and 8 times, respectively, the recommended human dose based on AUC (1). No evidence was found at these doses of impaired fertility or fetal harm. In male and female rats, rabeprazole caused gastric cell hyperplasia and, in female rats, gastric cell tumors, at all doses tested (1). In addition, positive results with the drug and its inactive metabolite were demonstrated in hamsters and mice with the *in vitro* Ames mutation assay and in some other mutagenicity tests (1).

It is not known if rabeprazole crosses the human placenta. The molecular weight (about 381 for the sodium salt) is low enough, however, that passage to the fetus should be expected. Another proton pump inhibitor, omeprazole, has a similar molecular weight and chemical structure and it is known to cross the human placenta (see Omeprazole).

No reports describing the use of rabeprazole during human pregnancy have been located. Human pregnancy experience with two other proton pump inhibitors (see Lansoprazole and Omeprazole) have not shown a causal relationship with congenital malformations. In some cases, for both agents, malformations may have been missed because of the design and size of the studies. The carcinogenic and mutagenic data are a potential concern, but the absence of follow-up studies prevents a risk assessment for exposed offspring. As with all drug therapy, avoidance of rabeprazole during pregnancy, especially during the 1st trimester, is the safest course. If rabeprazole is required or if inadvertent exposure does occur early in gestation, the known risk to the embryo/fetus for congenital defects, based on animal data for rabeprazole and the published experience with other proton pump inhibitors, appears to be low. Long-term follow-up of offspring exposed during gestation is warranted.

BREAST FEEDING SUMMARY

RECOMMENDATION: No Human Data - Potential Toxicity

No reports describing the use of rabeprazole during human lactation have been located. The drug is excreted into the milk of lactating rats (1). Moreover, the drug concentrated in rat milk, reaching levels 2–7 times concentrations found in the plasma. Decreased body weight gain of pups was observed when the drug was administered to rats in late gestation and during lactation at a dose 195 times the recommended human dose based on body surface area. The clinical significance of this in humans is unknown. The animal data and the relatively low molecular weight (about 381 for the sodium salt) suggests that rabeprazole will be excreted into human milk. Because of the mutagenicity shown in some animal tests, the carcinogenicity observed in female rats, and the potential for suppression of gastric acid secretion in the nursing infant, the use of rabeprazole during lactation should probably be avoided until clinical data are available.

Reference

1. Product information. Rabeprazole. Eisai, 2001.

Name:	**RAMIPRIL**	Risk Factor:	C_M*
Class:	**Antihypertensive**		

FETAL RISK SUMMARY

RECOMMENDATION: Human Data Suggest Risk in 2nd and 3rd Trimesters

Ramipril is an angiotensin-converting enzyme (ACE) inhibitor. Reproduction studies in rats, rabbits, and monkeys at doses 400, 2, and 400 times, respectively, the recommended human dose based on body surface area revealed no teratogenic effects (1).

No reports of the use of this agent in human pregnancy have been located, but this class of drugs should be used with caution, if at all, during gestation. Use of ACE inhibitors limited to the 1st trimester does not appear to present a significant risk to the fetus, but fetal exposure after this time has been associated with teratogenicity and severe toxicity in the fetus and newborn, including death. See Captopril or Enalapril for a summary of fetal and neonatal effects from these agents. If ramipril is used in pregnancy, healthcare professionals are encouraged to call the toll free number (800-670-6126) for information about patient enrollment in the Motherisk Study.

[**Risk Factor* D_M *if used in 2nd or 3rd trimesters.*]

BREAST FEEDING SUMMARY

RECOMMENDATION: No Human Data - Probably Compatible

No reports describing the use of ramipril during lactation have been located. The molecular weight (about 417) is low enough, however, that excretion into breast milk should be expected. Other ACE inhibitors are excreted into breast milk and the American Academy of Pediatrics classifies them as compatible with breast-feeding (see Captopril and Enalapril).

Reference

1. Product information. Altace. Monarch Pharmaceuticals, 2000.

Name: **RANITIDINE** Risk Factor: **B_M**

Class: **Gastrointestinal Agent (Antisecretory)**

FETAL RISK SUMMARY

RECOMMENDATION: Compatible

Ranitidine is a competitive, reversible inhibitor of histamine H_2-receptors used in treatment and maintenance of patients with duodenal or gastric ulcers, pathologic hypersecretory conditions such as Zollinger-Ellison syndrome, and gastroesophageal reflux disease (GERD).

Reproduction studies with ranitidine in rats and rabbits at doses up to 160 times the human dose have revealed no evidence of impaired fertility or fetal harm (1–3). In contrast to the controversy surrounding cimetidine, ranitidine apparently has no antiandrogenic activity in humans (4) or in animals (5,6) (see also Cimetidine).

Ranitidine crosses the placenta at term to produce mean fetal:maternal ratios after 50 mg IV and 150 mg orally of 0.9 and 0.38, respectively (7–9).

In a surveillance study of Michigan Medicaid recipients conducted between 1985 and 1992 involving 229,101 completed pregnancies, 516 newborns had been exposed to ranitidine during the 1st trimester (F. Rosa, personal communication, FDA, 1993). A total of 23 (4.5%) major birth defects were observed (22 expected). Specific data were available for six defect categories, including (observed/expected) 6/5 cardiovascular defects, 1/1 oral clefts, 1/0.5 spina bifida, 1/1 polydactyly, 0/1 limb reduction defects, and 1/1 hypospadias. These data do not support an association between the drug and congenital defects.

The drug has been used alone and in combination with antacids to prevent gastric acid aspiration (Mendelson's syndrome) before vaginal delivery or cesarean section (7–13). No effect was observed in the frequency and strength of uterine contractions, in fetal heart rate pattern, or in Apgar scores (7). Neonatal gastric acidity was not affected at 24 hours. No problems in the newborn attributable to ranitidine were reported in these studies.

Ranitidine has been studied for its effectiveness in alleviating the symptoms of gastroesophageal reflux (heartburn) during pregnancy (14–16). A twice-daily dosage regimen of ranitidine was effective for this indication (14–16), including in those cases resistant to antacids alone (16). Ranitidine was also effective in controlling acid secretion in pregnant women with Zollinger-Ellison syndrome (17).

A 1996 prospective cohort study compared the pregnancy outcomes of 178 women who were exposed during pregnancy to histamine H_2 blockers with 178 controls matched for maternal age, smoking, and heavy alcohol consumption (18). All of the women had contacted a Teratology Information Service concerning gestational exposure to H_2-receptor antagonists (subjects) or nonteratogenic or nonfetotoxic agents (controls). Among subjects (mean daily dose in parentheses), 71% took ranitidine (258 mg), 16% cimetidine (487 mg), 8% famotidine (32 mg), and 5% nizatidine (283 mg). There were no significant differences between the outcomes of subjects and controls in terms of live births, spontaneous and elective abortions, gestational age at delivery, delivery method, birth weight, infants small for gestational age, or major malformations. Among subjects, there were 3 birth defects (2.1%) among the 142 exposed to H_2 blockers in the 1st trimester: one each of atrial septal defect, ventricular septal defect, and tetralogy of Fallot. There were 5 birth defects (3.0%) among the 165 exposed anytime during pregnancy. For controls, the rates of defects were 3.5% (1st trimester) and 3.1% (anytime). There were also no differences between the groups in neonatal health problems and developmental milestones, but two children (one subject and one control) were diagnosed as developmentally delayed. The investigators concluded that 1st trimester exposure to histamine H_2 blockers did not represent a major teratogenic risk (18).

Data from the Swedish Medical Birth Registry were presented in 1998 (19). A total of 553 infants (6 sets of twins) were delivered from 547 women who had used acid-suppressing drugs early in pregnancy. A number of other pharmaceutical agents, identified only by drug category, were also used by these women. Seventeen infants with birth defects were identified (3.1%; 95% confidence interval [CI] 1.8–4.9) compared with the crude malformation rate of 3.9% in the Registry. The odds ration (OR) for a congenital malformation, stratified for birth year, maternal age, parity, and smoking was 0.72 (95% CI 0.41–1.24). The OR for malformations after proton pump blocker exposure was 0.91 (95% CI 0.45–1.84), compared with 0.46 (95% CI 0.17–1.20) for H_2-receptor antagonists (OR 0.86, 95% CI 0.33–2.23; $p = 0.13$). Of the 17 infants with birth defects, 10 had been exposed to proton pump blockers, 6 to H_2 antagonists, and 1 to both classes of drug. Ranitidine was the only acid-suppressing drug exposure for 156 infants. Twenty other offspring were exposed *in utero* to ranitidine combined either with famotidine (2 infants) or with omeprazole (18 infants). Six birth defects (3.8%) were observed in the group where ranitidine was the only acid-suppressing agent used. The defects were: cerebral arteriovenous malformation, unspecified cardiac defect, hydronephrosis, undescended testicle, hypospadias, and unstable hip. Hypospadias was observed in a newborn exposed to a combination of ranitidine and omeprazole (19).

Two databases, one from England and the other from Italy, were combined for a study published in 1999 that was designed to assess the incidence of congenital malformations in women who had received a prescription during the 1st trimester for an acid-suppressing drug (ranitidine, cimetidine, and omeprazole) (20). Nonexposed women were selected from the same databases to form a control group. Spontaneous abortions and elective abortions (except two cases for anomalies that were grouped with stillbirths) were excluded from the analysis. Stillbirths were defined as any pregnancy loss occurring at 28 weeks' gestation or later. Ranitidine was taken in 322 pregnancies, resulting in 330 live births (29 [8.8%] premature), 2 stillbirths, and 1 neonatal death. Twenty (6.1%) of the newborns had a congenital malformation (shown by system): central nervous system (spina bifida/hydrocephaly), craniofacial (cleft palate only; asymmetric skull/plagiocephaly; tongue tie), eye (Duane's eye syndrome), cardiac (septal defect; anomaly of cardiac valve), musculoskeletal (dysplastic hip/dislocation/clicking hip $N = 3$; syndactyly; sacral sinus), genital and urinary (undescended testes $N = 2$; congenital hydrocele/inguinal hernia $N = 2$; ovarian cyst), multiple (pyloric stenosis and talipes equinovarus), and two genetic anomalies (Hallermann-Streiff and Down's syndromes). In addition, two newborns were small for gestational age and nine had a small head circumference for gestational age. In comparison, the outcomes of 1547 nonexposed pregnancies included 1560 live births (115 [7.4%] premature), 15 stillbirths (includes 2 elective abortions for anomalies), and 10 neonatal deaths. Sixty-four (4.1%) of the newborns had malformations involving the following: central nervous system ($N = 2$), head/face ($N = 13$), eye ($N = 2$), heart ($N = 7$), muscle/skeletal ($N = 13$), genital/urinary ($N = 18$), gastrointestinal ($N = 2$), and those of polyformation ($N = 3$) or known genetic defects ($N = 4$). There were 21 newborns that were small for gestational age and 78 had a small head circumference for gestational age. The relative risk of malformation (adjusted for mother's age and prematurity) associated with ranitidine was 1.5 (95% CI 0.9–2.6), with cimetidine 1.3 (95% CI 0.7–2.6), and with omeprazole 0.9 (95% CI 0.4–2.4) (20).

In summary, the absence of teratogenicity or toxicity in animals and the available human pregnancy data indicate that ranitidine is not a major teratogen. Because it has no antiandrogenic activity in animals or nonpregnant humans, ranitidine may be a safer choice than cimetidine for chronic use during pregnancy. The antiandrogenic activity of cimetidine, however, has not been observed or studied following *in utero* exposure (see Cimetidine).

BREAST FEEDING SUMMARY

RECOMMENDATION: Limited Human Data - Probably Compatible

Following a single oral dose of 150 mg in six subjects, ranitidine milk concentrations increased with time, producing mean milk:plasma ratios at 2, 4, and 6 hours of 1.9, 2.8, and 6.7, respectively (21). The effect of these concentrations on the nursing infant is not known. Ranitidine decreases gastric acidity, but this effect has not been studied in nursing infants. However, cimetidine, an agent with similar activity, is classified as compatible during breast-feeding by the American Academy of Pediatrics (see Cimetidine).

References

1. Product information. Zantac. Glaxo Wellcome, 2000.
2. Higashida N, Kamada S, Sakanove M, Takeuchi M, Simpo K, Tanabe T. Teratogenicity studies in rats and rabbits. J Toxicol Sci 1983;8:101–50. As cited in Shepard TH. *Catalog of Teratogenic Agents*. 6th ed. Baltimore, MD: Johns Hopkins University Press, 1989:550.
3. Higashida N, Kamada S, Sakanove M, Takeuchi M, Simpo K, Tanabe T. Teratogenicity studies in rats and rabbits. J Toxicol Sci 1984;9:53–72. As cited in Shepard TH. *Catalog of Teratogenic Agents*. 6th ed. Baltimore, MD: Johns Hopkins University Press, 1989: 550.
4. Wang C, Wong KL, Lam KC, Lai CL. Ranitidine does not affect gonadal function in man. Br J Clin Pharmacol 1983;16:430–2.
5. Parker S, Udani M, Gavaler JS, Van Thiel DH. Pre- and neonatal exposure to cimetidine but not ranitidine adversely affects adult sexual functioning of male rats. Neurobehav Toxicol Teratol 1984;6:313–8.
6. Parker S, Schade RR, Pohl CR, Gavaler JS, Van Thiel DH. Prenatal and neonatal exposure of male rat pups to cimetidine but not ranitidine adversely affects subsequent adult sexual functioning. Gastroenterology 1984;86:675–80.
7. McAuley DM, Moore J, Dundee JW, McCaughey W. Preliminary report on the use of ranitidine as an antacid in obstetrics. Ir J Med Sci 1982;151:91–2.
8. McAuley DM, Moore J, McCaughey W, Donnelly BD, Dundee JW. Ranitidine as an antacid before elective caesarean section. Anaesthesia 1983;38:108–14.
9. McAuley DM, Moore J, Dundee JW, McCaughey W. Oral ranitidine in labour. Anaesthesia 1984;39:433–8.
10. Gillett GB, Watson JD, Langford RM. Prophylaxis against acid aspiration syndrome in obstetric practice. Anesthesiology 1984;60:525.
11. Mathews HML, Wilson CM, Thompson EM, Moore J. Combination treatment with ranitidine and sodium bicarbonate prior to obstetric anaesthesia. Anaesthesia 1986;41:1202–6.
12. Ikenoue T, Iito J, Matsuda Y, Hokanishi H. Effects of ranitidine on maternal gastric juice and neonates when administered prior to caesarean section. Aliment Pharmacol Ther 1991;5:315–8.
13. Rout CC, Rocke DA, Gouws E. Intravenous ranitidine reduces the risk of acid aspiration of gastric contents at emergency cesarean section. Anesth Analg 1993;76:156–61.
14. Larson J, Patatanian E, Miner P, Rayburn W, Robinson M. Double-blind, placebo controlled study of ranitidine (Zantac) for gastroesophageal reflux symptoms during pregnancy (abstract). Am J Obstet Gynecol 1997;176:S23.
15. Larson JD, Patatanian E, Miner PB Jr, Rayburn WF, Robinson MG. Double-blind, placebo-controlled study of ranitidine for gastroesophageal reflux symptoms during pregnancy. Obstet Gynecol 1997;90:83–7.
16. Rayburn W, Liles E, Christensen H, Robinson M. Antacids vs. antacids plus non-prescription ranitidine for heartburn during pregnancy. Int J Gynaecol Obstet 1999;66:35–7.
17. Stewart CA, Termanini B, Sutliff VE, Corleto VD, Weber HC, Gibril F, Jensen RT. Management of the Zollinger-Ellison syndrome in pregnancy. Am J Obstet Gynecol 1997;176:224–33.
18. Magee LA, Inocencion G, Kamboj L, Rosetti F, Koren G. Safety of first trimester exposure to histamine H_2 blockers. A prospective cohort study. Dig Dis Sci 1996;41:1145–9.
19. Kallen B. Delivery outcome after the use of acid-suppressing drugs in early pregnancy with special reference to omeprazole. Br J Obstet Gynaecol 1998;105:877–81.
20. Ruigomez A, Rodriguez LAG, Cattaruzzi C, Troncon MG, Agostinis L, Wallander MA, Johansson S. Use of cimetidine, omeprazole, and ranitidine in pregnant women and pregnancy outcomes. Am J Epidemiol 1999;150:476–81.
21. Riley AJ, Crowley P, Harrison C. Transfer of ranitidine to biological fluids: milk and semen. In Misiewicz JJ, Wormsley KG, eds. *Proceedings of the 2nd International Symposium on Ranitidine*. London. Oxford, UK: Medicine Publishing Foundation, 1981:78–81.

R

Name: **REMIFENTANIL** Risk Factor: **C_M***

Class: **Narcotic Agonist Analgesic**

FETAL RISK SUMMARY

RECOMMENDATION: Human Data Suggest Risk in 3rd Trimester

Remifentanil is a rapid-onset, short-acting, synthetic μ-opioid agonist analgesic that is administered intravenously, in combination with other agents, for the induction and maintenance of general anesthesia. The elimination half-life is approximately 3 to 10 minutes. Because remifentanil is extensively metabolized by nonspecific esterases, not plasma cholinesterase (pseudocholinesterase), a normal duration of action is expected in patients with atypical cholinesterase. Furthermore, remifentanil is not appreciably metabolized by the liver or lung (1), as are other opioid analgesics.

Fertility studies in male and female rats were conducted with IV doses 40 and 80 times, respectively, the maximum recommended human dose based on body surface area (MRHD) (1). Reduced fertility was observed in male rats when the dose was administered daily for more than 70 days. In contrast, no effect was observed on the fertility of female rats dosed daily for at least 15 days before mating. Reproduction studies conducted in pregnant rats and rabbits at doses up to 400 and 125 times, respectively, the MRHD revealed no evidence of teratogenicity (1). The timing of the exposures was not specified. When remifentanil was given to rats throughout late gestation and lactation at a dose about 400 times the MRHD, no significant effect on the survival, development, or reproductive performance was observed in the exposed offspring (1).

Placental transfer to the fetus has been demonstrated in pregnant animals (rats and rabbits) and humans (1–3). This is consistent with its relatively low molecular weight (about 413) and high lipid solubility. The manufacturer reported that in human clinical trials, the average maternal concentration was approximately twice the levels observed in the fetus (1). However, in some cases, the maternal:fetal ratios were similar. The umbilical artery:umbilical vein (UA:UV) ratio, however, was approximately 0.30 suggesting metabolism of the drug in the neonate (1).

In an abstract (2) and a full report (3), information was presented on the placental transfer of remifentanil in 16 healthy women who were delivered by nonemergent cesarean section. Anesthesia appropriate for cesarean section was established with a lidocaine/epinephrine epidural before starting an IV infusion of remifentanil (0.1 μg/kg/minute) that was continued until skin closure. The mean umbilical vein:maternal artery (UV:MA) and UA:UV ratios for remifentanil were 0.88 and 0.29, respectively (3). For remifentanil acid, the inactive primary metabolite, the mean UV:MA and UA:UV ratios were 0.56 and 1.23, respectively (3). These results suggested to the investigators that the narcotic rapidly crossed the placenta and was metabolized and redistributed in the fetus. The mean Apgar scores (ranges) at 1, 5, 10, and 20 minutes were 8 (4–9), 9 (8–9), 9 (9–10), and 9 (9–10), respectively. Neurobehavioral and Adaptive Capacity Scores noted at 30 and 60 minutes were 37 (range 35–39) and 35 (range 34–39), respectively, all within normal limits. Although there were no adverse effects in the newborns, sedative and respiratory depressant effects were noted in the mothers (3).

A 1998 report described the case of a woman at term with mixed mitral valve disease, marked obesity, asthma and preeclampsia who was delivered by an emergency cesarean section under general anesthesia, after receiving a bupivacaine/fentanyl epidural (4).

Rapid-sequence induction was conducted with remifentanil (2 μg/kg), etomidate (20 mg), and succinylcholine (100 mg). A male infant (birth weight not given) was delivered 3 minutes after induction of anesthesia. The Apgar scores were 6, 8, and 8 at 1, 5, and 10 minutes, respectively. No signs of respiratory depression were observed (4).

A 30-year-old woman was delivered by cesarean section at 36 weeks' gestation because of the need for surgical resection of a right acoustic neuroma (5). Remifentanil (0.1–0.2 μg/kg/minute) was infused for induction of general anesthesia followed by propofol and succinylcholine. A healthy 2,970-g female infant was delivered 7 minutes after the start of remifentanil. Apgar scores were 7 and 8 at 1 and 5 minutes, respectively. Although there were no clinical signs of respiratory distress, her initial room air oxygen saturation was 85%–91% and she was placed in a 40% oxygen tent for 1 hour. She was discharged home at 3 days of age (5).

A 23-year-old woman at 37 weeks' gestation whose condition was complicated by a recurrent aortic coarctation with 50% narrowing of the aortic arch was delivered by an elective cesarean section (6). Remifentanil infusion up to 0.2 μg/kg/minute was combined with etomidate, succinylcholine, and isoflurane. Delivery took place 7 minutes after induction of anesthesia. The newborn (sex and weight not specified) had Apgar scores of 6 and 9 at 1 and 5 minutes, respectively. The infant did well after birth with no need for naloxone or evidence of respiratory distress (6).

Three studies have been located that describe the use of remifentanil for labor pain (7–9). In one study, four laboring women with singleton term pregnancies were treated with remifentanil either from a patient-controlled analgesia (PCA) pump (0.25 μg/kg, 5-minute lockout duration) or with IV bolus doses (0.25–0.50 μg/kg every 2 minutes as needed) (7). Failure of the pain to respond to increased doses and adverse effects (sedation, oxygen desaturation episodes, respiratory depression, nausea and vomiting, and pruritus) resulted in removal of the patients from the study. Healthy newborns (sex and weight not specified) were delivered 4 to 6 hours after discontinuance of remifentanil. All had Apgar scores of 9 or 10 (7). A study published in 2000 described two women in labor who were treated with remifentanil administered by a PCA pump (8). The on-demand dose was 20 μg with a 3-minute lockout duration (no basal infusion). The total doses administered during labor were 740 and 940 μg. No adverse effects attributable to the analgesic were observed in the newborns. The effects of remifentanil PCA on 42 laboring women were described in a 2001 abstract (9). The technique used was thought to be safe for the mother and newborn (9).

A study published in 1999 concluded that remifentanil-based general anesthesia (combined with propofol or isoflurane but without nitrous oxide) was a suitable alternative to sedation (induced by midazolam, diazepam, or propofol) for oocyte retrieval in an *in vitro* fertilization program (10). In a comparison between the general anesthesia and sedation groups, no significant differences were observed in the number of fertilized oocytes, or in the cleavage and pregnancy rates. However, the number of collected oocytes was significantly higher in the general anesthesia group (10).

In summary, remifentanil was not teratogenic or toxic in animals, but the absence of reports in early gestation prevents an assessment of its risk to the human fetus. However, narcotic analgesics are not considered to be human teratogens. Neonatal respiratory depression and sedation immediately after birth are potential complications of all narcotics when administered to a woman during labor. The short duration of remifentanil and its apparent rapid metabolism by the fetus may lessen these potential effects, but additional studies are needed to demonstrate this benefit.

[**Risk Factor D if used for prolonged periods or in high doses at term.*]

BREAST FEEDING SUMMARY

RECOMMENDATION: No Human Data - Probably Compatible

No reports describing the use of remifentanil in a lactating woman have been located. The agent is excreted into the milk of lactating rats (1). The relatively low molecular weight (about 413) and high lipid solubility suggest that it will also be excreted into human milk. Other narcotic agents (e.g., codeine, fentanyl, and morphine) are excreted into human breast milk but are classified as compatible with breast-feeding by the American Academy of Pediatrics (see specific agents). The very short elimination time suggests that use of remifentanil during cesarean section or other surgery would not represent a significant risk to a newborn that started or continued breast-feeding a few hours later.

References

1. Product information. Ultiva. Abbott Laboratories, 2001.
2. Hughes SC, Kan RE, Rosen MA, Kessin C, Preston PG, Lobo EP, Johnson LR, Johnson JL. Remifentanil: ultra-short acting opioid for obstetric anesthesia (abstract). Anesthesiology 1996;85:A894.
3. Kan RE, Hughes SC, Rosen MA, Kessin C, Preston PG, Lobo EP. Intravenous remifentanil. Placental transfer, maternal and neonatal effects. Anesthesiology 1998;88:1467–74.
4. Scott H, Bateman C, Price M. The use of remifentanil in general anaesthesia for Caesarean section in a patient with mitral value disease. Anaesthesia 1998;53:691–701.
5. Bedard JM, Richardson MG, Wissler RN. General anesthesia with remifentanil for Cesarean section in a parturient with an acoustic neuroma. Can J Anesth 1999;46:576–80.
6. Manullang TR, Chun K, Egan TD. The use of remifentanil for Cesarean section in a parturient with recurrent aortic coarctation. Can J Anesth 2000;47:454–9.
7. Olufolabi AJ, Booth JV, Wakeling HG, Glass PS, Penning DH, Reynolds JD. A preliminary investigation of remifentanil as a labor analgesic. Anesth Analg 2000;91:606–8.
8. Thurlow JA, Waterhouse P. Patient-controlled analgesia in labour using remifentanil in two parturients with platelet abnormalities. Br J Anaesth 2000;84:411–3.
9. Evron S, Sadan O, Ezri T, Boaz M, Glezerman M. Remifentanil: a new systemic analgesic for labor pain and an alternative to dolestine (abstract). Am J Obstet Gynecol 2001;185:S210.
10. Hammadeh ME, Wilhelm W, Huppert A, Rosenbaum P, Schmidt W. Effects of general anaesthesia vs. sedation on fertilization, cleavage and pregnancy rates in an IVF program. Arch Gynecol Obstet 1999;263:56–59.

Name:	**REPAGLINIDE**	Risk Factor:	**C_M**
Class:	**Oral Hypoglycemic**		

FETAL RISK SUMMARY

RECOMMENDATION: No Human Data - Animal Data Suggest Moderate Risk

Repaglinide is a nonsulfonylurea oral hypoglycemic agent (meglitinide class) that is used, either alone or in combination with metformin, as an adjunct to diet and exercise in the management of type II diabetes (non-insulin dependent diabetes mellitus). It is an insulin secretagogue. After absorption from the gastrointestinal tract, repaglinide is rapidly metabolized to inactive metabolites.

In animal reproduction studies, repaglinide was not teratogenic in rats and rabbits at doses 40 and 0.8 times the human clinical exposure based on a body surface area (HCE), respectively (1). However, offspring of rat dams given doses 15 times the HCE in the latter part of gestation and during lactation developed skeletal deformities consisting of shortening, thickening, and bending of the humerus during the postnatal period. The no-effect doses were 2.5 times the HCE given throughout pregnancy (through day 22) or higher doses given through gestational day 16 (1). A study published in 2000 found effects similar to those above in pregnant rats (2). Because the toxic effects on long bone development were only observed after organogenesis and only with high doses, the investigators concluded that the toxicity was limited to effects on growth and that repaglinide was not teratogenic (2).

It is not known if repaglinide crosses the human placenta. The molecular weight (about 453) is low enough, however, that transfer to the fetus should be expected.

No reports describing the use of repaglinide during human pregnancy have been located. Insulin is the treatment of choice for pregnant diabetic patients because, in general, other hypoglycemic agents do not provide adequate glycemic control. Moreover, insulin, unlike most oral agents, does not cross the placenta to the fetus, thus eliminating the additional concern that the drug therapy itself will adversely effect the fetus. Carefully prescribed insulin therapy provides better control of the mother's glucose, thereby preventing the fetal and neonatal complications that occur with this disease. High maternal glucose levels, as may occur in diabetes mellitus, are closely associated with a number of maternal and fetal adverse effects, including fetal structural anomalies if the hyperglycemia occurs early in gestation. To prevent this toxicity, most experts, including the American College of Obstetricians and Gynecologists, recommend that insulin be used for types I and II diabetes occurring during pregnancy and, if diet therapy alone is not successful, for gestational diabetes (3,4).

BREAST FEEDING SUMMARY

RECOMMENDATION: No Human Data - Potential Toxicity

No reports describing the use of repaglinide during human lactation have been located. The molecular weight (about 453) is low enough that excretion into breast milk should be expected. Consistent with the relatively low molecular weight, repaglinide was detected in the milk of lactating rats (1). Skeletal deformities (see above) were produced in nursing pups that had not been exposed to the drug during gestation (1,2). Because of the unknown potentials for this toxicity and hypoglycemia in a nursing infant, repaglinide should not be used during breast-feeding (5).

References

1. Product information. Prandin. Novo Nordisk Pharmaceuticals, 2000.
2. Viertel B, Guttner J. Effects of the oral antidiabetic repaglinide on the reproduction of rats. Arzneimittelforschung 2000;50:425–40.
3. American College of Obstetricians and Gynecologists. Diabetes and pregnancy. *Technical Bulletin*. No. 200, December 1994.
4. Coustan DR. Management of gestational diabetes, Clin Obstet Gynecol 1991;34:558–64.
5. Guay DRP. Repaglinide, a novel, short-acting hypoglycemic agent for type 2 diabetes mellitus. Pharmacotherapy 1998;18:1195–1204.

Name:	**RESERPINE**	Risk Factor:	**C_M**
Class:	**Antihypertensive**		

FETAL RISK SUMMARY

RECOMMENDATION: Limited Human Data - No Relevant Animal Data

The Collaborative Perinatal Project monitored 50,282 mother-child pairs, 48 of whom had 1st trimester exposure to reserpine (1, p. 376). There were four defects with 1st trimester use. Although this incidence (8%) is greater than the expected frequency of occurrence, no major category or individual malformations were identified. For use anytime in pregnancy, 475 exposures were recorded (1, p. 441). Malformations included the following: microcephaly (7 cases), hydronephrosis (3 cases), hydroureter (3 cases), and inguinal hernia (12 cases) (1, p. 495).

Reserpine crosses the placenta. Use of reserpine near term has resulted in nasal discharge, retraction, lethargy, and anorexia in the newborn (2). Concern over the ability of reserpine to deplete catecholamine levels has appeared (3). The significance of this is not known.

In a surveillance study of Michigan Medicaid recipients conducted between 1985 and 1992 involving 229,101 completed pregnancies, 15 newborns had been exposed to reserpine during the 1st trimester (F. Rosa, personal communication, FDA, 1993). No major birth defects were observed (one expected).

BREAST FEEDING SUMMARY

RECOMMENDATION: Limited Human Data - Probably Compatible

Reserpine is excreted into breast milk (4). No clinical reports of adverse effects in the nursing infant have been located.

References

1. Heinonen OP, Slone D, Shapiro S. *Birth Defects and Drugs in Pregnancy*. Littleton, MA: Publishing Sciences Group, 1977.
2. Budnick IS, Leikin S, Hoeck LE. Effect in the newborn infant to reserpine administration ante partum. Am J Dis Child 1955;90:286–9.
3. Towell ME, Hyman AI. Catecholamine depletion in pregnancy. J Obstet Gynaecol Br Commonw 1966;73:431–8.
4. Product information. Serpasil. Ciba Pharmaceutical, 1993.

Name: **RETEPLASE** Risk Factor: C_M

Class: **Thrombolytic**

FETAL RISK SUMMARY

RECOMMENDATION: Compatible - Maternal Benefit >> Embryo/Fetal Risk

The enzyme reteplase is a nonglycosylated deletion mutein of tissue-plasminogen activator (tPA; see also Alteplase and Tenecteplase) produced by recombinant technology in *Escherichia coli*. It contains 355 of the 527 amino acids of natural human tPA. Reteplase is indicated for use in the management of acute myocardial infarction for the improvement of ventricular function, the reduction in the incidence of congestive heart failure, and the reduction of mortality. The effective half-life of reteplase is 13–16 minutes, based on the measurement of thrombolytic activity (1).

Reproduction studies have been conducted in rats and rabbits. In rats, doses up to 15 times the human dose (HD) (based on weight) revealed no evidence of impaired fertility or teratogenicity. In rabbits, a dose 3 times the HD administered in mid-gestation resulted in genital bleeding and abortions (1).

It is not known if reteplase crosses the human placenta. The molecular weight (39,571) and very short effective half-life suggest that the protein does not cross to the embryo or fetus.

No reports describing the use of reteplase in human pregnancy have been located. Bleeding appears to be the major risk in animals and humans. Pregnancy may increase this risk (1). However, if indicated, the maternal benefit probably outweighs the potential risk to the embryo or fetus.

BREAST FEEDING SUMMARY

RECOMMENDATION: No Human Data - Probably Compatible

No reports describing the use of reteplase during human lactation have been located. However, the indication for reteplase suggests that such reports will not be forthcoming. In addition, the molecular weight (39,571) and very short effective half-life (13–16 minutes) suggest that the protein will not be excreted in clinically significant amounts into breast milk. Therefore, breast-feeding should be initiated or resumed based on the mother's condition and not the drug therapy.

Reference

1. Product information. Retavase. Centocor, 2004.

Name:	**REVIPARIN**	Risk Factor:	**B**
Class:	**Anticoagulant**		

FETAL RISK SUMMARY

RECOMMENDATION: Compatible

Reviparin is a low-molecular-weight heparin prepared by depolymerization of heparin obtained from porcine intestinal mucosa (1). It is not available in the United States (see also Dalteparin and Enoxaparin). Reviparin has an average molecular weight of 3500–4500 (range 2000–8000) (1). Because this is a relatively large molecule, it probably does not cross the placenta and, thus, presents a low risk to the fetus.

An abstract published in 1997 described the use of reviparin and aspirin (100 mg/day) in 50 women with unexplained recurrent fetal loss and autoantibodies (2). Reviparin was administered either as 4900 units SC once daily or as 2800 units SC twice daily. The once daily injection produced comparable plasma anti-factor Xa levels to the twice daily regimen. No maternal bleeding, thrombocytopenia, or decreased bone density was noted and no placental pathology was found in the 43 women who had completed their pregnancies (7 pregnancies were still in progress). The outcomes of the 43 completed pregnancies were 35 normal newborns (no premature deliveries), 7 spontaneous abortions, and 1 ectopic pregnancy. No congenital malformations or low-birth-weight newborns were observed.

BREAST FEEDING SUMMARY

RECOMMENDATION: No Human Data - Probably Compatible

No reports describing the use of reviparin during human lactation have been located. Reviparin, a low-molecular-weight heparin, still has a relatively high molecular weight (average 3500–4500) and, as such, should not be expected to be excreted into human milk. Because reviparin would be inactivated in the gastrointestinal tract, the risk to a nursing infant from ingesting the drug is probably nil.

References

1. Reynold JEF, ed. *Martindale. The Extra Pharmacopoeia.* 30th ed. London, UK: The Pharmaceutical Press, 1993:232.
2. Laskin C, Ginsberg J, Farine D, Crowther M, Spitzer K, Soloninka C, Ryan G, Seaward G, Ritchie K. Low molecular weight heparin and ASA therapy in women with autoantibodies and unexplained recurrent fetal loss (U-RFL). Society of Perinatal Obstetricians abstracts. Am J Obstet Gynecol 1997;176:S125.

Name:	**RIBAVIRIN**	Risk Factor:	X_M
Class:	**Antiviral**		

FETAL RISK SUMMARY

RECOMMENDATION: Contraindicated

Ribavirin is available in oral, IV, and inhalation formulations. It has demonstrated dose-related teratogenicity or embryo lethality at doses well below the recommended human dose in all animal species tested (1–3). Malformations observed in the offspring of hamsters, rats, and rabbits included defects of the skull, palate, eye, jaw, limbs, skeleton, and gastrointestinal tract. The manufacturers of oral ribavirin warn that the drug should not be used by men with female partners of reproductive age unless effective contraception (two reliable forms) is used or if their female partner is pregnant (2,3). Effective contraception should be continued for 6 months after ribavirin therapy has been stopped.

A 34-year-old woman, at 33 weeks' gestation, was treated with ribavirin inhalation therapy for influenza pneumonia complicated by respiratory failure (4). Shortly after treatment, a cesarean section was performed because of worsening maternal cardiopulmonary function. A normal female infant was delivered, who was alive and well at 1 year of age (4).

In 1988, the Centers for Disease Control and Prevention stated the use of ribavirin during pregnancy is contraindicated (5). In a statement addressing the issue of inhaled ribavirin exposure among health care personnel, the CDC commented: "... health-care workers who are pregnant, or may become pregnant should be advised of the potential risks of exposure during direct patient care when patients are receiving ribavirin through oxygen tent or mist mask and should be counseled about risk-reduction strategies, including alternative job responsibilities" (5).

In 13 pregnant or postpartum women hospitalized because of measles, 10 were treated for pneumonitis and/or severe disease in the 2nd or 3rd trimesters with ribavirin aerosol therapy (6). One woman was treated for 5 days before an elective abortion for worsening pulmonary status at 21 weeks' gestation. The remaining nine women had normal newborns with Apgar scores of 7–9 and 8–10 at 1 and 5 minutes, respectively (6).

A 2001 case report described two men with chronic hepatitis C who were treated with a combination of ribavirin (800 and 1200 mg/day) and interferon alfa-2a (6 million units every other day) (7). After about 5 months of therapy, their wife's became pregnant and both delivered healthy infants at term. The infants were developing normally at 4 months of age (7).

A 2003 review summarized the developmental toxicity of ribavirin and interferon alfa-2b, a combination used for the treatment of hepatitis C (8). The authors lamented the lack of reported human pregnancy experience and the possibility that the labels overstated the risks of men passing a potentially toxic amount of ribavirin in their sperm to a pregnant woman. A brief case report in the same journal described a pregnancy outcome in which the father was treated with interferon alfa-2b (3 million units three times/week) and ribavirin (1000 mg/day) for 4 weeks before the last menstrual cycle and continued during pregnancy (9). A 3380-g, healthy male infant was delivered at term with no evidence of malformations. The authors noted the lack of information relating the amount of ribavirin in sperm and the lack of experimental or clinical evidence for birth defects after paternal exposure (9).

BREAST FEEDING SUMMARY

RECOMMENDATION: No Human Data - Potential Toxicity

No data are available.

References

1. Product information. Virazole. ICN Pharmaceuticals, 2000.
2. Product information. Copegus. Roche Laboratories, 2004.
3. Product information. Rebetol. Schering, 2004.
4. Kirshon B, Faro S, Zurawin RK, Samo TC, Carpenter RJ. Favorable outcome after treatment with amantadine and ribavirin in a pregnancy complicated by influenza pneumonia: a case report. J Reprod Med 1988;33:399–401.
5. CDC. Assessing exposures of health-care personnel to aerosols of ribavirin-California. MMWR 1988;37:560–3.
6. Atmar RL, Englund JA, Hammill H. Complications of measles during pregnancy. Clin Infect Dis 1992;14:217–26.
7. Hegenbarth K, Maurer U, Kroisel PM, Fickert P, Trauner M, Stauber RE. No evidence for mutagenic effects of ribavirin: report of two normal pregnancies. Am J Gastroenterol 2001;96:2286–7.
8. Polifka JE, Friedman JM. Developmental toxicity of ribarvirin/IFα combination therapy: is the label more dangerous than the drugs? Birth Defects Res Part A Clin Mol Teratol 2003;67:8–12.
9. Biana S, Ettore G. Male periconceptional ribavirin–interferon alpha-2B exposure with no adverse fetal effects. Birth Defects Res Part A Clin Mol Teratol 2003;67:77–8.

Name:	**RIBOFLAVIN**	Risk Factor:	**A***
Class:	**Vitamin**		

FETAL RISK SUMMARY

RECOMMENDATION: Compatible

Riboflavin (vitamin B_2), a water-soluble B complex vitamin, acts as a coenzyme in humans and is essential for tissue respiration systems (1). The National Academy of Sciences' recommended dietary allowance (RDA) for riboflavin in pregnancy is 1.6 mg (1).

The vitamin is actively transferred to the fetus, resulting in higher concentrations of riboflavin in the newborn than in the mother (2–12). The placenta converts flavin-adenine dinucleotide existing in the maternal serum to free riboflavin found in the fetal circulation (5,6). This allows retention of the vitamin by the fetus, because the transfer of free riboflavin back to the mother is inhibited (6,12). At term, mean riboflavin values in 174 mothers were 184 ng/mL (range 80–390 ng/mL) and in their newborns 318 ng/mL (range 136–665 ng/mL) (7). In a more recent study, the cord serum concentration was 158 nmol/L compared with 113 nmol/L in the maternal serum (11).

The incidence of riboflavin deficiency in pregnancy is low (7,13). In two studies, no correlation was discovered between the riboflavin status of the mother and the outcome of pregnancy even when riboflavin deficiency was present (14,15). A 1977 study found no difference in riboflavin levels between infants of low and normal birth weight (10).

Riboflavin deficiency is teratogenic in animals (16). Although human teratogenicity has not been reported, low riboflavin levels were found in six mothers who had given birth to infants with neural tube defects (17). Other vitamin deficiencies present in these women were thought to be of more significance (see Folic Acid and Vitamin B_{12}).

A mother has been described with multiple acylcoenzyme A dehydrogenase deficiency probably related to riboflavin metabolism (18). The mother had given birth to a healthy child followed by one stillbirth and six infants who had been breast-fed and died in early infancy after exhibiting a strong sweaty foot odor. In her 9th and 10th pregnancies, she was treated with 20 mg/day of riboflavin during the 3rd trimesters and delivered healthy infants. The authors thought the maternal symptoms were consistent with a mild form of acute fatty liver of pregnancy.

[**Risk Factor C if used in doses above the RDA.*]

BREAST FEEDING SUMMARY

RECOMMENDATION: Compatible

Riboflavin (vitamin B_2) is excreted into breast milk (19–23). Well-nourished lactating women were given supplements of a multivitamin preparation containing 2.0 mg of riboflavin (19). At 6 months postpartum, milk concentrations of riboflavin did not differ significantly from those in control patients not receiving supplements. In a study of lactating women with low nutritional status, supplementation with riboflavin in doses of 0.10–10.0 mg/day resulted in mean milk concentrations of 200–740 ng/mL (20). Milk concentrations were directly proportional to dietary intake. A 1983 English study measured riboflavin levels in pooled human milk obtained from preterm (26 mothers: 29–34 weeks) and term (35 mothers: 39 weeks or longer) patients (21). Milk obtained from preterm mothers rose from 276 ng/mL (colostrum) to 360 ng/mL (6–15 days) and then fell to 266 ng/mL (16–196 days). During approximately the same time frame, milk levels from term mothers were 288, 279, and 310 ng/mL. In a Finnish study, premature infants (mean gestational age 30.1 weeks) fed human milk, but without riboflavin supplementation, became riboflavin deficient by 6 weeks of age (24).

The National Academy of Sciences' RDA for riboflavin during lactation is 1.8 mg (1). If the diet of the lactating woman adequately supplies this amount, supplementation with riboflavin is not needed (22). Maternal supplementation with the RDA for riboflavin is recommended for those women with inadequate nutritional intake. The American Academy of Pediatrics classifies riboflavin as compatible with breast-feeding (25).

References

1. American Hospital Formulary Service. *Drug Information 1997*. Bethesda, MD: American Society of Health-System Pharmacists, 1997:2817–8.
2. Hill EP, Longo LD. Dynamics of maternal-fetal nutrient transfer. Fed Proc 1980;39:239–44.
3. Lust JE, Hagerman DD, Villee CA. The transport of riboflavin by human placenta. J Clin Invest 1954;33:38–40.
4. Frank O, Walbroehl G, Thomason A, Kaminetzky H, Kubes Z, Baker H. Placental transfer: fetal retention of some vitamins. Am J Clin Nutr 1970;23:662–3.
5. Kaminetzky HA, Baker H, Frank O, Langer A. The effects of intravenously administered water-soluble vitamins during labor in normovitaminemic and hypovitaminemic gravidas on maternal and neonatal blood vitamin levels at delivery. Am J Obstet Gynecol 1974;120:697–703.

6. Kaminetzky HA, Baker H. Micronutrients in pregnancy. Clin Obstet Gynecol 1977;20:363–80.
7. Baker H, Frank O, Thomason AD, Langer A, Munves ED, De Angelis B, Kaminetzky HA. Vitamin profile of 174 mothers and newborns at parturition. Am J Clin Nutr 1975;28:59–65.
8. Baker H, Frank O, Deangelis B, Feingold S, Kaminetzky HA. Role of placenta in maternal-fetal vitamin transfer in humans. Am J Obstet Gynecol 1981;141: 792–6.
9. Bamji MS. Enzymic evaluation of thiamin, riboflavin and pyridoxine status of parturient women and their newborn infants. Br J Nutr 1976;35:259–65.
10. Baker H, Thind IS, Frank O, DeAngelis B, Caterini H, Lquria DB. Vitamin levels in low-birth-weight newborn infants and their mothers. Am J Obstet Gynecol 1977;129:521–4.
11. Kirshenbaum NW, Dancis J, Levitz M, Lehanka J, Young BK. Riboflavin concentration in maternal and cord blood in human pregnancy. Am J Obstet Gynecol 1987;157:748–52.
12. Dancis J, Lehanka J, Levitz M. Placental transport of riboflavin: differential rates of uptake at the maternal and fetal surfaces of the perfused human placenta. Am J Obstet Gynecol 1988;158:204–10.
13. Dostalova L. Correlation of the vitamin status between mother and newborn during delivery. Dev Pharmacol Ther 1982;4(Suppl 1):45–57.
14. Vir SC, Love AHG, Thompson W. Riboflavin status during pregnancy. Am J Clin Nutr 1981;34:2699–2705.
15. Heller S, Salkeld RM, Korner WF. Riboflavin status in pregnancy. Am J Clin Nutr 1974;27:1225 30.
16. Shepard TH. *Catalog of Teratogenic Agents*. 6th ed. Baltimore, MD: Johns Hopkins University Press, 1989:557–8.
17. Smithells RW, Sheppard S, Schorah CJ. Vitamin deficiencies and neural tube defects. Arch Dis Child 1976;51:944–50.
18. Harpey JP, Charpentier C. Acute fatty liver of pregnancy. Lancet 1983;1:586–7.
19. Thomas MR, Sneed SM, Wei C, Nail PA, Wilson M, Sprinkle EE III. The effects of vitamin C, vitamin B_6, vitamin B_{12}, folic acid, riboflavin, and thiamin on the breast milk and maternal status of well-nourished women at 6 months postpartum. Am J Clin Nutr 1980;33:2151–6.
20. Deodhar AD, Rajalakshmi R, Ramakrishnan CV. Studies on human lactation. Part III. Effect of dietary vitamin supplementation on vitamin contents of breast milk. Acta Paediatr Scand 1964;53:42–8.
21. Ford JE, Zechalko A, Murphy J, Brooke OG. Comparison of the B vitamin composition of milk from mothers of preterm and term babies. Arch Dis Child 1983;58:367–72.
22. Nail PA, Thomas MR, Eakin R. The effect of thiamin and riboflavin supplementation on the level of those vitamins in human breast milk and urine. Am J Clin Nutr 1980;33:198–204.
23. Gunther M. Diet and milk secretion in women. Proc Nutr Soc 1968;27:77–82.
24. Ronnholm KAR. Need for riboflavin supplementation in small prematures fed human milk. Am J Clin Nutr 1986;43:1–6.
25. Committee on Drugs, American Academy of Pediatrics. The transfer of drugs and other chemicals into human milk. Pediatrics 2001;108:776–89.

Name: **RIFABUTIN** Risk Factor: B_M

Class: **Antibiotic**

R

FETAL RISK SUMMARY

RECOMMENDATION: No Human Data - Animal Data Suggest Low Risk

Rifabutin is an oral semi-synthetic ansamycin antibiotic that is derived from rifamycin S. It is indicated for the prevention of disseminated *Mycobacterium avium* complex (MAC) (*note:* MAC includes *M. avium* and *M. intracellulare*) disease in patients with advanced human immunodeficiency virus (HIV) infection. Five metabolites have been identified, one of which is active (contributes up to 10% of the antimicrobial activity). Rifabutin is moderately (about 85%) bound to plasma proteins and has a mean terminal half-life of 45 hours (1).

Rifabutin was not carcinogenic in mice and rats at doses about 32 and 12 times, respectively, the recommended human daily dose based on body weight (RHDD). In addition, no mutagenicity was observed in several assays (1).

Reproduction tests have been conducted in rats and rabbits. In rats, doses up to 40 times the RHDD were not teratogenic, but the highest dose caused a decrease in fetal viability. At 8 times the RHDD, an increase in fetal skeletal variants was observed. In rabbits, no teratogenic effects were observed with doses up to 40 times the RHDD. A dose

16 times the RHDD was maternal toxic and resulted in an increase in fetal skeletal anomalies (1).

It is not known if rifabutin or its active metabolite crosses the human placenta. The molecular weight of the parent compound (about 847), moderate plasma protein binding, high lipid solubility, and prolonged terminal half-life suggest that passage to the embryo/fetus will occur.

Rifabutin induces the metabolism of ethinyl estradiol and norethindrone, thereby decreasing the efficacy of oral contraceptives (1). Therefore, additional, nonhormonal methods of birth control should be used during treatment with this antibiotic.

No reports describing the use of rifabutin in human pregnancy have been located. The animal data are suggestive of low risk, but the absence of human pregnancy experience prevents an assessment of the embryo/fetal risk. However, the maternal benefit appears to outweigh the unknown risk to the embryo or fetus, so therapy should not be withheld because of pregnancy.

BREAST FEEDING SUMMARY

RECOMMENDATION: No Human Data - Potential Toxicity
Contraindicated (Patients with HIV Infection)

No reports describing the use of rifabutin during human lactation have been located. The molecular weight (about 847), moderate plasma protein binding, and prolonged terminal half-life suggest that excretion into milk should be expected. Milk may be stained a brown-orange color. The effects of this exposure on a nursing infant are unknown but serious toxicity (e.g., leukopenia, neutropenia, rash, etc.) is a potential complication. Moreover, rifabutin is indicated for the prevention of disseminated *Mycobacterium avium* complex (MAC) in patients with advanced human immunodeficiency virus (HIV) infections and women with HIV should not breast-feed. Therefore, rifabutin is contraindicated in this patient population.

Reference

1. Product information. Mycobutin. Pharmacia & Upjohn, 2004.

R

Name:	**RIFAMPIN**	Risk Factor:	C_M
Class:	**Antituberculosis Agent**		

FETAL RISK SUMMARY

RECOMMENDATION: Compatible

Reproduction studies with rifampin in mice and rats at doses greater than 150 mg/kg produced spina bifida in both species and cleft palates in the mouse fetuses (1). Teratogenicity in rodents has been reported with oral doses 15 to 25 times the human dose (2). Studies with pregnant rabbits revealed no evidence of teratogenicity (1).

In a surveillance study of Michigan Medicaid recipients conducted between 1985 and 1992 involving 229,101 completed pregnancies, 20 newborns had been exposed to

rifampin during the 1st trimester (F. Rosa, personal communication, FDA, 1993). No major birth defects were observed (one expected).

No controlled studies have linked the use of rifampin with congenital defects (3,4). One report described nine malformations in 204 pregnancies that went to term (5). This incidence, 4.4%, is similar to the expected frequency of defects in a healthy nonexposed population but higher than the 1.8% rate noted in other tuberculosis patients (5): anencephaly (1 case), hydrocephalus (2 cases), limb malformations (4 cases), renal tract defects (1 case), and congenital hip dislocation (1 case).

Several reviews have evaluated the available treatment of tuberculosis during pregnancy (6–8). All concluded that rifampin was not a proven teratogen and recommended use of the drug with isoniazid and ethambutol if necessary. Other reports on the use of the agent in pregnancy have observed no fetal harm (9,10).

Rifampin crosses the placenta to the fetus (11–13). At term, the cord:maternal serum ratio ranged from 0.12–0.33 (12). In a second case involving pregnancy termination at 13 weeks' gestation, the fetal:maternal ratio 4 hours after a 300-mg dose was 0.23 (11).

Rifampin has been implicated as one of the agents responsible for hemorrhagic disease of the newborn (14). In one of the three infants affected, only laboratory evidence of hemorrhagic disease of the newborn was present, but in the other two, clinically evident bleeding was observed. Prophylactic vitamin K_1 is recommended to prevent this serious complication (see Phytonadione).

Rifampin may interfere with oral contraceptives, resulting in unplanned pregnancies (see Oral Contraceptives) (15).

BREAST FEEDING SUMMARY

RECOMMENDATION: Compatible

Rifampin is excreted into human milk. In one report, the concentrations were 1–3 μg/mL with about 0.05% of the daily dose appearing in the milk (16). In another study, milk levels were 3.4–4.9 μg/mL, 12 hours after a single 450-mg oral dose (17). Maternal plasma samples averaged 21.3 μg/mL, indicating a milk:plasma ratio of about 0.20. These amounts were thought to represent a very low risk to the nursing infant (18). No reports describing adverse effects in nursing infants have been located. The American Academy of Pediatrics classifies rifampin as compatible with breast-feeding (19).

References

1. Tuchmann-Duplessis H, Mercier-Parot L. Influence d'un antibiotique, la rifampicine, sur le developpement prenatal des ronguers. C R Acad Sci (d) (Paris) 1969;269:2147–9. As cited in Shepard TH. *Catalog of Teratogenic Agents*. 6th ed. Baltimore, MD: Johns Hopkins University Press, 1989:558–9.
2. Product information. Rifadin. Hoechst Marion Roussel, 2000.
3. Reimers D. Missbildungen durch Rifampicin. Bericht ueber 2 faelle von normaler fetaler entwicklung nach rifampicin-therapie in der fruehsch wangerschaft. Munchen Med Wochenschr 1971;113: 1690.
4. Warkany J. Antituberculous drugs. Teratology 1979;20:133–8.
5. Steen JSM, Stainton-Ellis DM. Rifampicin in pregnancy. Lancet 1977;2:604–5.
6. Snider DE, Layde PM, Johnson MW, Lyle MA. Treatment of tuberculosis during pregnancy. Am Rev Respir Dis 1980;122:65–79.
7. American Thoracic Society. Treatment of tuberculosis and tuberculosis infection in adults and children. Am Rev Respir Dis 1986;134:355–63.
8. Medchill MT, Gillum M. Diagnosis and management of tuberculosis during pregnancy. Obstet Gynecol Surv 1989;44:81–4.
9. Shneerson JM, Frances RS. Ethambutol in pregnancy: foetal exposure. Tubercle 1979;60:167–9.
10. Kingdon JCP, Kennedy DH. Tuberculosis meningitis in pregnancy. Br J Obstet Gynaecol 1989;96:233–5.

11. Rocker I. Rifampicin in early pregnancy. Lancet 1977;2:48.
12. Kenny MT, Strates B. Metabolism and pharmacokinetics of the antibiotic rifampin. Drug Metab Rev 1981;12:159–218.
13. Holdiness MR. Transplacental pharmacokinetics of the antituberculosis drugs. Clin Pharmacokinet 1987;13:125–9.
14. Eggermont E, Logghe N, Van De Casseye W, Casteels-Van Daele M, Jaeken J, Cosemans I, Verstraete M, Renaer M. Haemorrhagic disease of the newborn in the offspring of rifampicin and isoniazid treated mothers. Acta Paediatr Belg 1976;29:87–90.
15. Gupta KC, Ali MY. Failure of oral contraceptives with rifampicin. Med J Zambia 1980,15:23.
16. Vorherr H. Drug excretion in breast milk. Postgrad Med J 1974;56:97–104.
17. Lenzi E, Santuari S. Preliminary observations on the use of a new semi-synthetic rifamycin derivative in gynecology and obstetrics. Atti Accad Lancisiana Roma 1969;13(Suppl 1):87–94. As cited in Snider DE Jr, Powell KE. Should women taking antituberculosis drugs breast-feed? Arch Intern Med 1984;144:589–90.
18. Snider DE Jr, Powell KE. Should women taking antituberculosis drugs breast-feed? Arch Intern Med 1984;144:589–90.
19. Committee on Drugs, American Academy of Pediatrics. The transfer of drugs and other chemicals into human milk. Pediatrics 2001;108:776–89.

Name: **RIFAPENTINE** Risk Factor: **C_M**
Class: **Antituberculosis Agent**

FETAL RISK SUMMARY

RECOMMENDATION: Limited Human Data - Animal Data Suggest Risk

The antibiotic rifapentine is a semi-synthetic cyclopentyl derivative of rifamycin and has a similar profile of microbiological activity to rifampin. It is indicated for the treatment of pulmonary tuberculosis. The antibiotic inhibits DNA-dependent RNA polymerase in *Mycobacterium tuberculosis*, but this effect does not occur in mammalian cells. The elimination half-lives of rifapentine and its active metabolite are each about 13 hours (1).

Reproduction studies with rifapentine in rats and rabbits produced teratogenic and toxic effects in both species. In rats, doses 0.6 times the human dose based on body surface area (HD) administered during organogenesis resulted in cleft palates, right aortic arch, an increased incidence of delayed ossification, and an increased number of ribs. Embryo and fetal toxic effects included increases in resorption rates, postimplantation losses, and stillbirths, and decreased fetal weight. Administration of doses 0.3 times the HD from day 15 of gestation through postpartum day 21 was associated with decreased pup weights and stillbirths. Major anomalies observed in the offspring of pregnant rabbits administered doses 0.3 to 1.3 times the HD included ovarian agenesis, pes varus (i.e., *talipes varus*), arhinia, microphthalmia, and irregularities of the ossified facial tissues. When doses 1.3 times the HD were given, increased incidences of postimplantation losses and stillbirths were observed (1).

It is not known if rifapentine crosses the human placenta. However, the molecular weight (about 877) is low enough that exposure of the embryo and/or fetus probably occurs. In addition, the prolonged elimination half-lives of the parent compound and its active metabolite increase the opportunity for passage of the agents into the fetal compartment.

In a clinical study by the manufacturer, three women became pregnant while receiving rifapentine (600 mg twice weekly [combined with isoniazid, ethambutol, pyrazinamide, and pyridoxine]) and three became pregnant during follow-up (1,2). The first patient had a positive serum pregnancy test at baseline and subsequently received a single 600-mg dose of rifapentine before being dropped from the study. An elective abortion was conducted to terminate the pregnancy. The second patient, with a history of alcohol abuse, received 10 doses of rifapentine 600 mg over 42 days before exclusion from the study. She had a

R

1st trimester spontaneous abortion 9 days after the last dose. The third woman had an HIV infection as well as tuberculosis. She was treated over 85 days with 22 rifapentine 600-mg doses and had a 1st trimester spontaneous abortion 16 days after the last dose. The investigator concluded that the abortion was secondary to the HIV infection. The outcomes of the three pregnancies in the follow-up stage of the study, which were not thought to have been exposed to the drug during gestation, were two normal deliveries and one lost to follow-up (1,2).

When taken in the last few weeks of pregnancy, rifapentine may cause hemorrhage in both the mother and newborn secondary to vitamin K deficiency (1). This effect is similar to that observed with rifampin. Prophylactic vitamin K_1 is recommended to prevent hemorrhage. (See also Phytonadione.)

Rifapentine may increase the metabolism and reduce the activity of oral or other systemic hormonal contraceptives (1). Unplanned pregnancies may result from this interaction. Patients receiving rifapentine should be advised to change to nonhormonal methods of birth control (1).

In summary, rifapentine induces toxicity and teratogenicity in two experimental animal species at doses close to those used in humans. Human pregnancy experience is limited to three cases, two of which ended in 1st trimester spontaneous abortions. Although comorbid conditions were present and may have caused the losses, the outcomes are sufficiently concerning to warrant caution in prescribing rifapentine early in pregnancy. Until additional data are forthcoming, rifapentine is best avoided during the 1st trimester.

Because active untreated tuberculosis represents a greater risk to the fetus than does treatment, immediate initiation of drug therapy is usually recommended, regardless of the gestational stage (3–6). The Centers for Disease Control and Prevention (CDC) recommends a combination of isoniazid (plus pyridoxine), rifampin, and ethambutol as the treatment of choice for pulmonary tuberculosis during pregnancy and breastfeeding (5). An earlier statement by the World Health Organization recommended a 6-month regimen of isoniazid (plus pyridoxine), rifampin, and pyrazinamide as first-line treatment in pregnancy (6). Ethambutol was recommended if a fourth drug was needed during the initial phase. Although the CDC did not recommend pyrazinamide, it classified this agent as probably safe in pregnancy (5). Moreover, the CDC stated that if pyrazinamide was not included in the initial treatment regimen, the minimum duration of therapy should be 9 months (39 weeks) instead of 6 months (26 weeks). Significantly, the CDC did not recommend rifapentine in pregnancy because of insufficient information (5).

BREAST FEEDING SUMMARY

RECOMMENDATION: No Human Data - Probably Compatible

No reports describing the use of rifapentine during lactation have been located. The molecular weight of rifapentine (about 877) and the prolonged half-lives of the parent compound and the active metabolite (both about 13 hours) suggest that these agents will be excreted into milk. Breast milk may be discolored because rifapentine produces a red-orange discoloration of body fluids. The effects of this exposure, if any, on a nursing infant are unknown. Rifampin, a closely related antibiotic with a similar molecular weight (about 823), is excreted in low amounts into breast milk. The American Academy of Pediatrics classifies rifampin as compatible with breast-feeding (see Rifampin).

References

1. Product information. Priftin. Aventis Pharmaceuticals, 2004.
2. Center for Drug Evaluation and Research. Food and Drug Administration. Approval Package: Priftin (Rifapentine) 150 mg tablets. Hoechst Marion Roussel, June 22, 1998.
3. Medchill MT, Gillum M. Diagnosis and management of tuberculosis during pregnancy. Obstet Gynecol Surv 1989;44:81–4.
4. American Thoracic Society. Treatment of tuberculosis and tuberculosis infection in adults and children. Am J Respir Crit Care Med 1994;149:1359–74.
5. Centers for Disease Control and Prevention. Treatment of tuberculosis. MMWR 2003;52(RR11):1–77.
6. World Health Organization. *Treatment of Tuberculosis: Guidelines for National Programs*. 2nd ed. Geneva, Switzerland: World Health Organization, 1997.

Name:	**RIMANTADINE**	Risk Factor:	C_M
Class:	**Antiviral**		

FETAL RISK SUMMARY

RECOMMENDATION: No Human Data - Animal Data Suggest Moderate Risk

Rimantadine is a synthetic antiviral agent used in the prophylaxis and treatment of influenza A virus infections. In nonpregnant patients, rimantadine shares the toxic profile of a similar antiviral agent, amantadine, which is also used for influenza A virus infections (see Amantadine) (1). It is not known whether rimantadine crosses the human placenta to the fetus, but the relatively low molecular weight (about 216) probably ensures that transfer occurs.

Rimantadine was embryotoxic (increased fetal resorption) in rats at a dose 11 times the recommended human dose based on body surface area (RHD) (2). This dose also produced maternal toxicity. No embryotoxicity was observed in rabbits given up to 5 times the RHD, but a developmental abnormality was observed as evidenced by an increase in the ratio of fetuses with 12–13 ribs from the normal litter distribution of 50:50 to 80:20 (2).

No reports describing the use of rimantadine during human pregnancy have been located. In addition, as of late 1996, the FDA had not received any reports of pregnancy exposure to rimantadine (F. Rosa, personal communication, FDA, 1996). Although the lack of human data does not allow an assessment of fetal risk, the absence of significant animal teratogenicity may indicate that rimantadine is a safer agent during pregnancy than the closely related drug, amantadine.

BREAST FEEDING SUMMARY

RECOMMENDATION: No Human Data - Potential Toxicity

Rimantadine is concentrated in the milk of lactating rats with milk levels approximately twice those measured in the serum 2–3 hours after a dose (2). No reports have described the use of rimantadine during human lactation, but passage of the antiviral agent into human milk should be anticipated because of its relatively low molecular weight (about 216). Because of adverse effects noted in nursing rats whose mothers were given rimantadine, the manufacturer recommends the drug not be administered to nursing women (2).

References

1. Morris DJ. Adverse effects and drug interactions of clinical importance with antiviral drugs. Drug Saf 1994;10:281–91.
2. Product information. Flumadine. Forest Pharmaceuticals, 2000.

Name:	**RISPERIDONE**	Risk Factor:	C_M
Class:	**Antipsychotic**		

FETAL RISK SUMMARY

RECOMMENDATION: Limited Human Data - Animal Data Suggest Moderate Risk

Risperidone, a benzisoxazole derivative, is indicated in the management of the manifestations of psychotic disorders, such as schizophrenia (1). Although not approved for this indication by the U.S. Food and Drug Administration, it is also used for the management of bipolar disorder and in patients with dementia-related psychotic symptoms.

The mechanism of the antipsychotic action of risperidone is unknown, but may be due to a combination of dopamine type 2 and serotonin type 2 receptor antagonism. The antagonism of dopamine type 2 receptors may account for the hyperprolactinemia observed with risperidone. The drug also has high affinity for and antagonizes α_1- and α_2-adrenergic and H_1-histaminergic receptors. Risperidone is metabolized to an active metabolite, 9-hydroxyrisperidone that is equi-effective with the parent drug in terms of receptor binding activity (1).

Reproduction studies have been conducted in pregnant rats and rabbits (1). No increase in the incidence of congenital malformations was observed in either species at doses 0.4 to 6 times the human dose based on body surface area (HD). At 1.5 times the HD, however, an increase in stillbirths was noted in rats. In addition, increased pup mortality during the first 4 days of lactation occurred at 0.1 to 3 times the HD. There was no no-effect dose for this toxicity. It was not known if the deaths were the result of a direct effect on the pups or toxicity in the dams (1). Risperidone caused a dose-related decrease in serum testosterone in Beagle dogs, as well as a decrease in sperm motility and concentration, at doses 0.6 to 10 times the HD (1).

Risperidone crosses the rat placenta, but this has not been studied in humans. The molecular weight (about 410), however, is low enough that passage to the fetus should be expected.

The outcomes of 10 pregnancies involving 9 women were described in a large postmarketing study involving 7,684 patients treated with risperidone (2). The outcomes were three elective terminations and seven live births. No congenital malformations were reported among the live births. The manufacturer has also reported an unpublished case of agenesis of the corpus callosum in an infant exposed to risperidone during gestation (1). The relationship between the drug and the defect is unknown.

A 1997 review of antipsychotic use in pregnancy concluded that the safety of risperidone in human pregnancy had not been established (3). The reviewers commented that although no teratogenicity or direct toxicity had been shown in animal studies, some indirect, prolactin- and central nervous system (CNS)-mediated effects had been observed (3).

In a comparison of drugs used in the treatment of schizophrenia during pregnancy, the American Academy of Pediatrics classified risperidone as high-potency (4). The classification was based on the potential for extrapyramidal reactions (e.g., acute dystonia, akathisia, parkinsonism, and tardive dyskinesia). The academy cautioned that large maternal doses of high-potency drugs could produce these effects in newborns. However, it did note that high-potency antipsychotics were preferred to minimize maternal anticholinergic, hypotensive, and antihistamine effects. No recommendation concerning the use of risperidone during pregnancy was made because of the lack of data (4).

In summary, risperidone is not an animal teratogen, but stillbirths, pup mortality, and toxicity have been associated with the drug at doses near the human dose. Only 11 cases are known to have been exposed to the antipsychotic during human pregnancy. This experience is too limited to assess, but if the mother's disease requires the use of risperidone, the benefits to her will probably outweigh any fetal risk.

BREAST FEEDING SUMMARY

RECOMMENDATION: Limited Human Data - Potential Toxicity

Risperidone and its active metabolite, 9-hydroxyrisperidone, are excreted into the milk of lactating animals (1) and humans (5). A 21-year-old mother with a 2-year history of bipolar disorder stopped all medication when her pregnancy was diagnosed (5). She did well during pregnancy and delivered a healthy infant at 38 weeks' gestation. After birth, she became increasingly depressed complicated by psychotic symptoms. She was admitted to the hospital 2.5 months after delivery and started on risperidone, eventually reaching a steady-state dose of 6 mg/day. She had been advised to stop breast-feeding because of the lack of information on the excretion of risperidone into milk. Concentrations of risperidone and the active metabolite were determined in the plasma and milk. The milk:plasma ratios for the parent drug and metabolite, based on 24-hour concentration time curves, were 0.42 and 0.24, respectively. Based on a daily milk intake of 150 mL/kg, the nursing infant would have received 0.84% of the mother's risperidone dose (mg/kg/day) and an additional 3.46% from the metabolite (as risperidone equivalents), or about 4.3% of the weight-adjusted maternal dose (5).

Although the combined amounts of risperidone and active metabolite measured in breast milk are probably too low to cause extrapyramidal effects, the above investigators expressed a concern for other effects, such as neuroleptic malignant syndrome, and effects on cognitive development (5). Moreover, the potential for drug accumulation in a nursing infant has not been addressed.

The American Academy of Pediatrics (AAP) classifies other antipsychotic drugs as agents for which the effect on nursing infants is unknown but may be of concern, especially when given for long periods (6). Although risperidone was not mentioned, the AAP noted that antipsychotics are excreted into breast milk and could conceivably alter both short-term and long-term CNS function.

R

References

1. Product information. Risperdal. Janssen Pharmaceutica Products, 2002.
2. Mackay FJ, Wilton LV, Pearce GL, Freemantle SN, Mann RD. The safety of risperidone: a post-marketing study on 7684 patients. Hum Psychopharmacol Clin Exp 1998;13:413–8.
3. Trixler M, Tenyi T. Antipsychotic use in pregnancy. What are the best treatment options? Drug Saf 1997;16:403–10.
4. Committee on Drugs, American Academy of Pediatrics. Use of psychoactive medication during pregnancy and possible effects on the fetus and newborn. Pediatrics 2000;105:880–7.
5. Hill RC, McIvor RJ, Wojnar-Horton RE, Hackett LP,

5. Ilett KF. Risperidone distribution and excretion into human milk: case report and estimated infant exposure during breast-feeding. J Clin Psychopharmacol 2000;20:285–6.
6. Committee on Drugs, American Academy of Pediatrics. The transfer of drugs and other chemicals into human milk. Pediatrics 2001;108:776–89.

Name:	**RITODRINE**	Risk Factor:	B_M
Class:	**Sympathomimetic (Adrenergic)**		

FETAL RISK SUMMARY

RECOMMENDATION: Compatible

Ritodrine is a β-sympathomimetic agent approved for the management of preterm labor. Although congenital malformations caused by ritodrine have not been observed, experience with the drug before the 20th week of gestation is very limited and no reports of 1st trimester use have been located. The manufacturer considers ritodrine to be contraindicated before the 20th week of gestation (1).

Ritodrine rapidly crosses the placenta, appearing in cord blood in amounts ranging from 26% to 117% of the maternal level (2–5). The mean cord:maternal venous blood ratio in eight of nine women delivering at a gestational length of 32 weeks or greater was 0.67 (2). In experiments using an *in vitro* perfused lobe of human placental tissue, ritodrine was shown to diffuse freely to the fetal side (3). Maternal and fetal plasma concentrations were determined in 28 woman-infant pairs who had been treated with IV ritodrine for preterm labor but who progressed to delivery in spite of the therapy (4). A mean cord:maternal venous ratio of 1.17 (range 0.79–2.24) was measured. In addition, ritodrine levels greater than 10 ng/mL in both maternal and fetal venous samples were present up to 5 hours after cessation of ritodrine therapy with detectable concentrations present up to 16.5 hours. Umbilical cord vein ritodrine levels up to 7 ng/mL were measured at this latter time. Fetal concentrations were closely correlated with maternal dose and the time interval between cessation of IV therapy and delivery (4). In a study of the placental passage of ritodrine using seven healthy women undergoing elective cesarean section at 39–40 weeks' gestation, ritodrine was infused at a rate of 72–149 μg/minute for 161–335 minutes (5). The mean cord:maternal venous blood ratio in this study was only 0.263 (range 0.066–0.544). The mean ritodrine concentrations (approximately 21–24 ng/mL) in umbilical vein, umbilical artery, and amniotic fluid were similar. In an investigation of the effects of ritodrine on fetal and placental blood flow, no significant changes in either intervillous or umbilical vein blood flows were noted at 1 hour in 14 women with premature uterine contractions at 31–36 weeks of gestation given ritodrine at 200 μg/minute (6). A comparison of the pharmacokinetics of orally administered ritodrine in pregnant and nonpregnant women has been published (7).

The effects of ritodrine on the mother, fetus, and the newborn have been the subject of several reviews (8–11). Maternal complications may occur frequently with IV therapy, especially when the dose is rapidly increased. The more serious adverse effects include tachycardia, pulmonary edema, myocardial ischemia, cardiac arrhythmias, hyperglycemia followed by a rise in serum insulin levels, and hypokalemia. Severe maternal hypoglycemia secondary to hyperinsulinemia has been reported in a woman following a cesarean section for triplets (12). The woman had been treated prophylactically with oral ritodrine from 15 to 32 weeks' gestation and then with IV ritodrine or high-dose oral therapy for another 12 days. Delivery occurred at approximately 34 weeks' gestation. Symptoms of hypoglycemia, including unconsciousness, occurred slightly more than 24 hours after delivery with blood glucose levels as low as 20 mg/dL and plasma insulin levels up to 19.4 mU/L. Normal glucose levels finally returned about 5 days later. Other causes of the hyperinsulinemia were excluded, and the investigators concluded that the condition was most likely caused by prolonged ritodrine therapy.

Severe fetal and neonatal complications of ritodrine therapy occur infrequently. Increases in fetal heart rate are the most commonly observed manifestation of toxicity. Fetal heart rates up to 200 beats/minute have been recorded (1,8–10). Neonatal cardiac arrhythmias have been reported in three newborns exposed *in utero* to IV ritodrine (13–15). One infant presented with paroxysmal supraventricular tachycardia involving short bursts up to 300 beats/minute with cyanosis and right cardiac failure occurring 10 minutes, 42 hours, and 60 hours after birth (13). The heart rate converted spontaneously to sinus rhythm a minute after each occurrence. Digitalization, continued until 2 months of age, may have prevented further episodes of the arrhythmia in this infant, but therapy was not required in a second case. In this newborn, the episodes of tachyarrhythmias first presented at 11 hours of age and then decreased in frequency until 24 hours of age, after which no further episodes were observed (14). A third case involved a newborn twin with hydrops fetalis who experienced atrial fibrillation at birth with tachycardia and congestive heart failure most likely caused by maternal treatment with IV ritodrine (15).

Disproportionate septal hypertrophy (DSH), defined as an interventricular septal thickness/posterior left ventricular wall thickness ratio (ST/PW) of greater than 1.3, was observed in infants exposed *in utero* to ritodrine for 2 weeks or longer (16). Compared with 22 control infants matched for gestational age, the mean ST/PW ratios for all ritodrine-exposed newborns ($N = 41$) and for a subset of infants exposed for 2 weeks or longer ($N = 22$) were significantly increased. Ritodrine exposure of less than 2 weeks did not cause DSH. However, significant posterior wall thinning was observed in all exposed infants (mean duration of therapy was 16.2 days (range 1–49 days). In those infants exposed for 2 weeks or longer, DSH was caused by an increasing interventricular septal thickness and a thinning posterior wall thickness. Both the ST/PW ratio and the septal thickness were highly correlated with duration of ritodrine exposure (16). The right systolic time interval was also significantly higher in the exposed infants compared with controls. The echocardiographic changes lasted for less than 3 months. Because there were no statistical differences in the mortality rates between the ritodrine and control groups, the clinical significance of these findings is unknown. Possible mechanisms for the defects were thought to include chronic fetal tachycardia, increased glycogen deposition, pulmonary hypertension, or genetic factors (16).

Use of ritodrine may result in transient maternal and fetal hyperglycemia followed by increases in levels of serum insulin. If delivery occurs before these effects have terminated (usually 48–72 hours), hypoglycemia in the newborn may occur (17). Severe maternal ketoacidosis with fetal death has been reported (18). An insulin-dependent diabetic was treated with IV ritodrine up to 0.3 mg/minute for preterm labor at 28 weeks of gestation. Fetal heart rate patterns were normal before therapy. Maternal hyperglycemia with ketoacidosis developed after 26 hours of therapy and 6 hours later fetal heart activity was undetectable. She was subsequently delivered of a stillborn 970-g fetus with cheilognathouranoschisis but with no other abnormalities in either the fetus or the placenta.

A 1989 study compared indomethacin, administered for 48 hours, with IV ritodrine (initiated at 50 μg/minute, then titrated, based on response, to a maximum of 350 μg/minute) in 106 women in preterm labor with intact membranes who were at a gestational age of 32 weeks or less (19). Fifty-four women received ritodrine and 52 received indomethacin. Thirteen (24%) of the ritodrine group developed adverse drug reactions severe enough to require discontinuance of the drug and a change to magnesium sulfate: cardiac arrhythmia (1), chest pain (2), tachycardia (3), and hypotension (7). None of the indomethacin cases developed drug intolerance. For all maternal adverse drug reactions, 39 (72%) of those treated with ritodrine had a side effect vs. 6 (11.5%) of the indomethacin group. The outcomes of the pregnancies were similar, regardless of whether delivery occurred close to or remote from therapy. Of those delivered within 48 hours of initiation of therapy, the mean glucose level in the ritodrine-exposed newborns ($N = 9$) was significantly higher than that in those exposed to indomethacin ($N = 8$), 198 vs. 80 mg/dL ($p < 0.05$), respectively. No cases of premature closure of the ductus arteriosus or pulmonary hypertension were observed. A reduction in amniotic fluid volume was noted in three (5.6%) of the ritodrine group and in six (11.5%) of those treated with indomethacin. On a cost basis, tocolysis with indomethacin was 17 times less costly than tocolysis with ritodrine (19).

Ritodrine-induced neonatal hypoglycemia appears to be related to the route of drug administration. In a double-blind comparison of 17 mothers treated with IV, followed by oral, ritodrine for a mean duration of 9 days vs. 18 control mothers treated with placebo for 10 days, no significant differences between the groups were measured up to 12 hours of age in terms of heart rate, blood pressure, blood volume (measured at 12–24 hours of age), arterial or venous pH, plasma insulin, or blood glucose (20). In contrast, neonatal hypoglycemia (defined as less than 45 mg/dL) was found in 32% (17 of 53) of newborns exposed to IV ritodrine within 12 hours of birth compared with 15% (8 of 54) of controls matched for gestational age and birth weight (21). The mean onset of hypoglycemia was at 1.0 hour of age. Neither gestational age nor maternal ritodrine dose nor the interval between cessation of therapy and delivery correlated well with the onset. Other parameters not significantly different between the groups were Apgar scores, neonatal pH, plasma bicarbonate, hypotension, respiratory distress syndrome, and neonatal mortality. This lack of neonatal toxicity (other than hypoglycemia) has been confirmed by other studies. In a report involving 82 infants whose mothers had been treated with parenteral ritodrine, with or without oral therapy, for an average of 28.5 days compared with a similar number of matched controls, umbilical pH, Apgar scores, head circumference, and neurologic condition were statistically similar (22). Five study infants had neonatal jaundice compared with none of the controls, but the groups were statistically similar in the number of infants with bilirubin values above 5.2 mg/dL (28 and 23, respectively) (22). The investigators were unable to determine whether ritodrine caused the increased incidence of jaundice.

Neonatal renal function was evaluated in 15 infants exposed *in utero* to ritodrine for at least 12 of the 24 hours before delivery compared with 15 matched controls (23). On day 1 (12–36 hours of age), exposed infants had significantly decreased glomerular filtration rates (as measured by inulin clearances), higher plasma renin activity, and higher urinary arginine vasopressin excretion than controls. These parameters were not statistically different between the groups on day 6. Both plasma renin activity and urinary arginine vasopressin excretion were statistically associated with plasma ritodrine levels (mean 16.6 ng/mL on day 1) but not inulin clearance. Correlations were not conducted on day 6 because of the low ritodrine levels (mean 1.0 ng/mL in six infants, less than 0.3 ng/mL in nine). The clinical significance of these findings is unknown because clinical signs of renal failure were not observed in any infant. Furthermore, serum and urine electrolyte values, osmolality, fractional sodium excretion, and urine flow rate were similar in treated and control infants.

In a 1988 review of 12 published and 4 unpublished "methodologically acceptable" controlled trials of β-sympatholytic tocolytic therapy, ritodrine was used in 12 (8 published/4 unpublished) (24). The total number of women involved in the ritodrine trials consisted of 412 treated and 329 controls. The outcomes analyzed, not all of which were available in each trial, were (a) delivery within 24 hours of trial entry; (b) delivery within 48 hours of trial entry; (c) delivery before 37 completed weeks; (d) birth weight below 2500 g; (e) respiratory distress syndrome or severe respiratory problems; and (f) perinatal death. The reviewers confirmed that ritodrine was effective in delaying delivery after preterm labor in comparison to placebo or other, nontocolytic therapy. The frequencies of both preterm birth and low birth weight were reduced. However, in contrast to the prevailing view that ritodrine does not decrease the incidence of neonatal death and respiratory distress syndrome (25–27), neither perinatal mortality nor severe neonatal respiratory problems were reduced. This raised important questions as to the clinical significance of the positive benefits (24). In attempting to explain their findings, the investigators speculated that the trials may have included too many women in whom tocolytic therapy was unlikely to benefit their fetuses. In addition, they concluded that only a small percentage of perinatal mortality resulted from pregnancies that might benefit from tocolytic therapy. The primary benefit of tocolytic therapy, in their opinion, was the attainment of short-term delay of delivery to allow transfer of the patient to medical centers with obstetric and neonatal intensive care facilities and to allow time for the beneficial effects of glucocorticoids on fetal lung development to appear.

Two-year follow-up studies of infants exposed *in utero* to ritodrine have failed to detect harmful effects on growth, incidence of disease, development, or functional maturation (28,29). Studies that are more recent have also failed to detect statistical evidence of adverse effects of ritodrine exposure (30,31). In a study of 20 children examined at 7–9 years of age who had been exposed between 24 and 34 weeks' gestation, no significant differences were found compared with controls in physical growth (height and weight), neurologic parameters (motor, sensory, and cerebellar function), and psychometric testing (30). However, scores and measurements were consistently poorer, although not significantly, in the exposed group, even after correction for socioeconomic status. Most of the controls, however, had not experienced preterm labor, which may have affected the findings (30). A group of 78 6-year-old children exposed *in utero* at a mean gestational age of 32.1 weeks (range 12–37 weeks) for a mean duration of 28.2 days (range 7–163 days) was compared with two control groups composed of 78 children each (31). No significant differences between the three groups were discovered in urinalysis (including no glucosuria in any child), body length and weight, head circumference, neurologic findings, and general behavior as judged by their parents and teachers. The teachers, however, believed that the exposed group did worse in school performance (motor and social skills, emotional and cognitive development). As in previous studies, the authors could not determine whether the latter assessment was caused by ritodrine exposure, an unfavorable obstetric situation, or other factors.

BREAST FEEDING SUMMARY

RECOMMENDATION: No Human Data - Probably Compatible

No data are available.

References

1. Product information. Yutopar, Astra Pharmaceutical Products, 1990.
2. Gandar R, de Zoeten LW, van der Schoot JB. Serum level of ritodrine in man. Eur J Clin Pharmacol 1980;17:117–22.
3. Sodha RJ, Schneider H. Transplacental transfer of beta-adrenergic drugs studied by an in vitro perfusion method of an isolated human placental lobule. Am J Obstet Gynecol 1983;147:303–10.
4. Gross TL, Kuhnert BR, Kuhnert PM, Rosen MG, Kazzi

NJ. Maternal and fetal plasma concentrations of ritodrine. Obstet Gynecol 1985;65:793–7.
5. Fujimoto S, Akahane M, Sakai A. Concentrations of ritodrine hydrochloride in maternal and fetal serum and amniotic fluid following intravenous administration in late pregnancy. Eur J Obstet Reprod Biol 1986;23: 145–52.
6. Jouppila P, Kirkinen P, Koivula A, Ylikorkala O. Ritodrine infusion during late pregnancy: effects on fetal and placental blood flow, prostacyclin, and thromboxane. Am J Obstet Gynecol 1985;151:1028–32.
7. Cartis SN, Venkataramanan R, Cotroneo M, Chiao J-P. Pharmacokinetics of orally administered ritodrine. Am J Obstet Gynecol 1989;161:32–5.
8. Barden TP, Peter JB, Merkatz IR. Ritodrine hydrochloride: a betamimetic agent for use in preterm labor. I. Pharmacology, clinical history, administration, side effects, and safety. Obstet Gynecol 1980;56:1–6.
9. Anonymous. Ritodrine for inhibition of preterm labor. Med Lett Drugs Ther 1980;22:89–90.
10. Finkelstein BW. Ritodrine (Yutopar, Merrell Dow Pharmaceuticals Inc.). Drug Intell Clin Pharm 1981;15:425–33.
11. Benedetti TJ. Maternal complications of parenteral β-sympathomimetic therapy for premature labor. Am J Obstet Gynecol 1983;145:1–6.
12. Caldwell G, Scougall I, Boddy K, Toft AD. Fasting hyperinsulinemic hypoglycemia after ritodrine therapy for premature labor. Obstet Gynecol 1987;70:478–80.
13. Brosset P, Ronayette D, Pierre MC, Lorier BLE, Bouquier JJ. Cardiac complications of ritodrine in mother and baby. Lancet 1982;1:1468.
14. Hermansen MC, Johnson GL. Neonatal supraventricular tachycardia following prolonged maternal ritodrine administration. Am J Obstet Gynecol 1984;149: 798–9.
15. Beitzke A, Winter R, Zach M, Grubbauer HM. Kongenitales vorhofflattern mit hydrops fetalis durch mutterliche tokolytikamedikation. Klin Paediatr 1979;191:410–7.
16. Nuchpuckdee P, Brodsky N, Porat R, Hurt H. Ventricular septal thickness and cardiac function in neonates after in utero ritodrine exposure. J Pediatr 1986;109:687–91.
17. Leake RD, Hobel CJ, Oh W, Thiebeault DW, Okada DM, Williams PR. A controlled, prospective study of the effects of ritodrine hydrochloride for premature labor (abstract). Clin Res 1980;28:90A.
18. Schilthuis MS, Aarnoudse JG. Fetal death associated with severe ritodrine induced ketoacidosis. Lancet 1980;1:1145.
19. Morales WJ, Smith SG, Angel JL, O'Brien WF, Knuppel RA. Efficacy and safety of indomethacin versus ritodrine in the management of preterm labor: a randomized study. Obstet Gynecol 1989;74:567–72.
20. Leake RD, Hobel CJ, Okada DM, Ross MG, Williams PR. Neonatal metabolic effects of oral ritodrine hydrochloride administration. Pediatr Pharmacol 1983;3:101–6.
21. Kazzi NJ, Gross TL, Kazzi GM, Williams TG. Neonatal complications following in utero exposure to intravenous ritodrine. Acta Obstet Gynecol Scand 1987;66:65–9.
22. Huisjes HJ, Touwen BCL. Neonatal outcome after treatment with ritodrine: a controlled study. Am J Obstet Gynecol 1983;147:250–3.
23. Hansen NB, Oh W, LaRochelle F, Stonestreet BS. Effects of maternal ritodrine administration on neonatal renal function. J Pediatr 1983;103:774–80.
24. King JF, Grant A, Keirse MJNC, Chalmers I. Betamimetics in preterm labour: an overview of the randomized controlled trials. Br J Obstet Gynaecol 1988;95:211–22.
25. Boog G, Ben Brahim M, Gandar R. Beta-mimetic drugs and possible prevention of respiratory distress syndrome. Br J Obstet Gynaecol 1975;82:285–8.
26. Merkatz IR, Peter JB, Barden TP. Ritodrine hydrochloride: a betamimetic agent for use in preterm labor. II. Evidence of efficacy. Obstet Gynecol 1980;56: 7–12.
27. Lauersen NH, Merkatz IR, Tejani N, Wilson KH, Roberson A, Mann LI, Fuchs F. Inhibition of premature labor: a multicenter comparison of ritodrine and ethanol. Am J Obstet Gynecol 1977;127:837–45.
28. Freysz H, Willard D, Lehr A, Messer J, Boog G. A long term evaluation of infants who received a betamimetic drug while in utero. J Perinat Med 1977;5: 94–9.
29. Product information and clinical summary of Yutopar. Merrell National Laboratories, Inc., 1980.
30. Polowczyk D, Tejani N, Lauersen N, Siddiq F. Evaluation of seven- to nine-year-old children exposed to ritodrine in utero. Obstet Gynecol 1984;64:485–8.
31. Hadders-Algra M, Touwen BCL, Huisjes HJ. Long-term follow-up of children prenatally exposed to ritodrine. Br J Obstet Gynaecol 1986;93:156–61.

Name:	**RITONAVIR**	Risk Factor:	B_M
Class:	**Antiviral**		

FETAL RISK SUMMARY

RECOMMENDATION: Compatible - Maternal Benefit >> Embryo/Fetal Risk

Ritonavir is an inhibitor of protease in human immunodeficiency virus type 1 (HIV-1) and 2 (HIV-2). Protease is an enzyme that is required for the cleavage of viral polyprotein precursors into active functional proteins found in infectious HIV. The mechanism of action is similar to four other protease inhibitors: amprenavir, indinavir, nelfinavir, and saquinavir (1).

Reproduction studies have been conducted in pregnant rats and rabbits. Maternal toxicity and fetal toxicity, but not teratogenicity, were observed in rats at dose exposures equivalent to approximately 30% of that achieved with the human dose. Fetal toxicity consisted of early resorptions, decreased body weight, ossification delays, and developmental variations. At a dose exposure equivalent to 22% of that achieved with the human dose, a slight increase in cryptorchidism was observed. Fetal toxicity (resorptions, decreased litter size, and decreased weights) and maternal toxicity were observed in rabbits at a dose 1.8 times the human dose based on body surface area (1).

Transplacental passage in rats has been demonstrated with fetal tissue:maternal serum ratios ≥1.0 at 24 hours after the dose in mid- and late-gestation (L. M. Mofenson, personal communication, NIH, 1997). A 1998 *in vitro* experiment using term perfused human placentas demonstrated that the placental transfer of ritonavir was concentration dependent and that the clearance index, at both maternal trough and peak concentrations, was very low (2). The investigators attributed the low transfer to the molecular weight (about 721) and solubility characteristics of ritonavir (2).

The Antiretroviral Pregnancy Registry reported, for the period January 1989 through January 2004, prospective data (reported to the Registry before the outcomes were known) involving 1537 live births that had been exposed during the 1st trimester to one or more antiretroviral agents (3). Forty-seven of the newborns had congenital defects (3.1%, 95% confidence interval [CI] 2.3–4.1). In the 2407 live births with earliest exposure in the 2nd/3rd trimesters, there were 56 infants with defects (2.3%, 95% CI 1.8–3.0). The prevalence rates for the two periods did not differ significantly. There were 103 infants with birth defects among 3944 live births with exposure anytime during pregnancy (2.6%, 95% CI 2.1–3.2). The prevalence rate did not differ significantly from the rate expected in a nonexposed population (3). There were 164 outcomes exposed to ritonavir (74 in the 1st trimester and 90 in the 2nd/3rd trimesters) in combination with other antiretroviral agents. There were three birth defects among the 1st trimester exposures and three in those exposed in the 2nd/3rd trimesters. In reviewing the birth defects of prospective and retrospective (pregnancies reported after the outcomes were known) registered cases, and clinical reports, the Registry concluded that there was no pattern of anomalies to suggest a common cause (3). (See Lamivudine for required statement.)

The experience of one perinatal center with the treatment of HIV infected pregnant women was summarized in a 1999 abstract (4). Of 55 women receiving ≥3 antiviral drugs, 39 were treated with a protease inhibitor (6 with ritonavir). The outcomes included 2 spontaneous abortions, 5 elective abortions, 27 newborns, and 5 ongoing pregnancies. One woman was taken off indinavir because of ureteral obstruction and another (drug therapy not specified) developed gestational diabetes. None of the newborns tested positive for HIV, had major congenital anomalies, or complications (4).

A public health advisory has been issued by the Food and Drug Administration (FDA) on the association between protease inhibitors and diabetes mellitus (5). Because pregnancy is a risk factor for hyperglycemia, there was concern that these antiviral agents would exacerbate this risk. An abstract published in 2000 described the results of a study involving 34 pregnant women treated with protease inhibitors (5 with ritonavir) compared to 41 controls that evaluated the association with diabetes (6). No association between protease inhibitors and an increased incidence of gestational diabetes was found.

A case of combined transient mitochondrial and peroxisomal β-oxidation dysfunction after exposure to nucleoside analog reverse transcriptase inhibitors (NRTIs) (lamivudine and zidovudine) combined with protease inhibitors (ritonavir and saquinavir) throughout gestation was reported in 2000 (7). A male infant was delivered at 38 weeks' gestation. He received postnatal prophylaxis with lamivudine and zidovudine for 4 weeks until the agents were discontinued because of anemia. Other adverse effects that were observed in the infant (age at onset) were hypocalcemia (shortly after birth), Group B streptococcal sepsis, ventricular extrasystoles, prolonged metabolic acidosis, and lactic acidemia (8 weeks), a mild elevation of long chain fatty acids (9 weeks), and neutropenia (3 months). The metabolic acidosis required treatment until 7 months of age, whereas the elevated plasma lactate resolved over 4 weeks. Cerebrospinal fluid lactate was not determined nor was a muscle biopsy conducted. Both the neutropenia and the cardiac dysfunction had resolved by 1 year of age. The elevated plasma fatty acid level was confirmed in cultured fibroblasts, but other peroxisomal functions (plasmalogen biosynthesis and catalase staining) were normal. Although mitochondrial dysfunction has been linked to NRTI agents, the authors were unable to identify the cause of the combined abnormalities in this case (7). The child was reported to be healthy and developing normally at 26 months of age.

A multicenter, retrospective survey of pregnancies exposed to protease inhibitors was published in 2000 (8). There were 92 live born infants delivered from 89 women (3 sets of twins) at six health care centers. One nonviable infant, born at 22 weeks' gestation, died. The surviving 91 infants were evaluated in terms of adverse effects, prematurity rate, and frequency of HIV-1 transmission. Most of the infants were exposed *in utero* to a single protease inhibitor, but a few were exposed to more than one because of sequential or double combined therapy. The number of newborns exposed to each protease inhibitor was indinavir ($N = 23$), nelfinavir ($N = 39$), ritonavir ($N = 5$), and saquinavir ($N = 34$). Protease inhibitors were started before conception in 18, and during the 1st, 2nd, or 3rd trimesters in 12, 44, and 14, respectively, and not reported in one. Other antiretrovirals used with the protease inhibitors included four NRTIs (didanosine, lamivudine, stavudine, and zidovudine). The most common NRTI regimen was a combination of zidovudine and lamivudine (65% of women). In addition, seven women were enrolled in the AIDS Clinical Trials Group Protocol 316 and, at the start of labor, received a single dose of either the non-nucleoside reverse transcriptase inhibitor nevirapine or placebo. Maternal conditions, thought possibly or likely to be related to therapy, were mild anemia in eight, severe anemia in one (probably secondary to zidovudine), and thrombocytopenia in one. Gestational diabetes mellitus was observed in three women (3.3%), a rate similar to the expected prevalence of 2.6% in a nonexposed population (8). One mother developed postpartum cardiomyopathy and died 2 months after birth of twins, but the cause of death was not known. For the surviving newborns, there was no increase in adverse effects over that observed in previous clinical trials of HIV-positive women, including the prevalence of anemia (12%), hyperbilirubinemia (6%; none exposed to indinavir), and low birth weight (20.6%). Premature delivery occurred in 19.1% of the pregnancies (close to the expected rate). The percentage of infants infected with HIV was 0 (95% CI 0%–3%) (8).

In summary, although the limited human data do not allow an assessment of the safety of ritonavir during pregnancy, the animal data suggests that the drug may represent a low risk to the developing fetus. Two reviews, one in 1996 and the other in 1997, concluded that all women currently receiving antiretroviral therapy should continue to receive therapy during pregnancy and that treatment of the mother with monotherapy should be considered inadequate therapy (9,10). In 1998, the Centers for Disease Control and Prevention (CDC) made a similar recommendation that antiretroviral therapy should be continued during pregnancy, but discontinuation of all therapy during the 1st trimester was a consideration (5). If indicated, therefore, protease inhibitors, including ritonavir, should not be withheld in pregnancy (with the possible exception of the 1st trimester) because the expected benefit to the HIV-positive mother probably outweighs the unknown risk to the fetus. Moreover, one review suggested that during pregnancy ritonavir was the drug of choice among the protease inhibitors (10). Pregnant women taking protease inhibitors should be monitored for hyperglycemia. The efficacy and safety of combined therapy in preventing vertical transmission of HIV to the newborn, however, are unknown, and zidovudine remains the only antiretroviral agent recommended for this purpose (9,10).

BREAST FEEDING SUMMARY

RECOMMENDATION: Contraindicated

No reports describing the use of ritonavir during lactation have been located. The molecular weight (about 721) is low enough that excretion into breast milk should be expected.

Reports on the use of ritonavir during human lactation are unlikely because the antiviral agent is used in the treatment of human immunodeficiency virus (HIV) infections. HIV-1 is transmitted in milk, and in developed countries, breast-feeding is not recommended (9–13). In developing countries, breast-feeding is undertaken, despite the risk, because there are no affordable milk substitutes available. Until 1999, no studies had been published that examined the effect of any antiretroviral therapy on HIV-1 transmission in milk. In that year, a study involving zidovudine was published that measured a 38% reduction in vertical transmission of HIV-1 infection in spite of breast-feeding when compared to controls (see Zidovudine).

References

1. Product information. Norvir. Abbott Laboratories, 2001.
2. Casey BM, Bawdon RE. Placental transfer of ritonavir with zidovudine in the ex vivo placental perfusion model. Am J Obstet Gynecol 1998;179:758–61.
3. Antiretroviral Pregnancy Registry Steering Committee, Antiretroviral Pregnancy Registry International Interim Report for 1 January 1989 through 31 January 2004. Wilmington, NC: Registry Coordinating Center; 2004.
4. Stek A, Kramer F, Fassett M, Khoury M. The safety and efficacy of protease inhibitor therapy for HIV infection during pregnancy (abstract). Am J Obstet Gynecol 1999;180:S7.
5. CDC. Public Health Service Task Force recommendations for the use of antiretroviral drugs in pregnant women infected with HIV-1 for maternal health and for reducing perinatal HIV-1 transmission in the United States. MMWR 1998;47:No. RR-2.
6. Fassett M, Kramer F, Stek A. Treatment with protease inhibitors in pregnancy is not associated with an increased incidence of gestational diabetes (abstract). Am J Obstet Gynecol 2000;182:S97.
7. Stojanov S, Wintergerst U, Belohradsky BH, Rolinski B. Mitochondrial and peroxisomal dysfunction following perinatal exposure to antiretroviral drugs. AIDS 2000;14:1669.
8. Morris AB, Cu-Uvin S, Harwell JI, Garb J, Zorrilla C, Vajaranant M, Dobles AR, Jones TB, Carlan S, Allen DY. Multicenter review of protease inhibitors in 89 pregnancies. J Acquir Immune Defic Syndr 2000;25:306–11.
9. Carpenter CCJ, Fischi MA, Hammer SM, Hirsch MS, Jacobsen DM, Katzenstein DA, Montaner JSG, Richman DD, Saag MS, Schooley RT, Thompson MA, Vella S, Yeni PG, Volberding PA. Antiretroviral therapy for HIV infection in 1996. JAMA 1996;276;146–54.
10. Minkoff H, Augenbraun M. Antiretroviral therapy for pregnant women. Am J Obstet Gynecol 1997;176:478–89.
11. Brown ZA, Watts DH. Antiviral therapy in pregnancy. Clin Obstet Gynecol 1990;33:276–89.
12. de Martino M, Tovo P-A, Pezzotti P, Galli L, Massironi E, Ruga E, Floreea F, Plebani A, Gabiano C, Zuccotti GV. HIV-1 transmission through breast-milk: appraisal of risk according to duration of feeding. AIDS 1992;6:991–7.
13. Van de Perre P. Postnatal transmission of human immunodeficiency virus type 1: the breast feeding dilemma. Am J Obstet Gynecol 1995;173:483–7.

Name:	**RIVASTIGMINE**	Risk Factor:	B_M
Class:	**Cholinesterase Inhibitor (CNS Agent)**		

FETAL RISK SUMMARY

RECOMMENDATION: No Human Data - Animal Data Suggest Low Risk

Rivastigmine is a reversible cholinesterase inhibitor that is indicated for the treatment of mild to moderate dementia of the Alzheimer's type. Rivastigmine penetrates the blood brain barrier with drug concentrations in the cerebral spinal fluid about 40% of those in the plasma. It is extensively metabolized to inactive metabolites. Protein binding is moderate (about 40%) and the plasma elimination half-life is about 1.5 hours (1).

Reproduction studies have been conducted in rats and rabbits. In rats, doses up to about two times the maximum recommended human dose based on body surface area (MRHD) were not teratogenic. Decreased fetal/pup weights were observed in rats at doses several-fold lower than the MRHD, usually at doses causing some maternal toxicity. No effects on fertility or reproductive performance were observed at doses about 0.9 times the MRHD. No evidence of teratogenicity was noted in rabbits given doses up to about four times the MRHD (1).

Rivastigmine and/or its metabolites cross the rabbit placenta producing an average fetal-to-placenta tissue ratio of 0.5 (2). It is not known if rivastigmine or its metabolites cross the human placenta. The molecular weight of the parent compound (about 250 for the free base), moderate protein binding, and the ability to cross the blood brain barrier and rabbit placenta suggest that the drug will cross to the fetal compartment. However, the very short elimination half-life will decrease the amount of drug available for transfer.

No reports describing the use of rivastigmine in human pregnancy have been located. Because of its indication, such reports should be rare. Moreover, the animal data suggest that the risk to the embryo and/or fetus is low. Therefore, inadvertent exposure to rivastigmine during pregnancy should not be a reason for pregnancy termination.

BREAST FEEDING SUMMARY

RECOMMENDATION: No Human Data - Potential Toxicity

No reports describing the use of rivastigmine during human lactation have been located. Because of its indication, such reports should be rare. The molecular weight (about 250 for the free base), moderate protein binding, and the ability to cross the blood brain barrier suggest that the drug will be excreted into breast milk. However, the very short elimination half-life will decrease the amount of drug available for excretion. The effects of this exposure on a nursing infant are unknown.

References

1. Product information. Exelon. Novartis Pharmaceuticals, 2004.
2. Habucky K, Tse FLS. Disposition of SDZ ENA 713, an acetylcholinesterase inhibitor, in the rabbit. Biopharm Drug Dispos 1998;19:285–90.

Name:	**RIZATRIPTAN**	Risk Factor:	C_M
Class:	**Antimigraine**		

FETAL RISK SUMMARY

RECOMMENDATION: Limited Human Data - Animal Data Suggest Risk

Rizatriptan, an oral, selective 5-hydroxytryptamine$_{1B/1D}$ receptor agonist, is indicated for the treatment of acute migraine attacks with or without aura in adults.

Reproduction studies have been conducted in rats and rabbits (1). Female rats were treated before and during mating, and throughout gestation and lactation with doses that produced maternal exposures (AUC) 15 and 225 times, respectively, the exposure in humans from the maximum recommended human dose of 30 mg (MRHD). These doses were not maternal toxic, but did cause decreased birth weight and reduced pre- and post-weaning weight gain in offspring. In a pre- and post-natal development toxicity study in rats, doses producing maternal exposures 225 to more than 500 times the MRHD caused toxicity in the offspring as shown by increased mortality at birth and for the first 3 days after birth, reduced pre- and post-weaning weight gain, and decreased learning capacity. The no-effect dose for all of these effects was approximately 7.5 times the MRHD. In embryo and fetal development studies, no teratogenic effects were observed in rats and rabbits given doses during organogenesis producing maternal exposures 225 and 115 times, respectively, the MRHD. Fetal weights were decreased at these doses, but maternal weight gain was also reduced. The developmental no-effect doses, in both species, were approximately 15 times the MRHD.

Rizatriptan crosses the placentas of rats and rabbits (1). The relatively low molecular weight of the free base (about 269) suggests that placental transfer of the drug will also occur in humans.

In the Merck Pregnancy Registry program, 41 women were prospectively enrolled after exposure to rizatriptan (2). The outcomes of these pregnancies were 7 lost to follow-up, 12 outcomes pending, 3 spontaneous abortions (SABs), 1 elective abortion (EAB) (chromosomal anomaly—partial replication of chromosome 3 in a 39-year-old woman), 1 fetal death (cord accident), 1 neonatal death (as a consequence of prematurity), and 16 healthy term infants. The rate of SABs (14.3%, 3 of 21 pregnancies) does not exceed the expected background rate in the United States. There were also four retrospective cases (reported after the outcome was known) that involved two infants with congenital malformations, one of whom had an abnormal karyotype possibly related to advanced maternal age. In clinical trials, there were 22 inadvertent exposures during pregnancy. The outcomes of these cases were 5 SABs (1 molar pregnancy), 5 EABs, 1 lost to follow-up, and 11 healthy newborns (1 set of twins). Two liveborns (male twins) were premature. Although no adverse outcomes were observed in liveborn offspring in the prospective registry or clinical trials, the limited number of exposures studied is not sufficient to detect a risk of rare disorders such as individual birth defects (2). Health care providers are encouraged to report prenatal exposures to rizatriptan by calling (800)-986-8999.

BREAST FEEDING SUMMARY

RECOMMENDATION: No Human Data - Probably Compatible

No reports describing the use of rizatriptan in human lactation have been located. The relatively low molecular weight of the free base (about 269) suggests that the drug will be excreted into breast milk. The effects of this exposure on a nursing infant are unknown.

References

1. Product information. Maxalt. Merck, 2001.
2. Fifth Annual Report from the Merck Pregnancy Registry for Maxalt (rizatriptan benzoate) covering the period from approval (June 1998) through July 31, 2003.

Name: **ROCURONIUM** Risk Factor: C_M

Class: **Skeletal Muscle Relaxant**

FETAL RISK SUMMARY

RECOMMENDATION: Limited Human Data - Animal Data Suggest Low Risk

Rocuronium (rocuronium bromide) is a competitive (nondepolarizing) neuromuscular blocking agent. Structurally, it is a quaternary ammonium compound that is an analogue of vecuronium. Rocuronium is indicated as an IV adjunct to general anesthesia to provide skeletal muscle relaxation during surgery or mechanical ventilation. In normal adult patients, the elimination half-life is about 2.4 hours. Approximately 30% is bound to plasma proteins (1).

Reproduction studies have been conducted in rats and rabbits. In these species, the maximum tolerated IV dose administered three times daily during organogenesis was not teratogenic. The doses were 15%–30% and 25%, respectively, of the human intubation dose of 0.6–1.2 mg/kg based on body surface area. In rats, the incidence of fetal death was increased, an effect that was thought to be due to oxygen deficiency that resulted from acute symptoms of respiratory dysfunction in the dams (1).

Consistent with the molecular weight (about 610 for rocuronium bromide) and the limitation placed on placental passage by ionization at physiologic pH, small amounts of rocuronium cross the placenta. In 32 patients from the study below, the mean maternal venous (MV) and umbilical venous (UV) blood was about 2412 ng/mL and 390 ng/mL, respectively. The UV:MV ratio was 0.16. In 12 patients, the mean drug concentration in umbilical arterial (UA) plasma was about 271 ng/mL, resulting in a UA/UV ratio of 0.62 (2).

In a 1994 prospective, non-randomized, multi-center study, 40 women undergoing cesarean section at term received anesthesia induction with rocuronium and thiopental, followed by isoflurane and nitrous oxide maintenance (2). No adverse effects on the newborns attributable to rocuronium were observed as evaluated by Apgar scores, time to sustained respiration, total and muscular neuroadaptive capacity scores, acid-base status, and blood-gas tensions in umbilical arterial and venous blood (2). This study generated a number of letters referring either to the doses used or to what was considered the drug of choice (succinylcholine) (3–7).

A 1996 report described the use of rocuronium in a 31-year-old patient at 28 weeks' gestation who presented with a penetrating injury of her left eye secondary to a motor vehicle accident (8). Prior to induction of anesthesia, she was started on IV magnesium sulfate to treat newly onset uterine contractions. Anesthesia was induced with rocuronium

(0.9 mg/kg), fentanyl (200 μg), and sodium thiopental (400 mg). The fetal heart rate (140–150 beats/minute) was monitored throughout the 6-hour surgical procedure. Except for a decrease in short-term variability attributable to anesthesia of the fetus, no other effects on the fetal heart rate were observed. Although the authors were aware of the interaction with magnesium, they chose a higher dose (usual dose is 0.6 mg/kg) to allow for more rapid intubation. As expected, the duration of paralysis was prolonged secondary to the high dose and interaction with magnesium, but the authors thought this was acceptable given the patient's condition. The woman was discharged from the hospital 6 days after surgery with an apparently normal ongoing pregnancy (8). Information on the pregnancy outcome was not provided. Later correspondence regarding this case report discussed the benefits and risks of the therapy and dose (9,10).

Rocuronium was used in a 35-year-old patient undergoing a combined cesarean section delivery and posterior fossa craniotomy at 37 weeks' gestation (11). The patient had von Hippel-Lindau disease and surgery was required for an enlarged hemangioblastoma. General anesthesia was induced with rocuronium (50 mg), fentanyl (200 μg), and sodium thiopental (300 mg). A male infant (weight not specified) was delivered with Apgar scores of 5, 7, and 9 at 1, 5, and 10 minutes, respectively. Naloxone was required because of weak respiratory efforts 2 minutes after delivery (11).

A 1997 study compared thiopental-rocuronium with ketamine-rocuronium (20 in each group) for rapid-sequence intubation in women undergoing cesarean section (12). The authors concluded that either drug combination was suitable. Based on 1- and 5-minute Apgar scores, no significant differences in neonatal condition was found between the two groups (12).

In summary, human pregnancy experience with rocuronium is limited to the 2nd and 3rd trimesters. Although the absence of exposures during organogenesis prevents a more thorough assessment, neuromuscular blocking agents generally do not appear to represent a significant risk for an embryo or fetus. The animal data for rocuronium suggest low embryo/fetal risk. Moreover, the agent contains a quaternary ammonium site in its structure that will limit its placental transfer. One review predicted that the maternal drug concentrations would always exceed fetal drug levels (13). Neuromuscular blockade in a newborn is probably a rare but potential toxicity (14). If indicated, rocuronium should not be withheld because of pregnancy.

BREAST FEEDING SUMMARY

R

RECOMMENDATION: No Human Data - Probably Compatible

No reports describing the use of rocuronium in a lactating woman have been located. Because of the indications for this agent, it is doubtful if such reports will be forthcoming. The molecular weight (about 610 for rocuronium bromide) is low enough for excretion into breast milk, but the amount excreted will be limited because the drug is ionized at physiologic pH. The effects of this exposure on a nursing infant are unknown, but are probably not clinically significant.

References

1. Product information. Zemuron. Organon USA, 2004.
2. Abouleish E, Abboud T, Lechevalier T, Zhu J, Chalian A, Alford K. Rocuronium (Org 9426) for caesarean section. Br J Anaesth 1994;73:336–41.
3. Kwan WF, Chen BJ, Liao KT. Rocuronium for caesarean section. Br J Anaesth 1995;74:347.
4. Abouleish E, Abboud T. Rocuronium for caesarean section. Br J Anaesth 1995;74:347–8.
5. McSiney M, Edwards C, Wilkins A. Rocuronium for caesarean section. Br J Anaesth 1995;74:348.
6. Swales HA, Gaylord DG. Rocuronium for caesarean section. Br J Anaesth 1995;74:348.

7. Abouleish E, Abboud T. Rocuronium for caesarean section. Br J Anaesth 1995;74:348.
8. Gaiser RR, Seem EH. Use of rocuronium in a pregnant patient with an open eye injury, receiving magnesium medication, for preterm labour. Br J Anaesth 1996;77:669–71.
9. James MFM. Use of rocuronium in a pregnant patient receiving magnesium medication. Br J Anaesth 1997;78:772.
10. Gaiser K. Use of rocuronium in a pregnant patient receiving magnesium medication (reply). Br J Anaesth 1997;78:772.
11. Boker A, Ong BY. Anesthesia for cesarean section and posterior fossa craniotomy in a patient with von Hippel-Lindau disease. Can J Anesth 2001;48:387–90.
12. Baraka AS, Sayyid SS, Assaf BA. Thiopental-rocuronium versus ketamine-rocuronium for rapid-sequence intubation in parturients undergoing cesarean section. Anesth Analg 1997;84:1104–7.
13. Guay J, Grenier Y, Varin F. Clinical pharmacokinetics of neuromuscular relaxants in pregnancy. Clin Pharmacokinet 1998;34:483–96.
14. Atherton DP, Hunter JM. Clinical pharmacokinetics of the newer neuromuscular blocking drugs. Clin Pharmacokinet 1999;36:169–89.

Name: **ROFECOXIB** Risk Factor: **C_M***
Class: **Nonsteroidal Anti-inflammatory**

FETAL RISK SUMMARY

RECOMMENDATION: Human Data Suggest Risk in 1st and 3rd Trimesters

Rofecoxib is a second-generation nonsteroidal anti-inflammatory drug (NSAID) that inhibits prostaglandin synthesis via the inhibition of cyclooxygenase-2 (COX-2). At therapeutic concentrations, it does not inhibit, as do first-generation NSAIDs, the cyclooxygenase-1 (COX-1) isoenzyme. It is indicated for the relief of the signs and symptoms of osteoarthritis, acute pain, and primary dysmenorrhea (1). Rofecoxib is in the same NSAID subclass (COX-2) as celecoxib and valdecoxib.

In animal reproduction studies with rats and rabbits, rofecoxib caused peri- and postimplantation losses and reduced embryo and fetal survival at doses approximately 9 and 2 times, respectively, the human exposure based on $AUC_{Ø-24\,Hours}$ (HE) at 25 mg/day, or 3 and <1 times, respectively, the HE at 50 mg/day (1). These effects are a natural consequence of inhibition of prostaglandin synthesis. No teratogenicity was observed in rats at doses 28 and 10 times the HE at 25 and 50 mg/day. In rabbits, a slight, nonstatistically significant increase in the incidence of vertebral malformations was seen at doses 1 and <1 times the HE at 25 and 50 mg/day. In pregnant rats administered a single dose of rofecoxib, a decrease in the diameter of the ductus arteriosus was seen at all doses used (lowest dose tested: 2 and <1 times the HE at 25 and 50 mg/day). At 10 and 3 times the HE at 25 and 50 mg/day, rofecoxib did not cause a significantly delayed labor or parturition in rats (1).

It is not known if rofecoxib crosses the human placenta. The molecular weight (about 314) is low enough that transfer to the fetus should be expected. Rofecoxib crosses the placenta in rats and rabbits (1).

A combined 2001 population-based observational cohort study and a case-control study estimated the risk of adverse pregnancy outcome from the use of NSAIDs (2). The use of NSAIDs during pregnancy was not associated with congenital malformations, preterm delivery, or low birth weight, but a positive association was discovered with spontaneous abortions (SABs). A similar study, also published in 2001, failed to find a relationship, in general, between NSAIDs and congenital malformations, but did find a significant association with cardiac defects and orofacial clefts (3). In addition, a 2003 study found a significant association between exposure to NSAIDs in early pregnancy and SABs (4). (See Ibuprofen for details on the three studies.)

R

Data from the Merck Pregnancy Registry for Vioxx (rofecoxib), as of October 31, 2003, include 16 pregnancies exposed in the 1st trimester to rofecoxib during clinical trials (5). In another three cases, the exposures remain blinded (the subjects may have received rofecoxib, placebo, or a comparative drug). Outcomes of the 16 exposed pregnancies were 4 SABs, 1 elective abortion (no reason given), and 11 liveborn infants. Among the latter group, there was one premature infant (35 weeks; otherwise healthy and normal), one infant with bilateral undescended testes, and one infant with patent ductus arteriosus vs. atrial septal defect (5). Thirty-two pregnancies were reported prospectively to the Registry. The outcomes in these cases were 14 liveborn infants (exposed in 1st trimester; 1 was premature at 35 weeks as a consequence of premature rupture of membranes and had a large nasal septum), 2 SABs (1st trimester), 10 lost to follow-up, and 6 unknown outcomes. Four pregnancies were reported retrospectively to the Registry (5). One 9-week-old infant had growth restriction in the area of the hips and buttocks. A second infant, born at 34 weeks' gestation that died, had multiple deformities (hydrocephalus, short femur, cardiac, tracheal, and intestinal defects). In this latter case, however, exposure had occurred 9 days after the first day of the last menstrual period (LMP), so a relationship with the anomalies is not possible. Moreover, there was a family history of similar defects (5). In addition to the above reports, the Registry also noted 59 prospective international reports, but 40 of these reports have unknown outcomes (5). Among the known cases, there were two adverse outcomes: one infant with bowel malrotation resulting in neonatal death due to bowel necrosis; and one fetal death at 26 weeks' gestation secondary to intrauterine growth retardation and oligohydramnios but no congenital anomalies (exposed from gestational weeks 14 to 18). Two retrospective international reports described pregnancies with oligohydramnios: one infant delivered at 31 weeks' was healthy and normal (exposed gestational weeks 30 to 31); and one infant that did not survive was delivered at 34 weeks' gestation with renal failure and complications of oligohydramnios (clubfoot, arm contractures, and pulmonary hypoplasia) (exposed from LMP to delivery). Finally, the Swedish Medical Birth Registry reported to the Merck Registry 35 pregnancies exposed to rofecoxib in the 1st trimester. Only one minor defect (a nevus) was noted in these cases (5).

A brief 2003 editorial on the potential for NSAID-induced developmental toxicity concluded that the NSAIDs, and specifically those with greater COX-2 affinity, had a lower risk of this toxicity in humans than aspirin (6).

A 2004 study compared the tocolytic effects of oral rofecoxib and IV magnesium sulfate in patients in preterm labor at 22–34 weeks' gestation (7). Patients were randomly assigned to receive 50 mg/day rofecoxib ($N = 105$) or magnesium sulfate ($N = 109$) for 48 hours. No difference in the arrest of preterm labor for 48 hours between the groups was observed, but the women in the magnesium group complained of more side effects. There was no difference between the groups in the incidence of neonatal adverse effects (7).

Constriction of the ductus arteriosus *in utero* is a pharmacologic consequence arising from the use of prostaglandin synthesis inhibitors during pregnancy (see also Indomethacin) (8). Persistent pulmonary hypertension of the newborn may occur if these agents are used in the 3rd trimester close to delivery (8,9). First-generation NSAIDs have been shown to inhibit labor and prolong gestation, both in humans (10) (see also Indomethacin) and in animals (11). Although animal studies with rofecoxib did not show this effect, it is not known if humans would be similarly unaffected. Women attempting to conceive should not use any prostaglandin synthesis inhibitor, including rofecoxib, because of the findings in a variety of animal models that indicate these agents block blastocyst implantation (12,13). Moreover, as noted above, NSAIDs have been associated with SABs and congenital malformations. If rofecoxib is used in pregnancy for the treatment of rheumatoid arthritis,

R

healthcare professionals are encouraged to call the toll-free number (877-311-8972) for information about patient enrollment in the OTIS Rheumatoid Arthritis study.

[**Risk Factor D if used in 3rd trimester or near delivery.*]

BREAST FEEDING SUMMARY

RECOMMENDATION: No Human Data - Potential Toxicity

No reports describing the use of rofecoxib during human lactation have been located. The molecular weight (about 314) is low enough that excretion into breast milk should be expected. The drug is excreted in the milk of lactating rats at concentrations similar to those in the plasma (1). At a maternal dose approximately 18 times the HE at 25 mg/day (6 times the HE at 50 mg/day), there was an increase in nursing pup mortality and a decrease in pup body weight.

The effects on a human nursing infant from exposure to rofecoxib in breast milk are unknown. Although several first-generation NSAIDs are considered low risk during nursing (e.g., see Diclofenac, Fenoprofen, Flurbiprofen, Ibuprofen, Ketoprofen, Ketorolac, and Tolmetin), the relatively long adult serum half-life of rofecoxib (about 17 hours) and the absence of clinical pharmacologic data in infants suggest that this agent should be avoided during nursing.

References

1. Product information. Vioxx. Merck, 2001.
2. Nielsen GL, Sorensen HT, Larsen H, Pedersen L. Risk of adverse birth outcome and miscarriage in pregnant users of non-steroidal anti-inflammatory drugs: population based observational study and case-control study. BMJ 2001;322:266–70.
3. Ericson A, Kallen BAJ. Nonsteroidal anti-inflammatory drugs in early pregnancy. Reprod Toxicol 2001; 15:371–5.
4. Li DK, Liu L, Odouli R. Exposure to non-steroidal anti-inflammatory drugs during pregnancy and risk of miscarriage: population based cohort study. BMJ 2003;327:368–71.
5. Fourth Annual Report on Exposure during Pregnancy from the Merck Pregnancy Registry for VIOXX (rofecoxib). May 1999 through October 5, 2003.
6. Tassinari MS, Cook JC, Hurtt ME. NSAIDs and developmental toxicity. Birth Defects Res Part B Dev Reprod Toxicol 2003;68:3–4.
7. McWhorter J, Carlan SJ, O'Leary TD, Richichi K, O'Brien WF. Rofecoxib versus magnesium sulfate to arrest preterm labor: a randomized trial. Obstet Gynecol 2004;103:923–30.
8. Levin DL. Effects of inhibition of prostaglandin synthesis on fetal development, oxygenation, and the fetal circulation. Semin Perinatol 1980;4:35–44.
9. Van Marter LJ, Leviton A, Allred EN, Pagano M, Sullivan KF, Cohen A, Epstein MF. Persistent pulmonary hypertension of the newborn and smoking and aspirin and nonsteroidal antiinflammatory drug consumption during pregnancy. Pediatrics 1996;97:658–63.
10. Fuchs F. Prevention of prematurity. Am J Obstet Gynecol 1976;126:809–20.
11. Powell JG, Cochrane RL. The effects of a number of non-steroidal anti-inflammatory compounds on parturition in the rat. Prostaglandins 1982;23:469–88.
12. Matt DW, Borzelleca JF. Toxic effects on the female reproductive system during pregnancy, parturition, and lactation. In Wilorsch RJ, ed. *Reproductive Toxicology*. 2nd ed. New York, NY: Raven Press, 1995:175–93.
13. Dawood MY. Nonsteroidal antiinflammatory drugs and reproduction. Am J Obstet Gynecol 1993;169:1255–65.

Name:	**ROPINIROLE**	Risk Factor:	**C_M**
Class:	**Antiparkinsonian Agent**		

FETAL RISK SUMMARY

RECOMMENDATION: No Human Data - Animal Data Suggest Risk

Ropinirole is a non-ergoline dopamine agonist that is indicated for the treatment of the signs and symptoms of idiopathic Parkinson disease. The drug has high specificity for the

D_2 and D_3 dopamine receptor subtypes. Ropinirole is metabolized to inactive compounds and eliminated renally with a half-life of about 6 hours. Up to 40% is bound to plasma proteins (1). The agent is commonly used in combination with levodopa.

Reproduction studies in pregnant rats and rabbits have revealed embryo-fetal toxicity and teratogenicity (1). In rats, decreased fetal weight, increased fetal deaths, and digital malformations were observed with doses 24, 36, and 60 times, respectively, the maximum recommended human clinical dose based on body surface area administered during organogenesis and later. In pregnant rabbits during organogenesis, no harmful fetal effects were observed when ropinirole was given at a maternal toxic dose 16 times the maximum recommended human dose based on body surface area (MRHD). However, when ropinirole (8 times the MRHD) was combined with levodopa (250 mg/kg/day), a greater incidence and severity of fetal malformations (primarily digit defects) occurred than when levodopa was used alone. In a 2-year carcinogenicity study in mice, ropinirole was associated with an increase in benign uterine endometrial polyps at a dose 10 times the MRHD (1).

It is not known if ropinirole can cross the placenta. The relatively low molecular weight (about 260 for the free base) and the moderate degree of protein binding providing free drug in the plasma, however, suggest that the drug will cross to the embryo and fetus.

No reports describing the use of ropinirole in human pregnancy have been located. The agent, when given alone, produced digital malformations in rats at embryo/fetal toxic doses. In rabbits, an increased incidence and severity of digital anomalies also were observed when ropinirole, at a dose 8 times the human dose, was combined with levodopa. The complete absence of human pregnancy experience, however, prevents an assessment of the human risk. Because Parkinson disease is relatively uncommon during the childbearing years, the use of ropinirole during pregnancy also will be uncommon. Until data on such use are available, the safest course is to avoid, if possible, the use of ropinirole during the 1st trimester.

BREAST FEEDING SUMMARY

RECOMMENDATION: No Human Data - Potential Toxicity

No reports describing the use of ropinirole during human lactation have been located (1). Ropinirole is excreted into the milk of lactating rats. This excretion is consistent with its low molecular weight (about 297; 260 for the free base) and its moderate degree of protein binding (up to 40%). Excretion into human breast milk should be expected. Because the milk is slightly acidic compared with the plasma, accumulation (ion trapping) in milk may occur. The effects of this exposure, if any, on a nursing infant are unknown. Infants should be monitored for adverse events commonly observed in adults, such as fatigue, syncope, somnolence, dizziness, dyspepsia, and nausea and vomiting. Ropinirole inhibits prolactin secretion and may inhibit lactation. Until data on its safe use are available, ropinirole should not be used during lactation.

Reference

1. Product information. Requip. GlaxoSmithKline, 2003.

Name: **ROPIVACAINE** Risk Factor: **B_M**
Class: **Local Anesthetic**

FETAL RISK SUMMARY

RECOMMENDATION: Compatible

Ropivacaine is a member of the amino amide class of local anesthetics. It is indicated for local or regional anesthesia for surgery and for acute pain management. Ropivacaine is a pure S-enantiomer that is structurally similar to bupivacaine. It has been used for local and regional anesthesia before cesarean section and during labor. Plasma protein binding (94%) is primarily to α_1-glycoprotein. The mean terminal half-life is 4.2 hours after epidural administration (1).

Reproduction studies have been conducted in rats and rabbits. In rats, daily SC doses up to about 0.33 times the maximum recommended human dose (epidural, 770 mg/24 hours) based on body surface area (MRHD) during organogenesis revealed no teratogenic effects. When rats were given daily SC doses from gestational day 15 through postpartum day 20, there were no treatment-related effects on late fetal development, parturition, lactation, neonatal viability, or growth of the offspring. In another study, female rats were given daily SC doses that were about 0.3 times the MRHD for 2 weeks before mating, then during mating, pregnancy, and lactation, up to day 42-post coitus. There was an increased loss of pups during the first 3 days postpartum, an effect thought to have occurred because of reduced maternal care due to maternal toxicity. In rabbits, SC doses up to about 0.33 times the MRHD during organogenesis revealed no teratogenicity (1).

Pregnant sheep were given a 60-minute IV infusion of a local anesthetic (ropivacaine, bupivacaine, or levobupivacaine) at a rate that obtained a maternal serum concentration equivalent to that obtained during routine epidural anesthesia for cesarean delivery (2). No significant changes (heart rate, mean arterial blood pressure, arterial blood pH, and arterial oxygenation) in the fetuses were observed. Maternal hemodynamic parameters also were not affected. All three anesthetics crossed the placenta to the fetus with varying concentrations measured in all fetal tissues tested (heart, brain. liver, lung, kidney, and adrenals). The ropivacaine fetal:maternal serum ratio was approximately 0.3 (2).

A 1999 study used a dual perfused, single cotyledon human placental model to compare the placental transfer of ropivacaine and bupivacaine (3). Simulation of the actual *in vivo* plasma protein concentration (using a 4% albumin solution) resulted in a 50% decrease in the amounts transferred compared to a 2% albumin solution. In addition, decreasing the pH on the fetal side resulted in a significant increase in placental transfer. The investigators concluded that the placental transfer of both anesthetics was highly influenced by the amount of maternal and fetal protein binding and fetal pH (3).

In another study, epidural ropivacaine was given to women for cesarean section (4). The umbilical:maternal (U:M) veins ratio of unbound drug at delivery was 0.72 (4). A 1997 report measured mean U:M vein ratios for total and unbound ropivacaine after epidural of 0.31 and 0.74, respectively (5). In a third study, total ropivacaine concentrations in the umbilical vein and artery were 0.13–0.52 mg/L and 0.12–0.41 mg/L, respectively, whereas the concentrations of unbound drug were 0.027–0.063 mg/L and 0.027–0.058 mg/L, respectively (6).

A number of studies have reported normal Apgar scores, umbilical acid-base values, and neurobehavioral assessments when ropivacaine epidurals were used in women in labor (4–11). In one study conducted at six different centers, fewer infants delivered vaginally from mothers receiving ropivacaine had abnormal neurological and adaptive capacity scores at 24 hours compared to those delivered vaginally from mothers receiving bupivacaine (11).

In summary, the human and animal data suggest that the risk to a human fetus from the use of ropivacaine in pregnancy is very low or nonexistent. However, there is no human pregnancy experience in the 1st trimester, usually the most vulnerable period in gestation. Nonetheless, the amounts measured in the maternal circulation are very low and do not appear to represent a significant embryo/fetal risk.

BREAST FEEDING SUMMARY

RECOMMENDATION: No Human Data - Probably Compatible

No reports describing the use of ropivacaine during human lactation have been located. As noted above, the primary use in pregnancy of this local anesthetic occurs during labor. Only very small amounts appear in the maternal circulation after epidural use and these concentrations would be cleared within 24 hours. In addition, only small amounts of ropivacaine have been measured in cord blood and these appear to be clinically in significant. Based on milk:plasma ratios determined in lactating rats, the estimated daily dose for a nursing pup was about 4% of the maternal dose (1). If a similar milk:plasma ratio exists in humans, the exposure to a nursing infant is far less than the exposure *in utero* in pregnant women at term (1). Therefore, there appears to be no risk to a nursing infant.

References

1. Product information. Naropin. AstraZeneca, 2001.
2. Santos AC, Karpel B, Noble G. The placental transfer and fetal effects of levobupivacaine, racemic bupivacaine, and ropivacaine. Anesthesiology 1999;90: 1698–703.
3. Johnson RF, Cahana A, Olenick M, Herman N, Paschall RL, Minzter B, Ramasubramanian R, Gonzalez H, Downing JW. A comparison of the placental transfer of ropivacaine versus bupivacaine. Anesth Analg 1999;89:703–8.
4. Datta S, Camann W, Bader A, VanderBurgh L. Clinical effects and maternal and fetal plasma concentrations of epidural ropivacaine versus bupivacaine for cesarean section. Anesthesiology 1995;82:1346–52.
5. Morton CPJ, Bloomfield S, Magnusson A, Jozwiak H, McClure JH. Ropivacaine 0.75% for extradural anaesthesia in elective caesarean section: an open clinical and pharmacokinetic study in mother and neonate. Br J Anaesth 1997;79:3–8.
6. Irestedt L, Ekblom A, Olofsson C, Dahlstrom AC, Emanuelsson BM. Pharmacokinetics and clinical effect during continuous epidural infusion with ropivacaine 2.5 mg/mL or bupivacaine 2.5 mg/mL for labour pain relief. Acta Anaesthesiol Scand 1998;42:890–6.
7. Gaiser RR, Venkateswaren P, Cheek TG, Persiley E, Buxbaum J, Hedge J, Joyce TH, Gutsche BB. Comparison of 0.25% ropivacaine and bupivacaine for epidural analgesia for labor and vaginal delivery. J Clin Anesthesia 1997;9:564–8.
8. McCrae AF, Jozwiak H, McClure JH. Comparison of ropivacaine and bupivacaine in extradural analgesia for the relief of pain in labour. Br J Anaesth 1995;74:261–5.
9. Eddleston JM, Holland JJ, Griffin RP, Corbett A, Horsman EL, Reynolds F. A double-blind comparison of 0.25% ropivacaine and 0.25% bupivacaine for extradural analgesia in labour. Br J Anaesth 1996;76: 66–71.
10. Irestedt L, Emanuelsson BM, Ekblom A, Olofsson C, Reventlid H. Ropivacaine 7.5 mg/ml for elective caesarean section. A clinical and pharmacokinetic comparison of 150 mg and 187.5 mg. Acta Anaesthesiol Scan 1997;41:1149–56.
11. Writer WDR, Stienstra R, Eddleston JM, Gatt SP, Griffin R, Gutsche BB, Joyce TH, Hedlund C, Heeroma K, Selander D. Neonatal outcome and mode of delivery after epidural analgesia for labour with ropivacaine and bupivacaine: a prospective meta-analysis. Br J Anaesth 1998;81:713–7.

R

Name:	**ROSIGLITAZONE**	Risk Factor:	C_M
Class:	**Oral Hypoglycemic**		

FETAL RISK SUMMARY

RECOMMENDATION: No Human Data - Animal Data Suggest Risk

Rosiglitazone, a thiazolidinedione antidiabetic agent, is used as an adjunct to diet and exercise to improve glycemic control in patients with type II diabetes (non-insulin-dependent diabetes mellitus). It is used either alone or in combination with metformin. Rosiglitazone is not an insulin secretagogue, but acts to decrease insulin resistance in the periphery and in the liver (i.e., decreases insulin requirements). Rosiglitazone undergoes extensive metabolism to inactive metabolites. The plasma half-life of rosiglitazone-related materials (parent drug and inactive metabolites ranges from 103–158 hours and the binding to plasma proteins, primarily albumin, is high (99.8%) (1).

Reproduction studies with rosiglitazone have been conducted in rats and rabbits at doses up to 20 and 75 times, respectively, the AUC at the maximum recommended human daily dose (MRHD). No teratogenicity or adverse effect on implantation or the embryo were observed in either species, but placental pathology was noted in rats. Moreover, dosing during mid- to late-gestation was associated with fetal death and growth retardation in both rats and rabbits. Treatment extending through the lactation period in rats was associated with reduced litter size and decreased neonatal viability and postnatal growth. Growth retardation was reversible after puberty. For effects on the placenta, embryo, fetus, and offspring, the no-effect dose levels were approximately 4 times the MRHD for both species (1).

It is not known if rosiglitazone crosses the human placenta, but the molecular weight of the free base (about 357) and prolonged elimination half-life of the parent drug and/or inactive metabolites suggest that transfer to the embryo/fetus will occur. However, the extensive metabolism and protein binding should limit the transfer of active drug.

A 2002 report described the use of rosiglitazone in early pregnancy (2). A 35-year-old woman with several diseases (hypertension, diabetes mellitus, hypercholesterolemia, anxiety disorder, epilepsia, and morbid obesity) who conceived while being treated with multiple drugs: rosiglitazone (4 mg/day), gliclazide (a sulfonylurea), atorvastatin, acarbose, spironolactone, hydrochlorothiazide, carbamazepine, thioridazine, amitriptyline, chlordiazepoxide, and pipenzolate bromide (an anti-spasmodic). Pregnancy was diagnosed in the 8th week of gestation and all medications were stopped. She was treated with methyldopa and insulin for the remainder of her pregnancy. At 36 weeks' gestation, a repeat cesarean section delivered a healthy, 3.5-kg female infant with Apgar scores of 7 and 8 at 1 and 5 minutes, respectively. The infant was developing normally after 4 months (2).

Rosiglitazone is sometimes used for the treatment of insulin resistance in women with polycystic ovarian syndrome. Spontaneous ovulation and enhancement of clomiphene-induced ovulation resulting in conception has been reported after the use of rosiglitazone (3–5). Because this treatment may result in pregnancy, appropriate contraception is advised (6).

Insulin is the treatment of choice for pregnant diabetic patients because, in general, other hypoglycemic agents do not provide adequate glycemic control. Moreover, insulin, unlike most oral agents, does not cross the placenta to the fetus, thus eliminating the additional concern that the drug therapy itself will adversely effect the fetus. Carefully prescribed insulin therapy provides better control of the mother's glucose, thereby preventing the fetal and neonatal complications that occur with this disease. High maternal glucose levels, as may occur in diabetes mellitus, are closely associated with a number of maternal and fetal adverse effects, including fetal structural anomalies if the hyperglycemia occurs early in gestation. To prevent this toxicity, most experts, including the American College of Obstetricians and Gynecologists, recommend that insulin be used for types I and II diabetes occurring during pregnancy and, if diet therapy alone is not successful, for gestational diabetes (7,8).

BREAST FEEDING SUMMARY

RECOMMENDATION: No Human Data - Probably Compatible

No reports describing the use of rosiglitazone during human lactation have been located. The molecular weight of the free base (about 357) is low enough, however, that excretion into breast milk should be expected. Rosiglitazone-related material (parent drug or metabolites) were detected in the milk of lactating rats (1). The effects on a nursing infant from exposure to the drug in milk are unknown.

References

1. Product information. Avandia. SmithKline Beecham Pharmaceuticals, 2000.
2. Yaris F, Yaris E, Kadioglu M, Ulku C, Kesim M, Kalyoncu NI. Normal pregnancy outcome following inadvertent exposure to rosiglitazone, gliclazide, and atorvastatin in a diabetic and hypertensive woman. Reprod Toxicol 2004;18:619–21.
3. Cataldo NA, Abbasi F, McLaughlin TL, Lamendola C, Reaven GM. Improvement in insulin sensitivity followed by ovulation and pregnancy in a woman with polycystic ovary syndrome who was treated with rosiglitazone. Fertil Steril 2001;76:1057–9.
4. Belli SH, Graffigna MN, Oneto A, Otero P, Schurman L, Levalle OA. Effect of rosiglitazone on insulin resistance, growth factors, and reproductive disturbances in women with polycystic ovary syndrome. Fertil Steril 2004;81:624–9.
5. Ghazeeri G, Kutteh WH, Bryer-Ash M, Haas D, Ke RK. Effect of rosiglitazone on spontaneous and clomiphene citrate-induced ovulation in women with polycystic ovary syndrome. Fertil Steril 2003;79:562–6.
6. O'Moore-Sullivan TM, Prins JB. Thiazolidinediones and type 2 diabetes: new drugs for an old disease. Med J Aust 2002;176:381–6.
7. American College of Obstetricians and Gynecologists. Diabetes and pregnancy. *Technical Bulletin*. No. 200, December 1994.
8. Coustan DR. Management of gestational diabetes, Clin Obstet Gynecol 1991;34:558–64.

R

S

Name:	**SACCHARIN**	Risk Factor:	**C**
Class:	**Artificial Sweetener**		

FETAL RISK SUMMARY

RECOMMENDATION: Limited Human Data - Animal Data Suggest Low Risk

Saccharin is a nonnutritive sweetening agent discovered accidentally in 1879 and used in the United States since 1901 (1). The agent is approximately 300 times sweeter than sucrose (1,2). Saccharin, a derivative of naphthalene, is absorbed slowly after oral ingestion and is rapidly and completely excreted, as the unmetabolized compound, by the kidneys (1). Although a large amount of medical research has been generated concerning saccharin, very little of this information pertains to its use by pregnant women or to its effect on the fetus (1,2).

In pregnant rhesus monkeys administered IV saccharin, fetal accumulation of the sweetener occurred after rapid, but limited, transfer across the placenta (3). Saccharin appeared to be uniformly distributed to all fetal tissues except the central nervous system. Fetal levels were still present 5 hours after the end of the infusion and 2 hours after maternal concentrations were undetectable. A study, published in 1986, documented that saccharin also crosses the placenta to the human fetus (4). Six diabetic women, consuming 25–100 mg/day of saccharin by history, were delivered at 36–42 weeks. Maternal serum saccharin concentrations, measured between 0.5 hour before and 2 hours after delivery, ranged from 20 to 263 ng/mL. Cord blood samples varied from 20 to 160 ng/mL.

Saccharin is not an animal teratogen (3,5,6). No increase in the incidence of spontaneous abortions among women consuming saccharin has been found (7). Concerns for human use focus on the potential carcinogenicity of the agent. In some animal species, particularly after second-generation studies, an increased incidence of bladder tumors was observed (2). However, epidemiologic studies have failed to associate the human use of saccharin with bladder cancer (2). Similarly, no evidence was found in a study of the Danish population that *in utero* saccharin exposure was associated with an increased risk of bladder cancer during the first 30–35 years of life (2,8). However, at least one investigator believes that these studies must be extended much further before they are meaningful, because bladder cancer is usually diagnosed in the elderly (9).

There is limited information available on the risk for humans following *in utero* exposure to saccharin. The Calorie Control Council believes the agent can be safely used by pregnant women (10). However, others recommended avoidance of saccharin or, at least, cautious use of it in pregnancy (1,2,9).

BREAST FEEDING SUMMARY

RECOMMENDATION: Compatible

Saccharin is excreted into human milk (11). In six healthy women, saccharin, 126 mg/12 fluid ounces, contained in two commercially available soft drinks, was given every 6 hours for nine doses. After single or multiple doses, median peak concentrations of saccharin occurred at 0.75 hour in plasma and at 2.0 hours in milk. Milk concentrations ranged from <200–1056 ng/mL after one dose to 1765 ng/mL after nine doses. The ratios of the concentration-time curves for milk and plasma averaged 0.542 on day 1 and 0.715 on day 3, indicating that accumulation in the milk occurred with time (11). The amounts of saccharin a nursing infant could consume from milk were predicted to be much less than the usual intakes of children less than 2 years old (11).

References

1. London RS. Saccharin and aspartame: Are they safe to consume during pregnancy? J Reprod Med 1988;33:17–21.
2. Council on Scientific Affairs, American Medical Association. Saccharin: review of safety issues. JAMA 1985;254:2622–4.
3. Pitkin RM, Reynolds WA, Filer LJ Jr, Kling TG. Placental transmission and fetal distribution of saccharin. Am J Obstet Gynecol 1971;111:280–6.
4. Cohen-Addad N, Chatterjee M, Bekersky I, Blumenthal HP. In utero exposure to saccharin: a threat? Cancer Lett 1986;32:151–4.
5. Fritz H, Hess R. Prenatal development in the rat following administration of cyclamate, saccharin and sucrose. Experientia 1968;24:1140–1.
6. Shepard TH. *Catalog of Teratogenic Agents*. 6th ed. Baltimore, MD: Johns Hopkins University Press, 1989:566–7.
7. Kline J, Stein ZA, Susser M, Warburton D. Spontaneous abortion and the use of sugar substitutes. Am J Obstet Gynecol 1978;130:708–11.
8. Jensen OM, Kamby C. Intra-uterine exposure to saccharin and risk of bladder cancer in man. Int J Cancer 1982;15:507–9.
9. London RS. Letter to the editors. J Reprod Med 1988;33(8):102.
10. Nabors LO. Letter to the editors. J Reprod Med 1988;33(8):102.
11. Collins Egan P, Marx CM, Heyl PS, Popick A, Bekersky I. Saccharin excretion in mature human milk (abstract). Drug Intell Clin Pharm 1984;18:511.

Name:	**SALMETEROL**	Risk Factor:	**C_M**
Class:	**Respiratory Drug (Bronchodilator)**		

FETAL RISK SUMMARY

RECOMMENDATION: Limited Human Data - Probably Compatible

Salmeterol is a selective β_2-adrenergic bronchodilator that is indicated in the management of asthma. It is administered as an aerosol or powder for oral inhalation. Because the drug acts locally in the lung, plasma levels are very low or undetectable and are a result of swallowed salmeterol.

Animal reproduction studies have been conducted in the rat and rabbit (1). In the rat, oral doses up to approximately 160 times the maximum recommended daily human inhalation dose based on body surface area (MRDHID-BSA) produced no evidence of impaired fertility or teratogenic effects. In pregnant Dutch rabbits, an oral dose about 10 times the maximum recommended daily human inhalation dose based on AUC (MRDHID-AUC) produced no fetal toxicity. When the dose was increased to about 20 times the MRDHID-AUC, fetal toxicity secondary to β-adrenoceptor stimulation was observed (precocious eyelid openings, cleft palate, sternebral fusion, limb and paw flexures, and delayed ossification of the frontal cranial bones) (1). However, New Zealand White rabbits were much less sensitive, exhibiting only delayed ossification of the frontal cranial bones at oral doses 1600 times the MRDHID-BSA (1). The fetal toxicity noted in rabbits was not thought to be relevant to humans because β-agonists characteristically induce these effects in animals (1).

In a study with pregnant rats, salmeterol concentrations in mammary tissue, placenta, and fetus after oral administration were comparable to those in maternal blood up to 6 hours after a dose (2). At 24 hours, the disposition of the drug in the fetus was primarily in the gastrointestinal tract.

It is not known if salmeterol crosses the placenta to the fetus. Although the molecular weight (about 604 for salmeterol xinafoate) is low enough, plasma levels after an inhaled therapeutic dose are very low or undetectable.

A 1998 non-interventional observational cohort study described the outcomes of pregnancies in women who had been prescribed one or more of 34 newly marketed drugs by general practitioners in England (3). Data were obtained by questionnaires sent to the prescribing physicians 1 month after the expected or possible date of delivery. In 831 (78%) of the pregnancies, a newly marketed drug was thought to have been taken during the 1st trimester with birth defects noted in 14 (2.5%) singleton births of the 557 newborns (10 sets of twins). In addition, two birth defects were observed in aborted fetuses. However, few of the aborted fetuses were examined. Salmeterol was taken during the 1st trimester in 65 pregnancies. The outcomes of these pregnancies included 7 spontaneous abortions, 2 ectopic pregnancies, 4 elective abortions, 5 unknown outcomes, and 47 births (3 premature). One full-term newborn was diagnosed with Aarskog syndrome (a male child with short stature, and facial, digital, and genital malformations; pectus excavatum, metatarsus adductus, and joint laxity are frequent skeletal features [4]) (3). The syndrome is thought to be secondary to X-linked recessive inheritance (4).

In summary, one review concluded that salmeterol was safe during human pregnancy (5), but others thought it should not be a first- line drug because of the lack of published human experience (6,7). Although human data have been published and no congenital malformations attributable to salmeterol were observed, the data are too limited to assess the safety of salmeterol. Moreover, the above study lacked the sensitivity to identify minor anomalies because of the absence of standardized examinations. Late-appearing major defects may also have been missed because of the timing of the questionnaires. However, if a patient with moderate or severe asthma had demonstrated a good therapeutic response before conception, this may favor the drug's continuation during pregnancy (6). Moreover, salmeterol is more effective than doubling the dose of inhaled corticosteroids and may have advantages over theophylline in terms of effectiveness and tolerability (6). In addition, the very low or undetectable maternal plasma levels that occur with therapeutic inhaled doses suggests that the risk to the fetus from the drug is probably minimal or nonexistent.

BREAST FEEDING SUMMARY

RECOMMENDATION: No Human Data - Probably Compatible

No reports describing the use of salmeterol during human lactation have been located. When given orally, salmeterol is excreted into the milk of lactating rats (1). The molecular weight (about 604 for salmeterol xinafoate) is low enough for excretion into breast milk, but maternal plasma levels after an inhaled therapeutic dose are very low or undetectable. Thus, it is unlikely that clinically significant amounts would be found in milk.

References

1. Product information. Serevent. Glaxo Wellcome, 2002.
2. Manchee GR, Barrow A, Kulkarni S, Palmer E, Oxford J, Colthup PV, Maconochie JG, Tarbit MH. Disposition of salmeterol xinafoate in laboratory animals and humans. Drug Metab Dispos 1993;21:1022–8.
3. Wilton LV, Pearce GL, Martin RM, Mackay FJ, Mann RD. The outcomes of pregnancy in women exposed to newly marketed drugs in general practice in England. Br J Obstet Gynaecol 1998;105:882–9.
4. Buyse ML, editor. *Birth Defects Encyclopedia*. Volume 1. Cambridge, MA: Blackwell Scientific Publications, 1990:1–2.
5. Anonymous. Drugs for asthma. Med Lett Drugs Ther 2000;42:19–24.
6. Position statement. The American College of Obstetricians and Gynecologists (ACOG) and the American College of Allergy, Asthma and Immunology (ACAAI). The use of newer asthma and allergy medications during pregnancy. Ann Allergy Asthma Immunol 2000;84:475–80.
7. Tan KS, Thomson NC. Asthma in pregnancy. Am J Med 2000;109:727–33.

Name:	**SAQUINAVIR**	Risk Factor:	B_M
Class:	**Antiviral**		

FETAL RISK SUMMARY

RECOMMENDATION: Compatible - Maternal Benefit >> Embryo/Fetal Risk

Saquinavir, a synthetic peptide-like substrate analogue, inhibits the activity of human immunodeficiency virus (HIV) protease, thus preventing the cleavage of viral polyproteins and the maturation of infectious virus. The mechanism of action is similar to four other protease inhibitors: amprenavir, indinavir, nelfinavir, and ritonavir (1).

In reproduction studies in rats and rabbits, embryotoxicity and teratogenicity were not observed at plasma concentrations up to approximately 50% and 40%, respectively, of the human exposure based on AUC achieved from the recommended clinical dose. There was also no evidence that at this dose the drug affected fertility or reproductive performance in rats. A similar lack of toxicity, as measured by survival, growth, and development of offspring to weaning, was found in rats treated during late pregnancy through lactation with doses producing the same plasma concentrations as those above (1).

It is not known if saquinavir crosses the human placenta. The molecular weight of the free base is low enough (about 671) that some degree of transfer should be anticipated. In rats and rabbits, placental transfer of saquinavir is low (less than 5% of maternal plasma concentrations) (1).

The Antiretroviral Pregnancy Registry reported, for the period January 1989 through January 2004, prospective data (reported to the Registry before the outcomes were known) involving 1537 live births that had been exposed during the 1st trimester to one or more antiretroviral agents (2). Forty-seven of the newborns had congenital defects (3.1%, 95% confidence interval [CI] 2.3–4.1). In the 2407 live births with earliest exposure in the 2nd/3rd trimesters, there were 56 infants with defects (2.3%, 95% CI 1.8–3.0). The prevalence rates for the two periods did not differ significantly. There were 103 infants with birth defects among 3944 live births with exposure anytime during pregnancy (2.6%, 95% CI 2.1–3.2). The prevalence rate did not differ significantly from the rate expected in a nonexposed population (2). There were 152 outcomes exposed to saquinavir (70 in the

S

1st trimester and 82 in the 2nd/3rd trimesters) in combination with other antiretroviral agents. There were four birth defects among the 1st trimester exposures and four in those exposed in the 2nd/3rd trimesters. In reviewing the birth defects of prospective and retrospective (pregnancies reported after the outcomes were known) registered cases, and clinical reports, the Registry concluded that there was no pattern of anomalies to suggest a common cause (2). (See Lamivudine for required statement.)

A study published in 1999 evaluated the safety, efficacy, and perinatal transmission rates of HIV in 30 pregnant women receiving various combinations of antiretroviral agents (3). Many of the women were substance abusers. Protease inhibitors (nelfinavir $N = 7$, indinavir $N = 6$, and saquinavir $N = 1$ in combination with nelfinavir) were used in 13 of the women. Antiretroviral therapy was initiated at a median of 14 weeks' gestation (range preconception to 32 weeks). In spite of previous histories of extensive antiretroviral experience and of vertical transmission of HIV, combination therapy was effective in treating maternal disease and in preventing transmission to the current newborns. The outcomes of the pregnancies treated with protease inhibitors appeared to be similar to the 17 cases that did not receive these agents, except that the birth weights were lower (3).

The experience of one perinatal center with the treatment of HIV infected pregnant women was summarized in a 1999 abstract (4). Of 55 women receiving $\geq$3 antiviral drugs, 39 were treated with a protease inhibitor (11 with saquinavir). The outcomes included 2 spontaneous abortions, 5 elective abortions, 27 newborns, and 5 ongoing pregnancies. One woman was taken off indinavir because of ureteral obstruction and another (drug therapy not specified) developed gestational diabetes. None of the newborns tested positive for HIV, had major congenital anomalies, or complications (4).

A public health advisory has been issued by the Food and Drug Administration (FDA) on the association between protease inhibitors and diabetes mellitus (5). Because pregnancy is a risk factor for hyperglycemia, there was concern that these antiviral agents would exacerbate this risk. An abstract published in 2000 described the results of a study involving 34 pregnant women treated with protease inhibitors (7 with saquinavir) compared to 41 controls that evaluated the association with diabetes (6). No relationship between protease inhibitors and an increased incidence of gestational diabetes was found.

A case of combined transient mitochondrial and peroxisomal β-oxidation dysfunction after exposure to nucleoside analog reverse transcriptase inhibitors (NRTIs) (lamivudine and zidovudine) combined with protease inhibitors (ritonavir and saquinavir) throughout gestation was reported in 2000 (7). A male infant was delivered at 38 weeks' gestation. He received postnatal prophylaxis with lamivudine and zidovudine for 4 weeks until the agents were discontinued because of anemia. Other adverse effects that were observed in the infant (age at onset) were hypocalcemia (shortly after birth), Group B streptococcal sepsis, ventricular extrasystoles, prolonged metabolic acidosis, and lactic acidemia (8 weeks), a mild elevation of long chain fatty acids (9 weeks), and neutropenia (3 months). The metabolic acidosis required treatment until 7 months of age, whereas the elevated plasma lactate resolved over 4 weeks. Cerebrospinal fluid lactate was not determined nor was a muscle biopsy conducted. Both the neutropenia and the cardiac dysfunction had resolved by 1 year of age. The elevated plasma fatty acid level was confirmed in cultured fibroblasts, but other peroxisomal functions (plasmalogen biosynthesis and catalase staining) were normal. Although mitochondrial dysfunction has been linked to NRTI agents, the authors were unable to identify the cause of the combined abnormalities in this case (7). The child was reported to be healthy and developing normally at 26 months of age.

A multicenter, retrospective survey of pregnancies exposed to protease inhibitors was published in 2000 (8). There were 92 live born infants delivered from 89 women (3 sets of twins) at six health care centers. One nonviable infant, born at 22 weeks' gestation, died. The surviving 91 infants were evaluated in terms of adverse effects, prematurity rate, and frequency of HIV-1 transmission. Most of the infants were exposed *in utero* to a single protease inhibitor, but a few were exposed to more than one because of sequential or double combined therapy. The number of newborns exposed to each protease inhibitor was indinavir ($N = 23$), nelfinavir ($N = 39$), ritonavir ($N = 5$), and saquinavir ($N = 34$). Protease inhibitors were started before conception in 18, and during the 1st, 2nd, or 3rd trimesters in 12, 44, and 14, respectively, and not reported in one. Other antiretrovirals used with the protease inhibitors included four NRTIs (didanosine, lamivudine, stavudine, and zidovudine). The most common NRTI regimen was a combination of zidovudine and lamivudine (65% of women). In addition, seven women were enrolled in the AIDS Clinical Trials Group Protocol 316 and, at the start of labor, received a single dose either of the non-nucleoside reverse transcriptase inhibitor, nevirapine, or placebo. Maternal conditions, thought possibly or likely to be related to therapy, were mild anemia in eight, severe anemia in one (probably secondary to zidovudine), and thrombocytopenia in one. Gestational diabetes mellitus was observed in three women (3.3%), a rate similar to the expected prevalence of 2.6% in a nonexposed population (8). One mother developed postpartum cardiomyopathy and died 2 months after birth of twins, but the cause death was not known. For the surviving newborns, there was no increase in adverse effects over that observed in previous clinical trials of HIV-positive women, including the prevalence of anemia (12%), hyperbilirubinemia (6%; none exposed to indinavir), and low birth weight (20.6%). Premature delivery occurred in 19.1% of the pregnancies (close to the expected rate). The percentage of infants infected with HIV was 0 (95% CI 0%–3%) (8).

In summary, although the limited human data do not allow an assessment of the safety of saquinavir during pregnancy, the animal data suggests that the embryo/fetal risk is low. Two reviews, one in 1996 and the other in 1997, concluded that all women currently receiving antiretroviral therapy should continue to receive therapy during pregnancy and that treatment of the mother with monotherapy was inadequate therapy (9,10). In 1998, the Centers for Disease Control and Prevention (CDC) made a similar recommendation that antiretroviral therapy should be continued during pregnancy, but discontinuation of all therapy during the 1st trimester was a consideration (5). If indicated, therefore, protease inhibitors, including saquinavir, should not be withheld in pregnancy (with the possible exception of the 1st trimester) because the expected benefit to the HIV-positive mother probably outweighs the unknown risk to the fetus. Pregnant women taking protease inhibitors should be monitored for hyperglycemia. Possibly because of the poor bioavailability of saquinavir, one review suggested that during pregnancy ritonavir (see Ritonavir) was the drug of choice among the protease inhibitors (10). The efficacy and safety of combined therapy in preventing vertical transmission of HIV to the newborn, however, are unknown and zidovudine remains the only antiretroviral agent recommended for this purpose (9,10).

S

BREAST FEEDING SUMMARY

RECOMMENDATION: Contraindicated

No reports describing the use of saquinavir during lactation have been located. The molecular weight of the free base (about 671) is low enough that excretion into breast milk should be expected.

Reports on the use of saquinavir during lactation are unlikely because the drug is indicated in the treatment of patients with HIV. HIV type 1 (HIV-1) is transmitted in milk, and in developed countries, breast-feeding is not recommended (9–13). In developing countries, breast-feeding is undertaken, despite the risk, because there are no affordable milk substitutes available. Until 1999, no studies had been published that examined the effect of any antiviral therapy on HIV-1 transmission in milk. In that year, a study involving zidovudine was published that measured a 38% reduction in vertical transmission of HIV-1 infection in spite of breast-feeding when compared to controls (see Zidovudine).

References

1. Product information. Invirase. Roche Laboratories, 2000.
2. Antiretroviral Pregnancy Registry Steering Committee. *Antiretroviral Pregnancy Registry International Interim Report for 1 January 1989 through 31 January 2004*. Wilmington, NC: Registry Coordinating Center, 2004.
3. McGowan JP, Crane M, Wiznia AA, Blum S. Combination antiretroviral therapy in human immunodeficiency virus-infected pregnant women. Obstet Gynecol 1999;94:641–6.
4. Stek A, Kramer F, Fassett M, Khoury M. The safety and efficacy of protease inhibitor therapy for HIV infection during pregnancy (abstract). Am J Obstet Gynecol 1999;180:S7.
5. CDC. Public Health Service Task Force recommendations for the use of antiretroviral drugs in pregnant women infected with HIV-1 for maternal health and for reducing perinatal HIV-1 transmission in the United States. MMWR 1998;47:No. RR-2.
6. Fassett M, Kramer F, Stek A. Treatment with protease inhibitors in pregnancy is not associated with an increased incidence of gestational diabetes (abstract). Am J Obstet Gynecol 2000;182:S97.
7. Stojanov S, Wintergerst U, Belohradsky BH, Rolinski B. Mitochondrial and peroxisomal dysfunction following perinatal exposure to antiretroviral drugs. AIDS 2000;14:1669.
8. Morris AB, Cu-Uvin S, Harwell JI, Garb J, Zorrilla C, Vajaranant M, Dobles AR, Jones TB, Carlan S, Allen DY. Multicenter review of protease inhibitors in 89 pregnancies. J Acquir Immune Defic Syndr 2000;25:306–11.
9. Carpenter CCJ, Fischi MA, Hammer SM, Hirsch MS, Jacobsen DM, Katzenstein DA, Montaner JSG, Richman DD, Saag MS, Schooley RT, Thompson MA, Vella S, Yeni PG, Volberding PA. Antiretroviral therapy for HIV infection in 1996. JAMA 1996;276:146–54.
10. Minkoff H, Augenbraun M. Antiretroviral therapy for pregnant women. Am J Obstet Gynecol 1997;176:478–89.
11. Brown ZA, Watts DH. Antiviral therapy in pregnancy. Clin Obstet Gynecol 1990;33:276–89.
12. de Martino M, Tovo P-A, Pezzotti P, Galli L, Massironi E, Ruga E, Floreea F, Plebani A, Gabiano C, Zuccotti GV. HIV-1 transmission through breast-milk: appraisal of risk according to duration of feeding. AIDS 1992;6:991–7.
13. Van de Perre P. Postnatal transmission of human immunodeficiency virus type 1: the breast feeding dilemma. Am J Obstet Gynecol 1995;173:483–7.

Name: **SARGRAMOSTIM** Risk Factor: **C_M**

Class: **Hematopoietic**

S

FETAL RISK SUMMARY

RECOMMENDATION: No Human Data - No Relevant Animal Data

The human granulocyte-macrophage colony-stimulating factor (GM-CSF) sargramostim is produced by recombinant DNA technology. Sargramostim differs slightly from the natural human GM-CSF. It has several specific indications: following induction chemotherapy in acute myelogenous leukemia; for mobilization and following transplantation of autologous peripheral blood progenitor cells; for myeloid reconstitution after allogeneic bone marrow transplantation; and for bone marrow transplantation failure or engraftment delay. The mean beta half-lives after IV and SC administration were 60 and 162 minutes, respectively. Animal reproduction studies have not been conducted with sargramostim (1).

Sargramostim is a 127-amino acid glycoprotein that is characterized by three primary molecular species with molecular weights of 19,500, 16,800, and 15,500. Although studies involving placental passage of sargramostim have not been conducted, endogenous

GM-CSF does cross the human placenta. In an *in vitro* experiment using term placentas, small amounts (about 2.4%) of GM-CSF crossed to the fetal side (2). Therefore, sargramostim also probably crosses the placenta, at least at term.

Endogenous GM-CSF promotes the growth and development of pre-implantation embryos (3). GM-CSF is synthesized in the uterus with the highest concentrations occurring around the interval when implantation would occur (4).

In a 2003 study, levels of endogenous free GM-CSF were measured in peripheral blood in pregnant and nonpregnant women and in women with recurrent spontaneous abortions (RSA) (5). In healthy women, a significant increase in GM-CSF levels was measured during pregnancy, but there was no increase in women with RSA. After an IV infusion of immunoglobulin, however, the GM-CSF levels almost doubled in women with RSA (5).

Other investigators have reached conflicting conclusions on the presence of endogenous GM-CSF in maternal blood and amniotic fluid. One study was unable to detect GM-CSF expression (using mRNA coding) in maternal serum at any stage of pregnancy or in nonpregnant women (6). Similarly, amniotic fluid GM-CSF was undetectable in laboring and non-laboring women at term in another study (7). In contrast, a third study found that amniotic fluid GM-CSF concentrations increased as a function of gestational age, the status of the membranes (intact or ruptured), and the presence of labor (8). In addition, a fourth study found a significant increase in placental and peripheral blood levels of GM-CSF in women with preeclampsia (9).

No reports describing the use of sargramostim in human pregnancy have been located. The absence of animal and human pregnancy data prevents an assessment of the risk from maternal administration that this cytokine presents to a human embryo or fetus. However, sargramostim differs only slightly from endogenous GM-CSF. In addition, maternal serum concentrations of natural GM-CSF increase throughout pregnancy with the highest levels occurring during term labor (10). Therefore, it is doubtful if recommended doses of sargramostim will cause direct toxicity to the embryo or fetus. Until human pregnancy data are available, however, the safest course is to avoid sargramostim during gestation. Planned or inadvertent pregnancy exposure appears to represent a low risk for the embryo and fetus.

BREAST FEEDING SUMMARY

RECOMMENDATION: No Human Data - Probably Compatible

No reports describing the use of sargramostim during human lactation have been located. Endogenous granulocyte-macrophage colony-stimulating factor (GM-CSF) is excreted into breast milk (11). Using an immunoradiometric assay, milk concentrations of GM-CSF (100 pg/mL) were much higher than the levels in the cord blood or maternal and infant serums. At 5 days of age, breast-fed infants had higher serum GM-CSF concentrations than formula-fed infants, but the difference was not significant. However, there was no difference in neutrophil chemotaxis between the groups suggesting that either GM-CSF was inactivated or not absorbed from the milk (11). In contrast, a study using an enzyme-linked immunosorbent assay (ELISA) was unable to detect GM-CSF (<10 pg/mL) in breast milk (12).

Whether sargramostim, a glycoprotein that is slightly different from the natural protein, is excreted into milk is not known, but its close similarity to native GM-CSF suggests that it also will be excreted into milk. The effect on a nursing infant from this exposure is unknown, but because endogenous GM-CSF is present in milk and appears to be inactivated or not absorbed, the risk from sargramostim is probably very low or nonexistent.

References

1. Product information. Leukine. Berlex Laboratories, 2004.
2. Gregor H, Egarter C, Levin D, Sternberger B, Heinze G, Leitich H, Reisenberger K. The passage of granulocyte-macrophage colony-stimulating factor across the human placenta perfused in vitro. J Soc Gynecol Investig 1999;6:307–10.
3. Sjöblom C, Wikland M, Robertson SA. Granulocyte-macrophage colony-stimulating factor (GM-CSF) acts independently of the beta common subunit of the GM-CSF receptor to prevent inner cell mass apoptosis in human embryos. Biol Reprod 2002;67:1817–23.
4. Salamonsen LA, Dimitriadis E, Robb L. Cytokines in implantation. Semin Reprod Med 2000;18:299–310.
5. Perricone R, De Carolis C, Giacomelli R, Guarino MD, De Sanctis G, Fontana L. GM-CSF and pregnancy: evidence of significantly reduced blood concentrations in unexplained recurrent abortion efficiently reverted by intravenous immunoglobulin treatment. Am J Reprod Immunol 2003;50:232–7.
6. Tranchot-Diallo J, Gras G, Parnet-Mathieu F, Benveniste O, Marcé D, Roques P, Milliez J, Chaquat G, Dormont D. Modulations of cytokine expression in pregnant women. Am J Reprod Immunol 1997;37:215–26.
7. Oláh KS, Vince GS, Neilson JP, Deniz G, Johnson PM. Interleukin-6, interferon-γ, interleukin-8, and granulocyte-macrophage colony-stimulating factor levels in human amniotic fluid at term. J Reprod Immunol 1996;32:89–98.
8. Bry K, Hallman M, Teramo K, Waffarn F, Lappalainen U. Granulocyte-macrophage colony-stimulating factor in amniotic fluid and in airway specimens of newborn infants. Pediatr Res 1997;41:105–9.
9. Hayashi M, Hamada Y, Ohkura T. Elevation of granulocyte-macrophage colony-stimulating factor in the placenta and blood in preeclampsia. Am J Obstet Gynecol 2004;190:456–61.
10. Vassiliadis S, Ranella A, Papadimitriou L, Makrygiannakis A, Athanassakis I. Serum levels of pro- and anti-inflammatory cytokines in non-pregnant women, during pregnancy, labour and abortion. Mediators Inflamm 1998;7:69–72.
11. Gasparoni A, Chirico G, Ciardelli L, Marchesi ME, Rondini G. Granulocyte-macrophage colony-stimulating factor in human milk. Eur J Pediatr 1996;155:69.
12. Srivastave MD, Srivastava A, Brouhard B, Saneto R, Groh-Wargo S, Kubit J. Cytokines in human milk. Res Commun Mol Pathol Pharmacol 1996;93:263–87.

Name:	**SCOPOLAMINE**	Risk Factor:	C_M
Class:	**Parasympatholytic (Anticholinergic)**		

FETAL RISK SUMMARY

RECOMMENDATION: Human Data Suggest Low Risk

S

Scopolamine is an anticholinergic agent. A scopolamine transdermal system is used to prevent nausea and vomiting associated with motion sickness and recovery from anesthesia and surgery.

Reproduction studies in rats with daily IV doses did not observe fetal harm. A marginal embryotoxic effect was seen in rabbits at daily IV doses that produced plasma concentrations approximately 100 times the level achieved in humans with the transdermal system (1).

The Collaborative Perinatal Project monitored 50,282 mother-child pairs, 309 of whom used scopolamine in the 1st trimester (2, pp. 346–353). For anytime use, 881 exposures were recorded (2, p. 439). In neither case was evidence found for an association with malformations. However, when the group of parasympatholytics was taken as a whole (2323 exposures), a possible association with minor malformations was found (2, pp. 346–353).

In a surveillance study of Michigan Medicaid recipients conducted between 1985 and 1992 involving 229,101 completed pregnancies, 27 newborns had been exposed to scopolamine during the 1st trimester (F. Rosa, personal communication, FDA, 1993). One (3.7%)

major birth defect was observed (one expected), but specific information on the malformation is not available. No anomalies were observed in six categories of defects, including cardiovascular defects, oral clefts, spina bifida, polydactyly, limb-reduction defects, and hypospadias.

Scopolamine readily crosses the placenta (3). When administered to the mother at term, fetal effects include tachycardia, decreased heart rate variability, and decreased heart rate deceleration (4–6). Maternal tachycardia is comparable to that with other anticholinergic agents, such as atropine or glycopyrrolate (7).

Scopolamine toxicity in a newborn has been described (8). The mother had received six doses of scopolamine (1.8 mg total) with several other drugs during labor. Symptoms in the female infant consisted of fever, tachycardia, and lethargy; she was also "barrel chested" without respiratory depression. Therapy with physostigmine reversed the condition.

In a clinical study in women undergoing cesarean section, a scopolamine transdermal system was used with epidural anesthesia and opiate analgesia and no evidence of central nervous system depression was observed in the newborns (1).

BREAST FEEDING SUMMARY

RECOMMENDATION: Limited Human Data - Probably Compatible

No reports of adverse effects secondary to scopolamine in breast milk have been located. The drug is excreted into human milk (1). The American Academy of Pediatrics classifies scopolamine as compatible with breast-feeding (9).

References

1. Product information. Transderm Scop. Novartis Consumer Health, 2000.
2. Heinonen OP, Slone D, Shapiro S. *Birth Defects and Drugs in Pregnancy*. Littleton, MA: Publishing Sciences Group, 1977.
3. Moya F, Thorndike V. The effects of drugs used in labor on the fetus and newborn. Clin Pharmacol Ther 1963;4:628–53.
4. Shenker L. Clinical experiences with fetal heart rate monitoring of one thousand patients in labor. Am J Obstet Gynecol 1973;115:1111–6.
5. Boehm FH, Growdon JH Jr. The effect of scopolamine on fetal heart rate baseline variability. Am J Obstet Gynecol 1974;120:1099–1104.
6. Ayromlooi J, Tobias M, Berg P. The effects of scopolamine and ancillary analgesics upon the fetal heart rate recording. J Reprod Med 1980;25:323–6.
7. Diaz DM, Diaz SF, Marx GF. Cardiovascular effects of glycopyrrolate and belladonna derivatives in obstetric patients. Bull N Y Acad Med 1980;56:245–8.
8. Evens RP, Leopold JC. Scopolamine toxicity in a newborn. Pediatrics 1980;66:329–30.
9. Committee on Drugs, American Academy of Pediatrics. The transfer of drugs and other chemicals into human milk. Pediatrics 2001;108:776–89.

Name:	SECOBARBITAL	Risk Factor:	D_M
Class:	Sedative/Hypnotic		

FETAL RISK SUMMARY

RECOMMENDATION: Limited Human Data - Probably Compatible

No reports linking the use of secobarbital with congenital defects have been located. The Collaborative Perinatal Project monitored 50,282 mother-child pairs, 378 of whom had 1st trimester exposure to secobarbital (1). No evidence was found to suggest a relationship to large categories of major or minor malformations or to individual defects. Hemorrhagic disease of the newborn and barbiturate withdrawal are theoretical possibilities (see also Phenobarbital).

An *in utero* study found no evidence of chromosomal changes on exposure to secobarbital (2).

BREAST FEEDING SUMMARY

RECOMMENDATION: Limited Human Data - Probably Compatible

Secobarbital is excreted into breast milk (3). The amount and effects on the nursing infant are not known. The American Academy of Pediatrics classifies secobarbital as compatible with breast-feeding (4).

References

1. Heinonen OP, Slone D, Shapiro S. *Birth Defects and Drugs in Pregnancy*. Littleton, MA: Publishing Sciences Group, 1977:336–7.
2. Stenchever MA, Jarvis JA. Effect of barbiturates on the chromosomes of human cells in vitro—a negative report. J Reprod Med 1970;5:69–71.
3. Wilson JT, Brown RD, Cherek DR, Dailey JW, Hilman B, Jobe PC, Manno BR, Manno JE, Redetzki HM, Stewart JJ. Drug excretion in human breast milk: principles, pharmacokinetics and projected consequences. Clin Pharmacokinet 1980;5:1–66.
4. Committee on Drugs, American Academy of Pediatrics. The transfer of drugs and other chemicals into human milk. Pediatrics 2001;108:776–89.

Name:	**SELEGILINE**	Risk Factor:	C_M
Class:	**Antiparkinsonian Agent**		

FETAL RISK SUMMARY

RECOMMENDATION: Limited Human Data - Animal Data Suggest Low Risk

Selegiline (*l*-deprenyl; MAO-B), a selective irreversible inhibitor of monoamine oxidase type B, is used as an adjunct in the management of parkinsonian patients being treated with levodopa/carbidopa. The drug has no beneficial effect when used alone (1,2).

Reproduction studies in pregnant rats and rabbits at doses up to 35 and 95 times the human therapeutic dose based on a body surface area (HTD), respectively, did not reveal any evidence of teratogenicity (1,2). At the highest doses tested, however, rat fetal body weight was decreased, and the number of resorptions and postimplantation losses in rabbits increased, resulting in fewer live fetuses. An increase in the number of stillbirths and decreases in pup survival and body weight (at birth and throughout the lactation period) were observed when rats were given doses up to 15 and 62 times the HTD during late gestation and throughout lactation (1,2). At 62 times the HTD, no pups born alive survived to day 4 postpartum.

In a 1994 study, rats were treated daily throughout gestation with a combination of SC selegiline (3 mg/kg) and clorgyline, a monoamine oxidase-A inhibitor (3 mg/kg) (3). In another treatment group, the same doses of the drugs were administered to pregnant females throughout gestation but, at birth, the daily injections of the drugs were administered to the pups until sacrifice. Saline control groups were used for comparison. Pregnancy duration was significantly longer in the treated groups than in controls, but the litter sizes were the same. Other developmental milestones (eye opening, incisor eruption, or

S

olfactory responses) were similar to that of controls. Pup weight gain in both treatment groups was significantly slower than their controls. The decreased weight gain may have been due to less frequent nursing, a condition that was not resolved even when the pups were cross-fostered with control dams. None of the exposed offspring had changes in the development of the dopamine system (as indicated by dopamine terminal density). Moreover, monoamine oxidase (MAO) activity in the brain tissue of pups exposed to the drugs only during gestation was not significantly different from that of controls at 5 days of age. In contrast, MAO activity in pups continually exposed to the drugs was significantly less than controls. Compared with controls, the treatment groups were very aggressive, frequently biting the investigators. In addition, significant deficits in passive avoidance were observed at 24 days of age, and open field activity was significantly increased at 30 days of age. These two results were thought to be a measure of impulsivity (3). Major alterations of the serotonin system were also observed (as indicated by serotonin terminal density) in the hippocampus (higher density), caudate (higher density), and cortex (less density at 5 and 30 days, but increased at 15 days). Seizures and visual impairment were noted in pups that received the drugs during pregnancy and after birth, but not in those exposed only *in utero*.

It is not known if selegiline crosses the placenta to the fetus. The low molecular weight (about 188 for the free base), however, suggests that passage to the fetus should be expected.

Human pregnancy experience with selegiline is limited. A 1998 report described a case involving a 34-year-old woman with an 8-year history of Parkinson's disease who became pregnant while under treatment with selegiline (10 mg/day), levodopa (450 mg/day), and benserazide (128.25 mg/day) (4). Because of insufficient pregnancy safety information, selegiline was discontinued (gestational time not specified). A normal healthy, 3050-g, 49-cm-long male infant was delivered at term with Apgar scores of 9, 10, and 10 at 1, 5, and 10 minutes, respectively.

In a second case, a 39-year-old woman with a 5-year history of Parkinson's disease took selegiline (10 mg/day), levodopa (400–600 mg/day), and benserazide (100–150 mg/day) throughout gestation (5). She was advised to stop selegiline but continued it against medical advice. She delivered a healthy 3800-g male infant at term with Apgar scores of 10 at 1 and 10 minutes. She breast-fed the infant for 3 days and then changed to bottle feeding out of concern over drug transfer into her breast milk. The boy, monitored closely by a pediatrician and a neurologist, was doing very well at 10 years of age with normal somatic and mental development, and was excelling at school and in sports.

In summary, only two cases of exposure to selegiline during human pregnancy have been located, and only one of them involved exposure throughout gestation. Although there is no indication of physical teratogenicity in animal studies or the two human cases, selegiline did result in significant neurological changes in rats when combined with another monoamine oxidase inhibitor. Until additional human data are available, the use of selegiline during pregnancy should be avoided if possible (4,5).

BREAST FEEDING SUMMARY

RECOMMENDATION: Limited Human Data - Potential Toxicity

Except for the one case above (breast-feeding for 3 days), no reports have described the use of selegiline during human lactation. The low molecular weight (about 188 for the free base) suggests that excretion into breast milk should be expected. The effects of this exposure on a nursing infant are unknown. However, significant neurotoxicity was observed in rat pups administered the combination of selegiline and clorgyline directly (see above) (3). Although, in that study, two MAO inhibitors were used and the dose of selegiline was high, the safest course is to avoid selegiline during nursing, at least until the amount of the drug in human milk has been determined.

References

1. Product information. Carbex. Endo Pharmaceuticals, 2000.
2. Product information. Eldepryl. Somerset Pharmaceuticals, 2000.
3. Whitaker-Azmitia PM, Zhang X, Clarke C. Effects of gestational exposure to monoamine oxidase inhibitors in rats: preliminary behavioral and neurochemical studies. Neuropsychopharmacology 1994;11:125–32.
4. Hagell P, Odin P, Vinge E. Pregnancy in Parkinson's disease: a review of the literature and a case report. Mov Disord 1998;13:34–8.
5. Kupsch A, Oertel WH. Selegiline, pregnancy, and Parkinson' disease. Mov Disord 1998;13:175–94.

Name: **SENNA** Risk Factor: **C**
Class: **Laxative**

FETAL RISK SUMMARY

RECOMMENDATION: Compatible

Senna, a naturally occurring laxative, contains the stereoisomeric glucosides sennosides A and B. These anthraquinone glucosides are prodrugs that are converted by bacterial enzymes in the colon to rhein-9-anthrone that is oxidized to rhein, the active cathartic agent of senna (1). Senna is not teratogenic in animals (2). No reports of human teratogenicity or other fetal toxicity have been located.

BREAST FEEDING SUMMARY

RECOMMENDATION: Compatible

S

Sennosides A and B are not excreted into breast milk. A 1973 study using colorimetric analysis (sensitivity limit 0.34 μg/mL) failed to detect the natural agents (3). The active metabolite, rhein, however, is excreted into milk in very small amounts (1). Lactating women administered 5 g of senna daily for 3 days excreted a mean 0.007% of the dose in their milk and no adverse effects were observed in the nursing infants. This is compatible with the fact that the anthraquinone laxatives are absorbed only slightly after oral administration (4). In addition to the study above (1), use of the laxative during lactation has been reported in three other studies (3,5,6). Although diarrhea occurred in some of the infants, this was probably related to other causes, not to senna. In one study, mothers who ingested a single 100-mg dose of senna (containing 8.6 mg of sennosides A and B) and whose infants developed diarrhea were later given a double dose of the laxative (3). No diarrhea was observed in the infants after the higher dose. The American Academy of Pediatrics classifies senna as compatible with breast-feeding (7).

References

1. Faber P, Strenge-Hesse A. Relevance of rhein excretion into breast milk. Pharmacology 1988;36(Suppl 1):212–20.
2. Shepard TH. *Catalog of Teratogenic Agents*. 6th ed. Baltimore, MD: Johns Hopkins University Press, 1989:574–5.
3. Werthmann MW Jr, Krees SV. Quantitative excretion of Senokot in human breast milk. Med Ann Dist Columbia 1973;42:4–5.
4. American Hospital Formulary Service. *Drug Information 1997*. Bethesda, MD: American Society of Health-System Pharmacists, 1997:2236–8.
5. Baldwin WF. Clinical study of senna administration to nursing mothers: assessment of effects on infant bowel habits. Can Med Assoc J 1963;89:566–8.
6. Greenhalf JO, Leonard HSD. Laxatives in the treatment of constipation in pregnant and breast-feeding mothers. Practitioner 1973;210:259–63.
7. Committee on Drugs, American Academy of Pediatrics. The transfer of drugs and other chemicals into human milk. Pediatrics 2001;108:776–89.

Name: **SERTRALINE** Risk Factor: **C_M**

Class: **Antidepressant**

FETAL RISK SUMMARY

RECOMMENDATION: Human Data Suggest Risk in 3rd Trimester

Although the mechanism of action of the antidepressant sertraline is unknown, it is a selective serotonin reuptake inhibitor (SSRI) similar to other drugs in this class. This effect of sertraline results in the potentiation of serotonin activity in the brain. The chemical structure of sertraline is unrelated to other antidepressants.

All the antidepressant agents in the SSRI class (citalopram, escitalopram, fluoxetine, fluvoxamine, paroxetine, and sertraline) are thought to share a similar mechanism of action, although they have different chemical structures. These differences could be construed as evidence against any conclusion that they share similar effects on the embryo, fetus, or newborn. In the mouse embryo, however, craniofacial morphogenesis appears to be regulated, at least in part, by serotonin. Interference with serotonin regulation by chemically different inhibitors produces similar craniofacial defects (1). Regardless of the structural differences, therefore, some of the potential adverse effects on pregnancy outcome may also be similar.

Reproductive studies in rats and rabbits, conducted with doses up to approximately 4 times the maximum recommended human dose based on body surface area (MRHD) did not reveal evidence of teratogenicity (2). Delayed ossification of rat and rabbit fetuses, however, occurred at doses during organogenesis of 0.5 and 4 times the MRHD, respectively. When female rats were dosed at 1 times the MRHD during the last third of gestation and throughout lactation, an increase in the number of stillbirths, decreased pup survival, and decreased pup weights were observed. The decreased pup survival was shown to be a result of *in utero* exposure to sertraline. The no effect dose for rat pup mortality was 0.5 times the MRHD (2).

Consistent with its low molecular weight (about 307 for the free base), sertraline crosses the human placenta. A 2003 study of the placental transfer of antidepressants found cord blood:maternal serum ratios for sertraline and its metabolite that ranged from 0.14–0.66 and 0.14–0.77, respectively (3). The dose-to-delivery interval was 7–35 hours with the highest ratio for the parent drug and metabolite occurring at 24 hours.

S

A 24-year-old woman (gravida 5, para 0, therapeutic abortion 4) was treated before and during the first few weeks of gestation with sertraline for depression and bulimia (K. Murray and D. Jackson, personal communication, Eugene, Oregon, 1994). Ultrasound revealed a single fetus with anencephaly and an abdominal wall defect. Chromosomal analysis performed after termination indicated that the fetus had trisomy 18 (47,XX,+18). Because trisomy 18 is a naturally occurring mutation, in the absence of any animal or other evidence for a causal relationship, it is doubtful that the drug therapy was related to the outcome of this pregnancy.

Fifteen diverse birth defects have been reported to the FDA as of December 1995 (F. Rosa, personal communication, FDA, 1996).

A 1995 report described the use of sertraline 100 mg/day and nortriptyline 125 mg/day in a woman with recurrent major depression (4). The patient ingested these drugs before and throughout gestation. Attempts to discontinue the agents in the 1st and 2nd trimesters were unsuccessful. She eventually gave birth at term to a healthy infant (sex and weight not specified) who, at age 3 months, was doing well and achieving the appropriate developmental milestones (see also Breast-Feeding section below) (4).

A brief 1995 report described a case of a 32-year-old woman who took sertraline 200 mg/day throughout pregnancy (5). Lithium and thioridazine were also taken during the first 6 weeks of gestation. She continued the same dose of sertraline for 3 weeks after delivery of a healthy, full term male infant. During this period, she breastfed the infant who was feeding and developing normally. One day after she stopped sertraline, the infant developed agitation, restlessness, poor feeding, constant crying, insomnia, and enhanced startle reaction. The infant's symptoms continued for another 48 hours before gradually resolving over several days. Similar symptoms were not observed in the mother. Because the same type of symptoms has been observed in adults after discontinuing sertraline (1), the authors attributed them to withdrawal (5).

A 1998 non-interventional observational cohort study described the outcomes of pregnancies in women who had been prescribed one or more of 34 newly marketed drugs by general practitioners in England (6). Data were obtained by questionnaires sent to the prescribing physicians 1 month after the expected or possible date of delivery. In 831 (78%) of the pregnancies, a newly marketed drug was thought to have been taken during the 1st trimester with birth defects noted in 14 (2.5%) singleton births of the 557 newborns (10 sets of twins). In addition, two birth defects were observed in aborted fetuses. However, few of the aborted fetuses were examined. Sertraline was taken during the 1st trimester in 51 pregnancies. The outcomes of these pregnancies included 1 ectopic pregnancy, 2 spontaneous abortions, 11 elective abortions, 1 intrauterine death, 26 normal, full-term newborns, 2 infants with birth defects, and 8 pregnancies lost to follow-up. The congenital malformations were one case each of congenital laryngeal stridor and a duplication cyst (gastrointestinal) (6).

A prospective, multicenter, controlled cohort study published in 1998 evaluated the pregnancy outcomes of 267 women exposed to one or more of three SSRI antidepressants during the 1st trimester: fluvoxamine ($N = 26$), paroxetine ($N = 97$), and sertraline ($N = 147$) (7). The women were combined into a study group without differentiation as to the drug they had consumed. All of the women had contacted a teratogen information service about their use of the drugs during pregnancy. A randomly selected control group ($N = 267$) was formed from women who had contacted one service after exposure to nonteratogenic agents. The pregnancy outcomes were determined, in most cases, 6–9 months after delivery. The study group was significantly more likely to smoke cigarettes and to have had a previous elective abortion but less likely to be a primigravid. Other characteristics, such as a previous spontaneous abortion, alcohol consumption, and maternal age at conception did not differ between the groups. As for pregnancy outcomes, no significant differences were measured in the number of live births, spontaneous or elective abortions, stillbirths, major malformations, birth weight, or gestational age at birth. Nine major malformations were observed in each group. The relative risk for major anomalies was 1.06 (95% confidence interval [CI] 0.43–2.62). No clustering of defects was apparent. In the study group, no differences were found in the pregnancy outcomes of smokers compared to nonsmokers. In addition, the outcomes of women who took an antidepressant throughout gestation were similar to those who took an antidepressant only during the 1st trimester (7). One of the investigators, in response to subsequent correspondence regarding the study (8,9), clarified that all of the 267 women in the study group had taken an antidepressant during embryogenesis (10). Other concerns relating to the outcomes and sample size were also addressed.

In 1999, the Swedish Medical Birth Registry published the results of a study on the use of antidepressants in early pregnancy and delivery outcome for the years 1995–1997 (11). During the period, 281,728 infants were registered, 531 of whom had been exposed *in utero* to SSRI antidepressants, 15 to SSRIs plus a non-SSRI antidepressant, and 423 to non-SSRI antidepressants. Of the 34 women who used sertraline, 32 used it alone and 2 used it in combination with another SSRI agent (citalopram and paroxetine). There were no significant differences in relative risk (RR = observed/expected) for birth defects between those exposed to any antidepressant (total 39; RR 1.13), SSRIs only (total 21; RR 1.12), and non-SSRIs only (total 18; RR 1.15) (specific defects were only given for those exposed to citalopram). Similarly, no significant differences in infant survival were observed among the groups. A shorter gestational duration (<37 weeks) was observed for exposure to any antidepressant (OR 1.43, 95% CI 1.14–1.80) but no difference between SSRI and non-SSRI antidepressants. Moreover, antidepressant exposure was not associated with an increased risk of low birth weight (defined as <2500 g) among singletons as the crude OR 1.32, 95% CI 0.96–1.80 decreased to 1.03 after adjustment for confounders (11).

A 1999 abstract detailed the prospectively ascertained outcomes of 112 pregnant women taking sertraline compared to 191 controls (12). All of the women had contacted a teratology information service. The rate of major congenital defects did not differ between subjects and controls (3.8% vs. 1.9%). In the sertraline group, the defects included: bilateral choanal atresia; valvular pulmonic stenosis with an atrial septal aneurysm; unilateral clubfoot; and Down syndrome (pregnancy terminated). No difference in the rate of minor congenital defects was seen in the 158 infants who received a dysmorphological examination. Infants exposed to sertraline in the 3rd trimester were more likely to be premature, to have neonatal transition difficulty, or to be admitted to a special care nursery. A dose response was noted for the latter two complications (12).

The effect of SSRIs on birth outcomes and postnatal neurodevelopment of children exposed prenatally was reported in 2003 (13). Thirty-one children (mean age 12.9 months) exposed during pregnancy to SSRIs (15 sertraline, 8 paroxetine, 7 fluoxetine, and 1 fluvoxamine) were compared to 13 children (mean age 17.7 months) of mothers with depression who elected not to take medications during pregnancy. All of the mothers had healthy lifestyles (i.e., took prenatal vitamins, no smoking, little alcohol use, and regular exercise). The timing of the exposures was 71% in the 1st trimester, 74% in the 3rd trimester, and 45% throughout. The average duration of breast-feeding in the subjects and controls was 6.4 and 8.5 months. Twenty-eight (90%) subjects nursed their infants, 17 of who took SSRIs (10 sertraline, 4 paroxetine, and 3 fluoxetine) compared to 11 (85%) controls, three of whom took sertraline. There were no significant differences between the groups in terms of gestational age at birth, premature births, birth weight and length or, at follow-up, in sex distribution or gain in weight and length (expressed at percentage). Seven (23%) of the exposed infants were admitted to a neonatal intensive care unit (6 respiratory distress, 4 meconium aspiration, and 1 cardiac murmur) compared to none of the controls ($p = 0.06$). Follow-up examinations were conducted by a pediatric neurologist, psychologist, and a dysmorphologist who were blinded as to the mother's mediations status. The mean Apgar scores at 1 and 5 minutes were lower in the exposed group than in controls, 7.0 vs. 8.2, and 8.4 vs. 9.0, respectively. There was one major defect in each group: small asymptomatic ventricular septal defect (exposed); bilateral lacrimal duct stenosis that required surgery (control). The test outcomes for mental development were similar in the groups, but significant differences in the subjects included a slight delay in psychomotor development and lower behavior motor quality (tremulousness and fine motor movements) (13).

A 2004 prospective study examined the effect of four SSRIs (citalopram, fluoxetine, paroxetine, and sertraline) on newborn neurobehavior, including behavioral state, sleep organization, motor activity, heart rate variability, tremulousness, and startles (14). Seventeen SSRI-exposed, healthy, full-birth-weight newborns and 17 nonexposed, full-birth-weight newborns were matched for maternal cigarette use, social class, and maternal age. A wide range of disrupted neurobehavioral outcomes were shown in the infants exposed *in utero* to SSRIs. After adjustment for gestational age, the exposed infants were found to differ significantly from controls in terms of tremulousness, behavioral states, and sleep organization. Although the effects observed on motor activity, startles, and heart rate variability were not significant after adjustment, the investigators thought they might be mediated through the effects of SSRI exposure on gestational age (14).

In summary, the limited animal and human data suggest that sertraline is not a major teratogen. A 1999 review of SSRI antidepressants concluded that if therapy were required during pregnancy, the SSRIs were a good choice because of their side-effect profile and safety in overdose (15). However, the studies cited above lack the sensitivity to identify minor anomalies because of the absence of standardized examinations. Late-appearing major defects might have been missed in one study because of the timing of the questionnaires. One study has demonstrated that an SSRI (see Fluoxetine) can induce long-term, perhaps permanent changes in the brains of *in utero* exposed rats. As described above, disrupted neurobehavior has been observed in human infants. Moreover, withdrawal symptoms have been reported with sertraline and other SSRIs (see Citalopram, Fluoxetine, and Paroxetine). Long-term studies of the neurobehavior of exposed infants are warranted.

S

BREAST FEEDING SUMMARY

RECOMMENDATION: Limited Human Data - Potential Toxicity

Six reports describing the use of sertraline during lactation have been located (4,16–20). In a 1995 case (described above), a woman with recurrent major depression consumed sertraline 100 mg/day and nortriptyline 125 mg/day throughout gestation and while breast-feeding her term infant (4). After 3 weeks of breast-feeding, milk levels (8 times during a 24-hour interval) and maternal and infant serum levels (12 hours after the dose) were measured. Serum sampling was repeated a second time after 7 weeks of exclusive breast-feeding. Maternal serum levels at 3 and 7 weeks were 48 and 47 ng/mL, respectively, while the serum levels in her fully breast-fed infant were below the test sensitivity (<0.5 ng/mL) at both samplings. Milk concentrations during the 24-hour period ranged from 8.8 to 43 ng/mL, with the highest concentrations in the samples obtained at 5 and 9 hours after the dose. Milk levels of nortriptyline were not analyzed nor were metabolites of either drug. At the 3-week sampling, serum levels of nortriptyline in the mother and child were 120 ng/mL and not detectable (test sensitivity 10 ng/mL), respectively. These tests were not repeated at 7 weeks. The infant was doing well at 3 months of age with normal weight and development (4).

A brief 1995 correspondence described a 32-year-old woman who was treated with sertraline 150 mg/day during the second half of gestation and while breast-feeding (16). She stopped nursing after 11 days. No adverse effects were noted in the normal healthy infant either during or after breast-feeding.

In four lactating women being treated for postpartum depression with maximum doses of either 50 mg/day ($N = 2$) or 100 mg/day ($N = 2$), whole blood 5-hydroxytryptamine (serotonin) levels in the mothers and infants were determined before and after 9–12 weeks of therapy (17). Sertraline and desmethylsertraline plasma levels were also measured at the time of post-exposure sampling. One infant in each dose group was fully breast-fed and the other two infants were breast-fed 3 or 4 times daily. The ages of the infants at the start of maternal treatment were 15 days, 26 days, 6 months, and 12 months. Sertraline and metabolite plasma levels in the infants were less than 2.5 ng/mL and 5 ng/mL, respectively, compared with maternal plasma levels ranging from 10.3 to 48.2 ng/mL and from 19.7 to 64.5 ng/mL, respectively. Little to no change was observed in the platelet (equivalent to whole-blood) levels of serotonin in the infants, in contrast to the marked decreases measured in the mothers. Although the authors could not exclude other possible pharmacologic effects in the infants, the lack of changes measured in serotonin levels was reassuring (17).

Milk samples were collected from 12 women after a sertraline dose at 4–6 hours for 24 hours (18). Additionally, maternal (24 hours after a dose) and infant serum levels (2–4 hours after nursing) were also determined in 11 mother-infant pairs. All of the subjects had been taking a fixed dose (25–200 mg/day) for 14 to 21 days. Three of the women had been treated with the antidepressant during pregnancy. Therapy was started in the postpartum period in the remaining nine subjects. Sertraline (range 17–173 ng/mL) and the relatively inactive metabolite, desmethylsertraline (range 22–294 ng/mL), were present in all milk samples. The first 10–20 mL of milk (foremilk) had approximately one-half of the drug concentrations of sertraline and metabolite as did the hindmilk. The mean milk:serum ratio for the parent drug was 2.3 ± 1.3 and 1.4 ± 0.8 for the metabolite. In maternal serum (doses 25–150 mg/day), the concentrations of sertraline and metabolite ranged from 9 to 92 ng/mL and 15 to 212 ng/mL, respectively. In contrast, only three infants had measurable serum sertraline levels (2.7–3.0 ng/mL) whereas six had measurable metabolite levels (1.6–10.0 ng/mL) (quantitative limit for both 1.0 ng/mL). The calculated sertraline and metabolite doses received by the infants from milk ranged from 0.019 to 0.124 mg/day and 0.023 to 0.181 mg/day, respectively (18).

In a 1998 study, the mean milk:plasma ratios of sertraline and the metabolite in eight lactating women (mean dose 1.05 mg/kg/day) were 1.93 and 1.64, respectively (19). The estimated infant doses were 0.2% and 0.3%, respectively, of the weight-adjusted maternal dose. Neither sertraline or desmethylsertraline was detected in the plasma samples obtained from four infants. No adverse effects from the drug exposure were noted in the infants. All had achieved normal development milestones (19).

In another 1998 study, serum levels of sertraline and desmethylsertraline were measured in nine nursing mother-infant pairs (20). The maternal serum levels ranged from 12 to 134 ng/mL and 28 to 285 ng/mL, respectively. In six infants, the serum concentration of sertraline was below the quantification limit (<2 ng/mL), not detectable in one, and 3 ng/mL in another. The metabolite serum levels in these eight infants ranged from nonquantifiable to 24 ng/mL. In the ninth infant, however, the serum sertraline concentration was 64 ng/mL, 55% of the mother's serum level (117 ng/mL). The metabolite serum concentrations in the infant and mother were 68 and 117 ng/mL, respectively. The mother's dose in this case was 100 mg/day. The serum samples from the mother and infant were drawn 2 hours after a dose. Because the levels were so unusual, the investigators checked the values twice. Although they speculated as to possible cause(s), they were unable to determine why the levels in this particular case were so high (20).

The effect of sertraline on serotonin (5-HT) reuptake in nursing infants was studied in 14 mother-infant pairs in a 2001 report (21). Preexposure levels of 5-HT were drawn from the infants at a mean age of 17.3 weeks, whereas postexposure levels were drawn at a mean age of 26.3 weeks. The mean maternal plasma levels of sertraline and the metabolite desmethylsertraline were 30.7 ng/mL and 45.3 ng/mL. In the mothers, sertraline (25–200 mg/day) caused marked declines (70%–96%) in whole blood (i.e., platelet) 5-HT levels. In contrast, 5-HT levels in nursing infant's whole blood (i.e., platelets) were not affected (preexposure 223.7 ng/mL vs. postexposure 227.0 ng/mL). Infant plasma levels of sertraline and the metabolite were below the level of detection (<2.5 ng/mL and <5.0 ng/mL, respectively). The results suggested that treatment of the mother with sertraline would not affect peripheral or central 5-HT transport in their nursing infants (21).

A 1999 review of SSRI agents concluded that if there were compelling reasons to treat a mother for postpartum depression, a condition in which a rapid antidepressant effect is important, the benefits of therapy with SSRIs would most likely outweigh the risks (22). However, because the long-term effects of exposure to SSRI antidepressants in breast milk on the infant's neurobehavioral development are unknown (no such adverse effects have been identified to date but research is needed), stopping or reducing the frequency of breast-feeding should be considered if therapy with these agents is required. Avoiding nursing around the time of peak maternal concentration (about 4 hours after a dose) may limit infant exposure. The American Academy of Pediatrics classifies sertraline as a drug for which the effect on nursing infants is unknown but may be of concern (23).

S

References

1. Shuey DL, Sadler TW, Lauder JM. Serotonin as a regulator of craniofacial morphogenesis: site-specific malformations following exposure to serotonin uptake inhibitors. Teratology 1992;46:367–78.
2. Product information. Zoloft. Pfizer, 2000.
3. Hendrick V, Stowe ZN, Altshuler LL, Hwang S, Lee E, Haynes D. Placental passage of antidepressant medications. Am J Psychiatry 2003;160:993–6.
4. Altshuler LL, Burt VK, McMullen M, Hendrick V. Breastfeeding and sertraline: a 24-hour analysis. J Clin Psychiatry 1995;56:243–5.
5. Kent LSW, Laidlaw JDD. Suspected congenital sertraline dependence. Br J Psychiatry 1995;167:412–3.
6. Wilton LV, Pearce GL, Martin RM, Mackay FJ, Mann RD. The outcomes of pregnancy in women exposed to newly marketed drugs in general practice in England. Br J Obstet Gynaecol 1998;105:882–9.
7. Kulin NA, Pastuszak A, Sage SR, Schick-Boschetto B, Spivey G, Feldkamp M, Ormond K, Matsui D, Stein-Schechman AK, Cook L, Brochu J, Rieder M, Koren G. Pregnancy outcome following maternal use of the new selective serotonin reuptake inhibitors. A prospective controlled multicenter study. JAMA 1998;279:609–10.
8. Grush LR. Risk of fetal anomalies with exposure to selective serotonin reuptake inhibitors. JAMA 1998;279:1873.
9. Witlin AG. Risk of fetal anomalies with exposure to selective serotonin reuptake inhibitors. JAMA 1998;279:1873.
10. Koren G. In reply. Risk of fetal anomalies with exposure to selective serotonin reuptake inhibitors. JAMA 1998;279:1873–4.
11. Ericson A, Kallen B, Wiholm BE. Delivery outcome

after the use of antidepressants in early pregnancy. Eur J Clin Pharmacol 1999;55:503–8.
12. Chambers CD, Dick LM, Felix RJ, Johnson KA, Jones KL. Pregnancy outcome in women who use sertraline (abstract). Teratology 1999;59:376.
13. Casper RC, Fleisher BE, Lee-Ancajas JC, Gilles A, Gaylor E, DeBattista A, Hoyme HE. Follow-up of children of depressed mothers exposed or not exposed to antidepressant drugs during pregnancy. J Pediatr 2003;142:402–8.
14. Zeskind PS, Stephens LE. Maternal selective serotonin reuptake inhibitor use during pregnancy and newborn neurobehavior. Pediatrics 2004;113:368–75.
15. Masand PS, Gupta S. Selective serotonin-reuptake inhibitors: an update. Harv Rev Psychiatry 1999;7:69–84.
16. Ratan DA, Friedman T. Antidepressants in pregnancy and breast-feeding. Br J Psychiatry 1995;167:824.
17. Epperson CN, Anerson GM, McDougle CJ. Sertraline and breast-feeding. N Engl J Med 1997;336:1189–90.
18. Stowe ZN, Owens MJ, Landry JC, Kilts CD, Ely T, Llewellyn A, Nemeroff CB. Sertraline and desmethylsertraline in human breast milk and nursing infants. Am J Psychiatry 1997;154:1255–60.
19. Kristensen JH, Ilett KF, Dusci LJ, Hackett LP, Yapp P, Wojnar-Horton RE, Roberts MJ, Paech M. Distribution and excretion of sertraline and *N*-desmethylsertraline in human milk. Br J Clin Pharmacol 1998;45:453–7.
20. Wisner KL, Perel JM, Blumer J. Serum sertraline and *N*-desmethylsertraline levels in breast-feeding mother-infant pairs. Am J Psychiatry 1998;155:690–2.
21. Epperson N, Czarkowski KA, Ward-O'Brien D, Weiss E, Gueorguieva R, Jatlow P, Anderson GM. Maternal sertraline treatment and serotonin transport in breast-feeding mother-infant pairs. Am J Psychiatry 2001;158:1631–7.
22. Edwards JG, Anerson I. Systematic review and guide to selection of selective serotonin reuptake inhibitors. Drugs 1999;57:507–33.
23. Committee on Drugs, American Academy of Pediatrics. The transfer of drugs and other chemicals into human milk. Pediatrics 2001;108:776–89.

Name:	**SEVELAMER**	Risk Factor:	C_M
Class:	**Antidote (Phosphate Binders)**		

FETAL RISK SUMMARY

RECOMMENDATION: No Human Data - Animal Data Suggest Low Risk

Sevelamer is a polymeric phosphate binder that is administered orally. It is used in patients with end-stage renal disease for the reduction of serum phosphorus. The drug inhibits intestinal phosphate absorption by binding phosphorus. Sevelamer is not absorbed into the systemic circulation (1).

Reproduction studies have been conducted in rats and rabbits. No evidence of impaired fertility was observed in male and female rats. In pregnant rats, doses about 15 times the human dose based on body weight (HD) or higher caused reduced or irregular ossification of fetal bones. The toxicity was thought to be due to reduced absorption of vitamin D. In rabbits, a dose about 10 times the HD caused an increased incidence of early resorptions resulting in a slight increase in prenatal mortality (1).

No reports describing the use of sevelamer in human pregnancy have been located. The limited animal data suggest a risk of toxicity that may be partially caused by a deficiency of fat-soluble vitamins, such as vitamin D. The effect of sevelamer on the absorption of vitamins in pregnant women has not been studied (1). However, supplementation with higher oral doses of vitamins, especially fat-soluble vitamins (except vitamin A), might be required or IV vitamins should be considered.

BREAST FEEDING SUMMARY

RECOMMENDATION: No Human Data - Probably Compatible

No reports describing the use of sevelamer during human lactation have been located. The drug is not absorbed into the systemic circulation, but it may cause vitamin deficiencies in the mother by preventing intestinal vitamin absorption, especially of fat-soluble vitamins. Because vitamins are excreted into breast milk, thereby further reducing maternal vitamin concentrations, women who are taking sevelamer might have to take higher oral doses of vitamins, especially fat-soluble vitamins (except vitamin A), or IV vitamin administration should be considered.

Reference

1. Product information. Renagel. Genzyme, 2004.

Name:	**SEVOFLURANE**	Risk Factor:	**C**
Class:	**General Anesthetic**		

FETAL RISK SUMMARY

RECOMMENDATION: Limited Human Data - Animal Data Suggest Low Risk

Sevoflurane, a noninflammable general anesthetic agent administered via vaporizer, is indicated for the induction and/or maintenance of anesthesia during surgery. Sevoflurane is in the same class of volatile liquid halogenated agents as desflurane, enflurane, halothane, isoflurane, and methoxyflurane. It has a lower solubility in lipids (oil:gas partition coefficient about 47–53) and blood (blood:gas partition coefficient 0.68) than halothane or isoflurane, but higher than desflurane (1). The anesthetic potency, based on the MAC (*note: the minimum alveolar anesthetic concentration [MAC] is the concentration that causes immobility in 50% of patients exposed to a noxious stimulus such as a surgical incision; it represents the* ED_{50} *[2]*) is about 50% less than that of isoflurane but about 30% more than that of desflurane (1).

In an animal reproduction study, mice were exposed for 8 hours to sevoflurane and enflurane combined with three different concentrations of oxygen (3). Both anesthetic agents caused cleft palate, but the incidence was lower than that observed with halothane. Increasing the concentrations of oxygen lowered the incidence of the defect (3).

The teratogenic potential of sevoflurane, enflurane, and isoflurane was studied by evaluating the effect of each agent on the proliferation and differentiation of cells exiting from the G1-phase of the cell cycle (4). The theory behind the study was that normal development during embryogenesis, organogenesis, and histogenesis depended upon the proliferation and differentiative processes of cell migration (4). For example, valproate, a known human teratogen, is a potent G1-phase inhibitor of the *in vitro* proliferation rate at concentrations less than two times the therapeutic plasma concentration. At anesthetic concentrations less than two times the MAC, the antiproliferative potency of the three agents was isoflurane = enflurane >> sevoflurane. However, in the growth-arrested cell population, there was no specific accumulation of any cell-cycle phase and no specific effect on the G1 phase. The investigators concluded that the three agents lacked the specific *in vitro* characteristics of valproate (4).

In an *in vitro* experiment with pregnant rats, sevoflurane, halothane, and isoflurane significantly inhibited oxytocin-induced contractions of uterine smooth muscle (5).

Two reviews have concluded that, in general, inhalational anesthetics are freely transferred to fetal tissues (6,7) and, in most cases, the maternal and fetal concentrations are equivalent (7). The low molecular weight (about 200) and the presence of sevoflurane in the maternal brain support this assertion.

A 1999 case report described the use of sevoflurane for maintenance of general anesthesia during non-obstetric surgery in a 25-year-old woman at 13 weeks' gestation (8). Six months later a cesarean section delivered a 2820-g female infant without abnormalities.

Two reports described the use of sevoflurane for emergency cesarean section (9,10). Although successful outcomes occurred in both cases, the former report generated several letters and a reply (11–16).

Chronic occupational exposure to anesthetic gases in operating rooms during pregnancy has raised concerns that such exposure could cause birth defects and spontaneous abortions (17). A 1988 review cited a number of studies investigating the possible association between occupational exposure to anesthetic gases and adverse pregnancy outcomes (6). The reviewer concluded that serious methodological weaknesses in these studies precluded arriving at a firm conclusion, but a slightly increased risk of miscarriage was a possibility. However, there was no evidence of an association between occupational exposure and congenital anomalies (6).

A 2004 study, however, found a significant association between maternal occupational exposure to waste anesthetic gases during pregnancy and developmental deficits in their children, including gross and fine motor ability, inattention/hyperactivity, and IQ performance (see Nitrous Oxide).

In summary, sevoflurane is teratogenic in mice, but no reports of its use in early human gestation have been located. The absence of human experience during organogenesis prevents an assessment of the risk for structural anomalies. In addition, general anesthesia usually involves the use of multiple pharmacological agents. Although no teratogenicity has been observed with other halogenated general anesthetic agents, only halothane has 1st trimester human exposure data (see Halothane). Sevoflurane has been used immediately prior to delivery but its effect on the newborn has not been studied. However, its affect on the newborn is probably no different from other general anesthetic agents. The uterine effects of sevoflurane (relaxation and increased blood loss) also appear to be similar to other agents in this class, but the low concentrations used clinically minimize these actions (see Enflurane). All anesthetic agents can cause depression in the newborn that may last for 24 hours or more but, again, this is lessened by the low doses. The potential reproductive toxicity (spontaneous abortion and infertility) of occupational exposure to halogenated general anesthetic agents has not been adequately studied.

BREAST FEEDING SUMMARY

RECOMMENDATION: No Human Data - Probably Compatible

Although sevoflurane has been administered during delivery, the effects of this exposure on the infant that begins nursing immediately after birth have not been described. Sevoflurane is probably excreted into colostrum and milk as suggested by its presence in the maternal blood and its low molecular weight (about 200), but the toxic potential of this exposure for the infant is unknown. However, the risk to a nursing infant from exposure to sevoflurane via milk is probably very low (18). Another halogenated inhalation anesthetic is classified as compatible with breast-feeding by the American Academy of Pediatrics (see Halothane).

References

1. Patel SS, Goa KL. Sevoflurane. A review of its pharmacodynamic and pharmacokinetic properties and its clinical use in general anaesthesia. Drugs 1996;51:658–700.
2. Trevor AJ, Miller RD. General anesthetics. In Katzung BG, ed. *Basic and Clinical Pharmacology*. 8th ed. New York: McGraw-Hill, 2001:426.
3. Natsume N, Miura S, Sugimoto S, Nakamura T, Horiuchi R, Kondo S, Furukawa H, Inagaki S, Kawai T, Yamada M, Arai T, Hosoda R. Teratogenicity caused by halothane, enflurane, and sevoflurane, and changes depending on O_2 concentration (abstract). Teratology 1990;42:30A.
4. O'Leary G, Bacon CL, Odumeru O, Fagan C, Fitzpatrick T, Gallagher HC, Moriarty DC, Regan CM. Antiproliferative actions of inhalational anesthetics: comparisons to the valproate teratogen. Int J Dev Neurosci 2000;18:39–45.
5. Yamakage M, Tsujiguchi N, Chen X, Kamada Y, Namiki A. Sevoflurane inhibits contraction of uterine smooth muscle from pregnant rats similarly to halothane and isoflurane. Can J Anesth 2002;49:62–6.
6. Friedman JM. Teratogen update: anesthetic agents. Teratology 1988;37:69–77.
7. Kanto J. Risk-benefit assessment of anaesthetic agents in the puerperium. Drug Saf 1991;6:285–301.
8. Kanazawa M, Kinefuchi Y, Suzuki T, Fukuyama H, Takiguchi M. The use of sevoflurane anesthesia during early pregnancy. Tokai J Exp Clin Med 1999;24:53–5.
9. Schaut DJ, Khona R, Gross JB. Sevoflurane inhalation induction for emergency cesarean section in a parturient with no intravenous access. Anesthesiology 1997;86:1392–4.
10. Que JC, Lusaya VO. Sevoflurane induction for emergency cesarean section in a parturient in status asthmaticus. Anesthesiology 1999;90:1475–6.
11. Klafta JM. The practice of using sevoflurane inhalation induction for emergency cesarean section and a parturient with no intravenous access. Anesthesiology 1998;88:275.
12. Bhavani-Shankar K, Camann WR. The practice of using sevoflurane inhalation induction for emergency cesarean section and a parturient with no intravenous access. Anesthesiology 1998;88:275–6.
13. Sitzman BT. The practice of using sevoflurane inhalation induction for emergency cesarean section and a parturient with no intravenous access. Anesthesiology 1998;88:276.
14. Gambling DR, Reisner LS. The practice of using sevoflurane inhalation induction for emergency cesarean section and a parturient with no intravenous access. Anesthesiology 1998;88:276–7.
15. Maltby JR. The practice of using sevoflurane inhalation induction for emergency cesarean section and a parturient with no intravenous access. Anesthesiology 1998;88:277–8.
16. Gross JB. The practice of using sevoflurane inhalation induction for emergency cesarean section and a parturient with no intravenous access. Anesthesiology 1998;88:278.
17. Corbett TH. Cancer and congenital anomalies associated with anesthetics. Ann N Y Acad Sci 1976;271:58–66.
18. Spigset O. Anaesthetic agents and excretion in breast milk. Acta Anaesthesiol Scand 1994;38:94–103.

Name: **SIBUTRAMINE** Risk Factor: **C_M**

Class: **Anorexiant**

FETAL RISK SUMMARY

S

RECOMMENDATION: No Human Data - Animal Data Suggest Low Risk

Sibutramine is indicated for the management of obesity. The drug and its two active metabolites (M1 and M2) inhibit the reuptake of norepinephrine, serotonin, and dopamine. They exhibit no anticholinergic or antihistaminergic actions. Because of extensive first-pass hepatic metabolism, sibutramine has a short half-life (1.1 hours). However, M2 has an elimination half-life of 17.2 hours in obese subjects and 22.7 hours in patients with moderate hepatic impairment. Similar data are not available for M1 (1).

Reproduction studies with sibutramine have been conducted in rats and rabbits. In rats, no evidence of teratogenicity or effects on fertility were observed with doses resulting in combined AUCs of M1 and M2 up to about 32 times those obtained after the human dose of 15 mg (HD-AUC). However, maternal toxicity (impaired nest-building behavior) was noted at 13 times the HD-AUC). The no-effect dose for maternal toxicity was approximately 4 times the HD-AUC. In rabbits, maternal toxicity was observed with doses approximately five or more times the HD-AUC. At markedly toxic maternal doses, fetuses of Dutch Belted rabbits had a slightly higher incidence of anomalies (broad short snout, short rounded pinnae, short tail and shorter thickened limb bones) than did controls. At these maternal toxic doses, New Zealand White rabbits had a slightly higher incidence of cardiovascular defects in one study, but a lower incidence in a second study (1).

Although low amounts of sibutramine are transferred to the fetus in rats (1), it is not known if the drug or its active metabolites cross the human placenta. The molecular weight of the parent compound (about 334) is low enough to cross the placenta but its short plasma half-life will limit the amount of drug at the maternal-fetal interface. In addition, the high protein binding of sibutramine and the two metabolites—97%, 94%, and 94%, respectively—also will limit the amounts of drug and metabolites available for transfer to the fetus. However, the M2 active metabolite has a prolonged elimination half-life (17.2 hours or more) that could promote exposure of the embryo/fetus.

A 2004 report described the outcomes of two pregnancies that were exposed to sibutramine early in gestation (2). Both women were taking 10 mg/day of sibutramine. The first pregnancy was exposed during gestational weeks 4–6, the second during weeks 4–8. Both delivered healthy infants at term. The infants were developing normally at 18 and 2 months, respectively, without evidence of major or minor anomalies (2).

In summary, two reports have described the use of sibutramine during early human pregnancy. The animal data suggest a low risk for congenital defects, but the human data are too limited to assess of the actual risk. In general, the use of any anorexiant in pregnancy would be inappropriate, but inadvertent exposures could occur. Women of reproductive age should be counseled to discontinue the drug if a pregnancy is planned. If pregnancy has occurred, the embryo/fetal risk probably is low, but the drug should be discontinued immediately. If sibutramine is used in pregnancy, healthcare professionals are encouraged to call the toll free number (800-670-6126) for information about patient enrollment in the Motherisk study.

BREAST FEEDING SUMMARY

RECOMMENDATION: No Human Data - Potential Toxicity

No reports describing the use of sibutramine during lactation have been located. Although the molecular weight of the parent compound (about 334) is low enough, the short plasma half-life (1.1 hours) and extensive protein binding (97%) argue against the excretion of clinically significant amounts of sibutramine into breast milk. However, there are two active metabolites. Although both are highly protein bound (94% each), the prolonged elimination half-life of one of them (17.2 hours or more) could allow excretion into milk and eventual accumulation in an infant with immature liver function. The effects of this exposure on a nursing infant are unknown, but there is a potential for significant toxicity (e.g., anorexia, constipation, tachycardia, and stimulation of the central nervous system). Therefore, women receiving sibutramine should not breast-feed.

References

1. Product information. Meridia. Abbott Laboratories, 2004.
2. Kadioglu M, Ulku C, Yaris F, Kesim M, Kalyoncu NI, Yaris E. Sibutramine use in pregnancy: report of two cases. Birth Defects Res Part A Clin Mol Teratol 2004;70:545–6.

S

Name:	**SILICONE BREAST IMPLANTS**	Risk Factor:	**C**
Class:	**Miscellaneous**		

FETAL RISK SUMMARY

RECOMMENDATION: Compatible

Silicone breast implants are composed of a shell of high-molecular-weight polydimethylsiloxane (PDMS, dimethicone) gum (i.e., elastomer or rubber) containing either saline, a silicone "oil" composed of unlinked polymers, or a lower viscosity PDMS gel (1,2). The difference in the viscosity of the organosiloxane shell and filler is dependent on the average molecular weight and molecular number distribution of the polymer (1). Leakage (bleeding) of the filler onto the surface of the shell may occur by simple diffusion and is associated with contracture of fibrous tissue around the implant, a foreign body response, or both (1). Gel bleeding may decrease the tensile strength of the shell and, by implication, may increase the incidence of implant rupture. The prevalence of implant rupture has been estimated to be 4%–6% (1).

Silicone breast implants have been generally available since the early 1980s, although they were first used experimentally in the 1940s (2). Several serious health concerns have been raised in relation to these implants, including silicone gel implant bleed, contracture (moderate degrees of contracture may be beneficial), implant rupture, carcinogenesis, immune disorders, and impaired breast cancer detection (1–3). However, a causal relationship between breast implants and connective-tissue and autoimmune disease seems unlikely based on the results of a meta-analysis described below.

A 2000 study conducted a meta-analysis of 20 studies (9 cohort, 9 case-control, and 2 cross-sectional) to determine if breast implants were associated with an increased risk of connective-tissue and autoimmune diseases (4). The study was part of a report prepared by a scientific panel formed to advise the federal judiciary on silicone breast implants (5). No evidence of an increase in individual connective-tissue diseases (rheumatoid arthritis, systemic lupus erythematosus, scleroderma or systemic sclerosis, and Sjögren's syndrome), all connective-tissue diseases combined, or other autoimmune or rheumatic conditions was found. Similarly, no evidence of a significantly increased risk was found specifically for silicone-gel-filled implants (4).

A study published in 1996 found no significant difference in the prevalence of autoantibodies between children ($N = 80$) born to mothers with silicone breast implants and control children ($N = 42$) born to mothers without implants (6). Moreover, no association between the clinical symptoms in the children and the presence of autoantibodies was found. Control children had been referred to the authors because of irritable bowel syndrome or lactose intolerance ($N = 21$) or fibromyalgia ($N = 21$), whereas the children in the study group had been referred because of concerns about adverse effects from the mother's implants. The authors concluded that determination of the antibodies was of limited clinical value in this patient population (6).

In a three-part study, investigators studied whether the immunogenicity of silicone, which appears to have been confirmed in humans and in at least one animal model, could be transferred from the mother to her offspring (7). In part 1 of the study, using silicon dioxide (silica), T lymphocyte cell-mediated immune responses were elicited in 21 of 24 children from 15 women with silicone breast implants. Subjects in part 2 of the study were the offspring of three women who gave birth to four children before they received their implants and to seven children after the implants. Five of the postimplant offspring were found to be positive to T-cell memory for silica compared with none of the preimplant offspring. Part 3 was a blinded study that evaluated 30 children of mothers with silicone implants compared with 10 control children of mothers without implants. A significant increase in T-cell stimulation was measured in the exposed children in comparison to the controls. Because not all of the above offspring were breast-fed, the investigators concluded that the results indicated either the transplacental passage of immunogens from silicone or transfer by maternal-fetal cellular exchange (7).

A 1998 epidemiologic cohort study conducted in Denmark examined the occurrence of esophageal disorders, connective tissue diseases, and congenital malformations in children (born during the period 1977 to 1992) of mothers with breast implants (8). A total of 939 children born from mothers with breast implants for cosmetic reasons (660 before the implant surgery and 279 after) were compared with 3906 children born from mothers who had undergone breast reduction surgery (1739 before surgery and 2167 after). The mean time from surgery to delivery for the two groups were 5.0 and 5.5 years, respectively. In the implant group, the observed/expected ratios (95% confidence intervals in parentheses) for various offspring outcomes before and after implants were as follows: esophageal disorders 2.7 (1.4–4.7) and 2.9 (0.8–7.4); rheumatic diseases 0.7 (0.0–4.1) and 0.0 (0.0–12.9); all types of congenital malformations 1.2 (0.9–1.5) and 1.3 (0.8–2.0); and defects of the digestive organs 1.4 (0.5–3.0) and 1.3 (0.2–4.6). Among the four children with an esophageal disorder who were born after the implants, three were hospitalized because of mild regurgitation that resolved without treatment. The fourth case involved a child with microcephaly, which was diagnosed as part of a genetic syndrome, and cerebral palsy. The results provided no evidence that silicone breast implants were associated with an increased risk of connective tissue diseases or malformations. Similar, nonsignificant differences for each of the categories were also found in the breast reduction group. The investigators concluded that women in both groups were more likely to seek professional medical care for problems normally solved outside the hospital (8).

Approximately 2 million women in the United States alone have received silicone implants (3), but no estimation of the number of pregnant women exposed to these devices has been located. Passage of PDMS to the fetus should not occur because of the high molecular weight of this polymer, and no evidence has been published that any of its multiple breakdown products cross the placenta. However, silicon, the second most abundant element in the earth's crust and a major component of biologic systems including the human skeleton (2), crosses to the fetus with concentrations in the amniotic fluid ranging from 34 to 800 ng/mL (mean 154.7 ng/mL) at 16–19 weeks' gestation (9). Transplacental passage of maternal immunoglobulin antibodies (IgG, IgA, or IgM) from silicone-induced immune disease is potentially possible, but this was not found in the study cited above. Moreover, some data presented in the Breast Feeding Summary argue against the clinical significance of this occurrence. Furthermore, a meta-analysis found no evidence that silicone implants are associated with connective-tissue or autoimmune diseases.

S

BREAST FEEDING SUMMARY

RECOMMENDATION: Compatible

Studies concerning the excretion of polydimethylsiloxane (PDMS) (see above) or the breakdown products of this macromolecule into milk have not been located, but two reports discussed below have described unusual disease symptoms in breast-fed infants of mothers with silicone breast implants (10,11). For the present, any association between the symptoms and the organosiloxane components of the implants is speculative and further studies are needed to establish a causal relationship.

A 1994 report described 67 (56 breast-fed, 11 bottle-fed) children born to mothers with silicone breast implants who had been self-referred because of concerns relating to implant-induced toxicity (10). Forty-three (35 breast-fed, 8 bottle-fed) of the children had complaints of recurrent abdominal pain, and 26 (20 breast-fed, 6 bottle-fed) of this group had additional symptoms, such as recurrent vomiting, dysphagia, decreased weight-height ratio, or a sibling with these complaints. Of these latter 26 children, 11 (8 breast-fed, 3 bottle-fed; mean age 6.0 years, range 1.5–13 years; 6 boys and 5 girls) agreed to undergo further evaluation. A group composed of 17 subjects (mean age 10.7 years; range 2–18 years; 11 boys and 6 girls) with abdominal pain who had not been exposed to silicone breast implants served as controls. No significant differences ($p > 0.05$) were found between the implant-exposed breast-fed and bottle-fed subjects, or between the total exposed group and controls (7 of the 17 were tested) in autoantibodies to eight antigens (nuclear, Sci-70, centromere, ribonucleoprotein, Sm, Ro, La, and phospholipid). Endoscopy was performed on all subjects, and no gross visual abnormalities were observed. Chronic esophagitis was discovered on biopsy specimens in 8 exposed (6 breast-fed, 2 bottle-fed) children (all graded as mild) and in 13 of 16 controls (1 not tested) (mild to moderate in 7, severe in 6). No granulomas or crystals were identified in the biopsy specimens. The histology of the specimens did not differ between the exposed children or between the exposed children and controls. When esophageal manometry was used to test the esophageal motility of the subjects, six of the eight breast-fed exposed children were found to have significantly abnormal motility with nearly absent peristalsis in the distal two-thirds of the esophagus. Esophageal sphincter pressure, esophageal wave propagation, and wave amplitude were measured and compared in the breast-fed exposed, bottle-fed exposed, and control groups by an investigator blinded to the clinical status of the children. The following results were obtained in the three groups: 13.1 ($p < 0.05$ compared with controls), 22.7, and 24.8 mm Hg, respectively; 14.7 ($p < 0.05$ compared with controls), 64.3, and 53.0%, respectively; and 42.3, 60.3, and 50.6 mm Hg, respectively. No improvement in the motility abnormalities was found in three of the breast-fed exposed subjects who were retested 10 months later after long-term ranitidine therapy had reduced the episodes of abdominal pain (10).

The symptoms present in the breast-fed exposed children were considered to be characteristic of systemic sclerosis, although the children did not meet the clinical criteria for the disease (10). Moreover, the investigators excluded the possibility that the abnormal motility was a consequence of chronic esophagitis. The blinded manometric findings suggested that the esophageal disorder might have been related to exposure to substances in breast milk because the bottle-fed exposed children had values similar to those of controls. The nature of these substances, if any, could not be determined by this study, but the investigators considered the possibilities to include silicone and other breakdown products of the implants that could be transferred across the immature intestinal barrier of the nursing infant and eventually lead to immunologically mediated damage (10).

In an accompanying editorial to the above report, several possible mechanisms for silicone-induced toxicity were explored (12). These included mother-to-child transmission of silicone products or maternal autoantibodies across the placenta or through breast milk. However, an argument against the latter mechanism is the usually short-term effects of passively acquired antibodies compared with the prolonged nature of the disorders in the affected children (12).

The second study, also published in 1994, described two female children, ages 2.67 and 9 years, who had long-standing, unusual, diffuse myalgias and arthralgias, not consistent with juvenile arthritis, and positive antinuclear antibodies (1:80 and 1:160, respectively; both speckled pattern) (11). The 9-year-old girl had a markedly elevated titer of antibodies against denatured human type II collagen. Both girls had been breast-fed, the youngest for 3 months and the other for 6 months, by mothers with silicone breast implants. The right implant in the mother of the youngest girl had ruptured during pregnancy, and a recent breast ultrasound of the other mother was suggestive for implant rupture, but the timing was unknown (11).

A number of comments were published in response to the above two studies (13–25). In one of the comments, the authors described the results of a study in which no silicone was detected (detection level 0.5 μg/mL) in two women with silicone breast implants (17). Two of the references stated that without more evidence, breast feeding by women with silicone breast implants should not be contraindicated (22) or should be recommended (23).

Macrophage activation was suggested from the results of a case-control study of 38 breast-fed children from mothers with silicone breast implants compared with 30 controls (healthy children $N = 10$, children with gastrointestinal symptoms similar to study patients $N = 10$, children with benign urinary abnormalities $N = 7$, and children with joint symptoms similar to study patients $N = 3$) (26). Researchers measured the urinary excretion of stable nitric oxide (NO) metabolites (NO_3^- plus NO_2^-) and neopterin, inflammatory mediators released by phagocytosis of foreign material by macrophages. Mean levels of NO metabolites in the study patients were higher than those in controls, but significantly higher only when compared with levels in the subgroup of healthy children. Mean neopterin excretion in study patients was higher than each of the four control subgroups, but significantly so only in comparison to the healthy, GI, and joint symptom subgroups. The investigators speculated that macrophage activation by silicone results in the release of NO and other substances with subsequent inhibition of esophageal peristalsis (26).

At follow-up (mean 2.1 years) of 11 children with esophageal dysmotility who had been breast-fed by mothers with silicone breast implants, 7 had subjective clinical improvement in their symptoms (27). Esophageal sphincter pressures (both lower and upper) and percent of wave propagation into the distal esophagus following swallowing were statistically similar to the values obtained at initial manometric testing. Wave amplitude in the distal esophagus, however, did increase significantly. Urinary neopterin decreased significantly, whereas urinary nitrates (NO_3^- plus NO_2^-) decreased but not significantly. The data suggested that the dysmotility had become a chronic condition in this group of children (27).

In a 1998 study, silicon concentrations in milk and blood of 15 women with bilateral silicone gel-filled implants were compared with similar samples in 34 women with no implants, store-bought cow's milk, and 26 brands of commercially available infant formula (28). Silicon was used as a "proxy" measure for silicone. Mean milk and blood silicon levels were statistically similar in the implant group compared with women without implants: 55.45 and 79.29 ng/mL vs. 51.05 and 103.76 ng/mL, respectively. Much higher mean silicon concentrations were found in cow's milk (708.94 ng/mL) and commercial infant formula (4402.5 ng/mL) (28).

In summary, two studies have described unusual signs and symptoms in children who had been breast-fed by mothers with silicone breast implants. Follow-up studies by the same investigators suggested that these effects may have been caused by the transfer of maternal mutagenicity to silicone to the fetuses or infants during pregnancy or breast feeding and that the pathogenesis in the offspring might be caused by macrophage activation. However, these conclusions are controversial (29–31) and have not been confirmed. Many experts recommend that women with silicone breast implants should be encouraged to breast-feed because the benefits of breast-feeding appear to far outweigh the potential, if any, risk to the nursing infant. Mothers with silicone breast implants should be fully informed of the current state of knowledge so that they are actively involved in the decision whether to breast-feed. The American Academy of Pediatrics concluded that the available evidence does not justify classifying silicone implants as a contraindication to breast-feeding (32).

References

1. Council on Scientific Affairs, American Medical Association. Silicone gel breast implants. JAMA 1993;270:2602–6.
2. Yoshida SH, Chang CC, Teuber SS, Gershwin ME. Silicon and silicone: Theoretical and clinical implications of breast implants. Regul Toxicol Pharmacol 1993;17:3–18.
3. Kessler DA, Merkatz RB, Schapiro R. A call for higher standards for breast implants. JAMA 1993;270: 2607–8.
4. Janowsky EC, Kupper LL, Hulka BS. Meta-analyses of the relation between silicone breast implants and the risk of connective-tissue diseases. N Engl J Med 2000;342:781–90.
5. Hulka BS, Kerkvliet NL, Tugwell P. Experience of a scientific panel formed to advise the federal judiciary on silicone breast implants. N Engl J Med 2000;342: 812–5.
6. Levine JJ, Lin H-C, Rowley M, Cook A, Teuber SS, Ilowite NT. Lack of autoantibody expression in children born to mothers with silicone breast implants. Pediatrics 1996;97:243–5.
7. Smalley DL, Levine JJ, Shanklin DR, Hall MF, Stevens MV. Lymphocyte response to silica among offspring of silicone breast implant recipients. Immunobiology 1996/1997:196:567–74.
8. Kjoller K, McLaughlin JK, Friis S, Blot WJ, Mellemkjaer L, Hogsted C, Winther JF, Olsen JH. Health outcomes in offspring of mothers with breast implants. Pediatrics 1998;102:1112–5.
9. Hall GS, Carr MJ, Cummings E, Lee M-L. Aluminum, barium, silicon, and strontium in amniotic fluid by emission spectrometry. Clin Chem 1983;29:1318.
10. Levine JJ, Ilowite NT. Sclerodermalike esophageal disease in children breast-fed by mothers with silicone breast implants. JAMA 1994;271:213–6.
11. Teuber SS, Gershwin ME. Autoantibodies and clinical rheumatic complaints in two children of women with silicone gel breast implants. Int Arch Allergy Immunol 1994;103:105–8.
12. Flick JA. Silicone implants and esophageal dysmotility. Are breast-fed infants at risk?. JAMA 1994;271: 240–1.
13. Bartel DR. Sclerodermalike esophageal disease in children of mothers with silicone breast implants. JAMA 1994;272:767.
14. Cook RR. Sclerodermalike esophageal disease in children of mothers with silicone breast implants. JAMA 1994;272:767–8.
15. Epstein WA. Sclerodermalike esophageal disease in children of mothers with silicone breast implants. JAMA 1994;272:768.
16. Placik OJ. Sclerodermalike esophageal disease in children of mothers with silicone breast implants. JAMA 1994;272:768–9.
17. Liau M, Ito S, Koren G. Sclerodermalike esophageal disease in children of mothers with silicone breast implants. JAMA 1994;272:769.
18. Levine JJ, Ilowite NT. Sclerodermalike esophageal disease in children of mothers with silicone breast implants. In reply. JAMA 1994;272:769–70.
19. Brody GS. Sclerodermalike esophageal disease in children of mothers with silicone breast implants. JAMA 1994;272:770.
20. Flick JA. Sclerodermalike esophageal disease in children of mothers with silicone breast implants. In reply. JAMA 1994;272:770.
21. Williams AF. Silicone breast implants, breast-feeding, and scleroderma. Lancet 1994;343:1043–4.
22. Berlin CM Jr. Silicone breast implants and breast-feeding. Pediatrics 1994;94:547–9.
23. Jordan ME, Blum RWM. Should breast-feeding by women with silicone implants be recommended? Arch Pediatr Adolesc Med 1996;150:880–1.
24. Epstein WA. Silicone breast implants and scleroderma-like esophageal disease in breast-fed infants. JAMA 1996;275:184.
25. Levine JJ, Ilowite NT. Silicone breast implants and sclerodermalike esophageal disease in breast-fed infants. JAMA 1996;275:184–5.
26. Levine JJ, Ilowite NT, Pettei MJ, Trachtman H. Increased urinary NO_3^- + NO_2^- and neopterin excretion in children breast-fed by mothers with silicone breast implants: evidence for macrophage activation. J Rheumatol 1996;23:1083–7.
27. Levine JJ, Trachtman H, Gold DM, Pettei MJ. Esophageal dysmotility in children breast-fed by mothers with silicone breast implants. Long-term follow-up and response to treatment. Dig Dis Sci 1996;41: 1600–3.
28. Semple JL, Lugowski SJ, Baines CJ, Smith DC, McHugh A. Breast milk contamination and silicone implants: preliminary results using silicon as a proxy measurement for silicone. Plast Reconstr Surg 1998;102: 528–33.
29. Epstein WA. Silicone breast implants and breast feeding. J Rheumatol 1997;24:1013.
30. Hoshaw SJ, Klykken PC, Abbott JP. Silicone breast implants and breast feeding. J Rheumatol 1997;24:1014.

S

31. Levine JL, Ilowite NT, Pettei MJ, Trachtman H. Silicone breast implants and breast feeding. J Rheumatol 1997;24:1014–5.

32. Committee on Drugs, American Academy of Pediatrics. The transfer of drugs and other chemicals into human milk. Pediatrics 2001;108:776–89.

Name: **SIMETHICONE** Risk Factor: **C**

Class: **Antiflatulent/Defoaming Agent**

FETAL RISK SUMMARY

RECOMMENDATION: Compatible

Simethicone is a nonabsorbable silicone product that is used as an antiflatulent. No published reports linking the use of this agent with congenital defects have been located.

In a surveillance study of Michigan Medicaid recipients conducted between 1985 and 1992 involving 229,101 completed pregnancies, 248 newborns had been exposed to simethicone during the 1st trimester (F. Rosa, personal communication, FDA, 1993). A total of 14 (5.6%) major birth defects were observed (11 expected). Specific data were available for six defect categories, including (observed/expected) 6/2 cardiovascular defects, 0/0.5 oral clefts, 0/0 spina bifida, 2/1 polydactyly, 0/.5 limb reduction defects, and 1/0.5 hypospadias. Only the cases of cardiovascular defects suggest a possible association with the drug. However, other factors, such as the mother's disease, concurrent drug use, and chance, are most likely involved because simethicone is not absorbed.

BREAST FEEDING SUMMARY

RECOMMENDATION: No Human Data - Probably Compatible

No reports describing the use of simethicone during human lactation have been located. The risk to a nursing infant from maternal use of the drug is negligible because the drug is not absorbed.

Name: **SIMVASTATIN** Risk Factor: **X_M**

Class: **Antilipemic Agent**

FETAL RISK SUMMARY

RECOMMENDATION: Contraindicated

Simvastatin (a "statin") is a lipophilic agent that is used to lower elevated levels of cholesterol. It has the same cholesterol-lowering mechanism (i.e., inhibition of hepatic 3-hydroxy-3-methylglutaryl-coenzyme A [HMG-CoA] reductase) as other agents in this class (atorvastatin, cerivastatin, fluvastatin, lovastatin, and pravastatin) and is structurally similar to lovastatin and pravastatin.

Simvastatin was not teratogenic in rats and rabbits at doses up to 3 times the human exposure based on body surface area (1). A decrease in fertility was observed in male rats dosed for 34 weeks at 4 times the maximum human exposure level based on area under the concentration curve (AUC), but this effect was not observed when the study was repeated for 11 weeks (1). Male dogs given 10 mg/kg/day (about 2 times the human exposure based on AUC at 80 mg/day) demonstrated a drug-related testicular atrophy, decreased spermatogenesis, spermatocytic degeneration, and giant cell formation (1).

Shepard reviewed four studies involving the administration of simvastatin to pregnant rats and rabbits (2–5). Although maternal weight was reduced compared with controls, no teratogenicity, adverse effects on fertility, or interference with postnatal behavior or fertility were observed.

Five cases of fetal loss were reported to the FDA in 1995, but additional data on these cases are not available (F. Rosa, personal communication, FDA, 1995).

A 1996 report described the outcomes of simvastatin-exposed pregnancies gathered from a worldwide postmarketing surveillance by the manufacturer (6). A total of 187 cases of inadvertent exposure to simvastatin had been identified, among which the outcomes of 15 (8%) were still pending, 46 (25%) had been lost to follow-up, and 40 (21%) underwent elective abortions. None of the products of conception from the elective abortions underwent morphologic and/or chromosomal evaluations (7). In the remaining 86 cases, there were 64 (74.4%) normal outcomes, 13 (15.1%) spontaneous abortions, 5 (5.8%) congenital malformations, 1 (1.2%) fetal death, and 3 (3.5%) miscellaneous adverse outcomes. In at least 59 (92%) of the 64 normal outcomes, the mother had been taking the drug before conception so that exposure had occurred from the start of the pregnancy. In three cases, exposure occurred from the 10th week through term, and in two cases the mother took the drug during the 1st trimester, but the exact timing during this period was unknown. The one fetal death occurred at 23 weeks' gestation in a pregnancy exposed to simvastatin (10 mg/day) during the first 3–4 weeks of gestation, but specific details on the case were not available. Congenital anomalies after 1st trimester exposure to simvastatin occurred in five infants, one of which was a twin. Four reports were prospective and one was retrospective. The defects were (maternal dose and exposure in weeks from last menstrual period) polydactyly with small, boneless, outgrowth from hand (10 mg/day, 3–5 weeks); unilateral cleft lip without cleft palate, amniocentesis normal (10 mg/day, 0–6 weeks); balanic hypospadias (10 mg/day, 0–6 weeks); trisomy 18, multiple malformations in a dead fetus, other twin normal (5 mg/day, 0–7 weeks); and club foot, mother also treated for hypertension (10 mg/day, 0–12 weeks). The cases of polydactyly and hypospadias were thought not to be drug-induced because the time of drug exposure in both cases occurred before the critical periods for these defects (6). The trisomy was also dismissed as drug-induced because of the lack of evidence that this defect could be caused by drugs. The miscellaneous adverse effects were patent ductus arteriosus in a 1814-g premature infant delivered from a hypertensive mother (10 mg/day, 0–10 weeks); respiratory distress, cardiac arrhythmia, anemia, and infection in a 1900-g premature infant delivered from a hypertensive mother (10 mg/day, 0–7 weeks); and bilateral hydrocele, hyperbilirubinemia in a 1720-g premature infant (20 mg/day, 0–9 weeks). All three cases were thought to be possibly related to prematurity (6).

A 2004 report described the outcomes of pregnancy that had been exposed to statins and reported to the FDA (see Lovastatin).

In summary, based on the animal data and limited human experience, exposure to simvastatin during early pregnancy does not appear to present a significant risk to the fetus. However, because the interruption of cholesterol-lowering therapy during pregnancy should have no apparent effect on the long-term treatment of hyperlipidemia, simvastatin should not be used during pregnancy. Women taking this agent before conception should ideally stop the therapy before becoming pregnant and certainly on recognition of pregnancy. Accidental use of the drug during gestation, though, apparently has no known consequences for the fetus. If simvastatin is used in pregnancy, healthcare professionals are encouraged to call the toll free number (800-670-6126) for information about patient enrollment in the Motherisk study.

BREAST FEEDING SUMMARY

RECOMMENDATION: Contraindicated

No published reports describing the use of simvastatin during lactation have been located. However, the passage of simvastatin into milk should be expected because at least two other similar agents (Fluvastatin and Pravastatin) appear in human milk. Because of the potential for adverse effects in the nursing infant, the drug should not be used during lactation.

References

1. Product information. Zocor. Merck, 2000.
2. Wise LD, Minsker DH, Robertson RT, Bokelman DL, Akutsu S, Fujii T. Simvastatin (mk-0733): oral fertility study in rats. Oyo Yakuri 1990;39:127–41. As cited in Shepard TH. *Catalog of Teratogenic Agents*. 7th ed. Baltimore, MD: Johns Hopkins University Press, 1992: 359–60.
3. Wise LD, Majka JA, Robertson RT, Bokelman DL. Simvastatin (mk-0733): oral teratogenicity study in rats pre- and postnatal observation. Oyo Yakuri 1990;39: 143–58. As cited in Shepard TH. *Catalog of Teratogenic Agents*. 7th ed. Baltimore, MD: Johns Hopkins University Press, 1992:359–60.
4. Wise LD, Prahalada S, Robertson RT, Bokelman DL, Akutsu S, Fujii T. Simvastatin (mk-0733): oral teratogenicity study in rabbits. Oyo Yakuri 1990;39:159–67. As cited in Shepard TH. *Catalog of Teratogenic Agents*. 7th ed. Baltimore, MD: Johns Hopkins University Press, 1992:359–60.
5. Minsker DH, Robertson RT, Bokelman DL. Simvastatin (mk-0733): oral late gestation and lactation study in rats. Oyo Yakuri 1990;39:169–79. As cited in Shepard TH. *Catalog of Teratogenic Agents*. 7th ed. Baltimore, MD: Johns Hopkins University Press, 1992:359–60.
6. Manson JM, Freyssinges C, Ducrocq MB, Stephenson WP. Postmarketing surveillance of lovastatin and simvastatin exposure during pregnancy. Reprod Toxicol 1996;10:439–46.
7. Manson JM. Postmarketing surveillance of lovastatin and simvastatin exposure during pregnancy (reply). Reprod Toxicol 1997;11:641–2.

Name:	**SODIUM IODIDE**	Risk Factor:	**D**
Class:	**Respiratory Drug (Expectorant)**		

See Potassium Iodide.

Name:	**SODIUM IODIDE ^{125}I**	Risk Factor:	**X**
Class:	**Radiopharmaceutical**		

See Sodium Iodide ^{131}I.

Name:	**SODIUM IODIDE ^{131}I**	Risk Factor:	**X**
Class:	**Radiopharmaceutical/Antithyroid**		

FETAL RISK SUMMARY

RECOMMENDATION: Contraindicated

Iodine-131–labeled sodium iodide ($Na^{131}I$) is a radiopharmaceutical agent used for diagnostic procedures and for therapeutic destruction of thyroid tissue. The diagnostic dose is approximately one-thousandth of the therapeutic dose. Like all iodides, the drug concentrates in the thyroid gland. ^{131}I readily crosses the placenta. The fetal thyroid is able to accumulate ^{131}I until after about 10–12 weeks of gestation (1–4). At term, the maternal serum: cord blood ratio is 1 (5).

As suggested by the above studies on uptake of ^{131}I in fetal thyroids, maternal treatment with radioiodine early in the 1st trimester should not pose a significant danger to the fetus. Two reports describing Na^{131}I therapy at 4 and 8 weeks' gestation resulting in normal infants seemingly confirmed the lack of risk (6,7). However, a newborn, who was exposed to Na^{131}I at about 2 weeks' gestation, has been described as having a large head, exophthalmia, and thick, myxedematous-like skin (8). The infant died shortly after birth. In another early report, exposure to a diagnostic dose of Na^{131}I during the middle of the 1st trimester was considered the cause of anomalies observed in the newborn, including microcephaly, hydrocephaly, dysplasia of the hip joints, and clubfoot (9). Finally, Na^{131}I administered 1–3 days before conception was suggested as the cause of a spontaneous abortion at the end of the 1st trimester (10). All three of these latter reports must be viewed with caution because of the uniqueness of the effects and the timing of the exposure. Factors other than radioiodine may have been involved.

Therapeutic doses of radioiodine administered near the end of the 1st trimester (12 weeks) or beyond usually result in partial or complete abolition of the fetal thyroid gland (11–21). This effect is dose-dependent, however, as one mother was treated at 19 weeks' gestation with 6.1 mCi of Na^{131}I apparently without causing fetal harm (2). In the pregnancies terminating with a hypothyroid infant, Na^{131}I doses ranged from 10 to 225 mCi (11–21). Clinical features observed at or shortly after birth in 10 of the 12 newborns were consistent with congenital hypothyroidism. One of these infants was also discovered to have hypoparathyroidism (21). In one child, exposed *in utero* to repeated small doses during a 5-week period (total dose 12.2 mCi), hypothyroidism did not become evident until 4 years of age (18). Unusual anomalies observed in another infant included hydrocephaly, cardiopathy, genital hypotrophy, and a limb deformity (16).

In a 1998 case report, a woman received 500 MBq of I^{131} in the 20th gestational week (22). Based on gamma camera examinations, the fetal thyroid gland uptake at 24 hours was estimated to be 10 MBq (2% of the dose) or an absorbed dose to the gland of 600 Gy (an ablative dose). The absorbed dose to the fetal body and brain was approximately 100 mGy, whereas the fetal gonads received about 40 mGy. At term, a hypothyroid, but otherwise healthy 3150-g male infant was delivered. Treatment with thyroxine was begun at 14 days of age. A neuropsychological examination at 8 years of age revealed normal mental performance, but with a low attention score and subnormal capacity regarding figurative memory. Plans were made for long-term surveillance of the infant because of the potential for thyroid cancer (22).

In summary, Na^{131}I is a proven human teratogen. Because the effects of even small doses are not predictable, the use of the drug for diagnostic and therapeutic purposes should be avoided during pregnancy. A 1999 reference reviewed the effects of ^{131}I on the fetal thyroid after administration to the mother in early gestation (4).

BREAST FEEDING SUMMARY

RECOMMENDATION: Hold Breast Feeding

Iodine-131–labeled sodium iodide (Na^{131}I) is concentrated in breast milk (23–26). Na^{125}I also appears in milk in significant quantities (27,28). Uptake of ^{131}I contained in milk by an infant's thyroid gland has been observed (23). The time required for elimination of radioiodine from the milk may be as long as 14 days. For iodine-123 (^{123}I) and iodine-125 (^{125}I), radioactivity may be present in milk for up to 36 hours and 12 days, respectively (29). Because exposure to radioactive iodine may result in damage to the nursing infant's thyroid, including an increased risk of thyroid cancer, breast-feeding should be stopped until radioactivity is no longer present in the milk (29).

References

1. Chapman EM, Corner GW Jr, Robinson D, Evans RD. The collection of radioactive iodine by the human fetal thyroid. J Clin Endocrinol Metab 1948;8:717–20.
2. Hodges RE, Evans TC, Bradbury JT, Keettel WC. The accumulation of radioactive iodine by human fetal thyroids. J Clin Endocrinol Metab 1955;15:661–7.
3. Shepard TH. Onset of function in the human fetal thyroid: biochemical and radioautographic studies from organ culture. J Clin Endocrinol Metab 1967;27:945–58.
4. Pauwels EKJ, Thomson WH, Blokland JAK, Schmidt ME, Bourguignon M, El-Maghraby TAF, Broerse JJ, Harding LK. Aspects of fetal thyroid dose following iodine-131 administration during early stages of pregnancy in patients suffering from benign thyroid disorders. Eur J Nucl Med 1999;26:1453–7.
5. Kearns JE, Hutson W. Tagged isomers and analogues of thyroxine (their transmission across the human placenta and other studies). J Nucl Med 1963;4:453–61.
6. Hollingsworth DR, Austin E. Observations following I^{131} for Graves' disease during first trimester of pregnancy. South Med J 1969;62:1555–6.
7. Talbert LM, Thomas CG Jr, Holt WA, Rankin P. Hyperthyroidism during pregnancy. Obstet Gynecol 1970;36:779–85.
8. Valensi G, Nahum A. Action de l'iode radio-actif sur le foetus humain. Tunisie med 1958;36:69. As cited in Nishimura H, Tanimura T. *Clinical Aspects of the Teratogenicity of Drugs*. New York, NY: American Elsevier, 1976:260.
9. Falk W. Beitrag zur Frage der menschlichen Fruchtschadigung durch kunstliche radioaktive Isotope. Medizinische 1959;22:1480. As cited in Nishimura H, Tanimura T. *Clinical Aspects of the Teratogenicity of Drugs*. New York, NY: American Elsevier, 1976:260.
10. Berger M, Briere J. Les dangers de la therapeutique par l'iode radioactif au debut d'une grossesse ignoree. Bull Med Leg Toxicol Med 1967;10:37. As cited in Nishimura H, Tanimura T. *Clinical Aspects of the Teratogenicity of Drugs*. New York, NY: American Elsevier, 1976:260.
11. Russell KP, Rose H, Starr P. The effects of radioactive iodine on maternal and fetal thyroid function during pregnancy. Surg Gynecol Obstet 1957;104:560–4.
12. Ray EW, Sterling K, Gardner LI. Congenital cretinism associated with I^{131} therapy of the mother. Am J Dis Child 1959;98:506–7.
13. Hamill GC, Jarman JA, Wynne MD. Fetal effects of radioactive iodine therapy in a pregnant woman with thyroid cancer. Am J Obstet Gynecol 1961;81:1018–23.
14. Fisher WD, Voorhess ML, Gardner LI. Congenital hypothyroidism in infant following maternal I^{131} therapy. J Pediatr 1963;62:132–46.
15. Pfannenstiel P, Andrews GA, Brown DW. Congenital hypothyroidism from intrauterine ^{131}I damage. In Cassalino C, Andreoli M, eds. *Current Topics in Thyroid Research*. New York, NY: Academic Press, 1965:749. As cited in Nishimura H, Tanimura T. *Clinical Aspects of the Teratogenicity of Drugs*. New York, NY: American Elsevier, 1976:260.
16. Sirbu P, Macarie E, Isaia V, Zugravesco A. L'influence de l'iode radio-actif sur le foetus. Bull Fed Soc Gynecol Obstet Franc 1968;20: Suppl 314. As cited in Nishimura H, Tanimura T. *Clinical Aspects of the Teratogenicity of Drugs*. New York, NY: American Elsevier, 1976:260.
17. Hollingsworth DR, Austin E. Thyroxine derivatives in amniotic fluid. J Pediatr 1971;79:923–9.
18. Green HG, Gareis FJ, Shepard TH, Kelley VC. Cretinism associated with maternal sodium iodide I 131 therapy during pregnancy. Am J Dis Child 1971;122:247–9.
19. Jafek BW, Small R, Lillian DL. Congenital radioactive iodine-induced stridor and hypothyroidism. Arch Otolaryngol 1974;99:369–71.
20. Exss R, Graewe B. Congenital athyroidism in the newborn infant from intra-uterine radioiodine action. Biol Neonate 1974;24:289–91.
21. Richards GE, Brewer ED, Conley SB, Saldana LR. Combined hypothyroidism and hypoparathyroidism in an infant after maternal ^{131}I administration. J Pediatr 1981;99:141–43.
22. Berg GEB, Nystrom EH, Jacobsson L, Lindberg S, Lindstedt RG, Mattsson S, Niklasson CA, Noren AH, Westphal OGA. Radioiodine treatment of hyperthyroidism in a pregnant woman. J Nucl Med 1998;39:357–61.
23. Nurnberger CE, Lipscomb A. Transmission of radioiodine (I^{131}) to infants through human maternal milk. JAMA 1952;150:1398–1400.
24. Miller H, Weetch RS. The excretion of radioactive iodine in human milk. Lancet 1955;2:1013.
25. Weaver JC, Kamm ML, Dobson RL. Excretion of radioiodine in human milk. JAMA 1960;173:872–5.
26. Karjalainen P, Penttila IM, Pystynen P. The amount and form of radioactivity in human milk after lung scanning, renography and placental localization by ^{131}I labelled tracers. Acta Obstet Gynecol Scand 1971;50:357–61.
27. Bland EP, Crawford JS, Docker MF, Farr RF. Radioactive iodine uptake by thyroid of breast-fed infants

S

after maternal blood-volume measurements. Lancet 1969;2:1039–41.
28. Palmer KE. Excretion of ^{125}I in breast milk following administration of labelled fibrinogen. Br J Radiol 1979;52:672–3.
29. Committee on Drugs, American Academy of Pediatrics. The transfer of drugs and other chemicals into human milk. Pediatrics 2001;108:776–89.

Name:	**SOMATOSTATIN**	Risk Factor:	**B**
Class:	**Pituitary Hormone**		

FETAL RISK SUMMARY

RECOMMENDATION: No Human Data - Probably Compatible

No data are available (see also Octreotide).

BREAST FEEDING SUMMARY

RECOMMENDATION: No Human Data - Probably Compatible

No data are available (see also Octreotide).

Name:	**SOTALOL**	Risk Factor:	**B_M***
Class:	**Antiarrhythmic**		

FETAL RISK SUMMARY

RECOMMENDATION: Human Data Suggest Risk in 2nd and 3rd Trimesters

Sotalol is a sympatholytic agent indicated for the treatment of cardiac arrhythmias. The antiarrhythmic action of the drug includes both Class II (β-adrenoreceptor blocking) and Class III (cardiac action potential duration prolongation) properties. It has also been used for hypertension. Sotalol is a racemic mixture of the *d*- and *l*-isomers. Only the *l*-isomer exhibits β-adrenergic blocking activity (without intrinsic sympathomimetic activity), but both isomers have Class III antiarrhythmic properties (1).

Sotalol was not teratogenic in rats and rabbits given doses 9 and 7 times the maximum recommended human dose on a body surface area basis (MRHD), respectively, during organogenesis (2). In rabbits, a dose 16 times the MRHD, but not 8 times, resulted in a slight increase in fetal death that was thought to be related to maternal toxicity. Fetal resorptions were observed in rats at 18 times the MRHD, but not at 2.5 times (2).

In a 1996 study, the embryotoxicity of *d*-sotalol in rats was shown to be gestational-age related and resulted from dose-dependent bradycardia in *in vitro* (rat embryo culture) and *in vivo* (pregnant rat) experiments (3). In embryo cultures, the minimum effective concentration (15 μg/mL) for causing significant bradycardia was about 5 times the human therapeutic plasma concentration (3 μg/mL) achieved in pregnant women after a 400-mg oral dose (3). In nine pregnant rats, a single oral dose (1000 mg/kg) was administered on gestational day 13. No malformations were observed, but a resorption rate of almost 14% was noted (3).

The pharmacokinetics of sotalol in the 3rd trimester (32–36 weeks' gestation) of pregnancy and in the postpartum (at 6 weeks) period was reported in 1983 (4).

Sotalol crosses the placenta to the fetus (5–8). Twelve hypertensive pregnant women were prescribed sotalol (final daily dose 200–800 mg) beginning at 10–31 weeks' gestation (5). The mean gestational age at delivery was 37.7 weeks (range 32–40 weeks). The mean maternal plasma concentration of sotalol at delivery was 1.8 μg/mL, nearly identical to the mean umbilical cord plasma level of 1.7 μg/mL. In six women, the mean amniotic fluid concentration of sotalol was 7.0 μg/mL. No data were provided on the time interval between the last sotalol dose and the collection of plasma samples. In a second study, eight women scheduled for elective cesarean section were given 80 mg of the drug orally 3 hours before the procedure (6). The mean maternal concentration of sotalol at surgery was 0.68 μg/mL, compared with the mean umbilical vein concentration of 0.32 μg/mL, a fetal:maternal ratio of 0.47. A 1990 report described the use of sotalol, 80 mg twice daily, in one woman throughout gestation (7). A cesarean section was performed at approximately 37 weeks' gestation, 11 hours after the last dose. Maternal plasma and umbilical cord sotalol concentrations were 0.95 and 1.35 μg/mL, respectively, a ratio of 1.42. Maternal and cord serum concentrations of sotalol at delivery from a woman treated with 80 mg 3 times daily throughout a 42 week gestation were 0.77 and 0.65 μg/mL (fetal:maternal ratio 0.84), respectively (8).

Sotalol was used in 12 pregnant women for the treatment of hypertension (dosage and gestational weeks when therapy was begun are detailed above) (5). No fetal adverse effects attributable to the drug were observed, but bradycardia (90–110 beats/minute), lasting up to 24 hours, was discovered in five of the six newborns with continuous heart rate monitoring. In a 1987 report, sotalol, in increasing doses up to 480 mg/day during a 12-day period, was combined with digoxin beginning at 31 weeks' gestation in an unsuccessful attempt to treat a hydropic fetus with supraventricular tachycardia (9). Therapy was eventually changed to amiodarone plus digoxin with return of a normal fetal heart rate and resolution of the fetal edema. A normal infant was delivered at 38 weeks' gestation that was alive and well at 10 months of age.

A 23-year-old woman was treated throughout gestation with sotalol and flecainide for bursts of ventricular tachycardia and polymorphous ventricular premature complexes associated with an aneurysm of the left ventricle (7). A normal infant was delivered at approximately 37 weeks' gestation by cesarean section. No adverse effects of drug exposure, including bradycardia, were noted in the newborn, which was growing normally at 1 year of age.

A 2000 retrospective study evaluated the use of sotalol for fetal tachycardia in 21 pregnant women (10). The fetal arrhythmias were atrial flutter (AF) ($N = 10$), supraventricular tachycardia (SVT) ($N = 10$), and ventricular tachycardia (VT) ($N = 1$). Hydrops fetalis was present in nine fetuses. Sinus rhythm was established in eight fetuses with AF and six with SVT, but four deaths (19%) occurred (one with AF and three with SVT). Two newborns (one each with AF and SVT), both successfully converted to a sinus rhythm *in utero*, had significant neurological morbidity consisting of intracranial hemorrhage in one and cerebral hypoxic ischemia in the other. The authors concluded that sotalol was effective in AF, but the mortality and low conversion rate in fetuses with SVT indicated that the risks of sotalol outweighed the benefits in this group (10).

Several reviews have examined the use of β-adrenergic blockers in human pregnancy, concluding that these agents are relatively safe for the fetus (11–14). However, some β-blockers may cause intrauterine growth retardation (IUGR) and reduced placental weight,

S

especially those lacking intrinsic sympathomimetic activity (ISA) (i.e., partial agonist). Treatment beginning early in the 2nd trimester results in the greatest weight reductions, whereas treatment restricted to the 3rd trimester primarily affects only placental weight. However, IUGR and reduced placental weight may potentially occur with all agents within this class. Although growth retardation is a serious concern, the benefits of maternal therapy with β-blockers, in some cases, might outweigh the risks to the fetus and must be judged on a case-by-case basis. Newborns exposed near delivery should be closely observed during the first 24–48 hours for signs and symptoms of β-blockade. Long-term effects of *in utero* exposure to this class of drugs have not been studied but warrant evaluation.

[**Risk Factor D if used in 2nd or 3rd trimesters.*]

BREAST FEEDING SUMMARY

RECOMMENDATION: Limited Human Data - Potential Toxicity

Sotalol is concentrated in human milk with milk levels 3–5 times those in the mother's plasma (5,7,8). Twenty paired samples of breast milk and maternal blood were obtained from 5 of the 12 women treated during and after pregnancy with sotalol for hypertension (dosage detailed above) (5). Specific details of dosage and the timing of sample collection in relationship to the last dose were not given. The mean concentrations in milk and plasma were 10.5 μg/mL (range 4.8–20.2 μg/mL) and 2.3 μg/mL (range 0.8–5.0 μg/mL), respectively. The mean milk:plasma ratio was 5.4 (range 2.2–8.8). No β-blockade effects were observed in the five nursing infants, including the one infant who had bradycardia at birth. The mother of this infant produced the highest concentrations of sotalol in milk (20.2 μg/mL) observed in the study (5).

A woman treated throughout gestation with sotalol (80 mg twice daily) and flecainide was continued on these drugs during the postpartum period (7). The infant was not breastfed. Simultaneous milk and plasma samples were drawn 3 hours after the second dose of the day on the 5th and 7th postpartum days. The milk and plasma concentrations on day 5 were 5 and 1.4 μg/mL, respectively, compared with 4.4 and 1.60 μg/mL, respectively, on day 7. The two milk:plasma ratios were 3.57 and 2.75, respectively.

Sotalol, 80 mg 3 times daily, was taken by a woman throughout a 42-week gestation and during the first 14 days of the postpartum period, at which time the dose was reduced to 80 mg twice daily (8). On the 5th postpartum day, milk and serum levels, approximately 6.5 hours after a dose (prefeeding), were 4.06 and 0.72 μg/mL, respectively, a ratio of 5.6. A postfeeding milk sample collected 0.7 hour later yielded a concentration of 3.65 μg/mL. The study was repeated on the 105th postpartum day, yielding prefeeding milk and serum concentrations 2.8 hours after the last dose of 2.36 and 0.97 μg/mL (ratio 2.4), respectively. A postfeeding milk level 0.5 hour later was 3.16 μg/mL. The authors calculated that the infant was consuming about 20%–23% of the maternal dose. No adverse effects were observed in the infant, who continued to develop normally throughout the study period.

Although symptoms of β-blockade, such as bradycardia and hypotension, were not observed in the nursing infants described above, these effects have been noted with other β-adrenergic blockers (see also Acebutolol, Atenolol, and Nadolol) and may occur with sotalol. Long-term effects of exposure to β-blockers from milk have not been studied but warrant evaluation. The American Academy of Pediatrics classifies sotalol as compatible with breast-feeding (15).

References

1. American Hospital Formulary Service. *Drug Information 2000*. Bethesda, MD: American Society of Health-System Pharmacists, 2000:1596–1600.
2. Product information. Betapace. Berlex Laboratories, 2001.
3. Webster WS, Brown-Woodman PDC, Snow MD, Danielsson BRG. Teratogenic potential of almokalant, dofetilide, and d-sotalol: drugs with potassium channel blocking activity. Teratology 1996;53:168–75.
4. O'Hare MF, Leahey W, Murnaghan GA, McDevitt DG. Pharmacokinetics of sotalol during pregnancy. Eur J Clin Pharmacol 1983;24:521–4.
5. O'Hare MF, Murnaghan GA, Russell CJ, Leahey WJ, Varma MPS, McDevitt DG. Sotalol as a hypotensive agent in pregnancy. Br J Obstet Gynaecol 1980;87:814–20.
6. Erkkola R, Lammintausta R, Liukko P, Anttila M. Transfer of propranolol and sotalol across the human placenta. Their effect on maternal and fetal plasma renin activity. Acta Obstet Gynecol Scand 1982;61:31–4.
7. Wagner X, Jouglard J, Moulin M, Miller AM, Petitjean J, Pisapia A. Coadministration of flecainide acetate and sotalol during pregnancy: lack of teratogenic effects, passage across the placenta, and excretion in human breast milk. Am Heart J 1990;119:700–2.
8. Hackett LP, Wojnar-Horton RE, Dusci LJ, Ilett KF, Roberts MJ. Excretion of sotalol in breast milk. Br J Clin Pharmacol 1990;29:277–8.
9. Arnoux P, Seyral P, Llurens M, Djiane P, Potier A, Unal D, Cano JP, Serradimigni A, Rouault F. Amiodarone and digoxin for refractory fetal tachycardia. Am J Cardiol 1987;59:166–7.
10. Oudijk MA, Michon MM, Kleinman CS, Kapusta L, Stoutenbeek P, Visser GHA, Meijboom EJ. Sotalol in the treatment of fetal dysrhythmias. Circulation 2000;101:2721–6.
11. Tamari I, Eldar M, Rabinowitz B, Neufeld HN. Medical treatment of cardiovascular disorders during pregnancy. Am Heart J 1982;104:1357–63.
12. Rotmensch HH, Elkayam U, Frishman W. Antiarrhythmic drug therapy during pregnancy. Ann Intern Med 1983;98:487–97.
13. Sandstrom B. Clinical trials of adrenergic antagonists in pregnancy hypertension. Acta Obstet Gynecol Scand 1984;Suppl 118:57–60.
14. Lubbe WF. Treatment of hypertension in pregnancy. J Cardiovasc Pharmacol 1990;16(Suppl 7):S110–3.
15. Committee on Drugs, American Academy of Pediatrics. The transfer of drugs and other chemicals into human milk. Pediatrics 2001;108:776–89.

Name: **SPARFLOXACIN** Risk Factor: C_M

Class: **Anti-infective (Quinolone)**

FETAL RISK SUMMARY

RECOMMENDATION: Human Data Suggest Low Risk

Sparfloxacin is an oral, synthetic, broad-spectrum antibacterial agent. As a fluoroquinolone, it is in the same class of agents as ciprofloxacin, enoxacin, levofloxacin, lomefloxacin, norfloxacin, and ofloxacin. Nalidixic acid is also a quinolone drug.

Reproduction studies, conducted in male and female rats, found no evidence of impaired fertility or reproductive performance at oral doses approximately 15 times the maximum human dose based on body surface area (MHD) (1). No teratogenic effects were observed in rats, rabbits, and monkeys at oral doses approximately 6, 4, and 3 times, respectively, the MHD, although maternal toxicity was evident at these dose levels. When the dose was increased to about 9 times the MHD or higher in pregnant rats, a dose-dependent increase in the number of fetuses with ventricular septal defects was observed. This effect did not occur in rabbits or monkeys.

In a prospective follow-up study conducted by the European Network of Teratology Information Services (ENTIS), data on 549 pregnancies exposed to fluoroquinolones (none to sparfloxacin) were described in a 1996 reference (see also Ciprofloxacin) (2). Data on another 116 prospective and 25 retrospective pregnancy exposures to the antibacterials were also included. Of the 666 cases with known outcome, 32 (4.8%) of the embryos, fetuses, or newborns had congenital malformations. Based on previous epidemiologic data, the authors concluded that the 4.8% frequency of malformations did not exceed the background rate (2). Finally, 25 retrospective reports of infants with anomalies, who had been exposed *in utero* to fluoroquinolones, were analyzed, but no specific patterns of major congenital malformations were detected.

The authors of the above study concluded that pregnancy exposure to quinolones was not an indication for termination, but that this class of antibacterials should still be considered contraindicated in pregnant women. Moreover, this study did not address the issue of cartilage damage from quinolone exposure, and the authors recognized the need for follow-up studies of this potential toxicity in children exposed *in utero*. Because of their own and previously published findings, they further recommended that the focus of future studies should be on malformations involving the abdominal wall and urogenital system, and on limb-reduction defects (2).

In summary, although no reports describing the use of sparfloxacin during human gestation have been located, the available evidence for other members of this class indicates that a causal relationship with birth defects cannot be excluded (see Ciprofloxacin, Norfloxacin, or Ofloxacin), although the lack of a pattern among the anomalies is reassuring. Because of these concerns and the available animal data, the use of sparfloxacin during pregnancy, especially during the 1st trimester, should be avoided, if possible. A 1993 review on the safety of fluoroquinolones concluded that these antibacterials should be avoided during pregnancy because of the difficulty in extrapolating animal mutagenicity results to humans and because interpretation of this toxicity is still controversial (3). The authors of this review were not convinced that fluoroquinolone-induced fetal cartilage damage and subsequent arthropathies were a major concern, even though this effect had been demonstrated in several animal species after administration to both pregnant and immature animals and in occasional human case reports involving children (3). Others have also concluded that fluoroquinolones should be considered contraindicated in pregnancy, because safer alternatives are usually available (2).

BREAST FEEDING SUMMARY

RECOMMENDATION: No Human Data - Probably Compatible

When first marketed, the administration of sparfloxacin during breast-feeding was not recommended because of the potential for arthropathy and other serious toxicity in the nursing infant (1). Phototoxicity has been observed with quinolones when exposure to excessive sunlight (i.e., ultraviolet [UV] light) has occurred (1). Well-differentiated squamous cell carcinomas of the skin has been produced in mice who were exposed chronically to some fluoroquinolones and periodic UV light (e.g., see Lomefloxacin), but studies to evaluate the carcinogenicity of sparfloxacin in this manner have not been conducted.

S

No reports describing the use of sparfloxacin during human lactation have been located. The manufacturer states that the antibacterial agent is excreted in human milk (1). Two other fluoroquinolones are classified as compatible with breast-feeding by the American Academy of Pediatrics (see Ciprofloxacin and Ofloxacin).

References

1. Product information. Zagam. Bertek Pharmaceuticals, 2000.
2. Schaefer C, Amoura-Elefant E, Vial T, Ornoy A, Garbis H, Robert E, Rodriguez-Pinilla E, Pexieder T, Prapas N, Merlob P. Pregnancy outcome after prenatal quinolone exposure. Evaluation of a case registry of the European Network of Teratology Information Services (ENTIS). Eur J Obstet Gynecol Reprod Biol 1996;69:83–9.
3. Norrby SR, Lietman PS. Safety and tolerability of fluoroquinolones. Drugs 1993;45(Suppl 3):59–64.

Name:	**SPECTINOMYCIN**	Risk Factor:	**C**
Class:	**Antibiotic**		

FETAL RISK SUMMARY

RECOMMENDATION: Human Data Suggest Low Risk

No reports linking the use of spectinomycin with congenital defects have been located. The drug has been used to treat gonorrhea in pregnant patients allergic to penicillin. Available data do not suggest a threat to mother or fetus (1,2).

BREAST FEEDING SUMMARY

RECOMMENDATION: No Human Data - Probably Compatible

No data are available.

References

1. McCormack WM, Finland M. Spectinomycin. Ann Intern Med 1976;84:712–6.
2. Anonymous. Treatment of syphilis and gonorrhea. Med Lett Drugs Ther 1977;19:105–7.

Name:	**SPIRAMYCIN**	Risk Factor:	**C**
Class:	**Antibiotic**		

FETAL RISK SUMMARY

RECOMMENDATION: Compatible

Spiramycin, a macrolide antibiotic available in the United States only as an orphan drug but widely used in Europe for more than 30 years, is used primarily in the treatment of the protozoal infections cryptosporidiosis and toxoplasmosis.

Infection of the mother with *Toxoplasmosis gondii* early in gestation may result in the birth of infants with a clinical syndrome whose characteristics may include hydrocephalus or microcephalus, hepatosplenomegaly, icterus, maculopapular rash, chorioretinitis, and cerebral calcifications (1,2). No evidence has been found that maternal infection before conception results in infection of the fetus or delivery of an infant with congenital toxoplasmosis (1).

Spiramycin crosses the placenta to the fetus (2). Concentrations of the antibiotic in maternal serum, cord blood, and the placenta after a dosage regimen of 2 g/day were 1.19, 0.63, and 2.75 μg/mL, respectively. When the maternal dose was increased to 3 g/day, the levels were 1.69, 0.78, and 6.2 μg/mL, respectively. Based on these results, the cord:maternal serum ratio is approximately 0.5. Moreover, at these doses, spiramycin is concentrated in the placenta with levels approximately 2–4 times those in the maternal serum.

No reports of adverse fetal outcome attributable to spiramycin have been located. According to two French investigators in 1974, the antibiotic had been used for more than 15 years in Europe without any evidence of fetal harm (3). Spiramycin, 2–3 g/day in divided dosage throughout the remainder of gestation, is the treatment of choice when primary

S

infection with toxoplasmosis occurs in the pregnant woman (3–10). If fetal infection is subsequently diagnosed, pyrimethamine, sulfadoxine or sulfadiazine, and folic acid are added to the spiramycin therapy (11–14). However, the belief that the addition of pyrimethamine and a sulfonamide to the treatment regimen has proven to reduce significantly the incidence of severe congenital toxoplasmosis is still controversial because of the potential added risk to the fetus from the combination drug therapy (15,16).

BREAST FEEDING SUMMARY

RECOMMENDATION: Limited Human Data - Probably Compatible

Spiramycin is excreted into breast milk. Nursing infants of mothers receiving 1.5 g/day for 3 days had spiramycin serum concentrations of 20 μg/mL (17). This concentration was bacteriostatic (17).

References

1. Shepard TH. *Catalog of Teratogenic Agents*. 6th ed. Baltimore, MD: Johns Hopkins University Press, 1989:627.
2. Remington JS, Desmonts G. Toxoplasmosis. In Remington JS, Klein JO, eds. *Infectious Diseases of the Fetus and Newborn Infant*. 2nd ed. Philadelphia, PA: WB Saunders, 1983:143–263.
3. Desmonts G, Couvreur J. Congenital toxoplasmosis: a prospective study of 378 pregnancies. N Engl J Med 1974;290:1110–6.
4. Desmonts G, Couvreur J. Toxoplasmosis in pregnancy and its transmission to the fetus. Bull N Y Acad Med 1974;50:146–59.
5. Russo M, Galanti B, Nardiello S. Treatment of toxoplasmosis: present knowledge and problems. Ann Sclavo 1980;22:877–88.
6. Fleck DG. Toxoplasmosis. Arch Dis Child 1981;56:494–5.
7. Desmonts G, Daffos F, Forestier F, Capella-Pavlovsky M, Thulliez PH, Chartier M. Prenatal diagnosis of congenital toxoplasmosis. Lancet 1985;1:500–4.
8. Ellis CJ. Antiparasitic agents in pregnancy. Clin Obstet Gynaecol 1986;13:269–75.
9. Carter AO, Frank JW. Congenital toxoplasmosis: epidemiologic features and control. CMAJ 1986;135:618–23.
10. Ghidini A, Sirtori M, Spelta A, Vergani P. Results of a preventive program for congenital toxoplasmosis. J Reprod Med 1991;36:270–3.
11. Daffos F, Forestier F, Capella-Pavlovsky M, Thulliez P, Aufrant C, Valenti D, Cox WL. Prenatal management of 746 pregnancies at risk for congenital toxoplasmosis. N Engl J Med 1988;318:271–5.
12. Couvreur J, Desmonts G, Thulliez PH. Prophylaxis of congenital toxoplasmosis: effects of spiramycin on placental infection. J Antimicrob Chemother 1988;22(Suppl B):193–200.
13. Garin JP, Mojon M, Piens MA, Chevalier-Nuttall I. Monitoring and treatment of toxoplasmosis in the pregnant woman, fetus and newborn. Pediatrie 1989;44:705–12.
14. Hohlfeld P, Daffos F, Thulliez P, Aufrant C, Courvreur J, MacAleese J, Descombey D, Forestier F. Fetal toxoplasmosis: outcome of pregnancy and infant follow-up after in utero treatment. J Pediatr 1989;115:765–9.
15. Wilson CB. Treatment of congenital toxoplasmosis during pregnancy. J Pediatr 1990;116:1003–4.
16. Hohlfeld P, Daffos F. Treatment of congenital toxoplasmosis during pregnancy (reply). J Pediatr 1990;116:1004–5.
17. Goisis M, Cavalli P. Variations of the organoleptic properties of human milk under treatment with antibiotics. Minerva Ginac 1959;11:794–804. As cited in Onnis A, Grella P. *The Biochemical Effects of Drugs in Pregnancy*. Vol 2. Chichester, UK: Ellis Horwood Limited, 1984:340–1.

Name: **SPIRONOLACTONE** Risk Factor: **C_M***
Class: **Diuretic**

FETAL RISK SUMMARY

RECOMMENDATION: Limited Human Data - Animal Data Suggest Risk

Spironolactone, a potassium-conserving diuretic, an action that results from its antagonism of aldosterone in the distal convoluted renal tubule. The diuretic action results in an antihypertensive effect. Spironolactone also has progestational and anti-androgenic activity. The latter activity may result in apparent estrogenic adverse effects in humans (1).

Reproduction studies in mice at 20 mg/kg/day, a dose substantially below the maximum recommended human dose on a body surface area basis (MRHD), revealed no embryo or fetal adverse effects (1). In rabbits dosed at 20 mg/kg/day (approximately the MRHD), an increased number of resorptions and lower number of live fetuses was observed. Because of spironolactone's anti-androgenic activity, feminization of male rat fetuses occurred at a dose of 200 mg/kg/day administered to the mothers during late embryogenesis and fetal development (1). In addition, rat offspring of both sexes exposed *in utero* in late gestation to 50 or 100 mg/kg/day exhibited permanent dose-related changes in their reproductive tracts (1).

No reports linking spironolactone with human congenital defects have been located. Some have commented, however, that spironolactone may be contraindicated during pregnancy based on the known anti-androgenic effects in humans and the feminization observed in male rat fetuses (2). Other investigators consider diuretics in general to be contraindicated in pregnancy, except for patients with cardiovascular disorders, because they do not prevent or alter the course of toxemia and they may decrease placental perfusion (3–5). In general, diuretics are not recommended for the treatment of gestational hypertension because of the maternal hypovolemia characteristic of this disease.

In a surveillance study of Michigan Medicaid recipients conducted between 1985 and 1992 involving 229,101 completed pregnancies, 31 newborns had been exposed to spironolactone during the 1st trimester (F. Rosa, personal communication, FDA, 1993). Two (6.5%) major birth defects were observed (one expected), one of which was an oral cleft (none expected). No anomalies were observed in five other categories of defects (cardiovascular defects, spina bifida, polydactyly, limb reduction defects, and hypospadias) for which specific data were available.

[**Risk Factor D if used in gestational hypertension.*]

BREAST FEEDING SUMMARY

RECOMMENDATION: Limited Human Data - Probably Compatible

It is not known whether unmetabolized spironolactone is excreted in breast milk. Canrenone, the principal and active metabolite, was found with milk:plasma ratios of 0.72 (2 hours) and 0.51 (14.5 hours) (6). These amounts would provide an estimated maximum of 0.2% of the mother's daily dose to the infant (6). The effects on the infant from this ingestion are unknown, but the amounts appear to be clinically insignificant. However, consideration should be given to the fact that spironolactone is tumorigenic in rats (1). The American Academy of Pediatrics classifies spironolactone as compatible with breastfeeding (7).

S

References

1. Product information. Aldactone. G.D. Searle, 2000.
2. Messina M, Biffignandi P, Ghiga E, Jeantet MG, Molinatti GM. Possible contraindication of spironolactone during pregnancy. J Endocrinol Invest 1979;2:222.
3. Pitkin RM, Kaminetzky HA, Newton M, Pritchard JA. Maternal nutrition: a selective review of clinical topics. Obstet Gynecol 1972;40:773–85.
4. Lindheimer MD, Katz AI. Sodium and diuretics in pregnancy. N Engl J Med 1973;288:891–4.
5. Christianson R, Page EW. Diuretic drugs and pregnancy. Obstet Gynecol 1976;48:647–52.
6. Phelps DL, Karim A. Spironolactone: relationship between concentrations of dethioacetylated metabolite in human serum and milk. J Pharm Sci 1977;66:1203.
7. Committee on Drugs, American Academy of Pediatrics. The transfer of drugs and other chemicals into human milk. Pediatrics 2001;108:776–89.

Name:	**STAVUDINE**	Risk Factor:	C_M
Class:	**Antiviral**		

FETAL RISK SUMMARY

RECOMMENDATION: Compatible - Maternal Benefit >> Embryo/Fetal Risk

Stavudine (2′,3′-didehydro-3′-deoxythymidine; d4T) inhibits viral reverse transcriptase and DNA synthesis. It is classified as a nucleoside reverse transcriptase inhibitor (NRTI) used for the treatment of human immunodeficiency virus (HIV) infections. Its mechanism of action is similar to that of five other nucleoside analogues: abacavir, didanosine, lamivudine, zalcitabine, and zidovudine. Stavudine is converted by intracellular enzymes to the active metabolite, stavudine triphosphate.

No evidence of teratogenicity was observed in pregnant rats and rabbits exposed to maximum plasma concentrations up to 399 and 183 times, respectively, of those produced by a human dose of 1 mg/kg/day (1). A dose-related increase in common skeletal variations, post-implantation loss, and early neonatal mortality was observed in one or both species.

Antiretroviral nucleosides have been shown to have a direct dose-related cytotoxic effect on preimplantation mouse embryos. A 1994 report compared this toxicity among zidovudine and three newer compounds, stavudine, didanosine, and zalcitabine (2). Whereas significant inhibition of blastocyst formation occurred with a 1 μmol/L concentration of zidovudine, stavudine and zalcitabine toxicity was not detected until 100 μmol/L, and no toxicity was observed with didanosine up to 100 μmol/L. Moreover, postblastocyst development was severely inhibited in those embryos that did survive exposure to 1 μmol/L zidovudine. As for the other compounds, stavudine, at a concentration of 10 μmol/L (2.24 μg/mL), inhibited postblastocyst development, but no effect was observed with concentrations up to 100 μmol/L of didanosine or zalcitabine. Although there are no human data, the authors of this study concluded that the three newer agents may be safer than zidovudine to use in early pregnancy.

Similar to other nucleoside analogues, stavudine appears to cross the human placenta by simple diffusion (3). The relatively low molecular weight (about 224) is in agreement with this. Stavudine also crosses the placenta in rats, resulting in a fetal:maternal ratio of approximately 0.5 (1). In near-term macaques, the steady-state fetal:maternal plasma ratio was approximately 0.8 (4). A related study found that zidovudine did not affect the placental transfer of stavudine in macaques (5). However, no reports in animals or humans have been located relating to the placental transfer of stavudine triphosphate (the active metabolite) or to the capability of the placenta or the fetus to metabolize stavudine.

Three experimental *in vitro* models using perfused human placentas to predict the placental transfer of NRTIs (didanosine, stavudine, zalcitabine, and zidovudine) were described in a 1999 publication (6). For each drug, the predicted fetal:maternal plasma drug concentration ratios at steady state with each of the three models were close to those actually observed in pregnant macaques. Based on these results, the authors concluded that their models would accurately predict the mechanism, relative rate, and the extent of *in vivo* human placental transfer of NRTIs (6).

The Antiretroviral Pregnancy Registry reported, for the period January 1989 through January 2004, prospective data (reported to the Registry before the outcomes were known) involving 1537 live births that had been exposed during the 1st trimester to one or more antiretroviral agents (7). Forty-seven of the newborns had congenital defects (3.1%, 95% confidence interval [CI] 2.3–4.1). In the 2407 live births with earliest exposure in the 2nd/3rd trimesters, there were 56 infants with defects (2.3%, 95% CI 1.8–3.0). The prevalence rates for the two periods did not differ significantly. There were 103 infants with birth defects among 3944 live births with exposure anytime during pregnancy (2.6%, 95% CI 2.1–3.2). The prevalence rate did not differ significantly from the rate expected in a nonexposed population (7). There were 512 outcomes exposed to stavudine (381 in the 1st trimester and 131 in the 2nd/3rd trimesters) in combination with other antiretroviral agents. There were 11 (2.9%, 95% CI 1.4–5.1) birth defects among the 1st trimester exposures and 5 (3.8%, 95% CI 1.3–8.7) in those exposed in the 2nd/3rd trimesters. In reviewing the birth defects of prospective and retrospective (pregnancies reported after the outcomes were known) registered cases, and clinical reports, the Registry concluded that there was no pattern of anomalies to suggest a common cause (7). (See Lamivudine for required statement.)

A 2000 case report described the adverse pregnancy outcomes, including neural tube defects (NTDs), of two pregnant women with HIV infection who were treated with the anti-infective combination, trimethoprim/sulfamethoxazole, for prophylaxis against *Pneumocystis carinii*, concurrently with antiretroviral agents (8). Exposure to stavudine occurred in one of these cases. A 31-year-old woman presented at 15 weeks' gestation. She was receiving trimethoprim/sulfamethoxazole, didanosine, stavudine, nevirapine, and vitamin B supplements (specific vitamins and dosage not given) that had been started before conception. A fetal ultrasound at 19 weeks' gestation revealed spina bifida and ventriculomegaly. The patient elected to terminate her pregnancy. The fetus did not have HIV infection. Defects observed at autopsy included ventriculomegaly, an Arnold-Chiari malformation, sacral spina bifida, and a lumbo-sacral meningomyelocele. The authors attributed the NTDs in both cases to the antifolate activity of trimethoprim (8).

A 1999 case report described a 26-year-old woman with a 5-year history of HIV infection (9). Two years before her current pregnancy, she had received monotherapy with zidovudine for 19 months followed by 6 months of monotherapy with zalcitabine. She stopped therapy during the first 19 gestational weeks, then started stavudine and lamivudine that was continued until vaginal delivery at term of a healthy 3560-g girl. The infant was not infected with HIV and was doing well at 9 months of age.

No data are available on the advisability of treating pregnant women who have been exposed to HIV via occupational exposure, but one author discourages this use (10).

In summary, the animal and human data suggest that stavudine represents a low risk to the embryo/fetus. Theoretically, exposure to stavudine at the time of implantation could result in impaired fertility because of embryonic cytotoxicity, but this has not been studied in humans. Stavudine peak serum concentrations achievable in humans with therapeutic doses, however, are in the same range that has been found to inhibit postblastocyst development in mice. Mitochondrial dysfunction in offspring exposed *in utero* or postnatally to NRTIs has been reported (see Lamivudine and Zidovudine), but these findings are controversial and require confirmation.

Two reviews, one in 1996 and the other in 1997, concluded that all women currently receiving antiretroviral therapy should continue to receive therapy during pregnancy and that treatment of the mother with monotherapy should be considered inadequate therapy (11,12). In 1998, the Centers for Disease Control and Prevention (CDC) made a similar recommendation that antiretroviral therapy should be continued during pregnancy, but discontinuation of all therapy during the 1st trimester was a consideration (13). If indicated, therefore, stavudine should not be withheld in pregnancy (with the possible exception of the 1st trimester) because the expected benefit to the HIV-positive mother probably outweighs the unknown risk to the fetus. The efficacy and safety of combined therapy in preventing vertical transmission of HIV to the newborn, however, are unknown, and zidovudine remains the only antiretroviral agent recommended for this purpose (11,12).

BREAST FEEDING SUMMARY

RECOMMENDATION: Contraindicated

No reports describing the use of stavudine during lactation have been located. The relatively low molecular weight (about 224), however, suggests that stavudine will be excreted into breast milk. The drug is excreted into the milk of lactating rats (1).

Reports on the use of stavudine during human lactation are unlikely because the antiviral agent is used in the treatment of human immunodeficiency virus (HIV) infections. HIV-1 is transmitted in milk, and in developed countries, breast-feeding is not recommended (11,12,14–16). In developing countries, breast-feeding is undertaken, despite the risk, because there are no affordable milk substitutes available. Until 1999, no studies had been published that examined the effect of any antiretroviral therapy on HIV-1 transmission in milk. In that year, a study involving zidovudine was published that measured a 38% reduction in vertical transmission of HIV-1 infection in spite of breast-feeding when compared to controls (see Zidovudine).

References

1. Product information. Zerit. Bristol-Myers Squibb, 2001.
2. Toltzis P, Mourton T, Magnuson T. Comparative embryonic cytotoxicity of antiretroviral nucleosides. J Infect Dis 1994;169:1100–2.
3. Bawdon RE, Kaul S, Sobhi S. The ex vivo transfer of the anti-HIV nucleoside compound d4T in the human placenta. Gynecol Obstet Invest 1994;38:1–4.
4. Odinecs A, Nosbisch C, Keller RD, Baughman WL, Unadkat JD. In vivo maternal-fetal pharmacokinetics of stavudine (2′,3′-didehydro-3′-deoxythymidine) in pigtailed macaques (*Macaca nemestrina*). Antimicrob Agents Chemother 1996;40:196–202.
5. Odinecs A, Nosbisch C, Unadkat JD. Zidovudine does not affect transplacental transfer or systemic clearance of stavudine (2′,3′-didehydro-3′-doxythymidine) in the pigtailed macaque (*Macaca nemestrina*). Antimicrob Agents Chemother 1996;40:1569–71.
6. Tuntland T, Odinecs A, Pereira CM, Nosbisch C, Unadkat JD. *In vitro* models to predict the *in vivo* mechanism, rate, and extent of placental transfer of dideoxynucleoside drugs against human immunodeficiency virus. Am J Obstet Gynecol 1999;180:198–206.
7. Antiretroviral Pregnancy Registry Steering Committee. *Antiretroviral Pregnancy Registry International Interim Report for 1 January 1989 through 31 January 2004*. Wilmington, NC: Registry Coordinating Center. 2004.
8. Richardson MP, Osrin D, Donaghy S, Brown NA, Hay, Sharland M. Spinal malformations in the fetuses of HIV infected women receiving combination antiretroviral therapy and co-trimoxazole. Eur J Obstet Gynecol Reprod Biol 2000;93:215–7.
9. Ristola M, Salo E, Ammala P, Suni J. Combined stavudine and lamivudine during pregnancy. AIDS 1999;13:285.
10. Gerberding JL. Management of occupational exposures to blood-borne viruses. N Engl J Med 1995;332:444–51.
11. Carpenter CCJ, Fischi MA, Hammer SM, Hirsch MS, Jacobsen DM, Katzenstein DA, Montaner JSG, Richman DD, Saag MS, Schooley RT, Thompson MA, Vella S, Yeni PG, Volberding PA. Antiretroviral therapy for HIV infection in 1996. JAMA 1996;276;146–54.
12. Minkoff H, Augenbraun M. Antiretroviral therapy for pregnant women. Am J Obstet Gynecol 1997;176:478–89.
13. CDC. Public Health Service Task Force recommendations for the use of antiretroviral drugs in pregnant women infected with HIV-1 for maternal health and for reducing perinatal HIV-1 transmission in the United States. MMWR 1998;47:No. RR-2.
14. Brown ZA, Watts DH. Antiviral therapy in pregnancy. Clin Obstet Gynecol 1990;33:276–89.
15. de Martino M, Tovo P-A, Tozzi AE, Pezzotti P, Galli L, Livadiotti S, Caselli D, Massironi E, Ruga E, Fioredda F, Plebani A, Gabiano C, Zuccotti GV. HIV-1 transmission through breast-milk: appraisal of risk according to duration of feeding. AIDS 1992;6:991–7.
16. Van de Perre P. Postnatal transmission of human immunodeficiency virus type 1: the breast-feeding dilemma. Am J Obstet Gynecol 1995;173:483–7.

S

Name:	**ST. JOHN'S WORT**	Risk Factor:	**C**
Class:	**Herb**		

FETAL RISK SUMMARY

RECOMMENDATION: Limited Human Data - No Relevant Animal Data

Hypericum perforatum (St. John's wort) is an aromatic, aggressive perennial weed that is native to Europe but also grows throughout the United States and parts of Canada (1). The plant is harvested for medicinal purposes during July and August (1). A large number of chemical constituents have been isolated from the plant, including hypericin, pseudohypericin, flavonoids, glycosides, phenols, tannins, volatile oils, and other compounds (1–8). Hypericin and pseudohypericin are considered to be the primary orally active ingredients (1,5–8).

Preparations made from *H. perforatum* have been used for medicinal purposes for thousands of years. These uses have included the management of anxiety, depression, insomnia, inflammation, and gastritis. They have also been used as a diuretic and, topically, for the treatment of hemorrhoids and to enhance wound-healing (1–5). More recently, hypericin has been investigated for activity against the human immunodeficiency virus (HIV) and other viruses (1,5,8). In addition, extracts and tinctures of hypericum have shown activity against gram negative and gram positive bacteria (1).

No data are available on the animal or human placental transfer of hypericin, pseudohypericin, or other constituents of St. John's wort.

The mechanism of antidepressant action is thought to be related to selected serotonin-reuptake inhibition, monoamine oxidase inhibitors, a combination of both, or other mechanisms (1–4,6–9). Adverse effects induced by hypericum preparations, relatively infrequent in nonpregnant humans but not studied in pregnant women, include gastrointestinal upset and constipation, allergic reactions, fatigue, dry mouth, dizziness, and confusion (1–10). Rare photosensitivity in fair-skinned individuals has also been observed.

Surprisingly, for a product that has been in use since ancient Greek and Roman times, only one report has been located that described its consumption during human pregnancy (see below). Moreover, there are few animal reproductive studies available for evaluation of its embryo and fetal safety. Aqueous extractions of *H. perforatum* demonstrated weak uterine tonus-enhancing activity in experiments using isolated rabbit and guinea pig uterine horns (11). Uterotonic activity or abortions, however, have apparently not been reported after consumption of the herb by animals or humans.

S

In a randomized, placebo-controlled reproductive study, adult female mice were fed either hypericum (180 mg/kg/day) or placebo for 2 weeks before mating and then throughout gestation (12). The dose, which has antidepressant efficacy in adult mice, was equivalent to the human dose on a kg/m^2 basis (12,13). The birth weights of all exposed pups were smaller than controls, but only the reduced birth weights of male pups reached statistical significance in comparison to controls (1.68 g vs. 1.75 g, $p<0.01$) (13). Moreover, successful performance on the negative geotaxis task, a measure of behavior during early development, was significantly lower in exposed male pups (but not female pups) on postnatal day 3 (13). Both the body weight and negative geotaxis task performance were comparable to controls by postnatal day 5 (13). No differences, regardless of gender, were observed between exposed and nonexposed pups in body length, head circumference, sexual maturation, or the attainment of developmental milestones up to adulthood (12).

Similarly, no differences were observed between the groups in pup-dam interactions, performance of locomotor, depression, and anxiety tasks during juvenile and adult periods, or in male sexual behavior and aggression. An evaluation of second-generation offspring found no differences between the groups in any measurement (12,13).

An aqueous ethanolic extract of hypericum was tested for mutagenic activity in a study published in 1990 (14). Using both *in vitro* and *in vivo* test systems (mice, hamsters, etc.), no evidence of mutagenic effects was observed.

In a sperm penetration assay, zona-free hamster oocytes were incubated for 1 hour with two concentrations of *H. perforatum*, 0.06 mg/mL and 0.6 mg/mL, dissolved in HEPES-buffered synthetic human tubal fluid (modified HTF) (15). Fresh human donor sperm was suspended in the modified HTF and then mixed with the oocytes for 3 hours. Modified HTF served as the control. At the 0.06 mg/mL concentration, all the oocytes were penetrated, whereas at 0.6 mg/mL, zero penetration occurred. The decrease in penetration was not associated with a decrease in sperm motility (15). In the second part of the study, sperm were incubated with the herbal solutions for 7 days (15). Both concentrations caused significant sperm DNA denaturation concomitant with decreases in sperm viability compared with controls. The higher concentration showed point mutation of a selected sperm sentinel gene, the BRCA1 exon 11 gene (15). Extrapolation of these data to the reproductive risk of hypericum in males is difficult, in part because the concentration of hypericum in semen or sperm has not been studied (15). Moreover, although the doses used in this study are small fractions of the actual recommended human dose, usually expressed in grams of hypericin, there is no published evidence that the adverse effects observed have occurred *in vivo*.

A brief 1998 case report described the use of St. John's wort by two pregnant women, but only one of the cases has outcome data (16). In the first case, a 38-year-old woman began taking 900 mg/day St. John's wort at 24 weeks' gestation for a major depressive disorder that had recurred during the 1st trimester. She continued the herbal medicine throughout the remainder of her pregnancy, taking her last dose 24 hours before delivery (gestational age not specified). Other than late onset thrombocytopenia (platelet count 88,000), the pregnancy was unremarkable (16). The woman delivered a healthy, 7 lb, 8 oz (about 3400 g) female infant with Apgar scores of 9 and 9 at both 1 and 5 minutes. The physical examination and laboratory results were normal. Neonatal jaundice developed on day 5 but responded to brief phototherapy. Behavioral assessment at 4 and 33 days of age was normal. The second case involved a 43-year-old woman who had been taking fluoxetine and methylphenidate for a recurrent major depressive disorder (16). After an unexpected conception, she discontinued these medications because of concerns about potential adverse fetal effects and began self-medicating with St. John's wort, 900 mg/day. Apparently, this pregnancy was ongoing, because no outcome data were presented.

In summary, only one report describing the use of St. John's wort (*H. perforatum*) during human pregnancy has been located, and only one of the two cases contained in the report has outcome data. Two animal studies apparently did not look for structural defects, but neither observed behavioral teratogenic effects. Moreover, no mutagenicity was found with various tests involving mammalian cells. Hypericum has demonstrated human sperm toxicity *in vitro*, but no reports describing this adverse effect after ingestion of the drug have been located. Similarly, the uterotonic action observed in an *in vitro* animal experiment has not been reported in animals or humans following consumption. This lack of reported toxicity is reassuring. Moreover, because the use of St. John's wort is widespread and dates back thousands of years, it is doubtful that a major teratogenic action or other reproductive toxicity would have escaped notice. More subtle or low-incidence effects, however, including structural and behavioral teratogenicity, the induction of abortions, and infertility may have escaped detection, and further study is required before human reproductive risk or safety can be assessed.

Because standardization of any herbal product as to its constituents, concentrations, and the presence of contaminants is generally lacking, consumption of these preparations during pregnancy may result in fetal exposure to unintended chemicals and doses. Furthermore, pregnant women should be counseled on the risks to themselves and their pregnancies that may result from self-medication or discontinuing prescribed therapy without first consulting their health care provider. If St. John's wort is used in pregnancy, healthcare professionals are encouraged to call the toll free number (800-670-6126) for information about patient enrollment in the Motherisk study.

BREAST FEEDING SUMMARY

RECOMMENDATION: Limited Human Data - Potential Toxicity

Only one report describing the use of St. John's wort (*H. perforatum*) during human lactation has been located. A 38-year-old mother had taken 900 mg/day St. John's wort from 24 weeks' gestation until delivery (16). (See case above.) She began breast-feeding her female infant after delivery and then resumed taking the herbal product 20 days after delivery. Neonatal jaundice was noted at 5 days of age but responded to brief phototherapy. Behavioral assessments of the nursing infant at 4 and 33 days of age were normal.

It is not known if any of the constituents and possible contaminants that may be found in preparations of St. John's wort are excreted into human milk or if exposure to them via the milk represents a risk to a nursing infant.

References

1. St. John's Wort. *The Review of Natural Products*. St. Louis, MO: Facts and Comparisons, November 1997.
2. Chavez ML, Chavez PI. Saint Johns' wort. Hosp Pharm 1997;32:1621–32.
3. Miller LG. Herbal medicinals. Selected clinical considerations focusing on known or potential drug-herb interactions. Arch Intern Med 1998;158:2200–11.
4. Klepser TB, Klepser ME. Unsafe and potentially safe herbal therapies. Am J Health Syst Pharm 1999;56:125–38.
5. Pepping J. St. Alternative therapies. St. John's wort: *Hypericum perforatum*. Am J Health Syst Pharm 1999;56:329.
6. Wong AHC, Smith M, Boon HS. Herbal remedies in psychiatric practice. Arch Gen Psychiatry 1998;55:1033–44.
7. Bennett DA Jr, Phun L, Polk JF, Voglino SA, Zlotnik V, Raffa RB. Neuropharmacology of St. John's wort (*Hypericum*). Ann Pharmacother 1998;32:1201–8.
8. Cupp MJ. Herbal remedies: adverse effects and drug interactions. Am Fam Physician 1999;59:1239–44.
9. Zink T, Chaffin J. Herbal "health" products: what family physicians need to know. Am Fam Physician 1998;58:1133–40.
10. Linde K, Ramirez G, Mulrow CD, Pauls A, Weidenhammer W, Melchart D. St. John's wort for depression—an overview and meta-analysis of randomised clinical trials. BMJ 1996;313:253–8.
11. Shipochliev T. Uterotonic action of extracts from a group of medicinal plants. Vet Med Nauki 1981;18:94–8.
12. Christensen HD, Rayburn WF, Coleman FH, Gonzalez CL. Effect of antenatal hypericum (St. John's wort) on growth and physical development of mice offspring (abstract). Teratology 1999;59:411.
13. Rayburn WF, Christensen HD, Gonzalez CL. Effect of antenatal exposure to Saint John's wort (*Hypericum*) on neurobehavior of developing mice. Am J Obstet Gynecol 2000;183:1225–31.
14. Okpanyi SN, Lidsba H, Scholl BC, Miltenburger HG. Genotoxicity of a standardized hypericum extract. Arzneimittelforschung 1990;40:851–5.
15. Ondrizek RR, Chan PJ, Patton WC, King A. An alternative medicine study of herbal effects on the penetration of zona-free hamster oocytes and the integrity of sperm deoxyribonucleic acid. Fertil Steril 1999;71:517–22.
16. Grush LR, Nierenberg A, Keefe B, Cohen LS. St. John's wort during pregnancy. JAMA 1998;280:1566.

Name:	**STREPTOKINASE**	Risk Factor:	C_M
Class:	**Thrombolytic**		

FETAL RISK SUMMARY

RECOMMENDATION: Compatible

No reports linking the use of streptokinase with congenital defects have been located. Animal reproductive studies have not been conducted with streptokinase (1).

Only minimal amounts cross the placenta and are not sufficient to cause fibrinolytic effects in the fetus (2–8). Although the passage of streptokinase is blocked by the placenta, streptokinase antibodies do cross to the fetus (6). This passive sensitization would have clinical importance only if the neonate required streptokinase therapy. A 1970 review briefly mentioned the use of streptokinase in 12 pregnant women with deep vein thrombosis and in one case of placental insufficiency, but no fetal or neonatal data were given (9).

Fetal death occurred in one case shortly after the start of streptokinase for massive pulmonary embolism in a 24-year-old multipara at 34 weeks' gestation (4). An autopsy found no evidence of fetal hemorrhage and the loss was attributed to maternal hypoxia.

In one study, 24 patients were treated in the 2nd and 3rd trimesters without fetal complications (6). Use in the 1st trimester for maternal thrombophlebitis has also been reported (7). No adverse effects were observed in the infant born at term.

A 1970 report described the use of streptokinase in a 35-year-old pregnant woman with recurrent embolism of the left middle cerebral artery (10,11). At 33 weeks' gestation, low-dose streptokinase was infused at 10,000 IU/hour for 2 hours, then 5000 IU/hour for 4 hours. Warfarin (50 mg IV) was given during the infusion and heparin was started following streptokinase. Complete resolution of carotid occlusion was documented on angiogram with improvement of the patient's symptoms. Rupture of the membranes occurred 9 hours after the start of streptokinase followed 1 hour later by delivery of premature triplets (1.7, 1.5, and 1.7 kg). No complications of streptokinase were observed in the mother or newborns, although one of the triplets died 5 days later of respiratory distress syndrome.

Two women were treated with streptokinase (60,000 IU for 30 minutes, then 100,000 IU/hour for approximately 3–7 days) for iliofemoral thrombi in the left leg at 3 and 6 months' gestation (12). No other specific data were given except that the women had no complications and both had normal deliveries.

S

An abstract published in 1981 briefly summarized the results of treating acute thrombotic occlusion of one or both iliofemoral veins in 122 pregnant women (13). Gestational ages varied between 14 and 38 weeks' gestation. Dosage was 1.0–1.5 million IU for 30 minutes followed by an hourly infusion of not more than 250,000 IU/hour for 24–48 hours. The complications included premature rupture of membranes (1), abruptio placentae (1) with fetal death, and severe maternal hemorrhage during treatment necessitating emergency delivery by cesarean section (2).

A 21-year-old woman presented in her 26th week of pregnancy with premature labor and a marginal placental abruption (without retroplacental clot) (14). She was treated with two courses of tranexamic acid (an antifibrinolytic agent) and started on terbutaline. At 28 weeks' gestation, the patient developed acute massive pulmonary embolism and was started on heparin therapy. She continued to deteriorate and, after 40 hours, therapy was changed to streptokinase, 100,000 IU for 30 minutes followed by an infusion of 100,000 IU/hour for 10 hours. Therapy was stopped at this time because of the return of regular uterine contractions. A spontaneous vaginal delivery of a breech, preterm, 1140-g male infant occurred 75 minutes later. No complications of therapy were noted in the infant. The mother, who was restarted on streptokinase 8 hours after delivery, had postpartum hemorrhage that required transfusion and eventual discontinuance of therapy after a total treatment time of 29 hours.

A 28-year-old patient at 28 weeks' gestation was treated with streptokinase, 250,000 IU for 30 minutes then 100,000 IU/hour for 24 hours, for prosthetic mitral valve obstruction secondary to a thrombus (15). Treatment resulted in the complete resolution of her symptoms and the return of normal valve function. Heparin infusion was started following streptokinase therapy and continued until the onset of labor 7 days later. A premature 1.4-kg infant was delivered vaginally who did well except for neonatal jaundice that responded to phototherapy.

A 1995 reference reviewed the treatment of 166 women with streptokinase (24 case reports including those described above, the majority of which have occurred in Germany), for deep vein thrombosis, pulmonary embolus, thrombosed prosthetic heart valve, axillary vein thrombosis, and cerebral arterial embolism (16). Gestational lengths varied from 9 to 38 weeks. Complications included maternal hemorrhage ($N = 13$), maternal death ($N = 2$), preterm delivery ($N = 6$), and pregnancy loss ($N = 9$) (16). The fetal and neonatal deaths included fetal loss because of maternal death ($N = 2$), spontaneous abortion and/or intrauterine fetal death without further details ($N = 3$), spontaneous abortion at 13 weeks' gestation ($N = 1$), neonatal death secondary to respiratory distress syndrome ($N = 1$), fetal death secondary to abruptio placentae during therapy ($N = 1$), and intrauterine fetal death occurring 8 hours after start of therapy ($N = 1$). No direct relationship between thrombolytic therapy and fetal death was apparent in seven of the losses, but a causal association cannot be excluded in the latter two cases (16). The theoretical concern that thrombolytic therapy before 14 weeks' gestation may interfere with placental implantation cannot be answered from the available reports. Four women were treated with streptokinase prior to 14 weeks, one of whom had a spontaneous abortion (16). No congenital anomalies were reported after streptokinase therapy, including the five cases in which treatment occurred during the 1st trimester.

In a 2004 report, massive subchorionic hematomas were observed in two women treated with streptokinase and other agents for thrombosed heart valves (17). The first case involved a 20-year-old woman with a history of rheumatic heart disease that required mitral valve replacement. She had been treated with oral anticoagulants starting at 13 weeks' gestation. At 26 weeks' gestation, she presented with a thrombosed mitral valve and heart failure. She was treated with streptokinase for a total of 64 hours (250,000 units over 30 minutes, then 100,000 U/hour). Ultrasonography showed large cystic lesions (the largest 9.3 cm by 2.2 cm) covering the entire fetal plate of the placenta. She was followed closely and was delivered at 34 weeks' because of worsening heart disease. The 2270-g female infant had Apgar scores of 9 and 10 at 1 and 5 minutes, respectively. The presentation and treatment in the second case was similar to the first woman. She was treated at 15 weeks' gestation for a thrombosed mitral valve with the same dose of streptokinase, but given over 36 hours. After streptokinase therapy, ultrasonography again revealed a massive hematoma. In this case, however, the hematoma had completely resolved by 34 weeks', and she eventually delivered a healthy 3500-g infant at term. Apgar scores were 8 and 10 at 1 and 5 minutes, respectively. No additional follow-up of the infants was reported (17).

In summary, streptokinase does not appear to present a major direct or indirect risk to the fetus, especially if treatment is withheld during the intrapartum period. Fetal losses have occurred that may have been related to therapy, but fetal hemorrhage and teratogenicity as a result of streptokinase have not been reported and are not expected because of the minimal placental transfer. Sensitization of the newborn to streptokinase from antibodies received *in utero* is a complication only if the neonate required therapy. The effect of thrombolytic therapy on placental implantation early in pregnancy has not been determined. Based on these data, streptokinase can be used during gestation if the mother's condition requires this therapy.

BREAST FEEDING SUMMARY

RECOMMENDATION: No Human Data - Probably Compatible

No reports describing the use of streptokinase during lactation have been located. Because of the nature of the indications for this agent and its very short half-life (approximately 23 minutes for the streptokinase-plasminogen complex), the opportunities for its use during lactation and potential exposure of the nursing infant are minimal.

References

1. Product information. Streptase. Astra USA, 1996.
2. Pfeifer GW. Distribution and placental transfer of ^{131}I streptokinase. Aust Ann Med 1970;19(Suppl):17–8.
3. Hall RJC, Young C, Sutton GC, Campbell S. Treatment of acute massive pulmonary embolism by streptokinase during labour and delivery. Br Med J 1972;4: 647–9.
4. McTaggart DR, Ingram TG. Massive pulmonary embolism during pregnancy treated with streptokinase. Med J Aust 1977;1:18–20.
5. Benz JJ, Wick A. The problem of fibrinolytic therapy in pregnancy. Schweiz Med Wochenschr 1973;103:1359–63.
6. Ludwig H. Results of streptokinase therapy in deep venous thrombosis during pregnancy. Postgrad Med J 1973;49(Suppl 5):65–7.
7. Walter C, Koestering H. Therapeutische thrombolyse in der neunten schwangerschalftswoche. Dtsch Med Wochenschr 1969;94:32–4.
8. Witchitz S, Veyrat C, Moisson P, Scheinman N, Rozenstajn L. Fibrinolytic treatment of thrombus on prosthetic heart valves. Br Heart J 1980;44:545–54.
9. Pfeifer GW. The use of thrombolytic therapy in obstetrics and gynaecology. Aust Ann Med 1970;19(Suppl):28–31.
10. Amias AG. Cerebral vascular disease in pregnancy. 2. Occlusion. J Obstet Gynaecol Br Commonw 1970;77:312–25.
11. Amias AG. Streptokinase, cerebral vascular disease - and triplets. Br Med J 1977;1:1414–5.
12. Johansson E, Ericson K, Zetterquist S. Streptokinase treatment of deep venous thrombosis of the lower extremity. Acta Med Scand 1976;199:89–74.
13. Ludwig H, Genz HJ. Thrombolytic treatment during pregnancy. Thromb Haemost 1981;46:438.
14. Fagher B, Ahlgren M, Åstedt B. Acute massive pulmonary embolism treated with streptokinase during labor and the early puerperium. Acta Obstet Gynecol Scand 1990;69:659–62.
15. Ramamurthy S, Talwar KK, Saxena A, Juneja R, Takkar D. Prosthetic mitral valve thrombosis in pregnancy successfully treated with streptokinase. Am Heart J 1994;127:446–8.
16. Turrentine MA, Braems G, Ramirez MM. Use of thrombolytics for the treatment of thromboembolic disease during pregnancy. Obstet Gynecol Surv 1995;50: 534–41.
17. Usta IM, Abdallah M, El-Hajj M, Nassar AH. Massive subchorionic hematomas following thrombolytic therapy in pregnancy. Obstet Gynecol 2004;103:1079–82.

S

Name: **STREPTOMYCIN**		Risk Factor: D_M
Class: **Antibiotic (Aminoglycoside)**		

FETAL RISK SUMMARY

RECOMMENDATION: Human Data Suggest Risk

Streptomycin is an aminoglycoside antibiotic. The drug rapidly crosses the placenta into the fetal circulation and amniotic fluid, obtaining concentrations that are usually less than 50% of the maternal serum level (1,2). Early investigators, well aware of streptomycin-induced ototoxicity, were unable to observe this defect in infants exposed *in utero* to the agent (3–5). Eventually, ototoxicity was described in a 2 1/2-month-old infant whose mother had been treated for tuberculosis with 30 g of streptomycin during the last month of pregnancy (6). The infant was deaf with a negative cochleopalpebral reflex. Several other case reports and small surveys describing similar toxicity followed this initial report (7,8). In general, however, the incidence of congenital ototoxicity, cochlear or vestibular, from streptomycin is low, especially with careful dosage calculations and if the duration of fetal exposure is limited (9).

Except for eighth cranial nerve damage, no reports of congenital defects caused by streptomycin have been located. The Collaborative Perinatal Project monitored 50,282 mother-child pairs, 135 of whom had 1st trimester exposure to streptomycin (10, pp. 297–301). For use anytime during pregnancy, 355 exposures were recorded (10, p. 435). In neither group was evidence found to suggest a relationship to large categories of major or minor malformations or to individual defects.

In a group of 1,619 newborns whose mothers were treated for tuberculosis during pregnancy with multiple drugs, including streptomycin, the incidence of congenital defects was the same as in a healthy control group (2.34% vs. 2.56%) (11). Other investigators had previously concluded that the use of streptomycin in pregnant tuberculosis patients was not teratogenic (12).

The population-based dataset of the Hungarian Case-Control Surveillance of Congenital Abnormalities, covering the period of 1980–1996, was used to evaluate the teratogenicity of aminoglycoside antibiotics (parenteral gentamicin, streptomycin, tobramycin, and oral neomycin) in a study published in 2000 (13). A case group of 22,865 women who had fetuses or newborns with congenital malformations were compared to 38,151 women who had no newborns with structural defects. A total of 38 cases and 42 controls were treated with the aminoglycosides. There was one case, but no controls, treated with streptomycin (odds ratio 5.0, 95% confidence interval 0.2–122.9). The investigators concluded that there was no detectable teratogenic risk for structural defects for any of the aminoglycoside antibiotics (13). They also concluded, although it was not investigated in this study, that the risk of deafness after *in utero* aminoglycoside exposure was small.

BREAST FEEDING SUMMARY

RECOMMENDATION: Compatible

Streptomycin is excreted into breast milk. Milk:plasma ratios of 0.5–1.0 have been reported (14). Because the oral absorption of this antibiotic is poor, ototoxicity in the infant would not be expected. However, three potential problems exist for the nursing infant: modification of bowel flora, direct effects on the infant, and interference with the interpretation of culture results if a fever workup is required. The American Academy of Pediatrics classifies streptomycin as compatible with breast-feeding (15).

S

References

1. Woltz J, Wiley M. Transmission of streptomycin from maternal blood to the fetal circulation and the amniotic fluid. Proc Soc Exp Biol Med 1945;60:106–7.
2. Heilman D, Heilman F, Hinshaw H, Nichols D, Herrell W. Streptomycin: absorption, diffusion, excretion and toxicity. Am J Med Sci 1945;210:576–84.
3. Watson E, Stow R. Streptomycin therapy: effects on fetus. JAMA 1948;137:1599–1600.
4. Rubin A, Winston J, Rutledge M. Effects of streptomycin upon the human fetus. Am J Dis Child 1951;82:14–6.
5. Kistner R. The use of streptomycin during pregnancy. Am J Obstet Gynecol 1950;60:422–6.
6. Leroux M. Existe-t-il une surdité congénitale acquise due à la streptomycine? Ann Otolaryngol 1950;67:194–6.

7. Nishimura H, Tanimura T. *Clinical Aspects of the Teratogenicity of Drugs*. New York, NY: Excerpta Medica, 1976:130.
8. Donald PR, Sellars SL. Streptomycin ototoxicity in the unborn child. S Afr Med J 1981;60:316–8.
9. Mann J, Moskowitz R. Plaque and pregnancy. A case report. JAMA 1977;237:1854–5.
10. Heinonen OP, Slone D, Shapiro S. *Birth Defects and Drugs in Pregnancy*. Littleton, MA: Publishing Sciences Group, 1977.
11. Marynowski A, Sianozecka E. Comparison of the incidence of congenital malformations in neonates from healthy mothers and from patients treated because of tuberculosis. Ginekol Pol 1972;43:713–5.
12. Lowe C. Congenital defects among children born under supervision or treatment for pulmonary tuberculosis. Br J Prev Soc Med 1964;18:14–6.
13. Czeizel AE, Rockenbauer M, Olsen J, Sorensen HT. A teratological study of aminoglycoside antibiotic treatment during pregnancy. Scand J Infect Dis 2000;32:309–13.
14. Wilson JT. Milk/plasma ratios and contraindicated drugs. In Wilson JT, ed. *Drugs in Breast Milk*. Balgowlah, Australia: ADIS Press, 1981:79.
15. Committee on Drugs, American Academy of Pediatrics. The transfer of drugs and other chemicals into human milk. Pediatrics 2001;108:776–89.

Name: **STREPTOZOCIN** Risk Factor: **D_M**
Class: **Antineoplastic**

FETAL RISK SUMMARY

RECOMMENDATION: Limited Human Data - Animal Data Suggest Risk

Streptozocin (streptozotocin) is an alkylating antineoplastic that is obtained from *Streptomyces acromogenes*. This nitrosourea agent belongs to the same group as carmustine (BCNU) and lomustine (CCNU). Streptozocin is indicated for the treatment of metastatic islet cell carcinoma of the pancreas but also is used in other cancers. It is rapidly cleared from the plasma and is distributed to tissues, primarily the kidneys, liver, intestines, and pancreas (1,2). Streptozocin undergoes extensive metabolism and, although it does not cross the blood-brain barrier, its metabolites are found in the cerebrospinal fluid (CSF) (1).

Streptozocin is mutagenic in bacteria, plants, and mammalian cells and is carcinogenic (renal, hepatic, stomach and pancreatic tumors) in various animal species such as mice, rats, and hamsters (2). The drug also is diabetogenic in laboratory animals (3).

Reproduction studies with streptozocin have been conducted in pregnant rats and rabbits. Although the doses and administration times were not specified, streptozocin was teratogenic (types of defects not specified) in rats and had abortifacient effects in rabbits (2). No mention was made of maternal toxicity in these studies.

S

Studies investigating the passage of streptozocin across the human placenta have not been located. The molecular weight (about 265) is low enough that exposure of the embryo or fetus should be expected. Moreover, in pregnant monkeys administered IV streptozocin, the agent appeared rapidly in the fetal circulation (2). However, the rapid clearance from the blood and the absence of the parent drug in the CSF suggest that the amount crossing the placenta, at least of unmetabolized drug, will be limited.

A 1984 report described a 21-year-old woman with diffuse histiocytic lymphoma treated before pregnancy with multiple courses of chemotherapy including cyclophosphamide, doxorubicin, vincristine, bleomycin, methotrexate, cytarabine, and etoposide, in addition to radiation therapy to the neck (4). Because of the failure of that therapy, she was changed to carmustine and procarbazine for 5 months before conception. The patient refused to terminate her pregnancy, and treatment with carmustine and procarbazine was continued during the first 24 weeks of pregnancy. Because of disease progression, her therapy was changed at 24 weeks' gestation to three courses of streptozocin, 800 mg IV/day for 3 days every 4 weeks. The last course was administered 2 weeks before delivery at 35 weeks' gestation. The normal-appearing male infant weighed 2.34 kg with a head circumference of 32.5 cm and a length of 51.5 cm. The Apgar scores were 7 and 9 at 1 and 5 minutes, respectively. Initial tests revealed normal hemoglobin, and white blood cell and platelet counts. All other clinical tests were within normal limits including electrolytes, multiple chemistry, urinalysis, renal ultrasound, and chromosome studies (2).

In summary, streptozocin is teratogenic or embryotoxic in several animal species, as well as possessing mutagenic and carcinogenic effects. The potential for human embryo/fetal injury is a concern, but because the animal reproduction data lacked dosage and time of exposure information and other data, the degree of risk is unknown. One report has described the use of this drug during the latter half of gestation without apparent fetal harm. Until additional data are forthcoming, streptozocin should be considered a potential human teratogen if exposure occurs during organogenesis.

BREAST FEEDING SUMMARY

RECOMMENDATION: Contraindicated

No reports describing the use of streptozocin during human lactation have been located. The relatively low molecular weight (about 265) suggests that the drug will be excreted in breast milk. The effects of this exposure on a nursing infant are unknown. Because of the potential for serious toxicity, women receiving streptozocin should not nurse.

References

1. Parfitt K. Editor. *Martindale. The Complete Drug Reference*. 32nd ed. London, UK: Pharmaceutical Press, 1999:562.
2. Product information. Zanosar. Pharmacia & Upjohn, 2000.
3. Schein PS, Winokur SH. Immunosuppressive and cytotoxic chemotherapy: long-term complications. Ann Intern Med 1975;82:84–95.
4. Schapira DV, Chudley AE. Successful pregnancy following continuous treatment with combination chemotherapy before conception and throughout pregnancy. Cancer 1984;54:800–3.

Name: **SUCCIMER** Risk Factor: **C_M**

Class: **Chelating Agent**

FETAL RISK SUMMARY

RECOMMENDATION: No Human Data - Animal Data Suggest Risk

The heavy metal chelating agent succimer (*meso*-2,3-dimercaptosuccinic acid; DMSA) is indicated for the treatment and prophylaxis of lead poisoning in pediatric patients. The drug has also been used as an antidote for the treatment of arsenic, mercury, and cadmium poisoning (2). Succimer has no significant effect on the urinary elimination of iron, calcium, or magnesium but doubles the excretion of zinc (1). After oral administration, approximately 60% is absorbed systemically from an initial dose of 30 mg/kg/day (1050 mg/m^2/day) with an apparent elimination half-life of approximately 2 days (1).

In addition to the animal reproductive data provided by the manufacturer (1), a number of published animal studies have described the effect of succimer on the fetus (2–11). In pregnant rats doses of 100–1000 mg/kg/day administered orally on gestational days 6–15 were not teratogenic but did produce maternal toxicity (decreased weight gain) (2). At pregnancy termination on day 20, fetal toxicity, characterized by increased early resorptions, post-implantation losses, and reduced fetal body weight per litter, was evident at all doses. The no-observable-effect level (NOEL) was <100 mg/kg/day (2).

In another portion of the above study, the concentrations of five minerals (calcium, magnesium, zinc, copper, and iron) were measured in maternal and fetal tissues (3). Marked alterations were observed on the mineral concentrations in the fetuses. These effects suggested that the fetal toxicity noted was partially caused by changes in mineral metabolism (3).

Succimer was teratogenic and fetotoxic when SC doses were given to pregnant mice during organogenesis (days 6–15 of gestation) at doses of 410 to 1640 mg/kg/day (1,4). At the maximum dose, maternal toxicity (reduced weight gain) was evident (4). Significant embryo and fetal toxicity as evidenced by an increased incidence of resorptions and stunting, and a decrease in the number of live fetuses per litter, were observed at 1640 mg/kg/day. At 820 mg/kg/day, significant decreases in fetal weight and length were noted (4). A dose relationship was found for structural defects including significant increases (compared with controls) in gross external defects (hematomas in the facial area, exencephaly, and micrognathia), internal soft-tissue defects (hydrocephaly, small thoracic cavities, and brain defects), and skeletal variations (decreased ossification, hypoplasia of the mandible, and irregular-shaped ribs). The no-effect dose for defects was 410 mg/kg/day (4).

In a continuation of the above study, pregnant mice were given oral succimer (200–800 mg/kg/day) from gestational day 14 through postnatal day 21 (weaning) (5). No maternal toxicity was observed at any dose. Adverse effects were observed only in the offspring exposed during lactation to the highest maternal dose. The effects observed in the nursing pups included significant decreases in body weight and a corresponding increase in relative brain weight (brain weight/body weight). The NOEL for adverse effects in the nursing pups was >400 mg/kg/day (5).

The type of developmental toxicity observed in mice suggested to some investigators that the toxicity may have been related to an interaction between succimer and zinc (4). However, in a subsequent report, no consistent changes could be demonstrated in mice fetal tissue levels of zinc, iron, calcium, or magnesium (6). Moreover, supplemental zinc did not protect the fetuses. Disturbance of maternal/fetal copper metabolism may have been related to the developmental toxicity because dose-dependent decreases in fetal liver copper levels were observed (6).

A 1991 report examined the efficacy of succimer to protect mice fetuses from the toxicity and teratogenicity of an intraperitoneal (IP) dose (12 mg/kg) of sodium arsenite administered to pregnant mice on day 10 of gestation (7). In the dose-finding portion of the study, succimer SC doses of 80, 160, and 320 mg/kg were given immediately after sodium arsenite injection. An increasing protective effect was noted with an increasing succimer dose. The effect of the time interval between IP injection of sodium arsenite and injection of succimer was then studied. A single SC dose of succimer (320 mg/kg) was given to pregnant mice at various times up to 12 hours after a dose of sodium arsenite. Significant reductions in arsenite-induced embryo toxicity and teratogenicity were achieved only when succimer was administered within 1 hour of the arsenite dose (7).

Using a similar study design, the above investigators examined the effect of succimer in protecting fetal mice from the toxicity and teratogenicity of dibasic sodium arsenate (8). Sodium arsenate is the most common form of inorganic arsenic in the environment and is less fetotoxic than sodium arsenite (7,8). As in the above study, the investigators demonstrated a dose-related protective effect of succimer at SC doses of 37.5, 75, and 150 mg/kg administered at four successive time intervals (2, 24, 48, and 72 hours) after IP injection of dibasic sodium arsenate (45 mg/kg) (8).

A 1978 study in pregnant rats demonstrated that daily administration of succimer was effective in reducing methylmercury concentrations in neonatal rat brains (9). A 40-mg oral dose was more effective (70% reduction in methylmercury) than a 20-mg dose (50% reduction). In a later study with pregnant mice, a dose-related protective effect from methylmercury-induced embryo lethality and teratogenicity was demonstrated with the maximum protection achieved with a SC dose of 320 mg/kg/day (10).

The effect on the immune function of female rats exposed to succimer *in utero* was described in a 1999 report (11). Pregnant rats were administered lead acetate (250 ppm) in drinking water from 2 weeks before mating until parturition. Succimer (60 mg/kg/day), given orally from days 6–21 of gestation, significantly lowered the blood lead levels in both the dams and embryos. Several lead-induced changes in 13-week-old female offspring were reversed by the chelating agent (succimer-induced changes in parentheses) including body weight (increased), relative spleen weight (decreased), interferon γ (increased), and interleukin-4 (decreased). However, succimer alone affected immune function in the female offspring by decreasing the delayed-type hypersensitivity response and increasing interleukin-2 production. Therefore, succimer treatment during gestation did reverse some of the lead-induced immunotoxicity but also causes subsequent adult immunomodulation (11).

It is not known if succimer crosses the human placenta. The molecular weight (about 182), however, is low enough that fetal exposure should be expected. The studies cited above suggest that succimer crosses the placenta in mice and rats.

In summary, no reports describing the use of succimer during human pregnancy have been located. The chelating agent produces fetotoxicity and teratogenicity in mice and fetotoxicity in rats. These toxic effects often occurred at oral doses at or less than 10 times the human dose (weight basis). In addition, succimer-induced modulation of adult female rat immune function has been demonstrated. The exact mechanism of the animal developmental toxicity is unknown but appears to result from disturbances in mineral metabolism, especially that of zinc and copper. Therefore, if succimer is used in human pregnancy, the effects on maternal and fetal mineral metabolism—in particular, of zinc and copper—should be evaluated (12).

BREAST FEEDING SUMMARY

RECOMMENDATION: Contraindicated

No studies describing the use of succimer during lactation have been located. The relatively low molecular weight (about 182), however, suggests that the drug will be excreted into milk. The effects of this exposure on a nursing infant are unknown. However, because the use of succimer implies poisoning with lead, or other heavy metals, these substances might also be excreted into milk and cause toxicity in a nursing infant. Therefore, breast-feeding is contraindicated in women receiving succimer.

S

References

1. Product information. Chemet. Sanofi-Synthelabo, 2002.
2. Domingo JL, Ortega A, Paternain JL, Llobet JM. Oral *meso*-2,3-dimercaptosuccinic acid in pregnant Sprague-Dawley rats: teratogenicity and alterations in mineral metabolism. I. Teratological evaluation. J Toxicol Environ Health 1990;30:181–90.
3. Paternain JL, Ortega A, Domingo JL, Llobet JM. Oral *meso*-2,3-dimercaptosuccinic acid in pregnant Sprague-Dawley rats: teratogenicity and alterations in mineral metabolism. II. Effect on mineral metabolism. J Toxicol Environ Health 1990;30:191–7.
4. Domingo JL, Paternain JL, Llobet JM, Corbella J. Developmental toxicity of subcutaneously administered meso-2,3-dimercaptosuccinic acid in mice. Fundam Appl Toxicol 1988;11:715–22.

5. Domingo JL, Bosque MA, Corbella J. Effects of oral *meso*-2,3-dimercaptosucinic acid (DMSA) administration on late gestation and postnatal development in the mouse. Life Sci 1990;47:1745–50.
6. Taubeneck MW, Domingo JL, Llobet JM, Keen CL. *Meso*-2,3-dimercaptosuccinic acid (DMSA) affects maternal and fetal copper metabolism in Swiss mice. Toxicology 1992;72:27–40.
7. Domingo JL, Bosque MA, Piera V. *meso*-2,3-dimercaptosuccinic acid and prevention of arsenite embryotoxicity and teratogenicity in the mouse. Fundam Appl Toxicol 1991;17:314–20.
8. Bosque MA, Domingo JL, Llobet JM, Corbella J. Effects of Meso-2,3-dimercaptosuccinic acid (DMSA) on the teratogenicity of sodium arsenate in mice. Bull Environ Contam Toxicol 1991;47:682–8.
9. Hughes JA, Sparber SB. Reduction of methylmercury concentration in neonatal rat brains after administration of dimercaptosuccinic acid to dams while pregnant. Res Commun Chem Pathol Pharmacol 1978;22:357–63.
10. Sanchez DJ, Gomez M, Llobet JM, Domingo JL. Effects of *meso*-2,3-dimercaptosuccinic acid (DMSA) on methyl mercury-induced teratogenesis in mice. Ecotoxicol Environ Saf 1993;26:33–9.
11. Chen S, Golemboski KA, Sander FS, Dietert RR. Persistent effect of in utero meso-2,3-dimercaptosuccinic acid (DMSA) on immune function and lead-induced immunotoxicity. Toxicology 1999;132:67–79.
12. Domingo JL. Developmental toxicity of metal chelating agents. Reprod Toxicol 1998;12:499–510.

Name: **SUCCINYLCHOLINE** Risk Factor: **C_M**

Class: **Skeletal Muscle Relaxant**

FETAL RISK SUMMARY

RECOMMENDATION: Compatible

Succinylcholine is a depolarizing neuromuscular blocking agent that is used as an adjunct to general anesthesia, to facilitate tracheal intubation, and to provide skeletal muscle relaxation during surgery or mechanical ventilation. Approximately 90% of the drug is rapidly hydrolyzed by plasma cholinesterase to succinylmonocholine, a metabolite that is clinically inactive, and then more slowly to succinic acid and choline. The remaining 10% is excreted unchanged in the urine (1).

According to the manufacturer, reproduction studies in animals with succinylcholine have not been conducted (1). A 1984 source, however, stated that studies conducted in the 1950s in rabbits and dogs did not observe embryo or fetal toxicity or teratogenicity (2). Succinylcholine has no direct action on the uterus or other smooth muscles and, because it is highly ionized and has low lipid solubility, does not readily cross the placenta (1).

A study published in 1961 noted the lack of quantitative data on the placental transfer of succinylcholine in animals and humans (3). Although published reports involving more than 1,800 deliveries had shown the drug to be safe for the fetus and newborn, there were anecdotal reports of flaccid, apneic infants whose condition was attributed to succinylcholine (3). The authors cited two studies in which doses less than 100 mg in pregnant rabbits had no adverse effect on the newborns, but in dogs, paralysis was demonstrated in pups when a 400-mg dose was administered to the mother immediately before delivery (3). They then studied 14 patients delivered by cesarean section under general anesthesia, in which a single 100-mg IV dose of succinylcholine was followed by a continuous infusion of a 0.2% succinylcholine solution (3). The patients received a total dose (IV plus infusion) of 100–600 mg. Three of the newborn infants had Apgar scores less than 7 (time when determined not specified). In an additional eight patients undergoing vaginal delivery, a single 100-mg IV dose was given within 4 minutes of birth. None of these infants had a depressed Apgar score. Of the total 22 newborns, no paralysis was observed. Placental transfer of succinylcholine as determined by a biologic test, however, could not be demonstrated in any of the cases (3).

In a second study by these same authors, pregnant rabbits at term were treated with a single IV dose of succinylcholine (0.25–570 mg/kg) with delivery of the fetuses 3–6 minutes later (4). A difference in vigor compared with that in controls was observed when the mother had received 340 mg/kg, about 600 times the human clinical dose based on weight. [The human clinical dose to facilitate tracheal intubation is 0.6 mg/kg IV, range 0.3–1.1 mg/kg (1)]. At 540 mg/kg, all rabbit fetuses were alive but paralyzed. In the human part of this study, 13 women at term who were about to undergo vaginal delivery were given a single 200- to 500-mg rapid IV dose, 1–5.25 minutes before delivery (4). Maternal blood levels varied from 0 to 11.6 μg/mL, whereas cord blood concentrations varied from 0 to 2.0 μg/mL. Cord blood levels of 1.1–2.0 μg/mL occurred in six of eight fetuses whose mothers had received doses of 300 mg/kg or more. No drug was found in the cord blood of five newborns after a 200-mg/kg maternal dose. None of the newborns appeared to be affected by succinylcholine, but all of the mothers were apneic at delivery and for periods up to 16 minutes.

The placental transfer of succinylcholine using radioactive tracers was studied in near-term *Macaca mulatta* monkeys, using IV doses of 2–3 mg/kg followed by repeated doses of 1.2 and 2 mg/kg (5). Rapid placental transfer occurred, reaching a peak fetal plasma concentration approximately 30% of the maternal plasma level 5–10 minutes after the dose. Fetal metabolism of succinylcholine to inactive succinylmonocholine was demonstrated, albeit at a slower rate than that which occurred in the mother, an indication that fetal cholinesterase (pseudocholinesterase) activity was lower than that in the mother (5). The authors concluded that the amount of active drug transferred to the fetus produced a slight effect on skeletal muscle activity and was unlikely to depress respiration in the newborn (5).

Atypical cholinesterase is an autosomal dominant inherited condition with a prevalence, for the dibucaine-resistant form, of 1:2000 to 1:4000 in various populations (6). The homozygote state is diagnosed by the onset of prolonged apnea (>10 minutes), in the absence of excessive amounts of other depressants, after succinylcholine (1–3 mg/kg) administration (6). Some of the anecdotal reports, mentioned in reference #3, of flaccid, apneic infants after succinylcholine administration may represent cases of this genetic trait. Four maternal cases of atypical cholinesterase with probable atypical homozygote infants in three are discussed below.

A study published in 1975 described respiratory depression and decreased muscular activity in a newborn whose mother had received succinylcholine, 80 mg IV followed by an IV infusion that delivered an additional 60 mg of drug, for cesarean section at term (7). Newborn ventilation support was required for 10 minutes after birth. Neuromuscular block in the mother continued for approximately 5.5 hours. Because the cholinesterase activity in the mother and that in the 2-day-old infant were 10% of normal, neither was able to rapidly metabolize the succinylcholine (7).

Low concentrations of plasma cholinesterase were thought to be responsible for transient respiratory depression in a newborn following the use of succinylcholine for cesarean section (8). The mother had received 200 mg thiamylal (a barbiturate similar to thiopental that is not currently available) and 100 mg succinylcholine IV for induction of general anesthesia 3 minutes prior to delivery. The onset of respiration and the development of an acceptable respiratory pattern in the newborn were slightly delayed with Apgar scores of 5 and 8 at 1 and 5 minutes, respectively. After recovery, the newborn did well. The mother required mechanical ventilation for 4 hours before return of spontaneous muscular activity and respiration (8). Cholinesterase activity in the mother was below the level of test sensitivity. Enzyme activity in the newborn was 410 U/L (normal 2436–4872 U/L) (8).

Three months later, the infant's pseudocholinesterase activity had risen to 910 U/L. Enzyme concentrations in the father (2420 U/L) were slightly low, normal in one sibling (2480 U/L), and markedly depressed in five other siblings (range 150–760 U/L).

A description of two mothers at term with atypical cholinesterase who were administered succinylcholine prior to elective cesarean section was reported in 1975 (9). The first mother received 100 mg IV succinylcholine 5 minutes before delivery of a male baby. Apnea in the mother persisted for 2.5 hours after delivery before return of spontaneous respirations. Her infant was flaccid, apneic, and unresponsive to stimulation. Respiratory assistance was required for 6 hours before occurrence of full recovery. In the second mother, who also received succinylcholine 100 mg IV, recovery from paralysis required 2 hours. Her infant, delivered 10 minutes after the dose, cried immediately and had Apgar scores of 8 and 10 at 1 and 5 minutes, respectively. Analysis of serum cholinesterase activity and dibucaine numbers in the mothers and infants revealed that the mothers and the affected infant were atypical homozygotes, whereas the unaffected infant was a heterozygote (9).

The Collaborative Perinatal Project monitored 50,282 mother-child pairs, 26 of whom had 1st-trimester exposure to succinylcholine (10). No congenital malformations were observed in any of the newborns.

In summary, succinylcholine is not embryotoxic or teratogenic in two animal species or, although the data are very limited, in humans. Succinylcholine has been routinely used in obstetrical patients prior to delivery since the 1950s and no reports of fetal toxicity have been located. Partial or complete newborn paralysis with resulting respiratory depression have been reported, however, when the drug was administered to women with the genetic trait for atypical cholinesterase. Prolonged newborn respiratory depression may occur when this trait has been inherited by the infant. The level of cholinesterase activity in the infant will determine the duration of paralysis. Women without the genetic trait for atypical cholinesterase rapidly metabolize the drug and, because clinically significant placental transfer is concentration-dependent, prevent toxicity in the newborn.

BREAST FEEDING SUMMARY

RECOMMENDATION: No Human Data - Probably Compatible

The passage of succinylcholine into breast milk has not been studied. Because the drug is rapidly hydrolyzed by plasma cholinesterase (pseudocholinesterase) to an inactive metabolite, it is doubtful that clinically significant amounts of active drug are transferred into milk (11). Women with the genetic trait for atypical cholinesterase will have high concentrations of succinylcholine, but the effects of the drug on the mother will preclude nursing.

S

References

1. Product information. Anectine. Glaxo Wellcome, 1998.
2. Onnis A, Grella P. *The Biochemical Effects of Drugs in Pregnancy*. Vol 1. West Sussex, England: Ellis Horwood Limited, 1984:230–1.
3. Moya F, Kvisselgaard N. The placental transmission of succinylcholine. Anesthesiology 1961;22:1–6.
4. Kvisselgaard N, Moya F. Investigation of placental thresholds to succinylcholine. Anesthesiology 1961;22:7–10.
5. Drabkova J, Crul JF, van der Kleijn E. Placental transfer of ^{14}C labelled succinylcholine in near-term *Macaca mulatta* monkeys. Br J Anaesthesia 1973;45:1087–96.
6. Donnell GN. Cholinesterase, atypical. In Buyse ML, editor-in-chief. *Birth Defects Encyclopedia*. Vol 1. Cambridge, MA: Blackwell Scientific Publications, 1990:316–7.
7. Owens WD, Zeitlin GL. Hypoventilation in a newborn following administration of succinylcholine to the mother: a case report. Anesth Analg 1975;54:38–40.
8. Cherala SR, Eddoe DN, Sechzer PH. Placental transfer of succinylcholine causing transient respiratory depression in the newborn. Anaesth Intensive Care 1989;17:202–4.
9. Baraka A, Haroun S, Bassili M, Abu-Haider G.

Response of the newborn to succinylcholine injection in homozygotic atypical mothers. Anesthesiology 1975;43:115–6.
10. Heinonen OP, Slone D, Shapiro S. *Birth Defects and Drugs in Pregnancy*. Littleton, MA: Publishing Sciences Group, 1977:358–60.
11. Spigset O. Anaesthetic agents and excretion in breast milk. Acta Anaesthesiol Scand 1994;38:94–103.

Name:	**SUCRALFATE**	Risk Factor:	B_M
Class:	**Gastrointestinal Agent (Antisecretory)**		

FETAL RISK SUMMARY

RECOMMENDATION: Compatible

Sucralfate is an aluminum salt of a sulfated disaccharide that inhibits pepsin activity and protects against ulceration. The drug is a highly polar anion when solubilized in strong acid solutions, which probably accounts for its poor gastrointestinal absorption. Its ulcer protectant and healing effects are exerted through local, rather than systemic, action (1). The small amounts that are absorbed, up to 2.2% of a dose in one study using healthy males (2), are excreted in the urine (1,2).

In mice, rats, and rabbits, sucralfate had no effect on fertility and was not teratogenic with doses up to 50 times those used in humans (1). Sucralfate is a source of bioavailable aluminum (3,4). Each 1-g tablet of sucralfate contains 207 mg of aluminum (3). The potential fetal toxicity of this drug relates to its aluminum content.

When administered parenterally to pregnant animals, aluminum accumulates in the fetus causing an increased perinatal mortality and impaired learning and memory (5,6). Teratogenic effects, however, were not observed (6). Prolonged exposure to the metal causes neurobehavioral and skeletal toxicity (7). A 1985 review of aluminum described these toxic effects on the brain and bone tissue as dialysis encephalopathy in patients with renal failure and a unique form of osteodystrophy in uremic patients (3). Aluminum received from IV fluids may also be related to osteopenia in premature infants (8). A 1991 report described the results of a study of 88 pregnancies in women exposed to high amounts of aluminum sulfate that had been accidentally added to the city's water supply (9). Except for an increased rate of talipes (clubfoot) (four cases, one control; $p = 0.01$), there was no evidence that the exposure was harmful to the fetuses. Several theoretical explanations for the four cases of clubfoot were offered by the investigators, including the possibility that the observed incidence occurred by chance (9).

In patients with end-stage chronic renal failure, the use of sucralfate to bind phosphate resulted in serum aluminum levels comparable to those obtained from the antacid aluminum hydroxide (4). Administration of sucralfate to normal subjects did not increase plasma aluminum concentrations, but evidence of tissue aluminum loading was found in experiments with animals (3).

Analysis of 97 amniotic fluid samples, mostly from women undergoing amniocentesis for advanced maternal age, found a mean aluminum concentration of 93.4 μg/L (range 37–149 μg/L) (10). The authors of this study did not mention whether the women were consuming aluminum-containing medications, and the measured levels are apparently the normal baseline for the patient population studied.

In a surveillance study of Michigan Medicaid recipients conducted between 1985 and 1992 involving 229,101 completed pregnancies, 183 newborns had been exposed to sucralfate during the 1st trimester (F. Rosa, personal communication, FDA, 1993). A total of five (2.7%) major birth defects were observed (eight expected). Specific data were available for six defect categories, including (observed/expected) 1/2 cardiovascular defects, 1/0 oral clefts, 0/0 spina bifida, 1/0.5 polydactyly, 0/0.5 limb reduction defects, and 1/0.5 hypospadias. These data do not support an association between the drug and congenital defects.

Although the toxicity of aluminum has been well documented, there is no evidence that normal doses of aluminum-containing medications, such as sucralfate, present a risk to the fetuses of pregnant women with normal renal function. Oral absorption of aluminum is poor with only an average of 12% retained in one study of six normal subjects ingesting 1–3 g of aluminum per day (3). Moreover, no evidence has been found to suggest that aluminum is actively absorbed from the gastrointestinal tract (3). Because of these characteristics and the lack of reports of adverse fetal effects in humans or animals attributable to sucralfate, the risk to the fetus is probably nil. A 1985 review on the use of gastrointestinal drugs during pregnancy and lactation by the American College of Gastroenterology classified sucralfate as an agent whose potential benefits outweighed any potential risks (11).

BREAST FEEDING SUMMARY

RECOMMENDATION: No Human Data - Probably Compatible

Minimal, if any, excretion of sucralfate into milk should be expected, because only small amounts of this drug are absorbed systemically.

References

1. Product information. Carafate. Hoechst Marion Roussel, 2000.
2. Giesing D, Lanman R, Runser D. Absorption of sucralfate in man (abstract). Gastroenterology 1982;82:1066.
3. Lione A. Aluminum toxicology and the aluminum-containing medications. Pharmacol Ther 1985;29: 255–85.
4. Leung ACT, Henderson IS, Halls DJ, Dobbie JW. Aluminum hydroxide versus sucralfate as a phosphate binder in uraemia. Br Med J 1983;286:1379–81.
5. Yokel RA. Toxicity of gestational aluminum exposure to the maternal rabbit and offspring. Toxicol Appl Pharmacol 1985;79:121–33.
6. McCormack KM, Ottosen LD, Sanger VL, Sprague S, Major GH, Hook JB. Effect of prenatal administration of aluminum and parathyroid hormone on fetal development in the rat (40493). Proc Soc Exp Biol Med 1979;161:74–7.
7. Yokel RA, McNamara PJ. Aluminum bioavailability and disposition in adult and immature rabbits. Toxicol Appl Pharmacol 1985;77:344–52.
8. Sedman AB, Klein GL, Merritt RJ, Miller NL, Weber KO, Gill WL, Anand H, Alfrey AC. Evidence of aluminum loading in infants receiving intravenous therapy. N Engl J Med 1985;312:1337–43.
9. Golding J, Rowland A, Greenwood R, Lunt P. Aluminum sulphate in water in north Cornwall and outcome of pregnancy. BMJ 1991;302:1175–7.
10. Hall GS, Carr MJ, Cummings E, Lee M. Aluminum, barium, silicon, and strontium in amniotic fluid by emission spectrometry. Clin Chem 1983;29: 1318.
11. Lewis JH, Weingold AB. The use of gastrointestinal drugs during pregnancy and lactation. Am J Gastroenterol 1985;80:912–23.

S

Name: **SUFENTANIL** Risk Factor: **C_M***
Class: **Narcotic Agonist Analgesic**

FETAL RISK SUMMARY

RECOMMENDATION: Human Data Suggest Risk in 3rd Trimester

Sufentanil is a potent narcotic drug that is used as an analgesic adjunct to, or primary anesthetic agent during, general anesthesia and in combination with bupivacaine for epidural anesthesia during labor and vaginal delivery.

No evidence of teratogenicity was observed in rats and rabbits, but the drug was embryocidal (most likely due to maternal toxicity) in both species when it was given for 10–30 days in a dose 2.5 times the upper human IV dose (1). No adverse reproductive (number of implantations and live fetuses, percent fetal wastage per litter, or mean fetal weight) or teratogenic effects (major or minor malformations) were observed in rats administered continuous infusions of sufentanil at doses of 10, 50, or 100 μg/kg/day from day 5 through day 20 of pregnancy (2).

The placental transfer of sufentanil was studied in an experiment using the dual-perfused, single-cotyledon human placental model at doses of 1, 10, 20, and 100 ng/mL (3). Sufentanil was shown to rapidly cross the placenta by passive diffusion, but high maternal protein binding significantly reduced this transfer, whereas progressive fetal acidemia (reduction in pH from 7.4 to 6.8 in 0.2 increments) significantly increased transfer. Placental tissues appeared to bind sufentanil, but this accumulation apparently did not affect the overall net drug transfer to the fetus (i.e., placenta accumulated sufentanil during periods of increasing maternal concentrations and then functioned as source to sustain fetal drug levels when maternal concentrations declined) (3).

In another *in vitro* study, a single-pass (open) placental perfusion model was used to assess the placental transfer of sufentanil (1 and 100 ng/mL) and the effect of maternal plasma proteins, placental metabolism, and fetal pH (7.4–6.8) on the transfer (4). The conclusions of this study were identical to those of the study above, in that sufentanil rapidly crossed the placenta by passive diffusion, the placenta acted as a depot for the narcotic, maternal protein binding (not albumin) decreased transfer, and fetal acidosis increased the amount reaching the fetus (4). The authors also concluded that because of its low initial transfer (umbilical vein concentration only 2% of maternal concentration at 5 minutes), sufentanil may be the narcotic of choice if delivery is imminent (<45 minutes) (4).

Sufentanil crosses the placenta to the fetal circulation following maternal epidural anesthesia (5,6). In a 1991 double-blind study, 60 women undergoing elective cesarean section at term were randomized to receive epidural anesthesia consisting of 0.5% bupivacaine with epinephrine (1:200,000) alone ($N = 20$), sufentanil 20 μg plus bupivacaine with epinephrine ($N = 20$), or sufentanil 30 μg plus bupivacaine with epinephrine ($N = 20$) (6). The mean plasma concentrations of sufentanil in the mother and newborn in the 20-μg group (14 subjects) were 0.030 and 0.025 ng/mL, respectively, whereas those in the 30-μg group (15 subjects) were 0.056 and 0.042 ng/mL, respectively. The fetal:maternal ratios in the two groups were 0.83 and 0.75, respectively. To evaluate the safety of the epidural solutions for the newborn, the Neurological and Adaptive Capacity Scoring System (NACS) was used to evaluate the infants at birth and between 1 and 2 hours. In each of the three groups, the percentage of neonates with a perfect score in each category of the NACS was statistically similar (6).

S

The placental transfer of sufentanil, fentanyl, and bupivacaine was studied in a double-blind, randomized trial involving 36 women at term who received epidural anesthesia during labor prior to vaginal delivery (6). Patients received a 12-mL bolus of either bupivacaine 0.25% alone ($N = 13$), bupivacaine 0.125% plus sufentanil 15 μg ($N = 9$), or bupivacaine 0.125% plus fentanyl 75 μg ($N = 14$), followed by a 10 mL/hour infusion of bupivacaine 0.125% alone, bupivacaine 0.125% plus sufentanil 0.25 μg/mL, or bupivacaine 0.125% plus fentanyl 1.5 μg/mL. The mean umbilical vein:maternal vein (UV:MV) ratios for bupivacaine in the three groups were 0.29, 0.43, and 0.33, respectively. The mean umbilical vein concentrations of the narcotics for sufentanil and fentanyl were 0.016 and 0.18 ng/mL, respectively, whereas the mean maternal vein concentrations were 0.019 and

0.52 ng/mL, respectively. The UV:MV ratios for sufentanil and fentanyl were 0.81 and 0.37, respectively. The NACS was used to assess the newborns in each group at delivery, 2 hours of age, and 24 hours of age (6). No statistical differences between the three groups were observed at delivery or at 2 hours of age, but at 24 hours, the bupivacaine-fentanyl group's NACS was significantly lower than that of the bupivacaine-sufentanil group, a result thought to reflect the continued presence of fentanyl in the neonate (6).

Intrathecal sufentanil (10 μg), followed at least 1 hour later with bupivacaine epidural analgesia ($N = 65$), was compared to bupivacaine epidural analgesia alone ($N = 64$) in a 1996 report comparing the effects of the two analgesic regimens on fetal heart rate changes during labor (7). No statistical differences were observed between the groups in the incidence of clinically significant fetal heart rate tracing abnormalities (recurrent late decelerations and/or bradycardia) or in maternal hypotension within the first hour of administration (7). In addition, there were no differences between the groups in arterial or venous cord pH or the number of 5-minute Apgar scores less than 7. No abnormal fetal heart rate patterns were observed in an earlier study that compared intrathecal sufentanil (10 μg) either alone ($N = 20$) or with 0.2 mg epinephrine ($N = 20$) (8). Epinephrine did not prolong analgesia but did increase the incidence of vomiting while decreasing the incidence and severity of pruritus. In a 1993 report, abnormal fetal heart rate changes were observed in 15% (11 of 73 tracings that were acceptable for analysis) among 108 women who received intrathecal sufentanil (10 μg) during active labor (9). Of the 11 abnormal tracings, 5 were of moderate but transient variable decelerations, 4 were of mild nonrepetitive late decelerations, 1 was of a single episode of bradycardia, and 1 was of an episode of decreased variability. None of 11 affected pregnancies required intervention for fetal compromise.

A number of studies have reported the successful use of sufentanil to produce adequate labor analgesia without fetal or newborn harm (10–19). A 1992 reference concluded that sufentanil 10 μg administered intrathecally produced faster and superior analgesia to that observed with epidural or IV administration of the same dose (10). Intermittent injections of intrathecal sufentanil (5 μg) were compared to intermittent injections of intrathecal fentanyl (10 μg) or meperidine (10 mg) in another 1992 report (11). In this study, meperidine provided better maternal analgesia once cervical dilation had progressed beyond 6 cm (11). No intergroup differences were observed in umbilical cord blood gasses and none of the newborns had a 5-minute Apgar score less than 7. No significant differences were observed in Apgar scores, umbilical cord blood pH levels, or NACS at 2 and 24 hours in a study comparing epidural sufentanil plus bupivacaine ($N = 30$) to epidural fentanyl plus bupivacaine ($N = 30$) (12). During labor, the patients received epidural infusions at 12 mL/hour of either sufentanil (0.25 μg/mL) or fentanyl (2.5 μg/mL), both in 0.0625% bupivacaine. The total narcotic doses of sufentanil or fentanyl were 15.9 and 139.8 μg, respectively. In seven other studies, spinal sufentanil either alone or combined with other various agents compared favorably with controls in efficacy and fetal and newborn safety (13–19).

A case of maternal respiratory depression following a 15-μg dose of intrathecal sufentanil during labor was described in 1994 (20). A marked decrease (to 89%) in the patient's hemoglobin oxygen saturation was noted that was treated with tactile stimulation and oxygen via face mask. A healthy, 3905-g male infant was delivered 2.5 hours later with Apgar scores of 7 and 8 at 1 and 5 minutes, respectively. No adverse effects were observed in the neonate during routine hospital follow-up.

In summary, the use of sufentanil during pregnancy with clinically used doses does not appear to present a significant risk to the fetus or newborn. Although no reports describing the use of the narcotic during the 1st trimester have been located, the lack of teratogenicity in animals and the general opinion that narcotic agents, in general, pose little risk of congenital malformations are reassuring. Sufentanil rapidly crosses the placenta to the fetus, even more so in the presence of fetal acidosis, and similar to all narcotics, dose-related depression of the fetus and newborn may occur. Both respiratory depression and adverse effects on neonatal neurobehavior are potential problems in the newborn.

[**Risk Factor D if used for prolonged periods or in high doses at term.*]

BREAST FEEDING SUMMARY

RECOMMENDATION: No Human Data - Probably Compatible

The use of sufentanil during lactation is unlikely because of its clinical indications. It is not surprising, therefore, that no reports describing the use of this agent during lactation have been located. The molecular weight (about 579) of sufentanil citrate, the commercial form of the drug, is low enough that passage into milk should be expected. The effects, if any, of this exposure on a nursing infant are unknown.

References

1. Product information. Sufenta. Janssen Pharmaceutica, 1998.
2. Fujinaga M, Mazze RI, Jackson EC, Baden JM. Reproductive and teratogenic effects of sufentanil and alfentanil in Sprague-Dawley rats. Anesth Analg 1988;67:166–9.
3. Johnson RF, Herman N, Arney TL, Johnson HV, Paschall RL, Downing JW. The placental transfer of sufentanil: effects of fetal pH, protein binding, and sufentanil concentration. Anesth Analg 1997;84:1262–8.
4. Krishna BR, Zakowski MI, Grant GJ. Sufentanil transfer in the human placenta during in vitro perfusion. Can J Anaesth 1997;44:996–1001.
5. Vertommen JD, Van Aken H, Vandermeulen E, Vangerven M, Devlieger H, Van Assche AF, Shnider SM. Maternal and neonatal effects of adding epidural sufentanil to 0.5% bupivacaine for cesarean delivery. J Clin Anesth 1991;3:371–6.
6. Loftus JR, Hill H, Cohen SE. Placental transfer and neonatal effects of epidural sufentanil and fentanyl administered with bupivacaine during labor. Anesthesiology 1995;83:300–8.
7. Nielsen PE, Erickson JR, Abouleish EI, Perriatt S, Sheppard C. Fetal heart rate changes after intrathecal sufentanil or epidural bupivicaine *[sic]* for labor analgesia: incidence and clinical significance. Anesth Analg 1996;83:742–60.
8. Camann WR, Minzter BH, Denney RA, Datta S. Intrathecal sufentanil for labor analgesia. Effects of added epinephrine. Anesthesiology 1993;78:870–4.
9. Cohen SE, Cherry CM, Holbrook RH Jr, El-Sayed YY, Gibson RN, Jaffe RA. Intrathecal sufentanil for labor analgesia - sensory changes, side effects, and fetal heart rate changes. Anesth Analg 1993;77:1155–60.
10. Camann WR, Denney RA, Holby ED, Datta S. A comparison of intrathecal, epidural, and intravenous sufentanil for labor analgesia. Anesthesiology 1992;77:884–7.
11. Honet JE, Arkoosh VA, Norris MC, Huffnagle HJ, Silverman NS, Leighton BL. Comparison among intrathecal fentanyl, meperidine, and sufentanil for labor analgesia. Anesth Analg 1992;75:734–9.
12. Russell R, Reynolds F. Epidural infusions for nulliparous women in labour. A randomised double-blind comparison of fentanyl/bupivacaine and sufentanil/bupivacaine. Anaesthesia 1993;48:856–61.
13. Phillips GH. Epidural sufentanil/bupivacaine combinations for analgesia during labor: effect of varying sufentanil doses. Anesthesiology 1987;67:835–8.
14. Van Steenberge A, Debroux HC, Noorduin H. Extradural bupivacaine with sufentanil for vaginal delivery. A double-blind trial. Br J Anaesth 1987;59:1518–22.
15. Le Polain B, De Kock M, Scholtes JL, Van Lierde M. Clonidine combined with sufentanil and bupivacaine with adrenaline for obstetric analgesia. Br J Anaesth 1993;71:657–60.
16. Grieco WM, Norris MC, Leighton BL, Arkoosh VA, Huffnagle HJ, Honet JE, Costello D. Intrathecal sufentanil labor analgesia: the effects of adding morphine or epinephrine. Anesth Anal 1993;77:1149–54.
17. D'Angelo R, Anderson MT, Philip J, Eisenach JC. Intrathecal sufentanil compared to epidural bupivacaine for labor analgesia. Anesthesiology 1994;80:1209–15.
18. Vertommen JD, Lemmens E, Van Aken H. Comparison of the addition of three different doses of sufentanil to 0.125% bupivacaine given epidurally during labour. Anaesthesia 1994;49:678–81.
19. Dahlgren G, Hultstrand C, Jakobsson J, Norman M, Eriksson EW, Martin H. Intrathecal sufentanil, fentanyl, or placebo added to bupivacaine for cesarean section. Anesth Analg 1997;85:1288–93.
20. Hays RL, Palmer CM. Respiratory depression after intrathecal sufentanil during labor. Anesthesiology 1994;81:511–2.

Name:	**SULBACTAM**	Risk Factor:	B_M
Class:	**Anti-infective**		

FETAL RISK SUMMARY

RECOMMENDATION: Compatible

Sulbactam is a semi-synthetic beta-lactamase irreversible inhibitor that is derived from the basic penicillin nucleus. When used alone, sulbactam does not have effective anti-infective activity (accept against the *Neisseriaceae*). However, sulbactam extends the activity of ampicillin when given in combination with this antibiotic (1).

Reproduction studies reported by the manufacturer involved mice, rats, and rabbits but only with the combination of sulbactam and ampicillin (1). There was no evidence of impaired fertility or fetal harm in each species at doses up to 10 times the human dose. Pregnant rats given IV sulbactam at doses up to 500 mg/kg/day at various times, including before mating and throughout gestation, showed no evidence of adverse reproductive effects (2).

Sulbactam crosses the human placenta to the fetus at term (3,4). Placental transfer studies early in gestation have not been located. An abstract from a 1983 symposium reported a linear relationship between fetal and maternal serum sulbactam concentrations when sulbactam/ampicillin was given as a single dose (either 0.5 g/1 g, or 1 g/1 g) just before cesarean section. The mean peak fetal serum level of sulbactam was less than 20 μg/mL (3). In an *in vitro* experiment with bidirectional perfused human placental lobules, sulbactam was demonstrated to cross by simple diffusion (4). The placental transfer is consistent with its low molecular weight (about 255).

A 1992 study compared the concentration of three antibiotics (sulbactam/ampicillin, ticarcillin/clavulanic acid, and cefotaxime) in maternal blood, placental tissue, and cord blood in 15 laboring women with chorioamnionitis at 37 weeks' gestation or greater (5). Five of the women received the sulbactam/ampicillin combination. The mean concentrations of sulbactam in maternal blood, placental tissue, and cord blood were 7.25, 3.75, and 9.68 μg/mL. The cord:maternal ratio was 1.3. The time interval between dosing and delivery and the dose used were not specified (5).

The pharmacokinetics of sulbactam at term were described in a 1993 study (6). The kinetics (area under drug versus time curve, elimination rate constant, half-life, volume of distribution, and clearance) of a 0.5-g dose of sulbactam (combined with 1 g ampicillin) administered intravenously at cord clamping were not significantly different from those in non-pregnant patients. Changes were noted but did not reach statistical significance (6).

S

The combination of sulbactam and ampicillin has been used frequently in the 2nd and 3rd trimesters of pregnancy (7–15). These studies involved prophylaxis, as in cases of preterm premature rupture of the membranes, and therapy for established infections. No cases of fetal or newborn direct harm from exposure to the combination were reported. However, indirect harm to the newborn from antibiotic-related superinfection with resistant bacteria is a concern (15).

Inadvertent intrauterine infusion of sulbactam (1 g) plus ampicillin (2 g) was reported in a brief 2000 communication (16). The antibiotic combination was being given for prophylaxis of preterm premature rupture of the membranes at 30 weeks' gestation. Apparently the error occurred when the antibiotic was infused into an intrauterine catheter instead of the intended IV catheter. A 1690-g infant (sex not specified) was delivered by cesarean section the next day. No adverse effects of the error were observed.

In summary, sulbactam is always given in combination with ampicillin. It has caused no harm in animal reproduction studies, but reports of human exposure in early gestation are lacking. However, none of the penicillins have been shown to be teratogenic. Sulbactam readily crosses the human placenta to the fetus. Although no direct adverse effects of this exposure on the fetus or newborn have been reported, use of the antibiotic combination near delivery may result in super-infection with resistant bacteria in the newborn.

BREAST FEEDING SUMMARY

RECOMMENDATION: Compatible

Sulbactam is excreted into the breast milk of animals (sheep and goats) and humans (17,18). Sulbactam (0.5 or 1.0 g) was infused either with cephalothin or ampicillin in four postpartum women 2 days after cesarean section (17). The milk concentrations obtained 10–21 hours after a dose ranged from 0.13 to 1.2 μg/mL (mean 0.52 μg/mL). No sulbactam was found in one sample obtained at 49 hours. The investigators did not state whether the infants were allowed to nurse. The potential effects of exposure to sulbactam on the nursing infant are unknown, but are probably similar to those that might occur with other antibiotics: modification of bowel flora, direct effects on the infant (e.g., allergy or sensitization), and interference with the interpretation of culture results if a fever workup is required. The American Academy of Pediatrics classifies sulbactam as compatible with breast-feeding (19).

References

1. Product information. Unasyn. Pfizer, 2002.
2. Horimoto M, Sakai T, Ohtsuki I, Noguchi Y. Reproduction studies with sulbactam and combinations of sulbactam and cefoperazone in rats. Chemotherapy 1984;32:108–15. As cited in Shepard TH. *Catalog of Teratogenic Agents*. 10th ed. Baltimore, MD: Johns Hopkins University Press, 2001:469.
3. Dubois M, Coibion M, Deco J, Delapierre D, Lambotte R, Dresse A. The transplacental transfer of sulbactam sodium when co-administered with ampicillin to healthy pregnant women in labor (abstract). In Spitzy KH, Karrer K, Breyer S, Lenzhofer R, Moser K, Pichler H, Rainer H, eds. 13th International Congress of Chemotherapy, Vienna, 28th August to 2 September, 1983. TOM 1, Antimicrobial Symposia. Verlag H. Egermann, Publ. Vienna, 1983.
4. Fortunato SJ, Bawdon RE, Baum M. Placental transfer of cefoperazone and sulbactam in the isolated in vitro perfused human placenta. Am J Obstet Gynecol 1988;159:1002–6.
5. Maberry MC, Trimmer KJ, Bawdon RE, Sobhi S, Dax JB, Gilstrap LC III. Antibiotic concentration in maternal blood, cord blood and placental tissue in women with chorioamnionitis. Gynecol Obstet Invest 1992;33:185–6.
6. Chamberlain A, White S, Bawdon R, Thomas S, Larsen B. Pharmacokinetics of ampicillin and sulbactam in pregnancy. Am J Obstet Gynecol 1993;168:667–73.
7. Smith LG Jr, Summers PR, Miles RW, Biswas MK, Pernoll ML. Gonococcal chorioamnionitis associated with sepsis: a case report. Am J Obstet Gynecol 1989;160:573–4.
8. Newton ER, Shields L, Ridgway LE III, Berkus MD, Elliott BD. Combination antibiotics and indomethacin in idiopathic preterm labor: a randomized double-blind clinical trial. Am J Obstet Gynecol 1991;165:1753–9.
9. Lewis DF, Fontenot MT, Brooks GG, Wise R, Perkins MB, Heyman AR. Latency period after preterm premature rupture of membranes: a comparison of ampicillin with and without sulbactam. Obstet Gynecol 1995;86:392–5.
10. Adair CD, Ernest JM, Sanchez-Ramos L, Burrus DR, Boles ML, Veille JC. Meconium-stained amniotic fluid-associated infectious morbidity: a randomized, double-blind trial of ampicillin-sulbactam prophylaxis. Obstet Gynecol 1996;88:216–20.
11. Lewis DF, Brody K, Edwards MS, Brouillette RM, Burlison S, London SN. Preterm premature ruptured membranes: a randomized trial of steroids after treatment with antibiotics. Obstet Gynecol 1996;88:801–5.
12. Cox SM, Bohman VR, Sherman ML, Leveno KJ. Randomized investigation of antimicrobials for the prevention of preterm birth. Am J Obstet Gynecol 1996;174:206–10.
13. Lovett SM, Weiss JD, Diogo MJ, Williams PT, Garite TJ. A prospective, double-blind, randomized, controlled clinical trial of ampicillin-sulbactam for preterm premature rupture of membranes in women receiving antenatal corticosteroid therapy. Am J Obstet Gynecol 1997;176:1030–8.

S

14. Perry KG Jr, Gebhart LD III, Turner KY, Martin RW. Ampicillin/sulbactam and corticosteroids in the management of preterm premature rupture of membranes (abstract). Am J Obstet Gynecol 1998;178:S201.
15. Carroll EM, Heywood PA, Besinger RE, Muraskas JK, Fisher SG, Gianopoulos JG. A prospective randomized double-blind trial of ampicillin with and without sulbactam in preterm premature rupture of the membranes (abstract). Am J Obstet Gynecol 2000;182:S61.
16. Sigg TR, Kuhn BR. Inadvertent intrauterine infusion of ampicillin-sulbactam. Am J Health-Syst Pharm 2000;57:215.
17. Escudero E, Espuny A, Vicente MS, Carceles CM. Comparative pharmacokinetics of an ampicillin/sulbactam combination administered intramuscularly in lactating sheep and goats. Vet Res 1996;27:201–8.
18. Foulds G, Miller RD, Knirsch AK, Thrupp LD. Sulbactam kinetics and excretion into breast milk in postpartum women. Clin Pharmacol Ther 1985;38:692–6.
19. Committee on Drugs, American Academy of Pediatrics. The transfer of drugs and other chemicals into human milk. Pediatrics 2001;108:776–89.

Name: **SULFASALAZINE** Risk Factor: B_M*

Class: **Gastrointestinal Agent/Immunologic Agent (Antirheumatic)**

FETAL RISK SUMMARY

RECOMMENDATION: Human Data Suggest Low Risk

Sulfasalazine is a compound composed of 5-aminosalicylic acid (5-ASA) joined to sulfapyridine by an azo linkage (refer to Sulfonamides for a complete review of this class of agents). Sulfasalazine is used for the treatment of ulcerative colitis, Crohn's disease, and rheumatoid arthritis. Reproduction studies in rats and rabbits at doses up to 6 times the human dose revealed no impairment of fertility or fetal harm (1).

No increase in human congenital defects or newborn toxicity has been observed from its use in pregnancy (2–12). However, three reports, involving five infants (two stillborn), have described congenital malformations after exposure to this drug (13–15). It cannot be determined whether the observed defects were related to the therapy, the disease, or a combination of these or other factors: bilateral cleft lip/palate, severe hydrocephalus, death (13); ventricular septal defect, coarctation of aorta (14); Potter-type IIa polycystic kidney, rudimentary left uterine cornu, stillborn (first twin) (14); Potter's facies, hypoplastic lungs, absent kidneys and ureters, talipes equinovarus, stillborn (second twin) (14); ventricular septal defect, coarctation of aorta, macrocephaly; gingival hyperplasia, small ears (both thought to be inherited) (15).

S

Sulfasalazine and its metabolite, sulfapyridine, readily cross the placenta to the fetal circulation (6,7). Fetal concentrations are approximately the same as maternal concentrations. Placental transfer of 5-ASA is limited because only negligible amounts are absorbed from the cecum and colon, and these are rapidly excreted in the urine (16).

At birth, concentrations of sulfasalazine and sulfapyridine in 11 infants were 4.6 and 18.2 μg/mL, respectively (7). Neither of these levels was sufficient to cause significant displacement of bilirubin from albumin (7). Kernicterus and severe neonatal jaundice have not been reported following maternal use of sulfasalazine, even when the drug was given up to the time of delivery (7,8). Caution is advised, however, because other sulfonamides have caused jaundice in the newborn when given near term (see Sulfonamides).

Sulfasalazine is a folic acid antagonist (dihydrofolate reductase inhibitor). In a 2000 case-control study, the affect of folic acid supplementation on the risks for certain congenital defects were examined (17). Supplementation reduced the teratogenic risk from sulfasalazine and similar acting folic acid antagonists. See Trimethoprim for details of this study.

Sulfasalazine may adversely affect spermatogenesis in male patients with inflammatory bowel disease (18,19). Sperm counts and motility are both reduced and require 2 months or longer after the drug is stopped to return to normal levels (18). If sulfasalazine is used in pregnancy for the treatment of rheumatoid arthritis, healthcare professionals are encouraged to call the toll free number (877-311-8972) for information about patient enrollment in the OTIS Rheumatoid Arthritis study.

[**Risk Factor D if administered near term.*]

BREAST FEEDING SUMMARY

RECOMMENDATION: Limited Human Data - Potential Toxicity

Sulfapyridine is excreted into breast milk (see also Sulfonamides) (6,16,20). Milk concentrations were approximately 40%–60% of maternal serum levels. One infant's urine contained 3–4 μg/mL of the drug (1.2–1.6 mg/24 hours), representing about 30%–40% of the total dose excreted in the milk. Unmetabolized sulfasalazine was detected in only one of the studies (milk:plasma ratio of 0.3) (6). Levels of 5-ASA were undetectable. No adverse effects were observed in the 16 nursing infants exposed in these reports (6,16,20). However, bloody diarrhea in an infant exclusively breast-fed, occurring first at 2 months of age, and then recurring 2 weeks later and persisting until 3 months of age, was attributed to the mother's sulfasalazine therapy (3 g/day) (21). The mother was a slow acetylator with a blood concentration of sulfapyridine of 42.4 μg/mL (therapeutic range 20–50 μg/mL). The acetylation phenotype of the infant was not determined, but his blood level of sulfapyridine was 5.3 μg/mL. A diagnostic workup of the infant was negative. The bloody diarrhea did stop, however, 48–72 hours after discontinuance of the mother's therapy. A repeat colonoscopy of the infant 1.5 months later was normal (21).

Based on the above report, the American Academy of Pediatrics classifies sulfasalazine as a drug that has been associated with significant effects on some nursing infants and should be given to nursing mothers with caution (22).

References

1. Product information. Azulfidine EN-tabs. Pharmacia & Upjohn, 2000.
2. McEwan HP. Anorectal conditions in obstetric practice. Proc R Soc Med 1972;65:279–81.
3. Willoughby CP, Truelove SC. Ulcerative colitis and pregnancy. Gut 1980;21:469–74.
4. Levy N, Roisman I, Teodor I. Ulcerative colitis in pregnancy in Israel. Dis Colon Rectum 1981;24:351–4.
5. Mogadam M, Dobbins WO III, Korelitz BI, Ahmed SW. Pregnancy in inflammatory bowel disease: effect of sulfasalazine and corticosteroids on fetal outcome. Gastroenterology 1981;80:72–6.
6. Azad Khan AK, Truelove SC. Placental and mammary transfer of sulphasalazine. Br Med J 1979;2:1553.
7. Jarnerot G, Into-Malmberg MB, Esbjorner E. Placental transfer of sulphasalazine and sulphapyridine and some of its metabolites. Scand J Gastroenterol 1981;16:693–7.
8. Mogadam M. Sulfasalazine, IBD, and pregnancy (reply). Gastroenterology 1981;81:194.
9. Fielding JF. Pregnancy and inflammatory bowel disease. J Clin Gastroenterol 1983;5:107–8.
10. Sorokin JJ, Levine SM. Pregnancy and inflammatory bowel disease: a review of the literature. Obstet Gynecol 1983;62:247–52.
11. Baiocco PJ, Korelitz BI. The influence of inflammatory bowel disease and its treatment on pregnancy and fetal outcome. J Clin Gastroenterol 1984;6:211–6.
12. Fedorkow DM, Persaud D, Nimrod CA. Inflammatory bowel disease: a controlled study of late pregnancy outcome. Am J Obstet Gynecol 1989;160:998–1001.
13. Craxi A, Pagliarello F. Possible embryotoxicity of sulfasalazine. Arch Intern Med 1980;140:1674.
14. Newman NM, Correy JF. Possible teratogenicity of sulphasalazine. Med J Aust 1983;1:528–9.
15. Hoo JJ, Hadro TA, Von Behren P. Possible teratogenicity of sulfasalazine. N Engl J Med 1988;318:1128.
16. Berlin CM Jr, Yaffe SJ. Disposition of salicylazosulfapyridine (Azulfidine) and metabolites in human breast milk. Dev Pharmacol Ther 1980;1:31–9.
17. Hernandez-Diaz S, Werler MM, Walker AM, Mitchell AA. Folic acid antagonists during pregnancy and the risk of birth defects. N Engl J Med 2000;343:1608–14.
18. Toovey S, Hudson E, Hendry WF, Levi AJ. Sulphasalazine and male infertility: reversibility and possible mechanism. Gut 1981;22:445–51.

19. Freeman JG, Reece VAC, Venables CW. Sulphasalazine and spermatogenesis. Digestion 1982;23:68–71.
20. Jarnerot G, Into-Malmberg MB. Sulphasalazine treatment during breast feeding. Scand J Gastroenterol 1979;14:869–71.
21. Branski D, Kerem E, Gross-Kieselstein E, Hurvitz H, Litt R, Abrahamov A. Bloody diarrhea-a possible complication of sulfasalazine transferred through human breast milk. J Pediatr Gastroenterol Nutr 1986;5:316–7.
22. Committee on Drugs, American Academy of Pediatrics. The transfer of drugs and other chemicals into human milk. Pediatrics 2001;108:776–89.

Name:	**SULFONAMIDES**	Risk Factor:	C_M*
Class:	**Anti-infective**		

FETAL RISK SUMMARY

RECOMMENDATION: Human Data Suggest Risk in 3rd Trimester

Sulfonamides are a large class of antibacterial agents. Although there are differences in their bioavailability, all share similar actions in the fetal and newborn periods, and they will be considered as a single group.

Sulfamethoxazole was teratogenic (primarily cleft palates) in rats given oral doses of 533 mg/kg (1). The highest dose that did not produce cleft palates was 512 mg/kg.

The sulfonamides readily cross the placenta to the fetus during all stages of gestation (2–10). Equilibrium with maternal blood is usually established after 2–3 hours, with fetal levels averaging 70%–90% of maternal. Significant levels may persist in the newborn for several days after birth when given near term. The primary danger of sulfonamide administration during pregnancy is manifested when these agents are given close to delivery. Toxicities that may be observed in the newborn include jaundice, hemolytic anemia, and, theoretically, kernicterus. Severe jaundice in the newborn has been related to maternal sulfonamide ingestion at term by several authors (11–16). Premature infants seem especially prone to development of hyperbilirubinemia (15). However, a study of 94 infants exposed to sulfadiazine *in utero* for maternal prophylaxis of rheumatic fever failed to show an increase in prematurity, hyperbilirubinemia, or kernicterus (17). Hemolytic anemia has been reported in two newborns and in a fetus following *in utero* exposure to sulfonamides (11,12,16). Both newborns survived. In the case involving the fetus, the mother had homozygous glucose-6-phosphate dehydrogenase deficiency (16). She was treated with sulfisoxazole for a urinary tract infection 2 weeks before delivery of a stillborn male infant. Autopsy revealed a 36-week gestation infant with maceration, severe anemia, and hydrops fetalis.

Sulfonamides compete with bilirubin for binding to plasma albumin. *In utero*, the fetus clears free bilirubin by the placental circulation, but after birth, this mechanism is no longer available. Unbound bilirubin is free to cross the blood-brain barrier and may result in kernicterus. Although this toxicity is well known when sulfonamides are administered directly to the neonate, kernicterus in the newborn following *in utero* exposure has not been reported. Most reports of sulfonamide exposure during gestation have failed to demonstrate an association with congenital malformations (10,11,18–24). Offspring of patients treated throughout pregnancy with sulfasalazine (sulfapyridine plus 5-aminosalicylic acid) for ulcerative colitis or Crohn's disease have not shown an increase in adverse effects (see also Sulfasalazine) (10,21,23). In contrast, a retrospective study of 1369 patients found that significantly more mothers of 458 infants with congenital malformations took sulfonamides than did mothers in the control group (25). A 1975 study examined the *in utero* drug exposures of 599 children born with oral clefts (26). A significant difference

($p < 0.05$), as compared with matched controls, was found with 1st and 2nd trimester sulfonamide use only when other defects, in addition to the clefts, were present.

As noted above, some sulfonamides are animal teratogens. Because of this, warnings of human teratogenicity have been published (27,28). In two reports, investigators associated *in utero* sulfonamide exposure with tracheoesophageal fistula and cataracts, but additional descriptions of these effects have not appeared (29,30). A mother treated for food poisoning with sulfaguanidine in early pregnancy delivered a child with multiple anomalies (31). The author attributed the defects to use of the drug, but a relationship is doubtful.

The Collaborative Perinatal Project monitored 50,282 mother-child pairs, 1455 of whom had 1st trimester exposure to sulfonamides (32, pp. 296–313). For use anytime during pregnancy, 5689 exposures were reported (32, p. 435). In neither group was evidence found to suggest a relationship to large categories of major or minor malformations. Several possible associations were found with individual defects after anytime use, but independent confirmation is required: ductus arteriosus persistens (8 cases); coloboma (4 cases); hypoplasia of limb or part thereof (7 cases); miscellaneous foot defects (4 cases); urethral obstruction (13 cases); hypoplasia or atrophy of adrenals (6 cases); and benign tumors (12 cases) (32, pp. 485–6).

In a surveillance study of Michigan Medicaid recipients conducted between 1985 and 1992 involving 229,101 completed pregnancies, 131 newborns had been exposed to sulfisoxazole, 1138 to sulfabenzamide vaginal cream, and 2296 to the combination of sulfamethoxazole-trimethoprim during the 1st trimester (F. Rosa, personal communication, FDA, 1993). For sulfisoxazole, eight (6.1%) major birth defects were observed (six expected), two cardiovascular defects (one expected) and one oral cleft (none expected). No anomalies were observed in four other categories of defects (spina bifida, polydactyly, limb reduction defects, and hypospadias) for which data were available. For sulfabenzamide, 43 (3.8%) major birth defects were found (44 expected), including 11/10 cardiovascular defects, 0/2 oral clefts, 0/0.5 spina bifida, 2/3 polydactyly, 1/2 limb reduction defects, and 1/3 hypospadias. The data for sulfisoxazole and sulfabenzamide do not support an association between the drug and congenital defects. In contrast, a possible association was found between sulfamethoxazole-trimethoprim and congenital defects (126 observed/98 expected; 5.5%) in general and for cardiovascular defects (37/23) in particular (see Trimethoprim for details).

Taken in sum, sulfonamides, as single agents, do not appear to pose a significant teratogenic risk. Because of the potential toxicity to the newborn, these agents should be avoided near term.

[**Risk Factor D if administered near term.*]

S

BREAST FEEDING SUMMARY

RECOMMENDATION: Limited Human Data - Potential Toxicity

Sulfonamides are excreted into breast milk in low concentrations. Milk levels of sulfanilamide (free and conjugated) are reported to range from 6 to 94 μg/mL (4,33–38). Up to 1.6% of the total dose could be recovered from the milk (33,36). Milk levels often exceeded serum levels and persisted for several days after maternal consumption of the drug was stopped. Milk:plasma ratios during therapy with sulfanilamide were 0.5–0.6 (37). Reports of adverse effects in nursing infants are rare. One author found reports of diarrhea and rash in breast-fed infants whose mothers were receiving sulfapyridine or sulfathiazole (7). (See Sulfasalazine for another report of bloody diarrhea.) Milk levels of sulfapyridine, the active metabolite of sulfasalazine, were 10.3 μg/mL, a milk:plasma ratio of 0.5 (10).

Based on these data, the nursing infant would receive approximately 3–4 mg/kg/day of sulfapyridine, an apparently nontoxic amount for a healthy neonate (17). Sulfisoxazole, a very water-soluble drug, was reported to produce a low milk:plasma ratio of 0.06 (39). The conjugated form achieved a ratio of 0.22. The total amount of sulfisoxazole recovered in milk during 48 hours after a 4-g divided dose was only 0.45%. Although controversial, breast-feeding during maternal administration of sulfisoxazole seems to represent a very low risk for the healthy neonate (40,41).

In summary, sulfonamide excretion into breast milk apparently does not pose a significant risk for the healthy, full-term neonate. Exposure to sulfonamides via breast milk should be avoided in ill, stressed, or premature infants and in infants with hyperbilirubinemia or glucose-6-phosphate dehydrogenase deficiency. With these latter precautions, the American Academy of Pediatrics classifies sulfapyridine, sulfisoxazole, and sulfamethoxazole (when combined with trimethoprim) as compatible with breast-feeding (42).

References

1. Product information. Bactrim. Roche Laboratories, 2000.
2. Barker RH. The placental transfer of sulfanilamide. N Engl J Med 1938;219:41.
3. Speert H. The passage of sulfanilamide through the human placenta. Bull Johns Hopkins Hosp 1938;63:337–9.
4. Stewart HL Jr, Pratt JP. Sulfanilamide excretion in human breast milk and effect on breast-fed babies. JAMA 1938;111:1456–8.
5. Speert H. The placental transmission of sulfanilamide and its effects upon the fetus and newborn. Bull Johns Hopkins Hosp 1940;66:139–55.
6. Speert H. Placental transmission of sulfathiazole and sulfadiazine and its significance for fetal chemotherapy. Am J Obstet Gynecol 1943;45:200–7.
7. von Freisen B. A study of small dose sulphamerazine prophylaxis in obstetrics. Acta Obstet Gynecol Scand 1951;31(Suppl):75–116.
8. Sparr RA, Pritchard JA. Maternal and newborn distribution and excretion of sulfamethoxypyridazine (Kynex). Obstet Gynecol 1958;12:131–4.
9. Nishimura H, Tanimura T. *Clinical Aspects of the Teratogenicity of Drugs*. New York, NY: Excerpta Medica, 1976:88.
10. Azad Khan AK, Truelove SC. Placental and mammary transfer of sulphasalazine. Br Med J 1979;2:1553.
11. Heckel GP. Chemotherapy during pregnancy. Danger of fetal injury from sulfanilamide and its derivatives. JAMA 1941;117:1314–6.
12. Ginzler AM, Cherner C. Toxic manifestations in the newborn infant following placental transmission of sulfanilamide. With a report of 2 cases simulating erythroblastosis fetalis. Am J Obstet Gynecol 1942;44:46–55.
13. Lucey JF, Driscoll TJ Jr. Hazard to newborn infants of administration of long-acting sulfonamides to pregnant women. Pediatrics 1959;24:498–9.
14. Kantor HI, Sutherland DA, Leonard JT, Kamholz FH, Fry ND, White WL. Effect on bilirubin metabolism in the newborn of sulfisoxazole administration to the mother. Obstet Gynecol 1961;17:494–500.
15. Dunn PM. The possible relationship between the maternal administration of sulphamethoxypyridazine and hyperbilirubinaemia in the newborn. J Obstet Gynaecol Br Commonw 1964;71:128–31.
16. Perkins RP. Hydrops fetalis and stillbirth in a male glucose-6-phosphate dehydrogenase-deficient fetus possibly due to maternal ingestion of sulfisoxazole. Am J Obstet Gynecol 1971;111:379–81.
17. Baskin CG, Law S, Wenger NK. Sulfadiazine rheumatic fever prophylaxis during pregnancy: Does it increase the risk of kernicterus in the newborn? Cardiology 1980;65:222–5.
18. Bonze EJ, Fuerstner PG, Falls FH. Use of sulfanilamide derivative in treatment of gonorrhea in pregnant and nonpregnant women. Am J Obstet Gynecol 1939;38:73–9.
19. Carter MP, Wilson F. Antibiotics and congenital malformations. Lancet 1963;1:1267–8.
20. Little PJ. The incidence of urinary infection in 5000 pregnant women. Lancet 1966;2:925–8.
21. McEwan HP. Anorectal conditions in obstetric patients. Proc R Soc Med 1972;65:279–81.
22. Williams JD, Smith EK. Single-dose therapy with streptomycin and sulfametopyrazine for bacteriuria during pregnancy. Br Med J 1970;4:651–3.
23. Mogadam M, Dobbins WO III, Korelitz BI, Ahmed SW. Pregnancy in inflammatory bowel disease: effect of sulfasalazine and corticosteroids on fetal outcome. Gastroenterology 1981;80:72–6.
24. Richards IDG. A retrospective inquiry into possible teratogenic effects of drugs in pregnancy. Adv Exp Med Biol 1972;27:441–55.
25. Nelson MM, Forfar JO. Association between drugs administered during pregnancy and congenital abnormalities of the fetus. Br Med J 1971;1:523–7.
26. Saxen I. Associations between oral clefts and drugs taken during pregnancy. Int J Epidemiol 1975;4:37–44.
27. Anonymous. Teratogenic effects of sulphonamides. Br Med J 1965;1:142.
28. Green KG. "Bimez" and teratogenic action. Br Med J 1963;2:56.
29. Ingalls TH, Prindle RA. Esophageal atresia with tracheoesophageal fistula. Epidemiologic and teratologic implications. N Engl J Med 1949;240:987–95.

S

30. Harly JD, Farrar JF, Gray JB, Dunlop IC. Aromatic drugs and congenital cataracts. Lancet 1964;1:472–3.
31. Pogorzelska E. A case of multiple congenital anomalies in a child of a mother treated with sulfaguanidine. Patol Pol 1966;17:383–6.
32. Heinonen OP, Slone D, Shapiro S. *Birth Defects and Drugs in Pregnancy*. Littleton, MA: Publishing Sciences Group, 1977.
33. Adair FL, Hesseltine HC, Hac LR. Experimental study of the behavior of sulfanilamide. JAMA 1938;111: 766–70.
34. Hepburn JS, Paxson NF, Rogers AN. Secretion of ingested sulfanilamide in breast milk and in the urine of the infant. J Biol Chem 1938;123:liv–lv.
35. Pinto SS. Excretion of sulfanilamide and acetylsulfanilamide in human milk. JAMA 1938;111:1914–6.
36. Hac LR, Adair FL, Hesseltine HC. Excretion of sulfanilamide and acetylsulfanilamide in human breast milk. Am J Obstet Gynecol 1939;38:57–66.
37. Foster FP. Sulfanilamide excretion in breast milk: report of a case. Proc Staff Meet Mayo Clin 1939;14:153–5.
38. Hepburn JS, Paxson NF, Rogers AN. Secretion of ingested sulfanilamide in human milk and in the urine of the nursing infant. Arch Pediatr 1942;59:413–8.
39. Kauffman RE, O'Brien C, Gilford P. Sulfisoxazole secretion into human milk. J Pediatr 1980;97:839–41.
40. Elliott GT, Quinn SI. Sulfisoxazole in human milk. J Pediatr 1981;99:171–2.
41. Kauffman RE. Sulfisoxazole in human milk (reply). J Pediatr 1981;99:172.
42. Committee on Drugs, American Academy of Pediatrics. The transfer of drugs and other chemicals into human milk. Pediatrics 2001;108:776–89.

Name: **SULINDAC** Risk Factor: **B***

Class: **Nonsteroidal Anti-inflammatory**

FETAL RISK SUMMARY

RECOMMENDATION: Human Data Suggest Risk in 1st and 3rd Trimesters

Sulindac is a nonsteroidal anti-inflammatory prodrug (NSAID) that is converted *in vivo* to the biologically active sulfide metabolite. It is used for the relief of the signs and symptoms of rheumatoid arthritis, osteoarthritis, gouty arthritis, ankylosing spondylitis, and acute painful shoulder (1). Sulindac is in the same NSAID subclass (acetic acids) as diclofenac, indomethacin, and tolmetin. However, sulindac, a derivative of indomethacin, is seven times more COX-2 selective than indomethacin and is sometimes referred to as a COX-2 selective agent (2).

When administered to pregnant rats, similar to other nonsteroidal anti-inflammatory agents, sulindac reduces fetal weight and pup survival (at doses 2.5 times or higher than the usual maximum human daily dose), prolongs the duration of gestation, and may cause dystocia (1,3).

Consistent with the molecular weight (about 356), sulindac and its active metabolite cross the human placenta to the fetus. Nine women at a mean gestational age of 31.8 weeks (24.3–36.4 weeks) were given a single 200-mg oral dose of the drug a mean 5.5 hours (4.4–6.7 hours) before cordocentesis (4,5). Maternal serum was obtained a mean 5.8 hours (3.5–7.3 hours) after the dose. The mean concentrations of sulindac in the mothers and fetuses were 0.59 and 0.98 μg/mL, respectively, and of the sulfide metabolite 1.42 and 0.68 μg/mL, respectively. The corresponding sulfide:sulindac ratios in the mother and fetal compartments were 2.32 and 0.53, respectively. The reduced amounts of metabolite in the fetus, compared with those in the mother, were thought to be caused by decreased placental transfer of the metabolite and slower metabolism of sulindac in the fetus (5). Because of these findings, the investigators theorized that, as a tocolytic, sulindac would be expected to cause less fetal toxicity than indomethacin.

Using a human term placental perfusion model, a 1999 study demonstrated that the sulfide metabolite reaches the fetus in higher concentrations than does sulindac or indomethacin (6). The fetal:maternal ratios after 2-hour perfusions were 0.34 (sulindac),

S

0.54 (sulfide metabolite), and 0.45 (indomethacin). Neither sulindac or indomethacin were metabolized by the placenta.

In a surveillance study of Michigan Medicaid recipients conducted between 1985 and 1992 involving 229,101 completed pregnancies, 69 newborns had been exposed to sulindac during the 1st trimester (F. Rosa, personal communication, FDA, 1995). Three (4.3%) major birth defects were observed (three expected), including one cardiovascular defect (one expected). No anomalies were observed in five other categories of defects (oral clefts, spina bifida, polydactyly, limb reduction defects, and hypospadias) for which specific data were available. For exposure during any trimester (102 newborns), two malformations of the eyeball (excludes oculomotor and ptosis) were observed (none expected), but no brain defects were recorded.

A combined 2001 population-based observational cohort study and a case-control study estimated the risk of adverse pregnancy outcome from the use of NSAIDs (7). The use of NSAIDs during pregnancy was not associated with congenital malformations, preterm delivery, or low birth weight, but a positive association was discovered with spontaneous abortions (SABs). A similar study, also published in 2001, failed to find a relationship, in general, between NSAIDs and congenital malformations, but did find a significant association with cardiac defects and orofacial clefts (8). In addition, a 2003 study found a significant association between exposure to NSAIDs in early pregnancy and SABs (9). (See Ibuprofen for details on these three studies.)

A brief 2003 editorial on the potential for NSAID-induced developmental toxicity concluded that NSAIDs, and specifically those with greater COX-2 affinity, had a lower risk of this toxicity in humans than aspirin (10).

An abstract and a full report, both published in 1992, described the use of sulindac in the treatment of preterm labor in comparison with indomethacin (11,12). The gestational ages at treatment for the groups were 29 and 30 weeks, respectively. The sulindac group ($N = 18$) received 200 mg orally every 12 hours for 48 hours, whereas those receiving indomethacin ($N = 18$) were given 100 mg orally once followed by 25 mg orally every 4 hours for 48 hours. Both groups received IV magnesium sulfate and some in both groups received subcutaneous terbutaline. The response to tocolysis was statistically similar for sulindac and indomethacin. However, the sulindac-treated women had significantly greater hourly fetal urine output, the deepest amniotic fluid pocket, and the largest amniotic fluid index. Patent ductus arteriosus was observed in 11% vs. 22%, respectively, and intraventricular hemorrhage in the newborn occurred in 11% of both groups. These differences were not significant. No cases of primary pulmonary hypertension in the newborns were observed (11,12).

S

A comparison between sulindac (200 mg orally every 12 hours times 4 days) and indomethacin (100 mg rectally on the 1st day, then 50 mg orally every 8 hours times 3 days) on fetal cardiac function was published in 1995 (13). Each group was composed of 10 patients with threatened premature labor between 28 and 32 weeks' gestation. Significant reductions in the mean pulsatility index of the fetal ductus arteriosus began 4 hours after the first indomethacin dose. The reduction increased with time and resolved 24 hours after the last dose. Other secondary changes in fetal cardiac function resulting from ductal constriction were also noted. In the sulindac group, a significant decrease in the mean pulsatility index, without secondary changes, was observed only at 24 hours (13).

A study comparing the fetal cardiovascular effects of sulindac (200 mg orally every 12 hours) and terbutaline (5 mg orally every 4 hours) for 68 hours at an approximate mean gestational age of 32 weeks was published in abstract form in 1996 (14) and in a full report in 1999 (15). Significant ductal constriction was noted only in the sulindac group. In contrast to the study cited above, therapy was stopped because of severe constriction in 2 (one at 12 hours and the other at 24 hours) of the 10 patients. The constriction of the fetal ductus arteriosus occurred within 5 hours of receiving sulindac and resolved within 48 hours of discontinuing the drug (14,15).

A 1994 abstract reported that the tocolytic effect of a 7-day course of sulindac, 200 mg orally every 12 hours, following arrest of labor with IV magnesium sulfate was no different from placebo and observation (16). The difference in prolongation of pregnancy between the sulindac (N = 13) and placebo (N = 15) groups, 33 ± 25 days vs. 26 ± 17 days, respectively, was not significant. No differences between the groups on days 0, 7, and 14 were found for hourly fetal urine production, amniotic fluid index, or ductus arteriosus velocity (16).

Two 1995 references from the same group of investigators, using a similar study design, concluded that sulindac did not reduce the rate of premature birth but did lengthen the interval to retocolysis in those patients who required retocolysis (17,18). No difference was found between sulindac and placebo in prolongation of pregnancy, delivery at >35 weeks' gestation, recurrent preterm labor, birth weight, or time spent in the neonatal intensive care unit. No adverse effects were observed in the exposed fetuses (17,18).

As demonstrated with other NSAIDs (see also Indomethacin), sulindac reduces amniotic fluid volume by decreasing fetal urine output in a dose-related manner (19). Sulindac, 200 mg twice daily, was given to the mothers of three sets of monoamniotic twins, diagnosed as having cord entanglement, beginning at 24, 27, and 29 weeks, respectively, and continued until elective cesarean section at 32 weeks' gestation. One of the twins had a preexisting heart defect (transposition of the great vessels and a ventricular septal defect). The dose was reduced in one patient to 200 mg/day to maintain an adequate amniotic fluid index. No significant changes in the umbilical artery or the ductus arteriosus Doppler waveforms were observed. All of the newborns had appropriate weights for gestation, had normal renal function during the first week of life, and none required ventilation (19).

A 2000 abstract described a retrospective case-cohort study that compared the neonatal effects of sulindac with indomethacin (20). The infants (born between 1994 and 1999) had been exposed to antenatal sulindac (N = 25) or indomethacin (N = 66) and weighed <1500 g. Those exposed to both drugs or with congenital abnormalities were excluded. There were no significant differences between the indomethacin and sulindac groups in intraventricular hemorrhage (IVH) 32% vs. 36%, grade III–IV IVH 14% vs. 12%, necrotizing enterocolitis 8% vs. 8%, serum creatinine >1.4 mg/dL 19% vs. 15%, patent ductus arteriosus 17% vs. 28%, and mortality 12% vs. 12%, respectively. However, there was a significant increase in the risk for bronchopulmonary dysplasia after exposure to indomethacin (adjusted odds ratio 4.9, 95% confidence interval 1.01–23.44) (20).

A 2003 review concluded that COX-2 selective drugs, such as sulindac, should only be used as tocolytics in randomized controlled trials (2). This conclusion was based on the uncertainty over whether the fetal toxicity observed with sulindac resulted from COX-2-dependent effects, or from fetal accumulation of drug levels sufficient to cause COX-1 inhibition (2).

Theoretically, sulindac, a prostaglandin synthesis inhibitor, could cause constriction of the ductus arteriosus *in utero*, as well as inhibition of labor, prolongation of pregnancy, and suppression of fetal renal function (21,22). Persistent pulmonary hypertension of the newborn should also be considered (23). Women attempting to conceive should not use any prostaglandin synthesis inhibitor, including sulindac, because of the findings in a variety of animal models that indicate these agents block blastocyst implantation (24,25). Moreover, as noted above, NSAIDs have been associated with SABs and congenital malformations.

[**Risk Factor D if used in the 3rd trimester or near delivery.*]

BREAST FEEDING SUMMARY

RECOMMENDATION: No Human Data - Potential Toxicity

No reports describing the use of sulindac during lactation have been located. The mean adult serum half-life of the biologically active sulfide metabolite is 16.4 hours (1). One reviewer concluded that because of the prolonged half-life, other agents in this class (diclofenac, fenoprofen, flurbiprofen, ibuprofen, ketoprofen, ketorolac, and tolmetin) were safer alternatives if a NSAID was required during nursing (26).

References

1. Product information. Clinoril. Merck, 2001.
2. Loudon JAZ, Groom KM, Bennett PR. Prostaglandin inhibitors in preterm labour. Best Pract Res Clin Obstet Gynaecol 2003;17:731–44.
3. Lione A, Scialli AR. The developmental toxicity of indomethacin and sulindac. Reprod Toxicol 1995;9:7–20.
4. Kramer W, Saade G, Belfort M, Ou C-N, Rognerud C, Knudsen L, Moise K Jr. Placental transfer of sulindac and its active metabolite in humans (abstract). Am J Obstet Gynecol 1994;170:389.
5. Kramer WB, Saade G, Ou C-N, Rognerud C, Dorman K, Mayes M, Moise KJ Jr. Placental transfer of sulindac and its active sulfide metabolite in humans. Am J Obstet Gynecol 1995;172:886–90.
6. Lampela ES, Nuutinen LH, Ala-Kkokko TL, Parikka RM, Laitinen RS, Jouppila PI, Vahakangas KH. Placental transfer of sulindac, sulindac sulfide, and indomethacin in a human placental perfusion model. Am J Obstet Gynecol 1999;180:174–80.
7. Nielsen GL, Sorensen HT, Larsen H, Pedersen L. Risk of adverse birth outcome and miscarriage in pregnant users of non-steroidal anti-inflammatory drugs: population based observational study and case-control study. BMJ 2001;322:266–70.
8. Ericson A, Kallen BAJ. Nonsteroidal anti-inflammatory drugs in early pregnancy. Reprod Toxicol 2001;15:371–5.
9. Li DK, Liu L, Odouli R. Exposure to non-steroidal anti-inflammatory drugs during pregnancy and risk of miscarriage: population based cohort study. BMJ 2003;327:368–71.
10. Tassinari MS, Cook JC, Hurtt ME. NSAIDs and developmental toxicity. Birth Defects Res Part B Dev Reprod Toxicol 2003;68:3–4.
11. Carlan SJ, O'Brien WF, O'Leary TD, Mastrogiannis DS. A randomized comparative trial of indomethacin and sulindac for the treatment of refractory preterm labor (abstract). Am J Obstet Gynecol 1992;166:361.
12. Carlan SJ, O'Brien WF, O'Leary TD, Mastrogiannis D. Randomized comparative trial of indomethacin and sulindac for the treatment of refractory preterm labor. Obstet Gynecol 1992;79:223–8.
13. Rasanen J, Jouppila P. Fetal cardiac function and ductus arteriosus during indomethacin and sulindac therapy for threatened preterm labor: a randomized study. Am J Obstet Gynecol 1995;173:20–5.
14. Kramer W, Saade G, Belfort M, Dorman K, Mayes M, Moise K Jr. Randomized double-blind study comparing sulindac to terbutaline: fetal cardiovascular effects (abstract). Am J Obstet Gynecol 1996;174:326.
15. Kramer WB, Saade GR, Belfort M, Dorman K, Mayes M, Moise KJ Jr. A randomized double-blind study comparing the fetal effects of sulindac to terbutaline during the management of preterm labor. Am J Obstet Gynecol 1999;180:396–401.
16. Carlan S, Jones M, Schorr S, McNeill T, Rawji H, Clark K. Oral sulindac to prevent recurrence of preterm labor (abstract). Am J Obstet Gynecol 1994;170:381.
17. Jones M, Carlan S, Schorr S, McNeill T, Rawji R, Clark K, Fuentes A. Oral sulindac to prevent recurrence of preterm labor (abstract). Am J Obstet Gynecol 1995;172:416.
18. Carlan SJ, O'Brien WF, Jones MH, O'Leary TD, Roth L. Outpatient oral sulindac to prevent recurrence of preterm labor. Obstet Gynecol 1995;85:769–74.
19. Peek MJ, McCarthy A, Kyle P, Sepulveda W, Fisk NM. Medical amnioreduction with sulindac to reduce cord complications in monoamniotic twins. Am J Obstet Gynecol 1997;176:334–6.
20. Sciscione A, Leef K, Vakili B, Paul D. Neonatal effects after antenatal treatment with indomethacin vs. sulindac (abstract). Am J Obstet Gynecol 2000;182:S66.
21. Levin DL. Effects of inhibition of prostaglandin synthesis on fetal development, oxygenation, and the fetal circulation. Semin Perinatol 1980;4:35–44.
22. Fuchs F. Prevention of prematurity. Am J Obstet Gynecol 1976;126:809–20.
23. Van Marter LJ, Leviton A, Allred EN, Pagano M,

S

Sullivan KF, Cohen A, Epstein MF. Persistent pulmonary hypertension of the newborn and smoking and aspirin and nonsteroidal antiinflammatory drug consumption during pregnancy. Pediatrics 1996;97:658–63.

24. Matt DW, Borzelleca JF. Toxic effects on the female reproductive system during pregnancy, parturition, and lactation. In Witorsch RJ, editor. *Reproductive Toxicology*. 2nd ed. New York, NY: Raven Press, 1995: 175–93.
25. Dawood MY. Nonsteroidal antiinflammatory drugs and reproduction. Am J Obstet Gynecol 1993;169:1255–65.
26. Anderson PO. Medication use while breast-feeding a neonate. Neonatal Pharmacol Q 1993;2:3–14.

Name: **SUMATRIPTAN** Risk Factor: **C_M**

Class: **Antimigraine**

FETAL RISK SUMMARY

RECOMMENDATION: Limited Human Data - Animal Data Suggest Moderate Risk

Sumatriptan (GR 43175) is a selective serotonin (5-hydroxytryptamine$_1$; 5-HT) receptor subtype agonist used for the acute treatment of migraine headaches. It has also been used for the treatment of cluster headaches. The compound is available in oral tablets and as a subcutaneous (SC) injection.

Sumatriptan was embryolethal in rabbits when given in daily IV doses approximately equivalent to the maximum recommended single human SC dose of 6 mg on a body surface area basis (MRHD) (1). The doses were at or close to those producing maternal toxicity. Fetuses of rabbits administered oral sumatriptan (at doses greater than 50 times the MRHD) during organogenesis had an increased incidence of cervicothoracic vascular and skeletal anomalies (1). In contrast, embryo or fetal lethality was not observed in pregnant rats treated throughout organogenesis with IV doses approximately 20 times the MRHD. Moreover, no rat embryo/fetal lethality or teratogenicity was observed with daily SC doses before and throughout gestation (1). Shepard described a study in which no fetal adverse effects were observed in rats given up to 1000 mg/kg orally during organogenesis (2).

No studies examining the placental transfer of sumatriptan in animals or humans have been located. The molecular weight of the drug (about 414) is low enough, however, to allow passage to the fetus.

Individual reports and data from Medicaid studies totaled 14 spontaneous abortions with the use of sumatriptan during early pregnancy (F. Rosa, personal communication, FDA, 1996). Seven birth defect case reports received by the FDA included two chromosomal anomalies (both of which could have been exposed before conception), one infant with an ear tag, one case of a phocomelia, a reduction defect of the lower limbs (tibial aplasia), a case of developmental retardation, and one unspecified defect (some of these defects appear to be also included in data from the Pregnancy Registry cited below).

In an interim report of the Sumatriptan Pregnancy Registry, covering the period of January 1, 1996, through April 30, 2004, the outcomes of 414 prospectively enrolled pregnancies (420 outcomes; 4 sets of twins and 1 set of triplets) exposed to sumatriptan were described (3). Some of the data were also reported in a 1997 abstract (4). There were 366 outcomes with earliest exposure in the 1st trimester, 41 with earliest exposure in the 2nd trimester, 9 in the 3rd trimester, and 4 were exposed at an unspecified time. In the 1st trimester group with no birth defects reported, there were 27 spontaneous abortions (<20 weeks' gestation), 11 elective abortions, 4 stillbirths ((20 weeks' gestation), and

S

310 live-born infants. All of the outcomes in the other three groups with no birth defects reported involved live births. From the four exposure groups, 17 infants had birth defects: 14 after earliest exposure in the 1st trimester, 2 with earliest exposure in the 2nd trimester, and 1 (elective abortion) with an unspecified earliest exposure time (details of the malformations are shown below).

Prospective Reports
Earliest exposure 1st trimester:
Hypertrophic pyloric stenosis
Stillbirth at 23 weeks, left hand anomaly (one digit missing and concretion and shortening of two others)
Odd cry, low ears, abnormal head circumference, single palmar crease, and soft systolic murmur
Cerebral abnormality with developmental delay
Diaphragmatic hernia at 18 months of age
Ventricular septal defect (VSD)—4 cases; one with small defect expected to close spontaneously
Anterior displacement of the anus
Polydactyly
Down's syndrome (induced abortion)—2 cases
Partial small cleft lip
Earliest exposure 2nd trimester:
Congenital hypothyroidism
Down's syndrome
Earliest exposure unknown:
Down's syndrome (induced abortion)

Although retrospective reports (reported after the pregnancy outcome was known) are often biased (only adverse outcomes are reported), there were 24 cases of birth defects reported to the Registry, 21 involving 1st trimester exposure to sumatriptan (3). Review of all birth defects from prospective and retrospective reports showed no signal or consistent pattern to suggest a common etiology (3).

A 1998 report (first published in 1997 as an abstract [5]) described the prospectively determined pregnancy outcomes of 96 women exposed to sumatriptan (95 exposed during 1st trimester) (6). No difference in the rate of major birth defects was found between the study patients and non-teratogen-exposed controls or disease-matched controls. One major birth defect was reported in a sumatriptan-exposed infant: vesicoureteral reflux requiring bilateral re-implant (6).

A 1998 non-interventional observational cohort study described the outcomes of pregnancies in women who had been prescribed one or more of 34 newly marketed drugs by general practitioners in England (7). Data were obtained by questionnaires sent to the prescribing physicians one month after the expected or possible date of delivery. In 831 (78%) of the pregnancies, a newly marketed drug was thought to have been taken during the 1st trimester with birth defects noted in 14 (2.5%) singleton births of the 557 newborns (10 sets of twins). In addition, two birth defects were observed in aborted fetuses. However, few of the aborted fetuses were examined. Sumatriptan was taken during the 1st trimester in 35 pregnancies. The outcomes of these pregnancies included 4 spontaneous abortions, 3 elective abortions, 5 pregnancies lost to follow-up, and 23 normal infants (2 premature) (7).

A 2004 case report described a 24-year-old woman who took sumatriptan (100 mg about once a week), naproxen (550 mg about twice a week), and bisoprolol (5 mg/day) for migraine headaches during the first 5 weeks of pregnancy (8). An elective cesarean section was performed at 37 weeks' for breech presentation to deliver a 3125-g male infant. The infant had a wide bilateral cleft lip/palate, marked hypertelorism, a broad nose, and bilateral but asymmetric toe abnormalities (missing and hypoplastic phalanges) (8).

In an *in vitro* study, only high concentrations of sumatriptan were capable of increasing uterine contractions (9). The findings suggested that therapeutic concentrations of the drug would not induce preterm labor.

In summary, although sumatriptan caused toxicity and malformations in one animal species, the drug does not appear to present a major teratogenic risk in humans. Moreover, except for the four cases of VSD, there was no consistent pattern among the reported birth defects to suggest a common cause. The above studies, however, lack the sensitivity to identify minor anomalies because of the absence of standardized examinations. In one study, late-appearing major defects may also have been missed as a consequence of the timing of the questionnaires. Thus, although the data are generally reassuring, the number and follow-up of exposed pregnancies are still too limited to assess, with confidence, the safety of the agent or its teratogenic potential.

Required statement: *Sumatriptan:* The number of exposed pregnancy outcomes accumulated to date represents a sample of insufficient size for reaching definitive conclusions regarding the possible teratogenic risk of sumatriptan. Specifically, the sample size to date remains too small for formal comparisons of the frequency of specific birth defects. If the baseline frequency of total birth defects is 3 in 100 live births, a sample size of 324 for first trimester exposure has an 80 percent chance (80% power) of correctly detecting at least a 1.9-fold increase from baseline in the frequency of birth defects. If the baseline frequency of specific birth defects is 1 in 1000 live births, a sample size of 324 for first trimester exposure has an 80 percent (80% power) of correctly detecting at least an 8.1-fold increase from baseline in the frequency of a specific birth defect.

Naratriptan: The data represent a sample of insufficient size for reaching definitive conclusions regarding the possible teratogenic risk of naratriptan. If the baseline frequency of total birth defects is 3 in 100 live births, a sample size of 31 for the first trimester exposure has an 80 percent chance (80% power) of correctly detecting at least a 4.6-fold increase from baseline in the frequency of total birth defects. If the baseline frequency for a specific birth defect is 1 in 1000 live births, a sample size of 31 for first trimester exposure has an 80 percent chance (80% power) of correctly detecting at least a 40.9-fold increase from baseline in the frequency of a specific birth defect.

The number of exposed pregnancy outcomes accumulated to date represents a sample of insufficient size for reaching definitive conclusions regarding the possible teratogenic risk of sumatriptan or naratriptan. It is expected that a teratogenic exposure in the first trimester would result in an increased frequency of one or a combination of individual defects or types of defects, but not necessarily in all defects.

As reporting of pregnancies to the Sumatriptan and Naratriptan Registry is voluntary, it is possible that even in prospectively reported pregnancies there could be bias in type of pregnancies reported. For example, differential reporting of low-risk or high-risk pregnancies may be a potential limitation to this type of registry. In addition, reporting of defects from maternal health care providers may limit detection of detects not immediately apparent at birth. Despite this, the Registry is intended both to supplement animal toxicology studies and other structured epidemiologic studies and clinical trial data, and to assist clinicians in weighing the risks and benefits of treatment for individual patients and circumstances.

BREAST FEEDING SUMMARY

RECOMMENDATION: Limited Human Data - Probably Compatible

Sumatriptan is excreted in the milk of experimental animals (1) and humans. Five women with a mean duration of lactation of 22.2 weeks (range 10.8–28.4 weeks) were administered a 6-mg SC dose of sumatriptan (10). Milk samples were obtained hourly for 8 hours by emptying both breasts of each subject with a breast pump. Frequent blood samples were also obtained from the women. The mean milk:plasma ratio was 4.9. The mean cumulative excretion of drug in milk during the 8-hour sampling period was 12.6 μg and, by extrapolation, a total recovery of only 14.4 μg after a 6-mg dose. Using this latter value, the authors estimated that the mean weight-adjusted dose (i.e., μg sumatriptan/kg of infant body weight as a percentage of the mother's dose in μg/kg) for the infants would have been 3.5% (10). The investigators considered the risk to a nursing infant from this exposure to be not significant.

In adults, the mean oral bioavailability of sumatriptan is 14%–15% (range 10%–26%) (1,11), indicating that absorption from the gastrointestinal tract is inhibited. Thus, although the oral absorption in infants may be markedly different from adults, the amount of sumatriptan reaching the systemic circulation of a breast-feeding infant is probably negligible. Discarding the milk for 8 hours after a dose, an interval during which about 88% of the amount excreted into milk can be recovered, would reduce even more the small amounts present in milk. The American Academy of Pediatrics classifies sumatriptan as compatible with breast-feeding (12).

References

1. Product information. Imitrex. Glaxo Wellcome, 1998.
2. Shepard TH. *Catalog of Teratogenic Agents*. 8th ed. Baltimore, MD: Johns Hopkins University Press, 1995:397.
3. The Sumatriptan and Naratriptan Pregnancy Registry. Interim Report. 1 January 1996 through 30 April 2004. Glaxo Wellcome, July 2004.
4. Eldridge RE, Ephross SA. Monitoring birth outcomes in the sumatriptan pregnancy registry (abstract). Teratology 1997;55:48.
5. Shuhaiber S, Pastuszak A, Schick B, Koren G. Pregnancy outcome following gestational exposure to sumatriptan (Imitrex) (abstract). Teratology 1997;55:103.
6. Shuhaiber S, Pastuszak A, Schick B, Matsui D, Spivey G, Brochu J, Koren G. Pregnancy outcome following first trimester exposure to sumatriptan. Neurology 1998;51:581–3.
7. Wilton LV, Pearce GL, Martin RM, Mackay FJ, Mann RD. The outcomes of pregnancy in women exposed to newly marketed drugs in general practice in England. Br J Obstet Gynaecol 1998;105:882–9.
8. Kajantie E, Somer M. Bilateral cleft lip and palate, hypertelorism and hypoplastic toes. Clin Dysmorphol 2004;13:195–6.
9. Gei A, Longo M, Vedernikov Y, Saade G, Garfield R. The effect of sumatriptan on the uterine contractility of human myometrium (abstract). Am J Obstet Gynecol 2001;184:S193.
10. Wojnar-Horton RE, Hackett LP, Yapp P, Dusci LJ, Paech M, Ilett KF. Distribution and excretion of sumatriptan in human milk. Br J Clin Pharmacol 1996;41: 217–21.
11. Fullerton T, Gengo FM. Sumatriptan: a selective 5-hydroxytryptamine receptor agonist for the acute treatment of migraine. Ann Pharmacother 1992;26:800–8.
12. Committee on Drugs, American Academy of Pediatrics. The transfer of drugs and other chemicals into human milk. Pediatrics 2001;108:776–89.

T

Name:	**TACROLIMUS**	Risk Factor:	C_M
Class:	**Immunologic Agent (Immunosuppressant)**		

FETAL RISK SUMMARY

RECOMMENDATION: Human and Animal Data Suggest Risk

Tacrolimus (FK506) is a macrolide immunosuppressant agent produced by *Streptomyces tsukubaensis* that acts similarly to cyclosporine but is a more potent immunosuppressant (1). It is used for the prophylaxis of organ rejection in patients receiving various allogeneic organ transplants, such as kidney, liver, heart, and pancreas.

Reproduction studies have been reported in rats, rabbits, and mice (2,3). In pregnant rabbits, tacrolimus given in oral doses about 0.5–1 and 1.6–3.3 times the recommended human dose based on body surface area (RHD) during organogenesis was associated with maternal toxicity and an increased incidence of abortions (2). At the higher dose, an increased incidence of malformations and developmental variations was also observed (type of defects was not specified). Pregnant rats dosed at 2.3–4.6 times the RHD exhibited maternal toxicity and an increase in late resorptions, decreased numbers of live births, and decreased pup weight and viability (2). Oral doses 0.7–1.4 and 2.3–4.6 times the RHD given after organogenesis and during lactation were associated with reduced pup weight (2).

Mice were treated with IM tacrolimus, 0.17 mg/kg/day or 1.37 mg/kg/day (relationship to human dose not specified), from day 1 through day 16 of gestation (3). No effects on maternal weight gain were observed in the low-dose group, but the number of resorptions was significantly increased over the number observed in controls. In contrast, none of the 13 pregnancies treated with high-dose tacrolimus was carried to term, and maternal weight gain was significantly less than that of controls. Except for the embryocidal action, low-dose tacrolimus, compared with untreated and saline controls, had no effect on mean placental or fetal weight and was not associated with an increase in malformations (3).

The molecular weight of tacrolimus (about 804 for the nonhydrated form) is low enough that the drug crosses the human placenta (2,4–6). In 12 pregnant women with liver transplants who were treated with tacrolimus (mean dose in 11 patients was about 10 mg/day; 1 patient treated with 48–64 mg/day), the mean cord:maternal plasma ratio of tacrolimus was 0.49 (median 0.36) (4). The placentas contained higher drug amounts (mean 4.30 ng/g) than that measured in maternal plasma (about 4 times) or cord plasma (2–56 times) and were thought to indicate a partial placental barrier to passage of the drug (4). A cord:maternal plasma ratio of 0.49 was also reported in another case (see below) (5). In two pregnancies (described below) under tacrolimus immunosuppression, the mothers were taking 15 mg/day and 10 mg/day, respectively (6). At delivery, umbilical cord blood concentrations were 13.2 ng/mL and 5.9 ng/mL, respectively, whereas the maternal venous blood concentrations were 11.8 and 31.2 ng/mL, respectively. The cord:maternal blood ratios were 1.12 and 0.19, respectively.

A number of reports have described the use of tacrolimus during human pregnancy. A 1993 letter reported a case of a woman with a liver transplant who was receiving tacrolimus (0.1 mg/kg/day with a target plasma level of <1.0 ng/mL) and who conceived about a year after her second transplant (5). At 28 weeks' gestation, a threatened acute graft rejection (tacrolimus plasma level <0.05 ng/mL) was successfully treated with bolus corticosteroids and an increase in the tacrolimus dose to 0.15 mg/kg/day. She delivered a healthy, 2860-g male infant at 36 weeks' gestation that was doing well at 12 months of age. The tacrolimus cord blood and maternal plasma concentrations at birth were 0.24 and 0.49 ng/mL, respectively, a ratio of 0.49 (5).

A woman who had received a combined kidney and pancreaticoduodenal graft conceived while receiving tacrolimus (12 mg/day) and prednisolone (7.5 mg/day) (6). She also received furosemide and methyldopa for hypertension that was well controlled throughout gestation. Her pregnancy was complicated by hyperemesis gravidarum, septicemia (*Escherichia coli*) and endocarditis, and esophagitis. At 38 weeks' gestation, she delivered a normal, 3410-g female infant with Apgar scores of 9 and 9 at 1 and 5 minutes, respectively. At delivery, the tacrolimus cord:maternal blood ratio was 1.12. In a second case, a woman conceived approximately 22 months after her second renal transplant. She received tacrolimus (10 mg/day), azathioprine (75 mg/day), and prednisolone (5 mg/day) for immunosuppression. Nifedipine and methyldopa were used to control her hypertension. Because of a possible placental abruption at 36 weeks' gestation, a normal, 2400-g female infant was delivered by cesarean section. Her Apgar scores were 9 and 9 at 1 and 5 minutes, respectively. The tacrolimus cord:maternal blood ratio was 0.19. Both of the above infants were doing well at 3 months of age (6).

In a 1993 letter, the pregnancy outcomes of nine liver transplant patients who had received tacrolimus (2–64 mg/day) immunosuppression throughout their gestation were detailed (7). Five of the women had also received corticosteroid therapy during pregnancy. None of the newborns was small for gestational age. Complications observed in the newborns included hyperkalemia in five (range 6.1–10.9 mEq/L; potassium levels measured in 7 of the 9 newborns), hypoxia in one who tested positive for cocaine (mother was taking cocaine), and anuria for 36 hours in one (thought to be secondary to high tacrolimus concentrations in the cord blood caused by the mother's renal impairment) who regained normal renal function in 1 week; death after delivery occurred in one at 22 weeks' gestation. In this latter case, the mother had conceived 1 month after transplantation and had cytomegalovirus in her blood and gastrointestinal tract that was being treated with ganciclovir. Of the eight surviving infants, all were alive and developing normally (7).

Some of the cases described in reference #7 above may have been included in a 1997 abstract that reported the outcomes of 14 pregnancies in 13 liver transplant patients receiving various immunosuppressant agents, including tacrolimus (8). Although the agent used in each of the pregnancies was not specified, the complications included maternal renal insufficiency ($N = 8$), early hypertension ($N = 5$), preeclampsia ($N = 4$), worsening hypertension ($N = 2$), pyelonephritis ($N = 2$), anemia ($N = 4$), prolonged premature rupture of the membranes ($N = 3$), and cytomegalovirus infection ($N = 3$). The mean gestational age at delivery was 32.6 weeks, and the mean birth weight was 1913 g. Three newborns died; all three deaths were associated with cytomegalovirus infection and prematurity. No structural birth defects were mentioned (8).

A third report, from the same medical center as references #7 and #8, was published in 1997 and detailed the outcomes of 27 pregnancies of 21 liver recipients who were treated with tacrolimus before and throughout gestation between October 1990 and April 1996 (4). The mean gestational age at delivery was 36.6 weeks, and the mean birth weight was 2638 g (50.2 percentile). Two infants died from prematurity after delivery at 23 and 24 weeks, respectively. The mean follow-up time of the infants was 39 months, and their mean growth weight percentile was 62. Unilateral nonfunctional cystic renal disease in one newborn was the only congenital anomaly observed in this series. In addition to the retarded growth and premature births in the total series, two other transient complications, noted among the first 13 infants born, were hyperkalemia in 10 and renal impairment in 7. Both adverse effects were thought to be caused by the drug (4).

Successful immunosuppression with tacrolimus following heart transplantation had been maintained for 2 years before conception occurred in a 39-year-old woman (9). She also took prophylactic trimethoprim-sulfamethoxazole before and throughout gestation, and her chronic hypertension was controlled with a long-acting calcium channel blocker (name not specified). Preeclampsia (rising blood pressure, proteinuria, and worsening renal impairment) was manifested between 26 and 31 weeks' gestation. An apparently normal, 2093-g female infant, who had Apgar scores of 9 and 9 at 1 and 5 minutes, respectively, was delivered by repeat cesarean section at 33 weeks. The newborn required, most likely because of prematurity, transient oxygen therapy, theophylline for apnea, and phototherapy for hyperbilirubinemia (9).

A 26-year-old renal transplant patient was treated with tacrolimus (10 mg/day) and prednisolone (10 mg/day) throughout a 33.5-week pregnancy (10). Conception had occurred about 25 months after transplantation. The target blood concentration was 10 ng/mL. Symmetrical intrauterine growth retardation (IUGR) was discovered after 20 weeks' gestation. Because of spontaneous rupture of the membranes and breech presentation, a 1312-g female infant was delivered by cesarean section. A physical and ultrasonic examination found no congenital malformations. Complications other than IUGR noted in the newborn, included mild hyperkalemia and a prolonged course of hyperbilirubinemia. Although not stated, the latter complication may have been secondary to prematurity.

A 1998 case report described the course and outcome of a pregnancy in a 32-year-old woman 17 months after renal transplantation for focal sclerosing glomerulonephritis (11). Tacrolimus, with a target plasma level of 5.0–11.5 ng/mL, was used alone throughout gestation after discontinuance of prednisolone (5 mg/day) early in gestation. Hypertension developed in the 22nd week of gestation and was treated with isradipine. A cesarean section was performed at 31 weeks' gestation because of severe hypertension, a progressive decline in graft function, and an abnormal Doppler assessment of blood velocity in the umbilical artery. No congenital malformations were noted in the 1140-g (3rd percentile) male infant who had Apgar scores of 8, 9, and 9 at 1, 5, and 10 minutes, respectively. The tacrolimus concentration in the umbilical vein was 8.1 ng/mL (maternal level at the time of delivery was not reported). At 2 days of age, the plasma drug level had decreased to 6.4 ng/mL, and at 8 days, the level was <5.0 ng/mL. Complications in the infant included mild hyperkalemia (6.4 mmol/L) on the 2nd day and transient renal impairment (serum creatinine 3.0 mg/dL at birth) that resolved completely over the next few weeks. A renal ultrasound examination was normal. Respiratory distress syndrome and a patent ductus arteriosus were successfully treated, and at a corrected age of 4 months, the healthy infant was developing normally (11).

A 1998 study examined the relationship between antenatal complications and various maternal factors in women who had undergone orthotopic liver transplantation (12). Of the 14 pregnancies studied, tacrolimus had been used in 5 (combined with prednisone in 3; with azathioprine and prednisone in 1), cyclosporine in 8 (combined with prednisone in 6; with azathioprine and prednisone in 2), and prednisone only in 1. Three of the complications—preeclampsia, worsening hypertension, and small for gestational age—occurred only in women with renal dysfunction (creatinine $\geq$1.3 mg/dL) at conception. Cyclosporine was more commonly associated ($p = 0.03$) with renal dysfunction than was tacrolimus (12).

A review of pregnancy outcomes after renal transplant was published in 1998 (13). The liveborn incidence among seven cases treated with tacrolimus was 71%.

In a 1999 case report, a woman with a history of renal transplant was treated throughout gestation with tacrolimus (10–12 mg/day), prednisone, amlodipine, and labetalol (14). Azathioprine was also used during the first 10 weeks. Her pregnancy was complicated by worsening renal function, but her hypertension was controlled until shortly before delivery. At 32 weeks' gestation, she delivered twin male infants who developed severe respiratory distress syndrome and congestive heart failure. Echocardiograms showed dilated heart chambers in both infants and only twin B survived. Autopsy of twin A revealed thrombotic cardiomyopathy with degeneration of cardiac muscle. Because animal studies had shown that tacrolimus could cause vasculitis in the cardiac muscle of baboons and dogs, the authors concluded that the cardiomyopathy seen in the twins might have been caused by tacrolimus (14).

Two case reports, one in 2001 and the other in 2004, detailed the use of tacrolimus and mycophenolate during pregnancies that involved adverse outcomes (see Mycophenolate).

A 2003 retrospective review detailed the outcomes of 38 pregnancies in 29 women who had undergone liver transplantation before pregnancy (15). Sixteen pregnancies (nine live births, seven elective abortions) had been exposed to tacrolimus combined with other agents. There were no fetal or neonatal deaths. Two tacrolimus-exposed infants had small membranous ventricular septal defects (15).

The pregnancies of 38 renal allograft recipients were reported in a 2003 study (16). Four of the patients were treated with tacrolimus (three combined with prednisone and one with prednisone and azathioprine). The outcomes of 73 pregnancies (48 live births) in the group were compared to 59 pregnancies (41 women; 48 live births) with primary renal disease not treated with immunosuppressive drugs. The study group had significantly more preterm deliveries, infants with intrauterine growth retardation, and infants requiring hospitalization in neonatal intensive care units. However, there was no difference in the incidence of either major (4.2% vs. 4.2%) or minor malformations (20.8% vs. 16.6%) (16).

In summary, tacrolimus has demonstrated abortifacient properties in three animal species and dose-related teratogenicity in one, but the use of this agent during human pregnancy has not been associated with either of these outcomes, although the number of exposed fetuses is small. Common complications in infants, however, are hyperkalemia, that usually resolves untreated within 24–48 hours, renal toxicity, IUGR, and premature delivery (because of hypertension, preeclampsia, and premature rupture of membranes). A causal association between tacrolimus and cardiomyopathy has not been established. No other reports of this adverse effect in relation to *in utero* tacrolimus exposure have been located. Based on one report, renal dysfunction is more common with cyclosporine than it is with tacrolimus. Moreover, IUGR and premature delivery are associated with the use of all immunosuppressant agents in pregnant transplant patients. Because of the risk of cytomegalovirus infection in the mother and fetus, two reviews advised waiting at least 6 months before conception is attempted following transplantation and during periods of rejection when high doses of immunosuppressant agents may be used (i.e., the periods when infection with the virus is most likely) (17,18).

BREAST FEEDING SUMMARY

RECOMMENDATION: Limited Human Data - Potential Toxicity

Tacrolimus is excreted into breast milk (4). Ten colostrum samples were obtained from six women in the immediate postpartum period (0–3 days) with a mean drug concentration of 0.79 ng/mL (range 0.3–1.9 ng/mL). The median milk:maternal plasma ratio was 0.5. The authors of this study did not mention if the women breast-fed their infants. Because the potential for adverse effects in a nursing infant from exposure to tacrolimus in milk are unknown, breast-feeding should be avoided if the mother requires immunosuppressant therapy with tacrolimus.

References

1. Peters DH, Fitton A, Plosker GL, Faulds D. Tacrolimus. A review of its pharmacology, and therapeutic potential in hepatic and renal transplantation. Drugs 1993;46:746 94.
2. Product information. Prograf. Fujisawa USA, 2000.
3. Farley DE, Shelby J, Alexander D, Scott JR. The effect of two new immunosuppressive agents, FK506 and didemnin B, in murine pregnancy. Transplantation 1991;52:106–10.
4. Jain A, Venkataramanan R, Fung JJ, Gartner JC, Lever J, Balan V, Warty V, Starzl TE. Pregnancy after liver transplantation under tacrolimus. Transplantation 1997;64:559–65.
5. Winkler ME, Niesert S, Ringe B, Pichlmayr R. Successful pregnancy in a patient after liver transplantation maintained on FK 506. Transplantation 1993;56:751–3.
6. Midtvedt K, Hartmann A, Brekke IB, Lyngdal PT, Bentdal O, Haugen G. Successful pregnancies in a combined pancreas and renal allograft recipient and in a renal graft recipient on tacrolimus treatment. Nephrol Dial Transplant 1997;12:2764–5.
7. Jain A, Venkataramanan R, Lever J, Warty V, Fung J, Todo S, Starzl T. FK506 and pregnancy in liver transplant patients. Transplantation 1993;56:751.
8. Casele H, Woelkers D, Laifer S. Pregnancy outcome after liver transplantation (abstract). Am J Obstet Gynecol 1997;176:S23.
9. Laifer SA, Yeagley CJ, Armitage JM. Pregnancy after cardiac transplantation. Am J Perinatol 1994;11: 217–9.
10. Yoshimura N, Oka T, Fujiwara Y, Ohmori Y, Yasumura T, Honjo H. A case report of pregnancy in a renal transplant recipient treated with FK506 (tacrolimus). Transplantation 1996;61:1552–3.
11. Resch B, Mache CJ, Windhager T, Holzer H, Leitner G, Muller W. FK 506 and successful pregnancy in a patient after renal transplantation. Transplant Proc 1998;30:163 4.
12. Casele HL, Laifer SA. Association of pregnancy complications and choice of immunosuppressant in liver transplant patients. Transplantation 1998;65:581–3.
13. Armenti VT, McGrory CH, Carter JR, Radomski JS, Moritz MJ. Pregnancy outcomes in female renal transplant recipients. Transplant Proc 1998;30:1732–4.
14. Vyas S, Kumar A, Piecuch S, Hidalgo G, Singh A, Anderson V, Markell MS, Baqi N. Outcome of twin pregnancy in a renal transplant recipient treated with tacrolimus. Transplantation 1999;67:490–2.
15. Nagy S, Bush MC, Berkowitz R, Fishbein TM, Gomez-Lobo V. Pregnancy outcome in liver transplant recipients. Obstet Gynecol 2003;102:121–8.
16. Bar J, Stahl B, Hod M, Wittenberg C, Pardo J, Merlob P. Is immunosuppression therapy in renal allograft recipients teratogenic? A single-center experience. Am J Med Genet 2003;116A:31–6.
17. Laifer SA, Guido RS. Reproductive function and outcome of pregnancy after liver transplantation in women. Mayo Clin Proc 1995;70:388–94.
18. Casele HL, Laifer SA. Pregnancy after liver transplantation. Semin Perinatol 1998;22:149–55.

Name: **TAMOXIFEN** Risk Factor: **D_M**
Class: **Antineoplastic/Antiestrogen**

FETAL RISK SUMMARY

RECOMMENDATION: Contraindicated

Tamoxifen, a triphenylethylene derivative that is structurally related to clomiphene, is a nonsteroidal, antiestrogen agent used in the treatment of breast cancer (1,2). In addition to its antiestrogen properties, it may also produce weak estrogenic and estrogenic-like activity at some sites. Unlabeled uses have included induction of ovulation and treatment of idiopathic oligospermia. Tamoxifen is thought to act by competing with estrogen for binding sites in target tissues (2). The parent drug has an elimination half-life of about 5–7 days (range 3–21 days) (1,2), whereas the elimination half-life of the major metabolite, *N*-desmethyltamoxifen, is approximately 9–14 days (1). Following prolonged treatment (e.g., 2 to 3 months), clearance of tamoxifen and its metabolites from the system may require 6–8 weeks (3).

Tamoxifen is carcinogenic, producing ovarian and testicular tumors in immature and mature mice and hepatocellular carcinoma in rats, at all doses tested (5, 20, and 35 mg/kg/day for up to 2 years) (2). The drug is also genotoxic in rat liver cells and in the human lymphoblastoid cell line. Tamoxifen, at a dose of 0.04 mg/kg/day (approximately 1/10th the human dose based on body weight) for 2 weeks before conception through day 7 of pregnancy, impaired the fertility of female rats causing a decreased number of implantations and 100% fetal mortality (2).

In reproductive studies reported by the manufacturer, no teratogenicity was observed with rats, rabbits, and marmosets, but fetal toxicity was common (2). In rats, however, reversible, nonteratogenic developmental skeletal changes were observed at doses equal to or below the human dose (2). An increased fetal death rate occurred in pregnant rats when tamoxifen, 0.16 mg/kg/day (human dose about 0.4–0.8 mg/kg/day), was administered from days 7 to 17 (2). When this dose was given from day 17 of pregnancy to 1 day before weaning, an increased number of dead pups were noted and some of the surviving pups demonstrated slower learning behavior. Moreover, *in utero* growth retardation was evident in some of the pups (2). Tamoxifen, 0.125 mg/kg/day administered to pregnant rabbits during days 6 through 18 of pregnancy, caused abortions and premature delivery (2). Higher doses produced fetal deaths. Abortions were observed in pregnant marmosets given 10 mg/kg/day either during organogenesis or in the last half of pregnancy (2).

A 1976 study administered oral tamoxifen, 2 mg/kg/day, to rabbits starting at either day 10 or day 20 of pregnancy (4). A significant increase in embryonic loss occurred in the first group, whereas treatment later in gestation resulted in premature delivery or abortion.

Several studies have described the effectiveness of tamoxifen as a post-coital contraceptive in animals (5–11). The action of tamoxifen as an antifertility agent appears to be a dose-related antiestrogen effect that prevents implantation in the uterus. In one report, however, a single, 5-mg/kg dose on day 4 after ovulation in macaques had no effect on fertility (12). No reports describing the use of tamoxifen as a contraceptive in humans have been located.

In rats and guinea pigs, tamoxifen produced significant, dose-related changes in the reproductive tract of the fetus and newborn (13–17). These changes, most pronounced in the guinea pig, involved trophic effects on the uterus and vagina similar to those produced by estrogens. Abnormalities in sexual differentiation of female offspring of guinea pigs have also been observed (18).

In a study published in 1987, the estrogenicity and potential teratogenicity of tamoxifen were demonstrated in genital tracts isolated from aborted 4- to 19-week-old human female fetuses grown for 1–2 months in mice (19). Some mice were used as controls, and others were treated with tamoxifen, clomiphene, or diethylstilbestrol (DES). In comparison with controls, abnormalities observed in the drug-treated mice included proliferation and maturation of the squamous vaginal epithelium, a decrease in the number of endometrial and cervical glands, impaired condensation and segregation of the uterine mesenchyme, and hyperplastic, disorganized epithelium and distorted mucosal plications in the fallopian tube. The abnormalities induced by tamoxifen and clomiphene were, in most instances, comparable to those of DES (19). A study published in 1979 examined the effects of tamoxifen administration on newborn female rats (5 μg on days 1, 3, and 5), observing several abnormalities of reproductive development, including early vaginal opening, absence of cycles, atrophic ovaries and uteri, vaginal adenosis, and severe squamous metaplasia of the oviducts (20). Gonad and genitourinary tract abnormalities, including uterine hypoplasia and vaginal adenosis, were also observed in newborn female mice given tamoxifen for 5 days (21). A 1997 report compared the uterotropic effects of tamoxifen (100 μg), DES (1 μg), or placebo administered SC daily to newborn female rat pups for 5 days (22). At postnatal day 6, both tamoxifen and DES produced significant epithelial hypertrophy and myometrial thickening, as well as other uterine changes that led the investigators to conclude that tamoxifen's estrogenic action on the developing uterus was similar to that produced by DES (22).

The clinical significance of the above studies demonstrating developmental changes in animals, three of which involved neonatal exposure to tamoxifen, is presently unknown, but some of the alterations observed in experiments, especially vaginal adenosis, are similar to those observed in young women following *in utero* exposure to DES (2). Moreover, too few women have been exposed *in utero* to tamoxifen and followed long enough (up to 20 years), to determine whether the drug presents a risk of clear-cell adenocarcinoma of the vagina or cervix similar to DES (about 1 in 1,000) (2) (see also Diethylstilbestrol). It should also be noted that long-term exposure of nonpregnant, adult humans to tamoxifen has been associated with an increased incidence of endometrial cancer (2).

Data pertaining to human fetal exposure to tamoxifen are limited. A 1993 letter cited a statement made by tamoxifen researchers that 85 women had become pregnant while receiving the drug and that no fetal abnormalities had been reported (23). A 1994 letter, however, citing data (oral and written) reported to the manufacturer, described the outcomes of 50 pregnancies associated with tamoxifen therapy (24). Of the total, there were 19 normal births, 8 elective abortions, 10 with a fetal or neonatal disorder (2 of which were congenital craniofacial defects), and 13 unknown outcomes. Although the number of adverse outcomes is suggestive of human teratogenicity, no mention was made whether the above cases represented prospective or retrospective reporting. The latter type frequently involves biased reporting in that adverse outcomes are much more likely to be communicated. Also included in this letter was the description of a case in which a 35-year-old woman, following breast cancer surgery, took tamoxifen, 20 mg/day, throughout an approximately 27-week pregnancy (24). Because of premature labor, chorioamnionitis, and an abnormal lie, a cesarean section was performed to deliver an 896-g, karyotypically normal infant (sex not specified). Malformations noted in the infant, consistent with a diagnosis of Goldenhar's syndrome, included right-sided microtia, preauricular skin tags, and hemifacial microsomia (24). Other exposures, in addition to tamoxifen, were cocaine and marijuana smoking (1 or 2 times/week) during the first 6 weeks of gestation and a bone scan performed using technetium-99m medronate. The causal relationship between tamoxifen and the defects in the infant was unknown (24), but in some reports of familial cases, the patterns of inheritance of Goldenhar's syndrome (oculoauriculovertebral anomaly) have been described as consistent with an autosomal dominant, autosomal recessive, and multifactorial inheritance (25).

Ambiguous genitalia in a female newborn exposed *in utero* to tamoxifen during the first 20 weeks of pregnancy was reported in 1997 (26). The 35-year-old mother had been treated with tamoxifen, 20 mg daily, for about 1 year for metastatic breast cancer. Because of the mother's deteriorating condition, the normal 46,XX karyotype, 1360-g infant was delivered at 29 weeks' gestation. Reproductive malformations included an enlarged, phallic-like clitoris (1.4 × 0.6 cm), a single perineal opening for the urethra and vagina, and fusion of the posterior portion of the rugated labioscrotal folds without palpable glands. An ultrasound examination revealed a normal uterus and ovaries without identifiable male structures. Congenital adrenal hyperplasia was excluded and a serum testosterone level was normal for a female infant. At 6 months of age, a reduction phalloplasty and vaginal reconstruction were performed without complications (26).

Two reports have described three successful pregnancies following chemotherapy with tamoxifen (27,28). In one of two cases described in a 1986 reference, a 26-year-old woman with a pituitary microadenoma and primary infertility was successfully treated with tamoxifen 20 mg/day and bromocriptine 10 mg/day (27). Combination therapy was used because she could not tolerate high-dose bromocriptine monotherapy. She ovulated and conceived approximately 7.5 months after combination therapy was begun. Tamoxifen was discontinued when pregnancy was confirmed (exact timing not specified), but bromocriptine was continued until 8 weeks' gestation. She delivered a normal, 3240-g female infant at term. In the second case, a 25-year-old woman with a pituitary macroadenoma and primary infertility was treated for about 3 months with the same combination therapy as in the first case, again because of intolerance to monotherapy (27). Combination therapy was stopped when pregnancy was confirmed (exact timing not specified) and she delivered a normal, 2600-g female infant at 37 weeks' gestation. The third pregnancy involved a 31-year-old woman with a diagnosis of well-differentiated adenocarcinoma of the endometrium who elected to receive 6 months of hormonal therapy with tamoxifen 30 mg/day and megestrol acetate 160 mg/day, combined with repeated hysteroscopy and uterine curettage, rather than undergo a hysterectomy (28). She was then placed on combination oral contraceptives for 3 months and conceived 1 month after they were discontinued. She eventually delivered a normal, 3340-g male infant at term.

A number of studies have examined the efficacy of tamoxifen, often in direct comparison with clomiphene, for ovulation induction in infertile women (29–35). Although no fetal anomalies were reported in these pregnancies following tamoxifen induction, a higher than expected occurrence of spontaneous abortion was noted in two studies (29,33). In contrast to clomiphene, however, tamoxifen induction did not appear to increase the frequency of multiple gestations (34).

In males, tamoxifen, like clomiphene, has been used for the treatment of idiopathic oligospermia (36–41). Tamoxifen appears to improve sperm density and the number of live spermatozoa, but conflicting results have been reported concerning the effect on sperm motility or morphology (37,40,41). A 1987 review, moreover, concluded that there was no convincing evidence that tamoxifen was effective in increasing the conception rate (41).

In summary, tamoxifen is an antiestrogen that has weak estrogenic activity in some tissues. Although tamoxifen is not considered an animal teratogen, it is carcinogenic in rodents and has been associated with intrauterine growth retardation, abortions, and premature delivery in some species. Uterine cancer has been reported in human adults treated with tamoxifen. Moreover, tamoxifen has produced toxic changes in the reproductive tracts of animals. Some of these changes were similar to those observed in humans exposed *in utero* to DES, but the risk of tamoxifen-induced clear cell adenocarcinoma of the vagina or cervix in exposed offspring is unknown because too few humans have been exposed during pregnancy or followed up long enough. Two adverse outcomes following inadvertent exposure to tamoxifen during gestation have been described. The relationship between tamoxifen and Goldenhar's syndrome in the first case is unknown, but, in the second case, a causal association between the drug and the ambiguous genitalia noted in the female infant appears to be more certain. In addition, a number of fetal and neonatal disorders and defects have been reported to the manufacturer, but it is not known whether this is the result of retrospective reporting. Because of the various toxicities noted in animals, the increased incidence of abortions noted in some patients when the drug was used for ovulation induction, and the possible human teratogenicity, the best course is to avoid use of tamoxifen during pregnancy. Moreover, because both the parent compound and the major metabolite have prolonged half-lives that may require up to 8 weeks to eliminate, women of child-bearing age should be informed that a pregnancy occurring within 2 months of tamoxifen therapy may expose the embryo and/or fetus to the drug. If an inadvertent pregnancy does occur, the potential fetal and newborn risks must be discussed with the patient. Offspring who have been exposed to tamoxifen during pregnancy require long-term (up to 20 years) follow-up to access the risk of carcinogenicity.

BREAST FEEDING SUMMARY

RECOMMENDATION: Contraindicated

Tamoxifen has been shown to inhibit lactation (42,43). In a double-blind, placebo-controlled trial, tamoxifen started within 2 hours after delivery was effective in preventing milk secretion and breast engorgement (42). Two treatment courses were studied: 30 mg twice daily × 2 days, then 20 mg twice daily × 2 days, then 10 mg twice daily × 2 days ($N = 50$); and 10 mg twice daily × 14 days ($N = 42$). Two groups of control patients ($N = 25$ and $N = 23$) received similar placebo tablets. The 6-day treatment course was "superior" (statistical analysis was not done) to the 14-day treatment course with 43 (86%) vs. 31 (74%) of the women having a "good" response (i.e., either no milk in their breasts or only slight to moderate milk secretion) (42). Only 6 (13%) of the control patients had a "good" response. No adverse effects or rebound engorgement were observed in the women who had received tamoxifen.

In a second, placebo-controlled, single blinded study, tamoxifen ($N = 60$, 10 mg 4 times daily) or placebo ($N = 20$) was started within 24 hours of delivery and continued for 5 days (43). Breast stimulation using a mechanical breast pump was used before the first dose, and then on days 3 and 5, followed by blood sampling for serum prolactin. By the 5th day, a significant decrease (compared with baseline) in serum prolactin concentration occurred in the tamoxifen group, but not in controls. Moreover, tamoxifen was effective in inhibiting lactation and preventing breast engorgement, and no rebound lactation was observed (43).

Because tamoxifen inhibits lactation and because of the adverse effects noted in newborn animals and human adults (see Fetal Risk Summary above) given the drug directly, the drug is contraindicated during nursing.

T

References

1. American Hospital Formulary Service. *Drug Information 1997*. Bethesda, MD: American Society of Health-System Pharmacists, 1997:861–6.
2. Product information. Nolvadex. Zeneca Pharmaceuticals, 1997.
3. Jordan VC. The role of tamoxifen in the treatment and prevention of breast cancer. Curr Probl Cancer 1992;16:129–76.
4. Furr BJA, Valcaccia B, Challis JRG. The effects of Nolvadex (tamoxifen citrate; ICI 46,474) on pregnancy in rabbits. J Reprod Fertil 1976;48:367–9.
5. Bloxham PA, Pugh DM, Sharma SC. An effect of tamoxifen (I.C.I. 46,474) on the surface coat of the late preimplantation mouse blastocyst. J Reprod Fertil 1975;45:181–3.
6. Watson J, Anderson FB, Alam M, O'Grady JE, Heald PJ. Plasma hormones and pituitary luteinizing hormone in the rat during the early stages of pregnancy and after post-coital treatment with tamoxifen (ICI 46,474). J Endocrinol 1975;65:7–17.
7. Pugh DM, Sumano HS. The anti-implantation action of tamoxifen in mice. Arch Toxicol 1982;5(Suppl):209–13.
8. Ravindranath N, Moudgal NR. Use of tamoxifen, an antioestrogen, in establishing a need for oestrogen in early pregnancy in the bonnet monkey (*Macaca radiata*). J Reprod Fertil 1987;81:327–36.

9. Bowen RA, Olson PN, Young S, Withrow SJ. Efficacy and toxicity of tamoxifen citrate for prevention and termination of pregnancy in bitches. Am J Vet Res 1988;49:27–31.
10. Majumdar M, Datta JK. Contraceptive efficacy of tamoxifen in female hamsters. Contraception 1990;41:93–103.
11. Hodgson BJ. Effects of indomethacin and ICI 46,474 administered during ovum transport on fertility in rabbits. Biol Reprod 1976;14:451–7.
12. Tarantal AF, Hendrickx AG, Matlin SA, Lasley BL, Gu Q-Q, Thomas CAA, Vince PM, Van Look PFA. Tamoxifen as an antifertility agent in the long-tailed macaque (*Macaca fascicularis*). Contraception 1993;47: 307–16.
13. Clark JH, McCormack SA. The effect of Clomid and other triphenylethylene derivatives during pregnancy and the neonatal period. J Steroid Biochem 1980;12:47–53.
14. Pasqualini JR, Gulino A, Sumida C, Screpanti I. Antiestrogens in fetal and newborn target tissues. J Steroid Biochem 1984;20:121–8.
15. Gulino A, Screpanti I, Pasqualini JR. Differential estrogen and antiestrogen responsiveness of the uterus during development in the fetal, neonatal and immature guinea pig. Biol Reprod 1984;31:371–81.
16. Nguyen BL, Giambiagi N, Mayrand C, Lecerf F, Pasqualini JR. Estrogen and progesterone receptors in the fetal and newborn vagina of guinea pig: biological, morphological, and ultrastructural responses to tamoxifen and estradiol. Endocrinology 1986;119: 978–88.
17. Pasqualini JR, Giambiagi N, Sumida C, Nguyen BL, Gelly C, Mayrand C, Lecerf F. Biological responses of tamoxifen in the fetal and newborn vagina and uterus of the guinea-pig and in the R-27 mammary cancer cell line. J Steroid Biochem 1986;24:99–108.
18. Hines M, Alsum P, Roy M, Gorski RA, Goy RW. Estrogenic contributions to sexual differentiation in the female guinea pig: influences of diethylstilbestrol and tamoxifen on neural, behavioral, and ovarian development. Horm Behav 1987;21:402–17.
19. Cunha GR, Taguchi O, Namikawa R, Nishizuka Y, Robboy SJ. Teratogenic effects of clomiphene, tamoxifen, and diethylstilbestrol on the developing human female genital tract. Hum Pathol 1987;18: 1132–43.
20. Chamness GC, Bannayan GA, Landry LA Jr, Sheridan PJ, McGuire WL. Abnormal reproductive development in rats after neonatally administered antiestrogen (tamoxifen). Biol Reprod 1979;21:1087–90.
21. Iguchi T, Hirokawa M, Takasugi N. Occurrence of genital tract abnormalities and bladder hernia in female mice exposed neonatally to tamoxifen. Toxicology 1986;42:1–11.
22. Poulet FM, Roessler ML, Vancutsem PM. Initial uterine alterations caused by developmental exposure to tamoxifen. Reprod Toxicol 1997;11:815–22.
23. Clark S. Prophylactic tamoxifen. Lancet 1993;342: 168.
24. Cullins SL, Pridjian G, Sutherland CM. Goldenhar's syndrome associated with tamoxifen given to the mother during gestation. JAMA 1994;271:1905–6.
25. Rollnick BR, Kaye CI. Oculo-auriculo-vertebral anomaly. In Buyse ML, editor-in-chief. *Birth Defects Encyclopedia*. Vol. II. Cambridge, MA: Blackwell Scientific Publications, 1990:1272–4.
26. Tewari K, Bonebrake RG, Asrat T, Shanberg AM. Ambiguous genitalia in infant exposed to tamoxifen in utero. Lancet 1997;350:183.
27. Koizumi K, Aono T. Pregnancy after combined treatment with bromocriptine and tamoxifen in two patients with pituitary prolactinomas. Fertil Steril 1986;46:312–4.
28. Lai C-H, Hsueh S, Chao A-S, Soong Y-K. Successful pregnancy after tamoxifen and megestrol acetate therapy for endometrial carcinoma. Br J Obstet Gynaecol 1994;101:547–9.
29. Ruiz-Velasco V, Rosas-Arceo J, Matute MM. Chemical inducers of ovulation: comparative results. Int J Fertil 1979;24:61–4.
30. Messinis IE, Nillius SJ. Comparison between tamoxifen and clomiphene for induction of ovulation. Acta Obstet Gynecol Scand 1982;61:377–9.
31. Fukushima T, Tajima C, Fukuma K, Maeyama M. Tamoxifen in the treatment of infertility associated with luteal phase deficiency. Fertil Steril 1982;37:755–61.
32. Tajima C, Fukushima T. Endocrine profiles in tamoxifen-induced ovulatory cycles. Fertil Steril 1983; 40:23–30.
33. Tsuiki A, Uehara S, Kyono K, Saito A, Hoshi K, Hoshiai H, Hirano M, Suzuki M. Induction of ovulation with an estrogen antagonist, tamoxifen. Tohoku J Exp Med 1984;144:21–31.
34. Weseley AC, Melnick H. Tamoxifen in clomiphene-resistant hypothalamic anovulation. Int J Fertil 1987; 32:226–8.
35. Suginami H, Yano K, Kitagawa H, Matsubara K, Nakahashi N. A clomiphene citrate and tamoxifen citrate combination therapy: a novel therapy for ovulation induction. Fertil Steril 1993;59:976–9.
36. Lunglmayr G. Potentialities and limitations of endocrine treatment in idiopathic oligozoospermia. Acta Eur Fertil 1983;14:401–4.
37. Schill WB, Schillinger R. Selection of oligozoospermic men for tamoxifen treatment by an antiestrogen test. Andrologia 1987;19:266–72.
38. Brake A, Krause W. Treatment of idiopathic oligozoospermia with tamoxifen—a follow-up report. Int J Androl 1992;15:507–8.
39. Breznik R, Borko E. Effectiveness of antiestrogens in infertile men. Arch Androl 1993;31:43–8.
40. Kotoulas I-G, Mitropoulos D, Cardamakis E, Dounis A, Michopoulos J. Tamoxifen treatment in male infertility. I. Effect on spermatozoa. Fertil Steril 1994;61: 911–4.
41. Sigman M, Vance ML. Medical treatment of idiopathic infertility. Urol Clin North Am 1987;14:459–69.
42. Shaaban MM. Suppression of lactation by an antiestrogen, tamoxifen. Eur J Obstet Gynecol Reprod Biol 1975;4:167–9.
43. Masala A, Delitala G, Lo Dico G, Stoppelli I, Alagna S, Devilla L. Inhibition of lactation and inhibition of prolactin release after mechanical breast stimulation in puerperal women given tamoxifen or placebo. Br J Obstet Gynecol 1978;85:134–7.

Name: **TAZAROTENE**
Class: **Dermatologic Agent**
Risk Factor: **X_M**

FETAL RISK SUMMARY

RECOMMENDATION: Contraindicated

Tazarotene is a retinoid prodrug that is rapidly converted *in vivo* to the active form, the cognate carboxylic acid of tazarotene ("tazarotenic acid"). The drug is indicated for the topical treatment of acne vulgaris and plaque psoriasis. The active drug is absorbed into the systemic circulation producing peak plasma levels up to approximately 2 ng/mL. In females treated for acne, doses applied to 15% of the body surface area produced peak plasma levels 12 times higher than those from applications to only the face (1.2 vs. 0.1 ng/mL). Peak plasma levels occurred on day 15 of treatment and the highest observed level was 1.91 ng/mL (1).

Reproduction studies have been conducted in rats and rabbits (1). Topical doses resulted in reduced fetal body weights and reduced skeletal ossification in rats and single incidents of retinoid malformations, including spina bifida, hydrocephaly, and heart defects in rabbits. The systemic exposures resulting from the doses used in rats and rabbits were 1.2 and 13 times, respectively, the exposure resulting from treating a psoriatic patient with 0.1% cream over 35% of the body surface area, and 4.0 and 44 times, respectively, the maximum systemic exposure of acne patients treated with 0.1% cream over 15% of the body surface area (1). Oral administration of tazarotene caused developmental delays in rats, and teratogenicity and resorptions in rats and rabbits at doses 1.1 and 26 times, respectively, the systemic exposure of a psoriatic patient and 3.5 and 85 times, respectively, the maximum systemic exposure of acne patients.

It is not known whether tazarotene or its active metabolite crosses the placenta to the fetus. The molecular weight (about 351) is low enough that transfer usually would be expected. However, the drug is highly bound to plasma protein (>99%) and maternal plasma concentrations are very low. Both of these factors should inhibit placental transfer.

The manufacturer has reports on nine pregnant women who were inadvertently exposed to tazarotene during clinical trials, two during studies involving acne patients and seven in other trials (1). One woman terminated her pregnancy, and healthy infants were delivered in the other eight cases. The timing of the exposures and the dosage used were not certain, so the significance of these findings is unknown (1).

In summary, tazarotene is a retinoid that causes retinoid-like malformations in experimental animals. Because of this and the experience with other retinoids (e.g., see Isotretinoin), the drug is contraindicated in women who are or who may become pregnant. A negative pregnancy test should be obtained within 2 weeks before starting therapy with this agent, which should begin during a normal menstrual period (1).

BREAST FEEDING SUMMARY

RECOMMENDATION: Limited Human Data - Potential Toxicity

Trace amounts of tazarotene are excreted into human milk (1). The risk to a nursing infant from this exposure is unknown.

Reference

1. Product information. Tazorac. Allergan, 2003.

Name:	**TAZOBACTAM**	Risk Factor:	B_M
Class:	**Anti-infective**		

FETAL RISK SUMMARY

RECOMMENDATION: No Human Data - Animal Data Suggest Low Risk

Tazobactam, a β-lactamase inhibitor, is combined with piperacillin to increase its antibacterial spectrum. It is not available as a single agent. Structurally, tazobactam is a derivative of the penicillin nucleus and is metabolized to an inactive metabolite. The plasma half-life ranges from 0.7 to 1.2 hours. Only 30% of tazobactam (and none of the metabolite) is bound to plasma proteins.

Reproduction studies with tazobactam have been conducted in mice and rats. No evidence of fetal harm was observed in these species at doses up to 6 and 14 times, respectively, the human dose based on body surface area. In rats, no effects on fertility were observed with doses up to 3 times the maximum recommended human daily dose based on body surface area.

Tazobactam crosses the rat placenta resulting in fetal concentrations equal to or less than 10% of those found in maternal plasma (1). This is consistent with its molecular weight (about 322) and its low protein binding. As expected, tazobactam also crosses the human placenta. A 1998 report described the pharmacokinetics of piperacillin-tazobactam in six women with gestations of 25 to 32 weeks (2). Because of the increase in renal clearance and other factors, a marked decrease in maternal serum concentrations of both agents was observed. In one of the women (samples were inadequate in the other five), the fetal:maternal serum ratio of tazobactam was 2 about 3 hours after a dose. In two other women, low concentrations of tazobactam, 2.3 and 3.7 μg/mL, respectively, were measured in the amniotic fluid and, in two others, low concentrations in fetal urine, 8.2 and 12.4 μg/mL, respectively.

In summary, although no other reports describing the use of tazobactam-piperacillin have been located, the combination appears to be relatively safe in human pregnancy. No fetal harm in animals was observed at doses very close to those used in humans. Moreover, there is substantial experience with penicillins in human pregnancy that has shown this class of anti-infectives to be safe for the embryo and fetus. Because tazobactam is a derivative of the penicillin nucleus, it also probably is safe in pregnancy.

BREAST FEEDING SUMMARY

RECOMMENDATION: Limited Human Data - Probably Compatible

Although specific details were lacking, the manufacturer states that tazobactam is excreted into breast milk in low concentrations (1). This is consistent with its relatively low molecular weight (about 322) and protein binding (30%). Piperacillin also is excreted into milk (see Piperacillin). The effects of this low exposure on a nursing infant probably are not clinically significant, but three potential problems exist for the nursing infant: modification of bowel flora, direct effects on the infant, and interference with the interpretation of culture results if a fever workup is required.

References

1. Product information. Zosyn. Wyeth Pharmaceuticals, 2004.
2. Bourget P, Sertin A, Lesne-Hulin A, Fernandez H, Ville Y, Van Peborgh P. Influence of pregnancy on the pharmacokinetic behaviour and the transplacental transfer of the piperacillin-tazobactam combination. Eur J Obstet Gynecol Reprod Biol 1998;76:21–7.

Name: **TELMISARTAN** Risk Factor: C_M*

Class: **Antihypertensive**

FETAL RISK SUMMARY

RECOMMENDATION: Human Data Suggest Risk in 2nd and 3rd Trimesters

Telmisartan is a selective angiotensin II receptor antagonist that is used, either alone or in combination with other antihypertensive agents, for the treatment of hypertension. Telmisartan blocks the vasoconstrictor and aldosterone-secreting effects of angiotensin II by preventing angiotensin II from binding to AT_1 receptors.

Reproduction studies have been conducted in pregnant rats and rabbits (1). No teratogenicity was observed in either species at oral doses up to approximately 6.3 and 6.4 times the maximum recommended human dose of 80 mg on a body surface area basis (MRHD), respectively, but embryo lethality was noted at the highest dose in rabbits. The highest doses were maternally toxic (reduced body weight gain and food consumption) in both species. In rats, an oral dose approximately 1.9 times the MRHD (also maternal toxic) during late gestation and lactation resulted in neonatal adverse effects, including reduced viability, low birth weight, delayed maturation, and decreased weight gain (1). The no-observed-effect doses for developmental toxicity in rats and rabbits were 0.64 and 3.7 times the MRHD. No adverse effects on reproductive performance were noted in male and female rats at a dose about 13 times the MRHD (1).

It is not known if telmisartan crosses the human placenta to the fetus. The drug is found in rat fetuses in late gestation (1). The molecular weight (about 515) is low enough that passage to the human fetus should be expected.

A 2003 case report described transient renal failure in a newborn secondary to maternal use of telmisartan (2). A 35-year-old woman with hypertension was treated with telmisartan throughout pregnancy. Oligohydramnios was diagnosed at 34 weeks' gestation and a 2.2-kg female infant was delivered by cesarean section. Apgar scores were 9, 10, and 10 at 1, 5, and 10 minutes, respectively. The infant was anuric until the third day of life, but renal function improved thereafter. Telmisartan plasma levels on day 10 and 13 were 20 and 13 ng/L, respectively. The infant's renal function had normalized by 1.5 months of age (2).

The antihypertensive mechanisms of action of telmisartan and angiotensin-converting enzyme (ACE) inhibitors are very close. That is, the former selectively blocks the binding of angiotensin II to AT_1 receptors, whereas the latter prevents the formation of angiotensin II itself. Therefore, use of this drug during the 2nd and 3rd trimesters may cause teratogenicity and severe fetal and neonatal toxicity that is identical to that seen with ACE inhibitors (e.g., see Captopril or Enalapril). Fetal toxic effects may include anuria, oligohydramnios, fetal hypocalvaria, intrauterine growth retardation, prematurity, and patent ductus arteriosus. Anuria-associated oligohydramnios may produce fetal limb contractures,

T

craniofacial deformation, and pulmonary hypoplasia. Severe anuria and hypotension that are resistant to both pressor agents and volume expansion, may occur in the newborn following *in utero* exposure to telmisartan. Newborn renal function and blood pressure should be closely monitored. If telmisartan is used in pregnancy, healthcare professionals are encouraged to call the toll free number (800-670-6126) for information about patient enrollment in the Motherisk study.

[**Risk Factor D_M if used in 2nd or 3rd trimesters.*]

BREAST FEEDING SUMMARY

RECOMMENDATION: No Human Data - Probably Compatible

No reports describing the use of telmisartan during human lactation have been located. The drug is excreted into the milk of lactating rats (1). Because the molecular weight (515) is low enough, excretion into human breast milk should also be expected. The effects of this exposure on a nursing infant are unknown. The American Academy of Pediatrics, however, classifies ACE inhibitors, a closely related group of antihypertensive agents, as compatible with breast-feeding (see Captopril or Enalapril).

References

1. Product information. Micardis. Boehringer Ingelheim Pharmaceuticals, 2000.
2. Pietrement C, Malot L, Santerne B, Roussel B, Motte J, Morville P. Neonatal acute renal failure secondary to maternal exposure to telmisartan, angiotension II receptor antagonist. J Perinatol 2003;23:254–5.

Name:	**TEMAZEPAM**	Risk Factor:	**X_M**
Class:	**Hypnotic**		

FETAL RISK SUMMARY

RECOMMENDATION: Limited Human Data - Animal Data Suggest Risk

Temazepam is a benzodiazepine that is used as a hypnotic for the short-term management of insomnia. Reproductive studies in rats revealed increased resorptions and an increased incidence of rudimentary ribs, which were considered skeletal variants (1). Exencephaly and fusion or asymmetry of ribs were observed in rabbits (1).

In a surveillance study of Michigan Medicaid recipients conducted between 1985 and 1992 involving 229,101 completed pregnancies, 146 newborns had been exposed to temazepam during the 1st trimester (F. Rosa, personal communication, FDA, 1993). Six (4.1%) major birth defects were observed (six expected), including one cardiovascular defect (one expected) and two oral clefts (none expected). No anomalies were observed in four other categories of defects (spina bifida, polydactyly, limb reduction defects, and hypospadias) for which specific data were available. Although the two oral clefts suggest a relationship with the drug, other factors, such as the mother's disease, concurrent drug use, and chance, may be involved.

A potential drug interaction between temazepam and diphenhydramine, resulting in the stillbirth of a term female infant, has been reported (2). The mother had taken diphenhydramine 50 mg for mild itching of the skin and approximately 1.5 hours later took 30 mg of temazepam for sleep. Three hours later, she awoke with violent intrauterine fetal movements, which lasted several minutes and then abruptly stopped. The stillborn infant was delivered approximately 4 hours later. Autopsy revealed no gross or microscopic anomalies. In an experiment with pregnant rabbits, neither of the drugs alone caused fetal mortality but when combined, 51 (81%) of 63 fetuses were stillborn or died shortly after birth (2). No definite mechanism could be established for the apparent interaction.

BREAST FEEDING SUMMARY

RECOMMENDATION: Limited Human Data - Potential Toxicity

Temazepam is excreted into breast milk. Ten mothers, within 15 days of delivery, were administered 10–20 mg of temazepam for at least 2 days as a bedtime hypnotic (3). Milk and plasma samples were obtained about 15 hours later corresponding to an infant feeding. Temazepam was detected (limit of detection 5 ng/mL) in the milk of only one woman with before and after feeding levels of 28 and 26 ng/mL, respectively. The milk:plasma ratio in this patient was 0.12. Although no adverse effects were observed in the nursling, nursing infants of mothers consuming temazepam should be closely observed for sedation and poor feeding. The American Academy of Pediatrics classifies temazepam as a drug for which the effect on nursing infants is unknown but may be of concern (4).

References

1. Product information. Restoril. Sandoz Pharmaceuticals Corp., 1993.
2. Kargas GA, Kargas SA, Bruyere HJ Jr, Gilbert EF, Opitz JM. Perinatal mortality due to interaction of diphenhydramine and temazepam. N Engl J Med 1985;313:1417.
3. Lepedevs TH, Wojnar-Horton RE, Yapp P, Roberts MJ, Dusci LJ, Hackett LP, Ilett KF. Excretion of temazepam in breast milk. Br J Clin Pharmacol 1992;33:204–6.
4. Committee on Drugs, American Academy of Pediatrics. The transfer of drugs and other chemicals into human milk. Pediatrics 2001;108:776–89.

Name: **TENECTEPLASE** Risk Factor: **C_M**

Class: **Thrombolytic**

FETAL RISK SUMMARY

RECOMMENDATION: Compatible - Maternal Benefit >> Embryo/Fetal Risk

Tenecteplase is a modified form of human tissue-plasminogen activator (tPA) that is produced by recombinant DNA technology using Chinese Hamster Ovary cells. It is a 527-amino-acid glycoprotein that is indicated for use in the reduction of mortality associated with acute myocardial infarction. Tenecteplase is cleared from the plasma with a half-life of 20–24 minutes, but the terminal phase half-life is 90–130 minutes (1).

In pregnant rabbits given multiple IV daily doses of 0.5, 1.5 mg, and 5.0 mg/kg/day, vaginal hemorrhage resulted in maternal deaths. No fetal anomalies were observed. Single IV doses (the recommended human dose is a single bolus injection) in rabbits did not cause maternal or embryo toxicity. The no-observable-effect level (NOEL) of a single IV dose was 5 mg/kg (about 8–10 times the human dose; *assumed to be based on weight*) (1).

It is not known if tenecteplase crosses the human placenta. Tenecteplase is a glycoprotein and, although some proteins do cross, the short plasma half-life will limit the exposure of the embryo/fetus to the enzyme.

No reports describing the use of tenecteplase in human pregnancy have been located. The limited animal data do not suggest a direct risk. Moreover, fetal toxicity has not been observed with limited pregnancy exposure to another, similar glycoprotein enzyme, alteplase.

Although maternal hemorrhage is a major risk, tenecteplase should not be withheld because of pregnancy if the maternal condition requires such therapy.

BREAST FEEDING SUMMARY

RECOMMENDATION: Hold Breast Feeding

No reports describing the use of tenecteplase during human lactation have been located. It is not known whether the glycoprotein is excreted into human milk. Because of the nature of the indication for this agent and its very short plasma and terminal half-life, the opportunities for its use during lactation or the possible exposure of a nursing infant are minimal.

Reference

1. Product information. TNKase. Genentech, 2004.

Name:	**TENIPOSIDE**	Risk Factor:	**D**
Class:	**Antineoplastic**		

FETAL RISK SUMMARY

RECOMMENDATION: Contraindicated - 1st Trimester

Teniposide, a podophyllin derivative, has been used in the 2nd and 3rd trimesters of one pregnancy (1). An apparently normal infant was delivered at 37 weeks of gestation.

Reproduction studies in rats given IV doses of 0.1–3 mg/kg (0.6–18 mg/m^2) every second day from day 6 to day 16 post coitum revealed dose-related embryotoxicity and teratogenicity (2). Congenital malformations consisted of spinal and rib defects, deformed extremities, anophthalmia, and celosomia.

Long-term studies of growth and mental development in offspring exposed to antineoplastic agents during the 2nd trimester, the period of neuroblast multiplication, have not been conducted (3).

Occupational exposure of the mother to antineoplastic agents during pregnancy may present a risk to the fetus. A position statement from the National Study Commission on Cytotoxic Exposure and a research article involving some antineoplastic agents are presented in the monograph for cyclophosphamide (see Cyclophosphamide).

BREAST FEEDING SUMMARY

RECOMMENDATION: No Human Data - Potential Toxicity

No data are available.

References

1. Lowenthal RM, Funnell CF, Hope DM, Stewart IG, Humphrey DC. Normal infant after combination chemotherapy including teniposide for Burkitt's lymphoma in pregnancy. Med Pediatr Oncol 1982;10:165–9.
2. Product information. Vumon. Bristol-Myers Squibb, 2000.
3. Dobbing J. Pregnancy and leukaemia. Lancet 1977;1:1155.

Name: **TENOFOVIR** Risk Factor: **B_M**
Class: **Antiviral**

FETAL RISK SUMMARY

RECOMMENDATION: Compatible - Maternal Benefit >> Embryo/Fetal Risk

Tenofovir is available as a prodrug, tenofovir disoproxil fumarate (PMPA), a fumaric acid salt of the ester derivative that is converted to tenofovir after oral administration (1). Tenofovir is an acyclic nucleoside analogue reverse transcriptase inhibitor in the same antiviral class as abacavir, didanosine, emtricitabine, lamivudine, stavudine, zalcitabine, and zidovudine. It has activity against HIV types 1 and 2 (2). Tenofovir is indicated in combination with other antiretroviral agents for the treatment of human immunodeficiency disease virus type 1 (HIV-1). About 1% and 7% of tenofovir is bound by plasma and serum proteins, respectively (1,2).

Reproduction studies have been conducted in rats and rabbits. In these species, doses up to 14 and 19 times the human dose based on body surface area (HD), respectively, revealed no evidence of impaired fertility or fetal harm. There were no effects on fertility or mating performance, or early embryonic development in male and female rats given doses up to 10 times the HD for several weeks prior to mating and, in female rats, through the first 7 days of gestation (1).

Tenofovir crosses the placentas of gravid rhesus monkeys (3). Tenofovir was given to the monkeys at a dose of 30 mg/kg SC once daily starting early in the 2nd trimester (gestational day 80) and continuing until delivery at term (gestational day 157). The fetal:maternal blood levels (based on $AUC_{U\text{-infinity}}$, μg/hour) were 49.2/117.3 (ratio 0.42; gestational day 120) and 39.1/87.0 (ratio 0.45; gestational day 140). Although normal fetal growth patterns were observed, the mean birth weight of tenofovir-exposed newborns was significantly less (about 381 g vs. 467 g) than nonexposed controls. In addition, the crown-rump, humerus, and femur lengths were significantly reduced (3).

In a follow-up to the above study, investigators gave rhesus monkeys tenofovir 30 mg/kg SC once daily from gestation days 20 to 150 (4). As in the study above, fetal development was normal but body weights and crown-rump lengths were significantly less than age-matched controls. In addition, fetal insulin-like growth factor was significantly reduced, as was fetal bone porosity, but alkaline phosphatase levels were increased. Transient alterations in maternal body weights and bone-related biomarkers and elevated alkaline phosphatase were observed during treatment (4).

The passage of tenofovir across the human placenta apparently has not been studied. However, the molecular weight (about 636 for the prodrug), and low plasma and serum protein binding, combined with the data from monkeys, suggest that the drug will cross to the human embryo and fetus.

The Antiretroviral Pregnancy Registry reported, for the period January 1989 through January 2004, prospective data (reported to the Registry before the outcomes were known) involving 1537 live births that had been exposed during the 1st trimester to one or more antiretroviral agents (2). Forty-seven of the newborns had congenital defects (3.1%, 95% confidence interval [CI] 2.3–4.1). In the 2407 live births with earliest exposure in the 2nd/3rd trimesters, there were 56 infants with defects (2.3%, 95% CI 1.8–3.0). The prevalence rates for the two periods did not differ significantly. There were 103 infants with birth defects among 3944 live births with exposure anytime during pregnancy (2.6%, 95% CI 2.1–3.2).

The prevalence rate did not differ significantly from the rate expected in a nonexposed population (2). There were 114 outcomes exposed to tenofovir (48 in the 1st trimester and 66 in the 2nd/3rd trimesters) in combination with other antiretroviral agents. There were no birth defects among the 1st trimester exposures and one in the 2nd/3rd trimester group. In reviewing the birth defects of prospective and retrospective (pregnancies reported after the outcomes were known) registered cases, and clinical reports, the Registry concluded that there was no pattern of anomalies to suggest a common cause (2). (See Lamivudine for required statement.)

No reports, other than the data above, describing the use of tenofovir in human pregnancy have been located. Although the animal data are suggestive of risk (decreased growth), the limited human experience suggests that the embryo/fetal risk is low, at least for structural anomalies. Past reviewers have concluded that all women currently receiving antiretroviral therapy should continue to receive therapy during pregnancy (5–7). Discontinuing all therapy, however, until after 10–12 weeks' gestation is an option (7,8). If indicated, therefore, tenofovir should not be withheld in pregnancy, except possibly in the 1st trimester, because the expected benefit for the HIV-positive mother appears to outweigh the unknown risks to the fetus. The efficacy and safety of combined therapy in preventing vertical transmission of HIV to the newborn, however, are unknown, and zidovudine remains the only antiretroviral agent recommended for this purpose (8).

BREAST FEEDING SUMMARY

RECOMMENDATION: Contraindicated

No reports describing the use of tenofovir during human lactation have been located. The molecular weight (about 636 for the prodrug) and low plasma (about 1% and serum (about 7%) protein binding suggest that the drug will be excreted into human breast milk. The effects of this exposure on a nursing infant are unknown. However, reports on the use of tenofovir during lactation are unlikely because the drug is indicated in the treatment of patient's with HIV. HIV type 1 (HIV-1) is transmitted in milk, and in developed countries, breast-feeding is not recommended (5,6,9–12). In developing countries, breast-feeding is undertaken, despite the risk, because there are no affordable milk substitutes available.

References

1. Product information. Viread. Gilead Sciences, 2004.
2. Antiretroviral Pregnancy Registry Steering Committee. *Antiretroviral Pregnancy Registry International Interim Report for 1 January 1989 through 31 January 2004*. Wilmington, NC: Registry Coordinating Center, 2004.
3. Tarantal AF, Marthas ML, Shaw JP, Cundy K, Bischofberger N. Administration of 9-[2-(R)-(phosphonomethoxy) propyl]adenine (PMPA) to gravid and infant rhesus macaques (*Macaca mulatta*): safety and efficacy studies. J Acquir Immune Defic Syndr Hum Retroviral 1999;20:323–33.
4. Tarantal AF, Castillo A, Ekert JE, Bischofberger N, Martin RB. Fetal and maternal outcome after administration of tenofovir to gravid rhesus monkeys (*Macaca mulatta*). J Acquir Immune Defic Syndrome 2002;29:207–20.
5. Carpenter CCJ, Fischi MA, Hammer SM, Hirsch MS, Jacobsen DM, Katzenstein DA, Montaner JSG, Richman DD, Saag MS, Schooley RT, Thompson MA, Vella S, Yeni PG, Volberding PA. Antiretroviral therapy for HIV infection in 1996. JAMA 1996;276:146–54.
6. Minkoff H, Augenbraun M. Antiretroviral therapy for pregnant women. Am J Obstet Gynecol 1997;176: 478–89.
7. Centers for Disease Control and Prevention. Public Health Service Task Force recommendations for the use of antiretroviral drugs in pregnant women infected with HIV-1 for maternal health and for reducing perinatal HIV-1 transmission in the United States. MMWR 1998;47:No. RR-2.
8. Public Health Service Task Force Perinatal HIV Guidelines Working Group. Summary of the updated recommendations from the Public Health Service Task Force to reduce perinatal human immunodeficiency virus-1 transmission in the United States. Obstet Gynecol 2002;99:1117–26.
9. Brown ZA, Watts DH. Antiviral therapy in pregnancy. Clin Obstet Gynecol 1990;33:276–89.

10. de Martino M, Tovo P-A, Pezzotti P, Galli L, Massironi E, Ruga E, Floreea F, Plebani A, Gabiano C, Zuccotti GV. HIV-1 transmission through breast-milk: appraisal of risk according to duration of feeding. AIDS 1992;6:991–7.
11. Van de Perre P. Postnatal transmission of human immunodeficiency virus type 1: the breast-feeding dilemma. Am J Obstet Gynecol 1995;173:483–7.
12. American College of Obstetricians and Gynecologists. Breastfeeding: maternal and infant aspects. *Educational Bulletin*. No. 258, July 2000.

Name:	**TERAZOSIN**	Risk Factor:	**C_M**
Class:	**Sympatholytic (Antiadrenergic)**		

FETAL RISK SUMMARY

RECOMMENDATION: No Human Data - Animal Data Suggest Low Risk

Terazosin is a peripherally acting α_1-adrenergic blocking agent used in the treatment of hypertension and symptomatic benign prostatic hyperplasia.

Reproduction studies in rats and rabbits at doses 280 and 60 times the recommended maximum human dose (RMHD) revealed no teratogenic effects, but an increased incidence of fetal resorptions occurred in both species (1). In addition, decreased fetal weight and an increased number of supernumerary ribs were observed in rabbit offspring. The embryo/fetal toxicity in both species was attributed to maternal toxicity (1). A significant increase in rat pup mortality was also seen at doses more than 75 times the RMHD in peri- and post-natal studies (1).

No reports describing the use of terazosin in human pregnancy have been located.

BREAST FEEDING SUMMARY

RECOMMENDATION: No Human Data - Probably Compatible

No reports describing the use of terazosin during lactation have been located. The molecular weight (about 424 for the free base) is low enough, however, that excretion into breast milk should be expected.

Reference

1. Product information. Hytrin. Abbott Laboratories, 2000.

Name:	**TERBINAFINE**	Risk Factor:	**B_M**
Class:	**Antifungal**		

FETAL RISK SUMMARY

RECOMMENDATION: No Human Data - Animal Data Suggest Low Risk

Terbinafine is a synthetic allylamine antifungal agent that is indicated for the treatment of onychomycosis of the toenail or fingernail caused by dermatophytes (tinea unguium) (1). No studies evaluating the placental transfer of terbinafine in humans have been located. The molecular weight (about 328) is low enough that transfer to the fetus should be expected.

Reproduction studies have been conducted in rats and rabbits (1). Oral doses in rats up to approximately 12 times the maximum recommended human dose based on body surface area (MRHD) had no effect on fertility or other reproductive parameters. In pregnant rabbits, intravaginal administration of terbinafine did not cause abortions, premature delivery, or affect fetal parameters. In pregnant rats and rabbits, no evidence of impaired fertility or fetal harm was seen with oral doses up to 12 and 9 times the MRHD, respectively (1).

Although the animal reproduction data are encouraging, the lack of human pregnancy data do not allow a full assessment of the fetal risk from terbinafine. If possible, therefore, waiting to begin treatment until after a pregnancy has been concluded would be the safest course. If terbinafine is used in pregnancy, healthcare professionals are encouraged to call the toll free number (800-670-6126) for information about patient enrollment in the Motherisk study.

BREAST FEEDING SUMMARY

RECOMMENDATION: Limited Human Data - Potential Toxicity

Terbinafine is excreted into human milk (1). No specific details were given, but the milk:plasma ratio in nursing women was 7:1. The effects of this exposure on a nursing infant are unknown. Because the duration of therapy is usually prolonged (6 or 12 weeks for patients with fingernail or toenail onychomycosis, respectively), the potential for serious toxicity in a nursing infant may be increased. Based on the accumulation in milk and the prolonged exposure, women taking terbinafine should probably not breast-feed.

Reference

1. Product information. Lamisil. Novartis Pharmaceuticals, 2001.

Name:	**TERBUTALINE**	Risk Factor:	**B_M**
Class:	**Sympathomimetic (Adrenergic)**		

FETAL RISK SUMMARY

RECOMMENDATION: Limited Human Data - Animal Data Suggest Low Risk

T

Terbutaline is a β-sympathomimetic indicated for the prevention and reversal of bronchospasm. During pregnancy, it is primarily used as a tocolytic agent. No reports linking the use of terbutaline with congenital defects have been located. However, the tocolytic use of this drug is confined to the late 2nd and early 3rd trimesters. Published reports describing the use of terbutaline as a bronchodilator during early pregnancy have not been found.

Reproduction studies in mice, rats, and rabbits at doses up to 1500 times the SC maximum recommended human daily dose of 0.1 mg/kg have revealed no evidence of impaired fertility or fetal harm (1).

In a surveillance study of Michigan Medicaid recipients conducted between 1985 and 1992 involving 229,101 completed pregnancies, 149 newborns had been exposed to terbutaline during the 1st trimester (F. Rosa, personal communication, FDA, 1993). Seven (4.7%) major birth defects were observed (six expected), including three cardiovascular defects (two expected) and one oral cleft (none expected). No anomalies were observed in four other categories of defects (spina bifida, polydactyly, limb reduction defects, and hypospadias) for which specific data were available. These data do not support an association between the drug and congenital defects.

Terbutaline rapidly crosses the placenta to the fetus (2). In seven women given 0.25 mg IV during the second stage of labor, cord blood levels 7–60 minutes after the dose ranged from 12% to 55% (mean 36%) of maternal serum.

Terbutaline has been used as a tocolytic agent since the early 1970s (3,4). The incidence of maternal side effects is usually low (e.g., 5% or less) but may be severe (3,5–9). A 1983 review listed the more serious side effects of parenteral β-sympathomimetic therapy (e.g., terbutaline, ritodrine) as pulmonary edema, myocardial ischemia, cardiac arrhythmias, cerebral vasospasm, hypotension, hyperglycemia, and miscellaneous metabolic alterations (hypokalemia, increased serum lactate, and a decrease in measured hemoglobin concentration) (10). The more serious adverse effects are seen with continuous infusions of these drugs. Avoidance of this route of administration as well as careful selection of patients, appropriate dosing, and close monitoring of patient status may help to prevent serious maternal effects.

Terbutaline may cause fetal and maternal tachycardia (3,5–7). Fetal rates are usually less than 175 beats/minute (6). As mentioned previously, maternal hypotension may occur, especially in the bleeding patient (10). More commonly, increases in systolic pressure and decreases in diastolic pressure occur with no reduction in mean arterial pressure and, thus, do not adversely affect the fetus (7,10,11).

Like all β-mimetics, terbutaline may cause transient maternal hyperglycemia followed by an increase in serum insulin levels (3,12,13). Sustained neonatal hypoglycemia may be observed if maternal effects have not terminated before delivery (12). Maternal glucose intolerance was observed at 1 hour in 19 of 30 patients receiving oral terbutaline for at least 1 week (14). Although macrosomia was not observed, the birth weights (after adjustment for gestational age) of infants from terbutaline-treated mothers had a tendency to be greater than those of babies from comparable controls (14).

Sudden, unexplained intrapartum death in a fetus at 30 weeks' gestation occurred 5 hours after the start of an IV infusion of terbutaline for premature labor (15). No evidence of uterine, placental, or fetal anomalies was discovered.

Myocardial necrosis in a newborn was reported in 1991 (16). A continuous SC infusion of terbutaline (initial dose 0.5 mg/hour) was started at 25 weeks' gestation for premature labor in a 22-year-old woman with gestational diabetes. Therapy was continued until delivery at 37 weeks' gestation of a 2850-g male infant. Tachypnea (80–100 breaths/minute) developed shortly after birth and chest radiography demonstrated mild cardiomegaly with increased pulmonary vascularity (16). A right ventricular biopsy obtained during cardiac catheterization showed marked myocardial fiber degeneration and focal bizarre nuclear dysmorphism (16). These findings were believed to be caused by catecholamine excess. Normal electrocardiogram and echocardiogram were found on examination at 1 month of age.

Maternal liver impairment was reported in a patient after 1 week of continuous IV administration of terbutaline (17). Therapy was stopped and 1 week later, a healthy newborn was delivered without signs of liver toxicity.

A paradoxical reaction to terbutaline was observed in a patient after 0.25 mg IV produced marked uterine hypertonus and subsequent severe fetal bradycardia (<50 beats/minute) (18). A healthy baby was delivered by emergency cesarean section.

Terbutaline has been used frequently to treat intrapartum fetal distress (19–23). The mechanism of the beneficial effects on fetal pH and heart rate are thought to be caused by relief of the ischemia produced by uterine contractions on the placental circulation.

Although maternal complications may occur, few direct adverse effects, other than transient tachycardia and hypoglycemia, and the single report of myocardial necrosis, have been observed in the fetus or newborn. In many studies, neonatal complications are minimal or nonexistent (24–28). Compared with controls, prophylactic terbutaline in low-risk patients with twin gestations has produced significant gains in birth weights caused by longer gestational times (27). In addition, terbutaline decreases the incidence of neonatal respiratory distress syndrome in a manner similar to other β-mimetics (29). Long-term evaluation of infants exposed to terbutaline *in utero* has been reported (30–32). No harmful effects in the infants (2–24 months) have been found.

In summary, terbutaline has been used as a tocolytic since the early 1970s. Only rare reports of serious toxicity in the fetus or newborn have appeared, and although maternal adverse effects are much more common, toxicity in both are no more frequent than with other β-mimetics used for the treatment of premature labor. Avoidance of continuous terbutaline infusions lessens the chance of serious maternal effects. The manufacturer has now categorized the drug as "not indicated for the management of preterm labor," but this was apparently done for regulatory concerns as published information does not support the reclassification.

BREAST FEEDING SUMMARY

RECOMMENDATION: Limited Human Data - Probably Compatible

Terbutaline is excreted into breast milk. In two mothers with chronic asthma about 6–8 weeks postpartum, 5 mg 3 times daily produced mean maternal plasma levels of 1.9–4.8 ng/mL, whereas milk concentrations ranged between 2.5 and 3.8 ng/mL (33). The nursing infants ingested approximately 0.2% of the maternal dose, and the drug could not be detected in their plasma. In the second report, two mothers, both at 3 weeks postpartum and both with chronic asthma, were treated with 2.5 mg 3 times a day (34). Plasma levels varied between 0.97 and 3.07 ng/mL, whereas mean milk levels were 2.76–3.91 ng/mL. Peak milk concentrations occurred at about 4 hours. The milk:plasma ratios of 1.4–2.9 are indicative of ionic trapping in the milk (34). Concentrations of terbutaline were highest in the fat fraction of the milk. Based on calculations, the infants were ingesting approximately 0.7% of the maternal dose.

No symptoms of adrenergic stimulation were observed in the four infants and all exhibited normal development. Long-term effects of this exposure, however, have not been studied. The American Academy of Pediatrics classifies terbutaline as compatible with breast-feeding (35).

References

T

1. Product information. Brethine. Novartis Pharmaceuticals, 2000.
2. Ingemarsson I, Westgren M, Lindberg C, Ahren B, Lundquist I, Carlsson C. Single injection of terbutaline in term labor: placental transfer and effects on maternal and fetal carbohydrate metabolism. Am J Obstet Gynecol 1981;139:697–701.
3. Haller DL. The use of terbutaline for premature labor. Drug Intell Clin Pharm 1980;14:757–64.
4. Ingemarsson I. Cardiovascular complications of terbutaline for preterm labor. Am J Obstet Gynecol 1982; 142:117.
5. Andersson KE, Bengtsson LP, Gustafson I, Ingemarsson I. The relaxing effect of terbutaline on the human uterus during term labor. Am J Obstet Gynecol 1975;121:602–9.
6. Ingermarrson I. Effect of terbutaline on premature labor. A double-blind placebo-controlled study. Am J Obstet Gynecol 1976;125:520–4.
7. Ravindran R, Viegas OJ, Padilla LM, LaBlonde P. Anesthetic considerations in pregnant patients receiving terbutaline therapy. Anesth Analg (Cleve) 1980;59:391–2.
8. Katz M, Robertson PA, Creasy RK. Cardiovascular complications associated with terbutaline treatment for preterm labor. Am J Obstet Gynecol 1981;139:605–8.
9. Ingemarsson I, Bengtsson B. A five-year experience with terbutaline for preterm labor: low rate of severe side effects. Obstet Gynecol 1985;66:176–80.
10. Benedetti TJ. Maternal complications of parenteral β-sympathomimetic therapy for premature labor. Am J Obstet Gynecol 1983;145:1–6.

11. Vargas GC, Macedo GJ, Amved AR, Lowenberg FE. Terbutaline, a new uterine inhibitor. Ginecol Obstet Mex 1974;36:75–88.
12. Epstein MF, Nicholls RN, Stubblefield PG. Neonatal hypoglycemia after beta-sympathomimetic tocolytic therapy. J Pediatr 1979;94:449–53.
13. Westgren M, Carlsson C, Lindholm T, Thysell H, Ingemarsson I. Continuous maternal glucose measurements and fetal glucose and insulin levels after administration of terbutaline in term labor. Acta Obstet Gynecol Scand Suppl 1982;108:63–5.
14. Main EK, Main DM, Gabbe SG. Chronic oral terbutaline tocolytic therapy is associated with maternal glucose intolerance. Am J Obstet Gynecol 1987;157:644–7.
15. Lenke RR, Trupin S. Sudden, unforeseen fetal death in a woman being treated for premature labor: a case report. J Reprod Med 1984;29:872–4.
16. Fletcher SE, Fyfe DA, Case CL, Wiles HB, Upshur JK, Newman RB. Myocardial necrosis in a newborn after long-term maternal subcutaneous terbutaline infusion for suppression of preterm labor. Am J Obstet Gynecol 1991;165:1401–4.
17. Suzuki M, Inagaki K, Kihira M, Matsuzawa K, Ishikawa K, Ishizuka T. Maternal liver impairment associated with prolonged high-dose administration of terbutaline for premature labor. Obstet Gynecol 1985;66:14S–15S.
18. Bhat N, Seifer D, Hensleigh P. Paradoxical response to intravenous terbutaline. Am J Obstet Gynecol 1985;153:310–1.
19. Tejani NA, Verma UL, Chatterjee S, Mittelmann S. Terbutaline in the management of acute intrapartum fetal acidosis. J Reprod Med 1983;28:857–61.
20. Barrett JM. Fetal resuscitation with terbutaline during eclampsia-induced uterine hypertonus. Am J Obstet Gynecol 1984;150:895.
21. Ingemarsson I, Arulkumaran S, Ratnam SS. Single injection of terbutaline in term labor. I. Effect on fetal pH in cases with prolonged bradycardia. Am J Obstet Gynecol 1985;153:859–65.
22. Ingemarsson I, Arulkumaran S, Ratnam SS. Single injection of terbutaline in term labor. II. Effect on uterine activity. Am J Obstet Gynecol 1985;153:865–9.
23. Mendez-Bauer C, Shekarloo A, Cook V, Freese U. Treatment of acute intrapartum fetal distress by β2-sympathomimetics. Am J Obstet Gynecol 1987;156:638–42.
24. Stubblefield PG, Heyl PS. Treatment of premature labor with subcutaneous terbutaline. Obstet Gynecol 1982;59:457–62.
25. Caritis SN, Carson D, Greebon D, McCormick M, Edelstone DI, Mueller-Heubach E. A comparison of terbutaline and ethanol in the treatment of preterm labor. Am J Obstet Gynecol 1982;142:183–90.
26. Kaul AF, Osathanondy R, Safon LE, Frigoletto FD Jr, Friedman PA. The management of preterm labor with the calcium channel-blocking agent nifedipine combined with the β-mimetic terbutaline. Drug Intell Clin Pharm 1985;19:369–71.
27. O'Leary JA. Prophylactic tocolysis of twins. Am J Obstet Gynecol 1986;154:904–5.
28. Arias F, Knight AB, Tomich PB. A retrospective study on the effects of steroid administration and prolongation of the latent phase in patients with preterm premature rupture of the membranes. Am J Obstet Gynecol 1986;154:1059–63.
29. Bergman B, Hedner T. Antepartum administration of terbutaline and the incidence of hyaline membrane disease in preterm infants. Acta Obstet Gynecol Scand 1978;57:217–21.
30. Wallace R, Caldwell D, Ansbacher R, Otterson W. Inhibition of premature labor by terbutaline. Obstet Gynecol 1978;51:387–93.
31. Svenningsen NW. Follow-up studies on preterm infants after maternal β-receptor agonist treatment. Acta Obstet Gynecol Scand Suppl 1982;108:67–70.
32. Karlsson K, Krantz M, Hamberger L. Comparison of various β-mimetics on preterm labor, survival and development of the child. J Perinat Med 1980;8:19–26.
33. Lonnerholm G, Lindstrom B. Terbutaline excretion into breast milk. Br J Clin Pharmacol 1982;13:729–30.
34. Boreus LO, de Chateau P, Lindberg C, Nyberg L. Terbutaline in breast milk. Br J Clin Pharmacol 1982;13:731–2.
35. Committee on Drugs, American Academy of Pediatrics. The transfer of drugs and other chemicals into human milk. Pediatrics 2001;108:776–89.

Name: **TERCONAZOLE** Risk Factor: **C_M**

Class: **Antifungal**

FETAL RISK SUMMARY

RECOMMENDATION: Limited Human Data - Animal Data Suggest Low Risk

Terconazole is available as either a vaginal cream or suppositories. The antifungal agent is absorbed into the systemic circulation in humans after vaginal administration (1). Fetal exposure to the drug is also possible by direct transfer of terconazole across the amniotic membranes after vaginal administration (1).

No evidence of teratogenicity was found after oral and SC administration of terconazole to rats and rabbits, but some embryotoxicity was observed at high doses (1).

No published reports describing the use of terconazole in human pregnancy have been located.

In a surveillance study of Michigan Medicaid recipients conducted between 1985 and 1992 involving 229,101 completed pregnancies, 1,167 newborns had been exposed to terconazole during the 1st trimester (F. Rosa, personal communication, FDA, 1993). A total of 34 (2.9%) major birth defects were observed (48 expected). Specific data were available for six defect categories, including (observed/expected) 14/12 cardiovascular defects, 0/2 oral clefts, 0/0.5 spina bifida, 3/3 polydactyly, 1/2 limb reduction defects, and 1/3 hypospadias. These data do not support an association between the drug and congenital defects.

BREAST FEEDING SUMMARY

RECOMMENDATION: No Human Data - Probably Compatible

No reports describing the use of terconazole during lactation have been located.

Reference

1. Product information. Terazol. Ortho Pharmaceutical, 1993.

Name:	**TERFENADINE**	Risk Factor:	C_M
Class:	**Antihistamine**		

FETAL RISK SUMMARY

RECOMMENDATION: Compatible

No reports linking this second-generation histamine H_1-receptor antagonist with congenital anomalies or other adverse fetal outcomes have been located. Similarly, no abnormalities or adverse fetal effects were observed in rats fed 300 mg/kg/day or in rabbits given 500 mg/kg/day (1).

One report described the use of terfenadine in a woman with hereditary angioedema and immunoglobulin A deficiency who was treated throughout most of her pregnancy with the drug. She eventually delivered a 2523-g male infant at 36 weeks' gestation (2). No details of the infant's condition were provided.

A 1994 abstract summarized the results of a prospective study that compared the outcomes of 134 women who took terfenadine during the 1st and early 2nd trimesters with 134 matched controls (3). Nine (6.7%) of the study patients were lost to follow-up. Among the remaining 125 study patients, there were 98 (78.4%) normal outcomes, 16 (12.8%) spontaneous abortions, 4 (3.2%) elective terminations, 1 (0.8%) stillbirth (cord accident), and 6 (4.8%) infants with congenital malformations. The malformations observed in the 6 infants were: trisomy 21 (maternal age 41 years), a chromosomal anomaly (45,X/46,XY), patent ductus arteriosus, hemangioma, underdeveloped earlobe, and dislocated hips. No differences were found in the outcomes between the study patients and the control group (3).

In a surveillance study of Michigan Medicaid recipients conducted between 1985 and 1992 involving 229,101 completed pregnancies, 1034 newborns had been exposed to terfenadine during the 1st trimester (F. Rosa, personal communication, FDA, 1993). A total of

51 (4.9%) major birth defects were observed (44 expected). Specific data were available for six defect categories, including (observed/expected) 13/10 cardiovascular defects, 2/2 oral clefts, 0/0.5 spina bifida, 12/3 polydactyly, 3/2 limb reduction defects, and 2/2 hypospadias. The suggested association of terfenadine with polydactyly remains to be confirmed in other studies.

A 2002 study found no increased risk of teratogenicity or other pregnancy or newborn complications for antihistamines when used in early pregnancy for the treatment of nausea and vomiting ($N = 12{,}394$) and allergy ($N = 5041$) (4). Terfenadine was used by 1164 women.

BREAST FEEDING SUMMARY

RECOMMENDATION: Limited Human Data - Probably Compatible

The excretion of terfenadine into human milk was described in a 1995 report (5). Four lactating women were given terfenadine (60 mg every 12 hours for 4 doses), and then milk and plasma samples were collected after the last dose at various times for 30 hours. None of the parent compound was detected in the milk or plasma. The maximum concentrations of the active metabolite in the plasma and milk were 309 and 41 ng/mL, respectively, both occurring approximately 4 hours after the last dose. Based on the 12-hour excretion, the mean milk:plasma ratio was 0.21. The maximum exposure of a nursing infant was estimated to be 0.45% of the recommended maternal weight-corrected dose (5).

Although the amounts of terfenadine measured in the above study appear to be clinically insignificant, there is still no reported experience of infants nursing while their mothers are being treated with the antihistamine. Thus, the clinical effects of exposure to terfenadine via the milk are still unknown. The American Academy of Pediatrics classifies terfenadine as compatible with breast-feeding (6).

References

1. Gibson JP, Huffman KW, Newborne JW. Preclinical safety studies with terfenadine. Arzneimittelforschung 1982;22:1179–84. As cited in Shepard TH. *Catalog of Teratogenic Agents*. 6th ed. Baltimore, MD: Johns Hopkins University Press, 1989:599.
2. Peters M, Ryley D, Lockwood C. Hereditary angioedema and immunoglobulin A deficiency in pregnancy. Obstet Gynecol 1988;72:454–5.
3. Schick B, Hom M, Librizzi R, Arnon J, Donnenfeld A. Terfenadine (Seldane) exposure in early pregnancy (abstract). Teratology 1994;49:417.
4. Kallen B. Use of antihistamine drugs in early pregnancy and delivery outcome. J Matern Fetal Neonatal Med 2002;11:146–52.
5. Lucas BD Jr, Purdy CY, Scarim SK, Benjamin S, Abel SR, Hilleman DE. Terfenadine pharmacokinetics in breast milk in lactating women. Clin Pharmacol Ther 1995;57:398–402.
6. Committee on Drugs, American Academy of Pediatrics. The transfer of drugs and other chemicals into human milk. Pediatrics 2001;108:776–89.

Name:	**TERPIN HYDRATE**	Risk Factor:	**D**
Class:	**Respiratory Drug (Expectorant)**		

FETAL RISK SUMMARY

RECOMMENDATION: Contraindicated (Significant Alcohol Content)

Although no longer approved as an expectorant, this agent has been used for a number of years and may still be available for this indication. At one time it was combined with codeine as an expectorant-antitussive proprietary mixture. No animal reproductive studies of terpin hydrate have been located.

The Collaborative Perinatal Project monitored 50,282 mother-child pairs, 146 of whom had 1st trimester exposure to terpin hydrate (1, pp. 378–9). Congenital malformations were observed in 13 (standardized relative risk [SRR] 1.29) of the newborns. For use anytime in pregnancy, 1,762 mother-child pairs were exposed (1, p. 442). Twenty-nine (30.6 expected) of the newborns had anomalies (SRR 0.95). Neither of the exposure periods indicates an increased fetal risk from the drug. Specific malformations or conditions identified following use of terpin hydrate anytime in pregnancy were any benign tumors 9 (SRR 1.9), clubfoot 11 (SRR 1.2), and inguinal hernia 34 (SRR 1.4) (1, p. 496). However, these data are uninterpretable without independent confirmation from other studies. Any positive or negative associations may have occurred by chance (1, p. 481). A 1964 study found no abnormalities in six infants exposed *in utero* to terpin hydrate (with or without codeine) during the 1st trimester (2). Neither of the above studies specified the doses consumed by the patients.

The recommended dose of terpin hydrate, which contains approximately 42% ethanol, is 5–10 mL 3 or 4 times daily. The maximum daily dose would therefore contain about 17 mL of absolute ethanol or about one-half of the amount that has been shown to produce mild fetal alcohol syndrome (see Ethanol). Because the minimum amount of ethanol exposure required to produce fetal developmental toxicity is unknown, this product should be avoided during pregnancy.

BREAST FEEDING SUMMARY

RECOMMENDATION: Contraindicated

No reports describing the use of terpin hydrate during lactation have been located. Because of the high ethanol content (about 42%) of terpin hydrate, frequent use of this product should be avoided during lactation (see also Ethanol).

References

1. Heinonen OP, Slone D, Shapiro S. *Birth Defects and Drugs in Pregnancy*. Littleton, MA: Publishing Sciences Group, 1977.
2. Mellin GW. Drugs in the first trimester of pregnancy and the fetal life of *Homo sapiens*. Am J Obstet Gynecol 1964;90:1169–80.

Name: **TESTOSTERONE**	Risk Factor: X_M
Class: **Androgenic Hormone**	

FETAL RISK SUMMARY

RECOMMENDATION: Contraindicated

Testosterone is a natural hormone with androgenic and anabolic properties. Testosterone and its derivatives (e.g., methyltestosterone) are primarily indicated as replacement therapy in male hypogonadal disorders secondary to various causes. Preparations of testosterone products are available for oral, buccal, topical, and IM administration. About 80% of testosterone is bound to sex-hormone binding globulin. Several metabolic pathways of testosterone have been identified, including aromatization to form estrogenic derivatives.

The plasma elimination half-life of testosterone is the range of 10 to 100 minutes (1). Testosterone rapidly crosses the human placenta to the embryo or fetus (2).

In a 1987 study, testosterone exposure of female rhesus monkeys *in utero* appeared to have induced irreversible changes in the pattern of luteinizing hormone secretion in adult life (3). Seventeen female pseudohermaphrodites (exposed *in utero*) and 24 normal females were studied at about 13–14 years of age. All subject and control animals demonstrated evidence of ovulatory menstrual cycles. The 17 monkeys with pseudohermaphroditism had been exposed *in utero* to testosterone that had resulted in external genital masculinization/obliteration of the external vaginal orifice or clitoromegaly alone (degree of genital masculinization was dependent on the timing of exposure). Compared to controls, significant increases in the ratio of luteinizing hormone to follicle-stimulating hormone in the luteal and follicular phases of the ovulatory menstrual cycles were measured in the pseudohermaphrodites (3).

A 1957 report cited a number of animal studies published in the late 1940s and early 1950s that had demonstrated that administration of testosterone or its derivatives to pregnant animals resulted in masculinization of female fetuses (4). A later report also reviewed the animal data and specifically evaluated the dose and fetal age associated with masculinization of female fetuses (2).

Testosterone and its derivatives are contraindicated in pregnancy because they cause virilization of female fetuses (4–15). Two case reports, one in 1953 and the other in 1955 (both in German), were the first to describe female pseudohermaphroditism in human infants after exposure to a testosterone derivative (methylandrostenediol; methandriol) (5) or testosterone/methyltestosterone/estradiol (6).

The first English language cases of nonadrenal human female pseudohermaphroditism secondary to maternal use of testosterone were published in 1957. A woman was treated with oral methyltestosterone 20 mg/day for alopecia starting in the 7th week of pregnancy and continuing irregularly until term (total dose 1.5 g) (4). During treatment, the woman noted a deepening voice, hirsutism, and a male-pattern of body hair, as well as partial resolution of her alopecia. Sex of the newborn, which initially appeared to be male, was not established until 7 months of age when the diagnosis of female pseudohermaphroditism was made (4). In the second case, a woman at 10 weeks' gestation was treated with two doses of testosterone (100 mg IM on day 1 and 3) and 51 days of oral methyltestosterone (30 mg/day) for nausea and vomiting of pregnancy (7). The therapy was discontinued because of the woman's deepening voice. A 3.4-kg infant was delivered at term that had cyanosis and bradycardia of short duration. Although the sex was ambiguous (small penis, undescended testes), the infant was raised as a male. Detailed examination at 6 months of age revealed the infant to be a female (7).

Other cases have described nonadrenal female pseudohermaphroditism secondary to exposures to methyltestosterone or testosterone, sometimes in combination with estradiol or other estrogens, in the 1st trimester (8–15). In each of these cases, examination of the newborn infant usually revealed a hypoplastic penis, cryptorchidism, and hypospadias. The actual diagnosis of female sex with clitoral hypertrophy, with or without fused labia, and an occasionally absent vagina, was made weeks to months after birth. Surgery was usually required to correct the genital abnormalities. In two cases, the infants had been exposed to methyltestosterone or testosterone during the first 12 or 16 weeks of pregnancy (12,13). They were later diagnosed as females and the genital abnormalities were corrected surgically. In their early 20s, both had normal pregnancies and gave birth to healthy infants (13,14). In another case, the mother received daily oral methyltestosterone from the 14th week until term for breast engorgement (2). In addition, she was given four IM doses

T

of testosterone (total dose 115 mg) between the 14th and 35th weeks of gestation). Except for clitoral hypertrophy, no other signs of virilization were observed in infant or the mother (2).

The only report of structural defects, other than genital, associated with the use of testosterone appeared in a 1953 article (16). Three infants with limb anomalies had been exposed during the 1st trimester to a combination of testosterone and progesterone (16).

The Collaborative Perinatal Project monitored 50,282 mother-child pairs, 26 of whom were exposed to a group of miscellaneous hormones during the 1st trimester (17). Among the 26 cases, three were exposed to testosterone, four to methandrostenolone, and one each to methyltestosterone, fluoxymesterone, and an unspecified male hormone. There were no congenital malformations observed in the 26 exposures (17).

In summary, 1st trimester *in utero* exposure of female fetuses to exogenous testosterone or its derivatives causes clitoral hypertrophy, fused or partial fused labia, and, possibly, absent vagina. These varying degrees of masculinization are referred to as nonadrenal female pseudohermaphroditism. Exposure to testosterone hormones at any gestational age is associated with clitoral hypertrophy (18). However, to cause labial-scrotal fusion, exposure must occur before the 10th or 11th fetal week when female differentiation of external genitalia is complete (18). Other than the genital abnormalities, testosterone and its derivatives do not appear to cause structural defects. Only one report of nongenital malformations after testosterone exposure has been published, but this association lacks confirmation. However, a study in monkeys has suggested that long-term, potentially permanent changes in the central nervous system of female offspring may result from *in utero* testosterone exposure. Apparently, this has not been studied in humans. Testosterone and its derivatives are contraindicated at any time during pregnancy.

BREAST FEEDING SUMMARY

RECOMMENDATION: Contraindicated

Testosterone, usually combined with an estrogen, has been used to suppress lactation and to treat postpartum breast pain and engorgement (19–29). Testosterone suppresses lactation apparently by prolactin inhibition (29). Although the amount of testosterone administered was very large, no cases of virilization or other adverse effects attributable to the androgen have been reported. The combination, however, is no longer used because the estrogen/testosterone combination was associated with frequent rebound lactation and an increased incidence of postpartum thromboembolic disease (29).

Although testosterone inhibits prolactin, suckling or any breast manipulation may antagonize the inhibitory effect (21). This has been shown in cases where a mother has received the testosterone/estrogen combination, then changed her mind and breast-fed her infant. The amounts of testosterone excreted into milk have apparently not been determined. The absence of reports of adverse effects in nursing infants probably indicates that the short-term exposure is benign. However, the effects from long-term maternal use of testosterone or its derivatives on a nursing infant have not been studied. Therefore, breast-feeding should be halted if these agents are required.

References

1. Parfitt K, editor. *Martindale. The Complete Drug Reference*. 32nd ed. London, UK: Pharmaceutical Press, 1999:1464–6.
2. Grumbach MM, Ducharme JR. The effects of androgens on fetal sexual development. Fertil Steril 1960;11:157–80.
3. Dumesic DA, Abbott DH, Eisner JR, Goy RW. Prenatal exposure of female rhesus monkeys to testosterone

propionate increases serum luteinizing hormone levels in adulthood. Fertil Steril 1997;67:155–63.
4. Hayles AB, Nolan RB. Female pseudohermaphroditism: report of case in an infant born of a mother receiving methyltestosterone during pregnancy. Proc Staff Meet Mayo Clin 1957;32:41–4.
5. Zander J, Muller HA. Uber die methylandrosteniolbehandlung wahrend emer schwangerschaft. Geburtschilfe Frauenheilkd 1953;13:216–4. As cited by Schardein JL. *Chemically Induced Birth Defects*. 3rd ed. New York, NY: Marcel Dekker, 2000:286.
6. Hoffman F, Overzier C, Uhde G. Zur frage der hormonanlen frzeugung fataler zwittenbildungen beim menschen. Geburtschilfe Frauenheilkd 1955; 15:1061–70. As cited by Schardein JL. *Chemically Induced Birth Defects*. 3rd ed. New York, NY: Marcel Dekker, 2000:286.
7. Grunwaldt E, Bates T. Nonadrenal female pseudohermaphrodism after administration of testosterone to mother during pregnancy. Pediatrics 1957;20. 503–5.
8. Nellhaus G. Artificially induced female pseudohermaphroditism. N Engl J Med 1958;258:935–8.
9. Gold AP, Michael AF Jr. Testosterone-induced female pseudohermaphrodism. J Pediatr 1958;52:279–83.
10. Moncrieff A. Non-adrenal female pseudohermaphroditism associated with hormone administration in pregnancy. Lancet 1958;2:267–8.
11. Black JA, Bentley JFR. Effect on the foetus of androgens given during pregnancy. Lancet 1959;1:21–4.
12. Dewhurst CJ, Gordon RR. Change of sex. Lancet 1963;2:1213–6.
13. Reschini E, Giustina G, D'Alberton A, Candiani GB. Female pseudohermaphroditism due to maternal androgen administration: 25-year follow-up. Lancet 1985; 1:1226.
14. Dewhurst J, Gordon RR. Fertility following change of sex: a follow-up. Lancet 1984;2:1461–2.
15. Bisset WH, Bain AD, Gauld IK. Female pseudohermaphrodite presenting with bilateral cryptorchidism. Br Med J 1966;1:279–80.
16. Martinie-Dubousquet J. Embryopathy entailed by administration of sex hormones to the mother. Rev Pathol Gen Comp 1953;53:1065–76. As cited by Schardein JL. *Chemically Induced Birth Defects*. 3rd ed. New York, NY: Marcel Dekker, 2000:289.
17. Heinonen OP, Slone D, Shapiro S. *Birth Defects and Drugs in Pregnancy*. Littleton, MA: Publishing Sciences Group, 1977:389–90.
18. Reilly WA. Hormone therapy during pregnancy: effects on the fetus and newborn. Q Rev Pediatr 1958;13:198–202.
19. Iliya FA, Safon L, O'Leary JA. Testosterone enanthate (180 mg.) and estradiol valerate (8 mg.) for suppression of lactation: a double-blind evaluation. Obstet Gynecol 1966;27:643–5.
20. Morris JA, Creasy RK, Hohe PT. Inhibition of puerperal lactation. Double-blind comparison of chlorotrianisene, testosterone enanthate and estradiol valerate and placebo. Obstet Gynecol 1970;36:107–14.
21. Vorherr H. Suppression of postpartum lactation. Postgrad Med 1972;52:145–52.
22. Ng KH, Lee KH. Inhibition of postpartum lactation with single-dose drugs. Aust N Z J Obstet Gynaecol 1972;12:59–61.
23. McNicol E, Struthers JO. A combined/oestrogen/progestogen/testosterone agent for the inhibition of lactation. Br J Clin Pract 1972;26:567–8.
24. Llewellyn-Jones D, Lawrenson K. A new method of inhibition of lactation. Med J Aust 1973;2:780–1.
25. Schwartz DJ, Evans PC, Garcia CR, Rickels K, Fisher E. A clinical study of lactation suppression. Obstet Gynecol 1973;42:599–606.
26. Louviere RL, Upton RT. Evaluation of Deladumone OB in the suppression of postpartum lactation. Am J Obstet Gynecol 1975;121:641–2.
27. Biggs JSG, Hacker N, Andrews E, Munro C. Bromocriptine, methyltestosterone and placebo for inhibition of physiologic lactation. Med J Aust 1978;2(3 Suppl): 23–5.
28. Welti H, Paiva F, Felber JP. Prevention and interruption of postpartum lactation with bromocriptine (Parlodel) and effect on plasma prolactin, compared with a hormonal preparation (Ablacton). Eur J Obstet Gynecol Reprod Biol 1979;9:35–9.
29. Kochenour NK. Lactation suppression. Clin Obstet Gynecol 1980;23:1045–59.

Name: **TETANUS/DIPHTHERIA TOXOIDS (ADULT)** Risk Factor: C_M

Class: **Toxoid**

T

FETAL RISK SUMMARY

RECOMMENDATION: Compatible - Maternal Benefit >> Embryo/Fetal Risk

Tetanus/diphtheria toxoids for adult use are the specific toxoids of *Clostridium tetani* and *Corynebacterium diphtheriae* adsorbed onto aluminum compounds. Reproduction studies in animals have not been conducted with this product (1).

In a 1999 study using the Hungarian Case-Control Surveillance of Congenital Abnormalities, 1980–1994, database, exposure to tetanus toxoid during pregnancy was examined in

21,563 women who had offspring with congenital defects (2). The control group consisted of 35,727 women who had infants without defects. Exposure to tetanus toxoid occurred in 25 (0.12%) case women (13 in the 1st trimester) compared to 33 (0.09%) control women (17 in the 1st trimester). The difference was not significant (2).

Tetanus and diphtheria produce severe morbidity in the mother with mortality rates of 30% and 10%, respectively (3,4). In neonates, the tetanus mortality rate is 60%. The risk to the fetus from tetanus/diphtheria toxoids is unknown (3,4). The American College of Obstetricians and Gynecologists *Technical Bulletin* No. 160 recommends the use of tetanus/diphtheria toxoids in pregnancy for those women at risk who lack the primary series of immunizations or in whom no booster has been given within the past 10 years (3).

BREAST FEEDING SUMMARY

RECOMMENDATION: No Human Data - Probably Compatible

No data are available.

References

1. Product information. Tetanus and Diphtheria Toxoids Adsorbed. Lederle Laboratories, 2000.
2. Czeizel AE, Rockenbauer M. Tetanus toxoid and congenital abnormalities. Int J Gynecol Obstet 1999;64:253–8.
3. American College of Obstetricians and Gynecologists. Immunization during pregnancy. *Technical Bulletin*, Number 160, October 1991.
4. Amstey MS. Vaccination in pregnancy. Clin Obstet Gynaecol 1983;10:13–22.

Name: **TETRABENAZINE** Risk Factor: **C**

Class: **Tranquilizer**

FETAL RISK SUMMARY

RECOMMENDATION: Limited Human Data - No Relevant Animal Data

Tetrabenazine has been used in pregnancy for the treatment of chorea gravidarum (1). Therapy was started late in the 2nd trimester in one patient. No drug-induced fetal or newborn effects were observed. A small ventricular septal defect was probably not related to tetrabenazine exposure.

BREAST FEEDING SUMMARY

RECOMMENDATION: No Human Data - Potential Toxicity

No reports describing the use of tetrabenazine during lactation have been located.

Reference

1. Lubbe WF, Walker EB. Chorea gravidarum associated with circulating lupus anticoagulant: Successful outcome of pregnancy with prednisone and aspirin therapy. Case report. Br J Obstet Gynaecol 1983;90:487–90.

Name:	TETRACYCLINE	Risk Factor:	D
Class:	Antibiotic (Tetracycline)		

FETAL RISK SUMMARY

RECOMMENDATION: Contraindicated - 2nd and 3rd Trimesters

Tetracyclines are a class of antibiotics that should be used with extreme caution, if at all, in pregnancy. The following discussion, unless otherwise noted, applies to all members of this class. Problems attributable to the use of the tetracyclines during or around the gestational period can be classified into four areas:

Adverse effects on fetal teeth and bones
Maternal liver toxicity
Congenital defects
Miscellaneous effects

Placental transfer of a tetracycline was first demonstrated in 1950 (1). The tetracyclines were considered safe for the mother and fetus and were routinely used for maternal infections during the following decade (2–5). It was not until 1961 that an intense yellow-gold fluorescence was observed in the mineralized structures of a fetal skeleton whose mother had taken tetracycline just before delivery (6). Following this report, a 2-year-old child was described whose erupted deciduous teeth formed normally but were stained a bright yellow because of tetracycline exposure *in utero* (7). Fluorescence under ultraviolet light and yellow-colored deciduous teeth that eventually changed to yellow-brown were associated with maternal tetracycline ingestion during pregnancy by several other investigators (8–22). An increase in enamel hypoplasia and caries was initially suspected but later shown not to be related to *in utero* tetracycline exposure (14,15,22). Newborn growth and development were normal in all of these reports, although tetracycline has been shown to cause inhibition of fibula growth in premature infants (6). The mechanism for the characteristic dental defect produced by tetracycline is related to the potent chelating ability of the drug (13). Tetracycline forms a complex with calcium orthophosphate and becomes incorporated into bones and teeth undergoing calcification. In the latter structure, this complex causes a permanent discoloration, as remodeling and calcium exchange do not occur after calcification is completed. Because the deciduous teeth begin to calcify at around 5 or 6 months *in utero*, use of tetracycline after this time will result in staining.

The first case linking tetracycline with acute fatty metamorphosis of the liver in a pregnant woman was described in 1963 (23), although two earlier papers reported the disease without associating it with the drug (24,25). This rare but often fatal syndrome usually follows IV dosing of more than 2 g/day. Many of the pregnant patients were being treated for pyelonephritis (24–37). Tetracycline-induced hepatotoxicity differs from acute fatty liver of pregnancy in that it is not unique to pregnant women and reversal of the disease does not occur with pregnancy termination (38). The symptoms include jaundice, azotemia, acidosis, and terminal irreversible shock. Pancreatitis and nonoliguric renal failure are often related findings. The fetus may not be affected directly, but as a result of the maternal pathology, stillborns and premature births are common. In an experimental study, increasing doses of tetracycline caused increasing fatty metamorphosis of the liver (39). The possibility that chronic maternal use of tetracycline before conception could result in fatal hepatotoxicity of pregnancy has been raised (36). The authors speculated that tetracycline deposited in the bone of a 21-year-old patient was released during pregnancy, resulting in liver damage.

In a surveillance study of Michigan Medicaid recipients conducted between 1985 and 1992 involving 229,101 completed pregnancies, a large number of newborns had been exposed to the tetracycline group of antibiotics during the 1st trimester (F. Rosa, personal communication, FDA, 1993). For four tetracyclines (T = tetracycline; D = doxycycline; O = oxytetracycline; M = minocycline), specific data were available for six defect categories, including (observed/expected):

	T	D	O	M
Number of exposures	1,004	1,795	26	181
Number of major defects	47	78	1	8
Percent	4.7%	4.3%	3.8%	4.4%
Number of major defects expected	43	76	1	7
Cardiovascular defects	12/10	20/18	0/0.3	2/2
Oral clefts	1/2	0/3	0/0	1/0.5
Spina bifida	0/0.5	2/1	0/0	0/0
Polydactyly	5/3	7/5	0/0	0/0.5
Limb-reduction defects	1/2	0/3	0/0	0/0.5
Hypospadias	1/2	4/4	0/0	0/0.5

These data do not support an association between the drugs and the specific malformations evaluated.

The Collaborative Perinatal Project monitored 50,282 mother-child pairs, 341 of whom had 1st trimester exposure to tetracycline, 14 to chlortetracycline, 90 to demeclocycline, and 119 to oxytetracycline (40, pp. 297–313). For use anytime in pregnancy, 1336 exposures were recorded for tetracycline, 0 for chlortetracycline, 280 for demeclocycline, and 328 for oxytetracycline (40, p. 435). The findings of this study were as follows:

Tetracycline: Evidence was found to suggest a relationship to minor, but not major, malformations. Three possible associations were found with individual defects, but independent confirmation is required: hypospadias (1st trimester only) (5 cases); inguinal hernia (25 cases); and hypoplasia of limb or part thereof (6 cases) (40, pp. 472, 485).

Chlortetracycline: No evidence was found to suggest a relationship to large categories of major or minor malformations or to individual defects. However, the sample size is extremely small, and safety should not be inferred from these negative results.

Demeclocycline: No evidence was found to suggest a relationship to large categories of major or minor malformations, but the sample size is small (40, pp. 297–313). Two possible associations were found with individual defects, but independent confirmation is required: clubfoot (1st trimester only) (3 cases); and inguinal hernia (8 cases) (40, pp. 472, 485).

Oxytetracycline: Evidence was found to suggest a relationship to large categories of major and minor malformations (40, pp. 297–313). One possible association was found with individual defects, but independent confirmation is required: inguinal hernia (14 cases) (40, pp. 472, 485).

In 1962, a woman treated with tetracycline in the 1st trimester for acute bronchitis delivered an infant with congenital defects of both hands (41,42). The mother had a history of minor congenital defects on her side of the family and doubt was cast on the role of the drug in this anomaly (43). A possible association between the use of tetracyclines in pregnancy or during lactation and congenital cataracts has been reported in four patients (44). The effects of other drugs, including several antibiotics, and maternal infection could not be determined, and a causal relationship to the tetracyclines seems remote. An infant with multiple anomalies whose mother had been treated for acne with clomocycline daily during the first 8 weeks of pregnancy has been described (45). Some of the defects, particularly the incomplete fibrous ankylosis and bone changes, made the authors suspect this tetracycline as the likely cause.

Doxycycline has been used for 10 days very early in the 1st trimester for the treatment of *Mycoplasma* infection in a group of previously infertile women (46). Dosage was based on the patient's weight, varying from 100–300 mg/day. All 43 of the exposed liveborns were normal at 1 year of age. Bubonic plague occurring in a woman at 22 weeks' gestation was successfully treated with tetracycline and streptomycin (47). Long-term evaluation of the infant was not reported.

A 1997 report examined the question of doxycycline-induced teratogenicity in the large population-based data set of the Hungarian Case-Control Surveillance of Congenital Abnormalities, 1980–1992 (48). Some mild defects were excluded, including hemangiomas and minor malformations. Moreover, although an extensive retrospective assessment of drug use during pregnancy was performed, a history of tobacco and alcohol exposure was not obtained because the accuracy of these data were believed to have low validity (48). Among the 32,804 women who had normal infants (controls), 63 (0.19%) had taken doxycycline, whereas 56 (0.30%) of the 18,515 women who delivered infants with congenital anomalies had taken the antibiotic ($p = 0.01$). A case-control pair analysis of exposures during the 2nd and 3rd months of gestation, however, did not show a significant difference among the groups in any of the malformation types.

A 2000 report, using the same database as above, but now for the years 1980–1996, examined the relationship between oral oxytetracycline and congenital malformations (49). Of 22,865 women who had offspring with a congenital defect, 216 (0.9%) had been treated with oxytetracycline, whereas of 38,151 women with offspring without defects, 214 (0.6%) had been treated (odds ratio [OR] 1.7, 95% confidence interval [CI] 1.4–2.0). Analysis of medically documented treatment in the second/third months of gestation revealed significant associations with neural tube defects (NTDs) (OR 9.7, 95% CI 2.0–47.1), cleft palate (OR 17.2, 95% CI 3.5–83.5), and multiple defects (mainly neural tube defects and cardiovascular malformations) (OR 12.9, 95% CI 3.8–44.3). However, these results were based on a very small number of cases: two NTD, two cleft palates, and four multiple defects. The number of cases, OR, and 95% CI occurring in the entire pregnancy for these outcomes were neural tube defects (7, 5.4, 2.4–12.1), cleft palate (3, 4.6, 1.4–15.0), and multiple defects (6, 3.3, 1.4–7.9) (49).

Under miscellaneous effects, two reports have appeared that, although they do not directly relate to effects on the fetus, do directly affect pregnancy. In 1974, a researcher observed that a 1-week administration of 500 mg/day of chlortetracycline to male subjects was sufficient to produce semen levels of the drug averaging 4.5 μg/mL (50). He theorized that tetracycline overdose could modify the fertilizing capacity of human sperm by inhibiting capacitation. Finally, a possible interaction between oral contraceptives and tetracycline resulting in pregnancy has been reported (51). The mechanism for this interaction may involve the interruption of enterohepatic circulation of contraceptive steroids by inhibiting gut bacterial hydrolysis of steroid conjugates, resulting in a lower concentration of circulating steroids.

BREAST FEEDING SUMMARY

RECOMMENDATION: Compatible

Tetracycline is excreted into breast milk in low concentrations. Milk:plasma ratios vary between 0.25 and 1.5 (4,52,53). In a 1996 case, black breast milk was reported in a woman taking minocycline, a semisynthetic derivative of tetracycline (54). She had stopped breast-feeding 18 months before she was treated with minocycline 150 mg/day and topical clindamycin for acne. Within 4 weeks of starting minocycline, milk expressed from her breasts was black. No other abnormalities were found on a diagnostic work-up. Analysis of the milk demonstrated black pigment particles within macrophages, as well as extracellular, that stained positive for iron. The milk contained a high iron concentration (11.9 μmol/g wet weight) (54).

Theoretically, dental staining and inhibition of bone growth could occur in breast-fed infants whose mothers were consuming tetracycline. However, this theoretical possibility seems remote, because tetracycline serum levels in infants exposed in such a manner were undetectable (<0.05 μg/mL) (4). Three potential problems may exist for the nursing infant even though there are no reports in this regard: modification of bowel flora, direct effects on the infant, and interference with the interpretation of culture results if a fever workup is required. The American Academy of Pediatrics classifies tetracycline as compatible with breast-feeding (55).

References

1. Guilbeau JA, Schoenbach EG, Schaub IG, Latham DV. Aureomycin in obstetrics: therapy and prophylaxis. JAMA 1950;143:520–6.
2. Charles D. Placental transmission of antibiotics. J Obstet Gynaecol Br Emp 1954;61:750–7.
3. Gibbons RJ, Reichelderfer TE. Transplacental transmission of demethylchlortetracycline and toxicity studies in premature and full term, newly born infants. Antibiot Med Clin Ther 1960;7:618–22.
4. Posner AC, Prigot A, Konicoff NG. Further observations on the use of tetracycline hydrochloride in prophylaxis and treatment of obstetric infections. In *Antibiotics Annual, 1954–55*. New York, NY: Medical Encyclopedia, 1955:594–8.
5. Posner AC, Konicoff NG, Prigot A. Tetracycline in obstetric infections. In *Antibiotics Annual, 1955–56*. New York, NY: Medical Encyclopedia, 1956: 345–8.
6. Cohlan SQ, Bevelander G, Bross S. Effect of tetracycline on bone growth in the premature infant. Antimicrob Agents Chemother 1961:340–7.
7. Harcourt JK, Johnson NW, Storey E. In vivo incorporation of tetracycline in the teeth of man. Arch Oral Biol 1962;7:431–7.
8. Rendle-Short TJ. Tetracycline in teeth and bone. Lancet 1962;1:1188.
9. Douglas AC. The deposition of tetracycline in human nails and teeth: a complication of long term treatment. Br J Dis Chest 1963;57:44–7.
10. Kutscher AH, Zegarelli EV, Tovell HM, Hochberg B. Discoloration of teeth induced by tetracycline. JAMA 1963;184:586–7.
11. Kline AH, Blattner RJ, Lunin M. Transplacental effect of tetracyclines on teeth. JAMA 1964;188: 178–80.
12. Macaulay JC, Leistyna JA. Preliminary observations on the prenatal administration of demethylchlortetracycline HCl. Pediatrics 1964;34:423–4.
13. Stewart DJ. The effects of tetracyclines upon the dentition. Br J Dermatol 1964;76:374–8.
14. Swallow JN. Discoloration of primary dentition after maternal tetracycline ingestion in pregnancy. Lancet 1964;2:611–2.
15. Porter PJ, Sweeney EA, Golan H, Kass EH. Controlled study of the effect of prenatal tetracycline on primary dentition. Antimicrob Agents Chemother 1965: 668–71.
16. Toaff R, Ravid R. Tetracyclines and the teeth. Lancet 1966;2:281–2.
17. Kutscher AH, Zegarelli EV, Tovell HM, Hochberg B, Hauptman J. Discoloration of deciduous teeth induced by administrations of tetracycline antepartum. Am J Obstet Gynecol 1966;96:291–2.
18. Brearley LJ, Stragis AA, Storey E. Tetracycline-induced tooth changes. Part 1. Prevalence in pre-school children. Med J Aust 1968;2:653–8.
19. Brearley LJ, Storey E. Tetracycline-induced tooth changes. Part 2. Prevalence, localization and nature of staining in extracted deciduous teeth. Med J Aust 1968;2:714–9.
20. Baker KL, Storey E. Tetracycline-induced tooth changes. Part 3. Incidence in extracted first permanent molar teeth. Med J Aust 1970;1:109–13.
21. Anthony JR. Effect on deciduous and permanent teeth of tetracycline deposition in utero. Postgrad Med 1970;48:165–8.
22. Genot MT, Golan HP, Porter PJ, Kass EH. Effect of administration of tetracycline in pregnancy on the primary dentition of the offspring. J Oral Med 1970;25:75–9.

T

23. Schultz JC, Adamson JS Jr, Workman WW, Normal TD. Fatal liver disease after intravenous administration of tetracycline in high dosage. N Engl J Med 1963;269:999–1004.
24. Bruno M, Ober WB. Clinicopathologic conference: jaundice at the end of pregnancy. N Y State J Med 1962;62:3792–800.
25. Lewis PL, Takeda M, Warren MJ. Obstetric acute yellow atrophy. Report of a case. Obstet Gynecol 1963;22:121–7.
26. Briggs RC. Tetracycline and liver disease. N Engl J Med 1963;269:1386.
27. Leonard GL. Tetracycline and liver disease. N Engl J Med 1963;269:1386.
28. Gough GS, Searcy RL. Additional case of fatal liver disease with tetracycline therapy. N Engl J Med 1964;270:157–8.
29. Whalley PJ, Adams RH, Combes B. Tetracycline toxicity in pregnancy. JAMA 1964;189:357–62.
30. Kunelis CT, Peters JL, Edmondson HA. Fatty liver of pregnancy and its relationship to tetracycline therapy. Am J Med 1965;38:359–77.
31. Lew HT, French SW. Tetracycline nephrotoxicity and nonoliguric acute renal failure. Arch Intern Med 1966;118:123–8.
32. Meihoff WE, Pasquale DN, Jacoby WJ Jr. Tetracycline-induced hepatic coma, with recovery. A report of a case. Obstet Gynecol 1967;29:260–5.
33. Aach R, Kissane J. Clinicopathologic conference: a seventeen year old girl with fatty liver of pregnancy following tetracycline therapy. Am J Med 1967;43: 274–83.
34. Whalley PJ, Martin FG, Adams RH, Combes B. Disposition of tetracycline by pregnant women with acute pyelonephritis. Obstet Gynecol 1970;36:821–6.
35. Pride GL, Cleary RE, Hamburger RJ. Disseminated intravascular coagulation associated with tetracycline-induced hepatorenal failure during pregnancy. Am J Obstet Gynecol 1973;115:585–6.
36. Wenk RE, Gebhardt FC, Behagavan BS, Lustgarten JA, McCarthy EF. Tetracycline-associated fatty liver of pregnancy, including possible pregnancy risk after chronic dermatologic use of tetracycline. J Reprod Med 1981;26:135–41.
37. King TM, Bowe ET, D'Esopo DA. Toxic effects of the tetracyclines. Bull Sloane Hosp Women 1964;10: 35–41.
38. Kaplan MM. Acute fatty liver of pregnancy. N Engl J Med 1985;313:367–70.
39. Allen ES, Brown WE. Hepatic toxicity of tetracycline in pregnancy. Am J Obstet Gynecol 1966;95:12–8.
40. Heinonen O, Slone D, Shapiro S. *Birth Defects and Drugs in Pregnancy*. Littleton, MA: Publishing Sciences Group, 1977.
41. Wilson F. Congenital defects in the newborn. Br Med J 1962;2:255.
42. Carter MP, Wilson F. Tetracycline and congenital limb abnormalities. Br Med J 1962;2:407–8.
43. Mennie AT. Tetracycline and congenital limb abnormalities. Br Med J 1962;2:480.
44. Harley JD, Farrar JF, Gray JB, Dunlop IC. Aromatic drugs and congenital cataracts. Lancet 1964;1:472.
45. Corcoran R, Castles JM. Tetracycline for acne vulgaris and possible teratogenesis. Br Med J 1977;2:807–8.
46. Horne HW Jr, Kundsin RB. The role of mycoplasma among 81 consecutive pregnancies: a prospective study. Int J Fertil 1980,25.315–7.
47. Coppes JB. Bubonic plague in pregnancy. J Reprod Med 1980;25:91–5.
48. Czeizel AE, Rockenbauer M. Teratogenic study of doxycycline. Obstet Gynecol 1997;89:524–8.
49. Czeizel AE, Rockenbauer M. A population-based case-control teratologic study of oral oxytetracycline treatment during pregnancy. Eur J Obstet Gynecol Reprod Biol 2000;88:27–33.
50. Briggs M. Tetracycline and steroid hormone binding to human spermatozoa. Acta Endocrinol 1974;75: 785–92.
51. Bacon JF, Shenfield GM. Pregnancy attributable to interaction between tetracycline and oral contraceptives. Br Med J 1980;1:283.
52. Knowles JA. Drugs in milk. Pediatr Curr 1972;21: 28–32.
53. Graf VH, Reimann S. Untersuchungen uber die Konzentration von Pyrrolidino-methyl-tetracycline in der Muttermilch. Dtsch Med Wochenschr 1959;84:1694.
54. Hunt MJ, Salisbury ELC, Grace J, Armati R. Black breast milk due to minocycline therapy. Br J Dermatol 1996;134:943–4.
55. Committee on Drugs, American Academy of Pediatrics. The transfer of drugs and other chemicals into human milk. Pediatrics 2001;108:776–89.

Name: **THALIDOMIDE**	Risk Factor: X_M
Class: **Immunologic Agent (Immunomodulator)**	

FETAL RISK SUMMARY

RECOMMENDATION: Contraindicated

Thalidomide is an immunomodulatory agent used for the acute treatment of erythema nodosum leprosum, a cutaneous manifestation of Hansen's disease (leprosy) (1). The agent was recently approved for use in the United States for the first time, making its debut in 1999. Thalidomide was one of the first drugs that was clearly shown to be a human teratogen and probably has caused more known severe malformations in humans than any other drug.

A large number (>30) of animal (mice, rats, rabbits, and monkeys) reproduction studies conducted with thalidomide were reviewed in a 1976 reference (2). Embryo lethality and teratogenicity (structural and/or functional abnormalities) were noted commonly in some species. Evidence of significant thalidomide teratogenicity was found in monkeys, but in mice and rats, limb reduction defects were not observed and, in some cases, there was no evidence of teratogenicity. Amelia and micromelia were noted in two mouse fetuses and a limb defect in another that closely resembled the defects observed in humans, but these reports were considered inconclusive (2). In a 1983 study with rats, however, increased rates of both embryo lethality and congenital defects involving the skeleton (ribs and spine) and eyes (ophthalmorrhexis and microphthalmia) were observed (3). The authors speculated that the difference in outcome between their study and previous experimental work with rats was possibly due to hydrolysis of the drug before administration, the use of toxic solvents that masked the teratogenic effect of thalidomide, or the low solubility of thalidomide in the solvent that prevented delivery of an effective dose to the target site (3). Experiments in rabbits have consistently revealed fetal limb malformations that are very similar to those seen in human infants exposed *in utero* to thalidomide (4–8). Other anomalies noted in rabbit fetuses included hemangioma of the nose and defects of the skull, nostril, external genitalia, and tail (6). Another study with rabbits observed limb anomalies, arthrogryposis, dysplasia of the kidneys and gallbladder, cleft palate, hernia, and gastric hypoplasia (8). Experiments with chick embryos demonstrated that thalidomide induced cardiovascular anomalies in this species (9).

Several reviews have described the various human systems affected by thalidomide-induced embryopathy (10–19). One of these reviews presented the pregnancy history of two children (twins), born in the United States, who had very different severity of thalidomide embryopathy (10). The first twin, 2211-g female, was born with duodenal atresia, a rectoperineal fistula, and hypoplastic, dislocated thumbs (right thumb worse than left). The other twin, a 2240-g male, had phocomelia of both upper extremities and a midline hemangioma on the forehead. Missing or hypoplastic digits were noted on both hands (10).

The critical period of fetal exposure to thalidomide is 34–50 days after the first day of the last menstrual period (LMP) (20 $\pm$ 1 days to 36 $\pm$ 1 days after conception) (13,16–18). Congenital malformations that have been associated with approximate time periods within this 17-day interval include (days after LMP; when two ranges are shown, the references cited disagreed): anotia (34–38 days); microtia (39–43 days); thumb duplication (35–38 days); thumb aplasia (35–43 days); thumb hypoplasia (38–40 days); thumb triphalangism (46–50 days); eye defects (35–42 days); cardiovascular defects (ductus, conotruncal defects, and septal defects) (36–45 days); duplication of the vagina (35–39 days); cranial nerve palsy (35–37 days); amelia of the arms (38–43 days); phocomelia of the arms (38–47 or 49 days); dislocation of the hip (38–48 days); amelia of the legs (41–45 days); phocomelia of the legs (40 or 42–47 days); choanal atresia (43–46 days); duodenal atresia (40–47 days); anal atresia (41–43 days); aplasia of gallbladder (42–43 days); pyloric stenosis (40–47 days); duodenal stenosis (41–48 days); rectal stenosis (49–50 days); ectopic kidney and hydronephrosis (38–43 days); other genitourinary defects (45–47 days); and abnormal lobulation of lungs (43–46 days) (13,17).

Perhaps the best description of the spectrum of congenital defects caused by thalidomide was written by Newman (16,17). The limb-reduction defects are bilateral, usually grossly symmetrical, and upper limb anomalies are commonly associated with lower-limb defects. Shoulder and hip malformations occur with increasing severity of upper-limb defects. Vertebral defects include an increased incidence of progressive ossification of the anterior spinal ligaments that converts the sacral and lumbar vertebral bodies into one bone mass, loss of distal segment of the sacrum, and spondylolisthesis. Spina bifida occulta and meningomyelocele occur with increased frequency. A nonspecific facial asymmetry may occur, as well as tooth hypoplasia and a deficiency in the number of teeth. There may be a hypoplastic nasal bridge with an expanded nasal tip, and choanal atresia can affect one or both nostrils. Laryngeal and tracheal anomalies and abnormal lobulation of the lungs have been observed. Ocular defects include refractive errors, pupillary abnormalities, muscle dysfunction, coloboma, microphthalmos, cataracts, and abnormalities of all three components of the oculomotor nerve. Ear defects are frequently associated with ocular malformations, as is facial nerve palsy. The defects of the ears include external, middle, and internal anomalies and are frequently associated with deafness (either conductive, neural, or both). A midline capillary hemangioma or nevus of the nose and philtrum have been described, but may fade as the child grows older. Cardiac defects, commonly of the conotruncal region, occur frequently and are a major cause of early death (30% at birth, 6% in survivors). Gastrointestinal tract defects include atresia and stenosis, and absence of the gallbladder and appendix. Inguinal hernias may be observed. Genitourinary malformations involve the kidneys (ectopic, horseshoe, hydronephrosis, and double ureter), double vagina, and cryptorchism (16,17).

Thalidomide was introduced into clinical medicine in West Germany in 1956 (20). Although a wide range of indications was promoted for the drug, it was primarily used as a sedative and tranquilizer. Because of the concern over birth defects, thalidomide was withdrawn from the market in most countries in late 1961 (21).

In 1961, two cases of congenital defects of the limbs were presented at a German pediatric meeting (22). At the meeting, Lenz proposed that thalidomide was the cause of the defects (23). A brief 1961 correspondence, however, was the first published English language article to describe birth defects that were suspected as being induced by thalidomide (24). McBride had noted an approximate 20% incidence of polydactyly, syndactyly, and limb reduction defects consisting of abnormally short femora and radii in infants exposed *in utero* to thalidomide (24). In early 1962, Lenz estimated that 2000–3000 thalidomide-exposed babies had been born in West Germany since 1959 (23).

A number of communications have been published that describe the types of congenital malformations caused by thalidomide (10,15–19,23–64,66–81,83):

Thalidomide Embryopathy

Limb Defects

upper and lower limbs (bilateral amelia or phocomelia, absence or hypoplasia of radius/ulna and/or tibia/fibula, femoral hypoplasia, preaxial aplasia upper and lower limbs, absence of the fingers and/or toes, thumb defects such as duplication, hypoplasia and triphalangism, duplication of big toe and triphalangism) (10,15–19,23–38,40,41, 45–47,49–51,54–59,61–64,66,67,69,71,72,75–81,83)

osteochondritis of femoral head (Legg-Calve-Perthes disease) (possibly a late complication that results from growth disturbance of the upper end of the femur; appeared in early childhood) (51)

knee joints (laxity of cruciate ligaments) (16,17,61)

Other Skeletal Defects
spine (ossification of sacral and lumbar vertebrae, loss of distal segment of sacrum, spondylolisthesis, scoliosis) (15–18,35–37,40,43,49,50,58,61,67,72,79,80)
shoulder (hypoplasia/dysplasia of glenoid cavity, dysplasia of neck of scapula, altered humeral head) (16,17,19,61)
hip/pelvis (dislocation, pelvic girdle hypoplasia) (16,17,19,35,51,59,61,67,79,80)
jaw (70,75)

Craniofacial
eye (refractive errors, pupil, motility, coloboma of the iris, uvea, lens, and choroid, microphthalmos, cataracts, glaucoma, crocodile-tear syndrome) (15–19,25,30,33,36,37,40,45–47,49,50,62,63,66,67,69,71–78)
ear (anotia, microtia, low-set, middle and internal ear, deafness) (15–19,23,25–27,29,30,33,35,37,39,41,43–45,48,53,56–58,61–64,66–69,71,74–78)
face/skull (face-asymmetrical; skull-rhomboid shape) (16,17,58,70) tongue (dysplasias of lingual frenulum in the form of an ankyloglossia [tongue-tie] or a shortened, sinew-shaped frenulum; grooved point of tongue [bifid tongue]) (16,70)
nose (hypoplastic nasal bridge with expanded nasal tip) (16,17,19,58,67)
choanal atresia (16–19,29,37,62,66,71,72,76)
teeth (hypodontia, hyperdontia, malformed crown, enamel hypoplasia, discoloring, malocclusion, missing teeth) (16–18,58,60,70,76)
midline hemangioma or nevus (nose, upper lip, frontal area) (10,16,17,23,25,30,33,35,45,46,57,58,60,66,67,72)

Central Nervous System
facial nerve palsy (often associated with eye and ear anomalies) (15–19,35,39,43,61,63,69,72,74,76–78)
hydrocephalus (37,57,66,74)
spina bifida occulta (16,17,79,80)
meningomyelocele (16,17,35)
autism (18,78)
epilepsy (15,16,77,78)
Marcus Gunn phenomenon or **jaw winking syndrome** (16,19)
Crocodile-tear syndrome (see **Eye**)

Major Organ Systems
respiratory system (laryngeal and tracheal abnormalities, abnormal lobulation of lungs) (16,17,19,29,33,36,37,49,62,66,67,75,76)
cardiovascular (ventricular septal defect, atrial septal defect, tetralogy of Fallot, cor triloculare, pericardial effusion, hypertrophy of atrium and ventricle, coarctation of aorta, systolic murmurs) (16–19,23,25,30,33,35–37,39,40,42,43,45,57,61,62,66,67,71,72,76,77)
gastrointestinal tract
esophageal atresia (23,29,30,37,75)
duodenal atresia (10,16,19,23,29,30,33,35,37,49,61,62,67,71)
common bile duct atresia (33,67)
anal atresia (16,18,19,23,29,30,33,35,37,44,61,62,67,76)
rectoperineal fistula (10)
malrotation (25,30,33,35,67)

stenosis (16–19,25,30,37,40,45,46,53,61,62,66,67,71,77)
abnormal lobulation of liver (33,37)
aplasia of appendix (16,17,19,23,29,30,33,37,40,46,52,53,59,66,67)
aplasia of cecum (33)
aplasia of gallbladder (16,17,19,23,30,33,36,49,57,66,67)
rectoperineal fistula (10)

genitourinary system
unspecified (25,30,33,37,76)
renal abnormalities (16–19,29,35–37,46,57,59,61,62,66,67,71,75,76,83)
defects and duplication of ureters (16,17,19,37,83)
aplasia of fallopian tube (62)
defects of uterus and/or vagina (16,17,19,33,37,55,62,66,67,81)
penile maldevelopment (66)
cryptorchism (16,17,19,25,36,61,66,67)

Other
excessive sweating (52,54)
inguinal hernias (16,17,19,61,67)

Cleft lip with or without cleft palate has occasionally been observed in newborns with thalidomide embryopathy (35,44,48,49,66,67,70–72), but it is not thought to be related to thalidomide exposure (19).

In 1962, Lenz and Knapp reviewed the fetal effects of thalidomide that were known at the time (62). Of 293 cases known to the authors or from published reports, the approximate percentage of each defect was arms only, 52%; arms and legs, 28%; arms, legs, and ears, 3%; arms and ears, 6%; ears only, 7%; legs only, 2%; and other malformations, 3%. The anomalies observed in the eight infants grouped as "other malformations" included one case each of a right polycystic kidney with aplasia of the left kidney; aplasia of left fallopian tube and left cornu of the uterus; multicystic kidneys; anal stenosis with hydronephrosis; fistula of the neck; congenital heart disease; choanal atresia; and anal atresia (62). In addition, malformations that accompanied those of the limbs and ears were pyloric stenosis, duodenal stenosis, duodenal atresia, cardiac defect, microphthalmos, anophthalmia, imperforate anus, and choanal atresia (62). Two additional review articles by Lenz, focusing on thalidomide-induced defects, appeared in 1966 (63) and 1971 (64), one with a commentary by Warkany (65).

In 1963, Japanese investigators reported phocomelia and other malformations in 10 cases (5 live infants and 5 stillbirths or early neonatal deaths) (66). Another investigator evaluated 160 cases of thalidomide embryopathy that occurred in Japan (67). Of the 160 cases, 99 had a well-documented history of thalidomide intake in early pregnancy. Of these, 70% had defects of the arms only, 14% of arms and legs, 5% of the arms, legs, and ears, 5% of the ears only, 3% of the arms and ears, and 3% of other organs (67). In 41 of the cases with malformations of the limbs and ears, an autopsy found multiple other defects of various organ systems that were similar to those reported by Lenz and Knapp (see reference 62) (67).

The importance of early examinations for ear anomalies, especially for resulting hearing impairment, was emphasized in a study published in 1965 (68). The author had observed 14 cases of bilateral congenital meatal atresia in thalidomide-exposed infants at his center, but he was aware of 50 such cases throughout England. Eleven of the cases (three were unsuitable for operation) underwent either bilateral or unilateral surgery to construct a sound conducting mechanism (68). Gross malformations determined by x-ray and tomographic examinations in the 14 cases (28 ears) involved the ossicles (32%), middle ear (21%), and labyrinth (25%).

A later study, published in 1976, evaluated the ear anomalies in 18 children, ages 12 to 16 years, who had thalidomide-induced malformations (69). Hearing impairment and vestibular hypofunction or absence of function were each found in 15 (83%) of the children. External and middle ear anomalies found in 11 of the 18 children included bilateral microtia (*N* = 5), bilateral microtia and bilateral atresia of the auditory canal (*N* = 5), and bilateral microtia and unilateral atresia of the auditory canal (*N* = 1). In one 13-year-old girl, surgical exploration revealed that the stapes and the oval and round windows had not developed, the long process of the incus was shaped like a string, and there was a nearly normal malleus. X-ray examination revealed inner ear malformations in 15 cases (83%) consisting of bilateral inner ear aplasia (*N* = 9), cystic deformity with the shape of the anterior semicircular canal (*N* = 4), large cystic defect of the inner ear (*N* = 1), and a narrow, internal auditory canal bilaterally (*N* = 1) (69). In addition to the ear defects, 12 children had eye-movement disturbances consisting of bilateral abducens palsy (*N* = 5), bilateral abducens palsy and bilateral adduction disturbance (*N* = 6), and unilateral abducens palsy (*N* = 1). Bilateral (*N* = 3) or unilateral (*N* = 3) facial palsy, and "crocodile-tear" syndrome (i.e., abnormal lacrimation that accompanies eating) (*N* = 7) were also observed (69).

A 1968 reference described the findings that resulted from clinical, orthodontic, and radiologic examinations of the face and jaws of children with thalidomide embryopathy (70). The findings in 127 children (approximate ages 4 to 6 years) with thalidomide embryopathy (group 1) were compared with 57 children with non-thalidomide-induced dysmelia (group 2), and 120 children without malformation of the limbs (group 3). Thalidomide exposure did not disturb either the shape or number of the deciduous or permanent teeth (70). However, in the 103 children of group 1 with complete deciduous dentition, there was an increase in the frequency of abnormalities of the maxilla and/or mandible. The other important findings were malformation at the base of the skull, asymmetry of the skull, and dysplasia of the point of the tongue and the frenum (70).

One investigator categorized the malformations found in 154 children with thalidomide embryopathy using a classification system of principal defects that he had designed (71). The type of defects were the same as those listed above for thalidomide embryopathy. In eight groups, limb defects were dominant but other defects were often present, whereas in two groups, limb defects were absent or minimal. The defect classifications and the number and approximate percentage of children in each group were: upper limb amelia or phocomelia with normal legs (*N* = 60, 39%); upper limb amelia or phocomelia with other leg defects (*N* = 18, 12%); forearm defects with normal legs (*N* = 17, 11%); four-limb phocomelia (*N* = 15, 10%); anomalies of the ears (*N* = 16, 10%); severe lower limb defects with less severe upper limb defects (*N* = 10, 6%); other limb defects (*N* = 9, 6%); forearm defects with defects of the lower limbs (*N* = 5, 3%); lower limb defects with normal upper limbs (*N* = 3, 2%); and other anomalies (*N* = 1, $<$1%). A discussion of the disabilities caused by the defects in each group was also included in the text (71).

The focus of eight studies was on thalidomide-induced ocular malformations (18,46,47,72–76). Four children with ocular defects and typical thalidomide embryopathy were described in a 1964 report (46). The eye defects thought to be thalidomide related were: left optic disc with a very deep physiologic cup; bilateral coloboma of the iris, unilateral coloboma of the choroid and retina involving the optic disc, and unilateral microphthalmos; unilateral coloboma of the choroid and retina; and bilateral coloboma of the

T

iris, choroid, and retina, involving the optic disc on one side, and unilateral microphthalmos (46). At one ophthalmology center, minor ocular abnormalities were found in some children consisting of pigmentary retinopathy, a high refractive error, and reduced visual acuity (47). A 1963 study evaluated 20 children with known or suspected thalidomide-induced limb malformations for ocular anomalies (72). Thirteen of the children had anatomically normal eyes with apparently normal function and seven (35%) had visual defects. Five of the seven had structural defects consisting of either unilateral or bilateral coloboma of the iris, choroid, or lens, sometimes involving the macular areas or the disc, and microphthalmos. The other two had anatomically normal eyes but abnormalities in visual function. The visual prognosis was rated as good in three cases, poor in two, and uncertain in two (72). A 1966 study from Sweden examined 38 children for ocular malformations who had thalidomide-induced defects (73). Abducens paralysis was found in 17 children, bilateral in 13 and unilateral in four. Bilateral oculomotor paralysis was present in two of these cases and unilateral in one (73). Other conditions, often concomitant with additional defects, included strabismus; unequal pupils (both reactive to light); non-reactive pupil; microphthalmos (both bilateral and unilateral); anophthalmos on one side and severe microphthalmos on the other; coloboma of the choroid; bilateral aplasia of macula with nystagmus; and bilateral epiphora (with free tear ducts and grossly normal drainage system) (73). Of note, more than half of the children had hearing impairment of varying severity. A 1967 report reviewed the previously published cases of ocular abnormalities induced by thalidomide and presented additional data on 21 Canadian children (ages 3 to 4.5 years) exposed *in utero* to the drug (74). Only four of these children had ocular malformations and none had a coloboma.

Ocular abnormalities associated with thalidomide embryopathy were reported in a 1991 study of 21 Swedish patients, ages 28 to 29 years (75). Horizontal incomitant strabismus, usually of the Duane syndrome type, was the most common ocular motility abnormality, but other motility abnormalities were also noted (75). Abnormal tearing, facial nerve (7th cranial nerve) palsy, and ear anomalies were also present in some cases. Citing previous studies, facial nerve palsy and ear anomalies were thought to have occurred from thalidomide exposure on days 20–29 after conception (75). This time period is consistent with the time intervals (34–43 days after LMP) given earlier. Two years later, these same authors reported the results of an ophthalmological study conducted in 86 of 100 Swedes with documented thalidomide embryopathy (76). The subjects, 49 males and 37 females, ranged in age from 27 to 30 years. Forty-six (54%) had one or more abnormal eye signs. The ocular abnormalities included the following: (a) motility defects ($N = 43$, 50%), including 37 with horizontal incomitant strabismus (26 with Duane syndrome, 4 with marked limitation of abduction, and 7 with gaze paresis), and 6 with horizontal comitant strabismus (all esotropia); (b) facial nerve palsy ($N = 17$, 20%); (c) abnormal lacrimation ($N = 17$, 20%); (d) coloboma of uvea and optic disc ($N = 1$, 1%) or optic disc only ($N = 2$, 2%); (e) microphthalmos ($N = 2$, 2%); and (e) one each of congenital glaucoma, conjunctival lipodermoid, and hypertelorism (76).

In a subsequent paper, the authors again reviewed the above ocular findings but also included the multiple other thalidomide-induced defects that were found in the 86 subjects (18). The defects and the number of cases for each were (note that all cases had more than one defect): thumbs (triphalangeal, absent, misplaced, hypoplastic, or extra digit) $N = 70$ (81%), upper limb excluding thumb $N = 59$ (69%), lower limb $N = 21$ (24%), ears/hearing $N = 33$ (38%), facial nerve palsy $N = 17$ (20%), kidney (absent, horseshoe, hydronephrosis, dysfunctional) $N = 12$ (14%), cardiovascular (VSD, arrhythmia, ductus botalli, murmur) $N = 7$ (8%), chest/lung (cardiovascular defects, pulmonary atresia, enlarged chest wall

T

or structural anomaly) $N = 4$ (5%), genitalia (absent uterus and vagina, double vagina) $N = 3$ (3%), anal atresia $N = 4$ (5%), choanal atresia $N = 2$ (2%), dental anomalies $N = 4$ (5%), mental retardation (moderate to severe) $N = 5$ (6%), and autism (all had mental retardation) $N = 4$ (5%) (18). The authors also expanded the type of ocular malformations listed in their previous study (reference 74) to include two cases of myelinated nerve fiber, two cases of ptosis, and one additional case each of coloboma (uveal or optic disc) and microphthalmos (18).

Neurologic complications of thalidomide embryopathy include epilepsy. In a study that appeared in 1976, the incidence of epilepsy was determined from a data base that included all surviving children ($N = 408$) with documented thalidomide embryopathy in the United Kingdom (77). Seven children (1.7%) met established criteria for the diagnosis of epilepsy and were classified into two groups: (a) children with normal ears (four had upper limb defects, two had mental impairment, and one had ocular anomalies, facial palsy, and "high intelligence") ($N = 4$); and (b) children with abnormal ears (in addition, one had ocular defects and facial palsy, one had defects of the thumbs, and one had facial palsy and bilateral sixth nerve palsies) ($N = 3$) (77). In a third group, those with cardiac abnormalities, the diagnosis of epilepsy was uncertain. The two children in this group also had other defects consisting of amelia of the upper limbs, pyloric stenosis, and ocular and ear defects in one, and upper limb defects in the other. These two cases were apparently excluded from the prevalence rate calculations below. The prevalence rates of epilepsy calculated for various ages were significant when compared to published rates in the population as a whole: active epilepsy-5 cases, 12.5/1000 vs. 2.7/1000 ($p < 0.01$); epilepsy between birth and nine years of age-7 cases, 17.2/1000 vs. 2.42/1000 ($p < 0.0001$); and new cases in first 7 years of life-6 cases, 2.1/1000 vs. 0.43/1000 ($p < 0.01$) (77). The types of epilepsy in the first group (normal ears) were thought to be consistent with structural defects of the cerebral cortex (77). Moreover, two of the children in this group had severe refractory epilepsy, a prevalence of 5/1000 vs. 0.5/1000 in the general population. The unlocalized or generalized seizures in the second group (abnormal ears) suggested abnormalities in the brainstem (77).

Five subjects, suspected of having a severe learning disorder (IQ scores <20 to 70–84), were identified from a group of 100 patients previously studied for ocular malformations (78). The five cases were then evaluated for the presence of autism. The ages of the subjects (three males, two females) ranged from 30 to 31 years. All had physical stigmata (i.e., ocular motility defects, other cranial nerve disorders, ear and upper-limb anomalies) characteristic of thalidomide embryopathy that had occurred from drug exposure approximately 20–24 days after conception (34–38 days after LMP). Four of the cases (two males, two females) met the criteria for autism. Based on an incidence of 4%, compared to a prevalence of about 0.08% in the general population, the investigators estimated that there was a 50-fold higher rate of autism in those with thalidomide embryopathy (78).

A 1977 report evaluated the spinal deformities in 28 children, ages 10–14 years, who had thalidomide embryopathy (79). The children's spinal defects had been first studied at 4–8 years of age (80), and the current study was part of a continuing evaluation of their status. The initial group contained 32 cases, but 4 were either lost to follow-up or had died. All of the subjects had characteristic limb defects. In both studies, the spinal abnormalities were classified into five types. The initial and current (shown in *italics*) findings for each group were: (i) local anomalies of bone development (spina bifida, $N = 3$; fusion of adjacent spinous processes, $N = 2$), *neural arch defect more obvious, increased number of minor changes*; (ii) scoliosis ($N = 18$), *20 children now had scoliosis;* (iii) wedge deformity of solitary vertebral bodies ($N = 4$), *worsened in four cases*; (iv) disc space calcification

($N = 3$); and (v) end-plate and disc defects ($N = 16$), *two additional cases of vertebral fusion, extension of fusion in two others, reduction in lumbar lordosis in 10 cases* (79).

The pregnancy outcomes of women with thalidomide embryopathy were presented in a 1988 publication (81), and also discussed in 1989 (82). The pregnancy of one woman was described in detail (81). This case involved a 24-year-old primigravida with upper limb amelia and lower limb phocomelia. Although there were many technical difficulties (e.g., blood pressure determination, blood sampling, and obesity), she eventually delivered a term, 3.4-kg healthy female infant without any apparent abnormalities. The baby was doing well at the first postnatal check. During the cesarean section, a left rudimentary uterine horn was noted that did not communicate with the uterine cavity (81). Supplementing their case history, the authors described the outcomes of 70 pregnancies in 35 women (includes the case history) who were living in England and who had thalidomide embryopathy (8 with absent upper and/or lower limbs; 27 with minor disabilities of the upper limbs and ears). Six miscarriages (9%) had occurred, but there were no congenital malformations in the 64 live births (81).

Renal failure complicated the fifth pregnancy of a 26-year-old woman with upper limb phocomelia and kidney and ureter malformations secondary to thalidomide (83). At 11 years of age, bilateral refluxing megaureters with dilated calices and thinning of the renal cortex were diagnosed because of chronic urinary tract infections and she underwent a bilateral antireflux procedure. Her first pregnancy, 7 years previously, had been normotensive but complicated by proteinuria, hematuria, and premature labor thought to have been precipitated by a urinary tract infection. She had delivered a 660-g female infant who was currently alive and well. Her next three pregnancies resulted in a spontaneous abortion and two elective terminations. At 24 weeks' gestation in the index pregnancy, complications included normochromic normocytic anemia, hypertension, proteinuria, hematuria, urinary tract infection, and renal failure (creatinine clearance 11 mL/minute). A renal ultrasound revealed small kidneys with diffuse caliceal clubbing, a very thin parenchyma, and dilated ureters to the bladder (83). Peritoneal dialysis, in addition to antihypertensive, antibiotic, and iron therapy, was initiated with ritodrine tocolysis. Two weeks later, however, ultrasound confirmed that no fetal growth had occurred and her hypertension and renal failure had worsened. A cesarean section was performed to deliver a 460-g male infant who died 6 hours after birth. Because of her continued renal failure, the patient eventually received a kidney transplant (83).

The mechanism of thalidomide-induced malformations is still unknown. The findings of many investigations have been discussed in reviews published in 1988 (84) and 2000 (85,86). Four other references (87–90) have developed additional hypotheses to explain how thalidomide causes structural defects.

A review published in 1988 listed 24 proposed mechanisms for thalidomide teratogenesis (84). Eight of the proposals were rejected by the author for various reasons. The remaining 16 proposed mechanisms were classified as those involving biochemical or molecular mechanisms ($N = 9$), cellular mechanisms ($N = 2$), or tissue-levels mechanisms ($N = 5$) (84). The absence of solid experimental evidence for the proposed mechanisms, however, led the author to the conclusion that none of the proposals could adequately account for thalidomide teratogenicity (84).

The role of a toxic arene oxide metabolite was thought to be involved in thalidomide teratogenicity according to a 1981 study (87). In an *in vitro* experiment, the human lymphocyte toxicity of a thalidomide metabolite was enhanced in the presence of epoxide hydrolase inhibitors and abolished by addition of the pure enzyme. The toxic thalidomide metabolite was not produced by rat liver microsomes, but was produced in hepatic preparations from maternal rabbits, and fetal rabbits, monkeys, and humans. These results were consistent with the lack of sensitivity to thalidomide teratogenesis in the rat versus the sensitivity of rabbits, monkeys, and humans (87). A decrease in ascorbic acid (vitamin C) levels has been suggested as a mechanism of thalidomide teratogenesis (88). Two important consequences of ascorbic acid deficiency in the fetus would be inhibition of collagen synthesis and disruption of the development of nerve ganglia innervating limb buds (88).

A 1996 research study used developing chick embryos to test the hypothesis that elimination of the mesonephros, in the absence of scarring, would produce limb abnormalities similar to those observed with thalidomide (89). Tantalum foil barriers were used at various levels of the intermediate mesoderm to prevent caudal elongation of the mesonephros. Limb-reduction defects were produced when the mesonephros was prevented from forming caudal to somite 14. The types and percentage of limb defects in the chick embryos were: upper limb only (57%), upper and lower limb (31%), and lower limb only (12%). In comparison, the corresponding percentages of limb reduction defects in 1,252 human cases of thalidomide embryopathy were 64%, 34%, and 2%, respectively (89). Based on these results and previous studies, the investigators concluded that disruption of the mesonephros (or factors produced in the mesonephros) results in limb-reduction defects and that the mechanism of thalidomide-induced limb anomalies probably also involves disruption of the mesonephros (89).

Whole-embryo culture was used in a study directly comparing thalidomide-resistant rats and thalidomide-sensitive rabbits (90). Various concentrations of thalidomide were shown to significantly decrease the concentration of glutathione in rabbit visceral yolk sacs, but not in the rat. Cysteine concentrations were not affected in either species, but the cysteine levels in control rabbits were 65% lower than those in control rats. Thus, a possible role for glutathione was suggested by the results (90).

In a study published in 1996, a highly teratogenic derivative of thalidomide (EM12) was used in an experiment with nonhuman primates (marmosets) (91). EM12 was chosen because it is a more potent teratogen than thalidomide, is more stable to hydrolysis, and produces a teratogenic incidence close to 100% in the marmoset. Moreover, the pattern of malformations produced in the marmoset are identical to those seen in humans after *in utero* exposure to thalidomide (91). The data indicated that thalidomide produced a statistically significant down-regulation (in some cases, complete disappearance) of several surface adhesion receptors found on early limb bud cells and other organs. The adhesion receptors identified were receptors of the integrin family (β_1-integrins, β_2-integrins, and β_3-integrins), the immunoglobulin family, and the selectin family. These receptors are involved in the development of the limbs, heart, head, and body. The down-regulation of these receptors, which was most pronounced in those involved with limb development, was expected to alter cell-cell and cell-extracellular matrix interactions (91).

A 1998 communication proposed that the mechanism of limb-reduction anomalies induced by thalidomide was related to the inhibition of mesenchymal proliferation in the limb bud (92). In the progress-zone model, the proximal and distal structures of the limb are specified sequentially by a continuous signal (thought to be fibroblast growth factor [FGF]) from the apical ectodermal ridge (92). The mesenchyme at the tip of the limb bud is respecified by FGF to produce distal structures, whereas those not receiving a continuous FGF signal develop into proximal structures. If thalidomide blocks mesenchymal cell growth, all of the progress-zone cells remain under the influence of FGF and are programmed only to form the distal most elements (i.e., a phocomelia) (92).

Two 2000 reviews by the same group of investigators evaluated 30 mechanistic hypotheses of thalidomide embryopathy (85,86). Fourteen of the proposals were rejected because they were either unsubstantiated or had been proven not to be viable. The 16 remaining hypotheses were grouped into six categories with thalidomide affecting: (a) DNA synthesis or transcription, synthesis and/or function of (b) growth factors (insulin-like growth factor and FGF) or (c) integrins (a subunit type v and β subunit type 3), (d) angiogenesis, (e) chondrogenesis, or (f) cell death or injury (85,86). The hypotheses were not thought to be necessarily mutually exclusive, but could eventually be fitted into a unified model (85,86). Citing evidence from the literature, they proposed that thalidomide, or a metabolite, intercalates into the DNA of specific promoter regions of genes that code for proteins involved in normal limb development. The binding of thalidomide would inhibit the transcription of these genes, resulting in interference with the development of new blood vessels and leading to truncation of the limb (85,86).

Although thalidomide was withdrawn from England and the European markets in late 1961, the agent has continued to be available in 8 of 10 South American countries for the treatment of leprosy (56,93). Thalidomide is manufactured in Argentina and Brazil and is available either through pharmacies (Brazil) or government health agencies (Brazil and Argentina) (93). A 1987 case report from Brazil described a 17-week-old fetus that was diagnosed by prenatal ultrasound with malformations secondary to thalidomide (56). After pregnancy termination, an autopsy revealed upper limb phocomelia, absent tibiae and fibulae (both feet connected directly to the femora), missing toes on both feet, and absent external ears (56). This case was apparently the first to report a prenatal diagnosis of thalidomide syndrome (56). In a second report, 34 children with thalidomide embryopathy who were born in South America after 1965 were identified by the Latin American Collaborative Study of Congenital Malformations (ECLAMC) in endemic areas for leprosy (93). Specific details of the typical thalidomide-induced malformations in 11 of these cases (including the case in reference 56) were presented.

A study published in 1988 reviewed the history of thalidomide embryopathy and cited 4,336 cases that had been identified in various countries (20). The number of cases was considered a minimal estimate, however, because stillborns and early deaths were underrepresented and the ascertainment of surviving cases in many countries was thought to be incomplete (20). The countries and the number of affected fetuses/infants are shown below. Note that none of the cases from the United States (resulting from thalidomide obtained elsewhere) were included.

Australia 26	Mexico 4
Austria 7	Netherlands 34
Belgium 35	Norway 11
Brazil 99	Portugal 8
Canada 122	Spain 5
Denmark 20	Sweden 153
Finland 8	Switzerland 12
Ireland 51	Taiwan 36
Italy 86	United Kingdom 271
Japan 299	West Germany 3,049

Seventeen years before the above report, a review on the medicolegal implications of the thalidomide tragedy estimated that a total of 5000 to 6000 babies had been affected, about 4000 of these in West Germany (94).

In summary, thalidomide is a potent teratogen in rats, rabbits, nonhuman primates, and humans. In humans, the severe malformations induced by thalidomide may involve defects of the limbs, axial skeleton, head and face, eyes, ears, tongue, teeth, central nervous, respiratory, cardiovascular, and genitourinary systems, and the gastrointestinal tract. The neurological complications may include severe mental retardation secondary to sensory deprivation. The critical period of exposure is 34–50 days after the LMP (20 ± 1 days to 36 ± 1 days after conception). The critical maternal dose is at least 100 mg (96). However, normal pregnancy outcomes have occurred, even when thalidomide was taken during the critical period (45,95). In addition, other causes of limb reduction defects and heart defects, such as Holt-Oram syndrome, may mimic thalidomide-induced malformations (19).

The risk of congenital malformations after exposure during the critical period has been estimated to be between 20% and 50% (17). The large degree of uncertainty in the estimated risk is a result of the lack of epidemiologic studies and any organized attempt to determine the number of normal, yet exposed children (17). Just as uncertain, because it is based on only four reports, the frequency of specific malformations is thought to be in the following order: arms only > arms and legs > ears only > arms and ears ≥arms, legs, and ears > legs only (62,67,71,89). The frequencies of the other malformations associated with thalidomide are unknown, partially because many of them were determined at autopsy, were only recognized later in life and in specialized groups, or have not been fully analyzed.

Although thalidomide had not been approved for use in the United States when thalidomide embryopathy was discovered, at least 17 such cases were delivered in this country, apparently from women who had received the drug elsewhere (10,94). Fortunately, thalidomide did not receive approval in the United States because of the alertness of the FDA (94,97).

Thalidomide is indicated (FDA approved) for the treatment of a leprosy skin complication (erythema nodosum leprosum) (1), but it may also have eventual application in other serious conditions, such as chronic graft-versus-host disease, rash caused by systemic lupus erythematosus, Behçet's syndrome, inflammatory bowel disease, prostate cancer, metastatic breast cancer, rheumatoid arthritis, uremic pruritus, severe atopic erythroderma, weight loss in tuberculosis, and in the complications of acquired immunodeficiency syndrome (aphthous ulcers, microsporidiosis diarrhea, macular degeneration, wasting, Kaposi's sarcoma, and human immunodeficiency virus replication) (85,98,99). The mechanism of action of thalidomide teratogenesis is unknown, but recent investigations have suggested that it involves disruption of specific genes involved in normal limb development. If the mechanism can be fully understood, development of nonteratogenic derivatives, that retain the ability to treat disease, may be possible (85,86).

Thalidomide is contraindicated during pregnancy and in women of childbearing age who are not receiving two reliable methods of contraception for 1 month prior to starting therapy, during therapy, and for 1 month after stopping therapy (1). In addition, it is contraindicated in women who do not meet the specific requirements of the STEPS program (System for Thalidomide Education and Prescribing Safety). The STEPS program was developed by the manufacturer to limit the prescribing and use of thalidomide to tightly controlled situations and to prevent inadvertent exposure of pregnant women (1,99). Any suspected fetal exposure to thalidomide should be reported to the FDA (MedWatch Program at 1-800-FDA-1088) and/or to the manufacturer (1).

BREAST FEEDING SUMMARY

RECOMMENDATION: No Human Data - Potential Toxicity

No reports describing the use of thalidomide during lactation have been located. The molecular weight (about 258) is low enough, however, that excretion into milk should be expected. Moreover, nothing is known about the excretion of thalidomide metabolites into breast milk. Women who are taking thalidomide should not nurse because the effects on an infant from exposure to thalidomide and its metabolites in breast milk are unknown.

References

1. Product information. Thalomid. Celgene Corporation, 2000.
2. Nishimura H, Tanimura T. *Clinical Aspects of The Teratogenicity of Drugs*. New York, NY: American Elsevier Publishing Company, 1976:292–7.
3. Parkhie M, Webb M. Embryotoxicity and teratogenicity of thalidomide in rats. Teratology 1983;27: 327–32.
4. Somers GF. Thalidomide and congenital abnormalities. Lancet 1962;1:912–3.
5. Spencer KEV. Thalidomide and congenital abnormalities. Lancet 1962;2:100.
6. Dekker A, Mehrizi A. The use of thalidomide as a teratogenic agent in rabbits. Bull Johns Hopkins Hosp 1964;115:223–30.
7. Vickers TH. Concerning the morphogenesis of thalidomide dysmelia in rabbits. Br J Exp Pathol 1967;48: 579–92.
8. Sterz H, Nothdurft H, Lexa P, Ockenfels H. Teratologic studies on the Himalayan rabbit: new aspects of thalidomide-induced teratogenesis. Arch Toxicol 1987;60:376–81.
9. Gilani SH. Cardiovascular malformations in the chick embryo induced by thalidomide. Toxicol Appl Pharmacol 1973;25:77–83.
10. Mellin GW, Katzenstein M. The saga of thalidomide. Neuropathy to embryopathy, with case reports of congenital anomalies. N Engl J Med 1962;267:1104–93.
11. Mellin GW, Katzenstein M. The saga of thalidomide (concluded). Neuropathy to embryopathy, with case reports of congenital anomalies. N Engl J Med 1962;267:1238–44.
12. Taussig HB. A study of the German outbreak of phocomelia. JAMA 1962;180:1106–14.
13. Nowack E. The sensitive period of thalidomide embryopathy (in German). Humangenetik 1965;1:516–36.
14. Smithells RW. The thalidomide legacy. Proc R Soc Med 1965;58:491–2.
15. Newman CGH. Clinical observations on the thalidomide syndrome. Proc R Soc Med 1977;70:225–7.
16. Newman CGH. Teratogen update: clinical aspects of thalidomide embryopathy—a continuing preoccupation. Teratology 1985;32:133–44.
17. Newman CGH. The thalidomide syndrome: risks of exposure and spectrum of malformations. Clin Perinatol 1986;13:555–73.
18. Miller MT, Stromland K. Teratogen update: thalidomide: a review, with focus on ocular findings and new potential uses. Teratology 1999;60:306–21.
19. Brent RL, Holmes LB. Clinical and basic science lessons from the thalidomide tragedy: what have we learned about the causes of limb defects? Teratology 1988;38:241–51.
20. Lenz W. A short history of thalidomide embryopathy. Teratology 1988;38:203–15.
21. Hayman DJ. Distaval. Lancet 1961;2:1262.
22. Kosenow W, Pfeiffer RA. Micromelia, haemangioma und duodenal stenosis exhibit. German Pediatric Society, Kassel, 1960. As cited by Taussig HB. A study of the German outbreak of phocomelia. JAMA 1962; 180:1106–14.
23. Lenz W. Thalidomide and congenital abnormalities. Lancet 1962;1:45.
24. McBride WG. Thalidomide and congenital abnormalities. Lancet 1961;2:1358.
25. Pfeiffer RA, Kosenow W. Thalidomide and congenital abnormalities. Lancet 1962;1:45–6.
26. Jones EE, Williamson DAJ. Thalidomide and congenital abnormalities. Lancet 1962;1:222.
27. Burley DM. Thalidomide and congenital abnormalities. Lancet 1962;1:271.
28. Lenz W. Thalidomide and congenital abnormalities. Lancet 1962;1:271–2.
29. Speirs AL. Thalidomide and congenital abnormalities. Lancet 1962;1:303–5.
30. Anonymous. Thalidomide and congenital malformations. Lancet 1962;1:307–8.
31. Kohler HG, Fisher AM, Dunn PM. Thalidomide and congenital abnormalities. Lancet 1962;1:326.
32. Willman A, Dumoulin JG. Thalidomide ("Distaval") and foetal abnormalities. Br Med J 1962;1:477.
33. Pliess G. Thalidomide and congenital abnormalities. Lancet 1962;1:1128–9.
34. Rodin AE, Koller LA, Taylor JD. Association of thalidomide (Kevadon) with congenital anomalies. Can Med Assoc J 1962;86:744–6.
35. Smithells RW. Thalidomide and malformations in Liverpool. Lancet 1962;1:1270–3.
36. Kajii T. Thalidomide and congenital deformities. Lancet 1962;2:151.
37. Leck IM, Millar ELM. Incidence of malformations since the introduction of thalidomide. Br Med J 1962;2: 16–20.
38. Jacobs J. Drugs and foetal abnormalities. Br Med J 1962;2:407.
39. Pfeiffer RA, Nessel E. Multiple congenital abnormalities. Lancet 1962;2:349–50.
40. Ward SP. Thalidomide and congenital abnormalities. Br Med J 1962;2:646–7.
41. Knapp K, Lenz W, Nowack E. Multiple congenital abnormalities. Lancet 1962;2:725.
42. Owen R, Smith A. Cor triloculare and thalidomide. Lancet 1962;2:836.
43. Rosendal T. Thalidomide and aplasia-hypoplasia of the otic labyrinth. Lancet 1963;1:724–5.
44. Kajii T, Goto M. Cleft lip and palate after thalidomide. Lancet 1963;2:151–2.
45. McBride WG. The teratogenic action of drugs. Med J Aust 1963;2:689–93.
46. Cullen JF. Ocular defects in thalidomide babies. Br J Ophthalmol 1964;48:151–3.
47. Cant JS. Minor ocular abnormalities associated with thalidomide. Lancet 1966;1:1134.
48. Fogh-Andersen P. Thalidomide and congenital cleft deformities. Acta Chir Scand 1966;131:197–200.
49. Kajii T, Kida M, Takahashi K. The effect of thalidomide intake during 113 human pregnancies. Teratology 1973;8:163–6.

T

50. Murphy R, Mohr P. Two congenital neurological abnormalities caused by thalidomide. Br Med J 1977;2:1191.
51. Stainsby GD, Quibell EP. Perthes-like changes in the hips of children with thalidomide deformities. Lancet 1967;2:242–3.
52. Smithells RW. Thalidomide, absent appendix, and sweating. Lancet 1978;1:1042.
53. Bremner DN, Mooney G. Agenesis of appendix: a further thalidomide anomaly. Lancet 1978;1:826.
54. McBride WG. Excessive sweating and reduction deformities. Lancet 1978;1:826.
55. McBride WG. Another, late thalidomide abnormality. Lancet 1981;2:368.
56. Gollop TR, Eigier A, Guidugli-Neto J. Prenatal diagnosis of thalidomide syndrome. Prenat Diagn 1987;7:295–8.
57. Hagen EO. Congenital malformations in a thalidomide baby: a postmortem anatomical study. Can Med Assoc J 1965;92:283–6.
58. Hammarstrom L, Henrikson CO, Larsson KS. Anomalies of the teeth in a child with upper phocomelia. Report of a case. Oral Surg 1970;29:191–6.
59. Shand JEG, Bremner DN. Agenesis of the vermiform appendix in a thalidomide child. Br J Surg 1977;64:203–4.
60. Axrup K, d'Avignon M, Hellgren K, Henrikson C-O, Juhlin I-M, Larsson KS, Persson GE, Welander E. Children with thalidomide embryopathy: odontologic observations and aspects. Dent Dig 1966;72:403–5,425.
61. Ruffing L. Evaluation of thalidomide children. Birth Defects Orig Artic Ser 1977;13:287–300.
62. Lenz W, Knapp K. Thalidomide embryopathy. Arch Environ Health 1962;5:100–5.
63. Lenz W. Malformations caused by drugs in pregnancy. Am J Dis Child 1966;112:99–106.
64. Lenz W. How can the teratogenic action of a factor be established in man? South Med J 1971;64(Suppl 1):41–7.
65. Warkany J. How can the teratogenic action of a factor be established in man? Comments. South Med J 1971;64(Suppl 1):48–50.
66. Tabuchi A, Yamada A, Umisa H, Shintani T, Horikawa M, Shirasuna K, Sawasaki M. Phocomelia-like deformity and thalidomide preparations. Hiroshima J Med Sci 1963;12:11–35.
67. Kajii T. Thalidomide experience in Japan. Ann Paediatr 1965;205:341–54.
68. Livingstone G. Congenital ear abnormalities due to thalidomide. Proc R Soc Med 1965;58:493–7.
69. Takemori S, Tanaka Y, Suzuki J-I. Thalidomide anomalies of the ear. Arch Otolaryngol 1976;102:425–7.
70. Stahl A. Clinical, orthodontic, and radiological findings in the jaws and face of children with dysmelia associated with thalidomide-embryopathy. Int Dent J 1968;18:631–8.
71. Smithells RW. Defects and disabilities of thalidomide children. Br Med J 1973;1:269–72.
72. Gilkes MJ, Strode M. Ocular anomalies in association with developmental limb abnormalities of drug origin. Lancet 1963;1:1026–7.
73. Zetterstrom B. Ocular malformations caused by thalidomide. Acta Ophthalmol 1966;44:391–5.
74. Rafuse EV, Arstikaitis M, Brent HP. Ocular findings in thalidomide children. Can J Ophthalmol 1967;2:222–5.
75. Miller MT, Stromland K. Ocular motility in thalidomide embryopathy. J Pediatr Ophthalmol Strabismus 1991;28:47–54.
76. Stromland K, Miller MT. Thalidomide embryopathy: revisited 27 years later. Acta Ophthalmol 1993;71:238–45.
77. Stephenson JBP. Epilepsy: a neurological complication of thalidomide embryopathy. Dev Med Child Neurol 1976;18:189–97.
78. Stromland K, Nordin V, Miller M, Akerstrom B, Gillberg C. Autism in thalidomide embryopathy: a population study. Dev Med Child Neurol 1994;36:351–6.
79. Edwards DH, Nichols PJR. The spinal abnormalities in thalidomide embryopathy. Acta Orthop Scand 1977;48:273–6.
80. Nichols PJR, Boldero JL, Goodfellow JW, Hamilton A. Abnormalities of the vertebral column associated with thalidomide-induced limb deformities. Orthop (Oxford) 1968;1:71–90. As cited by Edwards DH, Nichols PJR. The spinal abnormalities in thalidomide embryopathy. Acta Orthop Scand 1977;48:273–6.
81. Maouris PG, Hirsch PJ. Pregnancy in women with thalidomide-induced disabilities. Case report and a questionnaire study. Br J Obstet Gynecol 1988;95:717–9.
82. Chamberlain G. The obstetric problems of the thalidomide children. BMJ 1989;298:6.
83. Brown MA, Farrell C, Newton P, Child RP. Thalidomide, pregnancy and renal failure. Med J Aust 1990;152:148–9.
84. Stephens TD. Proposed mechanisms of action in thalidomide embryopathy. Teratology 1988;38:229–39.
85. Stephens TD, Fillmore BJ. Hypothesis: Thalidomide embryopathy-proposed mechanism of action. Teratology 2000;61:189–95.
86. Stephens TD, Bunde CJW, Fillmore BJ. Mechanism of action in thalidomide teratogenesis. Biochem Pharmacol 2000;59:1489–99.
87. Gordon GB, Spielberg SP, Blake DA, Balasubramanian V. Thalidomide teratogenesis: Evidence for a toxic arene oxide metabolite. Proc Natl Acad Sci U S A 1981;78:2545–8.
88. Vaisman B. To the editor. Teratology 1996;53:283–4.
89. Smith DM, Torres RD, Stephens TD. Mesonephros has a role in limb development and is related to thalidomide embryopathy. Teratology 1996;54:126–34.
90. Hansen JM, Carney EW, Harris C. Differential alteration by thalidomide of the glutathione content of rat vs. rabbit conceptuses in vitro. Reprod Toxicol 1999;13:547–54.
91. Neubert R, Hinz N, Thiel R, Neubert D. Down-regulation of adhesion receptors on cells of primate embryos as a probable mechanism of the teratogenic action of thalidomide. Life Sci 1996;58:295–316.
92. Tabin CJ. A developmental model for thalidomide defects. Nature 1998;396:322–3.
93. Castilla EE, Ashton-Prolla P, Barreda-Mejia E, Brunoni D, Cavalcanti DP, Correa-Neto J, Delgadillo JL, Dutra MG, Felix T, Giraldo A, Juarez N, Lopez-Camelo JS, Nazer J, Orioli IM, Paz JE, Pessoto MA, Pina-Neto JM, Quadrelli R, Rittler M, Rueda S, Saltos M, Sanchez O, Schuler L. Thalidomide, a current teratogen in South America. Teratology 1996;54:273–7.

T

94. Curran WJ. The thalidomide tragedy in Germany: the end of a historic medicolegal trial. N Engl J Med 1971;284:481–2.
95. Pembrey ME, Clarke CA. Normal child after maternal thalidomide ingestion in critical period of pregnancy. Lancet 1970;1:275–7.
96. Buyse ML, editor-in-chief. *Birth Defects Encyclopedia*. Volume 1. Dover, MA: Center for Birth Defects Information Services, 1990:726–7.
97. McFadyen RE. Thalidomide in America: a brush with tragedy. Clin Medica 1976;11:79–93.
98. Friedman JM, Kimmel CA. Teratology Society 1988 Public Affairs Committee symposium: The new thalidomide era: dealing with the risks. Teratology 1999;59:120–3.
99. Public Affairs Committee, Teratology Society. Teratology Society Public Affairs Committee position paper: thalidomide. Teratology 2000;62:172–3.

Name: **THEOPHYLLINE** Risk Factor: C_M

Class: **Respiratory Drug (Bronchodilator)**

FETAL RISK SUMMARY

RECOMMENDATION: Compatible

Theophylline is the bronchodilator of choice for asthma and chronic obstructive pulmonary disease in the pregnant patient (1–6). No published reports linking the use of theophylline with congenital defects have been located.

Reproduction studies in mice and rats at oral doses up to approximately 2.0 and 3.0 times, respectively, the recommended human dose based on body surface area (RHD) revealed no evidence of teratogenicity (7). At a slightly lower dose (about 2.5 times the RHD) in rats, embryo toxicity, but not maternal toxicity, was observed.

In a surveillance study of Michigan Medicaid recipients conducted between 1985 and 1992 involving 229,101 completed pregnancies, 1240 newborns had been exposed to theophylline and 36 to aminophylline during the 1st trimester (F. Rosa, personal communication, FDA, 1993). A total of 68 (5.5%) major birth defects were observed (53 expected) with theophylline and 1 (2.8%) major defect (2 expected) with aminophylline. For theophylline, specific data were available for six defect categories, including (observed/expected) 20/12 cardiovascular defects, 5/1 oral clefts, 2/0.5 spina bifida, 5/4 polydactyly, 0/2 limb reduction defects, and 2/3 hypospadias. Three of the defect categories, cardiovascular, oral clefts, and spina bifida, suggest an association with the drug, but other factors, such as the mother's disease, concurrent drug use, and chance, may be involved. For aminophylline, the single defect was a polydactyly.

The Collaborative Perinatal Project monitored 193 mother-child pairs with 1st trimester exposure to theophylline or aminophylline (8). No evidence was found for an association with malformations.

Theophylline crosses the placenta, and newborn infants may have therapeutic serum levels (9–13). Transient tachycardia, irritability, and vomiting have been reported in newborns delivered from mothers consuming theophylline (9,10). These effects are more likely to occur when maternal serum levels at term are in the high therapeutic range or above (therapeutic range 8–20 μg/mL) (11). Cord blood levels are approximately 100% of the maternal serum concentration (12,13).

In patients at risk for premature delivery, aminophylline (theophylline ethylenediamine) was found to exert a beneficial effect by reducing the perinatal death rate and the frequency of respiratory distress syndrome (14,15). In a nonrandomized study, aminophylline 250 mg IM every 12 hours up to a maximum of 3 days was compared with betamethasone, 4 mg IM every 8 hours for 2 days (15). Patients in the aminophylline group were excluded from receiving corticosteroids because of diabetes (4 patients), hypertension

(10 patients), and ruptured membranes for more than 24 hours (4 patients). The aminophylline and steroid groups were comparable in length of gestation (32.5 weeks vs. 32.1 weeks), male:female infant sex ratio (10:8 vs. 8:8), Apgar scores (7.6 vs. 7.7), birth weight (1720 g vs. 1690 g), and hours between treatment and delivery (73 vs. 68). Respiratory distress syndrome occurred in 11% (2 of 18) of the aminophylline group compared with 0% (0 of 16) of the corticosteroid group (*n.s.*). A significant difference ($p = 0.01$) was found in the incidence of neonatal infection with 8 of 16 (50%) of the betamethasone group having signs of infection and none in the aminophylline group. The mechanism proposed for aminophylline-induced fetal lung maturation is similar to that observed with betamethasone: enhancement of tissue cyclic AMP by inhibition of cyclic AMP phosphodiesterase and a corresponding increased production and/or release of phosphatidylcholine (15).

An IV infusion of aminophylline has been tested for its tocolytic effects on oxytocin-induced uterine contractions (16). A slight decrease in uterine activity occurred in the first 15 minutes, but this was related to the effect on contraction intensity, not frequency. The author concluded that aminophylline was a poor tocolytic agent. However, a more recent *in vitro* study examined the effect of increasing concentrations of aminophylline on pregnant human myometrium (17). Aminophylline produced a dose-related decrease in contraction strength and a non-dose-dependent lengthening of the period of contraction. In this study, the authors concluded that aminophylline may be a clinically useful tocolytic agent (17).

A reduction in the occurrence of preeclampsia among pregnant asthmatic women treated with theophylline has been reported (18). Preeclampsia occurred in 1.2% (1 of 85) of patients treated with theophylline compared with 8.8% (6/68) ($p < 0.05$) of asthmatic patients not treated with the drug. Although the results were significant, the small numbers indicate that the results must be interpreted cautiously (18). The authors proposed a possible mechanism for the protective effect, if indeed it does occur, involving the inhibition of platelet aggregation and the altering of vascular tone, two known effects of theophylline (18).

Concern over the depressant effects of methylxanthines on lipid synthesis in developing neural systems has been reported (19). Recent observations that infants treated for apnea with theophylline exhibit no overt neurologic deficits at 9–27 months of age are encouraging (20,21). However, the long-term effects of these drugs on human brain development are not known (19).

Frequent, high-dose asthmatic medication containing theophylline, ephedrine, phenobarbital, and diphenhydramine was used throughout pregnancy by one woman who delivered a stillborn girl with complete triploidy (22). Although drug-induced chromosomal damage could not be proven, theophylline has been shown in *in vitro* tests to cause breakage of chromosomes in human lymphocytes (23). However, the clinical significance of this breakage is doubtful.

Theophylline withdrawal in a newborn exposed throughout gestation has been reported (12). Apneic spells developed at 28 hours after delivery and became progressively worse over the next 4 days. Therapy with theophylline resolved the spells.

The pharmacokinetics of theophylline during pregnancy have been studied (24,25). One report suggested that plasma concentrations of theophylline fall during the 3rd trimester because of an increased maternal volume of distribution (24). However, a more recent study found a significantly lower clearance of theophylline during the 3rd trimester, ranging in some cases between 20% and 53% less (25). Two women had symptoms of toxicity requiring a dosage reduction.

BREAST FEEDING SUMMARY

RECOMMENDATION: Compatible

Theophylline is excreted into breast milk (26,27). A milk:plasma ratio of 0.7 has been measured (27). Estimates indicate that less than 1% of the maternal dose is excreted into breast milk (26,27). However, one infant became irritable secondary to a rapidly absorbed oral solution of aminophylline taken by the mother (26). Because very young infants may be more sensitive to levels that would be nontoxic in older infants, less rapidly absorbed theophylline preparations may be advisable for nursing mothers (10,28). Except for the precaution that theophylline may cause irritability in the nursing infant, the American Academy of Pediatrics classifies the drug as compatible with breast-feeding (29).

References

1. Greenberger P, Patterson R. Safety of therapy for allergic symptoms during pregnancy. Ann Intern Med 1978;89:234–7.
2. Weinstein AM, Dubin BD, Podleski WK, Spector SL, Farr RS. Asthma and pregnancy. JAMA 1979;241:1161–5.
3. Hernandez E, Angell CS, Johnson JWC. Asthma in pregnancy: current concepts. Obstet Gynecol 1980;55:739–43.
4. Turner ES, Greenberger PA, Patterson R. Management of the pregnant asthmatic patient. Ann Intern Med 1980;93:905–18.
5. Pratt WR. Allergic diseases in pregnancy and breast feeding. Ann Allergy 1981;47:355–60.
6. Lalli CM, Raju L. Pregnancy and chronic obstructive pulmonary disease. Chest 1981;80:759–61.
7. Product information. Theo-Dur. Key Pharmaceuticals, 2000.
8. Heinonen OP, Slone D, Shapiro S. *Birth Defects and Drugs in Pregnancy*. Littleton, MA: Publishing Sciences Group, 1977:367, 370.
9. Arwood LL, Dasta JF, Friedman C. Placental transfer of theophylline: two case reports. Pediatrics 1979;63:844–6.
10. Yeh TF, Pildes RS. Transplacental aminophylline toxicity in a neonate. Lancet 1977;1:910.
11. Labovitz E, Spector S. Placental theophylline transfer in pregnant asthmatics. JAMA 1982;247:786–8.
12. Horowitz DA, Jablonski W, Mehta KA. Apnea associated with theophylline withdrawal in a term neonate. Am J Dis Child 1982;136:73–4.
13. Ron M, Hochner-Celnikier D, Menczel J, Palti Z, Kidroni G. Maternal-fetal transfer of aminophylline. Acta Obstet Gynecol Scand 1984;63:217–8.
14. Hadjigeorgiou E, Kitsiou S, Psaroudakis A, Segos C, Nicolopoulos D, Kaskarelis D. Antepartum aminophylline treatment for prevention of the respiratory distress syndrome in premature infants. Am J Obstet Gynecol 1979;135:257–60.
15. Granati B, Grella PV, Pettenazzo A, Di Lenardo L, Rubaltelli FF. The prevention of respiratory distress syndrome in premature infants: efficacy of antenatal aminophylline treatment versus prenatal glucocorticoid administration. Pediatr Pharmacol (New York) 1984;4:21–4.
16. Lipshitz J. Uterine and cardiovascular effects of aminophylline. Am J Obstet Gynecol 1978;131:716–8.
17. Bird LM, Anderson NC Jr, Chandler ML, Young RC. The effects of aminophylline and nifedipine on contractility of isolated pregnant human myometrium. Am J Obstet Gynecol 1987;157:171–7.
18. Dombrowski MP, Bottoms SF, Boike GM, Wald J. Incidence of preeclampsia among asthmatic patients lower with theophylline. Am J Obstet Gynecol 1986;155:265–7.
19. Volpe JJ. Effects of methylxanthines on lipid synthesis in developing neural systems. Semin Perinatol 1981;5:395–405.
20. Aranda JV, Dupont C. Metabolic effects of methylxanthines in premature infants. J Pediatr 1976;89:833–4.
21. Nelson RM, Resnick MB, Holstrum WJ, Eitzman DV. Development outcome of premature infants treated with theophylline. Dev Pharmacol Ther 1980;1:274–80.
22. Halbrecht I, Komlos L, Shabtay F, Solomon M, Book JA. Triploidy 69,XXX in a stillborn girl. Clin Genet 1973;4:210–2.
23. Weinstein D, Mauer I, Katz ML, Kazmer S. The effect of methylxanthines on chromosomes of human lymphocytes in culture. Mutat Res 1975;31:57–61.
24. Sutton PL, Koup JR, Rose JQ, Middleton E. The pharmacokinetics of theophylline in pregnancy. J Allergy Clin Immunol 1978;61:174.
25. Carter BL, Driscoll CE, Smith GD. Theophylline clearance during pregnancy. Obstet Gynecol 1986;68:555–9.
26. Yurchak AM, Jusko WJ. Theophylline secretion into breast milk. Pediatrics 1976;57:518–25.
27. Stec GP, Greenberger P, Ruo TI, Henthorn T, Morita Y, Atkinson AJ Jr, Patterson R. Kinetics of theophylline transfer to breast milk. Clin Pharmacol Ther 1980;28:404–8.
28. Berlin CM. Excretion of methylxanthines in human milk. Semin Perinatol 1981;5:389–94.
29. Committee on Drugs, American Academy of Pediatrics. The transfer of drugs and other chemicals into human milk. Pediatrics 2001;108:776–89.

T

Name: **THIABENDAZOLE** Risk Factor: **C_M**
Class: **Anthelmintic**

FETAL RISK SUMMARY

RECOMMENDATION: Limited Human Data - Animal Data Suggest Low Risk

Thiabendazole is an anthelmintic agent. Reproduction studies in mice, rats, and rabbits at doses up to 2.5, 1, and 15 times, respectively, the usual human dose have revealed no evidence of fetal harm (1). When thiabendazole was prepared in an aqueous suspension, no defects were observed in mice given a dose 10 times the usual human dose. When the drug was suspended in olive oil at the same dose, however, cleft palate and axial skeletal defects were seen in mice offspring (1).

No reports of human teratogenicity caused by thiabendazole have been located. No adverse fetal effects were encountered when a single or divided dose of 50 mg/kg body weight was given to a group of pregnant women with intestinal parasites, although maternal side effects such as nausea and vomiting were common (2). The period of gestation was not specified in this report except that many of the pregnant patients received the drug just before delivery.

A 1985 review of intestinal parasites and pregnancy concluded that treatment of the pregnant patient should only be considered if the "parasite is causing clinical disease or may cause public health problems" (3). That review, and a similar article published in 1986 (4), recommended thiabendazole, when indicated, for the treatment of *Strongyloides stercoralis* infection occurring during pregnancy.

BREAST FEEDING SUMMARY

RECOMMENDATION: No Human Data - Probably Compatible

No reports describing the use of thiabendazole during lactation have been located. The molecular weight (about 201) is low enough, however, that excretion into breast milk should be expected.

References

1. Product information. Mintezol. Merck, 2000.
2. Chari MV, Hiremath RS. Thiabendazole (a new broad-spectrum anthelmintic) in intestinal helminthiasis. J Assoc Physicians India 1967;15:93–6.
3. D'Alauro F, Lee RV, Pao-In K, Khairallah M. Intestinal parasites and pregnancy. Obstet Gynecol 1985;66:639–43.
4. Ellis CJ. Antiparasitic agents in pregnancy. Clin Obstet Gynecol 1986;13:269–75.

T

Name: **THIAMINE** Risk Factor: **A***
Class: **Vitamin**

FETAL RISK SUMMARY

RECOMMENDATION: Compatible

Thiamine (vitamin B_1), a water-soluble B complex vitamin, is an essential nutrient required for carbohydrate metabolism (1). The National Academy of Sciences' recommended dietary allowance (RDA) for thiamine in pregnancy is 1.5 mg (1).

Thiamine is actively transported to the fetus (2–5). Like other B complex vitamins, concentrations of thiamine in the fetus and newborn are higher than in the mother (4–11).

Maternal thiamine deficiency is common during pregnancy (11–12). Supplementation with multivitamin products reduces the thiamine hypovitaminemia only slightly (9). Since 1938, several authors have attempted to link this deficiency to toxemia of pregnancy (13–16). A 1945 paper summarized the early work published in this area (14). All of the reported cases, however, involved patients with poor nutrition and pregnancy care in general. More recent investigations have failed to find any relationship between maternal thiamine deficiency and toxemia, fetal defects, or other outcome of pregnancy (8,17).

No association was found between low birth weight and thiamine levels in a 1977 report (7). One group has shown experimentally, though, that the characteristic intrauterine growth retardation of the fetal alcohol syndrome may be caused by ethanol-induced thiamine deficiency (18).

Thiamine has been used to treat hyperemesis gravidarum, although pyridoxine (vitamin B_6) was found to be more effective (see Pyridoxine) (19–21). In one early report, thiamine was effective in reversing severe neurologic complications associated with hyperemesis (19). A mother treated with frequent injections of thiamine and pyridoxine, 50 mg each/dose, for hyperemesis during the first half of two pregnancies delivered two infants with severe convulsions, one of whom died within 30 hours of birth (21). The convulsions in the mentally retarded second infant were eventually controlled with pyridoxine. Pyridoxine dependency-induced convulsions are rare. The authors speculated that the defect was caused by *in utero* exposure to high circulating levels of the vitamin. Thiamine was not thought to be involved (see Pyridoxine).

An isolated case report described an anencephalic fetus whose mother was under psychiatric care (22). She had been treated with very high doses of vitamins B_1, B_6, C, and folic acid. The relationship between the vitamins and the defect is unknown. Also unproven is the speculation by one researcher that an association exists between thiamine deficiency and Down's syndrome (trisomy 21) or preleukemic bone marrow changes (23).

[**Risk Factor C if used in doses above the RDA.*]

BREAST FEEDING SUMMARY

RECOMMENDATION: Compatible

Thiamine (vitamin B_1) is excreted into breast milk (24–27). One group of investigators supplemented well-nourished lactating women with a multivitamin preparation containing 1.7 mg of thiamine (24). At 6 months postpartum, milk concentrations of thiamine did not differ significantly from those of control patients not receiving supplements. In a study of lactating women with low nutritional status, supplementation with thiamine, 0.2–20.0 mg/day, resulted in mean milk concentrations of 125–268 ng/mL (25). Milk concentrations were directly proportional to dietary intake. A 1983 English study measured thiamine levels in pooled human milk obtained from preterm (26 mothers: 29–34 weeks) and term (35 mothers: 39 weeks or longer) patients (26). Milk obtained from preterm mothers rose from 23.7 ng/mL (colostrum) to 89.3 ng/mL (16–196 days) while milk from term mothers increased during the same period from a level of 28.4 to 183 ng/mL.

In Asian mothers with severe thiamine deficiency, including some with beriberi, infants have become acutely ill after-breast feeding, leading in some cases to convulsions and sudden death (28–31). Pneumonia was usually a characteristic finding. One author thought the condition was related to toxic intermediary metabolites, such as methylglyoxal, passing to the infant via the milk (28). Although a cause-and-effect relationship has not been

T

proven, one report suggested that thiamine deficiency may aggravate the condition (29). Indian investigators measured very low thiamine milk levels in mothers of children with convulsions of unknown cause (32). Mean milk thiamine concentrations in mothers of healthy children were 111 ng/mL, whereas those in mothers of children with convulsions were 29 ng/mL. The authors were unable to establish an association between the low thiamine content in milk and infantile convulsions (see Pyridoxine for correlation between low levels of vitamin B_6 and convulsions).

A 1992 case described the features of "Shoshin beriberi" in a 3-month-old breast-fed infant (33). Both the infant and the mother had biochemical evidence of thiamine deficiency. Clinical features in the infant included cardiac failure with vasoconstriction, hypotension, severe metabolic acidosis, and atypical grand mal seizures. He responded quickly to thiamine and made an unremarkable recovery.

The National Academy of Sciences' RDA for thiamine during lactation is 1.6 mg (1). If the diet of the lactating woman adequately supplies this amount, maternal supplementation with thiamine is not needed (27). Supplementation with the RDA for thiamine is recommended for those women with inadequate nutritional intake. The American Academy of Pediatrics classifies thiamine as compatible with breast-feeding (34).

References

1. American Hospital Formulary Service. *Drug Information 1997*. Bethesda, MD: American Society of Health-System Pharmacists, 1997:2818–20.
2. Frank O, Walbroehl G, Thomson A, Kaminetzky H, Kubes Z, Baker H. Placental transfer: fetal retention of some vitamins. Am J Clin Nutr 1970;23:662–3.
3. Hill EP, Longo LD. Dynamics of maternal-fetal nutrient transfer. Fed Proc 1980;39:239–44.
4. Kaminetzky HA, Baker H, Frank O, Langer A. The effects of intravenously administered water-soluble vitamins during labor in normovitaminemic and hypovitaminemic gravidas on maternal and neonatal blood vitamin levels at delivery. Am J Obstet Gynecol 1974;120:697–703.
5. Baker H, Frank O, Deangelis B, Feingold S, Kaminetzky HA. Role of placenta in maternal-fetal vitamin transfer in humans. Am J Obstet Gynecol 1981;141:792–6.
6. Slobody LB, Willner MM, Mestern J. Comparison of vitamin B_1 levels in mothers and their newborn infants. Am J Dis Child 1949;77:736–9.
7. Baker H, Thind IS, Frank O, DeAngelis B, Caterini H, Lquria DB. Vitamin levels in low-birth-weight newborn infants and their mothers. Am J Obstet Gynecol 1977;129:521–4.
8. Heller S, Salkeld RM, Korner WF. Vitamin B_1 status in pregnancy. Am J Clin Nutr 1974;27:1221–4.
9. Baker H, Frank O, Thomson AD, Langer A, Munves ED, De Angelis B, Kaminetzky HA. Vitamin profile of 174 mothers and newborns at parturition. Am J Clin Nutr 1975;28:59–65.
10. Tripathy K. Erythrocyte transketolase activity and thiamine transfer across human placenta. Am J Clin Nutr 1968;21:739–42.
11. Bamji MS. Enzymic evaluation of thiamin, riboflavin and pyridoxine status of parturient women and their newborn infants. Br J Nutr 1976;35:259–65.
12. Dostalova L. Correlation of the vitamin status between mother and newborn during delivery. Dev Pharmacol Ther 1982;4(Suppl 1):45–57.
13. Siddall AC. Vitamin B_1 deficiency as an etiologic factor in pregnancy toxemias. Am J Obstet Gynecol 1938;35:662–7.
14. King G, Ride LT. The relation of vitamin B_1 deficiency to the pregnancy toxaemias: a study of 371 cases of beriberi complicating pregnancy. J Obstet Gynaecol Br Emp 1945;52:130–47.
15. Chaudhuri SK, Halder K, Chowdhury SR, Bagchi K. Relationship between toxaemia of pregnancy and thiamine deficiency. J Obstet Gynaecol Br Commonw 1969;76:123–6.
16. Chaudhuri SK. Role of nutrition in the etiology of toxemia of pregnancy. Am J Obstet Gynecol 1971; 110:46–8.
17. Thomson AM. Diet in pregnancy. 3. Diet in relation to the course and outcome of pregnancy. Br J Nutr 1959;13:509–25.
18. Roecklein B, Levin SW, Comly M, Mukherjee AB. Intrauterine growth retardation induced by thiamine deficiency and pyrithiamine during pregnancy in the rat. Am J Obstet Gynecol 1985;151:455–60.
19. Fouts PJ, Gustafson GW, Zerfas LG. Successful treatment of a case of polyneuritis of pregnancy. Am J Obstet Gynecol 1934;28:902–7.
20. Willis RS, Winn WW, Morris AT, Newsom AA, Massey WE. Clinical observations in treatment of nausea and vomiting in pregnancy with vitamins B_1 and B_6: a preliminary report. Am J Obstet Gynecol 1942;44:265–71.
21. Hunt AD Jr, Stokes J Jr, McCrory WW, Stroud HH. Pyridoxine dependency: report of a case of intractable convulsions in an infant controlled by pyridoxine. Pediatrics 1954;13:140–5.
22. Averback P. Anencephaly associated with megavitamin therapy. Can Med Assoc J 1976;114:995.
23. Reading C. Down's syndrome, leukaemia and maternal thiamine deficiency. Med J Aust 1976;1:505.
24. Thomas MR, Sneed SM, Wei C, Nail P, Wilson M, Sprinkle EE III. The effects of vitamin C, vitamin B_6, vitamin B_{12}, folic acid, riboflavin, and thiamin on the breast

T

milk and maternal status of well-nourished women at 6 months postpartum. Am J Clin Nutr 1980;33:2151–6.
25. Deodhar AD, Rajalakshmi R, Ramakrishnan CV. Studies on human lactation. Part III. Effect of dietary vitamin supplementation on vitamin contents of breast milk. Acta Paediatr Scand 1964;53:42–8.
26. Ford JE, Zechalko A, Murphy J, Brooke OG. Comparison of the B vitamin composition of milk from mothers of preterm and term babies. Arch Dis Child 1983;58:367–72.
27. Nail PA, Thomas MR, Eakin R. The effect of thiamin and riboflavin supplementation on the level of those vitamins in human breast milk and urine. Am J Clin Nutr 1980;33:198–204.
28. Fehily L. Human-milk intoxication due to B_1 avitaminosis. Br Med J 1944;2:590–2.
29. Cruickshank JD, Trimble AP, Brown JAH. Interstitial mononuclear pneumonia: a cause of sudden death in Gurkha infants in the Far East. Arch Dis Child 1957;32:279–84.
30. Mayer J. Nutrition and lactation. Postgrad Med 1963;33:380–5.
31. Gunther M. Diet and milk secretion in women. Proc Nutr Soc 1968;27:77–82.
32. Rao RR, Subrahmanyam I. An investigation on the thiamine content of mother's milk in relation to infantile convulsions. Indian J Med Res 1964;52:1198–201.
33. Debuse PJ. Shoshin beriberi in an infant of a thiamine-deficient mother. Acta Paediatr 1992;81:723–4.
34. Committee on Drugs, American Academy of Pediatrics. The transfer of drugs and other chemicals into human milk. Pediatrics 2001;108:776–89.

Name: **THIOGUANINE** Risk Factor: **D_M**
Class: **Antineoplastic**

FETAL RISK SUMMARY

RECOMMENDATION: Human and Animal Data Suggest Risk

Thioguanine is a purine analogue that interferes with nucleic acid biosynthesis. The drug is potentially mutagenic, carcinogenic, and teratogenic (1).

Reproduction studies in rats at a dose 5 times the human dose caused resorptions and malformed or stunted offspring (1). Malformations observed included generalized edema, cranial defects, general skeletal hypoplasia, hydrocephalus, ventral hernia, situs inversus, and limb defects (1).

The use of thioguanine in pregnancy has been reported in 26 patients, four during the 1st trimester (2–19). An elective abortion, resulting in a normal fetus, was performed at 21 weeks' gestation in one pregnancy after 4 weeks of chemotherapy (17). Use in the 1st and 2nd trimesters has been associated with chromosomal abnormalities in one infant (relationship to antineoplastic therapy unknown), trisomy group C autosomes with mosaicism (2), and congenital malformations in another, two medial digits of both feet missing and distal phalanges of both thumbs missing with hypoplastic remnant of right thumb (3). In a third case, a fetus, who was not exposed to antineoplastic agents until the 23rd week, long after development of the affected extremity, was delivered at 42 weeks' gestation with polydactyly (six toes on the right foot), a condition that had occurred previously in this family (18).

Two cases of intrauterine fetal death have occurred after antineoplastic therapy with thioguanine and other agents (15,18). In one case, a mother, whose antileukemic chemotherapy was initiated at 15 weeks' gestation, developed severe pregnancy-induced hypertension in the 29th week of pregnancy (15). Before this time, fetal well-being had been continuously documented. One week after onset of the preeclampsia, intrauterine fetal death was confirmed by ultrasound. In the second case, a woman, with a history of two previous 1st trimester spontaneous abortions, was treated for acute myeloblastic leukemia and ulcerative colitis beginning at 15 weeks' gestation (18). Intrauterine fetal death occurred at 20 weeks. No congenital abnormalities were found at autopsy in either of the fetuses.

Data from one review indicated that 40% of the infants exposed to anticancer drugs were of low birth weight (20). This finding was not related to the timing of exposure. Long-term studies of growth and mental development in offspring exposed to thioguanine during the 2nd trimester, the period of neuroblast multiplication, have not been conducted (21). However, individual children have been followed for periods ranging from a few months to 5 years and, in each case, normal development was documented (14,15,17,18).

Although abnormal chromosomal changes were observed in one aborted fetus, the clinical significance of this observation and the relationship to antineoplastic therapy are unknown. In two other newborns, karyotyping of cultured cells did not show anomalies (2,5). Paternal use of thioguanine with other antineoplastic agents before conception has been suggested as a cause of congenital defects observed in three infants: anencephalic stillborn (22), tetralogy of Fallot with syndactyly of the first and second toes (22), and multiple anomalies (23). However, confirmation of these data has not been forthcoming, and any such relationship is probably tenuous at best. Exposed men have also fathered normal children (23,24).

Occupational exposure of the mother to antineoplastic agents during pregnancy may present a risk to the fetus. A position statement from the National Study Commission on Cytotoxic Exposure and a research article involving some antineoplastic agents are presented in the monograph for cyclophosphamide (see Cyclophosphamide).

BREAST FEEDING SUMMARY

RECOMMENDATION: Contraindicated

No reports describing the use of thioguanine during lactation have been located. It is not known if the drug is excreted into breast milk. Because of the potential for severe toxicity, including tumors, in a nursing infant, women receiving thioguanine should not breast-feed.

References

1. Product information. Thioguanine. Glaxo Wellcome, 2000.
2. Maurer LH, Forcier RJ, McIntyre OR, Benirschke K. Fetal group C trisomy after cytosine arabinoside and thioguanine. Ann Intern Med 1971;75:809–10.
3. Schafer AI. Teratogenic effects of antileukemic chemotherapy. Arch Intern Med 1981;141:514–5.
4. Au-Yong R, Collins P, Young JA. Acute myeloblastic leukaemia during pregnancy. Br Med J 1972;4:493–4.
5. Raich PC, Curet LB. Treatment of acute leukemia during pregnancy. Cancer 1975;36:861–2.
6. Gokal R, Durrant J, Baum JD, Bennett MJ. Successful pregnancy in acute monocytic leukaemia. Br J Cancer 1976;34:299–302.
7. Lilleyman JS, Hill AS, Anderton KJ. Consequences of acute myelogenous leukemia in early pregnancy. Cancer 1977;40:1300–3.
8. Moreno H, Castleberry RP, McCann WP. Cytosine arabinoside and 6-thioguanine in the treatment of childhood acute myeloblastic leukemia. Cancer 1977;40:998–1004.
9. Manoharan A, Leyden MJ. Acute non-lymphocytic leukaemia in the third trimester of pregnancy. Aust N Z J Med 1979;9:71–4.
10. Taylor G, Blom J. Acute leukemia during pregnancy. South Med J 1980;73:1314–5.
11. Tobias JS, Bloom HJG. Doxorubicin in pregnancy. Lancet 1980;1:776.
12. Pawliger DF, McLean FW, Noyes WD. Normal fetus after cytosine arabinoside therapy. Ann Intern Med 1971;74:1012.
13. Plows CW. Acute myelomonocytic leukemia in pregnancy: report of a case. Am J Obstet Gynecol 1982;143:41–3.
14. Lowenthal RM, Marsden KA, Newman NM, Baikie MJ, Campbell SN. Normal infant after treatment of acute myeloid leukaemia in pregnancy with daunorubicin. Aust N Z J Med 1978;8:431–2.
15. O'Donnell R, Costigan C, O'Connell LG. Two cases of acute leukaemia in pregnancy. Acta Haematol 1979;61:298–300.
16. Hamer JW, Beard MEJ, Duff GB. Pregnancy complicated by acute myeloid leukaemia. N Z Med J 1979;89:212–3.
17. Doney KC, Kraemer KG, Shepard TH. Combination chemotherapy for acute myelocytic leukemia during pregnancy: three case reports. Cancer Treat Rep 1979;63:369–71.
18. Volkenandt M, Buchner T, Hiddemann W, Van De Loo J. Acute leukaemia during pregnancy. Lancet 1987;2:1521–2.
19. Feliu J, Juarez S, Ordonez A, Garcia-Paredes ML,

T

Gonzalez-Baron M, Montero JM. Acute leukemia and pregnancy. Cancer 1988;61:580–4.
20. Nicholson HO. Cytotoxic drugs in pregnancy: review of reported cases. J Obstet Gynaecol Br Commonw 1968;75:307–12.
21. Dobbing J. Pregnancy and leukaemia. Lancet 1977;1:1155.
22. Russell JA, Powles RL, Oliver RTD. Conception and congenital abnormalities after chemotherapy of acute myelogenous leukaemia in two men. Br Med J 1976;1:1508.
23. Evenson DP, Arlin Z, Welt S, Claps ML, Melamed MR. Male reproductive capacity may recover following drug treatment with the L-10 protocol for acute lymphocytic leukemia. Cancer 1984;53:30–6.
24. Matthews JH, Wood JK. Male fertility during chemotherapy for acute leukemia. N Engl J Med 1980;303:1235.

Name: **THIOPROPAZATE** Risk Factor: **C**
Class: **Tranquilizer**

FETAL RISK SUMMARY

RECOMMENDATION: No Human Data - No Relevant Animal Data

Thiopropazate is a piperazine phenothiazine in the same group as prochlorperazine (see Prochlorperazine). Phenothiazines readily cross the placenta (1). No specific information on the use of thiopropazate in pregnancy has been located. Although occasional reports have attempted to link various phenothiazine compounds with congenital malformations, the bulk of the evidence indicates that these drugs are safe for the mother and low risk for the embryo/fetus (see Chlorpromazine).

BREAST FEEDING SUMMARY

RECOMMENDATION: No Human Data - Potential Toxicity

No data are available.

Reference

1. Moya F, Thorndike V. Passage of drugs across the placenta. Am J Obstet Gynecol 1962;84:1778–98.

Name: **THIORIDAZINE** Risk Factor: **C**
Class: **Tranquilizer**

FETAL RISK SUMMARY

RECOMMENDATION: Limited Human Data - No Relevant Animal Data

Thioridazine is a piperidyl phenothiazine. The drug is not teratogenic in animals (species not specified) (1).

The phenothiazines readily cross the placenta (2). Extrapyramidal symptoms were seen in a newborn exposed to thioridazine *in utero*, but the reaction was probably caused by chlorpromazine (3).

In a surveillance study of Michigan Medicaid recipients conducted between 1985 and 1992 involving 229,101 completed pregnancies, 63 newborns had been exposed to thioridazine during the 1st trimester (F. Rosa, personal communication, FDA, 1993). Two (3.2%)

major birth defects were observed (three expected), one of which was a cardiovascular defect (one expected). No anomalies were observed in five other categories of defects (oral clefts, spina bifida, polydactyly, limb-reduction defects, and hypospadias) for which specific data were available.

A case of a congenital heart defect was described in 1969 (4). However, one investigator found no anomalies in the offspring of 23 patients exposed throughout gestation to thioridazine (5). Twenty of the infants were evaluated for up to 13 years.

A brief 1993 report described a 31-year-old woman with depression, panic disorder, and migraine headaches who was exposed to a number of drugs in the first 6 weeks of pregnancy, including thioridazine, dihydroergotamine, citalopram, buspirone, and etilefrine (a sympathomimetic agent) (6). An elective abortion at 12 weeks' gestation revealed a normal fetus.

Although occasional reports have attempted to link various phenothiazine compounds with congenital malformations, the bulk of the evidence indicates that these drugs are safe for the mother and low risk for the embryo/fetus (see Chlorpromazine).

BREAST FEEDING SUMMARY

RECOMMENDATION: No Human Data - Potential Toxicity

No data are available.

References

1. Product information. Mellaril. Sandoz Pharmaceutical Corporation, 1993.
2. Moya F, Thorndike V. Passage of drugs across the placenta. Am J Obstet Gynecol 1962;84:1778–98.
3. Hill RM, Desmond MM, Kay JL. Extrapyramidal dysfunction in an infant of a schizophrenic mother. J Pediatr 1966;69:589–95.
4. Vince DJ. Congenital malformations following phenothiazine administration during pregnancy. Can Med Assoc J 1969;100:223.
5. Scanlan FJ. The use of thioridazine (Mellaril) during the first trimester. Med J Aust 1972;1:1271–2.
6. Seifritz E, Holsboer-Trachsler E, Haberthur F, Hemmeter U, Poldinger W. Unrecognized pregnancy during citalopram treatment. Am J Psychiatry 1993;150:1428–9.

Name:	**THIOTEPA**	Risk Factor:	**D_M**
Class:	**Antineoplastic**		

T

FETAL RISK SUMMARY

RECOMMENDATION: Contraindicated - 1st Trimester

Thiotepa is a polyfunctional cytotoxic agent that is related chemically and pharmacologically to nitrogen mustard (see Mechlorethamine).

The drug impairs fertility and is carcinogenic, mutagenic, and teratogenic in animals (1). Reproduction studies in mice and rats at intraperitoneal doses 1/8th and 1 times, respectively, the maximum recommended human dose based on body surface area (MRHD) revealed teratogenicity in both species. Embryo lethality was noted in rabbits at 2 times the MRHD (1).

Thiotepa has been used during the 2nd and 3rd trimesters in one patient without apparent fetal harm (2). Long-term studies of growth and mental development in offspring exposed to antineoplastic agents during the 2nd trimester, the period of neuroblast multiplication, have not been conducted (3).

Occupational exposure of the mother to antineoplastic agents during pregnancy may present a risk to the fetus. A position statement from the National Study Commission on Cytotoxic Exposure and a research article involving some antineoplastic agents are presented in the monograph for cyclophosphamide (see Cyclophosphamide).

BREAST FEEDING SUMMARY

RECOMMENDATION: Contraindicated

No reports describing the use of thiotepa during lactation have been located. The molecular weight (about 189) is low enough, however, that excretion into breast milk should be expected. Because of the potential for severe toxicity, including tumors, in a nursing infant, women receiving thiotepa should not breast-feed.

References

1. Product information. Thioplex. Immunex, 2000.
2. Gililland J, Weinstein L. The effects of cancer chemotherapeutic agents on the developing fetus. Obstet Gynecol Surv 1983;38:6–13.
3. Dobbing J. Pregnancy and leukaemia. Lancet 1977;1:1155.

Name:	**THIOTHIXENE**	Risk Factor:	**C**
Class:	**Tranquilizer**		

FETAL RISK SUMMARY

RECOMMENDATION: Limited Human Data - Animal Data Suggest Low Risk

Thiothixene is structurally and pharmacologically related to trifluoperazine and chlorprothixene (see Trifluoperazine). The drug is not teratogenic in mice, rats, rabbits, and monkeys (1–3).

In a surveillance study of Michigan Medicaid recipients conducted between 1985 and 1992 involving 229,101 completed pregnancies, 38 newborns had been exposed to thiothixene during the 1st trimester (F. Rosa, personal communication, FDA, 1993). One (2.6%) major birth defect (two expected), a cardiovascular defect (0.5 expected), was observed. No anomalies were observed in five other categories of defects (oral clefts, spina bifida, polydactyly, limb reduction defects, and hypospadias) for which specific data were available.

BREAST FEEDING SUMMARY

RECOMMENDATION: No Human Data - Potential Toxicity

No reports describing the use of thiothixene during lactation have been located. The molecular weight (about 444) is low enough, however, that excretion into breast milk should be expected. The effects on a nursing infant from exposure to the drug in milk are unknown.

References

1. Owaki Y, Momiyama H, Yokoi Y. Teratological studies on thiothixene in mice. (Japanese) Oyo Yakuri 1969;3:315–20. As cited in Shepard TH. *Catalog of Teratogenic Agents*. 6th ed. Baltimore, MD: Johns Hopkins University Press, 1989:618.
2. Owaki Y, Momiyama H, Yokoi Y. Teratological studies on thiothixene (Navane) in rabbits (Japanese). Oyo Yakuri 1969;3:321–4. As cited in Shepard TH. *Catalog of Teratogenic Agents*. 6th ed. Baltimore, MD: Johns Hopkins University Press, 1989;618.
3. Product information. Navane. Pfizer, 2000.

Name:	**THIPHENAMIL**	Risk Factor:	**C**
Class:	**Parasympatholytic (Anticholinergic)**		

FETAL RISK SUMMARY

RECOMMENDATION: No Human Data - No Relevant Animal Data

Thiphenamil is an anticholinergic agent used in the treatment of parkinsonism. No reports of its use in pregnancy have been located (see also Atropine).

BREAST FEEDING SUMMARY

RECOMMENDATION: No Human Data - Probably Compatible

No data are available.

Name:	**THYROGLOBULIN**	Risk Factor:	**A**
Class:	**Thyroid**		

See Thyroid.

Name:	**THYROID**	Risk Factor:	**A**
Class:	**Thyroid**		

FETAL RISK SUMMARY

RECOMMENDATION: Compatible

T

Thyroid contains the two thyroid hormones levothyroxine (T_4) and liothyronine (T_3) plus other materials peculiar to the thyroid gland. It is used during pregnancy for the treatment of hypothyroidism. Neither T_4 nor T_3 crosses the placenta when physiologic serum concentrations are present in the mother (see Levothyroxine and Liothyronine). In one report, however, two patients, each of whom had produced two cretins in previous pregnancies, were given huge amounts of thyroid, up to 1600 mg/day or more (1). Both newborns were normal at birth even though one was found to be athyroid. The authors concluded that sufficient hormone was transported to the fetuses to prevent hypothyroidism.

Congenital defects have been reported with the use of thyroid but are thought to be caused by maternal hypothyroidism or other factors (see Levothyroxine and Liothyronine).

In a surveillance study of Michigan Medicaid recipients conducted between 1985 and 1992 involving 229,101 completed pregnancies, 44 newborns had been exposed to thyroid during the 1st trimester (F. Rosa, personal communication, FDA, 1993). One (2.3%) major birth defect (two expected), a cardiovascular defect (0.5 expected), was observed.

Combination therapy with thyroid-antithyroid drugs was advocated at one time for the treatment of hyperthyroidism but is now considered inappropriate (see Propylthiouracil).

BREAST FEEDING SUMMARY

RECOMMENDATION: Compatible

See Levothyroxine and Liothyronine.

Reference

1. Carr EA Jr, Beierwaltes WH, Raman G, Dodson VN, Tanton J, Betts JS, Stambaugh RA. The effect of maternal thyroid function on fetal thyroid function and development. J Clin Endocrinol Metab 1959;19:1–18.

Name: **THYROTROPIN** Risk Factor: **C_M**
Class: **Thyroid**

FETAL RISK SUMMARY

RECOMMENDATION: Compatible

Thyrotropin (thyroid-stimulating hormone, TSH) does not cross the placenta (1). No correlation exists between maternal and fetal concentrations of TSH at any time during gestation (2).

BREAST FEEDING SUMMARY

RECOMMENDATION: Compatible

No reports describing the excretion of thyrotropin in human milk have been located. Serum levels of this hormone have been measured and compared in breast-fed and bottle-fed infants (3–7). Breast milk does not provide sufficient levothyroxine (T_4) or liothyronine (T_3) to prevent the effects of congenital hypothyroidism (see Levothyroxine and Liothyronine). As a consequence, serum levels of TSH in breast-fed hypothyroid infants are markedly elevated (3,4). In euthyroid babies, no differences in TSH levels have been discovered between breast-fed and bottle-fed groups (5–7).

T

References

1. Cohlan SQ. Fetal and neonatal hazards from drugs administered during pregnancy. N Y State J Med 1964; 64:493–9.
2. Feely J. The physiology of thyroid function in pregnancy. Postgrad Med J 1979;55:336–9.
3. Abbassi V, Steinour TA. Successful diagnosis of congenital hypothyroidism in four breast-fed neonates. J Pediatr 1980;97:259–61.
4. Letarte J, Guyda H, Dussault JH, Glorieux J. Lack of protective effect of breast-feeding in congenital hypothyroidism: report of 12 cases. Pediatrics 1980;65:703–5.
5. Mizuta H, Amino N, Ichihara K, Harada T, Nose O, Tanizawa O, Miyai K. Thyroid hormones in human milk and their influence on thyroid function of breast-fed babies. Pediatr Res 1983;17:468–71.
6. Hahn HB Jr, Spiekerman M, Otto WR, Hossalla DE. Thyroid function tests in neonates fed human milk. Am J Dis Child 1983;137:220–2.
7. Franklin R, O'Grady C, Carpenter L. Neonatal thyroid function: comparison between breast-fed and bottle-fed infants. J Pediatr 1985;106:124–6.

Name:	**TIAGABINE**	Risk Factor:	**C_M**
Class:	**Anticonvulsant**		

FETAL RISK SUMMARY

RECOMMENDATION: Limited Human Data - Animal Data Suggest Risk

The oral anticonvulsant tiagabine enhances the activity of gamma aminobutyric acid, the major inhibitory neurotransmitter in the central nervous system. It is not known if this relates to its anticonvulsant activity. Tiagabine is indicated as adjunctive therapy in the treatment of partial seizures. Its elimination half-life is 7–9 hours, but is decreased to 4–7 hours in patients who are concurrently receiving hepatic enzyme-inducing anticonvulsants (e.g., carbamazepine, phenytoin, primidone, and phenobarbital). A 1996 review stated that the elimination half-life was 4–13 hours (mean 7 hours) and decreased to 2–3 hours when combined with enzyme-inducing anticonvulsants (2). In plasma, 96% is bound to albumin and α_1-acid glycoprotein (1,2). Although not all of the metabolites have been identified, at least one is inactive (1). Of particular interest, a 1996 review stated that metabolism of tiagabine (based on data from a manufacturer) results in arene oxide metabolites (3). These intermediate free radicals have been associated with human teratogenicity (see Carbamazepine, Phenytoin, and Valproic Acid).

Reproduction studies with tiagabine have been conducted in rats and rabbits. In pregnant rats treated during organogenesis, maternal toxic (weight loss/reduced weight gain) doses approximately 16 times the maximum recommended human dose based on body surface area (MRHD) were associated with an increased incidence of fetal malformations (craniofacial, appendicular, and visceral defects) and growth retardation. When this dose was given during late gestation and throughout parturition and lactation, maternal toxicity (decreased weight gain), stillbirths, and decreased postnatal offspring viability and growth were observed. No maternal or fetal adverse effects were observed at three times the MRHD. In pregnant rabbits, a dose eight times the MRHD caused maternal toxicity (decreased weight gain), embryo death, and fetal variations. The no effect dose for maternal, embryo, and fetal toxicity was approximately equivalent to the MRHD (1).

In rats, high doses (36–100 times the plasma exposure [AUC] obtained with the maximum recommended human dose of 56 mg/day) for 2 years were carcinogenic (hepatocellular adenomas in females and Leydig cell tumors of the testis in males). In an *in vitro* test, tiagabine, in the absence of metabolic activation, caused increased structural chromosome aberration frequency in human lymphocytes. This toxicity, however, was not observed in the assay in the presence of metabolic activation. Similarly, no genetic toxicity was observed in several other *in vitro* or *in vivo* assays (1).

It is not known if tiagabine crosses the human placenta, but the molecular weight (376 for the free base) is low enough that exposure of the embryo and fetus should be expected. The moderately long elimination half-life will result in prolonged concentrations of the drug at the maternal blood-placenta interface, thus increasing the opportunity for embryo/fetal exposure.

Only one report has been located describing the outcomes of human pregnancies exposed to tiagabine (3). Among 23 pregnancies exposed in a preclinical trial, there was one maternal death (unrelated to therapy), four spontaneous abortions, eight elective abortions (including one blighted ovum and one ectopic pregnancy), eight normal outcomes, and one infant with unspecified malformations (also receiving other unspecified anticonvulsants). Specific data relating to the exposures (e.g., dose, duration, timing) were not provided.

The effect of tiagabine on folic acid levels and metabolism is unknown (3). Although not specifically referring to tiagabine, a 2003 review recommended that to reduce the risk of birth defects from anticonvulsants, women should start multivitamins with folic acid before conception (4). Although the recommendation did not specify the amount of folic acid, a recent study found that multivitamin supplements with folic acid (typically 0.4 mg) did not reduce the risk of congenital malformations from four first-generation anticonvulsants (see Carbamazepine, Phenytoin, Phenobarbital, or Primidone). Therefore, until further information is available, the best course is to start folic acid supplementation before conception. Although a specific dosage recommendation has not been determined for patients receiving anticonvulsants, 4 mg/day appears to be reasonable.

In summary, tiagabine was not teratogenic or embryo/fetal toxic in experimental animals at doses that did not cause maternal toxicity. The human data are too limited to determine the degree of risk this agent presents to human embryos or fetuses. Of concern, however, metabolism of tiagabine results in epoxide metabolites. As noted above, these intermediate arene oxide metabolites from other anticonvulsants have been associated with human teratogenicity. Therefore, the safest course is to avoid tiagabine, if possible, during the 1st trimester, but there is no evidence that exposure during organogenesis or at any other time during gestation will result in fetal harm. If tiagabine is required, monotherapy using the lowest effective dose is preferred, but because of its status as adjunctive therapy, this may not be possible.

BREAST FEEDING SUMMARY

RECOMMENDATION: No Human Data - Probably Compatible

No studies describing the use of tiagabine during human lactation have been located. The molecular weight (about 376 for the free base), however, is low enough that excretion into breast milk should be expected. The drug and/or its metabolites are excreted into the milk of lactating rats (1). The effects on the nursing infant from exposure to tiagabine in milk are unknown.

References

1. Product information. Gabitril. Cephalon, 2003.
2. Perucca E, Bialer M. The clinical pharmacokinetics of the newer antiepileptic drugs. Clin Pharmacokinet 1996;31:29–46.
3. Morrell MJ. The new antiepileptic drugs and women: efficacy, reproductive health, pregnancy, and fetal outcome. Epilepsia 1996;37(Suppl 6):S34–S44.
4. Yerby MS. Clinical care of pregnant women with epilepsy: neural tube defects and folic acid supplementation. Epilepsia 2003;44(Suppl 3):33–40.

T

Name:	**TICARCILLIN**	Risk Factor:	**B**
Class:	**Antibiotic (Penicillin)**		

FETAL RISK SUMMARY

RECOMMENDATION: Compatible

Ticarcillin is a penicillin antibiotic. Reproduction studies in mice and rats have revealed no evidence of impaired fertility or fetal harm (1).

Ticarcillin rapidly crosses the placenta to the fetal circulation and amniotic fluid (2). Following a 1-g IV dose, single determinations of the amniotic fluid from six patients, 15–76 minutes after injection, yielded levels ranging from 1.0 to 3.3 μg/mL. Similar measurements of ticarcillin in cord serum ranged from 12.6 to 19.2 μg/mL. In a study using *in vitro* perfused human placentas, the fetal:maternal ratio of ticarcillin was 0.91 (3).

No reports linking the use of ticarcillin with congenital defects have been located. The Collaborative Perinatal Project monitored 50,282 mother-child pairs, 3,546 of whom had 1st trimester exposure to penicillin derivatives (4, pp. 297–313). For use anytime during pregnancy, 7171 exposures were recorded (4, p. 435). In neither group was evidence found to suggest a relationship to large categories of major or minor malformations or to individual defects.

BREAST FEEDING SUMMARY

RECOMMENDATION: Compatible

Ticarcillin is excreted into breast milk in low concentrations. After a 1-g IV dose given to five patients, only trace amounts of drug were measured at intervals up to 6 hours (2). Although these amounts are probably not significant, three potential problems exist for the nursing infant: modification of bowel flora, direct effects on the infant (e.g., allergic response), and interference with the interpretation of culture results if a fever workup is required. The American Academy of Pediatrics classifies ticarcillin as compatible with breast-feeding (5).

References

1. Product information. Ticar. SmithKline Beecham Pharmaceuticals, 2000.
2. Cho N, Nakayama T, Vehara K, Kunii K. Laboratory and clinical evaluation of ticarcillin in the field of obstetrics and gynecology. Chemotherapy (Tokyo) 1977;25:2911–23.
3. Fortunato SJ, Bawdon RE, Swan KF, Bryant EC, Sobhi S. Transfer of Timentin (ticarcillin and clavulanic acid) across the in vitro perfused human placenta: comparison with other agents. Am J Obstet Gynecol 1992; 167:1595–9.
4. Heinonen OP, Slone D, Shapiro S. *Birth Defects and Drugs in Pregnancy*. Littleton, MA: Publishing Sciences Group, 1977.
5. Committee on Drugs, American Academy of Pediatrics. The transfer of drugs and other chemicals into human milk. Pediatrics 2001;108:776–89.

Name: **TICLOPIDINE** Risk Factor: **B_M**

Class: **Hematological Agent (Antiplatelet)**

T

FETAL RISK SUMMARY

RECOMMENDATION: Limited Human Data - Animal Data Suggest Low Risk

Ticlopidine is a direct, irreversible inhibitor of adenosine diphosphate (ADP)-induced platelet aggregation. The drug has at least 20 metabolites, all of which appear to be inactive. Reversible protein binding is extensive (98%), primarily to albumin and lipoproteins, but some (15%) also is bound to α_1-acid glycoprotein. Ticlopidine is indicated for the reduction of risk of thrombotic stroke in patients who have stroke precursors and in patients who have had a completed thrombotic stroke (1).

Reproduction studies have been conducted in mice, rats, and rabbits at doses up to 200, 400, and 200 mg/kg/day, respectively (1). There was no evidence of teratogenicity at these doses, but maternal and fetal toxicity was observed at 200, 400, and 100 mg/kg/day, respectively. In male and female rats, however, no effects on fertility were observed at the highest dose. The maximum doses in mice and rats were approximately 29 and 56 times, respectively, the human clinical dose (HCD) on a weight basis, or 3 and 8 times, respectively, the HCD on a body surface area basis. Ticlopidine was not carcinogenic in mice or rats, or mutagenic in *in vitro* or *in vivo* assays (1).

Whether ticlopidine crosses the placenta is not known, but the molecular weight (about 300) is low enough that transfer to the fetus should be expected. Of interest, a platelet aggregation study was conducted on cord blood from a term pregnancy of a woman who had been receiving ticlopidine and aspirin for 2 weeks (2). Complete inhibition of platelet aggregation to 20 micromoles of ADP was demonstrated.

A 1998 case report described the treatment of an acute myocardial infarction in a 30-year-old woman at 38 weeks' gestation (2). Her condition did not improve with aspirin, heparin, nitrates, or balloon angioplasty, so a stent was placed in the partially occluded left anterior descending coronary artery during abciximab (an antiplatelet agent) infusion. Adequate flow was reestablished in the artery. Postoperatively, she was treated with ticlopidine, aspirin, and an unspecified beta-blocker. Two weeks later, she delivered vaginally a healthy baby boy with a normal ductus arteriosus. No excessive maternal bleeding was observed (2).

A woman with a history of essential thrombocytopenia and an anterior wall myocardial infarction was treated with chemotherapy (details not specified) to normalize her platelet count (3). After cardiac bypass surgery, she conceived while taking ticlopidine (500 mg/day) and aspirin (300 mg/day). A spontaneous abortion occurred in the 2nd trimester, 6 months after surgery. The woman's therapy was changed to clopidogrel and intermittent low molecular weight heparin, and she eventually had a normal pregnancy outcome. The relationship between the abortion and the ticlopidine/aspirin combination is unknown (3).

A 24-year-old woman with a history of aortic valve replacement with a 21-mm St. Jude Medical mechanical valve and two spontaneous abortions was treated before and through the 36th week of pregnancy with ticlopidine (300 mg/day), dipyridamole (300 mg/day), and aspirin (81 mg/day) (4). At that time, oral therapy was replaced with continuous IV heparin until delivery of a healthy baby (sex not specified) by an elective cesarean section at 38 weeks' gestation. No maternal or fetal thrombotic or bleeding complications were observed. Other than being healthy, no other information was given about the newborn (4).

In summary, ticlopidine is not teratogenic in experimental animals, but the human pregnancy experience is too limited to assess the potential risk to the embryo or fetus. Only three case reports have described the use of ticlopidine in human pregnancy, one of which ended in a spontaneous abortion. Ticlopidine may cause life-threatening blood dyscrasias, including neutropenia/agranulocytosis, thrombotic thrombocytopenia purpura, and aplastic anemia (1). The peak incidence for these disorders is in the first 3 months of therapy. The adverse effects are not predictable by any known demographic or clinical characteristics (1). Theoretically, if ticlopidine crossed the placenta, the fetus or newborn could also be at risk, as well as the mother. Therefore, because other antiplatelet agents are available, ticlopidine should only be used during pregnancy if other agents are judged to be less effective for the mother's condition.

BREAST FEEDING SUMMARY

RECOMMENDATION: No Human Data - Potential Toxicity

No reports describing the use of ticlopidine during human lactation have been located. The molecular weight (about 300) is low enough that excretion into breast milk should be expected. Ticlopidine is excreted in the milk of lactating rats (1). The potential effects of this exposure on a nursing infant are unknown. However, the life-threatening hematological adverse reactions that have been reported with this drug (see above), especially in the first 3 months of therapy, suggest that ticlopidine should not used by the lactating woman.

References

1. Product information. Ticlid. Roche Pharmaceuticals, 2002.
2. Sebastian C, Scherlag M, Kugelmass A, Schechter E. Primary stent implantation for acute myocardial infarction during pregnancy: use of abciximab, ticlopidine, and aspirin. Cathet Cardiovasc Diagn 1998;45:275–9.
3. Klinzing P, Markert UR, Liesaus K, Peiker G. Case report: successful pregnancy and delivery after myocardial infarction and essential thrombocythemia treated with clopidogrel. Clin Exp Obstet Gynecol 2001;28:215–6.
4. Ueno M, Masuda H, Nakamura K, Sakata R. Antiplatelet therapy for a pregnant woman with a mechanical aortic valve: report of a case. Surg Today 2001;31:1002–4.

Name: **TIMOLOL** Risk Factor: **C_M***

Class: **Sympatholytic (Antihypertensive)**

FETAL RISK SUMMARY

RECOMMENDATION: Human Data Suggest Risk in 2nd and 3rd Trimesters

Timolol is a nonselective β-adrenergic blocking agent used for the treatment of hypertension, after myocardial infarction, for the prophylaxis of migraine headache, and topically for the treatment of glaucoma.

Reproductive studies in mice, rats, and rabbits at doses up to about 40 times the maximum recommended daily human dose based on patient weight of 50 kg (MRHD) found no evidence of teratogenicity (1). However, fetotoxicity (resorptions) was observed in rabbits at this dose and in mice exposed to 830 times the MRHD (a maternal toxic dose).

A study using an *in vitro* perfusion system of human placental tissue demonstrated that timolol crossed to the fetal side of the preparation (2). The placental transfer is consistent with the molecular weight of the compound (about 433 for timolol maleate).

A woman with glaucoma was treated throughout gestation with topical timolol, 0.5% two drops in each eye, pilocarpine, and oral acetazolamide (3). Within 48 hours of delivery at 36 weeks' gestation, the infant developed hyperbilirubinemia, hypocalcemia, hypomagnesemia, and metabolic acidosis. The toxic effects, attributed to the carbonic anhydrase inhibitor, acetazolamide (see Acetazolamide), quickly resolved on treatment. Mild hypertonicity was observed at examinations at 1, 3, and 8 months of age.

In a 1998 case report, a 37-year-old woman at 21 weeks' gestation was referred because of fetal bradycardia (74 beats/minute) with irregularity (4). There were no cardiac structural anomalies and no fetal hydrops. The mother had been taking timolol eye drops 0.5%, one drop in each eye once daily, for glaucoma for 3 years. Because no other cause of the bradycardia could be found, the dose was reduced to 0.25% in each eye once daily at about 25 weeks' gestation. Three days later, the fetal heart rate increased to 96 beats/minute, and then to 120 beats/minute 1 week later. After consulting with an ophthalmologist, timolol was stopped completely at about 30 weeks, and 3 days later the fetal heart rate was around 130 beats/minute. At term, a 3025-g female infant was delivered with Apgar scores of 8 and 10 at 1 and 5 minutes, respectively. After birth, a cardiac arrhythmia developed that was diagnosed as right ventricle tachycardia (200 beats/minute) with atrial extra systole. The condition required digitalization. The baby was doing well at 2 months of age (4).

A case report published in 1986 described the pregnancy of a 24-year-old woman at 30 weeks' gestation who was managed for recurrent pheochromocytoma with a combination of timolol, prazosin (an α_1-adrenergic blocker), and metyrosine (a tyrosine hydroxylase inhibitor) (5). Hypertension had been noted at her first prenatal visit at 12 weeks' gestation. Because of declines in fetal breathing, body movements, and amniotic fluid volume that began 2 weeks after the start of therapy, a cesarean section was conducted at 33 weeks. The 1450-g female infant had Apgar scores of 3 and 5 at 1 and 5 minutes, respectively. Mild metabolic acidosis was found on analysis of umbilical cord blood gases. Multiple infarcts were noted in the placenta but no evidence of metastatic tumor. The growth-retarded infant did well and was discharged home on day 53 of life (5).

Systemic use of some β-blockers may cause intrauterine growth retardation (IUGR) and reduced placental weight, especially those lacking intrinsic sympathomimetic activity (ISA) (i.e., partial agonist). Treatment beginning early in the 2nd trimester results in the greatest weight reductions, whereas treatment restricted to the 3rd trimester primarily affects only placental weight. Timolol does not possess ISA. However, IUGR and reduced placental weight may potentially occur with all agents within this class. Although growth retardation is a serious concern, the benefits of maternal therapy with β-blockers, in some cases, might outweigh the risks to the fetus and must be judged on a case-by-case basis.

The systemic use near delivery of some agents in this class has resulted in persistent β-blockade in the newborn (see Acebutolol, Atenolol, and Nadolol). Thus, newborns exposed *in utero* to timolol should be closely observed during the first 24–48 hours after birth for bradycardia and other symptoms. The long-term effects of *in utero* exposure to β-blockers have not been studied but warrant evaluation.

[**Risk Factor D if used systemically in 2nd or 3rd trimesters.*]

BREAST FEEDING SUMMARY

RECOMMENDATION: Limited Human Data - Potential Toxicity

Timolol is excreted into breast milk (6,7). In nine lactating women given 5 mg orally 3 times daily, the mean milk concentration of timolol 105–135 minutes after a dose was 15.9 ng/mL (6). When a dose of 10 mg 3 times daily was given to four patients, mean milk levels of 41 ng/mL were measured. The milk:plasma ratios for the two regimens were 0.80 and 0.83, respectively.

A woman with elevated intraocular pressure applied ophthalmic 0.5% timolol drops to the right eye twice daily, resulting in excretion of the drug in her breast milk (7). Maternal timolol levels in milk and plasma were 5.6 and 0.93 ng/mL, respectively, about 1.5 hours after a dose. A milk sample taken 12 hours after the last dose contained 0.5 ng/mL of timolol. Assuming that the infant nursed every 4 hours and received 75 mL at each feeding, the daily dose would be below that expected to produce cardiac effects in the infant (7).

No adverse reactions were noted in the nursing infants described in the above reports. However, infants exposed to timolol via breast milk should be closely observed for bradycardia and other signs or symptoms of β-blockade. Long-term effects of exposure to β-blockers from milk have not been studied but warrant evaluation. The American Academy of Pediatrics classifies timolol as compatible with breast-feeding (8).

References

1. Product information. Blocadren. Merck, 2000.
2. Schneider H, Proegler M. Placental transfer of β-adrenergic antagonists studied in an in vitro perfusion system of human placental tissue. Am J Obstet Gynecol 1988;159:42–7.
3. Merlob P, Litwin A, Mor N. Possible association between acetazolamide administration during pregnancy and metabolic disorders in the newborn. Eur J Obstet Gynecol Reprod Biol 1990;35:85–8.
4. Wagenvoort AM, Van Vugt JMG, Sobotka M, Van Geijn HP. Topical timolol therapy in pregnancy: is it safe for the fetus? Teratology 1998;58:258–62.
5. Devoe LD, O'Dell BE, Castillo RA, Hadi HA, Searle N. Metastatic pheochromocytoma in pregnancy and fetal biophysical assessment after maternal administration of alpha-adrenergic, beta-adrenergic, and dopamine antagonists. Obstet Gynecol 1986;68:15S–8S.
6. Fidler J, Smith V, DeSwiet M. Excretion of oxprenolol and timolol in breast milk. Br J Obstet Gynaecol 1983;90:961–5.
7. Lustgarten JS, Podos SM. Topical timolol and the nursing mother. Arch Ophthalmol 1983;101:1381–2.
8. Committee on Drugs, American Academy of Pediatrics. The transfer of drugs and other chemicals into human milk. Pediatrics 2001;108:776–89.

Name:	**TINZAPARIN**	Risk Factor:	**B**
Class:	**Anticoagulant**		

FETAL RISK SUMMARY

RECOMMENDATION: Compatible

Tinzaparin is a low-molecular-weight heparin prepared by depolymerization of heparin obtained from porcine intestinal mucosa (1). Tinzaparin has an average molecular weight of 4500 (range 1500–10,000) (1). Because this is a relatively large molecule, it probably does not cross the placenta and, thus, presents a low risk to the fetus.

In a 2004 report, 54 women (55 pregnancies) received tinzaparin, 12 for treatment of thrombosis and 42 for thrombolic prophylaxis (2). Four women required a dose increase during pregnancy to achieve the target anti-Xa activity. The pregnancy outcomes included three 1st trimester spontaneous abortions, one intrauterine death at 17 weeks' gestation (cord entanglement), and one intrauterine death at 30 weeks' gestation (no identifiable cause). The remaining 50 outcomes were live births with no neonatal adverse events related to tinzaparin (2).

BREAST FEEDING SUMMARY

RECOMMENDATION: No Human Data - Probably Compatible

T

No reports describing the use of tinzaparin during lactation have been located. Tinzaparin, a low-molecular-weight heparin, still has a relatively high molecular weight (average 4500) and, as such, should not be expected to be excreted into human milk. Because tinzaparin would be inactivated in the gastrointestinal tract, the risk to a nursing infant from ingestion of the drug from milk appears to be negligible.

References

1. Reynold JEF, ed. *Martindale. The Extra Pharmacopoeia*. 30th ed. London, UK: The Pharmaceutical Press, 1993:232.
2. Smith MP, Norris LA, Steer PJ, Savidge GF, Bonnar J. Tinzaparin sodium for thrombosis treatment and prevention during pregnancy. Am J Obstet Gynecol 2004;190:495–501.

Name:	**TIZANIDINE**	Risk Factor:	C_M
Class:	**Skeletal Muscle Relaxant**		

FETAL RISK SUMMARY

RECOMMENDATION: No Human Data - Animal Data Suggest Risk

Tizanidine is a centrally acting α_2-adrenergic agonist structurally related to clonidine that is used for the management of spasticity. Based on animal studies, tizanidine has no direct effect on skeletal muscle fibers or the neuromuscular junction. Although, in animals the drug has a small fraction (2%–10%) of the potency of clonidine in lowering blood pressure, dose-related hypotension has been observed in humans. The terminal elimination half-life is about 2.5 hours (1).

Reproduction studies have been conducted in rats and rabbits. In rats, a dose equal to the maximum recommended human dose based on body surface area (MRHD) revealed no evidence of teratogenicity. At doses up to eight times the MRHD, increased the duration of gestation, increased prenatal and postnatal pup mortality and retarded development. In rabbits, no evidence of structural defects was evident at a dose 16 times the MRHD. However, postimplantation loss was increased at a dose equal to or greater than 0.5 times the MRHD (1).

It is not known if tizanidine crosses the human placenta. The relatively low molecular weight (about 254 for the free base) and lipid solubility, however, suggest that passage to the embryo or fetus should be expected.

No reports describing the use of tizanidine in human pregnancy have been located. The animal data is suggestive of toxicity but not congenital defects. The absence of human pregnancy experience prevents an assessment of the embryo/fetal risk. However, dose-related hypotension has been observed in humans and this could be a potentially serious adverse effect in pregnancy woman. Single doses of the recommended dose (8 mg) have caused a 20% reduction in either the systolic or the diastolic blood pressure in two-thirds of patients. This effect may be minimized by titration of the dose, but close monitoring of the maternal blood pressure is required. In addition, if the drug must be used in pregnancy, avoidance of the 1st trimester is recommended.

BREAST FEEDING SUMMARY

RECOMMENDATION: No Human Data - Potential Toxicity

No reports describing the use of tizanidine during human lactation have been located. The relatively low molecular weight (about 254 for the free base) and lipid solubility, however, suggest that excretion into breast milk will occur. The effects of this exposure on a nursing infant are unknown, but serious toxicity (e.g., sedation, hypotension, liver injury, and hallucinations/psychotic-like symptoms as seen in adults) is a potential complication. Because of these potential adverse effects, breast-feeding is not recommended.

Reference

1. Product information. Zanaflex. Elan Biopharmaceuticals, 2004.

Name:	**TOBRAMYCIN**	Risk Factor:	**C***
Class:	**Antibiotic (Aminoglycoside)**		

FETAL RISK SUMMARY

RECOMMENDATION: Human Data Suggest Low Risk

Tobramycin is an aminoglycoside antibiotic. Renal toxicity was observed in pregnant rats and their fetuses after maternal administration of high doses of tobramycin, 30 or 60 mg/kg/day for 10 days, during organogenesis (1). The dose-related fetal renal toxicity consisted of granularity and swelling of proximal tubule cells, poor glomerular differentiation, and increased glomerular density (1).

Tobramycin crosses the placenta into the fetal circulation and amniotic fluid (2,3). Studies in patients undergoing elective abortions in the 1st and 2nd trimesters indicate that tobramycin distributes to most fetal tissues except the brain and cerebrospinal fluid (2). Amniotic fluid levels generally did not occur until the 2nd trimester. The highest fetal concentrations were found in the kidneys and urine (2). In a woman undergoing surgical termination of an ovarian gestation in a 22-week heterotopic pregnancy (intrauterine and ovarian), a single 2 mg/kg IV dose of tobramycin was administered for 10 minutes 5.6 hours before cesarean section (3). Tobramycin was found in all fluids and tissues of the 260-g ovarian fetus, with the highest concentrations occurring in the fetal spleen (1.53 μg/mL) and kidney (2.98 μg/mL). The intrauterine fetus developed normally and a healthy 2900-g girl was eventually delivered at 38 weeks' gestation. Reports measuring the passage of tobramycin in the 3rd trimester or at term are lacking.

No reports linking the use of tobramycin with congenital defects have been located. The antibiotic is not teratogenic in rats and rabbits (4). Ototoxicity, which is known to occur after tobramycin therapy, has not been reported as an effect of *in utero* exposure. However, eighth cranial nerve toxicity in the fetus is well known following exposure to other aminoglycosides (see Kanamycin and Streptomycin) and may potentially occur with tobramycin.

In a surveillance study of Michigan Medicaid recipients conducted between 1985 and 1992 involving 229,101 completed pregnancies, 81 newborns had been exposed to tobramycin during the 1st trimester (F. Rosa, personal communication, FDA, 1993). A total of three (3.7%) major birth defects were observed (three expected), one of which was a cardiovascular defect (one expected). No anomalies were observed in five other categories of defects (oral clefts, spina bifida, polydactyly, limb reduction defects, and hypospadias) for which specific data were available.

The population-based dataset of the Hungarian Case-Control Surveillance of Congenital Abnormalities, covering the period 1980–1996, was used to evaluate the teratogenicity of aminoglycoside antibiotics (parenteral gentamicin, streptomycin, tobramycin, and oral neomycin) in a study published in 2000 (5). A case group of 22,865 women who had fetuses or newborns with congenital malformations were compared to 38,151 women who had no newborns with structural defects. A total of 38 cases and 42 controls were treated with aminoglycosides. There were two cases and four controls treated with tobramycin (odds ratio 0.8, 95% confidence interval 0.2–3.9). The investigators concluded that there was no detectable teratogenic risk for structural defects for any of the aminoglycoside antibiotics (5). They also concluded, although it was not investigated in this study, that the risk of deafness after *in utero* aminoglycoside exposure was small.

A potentially serious drug interaction may occur in newborns treated with aminoglycosides who were also exposed *in utero* to magnesium sulfate (see Gentamicin).

[**Risk Factor D according to manufacturer, Eli Lilly, 2000.*]

BREAST FEEDING SUMMARY

RECOMMENDATION: Compatible

Tobramycin is excreted into breast milk. Following an 80-mg IM dose given to five patients, milk levels varied from a trace to 0.52 μg/mL over 8 hours (6). Peak levels occurred at 4 hours after injection. Because oral absorption of this antibiotic is poor, ototoxicity in the infant would not be expected. However, three potential problems exist for the nursing infant: modification of bowel flora, direct effects on the infant, and interference with the interpretation of culture results if a fever workup is required.

References

1. Mantovani A, Macri C, Stazi AV, Ricciardi C, Guastadisegni C, Maranghi F. Tobramycin-induced changes in renal histology of fetal and newborn Sprague-Dawley rats. Teratog Carcinog Mutagen 1992;12:19–30.
2. Bernard B, Garcia-Cazares S, Ballard C, Thrupp L, Mathies A, Wehrle P. Tobramycin: maternal-fetal pharmacology. Antimicrob Agents Chemother 1977;11:688–94.
3. Fernandez H, Bourget P, Delouis C. Fetal levels of tobramycin following maternal administration. Obstet Gynecol 1990;76:992–4.
4. Welles JS, Emmerson JL, Gibson WR, Nickander R, Owen NV, Anderson RC. Preclinical toxicology studies of tobramycin. Toxicol Appl Pharmacol 1973;25:398–409. As cited in Shepard TH. *Catalog of Teratogenic Agents*. 6th ed. Baltimore, MD: Johns Hopkins University Press, 1989:623.
5. Czeizel AE, Rockenbauer M, Olsen J, Sorensen HT. A teratological study of aminoglycoside antibiotic treatment during pregnancy. Scand J Infect Dis 2000;32:309–13.
6. Takase Z. Laboratory and clinical studies on tobramycin in the field of obstetrics and gynecology. Chemotherapy (Tokyo) 1975;23:1402.

Name: **TOCAINIDE** Risk Factor: **C_M**

Class: **Antiarrhythmic**

FETAL RISK SUMMARY

RECOMMENDATION: No Human Data - Animal Data Suggest Low Risk

Tocainide is indicated for the treatment of ventricular arrhythmias but has also been used in the treatment of myotonic dystrophy and trigeminal neuralgia.

In mice, tocainide and its metabolites cross the placenta to the fetus (T. P. Dowling, personal communication, Merck Sharpe & Dohme, 1987). The drug was not teratogenic in rats and rabbits exposed to doses up to 4 and 12 times the usual human dose, respectively (1). These doses were maternotoxic in both species. At maternotoxic doses 8–12 times the usual human dose in rats, dystocia, delayed parturition, an increased incidence of stillbirth, and reduced survival of the offspring in the first week after birth were noted (1). No reports describing the use of tocainide in human pregnancy have been located.

BREAST FEEDING SUMMARY

RECOMMENDATION: No Human Data - Probably Compatible

No reports describing the use of tocainide during lactation have been located. The low molecular weight (about 229), however, is low enough that passage into milk should be anticipated. The effect of this exposure on a nursing infant is unknown.

Reference

1. Product information. Tonocard. AstraZeneca, 2000.

Name:	**TOLAZAMIDE**	Risk Factor:	**C_M**
Class:	**Oral Hypoglycemic**		

FETAL RISK SUMMARY

RECOMMENDATION: Human Data Suggest Risk in 3rd Trimester

Tolazamide is a sulfonylurea used for the treatment of adult-onset diabetes mellitus. It is not indicated for the pregnant diabetic.

No reports describing the placental transfer of tolazamide have been located. The molecular weight (about 311) suggests, however, that transfer to the fetus probably occurs (see Chlorpropamide).

A 1991 report described the outcomes of pregnancies in 21 non-insulin-dependent diabetic women who were treated with oral hypoglycemic agents (17 sulfonylureas, 3 biguanides, and 1 unknown type) during the 1st trimester (1). The duration of exposure ranged from 3 to 28 weeks, but all patients were changed to insulin therapy at the first prenatal visit. Forty non-insulin-dependent diabetic women matched for age, race, parity, and glycemic control served as a control group. Eleven (52%) of the exposed infants had major or minor congenital malformations compared with six (15%) of the controls. Moreover, ear defects, a malformation that is observed, but uncommonly, in diabetic embryopathy, occurred in six of the exposed infants and in none of the controls (1). One infants with an ear defect (thickened curved pinnae and malformed superior helices) had been exposed *in utero* to tolazamide during the first 12 weeks of gestation. Sixteen live births occurred in the exposed group compared with 36 in controls. The groups did not differ in the incidence of hypoglycemia at birth (53% vs. 53%), but three of the exposed newborns had severe hypoglycemia lasting 2, 4, and 7 days even though the mothers had not used oral hypoglycemics (none of the three was exposed to tolazamide) close to delivery. The authors attributed this to irreversible β-cell hyperplasia that may have been increased by exposure to oral hypoglycemics (1). Hyperbilirubinemia was noted in 10 (67%) of 15 exposed newborns compared with 13 (36%) controls ($p < 0.04$), and polycythemia and hyperviscosity requiring partial exchange transfusions were observed in 4 (27%) of 15 exposed vs. 1 (3.0%) control ($p < 0.03$) (1 exposed infant was not included in these data because the infant was delivered after completion of the study).

In summary, although the use of tolazamide during human gestation does not appear to be related to structural anomalies, insulin is still the treatment of choice for this disease. Oral hypoglycemics are not indicated for the pregnant diabetic because they will not provide good control in patients who cannot be controlled by diet alone (2). Moreover, insulin, unlike tolazamide, does not cross the placenta and, thus, eliminates the additional concern that the drug therapy is adversely affecting the fetus. Carefully prescribed insulin therapy will provide better control of the mother's blood glucose, thereby preventing the fetal and neonatal complications that occur with this disease. High maternal glucose levels, as may occur in diabetes mellitus, are closely associated with a number of maternal and fetal adverse effects, including structural anomalies if the hyperglycemia occurs early in gestation. To prevent this toxicity, most experts, including the American College of Obstetricians and Gynecologists, recommend that insulin be used for types I and II diabetes occurring during pregnancy and, if diet therapy alone is not successful, for gestational diabetes (3,4). If tolazamide is used during pregnancy, therapy should be changed to insulin and tolazamide discontinued before delivery (the exact time before delivery is unknown) to lessen the possibility of prolonged hypoglycemia in the newborn.

BREAST FEEDING SUMMARY

RECOMMENDATION: No Human Data - Potential Toxicity

No reports describing the use of tolazamide during human lactation have been located. The molecular weight (about 311), however, is low enough that excretion in milk should be expected (see Chlorpropamide). The effects of tolazamide in milk on the nursing infant are unknown, but hypoglycemia is a potential toxicity.

References

1. Piacquadio K, Hollingsworth DR, Murphy H. Effects of *in utero* exposure to oral hypoglycaemic drugs. Lancet 1991;338:866–9.
2. Friend JR. Diabetes. Clin Obstet Gynaecol 1981;8:353–82.
3. American College of Obstetricians and Gynecologists. Diabetes and pregnancy. *Technical Bulletin*. No. 200. December 1994.
4. Coustan DR. Management of gestational diabetes. Clin Obstet Gynecol 1991;34:558–64.

Name:	**TOLAZOLINE**	Risk Factor:	**C**
Class:	**Vasodilator**		

FETAL RISK SUMMARY

RECOMMENDATION: Limited Human Data - No Relevant Animal Data

Tolazoline is structurally and pharmacologically related to phentolamine (see Phentolamine). Experience with tolazoline in pregnancy is limited. The Collaborative Perinatal Project monitored two 1st trimester exposures to tolazoline plus 13 other patients exposed to other vasodilators (1). From this small group of 15 patients, 4 malformed children were observed. It was not stated whether tolazoline was taken by any of the mothers of the affected infants.

The lack of animal pregnancy data and the very limited human pregnancy experience prevents an assessment of the embryo/fetal risk from tolazoline.

BREAST FEEDING SUMMARY

RECOMMENDATION: No Human Data - Probably Compatible

No data are available.

Reference

1. Heinonen OP, Slone D, Shapiro S. *Birth Defects and Drugs in Pregnancy*. Littleton, MA: Publishing Sciences Group, 1977:371–3.

Name:	**TOLBUTAMIDE**	Risk Factor:	C_M
Class:	**Oral Hypoglycemic**		

FETAL RISK SUMMARY

RECOMMENDATION: Human Data Suggest Risk in 3rd Trimester

Tolbutamide is a sulfonylurea used for the treatment of adult-onset diabetes mellitus. It is not the treatment of choice for the pregnant diabetic patient.

Shepard reviewed four studies that had reported teratogenicity in mice and rats, but not in rabbits (1). In a study using early-somite mouse embryos in whole embryo culture, tolbutamide produced malformations and growth retardation at concentrations similar to therapeutic levels in humans (2). The defects were not a result of hypoglycemia. In a similar experiment, but using tolbutamide concentrations 2–4 times the human therapeutic level, investigators concluded that tolbutamide had a direct embryotoxic effect on the rat embryos (3).

When administered near term, the drug crosses the placenta (4,5). Neonatal serum levels are higher than corresponding maternal concentrations. In one infant whose mother took 500 mg/day, serum levels at 27 hours were 7.2 mg/dL (maternal 2.7 mg/dL) (5).

In an abstract (6), and later in a full report (7), the *in vitro* placental transfer, using a single-cotyledon human placenta, of four oral hypoglycemic agents was described. As expected, molecular weight was the most significant factor for drug transfer, with dissociation constant (pKa) and lipid solubility providing significant additive effect. The cumulative percent placental transfer at 3 hours of the four agents and their approximate molecular weight (shown in parenthesis) were tolbutamide (270) 21.5%, chlorpropamide (277) 11.0%, glipizide (446) 6.6%, and glyburide (494) 3.9%.

Although teratogenic in animals, an increased incidence of congenital defects, other than those expected in diabetes mellitus, has not been found with tolbutamide in a number of studies (8–18). Four malformed infants have been attributed to tolbutamide but the relationship is unclear: right-sided preauricular skin tag, accessory right thumb, thrombocytopenia (nadir 19,000/mm^3 on 4th day) (5); hand and foot anomalies, finger and toe syndactyly, external ear defect, atresia of external auditory canal, gastrointestinal, heart, and renal anomalies (19); grossly malformed (20); and severe talipes, absent left toe (21).

The neonatal thrombocytopenia, persisting for about 2 weeks, was thought to have been induced by tolbutamide (5).

In a surveillance study of Michigan Medicaid recipients conducted between 1985 and 1992 involving 229,101 completed pregnancies, 4 newborns had been exposed to tolbutamide during the 1st trimester (F. Rosa, personal communication, FDA, 1993). One (25%) major birth defect was observed (none expected), but specific information on the defect is not available. No anomalies were observed in six categories of defects (cardiovascular defects, oral clefts, spina bifida, polydactyly, limb reduction defects, and hypospadias.

A 1991 report described the outcomes of pregnancies in 21 non-insulin-dependent diabetic women who were treated with oral hypoglycemic agents (17 sulfonylureas, 3 biguanides, and 1 unknown type) during the 1st trimester (22). The duration of exposure ranged from 3 to 28 weeks, but all patients were changed to insulin therapy at the first prenatal visit. Forty non-insulin-dependent diabetic women matched for age, race, parity, and glycemic control served as a control group. Eleven (52%) of the exposed infants had major or minor congenital malformations compared with six (15%) of the controls. Moreover, ear defects, a malformation that is observed, but uncommonly, in diabetic embryopathy, occurred in six of the exposed infants and in none of the controls. None of the infants with defects were exposed to tolbutamide. Sixteen live births occurred in the exposed group compared with 36 in controls. The groups did not differ in the incidence of hypoglycemia at birth (53% vs. 53%), but three of the exposed newborns had severe hypoglycemia lasting 2, 4, and 7 days, even though the mothers had not used oral hypoglycemics (none of the three was exposed to tolbutamide) close to delivery. The authors attributed this to irreversible β-cell hyperplasia that may have been increased by exposure to oral hypoglycemics. Hyperbilirubinemia was noted in 10 (67%) of 15 exposed newborns compared with 13 (36%) of controls ($p < 0.04$), and polycythemia and hyperviscosity requiring partial exchange transfusions were observed in 4 (27%) of 15 exposed vs. 1 (3.0%) control ($p < 0.03$) (1 exposed infant was not included in these data because the infant was delivered after completion of the study) (22).

A case of prolonged hypoglycemia in a premature infant whose mother was treated with tolbutamide for gestational diabetes was reported in 1998 (23). The mother was treated with tolbutamide starting from 23 weeks' gestation until deliver at 34 weeks. The male infant's weight and length were 3200 g and 49 cm, respectively, both values above 1 standard deviation of the mean for gestational age. Hypoglycemia was diagnosed 1 hour after birth and IV 20% glucose was required for the first 3 days of life. Subcutaneous octreotide was also administered for first 9 days of life. Serum tolbutamide concentrations decreased from 38 μg/mL (140.6 μmol/L) at 3 hours after birth to 2 μg/mL (7.4 μmol/L) at 90 hours. The decline in serum concentration showed zero-order kinetics with an initial half-life of 46 hours that declined to 6 hours. The change in tolbutamide elimination suggested immaturity of hepatic elimination during the first 2 days of life (23). The infant displayed normal psychomotor development without seizures and normal glucose values at 3 months of age.

In summary, although the use of tolbutamide during human gestation does not appear to be related to structural anomalies, insulin is still the treatment of choice for this disease. Oral hypoglycemics are not indicated for the pregnant diabetic because they will not provide good control in patients who cannot be controlled by diet alone (24). Moreover, insulin, unlike tolbutamide, does not cross the placenta and, thus, eliminates the additional concern that the drug therapy itself is adversely affecting the fetus. Because tolbutamide crossed the placenta, prolonged hypoglycemia occurred in a premature infant. Carefully prescribed insulin therapy will provide better control of the mother's blood glucose, thereby preventing the fetal and neonatal complications that occur with this disease. High maternal glucose levels, as may occur in diabetes mellitus, are closely associated with a number of maternal and fetal adverse effects, including fetal structural anomalies if the hyperglycemia occurs early in gestation. To prevent this toxicity, most experts, including the American College of Obstetricians and Gynecologists, recommend that insulin be used for types I and II diabetes occurring during pregnancy and, if diet therapy alone is not successful, for gestational diabetes (25,26). If tolbutamide is used during pregnancy, therapy should be changed to insulin and tolbutamide discontinued before delivery to lessen the possibility of prolonged hypoglycemia in the newborn. The timing when therapy should be changed to insulin is not certain but at least 4 days before delivery appears reasonable based on one case.

BREAST FEEDING SUMMARY

RECOMMENDATION: Limited Human Data - Potential Toxicity

Tolbutamide is excreted into breast milk. Following long-term dosing with 500 mg orally twice daily, milk levels 4 hours after a dose in two patients averaged 3 and 18 μg/mL (27). Milk:plasma ratios were 0.09 and 0.40, respectively. The effect on an infant from these levels is unknown, but hypoglycemia is a potential toxicity. The American Academy of Pediatrics, although noting the possibility of jaundice in the nursing infant, classifies tolbutamide as compatible with breast-feeding (28).

References

1. Shepard TH. *Catalog of Teratogenic Agents*. 8th ed. Baltimore, MD: Johns Hopkins University Press, 1995:417.
2. Smoak IW. Teratogenic effects of tolbutamide on early-somite mouse embryos in vitro. Diabetes Res Clin Pract 1992;17:161–7.
3. Ziegler MH, Grafton TF, Hansen DK. The effect of tolbutamide on rat embryonic development in vitro. Teratology 1993;48:45–51.
4. Miller DI, Wishinsky H, Thompson G. Transfer of tolbutamide across the human placenta. Diabetes 1962;11(Suppl):93–7.
5. Schiff D, Aranda J, Stern L. Neonatal thrombocytopenia and congenital malformation associated with administration of tolbutamide to the mother. J Pediatr 1970;77:457–8.
6. Elliott B, Schenker S, Langer O, Johnson R, Prihoda T. Oral hypoglycemic agents: profound variation exists in their rate of human placental transfer. Society of Perinatal Obstetricians Abstract. Am J Obstet Gynecol 1992;166:368.
7. Elliott BD, Schenker S, Langer O, Johnson R, Prihoda T. Comparative placental transport of oral hypoglycemic agents in humans: a model of human placental drug transfer. Am J Obstet Gynecol 1994;171:653–60.
8. Ghanem MH. Possible teratogenic effect of tolbutamide in the pregnant prediabetic. Lancet 1961; 1:1227.
9. Dolger H, Bookman JJ, Nechemias C. The diagnostic and therapeutic value of tolbutamide in pregnant diabetics. Diabetes 1962;11(Suppl):97–8.
10. Jackson WPU, Campbell GD, Notelovitz M, Blumsohn D. Tolbutamide and chlorpropamide during pregnancy in human diabetes. Diabetes 1962;11(Suppl):98–101.
11. Campbell GD. Chlorpropamide and foetal damage. Br Med J 1963;1:59–60.
12. Macphail I. Chlorpropamide and foetal damage. Br Med J 1963;1:192.
13. Jackson WPU, Campbell GD. Chlorpropamide and perinatal mortality. Br Med J 1963;2:1652.
14. Malins JM, Cooke AM, Pyke DA, Fitzgerald MG. Sulphonylurea drugs in pregnancy. Br Med J 1964;2:187.
15. Moss JM, Connor EJ. Pregnancy complicated by diabetes. Report of 102 pregnancies including eleven treated with oral hypoglycemic drugs. Med Ann Dist Col 1965;34:253–60.
16. Adam PAJ, Schwartz R. Diagnosis and treatment: should oral hypoglycemic agents be used in pediatric and pregnant patients? Pediatrics 1968;42:819–23.
17. Dignan PSJ. Teratogenic risk and counseling in diabetes. Clin Obstet Gynecol 1981;24:149–59.
18. Burt RL. Reactivity to tolbutamide in normal pregnancy. Obstet Gynecol 1958;12:447–53.
19. Larsson Y, Sterky G. Possible teratogenic effect of tolbutamide in a pregnant prediabetic. Lancet 1960;2:1424–6.
20. Campbell GD. Possible teratogenic effect of tolbutamide in pregnancy. Lancet 1961;1:891–2.
21. Soler NG, Walsh CH, Malins JM. Congenital malformations in infants of diabetic mothers. Q J Med 1976;45:303–13.
22. Piacquadio K, Hollingsworth DR, Murphy H. Effects of in-utero exposure to oral hypoglycaemic drugs. Lancet 1991;338:866–9.
23. Christesen HBT, Melander A. Prolonged elimination of tolbutamide in a premature newborn with hyperinsulinaemic hypoglycaemia. Eur J Endocrinol 1998;138:698–701.
24. Friend JR. Diabetes. Clin Obstet Gynaecol 1981;8: 353–82.
25. American College of Obstetricians and Gynecologists. Diabetes and pregnancy. *Technical Bulletin*. No. 200. December 1994.
26. Coustan DR. Management of gestational diabetes. Clin Obstet Gynecol 1991;34:558–64.
27. Moiel RH, Ryan JR. Tolbutamide (Orinase) in human breast milk. Clin Pediatr 1967;6:480.
28. Committee on Drugs, American Academy of Pediatrics. The transfer of drugs and other chemicals into human milk. Pediatrics 2001;108:776–89.

Name: **TOLCAPONE** Risk Factor: **C_M**

Class: **Antiparkinsonian Agent**

FETAL RISK SUMMARY

RECOMMENDATION: No Human Data - Animal Data Suggest Risk

Tolcapone is used as an adjunct to levodopa/carbidopa for the treatment of Parkinson's disease. The agent is a selective and reversible inhibitor of catechol-*O*-methyltransferase (COMT), an enzyme involved in the metabolism of levodopa. Inhibition of COMT by tolcapone allows for more sustained plasma levels of levodopa resulting in greater beneficial effects on the signs and symptoms of Parkinson disease. Because the drug may cause potentially fatal, acute fulminant liver failure, it is recommended that it should only be used in patients who are not appropriate candidates for other adjunctive therapies (1). Tolcapone is nearly completely metabolized to inactive metabolites before excretion in the urine. It has an elimination half-life of 2–3 hours with no evidence of accumulation after repeat dosing (1).

Reproduction studies with tolcapone alone have been conducted in rats and rabbits. In rats, doses up to 5.7 times the recommended human clinical dose of 600 mg/day based on body surface area (RHCD) had no effect on fertility or general reproductive performance. There was no evidence of teratogenicity with these doses during organogenesis, but the highest dose was associated with maternal toxicity (decreased weight gain, death). When tolcapone was given to rats in late gestation and throughout lactation, decreased litter size, and impaired growth and learning performance were observed in female pups. Because the initial dose (4.8 times the RHCD) was associated with a high rate of maternal mortality, the dose was reduced during late gestation to 2.9 times the RHCD (1).

Treatment of rabbits during organogenesis with doses up to 15 times the RHCD revealed no evidence of teratogenicity, but an increased rate of abortion was observed at 3.7 times the RHCD (plasma exposure 0.5 times the expected human exposure based on AUC). Maternal toxicity was evident at the highest dose (15 times the RHCD) (1).

Pregnant rabbits were also treated with a combination of tolcapone (0.5 times the expected human exposure based on AUC) and levodopa/carbidopa (6 times the expected human therapeutic exposure of levodopa based on AUC) during organogenesis. The three-drug regimen (tolcapone, levodopa and carbidopa) resulted in an increased incidence of fetal anomalies, primarily external and skeletal digit defects, compared with levodopa/carbidopa alone. The combination of levodopa/carbidopa is known to cause visceral and skeletal malformations in rabbits (1). The three-drug regimen in pregnant rats with tolcapone (0.5 times the expected human exposure or higher based on AUC) and levodopa/carbidopa (levodopa exposures 21 times the human exposure or higher) was associated with reduced fetal body weights. However, no effect on fetal body weight was observed when tolcapone (1.4 times the expected human exposure based on AUC) was used alone (1).

It is not known if tolcapone crosses the human placenta. The molecular weight (about 273) is low enough that embryo and fetal exposure should be expected. However, the nearly complete metabolism and relatively short elimination half-life should limit the amount of active parent drug available for distribution to the fetus.

In summary, no reports describing the use of tolcapone in human pregnancy have been located. Because the drug is always used concomitantly with levodopa/carbidopa, the increased incidence of fetal anomalies and reduced fetal weight observed in rats treated with combination therapy resulting in plasma exposures of tolcapone only one-half of the expected human exposure is noteworthy. Embryo and/or fetal toxicity were also observed in rats and rabbits with tolcapone doses ranging from less than to slightly above the typical human dose. The complete lack of human pregnancy experience, however, prevents an assessment of the potential embryo and fetal risk from tolcapone. The low incidence of Parkinson's disease in women of reproductive age and the risk of potentially fatal, acute fulminant liver failure should markedly limit the use of tolcapone in this patient population.

BREAST FEEDING SUMMARY

RECOMMENDATION: No Human Data - Potential Toxicity

No reports describing the use of tolcapone during human lactation have been located. The drug is excreted into the milk of lactating rats. The molecular weight (about 273) is low enough that excretion into breast milk should be expected. However, the complete metabolism and relatively short elimination half-life should limit the amount of active drug available for passage into milk. The effect on a nursing infant from exposure to tolcapone from milk is unknown. Because of the potential for severe toxicity (e.g., potentially fatal, acute fulminant liver failure as seen in adults), lactating women who are taking tolcapone should not breast-feed.

Reference

1. Product information. Tasmar. Roche Pharmaceuticals, 2003.

Name: **TOLMETIN** Risk Factor: **C_M***
Class: **Nonsteroidal Anti-inflammatory**

FETAL RISK SUMMARY

RECOMMENDATION: Human Data Suggest Risk in 1st and 3rd Trimesters

Tolmetin is a nonsteroidal anti-inflammatory drug (NSAID) used for the relief of the signs and symptoms of rheumatoid arthritis, juvenile arthritis, and osteoarthritis. It is the same subclass (acetic acids) as three other NSAIDs (diclofenac, indomethacin, and sulindac).

Tolmetin is not teratogenic in rats and rabbits (1,2). The doses used in some of the studies were up to 1.5 times the maximum clinical dose based on a body weight of 60 kg (2).

It is not known if tolmetin crosses the human placenta. The molecular weight of the sodium salt (about 315) is low enough, however, that passage to the fetus should be expected.

In a surveillance study of Michigan Medicaid recipients conducted between 1985 and 1992 involving 229,101 completed pregnancies, 99 newborns had been exposed to tolmetin during the 1st trimester (F. Rosa, personal communication, FDA, 1993). One (1.0%) infant had a major birth defect (four expected) consisting of a cardiovascular defect (one expected) and polydactyly (none expected).

A combined 2001 population-based observational cohort study and a case-control study estimated the risk of adverse pregnancy outcome from the use of NSAIDs (3). The use of NSAIDs during pregnancy was not associated with congenital malformations, preterm delivery, or low birth weight, but a positive association was discovered with spontaneous abortions (SABs). A similar study, also published in 2001, failed to find a relationship, in general, between NSAIDs and congenital malformations, but did find a significant association with cardiac defects and orofacial clefts (4). In addition, a 2003 study found a significant association between exposure to NSAIDs in early pregnancy and SABs (5). (See Ibuprofen for details on these three studies.)

A brief 2003 editorial on the potential for NSAID-induced developmental toxicity concluded that NSAIDs, and specifically those with greater COX-2 affinity, had a lower risk of this toxicity in humans than aspirin (6).

Constriction of the ductus arteriosus *in utero* is a pharmacologic consequence arising from the use of prostaglandin synthesis inhibitors during pregnancy (see also Indomethacin) (7). Persistent pulmonary hypertension of the newborn may occur if these agents are used in the 3rd trimester close to delivery (7,8). These drugs also have been shown to inhibit labor and prolong pregnancy, both in humans (9) (see also Indomethacin) and in animals (10). Women attempting to conceive should not use any prostaglandin synthesis inhibitor, including tolmetin, because of the findings in a variety of animal models that indicate these agents block blastocyst implantation (11,12). Moreover, as noted above, NSAIDs have been associated with SABs and congenital malformations.

[**Risk Factor D if used in 3rd trimester or near delivery.*]

BREAST FEEDING SUMMARY

RECOMMENDATION: Limited Human Data - Probably Compatible

Tolmetin is excreted into breast milk (2,13). In the 4 hours following a single 400-mg oral dose, milk levels varied from 0.06 to 0.18 μg/mL with the highest concentration occurring at 0.67 hour. Milk:plasma ratios were 0.005–0.007. The clinical significance of these levels to the nursing infant is unknown. The American Academy of Pediatrics classifies tolmetin as compatible with breast-feeding (14).

References

1. Nishimura K, Fukagawa S, Shigematsu K, Makumoto K, Terada Y, Sasaki H, Nanto T, Tatsumi H. Teratogenicity study of tolmetin sodium in rabbits. (Japanese) Iyakuhin Kenkyu 1977;8:158–64. As cited in Shepard TH. *Catalog of Teratogenic Agents*. 6th ed. Baltimore, MD: Johns Hopkins University Press, 1989:625.
2. Product information. Tolectin. Ortho-McNeil Pharmaceutical, 2001.
3. Nielsen GL, Sorensen HT, Larsen H, Pedersen L. Risk of adverse birth outcome and miscarriage in pregnant users of non-steroidal anti-inflammatory drugs: population based observational study and case-control study. BMJ 2001;322:266–70.
4. Ericson A, Kallen BAJ. Nonsteroidal anti-inflammatory drugs in early pregnancy. Reprod Toxicol 2001;15:371–5.
5. Li DK, Liu L, Odouli R. Exposure to non-steroidal anti-inflammatory drugs during pregnancy and risk of miscarriage: population based cohort study. BMJ 2003;327:368–71.
6. Tassinari MS, Cook JC, Hurtt ME. NSAIDs and developmental toxicity. Birth Defects Res Part B Dev Reprod Toxicol 2003;68:3–4.
7. Levin DL. Effects of inhibition of prostaglandin synthesis on fetal development, oxygenation, and the fetal circulation. Semin Perinatol 1980;4:35–44.
8. Van Marter LJ, Leviton A, Allred EN, Pagano M, Sullivan KF, Cohen A, Epstein MF. Persistent pulmonary hypertension of the newborn and smoking and aspirin and nonsteroidal antiinflammatory drug consumption during pregnancy. Pediatrics 1996;97:658–63.
9. Fuchs F. Prevention of prematurity. Am J Obstet Gynecol 1976;126:809–20.
10. Powell JG, Cochrane RL. The effects of a number of non-steroidal anti-inflammatory compounds on parturition in the rat. Prostaglandins 1982;23:469–88.
11. Matt DW, Borzelleca JF. Toxic effects on the female reproductive system during pregnancy, parturition, and lactation. In Witorsch RJ, editor. *Reproductive Toxicology*. 2nd ed. New York, NY: Raven Press, 1995: 175–93.
12. Dawood MY. Nonsteroidal antiinflammatory drugs and reproduction. Am J Obstet Gynecol 1993; 169:1255–65.
13. Sagraves R, Waller ES, Goehrs HR. Tolmetin in breast milk. Drug Intell Clin Pharm 1985;19:55–6.
14. Committee on Drugs, American Academy of Pediatrics. The transfer of drugs and other chemicals into breast milk. Pediatrics 2001;108:776–89.

T

Name: **TOLTERODINE** Risk Factor: **C_M**

Class: **Urinary Tract Agent (Antispasmodic)**

FETAL RISK SUMMARY

RECOMMENDATION: No Human Data - Animal Data Suggest Low Risk

Tolterodine is a competitive muscarinic receptor antagonist that is indicated for the treatment of overactive bladder with symptoms of urge urinary incontinence, urgency, and frequency. The drug is metabolized in the liver to a major active metabolite that has the same potency as tolterodine. Metabolism is mediated by the cytochrome P450 2D6 (CYP2D6). After multiple dosing, the elimination half-life is 2.2 hours in extensive metabolizers. In those persons lacking CYP2D6 (poor metabolizers; about 7% of the population), metabolism (to an inactive metabolite) is mediated by CYP3A4 and the elimination half-life of tolterodine is 9.6 hours. About 96% of tolterodine is bound in the plasma, primarily to α_1-glycoprotein, but the binding of the active metabolite is only 64% (1).

Reproduction studies have been conducted in mice and rabbits. In pregnant mice, oral doses producing systemic exposures about 14 times the human exposure (HE) revealed no evidence of teratogenicity. At doses 20 to 25 times the HE, embryo lethality, reduced fetal weight, and increased incidences of intra-abdominal hemorrhage and malformations (cleft palate and digital and various skeletal abnormalities) were seen. In pregnant rabbits, SC doses producing systemic exposures about three times the HE did not cause embryotoxicity or teratogenicity. Tolterodine is neither carcinogenic nor mutagenic in experimental systems (1).

Tolterodine crosses the placenta in mice (2). It is not known if tolterodine or its active metabolite crosses the human placenta. The molecular weight of tolterodine tartrate (about 476) is low enough, however, that placental transfer should be expected.

No reports describing the use of tolterodine in human pregnancy have been located. The limited animal data suggest low risk, but the complete lack of human pregnancy experience prevents an assessment of embryo/fetal risk. The safest course is to avoid the 1st trimester, but inadvertent exposure in early pregnancy does not appear to represent a major risk.

BREAST FEEDING SUMMARY

RECOMMENDATION: No Human Data - Potential Toxicity

No reports describing the use of tolterodine during human lactation have been located. The molecular weight of the parent compound (about 476) is low enough, however, that transfer into breast milk should be expected. Moreover, tolterodine has an equipotent metabolite that also might be excreted into milk. Tolterodine was excreted into the milk of lactating rats and caused slightly reduced body-weight gain in offspring (1). The amount transferred in mice was low (about 0.2% of the dose) (2).

References

1. Product information. Detrol. Pharmacia & Upjohn, 2004.
2. Pahlman I, d'Argy R, Nilvebrant L. Tissue distribution of tolterodine, a muscarinic receptor antagonist, and transfer into fetus and milk in mice. Arzneimittelforschung 2001;51:125–33.

Name: **TOPIRAMATE** Risk Factor: **C_M**
Class: **Anticonvulsant**

FETAL RISK SUMMARY

RECOMMENDATION: Limited Human Data - Animal Data Suggest Risk

Topiramate, a sulfamate-substituted monosaccharide, is an antiepileptic agent indicated as adjunctive therapy in patients with partial onset seizures, primary generalized tonic-clonic seizures, and seizures associated with Lennox-Gastaut syndrome. The drug undergoes partial metabolism to six metabolites, none of which constitutes more than 5% of the dose, with approximately 70% of the dose eliminated unchanged in the urine. Only 13%–17% is bound to human plasma proteins and the mean plasma elimination half-life is 21 hours. Topiramate is a weak carbonic anhydrase inhibitor, but this activity is not thought to be a major contributing factor to its antiepileptic action (1).

Reproduction studies with topiramate have been conducted in mice, rats, and rabbits (1). In pregnant mice, oral doses, 0.2–5 times the recommended human dose (400 mg/day) based on body surface area (RHD), administered during organogenesis increased the incidence of fetal malformations at all doses. The primary anomalies were craniofacial defects. At the highest dose (5 times the RHD), reduced fetal body weights and ossification were evident, but this dose also caused maternal toxicity (decreased body weight gain).

Topiramate at doses of 0.005 to 12.5 times the RHD was administered to pregnant rats during organogenesis (1). At 10 times the RHD or higher, the frequency of limb malformations (ectrodactyly, micromelia, and amelia) was increased. In addition, in the postnatal portion of the study, pups exposed to topiramate during organogenesis exhibited delayed physical development (doses 10 times the RHD) and persistent reductions in body weight gain (doses 1 times the RHD or higher). The teratogenic dose (10 times the RHD or higher) produced clinical signs of maternal toxicity. At 2.5 times the RHD or higher, reduced maternal weight gain was evident. However, fetotoxicity (reduced fetal body weight and increased incidence of structural variations) was observed at 0.5 times the RHD. Pregnant rats also were treated during the latter part of gestation and throughout lactation with doses ranging from 0.005 to 5 times the RHD. No drug-related effects on gestation length or parturition were observed at any studied dose. At 0.05 times the RHD or higher, reductions in pre- and/or post-weaning body weight gain were observed. At 5 times the RHD, offspring exhibited decreased viability and delayed physical development.

Pregnant rabbits were administered oral doses during organogenesis that were approximately 0.6–11 times the RHD (1). At 2 times the RHD and above, embryo and fetal mortality was observed, but maternal toxicity (decreased body weight gain, clinical signs, and/or mortality) were also evident. At 6 times the RHD, teratogenic effects, primarily rib and vertebral malformations, were observed.

Topiramate crosses the placenta to the fetus with cord and maternal plasma drug levels approximately equivalent at term (2,3). Diffusion across the placenta to the embryo early in gestation has not been studied. However, the low molecular weight (about 339), the relatively lack of protein binding and low metabolism, and the prolonged plasma elimination all favor transfer of the drug.

Human pregnancy experience with topiramate is limited. Postmarketing experience has been reported by the manufacturer (1). Without providing specific details, it stated that cases of hypospadias had been observed in male infants exposed *in utero* to the drug, with or without other anticonvulsants. However, a causal relationship with topiramate has not been established (1).

A 2003 reference cited details from pregnancy exposure during clinical trials (2). Among 28 pregnancies, all involving polytherapy (other anticonvulsants not specified), there was "one malformation and two children with anomalies." In addition, the outcomes of 139 pregnancies identified during postmarketing surveillance were 87 live births, 23 elective abortions, and 29 lost to follow-up. The patient's anticonvulsant therapy was not specified. Five cases of hypospadias were observed, presumably in the live births (2).

In cases reported in a 2002 publication, five women were treated with topiramate (100–400 mg/day) combined with either carbamazepine (four cases) or valproic acid (one case) throughout gestation (2). All five newborns were healthy, normal infants. Birth weights of three infants ranged from 3520 to 3855 g, whereas the other two, both delivered from smoking mothers, had lower weights: 3160 g (six cigarettes/day) and 2720 g (10 cigarettes/day), respectively. Cord blood levels of topiramate (average 8.1 μM) were nearly equivalent to the maternal plasma concentration at delivery (average 8.4 μM) (3).

A 2002 review cited a case of a pregnant patient who had been treated with topiramate (1400 mg/day) monotherapy throughout gestation (4). The growth-retarded newborn had several minor anomalies, including generalized hirsutism, a third fontanelle, short nose with anteverted nares, blunted distal phalanges and nails, and fifth nail hypoplasia (3). The similarity of some of these anomalies to those observed with other anticonvulsants suggested to the authors that genetic factors might have been involved (4).

A dose-related interaction between topiramate and a combined oral contraceptive (ethinylestradiol 35 μg/norethindrone 1 mg) been reported (1,5). At a dose of 400 mg/day, peak levels of the estrogen were decreased. At 800 mg/day, estrogen bioavailability was reduced and clearance increased. Norethindrone clearance was also increased at 800 mg/day (5). Thus, the concurrent use of these agents could reduce the efficacy of the contraceptive, possibly requiring a higher-dose contraceptive combination (5).

Topiramate is known to induce hepatic enzymes and may increase the incidence of early hemorrhagic disease of the newborn by depleting fetal vitamin K stores. Although vitamin K_1 (see Phytonadione) does not readily cross the placenta, 10 mg/day of the vitamin may be given orally to the mother in the last 4 weeks of pregnancy. In addition, 1 mg of vitamin K_1 should be given IV or IM at birth (6).

In summary, topiramate was teratogenic in three animal species, but in two of them, maternal toxicity was also observed at the teratogenic dose. In addition, fetal and pup toxicity was observed in rats. All of these adverse effects occurred at doses ranging from much less to slightly above the human dose based on body surface area. Experience in human pregnancy is too limited to assess the embryo/fetal risk. Although hypospadias has been observed in male infants exposed *in utero*, a causal association with the drug has not been established. Topiramate does not produce epoxide metabolites (7). Because these intermediate arene oxide metabolites have been associated with teratogenicity (see Carbamazepine, Phenytoin, and Valproic Acid), this may indicate a lower risk of teratogenicity with topiramate compared to the other agents. The effect of topiramate on folic acid levels or metabolism is unknown (7). Until this information is available, the safest course is to start folic acid supplementation before conception with topiramate, as is done with other antiepileptic agents. With the currently available human data, topiramate should probably be avoided, if possible, during the 1st trimester. If therapy is required, the lowest effective dose should always be prescribed.

BREAST FEEDING SUMMARY

RECOMMENDATION: Limited Human Data - Potential Toxicity

Topiramate is excreted into human breast milk. This is consistent with the low molecular weight (about 339), the relative lack of protein binding, the low metabolism, and the prolonged plasma elimination. It also was excreted into the milk of lactating rats and was associated with toxicity in the pups (1).

Three women who had been treated with topiramate throughout pregnancy (see above) and continued during nursing were studied (3). The maternal daily doses were 150, 200, and 200 mg/day. The mean milk:plasma ratio 3 weeks after delivery was 0.86 (range 0.67–1.1). In one case, the ratio was 0.69 3 months after delivery. The weight adjusted infant doses, based on 150 mL/kg of milk per day, were 3%–23% of the maternal doses. Plasma levels of topiramate in two infants at 3 weeks of age, before and after nursing, were 1.4 and 1.3 μM, and 1.6 and 1.9 μM, respectively. The latter infant had a topiramate plasma concentration of 2.1 μM at 3 months of age. *(Note: possible antiepileptic effects of topiramate on cultured neurons are concentration-dependent within the range of 1 μM to 200 μM [1].)* Plasma levels in the third infant were undetectable at 2 and 4 weeks postdelivery. No adverse effects of the exposure were observed (4).

In pediatric patients (ages 2–16 years), common adverse effects (most occurred twice as often or more than those in placebo-treated patients) associated with topiramate were fatigue, somnolence, difficulty with concentration/attention, aggressive reaction, confusion, difficulty with memory, ataxia, purpura, epistaxis, infections (viral and pneumonia), and anorexia and weight decrease (1). (Patients also were receiving one or two other anticonvulsants.) The potential for these or other adverse effects in a nursing infant cannot be assessed with the available data. Therefore, nursing women who are being treated with topiramate, particularly those receiving high doses, should be advised to monitor their infants for signs of toxicity and for changes in alertness, behavior, and feeding habits.

References

1. Product information. Topamax. Ortho-McNeil Pharmaceutical, 2003.
2. Yerby MS. Clinical care of pregnant women with epilepsy: neural tube defects and folic acid supplements. Epilepsia 2003;44(Suppl 3):33–40.
3. Ohman I, Vitols S, Luef G, Soderfeldt B, Tomson T. Topiramate kinetics during delivery, lactation, and in the neonate: preliminary observations. Epilepsia 2002;43:1157–60.
4. Palmieri C, Canger R. Teratogenic potential of the newer antiepileptic drugs. What is known and how should this influence prescribing? CNS Drugs 2002;16:755–64.
5. Crawford P. Interactions between antiepileptic drugs and hormonal contraception. CNS Drugs 2002;16: 263–72.
6. Bruno MK, Harden CL. Epilepsy in pregnancy women. Curr Treat Options Neurol 2002;4:31–40.
7. Morrell MJ. The new antiepileptic drugs and women: efficacy, reproductive health, pregnancy, and fetal outcome. Epilepsia 1996;37(Suppl 6):S34–S44.

Name:	**TRAMADOL**	Risk Factor:	C_M
Class:	**Central Analgesic**		

FETAL RISK SUMMARY

RECOMMENDATION: Human Data Suggest Risk in 3rd Trimester

Tramadol is a synthetic, centrally acting, analgesic analogue of codeine that has the potential to cause physical dependence similar to, but much less, than that produced by opiates.

Because of its low addiction potential, tramadol is not classified as a controlled substance. The drug is available only as an oral tablet in the United States but has been used both parenterally and rectally in other countries.

Oral doses up to 50 mg/kg in male rats and 75 mg/kg in female rats had no effects on fertility (1). Reproductive studies, conducted with tramadol in mice (120 mg/kg), rats (25 mg/kg or higher), and rabbits (75 mg/kg or higher), showed embryotoxic and fetotoxic effects at maternally toxic doses, 3–15 times the maximum human dose or higher, but no fetal toxicity was observed with lower doses that were not maternally toxic (1). No teratogenic effects were observed with any of the doses. The observed toxicity consisted of decreased fetal weights, skeletal ossification, and increased supernumerary ribs. Transient delays in developmental or behavioral parameters were seen in rat pups.

Shepard described a reproductive study using oral and SC tramadol in mice, at doses up to 120 mg/kg, and in rats, at doses up to 60 mg/kg, that observed no teratogenic effects (2). Schardein also cited the same study (3).

Tramadol has a molecular weight of about 300 and crosses the placenta to the fetus. In 40 women given 100 mg of tramadol during labor, the mean ratio of drug concentrations in the umbilical cord and maternal serum was 0.83 (4).

Several studies outside of the United States, some of which were reviewed in 1993 (5) and 1997 publications (4), have compared the use of tramadol with meperidine or morphine for labor analgesia (6–12). In five of these studies (6–10), the use of tramadol was associated with less neonatal respiratory depression than meperidine, but no difference was observed in two studies in comparison with meperidine or morphine (11,12). In one of these latter studies, no differences in maternal response, adverse effects, or newborn condition were observed between tramadol, meperidine, and morphine (11). In the other study, tramadol and meperidine were combined with triflupromazine, a phenothiazine tranquilizer added in an attempt to reduce the emetic effects of the analgesics, and compared with tramadol alone (12). No decrease or difference between the three groups in the incidence and severity of the side effects was observed.

The effects of tramadol and meperidine, 100 mg IV for each drug, were compared in laboring patients in a study conducted in Thailand (9). A second or third dose of 50 mg IV was given at 30-minute intervals if requested. A significant increase in the incidence of neonatal respiratory depression was observed in the offspring of the meperidine group, if delivery occurred 2–4 hours after the last dose. The respiratory depressant effects of meperidine are known to be time- and dose-related, increasing markedly after 60 minutes (see Meperidine).

A study from Singapore found that 100 mg IM of tramadol was equivalent in analgesic effect to 75 mg IM of meperidine for the control of labor pain (10). Meperidine was associated with a significantly higher frequency of adverse effects (nausea, vomiting, fatigue, drowsiness, and dizziness) in the mothers and a significantly lower respiratory rate in the newborns. However, the injection-delivery interval in the patients was 7–8 hours.

In a 1997 case report, a male infant developed withdrawal symptoms between 24 and 48 hours after birth (13). Symptoms consisted of trembling, tachypnea, tachycardia, hypertonic muscle tone, signs of tetany when touched, and a single mild convulsion. The mother admitted to taking tramadol 300 mg/day for 4 years. The infant was treated with diazepam and/or phenobarbital for 13 days until the symptoms had fully resolved. No long-term follow-up of the infant was reported. The authors concluded that the estimated elimination half life of 36 hours was consistent with the course of the withdrawal syndrome (13).

Only the one report above has described the use of tramadol early in human gestation and an assessment of the risk, if any, that the drug presents to the embryo and fetus cannot be determined. Based on that case, neonatal withdrawal is a potential complication after continuous use in the mother. Because dose-related embryo and fetal toxicity have been observed in animals, use of tramadol during early human gestation should probably be avoided until additional data are available. Moreover, the delays in development and behavior observed in newborn rats appear to lessen any clinically significant advantage the drug may have over traditional narcotic analgesics.

BREAST FEEDING SUMMARY

RECOMMENDATION: Limited Human Data - Probably Compatible

Both tramadol and its pharmacologic active metabolite are excreted into human milk (1). After a single 100-mg IV dose, the cumulative amounts of the parent drug and metabolite excreted into milk within 16 hours were 100 and 27 μg, respectively (1). The recommended dose of tramadol is 50–100 mg every 4–6 hours up to a maximum of 400 mg/day. Moreover, the mean absolute bioavailability of a 100-mg oral dose is 75%. Thus, ingestion of the recommended dose may produce drug amounts in breast milk that could exceed those reported above. The effects of this exposure on a nursing infant are unknown.

References

1. Product information. Ultram. McNeil Pharmaceutical, 1997.
2. Yamamoto H, Kuchii M, Hayano T, Nishino H. A study on teratogenicity of both CG-315 and morphine in mice and rats. Oyo Yakuri 1972,6:1055–69. As cited in Shepard TH. *Catalog of Teratogenic Agents*. 8th ed. Baltimore, MD: Johns Hopkins University Press, 1995:420.
3. Yamamoto H, Kuchii M, Hayano T, Nishino H. Teratogenicity of the new central analgesic 1-(m-methoxyphenyl)-2-(dimethylaminomethyl) cyclohexanol hydrochloride (Cg-315) in mice and rats. Oyo Yakuri 1972;6:1055–69. As cited in Schardein JL. *Chemically Induced Birth Defects*. 2nd ed. New York, NY: Marcel Dekker, 1993:133.
4. Lewis KS, Han NH. Tramadol: a new centrally acting analgesic. Am J Health Syst Pharm 1997;54:643–52.
5. Lee CR, McTavish D, Sorkin EM. Tramadol. A preliminary review of its pharmacodynamic and pharmacokinetic properties, and therapeutic potential in acute and chronic pain states. Drugs 1993;46:313–40.
6. Husslein P, Kubista E, Egarter C. Obstetrical analgesia with tramadol-results of a prospective randomized comparative study with pethidine. Z Geburtshilfe Perinatol 1987;191:234–7.
7. Bitsch M, Emmrich J, Hary J, Lippach G, Rindt W. Obstetrical analgesia with tramadol. Fortschr Med 1980;98:632–4.
8. Bredow V. Use of tramadol versus pethidine versus denaverine suppositories in labor-a contribution to noninvasive therapy of labor pain. Zentralbl Gynakol 1992;114:551–4.
9. Suvonnakote T, Thitadilok W, Atisook R. Pain relief during labour. J Med Assoc Thailand 1986;69: 575–80.
10. Viegas OAC, Khaw B, Ratnam SS. Tramadol in labour pain in primiparous patients. A prospective comparative clinical trial. Eur J Obstet Gynecol Reprod Biol 1993;49:131–5.
11. Prasertsawat PO, Herabutya Y, Chaturachinda K. Obstetric analgesia: comparison between tramadol, morphine, and pethidine. Curr Ther Res Clin Exp 1986;40:1022–8.
12. Kainz C, Joura E, Obwegeser R, Plockinger B, Gruber W. Effectiveness and tolerance of tramadol with or without an antiemetic and pethidine in obstetric analgesia. Z Geburtshilfe Perinatol 1992;196:78–82.
13. Meyer FP, Rimasch H, Blaha B, Banditt P. Tramadol withdrawal in a neonate. Eur J Clin Pharmacol 1997; 53:159–60.

T

Name: **TRANDOLAPRIL** Risk Factor: **C_M***
Class: **Antihypertensive**

FETAL RISK SUMMARY

RECOMMENDATION: Human Data Suggest Risk in 2nd and 3rd Trimesters

The prodrug trandolapril is rapidly metabolized to the active drug trandolaprilat. It is indicated in the management of hypertension either alone, or in combination with other antihypertensives (e.g., hydrochlorothiazide). Trandolapril is also indicated in the management of stable patients with heart failure or left-ventricular dysfunction after myocardial infarction. The active metabolite, trandolaprilat, is a competitive inhibitor of angiotensin I-converting enzyme (ACE inhibitor), thus preventing the conversion of angiotensin I to angiotensin II.

Reproduction studies have been conducted in rats, rabbits, and cynomolgus monkeys (1). No teratogenicity was observed in the three species at doses that were 2564, 3, and 108 times, respectively, the maximum projected human dose based on body surface area.

It is not known if trandolapril or trandolaprilat cross the human placenta. The molecular weights (about 431 for trandolapril; about 403 for trandolaprilat) are low enough that transfer to the fetus should be expected.

No reports describing the use of trandolapril during human pregnancy have been located. Based on the human pregnancy experience with other ACE inhibitors, trandolapril exposure during the 1st trimester would not be expected to represent a risk to the fetus. However, use of trandolapril during the 2nd and 3rd trimesters may cause teratogenicity and severe fetal and neonatal toxicity (see Captopril or Enalapril). Fetal toxic effects may include anuria, oligohydramnios, fetal hypocalvaria, intrauterine growth retardation, prematurity, and patent ductus arteriosus. Anuria-associated oligohydramnios may produce fetal limb contractures, craniofacial deformation, and pulmonary hypoplasia. Severe anuria and hypotension, that is resistant to both pressor agents and volume expansion, may occur in the newborn following *in utero* exposure to ACE inhibitors.

In cases in which the mother's disease requires trandolapril (or other ACE inhibitor), the lowest possible dose should be used. Close monitoring of amniotic fluid levels and fetal well-being should be conducted during gestation, followed by close observation of renal function and blood pressure in the newborn. If trandolapril is used in pregnancy, healthcare professionals are encouraged to call the toll free number (800-670-6126) for information about patient enrollment in the Motherisk study.

[**Risk Factor* D_M *if used in the 2nd and/or 3rd trimesters*]

BREAST FEEDING SUMMARY

RECOMMENDATION: No Human Data - Probably Compatible

No reports describing the use of trandolapril in human lactation have been located. The molecular weights (about 431 for trandolapril; about 403 for trandolaprilat) suggest that excretion into breast milk should be expected. The effect of this exposure on a nursing infant are unknown. However, other ACE inhibitors are excreted into breast milk and are considered compatible with breast-feeding by the American Academy of Pediatrics (see Captopril and Enalapril).

T

Reference

1. Product information. Mavik. Knoll Pharmaceutical, 2001.

Name: **TRANEXAMIC ACID** Risk Factor: **B_M**
Class: **Hemostatic**

FETAL RISK SUMMARY

RECOMMENDATION: Limited Human Data - Animal Data Suggest Low Risk

This hemostatic agent, a competitive inhibitor of plasminogen activation, is used to reduce or prevent hemorrhage in hemophilia and in other bleeding disorders. The drug blocks the action of plasminogen activators (e.g., tissue-plasminogen activator [alteplase; t-PA], streptokinase, and urokinase) by inhibiting the conversion of plasminogen to plasmin. No adverse fetal effects were observed in reproductive toxicity testing in mice, rats, and rabbits (1,2). Both Schardein (3) and Shepard (4) cited a 1971 study in which doses up to 1500 mg/kg/day were given to mice and rats during organogenesis without causing adverse fetal effects.

Tranexamic acid crosses the human placenta to the fetus (5). Twelve women were given an IV dose of 10 mg/kg just before cesarean section. Cord serum and maternal blood samples were drawn immediately following delivery, a mean of 13 minutes after the dose of tranexamic acid. The mean drug concentrations in the cord and maternal serum were 19 μg/mL (range <4–31 μg/mL) and 26 μg/mL (range 10–53 μg/mL), respectively, a ratio of 0.7.

Twelve women with vaginal bleeding between 24 and 36 weeks' gestation were treated with 7-day courses of tranexamic acid, 1 g orally every 8 hours (6). Additional courses were given if bleeding continued (number of patients with repeat courses not specified). Four women underwent cesarean section (placenta previa in three, breech in one) and the remainder had vaginal deliveries. One of the newborns was delivered at 30 weeks' gestation, but the gestational ages of the other newborns were not specified. All of the newborns were alive and well. Two of the mothers were receiving treatment at the time of delivery, and the drug concentrations in the cord blood were 9 and 12 μg/mL.

A pregnant woman with fibrinolysis was treated with tranexamic acid and fibrinogen for 64 days until spontaneous delivery of a normal 1400-g girl at 30 weeks' gestation (7). No adverse fetal or newborn effects attributable to the drug were reported. Tranexamic acid was used in a woman with abruptio placentae during her third pregnancy (8). She had a history of two previous pregnancy losses because of the disorder. Treatment with tranexamic acid (1 g IV every 4 hours for 3 days, then 1 g orally 4 times daily) was begun at 26 weeks' gestation and continued until 33 weeks' gestation, at which time a cesarean section was performed because of the risk of heavier bleeding. A healthy 1430-g male infant was delivered.

The use of tranexamic acid in a woman with Glanzmann's thrombasthenia disease was described in an abstract published in 1981 (9). Treatment was started at 24 weeks' gestation and continued until spontaneous delivery at 42 weeks' gestation of a healthy boy. A study published in 1980 described the use of tranexamic acid in 73 consecutive cases of abruptio placentae, 6 of which were treated for 1–12 weeks (10). Six (8.2%) of the newborns were either stillbirths ($N = 4$) or died shortly after delivery ($N = 2$), a markedly reduced mortality rate compared with the expected 33%–37% at that time (10). None of the deaths were attributed to the drug. No cases of increased hemorrhage, thromboses, or maternal deaths were observed.

Tranexamic acid (4 g/day) was used in a 21-year-old primigravida at 26 weeks' gestation for the treatment of vaginal bleeding (11). She also received terbutaline and betamethasone for premature labor. Tranexamic acid was administered as a single dose on admission, and 6 days later a 10-day course was initiated for continued bleeding. Acute massive pulmonary embolism occurred at the termination of tranexamic acid, and following 2–3 days of treatment with heparin and streptokinase, a preterm 1140-g male infant was spontaneously delivered. No adverse effects in the fetus or newborn attributable to the drug therapy were noted.

A retrospective study published in 1993 examined the question of whether tranexamic acid was thrombogenic when administered during pregnancy (12). Between 1979 and 1988 in Sweden, among pregnant women with various bleeding disorders, 256 had been treated with tranexamic acid (mean duration 46 days), whereas 1846 had not been treated (controls). Two patients (0.78%) in the treated group had pulmonary embolism compared with 4 (0.22%) (3 deep vein thromboses, 1 pulmonary embolism) (odds ratio 3.6, 95% confidence limits 0.7–17.8) in the control group. In the subgroups of those patients who were delivered by cesarean section (168 treated, 439 controls), the rates of thromboembolism were 1 (0.60%) and 4 (0.91%) (odds ratio 0.65, 95% confidence limits 0.1–5.8), respectively. Thus, no evidence was found indicating that the use of tranexamic acid during gestation was thrombogenic. Although the purpose of this study did not include examining the effects of the therapy on the fetus or newborn, the authors concluded that in the absence of a thrombogenic risk, there was no reason to change the indications for its use during pregnancy.

In summary, no adverse effects attributable to use of tranexamic acid during pregnancy, in either animals or humans, have been reported in the fetus or newborn. The drug crosses the placenta to the fetus, but its reported lack of effect on plasminogen activator activity in the vascular wall (10,12) (versus its known effect in the peripheral circulation) may protect the fetus and newborn from potential thromboembolic complications.

BREAST FEEDING SUMMARY

RECOMMENDATION: Limited Human Data - Probably Compatible

Tranexamic acid is excreted into human milk. One hour after the last dose following a 2-day treatment course in lactating women, the milk concentration of the agent was 1% of the peak serum concentration (13). In adults, approximately 30%–50% of an oral dose is absorbed (1). The amount a nursing infant would absorb is unknown, as is the effect of the small amount of drug present in milk.

References

1. Product information. Cyklokapron. Pharmacia, 1996.
2. Onnis A, Grella P, Lewis PJ. *The Biochemical Effects of Drugs in Pregnancy*. Volume 1. Chichester, England: Ellis Horwood, 1984:385.
3. Schardein JL. *Chemically Induced Birth Defects*. 2nd ed. New York, NY: Marcel Dekker, 1993:107.
4. Shepard TH. *Catalog of Teratogenic Agents*. 8th ed. Baltimore, MD: Johns Hopkins University Press, 1995:420.
5. Kullander S, Nilsson IM. Human placental transfer of an antifibrinolytic agent (AMCA). Acta Obstet Gynecol Scand 1970;49:241–2.
6. Walzman M, Bonnar J. Effects of tranexamic acid on the coagulation and fibrinolytic systems in pregnancy complicated by placental bleeding. Arch Toxicol Suppl 1982;5:214–20.
7. Storm O, Weber J. Prolonged treatment with tranexamic acid (Cyklokapron) during pregnancy. Ugeskr Laeg 1976;138:1781–2.
8. Åstedt B, Nilsson IM. Recurrent abruptio placentae treated with the fibrinolytic inhibitor tranexamic acid. Br Med J 1978;1:756–7.
9. Sundqvist S-B, Nilsson IM, Svanberg L, Cronberg S. Glanzmann's thrombasthenia: pregnancy and parturition (abstract). Thromb Haemost 1981;46:225.
10. Svanberg L, Åstedt B, Nilsson IM. Abruptio placentae–treatment with the fibrinolytic inhibitor tranexamic acid. Acta Obstet Gynecol Scand 1980;59:127–30.

11. Fagher B, Ahlgren M, Åstedt B. Acute massive pulmonary embolism treated with streptokinase during labor and the early puerperium. Acta Obstet Gynecol Scand 1990;69:659–62.
12. Lindoff C, Rybo G, Åstedt B. Treatment with tranexamic acid during pregnancy and the risk of thrombo-embolic complications. Thromb Haemost 1993;70:238–40.
13. Eriksson O, Kjellman H, Nilsson L. Tranexamic acid in human milk after oral administration of Cyklokapron to lactating women. Data on file, KabiVitrum AB, Stockholm, Sweden. (Data supplied by R. G. Leonardi, Ph.D., KabiVitrum, 1987.)

Name: **TRANYLCYPROMINE** Risk Factor: **C**

Class: **Antidepressant**

FETAL RISK SUMMARY

RECOMMENDATION: Limited Human Data - No Relevant Animal Data

Tranylcypromine is a monoamine oxidase inhibitor used in the treatment of major depressive episode without melancholia. The drug crosses the placenta to the fetus in rats (1).

The Collaborative Perinatal Project monitored 21 mother-child pairs exposed to monoamine oxidase inhibitors during the 1st trimester, 13 of whom were exposed to tranylcypromine (2). Three of the 21 infants had malformations (relative risk 2.26). Details of the 13 cases with exposure to tranylcypromine were not specified.

A brief 2000 abstract described two consecutive adverse pregnancy outcomes in a woman treated with tranylcypromine (3). In the first pregnancy, the 41-year-old woman with severe depression was treated with tranylcypromine (100 mg/day), pimozide (1 mg/day), and diazepam (5–10 mg/day). The woman delivered a stillborn fetus at 31 weeks' gestation. Examination of the macerated female fetus revealed hypertelorism, a large atrioventricular septal defect, single coronary ostium and right pulmonary isomerism. The placenta had multiple infarcts that were considered significant factors in the fetal death. In her second pregnancy (other drugs and doses not specified), an ultrasound at 19 weeks' gestation revealed a fetus with a head described as "lemon-shaped." A female infant (normal karyotype) was delivered at 38 weeks' gestation because of poor growth (weight not specified). The infant had multiple defects, including hypertelorism, low-set, overfolded ears, cleft palate, micrognathia, marked distal phalangeal hypoplasia, agenesis of the corpus callosum, and an atrioventricular septal defect (first detected at 26 weeks' gestation). The outcomes of both pregnancies were attributed to tranylcypromine, possibly as a result of reduced uterine and placental blood flow (3).

BREAST FEEDING SUMMARY

RECOMMENDATION: No Human Data - Potential Toxicity

No reports describing the use of tranylcypromine during lactation have been located. The molecular weight (about 365) is low enough, however, that excretion into breast milk should be expected. The drug is found in the milk of lactating dogs (1). The potential effects of exposure on a nursing infant are unknown.

References

1. Product information. Parnate. SmithKline Beecham Pharmaceuticals, 2000.
2. Heinonen OP, Slone D, Shapiro S. *Birth Defects and Drugs in Pregnancy*. Littleton, MA: Publishing Sciences Group, 1977:336–7.
3. Kennedy DS, Evans N, Wang I, Webster WS. Fetal abnormalities associated with high-dose tranylcypromine in two consecutive pregnancies (abstract). Teratology 2000;61:441.

T

Name:	TRASTUZUMAB	Risk Factor:	B_M
Class:	Antineoplastic		

FETAL RISK SUMMARY

RECOMMENDATION: No Human Data - Animal Data Suggest Low Risk

Trastuzumab, a recombinant DNA-derived humanized monoclonal antibody (an IgG_1 kappa), selectively binds with high affinity to the extracellular domain of the human epidermal growth factor receptor 2 protein (HER2). It is indicated, either alone or in combination with paclitaxel, for the treatment of patients with metastatic breast cancer whose tumors overexpress the HER2 protein. Trastuzumab is administered as an IV infusion. The mean elimination half-life, after a 4 mg/kg loading dose followed by a weekly maintenance dose of 2 mg/kg, was 5.8 days (range 1–32 days).

No evidence of impaired fertility or fetal harm were observed in female cynomolgus monkeys administered doses up to 25 times the weekly human dose of 2 mg/kg (HD). However, HER2 protein expression is high in many embryonic tissues, such as cardiac and neural tissues. Early death was observed in embryos of mutant mice that lacked this protein (1).

It is not known if trastuzumab crosses the human placenta. The antibody does cross the placentas of cynomolgus monkeys in both early (gestational days 20 and 50) and late (gestational days 120 and 150) gestation (1). The presence of trastuzumab in the serum of infant monkeys had no adverse effect on growth or development from birth to 3 months of age (1).

No reports describing the use of trastuzumab in human pregnancy have been located. Because of the very long elimination half-life, the antibody could be present in the maternal system for up to 5–6 months after the last dose. The lack of fetal harm in cynomolgus monkeys is reassuring but, as noted above, HER2 protein expression is critical to fetal development. Therefore, the embryo and/or fetal risk cannot be assessed until human pregnancy experience is available. One reviewer recommended that the use of growth factor pathway blockers, such as trastuzumab, in pregnancy should be limited until human pregnancy data are available (2). However, the reviewer also noted that compared to standard chemotherapy, the use of trastuzumab could improve the pregnancy outcome for both the mother and her fetus (2).

BREAST FEEDING SUMMARY

RECOMMENDATION: No Human Data - Potential Toxicity

No reports describing the use of trastuzumab during human lactation have been located. The antibody is excreted into the milk of lactating cynomolgus monkeys after a dose that was 25 times the HD (1). Human immunoglobulin G also is excreted into breast milk (2). The effects, if any, of exposure to trastuzumab from milk on a nursing infant are unknown. In women treated with the drug, adverse effects included congestive heart failure, cardiac dysfunction, anemia, leucopenia, diarrhea, and an increased incidence of infection. The manufacturer recommends that women receiving trastuzumab should not breast-feed for 6 months after the last dose of the antibody (1).

References

1. Product information. Herceptin. Genentech, 2000.
2. Leslie KK. Chemotherapy and pregnancy. Clin Obstet Gynecol 2002;45:153–64.

Name:	**TRAZODONE**	Risk Factor:	C_M
Class:	**Antidepressant**		

FETAL RISK SUMMARY

RECOMMENDATION: Limited Human Data - Animal Data Suggest Low Risk

Trazodone is an antidepressant. At high doses in some animal species, trazodone is fetal toxic and teratogenic. However, others have reported no teratogenicity in rats and rabbits (1).

One manufacturer has received several anecdotal descriptions concerning the use of trazodone in pregnancy (T. Donosky, personal communication, Mead Johnson Pharmaceutical Division, 1987). Included in these was a report of an infant born with an undefined birth defect after *in utero* exposure to the antidepressant. Another report described a normal infant exposed throughout gestation beginning with the 5th week. No confirmatory follow-up information was available for either of these cases. A third case from the manufacturer's files involved a woman who took trazodone, 50–100 mg/day, during the first 3 weeks of pregnancy and eventually delivered a normal infant. Finally, a woman was treated with trazodone for 8 days, at which time the drug was discontinued because of a positive pregnancy test. A spontaneous abortion occurred approximately 1.5 months later. No cause and effect relationship can be inferred between trazodone and any of the above adverse outcomes.

In a surveillance study of Michigan Medicaid recipients conducted between 1985 and 1992 involving 229,101 completed pregnancies, 100 newborns had been exposed to trazodone during the 1st trimester (F. Rosa, personal communication, FDA, 1993). One (1%) major birth defect was observed (four expected), but details are not available. No anomalies were observed in six defect categories (cardiovascular defects, oral clefts, spina bifida, polydactyly, limb-reduction defects, and hypospadias) for which specific data were available.

A prospective multicenter study evaluated the effects of lithium exposure during the 1st trimester in 148 women (2). One of the pregnancies was terminated at 16 weeks' gestation because of a fetus with the rare congenital heart defect, Ebstein's anomaly. The fetus had been exposed to lithium, trazodone, fluoxetine, and L-thyroxine during the 1st trimester. The defect was attributed to lithium exposure.

In a 1996 descriptive case series, the European Network of the Teratology Information Services (ENTIS) prospectively examined the outcomes of 689 pregnancies exposed to antidepressants (3). Multiple-drug therapy occurred in about two-thirds of the mothers. Trazodone was used in 13 pregnancies. The outcomes of these pregnancies were two elective abortions, eight normal newborns (includes one premature infant), and three normal infants that died after birth (after difficult delivery; twins delivered at 27 weeks' gestation; multiple other drugs) (3).

A 2003 prospective controlled study described the outcomes of 147 pregnancies exposed in the 1st trimester (52 used the drugs throughout gestation) to either trazodone or nefazodone, a closely related antidepressant (4). The data were gathered from five teratology information services in Canada (two sites), the United States (two sites), and Italy. The outcomes were compared to two control groups (one exposed to other antidepressants and one exposed to nonteratogens). There were no significant differences between the three groups in terms of spontaneous abortions, elective abortions, stillbirths, major malformations, gestational age at birth, or birth weights. In the study group, there were two (1.6%) major malformations: neural tube defect and Hirschsprung's disease (4).

BREAST FEEDING SUMMARY

RECOMMENDATION: Limited Human Data - Potential Toxicity

Trazodone is excreted into human milk. In six healthy lactating women, 3–8 months postpartum, a single 50-mg oral dose of trazodone was given after an overnight fast (5). Simultaneous serum and milk samples were collected at various times up to 30 hours after ingestion. The infants of the mothers were not allowed to breast-feed during the first 4 hours after the dose. The mean milk:plasma ratio, based on the concentration-time curves for the two fluids, was 0.142. Based on 500 mL of milk consumed during a 12-hour interval, the infants would have received a trazodone dose of 0.005 mg/kg. This study was unable to include a potentially active metabolite, 1-*m*-chlorophenylpiperazine, in the analysis (5).

Although the amount of trazodone in milk is very small, the American Academy of Pediatrics classifies trazodone as a drug for which the effect on nursing infants is unknown but may be of concern (6).

References

1. Schardein JL. Psychotropic drugs. *Chemically Induced Birth Defects*. 3rd ed. New York, NY: Marcel Dekker, 2000:252.
2. Jacobson SJ, Jones K, Johnson K, Ceolin L, Kaur P, Sahn D, Donnenfeld AE, Rieder M, Santelli R, Smythe J, Pastuszak A, Einarson T, Koren G. Prospective multicentre study of pregnancy outcome after lithium exposure during first trimester. Lancet 1992;339:530–3.
3. McElhatton PR, Garbis HM, Elefant E, Vial T, Bellemin B, Mastroiacovo P, Arnon J, Rodriguez-Pinilla E, Schaefer C, Pexieder T, Merlob P, Dal Verme S. The outcome of pregnancy in 689 women exposed to therapeutic doses of antidepressants. A collaborative study of the European Network of Teratology Information Services (ENTIS). Reprod Toxicol 1996;10:285–94.
4. Einarson A, Bonari L, Voyer-Lavigne S, Addis A, Matsui D, Johnson Y, Koren G. A multicentre prospective controlled study to determine the safety of trazodone and nefazodone use during pregnancy. Can J Psychiatry 2003;48:106–9.
5. Verbeeck RK, Ross SG, McKenna EA. Excretion of trazodone in breast milk. Br J Clin Pharmacol 1986;22:367–70.
6. Committee on Drugs, American Academy of Pediatrics. The transfer of drugs and other chemicals into human milk. Pediatrics 2001;108:776–89.

Name:	**TREPROSTINIL**	Risk Factor:	B_M
Class:	**Hematologic Agent (Antiplatelet)**		

FETAL RISK SUMMARY

RECOMMENDATION: No Human Data - Animal Data Suggest Low Risk

Treprostinil is an inhibitor of platelet aggregation. Its action includes direct vasodilation of pulmonary and systemic arterial vascular beds. Treprostinil is administered by continuous

SC infusion for the treatment of pulmonary arterial hypertension. The terminal elimination half-life is about 2–4 hours. Treprostinil is extensively metabolized in the liver but the biological activity of the metabolites is unknown (1).

Reproduction studies have been conducted in rats and rabbits. In pregnant rats during organogenesis, continuous SC infusions of doses up to about 117 times the recommended starting rate in humans based on body surface area (HD) and about 16 times the average rate achieved in clinical trials (AR) revealed no evidence of fetal harm. At doses up to about 8 times the AR, continuous SC infusions administered from implantation to the end of lactation had no effect on growth or development of offspring. In pregnant rabbits during organogenesis, a continuous SC infusion at 41 times the HD and about 5 times the AR produced fetal skeletal variations. However, maternal toxicity (decreased body weight and food consumption) was evident at this dose (1).

It is not known if treprostinil crosses the human placenta. The molecular weight (about 412) is low enough, however, that passage to the fetus should be expected. Moreover, the drug is administered as a continuous SC infusion that should result in relatively constant plasma drug concentrations at the placental maternal-fetal interface.

In summary, no reports describing the use of treprostinil during human pregnancy have been located. The animal data are suggestive of low risk, but the lack of human pregnancy experience prevents an assessment of the embryo/fetal risk. However, maternal hypotension, resulting in decreased placental perfusion and fetal hypoxia, is a potential risk

BREAST FEEDING SUMMARY

RECOMMENDATION: No Human Data - Potential Toxicity

No reports describing the use of treprostinil during lactation have been located. The molecular weight (about 412) and method of administration (continuous SC infusion) suggest that the drug will be excreted into breast milk. In adults, treprostinil undergoes extensive hepatic metabolism, but the biological activity of the metabolites has not been characterized. However, even if the metabolites are inactive, the neonatal immature hepatic function could allow systemic levels of the parent drug. Although the effects of this exposure on a nursing infant are unknown, treprostinil has caused clinically significant adverse effects in adults (e.g., headache, nausea/vomiting, restlessness, and anxiety). Therefore, women who are receiving treprostinil should not breast-feed.

Reference

1. Product information. Remodulin. United Therapeutics, 2002.

T

Name:	**TRETINOIN (SYSTEMIC)**	Risk Factor:	D_M
Class:	**Antineoplastic/Vitamin**		

FETAL RISK SUMMARY

RECOMMENDATION: Contraindicated - 1st Trimester

Tretinoin (all-*trans* retinoic acid; retinoic acid; vitamin A acid) is a retinoid and vitamin A (retinol) metabolite that is available both as a topical formulation (see Tretinoin [Topical]) and as an oral antineoplastic for the treatment of acute promyelocytic leukemia. Like other retinoids, all-*trans* retinoic acid is a potent teratogen when taken systemically during early pregnancy (see Etretinate, Isotretinoin, and Vitamin A), producing a pattern of birth defects termed retinoic acid embryopathy (central nervous system, craniofacial, cardiovascular, and thymic anomalies). The teratogenic effect of all-*trans* retinoic acid is dose-dependent because an endogenous supply of the vitamin is required for normal morphogenesis and differentiation of the embryo, including a role in physiologic developmental gene expression (1). Low serum concentrations or frank deficiency of vitamin A and all-*trans* retinoic acid is also teratogenic (see Tretinoin [Topical]).

The teratogenicity of all-*trans* retinoic acid in animals is summarized under the topical formulation as is the reported human pregnancy experience following topical use.

A number of reports have described the use of systemic tretinoin (45 mg/m^2/day in eight cases, 70 mg/day in one) for the treatment of acute promyelocytic leukemia during pregnancy (2–10). In one case treatment was started during the 6th week of gestation (about 36 days from the last menstruation) (2); in five cases (1 set of twins), treatment was started during the 2nd trimester (3–7); and in three cases, treatment was started during the 3rd trimester (8–10). No congenital abnormalities were observed in the 10 newborns, although 8 were delivered prematurely (4 by elective cesarean section at 32, 32, 32, and 30 weeks; and 4 [1 set of twins] by spontaneous vaginal delivery at 32, 32 and 33 weeks). The growth and development in eight of the infants (postnatal examinations not reported in two cases) were normal in the follow-up periods ranging up to 15 months.

BREAST FEEDING SUMMARY

RECOMMENDATION: No Human Data - Probably Compatible

Vitamin A and, presumably, tretinoin (all-*trans* retinoic acid) are natural constituents of human milk. There is no data available on the amount of all-*trans* retinoic acid excreted into breast milk following the doses used for the treatment of promyelocytic leukemia or the risk, if any, this may present to a nursing infant.

References

1. Morriss-Kay, G. Retinoic acid and development. Pathobiology 1992;60:264–70.
2. Simone MD, Stasi R, Venditti A, Del Poeta G, Aronica G, Bruno A, Masi M, Tribalto M, Papa G, Amadori S. All-*trans* retinoic acid (ATRA) administration during pregnancy in relapsed acute promyelocytic leukemia. Leukemia 1995;9:1412–3.
3. Stentoft J, Lanng Nielsen J, Hvidman LE. All-*trans* retinoic acid in acute promyelocytic leukemia in late pregnancy. Leukemia 1994;8(Suppl 2):S77–S80.
4. Harrison P, Chipping P, Fothergill GA. Successful use of all-trans retinoic acid in acute promyelocytic leukaemia presenting during the second trimester of pregnancy. Br J Haematol 1994;86:681–2.
5. Lin C-P, Huang M-J, Liu H-J, Chang IY, Tsai C-H. Successful treatment of acute promyelocytic leukemia in a pregnant Jehovah's Witness with all-trans retinoic acid, rhG-CSF, and erythropoietin. Am J Hematol 1996;51:251–2.
6. Incerpi MH, Miller DA, Posen R, Byrne JD. All-trans retinoic acid for the treatment of acute promyelocytic leukemia in pregnancy. Obstet Gynecol 1997;89:826–8.
7. Morton J, Taylor K, Wright S, Pitcher L, Wilson E, Tudehope D, Savage J, Williams B, Taylor D, Wiley J, Tsoris D, O'Donnell A. Successful maternal and fetal outcome following the use of ATRA for the induction APML late in the first trimester (abstract). Blood 1995;86(Suppl 1):772a.
8. Watanabe R, Okamoto S, Moriki T, Kizaki M, Kawai Y, Ikeda Y. Treatment of acute promyelocytic leukemia with all-*trans* retinoic acid during the third trimester of pregnancy. Am J Hematol 1995;48:210–1.
9. Nakamura K, Dan K, Iwakiri R, Gomi S, Nomura T. Successful treatment of acute promyelocytic leukemia in pregnancy with all-*trans* retinoic acid. Ann Hematol 1995;71:263–4.
10. Lipovsky MM, Biesma DH, Christiaens GCML, Petersen EJ. Successful treatment of acute promyelocytic leukaemia with all-*trans*-retinoic-acid during late pregnancy. Br J Haematol 1996;94:699–701.

Name:	TRETINOIN (TOPICAL)	Risk Factor:	C_M
Class:	**Dermatologic Agent**		

FETAL RISK SUMMARY

RECOMMENDATION: Human Data Suggest Low Risk

Tretinoin (all-*trans* retinoic acid; retinoic acid; vitamin A acid) is a retinoid and vitamin A (retinol) metabolite used topically for the treatment of acne vulgaris and other skin disorders and systemically in the treatment of acute promyelocytic leukemia (see Tretinoin [Systemic]). Like other retinoids, the drug is a potent teratogen after exposure in early pregnancy (see also Etretinate, Isotretinoin, and Vitamin A), producing a pattern of birth defects termed retinoic acid embryopathy (central nervous system [CNS], craniofacial, cardiovascular, and thymic anomalies). However, an endogenous supply of retinoic acid is required for normal morphogenesis and differentiation of the embryo, including a role in physiologic developmental gene expression. The teratogenic effect of retinoic acid is manifested when the levels are excessive (1).

Low serum concentration or frank deficiency of vitamin A and all-*trans* retinoic acid is also teratogenic. Recent studies have shown that inhibition of the conversion of retinol to retinoic acid or depletion of retinol may be involved in the teratogenic mechanisms of such agents as ethanol (2–6) and some anticonvulsants (7).

Two manufacturers have stated that reproduction studies with topical tretinoin in animals are equivocal (8,9). In pregnant rats, daily doses greater than 200 times the recommended human topical dose (RHTD) were associated with shortened or kinked tail. At 2000 times the RHTD, skeletal anomalies (humerus: short, bent; os parietale incompletely ossified) were observed. In rabbits, fetotoxicity was observed with doses 100 times the RHTD. Doses approximately 80 times the RHTD in pregnant rabbits were associated with domed head and hydrocephaly, anomalies that are typical of retinoid-induced malformations in this species (8,9). In addition, a dose 91 times the RHTD was also associated with an increased incidence of cleft palate (9). In contrast, other studies with topical tretinoin in rats and rabbits at doses 100–200 times the RHTD have not demonstrated a teratogenic effect (8,9).

A 1997 report described the developmental toxicity of topical and oral tretinoin in pregnant rats (10). Topical doses of 10 mg/kg/day (approximately 2000 times the RHTD) or more were not tolerated, causing severe local and systemic maternal toxicity. Maternal toxicity (reduced weight gain and food consumption) was also evident at doses of 2.5 mg/kg/day (approximately 500 times the RHTD) or more. A significant increase in the occurrence of supernumerary ribs was observed at this dose, a result thought to be nonspecific or maternally mediated (10). In contrast, oral tretinoin doses of 5 and 10 mg/kg/day were not maternally toxic, but were associated with an increased incidence of supernumerary ribs (5 mg/kg/day) and cleft palate (10 mg/kg/day). Based on these results, the investigators concluded that only the highest oral dose was teratogenic (10).

Dose-related maternal toxicity was observed in rabbits treated topically with tretinoin cream at dosages of 10 and 100 times the human clinical dose (500 mg of 0.05% cream in a 50-kg adult = 0.005 mg/kg/day) based on body weight (11). Maternal endogenous plasma tretinoin levels were below the detection level (5 ng/mL) in all animals. After treatment, however, a few rabbits had detectable concentrations of retinoic acid, 13-*cis*-retinoic acid, or their metabolites. The maternal toxicity was associated with an increased incidence

T

of abortions, resorptions, and reduced fetal body weight. Some significant ($p \leq 0.01$) increases in malformations (open eyelids and cleft palate) and variations (nasal ossification, fused sternebrae, and irregular-shaped scapular alae) were observed. However, these were not considered to be tretinoin-related because they were not dose-related, and the litter incidences either did not differ significantly from those of controls or were within expected ranges for the species (11).

Additional literature on the teratogenicity of both systemic and topical tretinoin in various animal species has been summarized in several sources (12–16). The latter reference has particular application to the study of the teratogenic effects of tretinoin because it examined the toxicity of very small oral doses of this compound at presomite stages in mouse embryos, thought to be the most sensitive period for retinoid-induced teratogenesis (16). An increasing incidence of severe microphthalmia, anophthalmia, and iridial colobomata was produced as the dose was increased from 0 to 1.25 mg/kg. These doses were much less than those typically used for reproductive toxicity testing at later gestational periods. Slightly higher threshold doses produced exencephaly (2.5 mg/kg) and marked craniofacial defects (7.5 mg/kg) representative of the holoprosencephaly-aprosencephaly spectrum (16).

When tretinoin is used topically, its teratogenic risk had been thought to be close to 0 (17). According to one source, no cases of toxicity had been reported after nearly 20 years of use (17). In support of this, it has been estimated that even if maximal absorption (approximately 33%) occurred from a 1-g daily application of a 0.1% preparation, this would result in only about one-seventh of the vitamin A activity received from a typical prenatal vitamin supplement (18). One source stated that 80% of a 0.1% formulation in alcohol remained on the skin's surface, but when a 0.1% ointment was applied to the back with a 16-hour occlusive dressing, only 50% of the drug remained on the skin surface and 6% was excreted in the urine within 56 hours (19).

Authors of a 1992 reference reviewed the teratogenicity of vitamin A and its congeners, including tretinoin, but did not derive a conclusion on the safety of the drug after topical use (20), most likely because of the lack of studies with the drug in pregnancy.

Five reports of congenital malformations in newborns whose mother's were using tretinoin during the 1st trimester have been located (21–25). The first case involved a woman who had used tretinoin cream 0.05% during the month before her last menstruation and during the first 11 weeks of pregnancy (21). Her term, growth-retarded (weight 2620 g, <3rd percentile; length 49 cm, 25th percentile; head circumference 32.5 cm, 3rd percentile) female infant had a crumpled right hypoplastic ear and atresia of the right external auditory meatus, a pattern of ear malformation identical with that observed with vitamin A congeners (21). The remainder of the examination was normal, including the eyes, cerebral computed tomography, and chromosomal analysis.

The second report described the female infant of a woman who had used an over-the-counter alcohol-based liquid preparation of 0.05% tretinoin for severe facial acne (22). The infant had multiple congenital defects consisting of supraumbilical exomphalos, a diaphragmatic hernia, a pericardial defect, dextroposition of the heart, and a right-sided upper limb-reduction defect.

A 1998 case report described the pregnancy outcome of a woman who had used, before conception and during the first 2 months of gestation, a topical alcohol-based preparation of tretinoin 0.05% combined with benzoyl peroxide 2.5% for facial acne (23). Except for doxycycline (200 mg/day) that had been taken for an unknown duration, she had no other exposures to medications or vitamins. An ultrasound examination at 5 months' gestation detected hand and heart malformations. The female infant (2800 g; length 48 cm; normal karyotype 46,XX) was delivered at term with coarctation of the aorta, hypoplastic left hand, and small ear canals. The authors noted the similarity of some of the anomalies to those observed in retinoic acid embryopathy and speculated that the keratolytic action of benzoyl peroxide may have enhanced the cutaneous absorption of tretinoin. However, they also noted that any association between tretinoin and the birth defects may have been fortuitous (23).

Severe malformations were reported in a term, female infant whose mother had used tretinoin 0.05% twice daily for facial acne before and throughout gestation (24). The defects were thought to be consistent with abnormal cranial neural crest cell migration. They included craniofacial defects (cleft palate and harelip, fused palpebral fissures, hypertelorism, a depressed nasal bridge, and deficient left naris), and CNS anomalies (disorganized rudimentary optic cup derivatives with optic tract dysgenesis, arrhinencephaly, agenesis of the corpus callosum, fornices and cingulate gyri, cerebellar hypoplasia, and aqueduct stenosis with hydrocephalus) (24).

The fifth case report involved a 4090-g term male infant who was born with absence of the right ear and external auditory canal (25). The mother had used tretinoin 0.025% topically on her face and over a large area of her back before conception and during the first 2–3 months of gestation. She took prenatal vitamins during pregnancy. The father was using isotretinoin before conception. Examinations at 16 and 20 months of age revealed a nonverbal infant with poor receptive language consistent with cognitive impairment. He had age-appropriate muscle strength, tone and bulk. There was a diminished optokinetic response and no oculovestibular response when rotating toward the right. Extensive examinations revealed cerebral calcification of the right posterior hemisphere, an overall reduction in the volume of the right cerebral hemisphere, a remote infarct in the deep basal ganglia, focal atrophy and encephalomalacia of the right parieto-occipital lobe (25). Marked abnormalities were noted in the posterior cerebral artery and some of its branches. Hypometabolism, sometimes severe, was observed in several regions of the brain, including the thalamus (25).

The results of a prospective survey involving 60 completed pregnancies exposed to tretinoin early in pregnancy were presented in a 1994 abstract (26). From these pregnancies there were 53 liveborns (1 set of twins), 3 lost to follow-up, 4 spontaneous abortions, and 1 elective termination. No major malformations characteristic of retinoic acid embryopathy were observed except for one case in which the mother had also taken isotretinoin.

Among 25 birth defect cases with 1st trimester exposure to tretinoin reported to the FDA from 1969 to 1993, 5 were cases of holoprosencephaly (27). Six other cases of holoprosencephaly involved other vitamin A derivatives: isotretinoin ($N = 4$), etretinate ($N = 1$), and megadose vitamin A ($N = 1$). In contrast, among 8700 non-retinoid-exposed birth defect reports to the FDA, only 19 involved suspected holoprosencephalies (27). Pregnancy outcomes from 1120 apparent 1st-trimester tretinoin exposures were also examined. Among the 49 birth defects observed (the expected incidence), no cases of holoprosencephaly were seen. Although it is speculation, the contrasting findings in the above two reports (26,27) on early pregnancy tretinoin exposure may reflect (a) fetal exposure to different doses of tretinoin at the critical times from the use of higher maternal doses or from enhanced systemic absorption, or (b) selective (biased) reporting of adverse pregnancy outcomes to the FDA.

A 1993 report summarized data gathered from the Group Health Cooperative of Puget Sound, Washington, involving 1st-trimester exposure to topical tretinoin and congenital malformations (28). A total of 215 women who had delivered live or stillborn infants and were presumed to have been exposed to the drug in early pregnancy were compared with

430 age-matched non-exposed controls of women whose live or stillborn infants were delivered at the same hospitals. A total of 4 (1.9%) infants in the exposed group had major anomalies compared with 11 (2.6%) among the controls, a relative risk of 0.7 (0.2–2.3) (28). The defects observed in the exposed infants were hypospadias, undescended or absent testicles, metatarsus adductus, and esophageal reflux. The three stillborn infants in the exposed group were all associated with umbilical cord accidents. The authors concluded that these data provided no evidence for a relationship between topical tretinoin and the congenital abnormalities normally observed with other vitamin A congeners or for an increased incidence of defects compared with data from women not using tretinoin (28). The findings of this study were summarized in a review article on retinoids and teratogenicity (29).

A brief 1997 report described a prospective, observational, controlled study that compared the pregnancy outcomes of 94 women who had used topical tretinoin during pregnancy with 133 women not exposed to topical tretinoin or other known human teratogens (30). Both groups were composed of pregnant women who had contacted a teratology information service in the years from 1988 to 1996. No differences between the groups were found for the number of live births, miscarriages, elective terminations, major malformations, duration of pregnancy, cesarean sections, birth weight (after exclusion of one baby weighing 5396 g in the control group), and low birth weight. Two live-born infants from the tretinoin-exposed group had major birth defects: a bicuspid aortic valve in one and dysplastic kidneys in one. Neither defect is consistent with retinoic-acid embryopathy (30). Malformations in the four infants from the control group were congenitally dislocated hip in two, aortic valvular stenosis in one, and imperforate anus in one.

Several comments concerning the above study were made in a 1999 letter (31). The primary concern expressed was that the number of subjects enrolled in the study was too small to derive any conclusions as to the safety of tretinoin in the 1st trimester. The authors thought that the risk of certain birth defects, specifically cardiac anomalies and microtia, could not be excluded, and that the use of tretinoin in pregnancy was contraindicated (31).

In summary, elevated serum concentrations of all-*trans* retinoic acid in early gestation are considered teratogenic in humans. Because of its relatively poor systemic absorption (if occlusive dressings are not used) after topical administration, tretinoin is not thought to present a significant fetal risk. Because some absorption does occur, however, it is not possible to exclude a teratogenic risk (32). Congenital malformations, some of which are consistent with those observed in retinoic acid embryopathy, have been reported after topical use, but a causal association has yet to be established. The reports may reflect (a) greater-than-normal fetal exposure from higher-than-usual maternal doses or enhanced systemic absorption, or (b) selective reporting of adverse outcomes that are not caused by tretinoin. Until more data are available, however, the safest course is to avoid the use of tretinoin during pregnancy, especially in the 1st trimester. But if inadvertent exposure does occur during early pregnancy, the fetal risk, if any, appears to be very low.

BREAST FEEDING SUMMARY

RECOMMENDATION: No Human Data - Probably Compatible

Vitamin A and, presumably, tretinoin (all-*trans* retinoic acid) are natural constituents of human milk. There is no data available on the amount of all-*trans* retinoic acid excreted into milk after topical use. Although other retinoids are excreted (see Vitamin A), the minimal absorption that occurs after topical application of tretinoin probably precludes the detection of clinically significant amounts in breast milk from this source. Thus, use of tretinoin while breast-feeding does not appear to represent a significant risk to a nursing infant.

References

1. Morriss-Kay G. Retinoic acid and development. Pathobiology 1992;60:264–70.
2. Keir WJ. Inhibition of retinoic acid synthesis and its implications in fetal alcohol syndrome. Alcohol Clin Exp Res 1991;15:560–4.
3. Pullarkat RK. Hypothesis: prenatal ethanol-induced birth defects and retinoic acid. Alcohol Clin Exp Res 1991;15:565–7.
4. Duester G. A hypothetical mechanism for fetal alcohol syndrome involving ethanol inhibition of retinoic acid synthesis at the alcohol dehydrogenase step. Alcohol Clin Exp Res 1991;15:568–72.
5. Dreosti IE. Nutritional factors underlying the expression of the fetal alcohol syndrome. Ann N Y Acad Sci 1993;678:193–204.
6. DeJonge MH, Zachman RD. The effect of maternal ethanol ingestion on fetal rat heart vitamin A: a model for fetal alcohol syndrome. Pediatr Res 1995;37:418–23.
7. Fex G, Larsson K, Andersson A, Berggren-Söderlund M. Low serum concentration of *all-trans* and *13-cis* retinoic acids in patients treated with phenytoin, carbamazepine and valproate. Possible relation to teratogenicity. Arch Toxicol 1995;69:572–4.
8. Product information. Avita. Bertek Pharmaceuticals, 2002.
9. Product information. Renova, Retin-A. Ortho Dermatological, 2002.
10. Seegmiller RE, Ford WH, Carter MW, Mitala JJ, Powers WJ Jr. A developmental toxicity study of tretinoin administered topically and orally to pregnant Wistar rats. J Am Acad Dermatol 1997;36:S60–6.
11. Christian MS, Mitala JJ, Powers WJ Jr, McKenzie BE, Latriano L. A developmental toxicity study of tretinoin emollient cream (Renova) applied topically to New Zealand white rabbits. J Am Acad Dermatol 1997;36:S67–S76.
12. Schardein JL. *Chemically Induced Birth Defects*. 2nd ed. New York, NY: Marcel Dekker, 1993:555–62.
13. Shepard TH. *Catalog of Teratogenic Agents*. 8th ed. Baltimore, MD: Johns Hopkins University Press, 1995:370–3.
14. Sanders DD, Stephens TD. Review of drug-induced limb defects in mammals. Teratology 1991;44:335–54.
15. Apgar J, Kramer T, Smith JC. Retinoic acid and vitamin A: effect of low levels on outcome of pregnancy in guinea pigs. Nutr Res 1994;14:741–51.
16. Sulik KK, Dehart DB, Rogers JM, Chernoff N. Teratogenicity of low doses of all-trans retinoic acid in presomite mouse embryos. Teratology 1995;51:398–403.
17. Kligman AM. Question and answers: is topical tretinoin teratogenic? JAMA 1988;259:2918.
18. Zbinden G. Investigations on the toxicity of tretinoin administered systemically to animals. Acta Derm Venereol Suppl (Stockh) 1975;74:36–40.
19. American Hospital Formula Service. *Drug Information 1996*. Bethesda, MD: American Society of Health-System Pharmacists, 1996:2608–10.
20. Pinnock CB, Alderman CP. The potential for teratogenicity of vitamin A and its congeners. Med J Aust 1992;157:804–9.
21. Camera G, Pregliasco P. Ear malformation in baby born to mother using tretinoin cream. Lancet 1992;339:687.
22. Lipson AH, Collins F, Webster WS. Multiple congenital defects associated with maternal use of topical tretinoin. Lancet 1993;341:1352–3.
23. Navarre-Belhassen C, Blanchet P, Hillaire-Buys D, Sarda P, Blayac JP. Multiple congenital malformations associated with topical tretinoin. Ann Pharmacother 1998;32:505–6.
24. Colley SMJ, Walpole I, Fabian VA, Kakulas BA. Topical tretinoin and fetal malformations. Med J Aust 1998;168:467.
25. Selcen D, Seidman S, Nigro MA. Otocerebral anomalies associated with topical tretinoin use. Brain Dev 2000;22:218–20.
26. Johnson KA, Chambers CD, Felix R, Dick L, Jones KL. Pregnancy outcome in women prospectively ascertained with Retin-A exposures: an ongoing study (abstract). Teratology 1994;49:375.
27. Rosa F, Piazza-Hepp T, Goetsch R. Holoprosencephaly with 1st trimester topical tretinoin (abstract). Teratology 1994;49:418–9.
28. Jick SS, Terris BZ, Jick H. First trimester topical tretinoin and congenital disorders. Lancet 1993;341:1181–2.
29. Jick H. Retinoids and teratogenicity. J Am Acad Dermatol 1998;39:S118–22.
30. Shapiro L, Pastuszak A, Curto G, Koren G. Safety of first-trimester exposure to topical tretinoin: prospective cohort study. Lancet 1997;350:1143–4.
31. Martinez-Frias ML, Rodriguez-Pinilla E. First-trimester exposure to topical tretinoin: its safety is not warranted. Teratology 1999;60:5.
32. Rothman KF, Pochi PE. Use of oral and topical agents for acne in pregnancy. J Am Acad Dermatol 1988;19:431–42.

Name:	**TRIAMCINOLONE**	Risk Factor:	C_M*
Class:	**Corticosteroid**		

FETAL RISK SUMMARY

RECOMMENDATION: Human and Animal Data Suggest Risk

Triamcinolone is a synthetic fluorinated corticosteroid that can be administered, depending on the preparation selected, orally, parenterally, topically, or by oral inhalation. In animal models of inflammation, triamcinolone is approximately 1–2 times as potent as prednisone, whereas triamcinolone acetonide is about 8 times more potent (1). Oral inhalation of usual therapeutic doses of the latter agent do not appear to suppress the hypothalamic-pituitary-adrenal axis (2).

Triamcinolone is teratogenic in animals. Cleft palate was induced in fetal mice and rats exposed *in utero* to triamcinolone, triamcinolone acetonide, or triamcinolone diacetate (3–5). In one study with mice, high dietary fat intake (48% compared with a low-fat diet of 5.6%) increased the frequency and severity of cleft palate (5). IM administration of nonlethal maternal doses (0.125–0.5 mg/kg/day) of triamcinolone acetonide in pregnant rats at various gestational ages produced fetal growth retardation at all doses tested (6). Higher doses were associated with resorption, cleft palate, umbilical hernias, undescended testes, and reduced ossification (6). A second report by these latter investigators compared the teratogenic potency, as measured by the induction of cleft palate, of triamcinolone, triamcinolone acetonide, and cortisol in rats (7). Triamcinolone acetonide was 59 times more potent than triamcinolone, which, in turn, was more potent than cortisol. Other anomalies observed with triamcinolone acetonide were umbilical hernias, resorption, and fetal death. All three agents produced fetal growth retardation.

Morphologically abnormal lungs and increased epithelial maturation were found in fetal rat whole-organ lung cultures exposed to triamcinolone acetonide (8). Similarly, accelerated fetal lung maturation was observed following administration of IM triamcinolone acetonide to pregnant rhesus macaques at various stages of gestation (9). However, treatment earlier in gestation produced growth retardation of some of the lung septa, as well as decreased body weight and length (9).

A series of studies described the teratogenic effects of single and multiple doses of IM triamcinolone acetonide administered early in gestation to nonhuman primates (bonnet monkeys, rhesus monkeys, and baboons) at doses ranging from approximately equivalent to the human dose up to 300 times the human dose (10–13). Resorption, intrauterine death, orocraniofacial anomalies, and defects of the thorax, hind limbs, thymus, adrenal, and kidney were observed. The most common malformations involved the central nervous system and cranium in all three species (11); growth retardation was also common in all species (10).

Published human pregnancy experience with triamcinolone is limited to 16 cases. The Collaborative Perinatal Project monitored 50,282 mother-child pairs, 56 of whom were exposed during the 1st trimester to a category of miscellaneous corticosteroids (14). Included in this group were 8 triamcinolone-exposed mother-child pairs. Two (3.6%; relative risk 0.47) newborns with malformations were observed in the total group, suggesting a lack of any relationship to large categories of major or minor malformations or to individual defects.

A 1966 reference described a woman with benign adrenogenital syndrome who took 4–8 mg of triamcinolone orally throughout gestation (15). She delivered a normal 2.61-kg male infant at 38 weeks without evidence of hypoadrenalism. A 1975 report included 5 patients treated with triamcinolone acetonide, presumably by oral inhalation, among 70 women with asthma who were treated with various corticosteroids throughout gestation (16). No adverse fetal outcomes were observed in the five triamcinolone-exposed cases, although one of the mothers delivered prematurely. None of the 70 newborns had evidence of adrenal insufficiency.

Symmetrical growth retardation was observed in a 700-g, small-for-gestational age newborn delivered via cesarean section at 31 weeks' gestation because of fetal distress, diminished amniotic fluid, and lack of growth (17). The Dubowitz evaluation was compatible with the menstrual dates. The normotensive, nonsmoking mother had applied 0.05% triamcinolone acetonide cream to her legs, abdomen, and extremities for atopic dermatitis from 12 to 29 weeks' gestation. The authors estimated her daily dose to be approximately 40 mg, but she had no signs or symptoms of adrenal insufficiency. The newborn was breathing room air within 12 hours without evidence of respiratory distress. Although not discussed, the apparent fetal lung maturity in a 31-week fetus may have been the result of chronic corticosteroid exposure. At 14 days of age, necrotizing enterocolitis occurred and, following multiple surgeries, the infant was alive at 10 months of age on total parenteral nutrition. In an addendum to their report, the authors noted that the mother had had a second pregnancy, this time without the use of triamcinolone, and delivered a 1660-g (10th percentile for gestational age) male infant at 34 weeks' gestation. The authors attributed the growth retardation in the first infant to triamcinolone because no other cause was discovered. The result of the second pregnancy, however, probably indicates that other factors were involved in addition to any effect of the corticosteroid.

Four large epidemiologic studies have associated the use of corticosteroids during the 1st trimester with orofacial clefts. The specific corticosteroid was not identified in three of these studies (see Hydrocortisone for details), but in a 1999 study described below, the corticosteroids were listed.

In a case-control study, the California Birth Defects Monitoring Program evaluated the association between selected congenital anomalies and the use of corticosteroids 1 month before to 3 months after conception (periconceptional period) (18). Case infants or fetal deaths diagnosed with orofacial clefts, conotruncal defects, neural tubal defects (NTDs), and limb anomalies were identified from a total of 552,601 births that occurred from 1987 through the end of 1989. Controls, without birth defects, were selected from the same data base. Following exclusion of known genetic syndromes, mothers of case and control infants were interviewed by telephone, an average of 3.7 years (cases) or 3.8 years (controls) after delivery, to determine various exposures during the periconceptional period. The number of interviews completed were orofacial cleft case mothers ($N = 662$, 85% of eligible), conotruncal case mothers ($N = 207$, 87%), NTD case mothers ($N = 265$, 84%), limb anomaly case mothers ($N = 165$, 82%), and control mothers ($N = 734$, 78%) (18). Orofacial clefts were classified into four phenotypic groups: isolated cleft lip with or without cleft palate (ICLP, $N = 348$), isolated cleft palate (ICP, $N = 141$), multiple cleft lip with or without cleft palate (MCLP, $N = 99$), and multiple cleft palate (MCP, $N = 74$). A total of 13 mothers reported using corticosteroids during the periconceptional period for a wide variety of indications. Six case mothers of infants with ICLP and three of infants with ICP used corticosteroids (unspecified corticosteroid $N = 1$, prednisone $N = 2$, cortisone $N = 3$, triamcinolone acetonide $N = 1$, dexamethasone $N = 1$, and cortisone plus prednisone $N = 1$). One case mother of an infant with NTD used cortisone and an

T

injectable unspecified corticosteroid, and three controls used corticosteroids (hydrocortisone $N = 1$ and prednisone $N = 2$). The odds ratio for corticosteroid use and ICLP was 4.3 (95% confidence interval 1.1–17.2), whereas the odds ratio for ICP and corticosteroid use was 5.3 (95% confidence interval 1.1–26.5). No increased risks were observed for the other anomaly groups. Commenting on their results, the investigators thought that recall bias was unlikely because they did not observe increased risks for other malformations, and it was also unlikely that the mothers would have known of the suspected association between corticosteroids and orofacial clefts (18).

[**Risk Factor D if used in 1st trimester.*]

BREAST FEEDING SUMMARY

RECOMMENDATION: No Human Data - Probably Compatible

No reports describing the use of triamcinolone during lactation have been located. The molecular weight (about 394) is low enough, however, that excretion into breast milk should be expected. Small amounts of other corticosteroids (see Hydrocortisone and Prednisone) are excreted into milk and do not appear to present a risk to a nursing infant. Similar excretion probably occurs following inhaled triamcinolone. At least one source states that inhaled corticosteroids used for asthma are not contraindicated during breast-feeding (19). No data are available to assess the potential risk to a nursing infant following systemic use of triamcinolone in a breast-feeding woman.

References

1. Product information. Azmacort. Rhône-Poulenc Rorer Pharmaceuticals, Inc., 1994.
2. American Hospital Formulary Service. *Drug Information 1997*. Bethesda, MD: American Society of Health-System Pharmacists, 1997:2368–70.
3. Walker BE. Cleft palate produced in mice by human-equivalent dosage with triamcinolone. Science 1965; 149:862–3.
4. Walker BE. Induction of cleft palate in rats with anti-inflammatory drugs. Teratology 1971;4:39–42.
5. Zhou M, Walker BE. Potentiation of triamcinolone-induced cleft palate in mice by maternal high dietary fat. Teratology 1993;48:53–7.
6. Rowland JM, Hendrickx AG. Teratogenicity of triamcinolone acetonide in rats. Teratology 1983;27: 13–8.
7. Rowland JM, Hendrickx AG. Comparative teratogenicity of triamcinolone acetonide, triamcinolone, and cortisol in the rat. Teratog Carcinog Mutagen 1983; 3:313–9.
8. Massoud EAS, Sekhon HS, Rotschild A, Thurlbeck WM. The in vitro effect of triamcinolone acetonide on branching morphogenesis in the fetal rat lung. Pediatr Pulmonol 1992;14:28–36.
9. Bunton TE, Plopper CG. Triamcinolone-induced structural alterations in the development of the lung of the fetal rhesus macaque. Am J Obstet Gynecol 1984;148:203–15.
10. Hendrickx AG, Sawyer RH, Terrell TG, Osburn BI, Hendrickson RV, Steffek AJ. Teratogenic effects of triamcinolone on the skeletal and lymphoid systems in nonhuman primates. Fed Proc 1975;34:1661–5.
11. Hendrickx AG, Pellegrini M, Tarara R, Parker R, Silverman S, Steffek AJ. Craniofacial and central nervous system malformations induced by triamcinolone acetonide in nonhuman primates: I. General teratogenicity. Teratology 1980;22:103–14.
12. Parker RM, Hendrickx AG. Craniofacial and central nervous system malformations induced by triamcinolone acetonide in nonhuman primates: II. Craniofacial pathogenesis. Teratology 1983;28:35–44.
13. Tarara RP, Cordy DR, Hendrickx AG. Central nervous system malformations induced by triamcinolone acetonide in nonhuman primates: pathology. Teratology 1989;39:75–84.
14. Heinonen OP, Slone D, Shapiro S. *Birth Defects and Drugs in Pregnancy*. Littleton, MA: Publishing Sciences Group, 1977:388–400.
15. Rolf BB. Corticosteroids and pregnancy. Am J Obstet Gynecol 1966;95:339–44.
16. Schatz M, Patterson R, Zeitz S, O'Rourke J, Melam H. Corticosteroid therapy for the pregnant asthmatic patient. JAMA 1975;233:804–7.
17. Katz VL, Thorp JM Jr, Bowes WA Jr. Severe symmetric intrauterine growth retardation associated with the topical use of triamcinolone. Am J Obstet Gynecol 1990;162:396–7.
18. Carmichael SL, Shaw GM. Maternal corticosteroid use and risk of selected congenital anomalies. Am J Med Genet 1999;86:242–4.
19. Report of the Working Group on Asthma and Pregnancy. *Management of Asthma During Pregnancy.* U.S. Department of Health and Human Services, NIH Publication No. 93-3279, 1993:19.

Name:	**TRIAMTERENE**	Risk Factor:	**C_M***
Class:	**Diuretic**		

FETAL RISK SUMMARY

RECOMMENDATION: Human Data Suggest Risk

Triamterene is a potassium-conserving diuretic. It is a weak folic acid antagonist. Reproduction studies in rats at doses up to 6 times the maximum recommended human dose based on body surface area found no evidence of fetal harm (1).

The drug crosses the placenta in animals (1). The molecular weight (about 253) is low enough that transfer to the human fetus should be expected.

No defects were observed in five infants exposed to triamterene in the 1st trimester (2, p. 372). For use anytime during pregnancy, 271 exposures were recorded without an increase in malformations (2, p. 441).

In a surveillance study of Michigan Medicaid recipients conducted between 1985 and 1992 involving 229,101 completed pregnancies, 318 newborns had been exposed to triamterene during the 1st trimester (F. Rosa, personal communication, FDA, 1993). A total of 15 (4.7%) major birth defects were observed (13 expected). Three cases of cardiovascular defects (three expected) and one case of polydactyly (one expected) were observed, but specific information was not available for the other defects. No anomalies were observed in four other categories of defects (oral clefts, spina bifida, limb reduction defects, and hypospadias) for which data were available. These data do not support an association between the drug and congenital defects.

The effects of exposure (at any time during the 2nd or 3rd month after the last menstrual period) to folic acid antagonists on embryo/fetal development were evaluated in a large, multicenter, case-control surveillance study published in 2000 (3). The report was based on data collected between 1976 and 1998 by the Slone Epidemiology Unit Birth Defects Study from 80 maternity or tertiary care hospitals in Boston, Philadelphia, Toronto, and Iowa. Mothers were interviewed within 6 months of delivery about their use of drugs during pregnancy. Folic acid antagonists were categorized into two groups: group I—dihydrofolate reductase inhibitors (aminopterin, methotrexate, sulfasalazine, pyrimethamine, triamterene, and trimethoprim); group II—agents that affect other enzymes in folate metabolism, impair the absorption of folate, or increase the metabolic breakdown of folate (carbamazepine, phenytoin, primidone, and phenobarbital) (3). The case subjects were 3,870 infants with cardiovascular defects, 1962 with oral clefts, and 1100 with urinary tract malformations. Infants with defects associated with a syndrome were excluded, as were infants with coexisting neural tube defects (NTDs; known to be reduced by maternal folic acid supplementation). Too few infants with limb-reduction defects were identified to be analyzed. Controls ($N = 8387$) were infants with malformations other than oral clefts and cardiovascular, urinary tract, and limb-reduction defects and NTDs, but included infants with chromosomal and genetic defects. The risk of malformations in control infants would not have been reduced by vitamin supplementation, and none of the controls used folic acid antagonists (3). For group I cases, the relative risks (RRs) of cardiovascular defects and oral clefts were 3.4 (95% confidence interval [CI] 1.8–6.4) and 2.6 (95% CI 1.1–6.1), respectively. For group II cases, the RRs of cardiovascular and urinary tract defects, and oral clefts were 2.2 (95% CI 1.4–3.5), 2.5 (95% CI 1.2–5.0), and 2.5 (95% CI 1.5–4.2), respectively. Maternal use of multivitamin supplements with folic acid (typically 0.4 mg) reduced the risks in group I cases, but not in group II cases (3).

Many investigators consider diuretics to be contraindicated in pregnancy, except for patients with heart disease, because they do not prevent or alter the course of toxemia, and they may decrease placental perfusion (4–6). In general, diuretics are not recommended for the treatment of gestational hypertension because of the maternal hypovolemia characteristic of this disease.

[**Risk Factor D if used in gestational hypertension.*]

BREAST FEEDING SUMMARY

RECOMMENDATION: No Human Data - Probably Compatible

No reports describing the use of triamterene during lactation have been located. The molecular weight (about 253) is low enough that excretion into breast milk should be expected. The diuretic is excreted in animal milk (1). The potential effects of this exposure on a nursing infant are unknown.

References

1. Product information. Dyrenium. WellSpring Pharmaceuticals, 2001.
2. Heinonen OP, Slone D, Shapiro S. *Birth Defects and Drugs in Pregnancy*. Littleton, MA: Publishing Sciences Group, 1977.
3. Hernandez-Diaz S, Werler MM, Walker AM, Mitchell AA. Folic acid antagonists during pregnancy and the risk of birth defects. N Engl J Med 2000;343:1608–14.
4. Pitkin RM, Kaminetzky HA, Newton M, Pritchard JA. Maternal nutrition: a selective review of clinical topics. Obstet Gynecol 1972;40:773–85.
5. Lindheimer MD, Katz AI. Sodium and diuretics in pregnancy. N Engl J Med 1973;288:891–4.
6. Christianson R, Page EW. Diuretic drugs and pregnancy. Obstet Gynecol 1976;48:647–52.

Name:	**TRIAZOLAM**	Risk Factor:	X_M
Class:	**Hypnotic**		

FETAL RISK SUMMARY

RECOMMENDATION: Limited Human Data - Animal Data Suggest Low Risk

Triazolam, a short-acting benzodiazepine, is used as a hypnotic for the treatment of insomnia. Although no congenital anomalies have been attributed to the use of triazolam during human pregnancies, other benzodiazepines (e.g., see Diazepam) have been suspected of producing fetal malformations after 1st-trimester exposure. In one report, the drug was not teratogenic in pregnant animals when administered in large oral doses (1).

T

No data have been located on the placental passage of triazolam. However, other benzodiazepines, such as diazepam, freely cross the placenta and accumulate in the fetus (see Diazepam). A similar distribution pattern should be expected for triazolam.

By the middle of 1988, the manufacturer had received more than 100 reports of *in utero* exposure to triazolam (J. H. Markillie, personal communication, Upjohn, 1989). Approximately one-seventh of these women were either lost to follow-up or further information was not available. Of the cases in which the outcome was known, more than one-half of the completed pregnancies ended with the delivery of a normal infant. Some of these exposures were reported in a 1987 correspondence that also included experience with alprazolam, another short-acting benzodiazepine (2). From these two sources, a total of five infants with congenital malformations have been described after *in utero* exposure to triazolam: extra digit on left foot and cleft uvula; incomplete closure of the foramen ovale (resolved spontaneously); small-for-gestational-age infant with left pelvic ectopic kidney; ventricular septal defect and possible coarctation of aorta (exposed to multiple drugs including triazolam); and premature, low-birth-weight infant with ventricular septal defect, pulmonary stenosis, intraventricular hemorrhage, hydrocephalus, apnea, bradycardia, anemia, jaundice, and seizure disorder (exposed to single 0.125-mg tablet at 1–2 weeks' gestation).

Single reports received by the manufacturer of defects in infants exposed *in utero* to either triazolam or alprazolam include pyloric stenosis, moderate tongue-tie, umbilical hernia and ankle inversion, and clubfoot (2).

Three cases of nonmalformation toxicities have been observed in infants exposed during gestation to triazolam: tachycardia, bradycardia, respiratory pauses, hypotonia and axial hypotony, impaired arachnoid reflexes, hypothermia, sleepy, and lifeless (symptoms resolved after infant received supportive care for several days; mother took multiple medications during pregnancy); fetal distress requiring emergency cesarean section and infant resuscitation, umbilical cord wrapped around neck, seizure activity, and generalized cortical atrophy (exposed to triazolam and a second [not identified] benzodiazepine early in pregnancy and during the last week of gestation; apparent recovery with no permanent disability by 6 months of age); bradycardia, malaise, cyanosis, leukopenia, and chewing movements at 4 days of age (exposed during 3rd trimester; symptoms resolved by 1 week of age) (2).

Based on the available information, a cause-and-effect relationship between triazolam and the various infant outcomes does not appear to exist. Moreover, these cases cannot be used to derive rate or incidence data, because of the probable bias involved in the reporting of pregnancy exposures to the manufacturer (2).

In a surveillance study of Michigan Medicaid recipients conducted between 1985 and 1992 involving 229,101 completed pregnancies, 138 newborns were exposed to triazolam during the 1st trimester (F. Rosa, personal communication, FDA, 1993). A total of seven (5.1%) major birth defects were observed (six expected). One cardiovascular defect (one expected) and one case of polydactyly (0.5 expected) were observed, but specific information on the other defects was not available. No anomalies were observed in four other categories of defects (oral clefts, spina bifida, limb reduction defects, and hypospadias) for which specific data were available. These data do not support an association between the drug and congenital defects.

A 1990 report evaluated the available published data to determine the fetal risk that occurs from exposure to various drugs (3). The risk for triazolam, based on poor data, was determined to be "none-minimal." This risk assignment was defined as ". . . a magnitude that patients and physicians would generally consider to be too small to influence the management of an exposed pregnancy" (3).

BREAST FEEDING SUMMARY

RECOMMENDATION: No Human Data - Potential Toxicity

Triazolam and its metabolites are excreted in milk of rats (4). No reports describing the use of triazolam during human lactation or measuring the amount, if any, excreted into milk have been located. The molecular weight (about 343), however, is low enough that passage into human milk should be anticipated. The effects of this exposure on a nursing infant are unknown, but closely related drugs are classified by the American Academy of Pediatrics as agents that may be of concern during breast-feeding (e.g., see Diazepam).

References

1. Matsuo A, Kast A, Tsunenari Y. Reproduction studies of triazolam in rats and rabbits. Iyakuhin Kenkyu 1979;10:52–67. As cited in Shepard TH. *Catalog of Teratogenic Agents*. 6th ed. Baltimore, MD: Johns Hopkins University Press, 1989:630.
2. Barry WS, St Clair SM. Exposure to benzodiazepines in utero. Lancet 1987;1:1436–7.
3. Friedman JM, Little BB, Brent RL, Cordero JF, Hanson JW, Shepard TH. Potential human teratogenicity of frequently prescribed drugs. Obstet Gynecol 1990;75:594–9.
4. Product information. Halcion. Pharmacia & Upjohn, 1998.

Name: **TRICHLORMETHIAZIDE**	Risk Factor: **C***
Class: **Diuretic**	

See Chlorothiazide.

[**Risk Factor D if used in gestational hypertension.*]

Name: **TRIDIHEXETHYL**	Risk Factor: **C**
Class: **Parasympatholytic (Anticholinergic)**	

FETAL RISK SUMMARY

RECOMMENDATION: Limited Human Data - No Relevant Animal Data

Tridihexethyl is an anticholinergic quaternary ammonium chloride. In a large prospective study, 2323 patients were exposed to this class of drugs during the 1st trimester, 6 of whom took tridihexethyl (1). A possible association was found between the total group and minor malformations, but the significance of this is unknown. Independent confirmation is required (1).

T

BREAST FEEDING SUMMARY

RECOMMENDATION: No Human Data - Probably Compatible

No data are available.

Reference

1. Heinonen OP, Slone D, Shapiro S. *Birth Defects and Drugs in Pregnancy*. Littleton, MA: Publishing Sciences Group, 1977:346–53.

Name:	**TRIENTINE**	Risk Factor:	**C_M**
Class:	**Chelating Agent**		

FETAL RISK SUMMARY

RECOMMENDATION: Limited Human Data - Animal Data Suggest Moderate Risk

Trientine is a chelating agent used for the removal of excess copper from the systems of patients with Wilson's disease who either cannot tolerate penicillamine or who have developed penicillamine resistance. The drug is available in the United States only as an orphan drug.

In studies with pregnant rats, trientine was teratogenic in doses similar to those used in humans (1–6). The frequency of fetal resorptions and malformations, including hemorrhage and edema, was directly related to the decrease in fetal copper concentrations.

Data on the human placental transfer of trientine have not been located, but the molecular weight of the compound (about 147 for the free base) suggests that drug in the maternal serum reaches the fetus.

Only one reference has been located that describes the use of trientine in human pregnancy (7). Seven women with Wilson's disease, treated with the chelating agent, were observed through 11 pregnancies. At the time of conception, the average duration of therapy had been 5 years (range 2–3 weeks to 9 years). Therapy was continued throughout pregnancy in seven cases, interrupted in the 2nd trimester of one because of inability to obtain the drug, and apparently was discontinued in the final few weeks of still another because of nausea not related to trientine (7). One woman underwent a therapeutic abortion at 10 weeks' gestation and one spontaneously aborted a normal male fetus, together with a copper contraceptive coil, at 14 weeks' gestation.

Of the pregnancies ending with a live infant, there were four males, four females, and one infant whose sex was not specified. The mean birth weight of the full-term infants was 3263 g. Two of the infants were delivered prematurely, one male at 36 weeks (2400 g) and one female at 31 weeks (800 g). The latter infant had an isochromosome X, but both parents had normal X chromosomes. No other abnormalities were observed in the infants at the time of birth. Because copper deficiency is thought to be teratogenic, the author concluded that the exposed fetuses did not become copper depleted (7). Evidence supporting this conclusion was obtained from the mean ceruloplasmin concentration of cord blood, 9.9 mg/dL, which was nearly identical to nontreated controls (10 mg/dL) (7). Additional studies, however, are needed before this conclusion can be accepted with confidence. Except for slow progress at 3 months in the infant with the isochromosome X, development in the other children was normal during follow-up evaluations ranging from 2 months–9 years.

BREAST FEEDING SUMMARY

RECOMMENDATION: No Human Data - Potential Toxicity

No reports describing the use of trientine during lactation have been located. The molecular weight (about 147 for the free base), however, is low enough that passage into milk should be anticipated. The effect of this exposure on a nursing infant is unknown.

References

1. March L, Fraser FC. Chelating agents and teratogenesis. Lancet 1973;2:846.
2. Keen CL, Mark-Savage P, Lonnerdal B, Hurley LS. Low tissue copper and teratogenesis in rats resulting from D-penicillamine (abstract). Fed Proc 1981; 40:917.
3. Keen CL, Cohen NL, Lonnerdal B, Hurley LS. Low tissue copper and teratogenesis in trientine-treated rats. Lancet 1982;1:1127.
4. Keen CL, Lonnerdal B, Cohen NL, Hurley LS. Drug-induced Cu deficiency: a model for Cu deficiency teratogenicity (abstract). Fed Proc 1982;41:944.
5. Cohen NL, Keen CL, Lonnerdal B, Hurley LS. Low tissue copper and teratogenesis in triethylenetetramine-treated rats (abstract). Fed Proc 1982;41:944.
6. Product information. Syprine. Merck, 2000.
7. Walshe JM. The management of pregnancy in Wilson's disease treated with trientine. Q J Med 1986;58;81–7.

Name: **TRIFLUOPERAZINE** Risk Factor: **C**

Class: **Tranquilizer**

FETAL RISK SUMMARY

RECOMMENDATION: Limited Human Data - Animal Data Suggest Low Risk

Trifluoperazine is a piperazine phenothiazine. The drug readily crosses the placenta (1). Trifluoperazine has been used for the treatment of nausea and vomiting of pregnancy, but it is primarily used as a psychotropic agent.

Reproduction studies with trifluoperazine have been conducted in rats, rabbits, and monkeys (2). In rats, doses over 600 times the human dose revealed an increased incidence of malformations and reduced litter size and weight associated with maternal toxicity. These effects were not observed when the dose was reduced in half (2). No fetal adverse effects were observed in rabbits or monkeys at doses of 700 and 25 times the human dose, respectively.

In 1962, the Canadian Food and Drug Directorate released a warning that eight cases of congenital defects had been associated with trifluoperazine therapy (3). This correlation was refuted in a series of articles from the medical staff of the manufacturer of the drug (4–6). In 480 trifluoperazine-treated pregnant women, the incidence of live-born infants with congenital malformations was 1.1%, as compared with 8472 nontreated controls with an incidence of 1.5% (5). Two reports of phocomelia appeared in 1962–1963 and a case of a congenital heart defect in 1969 (7–9): twins, both with phocomelia of all four limbs (7); phocomelia of upper limbs (8); and complete transposition of great vessels in heart (9).

In none of these cases is there a clear relationship between use of the drug and the defect. Extrapyramidal symptoms have been described in a newborn exposed to trifluoperazine *in utero*, but the reaction was probably caused by chlorpromazine (see Chlorpromazine) (10).

The Collaborative Perinatal Project monitored 50,282 mother-child pairs, 42 of whom had 1st trimester exposure to trifluoperazine (11). No evidence was found to suggest a relationship to malformations or an effect on perinatal mortality rate, birth weight, or intelligence quotient scores at 4 years of age.

In a surveillance study of Michigan Medicaid recipients conducted between 1985 and 1992 involving 229,101 completed pregnancies, 29 newborns had been exposed to trifluoperazine during the 1st trimester (F. Rosa, personal communication, FDA, 1993). One (3.4%) major birth defect (one expected), a cardiovascular malformation (0.5 expected), was observed.

Attempted maternal suicide at 31 weeks' gestation with trifluoperazine and misoprostol resulting in fetal death has been described (12). The adverse fetal outcome was attributed to tetanic uterine contractions caused by misoprostol (see Misoprostol).

In summary, although some reports have attempted to link trifluoperazine with congenital defects, the bulk of the evidence suggests that the drug is safe for the mother and low risk for the embryo/fetus. Other reviewers have also concluded that the phenothiazines are not teratogenic (13,14).

BREAST FEEDING SUMMARY

RECOMMENDATION: No Human Data - Potential Toxicity

No reports describing the use of trifluoperazine during lactation have been located. The molecular weight (about 408 for the free base) is low enough, however, that passage into milk should be anticipated. The American Academy of Pediatrics classifies trifluoperazine as a drug for which the effect on nursing infants is unknown but may be of concern (15).

References

1. Moya F, Thorndike V. Passage of drugs across the placenta. Am J Obstet Gynecol 1962;84:1778–98.
2. Product information. Stelazine. SmithKline Beecham Pharmaceuticals, 2000.
3. Canadian Department of National Health and Welfare, Food and Drug Directorate. Letter of notification to Canadian physicians. Ottawa, December 7, 1962.
4. Moriarity AJ. Trifluoperazine and congenital malformations. Can Med Assoc J 1963;88:97.
5. Moriarty AJ, Nance MR. Trifluoperazine and pregnancy. Can Med Assoc J 1963;88:375–6.
6. Schrire I. Trifluoperazine and foetal abnormalities. Lancet 1963;1:174.
7. Corner BD. Congenital malformations. Clinical considerations. Med J Southwest 1962;77:46–52.
8. Hall G. A case of phocomelia of the upper limbs. Med J Aust 1963;1:449–50.
9. Vince DJ. Congenital malformations following phenothiazine administration during pregnancy. Can Med Assoc J 1969;100:223.
10. Hill RM, Desmond MM, Kay JL. Extrapyramidal dysfunction in an infant of a schizophrenic mother. J Pediatr 1966;69:589–95.
11. Slone D, Siskind V, Heinonen OP, Monson RR, Kaufman DW, Shapiro S. Antenatal exposure to the phenothiazines in relation to congenital malformations, perinatal mortality rate, birth weight, and intelligence quotient score. Am J Obstet Gynecol 1977;128:486–8.
12. Bond GR, Zee AV. Overdosage of misoprostol in pregnancy. Am J Obstet Gynecol 1994;171:561–2.
13. Ayd FJ Jr. Children born of mothers treated with chlorpromazine during pregnancy. Clin Med 1964;71:1758–63.
14. Ananth J. Congenital malformations with psychopharmacologic agents. Compr Psychiatry 1975;16:437–45.
15. Committee on Drugs, American Academy of Pediatrics. The transfer of drugs and other chemicals into human milk. Pediatrics 2001;108:776–89.

Name: **TRIFLUPROMAZINE** Risk Factor: **C**

Class: **Tranquilizer**

T

FETAL RISK SUMMARY

RECOMMENDATION: Limited Human Data - No Relevant Animal Data

Triflupromazine is a propylamino phenothiazine in the same class as chlorpromazine. The phenothiazines readily cross the placenta (1). The Collaborative Perinatal Project monitored 50,282 mother-child pairs, 36 of which had 1st trimester exposure to triflupromazine (2). No evidence was found to suggest a relationship to malformations or an effect on perinatal mortality rates, birth weight, or intelligence quotient scores at 4 years of age. Although occasional reports have attempted to link various phenothiazine compounds with congenital defects, the bulk of the evidence indicates that these drugs are safe for the mother and low risk for the embryo/fetus (see also Chlorpromazine).

BREAST FEEDING SUMMARY

RECOMMENDATION: No Human Data - Potential Toxicity

No reports describing the use of triflupromazine during lactation have been located. The molecular weight (about 353 for the free base) is low enough, however, that excretion into breast milk should be expected. The potential effects of exposure on a nursing infant are unknown.

References

1. Moya F, Thorndike V. Passage of drugs across the placenta. Am J Obstet Gynecol 1962;84:1778–98.
2. Slone D, Siskind V, Heinonen OP, Monson RR, Kaufman DW, Shapiro S. Antenatal exposure to the phenothiazines in relation to congenital malformations, perinatal mortality rate, birth weight, and intelligence quotient score. Am J Obstet Gynecol 1977;128:486–8.

Name: **TRIHEXYPHENIDYL** Risk Factor: **C**
Class: **Parasympatholytic (Anticholinergic)**

FETAL RISK SUMMARY

RECOMMENDATION: Limited Human Data - No Relevant Animal Data

Trihexyphenidyl is an anticholinergic agent used in the treatment of parkinsonism. In a large prospective study, 2323 patients were exposed to this class of drugs during the 1st trimester, nine of whom took trihexyphenidyl (1). A possible association was found between the total group and minor malformations.

BREAST FEEDING SUMMARY

RECOMMENDATION: No Human Data - Probably Compatible

No data are available.

Reference

1. Heinonen OP, Slone D, Shapiro S. *Birth Defects and Drugs in Pregnancy*. Littleton, MA: Publishing Sciences Group, 1977:346–53.

Name: **TRIMEPRAZINE** Risk Factor: **C**
Class: **Antihistamine**

FETAL RISK SUMMARY

RECOMMENDATION: Limited Human Data - Probably Compatible

Trimeprazine is a phenothiazine antihistamine that is primarily used as an antipruritic. The Collaborative Perinatal Project monitored 50,282 mother-child pairs, 14 of whom had 1st trimester exposure to trimeprazine (1, p. 323). From this small sample, no evidence was found to suggest a relationship to large categories of major or minor malformations or to individual malformations. For use anytime in pregnancy, 140 exposures were recorded (1, p. 437). Based on defects in five children, a possible association with malformations was found, but the significance of this is unknown.

In a 1971 study, infants of mothers who had ingested antihistamines during the 1st trimester actually had significantly fewer abnormalities when compared with controls (2). Trimeprazine was the eighth most commonly used antihistamine.

BREAST FEEDING SUMMARY

RECOMMENDATION: Limited Human Data - Probably Compatible

Trimeprazine is excreted into human milk but the levels are too low to produce effects in the infant (3).

References

1. Heinonen OP, Slone D, Shapiro S. *Birth Defects and Drugs in Pregnancy*. Littleton, MA: Publishing Sciences Group, 1977.
2. Nelson MM, Forfar JO. Associations between drugs administered during pregnancy and congenital abnormalities. Br Med J 1971;1:523–7.
3. O'Brien TE. Excretion of drugs in human milk. Am J Hosp Pharm 1974;31:844–54.

Name: **TRIMETHADIONE** Risk Factor: **D**

Class: **Anticonvulsant**

FETAL RISK SUMMARY

RECOMMENDATION: Contraindicated - 1st Trimester

Trimethadione is an oxazolidinedione anticonvulsant used in the treatment of petit mal epilepsy. Several case histories have suggested a phenotype for a fetal trimethadione syndrome of congenital malformations (1–7). The use of trimethadione in nine families was associated with a 69% incidence of congenital defects—25 malformed children from 36 pregnancies. Three of these families reported five normal births after the anticonvulsant medication was stopped (1,4). The incidence of fetal loss in these families was also increased compared with that seen in the general epileptic population. Because trimethadione has demonstrated both clinical and experimental fetal risk greater than other anticonvulsants, its use should be abandoned in favor of other medications used in the treatment of petit mal epilepsy (8–11).

Features of Fetal Trimethadione Syndrome (25 cases)

Feature	*No.**	*%*	*Feature*	*No.**	*%*
Growth:			*Cardiac:*		
Prenatal deficiency	8	32	Septal defect	5	20
Postnatal deficiency	6	24	Not stated	4	16

(*continued*)

Features of Fetal Trimethadione Syndrome (25 cases) (*Continued*)

Feature	*No.**	*%*	*Feature*	*No.**	*%*
Performance (19 cases):			Patent ductus arteriosus	4	16
Mental retardation	7	28	*Limb:*		
Vision (myopia)	5	20	Simian crease	7	28
Speech disorder	4	16	Malformed hand	2	8
Impaired hearing	2	8	Clubfoot	1	4
Craniofacial:			*Genitourinary:*		
Low-set, cupped or abnormal ears	18	72	Kidney and ureter abnormalities	5	20
High arched or cleft lip and/or palate	16	64	Inguinal hernia(s)	3	12
			Hypospadias	3	12
Microcephaly	6	24	Ambiguous genitalia	2	8
Irregular teeth	4	16	Clitoral Hypertrophy	1	4
Epicanthic folds	3	12	Imperforate anus	1	4
Broad nasal bridge	3	12	*Other:*		
Strabismus	3	12	Tracheoesophageal fistula	3	12
Low hairline	2	8	Esophageal atresia	2	8
Facial hemangiomata	1	4			
Unusual facies (details not given)	3	12			

*Not mutually exclusive.

BREAST FEEDING SUMMARY

RECOMMENDATION: No Human Data - Probably Compatible

No data are available.

References

1. German J, Kowan A, Ehlers KH. Trimethadione and human teratogenesis. Teratology 1970;3:349–62.
2. Zackae EH, Mellman WJ, Neiderer B, Hanson JW. The fetal trimethadione syndrome. J Pediatr 1975;87:280–4.
3. Nichols MM. Fetal anomalies following maternal trimethadione ingestion. J Pediatr 1973;82:885–6.
4. Feldman GL, Weaver DD, Lourien EW. The fetal trimethadione syndrome. Report of an additional family and further delineation of this syndrome. Am J Dis Child 1977;131:1389–92.
5. Rosen RC, Lightner ES. Phenotypic malformations in association with maternal trimethadione therapy. J Pediatr 1978;92:240–4.
6. Zellweger H. Anticonvulsants during pregnancy: a danger to the developing fetus? Clin Pediatr 1974;13:338–45.
7. Rischbieth RH. Troxidone (trimethadione) embryopathy: case report with review of the literature. Clin Exp Neurol 1979;16:251–6.
8. Fabro S, Brown NA. Teratogenic potential of anticonvulsants. N Engl J Med 1979;300:1280–1.
9. National Institute of Health. Anticonvulsants found to have teratogenic potential. JAMA 1981;245:36.
10. Dansky L, Andermann E, Andermann F. Major congenital malformations in the offspring of epileptic patients. Genetic and environmental risk factors. In *Epilepsy, Pregnancy and the Child*. Proceedings of a Workshop held in Berlin, September 1980. New York, NY: Raven Press, 1981.
11. Nakane Y, Okuma T, Takahashi R, Sato Y, Wada T, Sato T, Fukushima Y, Kumashiro H, Ono T, Takahashi T, Aoki Y, Kazamatsuri H, Inami M, Komai S, Seino M, Miyakoshi M, Tanimura T, Hazama H, Kawahara R, Otsuki S, Hosokawa K, Inanaga K, Nakazawa Y, Yamamoto K. Multi-institutional study on the teratogenicity and fetal toxicity of antiepileptic drugs: a report of a collaborative study group in Japan. Epilepsia 1980;21:663–80.

Name:	**TRIMETHAPHAN**	Risk Factor:	**C**
Class:	**Antihypertensive**		

FETAL RISK SUMMARY

RECOMMENDATION: Contraindicated

No reports linking the use of trimethaphan with congenital defects have been located. Trimethaphan, a short acting ganglionic blocker that requires continuous infusion for therapeutic effect, has been studied in pregnant patients (1,2). It is not recommended for use in pregnancy, however, because of adverse hemodynamic effects (3). The drug is not effective in the control of hypertension in toxemic patients (1–3).

BREAST FEEDING SUMMARY

RECOMMENDATION: No Human Data - Potential Toxicity

No data are available.

References

1. Assali NS, Douglas RA Jr, Suyemoto R. Observations on the hemodynamic properties of a thiophanium derivative, Ro 2-2222 (Arfonad), in human subjects. Circulation 1953;8:62–9.
2. Assali NS, Suyemoto R. The place of the hydrazinophthalazine and thiophanium compounds in the management of hypertensive complications of pregnancy. Am J Obstet Gynecol 1952;64:1021–36.
3. Assali NS. Hemodynamic effects of hypotensive drugs used in pregnancy. Obstet Gynecol Surv 1954;9:776–94.

Name:	**TRIMETHOBENZAMIDE**	Risk Factor:	**C**
Class:	**Antiemetic**		

FETAL RISK SUMMARY

RECOMMENDATION: Human Data Suggest Low Risk

Trimethobenzamide is an antiemetic agent. Reproduction studies have been conducted in rats and rabbits and revealed no evidence of teratogenicity (1). An increased incidence of resorptions and stillborn pups were noted in rats (at 20 and 100 mg/kg) and an increased number of resorptions in rabbits (at 100 mg/kg), but these adverse effects occurred in only one or two dams in both species (1).

Trimethobenzamide has been used in pregnancy to treat nausea and vomiting (2,3). No adverse effects in the fetus were observed. In a third study, 193 patients were treated with trimethobenzamide in the 1st trimester (4). The incidences of severe congenital defects at 1 month, 1 year, and 5 years were 2.6%, 2.6%, and 5.8%, respectively. The 5.8% incidence was increased compared with nontreated controls (3.2%) ($p < 0.05$), but other factors, including the use of other antiemetics in some patients, may have contributed to the results. The authors concluded that the risk of congenital malformations with trimethobenzamide was low.

T

BREAST FEEDING SUMMARY

RECOMMENDATION: No Human Data - Probably Compatible

No reports describing the use of trimethobenzamide during lactation have been located. The molecular weight (about 389 for the free base) is low enough, however, that excretion into breast milk should be expected. The potential effects of this exposure on a nursing infant are unknown.

References

1. Product information. Tigan. Roberts Pharmaceutical, 2000.
2. Breslow S, Belafsky HA, Shangold JE, Hirsch LM, Stahl MB. Antiemetic effect of trimethobenzamide in pregnant patients. Clin Med 1961;8:2153–5.
3. Winters HS. Antiemetics in nausea and vomiting of pregnancy. Obstet Gynecol 1961;18:753–6.
4. Milkovich L, van den Berg BJ. An evaluation of the teratogenicity of certain antinauseant drugs. Am J Obstet Gynecol 1976;125:244–8.

Name: **TRIMETHOPRIM** Risk Factor: **C_M**
Class: **Anti-infective**

FETAL RISK SUMMARY

RECOMMENDATION: Human and Animal Data Suggest Risk

Trimethoprim is available as a single agent and in combination with various sulfonamides (see Sulfonamides). Because trimethoprim is a folate antagonist, caution has been advocated for its use in pregnancy (1–3). Published case reports and placebo-controlled trials involving several hundred patients, during all phases of gestation, have failed to demonstrate an increase in fetal abnormalities (4–13). However, other reports (14–19) and the unpublished data cited below are suggestive that trimethoprim use during the 1st trimester may result in structural defects. Maternal supplementation with multivitamins that contain folic acid may reduce this risk (16).

Trimethoprim (200 mg/kg) given to pregnant rats resulted in cleft palates (20). The no-effect dose was 192 mg/kg. When trimethoprim (88 mg/kg) was combined with sulfamethoxazole (355 mg/kg), cleft palates were observed in one litter out of nine. In two other rat studies, however, no teratogenic effects were seen at a combined dose of 128 and 512 mg/kg, respectively. In some studies with pregnant rabbits, a trimethoprim dose 6 times the human therapeutic dose was associated with resorptions, fetal death, and malformations (20).

Trimethoprim (molecular weight about 290) crosses the placenta, producing similar levels in fetal and maternal serum and in amniotic fluid (21–23). Using an *in vitro* perfused human cotyledon, both trimethoprim and sulfamethoxazole were shown to cross the placenta (24). After 1 hour in a closed system at maternal trimethoprim concentrations of 7.2 and 1.0 μg/mL, concentrations on the fetal side were 1.4 (19%) and 0.08 μg/mL (8%), respectively. Under similar conditions, maternal sulfamethoxazole levels of 29.6, 112.6, and 127.7 μg/mL produced fetal levels of 5.1 (17%), 9.6 (9%), and 14.8 μg/mL (12%). (Note: The mean steady state serum levels following 160 mg/800 mg trimethoprim/sulfamethoxazole orally twice daily are 1.72 and 68 μg/mL, respectively [20].)

A 27-year-old woman consumed a low-calorie (Nutra System) diet 10 months before conception through the 4th gestational week (14). Her pregnancy was complicated by otitis, treated with a combination of trimethoprim-sulfamethoxazole for 10 days beginning in the 3rd week, and the onset of hyperemesis gravidarum at 5–6 weeks' gestation that lasted until the 8th month. Dimenhydrinate was taken intermittently as an antiemetic from the 7th week through the 8th month. She gave birth at 38 weeks' gestation to a 3225-g, female infant with a lobar holoprosencephaly. The malformations included a median cleft lip and palate, a flat nose without nostrils, hypoplasia of the optic discs, and a single ventricle and midline fused thalami. The infant developed progressive hydrocephalus, myoclonic jerks, intractable seizures, and muscle tone that changed from hypotonic to hypertonic at 2 months of age. Although the critical period for development of holoprosencephaly was thought to be during the period of gastrulation (i.e., the 3rd week of pregnancy), the cause of the defects was unknown (14).

In a surveillance study of Michigan Medicaid recipients conducted between 1985 and 1992 involving 229,101 completed pregnancies, 2296 newborns had been exposed to the combination of trimethoprim-sulfamethoxazole during the 1st trimester (F. Rosa, personal communication, FDA, 1993). A total of 126 (5.5%) major birth defects were observed (98 expected). This incidence is suggestive of an association between the drug combination and congenital defects. Specific data were available for six defect categories, including (observed/expected) 37/23 cardiovascular defects, 3/4 oral clefts, 1/1 spina bifida, 7/7 polydactyly, 3/4 limb reduction defects, and 7/5 hypospadias. Only the cardiovascular defects are suggestive of an association among the six specific malformations, but other factors such as the mother's disease, concurrent drug use, and chance may be involved.

A 2000 case report described the adverse pregnancy outcomes, including neural tube defects (NTDs), of two pregnant women with human immunodeficiency virus (HIV) infection who were treated with the anti-infective combination, trimethoprim/sulfamethoxazole, for prophylaxis against *Pneumocystosis carinii*, concurrently with antiretroviral agents (15). In the first case, a 32-year-old woman with a 3-year history of HIV and recent diagnosis of acquired immunodeficiency syndrome was treated before and throughout gestation with the anti-infective combination plus zidovudine and zalcitabine. Folic acid 10 mg/day was added after the diagnosis of pregnancy (gestational age not specified). At term, a female infant was delivered by cesarean section without HIV infection, but with a bony mass in the lumbar spine (identified by ultrasound at 32 weeks' gestation). A diagnostic evaluation revealed that the second lumbar vertebra consisted of hemivertebrae and projected posteriorly into the spinal canal. A malformed and displaced first lumbar vertebra was also noted. Surgery was planned to correct the defect. The second case involved a 31-year-old woman who presented at 15 weeks' gestation. She was receiving trimethoprim/sulfamethoxazole, didanosine, stavudine, nevirapine, and vitamin B supplements (specific vitamins and dosage not given) that had been started before conception. A fetal ultrasound at 19 weeks' gestation revealed spina bifida and ventriculomegaly. The patient elected to terminate her pregnancy. The fetus did not have HIV infection. Defects observed at autopsy included ventriculomegaly, an Arnold-Chiari malformation, sacral spina bifida, and a lumbo-sacral meningomyelocele. The authors attributed the NTDs in both cases to the antifolate activity of trimethoprim (15).

The effects of exposure (at any time during the 2nd or 3rd month after the last menstrual period) to folic acid antagonists on embryo/fetal development were evaluated in a large, multicenter, case-control surveillance study published in 2000 (16). The report was based on data collected between 1976 and 1998 by the Slone Epidemiology Unit Birth Defects Study from 80 maternity or tertiary care hospitals in Boston, Philadelphia, Toronto, and Iowa. Mothers were interviewed within 6 months of delivery about their use of drugs during pregnancy. Folic acid antagonists were categorized into two groups: group I—dihydrofolate

T

reductase inhibitors (aminopterin, methotrexate, sulfasalazine, pyrimethamine, triamterene, and trimethoprim); group II—agents that affect other enzymes in folate metabolism, impair the absorption of folate, or increase the metabolic breakdown of folate (carbamazepine, phenytoin, primidone, and phenobarbital). The case subjects were 3870 infants with cardiovascular defects, 1962 with oral clefts, and 1100 with urinary tract malformations. Infants with defects associated with a syndrome were excluded, as were infants with coexisting NTDs known to be reduced by maternal folic acid supplementation). Too few infants with limb-reduction defects were identified to be analyzed. Controls ($N = 8{,}387$) were infants with malformations other than oral clefts and cardiovascular, urinary tract, and limb-reduction defects and NTDs, but included infants with chromosomal and genetic defects. The risk of malformations in control infants would not have been reduced by vitamin supplementation, and none of the controls used folic acid antagonists (16). For group I cases, the relative risks (RRs) of cardiovascular defects and oral clefts were 3.4 (95% confidence interval [CI] 1.8–6.4) and 2.6 (95% CI 1.1–6.1), respectively. For group II cases, the RRs of cardiovascular and urinary tract defects, and oral clefts were 2.2 (95% CI 1.4–3.5), 2.5 (95% CI 1.2–5.0), and 2.5 (95% CI 1.5–4.2), respectively. Maternal use of multivitamin supplements with folic acid (typically 0.4 mg) reduced the risks in group I cases. For cardiovascular defects, the RR and 95% CI without or with folic acid were 7.7 (2.8–21.7) and 1.5 (0.6–3.8), respectively. The same comparison for oral clefts could not be completed because only three case infants were exposed to folic acid during the second and third month. However, there were six (0.3%) cases of oral clefts without folic acid and three (0.2%) with folic acid. In contrast, in group II cases, folic acid did not reduce the risks of cardiovascular defects, oral clefts, or urinary tract defects (16).

Additional data related to the above study appeared in a reply to correspondence (17). Analysis for trimethoprim exposure resulted in a RR of 4.2 (95% CI 1.5–11.5) for cardiovascular defects based on 12 cases. Additional analysis for oral clefts (three cases) and urinary tract defects (one case) was not conducted because of the small number of exposures (17).

A 2001 case-control study, using the same database as in the above study, compared data on 1242 infants with NTDs (spina bifida, anencephaly, and encephalocele) to a control group of 6660 infants with congenital defects not related to vitamin supplementation (18). Based on five exposed cases, the adjusted odds ratio (OR) for trimethoprim was 4.8, 95% CI 1.5–16.1. For all folic acid antagonists (carbamazepine, phenobarbital, phenytoin, primidone, sulfasalazine, triamterene, and trimethoprim), based on 27 cases, the adjusted OR was 2.9, 95% CI 1.7–4.6 (18).

A 2002 review, briefly citing the above two studies, stated that the results were consistent with previous studies that folic acid supplementation early in pregnancy reduces the risk of cardiac defects, oral clefts, and NTDs (19). However, additional studies are needed to determine if early folic acid supplementation would also reduce the risk of these anomalies from trimethoprim (19).

A 2001 case-control study used the population-based data set of the Hungarian Case-Control Surveillance of Congenital Abnormalities, 1980–1996, to examine the teratogenic risk of trimethoprim in combination with either sulfamethoxazole or sulfamethazine (20). There were 22,865 case women that had delivered an infant with congenital malformations and 38,151 controls that had infants without malformations. In the cases and controls, 351 (1.5%) and 443 (1.2%) were treated with trimethoprim-sulfamethoxazole, respectively, in the 2nd/3rd months of pregnancy. For trimethoprim-sulfamethazine, 45 (0.2%) cases and 39 (0.1%) controls were treated, respectively, in the 2nd/3rd months of pregnancy. Since both combinations contained trimethoprim, the drugs were combined in the case-control pair analysis. Two congenital abnormalities had higher use of drug treatments: cardiovascular anomalies (29 vs. 10; adjusted OR 2.9, 95% CI 1.4–6.0) and multiple anomalies (mainly urinary tract and cardiovascular) (9 vs. 1; adjusted OR 9.0, 95% CI 1.1–71.0). For NTDs, analysis of trimethoprim-sulfamethoxazole in the 1st month revealed 9 cases (adjusted OR 4.3, 95% CI 2.1–8.6) and 7 cases in the 2nd/3rd months (adjusted OR 2.2, 95% CI 1.0–4.8) (20).

A case of Niikawa-Kuroki syndrome (i.e., Kabuki make-up syndrome) has been described in a non-Japanese girl whose mother had a viral and bacterial infection during the 2nd month of pregnancy (26). The bacterial infection was treated with trimethoprim-sulfamethoxazole. The syndrome is characterized by mental and growth retardation and craniofacial malformations (26). The cause of the defects in this patient, as in all cases of this syndrome, was unknown. Some have speculated, however, that the syndrome is caused by autosomal dominant inheritance (27).

Sulfonamide-trimethoprim combinations have been shown to cause a drop in the sperm count after 1 month of continuous treatment in males (28). Decreases varied between 7% and 88%. The authors theorized that trimethoprim deprived the spermatogenetic cells of active folate by inhibiting dihydrofolate reductase.

No interaction between trimethoprim-sulfamethoxazole and oral contraceptives was found in one study (29). Short courses of the anti-infective combination are unlikely to affect contraceptive control.

BREAST FEEDING SUMMARY

RECOMMENDATION: Compatible

Trimethoprim is excreted into breast milk in low concentrations. Following 160 mg twice daily for 5 days, milk concentrations varied between 1.2 and 2.4 μg/mL (average 1.8 μg/mL) with peak levels occurring at 2–3 hours (30). No adverse effects were reported in the infants. Nearly identical results were found in a study with 50 patients (31). Mean milk levels were 2.0 μg/mL, representing a milk:plasma ratio of 1.25. The authors concluded that these levels represented a negligible risk to the suckling infant. The American Academy of Pediatrics classifies the combination of trimethoprim-sulfamethoxazole as compatible with breast-feeding (32).

References

1. McEwen LM. Trimethoprim/sulphamethoxazole mixture in pregnancy. Br Med J 1971;4:490–1.
2. Smithells RW. Co-trimoxazole in pregnancy. Lancet 1983;2:1142.
3. Tan JS, File TM Jr. Treatment of bacteriuria in pregnancy. Drugs 1992;44:972–80.
4. Williams JD, Condie AP, Brumfitt W, Reeves DS. The treatment of bacteriuria in pregnant women with sulphamethoxazole and trimethoprim. Postgrad Med J 1969;45(Suppl):71–6.
5. Ochoa AG. Trimethoprim and sulfamethoxazole in pregnancy. JAMA 1971;217:1244.
6. Brumfitt W, Pursell R. Double-blind trial to compare ampicillin, cephalexin, co-trimoxazole, and trimethoprim in treatment of urinary infection. Br Med J 1972;2:673–6.
7. Brumfitt W, Pursell R. Trimethoprim/sulfamethoxazole in the treatment of bacteriuria in women. J Infect Dis 1973;128(Suppl):S657–63.
8. Brumfitt W, Pursell R. Trimethoprim/sulfamethoxazole in the treatment of urinary infection. Med J Aust 1973;1(Suppl):44–8.
9. Bailey RR. Single-dose antibacterial treatment for bacteriuria in pregnancy. Drugs 1984;27:183–6.
10. Soper DE, Merrill-Nach S. Successful therapy of penicillinase-producing *Neisseria gonorrhoeae* pharyngeal infection during pregnancy. Obstet Gynecol 1986;68:290–1.
11. Cruikshank DP, Warenski JC. First-trimester maternal *Listeria monocytogenes* sepsis and chorioamnionitis with normal neonatal outcome. Obstet Gynecol 1989;73:469–71.
12. Seoud M, Saade G, Awar G, Uwaydah M. Brucellosis in pregnancy. J Reprod Med 1991;36:441–5.
13. Frederiksen B. Maternal septicemia with *Listeria monocytogenes* in second trimester without infection of the fetus. Acta Obstet Gynecol Scand 1992;71:313–5.

T

14. Ronen GM. Holoprosencephaly and maternal low-calorie weight-reducing diet. Am J Med Genet 1992;42:139.
15. Richardson MP, Osrin D, Donaghy S, Brown NA, Hay, Sharland M. Spinal malformations in the fetuses of HIV infected women receiving combination antiretroviral therapy and co-trimoxazole. Eur J Obstet Gynecol Reprod Biol 2000;93:215–7.
16. Hernandez-Diaz S, Werler MM, Walker AM, Mitchell AA. Folic acid antagonists during pregnancy and the risk of birth defects. N Engl J Med 2000;343: 1608–14.
17. Hernandez-Diaz S, Mitchell AA. Folic acid antagonists during pregnancy and risk of birth defects. N Engl J Med 2001;344:934–5.
18. Hernandez-Diaz S, Werler MM, Walker AM, Mitchell AA. Neural tube defects in relation to use of folic acid antagonists during pregnancy. Am J Epidemiol 2001;153:961–8.
19. Shepard TH, Brent RL, Friedman JM, Jones KL, Miller RK, Moore CA, Polifka JE. Update on new developments in the study of human teratogens. Teratology 2002;65:153–61.
20. Czeizel AE, Rockenbauer M, Sorensen HT, Olsen J. The teratogenic risk of trimethoprim-sulfonamides: a population based case-control study. Reprod Toxicol 2001;15:637–46.
21. Product information. Septra. Monarch Pharmaceuticals, 2001.
22. Ylikorkala O, Sjostedt E, Jarvinen PA, Tikkanen R, Raines T. Trimethoprim-sulfonamide combination administered orally and intravaginally in the 1st trimester of pregnancy: its absorption into serum and transfer to amniotic fluid. Acta Obstet Gynecol Scand 1973;52:229–34.
23. Reid DWJ, Caille G, Kaufmann NR. Maternal and transplacental kinetics of trimethoprim and sulfamethoxazole, separately and in combination. Can Med Assoc J 1975;112:67s–72s.
24. Reeves DS, Wilkinson PJ. The pharmacokinetics of trimethoprim and trimethoprim/sulfonamide combinations, including penetration into body tissues. Infection 1979;7(Suppl 4):S330–41.
25. Bawdon RE, Maberry MC, Fortunato SJ, Gilstrap LC, Kim S. Trimethoprim and sulfamethoxazole transfer in the in vitro perfused human cotyledon. Gynecol Obstet Invest 1991;31:240–2.
26. Koutras A, Fisher S. Niikawa-Kuroki syndrome: a new malformation syndrome of postnatal dwarfism, mental retardation, unusual face, and protruding ears. J Pediatr 1982;101:417–9.
27. Niikawa N. Kabuki make-up syndrome. In Buyse ML, Editor-in-Chief. *Birth Defects Encyclopedia*. Volume 2. Dover, MA: Center for Birth Defects Information Services, 1990:998–9.
28. Murdia A, Mathur V, Kothari LK, Singh KP. Sulpha-trimethoprim combinations and male fertility. Lancet 1978;2:375–6.
29. Grimmer SFM, Allen WL, Back DJ, Breckenridge AM, Orme M, Tjia J. The effect of cotrimoxazole on oral contraceptive steroids in women. Contraception 1983;28:53–9.
30. Arnauld R, Soutoul JH, Gallier J, Borderon JC, Borderon E. A study of the passage of trimethoprim into the maternal milk. Quest Med 1972;25:959–64.
31. Miller RD, Salter AJ. The passage of trimethoprim/sulphamethoxazole into breast milk and its significance. In Daikos GK, ed. *Progress in Chemotherapy*, Proceedings of the Eighth International Congress of Chemotherapy, Athens, 1973. Athens, Greece: Hellenic Society for Chemotherapy, 1974:687–91.
32. Committee of Drugs, American Academy of Pediatrics. The transfer of drugs and other chemicals into human milk. Pediatrics 2001;108:776–89.

Name:	**TRIMETREXATE**	Risk Factor:	**D_M**
Class:	**Anti-infective/Antineoplastic (Orphan Drug)**		

FETAL RISK SUMMARY

RECOMMENDATION: No Human Data - Animal Data Suggest Risk

Trimetrexate is a synthetic, competitive inhibitor of the enzyme dihydrofolate reductase from bacterial, protozoan, and mammalian sources. Its mechanism of action is similar to another folate antagonist, trimethoprim. Trimetrexate is indicated, in combination with leucovorin, as an alternative therapy for the treatment of *Pneumocystis carinii* pneumonia in immunocompromised patients, such as those with acquired immunodeficiency syndrome. Leucovorin (folinic acid), an active derivative of folic acid, must be given with trimetrexate to protect normal host cells (1). Trimetrexate is also used, as an orphan drug, for the treatment of some metastatic cancers.

Reproduction studies with trimetrexate have been conducted in rats and rabbits (1). In pregnant rats and rabbits, IV doses greater than 1.5 and 2.5 mg/kg, respectively, caused fetal and maternal toxicity. At lower, nontoxic maternal IV doses (5%–50% of the equivalent human therapeutic dose based on body surface area), retarded fetal development and teratogenicity were observed. Teratogenic effects included skeletal, visceral, ocular, and cardiovascular malformations.

It is not known if trimetrexate crosses the human placenta. The molecular weight of the free base (about 369) is low enough that transfer to the fetus should be expected.

No reports describing the use of trimetrexate during human pregnancy have been located. Structural abnormalities and fetal toxicity (e.g., bone marrow depression and hepatotoxicity) are potential risks if this drug is used during pregnancy. Women of childbearing age who are receiving this drug should be advised to avoid becoming pregnant.

BREAST FEEDING SUMMARY

RECOMMENDATION: No Human Data - Potential Toxicity

No reports describing the use of trimetrexate in human lactation have been located. The molecular weight of the free base (about 369) is low enough that excretion into breast milk should be expected. Because of the potential for severe toxicity (e.g., bone marrow depression and hepatotoxicity), women receiving this drug should not breast-feed.

Reference

1. Product information. Neutrexin. MedImmune, 2001.

Name:	**TRIMIPRAMINE**	Risk Factor:	**C_M**
Class:	**Antidepressant**		

FETAL RISK SUMMARY

RECOMMENDATION: Human Data Suggest Low Risk

Trimipramine is a tricyclic antidepressant in the same class as amitriptyline, clomipramine, doxepin, and imipramine. It is indicated for the relief of symptoms of depression (1). Trimipramine has an elimination half-life of 9–11 hours and it is metabolized in the liver to an active metabolite (2).

Reproduction studies have been conducted in rats, rabbits, and mice. In rats and rabbits, evidence of embryotoxicity and/or increased incidence of major anomalies (type not specified) were observed at doses 20 times the human dose (*assumed to be based on weight*) (1). A single SC dose given to mice on day 9 of gestation resulted in exencephaly and other defects of the central nervous system (3). In the isolated rat uterus, trimipramine had greater antihistamine H_2 activity than cimetidine, amitriptyline or imipramine (4).

It is not known if trimipramine or its active metabolite crosses the human placenta. The molecular of the free base (about 294) and the long elimination half-life suggest that both compounds will cross to the embryo and/or fetus.

In a 1996 descriptive case series, the European Network of the Teratology Information Services (ENTIS) prospectively examined the outcomes of 689 pregnancies exposed to antidepressants (5). Multiple drug therapy occurred in about two-thirds of the mothers. There were nine exposures) to trimipramine. The outcomes of these pregnancies were eight normal newborns (includes three premature infants) and one normal infant with a neonatal disorder (bilateral metatarsus varus [possible positional]) (5).

The animal data suggest low risk but, if the comparison to the human dose had been based on body surface area, the toxic dose would have been close to the human dose. The human data are too limited to assess the risk to the embryo/fetus. In general, though, most tricyclic antidepressants do not have a known teratogenic effect in humans. In addition, of the tricyclic antidepressants, nortriptyline and desipramine are preferred during pregnancy because they have the least sedative action and maternal adverse effects (6).

BREAST FEEDING SUMMARY

RECOMMENDATION: No Human Data - Potential Toxicity

No reports describing the use of trimipramine during human lactation have been located. The molecular of the free base (about 294) and the long elimination half-life (9–11 hours) suggest that both compounds will be excreted into milk. The effects of this exposure on a nursing infant are unknown. However, the American Academy of Pediatrics classifies other tricyclic antidepressants as drugs whose effect on the nursing infant is unknown but may be of concern (see Amitriptyline).

References

1. Product information. Surmontil. Odyssey Pharmaceuticals, 2004.
2. Parfitt K, Editor. *Martindale. The Complete Drug Reference*. 32nd ed. London, UK: Pharmaceutical Press, 1999:310.
3. Jurand A. Malformations of the central nervous system induced by neurotropic drugs in mouse embryos. Develop Growth Differ 1980;22:61–78. As cited by Shepard TH. *Catalog of Teratogenic Agents*. 10th ed. Baltimore, MD: The Johns Hopkins University Press, 2001:510.
4. Alvarez FJ, Casas E, Franganillo A, Velasco A. Effects of antidepressants on histamine H_2 receptors in rat isolated uterus. J Pharmacol (Paris) 1986;17:351–4.
5. McElhatton PR, Garbis HM, Elefant E, Vial T, Bellemin B, Mastroiacovo P, Arnon J, Rodriguez-Pinilla E, Schaefer C, Pexieder T, Merlob P, Dal Verme S. The outcome of pregnancy in 689 women exposed to therapeutic doses of antidepressants. A collaborative study of the European Network of Teratology Information Services (ENTIS). Reprod Toxicol 1996;10:285–94.
6. Committee on Drugs, American Academy of Pediatrics. Use of psychoactive medication during pregnancy and possible effects on the fetus and newborn. Pediatrics 2000;105:880–7.

Name: **TRIPELENNAMINE** Risk Factor: **B**

Class: **Antihistamine**

FETAL RISK SUMMARY

RECOMMENDATION: Limited Human Data - Probably Compatible

The Collaborative Perinatal Project monitored 50,282 mother-child pairs, 100 of whom were exposed to tripelennamine in the 1st trimester (1, pp. 323–324). For use anytime during pregnancy, 490 exposures were recorded (1, pp. 436–437). In neither group was evidence found to suggest a relationship to major or minor malformations.

The illicit use of pentazocine and tripelennamine (T's and blue's) has been described in a number of cases (2–5). These cases are discussed in detail under the monograph for pentazocine (see Pentazocine).

BREAST FEEDING SUMMARY

RECOMMENDATION: No Human Data - Probably Compatible

Tripelennamine is excreted into bovine milk but human studies have not been reported (6). The manufacturer considers the drug to be contraindicated in the nursing mother, possibly because of the increased sensitivity of newborn or premature infants to antihistamines (7).

References

1. Heinonen OP, Slone D, Shapiro S. *Birth Defects and Drugs in Pregnancy*. Littleton, MA. Publishing Sciences Group, 1977.
2. Dunn DW, Reynolds J. Neonatal withdrawal symptoms associated with "T's and blue's" (pentazocine and tripelennamine). Am J Dis Child 1982;136:644–5.
3. Pastorek JG II, Plauche WC, Faro S. Acute bacterial endocarditis in pregnancy: a report of three cases. J Reprod Med 1983;28:611–4.
4. Chasnoff IJ, Hatcher R, Burns WJ, Schnoll SH. Pentazocine and tripelennamine ("T's and blue's"): effects on the fetus and neonate. Dev Pharmacol Ther 1983;6:162–9.
5. von Almen WF II, Miller JM Jr. "Ts and BLues" in pregnancy. J Reprod Med 1986;31:236–9.
6. O'Brien TE. Excretion of drugs in human milk. Am J Hosp Pharm 1974;31:844–54.
7. Product information. PBZ. Geigy Pharmaceuticals, 1990.

Name: **TRIPROLIDINE** Risk Factor: C_M

Class: **Antihistamine**

FETAL RISK SUMMARY

RECOMMENDATION: Compatible

Triprolidine is an antihistamine in the same class as brompheniramine, chlorpheniramine, and dexchlorpheniramine. The drug is used in a number of proprietary decongestant-antihistamine mixtures.

The Collaborative Perinatal Project monitored 50,282 mother-child pairs, 16 of whom had 1st-trimester exposure to triprolidine (1). From this small sample, no evidence was found to suggest a relationship to large categories of major or minor malformations or to individual malformations.

In a 1971 study, infants and mothers who had ingested antihistamines during the 1st trimester actually had fewer abnormalities when compared with controls (2). Triprolidine was the third most commonly used antihistamine. The manufacturer claims that in more than 20 years of marketing the drug no reports of triprolidine teratogenicity have been received (M. F. Frosolono, personal communication, Burroughs Wellcome, 1980). Their animal studies have also been negative.

Two studies, one appearing in 1981 (3) and the second in 1985 (4), described the 1st-trimester drug exposures of 6837 and 6509 mothers, respectively, treated by the Group Health Cooperative of Puget Sound and whose pregnancies terminated in a live birth. Both studies covered 30-month periods, 1977–1979, and 1980–1982, respectively. From the total of 13,346 mothers, 628 (4.7%) consumed during the 1st trimester (based on the filling of a prescription) a proprietary product containing triprolidine hydrochloride and pseudoephedrine (Actifed). Nine (1.4%) of the exposed infants had a major congenital abnormality (type not specified). Spontaneous or induced abortions, stillbirths, and many minor anomalies, such as clubfoot, syndactyly, polydactyly, clinodactyly, minor ear defects, coronal or first-degree hypospadias, and hernia, were excluded from the data.

In two surveillance studies of Michigan Medicaid recipients conducted between 1980 and 1983, and 1985 and 1992 involving 333,440 completed pregnancies, 910 newborns had been exposed to triprolidine during the 1st trimester (F. Rosa, personal communication, FDA, 1994). Of the 900 exposed newborns identified in the 1980–1983 group, 65 (7.2%) had major birth defects (59 expected), 10 of which were cardiovascular defects (8 expected). No cases of cleft lip and/or palate were observed. None of the 10 newborns included in the 1985–1992 data had congenital malformations.

BREAST FEEDING SUMMARY

RECOMMENDATION: Limited Human Data - Probably Compatible

Triprolidine is excreted into breast milk (5). Three mothers, who were nursing healthy infants, were given an antihistamine-decongestant preparation containing 2.5 mg of triprolidine and 60 mg of pseudoephedrine. The women had been nursing their infants for 14 weeks, 14 weeks, and 18 months. Triprolidine was found in the milk of all three subjects, with milk:plasma ratios in one woman at 1, 3, and 12 hours of 0.5, 1.2, and 0.7, respectively. Using AUCs in the other two women gave more reliable results of 0.56 and 0.50 (5). The authors calculated that a milk production of 1000 mL/24 hours would contain 0.001–0.004 mg of triprolidine base, or about 0.06%–0.2% of the maternal dose. The American Academy of Pediatrics classifies triprolidine as compatible with breastfeeding (6).

References

1. Heinonen OP, Slone D, Shapiro S. *Birth Defects and Drugs in Pregnancy*. Littleton, MA: Publishing Sciences Group, 1977:323.
2. Nelson MM, Forfar JO. Associations between drugs administered during pregnancy and congenital abnormalities of the fetus. Br Med J 1971;1:523–7.
3. Jick H, Holmes LB, Hunter JR, Madsen S, Stergachis A. First-trimester drug use and congenital disorders. JAMA 1981;246:343–6.
4. Aselton P, Jick H, Milunsky A, Hunter JR, Stergachis A. First-trimester drug use and congenital disorders. Obstet Gynecol 1985;65:451–5.
5. Findlay JWA, Butz RF, Sailstad JM, Warren JT, Welch RM. Pseudoephedrine and triprolidine in plasma and breast milk of nursing mothers. Br J Clin Pharmacol 1984;18:901–6.
6. Committee on Drugs, American Academy of Pediatrics. The transfer of drugs and other chemicals into human milk. Pediatrics 2001;108:776–89.

T

Name: **TROGLITAZONE**[§] Risk Factor: B_M
Class: **Oral Hypoglycemic**

FETAL RISK SUMMARY

RECOMMENDATION: Limited Human Data - Animal Data Suggest Moderate Risk

Troglitazone, a thiazolidinedione antidiabetic agent, is used as an adjunct to diet and exercise, either alone or in combination with a sulfonylurea, a sulfonylurea and metformin, or insulin, to improve glycemic control in type II diabetes (non-insulin-dependent diabetes mellitus) (1,2). Troglitazone decreases hepatic glucose output by inhibiting liver gluconeogenesis and improves target cell response to insulin. It is not an insulin secretagogue.

Reproduction studies with troglitazone have been conducted in rats and rabbits (1). Doses 3–9 times the human exposure from 400 mg/day based on AUC (HE) produced no adverse effects on fertility or reproduction in male and female rats. No evidence of teratogenicity was found in rats and rabbits given doses up to 9 and 3 times the HE, respectively. However, in rats, the highest dose was associated with decreased fetal and newborn pup weights. Much smaller doses given to rats late in gestation and during lactation caused delayed postnatal development that was attributed to decreased body weight. The no-effect dose was 1% of the maximum dose used above (1).

It is not known if troglitazone crosses the human placenta. The molecular weight (about 442) is low enough that transfer to the fetus should be expected.

Troglitazone (during days 1–28 of the menstrual cycle) was given either alone or in combination with clomiphene (during days 3–7 of the cycle) to induce ovulation in women with clomiphene-resistant polycystic ovary syndrome (all of the women had previously failed to ovulate with clomiphene 200 mg/day) (3). Ovulation was successfully induced in 15 of 18 patients and 7 of these women achieved pregnancy. Assuming that conception occurred in mid-cycle, then the last dose of troglitazone was taken on day 14 of gestation. The outcomes of the seven pregnancies were two 1st-trimester spontaneous abortions and five full-term healthy infants (3). In another case involving a woman with the hyperandrogenic, insulin-resistant acanthosis nigricans syndrome, troglitazone was discontinued when pregnancy was diagnosed (4). The outcome of the pregnancy was not mentioned.

Except for the reports of early pregnancy exposure noted above, no other cases describing the use of troglitazone during human pregnancy have been located. Insulin is the treatment of choice for pregnant diabetic patients because, in general, other hypoglycemic agents do not provide adequate glycemic control. Moreover, insulin, unlike most oral agents, does not cross the placenta to the fetus, thus eliminating the additional concern that the drug therapy itself will adversely affect the fetus. Carefully prescribed insulin therapy provides better control of the mother's glucose, thereby preventing the fetal and neonatal complications that occur with this disease. High maternal glucose levels, as may occur in diabetes mellitus, are closely associated with a number of maternal and fetal adverse effects, including fetal structural anomalies if the hyperglycemia occurs early in gestation. To prevent this toxicity, most experts, including the American College of Obstetricians and Gynecologists, recommend that insulin be used for types I and II diabetes occurring during pregnancy and, if diet therapy alone is not successful, for gestational diabetes (5,6). An additional concern is the severe idiosyncratic hepatocellular injury that has been reported in adults who were taking troglitazone (1,7).

[§*Withdrawn from the market in 2000.*]

T

BREAST FEEDING SUMMARY

RECOMMENDATION: No Human Data - Potential Toxicity

No reports describing the use of troglitazone in human lactation have been located. The drug has been detected in the milk of lactating rats (1). This is consistent with its relatively low molecular weight (about 442), and excretion into human breast milk should be expected. The effects of this exposure on a nursing infant are unknown. However, because of the severe idiosyncratic hepatocellular injury that has been reported in adults who were taking troglitazone, the drug should probably not be used during nursing.

References

1. Product information. Rezulin. Parke-Davis, 2000.
2. Sparano N, Seaton TL. Troglitazone in type II diabetes mellitus. Pharmacotherapy 1998;18:539–48.
3. Mitwally MFM, Kuscu NK, Yalcinkaya TM. High ovulatory rates with use of troglitazone in clomiphene-resistant women with polycystic ovary syndrome. Hum Reprod 1999;14:2700–3.
4. Elkind-Hirsch KE, McWilliams RB. Pregnancy after treatment with the insulin-sensitizing agent troglitazone in an obese woman with hyperandrogenic, insulin-resistant acanthosis nigricans syndrome. Fertil Steril 1999;71:943–7.
5. American College of Obstetricians and Gynecologists. Diabetes and pregnancy. *Technical Bulletin*. No. 200, December 1994.
6. Coustan DR. Management of gestational diabetes. Clin Obstet Gynecol 1991;34:558–64.
7. Rezulin labeling updated to recommend more frequent patient monitoring. JAMA 1998;279:9.

Name:	**TROLEANDOMYCIN**	Risk Factor:	**C**
Class:	**Antibiotic**		

Troleandomycin is the triacetyl ester of oleandomycin (see Oleandomycin).

Name:	**TROVAFLOXACIN**	Risk Factor:	**C_M**
Class:	**Anti-infective (Quinolone)**		

FETAL RISK SUMMARY

RECOMMENDATION: Human Data Suggest Low Risk

Trovafloxacin is a synthetic, broad-spectrum, fluoroquinolone antibacterial agent. It is in the same anti-infective class as ciprofloxacin, enoxacin, gatifloxacin, lomefloxacin, levofloxacin, moxifloxacin, norfloxacin, ofloxacin, and sparfloxacin. The injectable form of trovafloxacin is alatrofloxacin, the *L*-alanyl-*L*-alanyl prodrug that is rapidly hydrolyzed *in vivo* to trovafloxacin (1).

Neither trovafloxacin or alatrofloxacin affected the fertility of male and female rats at oral and IV doses that were approximately 2 times the maximum recommended human dose based on body surface area (MRHD) (1). At this dose, some dams experienced uterine dystocia. At oral doses 6 times the MRHD, an increased incidence of preimplantation loss occurred. In addition, oral doses greater than about 0.14 times the MRHD were associated with prolonged gestation (1).

When an oral dose of trovafloxacin 2 times the MRHD was administered during organogenesis, an increase in skeletal variations was seen in rat fetuses, but not at 0.4 times the MRHD. (1). Other signs of fetal toxicity observed at the higher dose were increased perinatal mortality and decreased body weights. No increase in the incidence of skeletal variations or malformations were observed in pregnant rabbits at 2.7 times the MRHD (1). In contrast, an increase in skeletal variations and malformations were seen in rats with daily IV doses of alatrofloxacin at ≥0.6 times the MRHD during organogenesis. Skeletal malformations were also seen in rabbits at an IV dose approximately equal to the MRHD during organogenesis. No skeletal variations or malformations were seen at IV doses that were 0.2 (rat) and 0.3 (rabbit) times, respectively, the MRHD.

It is not known if trovafloxacin crosses the human placenta. The molecular weight of about 512 is low enough that transfer to the fetus should be expected.

No reports describing the use of either the IV or oral forms of trovafloxacin during human pregnancy have been located. The animal toxicity observed at or near the maximum recommended human doses should be considered before this anti-infective is used in pregnant women. Moreover, because of severe hepatic toxicity in adults, trovafloxacin should not be used in any patient if safer alternatives will be effective (1). In addition, some reviewers have concluded that all fluoroquinolones should be considered contraindicated in pregnancy (e.g., see Ciprofloxacin and Norfloxacin), because safer alternatives are usually available.

BREAST FEEDING SUMMARY

RECOMMENDATION: Limited Human Data - Probably Compatible

Trovafloxacin is excreted into breast milk (1). The average milk concentration in three lactating women was 0.8 μg/mL (range 0.2–2.1 μg/mL) after a single IV alatrofloxacin dose (300 mg trovafloxacin equivalents) and repeated oral 200 mg doses (1). The effects of this exposure on a nursing infant are unknown.

Reference

1. Product information. Trovan. Pfizer, 2001.

Name:	**TYROPANOATE**	Risk Factor:	**D**
Class:	**Diagnostic**		

FETAL RISK SUMMARY

RECOMMENDATION: Human Data Suggest Risk in 2nd and 3rd Trimesters

Tyropanoate contains a high concentration of organically bound iodine. See Diatrizoate for possible effects on the fetus and newborn.

BREAST FEEDING SUMMARY

RECOMMENDATION: No Human Data - Probably Compatible

See Potassium Iodide.

U

Name:	**UREA**	Risk Factor:	**C**
Class:	**Diuretic**		

FETAL RISK SUMMARY

RECOMMENDATION: No Human Data - No Relevant Animal Data

Urea is an osmotic diuretic that is used primarily to treat cerebral edema. Topical formulations for skin disorders are also available. No reports of its use in pregnancy following IV, oral, or topical administration have been located. Urea, given by intra-amniotic injection, has been used for the induction of abortion (1).

BREAST FEEDING SUMMARY

RECOMMENDATION: No Human Data - Probably Compatible

No data are available.

Reference

1. Ware A, ed. *Martindale: The Extra Pharmacopoeia*. 27th ed. London: The Pharmaceutical Press, 1977:572.

Name:	**UROKINASE**	Risk Factor:	**B_M**
Class:	**Thrombolytic**		

FETAL RISK SUMMARY

RECOMMENDATION: Limited Human Data - Animal Data Suggest Low Risk

Urokinase, 100,000 IU/kg intraperitoneal, was not teratogenic in rats or mice (1). The manufacturer cites studies in which doses up to 1000 times the human dose did not impair fertility or produce fetal harm in rats and mice (2). Six reports of its use in human pregnancy have been located.

A woman, at 28 weeks' gestation, was treated with urokinase, 4,400 IU/kg for 10 minutes followed by 4,400 IU/kg/hour for 12 hours, for pulmonary embolism (3). Heparin therapy was then administered—first IV, then SC—for the remainder of the pregnancy. A healthy term infant was delivered 2 months after initiation of therapy.

A 1995 review briefly cited two reports of patients treated with urokinase, apparently without fetal or neonatal complications, for thrombosed prosthetic heart valves (4). A 36-year-old woman was treated at 14 and 32 weeks' gestation and had an uncomplicated cesarean delivery at 34 weeks (4,5). The second patient, a 32-year-old woman, was treated twice with different thrombolytics: first at 3 months' gestation with urokinase and second at 6 months' gestation with streptokinase (4,6). Minor uterine hemorrhage because of placental separation occurred at 3 months' gestation and a cesarean section was performed at 7 months' gestation. Maternal transfusion and surgical drainage were required following the delivery.

A 27-year-old woman, in premature labor, developed a massive pulmonary embolism at 31 weeks' gestation (7). She was initially treated with a bolus dose of urokinase (200,000 IU) and heparin. Dobutamine was also administered to maintain a stable hemodynamic state. Because her condition continued to deteriorate, she was treated with low-dose alteplase with eventual successful resolution of the embolism. A healthy, preterm, 2100-g male infant was delivered about 3 days after urokinase administration.

A 1994 report described a woman at 26 weeks' gestation who suffered a myocardial infarction (8). Following stabilization, she underwent cardiac catheterization, 9 days after the initial infarction, which revealed 90% occlusion of the proximal right coronary artery and mild narrowing of other cardiac arteries. A prolonged intracoronary infusion of urokinase, in preparation for a planned angioplasty, failed to improve the right coronary occlusion, and coronary stents were subsequently placed. A healthy female infant was eventually delivered at 39 weeks' gestation.

The treatment of massive pulmonary embolism, diagnosed in a 20-year-old woman at 21 weeks' gestation, with urokinase and heparin was described in a 1995 case report (9). The patient markedly improved after receiving two courses of urokinase, 4,400 IU/kg for 10 minutes followed by 4,400 IU/kg/hour continuous infusion for 12 hours, approximately 6 hours apart, followed by continuous heparin. No complications of therapy were observed in the fetus, and she eventually delivered a healthy, 3122-g male infant at term.

In summary, the use of urokinase during pregnancy does not appear to represent a major risk to the fetus. The drug is not fetotoxic or teratogenic in rodents. However, only one human case treated with this thrombolytic agent during the 1st trimester (at 3 months) has been reported. It is not known whether the drug crosses the placenta to the fetus, but placental tissue contains proteinase inhibitors that inactivate urokinase (10,11). Placental separation and hemorrhage is a potential complication and has been reported in one case.

BREAST FEEDING SUMMARY

RECOMMENDATION: No Human Data - Probably Compatible

No reports describing the use of urokinase during lactation have been located. Because of the nature of the indications for urokinase and its very short half-life (20 minutes or less), the opportunities for its use during lactation and the potential exposure of the nursing infant are minimal.

U

References

1. Shepard TH. *Catalog of Teratogenic Agents*. 8th ed. Baltimore, MD: Johns Hopkins University Press, 1995:437–8.
2. Product information. Abbokinase. Abbott Laboratories, 2000.
3. Delclos GL, Davila F. Thrombolytic therapy for pulmonary embolism in pregnancy: a case report. Am J Obstet Gynecol 1986;155:375–6.
4. Turrentine MA, Braems G, Ramirez MM. Use of thrombolytics for the treatment of thromboembolic disease during pregnancy. Obstet Gynecol Surv 1995;50:534–41.
5. Jimenez M, Vergnes C, Brottier L, Dequeker JL, Billes MA, Lorient Roudaut MF, Choussat A, Boisseau MR. Thrombose récidivante d'une prothèse valvulaire aortique chez une femme enceinte. Traitement par urokinase. J Mal Vasc 1988;13:46–9.
6. Tissot H, Vergnes C, Rougier P, Bricaud H, Dallay D.

Traitement fibrinolytique par urokinase et streptokinase d'une thrombose récidivante sur double prothèse valvulaire aortique mitrale au cours de la grossesse. J Gynecol Obstet Biol Reprod (Paris) 1991;20:1093–6.
7. Flossdorf Th, Breulmann M, Hopf H-B. Successful treatment of massive pulmonary embolism with recombinant tissue type plasminogen activator (rt-PA) in a pregnant woman with intact gravidity and preterm labour. Intensive Care Med 1990;16:454–6.
8. Sanchez-Ramos L, Chami YG, Bass TA, DelValle GO, Adair CD. Myocardial infarction during pregnancy: management with transluminal coronary angioplasty and metallic intracoronary stents. Am J Obstet Gynecol 1994;171:1392–3.
9. Kramer WB, Belfort M, Saade GR, Surani S, Moise KJ Jr. Successful urokinase treatment of massive pulmonary embolism in pregnancy. Obstet Gynecol 1995;86:660–2.
10. Holmberg L, Lecander I, Persson B, Åstedt B. An inhibitor from placenta specifically binds urokinase and inhibits plasminogen activator released from ovarian carcinoma in tissue culture. Biochem Biophys Acta 1978;544:128–37.
11. Walker JE, Gow L, Campbell DM, Ogston D. The inhibition by plasma of urokinase and tissue activator-induced fibrinolysis in pregnancy and the puerperium. Thromb Haemost 1983;49:21–3.

Name: **URSODIOL** Risk Factor: **B_M**

Class: **Gastrointestinal Agent (Gallstone Solubilizing Agent)**

FETAL RISK SUMMARY

RECOMMENDATION: Compatible

Ursodiol (ursodeoxycholic acid) is a naturally occurring bile acid used orally to dissolve gallstones. The drug has been used for the treatment of intrahepatic cholestasis of pregnancy.

No fetal adverse effects were observed when ursodiol (up to 200 mg/kg/day) was fed to pregnant rats (1). Embryotoxicity was observed in a rat study, but this was less than with another closely related bile acid, chenodiol, and no evidence of hepatotoxicity was observed at three dosage levels (2). Reproduction studies in rats with doses up to 22 times the recommended maximum human dose based on body surface area (RMHD), and in rabbits with doses up to 7 times the RMHD revealed no evidence of impaired fertility or fetal harm (3).

Ursodiol is absorbed from the small intestine and is extracted and conjugated by the liver. Although 30%–50% of a dose may enter the systemic circulation, continuous hepatic uptake keeps ursodiol blood levels low and uptake by tissues other than the liver are considered nil (4). These factors combined with tight binding to albumin probably indicate that placental passage to the fetus does not occur.

During clinical trials, inadvertent exposure during the 1st trimester to therapeutic doses of ursodiol in four women had no effect on their fetuses or newborns (3). Several reports, summarized below, have described the apparent safe use of ursodiol in the latter portion of human pregnancy for the treatment of intrahepatic cholestasis.

A brief 1991 report described the use of ursodiol in the treatment of late-onset intrahepatic cholestasis during pregnancy (5). A 30-year-old primigravida was given ursodiol 600 mg/day in two divided doses for 20 days starting at 34 weeks' gestation. No signs of fetal distress were observed during treatment. Labor was induced at 37 weeks' gestation and a 2670-g, healthy baby girl was delivered; her Apgar scores were 9 and 10 at 1 and 5 minutes, respectively (5).

A second letter, published in 1992, briefly described the successful outcome of eight pregnant women with intrahepatic cholestasis treated with ursodiol, 1 g/day for 3 weeks

(6). The full report of this study was also published in 1992 (7). Treatment began after 25 weeks' gestation in the eight women, five receiving 1 g/day in divided dosage for 20 consecutive days and the other three receiving the same dose for two 20-day treatment courses, separated by a 14-day drug-free interval (7). The mean dose was 14 mg/kg/day (range 12–17 mg/kg/day). All of the newborns had Apgar scores greater than 7 (at 1 and 5 minutes) and all were progressing normally at a 5-month follow-up (7).

A 1994 report described the use of ursodiol, 450 mg/day, in three pregnancies (singleton, twin, and quintuplet) for intrahepatic cholestasis (8). Ursodiol was started because of unsuccessful attempts to control the disease with cholestyramine or ademetionine (S-adenosyl-L-methionine; SAMe). The singleton pregnancy was treated from 29 weeks' gestation to delivery at 37 weeks' gestation, the twin pregnancy from 27 to 33 weeks' gestation, and the woman with quintuplets from 21 weeks' gestation to delivery at 30 weeks' gestation. No adverse effects were observed in the eight newborns (8).

A study published in 1995 described significant reductions in the perinatal mortality and morbidity associated with cholestasis of pregnancy following the use of ursodiol (9). Eight women with a history of 13 pregnancies affected by the disease were referred to a specialty clinic before conception. Expectant management had been used in 12 of the 13 pregnancies, with 11 experiencing adverse outcomes: 8 stillbirths, 2 premature deliveries with 1 death in the perinatal period, and 1 emergency cesarean section for fetal distress. Subsequently, three of the women became pregnant again and each suffered a recurrence of cholestasis. Therapy with ursodiol, 750 mg/day in two patients, and 1000 mg/day in one patient, was initiated at 31, 33, and 37 weeks' gestation, respectively. The first patient had been pretreated with ademetionine from 16 to 31 weeks' gestation in an unsuccessful attempt to prevent cholestasis. Each of the three women showed rapid clinical improvement and resolution of their abnormal liver tests following initiation of ursodiol. Normal infants, who were doing well, were delivered at 35, 35, and 38 weeks' gestation, respectively (9).

A double-blind, placebo-controlled trial in women with intrahepatic cholestasis of pregnancy compared the effect of ursodiol treatment ($N = 8$) with placebo ($N = 8$) (10). Significant decreases in the pruritus score and all liver biochemical parameters occurred in the ursodiol group, but only the pruritus score and alanine aminotransferase were significantly improved in controls. Moreover, the gestational age at delivery in the treated group was 38 weeks compared with 34 weeks in controls ($p < 0.01$), resulting in higher mean birth weights (2935 g vs. 2025 g). Apgar scores were also higher in the treated group. Fetal distress was observed in four of the control pregnancies (none in the study group) and these were delivered by cesarean section. In the treated group, six of the eight newborns were delivered vaginally. At a 5-month follow-up, all infants were developing normally (10). A number of other reports have found that ursodiol is safe and effective for the treatment of cholestasis of pregnancy (11–15).

BREAST FEEDING SUMMARY

RECOMMENDATION: No Human Data - Probably Compatible

No reports have been located that described the use of ursodiol during lactation. Because only small amounts of ursodiol appear in the systemic circulation and these are tightly bound to albumin, it is doubtful if clinically significant amounts are excreted into breast milk.

References

1. Toyoshima S, Fujita H, Sakurai T, Sato R, Kashima M. Reproduction studies of ursodeoxycholic acid in rats. II. Teratogenicity study. Oyo Yakuri 1978;15:931–45. As cited in Shepard TH. *Catalog of Teratogenic Agents*. 8th ed. Baltimore, MD: Johns Hopkins University Press, 1995:438.
2. Celle G, Cavanna M, Bocchini R, Robbiano L. Chenodeoxycholic acid (CDCA) versus ursodeoxycholic acid (UDCA): a comparison of their effects in pregnant rats. Arch Int Pharmacodyn Ther 1980;246:149–58.
3. Product information. Urso. Axcan Pharma U.S., 2000.
4. Bachrach WH, Hofmann AF. Ursodeoxycholic acid in the treatment of cholesterol cholelithiasis. Part I. Dig Dis Sci 1982;27:737–61.
5. Mazzella G, Rizzo N, Salzetta A, Iampieri R, Bovicelli L, Roda E. Management of intrahepatic cholestasis in pregnancy. Lancet 1991;338:1594–5.
6. Palma J, Reyes H, Ribalta J, Iglesias J, Gonzalez M. Management of intrahepatic cholestasis in pregnancy. Lancet 1992;339:1478.
7. Palma J, Reyes H, Ribalta J, Iglesias J, Gonzalez MC, Hernandez I, Alvarez C, Molina C, Danitz AM. Effects of ursodeoxycholic acid in patients with intrahepatic cholestasis of pregnancy. Hepatology 1992;15: 1043–7.
8. Floreani A, Paternoster D, Grella V, Sacco S, Gangemi M, Chiaramonte M. Ursodeoxycholic acid in intrahepatic cholestasis of pregnancy. Br J Obstet Gynaecol 1994;101:64–5.
9. Davies MH, da Silva RCMA, Jones SR, Weaver JB, Elias E. Fetal mortality associated with cholestasis of pregnancy and the potential benefit of therapy with ursodeoxycholic acid. Gut 1995;37:580–4.
10. Diaferia A, Nicastri PL, Tartagni M, Loizzi P, Iacovizzi C, Di Leo A. Ursodeoxycholic acid therapy in pregnant women with cholestasis. Int J Gynecol Obstet 1996;52:133–40.
11. Floreani A, Paternoster D, Melis A, Grella PV. S-adenosylmethionine versus ursodeoxycholic acid in the treatment of intrahepatic cholestasis of pregnancy: preliminary results of a controlled trial. Eur J Obstet Gynecol Reprod Biol 1996;67:109–13.
12. Palma J, Reyes H, Ribalta J, Hernandez I, Sandoval L, Almuna R, Liepins J, Lira F, Sedano M, Silva O, Toha D, Silva JJ. Ursodeoxycholic acid in the treatment of cholestasis of pregnancy: a randomized, double-blind study controlled with placebo. J Hepatol 1997;27:1022–8.
13. Brites D, Rodrigues CMP, Oliveira N, Cardoso MC, Graca LM. Correction of maternal serum bile acid profile during ursodeoxycholic acid therapy in cholestasis of pregnancy. J Hepatol 1998;28:91–8.
14. Brites D, Rodrigues CMP, Cardoso MC, Graca LM. Unusual case of severe cholestasis of pregnancy with early onset, improved by ursodeoxycholic acid administration. Eur J Obstet Gynecol Reprod Biol 1998;76:165–8.
15. Nicastri PL, Diaferia A, Taartagni M, Loizzi P, Fanelli M. A randomized placebo-controlled trial of ursodeoxycholic acid and S-adenosylmethionine in the treatment of intrahepatic cholestasis of pregnancy. Br J Obstet Gynaecol 1998;105:1205–7.

V

Name: **VACCINE, ANTHRAX** Risk Factor: **C**

Class: **Vaccine**

FETAL RISK SUMMARY

RECOMMENDATION: Compatible

Anthrax vaccine adsorbed (AVA) is prepared from a cell-free, noninfectious filtrate of *Bacillus anthracis* that contains a mix of cellular products adsorbed to aluminum hydroxide (1). This vaccine has replaced a previously available alum-precipitated vaccine. An avirulent, nonencapsulated strain (V770-NP1OR) of *B. anthracis* is used in the production of the vaccine, which contains no dead or live bacteria (1,2). The cellular products in the vaccine include, in unknown amounts, three proteins known as protective antigen (PA), lethal factor (LF), and edema factor (EF). Live *B. anthracis* forms combinations of these proteins resulting in two exotoxins known as lethal toxin (PA and LF) and edema toxin (PA and EF). The recommended vaccination schedule is 0.5 mL at 0, 2, and 4 weeks; three booster vaccinations at 6, 12, and 18 months; and then an annual booster injection (1).

Reproduction studies with anthrax vaccine have not been conducted in experimental animals (3). However, no plausible biological mechanism for an adverse effect on an embryo or fetus has been proposed (2).

The placental transfer of the three proteins contained in the vaccine has not been studied. Because of the very high molecular weight, however, simple diffusion does not appear to be possible for transfer.

Only one study has been located that examined the effects of anthrax vaccine, administered before conception, on pregnancy outcome (2). Women, age 17 to 44 years, assigned to two U.S. Army installations formed the study population. During the study period from January 1999 to March 2000, 3136 women received at least one dose of the vaccine (most received two or three doses), whereas 962 women were not vaccinated. Departure from the study sites was the most common reason for not receiving the vaccine. The only acceptable medical indications to defer or refuse the vaccine were pregnancy or immunity-compromising disease. There were 385 pregnancies after at least one dose of the vaccine. The annualized pregnancy rates in those vaccinated and not vaccinated were 159.5 and 160.0 per 1000 person-years, respectively. These rates were nearly identical to the pregnancy rates before the study. Compared with unvaccinated women, vaccinated women were 1.2 times as likely to give birth (95% confidence interval [CI] 0.8–1.8). Adjustment for marital status, race, and age did not change the odds ratio (OR). A total of 327 births (vaccinated and unvaccinated) were available for outcome analysis. Low birth weight (<2500 g) occurred in 11 cases (3.3%). After adjustment, the OR for vaccination and low birth weight was 1.3, 95% CI 0.2–6.4. Congenital malformations (specific details not provided) were observed in 15 cases, but no unusual patterns or clusters were noted. Only one malformation (polydactyly of the fingers) had multiple occurrences (three cases: two vaccinated, one unvaccinated). After adjustment, the OR for vaccination and structural anomalies was 0.7, 95% CI 0.2–2.3. The adjusted OR for vaccination and any adverse birth outcome was 0.9, 95% CI 0.4–2.4 (2).

In summary, although experimental animal reproduction studies with AVA have not been conducted, there appears to be no plausible biological mechanism for adverse pregnancy effects. Because of the absence of human pregnancy experience, however, the use of anthrax vaccine during gestation is not recommended. The human reproductive data, limited to vaccination before conception, do not appear to suggest a risk from vaccination to either a woman's subsequent fertility or a subsequent pregnancy outcome. However, the published study cited above lacked sufficient power to detect adverse birth outcomes (2). Moreover, there are no reports describing the effects of the vaccine on a current pregnancy. Until such data are available, the recommendation made by the Centers for Disease Control and Prevention (CDC) in 2000 (1) that "pregnant women should be vaccinated against anthrax only if the potential benefits outweigh the potential risks to the fetus" is still relevant. The American College of Obstetricians and Gynecologists *Committee Opinion* states that the vaccine is not routinely recommended unless the pregnant woman works directly with *B. anthracis*, imported animal hides, potentially infected animals in high incidence areas (not the United States), or military personnel deployed in high-risk exposure areas (4).

BREAST FEEDING SUMMARY

RECOMMENDATION: Compatible

No studies describing the use of anthrax vaccine in lactating women have been located. Because of the nature of anthrax vaccine, the potential for adverse effects in a nursing infant appear to be nil. The CDC states that there is no evidence to suggest a risk to the mother or nursing infant, and the administration of the vaccine during breast-feeding is not medically contraindicated (1).

References

1. CDC. Use of anthrax vaccine in the United States. Recommendations of the Advisory Committee on Immunization Practices (ACIP). MMWR 2000;49(No. RR15):11.
2. Wiesen AR, Little CT. Relationship between prepregnancy anthrax vaccination and pregnancy and birth outcomes among US Army women. JAMA 2002; 287:1556–60.
3. CDC. Notice to readers: Status of U.S. Department of Defense preliminary evaluation of the association of anthrax vaccination and congenital anomalies. MMWR 2002;51(06):127.
4. American College of Obstetricians and Gynecologists. Immunization during pregnancy. *Committee Opinion*. Number 282, January 2003.

Name:	**VACCINE, BCG**	Risk Factor:	C_M
Class:	**Vaccine**		

FETAL RISK SUMMARY

RECOMMENDATION: Compatible - Maternal Benefit >> Embryo/Fetal Risk

BCG vaccine is a live, attenuated bacteria vaccine used to provide immunity to tuberculosis (1,2). Animal reproduction studies have not been conducted with the vaccine.

The risk to the fetus from maternal vaccination is unknown. Because it is a live preparation, one reviewer thought the vaccine should probably not be used during pregnancy (2). A more recent publication cited the recommendation of the Immunization Practices Advisory Committee (ACIP) that BCG vaccine should only be used if there is an immediate, excessive risk of unavoidable exposure to infectious tuberculosis (2).

BREAST FEEDING SUMMARY

RECOMMENDATION: No Human Data - Probably Compatible

No data are available.

References

1. American Hospital Formulary Service. *Drug Information 1997*. Bethesda, MD: American Society of Health-System Pharmacists, 1997:2569–72.
2. Amstey MS. Vaccination in pregnancy. Clin Obstet Gynaecol 1983;10:13–22.

Name: **VACCINE, CHOLERA** Risk Factor: **C_M**

Class: **Vaccine**

FETAL RISK SUMMARY

RECOMMENDATION: Compatible

Cholera vaccine is a killed bacteria vaccine (1). Cholera during pregnancy may result in significant morbidity and mortality to the mother and the fetus, particularly during the 3rd trimester. The risk to the fetus from maternal vaccination is unknown because there is no specific information on the safety of the vaccine during pregnancy (2). The Centers for Disease Control and Prevention (CDC) recommends that the use of the vaccine in pregnancy should reflect actual need (2).

BREAST FEEDING SUMMARY

RECOMMENDATION: Compatible

Maternal vaccination with cholera vaccine has increased specific IgA antibody titers in breast milk (3). In a second study, cholera vaccine (whole cell plus toxoid) was administered to six lactating mothers, resulting in a significant rise in milk anticholera toxin IgA titers in five of the patients (5). Milk from three of these five mothers also had a significant increase in anti-cholera toxin IgG titers.

References

1. Amstey MS. Vaccination in pregnancy. Clin Obstet Gynaecol 1983;10:13–22.
2. CDC. Recommendations of the Immunization Practices Advisory Committee. Cholera vaccine. MMWR 1988;37 (No. 40):617–24.
3. Svennerholm AM, Holmgren J, Hanson LA, Lindblad BS, Quereshi F, Rahimtoola RJ. Boosting of secretory IgA antibody responses in man by parenteral cholera vaccination. Scand J Immunol 1977;6:1345–49.
4. Merson MH, Black RE, Sack DA, Svennerholm AM, Holmgren J. Maternal cholera immunisation and secretory IgA in breast milk. Lancet 1980;1:931–2.

Name: **VACCINE, *ESCHERICHIA COLI*** Risk Factor: **C**
Class: **Vaccine**

FETAL RISK SUMMARY

RECOMMENDATION: Limited Human Data - Probably Compatible

Escherichia coli (*E. coli*) vaccine is a nonpathogenic strain of bacteria used experimentally as a vaccine. Two reports of its use (strains O111 and 083) in pregnant women in labor or waiting for the onset of labor have been located (1,2). The vaccines were given to these patients in an attempt to produce antimicrobial activity in their colostrum. No adverse effects in the newborn were noted.

BREAST FEEDING SUMMARY

RECOMMENDATION: Compatible

Escherichia coli (*E. coli* strains O111 and 083) vaccines were given to mothers in labor or waiting for the onset of labor (1,2). Antibodies against *E. coli* were found in the colostrum of 7 of 47 (strain 0111) and 3 of 3 (strain 083) treated mothers but in only 1 of 101 controls. No adverse effects were noted in the nursing infants.

References

1. Dluholucky S, Siragy P, Dolezel P, Svac J, Bolgac A. Antimicrobial activity of colostrum after administering killed Escherichia coli O111 vaccine orally to expectant mothers. Arch Dis Child 1980;55:558–60.
2. Goldblum RM, Ahlstedt S, Carlsson B, Hanson LA, Jodal U, Lidin-Janson G, Sohl-Akerlund A. Antibody-forming cells in human colostrum after oral immunisation. Nature 1975;257:797–9.

Name: **VACCINE, GROUP B STREPTOCOCCAL** Risk Factor: **C**
Class: **Vaccine**

FETAL RISK SUMMARY

RECOMMENDATION: Compatible

Group B *Streptococcus* (GBS) capsular polysaccharides (CPS) vaccine has been used in pregnancy in an attempt to prevent infection in the newborn (1). Forty women at a mean gestational age of 31 weeks (range 26–36 weeks) were administered a single 50-μg dose of type III CPS of GBS (1). No adverse effects were observed in the 40 newborns. The overall response rate to the vaccine, which is not commercially available, was 63%. Twenty-five infants were born to mothers who had responded to the vaccine, and at 1 and 3 months of age, 80% and 64%, respectively, continued to have protective levels of antibody (1). Although the vaccine is considered safe (2), as are other bacterial vaccines (3), the clinical effectiveness of the vaccine has not been determined and its use remains controversial (4–7).

In an attempt to improve on the immunogenic response in adults, researchers designed a GBS type III CPS-tetanus toxoid conjugate vaccine (8). Although administered to

V

nonpregnant women, vaccination with the CPS-protein conjugate preparation resulted in enhanced immunogenicity compared with uncoupled vaccine. Although the results are encouraging, it is not known at the present time whether this vaccine will produce a similar response in pregnant women or whether it will prevent perinatal infection.

BREAST FEEDING SUMMARY

RECOMMENDATION: Compatible

No data are available.

References

1. Baker CJ, Rench MA, Edwards MS, Carpenter RJ, Hays BM, Kasper DL. Immunization of pregnant women with a polysaccharide vaccine of Group B streptococcus. N Engl J Med 1988;319:1180–5.
2. Faix RG. Maternal immunization to prevent fetal and neonatal infection. Clin Obstet Gynecol 1991;34:277–87.
3. CDC. Immunization Practices Advisory Committee. General recommendations on immunization. MMWR 1989;38:205–27.
4. Franciosi RA. Group B streptococcal vaccine in pregnant women. N Engl J Med 1989;320:807–8.
5. Baker CJ, Edwards MS. Group B streptococcal vaccine in pregnant women. N Engl J Med 1989;320:808.
6. Insel RA. Group B streptococcal vaccine in pregnant women. N Engl J Med 1989;320:808–9.
7. Linder N, Ohel G. In utero vaccination. Clin Perinatol 1994;21:663–74.
8. Kasper DL, Paoletti LC, Wessels MR, Guttormsen H-K, Carey VJ, Jennings HJ, Baker CJ. Immune response to type III Group B streptococcal polysaccharide-tetanus toxoid conjugate vaccine. J Clin Invest 1996;98:2308–14.

Name:	VACCINE, HAEMOPHILUS B CONJUGATE	Risk Factor:	C_M
Class:	Vaccine		

FETAL RISK SUMMARY

RECOMMENDATION: Compatible

Commercially available Haemophilus B conjugate vaccine is a combination of the capsular polysaccharides or oligosaccharides purified from *Haemophilus influenzae* type B bound with various proteins including tetanus toxoid, diphtheria toxoid, meningococcal protein, or diphtheria CRM_{197} (1). Two reports (2,3) and a review (4) have described the maternal immunization with the capsular polysaccharide vaccine of *H. influenzae* type B during the 3rd trimester of pregnancy to achieve passive immunity in the fetus and newborn. No adverse effects were observed in the newborns.

BREAST FEEDING SUMMARY

RECOMMENDATION: Compatible

Women who were vaccinated with Haemophilus B conjugate vaccine at 34–36 weeks' gestation had significantly higher antibody titers (>20-fold) in their colostrum than either nonimmunized women or those who were vaccinated before pregnancy (5). Breast milk antibody titers were also significantly higher (>20-fold) than the comparison groups at 3 and 6 months after delivery.

References

1. American Hospital Formulary Service. *Drug Information 1997*. Bethesda, MD: American Society of Health-System Pharmacists, 1997:2574–81.
2. Amstey MS, Insel R, Munoz J, Pichichero M. Fetal-neonatal passive immunization against *Haemophilus influenzae*, type B. Am J Obstet Gynecol 1985;153:607–11.
3. Glezen WP, Englund JA, Siber GR, Six HR, Turner C, Shriver D, Hinkley CM, Falcao O. Maternal immunization with the capsular polysaccharide vaccine for *Haemophilus influenzae* type B. J Infect Dis 1992;165(Suppl 1):S134–6.
4. Linder N, Ohel G. *In utero* vaccination. Clin Perinatol 1994;21:663–74.
5. Insel RA, Amstey M, Pichichero ME. Postimmunization antibody to the *Haemophilus influenzae* type B capsule in breast milk. J Infect Dis 1985;152:407–8.

Name: **VACCINE, HEPATITIS A** Risk Factor: **C_M**

Class: **Vaccine**

FETAL RISK SUMMARY

RECOMMENDATION: No Human Data - Probably Compatible

Hepatitis A virus vaccine inactivated is a noninfectious vaccine (1,2). Animal reproduction studies have not been conducted with the vaccine.

No reports describing the use of the vaccine in pregnant humans have been located, but based on similar vaccines, any risk to the fetus from maternal vaccination is probably minimal. The Centers for Disease Control and Prevention considers the theoretical risk to the developing fetus to be low (3). The American College of Obstetricians and Gynecologists recommends that the vaccine should given pre- or postexposure to pregnant women at risk for infection and international travelers (4).

Based on the experience with other inactivated viral vaccines, hepatitis A vaccine can be given to the pregnant woman at risk of infection (3,5).

BREAST FEEDING SUMMARY

RECOMMENDATION: No Human Data - Probably Compatible

No data are available, but based on other inactivated viral vaccines, hepatitis A vaccine does not appear to be contraindicated during nursing.

References

1. Product information. Havrix (Hepatitis A Vaccine, Inactivated). SmithKline Beecham, 2001.
2. Product information. Vaqta (Hepatitis A Vaccine, Inactivated). Merck, 2001.
3. CDC. Prevention of hepatitis A through active or passive immunization: recommendations of the Advisory Committee on Immunization Practices (ACIP). MMWR 1996;46(No. RR-15):1–30.
4. American College of Obstetricians and Gynecologists. Immunization during pregnancy. *Committee Opinion*. Number 282, January 2003.
5. Duff B, Duff P. Hepatitis A vaccine: ready for prime time. Obstet Gynecol 1998;91:468–71.

Name: **VACCINE, HEPATITIS B** Risk Factor: C_M
Class: **Vaccine**

FETAL RISK SUMMARY

RECOMMENDATION: Compatible

Hepatitis B virus vaccine inactivated (recombinant) is a noninfectious surface antigen (HBsAg) vaccine (1,2). Animal reproduction studies have not been conducted with the vaccine.

No risks to the fetus from maternal vaccination have been reported (1,2). One source recommends that administration after the 1st trimester, because of a theoretical risk of teratogenicity, is preferred (3). The Centers for Disease Control and Prevention (CDC) states that there is no apparent risk of fetal adverse effects (based on unpublished CDC data) and that pregnancy is not a contraindication to vaccination in women (1). Pre- and postexposure prophylaxis is indicated in pregnant women at high risk of infection (2,4). (See also Immune Globulin, Hepatitis B.) The American College of Obstetricians and Gynecologists recommends that the vaccine should given pre- or postexposure to pregnant women at risk for infection (5).

If hepatitis B vaccine is used in pregnancy, healthcare professionals are encouraged to call the toll free number (800-670-6126) for information about patient enrollment in the Motherisk study.

BREAST FEEDING SUMMARY

RECOMMENDATION: No Human Data - Probably Compatible

No data are available, but the vaccine can be used during lactation (1).

References

1. CDC. Hepatitis B virus: a comprehensive strategy for eliminating transmission in the United States through universal childhood vaccination. Recommendations of the Immunization Practices Advisory Committee (ACIP). MMWR 1991;40(No. RR-13):1–25.
2. American College of Obstetricians and Gynecologists. Immunization during pregnancy. *Technical Bulletin*. No. 160, October 1991.
3. Linder N, Ohel G. *In utero* vaccination. Clin Perinatol 1994;21:663–74.
4. Faix RG. Maternal immunization to prevent fetal and neonatal infection. Clin Obstet Gynecol 1991;34:277–87.
5. American College of Obstetricians and Gynecologists. Immunization during pregnancy. *Committee Opinion*. Number 282, January 2003.

Name: **VACCINE, INFLUENZA** Risk Factor: C_M
Class: **Vaccine**

FETAL RISK SUMMARY

RECOMMENDATION: Compatible

Influenza vaccine is an inactivated virus vaccine (1). Animal reproduction studies have not been conducted with the vaccine.

Influenza during pregnancy may potentially result in an increased rate of spontaneous abortions (1). The vaccine is considered safe during all stages of pregnancy (2–7). Neonatal passive immunization of short duration has been documented in some studies (4). The American College of Obstetricians and Gynecologists recommends that the vaccine be given to pregnant women in the 2nd and 3rd trimesters during the flue season (October–March) and to those at high risk for pulmonary complications regardless of trimester (1).

In 1999, the Advisory Committee on Immunization Practices (ACIP) recommended that the vaccine should be administered to women who would be in the 2nd and 3rd trimester (i.e., ≥14 weeks' gestation) during the influenza season (5). In addition, pregnant women who have medical conditions that increase their risk for complications from influenza should receive the vaccine regardless of the stage of pregnancy (5). Moreover, many experts consider influenza vaccine safe at any time in pregnancy, but vaccination during the 2nd trimester can avoid a coincidental association with spontaneous abortion that is common in the 1st trimester (5).

BREAST FEEDING SUMMARY

RECOMMENDATION: Compatible

Maternal vaccination is compatible with breast-feeding and presents no risk to the nursing infant (5).

References

1. American College of Obstetricians and Gynecologists. Immunization during pregnancy. *Committee Opinion*. Number 282, January 2003.
2. Philit F, Cordier J-F. Therapeutic approaches of clinicians to influenza pandemic. Eur J Epidemiol 1994;10:491–2.
3. Bandy U. Influenza: prevention and control. R I Med 1994;77:393–4.
4. Linder N, Ohel G. *In utero* vaccination. Clin Perinatol 1994;21:663–74.
5. CDC. Prevention and control of influenza: recommendations of the Advisory Committee on Immunization Practices (ACIP). MMWR 1999;48(No. RR-4):1–28.
6. Yeager DP, Toy EC, Baker B III. Influenza vaccination in pregnancy. Am J Perinatol 1999;16:283–6.
7. Kashyap S, Gruslin A. Influenza vaccination during pregnancy. Prim Care Update Ob/Gyns 2000;7:7–11.

Name:	**VACCINE, LYME DISEASE**	Risk Factor:	C_M
Class:	**Vaccine**		

FETAL RISK SUMMARY

RECOMMENDATION: No Human Data - Probably Compatible

Lyme disease vaccine (recombinant OspA) contains an outer surface protein of *Borrelia burgdorferi* sensu stricto (lipoprotein OspA) that is noninfectious (1,2). The recombinant OspA protein is expressed in *Escherichia coli* and then purified. Only the LYMErix vaccine is licensed for use in the United States (2). The vaccine (30 μg/0.5 mL) is administered IM on a three-dose schedule of 0, 1, and 12 months.

V

Lyme disease is a tickborne infection caused by the spirochete *B. burgdorferi*, with an incubation period from infection to onset of rash (erythema migrans) of 7–14 days (range 3–30 days) (2). The disease is characterized by rash, fever, malaise, fatigue, headache, myalgia, and arthralgia (2). Without adequate antibiotic treatment, chronic disease of the nervous system, musculoskeletal system, or the heart may occur.

No cases describing the use of Lyme disease vaccine in pregnancy have been located. Moreover, animal reproductive tests have not been conducted with the vaccine.

A 1985 case report described a woman who developed Lyme disease during the 1st trimester of pregnancy (3). She received no antibiotic therapy for her disease (3). She delivered a 3000-g, male infant at an estimated 35 weeks' gestation who developed respiratory distress shortly after birth. Studies revealed a dilated, poorly contractile left ventricle, aortic valvular stenosis, patent ductus arteriosus, and coarctation of the aorta (3). The infant died at age 39 hours. Cardiovascular malformations found at autopsy were tubular hypoplasia of the ascending aorta and aortic arch, marked endocardial fibroelastosis, and a persistent left superior vena cava draining into the coronary sinus (3). No signs of infection, such as inflammation, necrosis, or granuloma formation, were found in the heart or other organs, but a few spirochetes similar to the Lyme disease spirochete were found in the spleen, renal tubules, and bone marrow. Evaluation of the mother was consistent with Lyme disease, and she was successfully treated with tetracycline therapy.

A second case of fetal death associated with Lyme disease was published in 1987 (4). A 24-year-old woman with an apparent onset of infection (annular erythematous patch noted near her left knee followed by pain and swelling in the knee) near the time of conception delivered a 2500-g stillborn infant at term. Serologic studies of maternal blood were positive for *B. burgdorferi* in two of three samples. At autopsy, the only malformation found was an atrioventricular canal ventricular septal defect (4). Spirochetes immunologically consistent with *B. burgdorferi* were recovered from the fetal liver, myocardium, adrenal gland, and subarachnoid space of the midbrain. The authors concluded that the fetus had died near term of overwhelming spirochetosis (4).

The outcomes of 19 pregnancies of women with documented Lyme disease were described in 1986 (5). Eight of the pregnancies were followed prospectively, and 11 were identified retrospectively. Among the 17 women with erythema chronicum migrans (ECM), eight had the onset of disease in the 1st trimester, seven in the 2nd trimester, and two in the 3rd trimester. The onset of infection could not be determined in the remaining two, but one developed facial palsy in the 1st trimester and the other developed arthritis in the 3rd trimester. Normal outcomes occurred in 14 pregnancies, seven with onset of illness in the 1st trimester, four in the 2nd trimester, two in the 3rd trimester, and one with unknown time of onset. Six of the women (three in 1st trimester; one in 2nd trimester; one in 3rd trimester) did not receive antibiotic therapy, but all delivered apparently normal infants, although two had transient problems. One of these, a 2100-g infant delivered prematurely, developed hyperbilirubinemia at 4 days of age but has had otherwise normal development through 9 years of age. Another, delivered 7 days after onset of maternal ECM and meningitis, had hyperbilirubinemia and a generalized, petechial, vesicular rash at 5 days of age. Viral and bacterial blood and skin cultures were negative; tests for *B. burgdorferi* were not available at that time. The rash faded within 1 week during treatment with penicillin. The remaining three pregnancies had abnormal outcomes as described below (time of onset of maternal illness shown in parentheses):

(1st trimester) intrauterine fetal death at 16 weeks' gestation; no congenital abnormalities; no inflammation noted in fetal tissues; culture and indirect immunofluorescence assay of placenta and fetal tissues were negative

(2nd trimester) syndactyly (type 1) of second and third toes

(2nd trimester) full-term, healthy male infant at birth, developed cortical blindness and developmental delay at 8 months of age; diagnostic studies were negative; no serum antibodies to *B. burgdorferi* found at 1 year of age; mother had a previous child with trisomy 18

None of the five adverse outcomes described above can be directly attributed to maternal Lyme disease (5). At least one is known to be a fairly common genetic defect (i.e., syndactyly), and two were minor, transient adverse effects (5). Moreover, no cardiovascular anomalies were observed, but because only eight cases with ECM occurred in the 1st trimester, the power of this study to detect such defects is limited (5).

Two reports from the same group of investigators, one published in 1993 and the other in 1995, examined the effects of maternal exposure to Lyme disease and pregnancy outcome (6,7). A total of 2014 women were enrolled in the first study at their first prenatal visit (6). Of these, 11 were seropositive for Lyme disease, but information on the presence of congenital malformations was available for only 10 of their infants. Among these 10 newborns, 1 infant had a major defect (multiple major anomalies with VATER association [vertebral defects, imperforate anus, tracheoesophageal fistula, and radial and renal dysplasia]) (6). Two other infants had minor malformations: metatarsus adductus and stomach reflux. Other outcome data included no spontaneous abortions and a mean birth weight of 3650 g. None of these outcomes differed significantly from the group without Lyme disease exposure (i.e., with no significant titer and negative clinical history) (6).

In the second study, no difference in the incidence of total congenital malformations (odds ratio [OR] 0.87; 95% confidence interval [CI] 0.70–1.06) was observed in the infants of mothers in an endemic hospital cohort ($N = 2504$) compared with the infants of mothers in a control hospital ($N = 2507$) (7). The total number represented 81% of all eligible infants. However, the rate of cardiac malformations (most commonly ventricular septal defect [VSD]) was significantly higher in the endemic cohort (OR 2.40; 95% CI 1.25–4.59). Although the incidence of total minor malformations was no different between the groups, three minor defects (hemangiomas, polydactyly, and hydrocele) were significantly higher ($p < 0.05$) in the control group. Only the difference in polydactyly could be explained by demographic variations (7). Comparisons of mean birth weights between the cohorts found no significant differences.

In the endemic cohort, 22 of the mothers had Lyme disease before pregnancy (7). Among their 23 offspring (1 set of twins), there were two major malformations: multiple heart defects (infant died), and hydrocele and laryngomalacia. Six mothers contracted the disease during pregnancy and one of their infants had a major defect (hypospadias). Of the infants born to mothers ($N = 67$) who had reported a tick bite during pregnancy, three had major malformations (VSD, vesicoureteral block with reflux, and hypospadias) and five had minor defects (inguinal hernia, laryngomalacia, hemangioma, genu varum, and metatarsus adductus). Of the 20 infants born from mothers who had immunoglobulin G anti-*B. burgdorferi* antibodies in their cord blood (all infants were tested), one had a minor defect (cryptorchidism). Within the endemic cohort, there were no differences between those who had possible exposure to Lyme disease or who had positive cord serology compared with those who were not exposed and had negative serology in terms of mean birth weight or the rate of major or minor abnormalities (7).

A 1999 retrospective case-control study compared 796 children with a diagnosis of congenital cardiac anomaly with 704 children from the same region without cardiac defects (8). Records of all of the children were obtained from a medical center in a suburban area where Lyme disease is endemic. All had been born in the study area. No statistical differences in the frequencies of maternal conditions and exposures between the two groups were found for cigarette smoking, alcohol use, conception while using contraceptives, the use of fertility drugs, the use of electric blankets or heated waterbeds, vaginal bleeding during pregnancy, occupational exposure to video display terminals, asthma, upper respiratory tract infections, or thyroid disorders. More study mothers had high blood pressure (6.7% vs. 3.5%, $p = 0.007$), whereas more controls had occupational exposure to X-ray films or anesthesia (6.1% vs. 9.1%, $p = 0.03$). There were no statistical differences between the groups in Lyme disease during pregnancy (or 3 months, 1 year, or at anytime before conception) or in those who had received a tick bite during pregnancy (or 3 months, 1 year, or at anytime before conception). The authors concluded that there was no increased risk of congenital heart defects when maternal Lyme disease was contacted before or during pregnancy (8). However, their study could not exclude a risk to a fetus from undiagnosed and untreated Lyme disease (8).

Although there is concern that maternal Lyme disease may infect the fetus as other spirochetal infections (e.g., syphilis) do (5,9), the risk for this, based on the above studies, appears to be low. In addition, a survey published in 1994 found no cases of clinically significant nervous system disease attributable to transplacentally acquired Lyme disease that had been recognized among pediatric neurologists in regions of the United States in which Lyme disease was endemic (10). The regions surveyed included all or portions of Connecticut, Massachusetts, Minnesota, New Jersey, New York, Rhode Island, and Wisconsin. Some adult neurologists were also contacted in Connecticut. One pediatric neurologist was following three children with "congenital Lyme disease," but none of the mothers of these children met the Centers for Disease Control and Prevention's diagnostic criteria for Lyme disease (10). The authors concluded that either congenital neuroborreliosis was not occurring or that the incidence was extremely low in endemic areas (10).

In summary, the occurrence of Lyme disease during pregnancy presents a serious but apparently small risk to the fetus. The greatest fetal risk may be in cases where the mother does not receive appropriate antibiotic treatment. The data to support this conclusion are limited and controversial. Because there have been no reports on the use of Lyme disease vaccine during gestation, the fetal risk from the vaccine is unknown. However, because Lyme disease itself may cause fetal harm and the vaccine is noninfectious, vaccination of women of childbearing age who are at risk for acquiring the disease may be the safest course. Although the direct risk to a fetus appears to be low, the Advisory Committee on Immunization Practices recommends that pregnant women not receive the vaccine because its safety during pregnancy has not been established (2). If a pregnant woman receives the vaccine, health care professionals are encouraged to register the case with the SmithKline Beecham Pharmaceuticals vaccination pregnancy registry by calling (800) 366-8900, extension 5231 (1).

BREAST FEEDING SUMMARY

RECOMMENDATION: No Human Data - Probably Compatible

No reports describing the use of Lyme disease vaccine during lactation have been located. DNA of the spirochete *B. burgdorferi* has been detected in the breast milk of two women by polymerase chain reaction (PCR) (11). Breast milk samples from three healthy controls were nonreactive. Both women with reactive samples had Lyme disease as characterized by the presence of erythema migrans, and both had PCR-positive urine samples. One of the nursing infants was hospitalized at 6 months of age because of fever and vomiting. The cause of the symptoms was undetermined, but they resolved spontaneously after a few days. The urine of the infant and mother were tested 1 year later, and both were nonreactive.

References

1. Product information. LYMErix. SmithKline Beecham Pharmaceuticals, 2001.
2. CDC. Recommendations for the use of Lyme disease vaccine. Recommendations of the Advisory Committee on Immunization Practices (ACIP). MMWR 1999;48(RR-7):1–17.
3. Schlesinger PA, Duray PH, Burke BA, Steere AC, Stillman T. Maternal-fetal transmission of the Lyme disease spirochete, *Borrelia burgdorferi*. Ann Intern Med 1985;103:67–8.
4. MacDonald AB, Benach JL, Burgdorfer W. Stillbirth following maternal Lyme disease. N Y State J Med 1987;87:615–6.
5. Markowitz LE, Steere AC, Benach JL, Slade JD, Broome CV. Lyme disease during pregnancy. JAMA 1986;255:3394–6.
6. Strobino BA, Williams CL, Abid S, Chalson R, Spierling P. Lyme disease and pregnancy outcome: a prospective study of two thousand prenatal patients. Am J Obstet Gynecol 1993;169:367–74.
7. Williams CL, Strobino B, Weinstein A, Spierling P, Medici F. Maternal Lyme disease and congenital malformations: a cord blood serosurvey in endemic and control areas. Paediatr Perinat Epidemiol 1995;9:320–30.
8. Strobino B, Abid S, Gewitz M. Maternal Lyme disease and congenital heart disease: a case-control study in an endemic area. Am J Obstet Gynecol 1999;180:711–6.
9. Shapiro ED. Lyme disease in children. Am J Med 1995;98(Suppl 4A):69S–73S.
10. Gerber MA, Zalneraitis EL. Childhood neurologic disorders and Lyme disease during pregnancy. Pediatr Neurol 1994;11:41–3.
11. Schmidt BL, Aberer E, Stockenhuber C, Klade H, Breier F, Luger A. Detection of *Borrelia burgdorferi* DNA by polymerase chain reaction in the urine and breast milk of patients with Lyme borreliosis. Diagn Microbiol Infect Dis 1995;21:121–8.

Name: **VACCINE, MEASLES** Risk Factor: **C_M**

Class: **Vaccine**

FETAL RISK SUMMARY

RECOMMENDATION: Contraindicated

Measles (rubeola) vaccine is a live, attenuated virus vaccine (1–3). Animal reproduction studies have not been conducted with the vaccine.

Measles occurring during pregnancy may result in significant maternal morbidity, an increased abortion rate, stillbirth, prematurity, and congenital malformations (1,2). Although a fetal risk from the vaccine has not been confirmed, the vaccine should not be used during pregnancy because fetal infection with the attenuated viruses may occur (1–4). The manufacturer and the American College of Obstetricians and Gynecologists lists pregnancy as a contraindication (1,2). The manufacturer recommends that pregnancy should be avoided for 3 months following vaccination (2). A shorter interval is recommended by the Centers for Disease Control and Prevention (CDC) (5). They recommend that women avoid becoming pregnant for 30 days after vaccination (5). However, no cases of congenital malformations attributable to measles vaccine virus have been reported (5).

BREAST FEEDING SUMMARY

RECOMMENDATION: No Human Data - Probably Compatible

Measles (rubeola) vaccine can be given during breast-feeding (1).

References

1. American College of Obstetricians and Gynecologists. Immunization during pregnancy. *Committee Opinion*. Number 282, January 2003.
2. Product information. Attenuvax. Merck, 2004.
3. Amstey MS. Vaccination in pregnancy. Clin Obstet Gynaecol 1983;10:13–22.
4. Linder N, Ohel G. *In utero* vaccination. Clin Perinatol 1994;21:663–74.

5. CDC. Measles, mumps, and rubella—vaccine use and strategies for elimination of measles, rubella, and congenital rubella syndrome and control of mumps. Recommendations of the Advisory Committee on Immunization Practices (ACIP). MMWR 1998;47(No. RR-8): 1–57.

Name:	**VACCINE, MENINGOCOCCAL**	Risk Factor:	C_M
Class:	**Vaccine**		

FETAL RISK SUMMARY

RECOMMENDATION: Compatible

Meningococcal polysaccharide vaccine is a killed bacteria (cell wall) vaccine (1,2). Animal reproduction studies have not been conducted with the vaccine (1).

The risk to the fetus from vaccination during pregnancy is unknown. In one study, vaccination resulted in transfer of maternal antibodies to the fetus, but the transfer was irregular and was not dependent on maternal titer or the period in pregnancy when vaccination occurred (3).

A 1998 study evaluated the pregnancy outcomes of 34 women who received meningococcal vaccine during pregnancy (4). The trimesters of exposures were 4 (11.8%) in the 1st, 17 (50.0%) in the 2nd, and 13 (38.2%) in the 3rd. There were 34 singleton deliveries with a mean follow-up of the offspring of 13.2 months (range 1–24 months). Excluding one congenital malformation, there was no increase in the observed unusual birth events compared with the expected rates. In fact, there were significantly fewer cases of newborn cardiac murmurs and physiologic jaundice in offspring of vaccinated mothers. One birth defect observed in an infant of a mother vaccinated at 33 weeks' gestation was consistent with the oromandibular limb hypogenesis spectrum (Charlie M syndrome) (expected frequency <0.00002%). This pattern of defects would probably have occurred very early in gestation (4). The cause of Charlie M syndrome is unknown; it has not yet been identified as a genetic defect and it has not been associated with teratogens. All of the infants had normal growth and development in the follow-up period (4).

A 1994 review stated that the use of the vaccine during pregnancy is controversial (5). However, the American College of Obstetricians and Gynecologists states that indications for the vaccine are not altered by pregnancy and recommends that its use in unusual outbreak situations (6).

In a 1996 study, 75 mothers received meningococcal vaccine in the last trimester of pregnancy (7). No adverse effects in the newborns attributable to the vaccine were observed.

BREAST FEEDING SUMMARY

RECOMMENDATION: No Human Data - Probably Compatible

No data are available.

References

1. Product information. Menomune-A/C/Y/W-135. Aventis Pasteur, 2001.
2. Amstey MS. Vaccination in pregnancy. Clin Obstet Gynaecol 1983;10:13–22.
3. Carvalho ADA, Giampaglia CMS, Kimura H, Pereira OADC, Farhat CK, Neves JC, Prandini R, Carvalho EDS, Zarvos AM. Maternal and infant antibody response to meningococcal vaccination in pregnancy. Lancet 1977;2:809–11.
4. Letson GW, Little JR, Ottman J, Miller GL. Meningococcal vaccine in pregnancy: an assessment of infant risk. Pediatr Infect Dis 1998;17:261–3.

V

5. Linder N, Ohel G. In utero vaccination. Clin Perinatol 1994;21:663–74.
6. American College of Obstetricians and Gynecologists. Immunization during pregnancy. *Committee Opinion*. Number 282, January 2003.
7. O'Dempsey TJD, McArdle T, Ceesay SJ, Banya WAS, Demba E, Secka O, Leinonen M, Kayhty H, Francis N, Greenwood BM. Immunization with a pneumococcal capsular polysaccharide vaccine during pregnancy. Vaccine 1996;14:963–70.

Name: **VACCINE, MUMPS** Risk Factor: **C_M**
Class: **Vaccine**

FETAL RISK SUMMARY

RECOMMENDATION: Contraindicated

Mumps vaccine is a live attenuated virus vaccine (1–3). Animal reproduction studies have not been conducted with the vaccine.

Mumps occurring during pregnancy may result in an increased rate of 1st trimester spontaneous abortion (1,3). Although a fetal risk from the vaccine has not been confirmed, the vaccine should not be used during pregnancy because fetal infection with the attenuated viruses may occur (1–4). The manufacturer and the American College of Obstetricians and Gynecologists state that the vaccine is contraindicated during pregnancy (1,3). In addition, the manufacturer recommends avoiding pregnancy for 3 months following vaccination (3). A shorter interval is recommended by the Centers for Disease Control and Prevention (CDC) (5). They recommend that women who receive the mumps vaccine should avoid becoming pregnant for 30 days (5). However, no cases of congenital malformations attributable to infection with mumps vaccine virus have been reported (5).

BREAST FEEDING SUMMARY

RECOMMENDATION: No Human Data - Probably Compatible

No data are available.

References

1. American College of Obstetricians and Gynecologists. Immunization during pregnancy. *Committee Opinion*. Number 282, January 2003.
2. Amstey MS. Vaccination in pregnancy. Clin Obstet Gynaecol 1983;10:13–22.
3. Product information. Mumpsvax. Merck, 2001.
4. Linder N, Ohel G. *In utero* vaccination. Clin Perinatol 1994;21:663–74.
5. CDC. Measles, mumps, and rubella-vaccine use and strategies for elimination of measles, rubella, and congenital rubella syndrome and control of mumps. Recommendations of the Advisory Committee on Immunization Practices (ACIP). MMWR 1998;47(No. RR-8): 1–57.

V

Name: **VACCINE, PLAGUE** Risk Factor: **C_M**
Class: **Vaccine**

FETAL RISK SUMMARY

RECOMMENDATION: No Human Data - Probably Compatible

Plague vaccine is a killed bacteria vaccine (1). No risk to the fetus from vaccination during pregnancy has been reported.

BREAST FEEDING SUMMARY

RECOMMENDATION: No Human Data - Probably Compatible

No data are available.

Reference

1. Amstey MS. Vaccination in pregnancy. Clin Obstet Gynaecol 1983;10:13–22.

Name:	**VACCINE, PNEUMOCOCCAL POLYVALENT**	Risk Factor:	**C_M**
Class:	**Vaccine**		

FETAL RISK SUMMARY

RECOMMENDATION: Compatible

Pneumococcal vaccine polyvalent is a killed bacteria vaccine that contains a mixture of purified capsular polysaccharides from 23 types of *Streptococcus pneumoniae* (1,2). Animal reproduction studies have not been conducted with the vaccine (1,2).

The risk to the fetus from pneumococcal polysaccharide vaccine during the 1st trimester of pregnancy is unknown (1–4). However, the Immunization Practices Advisory Committee (ACIP) states that there are no reports of adverse consequences in newborns whose mothers were inadvertently vaccinated during pregnancy (4).

The American College of Obstetricians and Gynecologists states that the indications for the vaccine are not altered by pregnancy and recommends that the vaccine be used in pregnancy only for high-risk patients (3). A 1991 review stated that maternal antibodies induced by pneumococcal polyvalent vaccine cross the placenta and may offer significant protection to the newborn (5).

A study conducted in Bangladesh and published in 1995 described the administration of pneumococcal polyvalent vaccine to healthy women at 30–34 weeks' gestation (6). Meningococcal vaccine was administered to a control group. The immunologic response of the infants resulting from the maternal immunization was monitored from birth to 5 months of age. The results indicated that sufficient amounts of specific immunoglobulin G serum antibody passed to the fetus to provide passive immunity to invasive pneumococcal infection in early infancy. The authors concluded that, in geographic regions where such infections are a serious public health problem, maternal immunization would be a safe and inexpensive method to reduce the incidence of the disease, if subsequent studies did not show that passive immunity of the infants interfered with active immunization later in life (6).

In a 1996 study, pneumococcal polyvalent vaccine was administered in the 3rd trimester in an attempt to protect against pneumococcal disease in the infant during the first few months of life (7). The degree and duration of protection was uncertain because the pneumococcal antibodies in the infants disappeared rapidly. A 1998 reference noted that large studies are needed to determine if maternal administration of the vaccine can decrease infant mortality and morbidity (9). Because of the high cost of vaccinations with newly developed conjugate vaccines, one author thought that vaccination of pregnant women with the polysaccharide vaccine might be the most practical method for preventing pneumococcal sepsis in young infants in developing countries (9).

BREAST FEEDING SUMMARY

RECOMMENDATION: No Human Data - Probably Compatible

In a study conducted in Bangladesh (described above), marked increases of specific immunoglobulin A (IgA) antibody titers were measured in the colostrum of mothers who had received pneumococcal polyvalent vaccine at 30–34 weeks' gestation (6). Antibody titers remained higher than controls up to 5 months after delivery.

References

1. Product information. Pneumovax. Merck, 2001.
2. Product information. Pnu-Imune. Lederle Pharmaceutical, 2001.
3. American College of Obstetricians and Gynecologists. Immunization during pregnancy. *Committee Opinion*. Number 282, January 2003.
4. CDC. Prevention of pneumococcal disease: recommendations of the Advisory Committee on Immunization Practices (ACIP). MMWR 1997;46:(No. RR-8):1–24.
5. Faix RG. Maternal immunization to prevent fetal and neonatal infection. Clin Obstet Gynecol 1991;34: 277–87.
6. Shahid NS, Steinhoff MC, Hoque SS, Begum T, Thompson C, Siber GR. Serum, breast milk, and infant antibody after maternal immunisation with pneumococcal vaccine. Lancet 1995;346:1252–7.
7. O'Dempsey TJD, McArdle T, Ceesay SJ, Banya WAS, Demba E, Secka O, Leinonen M, Kayhty H, Francis N, Greenwood BM. Immunization with a pneumococcal capsular polysaccharide vaccine during pregnancy. Vaccine 1996;14:963–70.
8. Mulholland K. Maternal immunization for the prevention of bacterial infection in young infants. Vaccine 1998;16:1464–6.
9. Glezen WP. Pneumococcal polysaccharide vaccine in pregnancy. Pediatrics 1999;104:1417–8.

Name: **VACCINE, POLIOVIRUS INACTIVATED** Risk Factor: **C_M**

Class: **Vaccine**

FETAL RISK SUMMARY

RECOMMENDATION: Compatible

Poliovirus vaccine inactivated (Salk vaccine, IPV) is an inactivated virus vaccine administered by injection (1,2). Animal reproduction studies have not been conducted with the vaccine.

Although fetal damage may occur when the mother contracts the disease during pregnancy, the risk to the fetus from the vaccine is unknown (1). No adverse effects attributable to the use of the inactivated vaccine have been reported (2,3). Both the American College of Obstetricians and Gynecologists and the Immunization Practices Advisory Committee (ACIP) recommend use of the vaccine during pregnancy only if an increased risk of exposure exists (1,3). If immediate protection against poliomyelitis is needed, the ACIP states that either the inactivated or the oral vaccine may be used in accordance with the recommended schedules for adults (see reference for specific details) (3). The inactivated vaccine, however, was preferred over the oral form because of a lower risk of vaccine-associated paralysis.

The Collaborative Perinatal Project monitored 50,282 mother-child pairs, 6774 of whom had 1st-trimester exposure to the vaccine (4, p. 315). Congenital malformations were observed in 461 (standardized relative risk [SRR] 1.03). In general, no associations

(SRR >1.5) were found (4, p. 318). Specific malformations with SRR >1.5 were: craniosynostosis, 6 (SRR 2.1); atrial septal defect, 6 (SRR 4.0); cleft lip with or without cleft palate, 9 (SRR 1.6); omphalocele 5, (SRR 2.4); and any malignant tumors, 7 (SRR 3.3) (4, p. 473–474). For use anytime in pregnancy, 18,219 mother-child pairs were exposed (4, p. 436). A total of 374 newborns had anomalies (SRR 1.08). Specific malformations with SRR >1.5 were: hypoplasia of limb or part thereof, 24 (SRR 1.6); malformations of thoracic wall, 9 (SRR 2.4); anomalies of the teeth, 8 (SRR 2.0); corneal opacity, 5 (SRR 3.5); and central nervous system tumors, 7 (SRR 17.9) (4, p. 486–487). The authors of this study cautioned that these data are uninterpretable without independent confirmation from other studies and that any positive or negative association may have occurred by chance (4).

BREAST FEEDING SUMMARY

RECOMMENDATION: No Human Data - Probably Compatible

No data are available.

References

1. American College of Obstetricians and Gynecologists. Immunization during pregnancy. *Committee Opinion*. Number 282, January 2003.
2. Linder N, Ohel G. In utero vaccination. Clin Perinatol 1994;21:663–74.
3. CDC. Poliomyelitis prevention in the United States: introduction of a sequential vaccination schedule of inactivated poliovirus vaccine followed by oral poliovirus vaccine. Recommendations of the Advisory Committee on Immunization Practices (ACIP). MMWR 1997;46(No. RR-3):1–25.
4. Heinonen OP, Slone D, Shapiro S. *Birth Defects and Drugs in Pregnancy*. Littleton, MA: Publishing Sciences Group, 1977.

Name:	**VACCINE, POLIOVIRUS LIVE**	Risk Factor:	**C_M**
Class:	**Vaccine**		

FETAL RISK SUMMARY

RECOMMENDATION: Compatible

Poliovirus vaccine live (Sabin vaccine; OPV; TOPV) is a live, trivalent (types 1, 2, and 3) attenuated virus strain vaccine administered orally (1).

Although fetal damage may occur when the mother contracts the disease during pregnancy, the risk to the fetus from the vaccine is unknown (1). A brief 1990 report found no increase in spontaneous abortions or adverse effect on the placenta or embryo following 1st-trimester use of oral poliovirus vaccine (2).

Both the American College of Obstetricians and Gynecologists and the Immunization Practices Advisory Committee (ACIP) recommend use of the vaccine during pregnancy only if an increased risk of exposure exists (1,3). If immediate protection against poliomyelitis is needed, the ACIP states that either the inactivated or the oral vaccine may be used in accordance with the recommended schedules for adults (see reference for specific details) (3). The inactivated vaccine, however, was preferred over the oral form because of a lower risk of vaccine-associated paralysis.

The Collaborative Perinatal Project monitored 50,282 mother-child pairs, 1628 of whom had 1st-trimester exposure to oral live poliovirus vaccine (4, p. 315). Congenital malformations were observed in 114 (standardized relative risk [SRR] 1.11) of the newborns. Malformations identified with SRR >1.5 were gastrointestinal (GI) defects (SRR 1.67) and Downs' syndrome (SRR 1.60) (4, p. 319). Specific malformations with SRR >1.5 were omphalocele, 3 (SRR 5.4); malrotation of the GI tract, 5 (SRR 7.9); and any benign tumors, 7 (SRR 1.8) (4, p. 474). For use anytime in pregnancy, 3,059 mother-child pairs were exposed (4, p. 436). In this group, there were 44 malformed children (SRR 0.81) with the following specific malformations having SRR >1.5: Hirschsprung's disease, 4 (SRR 8.8); any benign tumors, 12 (SRR 1.7); and pectus excavatum, 8 (SRR 2.0) (4, p. 487). The authors of this study cautioned that these data are uninterpretable without independent confirmation from other studies and that any positive or negative association may have occurred by chance (4).

The death of a 3-month old male infant because of complications arising from bilateral renal dysplasia affecting predominantly the glomeruli was thought to be possibly caused by maternal vaccination with oral poliovirus vaccine during the 1st or 2nd month of pregnancy (5). A causal relationship, however, could not be established based on the pathologic findings.

A 19-year-old previously immune woman inadvertently received oral poliovirus vaccine at 18 weeks' gestation (6). For other reasons, she requested termination of the pregnancy at 21 weeks' gestation. Polio-like changes were noted in the small-for-dates female fetus (crown-rump and foot length compatible with 17.5–19 weeks' gestation) consisting of damage to the anterior horn cells of the cervical and thoracic spinal cord with more limited secondary skeletal muscle degenerative changes in the arm (6). Poliovirus could not be isolated from the placenta or fetal brain, lung, or liver. Specific fluorescent antibody tests for poliovirus types 2 and 3 were positive in the dorsal spinal cord but not at other sites.

In response to an outbreak of wild-type 3 poliovirus in Finland, a mass vaccination program of adults was initiated with trivalent oral poliovirus vaccine in 1985, with 94% receiving the vaccine during about a 1-month period (7). Because Finland has compulsory notification of all congenital malformations detected during the first year of life, a study was conducted to determine the effect, if any, on the incidence of birth defects from the vaccine. In addition to all defects, two indicator groups were chosen because of their high detection and reporting rates: central nervous system defects and orofacial clefts. No significant changes from the baseline prevalence were noted in the three groups, but the data could not exclude an increase in less common types of congenital defects (7).

A follow-up to the above report was published in 1993 and included all structural malformations that occurred during the 1st trimester (8). The outcomes of approximately 9000 pregnancies were studied, divided nearly equally between those occurring before, during, or after (i.e., one study and two reference cohorts) the vaccination program. Women in the study group had been vaccinated during the 1st trimester (defined as from conception through 15 weeks). A total of 209 cases (2.3%) were identified from liveborns, stillborns, and known abortions. There was no difference in outcomes between the cohorts (the study had a statistical power estimate to detect an increase greater than 0.5%) (8).

The analysis of Finish women receiving the oral poliovirus vaccine during gestation was expanded to anytime during pregnancy in a 1994 report (9). The outcomes of three study groups (about 3000 pregnant women vaccinated in each of the three trimesters of pregnancy) were compared with two reference cohorts (about 6000 pregnant women who delivered before the vaccination program and about 6000 who conceived and delivered afterward). No differences were found between the study and reference groups in terms of intrauterine growth or in the prevalences of stillbirth, neonatal death, congenital anomalies, premature birth, perinatal infection, and neurologic abnormalities (9). The authors concluded that the vaccination of pregnant women with the oral poliovirus vaccine, as conducted in Finland, appeared to be safe.

A 1993 report described the use of oral poliovirus vaccine in a nationwide (Israel) vaccination campaign, including pregnant women, after the occurrence of 15 cases of polio in the summer of 1988 (10). The investigators compared the frequency of anomalies and premature births in their area in 1988 (controls) with those in 1989 (exposed). In 1988, 15,021 live births occurred, with 204 malformed newborns (1.36%) and 999 (6.65%) premature infants. These numbers did not differ statistically from those in 1989; 15,696, 243 (1.55%), and 1,083 (6.87%), respectively. The authors concluded that oral poliovirus vaccine was preferred to the inactivated vaccine if vaccination was required during pregnancy (10).

In a follow up of the Israeli vaccination campaign, investigators measured the presence of neutralizing antibodies to the three poliovirus types in the sera of infants whose mothers had been vaccinated 2–7 weeks before delivery (11). In newborns, higher levels of protecting antibodies were found for poliovirus types 1 and 2 than for type 3, indicating less placental transfer and a greater risk of infection with poliovirus type 3.

BREAST FEEDING SUMMARY

RECOMMENDATION: Compatible

Human milk contains poliovirus antibodies in direct relation to titers found in the mother's serum. When oral poliovirus vaccine (Sabin vaccine, OPV) is administered to the breast-fed infant in the immediate neonatal period, these antibodies, which are highest in colostrum, may prevent infection and development of subsequent immunity to wild poliovirus (12–23). To prevent inhibition of the vaccine, breast feeding should be withheld 6 hours before and after administration of the vaccine, although some authors recommend shorter times (18–22).

In the United States, the ACIP and the Committee on Infectious Diseases of the American Academy of Pediatrics do not recommend vaccination before 6 weeks of age (4,24). At this age or older, the effect of the oral vaccine is not inhibited by breast-feeding and no special instructions or planned feeding schedules are required (4,24–28).

References

1. American College of Obstetricians and Gynecologists. Immunization during pregnancy. *Committee Opinion*. Number 282, January 2003.
2. Ornoy A, Arnon J, Feingold M, Ben Ishai P. Spontaneous abortions following oral poliovirus vaccination in first trimester. Lancet 1990;335:800.
3. CDC. Poliomyelitis prevention in the United States: introduction of a sequential vaccination schedule of inactivated poliovirus vaccine followed by oral poliovirus vaccine. Recommendations of the Advisory Committee on Immunization Practices (ACIP). MMWR 1997;46(No. RR-3):1–25.
4. Heinonen OP, Slone D, Shapiro S. *Birth Defects and Drugs in Pregnancy*. Littleton, MA: Publishing Sciences Group, 1977.
5. Castleman B, McNeely BU. Case records of the Massachusetts General Hospital. Case 47–1964. Presentation of Case. N Engl J Med 1964;271:676–82.
6. Burton AE, Robinson ET, Harper WF, Bell EJ, Boyd JF. Fetal damage after accidental polio vaccination of an immune mother. J R Coll Gen Pract 1984;34:390–4.
7. Harjulehto T, Aro T, Hovi T, Saxen L. Congenital malformations and oral poliovirus vaccination during pregnancy. Lancet 1989;1:771–2.
8. Harjulehto-Mervaala T, Aro T, Hiilesmaa VK, Saxen H, Hovi T, Saxen L. Oral polio vaccination during pregnancy: no increase in the occurrence of congenital malformations. Am J Epidemiol 1993;138:407–14.
9. Harjulehto-Mervaala T, Aro T, Hiilesmaa VK, Hovi T, Saxen H, Saxen L. Oral polio vaccination during pregnancy: lack of impact on fetal development and perinatal outcome. Clin Infect Dis 1994;18:414–20.
10. Ornoy A, Ben Ishai PB. Congenital anomalies after oral poliovirus vaccination during pregnancy. Lancet 1993;341:1162.
11. Linder N, Handsher R, Fruman O, Shiff E, Ohel G, Reichman B, Dagan R. Effect of maternal immunization with oral poliovirus vaccine on neonatal immunity. Pediatr Infect Dis J 1994;13:959–62.

V

12. Lepow ML, Warren RJ, Gray N, Ingram VG, Robbins FC. Effect of Sabin type I poliomyelitis vaccine administered by mouth to newborn infants. N Engl J Med 1961;264:1071–8.
13. Holguin AH, Reeves JS, Gelfand HM. Immunization of infants with the Sabin oral poliovirus vaccine. Am J Public Health 1962;52:600–10.
14. Sabin AB, Fieldsteel AH. Antipoliomyelitic activity of human and bovine colostrum and milk. Pediatrics 1962;29:105–15.
15. Sabin AB, Michaels RH, Krugman S, Eiger ME, Berman PH, Warren J. Effect of oral poliovirus vaccine in newborn children. I. Excretion of virus after ingestion of large doses of type I or of mixture of all three types, in relation to level of placentally transmitted antibody. Pediatrics 1963;31:623–40.
16. Warren RJ, Lepow ML, Bartsch GE, Robbins FC. The relationship of maternal antibody, breast feeding, and age to the susceptibility of newborn infants to infection with attenuated polioviruses. Pediatrics 1964;34:4–13.
17. Plotkin SA, Katz M, Brown RE, Pagano JS. Oral poliovirus vaccination in newborn African infants. The inhibitory effect of breast feeding. Am J Dis Child 1966;111:27–30.
18. Katz M, Plotkin SA. Oral polio immunization of the newborn infant; a possible method for overcoming interference by ingested antibodies. J Pediatr 1968;73:267–70.
19. Adcock E, Greene H. Poliovirus antibodies in breast-fed infants. Lancet 1971;2:662–3.
20. Anonymous. Sabin vaccine in breast-fed infants. Med J Aust 1972;2:175.
21. John TJ. The effect of breast-feeding on the antibody response of infants to trivalent oral poliovirus vaccine. J Pediatr 1974;84:307.
22. Plotkin SA, Katz M. Administration of oral polio vaccine in relation to time of breast-feeding. J Pediatr 1974;84:309.
23. Deforest A, Smith DS. The effect of breast-feeding on the antibody response of infants to trivalent oral poliovirus vaccine (reply). J Pediatr 1974;84:308.
24. Kelein JO, Brunell PA, Cherry JD, Fulginiti VA, eds. *Report of the Committee on Infectious Diseases*. 19th ed. Evanston, IL: American Academy of Pediatrics, 1982:208.
25. Kim-Farley R, Brink E, Orenstein W, Bart K. Vaccination and breast-feeding. JAMA 1982;248:2451–2.
26. Deforest A, Parker PB, DiLiberti JH, Yates HT Jr, Sibinga MS, Smith DS. The effect of breast-feeding on the antibody response of infants to trivalent oral poliovirus vaccine. J Pediatr 1973;83:93–5.
27. John TJ, Devarajan LV, Luther L, Vijayarathnam P. Effect of breast-feeding on seroresponse of infants to oral poliovirus vaccination. Pediatrics 1976;57:47–53.
28. Welsh J, May JT. Breast-feeding and trivalent oral polio vaccine. J Pediatr 1979;95:333.

Name:	**VACCINE, RABIES (HUMAN)**	Risk Factor:	C_M
Class:	**Vaccine**		

FETAL RISK SUMMARY

RECOMMENDATION: Compatible - Maternal Benefit >> Embryo/Fetal Risk

Rabies vaccine (human) is an inactivated virus vaccine (1,2). Animal reproduction studies have not been conducted with the vaccine.

Because rabies is nearly 100% fatal if contracted, the vaccine should be given for postexposure prophylaxis (1,2). The American College of Obstetricians and Gynecologists states that indications for prophylaxis are not altered by pregnancy (1). Three reports described the use of rabies vaccine (human) during pregnancy (3–5). Passive immunity was found in one newborn (titer >1:50) but was lost by 1 year of age (3). No adverse effects from the vaccine were noted in the newborn. The mother had not delivered at the time of the report in the second case (4).

A 1990 brief report described the use of rabies vaccine in 16 pregnant women, 15 using the human diploid cell vaccine and 1 receiving the purified chick embryo cell product (5). In 15 cases, the stage of pregnancy was known: nine 1st trimester, three 2nd trimester, and three 3rd trimester. Two women had spontaneous abortions, but the causes were probably not vaccine related. The remaining pregnancy outcomes were 12 full-term healthy newborns, 1 premature delivery at 36 weeks' gestation, and 1 newborn with grand-mal seizures on the 2nd day. In the latter case, no anti-rabies antibodies were detectable in the infant's serum, indicating that the condition was not vaccine related (5).

In two reports, duck embryo-cultured vaccine was used during pregnancy (6,7). In 1974, a report appeared describing the use of rabies vaccine (duck embryo) in a woman in her 7th month of pregnancy (6). She was given a 21-day treatment course of the vaccine. She subsequently delivered a healthy term male infant who was developing normally at 9 months of age. The second case was described in 1975 involving a woman exposed to rabies at 35 weeks' gestation (7). She was treated with a 14-day course of vaccine (duck embryo) followed by three booster injections. She gave birth at 39 weeks' gestation to a healthy male infant. Cord blood rabies neutralizing antibody titer was 1:30, indicative of passive immunity, compared with a titer of 1:70 in maternal serum. Titers in the infant fell to 1:5 at 3 weeks of age, then to <1:5 at 6 weeks. Development was normal at 9 months of age.

A 1989 report from Thailand described the use of purified Vero cell rabies vaccine for postexposure vaccination in 21 pregnant women (8). Equine rabies immune globulin was also administered to 12 of the women with severe exposures. One patient aborted 3 days after her first rabies vaccination, but she had noted vaginal bleeding on the day of rabies exposure. No congenital malformations were observed and none of the mothers or their infants developed rabies after a 1-year follow-up (8).

In a subsequent prospective study, the above researchers administered the purified Vero cell rabies vaccine (5-dose regimen) after exposure to 202 pregnant women (9). Some of these women also received a single dose of rabies immune globulin (human or equine). Follow-up of 1 year or greater was conducted in 190 patients; 12 patients were lost to follow-up following postexposure treatment. No increase in maternal (spontaneous abortion, hypertension, placenta previa, or gestational diabetes) or fetal (stillbirth, minor birth defect, or low birth weight) complications was observed in comparison with a control group of nonvaccinated, nonexposed women. The one minor congenital defect observed in the treated group was a type of clubfoot (talipes equinovalgus).

BREAST FEEDING SUMMARY

RECOMMENDATION: No Human Data - Probably Compatible

No data are available.

References

1. American College of Obstetricians and Gynecologists. Immunization during pregnancy. *Committee Opinion*. Number 282, January 2003.
2. Amstey MS. Vaccination in pregnancy. Clin Obstet Gynaecol 1983;10:13–22.
3. Varner MW, McGuinness GA, Galask RP. Rabies vaccination in pregnancy. Am J Obstet Gynecol 1982; 143:717–8.
4. Klietmann W, Domres B, Cox JH. Rabies post-exposure treatment and side-effects in man using HDC (MRC 5) vaccine. Dev Biol Stand 1978;40:109–13.
5. Fescharek R, Quast U, Dechert G. Postexposure rabies vaccination during pregnancy: experience from post-marketing surveillance with 16 patients. Vaccine 1990;8:409–10.
6. Cates W Jr. Treatment of rabies exposure during pregnancy. Obstet Gynecol 1974;44:893–6.
7. Spence MR, Davidson DE, Dill GS Jr, Boonthai P, Sagartz JW. Rabies exposure during pregnancy. Am J Obstet Gynecol 1975;123:655–6.
8. Chutivongse S, Wilde H. Postexposure rabies vaccination during pregnancy: experience with 21 patients. Vaccine 1989;7:546–8.
9. Chutivongse S, Wilde H, Benjavongkulchai M, Chomchey P, Punthawong S. Postexposure rabies vaccination during pregnancy: effect on 202 women and their infants. Clin Infect Dis 1995;20:818–20.

Name:	**VACCINE, RUBELLA**	Risk Factor:	C_M
Class:	**Vaccine**		

FETAL RISK SUMMARY

RECOMMENDATION: Contraindicated

Rubella (German measles) vaccine is a live, attenuated virus vaccine (1,2). Animal reproduction studies have not been conducted with the vaccine.

Rubella occurring during pregnancy may result in the congenital rubella syndrome (CRS). The greatest risk period for viremia and congenital defects is 1 week before to 4 weeks after conception (3). Moreover, rubella reinfection, most often presenting as a subclinical infection that can be detected by a rise in antibody titers, may occur in previously vaccinated patients and in those who are naturally immune (4,5). The fetal risk of infection in these cases is low but has not yet been quantified.

The Centers for Disease Control and Prevention (CDC) defines CRS as any two complications from list A or one complication from list A plus one from list B (3):

LIST A
Cataracts or congenital glaucoma
Congenital heart disease
Loss of hearing
Pigmentary retinopathy

LIST B
Purpura
Splenomegaly
Jaundice (onset within 24 hours of birth)
Microcephaly
Mental retardation
Meningoencephalitis
Radiolucent bone disease

Before April 1979, the CDC collected data on 538 women vaccinated within 3 months before or after conception with either the Cendehill or HPV-77 vaccines (3). A total of 149 of these women were known to be susceptible at the time of vaccination and the outcome of pregnancy was known for 143 (96%). No evidence of CRS or other maternal or fetal complication was found in any of these cases or in an additional 196 infants exposed during pregnancy (3). Eight infants had serologic evidence of intrauterine infection after maternal vaccination, but follow-up for 2–7 years revealed no problems attributable to CRS.

V

Since January 1979, only RA 27/3 rubella vaccine has been available in the United States. In the United States between January 1979 and December 1988, a total of 683 women vaccinated with RA 27/3 have been reported to the CDC (6). The outcomes of these pregnancies were:

Total vaccinated (1/79–12/88)	*683*
Susceptible at vaccination	*272*
Live births	212 (2 sets of twins)
Spontaneous abortions or stillbirths	13

Induced abortions	31
Outcome unknown	18
Immune or unknown at vaccination	411
Live births	350 (1 set of twins)
Spontaneous abortions or stillbirths	9
Induced abortions	24
Outcome unknown	29

Evidence of subclinical infection was found in 3 (2%) of the 154 liveborn infants from susceptible mothers who were serologically evaluated (6). However, no evidence of defects compatible with CRS was found in the total sample of 212 liveborn infants. Two infants did have asymptomatic glandular hypospadias, but both mothers had negative rubella-specific immunoglobulin M (IgM) titers in the cord blood at birth (6). In a 1985 evaluation of earlier CDC data, no defects compatible with CRS were found in any of the fetuses or infants in whom the outcome was known (7). Examinations up to 29 months after birth have revealed normal growth and development (6,7).

A 2000 report described six women who received rubella vaccine (live, attenuated vaccine strain RA27/3) either in the pre- or periconceptional periods (8). No evidence of fetal infection was observed in five of the women. In one case, however, vertical transmission of the virus was documented that resulted in persistent fetal infection. The 25-year-old woman, unaware of her pregnancy, received the vaccine 3 weeks after conception. Virus isolation and polymerase chain reaction (PCR) of amniotic fluid obtained by amniocentesis at 16 weeks' gestation confirmed the vertical transmission (8). Multiple maternal and fetal serologic and virologic testings were done throughout the pregnancy. Rising IgG titers and persistent IgM levels were measured in the fetus. At 39 weeks' gestation, a cord blood sample was positive for virus isolation and PCR. Although a persistent rubella viral infection was documented, frequent monitoring of the pregnancy revealed no pathological findings or complications and a healthy, 3450-g male infant was delivered at 40 weeks' gestation. Apgar scores were 9, 9, and 10 at 1, 5, and 10 minutes, respectively. At 23 weeks of age, IgM, PCR, and virus isolation in his peripheral blood were negative. His growth and development have been normal up to 14 months of age (8).

Although no defects attributable to rubella vaccine have been reported, the CDC calculates the theoretical risk of CRS following vaccination with the RA 27/3 vaccine to range from zero to 1.6%, or from zero to 1.2% if data from all rubella vaccines are included (9). These risks are considerably lower than the 20% or greater risk associated with wild rubella virus infection during the 1st trimester (6). Because a theoretical risk does exist, the use of the vaccine in pregnancy is contraindicated (1–3,6,7,9). Moreover, both the manufacturer and the CDC recommend that women should avoid becoming pregnant for 3 months after receiving the vaccine (2,9). However, if vaccination does occur within 3 months of conception or during pregnancy, the actual risk, as stated above, is considered to be negligible and, in itself, should not be an indication to terminate the pregnancy (3,6,7,10,11).

BREAST FEEDING SUMMARY

RECOMMENDATION: Compatible

Vaccination of susceptible women with rubella vaccine in the immediate postpartum period is recommended by the American College of Obstetricians and Gynecologists and the CDC

(1,9). A large number of these women will breast-feed their newborns. Although two studies failed to find evidence of the attenuated virus in milk, subsequent reports have demonstrated transfer (12–16).

In one case, the mother noted rash and adenopathy 12 days after vaccination with the HPV-77 vaccine on the 1st postpartum day (13). Rubella virus was isolated from her breast milk and from the infant's throat (14). A significant level of rubella-specific cell-mediated immunity was found in the infant, but there was no detectable serologic response as measured by rubella hemagglutination inhibition antibody titers (14). No adverse effects were noted in the infant. In a second case report, a 13-day-old breast-fed infant developed rubella about 11 days after maternal vaccination with HPV-77 (17). It could not be determined whether the infant was infected by virus transmission via the milk (18,19). Nine (69%) of 13 lactating women given either HPV-77 or RA 27/3 vaccine in the immediate postpartum period shed virus in their milk (15). In another report by these same researchers, 11 (68%) of 16 vaccinated women shed rubella virus or virus antigen in their milk (16). No adverse effects or symptoms of clinical disease were observed in the infants.

References

1. American College of Obstetricians and Gynecologists. Immunization during pregnancy. *Committee Opinion*. Number 282, January 2003.
2. Product information. Meruvax. Merck, 2001.
3. CDC. Rubella vaccination during pregnancy—United States, 1971–1982. MMWR 1983;32:429–32.
4. Burgess MA. Rubella reinfection—what risk to the fetus? Med J Aust 1992;156:824–5.
5. Condon R, Bower C. Congenital rubella after previous maternal vaccination. Med J Aust 1992;156:882.
6. CDC. Rubella vaccination during pregnancy—United States, 1971–1988. MMWR 1989;38:289–93.
7. Preblud SR, Williams NM. Fetal risk associated with rubella vaccine: implications for vaccination of susceptible women. Obstet Gynecol 1985;66:121–3.
8. Hofmann J, Kortung M, Pustowoit B, Faber R, Piskazeck U, Liebert UG. Persistent fetal rubella vaccine virus infection following inadvertent vaccination during early pregnancy. J Med Virol 2000;61:155–8.
9. CDC. Measles, mumps, and rubella—vaccine use and strategies for elimination of measles, rubella, and congenital rubella syndrome and control of mumps: recommendations of the Advisory Committee on Immunization Practices (ACIP). MMWR 1998;47(No. RR-8):1–57.
10. Burgess MA. Rubella vaccination just before or during pregnancy. Med J Aust 1990;152:507–8.
11. Linder N, Ohel G. *In utero* vaccination. Clin Perinatol 1994;21:663–74.
12. Isacson P, Kehrer AF, Wilson H, Williams S. Comparative study of live, attenuated rubella virus vaccines during the immediate puerperium. Obstet Gynecol 1971;37:332–7.
13. Grillner L, Hedstrom CE, Bergstrom H, Forssman L, Rigner A, Lycke E. Vaccination against rubella of newly delivered women. Scand J Infect Dis 1973;5:237–41.
14. Buimovici-Klein E, Hite RL, Byrne T, Cooper LZ. Isolation of rubella virus in milk after postpartum immunization. J Pediatr 1977;91:939–41.
15. Losonsky GA, Fishaut JM, Strussenberg J, Ogra PL. Effect of immunization against rubella on lactation products. I. Development and characterization of specific immunologic reactivity in breast milk. J Infect Dis 1982;145:654–60.
16. Losonsky GA, Fishaut JM, Strussenberg J, Ogra PL. Effect of immunization against rubella on lactation products. II. Maternal-neonatal interactions. J Infect Dis 1982;145:661–6.
17. Landes RD, Bass JW, Millunchick EW, Oetgen WJ. Neonatal rubella following postpartum maternal immunization. J Pediatr 1980;97:465–7.
18. Lerman SJ. Neonatal rubella following maternal immunization. J Pediatr 1981;98:668.
19. Bass JW, Landes RD. Neonatal rubella following maternal immunization (reply). J Pediatr 1981;98:668–9.

Name: **VACCINE, SMALLPOX** Risk Factor: **X**

Class: **Vaccine**

FETAL RISK SUMMARY

RECOMMENDATION: Human Data Suggest Risk

Smallpox vaccine is a live, attenuated virus vaccine (1,2). Although smallpox infection had a high mortality rate, the disease has been largely eradicated from the world (1,3).

Vaccination during pregnancy between 3 and 24 weeks has resulted in fetal death (2,3). A 1974 reference reviewed the published reports of smallpox vaccination during pregnancy and found 20 cases of fetal vaccinia among more than 8,500 maternal vaccinations (4). Of the 21 exposed fetuses (1 set of twins), only 3 of the 10 liveborns survived. There was only weak evidence, however, that vaccination during the 1st trimester increased fetal wastage compared with that occurring later in gestation (4).

In a 2004 review that documented the rarity of fetal vaccinia, only about 50 cases were found of fetal infection after smallpox vaccination during pregnancy or shortly before conception (5). Although the exact number of women given the vaccine during pregnancy was unknown, the number is probably large because, in past years, pregnant women were routinely vaccinated during outbreaks of smallpox. The 50 cases were documented in women who had received the vaccine at anytime in pregnancy, after primary vaccination and revaccination, and in nonvaccinated women who had contact with vaccines. The authors concluded that there was insufficient evidence to recommend prophylactic treatment with vaccinia immune globulin if the woman was pregnant or shortly before conception when she received the vaccine (5).

The Centers for Disease Control and Prevention (CDC) announced the establishment of the *National Smallpox Vaccine in Pregnancy Registry* in 2003 (6). The Registry was established to monitor pregnancy outcomes of women who had received the vaccine during pregnancy, or who became pregnant or were in close contact with a vaccinee within 28 days after vaccination. Healthcare providers and public health staff were encouraged to report cases by calling (877) 554-4625 or (404) 639-8253 (6).

Two months after the above announcement, the CDC reported, for the period of November 2001–April 2003, that 103 women had received the vaccine either during pregnancy or within 4 weeks of conception (7). The exposures occurred in military personnel, civilian healthcare and public health workers, and clinical studies. In the civilian group, two women conceived within 1 week before vaccination and four conceived within 28 days after vaccination. Two (timing of vaccination not specified) of the six women had early spontaneous abortions (7). Other pregnancy outcomes, other than these two, have apparently not yet been reported.

The CDC classifies smallpox vaccine as contraindicated during pregnancy, within 28 days of conception, and in persons who might have close contact with pregnant women within 28 days of their vaccination (7). Other sources also consider smallpox vaccine to be contraindicated during pregnancy (1–3,8). However, the vaccine should be given to pregnant women who have been exposed to smallpox or monkeypox (7,9). Because the risk for fetal vaccinia is low, inadvertent exposure to the vaccine during or before pregnancy should not be a reason for pregnancy termination (7).

BREAST FEEDING SUMMARY

RECOMMENDATION: Contraindicated

No reports of nursing women receiving smallpox vaccine have been located, In an unusual report, tertiary contact vaccinia transmission from a mother to her nursing infant through direct skin-to-skin and skin-to-mucous membrane contact was documented (10). The father, a soldier in the United States Army, had received smallpox vaccination, but had reportedly taken standard precautions to avoid spread to his family. Approximately 1–2 weeks later, his wife developed vesicles on both areolas. About 2 weeks later, a papule developed on the philtrum of the breast-feeding infant. Polymerase chain reaction and culture for vaccinia of the mother and infant confirmed contact vaccinia (10).

Because of the risk of contact vaccinia in a nursing infant, the CDC recommends that breast-feeding mothers should not be routinely vaccinated (10). However, based on the recommendations during pregnancy, if a nursing woman is exposed to smallpox or monkeypox, she should receive the vaccine but should probably stop breast-feeding.

References

1. Amstey MS. Vaccination in pregnancy. Clin Obstet Gynaecol 1983;10:13–22.
2. American Hospital Formulary Service. *Drug Information 1997*. Bethesda, MD: American Society of Health-System Pharmacists, 1997:2646–9.
3. Hart RJC. Immunization. Clin Obstet Gynaecol 1981;8: 421–30.
4. Levine MM. Live-virus vaccines in pregnancy. Risks and recommendations. Lancet 1974;2:34–8.
5. Napolitano PG, Ryan MAK, Grabenstein JD. Pregnancy discovered after smallpox vaccination: is vaccinia immune globulin appropriate? Am J Obstet Gynecol 2004;191:1863–7.
6. CDC. Notice to readers: National Smallpox Vaccine in Pregnancy Registry. MMWR 2003;52:256.
7. CDC. Women with smallpox vaccine exposure during pregnancy reported to the National Smallpox Vaccine in Pregnancy Registry - United States, 2003. MMWR 2003;52:386–88.
8. Linder N, Ohel G. *In utero* vaccination. Clin Perinatol 1994;21:663–74.
9. Jamieson DJ, Cono J, Richards CL, Treadwell TA. The role of the obstetrician-gynecologist in emerging infectious diseases: monkeypox and pregnancy. Obstet Gynecol 2004;103:754–6.
10. Garde V, Harper D, Fairchok M.P. Tertiary contact vaccinia in a breastfeeding infant. JAMA 2004;291: 725–7.

Name:	**VACCINE, TC-83 VENEZUELAN EQUINE ENCEPHALITIS**	Risk Factor:	**X**
Class:	**Vaccine**		

FETAL RISK SUMMARY

RECOMMENDATION: Contraindicated

A live, attenuated strain of Venezuelan equine encephalitis (VEE) virus, TC-83, is used as a vaccine (1). VEE, transmitted by mosquitoes, is primarily found in South America and Central America, but cases have occurred in Texas (1). Although many human cases of VEE are asymptomatic, some patients may have severe symptoms, including confusion, seizures, and nuchal rigidity (1).

VEE was embryo- and fetotoxic and teratogenic in rats inoculated with the virulent Guajira strain during the first 2 weeks of pregnancy (2). All embryos died within 3–4 days with evidence of necrosis and hemorrhage. Inoculation later in pregnancy resulted in similar outcomes, including infarcts of the placenta.

Fetal rhesus monkeys were administered TC-83 Venezuelan equine encephalitis virus vaccine via the intracerebral route at 100 days' gestation and then were allowed to proceed to term (159–161 days' gestation) (3). All of the infected fetuses were born alive. Some of the newborns were killed and examined within 24 hours of birth, others at 1 month, and the remainder at 3 months. Malformations evident in all of the offspring were microencephaly, hydrocephaly, and cataracts, and two-thirds had porencephaly.

A 1977 brief accounting of the 1962 outbreak of Venezuelan equine encephalitis in Venezuela cited the frequent abortion of women who were infected during the 1st trimester (4). In addition, the infection of seven pregnant women, between the 13th and 36th weeks of gestation, and the subsequent fatal fetal and newborn outcomes were discussed (4). All of the fetuses and newborns had destruction of the fetal cerebral cortex, the degree of which was determined by the interval between infection and delivery. In one of the cases, the mother had severe encephalitis at 13 weeks and eventually gave birth at 33 weeks' gestation. Microcephaly, microphthalmia, luxation of the hips, severe medulla hypoplasia, and the near absence of neural tissue in the cranium were evident in the stillborn fetus (4).

The fatal outcome of a case in which a 21-year-old laboratory worker became pregnant (against medical advice) after receiving the TC-83 vaccine was described in a 1987 report (1). The mother's VEE virus titers were 1:20 at 17 weeks' gestation and 1:10, 3 months later. Maternal serum α-fetoprotein and an ultrasound examination were normal at 17 weeks, but a lack of fetal movement was noted at 26 weeks. One week later, a stillborn, hydropic female fetus was delivered. Generalized edema, ascites, hydrothorax, and a large multilobulated cystic hygroma were noted on examination. Mononuclear infiltrate was found in the myocardium and pulmonary arterioles and an inflammatory cell infiltrate was noted in the trachea, intestinal adventitia, brain, uterus, and fallopian tubes (1). Marked autolysis of the brain had occurred. Abnormalities in the placenta included calcifications, infarcts, petechiae, and thrombosis in the decidua (1).

In summary, only a single case of human pregnancy exposure to TC-83 Venezuelan equine encephalitis vaccine has been reported, but the adverse fetal outcome combined with the animal data indicates that the vaccine should not be given to pregnant women. In the United States, routine immunization is not practiced, but some laboratory workers may require the vaccine because of potential exposure to the virus in their work (1). Based on the available data, pregnancy should be excluded before administration of the vaccine, and the woman warned against conception in the immediate future (in the case above, the woman was advised not to become pregnant for 1 month after vaccination, but references confirming this as a safe interval for this vaccine have not been located)

BREAST FEEDING SUMMARY

RECOMMENDATION: No Human Data - Probably Compatible

No data are available.

References

1. Casamassima AC, Hess LW, Marty A. TC-83 Venezuelan equine encephalitis vaccine exposure during pregnancy. Teratology 1987;36:287–9.
2. Garcia-Tamayo J, Esparza J, Martinez AJ. Placental and fetal alterations due to Venezuelan equine encephalitis virus in rats. Infect Immun 1981;32:813–21.
3. London WT, Levitt NH, Kent SG, Wong VG, Sever JL. Congenital cerebral and ocular malformations induced in rhesus monkeys by Venezuelan equine encephalitis virus. Teratology 1977;16:285–96.
4. Wenger F. Venezuelan equine encephalitis. Teratology 1977;16:359–62.

Name: **VACCINE, TULAREMIA** Risk Factor: **C**

Class: **Vaccine**

FETAL RISK SUMMARY

RECOMMENDATION: Compatible - Maternal Benefit >> Embryo/Fetal Risk

Tularemia vaccine is a live, attenuated bacteria vaccine (1,2). Tularemia is a serious infectious disease occurring primarily in laboratory personnel, rabbit handlers, and forest workers (1).

The risk to the fetus from the vaccine is unknown. One report described vaccination in a woman early in the 1st trimester with transplacental passage of antibodies (2,3). No adverse effects were observed in the term infant or at 1-year follow-up. Because tularemia is a severe disease, preexposure prophylaxis of indicated persons should occur regardless of pregnancy (1).

BREAST FEEDING SUMMARY

RECOMMENDATION: No Human Data - Probably Compatible

No data are available.

References

1. Amstey MS. Vaccination in pregnancy. Clin Obstet Gynaecol 1983;10:13–22.
2. Albrecht RC, Cefalo RC, O'Brien WF. Tularemia immunization in early pregnancy. Am J Obstet Gynecol 1980;138:1226–7.
3. Linder N, Ohel G. In utero vaccination. Clin Perinatol 1994;21:663–74.

Name: **VACCINE, TYPHOID** Risk Factor: **C_M**
Class: **Vaccine**

FETAL RISK SUMMARY

RECOMMENDATION: Compatible - Maternal Benefit >> Embryo/Fetal Risk

Three typhoid vaccines are available: typhoid Vi polysaccharide vaccine that is given IM (1); typhoid vaccine live attenuated oral Ty21a (2); and typhoid vaccine of inactivated (killed) bacteria that is given SC (3). No animal reproduction studies have been conducted with any of the vaccine types.

Typhoid is a serious infectious disease with high morbidity and mortality. The risk to the fetus from the vaccine is unknown (4). The American College of Obstetricians and Gynecologists recommends vaccination during pregnancy only for close, continued exposure or travel to endemic areas (5).

BREAST FEEDING SUMMARY

RECOMMENDATION: No Human Data - Probably Compatible

No data are available.

V

References

1. Product information. Typhim VI. Aventis Pasteur, 2001.
2. Product information. Vivotif Berna Vaccine. Berna Products, 2001.
3. Product information. Typhoid Vaccine. Wyeth-Ayerst Pharmaceuticals, 2001.
4. CDC. Typhoid immunization. Recommendations of the Advisory Committee on Immunization Practices (ACIP). MMWR 1994;43(No. RR-14):1–7.
5. American College of Obstetricians and Gynecologists. Immunization during pregnancy. *Committee Opinion*. Number 282, January 2003.

Name:	**VACCINE, VARICELLA VIRUS**	Risk Factor:	**C_M**
Class:	**Vaccine**		

FETAL RISK SUMMARY

RECOMMENDATION: Contraindicated

Varicella virus vaccine is prepared from the Oka/Merck strain of live, attenuated varicella-zoster virus (1,2). The vaccine became commercially available in May 1995. Animal reproductive studies have not been conducted with the vaccine.

The manufacturer considers vaccination of a woman within 3 months of conception and during pregnancy to be contraindicated because the effects of the vaccine on the fetus are unknown (1). Both the Advisory Committee on Immunization Practices (ACIP) and the American Academy of Pediatrics, however, recommend avoiding pregnancy for only 1 month following an immunization injection (2,3). The American College of Obstetricians and Gynecologists states the vaccine is contraindicated during pregnancy (4). Vaccination of a child is not contraindicated if the child's nonimmune mother or other nonimmune household member is pregnant (2,3).

A large number of references have described the effects of natural (wild) varicella infection during pregnancy on the fetus and newborn (3, 5–40). Infection with wild varicella zoster virus during the first 20 weeks of pregnancy is associated with a risk of congenital varicella syndrome (2,5–7). The syndrome is commonly characterized by low birth weight. Other clinical features, not all of which may be apparent in each case, are shown below (2,5–7):

Cutaneous: cicatricial skin lesions, denuded skin
Neurologic: microcephaly, cortical atrophy, myoclonic seizures, hypotonia, hyporeflexia, encephalomyelitis, dorsal radiculitis, Horner's syndrome, bulbar dysphagia, deafness, mental retardation
Ophthalmic: microphthalmia, chorioretinitis, cataracts, nystagmus, anisocoria, enophthalmos, hypoplasia of the optic discs, optic atrophy, squint
Skeletal: limb hypoplasia of bone and muscle (usually on same side as scarring), hypoplasia of mandible, clavicle, scapula, ribs, fingers and toes, club foot
Gastrointestinal: gastroesophageal reflux, duodenal stenosis, jejunal dilatation, microcolon, atresia of sigmoid colon, malfunction of anal sphincter
Genitourinary: neurogenic bladder

In addition, infection in the 2nd and 3rd trimesters (13 weeks' gestation to term) is associated with a risk of clinical varicella infection during the newborn period or with clinical zoster during infancy and early childhood (2). Severe neonatal varicella may occur in 17%–30% of newborns if the onset of maternal varicella infection is 5 days before to 2 days after delivery (2). Although based on small numbers, possibly affected by reporting bias and not reflective of modern treatment models (data reported in 1974), the death rate in neonates whose mothers had an onset of rash 0–4 days before delivery was 31% (2).

Data from five prospective studies indicate the risk of congenital varicella syndrome during the 1st trimester was 1.0% (6 of 617 infants) (range 0%–9.1%) (5,8–11). A higher risk, 2.0% (7 of 351 infants), was found if the infection occurred during 13–20 weeks' gestation (11). Based on these five studies, the overall incidence of congenital varicella syndrome from maternal infection during the first 20 weeks' gestation was 1.3% (13 of 968).

In addition to children 12 months of age or older who have not had varicella, the ACIP recommends vaccination for nonimmune adults because of the severity of chickenpox in this population (2,3). Vaccination is contraindicated in pregnancy because of the unknown effects of the vaccine on the fetus and because of the known fetal adverse effects of the natural (wild) varicella-zoster virus (1–3).

A 1996 report from the manufacturer's pregnancy registry for Varivax described seven pregnant women who had received the vaccine between June 1995 and late 1996 (41,42). The women, thought to be nonimmune, had been exposed to varicella and were inadvertently given the vaccine instead of the indicated varicella-zoster immune globulin (see also Immune Globulin, Varicella-Zoster [Human]). Moreover, one of the women received 5 times the recommended dose of the vaccine (41,42). None of the women had histories of varicella infection, but their immune status prior to the vaccine was not reported. Four of the seven women had a gestational age at vaccination of <20 weeks, and three had pregnancy durations in the range of >20 weeks to 31 weeks. Two women had delivered healthy children but the outcomes of the other five pregnancies were pending at the time of this report.

The eighth annual report from the Merck/CDC pregnancy registry covered the period from March 17, 1995, through March 16, 2003 (43). These data, which include the first seven pregnancy exposures discussed above, involved 847 reports of women vaccinated 3 months prior to or at any time during pregnancy. Fifty-six women had due dates after March 16, 2004, and were not included in the analysis. The number of enrolled women included 748 prospective cases (reported before the outcome was known) and 43 retrospective exposures (reported after the outcome was known). Thirty-five prospective and three retrospective cases electively terminated their pregnancies. In 498 cases, the timing of vaccine exposure was known: 177 were vaccinated before the last menstrual period (LMP); 318 were vaccinated in the 1st ($N = 294$) and 2nd ($N = 24$) trimesters (highest risk for congenital varicella syndrome); and 3 received the vaccine in the 3rd trimester. Among the 1st trimester exposures, 274 cases were in the period of highest risk for congenital defects (first 8 weeks). The outcomes of the 498 cases with known timing of exposure: Before LMP: spontaneous abortions (SABs) 20, live births 157; 1st trimester: 34 SABs, 1 later fetal death, 283 live births; 2nd trimester: 27 live births; and 3rd trimester: 3 live births. In prospectively reported cases, there were four congenital defects in pregnancies involving SABs (trisomy 13) or elective abortions (trisomy 18; trisomy 21; hydrocephalus) and 11 anomalies in live births (2.4%, 95% confidence interval 1.2–4.3). In none of the outcomes, life births or abortions, was there evidence of congenital varicella syndrome and none of the anomalies were consistent with the congenital varicella syndrome. There were six reports of adverse outcomes in retrospectively reported cases. The anomalies in both groups did not show a specific pattern or target organ and the exposure timing did not support a causative relationship. However, the registry does not have sufficient statistical power to detect an increased risk of rare disorders or individual birth defects (43).

V

A 1997 report described a well-documented case of child-to-mother transmission of varicella-vaccine virus (44). A 12-month-old boy received varicella vaccine and about 3 weeks later had approximately 30 generalized lesions without fever or feeling ill. The lesions were thought to be mild varicella. The 30-year-old mother had a serologic titer negative for varicella and a negative urine pregnancy test at that time. Neither the mother nor her child had any evidence (clinical or laboratory) of immunodeficiency. Sixteen days after appearance of the lesions on her child, she developed a papulovesicular rash diagnosed as varicella. A repeat urine pregnancy was now positive with an estimated gestational age of 5–6 weeks. Five days later, approximately 100 lesions were counted on the mother, who remained afebrile. On repeat test, seroconversion was documented with a positive varicella titer. Virus was isolated from three of the mother's lesions and identified as Oka strain varicella-zoster virus by polymerase chain reaction test, indicating that her lesions resulted from the vaccine administered to her child. She had an elective abortion during the 7th gestational week because of her concerns that the fetus could acquire the congenital varicella syndrome or other malformations. No varicella-zoster virus DNA was isolated from the fetal tissue. The authors, using a transmission rate of 17% reported for vaccinees with leukemia, estimated the risk of virus transmission from a healthy vaccinee with rash to a nonimmune household member to be about 0.85% (44).

In an editorial comment on the above case, the child's medical history before vaccination was thought to be compatible with a significant allergic diathesis (45). Moreover, at the time of the vaccination his eczema was being treated with the topical corticosteroid, desonide 0.05% (45). A combination of factors, including the number of postvaccination lesions on the child, the contribution of the child's eczema to viral expression, the immunosuppression produced by the corticosteroid, the close contact of the mother to the child resulting from the child's age and the application of the topical corticosteroid, and her pregnancy, were believed to account for the abundance of lesions on the mother. The author estimated the maximum theoretical risk for congenital varicella syndrome resulting from the transmission of varicella-vaccine virus to a nonimmune pregnant woman to be less than 1 in 10,000 (<0.01%). The actual risk, however, was thought to be "exponentially lower," possibly 0, because of the rarity of documented viremia in children after vaccination and the absence of reported embryopathy with attenuated varicella-zoster virus (45). Neither the author of the editorial (45) nor another correspondent (46) thought that vaccination of a child should be postponed if a nonimmune mother was pregnant or attempting to conceive.

In summary, the risk of congenital varicella syndrome with natural (wild) varicella virus is approximately 1%–2% during the first 20 weeks of gestation. Moreover, there is significant risk for infectious morbidity and possible mortality in the neonate and young child when maternal varicella infection occurs after the 1st trimester. The risk from the vaccine is thought to be much less, because the virulence of the attenuated virus used in the vaccine is less than that of the natural virus. Although varicella virus vaccine is contraindicated immediately before and during pregnancy because of unknown fetal effects, the potential for harmful fetal effects appears to be very low as estimated above. No cases of varicella vaccine-induced fetal harm have been identified to date. Because of this, the ACIP recommends that a decision to terminate a pregnancy should not be based on whether the vaccine was given during pregnancy (2). Health care professionals are encouraged to report patients who receive the vaccine 3 months before or at any time during pregnancy to the Varivax Pregnancy Registry by calling (800)-986-8999.

BREAST FEEDING SUMMARY

RECOMMENDATION: Compatible

V

In a 1986 study, no viruses were cultured from the breast milk of two women with varicella-zoster virus infections (47). One of the women had a herpes zoster dermatitis 6 months postpartum and was nursing. Direct lesion contact was prevented, and she continued to breast-feed. In the other case, the woman developed varicella pneumonia at 40 weeks' gestation and her infant was delivered by emergency cesarean section. The infant did not become infected after prophylactic treatment with immune globulin varicella-zoster (human) and parenteral acyclovir. In spite of the mother's serious postpartum condition, she maintained lactation with a breast pump. Although a varicella virus culture of the milk was negative, the milk was not given to her infant, nor was the infant allowed to breast-feed (47).

A 2003 study reported that varicella DNA was not detected in 217 postvaccination samples of breast milk from 12 women who had received two doses of vaccine (48). Because there was no evidence of varicella vaccine virus excretion into milk, the investigators concluded that there was no need to delay vaccination in breast-feeding women (48).

Both the Centers for Disease Control and Prevention (CDC) and the American Academy of Pediatrics consider the vaccination of a varicella-zoster virus-susceptible nursing mother to be appropriate if the risk of exposure to the natural virus is high (2,3).

References

1. Product information. Varivax. Merck, 2000.
2. CDC. Prevention of varicella. MMWR 1996;45(RR-11):1–36.
3. Committee on Infectious Diseases, American Academy of Pediatrics. Recommendations for the use of live attenuated varicella vaccine. Pediatrics 1995;95:791–6.
4. American College of Obstetricians and Gynecologists. Immunization during pregnancy. *Committee Opinion*. Number 282, January 2003.
5. Pastuszak AL, Levy M, Schick B, Zuber C, Feldkamp M, Gladstone J, Bar-Levy F, Jackson E, Donnenfeld A, Meschino W, Koren G. Outcome after maternal varicella infection in the first 20 weeks of pregnancy. N Engl J Med 1994;330:901–5.
6. Dickinson J, Gonik B. Teratogenic viral infections. Clin Obstet Gynecol 1990;33:242–52.
7. Birthistle K, Carrington D. Fetal varicella syndrome—a reappraisal of the literature. J Infect 1998;36(Suppl 1):25–9.
8. Siegel M. Congenital malformations following chickenpox, measles, mumps, and hepatitis. Results of a cohort study. JAMA 1973;226:1521–4.
9. Paryani SG, Arvin AM. Intrauterine infection with varicella-zoster virus after maternal varicella. N Engl J Med 1986;314:1542–6.
10. Balducci J, Rodis JF, Rosengren S, Vintzileos AM, Spivey G, Vosseller C. Pregnancy outcome following first-trimester varicella infection. Obstet Gynecol 1992;79:5–6.
11. Enders G, Miller E, Cradock-Watson J, Bolley I, Ridehalgh M. Consequences of varicella and herpes zoster in pregnancy: prospective study of 1739 cases. Lancet 1994;343:1547–50.
12. Laforet EG, Lynch CL Jr. Multiple congenital defects following maternal varicella. Report of a case. N Engl J Med 1947;236:534–7.
13. Harris RE, Rhoades ER. Varicella pneumonia complicating pregnancy. Report of a case and review of literature. Obstet Gynecol 1965;25:734–40.
14. Sever J, White LR. Intrauterine viral infections. Annu Rev Med 1968;19:471–86.
15. McKendry JBJ, Bailey JD. Congenital varicella associated with multiple defects. Can Med Assoc J 1973;108:66–8.
16. Savage MO, Moosa A, Gordon RR. Maternal varicella infection as a cause of fetal malformations. Lancet 1973;1:352–4.
17. Srabstein JC, Morris N, Larke RPB, DeSa DJ, Castelino BB, Sum E. Is there a congenital varicella syndrome? J Pediatr 1974;84:239–43.
18. Frey HM, Bialkin G, Gershon AA. Congenital varicella: case report of a serologically proved long-term survivor. Pediatrics 1977;59:110–2.
19. Bai PVA, John TJ. Congenital skin ulcers following varicella in late pregnancy. J Pediatr 1979;94:65–7.
20. Enders G. Varicella-zoster virus infection in pregnancy. Prog Med Virol 1984;29:166–96.
21. Landsberger EJ, Hager WD, Grossman JH III. Successful management of varicella pneumonia complicating pregnancy. A report of three cases. J Reprod Med 1986;31:311–4.
22. Hockberger RS, Rothstein RJ. Varicella pneumonia in adults: a spectrum of disease. Ann Emerg Med 1986;15:931–4.
23. Glaser JB, Loftus J, Ferragamo V, Mootabar H, Castellano M. Varicella-zoster infection in pregnancy. N Engl J Med 1986;315:1416.
24. Preblud SR, Cochi SL, Orenstein WA. Varicella-zoster infection in pregnancy. N Engl J Med 1986;315:1416–7.
25. Trlifajova J, Benda R, Benes C. Effect of maternal varicella-zoster virus infection on the outcome of pregnancy and the analysis of transplacental virus transmission. Acta Virol 1986;30:249–55.
26. Alkalay AL, Pomerance JJ, Rimoin DL. Fetal varicella syndrome. J Pediatr 1987;111:320–3.
27. Higa K, Dan K, Manabe H. Varicella-zoster virus infections during pregnancy: hypothesis concerning the mechanisms of congenital malformations. Obstet Gynecol 1987;69:214–22.
28. Hankins GDV, Gilstrap LC III, Patterson AR. Acyclovir treatment of varicella pneumonia in pregnancy. Crit Care Med 1987;15:336–7.
29. Eder SE, Apuzzio JJ, Weiss G. Varicella pneumonia during pregnancy. Treatment of two cases with acyclovir. Am J Perinatol 1988;5:16–8.
30. Boyd K, Walder E. Use of acyclovir to treat chickenpox in pregnancy. BMJ 1988;296:393–4.
31. Smego RA Jr, Asperilla MO. Use of acyclovir for

V

varicella pneumonia during pregnancy. Obstet Gynecol 1991;78:1112–6.
32. Broussard RC, Payne K, George RB. Treatment with acyclovir of varicella pneumonia in pregnancy. Chest 1991;99:1045–7.
33. Michie CA, Acolet D, Charlton R, Stevens JP, Happerfield LC, Bobrow LG, Kangro H, Gau G, Modi N. Varicella-zoster contracted in the second trimester of pregnancy. Pediatr Infect Dis J 1992;11:1050–3.
34. Pretorius DH, Hayward I, Jones KL, Stamm E. Sonographic evaluation of pregnancies with maternal varicella infection. J Ultrasound Med 1992;11:459–63.
35. Whitty JE, Renfroe YR, Bottoms SF, Isada NB, Iverson R, Cotton DB. Varicella pneumonia in pregnancy: clinical experience (abstract). Am J Obstet Gynecol 1993;168:427.
36. Martin KA, Junker AK, Thomas EE, Van Allen MI, Friedman JM. Occurrence of chickenpox during pregnancy in women seropositive for varicella-zoster virus. J Infect Dis 1994;170:991–5.
37. Jones KL, Johnson KA, Chambers CD. Offspring of women infected with varicella during pregnancy: a prospective study. Teratology 1994;49:29–32.
38. Andreou A, Basiakos H, Hatzikoumi I, Lazarides A. Fetal varicella syndrome with manifestations limited to the eye. Am J Perinatol 1995;12:347–8.
39. Figueroa-Damian R, Arredondo-Garcia JL. Perinatal outcome of pregnancies complicated with varicella infection during the first 20 weeks of gestation. Am J Perinatol 1997;14:411–4.
40. Nathwani D, Maclean A, Conway S, Carrington D. Varicella infections in pregnancy and the newborn. A review prepared for the UK Advisory Group on Chickenpox on behalf of the British Society for the Study of Infection. J Infect 1998;36(Suppl 1):59–71.
41. CDC. Unintentional administration of varicella virus vaccine—United States, 1996. MMWR 1996;45:1017–8.
42. CDC. Unintentional administration of varicella virus vaccine—United States, 1996. MMWR 1996;45:1017–8 as cited in JAMA 1996;276:1792.
43. Merck/CDC Pregnancy Registry for Varivax: the 8th annual report, 2003. Covering the period from approval (March 17, 1995) through March 16, 2003.
44. Salzman MB, Sharrar RG, Steinberg S, LaRussa P. Transmission of varicella-vaccine virus from a healthy 12-month-old child to his pregnant mother. J Pediatr 1997;131:151–4.
45. Long SS. Toddler-to-mother transmission of varicella-vaccine virus: how bad is that? J Pediatr 1997;131:10–2.
46. Wald ER. Transmission of varicella-vaccine virus: what is the risk? J Pediatr 1998;133:310.
47. Frederick IB, White RJ, Braddock SW. Excretion of varicella-herpes zoster virus in breast milk. Am J Obstet Gynecol 1986;154:1116–7.
48. Bohlke K, Galil K, Jackson LA, Schmid DS, Starkovich P, Loparev VN, Seward JF. Postpartum varicella vaccination: is the vaccine virus excreted in breast milk? Obstet Gynecol 2003;102:970–7.

Name:	**VACCINE, YELLOW FEVER**	Risk Factor:	**D**
Class:	**Vaccine**		

FETAL RISK SUMMARY

RECOMMENDATION: Compatible - Maternal Benefit >> Embryo/Fetal Risk

Yellow fever vaccine is a live, attenuated virus vaccine (1,2). Yellow fever is a serious infectious disease with high morbidity and mortality. The risk to the fetus from the vaccine is unknown (1,2). The American College of Obstetricians and Gynecologists states that the vaccine is contraindicated in pregnancy except if exposure is unavoidable (1).

The Collaborative Perinatal Project monitored 50,282 mother-child pairs, 3 of whom had 1st trimester exposure to yellow fever vaccine (3). There were no birth defects.

A 1993 report described the use of yellow fever vaccine (vaccine strain 17D) in 101 women at various stages of pregnancy during the 1986 outbreak of yellow fever in Nigeria (4). The women received the vaccine during gestation either because of an unknown pregnancy or because they feared acquiring the disease. The vaccine was administered to 4 women in the 1st trimester, 8 in the 2nd trimester, and 89 in the 3rd trimester, with the gestational ages ranging from 6 to 38 weeks. Serum samples were obtained before and after vaccination from the women as well as from 115 vaccinated, nonpregnant controls. Measurements of immunoglobulin M (IgM) antibody and neutralizing antibody in these samples revealed that the immune response of pregnant women was significantly lower than that of controls. One woman, with symptoms of acute yellow fever during the week before vaccination, suffered a spontaneous abortion 8 weeks after vaccination. Although the cause of the abortion was unknown, the investigators concluded that it was not caused by the vaccine. No evidence was found for transplacental passage of the attenuated virus. Nine of the mothers produced IgM antibody after vaccination, but the antibody was not detected in their newborns. Neutralizing antibody either crossed the placenta or was transferred via colostrum in 14 of 16 newborns delivered from mothers with this antibody. No adverse effects on physical or mental development were observed in the offspring during a 3- to 4- year follow-up period (4).

The first reported case of congenital infection following vaccination was described in a study in which attenuated yellow fever vaccine, in response to a threat of epidemic yellow fever, was administered to 400,000 people in Trinidad (5). Pregnant women, all of whom received the vaccine during the 1st trimester during pregnancies unrecognized at the time of vaccination, were identified retrospectively. Serum samples were collected from 47 women and 41 term infants, including 35 mother-child pairs. Women who delivered prematurely and those suffering spontaneous abortions were not sampled. One of the 41 infants had IgM and elevated neutralizing antibodies to yellow fever, indicating congenital infection. Natural exposure to the virus was thought to be unlikely because virus transmission during that period was limited to forest monkeys with no human cases reported. The infected, 2920-g infant, the product of a normal, full-term pregnancy, appeared healthy on examination and without observable effect on morphogenesis. However, because the neurotropism of yellow fever virus for the developing nervous system has been well documented (e.g., vaccine-induced encephalitis occurs almost exclusively in infants and young children), the authors considered this case as further evidence that the vaccine should be avoided during pregnancy (5).

A 1999 report from the European Network of Teratology Information Services described the prospectively ascertained outcomes in 58 of 74 pregnancies exposed to yellow fever vaccine (6). Timing of exposure was before the last menstrual period (LMP), in the 1st trimester, or in the 2nd trimester in 3, 69, and 2, respectively. Sixteen of the cases did not have complete follow-up data and were excluded from the analysis. The pregnancy outcomes included 7 spontaneous abortions, 5 induced abortions, and 46 live births. In the newborns, there were two major malformations: ureteral stenosis and triphalangeal hallux. There were also three cases of minor anomalies: bilateral pes varus, slight deviation of the nasal wall, and mild ventricular septal defect. Vaccination in all of these five cases occurred early in gestation. The rates of abortion and congenital malformations are within expected ranges. The investigators also found 4 cases exposed *in utero* to yellow fever vaccine among 23,925 cases of birth defects reported between 1980 and 1995 to the France/Central-East registry of malformations. The defects in these cases were (timing of exposure in parentheses) right ectromelia of upper limb (1st trimester), a VATER association (2nd trimester), stenosis of the aortic orificium (1st trimester), and hydrocephalus in an infant stillborn near term (2nd trimester). Two other cases of spontaneous abortion (respectively at 6 and 13 weeks after the LMP) were reported by a French manufacturer to the investigators. The authors concluded that although their sample was far too small to rule out a moderate increased risk of adverse outcome, their data do not support such an association and could be used to reassure pregnant women who have inadvertently received the vaccine (6).

A 1994 review concluded that pregnant women should be vaccinated, preferably after the 1st trimester, if exposure to a yellow fever epidemic is unavoidable (7).

BREAST FEEDING SUMMARY

RECOMMENDATION: No Human Data - Probably Compatible

No data are available.

References

1. American College of Obstetricians and Gynecologists. Immunization during pregnancy. *Committee Opinion*. Number 282, January 2003.
2. Amstey MS. Vaccination in pregnancy. Clin Obstet Gynaecol 1983;10:13–22.
3. Heinonen OP, Slone D, Shapiro S. *Birth Defects and Drugs in Pregnancy*. Littleton, MA: Publishing Sciences Group, 1977:315.
4. Nasidi A, Monath TP, Vandenberg J, Tomori O, Calisher CH, Hurtgen X, Munube GRR, Sorungbe AOO, Okafor GC, Wali S. Yellow fever vaccination and pregnancy: a four-year prospective study. Trans R Soc Trop Med Hyg 1993;87:337–9.
5. Tsai TF, Paul R, Lynberg MC, Letson GW. Congenital yellow fever virus infection after immunization in pregnancy. J Infect Dis 1993;168:1520–3.
6. Robert E, Vial T, Schaefer C, Arnon J, Reuvers M. Exposure to yellow fever vaccine in early pregnancy. Vaccine 1999;17:283–5.
7. Linder N, Ohel G. *In utero* vaccination. Clin Perinatol 1994;21:663–74.

Name:	**VALACYCLOVIR**	Risk Factor:	B_M
Class:	**Antiviral**		

FETAL RISK SUMMARY

RECOMMENDATION: Compatible

Valacyclovir is biotransformed to acyclovir and *L*-valine by first-pass intestinal and/or hepatic metabolism. The drug is active against herpes simplex virus types 1 and 2 and varicella-zoster virus. It is used in the treatment of herpes zoster (shingles) and recurrent genital herpes simplex.

Reproduction studies were conducted in rats and rabbits during organogenesis with doses producing concentrations 10 and 7 times human plasma levels, respectively (1). No teratogenic effects were observed with these doses.

The active metabolite, acyclovir, readily crosses the human placenta (see Acyclovir). An abstract and study, both published in 1998, compared the pharmacokinetics of valacyclovir and acyclovir in late pregnancy (2,3). Acyclovir accumulated in the amniotic fluid but not in the fetus. The mean maternal/umbilical vein plasma ratio at delivery was 1.7.

The Valacyclovir Pregnancy Registry listed 157 prospective reports of women exposed to the oral antiviral drug during gestation covering the period from January 1, 1995, through April 30, 1999 (4). Of the total, 47 (30%) pregnancies were lost to follow-up. Among the 111 (1 set of twins) known outcomes, 29 had earliest exposure in the 1st trimester and their outcomes were 5 spontaneous abortions, 2 induced abortions, 1 infant with a birth defect (talipes), and 21 infants (including the twins) without birth defects. When the earliest exposure was in the 2nd trimester, 31 pregnancies were enrolled and their outcomes were 2 stillbirths, 2 infants with birth defects (fingers and toes fused—extensive webbing; small cleft in front gum), and 27 without birth defects. In the remaining 51, the earliest exposure occurred in the 3rd trimester, with 1 infant with a dermal sinus tract and 50 without birth defects (4).

A total of 34 retrospective reports of valacyclovir exposure during pregnancy were submitted to the Registry (4). Two of the exposures occurred during an unspecified gestational time and both resulted in live births without defects. In 14 pregnancies, the earliest exposure occurred during the 1st trimester. The outcomes of these pregnancies were three spontaneous losses, eight induced abortions, and three infants without birth defects. For the pregnancies whose earliest exposure was in the 2nd trimester ($N = 4$) or 3rd trimester ($N = 14$), there was 1 birth defect (2nd trimester exposure) and 17 infants without defects.

A 1999 case report described a woman at 20 weeks' gestation that had a generalized herpes simplex virus infection that was treated with IV acyclovir for about 2 weeks followed by valacyclovir for the remainder of the pregnancy (5). She delivered a full-term, healthy female infant who was treated prophylactically with oral acyclovir for 1 month. No abnormalities were detected during a neurologic examination at 8 months of age.

Except for the above data, no other reports describing the use of valacyclovir during human pregnancy have been located. However, a large number of studies have reported the use of the active metabolite, acyclovir, during human pregnancy (see also Acyclovir). Based on the combined data, there does not appear to be any major risk to the human fetus from valacyclovir or acyclovir. Long-term follow-up of children exposed *in utero* to these agents is warranted.

BREAST FEEDING SUMMARY

RECOMMENDATION: Compatible

Valacyclovir is rapidly and nearly completely converted to acyclovir and the amino acid, *L*-valine. Acyclovir is concentrated in human milk with milk:plasma ratios in the 3–4 range (see Acyclovir).

In a 2002 study, five healthy postpartum women that were breast-feeding were given valacyclovir (500 mg twice daily for 7 days) (6). Maternal serum and milk samples were collected after the first dose, on day 5, and 24 hours after the last dose. Infant urine samples were collected on day 5. All samples were analyzed for acyclovir. The peak milk concentration occurred 4 hours after the first dose (milk:serum ratio 3.4), whereas the peak serum level occurred at 2 hours. At steady state, the milk:serum ratio was about 1.9. The median infant urine acyclovir concentration was 0.74 μg/mL. Twenty-four hours after the last dose the milk:serum ratio was 0.25. The estimated infant dose (based on a consumption of 750 mL/day of milk by a 2.75-kg infant) would be about 0.2% of the therapeutic dose for neonates (6).

Because acyclovir has been used to treat herpesvirus infections in the neonate, and because of the lack of adverse effects in reported cases in which acyclovir was used during breast-feeding, the American Academy of Pediatrics classifies acyclovir as compatible with breast-feeding (see Acyclovir). Valacyclovir is compatible with breast-feeding.

References

1. Product information. Valtrex. Glaxo Wellcome, 1997.
2. Kimberlin DF, Weller S, Andrews WW, Hauth JC, Whitley RJ, Lakeman F, Miller G, Lee C, Goldenberg RL. Valacyclovir pharmacokinetics in late pregnancy (abstract). Am J Obstet Gynecol 1998;178:S12.
3. Kimberlin DF, Weller S, Whitley RJ, Andrews WW, Hauth JC, Lakeman F, Miller G. Pharmacokinetics of oral valacyclovir and acyclovir in late pregnancy. Am J Obstet Gynecol 1998;179:846–51.
4. Acyclovir Pregnancy Registry and Valacyclovir Pregnancy Registry. Final study report. 1 June 1984 through 30 April 1999. Glaxo Wellcome, 1999.
5. Anderson R, Lundqvist A, Bergstrom T. Successful treatment of generalized primary herpes simplex type 2 infection during pregnancy. Scand J Infect Dis 1999;31:201–2.
6. Sheffield JS, Fish DN, Hollier LM, Cadematori S, Nobles BJ, Wendel GD Jr. Acyclovir concentrations in human breast milk after valacyclovir administration. Am J Obstet Gynecol 2002;186:100–2.

Name:	**VALDECOXIB**	Risk Factor:	C_M*
Class:	**Nonsteroidal Anti-inflammatory**		

FETAL RISK SUMMARY

RECOMMENDATION: Human Data Suggest Risk in 1st and 3rd Trimesters

Valdecoxib is a second-generation nonsteroidal anti-inflammatory agent (NSAID) that inhibits prostaglandin synthesis via the inhibition of cyclooxygenase-2 (COX-2). It is indicated for the relief of the signs and symptoms of osteoarthritis and adult rheumatoid arthritis, and for the treatment of primary dysmenorrhea. Valdecoxib is in the same NSAID subclass (COX-2 inhibitors) as celecoxib and rofecoxib. At therapeutic concentrations, it does not inhibit, as do the first-generation NSAIDs, the cyclooxygenase-1 (COX-1) isoenzyme. One active metabolite has been identified in plasma at about 10% the concentration of valdecoxib, but it is a less potent COX-2 inhibitor and is not thought to contribute significantly to the efficacy profile of valdecoxib. Plasma protein binding of valdecoxib is about 98% and the elimination half-life is about 8 hours (1).

Reproduction studies have been conducted in rats and rabbits. In rats, oral doses up to about 19 times the human exposure at 20 mg/day based on $AUC_{0-24hours}$ (HD) revealed no evidence of teratogenicity. At this dose during organogenesis, however, there was an increased incidence of pre- and post-implantation loss resulting in fewer live fetuses. Treatment throughout organogenesis and the lactation period with a dose seven times the HD resulted in decreased neonatal survival and neonatal body weight. In rabbits, a dose approximately 8 times the HD was not teratogenic, but increasing the dose to about 72 times the HD caused a slightly higher incidence of fetuses with skeletal malformations (semi-bipartite thoracic vertebra centra and fused sternebrae). The higher dose during organogenesis also resulted in an increased incidence of pre- and post-implantation loss resulting in fewer live fetuses (1).

Valdecoxib crosses the placenta in rats and rabbits (1). It is not known if the drug or its active metabolite cross the human placenta. The molecular weight (about 314), lipid solubility, and moderately long elimination half-life suggest that valdecoxib should cross the human placenta. The extensive plasma protein binding, however, should limit the amount of drug reaching the embryo or fetus.

A combined 2001 population-based observational cohort study and a case-control study estimated the risk of adverse pregnancy outcome from the use of NSAIDs (2). The use of NSAIDs during pregnancy was not associated with congenital malformations, preterm delivery, or low birth weight, but a positive association was discovered with spontaneous abortions (SABs). A similar study, also published in 2001, failed to find a relationship, in general, between NSAIDs and congenital malformations, but did find a significant association with cardiac defects and orofacial clefts (3). In addition, a 2003 study found a significant association between exposure to NSAIDs in early pregnancy and SABs (4). (See Ibuprofen for details on the three studies.)

No reports describing the use of valdecoxib in human pregnancy have been located. The animal data are suggestive of a low risk for congenital malformations. Moreover, a brief 2003 editorial on the potential for NSAID-induced developmental toxicity concluded that NSAIDs, and specifically those with greater COX-2 affinity, had a lower risk of this toxicity in humans than aspirin (5). However, the animal data are consistent with the human reports of early pregnancy loss.

The use of first-generation NSAIDs during the latter half of pregnancy has been associated with oligohydramnios and premature closure of the ductus arteriosus (e.g., see Indomethacin) (6). Persistent pulmonary hypertension of the newborn may occur if NSAIDs are used in the 3rd trimester close to delivery (6,7). These drugs also have been shown to inhibit labor and prolong pregnancy, both in humans (8) and in animals (9). Similar effects should be expected in valdecoxib is used during the 3rd trimester or close to delivery. Women attempting to conceive should not use any prostaglandin synthesis inhibitor, including valdecoxib, because of the findings in a variety of animal models that indicate these agents block blastocyst implantation (10,11). Moreover, as noted above, NSAIDs have been associated with SABs in humans. If valdecoxib is used in pregnancy for the treatment of rheumatoid arthritis, healthcare professionals are requested to call the toll free number (877)-311-8972 for information about patient enrollment in the OTIS Rheumatoid Arthritis study.

[**Risk Factor D if used in 3rd trimester or near delivery.*]

BREAST FEEDING SUMMARY

RECOMMENDATION: No Human Data - Potential Toxicity

No reports describing the use of valdecoxib during human lactation have been reported. Valdecoxib and its active metabolite are excreted in the milk of lactating rats (1). The molecular weight (about 314), lipid solubility, and relatively long elimination half-life (about 8 hours) suggest that valdecoxib will be excreted into breast milk. The extensive plasma protein binding, however, should limit the amount in milk. The effects of this exposure on a nursing infant are unknown. Although several first-generation NSAIDS are considered low-risk during nursing (e.g., see Diclofenac, Fenoprofen, Flurbiprofen, Ibuprofen, Ketoprofen, Ketorolac, and Tolmetin), the relatively long adult plasma half-life of valdecoxib and the absence of clinical pharmacologic data in infants suggest that this agent should be avoided during nursing.

References

1. Product information. Bextra. Pfizer, 2004.
2. Nielsen GL, Sorensen HT, Larsen H, Pedersen L. Risk of adverse birth outcome and miscarriage in pregnant users of non-steroidal anti-inflammatory drugs: population based observational study and case-control study. BMJ 2001;322:266–70.
3. Ericson A, Kallen BAJ. Nonsteroidal anti-inflammatory drugs in early pregnancy. Reprod Toxicol 2001;15:371–5.
4. Li DK, Liu L, Odouli R. Exposure to non-steroidal anti-inflammatory drugs during pregnancy and risk of miscarriage: population based cohort study. BMJ 2003;327:368–71.
5. Tassinari MS, Cook JC, Hurtt ME. NSAIDs and developmental toxicity. Birth Defects Res Part B Dev Reprod Toxicol 2003;68:3–4.
6. Levin DL. Effects of inhibition of prostaglandin synthesis on fetal development, oxygenation, and the fetal circulation. Semin Perinatol 1980;4:35–44.
7. Van Marter LJ, Leviton A, Allred EN, Pagano M, Sullivan KF, Cohen A, Epstein MF. Persistent pulmonary hypertension of the newborn and smoking and aspirin and nonsteroidal antiinflammatory drug consumption during pregnancy. Pediatrics 1996;97:658–63.
8. Fuchs F. Prevention of prematurity. Am J Obstet Gynecol 1976;126:809–20.
9. Powell JG, Cochrane RL. The effects of a number of non-steroidal anti-inflammatory compounds on parturition in the rat. Prostaglandins 1982;23:469–88.
10. Matt DW, Borzelleca JF. Toxic effects on the female reproductive system during pregnancy, parturition, and lactation. In Witorsch RJ, ed. *Reproductive Toxicology*. 2nd ed. New York, NY: Raven Press, 1995:175–93.
11. Dawood MY. Nonsteroidal antiinflammatory drugs and reproduction. Am J Obstet Gynecol 1993;169:1255–65.

Name:	**VALERIAN**	Risk Factor:	**B**
Class:	**Herb**		

FETAL RISK SUMMARY

RECOMMENDATION: Limited Human Data - No Relevant Animal Data

Valeriana officinalis, the plant most often used for medicinal purposes, is one species of approximately 200 of the genus *Valeriana*, an herbaceous perennial that grows widely in the temperate regions of North America, Europe, and Asia (1). A large number of preparations containing valerian are commercially available (2). The herb is used as a sedative and hypnotic for anxiety, restlessness, and sleep disturbances (1–5). Other pharmacologic claims that have been made for valerian include antispasmodic, anticonvulsive, antidepressant, and antihypertensive properties (1,3,4). The extracts and root oil have also been used as flavorings for foods and beverages (1).

Although the specific agents responsible for the effects of valerian are unknown, as is the mechanism of action, three classes of compounds have been identified: a volatile oil that contains sesquiterpenes; nonglycosidic iridoid esters (known as valepotriates); and alkaloids (1,3). Of these, the valepotriates, found primarily in the roots, are most likely responsible for the sedative action, but components from the other two classes probably contribute as well (1,3). Because these compounds produce central nervous system depression, they should not be used with other depressants, such as alcohol, benzodiazepines, barbiturates, or opiates (3–5). Moreover, nonpregnant adult human hepatotoxicity has been associated with short-term use (i.e., a few days to several months) of herbal preparations containing valerian (6). Long-term use in a male has also been associated with benzodiazepine-like withdrawal symptoms resulting in cardiac complications and delirium (7).

Reproductive studies in animals with valerian have not shown antiovulation, antifertilization, or embryotoxic effects (8). Furthermore, the valepotriates exhibit low toxicity in mice, producing no deaths in doses of up to 1600 mg/kg intraperitoneally or 4600 mg/kg orally (1). Toxicity in mice was characterized by ataxia, hypothermia, and increased muscle relaxation (1).

The cytotoxic activities of three valepotriate compounds, valtrate, didrovaltrate, and baldrinal (a degradation product of valtrate), in cultured rat hepatoma cells were described in a 1981 reference (9). Both valtrate and didrovaltrate demonstrated much greater cytotoxic activity than did baldrinal, with rapid and irreversible toxicity. In addition, the antitumor activity of didrovaltrate was demonstrated *in vivo* on female mice KREBS II ascitic tumors (9). Five surviving mice were then bred with normal male mice 50 days after treatment with didrovaltrate. Each had a normal pregnancy and produced normal offspring.

In a 1988 report, two cases of attempted suicide with valerian dry extract plus other drugs were described (10). In one case, a woman at 10 weeks' gestation ingested 2.5 g of valerian dry extract and 0.5 g of phenobarbital. An apparently normal, 4350-g female infant was delivered at 42 weeks' gestation. Examination of the child (age not specified) indicated an IQ in the range of 111 to 120. In the second case, the mother ingested a combination of valerian dry extract (3.0 g), phenobarbital (0.6 g), glutethimide (5.0 g), amobarbital (5.0 g), and promethazine (0.3 g) at 20 weeks' gestation. A mentally retarded, 2650-g male infant was born at 36 weeks' gestation. About 2 years later in her next pregnancy, this woman again attempted suicide at 20 weeks' gestation, by ingesting glutethimide (3.75 g), amobarbital (3.75 g), and promethazine (0.23 g). She delivered another mentally retarded,

2650-g male infant at 43 weeks' gestation. The infant also had a unilateral undescended testicle. Of interest, none of the woman's other 10 children is mentally retarded.

Two additional cases of self-poisoning with valerian were described in 1987 by the same group responsible for the above report (11). In both cases exposure occurred early in gestation, with ingestion of 5 g and 2 g of valerian at 3 and 4 weeks of fetal development, respectively. No congenital abnormalities were observed in the offspring.

In summary, the very limited animal and human data do not allow a conclusion as to the safety of valerian during pregnancy. Moreover, as a natural, unregulated product, the concentration, contents, and presence of contaminants in valerian preparations cannot be easily determined. Because of this uncertainty and the potential for cytotoxicity in the fetus and hepatotoxicity in the mother, the product should be avoided during pregnancy. Other authors have arrived at the same conclusion (3,4). The risk to a fetus from short-term or inadvertent use during any part of gestation, however, is probably low, if it exists at all.

BREAST FEEDING SUMMARY

RECOMMENDATION: No Human Data - Potential Toxicity

No reports describing the use of valerian during lactation have been located. For the reasons cited above, the use of this herbal product should be avoided during breast-feeding.

References

1. Valerian. The Lawrence review of natural products. *Facts and Comparisons*. St. Louis, MO: J. B. Lippincott, October 1991.
2. Reynolds JEF, editor. *Martindale. The Extra Pharmacopoeia*. 31st ed. London, England: Royal Pharmaceutical Society, 1996:1765–6.
3. Klepser TB, Klepser ME. Unsafe and potentially safe herbal therapies. Am J Health Syst Pharm 1999; 56:125–38.
4. Wong AHC, Smith M, Boon HS. Herbal remedies in psychiatric practice. Arch Gen Psychiatry 1998; 55:1033–44.
5. Miller LG. Herbal medicines. Selected clinical considerations focusing on known or potential drug-herb interactions. Arch Intern Med 1998;158:2200–11.
6. MacGregor FB, Abernethy VE, Dahabra S, Cobden I, Hayes PC. Hepatotoxicity of herbal remedies. BMJ 1989;299:1156–7.
7. Garges HP, Varia I, Doraiswamy PM. Cardiac complications and delirium associated with valerian root withdrawal. JAMA 1998;280:1566–7.
8. Randor S, Einarson TR, Pastuszak A, Koren G. Maternal-fetal toxicology of medicinal plants: a clinician's guide. In Koren G, editor. *Maternal-Fetal Toxicology. A Clinician's Guide*. 2nd ed. New York, NY: Marcel Dekker, 1994:495–6.
9. Bounthanh C, Bergmann C, Beck JP, Haag-Berrurier M, Anton R. Valepotriates, a new class of cytotoxic and antitumor agents. Planta Med 1981;41:21–8.
10. Czeizel A, Szentesi I, Szekeres H, Molnar G, Glauber A, Bucski P. A study of adverse effects on the progeny after intoxication during pregnancy. Arch Toxicol 1988;62:1–7.
11. Czeizel AE, Tomcsik M, Timar L. Teratologic evaluation of 178 infants born to mothers who attempted suicide by drugs during pregnancy. Obstet Gynecol 1997;90:195–201.

Name: **VALGANCICLOVIR** Risk Factor: **C_M**
Class: **Antiviral**

FETAL RISK SUMMARY

RECOMMENDATION: Compatible - Maternal Benefit >> Embryo/Fetal Risk

After oral administration, the prodrug valganciclovir is rapidly converted to ganciclovir by intestinal and hepatic enzymes. The antiviral effect, therefore, is identical to ganciclovir (see Ganciclovir). Valganciclovir is indicated for the treatment of cytomegalovirus (CMV) retinitis in patients with acquired immunodeficiency syndrome (AIDS). Plasma protein binding of valganciclovir is not relevant because of its rapid metabolism to ganciclovir, but binding of ganciclovir is very low (1%–2%). The elimination half-life of ganciclovir after valganciclovir administration is about 4.1 hours, compared to 3.8 hours when IV ganciclovir is administered (1). Ganciclovir crosses the human placenta (see Ganciclovir).

Reproduction studies have been conducted in animals with the active metabolite ganciclovir (1). (See Ganciclovir.)

No reports describing the use of valganciclovir in human pregnancy have been located. For ganciclovir, human pregnancy experience that has not shown toxicity, but the number of cases is very limited. The animal data for ganciclovir are suggestive of high embryo/fetal risk because carcinogenic, mutagenic, teratogenic, and embryotoxic effects have been observed. Primary CMV infections occurring in pregnancy have a high risk of transplacental passage of the virus to the fetus. Some of the embryos or fetuses exposed to the virus will be damaged and the development of later toxicity in childhood is an additional concern. However, the prevention of these *in utero* infections by ganciclovir has not been proven (see Ganciclovir).

BREAST FEEDING SUMMARY

RECOMMENDATION: Contraindicated

No reports describing the use of valganciclovir during human lactation have been located. Because the active metabolite, ganciclovir, has the potential to cause serious toxicity in a nursing infant, mothers taking this drug should not breast-feed. Furthermore, breast-feeding is contraindicated if the mother is infected with human immunodeficiency virus (HIV).

Reference

1. Product information. Valcyte. Roche Pharmaceuticals, 2004.

Name:	**VALPROIC ACID**	Risk Factor:	**D_M**
Class:	**Anticonvulsant**		

FETAL RISK SUMMARY

RECOMMENDATION: Human Data Suggest Risk

Valproic acid and its salt form, sodium valproate, are anticonvulsants used in the treatment of seizure disorders. The drugs readily cross the placenta to the fetus. At term, the range of cord blood:maternal serum ratios of total valproic acid (protein bound and unbound) has been reported to be 0.52–4.6 (1–13). Studies that are more recent have reported mean ratios of 1.4–2.4 (4,7,9–13). In contrast, the mean cord blood:maternal serum ratio of free (unbound) valproic acid was 0.82 (10). Two mechanisms have been proposed to account for the accumulation of total valproic acid in the fetus: partial displacement of the drug from maternal binding sites by increased free fatty acid concentrations in maternal blood at the time of birth (10) and increased protein binding of valproic acid in fetal serum (11). Increased unbound valproic acid in the maternal serum may also be partially a result

V

of decreased serum albumin (14). Although one study measured a mean serum half-life for valproic acid in the newborn of 28.3 hours (9), other studies have reported values of 43–47 hours, approximately 4 times the adult value (2,4,8,10,13). In agreement with these data, valproic acid has been shown to lack fetal hepatic enzyme induction activity when used alone and will block the enzyme induction activity of primidone when the two anticonvulsants are combined during pregnancy (15).

In published reports, doses of valproic acid in pregnancy have ranged from 300 to 3000 mg (1–3,8,12,16–28). Although a good correlation between serum levels and seizure control is not always observed, most patients will respond when levels are in the range of 50–100 μg/mL (29). In early pregnancy, high (i.e., >1000 mg) daily doses of valproic acid may produce maternal serum concentrations that are much greater than 100 μg/mL (8). However, as pregnancy progresses and without dosage adjustment, valproic acid levels fall steadily so that in the 3rd trimester, maternal levels are often less than 50 μg/mL (8). One study concluded that the decreased serum concentrations were a result of increased hepatic clearance and an increased apparent volume of distribution (8).

Fetal or newborn consequences resulting from the use of valproic acid and sodium valproate during pregnancy have been reported to include major and minor congenital abnormalities, intrauterine growth retardation, hyperbilirubinemia, hepatotoxicity (which may be fatal), transient hyperglycinemia, afibrinogenemia (one case), and fetal or neonatal withdrawal.

Before 1981, the maternal use of valproic acid was not thought to present a risk to the fetus. A 1981 editorial recommended sodium valproate or carbamazepine as anticonvulsants of choice in appropriate types of epilepsy for women who may become pregnant (30). Although the drug was known to be a potent animal teratogen (31), more potent than phenytoin and at least as potent as trimethadione (32), only a single unconfirmed case of human teratogenicity (in a fetus exposed to at least two other anticonvulsants) had been published between 1969 and 1976 (33). (An editorial comment in that report noted that subsequent investigation had failed to confirm the defect.) In other published cases, both before and after 1980, healthy term infants resulted after *in utero* exposure to valproic acid (1–3,12,19,27,28,32,34–38). Moreover, a committee of the American Academy of Pediatrics stated in 1982 that the data for a teratogenic potential in humans for valproic acid were inadequate and that recommendations for or against its use in pregnancy could not be given (39).

The first confirmed report of an infant with congenital defects after valproic acid exposure during pregnancy appeared in 1980 (16). The mother, who took 1000 mg of valproic acid daily throughout gestation, delivered a growth-retarded infant with facial dysmorphism and heart and limb defects. The infant died at 19 days of age. Since this initial report, a number of studies and case reports have described newborns with malformations after *in utero* exposure to either valproic acid monotherapy or combination therapy (4,17–26,36,40–60).

The most serious abnormalities observed with valproic acid (or sodium valproate) exposure are defects in neural tube closure. The absolute risk of this defect is approximately 1%–2%, about the same risk for a familial occurrence of this anomaly (37,40,61,62). No cases of anencephaly have been associated with valproic acid (21,62,63). Exposure to valproic acid between the 17th and 30th day after fertilization must occur before the drug can be considered a cause of neural tube defects (64). Other predominant defects involve the heart, face, and limbs. A characteristic pattern of minor facial abnormalities has been attributed to valproic acid (61). Cardiac anomalies and cleft lip and palate occur with most anticonvulsants and a causal relationship with valproic acid has not been established (37,46). In addition, almost all types of congenital malformations have been observed after treatment of epilepsy during pregnancy (see Janz 1982, Phenytoin). Consequently, the list below, although abstracting the cited references, is not meant to be inclusive and, at times, reflects multiple anticonvulsant therapy.

NEURAL TUBE DEFECTS
Defects in neural tube closure (includes entire spectrum from spina bifida occulta to meningomyelocele) (17,19,21,22,24,26,40–42,44–46,53–58)

CARDIAC DEFECTS
Multiple (not specified) (21,24,26,37,42,44,51)
Levocardia (16)
Anomalies of great vessels (51)
Patent ductus arteriosus (4,26,48,50,52)
Valvular aortic stenosis (23,48)
Ventricular septal defect (4,20,48)
Tetralogy of Fallot (18,51)
Partial right bundle branch block (16)

FACIAL DEFECTS
Facial dysmorphism (4,26,42,46,50,53,59)
Small nose (16,20,24,26,50,53,59)
Small nose (16,20,24,26,50,53,59)
Depressed nasal bridge (18,20,26,50,59)
Epicanthal folds (4,26,50,53,59)
Protruding eyes (16)
Hypertelorism (4,26)
Low-set/rotated ears (4,16,24,26,50)
Micrognathia/retrognathia (16,23,26)
Depigmentation of eyelashes and brow (16,25)
Thin upper vermilion border (24,26,48,50,53)
Down-turned angles of mouth (50,59)
High forehead (24,26)
Bulging frontal eminences (16,20)
Strabismus (50)
Nystagmus (50)
Flat orbits (26)
Coarsened facies (20)
Cleft lip/palate (18,37,42,44,51)
Microstomia (24,26,48,50)
Esotropia (50)
Long upper lip (26,50,59)
Short palpebral fissure (26,48,50)
Agenesis of lacrimal ducts (51)

HEAD/NECK DEFECTS
Brachycephaly (24,26)
Hydrocephaly (19,21,42,46)
Short neck (20)
Abnormal or premature stenosis of metopic suture (24,26,50)
Microcephaly (4,21,24,38,50,64,65)
Wide anterior fontanelle (18)
Craniostenosis (26)
Aplasia cutis (60)

UROGENITAL DEFECTS
Bilateral duplication of caliceal collecting systems (25)
Bilateral undescended testes (23)
Nonspecified (26)
Hypospadias (21,23,26,46,50)
Bilateral renal hypoplasia (23)

SKELETAL/LIMB DEFECTS
Aplasia of radius (23,26)
Dislocated hip (16,26,35)
Hypoplastic thumb (20)
Hemifusion of second and third lumbar vertebrae (25)
Arachnodactyly (24,26)
Overlapping fingers/toes (24,26)
Rib defects (24,26)
Foot deformity (17,23,24,50)
Abnormal digits (23,26,37,42)
Shortened fingers and toes (4,20)
Abnormal sternum (16,26)
Scoliosis (25)
Clinodactyly of fingers (26)

(*continued*)

V

Broad or asymmetric chest (16,26)	Tracheomalacia (53)
Multiple (not specified) (24)	Talipes equinovarus (53)
SKIN/MUSCLE DEFECTS	
Accessory, wide-spaced, or inverted nipples (20,26)	Cutis aplasia of scalp (50)
Diastasis recti abdominis (4,25)	Weak abdominal walls (4)
Syndactyly of toes (16,23,50)	Hirsutism (26)
Hyperconvex fingernails (24,26)	Abnormal palmar creases (16,18,50)
Hemangioma (4,25,26,50)	Hypoplastic nails (4,18)
Sacral dimple (43)	Umbilical hernias (4,26)
Telangiectasia (4)	Linea alba hernia (47)
Omphalocele (59)	Inguinal hernia (4,26,50)
OTHER DEFECTS	
Multiple defects (not specified) (24,51)	Withdrawal or irritation (4,50)
Duodenal atresia (25)	Mental retardation (4,20,50,51,53)
Single umbilical artery (50)	

Although a wide variety of minor anomalies, many of which are similar in nature, occurs in infants of epileptic mothers, three groups of investigators have concluded that the deformities associated with valproic acid are distinctly different from those associated with other anticonvulsants and may constitute a fetal valproate syndrome (FVS) (26,50,53). The combined features cited in the three reports were: (a) neural tube defects; (b) craniofacial: brachycephaly, high forehead, epicanthal folds, strabismus, nystagmus, shallow orbits, flat nasal bridge, small up-turned nose, hypertelorism, long upper lip, thin upper vermillion border, microstomia, down-turned angles of mouth, low-set/rotated ears; (c) digits: long, thin, partly overlapping fingers and toes, hyperconvex nails; (d) urogenital: hypospadias (in about 50% of males); and (e) other: retarded psychomotor development, low birth weight. Normal psychomotor development has been observed, however, in follow-up studies of children up to 4 years of age after *in utero* exposure to either mono- or combination therapy with valproic acid (3,34,65,66).

A 1995 review listed the facial features seen in the FVS as trigonocephaly, tall forehead with bifrontal narrowing, epicanthic folds, medial deficiency of eyebrows, flat nasal bridge, broad nasal root anteverted nares, shallow philtrum, long upper lip with thin vermilion border, thick upper lip, small, downturned mouth (67). The most common major congenital defects observed were neural tube defects, congenital heart disease, cleft lip and palate, genital anomalies, and limb defects. Other, less common abnormalities were tracheomalacia, abdominal wall defects, and strabismus. Dose-related withdrawal symptoms (irritability, jitteriness, hypotonia, and seizures) were considered to be very common, typically occurring 12–48 hours after birth (67).

A correlation between valproic acid dosage and the number of minor anomalies in an infant has been proposed (26). Such a correlation has not been observed with other anticonvulsants (26). The conclusion was based on the high concentrations of valproic acid that occur in the 1st trimester after large doses (i.e., 1500–2000 mg/day).

In a surveillance study of Michigan Medicaid recipients conducted between 1985 and 1992 involving 229,101 completed pregnancies, 26 newborns had been exposed to valproic acid during the 1st trimester (F. Rosa, personal communication, FDA, 1993). Five (19.2%) major birth defects were observed (one expected), one of which was a hypospadias. No anomalies were observed in five other categories of defects (cardiovascular, oral clefts, spina bifida, polydactyly, and limb reduction defects) for which specific data were available. Hypospadias has been associated with 1st trimester valproic acid exposure (see above).

A 2000 study, using data from the MADRE (an acronym for MAlformation and DRug Exposure) surveillance project, assessed the human teratogenicity of anticonvulsants (68). Among 8,005 malformed infants, cases were infants with a specific malformation, whereas controls were infants with other anomalies. Of the total group, 299 were exposed in the 1st trimester to anticonvulsants. Among these, exposure to monotherapy occurred in the following: valproic acid ($N = 80$), phenobarbital ($N = 65$), mephobarbital ($N = 10$), carbamazepine ($N = 46$), phenytoin ($N = 24$), and other agents ($N = 16$). Statistically significant associations (CI not overlapping 1 and $p \leq 0.05$) were found between valproic acid monotherapy and spina bifida ($N = 12$), hypospadias ($N = 10$), porencephaly/multiple cerebral cysts and other specified anomalies of brain ($N = 2$), microstomia, microcheilia, and other anomalies of face ($N = 2$), coarctation of aorta ($N = 2$), and limb reduction defects ($N = 5$). When all 1st trimester exposures (mono- and polytherapy) were evaluated, significant associations were found between valproic acid and spina bifida ($N = 14$), cardiac defects ($N = 26$), hypospadias ($N = 14$), porencephaly/multiple cerebral cysts and other specific anomalies of brain ($N = 2$), limb reduction defects ($N = 5$), and hypertelorism, localized skull defects ($N = 2$). Although the study confirmed some previously known associations, several new associations with anticonvulsants were discovered and require independent confirmation (see also Carbamazepine, Mephobarbital, Phenobarbital, and Phenytoin) (68).

The risk of valproic acid-induced limb deficiencies was estimated in a 2000 study that used data from the Spanish Collaborative Study of Congenital Malformations (ECEMC) collected between 1976 and 1997 (69). A total of 22,294 consecutive malformed infants (excluding genetic syndromes) were compared to 21,937 control infants. A total of 57 malformed infants and 10 controls were exposed to valproic acid during the 1st trimester (odds ratio [OR] 5.62, 95% confidence interval [CI] 2.78–11.71, $p < 0.0000001$). Among the 57 infants, 21 (36.8%) had congenital limb defects of different types (overlapping digits, talipes, clinodactyly, arachnodactyly, hip dislocation, pre- and postaxial polydactyly, and limb deficiencies). Five of the 21 cases, however, were thought to have resulted from immobility (e.g., talipes equinovarus) caused by spina bifida. After exclusion of these cases and their respective controls, the OR for congenital limb defects was 3.95, 95% CI 1.24–13.94, $p = 0.01$. Three of the malformed infants had limb deficiencies: hypoplasia of the left hand; unilateral forearm defect and hypoplastic first metacarpal bone in the left hand; and short hands with hypoplastic first metacarpal bone, absent and hypoplastic phalanges (this case also had retrognathia, facial asymmetry, hypospadias, telangiectatic angioma in the skull, and hypotonia). The case-control analysis showed a risk for limb deficiencies of OR 6.17, 95% CI 1.28–29.66, $p = 0.023$. In their population, the prevalence at birth of limb deficiencies was 6.88 per 10,000 live births. Based on this, they estimated that the risk of limb deficiencies after exposure to valproic acid in the 1st trimester would be about 0.42% (69).

A prospective study published in 1999 described the outcomes of 517 pregnancies of epileptic mothers identified at one Italian center from 1977 (70). Excluding genetic and chromosomal defects, malformations were classified as severe structural defects, mild structural defects, and deformations. Minor anomalies were not considered. Spontaneous ($N = 38$) and early ($N = 20$) voluntary abortions were excluded from the analysis, as were 7 pregnancies that delivered at other hospitals. Of the remaining 452 outcomes, 427 were exposed to anticonvulsants of which 313 involved monotherapy: valproate ($N = 44$), carbamazepine (*N* = 113), phenobarbital (*N* = 83), primidone (*N* = 35), phenytoin (*N* = 31), clonazepam (*N* = 6), and other (*N* = 1). There were no defects in the 25 pregnancies not exposed to anticonvulsants. Of the 42 (9.3%) outcomes with malformations, 24 (5.3%) were severe, 10 (2.2%) were mild, and 8 (1.8%) were deformities. There were eight malformations with valproic acid monotherapy: six (13.6%) were severe (spina bifida, hydrocephalus, pyloric stenosis, and cardiac defect), one (2.3%) was mild (inguinal hernia), and one was a deformation (arthrogryposis). The investigators concluded that the anticonvulsants were the primary risk factor for an increased incidence of congenital malformations (see also Carbamazepine, Clonazepam, Phenobarbital, Phenytoin, and Primidone) (70).

A 1997 case report described autism diagnosed in a 5.5-year-old boy who had typical clinical features of the FVS (71). The mother had taken valproic acid (2000 mg/day) during the first 5 months of pregnancy for the treatment of dizzy spells, possible absence seizures, and an abnormal EEG. Although his gross motor milestones were normal, both his speech and language development were delayed. Based on their review of the literature, the authors concluded that a possible relationship between autism and FVS existed (71).

The relationship between maternal anticonvulsant therapy, neonatal behavior, and neurological function in children was reported in a 1996 study (72). Among newborns exposed to maternal monotherapy, 18 were exposed to phenobarbital (including primidone), 13 to phenytoin, and 8 to valproic acid. Compared to controls, neonates exposed to phenobarbital had significantly higher mean apathy and optimality scores. Phenytoin-exposed neonates also had a significantly higher mean apathy score. However, the neonatal optimality and apathy scores did not correlate with neurological outcome of the children at 6 years of age. In contrast, those exposed to valproic acid had optimality and apathy scores statistically similar to controls but a significantly higher hyperexcitability score. Moreover, the hyperexcitability score correlated with minor and major neurological dysfunction at age 6 years (72).

Intrauterine growth retardation (IUGR) or small-for-gestational-age infants have been noted in several reports (4,16,19,23,24,47,48,50,65,73). Both monotherapy and combination therapy with valproic acid were involved in these cases. However, normal birth weights, heights, and head circumferences have been reported with valproic acid monotherapy (25,50,53,65). Growth impairment is a common problem with some anticonvulsant therapy (e.g., see Phenytoin), but the relationship between this problem and valproic acid needs further clarification.

A 1983 letter proposed that the mechanism for valproic acid-induced teratogenicity involved zinc deficiency (74). From *in utero* studies, the authors had previously shown that valproic acid readily binds zinc. Low zinc serum levels potentiated the teratogenicity of certain drugs in animals and produced adverse effects similar to valproic acid-induced human toxicity (74). Another proposed mechanism, especially when valproic acid is combined with other anticonvulsants, involves the inhibition of liver microsomal epoxide hydrolase, the enzyme responsible for the biotransformation of reactive epoxide metabolites (75). The inhibition of the detoxifying enzyme could result in enhanced fetal exposure to reactive epoxide metabolites, such as carbamazepine epoxide, by preventing its biotransformation to a *trans*-dihydrodiol metabolite. Based on these findings, the authors recommended that combination drug therapy with valproic acid be avoided during pregnancy (75).

Three reports have observed hyperbilirubinemia in nine newborns exposed *in utero* to valproic acid monotherapy and in one infant exposed to combination therapy (4,25,48). A causal relationship is uncertain because other studies have not reported this problem.

Liver toxicity has been observed in three infants after *in utero* exposure to valproic acid (47,48). In the first report, a growth-retarded female infant, exposed to valproic acid and phenytoin, had a linea alba hernia noted at birth but liver function tests were normal (47). The mother breast-fed the child for the first several weeks. At 2.5 months of age, the infant presented with an enlarged liver, slight icterus, vomiting, and failure to thrive. Liver function tests indicated a cholestatic type of hyperbilirubinemia, and liver biopsy specimen demonstrated fibrosis with ongoing necrosis of liver cells. Although they were unable to determine which anticonvulsant caused the injury, the authors concluded that valproic acid was the more likely offending agent. The second report described two siblings born of a mother treated with valproic acid monotherapy during two pregnancies (48). A male infant, exposed *in utero* to 300 mg/day, was normal at birth but died at age 5 months of liver failure. Autopsy revealed liver atrophy, necrosis, and cholestasis. The female infant, exposed *in utero* to 500 mg/day, died at age 6 weeks of liver failure. At birth, the infant was noted to have defects characteristic of valproic acid exposure (defects described in list above), IUGR, hyperbilirubinemia, hypoglycemia, hypocalcemia, and seizures. Liver atrophy and cholestasis were noted at autopsy (48).

Undetectable fibrinogen levels resulting in fatal hemorrhage in a full-term 2-day-old infant were attributed to *in utero* sodium valproate exposure (76). The mother had taken daily doses of sodium valproate 600 mg, phenytoin 375 mg, and lorazepam 1 mg throughout pregnancy. In a subsequent pregnancy, the measurement of slightly decreased maternal fibrinogen levels in late gestation caused the authors to discontinue the sodium valproate while continuing the other two agents. Oral vitamin K was also administered to the mother. A healthy infant without bleeding problems resulted (76).

Transient hyperglycinemia has been observed in two newborns exposed *in utero* to sodium valproate combination therapy (combined with phenytoin in one and phenytoin, carbamazepine, and clonazepam in the other) (3). Similar increases of glycine have been observed in epileptic adults treated with valproic acid. No adverse effects in the newborns resulted from the amino acid alteration (3).

Fetal distress during labor (late decelerations, silent or accelerated beat-to-beat variations) was observed in 6 (43%) of 14 cases exposed to valproic acid monotherapy (26). Two of the newborns with fetal distress plus two others had low Apgar scores (0–3 after 1 minute or 0–6 after 5 minutes). Maternal doses were 1500–1800 mg/day in 3 cases and 600 mg/day in 1 case. Low Apgar scores were not observed in 12 infants whose mothers had been treated with valproic acid combination therapy. Other studies and case reports have not mentioned this complication. The fetal and newborn depression was thought to have resulted from a 3-fold increase in the maternal serum of valproic acid free fraction (26). A similar increase had been measured in an earlier study (10).

No decreases in adrenocorticotropic hormone or cortisol levels were measured in a mother or her newborn after the use of valproic acid 3000 mg/day during the last 3 months of pregnancy (28). The mother had received combination anticonvulsant therapy during the first 6 months of gestation.

Valproic acid has been measured in the semen of two healthy males (77). Following oral doses of 500 mg, semen levels ranged from 0.53 to 3.26 μg/mL up to 39 hours after the dose. Simultaneous serum levels were 11–17 times those measured in the semen. No effect on sperm motility was suggested based on animal experiments.

In summary, valproic acid and the salt form, sodium valproate, are human teratogens. The absolute risk of producing a child with neural tube defects when these agents are used between the 17th and 30th days after fertilization is 1%–2%. A characteristic pattern of minor facial defects is apparently also associated with valproic acid. Two studies have suggested that a distinct constellation of defects may exist for infants exposed *in utero* to the anticonvulsant. These defects involve the head and face, digits, urogenital tract, and mental and physical growth. A correlation between maternal dose and major and minor anomalies has been reported, but additional studies are needed for confirmation. Other problems, such as IUGR, hyperbilirubinemia, hepatotoxicity, and fetal or newborn distress, also need additional investigation. Because of the risk for neural tube defects, women exposed during the critical period of gestation should consult their physician about prenatal testing (37,78,79).

BREAST FEEDING SUMMARY

RECOMMENDATION: Limited Human Data - Potential Toxicity

Valproic acid and its salt, sodium valproate, are excreted into human milk in low concentrations (1,2,4,5,8,10,12,80–82). Milk concentrations have been measured up to 15% of the corresponding level in the mother's serum. In two infants, serum levels of valproate were 1.5% and 6.0% of maternal values (81).

Only one report of adverse effects in a nursing infant attributable to valproate in breast milk has been located. Thrombocytopenia purpura, anemia, and reticulocytosis were observed in a 3-month-old male breast-fed infant whose mother was taking sodium valproate (monotherapy; 1200 mg/day) for epilepsy (82). The infant had a 2-week history of increasing petechiae and minor hematoma on the lower part of the legs. The infant's serum valproate level was 6.6 μg/mL. Breast-feeding was discontinued for 5 days but had no effect on the infant's low platelet count. The mother continued to nurse for another 2 weeks and again stopped. Twelve days later, valproate was undetectable in the infant's serum and 7 days later (19 days after nursing was stopped), the platelet count began to rise, reaching normal values sometime after 35 days. At about this same time, the petechiae had resolved. The blood hemoglobin and the reticulocytes normalized between 12 and 19 days after breast feeding was stopped (82).

The American Academy of Pediatrics classifies valproic acid as compatible with breastfeeding (83).

References

1. Alexander FW. Sodium valproate and pregnancy. Arch Dis Child 1979;54:240.
2. Dickinson RG, Harland RC, Lynn RK, Smith WB, Gerber N. Transmission of valproic acid (Depakene) across the placenta: half-life of the drug in mother and baby. J Pediatr 1979;94:832–5.
3. Simila S, von Wendt L, Hartikainen-Sorri A-L, Kaapa P, Saukkonen A-L. Sodium valproate, pregnancy, and neonatal hyperglycinaemia. Arch Dis Child 1979;54:985–6.
4. Nau H, Rating D, Koch S, Hauser I, Helge H. Valproic acid and its metabolites: placental transfer, neonatal pharmacokinetics, transfer via mother's milk and clinical status in neonates of epileptic mothers. J Pharmacol Exp Ther 1981;219:768–77.
5. Froescher W, Eichelbaum M, Niesen M, Altmann D, von Unruh GE. Antiepileptic therapy with carbamazepine and valproic acid during pregnancy and lactation period. In Dam M, Gram L, Penry JK, eds. *Advances in Epileptology: the XIIth Epilepsy International Symposium*. New York, NY: Raven Press, 1981;581–8. As cited in Froescher W, Gugler R, Niesen M, Hoffmann F. Protein binding of valproic acid in maternal and umbilical cord serum. Epilepsia. 1984;25:244–9.
6. Froescher W, Niesen M, Altmann D, Eichelbaum M, Gugler R, Hoffmann F, Penin H. Antiepileptika-Therapie wahrend Schwangerschaft und Geburt. In Remschmidt H, Rentz R, Jungmann J, eds. *Epilepsie 1980*. Stuttgart: Georg Thieme Publishers, 1981:152–63. As cited in Froescher W, Gugler R, Niesen M, Hoffman F. Protein binding of valproic acid in maternal and umbilical cord serum. Epilepsia 1984;25:244–9.
7. Iskizaki T, Yokochi K, Chiba K, Tabuchi T, Wagatsuma T. Placental transfer of anticonvulsants (phenobarbital, phenytoin, valproic acid) and the elimination from neonates. Pediatr Pharmacol 1981;1:291–303.
8. Nau H, Kuhnz W, Egger H-J, Rating D, Helge H. Anticonvulsants during pregnancy and lactation:

V

transplacental, maternal and neonatal pharmacokinetics. Clin Pharmacokinet 1982;7:508–43.
9. Kaneko S, Otani K, Fukushima Y, Sato T, Nomura Y, Ogawa Y. Transplacental passage and half-life of sodium valproate in infants born to epileptic mothers. Br J Clin Pharmacol 1983;15:503–6.
10. Nau H, Helge H, Luck W. Valproic acid in the perinatal period: decreased maternal serum protein binding results in fetal accumulation and neonatal displacement of the drug and some metabolites. J Pediatr 1984;104:627–34.
11. Froescher W, Gugler R, Niesen M, Hoffmann F. Protein binding of valproic acid in maternal and umbilical cord serum. Epilepsia 1984;25:244–9.
12. Philbert A, Pedersen B, Dam M. Concentration of valproate during pregnancy, in the newborn and in breast milk. Acta Neurol Scand 1985;72:460–3.
13. Nau H, Schafer H, Rating D, Jakobs C, Helge H. Placental transfer and neonatal pharmacokinetics of valproic acid and some of its metabolites. In Janz D, Bossi L, Dam M, Helge H, Richens A, Schmidt D, eds. *Epilepsy, Pregnancy, and the Child*. New York, NY: Raven Press, 1982:367–72.
14. Perucca E, Ruprah M, Richens A. Altered drug binding to serum proteins in pregnant women: therapeutic relevance. J R Soc Med 1981;74:422–6.
15. Rating D, Jager-Roman E, Koch S, Nau H, Klein PD, Helge H. Enzyme induction in neonates due to antiepileptic therapy during pregnancy. In Janz D, Bossi L, Dam M, Helge H, Richens A, Schmidt D, eds. *Epilepsy, Pregnancy, and the Child*. New York, NY: Raven Press, 1982:349–55.
16. Dalens B, Raynaud E-J, Gaulme J. Teratogenicity of valproic acid. J Pediatr 1980;97:332–3.
17. Gomez MR. Possible teratogenicity of valproic acid. J Pediatr 1981;98:508–9.
18. Thomas D, Buchanan N. Teratogenic effects of anticonvulsants. J Pediatr 1981;99:163.
19. Weinbaum PJ, Cassidy SB, Vintzileos AM, Campbell WA, Ciarleglio L, Nochimson DJ. Prenatal detection of a neural tube defect after fetal exposure to valproic acid. Obstet Gynecol 1986;67:31S–3S.
20. Clay SA, McVie R, Chen H. Possible teratogenic effect of valproic acid. J Pediatr 1981;99:828.
21. Robert E, Guibaud P. Maternal valproic acid and congenital neural tube defects. Lancet 1982;2:937.
22. Blaw ME, Woody RC. Valproic acid embryopathy? Neurology 1983;33:255.
23. Bailey CJ, Pool RW, Poskitt EME, Harris F. Valproic acid and fetal abnormality. Br Med J 1983;286:190.
24. Koch S, Jager-Roman E, Rating D, Helge H. Possible teratogenic effect of valproate during pregnancy. J Pediatr 1983;103:1007–8.
25. Bantz EW. Valproic acid and congenital malformations: a case report. Clin Pediatr 1984;23:353–4.
26. Jager-Roman E, Deichi A, Jakob S, Hartmann A-M, Koch S, Rating D, Steldinger R, Nau H, Helge H. Fetal growth, major malformations, and minor anomalies in infants born to women receiving valproic acid. J Pediatr 1986;108:997–1004.
27. Shakir RA, Johnson RH, Lambie DG, Melville ID, Nanda RN. Comparison of sodium valproate and phenytoin as single drug treatment in epilepsy. Epilepsia 1981;22:27–33.
28. Hatjis CG, Rose JC, Pippitt C, Swain M. Effect of treatment with sodium valproate on plasma adrenocorticotropic hormone and cortisol concentrations in pregnancy. Am J Obstet Gynecol 1985;152:315–6.
29. Product information. Depakene. Abbott Laboratories, 2000.
30. Anonymous. Teratogenic risks of antiepileptic drugs. Br Med J 1981;283:515–6.
31. Paulson GW, Paulson RR. Teratogenic effects of anticonvulsants. Arch Neurol 1981;38:140–43.
32. Brown NA, Kao J, Fabro S. Teratogenic potential of valproic acid. Lancet 1980;1:660–1.
33. Whittle BA. Pre-clinical teratological studies on sodium valproate (Epilim) and other anticonvulsants. In Legg NJ, ed. *Clinical and Pharmacological Aspects of Sodium Valproate (Epilim) in the Treatment of Epilepsy*. Tunbridge Wells, England: MCS Consultants, 1976:105–11.
34. Hiilesmaa VK, Bardy AH, Granstrom M-L, Teramo KAW. Valproic acid during pregnancy. Lancet 1980;1:883.
35. Nakane Y, Okuma T, Takahashi R, Sato Y, Wada T, Sato T, Fukushima Y, Kumashiro H, Ono T, Takahashi T, Aoki Y, Kazamatsuri H, Inami M, Komai S, Seino M, Miyakoshi M, Tanimura T, Hazama H, Kawahara R, Otsuki S, Hosokawa K, Inanaga K, Nakazawa Y, Yamamoto K. Multi-institutional study on the teratogenicity and fetal toxicity of antiepileptic drugs: a report of a collaborative study group in Japan. Epilepsia 1980;21:663–80.
36. Jeavons PM. Non-dose-related side effects of valproate. Epilepsia 1984;25(Suppl 1):S50–S5.
37. CDC. Valproate: a new cause of birth defects report from Italy and follow-up from France. MMWR 1983;32:438–9.
38. Bossi L, Battino D, Boldi B, Caccamo ML, Ferraris G, Latis GO, Simionato L. Anthropometric data and minor malformations in newborns of epileptic mothers. In Janz D, Bossi L, Dam M, Helge H, Richens A, Schmidt D, eds. *Epilepsy, Pregnancy, and the Child*. New York, NY: Raven Press, 1982:299–301.
39. Committee on Drugs, American Academy of Pediatrics. Valproic acid: benefits and risks. Pediatrics 1982;70:316–9.
40. Bjerkedal T, Czeizel A, Goujard J, Kallen B, Mastroiacova P, Nevin N, Oakley G Jr, Robert E. Valproic acid and spina bifida. Lancet 1982;2:1096,1172.
41. Stanely OH, Chambers TL. Sodium valproate and neural tube defects. Lancet 1982;2:1282.
42. Jeavons PM. Sodium valproate and neural tube defects. Lancet 1982;2:1282–3.
43. Castilla E. Valproic acid and spina bifida. Lancet 1983;2:683.
44. Robert E, Rosa F. Valproate and birth defects. Lancet 1983;2:1142.
45. Mastroiacovo P, Bertollini R, Morandini S, Segni G. Maternal epilepsy, valproate exposure, and birth defects. Lancet 1983;2:1499.
46. Lindhout D, Meinardi H. Spina bifida and in-utero exposure to valproate. Lancet 1984;2:396.
47. Felding I, Rane A. Congenital liver damage after treatment of mother with valproic acid and phenytoin? Acta Paediatr Scand 1984;73:565–8.
48. Legius E, Jaeken J, Eggermont E. Sodium valproate,

pregnancy, and infantile fatal liver failure. Lancet 1987;2:1518–9.
49. Rating D, Jager-Roman E, Koch S, Gopfert-Geyer I, Helge H. Minor anomalies in the offspring of epileptic parents. In Janz D, Bossi L, Dam M, Helge H, Richens A, Schmidt D, eds. *Epilepsy, Pregnancy, and the Child*. New York, NY: Raven Press, 1982:283–8.
50. DiLiberti JH, Farndon PA, Dennis NR, Curry CJR. The fetal valproate syndrome. Am J Med Genet 1984;19:473–81.
51. Lindhout D, Meinardi H, Barth PG. Hazards of fetal exposure to drug combinations. In Janz D, Bossi L, Dam M, Helge H, Richens A, Schmidt D, eds. *Epilepsy, Pregnancy, and the Child*. New York, NY: Raven Press, 1982:275–81.
52. Koch S, Hartmann A, Jager-Roman E, Rating D, Helge H. Major malformations in children of epileptic parents—due to epilepsy or its therapy? In Janz D, Bossi L, Dam M, Helge H, Richens A, Schmidt D, eds. *Epilepsy, Pregnancy, and the Child*. New York, NY: Raven Press, 1982:313–5.
53. Ardinger HH, Atkin JF, Blackston RD, Elsas LJ, Clarren SK, Livingstone S, Flannery DB, Pellock JM, Harrod MJ, Lammer EJ, Majewski F, Schinzel A, Toriello HV, Hanson JW. Verification of the fetal valproate syndrome phenotype. Am J Med Genet 1988;29: 171–85.
54. Staunton H. Valproate, spina bifida, and birth defect registries. Lancet 1989;1:381.
55. Oakeshott P, Hunt GM. Valproate and spina bifida. Br Med J 1989;298:1300–1.
56. Oakeshott P, Hunt G. Valproate and spina bifida. Lancet 1989;1:611.
57. Martinez-Frias ML, Rodriguez-Pinilla E, Salvador J. Valproate and spina bifida. Lancet 1989;1:611–2.
58. Carter BS, Stewart JM. Valproic acid prenatal exposure: association with lipomyelomeningocele. Clin Pediatr 1989;28:81–5.
59. Boussemart T, Bonneau D, Levard G, Berthier M, Oriot D. Omphalocele in a newborn baby exposed to sodium valproate *in utero*. Eur J Pediatr 1995; 154:220–1.
60. Hubert A, Bonneau D, Couet D, Berthier M, Oriot D, Larregue M. Aplasia cutis congenita of the scalp in an infant exposed to valproic acid *in utero*. Acta Paediatr 1994;83:789–90.
61. CDC. Valproic acid and spina bifida: a preliminary report - France. MMWR 1982;31:565–6.
62. Lammer EJ, Sever LE, Oakley GP Jr. Teratogen update: valproic acid. Teratology 1987;35:465–73.
63. Anonymous. Valproate and malformations. Lancet 1982;2:1313–4.
64. Lemire RJ. Neural tube defects. JAMA 1988;259: 558–62.
65. Jager-Roman E, Rating D, Koch S, Gopfert-Geyer I, Jacob S, Helge H. Somatic parameters, diseases, and psychomotor development in the offspring of epileptic parents. In Janz D, Bossi L, Dam M, Helge H, Richens A, Schmidt D, eds. *Epilepsy, Pregnancy, and the Child*. New York, NY: Raven Press, 1982:425–32.
66. Granstrom M-L. Development of the children of epileptic mothers: preliminary results from the prospective Helsinki study. In Janz D, Bossi L, Dam M, Helge H, Richens A, Schmidt D, eds. *Epilepsy, Pregnancy, and the Child*. New York, NY: Raven Press, 1982;403–8.
67. Clayton-Smith J, Donnai D. Fetal valproate syndrome. J Med Genet 1995;32:724–7.
68. Arpino C, Brescianini S, Robert E, Castilla EE, Cocchi G, Cornel MC, de Vigan C, Lancaster PAL, Merlob P, Sumiyoshi Y, Zampino G, Renzi C, Rosano A, Mastroiacovo P. Teratogenic effects of antiepileptic drugs: use of an international database on malformations and drug exposure (MADRE). Epilepsia 2000;41: 1436–43.
69. Rodriguez-Pinilla E, Arroyo I, Fondevilla J, Garcia MJ, Martinez-Frias ML. Prenatal exposure to valproic acid during pregnancy and limb deficiencies: a case-control study. Am J Med Genet 2000;90:376–81.
70. Canger R, Battino D, Canevini MP, Fumarola C, Guidolin L, Vignoli A, Mamoli D, Palmieri C, Molteni F, Granata T, Hassibi P, Zamperini P, Pardi G, Avanzini G. Malformations in offspring of women with epilepsy: a prospective study. Epilepsia 1999;40: 1231–6.
71. Williams PG, Hersh JH. A male with fetal valproate syndrome and autism. Dev Med Child Neurol 1997;39:632–4.
72. Koch S, Jager-Roman E, Losche G, Nau H, Rating D, Helge H. Antiepileptic drug treatment in pregnancy: drug side effects in the neonate and neurological outcome. Acta Paediatr 1996;84:739–46.
73. Granstrom M-L, Hiilesmaa VK. Physical growth of the children of epileptic mothers: preliminary results from the prospective Helsinki study. In Janz D, Bossi L, Dam M, Helge H, Richens A, Schmidt D, eds. *Epilepsy, Pregnancy, and the Child*. New York, NY: Raven Press, 1982:397–401.
74. Hurd RW, Wilder BJ, Van Rinsvelt HA. Valproate, birth defects, and zinc. Lancet 1983;1:181.
75. Kerr BM, Levy RH. Inhibition of epoxide hydrolase by anticonvulsants and risk of teratogenicity. Lancet 1989;1:610–1.
76. Majer RV, Green PJ. Neonatal afibrinogenaemia due to sodium valproate. Lancet 1987;2:740–1.
77. Swanson BN, Harland RC, Dickinson RG, Gerber N. Excretion of valproic acid into semen of rabbits and man. Epilepsia 1978;19:541–6.
78. Frew J. Valproate link to spina bifida. Med J Aust 1983;1:150.
79. Committee on Drugs, American Academy of Pediatrics. Valproate teratogenicity. Pediatrics 1983; 71:980.
80. Bardy AH, Granstrom M-L, Hiilesmaa VK. Valproic acid and breast-feeding. In Janz D, Bossi L, Dam M, Helge H, Richens A, Schmidt D, eds. *Epilepsy, Pregnancy, and the Child*. New York, NY: Raven Press, 1982: 359–60.
81. Wisner KL, Perel JM. Serum levels of valproate and carbamazepine in breast-feeding mother-infant pairs. J Clin Psychopharmacol 1998;18:167–9.
82. Stahl MMS, Neiderud J, Vinge E. Thrombocytopenic purpura and anemia in a breast-fed infant whose mother was treated with valproic acid. J Pediatr 1997;130:1001–3.
83. Committee on Drugs, American Academy of Pediatrics. The transfer of drugs and other chemicals into human milk. Pediatrics 2001;108:776–89.

Name: **VALSARTAN** Risk Factor: C_M*
Class: **Antihypertensive**

FETAL RISK SUMMARY

RECOMMENDATION: Human Data Suggest Risk in 2nd and 3rd Trimesters

Valsartan is a selective angiotensin II receptor antagonist that is used, either alone or in combination with other antihypertensive agents, for the treatment of hypertension. Valsartan blocks the vasoconstrictor and aldosterone-secreting effects of angiotensin II by preventing angiotensin II from binding to AT_1 receptors.

Reproduction studies have been conducted in pregnant mice, rats, and rabbits (1). No teratogenic effects were observed in these species at oral doses up to 9, 18, and 0.5 times the maximum recommended human dose of 320 mg/day based on body surface area (MRHD), respectively. The highest dose caused rat maternal toxicity (reduction in body weight gain and food consumption). At this dose, administration during organogenesis or late gestation and lactation resulted in significant decreases in fetal weight, pup birth weight, pup survival rate, and slight delays in developmental milestones (1). In rabbits, maternal toxic doses (0.25 and 0.5 times the MRHD) resulted in fetal resorptions, litter loss, abortions, and low fetal body weight as well as maternal mortality. The no-observed-adverse-effect doses in mice, rats, and rabbits were 9, 6, and 0.1 times the MRHD, respectively (1). No adverse effects on reproductive performance of male and female rats were noted at oral doses up to 6 times the MRHD (1).

It is not known if valsartan crosses the human placenta to the fetus. The molecular weight (about 436) is low enough that passage to the fetus should be expected.

A 2001 case report described the pregnancy outcome of a 40-year-old woman with well-controlled chronic hypertension and diet-controlled type 2 diabetes mellitus that was treated with valsartan (80 mg/day) and atenolol (75 mg/day) until presentation at 24 weeks' gestation (2). Anhydramnios (amniotic fluid index zero), most likely caused by valsartan, was diagnosed by ultrasound, but fetal growth was appropriate for gestational age. Valsartan was stopped and atenolol was continued at the same dose. The amniotic fluid volume normalized within 2 weeks. The blood pressure and the diabetes remained under adequate control and there was no evidence of toxemia. Intrauterine fetal death was diagnosed at 31 weeks' gestation. At autopsy, very small, hypoplastic lungs were found (weight 18 g/expected 44 g), as were heavy kidneys (31 g/expected 18 g). The placenta was below the 10th percentile for gestational age (148 g/expected weight for gestational age at the 10th percentile 311 g). No other anomalies were detected. The very small placenta was thought to be primarily caused by atenolol, but valsartan may have contributed to the condition. Death of the female fetus probably resulted from chronic placental insufficiency induced by the combination of valsartan and atenolol (2).

Three other case reports described the effects of valsartan on six pregnancy outcomes (3–5). In a 2001 report, three women were taking valsartan (80 mg/day) for hypertension at the time of conception (3). The drug therapy was stopped at 7, 10, and 18 weeks' gestation, respectively. No congenital defects or evidence of renal dysfunction were observed in the newborns delivered at 38, 38, and 32 weeks' gestation, respectively. However, growth retardation attributed to hypertension was observed in one infant (3). In the another 2001 case report, two women (one with type 2 diabetes) were taking valsartan (80 mg/day in one, dose not specified in the other) in combination with hydrochlorothiazide during pregnancy (4). Anhydramnios was noted at 24 and 28 weeks' gestation, respectively.

Although the anhydramnios resolved in both cases when valsartan was discontinued, the pregnancies were terminated. Both fetuses had foot and face deformities, hypoplastic skull bones with widely open sutures, and large kidneys that were microscopically abnormal. Neither fetus had pulmonary hypoplasia (4). In 2004, anhydramnios was observed in a woman at 20 weeks' gestation (5). She had been taking valsartan for chronic hypertension. The drug was stopped and complete recovery of the amniotic fluid was noted at 23.5 weeks' gestation. A healthy 3050-female infant was delivered at term and was developing normally at 6 months of age.

The antihypertensive mechanisms of action of valsartan and angiotensin-converting enzyme (ACE) inhibitors are very close. That is, the former selectively blocks the binding of angiotensin II to AT_1 receptors, whereas the latter prevents the formation of angiotensin II itself. Therefore, use of this drug during the 2nd and 3rd trimesters may cause teratogenicity and severe fetal and neonatal toxicity identical to that seen with ACE inhibitors (e.g., see Captopril or Enalapril). Fetal toxic effects may include anuria, oligohydramnios, fetal hypocalvaria, intrauterine growth retardation, prematurity, and patent ductus arteriosus. Anuria-associated oligohydramnios may produce fetal limb contractures, craniofacial deformation, and pulmonary hypoplasia. Severe anuria and hypotension, resistant to both pressor agents and volume expansion, may occur in the newborn following *in utero* exposure to valsartan. Newborn renal function and blood pressure should be closely monitored. If valsartan is used in pregnancy, healthcare professionals are encouraged to call the toll free number (800-670-6126) for information about patient enrollment in the Motherisk study.

[**Risk Factor* D_M *if used in 2nd or 3rd trimesters.*]

BREAST FEEDING SUMMARY

RECOMMENDATION: No Human Data - Probably Compatible

No reports describing the use of valsartan during human lactation have been located. The drug is excreted into the milk of lactating rats (1). Because the molecular weight (about 436) is low enough, excretion into breast milk should also be expected. The effects of this exposure on a nursing infant are unknown. The American Academy of Pediatrics, however, classifies ACE inhibitors, a closely related group of antihypertensive agents, as compatible with breast-feeding (see Captopril or Enalapril).

References

1. Product information. Diovan. Novartis Pharmaceuticals, 2001.
2. Briggs GG, Nageotte MP. Fatal fetal outcome with the combined use of valsartan and atenolol. Ann Pharmacother 2001;35:859–61.
3. Chung NA, Lip GYH, Beevers M, Beevers DG. Angiotensin-II-receptor inhibitors in pregnancy. Lancet 2001;357:1620–1.
4. Martinovic J, Benachi A, Laurent N, Daikha-Dahmane F, Gubler MC. Fetal toxic effects and angiotensin-II-receptor antagonists. Lancet 2001;358:241–2.
5. Berkane N, Carlier P, Verstraete L, Mathieu E, Heim N, Uzan S. Fetal toxicity of valsartan and possible reversible adverse side effects. Birth Defects Res Part A Clin Mol Teratol 2004;70:547–9.

Name: **VANCOMYCIN** Risk Factor: B_M

Class: **Antibiotic**

FETAL RISK SUMMARY

RECOMMENDATION: Compatible

Vancomycin is an antibiotic that is used for Gram-positive bacteria when either the organisms are resistant to less toxic anti-infectives (e.g., penicillins and cephalosporins) or the patient is sensitive to these agents.

Reproduction studies in rats and rabbits at doses up to 1 and 1.1 times the maximum recommended human dose based on body surface area MRHD), respectively, have revealed no teratogenic effects (1). No effects on fetal weight or development were seen with the same doses in rats or slightly lower doses in rabbits (0.74 times the MRHD).

No cases of congenital defects attributable to vancomycin have been located. The manufacturer has received reports on the use of vancomycin in pregnancy without adverse fetal effects (A. F. Crumley, personal communication, Eli Lilly, 1983).

The pharmacokinetics of vancomycin in a woman at 26.5 weeks' gestation were described in a 1991 reference (2). Accumulation of the antibiotic, administered as 1 g IV every 12 hours (15 mg/kg/dose), was demonstrated in amniotic fluid (1.02 μg/mL on day 1, 9.2 μg/mL on day 13). At delivery at 28 weeks' gestation, cord blood levels were 3.65 μg/mL (6 hours after the mother's maximum serum concentration), 76% of the mother's serum level. The newborn's serum level, 3.25 hours after birth, was 2.45 μg/mL, indicating a half-life in the infant of 10 hours (2).

Vancomycin was used for subacute bacterial endocarditis prophylaxis in a penicillin-allergic woman at term with mitral valve prolapse (3). One hour before vaginal delivery, a 1-g IV dose was given during 3 minutes (recommended infusion time is 60 minutes [1,4]). Immediately after the dose, maternal blood pressure fell from 130/74 to 80/40 mm Hg and then recovered in 3 minutes. Fetal bradycardia, 90 beats/minute, persisted for 4 minutes. No adverse effects of the hypotension-induced fetal distress were observed in the newborn. The Apgar scores were 9 and 10 at 1 and 5 minutes, respectively.

A 1989 report examined the effects of multiple-dose vancomycin on newborn hearing and renal function (5). Ten pregnant, drug-dependent women were treated with IV vancomycin (1 g every 12 hours for at least 1 week) for suspected or documented infections caused by methicillin-resistant *Staphylococcus aureus*. Four of the 10 women also received concomitant gentamicin. Two control groups, neither of which received antibiotics, were formed: 10 infants from non-drug-dependent mothers (group II), and 10 infants from drug-dependent mothers (group III). Auditory brainstem response testing was conducted on the infants at birth and at 3 months of age, and blood urea nitrogen and serum creatinine were measured at birth. The placental transfer of vancomycin was measured in two patients with cord blood levels of 16.7 and 13.2 μg/mL, 6 and 2.5 hours after infusion, respectively. At birth, abnormal auditory brainstem responses were measured in a total of six infants: two infants from the study group (neither was exposed to gentamicin), three from control group II, and one from control group III. The hearing defect in all six infants was an absent wave V at 40 dB (the average behavioral threshold of adult listeners) in one or both ears. Repeat testing at 3 months in five infants was normal, indicating that the initial tests were falsely positive (5). In the sixth infant (one from the study group), the tests at 3 months again showed no response in either ear at 40 dB. This infant's mother had received a 2-g vancomycin dose after initial dosing had produced low serum levels (<20 μg/mL) of the antibiotic. The peak serum level obtained following the double dose was 65.7 μg/mL, a potentially toxic level if it was maintained. Following this, the mother was treated with the same regimen as the other women. On further examination, however, reduced compliance was discovered in both ears and the loss of hearing was diagnosed as a conduction defect, rather than sensorineural. Tests at 12 months, following improved compliance in both ears, were normal. Renal function studies in all 30 infants were also normal, although this latter conclusion has been challenged (6) and defended (7).

BREAST FEEDING SUMMARY

RECOMMENDATION: Limited Human Data - Probably Compatible

Vancomycin is excreted into breast milk. In one woman treated with IV vancomycin (1 g every 12 hours for at least 1 week), a milk level 4 hours after a dose was 12.7 μg/mL (5). This value was nearly identical to the serum trough concentration measured at 12 hours in the mother during pregnancy. The effect on the nursing infant of vancomycin in milk is unknown. Vancomycin is poorly absorbed from the normal, intact gastrointestinal tract, and thus, systemic absorption would not be expected (4). However, three potential problems exist for the nursing infant: modification of bowel flora, direct effects on the infant (e.g., allergic response or sensitization), and interference with the interpretation of culture results if a fever workup is required.

References

1. Product information. Vancocin. Eli Lilly, 2000.
2. Bourget P, Fernandez H, Delouis C, Ribou F. Transplacental passage of vancomycin during the second trimester of pregnancy. Obstet Gynecol 1991;78:908–11.
3. Hill LM. Fetal distress secondary to vancomycin-induced maternal hypotension. Am J Obstet Gynecol 1985;153:74–5.
4. American Hospital Formulary Service. *Drug Information 1997*. Bethesda, MD: American Society of Health-System Pharmacists, 1997:403–8.
5. Reyes MP, Ostrea EM Jr, Cabinian AE, Schmitt C, Rintelmann W. Vancomycin during pregnancy: Does it cause hearing loss or nephrotoxicity in the infant? Am J Obstet Gynecol 1989;161:977–81.
6. Gouyon JB, Petion AM. Toxicity of vancomycin during pregnancy. Am J Obstet Gynecol 1990;163:1375–6.
7. Reyes MP, Ostrea EM Jr. Toxicity of vancomycin during pregnancy. Reply. Am J Obstet Gynecol 1990;163:1376.

Name: **VASOPRESSIN** Risk Factor: **B**

Class: **Pituitary Hormone**

FETAL RISK SUMMARY

RECOMMENDATION: Compatible

No reports linking the use of vasopressin with congenital defects have been located. Vasopressin and the structurally related synthetic polypeptides, desmopressin and lypressin, have been used during pregnancy to treat diabetes insipidus, a rare disorder (1–10). Desmopressin has also been used at delivery in three women for the management of von Willebrand disease (11). No adverse effects on the newborns were reported.

A 3-fold increase of circulating levels of endogenous vasopressin has been reported for women in the last trimester and in labor as compared with nonpregnant women (12). Although infrequent, the induction of uterine activity in the 3rd trimester has been reported after IM and intranasal vasopressin (13). The IV use of desmopressin, which is normally given intranasally, has also been reported to cause uterine contractions (4).

Two investigators speculated that raised levels of vasopressin resulted from hypoxemia and acidosis and could produce signs of fetal distress (bradycardia and meconium staining) (14).

A 1995 reference described the use of desmopressin during pregnancy in 42 women with diabetes insipidus, 29 of whom received the drug throughout the whole pregnancy (15). One patient, treated with vasopressin during the first 6 months and then changed to desmopressin, delivered an infant who had a ventricular septal defect, a patent ductus arteriosus, and simian lines. The child died at age 14 years because of hypophyseal disease. Three of the infants exposed throughout gestation to desmopressin had birth weights close to or outside of the 99% confidence interval (two low and one high). The authors concluded that the use of desmopressin throughout pregnancy did not constitute a major fetal risk (15).

Diabetes insipidus developed in a 14-year-old girl at 33 weeks' gestation with resulting oligohydramnios and an amniotic fluid index of 0 (16). She was treated with intranasal desmopressin, 10 μg twice daily, with rapid resolution of the oligohydramnios and eventual, spontaneous delivery of a healthy, 2700-g male infant at 38 weeks.

BREAST FEEDING SUMMARY

RECOMMENDATION: Compatible

Patients receiving vasopressin, desmopressin, or lypressin for diabetes insipidus have been reported to breast-feed without apparent problems in the infant (1,2). Experimental work in lactating women suggests that suckling almost doubles the maternal blood concentration of vasopressin (12).

References

1. Hime MC, Richardson JA. Diabetes insipidus and pregnancy. Obstet Gynecol Surv 1978;33:375–9.
2. Hadi HA, Mashini IS, Devoe LD. Diabetes insipidus during pregnancy complicated by preeclampsia. A case report. J Reprod Med 1985;30:206–8.
3. Phelan JP, Guay AT, Newman C. Diabetes insipidus in pregnancy: a case review. Am J Obstet Gynecol 1978;130:365–6
4. van der Wildt B, Drayer JIM, Eske TKAB. Diabetes insipidus in pregnancy as a first sign of a craniopharyngioma. Eur J Obstet Gynecol Reprod Biol 1980;10:269–74.
5. Ford SM Jr. Transient vasopressin-resistant diabetes insipidus of pregnancy. Obstet Gynecol 1986;68:288–9.
6. Ford SM Jr, Lumpkin HL III. Transient vasopressin-resistant diabetes insipidus of pregnancy. Obstet Gynecol 1986;68:726–8.
7. Rubens R, Thiery M. Case report: diabetes insipidus and pregnancy. Eur J Obstet Gynecol Reprod Biol 1987;26:265–70.
8. Hughes JM, Barron WM, Vance ML. Recurrent diabetes insipidus associated with pregnancy: pathophysiology and therapy. Obstet Gynecol 1989;73:462–4.
9. Goolsby L, Harlass F. Central diabetes insipidus: a complication of ventriculoperitoneal shunt malfunction during pregnancy. Am J Obstet Gynecol 1996;174:1655–7.
10. Stubbe E. Pregnancies in diabetes insipidus. Geburtshilfe Frauenheilkd 1994;54:111–3.
11. Swanbeck J, Baxi L, Hurlet AM. DDAVP in the management of Von Willebrand's disease in pregnancy (abstract). Am J Obstet Gynecol 1992;166:427.
12. Robinson KW, Hawker RW, Robertson PA. Antidiuretic hormone (ADH) in the human female. J Clin Endocrinol Metab 1957;17:320–2.
13. Oravec D, Lichardus B. Management of diabetes insipidus in pregnancy. Br Med J 1972;4:114–5.
14. Gaffney PR, Jenkins DM. Vasopressin: mediator of the clinical signs of fetal distress. Br J Obstet Gynaecol 1983;90:987.
15. Kallen BA, Carlsson SS, Bengtsson BKA. Diabetes insipidus and use of desmopressin (Minirin) during pregnancy. Eur J Endocrinol 1995;132:144–6.
16. Hanson RS, Powrie RO, Larson L. Diabetes insipidus in pregnancy: a treatable cause of oligohydramnios. Obstet Gynecol 1997;89:816–7.

Name: **VECURONIUM** Risk Factor: **C_M**

Class: **Autonomic (Skeletal Muscle Relaxant)**

FETAL RISK SUMMARY

RECOMMENDATION: Limited Human Data - No Relevant Animal Data

The muscle relaxant vecuronium bromide is a nondepolarizing neuromuscular blocking agent that acts by competing for cholinergic receptors at the motor end plate (1). This quaternary ammonium compound belongs to the same general subclass (aminosteroidal) of neuromuscular blockers as pancuronium, pipecuronium, rapacuronium and rocuronium

(2). Vecuronium is indicated as an adjunct to general anesthesia, to facilitate endotracheal intubation, and to provide skeletal muscle relaxation during surgery or mechanical ventilation (1). Reproduction studies of vecuronium in experimental animals have not been located.

The pharmacokinetics of vecuronium in pregnancy were summarized in a 1998 review (3). At term, the elimination half-life of a 0.04 mg/kg dose was 36 minutes, approximately twice as long as atracurium but half the time of pancuronium (3).

Although the molecular weight of vecuronium (about 638) is relatively low, it is ionized in the plasma and has relatively low lipid solubility. In spite of these latter two characteristics, small amounts of vecuronium cross the human placenta at term (4–8). In 20 women undergoing general anesthesia for cesarean section, vecuronium 60–80 μg/kg was administered between 5 and 21 minutes before delivery (4). The venous cord:maternal ratio averaged 0.11. No neonatal adverse effect was noted as evidenced by normal 1- and 5-minute Apgar scores (4). Others have reported an identical (0.11) umbilical vein:maternal vein ratio (5,6). In these studies, the mean vecuronium-to-delivery interval was 6 to 7 minutes. No adverse effects on the newborns were observed, as noted by the Apgar scores at 1 and 5 minutes, and the Neurologic and Adaptive Capacity Scores (NACS) determined at 15 minutes, 2 hours, and 24 hours after birth (6).

A 1990 report described the use of vecuronium in 21 patients who were delivered at 36–41 weeks' gestation by elective cesarean section (7). In one group, 11 women received a 0.01 mg/kg IV priming dose, followed 4 to 6 minutes later by a 0.1 mg/kg IV dose. The second group of 10 women received a single IV dose of 0.2 mg/kg. The mean induction to delivery time intervals in the two groups was 9 and 11 minutes, respectively. The mean umbilical (UV) and maternal (MV) venous plasma concentrations of vecuronium in group 1 were 73 and 515 ng/mL, respectively, a UV/MV ratio of 0.14, whereas in group 2 the values were 107 and 838 ng/mL, respectively, a ratio of 0.13. The mean birth weights in the two groups were 3443 and 3405 g, respectively. The percentage of newborns having Apgar scores greater than 7 in groups 1 and 2 at 1 minute were 70% and 50%, and at 5 minutes 100% and 90%, respectively. There were no significant differences between the two groups in the 1- and 24-hour NACS, or in individual tests of passive and active tone within the overall NACS profile. However, the data suggested that vecuronium caused residual effects in the infants (7). A number of other reports have discussed the safe use of vecuronium during cesarean section (8–12).

In a 1999 report, investigators concluded that a more accurate estimation of vecuronium placental transfer during cesarean section would be shown by the ratio of umbilical vein (UV) to maternal artery (MA) concentrations (13). Following an intubation dose of 0.11 mg/kg, the mean UV/MA ratio was 0.056 at an intubation-to-umbilical-cord clamping (I-D) interval of 280 seconds. As expected, the ratio decreased as the I-D interval shortened.

Vecuronium (1 to 10 mg) has been used as an adjunct to general anesthesia in gamete intrafallopian transfer (GIFT) procedures (14). No effect on the pregnancy rate following GIFT was noted.

In a 1983 study, 19 newborns of mothers who had received vecuronium before delivery by cesarean section were compared to 9 newborns whose mothers had not received the agent (15). No significant difference in the Apgar scores at 1 and 5 minutes were observed between the two groups. In addition, vecuronium had no effect on maternal plasma cholinesterase activity (15).

A 1988 case study described the direct fetal administration of vecuronium under ultrasound guidance for fetal magnetic resonance imaging at 33 weeks' gestation of a brain defect (16). The dose used was 0.2 mg (0.1 mg/kg). A 3540-g male infant was delivered at 39 weeks' with Apgar scores of 10 and 10 at 1 and 5 minutes, respectively. Examination at 9 day of age confirmed the defect (16).

The successful anesthetic management of a woman at 32 week's gestation with dextrocardia, situs inversus, a double-outlet right ventricle, ventricular septal defect, and severe pulmonary stenosis was described in a 1994 report (17). No adverse effects attributable to vecuronium (0.1 mg/kg) were observed in the growth retarded (0.94 kg) infant, who was doing well at 2 weeks of age. Vecuronium (10 mg) was used to assist mechanical ventilation in another case involving a woman at 36 weeks' gestation in labor that had developed severe respiratory distress secondary to myocardial infarction related to cocaine use (18). The mother also received fentanyl and midazolam. Four hours later, the woman delivered a live female infant. Specific information on the infant's condition was not given.

A 1998 case report described respiratory muscle rigidity in a newborn that was attributed to fentanyl (see Fentanyl) (19). In addition to other drugs, the mother had received vecuronium (7 mg) at 31 weeks' gestation.

Vecuronium was used to paralyze 14 fetuses during 17 intrauterine intravascular exchange transfusions (20). The mean gestational age was 29.2 weeks (range 22–35 weeks) and the mean estimated fetal weight was 1,610 g (range 500–2500 g). The dose used (0.1 mg/kg) resulted in a mean onset of paralysis of 97.6 seconds (range 45–150 seconds) with a mean duration, as determined by maternal perception of fetal movements, of 122 minutes (range 55–160 minutes). The duration of paralysis was not correlated with gestational age. No maternal or fetal adverse effects were noted. All fetuses were delivered alive at a mean 35.8 weeks' gestation (20). In another 1992 report, vecuronium (0.15 mg/kg IV or IM) was used in nine intrauterine procedures involving five fetuses (21). The authors noted that whereas vecuronium caused no fetal heart rate changes, pancuronium caused increased fetal heart rates and decreased beat-to-beat variability for 2.5 hours post-dose.

Two pregnant women undergoing general anesthesia for cesarean section developed difficulty with breathing after receiving IV priming doses of vecuronium (10 and 13.7 μg/kg) (22). Rapid sequence induction was initiated and healthy infants with normal Apgar scores were delivered.

In summary, vecuronium has been used as an adjunct to general anesthesia during GIFT procedures and cesarean sections. It has also been used in the 2nd and 3rd trimesters by direct IV and IM fetal dosing to produce paralysis during various procedures. No adverse effects attributable to vecuronium on pregnancy rates, the fetus, or the newborn have been reported in these studies. Small amounts of vecuronium cross the placenta, even though this transfer is inhibited by the drug's low lipid solubility and ionization at physiologic pH. However, animal reproduction studies have not been conducted with vecuronium, and no studies, animal or human, have reported its use during organogenesis. Based on this lack of information, the fetal risk from exposure to vecuronium during organogenesis cannot be determined. Use in later times of gestation, however, appears to carry little, if any, risk to the fetus or newborn.

BREAST FEEDING SUMMARY

RECOMMENDATION: No Human Data - Probably Compatible

No reports describing the use of vecuronium during lactation have been located. However, even if such use was reported, it is doubtful if clinically significant amounts of vecuronium would be excreted into breast milk. The molecular weight (about 638) is low enough, but the low lipid solubility and ionization at physiologic pH would inhibit its excretion into milk. These factors suggest that vecuronium represents no risk to a breast-feeding infant.

References

1. Product information. Norcuron. Organon, 2002.
2. Muscle relaxants. Parfitt K, editor. *Martindale*. 32nd ed. London, UK: Pharmaceutical Press, 1999:1302.
3. Guay J, Grenier Y, Varin F. Clinical pharmacokinetics of neuromuscular relaxants in pregnancy. Clin Pharmacokinet 1998;483–96.
4. Demetriou M, Depoix JP, Diakite B, Fromentin M, Duvaldestin P. Placental transfer of ORG NC45 in women undergoing Caesarean section. Br J Anaesth 1982;54:643–5.
5. Dailey PA, Fisher DM, Shnider SM, Baysinger CL, Shinohara Y, Miller RD, Abboud TK, Kim KC. Pharmacokinetics, placental transfer, and neonatal effects of vecuronium (ORG NC45) administered prior to delivery (abstract). Anesthesiology 1982;57:A391.
6. Dailey PA, Fisher DM, Shnider SM, Baysinger CL, Shinohara Y, Miller RD, Abboud TK, Kim KC. Pharmacokinetics, placental transfer, and neonatal effects of vecuronium and pancuronium administered during cesarean section. Anesthesiology 1984;60:569–74.
7. Hawkins JL, Johnson TD, Kubicek MA, Skjonsby BS, Morrow DH, Joyce TH III. Vecuronium for rapid-sequence intubation for Cesarean section. Anesth Analg 1990;71:185–90.
8. Baraka A, Jabbour S, Tabboush Z, Sibai A, Bijjani A, Karam K. Onset of vecuronium neuromuscular block is more rapid in patients undergoing caesarean section. Can J Anaesth 1992;39:135–8.
9. Teviotdale BM. Vecuronium-thiopentone induction for emergency caesarean section under general anaesthesia. Anaesth Intensive Care 1993;21:288–91.
10. Brimacombe J, Berry A. Vecuronium for emergency caesarean section. Anaesth Intensive Care 1994;22:119.
11. Teviotdate B. Vecuronium for emergency caesarean section. Reply. Anaesth Intensive Care 1994;22:119–20.
12. Das S, Bhattacharjee M, Maitra S. Study of neonatal status after use of vecuronium as a muscle relaxant in caesarean section. J Indian Med Assoc 1993;91:54–6.
13. Iwama H, Kaneko T, Tobishima S, Komatsu T, Watanabe K, Akutsu H. Time dependency of the ratio of umbilical vein/maternal artery concentrations of vecuronium in Caesarean section. Acta Anaesthesiol Scand 1999;43:9–12.
14. Pierce ET, Smalky M, Alper MM, Hunter JA, Amrhein RL, Pierce EC Jr. Comparison of pregnancy rates following gamete intrafallopian transfer (GIFT) under general anesthesia with thiopental sodium or propofol. J Clin Anesth 1992;4:394–8.
15. Baraka A, Noueihed R, Sinno H, Wakid N, Agoston S. Succinylcholine-vecuronium (ORG NC 45) sequence for Cesarean section. Anesth Analg 1983;62:909–13.
16. Daffos F, Forestier F, MacAleese J, Aufrant C, Mandelbrot L, Cabanis EA, Iba-Zizen MT, Alfonso JM, Tamraz J. Fetal curarization for prenatal magnetic resonance imaging. Prenat Diagn 1988;8:312–4.
17. Rowbottom SJ, Gin T, Cheung LP. General anaesthesia for Caesarean section in a patient with uncorrected complex cyanotic heart disease. Anaesth Intensive Care 1994;22:74–8.
18. Liu SS, Forrester RM, Murphy GS, Chen K, Glassenberg R. Anaesthetic management of a parturient with myocardial infarction related to cocaine use. Can J Anaesth 1992;39:858 6.
19. Lindemann R. Respiratory muscle rigidity in a preterm infant after use of fentanyl during Caesarean section. Eur J Pediatr 1998;157:1012–3.
20. Leveque C, Murat I, Toubas F, Poissonnier MH, Brossard Y, Saint-Maurice C. Fetal neuromuscular blockade with vecuronium bromide: studies during intravascular intrauterine transfusion in isoimmunized pregnancies. Anesthesiology 1992;76:642–4.
21. Watson WJ, Atchison SR, Harlass FE. Comparison of pancuronium and vecuronium for fetal neuromuscular blockade during invasive procedures. J Matern Fetal Med 1996;5:151–4.
22. Cherala S, Eddie D, Halpern M, Shevdi K. Priming with vecuronium in obstetrics. Anaesthesia 1987;42:1021.

Name: **VENLAFAXINE** Risk Factor: **C_M**

Class: **Antidepressant**

FETAL RISK SUMMARY

RECOMMENDATION: Human Data Suggest Risk in 3rd Trimester

Venlafaxine, an antidepressant structurally unrelated to other available antidepressants, was approved by the FDA in December 1993. Although the mechanism of action of this agent and its active metabolite is unknown, it is believed to be related to the potentiation of neurotransmitter activity in the brain. Venlafaxine is a potent inhibitor of neuronal reuptake of serotonin and norepinephrine, and a weak inhibitor of dopamine reuptake.

Reproduction studies in rats and rabbits at doses up to 2.5 and 4 times the maximum recommended human daily dose based on body surface area (MRHD), respectively, did not reveal teratogenicity (1). When rats were given the same maximum dose during pregnancy through weaning, however, there was a decrease in pup weight and an increased number of stillbirths and pup deaths during the first 5 days of lactation. The no-effect dose for pup mortality was 0.25 times the MRHD (1).

A 1994 review of venlafaxine included citations of data from the clinical trials of this drug involving its use during gestation in 10 women for periods ranging from 10 to 60 days (2), apparently during the 1st trimester. No adverse effects of the exposure were observed in four of the infants (information not provided for the other six exposed pregnancies).

The FDA had not received any reports of adverse pregnancy outcomes involving the use of the drug during gestation (F. Rosa, personal communication, FDA, 1996).

In a 2001 prospective controlled study, the pregnancy outcomes of 150 women exposed to venlafaxine were compared to 150 women exposed to other SSRI antidepressants and 150 women exposed to nonteratogenic agents (3). The data were collected from seven teratology information services: 2 in Canada, 2 in the United States, 2 in Italy, and 1 in Brazil. There were no significant differences in the outcomes in the three groups in terms of spontaneous abortions, elective abortions, gestational age at birth, live births, birth weights, and major malformations. In the cases exposed to venlafaxine, there were two infants with birth defects (hypospadias; neural tube defect and clubfoot). In the control groups, there were three defects in the other SSRI group (ventricular septal defect; pyloric stenosis; and absent corpus callosum) and one in the nonteratogen group (congenital heart defect). The results suggested that venlafaxine does not increase the rates of major congenital defects over that expected in a nonexposed population (3).

Although venlafaxine does not appear to cause structural malformations, use in the 3rd trimester may result in toxicity in the newborn infant. The product information was changed in 2004 to reflect this potential toxicity (4).

BREAST FEEDING SUMMARY

RECOMMENDATION: Limited Human Data - Potential Toxicity

Venlafaxine is excreted into breast milk. A 1998 study measured the excretion of venlafaxine and its active metabolite, *O*-desmethylvenlafaxine, in the milk of three breast-feeding women (5). The three mothers, started on the antidepressant after delivery, had been taking a stable dose (3.04–8.18 mg/kg/day) for 0.23–5 months. The age of the infants ranged from 0.37 to 6 months. The mean milk:plasma (M:P) ratio (in two cases based on area under the concentration curve [12 hours], in one on a single point) for the parent drug was 4.14 (range 3.26–5.18), whereas it was 3.06 (range 2.93–3.19) for the metabolite. The mean infant doses for venlafaxine and metabolite were 3.49% and 4.08% of the mother's weight-adjusted dose, respectively. Venlafaxine was not detected in infant plasma, but the median infant metabolite plasma concentration was 100 μg/L (range 23–225 μg/L). The mean total infant dose was 7.57% (range 4.74%–9.23%). No adverse effects in the

V

suckling infants were noted. Because of the relatively high infant dose in comparison to other antidepressants, it was recommended that close observation of the infant for short-term adverse effects (e.g., agitation, insomnia, poor feeding, or failure to thrive) was required (5).

A brief 2001 report described two postpartum women who were taking venlafaxine and exclusively breast-feeding their infants (6). One mother had started the drug (75 mg/day) at delivery, whereas the other had taken the antidepressant throughout pregnancy (150 mg/day). At 3–4 weeks of age, maternal and infant samples were drawn 2–3 hours after a dose. The concentrations of parent drug and metabolite in the two women were 31 and 148 ng/mL and 38 and 230 ng/mL, respectively. Parent drug was not detected in the infants, but the metabolite levels were 16 ng/mL and 21 ng/mL, respectively. No adverse effects were observed in the infants (6).

The long-term effects on neurobehavior and cognitive development from exposure to potent serotonin reuptake inhibitors during a period of rapid central nervous system development have not been adequately studied. The American Academy of Pediatrics classifies other antidepressants as drugs for which the effect on nursing infants is unknown but may be of concern (7).

References

1. Product information. Effexor. Wyeth-Ayerst Pharmaceuticals, 2000.
2. Ellingrod VL, Perry PJ. Venlafaxine: a heterocyclic antidepressant. Am J Hosp Pharm 1994;51:3033–46.
3. Einarson A, Fatoye B, Sarkar M, Voyer-Lavigne S, Brochu J, Chambers C, Mastroiacovo P, Addis A, Matsui D, Schuler L, Einarson TR, Koren G. Pregnancy outcome following gestational exposure to venlafaxine: a multicenter prospective controlled study. Am J Psychiatry 2001;158:1728–30.
4. Anonymous. Recent changes to FDA-approved labeling. Am J Health Syst Pharm 2004;61:1653.
5. Ilett KF, Hackett LP, Dusci LJ, Roberts MJ, Kristensen JH, Paech M, Groves A, Yapp P. Distribution and excretion of venlafaxine and *O*-desmethylvenlafaxine in human milk. Br J Clin Pharmacol 1998;45:459–62.
6. Hendrick V, Altshuler L, Wertheimer A, Dunn WA. Venlafaxine and breast-feeding. Am J Psychiatry 2001;158:2089–90.
7. Committee on Drugs, American Academy of Pediatrics. The transfer of drugs and other chemicals into human milk. Pediatrics 2001;108:776–89.

Name: **VERAPAMIL** Risk Factor: C_M

Class: **Calcium Channel Blocker**

FETAL RISK SUMMARY

RECOMMENDATION: Compatible

Verapamil is a calcium channel inhibitor used as an antiarrhythmic agent. Reproductive studies in rats and rabbits at oral doses up to 60 mg/kg/day (6 times the human oral dose) and 15 mg/kg/day (1.5 times the human oral dose) found no evidence of teratogenicity (1). In rats, however, this dose was embryocidal, and retarded fetal growth and development, probably because of maternal toxicity (1).

Placental passage of verapamil has been demonstrated in two of six patients given 80 mg orally at term (2). Cord levels were 15.4 and 24.5 ng/mL (17% and 26% of maternal serum) in two newborns delivered at 49 and 109 minutes after verapamil administration, respectively. Verapamil could not be detected in the cord blood of four infants delivered 173–564 minutes after the dose. IV verapamil was administered to patients in labor at a rate of 2 μg/kg/minute for 60–110 minutes (3). The serum concentrations of the infants averaged 8.5 ng/mL (44% of maternal serum).

A 33-week fetus with a tachycardia of 240–280 beats/minute was treated *in utero* for 6 weeks with β-acetyldigoxin and verapamil (80 mg 3 times daily) (2). The fetal heart rate returned to normal 5 days after initiation of therapy, but the authors could not determine whether verapamil had produced the beneficial effect. At birth, no signs of cardiac hypertrophy or disturbances in repolarization were observed. Several other reports have described successful *in utero* treatment of supraventricular tachycardia with verapamil in combination with other agents (4–6). In one case, indirect therapy via the mother with verapamil, digoxin, and procainamide failed to control the fetal arrhythmia and direct fetal digitalization was required (7). In another case, verapamil, 120 mg 3 times daily, and digoxin were used successfully to control a fetal supraventricular tachycardia at 32 weeks' gestation (8). At 36 weeks' gestation, after 4 weeks of therapy, ultrasound examination showed complete resolution of both the hydropic changes and polyhydramnios, but the fetus died within 2 days. No autopsy was permitted. The authors speculated that the drug combination may have caused complete heart block (8). Maternal supraventricular tachycardia occurring in the 3rd trimester has been treated with a single 5-mg IV dose of verapamil (9). Other than the single case of fetal death in which the cause is not certain, no adverse fetal or newborn effects attributable to verapamil have been noted in the above reports.

Verapamil has been used to lower blood pressure in a woman with severe gestational hypertension in labor (10). Fifteen milligrams were given by rapid IV injection followed by an infusion of 185 mg during 6 hours. Fetal heart rate increased from 60 to 110 beats/minute, and a normal infant was delivered without signs or symptoms of toxicity. Tocolysis with verapamil, either alone or in combination with β-mimetics, has also been described (11–13).

In a surveillance study of Michigan Medicaid recipients conducted between 1985 and 1992 involving 229,101 completed pregnancies, 76 newborns had been exposed to verapamil during the 1st trimester (F. Rosa, personal communication, FDA, 1993). One (1.3%) major birth defect was observed (three expected), a cardiovascular defect. These data do not support an association between the drug and congenital defects.

A prospective, multicenter cohort study of 78 women (81 outcomes; 3 sets of twins) who had 1st trimester exposure to calcium channel blockers, including 41% to verapamil, was reported in 1996 (14). Compared with controls, no increase in the risk of major congenital malformations was found. Moreover, the manufacturer has reports of patients treated with verapamil during the 1st trimester without production of fetal problems (M. S. Anderson, personal communication, GD Searle & Co., 1981). However, hypotension (systolic and diastolic) has been observed in patients after rapid IV bolus (15), and reduced uterine blood flow with fetal hypoxia is a potential risk. If verapamil is used in pregnancy, healthcare professionals are encouraged to call the toll free number (800-670-6126) for information about patient enrollment in the Motherisk study.

BREAST FEEDING SUMMARY

RECOMMENDATION: Limited Human Data - Probably Compatible

Verapamil is excreted into breast milk (16,17). A daily dose of 240 mg produced milk levels that were approximately 23% of maternal serum (16). Serum levels in the infant were 2.1 ng/mL but could not be detected (<1 ng/mL) 38 hours after treatment was stopped.

No effects of this exposure were observed in the infant. In a second case, a mother was treated with 80 mg 3 times daily for hypertension for 4 weeks before the determination of serum and milk concentrations (17). Steady-state concentrations of verapamil and the metabolite, norverapamil, in milk were 25.8 and 8.8 ng/mL, respectively. These values were 60% and 16% of the concentrations in plasma. The investigators estimated that the breast-fed child received less than 0.01% of the mother's dose. Neither verapamil nor the metabolite could be detected in the plasma of the child. The American Academy of Pediatrics classifies verapamil as compatible with breast-feeding (18).

References

1. Product information. Calan. G. D. Searle, 2000.
2. Wolff F, Breuker KH, Schlensker KH, Bolte A. Prenatal diagnosis and therapy of fetal heart rate anomalies: with a contribution on the placental transfer of verapamil. J Perinat Med 1980;8:203–8.
3. Strigl R, Gastroph G, Hege HG, Döring P, Mehring W. Nachweis von Verapamil in Mutterlichen und fetalen Blut des Menschen. Geburtshilfe Frauenheilkd 1980;40:496–9.
4. Lilja H, Karlsson K, Lindecrantz K, Sabel KG. Treatment of intrauterine supraventricular tachycardia with digoxin and verapamil. J Perinat Med 1984;12:151–4.
5. Rey E, Duperron L, Gauthier R, Lemay M, Grignon A, LeLorier J. Transplacental treatment of tachycardia-induced fetal heart failure with verapamil and amiodarone: a case report. Am J Obstet Gynecol 1985; 153:311–2.
6. Maxwell DJ, Crawford DC, Curry PVM, Tynan MJ, Allan LD. Obstetric importance, diagnosis, and management of fetal tachycardias. BMJ 1988;297:107–10.
7. Weiner CP, Thompson MIB. Direct treatment of fetal supraventricular tachycardia after failed transplacental therapy. Am J Obstet Gynecol 1988;158:570–3.
8. Owen J, Colvin EV, Davis RO. Fetal death after successful conversion of fetal supraventricular tachycardia with digoxin and verapamil. Am J Obstet Gynecol 1988;158:1169–70.
9. Klein V, Repke JT. Supraventricular tachycardia in pregnancy: cardioversion with verapamil. Obstet Gynecol 1984;63:16S–8S.
10. Brittinger WD, Schwarzbeck A, Wittenmeier KW, et al. Klinisch-Experimentelle Untersuchungen uber die Blutdruckendende Wirkung von Verapamil. Dtsch Med Wochenschr 1970;95:1871–7.
11. Mosler KH, Rosenboom HG. Neuere Moglichkeiten einer tokolytischen Behandlung in de Geburtschilfe. Z Geburtshilfe Perinatol 1972;176:85–96.
12. Gummerus M. Prevention of premature birth with nylidrin and verapamil. Z Geburtshilfe Perinatol 1975;179:261–6.
13. Gummerus M. Treatment of premature labor and antagonization of the side effects of tocolytic therapy with verapamil. Z Geburtshilfe Perinatol 1977; 181:334–40.
14. Magee LA, Schick B, Donnenfeld AE, Sage SR, Conover B, Cook L, McElhatton PR, Schmidt MA, Koren G. The safety of calcium channel blockers in human pregnancy: a prospective, multicenter cohort study. Am J Obstet Gynecol 1996;174:823–8.
15. Rotmensch HH, Rotmensch S, Elkayam U. Management of cardiac arrhythmias during pregnancy: current concepts. Drugs 1987;33:623–33.
16. Andersen HJ. Excretion of verapamil in human milk. Eur J Clin Pharmacol 1983;25:279–80.
17. Anderson P, Bondesson U, Mattiasson I, Johansson BW. Verapamil and norverapamil in plasma and breast milk during breast feeding. Eur J Clin Pharmacol 1987;31:625–7.
18. Committee on Drugs, American Academy of Pediatrics. The transfer of drugs and other chemicals into human milk. Pediatrics 2001;108:776–89.

Name: **VIDARABINE** Risk Factor: **C_M**
Class: **Antiviral**

FETAL RISK SUMMARY

RECOMMENDATION: Limited Human Data - Animal Data Suggest High Risk

Vidarabine is a potent teratogen in mice, rats, and rabbits after topical and IM administration (1,2). Daily instillations of a 10% solution into the vaginas of pregnant rats in late gestation had no effect on the offspring (2).

Vidarabine was used for disseminated herpes simplex in one woman at about 28 weeks' gestation (3,4). Spontaneous rupture of the membranes occurred 48 hours after initiation of therapy, and a premature infant was delivered. The infant died on the 13th day of life of complications of prematurity. In a second case, a woman at 32 weeks' gestation with herpes simplex type II encephalitis was treated with vidarabine, 10 mg/kg/day, and acyclovir (5). A female infant with culture-documented herpes neonatorum was delivered by cesarean section 13 days later. The infant responded to further treatment with acyclovir and was alive and well at 2 months of age, but the mother died 2 days after delivery.

Vidarabine, 10 mg/kg/day (800 mg/day), was administered to a woman at 26 weeks' gestation with varicella pneumonitis (6). Peak and trough levels of the agent were 12.8 and 2.7 μg/mL, respectively. She delivered a healthy female infant at 38 weeks' gestation that was developing normally at 12 months of age. In a similar case, another woman with varicella pneumonitis at 27 weeks' gestation was treated with vidarabine (6). Except for a delay in speech at age 3 years that responded to special education, the child has done well and was considered normal at 5 years.

BREAST FEEDING SUMMARY

RECOMMENDATION: No Human Data - Probably Compatible

No reports involving the use of vidarabine in lactating women have been located. It is not known whether the drug is excreted into milk.

References

1. Pavan-Langston D, Buchanan RA, Alford CA Jr, eds. *Adenine Arabinoside: An Antiviral Agent*. New York, NY: Raven Press, 1975:153.
2. Schardein JL, Hertz DL, Petretre JA, Fitzgerald JE, Kurtz SM. The effect of vidarabine on the development of the offspring of rats, rabbits and monkeys. Teratology 1977;15:213–42.
3. Hillard P, Seeds J, Cefalo R. Disseminated herpes simplex in pregnancy: two cases and a review. Obstet Gynecol Surv 1982;37:449–53.
4. Peacock JE Jr, Sarubbi FA. Disseminated herpes simplex virus infection during pregnancy. Obstet Gynecol 1983;61:13S–8S.
5. Berger SA, Weinberg M, Treves T, Sorkin P, Geller E, Yedwab G, Tomer A, Rabey M, Michaeli D. Herpes encephalitis during pregnancy: failure of acyclovir and adenine arabinoside to prevent neonatal herpes. Isr J Med Sci 1986;22:41–4.
6. Landsberger EJ, Hager WD, Grossman JH III. Successful management of varicella pneumonia complicating pregnancy: a report of three cases. J Reprod Med 1986;31:311–4.

Name: **VINBLASTINE** Risk Factor: **D_M**

Class: **Antineoplastic**

FETAL RISK SUMMARY

RECOMMENDATION: Limited Human Data - Animal Data Suggest High Risk

Vinblastine is an antimitotic antineoplastic agent. The drug is embryocidal and teratogenic in laboratory animals (no details provided) (1).

The drug has been used in pregnancy, including the 1st trimester, without producing malformations (2–10). Two cases of malformed infants have been reported following 1st trimester exposure to vinblastine (10,11). In 1974, a case of a 27-year-old woman with Hodgkin's disease who was given vinblastine, mechlorethamine, and procarbazine during the 1st trimester was described (11). At 24 weeks' gestation, she spontaneously aborted a male fetus with oligodactyly of both feet with webbing of the third and fourth toes. These defects were attributed to mechlorethamine therapy. A mother with Hodgkin's disease treated with vinblastine, vincristine, and procarbazine in the 1st trimester (3 weeks after the last menstrual period) delivered a 1900-g male infant at about 37 weeks of gestation (12). The newborn developed fatal respiratory distress syndrome. At autopsy, a small secundum atrial septal defect was found.

Vinblastine in combination with other antineoplastic agents may produce gonadal dysfunction in men and women (13–16). Alkylating agents are the most frequent cause of this problem (15). Although total aspermia may result, return of fertility has apparently been documented in at least two cases (16). Ovarian function may return to normal with successful pregnancies possible, depending on the patient's age at the time of therapy and the total dose of chemotherapy received (14,17). The long-term effects of combination chemotherapy on menstrual and reproductive function were described in a 1988 report (18). Only 5 of 40 women treated for malignant ovarian germ cell tumors received vinblastine. The results of this study are discussed in the monograph for cyclophosphamide (see Cyclophosphamide).

In 436 long-term survivors treated with chemotherapy for gestational trophoblastic tumors between 1958 and 1978, 11 (2.5%) received vinblastine as part of their treatment regimens (19). Of the 11 women, 2 (18%) had at least one live birth (mean and maximum vinblastine dose 20 mg), and 9 (82%) did not try to conceive (mean dose 37 mg, maximum dose 80 mg). Additional details, including congenital anomalies observed, are described in the monograph for vincristine (see Vincristine).

Data from one review indicated that 40% of infants exposed to anticancer drugs were of low birth weight (20). This finding was not related to the timing of exposure. Long-term studies of growth and mental development in offspring exposed to vinblastine during the 2nd trimester, the period of neuroblast multiplication, have not been conducted (21). However, two children, exposed throughout gestation, beginning with the 3rd–4th week of gestation, were normal at 2 and 5 years of age, respectively (10).

Occupational exposure of the mother to antineoplastic agents during pregnancy may present a risk to the fetus. A position statement from the National Study Commission on Cytotoxic Exposure and a research article involving some antineoplastic agents are presented in the monograph for cyclophosphamide (see Cyclophosphamide).

BREAST FEEDING SUMMARY

RECOMMENDATION: Contraindicated

No reports describing the use of vinblastine during lactation have been located. Because of the potential for severe toxicity in a nursing infant, women who require this agent should not breast-feed.

References

1. Product information. Velban. Eli Lilly, 2000.
2. Armstrong JG, Dyke RW, Fouts PJ, Jansen CJ. Delivery of a normal infant during the course of oral vinblastine sulfate therapy for Hodgkin's disease. Ann Intern Med 1964;61:106–7.
3. Rosenzweig AI, Crews QE Jr, Hopwood HG. Vinblastine sulfate in Hodgkin's disease in pregnancy. Ann Intern Med 1964;61:108–12.
4. Lacher MJ. Use of vinblastine sulfate to treat Hodgkin's disease during pregnancy. Ann Intern Med 1964;61:113–5.
5. Lacher MJ, Geller W. Cyclophosphamide and vinblastine sulfate in Hodgkin's disease during pregnancy. JAMA 1966;195:192–4.
6. Nordlund JJ, DeVita VT Jr, Carbone PP. Severe vinblastine-induced leukopenia during late pregnancy with delivery of a normal infant. Ann Intern Med 1968;69:581–2.
7. Goguei A. Hodgkin's disease and pregnancy. Nouv Presse Med 1970;78:1507–10.
8. Johnson IR, Filshie GM. Hodgkin's disease diagnosed in pregnancy: case report. Br J Obstet Gynaecol 1977;84:791–2.
9. Nisce LZ, Tome MA, He S, Lee BJ III, Kutcher GJ. Management of coexisting Hodgkin's disease and pregnancy. Am J Clin Oncol 1986;9:146–51.
10. Malone JM, Gershenson DM, Creasy RK, Kavanagh JJ, Silva EG, Stringer CA. Endodermal sinus tumor of

V

the ovary associated with pregnancy. Obstet Gynecol 1986;68(Suppl):86S–9S.

11. Garrett MJ. Teratogenic effects of combination chemotherapy. Ann Intern Med 1974;80:667.
12. Thomas RPM, Peckham MJ. The investigation and management of Hodgkin's disease in the pregnant patient. Cancer 1976;38:1443–51.
13. Morgenfeld MC, Goldberg V, Parisier H, Bugnard SC, Bur GE. Ovarian lesions due to cytostatic agents during the treatment of Hodgkin's disease. Surg Gynecol Obstet 1972;134:826–8.
14. Ross GT. Congenital anomalies among children born of mothers receiving chemotherapy for gestational trophoblastic neoplasms. Cancer 1976;37:1043–7.
15. Schilsky RL, Lewis BJ, Sherins RJ, Young RC. Gonadal dysfunction in patients receiving chemotherapy for cancer. Ann Intern Med 1980;93:109–14.
16. Rubery ED. Return of fertility after curative chemotherapy for disseminated teratoma of testis. Lancet 1983;1:186.
17. Shalet SM, Vaughan Williams CA, Whitehead E. Pregnancy after chemotherapy induced ovarian failure. Br Med J 1985;290:898.
18. Gershenson DM. Menstrual and reproductive function after treatment with combination chemotherapy for malignant ovarian germ cell tumors. J Clin Oncol 1988;6:270–5.
19. Rustin GJS, Booth M, Dent J, Salt S, Rustin F, Bagshawe KD. Pregnancy after cytotoxic chemotherapy for gestational trophoblastic tumours. Br Med J 1984;288:103–6.
20. Nicholson HO. Cytotoxic drugs in pregnancy: review of reported cases. J Obstet Gynaecol Br Commonw 1968;75:307–12.
21. Dobbing J. Pregnancy and leukaemia. Lancet 1977;1:1155.

Name: **VINCRISTINE** Risk Factor: **D_M**

Class: **Antineoplastic**

FETAL RISK SUMMARY

RECOMMENDATION: Limited Human Data - Animal Data Suggest High Risk

Vincristine is an antimitotic antineoplastic agent. The drug is embryocidal and teratogenic in mice, hamsters, and monkeys (1). Doses that produced these effects were nontoxic to the pregnant animal.

The use of vincristine has been described in at least 36 pregnancies (1 with twins), 9 during the 1st trimester (2–31).

A mother with Hodgkin's disease treated with vincristine, vinblastine, and procarbazine in the 1st trimester (3 weeks after the last menstrual period) delivered a 1900-g male infant at about 37 weeks' gestation (10). Neonatal death occurred because of respiratory distress syndrome. At autopsy, a small secundum atrial septal defect was found. In a Hodgkin's case treated with vincristine, mechlorethamine, and procarbazine during the 1st trimester, the electively aborted fetus had malformed kidneys (markedly reduced size and malpositioned) (16). Other adverse fetal outcomes observed following vincristine use include a 1000-g male infant born with pancytopenia who was exposed to six different antineoplastic agents in the 3rd trimester (2) and transient severe bone marrow hypoplasia in another newborn that was most likely caused by mercaptopurine (19). Intrauterine fetal death occurred in a 1200-g female fetus 36 hours after maternal treatment with vincristine, doxorubicin, and prednisone for diffuse, undifferentiated lymphoma of T-cell origin at 31 weeks' gestation (22). The fetus was macerated, but no other abnormalities were observed at autopsy. In another case, a 34-year-old woman with acute lymphoblastic leukemia was treated with multiple antineoplastic agents from 22 weeks' gestation until delivery of a healthy female infant 18 weeks later (25). Vincristine was administered 4 times between 22 and 25 weeks' gestation. Chromosomal analysis of the newborn revealed a normal karyotype (46,XX) but with gaps and a ring chromosome. The clinical significance of these findings is unknown, but because these abnormalities may persist for several

V

years, the potential existed for an increased risk of cancer, as well as for a risk of genetic damage in the next generation (25).

A 1999 report from France described the outcomes of pregnancies in 20 women with breast cancer who were treated with antineoplastic agents (31). The first cycle of chemotherapy occurred at a mean gestational age of 26 weeks with delivery occurring at a mean 34.7 weeks. A total of 38 cycles were administered during pregnancy with a median of two cycles per woman. None of the women received radiation therapy during pregnancy. The pregnancy outcomes included two spontaneous abortions (SABs) (both exposed in the 1st trimester), one intrauterine death (exposed in the 2nd trimester), and 17 live births, one of whom died at 8 days of age without apparent cause. The 16 surviving children were developing normally at a mean follow-up of 42.3 months (31). Vincristine (V), in combination with doxorubicin (D), epirubicin (E), and/or methotrexate (M), was administered to two women at a mean dose of 2 mg/m^2. The outcomes were one SAB (VEM; exposed at 6 weeks' gestation) and one surviving liveborn infant (exposed to VD in the 2nd trimester) (31).

Data from one review indicated that 40% of the infants exposed to anticancer drugs were of low birth weight (32). This finding was not related to the timing of exposure. Long-term studies of growth and mental development in offspring exposed to these drugs during the 2nd trimester, the period of neuroblast multiplication, have not been conducted (33). However, individual infants have been evaluated for periods ranging from a few weeks up to 7 years and all have had normal growth and development (17–20,22–24,26,27,29).

Vincristine, in combination with other antineoplastic agents, may produce gonadal dysfunction in men and women (34–41). Alkylating agents are the most frequent cause of this problem (38). Ovarian and testicular function may return to normal with successful pregnancies possible, depending on the patient's age at time of treatment and the total dose of chemotherapy received (34). In a 1989 case report, a woman with an immature teratoma of the ovary was treated with conservative surgery and chemotherapy consisting of six courses of vincristine, dactinomycin, and cyclophosphamide (42). She conceived 20 months after her last chemotherapy and eventually delivered a normal 3340-g male infant. The long-term effects of combination chemotherapy on menstrual and reproductive function have been described in a 1988 report (43). Twenty-nine of 40 women treated for malignant ovarian germ cell tumors received vincristine. The results of this study are discussed in the monograph for cyclophosphamide (see Cyclophosphamide).

In 436 long-term survivors treated with chemotherapy between 1958 and 1978 for gestational trophoblastic tumors, 132 (30%) received vincristine in combination with other antineoplastic agents (44). The mean duration of chemotherapy was 4 months with a mean interval from completion of therapy to the first pregnancy of 2.7 years. Conception occurred within 1 year of therapy completion in 45 women (antineoplastic agents used in these women were not specified), resulting in 31 live births, 1 anencephalic stillbirth, 7 SABs, and 6 elective abortions. Of the 132 women treated with vincristine, 37 (28%) had at least one live birth (numbers in parentheses refer to mean/maximum vincristine dose in milligrams) (7.4/17.0), 8 (6%) had no live births (7.1/22.0), 4 (3%) failed to conceive (7.3/18.0), and 83 (63%) did not try to conceive (11.3/46.0). The average ages at the end of treatment in the four groups were 24.9, 24.4, 24.4, and 31.5 years, respectively. Congenital abnormalities noted in the total group (368 conceptions) were two cases of anencephaly, and one case each of spina bifida, tetralogy of Fallot, talipes equinovarus, collapsed lung, umbilical hernia, desquamative fibrosing alveolitis, asymptomatic heart murmur, and mental retardation. Another child had tachycardia but developed normally after treatment. One case of sudden infant death syndrome occurred in a female infant at 4 weeks of age. None of these outcomes differed statistically from that expected in a normal population (44).

Occupational exposure of the mother to antineoplastic agents during pregnancy may present a risk to the fetus. A position statement from the National Study Commission on Cytotoxic Exposure and a research article involving some antineoplastic agents are presented in the monograph for cyclophosphamide (see Cyclophosphamide).

BREAST FEEDING SUMMARY

RECOMMENDATION: Contraindicated

No reports describing the use of vincristine during lactation have been located. Because of the potential for severe toxicity in a nursing infant, women who require this agent should not breast-feed.

References

1. Product information. Oncovin. Eli Lilly, 2000.
2. Pizzuto J, Aviles A, Noriega L, Niz J, Morales M, Romero F. Treatment of acute, leukemia during pregnancy: presentation of nine cases. Cancer Treat Rep 1980;64:679–83.
3. Colbert N, Najman A, Gorin NC, Blum F, Treisser A, Lasfargues G, Cloup M, Barrat H, Duhamel G. Acute leukaemia during pregnancy: favourable course of pregnancy in two patients treated with cytosine arabinoside and anthracyclines. Nouv Presse Med 1980;9:175–8.
4. Daly H, McCann SR, Hanratty TD, Temperley IJ. Successful pregnancy during combination chemotherapy for Hodgkin's disease. Acta Haematol (Basel) 1980;64:154–6.
5. Tobias JS, Bloom HJG. Doxorubicin in pregnancy. Lancet 1980;1:776.
6. Garcia V, San Miguel J, Borrasea AL. Doxorubicin in the first trimester of pregnancy. Ann Intern Med 1981;94:547.
7. Dara P, Slater LM, Armentrout SA. Successful pregnancy during chemotherapy for acute leukemia. Cancer 1981;47:845–6.
8. Burnier AM. Discussion. In Plows CW. Acute myelomonocytic leukemia in pregnancy: report of a case. Am J Obstet Gynecol 1982;143:41–3.
9. Lilleyman JS, Hill AS, Anderton KJ. Consequences of acute myelogenous leukemia in early pregnancy. Cancer 1977;40:1300–3.
10. Thomas PRM, Peckham MJ. The investigation and management of Hodgkin's disease in the pregnant patient. Cancer 1976;38:1443–51.
11. Pawliger DF, McLean FW, Noyes WD. Normal fetus after cytosine arabinoside therapy. Ann Intern Med 1971;74:1012.
12. Lowenthal RM, Funnell CF, Hope DM, Stewart IG, Humphrey DC. Normal infant after combination chemotherapy including teniposide for Burkitt's lymphoma in pregnancy. Med Pediatr Oncol 1982;10:165–9.
13. Sears HF, Reid J. Granulocytic sarcoma: local presentation of a systemic disease. Cancer 1976;37:1808–13.
14. Durie BGM, Giles HR. Successful treatment of acute leukemia during pregnancy: combination therapy in the third trimester. Arch Intern Med 1977;137:90–1.
15. Newcomb M, Balducci L, Thigpen JT, Morrison FS. Acute leukemia in pregnancy: successful delivery after cytarabine and doxorubicin. JAMA 1978;239:2691–2.
16. Mennuti MT, Shepard TH, Mellman WJ. Fetal renal malformation following treatment of Hodgkin's disease during pregnancy. Obstet Gynecol 1975;46:194–6.
17. Coopland AT, Friesen WJ, Galbraith PA. Acute leukemia in pregnancy. Am J Obstet Gynecol 1969;105:1288–9.
18. Doney KC, Kraemer KG, Shepard TH. Combination chemotherapy for acute myelocytic leukemia during pregnancy: three case reports. Cancer Treat Rep 1979;63:369–71.
19. Okun DB, Groncy PK, Sieger L, Tanaka KR. Acute leukemia in pregnancy: transient neonatal myelosuppression after combination chemotherapy in the mother. Med Pediatr Oncol 1979;7:315–9.
20. Weed JC Jr, Roh RA, Mendenhall HW. Recurrent endodermal sinus tumor during pregnancy. Obstet Gynecol 1979;54:653–6.
21. Kim DS, Park MI. Maternal and fetal survival following surgery and chemotherapy of endodermal sinus tumor of the ovary during pregnancy: a case report. Obstet Gynecol 1989;73:503–7.
22. Karp GI, von Oeyen P, Valone F, Khetarpal VK, Israel M, Mayer RJ, Frigoletto FD, Garnick MB. Doxorubicin in pregnancy. possible transplacental passage. Cancer Treat Rep 1983;67:773–7.
23. Haerr RW, Pratt AT. Multiagent chemotherapy for sarcoma diagnosed during pregnancy. Cancer 1985;56:1028–33.
24. Volkenandt M, Buchner T, Hiddemann W, Van De Loo J. Acute leukaemia during pregnancy. Lancet 1987;2:1521–2.
25. Schleuning M, Clemm C. Chromosomal aberrations in a newborn whose mother received cytotoxic treatment during pregnancy. N Engl J Med 1987;317:1666–7.
26. Feliu J, Juarez S, Ordonez A, Garcia-Paredes ML,

Gonzalez-Baron M, Montero JM. Acute leukemia and pregnancy. Cancer 1988;61:580–4.
27. Turchi JJ, Villasis C. Anthracyclines in the treatment of malignancy in pregnancy. Cancer 1988;61:435–40.
28. Weinrach RS. Leukemia in pregnancy. Ariz Med 1972;29:326–9.
29. Ortega J. Multiple agent chemotherapy including bleomycin of non-Hodgkin's lymphoma during pregnancy. Cancer 1977;40:2829–35.
30. Jones RT, Weinerman ER. MOPP (nitrogen mustard, vincristine, procarbazine, and prednisone) given during pregnancy. Obstet Gynecol 1979;54:477–8.
31. Giacalone PL, Laffargue F, Benos P. Chemotherapy for breast carcinoma during pregnancy. Cancer 1999;86:2266–72.
32. Nicholson HO. Cytotoxic drugs in pregnancy: review of reported cases. J Obstet Gynaecol Br Commonw 1968;75:307–12.
33. Dobbing J. Pregnancy and leukaemia. Lancet 1977;1:1155.
34. Schilsky RL, Sherins RJ, Hubbard SM, Wesley MN, Young RC, DeVita VT Jr. Long-term follow-up of ovarian function in women treated with MOPP chemotherapy for Hodgkin's disease. Am J Med 1981;71:552–6.
35. Schwartz PE, Vidone RA. Pregnancy following combination chemotherapy for a mixed germ cell tumor of the ovary. Gynecol Oncol 1981;12:373–8.
36. Estiu M. Successful pregnancy in leukaemia. Lancet 1977;1:433.
37. Johnson SA, Goldman JM, Hawkins DF. Pregnancy after chemotherapy for Hodgkin's disease. Lancet 1979;2:93.
38. Schilsky RL, Lewis BJ, Sherins RJ, Young RC. Gonadal dysfunction in patients receiving chemotherapy for cancer. Ann Intern Med 1980;93:109–14.
39. Sherins RJ, DeVita VT Jr. Effect of drug treatment for lymphoma on male reproductive capacity. Ann Intern Med 1973;79:216–20.
40. Sherins RJ, Olweny CLM, Ziegler JL. Gynecomastia and gonadal dysfunction in adolescent boys treated with combination chemotherapy for Hodgkin's disease. N Engl J Med 1978;299:12–6.
41. Lendon PRM, Peckham MJ. The investigation and management of Hodgkin's disease in the pregnant patient. Cancer 1976;38:1944–51.
42. Lee RB, Kelly J, Elg SA, Benson WL. Pregnancy following conservative surgery and adjunctive chemotherapy for stage III immature teratoma of the ovary. Obstet Gynecol 1989;73:853–5.
43. Gershenson DM. Menstrual and reproductive function after treatment with combination chemotherapy for malignant ovarian germ cell tumors. J Clin Oncol 1988;6:270–5.
44. Rustin GJS, Booth M, Dent J, Salt S, Rustin F, Bagshawe KD. Pregnancy after cytotoxic chemotherapy for gestational trophoblastic tumours. Br Med J 1984;288:103–6.

Name: **VINORELBINE** Risk Factor: D_M
Class: **Antineoplastic**

FETAL RISK SUMMARY

RECOMMENDATION: Limited Human Data - Animal Data Suggest Risk

Vinorelbine is a semisynthetic vinca alkaloid that is used in the treatment of cancer. It is related to two other vinca alkaloids—vinblastine and vincristine.

Reproduction studies in mice and rabbits at one-third the human dose (HD) and one-fourth the HD have shown embryo and/or fetal toxicity (1). At maternal nontoxic doses, intrauterine growth retardation and delayed ossification were observed. Vinorelbine did not affect fertility when administered to rats at weekly doses that were one-third the HD or alternate-day doses that were one-seventh the HD before and during mating (1). The agent did reduce spermatogenesis and prostate/seminal vesicle secretion in male rats given biweekly doses about one-fifteenth and one-fourth the HD, respectively, for 13 or 26 weeks (1).

V

It is not known if vinorelbine crosses the placenta to the fetus. The relatively high molecular weight (about 1079) suggests that placental transfer of the drug to the embryo or fetus would be inhibited.

In a brief 1997 report, three pregnant women with breast cancer were successfully treated with two or three courses of vinorelbine (20–30 mg/m^2) and fluorouracil (500–750 mg/m^2) at 24, 28, and 29 weeks' gestation, respectively (2). Delivery occurred at 34, 41, and 37 weeks' gestation, respectively. One patient also required six courses of epidoxorubicin and cyclophosphamide. Her infant developed transient anemia at 21 days of age that resolved spontaneously. No adverse effects were observed in the other two newborns. All three infants were developing normally at about 2–3 years of age (2).

A 1999 report from France described the outcomes of pregnancies in 20 women with breast cancer who were treated with antineoplastic agents (3). The first cycle of chemotherapy occurred at a mean gestational age of 26 weeks with delivery occurring at a mean 34.7 weeks. A total of 38 cycles were administered during pregnancy with a median of two cycles per woman. None of the women received radiation therapy during pregnancy. The pregnancy outcomes included two spontaneous abortions (both exposed in the 1st trimester), one intrauterine death (exposed in the 2nd trimester), and 17 live births, one of whom died at 8 days of age without apparent cause. The 16 surviving children were developing normally at a mean follow-up of 42.3 months (3). Vinorelbine, in combination fluorouracil, was administered to four women at a mean dose of 37 mg/m^2 (range 20–50 mg/m^2) during the 2nd or 3rd trimesters. The outcomes were four surviving live-born infants (3).

BREAST FEEDING SUMMARY

RECOMMENDATION: Contraindicated

No reports describing the use of vinorelbine during lactation have been located. Because of the potential for severe toxicity (e.g., bone marrow depression as seen in adults) in a nursing infant, women who require this agent should not breast-feed.

References

1. Product information. Navelbine. Glaxo Wellcome, 1999.
2. Cuvier C, Espie M, Extra JM, Marty M. Vinorelbine in pregnancy. Eur J Cancer 1997;33:168–9.
3. Giacalone PL, Laffargue F, Benos P. Chemotherapy for breast carcinoma during pregnancy. Cancer 1999;86:2266–72.

Name: **VITAMIN A** Risk Factor: **A***
Class: **Vitamin**

FETAL RISK SUMMARY

RECOMMENDATION: Compatible
Contraindicated (Doses above U.S. RDA)

Vitamin A (retinol; vitamin A_1) is a fat-soluble essential nutrient that occurs naturally in a variety of foods. Vitamin A is required for the maintenance of normal epithelial tissue and for growth and bone development, vision, and reproduction (1). Two different daily intake recommendations for pregnant women in the United States have been made for vitamin A. The National Academy of Sciences' recommended dietary allowance (RDA) for normal pregnant women, published in 1989, is 800 retinol equivalents/day (about 2700 IU/day of vitamin A) (1,2). The FDA's RDA (i.e., U.S. RDA) for pregnant women, a recommendation made in 1976, is 8000 IU/day (3,4). The U.S. RDA of 8000 IU/day should be considered the maximum dose (4), although the difference between the two recommendations is probably not clinically significant.

The teratogenicity of vitamin A in animals is well known. Both high levels and deficiency of the vitamin have resulted in defects (5–13). In the past, various authors have speculated on the teratogenic effect of the vitamin in humans (5,14–16). A 1983 case report suggested that the vitamin A contained in a multivitamin product may have caused a cleft palate in one infant; however, the mother had a family history of cleft palate and had produced a previous infant with a malformation (16). Another case report, this one published in 1987, described an infant with multiple defects whose mother had consumed a vitamin preparation containing 2000 IU/day of vitamin A (17). The authors thought the phenotype of their patient was similar to the one observed with isotretinoin, but they could not exclude other causes of the defect, including a phenocopy of the isotretinoin syndrome (17). Therefore, in both cases, no definite association between the defects and vitamin A can be established, and the possibility that other causes were involved is high.

In response to the 1983 case report cited above, one investigator wrote in 1983 that there was no acceptable evidence of human vitamin A teratogenicity and none at all with doses less than 10,000 IU/day (18). Since that time, however, two synthetic isomers of vitamin A, isotretinoin and etretinate, have been shown to be powerful human teratogens (see Isotretinoin and Etretinate). In addition, recent studies have revealed that high doses of preformed vitamin A are human teratogens. These and the other reports are summarized below. Because of the combined animal and human data for vitamin A, and because of the human experience with isotretinoin and etretinate, large doses or severe deficiency of vitamin A must be viewed as harmful to the human fetus.

Severe human vitamin A deficiency has been cited as the cause of three malformed infants (19–21). In the first case, a mother with multiple vitamin deficiencies produced a baby with congenital xerophthalmia and bilateral cleft lip (19). The defects may have been caused by vitamin A deficiency because of their similarity to anomalies seen in animals deprived of this nutrient. The second report involved a malnourished pregnant woman with recent onset of blindness whose symptoms were the result of vitamin A deficiency (20). The mother gave birth to a premature male child with microcephaly and what appeared to be anophthalmia. The final case described a blind, mentally retarded girl with bilateral microphthalmia, coloboma of the iris and choroid, and retinal aplasia (21). During pregnancy, the mother was suspected of having vitamin A deficiency manifested by night blindness.

In 1986, investigators from the FDA reviewed 18 cases of suspected vitamin A-induced teratogenicity (22). Some of these cases had been reviewed in previous communications by an FDA epidemiologist (23,24). Six of the cases (25–30) had been previously published and 12 represented unpublished reports. All of the cases, except one, involved long-term, high-dose (>25,000 IU/day) consumption continuing past conception. The exception involved a woman who accidentally consumed 500,000 IU, as a single dose, during the 2nd month of pregnancy (29). Twelve of the infants had malformations similar to those seen in animal and human retinoid syndromes (i.e., central nervous system and cardiovascular anomalies, microtia, and clefts) (22). The defects observed in the 18 infants were microtia ($N = 4$), craniofacial ($N = 4$), brain ($N = 4$), facial palsy ($N = 1$), micro-/anophthalmia ($N = 2$), facial clefts ($N = 4$), cardio-aortic ($N = 2$), limb reduction ($N = 4$), gastrointestinal atresia ($N = 1$), and urinary ($N = 4$) (22).

The Centers for Disease Control and Prevention (CDC) reported in 1987 the results of an epidemiologic study conducted by the New York State Department of Health from April 1983 through February 1984 (3). The mothers of 492 live-born infants without congenital defects were interviewed to obtain their drug histories. Vitamin A supplements were taken by 81.1% (399 of 492) of the women. Of this group, 0.6% (3 of 492) took 25,000 IU/day or more, and 2.6% (13 of 492) consumed 15,000–24,999 IU/day (3). In an editorial comment, the CDC noted that the excessive vitamin A consumption by some of the women was a public health concern (3).

Results of a epidemiologic case-control study conducted in Spain between 1976 and 1987 were reported in preliminary form in 1988 (31) and as a full report in 1990 (32). A total of 11,293 cases of malformed infants were compared with 11,193 normal controls. Sixteen of the case mothers (1.4/1000) used high doses of vitamin A either alone or in combination with other vitamins during their pregnancies, compared with 14 (1.3/1000) of the controls, an odds ratio (OR) of 1.1 (*n.s.*). Five of the case infants and 10 of the controls were exposed to doses less than 40,000 IU/day (OR 0.5, $p = 0.15$). In contrast, 11 of the case infants and 4 controls were exposed to ≥40,000 IU (OR 2.7, $p = 0.06$). The risk of congenital anomalies, although not significant, appeared to be related to gestational age as the highest risk in those pregnancies exposed to ≥40,000 IU/day occurred during the first 2 months (32). The data suggested a dose-effect relationship and provided support for earlier statements that doses lower than 10,000 IU were not teratogenic (31,32).

Data from a case-control study was used to assess the effects of vitamin A supplements (daily use for at least 7 days of vitamin A either alone or with vitamin D, or of fish oils) and vitamin A-containing multivitamin supplements (33). Cases were 2,658 infants with malformations derived, at least in part, from cranial neural crest cells (primarily craniofacial and cardiac anomalies). Controls were 2609 infants with other malformations. Case mothers used vitamin A supplements in 15, 14, and 10 pregnancies during lunar months 1, 2, and 3, respectively, compared with 6 control mothers in each period (33). Although not significant, the OR in each period was 2.5 (95% confidence interval [CI] 1.0–6.2), 2.3 (95% CI 0.9–5.8), and 1.6 (95% CI 0.6–4.5), respectively. The authors cautioned that their data should be considered tentative because of the small numbers and lack of dosage and nutrition information (33). Even a small increased risk was excluded for vitamin A-containing multivitamins (33).

A congenital malformation of the left eye was attributed to excessive vitamin A exposure during the 1st trimester in a 1991 report (34). The mother had ingested a combination of liver and vitamin supplements that provided an estimated 25,000 IU/day of vitamin A. The unusual eye defect consisted of an "hourglass" cornea and iris with a reduplicated lens.

A brief 1992 correspondence cited the experience in the Hungarian Family Planning Program with a prenatal vitamin preparation containing 6000 IU of vitamin A (35). Evaluating their 1989 data base, the authors found no relationship, in comparison with a nonexposed control group, between the daily intake of the multivitamin at least 1 month before conception through the 12th week of gestation and any congenital malformation.

A study published in 1995 examined the effect of preformed vitamin A, consumed from vitamin supplements and food, on pregnancy outcomes (36). Vitamin A ingestion, from 3 months before through 12 weeks from the last menstrual period, was determined for 22,748 women. Most of the women were enrolled in the study between week 15 and week 20 of pregnancy. From the total group, 339 babies met the criteria for congenital anomalies established by the investigators. These criteria included malformations in four categories (number of defects of each type shown: *cranial-neural-crest defects* (craniofacial, central nervous system, and thymic $N = 69$; heart defects $N = 52$); *neural tube defects (NTDs)* (spina bifida, anencephaly, and encephalocele $N = 48$); *musculoskeletal* ($N = 58$) and *urogenital* ($N = 42$) *defects*; and *other defects* (gastrointestinal defects $N = 24$; agenesis or hypoplasia of the lungs, single umbilical artery, anomalies of the spleen, and cystic hygroma $N = 46$)

(36). The 22,748 women were divided into four groups based on their total (supplement plus food) daily intake of vitamin A: 0–5,000 IU ($N = 6{,}410$), 5,001–10,000 IU ($N = 12{,}688$), 10,001–15,000 IU ($N = 3{,}150$), and ≥15,001 IU ($N = 500$). Analysis of this grouping revealed that the women who took ≥15,001 IU daily had a higher prevalence ratio for defects associated with cranial-neural-crest tissue compared with those in the lowest group, 3.5 (95% CI 1.7–7.3). A slightly higher ratio was found for musculoskeletal and urogenital defects, no increase for neural tube defects or other defects, and for all birth defects combined, a ratio of 2.2 (95% CI 1.3–3.8) (36). Analysis of three groups (0–5000 IU, 5001–10,000 IU, and ≥10,001 IU) of vitamin A ingestion levels from food alone was hampered by the small number of women and, although some increased prevalence ratios were found in the highest groups, the small numbers made the estimates imprecise (36). A third analysis was then conducted based on four groups (0–5000 IU, 5001–8000 IU, 8001–10,000 IU, and (10,001 IU) of vitamin A ingestion levels from supplements. Compared with the lowest group, the prevalence ratio for all birth defects in the highest group was 2.4 (95% CI 1.3–4.4) and for defects involving the cranial-neural crest tissue, the ratio was 4.8 (95% CI 2.2–10.5). Of interest, the mean vitamin A intake in the highest group was 21,675 IU. Based on these data, the investigators concluded that following *in utero* exposure to more than 10,000 IU of vitamin A from supplements, about 1 infant in 57 (1.75%) had a vitamin A-induced malformation.

In response to the above study, a note of caution was sounded by two authors from the CDC (37). Citing results from previous studies, these authors concluded that without more data, they could not recommend use of the dose-response curve developed in the above study for advising pregnant women of the specific risk of anomalies that might arise from the ingestion of excessive vitamin A. Although they agreed that very large doses of vitamin A might be teratogenic, the question of how large a dose remained (37). A number of correspondences followed publication of the above study, all describing perceived methodologic discrepancies that may have affected the conclusions (38–42) with a reply by the authors supporting their findings (43).

Using case-control study data from California, a paper published in 1997 examined the relationship between maternal vitamin A ingestion and the risk of NTDs in singleton live-born infants and aborted fetuses (44). Although the number of cases was small, only 16 exposed to ≥10,000 IU/day and 6 to ≥15,000 IU/day, the investigators did not find a relationship between these levels of exposure and NTDs.

Referring to the question on the teratogenic level of vitamin A, a 1997 abstract reported the effects of increasing doses of the vitamin in the cynomolgus monkey, a species that is a well-documented model for isotretinoin-induced teratogenicity (45). Four groups of monkeys were administered increasing doses of vitamin A (7500–80,000 IU/kg) in early gestation (day 16–27). A dose-related increase in abortions and typical congenital malformations was observed in the offspring. The NOAEL (no-observed-adverse-effect level) was 7,500 IU/kg, or 30,000 IU/day based on an average 4-kg animal. A human NOAEL extrapolated from the monkey NOAEL would correspond to >300,000 IU/day (45).

A brief 1995 report described the outcomes of 7 of 22 women who had taken very large doses of vitamin A during pregnancy, 20 of whom had taken the vitamin during the 1st trimester (46). The mean daily dose was 70,000 IU (range 25,000–90,000 IU) for a mean of 44 days (range 7–180 days). None of the offspring of the 7 patients available at follow-up had congenital malformations. Data on the other 15 women were not available.

Two abstracts published in 1996 examined the issue of vitamin A supplementation in women enrolled in studies in Atlanta, Georgia, and in California, both during the 1980s

(47,48). In the first abstract, no increase in the incidence of all congenital defects or those classified as involving cranial-neural crest-derived was found for doses <8000 IU/day, or for those who took both a multivitamin and a vitamin A supplement (47). In the other abstract, subjects took amounts thought likely to exceed 10,000 IU/day and, again, no association with the major anomalies derived from cranial-neural crest cells (cleft lip, cleft palate, and conotruncal heart defects) was discovered (48).

Using data collected between 1985 and 1987 in California and Illinois by the National Institute of Child Health and Human Development Neural Tube Defects Study, a case-control study published in 1997 examined whether periconceptional vitamin A exposure was related to NTDs or other major congenital malformations (49). Three study groups of offspring were formed shortly after the pregnancy outcome was known (prenatally and postnatally): those with NTDs ($N = 548$), those with other major malformations ($N = 387$), and normal controls ($N = 573$). The latter two groups were matched to the NTDs group. A subgroup, formed from those with other major malformations, involved those with cranial-neural crest malformations ($N = 89$), consisting mainly of conotruncal defects of the heart and great vessels, including ventricular septal defects, and defects of the ear and face (49). The vitamin A (supplements and fortified cereals) exposure rates by group for those ingesting a mean >8000 IU/day or >10,000 IU/day were NTDs (3.3% and 2.0%), other major malformations (3.6% and 1.6%), cranial-neural crest malformations (3.4% and 2.2%), and controls (4.5% and 2.1%), respectively. None of the values were statistically significant, thus, no association between moderate consumption of vitamin A and the defect groups was found (49).

Several investigators have studied maternal and fetal vitamin A levels during various stages of gestation (5,50–61). Transport to the fetus is by passive diffusion (61). Maternal vitamin A concentrations are slightly greater than those found in either premature or term infants (50–52). In women with normal levels of vitamin A, maternal and newborn levels were 270 and 220 ng/mL, respectively (51). In 41 women not given supplements of vitamin A, a third of whom had laboratory evidence of hypovitaminemia A, mean maternal levels exceeded those in the newborn by almost a 2:1 ratio (51). In two reports, maternal serum levels were dependent on the length of gestation with concentrations decreasing during the 1st trimester, then increasing during the remainder of pregnancy until about the 38th week when they began to decrease again (5,53). A more recent study found no difference in serum levels between 10 and 33 weeks' gestation, even though amniotic fluid vitamin A levels at 20 weeks onward were significantly greater than at 16–18 weeks (54). Premature infants (36 weeks or less) have significantly lower serum retinol and retinol-binding protein concentrations than do term neonates (50,55–57).

Mild to moderate deficiency is common during pregnancy (51,58). A 1984 report concluded that vitamin A deficiency in poorly nourished mothers was one of the features associated with an increased incidence of prematurity and intrauterine growth retardation (50). An earlier study, however, found no difference in vitamin A levels between low-birth-weight (<2500 g) and normal-birth-weight (>2500 g) infants (52). Maternal vitamin A concentrations of the low-birth-weight group were lower than those of normals, 211 vs. 273 ng/mL, but not significantly. An investigation in premature infants revealed that infants developing bronchopulmonary dysplasia had significantly lower serum retinol levels as compared with infants who did not develop this disease (57).

Relatively high liver vitamin A stores were found in the fetuses of women younger than 18 and older than 40 years of age, two groups that produce a high incidence of fetal anomalies (5). Low fetal liver concentrations were measured in 2 infants with hydrocephalus and high levels in 14 infants with NTDs (5). In another report relating to NTDs, a high liver concentration occurred in an anencephalic infant (59). Significantly, higher vitamin A amniotic fluid concentrations were discovered in 12 pregnancies from which infants with NTDs were delivered as compared with 94 normal pregnancies (60). However, attempts to use this measurement as an indicator of anencephaly or other fetal anomalies failed because the values for abnormal and normal fetuses overlapped (54,60).

The effect of stopping oral contraceptives shortly before conception on vitamin A levels has been studied (61). Because oral contraceptives had been shown to increase serum levels of vitamin A, it was postulated that early conception might involve a risk of teratogenicity. However, no difference was found in early pregnancy vitamin A levels between users and nonusers. The results of this study have been challenged based on the methods used to measure vitamin A (63).

Vitamin A is known to affect the immune system (64). Three recent studies (65–67) and an editorial (68) have described or commented on the effect that maternal vitamin A deficiency has on the maternal-fetal transmission of human immunodeficiency virus (HIV). In each of the studies, a low maternal level of vitamin A was associated with HIV transmission to the infant. In the one study conducted in the United States, severe maternal vitamin A deficiency (<0.70 μmol/L) was associated with HIV transmission with an adjusted OR of 5.05 (95% CI 1.20–21.24) (67). In a related study, maternal vitamin A deficiency during pregnancy in women infected with HIV was significantly related to growth failure (height and weight) during the first year of life in their children, after adjustment for the effects of body mass index, child gender, and child HIV status (69).

In summary, excessive doses of preformed vitamin A are teratogenic, as may be marked maternal deficiency. In addition, recent evidence has demonstrated that severe maternal vitamin A deficiency may increase the risk of mother-to-child HIV transmission and reduced infant growth during the first year. β-Carotene, a vitamin A precursor, has not been associated with either human or animal toxicity (see β-Carotene). Doses exceeding the U.S. RDA (8000 IU/day) should be avoided by women who are, or who may become, pregnant. Moreover, the U.S. RDA established by the FDA should be considered the maximum dose (4). Although the minimum teratogenic dose has not yet been defined, doses of 25,000 IU/day or more, in the form of retinol or retinyl esters, should be considered potentially teratogenic (3,4,22), but based on one study, smaller doses than this may be teratogenic (36). One of the recommendations of the Teratology Society, published in a 1987 position paper, states: "Women in their reproductive years should be informed that the excessive use of vitamin A shortly before and during pregnancy could be harmful to their babies" (4). The Teratology Society also noted that the average balanced diet contains approximately 7000–8000 IU of vitamin A from various sources, and this should be considered prior to additional supplementation (4).

[**Risk Factor X if used in doses above the U.S. RDA.*]

BREAST FEEDING SUMMARY

RECOMMENDATION: Compatible

Vitamin A is a natural constituent of breast milk. Deficiency of this vitamin in breast-fed infants is rare (70). The RDA of vitamin A during lactation is approximately 4000 IU (1). It is not known whether high maternal doses of vitamin A represent a danger to the nursing infant or whether they reduce HIV transmission via the milk.

References

1. American Hospital Formulary Service. *Drug Information 1997*. Bethesda, MD: American Society of Health-System Pharmacists, 1997:2806–9.
2. National Research Council. *Recommended Dietary Allowances*, 10th ed. Washington, DC: National Academy Press, 1989.
3. CDC. Use of supplements containing high-dose vitamin A—New York State, 1983–1984. MMWR 1987;36:80–2.
4. Public Affairs Committee, Teratology Society. Position paper: recommendations for vitamin A use during pregnancy. Teratology 1987;35:269–75.
5. Gal I, Sharman IM, Pryse-Davies J. Vitamin A in relation to human congenital malformations. Adv Teratol 1972;5:143–59.
6. Cohlan SQ. Excessive intake of vitamin A as a cause of congenital anomalies in the rat. Science 1953;117:535–6.
7. Muenter MD. Hypervitaminosis A. Ann Intern Med 1974;80:105–6.
8. Morriss GM. Vitamin A and congenital malformations. Int J Vitam Nutr Res 1976;46:220–2.
9. Fantel AG, Shepard TH, Newell-Morris LL, Moffett BC. Teratogenic effects of retinoic acid in pigtail monkeys (*Macaca nemestrina*). Teratology 1977;15:65–72.
10. Vorhees CV, Brunner RL, McDaniel CR, Butcher RE. The relationship of gestational age to vitamin A induced postnatal dysfunction. Teratology 1978;17:271–6.
11. Ferm VH, Ferm RR. Teratogenic interaction of hyperthermia and vitamin A. Biol Neonate 1979;36:168–72.
12. Geelen JAG. Hypervitaminosis A induced teratogenesis. CRC Crit Rev Toxicol 1979;6:351–75.
13. Kamm JJ. Toxicology, carcinogenicity, and teratogenicity of some orally administered retinoids. J Am Acad Dermatol 1982;6:652–9.
14. Muenter MD. Hypervitaminosis A. Ann Intern Med 1974;80:105–6.
15. Read AP, Harris R. Spina bifida and vitamins. Br Med J 1983;286:560–1.
16. Bound JP. Spina bifida and vitamins. Br Med J 1983;286:147.
17. Lungarotti MS, Marinelli D, Mariani T, Calabro A. Multiple congenital anomalies associated with apparently normal maternal intake of vitamin A: A phenocopy of the isotretinoin syndrome? Am J Med Genet 1987;27:245–8.
18. Smithells RW. Spina bifida and vitamins. Br Med J 1983;286:388–9.
19. Houet R, Ramioul-Lecomte S. Repercussions sur l'enfant des avitaminoses de la mere pendant la grossesse. Ann Paediatr 1950;175:378. As cited in Warkany J. *Congenital Malformations. Notes and Comments*. Chicago, IL: Year Book Medical Publishers, 1971:127–8.
20. Sarma V. Maternal vitamin A deficiency and fetal microcephaly and anophthalmia. Obstet Gynecol 1959;13:299–301.
21. Lamba PA, Sood NN. Congenital microphthalmos and colobomata in maternal vitamin A deficiency. J Pediatr Ophthalmol 1968;115–7. As cited in Warkany J. *Congenital Malformation. Notes and Comments*. Chicago, IL: Year Book Medical Publishers, 1971:127–8.
22. Rosa FW, Wilk AL, Kelsey FO. Teratogen update: vitamin A congeners. Teratology 1986;33:355–64.
23. Rosa FW. Teratogenicity of isotretinoin. Lancet 1983;2:513.
24. Rosa FW. Retinoic acid embryopathy. N Engl J Med 1986;315:262.
25. Pilotti G, Scorta A. Ipervitaminosi A gravidica e malformazioni neonatali dell'apparato urinaria. Minerva Ginecol 1965;17:1103–8. As cited in Nishimura H, Tanimura T. *Clinical Aspects of the Teratogenicity of Drugs*. New York, NY: American Elsevier, 1976: 251–2.
26. Bernhardt IB, Dorsey DJ. Hypervitaminosis A and congenital renal anomalies in a human infant. Obstet Gynecol 1974;43:750–5.
27. Stange L, Carlstrom K, Eriksson M. Hypervitaminosis A in early human pregnancy and malformations of the central nervous system. Acta Obstet Gynecol Scand 1978,57:289–91.
28. Morriss GM, Thomson AD. Vitamin A and rat embryos. Lancet 1974;2:899–900.
29. Mounoud RL, Klein D, Weber F. A propos d'un cas de syndrome de Goldenhar: intoxication aigue a la vitamine A chez la mere pendant la grossesse. J Genet Hum 1975;23:135–54.
30. Von Lennep E, El Khazen N, De Pierreux G, Amy JJ, Rodesch F, Van Regemorter N. A case of partial sirenomelia and possible vitamin A teratogenesis. Prenat Diagn 1985;5:35–40.
31. Martinez-Frias ML, Salvador J. Megadose vitamin A and teratogenicity. Lancet 1988;1:236.
32. Martinez-Frias ML, Salvador J. Epidemiological aspects of prenatal exposure to high doses of vitamin A in Spain. Eur J Epidemiol 1990;6:118–23.
33. Werler MM, Lammer EJ, Rosenberg L, Mitchell AA. Maternal vitamin A supplementation in relation to selected birth defects. Teratology 1990;42:497–503.
34. Evans K, Hickey-Dwyer MU. Cleft anterior segment with maternal hypervitaminosis A. Br J Ophthalmol 1991;75:691–2.
35. Dudas I, Czeizel AE. Use of 6000 IU vitamin A during early pregnancy without teratogenic effect. Teratology 1992;45:335–6.
36. Rothman KJ, Moore LL, Singer MR, Nguyen U-SDT, Mannino S, Milunsky A. Teratogenicity of high vitamin A intake. N Engl J Med 1995;333:1369–73.
37. Oakley GP Jr, Erickson JD. Vitamin A and birth defects. Continuing caution is needed. N Engl J Med 1995;333:1414–5.
38. Werler M, Lammer EJ, Mitchell AA. Teratogenicity of high vitamin A intake. N Engl J Med 1996;334:1195.
39. Brent RL, Hendrickx AG, Holmes LB, Miller RK. Teratogenicity of high vitamin A intake. N Engl J Med 1996;334:1196.
40. Watkins M, Moore C, Mulinare J. Teratogenicity of high vitamin A intake. N Engl J Med 1996;334:1196.
41. Challem JJ. Teratogenicity of high vitamin A intake. N Engl J Med 1996;334:1196–7.
42. Hunt JR. Teratogenicity of high vitamin A intake. N Engl J Med 1996;334:1197.
43. Rothman KJ, Moore LL, Singer MR, Milunsky A. Teratogenicity of high vitamin A intake. N Engl J Med 1996;334:1197.

44. Shaw GM, Velie EM, Schaffer D, Lammer EJ. Periconceptional intake of vitamin A among women and risk of neural tube defect-affected pregnancies. Teratology 1997;55:132–3.
45. Hendrickx AG, Hummler H, Oneda S. Vitamin A teratogenicity and risk assessment in the cynomolgus monkey (abstract). Teratology 1997;55:68.
46. Bonati M, Nannini S, Addis A. Vitamin A supplementation during pregnancy in developed countries. Lancet 1995;345:736–7.
47. Khoury MJ, Moore CA, Mulinare J. Do vitamin A supplements in early pregnancy increase the risk of birth defects in the offspring? A population-based case-control study (abstract). Teratology 1996;53:91.
48. Lammer EJ, Shaw GM, Wasserman CR, Block G. High vitamin A intake and risk for major anomalies involving structures with an embryological cranial neural crest cell component (abstract). Teratology 1996;53:91–2.
49. Mills JL, Simpson JL, Cunningham GC, Conley MR, Rhoads GG. Vitamin A and birth defects. Am J Obstet Gynecol 1997;177:31–6.
50. Shah RS, Rajalakshmi R. Vitamin A status of the newborn in relation to gestational age, body weight, and maternal nutritional status. Am J Clin Nutr 1984;40:794–800.
51. Baker H, Frank O, Thomson AD, Langer A, Munves ED, De Angelis B, Kaminetzky HA. Vitamin profile of 174 mothers and newborns at parturition. Am J Clin Nutr 1975;28:59–65.
52. Baker H, Thind IS, Frank O, DeAngelis B, Caterini H, Lquria DB. Vitamin levels in low-birth-weight newborn infants and their mothers. Am J Obstet Gynecol 1977;129:521–4.
53. Gal I, Parkinson CE. Effects of nutrition and other factors on pregnant women's serum vitamin A levels. Am J Clin Nutr 1974;27:688–95.
54. Wallingford JC, Milunsky A, Underwood BA. Vitamin A and retinol-binding protein in amniotic fluid. Am J Clin Nutr 1983;38:377–81.
55. Brandt RB, Mueller DG, Schroeder JR, Guyer KE, Kirkpatrick BV, Hutcher NE, Ehrlich FE. Serum vitamin A in premature and term neonates. J Pediatr 1978;92: 101–4.
56. Shenai JP, Chytil F, Jhaveri A, Stahlman MT. Plasma vitamin A and retinol-binding protein in premature and term neonates. J Pediatr 1981:99:302–5.
57. Hustead VA, Gutcher GR, Anderson SA, Zachman RD. Relationship of vitamin A (retinol) status to lung disease in the preterm infant. J Pediatr 1984;105:610–5.
58. Kaminetzky HA, Langer A, Baker H, Frank O, Thomson AD, Munves ED, Opper A, Behrle FC, Glista B. The effect of nutrition in teen-age gravidas on pregnancy and the status of the neonate. I. A nutritional profile. Am J Obstet Gynecol 1973;115:639–46.
59. Gal I, Sharman IM, Pryse-Davies J, Moore T. Vitamin A as a possible factor in human teratology. Proc Nutr Soc 1969;28:9A–10A.
60. Parkinson CE, Tan JCY. Vitamin A concentrations in amniotic fluid and maternal serum related to neural-tube defects. Br J Obstet Gynaecol 1982;89:935–9.
61. Wild J, Schorah CJ, Smithells RW. Vitamin A, pregnancy, and oral contraceptives. Br Med J 1974;1: 57–9.
62. Hill EP, Longo LD. Dynamics of maternal-fetal nutrient transfer. Fed Proc 1980;39:239–44.
63. Bubb FA. Vitamin A, pregnancy, and oral contraceptives. Br Med J 1974;1:391–2.
64. Bates C. Vitamin A and infant immunity. Lancet 1993;341:28.
65. Semba RD, Miotti PG, Chiphangwi JD, Saah AJ, Canner JK, Dallabetta GA, Hoover DR. Maternal vitamin A deficiency and mother-to-child transmission of HIV-1. Lancet 1994;343:1593–7.
66. Semba RD, Miotti PG, Chiphangwi JD, Liomba G, Yang L-P, Saah AJ, Dallabetta GA, Hoover DR. Infant mortality and maternal vitamin A deficiency during human immunodeficiency virus infection. Clin Infect Dis 1995;21:966–72.
67. Greenberg BL, Semba RD, Vink PE, Farley JJ, Sivapalasingam M, Steketee RW, Thea DM, Schoenbaum EE. Vitamin A deficiency and maternal-infant transmission of HIV in two metropolitan areas in the United States. AIDS 1997;11:325–32.
68. Bridbord K, Willoughby A. Vitamin A and mother-to-child HIV-1 transmission. Lancet 1994;343:1585–6.
69. Semba RD, Miotti P, Chiphangwi JD, Henderson R, Dallabetta G, Yang L-P, Hoover D. Maternal vitamin A deficiency and child growth failure during human immunodeficiency virus infection. J Acquire Immune Defic Syndr Hum Retrovirol 1997;14:219–22.
70. Committee on Nutrition, American Academy of Pediatrics. Vitamin and mineral supplement needs in normal children in the United States. Pediatrics 1980;66:1015–21.

Name: **VITAMIN B_{12}** Risk Factor: **A***
Class: **Vitamin**

V

FETAL RISK SUMMARY

RECOMMENDATION: Compatible

Vitamin B_{12} (cyanocobalamin), a water-soluble B complex vitamin, is an essential nutrient required for nucleoprotein and myelin synthesis, cell reproduction, normal growth, and the maintenance of normal erythropoiesis (1). The National Academy of Sciences' recommended dietary allowance (RDA) for vitamin B_{12} in pregnancy is 2.2 μg (1).

Vitamin B_{12} is actively transported to the fetus (2–6). This process is responsible for the progressive decline of maternal levels that occurs during pregnancy (6–14). Fetal demands for the vitamin have been estimated to be approximately 0.3 μg/day (0.2 nmol/day) (15). Similar to other B complex vitamins, higher concentrations of B_{12} are found in the fetus and newborn than in the mother (5–9,16–24). At term, mean vitamin B_{12} levels in 174 mothers were 115 pg/mL and in their newborns 500 pg/mL, a newborn:maternal ratio of 4.3 (16). Comparable values have been observed by others (5,7,21–23). Mean levels in 51 Brazilian women, in their newborns, and in the intervillous space of their placentas were approximately 340, 797, and 1074 pg/mL, respectively (24). The newborn:maternal ratio in this report was 2.3. The high levels in the placenta may indicate a mechanism by which the fetus can accumulate the vitamin against a concentration gradient. This study also found a highly significant correlation between vitamin B_{12} and folate concentrations. This is in contrast to an earlier report that did not find such a correlation in women with megaloblastic anemia (25).

Maternal deficiency of vitamin B_{12} is common during pregnancy (16,17,26,27). Tobacco smoking reduces maternal levels of the vitamin even further (28). Megaloblastic anemia may result when the deficiency is severe, but it responds readily to therapy (29–32). On the other hand, tropical macrocytic anemia during pregnancy responds erratically to vitamin B_{12} therapy and is better treated with folic acid (32,33).

Megaloblastic (pernicious) anemia may be a cause of infertility (30,31,34). One report described a mother with undiagnosed pernicious anemia who had lost her 3rd, 9th, and 10th pregnancies (30). A healthy child resulted from her 11th pregnancy following treatment with vitamin B_{12}. In another study, eight infertile women with pernicious anemia were treated with vitamin B_{12} and seven became pregnant within 1 year of therapy (31). One of three patients in still another report may have had infertility associated with very low vitamin B_{12} levels (34).

Vitamin B_{12} deficiency was associated with prematurity (as defined by a birth weight of 2500 g or less) in a 1968 paper (9). However, many of the patients who delivered prematurely had normal or elevated vitamin B_{12} levels. No correlation between vitamin B_{12} deficiency and abruptio placentae was found in two studies published in the 1960s (35,36). Two reports found a positive association between low birth weight and low vitamin B_{12} levels (21,37). In both instances, however, folate levels were also low and iron was deficient in one. Others could not correlate low vitamin B_{12} concentrations with the weight at delivery (11,26). Based on these reports, it is doubtful whether vitamin B_{12} deficiency is associated with any of the conditions.

In experimental animals, vitamin B_{12} deficiency is teratogenic (7,38). Investigators studying the cause of neural tube defects measured very low vitamin B_{12} levels in three of four mothers of anencephalic fetuses (39). Additional evidence led them to conclude that the low vitamin B_{12} resulted in depletion of maternal folic acid and involvement in the origin of the defects. In contrast, two other reports have shown no relationship between low levels of vitamin B_{12} and congenital malformations (9,19).

No reports linking high doses of vitamin B_{12} with maternal or fetal complications have been located. Vitamin B_{12} administration at term has produced maternal levels approaching 50,000 pg/mL with corresponding cord blood levels of approximately 15,000 pg/mL (4,5). In fetal methylmalonic acidemia, large doses of vitamin B_{12}, 10 mg orally initially then changed to 5 mg IM, were administered daily to a mother to treat the affected fetus (40). On this dosage regimen, maternal levels rose as high as 18,000 pg/mL shortly after a dose. This metabolic disorder is not always treatable with vitamin B_{12}: one study reported a newborn with the vitamin B_{12}-unresponsive form of methylmalonic acidemia (41).

In summary, severe maternal vitamin B_{12} deficiency may result in megaloblastic anemia with subsequent infertility and poor pregnancy outcome. Less severe maternal deficiency apparently is common and does not pose a significant risk to the mother or fetus. Ingestion of vitamin B_{12} during pregnancy up to the RDA either via the diet or by supplementation is recommended.

[**Risk Factor C if used in doses above the RDA.*]

BREAST FEEDING SUMMARY

RECOMMENDATION: Compatible

Vitamin B_{12} is excreted into breast milk. In the first 48 hours after delivery, mean colostrum levels were 2431 pg/mL and then fell rapidly to concentrations comparable to those of normal serum (42). One group of investigators also observed very high colostrum levels ranging from 6 to 17.5 times that of milk (2). Milk:plasma ratios are approximately 1.0 during lactation (19). Reported milk concentrations of vitamin B_{12} vary widely (43–46). Mothers supplemented with daily doses of 1–200 μg had milk levels increase from a level of 79 to a level of 100 pg/mL (43). Milk concentrations were directly proportional to dietary intake. In a study using 8-μg/day supplements, mean milk levels of 1650 pg/mL at 1 week and 1100 pg/mL at 6 weeks were measured (44). Corresponding levels in unsupplemented mothers were significantly different at 1220 and 610 pg/mL, respectively. Other investigators also used 8-μg/day supplements and found significantly different levels compared with women not receiving supplements: 910 vs. 700 pg/mL at 1 week and 790 vs. 550 pg/mL at 6 weeks (45). In contrast, others found no difference between supplemented and unsupplemented well-nourished women with 5–100 μg/day (46). The mean vitamin B_{12} concentration in these latter patients was 970 pg/mL. A 1983 English study measured vitamin B_{12} levels in pooled human milk obtained from preterm (26 mothers: 29–34 weeks) and term (35 mothers: 39 weeks or longer) patients (47). Milk from preterm mothers decreased from 920 pg/mL (colostrum) to 220 pg/mL (16–196 days), whereas milk from term mothers decreased over the same period from a level of 490 to a level of 230 pg/mL.

Vitamin B_{12} deficiency in the lactating mother may cause severe consequences in the nursing infant. Several reports have described megaloblastic anemia in infants exclusively breast-fed by vitamin B_{12}-deficient mothers (48–52). Many of these mothers were vegetarians whose diets provided low amounts of the vitamin (49–52). The adequacy of vegetarian diets in providing sufficient vitamin B_{12} has been debated (53–55). However, a recent report measured only 1.4 μg of vitamin B_{12} intake/day in lactovegetarians (56). This amount is approximately 54% of the RDA for lactating women in the United States (1). Moreover, a 1986 case of vitamin B_{12}-induced anemia supports the argument that the low vitamin B_{12} intake of some vegetarian diets is inadequate to meet the total needs of a nursing infant for this vitamin (57). The case involved a 7-month-old male infant, exclusively breast-fed by a strict vegetarian mother, who was diagnosed as suffering from macrocytic anemia. The infant was lethargic, irritable, and failing to thrive. His vitamin B_{12} level was less than 100 pg/mL (normal 180–960 pg/mL), but iron and folate levels were both within normal limits. The anemia responded rapidly to administration of the vitamin, and he was developing normally at 11 months of age (57).

The National Academy of Sciences' RDA for vitamin B_{12} during lactation is 2.6 μg (1). If the diet of the lactating woman adequately supplies this amount, maternal supplementation with vitamin B_{12} is not needed. Supplementation with the RDA for vitamin B_{12} is recommended for those women with inadequate nutritional intake. The

American Academy of Pediatrics classifies vitamin B_{12} as compatible with breast-feeding (58).

References

1. American Hospital Formulary Service. *Drug Information 1997*. Bethesda, MD. American Society of Health-System Pharmacists, 1997:2820–3.
2. Luhby AL, Cooperman JM, Donnenfeld AM, Herrero JM, Teller DN, Wenig JB. Observations on transfer of vitamin B_{12} from mother to fetus and newborn. Am J Dis Child 1958;96:532–3.
3. Hill EP, Longo LD. Dynamics of maternal-fetal nutrient transfer. Fed Proc 1980;39:239–44.
4. Kaminetzky HA, Baker H, Frank O, Langer A. The effects of intravenously administered water-soluble vitamins during labor in normovitaminemic and hypovitaminemic gravidas on maternal and neonatal blood vitamin levels at delivery. Am J Obstet Gynecol 1974;120:697–703.
5. Frank O, Walbroehl G, Thomson A, Kaminetzky H, Kubes Z, Baker H. Placental transfer: fetal retention of some vitamins. Am J Clin Nutr 1970;23:662–3.
6. Luhby AL, Cooperman JM, Stone ML, Slobody LB. Physiology of vitamin B_{12} in pregnancy, the placenta, and the newborn. Am J Dis Child 1961;102:753–4.
7. Baker H, Ziffer H, Pasher I, Sobotka H. A Comparison of maternal and foetal folic acid and vitamin B_{12} at parturition. Br Med J 1958;1:978–9.
8. Boger WP, Bayne GM, Wright LD, Beck GD. Differential serum vitamin B_{12} concentrations in mothers and infants. N Engl J Med 1957;256:1085–7.
9. Temperley IJ, Meehan MJM, Gatenby PBB. Serum vitamin B_{12} levels in pregnant women. J Obstet Gynaecol Br Commonw 1968;75:511–6.
10. Boger WP, Wright LD, Beck GD, Bayne GM. Vitamin B_{12}: correlation of serum concentrations and pregnancy. Proc Soc Exp Biol Med 1956;92:140–3.
11. Martin JD, Davis RE, Stenhouse N. Serum folate and vitamin B_{12} levels in pregnancy with particular reference to uterine bleeding and bacteriuria. J Obstet Gynaecol Br Commonw 1967;74:697–701.
12. Ball EW, Giles C. Folic acid and vitamin B_{12} levels in pregnancy and their relation to megaloblastic anaemia. J Clin Pathol 1964;17:165–74.
13. Izak G, Rachmilewitz M, Stein Y, Berkovici B, Sadovsky A, Aronovitch Y, Grossowicz N. Vitamin B_{12} and iron deficiencies in anemia of pregnancy and puerperium. Arch Intern Med 1957;99:346–55.
14. Edelstein T, Metz J. Correlation between vitamin B_{12} concentration in serum and muscle in late pregnancy. J Obstet Gynaecol Br Commonw 1969;76:545–8.
15. Herbert V. Recommended dietary intakes (RDI) of vitamin B-12 in humans. Am J Clin Nutr 1987;45:671–8.
16. Baker H, Frank O, Thomson AD, Langer A, Munves ED, De Angelis B, Kaminetzky HA. Vitamin profile of 174 mothers and newborns at parturition. Am J Clin Nutr 1975;28:59–65.
17. Kaminetzky HA, Baker H. Micronutrients in pregnancy. Clin Obstet Gynecol 1977;20:363–80.
18. Lowenstein L, Lalonde M, Deschenes EB, Shapiro L. Vitamin B_{12} in pregnancy and the puerperium. Am J Clin Nutr 1960;8:265–75.
19. Baker SJ, Jacob E, Rajan KT, Swaminathan SP. Vitamin-B_{12} deficiency in pregnancy and the puerperium. Br Med J 1962;1:1658–61.
20. Killander A, Vahlquist B. The vitamin B_{12} concentration in serum from term and premature infants. Nord Med 1954;51:777–9.
21. Baker H, Thind IS, Frank O, DeAngelis B, Caterini H, Lquria DB. Vitamin levels in low-birth-weight newborn infants and their mothers. Am J Obstet Gynecol 1977;129:521–4.
22. Okuda K, Helliger AE, Chow BF. Vitamin B_{12} serum level and pregnancy. Am J Clin Nutr 1956;4:440–3.
23. Baker H, Frank O, Deangelis B, Feingold S, Kaminetzky HA. Role of placenta in maternal-fetal vitamin transfer in humans. Am J Obstet Gynecol 1981;141:792–6.
24. Giugliani ERJ, Jorge SM, Goncalves AL. Serum vitamin B_{12} levels in parturients, in the intervillous space of the placenta and in full-term newborns and their interrelationships with folate levels. Am J Clin Nutr 1985;41:330–5.
25. Giles C. An account of 335 cases of megaloblastic anaemia of pregnancy and the puerperium. J Clin Pathol 1966;19:1–11.
26. Roberts PD, James H, Petrie A, Morgan JO, Hoffbrand AV. Vitamin B_{12} status in pregnancy among immigrants to Britain. Br Med J 1973;3:67–72.
27. Dostalova L. Correlation of the vitamin status between mother and newborn during delivery. Dev Pharmacol Ther 1982;4(Suppl 1):45–57.
28. McGarry JM, Andrews J. Smoking in pregnancy and vitamin B_{12} metabolism. Br Med J 1972;2:74–7.
29. Heaton D. Another case of megaloblastic anemia of infancy due to maternal pernicious anemia. N Engl J Med 1979;300:202–3.
30. Varadi S. Pernicious anaemia and infertility. Lancet 1967;2:1305.
31. Jackson IMD, Doig WB, McDonald G. Pernicious anaemia as a cause of infertility. Lancet 1967;2:1059–60.
32. Chaudhuri S. Vitamin B_{12} in megaloblastic anaemia of pregnancy and tropical nutritional macrocytic anaemia. Br Med J 1951;2:825–8.
33. Patel JC, Kocher BR. Vitamin B_{12} in macrocytic anaemia of pregnancy and the puerperium. Br Med J 1950;1:924–7.
34. Parr JH, Ramsay I. The presentation of osteomalacia in pregnancy. Case report. Br J Obstet Gynaecol 1984;91:816–8.
35. Streiff RR, Little AB. Folic acid deficiency as a cause of uterine hemorrhage in pregnancy. J Clin Invest 1965;44:1102.
36. Streiff RR, Little AB. Folic acid deficiency in pregnancy. N Engl J Med 1967;276:776–9.
37. Whiteside MG, Ungar B, Cowling DC. Iron, folic acid and vitamin B_{12} levels in normal pregnancy, and their influence on birth-weight and the duration of pregnancy. Med J Aust 1968;1:338–42.
38. Shepard TH. *Catalog of Teratogenic Agents*. 3rd ed. Baltimore, MD: Johns Hopkins University Press, 1980:348–9.

V

39. Schorah CJ, Smithells RW, Scott J. Vitamin B_{12} and anencephaly. Lancet 1980;1:880.
40. Ampola MG, Mahoney MJ, Nakamura E, Tanaka K. Prenatal therapy of a patient with vitamin-B_{12}-responsive methylmalonic acidemia. N Engl J Med 1975;293:313–7.
41. Morrow G III, Schwarz RH, Hallock JA, Barness LA. Prenatal detection of methylmalonic acidemia. J Pediatr 1970;77:120–3.
42. Samson RR, McClelland DBL. Vitamin B_{12} in human colostrum and milk. Acta Paediatr Scand 1980;69:93–9.
43. Deodhar AD, Rajalakshmi R, Ramakrishnan CV. Studies on human lactation. Part III. Effect of dietary vitamin supplementation on vitamin contents of breast milk. Acta Paediatr Scand 1964;53:42–8.
44. Thomas MR, Kawamoto J, Sneed SM, Eakin R. The effects of vitamin C, vitamin B_6, and vitamin B_{12} supplementation on the breast milk and maternal status of well-nourished women. Am J Clin Nutr 1979;32:1679–85.
45. Sneed SM, Zane C, Thomas MR. The effects of ascorbic acid, vitamin B_6, vitamin B_{12}, and folic acid supplementation on the breast milk and maternal nutritional status of low socioeconomic lactating women. Am J Clin Nutr 1981;34:1338–46.
46. Sandberg DP, Begley JA, Hall CA. The content, binding, and forms of vitamin B_{12} in milk. Am J Clin Nutr 1981;34:1717–24.
47. Ford JE, Zechalko A, Murphy J, Brooke OG. Comparison of the B vitamin composition of milk from mothers of preterm and term babies. Arch Dis Child 1983;58:367–72.
48. Lampkin BC, Shore NA, Chadwick D. Megaloblastic anemia of infancy secondary to maternal pernicious anemia. N Engl J Med 1966;274:1168–71.
49. Jadhav M, Webb JKG, Vaishnava S, Baker SJ. Vitamin-B_{12} deficiency in Indian infants: a clinical syndrome. Lancet 1962;2:903–7.
50. Lampkin BC, Saunders EF. Nutritional vitamin B_{12} deficiency in an infant. J Pediatr 1969;75:1053–5.
51. Higginbottom MC, Sweetman L, Nyhan WL. A syndrome of methylmalonic aciduria, homocystinuria, megaloblastic anemia and neurologic abnormalities in a vitamin B_{12}-deficient breast-fed infant of a strict vegetarian. N Engl J Med 1978;299:317–23.
52. Frader J, Reibman B, Turkewitz D. Vitamin B_{12} deficiency in strict vegetarians. N Engl J Med 1978;299:1319.
53. Fleiss PM, Douglass JM, Wolfe L. Vitamin B_{12} deficiency in strict vegetarians. N Engl J Med 1978;299:1319.
54. Hershaft A. Vitamin B_{12} deficiency in strict vegetarians. N Engl J Med 1978;299:1319–20.
55. Nyhan WL. Vitamin B_{12} deficiency in strict vegetarians. N Engl J Med 1978;299:1320.
56. Abdulla M, Aly KO, Andersson I, Asp NG, Birkhed D, Denker I, Johansson CG, Jagerstad M, Kolar K, Nair BM, Nilsson-Ehle P, Norden A, Rassner S, Svensson S, Akesson B, Ockerman PA. Nutrient intake and health status of lactovegetarians: chemical analyses of diets using the duplicate portion sampling technique. Am J Clin Nutr 1984;40:325–38.
57. Sklar R. Nutritional vitamin B_{12} deficiency in a breast-fed infant of a vegan-diet mother. Clin Pediatr 1986;25:219–21.
58. Committee on Drugs, American Academy of Pediatrics. The transfer of drugs and other chemicals into human milk. Pediatrics 2001;108:776–89.

Name:	**VITAMIN C**	Risk Factor:	**A***
Class:	**Vitamin**		

FETAL RISK SUMMARY

RECOMMENDATION: Compatible

Vitamin C (ascorbic acid) is a water-soluble essential nutrient required for collagen formation, tissue repair, and numerous metabolic processes including the conversion of folic acid to folinic acid and iron metabolism (1). The National Academy of Sciences' recommended dietary allowance (RDA) for vitamin C in pregnancy is 70 mg (1).

V

Vitamin C is actively transported to the fetus (2–5). When maternal serum levels are high, placental transfer changes to simple diffusion (5). During gestation, maternal serum vitamin C progressively declines (6,7). As a consequence of this process, newborn serum vitamin C (9–22 μg/mL) is approximately 2–4 times that of the mother (4–10 μg/mL) (4–19).

Maternal deficiency of vitamin C without clinical symptoms is common during pregnancy (18–20). Most studies have found no association between this deficiency and maternal or fetal complications, including congenital malformations (11,12,21–24). When low vitamin C levels were found in women or fetuses with complications, it was a consequence of the condition and not a cause. However, a 1971 retrospective study of 1,369 mothers found that deficiency of vitamin C may have a teratogenic effect, although the authors advised caution in the interpretation of their results (25). In a later investigation, low 1st-trimester white blood cell vitamin C levels were discovered in six mothers giving birth to infants with neural tube defects (26). Folic acid, vitamin B_{12}, and riboflavin were also low in serum or red blood cells. The low folic acid and vitamin B_{12} levels were thought to be involved in the etiology of the defects (see also Folic Acid, Vitamin B_{12}, and Riboflavin).

A 1965 report suggested that high daily doses of vitamin C during pregnancy might have produced a "conditioned" scurvy in two infants (27). The mothers had apparent daily intakes of vitamin C in the 400-mg range throughout pregnancy, but both of their offspring had infantile scurvy. To study this condition, laboratory animals were given various doses of vitamin C throughout gestation. Two of 10 offspring exposed to the highest doses developed symptoms and histologic changes compatible with scurvy (27). The investigators concluded that the high *in utero* exposure may have induced ascorbic acid dependency. More recent reports of this condition have not been located; thus, the clinical significance is unknown.

Only one report has been found that potentially relates high doses of vitamin C with fetal anomalies. This was in a brief 1976 case report describing an anencephalic fetus delivered from a woman treated with high doses of vitamin C and other water-soluble vitamins and nutrients for psychiatric reasons (28). The relationship between the defect and the vitamins is unknown. In another study, no evidence of adverse effects was found with doses up to 2000 mg/day (29).

In summary, mild to moderate vitamin C deficiency or excessive doses do not seem to pose a major risk to the mother or fetus. Because vitamin C is required for good maternal and fetal health and an increased demand for the vitamin occurs during pregnancy, intake up to the RDA is recommended.

[**Risk Factor C if used in doses above the RDA.*]

BREAST FEEDING SUMMARY

RECOMMENDATION: Compatible

Vitamin C (ascorbic acid) is excreted into breast milk. Reported concentrations in milk vary from 24 to 158 μg/mL (30–38). In lactating women with low nutritional status, milk vitamin C is directly proportional to intake (31,32). Supplementation with 4–200 mg/day of vitamin C produced milk levels of 24–61 μg/mL (31). Similarly, in another group of women with poor vitamin C intake, supplementation with 34–103 mg/day resulted in levels of 34–55 μg/mL (32). In contrast, studies in well-nourished women consuming the RDA or more of vitamin C in their diets indicate that ingestion of greater amounts does not significantly increase levels of the vitamin in their milk (33–34). Even consumption of total vitamin C exceeding 1000 mg/day, 10 times the RDA, did not significantly increase milk concentrations or vitamin C intake of the infants (36). However, maternal urinary excretion of the vitamin did increase significantly. These studies indicate that vitamin C excretion into milk is regulated to prevent exceeding a saturation level (36).

Storage of human milk in the freezer for up to 3 months did not affect vitamin C concentrations of milk obtained from preterm mothers but resulted in a significant decrease in vitamin C concentrations in milk from term mothers (39). Both types of milk, however, maintained sufficient vitamin C to meet the RDA for infants.

The RDA for vitamin C during lactation is 95 mg (1). Well-nourished lactating women consuming the RDA of vitamin C in their diets normally excrete sufficient vitamin C in their milk to reach a saturation level and additional supplementation is not required. Maternal supplementation up to the RDA is needed only in those women with poor nutritional status.

References

1. American Hospital Formulary Service. *Drug Information 1997*. Bethesda, MD: American Society of Health-System Pharmacists, 1997:2823–5.
2. Hill EP, Longo LD. Dynamics of maternal-fetal nutrient transfer. Fed Proc 1980;39:239–44.
3. Streeter ML, Rosso P. Transport mechanisms for ascorbic acid in the human placenta. Am J Clin Nutr 1981;34:1706–11.
4. Hamil BM, Munks B, Moyer EZ, Kaucher M, Williams HH. Vitamin C in the blood and urine of the newborn and in the cord and maternal blood. Am J Dis Child 1947;74:417–33.
5. Kaminetzky HA, Baker H, Frank O, Langer A. The effects of intravenously administered water-soluble vitamins during labor in normovitaminemic and hypovitaminemic gravidas on maternal and neonatal blood vitamin levels at delivery. Am J Obstet Gynecol 1974;120:697–703.
6. Snelling CE, Jackson SH. Blood studies of vitamin C during pregnancy, birth, and early infancy. J Pediatr 1939;14:447–51.
7. Adlard BPF, De Souza SW, Moon S. Ascorbic acid in fetal human brain. Arch Dis Child 1974;49:278–82.
8. Braestrup PW. Studies of latent scurvy in infants. II. Content of ascorbic (cevitamic) acid in the blood-serum of women in labour and in children at birth. Acta Paediatr 1937;19:328–34.
9. Braestrup PW. The content of reduced ascorbic acid in blood plasma in infants, especially at birth and in the first days of life. J Nutr 1938;16:363–73.
10. Slobody LB, Benson RA, Mestern J. A comparison of the vitamin C in mothers and their newborn infants. J Pediatr 1946;29:41–4.
11. Teel HM, Burke BS, Draper R. Vitamin C in human pregnancy and lactation. I. Studies during pregnancy. Am J Dis Child 1938;56:1004–10.
12. Lund CJ, Kimble MS. Some determinants of maternal and plasma vitamin C levels. Am J Obstet Gynecol 1943;46:635–47.
13. Manahan CP, Eastman NJ. The cevitamic acid content of fetal blood. Bull Johns Hopkins Hosp 1938;62:478–81.
14. Raiha N. On the placental transfer of vitamin C. An experimental study on guinea pigs and human subjects. Acta Physiol Scand 1958;45:Suppl 155.
15. Khattab AK, Al Nagdy SA, Mourad KAH, El Azghal HI. Foetal maternal ascorbic acid gradient in normal Egyptian subjects. J Trop Pediatr 1970;16:112–5.
16. McDevitt E, Dove MA, Dove RF, Wright IS. Selective filtration of vitamin C by the placenta. Proc Soc Exp Biol Med 1942;51:289–90.
17. Sharma SC. Levels of total ascorbic acid, histamine and prostaglandins E2 and F2α in the maternal antecubital and foetal umbilical vein blood immediately following the normal human delivery. Int J Vitam Nutr Res 1982;52:320–5.
18. Dostalova L. Correlation of the vitamin status between mother and newborn during delivery. Dev Pharmacol Ther 1982;4(Suppl 1):45–57.
19. Baker H, Frank O, Thomson AD, Langer A, Munves ED, De Angelis B, Kaminetzky HA. Vitamin profile of 174 mothers and newborns at parturition. Am J Clin Nutr 1975;28:59–65.
20. Kaminetzky HA, Langer A, Baker H, Frank O, Thomson AD, Munves ED, Opper A, Behrle FC, Glista B. The effect of nutrition in teen-age gravidas on pregnancy and the status of the neonate. I. A nutritional profile. Am J Obstet Gynecol 1973;115:639–46.
21. Martin MP, Bridgforth E, McGanity WJ, Darby WJ. The Vanderbilt cooperative study of maternal and infant nutrition. X. Ascorbic acid. J Nutr 1957;62:201–24.
22. Chaudhuri SK. Role of nutrition in the etiology of toxemia of pregnancy. Am J Obstet Gynecol 1971;110:46–8.
23. Wilson CWM, Loh HS. Vitamin C and fertility. Lancet 1973;2:859–60.
24. Vobecky JS, Vobecky J, Shapcott D, Munan L. Vitamin C and outcome of pregnancy. Lancet 1974;1:630.
25. Nelson MM, Forfar JO. Associations between drugs administered during pregnancy and congenital abnormalities of the fetus. Br Med J 1971;1:523–7.
26. Smithells RW, Sheppard S, Schorah CJ. Vitamin deficiencies and neural tube defects. Arch Dis Child 1976;51:944–50.
27. Cochrane WA. Overnutrition in prenatal and neonatal life: a problem? Can Med Assoc J 1965;93:893–9.
28. Averback P. Anencephaly associated with megavitamin therapy. Can Med Assoc J 1976;114:995.
29. Korner WF, Weber F. Zur toleranz hoher Ascorbinsauredosen. Int J Vitam Nutr Res 1972;42:528–44.
30. Ingalls TH, Draper R, Teel HM. Vitamin C in human pregnancy and lactation. II. Studies during lactation. Am J Dis Child 1938;56:1011–19.
31. Deodhar AD, Rajalakshmi R, Ramakrishnan CV. Studies on human lactation. Part III. Effect of dietary vitamin supplementation on vitamin contents of breast milk. Acta Paediatr 1964;53:42–8.
32. Bates CJ, Prentice AM, Prentice A, Lamb WH, Whitehead RG. The effect of vitamin C supplementation on lactating women in Keneba, a West African rural community. Int J Vitam Nutr Res 1983;53:68–76.
33. Thomas MR, Kawamoto J, Sneed SM, Eakin R. The effects of vitamin C, vitamin B_6, and vitamin B_{12} supplementation on the breast milk and maternal status of well-nourished women. Am J Clin Nutr 1979;32:1679–85.
34. Thomas MR, Sneed SM, Wei C, Nail PA, Wilson M, Sprinkle EE III. The effects of vitamin C, vitamin B_6, vitamin B_{12}, folic acid, riboflavin, and thiamin on the breast milk and maternal status of well-nourished women at 6 months postpartum. Am J Clin Nutr 1980;33:2151–6.
35. Sneed SM, Zane C, Thomas MR. The effects of ascorbic acid, vitamin B_6, vitamin B_{12}, and folic acid

supplementation on the breast milk and maternal nutritional status of low socioeconomic lactating women. Am J Clin Nutr 1981;34:1338–46.
36. Byerley LO, Kirksey A. Effects of different levels of vitamin C intake on the vitamin C concentration in human milk and the vitamin C intakes of breast-fed infants. Am J Clin Nutr 1985;41:665–71.
37. Salmenpera L. Vitamin C nutrition during prolonged lactation: optimal in infants while marginal in some mothers. Am J Clin Nutr 1984;40:1050–6.
38. Grewar D. Infantile scurvy. Clin Pediatr 1965;4:82–9.
39. Bank MR, Kirksey A, West K, Giacoia G. Effect of storage time and temperature on folacin and vitamin C levels in term and preterm human milk. Am J Clin Nutr 1985;41:235–42.

Name:	**VITAMIN D**	Risk Factor:	**A***
Class:	**Vitamin**		

FETAL RISK SUMMARY

RECOMMENDATION: Compatible

Vitamin D analogues are a group of fat-soluble nutrients essential for human life with antirachitic and hypercalcemic activity (1). The National Academy of Sciences' recommended dietary allowance (RDA) for normal pregnant women in the United States is 400 IU (1).

The two natural biologically active forms of vitamin D are 1,25-dihydroxyergocalciferol and calcitriol (1,25-dihydroxyvitamin D_3) (1). A third active compound, 25-hydroxydihydrotachysterol, is produced in the liver from the synthetic vitamin D analogue, dihydrotachysterol.

Ergosterol (provitamin D_2) and 7-dehydrocholesterol (provitamin D_3) are activated by ultraviolet light to form ergocalciferol (vitamin D_2) and cholecalciferol (vitamin D_3), respectively. These, in turn, are converted in the liver to 25-hydroxyergocalciferol and calcifediol (25-hydroxyvitamin D_3), the major transport forms of vitamin D in the body. Activation of the transport compounds by enzymes in the kidneys results in the two natural active forms of vitamin D.

The commercially available forms of vitamin D are ergocalciferol, cholecalciferol, calcifediol, calcitriol, and dihydrotachysterol. Although differing in potency, all of these products have the same result in the mother and fetus. Thus, only the term *vitamin D*, unless otherwise noted, will be used in this monograph.

High doses of vitamin D are known to be teratogenic in experimental animals, but direct evidence for this is lacking in humans. Because of its action to raise calcium levels, vitamin D has been suspected in the pathogenesis of the supravalvular aortic stenosis syndrome, which is often associated with idiopathic hypercalcemia of infancy (2–4). The full features of this rare condition are characteristic elfin facies, mental and growth retardation, strabismus, enamel defects, craniosynostosis, supravalvular aortic and pulmonary stenosis, inguinal hernia, cryptorchidism in males, and early development of secondary sexual characteristics in females (2). Excessive intake or retention of vitamin D during pregnancy by mothers of infants who develop supravalvular aortic stenosis syndrome has not been consistently found (2,3,5). Although the exact cause is unknown, it is possible that the syndrome results from abnormal vitamin D metabolism in the mother, the fetus, or both.

Very high levels of vitamin D have been used to treat maternal hypoparathyroidism during pregnancy (6–9). In two studies, 15 mothers were treated with doses averaging 107,000 IU/day throughout their pregnancies to maintain maternal calcium levels within the normal range (6,7). All of the 27 children were normal at birth and during follow-up examinations ranging up to 16 years. Calcitriol, in doses up to 3 μg/day, was used to treat

V

another mother with hypoparathyroidism (8). The high dose was required in the latter half of pregnancy to prevent hypocalcemia. The infant had no apparent adverse effects from this exposure. In a similar case, a mother received 100,000 IU/day throughout gestation, resulting in a healthy, full-term infant (9). In contrast, a 1965 case report described a woman who received 600,000 IU of vitamin D and 40,000 IU of vitamin A daily for 1 month early in pregnancy (10). The resulting infant had a defect of the urogenital system, but this was probably caused by ingestion of excessive vitamin A (see Vitamin A).

Vitamin D deficiency can be induced by decreased dietary intake or lack of exposure to sunlight. The conversion of provitamin D_3 to vitamin D_3 is catalyzed by ultraviolet light striking the skin (1). Severe deficiency during pregnancy, resulting in maternal osteomalacia, leads to significant morbidity in the mother and fetus (11–21). Pitkin, in a 1985 article, reviewed the relationship between vitamin D and calcium metabolism in pregnancy (22).

Although rare in the United States, the peak incidence of vitamin D deficiency occurs in the winter and early spring when exposure to sunlight is at a minimum. Certain ethnic groups, such as Asians, seem to be at greater risk for developing this deficiency because of their dietary and sun exposure habits (11–21). In the pregnant woman, osteomalacia may cause, among other effects, decreased weight gain and pelvic deformities that prevent normal vaginal delivery (11,12). For the fetus, vitamin D deficiency has been associated with the following:

Reduced fetal growth (11,12)
Neonatal hypocalcemia without convulsions (12–14,20)
Neonatal hypocalcemia with convulsions (tetany) (15–17)
Neonatal rickets (18,19)
Defective tooth enamel (21,23)

Long-term use of heparin may induce osteopenia by inhibiting renal activation of calcifediol to the active form of vitamin D_3 (calcitriol or 1,25-dihydroxyvitamin D_3) (22). The decreased levels of calcitriol prevent calcium uptake by bone and result in osteopenia (see reference 23 for detailed review of calcium metabolism in pregnancy). One investigator suggests that these patients may benefit from treatment with supplemental calcitriol (22).

A number of investigators have measured vitamin D levels in the mother during pregnancy and in the newborn (24–34). Although not universal, most studies have found a significant correlation between maternal serum and cord blood levels (24–28). In one study, a close association between both of the transport vitamin D forms in maternal and cord serum was discovered (29). No significant correlation could be demonstrated, however, between the two biologically active forms in maternal and cord blood.

Using a perfused human placenta, a 1984 report confirmed that calcifediol and calcitriol were transferred from the mother to the fetus, although at a very slow rate (35). Binding to vitamin D_3-binding protein was a major rate-limiting factor, especially for calcifediol, the transport form of vitamin D_3. The researchers concluded that placental metabolism of calcifediol was not a major source of fetal calcitriol (35).

V

Maternal levels at term are usually higher than those in the newborn because the fetus has no need for intestinal calcium absorption (24–30). Maternal levels are elevated in early pregnancy and continue to increase throughout pregnancy (32). During the winter months a weak correlation may exist between maternal vitamin D intake and serum levels, with exposure to ultraviolet light the main determinant of maternal concentrations (33,34). A Norwegian study, however, was able to increase maternal concentrations of active vitamin D significantly during all seasons with daily supplementation of 400 IU (29).

[*_Risk Factor D if used in doses above the RDA._]

BREAST FEEDING SUMMARY

RECOMMENDATION: Compatible

Vitamin D is excreted into breast milk in limited amounts (36). A direct relationship exists between maternal serum levels of vitamin D and the concentration in breast milk (37). Chronic maternal ingestion of large doses may lead to greater than normal vitamin D activity in the milk and resulting hypercalcemia in the infant (38). In the lactating woman who is not receiving supplements, there is considerable controversy about whether her milk contains sufficient vitamin D to protect the infant from vitamin deficiency. Several studies have supported the need for infant supplementation during breast feeding (12,36, 39–41). Other investigators have concluded that supplementation is not necessary if maternal vitamin D stores are adequate (28,42–44).

A study published in 1977 measured high levels of a vitamin D metabolite in the aqueous phase of milk (45). Although two other studies supported these findings, the conclusions were in direct opposition to previous measurements and have been vigorously disputed (46,47). The argument that human milk is low in vitamin D is supported by clinical reports of vitamin D deficiency-induced rickets and decreased bone mineralization in breast-fed infants (40,41,48–50). Moreover, one investigation measured the vitamin D activity of human milk and failed to find any evidence for significant activity of water-soluble vitamin D metabolites (51). Vitamin D activity in the milk was 40–50 IU/L, with 90% of this accounted for by the usual fat-soluble components.

The National Academy of Sciences' RDA for vitamin D in the lactating woman is 400 IU (1). The Committee on Nutrition, American Academy of Pediatrics, recommends vitamin D supplements for breast-fed infants if maternal vitamin D nutrition is inadequate or if the infant lacks sufficient exposure to ultraviolet light (52). A second committee of the American Academy of Pediatrics classifies vitamin D as compatible with breast-feeding (53). However, the serum calcium levels of the infant should be monitored if the mother is receiving pharmacologic doses (53).

References

1. American Hospital Formulary Service. *Drug Information 1997*. Bethesda, MD: American Society of Health-System Pharmacists, 1997:2826–8.
2. Friedman WF, Mills LF. The relationship between vitamin D and the craniofacial and dental anomalies of the supravalvular aortic stenosis syndrome. Pediatrics 1969;43:12–8.
3. Rowe RD, Cooke RE. Vitamin D and craniofacial and dental anomalies of supravalvular stenosis. Pediatrics 1969;43:1–2.
4. Taussig HB. Possible injury to the cardiovascular system from vitamin D. Ann Intern Med 1966;65:1195–1200.
5. Anita AU, Wiltse HE, Rowe RD, Pitt EL, Levin S, Ottesen OE, Cooke RE. Pathogenesis of the supravalvular aortic stenosis syndrome. J Pediatr 1967;71:431–41.
6. Goodenday LS, Gordan GS. Fetal safety of vitamin D during pregnancy. Clin Res 1971;19:200.
7. Goodenday LS, Gordan GS. No risk from vitamin D in pregnancy. Ann Intern Med 1971;75:807–8.
8. Sadeghi-Nejad A, Wolfsdorf JI, Senior B. Hypoparathyroidism and pregnancy: treatment with calcitriol. JAMA 1980;243:254–5.
9. Greer FR, Hollis BW, Napoli JL. High concentrations of vitamin D2 in human milk associated with pharmacologic doses of vitamin D_2. J Pediatr 1984;105:61–4.
10. Pilotti G, Scorta A. Ipervitaminosi A gravidica e malformazioni neonatali dell'apparato urinaria. Minerva Ginecol 1965;17:1103–8. As cited in Nishimura H, Tanimura T. *Clinical Aspects of the Teratogenicity of Drugs*. New York, NY: American Elsevier, 1976: 251–2.
11. Parr JH, Ramsay I. The presentation of osteomalacia in pregnancy. Case report. Br J Obstet Gynaecol 1984;91:816–8.
12. Brooke OG, Brown IRF, Bone CDM, Carter ND, Cleeve HJW, Maxwell JD, Robinson VP, Winder SM. Vitamin D supplements in pregnant Asian women: effects on calcium status and fetal growth. Br Med J 1980;280: 751–4.
13. Rosen JF, Roginsky M, Nathenson G, Finberg L. 25-Hydroxyvitamin D: plasma levels in mothers and their premature infants with neonatal hypocalcemia. Am J Dis Child 1974;127:220–3.
14. Watney PJM, Chance GW, Scott P, Thompson JM. Maternal factors in neonatal hypocalcaemia: a study in three ethnic groups. Br Med J 1971;2:432–6.
15. Heckmatt JZ, Peacock M, Davies AEJ, McMurray J, Isherwood DM. Plasma 25-hydroxyvitamin D in pregnant Asian women and their babies. Lancet 1979;2: 546–9.

16. Roberts SA, Cohen MD, Forfar JO. Antenatal factors associated with neonatal hypocalcaemic convulsions. Lancet 1973;2:809–11.
17. Purvis RJ, Barrie WJM, MacKay GS, Wilkinson EM, Cockburn F, Belton NR, Forfar JO. Enamel hypoplasia of the teeth associated with neonatal tetany: a manifestation of maternal vitamin-D deficiency. Lancet 1973;2:811–4.
18. Ford JA, Davidson DC, McIntosh WB, Fyfe WM, Dunnigan MG. Neonatal rickets in Asian immigrant population. Br Med J 1973;3:211–2.
19. Moncrieff M, Fadahunsi TO. Congenital rickets due to maternal vitamin D deficiency. Arch Dis Child 1974;49:810–1.
20. Watney PJM. Maternal factors in the aetiology of neonatal hypocalcaemia. Postgrad Med J 1975; 51(Suppl 3):14–7.
21. Cockburn F, Belton NR, Purvis RJ, Giles MM, Brown JK, Turner TL, Wilkinson EM, Forfar JO, Barrie WJM, McKay GS, Pocock SJ. Maternal vitamin D intake and mineral metabolism in mothers and their newborn infants. Br Med J 1980;2:11–4.
22. Pitkin RM. Calcium metabolism in pregnancy and the perinatal period: a review. Am J Obstet Gynecol 1985;151:99–109.
23. Stimmler L, Snodgrass GJAI, Jaffe E. Dental defects associated with neonatal symptomatic hypocalcaemia. Arch Dis Child 1973;48:217–20.
24. Hillman LS, Haddad JG. Human perinatal vitamin D metabolism. I: 25-hydroxyvitamin D in maternal and cord blood. J Pediatr 1974;84:742–9.
25. Dent CE, Gupta MM. Plasma 25-hydroxyvitamin-D levels during pregnancy in Caucasians and in vegetarian and non-vegetarian Asians. Lancet 1975;2:1057–60.
26. Weisman Y, Occhipinti M, Knox G, Reiter E, Root A. Concentrations of 24,25-dihydroxyvitamin D and 25-hydroxyvitamin D in paired maternal-cord sera. Am J Obstet Gynecol 1978;130:704–7.
27. Steichen JJ, Tsang RC, Gratton TL, Hamstra A, DeLuca HF. Vitamin D homeostasis in the perinatal period: 1,25-dihydroxyvitamin D in maternal, cord, and neonatal blood. N Engl J Med 1980;302:315–9.
28. Birkbeck JA, Scott HF. 25-Hydroxycholecalciferol serum levels in breast-fed infants. Arch Dis Child 1980;55:691–5.
29. Markestad T, Aksnes L, Ulstein M, Aarskog D. 25-Hydroxyvitamin D and 1,25-dihydroxyvitamin D of D_2 and D_3 origin in maternal and umbilical cord serum after vitamin D_2 supplementation in human pregnancy. Am J Clin Nutr 1984;40:1057–63.
30. Kumar R, Cohen WR, Epstein FH. Vitamin D and calcium hormones in pregnancy. N Engl J Med 1980;302:1143–5.
31. Hillman LS, Haddad JG. Perinatal vitamin D metabolism. II. Serial 25-hydroxyvitamin D concentrations in sera of term and premature infants. J Pediatr 1975;86:928–35.
32. Kumar R, Cohen WR, Silva P, Epstein FH. Elevated 1,25-dihydroxyvitamin D plasma levels in normal human pregnancy and lactation. J Clin Invest 1979;63:342–4.
33. Hillman LS, Haddad JG. Perinatal vitamin D metabolism. III. Factors influencing late gestational human serum 25-hydroxyvitamin D. Am J Obstet Gynecol 1976;125:196–200.
34. Turton CWG, Stanley P, Stamp TCB, Maxwell JD. Altered vitamin-D metabolism in pregnancy. Lancet 1977;1:222–5.
35. Ron M, Levitz M, Chuba J, Dancis J. Transfer of 25-hydroxyvitamin D_3 and 1,25-dihydroxyvitamin D_3 across the perfused human placenta. Am J Obstet Gynecol 1984;148:370–4.
36. Greer FR, Hollis BW, Cripps DJ, Tsang RC. Effects of maternal ultraviolet B irradiation on vitamin D content of human milk. J Pediatr 1984;105:431–3.
37. Rothberg AD, Pettifor JM, Cohen DF, Sonnendecker EWW, Ross FP. Maternal-infant vitamin D relationships during breast-feeding. J Pediatr 1982;101: 500–3.
38. Goldberg LD. Transmission of a vitamin-D metabolite in breast milk. Lancet 1972;2:1258–9.
39. Greer FR, Ho M, Dodson D, Tsang RC. Lack of 25-hydroxyvitamin D and 1,25-dihydroxyvitamin D in human milk. J Pediatr 1981;99:233–5.
40. Greer FR, Searcy JE, Levin RS, Steichen JJ, Steichen-Asch PS, Tsang RC. Bone mineral content and serum 25-hydroxyvitamin D concentration in breast-fed infants with and without supplemental vitamin D. J Pediatr 1981;98:696–701.
41. Greer FR, Searcy JE, Levin RS, Steichen JJ, Steichen-Asche PS, Tsang RC. Bone mineral content and serum 25-hydroxyvitamin D concentrations in breast-fed infants with and without supplemental vitamin D: one-year follow-up. J Pediatr 1982;100:919–22.
42. Fairney A, Naughten E, Oppe TE. Vitamin D and human lactation. Lancet 1977;2:739–41.
43. Roberts CC, Chan GM, Folland D, Rayburn C, Jackson R. Adequate bone mineralization in breast-fed infants. J Pediatr 1981;99:192–6.
44. Chadwick DW. Commentary. Water-soluble vitamin D in human milk: a myth. Pediatrics 1982;70: 499.
45. Lakdawala DR, Widdowson EM. Vitamin-D in human milk. Lancet 1977;1:167–8.
46. Greer FR, Reeve LE, Chesney RW, DeLuca HF. Water-soluble vitamin D in human milk: a myth. Pediatrics 1982;69:238.
47. Greer FR, Reeve LE, Chesney RW, DeLuca HF. Commentary. Water-soluble vitamin D in human milk: a myth. Pediatrics 1982;70:499–500.
48. Bunker JWM, Harris RS, Eustis RS. The antirachitic potency of the milk of human mothers fed previously on "vitamin D milk" of the cow. N Engl J Med 1933;208:313–5.
49. O'Connor P. Vitamin D-deficiency rickets in two breast-fed infants who were not receiving vitamin D supplementation. Clin Pediatr (Phila) 1977;16: 361–3.
50. Little JA. Commentary. Water-soluble vitamin D in human milk: a myth. Pediatrics 1982;70:499.
51. Reeve LE, Chesney RW, DeLuca HF. Vitamin D of human milk: identification of biologically active forms. Am J Clin Nutr 1982;36:122–6.
52. Committee on Nutrition, American Academy of Pediatrics. Vitamin and mineral supplement needs in normal children in the United States. Pediatrics 1980;66:1015.
53. Committee on Drugs, American Academy of Pediatrics. The transfer of drugs and other chemicals into human milk. Pediatrics 2001;108:776–89.

Name: **VITAMIN E** Risk Factor: **A***
Class: **Vitamin**

FETAL RISK SUMMARY

RECOMMENDATION: Compatible

Vitamin E (tocopherols) comprises a group of fat-soluble vitamins that are essential for human health, although their exact biologic function is unknown (1). The National Academy of Sciences' recommended dietary allowance (RDA) for vitamin E in pregnancy is 10 mg (1).

Vitamin E concentrations in mothers at term are approximately 4–5 times that of the newborn (2–8). Levels in the mother rise throughout pregnancy (3). Maternal blood vitamin E usually ranges between 9 and 19 μg/mL with corresponding newborn levels varying from 2 to 6 μg/mL (2–9). Supplementation of the mother with 15–30 mg/day had no effect on either maternal or newborn vitamin E concentrations at term (4). Use of 600 mg/day in the last 2 months of pregnancy produced about a 50% rise in maternal serum vitamin E (+8 μg/mL) but a much smaller increase in the cord blood (+1 μg/mL) (7). Although placental transfer is by passive diffusion, passage of vitamin E to the fetus is dependent on plasma lipid concentrations (8–10). At term, cord blood is low in β-lipoproteins, the major carriers of vitamin E, in comparison with maternal blood; as a consequence, it is able to transport less of the vitamin (8). Because vitamin E is transported in the plasma by these lipids, recent investigations have focused on the ratio of vitamin E (in milligrams) to total lipids (in grams) rather than on blood vitamin E concentrations alone (9). Ratios above about 0.6–0.8 are considered normal depending on the author cited and the age of the patients (9,11,12).

Vitamin E deficiency is relatively uncommon in pregnancy, occurring in less than 10% of all patients (3,4,13). No maternal or fetal complications from deficiency or excess of the vitamin have been identified. Doses far exceeding the RDA have not proved to be harmful (7,14,15). Early studies used vitamin E in conjunction with other therapy in attempts to prevent abortion and premature labor, but no effect of the vitamin therapy was demonstrated (16,17). Premature infants born with low vitamin E stores may develop hemolytic anemia, edema, reticulocytosis, and thrombocytosis if not given adequate vitamin E in the first months following birth (15,18,19). In two studies, supplementation of mothers with 500–600 mg of vitamin E during the last 1–2 months of pregnancy did not produce values significantly different from controls in the erythrocyte hemolysis test with hydrogen peroxide, a test used to determine adequate levels of vitamin E (7,15).

In summary, neither deficiency nor excess of vitamin E has been associated with maternal or fetal complications during pregnancy. In well-nourished women, adequate vitamin E is consumed in the diet and supplementation is not required. If dietary intake is poor, supplementation up to the RDA for pregnancy is recommended.

[**Risk Factor C if used in doses above the RDA.*]

V

BREAST FEEDING SUMMARY

RECOMMENDATION: Compatible

Vitamin E is excreted into breast milk (11,12,20,21). Human milk is more than 5 times richer in vitamin E than cow's milk and is more effective in maintaining adequate serum vitamin E and vitamin E:total lipid ratio in infants up to 1 year of age (11,21). A 1985 study measured 2.3 μg/mL of the vitamin in mature milk (20). Milk obtained from preterm mothers (gestational age 27–33 weeks) was significantly higher, 8.5 μg/mL, during the 1st week and then decreased progressively over the next 6 weeks to 3.7 μg/mL (20). The authors concluded that milk from preterm mothers plus multivitamin supplements would provide adequate levels of vitamin E for very-low-birth-weight infants (<1500 g and appropriate for gestational age).

Japanese researchers examined the pattern of vitamin E analogues (α-, γ-, δ-, and β-tocopherols) in plasma and red blood cells from breast-fed and bottle-fed infants (22). Several differences were noted, but the significance of these findings to human health is unknown.

Vitamin E applied for 6 days to the nipples of breast-feeding women resulted in a significant rise in infant serum levels of the vitamin (23). The study group, composed of 10 women, applied the contents of one 400-IU vitamin E capsule to both areolae and nipples after each nursing. Serum concentrations of the vitamin rose from 4 to 17.5 μg/mL and those in a similar group of untreated controls rose from 3.4 to 12.2 μg/mL. The difference between the two groups was statistically significant ($p < 0.025$). Although no adverse effects were observed, the authors cautioned that the long-term effects were unknown.

The National Academy of Sciences' RDA of vitamin E during lactation is 12 mg (1). Maternal supplementation is recommended only if the diet does not provide sufficient vitamin E to meet the RDA.

References

1. American Hospital Formulary Service. *Drug Information 1997*. Bethesda, MD: American Society of Health-System Pharmacists, 1997:2832–3.
2. Moyer WT. Vitamin E levels in term and premature newborn infants. Pediatrics 1950;6:893–6.
3. Leonard PJ, Doyle E, Harrington W. Levels of vitamin E in the plasma of newborn infants and of the mothers. Am J Clin Nutr 1972;25:480–4.
4. Baker H, Frank O, Thomson AD, Langer A, Munves ED, De Angelis B, Kaminetzky HA. Vitamin profile of 174 mothers and newborns at parturition. Am J Clin Nutr 1975;28:59–65.
5. Dostalova L. Correlation of the vitamin status between mother and newborn during delivery. Dev Pharmacol Ther 1982;4(Suppl 1):45–57.
6. Kaminetzky HA, Baker H. Micronutrients in pregnancy. Clin Obstet Gynecol 1977;20:363–80.
7. Mino M, Nishino H. Fetal and maternal relationship in serum vitamin E level. J Nutr Sci Vitaminol 1973;19:475–82.
8. Haga P, Ek J, Kran S. Plasma tocopherol levels and vitamin E/B-lipoprotein relationships during pregnancy and in cord blood. Am J Clin Nutr 1982;36:1200–4.
9. Martinez FE, Goncalves AL, Jorge SM, Desai ID. Vitamin E in placental blood and its interrelationship to maternal and newborn levels of vitamin E. J Pediatr 1981;99:298–300.
10. Hill EP, Longo LD. Dynamics of maternal-fetal nutrient transfer. Fed Proc 1980;39:239–44.
11. Martinez FE, Jorge SM, Goncalves AL, Desai ID. Evaluation of plasma tocopherols in relation to hematological indices of Brazilian infants on human milk and cows' milk regime from birth to 1 year of age. Am J Clin Nutr 1984;39:969–74.
12. Mino M, Kitagawa M, Nakagawa S. Red blood cell tocopherol concentrations in a normal population of Japanese children and premature infants in relation to the assessment of vitamin E status. Am J Clin Nutr 1985;41:631–8.
13. Kaminetzky HA, Langer A, Baker O, Frank O, Thomson AD, Munves ED, Opper A, Behrle FC, Glista B. The effect of nutrition in teen-age gravidas on pregnancy and the status of the neonate. I. A nutritional profile. Am J Obstet Gynecol 1973;115:639–46.
14. Hook EB, Healy KM, Niles AM, Skalko RG. Vitamin E: teratogen or anti-teratogen? Lancet 1974;1:809.
15. Gyorgy P, Cogan G, Rose CS. Availability of vitamin E in the newborn infant. Proc Soc Exp Biol Med 1952;81:536–8.
16. Kotz J, Parker E, Kaufman MS. Treatment of recurrent and threatened abortion. Report of two hundred and twenty-six cases. J Clin Endocrinol 1941;1:838–49.
17. Shute E. Vitamin E and premature labor. Am J Obstet Gynecol 1942;44:271–9.
18. Oski FA, Barness LA. Vitamin E deficiency: a previously unrecognized cause of hemolytic anemia in the premature infant. J Pediatr 1967;70:211–20.
19. Ritchie JH, Fish MB, McMasters V, Grossman M. Edema and hemolytic anemia in premature infants. A vitamin E deficiency syndrome. N Engl J Med 1968;279:1185–90.
20. Gross SJ, Gabriel E. Vitamin E status in preterm infants fed human milk or infant formula. J Pediatr 1985;106:635–9.

21. Friedman Z. Essential fatty acids revisited. Am J Dis Child 1980;134:397–408.
22. Mino M, Kijima Y, Nishida Y, Nakagawa S. Difference in plasma- and red blood cell-tocopherols in breast-fed and bottle-fed infants. J Nutr Sci Vitaminol 1980;26:103–12.
23. Marx CM, Izquierdo A, Driscoll JW, Murray MA, Epstein MF. Vitamin E concentrations in serum of newborn infants after topical use of vitamin E by nursing mothers. Am J Obstet Gynecol 1985;152:668–70.

Name: **VITAMINS, MULTIPLE** Risk Factor: **A***
Class: **Vitamins**

FETAL RISK SUMMARY

RECOMMENDATION: Compatible

Vitamins are essential for human life. Preparations containing multiple vitamins (multivitamins) are routinely given to pregnant women. A typical product will contain the vitamins A, D, E, and C, plus the B complex vitamins thiamine (B_1), riboflavin (B_2), niacin (B_3), pantothenic acid (B_5), pyridoxine (B_6), B_{12}, and folic acid. Miscellaneous substances that may be included are iron, calcium, and other minerals. The practice of supplementation during pregnancy with multivitamins varies from country to country but is common in the United States. The National Academy of Sciences' recommended dietary allowance (RDA) for pregnant women, as of 1989, is as follows (1):

Vitamin A	800 RE	Niacin (B_3)	17 mg
Vitamin D	400 IU	Pyridoxine (B_6)	2.2 mg
Vitamin C	70 mg	Folic acid	0.4 mg
Thiamine (B_1)	1.5 mg	Vitamin B_{12}	2.2 μg
Riboflavin (B_2)	1.6 mg	Vitamin E	10 mg

Although essential for health, vitamin K is normally not included in multivitamin preparations because it is adequately supplied from natural sources. The fat-soluble vitamins, A, D, and E, may be toxic or teratogenic in high doses. The water-soluble vitamins, C and the B complex group, are generally considered safe in amounts above the RDA, but there are exceptions. Deficiencies of vitamins may also be teratogenic (see individual vitamin monographs for further details).

The role of vitamins in the prevention of certain congenital defects continues to be a major area of controversy. Two different classes of anomalies, cleft lip and/or palate (CLP) and neural tube defects (NTDs), have been the focus of numerous investigations with multivitamins. An investigation into a third class of anomalies, limb-reduction defects, has also appeared. The following sections will summarize the published work on these topics.

Animal research in the 1930s and 1940s had shown that both deficiencies and excesses of selected vitamins could result in fetal anomalies, but it was not until two papers in 1958 (2,3) that attention was turned to humans. These investigations examined the role of environmental factors, in particular the B complex vitamins, as agents for preventing the recurrence of CLP. In that same year, a study was published that involved 87 women who had previously given birth to infants with CLP (4). Although the series was too small to draw statistical conclusions, 48 women given no vitamin supplements had 78 pregnancies, resulting in 4 infants with CLP. The treated group, composed of 39 women, received multivitamins plus injectable B complex vitamins during the 1st trimester. This group had 59 pregnancies with none of the infants having CLP. A similar study found a CLP incidence of 1.9% (3 of 156) in treated pregnancies compared with 5.7% (22 of 383) in controls (5). The difference was not statistically significant. However, other researchers, in a 1964 survey, found no evidence that vitamins offered protection against CLP (6). Also in 1964, research was published involving 594 pregnant women who had previously given birth to an infant with CLP (7). This work was further expanded, and the total group involving 645 pregnancies was presented in a 1976 paper (8). Of the total group, 417 women were not given supplements during pregnancy, and they gave birth to 20 infants (4.8%) with CLP. In the treated group, 228 women were given B complex vitamins plus vitamin C before or during the 1st trimester. From this latter group, 7 infants (3.1%) with CLP resulted. Although suggestive of a positive effect, the difference between the two groups was not significant. Another investigator found only one instance of CLP in his group of 85 supplemented pregnancies (9). These patients were given daily multivitamins plus 10 mg of folic acid. In 206 pregnancies in women not given supplements in which the infants or fetuses were examined, 15 instances of CLP resulted. The difference between the two groups was significant ($p = 0.023$). In contrast, one author suggested that the vitamin A in the supplements caused a cleft palate in his patient (10). However, the conclusion of this report has been disputed (11). Thus, the published studies involving the role of multivitamins in the prevention of cleft lip and/or palate are inconclusive. No decisive benefit (or risk) of multivitamin supplementation has emerged from any of the studies.

The second part of the controversy surrounding multivitamins and the prevention of congenital defects involves their role in preventing NTDs. (Three excellent reviews on the pathophysiology and various other aspects of NTDs, including discussions on the role that multivitamins might play in the cause and prevention of these defects, have been recently published [12–14].) In a series of articles from 1976 to 1983, British investigators examined the effect of multivitamin supplements on a group of women who had previously given birth to one or more children with NTDs (15–19). For the purpose of their study, they defined NTDs to include anencephaly, encephalocele, cranial meningocele, iniencephaly, myelocele, myelomeningocele, and meningocele but excluded isolated hydrocephalus and spina bifida occulta (17). In their initial publication, they found that, in six mothers who had given birth to infants with NTDs, there were lower 1st-trimester levels of serum folate, red blood cell folate, white blood cell vitamin C, and riboflavin saturation index (15). The differences between the case mothers and the controls were significant for red blood cell folate ($p < 0.001$) and white blood cell vitamin C ($p < 0.05$). Serum vitamin A levels were comparable with those of controls. Based on this experience, a multicenter study was launched to compare mothers receiving full supplements with control patients not receiving supplements (16–19). The supplemented group received a multivitamin-iron-calcium preparation from 28 days before conception to the date of the second missed menstrual period, which is after the time of neural tube closure. The daily vitamin supplement provided:

Vitamin A	4000 IU	Nicotinamide	15 mg
Vitamin D	400 IU	Pyridoxine	1 mg
Vitamin C	40 mg	Folic acid	0.36 mg
Thiamine	1.5 mg	Ferrous sulfate	75.6 mg (as Fe)
Riboflavin	1.5 mg	Calcium phosphate	480 mg

Their findings, summarized in 1983, are shown below for the infants and fetuses who were examined (19):

One Previous NTD	
Supplemented	385
Recurrences	2* (0.5%)
Not supplemented	458
Recurrences	19* (4.1%) *$p = 0.0004$
Two or More Previous NTDs	
Supplemented	44
Recurrences	1* (2.3%)
Not supplemented	52
Recurrences	5* (9.6%) *$p = 0.145$
Total	
Supplemented	429
Recurrences	3 (0.7%)
Not supplemented	510
Recurrences	24 (4.7%)

Although the numbers were suggestive of a protective effect offered by multivitamins, at least three other explanations were offered by the investigators (16):

1. A low-risk group had selected itself for supplementation.
2. The study group aborted more NTD fetuses than did controls.
3. Other factors were responsible for the reduction in NTDs.

A 1980 report found that women receiving well-balanced diets had a lower incidence and recurrence rate of infants with NTDs than did women receiving poor diets (20). Although multivitamin supplements were not studied, it was assumed that those patients who consumed adequate diets also consumed more vitamins from their food compared with those with poor diets. This study, then, added credibility to the thesis that good nutrition can prevent some NTDs. Other researchers, using Smithells' protocol, observed that fully supplemented mothers ($N = 83$) had no recurrences whereas an unsupplemented group ($N = 141$) had four recurrences of NTDs (21,22). Interestingly, a short report that appeared 6 years before Smithells' work found that both vitamins and iron were consumed more by mothers who gave birth to infants with anencephalus and spina bifida (23).

The above investigations have generated a number of discussions, criticisms, and defenses (24–57). The primary criticism centered on the fact that the groups were not randomly assigned but were self-selected for supplementation or no supplementation. A follow-up study, in response to some of these objections, was published in 1986 (58). This study examined six factors that may have influenced the earlier results by increasing the risk of recurrence of NTDs: (a) two or more previous NTDs, (b) residence in Northern Ireland, (c) spontaneous abortions immediately before the studied pregnancy, (d) less than 12 months between studied pregnancy and abortion, (e) social class, and (f) therapeutic abortion immediately before the studied pregnancy. The relative risk was increased only for the first four factors, and only in those cases with two or more previous NTDs was the increase significant. In addition, none of the four factors would have predicted more than a 4% increase in the recurrence rate in unsupplemented mothers compared with those supplemented. The results indicated that none of these factors contributed significantly to the differential risk between supplemented and unsupplemented mothers, thus leading to the conclusion that the difference in recurrence rates was caused by the multivitamin (58).

Several recent studies examining the effect of multivitamins on NTDs have been published. A case-control, population-based study evaluated the association between periconceptional (3 months before and after conception) multivitamin use and the occurrence of NTDs (59). The case group involved either live-born or stillborn infants with anencephaly or spina bifida born during the years 1968–1980 in the Atlanta area. A total of 347 infants with NTDs were eligible for enrollment and became the case group, whereas 2,829 infants without birth defects served as controls. Multivitamin usage and other factors were ascertained by interview 2–16 years after the pregnancies. This long time interval might have induced a recall problem into the study, even though the authors did take steps to minimize any potential bias (59). A protective effect of periconceptional multivitamin usage against having an infant with an NTD was found in comparison with controls with an estimated relative risk for all NTDs of 0.41 (95% confidence interval [CI] 0.26–0.66), anencephaly 0.47 (95% CI 0.25–0.91), and spina bifida 0.37 (95% CI 0.19–0.70). The odds ratios for whites, but not for other races, were statistically significant. Except for anencephaly among whites (odds ratio [OR] 0.68, 95% CI 0.35–1.34), similar results were obtained when infants with congenital defects other than NTDs were used as controls. Although the results indicated that periconceptional use of multivitamins did protect against NTDs, the authors could not determine whether the effect was related to vitamins or to some unknown characteristic of vitamin users (59). In commenting on this study, one investigator speculated that if the lack of a statistical effect observed in black women was confirmed, it may be related to a different genetic makeup of the population (60). In other words, the gene(s) that cause NTDs are responsive to periconceptional multivitamins only in whites (60).

Three brief letter communications examined the effects of gastric or intestinal bypass surgery, performed for obesity, on the incidence of NTDs (61–63). The first report appeared in 1986 and described three births with NTDs occurring in Maine (61). During the interval 1980–1984, 261 gastric bypass procedures were performed in Maine, but only 133 were in women under the age of 35. One woman delivered an anencephalic fetus 2 years after her surgery. A second suffered a spontaneous abortion at 16 weeks' gestation, 6 years after a gastrojejunostomy. Her serum α-fetoprotein level 10 days before the abortion was 4.8 times the median. She became pregnant again 2 years later and eventually delivered a stillborn infant in the 3rd trimester. The infant had a midthoracic meningomyelocele, iniencephaly, absence of diaphragms, and hypoplastic lungs. During this latter pregnancy, she had intermittent heavy alcohol intake. In the third case, a woman, whose surgery had been done 7 years earlier, had an anencephalic fetus associated with a lumbar rachischisis diagnosed at 6 months' gestation. In response to this report, investigators in Denmark and Sweden could find no cases of NTDs in 77 infants born after their mothers had bypass operations for obesity (62). However, the procedures in these cases involved intestinal bypass, not gastric. Low birth weight and growth retardation were increased in 64 liveborn infants. Gastric bypass surgery is known to place recipients at risk for nutritional deficiencies, especially for iron, calcium, vitamin B_{12}, and folate (61,63). In the third report, of a total of 908 women who underwent the procedure, 511 (57%) responded to a questionnaire (63). Of these, 87 (17%) had been pregnant at least once after the surgery. The 87 women had 73 pregnancies (more than 20 weeks' gestation) before the operation with no cases of NTDs. After the surgery, these women had 110 pregnancies with two cases of NTDs. This represented a 12-fold increase in the risk for NTDs compared with the general population (incidence 0.15%) (63). A third case of an infant with an NTD born from a mother who had undergone the operation was identified later, but the mother was not part of the original group. In each of the three cases, the birth of the infant with an NTD had occurred more than 4 years after the bypass surgery. Moreover, the three mothers had not consumed vitamin supplements as prescribed by their physicians. Because of these findings, the authors recommended pregnancy counseling for any woman who has undergone this procedure and who then desires to become pregnant (63).

In another brief reference, the final results of a British clinical trial were presented in 1989 (64). Women who resided in the Yorkshire region were enrolled in the study if: (a) they had one or more previous NTD infants, (b) they were not pregnant at the time of enrollment, and (c) they were considering another pregnancy. Mothers were requested to take the vitamin formulation described above for at least 4 weeks before conception and until they had missed two menstrual periods (i.e., same as previously). The results of the study included three reporting intervals: 1977–1980, 1981–1984, and 1985–1987. The 148 fully supplemented mothers (those who took vitamins as prescribed or only missed taking vitamins on 1 day) had 150 infants or fetuses, only 1 (0.7%) of whom had an NTD. In contrast, 315 unsupplemented mothers had 320 infants or fetuses among which there were 18 (5.6%) cases of NTDs. The difference between the groups was significant ($p = 0.006$). In addition, 37 partially supplemented (defined as mothers who took the prescribed vitamin for a shorter period of time than the fully supplemented group) women had 37 pregnancies with no cases of NTDs. The investigators concluded that the difference between the groups could not be attributed to declining NTD recurrence rates or to selection bias. Summarizing these and previously published results, only 1 NTD recurrence had been observed in 315 infants or fetuses born to 274 fully supplemented mothers, and no recurrences had been observed among 57 examined infants or fetuses born to 58 partially supplemented women (64).

A 1989 study conducted in California and Illinois examined three groups of patients to determine whether multivitamins had a protective effect against NTDs (65). The groups were composed of women who had a conceptus with an NTD ($N = 571$) and two control groups: those who had a stillbirth or other defect ($N = 546$), and women who had delivered a normal child ($N = 573$). In this study, NTDs included anencephaly, meningocele, myelomeningocele, encephalocele, rachischisis, iniencephaly, and lipomeningocele. The periconceptional use of multivitamins, both in terms of vitamin supplements only and when combined with fortified cereals, was then evaluated for each of the groups. The outcome of this study, after appropriate adjustment for potential confounding factors, revealed an OR of 0.95 (95% CI 0.78–1.14) for NTD-supplemented mothers (i.e., those who received the RDA of vitamins or more) compared with unsupplemented mothers of abnormal infants, and an OR of 1.00 (95% CI 0.83–1.20) when the NTD group was compared with unsupplemented mothers of normal infants. Only slight differences from these values occurred when the data were evaluated by considering vitamin supplements only (no fortified cereals) or vitamin supplements of any amount (i.e., less than the RDA). Similarly, examination of the data for an effect of folate supplementation on the occurrence of NTDs did not change the results. Thus, this study could not show that the use of either multivitamin or folate supplements reduced the frequency of NTDs. However, the investigators cautioned that their results could not exclude the possibility that vitamins might be of benefit in a high-risk population. Several reasons were proposed by the authors to explain why their results were different than those obtained in the Atlanta study cited above: (a) recall bias, (b) a declining incidence of NTDs, (c) geographic differences such that a subset of vitamin-preventable NTDs was in the Atlanta region but not in the areas of the current study, and (d) the Atlanta study did not consider the vitamins contained in fortified cereals (65). However, others concluded that this study lead to a null result because: (a) the vitamin consumption history was obtained after delivery, (b) the history was obtained after the defect was identified, or (c) the study excluded those women taking vitamins after they knew they were pregnant (66).

In contrast to the above report, a Boston study published in 1989 found a significant effect of folic acid-containing multivitamins on the occurrence of NTDs (66). The study population comprised 22,715 women for whom complete information on vitamin consumption and pregnancy outcomes was available. Women were interviewed at the time of a maternal serum α-fetoprotein screen or an amniocentesis. Thus, in most cases, the interview was conducted before the results of the tests were known to either the patient or the interviewer. A total of 49 women had an NTD outcome (2.2/1000). Among these, 3 cases occurred in 107 women with a history of previous NTDs (28.0/1000), and 2 in 489 women with a family history of NTDs in someone other than an offspring (4.1/1000). After excluding the 87 women whose family history of NTDs was unknown, the incidence of NTDs in the remaining women was 44 cases in 22,093 (2.0/1000). Among the 3,157 women who did not use a folic acid-containing multivitamin, 11 cases of NTD occurred, a prevalence of 3.5/1000. For those using the preparation during the first 6 weeks of pregnancy, 10 cases occurred from a total of 10,713 women (prevalence 0.9/1000). The prevalence ratio estimate for these two groups was 0.27 (95% CI 0.12–0.59). For mothers who used vitamins during the first 6 weeks that did not contain folic acid, the prevalence was 3 cases in 926, a ratio of 3.2. The ratio, when compared with that of nonusers, was 0.93 (95% CI 0.26–3.3). When vitamin use was started in the 7th week of gestation, there were 25 cases of NTD from 7,795 mothers using the folic acid-multivitamin supplements (prevalence 3.2/1,000; prevalence ratio 0.92) and no cases in the 66 women who started consuming multivitamins without folate. This study, then, observed a markedly reduced risk of NTDs when folic acid-containing multivitamin preparations were consumed in the first 6 weeks of gestation.

A recent investigation into a third class of anomalies, limb reduction defects, was opened by a report that multivitamins may have caused this malformation in an otherwise healthy boy (52). The mother was taking the preparation because of a previous birth of a child with an NTD. A retrospective analysis of Finnish records, however, failed to show any association between 1st-trimester use of multivitamins and limb-reduction defects (67).

In summary, the use of multivitamins up to the RDA for pregnancy is recommended for the general good health of the mother and the fetus. There is no strong evidence to suggest that vitamin supplementation can prevent CLP. However, a body of evidence has accumulated that supplementation during the first few weeks of gestation, especially with folic acid, may reduce the risk of NTDs (see Folic Acid). The evidence appears particularly strong for the prevention of NTD recurrences in England. Additional studies will be needed to establish whether the protective effect includes only certain types of patients. Until that time, it seems prudent to recommend that folate-containing multivitamin preparations should be used immediately before and during at least the first few months of pregnancy. Women who have had gastric bypass surgery for obesity may be at increased risk for delivering offspring with NTDs, and pregnancy counseling to ensure adequate nutritional intake may be of benefit.

[*Risk Factor varies for amounts exceeding RDA. See individual vitamins.*]

BREAST FEEDING SUMMARY

RECOMMENDATION: Compatible

Vitamins are naturally present in breast milk (see individual vitamins). The recommended dietary allowance of vitamins and minerals during lactation (1st 6 months) are as follows (1):

Vitamin A 1300 RE
Vitamin D 400 IU
Vitamin E 12 mg
Vitamin C 95 mg
Folic acid 280 μg
Thiamine (B_1) 1.6 mg
Riboflavin (B_2) 1.8 mg
Niacin (B_3) 20 mg
Pyridoxine (B_6) 2.1 mg
Vitamin B_{12} 2.6 μg
Calcium 1200 mg
Phosphorus 1200 mg
Iodine 200 μg
Iron 15 mg
Magnesium 355 mg
Zinc 19 mg
Selenium 75 μg

References

1. American Hospital Formulary Service. *Drug Information 1997*. Bethesda, MD: American Society of Health-System Pharmacists, 1997:2805.
2. Douglas B. The role of environmental factors in the etiology of "so-called" congenital malformations. I. Deductions from the presence of cleft lip and palate in one of identical twins, from embryology and from animal experiments. Plast Reconstr Surg 1958;22:94–108.
3. Douglas B. The role of environmental factors in the etiology of "so-called" congenital malformations. II. Approaches in humans; study of various extragenital factors, "theory of compensatory nutrients," development of regime for first trimester. Plast Reconstr Surg 1958;22:214–29.
4. Conway H. Effect of supplemental vitamin therapy on the limitation of incidence of cleft lip and cleft palate in humans. Plast Reconstr Surg 1958;22:450–3.
5. Peer LA, Gordon HW, Bernhard WG. Experimental production of congenital deformities and their possible prevention in man. J Int Coll Surg 1963;39:23–35.
6. Fraser FC, Warburton D. No association of emotional stress or vitamin supplement during pregnancy to cleft lip or palate in man. Plast Reconstr Surg 1964;33:395–9.
7. Peer LA, Gordon HW, Bernhard WG. Effect of vitamins on human teratology. Plast Reconstr Surg 1964;34:358–62.
8. Briggs RM. Vitamin supplementation as a possible factor in the incidence of cleft lip/palate deformities in humans. Clin Plast Surg 1976;3:647–52.
9. Tolarova M. Periconceptional supplementation with vitamins and folic acid to prevent recurrence of cleft lip. Lancet 1982;2:217.
10. Bound JP. Spina bifida and vitamins. Br Med J 1983;286:147.
11. Smithells RW. Spina bifida and vitamins. Br Med J 1983;286:388–9.
12. Main DM, Mennuti MT. Neural tube defects: issues in prenatal diagnosis and counseling. Obstet Gynecol 1986;67:1–16.
13. Rhoads GG, Mills JL. Can vitamin supplements prevent neural tube defects? Current evidence and ongoing investigations. Clin Obstet Gynecol 1986;29:569–79.
14. Lemire RJ. Neural tube defects. JAMA 1988;259:558–62.
15. Smithells RW, Sheppard S, Schorah CJ. Vitamin deficiencies and neural tube defects. Arch Dis Child 1976;51:944–50.
16. Smithells RW, Sheppard S, Schorah CJ, Seller MJ, Nevin NC, Harris R, Read AP, Fielding DW. Possible prevention of neural-tube defects by periconceptional vitamin supplementation. Lancet 1980;1:339–40.
17. Smithells RW, Sheppard S, Schorah CJ, Seller MJ, Nevin NC, Harris R, Read AP, Fielding DW. Apparent prevention of neural tube defects by periconceptional vitamin supplementation. Arch Dis Child 1981;56:911–8.
18. Smithells RW, Sheppard S, Schorah CJ, Seller MJ, Nevin NC, Harris R, Read Ap, Fielding DW, Walker S. Vitamin supplementation and neural tube defects. Lancet 1981;2:1425.
19. Smithells RW, Nevin NC, Seller MJ, Sheppard S, Harris R, Read AP, Fielding DW, Walker S, Schorah CJ, Wild J. Further experience of vitamin supplementation for prevention of neural tube defect recurrences. Lancet 1983;1:1027–31.
20. Laurence KM, James N, Miller M, Campbell H. Increased risk of recurrence of pregnancies complicated by fetal neural tube defects in mothers receiving poor diets, and possible benefit of dietary counselling. Br Med J 1980;281:1592–4.
21. Holmes-Siedle M, Lindenbaum RH, Galliard A, Bobrow M. Vitamin supplementation and neural tube defects. Lancet 1982;1:276.
22. Holmes-Siedle M. Vitamin supplementation and neural tube defects. Lancet 1983;2:41.
23. Choi NW, Klaponski FA. On neural-tube defects: an

epidemiological elicitation of etiological factors. Neurology 1970;20:399–400.
24. Stone DH. Possible prevention of neural-tube defects by periconceptional vitamin supplementation. Lancet 1980;1:647.
25. Smithells RW, Sheppard S. Possible prevention of neural-tube defects by periconceptional vitamin supplementation. Lancet 1980;1:647.
26. Fernhoff PM. Possible prevention of neural-tube defects by periconceptional vitamin supplementation. Lancet 1980;1:648.
27. Elwood JH. Possible prevention of neural-tube defects by periconceptional vitamin supplementation. Lancet 1980;1:648.
28. Anonymous. Vitamins, neural-tube defects, and ethics committees. Lancet 1980;1:1061–2.
29. Kirke PN. Vitamins, neural tube defects, and ethics committees. Lancet 1980;1:1300–1.
30. Freed DLJ. Vitamins, neural tube defects, and ethics committees. Lancet 1980;1:1301.
31. Raab GM, Gore SM. Vitamins, neural tube defects, and ethics committees. Lancet 1980;1:1301.
32. Hume K. Fetal defects and multivitamin therapy. Med J Aust 1980;2:731–2.
33. Edwards JH. Vitamin supplementation and neural tube defects. Lancet 1982;1:275–6.
34. Renwick JH. Vitamin supplementation and neural tube defects. Lancet 1982;1:748.
35. Chalmers TC, Sacks H. Vitamin supplements to prevent neural tube defects. Lancet 1982;1:748.
36. Stirrat GM. Vitamin supplementation and neural tube defects. Lancet 1982;1:625–6.
37. Kanofsky JD. Vitamin supplements to prevent neural tube defects. Lancet 1982;1:1075.
38. Walsh DE. Vitamin supplements to prevent neural tube defects. Lancet 1982;1:1075.
39. Meier P. Vitamins to prevent neural tube defects. Lancet 1982;1:859.
40. Smith DE, Haddow JE. Vitamins to prevent neural tube defects. Lancet 1982;1:859–60.
41. Smithells RW, Sheppard S, Schorah CJ, Seller MJ, Nevin NC, Harris R, Read AP, Fielding DW. Vitamin supplements and neural tube defects. Lancet 1982;1:1186.
42. Anonymous. Vitamins to prevent neural tube defects. Lancet 1982;2:1255–6.
43. Lorber J. Vitamins to prevent neural tube defects. Lancet 1982;2:1458–9.
44. Read AP, Harris R. Spina bifida and vitamins. Br Med J 1983;286:560–1.
45. Rose G, Cooke ID, Polani, Wald NJ. Vitamin supplementation for prevention of neural tube defect recurrences. Lancet 1983;1:1164–5.
46. Knox EG. Vitamin supplementation and neural tube defects. Lancet 1983;2:39.
47. Emanuel I. Vitamin supplementation and neural tube defects. Lancet 1983;2:39–40.
48. Smithells RW, Seller MJ, Harris R, Fielding DW, Schorah CJ, Nevin NC, Sheppard S, Read AP, Walker S, Wild J. Vitamin supplementation and neural tube defects. Lancet 1983;2:40.
49. Oakley GP Jr, Adams MJ Jr, James LM. Vitamins and neural tube defects. Lancet 1983;2:798–9.
50. Smithells RW, Seller MJ, Harris R, Fielding DW, Schorah CJ, Nevin NC, Sheppard S, Read AP, Walker S, Wild J. Vitamins and neural tube defects. Lancet 1983;2:799.
51. Elwood JM. Can vitamins prevent neural tube defects? Can Med Assoc J 1983;129:1088–92.
52. David TJ. Unusual limb-reduction defect in infant born to mother taking periconceptional multivitamin supplement. Lancet 1984;1:507–8.
53. Blank CE, Kumar D, Johnson M. Multivitamins and prevention of neural tube defects: a need for detailed counselling. Lancet 1984;1:291.
54. Smithells RW. Can vitamins prevent neural tube defects? Can Med Assoc J 1984;131:273–6.
55. Wald NJ, Polani PE. Neural-tube defects and vitamins: the need for a randomized clinical trial. Br J Obstet Gynecol 1984;91:516–23.
56. Seller MJ. Unanswered questions on neural tube defects. Br Med J 1987;294:1–2.
57. Harris R. Vitamins and neural tube defects. Br Med J 1988;296:80–1.
58. Wild J, Read AP, Sheppard S, Seller MJ, Smithells RW, Nevin NC, Schorah CJ, Fielding DW, Walker S, Harris R. Recurrent neural tube defects, risk factors and vitamins. Arch Dis Child 1986;61:440–4.
59. Mulinare J, Cordero JF, Erickson JD, Berry RJ. Periconceptional use of multivitamins and the occurrence of neural tube defects. JAMA 1988;260:3141–5.
60. Holmes LB. Does taking vitamins at the time of conception prevent neural tube defects? JAMA 1988;260:3181.
61. Haddow JE, Hill LE, Kloza EM, Thanhauser D. Neural tube defects after gastric bypass. Lancet 1986;1:1330.
62. Knudsen LB, Kallen B. Gastric bypass, pregnancy, and neural tube defects. Lancet 1986;2:227.
63. Martin L, Chavez GF, Adams MJ Jr, Mason EE, Hanson JW, Haddow JE, Currier RW. Gastric bypass surgery as maternal risk factor for neural tube defects. Lancet 1988;1:640–1.
64. Smithells RW, Sheppard S, Wild J, Schorah CJ. Prevention of neural tube defect recurrences in Yorkshire: final report. Lancet 1989;2:498–9.
65. Mills JL, Rhoads GG, Simpson JL, Cunningham GC, Conley MR, Lassman MR, Walden ME, Depp OR, Hoffman HJ. The absence of a relation between the periconceptional use of vitamins and neural-tube defects. N Engl J Med 1989;321:430–5.
66. Milunsky A, Jick H, Jick SS, Bruell CL, MacLaughlin DS, Rothman KJ, Willett W. Multivitamin/folic acid supplementation in early pregnancy reduces the prevalence of neural tube defects. JAMA 1989;262:2847–2852.
67. Aro T, Haapakoski J, Heinonen OP, Saxen L. Lack of association between vitamin intake during early pregnancy and reduction limb defects. Am J Obstet Gynecol 1984;150:433.

Name: **VORICONAZOLE** Risk Factor: **D_M**
Class: **Antifungal**

FETAL RISK SUMMARY

RECOMMENDATION: No Human Data - Animal Data Suggest Risk

The antifungal drug voriconazole is indicated for the treatment of various systemic fungal infections. It is a triazole antifungal in the same class as fluconazole and itraconazole. The mechanism of action involves the inhibition of an essential fungal cytochrome P450 function. This inhibition is more selective for fungal cytochrome P450 enzymes than for those in mammalian cells (1).

Reproduction studies with voriconazole have been conducted in rats and rabbits. In pregnant rats, a dose 0.3 times than the recommended human maintenance dose or higher on a body surface area basis (RHMD) was teratogenic (cleft palates, hydronephrosis and hydroureter). Toxic effects observed at this dose were reduced ossification of sacral and caudal vertebrae, skull, and pubic and hyoid bones, super numerary ribs, anomalies of the sternebrae and dilatation of the ureter/renal pelvis. Treatment later in gestation resulted in increased gestational length and dystocia with a subsequent increase in perinatal pup mortality. Plasma estradiol in pregnant rats was reduced at all dose levels.

In pregnant rabbits, toxic effects, noted at 6 times the RHMD, consisted of increased embryo mortality, reduced fetal weight, and increased incidences of skeletal variations, cervical ribs and extra sternebrae ossification sites (1).

In 2-year studies, hepatocellular adenomas were observed in female rats at an oral dose 1.6 times the RHMD and hepatocellular carcinomas were seen in male rats at oral doses 0.2 and 1.6 times the RHMD. In mice, hepatocellular adenomas were observed in male and female mice and hepatocellular carcinomas in male mice at oral doses that were 1.4 times the RHMD. Voriconazole was clastogenic in an *in vitro* assay with human lymphocytes, but was not genotoxic in four other assays (1).

It is not known if voriconazole crosses the placenta to the fetus. The molecular weight (about 349), however, is low enough that exposure of the embryo and/or fetus should be expected.

In summary, no reports describing the use of voriconazole in human pregnancy have been located. The animal data are suggestive for a risk of toxicity and teratogenicity. However, inhibition of estrogen synthesis was observed in rats. This effect also has been noted in rats treated with another triazole agent, fluconazole. In those studies, the anti-estrogen action was thought to be responsible for the observed cleft palate and bone abnormalities. (See Fluconazole.) Whether this mechanism also applies to voriconazole is unknown. Nevertheless, based only on the animal data, one review concluded that voriconazole should be avoided in pregnancy (2). Although there are currently no human data, the close relationship with fluconazole, a suspected teratogen in high doses, is reason enough to avoid voriconazole in the 1st trimester. If inadvertent exposure has occurred, the patient should be advised of the potential but unknown risk to the embryo.

BREAST FEEDING SUMMARY

RECOMMENDATION: No Human Data - Potential Toxicity

No reports describing the use of voriconazole during lactation have been located. The relatively low molecular weight (about 349) suggests that the agent will be excreted into breast milk. There is potential for toxicity in nursing infants, especially during the neonatal period when hepatic function is immature. Therefore, women taking this drug should not breast-feed.

References

1. Product information. Vfend. Pfizer, 2004.
2. Moudgal VV, Sobel JD. Antifungal drugs in pregnancy: a review. Expert Opin Drug Saf 2003;2:475–83.

V

W

Name:	**WARFARIN**	Risk Factor:	**D***
Class:	**Anticoagulant**		

See Coumadin Derivatives.

[**Risk Factor X according to manufacturer-DuPont Pharma, 2000.*]

Z

Name:	ZAFIRLUKAST	Risk Factor:	B_M
Class:	Respiratory Agent		

FETAL RISK SUMMARY

RECOMMENDATION: No Human Data - Animal Data Suggest Low Risk

Zafirlukast is an oral selective peptide leukotriene receptor antagonist that is indicated for the prophylaxis and chronic treatment of asthma. Reproduction studies conducted in mice, rats, and monkeys with oral doses up to 160, 400, and 800 times the maximum recommended human oral dose based on body surface area, respectively, did not observe any evidence of impaired fertility (only rats tested) or teratogenicity (1). The maximum doses in rats and monkeys were maternal toxic, resulting in maternal deaths in some cases, fetal resorptions (rats), and spontaneous abortions (monkeys).

It is not known if zafirlukast crosses the human placenta. The molecular weight (about 576) is low enough, however, that passage to the fetus should be expected.

No reports describing the use of zafirlukast during human pregnancy have been located. One source states that zafirlukast may be safe to use during pregnancy, but this conclusion is based solely on animal studies (2). If zafirlukast is used in pregnancy, healthcare professionals are encouraged to call the toll free number (800-670-6126) for information about patient enrollment in the Motherisk study.

BREAST FEEDING SUMMARY

RECOMMENDATION: Limited Human Data - Potential Toxicity

The manufacturer reports that zafirlukast is excreted into breast milk (1). In healthy women taking 40 mg orally twice daily, the average steady-state concentration of zafirlukast in milk was 50 ng/mL compared with 255 ng/mL in the plasma (milk:plasma ratio 0.2). The effects in a nursing infant from exposure to the drug in milk are unknown. However, the manufacturer recommends against breast-feeding because of the potential for tumorigenicity noted in mice and rats, and the enhanced sensitivity to the adverse effects of the drug in neonatal rats and dogs (1).

References

1. Product information. Accolate. AstraZeneca, 2000.
2. Anonymous. Drugs for asthma. Med Lett Drugs Ther 2000;42:19–24.

Name:	**ZALCITABINE**	Risk Factor:	C_M
Class:	**Antiviral**		

FETAL RISK SUMMARY

RECOMMENDATION: Compatible - Maternal Benefit >> Embryo/Fetal Risk

Zalcitabine (2′,3′-dideoxycytidine; ddC) is a reverse transcriptase inhibitor that also inhibits viral DNA synthesis. It is classified as a nucleoside reverse transcriptase inhibitor (NRTI) used for the treatment of human immunodeficiency virus (HIV) infections. Its mechanism of action is similar to that of five other nucleoside analogues: abacavir, didanosine, lamivudine, stavudine, and zidovudine. Zalcitabine is converted *in vivo* to the active metabolite, dideoxycytidine 5′-triphosphate (ddCTP), by cellular enzymes (1).

Zalcitabine was teratogenic in mice given doses 1365 and 2730 times the maximum recommended human dose based on AUC measurements (MRHD) (1). A significant decrease in fetal weight was observed at both doses, and decreased embryo survival occurred at the highest dose. In rats, a dose 485 times the MRHD was not teratogenic, but doses greater than this were associated with reduced embryo survival, and a high incidence of hydrocephalus was observed at 1,071 times the MRHD (1). A significant number of rat offspring also had impaired learning and memory, and longer durations of hyperactivity. These findings were considered to result from extensive damage to or gross underdevelopment of the brain, consistent with hydrocephalus. Doses 2142 times the MRHD were teratogenic in rats and resulted in a significant decrease in fetal weight (1).

In a 1990 report, pregnant mice were given zalcitabine during gestational days 6–15 in doses of 0, 200, 400, 1000, and 2000 mg/kg/day (2). The highest doses, 1000 and 2000 mg/kg/day, were significantly associated with a variety of congenital malformations, reduced fetal weight, and increased resorption (reduced embryo survival).

The reproductive toxicity of zalcitabine in rats was compared in a combined *in vitro/in vivo* experiment with four other nucleoside analogues (vidarabine-phosphate, ganciclovir, 2′,3′-dideoxyadenosine [ddA; unphosphorylated active metabolite of didanosine], and zidovudine), and these results were then compared with previous data obtained under identical conditions with acyclovir (3). Using various concentrations of the drug in a whole-embryo culture system and direct administration to pregnant females (200 mg/kg SC every 4 hours × 3 doses) during organogenesis, *in vitro* vidarabine showed the highest potential to interfere with embryonic development, whereas *in vivo* acyclovir had the highest teratogenic potential. In this study, the *in vitro* reproductive toxicity of zalcitabine was less than that of vidarabine and acyclovir, but greater than that of the other three agents. The *in vivo* toxicity of zalcitabine was less than that of acyclovir, vidarabine, and ganciclovir, and equal to that observed with ddA and zidovudine (3).

Antiretroviral nucleosides have been shown to have direct dose-related cytotoxic effects on preimplantation mouse embryos. A 1994 report compared this toxicity among zidovudine and three newer compounds, zalcitabine, didanosine, and stavudine (4). Whereas significant inhibition of blastocyst formation occurred with a 1- μmol/L concentration of zidovudine, zalcitabine and stavudine toxicity was not detected until 100 μmol/L, and no toxicity was observed with didanosine up to 100 μmol/L. Moreover, postblastocyst development was severely inhibited in those embryos that did survive exposure to 1 μmol/L zidovudine. As for the other compounds, stavudine, at a concentration of 10 μmol/L, inhibited postblastocyst development, but no effect was observed with concentrations up to

100 μmol/L of zalcitabine or didanosine. Although there are no human data, the authors of this study concluded that the three newer agents might be safer than zidovudine to use in early pregnancy (4).

Zalcitabine crosses the placenta to the fetus (5–8). Using a perfused term human placenta, investigators concluded in a 1992 publication that the placental transfer of zalcitabine was most likely a result of simple diffusion (5). In near-term rhesus monkeys, a single IV bolus (0.6 mg/kg) of zalcitabine produced ratios of fetal:maternal area under the plasma concentration-time curves from 0 to 3 hours of 0.5 (6) and 0.32 (7). Concentrations of zalcitabine in the fetal brain were 20% of those in the fetal plasma by 3 hours (6,7). However, only very small amounts of the inactive monophosphorylated metabolite of zalcitabine (ddCMP), and none of the active triphosphate metabolite (ddCTP), were detected in fetal tissues (7).

Simple diffusion of zalcitabine across the placenta of near-term pigtailed macaques (*Macaca nemestrina*) was reported in a 1994 abstract (8). A continuous IV infusion (1.28 μg/minute/kg) resulted in a mean fetal:maternal plasma concentration at steady state of 0.58.

Three experimental *in vitro* models using perfused human placentas to predict the placental transfer of NRTIs (didanosine, stavudine, zalcitabine, and zidovudine) were described in a 1999 publication (9). For each drug, the predicted fetal:maternal plasma drug concentration ratios at steady state with each of the three models were close to those actually observed in pregnant macaques. Based on these results, the authors concluded that their models would accurately predict the mechanism, relative rate, and extent of *in vivo* human placental transfer of NRTIs (9).

The Antiretroviral Pregnancy Registry reported, for the period January 1989 through January 2004, prospective data (reported to the Registry before the outcomes were known) involving 1537 live births that had been exposed during the 1st trimester to one or more antiretroviral agents (10). Forty-seven of the newborns had congenital defects (3.1%, 95% confidence interval [CI] 2.3–4.1). In the 2407 live births with earliest exposure in the 2nd/3rd trimesters, there were 56 infants with defects (2.3%, 95% CI 1.8–3.0). The prevalence rates for the two periods did not differ significantly. There were 103 infants with birth defects among 3944 live births with exposure anytime during pregnancy (2.6%, 95% CI 2.1–3.2). The prevalence rate did not differ significantly from the rate expected in a nonexposed population (10). There were 33 outcomes exposed to zalcitabine (28 in the 1st trimester and 5 in the 2nd/3rd trimesters) in combination with other antiretroviral agents. There were two birth defects among the 1st trimester exposures and none in those exposed in the 2nd/3rd trimesters. In reviewing the birth defects of prospective and retrospective (pregnancies reported after the outcomes were known) registered cases, and clinical reports, the Registry concluded that there was no pattern of anomalies to suggest a common cause (10). (See Lamivudine for required statement.)

A case of life-threatening anemia following *in utero* exposure to antiretroviral agents was described in 1998 (11). A 30-year-old woman with HIV infection was treated with zidovudine, didanosine, and trimethoprim/sulfamethoxazole (3 times weekly) during the 1st trimester. Vitamin supplementation was also given. Because of an inadequate response, didanosine was discontinued and lamivudine and zalcitabine were started in the 3rd trimester. Two weeks before delivery the HIV viral load was undetectable. At term, a pale, male infant was delivered who developed respiratory distress shortly after birth. Examination revealed a hyperactive precordium and hepatomegaly without evidence of hydrops. The hematocrit was 11% with a reticulocyte count of zero. An extensive work-up of the mother and infant failed to determine the cause of the anemia. Bacterial and viral infections, including

HIV, parvovirus B19, cytomegalovirus, and others, were excluded. The infant received a transfusion and was apparently doing well at 10 weeks of age. Because no other cause of the anemia could be found, the authors attributed the condition to bone marrow suppression, most likely to zidovudine (11). A contribution of the other agents to the condition, however, could not be excluded.

A 2000 case report described the adverse pregnancy outcomes, including neural tube defects (NTDs), of two pregnant women with HIV infection who were treated with the anti-infective combination, trimethoprim/sulfamethoxazole, for prophylaxis against *Pneumocystis carinii*, concurrently with antiretroviral agents (12). Exposure to zalcitabine occurred in one of these cases. A 32-year-old woman with a 3-year history of HIV and recent diagnosis of acquired immunodeficiency syndrome was treated before and throughout gestation with the anti-infective combination plus zidovudine and zalcitabine. Folic acid 10 mg/day was added after the diagnosis of pregnancy (gestational age not specified). At term, a female infant was delivered by cesarean section without HIV infection, but with a bony mass in the lumbar spine (identified by ultrasound at 32 weeks' gestation). A diagnostic evaluation revealed that the second lumbar vertebra consisted of hemivertebrae and projected posteriorly into the spinal canal (12). A malformed and displaced first lumbar vertebra was also noted. Surgery was planned to correct the defect. The authors attributed the NTDs in both cases to the antifolate activity of trimethoprim (12).

No data are available on the advisability of treating pregnant women who have been exposed to HIV via occupational exposure, but one author discourages this use (13).

In summary, although the limited human data do not allow an assessment as to the safety of zalcitabine during pregnancy, the reproductive toxicity observed in animals is a concern. Theoretically, exposure to zalcitabine at the time of implantation could result in impaired fertility as a consequence of embryonic cytotoxicity, but this has not been studied in humans. Mitochondrial dysfunction in offspring exposed *in utero* or postnatally to NRTIs has been reported (see Lamivudine and Zidovudine), but these findings are controversial and require confirmation.

Two reviews, one in 1996 and the other in 1997, concluded that all women currently receiving antiretroviral therapy should continue to receive therapy during pregnancy and that treatment of the mother with monotherapy should be considered inadequate therapy (14,15). In 1998, the Centers for Disease Control and Prevention (CDC) made a similar recommendation that antiretroviral therapy should be continued during pregnancy, but discontinuation of all therapy during the 1st trimester was a consideration (16). If indicated, therefore, zalcitabine should not be withheld in pregnancy (with the possible exception of the 1st trimester) because the expected benefit to the HIV-positive mother probably outweighs the unknown risk to the fetus. The efficacy and safety of combined therapy in preventing vertical transmission of HIV to the newborn, however, are unknown, and zidovudine remains the only antiretroviral agent recommended for this purpose (14,15).

BREAST FEEDING SUMMARY

RECOMMENDATION: Contraindicated

No reports describing the use of zalcitabine during lactation have been located. The relatively low molecular weight (about 211) is low enough that excretion into milk should be expected.

Reports on the use of zalcitabine during human lactation are unlikely because the antiviral agent is used in the treatment of HIV infections. HIV-1 is transmitted in milk, and in developed countries, breast-feeding is not recommended (14,15,17–19). In developing countries, breast-feeding is undertaken, despite the risk, because there are no affordable milk substitutes available. Until 1999, no studies had been published that examined the effect of any antiretroviral therapy on HIV-1 transmission in milk. In that year, a study involving zidovudine was published that measured a 38% reduction in vertical transmission of HIV-1 infection in spite of breast-feeding when compared to controls (see Zidovudine).

References

1. Product information. Hivid. Roche Laboratories, 2001.
2. Lindstrom P, Harris M, Hoberman AM, Dunnick JK, Morrissey RE. Developmental toxicity of orally administered 2′,3′-dideoxycytidine in mice. Teratology 1990;42:131–6.
3. Klug S, Lewandowski C, Merker H-J, Stahlmann R, Wildi L, Neubert D. *In vitro* and *in vivo* studies on the prenatal toxicity of five virustatic nucleoside analogues in comparison to acyclovir. Arch Toxicol 1991;65:283–91.
4. Toltzis P, Mourton T, Magnuson T. Comparative embryonic cytotoxicity of antiretroviral nucleosides. J Infect Dis 1994;169:1100–2.
5. Bawdon RE, Sobhi S, Dax J. The transfer of anti-human immunodeficiency virus nucleoside compounds by the term human placenta. Am J Obstet Gynecol 1992;167:1570–4.
6. Slikker W Jr, Lipe G, Parker W, Rose L, Ali S, Schmued L, Scallet A, Binienda Z. Disposition of ^{3}H-ddC in the pregnant rhesus monkey (abstract). Placenta 1992;13:A.59.
7. Sandberg JA, Binienda Z, Lipe G, Rose LM, Parker WB, Ali SF, Slikker W Jr. Placental transfer and fetal disposition of 2′,3′-dideoxycytidine and 2′,3′-dideoxyinosine in the rhesus monkey. Drug Metab Dispos 1995;23:881–4.
8. Tuntland T, Nosbisch C, Baughman WL, Pereira CM, Unadkat JD. The transplacental transfer of dideoxycytidine is passive in *Macaca nemestrina* (abstract). Teratology 1994;49:415.
9. Tuntland T, Odinecs A, Pereira CM, Nosbisch C, Unadkat JD. *In vitro* models to predict the in vivo mechanism, rate, and extent of placental transfer of dideoxynucleoside drugs against human immunodeficiency virus. Am J Obstet Gynecol 1999;180:198–206.
10. Antiretroviral Pregnancy Registry Steering Committee. *Antiretroviral Pregnancy Registry International Interim Report for 1 January 1989 through 31 January 2004*. Wilmington, NC: Registry Coordinating Center, 2004.
11. Watson WJ, Stevens TP, Weinberg GA. Profound anemia in a newborn infant of a mother receiving antiretroviral therapy. Pediatr Infect Dis J 1998;17:435–6.
12. Richardson MP, Osrin D, Donaghy S, Brown NA, Hay, Sharland M. Spinal malformations in the fetuses of HIV infected women receiving combination antiretroviral therapy and co-trimoxazole. Eur J Obstet Gynecol Reprod Biol 2000;93:215–7.
13. Gerberding JL. Management of occupational exposures to blood-borne viruses. N Engl J Med 1995;332:444–51.
14. Carpenter CCJ, Fischi MA, Hammer SM, Hirsch MS, Jacobsen DM, Katzenstein DA, Montaner JSG, Richman DD, Saag MS, Schooley RT, Thompson MA, Vella S, Yeni PG, Volberding PA. Antiretroviral therapy for HIV infection in 1996. JAMA 1996;276;146–54.
15. Minkoff H, Augenbraun M. Antiretroviral therapy for pregnant women. Am J Obstet Gynecol 1997;176:478–89.
16. CDC. Public Health Service Task Force recommendations for the use of antiretroviral drugs in pregnant women infected with HIV-1 for maternal health and for reducing perinatal HIV-1 transmission in the United States. MMWR 1998;47:No. RR-2.
17. Brown ZA, Watts DH. Antiviral therapy in pregnancy. Clin Obstet Gynecol 1990;33:276–89.
18. de Martino M, Tovo P-A, Tozzi AE, Pezzotti P, Galli L, Livadiotti S, Caselli D, Massironi E, Ruga E, Fioredda F, Plebani A, Gabiano C, Zuccotti GV. HIV-1 transmission through breast-milk: appraisal of risk according to duration of feeding. AIDS 1992;6:991–7.
19. Van de Perre P. Postnatal transmission of human immunodeficiency virus type 1: the breast-feeding dilemma. Am J Obstet Gynecol 1995;173:483–7.

Name:	**ZALEPLON**	Risk Factor:	C_M
Class:	**Hypnotic**		

FETAL RISK SUMMARY

RECOMMENDATION: No Human Data - Animal Data Suggest Low Risk

The oral hypnotic zaleplon is chemically unrelated to benzodiazepines, barbiturates, and other known hypnotic agents, but it is a benzodiazepine receptor agonist. It is indicated for the short-term (e.g., 7–10 days) treatment of insomnia. Zaleplon undergoes substantial presystemic metabolism that significantly reduces its absolute bioavailability. Nearly all of zaleplon is metabolized to inactive metabolites. Plasma protein binding is moderate (about 60%) and the terminal-phase elimination half-life is short (about 1 hour). Zaleplon has an abuse potential similar to benzodiazepines and benzodiazepine-like hypnotics (1).

Reproduction studies have been conducted in rats and rabbits. No evidence of teratogenicity was observed in rats treated throughout organogenesis with doses up to about 49 times the maximum recommended human dose of 20 mg based on body surface area (MRHD). At the maximum dose, pre- and postnatal growth was decreased in rat offspring, but this dose was also maternal toxic (clinical signs and reduced body weight). Fertility and reproductive performance in female rats was also impaired at the maximum dose. The no-effect dose during organogenesis for reduced growth in offspring was 5 times the MRHD. However, treatment of pregnant rats in late gestation and during lactation, with a dose that did not cause maternal toxicity (about 3.4 times the MRHD or greater), did result in an increased incidence of stillbirth and postnatal death, and decreased growth and physical development. The toxicity was thought to have resulted from both *in utero* and lactational exposure to the drug. For exposure in late gestation and during lactation, the no-effect dose was about 0.5 times the MRHD. In rabbits, no evidence of teratogenicity or embryo/fetal toxicity was observed at doses up to 48 times the MRHD given throughout organogenesis (1).

It is not known if zaleplon crosses the human placenta. The molecular weight (about 305) is low enough for placental transfer, but the short elimination half-life will limit the amount drug available at the maternal:fetal interface.

No reports describing the use of zaleplon in human pregnancy have been located. The agent does compare favorably to other hypnotic benzodiazepine receptor agonists due to its rapid onset (15 minutes), short elimination half-life, and the absence of active metabolites (2). The drug is not an animal teratogen and the risk of human teratogenicity is probably very low. However, information from studies in one of the animal species suggests that long-term use could potentially result in human embryo/fetal toxicity. Therefore, use of zaleplon in pregnancy should be restricted to occasional, short-term (e.g., 7–10 days).

BREAST FEEDING SUMMARY

RECOMMENDATION: Limited Human Data - Probably Compatible

Small amounts of zaleplon are excreted into breast milk (1,3). In a study by the manufacturer, the peak drug concentrations in milk occurred about 1 hour after a 10-mg dose. The mean plasma elimination half-life in five lactating women (mean weight 65.1 kg) was about 1 hour, similar to nonlactating women (1,3). The average milk:plasma ratio was 0.5 (3). The investigators estimated the maximum infant exposure during a feeding at peak milk concentrations to be in the range of 1.28–1.66 μg (3). As the women did not breast-feed during the study, the effects of this exposure on a nursing infant are unknown. For a 65.1-kg woman nursing a 4-kg infant, the maximum estimated infant dose, as a percentage of the mother's dose, is 0.27%. It is doubtful if this amount from a 10-mg dose would have a clinically significant effect on a nursing infant. In addition, within 5 hours of a dose, about 97% of the drug will be eliminated from the maternal plasma and milk.

References

1. Product information. Sonata. Monarch Pharmaceuticals, 2004.
2. Hunt CE, Editor. Sleep problems and sleep disorders. *Clinical Updates in Women's Health Care*. American College of Obstetricians and Gynecologists. 2004;3(April):66–7.
3. Darwish M, Martin PT, Cevallos WH, Tse S, Wheeler S, Troy SM. Rapid disappearance of zaleplon from breast milk after oral administration to lactating women. J Clin Pharmacol 1999;39:670–4.

Name:	**ZANAMIVIR**	Risk Factor:	**C_M**
Class:	**Antiviral**		

FETAL RISK SUMMARY

RECOMMENDATION: No Human Data - Animal Data Suggest Low Risk

Zanamivir is formulated as a powder to be administered by oral inhalation. The agent is thought to act by inhibiting influenza virus neuraminidase with the possibility of alteration of virus particle aggregation and release. Zanamivir is indicated for the treatment of uncomplicated acute illness caused by influenza A and B virus in patients who have been symptomatic for no more than 3 days. The systemic bioavailability of the drug is approximately 4%–17%, plasma protein binding is <10%, and it is excreted unchanged (no metabolites have been detected) in the urine with a serum elimination half-life of 2.5–5.1 hours (1).

Reproduction studies with IV or SC zanamivir have been conducted in rats and rabbits. In pregnant rats, the highest IV daily doses administered produced exposures that were greater than 300 times the human exposure from the clinical dose based on AUC (HEAUC). Drug administration, during gestational days 6–15 or during gestational day 16 until litter day 21 to 23, revealed no evidence of malformations, embryotoxicity or maternal toxicity. In a different strain of rats administered SC zanamivir three times daily during gestational days 7 to 17, the highest SC dose produced exposures that were greater than 1000 times the HEAUC. In this study, minor skeletal alterations and variations were observed in the exposed offspring, but the incidence of these effects was within the background rates for the strain studied. In pregnant rabbits, IV doses (identical to the rat doses, but relationship to human dose not specified) administered during gestational days 7–19 revealed no evidence of malformations, embryotoxicity or maternal toxicity (1).

It is not known if zanamivir crosses the human placenta. The antiviral agent does cross the rat and rabbit placentas resulting in fetal blood levels significantly lower than levels in the maternal blood (1). The molecular weight (about 332), combined with the lack of metabolism and plasma protein binding, and the moderately long elimination half-life, suggest that the drug will cross the human placenta. However, the low systemic bioavailability after oral inhalation should limit the amount of drug available for transfer at the maternal:fetal interface.

No reports describing the use of zanamivir during human pregnancy have been located. Although the animal data suggest a low risk, the absence of human pregnancy experience prevents an assessment of the risk for the embryo/fetus.

BREAST FEEDING SUMMARY

RECOMMENDATION: No Human Data - Probably Compatible

No reports describing the use of zanamivir during human lactation have been located. The antiviral agent is excreted into the milk of lactating rats. The molecular weight (about 332), moderately long elimination half-life, and the lack of metabolism and plasma protein binding suggest that the drug will be excreted into breast milk. However, the low systemic bioavailability after oral inhalation should limit the amount of drug excreted into breast milk. The effects, if any, of this exposure on a nursing infant are unknown, but the risk of harm appears to be low.

Reference

1. Product information. Relenza. GlaxoSmithKline, 2004.

Name:	**ZIDOVUDINE**	Risk Factor:	**C_M**
Class:	**Antiviral**		

FETAL RISK SUMMARY

RECOMMENDATION: Compatible - Maternal Benefit >> Embryo/Fetal Risk

The thymidine analogue zidovudine (AZT) is a nucleoside reverse transcriptase inhibitor (NRTI) that is used for the treatment of human immunodeficiency virus (HIV) disease. Other drugs in this class are abacavir, didanosine, lamivudine, stavudine, and zalcitabine.

AZT was not teratogenic in pregnant rats or rabbits at oral doses up to 500 mg/kg/day (1). These doses resulted in peak plasma concentrations in rats 66–226 times, and in rabbits 12–87 times, the mean steady-state peak human plasma levels obtained with the recommended human dose (100 mg every 4 hours). At 150 or 450 mg/kg/day (rats) and 500 mg/kg/day (rabbits), embryo/fetal toxicity was observed as evidenced by an increased incidence of fetal resorptions (1). At a dose of 3000 mg/kg/day in rats (near the median lethal dose), marked maternal toxicity and an increased incidence of fetal malformations were observed (1). This dose produced peak plasma concentrations 350 times the peak human plasma levels (1). In an *in vitro* study, a dose-related reduction in blastocyst formation was noted in fertilized mouse oocytes (1).

A 1991 study in rats compared the *in vitro* and *in vivo* toxicity of five virustatic nucleoside analogues in whole-embryo cultures and on the 10th day of gestation (2). Among the agents tested (vidarabine, ganciclovir, zalcitabine, 2′3′-dideoxyadenosine [ddA], and AZT), AZT had the lowest teratogenic potential.

In an investigation conducted by the manufacturer, a split-dose regimen of 300 mg/kg on gestational day 10 in rats had no adverse effect on the mothers or offspring (3). The AZT concentration in the embryos was approximately one-third of that in the mother, 21.1 μg/g vs. 62.6 μg/g, respectively. However, another study administered AZT to pregnant mice from days 1 to 13 of gestation and observed dose-related fetal toxicity (decrease in the number of fetuses and fetal growth) (4). Concomitant treatment with erythropoietin, vitamin E, or interleukin-3 lessened the fetal toxicity. The adverse effects were thought most likely to be caused by a direct toxic effect on fetal cells, although a partial effect of maternal bone marrow depression could not be excluded.

Four studies have confirmed a direct dose-related toxic effect of AZT on preimplantation mouse embryos (5–8). The doses tested ranged from 1 to 20 times the concentrations obtainable with therapeutic human doses. Using an *in vitro* model, investigators demonstrated that exposure to AZT was highly correlated with failure to develop to the blastocyst stage (5). Similar developmental arrest, possibly caused by inhibition of DNA synthesis in blastomeres, was observed in a second study of preimplantation mouse embryos exposed *in vitro* to zidovudine (6). During the postimplantation portion of this investigation, no adverse fetal effects were observed with doses up to 300 mg/kg/day through all or part of gestation. A third study demonstrated that, when preimplantation mouse embryos were exposed to AZT either *in vivo* or *in vitro*, development was unable to proceed beyond the blastocyst stage (7). Exposure at the blastocyst and postblastocyst stages resulted in a lower degree of retarded cell division, indicating that the critical period of toxicity in mouse embryos is between ovulation and implantation. The comparative mouse embryo cytotoxicity of four antiretroviral nucleosides (AZT, didanosine, stavudine, and zalcitabine) was reported in a 1994 study (8). All of the agents showed dose-related inhibition of blastocyst formation, but AZT was the most toxic of the drugs. Cytotoxicity of the other agents was only evident at concentrations equal to the highest obtainable after therapeutic human doses (stavudine) or much higher (didanosine and zalcitabine).

AZT (1.5 mg/kg/dose every 4 hours) was administered via gastric catheter at least 10 days before and throughout gestation to pigtailed macaques (*Macaca nemestrina*) (9,10). Mean plasma concentrations (area under the plasma concentration-time curve [AUC]) of the drug were comparable to those obtained in human studies. Twelve pregnancies were brought to term (6 AZT, 6 controls), but significantly more matings (17 vs. 9, $p = 0.007$) were required to achieve pregnancy in the AZT-treated primates. A significant decrease in maternal hemoglobin was observed in the AZT-treated animals, but no differences in the mean hematocrit of the drug-exposed newborns or in fetal growth were found in comparison with controls. Moreover, no adverse effects were discovered in neurologic, perceptual, or motor development during a 9- to 10-month follow-up.

The authors of the above investigation speculated that the retarded macaque fertility might have been related to AZT blockage of progesterone synthesis. However, the following two studies on human trophoblast growth and function indicate that inhibition of cell division before blastocyst formation, as demonstrated in the previously described murine studies (5–8), must also be considered (11,12). Human trophoblasts were isolated from 1st-trimester and term pregnancies and maintained in culture (11). Using relatively high drug concentrations (20 μmol/L vs. recommended therapeutic concentrations of 3–5 μmol/L) for prolonged periods (2–11 days), no significant effects on trophoblast function, as measured by human chorionic gonadotropin secretion, protein synthesis, and glucose consumption, were observed. In one of the five term placentas, AZT exposure resulted in a significant decrease (20% of the control value) in progesterone secretion, but the secretion rate (17.2 ng/hour/10^6 cells) was still much higher than the control values of the other placentas (3.26–15.63 ng/hour/10^6 cells).

A 1999 study investigated the effects of a single 24-hour exposure of AZT or didanosine (ddI) on human trophoblast cells using a human choriocarcinoma cell line that exhibited many characteristics of the early placenta (12). Two drug concentrations (7.6 mM or 0.076 mM) were studied for their effects on trophoblast cell proliferation and hormone production (human chorionic gonadotropin [hCG], estradiol [E_2], and progesterone [P_4]).

The higher concentrations of AZT or ddI resulted in significant decreases in cell numbers and growth rate (38% and 51% of control values, respectively), but increased production of hCG, E_2, and P_4. The decrease in trophoblast cell proliferation may have been the mechanism for the increased incidence of rodent embryo loss observed with AZT (12). In contrast, the lower concentrations of AZT and ddI did not cause changes in cell numbers, producing only significant increases in E_2 production. Because of these findings, the researchers concluded that high therapeutic doses of either AZT or ddI during early human gestation were potentially embryotoxic (12).

Adverse effects on neurobehavior development in mice offspring resulting from a combination of AZT and lamivudine were described in a 2001 study (13). Pregnant mice received both drugs from day 10 of gestation to delivery. The effects on somatic and sensorimotor development were minor but more marked in exposed offspring than when either drugs was given alone (13). Both development endpoints were delayed with respect to control animals. Further, alterations of social behavior were observed in both sexes of exposed offspring (13).

AZT crosses the placenta to the fetus in both animals (14–16) and humans (1,17–27). Placental transfer of the drug is rapid and is by simple diffusion (17–19). Seven pregnant HIV-seropositive women with gestational lengths between 14 and 26 weeks were scheduled for therapeutic abortions (20) The women were given AZT, 200 mg orally every 4 hours for five doses, 1–2.75 hours before pregnancy termination. Fetal blood concentrations of the parent compound and its inactive glucuronide metabolite ranged from 100 to 287 ng/mL and from 346 to 963.5 ng/mL, respectively. In six patients (one woman had blood levels below the level of detection), mean AZT concentrations in the maternal blood, amniotic fluid, and fetal blood were 143, 168, and 205 ng/mL, respectively.

In a 1990 study, the pregnancy of an HIV-seropositive woman was terminated at 13 weeks' gestation (21). She had been taking AZT, 100 mg 4 times daily, for 6 weeks, with her last dose consumed approximately 4 hours before the abortion. Both AZT and the glucuronide metabolite were found in the amniotic fluid and various fetal tissues. The lower limit of detection for the assay was 0.01 μmol/L (0.01 nmol/g). The concentrations of the parent compound and the metabolite in maternal plasma were 0.35 and 0.90 μmol/L, respectively. In comparison, the fetal concentrations of AZT (corresponding levels of the metabolite are shown in parentheses) were: amniotic fluid, 0.31 μmol/L (1.16 μmol/L); liver, 0.14 nmol/g (0.16 nmol/g); muscle, 0.26 nmol/g (0.50 nmol/g); and central nervous system, 0.01 nmol/g (0.05 nmol/g). The low levels of AZT in the latter system probably indicate that transplacental passage of the drug, at this dose, may be insufficient to treat HIV infection of the fetal central nervous system (21). The significance of this result is increased by the finding that neurologic and neuropsychologic morbidity in infants exposed to HIV *in utero* is high (21,28).

A 1989 report described the treatment of a 30-year-old HIV-seropositive woman who was treated before and throughout gestation with AZT, 1200 mg/day (22). IV AZT, 0.12 mg/kg/hour, was infused 24 hours before labor induction at 39 weeks' gestation. An uncomplicated vaginal delivery occurred resulting in the birth of a normal male infant weighing 3110 g, with a height and head circumference of 48.5 and 35 cm, respectively. The newborn's renal and hepatic functions were normal, and no other toxicity, such as anemia or macrocytosis, was noted. At birth, concentrations of AZT in the maternal blood, amniotic fluid, and cord blood were 0.28, 3.82, and 0.47 μg/mL, respectively. AZT concentrations in the infant's blood at 6, 24, 36, and 48 hours were 0.46, 0.51, 0.44, and 0.27 μg/mL, respectively, indicating that in the first 24 hours elimination of the drug from the newborn was negligible (22). Levels of the inactive metabolite were also determined

Z

concurrently; in each sample, the metabolite concentration was higher than that of the parent compound. The infant was doing well and growing normally at 6 months of age.

Two HIV-positive women at 18 and 21 weeks' gestation were treated with AZT (1000 mg/day) for 3 days before elective abortion (23). The final 200-mg dose was consumed 2–3 hours before abortion. Both AZT and its metabolite were found in the two women and in amniotic fluid and fetal blood, with fetal:maternal ratios for AZT of 1.10 and 6.00, respectively, and for the metabolite of 0.84 and 3.75, respectively.

Three experimental *in vitro* models using perfused human placentas to predict the placental transfer of NRTIs (didanosine, stavudine, zalcitabine, and AZT) were described in a 1999 publication (29). For each drug, the predicted fetal:maternal plasma drug concentration ratios at steady state with each of the three models were close to those actually observed in pregnant macaques. Based on these results, the authors concluded that their models would accurately predict the mechanism, relative rate, and extent of *in vivo* human placental transfer of NRTIs (29).

The pharmacokinetics of AZT during human and nonhuman primate pregnancies have been determined in a number of studies (24,26,27,30–33). AZT was administered to seven HIV-positive women beginning at 28–35 weeks' gestation with a 200-mg IV dose on day 1, followed by 200 mg orally 5 times a day from day 2 until labor (24). The mean maternal plasma concentrations of AZT and its inactive glucuronide metabolite at delivery were 0.29 and 0.87 μg/mL, respectively. Similar amounts were measured in umbilical cord venous blood, with mean concentrations of 0.28 and 1.01 μg/mL, respectively, suggesting that the fetuses and newborns were unable to metabolize AZT (24). No significant drug-induced adverse effects were observed in the women or their newborns and no congenital malformations were noted. Fetal growth was normal in six and accelerated in one, and the slightly lower than normal hemoglobin values were not considered clinically significant (24).

In pregnant macaques or humans, the pharmacokinetics of AZT were not affected by pregnancy (macaques) (30), nor did AZT affect the transplacental pharmacokinetics of didanosine (macaques) (31), lamivudine (humans) (32), or stavudine (macaques) (33). Two other studies involving four women infected with HIV measured peak AZT maternal serum levels and elimination half-lives that were statistically similar to those of nonpregnant adults (26,27). However, in three women, the AUC during pregnancy was significantly less than after pregnancy (4.5 μmol/L vs. 6.8 μmol/L, $p = 0.02$), and the apparent total body clearance was significantly greater (2.5 L/hour/kg vs. 1.7 L/hour/kg, $p = 0.05$) (26). Moreover, the difference in the apparent volume of distribution during and after pregnancy reached near significance (3.9 L/kg vs. 2.6 L/kg, $p = 0.07$) (26).

The effect of AZT on the transplacental passage of HIV is unknown. A 1990 review of AZT in pregnancy focused on the issue of whether the drug prevented HIV passage to the fetus and concluded that available data were insufficient to provide an answer to this question (22). However, a 1993 study observed that, although AZT is transferred to the fetus relatively intact, the approximately 50% retained by the placenta is extensively metabolized, with one of the metabolites being zidovudine triphosphate, the product responsible for the antiviral activity of the parent drug (34). The effect of this may be a reduction in the risk of HIV transmission to the fetus (34).

Brief descriptions of the treatment and pregnancy outcome of 12 HIV-seropositive women were provided in a 1991 abstract (35). AZT therapy was started before conception in 4 women and between 21 and 34 weeks' (mean 25 weeks') gestation in 8. The mean duration of therapy was 8 weeks (range 1–24 weeks). Three of the women who had conceived while taking AZT underwent therapeutic abortions of grossly normal fetuses between 10 and 12 weeks' gestation. Five women had delivered grossly normal infants with a mean birth weight of 2900 g, and the infants of the remaining four women were undelivered between 24 and 36 weeks. Three other abstracts that appeared in 1992 and 1993 described 46 pregnant women treated with AZT without producing toxic effects or anomalies in their fetuses (36–38).

In a surveillance study of Michigan Medicaid recipients conducted between 1985 and 1992 involving 229,101 completed pregnancies, 2 newborns had been exposed to AZT during the 1st trimester (F. Rosa, personal communication, FDA, 1993). No major birth defects were observed.

Data on 45 newborns (2 sets of twins) of 43 pregnant women, enrolled in studies conducted by 17 institutions participating in acquired immunodeficiency syndrome (AIDS) Clinical Trial Units and who had been treated with AZT, were described in 1992 (39). AZT dosage ranged from 300 to 1200 mg/day, with 24 of the women taking the drug during at least two trimesters. All the infants were born alive. No congenital abnormalities were observed in 12 infants who had been exposed *in utero* to AZT during the 1st trimester, although one newborn with elevated 17α-hydroxyprogesterone levels had clitoral enlargement. Normal levels of the hormone were measured in this infant at 4 months of age. Two term infants were growth retarded, but 38 other singleton term infants had a mean birth weight of 3287 g. Seven infants had hemoglobin values less than 13.5 g/dL; three of these were delivered prematurely. The authors concluded that the few cases of anemia and growth retardation might have been, at least partially, caused by maternal AZT therapy (39). Another report involving 29 pregnant patients treated with AZT at government-sponsored AIDS clinical trial centers appeared in 1992, but no data on the outcome of these pregnancies were given (40).

The outcomes of 104 pregnancies in which AZT was used were described in a 1994 report (41). Sixteen of the pregnancies terminated during the 1st trimester—8 spontaneous and 8 elective abortions. Among the remaining 88 cases, 8 infants had birth defects, 4 after 1st-trimester exposure and 4 after exposure during the 2nd or 3rd trimesters. None of the defects could be attributed to AZT exposure (41): multiple minor anomalies (low-set ears, retrognathia, hirsutism, triangular face, blue sclera, prominent sacral dimple)*; multiple minor anomalies (type not specified)*; extra digits on both hands, hare lip (central), cleft palate; fetal alcohol syndrome; atrial septal defect (asymptomatic) with pectus excavatum*; microcephaly, chorioretinitis (*Toxoplasma gondii* infection); pectus excavatum*; and albinism with congenital ptosis, growth retardation, and oligohydramnios (* indicates chromosomal analysis normal) (41).

The Antiretroviral Pregnancy Registry reported, for the period January 1989 through January 2004, prospective data (reported to the Registry before the outcomes were known) involving 1537 live births that had been exposed during the 1st trimester to one or more antiretroviral agents (42). Forty-seven of the newborns had congenital defects (3.1%, 95% confidence interval [CI] 2.3–4.1). In the 2407 live births with earliest exposure in the 2nd/3rd trimesters, there were 56 infants with defects (2.3%, 95% CI 1.8–3.0). The prevalence rates for the two periods did not differ significantly. There were 103 infants with birth defects among 3944 live births with exposure anytime during pregnancy (2.6%, 95% CI 2.1–3.2). The prevalence rate did not differ significantly from the rate expected in a nonexposed population (42). There were 3361 outcomes exposed to zidovudine (1088 in the 1st trimester and 2573 in the 2nd/3rd trimesters) in combination with other antiretroviral agents. There were 34 (3.1%, 95% CI 2.2–4.3) birth defects among the 1st trimester exposures and 65 (2.5%, 95% CI 2.0–3.2) in those exposed in the 2nd/3rd trimesters. In reviewing the birth defects of prospective and retrospective (pregnancies reported after the outcomes were known) registered cases, and clinical reports, the Registry concluded that there was no pattern of anomalies to suggest a common cause (42). (See Lamivudine for required statement.)

The failure of maternal AZT therapy to prevent the transmission of HIV type 1 (HIV-1) infection to one of the mother's female twins was described in a 1990 report (43). The woman was treated with AZT, 400 mg/day, from 18 weeks' gestation until delivery. A cesarean section was performed at 27 weeks' gestation because of premature labor that was not responsive to tocolytic therapy. Twin A was diagnosed with culture-proven HIV-1 and cytomegalovirus infection. At the time of the report, the child was 9 months old with limited sight, severe failure to thrive, and encephalopathy. An HIV-1 culture in twin B was negative, but analysis for HIV-1 antigens continued to be positive through 20 weeks of age. A number of possible explanations were proposed by the authors concerning the failure of AZT to protect twin A from infection. Included among these were passage of the virus before the onset of treatment at 18 weeks' gestation, intrauterine transfer of the virus via an amniocentesis performed at 14 weeks' gestation, viral resistance to the drug, low fetal tissue drug levels, maternal noncompliance (doubtful), and acquisition of the virus during birth.

A 1992 review on the treatment of HIV-infected pregnant women stated that most obstetric experts offered AZT therapy in cases of AIDS, AIDS-related complex, or when the CD4+ cell counts were below 200 cells/μL (44). Although no fetal toxicity secondary to AZT had been reported, the author recommended caution with 1st-trimester use of the agent and noted the potential for fetal bone marrow depression and resulting anemia.

A clinical trial, the subject of several reviews and editorials (45–51), conducted from 1991 to 1993 and published in 1994, found that the risk of maternal-infant transmission of HIV disease could be decreased by 67.5% by treatment of pregnant women (who had mildly symptomatic HIV disease) with AZT (52). The randomized, double-blind, placebo-controlled trial enrolled untreated HIV-infected pregnant women, at 14–34 weeks' gestation, which had CD4+ T-lymphocyte counts above 200 cells/mm^3 and no clinical indications for antenatal antiretroviral therapy. The maternal AZT treatment regimen consisted of antepartum oral therapy (100 mg orally 5 times daily) and intrapartum IV dosing (2 mg/kg for 1 hour, then 1 mg/kg/hour until delivery). The newborns were treated with oral AZT (2 mg/kg every 6 hours) for 6 weeks. A total of 477 women were enrolled, 409 of whom delivered 415 liveborn infants during the study period. Among those with known HIV-infection status were 180 infants from the AZT-treated group and 183 placebo-treated controls. The authors of this study used statistical methods to predict the number of infants who would be HIV-infected at 18 months of age, thus allowing a faster analysis of their data. They estimated that the number of HIV-infected children would be 8.3% (95% CI 3.9%–12.8%) in the AZT group, and 25.5% (95% CI 18.4%–32.5%) in the placebo group (52). This was a 67.5% (95% CI 40.7%–82.1%) reduction in the risk of HIV transmission ($p = 0.00006$). No differences in growth, prematurity, or the number and patterns of major or minor congenital abnormalities were observed between the two groups. Thirty-three live-born infants had congenital defects, 17 of 206 (8.3%) in the treatment group and 16 of 209 (7.7%) in the nontreated controls. Cardiac malformations were observed in 10 infants (5 in each group), central nervous system defects in five (3 in the AZT group, 2 in controls), and 9 unspecified defects in each group. The total incidence of congenital malformations is higher than expected in the general population, but this probably reflects the population studied. The only drug-related adverse effect observed in the newborns was a decrease in hemoglobin concentration in those exposed to AZT *in utero*. The maximum difference in hemoglobin concentration between the groups, 1 g/dL, occurred at 3 weeks of age, but by 12 weeks of age, the hemoglobin values were similar.

Although AZT appeared to be effective in reducing transmission of HIV-1 to the fetus, some infants became infected despite treatment. Possible reasons proposed for these failures included (a) virus transmission before treatment began, (b) ineffective suppression of maternal viral replication, (c) poor maternal compliance with the drug regimen, and (d) virus resistance to AZT (52).

Recommendations for the treatment of pregnant women infected with HIV were updated by the U.S. Public Health Service in 1998 (53). Although the choice of antiretroviral therapy should be based on the same considerations as used for nonpregnant patients, the inclusion of AZT was considered an important component of all treatment plans. However, waiting to initiate therapy until after 10–12 weeks' gestation was an option. The recommendations also stated that AZT was the only drug that had been demonstrated to reduce the risk of perinatal HIV-1 transmission (53). Because of this, AZT should be given to the mother during the intrapartum period and to the newborn for 6 weeks, regardless of the antepartum antiretroviral regiment (53). (See publication for other specific recommendations.)

A series of studies and editorials appeared in 1998 through 2000 that evaluated or discussed the effect of short courses of AZT on the perinatal transmission of HIV in various populations (54–60). The most effective therapy, however, involved starting treatment of the mother at 28 weeks' gestation, with 6 weeks of treatment in the infant (59,60).

A 2000 review described seven clinical trials that have been effective in reducing perinatal transmission, five with AZT alone, one with AZT plus lamivudine, and one with nevirapine (61). Six of the trials were in less-developed countries. Prolonged use of AZT in the mother and infant was the most effective for preventing vertical transmission of HIV, but also the most expensive. The combination of AZT and lamivudine, consisting of antepartum, intrapartum, and postpartum maternal therapy with continued therapy in the infant for 1 week, may have been as effective as prolonged AZT (61). More data are needed, however, before the efficacy and safety of combined therapy in preventing vertical transmission of HIV to the newborn can be assessed.

A study published in 1999 evaluated the safety, efficacy, and perinatal transmission rates of HIV in 30 pregnant women receiving various combinations of antiretroviral agents (62). Many of the women were substance abusers. AZT was used by 26 women in various combinations that included didanosine, lamivudine, indinavir, nelfinavir, nevirapine, saquinavir, and delavirdine. Antiretroviral therapy was initiated at a median of 14 weeks' gestation (range preconception to 32 weeks). In spite of previous histories of extensive antiretroviral experience and of vertical transmission of HIV, combination therapy was effective in treating maternal disease and in preventing transmission to the current newborns. The outcomes of the pregnancies included one stillbirth, one case of microcephaly, and five infants with birth weights less than 2500 g, two of which were premature (62).

In another 1999 study, the safety and efficacy of a short-course of nevirapine was compared to AZT for the prevention of perinatal transmission of HIV-1 (63). At the onset of labor, women were randomly assigned to receive either a single dose of nevirapine (200 mg) plus a single dose (2 mg/kg) to their infants within 72 hours of birth ($N = 310$) or AZT (600 mg then 300 mg every 3 hours until delivery) plus 4 mg/kg twice daily for 7 days to their infants ($N = 308$). Nearly all (98.8%) of the women breast-fed their infants immediately after birth. Up to age 14–16 weeks, significantly fewer infants in the nevirapine group were HIV-1 infected, lowering the risk of infection or death, compared with AZT, by 48% (95% CI 24%–65%) (63). The prevalence of maternal and infant adverse effects were similar in the two groups. In an accompanying study, the nevirapine regimen was shown to be cost-effective in various seroprevalence settings (64).

In an unusual case, a woman was exposed to HIV through self-insemination with fresh semen obtained from a man with a high HIV ribonucleic acid viral load (>750,000 copies/mL plasma) (65). Ten days later, she was started on a prophylactic regimen of AZT (600 mg/day), lamivudine (300 mg/day), and indinavir (2400 mg/day). Pregnancy was confirmed 14 days after insemination. The indinavir dose was reduced to 1800 mg/day 4 weeks after the start of therapy because of the development of renal calculi. All antiretroviral therapy was stopped after 9 weeks because of negative tests for HIV. She gave birth at 40 weeks' gestation to a healthy 3490-g male infant, without evidence of HIV disease, who was developing normally at 2 years of age (65).

A case of life-threatening anemia following *in utero* exposure to antiretroviral agents was described in 1998 (66). A 30-year-old woman with HIV infection was treated with AZT, didanosine, and trimethoprim/sulfamethoxazole (3 times weekly) during the 1st trimester. Vitamin supplementation was also given. Because of an inadequate response, didanosine was discontinued and lamivudine and zalcitabine were started in the 3rd trimester. Two weeks before delivery the HIV viral load was undetectable. At term, a pale, male infant was delivered who developed respiratory distress shortly after birth. Examination revealed a hyperactive precordium and hepatomegaly without evidence of hydrops. The hematocrit was 11% with a reticulocyte count of zero. An extensive work-up of the mother and infant failed to determine the cause of the anemia. Bacterial and viral infections, including HIV, parvovirus B19, cytomegalovirus, and others, were excluded. The infant received a transfusion and was apparently doing well at 10 weeks of age. Because no other cause of the anemia could be found, the authors attributed the condition to bone marrow suppression, most likely to AZT (66). A contribution of the other agents to the condition, however, could not be excluded.

A study of the inhibitory effects of AZT on hematopoiesis was published in 1996 (67). The researchers compared the effect of increasing concentrations of AZT on hematopoietic progenitors from women of childbearing age (from bone marrow aspirates), mid-trimester aborted fetuses (from bone marrow and liver), and term newborns (from cord blood). The inhibitory effect of AZT was more pronounced on fetal and neonatal erythroid progenitors than those from the bone marrow of the women. AZT had no effect on granulocyte colony-stimulating factor or erythropoietin. The authors concluded that neonatal anemia after *in utero* exposure to AZT was due to reduced clonal maturation of erythroid progenitors (67).

A 1999 report from France described the possible association of AZT and lamivudine (NRTIs) use in pregnancy with mitochondrial dysfunction in the offspring (68). Mitochondrial disease is relatively rare in France (estimated prevalence: 1 in 5000–20,000 children) (68). From an ongoing epidemiological survey of 1754 mother-child pairs exposed to AZT and other agents during pregnancy, however, 8 children with possible mitochondrial dysfunction were identified. None of the eight infants were infected with HIV, but all received prophylaxis for up to 6 weeks after birth with the same antiretroviral regimen as given during pregnancy. Four of the cases were exposed to AZT alone and four to a combination of AZT and lamivudine. Two from the combination group died at about 1 year of age. All eight cases had abnormally low respiratory-chain enzyme activities. The authors concluded that their results supported the hypothesis of a causative association between mitochondrial respiratory-chain dysfunction and NRTIs. Moreover, the toxicity may have been potentiated by combination of these agents (68).

In a paper following the above study, investigators noted that NRTIs inhibit DNA polymerase γ, the enzyme responsible for mitochondrial DNA replication (69). They then hypothesized that this inhibition would induce depletion of mitochondrial DNA and mitochondrial DNA-encoded mitochondrial enzymes, thus resulting in mitochondrial dysfunction (69). Moreover, they stated that support for their hypothesis was suggested by the closeness of the clinical manifestations of inherited mitochondrial diseases with the adverse effects attributed to NRTIs. These adverse effects included polyneuropathy, myopathy, cardiomyopathy, pancreatitis, bone marrow suppression, and lactic acidosis. They also postulated this mechanism was involved in the development of a lipodystrophy syndrome of peripheral fat wasting and central adiposity, a condition that has been thought to be related to protease inhibitors (69).

A commentary on the above two studies concluded that the evidence for NRTI-induced mitochondrial dysfunction was equivocal (70). First, the clinical presentations in the infants were varied and not suggestive of a single cause; indeed, three of the infants were symptom-free and one had Leigh's syndrome, a classic mitochondrial disease (70). Second, the clinical features, in some cases, were not suggestive of mitochondrial dysfunction. Although three had neurologic symptoms, none had raised levels of lactate in the cerebrospinal fluid. Moreover, histologic or histochemical features of mitochondrial disease were only found in two cases. Finally, low mitochondrial DNA, that would have been direct evidence of NRTI toxicity, was not found in the three cases in which it was measured (70).

A case of combined transient mitochondrial and peroxisomal β-oxidation dysfunction after exposure to NRTIs (AZT and lamivudine) combined with protease inhibitors (ritonavir and saquinavir) throughout gestation was reported in 2000 (71). A male infant was delivered at 38 weeks' gestation. He received postnatal prophylaxis with AZT and lamivudine for 4 weeks until the drugs were discontinued because of anemia. Other adverse effects that were observed in the infant (age at onset) were hypocalcemia (shortly after birth), group B streptococcal sepsis, ventricular extrasystoles, prolonged metabolic acidosis, and lactic acidemia (8 weeks), a mild elevation of long chain fatty acids (9 weeks), and neutropenia (3 months). The metabolic acidosis required treatment until 7 months of age, whereas the elevated plasma lactate resolved over 4 weeks. Cerebrospinal fluid lactate was not determined nor was a muscle biopsy conducted. Both the neutropenia and the cardiac dysfunction had resolved by 1 year of age. The elevated plasma fatty acid level was confirmed in cultured fibroblasts, but other peroxisomal functions (plasmalogen biosynthesis and catalase staining) were normal. Although mitochondrial dysfunction has been linked to NRTI agents, the authors were unable to identify the cause of the combined abnormalities in this case (71). The child was reported to be healthy and developing normally at 26 months of age.

A study involving *Erythrocebus patas* monkeys exposed *in utero* to AZT was thought to be relevant to the reports of mitochondrial dysfunction in humans (72). Ten pregnant monkeys in the last half of gestation were given daily oral doses of AZT (1.5 mg/kg/day [$N = 3$] or 6 mg/kg/day [$N = 3$]) or no AZT (controls [$N = 4$]). The doses of AZT were 21% and 86% of the human dose, respectively, based on body weight for a 70-kg pregnant woman. All fetuses were delivered by cesarean section 24 hours after the last AZT dose and 3–5 days before term. No gross defects were evident in the heart left ventricle tissue or skeletal muscle tissue from AZT-exposed or control fetuses. Mitochondria observed by electron microscopy in the two tissue sites were similar in the AZT low-dose and control groups. In contrast, numerous abnormalities were observed in both heart and muscle tissue mitochondria from fetuses exposed to the AZT high-dose group. Moreover, there were dose-dependent alterations in oxidative phosphorylation enzyme assays, in the

Z

specific activities of NADH dehydrogenase (complex I), succinate dehydrogenase (complex II), and cytochrome-*c* oxidase (complex IV), and a dose-dependent depletion of mitochondrial DNA levels. The data were consistent with AZT-induced cardiac and skeletal muscle mitochondrial myopathy (72).

Based on the findings of the above research, a prospective study of the left ventricular structure and function of 382 noninfected (36 exposed to AZT) and 58 HIV-infected (12 exposed to AZT) infants born to HIV-infected women was published in 2000 (73). The median length of *in utero* exposure to AZT was 103 days (105 days for those not infected and 68 days for those infected at birth). Echocardiographic studies (mean left ventricular fractional shortening, contractility, end-diastolic dimension, and left ventricular mass) were conducted every 4–6 months during the first 14 months of life. All echocardiograms were examined without knowledge of the child's clinical status or medications. No statistical differences were found among the four echocardiographic measures in the four groups of children. The investigators identified at least four limitations of their study, including a small sample size that was unable to estimate the frequency of an uncommon toxic effect, the lack of an assessment of a possible dose-effect, the possibility that the sickest children were missed because they were unable to attend follow-up visits, and the effects of other drug therapy in the HIV-infected subgroup that could obscure the effects of AZT (73). Nonetheless, they concluded that perinatal exposure to AZT was not associated with acute or chronic abnormalities in left ventricular structure or function (73).

A 2000 case report described the adverse pregnancy outcomes, including neural tube defects (NTDs), of two pregnant women with HIV infection who were treated with the anti-infective combination trimethoprim/sulfamethoxazole for prophylaxis against *Pneumocystis carinii*, concurrently with antiretroviral agents (74). Exposure to AZT occurred in one of these cases. A 32-year-old woman with a 3-year history of HIV and recent diagnosis of AIDS was treated before and throughout gestation with the anti-infective combination plus AZT and zalcitabine. Folic acid 10 mg/day was added after the diagnosis of pregnancy (gestational age not specified). At term, a female infant was delivered by cesarean section without HIV infection, but with a bony mass in the lumbar spine (identified by ultrasound at 32 weeks' gestation). A diagnostic evaluation revealed that the second lumbar vertebra consisted of hemivertebrae and projected posteriorly into the spinal canal (74). A malformed and displaced first lumbar vertebra was also noted. Surgery was planned to correct the defect. The authors attributed the NTDs in both cases to the antifolate activity of trimethoprim (74).

The case of a 6-month-old male infant who was diagnosed with acute lymphoblastic leukemia (ALL) was described in a 2000 case report (75). His mother had been diagnosed with HIV infection during the 5th month of gestation. She had been treated with oral AZT for the last 3 months of pregnancy. The 3.5-kg infant had been delivered by cesarean section and treated with AZT prophylaxis (2 mg/kg 4 times a day) for 6 weeks. All tests for HIV in the infant were negative. He achieved complete remission after chemotherapy for the ALL and was currently receiving the maintenance phase of chemotherapy at age 16 months. The relationship between AZT exposure and the ALL was unknown (75).

Because of the AZT-induced carcinogenicity observed in animal studies, a 1999 study evaluated the short-term risk for tumors in a total of 727 children who had been exposed *in utero* (antepartum) and/or during the neonatal period to HIV and AZT (76). The children were participants in one of two multi-center clinical studies: Pediatric AIDS Clinical Trials Group (PACTG) 076/219 ($N = 115$) or the Women and Infants Transmission Study (WITS) ($N = 612$). The mean infant follow-up in the PACTG 076/219 group was 38.3 months (366.9 person-years follow-up) whereas it was 14.5 months (743.7 person-years follow-up) for WITS participants. The range for all children was 1 month to 6 years. No tumors of any nature were reported in the children (relative risk 0, 95% CI 0–17.6) (76).

The long-term effects of *in utero* exposure to AZT were the subject of a study published in 1999 (77). HIV-uninfected children ($N = 234$) born to 231 HIV-infected women enrolled in the PACTG 076 were evaluated under the PACTG 219 protocol (122 exposed to AZT, 112 in the placebo group). The main outcome measures included physical growth, immunologic parameters, cognitive/developmental function, tumors, and mortality data. Children were evaluated every 6 months up to 24 months, then yearly thereafter or as clinically indicated. The median age at the time of last follow-up was 4.2 years (range 3.2–5.6 years). There were no significant differences between those exposed to AZT and those not exposed in terms of the sequential outcome measurements. In addition, there were no deaths or malignancies. In the 137 (59%) children who had at least one ophthalmologic examination, 72 were in the AZT group and 65 were in the placebo group. Although there was no significant difference ($p = 0.99$) between the groups in abnormal ophthalmic findings, astigmatism was noted in two (AZT group), ptosis in one (AZT group), and epicanthal folds in one (placebo group). Two other AZT-exposed children had ophthalmic abnormalities: bilateral "thinned vessels; discs look slightly pale" in one with normal vision; and one with a fundus reported as "copper beaten look" that was not thought to be related to metabolic disease (77). One other asymptomatic, healthy 4-year-old child in the AZT group had a mild cardiomyopathy on echocardiogram (77).

New York Medicaid data were used in a study published in 2000 to determine if there was an association between prenatal zidovudine use and congenital anomalies (78). The study cohort included 1932 liveborn infants delivered from 1993 to 1996 to HIV-infected women in the state of New York, 29.5% of who were exposed *in utero* to AZT. The prevalence of any anomaly in the study cohort was 2.76 (95% CI 2.36–3.17) compared to the general New York state population. When AZT-exposed outcomes were compared to those not exposed, the adjusted odds ratios (OR) for major congenital malformations by trimester of first prescription were: 1.20 (95% CI 0.58–2.51) (1st trimester), 1.47 (95% CI 0.85–2.55) (2nd trimester), and 1.84 (95% CI 1.04–3.25) (3rd trimester). There was an increased unadjusted OR for central nervous system defects when compared to those not exposed to AZT (7.98 [95% CI 1.56–37.46]). However, this finding was based on only four such defects and must be interpreted cautiously (78).

High semen levels of AZT have been reported (79). Six males with HIV disease were treated with 200 mg of the antiviral agent orally every 4–6 hours. AZT concentrations in semen 3.0–4.5 hours after a dose ranged from 1.68 to 6.43 μmol/L, representing semen:serum ratios of 1.3–20.4. The semen levels were above the *in vitro* minimum inhibitory concentration for HIV-1. A 1994 study reported that AZT reversed the effects of HIV-1 disease progression on semen quality, including ejaculate volume, sperm concentration and total count, and the number of abnormal sperm forms (80). Moreover, AZT therapy significantly reduced the semen white blood cell count, the principal HIV-1 host cells in ejaculates of HIV-1-infected males. The researchers concluded that this might explain why infected males treated with AZT have a reduced viral load in their semen and a lower rate of sexual transmission (80).

In summary, AZT is effective for the reduction of maternal-fetal transmission of HIV-1 infection with few, if any, adverse effects in the newborns. However, neonatal anemia, a known toxic effect of AZT, may occur and requires monitoring. Although yet unproven, AZT may be effective in reducing the transmission of HIV-1 from semen, thereby lessening the chance of infection in a woman who, when pregnant, could transmit the virus to her offspring. The drug is not teratogenic in animals, except at very high doses, and the experience in humans shows no pattern of birth defects. Experimental evidence, however, indicates that AZT is toxic to rodent embryos, preventing blastocyst development when administered before implantation. In addition, evidence has also been published that AZT may affect human trophoblast cell growth and function in a dose-related manner. This cytotoxicity may have resulted in the reduced fertility observed in nonhuman primates. Thus, impaired human fertility is a concern if AZT is administered in high therapeutic doses during early pregnancy. Additionally, there are unanswered questions relating to the potential for long-term toxicity, such as mutagenesis, carcinogenesis, liver disease, heart disease, and reproductive system effects. One study cited, however, found no cancer in AZT-exposed children, some of whom were followed up to 6 years of age. Mitochondrial dysfunction in offspring exposed *in utero* to AZT and other NRTIs has been reported. Moreover, evidence of dose-dependent mitochondrial dysfunction was demonstrated in monkey fetuses whose mothers were given a human equivalent AZT dose. However, a recent study did not find cardiac toxicity in a small sample of children exposed to AZT during the perinatal period. The incidence and clinical significance of mitochondrial dysfunction after *in utero* exposure to AZT is, therefore, still unknown and requires further study.

Two reviews, one in 1996 and the other in 1997, concluded that all women currently receiving antiretroviral therapy should continue to receive therapy during pregnancy and that treatment of the mother with monotherapy should be considered inadequate therapy (81,82). In 1998, the Centers for Disease Control and Prevention (CDC) made a similar recommendation that antiretroviral therapy should be continued during pregnancy, but discontinuation of all therapy during the 1st trimester was a consideration (53). However, AZT should be given to the mother during the intrapartum period and to the newborn for 6 weeks, regardless of the antepartum antiretroviral regimen (53). If indicated, therefore, the benefits of maternal AZT treatment to the infant outweigh the risks of AZT-induced toxicity (73,77,78,83). Children exposed *in utero* to AZT should be monitored for long periods to answer these concerns fully.

BREAST FEEDING SUMMARY

RECOMMENDATION: Contraindicated

Only one report describing the excretion of zidovudine (AZT) in breast milk has been located (84). Six HIV-seropositive women were given a single 200-mg dose of AZT, and serum and breast milk samples were collected 1, 2, 4, and 6 hours later. Peak serum and milk concentrations, ranging between 422.1 and 1019.3 ng/mL and 472.1 and 1043.0 ng/mL, respectively, were measured at approximately 1–2 hours after the dose. The milk:serum ratio (based on AUC) ranged between 1.11 and 1.78. The authors speculated that the milk concentrations were sufficiently high to decrease the viral load in milk, thereby reducing the potential for maternal-infant HIV transmission (84).

Breast-feeding is not recommended in women with HIV infection because HIV-1 is transmitted in milk (85–87). Until 1999, no studies had been published that examined the effect of any antiretroviral therapy on HIV-1 transmission in milk. In that year, a double-blind placebo-controlled trial investigated the effect of oral AZT in the postpartum period on the transmission of HIV-1 to the breast-feeding infant (57). Infants (at 6 months of age) of women who had received an oral AZT regimen of 300 mg twice daily until labor, 600 mg at beginning of labor, then 300 mg twice daily for 7 days postpartum, had a 38% reduction (relative efficacy 0.38, 95% CI 0.05–0.60; $p = 0.027$) in vertical transmission of HIV-1 infection despite breast-feeding when compared to controls. Further, no excess of major adverse biological or clinical events were observed in the AZT group compared to controls (57).

References

1. Product information. Retrovir. Glaxo Wellcome, 2001.
2. Klug S, Lewandowski C, Merker H-J, Stahlmann R, Wildi L, Neubert D. In vitro and in vivo studies on the prenatal toxicity of five virustatic nucleoside analogues in comparison to acyclovir. Arch Toxicol 1991;65:283–91.
3. Greene JA, Ayers KM, De Miranda P, Tucker WE Jr. Postnatal survival in Wistar rats following oral dosage with zidovudine on gestation day 10. Fund Appl Toxicol 1990;15:201–6.
4. Gogu SR, Beckman BS, Agrawal KC. Amelioration of zidovudine-induced fetal toxicity in pregnant mice. Antimicrob Agents Chemother 1992;36:2370–4.
5. Toltzis P, Marx CM, Kleinman N, Levine EM, Schmidt EV. Zidovudine-associated embryonic toxicity in mice. J Infect Dis 1991;1212–8.
6. Sieh E, Coluzzi ML, Cusella de Angelis MG, Mezzogiorno A, Floridia M, Canipari R, Cossu G, Vella S. The effects of AZT and DDI on pre- and postimplantation mammalian embryos: an in vivo and in vitro study. AIDS Res Hum Retroviruses 1992;8:639–49.
7. Toltzis P, Mourton T, Magnuson T. Effect of zidovudine on preimplantation murine embryos. Antimicrob Agents Chemother 1993;37:1610–3.
8. Toltzis P, Mourton T, Magnuson T. Comparative embryonic cytotoxicity of antiretroviral nucleosides. J Infect Dis 1994;169:1100–2.
9. Nosbisch C, Ha JC, Sackett GP, Conrad SH, Ruppenthal GC, Unadkat JD. Fetal and infant toxicity of zidovudine in *Macaca nemestrina* (abstract). Teratology 1994;49:415.
10. Ha JC, Nosbisch C, Conrad SH, Ruppenthal GC, Sackett GP, Abkowitz J, Unadkat JD. Fetal toxicity of zidovudine (azidothymidine) in *Macaca nemestrina*: preliminary observations. J Acquir Immune Defic Syndr 1994;7:154–7.
11. Esterman AL, Rosenberg C, Brown T, Dancis J. The effect of zidovudine and 2′3′-dideoxyinosine on human trophoblast in culture. Pharmacol Toxicol 1995;76:89–92.
12. Plessinger MA, Miller RK. Effects of zidovudine (AZT) and dideoxyinosine (ddI) on human trophoblast cells. Reprod Toxicol 1999;13:537–46.
13. Venerosi A, Valanzano A, Alleva E, Calamandrei G. Prenatal exposure to anti-HIV drugs: neurobehavioral effects of zidovudine (AZT) + lamivudine (3TC) treatment in mice. Teratology 2001;63:26–37.
14. Unadkat JD, Lopez AA, Schuman L. Transplacental transfer and the pharmacokinetics of zidovudine (ZDV) in the near term pregnant macaque. In *Program and Abstracts of the Twenty-eighth Interscience Conference on Antimicrobial Agents and Chemotherapy, Los Angeles, October 1988*. Los Angeles, CA: American Society for Microbiology, 1988:372. As cited in Hankins GDV, Lowery CL, Scott RT, Morrow WR, Carey KD, Leland MM, Colvin EV. Transplacental transfer of zidovudine in the near-term pregnant baboon. Am J Obstet Gynecol 1990;163:728–32.
15. Lopez-Anaya A, Unadkat JD, Schumann LA, Smith AL. Pharmacokinetics of zidovudine (azidothymidine). I. Transplacental transfer. J Acquir Immune Defic Syndr 1990;3:959–64.
16. Hankins GDV, Lowery CL Jr, Scott RT, Morrow WR, Carey KD, Leland MM, Colvin EV. Transplacental transfer of zidovudine in the near-term pregnant baboon. Am J Obstet Gynecol 1990;163:728–32.
17. Liebes L, Mendoza S, Wilson D, Dancis J. Transfer of zidovudine (AZT) by human placenta. J Infect Dis 1990;161:203–7.
18. Bawdon RE, Sobhi S, Dax J. The transfer of anti-human immunodeficiency virus nucleoside compounds by the term human placenta. Am J Obstet Gynecol 1992;167:1570–4.
19. Schenker S, Johnson RF, King TS, Schenken RS, Henderson GI. Azidothymidine (zidovudine) transport by the human placenta. Am J Med Sci 1990;299:16–20.
20. Gillet JY, Garraffo R, Abrar D, Bongain A, Lapalus P, Dellamonica P. Fetoplacental passage of zidovudine. Lancet 1989;2:269–70.
21. Lyman WD, Tanaka KE, Kress Y, Rashbaum WK, Rubinstein A, Soeiro R. Zidovudine concentrations in human fetal tissue: implications for perinatal AIDS. Lancet 1990;335:1280–1.
22. Chavanet P, Diquet B, Waldner A, Portier H. Perinatal pharmacokinetics of zidovudine. N Engl J Med 1989;321:1548–9.
23. Pons JC, Taburet AM, Singlas E, Delfraissy JF, Papiernik F. Placental passage of azathiothymidine (AZT) during the second trimester of pregnancy: study by direct fetal blood sampling under ultrasound. Eur J Obstet Gynecol Reprod Biol 1991;40:229–31.
24. O'Sullivan MJ, Boyer PJJ, Scott GB, Parks WP, Weller S, Blum MR, Balsley J, Bryson YJ, Zidovudine Collaborative Working Group. The pharmacokinetics and safety of zidovudine in the third trimester of pregnancy for women infected with human immunodeficiency virus and their infants: Phase I Acquired Immunodeficiency Syndrome Clinical Trials group study (protocol 082). Am J Obstet Gynecol 1993;168:1510–6.
25. Unadkat JD, Pereira CM. Maternal-fetal transfer and fetal toxicity of anti-HIV drugs. A review. Trophoblast Res 1994;8:67–82.
26. Watts DH, Brown ZA, Tartaglione T, Burchett SK, Opheim K, Coombs R, Corey L. Pharmacokinetic disposition of zidovudine during pregnancy. J Infect Dis 1991;163:226–32.
27. Sperling RS, Roboz J, Dische R, Silides D, Holzman I, Jew E. Zidovudine pharmacokinetics during pregnancy. Am J Perinatol 1992;9:247–9.
28. Tindall B, Cotton R, Swanson C, Perdices M, Bodsworth N, Imrie A, Cooper DA. Fifth International Conference on the Acquired Immunodeficiency Syndrome. Med J Aust 1990;152:204–14.
29. Tuntland T, Odinecs A, Pereira CM, Nosbisch C, Unadkat JD. In vitro models to predict the in vivo mechanism, rate, and extent of placental transfer of dideoxynucleoside drugs against human immunodeficiency virus. Am J Obstet Gynecol 1999;180:198–206.

Z

30. Lopez-Anaya A, Unadkat JD, Schumann LA, Smith AL. Pharmacokinetics of zidovudine (azidothymidine). III. Effect of pregnancy. J Acquir Immune Defic Syndr 1991;4:64–8.
31. Pereira CM, Nosbisch C, Baughman WL, Unadkat JD. Effect of zidovudine on transplacental pharmacokinetics of ddI in the pigtailed macaque (*Macaca nemestrina*). Antimicrob Agents Chemother 1995;39:343–5.
32. Moodley J, Moodley D, Pillay K, Coovadia H, Saba J, van Leeuwen R, Goodwin C, Harrigan PR, Moore KHP, Stone C, Plumb R, Johnson MA. Pharmacokinetics and antiretroviral activity of lamivudine alone or when coadministered with zidovudine in human immunodeficiency virus type 1-infected pregnant women and their offspring. J Infect Dis 1998;178:1327–33.
33. Odinecs A, Nosbisch C, Unadkat JD. Zidovudine does not affect transplacental transfer or systemic clearance of stavudine (2′,3′-didehydro-3′-deoxythymidine) in the pigtailed macaque (*Macaca nemestrina*). Antimicrob Agents Chemother 1996;40:1569–71.
34. Liebes L, Mendoza S, Lee JD, Dancis J. Further observations on zidovudine transfer and metabolism by human placenta. AIDS 1993;7:590–2.
35. Viscarello RR, DeGennaro NJ, Hobbins JC. Preliminary experience with the use of zidovudine (AZT) during pregnancy. Society of Perinatal Obstetricians Abstracts. Am J Obstet Gynecol 1991;164:248.
36. Cullen MT, Delke I, Greenhaw J, Viscarello RR, Paryani S, Sanchez-Ramos L. HIV in pregnancy: factors predictive of maternal and fetal outcome. Society of Perinatal Obstetricians Abstracts. Am J Obstet Gynecol 1992;166:386.
37. Taylor U, Bardeguez A. Antiretroviral therapy during pregnancy and postpartum. Society of Perinatal Obstetricians Abstracts. Am J Obstet Gynecol 1992;166:390.
38. Delke I, Greenhaw J, Sanchez-Ramos L, Roberts W. Antiretroviral therapy during pregnancy. Society of Perinatal Obstetricians Abstracts. Am J Obstet Gynecol 1993;168:424.
39. Sperling RS, Stratton P, O'Sullivan MJ, Boyer P, Watts DH, Lambert JS, Hammill H, Livingston EG, Gloeb DJ, Minkoff H, Fox HE. A survey of zidovudine use in pregnant women with human immunodeficiency virus infection. N Engl J Med 1992;326:857–61.
40. Stratton P, Mofenson LM, Willoughby AD. Human immunodeficiency virus infection in pregnant women under care at AIDS Clinical Trials centers in the United States. Obstet Gynecol 1992;79:364–8.
41. Kumar RM, Hughes PF, Khurranna A. Zidovudine use in pregnancy: a report of 104 cases and the occurrence of birth defects. J Acquir Immune Defic Syndr 1994;7:1034–9.
42. Antiretroviral Pregnancy Registry Steering Committee. *Antiretroviral Pregnancy Registry International Interim Report for 1 January 1989 through 31 January 2004*. Wilmington, NC: Registry Coordinating Center, 2004.
43. Barzilai A, Sperling RS, Hyatt AC, Wedgwood JF, Reidenberg BE, Hodes DS. Mother to child transmission of human immunodeficiency virus 1 infection despite zidovudine therapy from 18 weeks of gestation. Pediatr Infect Dis J 1990;9:931–3.
44. Sperling RS, Stratton P, Obstetric-Gynecologic Working Group of the AIDS Clinical Trials Group of the National Institute of Allergy and Infectious Diseases. Treatment options for human immunodeficiency virus-infected pregnant women. Obstet Gynecol 1992;79:443–8.
45. Rogers MF, Jaffe HW. Reducing the risk of maternal-infant transmission of HIV: a door is opened. N Engl J Med 1994;331:1222–3.
46. CDC. Zidovudine for the prevention of HIV transmission from mother to infant. MMWR 1994;43:285–7.
47. CDC. Zidovudine for the prevention of HIV transmission from mother to infant. JAMA 1994;271:1567, 1570.
48. Cotton P. Trial halted after drug cuts maternal HIV transmission rate by two thirds. JAMA 1994;271:807.
49. Anonymous. Zidovudine for mother, fetus, and child: hope or poison? Lancet 1994;344:207–9.
50. Spector SA. Pediatric antiretroviral choices. AIDS 1994;4(Suppl 3):S15–8.
51. Murphy R. Clinical aspects of human immunodeficiency virus disease: clinical rationale for treatment. J Infect Dis 1995;171(Suppl 2):S81–7.
52. Connor EM, Sperling RS, Gelber R, Kiselev P, Scott G, O'Sullivan MJ, VanDyke R, Bey M, Shearer W, Jacobson RL, Jimenez E, O'Neill E, Bazin B, Delfraissy J-F, Culnane M, Coombs R, Elkins M, Moye J, Stratton P, Balsley J, for the Pediatric AIDS Clinical Trials Group Protocol 076 Study Group. Reduction of maternal-infant transmission of human immunodeficiency virus type 1 with zidovudine treatment. N Engl J Med 1994;331:1173–80.
53. CDC. Public Health Service Task Force recommendations for the use of antiretroviral drugs in pregnant women infected with HIV-1 for maternal health and for reducing perinatal HIV-1 transmission in the United States. MMWR 1998;47:No. RR-2.
54. Wade NA, Birkhead GS, Warren BL, Charbonneau TT, French PT, Wang L, Baum JB, Tesoriero JM, Savicki R. Abbreviated regimens of zidovudine prophylaxis and perinatal transmission of the human immunodeficiency virus. N Engl J Med 1998;339:1409–14.
55. Shaffer N, Chuachoowong R, Mock PA, Bhadrakom C, Siriwasin W, Young NL, Chotpitayasunondh T, Chearskul S, Roongpisuthipong A, Chinayon P, Karon J, Mastro TD, Simonds RJ, on behalf of the Bangkok Collaborative Perinatal HIV Transmission Study Group. Short-course zidovudine for perinatal HIV-1 transmission in Bangkok, Thailand: a randomised controlled trial. Lancet 1999;353:773–80.
56. Wiktor SZ, Ekpini E, Karon JM, Nkengasong J, Maurice C, Severin ST, Roels TH, Kouassi MK, Lackritz EM, Coulibaly IM, Greenberg AE. Short-course oral zidovudine for prevention of mother-to-child transmission of HIV-1 in Abidjan, Côte d'Ivoire: a randomised trial. Lancet 1999;353:781–5.
57. Dabis F, Msellati P, Meda N, Welffens-Ekra C, You B, Manigart O, Leroy V, Simonon A, Cartoux M, Combe P, Ouangre A, Ramon R, Ky-Zerbo O, Montcho C, Salamon R, Rouzioux C, Van de Perre P, Mandelbrot L, for the DITRAME Study Group. 6-month efficacy, tolerance, and acceptability of a short regimen of oral zidovudine to reduce vertical transmission of HIV in breastfed children in Côte d'Ivoire and Burkina Faso: a double-blind placebo-controlled multicentre trial. Lancet 1999;353:786–92.
58. Mofenson LM. Short-course zidovudine for prevention of perinatal infection. Lancet 1999;353:766–7.

59. Lallemant M, Jourdain G, Le Coeur S, Kim S, Koetsawang S, Comeau AM, Phoolcharoen W, Essex M, McIntosh K, Vithayasai V, for the Perinatal HIV Prevention Trial (Thailand) investigators. A trial of shortened zidovudine regimens to prevent mother-to-child transmission of human immunodeficiency virus type 1. N Engl J Med 2000;343:982–91.
60. Peckham C, Newell ML. Preventing vertical transmission of HIV infection. N Engl J Med 2000;343:1036–7.
61. Mofenson LM, McIntyre JA. Advances and research directions in the prevention of mother-to-child HIV-1 transmission. Lancet 2000;355:2237–44.
62. McGowan JP, Crane M, Wiznia AA, Blum S. Combination antiretroviral therapy in human immunodeficiency virus-infected pregnant women. Obstet Gynecol 1999;94:641–6.
63. Guay LA, Musoke P, Fleming I, Bagenda D, Allen M, Nakabiito C, Sherman J, Bakaki P, Ducar C, Deseyve M, Emel L, Mirochnick M, Fowler MG, Mofenson L, Miotti P, Dransfield K, Bray D, Mmiro F, Jackson JB. Intrapartum and neonatal single-dose nevirapine compared with zidovudine for prevention of mother-to-child transmission of HIV-1 in Kampala, Uganda: HIVNET 012 randomised trial. Lancet 1999;354:795–802.
64. Marseille E, Kahn JG, Mmiro F, Guay L, Musoke P, Fowler MG, Jackson JB. Cost effectiveness of single-dose nevirapine regimen for mothers and babies to decrease vertical HIV-1 transmission in sub-Saharan Africa. Lancet 1999;354:803–9.
65. Loch M, Carr A, Vasak E, Cunningham P, Smith D. The use of human immunodeficiency virus postexposure prophylaxis after successful artificial insemination. Am J Obstet Gynecol 1999;181:760–1.
66. Watson WJ, Stevens TP, Weinberg GA. Profound anemia in a newborn infant of a mother receiving antiretroviral therapy. Pediatr Infect Dis J 1998;17: 435–6.
67. Shah MM, Li Y, Christensen RD. Effects of perinatal zidovudine on hematopoiesis: a comparison of effects on progenitors from human fetuses versus mothers. AIDS 1996;10:1239–47.
68. Blanche S, Tardieu M, Rustin P, Slama A, Barret B, Firtion G, Ciraru-Vigneron N, Lacroix C, Rouzioux C, Mandelbrot L, Desguerre I, Rotig A, Mayaux MJ, Delfraissy JF. Persistent mitochondrial dysfunction and perinatal exposure to antiretroviral nucleoside analogues. Lancet 1999;354:1084–9.
69. Brinkman K, Smeitink JA, Romijn JA, Reiss P. Mitochondrial toxicity induced by nucleoside-analogue reverse-transcriptase inhibitors is a key factor in the pathogenesis of antiretroviral-therapy-related lipodystrophy. Lancet 1999;354:1112–15.
70. Morris AAM, Carr A. HIV nucleoside analogues: new adverse effects on mitochondria? Lancet 1999;354: 1046–7.
71. Stojanov S, Wintergerst U, Belohradsky BH, Rolinski B. Mitochondrial and peroxisomal dysfunction following perinatal exposure to antiretroviral drugs. AIDS 2000;14:1669.
72. Gerschenson M, Erhart SW, Paik CY, St. Claire MC, Nagashima K, Skopets B, Harbaugh SW, Harbaugh JW, Quan W, Poirier MC. Fetal mitochondrial heart and skeletal muscle damage in *Erythrocebus patas* monkeys exposed *in utero* to 3′-azido-3′-deoxythymidine. AIDS Res Hum Retroviruses 2000;16:635–44.
73. Lipshultz SE, Easley KA, Orav EJ, Kaplan S, Starc TJ, Bricker JT, Lai WW, Moodie DS, Sopko G, McIntosh K, Colan SD, for the Pediatric Pulmonary and Cardiac Complications of Vertically Transmitted HIV Infection Study Group. Absence of cardiac toxicity of zidovudine in infants. N Engl J Med 2000;343:759–66.
74. Richardson MP, Osrin D, Donaghy S, Brown NA, Hay, Sharland M. Spinal malformations in the fetuses of HIV infected women receiving combination antiretroviral therapy and co-trimoxazole. Eur J Obstet Gynecol Reprod Biol 2000;93:215–7.
75. Moschovi M, Theodoridou M, Papaevangelou V, Tzortzatou Stathopoulou F. Acute lymphoblastic leukaemia in an infant exposed to zidovudine *in utero* and early infancy. AIDS 2000;14:2410–1.
76. Hanson IC, Antonelli TA, Sperling RS, Oleske JM, Cooper E, Culnane M, Fowler MG, Kalish LA, Lee SS, McSherry G, Mofenson L, Shapiro DE. Lack of tumors in infants with perinatal HIV-1 exposure and fetal/neonatal exposure to zidovudine. J Acquir Immune Defic Syndr Hum Retrovirol 1999;20:463–7.
77. Culnane M, Fowler MG, Lee SS, McSherry G, Brady M, O'Donnell K, Mofenson L, Gortmaker SL, Shapiro DE, Scott G, Jimenez E, Moore EC, Diaz C, Flynn P, Cunningham B, Oleske J, for the Pediatric AIDS Clinical Trials Group Protocol 219/076 Teams. Lack of long-term effects of in utero exposure to zidovudine among uninfected children born to HIV-infected women. JAMA 1999;281:151–7.
78. Newschaffer CJ, Cocroft J, Anderson CE, Hauck WW, Turner BJ. Prenatal zidovudine use and congenital anomalies in a Medicaid population. J Acquir Immune Defic Syndr 2000;24:249–56.
79. Henry K, Chinnock BJ, Quinn RP, Fletcher CV, de Miranda P, Balfour HH Jr. Concurrent zidovudine levels in semen and serum determined by radioimmunoassay in patients with AIDS or AIDS-related complex. JAMA 1988,259.3023–6.
80. Politch JA, Mayer KH, Abbott AF, Anderson DJ. The effects of disease progression and zidovudine therapy on semen quality in human immunodeficiency virus type 1 seropositive men. Fertil Steril 1994;61; 922–8.
81. Carpenter CCJ, Fischi MA, Hammer SM, Hirsch MS, Jacobsen DM, Katzenstein DA, Montaner JSG, Richman DD, Saag MS, Schooley RT, Thompson MA, Vella S, Yeni PG, Volberding PA. Antiretroviral therapy for HIV infection in 1996. JAMA 1996;276: 145–54.
82. Minkoff H, Augenbraun M. Antiretroviral therapy for pregnant women. Am J Obstet Gynecol 1997;176: 478–89.
83. Mofenson LM. Perinatal exposure to zidovudine—benefits and risks. N Engl J Med 2000;343:803–5.
84. Ruff A, Hamzeh, Lietman P, Siberry G, Boulos R, Bell K, McBrien M, Davis H, Coberly J, Joseph D, Halsey N. Excretion of zidovudine (ZDV) in human breast milk. (abstract). Presented at the 34th Interscience Conference on Antimicrobial Agents and Chemotherapy, American Society for Microbiology, Orlando, Florida, October, 1994.
85. Brown ZA, Watts DH. Antiviral therapy in pregnancy. Clin Obstet Gynecol 1990;33:276–89.

86. de Martino M, Tovo P-A, Tozzi AE, Pezzotti P, Galli L, Livadiotti S, Caselli D, Massironi E, Ruga E, Fioredda F, Plebani A, Gabiano C, Zuccotti GV. HIV-1 transmission through breast-milk: appraisal of risk according to duration of feeding. AIDS 1992;6:991–7.
87. Van de Perre P. Postnatal transmission of human immunodeficiency virus type 1: the breast-feeding dilemma. Am J Obstet Gynecol 1995;173:483–7.

Name: **ZILEUTON** Risk Factor: C_M

Class: **Respiratory Agent**

FETAL RISK SUMMARY

RECOMMENDATION: No Human Data - Animal Data Suggest Risk

Zileuton, a specific inhibitor of the enzyme (5-lipoxygenase) that catalyzes the formation of leukotrienes (LTB_4, LTC_4, LTD_4, and LTE_4) from arachidonic acid, is given orally for the prophylaxis and chronic treatment of asthma.

Reproduction studies have been conducted in rats and rabbits (1). No effects on fertility were observed in male and female rats given oral doses approximately 8 and 18 times the systemic exposure (AUC) achieved at the maximum recommended human daily oral dose (MRHD), respectively. However, at doses 9 or more times the MRHD-AUC, a reduction in fetal implants was observed. At 4 or more times the MRHD-AUC, increases in gestation length and the number of stillbirths were noted. In addition, offspring of pregnant rats given 18 times the MRHD-AUC had reduced body weight and increased skeletal variations. A decrease in rat pup survival and growth occurred at this same dose in perinatal and postnatal studies. In pregnant rabbits given oral doses equivalent to the MRHD (based on body surface area), 3 (2.5%) of 118 fetuses had cleft palates (1).

It is not known if zileuton crosses the human placenta to the fetus, but the molecular weight (about 236) is low enough that transfer should be expected. The drug and/or its metabolites cross the rat placenta (1).

No reports on the use of zileuton in human pregnancy have been found. One source, based solely on animal data, recommends that the drug be avoided during gestation (2).

BREAST FEEDING SUMMARY

RECOMMENDATION: No Human Data - Probably Compatible

No reports describing the use of zileuton during human lactation have been located. The drug and/or its metabolites are excreted into rat milk (1). The molecular weight (about 236) is low enough that passage into human breast milk should be expected. The effects on a nursing infant from this exposure are unknown.

References

1. Product information. Zyflo. Abbott Laboratories, 2000.
2. Anonymous. Drugs for asthma. Med Lett Drugs Ther 2000;42:19–24.

Name: **ZOLMITRIPTAN** Risk Factor: **C_M**
Class: **Antimigraine**

FETAL RISK SUMMARY

RECOMMENDATION: No Human Data - Animal Data Suggest Low Risk

Zolmitriptan is an oral selective serotonin (5-hydroxytryptamine; 5-HT) receptor agonist that has high affinity for 5-HT_{1B} and 5-HT_{1D} receptors. The drug is closely related to almotriptan, eletriptan, frovatriptan, naratriptan, rizatriptan, and sumatriptan (see individual agents). It is indicated for the acute treatment of migraine with or without aura in adults. Protein binding is minimal (about 25%). Zolmitriptan has a several metabolites, one of which is 2 to 6 times more potent for the 5-$HT_{1B/1D}$ receptors than is the parent compound. The active metabolite contributes a substantial portion of the pharmacologic effect because its concentrations are about two-thirds that of zolmitriptan (1). The terminal elimination half-life of zolmitriptan is apparently unknown.

Reproduction studies have been conducted in rats and rabbits. In rats, zolmitriptan was given during organogenesis at oral doses resulting in maternal exposures ranging from 280 to 5000 times the exposure in humans receiving the maximum recommended total daily dose of 10 mg (MRHD). A dose-related increase in embryo lethality was observed, which became statistically significant at the high dose, but maternal toxicity (decreased weight gain during gestation) was also noted. When pregnant rats were treated throughout gestation and lactation, an increased incidence of hydronephrosis was seen in the offspring at a dose 1100 times the MRHD. This dose was also maternally toxic. In pregnant rabbits treated during organogenesis, an increased incidence of embryo lethality was observed at maternally toxic doses 11 or more times the MRHD. At 42 times the MRHD, increased incidences of fetal malformations (fused sternebrae, rib anomalies) and variations (blood vessels, rib ossification) were observed. The no-effect dose was equivalent to the MRHD (1).

It is not known if zolmitriptan or its active metabolite crosses the human placenta to the fetus. However, the relatively low molecular weight of the parent compound (about 287) and the minimal plasma protein binding suggest that the drug will transfer to the fetus.

In summary, no reports describing the use of zolmitriptan in human pregnancy have been located. The animal data are suggestive of low risk, but an assessment of the actual risk cannot be determined until human pregnancy experience is available.

BREAST FEEDING SUMMARY

RECOMMENDATION: No Human Data - Probably Compatible

No reports describing the use of zolmitriptan during human lactation have been located. In lactating rats, the agent is concentrated in milk with the concentration at 4 hours about four times higher than that measured in the blood (1). The relatively low molecular weight (about 287) and low plasma protein binding suggest that the drug, and possibly its active metabolite, will be excreted into breast milk. The effects of this exposure on a nursing infant are unknown.

Reference

1. Product information. Zomig. AstraZeneca, 2004.

Name:	**ZOLPIDEM**	Risk Factor:	B_M
Class:	**Hypnotic**		

FETAL RISK SUMMARY

RECOMMENDATION: Limited Human Data - Animal Data Suggest Low Risk

Zolpidem is a nonbenzodiazepine hypnotic of the imidazopyridine class. In subjects with normal liver function, a single 5-mg dose zolpidem had a relatively short elimination half-life (2.6 hours, range 1.4–4.5 hours) (1).

In reproductive studies in rats no teratogenic effects were observed, but dose-related toxicity was observed in the fetuses (delayed maturation as characterized by incomplete ossification of the skull) at doses about 25 and 125 times the maximum human dose based on body surface area (MHD) (1). The no-effect dose was 5 times the MHD. In rabbits, increased postimplantation fetal loss and incomplete ossification of the sternum in surviving fetuses were observed at about 28 times the MHD, both possibly related to maternal toxicity (decreased weight gain) (1). The no-effect dose in rabbits was 7 times the MHD. No teratogenic effects of the drug were observed. Shepard reviewed a reproductive toxicity study in rats during organogenesis that found no teratogenicity, but did observe a decrease in fetal weight at doses ranging from 5 to 125 mg/kg and an increase in wavy ribs at the highest dose (2).

It is not known if zolpidem crosses the human placenta. The molecular weight (about 765 for the tartrate salt) is low enough, however, that embryo/fetal exposure to the drug should be expected.

The FDA did not receive any reports of adverse fetal or newborn outcomes from pregnancy exposures to zolpidem between its approval in December 1992 and 1996 (personal communication, F. Rosa, FDA, 1996).

A 1998 noninterventional observational cohort study described the outcomes of pregnancies in women who had been prescribed one or more of 34 newly marketed drugs by general practitioners in England (3). Data were obtained by questionnaires sent to the prescribing physicians 1 month after the expected or possible date of delivery. In 831 (78%) of the pregnancies, a newly marketed drug was thought to have been taken during the 1st trimester with birth defects noted in 14 (2.5%) singleton births of the 557 newborns (10 sets of twins). In addition, two birth defects were observed in aborted fetuses. However, few of the aborted fetuses were examined. Zolpidem was taken during the 1st trimester in 18 pregnancies. The outcomes of these pregnancies included two spontaneous abortions, six elective abortions and 11 normal, term infants (one set of twins) (3).

Although no congenital malformations were observed in the above study, the data are too limited to assess the safety of zolpidem in the human embryo or fetus. Moreover, the study lacked the sensitivity to identify minor anomalies because of the absence of standardized examinations. Late-appearing major defects may also have been missed because of the timing of the questionnaires. Further, chronic maternal use of sedatives/hypnotics has been associated with withdrawal symptoms in newborns.

BREAST FEEDING SUMMARY

RECOMMENDATION: Limited Human Data - Probably Compatible

Zolpidem is excreted into breast milk, but the effects, if any, on a nursing infant have not been studied. In a 1989 report, five lactating women were administered a single 20-mg dose 3–4 days after delivery of a full-term infant (4). Breast-feeding was halted for 24 hours after drug administration. Milk and serum samples were collected before and 1.5 (serum only), 3, 13, and 16 hours after the dose. The total amount of zolpidem in milk at 3 hours (both breasts emptied with an electric breast pump and the milk pooled for each woman) ranged from 0.76 to 3.88 μg, representing 0.004%–0.019% of the dose. The drug was not detected in milk (detection level 0.5 ng/mL) at the other sampling times. The dose used in this study is twice the current maximum recommended human hypnotic dose.

In healthy adult patients, zolpidem has a relatively short serum half-life (about 2.6 hours) and accumulation is not expected to occur. The small amount of drug measured in milk after a dose that was twice the recommended human dose probably indicates that few, if any, adverse effects would occur in a nursing infant whose mother was consuming this hypnotic. In those instances in which the mother is taking zolpidem, however, she should observe her nursing infant for increased sedation, lethargy, and changes in feeding habits. Based on the one study above, the American Academy of Pediatrics classifies zolpidem as compatible with breast-feeding (5).

References

1. Product information. Ambien. G. D. Searle, 2000.
2. Shepard TH. *Catalog of Teratogenic Agents*. 8th ed. Baltimore, MD: Johns Hopkins University Press, 1995: 231.
3. Wilton LV, Pearce GL, Martin RM, Mackay FJ, Mann RD. The outcomes of pregnancy in women exposed to newly marketed drugs in general practice in England. Br J Obstet Gynaecol 1998;105:882–9.
4. Pons G, Francoual C, Guillet Ph, Moran C, Hermann Ph, Bianchetti G, Thiercelin J-F, Thenot J-P, Olive G. Zolpidem excretion in breast milk. Eur J Clin Pharmacol 1989;37:245–8.
5. Committee on Drugs, American Academy of Pediatrics. The transfer of drugs and other chemicals into human milk. Pediatrics 2001;108:776–89.

Name:	**ZONISAMIDE**	Risk Factor:	C_M
Class:	**Anticonvulsant**		

FETAL RISK SUMMARY

RECOMMENDATION: Limited Human Data - Animal Data Suggest High Risk

Zonisamide, a sulfonamide derivative, is indicated as adjunctive therapy in the treatment of partial seizures. Its anticonvulsant mechanism of action is unknown. The drug is bound extensively to erythrocytes with concentrations in red blood cells eight times higher than in plasma. Approximately 40%–60% is bound to plasma proteins, mainly albumin (1,2). After single oral doses, the elimination half-lives from erythrocytes and from plasma are 105 and 50–68 hours, respectively (1,2). The plasma elimination half-life is decreased to about 25–35 hours if the patient is receiving concurrent treatment with hepatic enzyme-inducing anticonvulsants (carbamazepine, phenytoin, phenobarbital, or primidone) (2).

Reproduction studies with zonisamide have been conducted during organogenesis in mice, rats, dogs and cynomolgus monkeys. In pregnant mice, doses approximately 1.5–6.0 times the maximum recommended human dose of 400 mg/day based on body surface area (MRHD-BSA) were associated with increased rates of fetal malformations (skeletal and/or craniofacial defects). In rats, increased frequencies of malformations (cardiovascular defects) and variations (persistent cords of thymic tissue and decreased skeletal ossification) were observed at all doses tested (0.5–5.0 times the MRHD-BSA). Perinatal deaths resulted when a dose 1.4 times the MRHD-BSA was given in the latter part of gestation up to weaning. The no-effect level for this toxicity was 0.7 times the MRHD-BSA (1).

In pregnant dogs, doses that produced peak maternal plasma levels (25 μg/mL) about 0.5 times the highest plasma levels measured in humans receiving the maximum recommended human dose of 400 mg/day (MRHD-PL) resulted in an increased incidence of fetal cardiovascular defects (ventricular septal defects, cardiomegaly, and valvular and arterial anomalies). At doses that produced plasma levels (44 μg/mL), approximately equal to the MRHD-PL, about 50% of the fetuses had cardiovascular malformations as well as increased incidences of skeletal malformations. Fetal growth retardation and increased rates of skeletal variations were observed with peak maternal dog plasma levels produced by all doses tested (0.25–1.0 times the MRHD-PL). When zonisamide was given to pregnant monkeys at doses approximately 0.1 times the MRHD-PL or higher, embryo-fetal deaths were observed. The cause of the deaths was unknown, but the possibility that they were due to malformations could not be excluded (1).

Zonisamide was not carcinogenic in mice and rats after 2 years of dietary administration. The agent was mutagenic in one test, but not mutagenic or clastogenic in other tests (1).

No reports describing the placental crossing of zonisamide early in gestation have been located. However, at term delivery of one newborn, the cord blood and maternal blood concentrations were 14.4 and 15.7 μg/mL (ratio 0.92), respectively (3). A comparable amount of drug was found in a second full-term newborn, but specific data were not given. Zonisamide probably also crosses the placenta early in gestation because of its low molecular weight (about 212). In addition,, the long elimination half-life from red blood cells and plasma will result in prolonged concentrations of the drug at the maternal blood - placenta interface, thus increasing the opportunity for embryo/fetal exposure.

A 1996 report described the outcomes of 26 offspring whose mothers had been treated with zonisamide during pregnancy (22 women; 25 pregnancies; 1 set of twins). The offspring were exposed to zonisamide either alone (4 cases) or combined with other anticonvulsants (22 cases) (4). Doses ranged from 100–600 mg per day. There were two elective abortions and 24 live-born infants (one set of twins). Two offspring (7.7%), both exposed to combination anticonvulsants, had major malformations. Neither of the mothers experienced seizures during pregnancy. The first case, electively terminated at 16 weeks' gestation, involved an anencephalic fetus (sex unknown) exposed to zonisamide (100 mg/day) and phenytoin (275 mg/day) throughout gestation. The second infant, a 2022-g female, was delivered by cesarean section at 37 weeks' gestation. She had an atrial septal defect. Combination therapy throughout gestation included zonisamide (200 mg/day), phenytoin (200 mg/day), and valproic acid (400 mg/day) (4).

In a 2002 case report, two women took multiple anticonvulsants throughout gestation and delivered apparently normal infants at about 40 weeks' gestation (3). One woman took zonisamide (400 mg/day), carbamazepine (1000 mg/day) and clonazepam (1 mg/day), whereas the other took zonisamide (400 mg/day) and carbamazepine (800 mg/day). Both newborns had Apgar scores at 1 and 5 minutes of 8 and 9, respectively. Birth weights were 3094 g and 3164 g, respectively.

The effect of zonisamide on folic acid levels and metabolism is unknown. A 2003 review recommended that to reduce the risk of birth defects from anticonvulsants, women should start multivitamins with folic acid before conception (5). Although the recommendation did not specify the amount of folic acid, a recent study found that multivitamin supplements with folic acid (typically 0.4 mg) did not reduce the risk of congenital malformations from four first-generation anticonvulsants (see Carbamazepine, Phenytoin, Phenobarbital, or

Primidone). Therefore, until further information is available, the best course is to start folic acid supplementation before conception. Although a specific dosage has not been recommended for patients receiving anticonvulsants, 4 mg/day appears to be reasonable.

In summary, zonisamide is teratogenic in three animal species and embryo lethal in a fourth at doses or exposures very near or less than doses and systemic concentrations used or obtained clinically. Human pregnancy experience is limited to 27 pregnancies (28 outcomes). Among these outcomes, two infants with congenital anomalies have been observed, but in both cases, other anticonvulsants known to be human teratogens also were used. However, the data are too limited to determine the embryo and fetal risk of zonisamide. The drug probably should be avoided, if possible, during the 1st trimester. If treatment with zonisamide is required, monotherapy using the lowest effective dose is preferred, but because of its status as adjunctive therapy, this may not be possible.

BREAST FEEDING SUMMARY

RECOMMENDATION: Limited Human Data - Potential Toxicity

Zonisamide is excreted into breast milk. A woman took 300 mg/day (100 mg three times daily) during pregnancy and continued the anticonvulsant while breast-feeding (6). The cord plasma drug concentration at delivery was 6.72 μg/mL, 2.5 hours after a dose. Milk and maternal plasma levels were determined on postpartum days 3, 6, 14, and 30 (1.5 to 2.5 hours after a dose). Milk concentrations ranged from 8.25 μg/mL (day 3) to 10.5 μg/mL (day 30), whereas maternal plasma levels ranged from 9.52 μg/mL (day 14) to 10.6 μg/mL (day 3). The milk:plasma (M:P) ratio consistently increased at each sampling. The average M:P ratio was 0.93 (range 0.81–1.03). No neonatal behavior problems were observed (6).

In another report, two mothers receiving zonisamide (400 mg/day) and other anticonvulsants (mother #1: carbamazepine and clonazepam; mother #2: carbamazepine) throughout gestation, as well as postpartum, breast-fed their apparently normal infants (see above) (3). Zonisamide concentrations were determined in the breast milk of mother #1. From delivery to postpartum day 9, the unbound maternal plasma zonisamide concentration ranged from 10.7–13.3 μg/mL, whereas the total zonisamide level ranged from 17.5–25.2 μg/mL. During the same interval, the drug concentrations in the watery portion of the milk (i.e., the whey) ranged from 8.9–10.9 μg/mL. The breast milk transfer rate was 41%–57%. The plasma zonisamide level in the infant on day 24 was 3.9 μg/mL (15% of the mother's level on postpartum day 9). No adverse effects in either nursing infant were mentioned (3).

In summary, zonisamide is excreted into breast milk. No adverse effects were noted in four nursing infants, but the milk concentrations were high enough that clinically significant doses appear to have been ingested. The relatively high plasma level found in one infant supports this assessment. Therefore, if a woman under treatment with zonisamide chooses to breast-feed, close clinical monitoring of her infant is recommended as well as the measurement of infant plasma drug levels. The long-term effects on nursing infants from this exposure are unknown but warrant investigation.

References

1. Product information. Zonegran. Elan Biopharmaceuticals, 2003.
2. Percucca E, Bialer M. The clinical pharmacokinetics of the newer antiepileptic drugs. Clin Pharmacokinet 1996;31:29–46.
3. Kawada K, Itoh S, Kusaka T, Isobe K, Ishii M. Pharmacokinetics of zonisamide in perinatal period. Brain Dev 2002;24:95–7.
4. Kondo T, Kaneko S, Amano Y, Egawa I. Preliminary report on teratogenic effects of zonisamide in the

offspring of treated women with epilepsy. Epilepsia 1996;37:1242–4.
5. Yerby MS. Clinical care of pregnant women with epilepsy: neural tube defects and folic acid supplementation. Epilepsia 2003;44(Suppl 3):33–40.
6. Shimoyama R, Ohkubo T, Sugawara K. Monitoring of zonisamide in human breast milk and maternal plasma by solid-phase extraction HPLC method. Biomed Chromatogr 1999;13:370–2.

Name:	**ZUCLOPENTHIXOL**	Risk Factor:	**C**
Class:	**Tranquilizer**		

FETAL RISK SUMMARY

RECOMMENDATION: No Human Data - No Relevant Animal Data

Zuclopenthixol is a thioxanthene tranquilizer with properties similar to those of chlorpromazine. No reports of the use of zuclopenthixol in pregnancy have been located.

BREAST FEEDING SUMMARY

RECOMMENDATION: Limited Human Data - Potential Toxicity

Zuclopenthixol is excreted into human milk. In six women treated with the agent between 3 days and 10 months after delivery, the mean milk:serum ratio was 0.29 (range 0.12–0.56) (1). Maternal dosages were 72 mg (IM depot injection) every 2 weeks in one patient and 4–50 mg/day orally in the other five women (time interval between oral dosing and sampling not specified). The milk concentrations were all less than 4 ng/mL, with the highest level occurring in the woman who received the injectable form. The authors estimated that an infant consuming 600 mL/day of milk would ingest 0.5–5 μg/day of zuclopenthixol. None of the nursing infants showed signs of sedation or other adverse effects.

In a 1988 study, zuclopenthixol was also measured in the milk of a woman who was being treated for puerperal psychosis 2 weeks after delivery of her first child (2). The mother was given 24 mg/day orally for 4 days, then 14 mg/day. Milk and serum samples were obtained on days 2, 3, 6, and 8 of therapy. The mean milk concentration while the mother was receiving 24 mg/day was 20 ng/mL (milk:serum ratio 0.71–2.20); it fell to 5 ng/mL while she was receiving 14 mg/day (ratio of 0.24–0.66) (the time interval between dosing and sampling was not specified). No adverse effects were observed in the nursing infant.

Although no adverse effects were observed in the seven infants exposed via the milk to zuclopenthixol, the long-term effects of this exposure have not been studied. Caution is advised, especially during prolonged therapy, until additional studies have been conducted (2).

References

1. Aaes-Jorgensen T, Bjorndal F, Bartels U. Zuclopenthixol levels in serum and breast milk. Psychopharmacology 1986;90:417–8.
2. Matheson I, Skjaeraasen J. Milk concentrations of flupenthixol, nortriptyline and zuclopenthixol and between-breast differences in two patients. Eur J Clin Pharmacol 1988;35:217–20.

APPENDIX

Classification of Drugs by Pharmacologic Category

[See drug generic name in Index for location of drug in this Appendix.]

1. ANESTHETICS

A. Local
Camphor (C)
Lidocaine (B_M)
Pramoxine (C_M)
Ropivacaine (B_M)

B. General
Desflurane (B_M)
Enflurane (B)
Halothane (B)
Isoflurane (B)
Ketamine (B)
Nitrous Oxide (C)
Sevoflurane (C)

2. ANTIDOTES
Acetylcysteine (B_M)
Deferoxamine (C_M)
Digoxin Immune FAB (Ovine) (C_M)
Dimercaprol (C_M)
Edetate Calcium Disodium (B_M)
Flumazenil (C_M)
Fomepizole (C_M)
Pralidoxime (C_M)
Sevelamer (C_M)

3. ANTIHISTAMINES
Antazoline (C)
Astemizole (C_M)
Azatadine (B_M)
Azelastine (C_M)
Bromodiphenhydramine (C)
Brompheniramine (C_M)
Buclizine (C)
Carbinoxamine (C)
Cetirizine (B_M)
Chlorcyclizine (C)
Chlorpheniramine (B)
Cinnarizine (C)
Clemastine (C)
Cyclizine (B)
Cyproheptadine (B_M)
Dexbrompheniramine (C)
Dexchlorpheniramine (B_M)
Dimenhydrinate (B_M)
Dimethindene (B)
Dimethothiazine (C)
Diphenhydramine (B_M)
Doxylamine (A)
Fexofenadine (C_M)
Hydroxyzine (C)
Loratadine (B_M)
Meclizine (B_M)
Methdilazine (C)
Pheniramine (C)
Phenyltoloxamine (C)
Promethazine (C)
Pyrilamine (C)
Terfenadine (C_M)
Trimeprazine (C)
Tripelennamine (B)
Triprolidine (C_M)

4. ANTI-INFECTIVES

A. Amebicide
Carbarsone (D)
Iodoquinol (C)
Metronidazole (B_M)
Paromomycin (C)

B. Aminoglycosides
Amikacin (C/D_M)
Gentamicin (C)

Kanamycin (D)
Neomycin (C)
Paromomycin (C)
Streptomycin (D_M)
Tobramycin (C/D_M)

C. Anthelmintics
Albendazole (C_M)
Gentian Violet (C)
Ivermectin (C_M)
Mebendazole (C_M)
Piperazine (B)
Praziquantel (B_M)
Pyrantel Pamoate (C)
Pyrvinium Pamoate (C)
Quinacrine (C)
Thiabendazole (C_M)

D. Antibiotics/Anti-infectives
Azithromycin (B_M)
Aztreonam (B_M)
Bacitracin (C)
Chloramphenicol (C)
Chlorhexidine (B)
Clarithromycin (C_M)
Clavulanate Potassium (B_M)
Clindamycin (B_M)
Colistimethate (C_M)
Dirithromycin (C_M)
Ertapenem (B_M)
Erythromycin (B_M)
Fosfomycin (B_M)
Furazolidone (C)
Hexachlorophene (C_M)
Imipenem-Cilastatin Sodium (C_M)
Lincomycin (B)
Linezolid (C_M)
Meropenem (B_M)
Metronidazole (B_M)
Novobiocin (C)
Oleandomycin (C)
Polymyxin B (B)
Quinupristin/Dalfopristin (B_M)
Rifabutin (B_M)
Spectinomycin (C)
Sulbactam (B_M)
Tazobactam (B_M)
Trimethoprim (C_M)
Trimetrexate (D_M)
Troleandomycin (C)
Vancomycin (B_M)

E. Antifungals
Amphotericin B (B_M)
Butoconazole (C_M)
Caspofungin (C_M)
Ciclopirox (B_M)
Clotrimazole (B_M)
Econazole (C_M)
Fluconazole (C_M)
Flucytosine (C_M)
Griseofulvin (C)
Itraconazole (C_M)
Ketoconazole (C_M)
Miconazole (C_M)
Nystatin (C_M)
Terbinafine (B_M)
Terconazole (C_M)
Voriconazole (D_M)

F. Antimalarials
Chloroquine (C)
Dapsone (C_M)
Hydroxychloroquine (C)
Mefloquine (C_M)
Primaquine (C)
Proguanil (B)
Pyrimethamine (C_M)
Quinacrine (C)
Quinidine (C_M)
Quinine (D/X_M)

G. Antiprotozoal
Atovaquone (C_M)
Nitazoxanide (B_M)
Pentamidine (C_M)
Spiramycin (C)

H. Antituberculosis
para-Aminosalicylic Acid (C)
Capreomycin (C_M)
Cycloserine (C_M)
Ethambutol (B)
Ethionamide (C_M)
Isoniazid (C)
Pyrazinamide (C_M)
Rifampin (C_M)
Rifapentine (C_M)

I. Antiretroviral Agents

i. Nucleoside Reverse Transcriptase Inhibitors

Abacavir (C_M)
Adefovir (C_M)
Didanosine (B_M)
Emtricitabine (B_M)
Lamivudine (C_M)
Stavudine (C_M)
Tenofovir (B_M)
Zalcitabine (C_M)
Zidovudine (C_M)

ii. Non-Nucleoside Reverse Transcriptase Inhibitors

Delavirdine (C_M)
Efavirenz (C_M)
Nevirapine (C_M)

iii. Protease Inhibitors

Amprenavir (C_M)
Atazanavir (B_M)
Fosamprenavir (C_M)
Indinavir (C_M)
Lopinavir (C_M)
Nelfinavir (B_M)
Ritonavir (B_M)
Saquinavir (B_M)

iv. Fusion Inhibitor

Enfuvirtide (B_M)

J. Other Antivirals

Acyclovir (B_M)
Adefovir (C_M)
Amantadine (C_M)
Cidofovir (C_M)
Famciclovir (B_M)
Foscarnet (C_M)
Ganciclovir (C_M)
Idoxuridine (C)
Oseltamivir (C_M)
Ribavirin (X_M)
Rimantadine (C_M)
Valacyclovir (B_M)
Valganciclovir (C_M)
Vidarabine (C_M)
Zanamivir (C_M)

K. Cephalosporins

Cefaclor (B_M)
Cefadroxil (B_M)
Cefamandole (B_M)
Cefatrizine (B)
Cefazolin (B_M)
Cefdinir (B_M)
Cefditoren (B_M)
Cefepime (B_M)
Cefixime (B_M)
Cefmetazole (B)
Cefonicid (B_M)
Cefoperazone (B_M)
Ceforanide (B_M)
Cefotaxime (B_M)
Cefotetan (B_M)
Cefoxitin (B_M)
Cefpodoxime (B_M)
Cefprozil (B_M)
Ceftazidime (B_M)
Ceftibuten (B_M)
Ceftizoxime (B_M)
Ceftriaxone (B_M)
Cefuroxime (B_M)
Cephalexin (B_M)
Cephalothin (B_M)
Cephapirin (B_M)
Cephradine (B_M)
Loracarbef (B_M)
Moxalactam (C_M)

L. Iodine

Iodine (D)
Povidone-Iodine (D)

M. Leprostatics

Clofazimine (C_M)
Dapsone (C_M)

N. Penicillins

Amoxicillin (B_M)
Ampicillin (B)
Bacampicillin (B_M)
Carbenicillin (B)
Cloxacillin (B_M)
Cyclacillin (B_M)
Dicloxacillin (B_M)
Hetacillin (B)
Methicillin (B_M)
Nafcillin (B)
Oxacillin (B_M)
Penicillin G (B_M)
Penicillin G, Benzathine (B_M)

Penicillin G, Procaine (B_M)
Penicillin V (B)
Piperacillin (B_M)
Ticarcillin (B)

O. Quinolones

Cinoxacin (C_M)
Ciprofloxacin (C_M)
Enoxacin (C_M)
Gatifloxacin (C_M)
Gemifloxacin (C_M)
Levofloxacin (C_M)
Lomefloxacin (C_M)
Moxifloxacin (C_M)
Nalidixic Acid (C_M)
Norfloxacin (C_M)
Ofloxacin (C_M)
Sparfloxacin (C_M)
Trovafloxacin (C_M)

P. Scabicide/Pediculicide

Lindane (B_M)
Permethrin (B_M)
Pyrethrins with Piperonyl Butoxide (C)

Q. Sulfonamides

Sulfonamides (C_M/D)

R. Tetracyclines

Chlortetracycline (D)
Clomocycline (D)
Demeclocycline (D)
Doxycycline (D_M)
Methacycline (D)
Minocycline (D)
Oxytetracycline (D)
Tetracycline (D)

S. Trichomonacides

Metronidazole (B_M)

T. Urinary Germicides

Cinoxacin (C_M)
Mandelic Acid (C)
Methenamine (C_M)
Methylene Blue (C_M/D)
Nalidixic Acid (C_M)
Nitrofurantoin (B_M)

5. ANTILIPEMIC AGENTS

Atorvastatin (X_M)
Cerivastatin (X_M)
Cholestyramine (B)
Clofibrate (C_M)
Colesevelam (B_M)
Colestipol (B)
Dextrothyroxine (C)
Ezetimibe (C_M)
Fenofibrate (C_M)
Fluvastatin (X_M)
Gemfibrozil (C_M)
Lovastatin (X_M)
Niacin (A/C)
Pravastatin (X_M)
Probucol (B_M)
Simvastatin (X_M)

6. ANTINEOPLASTICS

Aminopterin (X)
Asparaginase (C_M)
Bexarotene (X_M)
Bleomycin (D_M)
Busulfan (D_M)
Carboplatin (D_M)
Carmustine (D_M)
Chlorambucil (D_M)
Cisplatin (D_M)
Cyclophosphamide (D_M)
Cytarabine (D_M)
Dacarbazine (C_M)
Dactinomycin (C_M)
Daunorubicin (D_M)
Doxorubicin (D_M)
Epirubicin (D_M)
Etoposide (D_M)
Fluorouracil (D/X_M)
Hydroxyurea (D)
Idarubicin (D_M)
Ifosfamide (D_M)
Interferon Alfa (C_M)
(includes Interferon Alfa -n3, -NL, -2a, and -2b)
Laetrile (C)
Leuprolide (X_M)
Mechlorethamine (D_M)
Melphalan (D_M)
Mercaptopurine (D_M)
Methotrexate (X_M)
Mitoxantrone (D_M)
Paclitaxel (D_M)
Plicamycin (Mithramycin) (X_M)

Procarbazine (D_M)
Streptozocin (D_M)
Tamoxifen (D_M)
Teniposide (D)
Thioguanine (D_M)
Thiotepa (D_M)
Trastuzumab (B_M)
Tretinoin (Systemic) (D_M)
Trimetrexate (D_M)
Vinblastine (D_M)
Vincristine (D_M)
Vinorelbine (D_M)

A. Cytoprotective Agent
Mesna (B_M)

7. ARTIFICIAL SWEETENERS
Aspartame (B/C)
Cyclamate (C)
Saccharin (C)

8. AUTONOMICS

A. Parasympathomimetics (Cholinergics)
Acetylcholine (C)
Ambenonium (C)
Bethanechol (C_M)
Carbachol (C)
Cevimeline (C_M)
Demecarium (C/X_M)
Echothiophate (C)
Edrophonium (C)
Isoflurophate (C)
Neostigmine (C_M)
Physostigmine (C)
Pilocarpine (C_M)
Pyridostigmine (C)

B. Parasympatholytics (Anticholinergics)
Anisotropine (C)
Atropine (C)
Belladonna (C)
Benztropine (C)
Biperiden (C_M)
Clidinium (C)
Cycrimine (C)
Dicyclomine (B_M)
Diphemanil (C)
Ethopropazine (C)
Glycopyrrolate (B_M)
Hexocyclium (C)
Homatropine (C)
l-Hyoscyamine (C_M)
Ipratropium (B_M)
Isopropamide (C)
Mepenzolate (C)
Methantheline (C)
Methixene (C)
Methscopolamine (C)
Oxyphencyclimine (C)
Oxyphenonium (C)
Piperidolate (C)
Procyclidine (C)
Propantheline (C_M)
Scopolamine (C_M)
Thiphenamil (C)
Tridihexethyl (C)
Trihexyphenidyl (C)

C. Skeletal Muscle Relaxants
Atracurium (C_M)
Baclofen (C)
Carisoprodol (C)
Chlorzoxazone (C)
Cyclobenzaprine (B_M)
Dantrolene (C_M)
Decamethonium (C)
Metaxalone (B)
Methocarbamol (C)
Orphenadrine (C)
Pancuronium Bromide (C)
Rocuronium (C_M)
Succinylcholine (C_M)
Tizanidine (C_M)
Vecuronium (C_M)

D. Sympatholytics
Acebutolol (B_M/D)
Atenolol (D_M)
Betaxolol (C_M/D)
Bisoprolol (C_M/D)
Carteolol (C_M/D)
Carvedilol (C_M/D)
Celiprolol (B/D)
Dihydroergotamine (X_M)
Doxazosin (C_M)
Ergotamine (X_M)
Esmolol (C_M)
Guanabenz (C_M)

Guanadrel (B_M)
Guanethidine (C_M)
Guanfacine (B_M)
Labetalol (C_M/D)
Mepindolol (C/D)
Metoprolol (C_M/D)
Nadolol (C_M/D)
Oxprenolol (C/D)
Penbutolol (C_M/D)
Pindolol (B_M/D)
Prazosin (C_M)
Propranolol (C_M/D)
Sotalol (B_M/D)
Terazosin (C_M)
Timolol (C_M/D)

E. Sympathomimetics (Adrenergics)

Albuterol (C_M)
Cocaine (C_M/X)
Dobutamine (B_M)
Dopamine (C)
Ephedrine (C)
Epinephrine (C)
Fenoterol (B)
Hexoprenaline (C)
Isoetharine (C)
Isometheptene (C)
Isoproterenol (C)
Isoxsuprine (C)
Mephentermine (C)
Metaproterenol (C_M)
Metaraminol (C_M)
Methoxamine (C_M)
Midodrine (C_M)
Norepinephrine (D)
Oxymetazoline (C)
Phenylephrine (C)
Phenylpropanolamine (C)
Pseudoephedrine (C)
Ritodrine (B_M)
Terbutaline (B_M)

9. BISPHOSPHONATES

Alendronate (C_M)

10. CARDIOVASCULAR DRUGS

A. Antihypertensives

i. Angiotensin Converting Enzyme Inhibitors
Benazepril (C_M/D_M)
Captopril (C_M/D_M)
Enalapril (C_M/D_M)
Fosinopril (C_M/D_M)
Lisinopril (C_M/D_M)
Moexipril (C_M/D_M)
Perindopril (C_M/D_M)
Quinapril (C_M/D_M)
Ramipril (C_M/D_M)
Trandolapril (C_M/D_M)
ii. Angiotensin II Receptor Antagonists
Candesartan Celexetil (C_M/D_M)
Eprosartan (C_M/D_M)
Irbesartan (C_M/D_M)
Losartan (C_M/D_M)
Olmesartan (C_M/D_M)
Telmisartan (C_M/D_M)
Valsartan (C_M/D_M)
iii. Other Antihypertensives
Acebutolol (B_M/D)
Atenolol (D_M)
Betaxolol (C_M/D)
Bisoprolol (C_M/D)
Carteolol (C_M/D)
Carvedilol (C_M/D)
Celiprolol (B/D)
Clonidine (C_M)
Diazoxide (C_M)
Doxazosin (C_M)
Epoprostenol (B_M)
Esmolol (C_M)
Fenoldopam (B_M)
Guanabenz (C_M)
Guanadrel (B_M)
Guanethidine (C_M)
Guanfacine (B_M)
Hexamethonium (C)
Hydralazine (C_M)
Labetalol (C_M/D)
Mecamylamine (C_M)
Mepindolol (C/D)
Methyldopa (B_M)
Metoprolol (C_M/D)
Metyrosine (C_M)
Minoxidil (C_M)
Nadolol (C_M/D)
Nitroprusside (C)
Oxprenolol (C/D)

Pargyline (C_M)
Penbutolol (C_M/D)
Phenoxybenzamine (C_M)
Phentolamine (C_M)
Pindolol (B_M/D)
Prazosin (C_M)
Propranolol (C_M/D)
Reserpine (C_M)
Terazosin (C_M)
Sotalol (B_M/D)
Timolol (C_M/D)
Trimethaphan (C)

B. Calcium Channel Blockers
Amlodipine (C_M)
Bepridil (C_M)
Diltiazem (C_M)
Felodipine (C_M)
Isradipine (C_M)
Nicardipine (C_M)
Nifedipine (C_M)
Nimodipine (C_M)
Nisoldipine (C_M)
Verapamil (C_M)

C. Cardiac Drugs
Acetyldigitoxin (C)
Adenosine (C_M)
Amiodarone (D_M)
Amrinone (C_M)
Bretylium (C)
Deslanoside (C)
Digitalis (C)
Digitoxin (C_M)
Digoxin (C_M)
Disopyramide (C_M)
Dofetilide (C_M)
Encainide (B_M)
Flecainide (C_M)
Gitalin (C)
Ibutilide (C_M)
Lanatoside C (C)
Lidocaine (B_M)
Mexiletine (C_M)
Milrinone (C_M)
Moricizine (B_M)
Ouabain (B)
Procainamide (C_M)
Propafenone (C_M)
Quinidine (C_M)
Sotalol (B_M/D)
Tocainide (C_M)

D. Vasodilators
Amyl Nitrite (C)
Bosentan (X_M)
Cyclandelate (C)
Dioxyline (C)
Epoprostenol (B_M)
Erythrityl Tetranitrate (C_M)
Flosequinan (C_M)
Hydralazine (C_M)
Isosorbide Dinitrate (C_M)
Isosorbide Mononitrate (C_M)
Isoxsuprine (C)
Minoxidil (C_M)
Nicotinyl Alcohol (C)
Nitroglycerin (B/C_M)
Nylidrin (C_M)
Pentaerythritol Tetranitrate (C)
Tolazoline (C)

11. CENTRAL NERVOUS SYSTEM DRUGS

A. Analgesics and Antipyretics
Acetaminophen (B)
Antipyrine (C)
Ethoheptazine (C)
Methotrimeprazine (C)
Phenacetin (B)

B. Anticonvulsants
Aminoglutethimide (C_M)
Bromides (D)
Carbamazepine (D_M)
Clonazepam (D_M)
Ethosuximide (C)
Ethotoin (D)
Felbamate (C_M)
Gabapentin (C_M)
Lamotrigine (C_M)
Levetiracetam (C_M)
Magnesium Sulfate (B)
Mephenytoin (C)
Mephobarbital (D)
Metharbital (B)
Methsuximide (C)
Oxcarbazepine (C_M)
Paramethadione (D_M)

Phenobarbital (D)
Phensuximide (D)
Phenytoin (D)
Primidone (D)
Tiagabine (C_M)
Topiramate (C_M)
Trimethadione (D)
Valproic Acid (D_M)
Zonisamide (C_M)

C. Antidepressants

Amitriptyline (C_M)
Amoxapine (C_M)
Bupropion (B_M)
Butriptyline (C)
Citalopram (C_M)
Clomipramine (C_M)
Desipramine (C)
Dibenzepin (C)
Dothiepin (C)
Doxepin (C)
Escitalopram (C_M)
Fluoxetine (C_M)
Fluvoxamine (C_M)
Imipramine (C)
Iprindole (C)
Iproniazid (C)
Isocarboxazid (C)
Maprotiline (B_M)
Mebanazine (C)
Mirtazapine (C_M)
Nefazodone (C_M)
Nialamide (C)
Nortriptyline (C)
Opipramol (C)
Paroxetine (C_M)
Phenelzine (C)
Protriptyline (C)
Sertraline (C_M)
Tranylcypromine (C)
Trazodone (C_M)
Trimipramine (C_M)
Venlafaxine (C_M)

D. Antimigraine Agents

Almotriptan (C_M)
Dihydroergotamine (X_M)
Eletriptan (C_M)
Ergotamine (X_M)
Frovatriptan (C_M)
Naratriptan (C_M)
Rizatriptan (C_M)
Sumatriptan (C_M)
Zolmitriptan (C_M)

E. Antiparkinsonian Agents

Amantadine (C_M)
Carbidopa (C_M)
Entacapone (C_M)
Levodopa (C_M)
Pergolide (B_M)
Pramipexole (C_M)
Ropinirole (C_M)
Selegiline (C_M)
Tolcapone (C_M)

F. Cholinesterase Inhibitors

Donepezil (C_M)
Galantamine (B_M)
Rivastigmine (B_M)

G. Hallucinogens

Lysergic Acid Diethylamide (C)
Marijuana (X)
Phencyclidine (X)

H. Narcotic Agonist Analgesics

Alfentanil (C_M/D)
Alphaprodine (C_M/D)
Anileridine (B/D)
Codeine (C/D)
Dihydrocodeine Bitartrate (B/D)
Fentanyl (C_M/D)
Heroin (B/D)
Hydrocodone (C/D)
Hydromorphone (B/D)
Levorphanol (C_M/D)
Meperidine (B/D)
Methadone (B/D)
Morphine (C_M/D)
Oxycodone (B_M/D)
Oxymorphone (B/D)
Phenazocine (C/D)
Propoxyphene (C/D)
Remifentanil (C_M/D)
Sufentanil (C_M/D)

I. Narcotic Agonist-Antagonist Analgesics

Buprenorphine (C_M)
Butorphanol (C_M/D)

Nalbuphine (B_M/D)
Pentazocine (C/D)

J. Central Analgesics
Clonidine (C)
Tramadol (C_M)

K. Narcotic Antagonists
Cyclazocine (D)
Levallorphan (D)
Nalorphine (D)
Naloxone (B_M)
Naltrexone (C_M)

L. Nonsteroidal Anti-inflammatory Drugs
Aspirin (C/D)
Celecoxib (C_M/D)
Diclofenac (B_M/D)
Diflunisal (C_M/D)
Etodolac (C_M/D)
Fenoprofen (B/D)
Flurbiprofen (B_M/D)
Ibuprofen (B_M/D)
Indomethacin (B/D)
Ketoprofen (B_M/D)
Ketorolac (C_M/D)
Meclofenamate (B/D)
Mefenamic Acid (C_M/D)
Meloxicam (C_M/D)
Nabumetone (C_M/D)
Naproxen (B_M/D)
Oxaprozin (C_M/D)
Oxyphenbutazone (C)
Phenylbutazone (C_M/D)
Piroxicam (C_M/D)
Rofecoxib (C_M/D)
Sulindac (B/D)
Tolmetin (C_M/D)
Valdecoxib (C_M/D)

M. Physical Adjunct
Botulinum Toxin Type A (C_M)

N. Psychotherapeutics (Miscellaneous)
Atomoxetine (C_M)

O. Sedatives and Hypnotics
Alprazolam (D_M)
Amobarbital (D/B_M)
Aprobarbital (C)
Bromides (D)
Buspirone (B_M)
Butalbital (C/D)
Chloral Hydrate (C_M)
Chlordiazepoxide (D)
Clorazepate (D)
Diazepam (D)
Dichloralphenazone (B)
Estazolam (X_M)
Ethanol (D/X)
Ethchlorvynol (C_M)
Ethinamate (C_M)
Flunitrazepam (D)
Flurazepam (X_M)
Lorazepam (D_M)
Mephobarbital (D_M)
Meprobamate (D)
Methaqualone (D)
Metharbital (D)
Methotrimeprazine (C)
Midazolam (D_M)
Oxazepam (D)
Pentobarbital (D_M)
Phenobarbital (D)
Propofol (B_M)
Quazepam (X_M)
Secobarbital (D_M)
Temazepam (X_M)
Triazolam (X_M)
Zaleplon (C_M)
Zolpidem (B_M)

P. Stimulants and/or Anorexiants
Amphetamine (C_M)
Benzphetamine (X_M)
Caffeine (B)
Cigarette Smoking (X)
Dexfenfluramine (C_M)
Dexmethylphenidate (C_M)
Dextroamphetamine (C_M)
Diethylpropion (B)
Doxapram (B_M)
Ecstasy (C)
Fenfluramine (C_M)
Mazindol (C)
Methamphetamine (C_M)
Methylphenidate (C_M)
Modafinil (C_M)
Pemoline (B_M)

Phendimetrazine (C)
Phentermine (C_M)
Sibutramine (C_M)

Q. Tranquilizers/Antipsychotics
Acetophenazine (C)
Aripiprazole (C_M)
Butaperazine (C)
Carphenazine (C)
Chlorpromazine (C)
Chlorprothixene (C)
Clozapine (B_M)
Droperidol (C_M)
Flupenthixol (C)
Fluphenazine (C)
Haloperidol (C_M)
Lithium (D)
Loxapine (C)
Mesoridazine (C)
Molindone (C)
Olanzapine (C_M)
Perphenazine (C)
Pimozide (C_M)
Piperacetazine (C)
Prochlorperazine (C)
Promazine (C)
Quetiapine (C_M)
Risperidone (C_M)
Tetrabenazine (C)
Thiopropazate (C)
Thioridazine (C)
Thiothixene (C)
Trifluoperazine (C)
Triflupromazine (C)
Zuclopenthixol (C)

12. CHELATING AGENTS
Deferoxamine (C_M)
Penicillamine (D)
Succimer (C_M)
Trientine (C_M)

13. DERMATOLOGIC AGENTS
Adapalene (C_M)
Anthralin (C_M)
Etretinate (X_M)
Isotretinoin (X_M)
Tazarotene (X_M)
Tretinoin (Topical) (C_M)

14. DIAGNOSTIC AGENTS
Diatrizoate (D)
Ethiodized Oil (D/C_M)
Evans Blue (C)
Fluorescein Sodium (B)
Gadopentetate Dimeglumine (C_M)
Indigo Carmine (B)
Iocetamic Acid (D)
Iodamide (D)
Iodipamide (D)
Iodoxamate (D)
Iohexol (D)
Iopanoic Acid (D)
Iothalamate (D)
Ipodate (D)
Methylene Blue (C_M/D)
Metrizamide (D)
Metrizoate (D)
Tyropanoate (D)

15. DIURETICS
Acetazolamide (C)
Amiloride (B_M/D)
Bendroflumethiazide (C_M/D)
Benzthiazide (C/D)
Bumetanide (C_M/D)
Chlorothiazide (C_M/D)
Chlorthalidone (B_M/D)
Cyclopenthiazide (C/D)
Cyclothiazide (C/D)
Dichlorpenamide (C_M)
Ethacrynic Acid (B_M/D)
Furosemide (C_M/D)
Glycerin (C)
Hydrochlorothiazide (B_M/D)
Hydroflumethiazide (C_M/D)
Indapamide (B_M/D)
Isosorbide (C)
Mannitol (C)
Methazolamide (C)
Methyclothiazide (B_M/D)
Metolazone (B_M/D)
Polythiazide (C/D)
Quinethazone (C/D)
Spironolactone (C_M/D)
Triamterene (C_M/D)
Trichlormethiazide (C/D)
Urea (C)

16. ELECTROLYTES

Potassium Chloride (A)
Potassium Citrate (A)
Potassium Gluconate (A)

17. GASTROINTESTINAL AGENTS

A. Antidiarrheals

Alosetron (B_M)
Bismuth Subsalicylate (C)
Diphenoxylate (C_M)
Kaolin/Pectin (C)
Loperamide (B_M)
Opium (B/D)
Paregoric (B/D)

B. Antiemetics

Alosetron (B_M)
Buclizine (C)
Cyclizine (B)
Dimenhydrinate (B_M)
Dolasetron (B_M)
Domperidone (C)
Doxylamine (A)
Droperidol (C_M)
Granisetron (B_M)
Meclizine (B_M)
Metoclopramide (B_M)
Ondansetron (B_M)
Prochlorperazine (C)
Promethazine (C)
Trimethobenzamide (C)

C. Antiflatulents

Simethicone (C)

D. Anti-inflammatory Bowel Disease Agents

Balsalazide (B_M)
Infliximab (B_M)
Mesalamine (B_M)
Olsalazine (C_M)
Sulfasalazine (B/D)

E. Antisecretory Agents

Cimetidine (B_M)
Famotidine (B_M)
Lansoprazole (B_M)
Misoprostol (X_M)
Nizatidine (B_M)
Omeprazole (C_M)
Pantoprazole (B_M)
Rabeprazole (B_M)
Ranitidine (B_M)
Sucralfate (B_M)

F. Gallstone Solubilizing Agents

Chenodiol (X_M)
Ursodiol (B_M)

G. Laxatives/Purgatives

Casanthranol (C)
Cascara Sagrada (C)
Danthron (C)
Docusate Calcium (C)
Docusate Potassium (C)
Docusate Sodium (C)
Lactulose (B_M)
Magnesium Sulfate (B)
Mineral Oil (C)
Phenolphthalein (C)
Senna (C)

H. Lipase Inhibitors

Orlistat (B_M)

I. Stimulants

Cisapride (C_M)
Domperidone (C)
Metoclopramide (B_M)

18. HEMATOLOGICAL AGENTS

A. Anticoagulants

Anisindione (D)
Coumarin Derivatives (D/X_M)
Dalteparin (B_M)
Danaparoid (B_M)
Dicumarol (D)
Diphenadione (D)
Enoxaparin (B_M)
Ethyl Biscoumacetate (D)
Fondaparinux (B_M)
Heparin (C_M)
Nadroparin (B)
Nicoumalone (D)
Parnaparin (B)
Phenindione (D)
Phenprocoumon (D)
Reviparin (C)
Tinzaparin (B)
Warfarin (D/X_M)

B. Antiheparin
Protamine (C_M)

C. Antiplatelet
Abciximab (C_M)
Anagrelide (C_M)
Cilostazol (C_M)
Clopidogrel (B_M)
Dipyridamole (B_M)
Eptifibatide (B_M)
Ticlopidine (B_M)
Treprostinil (B_M)

D. Antithrombin
Antithrombin III (Human) (B_M)

E. Hematopoietic
Darbepoetin Alfa (C_M)
Epoetin Alfa (C_M)
Filgrastim (C_M)
Hemin (C_M)
Oprelvekin (C_M)
Pegfilgrastim (C_M)
Sargramostim (C_M)

F. Hemorrheologic
Pentoxifylline (C_M)

G. Hemostatics
Aminocaproic Acid (C_M)
Aprotinin (B_M)
Tranexamic Acid (B_M)

H. Thrombin Inhibitor
Argatroban (B_M)
Bivalirudin (B_M)
Lepirudin (B_M)

I. Thrombolytics
Alteplase (C_M)
Drotrecogin Alfa (Activated) (C_M)
Reteplase (C_M)
Streptokinase (C_M)
Tenecteplase (C_M)
Urokinase (B_M)

19. HERBS
Blue Cohosh (C)
Echinacea (C)
Garlic (C)
Ginger (C)
Ginkgo Biloba (C)
Ginseng (B)
Nutmeg (C)
Passion Flower (C)
St.John's Wort (C)
Valerian (B)

20. HORMONES

A. Adrenal
Beclomethasone (C_M)
Betamethasone (C/D)
Budesonide (B_M/C_M)
Cortisone (C/D)
Dexamethasone (C/D)
Hydrocortisone (C/D)
Prednisolone (C/D)
Prednisone (C/D)
Triamcinolone (C_M/D)

B. Antiadrenal
Aminoglutethimide (C_M)

C. Androgens
Danazol (X_M)
Fluoxymesterone (X_M)
Methyltestosterone (X_M)
Testosterone (X_M)

D. Antidiabetic Agents
Acarbose (B_M)
Acetohexamide (C)
Chlorpropamide (C_M)
Glimepiride (C_M)
Glipizide (C_M)
Glyburide (C_M)
Insulin (B)
Metformin (B_M)
Miglitol (B_M)
Nateglinide (C_M)
Pioglitazone (C_M)
Repaglinide (C_M)
Rosiglitazone (C_M)
Tolazamide (C_M)
Tolbutamide (C_M)
Troglitazone (B_M)

E. Antiestrogens
Tamoxifen (D_M)

F. Antiprogestogen
Mifepristone (X)

G. Antithyroid
Carbimazole (D)
Methimazole (D)
Propylthiouracil (D)
Sodium Iodide ^{131}I (X)

H. Calcium Regulation Hormone
Calcitonin-Salmon (C_M)

I. Estrogens
Chlorotrianisene (X_M)
Clomiphene (X_M)
Dienestrol (X_M)
Diethylstilbestrol (X_M)
Estradiol (X_M)
Estrogens, Conjugated (X_M)
Estrone (X)
Ethinyl Estradiol (X_M)
Hormonal Pregnancy Test Tablets (X)
Mestranol (X_M)
Oral Contraceptives (X_M)

J. Pineal Gland
Melatonin (C)

K. Pituitary
Corticotropin/Cosyntropin (C)
Desmopressin (B_M)
Leuprolide (X_M)
Lypressin (C_M)
Somatostatin (B)
Vasopressin (B)

L. Progestogens
Ethisterone (D)
Ethynodiol (D)
Hormonal Pregnancy Test Tablets (X)
Hydroxyprogesterone (D)
Lynestrenol (D)
Medroxyprogesterone (D_M)
Norethindrone (X_M)
Norethynodrel (X_M)
Norgestrel (X_M)
Oral Contraceptives (X_M)

M. Thyroid Agents
Iodothyrin (A)
Levothyroxine (A_M)
Liothyronine (A_M)
Liotrix (A)
Protirelin (C_M)
Thyroglobulin (A)
Thyroid (A)
Thyrotropin (C_M)

21. IMMUNOLOGIC AGENTS

A. Immunosuppressants
Azathioprine (D_M)
Cyclosporine (C_M)
Glatiramer (B_M)
Mycophenolate Mofetil (C_M)
Tacrolimus (C_M)

B. Immunomodulators
Adalimumab (B_M)
Anakinra (B_M)
Etanercept (B_M)
Interferon Alfa (C_M) (includes interferon Alfa-n3, -NL, -2a, and -2b)
Interferon Beta-1b (C_M)
Interferon Gamma-1b (C_M)
Thalidomide (X_M)

C. Antirheumatic Agents
Aurothioglucose (C_M)
Gold Sodium Thiomalate (C_M)
Hydroxychloroquine (C)
Infliximab (B_M)
Leflunomide (X_M)
Methotrexate (D)
Sulfasalazine (B/D)

22. KERATOLYTIC AGENTS
Podofilox (C_M)
Podophyllum (C)

23. NUTRIENTS/NUTRITIONAL SUPPLEMENTS
Hyperalimentation, Parenteral (C)
Lipids (C)
L-Lysine (C)
Melatonin (C)

24. OXYTOCIC
Methylergonovine Maleate (C)

25. PSORALENS
Acitretin (X_M)
Etretinate (X_M)
Methoxsalen (C_M)

26. RADIOPHARMACEUTICALS

Sodium Iodide ^{125}I (X)
Sodium Iodide ^{131}I (X)

27. RESPIRATORY DRUGS

A. Anti-inflammatory (Inhaled)

Cromolyn Sodium (B_M)
Nedocromil Sodium (B_M)

B. Antitussives

Codeine (C/D)
Dextromethorphan (C)
Hydrocodone (C/D)

C. Bronchodilators

Aminophylline (C)
Dyphylline (C_M)
Oxtriphylline (C)
Salmeterol (C_M)
Theophylline (C_M)

D. Corticosteroids (Inhaled)

Beclomethasone (C_M)
Budesonide (C_M)
Triamcinolone (C)

E. Expectorants

Ammmonium Chloride (B)
Guaifenesin (C)
Hydriodic Acid (D)
Iodinated Glycerol (X_M)
Potassium Iodide (D)
Sodium Iodide (D)
Terpin Hydrate (D)

F. Leukotriene Receptor Antagonists

Montelukast (B_M)
Zafirlukast (B_M)

G. Leukotriene Formation Inhibitor

Zileuton (B_M)

H. Mucolytic

Acetylcysteine (B_M)

28. SERUMS AND TOXOIDS

A. Serums

Immune Globulin, Hepatitis B (C_M)
Immune Globulin Intramuscular (C_M)
Immune Globulin Intravenous (C_M)
Immune Globulin, Rabies (C_M)
Immune Globulin, Tetanus (C_M)
Immune Globulin, Varicella Zoster (Human) (C)

B. Toxoids

Tetanus/Diphtheria Toxoids (Adult) (C_M)

29. VACCINES

Anthrax (C)
BCG (C_M)
Cholera (C_M)
Escherichia coli (C)
Group B Streptococcal (C)
Haemophilus b Conjugate (C_M)
Hepatitis A (C_M)
Hepatitis B (C_M)
Influenza (C_M)
Lyme Disease (C_M)
Measles (X/C_M)
Meningococcal (C_M)
Mumps (X/C_M)
Plague (C_M)
Pneumococcal Polyvalent (C_M)
Poliovirus Inactivated (C_M)
Poliovirus Live (C_M)
Rabies (Human) (C_M)
Rubella (X/C_M)
Smallpox (X)
TC-83 Venezuelan Equine Encephalitis (X)
Tularemia (C)
Typhoid (C_M)
Varicella Virus (C_M)
Yellow Fever (D)

30. TOXINS

Ciguatoxin (X)

31. URINARY TRACT AGENTS

A. Analgesic

Phenazopyridine (B_M)

B. Antispasmodic

Flavoxate (B_M)
Oxybutynin (B_M)
Tolterodine (C_M)

C. Urinary Acidifier

Ammonium Chloride (B)

D. Urinary Germicides

(see Anti-Infectives, Section R)

32. VAGINAL SPERMICIDES

Nonoxynol-9/Octoxynol-9 (C)

33. VITAMINS

Acitretin (X_M)
β-Carotene (C)
Calcifediol (C/D)
Calcitriol (C_M/D)
Cholecalciferol (C/D)
Dihydrotachysterol (A/D)
Ergocalciferol (A/D)
Etretinate (X_M)
Folic Acid (A/C)
Isotretinoin (X_M)
Leucovorin (C_M)
Menadione (C_M/X)
Niacin (A/C_M)
Niacinamide (A/C)
Pantothenic Acid (A/C)
Phytonadione (C_M)
Pyridoxine (A)
Riboflavin (A/C)
Thiamine (A/C)
Tretinoin (Systemic) (D_M)
Vitamin A (A/X)
Vitamin B_{12} (A/C)
Vitamin C (A/C)
Vitamin D (A/D)
Vitamin E (A/C)
Vitamins, Multiple (A)

34. MISCELLANEOUS

Allopurinol (C)
Bromocriptine (B_M)
Cabergoline (B_M)
Colchicine (D_M)
Disulfiram (C)
Electricity (D)
Octreotide (B_M)
Probenecid (C)
Silicone Breast Implants (C)

Index

Generic names are shown in **bold** with two sets of page numbers. The first set, also shown in **bold**, refers to the page number in the text where the monograph is located. The second set, shown in parentheses, refers to the page number in the Appendix where the drug is located by pharmacologic class. The trade names and synonyms are shown with one set of page numbers. These refer to their location in the text.